*(Continuation)*

| STD Agent | Interacting Drug | Interaction/Mechanism | Clinical Significance |
|---|---|---|---|
| *Sulfonamide* | Cyclosporine | Additive nephrotoxicity and/or reduced efficacy of cyclosporine; increased cyclosporine metabolism | Monitor levels |
| | Phenytoin | Increased phenytoin levels; inhibition of phenytoin metabolism | Monitor phenytoin levels |
| | Sulfonylureas | Enhanced hypoglycemic effects; uncertain | Monitor for hypoglycemia |
| *Tetracycline* | Antacids | Decreased absorption of tetracycline; chelation | Important with divalent or trivalent cation-containing antacids |
| | Carbamazepine | Doxycycline serum concentration may be decreased; stimulation of hepatic metabolism | Monitor patient's clinical response |
| | Digoxin | Decreased digoxin concentration; decreased bioavailability, mechanism unclear | Monitor digoxin levels |
| | Iron salts | Decreased absorption of tetracycline; chelation | Important if high doses of iron are taken concomitantly |
| | Oral contraceptives | Break-through bleeding and pregnancy; alteration of gut flora with decreased enterohepatic recycling and elimination of estrogen body stores | Use alternative birth control |
| | Penicillins | Antagonism; masks bactericidal effect | Little with therapeutic doses |
| | Phenobarbital | Doxycycline serum concentration may be decreased; stimulation of hepatic metabolism | Monitor patient's clinical response |
| | Warfarin | Enhanced anticoagulant effect; competition for protein-binding sites and/or decreased vitamin-K-producing bacteria | Monitor PTs |
| *Zidovudine (AZT)* | Acyclovir | *See* Acyclovir | *See* Acyclovir |
| | Dapsone | Increased risk of zidovudine toxicity; additive bone marrow suppression | Avoid concomitant use |
| | Flucytosine | Increased risk of zidovudine toxicity; additive bone marrow suppression | Avoid concomitant use |
| | Indomethacin | Increased zidovudine and/or indomethacin toxicity; competitive inhibition of glucuronidation | Avoid concomitant use |
| | Pentamidine | Increased risk of zidovudine toxicity; inhibition of glucuronidation and/or reduced renal excretion of zidovudine | Avoid concomitant use |
| | Probenecid | Increased zidovudine toxicity; inhibition of glucuronidation and/or reduced renal excretion of zidovudine | Avoid concomitant use |
| | Vincristine | Increased risk of zidovudine toxicity; additive bone marrow suppression | Avoid concomitant use |

# SEXUALLY TRANSMITTED DISEASES

# SEXUALLY TRANSMITTED DISEASES

SECOND EDITION

**Editors**

**King K. Holmes, M.D., Ph.D.**
Director, University of Washington Center for AIDS and STD, Professor of Medicine, Adjunct Professor of Epidemiology and Microbiology, University of Washington, Seattle, Washington

**Per-Anders Mårdh, M.D., Ph.D.**
Professor, Institute of Clinical Microbiology, University of Uppsala, Uppsala, Sweden

**P. Frederick Sparling, M.D.**
Chairman of the Department of Medicine, J. Herbert Bate Professor of Microbiology and Immunology and Medicine, University of North Carolina School of Medicine, Chapel Hill, North Carolina

**Paul J. Wiesner, M.D.**
Director, DeKalb County Health Department, Decatur, Georgia

**Associate Editors**

**Willard Cates, Jr., M.D., M.P.H.**
Director, Division of Sexually Transmitted Diseases, Centers for Disease Control, Atlanta, Georgia

**Stanley M. Lemon, M.D.**
Chief, Division of Infectious Diseases, Professor of Medicine and Microbiology and Immunology, University of North Carolina School of Medicine, Chapel Hill, North Carolina

**Walter E. Stamm, M.D.**
Professor of Medicine, Head, Infectious Diseases Division, Harborview Medical Center, Seattle, Washington

**McGraw-Hill, Inc.**
**HEALTH PROFESSIONS DIVISION**

New York St. Louis San Francisco Auckland Bogotá
Caracas Lisbon London Madrid Mexico Milan Montreal
New Delhi Paris San Juan Singapore Sydney Tokyo Toronto

**SEXUALLY TRANSMITTED DISEASES**



34567890 HDHD 998765432

ISBN 0-07-029677-4

This book was set in Sabon Roman by Waldman Graphics, Inc.; the editors were Avé McCracken and Peter McCurdy; the production supervisor was Bob Laffler; the cover designer and color insert designer was Edward R. Schultheis. Halliday Lithograph Corporation was printer and binder.

**Library of Congress Cataloging in Publication Data**

Sexually transmitted diseases.

Includes bibliographies and index.
1. Sexually transmitted diseases. I. Holmes, King K.
[DNLM: 1. Sexually Transmitted Diseases.
WC 140 S5174]
RC200.S49 1990 616.95′1 89-12465
ISBN 0-07-029677-4

# CONTRIBUTORS*

**Michael W. Adler, M.D.** [85]
Professor of Genito-Urinary Medicine, Academic Department of Genito-Urinary Medicine, James Pringle House, University College and Middlesex School of Medicine, London, England

**William Albritton, M.D.** [24]
Professor and Chair, Department of Microbiology, University of Saskatchewan, Saskatoon, Canada

**E. Russell Alexander, M.D.** [66]
Chief, Epidemiology Research Branch, Division of Sexually Transmitted Diseases, Center for Preventive Services, Centers for Disease Control, Atlanta, Georgia

**Sevgi O. Aral, Ph.D., M.A., M.S.** [2]
Sociologist/Demographer, Division of Sexually Transmitted Diseases, Centers for Disease Control, Atlanta, Georgia

**Timothy Baker** [88]
Office of the Deputy Director (AIDS), Centers for Disease Control, Atlanta, Georgia

**Sharon Baker, Ph.D.** [89]
Counseling Psychologist, Harborview Medical Center STD Clinic, University of Washington, Seattle, Washington

**Alfred O. Berg, M.D., M.P.H.** [93]
Associate Professor and Director of Research, Department of Family Medicine, University of Washington, Seattle, Washington

**Richard E. Berger, M.D.** [53]
Associate Professor of Urology, University of Washington; Director, Reproductive and Sexual Medicine Clinic, University of Washington, Seattle, Washington

**Stephan A. Billstein, M.D., M.P.H.** [41]
Director, Medical Marketing, Roche Laboratories, Hoffmann-La Roche, Inc., Nutley, New Jersey

**William R. Bowie, M.D.** [52]
Professor of Medicine, Faculty of Medicine, Division of Infectious Diseases, University of British Columbia, Vancouver, British Columbia, Canada

**Richard R. Brookman, M.D.** [8]
Associate Professor of Pediatrics, Chairman, Division of Adolescent Medicine, Children's Medical Center, Medical College of Virginia/Virginia Commonwealth University, Richmond, Virginia

*The numbers in brackets following the contributor name refer to chapter(s) authored or co-authored by the contributor.

**Donald C. Bross, J.D., Ph.D.** [94]
Associate Professor in Pediatrics (Family Law), University of Colorado School of Medicine, C. Henry Kempe National Center for the Prevention and Treatment of Child Abuse and Neglect, (Legal Counsel), Denver, Colorado

**Robert C. Brunham, M.D.** [64]
Professor and Head, Department of Medical Microbiology, University of Manitoba, Winnipeg, Manitoba, Canada

**James R. Carlson, Ph.D.** [80]
Assistant Professor of Pathology and Internal Medicine, Director, AIDS Virus Diagnostic Laboratory, Department of Pathology, School of Medicine, University of California, Davis, California

**William B. Carter, Ph.D.** [89]
Associate Professor, Associate Director of Health Services, University of Washington, Health Services Research and Development, Seattle VA Medical Center, Seattle, Washington

**Willard Cates, Jr., M.D., M.P.H.** [63,84,86,92]
Director, Division of Sexually Transmitted Diseases, Centers for Disease Control, Atlanta, Georgia

**Richard E. Chaisson, M.D.** [57]
Assistant Professor, Departments of Medicine and Epidemiology, The Johns Hopkins Schools of Medicine and Hygiene and Public Health; Director, AIDS Service, The Johns Hopkins Hospital, Baltimore, Maryland

**Thomas J. Coates, Ph.D.** [90]
Division of General Internal Medicine, and Center for AIDS Prevention Studies, University of California School of Medicine, San Francisco, San Francisco, California

**Myron S. Cohen, M.D.** [12]
Associate Professor of Medicine, Microbiology and Immunology, University of North Carolina at Chapel Hill, Chapel Hill, North Carolina

**Stig Colleen, M.D., Ph.D.** [54]
Associate Professor of Urology, University Hospital, Lund, Sweden

**Lawrence Corey, M.D.** [35,77]
Professor of Laboratory Medicine, Medicine and Microbiology, University of Washington School of Medicine, Seattle, Washington

**Ernest T. Creighton, M.P.H.** [75]
Division of Training, Public Health Practice Program Office, Centers for Disease Control, Atlanta, Georgia

**James W. Curran, M.D., M.P.H.** [31]
Director, AIDS Program, Centers for Disease Control, Atlanta, Georgia

**Dan Danielsson, M.D., Ph.D.** [73]
Professor and Chairman, Department of Microbiology and Immunology, Orebro Medical Center Hospital, Orebro, Sweden

**William W. Darrow, Ph.D.** [9]
AIDS Program, Center for Infectious Diseases, Centers for Disease Control, Atlanta, Georgia

**Jack A. DeHovitz, M.D., M.P.H.** [81]
Assistant Professor of Preventive Medicine and Community Health, Department of Medicine; Director, AIDS Preventive Center, SUNY Health Science Center at Brooklyn, Brooklyn, New York

**John Munroe Douglas, Jr., M.D.** [39]
Assistant Professor of Medicine, University of Colorado Health Sciences Center; Assistant Director of Disease Control, Denver Department of Public Health, Denver, Colorado

**D. Peter Drotman, M.D.** [88]
AIDS Program, Center for Infectious Diseases, Centers for Disease Control, Atlanta, Georgia

**Joanne E. Embree, M.Sc., M.D.** [64]
Assistant Professor, Department of Pediatrics and Medical Microbiology, University of Manitoba, Winnipeg, Manitoba, Canada

**David A. Eschenbach, M.D.** [51]
Professor of Obstetrics and Gynecology, University of Washington School of Medicine, Seattle, Washington

**M. Essex, D.V.M., Ph.D.** [33]
Professor and Chairman, Department of Cancer Biology, Harvard School of Public Health; Chairman, Harvard AIDS Institute, Boston, Massachusetts

**Karin Esteves** [88]
Division of Communicable Diseases, World Health Organization, Geneva, Switzerland

**Anthony S. Fauci, M.D.** [29]
Director, National Institute of Allergy and Infectious Diseases, National Institutes of Health, Bethesda, Maryland

**Kenneth H. Fife, M.D., Ph.D.** [77]
Associate Professor of Medicine, Microbiology, and Immunology, Indiana University School of Medicine, Indianapolis, Indiana

**Terence C. Gayle, M.D.** [89]
Clinical Assistant Professor of Psychiatry and Behavioral Science, University of Washington, Seattle, Washington

**J. Louise Gerberding, M.D.** [57]
Assistant Professor, Department of Medicine, University of California, San Francisco School of Medicine, San Francisco, California

**Mary R. Gillmore, Ph.D.** [4]
Research Assistant Professor, School of Social Work and Department of Sociology, University of Washington, Seattle, Washington

**Aaron Eli Glatt, M.D.** [26]
Assistant Chief, Division of Infectious Diseases, Nassau County Medical Center, East Meadow, New York; Assistant Professor of Medicine, SUNY Health Science Center, Stony Brook, New York

**Lynn Goldstein, M.D.** [79]
Vice President, Research, Genetic Systems Corporation, Seattle, Washington

**Matthew Goodstein, M.D.** [71]
Resident, Department of Otolaryngology-Head and Neck Surgery, The Johns Hopkins Hospital, Baltimore, Maryland

**Daniel O. Graney, Ph.D.** [10, 11]
Associate Professor of Biological Structure, School of Medicine, University of Washington, Seattle, Washington

**Ruth M. Greenblatt, M.D.** [90]
Assistant Professor of Medicine, Division of Infectious Diseases, University of California School of Medicine, San Francisco, California

**David A. Grimes, M.D.** [92]
Departments of Obstetrics and Gynecology and Preventive Medicine, University of Southern California School of Medicine, Women's Hospital, Los Angeles, California

**Richard L. Guerrant, M.D.** [44]
Professor of Medicine, Head, Division of Geographic Medicine, Department of Internal Medicine, University of Virginia School of Medicine, Charlottesville, Virginia

**Laura T. Gutman, M.D.** [65]
Associate Professor, Departments of Pediatrics and Pharmacology, Duke University Medical Center, Durham, North Carolina

**Ashley T. Haase, M.D.** [28]
Professor and Head, Department of Microbiology, University of Minnesota Medical School, Minneapolis, Minnesota

**H. Hunter Handsfield, M.D.** [14,61]
Professor of Medicine, University of Washington School of Medicine; Director, Sexually Transmitted Disease Control Program, Seattle-King County Department of Public Health, Seattle, Washington

**H. Robert Harrison, D. Phil., M.D., M.P.H.** [66]
Clinical Associate Professor of Pediatrics, Emory University School of Medicine, Atlanta, Georgia

**Gavin Hart, M.D., M.P.H.** [25,85]
Director, STD Services Branch, South Australian Health Commission; Clinical Associate Professor, School of Medicine, Flinders University, South Australia

**Bernadine P. Healy, M.D.** [22]
Chairman, Research Institute, The Cleveland Clinic Foundation, Cleveland, Ohio

**Harry R. Hill, M.D.** [69]
Professor of Pediatrics and Pathology; Head, Division of Clinical Immunology and Allergy, University of Utah, Salt Lake City, Utah

**Sharon L. Hillier, Ph.D.** [47]
Research Assistant Professor, Department of Obstetrics and Gynecology, University of Washington, Seattle, Washington

**Martin S. Hirsch, M.D.** [30]
Professor of Medicine, Harvard Medical School, Infectious Disease Unit, Massachusetts General Hospital, Boston, Massachusetts

**Scott D. Holmberg, M.D.** [31]
AIDS Program, Centers for Disease Control, Atlanta, Georgia

**King K. Holmes, M.D., Ph.D.** [2,16,46,47,50,64]
Director, University of Washington Center for AIDS and STD, Professor of Medicine, Adjunct Professor of Epidemiology and Microbiology, University of Washington, Seattle, Washington

**Edward W. Hook III, M.D.** [14]
Associate Professor of Medicine, The Johns Hopkins University School of Medicine; Chief, STD Clinical Services, Baltimore City Health Department, Baltimore, Maryland

**Eng-Shang Huang, Ph.D.** [36]
Professor of Medicine and Microbiology and Immunology, University of North Carolina at Chapel Hill, Chapel Hill, North Carolina

**Elizabeth F. Hunter, M.S.** [75]
Pathogenesis and Immunology Branch, Treponemal Sexually Transmitted Diseases Laboratory Program, Center for Infectious Diseases, Center for Disease Control, Atlanta, Georgia

**Michael S. Insler, M.D., J.D.** [62]
LSU Eye Center, LSU Medical Center School of Medicine, New Orleans, Louisiana

**Harold W. Jaffe, M.D.** [76]
Assistant Director for Science, AIDS Program, Centers for Disease Control, Atlanta, Georgia

**Myra B. Jennings, Ph.D.** [80]
Research Virologist, Associate Director, AIDS Virus Diagnostic Laboratory, Department of Pathology, School of Medicine, University of California, Davis, California

**Carole Jenny, M.D., M.B.A.** [72,95]
Assistant Professor, Department of Pediatrics, University of Washington School of Medicine; Medical Director, Harborview Sexual Assault Center, Seattle, Washington

**Franklyn N. Judson, M.D.** [87]
Director, Division of Public Health, Denver Department of Health and Hospitals; Professor, Departments of Medicine and Preventive Medicine, University of Colorado, Denver, Colorado

**Rudolph H. Kampmeier, M.D.** [23]
Professor Emeritus of Medicine, Vanderbilt University School of Medicine, Nashville, Tennessee

**Haskins K. Kashima, M.D.** [71]
Professor, Department of Otolaryngology—Head and Neck Surgery, The Johns Hopkins Hospital, Baltimore, Maryland

**Gerald T. Keusch, M.D.** [27]
Professor of Medicine; Chief, Division of Geographic Medicine and Infectious Diseases, New England Medical Center, Tufts University School of Medicine, Boston, Massachusetts

**Philip Kirby, M.D.** [58]
Assistant Professor of Medicine, University of Washington, Seattle, Washington

**Nancy Kiviat, M.D.** [48,50]
Associate Professor of Pathology, University of Washington, Seattle, Washington

**Scott Koenig, M.D.** [29]
Laboratory of Immunoregulation, National Institute of Allergy and Infectious Diseases, National Institutes of Health, Bethesda, Maryland

**Laura A. Koutsky, Ph.D.** [48]
Acting Instructor, Department of Epidemiology, University of Washington, Seattle, Washington

**John N. Krieger, M.D.** [10]
Associate Professor of Urology, University of Washington, School of Medicine, Seattle, Washington

**Sheldon H. Landesman, M.D.** [81]
Associate Professor of Medicine; Medical Director, AIDS Study Group, Kings County Hospital Center, SUNY Health Science Center at Brooklyn, Brooklyn, New York

**Sandra A. Larsen, Ph.D.** [75]
Chief, Treponemal Pathogenesis and Immunology Branch, Sexually Transmitted Diseases Laboratory Program, Center for Infectious Diseases, Centers for Disease Control, Atlanta, Georgia

**Stanley M. Lemon, M.D.** [40]
Chief, Division of Infectious Diseases, Professor of Medicine and Microbiology and Immunology, The University of North Carolina at Chapel Hill, Chapel Hill, North Carolina

**Attila T. Lörincz, Ph.D.** [78]
Section Head, Molecular Diagnostics Research, Life Technologies, Inc., Gaithersburg, Maryland

**Howard Maibach, M.D.** [42]
Professor of Dermatology, University of California, San Francisco, School of Medicine, San Francisco, California

**Per-Anders Mårdh, M.D., Ph.D.** [12,49,54,73,74]
Professor, Institute of Clinical Microbiology, University of Uppsala, Sweden

**Richard Marlink, M.D.** [33]
Lecturer, Department of Cancer Biology, Harvard School of Public Health, Cambridge, Massachusetts

**William M. McCormack, M.D.** [26]
Chief of ID, Downstate Medical Center; Professor of Medicine, SUNY Health Science Center, Brooklyn, New York

**André Z. Meheus, M.D., D.P.H.** [67,84,86]
Programme Manager, Sexually Transmitted Diseases, World Health Organization, Geneva, Switzerland

**Henk E. Menke, M.D.** [60]
Dermato-venereologist, St. Fransiscus Gasthuis, Kleiveg, National Institute of Public Health, Bilthoven, The Netherlands

**Donald E. Moore, M.D.** [63]
Associate Professor, Division of Reproductive Endocrinology, Department of Obstetrics and Gynecology, University of Washington, Seattle, Washington

**Tomasz F. Mroczkowski, M.D.** [85]
Visiting Professor, Department of Dermatology, Tulane University School of Medicine and Department of Medicine, Section of Infectious Diseases, Louisiana State University, New Orleans, Louisiana

**Miklós Müller, M.D.** [43]
Associate Professor of Biochemical Parasitology, The Rockefeller University, New York, New York

**F. Kevin Murphy, M.D.** [67]
Infectious Disease and Tropical Medicine, Private Practice; Clinical Associate Professor, Internal Medicine, University of Texas, Southwestern Medical Center, Dallas, Texas

**Daniel M. Musher, M.D.** [18,76]
Chief, Infectious Disease Section, Veterans Administration Hospital, Houston; Professor of Medicine, Professor of Immunology, Baylor College of Medicine, Houston, Texas

**John E. Newbold, Ph.D.** [40]
Assoicate Professor of Microbiology and Immunology, The University of North Carolina at Chapel Hill, Chapel Hill, North Carolina

**Elizabeth N. Ngugi, M.D.** [7]
Department of Medical Microbiology, University of Nairobi, Nairobi, Kenya

**Linda C. Novak, M.D.** [62]
LSU Eye Center, LSU Medical Center School of Medicine, New Orleans, Louisiana

**David Oriel, M.D.** [38]
Consultant Physician in Genito-Urinary Medicine, University College Hospital, London; Honorary Senior Clinical Lecturer, Department of Medicine, University College, London, Recognized Teacher of Venereal Disease, University of London, London, England

**Milton Orkin, M.D.** [42]
Clinical Professor, Department of Dermatology, University of Minnesota, Minnesota

**A. Olu Osoba, M.D.** [17]
Professor of Medical Microbiology, University College Hospital, Ibadan, Nigeria

**David G. Ostrow, M.D., Ph.D.** [6]
Director of Psychobiology Research, University of Michigan, Ann Arbor, Michigan

**Jorma Paavonen, M.D., Ph.D.** [48]
Associate Professor, Department of Obstetrics and Gynecology, University Central Hospital, Helsinki, Finland

**William Parra** [88]
Assistant Deputy Director for Operations (HIV), Office of the Deputy Director (HIV), Centers for Disease Control, Atlanta, Georgia

**Pisespong Patamasucon, M.D.** [67]
Assistant Professor of Pediatrics, Faculty of Medicine, Prince of Songkla University, Haadyai, Songkla, Thailand

**Peter L. Perine, M.D., M.P.H.** [17]
Professor and Director of Tropical Public Health and of Medicine, F. Edward Hebert School of Medicine, Uniformed Services University of the Health Sciences, Bethesda, Maryland

**Peter Piot, M.D., Ph.D.** [59]
Institute of Tropical Medicine, Antwerp, Belgium

**Francis A. Plummer, M.D.** [7,59]
Associate Professor, Departments of Medical Microbiology and Internal Medicine, University of Manitoba, Winnipeg, Manitoba, Canada

**P. Scott Pollock, M.D.** [61]
Clinical Assistant Professor, University of Washington School of Medicine, Seattle, Washington

**John J. Potterat** [91]
Director, Venereal Disease Control, El Paso County Health Department, Colorado Springs, Colorado

**Thomas C. Quinn, M.D.** [32,55]
Senior Investigator, Laboratory of Immunoregulation, National Institute of Allergy and Infectious Diseases, National Institutes of Health, Bethesda, Maryland;

Associate Professor of Medicine, The Johns Hopkins University School of Medicine, Baltimore, Maryland

**Jonathan I. Ravdin, M.D.** [44]
Associate Professor of Medicine and Pharmacology, Department of Internal Medicine, University of Virginia School of Medicine, Charlottesville, Virginia

**Michael F. Rein, M.D.** [43]
Associate Professor of Medicine, Division of Infectious Diseases, University of Virginia School of Medicine, Charlottesville, Virginia

**Edward P. Richards III, J.D., M.P.H.** [94]
Visiting Associate Professor, University of Denver College of Law, Research Fellow, National Center for Preventive Law

**Allan R. Ronald, M.D.** [24]
Professor and Chair, Department of Medicine, University of Manitoba, Winnipeg, Canada

**Michael W. Ross** [5]
Director, Research, Evaluation and Epidemiology, AIDS-STD Services, South Australian Health Commission; Clinical Senior Lecturer in Psychiatry and Primary Health Care, Flinders University Medical School, Adelaide, Australia

**Richard B. Rothenberg, M.D.** [3,91]
Assistant Director for Science, Center for Chronic Lesion Prevention, CDC, Atlanta, Georgia

**Arye Rubenstein, M.D.** [68]
Professor of Pediatrics, Microbiology and Immunology, Albert Einstein College of Medicine, Bronx, New York

**Mary E. Russo, Pharm.D.** [83]
Director, Product Development, Standard Products, Lederle Laboratories, Pearl River, New York

**Merle A. Sande, M.D.** [57]
Professor and Vice Chairman, Department of Medicine, University of California School of Medicine; Chief, Medical Service, San Francisco General Hospital, San Francisco, California

**Eric Sandström, M.D., Ph.D.** [58]
Assistant Professor, Department of Dermatology, University of Stockholm, Stockholm, Sweden

**Julius Schachter, Ph.D.** [15]
Professor of Epidemiology, Department of Laboratory Medicine, University of California at San Francisco, San Francisco, California

**Kenneth F. Schulz, M.B.A.** [67,86]
Associate Director for Quantitative Methods, Division of Sexually Transmitted Diseases, Center for Preventive Services, Centers for Disease Control, Atlanta, Georgia

**Pepper Schwartz, Ph.D.** [4]
Professor, Department of Sociology, University of Washington, Seattle, Washington

**Keerti V. Shah, Dr.P.H.** [37,71]
Professor, Department of Immunology and Infectious Diseases, The Johns Hopkins School of Hygiene and Public Health, Baltimore, Maryland

**Karolynn Siegel, Ph.D.** [9,88]
Director of Research, Department of Social Work, Memorial Sloan-Kettering Cancer Center; Associate Professor of Sociology in Public Health, Cornell University Medical College, Ithaca, New York

**Lynn Smiley, M.D.** [36]
Senior Clinical Research Scientist, Antimicrobial Therapy, Burroughs Wellcome Company, University of North Carolina at Chapel Hill, Chapel Hill, North Carolina

**Ewe-Hui Sng, MBBS** [82]
Medical Director, Department of Pathology, Ministry of Health, Singapore, Republic of Singapore

**Jack D. Sobel, M.D.** [45]
Chief, Division of Infectious Diseases; Professor of Medicine, Adjunct Professor of Microbiology and Immunology, Department of Medicine, Wayne State University School of Medicine, Detroit, Michigan

**P. Frederick Sparling, M.D.** [13,19]
Chairman of the Department of Medicine, J. Herbert Bate Professor of Microbiology and Immunology and Medicine, University of North Carolina at Chapel Hill, Chapel Hill, North Carolina

**Patricia G. Spear, Ph.D.** [34]
Professor and Chairman, Department of Microbiology and Immunology, The Medical and Dental Schools, Northwestern University, Chicago, Illinois

**Sergio Stagno, M.D.** [70]
Professor and Acting Chairman, Director of Resident Training Program, Department of Pediatrics, University of Alabama at Birmingham, Birmingham, Alabama

**Walter E. Stamm, M.D.** [16,55,74]
Professor of Medicine; Head, Infectious Disease Division, Harborview Medical Center, Seattle, Washington

**Andrezj Stapinski, M.D.** [85]
Professor of Medicine; Director, Institute of Venereology, Warsaw Medical Academy, Warsaw, Poland

**Ernst Stolz, M.D.** [60]
Professor, Dermato-venereology, Faculty of Medicine, Erasmus University, Rotterdam, The Netherlands

**Morton N. Swartz, M.D.** [21]
Professor of Medicine, Harvard Medical School; Chief, Infectious Diseases Unit, Massachusetts General Hospital, Boston, Massachusetts

**Teresa A. Tartaglione, Pharm.D.** [83]
Assistant Professor, Department of Pharmacy Practice, School of Pharmacy, University of Washington, Seattle, Washington

**David Taylor-Robinson, M.D.** [26]
Head, Division of Sexually Transmitted Diseases, Clinical Research Centre, Harrow, England

**R. N. Thin, M.D.** [20]
Consultant Physician, Department of Genitourinary Medicine, St. Thomas' Hospital, London, England

**Paul A. Volberding, M.D.** [56]
Associate Professor of Medicine, University of California, San Francisco; Chief, Medical Oncology and AIDS Activities Division, San Francisco General Hospital, San Francisco, California

**Louis A. Vontver, M.D.** [11]
Professor, Director, Division of Medical Education, Department of Obstetrics and Gynecology, School of Medicine, University of Washington, Seattle, Washington

**V. D. Vuzevski, M.D., Ph.D.** [60]
Associate Professor of Pathology, Erasmus University, Rotterdam, The Netherlands

**Michael Anthony Waugh, M.B. DHMSA.Dip. Ven.** [1]
Consultant Genito-urinary Physician, General Infirmary, Leeds, England

**Robert D. Weber, M.D.** [12]
University of North Carolina at Chapel Hill, Clinical Institute in Medicine, Chapel Hill, North Carolina

**Cynthia S. Weikel, M.D.** [44]
Assistant Professor of Medicine, Division of Gastroenterology and Infectious Diseases, Department of Internal Medicine, The Johns Hopkins School of Medicine, Baltimore, Maryland

**Lars Weström, M.D.** [49]
Associate Professor and Clinical Lecturer, Institute of Obstetrics and Gynecology, University of Lund, Lund, Sweden

**Richard J. Whitley, M.D.** [70]
Departments of Pediatrics, Microbiology, and Medicine, University of Alabama at Birmingham, Birmingham, Alabama

**Paul J. Wiesner, M.D.** [85]
Director, DeKalb County Health Department, Decatur, Georgia

**Catherine M. Wilfert, M.D.** [65]
Professor, Department of Pediatrics and Allergy, Immunology and Microbiology, Duke University Medical Center, Department of Pediatrics and Microbiology, Durham, North Carolina

**Pål Wølner-Hanssen, M.D. Med.Dr.** [50,51]
Assistant Professor, Department of Obstetrics and Gynecology, University of Washington School of Medicine, Seattle, Washington

# PREFACE

The subject of this text has changed enormously since the first edition was published 5 years ago. Major new fields of study have arisen dealing with human immunodeficiency virus (HIV) infections, human papillomavirus (HPV) infections, and behavioral intervention strategies to prevent the spread of sexually transmitted disease. Some of the most important fundamental advances in biomedical research are being made in studies of the immunology of AIDS, the molecular virology of HIV and HPV, and the pathogenicity of *Neisseria gonorrhoeae*. Newer diagnostic techniques, based on use of the polymerase chain reaction, offer previously unimaginable levels of sensitivity for the detection of sexually transmitted viruses. The theoretical tenets of health education and behavioral intervention, developed in programs for prevention of unhealthy behaviors that result in heart disease, cancer, teenage pregnancy, and addictions, are now being challenged and tested as never before in efforts to prevent high risk sexual behaviors. The continued epidemic spread of HIV and many other STDs in selected indigent and poorly educated populations now far exceeds the capacity of public clinics and public health systems to cope with all aspects of the problem. This situation dictates continuing re-prioritization of public health programs, reevaluation of the efficacy of traditional approaches to disease intervention, and development of innovative cost-effective approaches to STD prevention, diagnosis, and treatment. This is especially true in developing countries, which represent three quarters of the world's population, where the focus must be on health education and on development and use of appropriate, inexpensive technologies for STD control. The hope must be that continued investigation into the molecular pathogenesis of HIV and other STDs will lead ultimately to the development of inexpensive and effective vaccine strategies.

The goal of this text is to present a comprehensive and thoroughly referenced analysis of the sexually transmitted diseases by internationally recognized leaders in this field. We have encouraged authors to present a global perspective which considers the STD problem in both the industrial and the developing world. Thirty entirely new chapters have been added to the contents of the first edition; all of the chapters retained from the first edition have been updated, and most have been extensively revised. New or reorganized sections include a section containing 10 chapters dealing with STDs and reproductive health and pediatrics; 10 chapters dealing with guidelines for clinicians for diagnostic testing for STDs; and 12 new chapters concerning HIV infection. The color section and illustrations have also been considerably expanded. The book is intended to meet the needs of basic scientists, clinicians, and public health professionals who deal with STDs and AIDS.

# CONTENTS

# Part V SEXUALLY TRANSMITTED AGENTS

## Section 1: Bacteria, Chlamydia, and Mycoplasma



## Section 2: Viral Infections

## Part VIII DIAGNOSTIC TESTING FOR SELECTED SEXUALLY TRANSMITTED DISEASES: GUIDELINES FOR CLINICIANS



## Part IX PHARMACOLOGY



## Part X CONTROL OF SEXUALLY TRANSMITTED DISEASES

# SEXUALLY TRANSMITTED DISEASES

# PART I HISTORY OF SEXUALLY TRANSMITTED DISEASES

# Chapter 1

# History of clinical developments in sexually transmitted diseases

Michael Anthony Waugh

## DEFINING SEXUALLY TRANSMITTED DISEASES AS A SPECIALTY

The specialty of sexually transmitted diseases encompasses the complete study of sexually transmitted diseases, including: (a) pathogenesis and pathology of those conditions; their presentation, treatment, and management; (b) research and their sequelae; (c) those aspects of obstetrics and gynecology, pediatrics, and psychological medicine which are relevant to it, and (d) public health care and community medicine.

In the United Kingdom specialists have practiced venereology since the Royal Commission on Venereal Diseases in 1916.[1] Their numbers have greatly increased since the advent of the National Health Service in 1948. In continental Europe, however, venereology is a subspecialty of dermatology, dermato-venereology. In other countries it is even more fragmented. Urologists treat men with a urethral discharge, gynecologists treat females, and dermatologists treat anyone with the skin manifestations of sexually transmitted diseases. Elsewhere, notably in the United States of America, the specialty of sexually transmitted diseases is still developing from infectious diseases.

## WHY STUDY THE HISTORY OF STDs?

During the last twenty years, there have been enormous changes in the specialty of sexually transmitted diseases. No longer is it a narrow specialty whose purpose is to treat the classic venereal diseases, of which syphilis was foremost. But for many reasons, especially the predominance of viral STDs, the specialty now includes diverse sections of medicine and science. Those who practice this specialty of STDs hopefully learn from the past and are humbled by knowledge once known but often forgotten. A knowledge of the history of STDs is important because it is essentially a study of the events in cultures in which venereal diseases flourish and which in turn encourage the specialty to continue.

The history of STDs encompasses the development of medicine, moving from the province of surgeons, healers of external disease, to that of the physicians who discovered its constitutional effects. In the nineteenth century, the scientific foundations of medicine were laid down as well as the organization of organic chemistry, the development of the microscope and its use in medicine, and the understanding of physiology, epidemiology, and pathology. From pathology came bacteriology and its amazing application to the history of STDs at the turn of the present century. Immunology and serology were also established then. All of these are components in genitourinary medicine and therefore part of the study of the history of sexually transmitted diseases. At the same time other specialties grew, especially gynecology, dermatology, public health, urology, and psychiatry, all of which have a large part to play in the growth of venereology.

## ANCIENT EGYPT

At the end of the nineteenth century, important archaeologic discoveries brought to light medical artifacts, hieroglyphics, papyri, and mummies that elucidate the role of STDs in ancient Egypt. The Edwin Smith papyrus, with its surgical descriptions, was discovered at Thebes in 1862, and the papyrus of George Ebers of 1872, dating to about 1550 B.C., includes descriptions of a disease "which causes stricture in the flesh [genitalia] of a man or a woman" and "treatment for vaginitis and inflammation of the vulva and upper area of the thighs."[1a] It also notes remedies against lice infestation.

The anthropological and pathological phases of the paleopathology of Egypt were studied extensively between 1907 and 1911 by G. Elliot Smith and F. Wood Jones,[2] who investigated skeletal remains taken from that part of Nubia later flooded by the raising of the Aswan dam. Extensive studies of bones from the pre-Dynastic to Byzantine eras showed that syphilis was unknown. Subsequent studies have not shown any definite cases of syphilis in x-ray examinations of Egyptian mummies.

## OLD TESTAMENT

Some nineteenth century writers, notably Rosenbaum (1839), Buret (1891), and Proksch (1895), regarded certain passages in the Bible as references to syphilis, the most notable being the plague of Egypt (Exod. 11:1), the plague of Baal-peor (Num. 25:8), and the disease which attacked the Philistines (1 Sam. 5 and 6). Scholars of Hebrew such as Preuss[3] in 1911 refuted these views. Preuss points out that *magepha* as used in the text means an epidemic (plague). It is highly unlikely that the plague of Baal-peor, which included 24,000 victims, refers to epidemic syphilis. A later commentator[4] disagreed with Preuss and argued that the Israelites, uncircumcised at that time, had a disease like syphilis after behaving promiscuously with the Midianite women at the shrine of Baal-peor. A noted student of venereal reference in literature, Rolleston (1934)[5] argued that as prostitution and harlotry are mentioned so often in the Bible, surely if syphilis had been present at that time it would have been mentioned.

Whatever misgivings there are about syphilis, there is no doubt that urethritis, but not definitely gonorrhea, is noted in the Bible, notably in Leviticus 15. Not only is discharge in both men and women well described, but measures taken to isolate the sufferer and prevent contamination to others are thoroughly gone into. According to Brim[4] a man with a discharge from his penis, *Bosar*, was to be segregated, for the discharge made him contagious. *Tomeh* is the Hebrew word for pathological discharge. The pathological discharge *Zivo* is as thin as watery dough and is the color of the white of an egg. *Hechtim* means the discharge dries and forms a thick adherent cover, closing up the meatus of the penis.

After the discharge has ceased, the patient was to count seven successive clear days (rules were also laid down should symptoms recur). If there was no recurrence, he was to wash himself and his clothes in running water, and then he would be considered noncontagious. On the eighth day he was to make a sacrifice. Leviticus also makes the distinction between pathological discharge *Zov* and spermatorrhoea or pollution, *Schichvos zera*, "not so grave a sin," with not such a long period of segregation and less severe punishments. Washing and rinsing in water is recommended. If a man contaminates himself as a result of nocturnal emission, *Mikreh loyla*, he need only be isolated from the community for one day.

Pathological female vaginal discharges are discussed in Leviticus 15:19–33. A period of isolation for 7 days was advised. Again on the eighth day sacrifice was ordered.

Lice (Hebrew, *Kinim*) are not forgotten. They are the third of the ten scourges of Egypt enumerated in the ritual of the Passover.

## CLASSICAL ANTIQUITY

Hippocrates (460–370 B.C.) is sometimes credited with having described gonorrhea. In his *Aphorisms*, however, although there is much about urination (the flow of urine, stranguary in old men, clots in the urine, and other abnormalities) and the diseases of women, nothing really suggests gonorrhea. For example, in *Epidemics III–IV* the following description may or may not pertain to venereal matters: "Many had apththae and sores in the mouth. Fluxes about the genitals were copious, sores, tumors external and internal; the swellings which appear in the groin; watery inflammation of the eyes, chronic and painful. Growths of the eyelids, external and internal, in many cases destroying the sight which are called figs. There were also often growths and other sores, particularly in the genitals."[1b]

Later Greek and Roman writers more aptly described gonorrhea. Herodotus wrote that the Scythians who violated the shrine of Venus-Urania were attacked by the *morbus femineus*. Celsus, about A.D. 30, mentioned ulcers on the glans and prepuce and inside the urethra as well as the discharge of bloody purulent matter from the matter from the canal and ulcers of the mouth, nose, and tonsils. Since then other authors have given this different interpretations: Lancereaux (1866)[6], for instance, thought Celsus was alluding to hard chancres (syphilis) and soft sore (chancroid).

There are frank descriptions of both heterosexual and homosexual physical relationships in Roman erotic poems and epigrams in the second century but nothing adequately fits a knowledge of syphilis. Several passages in the writing of the poets Juvenal (II, 12), Martial (VI 49, VII 71, XI 15), and Carmina Priapeia (37) relate to lesions of the penis and anus, but they are of an exclusively local character and may be regarded as examples of herpes genitalis, chancroid, or lymphogranuloma venereum. Popular belief by that time had attributed anal warts (ficus) to sodomy. Oriel[7] found a possible early allusion to anal warts in Juvenal's writings.

Some nineteenth century writers tended to regard any description of skin disease in Roman times as syphilis. More modern medical historians have a more temperate view and suspect other diseases were involved. Galen (A.D. 131–201) is remembered in particular for describing satyriasis (the escape of semen without erection). In Pompeii urethral sounds have been found. Arateus the Cappadocian distinguished pathological vaginal discharge from fluor and recommended the use of simple remedies.

## EVIDENCE FOR TREPONEMAL DISEASE FROM PALEOPATHOLOGY

Some evidence for pre-Columbian syphilis in the New World has been documented. Williams (1932)[8] stated that relics have been found throughout the Americas with changes in the bones of the forehead which could be due to syphilis. Henschen (1966)[9] maintained that photographs of crania found in the Calendaria cave of Mexico had indications of tertiary syphilis and that syphilitic bone lesions have never been found in remains in Europe prior to 1493.

Yaws caused by *Treponema pertenue* is widespread in equatorial regions. It is closely related to syphilis, and infection with yaws may give some immunity to syphilis. Stewart and Spoehr (1952),[10] using carbon dating methods, described cranial periostitis probably due to yaws dated about A.D. 834 from the Mariana Islands in the western Pacific. Similar skulls have been found in Iraq dating from the first 500 years A.D. It even seems that the Persian physician Avicenna may have described a condition like yaws or bejel that still exists today in the margins of Arabia.

## THE MIDDLE AGES

Avicenna of Baghdad (980–1037), whose writings influenced so much medieval medicine, wrote at length on urethral discharge. Moses Maimonides (1135–1204), the Hispano-Jewish physician of Cordoba, described gonorrhea even more clearly: "fluid escaping without erection and without feeling of pleasure," the disease resulting from "amorousness and excesses."[1c] Descriptions of gonorrhea in the Middle Ages in Europe add little to knowledge gained from earlier times. John of Gaddesden (1320) is credited with the recognition of epididymitis and the introduction of the suspensory bandage. John of Arderne (1378) used the term "clap" to define the "certain inward heat and excoriation of the urethra,"[1c] a term still in use today.

More important descriptions of disease are records of measures taken to control gonorrhea and prostitution. In 1162 an edict was issued concerning the "Winchester Stews," the brothels of Southwark, a suburb of London which was controlled by the Bishop of Winchester: "No Stew holder to keep any women that hath the perilous infirmity of burning."[1c] (The terms *brenning, burning, ardor, ursuria, chaude pisse,* and *the hidden disease* were all used for gonorrhea in those times.) Another public edict issued in Avignon in 1347 stated that "a surgeon appointed by the authorities examine every Saturday all the whores in the house of prostitution and if one is found, who has contracted a disease from coitus, she shall be separated from the rest and live apart in order that she may not distribute her favours and may thus be prevented from conveying the disease to the youth."[1c]

It has been argued[5] that if syphilis had existed in the latter Middle Ages it would have been described by Chaucer in *The Canterbury Tales*, especially in the section of the Parson's Tale concerning "leccherie."

Similarly, there is no reference to venereal disease in Boccaccio's *Decameron* of 1353 or in the *Arabian Nights*, which was written about 50 years after Chaucer's death. It is also interesting that in the vast quantity of medieval sermon literature which deals with sexual immorality there is no indication of the likelihood of venereal disease as a consequence.

## THE OUTBREAK OF SYPHILIS IN EUROPE IN THE FIFTEENTH CENTURY

Syphilis is among the most interesting of diseases from a historical standpoint, not only because of conflicting views about its origin in Europe but because of its influence on morality and on public health and hygiene measures. The pre-Columbian (Europeanist) theory is that syphilis was somehow endemic in Europe throughout the Middle Ages, becoming pandemic at the end of the fifteenth century and venereally acquired. The Columbian (Americanist) theory is that in 1493 after the return of Christopher Columbus from the New World to Spain, his sailors brought back this new disease with them. Rodrigo Ruiz Diaz de Isla (1539), then nearly 80, wrote that as a young physician of 30 he had seen the first outbreak of this new serpentine malady, intimating that he had treated some of the crew. Of course by that time there was a considerable literature on syphilis.

The unitarian theory of E. Hudson[11] (1946) concerns yaws, a treponemal infection. Widespread in equatorial regions, it has many similarities to syphilis in its manifestations. Hudson emphasized the evolutionary relationship of yaws, pinta, endemic syphilis, and sporadic syphilis, regarding them all as varieties of one disease caused by one organism, *Treponema pallidum*. This concept considers sub-Saharan Africa to be the area where treponematosis originated.

Whatever the origin of syphilis, its passage was well described following 1495. In that year the French King Charles VIII took an army of mercenaries drawn from all the European countries and besieged Naples, which was held by Neapolitans and Spaniards under Ferdinand II. Fallopius (1523–1562) related that the Neapolitan harlots were driven out to the welcoming arms of the besiegers and before long Charles VIII had to withdraw and disband after his army became afflicted with the pox. The new disease soon appeared throughout Europe.

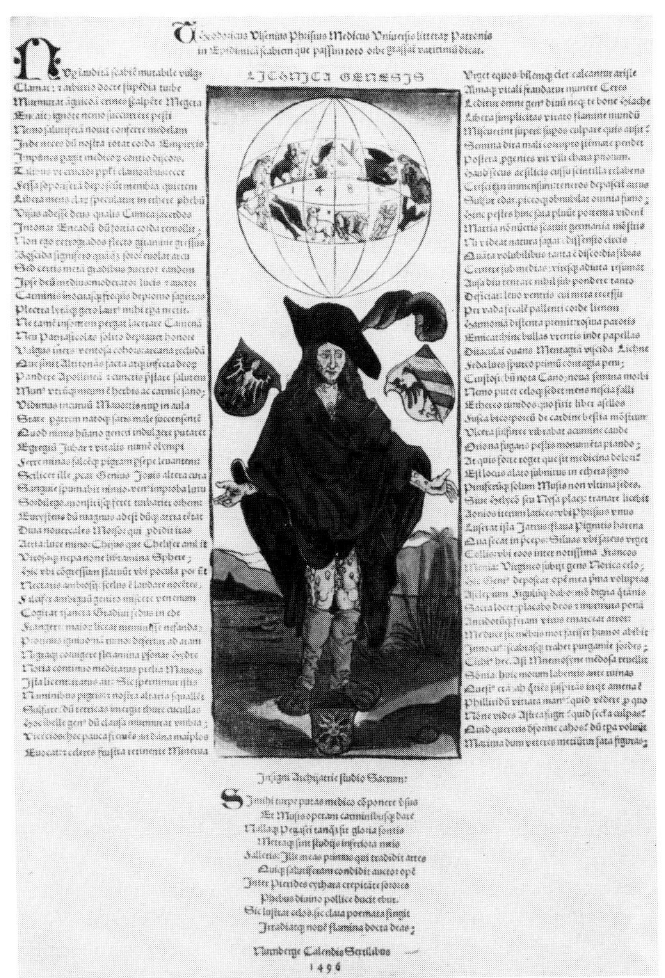

**Fig. 1-1.** *Syphilitic Man,* 1496, attributed to Albrecht Dürer, in a poem by Ulsenius.

A Malafrantzos morbo gallorum preseruatio ac Cura a Bartholomeo Stëbër Viennensi artium & medicine doctore nuper edita.

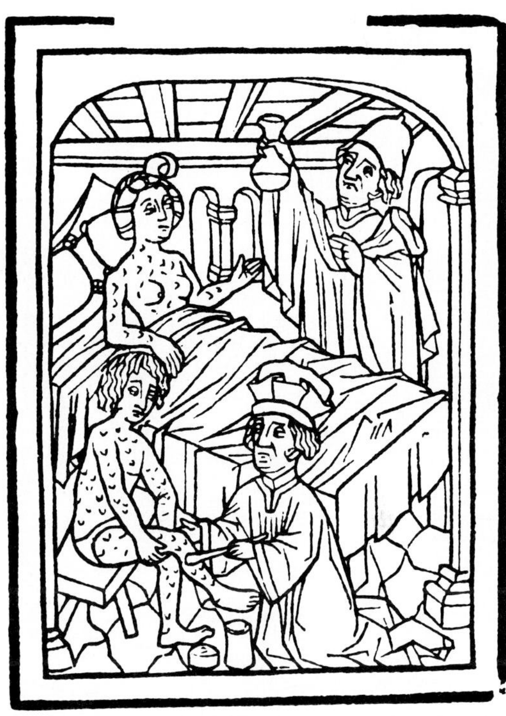

**Fig. 1-2.** Bartholomeus Steber, title page of *Malafrantzos Morbus Gallorum,* 1498. The woodcut shows treatment with mercury.

Much was written following the outbreak of 1495. In Italy, Caspare Torella (1497) called it *pudendagra* and cited its source from a chancre with inguinal lymphadenopathy through the primary and secondary stages, including osteoscopic pains and characteristic eruption, as aptly portrayed by Dürer in 1496 (Sudhoff, 1912[12]) (Fig. 1-1). Torella recommended mercury ointment (*Unguentum Saracenicum*), formerly used in various skin diseases, including leprosy, as did Steber (1498) of Vienna, who gave its differential diagnosis (Fig. 1-2). In the early days, the connection between sexual intercourse and the early stages of syphilis was not clearly understood. Perhaps it was a punishment sent by God (Gruenpeck, 1496). Or perhaps the conjunction between Saturn and Jupiter, or Saturn and Mars should be credited. Eventually its causation was well recognized. "But especially it is taken when one pocky person doth synne in lechery the one with another. All the kyndes of the pockes be infectiouse" (Andrew Boord, 1547) (Fig. 1-3).

John of Vigo (1514) in his great work on surgery described the course of the disease, recommended mercury, and gave descriptions of gummata. In 1519, Ulrich von Hutten, a young German humanist, wrote of the blessed relief he got from the effects of syphilis treated with mercury when he took *guaiacum*. Derived from a South American wood resin, it had a sudorific action. Despite his self-acclaimed cure, he died miserably of tertiary syphilis at an early age. In 1527 Jacques de Bethencourt of Rouen was the first to use the term venereal disease (*lues venerea*). In 1530 Fracastoro of Verona[13] (1484–1553) wrote the cele-

¶ Ein hübscher Tractat von dem vrsprung des Bösen Franzos. das man nennet die Wylden wärtzen. Auch ein Regiment wie man sich regiren soll in diser zeyt.

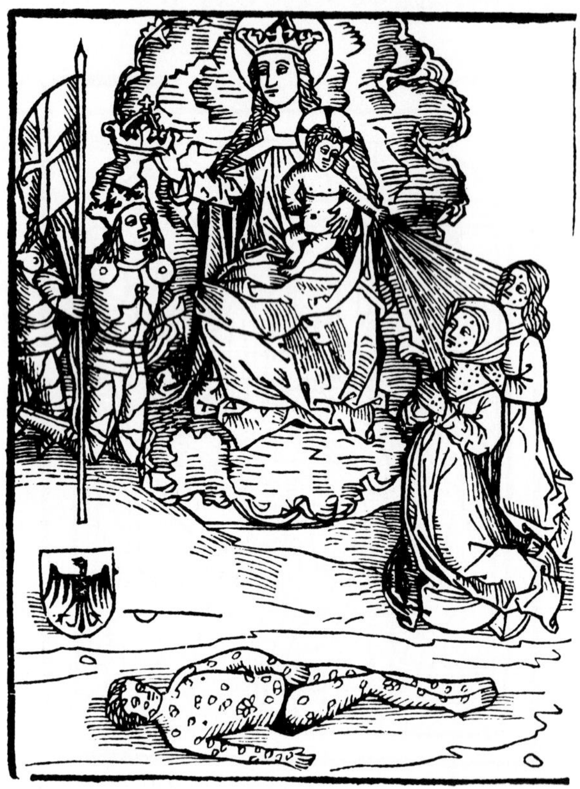

Fig. 1-3. Sebastian Brandt, title page of Gruenpeck's *De Pestilentiali Scorra sive Mala de Franczos,* Basle, 1496. The woodcut shows the Virgin and Child with two afflicted women praying and a corpse covered with syphilitic eruptions at their feet.

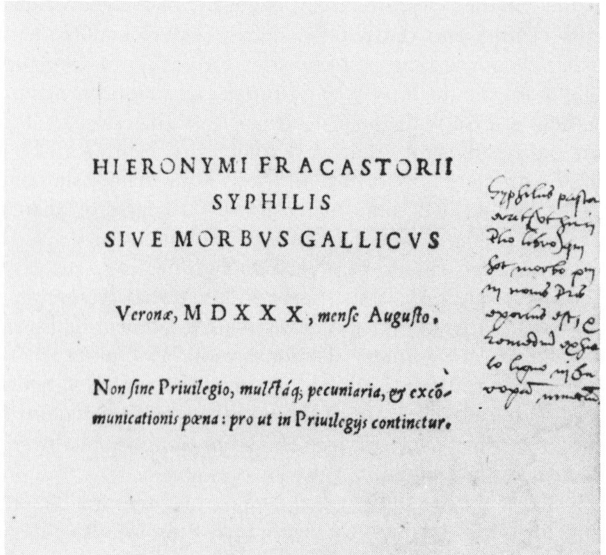

HIERONYMI FRACASTORII
SYPHILIS
SIVE MORBVS GALLICVS

*Veronæ,* M D X X X, *mense Augusto.*

*Non sine Priuilegio, mulctáq; pecuniaria, & excõmunicationis pœna: pro ut in Priuilegijs continetur.*

Fig. 1-4. The title page of Girolamo Fracastoro's *Syphilis sive Morbus Gallicus,* Verona, 1530.

brated poem "Syphilis sive Morbus Gallicus" (Fig. 1-4). Syphilis, a swineherd, was smitten by Apollo when he refused to make sacrifices to him. The term syphilis was not used in English literature until 1686, when the dramatist Nahum Tate translated Fracastoro's work. In English medical writing it was first used by Daniel Turner (1667–1740) in *Syphilis* (1717).

## CONFUSION BETWEEN SYPHILIS AND GONORRHEA

Gonorrhea and syphilis were not always regarded as different diseases. The confusion began with Bethencourt and was compounded by Paracelsus von Hohenheim (1553), who called *Morbus Gallicus* French gonorrhea and divided the disease into simple gonorrhea and virulent gonorrhea. For the next 300 years, until the French physician Philippe Ricord[14] (1838) offered the final proof, the medical world was split on the pathology of these venereal diseases. Even the celebrated English physician Thomas Sydenham (1624–1689) believed syphilis and gonorrhea were one and the same disease. The frequent association of gonorrhea with syphilis as well as the discharge due to a urethral chancre doubtless explains the tendency of the old writers to regard "clap" as the early stage and syphilis as the late stage of "the pox."

## LATER DEVELOPMENTS IN THE SIXTEENTH CENTURY

To understand the development of venereology requires an appreciation of important discoveries and progress in the field in the last 400 years.

In his posthumous work Fallopius (1564) described the indurated primary penile sore of syphilis as being typical of that disease. He differentiated between syphilitic condylomata lata and condylomata acuminata of genital warts. He also advised the use of the condom as a prophylaxis against venereal disease.

William Clowes (1543–1604) could be called the founder of English venereology. Although influenced by John of Vigo (1460–1520), he preferred the term *lues venerea* to *morbus Gallicus.* As the Master of the Barber Surgeons, he had considerable experience treating syphilis, and is quoted in 1579 as follows: "In the house of St. Bartholomew [one of the old London hospitals] very seldom but that among every twentye diseases persons are taken in, fiftene of them have the pocks."[1d] In 1579 Fernel (1506–1588) stated that the "virus" of syphilis could not pass through intact skin and introduced the concept of syphilis insontium.

An early treatment of syphilis was inunction with mercury ointment (*Unguentum Saracenicum*), as shown in Fig. 1-5. Mercury was also given by inhalation and fumigation. Fumigation was carried out in the sweating tub, or the "spital."

## SYPHILIS IN THE SEVENTEENTH AND EIGHTEENTH CENTURIES

The history of syphilis advanced slowly in the seventeenth century. Lancisi (1654–1720) in his posthumous work "De motu cordis et aneurysmatibus," (1728) correlated dilation of the heart with syphilis/aneurysma gallicum. In the same year Herman Boerhaave (1668–1738) also implicated syphilis as a cause of cardiovascular disease.

In France, Jean Astruc (1684–1766),[15] physician to Louis XV,

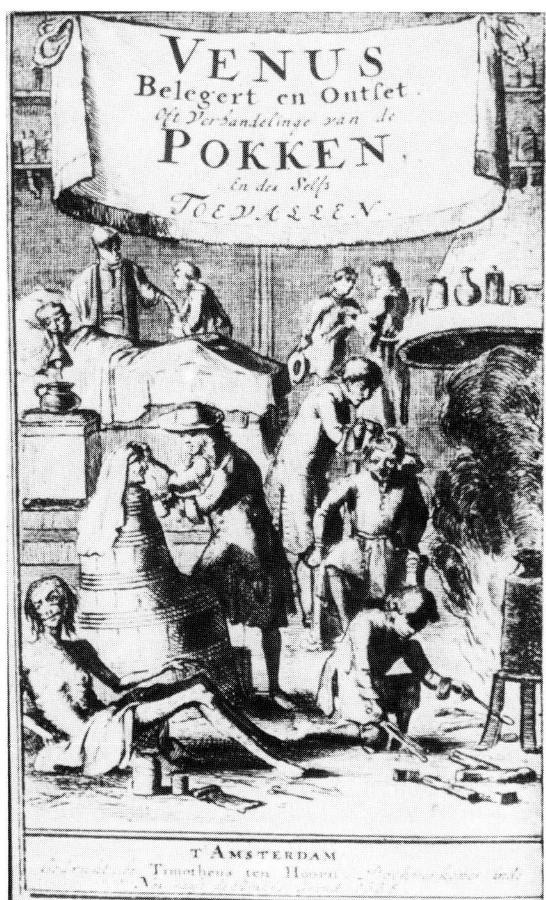


**Fig. 1-5.** The frontispiece of Stephen Blankaart's *Venus Belegert en Ontset,* Amsterdam, 1684. The drawing shows treatment of "the pox" by inhalations and inunctions.

summarized the whole corpus of knowledge on venereal disease including a bibliography in *De Morbis Venereis* (1736) favoring the Columbian origin for syphilis. Astruc was a monist, dividing venereal disease into purely local conditions and the more serious form which caused constitutional symptoms. In fact, apart from general paralysis of the insane and tabes dorsalis, he recognized all that is now known on the symptomatology of syphilis. In his book are descriptions which cannot be bettered in our own times, of condyloma acuminata, phimosis, paraphimosis, and herpes genitalis, including homosexually contracted anal herpes. Astruc was an advocate of mercury, and his influence spread throughout Europe during the next hundred years.

Gerhard Van Swieten (1700–1772), a pupil of Boerhaave, reinvigorated medicine in Vienna after 1749 under the patronage of the Empress Maria Theresa. In venereology he popularized Sanchez's mercury sublimate taken in small doses in brandy—thus preventing indiscriminate ptyalisation. He taught that no organ escaped the influence of the venereal poison, being a cause of "gummy tumours, exostoses, deep seated pains, apoplexy, epilepsy, blindness, deafness and paralysis" (Van Swieten, 1742).

In medieval times, lazar houses or locks came into being for the treatment of leprosy. As fewer people succumbed to that disease, the locks were turned over for the cure of venereal disease. In the 1600s St. Bartholomew's had seven scattered on the outskirts of London, but by 1760 the last two were closed. The administrators of new voluntary hospitals such as the Westminster and the Middlesex forbade the admission of patients with syphilis. In 1746 a philanthropic surgeon of St. George's Hospital, William Bromfield, founded the London Lock Hospital, an institution which existed for the treatment of venereal disease until the advent of the National Health Service in 1948. Almost every major European city had such special hospitals from the middle of the eighteenth century on.

## MONISTS VS. DUALISTS

When John Hunter (1728–1793) wrote *A Treatise on the Venereal Disease* (1786), it was not his greatest work, but his eminence was such that a great deal of importance was attached to it. He described the venereal sore characterized by indolent induration (and named after him), but he failed to appreciate the soft sore (later chancroid). He did not believe in the contagiousness of secondary syphilis, a view later held by Philippe Ricord. He also denied the hereditary transmission of the disease which had been previously believed, although in the last part of his work *Disease Resembling Syphilis,* he recorded not only yaws but several examples of probable congenital syphilis.

As a disciple of Astruc, Hunter's most important error was adhesion to the monist (unity) doctrine. In a famous experiment in 1767, Hunter, to prove the single identity of gonorrhea and syphilis, is supposed to have inoculated himself with the matter of gonorrhea with a stylet onto his prepuce and glans. Unfortunately, he chose the inoculum from a patient suffering from both syphilis and gonorrhea—and it has been suggested that he actually contracted syphilis. Recently, Qvist[16] and Dempster[17] argue that since the experiment is described in the third person, it may have been done to a patient. Hunter thought that the only difference between the two diseases depended on the nature of the surface to which the poison was applied: that it caused ulceration when it acted on a cutaneous surface, but only a purulent discharge without breach of surface when applied to a mucous membrane; and that the morbid secretions in either case might give rise to either set of symptoms according to the structure with which they come in contact.

In Edinburgh, Benjamin Bell (1749–1806) in "A Treatise on Gonorrhea virulenta and Lues venerea" (1793)—following the work of a dissertation by Francis Balfour (1767), who was much influenced by the pathologist Giovanni Morgagni (1682–1771)—presented strong arguments for the duality theory. A major point was that syphilis required mercury for a cure while gonorrhea did not (Fig. 1-6). The symptoms and consequences of the two diseases were different: gonorrhea was a local disease while syphilis was not; the inoculation of gonorrhea and syphilis between persons did not produce the other disease, and even in severe cases of gonorrhea no lues ensued; and no stage of pox had ever produced gonorrhea. Bell carried out experiments on three medical students to prove his arguments!

Without elaborating on the ethics of endangering human lives, the witty American-born Philippe Ricord (1800–1889) was able to show conclusively, by experiments in 1838 in Paris on 667 mental hospital patients, that gonorrhea and syphilis were different diseases.[14] Ricord also classified syphilis into three stages: primary, secondary, tertiary. Founder of a remarkable School of Venereology of France, he was once described as "the Voltaire of pelvic literature—a sceptic as to the morals of the race in general, who would have submitted Diana to treatment with his mineral specifics and ordered a course of blue pills (mercurials) to the vestal virgins."[17a]

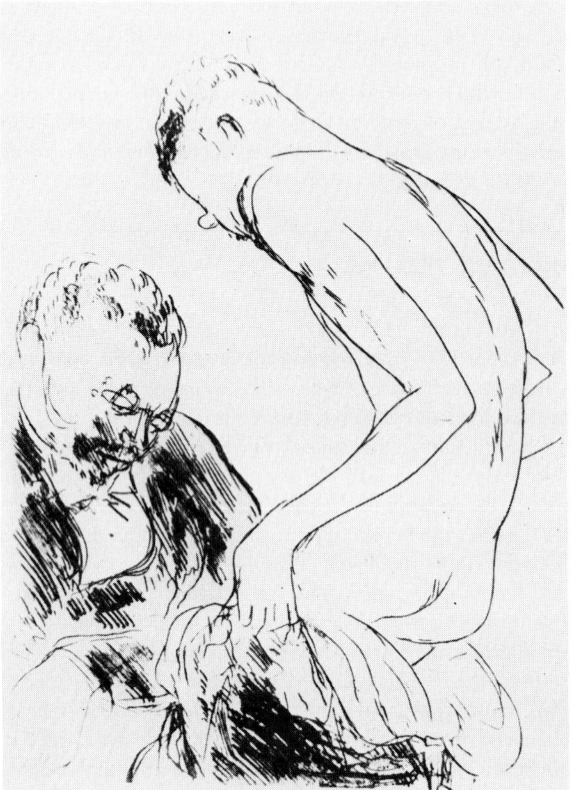

**Fig. 1-6.** André Dunoyer de Segonzac (b. 1884, d. 1974), *Medical Examination in the Hôpital Saint Louis. (From Vogt H: Medizinische Karaikature von 1800 bis zur Gegenwart. Munich, Lehmann, 1960.)*

## THE DECLINE OF MERCURY

That many doctors in Britain in the period between Bell and Ricord still accepted the old doctrine is shown by the warning which Sir Astley Cooper (1768–1841) gave in his lectures on venereal diseases at St. Thomas' Hospital in 1824. He declared that "a man who gives mercury in gonorrhea deserves to be flogged out of the profession because he must be quite ignorant of the principle in which the disease is cured."[17b]

Emphasis on the dangers of mercury, which meant that some surgeons forbade its use, led to a search for other drugs. Robert Williams of St. Thomas' Hospital, London, had used potassium iodine in secondary syphilis from 1831, but it was left to William Wallace (1791–1837) of Dublin in 1835 to popularize its use in tertiary syphilis. The ethical standards of that time are again illustrated by the fact that Wallace deliberately inoculated his healthy outpatients with the secondary eruptions of syphilitic cases in order to prove that Ricord was wrong in teaching that these cases were not infected. Another Dublin doctor, Abraham Colles (1773–1843) in 1837 stated the principle later known as Colles' law, that is, that a syphilitic child cannot infect its mother.

## PROGRESS IN THE NINETEENTH CENTURY

Descriptions of congenital syphilis have been cited by Torella (1497) and Pietro Mattioli (1533). There had been much controversy over its manifestations. Boerhave had described different sources of infection. Astruc[15] proposed complicated theories as to how much the father and mother contributed to the progeny. Rosen von Rosenstein (1764) had classified its symptoms and signs.

In 1854 Paul Diday[18] codified the whole of congenital syphilis to that time, with excellent descriptions of clinical features and discussions on prognosis and therapy. In this view, the mother of a syphilitic child was usually but not always syphilitic. He advocated treatment of the apparently healthy child born to syphilitic parents. From 1857 to 1863 Jonathan Hutchinson (1828–1913)[19] described in detail all the entities that came to be known as Hutchinson's triad (interstitial keratitis, notched teeth, labyrinthine disease). It was actually Alfred Fournier (Fig. 1-7) (1832–1914) in "La syphilis héréditaire tardive" (1886)[20] who coined the phrase "the triad of Hutchinson." H. Clutton of St. Thomas' Hospital described the rare symmetrical painless knee joints in older children in 1886.

From the time of Boerhaave (1728) it was known that syphilis had an effect on the constitution, especially the central nervous system. Moritz Romberg's great work on the nervous system of 1846, translated into English by the physician E. Sieveking in 1853, contains a classic description of tabes dorsalis, diminution of muscular sense, numbness of feet, swaying on standing with eyes closed (Romberg's sign), insecurity of gait, especially in the dark, urinary difficulties, girdle sensation, and lightning pains in the legs. The Victorian neurologist Sir William Gowers (1892) credits Argyll Robertson (1869) of Edinburgh with noticing the pupils of the eyes peculiar to tabes dorsalis. Even so, an eminent neurologist, Jean Martin Charcot (1825–1893), described tabetic arthropathy in frank locomotor ataxia in 1869—and stated that syphilis had nothing to do with the disease.

Eventually Fournier proposed in 1875[21] that syphilis was the cause of the symptoms of paralysis, motor incoordination, and progressive locomotor ataxia. Fournier formed the concept of parasyphilis: "those diseases of which syphilis is essentially the

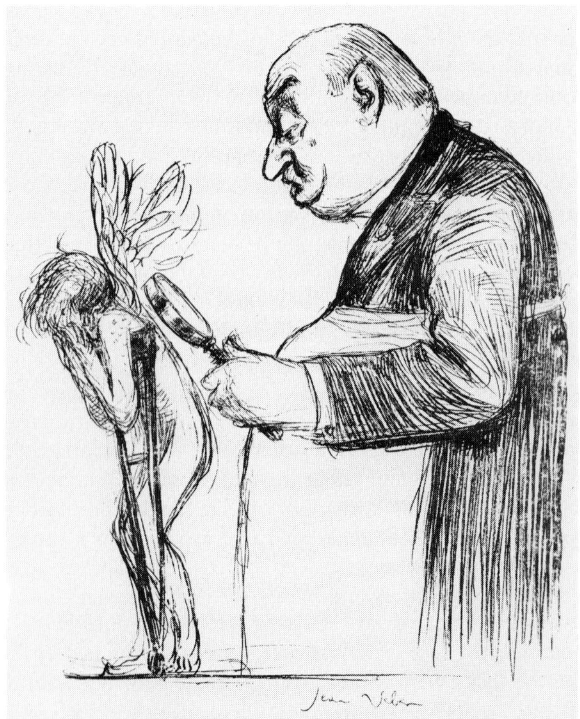

**Fig. 1-7.** Caricature by Alfred Fournier (1832–1914), *Looking through a magnifying glass at a little winged girl on crutches.* From Le Gotha Medical, not dated (probably from the early twentieth century).

cause, but which are not directly the result of the syphilitic virus, namely general paralysis, tabes dorsalis, tabo paresis and primary optic atrophy."[21a]

In the treatment of syphilis, subcutaneous injections of mercury were introduced in 1864 by Angelo Scrarenzio of Pavia, being taken up in London by Berkeley Hill in 1866. Adolf Jarisch (1850–1902), a pupil of Hebra, described the reaction now known as Jarisch-Herxheimer (the latter working on it with Krause in 1902) in 1895, "the observation of a reaction whereby in the first days of mercurial inunctions for syphilitic roseola there is an exaggeration of the clinical manifestations."[22]

The treatment of venereal diseases in Britain for most of the nineteenth century was in the hands of surgeons. Such was John Hunter's influence that even after Ricord had differentiated gonorrhea from syphilis in 1838 his views took a long time to be accepted by medical men treating venereal disease, with few exceptions. As late as 1876 James R. Lane, a surgeon at the London Lock Hospital, stated "There is no such thing as a specific gonorroheal poison."[22a]

Finally in 1879, Albert Neisser (1854–1916) working as an assistant in the dermatology section at Breslau, used Koch's staining methods to conclusively describe the causal agent of gonorrhea, and the concept of one microbe for that disease was generally accepted. Neisser[23] (1879) found the characteristic organism in 35 cases of gonorrhea but failed to find it in pus from chancres or simple vaginal discharges; he also made the important discovery that the gonococcus could be found in ophthalmia neonatorum.

The realization of any cause of urethritis other than gonococcal came slowly. The introduction of Gram's stain[24] (1884), culture of the gonococcus by Leo Leistikow[25] (1862) and Ernst von Bumm[26] (1885) and the fermentation tests of W. Elser and F. Huntoon[27] in 1909 for the differentiation of other *Neisseria,* aided in the realization of nongonococcal urethritis. Meanwhile, in the field of gonorrhea progress was being made. In 1881 Karl Credé[28] (1819–1892) of Leipzig, who began research on neonatal eye disease in those born to mothers with vaginal discharge in 1854, introduced instillation of silver nitrate into the eyes of the newborn to prevent gonococcal ophthalmia, in those days a common cause of blindness. In 1885 Eugen Fraenkel[29] showed gonococcus to be a cause of vulvo-vaginitis in children. In 1888 Ernst Finger[30] of Vienna, in a monograph which ran into many editions and was translated into English, summarized all the known knowledge on gonorrhea in women. Ernst Wertheim[31] in the 1890s demonstrated the gonococcus in the Fallopian tubes in acute salpingitis and brought to attention the difficulty of diagnosis of gonorrhea in women. To end the century, William S. Thayer[32] and George Blumer in 1896 found the organism in gonococcal endocarditis.

F. X. Swediaur[33] (1784) found that injection of ammonia into the urethra would produce a urethritis, and other authors, such as Carmichael[34] (1842), in Dublin and even Alfred Fournier[35] (1866) realized that there was a form of urethritis that did not resemble venereal clap in its true sense. After the finding of the gonococcus by Neisser[23] in 1879 it was presumed at first that all cases of urethritis must be gonococcal. Improved laboratory methods disproved this.

In 1907 L. Halberstaedter[36] and S. von Prowazek found inclusions in the eye in infants with neonatal conjunctivitis and then from genital discharge in the mothers. Finally K. Linder[37] (1909) made a great advance into the etiology of nongonococcal urethritis when he demonstrated initial bodies and elementary bodies morphologically indistinguishable from those seen in inclusion blenorrhea in urethral discharge.

## MINOR STDS IN THE NINETEENTH CENTURY

During the nineteenth century the recognition and importance of other sexually transmitted diseases emerged. Thomas Bateman (1778–1821),[38] in the fourth edition of *A Practical Synopsis of Cutaneous Disease* (1814), described herpes praeputalis (genitalis): "It occurs in a situation where it is liable to occasion a practical mistake of serious consequences to the patient. The progress of the herpetic clusters when seated on the prepuce, so closely resembles that of chancre, that it may be doubted whether it hasn't been frequently confounded with the latter."[38] He described the prodromal itching, formation, and breakdown of vesicles.

The eminent surgeon Jonathan Hutchinson, apart from having a great knowledge of syphilis, showed how well the problem of herpes genitalis was recognized in those days without modern diagnostic facilities. He wrote in 1887, "Herpetic vesicles may occur on the genitals of either sex quite independently of any venereal cause, and if they have occurred once they are very prone to occur again." And his comment—"yet it is certain that those who have so suffered are infinitely more prone to syphilis"[19] is worthy of attention.

Benjamin Brodie (1783–1862) in 1818 in his textbook on diseases of the joints described what is now considered to be Reiter's syndrome. His case was a man of 45 with urethral discharge, fever, recurrent joint swellings, and conjunctivitis. He mentioned similar cases he had seen in practice at the time, as did Astley Cooper in 1824. Hans Reiter's[39] case of 1916 would now be considered more likely to be more postdysenteric arthritis.

Alfred F. Donné[40] (1801–1878), an ardent advocate of the microscope in medicine, was able to describe in 1836 trichomonas vaginalis, thinking at first that it was the causal agent of gonorrhea. He was the first to describe a living organism in a pathological condition.

The French- and German-speaking countries vie for landmarks in the history of discoveries in scabies. Among the beneficial results of the French Revolution was the reorganization of medical education in Paris. In 1801 the Hôpital Saint Louis became a center specializing in skin diseases. Jean Louis Alibert (1768–1837), the teacher of Ricord and father of modern French dermatology, developed his polyclinic for research. He held out for an animalcular origin of scabies and was proved correct by one of his students, S. F. Renucci, in 1834. Johann Ernst Wichmann of Hanover, in 1786, and E. von Lobes in Prague, 1791, had described the acarus. But in German-speaking countries the belief in a psoric dyscaria as the cause of scabies persisted.

From about 1840, under the leadership of Josef Skoda (1805–1881) and Karl von Rokitansky (1804–1878), the Vienna Medical School became the foremost in central Europe. Ferdinand von Hebra (1816–1880) was appointed to the lowly post in charge of the Kratzestation (scabies station). Using the microscope and by autoinoculation ("I was plagued by a strong itch that spread over my entire body"), he was able to show conclusively in 1844 that the mite was the cause of scabies.[41] Hebra was the foremost influence in dermatology in German-speaking countries, classifying skin disease on the basis of underlying pathology. An advocate of mercury for syphilis, he founded a clinic for syphilis in Vienna. It was placed under the charge of Sigmund von Ilanor (1810–1883), a refuter of the unitarian views on venereal disease, who also recognized the dangers of gonococcal infection for both sexes—a new idea at that time.

J. Wilkinson[42] (1849) in England observed that vaginal thrush depended on a mycotic etiology. Later work by Robin and Haussmann in France in the 1860s and 1870s confirmed this.

Ricord, great man that he was, did not recognize at first the difference between simple (soft) sore and syphilitic chancres. Indeed it was not until 1859[43] that he realized that secondary syphilitic lesions were contagious. Ricord, however, had realized that if matter from a soft sore was inoculated, it did not produce constitutional symptoms but could be cured by topical application. He still insisted that it was syphilis. It was left to Leon Bassereau[44] (1811–1888) in 1852 to establish soft sore as a separate entity. Joseph Pierre Rollet (1824–1894)[45] in 1866 pointed out that a mixed sore could exist both syphilitic and chancroidal. Finally in Italy, Augusto Ducrey (1860–1940)[46] in 1888 was able to demonstrate a causal organism for chancroid (*Haemophilus ducreyi*).

The development of the recognition of chancroid led to a curious line of treatment called syphilization. It was stated that smallpox could be prevented by vaccinating with cowpox. Why not try to cure syphilis by inoculation with pus from a soft sore (erroneously thought to be a form of syphilis)? Auzias-Turenne about 1850 started patients on a course of multiple inoculations with pus from a soft sore, reinoculating so that the whole body was covered. It had its vogue but was soon given up as dangerous and useless.

## PROSTITUTION AND VENEREAL DISEASE IN THE NINETEENTH CENTURY

Prostitution can be traced from earliest times. It is recorded in the Old and New Testaments, and the history of ancient Greece and Rome is replete with its instances. Mention has been made in previous parts of this chapter of attempts at its control in earlier times.

By the nineteenth century, with the concept of the nation-state and the regulation by the state of various aspects of a citizen's life, the relationship of prostitution to venereal disease takes on new importance. In Paris, registration with the police was required. The number of prostitutes was probably underestimated at about 30,000. Alexandre J.-B. Parent-Duchatelet (1790–1836)[47], a pioneer in epidemiology, not only tabulated the social origins of prostitutes—where they came from, their former trades, and where they lived—but noted that syphilis, scabies, gonorrhea, and tumors of the uterus were all much more frequent among them than in the average woman in Paris.

Throughout Europe only a fine line divided the activities of some domestic servants and casual prostitution. As might be expected, a high incidence of syphilis was noted. Both herpes genitalis and pelvic inflammatory disease were common.

Rules were instituted in 1792 in Berlin to regulate prostitution but they still did not stop its growth. By 1840 Berlin's total population was approximately 350,000. Being a garrison town, police estimated its large population of unmarried men were serviced by at least 26 brothels. The Chârité became the main hospital dealing with syphilitics.

As London grew, it was thought that by the mid-century there were 50,000 venereal patients per annum. It was estimated that at any one time 500 of the 50,000 prostitutes in that city would have syphilis. The extent of venereal disease in the British Army was thought to be 1 in 5, and in the British Navy, 1 in 7.

In New York,[48] by midcentury, a great deal was written on prostitution and venereal disease. Prostitutes were not only native-born but immigrants. The population in 1855 was 630,000 and it was thought that prostitutes were 1 in 200 of the population. All the major hospitals, such as New York and Bellevue, as well as a number of street dispensaries every year recorded increasing cases of syphilis.

In 1914 Abraham Flexner[49] at the instigation of John D. Rockefeller wrote his masterly work *Prostitution in Europe*, which summed up all there was to know, not only about facts and figures of prostitution, regulations and orders on prostitution, but about prostitution and disease. Flexner noted that even when regulation occurred, examination of prostitutes was often badly performed, in unhygienic conditions, with little emphasis on the recent advances in the knowledge and treatment of gonorrhea or syphilis of the time. Only the clinics for the surveillance of venereal disease in Cologne, Hamburg, Frankfurt, Stockholm, and Budapest were commended. In centers in Vienna and Paris, facilities were antiquated, shocking, and often more like prisons. The same speculum was frequently used on every patient, and inspections were rushed.

## THE MODERN PERIOD OF SYPHILIS

After the 1850s enormous progress was made in the clinical observations of syphilis, not only by the doctors who spent most of their time studying venereology—Hutchinson of the London Hospital, Fournier in Paris, Friedrich W. von Baerensprung in Berlin, Sigmund von Ilanor and Isidor Neumann in Vienna—but by the physicians who were interested in the systemic aspects of syphilis—Samuel Wilks of Guy's Hospital or Hughlings Jackson at the London Hospital, for example. At the same time the new science of microbiology was making enormous progress in Europe. New scientific methods began to bring the knowledge of syphilis from mere clinical observation to exact diagnosis and rational treatment.

Between 1875 and 1877 Edwin Klebs (1834–1914)[50] of Prague had observed spirochetes in human syphilitic material and may have transmitted the disease to monkeys. Spiral organisms had also been described in erosive balanoposthitis by Berdal[51] and Bataille in Paris (1891). Experimental syphilis was reborn when Elie Metchnikoff[52] and Pierre P. E. Roux (1903) showed that syphilis could be consistently transmitted to chimpanzees. At that time it was thought that syphilis might be caused by a protozoon. Fritz R. Schaudinn (1871–1906), a protozoologist, collaborated with Erich Hoffman (1868–1959) in examining specimens of preparations of primary and secondary syphilis stained with aniline dye. On March 3, 1905, in Chârité Berlin, Schaudinn was able to demonstrate spirochetes in one of Hoffman's slides, a specimen taken from a papule of the right labia in a 25-year-old patient with secondary syphilis.[53] In the same year Aldo Castellani (1877–1971), working in Ceylon, described the spirochete (now *T. pertenue*) in yaws.[54] By 1906 Karl Landsteiner (1868–1943)[55] and Viktor Mucha were able to demonstrate *T. pallidum* by dark field methods. Although it had been felt for many years that general paralysis of the insane was a manifestation of syphilis, it was not until 1913 that Hideyo Noguchi (1876–1928)[56] and Joseph Moore (1879), using a silver method, were able to demonstrate *T. pallidum* in the brains of 12 cases of general paralysis of the insane.

The science of immunology was also born in the latter years of the nineteenth century. Jules Bordet (1870–1961) and Octave Gengou (1875–1957)[57] defined the complement fixation test in 1901, by means of which an infection could be diagnosed by finding its antibody in the serum. August von Wassermann

(1866–1925),[58] using a crude extract of the liver of a syphilitic infant, was able to show in 1906 the value of the complement fixation test in the diagnosis of syphilis. It was not, however, until 1907 that Karl Landsteiner and Rudolf Müller[59] in Vienna could explain the principle underlying the Wassermann reaction. Although many different serologic tests for syphilis were devised, it was not until the early 1940s that it was fully realized that many diseases could be responsible for a positive Wassermann reaction. The introduction of the first test for specific antibody, the treponemal immobilization test by Robert A. Nelson and Manfred M. Mayer[60] (1949), started an era of more accurate serologic diagnosis.

From the first epidemic manifestations of syphilis at the end of the fifteenth century the armamentarium of treatment had mainly depended on mercury, which at the most has a very weak treponemacidal activity in vivo. Iodines had been used especially in gummatous syphilis from 1936 onward. In 1891 Paul Ehrlich (1854–1915) reported the successful treatment of malaria with methylene blue, and from 1904 until his death in 1915 he worked continuously to produce synthetic agents which would cure infections. His work showed arsenicals to be promising, especially in trypanosomal infections. In 1907 Ehrlich patented the 606th compound synthesized, which was named Salvarsan, and later arsphenamine. By 1909 it was found to be largely effective in syphilis in animals, and on April 19, 1910, Ehrlich[61] announced that arsphenamine could cure syphilis in humans. He was besieged by doctors from all over the world for his "magic bullet," *therapeutica magnans*. Ehrlich refused to supply the drug unless the recipient was a trained syphilologist and had adequate laboratory and clinical facilities.

In 1887 Julius W. von Jauregg (1857–1940) suggested that therapeutically induced fever might be useful in the treatment of psychotic patients[62]. He advocated malaria and erysipelas but the latter proved unsatisfactory. In 1912 his satisfactory results for treating paresis with mercury-iodine combined with Koch's old tuberculin were published.[63] In 1917,[64] while looking after soldiers invalided from Macedonia, a man with malaria was accidentally admitted to one of Von Jauregg's beds. Instead of being given quinine straight away, drops of his malarial blood were scarified into the skin of three paretics. The successful results were published in 1921. Malaria therapy became the main method of treating general paralysis of the insane until it was superseded by penicillin 25 years later.

While not as active as arsenicals, bismuth, first suggested for use in syphilis in the nineteenth century, was found to be effective by R. Sazerac and Constantin Levaditi (1874–1953) in 1922.[65] Until the advent of penicillin, the alternative use of arsenicals and bismuth became a popular treatment for syphilis. Bismuth is hardly ever used now.

After the discovery in 1932 by Gerhard Domagk that the azodye, prontosil, could protect mice from death due to streptococcal septicemia,[66] the sulphonamides were rapidly developed. They were soon successfully used in the treatment of gonorrhea, which, however, became resistant to sulphonamides during the Second World War—luckily just about the time penicillin was being developed. The use of penicillin in the treatment of syphilis was first reported by John F. Mahoney (1889–1957) and coworkers; "Four patients with primary lesions were treated with 25,000 units of the drug intramuscularly at 4-hour intervals night and day for 8 days. The chancres all became darkfield negative within sixteen hours."[67] Penicillin still remains the main antibiotic in the treatment of syphilis. Its use and the advent of other antimicrobials in succeeding years has altered our conception of control of venereal diseases, not least in the attitudes of the public to those once taboo infections.

## VENEREOLOGY IN THE UNITED KINGDOM IN THE TWENTIETH CENTURY

The first ten years of the century were marked by amazing discoveries in the field of syphilis, all from Germany: the discovery of the spirochete (1905),[53] the Wassermann reaction (1906),[58] and the discovery of Salvarsan by Ehrlich (1909).[61] Characteristically the British reaction was makeshift.

The Lock (venereal disease) Hospitals did sterling work often with very limited means. Poor law (public charity) institutions were on the whole quite appalling in their treatment of venereal disease.

A Royal Commission[1] on Venereal Diseases was set up in 1913 to consider parliamentary acts concerned with venereal disease since 1864, review the prevalence and effects together with means of alleviation and prevention, and recommend action to be taken. Its report, published in 1916, revealed some startling facts, including the high mortality rate from late syphilis and such morbidity statistics for syphilis as 10 percent of London working class males and 25 percent of infantile blindness due to gonococcal ophthalmia.

Very few royal commissions have had such widespread effects as that of 1916. Sir William Osler (1914), one of the witnesses, had stated that "each medical student should pass through a venereal or genito-urinary clinic. . . . A great many people who would not go to a special venereal clinic would go willingly to a genito-urinary clinic." His evidence has become generally accepted.

Despite the stringencies of the Great War, the Public Health (Venereal Diseases) Regulations of 1916 recommended that county and borough councils organize free and confidential treatment for sufferers at convenient hours, duties taken over by the National Health Service in 1948. In 1917, the Venereal Diseases Act prohibited, under penalty, unqualified persons from treating these diseases, and forbade advertisements by persons other than local authorities concerning their treatment or prevention. The same act defined venereal disease as syphilis, gonorrhea, and soft sore (chancroid).

From 1942 to 1947 a wartime emergency measure was taken: Defense Regulation 33B, whereby a Medical Officer of Health could require a person to be compulsorily examined—and if found to be infected, treated—if reported as being the source of infection by two others.

A little-known statutory instrument is the National Health Service (Venereal Diseases) Regulation in 1974. Confidentiality is reinforced with respect to persons examined or treated for any sexually transmitted disease and also extends the scope of the service so as to include *all* sexually transmitted diseases.

Since 1917 the clinic system under the control of specialists in venereal diseases came into being. From 1925 on, national statistics for syphilis and gonorrhea have been collected from throughout the country. Statistics have also been obtained for nongonococcal urethritis, now called nonspecific genital infection, from 1951 on, and for a variety of other sexually transmitted infections since 1971.

The Medical Society for the Study of Venereal Diseases was founded in 1922. Many other countries have societies for the study of sexually transmitted diseases. In some European countries the professional organizations for the study of venereal diseases are combined with national societies for the study of dermatovenereology.

International cooperation within the medical profession in the field of venereology has a long history. The International Union Against the Venereal Diseases and Treponematoses was founded in 1923 and meets regularly throughout the world, not only to discuss new advances in this field but to formulate policies and advise governments and international organizations, such as the World Health Organization, about the control of sexually transmitted diseases. Recently many other international conferences have been convened to study problems caused by viral sexually transmitted diseases and AIDS.

## STDS IN THE UNITED STATES

The recorded history of venereal diseases in the United States is of fairly recent origin. In 1778 Congress decreed that any officer would be fined 10 dollars and any enlisted man, 4 dollars who was admitted to a hospital with a venereal disease.[68] Unfortunately, this encouraged stigmatization where venereal diseases were concerned and adversely affected the regulation of these diseases over the next 150 years in the services. Data on venereal disease incidence in the U.S. Army go back to 1820. In the Mexican, Civil, and Spanish wars and in the years between them no special measures for venereal disease control were undertaken. The rates for the U.S. Army in peacetime were between 50 and 75 per 1000 strength, doubling or trebling at time of war.[69]

In the nineteenth century, prostitution and venereal disease was an enormous problem, especially in New York. Half of all prostitutes were thought to have been infected with syphilis. By the 1890s there were six venereal disease wards in the New York City Hospital.[48]

As early as 1874[70] it was estimated that 1 in 20 of the U.S. population was infected with syphilis and that the life expectancy of a prostitute was at the most 5 years, the problem being compounded by alcoholism. Gonorrhea was also recognized as a serious cause of chronic morbidity. Emil Noeggerath[71] in 1872 wrote that about 90 percent of sterile women were married to husbands who had contracted gonorrhea either before or during their marriages.

An eminent contemporary authority was Prince Albert Morrow (1846–1913). After graduation, like many of his peers, he studied further in Europe and translated Fournier's classic *Syphilis and Marriage*[72] in 1880. In 1882 he was appointed clinical lecturer at New York University and in 1884 became Professor of Genito-urinary Diseases. An early epidemiologist and a scathing critic of those in the medical profession who were complacent about the problem of venereal disease, he recognized the underestimation of syphilis and gonorrhea in the population.

Louis Duhring (1845–1913) of Philadelphia, a dermatologist who studied in Vienna, Paris, and London, also wrote on clinical aspects of syphilis, especially its congenital effects. Like most physicians of that time, he recommended mercury salts in a syrup together with inunction with mercury. Another physician of the pre-Salvarsan era, Charles M. Smith (1867–1938) of the Massachusetts General Hospital, not only used mercury but was an exponent of potassium iodine, especially in tertiary syphilis. Philadelphia was blessed with good dermato-venereologists, another notable being Henry Wile (1857–1887),[73] who in the 1880s visited and reported on the skin clinic of Hebra in Vienna and the treatment of syphilis at the Chârité in Berlin, further emphasizing the close links between European training and the development of medical learning in the United States.

During this time the Social Hygiene Movement, which tried to motivate public opinion about syphilis, had been growing. The dangers of venereal disease were being recognized in the armed forces and in prostitutes as well as the public as a whole. In 1905 P. A. Morrow[74] founded the American Society for Sanitary and Moral Prophylaxis. In 1910 the Mann Act forbade the transportation of women across state lines for immoral purposes, i.e., prostitution.

As early as 1876 the American Medical Association had considered extending public health control techniques to the treatment of venereal disease. It had to wait till 1912 when California extended its contagious disease reporting to venereal diseases. By 1917 only nine states had started similar reporting.

## WORLD WAR I AND BEYOND

All the nations involved in World War I took measures to control venereal diseases among their troops, to a lesser extent by regulating the prostitutes to whom they resorted. At various times up to one quarter of some British and French regiments were noneffective from venereal disease. The U.S. Army had learned a few lessons by the time it went into the war of 1917. In the American Expeditionary Force in France, 246 venereal disease control officers were employed, 1 to each 10,000 troops. As a result, after an initial rise the incidence rate of venereal disease fell to below peacetime figures. There were enormous problems between the active approach to the control and the cure of syphilis by the American military medical authorities and the laissez-faire attitude of their French counterparts. H. H. Young[74] of Johns Hopkins Hospital observed that of the allied armies in France the policies of the New Zealand Expeditionary Force were the best. Condoms and chemical prophylaxis were provided and there were continued medical inspections.

Although the venereal disease corps was disbanded between the two world wars, the incidence of venereal disease in both the army and the navy continued to fall until 1940. By the beginning of World War II,[68] it was noticed that the greatest syphilis rates were in the southern states—in the army at home. In the navy, the West Indies, Panama Canal Zone, and the Philippines stations all had a high incidence of venereal disease.

## CIVILIAN PROGRESS AFTER WORLD WAR I

After demobilization, the U.S. Congress in the 1920s cut funding for venereal disease services and by 1922 discontinued appropriations for the state diagnosis and treatment clinics—because of the erroneous assumption that the problem had disappeared. Meanwhile in Europe the League of Red Cross Societies founded a division of social hygiene concerned with control of venereal disease. By 1923 the International Union Against the Venereal Diseases and Treponematoses evolved from this division, the first international voluntary organization to encourage official and voluntary efforts against syphilis and gonorrhea. The Union took a major role in the negotiations of the 1924 Brussels Agreement, under which signatory nations pledged to provide facilities for the diagnosis and treatment of venereal disease among merchant seamen in a number of large international ports.

With the onset of the Great Depression, funding for venereal disease control dropped even further. Thomas Parran (1892–1968) who had been Chief of the Venereal Disease Division of the Public Health Service and in 1930 State Health Commissioner for New York, realized the enormous problems which would be encountered if funding was not forthcoming for venereal disease control in all its forms.

In November 1934 Columbia Broadcasting Corporation arranged for Parran to speak on a radio program about future goals in public health and major problems in that field. When the powers-that-be realized that Parran planned to mention syphilis and gonorrhea, he was not allowed to go on the air. Parran pointed out in a press release the hypocrisy inherent in standards which allowed programs with various degrees of sexual innuendo to go on but which censored plain facts.

Thomas Parran instigated a public health campaign to make the public more aware of the dangers of venereal disease. In 1937 he wrote *Shadow on the Land: Syphilis*[75] in which he attacked the American medical and public health communities for a conspiracy of silence. There were no accurate estimates of prevalence or incidence. Cases of venereal disease were frequently not reported as required by law. Death certification as to venereal disease was tardy. Parran estimated in the late 1930s that 1 million potential mothers had previously had syphilis and that 60,000 children were born each year with congenital syphilis. He warned that the prevalence in the black population, especially in the south, was much higher than in the white population. He tried to dispel the public belief that syphilis and gonorrhea occurred only in prostitutes, and argued that extramarital liaisons were just as responsible.

Parran and Raymond Vonderlehr (Assistant Surgeon General) advocated a plan for a federally and state financed venereal disease program whereby control would be primarily a state and not a federal function, as it had been in the past. The Public Health Service must be involved—both to fund state treatment and diagnostic facilities and to undertake basic research—but the states would provide direct medical care to the patient through the appointment of district or county health officers and supervise local health care and delivery.

One of the greatest problems encountered was resistance by established medical societies to any move that would divert paying patients from doctors' offices to public clinics. P. S. Pelouze,[76] writing on gonorrhea in that period, noted that physicians and surgeons were unwilling to call in venereal disease specialists, even when it was the likely diagnosis. He also maintained there were a large number of very poorly controlled public dispensaries.

Under Parran, cooperative clinics were formed in most of the large cities of the United States. A central filing system was established, and a statistical system for the integration of findings in different clinics was begun.

## THE TUSKEGEE STUDY

From 1929 to 1932 the Julius Rosenwald Fund cooperated with the U.S. Public Health Service to conduct a study intended to detect and treat syphilis in the black population in some of the southern states, meeting with only limited success. Out of that study under the aegis of the Public Health Service grew the Tuskegee Study[77] in Macon County, Alabama. Four hundred black syphilitic men were told they were ill and promised free care. The purpose of the study was to determine the natural course and complications of untreated latent syphilis in black males and to ascertain whether it differed from the course of syphilis in whites. Among the multitude of ethical considerations ignored in the study, possibly the least was the failure to deliver appropriate therapy, especially penicillin, when in time it became available. It was not until 1972, when accounts of the study and its unfairness appeared in the press, that officialdom finally halted the experiment.

In the late 1930s a number of states began to require premarital blood tests for syphilis, then antenatal screening, together with reporting of syphilis and gonorrhea figures. In 1938 the La Follette-Bulwinkle Act was passed, which authorizes grants and aid for states for the expansion of venereal disease control activities and raised funding for the Venereal Disease Control Division.

## SECOND WORLD WAR

The United States entered the Second World War better equipped to fight venereal diseases than previously, largely due to experience drawn from public health knowledge. It was realized that high levels of syphilis were to be found in both civilian and military populations. Faster methods of delivery of salvarsan (arsphenamine) given by intravenous therapy in 5 to 10 days were made. Over 300,000 draftees found to have syphilis were treated by this method.

The problem of early syphilis was of paramount importance to the armed forces, seeking to conserve manpower. Combining research in the services, together with 25 civilian clinics in large centers, penicillin after 1943 was found to be effective, with almost complete lack of toxic effects. Rapid treatment centers were established and the results pooled in a central Statistical Unit under the direction of Joseph E. Moore (1892–1957) at Johns Hopkins Hospital. By 1949 Evan W. Thomas was able to state that in the future penicillin was the drug choice in syphilis and there were no longer good reasons for prescribing arsenic or bismuth in syphilis.[78]

As happened after the First World War, federal funding for venereal diseases dropped enormously in the 10 years after the Second World War. It was erroneously believed, not only in America, that penicillin wiped out the problems of venereal disease control. Public attitudes about sexuality had changed greatly, and mass testing for syphilis was becoming less desirable from a cost-effectiveness view. In the 1950s the U.S. Public Health Service advocated speed-zone epidemiology based on case finding in not only syphilis but gonorrhea.

By 1970 the prevalence of syphilis and gonorrhea approached epidemic levels again. The Department of Health, Education and Welfare convened a National Commission on Venereal Diseases,[79] assisted by a WHO[80] traveling seminar. The commission reported that clinics were run-down, medical standards were out of date, and legislation needed to be revised.

Federal responsibility for venereal disease control today devolves on the Division of Sexually Transmitted Diseases of the Centers for Disease Control. The Division offers aid for states, develops guidelines, makes recommendations for treatment uniformly throughout the United States, undertakes fundamental and operational research, and encourages coordinated training for all grades of health workers in the service.

In recent years, standardization of serology for syphilis, observation and reporting of resistance to various antibiotics by *Neisseria gonorrhea,* and, since 1981, the reporting on AIDS, exemplify how these issues should be addressed.

## WOMEN AND STDS

No advance in medicine takes place as an event by itself. The importance of women's interest in their own bodies, particularly as they see how sexually transmitted diseases affects them, whether personally or collectively, probably arises from the great changes brought about in the Paris Medical School during the 1850s. The reforms which had taken place after the Revolution of 1789 and the concept of equality of the sexes date from that time.

While dermatology had flowered under Alibert, it was left to his pupil, the witty Ricord, to influence the training and teaching of venereology in Paris from 1833 onward. His contemporary, Parent-Duchatelet, in his work of 1837 "Prostitution dans la ville de Paris," noted that in prostitutes not only were syphilis and scabies common but so was cancer of the uterus.[47] It was an early cause of death in such women, unlike nonprostitutes. So it seems that Rigoni-Stern, who noted in 1842 that cancer of the uterus was more common in married women than in nuns,[81] was not the first to associate sexual activity with uterine cancer. Ricord[14] noticed in 1838 the frequent occurrence of gonorrhea with trichomoniasis following Donné's[40] work on the latter. He also reintroduced examination by vaginal speculum in venereal diseases. His successor, Fournier, was the first advocate of the innocent female victim of syphilis, and from his time in charge of the wards for prostitutes at the Lourcine Hospital he commented on the awful inflictions caused by syphilis on the wives and children of male sufferers.[92]

His campaign was taken up in the United States by P. A. Morrow, who in 1905 founded the American Society for Sanitary and Moral Prophylaxis to fight the conditions that caused sexually transmitted disease.

Beginning in 1864, the Contagious Diseases (Women) Acts were made law in the United Kingdom. These acts applied the continental system of regulated prostitution in British garrison towns to control the so-called sexually immorality of soldiers and sailors. Any woman living in these towns might be declared on police say-so to be a common prostitute and forced to undergo medical examination, often from unsympathetic doctors.

The Women's Movement in Britain campaigned vigorously against these laws, led by Josephine Butler (1828–1906), a clergyman's wife of aristocratic background. The movement had hoped to get Elizabeth Garrett Anderson (1836–1917),[83] then the first and only woman doctor who qualified in 1865 practicing in the United Kingdom, to give her support. Anderson did not agree with the campaign. She believed compulsory, not voluntary, treatment necessary and thought powers of arrest a useful check, especially in the case of teenagers. Influenced by the surgeon James Paget (1814–1899), she thought compulsory hospital care of prostitutes was their only hope, and aligned herself with the traditional male outlook about female venereal disease. The campaign was successful, nonetheless, and the laws were repealed in 1886.[82]

Other women doctors, notably Elizabeth Blackwell, had qualified earlier (beginning in 1859) in the United States. Dr. Lucy Sewell of the New England Hospital for Women and Children at Boston was a teacher who greatly influenced Sophia Jex-Blake, the founder of the London School of Medicine for Women.

Although an article on venereal diseases was finally published in the *Ladies Home Journal* in 1937[84] and premarital and antenatal blood tests were being given to women routinely just before the Second World War, a chauvinistic attitude still prevailed. "Fighting men" were warned to beware of the perils of venereal disease which "scarlet women," whether amateur or professional, were just waiting to inflict on them.

In 1953 Alfred Kinsey[85] found that one-fifth of college-educated women had engaged in premarital coitus. Oral contraceptives became available in 1965. By the late 1960s about half of the college-educated women had premarital experience. Thus freer acceptance of sexuality outside marriage, coupled with ease of contraception, changing of established moral views on sexuality, rising disposable income in women, and greater personal freedom meant that sexually transmitted diseases by the 1960s were again increasing in young persons, especially in women, even if they had relatively few partner changes.

At the same time women were beginning not to accept male dominance in matters of health. They wanted to be better educated about their bodies and, in the course of events, about sexually transmitted diseases and contraception techniques. They have been fairly successful in most Western countries, not least in ensuring that physicians as a group have been prompted to be more considerate of the needs of their female patients. Women's groups, with the backing of concerned physicians, have campaigned for Well Women Clinics, family planning clinics, and facilities to determine breast and cervical cancer and sexually transmitted diseases.

## GAY RIGHTS AND STDS

In the last 30 years, there has been increasing awareness of the part played by homosexual behavior in the spread of venereal diseases. Some European countries whose laws were based on the Napoleonic Code of 1810, in which questions of fornication and homosexuality were left to the conscience of the individual, may have recognized early the phenomenon of variations from heterosexual behavior. However, with the Second World War and the movement of many young men during wartime, the part played in the spread of venereal disease by homosexual intercourse began to be acknowledged. Josephine Hinrichsen[86] wrote a comprehensive paper about the importance of knowledge of sexual habits in the diagnosis and control of venereal disease, with special reference to homosexual behavior. This covered most aspects of homosexually acquired venereal disease in the United States and Europe to that date. The importance of Kinsey[87] and his coworkers' study of 1948, and their findings on the prevalence of adult male homosexuality, increased the spotlight on the subject in America.

James Jefferiss[88] showed that in Britain, especially London, a significant proportion of male venereal disease patients were homosexuals. From 1956 onward, many reports on sexually transmitted diseases in gay men can be found in the literature from all European countries. After the relaxation of restrictions, and with the lifting of the criminal label from male homosexuality in 1967 in England, a far greater proportion of men were willing to admit to their sexuality in the causation of their presenting sexually transmitted diseases. The upsurge of the gay rights movement and increased sexual activity within the homosexual community has meant that STDs have been seen far more frequently.[89] Not only were syphilis and gonorrhea more often diagnosed but, especially in the early 1970s, various other diseases became more commonly recognized and associated with penile-anal and oral-anal sexual activity. Collectively termed in 1976 the "gay bowel syndrome,"[90] it referred to a constellation of diseases with proctologic complications occurring more frequently in homosexual men. During the same period viral STDs, especially hepatitis B, gained prominence in this group.

AIDS was first seen in the United States, probably in 1978 but was first recorded in 1981[91] and in Europe since 1982. It has meant that some gay men have to change their sexual practices if they are to survive. A decrease in homosexual activity has been noted in London since 1982.[93] A large proportion will have already been infected with HIV virus. Gay rights advocates—including the Gay Men's Health Crisis, and concerned physicians throughout the Western world—continue to champion gay men in their battle against sexually transmitted diseases, to make them aware of the dangers, and to stimulate compassion in the general populations.

## References


1 Final Report of the Commissioners: Royal Commission on Venereal Diseases. London, HMSO, 1916.

1a Reinhard F: *Arch Gesch Med,* Leipzig, 1915, vol 9, p 315; 1916, vol 10, p 124.

1b Morton RS: *Gonorrhoea.* Philadelphia, Saunders, 1977.

1c Finger EAF: *Gonorrhoea.* New York, Wm Wood, 1894.

1d Clowes W: "A Short and Profitable Treatise Touching the Cure of the Disease Called Morbus Gallicus by Unctions." London, 1579.

2 Smith GE et al: *The Archaelogical Survey of Nubia.* Ministry of Finance, Survey Department. Cairo, 1910.

3 Preuss J: *Biblical and Talmudic Medicine 1911.* F Rosner (trans). New York, Sanhedrin Press, 1978.

4 Brim CJ: *Medicine in the Bible.* New York, Froben Press, 1936.

5 Rolleston JD: Venereal disease in literature. *Br J Vener Dis* 10: 147, 1934.

6 Lancereaux E: *A Treatise on Syphilis. Historical and Practical (1866).* G. Whitley (trans). London, The New Sydenham Society, 1868.

7 Oriel JD: Anal warts and anal coitus. *Br J Vener Dis* 47: 373, 1971.

8 Williams HU: The origin and antiquity of syphilis. The evidence from diseased bones. *Arch Pathol (Chicago).* 13: 779, 1932.

9 Henschen F: *The History of Diseases.* London, Longmans Green, 1966.

10 Stewart TD et al: Evidence on the paleopathology of yaws. *Bull Hist Med* 26: 538, 1952.

11 Hudson EH: *Treponematosis. Oxford Medicine.* Oxford University Press, 1946.

12 Sudhoff K: Graphische und Typographische Erstlinge der Syphilis Literatur aus den Jahren 1495 und 1496. "Der Nurnberger Druch aus Ulsenius Gedichtes: bei Hans Mair." Now attributed to A. Dürer. Munich, Kuhn, 1912.

13 Fracastoro G: *Syphilis sive morbus gallicus.* Verona, S. Nicolini da Sabbio, 1530.

14 Ricord P: *Traité pratique des maladies vénériennes.* Paris, De Just Rouvier and le Bouvier, 1838.

15 Astruc J: *De morbis venereis.* Paris, G Cavalier, 1736.

16 Qvist G: John Hunter's alleged syphilis. *Ann R Coll Surg Engl* 59: 205, 1977.

17 Dempster WJ: Towards a new understanding of John Hunter. *Lancet* 1: 316, 1978.

17a Holmes OW: *Medical Essays 1842–1882.* London, Sampson Low, 1891.

17b Cooper A: Report of a lecture given on April 18, 1824. *Lancet* May 18, 1824.

18 Diday CJPE: *Traité de la Syphilis des nouveau-nés et des enfants à la mamelle.* Paris, V Masson, 1854.

19 Hutchinson J: *Syphilis.* London, Cassell, 1887.

20 Fournier A: *La syphilis héréditaire tardive.* Paris, G Masson, 1886.

21 Fournier A: De l'ataxie locomotrice d'origine syphilitique. *Ann Dermatol Syphiligraph* 1: 7, 1875.

21a Mott, FW: In *A System of Syphilis,* D Power, JK Murphy (eds). London, Oxford University Press, 1910, vol 4.

22 Jarisch A: Therapeutische versuche bei syphilis. *Wien Med Wochenschr* 45: 720, 1895.

22a Lane JR: Lectures on Syphilis Delivered at the Harveian Society, December 1876, 2d ed. London, Churchill, 1881.

23 Neisser ALS: Ueber eine der Gonorrhoe eigen-tümliche Microccusform. *Zentralb Med Wissenschaften.* 17: 497, 1879.

24 Gram HCJ: Ueber die isolirte Färburg der Schizomycetin in Schmitt und Trocken. *Prapareten Fortschritte der Medizin.* Halle. 2: 185, 1884.

25 Leistikow L: Ueber Bacterien bei den venerischen Krankheiten. *Chârité Ann* 7: 750, 1880.

26 Bumm E von: Der Mikro-Organismus der gonorrhoischen Schleim hauterkrankungen gonococcus Neisser. *Dtsch Med Wochenschr* 11: 508, 1885.

27 Elser WJ et al: Studies of Meningitis. *J Med Res* 21: 371, 1909.

28 Credé KSF: Die Verhütung der Augentzündung der Neugebarenen. *Arch Gynaekol* 17: 50, 1881.

29 Fraenkel E: Bericht über eine bei kindern beobachtete Endemie infectioser Colpitis. *Virchows Arch (A)* 99: 251, 1885.

30 Finger EAF: *Die Blenorrhoea der Sexual Organen und ihre Complicationen.* Leipzig, F. Deuticke, 1888.

31 Wertheim E: Ueber Uterus-Gonorrhoe. Leipzig, Verhandlungen der Deutschen Gesellschaft für Gynäkologie. 6: 199, 1895.

32 Thayer WS et al: Ulcerative endocarditis due to the gonococcus gonorrheal septicaemia. *Johns Hopkins Hospital Bull* 7: 57, 1896.

33 Swediaur FX: *Practical Observations on the More Obstinate and Inveterate Venereal Complaints.* London, J Johnson, 1784.

34 Carmichael R: *Clinical Lectures on Venereal Diseases.* Dublin, Hodges and Smith, 1842.

35 Fournier A: *Note pour servir à l'histoire du rhumatisme uréthral.* Paris, Malteste, 1866.

36 Halberstaedter L et al: Zur Atiologie des Trachoms. *Dtsch Med Wochenschr* 33: 1285, 1907.

37 Lindner K: Uebertragungsversuche von gonokokken freier Blennorrhoea neonatorum auf Affen. *Wien Klin Wochenshr* 22: 1554, 1909.

38 Bateman T: *A Practical Synopsis of Cutaneous Diseases,* 4th ed. London, Longman, Hurst, Rees, Orme and Brown, 1814.

39 Reiter H: Ueber eine bisher unerkannte Spirochäteninfektion. (Spirochaetosis arthritica). *Dtsch Med Wochenschr* 42: 1535, 1916.

40 Donné A: Animalcules observés dan les matières purulentes et le produit des sécretions des organes génitaux de l'homme et de la femme. *CR Acad Sci Paris* 3: 385, 1836.

41 Hebra F: Ueber Krätze. Medicinische Jahrbucher des kaiserlich-koniglichen österreichischen Staates. 42: 286, 47: 163, 1844.

42 Wilkinson JS: Some remarks upon the development of epiphytes with the destruction of new vegetable fermentation found in connection with the human uterus. *Lancet* 2: 448, 1849.

43 Ricord P: Contagion de la syphilis. *Gazette médicale de Paris.* 3: 14, 354, 1859.

44 Bassereau L: *Traité des affections de la peau symptomatiques de la syphilis.* Paris, JB Ballière, 1852.

45 Rollet JP: Coincidence de chancre syphilitique primitif avec la gale, la blénorrhagie, le chancre simple et la vaccine. *Gazette medicale de Lyon* 18: 160, 1866.

46 Ducrey A: Richerche experimentali sulla natura intima del contagio dell' ulcera venerea el sulla patogensi dele bubbone venerea. *Giornale italiano delle malattie Venereae della Pelle* 30: 377, 1889.

47 Parent-Duchatelet AJB: *De la prostitution dans la ville de Paris.* Brussels. Etablissement Encyclographique. 1837, p 80.

48 Sanger WW: *The History of Prostitution.* New York, The Medical Publishing Co., 1919.

49 Flexner A: *Prostitution in Europe.* New York, The Century Co, 1914.

50 Klebs E: Ueber syphilis-impfung bei Thieren und über die Natur des syphilischen contagiums. *Prager Med Wochenschr* 3: 409, 1878.

51 Berdal H et al: La balano-posthite érosive circinée. *La Médicine Moderne (Paris)* 2: 340, 1891.

52 Metchnikoff E et al: Études experimentales sur la syphilis. *Annales de l'Institut Pasteur (Paris)* 17: 809, 1903; 18: 1, 1904.

53 Schaudinn FR, Hoffman E: Vorlaufiger Bericht über das Vorkommen von Spirochaeten in Syphilitschen Krankheitsprodukten und bei papillomen. *Arbeiten aus dem Kaiserlichen Gesundheitsamte* 22: 527, 1905.

54 Castellani A: On the presence of spirochaetes in 2 cases of ulcerated parangi (yaws). *Br Med J* 1: 1280, 1905.

55 Landsteiner K et al: Technik der Spirochaetenunt-erschung. *Wien Klin Wochenschr* 19: 1349, 1906.

56 Noguchi H et al: A Demonstration of *T. pallidum* in the brain in cases of general paralysis. *J Exp Med* 17: 232, 1913.

57 Bordet J et al: Sur l'existence de substances sensibilatrices dans la plupart des sérum antimicrobiens. *Annales de l'Institut Pasteur.* 15: 289, 1901.

58 Wassermann A et al: Eine Serodiagnostische Reaktion bei Syphilis. *Dtsche Med Wochenschr* 32: 745, 1906.

59 Landsteiner K et al: Zur Technik der Spirochaenunterschung. *Wein Klin Wochenschr* 20: 1565, 1907.

60 Nelson RA et al: Immobilization of T. pallidum in vitro by antibody produced in syphilitic infection. *J Exp Med* 89: 369, 1949.

61 Ehrlich P et al: *Die experimentelle Chemotherapie der Spirillosen.* Berlin, J Springer, 1910.

62 von Jauregg RW: Ueber die Einwirkung fieber hafter Erkrankungen auf Psychosen. *Jahrbuch für Psychiatrie und Neurologie.* 7: 94, 1887.

63 von Jauregg JW: Ueber Behandlung der progressiven Paralyse mit Bakterien toxinen. *Wien Klin Wochenschr* 25: 61, 1912.

64 von Jauregg JW: Die Behandlung der progressiven Paralyse und Tabes. *Wien Klin Wochenschr* 34: 171, 1921.

65 Sazerac R et al: Traitement de la Syphilis par le bismuth. *CR Acad Sci Paris* 173: 338, 1921.

66 Domagk G: Ein Beitrag zur Chemotherapie der bakterielle Infekionen. *Dtsch Med Wochenschr* 61: 250, 1935.

67 Mahoney JF et al. Penicillin Treatment of Early Syphilis. A preliminary report. *Vener Dis Inf* 24: 355, 1943.

68 Moore JE: *The Modern Treatment of Syphilis,* 2d ed. Springfield, CC Thomas, 1947, p 619.

69 Stokes JH et al: *Modern Clinical Syphilology.* Philadelphia, Saunders, 1944, p 1237.

70 Gross SD: Syphilis in its relation to the national health. *Trans AMA* 25: 1874.

71 Noeggerath E: Latent gonorrhoea, especially with regard to its influence on fertility in women. *Trans Am Gynaecol Assoc* 1: 292, 1876.

72 Fournier A: *Syphilis and Marriage.* PA Morrow (trans), New York, 1880.

73 Wile H: The Vienna school of dermatology. *Philadelphia Med Times.* 13: 756, 1883.

74 Brandt AM: *No Magic Bullet. A Social History of Venereal Disease in the United States since 1880.* New York, Oxford University Press, 1987.

75 Parran T: *Shadow on the Land: Syphilis.* New York, Reynal and Hitchcock, 1937.

76 Pelouze PS: *Gonorrhoea in the Male and Female.* Philadelphia, Saunders, 1944.

77 Jones JH: *Bad Blood. The Tuskegee Syphilis Experiment.* New York, Free Press, 1981.

78 Thomas EW et al: *Syphilis: Its Course and Management.* New York, Macmillan, 1949.

79 Report of the National Commission on Venereal Disease. U.S. Department of Health, Education and Welfare. Publication No. (HSM) 72-8125. 1972.

80 Report of the International Travelling Seminar on Venereal Diseases in the United States of America. Washington, Pan American Health Office, 1974.

81 Briggs RM et al: Cervical intraepithelial neoplasia, in *Sexually Transmitted Diseases,* KK Holmes, PA Mardh, PF Sparling, PJ Wiesner (eds). New York, McGraw-Hill, 1984, p 589.

82 Petrie G: *A Singular Iniquity.* London, Macmillan. 1971.

83 Manton J: *Elizabeth Garett Anderson.* London, Methuen, 1965, p 179.

84 Parran T et al: We can end this sorrow. *Ladies Home Journal* 54: 23, August 1937.

85 Kinsey AL et al: *Sexual Behaviour in the Human Female.* Philadelphia, Saunders, 1953.

86 Hinrichsen J: The Importance of a knowledge of sexual habits in the diagnosis and control of venereal disease with special reference to homosexual behavior. *Urol Cutan Rev* 48: 469, 1944.

87 Kinsey AL et al: *Sexual Behavior in the Human Male.* Philadelphia, Saunders, 1948.

88 Jefferiss FJG: Venereal disease and the homosexual. *Br J Vener Dis* 32: 17, 1956.

89 Darrow WW et al: The gay report on sexually transmitted diseases. *Am J Public Health* 71: 1004, 1981.

90 Kazal HL et al: The gay bowel syndrome: Clinicopathologic correlation in 260 cases. *Ann Clin Lab Sci* 6: 184, 1976.

91 Pneumocystis pneumonia—Los Angeles. *MMWR* 30: 250, 1981.

92 Fournier A: *Clinique de l'Hôpital de Lourcine. Leçons sur la syphilis étudiée plus particulièrement chez la femme.* Paris, Delahaye, 1873.

93 Weller P, Hindley D, Adler M, Meldrum J: Gonorrhoea in homosexual men and media coverage of the acquired immune deficiency syndrome in London, 1982–1983. *Br Med J* 289: 1041, 1984.

# PART II EPIDEMIOLOGY OF SEXUALLY TRANSMITTED DISEASES

# Chapter 2

# Epidemiology of sexual behavior and sexually transmitted diseases

Sevgi O. Aral
King K. Holmes

## INTRODUCTION

This chapter concerns the incidence, distribution, and trends in STDs and related complications, and their determinants, throughout the world. The incidence and distribution of STDs show considerable variation across space and time, which reflects the distribution and trends in their determinants. These determinants include aspects of population composition, patterns of behavior and susceptibility of individuals, changing properties of the pathogens, societal efforts at primary prevention and disease control, and the complex interactions among these factors.

Our goal is not to summarize the epidemiology of the various STDs but rather to identify patterns which cut across several of the STDs, or patterns which differentiate them, to develop an overall perspective of the epidemiology of STDs. We are particularly interested in the importance of demographic and sociocultural change, the apparent reemergence of sex with prostitutes as a major factor in the epidemiology of STDs in many settings, the impact of AIDS on sexual behaviors, differences in the behavioral determinants of curable as compared with incurable STDs, and the growing importance and improved understanding of the epidemiology of viral STDs. In revising this chapter, we have modified and reorganized our material to reflect the major changes in our understanding of the epidemiology of STDs which occurred during the 1980s.

A prominent theme today is the influence of dynamically changing demographic and sociocultural forces on the spread of STDs. In most industrialized countries the incidence of classical STDs such as gonorrhea and syphilis has been declining rapidly during the AIDS era among educated middle and upper classes; while in North America, the incidence of the same STDs has been stable or actually increasing within selected population groups of lower socioeconomic status, perhaps among those least likely to modify behavior. Thus, in the United States both a relative and absolute increase of STD rates has occurred among urban, poor, and minority populations, particularly among adolescents, with highest rates among adolescent females. Prostitution has reemerged as a multiplier of STD, and the relatively new phenomenon of sex in exchange for drugs is contributing to epidemic spread of gonorrhea, syphilis, and chancroid in North America. The impact of social disintegration on the hyperendemic spread of STDs is seen not only in cities of developing countries but also in rapidly growing inner-city populations in North America.

Our understanding of the epidemiology of viral STDs has changed markedly from the mid-seventies to the mid-eighties. Epidemic increases in symptomatic genital herpes and genital warts were followed by the current AIDS epidemic. As dramatic as these three epidemics of symptomatic viral STDs seemed when first recognized, the development of improved diagnostic tests has led to recognition of much more widespread reservoirs of subclinical infection with each of these incurable sexually transmitted viral infections. This is forcing a reappraisal of the relative importance of sexual behavior, contraceptive (or barrier prophylaxis) behavior, and health care behavior, in the epidemiology of STDs. The incidence, trends, and distribution of incurable viral STDs differ in important ways from those of curable, mostly bacterial STDs. The determinants of the epidemiology of curable and incurable STDs also differ somewhat. Health-seeking behaviors and the extent and effectiveness of disease control strategies based on early diagnosis and treatment are important determinants of the incidence of curable STDs. These health-seeking behaviors are less important (though not negligible) in the epidemiology of the incurable viral STDs, however. Thus, strategies for control of viral STDs depend to a greater extent on societal efforts at primary prevention through health education of the general public, and individualized counseling of the clinically infected carrier. Moreover, not all curable STDs appear to be equally controllable; some, for example, chancroid and to a large extent syphilis, are more effectively controlled by existing strategies than are others like gonorrhea and chlamydia. This is especially true in developing countries, where the absence of resources needed for diagnosis of chlamydial infection or gonorrhea in women makes these diseases analogous to the incurable viral STDs, such that control is currently more dependent on societal efforts at health education and behavior change than on diagnosis and treatment. Behavioral intervention has again, for the first time since penicillin, become the most important approach to STD control.

As research proceeds to measure demographic and behavioral determinants of risk of individual STDs, and to define cofactors for transmission or for progression to certain complications such as AIDS or cervical cancer, it is necessary to carefully attempt to separate true risk factors directly involved in the causal chain leading to transmission or complications, from risk markers (risk indicators), which are simply covariates with true risk factors such as sexual behavior. This is particularly true for possible interactions between individual sexually transmitted diseases, e.g., the role of genital ulcers, chlamydial infection, or gonorrhea as risk factors for transmission or acquisition of HIV infection. This is also true for other important putative risk factors or protective factors for certain STDs or STD complications, such as contraceptive methods, male circumcision, and douching.

Data concerning the frequency and distribution of STDs are limited in several ways. Not all STDs are reportable, and even reportable diseases are seldom reported completely. Data from most of the world are sketchy, at times anecdotal. The frequency of STDs in developing societies has mostly been measured through sample populations attending STD clinics, which are not necessarily representative of the total population. Data from North America and Europe have shown steady increases in the incidence of viral STDs and genital chlamydial infections during the 1970s and 1980s, declines in the incidence of gonorrhea and syphilis, which differ greatly from country to country in terms of the time of the onset and rate of decline, and similar major declines in the sex ratio of males to females with bacterial STDs.

In the United States, morbidity rates for gonorrhea, PID, and infertility have varied markedly by age, race, and socioeconomic status. During the 1960s and 1970s, race differentials decreased as rates first increased most rapidly among white women, then declined most rapidly among nonwhites. However, during the

AIDS era, some communities are seeing a rapid decline in gonorrhea among whites with stable or even increasing rates among blacks. Findings from important seroepidemiological analyses based on data from samples representative of the total United States population are now available for the first time. These data provide direct estimates regarding the distribution across population subgroups of three STDs: syphilis, type 2 herpes simplex virus (HSV-2) infection, and hepatitis B. Unfortunately, these seroprevalence estimates reflect the cumulative STD experience of earlier decades, rather than current experience. In this chapter, we analyze the distribution of selected STDs within various populations, analyze trends in these distributions, and discuss implications for future research and control efforts.

## THE CURABLE BACTERIAL STDs

### GONORRHEA

The major bacterial STDs include gonorrhea, chlamydial infection, syphilis, and in many developing countries, chancroid. Data from Sweden (Fig. 2-1) are particularly intriguing, showing a steady fall in the male:female sex ratio extending more or less continuously from 1912 through 1973, then rising slowly thereafter; epidemics of gonorrhea during World War I and World War II, with discernible peaks in the late twenties, the early fifties, and a sustained epidemic beginning in 1958 and peaking in 1970; and an extraordinary decline in gonorrhea incidence from 1970 through 1987, amounting to more than a 15-fold decline from a total of 487 cases per 100,000 for 1970 to 31 cases per 100,000 for 1987. Gonorrhea has become a rare disease in Sweden. Factors often held responsible for the declining male:female sex ratio for gonorrhea have included improved detection of female cases resulting from use of selective culture media for isolation of *Neisseria gonorrhoeae* and partner notification, both of which came into increasing use during the 1960s and 1970s; and the "sexual liberation" of women coinciding with the advent of oral contraception in the 1960s. However, it is apparent from Fig. 2-1 that this declining sex ratio dates back at least to 1912 in Sweden.

In the United Kingdom, a similar increase occurred in the number of reported cases of gonorrhea from 1960, peaking in 1973 for men and in 1977 for women (Fig. 2-2). Note the declining male:female sex ratio from a peak of 4:1 in 1962 to about 1.5:1 in 1986. The rate of decline in reported gonorrhea among men has fallen more and more rapidly since 1982.

In the United States (Fig. 2-3), gonorrhea morbidity rates reached a peak in 1946 following World War II, then decreased until 1957 and increased again for nearly two decades.[1,2] From 1962 through 1975, the reported incidence of gonorrhea increased steadily at about 15 percent per year, peaking at 473 per 100,000 in 1975, then declining at an accelerating pace to 324 per 100,000 in 1987 (Fig. 2-3). The male:female ratio of reported incidence initially increased to over 3:1 by 1966, then declined rapidly to about 1.5:1 by 1973, and remained rather constant at that level thereafter. In 1987, the number of cases reported from public clinics (526,000) was nearly twice as high as the number reported by private providers (255,000). In Canada, the reported incidence of gonorrhea peaked later than in the United States, at 231 per 100,000 in 1981, falling steadily since then to 138 per 100,000 during 1986. In Asia, data from Singapore are among the most representative. The incidence of gonorrhea per 100,000 population in Singapore peaked at 684 cases in 1979, falling steadily since then to 318 cases in 1985.

Further analysis of reported gonorrhea cases in the United States reveals important differences in the incidence and trends in incidence by racial group. Between 1975 and 1984, the annual gonorrhea incidence rate declined less among white women (8.9 percent) and white men (13.6 percent) than among men and

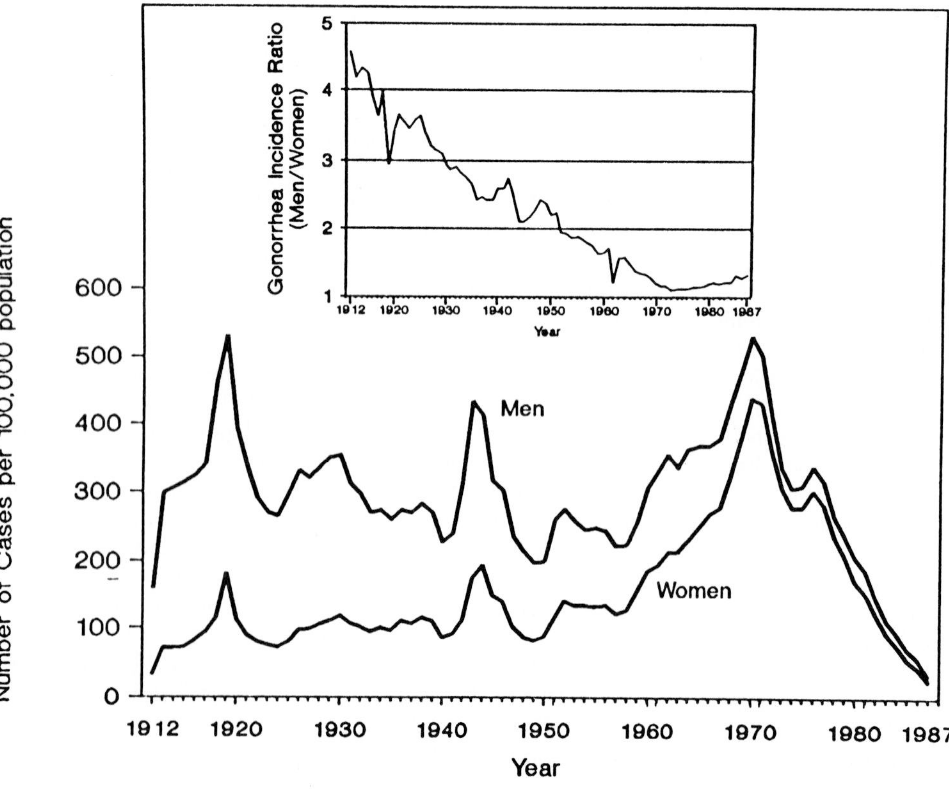


**Fig. 2-1.** Trends in the incidence of reported gonorrhea in men and women, and the ratio of male:female incidence, in Sweden, 1912–1987. Note the steady decline in the ratio of male:female cases during most of this period, and the precipitous drop in incidence in both sexes, beginning in 1970. (*Data provided by M. Bottiger and D. Danielsson.*)

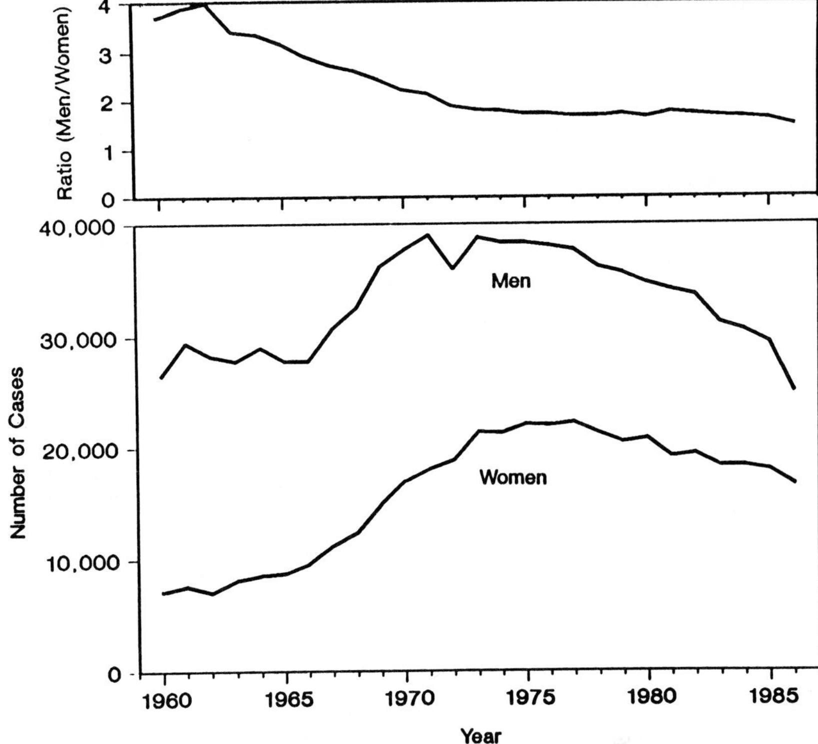


**Fig. 2-2.** Trends in the number of cases of reported gonorrhea in men and women, and the ratios of male:female cases, in England and Wales, 1960–1986. (*Data provided by M. Adler.*)

women of other races (19.2 and 18.3 percent, respectively). Thus, the race differential between whites and other races in the gonorrhea incidence rate became smaller.[3] Trends since 1984 have reversed this picture; the race differential between whites and blacks has grown between 1984 and 1987 (Fig. 2-4).

The pooling of data from all nonwhites may obscure differences in gonorrhea rates and trends among racial minorities. For example, in King County, Washington, during 1986 and 1987, the overall incidence of gonorrhea per 100,000 population was 3033 for blacks, 843 for Native Americans, 617 for Hispanics, 190 for Asians, and 121 for Caucasians (R. Rice, unpublished data). The incidence in King County was also independently correlated with low socioeconomic status, as determined by census tract of residence. Similarly, pooling of data by broad age groupings can obscure large differences in incidence of gonorrhea by age, gender, and race.

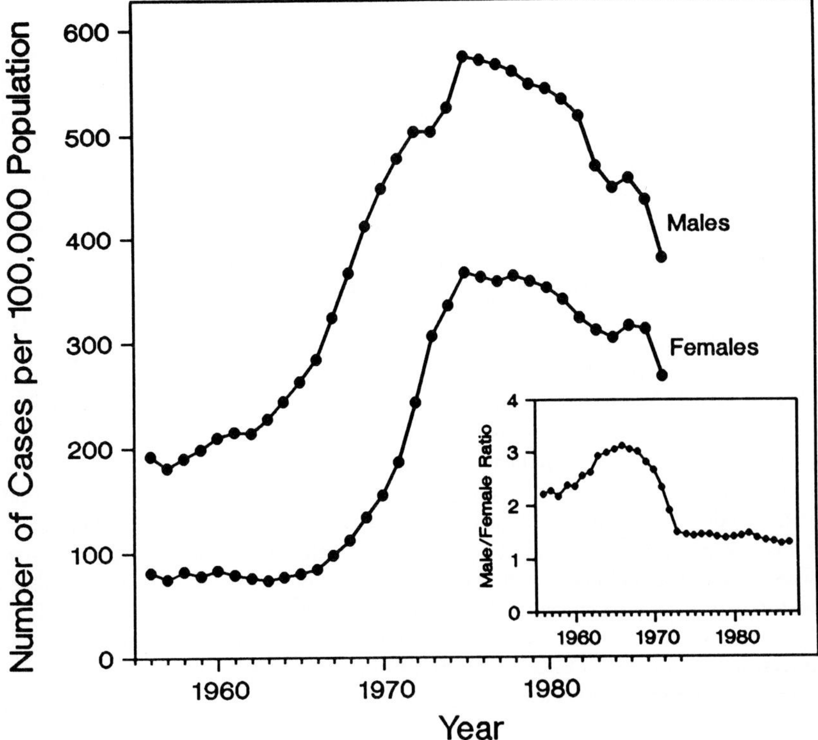


**Fig. 2-3.** Trends in the incidence of reported gonorrhea in men and women, and the ratio of male:female cases, in the United States, 1956–1987.

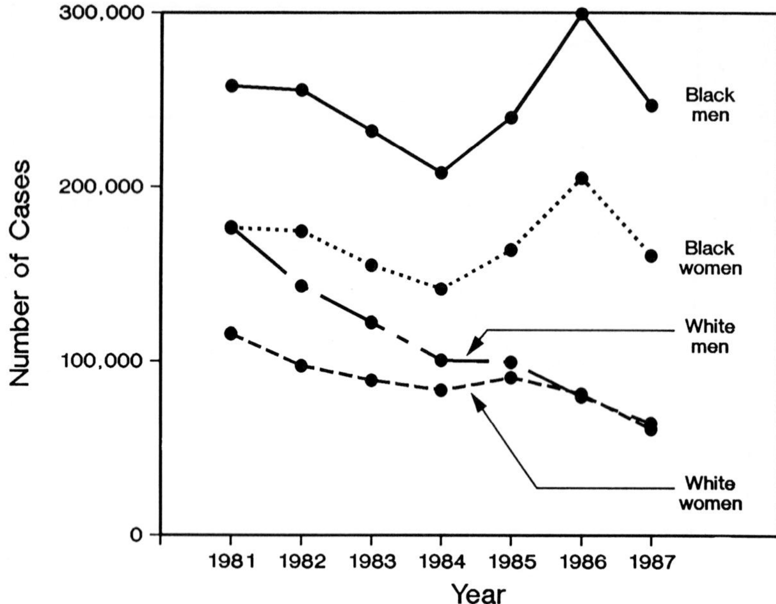


**Fig. 2-4.** Recent trends in reported cases of gonorrhea by race and gender, United States, 1981–1987. This figure shows reported cases to illustrate trends. It does not show the marked difference by race since the population size differences are not reflected here. For example, in 1988 the estimated population size was 81,563,000 white females and 12,106,000 black females, the rates therefore were 67 per 100,000 for white women and 1400 per 100,000 for black women—a 21:1 black/white ratio. Trends in reported cases in part reflect trends in reporting. Reporting by private sources is less complete than that by public sources. Shifts in health care utilization from public to private sources may mask increases or cause apparent decreases in disease incidence.

While in recent years the overall trend in gonorrhea morbidity in the United States and other developed countries has been encouraging,[4] problems with gonococcal antibiotic resistance have been increasingly discouraging.[5] Beta-lactamase-producing strains of *N. gonorrhoeae* were first isolated in the United States in 1976. Over the next several years, the reported numbers of such strains remained stable at less than 100 cases per year, and most cases were linked to overseas travel or military importation. In 1980, beta-lactamase-producing strains started to increase; the total number of reported cases was over 4500 by 1982. This early increase was accounted for by continued importation from endemic areas like Korea, the Philippines, and Africa, improved laboratory surveillance, documented role of prostitutes in "core" transmission, and finally, sustained domestic transmission produced by entrenchment of beta-lactamase-producing gonococci in some communities.[6] The number of reported cases began to increase sharply after 1984. By 1987 the number of reported beta-lactamase-positive isolates had reached 16,608 per year. In 1987, such strains accounted for 1.8 percent of all reported gonorrhea: 64 percent of cases occurred in the three areas previously identified as hyperendemic—Florida, New York City, and Los Angeles.[7,8] As the incidence of infections with beta-lactamase-producing strains of *N. gonorrhoeae* increased, the epidemiology changed: overseas travel and prostitute contact were identified as important risk factors in early outbreaks;[9] but once beta-lactamase-producing gonococci become endemic, they appear to have the same distribution as endemic, antibiotic-sensitive gonorrhea,[8] predominantly involving inner-city residents, members of ethnic minority groups, and heterosexuals. An outbreak of approximately 200 cases of gonorrhea was caused by a unique beta-lactamase-positive strain of *N. gonorrhoeae* in Seattle. The first cases predominantly involved Caucasian and Hispanic men with a history of prostitute contact; after a few months, most cases were in heterosexual black men and women, most of whom gave histories of prostitution, sex with prostitutes, or illegal drug use. Even though homosexual men are at high risk for gonococcal infections, outbreaks of beta-lactamase-producing strains among homosexual men have been rare.

## SYPHILIS

Syphilis has long been the classical example of an STD which can be successfully controlled by public health measures. The incidence of syphilis in Western countries apparently declined during the latter half of the nineteenth century, probably reflecting socioeconomic changes, because specific intervention other than use of mercurials was not available. In Sweden, a sharp rise in the incidence of syphilis in both sexes occurred during World Wars I and II (Fig. 2-5). Following World War I, the incidence of syphilis fell rapidly, coinciding with the availability of improved diagnostic tests and the arsenicals. After a brief rise in incidence during World War II, the incidence of syphilis began to fall again, coinciding with the introduction of penicillin. The incidence of syphilis, like that of gonorrhea, began to increase during the early 1960s; but unlike gonorrhea, the incidence of syphilis did not begin to fall in 1970, and in fact did not begin to fall again until 1982. Another striking difference in the epidemiology of gonorrhea and syphilis in Sweden concerns the trends in male:female ratios for the incidence of these diseases. The decline in the male:female ratio was much less for syphilis than for gonorrhea, though the ratio for syphilis did decline from a range of about 2.5:1 in the early 1900s to a range of about 1.5 to 1 from the mid-forties to the mid-fifties. Thereafter, a dramatic increase in the male:female ratio for syphilis occurred, reaching a peak of 6.5:1 in 1982, then falling sharply after the recognition of the AIDS epidemic.

In the United States, the incidence of primary and secondary syphilis rose during World War II, reached a peak at 76 cases per 100,000 in 1947, and then began to fall, to a nadir of about 4 per 100,000 for 1955–1958.[10] In 1959 the trend reversed, and the incidence rose rapidly in men and women, to 12 per 100,000 in 1965—triple the level of a decade earlier. Factors considered responsible at the time included declining federal, state, and local appropriations for venereal disease control (federal appropriations alone dropped from 17 million to 3 million annually in 1955); to a deemphasis on syphilis in medical teaching (e.g., in 1955, the phrase "and syphilology" was dropped from the

Fig. 2-5. Trends in the incidence of reported primary and secondary syphilis in men and women, and the ratio of male:female incidence in Sweden, 1912–1987. (*Data provided by M. Bottiger and D. Danielsson.*)

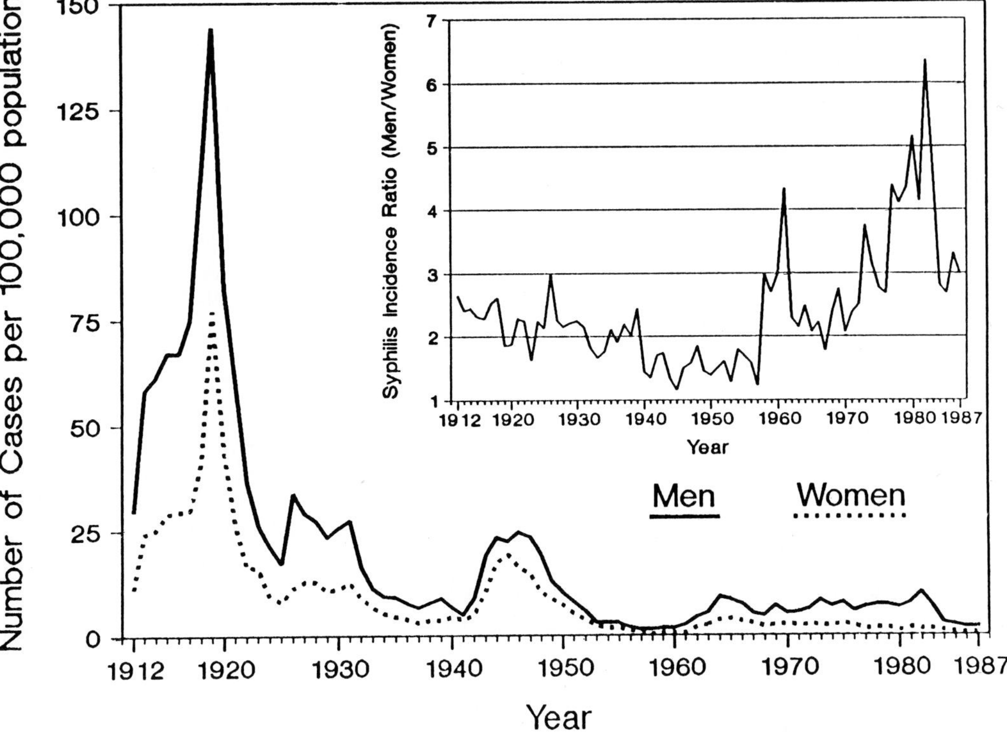


"AMA Archives of Dermatology and Syphilology"); and to a shift in management of syphilis from the public health clinic to the private office, with the availability of penicillin." From 1965 through 1980, the total incidence of primary and secondary syphilis changed very little, although the ratio of male:female cases increased steadily from about 1.5:1 up to about 3.5:1 in 1980 (Fig. 2-6).[12] Rates among white men were the only category to show sharp increases (true for cases seen in public clinics and by private practitioners), but the highest rates occurred in men of other races. As of 1982, all the morbidity trend data and the increasing percentage of men who reported at least one male partner clearly pointed to the increasing relative importance of homosexual practices among young white men in the epidemiology of syphilis. After 1982 trends in syphilis strongly reflected changes in the sexual behavior of homosexual men in response to the HIV epidemic.

Further analysis of these trends by race and by sex preference shows two striking changes in the epidemiology of syphilis in the United States. Data on sex preference were available on a national basis only through 1982. The proportion of men with primary and secondary syphilis who named other men as sex partners had increased from 23 percent in 1969 to 42 percent in 1982. Data from the state of Washington also reflect the increase in the proportion of men with primary and secondary syphilis who named men as sex partners from the mid-1960s through the mid-1980s; and in addition, they show the drastic decline in this proportion from about 50 percent of those with early syphilis in 1983–1984 to 8 percent in 1988 (Table 2-1). The basic patterns of declining primary and secondary syphilis among homosexual men and increase among women has continued through 1987. The sex ratio of reported primary and secondary syphilis cases had increased between 1977 and 1982 but has been declining since then (Fig. 2-6). From 1982 through 1986, the reported national primary and secondary syphilis incidence men had dropped steadily from 22.5 cases per 100,000 to 16.2 per 100,000, while rates in females remained unchanged.

However, during 1987, the incidence increased sharply in both men and women, with an overall 27 percent increase in the number of cases of syphilis. A sharp rise in the number of reported

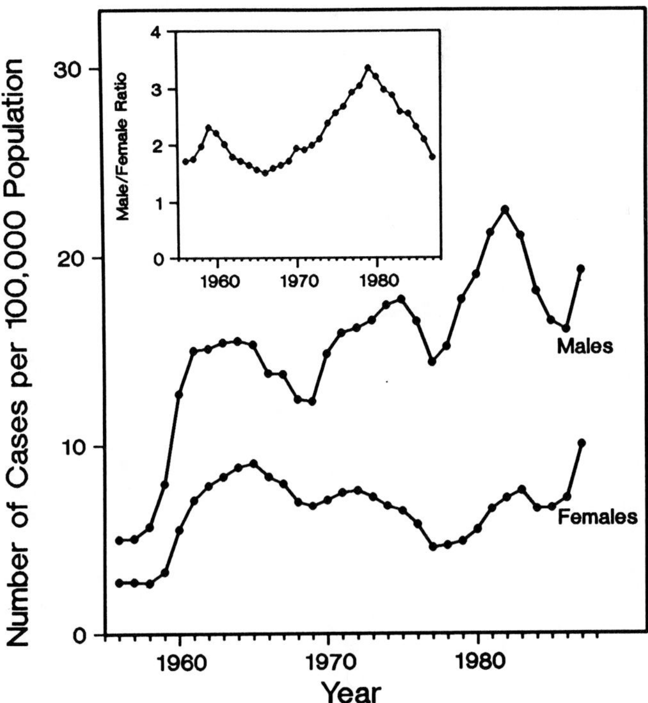


Fig. 2-6. Trends in the incidence of reported primary and secondary syphilis in men and women, and the ratio of male:female incidence, United States, 1956–1987.

**Table 2-1. Percentage of Early Syphilis Cases Involving Homosexual Men, State of Washington, 1960–1987**

| Year | Total number of cases of early syphilis* | Number of male cases (% of total) | Percent of male cases naming male partners | Percent of total cases involving homosexual men |
|---|---|---|---|---|
| 1960 | 161 | 120 (75) | 42 | 32 |
| 1969 | 61 | 50 (82) | 56 | 46 |
| 1970 | 63 | 56 (89) | 68 | 61 |
| 1971 | 142 | 126 (89) | 64 | 57 |
| 1972 | 129 | 115 (89) | 81 | 72 |
| 1973 | 156 | 137 (88) | 81 | 71 |
| 1974 | 138 | 118 (86) | 74 | 64 |
| 1983 | 311 | 246 (79) | 62 | 49 |
| 1984 | 229 | 186 (81) | 66 | 53 |
| 1985 | 175 | 120 (69) | 44 | 30 |
| 1986 | 293 | 195 (67) | 18 | 12 |
| 1987 | 293 | 176 (60) | 13 | 8 |

*Data for 1960–1974 [Blount JH, Holmes KK: Epidemiology of syphilis and the non-venereal treponematoses, in *The Biology of Parasitic Spirochetes,* Johnson RC (ed). New York, Academic, 1976, p 157] include only primary and secondary syphilis. Data for 1983–1987 also include early latent syphilis (under 1 year duration), and were kindly provided by Larry Klopfenstein, state of Washington, Department of Social and Health Services.

cases of primary and secondary syphilis among black men and women accounts for most of the recent increase (Fig. 2-7). In recent years sporadic, local syphilis outbreaks have emerged and contribute substantially to the national increase. Interestingly, these outbreaks have occurred in New York, Los Angeles, some areas in Texas, and in south Florida, areas where the recent outbreaks of chancroid have occurred and where heterosexual HIV seropositivity rates are highest.

Trends in the incidence of congenital syphilis reflect the incidence of primary and secondary syphilis among women of childbearing age, as well as the proportion of such cases in pregnant women that are detected and treated in prenatal care programs. Following 8 years of steady decline, the number of reported congenital syphilis cases among persons under 1 year of age in the United States rose during the period 1978–1987 from 108 to 449.[13] While part of this increase could be attributed to improved surveillance, increases in primary and secondary syphilis among women of reproductive age have also played a role in the rise of congenital syphilis. For example, the incidence of primary and secondary syphilis per 100,000 among women 20 to 24 years of age increased from 16.0 to 42.6 during this period.

## INFECTIONS DUE TO *CHLAMYDIA TRACHOMATIS*

During the late 1980s *Chlamydia trachomatis* has become the most prevalent sexually transmitted bacterial infection in North America and Europe.[14–17] The true incidence of *C. trachomatis* infections is difficult to determine in the United States, where the clinical syndromes caused by *C. trachomatis* are not uniformly reportable by the states and laboratory testing for *C. trachomatis* is not widely used at this time.

Indirect estimates based on the incidence of syndromes associated with *C. trachomatis* as determined by visits to private physicians, or on the case ratio of *C. trachomatis* to *N. gonorrhoeae* infections, indicate over 4 million infections per year in the United States, as of 1986.[17,18] The number of infections among women (2.6 million) was estimated to be greater than the number of

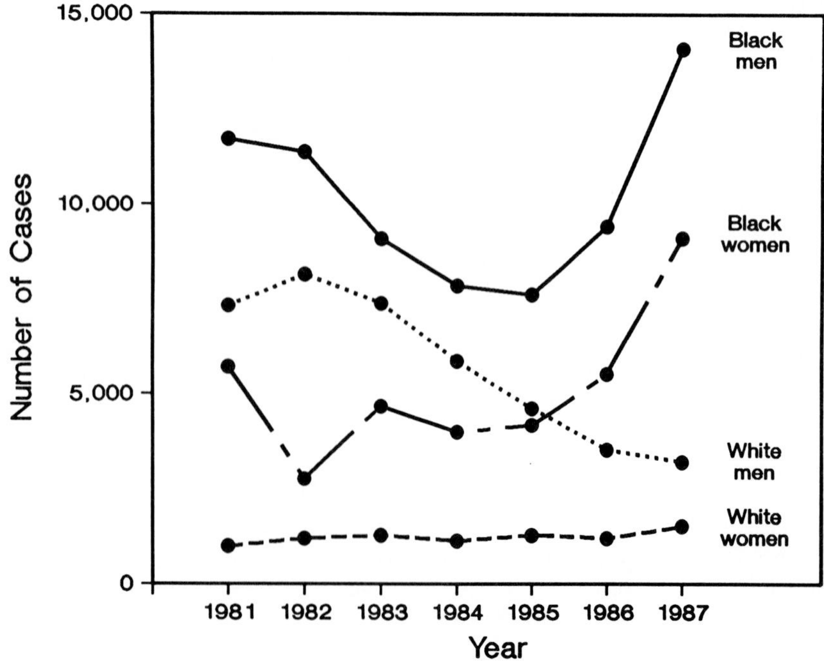


**Fig. 2-7.** Number of reported cases of primary syphilis by gender and race (black or white), United States, 1981–1987.

infections among men (1.8 million).[18,19] The distribution of chlamydia to gonorrhea ratios across population subgroups indicates a higher proportion of chlamydial infection (relative to gonorrhea) among whites, the young, and women using oral contraceptives, and individuals of higher socioeconomic status.

Although accurate national time trends in incidence of proved *C. trachomatis* infections cannot yet be defined because of lack of reporting and slowly increasing laboratory surveillance, trends of nongonococcal urethritis (NGU) incidence in men provide a reasonable approximation. The proportion of NGU attributable to *C. trachomatis* has remained fairly consistent at about 40 percent since the early 1970s.[19,20] Based on the estimated number of visits by men to private physicians' offices, the incidence of NGU has been increasing since the mid-1960s in the United States as well as in the United Kingdom. In 1972 in the United States, the number of visits to private physicians' offices for nongonococcal urethritis surpassed the number for gonococcal urethritis for the first time (Fig. 2-8), and by 1987 NGU was more than twice as common as gonococcal urethritis. The increase in office visits for NGU relative to office visits for gonococcal urethritis has been due mainly to a decline in the latter since 1971, rather than an increase in NGU. However, in England and Wales, the reported number of cases of NGU has continued to increase steadily, even as the reported number of cases of gonococcal urethritis has declined (see Chap. 16). Trends in other developed countries also fit this pattern of decreasing gonococcal urethritis contrasted with increasing NGU.[4] Other indicators for incidence of chlamydial infection, especially in women, are mucopurulent cervicitis,[21] pelvic inflammatory disease (PID), and the prevalence of perinatal chlamydial infection.[22]

The number of cases of chlamydial infection reported in Sweden rose from 20,000 in 1983 to 38,000 in 1987, at which time it was nearly equal to the number of cases of gonorrhea (40,000) reported in that country in 1970. The number of reported cases of chlamydial infection in Sweden in 1987 was nearly half the total number of cases of infection reported in 1987 in the United States—a country with 25 times the population of Sweden.[23] These data emphasize the extent of underreporting of chlamydial infections in the United States.

Why has chlamydial infection continued to increase in developed countries, while gonorrhea and syphilis generally decline? The data cited from the United States, Sweden, and England and Wales suggest public health efforts to control gonorrhea and syphilis have been effective, in contrast to the lack of effective control programs for chlamydial infection. The rise in reported chlamydial infection in Sweden, and in NGU in England and Wales, although probably influenced by increased surveillance, does suggest that the decline in gonorrhea and syphilis in those countries is not solely attributable to changing sexual behavior but also reflects the impact of gonorrhea and syphilis control programs. Finally, in selected U.S. cities where public health programs for controlling chlamydia have been in place for several years, the number of chlamydial infections has been declining. For example, at the Seattle STD Clinic, from 1982 to 1987 a decline occurred in the number of visits for NGU, in the percent of NGU cases with positive cultures for *C. trachomatis*, and in the percent of female cervical cultures that were positive for *C. trachomatis* (from a peak of 14 percent in 1983 to 8.6 percent in 1988) (H. Handsfield, W. Stamm, personal communication).

## CHANCROID

In the past decade most reported cases of chancroid in the United States have occurred in sporadic outbreaks.[24,25] The increased frequency of these outbreaks within recent years has led to a net increase in the incidence of these infections. Because chancroid may facilitate HIV transmission[26–28] and because recent U.S. outbreaks of chancroid are in metropolitan areas and heterosexual populations of high HIV prevalence, such increased incidence may be of great public health importance. Between 1984 and 1987, chancroid outbreaks occurred in Los Angeles, Dallas, Boston, New York City, and several Florida cities.[25,29] Chancroid is recognized far more frequently among men than among women. For example, in the United States during 1987, the male:female sex ratio was 5.8:1 for reported cases of chancroid, compared with 0.94:1 for genital herpes. Lack of circumcision is now well established in case-control studies as a risk factor for chancroid,

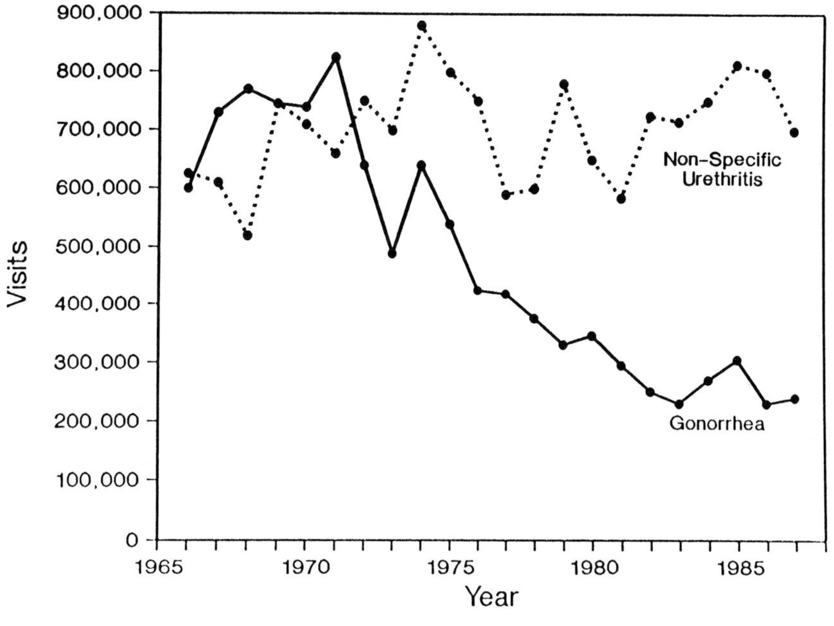

**Fig. 2-8.** Nongonococcal urethritis and gonococcal urethritis in men. Number of visits to private physicians' offices, United States, 1966–1987. (*Source: IMS, America.*)

Visits
900,000
800,000
700,000
600,000
500,000
400,000
300,000
200,000
100,000
0
1965 1970 1975 1980 1985
Year
Non-Specific Urethritis
Gonorrhea

and cultural circumcision practices probably also have an important influence on the incidence of chancroid in different ethnic groups.

Prostitute contact is repeatedly implicated in outbreaks of chancroid and is important in explaining the high male:female sex ratio, not only in recent U.S. outbreaks but in many developing countries of Africa, Asia, and Latin America where chancroid is endemic. For example, the prevalence of genital ulcers in prostitutes in a poor neighborhood of Nairobi, Kenya, was an extraordinary 42 percent,[30] and the majority were culture-positive for *Hemophilus ducreyi.* As discussed below, lack of circumcision is now well established in case-control studies as a risk factor for chancroid, and cultural circumcision practices probably also have an important influence on the incidence of chancroid in different ethnic groups.

## THE INCURABLE VIRAL STDs

During the 1980s, improved tests have been developed for type-specific serum antibody to HSV-2, and for detection of type-specific HPV DNA in epithelial cells. These new tests, together with development of tests for HIV antibody and antigen, have led to epidemiologic studies that disclose a greatly expanded scope of the problem of infection with these incurable viral STDs. Such studies are just now beginning to give a clearer picture of the distribution and determinants of these infections.

### GENITAL HERPES

Genital herpes simplex virus infection was the STD with the fastest documented increase from the mid-1960s until the onset of the AIDS epidemic. The annual number of private physician-patient consultations for symptomatic genital herpes in the United States increased from 30,000 in 1966 to over 450,000 by 1985, then declined slightly through 1987 (Fig. 2-9).[31–33] The number of office visits for newly diagnosed infections increased 8.8-fold, from 18,000 in 1966 to 157,000 in 1984, then declined through 1987. People 20 to 29 years of age had more office visits than other age groups. A comprehensive population-based 15-year prospective study of genital herpes in Rochester, Minnesota, found similar trends.[34] While women outnumbered men in genital herpes–related physician consultations, it is difficult to determine the extent to which this pattern reflects true differentials in genital herpes epidemiology rather than in health care–seeking behavior.

Data concerning physician consultation for genital herpes could be biased toward underestimation of total genital herpes infections because some symptomatic individuals do not seek health care, or seek health care through public clinics, and because asymptomatic infections are not represented in these data. Conversely, a bias toward overestimation could arise because media attention may have increased both physicians' and patients' awareness of the signs and symptoms of genital herpes, increasing the proportion of patients with genital herpes who seek physician consultations and receive a correct diagnosis.[19]

Based on the percentage of adults with serum antibody, the true annual incidence of new HSV-2 infections in the United States clearly exceeds the number of physician consultations for newly diagnosed symptomatic infections by several-fold. Recent analyses of serologic data have changed our view of herpes epidemiology: (1) Symptomatic genital herpes infections represent only a small proportion of all herpes infections. In Georgia only one-fourth of individuals with HSV-2 antibodies gave a history consistent with genital herpes infection.[35,36] In a female STD clinic population in Seattle, only one-third of those with HSV-2 antibody gave such a history even after careful interview.[37] (2) Women are more likely to have HSV-2 antibodies than men.[38] (3) HSV-2 antibody prevalence is higher among blacks than among whites,[35,36] by approximately threefold[39] (Fig. 2-10). (4) Antibodies to HSV-2 are also more prevalent among lower socioeconomic status individuals[38,39] and inner-city residents,[39,40] and were found to be approximately five times more prevalent among female STD clinic attendees than among female college students undergoing routine annual examination.[37] The prevalence of antibody increases sharply from ages 15 to 39, then tends to level off.

### GENITAL HUMAN PAPILLOMAVIRUS INFECTIONS

In recent years, the association between HPV (especially subtypes 16 and 18) and precancerous or invasive lesions of the cervix, vagina, vulva, anus, and penis has been clearly documented,[41] and as a result, interest in and physician awareness of genital HPV infections have increased (see also Chap. 48). Presently, genital and anal HPV infections and HSV appear to be the most prevalent STDs in the United States. The epidemiology of genital

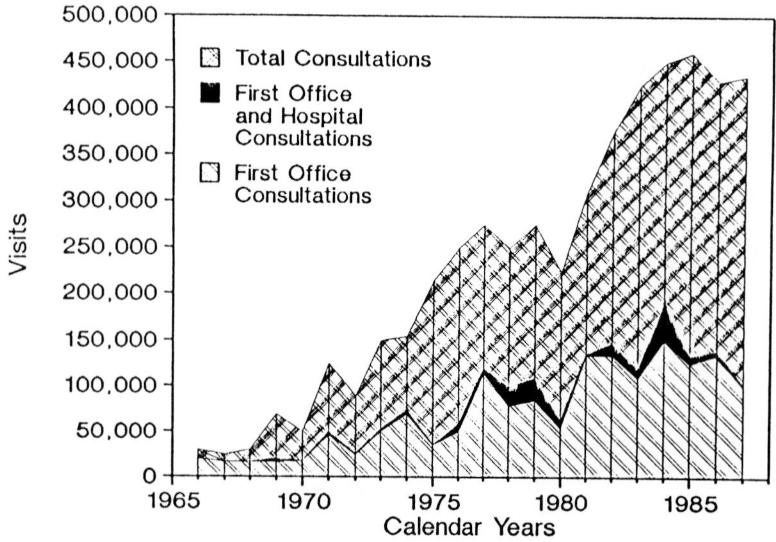


**Fig. 2-9.** Genital herpes simplex virus infections. Number of visits to private physicians' offices, United States, calendar years 1966–1987. (*Source: IMS, America.*)

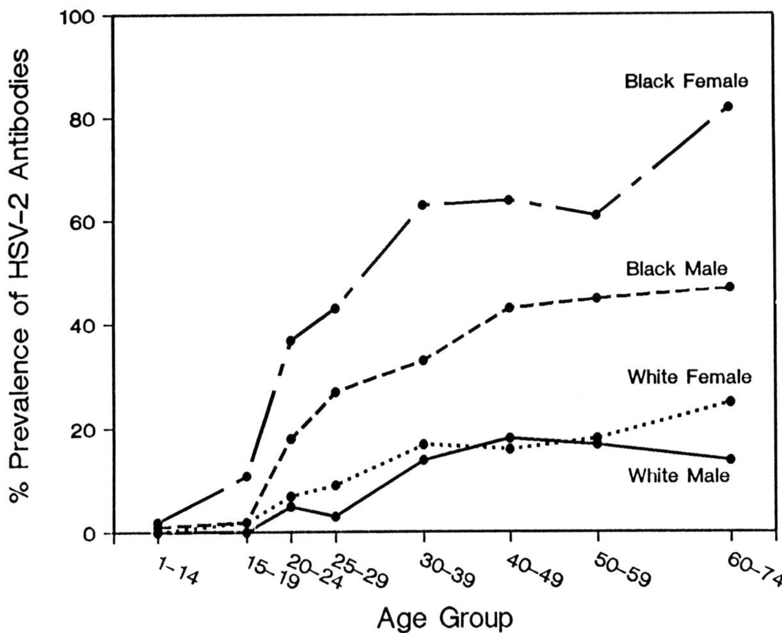


Fig. 2-10. Percent prevalence of serum antibody to HSV-2 by age group.

HPV infections is analogous to that of genital HSV infections, in that subclinical HPV infections are more prevalent than clinically evident genital warts. By screening for HPV DNA, antigen, or koilocytosis in the cervix, as well as for genital warts, the prevalence of genital HPV infections has ranged from 5 to 19 percent among women seeking health care at family planning and university student health clinics, to as high as 27 percent among women attending STD clinics.[42,43] However, as more sensitive methods for detection of HPV DNA are used, repeated sampling is performed, and multiple anatomic sites are tested, these appear to be underestimates of the true prevalence.[44] The advent of yet more sensitive tests for detection of HPV (i.e., DNA amplification by polymerase chain reaction) could serve to revise upward still further these estimates of prevalence of genital HPV infection. Serologic tests for antibody to those types of HPV found in the genital tract could eventually help to clarify the epidemiology of genital HPV infection in the same way that newer serologic tests are elucidating the epidemiology of HSV-2 infection.

While external genital warts do not represent all genital HPV infections, physician-patient consultation for this condition is the best available indicator of trends in the incidence of genital HPV infections. Such data best reflect trends in HPV which are most closely associated with genital warts, such as types 6 and 11. Consultations for genital warts increased from 169,000 in 1966 to over 1,800,000 in 1987, more than a 10-fold increase[33,45,46] (Fig. 2-11). In the United Kingdom, the incidence of genital warts increased by more than 250 percent between 1971 and 1982.[41] Similar increases have been found when studies have been conducted at the local level in STD clinics.[47] As with genital herpes–related consultations, consultations for genital warts were most common for individuals between 20 and 24 years of age, and more common for women than for men.

Among sexually active women, the prevalence of cervical HPV DNA and/or antigen has been highest for teenagers and those in the early twenties, and lower for older women.[43] Similarly, among normal male blood donors and dermatology clinic pa-

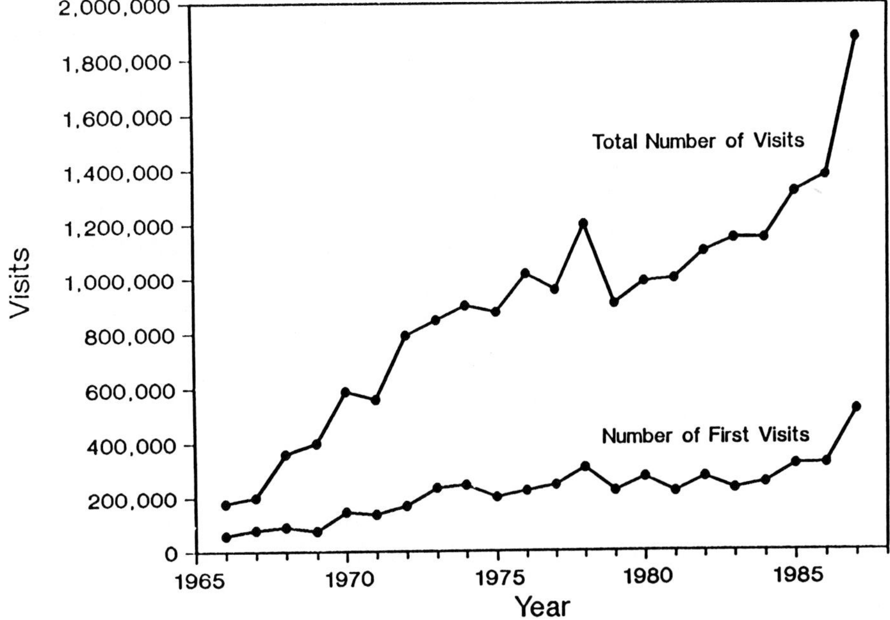


Fig. 2-11. Genital warts. Number of visits to private physicians' offices, United States, calendar years 1966–1987. (*Source: IMS, America.*)

tients in Germany,[48] HPV DNA was detected in cells swabbed from the penis in 8 percent of 365 men 16 to 35 years of age, and in 2 percent of 174 men 36 to 85 years of age. Although these data suggest that HPV DNA and antigen may disappear from cervical and penile epithelium over time, the declining prevalence with increasing age could represent a cohort effect (i.e., older individuals may have had less exposure than younger individuals to HPV infection). The natural history of genital HPV infection in men and women remains largely undefined.

Among college women undergoing routine pelvic examination, subclinical cervical infection, as defined by the presence of HPV DNA or antigen in the cervix, was more than 8 times more common than visible genital warts.[43] With a population of 122 million between ages 15 and 49 in the United States, if it is assumed that 1 percent have genital warts, 2 percent have subclinical lesions visible only with colposcopy, and 7 percent have clinically inapparent infections, then the number of individuals with HPV infection detectable by unaided examination, by colposcopy, and by laboratory tests could be over 12 million (Fig. 2-12).[41] The above discussion would suggest that even these are minimum estimates.

Health care behavior can be regarded as less important in the epidemiology of incurable viral STDs than in the epidemiology of curable bacterial STDs, as discussed below. However, one exception is cervical carcinoma, a possible complication of cervical HPV infection. Among individuals with cervical HPV infection, women who obtain regular cervical cytologic screening demonstrate a health care behavior that does allow early detection and treatment of cervical dysplasia, resulting in effective secondary prevention of invasive cervical carcinoma. Thus, as discussed in Chap. 48, the incidence of cervical cancer is considered to be exceptionally high in developing countries which lack programs for preventing cervical cancer; and it has been rising in some countries where the recommended frequency for cytology screening is relatively low. The higher incidence of cervical cancer in blacks than in whites in the United States could be attributable either to more frequent cervical HPV infection or to less frequent cytology screening or to both factors. Similarly, as discussed in Chap. 48, if early diagnosis and treatment of invasive cancer—tertiary intervention to prevent death—reflects health care behavior (partly determined by access to care), then the higher mortality rate for cervical cancer in black women than in white women could also reflect differences in health care behavior.

## HUMAN IMMUNODEFICIENCY VIRUS

The rapid accumulation of information on the epidemiology of HIV infection helps build a paradigm useful for the epidemiology of STDs. Although Chaps. 31 and 32 deal specifically with the overall epidemiology of HIV infections, we will review here selected aspects of sexually transmitted HIV infection.

### HIV infection as an STD

On a global basis, the overwhelming majority of HIV infections are sexually transmitted. Of sexually transmitted HIV infections, most of those occurring in North America are transmitted homosexually to men who practice receptive anorectal intercourse, whereas most of those occurring in Africa are transmitted heterosexually to men and women during vaginal intercourse. Intermediate patterns, where both homosexual and heterosexual transmission are common, have been seen in some European countries (where heterosexual transmission can nearly always be traced to individuals born in Africa or returning from Africa) and in the Caribbean. In North America and Latin America, homosexual transmission predominates among men, but heterosexual transmission is increasing, and accounts for virtually all sexually transmitted HIV infection among adult females. During 1988, approximately 5 percent of newly diagnosed cases of AIDS in the United States[49] and 10 percent of cases in Brazil[50] were attributed to heterosexual acquisition. Data are lacking on the proportion of new HIV infections occurring today in the United States which are heterosexually transmitted.

In sub-Saharan African countries, where AIDS is now epidemic and where over 90 percent of all cases are attributed to heterosexual transmission, the major demographic and sexual behavioral determinants of HIV infection have included urban residence, prostitution or sex with prostitutes, age, and gender. The age distribution of HIV seropositivity among asymptomatic individuals in Kinshasa, Zaire, appears to be markedly different for males and females, with the prevalence of antibody being

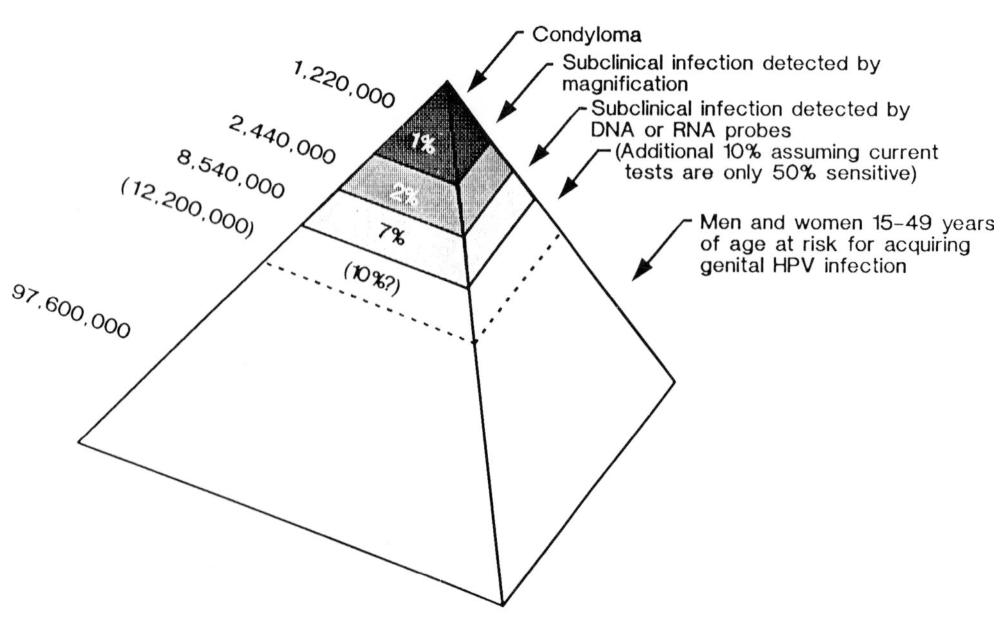


Fig. 2-12. Estimated prevalence of genital human papillomavirus infection among men and women between the ages of 15 and 49 years in the United States in 1987. (*From Ref. 41.*)

highest in adolescent and young adult women. Only among older adults was the prevalence higher among men than among women. Similar results have been obtained in a survey of hospitalized individuals throughout Uganda.[51] In a more recent study conducted in Kinshasa,[52] the rate of seropositivity for persons 15 to 29 years of age was 4 times higher for females than for males. High socioeconomic status has been correlated with seropositivity in some African studies.

The leading theories concerning the epidemic spread of HIV in sub-Saharan Africa are either that the virus itself was recently introduced into the human population; that it acquired enhanced virulence and infectivity by genetic change; or that the virus had been present in humans for a long time but began to spread at epidemic rates because of rapid urbanization, weakening of traditional culture, and other socioeconomic changes which have led to patterns of sexual behavior that promote epidemic spread of STDs, including HIV infection.

The epidemiologic features of sexual transmission of HIV infection in developed countries are much different. The appearance and spread of HIV among homosexual men can be traced to the late 1970s in the United States and, again, may represent initial introduction of the virus into this group of men or increasing levels of high-risk sexual activity among men during the 1960s and 1970s. Although longitudinal data on sexual behavior of representative samples of homosexually active men are not available prior to the mid-1980s, the increasing proportion of cases of early syphilis involving homosexual or bisexual men in the United States, and the increasing ratio of male:female cases of syphilis beginning in Sweden in the late fifties and in the United States in the late sixties, offer strong support for the latter hypothesis. Thus, increasing high-risk sexual activity among homosexual men in the United States may have played the major role in the epidemic spread of HIV in this group, just as increasing prostitution and sex with prostitutes may have been most responsible for the epidemic spread of HIV in sub-Saharan African cities. Further, the resulting epidemic spread of other STD, such as syphilis, HSV-2, and chancroid, in homosexual men of developed countries and in urban populations of developing countries may have reinforced the rapid spread of HIV in these groups.

In the United States, cases of AIDS ascribed to heterosexual transmission of HIV have disproportionately involved urban minority populations along the East Coast. For example, among U.S. women, the incidence of heterosexually acquired AIDS is approximately 20 times greater for blacks and 4 times greater for Hispanics than for whites.[53] The higher incidence of heterosexually acquired AIDS among U.S. blacks and Hispanics has several potential explanations. The incidence of HIV infection transmitted by intravenous-drug abuse is higher among blacks and Hispanics, providing a reservoir for heterosexual transmission. The incidence of other STDs is also higher among blacks and Hispanics, presumably reflecting differences in sexual and health care behavior that undoubtedly also make an important contribution to differences in heterosexual transmission of HIV. The extent to which this is influenced by social status and economic markers[54] has not been adequately examined. To the extent that certain STDs are risk factors for sexual transmission of HIV, the higher incidence of such STDs in racial minorities also may contribute to a higher incidence of HIV in minority groups.

### Interaction of other STDs with HIV infection

Evidence for bidirectional interactions of HIV infection with other STDs is intriguing and could have an important impact on the epidemiology of these conditions. The correlation of HIV-1 infection in homosexual men with serum antibody to HSV-2 and antibody to *Treponema pallidum* (Chap. 31) suggests that genital or anorectal herpes or syphilis may increase transmissibility of or susceptibility to HIV infection, although possible alternative explanations exist. Similarly, genital ulcers (usually due to chancroid) have been correlated with acquisition of HIV-1 in heterosexual African men and women in Kenya,[55] Zaire,[52] and Uganda[51] (Chap. 32). Conversely, HIV infection leads to altered manifestations of HSV infection, including chronic anorectal herpetic ulcers,[56–58] and increases the risk of single-dose quinolone treatment failure in chancroid.[57–60] Anecdotal evidence exists for failure of treatment for syphilis or altered manifestations thereof in HIV-positive individuals.[60–63] Thus, a positive reinforcement feedback can be postulated, in which syphilis, chancroid, and genital herpes promote spread of HIV; while conversely HIV infection and immunosuppression might promote spread of HSV-2, chancroid, and perhaps even syphilis. The influence of other STDs, such as gonorrhea, chlamydial infection, vaginitis, and HPV and CMV infections, on susceptibility to HIV and on the natural history of HIV infection requires further study, as does the influence of HIV infection on these other STDs.

## RISK FACTORS AND RISK MARKERS

In STD epidemiology the terms risk factor, risk marker (or indicator), and determinant have been used interchangeably without much attention to the existence of a *causal* link between the relevant attribute or exposure and the disease or disease outcome. Similarly, no differentiation has been made between modifiable and nonmodifiable risk factors, an important distinction within the context of prevention.

Many of the traditional STD risk factors appear to be correlates of the probability of encountering an infected partner, whereas others may influence the probability of infection if exposed, or the probability of disease if infected (Table 2-2). While the causal link between demographic variables and STDs can probably be explained in terms of coincidental differences in sexual behavior and/or disease prevalence, such variables may be most accurately referred to as risk markers or risk indicators. For example, single marital status and inner-city residence fall into this category.

Other variables, such as sexual behaviors and health care behaviors, are directly related to the probability of exposure to STDs, to infection following exposure, or to complications if infected, and can be referred to as true risk factors. Sexual behavior is the key determinant for incidence of incurable viral STDs, whereas both sexual and health care behaviors are important determinants of the incidence of bacterial STDs. In spite of the improvements in the measurement of sexual behavior, its various aspects are still not clearly defined.

At the present time, the major sexual behavioral risk factors for STDs appear to include a large number of sexual partners, high rates of acquiring new sexual partners within specific time periods, high rates of partner change, contact with casual sexual partners, sex preference, and specific sexual practices. All but the last of these really represent attempts to measure the probability of exposure to an infected partner. It is likely that not all infected partners are equally infectious. For example, a male with gonococcal urethritis may be more infectious than a female with chronic endocervical gonococcal infection who sheds low numbers of gonococci in cervical secretions. Individuals with HIV

**Table 2-2. Risk Markers and Risk Factors for Sexually Transmitted Diseases**

| Risk markers | Risk markers or risk factors | Risk factors |
|---|---|---|
| Marital status | Age | Sexual behaviors* |
| Race | Gender | Number of partners |
| Residence | Smoking | Rate of acquiring new partners |
| Rural/urban | Alcohol | Casual partners |
| SES | Drug abuse | Sex preference |
| | Other STDs | Sexual practices |
| | Lack of circumcision | Health care behaviors† |
| | Contraceptive method | No use of barriers and microbicidal agents |
| | | Late consultation for diagnosis, treatment |
| | | Nonreferral of partners |
| | | Noncompliance with therapy |
| | | Douching |

*The essential risk factor for acquiring an STD is exposure to an STD; some of these risk factors are current surrogates for such exposure. Better surrogates are needed. Several practices (e.g., rectal intercourse) can be additional risk factors for infection, given exposure.

†Poor health care behaviors are risk factors either for acquiring an STD or for developing complications of an STD.

infection may become more infective with time. We would expect a greater convergence of findings in this area as sexual behavior, as a proxy for exposure, is measured with greater precision and accuracy, and the design of epidemiological studies focusing on behavioral risk factors improves.

Health care behaviors which can reduce the risk of acquiring STDs or prevent complications include use of condoms for prophylaxis, early consultation for diagnosis and treatment, compliance with therapy, and partner referral (see Chap. 9). Absence of such behaviors can be regarded as risk factors for STDs. Douching represents a particular behavior which, though undertaken for "feminine hygiene," may actually increase the risk of PID and its sequelae.[64,65]

Several other variables could function both as risk markers and as risk factors, or are difficult to classify as one or the other at present (Table 2-2). For example, young age and gender are certainly risk indicators, indirectly related to risk of STDs as correlates of sexual behavior and of disease prevalence in sex partners. However, age and gender may also directly influence host susceptibility. For example, the prevalence of cervical ectopy is higher in young women than in older women, and ectopy may influence susceptibility to certain STD pathogens such as *C. trachomatis*.[66] Older individuals may have acquired immunity to STD pathogens, resulting in fewer infections per exposure. Regarding gender-specific risk, the risk of infection per exposure during vaginal intercourse may be greater for the female than for the male with respect to several STD pathogens such as *N. gonorrhoeae*,[67] *C. trachomatis*,[68] hepatitis B virus, and perhaps HIV,[49,69] although available evidence remains inconclusive. Some behavioral factors, like smoking and young age at sexual debut, which were generally assumed to be indicators of risk rather than causally related to disease outcome, have been linked to specific infections or related syndromes like genital HPV infections and cancer of the cervix even when other risk indicators and sexual behaviors are adjusted for in statistical analyses. Further empirical evidence is needed to conclusively determine whether these variables and others like them operate as true causal risk factors or are simply coincidental markers of high-risk sexual behaviors. Alcohol and drug abuse can perhaps be referred to as "risk modifiers," since they produce situational modification of sexual behavior or health care behavior.

## STDs AS RISK FACTORS FOR OTHER STDs

Many known interactions occur among different infectious diseases. For example, influenza increases host susceptibility to pneumococcal and staphylococcal pneumonia; schistosomiasis and bartonellosis increase the risk of *Salmonella* bacteremia; measles predisposes to bacterial otitis media, bacterial pneumonia, and reactivation of tuberculosis; bacterial endocarditis predisposes to fungal endocarditis; varicella predisposes to bacterial pyodermas; and so on. Mechanisms for these interactions vary. Until recently, interactions between STD pathogens in genitourinary infections have not been well studied.

The growing evidence that certain STDs function as risk factors for transmission of HIV infection is extremely important in and of itself but raises other questions about potential interactions, which at this point can be best posed as questions for further study rather than as questions that have been answered. For example:

1. *N. gonorrhoeae and C. trachomatis.* Does gonorrhea reactivate latent chlamydial infection in either sex? How do the manifestations of dual infections differ from infections with either agent alone?
2. *HSV, C. trachomatis, and HPV.* Is genital HSV-2 infection or *C. trachomatis* infection a cofactor with HPV 16, 18, or 31 for producing invasive cervical cancer or other genital cancer?
3. *HIV and HPV.* Does HIV infection "reactivate" genital or anal HPV infection? Does HIV infection increase the risk of genital or anal dysplasia or cancer among those with HPV infection? If so, is this related to or independent of level of immunosuppression?
4. *HIV, syphilis, and chancroid.* Does HIV infection alter the manifestations of syphilis and chancroid as it clearly alters the clinical manifestations of anorectal herpes?[56] Does HIV infection increase the risk of failure of standard treatments for syphilis,[60] as it reportedly increases the risk of failure of treatment for chancroid? Does syphilis influence progression of HIV infection to AIDS?
5. *T. vaginalis and N. gonorrhoeae.* Is the frequently observed association of vaginal trichomoniasis with cervical gonorrhea coincidental, or does this have a biological explanation? Does trichomoniasis increase the risk of failure of treatment for gonorrhea?[70]
6. *Vaginal flora and other STDs.* Is the normal lactobacillus-dominated vaginal flora protective against other STD pathogens? Does bacterial vaginosis increase susceptibility to other genital infections?
7. *N. gonorrhoeae, C. trachomatis, and "polymicrobial PID."* Does gonococcal or chlamydial salpingitis "pave the way" for tubal infection by vaginal organisms of lesser virulence?
8. *HSV and other genital ulcers.* Does HSV, by producing recurrent genital epithelial ulceration, present a risk factor for acquiring other genital epithelial infection, such as chancroid?

Assessing one STD as a cofactor for another STD presents unique problems, since the sexual exposures leading to one STD are those which directly lead to exposures to the other STDs. Case-control studies which will adequately adjust for such confounders as sexual behaviors are difficult to design. Cohort studies which allow assessment of the temporal relationships between a first and second STD, and intervention trials (e.g., prevention of one STD to reduce the risk of another STD) represent possible ways to assess such interactions.

## MALE CIRCUMCISION

Lack of circumcision was implicated as a major independent risk factor for HIV infection among men attending an STD clinic in Nairobi.[28,55] This potentially important observation raises the question of whether circumcision may influence the risk of other STDs, and if so, why. Several studies have found a correlation of lack of circumcision with chancroid (or with undifferentiated genital ulcers in chancroid-endemic areas).[26,28,55,71,72] Although lack of circumcision has also been correlated with syphilis in some studies,[73,74] and with genital herpes in another,[75] these observations require confirmation in studies designed to control for confounding variables. The incidence of gonorrhea was found to be higher in uncircumcised men than in circumcised men in a study of military personnel, although the effect was seen only in whites.[67] Lack of circumcision has been held to be a risk factor for penile warts and penile cancer,[76–78] but these associations appear not to have been adequately studied. Finally, both candidal[74] and nonspecific balanitis appear to be more common among uncircumcised men.[79]

Biologically plausible hypotheses exist to explain such associations. The recesses of the preputial sac are said to be "nonkeratinized" (i.e., like the vaginal and buccal epithelium, not covered by a layer of nonnucleated, keratin-dense squamous cells),[79] which might predispose to physical trauma or microbial infection. Similarly, balanitis per se might predispose to invasion by microbial pathogens. The preputial sac might serve as a reservoir for STD pathogens acquired during intercourse, from which invasion of the urethra or squamous epithelium might proceed. Clinical manifestations of urethritis, warts, or genital ulcers might go undetected longer in an uncircumcised man, which could increase transmission or complications of STDs.

However, despite such plausibility, circumcision practices are clearly related to religion, ethnicity and tribal culture, and economic status, all factors which are also strongly correlated with sexual behavior. Thus, the relationship of HIV infection and other STDs to lack of circumcision clearly requires cross-cultural analysis, with efforts to carefully adjust for confounders such as sexual behavior and socioeconomic status.

## PROSTITUTION

During the 1980s prostitute contact has been implicated as an important risk factor. The contribution of prostitution to the spread of STDs has been assessed by monitoring the incidence or prevalence of STDs in prostitutes and the proportion of male patients with STDs who acknowledge recent sex with a prostitute (see Chap. 7). Recent studies have focused on specific outbreaks of syphilis, chancroid, and resistant gonorrhea.[80,81]

The sociodemography of the men involved in these outbreaks has often (but not always) involved some form of transiency, as in the case of foreigners, servicemen, and migrant laborers. Transient populations are by definition not integrated into the community; their only sexual, and sometimes social, interaction with the main community may be through prostitute contact. The gender-selective nature of most international migration (especially initially), and of temporary unskilled and semiskilled labor reinforce, through the unavailability of women, the demand for prostitute contact. The social profiles of both the men and the women involved in some of the recent outbreaks have involved the exchange of drugs for sex and vice versa.[80,81] While such exchange is not a new epidemiologic factor, the specifics of the recent pattern may reflect increased use of new drugs (like crack cocaine) with characteristics more conducive to STD transmission. Recent evidence suggests that in some urban areas in the United States, exchange of sex for drugs such as crack has been correlated with gonorrhea,[80] syphilis,[81] and chancroid. Women, particularly adolescents, sometimes engage in large numbers of sexual contacts to support their addictions. In a 1986–1987 Seattle outbreak of a unique strain of PPNG, within a few months after the strain had been introduced into the community, approximately 80 percent of infections with this strain occurred in individuals who had sex with prostitutes or were themselves prostitutes, or who had used illicit drugs around the time that infection occurred.

On a global basis, prostitution has been most common in settings characterized by poverty, social disintegration, and a double standard of sexual behavior (e.g., Latin American countries). Where many of these factors coincide, prostitution is most prevalent.[82] Prostitution and prostitute contact are clearly major factors in the epidemiology of HIV and other STDs in many developing countries of Africa, Asia, and Latin America.[83] In such settings, the great majority of STD clinic attendees are male, and the majority of those with gonorrhea, syphilis, or chancroid identify the suspected source contact as a prostitute. The role of sex with prostitutes in the epidemiology of these STDs now requires close analysis, particularly in disadvantaged populations in developed countries, where the occurrence of bacterial STDs is contracting around an expanding core of inner-city minority populations, and in developing countries.

## CONTRACEPTION

Patterns of contraception usage markedly influence the transmission and sequelae of STDs. Barrier methods such as the diaphragm with spermicide probably offer some protection, particularly against organisms transmitted mainly between the columnar or transitional epithelium of the urethra and cervix (e.g., *C. trachomatis, N. gonorrhoeae*). Condoms, used properly, offer strong protection against organisms like *C. trachomatis* and *N. gonorrhoeae* and partial protection against those which commonly infect stratified squamous epithelium such as herpes simplex virus and human papilloma virus.[83a] Oral contraceptive usage has been associated with decreased risk of severe PID,[84] with increased risk of cervical infection with *C. trachomatis*,[85–88] and perhaps with increased risk of cervical infection with *N. gonorrhoeae*[89] (see Chap. 92).

Interest in patterns of contraceptive use has increased in recent years in part as a result of the rising incidence of STDs, including AIDS. Available data indicate that contraceptive attitudes and usage patterns have also changed, at least in the United States.[90] Between 1982 and 1987, favorable opinion of the pill increased among American women from 65 to 76 percent; favorable opinion of the condom increased even more, from 38 to 60 percent. During the same period approval of the IUD dropped from 26 to 19 percent. While overall level of contraceptive use remained stable at about 33 percent, use of the more effective methods, i.e., sterilization, pill, and IUD, increased from 68 to 71 percent. Pill use rose among married women from 17 to 22 percent, and among unmarried women from 43 to 48 percent. Use of sterilization went up from 46 to 51 percent among married women.

Condom use remained steady among married women, at about 15 percent, while among the unmarried it increased markedly from 9 to 16 percent. These recent trends in the United States, particularly the increased use of condoms among unmarried women, are encouraging.

Patterns of knowledge and use of condoms in most other parts of the world are less well known. During the 1970s in developed countries, the proportion of currently married females of child-bearing age who reported current use of condoms ranged from a low of 2 to 3 percent in Yugoslavia, Bulgaria, and Romania to a high of 50 percent in Japan; this percentage was 32 in Finland, 25 in Denmark, 18 in the United Kingdom, 16 in Norway, and 13 in Italy. More recent data are unavailable from most of these countries.

Survey data from around the developing world on prevalence of knowledge and use of condoms among reproductive-age women have recently been compiled.[91] These data reveal a wide range in knowledge of condoms, with the least knowledge in sub-Saharan Africa, including those countries with high HIV prevalence. Knowledge of condoms was most widespread in Latin America and the Caribbean, where over 80 percent of currently married women of reproductive age were familiar with condoms. Countries in Asia tended to report lower levels of knowledge of condoms. In the Middle East and North Africa, the proportion of women reporting knowledge of condoms ranged from 26 to 61 percent. Least knowledge of condoms was reported for Nigeria, Benin, and Mali.

Use of condoms is also highest among people living in and around the Caribbean: Costa Rica (13 percent), Trinidad and Tobago (12 percent), Jamaica (8 percent), Barbados and Venezuela (5 percent). Prevalence of reported condom use was 2 to 4 percent in India, Bangladesh, Mexico, Brazil, Malaysia, Turkey, and Tunisia. In a majority of developing countries with available data less than 1 percent of couples reported condom use. This pattern was observed in all of mainland sub-Saharan Africa, including countries like Zimbabwe and Botswana which have relatively high overall contraceptive prevalence; and in most of North Africa and the Middle East and in some Latin American nations such as Haiti, El Salvador, Honduras, and Bolivia. Past efforts by family planning groups have emphasized condom use for contraception, rather than for STD prophylaxis. Some family planning workers now express concern that condom promotion for disease prophylaxis may stigmatize condom use and undo the results of past efforts to promote condom acceptability.

Current global public health efforts to increase condom use to prevent transmission of STDs including HIV are targeted at large proportions of the sexually active population which do not use condoms, particularly in developing countries. However, interest is growing in targeted promotion of condom use for those at highest risk of STD (e.g., prostitutes, customers of prostitutes, etc.), which may be a more practical and cost-effective approach to STD prevention.

## DIMENSIONS OF SEXUAL BEHAVIOR

While sexual behavior has been recognized as a major risk factor for STDs all along, our understanding of its relevant components has changed considerably over the past two decades. A better understanding of the epidemiology of specific STDs, and the greater need for primary prevention in the context of increasing viral STDs, initiated such changes in the early 1980s. However, the AIDS epidemic has been the single most important factor to both highlight the need for more systematic information on sexual behavior and facilitate an unprecedented increase in infection-related studies of sexual behavior. The viral STDs are incurable, and sexual behavior remains the major determinant of disease prevalence and the major point of intervention.

The term "sexual behavior" involves many components: sexual experience and activity, age at sexual debut or "coitarche," current and lifetime number of sex partners, frequency of sexual intercourse, consistency of sexual activity, mode of recruitment of sexual partners and duration of sexual unions, and types of sexual practice.[92] While the conjoint distribution of these component variables in the population determines aggregate exposure to the risk of STDs, the specific relationship between each of these variables and STD risk, and the distribution of these variables across population subgroups, have not yet been determined.

The population at risk for STDs has, in its crudest form, been defined in terms of age groups, assuming those between ages 15 and 45 engage in sexual intercourse with new partners. Further refinements of this concept have included in the population at risk only the sexually experienced, defined as persons who have ever had sexual intercourse.[93,94] However, current sexual activity, rather than sexual experience per se, is a more accurate measure of exposure to the risk of STDs.[95]

In 1982, overall, 86 percent of 15- to 44-year-old women in the United States were sexually experienced. This proportion increased with increasing age. Among those ages 15 to 19, only 45 percent of white women and 56 percent of women of other races had ever had sexual intercourse. Teenagers were also the least currently sexually active. Sexual activity among teens ranged from 40 percent reporting sexual intercourse in the 3 months prior to interview to just one in seven having had regular intercourse every month in the preceding year.[92] Large proportions of teenagers were sexually experienced but abstainers; although they had had sexual intercourse at least once in their lives, they were not currently sexually active. Teenagers and older women of other races are similar in two respects: first, their sexual activity is marked by sporadicity; and second, relatively high levels of sexual activity occur in a relatively small subset of these groups.

One of the most frequent used risk markers in STD research is age at first sexual intercourse. This variable has often been employed to describe sexual activity levels of populations and to monitor the so-called sexual revolutions and evolutions. Age at sexual debut has two epidemiological functions: first as a true risk factor, causally related to disease outcome, and second as an indicator of other aspects of sexual activity. Etiologically, age at sexual debut has been associated with the development of cervical cancer in some studies, perhaps owing to the biological development of the female cervix during the teenage years. As a risk indicator, age at sexual debut is correlated with sociodemographic factors such as race and socioeconomic status, sexual behavior variables, number of sexual partners, and specific STDs.

Age at sexual debut together with age at first marriage has been the primary variable documenting the sexual revolution of the 1970s.[96] Data from national surveys conducted in 1971, 1976, 1979, and 1982 suggest that premarital sexual activity (defined in terms of sexual experience and number of sexual partners) increased among white teenagers during the 1970s and leveled off between 1979 and 1982. Among black teenagers, sexual activity rose during the early 1970s, leveled off between 1976 and 1979, and declined between 1979 and 1982.

Risk of exposure to an STD is directly associated with number of sexual partners within sex partner pools, where prevalence is constant. The number of sex partners within a specific time period, often 1 or 3 months, has been shown to be a risk factor for the transmission of gonorrhea,[97] chlamydia,[98,99] genital herpes, and human papillomavirus infections.[100] Lifetime number of sex partners is associated with the risk of cervical and other genital cancers.[101] However, the relationship between number of sex partners and STD risk is not simple; it is complicated by the partner's sexual behavior, the varying infectiousness of infected partners, and the "nonlinearity" of the increase in risk with increased numbers of sexual partners.

Some individuals are at risk for STDs because of their own sexual behaviors; these persons have a relatively high likelihood of being infected and perhaps are best described by the term "high-frequency transmitters." Poor health care behavior (e.g., failure to seek treatment while remaining sexually active with symptoms of STD) is another important feature of high-frequency transmitters. Other individuals are at risk for STDs because of the sexual behaviors of their partners; while the likelihood of their getting infected could be high, since they do not have many sexual partners their likelihood of infecting others is relatively low. This second category can be described as "receivers." Although systematically collected data on this typology are scarce, it appears that women are more likely to be receivers.

The nonlinear increase in STD risk with increasing numbers of sexual partners is increasingly well documented.[102–104] The marginal increase in STD risk suddenly multiplies as the number of sex partners reaches certain threshold levels. The possibility of STD risk due to one's partner's behavior and the nonlinear nature of the relationship between number of sex partners and STD risk point to the importance of two other dimensions of sexual behavior: choice of partners and contact with core groups of high-STD-risk individuals.

Whether one has sexual relationships with high-frequency transmitters is determined by who one's sex partners are and, indirectly, by how one chooses one's sex partners. The nature of sex partner recruitment has only recently emerged as a research topic, and very few data are available on it. However, the limited evidence we have suggests that both in the general population and among STD clinic attendees, marked gender differentials exist in the recruitment of sex partners. Compared with men, women tend to meet their potential partners through less casual associations and know them better and for longer periods of time prior to becoming sexually involved with them.[105,106] A nondiscriminating approach to sex partner recruitment increases the probability of sexual contact with members of high-risk core groups and thus of exposure to STDs. Better understanding of the prevalent modes of partner recruitment in population subgroups will help explain some of the variability in STD risk.

## DEMOGRAPHIC AND SOCIAL CORRELATES OF STDs

At the end of the 1980s, inner-city, poor, minority populations of developed countries, particularly the United States, and the populations of developing countries (especially their urban populations) appear to have similar profiles, vis-à-vis STD as a public health problem. Interestingly, these populations are also alike with respect to several demographic, sociopolitical, and economic characteristics which are associated with high levels of STD incidence.

First, both developing countries and inner-city minority populations have a youthful population composition marked by relatively high and increasing proportions of sexually active adolescents and young adults. In the United States the proportion of the white population in the sexually active age groups has started declining during the mid-1980s; the proportion of the nonwhite population in these age groups is still increasing, however. Thus, the minority population of the United States, unlike the white population, has an age pyramid which is similar to that of developing country populations and conducive to increasing STD incidence.

Second, both developing countries and inner-city minority populations are characterized by rapid demographic change. Developing countries in general have high population growth rates resulting from the combination of high fertility rates and low and/or declining mortality rates. In addition, these populations have high rates of urbanization, and population movement of all types including permanent or temporary rural-rural migration, rural-urban migration, or urban-urban migration.[107,108] Inner-city urban populations of developed countries are also marked by high physical mobility.[109,110] Rapid economic change is another characteristic which similarly marks the diverse populations of inner cities of the developed world and whole societies of the underdeveloped world. The transition from agricultural self-sufficiency to dependence on income from wage labor, which properly describes the economic state of most underdeveloped countries, is one of the best-known periods of rapid economic change in society; it involves structural transformations of the most basic kind.[111] The changes being introduced into the inner-city minority communities of the United States through the sale of drugs, especially crack cocaine, are described by observers in similar terms. Large sums of money change hands very rapidly in the course of drug trade; are suddenly introduced into the daily lives of inner-city communities, often through very young teenagers; and radically alter the existing social structure of these communities.

Third, developing countries and inner-city minority populations both have unstable power hierarchies and are thus marked by rapid political change. The frequency of civil wars, coups, and border disturbances, and the extensive need for police and military presence to assure peace in everyday life, are indicators of lack of political stability in many countries of the third world. Similarly, more frequent violence in inner-city communities in the United States is an indicator of the tentative nature of power hierarchies existing in these communities. The disruptive effects of drug use and drug trade on the stability of these communities are visible.

The rapid demographic, economic, and political changes in these populations result in a social situation where levels of transience and marginality are high, the normative structure is destabilized, and social disintegration reigns.[110] In these social systems, the basic patterning of need, dependency, and opportunity structures is such as to reinforce inequality-based social exchanges. Institutions like prostitution and drug trade actually emerge as adaptive responses to the existing sociopolitical structures and function as social factors which enhance the spread of STDs.

## SUMMARY AND IMPLICATIONS FOR THE FUTURE

Although efforts at individual and societal behavior change may seem inconsequential in the face of the above macrosocietal issues, the evidence for changing sexual behaviors of homosexual men stands as testimony to the actual power of efforts to change these behaviors. Trends in the epidemiology of syphilis, beginning in the mid-sixties and culminating in 1982, undoubtedly reflect a real but poorly documented increase in high-risk sexual behaviors that contributed to—and may have been solely responsible for—the epidemic sexual spread of HIV infection within the population. The ability of HIV to reproduce itself and spread within a population is related to both the efficiency of sexual transmission per encounter and the number of sex partners encountered per unit time by an infected individual.[112–114] Receptive anorectal intercourse is the most efficient method of sexual transmission of HIV, and genital and anorectal ulcers (caused by syphilis and HSV-2) are cofactors for homosexual acquisition of HIV. Perhaps the epidemic increase of syphilis among gay men during the seventies—and the less well documented epidemic increases of other infectious causes of epidemic proctitis during the same period—served to increase the efficacy of transmission concurrently with the increase in the frequency of encountering new partners.

The steady decrease in incidence of gonorrhea and syphilis among adult white heterosexuals in the United States and other countries is consistent with effective public health control measures, and with a decrease in unsafe sexual behaviors in this group, as in homosexual men. However, now we are beginning to see the reemergence of syphilis, chancroid, and gonorrhea in young, black, and Hispanic inner-city poor populations, in association with a reemergence of prostitution and sex with prostitutes, and in association with illegal drug use. These increases, coupled with the continuing increased incidence of viral STDs, decrease the accessibility of public health care for STDs. Persons who can afford them utilize private sources for STD care. Among poor minority populations, which cannot afford private health care, treatment is delayed and a longer duration of untreated infection contributes to further increases in bacterial STDs. Will this pattern, which is just coming into focus, be borne out with time and further study? If so, will the underlying changes of sexual behavior, together with the emerging epidemic of other STDs in such inner-city populations, be sufficient to sustain an epidemic of heterosexual spread of HIV, analogous to what has been seen in Africa?

As the reservoir of bacterial STDs retrenches to specific high-risk heterosexual populations—so-called core groups—in developed countries, innovative programs are needed to focus traditional STD control efforts on these groups. Such efforts not only could contain the spread of bacterial STD but could be highly effective in limiting the spread of HIV. However, traditional efforts involving diagnosis, treatment, and partner notification are less effective for the incurable viral STDs and, in some developing countries, have limited effectiveness even for certain of the bacterial STDs that are hard to diagnose, such as gonorrhea and chlamydial infection. Here, behavioral interventions are relatively more important, but again the group targeted for behavioral intervention should be selected on the basis of a clear understanding of the epidemiology of the diseases to be prevented.

## References


1 Centers for Disease Control: Gonorrhea annual survey 1983. *MMWR* 32:22, 1984.
2 Centers for Disease Control: Gonorrhea—United States, 1983. *MMWR* 33:361, 1984.
3 Rice RR et al: Gonorrhea in the United States 1975–1984: Is the giant only sleeping? *Sex Transm Dis* 14:83, 1987.
4 Cates W Jr, Holmes KK: Sexually transmitted diseases, in *Maxey-Rosenau Public Health and Preventive Medicine*, 12th ed, JM Last et al (eds). East Norwalk, Connecticut, Appleton-Century Crofts, 1986, p 257.
5 Barnes RC, Holmes KK: Epidemiology of gonorrhea-current perspectives. *Epidemiol Rev* 6:1, 1984.
6 Handsfield HH et al: Epidemiology of penicillinase-producing *Neisseria gonorrhoeae* infections: Analysis by auxityping and serotyping. *N Engl J Med* 306:950, 1982.
7 Centers for Disease Control: Penicillinase-producing *Neisseria gonorrhoeae*—United States, Florida. *MMWR* 35:12, 1986.
8 Centers for Disease Control: Penicillinase-producing *Neisseria gonorrhoeae*—United States, 1986. *MMWR* 36:107, 1987.
9 Jaffe HW et al: Infections due to penicillinase-producing *Neisseria gonorrhoeae* in the United States: 1976–1980. *J Infect Dis* 144:191, 1981.
10 Fleming WL: Syphilis through the ages. *Med Clin North Am* 48:587, 1964.
11 Fichtner RR et al: Syphilis in the United States, 1967–1979. *Sex Transm Dis* 10:77, 1983.
12 Centers for Disease Control: Syphilis—United States, 1983. *MMWR* 33:433, 1984.
13 Centers for Disease Control: Syphilis—United States, 1983–1985. *MMWR* 35:625, 1986.
14 Wienmeier E et al: Detection of chlamydia cervicitis with Papanicolaou-stained smears and cultures in a university study population. *J Reprod Med* 32:251, 1987.
15 Thompson SE, Washington AE: Epidemiology of sexually transmitted *Chlamydia trachomatis* infections. *Epidemiol Rev* 5:96, 1983.
16 Stamm WE, Holmes KK: Measures to control *Chlamydia trachomatis* infections: An assessment of new national policy guidelines. *JAMA* 256:1178, 1986.
17 Washington AE et al: *Chlamydia trachomatis* infections in the United States. What are they costing us? *JAMA* 257:2070, 1987.
18 Washington AE et al: Incidence of *Chlamydia trachomatis* infections in the United States: Using reported *Neisseria gonorrhoeae* as a surrogate, in *Chlamydial Infections*, D Oriel et al (eds). Cambridge, England, Cambridge University Press, 1986, p 487.
19 Cates W Jr: Epidemiology and control of sexually transmitted diseases: Strategic evolution, in *Infectious Disease Clinics of North America*, 1987, vol 1, no 1, p 1.
20 Judson FN: Epidemiology and control of nongonococcal urethritis and genital chlamydial infections: A review. *Sex Transm Dis* 8(suppl): 117, 1981.
21 Brunham RC et al: Mucopurulent cervicitis—The ignored counterpart in women of urethritis in men. *N Engl J Med* 311:1, 1984.
22 Alexander ER et al: Role of *Chlamydia trachomatis* in perinatal infection. *Rev Infect Dis* 5:713, 1983.
23 Danielsson D: Data presented at the International Symposium on Pathogenic Neisserai, Calloway Gardens, Georgia, 1988.
24 D'Costa LJ et al: Advances in the diagnosis and management of chancroid. *Sex Transm Dis* 13(suppl): 189, 1986.
25 Krockta WR et al: Genital ulceration with regional adenopathy. *Infect Dis Clin North Am* 1:217, 1987.
26 Greenblatt RM et al: Genital ulceration as a risk for human immunodeficiency virus infection. *AIDS* 2:47, 1988.
27 Plummer F et al: Cofactors in male-female transmission of HIV. IV International Conference on AIDS, Stockholm, June 13–16, 1988.
28 Simonsen JN et al: Human immunodeficiency virus infection among men with sexually transmitted diseases. *N Engl J Med* 319:274, 1988.
29 Centers for Disease Control: Chancroid—Massachusetts. *MMWR* 34:711, 1985.
30 Kreiss JK et al: AIDS virus infection in Nairobi prostitutes: Spread of the epidemic to East Africa. *N Engl J Med* 314:414, 1986.
31 Becker TM et al: Epidemiology of genital herpes infections in the United States: The current situation. *J Reprod Med* 31:359, 1986.
32 Centers for Disease Control: Genital herpes infections—United States, 1966–1984. *MMWR* 35:402, 1986.
33 Centers for Disease Control: Sexually Transmitted Disease Statis-

tics—1987. Issue 136. US Department of Health and Human Services, 1988.

34 Chuang T et al: Incidence and trends of herpes progenitalis: A 15-year population study. *Mayo Clin Proc* 58:436, 1983.

35 Lee R et al: New type-specific antigens for detecting antibodies to herpes simplex viruses type 1 (HSV-1) and type 2 (HSV-2). Presented at International Society for STD Research, Brighton, England, August 2, 1985.

36 Nahmias AJ et al: Prevalence of herpes infections in a health maintenance organization. Presented at The International Society for STD Research, Brighton, England, August 2, 1985.

37 Koutsky L et al: Unpublished data.

38 Stvrasky KM et al: Sexual and socioeconomic factors affecting the risk of past infections with herpes simplex virus type 2. *Am J Epidemiol* 118:109, 1983.

39 Johnson RE et al: Distribution of antibodies to herpes simplex virus type-2 in the United States as measured by a new antibody type-specific assay. *N Engl J Med* 1989 (in press).

40 Hahn RA et al: Race and the prevalence of syphilis infection in the U.S. population. A national sero-epidemiologic study. *Am J Public Health* 1989 (in press).

41 Koutsky L et al: Epidemiology of genital human papillomavirus. *Epidemiol Rev* 10:122, 1988.

42 Becker TM et al: Genital human papillomavirus infection: A growing concern. *Clin Obstet Gynecol* 1989 (in press).

43 Kiviat N et al: Prevalence of genital papillomavirus infection among women attending a college student health clinic or an STD clinic. *J Infect Dis* February 1989.

44 Kiviat N et al: Unpublished data.

45 Centers for Disease Control: Condyloma acuminata, 1966–1983. *MMWR* 33:81, 1986.

46 Becker TM: Genital warts—A sexually transmitted disease epidemic. *Colposc Gynecol Laser Surg* 1:47, 1985.

47 Stone KM et al: The epidemiology of genital warts in an STD clinic. Presented at The Second International Conference on Human Papillomavirus and Squamous Carcinoma, Chicago, Illinois, October 27, 1986.

48 Grussendorf-Conen E-S et al: Human papillomavirus genomes in penile smears of healthy men (letter). *Lancet* 1:1092, 1986.

49 Holmes KK, Kreiss J: Heterosexual transmission of human immunodeficiency virus: Overview of a neglected aspect of the AIDS epidemic. *AIDS* 1989 (in press).

50 Rodriguez L: Epidemiology of AIDS in Brazil. Presented at The 2nd International Pan American Health Organization on AIDS Teleconference. Rio de Janeiro, December 1988.

51 Berkley S et al: Risk factors associated with HIV infection in Uganda. *J Infect Dis* 1989 (in press).

52 Nzila N et al: Married couples in Zaire with discordant HIV serology. Fourth International Conference on AIDS, Stockholm, June 1988.

53 Holmes K et al: Perspectives on the increasing percentage of domestic cases of AIDS attributable to heterosexual transmission. Unpublished data.

54 Liberatos P et al: The measurement of social class in epidemiology. *Epidemiol Rev* 10:87, 1988.

55 Cameron DW et al: Incidence and risk factors for female to male transmission of HIV. IVth International Conference on AIDS, Stockholm, Sweden, June 1988.

56 Siegal FP et al: Severe acquired immunodeficiency in male homosexuals, manifested by chronic perianal ulcerative herpes simplex lesions. *N Engl J Med* 305:1439, 1981.

57 Dix RD et al: Herpes simplex virus type 2 encephalitis in two homosexual men with persistent lymphadenopathy. *Ann Neurol* 17:203, 1985.

58 Britton CB et al: A new complication of AIDS: Thoracic myelitis caused by herpes simplex virus. *Neurology* 25:1071, 1985.

59 MacDonald KS et al: Evaluation of fleroxacin (RO23-6240) as single oral dose therapy of culture-proven chancroid in Nairobi, Kenya. *AAC* 1989 (in press).

60 Berry CD et al: Neurologic relapse after benzathine penicillin therapy for secondary syphilis in a patient with HIV infection. *N Engl J Med* 316:1587, 1988.

61 Hicks CB et al: Seronegative secondary syphilis in a patient infected with the human immunodeficiency virus (HIV) with Kaposi sarcoma: A diagnostic dilemma. *Ann Intern Med* 107:492, 1987.

62 Radolf JD, Kaplan RP: Unusual manifestations of secondary syphilis and abnormal humoral immune response to *Treponema pallidum* antigens in a homosexual man with asymptomatic human immunodeficiency virus infection. *J Am Acad Dermatol* 18:432, 1988.

63 Johns DR et al: Alteration in the natural history of neurosyphilis by concurrent infection with the human immunodeficiency virus. *N Engl J Med* 316:1569, 1988.

64 Wølner-Hanssen P et al: Association between vaginal douching and acute pelvic inflammatory disease. Unpublished data.

65 Chow WH et al: Vaginal douching as a potential risk factor for tubal ectopic pregnancy. *Am J Obstet Gynecol* 153:72, 1985.

66 Harrison R et al: Cervical *Chlamydia trachomatis* infection in university women: Relationship to history, contraception, ectopy, and cervicitis. *Am J Obstet Gynecol* 153:244, 1985.

67 Hooper RR et al: Cohort study of venereal disease: I: The risk of gonorrhea transmission from infected women to men. *Am J Epidemiol* 108:136, 1978.

68 Lycke E et al: The risk of transmission of genital chlamydia trachomatis infection is less than that of genital *Neisseria gonorrhoeae* infection. *Sex Transm Dis* 7:6, 1980.

69 Peterman T et al: Risk of HIV transmission from heterosexual adults with transfusion-associated infections. *JAMA* 259:55, 1988.

70 Ovcinnikov NM, Delektorskij VV: Phagocytosis in the urethral discharge from patients with gonorrhea, in *Gonorrhea: Epidemiology and Pathogenesis,* FA Skinner et al (eds). London, Academic, 1977, p 158.

71 Hart G: Venereal disease in a war environment: Incidence and management. *Med J Aust* 1:808, 1975.

72 Fischl M: Seroprevalence and risks of HIV infections in spouses of persons infected with HIV. IV International Conference on AIDS, Stockholm, June 1988.

73 Wilson RA: Circumcision and venereal disease. *Can Med Assoc J* 56:54, 1947.

74 Parker SW et al: Circumcision and sexually transmissible disease. *Med J Aus* 2:288, 1983.

75 Taylor PK, Rodin P: Herpes genitalis and circumcision. *Br J Vener Dis* 51:274, 1975.

76 Dodge OG, Kavati JN: Male circumcision among the peoples of East Africa and the incidence of genital cancer. *East Afr Med J* 42:98, 1965.

77 Boczko S, Freed S: Penile carcinoma in circumcised males. *NY St J Med,* November 1979:1903.

78 Hosze K, McCurdy S: Circumcision and the risk of cancer of the penis. *Am J Dis Child* 134:484, 1980.

79 Fink AJ: *Circumcision: A Parent's Decision for Life.* Mountain View, CA, Kavanah Publishing Co., 1988.

80 Handsfield HH et al: *JAMA* 1989 (in press).

81 Rolfs R, Cates W Jr: The perpetual lessons of syphilis. *Arch Dermatol* 125:107, 1989.

82 Day S: Prostitute women and AIDS: Anthropology. *AIDS* 2:421, 1988.

83 Padian NS: Prostitute women and AIDS: Epidemiology. *AIDS* 2: 413, 1988.

83a Stone K et al: Personal protection against STD. *Am J Obstet Gynecol* 155:180, 1986.

84 Senanayake P et al: Contraception and the etiology of pelvic inflammatory disease: New perspectives. *Am J Obstet Gynecol* 138:852, 1980.

85 Kinghorn GR, Waugh MA: Oral contraceptive use and prevalence of infection with *Chlamydia trachomatis* in women. *Br J Vener Dis* 57:187, 1981.

86 Brunham R et al: Epidemiological and clinical correlates of *Chlamydia trachomatis* and *Neisseria gonorrhoeae* infection among

women attending a clinic for sexually transmitted diseases. *Clin Res* 29:47a, 1981.
87 Fraser JJ et al: Prevalence of cervical *Chlamydia trachomatis* and *Neisseria gonorrhoeae* infections in female adolescents. *Pediatrics* 71:333, 1983.
88 Kols A et al: Oral contraceptives in the 1980s. *Popul Rep [A]* 10:189, May–June 1982.
89 Washington et al: Oral contraceptives, *Chlamydia trachomatis* infection and pelvic inflammatory disease. A word of caution about protection. *JAMA* 253:2266, 1985.
90 Forrest JE et al: U.S. women's contraceptive attitudes and practice: How have they changed in the 1980s? *Fam Plann Perspect* 20:112, 1988.
91 Goldberg et al: Knowledge and use of condoms in less developed countries during the rise of AIDS. *WHO Bull* 1989 (in press).
92 Aral SO, Cates W Jr: Sexual behavior as risk factor for sexually transmitted disease: Sexually experienced are not necessarily sexually active. *Sex Transm Dis* 1989 (in press).
93 Weström L, Mårdh P-A: Pelvic inflammatory disease: Epidemiology, diagnosis, clinical manifestations, and sequelae, in *International Perspectives on Neglected Sexually Transmitted Diseases; Impact on Venereology, Infertility, and Maternal and Infant Health,* KK Holmes et al (eds). New York, McGraw-Hill, 1983, p 235.
94 Bell TA, Holmes KK: Age-specific risks of syphilis, gonorrhea, and hospitalized pelvic inflammatory disease in sexually experienced U.S. women. *Sex Transm Dis* 22:291, 1984.
95 Aral SO et al: Gonorrhea rates: What denominator is most appropriate? *Am J Public Health* 78:702, 1988.
96 Hofferth SL et al: Premarital sexual activity among U.S. teenage women over the past three decades. *Fam Plann Perspect* 19:46, 1987.
97 D'Costa LJ et al: Prostitutes are a major reservoir of sexually transmitted diseases in Nairobi, Kenya. *Sex Transm Dis* 12:64, 1985.
98 Handsfield HH et al: Criteria for selective screening for *Chlamydia trachomatis* infection in women attending family planning clinics. *JAMA* 255:1730, 1986.
99 Schachter J et al: Screening for chlamydial infections in women attending family planning clinics. *West J Med* 1387:375, 1983.
100 Syrjanen K et al: Sexual behavior of women with human papillomavirus (HPV) lesions of the uterine cervix. *Br J Vener Dis* 60:243, 1984.
101 Harris RWC et al: Characteristics of women with dysplasia or carcinoma in situ of the cervix uteri. *Br J Cancer* 42:360, 1980.
102 Schreeder MT et al: Hepatitis B in homosexual men: Prevalence of infection and factors related to transmission. *J Infect Dis* 146:7, 1982.
103 Alter MJ et al: Hepatitis B virus transmission between heterosexuals. *JAMA* 256:1307, 1986.
104 Dan B: Sex and the singles whirl: The quantum dynamics of hepatitis B. *JAMA* 256:1344, 1986.
105 Research and Forecasts, Inc: *The Abbott Report: STD's and Sexual Mores in the 1980's.* New York, July 14, 1987.
106 Aral SO et al: Unpublished data.
107 Sly DF: Lifetime migration patterns in Kenya, 1963, in *Advancing Agricultural Production in Africa.* Nairobi, Heinemann Educational Books, 1984, p 68.
108 Painter TM: Migrations, social reproduction and development in Africa: Critical notes from a case study in the West African Sahel. Development Policy and Practice Research Group Working Paper 7. Milton Keynes, UK: The Open University.
109 Wallace R: A synergism of plagues: "Planned shrinkage," contagious housing destruction and AIDS in the Bronx. *Environ Res* 47:1, 1988.
110 Harris FR, Wilkins RW: Quiet Riots: Race and Poverty in the United States. New York, Pantheon, 1988.
111 Martin CJ. The agrarian question and migrant labor: The case of Western Kenya. *J Afr Stud* 11:164, 1985.
112 Anderson RM et al: Possible demographic consequences of AIDS in developing countries. *Nature* 332:228, 1988.
113 May RM, Anderson RM: Transmission dynamics of HIV infection. *Nature* 326:137, 1988.
114 Anderson RM: The epidemiology of HIV infection: Variable incubation plus infectious periods and heterogeneity in sexual activity. *J R Stat Soc* 151:66, 1988.

Chapter 3

# Analytic approaches to the epidemiology of sexually transmitted diseases

Richard B. Rothenberg

Sexually transmitted diseases provide a unique environment for the application of epidemiologic methods. In the traditional transmission tetrahedron (Fig. 3-1), the agent may be represented by 30 or more venereal pathogens; the host, by a human immunologic system which responds in differing ways to different pathogens; the vector, by the varieties of sexual experience; and the environment, by the social and ethical system which affects individual sexuality. This complex interaction of microbiology, host factors, personal behavior, and social constraints provides a rich backdrop for application of analytic epidemiology. This chapter will focus on several such applications and their relevance to STD.

## HISTORICAL ASPECTS

The power of analytic epidemiology and knowledge about STDs have both grown at increasing rates in the past decades. Their concurrent history furnishes some interesting parallels in the development of tools to deal with sexually transmitted illness.

In the 1940s and 1950s, at a time when the early foundations for modern epidemiologic analysis were being laid down,[1–4] venereology in the United States dealt primarily with the "major" venereal diseases—syphilis and gonorrhea—and to a lesser extent with the "minor" ones—chancroid, lymphogranuloma venereum, and granuloma inguinale. Though other pathogens were recognized as transmissible sexually, the field had limited scope.

During the 1960s and 1970s, considerable theoretical development of epidemiologic methods took place, notably multivariate logistic regression,[5,6] proportional hazards models in survival analysis,[7] and measures of association and the assessment of confounding.[8,9] For venereology in those same years, the importance of "newer" agents, such as herpesvirus (Chaps. 34, 35), chlamydia (Chaps. 15, 16), and human papillomavirus (Chaps. 37, 38), burgeoned. The term "sexually transmitted" replaced "venereal" in the late 1970s, and a cadre of STD clinical specialists developed.

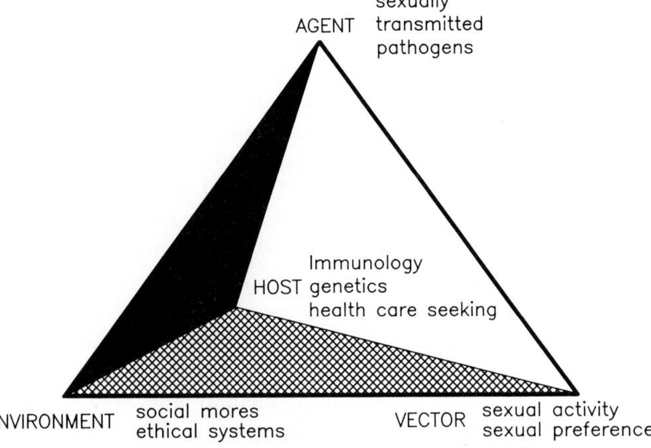


Fig. 3-1. The disease transmission tetrahedron of sexually transmitted diseases.

In the current decade, a major epidemiologic advance has been access to complex methods. Though the algorithms required for multivariate analysis were well understood, they were computationally intense and not widely available. Since 1980, extraordinary advances in computer technology have made analytic methods generally accessible. While ill-considered use of sophisticated techniques is a risk, it is far outweighed by the quantum advance in available analytic power.

The major STD event of the 1980s has been, of course, the onset of the AIDS epidemic. AIDS has provided enormous impetus to research in molecular biology, immunology, and sexual behavior. It is also an area in which the newer analytic methods are being applied.

## METHODS OF ANALYSIS

### DESCRIPTIVE EPIDEMIOLOGY

The traditional descriptors of time, place, and person are shown in Table 3-1 and are discussed in detail in several texts.[10–12] The STDs vary markedly in their descriptive characteristics,[13] a point that may be a source of confusion in analytic studies. Gonorrhea, for example, is a disease of high incidence, short duration, and hence, low prevalence. "Having gonorrhea" is a transient characteristic, and the study of gonorrhea patients must make the careful distinction between those who have been infected in the past, those who are infected at present, and those with a high risk of infection in the future. The extent to which these three groups differ may predetermine the outcome of studies of, for example, sexual behavior. In addition, the lack of effective natural immunity against gonorrhea leads to repeated episodes of disease for some individuals. Counting cases thus poses special problems,[14] since a single individual may serve as a "sexual node" connecting otherwise unrelated clusters of infection. Traditional concepts of incidence and prevalence, when applied to the microepidemiology of gonorrhea, require some modification.

Herpesvirus infection, on the other hand, is a disease of lower incidence (though population-based estimates of incidence comparable with those for gonorrhea are not available), but of higher prevalence, since the individual is presumably infected for life. This can lead to considerable variation in the estimates of disease occurrence[15] and bias in the determination of the clinical status of the individual patient. Other STDs, which occupy different places in the incidence/duration/prevalence spectrum, pose similar problems for descriptive epidemiology.

### MEASUREMENT OF RISK

One of the major epidemiologic rediscoveries in recent years has been the more precise distinction among rates, risks, proportions, and ratios.[16,17] In the first half of the nineteenth century, William Farr[18] first distinguished between two fundamental methods for describing incidence. In one, a true *rate* is calculated—that is, the numerator and denominator change simultaneously, since, when a case occurs, it must leave the denominator and enter the numerator. The appropriate measure of *risk* is not the individual

**Table 3-1. Epidemiologic Descriptors**

| Measure | Description |
|---|---|
| Incidence | 1. Events per person-time; terms incidence-diversity or "true" incidence rate<br>2. Cases per population accumulated over period of observation; termed cumulative incidence and synonymous with "risk" |
| Prevalence | 1. The number of cases at a theoretical "instant" in time divided by the population; *incorrectly* termed prevalence rate<br>2. The number of cases ascertained over a fixed (usually short) period of time; often termed "period prevalence" and the measure usually used for most purposes |
| Crude rate | The total number of cases divided by total person-years |
| Specific rate | The crude rate in a specific group, i.e., where both numerator and denominator have the same characteristics (e.g., gonorrhea cases in 20- to 24-year-old white men divided by person-years of exposure of 20- to 24-year-old white men) |
| Adjusted standardized rate | Using a reference standard to permit comparability among diverse populations (typically, to provide comparability among populations with different age structures)<br>1. Direct standardization—application of observed specific rates to a standard population; produces an (age/sex/race/etc.) adjusted rate<br>2. Indirect standardization—application of a standard set of rates to the population of interest; produces an "expected" rate, which, when divided by the observed rate, gives a standard morbidity (or mortality) ratio (SMR) |
| Trend | A series of rates (crude, adjusted, specific) arranged chronologically to demonstrate potential changes over time |
| Clustering | Specific rates, where the specific variable is a defined geographic area, permitting the demonstration of the geographic aggregation of cases |

per se but rather the length of time that the individual remains well and at risk (that is, remains in the denominator). This is usually measured as "person-time," and all equal combinations of "persons" multiplied by "time" are equivalent: 10 person-years are provided by 10 people at risk for 1 year, or 1 person at risk for 10 years. A true incidence rate, then, is calculated by dividing the number of cases by the number of person-years at risk, and is usually expressed as cases per population per year. For convenience, some preset population size is often used (e.g., cases per 100,000 per year).

Another approach to incidence simply divides the number of cases by the total population at risk at the start of the period of observation (i.e., the period during which the cases occurred). This *proportion* (cases divided by cases plus noncases) is usually synonymous with "risk." Finally, a *ratio* is, in the broadest sense, one quantity divided by another and usually implies that the numerator is not included in the denominator. It is clearly neither a risk, nor a rate, nor a measure of incidence, but is, as discussed later, used to compare these quantities.

Some of these distinctions have received little attention in STD research, in part because of the volumes of data available. A true rate, proportion, and ratio will not differ greatly when the denominator is large, the numerator is small, and the period of observation is sufficiently long. In the "microepidemiology" of disease transmission, however, their misuse may be a source of confusion. For example, the ratio of STD cases among men to STD cases among women (the male:female ratio) has long been used as an epidemiologic descriptor, whose presumed value "should be" in the region of 1. Clearly, however, the observed value is influenced by the assiduousness of case-finding activity, by the relative size of the male and female populations actually at risk, and by the extent of homosexual transmission. An unannotated ratio is not readily interpretable. On the other hand, a comparison of age-, gender-, and sex preference-specific rates in a small, defined geographic area (e.g., census tract) might provide insight into transmission. In New York State[19] a comparison of specific rates demonstrates that heterosexual transmission of syphilis is of increasing importance with increasing distances from urban centers. Further, homosexual black men are actually at greatest risk for syphilis, despite the predominance of cases among whites. Refining the denominators needed to calculate such rates will make it possible to specify ratios of both true rates and true risks more precisely.

## STUDY DESIGNS AND MEASURES OF ASSOCIATION

The distinctions among rates, risks, and ratios determine the accuracy of the measures of association generated by different study designs. In general, two types of approaches are used to assess the relationship between an exposure and an outcome: the difference between two measures or the ratio of two measures. Though the former, often termed "risk difference," has received some attention of late,[11] more epidemiologic emphasis has been placed on estimating the ratio of two risks, perhaps because this dimensionless number is not a function of the actual size of the risk. An unfortunate concomitant of the improvement in concepts has been a proliferation of terms to describe the ratio of two risks. The generic expression is "relative risk," which can be most simply defined as the ratio of the occurrence of the disease in people who are exposed to the occurrence of disease in those who are not exposed, or as the ratio of incidences. In 1951, Cornfield[1] noted that the relative risk could be approximated by the ratio of the relative odds of exposure among diseased persons to the relative odds of exposure among nondiseased persons (also called the odds ratio or cross-product ratio). He noted the necessity of assuming that the disease in question was "rare."

Since then the distinction between a relative risk that compares incidence rates (rate ratio, or incidence density ratio) and a relative risk that compares proportions (risk ratio or cumulative incidence ratio) has become clear. The term "relative risk" has been applied to both comparisons and in addition has been used in place of odds ratio, particularly in the setting of logistic regression.

The method of sampling cases and controls in a case-control study determines the type of measure of association and the validity of that measure as an estimate of the "true" relative risk. In classic terminology, the "cohort" study follows two groups of individuals, exposed and unexposed, prospectively to determine the frequency with which disease develops. This permits direct calculation of the true incidence rate (here, the number of cases per person-time of follow-up in exposed and unexposed groups). This approach was long assumed to provide the standard for validity. The case-control approach, which in its classic form selected cases from a defined population and controls from among those in the same population who were disease-free at the end of the study period, provided reasonable estimates of risk if the disease was rare, but this approach was considered less valid.

**Table 3-2. Types of Case-Control Studies**

| Design[9,19–23] | Source of control | Measure of association* | Required assumptions: Rare disease | Population†: Fixed | Population†: Stable |
|---|---|---|---|---|---|
| Classic | A sample of the population remaining at the end of the period of observation | OR = IDR | No | No | Yes |
| | | OR = IOR | No | Yes | No |
| | | OR = CIR | Yes | Yes | No |
| Case-base‡ or case-cohort | A sample of the population at the beginning of this period of risk excluding prevalent cases | OR = CIR | No | Yes | No |
| | | OR = IDR | No | Yes | No |
| Incidence density‡ | Sampled longitudinally throughout the risk period, excluding prevalent cases | OR = IDR | No | No | Yes |

* OR = odds ratio generated by the study design
IDR = incidence density ratio, or the ratio of the true incidence rates
IOR = incidence-odds ratio, or the odds ratio computed by using the cumulative incidence (i.e., the proportion affected at the end of the study period)
CIR = cumulative incidence ratio, or the ratio of the proportions affected at the end of the study period
†A "stable" population is one in which the variables of interest, including exposure, do not change over the risk period. A "fixed" population is one with no in-migration.
‡In both these studies, if disease develops in a control subject during the risk period, that subject is counted as both a case and a control.

Modifications of the classic case-control approach (Table 3-2) provide alternative ways of selecting cases and controls. Under the stipulated circumstances, the odds ratio can be shown to be an unbiased estimator of the incidence density ratio (the ratio of the true incidence rates).[20–24] Algebraic details aside, the case-control approach provides results that are, in principle, as valid as those of a prospective cohort study. The primary barriers to validity, then, are not issues of study design, but of the bias,[25] misclassification,[26] and confounding[27,28] that may be present. These issues relate to (1) methods of selecting and classifying cases and controls, (2) the accuracy with which important variables are measured, and (3) the extent to which extraneous factors may distort the observed results.

The use of appropriate study design and analysis is illustrated by the evolution of treatment studies for genital herpes infection. Original observations in an uncontrolled case series[29] suggested that photoactive dyes and light may help to prevent the recurrence of clinical herpes. A subsequent case-control study of the incidence density type[30] compared individuals with herpes for response to the new therapy versus placebo and demonstrated the lack of clinical efficacy. Use of alternative study designs (Table 3-2) may be increasing. Though many of the larger groups followed to determine the natural history of AIDS are referred to as "cohorts," in fact they represent defined populations from which "cases" emerge (either seropositive or clinically ill individuals), thus permitting the "nesting" of a case-control study within the cohort.[31] These cases may be compared with controls who were selected at the time of identification of the group (case-base), or in conjunction with the appearance of a case (incidence density). The San Francisco study of gay men,[32] identified through its participation in a study of hepatitis vaccine, and the San Francisco Men's Health Study group,[33] selected as a multistage probability sample, utilize both approaches. The Multicenter AIDS Cohort Study (MACS),[34] discussed later, is an example of the incidence density approach.

## ANALYTIC METHODS AND TESTS OF SIGNIFICANCE

As noted, computer algorithms are now available to perform the often tedious computations needed for epidemiologic analysis. Procedures are available for personal computers,[35] and mainframe algorithms are now accessible to perform two major analytic procedures—logistic regression and proportional hazards modeling.

The *logistic regression approach* creates a model to predict the probability of a dichotomous outcome as a function of variables that may influence that outcome. The relative odds of the outcome, not the outcome itself, is the dependent variable. With the appropriate formulation, the coefficient which is generated for each variable represents the logarithm of the odds ratio associated with that variable, controlling for other variables in the equation. The MACS study,[34] which follows a large group of men at risk for AIDS, provides a good illustration of this analytic approach. First, the potential association between the outcome (development of AIDS after HIV infection) and a large number of variables was examined by calculating the crude odds ratios. Those ORs that appeared important were included in a linear logistic model. The results suggest that the development of AIDS is less related to continued exposure (e.g., receptive anal intercourse) than to immunologic function and the possible presence of coinfection.

The *proportional hazards model,* a method for survival analysis, helps detect the relative risk for a dichotomous outcome in which time plays a major role. If survival can be thought of as "time to outcome," a number of variables can influence survival (time to disease development, time to death, etc.) in complicated ways. This method creates a model wherein the coefficients for each variable represent the logarithm of the odds ratio associated with that variable unconfounded by the others in the equation. In studies of AIDS, the survival analysis has been used to determine the probability of developing disease, given the presence of HIV infection.[36,37] The proportional hazards model has been employed to determine the probability of survival with AIDS as a function of the major demographic variables.[38]

The reporting of measures of association in epidemiologic studies has recently come under scrutiny.[39–41] Traditionally, a point estimate (such as an odds ratio or any of its congeners) is reported along with a *p value,* or the probability that the observed point estimate might have occurred by chance alone. For the odds ratio, the *p* value results from a test of the null hypothesis that the observed estimate is not different from 1. An alternative method of presentation gives the point estimate and a set of confidence limits (usually 90 or 95 percent) for the estimate. Examination of the point estimate and its confidence limits provides an immediate visual sense of the magnitude of the odds ratio and the probability space which surrounds it (i.e., the space that might contain 90 or 95 percent of the values which might have occurred by chance alone). Obviously, confidence limits convey whether or not this probability space contains the null value of 1. The two alternatives—$p$ values vs. confidence limits—thus take a different approach to presenting the same information. Confidence limits provide flexibility, whereas $p$ values are more precise; however, the latter can be interpreted too stringently.

## ANALYTIC METHODS FOR DECISION MAKING

### CAUSAL INFERENCE

Considerable epidemiologic thought has been devoted to the meaning of causation in epidemiologic research.[42–45] Much of this is directed to the relationship between epidemiologic methods and the establishment of causality—that is, how measures of association, confounding, and effect modification can help sort out the etiologic role of a given exposure with a given disease. Perhaps the most important point to emerge is that causal inference is distinctly different from statistical inference. The judgment that the association of a given exposure with a particular disease is causal rests on a number of interrelated attributes of that association, many of which may not be susceptible to formal statistical testing. As summarized by Hill,[46] these attributes include:

1. The strength of the association;
2. Its consistency, i.e., the repeated observation in a variety of settings;
3. The specificity of the association;
4. The logic of the temporal sequence connecting exposure and disease;
5. The presence of a biologic gradient, or dose-response curve;
6. The biological plausibility of the causative role;
7. The general coherence of the association with other epidemiologic phenomena;
8. The ability of the association to withstand an experimental test, such as cessation of the exposure and subsequent diminution of disease occurrence; and
9. The analogy of the disease-exposure relationship with some other known relationship.

This approach to causality should hold for all risk factors, including infectious agents. In fact, one might view Koch's postulates as a subset of those enumerated by Hill (3, 4, and 8, for example). In his landmark paper in 1976, Evans "updated" Koch's postulates to reflect modern thinking in microbial genetics and a different ethical environment.[47] He suggested groups of postulates to be used for acceptance of causality in different settings. One application for STDs involves the role of viruses in sexually transmitted cancer. For example, herpesvirus and human papillomavirus satisfy the criteria for causation of cervical cancer to different degrees (Table 3-3). Current thinking suggests that human papillomavirus may be the more important agent, particularly because viral genome has been demonstrated in affected tissue, but further work is still required for rigorous demonstration. In the future, the application of causal criteria is likely to have increasing importance in STD research, particularly with regard to analogues and variants of HIV.

**Table 3-3. Criteria for Viral Causation in Cervical Cancer**

| | Herpesvirus | Human papillomavirus |
|---|---|---|
| Seroepidemiologic criteria | | |
| 1. Antibody is present more often in cases than in controls | Yes | ? |
| 2. Antibody levels are significantly increased in cases over controls | Yes | ? |
| 3. Antibody to early antigen should be present in cases vs. controls | Yes | ? |
| 4. Antibody should be specific | +/− | ? |
| 5. Antibody should be absent before onset and should precede disease | ? | ? |
| 6. If association is variable, the presence of cofactors should be sought | Yes | Yes |
| Virologic criteria | | |
| 1. There is evidence of viral multiplication e.g., viral excretion | No | No |
| 2. Virus or viral genome is present in affected genome | No | Yes |
| 3. Virus can induce malignant transformation of cells in vitro | Yes | Yes |
| 4. Disease can be produced in animal models with purified virus | ? | ? |

### DECISION ANALYSIS

Decision theory is an important and complex branch of mathematics that deals with, among other things, choices under conditions of uncertainty. From such theory, a number of practical applications have been developed,[48] and it may be argued that the field of cost-benefit and cost-effectiveness analysis has grown from this theoretical base.[49,50] Decision theory has become a major tool in public health because of the need to make population-based decisions with limited resources. The critical distinction must be made between the individual clinical decision and the aggregate public health decision. Aggregate benefits may mitigate against adopting certain maneuvers, such as a yearly Pap smear[51] or routine syphilis serology testing,[52] as population-based public health policy. But the individual physician may still choose to perform these tests under circumstances that warrant it.

In using decision analysis, it is important to distinguish between cost-benefit and cost-effectiveness analysis.[49] This hinges in part—like the use of risk difference and risk ratio in epidemiologic studies—on the use of the difference between benefits and costs, or their ratio. Cost-benefit analysis determines whether there is a positive difference between benefits and costs. Investigators assign a monetary value to all outcomes of the maneuver, including human disease, disability, and death. Cost-effectiveness analysis sets priorities for alternative allocations of resources (frequently, alternative ways of achieving the same goal). These are examined for the ratio of benefits to costs, and the choice is based, in theory, on the size of the ratio. In this context, valuation of human life in monetary terms may not be necessary, since the same outcomes are being considered or some nonmonetary standard (e.g., "quality adjusted years of life") may be used.

The methods of cost-benefit and cost-effectiveness analysis are deceptively simple.[49] The critical first step is accurately to define the maneuver to be studied. The investigator then attempts to define four major types of associated costs: (1) the direct costs of medical care, (2) the costs of adverse effects of treatment, (3) the savings in health care costs that accrue because of prevention, and (4) the costs of treating illness that would occur because of gains in longevity that result from the prevention. Net benefits may be represented as the net increase in quality-adjusted years of life which result from prevention.

Performing such analysis is not simple. One must specify the elements to include in estimating costs, determine the valuation placed on these elements, calculate discounted future value, and create an overall model. In addition, each value is subject to variation and the model may be particularly sensitive to some of the estimates used. An overall sensitivity analysis is usually required as an adjunct to the major analysis.

Cost-benefit analysis has been widely applied in the STD field, with emphasis on such areas as the economic issues of chlamydia control,[53,54] screening,[55–57] and the treatment of sexual partners.[58,59] Specific results are less important in this context than recognizing the widespread usefulness of this technique. Note, however, that the typical cost-benefit or cost-effectiveness study, even with a sensitivity analysis, considers only a small proportion of the outcomes available.[60] Since some subjectivity is involved in selecting variables of interest and in assigning costs, a probabilistic approach may be appropriate in some instances. This entails an assessment of all possible outcomes, given certain reasonable limits to the variables, and determination of the probability that costs are greater than, less than, or equal to benefits.

## OTHER METHODS AND FUTURE DIRECTIONS

A variety of other analytic techniques have found application in the field of STD. Models for the dynamics of disease transmission, using the methods of population biology, have been developed for several STDs.[61,62] Analysis of sensitivity, specificity, and prevalence, with application of Bayes' theorem for determination of predictive value, has been applied to laboratory testing for STDs.[63,64] The receiver-operating characteristics curve, an offshoot of this technique wherein true positives are plotted against false positives, has been applied to determine the efficacy of clinical diagnosis.[65] Techniques for demonstrating disease clustering have been used to determine foci for transmission of beta-lactamase producing *Neisseria gonorrhoeae*.[66] The methods discussed here represent only a portion of the available technology.

The limits to investigation are not now imposed by analytic techniques but by the context for their application. In the 1980s access to computers and the onset of AIDS are two major epidemiologic events. Each has probably altered our world view, particularly concerning the relationship between the individual and society. Because of computer advances, individuals (or investigators) have greater access to information—but society has greater access to individuals. The AIDS epidemic has underscored the delicate balance between the privacy of individuals and the protection of groups. Analytic technology offers enormous potential, not yet fully realized, for studying STD problems. What is now required is commensurate social technology to avoid violating the balance.

## References


1 Cornfield J: A method of estimating comparative rates from clinical data applications to cancer of the lung, breast, and cervix. *J Natl Cancer Inst* 11:1269, 1951.

2 Cornfield J: A statistical problem arising from retrospective studies. *Proceedings of the Third Berkeley Symposium on Mathematical Statistics and Probability*. 4:135, 1956.

3 Levin M: The occurrence of lung cancer in man. *Acta Univ Intern Cancer* 9:1531, 1953.

4 Mantel N, Haenszel W: Statistical aspects of the analysis of data from retrospective studies of disease. *J Natl Cancer Inst* 22:719, 1959.

5 Cornfield J: Joint dependence of risk of coronary heart disease on serum cholesterol and systolic blood pressure: A discriminant function analysis. *Fed Proc* 2:58, 1962.

6 Truett J et al: A multivariate analysis of the risk of coronary artery disease in Framingham. *J Chronic Dis* 20:511, 1967.

7 Cox DR: Regression models and life tables (with discussion). *J R Stat Soc Ser B* 34:187, 1972.

8 Miettinen OS: Components of the crude risk ratio. *Am J Epidemiol* 96:168, 1972.

9 Miettinen OS: Estimability and estimation in case-referrent studies. *Am J Epidemiol* 103:226, 1976.

10 MacMahn B, Pugh TF: *Epidemiology: Principles and Methods*. Boston, Little, Brown, 1970.

11 Rothman KJ: *Modern Epidemiology*. Boston, Little, Brown, 1986.

12 Kleinbaum SG et al: *Epidemiologic Research Principles and Quantitative Methods*. Belmont, CA, Lifetime Learning, 1982.

13 STD Statistics No. 135. U.S. Department of Health and Human Services. Public Health Services, Centers for Disease Control, 1985.

14 Potterat JJ et al: Gonorrhea as a social disease. *Sex Trans Dis* 12:25, 1985.

15 Guinan ME et al: Epidemiology of genital herpes simplex infection. *Epidemiol Rev* 7:127, 1985.

16 Elandt-Johnson RC: Definition of rates: Some remarks on their use and misuse. *Am J Epidemiol* 102:267, 1975.

17 Morgenstern H et al: Measures of disease incidence used in epidemiologic research. *Int J Epidemiol* 9:97, 1980.

18 Vandenbrouek JP: On the rediscovery of a distinction. *Am J Epidemiol* 121:627, 1985.

19 Rothenberg RB: The geography of syphilis: A demonstration of epidemiologic diversity, in *Advances in Sexually Transmitted Diseases*, Morriset R, Kurstak E (eds). Utrecht, Netherlands, Elsevier, 1986, pp 125–133.

20 Greenland S, Thomas DC: On the need for the rare disease assumption in case-control studies. *Am J Epidemiol* 116:547, 1982.

21 Hogue CJR et al: Estimators of relative risk for case-control studies. *Am J Epidemiol* 118:396, 1983.

22 Prentice RL: A case-cohort design for epidemiologic cohort studies and disease prevention trials. *Biometrika* 783:1, 1986.

23 Greenland S et al: The rare-disease assumption revisited. *Am J Epidemiol* 124:869, 1986.

24 Hogue CJR et al: The case-exposure study. *Am J Epidemiol* 124:877, 1986.

25 Copeland KT et al: Bias due to misclassification in the estimation of relative risk. *Am J Epidemiol* 105:488, 1977.

26 Greenland S: The effect of misclassification in the presence of covariates. *Am J Epidemiol* 112:564, 1980.

27 Greenland S, Robins JM: Confounding and misclassification. *Am J Epidemiol* 122:495, 1985.

28 Miettinen OS, Cook EF: Confounding: essence and detection. *Am J Epidemiol* 114:593, 1981.

29 Friederich EG: Relief of herpes vulvitis. *Obstet Gynecol* 41:74, 1973.

30 Myers MG et al: Failure of neutral red photodynamic inactivation in recurrent herpes simplex virus infections. *N Engl J Med* 293:945, 1975.

31 Flanders WD, Louv WC: The exposure odds ratio in nested case-control studies with competing risks. *Am J Epidemiol* 124:684, 1986.

32 Hadler SC et al: Long-term immunogenicity and efficacy of hepatitis B vaccine in homosexual men. *N Engl J Med* 315:209, 1986.

33 Winkelstein W et al: Sexual practices and risk of infection by human immunodeficiency virus. *JAMA* 257:321, 1987.

34 Polk BF et al: Predictors of acquired immunodeficiency syndrome developing in a cohort of seropositive homosexual men. *N Engl J Med* 316:61, 1987.

35 Rothman KJ, Boice JD: *Epidemiologic Analysis with a Programmable Calculator*. Chestnut Hill, MA, Epidemiologic Resources, 1982.
36 Goedert JJ et al: Three-year incidence of AIDS in five cohorts of HTLV-III-infected risk group members. *Science* 231:992, 1986.
37 Curran JW: Unpublished data.
38 Rothenberg RB et al: Survival with AIDS: Experience in New York City with 5,883 cases. *N Engl J Med* 317:1297, 1987.
39 Poole C: Beyond the (confidence) interval. *Am J Public Health* 77:195, 1987.
40 Thompson WD: Statistical criteria in the interpretation of epidemiologic data. *Am J Public Health* 77:191, 1987.
41 Walker AM: Reporting the results of epidemiologic studies. *Am J Public Health* 76:556, 1986.
42 Rothman KJ: Causes. *Am J Epidemiol* 104:587, 1976.
43 Koopman JS: Causal models and sources of interaction. *Am J Epidemiol* 106:439, 1977.
44 Susser M: Judgment and causal inference: Criteria in epidemiologic studies. *Am J Epidemiol* 105:1, 1977.
45 Greenland S (ed): *Evolution of Epidemiologic Ideas*. Chestnut Hill, MA, Epidemiology Resources, 1987.
46 Hill AB: The environment and disease: Association or causation. *Proc R Soc Med* 58:295, 1965.
47 Evans AS: Causation and disease: The Henle-Koch postulates revisited. *Yale J Biol Med* 49:175, 1976.
48 Raiffa H: *Decision Analysis*. Reading, MA, Addison-Wesley, 1968.
49 Weinstein MC, Stason WB: Foundation of cost-effectiveness analysis for health and medical practices. *N Engl J Med* 296:716, 1977.
50 Machina M: Decision-making in the presence of risk. *Science* 236:537, 1987.
51 Foltz AM, Kelsey JJ: The annual Pap test: A dubious policy success. *Milbank Q* 56(4):426, 1978.
52 Hart G: Screening to control infectious diseases: Evaluation of control programs for gonorrhea and syphilis. *Rev Infect Dis* 2(5):701, 1980.
53 Nettlman MD et al: Cost-effectiveness of culturing patients attending a sexually transmitted disease clinic for chlamydia trachomatis. *Ann Intern Med* 105:189, 1986.
54 Washington AE et al: Economic cost of pelvic inflammatory disease including associated ectopic pregnancy and infertility. *JAMA* 255:1735, 1986.
55 Goddeeris JH, Bronken TP: Benefit-cost analysis of screening: A comparison of tests for gonorrhea. *Med Care* 23(11):1242, 1985.
56 William K: Screening for syphilis in pregnancy: An assessment of the costs and benefits. *Community Med* 7(1):37, 1985.
57 Tarrell BG et al: Cost-yield of routine Papanicolaou smear screening in a clinic for sexually transmitted diseases. *Sex Transm Dis* 12(3):110, 1985.
58 Tueshen H et al: Decision analytic approach to the management of gonorrhea contacts. *Sex Transm Dis* 11(3):137, 1984.
59 Johnson RE: Epidemiologic and prophylactic treatment of gonorrhea. *Sex Transm Dis* 6:159, 1979.
60 Rothenberg RB: Cost benefit analysis: Probabilities and provisos. *Sex Transm Dis* 10:216, 1983.
61 May RM, Anderson RM: Transmission dynamics of HIV infection. *Nature* 326:137, 1987.
62 Hethcote HW, Yorke JA: *Gonorrhea Transmission Dynamics and Control*. Lecture Notes in Biomathematics No. 56. Berlin, Springer-Verlag, 1984.
63 Rothenberg RB et al: Efficacy of selected diagnostic tests for sexually transmitted disease. *JAMA* 235:49, 1976.
64 Dans PE et al: Gonococcal serology: How much, how useful, how soon? *J Infect Dis* 135:330, 1977.
65 Rothenberg RB, Judson FN: The clinical diagnosis of urethral discharge. *J Am Dis Assoc* 10:24, 1983.
66 Zenilman JM et al: Penicillinase-producing *Neisseria gonorrheae* in Dade County, Florida: Evidence of coregroup transmitters and the impact of illicit antibiotics. *Sex Transm Dis* 15:45, 1988.

# PART III BEHAVIORAL ASPECTS OF SEXUALLY TRANSMITTED DISEASES

# Chapter 4

# Sociological perspectives on human sexuality

Pepper Schwartz
Mary Rogers Gillmore

Sociologists, though mindful of our biological heritage, maintain that human behavior cannot be understood without reference to the cultural, historical, and social context in which individual lives are enacted. We assume that as social history changes, people change. That is why Barzum and Graff (quoted in C. Wright Mills[1]) remarked that: "The title of Dr. Kinsey's famous book *Sexual Behavior in the Human Male* is a striking instance of a hidden—and in this case false—assumption: the book is not about human males, but about men in the United States in the mid-twentieth century." The social circumstances which affect sexual behavior may vary from large-scale socioeconomic conditions such as the greatly increasing numbers of women in the labor force to intimate interactions between two people. In the final analysis, sociologists assert not only that human *behavior* is socially patterned but that human character, personality, identities—indeed human thought—are affected by those same social forces that affect behavior. A sociological analysis seeks to identify the social factors which produce variation in sexual behavior and to explain why and how these factors influence sexual behavior.

We begin this chapter with an examination of postwar social trends and suggest how these social changes affected sexuality. We then describe current patterns of sexual behavior for heterosexuals: teenagers, single adults, and married adults. Next we look at patterns of sexual behavior among homosexual men and women. But even as we write, patterns of sexual behavior for gay men are changing in response to the AIDS threat. It remains to be seen whether this is true for other segments of the population. Although we have not included a separate section on bisexuality, we have incorporated findings on bisexuals in each of the major sections below. This choice reflects the fact that there is a paucity of research on bisexuals, and that many studies purporting to focus on homosexuals have included respondents who also engage in heterosexual activities. The chapter concludes with some speculation about future trends in sexual behavior based on current trends in the social and sexual scene.

## POSTWAR SOCIAL AND SEXUAL TRENDS: EVOLUTION AND REVOLUTION

The trends in sexual behavior which troubled Americans in the late sixties and early seventies were not apparent in 1945, though they had probably been slowly evolving throughout much of the century. These changes in sexual behavior were accompanied by, and related to, other social changes that were also occurring during the postwar period. Divorce rates, which had been rising very slowly since the turn of the century, briefly zoomed upward toward the end of the war but soon dropped to rates only slightly higher than the prewar figures (Fig. 4-1). Young men and women were marrying at the youngest ages on record and rates of first marriage were the highest ever as young men returned from the service. As a consequence, women were having their first babies at a younger age than during the war years, and had larger families (typically four children) than would have been predicted on the basis of the decline in fertility rates that had occurred during the first half of the century. These postwar changes fostered the baby boom, but the dramatic consequences of this seemingly innocuous "population bulge" would not become apparent until much later.

The Kinsey studies,[2,3] published in this postwar era, suggested that Americans not only were engaging in a wider variety of sexual activities both in and outside of marital relationships than would be expected on the basis of the prevailing moral attitudes of the time, but also, and most shocking, that such behaviors were increasing. Three of Kinsey's findings were deeply disturbing to the public: the frequent use of prostitutes by men, both married (10 to 20 percent) and unmarried (70 percent), the prevalence of homosexual activities—Kinsey estimated that 37 percent of all American males and 13 percent of females had at least one homosexual experience in their lifetimes—and the substantial rate of extramarital "affairs."[2,3]

These data suggest that significant changes in sexual behavior had been happening at least since World War II and perhaps even since the turn of the century. What the sixties ushered in was not a *revolution* in sexual behavior but rather an acceleration in rates of changes which were already occurring. Given the dramatic increase in the adolescent population in the sixties, due to the baby boom, along with the trend toward increased premarital sexuality among teenagers which had been occurring for quite some time, it is not surprising that Americans leapt to the conclusion that society was in moral decay. What were the major social trends which occurred after World War II, and how might they have influenced sexual behavior?

There was a movement of large numbers of young Americans into colleges, and this produced dramatic changes in the lives of many young men and women. Marriage began to be delayed in order to pursue educations, and these young people were removed from the direct supervision of their families. The rising age at first marriage left more years between puberty and marriage. These changes meant that larger numbers of young unmarried men and women had more time and freedom to explore their sexuality.

At the same time, dramatic changes were occurring in female labor force participation. Although female labor force participation rates had been slowly creeping up since the 1920s when 23.7 percent of American women were in the labor force, a dramatic increase occurred in the two decades between 1960 and 1980. By 1986, over half the married and separated women, and 74 percent of the divorced women, with children under the age of 6 were in the labor force.[4] This transition from homemaking to paid labor force participation greatly increased women's autonomy and provided opportunities for sexual liaisons that had not existed previously for the majority of American women. During this two-decade period of rapid change, the divorce rate made a quantum leap (Fig. 4-1), thus placing a large number of sexually experienced but newly single persons in the sexual marketplace. That they continued to be sexually active, though no longer married, is hardly surprising.

Most people did not remain unmarried for long, however. Although the divorce rate soared, remarriage was also commonplace. About four out of five divorced men and three out of four divorced women remarried within 3 years. This fostered the appearance that the institution of marriage had been reaffirmed,

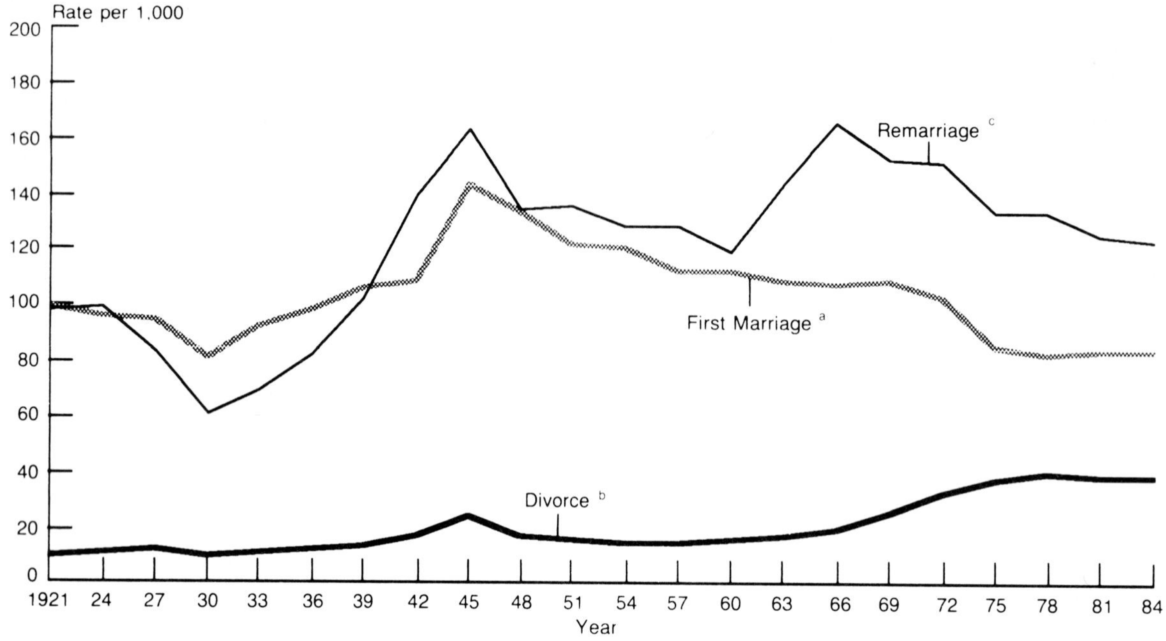


Source: U.S. National Center for Health Statistics, 1985a.
[a]First marriages per 1,000 single women 14 to 44 years old.
[b]Divorces per 1,000 married women 14 to 44 years old.
[c]Remarriages per 1,000 widowed and divorced women 14 to 54 years old.

**Fig. 4-1.** Rates of first marriage, divorce, and remarriage for women. *(From Norton and Moorman.[5] Copyrighted 1987 by the National Council on Family Relations, 1910 W County Rd B, Suite 147, St Paul, MN 55113. Reprinted by permission.)*

but it had changed radically in two important ways. First, the permanence of the marital union could no longer be taken for granted. This became more apparent as divorce rates for second marriages proved to be even higher than for first marriages. Second, not everyone remarried—the proportion of unmarried persons in the population has been rising[5]—and this small but significant trend produced profound changes in the sexual choices of men and women.

These same social trends gave impetus to the women's liberation movement, and with it a revised ideology about female sexuality. A new literature articulated women's concerns, differentiated female from male sexual needs, and called for a redefinition of sexuality which took both men's and women's preferences into account [cf. Ref. 6]. The marriage literature became more focused on sexual problems in marriage and courtship which were caused by *male* rather than female inadequacies, and guides to better lovemaking, such as *The Joy of Sex,* became best sellers. The pressure on men to become competent lovers, for women to be orgasmic and assertive in their sexual desires changed the meaning and experience of sex for both men and women. This new ideology was accompanied by increasingly more permissive attitudes about sexuality.[7,8] The emergence of women as sexually independent actors and the liberalization of attitudes about female sexuality represent a truly new phase of American sexual history.

The sixties were the culmination of this sexual evolution. Trends in sexual behavior which had been occurring for decades became more prominent as a result of the sheer numbers of the baby boom generation. In a period of just three decades, the lives of American women, and the meaning of marriage and family, has been inexorably altered. This, and not changes in sexual behavior, is the real "revolution" in American society.

## THE 1980S: A NEW CONSERVATISM?

After a period of at least two decades in which Americans experienced tremendous changes in marriage and divorce patterns, labor force participation by women, and social attitudes, some stabilization of these trends is evident in the 1980s. The divorce rate, after two decades of rapid increase, has begun to stabilize, though it remains at the highest level ever recorded.[5,9] It appears that the aging of the baby boom will naturally flatten the divorce rate, but the divorce rate is *not* just an artifact of that cohort's unique instability. Census experts estimate that approximately 50 percent of all marriages now taking place will end in divorce. The rate of first marriage, declining since the 1940s, and the rate of remarriage, declining since the early 1960s, also appear to be leveling off.[5]

Other social changes appear to be continuing. Median age at first marriage continues to increase as large numbers of young men and women seek additional education and experience in the work force before marriage.[10] Relative to the mid-1970s, a higher percentage of American women in 1985 have never married, and this is especially so among black women.[5] Although about three-fourths of the women who divorced in the past remarried, current trends suggest that the rate is dramatically lower today.[5,9]

These social trends suggest that there are likely to be more adult women in the 1980s who are unmarried than in the recent past. Based on Zelnik and Kantner's[11] findings regarding premarital sexuality, we anticipate that the majority of these women will be sexually experienced. Further, they are likely to have more partners than did women in the past. This is because, as Zelnik et al.[12] have shown, the longer the interval between first intercourse and first marriage, the more partners a sexually active woman has.

The AIDS epidemic also appears to have influenced sexual behavior, at least in the case of gay men. However, heterosexuals appear to be slow to change their behavior, perhaps because AIDS was mistakenly defined as a disease of gay men or because it is not yet perceived as a threat. Although contraceptive use is more prevalent than ever among adult heterosexuals—75 percent of females in their twenties who were queried in a recent national survey reported using a contraceptive at last intercourse[13]—condoms, which may afford protection against AIDS as well as against unwanted pregnancies, are not the contraceptive of choice, though their use may be increasing.[14] Moreover, teenagers, especially younger ones, are much less likely to use contraceptives.[12]

This vision of the 1980s is based on empirical studies of sexuality as well as on recent census data and epidemiological evidence. In the rest of this chapter we describe and interpret these studies. Before turning to this data, however, we alert the reader to the limitations of the available research.

## RESEARCH ON SEXUAL BEHAVIOR: A CAUTION

Unlike the U.S. census, which has provided regular population-based information on a number of social factors such as marriage and divorce for more than a century, there has not been a population-based survey of adult sexual behavior which employed representative sampling. In the absence of such data, drawing conclusions about general trends and patterns of sexual behavior is necessarily a tenuous undertaking. In contrast, adolescent (heterosexual) sexual behavior has been well documented in the national surveys conducted by Zelnik and Kantner in 1971, 1976, and 1979.[11,12]

Most studies of adult sexual behavior have been based on convenience samples. The volunteer respondents in such studies tend to be younger, white, middle class, better educated, and from somewhat higher socioeconomic levels than the general population. Refusal rates are very high (70 to 90 percent nonresponse rates are not unusual), adding another source of possible bias. Further, several major studies of sexual behavior have been conducted at different periods in American history leaving us in a quandary as to whether differences in findings are due to the uniqueness of the particular (nonrepresentative) sample or whether they represent changes over time in sexual behavior. We suspect, however, that when the data show a *consistent* pattern (e.g., increasing prevalence of premarital intercourse), the general trend, if not the exact figures, is probably accurately charted.

Additional caution is warranted because much of the literature on sexuality classifies individuals as *either* homosexual *or* heterosexual. This position implicitly assumes that (1) behavior and sexual orientations are congruent, (2) sexual orientations—like biological sex—are discrete categories, and less obviously, (3) sexual orientation is immutable.

There are ample data to show that the first two assumptions are false. From the early studies of Kinsey et al.[2,3] to the more recent research on sexuality,[15–17] the clear and consistent message is that few people are *exclusively* homosexual or heterosexual—in either sexual orientation or behavior—throughout their lives. Moreover, some persons define themselves as *exclusively* homosexual even though they have *never* had even a single sexual contact with a member of the same sex.[17] Analogously, some persons define themselves as *exclusively* heterosexual, even though they have sexual relations with members of the same sex (e.g., "swingers" or men and women incarcerated in prisons).

The third assumption, regarding the immutability of sexual orientation, represents the school of thought espoused by some researchers, as well as by some activist gay groups, that sexual preferences are biologically determined and hence unalterable. From a sociological point of view, homosexuality (or heterosexuality) is a process, not a state of being. Sexual preferences, orientations, and behaviors are seen as fluid, not discrete, and potentially malleable. The task of a sociological analysis is to understand the social factors that give rise to and foster the maintenance of particular forms of sexual expression.

We cannot settle the "nature vs. nurture" debate here; indeed it can never be settled definitively because biological and social factors are confounded. Much existing research on sexuality classifies people into these discrete categories, despite evidence to the contrary, and we have therefore used them as an organizing principle for this chapter. However, we think it is in the scientific community's best interests to keep in mind that actors, single, married, divorced, heterosexual, and homosexual, will inhabit more than one category in their lifetime and that the aware observer will keep these complications of human sexual behavior in mind.

## SEXUAL BEHAVIOR OF HETEROSEXUALS

### PREMARITAL SEX AMONG TEENAGERS

Perhaps no trend in sexual behavior has been better documented than the increase in premarital intercourse, especially among teenagers. Data from the Kinsey studies[3,18] suggest that this trend may have been occurring since the turn of the century.

Zelnik and Kantner's[11] data from national probability samples of metropolitan women ages 15 to 19 show a consistent increase over time in the prevalence of premarital intercourse throughout the 1970s (Table 4-1). Though the increase is evident among both blacks and whites, the rate of increase has been greater for white teenagers. However, recent data from the National Survey of Family Growth[19] suggest that this trend plateaued by 1982 (Table 4-1). Zelnik and Kantner's[11] 1979 survey of metropolitan teenagers, their first survey to include males, showed that 70 percent of the white males and 75 percent of the black males ages 17 to 21 had experienced premarital intercourse. These race and sex differences in premarital intercourse have been found by others as well.[2,3,15] Taken as a whole, the available data on premarital intercourse suggest that a sizable majority of teenagers experience sex before the age of 20.

Similar trends toward increasing sexuality among teenagers are apparent for age at first intercourse. Zelnik and Kantner's[11] data indicate that age at first intercourse for females, both black and white, has been falling over the page decade. Males, both black and white, on average initiate sexual intercourse about 1½ years earlier than females, and blacks of both sexes tend to have first intercourse at younger ages than whites (Table 4-1). However, contrary to the popular image of teenage promiscuity, the data suggest that the majority of white teenage women and over 40 percent of black teenage women have had, on average, only one partner.[12]

From 1971 to 1976 there appears to be a slight increase in the number of sexual partners teenagers have had (Table 4-1). This is probably related to the fact that teenage women became sexually active at a younger age in 1976 but married no younger and therefore had more years "at risk" of sexual activity. Indeed,

**Table 4-1. Changes over Time in Sexual Activities of Adolescent Females**

| | Percent Never-Married Women, Ages 15–19, Who Have Had Premarital Intercourse | | | |
|---|---|---|---|---|
| | 1971 | 1976 | 1979 | 1982 |
| White | 23.2 | 33.6 | 42.3 | 40.2 |
| Black | 52.4 | 64.3 | 64.8 | 57.8 |
| Total | 27.6 | 39.2 | 46.0 | 42.8 |
| | **Mean Age at First Intercourse** | | | |
| | 1971 | 1976 | 1979 | 1982 |
| White | 16.6 | 16.3 | 16.4 | — |
| Black | 15.9 | 15.6 | 15.5 | — |
| Total | 16.4 | 16.1 | 16.2 | 16.0* |
| | **Percent Sexually Active Females, Ages 15–19, Who Have Had Only One Sexual Partner** | | | |
| | 1971 | 1976 | | |
| White | 60.6 | 57.3 | | |
| Black | 61.6 | 43.2 | | |
| Total | 60.9 | 54.3 | | |
| | **Mean Frequency of Intercourse Month Prior to Interview: Never Married Females, Ages 15–19** | | | |
| | 1971 | 1976 | | |
| White | 3.1 | 3.0 | | |
| Black | 2.1 | 1.7 | | |
| Total | 2.9 | 2.6 | | |

*Figure is the mode.

SOURCE: 1982 data from Pratt et al.;[19] 1971–1979 data from Zelnik and Kantner, reprinted with permission from the Alan Guttmacher Institute, Family Planning Perspectives, vol 12, no 5, 1980; and from Zelnik, Kantner, and Ford, Sex and Pregnancy in Adolescence, pp 79, 86. Copyright © 1981 by Sage Publications. Reprinted by permission of Sage Publications, Inc.

Zelnik et al.[12] have shown that years at risk for premarital sexual activity is positively related to number of partners.

The females Zelnik et al.[12] surveyed in 1976 reported an average frequency of intercourse of just a little more than 2.5 times per month, with the modal frequency of intercourse during the 4 weeks prior to being surveyed at zero! Contrary to prevailing stereotypes, whites reported a higher frequency of intercourse than did blacks (Table 4-1).

In conclusion, while premarital intercourse is more prevalent than ever among teenagers, and adolescents are initiating sex at younger and younger ages, they are not very sexually active compared with single adults. The differential levels of sexual activity of teenagers and adult singles underscore the importance of social factors in predicting sexual activities. Most teenagers are still ensconced in their families and other social institutions which exert a conservative influence on their social (including sexual) behaviors. The real problem teenagers pose, in terms of social and public health concerns, is their failure to protect themselves against unwanted pregnancies and sexually transmitted diseases.

## SEXUALITY AMONG SINGLE ADULTS

Kinsey et al.[2,3] found that by the age of 25, 71 percent of males but only 33 percent of females had experienced intercourse. By 1974, virtually all the men and two-thirds of the women Hunt[15] studied were sexually experienced by this age. Based on the available data, it is probably safe to assume that nearly all of the population is sexually experienced by the age of 25. Although frequency rates for intercourse between singles are not reported in many studies, *Playboy* magazine[20] respondents reported rates of 2 to 3 times per week. (This figure includes some married respondents; however, most were single.)

DeLamater and MacCorquodale's[21] data indicated that about 70 percent of the non-college-educated men they randomly sampled in a university community had engaged in oral sex while closer to 60 percent of the college men had done so. Over half the college women and close to two-thirds of the non-college-educated women reported engaging in oral sex. Similar or somewhat higher rates of oral sex among single adults have been reported by others.[15,20]

Few studies have inquired about anal intercourse among heterosexuals. Hunt[15] found that more than one-sixth of the single males and females under age 25 had tried anal intercourse at least once, but less than 10 percent had engaged in it even occasionally within the past year. The more sexually adventuresome respondents to the *Playboy*[20] survey had much higher rates of anal intercourse; about 47 percent of the men and 61 percent of the women had tried it at least once. Over one-third had also engaged in anal-oral contact.

Although absolute estimates of the lifetime number of partners of single persons vary from study to study, it has been consistently found that males have more partners than females. However, the male-female differences are not always as great as might be expected. DeLamater and MacCorquodale,[21] for example, found that the college men in their study had a median of 6 partners, while the college women had 4.6 partners. Non-college-educated respondents, both male and female, reported even more partners (10 and 5.2, respectively). Studies[15,22] indicate, however, that a significant proportion of female respondents report having had only one premarital sex partner—often their fiancés, just as found in Kinsey's data.[3]

Divorced men and women tend to be more sexually active than sexually experienced never marrieds. Hunt's[15] data showed that divorced men had a median frequency of intercourse of more than twice a week, while for divorced women the rate was almost as high. Similar findings were obtained by Spanier and Thompson.[23] These frequencies are about the same as those reported by married respondents. Moreover, divorced males typically had sex with 8 partners per year while divorced women had a median of 4 partners per year. The overwhelming majority had engaged in oral sex during the past year.[15] Based on such data, Hunt[15] concluded that the divorced tend to be sexually liberated, not only relative to the previously married of Kinsey's day, but also relative to sexually active never married adults.

## SEXUALITY AMONG UNMARRIED COHABITING COUPLES

Although exact rates of cohabitation are not available, there is consensus among researchers that a dramatic rise in cohabitation rates occurred after 1960, and this increase became especially noticeable in the late 1970s.[24–28] In 1970, the number of cohabitating couples was estimated to be 523,000; in 1978, it had risen to 1.1 million.[25] Census experts project that the rate will continue to rise dramatically into the 1990s.[9]

The increased prevalence of cohabitation has been attributed to several factors including the liberalization of attitudes about alternative lifestyles, the increase in age at first marriage, an increase in sexual freedom so that marriage is not as necessary a prerequisite to gain access to a sexual partner, and more honesty in reporting as the social disapproval of such arrangements declines.

Cohabitation has always been more common among blacks than among whites, and this remains true today.[27] Rates of cohabitation are also higher for previously married persons than for the never married.[27] Both Croake et al.,[29] and Johnson[30] found that cohabiting couples are more permissive and more sexually active than the general population. By the age of 18, 94 percent of the males and 86 percent of the females in Croake et al.'s study were sexually experienced. These rates are higher than those reported for teenagers as a whole. Similarly, Newcomb,[31] comparing cohabiting couples with noncohabitors, found that cohabitors had had earlier and greater sexual experience than did noncohabiting single persons.

The cohabitors in Croake et al.'s[29] study reported from 4 to 10 lifetime sexual partners. However, for about one-fourth of the females, the current partner was the only sexual partner they had ever had. About 21 percent of the males, on the other hand, reported that they had had more than 20 lifetime sexual partners.

Blumstein and Schwartz[32] found that cohabitors, both males and females, were much more likely than married couples to engage in sex outside of their relationships. As might be expected, male cohabitors were slightly more likely than female cohabitors to have sex outside the relationship, but the difference was small (33 vs. 30 percent, respectively). The modal number of partners outside the relationship varied from two to five for male cohabitors, while the mode was only one for female cohabitors. A significant minority of female cohabitors (41 percent), however, reported that they had from two to five outside partners.

Taken as a whole, the data on cohabiting heterosexuals suggest that relative to single noncohabitors, cohabitors are more sexually active, more sexually experienced, and may have become sexually active at an earlier age.

In conclusion, there appear to have been four significant changes in the sexual behavior of heterosexual single persons since Kinsey's day. Clearly, the prevalence of premarital intercourse has greatly increased and the age at first intercourse has declined. In addition, the tremendous growth of cohabitation among heterosexuals in the 1970s and 1980s, especially among middle-class whites, represents an arrangement in which premarital and nonmarital sex is explicit, indeed taken for granted. Finally, the growth of the divorce rate has resulted in a population of sexually active but single persons who display relatively high rates of sexual activity, compared with never-married or widowed singles, despite the loss of a regular partner. The implication is that there is a large and growing segment of the adult heterosexual population who are not married but nevertheless are sexually active and are quite likely to have several partners over a year's time. Further, in view of the fact that the proportion of divorced persons who remarry is declining, we expect that the prevalence of nonmarital sex and the number of partners single persons have over the course of their lives is likely to increase.

## SEXUALITY OF MARRIED PERSONS

### Sex within the marital relationship

The frequency of intercourse among married couples depends on a number of factors including age, social class, and duration of marriage. The overall rate of intercourse typically reported is about twice a week,[22,32,33] though Hunt's[15] figures are slightly higher. The range is from no sex at all to intercourse at least once a day.[22] Studies consisently show an inverse relationship between the frequency of intercourse within the marital relation and duration of marriage.[2,3,15,32–35] The data also indicate that the frequency of marital intercourse declines with age of the partners, though Blumstein and Schwartz's[32] data suggest that marital duration is the more important factor. We suspect that the decline in rates of intercourse over time in a marriage are a function of both familiarity and the exigencies of child rearing. Nonetheless, despite the decline in the frequency of intercourse with age and/or marital duration, the data indicate that regardless of years of marriage, the majority of married couples engage in sex no less than once a week.

Although both Hunt[15] and Westoff[33] claimed that the frequency of marital coitus has increased over time, we find remarkably similar rates across studies (cf. Greenblat[34]). What may have changed for married couples, if anything, is the prevalence of sexual activities other than intercourse. Oral sex, for example, has become a common part of marital sexuality.[15,22,32] Anal sex among married couples is less commonly reported, though it does not appear to be rare. Hunt,[15] indicated that about 25 percent of the married respondents in his study had tried anal sex at some time in their lives, though few performed it regularly. Similarly, Tavris and Sadd[22] found that 43 percent of the married women who responded to the *Redbook* survey had tried anal sex, but only 2 percent engaged in it regularly.

### Nonmonogamy among married couples

Rates of nonmonogamy vary somewhat from study to study (see Table 4-2). Kinsey et al.[2,3] found somewhat higher rates of nonmonogamy among the better educated, women over age 25, and those from "white collar" backgrounds. Although the overall rates of nonmonogamy appear unchanged since Kinsey's day,[15] nonmonogamy appears to have increased among younger persons. Both Hunt's[15] and Blumstein and Schwartz's[32] data showed that younger married persons have higher rates of nonmonogamy than do older persons. Moreover, we suspect that rates of nonmonogamy have increased for women, although reliable data do not exist regarding such a trend. We think this is because of trends toward increased premarital sexuality, increased opportunities, the availability of contraceptives, and the acceptance by women, as well as the larger society, of the notion that women have sexual needs and rights that are similar to men's.

The majority of nonmonogamous women, according to the *Redbook* survey,[22] confined sexual relations to one partner; how-

**Table 4-2. Incidence of Nonmonogamy among Married Couples Reported in Studies over Time, Percent**

| Study | Men | Women |
|---|---|---|
| Kinsey (1948, 1953) | 50 | 26 |
| Johnson (1970) | 20 | 10 |
| Hunt (1974) | 41 | 18 |
| Bell, Turner, and Rosen (1975) | — | 26 |
| Maykovich (1976) | — | 32 |
| Tavris and Sadd (1977) | — | 29 |
| Yablonsky (1979) | 47 | — |
| *Playboy* survey (1982) | 48 | 38 |
| Blumstein and Schwartz (1983) | 26 | 21 |

SOURCE: Thompson;[36] Petersen;[20] Blumstein and Schwartz.[32]

ever, a significant minority (40 percent) reported extramarital sexual liaisons with 2 to 5 partners. The modal number of extramarital partners reported by married men in Blumstein and Schwartz's[32] study was from 2 to 5 while for wives it was 1.

Although the overall rate of nonmonogamy among married couples may not be increasing, it occurs in a sizable minority, and that fact should signal concern about STDs among married persons. Further, as others have also pointed out (cf. Thompson[36]), reported rates are likely to *underestimate* the true incidence since nonmonogamy is still widely disapproved of despite the liberalization of attitudes toward premarital sex.

### Mate swapping, group sex, and "swinging"

Only a few studies have examined other forms of nonmonogamy among married persons such as group sex, "swinging," or mate swapping. Those that have report similar incidences of about 1 to 3 percent of married couples who have ever tried it and a much lower proportion who are regular participants.[15,22,37] Studies suggest that married couples who participate in swinging or group sex are typically white collar college-educated couples in their thirties who appear to be quite conventional, even conservative, in other areas of their lives.[37–41]

Although sexual contact between females is usually acceptable among swingers, homosexual contact among males is forbidden and homosexuals are typically excluded from such groups. Anecdotal evidence suggests that this is especially true since AIDS has become well publicized. Indeed, many swinging groups allegedly require evidence that members are seronegative. However, despite the outbreak of AIDS, there is no evidence to suggest that these forms of nonmonogamy have begun to disappear.

### Married persons engaged in same sex contacts

Laud Humphries[42] shocked both researchers and lay people with his report that 54 percent of the respondents he observed in homosexual encounters in "tearooms" (public restrooms) were married and leading double lives. More recent studies, however, suggest that while many homosexual men and women have had heterosexual contacts at some point in their lives, only a tiny proportion of married men and women also engage in homosexual contacts. Saghir and Robins[43] found that although 18 percent of the 89 gay men they studied had been married, only 2 percent were currently married—a figure similar to that reported in the Kinsey studies.[2]

Studies suggest that a substantial minority of gay men—17 to 20 percent is the range typically reported (rates are higher among bisexuals)—have been married at some time during their lives.[6,16,44,45] Further, an even greater proportion have engaged in heterosexual sex after puberty. For example, three-quarters of the 156 gay male couples studied by McWhirter and Mattison[46] had sexual experience with women beyond puberty.

Lesbians have been studied far less than gay males. Perhaps as a result, the prevalence rates for marriages in this group varies more from study to study than does the rate for gay males. Bell and Weinberg[16] reported that about 35 percent of the lesbians they studied had had at least one marriage, whereas Schaefer[47] reported a marriage rate of only 14 percent. Gundlach and Reiss[48] found a 29 percent marriage rate among the lesbians they studied.

Lesbians report much more heterosexual intercourse. For example, Peplau et al.[49] reported that 80 percent of the 127 lesbians they studied had had sexual intercourse with a man at some time in their lives. In fact, the median number of men with whom these respondents engaged in sex was five. Similar rates of heterosexual coitus were reported by Schaefer.[47]

Clearly, many gay men and lesbian women have had sex, sometimes a substantial amount, with members of the opposite sex. Similarly, members of married couples—how many it is impossible to say—have extramarital sexual relations with members of their own sex. Thus, it is not safe to assume that a person who defines him- or herself as exclusively heterosexual is in fact behaviorally exclusively heterosexual. These persons are not necessarily "closeted" homosexuals but rather may not define the experience of sex with a person of the same sex as homosexuality, for example, "swingers" or bisexuals (cf. Blumstein and Schwartz[50,51]).

In conclusion, the data on sexuality among married couples have two important implications. First, a significant minority of married persons engage in extramarital sexual relations, and most, though not all, do so without their spouse's consent. Second, in a small proportion of these extramarital sexual relations, how many it is difficult to say, the spouse's extramarital partner is likely to be a member of the same sex. These findings suggest not only that the clinician would be wise to ask about behavior rather than sexual orientation but also that some married persons will perceive themselves to be at no (or low) risk of STDs when in fact their spouse's extramarital sexual activities may place them at risk.

## SEXUAL BEHAVIOR OF HOMOSEXUAL MEN AND WOMEN

Most (pre-AIDS) studies have found higher rates of sexual activity among homosexual males than among heterosexual males.[43,44] Bell and Weinberg[16] reported that the modal frequency of sex among both black and white homosexual males was two to three times a week, although overall blacks reported higher frequencies than did whites. Weinberg and Williams[44] reported that 50 percent of male homosexuals had sex at least once a week, while about two-thirds of Bell and Weinberg's respondents reported this frequency. About 20 percent of the white female homosexual respondents studied by Bell and Weinberg reported engaging in sex about once a week, while the majority of black homosexual women engaged in sex two or more times a week. However, this racial difference disappeared when controlling for age. These rates of sexual frequency for lesbians are similar to those reported by others.[49]

Homosexual males, studied before the outbreak of AIDS, had on average more lifetime sexual partners than heterosexual males.[43,52] Bell and Weinberg[16] found that over 40 percent of white males and one-third of black males had at least 500 partners during their homosexual careers, and an additional one-fourth reported between 100 and 500 partners. Further, over 90 percent of the homosexual male respondents reported at least 25 lifetime partners. Most whites, and fewer but still the majority of blacks, said that more than half of their partners had been strangers before the sexual encounters. A higher proportion of whites relative to blacks had sex only once with a given partner.

The majority of homosexual females Bell and Weinberg[16] studied reported fewer than five partners in the past year. In sharp contrast to the male homosexuals, few of the sexual partners of the lesbians were strangers. In fact, 62 percent reported that they had never engaged in sex with strangers.

As is true of heterosexuals, oral sex among both male and

female homosexuals, whether black or white, is extremely common, and males have higher rates than females.[16] The majority of both black and white males in Bell and Weinberg's[16] study reported engaging in oral sex at least once a week, but just 28 percent of the white females and 42 percent of the black females reported this frequency.

Among both black and white homosexual males in Bell and Weinberg's study,[16] fellatio was the most commonly reported sexual activity. For white males, mutual masturbation was the second most common activity, whereas for blacks it was anal sex. In Hunt's[15] sample of homosexuals, only 20 percent had performed anal sex and even fewer (18 percent) had engaged in receptive anal intercourse. Among female homosexuals, mutual masturbation was the most frequently reported sexual activity, followed by oral sex.[16]

Studies consistently show age differences in the sexual activities of gay men. Younger men have more partners, a greater frequency of sex, "cruise" more, and have shorter relationships than older men,[16,43,44,53] while older men are more likely to pay for sex.[16] Comparing data from the Kinsey studies with data from more recent (pre-AIDS) studies, Kaplan et al.[54] concluded that increases in anal sex, casual sex, and sexual contact with strangers have occurred among male homosexuals. These changes in sexual behavior parallel those occurring in the heterosexual population.

At present several ongoing research projects are focusing on the changes in sexual behaviors of gay and bisexual males in response to the AIDS threat. These studies have consistently shown decreases in both the overall number of sexual partners and the number of partners not previously known (i.e., anonymous partners) reported by gay men.[55–58] The evidence also suggests that receptive anal intercourse without a condom and oral sex in which semen is swallowed have also declined.[56–58] Although these studies suggest significant changes in the sexual behaviors of gay men since the AIDS crisis became evident, it is important to note that they are being conducted in areas of the country which have large and well-integrated gay communities and high incidences of AIDS (San Francisco, New York, and Chicago). Whether such change is evident elsewhere remains to be demonstrated. Furthermore, a significant minority of gay men continue to engage in high-risk sexual activities despite knowledge of the risks involved.[59,60] This phenomenon clearly warrants further research and explanation.

## COUPLED HOMOSEXUALS

Although the data suggest that homosexual men tend to have more partners, somewhat greater frequency of sex, and relationships of shorter duration than heterosexuals, many gay men have long-term relationships with a primary partner—perhaps as many as 50 percent.[61] A good deal of pre-AIDS evidence suggests, however, that monogamy is the exception rather than the rule in such relationships.[16,32,43,61,62] In contrast, lesbian couples tend to be monogamous.[32,49,63] The incidence of nonmonogamy for homosexual couples varies somewhat from study to study. Blumstein and Schwartz[32] found that over 80 percent of their gay male couples but only 28 percent of the lesbian couples they studied had been nonmonogamous, rates similar to those reported by others.

Of those respondents who had been nonomonogamous at some time throughout the course of their relationships, Blumstein and Schwartz[32] found that the majority of lesbians (53 percent) had had sex with only one other partner. In marked contrast, 43 percent of the gay men studied had more than 20 partners outside their primary relationship, and an additional 30 percent had had sex with 6 to 20 outside partners. The incidence of nonmonogamy among both lesbian and gay couples increased with relationship duration, especially after the first few years.

In the initial stages of their relationships, gay male couples have sex far more frequently than do heterosexual or lesbian couples, but they experience a sharper decline in sexual frequency over time relative to married couples.[32] This apparent decline in frequency must be interpreted in the light of the nonmonogamy rates for gay males which suggest that interest in sex has not declined over time. Blumstein and Schwartz[32] found that lesbian couples not only had a lower frequency of sex than any other couple type, they apparently were not compensating for this with outside partners.

Oral sex is a common and accepted sexual activity for gay male and lesbian couples, but it is considerably less common for lesbians. Both Blumstein and Schwartz[32] and McWhirter and Mattison[46] found oral sex to be more common than anal sex among gay couples. For example, only 4 percent of the gay men Blumstein and Schwartz studied rarely or never engaged in oral sex with their partners, while 30 percent said that they rarely or never have anal sex. This does indicate, however, that over two-thirds of the gay men engaged in anal sex regularly.

In conclusion, the results of pre-AIDS studies of homosexually oriented men consistently show greater intensity of sexual activities (i.e., greater frequency, greater number of partners, more nonmonogamy), regardless of whether the gay man is "single" or in a relationship, relative to persons of other sexual orientations. However, as noted above, the sexual activities of gay men are changing in response to the AIDS threat, and whether these differences in intensity of sexual activity will persist we do not know. Compared with homosexual men, lesbians engage in sex less frequently, have fewer partners, engage in casual sex less often, and have longer relationships with lower rates of nonmonogamy.

## CONCLUSIONS AND A LOOK AT THE FUTURE

By organizing this chapter by sexual orientation and by single vs. coupled persons, we have implicitly suggested two social factors that are related to the prevalence and intensity of sexual behaviors. But even within types of relationships there is considerable variation. Marriages, for example, can be either monogamous or nonmonogamous. Perhaps even more dramatic is the strong effect of gender on sexual behavior. The sexual behaviors of heterosexual and homosexual men look more similar than different when compared with the sexual behaviors of women, whether homosexual or heterosexual. Men become sexually active earlier, have a greater prevalence of premarital sex, have more partners, have a greater frequency of sex, are more likely to engage in casual sex, and are more likely to be nonmonogamous than are women. While many researchers would claim that this difference is inherent in the "beast," we are less confident that such differences can be so easily attributed to biology. As Ford and Beach[64] have pointed out, there is considerable variation cross-culturally in the sexual behaviors of men and women. Moreover, the sexual behaviors of men and women in our culture are becoming more and more alike over time. We can also see differences in sexual behavior by class and race. What these differences imply is that one's social location (e.g., class, race) carries with it a set of meanings and expectations regarding sexual activities just as it shapes speech, values, attitudes, and a host of other social behaviors.

We have attempted to give the reader an overview of sexual behavior in the last 20 years, but even as we write society is changing. The rise in premarital sexual behavior that has been occurring at least since World War II, and probably since the turn of the century, was enabled in part by the technological advances of birth control, the development of the modern women's liberation movement, and the social conditions and ideologies that promoted later marriage, women's entry into the labor force, and a high divorce rate. There is no reason to believe that all the present sexual practices and beliefs would stay in place if society changed drastically.

We have not yet seen evidence of the "sexual conservatism" that some writers have proclaimed. However, if the economy fails, if women encounter serious difficulties supporting themselves—which is not inconceivable given the increasing number of households headed by women, if AIDS invades the heterosexual world as disastrously as it has affected the gay community, we could see major changes in sexual behavior toward greater conservatism. Indeed, some change in this direction is already occurring among gay men. Nonetheless, the literature on changes in sexual behavior among gay and bisexual men in response to the AIDS threat shows that even in the face of death, old habits are hard to change. Part of the reason, we suspect, lies in the gay male culture which, given society's refusal to sanction gay marriages and relationships, is organized around being single and maintaining one's sexual marketability.

At present we are hearing about the worries of the sexually active heterosexual population, but changes in behavior appear to be modest, if gonorrhea rates among heterosexuals are any indication.[65] Continuing late age at first marriage and the recycling of divorced people back into dating at various time in their lives means that sex outside of marriage is likely to continue long into the foreseeable future. On the other hand, there is no indication that values about extramarital sex are changing, and so whatever nonmonogamy occurs will probably continue to be clandestine. The diseases confronting nonmonogamous married men and women might motivate them to take precautions, but until AIDS becomes even more common among heterosexuals, it is unlikely that much change will be evident. This is likely to be even more true for married homosexuals and bisexuals. Since they cannot satisfy homosexual desires within marriage, the impetus for concealed, discreet sexual contact will continue unless AIDS proves to be a more powerful deterrent than it has heretofore.

The very nature of teenage sexuality—erratic and ambivalent—indicates continued, if irregular, sexual activity. Everything we know about teenage sexuality indicates that it is impulsive, embarrassed, and narcissistic enough to imply a belief in a kind of divine protection from the consequences of one's acts. It seems as if the consequences must be more likely and more immediate to produce major change. While an education campaign is finally being mounted to tell children and adolescents about AIDS, sex education efforts to date have been scattered and uneven. Further, while education is clearly necessary for behavior change, it may not be sufficient to produce major behavioral changes toward safer sex in the case of teenagers.

Assuming that the AIDS epidemic is contained and that cataclysmic social changes do not occur, we expect the sexual landscape of the near future to look much the same as it has in the recent past. We feel this way because the conditions which brought about the evolution of sexual liberalism are still in place and the trend seems to be more of the same. If anything, we should see somewhat more liberal behavior because men and women are becoming more and more alike in attitudes and behavior. Moreover, the unique experience of the baby boom generation, most of whom are now in their thirties, is likely to continue to be evident as this cohort soon passes through middle age. This generation was more sexually active at an earlier age than previous generations. We suspect that they will continue to be sexually active for quite some time. This may produce the appearance of a "revolutionary" upswing in the sexual activities of older persons, just as it produced the appearance of a "revolution" in the sexuality of teenagers when this cohort entered adolescence in the sixties.

One caveat here is that older heterosexual women of the baby boom generation who are disadvantaged demographically (having fewer men available the older they become) may have a less active sex life than would be expected given the sexually liberated attitudes and behaviors they display. On the other hand, to the extent that marrige (or remarriage after divorce or loss of a spouse through death) appears unlikely for many in this cohort, the *only* sex available is out of wedlock. We expect, therefore, that a certain percentage will accept serendipitous sexual encounters or affairs with married men because it may be their only opportunity for physical intimacy. Given that at least 8 percent of women are expected to be single throughout the life cycle and 28 percent of all households are presently headed by single women, and including the fact that the majority of women will be single for at least several years in adulthood, sex outside of marriage seems to be a continuing part of the American way of life.

But just because a society has removed the necessity of having sex within the confines of marrige does not mean that we are sexually "sophisticated." Men and women, homosexual and heterosexual, married and single, still do not easily discuss or plan their sexual conduct with one another. Ultimately we must recognize the limits of people's ability to approach their sexuality in a rational manner.

The "social accounting"—prevalence, incidence, frequency rates, etc.—that we have presented is, we believe, a necessary first step toward understanding human sexual behavior. But it is no more than a point of departure. In order to make further inroads, we need to understand how the conditions of people's lives structure the choices that they make. There are reasons for the differences in sexual behavior between blacks and whites, young and old, gay and straight, males and females, upper and lower classes. Once we have a better understanding of why these and other factors predict differences in sexual behaviors, individuals, practitioners, and those making public policy will be in a much better position to design and implement more effective strategies in the interest of public health.

## References

1 Mills CW: *The Sociological Imagination.* New York, Oxford University Press, 1959.

2 Kinsey AC et al: *Sexual Behavior in the Human Male.* Philadelphia, Saunders, 1948.

3 Kinsey AC et al: *Sexual Behavior in the Human Female.* Philadelphia, Saunders, 1953.

4 *Statistical Abstracts of the United States,* 107th ed. U.S. Department of Commerce, 1987.

5 Norton AJ, Moorman JE: Current trends in marriage and divorce among American women. *J Marriage Fam* 49:3, 1987.

6 Masters WH, Johnson VE: *Human Sexual Response*. Boston, Little, Brown, 1966.
7 Reiss IL: *Premarital Sexual Standards in America*. New York, Free Press, 1960.
8 Glenn ND, Weaver CN: Attitudes toward premarital, extramarital, and homosexual relations in the U.S. in the 1970s. *J Sex Res* 15:108, 1979.
9 Glick PC: Marriage, divorce, and living arrangements: Prospective changes. *J Fam Issues* 5:7, 1984.
10 Rodgers WL, Thornton A: Changing patterns of first marriage in the United States. *Demography* 22:265, 1985.
11 Zelnik M, Kantner J: Sexual activity, contraceptive use and pregnancy among metropolitan-area teenagers: 1971–1979. *Fam Plann Perspect* 12:230, 1980.
12 Zelnik M et al: *Sex and Pregnancy in Adolescence*. Beverly Hills, Sage, 1981.
13 Tanfer K, Horn MC: Contraceptive use, pregnancy and fertility planning among single women in their 20s. *Fam Plann Perspect* 17:10, 1985.
14 Jones EF et al: *Teenage Pregnancy in Industralized Countries*. New Haven, Yale University Press, 1986.
15 Hunt M: *Sexual Behavior in the 1970s,* Chicago, Playboy Press, 1974.
16 Bell AP, Weinberg MS: *Homosexualities*. New York, Simon & Schuster, 1978.
17 Ponse B: *Identities in the Lesbian World: The Social Construction of Self*. Westport, CT, Greenwood, 1978.
18 Downy L: Intergenerational changes in sex behavior: A belated look at Kinsey's males, *Arch Sex Behav* 9:267, 1980.
19 Pratt WF et al: Understanding U.S. fertility: Findings from the national survey of family growth, cycle III. *Popul Bull* 39(5): 1984.
20 Peterson JR: The Playboy readers' sex survey. *Playboy* January, 1983, p. 12.
21 DeLamater J, MacCorquodale P: *Premarital Sexuality*. Madison, University of Wisconsin Press, 1979.
22 Tavris C, Sadd S: *Redbook Report on Female Sexuality*. New York, Dell, 1977.
23 Spanier GB, Thompson L: *Parting: The Aftermath of Separation and Divorce*. Beverly Hills, Sage, 1984.
24 Macklin ED: Nonmarital heterosexual cohabitation. *Marriage Fam Rev* 12:1, 1978.
25 Glick PC, Spanier GB: Married and unmarried cohabitation in the U.S. today. *J Marriage Fam* 42:19, 1980.
26 Glick PC, Norton RJ: Marrying, divorcing and living together in U.S. today. *Popul Bull* 32:36, 1977.
27 Clayton RR, Voss HL: Shacking up: Cohabitation in the 1970s. *J Marriage Fam* 39:273, 1977.
28 Bower DW, Christopherson V: University student cohabitation: A regional comparison of selected attitudes and behavior. *J Marriage Fam* 39:447, 1977.
29 Croake JW et al: *Unmarrieds Living Together: It's Not all Gravy!* Dubuque, Iowa, Kendall/Hunt, 1974.
30 Johnson P: Courtship and commitment: A study of cohabitation on a university campus. Unpublished master's thesis. Iowa City, IA, University of Iowa, 1969.
31 Newcomb MD: Sexual behavior of cohabitors: A comparison of three independent samples. *J Sex Res* 22:492, 1986.
32 Blumstein P, Schwartz P: *American Couples*. New York, Morrow, 1983.
33 Westoff CF: Coital frequency and contraception. *Fam Plann Perspect* 6:135, September–October 1974.
34 Greenblat CS: The salience of sexuality in the early years of marriage. *J Marriage Fam* 45:289, 1983.
35 Udry JR: Changes in the frequency of marital intercourse from panel data. *Arch Sex Behav* 9:319, 1980.
36 Thompson AP: Extramarital sex: A review of the research literature. *J Sex Res* 19:1, 1983.
37 Gilmartin B: *The Gilmartin Report*. Secaucus, NJ, Citadel Press, 1978.
38 Jenks RJ: Swinging: A test of two theories and a proposed new model. *Arch Sex Behav* 14:517, 1985.
39 O'Neill G, O'Neill N: Patterns in group sexual activity. *J Sex Res* 6:101, 1970.
40 Smith JR, Smith LG: Co-marital sex and the sexual freedom movement. *J Sex Res* 6:131, 1970.
41 Varni CA: An exploratory study of spouse swapping, in *Beyond Monogamy,* JR Smith, LG Smith (eds). Baltimore, Johns Hopkins University Press, 1974, p 246.
42 Humphreys L: *Tearoom Trade*. Chicago, Aldine, 1970.
43 Saghir MT, Robins E: *Male and Female Homosexuality: A Comprehensive Investigation*. Baltimore, Williams & Wilkins, 1973.
44 Weinberg MS, Williams CJ: *Male Homosexuals*. London, Oxford University, 1974.
45 Harry J: *Gay Couples*. New York, Praeger, 1984.
46 McWhirter DP, Mattison AM: *The Male Couple*. Englewood Cliffs, NJ, Prentice-Hall, 1984.
47 Schaefer S: Sexual and social problems of lesbians. *J Sex Res* 12:50, 1976.
48 Gundlach R, Reiss BF: Self and sexual identity in the female, in *New Directions in Mental Health,* BF Reiss (ed). New York, Grune & Stratton, 1968.
49 Peplau LA et al: Loving women: Attachment and autonomy in lesbian relationships. *J Soc Issues* 34:7, 1978.
50 Blumstein P, Schwartz P: Bisexuality: Some social psychological issues. *J Soc Issues* 33:30, 1977.
51 Blumstein PW, Schwartz P: Bisexuality in women. *Arch Sex Behav* 5:171, 1976.
52 Schofield MG: *Sociological Aspects of Homosexuality: A Comparative Study of Three Types of Homosexuals*. Boston, Little, Brown, 1965.
53 Harry J, DeVall, WB: *The Social Organization of Gay Males*. New York, Praeger, 1978.
54 Kaplan HB et al: The sociological study of AIDS: A critical review of the literature and suggested research agenda. *J Health Soc Behav* 28:140, 1987.
55 Ostrow DG et al: Sexual behavior change and persistence in homosexual men. Paper presented at the International Conference on AIDS, Atlanta, GA, Apr 14–17, 1985.
56 Siegel K, Hirsch, DA: Modifications in sexual practices among asymptomatic gay men in New York City. Paper presented at the International Conference on AIDS, Atlanta, GA, Apr 14–17, 1985.
57 Martin JL: The impact of AIDS on New York City gay men: Changes in sexual behavior patterns. Paper presented at the 113th annual meeting of the American Public Health Association, Washington, DC, Nov 21, 1985.
58 McKusick L et al: Reported changes in the sexual behavior of men at risk for AIDS, San Francisco, 1982–84. *Public Health Rep* 100:622, 1985.
59 Coates TJ et al: AIDS: A psychosocial research agenda. *Ann Behav Med* 9:21, 1987.
60 Roffman R et al: AIDS Risk Reduction Project: A Report to the King County Department of Public Health, Seattle, WA, June 1987.
61 Peplau LA, Gordon SL: The intimate relations of lesbians and gay men, in *Gender Roles and Gender Behavior,* ER Allgeier, NB McCormick (eds). Palo Alto, CA, Mayfield, 1983.
62 Peplau LA, Cochran S: Value orientations in the intimate relationships of gay men. *J Homosex* 6:1, 1981.
63 Cotton WI: Social and sexual relationships of lesbians. *J Sex Res* 11:139, 1975.
64 Ford CS, Beach FA: *Patterns of Sexual Behavior*. New York, Harper & Row, 1951.
65 Handsfield H: King County Health Dept. Report, Seattle, WA, 1987.

# Chapter 5

# Psychological perspectives on sexuality and sexually transmitted diseases*

Michael W. Ross

Psychological variables are intimately associated with sexually transmitted diseases (STDs) in both immediate (social psychology of situational pressures to engage in sex which may lead to higher risk of infection) and more distant (personality styles or attitudes to sex and sexuality which may put an individual at greater risk of STD infection) senses. This chapter focuses on psychological aspects of sexuality as they may affect both risk of STD infection and presentation for and response to treatment. A third area of psychology associated with the acquired immunodeficiency syndrome (AIDS) and other STDs is clinical psychology or psychiatry, in which maladaptive or pathological responses to infection (or fear of infection) may occur. A brief review of theories of sexual behavior accompanies these observations.

## PSYCHOLOGICAL THEORIES OF HUMAN SEXUALITY

Sexual behavior is an inborn drive in humans; even infants show signs of sexual behavior. Sex drive may be markedly modified by cultural, social, and interpersonal factors. Freud termed the energy of sex the libido and believed that, along with hostility and aggression, it accounted for most of the motivation behind human behavior. He postulated that the individual was born potentially able to respond to any individual sexually but that socialization through a series of stages directed the sexual urge toward heterosexual contact. Freud's stages included the oral stage, the anal stage, the genital stage, the latency stage, and the reawakening of sexual impulses at puberty. Major studies of children's sexual thinking[1] show that sexual understanding follows three Piagetian stages of nonsexual, transition sexual, and fully sexual stages of cognition rather than Freud's stages, and these depend strongly upon the cultural and educational information on sexuality available to children and adolescents.

There is general agreement that a fundamental propensity to act sexually exists but that it may be modified by learning. Ford and Beach[2] note that cultural conditioning accounts for the extent and type of sexual expression but falls short of accounting for what is biologically possible in humans. The psychological process of molding sexual expression is through conditioning. Modeling, in which individuals learn roles or behaviors through observing the behavior of others, is also involved.[3] Nevertheless, little is understood about the specific development of heterosexual or homosexual behavior.

Sexuality has a number of different aspects and meanings depending on variation in person, time, culture, age, and situation. Table 5-1 indicates that multiple meanings of sexual expression are certainly learned.[4] Sexuality is not a unitary phenomenon but part of social interaction and is best explained by contingencies of reinforcement acting upon a basic biological drive.

**Table 5-1. Theoretical Aspects and Meanings of Sexual Relationships**

| Aspects | Meanings |
|---|---|
| Reproduction | Continuation of species |
| Religious | Symbolic of union |
| Emotional | Extension of love for partner |
| Release of sexual urge | Release of frustration or libido |
| Financial | Prostitution |
| Duty | Socially expected, as in some marriages |
| Antisocial statement | Rejection of parental/social values |
| Ritual | During particular ceremonies; symbolic |
| Hedonistic (recreational) | Enjoyment |
| Experimental | Exploration of sexual feelings and behaviors |
| Relational | As part of wider social and attitudinal affinities |
| Dominance | Rape; expression of difference in relative power |
| Peer-sanctioned | Normative; status-associated |
| Forbidden or taboo | Associated with guilt or punishment |
| Dynastic | Cementing relations between families or groups |
| Mentor | Teaching sexuality to younger individuals |

SOURCE: Ross.[4]

## PSYCHOLOGICAL VARIABLES ASSOCIATED WITH RISK OF STD INFECTION

The psychological variables associated with increased risk of contracting STDs include those which are associated with behaviors which carry an increased risk of infection. In addition to specific behaviors such as high partner numbers, specific sexual practices, and the context in which the sex occurs, I review the variables generally which have been associated with STD infection. Where psychosocial factors are associated with risk of STD infection, such factors may be modified to decrease the probability of infection as well as to develop information on which education strategies may be based.

## PERSONALITY AND ATTITUDINAL VARIABLES

Hart[5] has argued not only that venereal disease is increasingly recognized as a behavioral disease but that all sociological variables implicated in venereal disease are primarily related to the personality of the individual. For his heterosexual sample he reported an increase in extroversion and to a lesser extent neuroticism, as measured by the Eysenck Personality Inventory,[6] associated with increased STD infection. Similar findings are reported by other researchers. Eysenck found that extroverts will have intercourse earlier, more frequently, with more different partners, and in more different positions than introverts; they will also engage in more varied sexual behavior outside intercourse and engage in longer foreplay.[7] Measuring attitudes on Eysenck's Sexual Attitudes Inventory (ESAI), Fulford et al.[8] found clinic subjects to be less interested than Eysenck's controls in physical sex and pornography, to have less sexual excitement and greater prudishness, sexual disgust, and neurotic sexual attitudes. Homosexual patients did not differ from heterosexual patients, and bisexual patients accounted for most of the differences found. Familial variables have also been implicated: Hart[9]

*There is a lack of current literature dealing with the psychological perspective on sexually transmitted diseases among heterosexual individuals, which explains any unintentional emphasis on homosexual men in this chapter.

has reported that soldiers coming from large (four or more children) families are significantly more at risk for STD infection, and I[10,11] reported that the extremes of rejecting and overly supportive parental relationships were significant predictors of multiple STD infections in the four western countries I studied.

Personality and attitudinal variables may be associated with increased risk of STD infection in homosexual men. Beliefs about the meaning of sexuality and its social and political implications predicted sexual behavior in Swedish homosexual men.[12] High psychoticism scorers (those who tend to be isolated, affectless, and aggressive) were also more sexually curious, more accepting of premarital sex, more promiscuous, and more hostile.[13] Extroverts scored high on the promiscuity scales and low on the nervousness scale (more promiscuous and less sexually nervous), while high scorers on the neuroticism scale had significantly lower scores on sexual satisfaction and significantly higher scores on excitement, nervousness, sexual hostility, sexual guilt, and sexual inhibition. High neuroticism scores are also closely associated with venereoneurosis: Hart[5] noted that certain sociological parameters to veneral infection may be of a secondary nature, in that all are primarily related to the personality of the individual.

The study done by Fulford et al.[8] using the ESAI found that while neuroticism correlated positively with syphilis and gonorrhea infections, extroversion correlated negatively with the diagnosis of syphilis.[8] Another study[12] refactored the ESAI after rewording it to make it appropriate for homosexual men, and derived nine interpretable dimensions. As anticipated, sexual attitudes did seem to underlie sexual behaviors. In fact, six of the nine scales were predictors of partner numbers, five were predictors of particular sexual practices, and six were predictors of places of partner contact. All these scales were related in a curvilinear rather than a linear fashion to partner numbers, with those with zero and high partner numbers having greater sexual prudishness, fear of sexual relationships, and lower interest in pornography, degree of sexual excitability, and sexual permissiveness. Those with higher partner numbers are highest on the scale for lack of control of libido.

## PSYCHOSOCIAL VARIABLES

The environmental stresses of war and immigration produce behavior patterns which many would not otherwise experience.[5,14] Half of the men with gonorrhea in the United Kingdom in the 1960s were immigrants. Single migrants may have numerous sexual encounters until they settle into their new cultural background.[15] This holds for nonwestern societies: Hart[16] reported that in single laborers and married immigrants in Papua, New Guinea, recourse to prostitutes and, to a lesser extent, homosexual behavior are more common outlets and venereal disease a prominent sequel. STD incidence rates in immigrants and soldiers increase markedly (in comparison with baseline rates prior to immigration or war) and instability and insecurity are associated with lack of discrimination and increase in frequency of sexual contacts. However, Kelus[17] took random samples of STD clinic attenders and inhabitants in a Polish town and found no differences between them apart from a tendency for patients to be more urbanized and less religious. Hooker[18] has suggested that for some, seeking sexual contacts is an activity isolated from all other aspects of their lives. We cannot assume that psychological factors which influence sexual contacts will be obvious in other areas of the individual's life.

## PSYCHOLOGICAL CONCOMITANTS OF PARTNER NUMBERS

Partner numbers are an important determinant of STD infection, as on the average they increase the probability of infection. If sexual practices which do not transfer body fluids are utilized, partner numbers are immaterial, and if all partners are monogamous, there is no risk. One report[19] found that partner numbers were not invariably associated with risk of STD infection in homosexual men. Schofield[20] reports little evidence that individuals with high partner numbers have personality defects, are emotionally damaged, or come from a less than adequate social milieu. Goode and Troiden[21] found that homosexual men with higher partner numbers tended to prefer emotionally superficial sex and were less well educated. Partner numbers are often depressed during dysphoric mood states (confusion, fatigue, and distress).[12] High partner numbers may also protect from psychological decompensation through their effect on increasing self-esteem. Depression increased in homosexual men who reduced their risk of contracting human immunodeficiency virus,[22] which suggests that there is some association between mood and partner numbers.

The homosexual male with high partner numbers sees himself as conventionally masculine, prefers a more feminine partner, and has high alcohol consumption. He will have had a more negative parental rearing pattern and will be under less stress than men with low partner numbers, be more involved in the homosexual subculture, see his homosexuality as more central to his lifestyle, and have had more STD infections.[12] These data illustrate the multifactorial nature of the variables associated with high partner numbers, variables that are internally consistent across white western cultures.

## PSYCHOLOGICAL CONCOMITANTS OF PARTICULAR SEXUAL PRACTICES

Practices that involve the transmission of body fluids, including unprotected anal or vaginal intercourse, brachioproctic ("fist fornication") activities, and fellatio may transmit pathogens; mutual masturbation and frottage (rubbing bodies together) will not. Haist and Hewitt[23] noted that homosexual men who preferred the anal insertee role also tended to prefer the oral insertee role in fellatio. However, Hooker[24] reported no relationship between sexual activity preferences and sex role. I[12] found that homosexual men who preferred oral activities, including both fellatio and analingus, appear to be differentiated from those with no such preference by negative maternal rearing patterns and by euphoric mood states, suggesting that they may be related both to gratification of oral dependency needs and to hedonism. Preference for insertor and insertee roles in both fellatio and anal intercourse appeared to be strongly related to conventional masculine and feminine sex roles, and activities such as full-body contact and mutual masturbation appear to be non-sex-role-related. The last two activities appear to occur when there is emphasis on emotional as well as physical closeness, and they are associated with decreased frequencies of STD infection. My data also suggest that sexual socialization into homosexual subcultures and, to a lesser extent, parental and peer models have a major influence on the type of sexual activities indulged in; increased time and degree of socialization into the homosexual subculture increases preference for specific roles, as does degree of organization of the homosexual subculture within which that socialization occurs.

Preference for particular practices appears to be more a function of increasing sexual experience, although the influence of masculine and feminine sex roles is significant. There is no literature on heterosexual concomitants of particular sexual practices.

## PSYCHOLOGICAL CONCOMITANTS OF PARTNER ANONYMITY AND PLACES OF SEXUAL CONTACT

Partner anonymity and place of sexual contact play an important part in STD infection; the links are threefold. First, contact tracing of anonymous partners is virtually impossible. Second, in some places of anonymous contact such as gay bathhouses, there are opportunities for multiple contacts with multiple partners within a short time. Third, such places may generate their own demands, which may lead to person-situation interactions in which the effect of being in the situation is significant. Apart from the classic study of Humphreys,[25] which classified men using public conveniences as places for sexual gratification into four groups—"trade," ambisexuals, gays, and closet queens—there is little data on places of sexual contact. Humphreys' "trade" group comprised working-class married men. Two-thirds took an insertor role in fellatio in sexual encounters. Ambisexuals were married men with high income: two-thirds of this group were insertees in fellatio, and saw themselves as bisexual. The gay group were individuals who were unmarried, had no preference for sexual roles, and had independent occupations. The "closet queens" were also unmarried but in lower middle-class occupations in which they were dependent on others for employment, and they avoided the homosexual subculture. They preferred to play the insertor role, at least until they lost their attractiveness.

I[12] demonstrated differences between those preferring particular places of meeting sexual partners. Those meeting in bars tended to prefer social as well as emotional contacts but had a history of overinvolved parents that may have made extended interaction difficult, and those making contacts through friends preferred homosocial as well as homosexual contacts with friends. Contrary to expectations, those meeting partners through cruising have more positive mood states and higher self-esteem than others and differed markedly from those who frequented bathhouses, who appear to be more depressed, avoiding close emotional contacts, probably as a result of much more negative parental relationship models. Psychological variables, particularly mood states, appear to be strongly associated with the drive for partners and the context in which they are sought, with a relationship between mood and partner seeking.

## THE PSYCHOLOGY OF STD INFECTIONS

A second area of importance is the psychological aspects of STD infection, such as reactions and abnormal behavior in those infected. This section considers the presentation and management of the psychosocial manifestations and psychopathology of STDs. Psychological sequelae to STD exposure are poorly understood, frequently unrecognized, and inadequately managed, despite being among the most common conditions encountered in STD practice.[5] Psychological and psychiatric problems in STD practice may be divided into three categories: the normal range of psychological reactions to STDs; abnormal reactions to STD infection (or belief in infection); and sexual dysfunctions which may become apparent in the course of consultation or present initially to STD clinics.

## PSYCHOSOCIAL RESPONSES TO STD INFECTION

Over 40 percent of cases attending public STD clinics are classified as psychiatric cases on the basis of screening tests.[26] Recent studies note that the anxiety caused by the presenting problem was probably the cause of such a high figure, since less than 5 percent had a sufficiently abnormal level of distress to justify calling it psychopathological.[27] Other studies report that less than 5 percent of STD patients required psychiatric referral.[28] It is therefore important to differentiate the normal range of reactions to STD infection from psychopathological ones.

One model concerning the meaning of STDs to the individual explains the beliefs underlying psychological reactions to STDs and the reasons for psychopathology when it occurs.[12] In discussing the meaning of STDs to the individual, there are at least four separate attributions:

1. STDs are a deserved outcome of indiscriminate sexual behavior and punishment for sexual sins.
2. STDs are a consequence of individual inadequacy that leads to sexually indiscriminate behavior.
3. STDs are a consequence of a breakdown in traditional social values and rapid social change.
4. STDs are solely the result of an individual's coming into intimate contact with a virulent pathogen.

There is a hierarchy of blame from attributions 1 to 4. Concomitant is a similar hierarchy of the degree to which individuals see themselves responsible for the infection. The degree of psychological investment in sexual behavior is also important. The meaning of STDs to the patient and to a lesser degree the attending health professional will affect not only the compliance with treatment but also the psychological sequelae and the subsequent risks the individual takes of exposure to STDs. The interaction between patients and physicians who hold conflicting attributions for STDs may lead to tension, anger, transference, and countertransference issues and resistance to taking advice or treatment, particularly where more divergent attributions are held. One should ascertain one's own position and make some estimate of the position of one's patient before seeking to educate or to modify risky behaviors.

## ABNORMAL REACTION TO STD INFECTION

Abnormal reactions to STD infection may arise from any of the four attitudes toward STDs noted above. These reactions may be further classified into abnormal illness behavior and venereoneuroses. Psychotic reactions which are either triggered by STD or have major venereological components are recognizable by such classic psychotic features as delusional thought patterns and the inability of patients to be convinced by rational discussion. Such patients with psychotic reactions will generally also have a history of psychotic illness.

### Abnormal illness behavior

Abnormal illness behavior has important implications for treatment. In individuals with an erroneous conviction that they have an STD, there is abnormal illness behavior in terms of both general hypochondriasis and a strong disease conviction without demonstrable pathology. Patients may also believe they "deserve" the infection, as noted above. Perhaps more common is seeing STD not as an illness but perhaps as only a minor nonsignificant risk of a particular lifestyle. In the absence of any illness behavior, patients may frequently compromise treatment by discontinuing medication after symptoms have resolved, continuing sexual activity after symptom resolution but before clearance, or not returning for proof of cure. Thus, both extreme illness behavior and lack of illness behavior can be abnormal and may have implications for the management of STDs. The repeated STD attenders rather than the first attenders seem to display the greatest anxiety and hypochondriasis over STD infection.[29] Those with higher previous numbers of infections also tended to deny life stresses more and to attribute their problems solely to the episode of illness. Such individuals also displayed significantly higher disease conviction and symptom preoccupation, and higher levels of symptom exaggeration. In comparison, first attenders tended to deny that an STD was an illness (denial of the contraction of a stigmatizing illness). Compared with other illnesses, in which there may be substantial secondary gain through sympathy, illness behavior appears to be different in STDs and to develop as a function of repeated infections. STD infection tends to be seen as a chance event until after several infections, when it is seen not only as an illness but also as a result of particular behaviors. I also found few differences in illness behavior with STD infections between heterosexual and homosexual men, apart from a less negative reaction to STD infection in gay men. The STD clinic population was closer in illness behavior scores to a psychiatric outpatient population than to a general practice one. It is unclear whether the disturbance was a function of having a stigmatized illness like an STD or was inherent in STD clinic attenders.

Another study[30] found that in STD clinics the proportion of individuals who admitted to being homosexual varied from 20 to 53 percent in Sweden, Finland, Australia, and Ireland—and there was no significant difference in the proportion of those admitting to being homosexual between public and private clinics in each country. The variables predictive of whether the respondent reveals his homosexual orientation when presenting to an STD clinic or medical practitioner are coherent. Nonadmitters are likely to conceal their homosexuality from most people, to expect the most negative social reaction to their homosexuality from significant others and society in general, and to believe in much more rigid and conservative sex roles for men and women. Compared with those who admit to homosexual contact, nonadmitters are more likely to report themselves as being more bisexual than exclusively homosexual, to have had no previous STD, and to have had poor relationships with their mother during adolescence. They are also more likely to be unassertive.

The lack of previous sexually transmitted infections in nonadmitters suggests that the clinic situation will be a new and potentially frightening one, in which condemnation is expected; in subsequent clinic visits the patient will tend to be more open if the clinician's approach has been nonjudgmental. When clinicians take histories in a manner that implies that any sexual contact was heterosexual, the patient may not have the courage to make a correction. These data suggest that significant and consistent psychological factors operate to prevent some homosexual men from revealing same-sex contacts in the context of STD clinics. However, these psychological factors clearly operate in interaction with environmental factors such as the clinic, the clinician, and the legal and social climate regarding homosexuality. The imposition of shame and guilt upon sexual interactions by religious and other traditional moralities is the single most important cause of psychological problems in STD treatment, and if the physician is able to assess and deal with this early in the treatment process, many difficulties may be prevented or minimized. To fail to do so may even introduce or reinforce shame or guilt and produce an iatrogenically strengthened psychopathology. A high index of suspicion for psychosocial problems attendant on STD infection or reported infection is mandatory to ensure maximal compliance with treatment, contact tracing, prevention, and preventive education, and the possible contribution of psychosocial factors to relapse or reinfection should not be underestimated.

## VENEREONEUROSES

Venereoneuroses may be divided into neuroses which manifest with exposure to infection and include overreaction to infection, and venereophobias and abnormal disease convictions, as well as factitious STDs and AIDS.

### Venereal overreaction and hypochondriasis

Individuals abnormally preoccupied with bodily processes can manifest a genitally focused hypochondriasis.[5] Irrational, sometimes obsessional, concern is focused on urethral, anal, or vaginal discharge or the appearance and sensations of the genitalia. Compulsive genital examination may itself cause irritation or discharge. Acceptance of these symptoms (or the patient's description of these symptoms) without objective evidence of infection or relapse may promote venereoneurosis and aggravation of the neurotic tendencies of the patient. Hart[5] has also reported that penile manipulation to produce discharge (often including vigorous squeezing of the glans and shaft, in contrast to the cautious manipulation by other patients) is a feature of such patients. In other manifestations, abnormal attention may be paid to irregularities in pigmentation or skin surface, skin tags, sebaceous cysts and hair follicles, and pearly penile papules. Demands for treatment, in the absence of demonstrable infection or pathology, are one indication of the presence of venereoneurosis, and Hart believes that such patients tend to be more severely disturbed.

Miller et al.[31] have reported individuals who focus on the nonspecific nature of the symptoms of HIV infection and attend for minor changes in skin pigmentation which they believe is Kaposi's sarcoma or for minor changes in respiratory function which they believe indicative of an opportunistic pulmonary infection. Obsessional palpation of cervical and axillary lymph nodes may lead to local irritation which may be interpreted as lymphadenopathy. Management involves discussing the patient's specific anxieties, and the opportunity to talk about these may in itself provide considerable relief. For those who have been infected with HIV and are worried about AIDS, it is important to focus on the patient's specific concerns, including fear of exposure, stigmatization, pain, death, and the uncertainty associated with the diagnosis of HIV infection and likelihood of progression.

### Venereophobias

Venereophobias have been recognized for most of this century, with syphilophobia as the earliest manifestation reported.[32] At present, AIDS phobias are more commonly reported,[33] probably because of the increased publicity surrounding AIDS and the perceived mortality and morbidity associated with it. With syphilophobia and AIDS phobias, individuals at no or low risk of contracting the disease believe that they are infected. While more accurately described as an abnormal disease conviction than a phobia, there may also be irrational precautions to avoid catching AIDS and fear or avoidance of situations in which there is a perceived risk of catching AIDS. AIDS-phobic patients differ from venereoneurotics in that symptoms are not usually genitally focused and often cannot be traced to a specific sexual episode. Underlying conflicts and life stresses are also likely to be major contributors and such presentations are usually associated with guilt over sexual behavior (commonly sexual activity outside a primary relationship or bisexual or homosexual contact).[33] The trigger is usually life stresses, often relationship-related, or media publicity on AIDS. The belief in infection may sometimes be near delusional, with patients refusing to believe the results of HIV tests or going from clinic to clinic in search of a test result that confirms their worst fears.

Management of venereophobias must encompass more than just reassurance of noninfection, which the patient may interpret as not being taken seriously. Excessive physical intervention, beyond that necessary to exclude disease, reinforces the patient's belief in the existence of disease. Taking a brief sexual history and noting current concerns, stresses, and conflicts will frequently bring out the underlying issues of guilt or concern over moral self-image or sexual orientation. Brief interpretive counseling focusing on the conflicts underlying the phobia and on the stresses which promote such conflicts, with emphasis on giving the patient a degree of insight into the processes which lead them to present with an abnormal disease conviction , will often resolve the problem. However, referral to appropriate mental health professionals should be considered and not delayed if resolution does not occur.

### Factitious illness

Several cases of factitious AIDS have been reported.[34,35] The individuals may present stating that they have been diagnosed as having full AIDS at another center but findings on examination do not agree with this. Immediate professional consultation with the center of previous treatment usually confirms that the claim of illness is incorrect. Individuals who have been confirmed to have factitious AIDS may be either seeking the secondary gain of sympathy and hospitalization or seeking to come to terms with the death of a significant other from AIDS. In the few cases reported, individuals usually strongly deny the diagnosis of factitious illness ("Munchausen syndrome") and may present in the future with other factitious illnesses with substituted symptoms. Such individuals are frequently quite medically sophisticated and may present plausible histories. Referral for psychiatric assessment is strongly recommended in such cases.

## ACQUIRED IMMUNODEFICIENCY SYNDROME AND HIV INFECTION

Reactions to HIV infection may be more extreme than reactions to other STDs for four reasons. First, the fully developed disease is fatal. Second, in western societies AIDS is commonly associated with stigmatized minority groups (homosexual and bisexual men, illicit intravenous drug users, and prostitutes) and a substantial component of attitudes toward AIDS comprises antihomosexual and antiminority beliefs and attribution of blame.[36] Third, such attitudes may be internalized in those infected and may lead to guilt and self-blame. Fourth, medical attendants may also contribute to stigmatization through overprecautions or avoidance of contact.[37] Consequently, the emotional impact on the patient of informing them they are infected with HIV is not significantly different from the news they have AIDS-related symptoms of full AIDS.[38]

Psychological complications of HIV infection may be exogenous or endogenous. Exogenous complications arise from the psychosocial stresses resulting from negative societal and interpersonal reactions to AIDS. Faulstich[39] notes that the "worried well" (whether infected or not) may exhibit generalized anxiety and panic attacks, along with excessive somatic preoccupation and fear of the disease. On diagnosis of HIV infection or AIDS, individuals may exhibit disbelief and denial, followed by depressive and anxiety symptoms. Emotional distress may commonly lead to adjustment disorders with depressed mood or major depression. Recurrent psychological themes include uncertainty about disease progression, social isolation (imposed or adopted), dealing with terminal illness, and guilt or blame over lifestyle. Suicidal ideation is often present.

Endogenous complications result from the neuropsychiatric sequelae of HIV infection, from either the direct effect of HIV neural infection, opportunistic CNS infections, or CNS neoplasia. Up to half of patients with AIDS present signs and symptoms of CNS infection, including subacute encephalitis characterized by malaise, social withdrawal, lethargy, and reduced sexual drive (these may also be signs and symptoms of depressed mood). Subsequently, signs of progressive dementia may appear. Neuropsychiatric deficits may typically involve impaired language, memory, and integrative abilities, and occasionally depressed mood, and their insidious onset makes it important to maintain a high index of suspicion that psychological symptoms may indicate onset of neurological involvement.

The potential for depressive reactions, sexual acting out, and further discrimination and stigmatization and loss of social supports makes informed consent and adequate pre- and post-HIV test counseling mandatory.[40] Where individuals are infected with HIV, frequent psychological support (or referral to appropriate agencies) and attention to patient's genuine fears of exposure, pain, discrimination, abandonment, and death is indicated, rather than general reassurance, which may be interpreted as being dismissive. In cases of chronic depressed mood, pharmacotherapy or referral for psychotherapeutic treatment are indicated.

## PSYCHOSEXUAL PROBLEMS

Studies in both Europe and India[26,41] note that sexual dysfunctions may present to STD clinics or be detected in STD clinics. Over 13 percent of STD clinic presentations are for sexual dysfunctions in India, compared with only 4 percent in psychiatric clinics. Of these, over 80 percent are males with concerns over the effect of masturbation, erectile dysfunction, and premature ejaculation. Generally, presenting dysfunctions in males include premature ejaculation, retarded ejaculation, and erectile dysfunction ("impotence"); in females, anorgasmia, general dysfunction ("frigidity"), and rarely vaginismus (spasm of the muscles of the vaginal introitus preventing penetration). Psychosexual problems usually occur in STD patients secondary to pain from infection or trauma, or from fear of infection, reinfection, or infecting others.

In mild or transient dysfunctions, the STD clinician will be able to provide reassurance that such transient dysfunctions are not unusual and are often limited to particular partners, situations, and times, and information or education to correct misapprehensions which affect sexual performance is appropriate. However, specific therapy for chronic psychosexual problems which are not a result of physical pathology should be referred to sex therapists. It is not uncommon to detect psychosexual dysfunctions in the course of history taking or treatment, and for some individuals the STD clinic will be the point of primary attendance. While it is estimated that most sexual dysfunctions are mild and transient and may resolve with adequate information and encouragement, the six major dysfunctions in males and females listed above will need more specific therapy from specialists in psychosexual dysfunctions.

In summary, psychological variables may be determinants of STD infection, and psychological problems are commonly associated with STD treatment. The physician should be aware of the range, nature, and presentations of these disorders, which may adversely affect attendance, compliance, and treatment as well as the psychological state of the individual.

## References


1 Goldman R, Goldman J: *Children's Sexual Thinking.* London, Routledge & Kegan Paul, 1984.
2 Ford CS, Beach FA: *Patterns of Sexual Behavior.* New York, Harper & Row, 1951.
3 Shope DF: *Interpersonal Sexuality.* Philadelphia, Saunders, 1975.
4 Ross MW: A theory of normal homosexuality, in *Male and Female Homosexuality: Psychological Approaches,* L Diamant (ed). New York, Hemisphere, 1987, pp 237–59.
5 Hart G: *Sexual Maladjustment and Disease: An Introduction to Modern Venereology.* Chicago, Nelson-Hall, 1977.
6 Eysenck HJ, Eysenck SBG: *Manual of the EPI.* London, London University Press, 1964.
7 Eysenck HJ, Wilson G: *The Psychology of Sex.* London, Dent, 1979.
8 Fulford KWM et al: Social and psychological factors in the distribution of STD in male clinic attenders. II. Personality disorders, psychiatric illness and abnormal sexual attitudes. *Br J Vener Dis* 59:381, 1983.
9 Hart G: Factors influencing venereal infection in a war environment. *Br J Vener Dis* 50:68, 1974.
10 Ross MW: Sexually transmitted diseases in homosexual men: a study of four societies. *Br J Vener Dis* 60:52, 1984.
11 Ross MW: Sociological and psychological predictors of STD infection in homosexual men. *Br J Vener Dis* 60:110, 1984.
12 Ross MW: *Psychovenereology: Personality and Lifestyle Factors in Sexually Transmitted Diseases in Homosexual Men.* New York, Praeger, 1986.
13 Eysenck HJ: *Sex and Personality.* London, Abacus, 1978.
14 Armytage WHG: Changing incidence and patterns of sexually transmitted diseases. *Proc 15th Annu Symp Eugenics Soc* 15:159, 1980.
15 Oriel JD: The global pattern of sexually transmitted diseases. *S Afr Med J* 61:993, 1982.
16 Hart G: Social and psychological aspects of venereal disease in Papua New Guinea. *Br J Vener Dis* 50:453, 1974.
17 Kelus J: Social and behavioural aspects of venereal disease. *Br J Vener Dis* 49:167, 1973.
18 Hooker E: Male homosexual lifestyles and venereal disease, in *Proceedings of the World Forum on Syphilis and Other Trepanemotoses.* Public Health Service Publication 977. Washington DC, Government Printing Office, 1964.
19 Ross MW: Predictors of partner numbers in homosexual men: Psychosocial factors in four societies. *Sex Transm Dis* 11:119, 1984.
20 Schofield M: *Promiscuity.* London, Victor Gollancz, 1976.
21 Goode E, Troiden RR: Correlates and accompaniments of promiscuous sex among male homosexuals. *Psychiatry* 43:51, 1980.
22 McKusick L et al: Prevention of HIV infection among gay and bisexual men: Two longitudinal studies. *Abstracts Second International Conference on AIDS.* Washington DC, Government Printing Office, 1987, p 213.
23 Haist M, Hewitt J: The butch-fem dichotomy in male homosexual behavior. *J Sex Res* 10:68, 1974.
24 Hooker E: An empirical study of some relations between sexual patterns and gender identity in male homosexuals. in *Sex Research: New Developments,* J Money (ed). New York, Holt, Rinehart & Winston, 1965, pp 24–52.
25 Humphreys RAL: *Tearoom Trade: A study of Impersonal Sex in Public Places.* London, Duckworth, 1970.
26 Catalan J et al: Sexual dysfunction and psychiatric morbidity in patients attending a clinic for sexually transmitted diseases. *Br J Psychiatry* 138:292, 1981.
27 Fitzpatrick R et al: Survey of psychological disturbance in patients attending a sexually transmitted diseases clinic. *Genitourin Med* 62:111, 1986.
28 Bhanji S, Mahony JDH: The value of a psychiatric service within the venereal disease clinic. *Br J Vener Dis* 54:566, 1978.
29 Ross MW: Illness behavior among patients attending a sexually transmitted disease clinic. *Sex Transm Dis* 14:174, 1987.
30 Ross MW: Psychosocial factors in admitting to homosexuality in sexually transmitted disease clinics. *Sex Transm Dis* 12:83, 1985.
31 Miller JD et al: A "pseudo-AIDS" syndrome following from fear of AIDS. *Br J Psychiatry* 146:550, 1985.
32 MacAlpine I: Syphilophobia. *Br J Vener Dis* 33:92, 1957.
33 Ross MW: AIDS phobias: A study of four cases. *Psychopathology 21:* 1988, in press.
34 Miller F et al: Two cases of factitious Acquired Immune Deficiency Syndrome. *Am J Psychiatry* 143:1483, 1986.
35 Robinson EN, Latham RH: A factitious case of Acquired Immune Deficiency Syndrome. *Sex Transm Dis* 14:54, 1987.
36 Ross MW: Measuring attitudes toward AIDS: Their structure and interactions. *Hosp Community Psychiatry 39:* 1988, in press.
37 Amchin J, Polan HJ: A longitudinal account of staff adaptation to AIDS patients on a psychiatric ward. *Hosp Community Psychiatry* 37:1235, 1986.
38 Rosser BRS, Ross MW: Emotional and life change impact of AIDS on homosexual men. *Psychology and Health 2:* 1988, in press.
39 Faulstich ME: Psychiatric aspects of AIDS. *Am J Psychiatry* 144:551, 1987.
40 Ross MW, Rosser BRS: Pretest counselling for AIDS screening: A guide for clinicians. *Patient Management* 11(7):93.
41 Rao RVR: Prevalence of psychosexual problems in patients attending the STD clinic. *Indian J Sex Transm Dis* 7:67, 1986.

# Chapter 6

# Homosexual behavior and sexually transmitted diseases

David G. Ostrow

## HOMOSEXUAL BEHAVIOR

A growing body of information implicates specific sexual practices common among homosexual males in the emergence of "new" STDs. Since detailed information regarding these illnesses is provided elsewhere (see Chapters 31, 36, 40, and 55), this chapter reviews those aspects of homosexual behavior relevant to the general practice of medicine and STD diagnosis and treatment. In addition, I include information useful to the provider of primary care to homosexually active patients and a description of information and treatment resources which are specifically designed to meet the needs of that population. Finally, information regarding efforts to control the spread of AIDS and STDs within the various gay communities is provided.

The homosexually active male has specific sexual practices that are most clearly related to the incidence and treatment of STDs. Little if any evidence links lesbian sexual practices to specific STDs,[1] and lesbians appear to be at decreased risk for most STDs, including AIDS.

The prevalence of homosexuality in modern western civilizations has been variously estimated to be anywhere from 2 to 10 percent of the adult male population. However, we must differentiate between the prevalence of homosexuality as a pattern of exclusive or nearly exclusive choice of same-gender partners for sexual activities and the practice of specific homosexual acts. In their landmark study, Kinsey et al. defined a spectrum of adult sexual gender preference ranging from exclusive heterosexuality to exclusive homosexuality.[2] Those same studies revealed that the occurrence of same-sex activities at some time in an individual's lifetime was the rule rather than the exception. They also found that a significant portion of the adult heterosexual male population continued to have occasional homosexual activities.

Thus, physicians must not only determine the predominant gender preference, homosexual or heterosexual, of a patient, but also they must be aware of the full range of specific sexual practices and their relative frequencies for that patient. Many physicians may find it difficult to inquire about some specific sexual practices and may be content with a patient's verbal or nonverbal acquiescence to a statement such as: "You don't do any of that stuff!" Such an approach to sexual-practices history taking will result in incomplete and potentially dangerous omissions in the examinations and workup of a significant number of patients. If we assume that at least 5 to 10 percent of male patients are either primarily homosexual in orientation or occasionally participate in same-gender sexual relations, then we are dealing with a relatively important segment of the patient population. In many large urban centers and clinics specializing in the treatment of STDs, the percentage may be considerably higher. If the clinician is so self-conscious as to be unable to inquire adequately into these aspects of a patient's history, then that practitioner should not hesitate to refer any patient with real or suspected STD problems to a colleague or service organization where such patients can receive nonjudgmental treatment.

Several recent population-based surveys[3] have attempted to define more valid patterns of male homosexual behavior than the stereotyped versions so visible in our culture. No single behavioral parameter can adequately be used to describe groups or typologies, but rather a number of criteria are important, including the level of sexual activity, the stability and types of coupling, the degree of functional and physical problems encountered in sexual activities, and the individual's acceptance of his or her homosexuality. Applying cluster analysis to the respondents interviewed in the San Francisco area during the mid-1960s, Bell and Weinberg[3] arrived at five general clusters of male homosexual behavior: close coupled, open-coupled, funtional, dysfunctional, and asexual.

## CLOSE-COUPLED

Accounting for approximately 10 percent of all respondents, *close-coupled* homosexuals are men living in a stable "marriage" with a sexual partner. Their standard scores on number of sexual problems, number of sexual partners, and amount of casual sexual activity were low. The respondents had fewer difficulties in finding a suitable partner, were better able to maintain an affectionate relationship with that partner, had less regret about their homosexuality, and had a generally higher level of sexual activity than the typical respondent.

## OPEN-COUPLED

Eighteen percent of the respondents were clustered in the category called *open-coupled.* The men were involved in a "marital" relationship with other men but had high scores on one or more of the following variables: number of sexual partners, number of sexual problems, and amount of cruising. Thus, although coupled, these individuals could not be classified as "fulfilled romantics" in whom a special relationship with another male had reduced their sexual problems or their interest in having a variety of contacts. Persons classified according to the above criteria tended to be exclusively homosexual, to worry in connection with their cruising, to report somewhat high levels of sexual activity, to have engaged in a wide variety of sexual techniques, and to have regrets about their homosexuality. Their partner's failure to respond to their sexual requests is the most prevalent sexual problem for the open-coupled respondents. Our own studies have substantiated and updated the concept of open-coupled gay men being diverse in their sexual practices and numbers of partners, similar to single functional men.[4]

## FUNCTIONAL

Fifteen percent of respondents made up the *functional* category. They were "single" and had high scores on number of sexual partners and level of sexual activity and low scores on regret over homosexuality and sexual problems. In addition, persons meeting these criteria did more cruising than the typical respondent, were less apt to worry about being exposed through sexual activity, and were apt to be more overt, to have a high level of sexual interest, and to rate their sex appeal as high. They were less likely to experience feelings of insufficiency in relation to sexual activity, of sexual inadequacy, or of worry about the morality of their homosexual activity. On demographic variables, the functional group tended to be younger and to include a higher percentage of black respondents.

## DYSFUNCTIONAL

The *dysfunctional* cluster comprised 12 percent of respondents who were single and sexually active but had high scores on number of sexual problems and on regret over their homosexuality. These concerns had to do chiefly with feelings of sexual inadequacy and difficulties in reaching orgasm, finding a suitable partner, and maintaining affection for that partner. They also tended to have more formal education than the typical respondent.

## ASEXUAL

Approximately 16 percent of respondents neither were coupled nor attained average scores on level of sexual activity or number of partners. In addition, this "asexual" group tended to have more sexual problems (difficulties in finding a partner and infrequent sexual activity), lower levels of sexual interest, less extensive sexual repertoires, and more regret over their homosexuality. The asexual respondent also tended to be less exclusively homosexual and more covert than other respondents. Members of this group tended to be older, and blacks were underrepresented in this classification.

Approximately 28 percent of respondents did not fit one of the above "pure" typologies. These "mixed" respondents did not differ from the average respondent in terms of any demographic characteristics except for their being somewhat younger.

Whatever the limitations of descriptive clusters based on a selected population of respondents, the classification of homosexual male behavior based on general characteristics of sexual and psychological functioning can be useful. Such classification can be utilized in delineating general levels of risk for STDs and in designing education and control measures aimed at reducing the incidence of STDs in gay men. We have found similar typologies to be useful for the evaluation of educational programs in reducing behaviors known to transmit the human immunodeficiency virus (HIV).[4,5]

## MYTHS AND ATTITUDES ABOUT HOMOSEXUALITY THAT INTERFERE WITH PRIMARY HEALTH CARE

The description of different homosexual categories based on differing patterns of sexual behavior challenges the notion of a stereotypical homosexual male. Thus, simplistic notions for dealing with homosexual male patients based on such a stereotype qualify for the status of "myths." By limiting the effectiveness of primary practitioners in dealing with gay male patients, these myths perpetuate the gay community's perception of the health care system as being nonresponsive and prejudiced.

1. "You can easily tell who your homosexual patients are from their appearance or mannerisms." No single pattern of behavior will allow you to determine which patients are homosexual or bisexual. Yet many private practitioners will categorically state that they know the sexual preference of their patients without specifically inquiring. The problem is further compounded by the fact that primary sexual preference alone will not provide the essential data on types, frequency, and anatomical sites of the specific sexual practices that determine an individual's risk for specific STDs. Only a complete history of sexual practices obtained from each patient can provide this essential information.[6]
2. "Being married indicates that a person is heterosexual." "A person in a marital relationship has a negligible risk of acquiring an STD." The distortions introduced into the doctor-patient relationship by the above assumptions exist for both homosexual and heterosexual patients. Furthermore, if we accept the notion that people can perceive themselves as heterosexual yet engage in same-gender sexual activities, we conclude that even if a patient explicitly declares a heterosexual orientation, it still is necessary to inquire about specific sexual practices which we otherwise associate with homosexuality. Out of desire for either societal acceptance or family life, many homosexual males enter into marital relationships with members of the opposite sex. Such individuals frequently continue to engage in homosexual activities, either surreptitiously or with the knowledge and consent of their marital partner. Similarly, the open-coupled homosexual male will perceive himself as being in a marital relationship yet may have the same variety of sexual partners and experiences as his single counterpart. While AIDS has increased the popularity of monogamy in both homosexual and heterosexual relationships, the extremely long latency period between infection and illness[7] requires examination of sexual history during the past 7 years to assess adequately the risk of HIV infection.
3. "Homosexual males assume either passive or active roles in their sexual relationship." This myth is related to myth number 1, and assumes that outward appearance corresponds to a stereotypical role in sexual relationships. Part of the gay liberation movement's contribution to our understanding of sexuality in general has been the destruction of this myth and the underlying assumption that there are passive or active roles in sexual or nonsexual behavior. Prior to 1984, it had become rare to find homosexual male patients who engaged in only one type of sexual activity or who assumed the "receptive" role in all sexual activities. More recently, however, the emphasis on "safer sex" education in the gay community has resulted in more limited sexual repertoires for the majority of gay men.[5,8]
4. "All homosexual males are promiscuous and have a large number of sexual partners." While certainly many single or open-coupled gay men will report having a large number of sexual partners, at least 10 percent of respondents reported monogamous relationships with a mate and little or no "extramarital" sexual activity. The proportion of gay men in stable monogamous relationships has increased significantly in recent years, apparently in response to the AIDS epidemic.[5,8]
5. "A person's pattern of sexual behavior is stable and unchanging." Any assessment of sexual practices must be viewed as valid only for the current period and must be updated at regular intervals. The concept of dynamic assessment of sexual practices is applicable to all patients, regardless of primary sexual orientation. In the phase known as "coming out," many gay men enter a period of increased sexual activity soon after accepting their homosexual orientation.[9] Similarly, an individual's pattern and variety of sexual activities will differ depending on the type of primary relationship, whether open-coupled or close-coupled, and the current degree of sexual and emotional satisfaction with that primary relationship.[3]

6. "People, whether gay or straight, are sexually inactive past a certain age." This myth is based not on erroneous assumptions about homosexuality but rather on our cultural biases concerning aging and the aged. A growing body of knowledge concerning human aging has validated the perspective that sexual activity does not abruptly end at any specific point; sexual activity can be an important part of an individual's life at any age.[10] Indeed, the gay community has developed social programs specifically aimed at older individuals. Such programs as Senior Action in a Gay Environment (SAGE) attempt to provide social settings for older gay men and women which can serve as alternatives to bars and other milieus geared to younger persons.
7. "The physician cannot significantly influence the patient's behavior without the use of counterproductive judgmental or coercive methods." In fact, it is the physician's responsibility to counsel patients at risk for STDs on ways in which they can reduce that risk. Such educational information can be given to patients in a positive, nonjudgmental, and noncoercive manner. At the very least, sexually active patients with multiple partners need to be counseled on the importance of periodic STD checkups, the value of self-examinations for lesions and discharges, and the importance of sexual abstinence during the symptomatic or treatment period in order to prevent spread or reinfection. The epidemic of AIDS makes physician counseling of "safer sex" guidelines imperative. A recent survey has shown that patients are more accepting of physician advice in sexual matters if it is provided in a nonjudgmental and concerned manner.[11]

The existence of legal and cultural biases against homosexual persons distorts the doctor-patient relationship from one of open communication to one of subtle denials. Although a complete sexual-practices history is an essential part of the STD workup, some patients will inevitably view such questioning as unnecessarily intrusive or even insulting. In large part this will depend on both the patient's and the clinician's own comfort in dealing with sexuality and, in particular, homosexuality. Most medical texts either omit discussion of homosexuality and homosexual behavior altogether or refer to the subject under the categories of sexual dysfunction, deviancy, or perversions. Likewise, medical professionals are no more comfortable with sexuality and homosexuality than are members of the general population,[12] and homosexual patients will often assume that the physician or health care worker is negatively biased against homosexuality. The term *homophobia*[13] was coined to describe the total body of individual and cultural bias against homosexuality that is the basis for many of the misconceptions described above as well as for the legal and cultural sanctions against homosexuality and homosexual persons. Under the guise of preventing the spread of AIDS, existing antisodomy laws are being more stringently enforced and reintroduced in states where they had previously been repealed. This results in the withholding of information regarding sexual experiences important to an accurate diagnostic workup or treatment plan. Moreover, medical problems are sometimes hidden from the health care system by the doctor for fear that the nature of the problem will reveal the individual's sexual orientation and adversely affect future medical treatment. In terms of the HIV antibody test, calls for routine testing and reporting to public health authorities of seropositive persons may well discourage individuals at risk of infection from seeking health care.[14]

These impediments to treatment are magnified for the young individual who has not yet come out, especially if a minor is still in the care of a pediatrician or family physician. Individuals may assume that revealing their sexual orientation to their physician will result in their parents' discovering their homosexuality. Frequently, such patients seek treatment at board of health STD clinics, gay community clinics, or hospital emergency rooms, precisely because of the relative anonymity such services provide. In addition, minors will often assume that any medical service will automatically report the visit to their parents; thus, they may delay seeking diagnosis and treatment of STD problems. Many gay patients arbitrarily split their medical care between a private practitioner and a gay community clinic.

No simple solutions exist either to the above problems or to homophobic attitudes and myths about homosexuality. Some states and communities have passed ordinances and regulations that allow health care providers to treat minors for STDs without reporting to or obtaining consent from the patient's parents. The existence of such laws and ordinances, however, does not automatically ensure enough trust in the health care provider to produce an open and truthful relationship. Ironically, to protect their patient's anonymity, many private physicians customarily do not report a patient's STD to the local board of health. This has resulted in a significant underreporting of STD information and has hindered the development of adequate diagnostic and treatment regimens.[15] We can expect a similar pattern with AIDS and HIV seropositivity as reporting and contact tracing are made mandatory.

To provide confidential and dignified STD diagnostic and treatment services to the gay community, community-sponsored STD clinics have been formed. Such clinics have developed systems that ensure confidentiality by utilizing clinic visit numbers rather than names when reporting STD incidence statistics to the local health department. These systems have enabled gay community clinics to optimize STD services through establishing a high level of trust with their gay patients. This has occurred at the cost of establishing burdensome confidentiality and record-keeping procedures as well as separate health care systems. Because of the high level of concern regarding the potential for discrimination relating to HIV antibody status and the proliferation of public health regulations mandating the reporting of HIV seropositivity to public health authorities, similar "shadow chart" practices are being adopted by many "mainstream" health care institutions. The ability of health care professionals to provide AIDS prevention education outreach and HIV antibody testing for at-risk individuals may be severely jeopardized by the growth of HIV reporting legislation and the accompanying movement "underground" of information and persons in need of counseling.

## THE SEXUAL-PRACTICES HISTORY

The most difficult part of taking a sexual-practices history is introducing the subject in the course of a general medical history in a way that will prompt the most truthful response from the patient. Obviously, the attitude of the health care provider will affect the ability to establish such a setting. The sexual-practices history is sometimes avoided until the very end of the history-taking process. In so doing, the clinician signals the patient that the examiner is uncomfortable with the subject. Close-ended questions such as "I assume that you are only having sex with your wife?" will severely limit the accuracy of sexual-practices information. The best approach is to obtain the sexual-practices history in the context of the overall social history. Thus, you can begin with a statement to the effect that: "In order to provide you with optimal care, there are a number of areas of your personal habits and practices that I need to understand and be aware of. These include the use of any nonprescription drugs or alcohol, any special diets you have been on, sexual practices, and foreign travel." Such an introductory statement alerts your patient to your interest in his or her sexual practices and places that concern within the overall context of an open and honest doctor-patient relationship.

Several sources describe the various sexual practices that need to be covered in a sexual-practices questionnaire.[6,16] As stressed above, it is usually necessary to inquire about specific practices as well as the broad categories of homo- and heterosexual orientation. Asking, "Do you have sex only with men, only with

**Table 6-1. Specific Sexual Practices and Possible Associated Disease Problems**

| Sexual practice (street terms) | Disease problems listed in approximate order of frequency |
|---|---|
| Close body contact | Pediculosis pubis<br>Scabies<br>Fungal infections |
| Masturbation (jacking off, beating off) | Physical abrasions<br>Conjunctivitis |
| Douches, lubricants | Allergic reactions<br>Rectal fatty tumors |
| Amyl nitrite, butyl nitrite (poppers) | Amyl and butyl nitrite burns; contact dermatitis |
| Fellatio, receptive (Do you suck your partner's penis?) | Physical abrasions<br>Oral gonorrhea<br>Oral herpes simplex virus (especially type 2)<br>Nongonococcal pharyngitis (chlamydia and others)<br>Oral condylomata, acuminata<br>Syphilis<br>Hepatitis B<br>Enteric infections<br>Lymphogranuloma venereum<br>Oral donovanosis (granuloma inguinale)<br>Oral chancroid |
| Fellatio, insertive (Does your partner suck your penis?) | Physical abrasions<br>Bites<br>Genital herpes simplex virus (especially type 1)<br>Nongonococcal urethritis<br>Gonococcal urethritis<br>Meningococcal urethritis |
| Anal intercourse, insertive (Do you put your penis into your partner's rectum?) | NGU<br>Gonococcal urethritis<br>Genital herpes simplex virus<br>Molluscum contagiosum<br>Condylomata acuminata<br>Syphilis<br>Trichomoniasia<br>Epididymitis and/or prostatitis<br>Fungal infections<br>Lymphogranuloma venereum<br>Donovanosis (Granuloma inguinale)<br>Chancroid<br>Cytomegalovirus (?)<br>Hepatitis B<br>HIV/AIDS |
| Anal intercourse, receptive (Does your partner put his penis into your rectum?) | Traumatic proctitis<br>Rectal gonorrhea<br>Anal condylomata, acuminata<br>HIV/AIDS<br>Molluscum contagiosum (rare)<br>Nonspecific proctitis (chlamydia and others)<br>Anorectal herpes simplex virus<br>Anorectal syphilis<br>Hepatitis B<br>Rectal trichomoniasis (?)<br>Lymphogranuloma venereum<br>Anorectal granuloma inguinale<br>Anorectal chancroid<br>Cytomegalovirus infection<br>Anorectal candidiasis |
| Anilingus (oral-anal intercourse) (Do you rim or do scat?) | Enteric infections<br>Shigellosis<br>Campylobacter fetus<br>Enterotoxigenic *Escherichia coli*<br>Hepatitis A, B, non-A non-B<br>Amebiasis<br>Giardiasis<br>Salmonellosis<br>*Enterobius vermicularis*<br>*Strongyloides stercoralis*<br>Oral infections<br>Oral warts<br>Oral gonorrhea<br>Syphilis<br>Lymphogranuloma venereum<br>Oral donovanosis<br>Oral chancroid<br>Oral or rectal HIV/AIDS (?)<br>Herpes simplex virus<br>Anorectal meningococcal infection |
| Fist and/or finger fornication, receptive (Have you been fist-fucked?) | Enteric infections |
| Toys and/or apparatus (cock rings, dildoes, leather, tit clamps, etc.) | Allergic reactions to metal, plastic, rubber<br>Friction dermatitis<br>Physical torsions<br>Varicoceles<br>Peyronie's disease<br>Fungal infections<br>Lost rectal foreign bodies<br>Testicular strangulation |
| Sadomasochism (piercing, bondage) (Are you into S/M, piercing, or bondage?) | Lacerations<br>Cutaneous infections<br>Trauma<br>HIV/AIDS |
| Group sex | *See* Anilingus (above) |

SOURCE: After Ostrow and Obermaier.[6]

**Table 6-2. Characteristics of Three Samples of Homosexual Males Attending Sexually Transmitted Disease Screening Sites**

| Screening site | N | Age mean (SD) | Race | | | Education, years (SD) | No. partners mean (SD)* |
|---|---|---|---|---|---|---|---|
| | | | %W | %B | %O | | |
| Van | 492 | 30.9 (8.4) | 79 | 10 | 11 | 14.9 (2.8) | 12.7 (20.2) |
| Clinic | 309 | 30.1 (7.4) | 95 | 3 | 2 | 15.8 (2.3) | 22.7 (22.9) |
| Baths | 212 | 31.2 (8.3) | 81 | 11 | 8 | 15.2 (2.8) | 26.2+ (27.4) |

*Defined as number of nonsteady same-sex partners patient has had contact with during prior 4-month period.
+When measured by detailed questioning of number of sexual contacts per bathhouse visit and frequency of visits, found to be a significant underestimate by factor of 1.5 to 2.0.

women, or with both?" will establish the presence or absence of same-sex activity. Questions regarding specific sexual practices with same- and/or opposite-sex partners should follow. Specific male homosexual practices may be associated with specific infections or traumatic problems (Table 6-1). Because patients will frequently use the vernacular terms and be unfamiliar with medical terminology, the lay term(s) for each practice is included in parentheses.

## INTERRELATIONSHIP BETWEEN SEXUAL BEHAVIOR AND STD TRANSMISSION AND PRESENTATION IN HOMOSEXUAL MALES

Certain sexual practices have greater associated STD risks than others (Table 6-1). Moreover, for each specific sexual practice, the number and type of partners (anonymous or known) and the setting in which the practice occurred will significantly affect the actual risk associated with that practice.[17] For example, the risk of acquiring amebiasis from fecal-oral contact, as in anilingus, depends on whether the sexual partner is infected and, if so, on the frequency and extent of contact, stage of infection, personal hygiene, etc. Using data from a hepatitis B cohort study, specific sexual practices added independently to the prospective risk of acquiring infection in order of relative importance:

1. Receptive (passive) anal-genital intercourse
2. Oral-anal intercourse (anilingus)
3. Insertive (active) anal-genital intercourse
4. Rectal douching in association with receptive anal-genital intercourse
5. Receptive manual-anal intercourse (passive partner in anal insertion of finger or fist)

These observations were extended to the other STDs frequently seen in homosexual males (syphilis, hepatitis B, and gonorrhea) in Chicago's gay male community.[18] Mean number of nonsteady homosexual partners in the last 4 months was quite different among three screening sites, with the bathhouse group being higher than the clinic group and the van group being lowest (Table 6-2). This same relative ordering (baths, highest; van, lowest) was observed for prevalence rates for the three STDs.

Combining patients from all three screening sites showed that those with a positive serology or those reporting a past history of one of the STDs had a significantly higher mean number of partners than those with nonreactive serologic tests or no history of an STD (Table 6-3). As expected, past history of one STD (particularly hepatitis B) was correlated with past history or positive serology for the other two STDs.

At least two conclusions can be drawn from these studies. First, in 1979–1980, number of nonsteady sexual partners was the most important risk factor for any of the major STDs seen in gay men. Since bathhouse patrons had the greatest opportunity for multiple anonymous partners and had significantly higher numbers of partners than respondents questioned at either the clinic or van,[18] bathhouse patrons are an especially high-risk group for STD infection. Accordingly, screening and education programs should be targeted to this group as well as to patients discovered currently to have an STD. Second, it appeared that specific sexual practices such as anal-genital intercourse and anilingus were responsible for the introduction into the STD catalog of a large number of enteric pathogens, including hepatitis B, *Giardia lamblia, Entamoeba histolytica,* and shigellosis. The full implication of these epidemiologic findings was not realized, however, until the appearance of AIDS and the subsequent discovery of the primary etiologic agent, HIV, and its routes of transmission.

**Table 6-3. Number of Partners and Years of Homosexual Activity as Predictors of Sexually Transmitted Disease History and Serology**

| Survey item | Mean no. partners* | | | | Mean no. years† | | | |
|---|---|---|---|---|---|---|---|---|
| | No | Yes | t | p | No | Yes | t | p |
| Hepatitis | 17.4 | 22.7 | 3.1 | $<0.01$ | 10.8 | 12.6 | 2.4 | $<0.01$ |
| Syphilis | 17.2 | 24.6 | 3.7 | $<0.01$ | 10.4 | 14.9 | 5.3 | $<0.01$ |
| Oral gonorrhea | 18.3 | 24.4 | 2.2 | $<0.05$ | 7.5 | 10.3 | N.S. | |
| Urethral gonorrhea | 17.5 | 20.7 | N.S. | — | 10.5 | 12.8 | 5.9 | $<0.001$ |
| Rectal gonorrhea | 16.5 | 26.4 | 5.0 | $<0.001$ | 8.6 | 10.5 | N.S. | |
| Hepatitis B seropositive‡ | 14.6 | 22.5 | 4.7 | $<0.001$ | 8.7 | 12.8 | 5.9 | $<0.001$ |
| VDRL reactive | 18.6 | 26.8 | 1.8 | $<0.05$ | 10.8 | 16.0 | 3.0 | $<0.001$ |

*Defined as number of nonsteady same-sex partners patient has had contact with during prior 4-month period.
+Defined as number of years patient had been homosexually active on a regular basis (at least one contact per month).
‡Defined as HBsAg and/or anti-HBs and/or anti-HBc.

## PREVENTION OF THE SEXUAL SPREAD OF AIDS IN THE GAY COMMUNITY

The early education of existing gay community clinics and newly organized AIDS educational projects met with considerable resistance from the target community. This resistance took the form of denial ("I'm not *that* promiscuous!"), lack of concern ("I'd rather die of AIDS than give up sex"), reliance on medical technology ("There will be a cure or vaccine before I come down with it"), and refusal to accept the sexually transmitted nature of the epidemic ("It's caused by drugs or the hepatitis B vaccine, so I'm staying away from them."). The reluctance of individuals, as well as the government and health officials, to take the threat of AIDS seriously before 1983 is poignantly portrayed in Larry Kramer's play *The Normal Heart*.[19] Since 1983, both scientific and prevention efforts have been able to move forward owing to increased funding and recognition of the potential of HIV infection and AIDS to move beyond the initial so-called high-risk groups of gay men and intravenous drug users. Focusing on actual specific behaviors rather than group labels appears to offer the combined benefits of piercing denial based on stereotypical concepts and reducing group stigmatization based on AIDS fears.

Another factor which has contributed to the impact of the AIDS epidemic on the gay male community is the propensity for infectious carriers to be relatively healthy for extended periods of time, during which sexual spread of the virus is most probable. Unfortunately, the development of an infectious chronic HIV carrier state is much more likely, possibly approaching 100 percent of persons infected,[20] than the 10 percent or so rate of chronic infection with HBV.[21] Although a recent epidemiologic study of HIV transmission between hemophiliacs and their sexual partners suggested increasing heterosexual transmission in the later stages of immunodeficiency,[22] there is ample epidemiologic evidence supporting prolonged transmittability from healthy seropositive men to their sexual contacts.[23] Apparently more restricted sexual modes of transmission affect HIV than other STDs. We[24] and others[25,26] have reported the lack of significant risk of HIV infection through oral exposure to the virus, in contrast to the well-documented risk of anal exposure. While the relative low infectivity via homosexual oral-genital intercourse may not hold for heterosexual intercourse, it does provide the scientific support for the commonly used trilevel hierarchy of sexual activities which forms the basis of most "safer sex" educational materials currently being distributed by gay community organizations (Table 6-4).

Safer sex education is based on the well-proved assumption that celibacy is not an easily adopted lifestyle for sexually active

**Table 6-4. Safer Sex Guidelines for Homosexual Men**

| Safe | Possibly safe | Unsafe |
|---|---|---|
| Mutual masturbation (male or female) | Anal intercourse with a condom | Receptive anal intercourse without condom |
| Social kissing (dry) | Fellatio interruptus | Insertive anal intercourse without a condom |
| Body massage, hugging | Mouth-to-mouth kissing | Manual-anal intercourse |
| Body-to-body rubbing (frottage) | Urine contact | Fellatio |
| Light S/M activities (without bruising or bleeding) | Vaginal intercourse with a condom | Oral-anal contact |
| Using one's own sex toys | Oral-vaginal contact (cunnilingus) | Vaginal intercourse without condom |

**Table 6-5. Reductions in HIV Seroconversion Rates Among Two Cohorts of Homosexually Active Men**

| | Seroconversion rates (annualized), % | |
|---|---|---|
| Time period | San Francisco cohort* | Chicago cohort+ |
| 7/82–12/84 | 18.4 (estimated) | N.A. |
| 4/84–12/84 to 1/85–6/85 | 5.4 | 9.4 |
| 1/85–6/85 to 7/85–12/85 | 3.1 | 5.0 |
| 7/85–12/85 to 1/86–7/86 | 4.2 | 2.4 |
| 1/86–7/86 to 7/86–1/87 | N.A. | 0.6 |

*After Winkelstein et al.[27] from the San Francisco Men's Health Study.
+From the Chicago cohort of the Multicenter AIDS Cohort Study (MACS).[42]

persons at risk for AIDS and that replacement of so-called high-risk activities, such as unprotected anal intercourse, with substantially lower-risk activities (e.g., anal intercourse with condoms or oral-genital intercourse without ejaculation) is the education message most likely to succeed in reducing the rate of transmission of HIV in the gay community. Another fundamental tenet of safer sex education is that except for long-term monogamous couples, it is impossible for either sexual partner to be absolutely sure of their own or their partner's HIV serostatus, thus requiring low-risk activities at all times. It is now clear from longitudinal cohort studies in both San Francisco[27] and Chicago[28] that the educational message of safer sex is being widely adopted by men participating in the studies, with a resulting sharp decline in HIV seroconversion rates (Table 6-5).

To what extent can these dramatic changes in behavior and HIV transmission, which have been demonstrated in limited cohorts of predominantly white and well-educated gay men, be generalized to the broader population of men at risk for AIDS due to homosexual activities? For a variety of reasons, including our inability to separate the effects of being involved in an intensive longitudinal study from the effects of communitywide education programs and the long lag time between HIV exposure and the development of reportable disease, this is a question which cannot be answered. What has been addressable, however, has been the individual and target group attributes which have contributed to the successful modification of sexual behavior by persons participating over the past 3 years (1984–1987) in several gay male cohort studies. As these findings are likely to be useful both for the design of effective AIDS educational programs elsewhere and for indicating where more intensively targeted outreach programs are most needed, they are summarized here.

1. *Knowledge about AIDS and high-risk behaviors:* Knowledge about AIDS has been shown to be most important in motivating initial behavioral change, particularly in persons who see themselves as being at relatively low risk and are initially less informed about the disease and the routes of transmission of HIV.[4] Knowledge alone, however, does not promote long-term sexual behavior change, as has been observed for other sexually transmitted conditions including genital herpes.[29]
2. *Perception of personal risk* appears to be more important than objective knowledge in motivating behavioral change.[30] This may be related to the frequently observed "optimistic bias,"[31] which was expressed in the Chicago cohort study by persons stating that they felt that they could choose safe sexual part-

ners or that "it won't happen to me."[5] This would appear to be an important area of potential intervention by mental health professionals who are in a position to help patients realistically assess their behavior and risk of HIV infection.

3. An individual's *perceived efficacy of behavioral change* in reducing their chances of developing AIDS appears to play an important role, except in persons perceiving themselves to be at the highest risk of infection.[32,33] This suggests that persons perceiving themselves to be at highest risk of infection may believe that it is "too late" in their own case because of the extremely long latency period between infection and disease and the lack of lifestyle changes proven to reduce the likelihood of developing illness once infected. In order to overcome this major obstacle to behavioral risk reduction, vigorous research efforts aimed at pinpointing potential lifestyle or psychosocial cofactors of disease progression in HIV infected individuals are needed. Similarly, the role of widespread HIV antibody testing in prevention remains controversial, as some persons will react to a positive test result with an increased sense of futility, while others will experience increased stress, both of which might compromise behavioral risk-reduction efforts.[34]
4. *Belief that science will provide a cure or prevention* was found to be directly correlated with increased numbers of partners and persistence of high-risk sexual practices in both the Chicago and San Francisco cohort studies.[32,33] Osborn has written about the negative impact that premature reports of vaccine or chemotherapy breakthroughs can have on both health behaviors and public attitudes regarding AIDS.[35] Overconfidence in technological solutions to the control of AIDS and HIV transmission may reflect incorrect knowledge or be a form of denial of individual risk perception.
5. *Demographic variables* which have been consistently related to health behavior change *in general* have been *geographical, financial, racial,* and *age.* In the case of AIDS risk behaviors, geographical differences have been related to the prevalence of the infection and likelihood of having a close friend or lover with AIDS.[33] Of particular interest is the consistent finding that increased age and years of homosexual activity are related to persistence of high-risk activity. This was also demonstrated prior to the recognition of AIDS for gay men at risk of hepatitis B infection,[36] and suggests that sexual behavior patterns become increasingly resistant to change over time. Little is known about racial and financial variables as related to AIDS risk reduction in homosexual/bisexual men as the vast majority of the cohorts studied to date have been white, middle-class, and well educated. There may well be important differences between whites, blacks, and Hispanics as regard factors motivating or retarding risk-reducing behavioral change. The few studies which have looked at racial differences in health-related behaviors have suggested the existence of significant differences not entirely explainable on the basis of economic or educational factors.[37]
6. While earlier studies consistently demonstrated that *adequate social support networks* facilitated positive health behavioral change, the findings of the Chicago cohort study suggest a complex relationship between social support, peer norms, and behavioral risk reduction,[4,32] While membership in a gay social support network in itself was not predictive of behavioral change, the presence of peer norms supportive of risk reduction was the variable most consistently and positively associated with multiple measures of sexual risk reduction over time. These findings suggest specific elements of peer support for "safer sex" practices need to be addressed in any community-based risk-reduction program. Similar findings are beginning to emerge in studies of intravenous drug use behaviors, such as the use of bleach to clean syringes.[38]
7. *Sexual impulse control* is a complex variable related to a broad set of biobehavioral factors including personality traits, setting, psychoactive substance use, partnership status, and affect.[39] The Chicago research group has directly assessed the perceived ability to control sexual impulses as a means of measuring the compulsive aspect of sexual behavior and change. Not surprisingly, reported ability to control sexual impulses was found to be significantly related to both reduction in number of sexual partners and modification (via condom use or withdrawal) of anal intercourse.[4,30,32]
8. The recent finding that *alcohol and recreational drug use patterns* are significantly related to the ability of gay men to reduce levels of sexual exposure to HIV is not surprising. However, in view of the extensive and complex relationships thought to exist between psychoactive substance use and sexual arousal, it is surprising that a consistent finding in both the San Francisco and Chicago cohort studies has been a uniformly positive correlation between all classes of drug and alcohol abuse and the persistence of high-risk sexual behaviors.[40,41] That these findings were not related to *absolute numbers* of sexual partners but were related to the use of drugs *with* sexual partners in both cohorts supports the notion that the disinhibiting effect of the drugs is an important mediator of the association. However, research aimed at further understanding of the relationship between psychoactive substance use and persistent high-risk sexual behaviors is impeded by scientific and social restrictions on sexual behavior research. Regardless of the mechanism of the association, the significance of these findings to behavioral interventions is clear: A complete assessment of drug and alcohol use patterns is a necessary part of any evaluation and explicit counseling regarding the role of substance use in impeding risk-reduction behavioral change is warranted for all patients reporting drug or alcohol use.

## CONCLUSIONS

The interval between the publication of the first and second editions of this text (1983 and 1988) has witnessed a dramatic change in homosexual behavior and the types of sexually transmitted diseases seen in homosexually active men. Much, if not all, of this change can be attributed to the emergence of AIDS as a major STD and the high prevalence of HIV infection among urban gay men in the United States. That change has taken place within the context of an epidemic which has preferentially stressed the gay male population, both directly in terms of illness and death due to AIDS, and indirectly in terms of the increased stigmatization and decreased social acceptance of homosexuality resulting from the general public's fears and misconceptions about AIDS. Although the early concept that AIDS was a "gay disease" has been vigorously countered by both community leaders and epidemiologic evidence, the necessary emphasis on AIDS information, education, and service delivery in the gay community has definitely influenced all aspects of gay life. Community STD clinics have, for the most part, become AIDS service providers. As we predicted in the first edition, the increasing emphasis on more serious and chronic illnesses among men seeking care at gay community-based facilities has led to increased interdependence between those community-based organizations and the mainstream medical establishment. In Chicago, the AIDS natural history and psychosocial research projects are performed as collaborative efforts between the Howard Brown Memorial Clinic and two major universities. In Washington, D.C., the medical director of the Whitman-Walker Clinic is a staff member at a nearby university medical center. And increasing proportions of the funding for community-based STD and AIDS treatment and prevention efforts are coming from governmental sources.

The future of homosexuality as a lifestyle is clearly linked to how the community and society deals with the AIDS epidemic. Denial of the seriousness of AIDS is no longer medically, socially, or politically tenable. Will our society treat AIDS as a health problem requiring compassionate and comprehensive care for both persons with HIV infection and those fearful of being exposed or will it seek punitive measures with moralistic overtones? And will the gay community find ways to preserve and enlarge institutions and traditions which maintain a sense of community while responsibly supporting the extensive long-term behavioral changes required to control the spread of HIV infection and AIDS? The two questions are obviously linked to one another, as actions by the majority society can clearly influence its subcultures and vice versa.

By the time the next edition of this chapter is written, a clearer vision of homosexual behavior in the "AIDS era" will be available. The full effects of HIV infection and disease will not be felt until the 1990s, as will the consequences of AIDS-related behavioral change upon the full spectrum of STDs within the gay community. It is safe to predict that the health care system will not be concerned much about the "traditional" STDs in the 1990s, concern about AIDS having eliminated or driven underground those behaviors recognized as transmitting gonorrhea, syphilis, hepatitis B, etc. But STDs will continue to exist, perhaps concentrated in disadvantaged and minority subpopulations of both the homosexual and heterosexual populations. Homophobic attitudes may be increasingly flavored by prejudices toward racial, ethnic, and economically disadvantaged groups. Already, within urban gay communities, barriers are developing between individuals seeing others as less sexually responsible vs. too easily acquiescing to demands seen as coming from an oppressive society. AIDS prevention education has to be increasingly attuned to these negative reverberations of the epidemic if it is to repair the social damage caused by AIDS rather than further it.

## References


1 Robertson P, Schachter J: Failure to identify venereal disease in a lesbian population. *Sex Transm Dis* 8:75, 1981.

2 Kinsey AC et al: *Sexual Behavior in the Human Male.* Philadelphia, Saunders, 1948.

3 Bell AP, Weinberg MS: Homosexualities: *A Study of Diversity among Men and Women.* New York, Simon and Schuster, 1978.

4 Emmons C et al: Psychosocial predictors of reported behavior change in homosexual men at risk for AIDS. *Health Educ Q* 13:331, 1986.

5 Ostrow DG et al: Multicenter AIDS Cohort Study (MACS). Psychosocial aspects of AIDS risk. *Psychopharmacol Bull* 22:678, 1986.

6 Ostrow DG, Obermaier A: Sexual practices history, in *Sexually Transmitted Diseases in Homosexual Men,* DG Ostrow (ed). New York, Plenum, 1983.

7 Ho DD et al: Pathogenesis of infection with human immunodeficiency virus. *N Engl J Med* 317:278, 1987.

8 Winkelstein W et al: Sexual practices and risk of infection by human immunodeficiency virus. *JAMA* 257:321, 1987.

9 Martin, DA, Hetrick ES: Designing an AIDS risk reduction program for gay teenagers: Problems and proposed solutions, in *Biobehavioral Control of AIDS,* DG Ostrow (ed). New York, Irvington Publishers, 1987.

10 Masters WH, Johnson VE: *Human Sexual Response.* Boston, Little, Brown, 1966.

11 Ross MW: Psychosocial factors in admitting to homosexuality in sexually transmitted disease clinics. *Sex Transm Dis* 12:83, 1985.

12 Sandholzer TA: Factors affecting the incidence and management of sexually transmitted disease in homosexual men, in *Sexually Transmitted Diseases in Homosexual Men,* Ostrow et al (eds). New York, Plenum, 1983.

13 Weinberg G: *Society and the Healthy Homosexual.* New York, St Martin's, 1972.

14 Ostrow DG et al: Epidemic control measures for AIDS: A psychosocial and historical discussion of policy alternatives, in *AIDS: Principles, Practices, and Politics,* I Corless (ed). New York, Harper & Row, 1987.

15 Darrow WW: Social and psychologic aspects of the sexually transmitted diseases: A different view. *Cutis* 27:307, 1981.

16 Owens WF: The clinical approach to the male homosexual patient. *Med Clinic North Am* 70:499, 1986.

17 Schreeder MT et al: Hepatitis B in homosexual men: Prevalence of the infection and factors related to transmission. *J Infect Dis* 146:7, 1982.

18 Ostrow DG, Altman NL: Sexually transmitted diseases and homosexuality. *Sex Transm Dis* 10:208, 1983.

19 Kramer L: *The Normal Heart.* New York, St. Martin's, 1983.

20 Gallo RC et al: The etiology of AIDS, in *AIDS: Etiology, Diagnosis, Treatment, and Prevention,* VT DeVita et al (eds). Philadelphia, Lippincott, 1985.

21 Shah N et al: Evolution of acute hepatitis B in homosexual men to chronic hepatitis B. *Arch Intern Med* 145:881, 1985.

22 Goedert et al: Heterosexual transmission of human immunodeficiency virus (HIV): Association with severe T4-cell depletion in male hemophiliacs. *Proc III Int Conf AIDS,* Washington, DC, 1987, p 106.

23 Feorino PM et al: Transfusion-associated acquired immunodeficiency syndrome. *N Engl J Med* 312:1293, 1985.

24 Kingsley LA et al: Risk factors for seroconversion to human immunodeficiency virus among male homosexuals. *Lancet* i:345, 1987.

25 Schechter MT et al: The Vancouver lymphadenopathy-AIDS study:6. HIV seroconversion in a cohort of homosexual men. *Can Med Assoc J* 135:1355, 1986.

26 Winkelstein W et al: Sexual practices and risk of infection by the human immunodeficiency virus. *JAMA* 257:321, 1987.

27 Winkelstein W et al: The San Francisco men's health study: III. Reduction in human immunodeficiency virus transmission among homosexual/bisexual men, 1982–1986. *Am J Public Health* 76:685, 1987.

28 Joseph JG et al: Coping and change: A summary of major psychosocial findings. *Proc Am Psychiatric Assoc Annu Meeting.* Chicago, IL, 1987, p 101.

29 Aral S et al: Herpes: Does knowledge lead to action? *Am J Public Health* 75:69, 1985.

30 Joseph JG et al: Perceived risk of AIDS: Assessing the behavioral and psychosocial consequences in a cohort of gay men. *J Appl Soc Psychol* 17:231, 1987.

31 Weinstein N: Reducing unrealistic optimism about illness susceptibility. *Health Psychol* 2:11, 1983.

32 Joseph JG et al: Magnitude and determinants of behavioral risk reduction: Longitudinal analysis of a cohort at risk for AIDS. *Psychol Health* 1:73, 1987.

33 McKusick M et al: Reported changes in the sexual behavior of men at risk for AIDS, San Francisco, 1982–1984; the AIDS Behavioral Research Project. *Public Health Rep* 100:622, 1985.

34 Ostrow DG: Medical and psychological implications of HTLV-III antibody testing, in *Biobehavioral Control of AIDS,* DG Ostrow (ed). New York, Irvington Publishers, 1987, p 19.

35 Osborn J: AIDS, social sciences, and health education: A personal perspective. *Health Educ Q* 13:287, 1986.

36 Ostrow DG, Altman NL: Sexually transmitted diseases and homosexuality. *Sex Transm Dis* 10:208, 1983.

37 Kessler R, Neighbors H: A new perspective on the relationships among race, social class, and psychological distress. *J Health Soc Behav* 27:107, 1986.

38 Waters J, Newmeyer J: AIDS risk-factors among IV drug users: Needle use and sexual practices. *Program and Abstracts 114th Annual Meeting of the American Public Health Association,* Las Vegas, 1986.

39 Levine S: A modern perspective on nymphomania. *J Sex Marital Ther* 8:316, 1982.

40 Stall R et al: Alcohol and drug use during sexual activity and compliance with safe sex guidelines for AIDS: The AIDS Behavioral Research Project. *Health Educ Q* 13:359, 1986.

41 Ostrow DG et al: Sexual and drug use behavior change in men at risk for AIDS. *Program and Abstracts, 114th Meeting of the American Public Health Association* 114:96 Ab, 1986.

42 Phair JP et al: The Chicago natural history study of HIV infection. *Proceedings 1987 Annual Meeting American Psychiatric Association* 140:101, 1987.

Chapter 7

# Prostitutes and their clients in the epidemiology and control of sexually transmitted diseases

Francis A. Plummer
Elizabeth N. Ngugi

## INTRODUCTION

For a communicable disease to continue to exist or even spread in a population, an infected individual must, on average, infect more than one susceptible individual. In the mathematics of epidemic theory, the basic reproductive rate of the disease must be greater than 1 for continued endemicity or an epidemic to occur. For diseases transmitted by sexual acts, since most members of a population are monogamous over short periods of time, this requirement is achieved through some members of the population having sex with multiple partners.[1] These "high-frequency transmitters" are at highest risk of acquiring and transmitting a sexually transmitted disease (STD); thus, they are, in essence, a dynamic *reservoir* of all STDs. Given the central role of these high-frequency-transmitter groups in the epidemiology of STDs, these groups should also have a major role in efforts to control STDs.

Prostitutes and their clients are one component of this dynamic reservoir of high-frequency transmitters. In this chapter, we consider the role of prostitution in the epidemiology and control of sexually transmitted diseases. Several recent authoritative discussions of the sociology of prostitution are available, and these topics are discussed here only as relevant to epidemiology and control of STDs.[2–6] In addition, this discussion will focus on female prostitution since most available data come from studies of women.

## DEFINITION OF PROSTITUTION

Society offers many definitions of prostitution, none of which is entirely satisfactory. It is difficult to define adequately an activity which takes so many forms in so many different parts of the world. The pejorative connotation of the term *prostitute* also causes some to take exception to any definition. The definition used here is a person—woman, man, or child—who exchanges sexual services for an immediate cash or in-kind return. In this chapter, we do not intend to blame those on one side of the prostitute-client relationship, but to point out the importance of prostitution in the epidemiology of STDs and how control of STDs might be achieved through intervention directed at them. Many of the observations about prostitutes apply directly to their clients as well.

## MOTIVATIONS FOR PROSTITUTION

Prostitution takes many forms in different social strata, societies, and nations and encompasses New York call girls, Nairobi slum prostitutes, and Japanese geishas. The common denominator of these groups is the sale of sex. However, viewing prostitution purely as a result of economic necessity is oversimplified for those concerned with the interaction of STDs and prostitutes. For impoverished women in a developing country, urban slum prostitution may be the only means of survival for themselves and their families;[6] for others, it is a means of supporting drug addiction; for others, it is a means of achieving an income sufficient for their expectations; and for still others, it is a part-time job, the source of supplemental income. Distinguishing necessity or compulsion from choice—that is, the degree of economic need—is important to the approach to control of STDs and to the success of interventions. A relatively educated woman who has another profession to turn to, or one who has a family to consider, may be more receptive to the idea of an intervention program than one who sells sex to support a drug addiction. Similarly, women who are prostitutes who are involved in other legally proscribed activities such as drug abuse are more difficult to reach through programs related to any figure of authority.[7,8]

Although few data are available, it seems a reasonable assumption that a minority of men would preferentially obtain sex from prostitutes if another source were available. When sex is hard to obtain, it becomes a commodity. When the demand for sex or a particular type of sexual encounter is unmet, prostitution flourishes.[2] In Nairobi, clients of prostitutes consist of single men, and married men whose wives reside in rural areas or whose wives are pregnant (F. A. Plummer et al., unpublished data). Scarcity of sex also existed in North America and Europe prior to the sexual revolution, continues to exist in Latin America[9] as a result of the stricter sexual morals for women, and exists in populations in which the number of unattached males greatly exceeds the number of females, for example, in African cities as a result of selective male migration to urban areas,[6] in seaports and around military bases, and in some areas during wars.

When a small number of women are having sex with a large number of men,[2,9] prostitution becomes extremely important in the epidemiology of STDs. Prostitutes may epidemiologically dominate transmission of some or all STDs. Studies from Nairobi illustrate this point in that one-third to two-thirds of men seen at an STD clinic report a prostitute as their source contact.[10]

## THE ROLE OF PROSTITUTES IN THE EPIDEMIOLOGY OF SPECIFIC SEXUALLY TRANSMITTED DISEASES

The relative importance of the prostitute-client component o high-frequency transmitters to the epidemiology of a particular STD is, in part, dependent on the relative role of prostitutes in providing sex in a community and on the specific STD. When a large segment of the male population has sex with prostitutes, the role will obviously be large. Some diseases such as chancroid are characteristically associated with prostitution.

## GONOCOCCAL INFECTION

The association of STDs and prostitutes was recognized before the agents of disease were known. However, by 1958, Rosenthal and Vandow, finding a decline in the prevalence of gonococcal cervicitis in prostitutes from 23.6 percent in 1946 to 5.2 percent in 1956, stated that "the prostitute is no longer the major vector of venereal disease" and that "the promiscuous amateur" was then fulfilling that role.[11]

The prevalence of gonococcal infection in prostitute populations is high (Table 7-1), varying from 10 percent in Groningen, Netherlands,[12] to 50 percent in one group of Nairobi prostitutes.[10] The incidence of gonococcal cervicitis is also extremely high in some prostitute populations. In Nairobi, a group of lower-socioeconomic-strata prostitutes had an 11 percent weekly incidence of gonococcal cervicitis.[10] These data on prevalence and incidence suggest that, in many areas of the world, a substantial fraction of gonococcal transmission may be attributed to prostitutes and their clients.

However, few data address what proportion of the total burden of gonococcal infection results from prostitutes. In Nairobi, 90 percent of men reported acquiring gonococcal urethritis from a prostitute (F. Plummer, unpublished). Since many of the non-prostitute-acquired infections were likely acquired from secondary prostitute-acquired infections, successful intervention in the prostitute component of the high-frequency-transmitter group is crucial to gonorrhea control in Nairobi. Using a simple model, it can be predicted that such intervention in Nairobi would be a cost-effective means of decreasing gonococcal morbidity.[10] In Sheffield, England, during the years 1969 to 1972, between 24 and 75 percent of male gonococcal infections were directly acquired from prostitutes.[19] In Colorado Springs, Colorado,[14] and Fresno, California,[13] programs of screening or mass treatment for gonococcal infection in prostitutes resulted in declines in the incidence of gonococcal infections in the community, suggesting that the role of prostitution in gonococcal epidemiology may be substantial in the United States as well. In the search for new strategies for control of gonococcal infection, the role of prostitutes and their clients in the epidemiology of *Neisseria gonorrhoeae* should be examined more fully.

Prostitutes using prophylactic antibiotics have played, and possibly continue to play, an important role in the development and dissemination of *N. gonorrhoeae* resistant to antimicrobial agents. Although prostitutes cannot be directly linked to the acquisition of β-lactamase plasmids by *N. gonorrhoeae*, the practice of taking prophylactic penicillin[20,21] seems to have selected for a higher prevalence of penicillinase-producing *N. gonorrhoeae* (PPNG) in prostitutes in the Far East during the initial phases of the PPNG pandemic.[22] Sexual contact of travelers with PPNG-infected prostitutes in other countries may have been responsible for the importation of PPNG to the United States.[23] Although the role of prostitutes who use prophylactic antibiotics in the development of chromosomally mediated resistance to penicillin and resistance to other antimicrobial agents is unknown, we can state with conviction that ideal circumstances for the selection of resistant organisms are thus created.

It is likely that the same is potentially true for other bacterial STDs such as chancroid, syphilis, and chlamydial infection.

**Table 7-1. Prevalence of Gonococcal Infection in Populations of Prostitutes**

| Countries | Year | Prevalence, % | Reference |
|---|---|---|---|
| *Industrialized* | | | |
| Fresno | 1979 | 22 | 13 |
| Colorado Springs | 1979 | 22 | 14 |
| Atlanta | 1981 | 17 | 15 |
| Groningen | 1988 | 10 | 8 |
| *Developing* | | | |
| Nairobi, Kenya | | | |
| Upper social strata | 1985 | 16 | 10 |
| Middle social strata | 1985 | 28 | 10 |
| Lower social strata | 1985 | 46 | 10 |
| Butare, Rwanda | 1974 | 51 | 16 |
| Philippines | 1969 | 15 | 17 |
| Singapore | 1977 | 9 | 18 |

## SYPHILIS

The eighteenth-century image of the "poxed" London prostitute illustrates that syphilis and prostitution have long been associated. At the height of the syphilis epidemic in the United States, prostitutes were estimated to be directly responsible for the transmission of 25 percent of all cases of syphilis.[24] Currently, syphilis is on the rise in the United States, and syphilis among heterosexuals is increasing for the first time in several decades.[25] At least a part of this increase is due to prostitution in association with "crack" cocaine use.[25] Epidemics of syphilis in heterosexuals have been described in Fresno, California,[13] and Winnipeg, Manitoba.[26] Each has been associated with prostitution in urban core areas. Moreover, since the prevalence of syphilis in the general heterosexual population is extremely low, it seems possible that much syphilis in heterosexuals in North America and Europe is ultimately derived from prostitutes.

Syphilis remains a frequent STD in many developing countries. In Lusaka, Zambia, 12.5 percent of pregnant women have positive serologic tests for syphilis.[27] The role of prostitutes as a reservoir of syphilis in developing countries has not been studied. From the experience with other STDs, one could conclude that it is likely to be major.

## CHANCROID AND *Haemophilus ducreyi*

Chancroid has been highly associated with prostitution, particularly lower-socioeconomic prostitution, in every major outbreak reported. During war, chancroid has been a serious health problem in military personnel. In several modern epidemics of chancroid—Winnipeg, Manitoba,[28] Orange County, California,[29] and south Florida[30]—prostitutes proved to be responsible for much of the transmission of *Haemophilus ducreyi*. The current epidemic of chancroid in New York is linked to prostitution.[31] Reported cases of chancroid are dramatically increasing in the United States, and at least some of the increase is directly attributable to prostitution.[32] In Nairobi, the best-studied area of chancroid endemicity, 66 percent of men with chancroid reported a paid sex partner as the source contact.[33] In one group of Nairobi prostitutes, the prevalence of culture-proven chancroid was 13 percent.[34]

The reasons for the association of chancroid and lower-socioeconomic-strata prostitution are not entirely clear. As the epidemiology of chancroid is currently understood, most female transmitters of *H. ducreyi* have genital ulcers.[33] It may be that poor women, in need of money and with restricted access to health care, must ignore symptoms rather than forego income for several days. Certainly in the Nairobi prostitute cohort, women continue to have sex in spite of severe genital ulcerations. Genital hygiene in men may also be a factor predisposing men to chancroid, thus adding a factor in the association of chancroid with lower-socioeconomic-strata prostitution.

Control of several urban North American epidemics of chancroid has been achieved with relative ease as compared with control of other STDs. In the epidemics of Winnipeg and Orange County, once the affected population of prostitutes was identified and treated, the disease disappeared.[28,29] Recently, control has proved more difficult in areas such as New York City and south Florida, where prostitution and drug abuse are intimately linked.[32]

## HUMAN IMMUNODEFICIENCY VIRUS INFECTION

Human immunodeficiency virus (HIV) infection is the most important STD associated with prostitution. Throughout the world, prostitutes and their clients are a major group at risk of HIV infection and acquired immunodeficiency syndrome (AIDS). They also form the major reservoir of HIV in many countries in Africa and a potential source for heterosexual spread in North America and Europe.

Prostitutes were first identified with HIV infection after studies of AIDS in Zaire and Rwanda showed the disease to be occurring in heterosexual men and women with multiple sexual partners. Initial studies showed an extremely high prevalence of HIV infection in women professing prostitution. Kigali prostitutes had an HIV prevalence of 88 percent.[35] In Nairobi the prevalence of HIV was 66 percent in 64 lower-socioeconomic-strata prostitutes and 31 percent in 26 higher-socioeconomic-strata prostitutes.[36] Subsequent studies in Uganda and Zaire have yielded similar results.[37,38]

Prostitutes in Africa also have an extremely hgh incidence of HIV infection. In a prospective 30-month study of HIV-seronegative prostitutes, the cumulative incidence of HIV seroconversion was 67 percent.[39] Prostitutes who had chancroid, had *Chlamydia trachomatis* infection, or used oral contraceptives had an independently increased risk of incident HIV infections.

In addition to being at extremely high risk of HIV infection, prostitutes in Africa are important disseminators of HIV infection. The concentration of HIV infection in urban areas and along major overland routes indirectly implicates prostitution in the spread of HIV throughout East Africa.[40] In Rwanda, the combination of late marriage in men and prized virginity in brides results in frequent prostitute contact in unmarried men, which has been invoked to explain the high HIV prevalence. Male STD clinic patients who had frequent prostitute contact and past and current genital ulcer disease (both of which are highly prostitute-associated) were more likely to have HIV infection.[41] An incidence of HIV infection of 8 percent followed a single sexual encounter with an HIV-infected prostitute.[42] A study in Nairobi estimated that 3750 men per day are exposed to HIV through sexual contact with one group of prostitutes.[43]

The emerging understanding of the role of cofactors in sexual transmission of HIV in Africa increases understanding of the importance of prostitutes in the transmission of HIV infection. Genital ulcers probably increase HIV shedding in the genital tract, rendering a woman more infectious to a sexual partner. Thus, prostitutes are probably more efficient transmitters of HIV because of their high prevalence of genital ulcers and perhaps other STDs. Additional factors serving to amplify transmission are that an immunosuppressed host more frequently has genital ulcers, and the ulcers are more refractory to treatment (F. Plummer, unpublished data).

The prevalence of HIV infection has also been studied in North American and European prostitutes. Studies in London, Paris, and Nuremberg found none of 50, 56, and 399 prostitutes tested respectively to be infected with HIV-1.[44–46] In Athens, 6 percent of 200 prostitutes who did not abuse intravenous drugs were found to be HIV-1 positive.[47] The prevalence of HIV-1 is somewhat higher in intravenous-drug-abusing prostitutes. Ten of 14 such women in Paderome, Italy, and 14 of 18 such women in Zurich, Switzerland, were positive for HIV-1.[48,49] In a large study of registered prostitutes in West Germany, half of 17 HIV-1 positive women among 2000 tested were intravenous drug abusers.[50] The prevalence of HIV-1 infection in prostitutes in south Florida was 41 percent.[51] Although the prevalence of HIV-1 antibody was somewhat higher in intravenous-drug-abusing prostitutes (46 percent), 8 of 27 (30 percent) women who denied intravenous-drug abuse were HIV-1 infected. Similarly, a prevalence of HIV-1 infection of 58 percent in intravenous-drug-abusing prostitutes, 84 percent in users of nonintravenous drugs, and 31 percent in non-drug users was found in New York and New Jersey.[52] In a multicenter study from the United States, the prevalence of HIV-1 infection in prostitutes ranged from zero in Nevada women to 57 percent in Newark–Jersey City–Paterson women.[53]

Most western prostitutes currently acquire HIV infection through intravenous drug abuse or from intravenous-drug-abusing sex partners rather than from clients.[53] Probable exceptions to this in the United States may be occurring in Florida and New Jersey.[51,52] The substantial numbers of prostitutes infected with HIV-1 create considerable potential for transmission of the virus to the general heterosexual population in North America and Europe. That this has not already occurred may be a result of condom use by clients or the relative absence of genital ulcers in these women. In three areas of the United States with current epidemics of chancroid (New York, Los Angeles, and southern Florida), significant numbers of heterosexually acquired AIDS cases are reported.

Intervention directed at prostitutes and their clients could prove to be a key strategy in the control of HIV infection. Increasing condom use and the control of factors which increase transmission, such as genital ulcers, may prove to be an important adjunct to general education measures in an effort to control HIV transmission.[54]

## INTERVENTIONS

Given the importance of prostitutes and their clients as transmitters of STDs in some areas of the world, STD-control strategies must be based on intervention in this group. Two general approaches are possible. First, strategies may focus on the control of prostitution itself by (1) criminalizing the practice of prostitution, (2) penalizing clients of prostitutes, (3) regulating legalized prostitution, (4) reducing the willingness of women to become prostitutes, and (5) reducing the demand of men for sexual services. Second, they may concentrate on STDs alone by (1) reducing the prevalence of STDs in prostitutes and (2) reducing the rate of acquisition and transmission of STDs (Table 7-2).

## PUNITIVE INTERVENTIONS

The legal approach to prostitution assumes that prostitution is an undesirable activity. Moral reasons or the association of prostitution with other crime is often the motivation for the legal

**Table 7-2. Strategies for Control of STDs through Interventions Directed at Prostitutes and Their Clients**

| | |
|---|---|
| Controlling Prostitution: | Criminalizing prostitution |
| | Penalizing clients of prostitutes |
| | Regulating legalized prostitution |
| | Reducing the supply of prostitutes |
| | Reducing the demand for prostitutes |
| Controlling STDs: | Reducing prevalence of STDs in prostitutes |
| | Reducing the incidence and transmission of STDs by prostitutes |

approach. It would seem that at least part of the association of prostitution with other crime is begotten by the criminality of prostitution.

Modern efforts to control prostitution by legal means (Chap. 1) began with the great social reform movements in the nineteenth and twentieth centuries.[2,5] In North America, these efforts have gradually lapsed into an attitude of partial unofficial tolerance of prostitution despite continued illegality. Periodic modern crusades against prostitutes probably do little to control STDs.[7,8] Prostitution is officially illegal in many developing countries of Africa but flourishes because of the enormity of the problem, the "victimless" nature of prostitution, and official corruption. Again, a situation of unofficial tolerance with periodic "swoops" to arrest prostitutes has evolved.

Many European countries have evolved a system of regulation of prostitution whereby prostitution is legal and prostitutes must submit to periodic examination and testing for STDs. These systems are more practical, humane, and likely to have an important effect on controlling STDs than repressive systems.

## CONSTRUCTIVE INTERVENTIONS

Interventions may be directed at the supply side of the prostitute-client equation. Two broad category strategies can be envisioned: reducing the necessity or reducing the willingness of women to become prostitutes. These approaches need not pass moral judgment on prostitution but may approach it purely as a health problem. The first addresses the root causes—poverty, drug addiction—and can only be achieved through great societal change. Schemes for providing alternative sources of income are labor-intensive and, we believe, of marginal impact. While they may have a major benefit for individuals, the effect on the problem at the level of society is small. This is particularly true in developing countries where an unlimited supply of poor women is available to replace women choosing other occupations. The second relies upon identifying motivations for not being a prostitute which are stronger than the motivation to become a prostitute. One of these may be the health risks of STDs. Pelvic inflammatory disease, infertility, repeated genital ulcers, cancer of the cervix, and AIDS are good reasons for women not to be prostitutes. If properly conveyed, such health information may reduce the supply of prostitutes somewhat. However, in Nairobi, in discussing these issues with lower-socioeconomic-strata prostitutes, one finds that the most frequent response is that they have no other option. Perhaps directing efforts at young women before they become prostitutes would be more effective.

Interventions can also be directed at the clients of prostitutes—operating on the demand side. One can work to decrease the willingness of men to seek sexual gratification from a prostitute through education regarding the health risks to the men themselves, their regular sexual partners, and their children. The effectiveness of this approach is uncertain. The program in Nairobi has found it very difficult to reach the clients of prostitutes except through STD clinics.

## STD-BASED INTERVENTION

Interventions can be directed solely at STDs, ignoring the issues of supply of prostitutes, demand for sexual gratification in men, and morality. Two approaches have been taken in the past: (1) decreasing the prevalence of STDs in prostitutes and (2) attempting to decrease the incidence of STDs in prostitutes and in clients. A number of programs have attempted to reduce the prevalence of several STDs in prostitutes. This is essentially the approach used in controlling chancroid and syphilis in Winnipeg, Fresno, and Orange County.[13,28,29] Several other programs have attempted to control gonococcal infections in this way.[10,14]

This strategy tries to eradicate or dramatically reduce the reservoir of an STD in one-half of the prostitute-client population. It has worked extremely well for chancroid and syphilis in North American cities during the epidemic phases of these diseases, presumably because the reservoirs were relatively discrete. The effect of such programs on gonococcal infection is not well documented. Gonococcal infections have a much broader reservoir, and the rates of reinfection may be extremely high. In Nairobi, in a prospective study of gonococcal infection in prostitutes, the mean time to reinfection was 12 days and the weekly incidence of gonococcal infection was 11 percent.[10] In this program, although screening and treatment undoubtedly resulted in fewer secondary cases of gonococcal infection and a lowering of gonococcal morbidity among the prostitutes, the time to reinfection was so short that a long-term screening program would need to be very frequent to be effective. In other situations, in which the incidence of infection is lower, this type of program may be more effective. Of course, strategies to reduce prevalence in prostitute populations are not useful for STDs for which no curative therapy exists or for which compliance with therapy is difficult.

Among high-incidence groups and for some STDs, screening programs appear to be futile. An additional strategy must be considered—preventing the transmitters from becoming infected or infecting their clients. A comprehensive approach combining health education, promotion of condoms (and perhaps other barrier methods of contraception and spermicides), screening and treatment of STDs, and promotion of alternative occupations is the model we recommend.

One such program has been operating in Nairobi since 1985.[43] The program is a community health project involving the community of prostitutes in the organization of the project and in decision making. Volunteer community health workers, themselves prostitutes, were organized, and a community-based STD clinic was established. Health education has been a major component of the program from the outset. A variety of media—lectures, public meetings, role-playing skits, songs, and individual counseling—have been used in health education. Community health workers serve as links to the community, health educators, and tracers of women defaulting. The program has also become a major distribution center for condoms, as HIV was recognized as a problem in this community.

The program successfully increased condom use in a culture in which condoms were anathema to men (Fig. 7-1). Currently, over 90 percent of women report some condom use (F. Plummer, un-

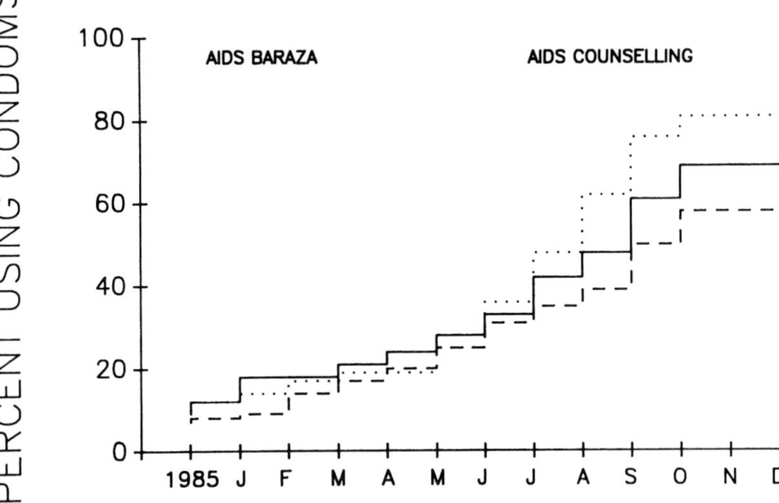


**Fig. 7-1.** Onset of condom use in response to AIDS education in a cohort of prostitutes in Nairobi. The first health education programs on AIDS were initiated in November 1985. AIDS counseling was initiated in May 1986, and condom distribution began in June 1986. Dotted line represents those who received the most health education, the solid line those who received an intermediate level of education, and the dashed line those who had received little or no education. (*From EN Ngugi et al, Lancet, in press.* Used with permission.)

published). The effect of this program on even the first-generation HIV transmission may be large. A simple model of HIV-transmission prevention demonstrates a large reduction in HIV infections (Table 7-3). Such a program would probably have an effect beyond the direct reduction of HIV transmission by decreasing the prevalence and incidence of other STDs which act to enhance HIV transmission.[34]

## DEVELOPMENT OF PROGRAMS

No blueprint exists for the development of programs for STD control in prostitutes. Of necessity, the approach will vary with the legal system, culture, society, and resources. However, some general principles derived from our experience in Nairobi can be stated. Prostitutes themselves should be involved from the early stages in development of the program. If possible, a primary health care approach—involvement of communities in their own health care—should be used. People are better motivated when they perceive themselves to be acting for themselves rather than acting in response to external authority. An obvious immediate benefit to program participants is convenient access to health care.

Programs must be implemented in a nonjudgmental and humane manner. If people feel stigmatized by participation in the program, it will fail. Finally, constant communication with participants (listening to their concerns and informing them of results of the program) is crucial to continued success.

**Table 7-3. A Simple Model of Reduction of HIV Transmission through Intervention in a Group of Prostitutes**

| | HIV-Exposed men/day | HIV-Infected men/day | % Reduction |
|---|---|---|---|
| No intervention | 1800 | 90 | |
| 50% condom use | 990 | 50 | 45 |
| 90% condom use | 342 | 17 | 81 |

Assumptions: 500 prostitutes
4 clients per day
90% prevalence of HIV in prostitutes
5% transmission rate with one sexual exposure
90% efficacy of condoms

## POTENTIAL DIFFICULTIES

While it is relatively easy to design a program for intervention, implementing the program and successfully continuing it may present great difficulty. The first difficulty is convincing decision makers of the need. Such programs are often viewed superficially as operating mainly to the benefit of prostitutes and, because of the limited constituency, are easy to cut during budget time. However, a compelling logic argues that the objective of the program is not to make life easier for prostitutes (although it undoubtedly has this effect) but to prevent them from transmitting STDs. Potential savings in cost may also be great, and arguments based upon cost-effectiveness can effectively convince authorities.

The second difficulty is how to find prostitutes and gain their participation. Women or men involved in an activity which is so stigmatized, often illegal, and often associated with other illegal activities are distrustful of authority. The initial approach must be carefully thought out. It may be best to approach an already organized group or a community. It may mean approaching bar or brothel management. Where no formal organization of prostitutes exists, initial efforts may have to reach individual women in bars or on streets and develop an organization later.

Maintaining the program may present problems of continued funding, rifts within the community of prostitutes, and pressure from outside groups. All these require commitment from program personnel, skillful management of people, and continued emphasis on the goal of the program—control of STDs.

## SUMMARY AND CONCLUSIONS

Prostitutes and their clients are one component of high-frequency transmitter populations in many societies. The magnitude of their role as reservoirs and transmitters of STDs varies with the particular setting. Their overall importance is probably greatest in developing countries where poverty, lack of opportunities for women, selective male migration to cities, and insufficient health resources create a high prevalence of prostitution and high rate of transmission of STDs. However, even in modern industrialized countries, prostitution may be central to the epidemiology of an STD, such as AIDS, for which there is no effective treatment. Focal outbreaks of certain STDs (chancroid, syphilis, PPNG) have emerged from foci of prostitution in industrialized countries.

HIV infection, chancroid, syphilis, and gonococcal infection are the diseases for which the role of prostitution is best ascertained. Control of sexual transmission of these diseases is best achieved through interventions directed at the reservoir—high-frequency transmitters—of which prostitutes and their clients are one important component. Programs developed in conjunction with prostitutes and their clients directed at preventing them from becoming infected and detecting and treating infections which occur can be an effective means of reducing the burden of STDs in the population as a whole.

## References


1 Yorke JA et al: Dynamics and control of the transmission of gonorrhea. *Sex Tramsm Dis* 5:51, 1987.

2 Hart G: *Sexual Maladjustment and Disease.* Chicago, Nelson Hall, 1977.

3 James J: Prostitutes and prostitution, in *Deviants: Voluntary Actors in a Hostile World,* E Sagarin, F Montanino (eds). Morristown, N.J., General Learning Press, 1977, p. 368.

4 Bess BE, James SS: Prostitution, in *The Sexual Experience,* BJ Sadock et al (eds), Baltimore, Williams & Wilkins, 1976, p. 594.

5 White L: Prostitutes, reformers and historians. *Crim Just Hist* 4:201, 1985.

6 Muga E: *Studies in prostitution (East, West and South Africa, Zaire and Nevada).* Nairobi, Kenya Literature Bureau, 1980.

7 Barton SE et al: Female prostitutes and sexually transmitted diseases. *Br J Hosp Med* 38:34, 1987.

8 Rosenberg MJ, Weiner JM: Prostitutes and AIDS: A health department priority? *Am J Public Health* 78:418, 1988.

9 Skegg DCG et al: Importance of the male factor in cervical cancer. *Lancet* 2:581, 1982.

10 D'Costa LJ et al: Prostitutes are a major reservoir of sexually transmitted diseases in Nairobi, Kenya. *Sex Transm Dis* 12:64, 1985.

11 Rosenthal T, Vandow J: Prevalence of venereal disease in prostitutes. *Br J Vener Dis* 34:94, 1959.

12 Ruijs GJ et al: Prevalence, incidence and risk of acquiring urogenital gonococcal or chlamydial infection in prostitutes working in brothels. *Genitourin Med* 64:49, 1988.

13 Jaffe HW et al: Selective mass treatment in a venereal disease control program. *Am J Public Health* 69:1181, 1979.

14 Potterat JJ et al: Gonorrhea in street prostitutes: Epidemiologic and legal implications. *Sex Transm Dis* 5:58, 1979.

15 Conrad GL et al: Sexually transmitted diseases among prostitutes and other sexual offenders. *Sex Transm Dis* 8:241, 1981.

16 Meheus A et al: Prevalence of gonorrhoea in prostitutes in a central African town. *Br J Vener Dis* 58:50, 1974.

17 Johnson DW et al: An evaluation of gonorrhea case finding in the chronically infected female. *Am J Epidemiol* 90:438, 1969.

18 Khoo R et al: A stud of sexually transmitted diseases in 200 prostitutes in Singapore. *Asian J Infect Dis* 1:77, 1977.

19 Turner EB, Morton RS: Prostitution in Sheffield. *Br J Vener Dis* 52:197, 1976.

20 Perine PL et al: Epidemiology and treatment of penicillinase-producing *Neisseria gonorrhoeae. Sex Transm Dis* 6:152, 1979.

21 Rajan VS et al: Epidemiology of penicillinase-producing *Neisseria gonorrhoeae* in Singapore. *Br J Vener Dis* 57:158, 1981.

22 Goh CL et al: Chemoprophylaxis and gonococcal infection in prostitutes. *Int J Epidemiol* 13:3446, 1984.

23 Handsfield HH et al: Epidemiology of penicillinase-producing *Neisseria gonorrhoeae* infections. *N Engl J Med* 306:950, 1982.

24 Parran T: Shadow on the land, in *Syphilis.* New York, Regnal/Hitchcock, 1937.

25 Centers for Disease Control: Continuing increase in infectious syphilis—United States. *MMWR* 37:35, 1988.

26 Lee C et al: Epidemiology of an outbreak of infectious syphilis in Manitoba. *Am J Epidemiol* 125:277, 1987.

27 Ratnam AV et al: Syphilis in pregnant women in Zambia. *Br J Vener Dis* 58:355, 1982.

28 Hammond GW et al: Epidemiologic, clinical, laboratory and therapeutic features of an urban outbreak of chancroid in North America. *Rev Infect Dis* 2:867, 1980.

29 Blackmore CA et al: An outbreak of chancroid in Orange County, California: Descriptive epidemiology and disease control measures. *J Infect Dis* 151:840, 1985.

30 Becker TM et al: *Haemophilus ducreyi* infection in South Florida: A rare disease on the rise? *South Med J* 80:182, 1987.

31 Centers for Disease Control: Chancroid—New York City, Dallas. *MMWR* (in press).

32 Schmid GP et al: Chancroid in the United States: Re-establishment of an old disease. *JAMA* 258:3265, 1987.

33 Plummer FA et al: Epidemiology of chancroid and *Haemophilus ducreyi* in Nairobi, Kenya. *Lancet* 2:1293, 1983.

34 Simonsen JN et al: Human immunodeficiency virus infection among lower socioeconomic strata prostitutes in Nairobi. *J Infect Dis* (submitted).

35 Van de Perre P et al: Female prostitutes: A risk group for infection with human T-cell lymphotropic virus type III. *Lancet* 2:524, 1985.

36 Kreiss JK et al: AIDS virus infection in Nairobi prostitutes: Extension of the epidemic to East Africa. *N Engl J Med* 314:414, 1986.

37 Carswell JW: HIV infection in healthy persons in Uganda. *AIDS* 1:223, 1987.

38 Mann JM et al: Sexual practices associated with LAV/HTLV-III seropositivity among female prostitutes in Kinshasa, Zaire. *AIDS* (in press).

39 Plummer FA et al: Co-factors in male-female sexual transmission of HIV. *N Engl J Med* (submitted).

40 Piot P et al: Retrospective seroepidemiology of AIDS virus infection in Nairobi populations. *J Infect Dis* 155:1108, 1987.

41 Simonsen JN et al: Human immunodeficiency virus infection among men with sexually transmitted diseases. Experience from a center of Africa. *N Engl J Med* 319:274, 1988.

42 Cameron DW et al: Genital ulcer disease and lack of circumcision are cofactors in female to male sexual transmission of human immunodeficiency virus. *N Engl J Med* (submitted).

43 Ngugi EN et al: Prevention of HIV transmission in Africa: The effectiveness of condom promotion and health education among high risk prostitutes. *Lancet* 2:887, 1988.

44 Barton SE et al: HTLV-III antibody in prostitutes, letter. *Lancet* 2:1424, 1985.

45 Brenky-Faudeux D, Fribourg-Blanc A: HTLV-III antibody in prostitutes, letter. *Lancet* 2:1424, 1985.

46 Smith GL, Smith KF. Lack of HIV infection and condom use in licensed prostitutes, letter. *Lancet* 2:1392, 1986.

47 Papaevangelou G et al: LAV/HTLV-III infection in female prostitutes, letter. *Lancet* 2:1018, 1985.

48 Tirelli U et al: HTLV-III antibody in prostitutes, letter. *Lancet* 2:1424, 1985.

49 Luthy R et al: Prevalence of HIV antibodies among prostitutes in Zurich, Switzerland. *Klin Wochenschr* (in press).

50 Schultz S et al: Female-to-male transmission of HTLV-III, letter. *JAMA* 255:1703, 1986.

51 Fischl MA et al: Human immunodeficiency virus infection (HIV) among female prostitutes in South Florida, abstracted. 3rd International Conference on AIDS, Washington, DC, 1987.

52 Sterk C: Cocaine and HIV seropositivity, letter. *Lancet* 1:1052, 1988.

53 Centers for Disease Control: Antibody to human immunodeficiency virus in female prostitutes. *MMWR* 36:157, 1987.

54 Plummer FA et al: Strategies for control of AIDS in Africa, in *Bailliere's Clinical Tropical Medicine and Communicable Diseases. International Practice and Research. April 1988—AIDS and HIV Infection in the Tropics*, P Piot, JM Mann (eds). London, Bailliere Tindall, 1988, vol 3, Chapter 11.

# Chapter 8
# Adolescent sexual behavior

Richard R. Brookman

Sexual thoughts, feelings, and behaviors, present throughout life, often are accentuated during adolescence. Puberty provides visible, undeniable evidence of physical maturity, obvious maleness or femaleness, and ability to reproduce. The normal developmental task of establishing an adult sexual identity and the capacity for intimacy may be frustrated by the prolonged interval between attainment of reproductive maturity and social permission to express one's sexuality as an adult.

Numerous surveys have suggested increased sexual experimentation by increasing numbers of teenagers at younger ages each year.[1–3] The discrepancy between traditional standards of premarital chastity and the sexually stimulating messages omnipresent in contemporary society may confuse teenagers and increase their risk of irresponsible or unwise behavior. Most professionals are concerned with the health consequences of adolescent sexual behavior: ill-timed pregnancy, infections, and potential psychosexual maladjustment. Parents and the general public fear these outcomes but extend their concerns to the existence and variety of any expressions of human sexuality among youth.

This chapter reviews from an American perspective adolescent development, adolescent sexual behavior and concerns, and features of puberty and adolescence which increase the risk of sexually transmitted infections and their complications. It also gives guidance on reproductive health care for adolescents.

## PUBERTY

Puberty results in a physically mature individual whose body habitus and secondary sexual characteristics usually testify unmistakably to maleness or femaleness and who is able to reproduce. The sequence of pubertal events is remarkably similar for most individuals despite broad variation in the timing and duration of the process. The onset of puberty is believed due to decreasing sensitivity of the hypothalamic-pituitary-gonadal axis to feedback inhibition by gonadal steroids, triggered by genetic potential with environmental factors. Increased secretion of gonadotropins stimulates gonadal growth and increased levels of circulating gonadal steroids, estrogens and androgens, which stimulate end organ responses such as growth of sexual hair, skeletal maturation, and development of reproductive organs.[4]

The average age of onset of male puberty is 11 to 12 years, range 9 to 14 years[5]. The first evidence is increased testicular size followed within a few months by the growth of pubic hair. During the next 4 to 5 years, testicular growth continues, the scrotum becomes larger, darker, and more rugated, and the penis enlarges in length and circumference. Pubic hair becomes dark, curled, and dense, filling the pubic triangle and extending up the abdomen, to the perineum and to the inner thighs. The peak height velocity is reached in mid to late puberty. Spontaneous erections occur with increasing frequency. Sperm may be found in the urine and seminal emissions begin, usually in midpuberty, as spontaneous nocturnal emissions ("wet dreams") or in response to masturbation or sexual intercourse. The average male adolescent may be fertile by age 15, physically mature by 16 to 17, and full-grown by 18 to 20 years. Those who have early onset of puberty may be fertile as they enter their teens.

Females begin puberty at an average age of 10 to 11 years, slightly earlier than males, with a normal range of 8 to 13 years.[6] The first sign is breast tissue enlargement beneath the nipple and areola, extending beyond the areola and maturing in size and consistency over several years. Pubic hair appears within a few months of breast buds and progresses as in males, but usually more rapidly than breast maturation. The peak height velocity is early in female puberty, often 2 to 3 years ahead of males. The first menstrual period usually occurs 2 to 3 years after onset of puberty, as the growth rate is slowing. It may take months to years to achieve mature menstrual cycles with consistent monthly ovulation. It is believed that many young women are not fertile—sufficiently mature to ovulate and sustain an implanted embryo—until the late teens.[7] However, early teenaged pregnancies attest to early fertility in some, usually girls who had early puberty with menarche at 10 to 11 years.

Variations in pubertal timing or events, rarely due to serious underlying disorders, may have major psychosexual implications for adolescents.[8,9] Late onset of puberty evokes fears of never attaining adulthood and creates embarrassment in situations requiring group showers or clothing changes. The late-maturing adolescent may be treated as a younger child by adults and age peers, resulting in social and emotional immaturity. Early onset of puberty also produces social discomfort. The child who appears physically mature elicits adult expectations that may be quite inappropriate for the level of emotional and cognitive development. This may include pressures from peers or even adults for sexual involvement beyond the adolescent's ability to comprehend or fully control.

Many young males have some degree of gynecomastia or breast development in midpuberty, usually regressing in 1 to 2 years, rarely requiring corrective surgery. However, this may stimulate fears of turning into a female, especially in those with insecure sexual identity. Hirsute females likewise may wonder if they are turning into males. Young males may be embarrassed by spontaneous, uncontrollable erections.

## ADOLESCENCE

Adolescence is the period of psychosocial development beginning in the preteen years, usually in conjunction with pubertal onset, and extending until the individual assumes an adult role in society.[10] The stage of psychosocial development and the level of cognitive maturation strongly influence each adolescent's response to any health concern, including those related to sexuality.

Early adolescence corresponds to ages 10 to 15 years, when most youth are in middle or junior high school. Most early adolescents are progressing through puberty, intensely aware of physical changes, and concerned about any changes which they perceive as "abnormal." They tend to exaggerate and worry about physical symptoms, although they may have difficulty verbalizing their concerns. Early adolescents are beginning to separate from childhood and their parents but tend to vacillate between adultlike and childlike behavior. They have rapid wide mood swings, become easily upset and emotional, and alternate between extreme cooperation and extreme resistance to adult guidance.

Early adolescents have a strong sense of invulnerability, the phenomenon of the "personal fable." They sincerely believe that adverse events will not happen to them or will be easily resolved. They persist in "magical thinking" where all things are possible despite any personal limitations or societal constraints. Early adolescents believe that "the whole world is watching or listening to them" at all times—the concept of the "imaginary audience." This sensitivity necessitates careful attention to privacy for interviews and examinations in any health care settings.

Sexually, as pubertal events occur, early adolescents may (re)discover masturbation and other pleasurable self-stimulation. They form close friendships with same-sex peers and may experiment sexually with them, usually to satisfy curiosity. Relationships with the opposite sex often occur at a distance, especially by telephone or in mixed sex groups in various youth settings. Early adolescents begin separating from parents by shifting their emotional ties to other adults, often developing "crushes" on teachers, coaches, and/or nationally known figures in sports, entertainment, or politics. There is much sexual content and innuendo in jokes, songs, and conversations away from adults. Sexual activity is uncommon; however, 18 percent of boys and 6 percent of girls claim to have had their first sexual intercourse by age 14.[11]

Middle adolescence, typically ages 14 to 18 years, finds most youth in high school or its equivalent. Puberty usually is complete, adult size is approaching, and fertility often is a reality. Adult appearance evokes from adults expectations of corresponding adult thinking and behavior, although the physically mature adolescent may be far from psychosocial maturity. Middle adolescents tend to show off their "new" adult bodies, even accentuating their physical attributes with padding, rather immodest dress, and suggestive postures. Strong sexual content in their language may be designed to impress peers, convey "adulthood," or even shock or anger adults.

Middle adolescents struggle the most with the development of self-identity, sexual identity, and autonomy. Separation conflicts are common, although neither disruptive nor destructive in most families. Middle adolescents seek peer group approval and may adopt styles of dress, hair, speech, and social behaviors to identify with a chosen peer group, however foreign those styles to the family. Research suggests that adolescents tend to affiliate with peers whose values, beliefs, attitudes, and behaviors are similar to those which the adolescent learned and observed within his or her own family. Peers thus reinforce behaviors learned from parents and other adult role models.[12,13] Peers may have an independent influence when there has been a lack of clearly expressed values within the family, when parental behaviors are inconsistent with their stated values, or when parental values are inflexible and so strictly enforced that they inhibit the normal questioning of values that accompanies development of autonomy.

Middle adolescents continue to feel invulnerable but now have increased mobility and independence and less adult presence and protection. Risk-taking behavior involving driving, substance use, and/or sexual activity may have harmful consequences which the adolescent is unable to anticipate or effectively prevent. Experimentation seems to be a normal, even necessary part of adolescent development. Contemporary society often tolerates and even promotes adolescent experimentation with smoking, drinking, and sex yet hesitates to provide adolescents with the knowledge and means of avoiding consequences.

Sexually, most middle adolescents have discovered masturbation and practice it with varying frequency. By age 17, approximately half of all adolescents have experienced sexual intercourse, some before puberty, many first at age 15 to 16.[11]. Coital frequency ranges from only once to several times a week. Sexual activity may include oral-genital or anal sex, especially as more adolescents learn about these varieties of sexual expression. Most adolescents have heterosexual relationships, although many have experimented with homosexual intimacy.

Late adolescence refers to the years past high school, from age 17 or 18 into the early twenties. Most late adolescents are physically adult, accepted as adults in their environment, and fertile. They are self-supporting or pursuing educational or vocational training to become able to support both self and a family. Their self-identity is consistent with the realities of their size, shape, and abilities and with societal limits and expectations. Late adolescents have a well-established sexual identity, usually heterosexual, and the ability to have intimate relationships that satisfy the emotional and sexual needs of both partners. Many have achieved parenthood one or more times, some are married, with or without children, and some have been divorced. Yet many have not yet reached the level of psychosocial maturity that would facilitate a healthy family life for themselves, their partners, and their children.

Cognitive development is closely linked with psychosocial development. Early adolescents progress from the stage of concrete, less mature thinking to the capacity for abstract, complex, more mature thinking. They gradually become able to understand complex causal relationships where multiple effects could result from subtle changes in causal factors. Their orientation shifts from the near present (days to weeks) to the future (months to years), enabling them to anticipate distant effects of present behaviors. By middle to late adolescence, most individuals have attained their highest level of cognitive ability, although they continue to gain experience in the use of their cognitive functions.[14]

## SEXUALITY CONCERNS

Adolescents and the adults responsible for them share many concerns about emerging adolescent sexuality as puberty and adolescence lead to more intense and obvious expressions of psychosexual development. Adolescents mainly worry about the normality of sexual thoughts, feelings, impulses, and behaviors. Adults, in contrast, focus on whether the adolescent attitudes or behaviors are a symptom of abnormality and/or whether they may lead to harmful consequences.

## MASTURBATION

Most adolescents have masturbated, some with regularity.[15,16] Cultural and religious opposition to masturbation coupled with remnants of the historical myths that masturbation may cause a variety of physical and mental disorders may create significant feelings of guilt and fears for adolescents. Physical symptoms of genital disorders, including infections, may be attributed by an adolescent to this "forbidden" act and intense guilt or embarrassment may inhibit the seeking of appropriate medical attention. Unfortunately, this safe, developmentally normal form of sexual expression often is rejected in favor of sexual intercourse, especially when adults are ambivalent or even intolerant about masturbation. Masturbation may be quite helpful in learning about one's own sexual responses and in relieving sexual urges while postponing sexual intercourse.

## DATING BEHAVIOR

Adolescents begin dating in the United States because peers, parents, and society expect and encourage this, beginning even in elementary school, with flowers and formal wear for class social events. By middle adolescence, most adolescents date for companionship and the physical and emotional closeness no longer sought from parents.[17] The interpersonal commitment which develops may be quite intense and should be respected by adults as quite serious to the teenagers. Physical intimacy within a dating relationship may range from hand holding to kissing, hugging, petting with and without clothing, and often coitus. In some sociocultural groups, intercourse may be an early event, bypassing less intimate expressions of affection.[18] Few adolescents are promiscuous, but relationships may last only weeks to months. Over a year, some adolescents will have several relationships with varying degrees of commitment and intimacy, including sexual intercourse.

Sexual intimacy serves the same spectrum of purposes for adolescents as for adults, although for youth the benefits more often are self-directed. Intimacy satisfies sexual urges, providing physical and emotional pleasure. It is an important nonverbal communication of commitment. It expresses one's maturity and affirms one's sexual identity as male or female to peers, parents, and oneself. It conforms to the expectations and challenges of peers and may result from the ambivalent expectations of parents. Continuing to follow a double standard, many parents fear the sexual development of daughters and the risk of pregnancy yet congratulate the sexual initiation of sons. Some parents may subtly or even overtly encourage sexual activity by expressing desire for and willingness to accept responsibility for grandchildren.

Sexual intimacy may be used by the adolescent as rebellion, as a means of coping with stress or loss, or in an attempt to hold onto a partner who is threatening to discontinue the relationship. Some adolescents engage in sexual intimacy for reward, especially those who are runaways supporting themselves or exchanging sex for drugs or money to buy drugs.

## SEXUAL PERFORMANCE

Adults reluctant to accept the fact of adolescent sexual activity may never consider the possibility that adolescents worry about their sexual performance. Adolescents seldom complain about sexual dysfunction.[19] They may be too embarrassed to reveal a personal failure, afraid of adult responses to knowledge that they are sexually active, or unaware of the range of normal human sexual responses and the frequency among adults of less than completely satisfactory sexual encounters. Adolescent males, if not yet biologically mature or sexually experienced, may have premature ejaculation or even lack of erection. Females may experience painful intercourse and lack of orgasm, often associated with inadequate lubrication. Hasty intercourse, perhaps due to fear of discovery, increases the chance of performance failures. Having failed once, the teenaged male especially may so fear failure that he repeatedly has difficulty with erection and/or ejaculation. Some may be devastated by worries about permanent dysfunction and inability to reproduce or attract a mate.

## SEXUAL ORIENTATION

Surveys of adults indicate that homosexual experience, even to the point of orgasm, is common during psychosexual development, although a minority of adults are exclusively homosexual or bisexual.[20,21] Society's yet unresolved perception of homosexuality and its meaning and the continuing stigma attached to homosexual behavior by some segments of the population may produce extreme guilt and anxiety in the adolescent who even thinks about or fantasizes a homosexual experience. The adolescent who feels attracted exclusively to the same sex or who has had homosexual intimacy may be extremely reluctant to disclose this to anyone, even when there is a health care problem.

The development of adult sexual orientation is believed to result from a complex interaction of each child's sex of rearing, the positive and negative reactions of adults to expressions of sexuality throughout childhood, and the hormonal milieu of fetal life.[22] Occasional dressing or behaving like the opposite sex during childhood does not necessarily predict adult sexual identity confusion or homosexuality. Persistent behavior inappropriate for gender may be more predictive. In early adolescence, strong emotional attachment to same-sex adults is a normal displacement of such feelings from the same-sex parent, as is strong attachment to same-sex peers. Especially among young boys, ages 8 to 13, genital exhibition, group masturbation, mutual masturbation, and more intimate sexual activity reportedly are common and represent varieties of sexual learning and satisfaction of curiosity. By mid to late adolescence, most youth are past this stage of experimentation and are forming close attachments to the opposite sex.

The homosexual or bisexual adolescent may have difficulty obtaining as well as seeking medical and counseling services, despite the increased health risks.[23] The entire spectrum of sexually transmitted infections, including AIDS and hepatitis B, are risked by gay adolescents, especially those with multiple partners or with promiscuous adult partners, or those who prostitute. Gay adolescents face more than the usual developmental stresses. They must define and accept a sexual identity unacceptable to much of society, often with little exposure during the educational process to this variety of sexual identity and lifestyle. They must adapt to the social consequences of minority group status with limited opportunities and rights—a double stress for gay adolescents who belong to ethnocultural minorities. Gay adolescents must resolve difficult decisions about telling family and friends and even must determine the extent of their visibility in gay political or social activities.

## GENDER DISORDERS

Cross dressing in adolescents may represent transvestism or fetishism, often a symptom of deep-rooted psychosexual disturbance requiring careful assessment and therapy. At times, it may indicate immature or regressed behavior with a lack of appropriate internal or external controls. Occasionally an adolescent will present as a transsexual, requesting a sex change. Such an adolescent often has serious sex role confusion or intense fear of homosexual thoughts but rarely the firm belief that he or she is "trapped" in the wrong sex. Adolescents who express strong conviction that they are of the wrong gender deserve referral to a center equipped for comprehensive evaluation and the necessary treatment of transsexualism.[24]

A serious manifestation of gender orientation disorders is the sexual asphyxiation syndrome, self-strangulation during autoerotic activity.[25] The practice consists of arranging a belt or rope to compress the neck, often also binding the extremities and/or wearing female clothing, viewing sexually explicit materials, and masturbating, with neck compression to enhance orgasm. The practice can be fatal. The most frequent victims are adolescent males, possibly due to ignorance or denial of the lethal potential. Surviving adolescent practitioners usually describe themselves as heterosexual and deny depression or suicidal thinking. The behavior is private, often repeated by those who avoid death, and, in time, may involve a partner of the same sex and a shift to homosexual orientation. Any adolescent who seems preoccupied with ropes or bondage or who has attempted self-hanging should be assessed for abnormal psychosexual development.

## DELINQUENT SEXUAL BEHAVIOR

Provocative sexual behavior among adolescents includes public use of sexually explicit language and gestures, flirtation with peers and/or adults, preference for highly revealing clothing, and public displays of affection such as exaggerated kissing, hugging, or petting. Adults may interpret such behavior as a symptom of sexual or emotional disturbance, an act of delinquency, or at least as proof that the adolescent is sexually experienced. However, this provocative behavior may be a means of testing the response of others, a form of nonverbal communication of sexuality-related anxieties, or a reaction to feelings of depression, poor self-image, or identity confusion. Clothing and behavior termed "seductive" by adults often are typical for the peer group and reflect the display of new physical development and affirmation of sexual identity characteristic of middle adolescence. Flirting is a means of experimenting with interpersonal relationships and testing one's ability to appeal to the opposite sex and impress one's peers. Adolescents who are restricted by chronic illness, disability, or hospitalization especially may use sexually provocative language or behavior to reassure themselves and others that they are normal teenagers.

Adolescent "sex offenses" may represent developmental sex play or peer-encouraged experimentation that is brought to public and/or police attention. Given the sexually explicit messages prevalent in society and the degree of open sexual behavior in some families, the unsophisticated adolescent may be unaware that such behavior is inappropriate for age or meant only for private settings. Mentally retarded adolescents are at risk of delinquency charges as sex offenders for behavior consistent with their psychointellectual development but incongruous with their age and physical maturity. Obscene phone calls, exhibitionism, and voyeurism ("peeping") are more extreme, less developmentally appropriate behaviors that may result in juvenile court action. These behaviors may be symptomatic of abnormal psychosexual development or of intense curiosity in adolescents whose environments have provided sexual titillation but no information about sexuality.[26]

Prostitution often is part of a constellation of problem behaviors including truancy, shoplifting, and substance abuse, typically beginning in middle adolescence.[27] Many young prostitutes seek escape from an intolerable home situation, often with long-standing physical, emotional, and/or sexual abuse. Prostitution may be a survival adaptation of male and female runaways and drug users to secure food, shelter, protection, or companionship. Sexual promiscuity outside the context of prostitution, repeated sexual offenses, and rape of either sex suggest a serious psychosexual disorder. Chronic sexual offenders often have a history of incest, rape victimization, limited educational achievement, unstable home life, and/or parental substance abuse.

## SEXUAL ASSAULT

Approximately half of female rape victims are adolescents. Any rape may produce serious physical and/or emotional trauma, immediate or long-term, even for those who are sexually experienced and who may know the assailant. Initial responses range from stoicism and denial to panic and hysteria. Later, phobias, sexual disorders, and multiple psychosomatic symptoms are common, in both male and female victims[28]. Recent attention has been drawn to the frequency of "date rape," forced sexual intercourse in a relationship when one partner chooses not to be so intimate at a particular time, perhaps having been more agreeable at other times. The added element of exploitation or betrayal may be especially upsetting.[29]

Sexual abuse may be involved in as many as half the cases of child abuse involving older children and adolescents.[30] Single episodes by strangers, especially when nonviolent and when a child is young, may have little adverse effect on psychosexual development. Violent abuse at any age and any sexual abuse at older ages have more serious consequences. The spectrum of sexual child abuse ranges from adult display of genitals to minors to manipulation of breasts or genitals by adult or minor to genital apposition and attempted or completed penetration of vagina, anus, and/or mouth. Terminology varies among legal jurisdictions (e.g., "molestation," "sexual misuse," "sodomy"). All terms imply the use of force, deception, or strong persuasion to involve a minor in sexual activity to which he or she cannot legally consent and which he or she may be unable to understand or resist.

Incest is sexual abuse by family members.[31] The most frequent reported incest involves girls and fathers or father substitutes, but it may involve mother and son, father and son, or any combination of relatives, even multiple generations. Sexual activity among siblings may be quite common, perhaps within the broad range of childhood sex play, and produces the least emotional consequences—unless adults also become involved and the incidences become a family secret. Often, incest develops within a disturbed family where a parent has psychosexual maturation deficits, poor impulse control, marital estrangement, yet reluctance to seek external sexual outlets. Incest often begins in late childhood and may decrease when menarche occurs because the father fears pregnancy or because the physically mature daughter is able to resist and is seeking sexual attention from peers. A younger sibling may replace the older as the object of incest. Incest continues because the father threatens abandonment or punishment, promises rewards, or uses physical force. Mother, frequently also a victim of incest, condones the act and condemns the daughter, often discrediting the daughter's reports.

Incest may be discovered when a child has a sexually transmitted infection or unexplained genital injury or when a young adolescent is found to be pregnant or infected despite a denial of sexual activity. Often, past or continuing incest is revealed in the context of individual or family therapy. Incest history is frequent in adolescents and adults with sexual dysfunctions, sexual promiscuity and prostitution, severe phobias, conversion disorders, delinquency, and suicidal behavior. Incest behavior or threats should be suspected in families when adolescents rebel to extreme against the opposite sex parent, show marked estrangement from the same sex parent, or act as a parent substitute in conjunction with any of the behaviors described above or unintended pregnancy or infection.

## ADOLESCENTS AND SEXUALLY TRANSMITTED DISEASES

Puberty and adolescence contribute to the incidence and clinical features of STDs in youth.[32] During puberty, genital maturation increases the capacity for intercourse and the internal genital tract becomes fully patent in both sexes, allowing any acquired infections to spread. In females, estrogenization decreases the susceptibility of the vulva and anterior vagina to most infections, alters vaginal flora and pH, and facilitates the growth of trichomonas if acquired. Until several years after menarche, the squamocolumnar junction is located on the exposed vaginal surface of the cervix, gradually progressing to the endocervical canal as thin columnar cells are transformed to layers of thick squamous cells.[33] The exposed columnar epithelium is especially likely to become infected with gonorrhea or chlamydia if there is contact with an infected partner. The transition zone itself is susceptible to carcinogenic factors, including various infectious organisms. Women who have the earliest sexual intercourse have the highest risk of developing cervical cancer, often detected 6 to 20 years after the first coitus.[34]

Denying the possibility of harm, early and middle adolescents are less likely than others to use preventive methods when engaging in sexual intimacy and more likely to deny symptoms of infection. Excessive attention to genital hygiene, such as frequent douching, or excessive neglect of perineal hygiene may complicate the clinical appearance of any infection. Adolescents who do suspect an infection may be embarrassed or frightened and delay seeking treatment for days to weeks. Once diagnosed, they may fail to complete therapy, especially if symptoms diminish, and/or may fail to appear for test of cure. They may fail to inform partners, because of anger, shame, or fear of accusations of infidelity. Adolescents who have a series of short-lived relationships each of which includes intercourse increase their risk of exposure to infection and complicate the task of contact treatment.

Adolescent contraceptive practices affect the risk of infections.[35,36] Many adolescents never use a method or rely solely on the oral contraceptive. Whether or not oral contraceptives increase susceptibility to certain infections, they clearly reduce the impetus to use a barrier method or to involve males in prevention. Adolescents who decide or can be persuaded to use barrier methods seldom use them consistently and often use them incorrectly. IUDs rarely are advised for adolescents and should never be considered for those at high risk for infection or for poor compliance with close follow-up.

STD control in adolescents, as in other age groups, may be frustrated by the high frequency of asymptomatic states, the presence of antibiotic-resistant strains, and the adolescent practice of partial treatment with self-prescribed antibiotics obtained from friends. Health professionals, inadequately trained about STDs, may miss the correct diagnosis in an adolescent whose presentation is atypical or whose range of sexual behaviors is never addressed. Limited accessibility of services, costs, and staff attitudes provide additional barriers to health care.

## REPRODUCTIVE HEALTH CARE FOR ADOLESCENTS

As normal psychosexual development occurs, some adolescents risk pregnancy, sexually transmitted infections, including AIDS, and factors which predispose to reproductive tract malignancies. Adolescents engaged in a variety of problem behaviors tend to be at greatest risk for these consequences. High index of suspicion, comprehensive assessment, and thorough treatment as well as preventive education are essential to reduce these risks.

## HISTORY

Routine health care of children and adolescents should include questions about sexual development and sexuality concerns. Knowledge and understanding about puberty and human reproduction should be assessed and misinformation corrected. "Am I normal" is a question common to most adolescents, even if not readily verbalized to parents or health professionals, and reassurance is greatly appreciated. Depending on age, the context of the visit, and any pertinent symptoms, girls should be asked about menstrual periods, always noting the date of the last and previous periods. Adolescents should be allowed to express any concerns about physical developmental changes, masturbation, dating behavior, sexual feelings, and pressures related to intimacy. Usual sources of sexuality information, extent of communication about sexuality within the family, and opportunities for formal sex education should be determined.

Adolescents should be asked if they ever have had sexual intercourse. Those who have should be asked about frequency and variety of intimate sexual behaviors, possible exposures to infection, knowledge and use of any preventive measures, and history of any health consequences such as infection, pregnancy, genital injury, or abuse. Those who have had any consequences should be asked about treatment, outcome, and their and their parents' response to the problem. It is helpful to ensure that interviewing about sexuality be done in private, after some degree of rapport has been established, and that both the adolescent and the interviewer understand the terminology each uses, including "street language" and ethnocultural variations in definitions.

Assurance of confidentiality often is necessary to initiate health care with an adolescent, especially when there is significant alienation from the family and/or distrust of professionals and institutions. In all states, parental consent is not required to evaluate and treat minors for STDs and usually is not required to provide a minor with family planning services.[37] In granting minors the right to consent to reproductive health care, state laws assume the capacity for informed consent in those minors. Generally, state laws neither require nor prohibit notification of parents when the minor is treated on his or her own consent. Rather than promise unconditional confidentiality, most clinicians will assure adolescents that information will not be shared with others without first discussing this with the adolescent. Clinicians must use their best judgment about confidentiality based on the developmental maturity of the adolescent, the severity of the problem, and the likelihood that the adolescent will need adult assistance to obtain proper medical care.[38] The goal usually is to aid the adolescent in communicating with parents and to enlist parental support for the adolescent.

## PHYSICAL EXAMINATION

The routine physical examination of any child or adolescent should include inspection of the genitalia, breasts, and axillae for normal development and observation of the onset and normal progression of puberty. When sexual activity is reported or suspected, a more complete genital-perineal examination should be done. The reasons for and nature of the examination should be explained while the adolescent is dressed and seated. Every effort should be made to ensure privacy and comfort, to preserve modesty with adequate coverage, to allow a chaperone if requested by either sex, and to provide a same-sex examiner when requested, if staffing permits. The examiner should maintain eye contact and avoid joking or any signs of discomfort during the exam.

Examination of sexually active adolescent males should include careful inspection of the pubic hair, penis, and scrotum for lesions, excoriations, or discharge. Testes should be palpated for size, consistency, and tenderness and may be measured if there is concern about pubertal development. Testicular self-examination should be taught. The inguinal regions should be palpated for adenopathy and hernias and the anus inspected for lesions or discharge. If homosexual activity is reported, anoscopy may be considered. A rectal examination should be done based on clinical indications, such as history of blood on the stool or symptoms of prostatitis.

Some adolescent medicine specialists recommend routine screening of all sexually active male adolescents for STDs while others screen based on symptoms or known or suspected exposure to infection.[39,40] Gram stain of urethral swab, culture or rapid test for chlamydia, and culture for gonorrhea always should be part of the screen for STDs with serologic testing for syphilis, hepatitis B, and possibly AIDS in those believed to be at risk. Use of spun sediment of the first 5 ml of freshly voided urine has been recommended as an alternative to urethral swabs for cultures and Gram stain.[41]

Sexually active adolescent females require inspection of the breasts, pubic hair, and external genitalia for lesions, excoriations, and obvious discharge. The urethra, periurethral glands, and Bartholin's glands should be closely examined for swelling or discharge. Inguinal regions should be palpated for adenopathy. Pelvic examination is indicated in all sexually active females with symptoms suggesting infection, known or suspected exposure to infection, other gynecologic symptoms, or lack of screening since beginning sexual activity. Many adolescents have a first pelvic examination when they request contraception, frequently months to years after first intercourse, or when they have been sexually assaulted. There is debate whether all females should have a first pelvic examination by a certain age such as 16 or 18, even if virginal, but most adolescent medicine specialists tend to wait for specific clinical indications.[42]

The speculum exam should be done using warm water lubrication. For a first examination or with a very anxious patient, if there is low suspicion for infection, a lubricated finger may be inserted first and the speculum introduced over the finger in the correct plane to locate the cervix easily. The cervix should be examined for discharge, friability, and any unusual appearance. Endocervical swabs should be obtained for gonorrhea culture, test for chlamydia, and Gram stain. At least yearly, a specimen should be obtained for Papanicolaou smear. Secretions from the posterior vagina should be obtained for wet-mount detection of trichomonads, hyphae, or "clue" cells and a KOH preparation for the "whiff" test for bacterial vaginosis. Following the speculum examination, a bimanual exam should be done, noting size and consistency of the cervix and uterine fundus, any pain on cervical motion, and any tenderness or swelling in the adnexae. A rectovaginal examination is recommended to fully appreciate any pelvic region pathology. Serology for syphilis, hepatitis B, and possibly AIDS should be considered in those felt to be at risk.

## TREATMENT CONSIDERATIONS

Adolescents found to be infected with any STD should be counseled about the infection(s), the possible complications, the importance of informing partner(s) to seek diagnosis and treatment, and the critical importance of completing therapy as recommended and returning for test of cure. The clinician should offer to screen, treat, and educate the sexual partner(s) whenever practical. Single-dose treatment on site is strongly recommended for adolescents. When there is no single-dose treatment, adolescents may comply best with twice daily oral antibiotics. Inpatient treatment of complicated infections, especially pelvic inflammatory disease or disseminated gonorrhea, is advisable, especially when compliance is uncertain.[43]

Infected adolescents may have questions about the source of infection and ultimately about the fidelity of their partners. They must be informed that STDs rarely occur from nonsexual transmission, that STDs may be present without symptoms for prolonged periods, and that partners are not always honest because of embarrassment or ignorance, not necessarily deceit. Information can be provided in printed form appropriate for intellectual level. Most adolescents benefit from repeated verbal education at subsequent visits. Follow-up should include observation of adverse effects on self-esteem, emotional adjustment, and interpersonal relationships with peers and family.

Because adolescent women may not indicate concerns about pregnancy or provide an accurate menstrual history, pregnancy testing is recommended prior to treating STD in adolescents. Conversely, whenever pregnancy is diagnosed in a teenager, screening for all possible STDs should be done at that same visit. Ambivalence about pregnancy, fear of revelation, and previously described barriers to health care may delay the teenager's decision and resolution of the pregnancy for weeks to months. Undetected, untreated infections increase the risk of adverse pregnancy outcome and, unfortunately, are common features of adolescent pregnancies.[44,45]

## EDUCATION FOR PREVENTION

Adolescent reproductive health care is best served by prevention of biopsychosocial consequences. Many adults believe that adolescents should refrain from sexual intercourse until marriage or at least until they have a mature committed relationship in which both partners are able and willing to take responsibility for any consequences. Many professionals believe that first intercourse should be postponed at least until the reproductive system is fully mature (late teens) and until there is sufficient psychosocial maturity for responsible behavior. If adolescents are willing to postpone first coitus, they remain at risk for transmission of STDs through noncoital intimate behaviors; however, it may be unrealistic to expect adolescents to abstain from all physical expressions of sexuality, especially if marriage is unlikely until the mid- to late twenties.

Adolescents who will not be persuaded to abstain from intercourse must be well informed about the risks of all forms of sexual intimacy and provided with the knowledge and methods for prevention of infection and pregnancy. Teenagers should be encouraged to use barrier contraceptives, especially both condom and vaginal spermicide, with every coital act, whether or not the female is using the oral contraceptive. Adolescents should be instructed about "safe sex" which may require description or at least mention of practices such as anal intercourse which increase the risk of serious infections or injuries. Sexually active teenagers, even those consistently using barrier methods and having a single partner, should be screened yearly for infections. More frequent screening should be considered for high-risk adolescents such as gay youth, runaways, drug abusers, and delinquents.

Sex education or family life education does not guarantee prevention of consequences, will not ensure abstinence, and has not been shown to increase sexual experimentation.[46] Teenagers who have been exposed to appropriate sex education tend to delay first intercourse, to use contraception when they have intercourse, and to avoid pregnancy.[47] Family life education of children and adolescents is a responsibility shared by parents, schools, health professionals, and other adults who provide services to youth. All contribute positively or negatively to each young person's understanding about and attitude toward human sexuality. Parents and other family members begin this process at childbirth and provide the major influence in the development of personal values and beliefs. Society's unresolved debate about the content and timing of sexuality education and parental reluctance to discuss sexuality topics often leave youth uninformed or misinformed. Incomplete or inaccurate sexual information tends to be derived from friends, the media, and available written materials ranging from dictionaries to sex-oriented adult magazines

As children reach adolescence, the normal distancing from parents may interfere with open communication and effective education even in the most enlightened and comfortable families. Health professionals can be important allies of parents and schools in providing scientific information and latest technical advances, in supporting developmentally appropriate communication within families, and in helping the community accept the importance of lifelong comprehensive family life education for all families. Professionals can be available to assist individual parents in educating their children and themselves and to assist in planning and promoting family life education curricula and opportunities in schools, churches, and other community settings.[48,49,50]

## References


1 Hofferth SL et al: Premarital sexual activity among U.S. teenage women over the past three decades. *Fam Plann Perspect* 19:46, 1987.

2 Coles R, Stokes G: *Sex and the American Teenager.* New York, Harper & Row, 1985.

3 Meikle S et al: *Teenage Sexuality.* San Diego, College-Hill Press, 1985.

4 Slap GB: Normal physiological and psychosocial growth in the adolescent. *J Adolesc Health Care* 7:13S, 1986.

5 Lee PA: Normal ages of pubertal events among American males and females. *J Adolesc Health Care* 1:26, 1980.

6 Moscicki A-B, Shafer MB: Normal reproductive development in the adolescent female. *J Adolesc Health Care* 7:41S, 1986.

7 Montagu MFA: *The Reproductive Development of the Female. A Study in the Comparative Physiology of the Adolescent Organism,* 3d ed. Littleton, MA, PSG Publishing, 1979.

8 Gross RT, Duke PM: The effect of early versus late maturation on adolescent behavior. *Pediatr Clin North Am* 27:71, 1980.

9 Nottelmann ED et al: Developmental processes in early adolescence: Relationships between adolescent adjustment problems and chronologic age, pubertal stage, and puberty-related serum hormone levels. *J Pediatr* 110:473, 1987.

10 Kreipe RE, McAnarney ER: Psychosocial aspects of adolescent medicine. *Semin Adolesc Med* 1:33, 1985.

11 Alan Guttmacher Institute: *Teenage Pregnancy: The Problem That Hasn't Gone Away.* New York, Alan Guttmacher Institute, 1981.

12 Shah F, Zelnik M: Parent and peer influence on sexual behavior, contraceptive use, and pregnancy experience of young women. *J Marr Fam* 43:339, 1981.

13 Nathanson CA, Becker MH: Family and peer influence on obtaining a method of contraception. *J Marr Fam* 48:513, 1986.

14 Blum RW, Stark T: Cognitive development in adolescence. Clinical cues and implication. *Semin Adolesc Med* 1:25, 1985.

15 Greydanus DE, Geller B: Masturbation. Historical perspective. *NY State J Med* 80:1892, 1980.

16 Wagner CA. Sexuality of American adolescents. *Adolescence* XV:567, 1980.

17 Diepold J, Young RD: Empirical studies of adolescent sexual behavior: A critical review. *Adolescence* XIV:45, 1979.

18 Smith EA, Udry JR: Coital and non-coital sexual behaviors of white and black adolescents. *Am J Public Health* 75:1200, 1985.

19 Greydanus DE et al: Sexual dysfunction in adolescents. *Semin Adolesc Med* 1:177, 1985.

20 Remafedi G: Homosexual youth. *JAMA* 258:222, 1987.

21 Bell AP et al: *Sexual Preference. Its Development in Men and Women.* Bloomington, Indiana University Press, 1981.

22 Greydanus DE, Dewdney D: Homosexuality in adolescence. *Semin Adolesc Med* 1:117, 1985.

23 Remafedi G: Adolescent homosexuality: Psychosocial and medical implications. *Pediatrics* 79:331, 1987.

24 Money J: *Love and Love Sickness. The Science of Sex, Gender Difference, and Pair-bonding.* Baltimore, Johns Hopkins Press, 1980.

25 Hazelwood RR et al: *Autoerotic Fatalities.* Lexington, MA, DC Heath, 1983.

26 Fehrenbach PA et al: Adolescent sexual offenders: Offender and offense characteristics. *Am J Orthopsychiatry* 56:225, 1986.

27 Nightingale R: Adolescent prostitution. *Semin Adolesc Med* 1:165, 1985.

28 Committee on Adolescence, AAP: Rape and the adolescent. *Pediatrics* 72:738, 1983.

29 Carlson BE: Dating violence: A research review and comparison with spouse abuse. *Soc Casework* 68:16, 1987.

30 Hibbard RA, Orr DP: Incest and sexual abuse. *Semin Adolesc Med* 1:153, 1985.

31 Renshaw DC: *Incest. Understanding and Treatment.* Boston, Little, Brown, 1982.

32 O'Reilly KR, Aral SO: Adolescence and sexual behavior. Trends and implications for STD. *J Adolesc Health Care* 6:262, 1985.

33 Gottardi G et al: Colposcopic findings in virgin and sexually active teenagers. *Obstet Gynecol* 63:613, 1984.

34 Sadeghi et al: Prevalence of cervical intraepithelial neoplasia in sexually active teenagers and young adults. *Am J Obstet Gynecol* 148:726, 1984.

35 Morrison DM. Adolescent contraceptive behavior: A review. *Psychol Bull* 98:538, 1985.

36 Zelnik M, Kantner JF: Reasons for nonuse of contraception by sexually active women aged 15–19. *Fam Plann Perspect* 11:289, 1979.

37 Holder AR: Minors' rights to consent to medical care. *JAMA* 257:3400, 1987.

38 Morrison JM et al: *Consent and Confidentiality in the Health Care of Children and Adolescents. A Legal Guide.* New York, Free Press, 1986.

39 Marks A, Fisher M: Health assessment and screening during adolescence. *Pediatrics* 80:135, 1987.

40 Brookman RR: Reproductive health assessment of the adolescent, in *Adolescent Medicine*, 2d ed., AD Hofmann, DE Greydanus (eds). New York, Appleton-Lange, 1988.

41 Adger H et al: Screening for *Chlamydia trachomatis* and *Neisseria gonorrhoeae* in adolescent males: Value of first-catch urine examination. *Lancet* II:944, 1984.

42 Emans SJ: Pelvic examination of the adolescent patient. *Pediatr Rev* 4:307, 1983.

43 Martien K, Emans SJ: Treatment of common genital infections in adolescents. *J Adolesc Health Care* 8:129, 1987.

44 Pitegoff JG, Cathro DM: Chlamydial infections and other sexually

transmitted diseases in adolescent pregnancy. *Semin Adolesc Med* 2:215, 1986.

45 Hardy PH et al: Prevalence of six sexually transmitted disease agents among pregnant inner-city adolescents and pregnancy outcome. *Lancet* II:333, 1984.

46 Kirby D: Sexuality education: A more realistic view of its effects. *J School Health* 55:421, 1985.

47 Marsiglio W, Mott FL: The impact of sex education on sexual activity, contraceptive use and premarital pregnancy among American teenagers. *Fam Plann Perspect* 18:151, 1986.

48 Haffner D, Casey S: Approaches to adolescent pregnancy prevention. *Semin Adolesc Med* 2:259, 1986.

49 Irwin CE, Millstein SG: Biopsychosocial correlates of risk-taking behaviors during adolescence. Can the physician intervene? *J Adolesc Health Care* 7:82S, 1986.

50 Brookman RR: Sexually transmitted diseases, in *Early Adolescent Transitions*, M Levine, ER McAnarney (eds). Lexington, MA, DC Heath, 1988.

Chapter 9

# Preventive health behavior and STD

William W. Darrow
Karolynn Siegel

This chapter focuses on health behavior as it relates to sexually transmitted disease (STD). Health behavior refers to everything a person does to prevent disease or to detect it in an asymptomatic stage.[1] Because STDs have been identified for which there are no effective treatments, increasing emphasis has been placed on encouraging at-risk persons to modify sexual behavior as a strategy for STD control.[2]

## MODELS OF HEALTH BEHAVIOR

A variety of sociopsychologic models attempts to explain the adoption of health behaviors. The most widely applied of these has been the Health Belief Model (HBM).[3] According to the HBM, the principal factors that influence adoption of a preventive health action are:

1. Perception of vulnerability or susceptibility to a disease
2. Perception of the severity of the disease
3. Belief in the efficacy of recommended health actions
4. Evaluation of the costs of adopting the behavior
5. The presence of a stimulus or cue to action (such as a health communication or a symptom)

A review[4] of the literature to 1984 for reports of attempts to test empirically the HBM (or elements of it) showed that separate dimensions of the HBM were frequently associated with whether persons had engaged in health-related behaviors. A perceived barrier was most often associated with a failure to adopt health actions in both retrospective and prospective studies. However, while the HBM has been useful in describing personal experiences with specific health practices, it has been considerably less useful in predicting the continuation of preventive behaviors over an extended period of time.[5,6]

Although other paradigms have been proposed,[7] the behaviors explained, the terms assigned to the categories of determinants, and the general factors included are similar. Cummings et al.[8] reduced 109 distinctly named variables in the various models to six factors:

1. Accessibility to care
2. Evaluation of health services
3. Perception of symptoms and threat of disease
4. Social network characteristics
5. Knowledge of the disease
6. Demographic factors

These factors have been used to explain a wide range of health behaviors including participation in cancer screening programs, vaccinations, breast self-examination, checkups for asymptomatic STD, and genetic screening.[4,9,10] However, the ability of these factors to predict effective health behavior related to STDs has not been consistently demonstrated.

Perceptions of susceptibility, benefits, and barriers were associated with self-reports of actions to prevent STDs and having checkups for STDs in a cross-sectional study of undergraduate students in New York City;[9] but clinic patients in Sacramento, California, who believed they were susceptible to future infections, that STDs were serious, and that condoms could prevent disease transmissions were no more likely to accept free samples of condoms than were clinic patients who did not hold these beliefs.[11]

Existing models may be severely limited in their ability to predict preventive practices in relation to STDs because they do not take into account two important features of the problem that may significantly influence behavior: the stigma associated with STDs and the interpersonal nature of sexual decision making.

## STD AND STIGMA

Illness is a social state as well as a physical condition. The assignment of a diagnosis affects both the behavior of the person labeled as sick and the actions of others toward "the patient."[12] Attributions of responsibility for a person's illness greatly influence how others behave toward him or her. Although American society has undergone major changes in its sexual standards, attitudes, and patterns of behavior, the traditional association of STDs with sin and moral depravity has remained relatively unchanged. Thus, STD "victims" must either deny their condition (e.g., "I never had it") or assert their innocence (e.g., "I got it from a toilet seat"). Brandt[13] noted in his social history of STDs,

> Since the late nineteenth century, venereal disease has been used as a symbol for society characterized by a corrupt sexuality. . . . Venereal disease makes clear the persistent association of disease with dirt and uncleanliness as well, revealing pervasive cultural attitudes and values. . . . The very term which the venereal disease control movement took for itself in the twentieth century—social hygiene—makes explicit this association" (p.5).

Because of the stigma associated with STDs, persons are inclined to deny their own susceptibility; in the absence of a sense of vulnerability, they are not sufficiently motivated to adopt preventive measures.

## INTERPERSONAL NATURE OF SEXUAL BEHAVIOR

Any conceptual model that attempts to explain health behavior in relation to STD must take into account the behavior of two (or more) persons. Unlike health behaviors for most medical conditions, decisions regarding precautions against STDs are usually made jointly by a couple. Obstacles in obtaining the consent of a potential sex partner complicate STD prevention.

Because of the interpersonal nature of sexual decision making, it is much more difficult to predict condom use, for example, than to predict vaccine acceptance. This point was noted in a study of factors associated with modification of high-risk sexual behavior in homosexual (gay) men at risk for acquired immunodeficiency syndrome (AIDS). Gay men who reported being more comfortable with negotiating limits with their partners were more likely to adopt "safer safe" practices.[14]

## BEING SICK AND BEING AT RISK

Persons at risk for particular illnesses are usually encouraged to engage in health behaviors designed to reduce rates of disease.

From an epidemiologic perspective, being at risk means that a person has a higher-than-average statistical probability of experiencing some adverse outcome (e.g., disease) because of some attribute or potential exposure. Persons who share common risk factors constitute a "risk group" for a disease. The epidemiologic concept of risk, however, applies to a population; it does not determine the precise risk for any particular person within a risk group.

## THE "SICK" ROLE

As long as persons can carry on the routine tasks associated with their social roles, they tend to define themselves as normal and healthy. When something interferes with their usual performance or they experience a specific sign or symptom of disease, they might suspect they are ill and seek the confirmation of others. If others, particularly physicians, confirm the illness, they are expected to adopt a special role—the "sick" role.[15]

The sick role is well established in our society and is supported by the medical profession. It clarifies the social expectations that exist once a person has been labeled as ill; ill persons are exempt from their usual tasks and social obligations and are entitled to certain privileges, such as unusual support or assistance from others. In return, ill persons must assume certain responsibilities: they must recognize that being ill is inherently undesirable, they must seek competent help, and they must cooperate with others in therapy.

## THE "AT-RISK" ROLE

The "at risk" role, unlike the "sick" role, does not have widely shared expectations attached to it and differs from the sick role in several significant ways.[16] For example, while the latter carries responsibilities and privileges, the at-risk role carries only obligations to avoid infection. The person at risk is expected to modify his or her behavior to reduce his or her risk but receives no special rights or privileges.

The sick role, especially with acute illness, is temporary.[15] The patient may anticipate resuming his or her usual role after convalescence; in contrast, the at-risk role may be constant. Because the sick role is well established, those accepting their obligations receive consistent reinforcement for meeting the expectations associated with the role; the at-risk role is not well established and does not carry with it such reinforcement.[16] In fact, at times, the social environment facilitates the very behavior that places persons at risk.

A final difference between the two roles concerns the assignment of responsibility. Once labeled ill by a physician, people can transfer most of the responsibility for their fate to the medical profession, which will be held accountable if they do not recover. The people at risk, however, must retain responsibility for their condition, especially when, as with STDs, they are at risk because of a chosen behavior or lifestyle. The risk taker who becomes sick may be held accountable for the outcome.

Because of these circumstances, most healthy persons are unwilling to assume the at-risk role. If members of the medical profession and society would legitimate the at-risk role, norms would develop to regulate social expectations associated with it,[16] which might cause friends and associates to exert social pressure on the risk taker to comply with preventive recommendations.

## CHANGING PERCEPTIONS OF STD

Most models of health behavior assume that a feeling of personal vulnerability or susceptibility to a disease is necessary for any person to consider adopting a preventive health behavior. Because the STD carrier has been stereotyped as a sexually promiscuous person of low moral character, most persons view themselves as unlikely victims and, therefore, presume themselves to be at low or no risk. Recently, attempts have been made in public health campaigns to debunk these stereotypes by educating the public that "even nice people get STDs."

## POTENTIAL SUSCEPTIBILITY

The publicity regarding genital herpes in the 1970s played an important part in raising awareness of susceptibility. The widespread media coverage of this epidemic alerted many to the fact that STDs are a potential, not necessarily rare, threat associated with casual or unprotected sexual exposures. Media reporting of herpes victims who did not fit the traditional stereotypes may have aided more widespread identification with STD patients, thereby enhancing many persons' feelings of susceptibility.

Additionally, because no effective treatment existed for herpes, persons recognized that the consequences of contracting the disease might have to be endured for a lifetime. Herpes differed from syphilis or gonorrhea and other well-known STDs for which safe, effective treatment was usually readily available and easy to administer. It was precisely the awareness (before herpes and later AIDS) that these diseases could be treated easily that made many sexually active persons unwilling to use condoms or limit their sexual freedom. They regarded the risk of acquiring an STD as acceptable given what they judged to be relatively insignificant consequences.

## SERIOUS CONSEQUENCES

To be motivated to take preventive action, a person must perceive a disease as having serious consequences. In a national telephone survey regarding genital herpes,[17] about 75 percent of respondents said they were familiar with the disease. That they felt it was serious was evident in the fact that 81 percent indicated they would favor an obligatory premarital test for herpes if one were available. Nineteen percent perceived themselves to be at risk of getting herpes. Yet only 45 percent of those at risk reported they had altered their sexual behavior to reduce their chances of contracting the disease.

These data indicate that raising the public's awareness of the prevalence of STDs and their potentially serious consequences can influence perceptions of vulnerability and lead to behavior change. However, they also suggest that social and psychological barriers may prevent behavior modification despite feelings of vulnerability and perceptions of the disease as serious.

If genital herpes made the public aware that STDs can be "forever," AIDS made them aware that STDs can kill. The threat of AIDS has already started to alter the sex practices of persons at relatively low risk. Very significant increases in the sales of condoms have been reported in New York City and San Francisco.[18] Women accounted for 40 percent of all retail condom sales in 1985, up from about 10 percent in 1975.

The implication of a sexually transmitted viral agent in the etiology of cervical cancer[19] has dramatized further the potentially serious consequences of STD. The venereal nature of this neoplasm may not be widely recognized, but as awareness grows, fear of a sexually transmitted cancer is likely to motivate more widespread preventive behavior.

## BARRIERS TO PERSONAL PROPHYLAXIS

Given the growing public recognition that STDs can have very serious long-term—and sometimes fatal—consequences, what prevents more widespread acceptance of prophylactic measures?

### MISCONCEPTIONS

Several surveys have been conducted to assess levels of knowledge concerning STDs. Most have centered on high school and college students or adolescents attending family planning clinics. Levels of knowledge about STDs are generally high,[20,21] but widespread misconceptions or specific gaps in information have been identified.[22–24] Unfortunately, findings from these studies cannot be meaningfully compared because they focus on populations that differ on such characteristics as sex composition, geographic locations, and sexual experience. The content and complexity of the questions used to assess knowledge also vary considerably.

Two surveys of high school students' knowledge about AIDS have been conducted.[24,25] From one-third to two-thirds of the respondents knew little about the risk groups, the consequences and treatment for disease, detection of AIDS, and lack of transmissibility of the AIDS virus through casual contact.

Few studies have been reported regarding the efficacy of STD education. These studies have focused on the correlation between such education and incidence of disease in a community, an outcome that cannot be significantly affected by education alone; or they measure only changes in attitudes and knowledge that may not predict health behavior.[26] Research that could provide a basis for rejecting or endorsing STD education has yet to be conducted.

Despite the lack of evidence demonstrating the potential efficacy of education as a strategy for STD control, its importance continues to be stressed. Knowledge is assumed to be a prerequisite of preventive health behavior. Accordingly, among the national STD objectives for 1990 established in 1979 by the U.S. Department of Health and Human Services was that "every junior and high school student in the United States should receive accurate, timely STD education.[27]

### UNPROTECTED EXPOSURES

The use of barrier methods—particularly condoms—appears to offer the greatest potential for reducing the prevalence of STDs. The advantages of the condom over other methods of protection are its

1. Demonstrated effectiveness in preventing STD[28–30]
2. Availability without a prescription or physical examination[31]
3. Relatively low unit cost, which makes it financially accessible to most at-risk persons[30]
4. Absence of unwanted side effects[31]
5. Ease of initiation by either partner[31]

Yet despite the efficacy and safety of the condom as a technique for STD control,[32] estimates of its use by STD clinic patients range only from 3 to 20 percent. In the general male population, condom use does not exceed 25 percent.[28]

While epidemics of genital herpes and AIDS have apparently renewed interest in the condom, certain barriers against its use persist, including:

1. The belief that condom use compromises the pleasure of intercourse[28,33–36]
2. The tendency to view the condom primarily as a contraceptive device rather than as an STD prophylactic[36]
3. The belief that its use is unnatural[33,34]
4. The tendency to underestimate the personal risk of infection present in a situation[28,36,37]
5. The belief that one's partner would be offended if a condom were used[36,38,39]

However, in the Sacramento Special Study, STD clinic patients who cited the most reasons for not using condoms were also the most likely to accept an offer of free condom samples.[33] It appeared that persons most aware of their potential disadvantages were also most informed about their potential benefits.

### TREATMENT BARRIERS

In a study of callers to an STD hotline,[40] self-proclaimed infected and exposed callers expressed concerns that might have hindered their seeking prompt medical assistance. The most common concerns were confidentiality, anxiety about diagnostic and therapeutic procedures, fear of humiliation and being handled with disdain, and concern about the long-term consequences of infection.[40] Many adolescents appear to believe they cannot be treated for STDs without parental consent,[20] and many know their parents would disapprove of their participation in premarital sex. Homosexual men also perceive barriers to using STD treatment facilities,[41] including (1) the need to reveal their sexual orientation[42] and (2) their reluctance to trust their health to public officials who might discriminate against them.[43] Practitioner awareness of the patients' sexual preference is essential to proper diagnosis and management.[41] Nevertheless, anxiety about sexual preference may deter practitioners from approaching the subject and inhibit patients from volunteering such information.

### SOCIAL OBSTACLES

While sociodemographic characteristics have been associated with a variety of health behaviors, the findings have been inconsistent, especially regarding social class (income and education) and race and ethnicity.[44–47] There is also disagreement about whether social characteristics directly contribute to health behaviors or only indirectly affect them through their influence on health beliefs and attitudes and the accessibility of services.[44,48]

Reported cases of syphilis, gonorrhea, and other STDs tend to be concentrated in inner city areas and occur most frequently in unmarried black males and their partners. Often it is assumed that these areas and populations have higher rates of STDs because social controls are weak and promiscuity prevails. However, surveys of adolescent sexual behavior indicate that differences between blacks and whites in sexual activity have narrowed.[49,50]

Differences in health behavior may be more important than differences in sexual behavior in explaining racial and ethnic variability in rates of STD. Teenaged and young adult blacks and Hispanics residing in lower socioeconomic urban areas may be less likely than their more affluent white peers to detect and respond to symptoms, seek prompt and effective medical care, and comply with directions for successful treatment and follow-up. In a study of STD clinic patients in Sacramento, California, conducted in 1971,[51] blacks were more likely than whites to have gonorrhea, and black men with symptoms delayed significantly longer than white men with symptoms before seeking treatment.

STD education directed at social obstacles may have prompted effective behavioral changes in some communities. In a study of patients attending an STD clinic in Columbus, Ohio, blacks sought care sooner after symptom onset than whites.[52] They were also more likely to curtail sexual activity after noticing symptoms. In the survey of public awareness of genital herpes cited earlier,[17] blacks who perceived themselves to be at risk for the disease were more likely than whites to report having changed their behavior in an effort to prevent contracting herpes. Regarding condoms, one study found that white adolescent girls were more likely to express resistance to using condoms than their black peers.[22]

Historically, males have been more willing than females to introduce the use of condoms. In Sacramento, about half as many female as male clinic patients accepted free samples of condoms.[33] In a study of college students in the middle west, women were less likely than men to agree that they did not (or would not) mind using a condom during intercourse.[21] They were also less likely than men to agree that it is acceptable both for a man to carry a condom in his wallet and a woman to carry one in her purse. When the same attitude items were asked of a sample of adolescent girls in Indianapolis, nearly twice as many respondents felt that it was more acceptable for a boy to carry a condom in his wallet than for a girl to carry one in her purse.[22]

Data from a study of undergraduates in California revealed that while both men and women were aware of the importance and favored the use of STD prevention methods, men were more likely to say they favored the use of condoms if they were available at no cost.[39] Interestingly, less favorable attitudes among women toward condom use coexisted with considerably higher levels of knowledge about STDs, suggesting that increasing knowledge does not necessarily overcome attitudinal barriers to preventive behavior. In the same study, respondents were asked to indicate their preference for five different STD prevention methods by ranking them in terms of how they felt about using them. Men rated "selection of partners" highest, followed by "condom," "washing," "abstinence," and "urination after intercourse." Women rated "abstinence" first, followed by "selection of partners," "condom," "washing," and "urination."

## PERSONALITY PROBLEMS

A psychological analysis of personality problems as they relate to STD is presented in Chap. 5. Rather than looking for an association between psychological disorders and contracting or spreading STDs, some researchers have tried to determine whether certain personality traits are associated with a greater tendency to take prophylactic actions. The personality construct most consistently linked to health-promoting behavior is "locus of control"—the extent to which persons perceive events in their lives to be within (or outside of) their personal control. Persons who hold internal expectations are more likely to assume active responsibility for maintaining their health. Presumably "internals" would be more likely than "externals" to practice effective prophylaxis against STDs.

In the Sacramento study, internally oriented clinic patients were not significantly more likely to accept free samples of condoms for gonorrhea prevention.[11] Externals were more responsive to the clinic staff's encouragement to take free samples during the pretest period. Thus, externals seemed more likely than internals to follow the directions of medical authorities. However, externally oriented women were significantly less likely than internally oriented women to return for examinations as requested by clinic staff members.

Some investigators have attempted to identify characteristics that separate persons with a single episode of STD from those with repeat infections. One study found no significant differences between STD clinic patients with and without previous infections.[53] Similarly, another observed no difference between patients attending an STD clinic for repeat infections and those attending for a first infection.[54] In a sample of black men attending an STD clinic, social characteristics, knowledge about gonorrhea, and personality characteristics were associated with number of lifetime infections but not with the number in a 3-month or 1-year period.[55] Other researchers found sociodemographic differences: persons attending an STD clinic for repeat gonorrheal infections were more likely than those with first infections to be younger, male, black, and residents of areas of lower socioeconomic status.[56]

## MODIFICATION OF SEXUAL BEHAVIOR

### HOMOSEXUAL AND BISEXUAL MEN

Although many changes in sexual behavior have been adopted by gay men in response to the AIDS epidemic,[14,57–60], some gay men still engage in high-risk sex practices. A variety of barriers to more widespread adoption of risk-reduction guidelines exist.

#### Gay identity

Some gay men regard participation in certain sex practices (e.g., unprotected anal intercourse and anonymous sex partners) as an expression of their gay identity. In their view, refraining from such practices is tantamount to abnegating their homosexuality and the principles of gay liberation. Their sexual activities represent important social behaviors that integrate them into a community. Changing partners or modifying sex practices may interfere with affiliations and acceptance. Recommendations for "safer sex" may conflict with values derived from years of struggle for the right to choose sexual options without externally imposed constraints.[61]

Early in the AIDS epidemic, some segments of the gay community charged that the labeling by epidemiologists of predominantly homosexual practices (such as anal intercourse) as high-risk behavior was part of an organized effort to suppress homosexual behavior and discredit homosexuality as an acceptable alternative lifestyle. Now the gay community generally acknowledges that certain of their preferred sex practices may legitimately be regarded as more efficient modes of AIDS virus transmission than heterosexually preferred practices. Yet the earlier suspicions remain and reflect the extent to which certain practices are inextricably tied to a homosexual identity for some men.

#### Misperception of risk

In a study of asymptomatic gay men in New York City, about 83 percent of those who engaged in unsafe sex practices probably underestimated the degree of risk for AIDS associated with their behavior despite high levels of awareness of safer sex guidelines.[62]

Although respondents were able to report which practices were generally considered safe and which risky, they were unable to interpret the implications of this knowledge for their own risky behavior.

Because these men perceived themselves to be complying with "safer sex" guidelines that advised them to "know their partners," they felt they had significantly reduced their risk of contracting AIDS. However, given the potentially long incubation period of AIDS, one would have to take an extensive sexual history of a potential partner to realistically assess the risk of infection associated with an unsafe sexual encounter with him; very few men probably ever undertake such an inquiry. (It should be noted that most of the data for this study were gathered before antibody testing for human immunodeficiency virus [HIV], the virus that causes AIDS, became widely available, so few partners of the respondents engaging in risky sex were likely to have known their HIV-antibody status).

These findings are important because a perception of personal vulnerability is generally regarded as a prerequisite to undertaking modifications in behavior to prevent a disease. If gay men engaging in risky practices consistently underestimate the risk associated with their behavior, and by extension their vulnerability to AIDS, they are not likely to change their behavior.

### Discounting risks

Persons create their own health schema or explanatory models to explain why certain people develop an illness or disease.[63] These schema influence their sense of susceptibility and consequently their likelihood of modifying their behavior. For example, two such cognitive schemes were identified in gay men who had persisted in "fast lane" sexual behavior despite the AIDS epidemic.[64]

The first group subscribed to a theory of "the holistic well-being of the human system." They believed that one could defend oneself against infection while engaging in risky practices by maintaining general overall good health through regular visits to a physician, exercise, sufficient sleep, and stress management. While such advice is often promoted and seems to make sense, it does not confer protection if one continues to engage in unsafe sex practices. Gay men must be informed that there is no scientific evidence to support this holistic theory.

The second group held a fatalistic attitude. Some of the men believed those vulnerable to AIDS had a genetic predisposition that could not be altered by behavior. Others believed that the risk of developing diseases like AIDS was endemic to being a homosexual and represented risks unavoidable to men participating in a gay lifestyle. Evidence of the long incubation period for AIDS contributed to this sense of fatalism. Some men have reasoned that because the incubation period might be 7 or more years, they were probably already infected; or if they had avoided infection, they presumed they probably possessed a natural immunity to HIV.

## HETEROSEXUAL MEN AND WOMEN

Most cases of AIDS in heterosexuals and infants in the United States have been traced to intravenous (IV)-drug use.[65] Women infected with HIV through needle sharing or by heterosexual exposure can in turn infect their children perinatally. About 79 percent of pediatric AIDS cases occur in families in which one or both parents have AIDS or are at increased risk for developing it because of IV-drug use.[66] Preventing the spread of HIV infection through needle sharing and by unprotected sexual exposures with IV-drug users is critical to slowing the epidemic.

## IV-DRUG USERS

Research on IV-drug users has focused on needle sharing to a greater extent than on sexual behavior. While some modifications in behavior have occurred, a very substantial proportion of IV-drug users continue to engage in activities that can result in HIV transmission. Of 261 IV-drug-user respondents from a methadone maintenance program and a major detention facility in New York City, 48 percent reported in 1986 they had not changed their sexual behavior in response to the threat of AIDS.[67] Of those who did report changes, 5 percent reported becoming monogamous or celibate, while 14 percent indicated using condoms or adopting other hygienic measures, such as washing before or after sex. (Although some "safer sex" guidelines recommend showering before or after sex, such activities probably confer no protection against HIV infection if one engages in risky sex practices).

The paucity of data on the sexual behavior of IV-drug users makes it difficult to identify barriers to change. Unlike gay men, IV-drug users are not a formally organized community; thus, it is difficult to reach them and educate them about the necessity of practicing prevention. While many IV-drug users can be identified through substance-abuse programs and the criminal justice system, some are not regular users of drugs and cannot be reached through these channels. Also, many IV-drug users support their habits through prostitution, and adopting condom use might communicate a fear of contracting (or transmitting) AIDS to potential clients.

### Vulnerability

While bidirectional transmission of HIV has been demonstrated,[68,69] most heterosexuals probably perceive themselves at very low risk of becoming infected. A tendency to underestimate the degree to which one is at risk of experiencing negative events, including contracting or dying from a variety of diseases,[70–72] helps avoid the anxiety accompanying a realistic appraisal of susceptibility.[73] Negative events within the person's control are particularly subject to "unrealistic optimism"[71,72] because in assessing their own risks, persons are likely to recall the precautions they undertook to avoid an event, while assuming that others undertook fewer preventive actions.

Persons also evaluate their risks of experiencing a negative life event by employing stereotypes (the "representativeness" heuristic[74]). That is, people tend to have a preconception of the typical person who experiences a particular kind of negative outcome—such as acquiring an STD. They appraise their own vulnerability based on their evaluation of how much or little they resemble their mental representation. Because the victims they imagine tend to be stereotypes, they generally judge themselves to be very different and therefore at low risk. This attitude provides another reason for public health campaigns to break down traditional stereotypes of the persons who acquire STDs and more recent stereotypes of persons at risk for AIDS.

### Negotiations

Because of the interpersonal nature of sexual intercourse, decisions to engage in or refrain from risky sex practices must be

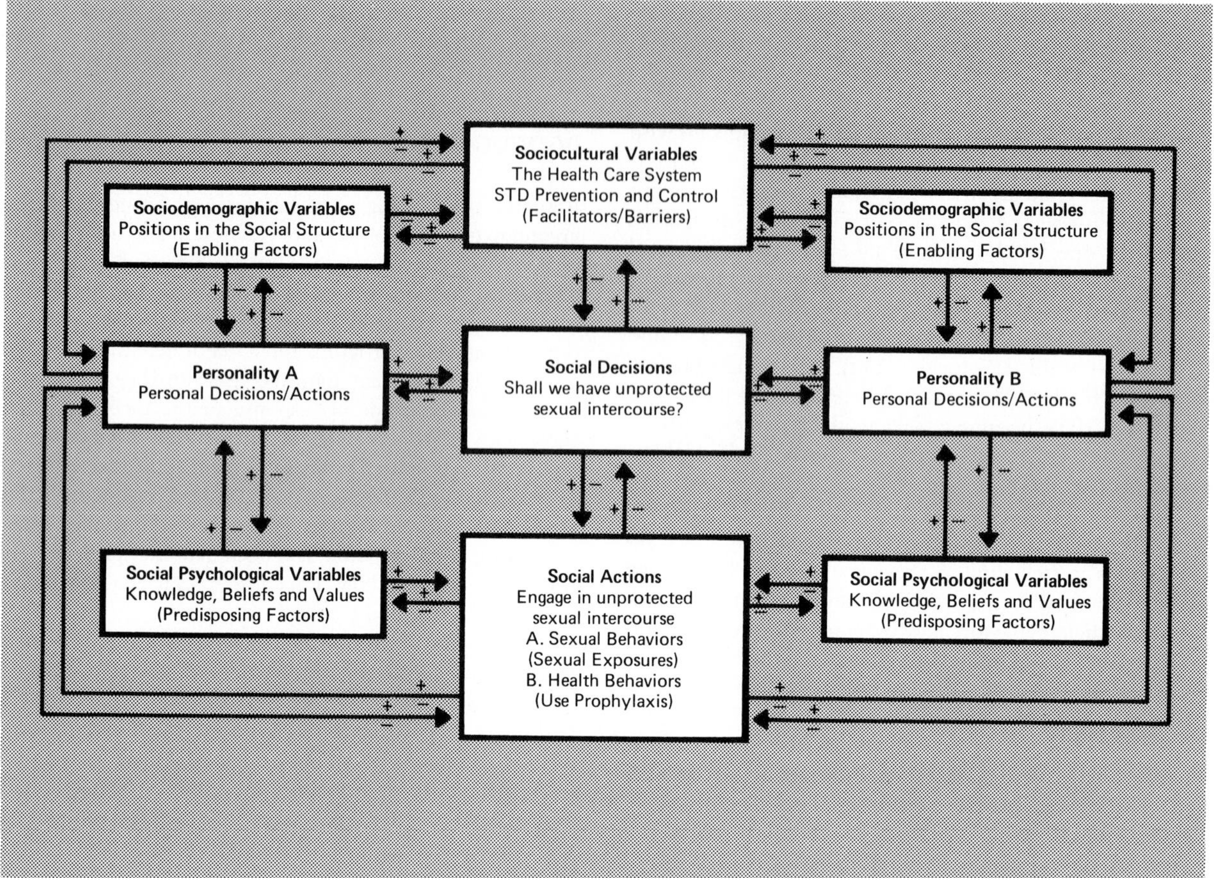


**Fig. 9-1.** A conceptual model of the relationships among sociocultural variables, sociodemographic variables, social-psychological variables, and health behaviors designed to prevent sexually transmitted diseases.

"negotiated." To practice safe sex effectively, both partners must agree on limits or to use condoms whenever the opportunity for the exchange of possibly infectious semen or blood exists. One partner who is not motivated to practice safer sex may not cooperate with the other partner, may undercut the other partner's resolve, or may refuse to use condoms properly. Social skills in resolving these problems must be learned.

## A CONCEPTUAL MODEL OF SEXUAL DECISIONS

The conceptual model shown in Fig. 9-1 indicates that sexual decision making occurs in the context of a sociocultural system. The sociocultural system that persons live in includes facilitators and barriers to health behavior that may affect different members of society differently. Thus, both positive and negative influences affect various persons who must make certain decisions and take actions, and most importantly, a specific decision and course of action that is central to the topic of this chapter, "Shall we have unprotected sexual intercourse?"

The conceptual model begins at the broadest level of social behavior to show that the prevention and early detection of STDs must be considered in the context of a changing society and an evolving sociocultural system. Actions and decisions regarding policies aimed at controlling and eventually eradicating STDs emerge out of a sociopolitical process influenced by many factors, including the prejudices of influential interest groups.[75,76] Different diseases are regarded differently by different social groups.[77] The dimensions of good and evil, clean and dirty, and socially acceptable and unacceptable will direct national and local interests, govern the distribution of resources, and limit the kinds of interventions that community leaders will tolerate and public agencies can implement at the local level.

The conceptual model also suggests that the differential placement of persons into various statuses and their accompanying roles channels their choices and affects their actions. For example, a 45-year-old executive will have more resources at his or her disposal to prevent STD than an 18-year-old high school student. However, these two statuses could be occupied by the same person during a lifetime.

Just as important as the structural variables that serve to facilitate or impede certain responses are the sociopsychologic variables that promote or deter certain responses and change over time. Similar structural and social psychologic variables may affect different persons differently; so the model requires that at least two persons be present. Person A must take into account the actions of person B, and vice versa. Each will presumably try to make rational decisions based on available information. Each will weigh the possible benefits of doing something against the attendant risks, sometimes deciding more carefully and proceeding more cautiously than at others.[78]

Most decision-making models for health-protective behavior have been constructed with one person, not a couple, in mind.[16,79] A counterproposal maintains that public health models for intervention should treat the community as the patient[80] and that prevailing sociocultural conditions, not risk takers, should be changed.[81] The model suggests that different units of analysis be studied at different levels of conceptualization. At the broadest level, the sociocultural environment is the proper unit of analysis. At the narrowest level, the individual risk taker is the appropriate subject. In the final analysis, the dyad should be selected as the most suitable unit, and those factors that influence sociosexual exchanges must be critically examined.

Central to the conceptual model is the interpersonal level of analysis where a specific question must be answered by the couple: "Shall we have unprotected sex?" Investigations have consistently shown that it is very easy to increase knowledge about STD in various groups; it is more difficult to alter attitudes (especially in high-risk groups), and it is most difficult to change behaviors. Few behavior-modification efforts have seriously attempted to define and measure behavioral objectives[82] or to employ the promising strategies of social learning or operant conditioning. Most importantly, none have accepted the fact that persons must take into account the behaviors of potential sex partners when they try to protect themselves from acquiring STDs. Although inexperienced teenagers may know that gonorrhea is spread by sexual intercourse, believe that condoms prevent STDs, and place a high value on their reproductive capacity in marriage, they may still have unprotected sex and subsequently develop gonococcal salpingitis because they are unable to convince their partners to use condoms properly. Our conceptual model calls for more systematic research at the interpersonal as well as personal level of behavior.

Finally, the model considers two different aspects of the crucial question regarding health behaviors and STD. STD can be prevented either by avoiding sexual exposures with infected partners or by properly using safe and effective prophylactic products (including immunizing agents). Thus, two messages should be delivered to the couple considering sexual intercourse: (1) Don't have sexual intercourse if either is infected with an STD and (2) if you have any doubts about infectiousness, don't have sex unless you properly use a safe and effective prophylactic agent. Since it is difficult to determine whether a person is infectious and the use-effectiveness of available prophylactics remains uncertain,[83] the ambiguity of these messages to couples considering unprotected sexual intercourse is confusing. The messages the public health community sends out to adolescents and young adults, and their interpretations of those messages, should be among the principal topics of future research.

## References


1 Kasl SV, Cobb S: Health behavior, illness behavior and sick role behavior, I: Health and illness behavior. *Arch Environ Health* 12:246, 1966.

2 Cates W: Priorities for sexually transmitted diseases in the late 1980s and beyond. *Sex Transm Dis* 13:114, 1986.

3 Rosenstock IM: Prevention of illness and maintenance of health, in *Poverty and Health*, J Kosa et al (eds). Cambridge, Harvard University Press, 1969.

4 Janz NK, Becker MH: The health belief model: A decade later. *Health Educ Q* 11:1, 1984.

5 Kasl SV: A social psychological perspective on successful community control of high blood pressure. *J Behav Med* 1:347, 1978.

6 Dishman R: Compliance/adherence in health-related exercise. *Health Psychol* 1:237, 1982.

7 Kirscht JP: Preventive health behavior: A review of research and issues. *Health Psychol* 2:277, 1983.

8 Cummings KM et al: Bringing the models together: An empirical approach to combining variables used to explain health actions. *J Behav Med* 3:123, 1980.

9 Simon KH, Das A: An application of the health belief model toward educational diagnosis of VD education. *Health Educ Q* 11:403, 1984.

10 Becker MH (ed): The health belief model and personal health. *Health Educ Monogr* 2:324, 1974.

11 Darrow WW: Innovative Health Behavior. Doctoral dissertation, Emory University, Department of Sociology, Atlanta, GA, 1973.

12 Freidson E: *The Profession of Medicine*. New York, Dodd Mead, 1970.

13 Brandt AM: *No Magic Bullet: A Social History of Venereal Diseases in the United States since 1880*. New York, Oxford University Press, 1985.

14 Siegel K, Bauman LB: Sexual behavior among gay men in New York City. Paper presented at the annual meeting of the American Sociological Association, New York City, August 1986.

15 Parsons T: Social structure and dynamic processes: The case of modern medical practice, in *The Social System*, T Parsons (ed). Glencoe, IL, Free Press, 1951.

16 Baric L: Recognition of the "at-risk" role: A means of influence health behavior. *Int J Health Educ* 12:24, 1969.

17 Aral SO et al: Genital herpes: Does knowledge lead to action? *Am J Public Health* 75:69, 1985.

18 Menzies HD: Back to a basic contraceptive. *New York Times*, Section 3, Jan 5, 1986.

19 Kessler II: Human cervical cancer as a venereal disease. *Cancer Res* 36:783, 1976.

20 Armonker RG: What do teens know about the facts of life? *J School Health* 50:527, 1980.

21 Yarber WL, Williams CE: Venereal disease prevention and a selected group of college students. *J Am Vener Dis Assoc* 2:17, 1975.

22 Yarber YL: Teenage girls and venereal disease prophylaxis. *Br J Vener Dis* 53:135, 1977.

23 Benell F: Drug abuse and venereal disease misconceptions of a selected group of college students. *J School Health* 43:584, 1973.

24 Price JH et al: High school students' perceptions and misperceptions about AIDS. *J School Health* 55:107, 1985.

25 DiClemente RJ et al: Adolescents and AIDS: A survey of knowledge, attitudes and beliefs about AIDS in San Francisco. *Am J Public Health* 76:1443, 1986.

26 Kroger F, Wiesner PJ: STD education: Challenge for the 80s. *J School Health* 51:242, 1981.

27 Parra WC, Cates W: Progress toward the 1990 objectives for sexually transmitted diseases: Good news and bad. *Public Health Rep* 100:261, 1985.

28 Hart G: Role of preventive methods in the control of venereal disease. *Clin Obstet Gynecol* 18:243, 1975.

29 Curran JW: Prevention of sexually transmitted disease, in *Sexually Transmitted Diseases*, KK Holmes et al (eds). New York, McGraw-Hill, 1984.

30 Stone KM et al: Personal protection against sexually transmitted diseases. *Am J Obstet Gynecol* 155:180, 1986.

31 Felman YM: A plea for the condom, especially for teenagers. *JAMA* 241:2517, 1979.

32 Conant M et al: Condoms prevent transmission of AIDS-associated retrovirus. *JAMA* 255:1706, 1986.

33 Darrow WW: Attitudes toward condom use and the acceptance of venereal disease prophylactics, In *The Condom: Increasing Utilization in the United States*, MH Redford et al (eds). San Francisco, CA, San Francisco Press, 1974, p 173.

34 Felman YM, Santora FJ: The use of condoms by VD clinic patients: A survey. *Cutis* 27:330, 1981.

35 Condoms. *Consumer Rep* 44:583, 1979.

36 Arnold CB: The sexual behavior of inner city adolescent condom users. *J Sex Res* 8:298, 1972.

37 Wittkower ED, Cowan J: Some psychological aspects of promiscuity. *Psychosom Med* 6:287, 1944.

38 Fiumara NJ: Effectiveness of condoms in preventing venereal disease. *Med Aspects Hum Sex* 6:146, 1972.

39 Yacenda JA: Knowledge and attitudes of college students about venereal disease and its prevention. *Health Serv Rep* 89:170, 1974.

40 Knox SR et al: Profile of callers to the VD national hotline. *Sex Transm Dis* 8:245, 1981.

41 Ostrow DG, Altman NL: Sexually transmitted diseases and homosexuality. *Sex Transm Dis* 10:208, 1983.

42 Felman Y, Morrison J: Examining the homosexual man for sexually transmitted diseases. *JAMA* 238:2046, 1977.

43 Judson F et al: Screening for gonorrhea and syphilis in the gay baths—Denver, Colorado. *Am J Public Health* 71:989, 1981.

44 Rosenstock IM: The health belief model and preventive health behavior. *Health Educ Monogr* 2:354, 1974.

45 Coburn D, Pope CR: Socioeconomic status and preventive health behavior. *J Health Soc Behav* 15:67, 1974.

46 Slesinger DP et al: The effects of social characteristics on the utilization of preventive medical services in contrasting health care programs. *Med Care* 14:392, 1976.

47 McCusker J, Morrow GR: Factors related to use of cancer early detection techniques. *Prev Med* 9:388, 1980.

48 Rosenstock IM: Why people use health services. *Milbank Mem Fund Q* 44:104, 1966.

49 Zelnick M, Kanter JF: Sexual activity, contraceptive use and pregnancy among metropolitan area teenagers: 1972–1979. *Fam Plann Perspect* 12:230, 1980.

50 O'Reilly KR, Aral SO: Adolescence and sexual behavior: Trends and implications for STD. *J Adolesc Health Care* 6:262, 1985.

51 Darrow WW: Venereal infections in three ethnic groups in Sacramento. *Am J Public Health* 66:446, 1976.

52 Kramer MA et al: Self-reported behavior patterns of patients attending a sexually transmitted disease clinic. *Am J Public Health* 70:997, 1980.

53 Hayes J, Prokop CK: Sociopsychiatric characteristics of clinic patrons with repeat gonorrhea infections. *J Am Vener Dis Assoc* 3:43, 1976.

54 Pedder JR, Goldberg DP: A survey by questionnaire of psychiatric disturbance in patients attending a venereal diseases clinic. *Br J Vener Dis* 46:58, 1970.

55 Glass LJ: An analysis of some characteristics of males with gonorrhea. *Br J Vener Dis* 43:128, 1967.

56 Brooks GF et al: Repeat gonorrhea: An analysis of importance and risk factors. *J Infect Dis* 137:161, 1978.

57 McKusick L et al: Reported changes in sexual behavior by men in San Francisco, 1982–1984—The AIDS behavioral research project. *Public Health Rep* 100:622, 1985.

58 Research and Decisions Corporation: Designing an effective AIDS prevention campaign strategy for San Francisco: Results from the second probability sample of an urban gay male community. San Francisco, CA, San Francisco AIDS Foundation, 1985.

59 Feldman DA: AIDS health promotion and clinically applied anthropology, in *The Social Dimensions of AIDS: Method and Theory,* DA Feldman, TM Johnson (eds). New York, Praeger, 1986, p 145.

60 Centers for Disease Control: Self-reported changes in sexual behaviors among homosexual and bisexual men from the San Francisco cohort. *MMWR* 36:187, 1987.

61 McKusick L et al: The AIDS epidemic: A model for developing intervention strategies for reducing high risk behavior in gay men. *Sex Transm Dis* 12:229, 1985.

62 Bauman LJ, Siegel K: Misperception among gay men of the risk for AIDS associated with their sexual behavior. *J Appl Soc Psychol* 17:329, 1987.

63 Morgan DL, Spanish MT: Social interaction and the cognitive organization of health-relevant knowledge. *Soc Health Illness* 7:401, 1985.

64 Kotarba JA, Lang NG: Gay lifestyle change and AIDS: Preventive health care, in *The Social Dimensions of AIDS: Methods and Theory,* DA Feldman, TM Johnson (eds). New York, Praeger, 1986, p 127.

65 DesJarlais DC, Friedman SR: HIV infection among intravenous drug users: Epidemiology and risk reduction. *AIDS* 1:67, 1987.

66 Centers for Disease Control: Update: Acquired immunodeficiency syndrome—United States. *MMWR* 35:757, 1986.

67 Selwyn PA et al: Knowledge about AIDS and high-risk behavior among intravenous drug abusers in New York City. *AIDS* 1:247, 1987.

68 Redfield R et al: Heterosexually acquired HTLV-III/LAV disease (AIDS-related complex and AIDS): Epidemiologic evidence for female-to-male transmission. *JAMA* 254:2094, 1985.

69 Calabrese LH, Gopalakrishna KV: Transmission of HTLV-III infection from man to woman to man. *N Engl J Med* 314:987, 1986.

70 Slovic et al: Cognitive processes and societal risk taking, in *Cognition and Social Behavior,* JS Carroll, JW Payne (eds). Hillsdale, NJ, Erlbaum, 1976.

71 Weinstein ND: Unrealistic optimism about future events. *J Pers Soc Psychol* 39:806, 1980.

72 Weinstein ND: Why it didn't happen to me: Perceptions of risk factors and susceptibility. *Health Psychol* 3:431, 1984.

73 Perloff LS: Social comparisons and illusions of invulnerability to negative life events, in *Clinical Social Psychological Perspectives on Negative Life Events,* CR Snyder, C Ford (eds). New York, Plenum, in press.

74 Tversky A, Kahneman D: Judgment under uncertainty: Heuristics and biases. *Science* 185:1124, 1974.

75 Kristein MM et al: Health economics and preventive care. *Science* 195:457, 1977.

76 Polonoff DB, Garland MJ: Oregon's premarital blood test. *Hastings Cent Rep* 9:5, 1979.

77 Jenkins CD, Zyzanski SJ: Dimensions of belief and feeling regarding three diseases. *Behav Sci* 13:372, 1968.

78 Luker K: *Taking Chances.* Berkeley, University of California Press, 1975.

79 Warnecke RB et al: Social and psychological correlates of smoking behavior among black women. *J Health Soc Behav* 19:397, 1978.

80 Barry PZ: Individual versus community orientation in the prevention of injuries. *Prev Med* 4:47, 1975.

81 Brown ER, Margo GE: Health education: Can the reformers be reformed? *Int J Health Serv* 8:3, 1978.

82 Bandura A: *Principles of Behavior Modification.* New York, Holt, Rinehart and Winston, 1969.

83 Harrison WO: Prophylaxis against gonorrhea. *Milit Med* 146:9, 1981.

# PART IV STRUCTURE, PHYSIOLOGY, AND EXAMINATION OF THE NORMAL GENITALIA

Chapter 10

# Anatomy and physical examination of the male genital tract

Daniel O. Graney
John N. Krieger

## INTRODUCTION

Any area of the body may be involved in sexually transmitted disease syndromes or in the differential diagnosis of these conditions. Clearly there is no single, optimal method for conducting the history and physical examination. The critical areas of interest are determined by the history, other physical findings, and conditions considered in the differential diagnosis. There are as many correct ways of eliciting historical data and physical findings as there are clinicians. Similarly, there are many critical anatomical points that may be important in some contexts yet irrelevant in others. Thus, this chapter reflects our bias and represents an attempt to succinctly present one approach to "the routine examination." Pertinent genitourinary tract anatomy will be presented in the context of this examination. This approach is selective in the extreme, but it is based on our own clinical experience in developing an efficient method for evaluating a large number of patients in a timely manner.

Most often, the standard examination of a patient in our clinic proceeds according to an orderly sequence. The pertinent portions of the examination usually follow the outline in Table 10-1. Proceeding in this fashion has two advantages. First, there is an orderly sequence to the examination that limits the opportunity for errors of omission in a busy clinical situation. Second, there is a minimal need for the patient to move. Ordinarily, we initiate the examination by having the patient sit on the examining table. If necessary, head and neck examination and percussion and auscultation of the chest may be done in this position. Next, the patient is asked to lie supine. Cardiovascular examination may be conducted in this position, if indicated, and attention is directed to the abdominal examination. The patient is then asked to stand for examination of the groin and genitalia. Finally, the patient is asked to turn and bend over, placing his elbows on the examining table, for the rectal and prostate examination. In sum, there is minimal need for the patient to move from position to position if the examination is done in this order.

The remainder of this chapter is organized to follow this suggested pattern of evaluation. The relevant considerations in routine examination of the male are presented for each section of the physical examination, and critical anatomical principles are considered for that area. Throughout, we emphasize a practical approach and minimize use of Latin terms. This means that we present the anatomy according to our own opinions, recognizing that some of these opinions are controversial and that other anatomists and/or clinicians may hold alternative, equally valid, viewpoints.

There are two major differences in anatomy and examination between male and female patients. First, in the male we are talking about genitourinary tract examination. In the female there is a urinary tract and a separate genital tract. These two functions are combined in the male lower genitourinary tract, in which the urethra serves as a common conduit for the excretory functions of the urinary tract and for the reproductive functions of delivery of semen. The second major difference is that the critical reproductive organs in the male are all easily palpable. In contrast, the reproductive organs in the female are located in the pelvis and therefore may be examined less readily than the comparable structures in the male. The clinical implication is that examination of the male lower urinary tract and the entire male genital tract is readily accomplished and is straightforward in most patients.

**Table 10-1. Routine STD Examination of the Male**

- General appearance
- Skin
- Abdominal examination
- Groin
  - Hernia
  - Adenopathy
- Genitalia
  - Penis
    - Prepuce
    - Urethral meatus
    - Shaft
  - Scrotum
    - Testis
    - Vas
    - Epididymis
- Rectal examination
  - Tone
  - Fissure, hemorrhoids, or mass lesions
  - Prostate examination
- Laboratory studies
  - Stool guaiac
  - Urethral smear
  - Urinalysis
  - Other

## EXAMINATION OF THE ABDOMEN AND GROIN

### ABDOMEN

Complete details of the abdominal examination are beyond the scope of this chapter. However, brief mention is necessary of the pelvic organs, specifically the urinary bladder. This may be distended in patients with bladder outflow obstruction caused by an enlarged prostate or urethral stricture, and occasionally in patients with neurological dysfunction, as may occur with herpetic infections. The normal bladder is not palpable or percussible when it is empty or nearly empty because of its location in the pelvis. As the volume increases to approximately 125 to 150 ml, the dome of the bladder rises out of the pelvis into the lower abdomen and may project above the symphysis pubis. As it continues to fill, the bladder rises progressively toward the umbilicus. When the bladder contains 400 ml or more, it may be identifiable by observation as a bulge in the lower abdomen. Percussion over a distended bladder may cause the patient to experience a desire to void and may result in a change of the normal resonance of the lower abdomen on percussion to a dull note. The distended bladder may be palpated as a firm, round, and tender mass in the lower abdomen.

## GROIN

The groin, or inguinal region, should be examined for the presence of adenopathy while the patient is lying supine on the examining table. The patient is then asked to stand and the inguinal area is again examined for the presence of hernia by direct palpation of the area and again by insertion of the index finger through the neck of the scrotum following the spermatic cord. Both examinations are done with the patient standing quietly and again while he is straining.

## GENITALIA

## PENIS

### Examination

It is critical that the clinic staff instruct patients to refrain from voiding, if at all possible, prior to examination because signs of urethritis may not be apparent if the patient has recently voided. In fact, in symptomatic patients who do not have objective evidence of urethritis on examination or on the urethral smear, it is our practice to repeat the examination prior to the first urination of the day. Initially, attention is directed to examination of the skin. Use of a good light source and a hand lens is strongly recommended. In patients undergoing evaluation for condylomata or sexual contacts of patients with condylomata, including women with dysplasia or carcinoma of the cervix, an acid "wash" is applied after the initial evaluation. This is done by soaking gauze pads in 3 to 5% acetic acid. The gauze is then applied to the skin of the scrotum and penis and left in place for 5 min prior to repeating the examination. This examination should be carried out with use of magnification looking for "flat warts."

Attention is then directed to examination of the penis. In uncircumcised patients, the foreskin should be retracted to rule out phimosis with an obstructing small opening. This maneuver may reveal balanitis, condylomata, and, occasionally, tumor, as the cause of a foul discharge. The glans and inner surface of the foreskin should be inspected to rule out presence of ulcers, vesicles, or warts. The location of the meatus is determined and the urethra is examined for presence of spontaneous discharge. If the location of the urethral meatus is abnormal, it can usually be found by following the midline along the undersurface of the penis. This is the most common location for an abnormal orifice and is termed *hypospadias*. Hypospadias is associated with a prepuce that does not completely encircle the glans but is incomplete on the lower surface. This is commonly termed a "hooded prepuce." Patients with more severe degrees of hypospadias, in which the urethral opening is located at the base of the penis or on the perineum, often have bifid, or split, scrotums. Rarely, the location of the urethral meatus may be on the upper surface of the phallus, a condition termed *epispadias*. In either hypospadias or epispadias, there is apt to be chordee, or an abnormal curvature of the phallus. Partial or complete duplication of the urethra may be noted. Commonly, patients with urethral duplications who present with urethritis have involvement of the accessory urethral meatus. The urethral meatus is examined by pinching the glans between the thumb and the forefinger at the 6 and 12 o'clock positions. This is important to exclude presence of meatal stenosis or intraurethral lesions, such as condylomata.

The shaft of the penis is palpated, looking for firm fibrosis plaques (characteristic of Peyronie's disease) and the urethra is palpated for evidence of induration. Induration is often secondary to infection, stricture (or scarring), or, rarely, tumor, abscess, or foreign body inserted by the patient. At this point, the urethra should be "milked" or stripped, beginning at the bulbous urethra (located at the perineal body, behind the scrotum in the midline) and proceeding to the meatus. This is necessary for evaluation for urethritis and may result in an expression of discharge at the meatus.

### Anatomy

**Major Divisions.** There are two parts of the penis, the base, which is attached to the pubis, and the pendular portion. Underlying the penile skin there are three cavernous erectile bodies, the paired corpora cavernosa that are primarily concerned with erection, and the corpus spongiosum which contains the urethra. These erectile bodies are separate structures at the base of the penis but become bound by fascia along the shaft of the penis (Fig. 10-1). The corpora cavernosa are cylindrical bodies in the shaft region but taper markedly at the base where they attach to the pubic ramus and perineal membrane. The corpus spongiosum has three parts; beginning at the perineum these are the bulb of the penis, the spongy portion, and the glans at the tip of the penis.

The base and proximal portion of the penile shaft are covered by thin muscles (Fig. 10-1). The paired ischiocavernosus muscles overlie the crura and corpora cavernosa. Another pair of muscles, the bulbospongiosus, overlies the corpus spongiosum.

**Urethra and Glans.** The urethra is named according to the part of the penis that it is traversing. Thus, in the penis the urethra is divided into bulbous, spongy, and glandular portions. The bulbous and spongy parts of the urethra are lined by a pseudostratified columnar epithelium, except at the tip of the penis, termed the *fossa navicularis*, which is lined by stratified squamous epithelium. The epithelium contains small acini of mucous cells (glands of Littré) as well as mucosal and submucosal glands termed *urethral* or *periurethral glands* (Figs. 10-2 and 10-3). These glands become infected and form abscesses.

On the superior surface of the corona of the glans penis, as well as on the undersurface near the frenulum, there are sebaceous glands, the glands of Tyson. These glands secrete a white cheesy type of material which with desquamating epithelial cells forms the smegma, a substance that accumulates between the prepuce and glans of uncircumcised men.

## SCROTUM

### Examination

**Skin.** The scrotum and its contents are examined next. Palpation of the scrotal skin may reveal small sebaceous cysts. These structures may be multiple and, on occasion, become quite large or develop infections. Malignant tumors of the scrotum are rare. In contrast, scrotal hemangiomas, bluish, vascular malformations, are common, and they may bleed spontaneously or following sexual activity. After the skin and subcutaneous tissues of the scrotum and perineum have been palpated, attention is directed to the intrascrotal contents.

**Scrotal Compartments.** The scrotum has two compartments which are divided in the midline. Each side is the mirror image of the other, and an identical examination is carried out for each

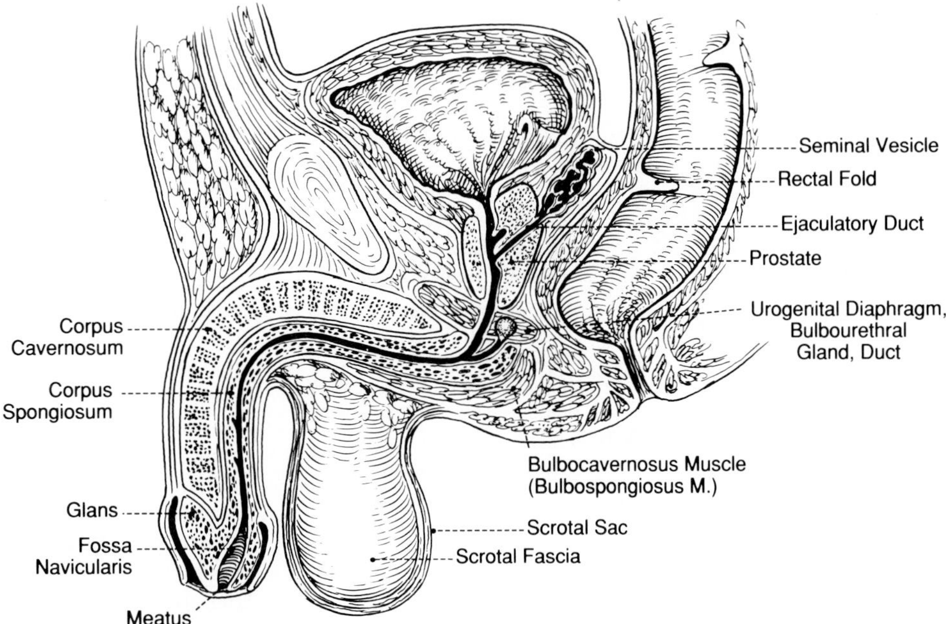


**Fig. 10-1.** Sagittal section of pelvis and male reproductive system.

scrotal compartment. The testis is the most anterior intrascrotal structure and must be examined carefully. The second most important structure in the scrotum is the epididymis, which lies immediately posterior to the testis.

**Testis.** Each testis should be palpated using two hands. Hard areas within the testicular parenchyma must be regarded as potentially malignant until proved otherwise. Testicular tumors are the most common genital urinary tract malignancy in men 20 to

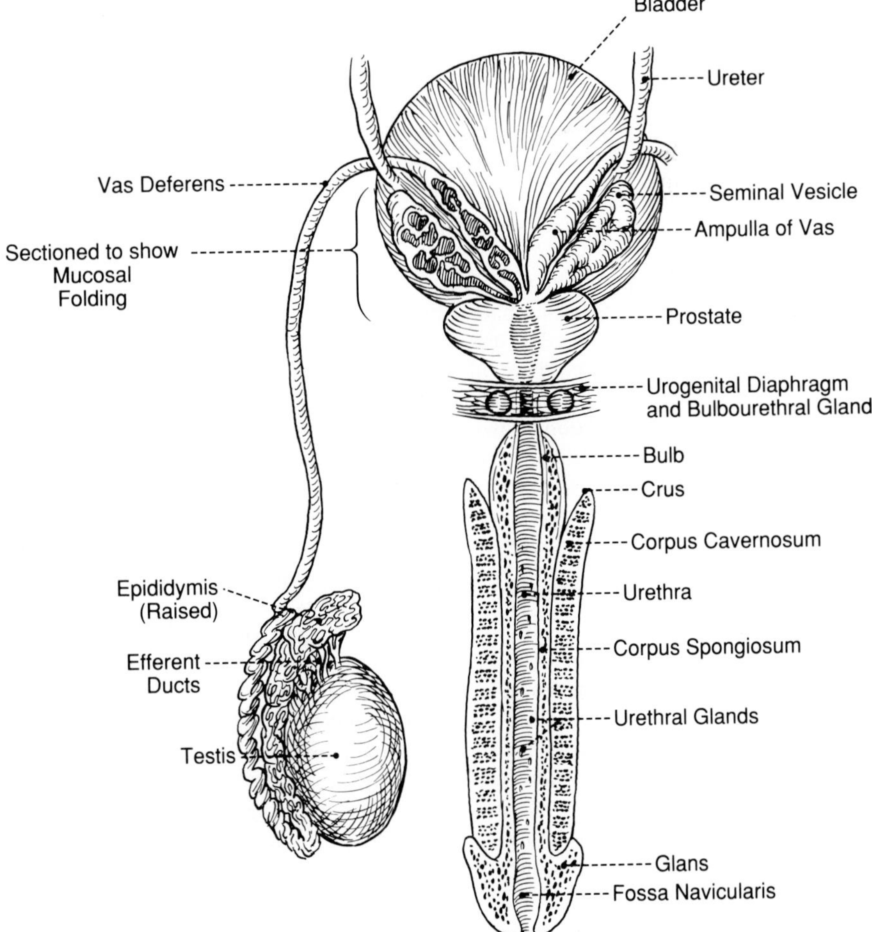


**Fig. 10-2.** Coronal section of male pelvis and urethra viewed posteriorly.

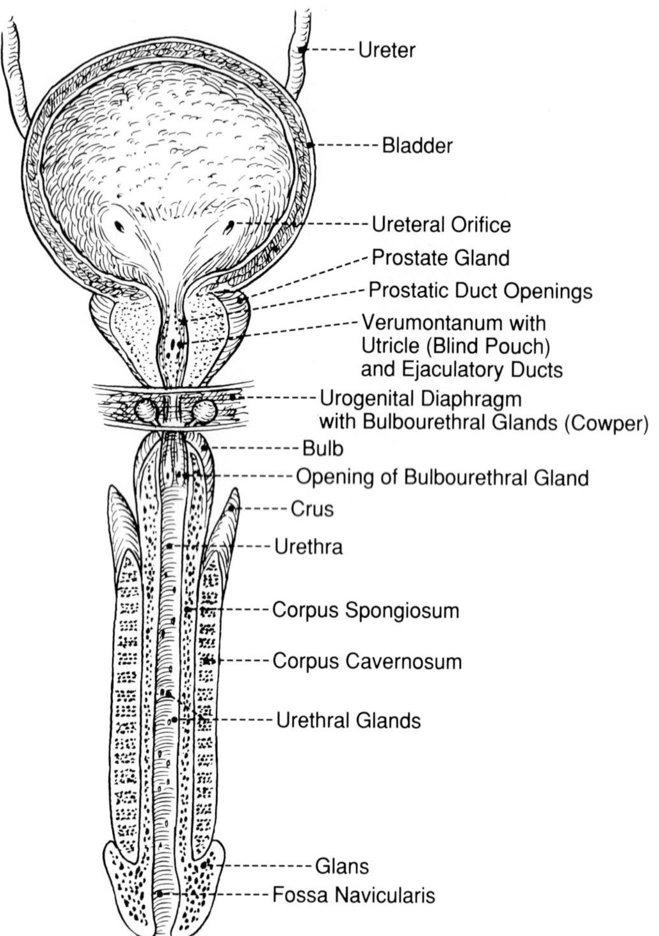


Fig. 10-3. Coronal section of male pelvis and urethra viewed anteriorly.

40 years old. Transillumination of all scrotal masses should be routine. The patient is placed in a dark room and a strong light is applied to the back of the scrotum. Light is transmitted well through benign cystic structures, such as hydroceles or spermatoceles, but not through solid mass lesions, such as testicular tumors. Tumors may be nodular in consistency but are often smooth. The testis that has been replaced by tumor or damaged by a gumma is often insensitive to pressure, and the usual sick sensation produced by firm pressure on the testis is absent. The testis may be absent from the scrotum as a result of maldescent during development, a condition known as *cryptorchidism,* or as the result of abnormal mobility within the scrotal sac and inguinal ring, a condition known as *retractile testis.* An atrophic testis is small and flabby in consistency and may be hypersensitive. This may be congenital; following treatment of an undescended testes; the result of previous infection, such as mumps orchitis; or may follow torsion or previous surgery, such as hernia repair. Although sperm production may not occur in these organs, hormone production may continue. Very small (1.5 × 1 × 1 cm), abnormally firm testes in a young adult usually are attributable to Klinefelter's syndrome, a relatively common condition present in 0.2 percent of men and is usually associated with infertility. Klinefelter's syndrome is associated with one Y and two X chromosomes. On occasion, the testis may twist within the scrotum, compromising its blood supply. This is termed *testicular torsion* and is one cause of acute scrotal pain and swelling.

**Epididymis.** The epididymis is a comma-shaped organ, that is usually applied closely to the posterior aspect of the testis. On occasion, however, the epididymis may be loosely applied to the testis. The epididymis should be carefully palpated for size, tenderness, and induration. Induration of the epididymis usually results from infection, as primary epididymal tumors are rare. It is often possible to feel the groove between the testis and the epididymis everywhere except superiorly, where the two structures are joined. During acute infections, the testis and epididymis are often indistinguishable, as both structures are involved in the inflammatory process. Tenderness is exquisite; swelling may be impressive and accompanied by an acute inflammatory hydrocele. In many men a small, ovoid mass, representing the appendix testis, a vestigial embryological structure, may be palpated near the groove between the upper pole of the testis and the epididymis. Occasionally, the appendix testis may twist, producing acute tenderness and swelling of the scrotum.

**Spermatic Cord.** The cord structures at the neck of the scrotum should be palpated between the thumb and index finger. The solid, ropelike vas is usually identified easily and may be followed to its junction with the tail of the epididymis. Other soft, stringy structures in the spermatic cord may be palpable but are usually not clearly defined. Swellings in the cord are usually cystic in nature (e.g., hydrocele or hernia) and are rarely solid (e.g., connective tissue tumor). Varicoceles represent collections of dilated veins, are usually present on the left side of the scrotum, are best demonstrated with the patient standing, and feel "like a bag of worms."

## Anatomy

**Testis.** The testis fulfills two main functions: it produces sperm and it secretes male hormones. Production of sperm takes place in the seminiferous tubules, whereas the production of testosterone, the major male hormone, takes place in the tissue located between the tubules. Each testis contains approximately 400 to 600 seminiferous tubules. Individual tubules are up to 70 cm in length and are coiled along most of their length in order to be accommodated in a fascial compartment of the testis. These compartments are extensions of the outer fibrous capsule of the testis, the tunica albuginea. The seminiferous tubules join to form the rete testis, which is the connection to the excretory duct system. The lining of the seminiferous tubules contains two main types of cells, the developing sperm cells and the Sertoli cells, which support and presumably "nurse" the sperm cells during their development process. Sperm are continuously produced in the testis from puberty to senility following an orderly sequence of events. In the testis this process takes about 64 days. However, when they leave the testis, the sperm cells are immature and are unable to fertilize an egg.

**Excretory Ducts.** The excretory ducts transport sperm from the testis to the end of the male reproductive tract. The excretory ducts are composed of five elements, beginning from the testis: the efferent ducts, epididymis, vas, ejaculatory duct, and urethra.

*Efferent ducts.* There are approximately twelve efferent ducts, which are convoluted tubules connecting the rete testis to the epididymis. The epithelium lining the ductules contains both ciliated and nonciliated cells. Ciliary movement helps propel sperm toward the epididymis. On electron microscopy, the nonciliated cells are found to be lined by tall microvilli. Surrounding the epithelium is a thin basal lamina, lamina propria, and smooth muscle fibers oriented circularly.

*Epididymis.* The epididymis receives the sperm and seminal fluid from each of the efferent ducts. The epididymis has three parts, the head, the body, and the tail. The initial segment of the epididymis is the head which fuses with the efferent ductules. The epididymis continues inferiorly along the posterior surface of the testis as the body of the epididymis (Fig. 10-2). At the inferior pole of the testis the epididymis thickens to form the tail.

Throughout its course the epididymis is lined by tall, thin columnar cells with nonmotile sterocilia. In electron micrographs the sterocilia are found to be exceptionally long filamentous microvilli. In addition, the fine structure of these cells is typical of a cell that is both secretory (abundant rough endoplasmic reticulum and Golgi cisternae) and absorptive (apical vesicles and tubules).

Within the epididymis, sperm undergo progressive maturation during their movement from the head to the tail. As sperm emerge from the testis they are infertile and relatively nonmotile. By the time they reach the tail of the epididymis, they are both motile and fertile. The average time of sperm transit through the epididymis is 12 days. The sperm and epididymal fluid together contribute about 10 percent of the ejaculate.

*Vas.* The vas is the continuation of the epididymal duct, with only slight modification of the epithelial surface but substantial thickening of the outer muscle coat. The thickness of the muscle coat produces the "whipcord" sensation when the vas is rolled between the thumb and forefinger during physical examination of the cord.

From the inferior pole of the testis, the vas ascends in the spermatic cord within the scrotum, until it reaches the superficial inguinal ring. After traversing the inguinal canal, the vas enters the preperitoneal space at the internal inguinal ring, where it courses inferiorly into the pelvis lying between the pelvic fascia and peritoneum. The terminal portion, or ampulla, of the vas is more dilated and fuses with the seminal vesicle to form the ejaculatory duct.

*Ejaculatory duct.* Traversing the substance of the posterior wall of the prostate, the ejaculatory duct opens into the prostatic urethra at the verumontanum, an oval-shaped mucosal excrescence.

## RECTUM AND PELVIC ORGANS

## EXAMINATION

Inspection may reveal presence of external hemorrhoids, rectal fissures, or fistulas. Internal examination is then carried out by inserting a well lubricated, gloved index finger into the anal canal. The sphincter tone is evaluated and the canal is examined for undue tenderness or induration. Presence of induration, rectal stenosis, or mass lesions may indicate the need for additional studies, such as anoscopy or proctoscopy.

With the patient bent over the examining table, the prostate and seminal vesicles are palpated through the anterior rectal wall. The normal prostate is about 4 cm in length and in width, about the size of the terminal segment of the thumb. The prostate is widest superiorly at the bladder neck. Two distinct "lobes" of the prostate are palpable, separated by a median sulcus, or indentation. Normally, the prostate gland is smooth, somewhat mobile, and nontender. The consistency is rubbery and resembles the tip of the nose.

One major problem in the prostate examination lies in differentiating firm areas. Differential diagnosis of a firm area in the prostate includes cancer: calculi, infarction, granulomatous prostatitis, and nodular, benign hyperplasia. Even the most experienced examiner may have difficulty distinguishing among these possibilities on digital rectal examination.

Above the prostate it may be possible to feel soft, tubular seminal vesicles extending obliquely beneath the base of the bladder (Fig. 10-2). Usually, clear presence of seminal vesicles on rectal examination indicates a pathological process. Most commonly, these patients have pelvic tumors such as prostate cancer or acute infectious processes.

## ANATOMY

### Rectum

In the rectum, there are two to four permanent semicircular transverse folds of the mucosa, which are termed rectal valves. They neither serve as valves nor support the feces, as suggested by some investigators. These valves are readily observed during endoscopy but may be lacerated during blind instrumentation of the rectum.

Microscopically, the mucosa of the rectum is composed of columnar absorptive cells, although goblet-type mucous cells are interspersed among the absorptive cells. Invaginations of the epithelial surface form straight, tubular colonic glands equivalent to the glands of Lieberkühn seen in the small intestine.

### Rectoanal junction

The rectoanal junction is not a discrete point but a region of longitudinal mucosal folds extending superiorly from a zone of mucosa that is paler and flatter (Fig. 10-4). This gives the appearance of a horizontal band with teeth, hence the term *pectinate line* (Latin *pecten,* "comb"). The mucosal ridges forming the toothlike character of the line are termed *anal folds* or *columns* (of Morgagni). At the pectinate line between the base of the anal columns, the mucosa is redundant and outpockets to form the anal crypts. The epithelium of the anus, i.e., distal to the pectinate line, is characterized by stratified squamous cells of the nonkeratinizing type.

### Accessory sex glands

The male accessory sex glands include the seminal vesicles, prostate, and bulbourethral glands (Cowper's glands).

**Seminal Vesicles.** The seminal vesicles are paired, saccular glands with multiple foldings of their mucous membrane (Figs. 10-1 and 10-2). Embryologically they begin as tubular buds from the vas. Hence, the seminal vesicles join with the vas, forming a common ejaculatory duct.

The seminal vesicles are lined by columnar epithelial cells with abundant Golgi, rough endoplasmic reticulum, and secretory granules in the apical cytoplasm. The mucosal folds of the seminal vesicles are supported by a moderate lamina propria, containing collagen and elastic fibers. There is also a substantial muscular coat, which is important in the emission of secretions.

The seminal vesicles secrete an alkaline, slightly yellowish viscid fluid which constitutes 60 to 70 percent of the ejaculate vol-

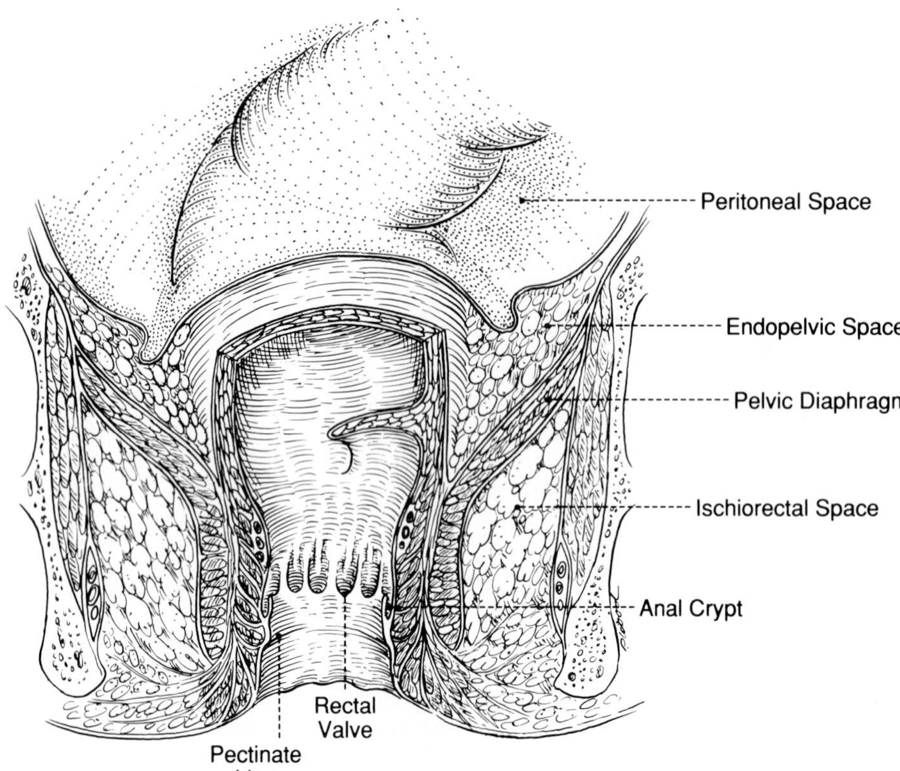


**Fig. 10-4.** Coronal section of male pelvis and rectoanal junction.

ume. Fractionation by "split-ejaculate" techniques shows that the semen consists of a presperm prostatic fraction, a sperm-rich fraction, and a postsperm vesicular fraction. Fructose and a variety of prostaglandins appear to be formed specifically by the seminal vesicle. Fructose is the principal energy source for sperm motility, but the role of prostaglandins in male fertility is uncertain.

**Prostate.** The prostate gland is located between the bladder neck and the urogenital diaphragm (Figs. 10-1, 10-2, and 10-3). The prostate completely encircles the urethra.

*Zones.* The prostate gland is composed of three zones of tissue: a periurethral zone, surrounding the urethra; a wedge-shaped central zone, bounded by the ejaculatory duct, urethra, and base of the bladder; and a peripheral zone, composed of all remaining glandular tissue.

The periurethral zone is composed of mucosal and submucosal glands penetrating the smooth muscle of the proximal urethra. Benign hyperplasia originates in this region and may lead to obstruction of urinary outflow from the bladder.

The central zone of the prostate is located between the urethra and ejaculatory duct. This area appears to be least susceptible to development of inflammatory, hyperplastic, or neoplastic disease.

The peripheral, or outer, zone is the portion of the prostate that is palpable on rectal examination. The peripheral zone is also the region of the prostate that is most frequently involved in carcinoma and inflammation.

*Prostatic secretions.* The prostate contributes approximately 30 percent of the ejaculate volume, in the form of a thin, slightly opaque fluid. The prostate gland appears to be important in protecting the male lower urogenital tract against infection, in providing enzymes for "liquefying" the semen after ejaculation, and in providing other components of the seminal fluid. Normally the pH of prostatic fluid is around 7. However, in men with well documented bacterial prostatitis, the secretions alkalinize and may reach or exceed pH 8. Zinc, magnesium, citric acid, and acid phosphatase in the ejaculate appear to originate in the prostatic secretions.

**Bulbourethral Glands (Cowper's glands).** These paired, pea-sized glands are located in the urogenital diaphragm (Fig. 10-2). Their excretory ducts drain into the posterior urethra. The glands secrete a thin mucoid material during the excitatory stage of sexual response, but the bulbourethral glands contribute only a minimal amount to the ejaculate. These glands are relatively immune to hyperplastic and neoplastic disease, although they can be involved in infections.

## BLOOD SUPPLY

### ARTERIAL PATHWAYS (INTERNAL ILIAC ARTERY)

The pelvic organs in the male all receive their blood supply from the internal iliac artery. The internal iliac artery arises at the pelvic brim from the common iliac artery and immediately divides into an anterior and posterior division.

#### Posterior division

The posterior division of the internal iliac artery provides small branches to the pelvic sidewall and has three branches which leave the pelvis, including the pudendal arteries.

The internal pudendal artery supplies the perineum (Fig. 10-5). This includes all structures located in the ischiorectal fossa and superficial and deep pouches. As it leaves the pelvis via the greater sciatic notch, the pudendal artery gives off the inferior rectal artery and then enters the pudendal canal. The pudendal arteries have three areas of distribution: the anal canal, the perineum, and the phallus.

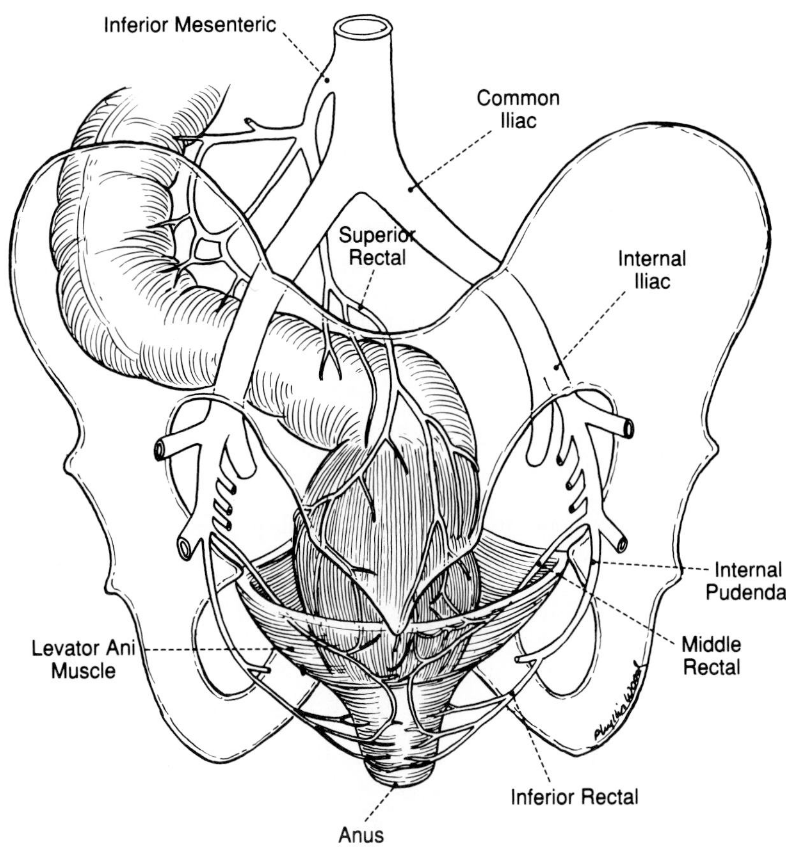


**Fig. 10-5.** Branches of the internal iliac artery and the distribution of the internal pudendal artery.

### Anterior division

The anterior division of the internal iliac courses on the sidewall of the pelvis until it reaches the symphysis pubis, where it ascends the anterior abdominal wall. As it turns superiorly, the lumen of the vessel disappears and the vessel becomes a fibrous cord, the medial umbilical ligament. The internal iliac branches to form the middle rectal, superior, and inferior vesical arteries. The middle rectal artery supplies the rectum and has anastomosing branches with the superior rectal artery from the sigmoid. The superior vesicle artery supplies the fundus of the bladder whereas the inferior vesicle artery supplies the bladder neck, seminal vesicle, vas deferens, and prostate. All these vessels anastomose with their members from the opposite side.

## VENOUS AND LYMPHATIC PATHWAYS

### Pelvic organs

**Venous Drainage.** The pelvic organs have abundant venous plexuses which give rise to larger veins that parallel the arterial pattern. These veins return blood from the pelvic organs to the internal iliac vein which merges with the external iliac vessel to form the common iliac vein. This pathway joins the caval system of veins. Some blood in the perirectal region enters anastomotic channels in the mucosal plexus and ascends via the superior rectal vein to enter the portal drainage system.

**Lymphatic Drainage.** The lymphatic pathways from the pelvic organs follow the venous pattern. The first series of regional nodes are along the proximal parts of the internal iliac artery. From these nodes, lymphatic channels ascend to the aorta and the paraaortic lymphatic chain before entering the thoracic duct. The sigmoid lymphatics follow the superior rectal veins to inferior mesenteric lymph nodes near the aorta.

### Perineal structures

**Venous Drainage.** Most structures supplied by the pudendal artery are drained by veins that enter the internal pudendal vein. This vessel returns along a similar route to enter the internal iliac vein. There are two exceptions to this pattern: the anorectal region and the dorsum of the penis.

In the anorectal region blood may return via veins in the endopelvic space and eventually reach the vena cava through internal iliac tributaries or may continue superiorly to reach the superior rectal tributaries of the portal system. Increased venous pressure in this region, due to increased venous resistance in either the portal system or the caval system, can result in anorectal hemorrhoids. The anorectal submucosal venous plexus is also a pathway for the spread of infection from the perianal and rectal areas to the endopelvic space.

The second nonpudendal venous pathway from the perineum is via the dorsal vein of the penis to the prostatic venous plexus at the neck of the bladder. These veins cross the urogenital diaphragm from the perineum to enter the endopelvic space. The prostatic veins are tributaries of the internal iliac system.

**Lymphatic Drainage.** The lymphatic drainage of the perineum differs from its venous drainage. In essence, all the skin and superficial structures of the perineum have lymphatics which course via the medial aspect of the thigh to the superficial inguinal nodes. Thus, anal and perianal ulcers caused by syphilis, chancroid, herpes simplex virus, or lymphogranuloma venereum cause inguinal lymphadenopathy. Channels from these nodes penetrate the fascia of the thigh at the saphenous opening to join the lymphatics from the leg. These lymphatic vessels course superiorly along the external iliac vein, then merge with paraaortic lymphatics.

An important exception is the lymphatic drainage of the testis, which does not follow the pattern described above. These lymphatics course superiorly in the spermatic cord, traverse the inguinal canal, and then ascend in the retroperitoneum with the testicular vein. In this manner the lymphatics reach the paraaortic lymph chain at the level of the renal vessels. This point is important clinically because metastases from testicular tumors do not cause inguinal adenopathy.

## NERVE SUPPLY OF THE PERINEUM AND PELVIC ORGANS

The three neural components which must reach the perineal and pelvic structures are the somatic, parasympathetic, and sympathetic nerves.

### SOMATIC NERVE SUPPLY

Only the perineum is supplied by somatic fibers. These arise in spinal cord segments S-2, -3, and -4 and travel via the pudendal nerve to all the skin and structures of the anal and urogenital triangles (Fig. 10-6). The pudendal nerve leaves the pelvis along with the pudendal vessels, entering the pudendal canal after giving off the inferior rectal nerves. These supply the perineal skin, external anal sphincter, and the skin of the anal canal. The pudendal nerve then divides into a perineal branch, supplying the deep and superficial pouch structures, and the dorsal nerve of the penis, supplying the skin of the penis. Branches of the perineal division supply the urogenital diaphragm, superficial perineal muscle, and skin of the scrotum.

### PARASYMPATHETIC NERVE SUPPLY

The parasympathetic innervation of the pelvic organs is also derived from spinal segments S-2, -3, and -4. However, these fibers

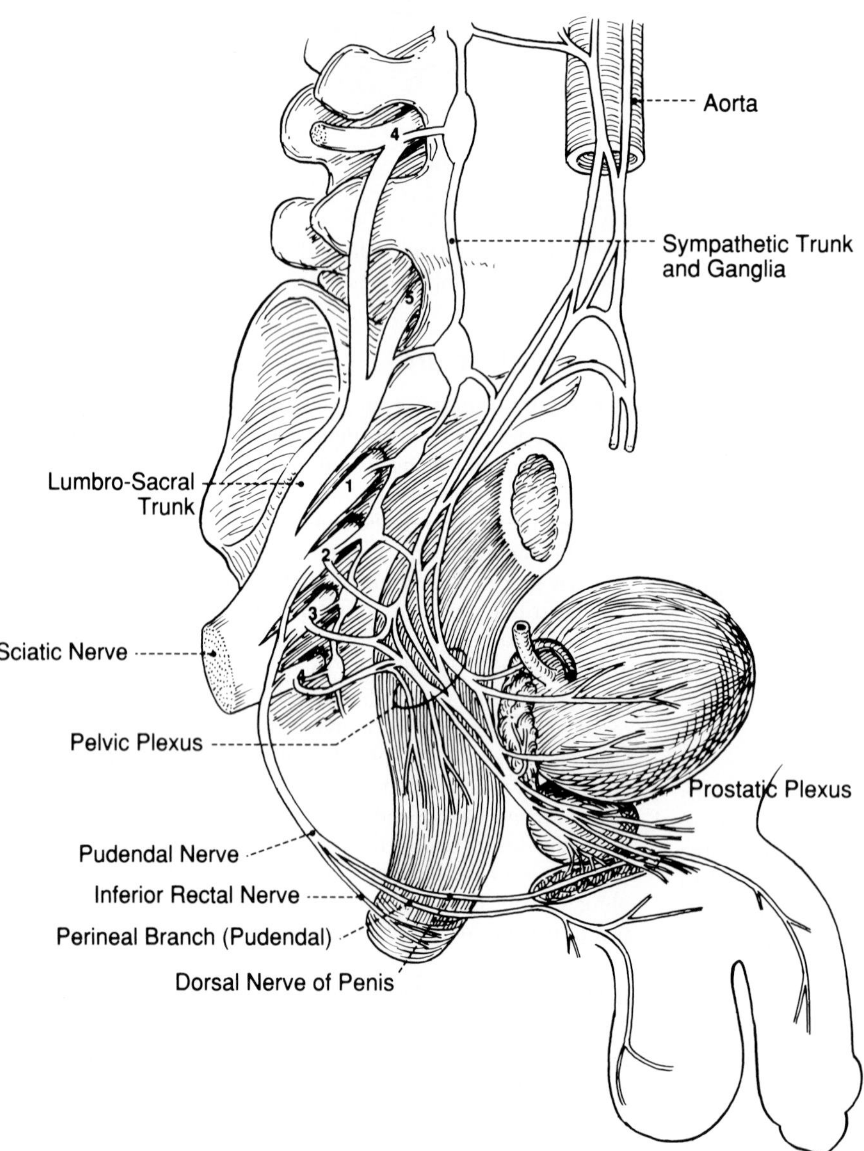


**Fig. 10-6.** Innervation of the pelvic viscera.

originate from neurons in the intermediolateral gray rather than the ventral gray, which is the origin for fibers in the pudendal nerve. After these fibers leave the anterior sacral foramina, they join to form the pelvic splanchnic nerve (nervi erigentes), which contributes these fibers to the plexus surrounding the viscera. This is termed the pelvic plexus. These fibers traverse the plexus without synapsing and enter the walls of the pelvic organs, rectum, bladder, and prostate, where they synapse in intramural ganglia. Short postganglionic fibers are then relayed to the muscle fibers.

## SYMPATHETIC NERVE SUPPLY

Sympathetic fibers to the pelvic viscera are believed to originate in the intermediolateral gray of the spinal segments T-12 to L-2. After joining a spinal nerve, they enter a sympathetic ganglion for that segment but do not synapse in the ganglion. The fibers descend briefly in the sympathetic chain, then course medially to enter the superior hypogastric plexus anterior to the aorta. The preganglionic fibers descend in the plexus to the inferior hypogastric plexus, which divides around the lateral sides of the pelvic organs and becomes the pelvic plexus (rectal, vesical, or prostatic). Synapses occur in the plexus or in the capsule of the organ innervated.

The pelvic plexus, therefore, is a mixture of parasympathetic and sympathetic fibers. In the region of the prostate, there is a group of fibers which course anteriorly at the upper edge of the urogenital diaphragm and supply the cavernous tissues of the penis (cavernous nerve). These fibers contain both parasympathetic and sympathetic components.

## Chapter 11

# Anatomy and physical examination of the female genital tract

Daniel O. Graney
Louis A. Vontver

## INTRODUCTION

Any area of the body may be involved in sexually transmitted disease syndromes or in the differential diagnosis of these conditions. Clearly there is no single, optimal method for conducting the history and physical examination. The critical areas of interest are determined by the history, other physical findings, and conditions considered in the differential diagnosis. Many critical anatomical points may be important in some contexts yet irrelevant in others. Thus, this chapter is an attempt to present succinctly one approach to "the routine examination." This approach is selective but is based on clinical experience in developing an efficient method for evaluating a large number of patients in a timely manner.

There are two major differences in the anatomy and the examination between male and female patients. First, in the female there is a genital tract and a separate urinary tract. In the male we conduct a single genitourinary tract examination. The second major difference is that the critical reproductive organs in the female are located in the pelvis, and are therefore less accessible and less easily palpated.

In the female patient who presents to the STD clinic, few portions of the physical examination will yield as much information as the pelvic examination. Symptomatic pathology abounds and unsuspected pathology is found in a significant proportion of relatively asymptomatic women.

Rapport with the patient is always important in the physical examination but is especially critical in the female pelvic exam. Evidence of concern for a woman's problems at the initial interview will help provide needed rapport. The woman worried about sexually transmitted disease expects to have a pelvic examination and is understandably concerned about the findings. For the most part such a woman will be very cooperative. A little effort on the part of the examiner in regard to her well-being and comfort during the pelvic examination will maintain that cooperation and enhance the diagnostic yield.

Some specific suggestions to establish and maintain rapport are as follows. Prior to the examination always wash your hands where the patient can see you. Unless you are checking for incontinence, have the patient void before the examination, as a full bladder is uncomfortable and inhibits the examination. Obtain urine for analysis and/or culture if indicated. Recognize that the dorsal lithotomy position is one of vulnerability. The patient's comfort may be improved by elevating the backrest, suggestng the patient wear her shoes so that the stirrups do not cause discomfort, and providing a drape if desired but allowing no draping if that is the desire of the patient. The speculum should be kept warm in a warming drawer or warmed with water just before the examination. All the equipment necessary for the examination should be present in the examination room, which should be private and quiet.

You should tell the patient what you are doing at each step. It will help the patient's anxiety if she is told of normal structures and normal findings during the examination. A mirror should be available to demonstrate specific findings to the patient, as the more involved the patient becomes in her own care the more apt she is to return for subsequent visits and necessary treatments. The pelvic examination is an opportunity to teach the patient about her anatomy and about the transmission of infectious disease.

The comfort of the examiner should not be overlooked. Equipment should be readily available, lighting should be good, and the examination table and stool should be at the right height. Most often, the standard examination of a patient in our clinic proceeds according to an orderly sequence. Proceeding in this fashion has two advantages. First, the sequence of the examination limits the opportunity for errors of omission in a busy clinical situation. Second, there is minimal need for the patient to move. During the examination any needed specimens should be obtained, and following the exam the findings should be recorded and correlated with the patient's history and complaints. The remainder of this chapter is organized to follow this suggested pattern of evaluation. The relevant considerations in routine examination of the female will be presented for each section of the physical examination, and critical anatomical principles will be considered for that area. We will present the examination and anatomical descriptions according to our own opinions, recognizing that some of these opinions are controversial and that other anatomists and/or clinicians may hold alternative, equally valid viewpoints.

## THE EXTERNAL GENITALIA AND PERINEUM

### PHYSICAL EXAMINATION

Ordinarily, we initiate the examination by having the patient sit on the examining table. If indicated, head and neck examination, inspection, palpation, percussion, and auscultation of the chest and breast may be done in this position. Next, the patient is asked to lie supine. Skin, extremity, breast, cardiovascular, and abdominal examination may be conducted in this position, if indicated. Attention is then directed to the pelvic examination.

The examination begins with palpation of the inguinal nodes and inspection of the mons pubis and the external genitalia. The quantity and location of pubic hair is noted. The amount of pubic hair varies greatly in different racial groups. What is normal for a southern European would imply hirsutism from androgen excess in an oriental. Nits on the shaft of the pubic hair are indicative of lice infestation. Freckles that move are probably lice.

The labia are separated and the vaginal introitus is inspected. Redness or erythema signifies an irritation which may be due to infection with Candida, *Trichomonas vaginalis*, herpes simplex virus (HSV), or certain bacteria (e.g., toxic shock syndrome, streptococcal cellulitis). A homogeneous white or gray discharge at the introitus is suggestive of bacterial vaginosis. Small tender fissures in the mucous membrane should arouse suspicion of genital herpes, as many genital HSV occurrences do not form classic ulcerations. Pigmented or nodular areas on the vulva may be due to human papilloma virus infection or carcinoma in situ. Multifocal carcinoma in situ (i.e., involving more than one site on the cervix, vagina, and/or vulva) is being found more frequently in young women, and biopsies of suspicious areas of the vulva are important to rule out this disease. Pigmented areas may also be benign nevi or malignant melanomas (see Chap. 60). A suspicious area which is darkly pigmented with irregular borders should be removed by excisional biopsy for histologic inspection. The inspection for such lesions should include the frenulum and clitoris.

While the vulva are held apart, the woman should be asked to strain, cough, or otherwise perform a Valsalva maneuver. This will allow observation of any vaginal relaxation or stress incontinence. At this time the urethra with its associated periurethral (Skene's) glands should be palpated and milked by gentle finger pressure from above downward. If infection or a urethral diverticulum is present, a small amount of discharge may be evident at the urethral meatus or at the orifices of Skene's glands.

The greater vestibular glands (of Bartholin) are located at approximately 5 and 7 o'clock on the face of the posterior fourchette (Fig. 11-1). When these regions are explored with gentle pressure between the thumb and forefinger, the normal gland cannot be palpated and the region is not tender. However, an infected gland is extremely tender. Occasionally a small asymptomatic Bartholin's duct cyst can be seen as a convexity of the posterior fourchette and felt as a discrete cystic nodule in the position of the Bartholin's gland. If any palpable mass is discovered in this area in a perimenopausal or menopausal woman, it should be removed for histologic examination, as the incidence of carcinoma increases with age.

## ANATOMY OF THE PERINEUM AND EXTERNAL GENITALIA

The strict anatomical definition of the perineum is a diamond-shaped region bounded by the symphysis pubis anteriorly, coccyx posteriorly, and ischial tuberosities laterally. Projecting a line between the ischial tuberosities divides the diamond space into two triangles, the urogenital triangle anteriorly and the anal triangle posteriorly. Thus, both triangles share a common base with the apex of the urogenital triangle pointing anterosuperiorly and the anal triangle pointing posterosuperiorly. In lateral profile the floor of the perineum is shaped like a shallow V rather than appearing flat as implied by a two-dimensional drawing. The plane of the anal triangle is open and is filled only with fatty tissue. The plane of the urogenital triangle is closed or occupied by a thick triangular membrane, the urogenital diaphragm. The diaphragm closes the anterior floor of the perineum and defines the anterior wall of the ischiorectal fossa.

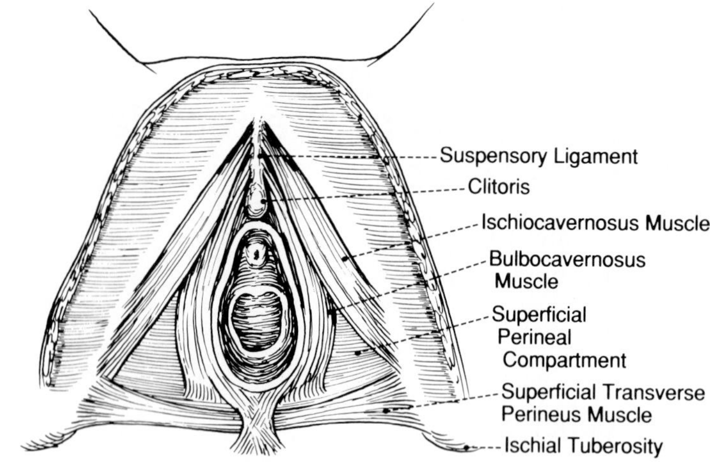


Fig. 11-2. Contents of the superficial perineal pouch.

The region of the urogenital triangle contains two spaces, the superficial and deep perineal spaces (Figs. 11-2, 11-3, 11-4). The superficial space can be imagined as a pair of spaces lying between the urogenital diaphragm and the skin of the labia majora. In fact, the two spaces are connected above the clitoris so that the space resembles an inverted U. It is bounded by the perineal fascia of the urogenital diaphragm which continues from the base of the diaphragm and reflects superiorly under the labial skin to join the membranous layer of superficial fascia of the abdomen above the symphysis pubis (Figs. 11-2, 11-3, 11-4). Because of these fascial attachments, a hematoma in the labia majora, i.e., superficial pouch, expands superiorly into the abdominal wall but neither laterally to the thigh nor posteriorly to the ischiorectal fossa.

The contents of the superficial perineal pouch include the greater vestibular glands (Bartholin's), crura of the clitoris, bulbs of the vestibule, which are composed of elongated erectile tissue (Fig. 11-3), and the overlying superficial perineal muscles (Fig. 11-2).

The deep perineal space is a potential space within the urogenital diaphragm. It is formed by the superior and inferior fascia

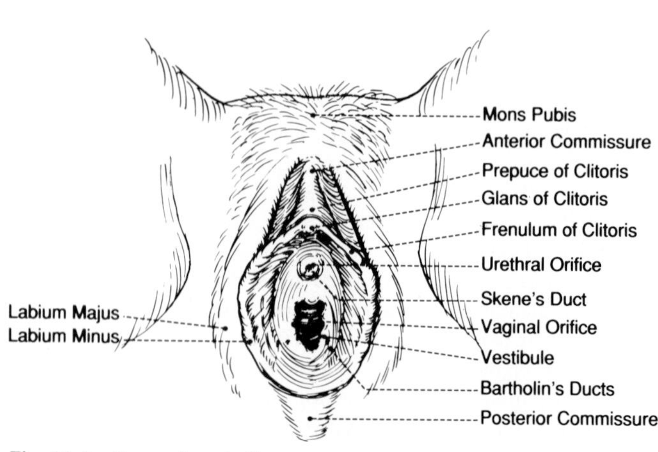


Fig. 11-1. External genitalia.

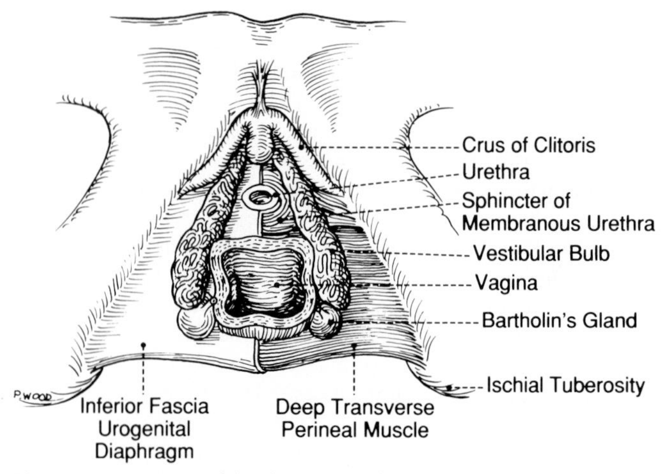


Fig. 11-3. Contents of the deep perineal pouch.

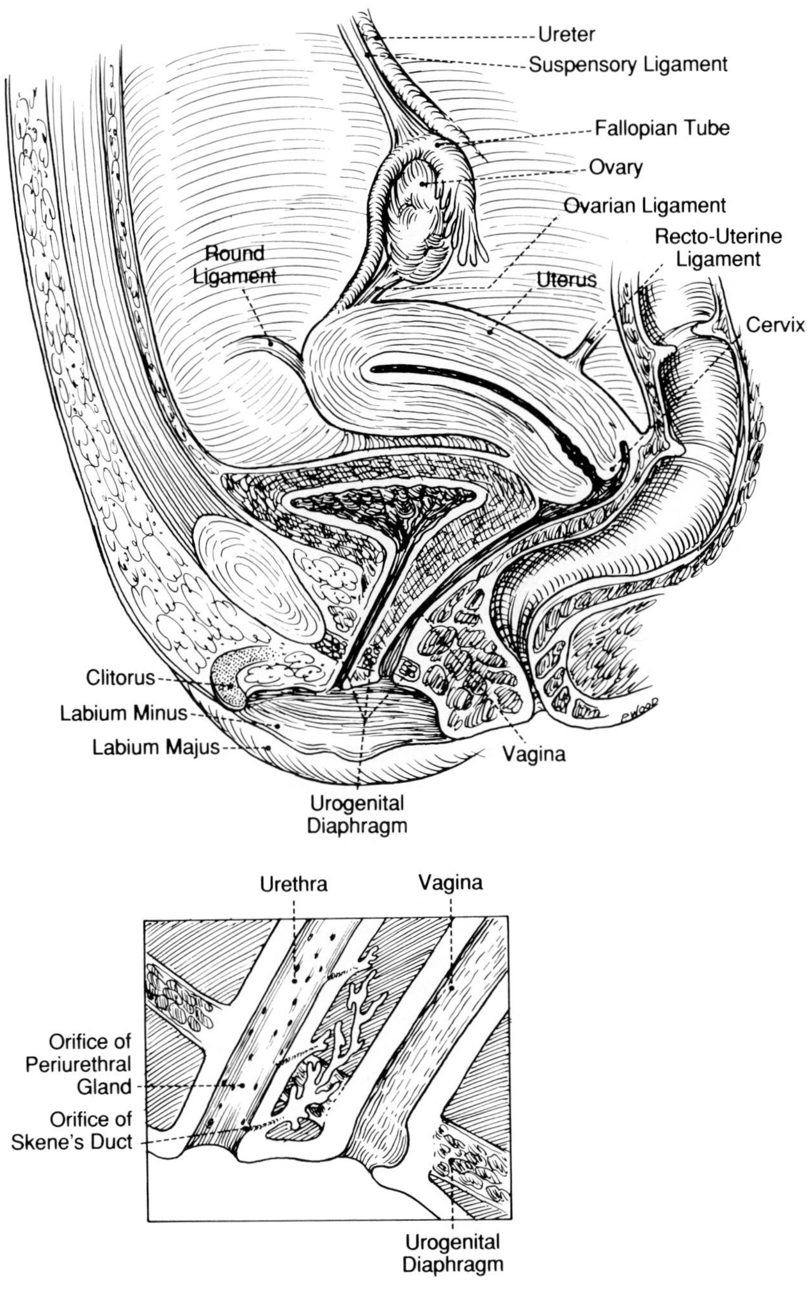

**Fig. 11-4.** Sagittal section of female pelvis. Inset shows magnification of urethra and urethral glands.

(perineal membrane) of the deep transverse perineal muscle which occupies the space. Together, the muscle and fascia form the urogenital diaphragm (Figs. 11-3, 11-4).

In the female, the contents of the deep perineal space include the deep transverse perineal muscle, and circular muscle fibers surrounding the urethra and vagina as these structures pierce the urogenital diaphragm.

**Female Urethra.** The female urethra measures 3 to 4 cm in length from the bladder neck to the meatus in the anterior vestibule of the vagina. Proximally the mucosa is composed of transitional epithelium gradually becoming stratified squamous as it courses distally. The lumen appears stellate in cross section because of extensive longitudinal folding of the mucosa. Beneath the mucosa is the lamina propria, rich in vascular and neural plexuses. The muscular coat, similar to other body tubes, is composed of a double layer of smooth muscle, with the inner fibers circularly arranged and the outer layer disposed longitudinally. As the urethra traverses the urogenital diaphragm, circularly arranged striated muscle fibers form an external sphincter of the urethra. These fibers are innervated by the internal pudendal nerve (somatic) in contrast to the internal urethral sphincter at the bladder neck which is innervated by the pelvic splanchnic nerve (parasympathetic).

In essence, the entire length of the female urethra is paralleled by paraurethral glands which are tubuloalveolar outgrowths of the mucosa. Located in the lamina propria, these glands have their openings on the posterior and posterolateral wall of the urethra (Fig. 11-4). At the distal end of the urethra there are usually two larger glands commonly identified as Skene's glands whose ducts are visible on the posterior wall. Both Skene's glands and the paraurethral glands are vulnerable to infection.

## VAGINA, CERVIX, UTERUS, AND ADNEXAL STRUCTURES

### PHYSICAL EXAMINATION

**Speculum Examination and Collection of Specimens for Microscopy and Culture.** A warm speculum should be inserted into the vagina and opened to reveal the cervix. It should be inserted at an angle directed toward the hollow of the sacrum (Fig. 11-5). Care should be taken not to apply pressure against the urethra and anterior bony arch of the pubis. With the speculum in place, specimens may be obtained for pH determination and wet mount examination of vaginal fluid; vaginal fluid Gram stain and selected cultures, if indicated; and endocervical Gram stain and cultures and Pap smear. If there are no symptoms or signs of vaginal discharge or inflammation, no tests of vaginal fluid are usually done. If such symptoms or signs exist, a specimen of the vaginal discharge should be tested on pH paper to ascertain the vaginal pH, which is normally 4.5 or below. If the vaginal pH is above 4.5, it is suggestive of bacterial vaginosis or of trichomoniasis. Care should be taken to avoid mixing vaginal discharge with cervical mucus for determination of vaginal fluid pH, since cervical mucus has a pH of about 7.0. Vaginal discharge should also be mixed with saline for microscopic examination for motile trichomonads and clue cells; and with 10% potassium hydroxide for detection of a fishy, amine-like odor, characteristic of bacterial vaginosis, and for microscopic detection of fungal elements (see Chap. 46). A Gram stain of a thinly smeared slide of vaginal discharge is useful for confirming the diagnosis of bacterial vaginosis. With rare exceptions (e.g., toxic shock syndrome), bacterial cultures of vaginal fluid are not useful. However, for detection of *Candida* or *Trichomonas vaginalis*, vaginal cultures are more sensitive than microscopic examination of vaginal fluid, especially in the absence of abnormal vaginal discharge.

For Pap smear, separate samples should be obtained from the ectocervix including the transformation zone, using an Ayre's spatulum; and from the endocervix, using a cytobrush (see Chap. 48). We recommend annual cervical cytologic screening for sexually active women. Specimens for culture for gonorrhea and for diagnosis of chlamydia by culture or antigen detection test are next taken from the endocervix. A cytobrush may provide a better endocervical sample for detection of chlamydia than is provided by a Dacron or cotton swab, but this requires further study. A specimen of the endocervical mucus can also be obtained at this time, inspected for color (yellow color indicates increased numbers of PMN leukocytes), and used to prepare a Gram-stained smear for microscopic enumeration of PMN leukocytes in cervical mucus and for detection of gonococci. Nabothian cysts are a normal finding on the cervix (Fig. 11-6). They develop when squamous epithelium covers mucus-secreting columnar epithelium and the secretions cause a small cyst to form. These cysts rupture and reform throughout the reproductive years. While the speculum is still in place, colposcopy can be performed before and after applying dilute (3%) acetic acid and/or dilute lugol solution to the cervix. Colposcopy enables one to better visualize cervical, vaginal, and vulvar abnormalities such as dysplasia or infection with human papilloma virus, as well as cervical ulcers caused by HSV, or "strawberry cervix" caused by *T. vaginalis*. Colposcopy is clearly essential for evaluating the cervix when Pap smears have shown dysplasia, to select lesions for biopsy. The role of colposcopy as an initial screening procedure is debated, and requires further evaluation.

**Bimanual Examination.** After removal of the speculum, the first two fingers of the vaginal examining hand are lubricated and inserted into the vagina. The bladder should be compressed. This should cause no discomfort other than the sensation of needing to void. The cervix should be palpated and moved. Both it and the attached uterine body should be freely mobile without pain. The body of the uterus is next located by providing suprapubic pressure with the abdominal hand to keep the uterus in the pelvic cavity. The two fingers of the examining vaginal hand should outline the uterus in its entirety. This is usually easy if the uterus is anterior. If it is in a mid or posterior retroflexed position, it will be more difficult to locate and may be best palpated on rectovaginal examination (Fig. 11-7). After noting the size, shape, position, mobility, consistency, and contour of the uterus, it is moved to the one side and the fingers of the examining hand are inserted into the right lateral vaginal fornix as far as possible (Fig. 11-8). The abdominal hand produces pressure on the right lower abdomen and the fingers of the vaginal hand are swept to the side to evaluate the adnexal structures consisting of the tube, ovary, round and cardinal ligaments, and the pelvic sidewall (Fig. 11-9). The same procedure is followed on the opposite side.

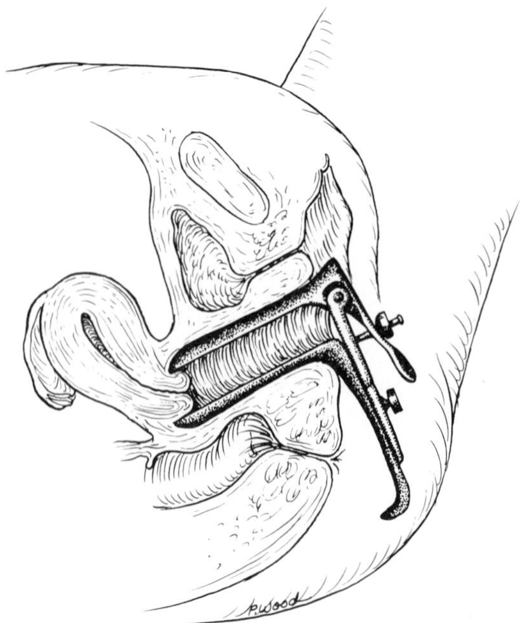

Fig. 11-5. Position of vaginal speculum.

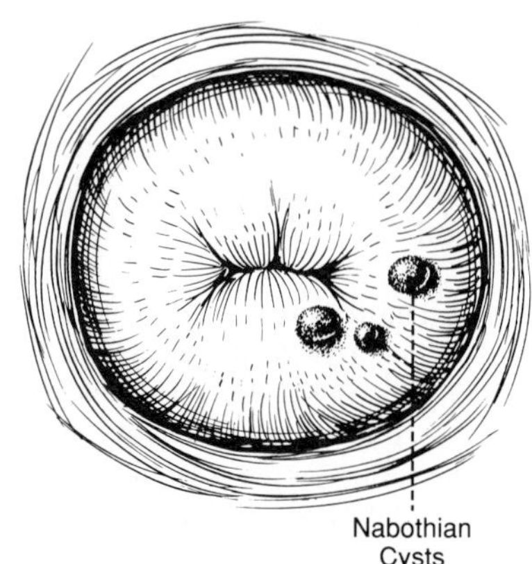


Fig. 11-6. Cervix, illustrating Nabothian cysts.

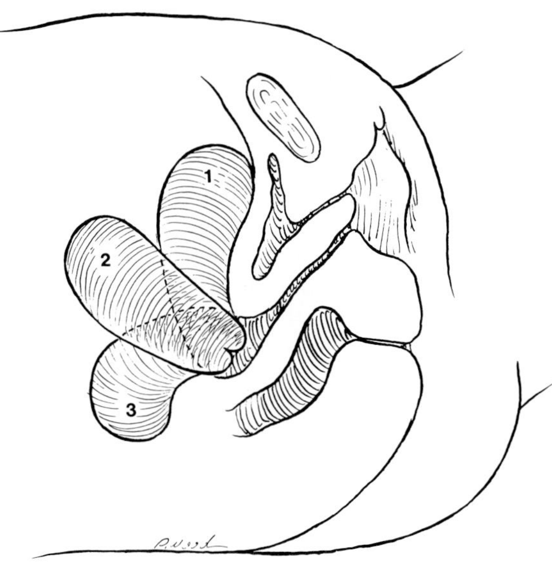


**Fig. 11-7.** Positions of the uterus: (1) anteverted, (2) midposition, and (3) retroflexed.

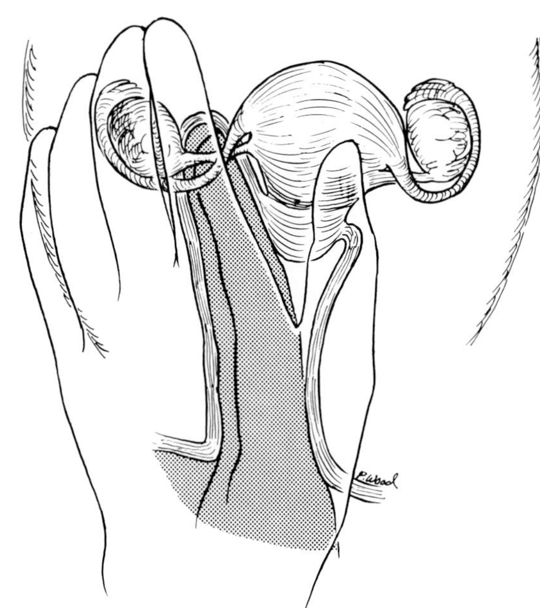

**Fig. 11-9.** Bimanual examination: comparing position of vaginal fingers (shaded) and abdominal hand.

(Some people prefer to change hands, using the left hand to examine the left side of the pelvis.) Only the ovaries should be palpable in the normal examination. Often they are not felt, especially if the patient is on birth control pills, which suppress the ovaries and decrease their size. A normal ovary in a menstruating nonsuppressed woman measures approximately 3 × 3 × 2 cm. Any enlargement above 5 to 6 cm is an abnormal finding. Both pelvic sidewalls should be evaluated for enlargements of the lymph nodes. Tenderness of any of the pelvic structures is noted. The examination is concluded with a rectovaginal exam.

**Rectovaginal Examination.** After the patient is informed of the procedure, a well-lubricated middle finger is placed in the rectum and the index finger is simultaneously placed in the vaginal vault. The patient can often facilitate the rectal examination by relaxing the pelvic muscles during insertion of the fingers. The rectal finger carefully evaluates the entire rectal wall for nodularity or polyps. It is then placed against the cervix, which is felt through the rectal and vaginal wall. Pressure from the abdominal hand brings the uterus down so its entire posterior surface can be palpated with the rectal finger. This is the best method to examine the posterior wall of the uterus if it is in the mid or posterior position in the pelvis. The uterosacral and cardinal ligament can be put on tension by elevating the cervix and palpated for nodularity such as may be found with endometriosis. The posterolateral sidewalls of the pelvis should be swept with the rectal finger, and a stool specimen can be obtained if indicated for evaluation of occult bleeding. The American Cancer Society recommends annual testing for gastrointestinal bleeding beginning at age 50.

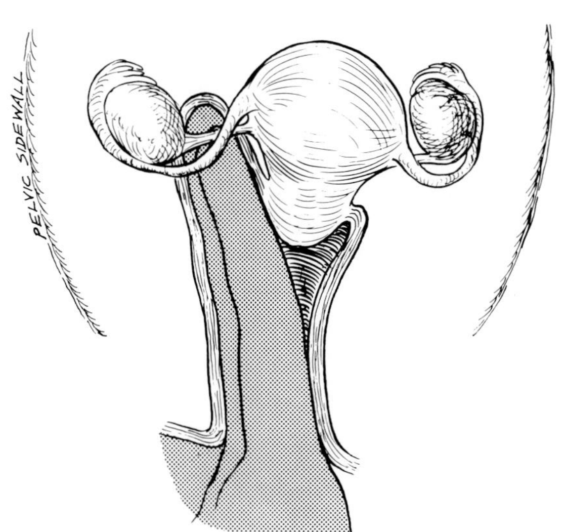


**Fig. 11-8.** Preparation for bimanual pelvic examination: placement of vaginal fingers (shaded).

Throughout the pelvic examination a mental image of the pelvic organs should be formed, noting size, shape, consistency, mobility, contour, and tenderness. These observations should be accurately documented in the record. Correlation of the patient's complaints or historical data with the physical findings and the laboratory evaluation will often resolve the concerns of the patient and the questions of the examining physician.

## ANATOMY

### Vagina

The vagina is a fibromuscular tube whose anterior and posterior walls are normally in contact with one another. A longitudinal ridge is present along the mucosal surface of both the anterior and posterior walls; from these ridges, secondary elevations called rugae extend laterally. The vaginal wall consists of three layers: (1) the mucous membrane, composed of stratified squamous nonkeratinized epithelium and an underlying lamina propria of connective tissue; (2) the muscular layer, composed of smooth muscle fibers disposed both longitudinally and circularly; (3) the adventitia, a dense connective tissue that blends with the surrounding fascia.

There are no glands in the vaginal wall. During sexual stimulation the marked increase in fluid production in the vagina is believed to be due to transudation across the vaginal wall.

The stratified squamous epithelium of the adult vagina is several layers thick. The basal layer is a single layer of cylindrical cells with oval nuclei. Above this area are several layers of polyhedral cells that appear to be connected together much like those of the stratum spinosum of the epidermis. Above these are several more layers of cells which are more flattened in appearance and accumulate glycogen in their cytoplasm, the significance of which is discussed below. They also exhibit keratohyalin granules intracellularly. This tendency toward keratinization, however, is not normally completed in the vaginal epithelium, and the surface cells always retain their nuclei.

The most superficial cells are desquamated into the vaginal lumen where their intracellular glycogen is converted into lactic acid, probably by the bacteria normally resident in the vagina. The resulting acidity is believed to be important in protecting the female reproductive system from infection by most pathogenic bacteria (Chap. 12).

Estrogen stimulates the production of glycogen and maintains the thickness of the entire epithelium. Before puberty and after menopause, when estrogen levels are relatively low, the epithelium is thin and the pH is higher than in the reproductive years (neutral before puberty and 6.0 or higher after the menopause). The thinness of the epithelium and the relatively high pH of the vaginal milieu are among the factors that are thought to render females in these age groups more susceptible to vaginal infections.

## Uterus

The uterus has two major components: (1) the expanded upper two-thirds of the organ, the body of the uterus; (2) the cylindrical lower one-third, the cervix (Figs. 11-10, 11-11). The fundus is the rounded upper part of the body, superior to the points of entry of the uterine tubes. The isthmus is the short, slightly constricted zone between the body and the cervix.

The two main components of the uterus are rather different from one another in their structure and function.

**The Cervix.** The cervix consists primarily of dense collagenous connective tissue. Only about 15 percent of its substance is smooth muscle. In the isthmus, the uterine lumen narrows down to form the internal os. Below this point the lumen widens slightly to form the cervical canal (or endocervical canal). Finally, a constricted opening, the external os, at the lower end of the cervix provides communication between the lumen of the cervix and that of the vagina.

Inside the cervix, the endocervical mucosa is arranged in a series of folds and ridges. A longitudinal ridge runs down the anterior wall and another down the posterior wall; from each of these, small folds (the *plicae palmatae*) run laterally. The resemblance of this arrangement to a tree trunk with upward-spreading branches has given rise to the term *arbor vitae uterina* to describe the endocervical mucosa.

The part of the cervix that projects into the vagina (the *portio vaginalis*, or ectocervix) is covered by stratified squamous, nonkeratinizing epithelium. Usually, in older women, this type of epithelium extends for a very short distance into the cervical canal, where it forms a rather abrupt junction with the simple columnar epithelium lining the rest of the canal. The site of the squamocolumnar junction varies, however. It may occur higher up in the cervical canal, or the columnar epithelium may actually extend out beyond the external os where it forms small patches known as physiologic eversion, or ectopy, on the vaginal surface of the cervix. Ectopy is usually present in adolescents, and decreases during the third and fourth decades of life.

The mucosa contains large branched endocervical glands. In reality, they are not true glands but are merely deep grooves or clefts (sometimes called crypts) which serve to increase the surface area of the mucosa tremendously. The epithelium of both the

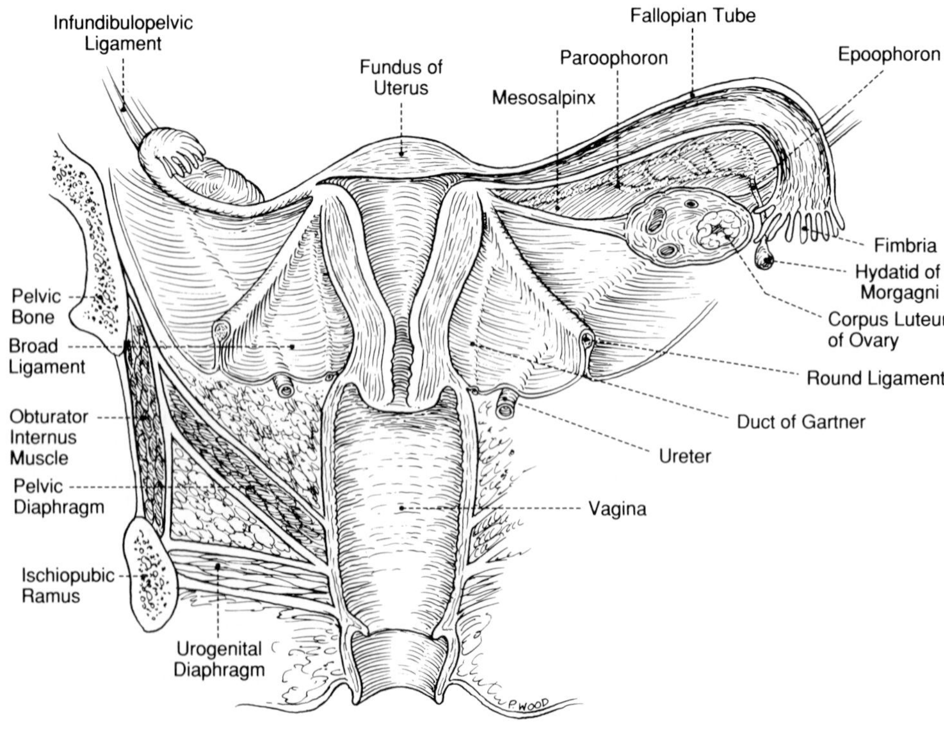


**Fig. 11-10.** Coronal section of pelvis illustrating broad ligament, endopelvic space, pelvic diaphragm, and urogenital diaphragm.

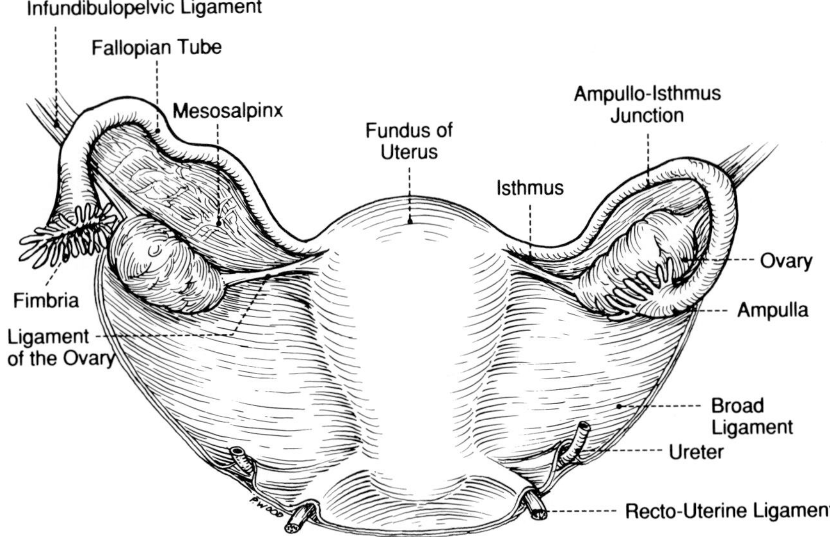


Fig. 11-11. Posterior view of broad ligament and female reproductive organs.

mucosal surface and the "glands" is of the simple columnar type in which almost all the cells are mucus-secreting cells. A few ciliated cells are present. If the ducts of the glands become blocked, mucous secretion accumulates inside them to form small lumps just under the surface (Nabothian cysts, Fig. 11-6).

Unlike the mucous membrane of the body of the uterus, the endocervical mucosa does not slough off at menstruation. It does, however, respond to cyclic changes in the levels of the ovarian hormones, estrogen and progesterone. It secretes up to 60 mg of mucus a day throughout much of the cycle, but near the time of ovulation (midcycle), when estrogen secretion reaches a peak, the secretion rate increases 10-fold and the abundant, clear mucus fills the cervical canal. It is less viscous than at other times during the cycle, and is easily penetrated by spermatozoa.

The production of progesterone by the corpus luteum after ovulation (or during pregnancy) changes the quantity and properties of mucus produced. It becomes more viscous, less abundant, and much less penetrable by spermatozoa. It acts as a plug to seal off the uterine cavity.

**The Body of the Uterus.** The wall of the body of the uterus is composed of three layers: (1) the endometrium, a glandular mucous membrane; (2) the myometrium or smooth muscle layer; (3) the serosa.

**Endometrium.** The function of the endometrium is to provide a suitable environment for the implantation and subsequent growth of the developing embryo. As such, it is a luxuriant mucosa with a large population of glycogen-secreting glands and a rich vascular network. However, if there is no developing embryo, most of the endometrium is sloughed off (causing the menstrual flow) and is regenerated again in the next menstrual cycle. This cyclic shedding and regeneration of the endometrium is under the control of the ovarian hormones, estrogen and progesterone. The rise and fall in ovarian hormone levels determine the rise and fall of the growth and shedding of the endometrium.

The endometrium varies from 0.5 mm to approximately 5 mm in thickness, depending upon the stage of the menstrual cycle. It is at its greatest height a few days after ovulation, at about the time of expected implantation. It consists of a simple columnar epithelium and a highly cellular lamina propria (the endometrial stroma) in which there are large numbers of tubular uterine glands. The epithelium contains both ciliated and secretory cells.

The endometrium can be subdivided into a rather narrow, deeper layer next to the myometrium, the basalis, and a much thicker, more superficial layer, the functionalis. The latter receives its name because it is the portion that is shed during menstruation.

The arteries that supply the endometrium play an important role in the onset of menstruation. Circumferentially oriented arteries in the myometrium give off numerous branches toward the endometrium. As they enter this region, small basal arteries branch off to supply the basalis. The arteries then become highly contorted as they enter the functionalis and are known as coiled or spiral arteries. These arteries spasmodically contract late in the menstrual cycle which induces ischemia, necrosis, and eventually sloughing of the functionalis.

During the menstrual cycle, the endometrium passes through a number of phases. In the menstrual phase (approximately days 1 to 4 of a typical 28-day cycle) the functionalis is sloughed off; cellular debris and blood are discharged into the vagina. From day 5 until the time of ovulation (approximately day 14) the endometrium is in its proliferative phase. Epithelium in the persisting portions of uterine glands in the basalis grows out and covers the denuded surface. Estrogen from the growing follicles in the ovary promotes rapid proliferation of the epithelium, glands, and stroma. The endometrium may thicken by 2 to 3 mm at this time. Progesterone and estrogen from the corpus luteum stimulate the secretory phase (days 15 to 28), in which the epithelial cells begin to secrete. Accumulation of secretory products in the lumina of the glands, together with some edema of the stroma, causes the endometrium to increase further in height.

Late in the secretory phase, ovarian hormone levels drop and the changes that herald menstruation occur. Intermittent constrictions in the spiral arteries cause stasis of blood and ischemia of vessels and tissues in the area of supply. During the intervening periods of relaxation blood escapes from the weakened vessels, promoting menstrual hemorrhage.

**Myometrium.** The myometrium consists of bundles of smooth muscle fibers separated by strands of connective tissue. Four layers of smooth muscle have been distinguished, but their boundaries are poorly defined owing to overlap between adjacent layers. In the innermost and outermost layers, most of the muscle fibers are disposed longitudinally, whereas in the middle layers there are rather more circular fibers.

Estrogen is essential for the maintenance of normal size and function in myometrial smooth muscle cells.

**Serosa.** The serosa is the peritoneal covering of the uterus; hence only the pelvic portion of uterus has a serosa. The cervix has no serosa. The peritoneal reflections are discussed later in the chapter in the section on the broad ligament.

## Uterine Tubes

Fertilization and the earliest steps in development occur within the uterine tube. These tubes must therefore perform a number of tasks. As well as providing a suitable milieu for the gametes and transporting them to the site of fertilization in the midsection of the duct, they must also provide the nutritional support necessary for the embryo during segmentation and morula formation. In addition, transport mechanisms in the proximal portion of the oviduct must be such that the embryo arrives in the uterus at the appropriate time, both in terms of its own development and in terms of uterine receptivity.

**General Structure.** The uterine tubes lie in the upper margins of the broad ligament. Each is composed of four parts. Beginning at the distal end these are: (1) the infundibulum, the funnel-shaped end of the uterine tube which bears numerous delicate processes, the fimbriae, around the abdominal ostium; (2) the ampulla, or longest portion; it accounts for slightly more than half of the total length; (3) the isthmus, a narrow portion leading to the uterus; and (4) the intramural (or interstitial) portion—that part of the duct that extends through the wall of the uterus. At its end there is a minute ostium that connects the cavities of the uterus and uterine tube.

Three layers form the wall of the uterine tube: (1) The mucous membrane, characteristically composed of epithelium and lamina propria. The epithelium is of the simple columnar variety and contains two types of cells, ciliated and secretory. The lamina propria is loose connective tissue. (2) The muscular layer consists typically of two layers of smooth muscle, an inner circular and an outer longitudinal, but the boundary between the two is not distinct. In the intramural portion another longitudinal layer has been described, internal to the circular layer. (3) The serosa, which is typical of serosa elsewhere.

The mucous membrane and the muscular layer vary from one region of the duct to another. The structure and function of the various regions will now be discussed in more detail.

**Infundibulum.** When the oocyte leaves the ruptured follicle at ovulation, it is still surrounded by a mass of follicular cells that made up the bulk of the cumulus oophorus. The oocyte and its surrounding cells are now called the cumulus mass. The fimbriae of the infundibulum have the task of removing the cumulus mass from the site of follicular rupture on the ovary and transporting it into the ostium. Once contact is made, the cumulus mass begins to be transported over the fimbrial surface by ciliary action. The surface is richly ciliated and all the cilia beat toward the ostium. Since oocytes freed of cumulus cells are easily dislodged and are transported rather poorly, it is believed that the cumulus cells are essential for normal "pickup" and transport.

The epithelium of the fimbriae (and indeed, of the entire uterine tube) is sensitive to ovarian hormones. As estrogen concentration rises during the follicular phase of the cycle, the epithelium increases in height and reaches a maximum at midcycle. During the late luteal phase, cell height decreases. There is little evidence for deciliation and reciliation during the menstrual cycle in the human, but there is no doubt that withdrawal of estrogen will result in deciliation. The fimbriae of postmenopausal uterine tubes are largely devoid of cilia, whereas these from postmenopausal women who are on estrogen therapy are richly ciliated.

**Ampulla.** The mucous membrane of the ampulla is thrown up into an elaborate system of longitudinal folds. Most of the lumen is thus reduced to a system of fine channels between the folds. Less than half of the epithelial cells are ciliated and they beat toward the isthmus.

Fertilization occurs in the proximal portion of the ampulla. There are potentially two mechanisms for transporting the cumulus mass to this site, ciliary activity and smooth muscle contraction.

Although the role of the ciliated cells in the ampulla is fairly clear, the function of the secretory cells is less certain. Loss of cilia may be caused by infection leading to poor gamete transport with resultant infertility or ectopic pregnancy. Infection may also occlude the tube and persisting secretion may result in hydrosalpinx.

**Isthmus.** The elaborate mucosal folds of the ampulla give way rather abruptly to simpler, lower folds in the isthmus. Concomitant with a decrease in complexity of the mucosal folds is a marked increase in the thickness of the muscle layer. The ciliated cells of the mucosa beat toward the uterus.

The isthmus is perhaps the least understood portion of the uterine tube. It has the capacity of transporting spermatozoa distally toward the site of fertilization and later, conducting the developing embryo proximally. It is not known how the isthmus (or perhaps the intramural portion) controls the passage of cleaving eggs into the uterus.

**Intramural Portion.** The lumen of the uterine tube becomes extremely narrow in the proximal isthmus and intramural portions. The mucosal folds are reduced to low ridges. The muscular layer, on the other hand, becomes thicker than in any other part of the tube. The large amount of muscle in this region might suggest that a sphincter exists which could close off the uterine tube and help to prevent the spread of infection. However, there are no reported observations documenting the existence of an anatomical sphincter.

**Broad Ligament.** The broad ligament represents a transverse double fold of peritoneum containing the uterus and the uterine adnexa (uterine tube and ligaments) as well as nerves, vessels, and lymphatics (Figs. 11-4, 11-5). Inferior to the sacral promontory the peritoneum covers the anterior surface of the sigmoid colon and dips to its lowest point overlying the posterior vaginal fornix. From this position it reflects superiorly over the fundus and body of the uterus and then anteriorly to cover the dome of the bladder. At the level of the pubic symphysis it reflects superiorly again onto the anterior abdominal wall. From either side of the body of the uterus the folded peritoneum is carried laterally to the wall of the pelvis, forming a transverse vertical partition, the broad ligament. This divides the inferior peritoneal cavity into an anterior vesicouterine (pouch of Douglas) and posterior rectouterine space.

**Suspensory Ligament of the Ovary.** The suspensory ligament (infundibulopelvic ligament) is an extension of the most superior and lateral part of the broad ligament. It is misnamed, as it provides no support for the ovary or uterus. In reality, it is merely a fold of peritoneum raised by the underlying ovarian vessels, nerves, and lymphatics as they course between the ovary and the retroperitoneum. It provides a potential route for the spread of infection from adnexal structures to the retroperitoneum and paraaortic nodes.

**Ovary.** The ovaries have two major functions: to nurture and release the female gametes, and to produce the female sex hormones, estrogen and progesterone. These functions entail considerable changes in ovarian structure, both cyclic changes during the reproductive years and long-term changes over the individual's lifetime.

The ovary is covered by a single layer of cells known as the germinal epithelium. This is actually a misnomer, since it does not give rise to germ cells, as was originally believed. The cells are cuboidal in the young individual but tend to become squamous with age. This epithelium is the source of most ovarian neoplasms. These masses may be detected on bimanual examination and can be confused with hydrosalpinx or more acute infectious processes, especially if the neoplasm undergoes torsion.

The substance of the ovary may be divided into an outer cortex and an inner medulla. The connective tissue stroma of the cortex contains many spindle-shaped cells that resemble fibroblasts and intercellular substance. In the outermost zone of the cortex, just under the epithelium, the ratio of intercellular material to cells is higher than elsewhere. The fibrous nature and relatively poor vascularity of this zone give it a whitish appearance which accounts for its name, the tunica albuginea. The stroma of the medulla is a loose connective tissue containing some smooth muscle cells, many elastic fibers, and large, tortuous blood vessels. The presence of elastic fibers and the convoluted nature of the blood vessels permit the ovary to adapt fairly readily to the large structural changes that occur in the organ during each menstrual cycle.

## BLOOD SUPPLY, LYMPHATIC DRAINAGE, AND INNERVATION OF THE PERINEUM AND EXTERNAL GENITALIA

### BLOOD SUPPLY

The internal pudendal artery is an arterial trunk providing blood to all the perineal structures inferior to the pelvic diaphragm (Figs. 11-10, 11-12). It begins as a branch of the internal iliac artery located subperitoneally in the lateral pelvis. It exits the bony pelvis, crosses the sacrospinous ligament, and enters the

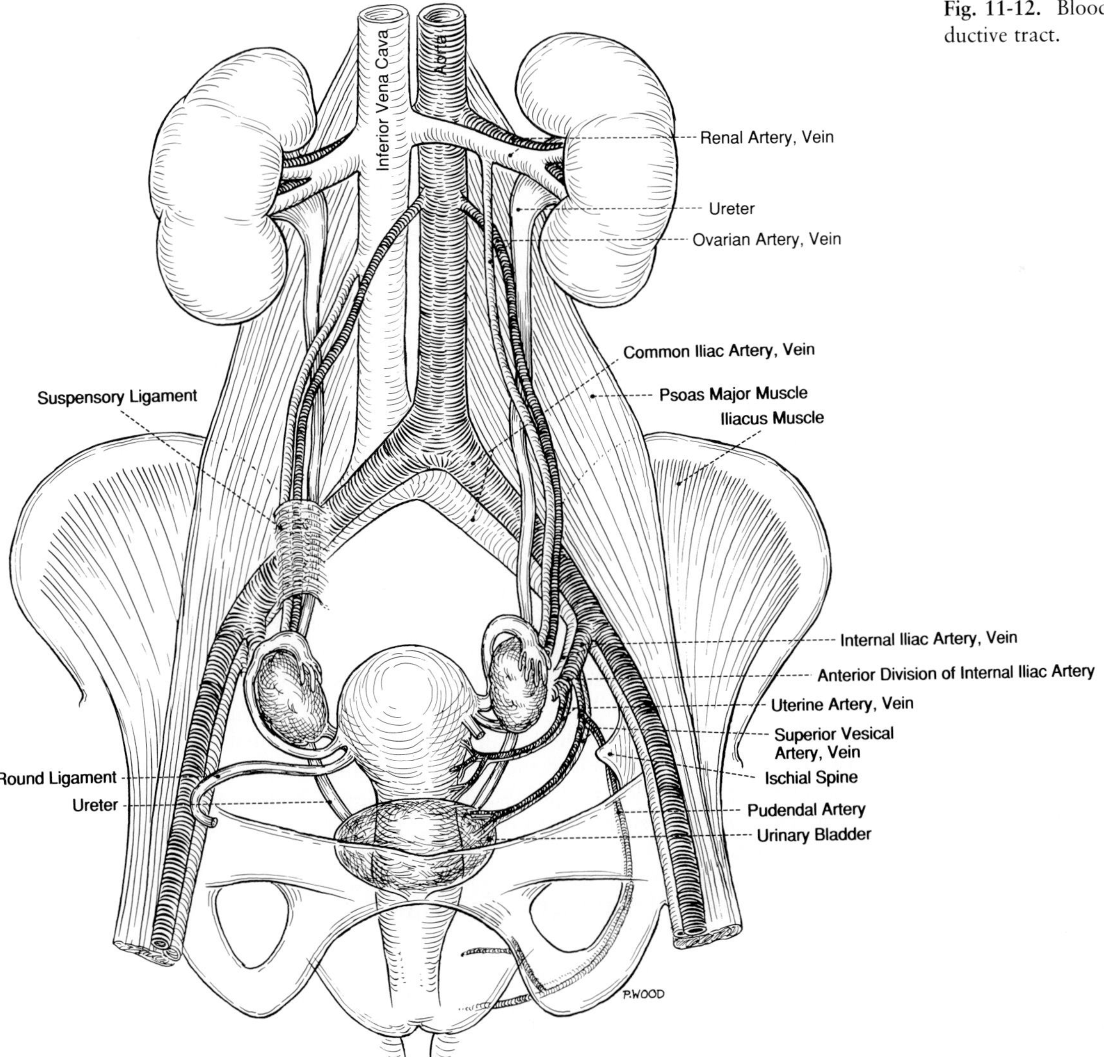


Fig. 11-12. Blood supply of female reproductive tract.

ischiorectal fossa. At this point the artery along with the internal pudendal vein and nerve becomes enclosed by the obturator fascia forming the pudendal canal (of Alcock). As the artery enters the pudendal canal it gives off an inferior rectal artery which supplies the anorectal junction. The remaining portion of the internal pudendal artery reaches the base of the urogenital diaphragm and gives off a series of perineal branches. These supply the contents of both superficial and deep perineal spaces, including the vagina and urethra and clitoris.

The venous drainage of both perineal triangles parallels the arterial supply. There is also a rich submucosal venous plexus in the distal vagina. Distension of these submucosal veins can produce vaginal or vulvar varices. The inferior rectal veins join the internal pudendal vein just as it leaves the ischiorectal fossa at the lesser sciatic foramen. Both the rectal and vaginal submucosal plexuses penetrate the pelvic diaphragm to communicate with the endopelvic space. Here, vaginal veins may anastomose with uterine veins and inferior rectal veins with middle rectal veins.

## LYMPHATIC DRAINAGE

As a general rule, lymphatic drainage follows the blood supply of a region. The lymphatic drainage of the perineum differs in this respect because there is a dual pathway. Deep lymphatics course upward following the pudendal veins, draining the deep parts of both urogenital and anal triangles. However, superficial lymphatics from the skin overlying the vulvar and anal areas course to the medial thigh where they communicate with superficial inguinal lymph nodes. Adenopathy of superficial inguinal nodes is well known in many vulvar and anal infections as well as in carcinoma of these regions.

## INNERVATION

The motor and sensory innervation of the perineum is via fibers from sacral roots S2, 3, and 4 forming the pudendal nerve (Fig. 11-13). Originating from the sacral plexus in the presacral region, the pudendal nerve exits the pelvis via the greater sciatic notch, crosses the sacrospinous ligament, enters the pudendal canal, and accompanies the pudendal vessels. The branches of the internal pudendal nerve are the inferior rectal, perineal, and dorsal clitoral nerves, supplying these respective areas.

# BLOOD SUPPLY, LYMPHATIC DRAINAGE, AND INNERVATION OF UTERUS AND VAGINA

## BLOOD SUPPLY

The uterus and upper vagina lie within the endopelvic space, that is, between the pelvic peritoneum and the pelvic diaphragm. These structures as well as the adjacent, rectum, bladder, etc., are all supplied by a single arterial trunk, the internal iliac artery (Fig. 11-12). It arises by division of the common iliac artery at the junction of the sacrum and the ilium. Descending in the lateral pelvis subperitoneally it gives off a series of visceral branches including rectal, uterine, and vesical. These course medially to enter the endopelvic space, at the base of the broad ligament. Before reaching the isthmus of the uterus the uterine artery crosses superior to the ureter, and gives branches to the vaginal fornix and cervix. Turning superiorly in the parametrial

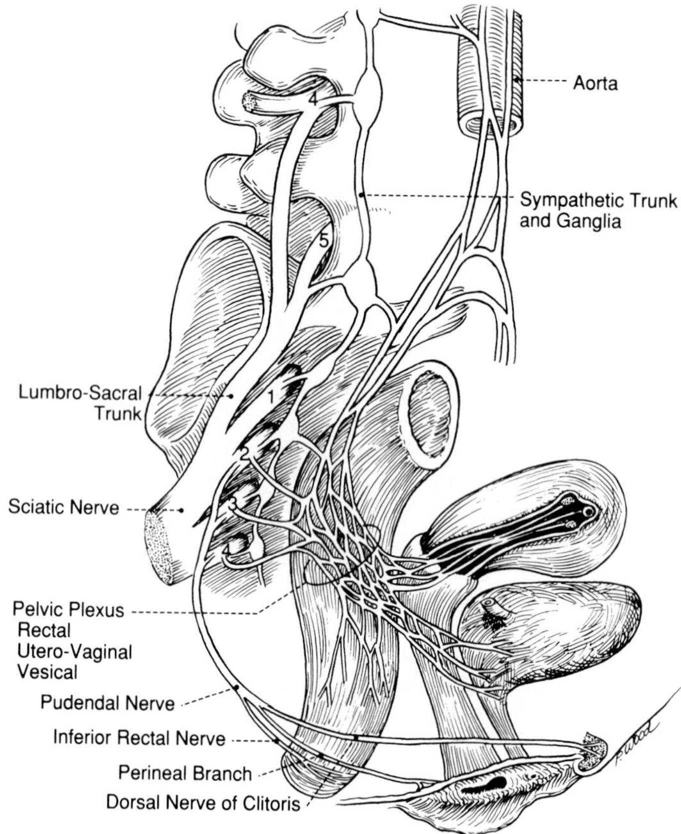


**Fig. 11-13.** Innervation of female reproductive tract.

space of the board ligament, a series of arterial branches is given to the body of the uterus until the artery anastomoses with the ovarian artery at the uterotubal junction.

The uterine vein is usually plexiform, coursing laterally in the base of the broad ligament before reaching the lateral pelvic wall. Here the plexus of veins forms a series of tributaries entering the internal iliac vein, which in turn empties into the inferior vena cava. Other veins in the endopelvic space include middle rectal veins draining the rectum.

The normal route of rectal venous flow is into the internal iliac vein. During pregnancy, the fetus may partially occlude the inferior vena cava when the woman is recumbent, increasing venous resistance and diminishing pelvic venous flow into the inferior vena cava. Because the middle rectal veins also communicate with the superior rectal branches of the inferior mesenteric vein, there is the potential that pelvic blood can ascend via the portal circulation. None of the pelvic veins contains valves, allowing blood to take the pathway of least resistance. Middle rectal veins also communicate with inferior rectal veins; these veins are tributaries of the internal pudendal vein which drains into the iliac veins before entering the inferior vena cava. Increased blood flow in these vessels, particularly in the last trimester of pregnancy, is a well-known cause of hemorrhoids.

## LYMPHATIC DRAINAGE

A plexus of uterine lymphatics parallels the course of uterine veins, entering regional lymph nodes along the internal iliac artery. From these nodes lymph trunks ascend to paraaortic nodes in the retroperitoneum.

### INNERVATION

The endopelvic space is the primary pathway for both motor and sensory nerve fibers supplying the uterus (Fig. 11-13). Sensory fibers from the uterine body descend in the parametrial space of the broad ligament to join other fibers from the cervix. These form a large plexus in the paracervical region termed the uterovaginal plexus or Frankenhauser's ganglion. In the endopelvic space these fibers commingle with visceral afferents from other pelvic viscera, before entering the inferior hypogastric plexus. Ascending the sacral promontory the fibers join the superior hypogastric plexus and enter the sympathetic trunk via lumbar splanchnic nerves.

From sympathetic ganglia white rami communicans conduct fibers to the dorsal roots of spinal nerves T10 to 12.

The uterovaginal plexus also includes parasympathetic motor fibers from sacral roots which enter the endopelvic space directly, as well as sympathetic motor fibers which enter from the sympathetic trunk. Concentration of uterine sensory fibers in the uterovaginal plexus is the anatomical basis for a regional anesthetic procedure, paracervical block. It is accomplished by inserting the needle of a syringe into each lateral vaginal fornix and infiltrating the paracervical area with a local anesthestic. This will often provide adequate anesthesia for instrumentation of the cervix and uterus.

## BLOOD SUPPLY, LYMPHATIC DRAINAGE, AND INNERVATION OF THE OVARY AND UTERINE TUBE

### BLOOD SUPPLY

The ovarian arteries arise as lateral branches from the abdominal aorta, descend in the retroperitoneal space, cross the ala of the sacrum, and enter the suspensory ligament of the ovary (Fig. 11-12). As the ovarian artery enters the lateral edge of the broad ligament it courses medially between the two layers of the ligament, giving branches to the ovary and uterine tube.

The venous drainage of the structures in the superior part of the broad ligament is via the ovarian vein, which parallels the ovarian artery as the vein ascends in the retroperitoneal space. On the right side the ovarian vein is a tributary of the inferior vena cava, whereas on the left side it drains into the left renal vein.

### LYMPHATIC DRAINAGE

Afferent lymphatics from the ovarian and uterine tube accompany ovarian vessels to paraaortic lymph nodes in the retroperitoneum. The fundus of the uterus is drained in part by this same route but also sends lymphatic vessels anteriorly paralleling the course of the round ligaments of the uterus. This bilateral course carries afferent lymphatics to inguinal lymph nodes on both sides of the pelvis.

### INNERVATION

The suspensory ligament of the ovary is also the afferent neural pathway for the ovary and uterine tube (Fig. 11-8). After reaching the retroperitoneum, these fibers join the superior hypogastric plexus, ascend briefly, and then enter a lumbar splanchnic to reach the sympathetic trunk. Ascending fibers leave the sympathetic trunk via rami communicantes to enter spinal sensory roots T10 to 12.

Chapter 12

# Genitourinary mucosal defenses

Myron S. Cohen
Robert D. Weber
Per-Anders Mårdh

The epidermal and mucosal surfaces provide an area wherein lower forms of life have an opportunity to parasitize a more sophisticated host. In this chapter we discuss the interaction between microbial pathogens and the host surfaces. This discussion also includes (1) a brief review of mucosal histology, (2) microbial adherence to the mucosa and possible microbial penetration of epidermis, (3) the interaction between microorganisms at the mucosal surface, (4) nonspecific mucosal defense mechanisms that help to prevent infection, and (5) humoral and cellular immunity at the mucosal surface. Effects of age, sexual activity, and hormonal and pharmacological influence are considered where relevant.

## THE STRUCTURE OF MUCOSA

Mucosa and epidermis are epithelial tissues which are protective barriers to underlying structures. Both mucosa tissue structures are separated from the underlying dermis by a basement membrane and have glandular structures which project deep into the dermis. In the epidermis, a layer of basal germinative cells undergo mitosis and exit toward the surface. During their migration these cells ultimately undergo changes in shape, and they extrude their nuclei (cornification) to form an outer horny layer (stratum corneum and granulosum); the formation of the stratum corneum is termed keratinization.[1] Mucosal epithelial surfaces can be distinguished from the epidermis by the fact that they do not form this horny layer of cornified cells; furthermore, mucosa is devoid of hair follicles.[2] Whereas the epidermis maintains an irregular, hard surface by virtue of the formation of the horny layer, the mucosa is shiny and smooth. Moisture is provided to the mucosa in two ways. First, a hydrophilic surface layer of glycoproteins and glycolipids is formed by epithelial cells, called the glycocalyx.[3] Second, goblet-shaped epithelial cells secrete a thick hydrophilic glycoprotein gel (mucus). Both the glycocalyx and mucus act as mucosal barriers.

Mucosa can be further defined by the morphology of the outermost layer (apical) cells and by the orientation of these cells.[2] Cellular morphology allows epithelial cells to be categorized as squamous or columnar. If a single layer is present, the epithelium is called *simple;* if several layers are present, it is labeled *stratified.* If only a single layer of cells is present, but the mucosa is folded so as to suggest multiple layers, it is called *pseudostratified.* Special mention should be made of "transitional" epithelium which is associated with the urogenital mucosa. In this tissue both squamous and columnar cells are present; because of the motion stresses to which it is subjected, the morphology may change.

The mucosa of the male and female urethra and of the female vagina and cervix is composed of all three morphogenic types of epithelium (columnar, squamous, and transitional). In addition, cornification of some cells occurs in the vaginal epithelium in response to maternal or postpubertal hormones. Local differences in the nature of epithelium within the same organ may influence susceptibility to sexually transmitted diseases, as has been reported with respect to adherence of bacteria in the oropharynx[4] and the urinary tract. Also, differences in microbial adherence to histologically indistinguishable cells are seen.[7,12]

The structure of the mucosa allows for the transport of substances from outside to the inside of the body (such as fluids and electrolytes in the gastrointestinal tract). In addition, the moisture provided by the mucosa facilitates transport of substances (such as semen) to the outside. On the other hand, loss of the protective horny layer of the epidermis increases risk of mucosal infection.[5]

Comment should be made regarding those pathogens which produce ulcers on the penile shaft or pudendal epidermis (e.g., herpes simplex, *Treponema pallidum, Haemophilus ducreyi*). Although a few fungi produce proteolytic enzymes which allow them to enter an unbroken stratum corneum,[5] penetration of this barrier by genital pathogens has not been demonstrated. It is widely speculated that sexual activity abrades the horny layer, thus allowing access to underlying epithelial cells.

## ACQUISITION OF MICROBIAL FLORA IN THE GENITAL TRACT

### ADHERENCE

Many microorganisms occur on genitourinary mucosal surfaces as transient organisms (e.g., in the vagina after sexual intercourse) and do not attach to the underlying tissue. Adherence of organisms to the mucosa represents a critical point of interaction. Organisms which are unable to attach and are swept away by mucociliary activity (e.g., in the cervix) and the mucus stream will generally not be able to efficiently damage underlying structures. Attachment may be followed by bacterial division without evidence of inflammation (colonization); this process leads to the formation of so-called normal, indigenous, or autochthonous microflora.[6,7] Alternatively, attachment may be associated with tissue damage and local inflammatory response (e.g., uncomplicated chlamydial and gonococcal infections) or disseminated disease (e.g., syphilis, disseminated gonococcal infection). Studies of human male and female urethral mucosa have demonstrated a very skewed distribution in bacterial attachment. That is, only a minority of urethral mucosal cells carry attached bacteria, but multiple bacteria attach to individual mucosal cells[6] (Figs. 12-1 and 12-2). This suggests the presence of differences in surface characteristics of urogenital mucosal cells.

The process by which bacteria attach to the mucosa can be summarized as follows. First, it is likely that microbes "sense" chemoattractant stimuli which lead them to bind to epithelial tissue (toxins).[8] At this point the organisms must find a suitable environment for the formation of flagellae and/or surfact factors (adhesins) which will ultimately enhance their attachment. There is increasing evidence that some bacteria have genetic mechanisms which allow rapid adaptation to different environments. For example, fimbriated (piliated) *Escherichia coli* attach efficiently to mucosa (see below),[9] but nonfimbriated cells are better adapted to disseminated disease because they are less likely than fimbriated cells to attach to neutrophils.[10] Pathogenic *E. coli* are programmed to undergo a frequent switch between the fimbriated and nonfimbriated states, which allows survival of the fittest organisms.[11]

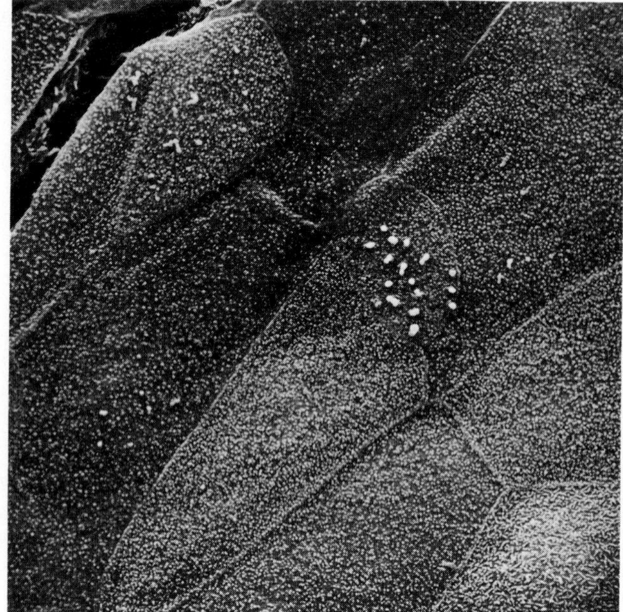

**Fig. 12-1.** Scanning electron micrograph of explant of male urethral mucosa, demonstrating skewed distribution in attachment of colonizing bacteria to mucosal cells.

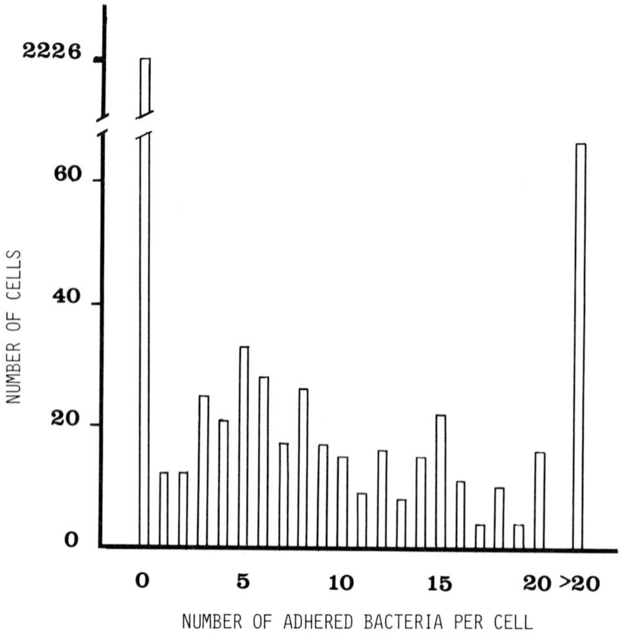

2226
60
40
20
0
NUMBER OF CELLS
0 5 10 15 20 >20
NUMBER OF ADHERED BACTERIA PER CELL

**Fig. 12-2.** Plot of numbers of adherent bacteria per mucosal cell, from an experiment similar to that described in Fig. 12-1. Most cells have no adherent bacteria, but a few cells have large numbers of adherent bacteria. *(From S Colleen et al, Scand J Urol Nephrol 14:9, 1980.)*

Subsequent to achieving the proper morphological state, a pathogen must overcome repelling physicochemical forces and penetrate the mucous gel which overlies the epithelium.[12] The physical characteristics of this gel vary dramatically in response to hormones as well as to other pharmacological stimuli[13,14] (see below). The mucous gel may act as a comfortable environment (rich in nutrients to support bacterial growth) or may in fact harbor specific and nonspecific defense mechanisms, compounds with antimicrobial activity produced by organisms colonizing the mucosal surfaces, and other factors which could impede the ability of the pathogen to reach the mucosa.[15] The antipathogenic activity of mucus will be discussed in more detail below.

## Biophysical factors which affect adherence

A wide variety of pathogens which have the ability to adhere to isolated epithelial cells or to intact mucosal tissue in vitro have been identified. The physicochemical characteristics which allow adherence of Enterobacteriaceae, different gram-positive cocci (e.g., *Staphylococcus epidermidis* and *S. saprophyticus*),[17] and *Neisseria gonorrhoeae*[16] have received attention. For the purposes of this discussion, the gonococcus will be used as a primary example.

It has been suggested that adherence depends on the outcome of specific and nonspecific interactions which must take place over both long and short distances.[12,16] Epithelial cells as well as bacterial pathogens have a net negative charge which results in an electrostatic repulsive force and therefore acts to prevent adherence. The eukaryotic cell surface charge is regulated by the ionized carboxylic groups of *N*-acetylneuraminic acid (which constitutes the bulk of the glycocalyx) as well as other anionic groups including alkaline phosphatase and ribonuclease-susceptible phosphate groups, and the beta- and gamma-carboxy groups of aspartic and glutamic acid.[12] The surface charge of bacteria is affected by the characteristics of the cell envelope and the formation of fimbriae or other adhesins.[16]

A theoretical explanation for the adherence of species that should be frankly repulsive is essential. One hypothesis which has gained attention is the notion of long-range attraction (at distances greater than 4 angstroms) between bacteria and mucosal cells. In the early 1940s Derjaquin, Landau, Verwey, and Ovherbeek advanced a theory, the DLVO hypothesis, to explain the paradoxical attraction between negatively charged hydrophobic colloid particles.[18] Experimental evidence provided by these investigators showed that the attraction or repulsion of particles is dependent on the distance at which this interaction is evaluated. Because repulsive energy decreases more rapidly than attractive force, a curve can be drawn which indicates a distance where bacterial-cell adhesion might actually be favored. Evidence to support this interaction has been summarized by Watt and Ward.[19] Furthermore, surface charge becomes less negative as pH is reduced because of a decrease in the dissociation of charged groups at anionic sites. Not surprisingly, if binding of bacteria to vaginal cells is measured at a reduced pH, a dramatic increase in binding can be documented.[20] In addition, if surface charge is raised by blocking anionic sites with compounds such as 1-ethyl-3-(dimethyl-aminopropyl) carbodilimide, a similar increase in binding of bacteria can be shown.[21]

These electrochemical forces are nonspecific. Another nonspecific variable is the hydrophobic-hydrophilic interaction between the pathogen and the cell; this interaction seems most important at close distances (short-range interaction).[16] Several groups have reported that those Enterobacteriaceae which are more hydrophobic display increased adherence to tissue culture cells relative to organisms which are less hydrophobic.[22–24] The importance of the hydrophobic interaction is less clear for the binding of gonococci.[19] Van Oss has suggested that a hydrophobic interaction may also be important for the binding of organisms to neutrophils[25] (see below).

### Bacterial adhesins

Once close interaction becomes possible, one or more bacterial cell surface characteristics (adhesins) probably mediate binding to specific cell receptors.[4,6,15,16] Ofek, Beachey, and several of their coworkers have demonstrated that a mannose-binding (type I pilus) protein in many strains of *E. coli* allows the attachment of such organisms to buccal epithelial cells.[9,10,16,26,27] It seems more than likely that this bacterial ligand is located in fimbriae.[9,10,28–30] A mannose resistant, type II, "P-fimbria" also allows attachment to uroepithelial cells glycolipid receptors which share the disaccharide gal-alpha-1-4-gal-beta,[31] and a unique helper region at the tip of the pilus has recently been described.[31] Attachment to these and other receptors[31–33] has a major impact on the pathogenesis of urinary tract infections. However, individuals lacking the P antigen can also develop pyelonephritis, and non-P-fimbriated *E. coli* strains are common among isolates from pyelonephritis cases. Neither has any difference in the density of receptors with P-antigen activity been found between persons who do and do not develop recurrent episodes of pyelonephritis. In many infections the adherence process is likely to be critical. For example, K88 *E. coli*, which cause piglet diarrhea, do not cause infection in animals lacking receptors for the K88 adhesin.[34]

With respect to gonococci, a clear advantage in binding to human cells exfoliated from the urogenital tract and human cells in tissue cell culture including fallopian tube explants can be demonstrated among fimbriated bacteria (T1 and T2 colony types).[19,35,36] The precise nature of the mucosal receptor(s) for binding of gonococcal pili is still under investigation, but carbohydrates are apparently involved.[19] Nonfimbriated gonococci are also able to bind to eukaryotic cells, although less efficiently. Several investigators have described outer membrane protein(s) (in the protein II group) which increase attachment of gonococci to mucosal cells as well as polymorphonuclear neutrophils (PMN)[37,38] (see below). The relative importance of fimbriae and outer-membrane proteins to adherence remains to be determined. In addition, binding of gonococci is influenced by the ionic concentration, pH, and temperature of the experimental medium.[19] Energy metabolism may also play an important role in adherence (see below).

Attachment of the bacterial species that do not form fimbriae deserves special attention. Gram-positive cocci may associate by virtue of surface lipoteichoic acids.[16] An attachment protein of mycoplasmas has been described which allows the binding of this organism to tracheal epithelium;[39] no data are available for the binding of mycoplasmas to genital mucosa.

With regard to *Candida albicans*, person-to-person variation in the ability of the yeast fungi to adhere to vaginal and buccal epithelial cells has been described.[40] While little variation between the two cell types have been demonstrated, *C. albicans* cells adhere in greater number per cell than other species of *Candida*, i.e., species less often encountered as vaginal pathogens.[41] *Candida* cells do not adhere better to vaginal cells from patients with recurrent vulvovaginal candidiasis than to such cells from healthy subjects.[42] (See also Chap. 45).

Microbial interaction may be important to keep *Candida* spp. in the vagina at a low number. In case the indigenous vaginal flora is disturbed as in patients treated with broad-spectrum antibiotics, such yeast fungi may increase dramatically in number.[43] It is thought that the disappearance of the production of compounds, e.g., bacteriocins, with antibacterial effect produced by bacteria of the normal vaginal flora may contribute to the expanding yeast flora.

The attachment and penetration of viral pathogens has been discussed in detail elsewhere.[44]

## NORMAL FLORA OF THE GENITAL TRACT

Organisms which cause an inflammatory response are pathogens; those which merely colonize the mucosa of normal hosts are designated normal flora.[6] The normal flora play a significant role in defense against infection by genital pathogens. The composition of the normal flora of the genital tract has been studied in great detail and will not be reviewed in this chapter. In males, the urethra normally contains comparatively few microorganisms (e.g., *S. epidermidis*, alpha-streptococci, corynebacteria). On the other hand, the female genital tract, especially the vaginal secretions, contains $10^8$ to $10^9$ bacteria per gram of fluid examined.[45] Both facultative (e.g., *S. epidermidis*, streptococci, and *E. coli*) and anaerobic (e.g., peptococci, lactobacilli, and *Bacteroides* spp.) bacteria can be isolated.[42,45–48] Facultative aerobic bacteria decrease in number in premenstrual specimens, whereas anaerobes tend to remain constant.[45] *Ureaplasma urealyticum* is often found in the genital tract of both males and females.[49] *Mycoplasma hominis* occurs in a proportion of healthy women. Although *M. hominis* is more commonly found in women with genital infections, its etiologic role in vaginitis and cervicitis is uncertain.[50] A co-occurrence of *M. hominis* and bacteria associated with bacterial vaginosis can be demonstrated.[42] Acquisition of *U. urealyticum* and *M. hominis* is directly related to sexual activity (see Chap. 26). Isolation of chlamydiae[51] or viruses[52] in the absence of signs of disease is less common, although the majority of infected areas are asymptomatic. Neither chlamydiae nor viruses are considered part of the normal flora.

A few additional points should be made about the normal flora of the genital tract. The organisms involved are often highly susceptible to the local environment and hormonal influence. The most traditional and well-studied view implies that glycogen is deposited in the vaginal epithelium in response to estrogenic hormones, and that glycogen is an optimal substrate for the growth of lactobacilli.[53] The vaginal flora has been believed to be restricted to those organisms that do well in an acidic environment.[53] More recent studies have explored the possibility that lactobacilli may produce substrates and enzymes that interact with other organisms in the female genital tract[54,55] (see below). L(+)-lactate, donated by lactobacilli or human cells (including phagocytes), appears to be a particularly important substrate for *N. gonorrhoeae*.[56] However, several observations challenge the importance of lactobacilli:

1. A decrease in vaginal lactobacilli does not always lead to an increase in pH.
2. In estrogen-treated patients the vaginal pH increases without relation to lactobacilli concentration.
3. Many lactobacilli do not metabolize glycogen.

The low level of lactobacilli in the vagina during menopause cannot be attributed to glycogen deficiency.[57] Experiments in rats[58] indicate that release of nutrients during vaginal epithelial proliferation and exfoliation has the most profound effects on the vaginal flora.

It has also been suggested that estrogen per se (independent of the deposition of glycogen) may have a direct effect on the number of organisms and composition of the bacterial flora.[57,59] Gonococci possess steroid receptors and progesterone suppresses their energy metabolism;[60] L(+)-lactate metabolism is least susceptible to the effects of progesterone (Lysko and Morse, unpublished data).

The virulence of microorganisms may differ depending on a variety of factors. For instance, a large body of literature suggests that urinary tract infections in females arise from the establishment of gram-negative rods in the vaginal vestibule and the periurethral areas,[33,48,61] from where they spread.[61] *S. saprophyticus* might also cause such infections[62] and is, next to *E. coli,* the most common cause of urinary tract infections in both males and females. *S. saprophyticus* adhere to epithelial cells and cast which can be demonstrated in urine sediments. Increased capacity for bacterial adherence to uroepithelial cells (either because of unusual properties of the bacterial isolates, epithelial cells, or mucosal secretions) may contribute to development of urinary tract infection.[61,63]

When high-absorbency tampons are used during menses, *S. aureus* may proliferate and produce a toxin(s) responsible for some or all of the manifestations of the toxic shock syndrome.[64,65] Such proliferation can also occur under other clinical circumstances.[66]

In addition, the genital tract represents an area of special concern because of its obvious importance to the fetus, which must pass through it during birth. Group B streptococci, chlamydiae, and viruses of the herpes group (herpes simplex virus types 1 and 2, cytomegalovirus) are major sources of disease for neonates;[67] isolation of these pathogens in the genital tract deserves special attention, even when the host suffers no immediate adverse consequences.

## MICROBIAL INTERACTIONS

There is a complicated interaction between pathogenic organisms and the indigenous bacterial flora[6] as well as between organisms of these two categories. This interaction may result in either synergy or antagonism of the genital pathogen. Vaginal lactobacilli in vitro can inhibit the growth of a wide variety of bacterial species that can grow on the genital mucosal surfaces, including genital pathogens.[54] Lactobacilli produce a number of compounds with antibacterial activity including lactocidin, acidolin, acidophilin, and lactacin B as well as lactic acid and hydrogen peroxide.[55] On the other hand, some of these organisms can inhibit lactobacilli.[54] Growth of gonococci is inhibited in vitro, e.g., by *Aeromonas* spp., lactobacilli, staphylococci, streptococci, vibrios, a variety of gram-negative rods, and *Candida* spp.[68–71] The contribution of the microflora to defense of the gastrointestinal tract mucosa is obvious, particularly in patients with severe neutropenia.[72] The clinical relevance of microbial interaction in the genital tract is far less certain and is an area that requires further evaluation. The rate of gonorrhea in women exposed to men with *N. gonorrhoeae* was not noticeably affected by the quantity or quality of the cervical-vaginal flora.[73] Sixbey and coworkers reported that superinfection of cervical explants with gonococci markedly increased formation of chlamydial inclusions.[74] This is nicely correlated with coinfection observed clinically.[75] Although gonococci have generally been considered aerobic, they are able to use nitrite as a terminal electron acceptor.[76] Gonococci grown under anaerobic conditions express new outer membrane proteins recognized by antibodies from patients recovering from PID or DGI.[77] L(+)-lactate metabolism greatly enhances gonococcal $O_2$ consumption,[56] and could facilitate the anaerobic microenvironment of the vagina.[78]

Interactions between staphylococci and other genital flora have also been studied. As early as 1899, Grosz and Kraus showed that staphylococci inhibited the growth of gonococci,[79] presumably through the production of extracellular antibacterial substances such as beta-acetylglucosaminidase. *S. aureus* produces lysostaphin interacting with bacterial cells of the same species. Coagulase-negative staphylococci, which are normal genital flora, also excrete inhibitory substances limiting growth of a variety of gram-negative (e.g., gonococci) and gram-positive competitors.[79–81] Some of these antibacterial products are most active at pH 5.5 to 6.5, consistent with the vaginal environment.[81] A low-molecular-weight polypeptide produced by coagulase-negative staphylococci was found to inhibit streptococci.[80] Staphylococcal products can protect embryonated hen's eggs from otherwise lethal staphylococcal infection.[82] Whether such a protective effect exists in vivo against staphylococcal colonization or clinical infection by *S. aureus* remains to be established.

## PROTECTION FROM INFECTION: NONSPECIFIC FACTORS

### Mucus

Mucus consists primarily of glycoproteins.[83] Once mucus has been secreted onto an epithelial surface, it provides a variety of functions, certainly the most important of which include lubrication and acting as a selective barrier to exogenous macromolecules.[84] Human semen and vaginal secretions are rich in mucus.[13,85] Mucus in the female genital tract is derived primarily from the cervix.[85] The secretion and structure of mucus are susceptible to a variety of pharmacological stimuli. Mucus in the female genital tract is quite clearly under hormonal control, and dramatic changes in viscosity can be demonstrated during the menstrual cycle.[13,85] Interestingly these rheological changes are associated with very minor alterations in protein structure.[13] Mucus in the genital tract is of paramount importance to conception,[85] and it may also play a role in host defenses in a variety of ways.[15] First, mucus may act to exclude a variety of pathogens or antigens. The altered flora and increased inflammation which are associated with atrophic vaginitis (where mucus content is decreased for a variety of reasons) may be viewed as a clue to the importance of this secretion. Second, since mucus is rich in carbohydrates, it has been suggested that one or more sugar moieties may be offered to the invading pathogen and occupy a critical bacterial ligand, thereby interfering with the adherence of the pathogen to the epithelial layer.[15,86] Carbohydrate residues in mucus may also act as receptors for the bacteria constituting the indigenous flora.

Mucus plays an indirect role in host defenses by providing an appropriate support medium for other defenses (e.g., lactoferrin, lysozyme, antibody) or by providing an appropriate environment in which phagocytic cells can engulf and kill invading pathogens. The hypothesis that mucus may act as an immunological defense is supported by the observation that the oral presentation of antigen-antibody complexes in the rodent gut directly stimulates the secretion of mucus by epithelial cells in response to antigen challenge.[87]

Alternatively, it is possible that mucus or one of its components interferes with host defenses. Using a mouse model of disseminated gonococcal infection, Corbeil and coworkers found that a mucin-hemoglobin mixture interfered with the animals' ability to limit gonococci injected into the peritoneal cavity, presumably by disrupting normal white cell function.[88] Brooks and his colleagues have identified a substance in seminal plasma which interferes with serum and PMN bactericidal activity, apparently through the action of a factor or factors which interfere with complement activation.[89]

### Other antimicrobial secretions

Both lysozyme and lactoferrin have been isolated in genital secretions. Lysozyme hydrolyzes beta-1,4 linkages of microorganisms in which this enzymatic site is available, and thereby allows osmotic lysis or the formation of spheroplasts in vivo.[90] It has also been suggested that lysozyme may inhibit bacterial adherence by stearic hindrance. In tissue cell cultures lysozyme had no inhibitory effect on chlamydiae, and at certain concentrations it actually stimulated the formation of intracytoplasmic chlamydial inclusions.[91] Lysozyme may act most effectively in concert with other antimicrobial defenses[92] (see below).

Lactoferrin is an iron-binding protein which may slow bacterial growth by competing for this essential element.[93] Payne and her colleagues have suggested that bacterial strains (e.g., *N. gonorrhoeae*) which produce uncomplicated mucosal infections are relatively poor in their ability to obtain iron in competition with the host, whereas those strains that produce disseminated infection have an enhanced ability to acquire iron.[94] More recently, Mickelsen et al.[95] have reported that gonococcal auxotrophs which are most commonly associated with asymptomatic infection (Arg-Hyx-Ura-strains) are poor in their ability to acquire iron from lactoferrin relative to other strains. It was suggested that these strains might fail to produce local disease because they do not multiply effectively when forced to compete with lactoferrin for iron. Under these circumstances the inception of disseminated gonococcal infection with menses might be due in part to the provision of iron in the form of hemin and transferrin, which would then abolish the limitations imposed by lactoferrin at the mucosal surface. More work is required to prove the importance of lactoferrin to defense against gonococci. Little, if any, information is available regarding the iron utilization of other genital pathogens. The lactoferrin concentration in vaginal secretions ranges between 3.8 and 218 μg/mg of protein.[96] Lactoferrin concentration is greatest just after menses, and falls off sharply during the latter (secretory) phase of the menstrual cycle. Women receiving estrogen/progesterone oral contraceptive pills were found to have persistently low levels of lactoferrin, emphasizing the hormonal regulation of this compound.

Another element that may play an important role at the mucosal surface is zinc.[97–99] Zinc is found in high concentration in prostatic tissue and secretions[97,98] (see also Chap. 54), and it is believed to be the active ingredient of "prostatic antibacterial factor" described by Fair and his coworkers.[97] Zinc inhibits the growth of a variety of urinary pathogens,[97] *Chlamydia trachomatis*,[91] *Candida* spp.,[100] herpes simplex,[101] and *Trichomonas vaginalis*.[102] Although patients with prostatic disease generally have a depressed concentration of zinc,[99] the concentrations encountered are generally higher than those required to inhibit most pathogens which have been examined. Cohen and coworkers have reported that the concentration of zinc in vaginal mucus ranges between 7.95 and 62 mg/mg of protein.[103] Other metal ions, e.g., $Cu^{2+}$, inhibit the formation of chlamydial inclusions in tissue cell cultures.[91]

Polyamines such as spermine found in high concentrations in prostatic fluid have a cidal effect on many bacteria.[98] Spermidine and spermine also have been demonstrated to interfere with *C. trachomatis* in tissue cell culture.[91]

## SPECIFIC IMMUNE MECHANISMS AT THE MUCOSAL SITES

### Humoral immunity

Antibody is readily identified in mucosal secretions.[104] Antibody molecules can act directly to interfere with attachment of bacteria or to neutralize viruses; they can act in concert with complement components to exert bactericidal activity; or, with the help of complement, they can opsonize pathogens to enhance their interaction with phagocytic cells or make them more susceptible to intracellular lysis.[105]

Over the last 15 years vigorous investigation into the nature of mucosal antibody secretion has revealed a remarkably complex system. This information has been compiled in reviews by Tomasi and his colleagues,[106–108] and more recently by Strober and coworkers.[109] To briefly summarize, the concentration of IgA in genital mucosal secretions generally exceeds the concentration of IgG or IgM.[110,111] Antibody is produced locally by plasma cells in the submucosal tissue, which lie in close proximity to the epithelium.[94] The IgA in genital secretions is strikingly different from IgA found in serum. It is composed of 10-S dimer (300,000 daktibs), a J chain, and a secretory component. The J chain is made by plasma cells and appears to polymerize 7-S IgA monomers (the IgA normally found in serum) into 10-S dimers. The secretory component is formed by the mucosal cells and binds to the polymeric immunoglobulin molecule as it is transported to the mucosal surface; secretory component may render IgA less susceptible to proteolytic substances found in genital secretions.[112] IgA consists of two subclasses ($IgA_1$ and $IgA_2$) which can be identified on the basis of structural and antigenic differences.[113] The relative concentrations of $IgA_2$ in genital secretions have not been determined.

The formation and secretion of IgA is clearly susceptible to external stimuli. IgA directed at specific gonococcal antigens can be detected after infection and lasts for at least several weeks.[112] Furthermore, McChesney and colleagues have recently shown that systemic (intramuscular) presentation of antigen (gonococcal pili) leads to an increased concentration of antibody in vaginal or urethral secretions.[114] This antibody may arise by the migration of responsive immunocytes to target tissues or by leakage of serum antibodies. The former theory is favored because a disproportionately high concentration of secretory IgA (SIgA) relative to IgG or IgM has been recovered in the genital secretions examined,[114] and by the literature surrounding gut immunity.[109]

A variety of specific biological functions for SIgA have been demonstrated. Using gut mucosa, Walker and his colleagues were able to show that SIgA interfered with absorption of some antigens.[115] Antigen-SIgA complexes stimulate mucus production, which may then impede the access of pathogens to the mucosa.[87] The ability of SIgA to interfere with the adherence of a wide variety of bacteria to mucosal surfaces has been repeatedly demonstrated.[106] Tramount and his colleagues[112] have shown that both IgG and IgA inhibit the attachment of *N. gonorrhoeae* to epithelial cells and that antibodies isolated in genital secretions subsequent to natural infection are strain-specific and last for several weeks. Binding of SIgA to different gram-negative rods alters the bacteria to make them hydrophilic, which might then interfere with their attachment to epithelial cells (see above);[114,115] paradoxically, however, SIgA reduces net negative surface charge which might be expected to make the bacteria less "repulsive" to the cell surface layer.[17] Furthermore, in general no advantage in phagocytosis by neutrophils can be demonstrated when bacteria are opsonized with IgA.[116–118] Bisno and coworkers,[119] however, reported enhanced phagocytosis of virulent gonococci opsonized by serum IgA isolated from a patient recovering from a disseminated gonococcal infection.

Although SIgA antibodies are able to agglutinate bacteria, they do not have innate bactericidal activity;[120,121] SIgA antibody may activate the alternative pathway of complement and thereby stimulate a lytic complex.[122] Several groups have suggested that the combination of lysozyme, SIgA, and complement may form a bactericidal defense.[120,121] At present the complement concentration of genital secretions is not well appreciated, although Price and Boettcher have reported that the hemolytic complement levels of cervical mucus are 11.5 percent of those of serum.[123] The biological relevance of the bactericidal activity of secretory antibody is not known. Several bacterial species (including gonococci) have evolved mechanisms to evade the bactericidal activity of serum.[124,125] Joiner et al. showed that blocking immunoglobulin G directed against the outer membrane protein PIII competes with bactericidal antibody for binding to gonococci.[126] There was enhanced complement activation but decreased killing in the presence of this antibody.[126] The observation that many gonococci isolated in mucosal surfaces are sensitive to the complement-mediated action of serum[127] raises serious doubt about the importance of the complement-mediated bactericidal mechanism as a mucosal defense.

Secretory antibodies are of undoubted importance in defense against a variety of viruses, as demonstrated by the ablation of the mucosal carriage of poliovirus after oral (Sabin) vaccine[128] and the clear protection offered against certain rhinoviruses by nasal immunization capable of eliciting SIgA.[129] Little or no information is available concerning the role of secretory antibody in defense against viruses of the herpes group or the human immunodeficiency virus (HIV), although systemic antibody response has been studied.[130–132] Likewise, the interaction between secretory immunoglobulin and toxins liberated by bacteria such as the staphylococci associated with the toxic shock syndrome has not been evaluated; host defense mechanisms which may be of importance in the toxic shock syndrome have recently been reviewed.[133]

A variety of microorganisms elaborate a protease which cleaves IgA at the hinge, thereby rendering SIgA subclass 1 inactive.[134,135] Mulks and Plaut[136] have reported that only pathogenic species of *Neisseria* produce IgA protease, implying that the protease is a major virulence factor in gonococcal infection. The relative importance, however, of SIgA in defense against gonococci remains poorly understood; the presence of SIgA in urethral secretion does not seem to prevent recurrent infection.[137] On the other hand, SIgA may help to prevent symptomatic salpingitis in patients who develop local endocervical gonococcal infection.[114,138]

## Phagocytic cells

Professional phagocytic cells (PMNs and monocytes) are critical for survival and most probably play an important defensive role at the mucosal surface. The interaction between gonococci and PMNs has been extensively studied (see below), and a growing body of literature is developing concerned with the interaction of phagocytes and chlamydiae,[139] group B streptococci,[140] trichomonads,[141,142] and viruses including HIV-1.[132] A discussion of this subject is most easily divided according to the essential functions of the phagocytic cell.

### Chemotaxis

Phagocytic cells must be signaled to migrate to areas of bacterial invasion. The necessary signals may actually emanate from the microbial pathogen involved or by the generation of complement components (C5a) when the pathogen is allowed to interact with serum.[103] There is disagreement about whether gonococci release soluble chemoattractants into the culture supernatant.[143,144] Densen and coworkers[145] have provided evidence that gonococci isolated from mucosal surfaces (in uncomplicated infections) generate complement-derived chemoattractants significantly more rapidly than gonococci isolated from patients with disseminated infection, implying that a rapid inflammatory response may help to prevent invasion or dissemination of gonococci. No information is available to explain the absence of an inflammatory response in the urethra of those men who harbor gonococci in the absence of symptoms. Poisson and Rein have reported that *T. vaginalis* may also interact with serum to form soluble chemoattractants.[142]

### Attachment and ingestion

Attachment of bacteria to phagocytic cells results from nonspecific factors, ligand-receptor interactions,[16] and opsonization with serum-derived immunoglobulin and complement.[105] All three components of this system are probably important. There is strong evidence that one or more surface factors (perhaps outer-membrane proteins) of the gonococcus mediate attachment to neutrophils in the absence of serum.[35,37,146,147] Alternatively, studies using both visual and metabolic assays support the notion that serum may enhance the cellular association of some types of gonococci.[119,148–152,153] Cohen and coworkers[154] have recently reported that interference with bacterial energy metabolism prevents maximal attachment of gonococci to phagocytic cells, presumably by interfering with charge derived from the proton motive force. Also, growth of gonococci in physiologic media such as serum allows expression of new outer membrane proteins and decreases attachment to polymorphonuclear leukocytes.[155] Attachment to phagocytic cells must be carefully separated from ingestion, but a variety of methodological problems make experimentation in this area difficult. Studies designed to investigate the ingestion of gonococci have found that fimbriae[147,148,156] as well as other surface factors[157] may be antiphagocytic. There is disagreement about whether serum is necessary to enhance the ingestion of nonfimbriated gonococci.[147,152]

Whereas cellular association with phagocytic cells is generally looked upon as a distinct disadvantage to the pathogen, special mention should be made of situations in which phagocytic cells may act as a reservoir of infection. Cytomegalovirus is associated with blood leukocytes,[158] and it is possible that cellular association may also be found with other herpes viruses as well. After ingestion of chlamydiae by monocytic phagocytes, the chlamydiae inhibit the fusion of lysosomes with the phagocytic vacuole and are then able to resist intracellular killing.[159] The tropism of HIV-1 for macrophages has been well documented,[132] and infection of this cell type allows viral replication, which may prove critically important to the biology of this infection (see below).

### Microbicidal metabolism

Phagocytic cells are uniquely designed to use their oxygen and glucose metabolism (the respiratory burst) to make toxic oxygen-reduction products such as superoxide and hydrogen peroxide and to employ prepackaged bactericidal granule enzymes.[92] Microbicidal metabolism is triggered by the perturbation of the phagocyte membrane, regardless of whether or not ingestion actually occurs (reviewed in Ref. 92). The interaction of gonococci and neutrophils has attracted special attention because of the observation that fimbriated gonococci activate neutrophil oxygen metabolism in the absence of ingestion.[148] Recent studies have demonstrated a role for both oxygen-dependent[149,150] and oxygen-independent mechanisms[151] in killing of chlamydiae in vitro. Interestingly, several authors have noted that phagocytic cells infected with viruses are impaired in their ability to use oxygen, form oxygen-reduction products, and kill bacterial pathogens.[160,161]

The available evidence supports the concepts that PMNs and monocytes are competent to kill ingested gonococci,[148,153,158,162] although some authors have suggested that gonococci are capable of intracellular survival, perhaps related to unique "resistance proteins."[163,164] Recently, Ross and Densen reported that serum-sensitive gonococcal isolates are more susceptible to neutrophil killing them are serum-resistant organisms, perhaps because of enhanced opsonization by the early components of complement.[165]

The mechanisms employed by PMNs to kill bacteria have been the subject of intense investigation. Rest and coworkers[153] reported that neutrophils incapable of using molecular oxygen (cells from patients with chronic granulomatous disease) were competent to kill gonococci. Daly and coworkers observed that gonococcal isolates differ in their susceptibility to nonoxidative killing by azurophilic PMN granule contents;[166] these differences seem to be based on minor variations in peptidoglycan cross-linking. Strains of gonococci which are likely to cause gonococcal bacteremia (penicillin-sensitive isolates) seem to be more resistant to killing by PMN granules than penicillin-resistant strains which rarely cause gonococcal bacteremia.[166] Gonococci in the presence of serum or phagocytic cells demonstrate enhanced metabolism which can be ascribed to L(+)-lactate oxidation.[56] Under some conditions incubation-stimulated bacterial respiration can completely eliminate the formation of reactive oxygen derivatives by neutrophils.[78]

Little is known about the mechanisms employed by phagocytic cells to kill other sexually transmitted pathogens. PMNs are certainly competent to kill trichomonads by oxygen-dependent mechanisms.[141] In fascinating phase-contrast microscopy of these events, Rein and coworkers showed that neutrophils surround, attack, and fragment the trichomonads, and that the trichomonad can subsequently be ingested in pieces.[141]

### Cell-mediated immunity and sexually transmitted diseases

It is difficult to study the role that lymphocyte-monocyte interactions play in mucosal defense. Investigators have shown the lymphocyte transformation of blood leukocytes in response to a variety of pathogens, including uncomplicated gonorrhea,[137,167] uncomplicated[168] and complicated[169] (e.g., salpingitis) chlamydial infection, *T. pallidum,* [170] and viruses of the herpes group.[130] In general, patients who have experienced one or more of these infections can be expected to have a lymphocytic response in vitro, although these responses may be susceptible to a variety of factors and generally are not protective against recurrent infection. Alternatively, it is possible that mucosal infection may adversely affect local and systemic immunity; for example, one or more of the staphylococcal toxins associated with toxic shock syndrome may modulate the activity of circulating lymphocytes.[133]

The acquired immunodeficiency syndrome (AIDS) predisposes one to a broad variety of "opportunistic infections" and neoplasms, clinical manifestations considered unusual in individuals not infected with HIV-1 (see Chaps. 30, 56, 57).[171] The virus has been isolated from tears, saliva, vaginal secretions, semen, urine, and serum (see Chaps. 28, 80).[172–176] Cervical secretions of women have been shown to contain the virus throughout the menstrual cycle.[177] There was no identifiable pattern to the shedding, and it occurred when simultaneous blood cultures for the virus tested negative. Blood cultures commonly became positive earlier than cultures of cervical secretions, suggesting a higher titer of virus in the blood. Certain individuals deviated from this pattern, however, suggesting rather high levels of virus in their cervical secretions. The source of HIV-1 in cervical secretions is not known, but it appears not to be solely due to menstrual bleeding.[177] HIV-1 is rarely found in cell-free filtrates, implying that it is cell-associated.[177,178] Similarly, it has been suggested that semen may contain HIV-1 more frequently than the peripheral blood.[156] Recent work has suggested that the sperm may play a role in the entry of HIV-1 into the host (Ref. 180 and V.L. Scofield, personal communication).

Certain sexual practices are associated with higher risk of HIV-1 infection, even when one controls for the number of sexual contacts. Sexual contact with IV drug users[181,182] or with prostitutes[183,184] confers a greater risk of HIV-1 infection, probably because these groups have a high risk of being seropositive. Anal receptive intercourse and anal insertive intercourse are also associated with a higher risk of infection.[185] This is presumably due to the mucosal trauma resulting from such behavior. Debate exists about the risk of sex during menses, with one report finding an increased risk[186] and another finding no increased risk.[185] Studies in Africa have suggested that a past history of genital ulcer disease confers a risk for HIV-1 infection as well.[187] This seems to be independent of the etiology of the genital ulcers, again inferring that the break in mucosal integrity is important. Presently little is known about the ability of HIV-1 to penetrate intact mucosa or the mechanisms whereby it might effect this. In the chimpanzee model, it has been possible to transmit HIV-1 infection by placing the virus on the vaginal mucosa but not the oral mucosa.[188]

In addition to the direct interaction between HIV-1 and the host mucosa, the presence of this infection has an indirect effect on the mucosal defenses. This is mediated through the effects of other infecting organisms such as *Candida* (e.g., oral, esophageal, rectal, or vaginal) or herpes simplex virus (types 1 or 2). Such organisms can cause ulcerations leading to a break in the mucosal barrier. Some attention has also been devoted to the role of HIV-1 in predisposing patients to periodontal disease that is quite severe in certain cases.[189] Women who are HIV-1 infected have a higher prevalence of vaginal or cervical squamous atypia than controls.[190]

## CONCLUSION

Sexually transmitted diseases represent a major and growing health hazard. In the last 10 years remarkable research efforts have provided a framework for understanding natural resistance to common pathogens such as *N. gonorrhoeae*, and similar data are being gathered for *C. trachomatis*. This research has gradually narrowed to a clear focus on mucosal defenses. The importance of understanding these defenses has been emphasized by frantic attempts to develop a vaccine for HIV-1 infection. It may ultimately prove essential to interrupt infection of one or more vaginal cell types to prevent transmission. Therefore, mucosal defenses will be subjected to even greater scrutiny in the coming years, and the information gained (although perhaps esoteric in title or description) can be expected to be of critical importance in the control and management of a variety of important disease processes.

## References


1 Breathnach AS, Wolff K: Structure and development of the skin, in *Dermatology in General Medicine,* TB Fitzpatrick et al (eds). New York, McGraw-Hill, 1979, p 41.

2 Lever WF, Schaumberg-Lever G: *Histopathology of the Skin*. Philadelphia, Lippincott, 1975, p 13.

3 Bennett HS: Morphological aspects of extracellular polysaccharides. *J Histochem Cytochem* 11:14, 1963.

4 Gibbons RJ, van Houte J: Bacterial adherence in oral microbial ecology. *Annu Rev Microbiol* 29:19, 1975.

5 Blank IH: The skin as an organ of protection against the external environment, in *Dermatology in General Medicine,* TB Fitzpatrick et al (eds). New York, McGraw-Hill, 1979, p 102.

6 Colleen S et al: Bacterial colonization of human urethral mucosa. I: Scanning electron microscopy. *Scand J Urol Nephrol* 14:9, 1980.

7 Savage DC: Adherence of normal flora to mucosal surfaces, in *Bacterial Adherence,* EH Beachey (ed). London, Chapman & Hall, 1980, p 33.

8 Adler J et al: Chemotaxis toward sugars in *Escherichia coli. J Bacteriol* 115:824, 1973.

9 Ofek I, Beachey EH: Mannose binding and epithelial cell adherence of *Escherichia coli. Infect Immun* 22:247, 1978.

10 Bar-Shavit Z et al: Mannose residues on phagocytes as receptors for the attachment of *Escherichia coli* and *Salmonella typhi. Biochem Biophys Res Comm* 78:455, 1977.

11 Eisenstein B: Phase variation of type 1 fimbriae in *Escherichia coli* is under transcriptional control. *Science* 214:337, 1981.

12 Colleen S: The human urethral mucosa: An experimental study with emphasis on microbial attachment. *Scand J Urol Nephrol* (suppl) 68:14, 1982.

13 Gibbons RA: Mucus of the mammalian genital tract. *Br Med Bull* 34:34, 1978.

14 Parke DV: Pharmacology of mucus. *Br Med Bull* 34:89, 1978.

15 Freter R: Prospects for preventing the association of harmful bacteria with host mucosal surfaces, in *Bacterial Adherence,* EH Beachey (ed). London, Chapman & Hall, 1980, p 441.

16 Beachey EH: Bacterial adherence in animals and man, in *Bacterial Adherence,* EH Beachey (ed). London, Chapman & Hall, 1980, p 3.

17 Colleen S et al: Physico-chemical properties of *Staphylococcus epidermidis* and *Staphyloccoccus saprophyticus* as studied by aqueous polymer two-phase systems. *Scand J Infect Dis* 24:165, 1980.

18 Verwey EJW, Ovherbeek TG: *The Theory of Stability of Lymphophobic Colloids*. Amsterdam, Elsevier, 1948.

19 Watt PU, Ward ME: Adherence of *Neisseria gonorrhoeae* and other *Neisseria* species to mammalian cells, in *Bacterial Adherence,* EH Beachey (ed). London, Chapman & Hall, 1980, p 253.

20 Mårdh P-A, Weström L: Adherence of bacteria to vaginal epithelial cells. *Infect Immun* 13:661, 1976.

21 Heckels JE et al: The influence of surface change on the attachment of *Neisseria gonorrhoeae* to human cells. *J Gen Microbiol* 96:359, 1976.

22 Perens L et al: Association of some enterobacteria with the intestinal mucosa of mouse in relation to their partition in aqueous polymer two-phase systems. *Acta Pathol Microbiol Scand* [B]:308, 1977.

23 Smythe CJ et al: Differences in hydrophobic surface characteristics of porcine enteropathogenic *Escherichia coli* with or without K88 antigen as revealed by hydrophobic interaction chromatography. *Infect Immun* 22:462, 1978.

24 Kihlström E, Edebo L: Association of viable and inactivated *Salmonella typhimurium* 395 MS and MR 10 with HeLa cells. *Infect Immun* 14:851, 1976.

25 Van Oss CJ, Gillman CF: Phagocytosis as a surface phenomenon: II. Contact angles and phagocytosis of encapsulated bacteria before and after opsonization by specific antiserum and complement. *J Reticuloendothel Soc* 12:492, 1972.

26 Ofek I et al: Adherence of *Escherichia coli* to human mucosal cells mediated by mannose receptors. *Nature* 265:623, 1977.

27 Ofek I et al: Surface sugars of animal cells as determinants of recognition in bacterial adherence. *Trends Biochem Sci* 3:159, 1978.

28 Salit IE, Gotschlich EC: Hemagglutination by purified type I *Escherichia coli* pili. *J Exp Med* 146:1169, 1977.

29 Salit IE, Gotschlich EC: Type I *Escherichia coli* pili: Characterization of binding to monkey kidney cells. *J Exp Med* 146:1182, 1977.

30 Issacson RE et al: In vitro adhesion of *Escherichia coli* to porcine small intestinal epithelial cells: Pili as adhesive factors. *Infect Immun* 21:392, 1978.

31 Lomberg H et al: Influence of blood group on the availability of receptors for attaching *E. coli. Infect Immun* 51:919, 1986.

32 Lindberg F et al: Localization of the receptor-binding protein adhesin at the tip of the bacterial pilus. *Nature* 328:84.

33 Kunin CM: *Detection, Prevention and Management of Urinary Tract Infections*. Philadelphia, Lea & Febiger, 1987, p 140.

34 Sellwood R et al: Adhesion of enteropathogenic *E. coli* to pig intestinal brush borders: The existence of two pig phenotypes. *J Med Microbiol* 8:405, 1975.

35 Swanson J: Studies on gonococcus infection. IV: Pili: Their role in attachment of gonococci to tissue culture cells. *J Exp Med* 137:571, 1973.

36 Mårdh P-A et al: Attachment of bacteria to exfoliated cells from the urogenital cells. *Invest Urol* 16:322, 1979.

37 Lambden PR et al: Variations in surface protein composition associated with virulence proteins in opacity types of *Neisseria gonorrhoeae. J Gen Microbiol* 114:305, 1979.

38 Swanson J: Adhesion and entry of bacteria into cells: A model for the pathogenesis of gonorrhoea, in *The Molecular Basis of Microbial Pathogenicity,* H Smith et al (eds). Weinheim, Verlag Chemie, 1980, p 17.

39 Hu PC et al: *Mycoplasma pneumoniae* infections: Role of a surface protein in the attachment organelle. *Science* 216:313, 1982.

40 Sobel JD et al: *C. albicans* adherence to vaginal epithelial cells. *J Infect Dis* 143:76, 1981.

41 King RD et al: Adherence of *C. albicans* and other candida species to mucosal epithelial cells. *Infect Immun* 27:667, 1980.

42 Holst E et al: Bacterial vaginosis: Microbiology and clinical findings. *Eur J Clin Bacteriol* 6:536, 1987.

43 Fleury FJ: Adult vaginitis. *Clin Obstet Gynecol* 24:407, 1981.

44 Dales S: Early events in cell-animal virus interactions. *Bacteriol Rev* 37:103, 1973.

45 Bartlett JG et al: Quantitative bacteriology of the vaginal flora. *J Infect Dis* 136:271, 1977.

46 Ohm MJ, Galask RP: Bacterial flora of the cervix from 100 prehysterectomy patients. *Am J Obstet Gynecol* 122:683, 1975.

47 Pfau A, Jacks T: The bacterial flora of the vaginal vestibule, urethra, and vagina in the normal premenopausal woman. *J Urol* 118:292, 1976.

48 Fair WR et al: Bacteriologic and hormonal observations of the urethra and vaginal vestibule in normal, premenopausal women. *J Urol* 104:426, 1970.

49 Mårdh P-A, Weström L: T-mycoplasmas in the genito-urinary tract of the female. *Acta Pathol Microbiol Scand* [B] 78:367, 1970.

50 McCormack WR, Taylor-Robinson D: Genital mycoplasmas. *N Engl J Med* 302:1003, 1980.

51 Schachter J: Chlamydial infections. *N Engl J Med* 298:428, 1978.

52 Rawls WE, Campione-Piccardo J: Epidemiology of herpes simplex virus type I and type II infections, in *The Human Herpesviruses: An Interdisciplinary Perspective,* AJ Nahmias et al (eds). New York, Elsevier, 1980, p 32.

53 Cruickshank R, Sharman A: The biology of the vagina in the human subject II: The bacterial flora and secretion of the vagina in relation to glycogen in the vaginal epithelium. *J Obstet Gynecol Br Emp* 41:208, 1939.

54 Mårdh P-A, Soltesz LV: In vitro interactions between lactobacilli and other microorganisms occurring in the vaginal flora. *Scand J Infect Dis Suppl* 40:47, 1983.

55 Metha AM et al: Isolation and purification of an inhibitory protein from *Lactobacillus acidophilus. AC Microbes* 37:37, 1983.

56 Britigan BE et al: Neutrophil derived lactate stimulates the metabolism of *Neisseria gonorrhoeae:* An unappreciated aspect of the phagocytic respiratory burst. *J Clin Invest* 88:318, 1988.

57 Gregoire AT et al: The glycogen content of the human vaginal epithelial tissue. *Fertil Steril* 22:64, 1971.

58 Larsen B, Galask RP: Vaginal microbial flora: Practical and theoretic relevance. *Obstet Gynecol* 55:100S, 1980.

59 Larsen B et al: Role of estrogen in controlling the genital microflora of female rats. *Appl Environ Microbiol* 34:534, 1977.

60 Morse SA, Fitzgerald TJ: Effect of progesterone on *Neisseria gonorrhoeae. Infect Immun* 10:1370, 1974.

61 Stamey TA: *Pathogenesis and Treatment of Urinary Tract Infections: Some Observations of the Pathogenesis of Recurrent Bacteriuria in Women and Children.* Baltimore, Williams & Wilkins, 1980, p 219.

62 Hovelius B et al: *Staphylococcus saprophyticus* in the aetiology of nongonococcal urethritis. *Br J Vener Dis* 55:369, 1979.

63 Svanborg-Eden C et al: Adhesion of *Escherichia coli* to human uroepithelial cells in vitro. *Infect Immun* 18:767, 1977.

64 Schlievert PM et al: Identification and characterization of an exotoxin from *Staphylococcus aureus* associated with toxic shock syndrome. *J Infect Dis* 143:569, 1981.

65 Bergdoll MS et al: A new staphylococcal enterotoxin, enterotoxin F, associated with toxic-shock syndrome *Staphylococcus aureus* isolates. *Lancet* 1:1017, 1981.

66 Todd JK: Toxic shock syndrome: A perspective through the looking glass. *Ann Intern Med* 96:839, 1982.

67 Remington JS, Klein JO: *Infectious Diseases of the Fetus and Newborn Infant.* Philadelphia, Saunders, 1976.

68 Kaye D, Levinson ME: In vitro inhibition of growth of *Neisseria gonorrhoeae* by genital microorganisms. *Sex Transm Dis* 4:1, 1977.

69 Hipp SS et al: Inhibition of *Neisseria gonorrhoeae* by a factor produced by *Candida albicans. Appl Microbiol* 27:192, 1974.

70 Shtibel R: Inhibition of growth of *Neisseria gonorrhoeae* by bacterial interference. *Can J Microbiol* 22:1430, 1976.

71 Saig JH et al: Inhibition of *Neisseria gonorrhoeae* by aerobic and facultatively anaerobic components of the endocervical flora. Evidence for a protective effect against infection. *Infect Immun* 19:704, 1978.

72 Schimpff SC et al: Origin of infection in acute nonlymphocytic leukemia: Significance of hospital acquisition of potential pathogens. *Ann Intern Med* 77:707, 1972.

73 Meck L, Sparling PF: Personal communication.

74 Sixbey JW et al: Growth of *Chlamydia trachomatis* in human cervical epithelial cell monolayers. *Clin Res* 30:379A, 1982.

75 Sweet RL et al: The occurrence of chlamydial and gonococcal salpingitis during the menstrual cycle. *JAMA* 255:2062, 1986.

76 Clark VL et al: Induction of and repression of outer membrane proteins by anaerobic growth of *Neisseria gonorrhoeae. Infect Immun* 55:1359, 1987.

77 Clark VL, Klimpel KW: Sera from UGI anaerobically expressed gonococcal outer membrane protein. *87th Annual meeting of the American Society of Microbiology.* 1987, p 16.

78 Britigan BE, Cohen MS: Effects of human serum on bacterial competition for molecular oxygen. *Infect Immun* 52:657, 1986.

79 Grosz S, Kraus R: Bacteriologische Studien über den Gonococcus. *Arch Dermatol Syph Wien* 45:329, 1899.

80 Loeb LJ et al: An antibiotic produced by *Micrococcus epidermidis. Can J Res* (E) 28:212, 1950.

81 Soltesz LV, Mårdh P-A: Antibiosis caused by bacteriolytic enzymes of coagulase-negative staphylococci with special reference to *Staphylococcus saprophyticus,* in *Coagulase-negative Staphylococci,* P-A Mårdh, KH Schleiffer (eds). Almquist & Wiksell International Stockholm, 1986, p 59.

82 Soltez LV, Mårdh P-A: Lethal effect of *Staphylococcus aureus* in embryonated hen's eggs inhibited by coagulase-negative staphylococci, in *Coagulase-negative Staphylococci,* P-A Mårdh, KH Schleifer (eds). Almquist & Wiksell International Stockholm, 1986, p 75.

83 Reid L, Clamp JR: The biochemical and histochemical nomenclature of mucus. *Br Med Bull* 34:5, 1978.

84 Edward PAW: Is mucus a selective barrier to macromolecules? *Br Med Bull* 39:55, 1978.

85 Elstein M: Functions and physical properties of mucus in the female genital tract. *Br Med Bull* 34:83, 1978.

86 Williams RC, Gibbons RJ: Inhibition of streptococcal attachment to receptors on human buccal epithelial cells by antigenically similar salivary glycoproteins. *Infect Immun* 11:711, 1975.

87 Lake AM et al: Intestinal goblet cell mucus release. II: In vivo stimulation by antigen in the immunized rat. *J Immunol* 122:834, 1979.

88 Corbeil LB et al: Disseminated gonococcal infection in mice. *Infect Immun* 26:984, 1979.

89 Brooks GF et al: Human seminal plasma inhibition of antibody complement-mediated killing and opsonization of *Neisseria gonorrhoeae* and other gram-negative organisms. *J Clin Invest* 67:1523, 1981.

90 Strominger JL, Ghuysen JM: Mechanisms of enzymatic bacteriolysis. *Science* 156:213, 1967.

91 Mårdh PA et al: Inhibitory effect on the formation of chlamydial inclusions in McCoy cells by seminal fluid and some of its components. *Invest Urol* 17:510, 1980.

92 Root RK, Cohen MS: The microbicidal mechanisms of human neutrophils and eosinophils. *Rev Infect Dis* 3:565, 1981.

93 Oram JD, Reiter B: Inhibition of bacteria by lactoferrin and other iron-chelating agents. *Biochim Biophys Acta* 170:351, 1968.

94 Payne SM, Finkelstein RA: The critical role of iron in host bacterial interactions. *J Clin Invest* 61:1428, 1978.

95 Mickelsen PA et al: Ability of *Neisseria gonorrhoeae, Neisseria meningitidis,* and commensal *Neisseria* species to obtain iron from lactoferrin. *Infect Immun* 35:915, 1982.

96 Cohen MS et al: Preliminary observations on lactoferrin secretion in human vaginal mucus: Variation during the menstrual cycle and evidence of hormonal regulation, and implications for infection with *N. gonorrhoeae. Am J Obstet Gynecol* (in press).

97 Fair WR et al: Prostatic antibacterial factor: Identity and significance. *Urology* 7:169, 1976.

98 Mårdh P-A, Colleen S: Antimicrobial activity of human semen. *Scand J Urol Nephrol* 9:17, 1975.

99 Colleen S et al: Magnesium and zinc in seminal fluid of healthy males and patients with non-acute prostatis with and without gonorrhoeae. *Scand J Urol Nephrol* 9:192, 1975.

100 Soll DR et al: Zinc and regulation of growth and phenotype in the infectious yeast *Candida albicans. Infect Immun* 32:1139, 1981.

101 Fridlender B et al: Selective inhibition of herpes simplex virus type I DNA polymerase by zinc ions. *Virology* 89:551, 1978.

102 Krieger JN, Rein MF: Canine prostatic secretions kill *Trichomonas vaginalis. Infect Immun* 37:77, 1982.

103 Cohen MS et al: Host defenses and vaginal mucosa: A reevaluation. *Scand J Urol Nephrol* 86:13, 1985.

104 Hulka JF, Omran K: The uterine cervix as a potential local antibody secretor. *Am J Obstet Gynecol* 104:440, 1969.

105 Root RK: Humoral immunity and complement, in *Principles and Practice of Infectious Diseases,* GL Mandell et al (eds). New York, Wiley, 1979, p 21.

106 McNabb PC, Tomasi TB: Host defense mechanisms at mucosal surfaces. *Annu Rev Microbiol* 35:477, 1981.

107 Tomasi TB, Grey HM: Structure and function of immunoglobulin A. *Prog Allergy* 16:136, 1972.

108 Tomasi TB: Secretions, in *The Immune System of Secretions,* AG Osler, L Weiss (eds). Englewood Cliffs, N.J., Prentice-Hall, 1976.

109 Strober W et al: *Recent Advances in Mucosal Immunity.* New York, Raven Press, 1982.

110 Waldman RH et al: Immunoglobulin levels and antibody to *Candida albicans* in human cervicovaginal secretions. *Clin Exp Immunol* 9:427, 1971.

111 Chipperfield EJ, Evans BA: Effect of local infection and oral contraception on immunoglobulin levels in cervical mucus. *Infect Immun* 11:215, 1975.

112 Tramont EC: Inhibition of adherence of *Neisseria gonorrhoeae* by human genital secretions. *J Clin Invest* 59:117, 1977.

113 Vaerman JP, Heremans JF: Subclasses of human immunoglobulin A based on differences in the alpha polypeptide chain. *Science* 153:647, 1966.

114 McChesney D et al: Genital antibody response to a parenteral gonococcal pilus vaccine. *Infect Immun* 36:1006, 1982.

115 Walker WA et al: Intestinal uptake of macromolecules: Effect of oral immunization. *Science* 177:608, 1972.

116 Magnusson K-E et al: Reduction of phagocytosis, surface hydrophobicity and charge of *Salmonella typhimurium* 395 MR10 by reaction with secretory IgA (SIgA). *Immunology* 36:439, 1979.

117 Magnusson K-E et al: The effect of colostrum and colostral antibody SIgA on the physico-chemical properties and phagocytosis of *Escherichia coli* 086. *Acta Pathol Microbiol Scand* [B] 86:113, 1978.

118 Que PG et al: Phagocytosis in subacute bacterial endocarditis: Localization of the primary opsonic site to Fc fragment. *J Exp Med* 128:553, 1968.

119 Bisno AL et al: Human immunity to *Neisseria gonorrhoeae* acquired serum opsonic antibodies. *J Lab Clin Med* 86:221, 1975.

120 Adinolfi M et al: Serological properties of A antibodies to *Escherichia coli* present in human colostrum. *Immunology* 10:517, 1966.

121 Hill IR, Porter P: Studies of bactericidal antibody to *Escherichia coli* of porcine serum and colostral immunoglobulins and the role of lysozyme with secretory IgA. *Immunology* 26:1239, 1974.

122 Gotze O, Muller-Eberhard HJ: The C3-activator system: An alternate pathway of complement activation. *J Exp Med* 134:90S, 1971.

123 Price RJ, Boettcher B: The presence of complement in human cervical mucus and its possible relevance to infertility in women with complement-dependent sperm immobilizing antibodies. *Fertil Steril* 32:61, 1979.

124 McCutchan JA et al: Role of blocking antibody in disseminated gonococcal infection. *J Immunol* 121:1884, 1978.

125 Shafer WM et al: Serum sensitivity of *Neisseria gonorrhoeae:* Role of lipopolysaccharide. *J Infect Dis* 149:175, 1984.

126 Joiner KA et al: Mechanism of action of blocking immunoglobulin G for *Neisseria gonorrhoeae. J Clin Invest* 76:1765, 1985.

127 Brooks GF, Ingwer I: Studies on the relationships between serum bactericidal activity and uncomplicated genital infections due to *Neisseria gonorrhoeae. J Infect Dis* 138:333, 1978.

128 Ogra PL et al: Immunoglobulin response in serum and secretions after immunization with live and inactivated polio vaccine and natural infection. *N Engl J Med* 279:893, 1968.

129 Perkins JC et al: Evidence for protective effect of an inactivated rhinovirus vaccine administered by the nasal route. *Am J Epidemiol* 90:319, 1969.

130 Shore SL, Feorino PM: Immunology of primary herpes virus infection in humans, in *The Human Herpesviruses: An Interdisciplinary Perspective,* AJ Nahmias et al (eds). New York, Elsevier, 1980, p 267.

131 Friedman MG, Kimmel N: Herpes simplex virus-specific serum immunoglobulin A: Detection in patients with primary or recurrent herpes infections and healthy contacts. *Infect Immun* 37:374, 1982.

132 Levy JA et al: Aids associated retroviruses can productively infect other cells besides human T helper cells. *Virology* 147:441, 1985.

133 David JP et al: Possible host-defense mechanisms in toxic shock syndrome. *Ann Intern Med* 96:986, 1982.

134 Plaut AG et al: Differential susceptibility of human IgA immunoglobulins to streptococcal IgA protease. *J Clin Invest* 54:1295, 1974.

135 Plaut AG et al: *Neisseria gonorrhoeae* and *Neisseria meningiditis:* Extracellular enzyme cleaves human immunoglobulin A. *Science* 190:1103, 1975.

136 Mulks MH, Plaut AG: IgA protease production as a characteristic distinguishing pathogenic from harmless *Neisseriaceae. N Engl J Med* 299:973, 1978.

137 Kearns DH et al: Paradox of the immune response to uncomplicated gonococcal urethritis. *N Engl J Med* 289:1170, 1973.

138 O'Reilly RJ et al: Secretory IgA antibody responses to *Neisseria gonorrhoeae* in the genital secretions of infected females. *J Infect Dis* 133:113, 1976.

139 Wyrick PB, Brownridge EA: Growth of *Chlamydia psittaci* in macrophages. *Infect Immun* 19:1054, 1978.

140 Anderson DC et al: Luminol-enhanced chemiluminescence for evaluation of type III group B streptococcal opsonins in human sera. *J Infect Dis* 141:320, 1980.

141 Rein MF et al: Trichomonacidal activity of human polymorphonuclear neutrophils: Killing by disruption and fragmentation. *J Infect Dis* 142:575, 1980.

142 Poisson MA, Rein MF: Chemoattractiveness of vaginal pathogens. *Twenty-first Conference on Antimicrobial Agents and Chemotherapy,* Chicago, abstract 573. 1981.

143 James AN, Williams RP: Chemotactic factor(s) of *Neisseria gonorrhoeae. Curr Microbiol* 1:341, 1978.

144 Watt PJ, Medlen AR: Generation of chemotaxins by gonococci, in *Immunobiology of Neisseria Gonorrhoeae,* GF Brooks et al (eds). Washington, DC, American Society for Microbiology, 1978, p 239.

145 Densen P et al: Gonococci causing uncomplicated gonorrhea or disseminated gonococcal infection differ in stimulation of neutrophil chemotaxis and phagocytosis, in *Genetics and Immunobiology of Pathogenic Neisseria,* S Normark, D Danielsson (eds). Hemavan, Sweden, EMBO Workshop, 1980.

146 King GJ, Swanson J: Studies on the gonococcus infection: Identification of surface proteins of *Neisseria gonorrhoeae* correlated with leukocyte association. *Infect Immun* 21:575, 1978.

147 Dilworth JA et al: Attachment and ingestion of gonoccocci by human neutrophils. *Infect Immun* 11:512, 1975.

148 Densen P, Mandell GL: Gonococcal interactions with polymorphonuclear neutrophils: Importance of the phagosome for bactericidal activity. *J Clin Invest* 62:1161, 1978.

149 Yong EC et al: Toxic effect of human polymorphonuclear leukocytes on *Chlamydia trachomatis. Infect Immun* 37:422, 1982.

150 Yong EC, Chi EY et al: Degradation of *Chlamydia trachomatis* in human polymorphonuclear leukocytes: An ultrastructural study of peroxidase-positive phagolysosomes. *Infect Immun* 53:427, 1986.

151 Register KB et al: Nonoxidative antimicrobial effects of human polymorphonuclear leukocyte granule proteins on *Chlamydia* spp. in vitro. *Infect Immun* 55:2420, 1987.

152 Schiller NL et al: The role of natural IgG and complement in phagocytosis of type 4 *Neisseria gonorrhoeae* by human polymorphonuclear leukocytes. *J Infect Dis* 140:698, 1979.

153 Rest RK et al: Interactions of *Neisseria gonorrhoeae* with human neutrophils: Effects of serum and gonococcal opacity on phagocyte killing and chemiluminescence. *Infect Immun* 36:737, 1982.

154 Cohen MS et al: Gonococcal energy is required for their association with human neutrophils. *Program and Abstracts of the Twenty-Seventh Interscience Conference on Antimicrobial Agents and Chemotherapy,* October 4–7, 1987, p 192.

155 Britigan BE et al: Effects of human serum on the growth and metabolism of *Neisseria gonorrhoeae:* An alternative view of serum. *Infect Immun* 50:738, 1985.

156 Punsalang AP Jr, Sawyer WD: Role of pili in the virulence of *Neisseria gonorrhoeae. Infect Immun* 8:255, 1973.

157 Rosenthal RS et al: Ethylenediaminetetraacetic acid-sensitive antiphagocytic activity of *Neisseria gonorrhoeae*. *Infect Immun* 15:817, 1977.
158 Winston DJ et al: Prophylactic granulocyte transfusions during human bone marrow transplantation. *Am J Med* 68:893, 1980.
159 Eisenberg LG, Syrick PB: Inhibition of phagolysosome fusion is localized to *Chlamydia psittaci*-laden vacuoles. *Infect Immun* 32:889, 1981.
160 Sawyer WD: Interaction of influenzae virus with leukocytes and its effect on phagocytosis. *J Infect Dis* 119:541, 1969.
161 Faden H et al: Effect of viruses on luminol dependent chemiluminescence of human neutrophils. *Infect Immun* 24:673, 1979.
162 Drutz DJ: Intracellular fate of *Neisseria gonorrhoeae*, in *Immunobiology of Neisseria gonorrhoeae*, GF Brooks et al (eds). Washington, DC, American Society for Microbiology, 1978, p 232.
163 Witt K et al: Resistance of *Neisseria gonorrhoeae* grown in vivo in ingestion and digestion by phagocytes of human blood. *J Gen Microbiol* 96:341, 1976.
164 Parsons NJ et al: A determinant of resistance of *Neisseria gonorrhoeae* to killing by human phagocytes: An outer membrane lipoprotein of about 20 kDa with a high content of glutamic acid. *J Gen Microbiol* 1323:3277, 1986.
165 Ross SG, Densen P: Local and disseminated gonococcal isolates differ in opsonic requirements and efficiency of phagocytosis by neutrophils. *Clin Res* 30:378A, 1982.
166 Daly JA et al: Gonococci with mutations to low-level penicillin resistance exhibit increased sensitivity to the oxygen-independent bactericidal activity of polymorphonuclear leukocyte granule extracts. *Infect Immun* 35:826, 1982.
167 Kraus SJ et al: Lymphocyte transformation in repeated gonococcal urethritis. *Infect Immun* 2:655, 1970.
168 Hanna L et al: Human cell-mediated immune response to chlamydial antigens. *Infect Immun* 23:412, 1979.
169 Hallberg T et al: Pelvic inflammatory disease in patients, infected with *Chlamydia trachomatis:* In vitro cell mediated immune response to chlamydial antigens. *Genitourin Med* 61:247, 1985.
170 Pavia CS et al: Selective in vitro response of thymus-derived lymphocytes from *Treponema pallidum*-infected rabbits. *Infect Immun* 18:603, 1977.
171 Masur H et al: An outbreak of community-acquired *Pneumocystis carinii* pneumonia: Initial manifestations of cellular immune dysfunction. *N Engl J Med* 305:1431, 1981.
172 Fujikawa LS et al: Isolation of human T-lymphotropic virus type III from the tears of a patient with the acquired immunodeficiency syndrome. *Lancet* 2:529, 1985.
173 Ho D et al: Infrequency of isolation of LTLV-III virus from saliva in AIDS. *N Engl J Med* 313:1606, 1985.
174 Groopman JE et al: HTLV-III in saliva of people with AIDS-related complex and healthy homosexual men at risk for AIDS. *Science* 226:447, 1984.
175 Vogt MW et al: Isolation of HTLV-III/LAV from cervical secretions of women at risk for AIDS. *Lancet* 1:525, 1986.
176 Wofsy CB et al: Isolation of AIDS-associated retrovirus from genital secretions of women with antibodies to the virus. *Lancet* 1:527, 1986.
177 Vogt MW et al: Isolation patterns of the human immunodeficiency virus from cervical secretions during the menstrual cycle of women at risk for the acquired immunodeficiency syndrome. *Ann Intern Med* 106:380, 1987.
178 Wofsy CB et al: Isolation of AIDS-associated retrovirus from genital secretions of women with antibodies to the virus. *Lancet* 1:527, 1986.
179 Lafleur FL et al: Prevalence of HTLV-III infection in peripheral blood, seminal mononuclear cells and cell free semen of AIDS-related complex and AIDS associated Kaposi's sarcoma patients: Preliminary analysis (Abstract 624), in *Program and Abstracts of the Second International Conference on AIDS, Paris, June 23–25, 1986*. Paris, L'association pour la Recherché sur les Deficits immunitaires Viro-Induits; p 143, 1986.
180 Ashida ER, Scofield VA: Lymphocyte major histocompatibility complex-encoded class II structures may act as sperm receptors. *Proc Natl Acad Sci USA* 84:3395, 1987.
181 Acquired immunodeficiency syndrome (AIDS) among blacks and Hispanics—United States. *MMWR* 35:655, 1986.
182 Guinan ME, Hardy A: Epidemiology of STDS in women in the United States: 1981 through 1986. *JAMA* 257:2039, 1987.
183 Clumeck N et al: Heterosexual promiscuity among African patients with AIDS. *N Engl J Med* 313:182, 1985.
184 Van de Perre P et al: Female prostitutes: A risk group for infection with human T-cell lymphotropic virus type III. *Lancet* 2:524, 1985.
185 Steigbigel NH et al: Heterosexual transmission of infection and disease by the human immunodeficiency virus (HIV). *III International Conference on AIDS, Washington, DC.* Abstracts, Volume, W.2.5, 1987.
186 Cohen JB et al: Sexual and other practices and risk of HIV infection in a cohort of 450 sexually active women in San Francisco. *III International Conference on AIDS*, Washington, DC. Abstracts, Volume, WP.57, 1987.
187 Greenblatt RM et al: Genital ulceration as a risk factor for human immunodeficiency virus infection in Kenya. *III International Conference on AIDS*, Washington, DC. Abstracts, Volume, THP.67, 1987.
188 Fultz PN et al: Vaginal transmission of human immunodeficiency virus (HIV) to a chimpanzee. *J Infect Dis* 154:896, 1986.
189 Wright DC et al: Chemoprophylaxis prevents recurrence of *Pneumocystis carinii* pneumonia (PCP) in retrovirus induced immunodeficiency (AIDS). *III International Conference on AIDS*, Washington, DC. Abstracts, Volume, TP. 166, 1987.
190 Schrager L et al: Increased risk of cervical and/or vaginal squamous atypia in women infected with HIV. *III International Conference on AIDS*, Washington, DC. Abstracts, Volume, TP.143, 1987.

# PART V SEXUALLY TRANSMITTED AGENTS

# Chapter 13
# Biology of *Neisseria gonorrhoeae*

P. Frederick Sparling

## DEFINITIONS

*Neisseria gonorrhoeae* (gonococci) are the etiologic agent of gonorrhea and its related clinical syndromes (urethritis, cervicitis, salpingitis, bacteremia, arthritis, and others). It is closely related to *N. meningitidis* (meningococci), the etiologic agent of one form of bacterial meningitis, and relatively closely to *N. lactamica,* an occasional human pathogen. The genus *Neisseria* includes a variety of other relatively or completely nonpathogenic organisms which are principally important because of their occasional diagnostic confusion with gonococci and meningococci.

This chapter is concerned principally with the microbiology, genetics, and pathogenicity of gonococci. Chapter 14 is concerned with the clinical syndromes caused by gonococci and their treatment. A detailed discussion of diagnostic methods for gonococcal infections is found in Chap. 73.

## HISTORY

Gonorrhea is one of the oldest known diseases of humans. There have been many reviews of the history of this disease of which one of the best is the monograph by R. S. Morton.[1] Gonorrhea undoubtedly was known to the authors of the Bible. The Book of Leviticus describes a person with urethral discharge. Proclamations that infected persons were to keep themselves from others for 7 days may indicate that they already knew the mean incubation period was 7 days. Biblical authors cautioned about transmission to social contacts and also about women copulating with afflicted men.

Hippocrates wrote extensively of gonorrhea in the fourth and fifth centuries B.C. He called acute gonorrhea "strangury" and understood that it resulted from "the pleasures of Venus." The Roman physician Celsus, who lived at about the time of Christ, was well aware of gonorrhea and its complications and was known to catheterize patients suffering from urethral stricture. Galen in the second century coined the word *gonorrhea,* by which he meant "flow of semen." Other early Greco-Roman physicians prescribed various treatments for gonorrhea including sexual abstinence and the washing of the eyes of the newborn.

Knowledge of gonorrhea and other sexually transmitted diseases in Europe was scant until near the end of the Dark Ages. The term *clap* which is still commonly used to refer to this disease, first appeared in print in 1378. The derivation of the word *clap* is unclear but possibly refers to the *Les Clapier* district of Pairs in which prostitutes were housed in the Middle Ages. Other origins for the term *clap* are possible, but regardless it was clear in European writings of the late Middle Ages that the disease was associated with sexual intercourse.

After the arrival of syphilis in Europe in the late fifteenth century, considerable confusion existed regarding the relation between gonorrhea and syphilis. Great surgeons such as Ambroise Paré (sixteenth century) and John Hunter (eighteenth century) considered syphilis and gonorrhea to be different manifestations of a single disease. Hunter's conclusions were the result of a famous experiment in which he inoculated himself with material from a patient with gonorrhea with the result that he acquired syphilis. Distinction between these diseases was first clearly achieved by Philippe Ricord, but real understanding was only achieved after Neisser's description of *N. gonorrhoeae* in 1879, and Leistikow's and Löffler's cultivation of the organism in 1882.

The twentieth century is remarkable for the introduction of new, safe, highly effective therapy for gonorrhea, replacing the sometimes horrific therapies used for centuries including urethral astringents, soundings, and other mechanical devices. Sulfonamides were first introduced for gonorrhea therapy in 1936 and penicillin in 1943. The second great development of this century concerns the revolution in our understanding of the pathogenic mechanisms of this fascinating organism, which started with the demonstration by Kellogg and his colleagues in 1963 that there are differences in virulence of gonococci with different colonial morphology.[2] These developments enable better understanding of how gonococci cause repeated infections in the same individual (Boswell, Samuel Johnson's famous biographer, had at least 19 separate bouts of urethritis), and may lead to development of an effective vaccine.

## EPIDEMIOLOGY

### TRANSMISSION

Humans are the only natural host for gonococci. Gonococci survive only a short time outside the human body. Although gonococci can be cultured from a dried environment such as a toilet seat up to 24 h after being artificially inoculated in large numbers onto such a surface, there is virtually no evidence that natural transmission occurs from toilet seats or similar objects. Gonorrhea is a classic example of an infection spread by contact: immediate physical contact with the mucosal surfaces of an infected person, usually a sexual partner, is required for transmission. (The single exception is the occasional epidemic among prepubescent females living together and sharing bath towels and similar objects.) Although meningococci can be spread by air droplet transmission over short distances, there is no evidence that gonorrhea is ever transmitted by such a mechanism.

### STRAIN TYPING

For epidemiologic studies it is useful to differentiate one strain from another. Several techniques have been developed that can be used successfully for this purpose.

#### Auxotypes

A relatively cumbersome system for differentiating gonococcal strains based on their ability to grow on chemically defined media has been developed. This system was originally developed by B. W. Catlin,[3] and classifies strains as to whether they can grow without certain amino acids, purines or pyrimidines, or other specific nutrients. A strain unable to grow on chemically defined media lacking proline is designated Pro$^-$, and a strain unable to grow without arginine is Arg$^-$. Naturally occurring gonococcal isolates exhibit remarkable diversity in their biosynthetic capacities, probably reflecting the biochemically rich environment of their human host, which provides the organisms with most of the compounds needed for growth. Genetic studies have shown that strains with a similar nutritional phenotype (e.g., Arg$^-$) may have multiple mutations in a single biochemical pathway.[4] The auxotyping system has been used successfully in a variety of epidemiologic studies.[5] Certain auxotypes are biologically and epidemiologically important. For instance, the Arg$^-$ Hyx$^-$ (hypoxanthine$^-$) Ura$^-$ (uracil$^-$), or AHU$^-$, auxotype typically is associated with multiple other properties, including resistance to killing by normal human serum; propensity for causing asymptomatic male urethral infection; increased likelihood for causing bacteremia, and others.[6] Because of the complexity of preparing the chemically defined media, and the short storage life of the media, the auxotyping technique is not widely used in clinical laboratories.

## Serotyping

Investigators tried for decades to develop a practical serotyping scheme. The most useful and widely available technique for this purpose at present is based on monoclonal antibodies specific for various epitopes on outer membrane protein I (P.I).[7] P.I occurs in two immunochemically distinct serogroups: P.IA and P.IB. By employing a set of monoclonal antibodies against serogroup P.IA strains and another set against P.IB strains, one can subdivide each of the serogroups into a wide variety of serovars (e.g., P.IA-6, P.IB-1) differing in their ability to react with certain members of the panel of monoclonal antibodies. Many dozens of specific serovars have been defined by these techniques.[5,7] By a combination of auxotyping and serotyping with anti-P.I monoclonal antibodies, gonococci can be divided into over 70 different strains; the number may turn out to be much larger. Techniques for use of monoclonal antibodies in serotyping are discussed more fully in Chap. 73. These reagents are widely available in the United States and can be stored for years.

A second scheme for serotyping is based on the known variability of the gonococcal lipooligosaccharides (LOSs). A variety of monoclonal antibodies against LOS epitopes have been isolated by Apicella and his colleagues, and at least four classes of LOS epitopes have been identified.[8] However, the utility of this system is compromised somewhat by the variability of expression of LOS epitopes in vivo and in vitro,[9–11] unlike P.I epitopes, which are expressed stably in vitro.

## Antimicrobial susceptibilities

A third method to strain type gonococci is based on antimicrobial susceptibilities. This once was used widely and still may be employed as a useful adjunct to the auxotyping and serotyping schemes,[12] but the ability of gonococci to transfer antibiotic resistance between strains seriously compromises the utility of this method for long-term epidemiologic studies.

# BIOLOGY

## MORPHOLOGY

Gonococci are gram-negative diplococci, nonmotile and non-spore-forming, which characteristically grow in pairs (diplococci) with adjacent sides flattened. In 1963 Kellogg showed that gonococci occur in multiple colony types when grown on a clear agar medium and viewed with obliquely transmitted light.[2] Small convex glistening type 1 and type 2 colonies were easily distinguished from the larger, flatter type 3 and type 4 colonies. The small colonies are now known to be piliated, and are designated P$^+$ or P$^{++}$, depending on their morphology; large colonies are nonpiliated (P$^-$) (Fig. 13–1). Colony types are variable, and although fresh isolates from patients usually are P$^+$ or P$^{++}$,[13] unselected transfer in vitro usually results in conversion to P$^-$.[2] Some P$^-$ colonies are capable of subsequent reversion to P$^+$. Using human male prison volunteers as experimental subjects, Kellogg and his coworkers showed that after 69 in vitro passages, P$^+$ "type 1" colonies retained virulence but the P$^-$ "type 4" colonies did not.[2]

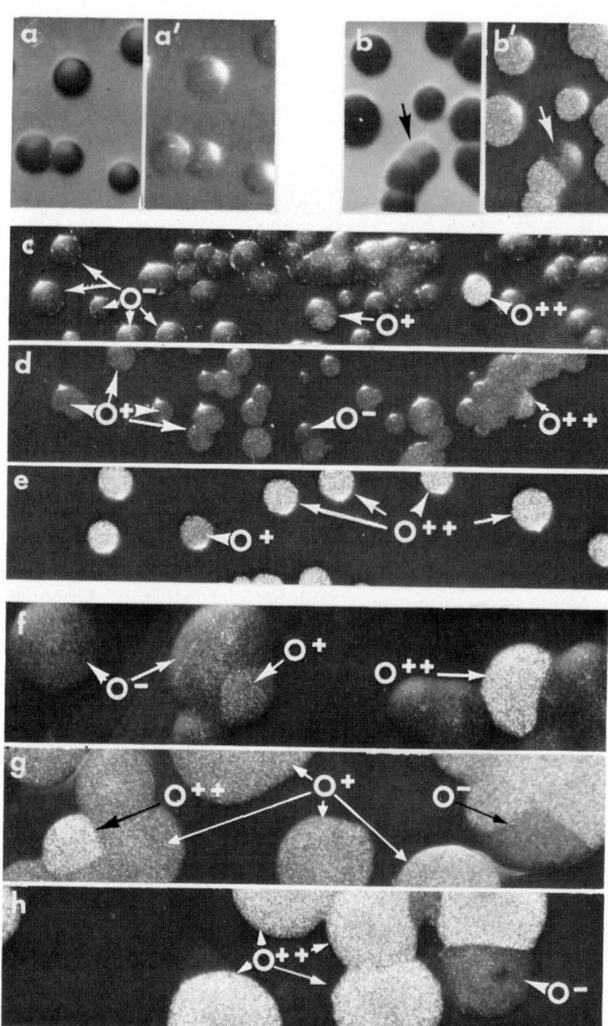


Fig. 13-1. Gonococcal colonial morphologies. A variety of sizes and forms are present in gonococci cultivated on clear medium, in vitro. Small colonies with darkly rimmed borders (*a–e*) contain heavily piliated organisms, whereas large colonies (*f–h*) are constituted of nonpiliated gonococci. Colonies of both piliated and nonpiliated organisms display variation in their color and opacity characteristics. Use of a diffusing substage reflector allows visualization of colony color (*a* and *b*) and is depicted here for very light (*a*) and very dark (*b*) colonies. Use of a polished substage mirror allows differentiation of colonial opacity variants (*a′*, *b′*, *c–h*). Transparent colony (O$^-$) populations are regularly "contaminated" by variances of intermediate (O$^+$) or marked (O$^{++}$) colonial opacities (*c*). Similarly, O$^-$ and O$^{++}$ colonies are found in O$^+$ preparations (*d*), and colonies of lesser opacity (O$^-$ or O$^+$) appear in O$^{++}$ colony populations (*e*). These variants can also be found in otherwise homogeneous O$^-$ (*f*), O$^+$ (*g*), and O$^{++}$ (*h*) populations of nonpiliated gonococcal colonies. (*Courtesy of J Swanson and L Mayer.*)

A second type of variation concerns relative opacity of the colonies when viewed through a low-power microscope on clear media in appropriate lighting.[14,15] Opaque (Op) colonies are darker and more granular than transparent (Tr) colonies (Fig. 13-1). The Op and Tr colony types undergo rapid reversible variations in vitro. The biochemical basis of the opaque-transparent colony variation is due to variation in expression of a family of outer membrane proteins designated protein II (P.II): Op colonies contain cells expressing P.II ($P.II^+$) whereas most transparent colonies contain cells that are not expressing P.II ($P.II^-$).[14–16]

## Membrane structure

When gonococci are viewed in cross section by transmission electron microscopy (TEM), they are seen to have a typical gram-negative outer membrane overlying a relatively thin peptidoglycan layer and cytoplasmic membrane. Meningococci contain a true polysaccharide capsule that is important to virulence, whereas gonococci lack such a structure in most studies. Frequently small blebs of outer membrane may be seen in TEM. Unlike *Escherichia coli* and many other enteric bacteria, gonococci are prone to release fragments of membrane into their surrounding environment; this may deliver toxic membrane components to distant sites and antigenic fragments that bind host antibodies.

## PILI

The most important parts of the gonococcus from the pathogenic point of view concern surface molecules that are involved in attachment to, or invasion or injury of, the host, or that serve as targets for host immune defenses. Because of the surge in research data of the past two decades, much is known about important surface molecules of gonococcus, particularly pili. Viewed by electron microscopy, pili are arranged in individual fibrils or fibrillar aggregates and cover virtually the entire outer cell surface of the organism (Fig. 13-2). Fibrillar pili actually are polymers composed of perhaps thousands of a subunit of about 18 kilodaltons.[17] A great deal is now known about the structure of the pilin subunit, but the full three-dimensional structure of the assembled pilus fibril has not yet been solved by x-ray crystallography. Pili are known to increase adhesion to host tissues,[18] but by electron microscopy no special structures such as a "tip adhesin" are visible on the pilus.

## Antigenic and phase variation

Pili undergo two types of variations, at relatively high frequency: antigenic variation, in which strains shift the antigenic type of their pilus; and phase variation, in which strains switch between $P^+$ and $P^-$ states. Immune sera raised in animals against a single purified pilus react relatively weakly with pili prepared from unrelated clinical isolates.[17] The pilus expressed by a single gonococcal strain is known to be able to undergo extensive antigenic variation, either during passage on agar plates, during growth in subcutaneous chambers implanted into experimental animals, or during natural infection of humans.[19–23] By both protein-sequencing and DNA-sequencing techniques, the complete structure of a number of pilin variants from three gonococcal strains (MS11, P9, and a recent clinical isolate) is well established.[23–26] There is a common N-terminal region of the pilin protein, and several variable domains in the midportion or carboxy terminus

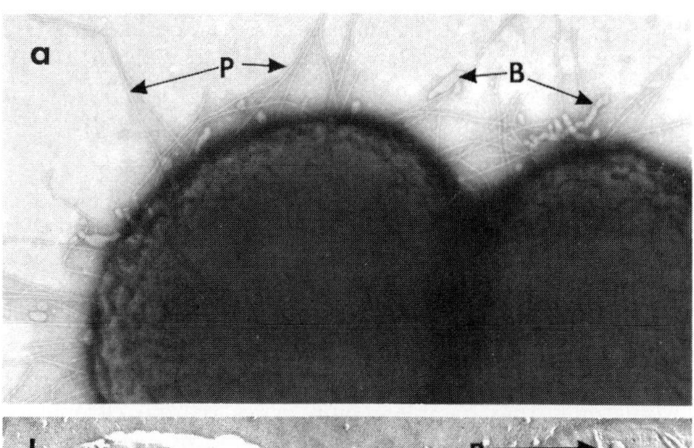


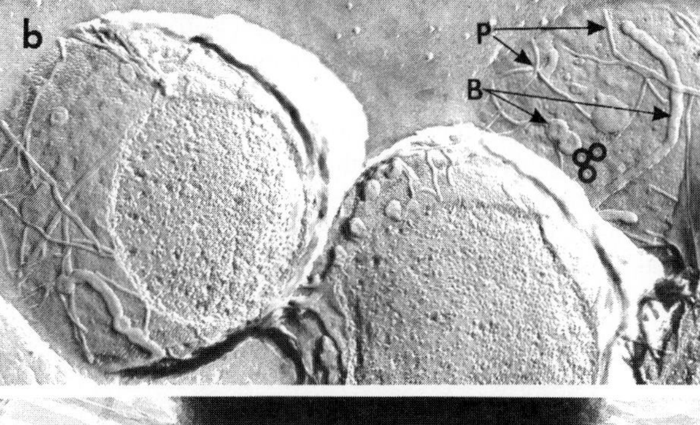


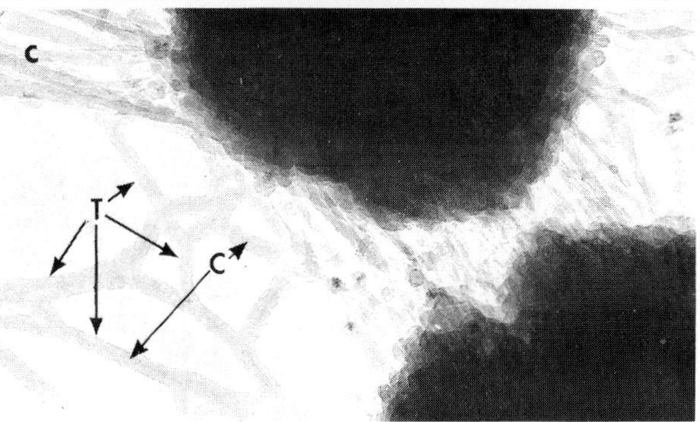


Fig. 13-2. Electron microscopic appearances of gonococcal surface constituents. Different methods of preparing gonococci for electron microscopic examination yield strikingly different views of these organisms' surface constituents. In negatively stained preparations (*a*), pili (*P*) appear as thin (approximately 8-nm) structures that are clearly differentiated from evaginated *blebs* (*B*) of the outer membrane. These blebs occur as elongated, sausagelike forms or as small vesicles. The actual surfaces of gonococci have a rugose appearance that is poorly resolved in this micrograph. After freeze-fracture freeze-etching (*b*), both pili (*P*) and outer-membrane blebs (*B*) are seen lying against the organisms' surfaces. Pili have diameters very similar to those found by negative staining. The "pebbled" appearance of the gonococcal surface is punctuated by *pits* (examples encircled). (*Courtesy of J Swanson and L Mayer.*)

of the protein (Fig. 13-3). Several relatively invariant or common regions are scattered amidst the variable domains, including two cysteines at amino acids 121 and 151 that form a disulfide bridge. The amino terminus is nearly identical in gonococci, meningococci, and several other organisms including *Bacteroides nodosus*, *Moraxella bovis*, and *Pseudomonas aeruginosa*.

**Molecular Mechanisms.** The mechanisms of pilus phase ($P^+ \rightleftarrows P^-$) and antigenic ($P^+_\alpha \rightarrow P^+_\beta$) variation have been studied extensively by molecular biological techniques. Studies by Meyer, Mlawer, and So[27] provided the initial leap in understanding. By cloning and subsequently sequencing the pilin structural gene and using it to probe restriction endonuclease digests of gonococcal

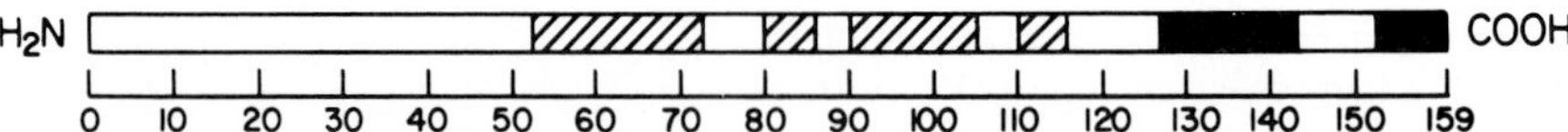


**Fig. 13-3.** Schematic diagram of variability of pilin structure as revealed by primer-extension DNA sequencing of expressed *pil* genes in multiple clinical isolates of a single epidemic strain. In the semivariable regions (*hatched*), single amino acid substitutions were found. In the hypervariable regions (*black*), there frequently were insertions or deletions of one to several amino acids. White areas are constant regions. Results are typical of those found in vitro in three laboratory strains. Numbers refer to amino acid residues of mature pilins. (*From PF Sparling et al, J Infect Dis 153:196, 1986.*)

chromosome, they and others[23,25,28–32] showed that there are one or sometimes two complete pilin genes on the chromosome. These "expression sites" contain an intact promoter region and ribosome binding site and encode the unusual short 7 amino acid signal sequence and the 159 to 160 amino acid mature pilin subunit. In addition there are six to eight "silent" regions scattered at various locales around the chromosome. Each silent locus contains various amounts of pilin sequences, but without a promoter region, signal peptide, or the 5′ end of the pilin structural gene. In some of these silent sites there are many different copies of incomplete pilin gene sequences arranged in a head-to-tail tandem repeat order, and many of these variant copies of pilin sequences are slightly different from each other (reviewed in Ref. 33). Nonreciprocal recombination events may move one of these silent variant copies of pilin sequence into the expression site, resulting in expression of an antigenically variant but fully functional pilus (antigenic variation). On occasion the variant copy of silent pilin DNA encodes a faulty peptide that when expressed results in a pilin that cannot be processed, assembled, or anchored into a mature pilus, and the cell becomes $P^-$ as a result. Reversion back to a $P^+$ state in these instances occurs when a functional pilin sequence is moved from another variant silent copy into the expression site, replacing the faulty pilin sequences (phase variation) (Fig. 13-4).

These movements of pilin sequences between the silent and the expression sites are mediated by the homologous sequences that flank or are located at intervals within the pilin DNA at the silent and the expression sites.[33] Movements of pilin DNA from the silent sites into the expression sites depend on a functional recombination system.[34] Occasionally a recombinational event results in deletion of the entirety of the 5′ and upstream regions of the structural gene in the expression site.[35] When this happens the organism becomes permanently nonpiliated since the necessary information to restore the pilus expression site is not contained within any of the silent copies.[31–33]

## PROTEIN I (P.I)

When outer membranes are purified from gonococci and proteins are solubilized and examined by the technique of sodium dodecyl sulfate–polyacrylamide gel electrophoresis (SDS-PAGE), a number of proteins are visualized.[36,37] Ordinarily the most prominent protein on such SDS-PAGE is a 34- to 36-kilodalton protein designated P.I. P.I is exposed on the surface of the outer membrane and in its native state in the membrane undoubtedly exists as a trimer.[38] In the outer membrane it is physically proximate to the LOS[39] and also to protein III.[40,41] P.I undoubtedly fulfills many

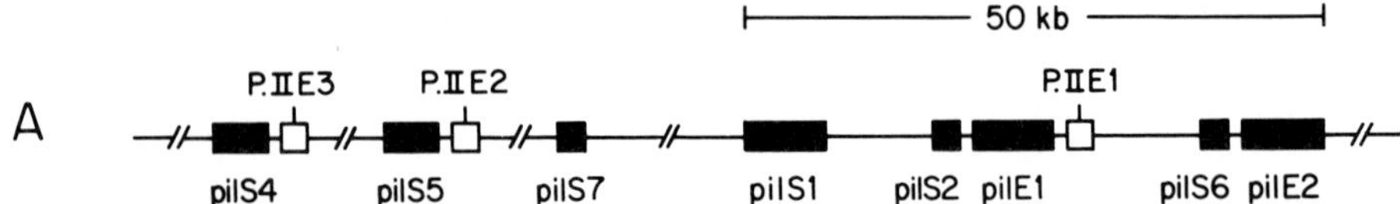


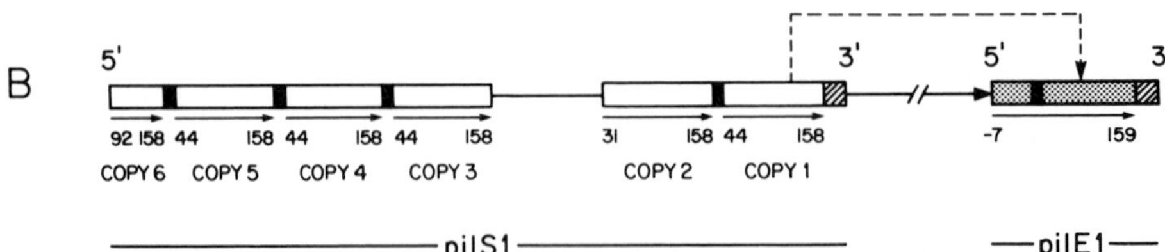


**Fig. 13-4.** Molecular basis of pilus variations. In (*a*) the approximate chromosomal organization of known loci for pilin (*pil*) or opacity proteins (P.II) is shown. In strain MS11 there are two complete ("expression") *pil* genes (*pil*E1, *pil*E2) and multiple incomplete ("silent") loci (e.g., *pil*S1) containing copies of the 3′ end of *pil* genes. In some instances, P.II genes are adjacent to *pil* loci (e.g., P.II E1), each encoding a complete P.II protein. There is no obvious rationale for the evident grouping of *pil* and P.II genes. In (*b*) is shown the organization of one silent locus (*pil*S1), which contains six slightly variant copies of the 3′ end of *pil* genes. Numbers below the bars indicate pilin amino acids encoded by the DNA. Solid bars or striped areas indicate constant regions in or around the *pil* genes; other constant DNA regions are omitted for simplicity. The dotted line and arrow refer to movement by recombination of DNA from one silent copy into an expression locus (*pil*E1), which is facilitated by homology between the constant regions. This may result in phase or antigenic variation, as described in the text. (*Adapted principally from data of R Haas and TF Meyer, Cell 44:107, 1986.*)

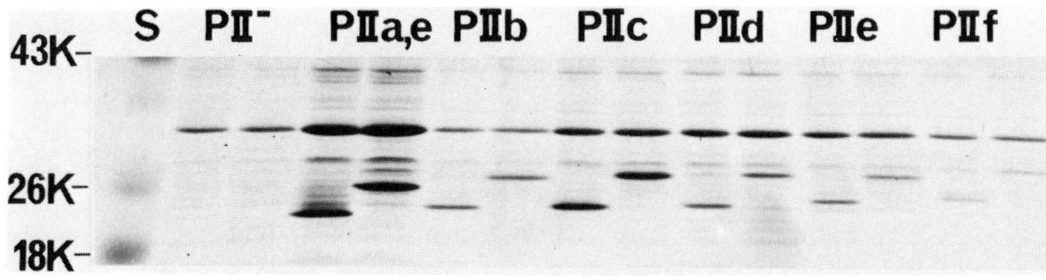


**Fig. 13-5.** Demonstration of the P.II family of outer-membrane proteins in gonococcal strain FA1090 by Coomassie Blue staining of proteins separated by SDS-PAGE. Pairs of lanes represent identical membrane protein preparations from a transparent (P.II$^-$) or various P.II$^+$ (expressing) variants, solubilized at either 37°C (*left lane in each pair*) or 100°C (*right lane in each pair*) prior to SDS-PAGE. A prominent protein of 24 to 28 kilodaltons that varies in $M_r$ depending on temperature of solubilization is seen in every pair except the P.II$^-$ isolate. The 36-kilodalton invariant protein is P.I. (*Courtesy of J Cannon.*)

functions for the gonococcus including forming an anion-specific channel through the lipid-rich outer membrane.[42,43] P.I exists in two major chemically and immunologically distinct classes designated P.IA and P.IB. A given strain possesses either P.IA or P.IB but never both. As indicated above, monoclonal antibody serotyping schemes based on P.I have been developed, and they have defined a number of antigenic variants of these two major families of porin protein.[7]

Recently the primary structures of one P.IA and two P.IB proteins have been determined by DNA sequencing.[44,45] Their structure is similar to that of porin proteins in other gram-negative bacteria. Comparison of the sequence of P.IA and P.IB proteins reveals certain regions that are common to both proteins and others where there is considerable variation.[44–46] The regions of variability probably represent areas of antigenic diversity. The P.IA and P.IB genes are alleles of a single locus previously designated *nmp* (for *n*ew *m*embrane *p*rotein). Hybrid P.IA/P.IB proteins can be constructed in the laboratory, but such hybrids virtually never occur in nature. The hybrids are useful to map epitopes on P.IA or P.IB.[46]

## PROTEIN II (P.II)

The opacity-associated protein family designated P.II comprises a set of closely related proteins involved in cell adhesion that share the property of heat modifiability.[14–16] These proteins vary in size from about 24 to about 28 kilodaltons and when heated to 100°C take on a different conformation and exhibit a higher apparent molecular weight in SDS-PAGE. A given strain has the capacity to produce at least six different variants of the P.II family, as judged by sizes and antigenic properties of the expressed P.II proteins[47] (Fig. 13–5). A strain may express none of these, or up to three different members of the P.II family simultaneously.[47] The P.II family undergoes both phase variations (P.II$^+ \rightleftarrows$P.II$^-$) and antigenic variation (P.IIA→P.IIB→P.IIC→ · · ·), analogous to pilus variations.

Some P.II proteins promote adherence of cells in a colony and also promote adhesion of gonococci to epithelial cells[48,49] (reviewed in Ref. 50). Most P.II proteins result in increased colony opacity, whereas all P.II$^-$ clones are transparent. The very high frequencies in variation of P.II proteins can easily be seen by examining colony morphologies under appropriate lighting; many colonies exhibit sectors varying in opacity, which reflects the variability in expression of P.II (Fig. 13-1).

### Mechanisms of P.II variations

The genetic basis for phase and antigenic variation of the P.II family is now quite well understood and is different from that used to control the expression of pilus proteins. Several P.II structural genes have been cloned and sequenced.[51–54] When Southern hybridizations are performed with the cloned P.II gene, up to 12 P.II-related restriction fragments of chromosomal DNA are visualized,[33,51–53] indicating that there is a family of P.II genes in the chromosome (Fig. 13–6). Each of the P.II genes is a complete gene with its own signal peptide and promoter, and each is transcribed into RNA at all times.[52,53] Variation in expression of these genes is achieved by varying the number of an identical

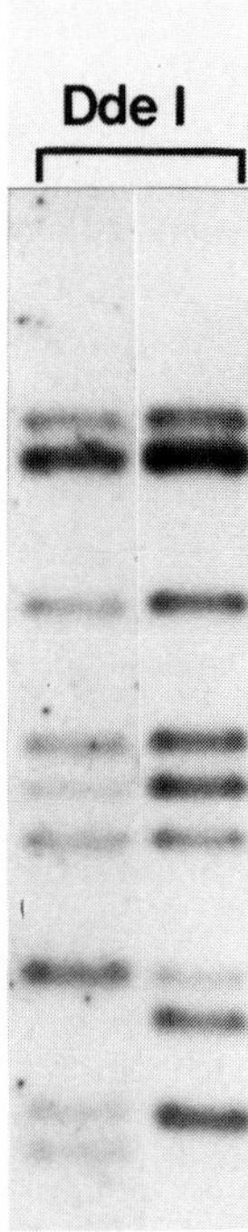


**Fig. 13-6.** Demonstration of the P.II gene family by hybridization of P.II-specific DNA probes to a DdeI digest of FA1090 genomic DNA in a Southern blot. Fragments containing P.II-specific DNA were detected by autoradiography. (*Left lane*) Probe was a P.II-specific synthetic oligonucleotide from a nonvariable domain in P.II. (*Right lane*) Probe was a cloned P.II gene. Multiple bands indicate there is a family of P.II-related genes. Variable intensity of bands suggests that some DdeI fragments might contain multiple P.II genes. (*Courtesy of J Cannon.*)

pentameric (CTCTT) repeat unit located immediately downstream from the ATG start codon, within the hydrophobic signal sequence, and upstream from the sequences coding for the mature structural protein.[52–54] When the number of these repeat units is evenly divisible by three (e.g., 9, 12, 15 . . . ), the gene is translationally in-frame and a P.II protein is expressed. Any other number of the pentameric repeat (e.g., 8, 10, 11, 13, 14 . . . ) results in transcription of a gene which is translationally out-of-frame, and no P.II is expressed. The number of the pentameric repeat undegoes high frequency variation, and this results in regulation of expression at the level of translation rather than the usual method for most genes of regulation at the level of transcription. Variable expression of P.II genes results in antigenic variation, because of differences in structures encoded by different P.II genes. In addition, there are hypervariable (HV) areas within the P.II genes, and recombination between HV regions results in increased variability in expressed P.II proteins.[54]

## PROTEIN III (P.III)

All pathogenic *Neisseria,* including all gonococci, contain an antigenically conserved protein designated P.III, a protein of about 30 to 31 kilodaltons which is characterized by its altered apparent molecular weight on SDS-PAGE under reducing conditions. The structural gene for P.III also has been cloned.[55] This protein is of interest in pathogenesis because many blocking antibodies that prevent serum bactericidal activity are directed against this antigen, as discussed below.

## H.8 PROTEINS

A monoclonal antibody (MAb) designated H.8 reacts with a conserved antigen found on all gonococci and meningococci, and on *N. lactamica* and *N. cinerea,* but not on other nonpathogenic *Neisseria.*[56] In gonococci and meningococci there are at least two proteins containing an H.8 MAb-binding epitope. One is a lipoprotein containing five imperfect repeats of the peptide Ala-Ala-Glu-Ala-Pro (AAEAP) at the N-terminal region, and an azurin-like sequence at the C-terminal region.[57,58] The azurins are copper-containing proteins that may be involved in electron transport. The function of the gonococcal azurin-like protein is not yet known. The second H.8 MAb-binding protein does not contain azurin-related sequences and is made up primarily of 13 imperfect repeats of the AAEAP peptide. The epitope for H.8 MAb is contained within the AAEAP repeating peptides.[58] During convalescence from gonorrhea humans make antibodies against the H.8 proteins,[59] but the role of H.8 in pathogenesis is unknown.

## IRON OR OXYGEN-REPRESSIBLE PROTEINS

The outer membrane contains a number of other proteins, many of which have not been completely characterized as to structure or function. One of these is an antigenically conserved very high molecular weight protein (about 800 kilodaltons), composed of 76-kilodalton subunits, that is found in every gonococcal strain; it was designated OMP-MC by Wilde et al.[60,61] A variety of other proteins are expressed only under certain conditions including iron starvation, anaerobic growth, or other limited-growth situations.[62–65] These iron-repressible proteins (FeRPs) include a 37-kilodalton protein[66] and several in the approximate range of 65 to over 100 kilodaltons.[62,63] The 37-kilodalton FeRP has been chemically purified and contains iron,[67] suggesting that it may be involved in iron transport. Virtually all gonococci and meningococci express an antigenically related 37-kilodalton FeRP.[68] A 70-kilodalton FeRP on the outer membrane also is common to virtually all gonococci and meningococci.[69] Since a meningococcal mutant that lacks the 70-kilodalton FeRP is unable to transport iron from a number of sources including transferrin and lactoferrin,[70] this protein also may be involved in iron transport. Several other proteins are expressed in considerable quantity during anaerobic growth.[64] Many of these growth-regulated proteins are expressed in vivo as evidenced by the ability of convalescent human sera to react with them in Western blots[71] (also from unpublished data of W. R. McKenna, D. W. Dyer, and P. F. Sparling).

## $IgA_1$ PROTEASES

All gonococci and meningococci but not other, nonpathogenic *Neisseria* produce a protease that recognizes both serum and secretory $IgA_1$ as its only known substrate.[72] There are two genetically and biochemically distinct variants of the gonococcal $IgA_1$ protease, and there is a correlation between auxotype, P.I serogroup, and the class of $IgA_1$ protease expressed by the strain.[73] Each of the $IgA_1$ proteases cleaves IgA at the hinge region,[72] resulting in release of Fab and Fc fragments. Since secretory IgA is the principal arm of antibody-mediated defenses at mucosal surfaces, the neisserial IgA protease may be important in inactivation of mucosal immune defenses, but unfortunately no firm data are available to confirm this intuitively obvious conclusion.

One particularly interesting feature of the gonococcal IgA protease was revealed by cloning and sequencing the entire structural gene for this protein.[74] Surprisingly the DNA sequence predicted a protein of over 169 kilodaltons, whereas the isolated, purified IgA protease prepared from gonococcal cells was only about 106 kilodaltons. It appears that the cell synthesizes a precursor protein of about 169 kilodaltons which then is proteolytically cleaved twice to create a 45-kilodalton membrane protein and the mature 106-kilodalton IgA protease molecule. The 45-kilodalton protein is thought to form a channel through the membrane which allows export of the IgA protease to the exterior.[74]

## LIPOOLIGOSACCHARIDE (LOS)

On their cell surface, all gonococci express LOS, similar to the lipopolysaccharide (LPS) of other gram-negative bacteria. Gonococcal LOS contains a lipid A moiety, and a core polysaccharide consisting of ketodeoxyoctanoic acid (KDO), heptose, glucose, galactose, and glucosamine and/or galactosamine.[8] Unlike other gram-negative bacteria, however, gonococci do not express a long polymeric sugar attached to this core, and thus the gonococcal LOS is considerably smaller than typical LPS of other bacteria. By both chemical and immunologic criteria there is intrastrain and interstrain variation in the nature of the core sugar antigens of LOS,[8–11] and this variation forms the basis for the serotyping scheme of Apicella. Phenotypic variation of LOS molecules occurs in vitro, depending on conditions of growth;[9–11] a single strain may make up to six variants of LOS, varying in apparent molecular mass from 3 to 7 kilodaltons. Since the core sugars of LOS form antigens that are important in immune bactericidal reactions,[75–78] phenotypic variation of these antigens may be pathogenically important. The biochemical and genetic mechanisms for phenotypic variation of gonococcal LOS have not been elucidated. Recent work suggests that the terminal sugars on gonococcal LOS may mimic the structure of certain human glycosphingolipids.[8]

## OTHER SURFACE STRUCTURES

Gonococcal peptidoglycan is similar to that of other gram-negative bacteria, containing a backbone of muramic acid and *N*-acetylglucosamine, but is rather unusual in the degree of its *O*-acetylation.[79] This may be relevant to the susceptibility of peptidoglycan fragments to biodegradation, and to its inflammatory and other biological properties.[80]

Gonococci do not express a true polysaccharide capsule despite several early reports to the contrary. (If they do produce a capsule, no one has succeeded in chemically isolating it to date.) Gonococci do produce a surface polyphosphate, however, which may serve some of the functions of a polysaccharide capsule, including provision of a hydrophilic and negatively charged cell surface.[81] The role of the polyphosphate "pseudocapsule" in gonococcal biology and pathogenesis presently is unknown. Gonococcal structures involved in pathogenesis are summarized in Table 13-1.

**Table 13-1. Some Gonococcal Structures Involved in Pathogenesis**

| Structure (abbreviation) | Function in infection |
|---|---|
| Protein I (P.I) | (?) Insertion into host cell membranes<br>Target for bactericidal, opsonic antibodies |
| Protein(s) II (P.II) | Adherence |
| Protein III (P.III) | Target for blocking antibodies |
| Pili ($P^+$) | Adherence<br>Resistance to neutrophils |
| Lipooligosaccharide (LOS) | Tissue toxin<br>Target for bactericidal, chemotactic antibodies |
| Peptidoglycan | Tissue toxin |
| Iron-repressible proteins (FeRPs) | (?) Iron uptake from transferrin, lactoferrin |
| H.8 protein | Unknown; found preferentially in pathogenic *Neisseria* |

## METABOLISM

Gonococci have complex growth requirements.[3] They utilize glucose, lactate, or pyruvate as sole sources of required carbon but cannot use other carbohydrates.[3] This forms the basis for the carbohydrate utilization tests used for decades to speciate neisserial organisms (Chap. 73). When grown in media supplemented with serum, they exhibit different outer membrane proteins and altered attachment to human neutrophils.[82] The factor that seems to stimulate these phenotypic variations is lactate.[83] Human neutrophils release lactate as an end product of metabolism, with the result that gonococci growing in vivo might encounter lactate as a principal carbon source.[83] All gonococci (as well as other *Neisseria*) rapidly oxidize dimethyl- or tetramethyl-phenylenediamine, and this turns colonies pink and then black, forming the basis of the oxidase test.

Gonococci are capable of growth under anaerobic conditions if nitrite is provided as an electron acceptor.[84] Their growth is stimulated by 5% gaseous $CO_2$ or if additional bicarbonate is added to liquid or solid growth media. They produce abundant catalase, which undoubtedly helps to promote growth in the presence of otherwise toxic peroxides, but unlike most aerobes they do not produce appreciable amounts of superoxide dismutase. It has been postulated that they grow in vivo under relatively anaerobic conditions,[64] although they ordinarily are grown in vitro under aerobic conditions.

Gonococci have an absolute requirement for iron for growth. In humans the principal sources of iron for gonococci are the serum glycoprotein transferrin and the mucosal glycoprotein lactoferrin. Gonococci possess an energy-requiring, iron-repressible system for scavenging iron from transferrin and lactoferrin; this is accomplished without evident synthesis of an iron-chelating siderophore.[63,85] Iron uptake from transferrin or lactoferrin is mediated by binding of the host protein to a specific gonococcal receptor, possibly one of the 75- to 90-kilodalton FeRPs (unpublished data of K. Blanton, J. Tsai, D. Dyer, P. F. Sparling, et al.). Many aspects of iron uptake in gonococci are unusual, in comparison with those of most other bacteria (no siderophores, presence of specific transferrin or lactoferrin receptors).

## GROWTH

Gonococci do not tolerate drying and ordinarily must be plated onto appropriate media immediately upon sampling patient secretions. As an alternative, gonococci may be put into one of several available transport media, in which they survive for up to 24 hs prior to being plated on definitive culture media. Growth is optimal at 35 to 37°C in a 5% $CO_2$ atmosphere, at a pH of about 6.5 to 7.5. When grown at relatively low pH (6.0 to 6.5), outer membrane composition is altered; below pH 6.0, no gonococci survive. (Vaginal secretions are quite acidic, but gonococci grow in the endocervix, where the pH is neutral.) Although certain nonpathogenic *Neisseria* grow at room temperature, gonococci do not grow well below 30°C, and they do not survive above 40°C

A complex growth medium is required. Ordinarily this is in the form of either chocolate agar or similar complex agar containing inorganic iron and supplemental glucose, vitamins, and cofactors. Many less fastidious microorganisms also found in the same ecological niches (pharynx, cervix, and rectum) grow more readily than gonococci, and relatively selective media have been devised which utilize antibiotics to inhibit growth of nonpathogenic *Neisseria*. Vancomycin, colistin, and nystatin were widely used for this purpose, but some gonococci are quite sensitive to the concentrations of vancomycin used in the selective media. Other formulations now have been developed in which vancomycin is replaced with lincomycin or other antibiotics. Diagnostic culture media and their use are discussed in Chap. 73.

## GENETIC SYSTEMS

There are two principal systems for performing genetic analysis of gonococci: transformation and conjugation. There are no known bacteriophages for gonococci (or meningococci), and a drug-resistance transposon system that functions within the pathogenic *Neisseria* has not been discovered. Siefert, So, and colleagues have developed a shuttle mutagenesis system that is extremely useful for genetic studies, in which the chloramphenicol acetyltransferase gene *cat* replaces β-lactamase (penicillinase) in a derivative of the transposon Tn3. The shuttle mutagenesis system is excellent for placing *cat* in a piece of cloned gonococcal DNA in *E. coli*, and for moving the cloned DNA containing *cat* back into the gonococcal chromosome by transformation[46] (also from personal communication from M. So), but these maneuvers require prior cloning of the gene of interest in an *E. coli* host.

## TRANSFORMATION

Gonococci are quite unusual in their constitutive expression of competence for transformation by exogenous DNA. Of over 50 strains examined in my laboratory over the years, only one has been noncompetent for transformation. In competent gonococci, virtually every cell is competent at all stages of growth, quite unlike many other transformable species in which competence is restricted to certain phases of the growth cycle. However, only piliated ($P^+$) gonococci are competent for transformation; $P^-$ derivatives are unable to take up transforming DNA into the cell and thus cannot be transformed.[86] The association between competence for transformation and expression of pili suggests that pili might be involved directly in recognition or entry of transforming DNA, but to date there are no experimental data to support this hypothesis. Pili may be merely a convenient morphologic marker for a complicated phenotypic state which includes the ability to take up and be transformed by DNA.

Although most $P^+$ gonococci are highly competent, they only take up their own (homologous) DNA into the cell.[87–88] The structural basis for specificity in recognition of homologous DNA is uncertain. Recently, a 10-base pair sequence was described that may be responsible for selective entry.[89]

Because gonococci are piliated (competent) in vivo and are highly autolytic and release transforming DNA in a biologically active form,[90] transformation may be used in nature to transfer genes between different gonococcal strains. This might be important in transfer of chromosomal antibiotic resistance genes or pilin silent genes, among others. Transformation has been used extensively in the research laboratory to map gonococcal genes (reviewed in Ref. 91), although the genetic map of the gonococcal genome is still primitive.

## CONJUGATION

May gonococci contain a 36-kilobase conjugal plasmid which efficiently mobilizes sexual transfer of certain other non-self-mobilizable plasmids such as the 4.5- or 7.2-kilobase penicillinase ($Pc^r$) plasmids.[92,93] The 36-kilobase conjugative plasmids also mobilize their own transfer with high efficiency, but they do not detectably mobilize chromosomal genes for transfer between gonococci,[94] despite some reports to the contrary. Conjugation undoubtedly is important for exchange of plasmids between gonococci in nature.

## MUTAGENESIS

Although gonococci are highly variable in certain properties (particularly expression of pilus, P.II, or LOS antigens), they are relatively nonmutagenic. They are very susceptible to ultraviolet light but lack photoreactivation and error-prone repair systems and do not undergo ultraviolet mutagenesis under ordinary conditions.[95] The recombination systems of the gonococcus are not fully characterized yet. A gonococcal homologue of the *E. coli recA* gene has been cloned, and isogenic gonococci have been constructed lacking RecA function;[96] the gonococcal *recA* mutants are hypersusceptible to ultraviolet light and show reduced frequencies of chromosomal transformation and of pilin antigenic variation.[34]

## RESTRICTION AND MODIFICATION SYSTEMS

Gonococci are known to contain at least three restriction endonucleases and their corresponding methylases.[97] Transformation by plasmid DNA is markedly reduced when plasmids are introduced into gonococci across restriction barriers, but chromosomal transformation seems to be little influenced by restriction barriers.[98] Gonococci have DNA methylases for which there is no corresponding restriction endonuclease (see Ref. 97 and references therein), which suggests that DNA methylation might be important to other biological functions including gene regulation.

## PLASMIDS

As indicated, many gonococci contain a 36-kilobase conjugal plasmid. Recently, slightly larger derivatives of the 36-kilobase plasmid have been isolated that contain the tetracycline resistance ($Tc^r$) *tetM* transposon.[99] A variety of gonococcal β-lactamase (penicillin resistant, $Pc^r$) plasmids have been isolated and characterized. The two most frequent plasmids are either about 5.3 or 7.2 kilobase.[100] The $Tc^r$ and $Pc^r$ plasmids are discussed below under Antimicrobial Susceptibility.

Most gonococci also contain a 4.2-kilobase plasmid of unknown function (*cryptic plasmid*).[101] The DNA sequence of this plasmid has been determined;[102] there are multiple open reading frames predicted from the DNA sequence, but the putative protein products of the plasmid have not been identified. All studied gonococci also contain a 1.6-kilobase chromosomal HindIII fragment that is partially homologous with the cryptic plasmid.[103] Occasional gonococci can be isolated that do not contain the freely replicating (cytoplasmic) 4.2-kilobase cryptic plasmid, but they appear biologically normal.[103]

# PATHOGENESIS

## CLINICAL CORRELATIONS

Consideration of clinical manifestations of gonorrhea suggests many facets of the pathogenesis of the infection. Since gonococci persist in the male urethra despite hydrodynamic forces which would tend to wash the organisms from the mucosal surface, they must be able to adhere effectively to mucosal surfaces. Similarly, since gonococci survive in the urethra despite close attachment to large numbers of neutrophils, they must have mechanisms that help them to survive interactions with polymorphonuclear neutrophils. Since some gonococci are able to invade and persist in the bloodstream for many days at least, they must be able to evade killing by normal defense mechanisms of plasma including antibodies, complement, and transferrin. Invasion of the bloodstream also implies that gonococci are able to invade mucosal barriers in order to gain access to the bloodstream. Repeated reinfections of the same patient by one strain[104] strongly suggest that gonococci are able to change surface antigens frequently and/or are able to escape local immune mechanisms (Table 13-2). The considerable tissue damage of fallopian tubes consequent to gonococcal salpingitis suggests that gonococci make at least one tissue toxin, or that gonococci trigger an immune response that results in damage to host tissues. There is evidence to support many of these inferences.

**Table 13-2. Mechanisms for Evasion of Host Defenses**

1. Antigenic variation
   - Pili
   - Protein II
   - Lipooligosaccharide
2. Blocking antibodies
   - Protein III
3. Antibody cleavage
   - $IgA_1$ protease
4. Antigen release
   - Membrane blebs
5. Intracellular growth
   - Nonciliated cells of fallopian tube
   - (?) Others

## MODEL SYSTEMS

Studies of pathogenesis are complicated by the absence of a suitable animal model. A variety of animal models have been developed, each of which has certain utility, but no model faithfully reproduces the full spectrum of naturally acquired disease of humans. Considerable evidence about antigenic variation and interactions with neutrophils has been obtained from inoculation of subcutaneous chambers in guinea pigs or other animals. A few investigators have recently utilized male human volunteers for critical studies of vaccines and pathogenesis, but only limited numbers of human volunteer studies are possible. The best model system for many in vitro studies is organ culture of human tissues, particularly the fallopian tube system exploited successfully by McGee and colleagues.[105]

## ADHERENCE

Two adherence ligands are well documented to be important: pili and protein II. Piliated gonococci adhere better to human columnar epithelial cells than to squamous cells, and to human cells better than to nonhuman cells. Isolated pili adhere in vitro,[18] and certain pilus antigenic variants exhibit selective ability to attach to particular cells under defined conditions in vitro.[106] Antibodies against pili decrease adherence of piliated gonococci to epithelial cells and red blood cells.[107–109] Similar evidence supports the role of P.II proteins in adherence: gonococci expressing certain P.II proteins adhere better than P.II$^-$ (transparent) gonococci to various cells,[49,110] and a monoclonal antibody raised against one P.II protein inhibits adherence.[48] Antigenic variation of both pili and P.II may be biologically advantageous not only for escape from specific immune responses but also by providing specific adherence ligands for attaching to different niches in vivo.

### Pilus adhesins

Many studies have attempted to identify the portion of pilus protein involved in adhesion, and the cell receptor to which the pilus binds, without clear answers. Using conveniently available human red blood cells as a model cell, several laboratories showed that a cyanogen bromide cleavage fragment of pilin from amino acids 8 to 96 inhibits binding of whole pili, whereas other pilin fragments would not.[108] The thesis was advanced that a relatively invariant and immunorecessive pilus domain contains the ligand for cell binding.[108] Polyclonal sera raised against synthetic pilin peptides were studied for ability to block adherence of two unrelated P$^+$ gonococci to epithelial cells, and only sera against pilin peptides from amino acids 41 to 50 and 69 to 84 were effective.[111] These peptides are from relatively invariant regions of pilin.[25–27,112] However, many monoclonal antibodies that recognize specific or unique epitopes on pilin are more active in blocking adherence than monoclonal antibodies directed at common epitopes,[109] which suggests that the pilin domain(s) involved in adherence actually are in variable region(s). This is consistent with pilus vaccination studies of human volunteers, in whom protection extended only to the homologous isolate from which the pilus vaccine was prepared.[113]

In *E. coli* and other gram-negative bacteria, pili (or fimbriae) are associated with increased adherence, but the adhesin is not the pilin subunit but rather is a minor pilus-related protein.[114] Difficulties in identifying the gonococcal pilus adhesin might be due to focusing research efforts entirely on pilin subunits. Gonococci contain several pilus-related proteins other than pilin based on chemical and antigenic criteria,[115] but there are no data currently (1988) regarding the roles of these proteins in pilus biology or in cell adhesion.

### P.II adhesin

The P.II adhesins undoubtedly are important in infection since almost all isolates taken from patients are opaque or P.II expressing; the only exception is isolates taken from the female cervix near menses when most isolates are transparent.[116] The nature of the P.II-related adhesin both for intergonococcal adherence and for gonococcal-epithelial cell adherence has not been elucidated. The one monoclonal antibody against P.II that is known to inhibit adherence recognizes a specific rather than a common P.II epitope.[48] The cell receptor for P.II-mediated binding also is unknown, although some evidence suggests it may be a complex glycoprotein.[110]

### Other adhesins

Recently whole P$^-$, P.II$^-$ gonococci were shown to adhere selectively to certain glycolipids in vitro.[117] Further work is needed to confirm this finding and to determine whether the putative third adhesin (nonpilus, non-P.II) is biologically (clinically) relevant.

## INTERACTIONS WITH LEUKOCYTES

Gonococci were formerly referred to as "*Neisseria intracellulare*" because Gram-stain smears from human infections sometimes showed neutrophils covered with gonococci, which were assumed to be inside the cell. Pili are known to increase adherence of gonococci to human polymorphonuclear neutrophils, but they also increase resistance to phagocytosis and killing. In contrast to nonpiliated gonococci, which are readily ingested and killed by neutrophils, piliated gonococci attach well but are ingested relatively poorly.[118,119] Antipilus antibodies increase phagocytosis ("opsonization").[120,121] Thus pili increase epithelial cell adherence and decrease neutrophilic killing, and antipilus antibodies block epithelial adherence and increase phagocytic killing. Attachment to neutrophils is also increased by certain members of the P.II family. The protein designated *leukocyte associated factor* by Swanson undoubtedly is similar to the P.II proteins involved in neutrophilic adherence.[122]

The majority of gonococci taken up by neutrophils are killed. There is some controversy over the relative survival of gonococci after phagocytic attack, but apparently up to 2 percent of gonococci survive ingestion by neutrophils.[123] Work in Smith's laboratory has identified a 20-kilodalton gonococcal protein that seems to play an important role in resistance to intracellular killing by neutrophils.[124]

Neutrophils possess both oxidative and nonoxidative methods for killing intracellular bacteria. Oxidative killing depends on enzymes contained within the specific and nonspecific granules of neutrophils, whereas the nonoxidative mechanisms depend on a variety of cationic or basic lysosomal proteins. Gonococci are sensitive to damage by the oxidative products generated intracellularly during the neutrophilic respiratory burst but also are killed efficiently by neutrophils from patients with chronic granulomatous disease which lack the oxidative killing mechanism.[125] One neutrophilic protein involved in nonoxidative killing of gonococci is cathepsin G.[126] Gonococci containing certain alterations in penicillin-binding proteins show increased susceptibility to cathepsin G,[126] which may explain the clinical observation that gonococci with low-level chromosomal resistance to penicillin are uncommonly isolated from the bloodstream.[6]

## INVASION

Biopsies from patients with gonorrhea show gonococci attached to host cells, frequently partially imbedded within the cell surface (Fig. 13-7). Gonococci also can be seen within the epithelial cell, sometimes surrounded by cellular membranes. Recently Shaw and Falkow employed a continuous culture of a human endometrial carcinoma cell to study variables affecting gonococcal invasion in vitro and found that invasion was increased when gonococci were grown in an iron-supplemented medium.[127] Studies with human fallopian tubes in organ culture have contributed significantly to understanding of the mechanisms of both adherence and invasion. Gonococci adhere selectively to mucus-secreting nonciliated cells of the fallopian tube and are gradually enfolded by pseudopods and engulfed by the host epithelial cell.[105] Gonococci appear to be able to multiply and divide intracellularly, although they do not invade laterally between cells.[105,128] Eventually some gonococci exit from the basal surface of the cell by a process termed *exocytosis*.[128] Once inside the epithelial cell, gonococci are immune to attack by antibody, complement, or neutrophils; their ability to survive to some degree inside epithelial cells suggests that they might be considered facultative intracellular parasites.

### Is P.I a "trigger" for invasion?

The molecular mechanisms for invasion of epithelial cells are unknown. Several observations suggest that P.I may play a role in invasion. Incubation of radiolabeled gonococcal membranes or whole bacteria with red blood cells results in transfer of the gonococcal porin protein (P.I) from the bacterial cell surface into the red cell membrane.[37] No other protein is translocated into the red cell membrane. Using phospholipid bilayers or so-called black lipid membranes to quantitate rates of transfer of porin protein, Lynch et al.[43] showed that gonococci containing P.IA transfer P.I into membranes more readily than gonococci containing P.IB. Since gonococci with P.IA are more likely to cause disseminated disease than gonococci with P.IB (see Chap. 14), these results are consistent with the hypothesis that translocation or spiking of host cells by P.I may be an important step in invasion of the host cell. Possibly gonococci are bound closely to mucus-secreting nonciliated cells by adhesins such as pili or P.II, and after tight attachment might initiate penetration of the cell by spiking it with P.I. These attractive ideas are still quite speculative, however. To date, it has not been demonstrated that gonococcal P.I translocates into epithelial cells, and it has not been shown that antibodies or peptides based on P.I block gonococcal attachment or invasion.

## TISSUE DAMAGE

Gonococci produce a variety of extracellular products that might damage host cells including enzymes (phospholipase, peptidases, and others), but no true extracellular protein toxin has been identified. Tissue damage appears to be due to two structural components of the cell surface: LOS and peptidoglycan.

Although gonococci do not attach to ciliated cells of fallopian tubes in organ culture, diminished beating of cilia is evident within hours after infection.[105] Electron micrographs demonstrate extrusion of ciliated cells, even though attached gonococci are only visible on adjacent nonciliated cells (Fig. 13-8). Similar effects are evident after purified gonococcal LOS is added to the fallopian tube model.[129] The toxic portion of LOS almost certainly is the lipid A portion,[129] as would be expected. Perhaps damage to ciliated cells results when membrane blebs containing lipid A are released from gonococci attached to nonciliated cells.

In addition to the unequivocal evidence that lipid A is a tissue toxin for gonococcal infections, there is also excellent evidence that fragments of the cell wall or peptidoglycan are capable of inducing damage in the human fallopian tube organ culture model.[130] Gonococcal peptidoglycan fragments also may be involved in the pathogenesis of inflammatory arthritis after bacteremic disease[131] similar to the role of peptidoglycan fragments in a well-studied animal model of poststreptococcal arthritis.[132]

## DISSEMINATION

### Serum resistance

The ability to resist the killing activity of antibodies and complement in normal human serum is closely related to the ability of gonococci to cause bacteremic illness with or without septic arthritis. A complex literature has evolved relating to the mechanisms of gonococcal resistance to serum antibodies and complement.

Most gonococci isolated from the bloodstream of patients are resistant to killing by serum from normal previously uninfected volunteers, whereas approximately two-thirds of isolates from mucosal infections are sensitive to killing by normal human serum.[6] Presumably the bactericidal activity of normal human

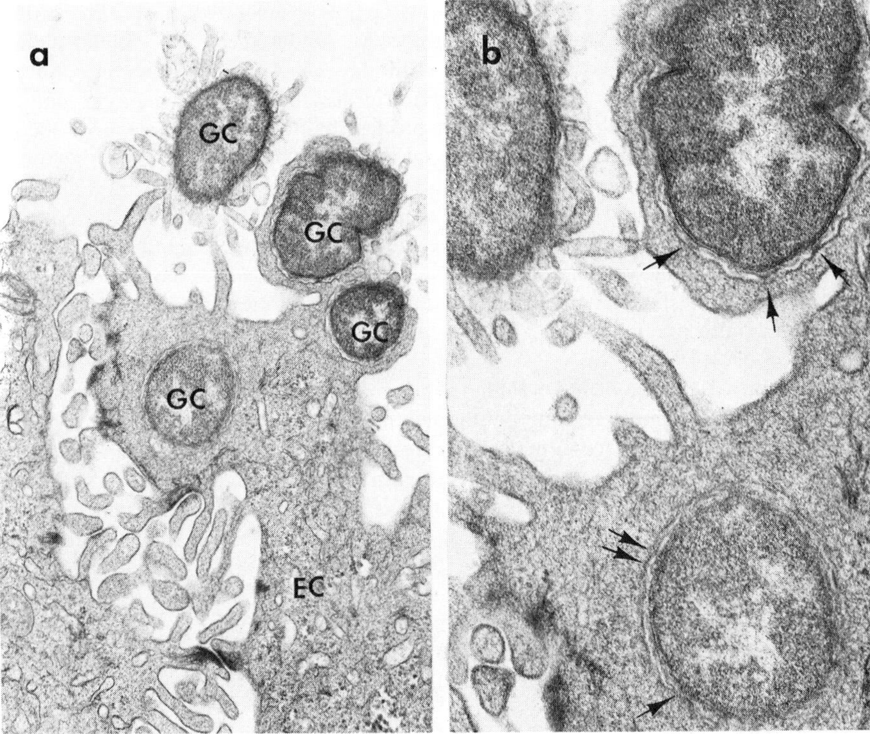


**Fig. 13-7.** Gonococcal–epithelial cell relation in cervical biopsies from a woman with acute gonorrhea. One of the exocervical epithelial cells (*EC*) seen in this electron micrograph (*b* is an enlarged portion of *a*) has closely adherent gonococci (*GC*). Some of the bacteria appear to be partially or completely endocytosed by the epithelial cells. Pili are not visible in this thin section and, in general, are usually difficult to visualize in thin-section preparations. Note the close apposition of gonococcal outer membrane and epithelial cell plasmalemma (*arrows*) and the apparent enfolding of the bacteria by the host's cervical cells. (*Courtesy of D Eschenbach and K Holmes.*)

serum for many gonococci results from previous exposure to common antigens shared by gonococci and other commensal bacteria. The nature of these common antigens and the bacteria on which they are carried are unknown.

**Unstable Serum Resistance.** Some gonococcal isolates are resistant to normal human serum upon first isolation from mucosal surfaces but rapidly lose serum resistance upon in vitro cultivation. Nearly every isolate from patients with bacteremic disease exhibits stable serum resistance in vitro,[6] which strongly suggests that unstable (phenotypically reversible) serum resistance is not biologically relevant to clinical gonococcal bacteremia. The remainder of this discussion refers to stable (genotypic) serum resistance or serum sensitivity.

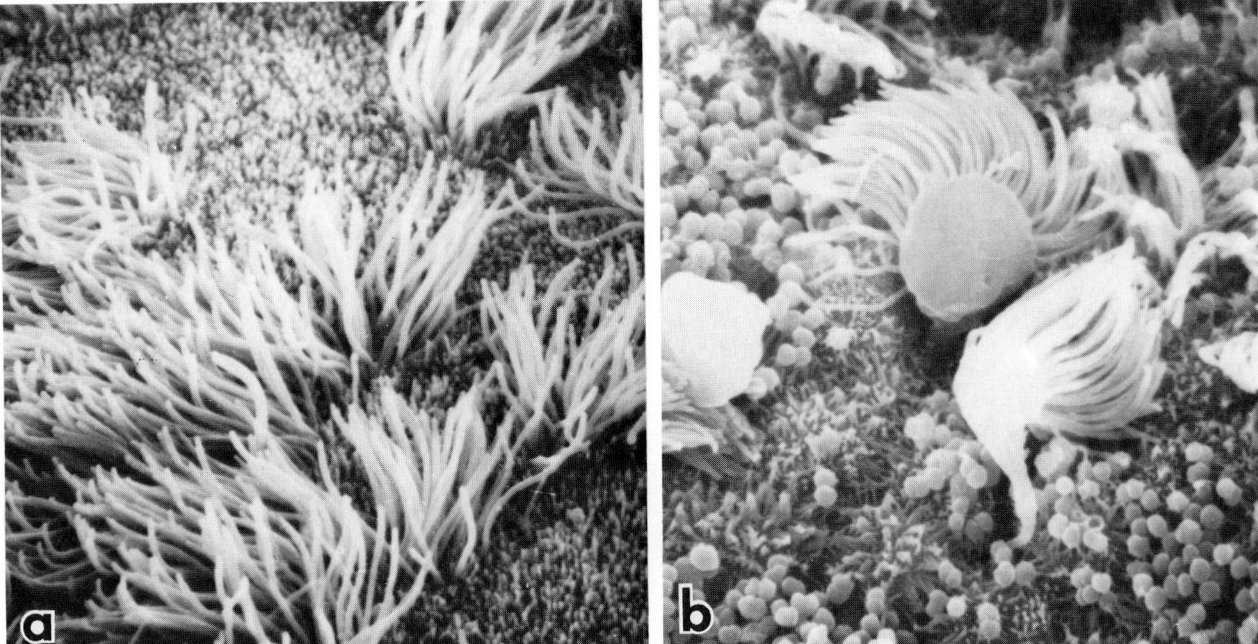


**Fig. 13-8.** Scanning electronic microscopy studies of normal, uninfected human fallopian tube mucosa showing (*a*) ciliated cells and nonciliated cells (the latter are covered with microvilli) and (*b*) human fallopian tube mucosa 20 h after infection with a piliated clone of *N. gonorrhoeae*. In (*b*) note morphologically intact ciliated cells (*far right* and *top*), two sloughing ciliated cells (*center*), and gonococci attached almost exclusively to the microvilli of nonciliated cells but not attached to a sloughing ciliated cells. ×4000 magnification. (*From ZA McGee et al, J Infect Dis 143:413, 1981.*)

**Immunochemistry.** In normal human serum the principal bactericidal activity against serum-sensitive gonococci is found in the IgM fraction.[76,133] Bactericidal antibodies of the IgG class also occur in pooled human serum globulins, or in convalescent sera. The antigens against which bactericidal complement-fixing antibodies are directed include LOS, although IgM and IgG bactericidal antibodies apparently recognize different epitopes on LOS.[76] Equal amounts of the complement "attack complex" are bound to the surface of both serum-sensitive and serum-resistant gonococci,[134,135] suggesting that serum-resistant gonococci somehow are able to resist the otherwise lethal action of a fully-formed complement attack complex.

**Blocking Antibodies: Role of P.III.** The interaction between serum antibodies, complement, and antigenic targets on LOS is complicated by the presence in many individuals of other non-complement-fixing IgG antibodies that recognize epitopes on P.III. These *blocking antibodies* sterically inhibit the ability of otherwise bactericidal IgM antibodies in normal human sera to recognize their target on LOS.[133,136] The killing activity of sera frequently depends on the balance between non-complement-fixing blocking antibodies and complement-fixing bactericidal antibodies. Presumably the close physical proximity between P.III and LOS accounts for the ability of anti-P.III antibodies to block access of other antibodies to LOS.

The genetics of gonococcal resistance to normal human serum has been studied extensively, and two loci designated *sac-1* and *sac-3* (*s*erum *a*ntibody *c*omplement) have been identified.[137] These loci are closely linked to each other and also to the structural gene *nmp* for P.I.[137] The *sac-3* gene product results in altered LOS apparent molecular weight and antigenicity, as determined by ability to react with a monoclonal antibody specific for an epitope on LOS.[78] This suggests that there is a cluster of genes on the gonococcal chromosome that affects either P.I or LOS structure. Recently recombinant DNA techniques have been used to clone a gene that encodes a 29-kilodalton protein that results in resistance to normal human serum.[138] The function of the 29-kilodalton protein in serum resistance is unknown; it does not appear to be identical to P.III.

**Chemotaxis.** Serum resistance of gonococci also may relate to the pathobiological potential of infection at mucosal sites. Serum-resistant gonococci that cause bacteremia frequently cause asymptomatic relatively noninflammatory infections at the mucosal surface (see Chap. 14); this correlates with their relative inability to trigger a chemotactic response for neutrophils.[130] In contrast, serum-sensitive isolates which rarely cause bacteremic disease but which frequently cause a marked inflammatory response at the mucosal surface elicit a much stronger chemotactic response in vitro.[139] Antibodies that elicit the C5a-dependent chemotactic response are directed against LOS antigens.[139] Since severe pelvic inflammatory disease is correlated with relatively high level sensitivity to serum killing in vitro,[140] local tissue damage may reflect the ability of some gonococci to trigger a chemotactic response, resulting in increased local inflammation and tissue damage.

## DIAGNOSIS

The details of diagnostic procedures are discussed fully in Chap. 73. The principles, however, can be outlined briefly here.

The standard procedure for diagnosing symptomatic disease in men with urethritis is the Gram stain. In asymptomatic men or in women with genital infection, the Gram stain is less useful, however, and cultures are necessary. Cultures also are useful whenever one is considering the possibility of an antibiotic-resistant gonococcal strain. A variety of tests have been developed to detect gonococcal antigen in genital secretions. These include enzyme immunoassays with polyclonal sera against gonococcal antigens, monoclonal antibodies against gonococcal antigens, and a *Limulus* amoebocyte gelation test for lipid A. The enzyme immunoassays have achieved the most widespread use, but the gold standard still is culture. DNA-DNA hybridization has potential for rapid diagnosis of gonorrhea but is not practical yet. See Chap. 73 for details.

Unfortunately, good diagnostic serologic tests have never been developed. Approximately one-half of infected persons develop antipilus antibodies in serum during convalescence, but the sensitivity of the test is not sufficiently high for its use in high-prevalence populations, and the specificity is too low to use as a screening test in low-prevalence populations. Serologic testing for diagnosing gonorrhea is still a problem for research.

A unique test that has clinical promise uses competent piliated gonococci as a test system to detect gonococcal transforming DNA in patient secretions.[141] The principle of this test is that gonococci can be transformed only by their own DNA and that virtually every gonococcal infection leaves residual amounts of biologically active transforming DNA in the environment. Since very small amounts of DNA are sufficient to elicit transformation of an appropriate test strain in vitro and gonococci are very specific in recognition of their own transforming DNA, this test is both sensitive and specific. It has not yet been widely utilized in practice, however.

## ANTIMICROBIAL SUSCEPTIBILITY

Gonococci are inherently quite sensitive to antimicrobial agents, compared with many other gram-negative bacteria. However, there has been a gradual selection for antibiotic-resistant mutants in clinical practice over the past several decades, and recently several different plasmids that mediate relatively high level antibiotic resistance have appeared. The consequence of these events has been to make penicillin therapy ineffective in some areas, and to threaten the clinical utility of tetracycline. Effective therapy is readily available for all resistant gonococcal strains, but new potent antibiotics such as spectinomycin and ceftriaxone are more expensive than penicillin G and tetracycline. The epidemiologic trends in prevalence of antibiotic-resistant gonococci, and proper modes for treatment of antibiotic-susceptible and antibiotic-resistant gonococcal infections, are discussed in Chap. 14. The biochemical and genetic basis for antibiotic resistance is discussed in this chapter.

## PENICILLIN

Isolates obtained in the 1940s typically were inhibited by 0.01 μg/ml penicillin G or less. A gradual increase in prevalence and extent of resistance to penicillin occurred over the subsequent several decades; this was shown to be due to the accumulation of several independent chromosomal mutations which affect cell surface structure. Three genetic loci resulting in low-level resistance to penicillin have been well studied, and results are reviewed in Ref. 91. One of them (*penA*) results in alteration of penicillin-binding protein two (PBP2), decreasing the affinity of PBP2 for penicillin. The gene for altered gonococcal PBP2 recently was cloned and sequenced, with the interesting suggestion that it might be the result of gene transfer from another related species in nature, leading to a hybrid PBP2.[142] The other loci (*mtr* and *penB*) result in low-level resistance to many antibiotics in addition to penicillins, probably by altering the outer membrane such that it is less permeable to entry by various compounds including penicillin. Introduction of *penA, mtr,* and *penB* into a sensitive gonococcal strain results in an increase in the minimum inhibitory concentration (MIC) of penicillin G from 0.01 to about 1.0 μg/ml. Recently there have been a number of reports of gonococci with chromosomally mediated resistance to penicillin in which the MIC for penicillin is 2 to 4 μg/ml.[104] The genetic and biochemical basis for increased resistance is unknown.

In 1976 a new type of gonococcal resistance to penicillin was first documented: the production of β-lactamase due to the presence of plasmids that encoded production of a TEM-1 type of β-lactamase.[143] The first $Pc^r$ (penicillinase-producing) gonococci contained either a 5.3 or a 7.2-kilobase plasmid. These two $Pc^r$ plasmids are very closely related, and each carries approximately 40 percent of the common gram-negative β-lactamase transposon Tn2.[144,145] Based on the molecular structure of the gonococcal and *Haemophilus ducreyi* $Pc^r$ plasmids, there is strong suspicion that gonococci acquired the $Pc^r$ plasmids from *H. ducreyi.*[146,147] Since the gonococcal $Pc^r$ plasmids can be mobilized efficiently for sexual transfer between gonococci by the 36-kilobase gonococcal conjugal plasmid, and between *H. ducreyi* and gonococci,[148] it is not surprising that there apparently has been spread of the $Pc^r$ plasmids to new gonococcal strains in the years since 1976.

## TETRACYCLINE

Resistance to tetracycline (Tc) also has increased in recent years and is due either to the additive effects of several chromosomal mutations or to acquisition of a previously undescribed tetracycline-resistance plasmid. Chromosomal loci mediating low-level resistance to tetracycline have been designated *mtr, penB,* and *tet* (see Ref. 91); two of these also are involved in low-level, non-β-lactamase-mediated penicillin resistance. In aggregate these three loci result in an increase in the tetracycline MIC from about 0.25 to 2–4 μg/ml. Much higher levels of resistance (tetracycline MIC $\geq$ 64 μg/ml) are found in gonococci containing a newly described 38-kilobase tetracycline-resistance ($Tc^r$) plasmid, which is a derivative of the 36-kilobase conjugal plasmid. Hybridization studies show that the $Tc^r$ plasmid contains *tetM,* which is carried on a transposon found in a variety of gram-positive and gram-negative microorganisms including many genital pathogens (*Gardnerella, Ureaplasma*).[99] The $Tc^r$ plasmids contain *tetM* in a position that does not inactivate conjugal function, and $Tc^r$ gonococci can transfer this plasmid as well as $Pc^r$ plasmids efficiently into other antibiotic-sensitive gonococci. The mechanism of resistance mediated by *tetM* involves production of a cytoplasmic protein that protects ribosomes from the action of tetracycline.

## SPECTINOMYCIN

For many years there were only rare reports of gonococci exhibiting high-level resistance to spectinomycin (Spc), but in areas where this antibiotic has been used frequently because of the prevalence of $Pc^r$ gonococci, $Spc^r$ isolates are becoming more common.[149] Single-step high-level resistance to Spc can be obtained relatively easily in the laboratory, and biochemical and genetic studies of $Spc^r$ mutants and of naturally occurring $Spc^r$ isolates show that they are virtually identical (see Ref. 91). The genetic locus *spc* maps within a cluster of chromosomal ribosomal genes and results in alteration of the 30-S ribosomal target on which Spc acts (see Ref. 91).

## OTHER ANTIBIOTICS

Streptomycin (Str) is not frequently used for therapy of gonorrhea at present, but many gonococci exhibit high-level resistance to Str. A locus for resistance to Str (*str*) maps near *spc* (see Ref. 91), and both are closely linked to those for resistance to tetracycline (*tet*), rifampin (*rif*), and others.

Resistance to nalidixic acid and related DNA gyrase inhibitors is obtained easily in the laboratory with mutation frequencies of approximately $1 \times 10^{-8}$. In contrast, $Spc^r$ mutants arise with a frequency of about $1 \times 10^{-10}$ to $1 \times 10^{-11}$. Resistance to several tested new quinolone inhibitors of DNA gyrase also occurs at about $1 \times 10^{-8}$ in vitro, but the levels of resistance are very low and probably would not immediately compromise therapy.

## HOST RESPONSE

Naturally acquired gonococcal infection results in serum antibodies against many gonococcal antigens including pili, P.I, P.II, and LOS.[150,151] As would be expected, serum antibody responses are greater in patients who have bacteremia or salpingitis than in those who have uncomplicated mucosal infection. Studies of mucosal secretions demonstrate that uncomplicated genital infection often results in IgA and IgG antibodies against the homologous isolate.[152,153] The duration of the local mucosal antibody response after natural infection may be quite brief, however, with antibodies disappearing in one study within a matter of a few months after therapy.[152] There also is a cellular immune response to natural gonococcal infection, although the cellular immunology of gonorrhea has been studied much less extensively than the humoral response.

## VACCINES

The principal efforts to stimulate protective immunity to date have focused on use of gonococcal pili as an antigen. Intramuscular or subcutaneous inoculation with purified pili results in both serum and mucosal antibodies that have antiadherence and opsonizing properties.[107,113,120] Limited in vitro studies of male volunteers vaccinated with a single antigenic type of pilus showed that there was partial protection against urethral challenge with the homologous strain.[154] Although the level of protection was modest, with only a 10- to 30-fold increase in the 50 percent infectious dose, this conceivably could result in clinically significant protection. Unfortunately challenge of vaccinated volunteers with a heterologous strain resulted in no protection (C. C. Brinton, presented at the International Pathogenic Neisseria Meeting, Montreal, 1982). A single antigenic type of pilus was used to vaccinate American military in a clinical trial, with the perhaps expected result that there was no protection against the diverse antigenic types of gonococci found in clinical practice.[113] It remains possible that a polyvalent pilus vaccine would be more effective, or that a common pilin domain or pilus-related protein antigen will be discovered that is more broadly protective against mucosal and/or systemic gonococcal infection.

Other vaccines are also under active investigation. These include P.I, which has been cloned and expressed in *E coli*[45] (also from unpublished data of N. Carbonetti, V. Simnad, and P. F. Sparling). The advantages of the recombinant P.I vaccine include its ability to be purified from *E. coli* without contamination by other potentially confounding antigens such as the blocking antigen P.III. Genital infection does not totally protect against reinfection by the same strain even within a few weeks of treatment,[104] but partial protection against reinfection by the same P.I serovar was demonstrated in a large study in Africa.[155] Reinfection by the same P.I serovar is rare in women with salpingitis.[156] These observations indicate there is some hope for vaccines based on P.I antigens. No published studies are available to evaluate the efficacy of P.I vaccines in volunteers.

Understanding of the pathogenesis of gonorrhea is now quite extensive. There is reason for some hope that this new information can be translated into protection against this common and sometimes serious infection. It remains for the future to determine whether this hope can be realized.

## References


1 Morton RS (ed): *Gonorrhoea* [vol. 9 in the series *Major Problems in Dermatology*. A Rook (consulting ed)]. London, Saunders, 1977.
2 Kellogg DS et al: *Neisseria gonorrhoeae:* I. Virulence genetically linked to clonal variation. *J Bacteriol* 85: 1274, 1963.
3 Catlin BW: Nutritional profiles of *Neisseria gonorrhoea, Neisseria meningitidis,* and *Neisseria lactamica* in chemically defined media and the use of growth requirements for gonococcal typing. *J Infect Dis* 128: 178, 1973.
4 Shinners EN, Catlin BW: Arginine and pyrimidine biosynthetic defects in *Neisseria gonorrhoeae* strains isolated from patients. *J Bacteriol* 151: 295, 1982.
5 Hook EW III et al: Auxotype/serovar diversity and antimicrobial resistance of *Neisseria gonorrhoeae* in two mid-sized American cities. *Sex Transm Dis* 14: 141, 1987.
6 Eisenstein BI et al: Penicillin sensitivity and serum resistance are independent attributes of strains of *Neisseria gonorrhoeae* causing disseminated gonococcal infection. *Infect Immun* 15: 834, 1977.
7 Knapp JS et al: Serological classification of *Neisseria gonorrhoeae* with use of monoclonal antibodies to gonococcal outer membrane protein I. *J Infect Dis* 150: 44, 1984.
8 Griffiss JM et al: Lipooligosaccharides: The principal glycolipids of the neisserial outer membrane. *Rev Infect Dis* 10: S287, 1988.
9 Morse SA et al: Effect of dilution rate on lipopolysaccharide and serum resistance of *Neisseria gonorrhoeae* grown in continuous culture. *Infect Immun* 41: 74, 1983.
10 Demarco de Hormaeche R et al: Gonococcal variants selected by growth *in vivo* or *in vitro* have antigenically different LPS. *Microbial Pathogenesis* 4: 289, 1988.
11 Apicella MA et al: Phenotypic variation in epitope expression of the *Neisseria gonorrhoeae* lipooligosaccharide. *Infect Immun* 55: 1755, 1987.
12 Dillon JR et al: Serological ecology of *Neisseria gonorrhoeae* (PPNG and non-PPNG) strains: Canadian perspective. *Genitourin Med* 63: 160, 1987.
13 Sparling PF, Yobs AR: Colonial morphology of *Neisseria gonorrhoeae* isolated from males and females. *J Bacteriol* 93: 513, 1967.
14 Walstad DL et al: Altered outer membrane protein in different colonial types of *Neisseria gonorrhoeae. J Bacteriol* 129: 1623, 1977.
15 Swanson J: Studies on gonococcus infection: XIV. Cell wall protein differences among color/opacity colony variants of *Neisseria gonorrhoeae: Infect Immun* 21: 292, 1978.
16 Swanson J: Colony opacity and protein II compositions of gonococci. *Infect Immun* 37: 359, 1982.
17 Buchanan TM: Antigenic heterogeneity of gonococcal pili. *J Exp Med* 151: 1470, 1975.
18 Pearce WA, Buchanan TM: Attachment role of gonococcal pili: Optimum conditions and quantitation of adherence of isolated pili to human cells in vitro. *J Clin Invest* 61: 931, 1978.
19 Brinton CC et al: Uses of pili in gonorrhoea control: Role of bacterial pili in disease, purification and properties of gonococcal pili, and progress in the development of a gonococcal pilus vaccine for gonorrhea, in *Immunobiology of Neisseria gonorrhoeae,* GF Brooks et al (eds). Washington, American Society for Microbiology, 1978, p 155.
20 Lambden PR et al: The identification and isolation of novel pilus types produced by isogenic variants of *Neisseria gonorrhoeae* P9 following selection *in vivo. FEMS Microbiol Lett* 10: 339, 1981.
21 Swanson J, Barrera O: Gonococcal pilus subunit size heterogeneity correlates with transitions in colony piliation phenotype, not with changes in colony opacity. *J Exp Med* 158: 1459, 1983.
22 Zak K et al: Antigenic variation during infection with *Neisseria gonorrhoeae:* Detection of antibodies to surface proteins in sera of patients with gonorrhea. *J Infect Dis* 149: 166, 1984.
23 Hagblom P et al: Intragenic recombination leads to pilus antigenic variation in *Neisseria gonorrhoeae. Nature* 315: 156, 1985.
24 Schoolnik GK et al: Gonococcal pili: Primary structure and receptor binding domain. *J Exp Med* 159: 1351, 1984.
25 Meyer TF et al: Pilus genes of *Neisseria gonorrhoeae:* Chromosomal organization and DNA sequence. *Proc Natl Acad Sci USA* 81: 6110, 1984.
26 Nicolson IJ et al: Localization of antibody-binding sites by sequence analysis of cloned pilin genes from *Neisseria gonorrhoeae. J Gen Microbiol* 133: 825, 1987.
27 Meyer TF et al: Pilus expression in *Neisseria gonorrhoeae* involves chromosomal rearrangement. *Cell* 30: 45, 1982.
28 Haas R, Meyer TF: The repertoire of silent pilus genes in *Neisseria gonorrhoeae:* Evidence for gene conversion. *Cell* 44: 107, 1986.
29 Segal E et al: Antigenic variation of gonococcal pilus involves assembly of separated silent gene segments. *Proc Natl Acad Sci USA* 83: 2177, 1986.
30 Swanson J et al: Gene conversion variations generate structurally distinct pilin polypeptides in *Neisseria gonorrhoeae. J Exp Med* 165: 1016, 1987.
31 Bergstrom S et al: Piliation control mechanisms in *Neisseria gonorrhoeae. Proc Natl Acad Sci USA* 83: 3890, 1986.
32 Swanson J et al: Gene conversion involving the pilin structural gene correlates with pilus$^+$ ⇄ pilus$^-$ changes in *Neisseria gonorrhoeae. Cell* 47: 267, 1986.
33 Meyer TF: Molecular basis of surface antigen variation in *Neisseria. Trends in Genetics* 3: 319, 1987.
34 Koomey M et al: Effects of *recA* mutations on pilus antigenic variation and phase transitions in *Neisseria gonorrhoeae. Genetics* 117: 391, 1987.
35 Segal E et al: Role of chromosomal rearrangement in *N. gonorrhoeae* pilus phase variation. *Cell* 40: 293, 1985.
36 Blake MS: Functions of the outer membrane proteins of *Neisseria gonorrhoeae,* in Bayer Symposium VIII, *The Pathogenesis of Bacterial Infections,* Berlin, Springer-Verlag, 1985, p 51.
37 Blake MS, Gotschlich EC: Gonococcal membrane proteins: Speculation on their role in pathogenesis. *Prog Allergy* 33: 298, 1983.
38 Blake MS, Gotschlich EC: Purification and partial characterization of the major outer membrane protein of *Neisseria gonorrhoeae. Infect Immun* 36: 277, 1982.
39 Hitchcock PJ: Analyses of gonococcal lipopolysaccharide in whole-cell lysates by sodium dodecyl sulfate–polyacrylamide gel electrophoresis: Stable association of lipopolysaccharide with the major outer membrane protein (Protein I) of *Neisseria gonorrhoeae. Infect Immun* 46: 202, 1984.

40 Newhall WJ et al: Crosslinking analysis of the outer membrane proteins of *Neisseria gonorrhoeae*. *Infect Immun* 28: 785, 1980.

41 Swanson J et al: Antigenicity of *Neisseria gonorrhoeae* outer membrane protein(s) III detected by immunoprecipitation and Western blot transfer with a monoclonal antibody. *Infect Immun* 38: 668, 1982.

42 Young JD-E et al: Properties of the major outer membrane protein from *Neisseria gonorrhoeae* incorporated into model lipid membranes. *Proc Natl Acad Sci USA* 80: 3831, 1983.

43 Lynch EC et al: Studies of porins: Spontaneously transferred from whole cells and reconstituted from purified proteins of *Neisseria gonorrhoeae* and *Neisseria meningitidis*. *Biophys J* 45: 104, 1984.

44 Gotschlich EC et al: Porin protein of *Neisseria gonorrhoeae:* Cloning and gene structure. *Proc Natl Acad Sci USA* 84: 8135, 1987.

45 Carbonetti NH, Sparling PF: Molecular cloning and characterization of the structural gene for protein I, the major outer membrane protein of *Neisseria gonorrhoeae*. *Proc Natl Acad Sci USA* 84: 9084, 1987.

46 Carbonetti NH et al: Genetics of protein I of *Neisseria gonorrhoeae:* construction of hybrid porins. *Proc Natl Acad Sci USA* 85: 6841, 1988.

47 Black WJ et al: Characterization of *Neisseria gonorrhoeae* protein II phase variation by use of monoclonal antibodies. *Infect Immun* 45: 453, 1984.

48 Sugasawara FJ et al: Inhibition of *Neisseria gonorrhoeae* attachment to HeLa cells with monoclonal antibody directed against a protein II. *Infect Immun* 42: 908, 1983.

49 Fischer SH, Rest RF: Gonococci possessing only certain P.II outer membrane proteins interact with human neutrophils. *Infect Immun* 56: 1574, 1988.

50 Sparling PF: Adherence of *Neisseria gonorrhoeae:* How little we really know, in *Surface Structures of Microorganisms and Their Interactions with the Mammalian Host,* E Schrinner et al (eds.). New York, VCH, 1988, p 197.

51 Stern A et al: Opacity determinants of *Neisseria gonorrhoeae:* Gene expression and chromosomal linkage to the gonococcal pilus gene. *Cell* 37: 447, 1984.

52 Stern A et al: Opacity genes in *Neisseria gonorrhoeae:* Control of phase and antigenic variation. *Cell* 47: 61, 1986.

53 Stern A, Meyer TF: Common mechanism controlling phase and antigenic variation in pathogenic *Neisseriae*. *Molecular Microbiol* 1: 5, 1987.

54 Connell TD et al: Recombination among protein II genes of *Neisseria gonorrhoeae* generates new coding sequences and increases structural variability in the protein II family. *Molecular Microbiol* 2: 227, 1988.

55 Gotschlich EC et al: Cloning of the structural genes of three H8 antigens and of protein III of *Neisseria gonorrhoeae*. *J Exp Med* 164: 868, 1986.

56 Cannon JG et al: Monoclonal antibody that recognizes an outer membrane antigen common to the pathogenic *Neisseria* species but not to most nonpathogenic *Neisseria* species. *Infect Immun* 43: 994, 1984.

57 Gotschlich EC, Seiff ME: Identification and gene structure of an azurin-like protein with a lipoprotein signal peptide in *Neisseria gonorrhoeae*. *FEMS Microbiol Lett* 43: 253, 1987.

58 Kawula TH et al: Localization of a conserved epitope and an azurin-like domain in the H.8 protein of pathogenic *Neisseria*. *Molecular Microbiol* 1: 179, 1987.

59 Black JR et al: Neisserial antigen H.8 is immunogenic in patients with disseminated gonococcal and meningococcal infections. *J Infect Dis* 151: 650, 1985.

60 Newhall V WJ et al: High-molecular-weight antigenic protein complex in outer membrane of *Neisseria gonorrhoeae*. *Infect Immun* 27: 475, 1980.

61 Hansen NW, Wilde CE III: Conservation of peptide structure of outer membrane protein–macromolecular complex from *Neisseria gonorrhoeae*. *Infect Immun* 43: 839, 1984.

62 Norqvist A et al: The effect of iron starvation on the outer membrane protein composition of *Neisseria gonorrhoeae*. *FEMS Microbiol Lett* 4: 71, 1978.

63 West SEH, Sparling PF: Response of *Neisseria gonorrhoeae* to iron limitation: Alterations in expression of membrane proteins without apparent siderophore production. *Infect Immun* 47: 388, 1985.

64 Clark VL et al: Induction and repression of outer membrane proteins by anaerobic growth of *Neisseria gonorrhoeae*. *Infect Immun* 55: 1359, 1987.

65 Keevil W et al: Physiology and virulence determinants of *Neisseria gonorrhoeae* grown in glucose-, oxygen- or cystine-limited continuous culture. *J Gen Microbiol* 132: 3289, 1986.

66 Mietzner TA et al: Identification of an iron-regulated 37,000-dalton protein in the cell envelope of *Neisseria gonorrhoeae*. *Infect Immun* 45: 410, 1984.

67 Mietzner TA et al: Purification and characterization of the major iron-regulated protein expressed by pathogenic *Neisseriae*. *J Exp Med* 165: 1041, 1987.

68 Mietzner TA et al: Distribution of an antigenically related iron-regulated protein among the *Neisseria* spp. *Infect Immun* 51: 60, 1986.

69 Black JR et al: Human immune response to iron-repressible outer membrane proteins of *Neisseria meningitidis*. *Infect Immun* 54: 710, 1986.

70 Dyer DW et al: A pleiotropic iron-uptake mutant of *Neisseria meningitidis* lacks a 70 kilodalton iron-regulated protein. *Infect Immun* 56: 977, 1988.

71 Fohn MJ et al: Human immunoglobulin G antibody response to the major gonococcal iron-regulated protein. *Infect Immun* 55: 3065, 1987.

72 Mulks MH, Plant AG: IgA protease production as a characteristic distinguishing pathogenic from harmless *Neisseriaceae*. *N Engl J Med* 299: 973, 1978.

73 Mulks MH, Knapp JS: Immunoglobulin $A_1$ protease types of *Neisseria gonorrhoeae* and their relationship to auxotype and serovar. *Infect Immun* 55: 931, 1987.

74 Pohlner J et al: Gene structure and extracellular secretion of *Neisseria gonorrhoeae* IgA protease. *Nature* 325: 458, 1987.

75 Schneider H et al: Immunological basis of serum resistance of *Neisseria gonorrhoeae*. *J Gen Microbiol* 128: 13, 1982.

76 Apicella MA et al: Bactericidal antibody response of normal human serum to the lipooligosaccharide of *Neisseria gonorrhoeae*. *J Infect Dis* 153: 520, 1986.

77 Griffiss JM et al: Physical heterogeneity of neisserial lipooligosaccharides reflects oligosaccharides that differ in apparent molecular weight, chemical composition, and antigenic expression. *Infect Immun* 55: 1792, 1987.

78 Stephens DS, Shafer WM: Evidence that the serum resistance genetic locus *sac-3* of *Neisseria gonorrhoeae* is involved in lipopolysaccharide structure. *J Gen Microbiol* 133: 2671, 1987.

79 Rosenthal RS et al: Strain-related differences in lysozyme sensitivity and extent of O-acetylation of gonococcal peptidoglycan. *Infect Immun* 37: 826, 1982.

80 Melly MA et al: Ability of monomeric peptidoglycan fragments from *Neisseria gonorrhoeae* to damage human fallopian-tube mucosa. *J Infect Dis* 149: 378, 1984.

81 Noegel A, Gotschlich EC: Isolation of a high molecular weight polyphosphate from *Neisseria gonorrhoeae*. *J Exp Med* 157: 2049, 1983.

82 Britigan B, Cohen MS: Effect of growth in serum on uptake of *Neisseria gonorrhoeae* by human neutrophils. *J Infect Dis* 152: 330, 1985.

83 Britigan BE et al: Phagocyte-derived lactate stimulates oxygen consumption by *Neisseria gonorrhoeae*. *J Clin Invest* 81: 318, 1988.

84 Knapp JS, Clark VL: Anaerobic growth of *Neisseria gonorrhoeae* coupled to nitrite reduction. *Infect Immun* 46: 176, 1984.

85 McKenna WR et al: Iron uptake from lactoferrin and transferrin by *Neisseria gonorrhoeae*. *Infect Immun* 56: 785, 1988.

86 Biswas GD et al: Factors affecting genetic transformation of *Neisseria gonorrhoeae*. *J Bacteriol* 129: 983, 1977.

87 Dougherty TJ et al: Specificity of DNA uptake in genetic transformation of gonococci. *Biochem Biophys Res Comm* 86: 97, 1979.

88 Graves JF et al: Sequence-specific DNA uptake in transformation of *Neisseria gonorrhoeae*. *J Bacteriol* 152: 1071, 1982.

89 Goodman SD, Scocca JJ: Identification and arrangement of the DNA sequence recognized in specific transformation of *Neisseria gonorrhoeae*. *Proc Natl Acad Sci USA* 85: 6982, 1988.
90 Sarubbi FA, Sparling PF: Transfer of antibiotic resistance in mixed cultures of *Neisseria gonorrhoeae*. *J Infect Dis* 130: 660, 1974.
91 Cannon JG, Sparling PF: The genetics of the gonococcus. *Ann Rev Microbiol* 38: 111, 1984.
92 Robert M, Falkow S: Conjugal transfer of R plasmids in *Neisseria gonorrhoeae*. *Nature* 266: 630, 1977.
93 Eisenstein BI et al: Conjugal transfer of the gonococcal penicillinase plasmid. *Science* 195: 998, 1977.
94 Biswas GD et al: High-frequency conjugal transfer of a gonococcal penicillinase plasmid. *J Bacteriol* 143: 1318, 1980.
95 Campbell LA, Yasbin RE: Mutagenesis of *Neisseria gonorrhoeae:* Absence of error-prone repair. *J Bacteriol* 160: 288, 1984.
96 Koomey JM, Falkow S: Cloning of the *recA* gene of *Neisseria gonorrhoeae* and construction of gonococcal *recA* mutants. *J Bacteriol* 169: 790, 1987.
97 Sullivan KM et al: Characterization of DNA restriction and modification activities in *Neisseria* species. *FEMS Microbiol Lett* 44: 389, 1987.
98 Stein DC et al: Restriction of plasmid DNA during transformation but not conjugation in *Neisseria gonorrhoeae*. *Infect Immun* 56: 112, 1988.
99 Morse SA et al: High-level tetracycline resistance in *Neisseria gonorrhoeae* is result of acquisition of streptococcal *tetM* determinant. *Antimicrob Agents Chemother* 30: 664, 1986.
100 Perine PL et al: Evidence for two distinct types of penicillinase-producing *Neisseria gonorrhoeae*. *Lancet* 2: 993, 1977.
101 Robert M et al: The ecology of gonococcal plasmids. *J Gen Microbiol* 114: 491, 1979.
102 Korch C et al: Cryptic plasmid of *Neisseria gonorrhoeae:* Complete nucleotide sequence and genetic organization. *J Bacteriol* 163: 430, 1985.
103 Biswas GD et al: Construction of isogenic gonococcal strains varying in the presence of a 4.2-kilobase cryptic plasmid. *J Bacteriol* 167: 685, 1986.
104 Faruki H et al: A community-based outbreak of infection with penicillin-resistant *Neisseria gonorrhoeae* not producing penicillinase (chromosomally mediated resistance). *N Engl J Med* 313: 607, 1985.
105 McGee ZA et al: Pathogenic mechanisms of *Neisseria gonorrhoeae:* Observations on damage to human fallopian tubes in organ culture by gonococci of colony type 1 or type 4. *J Infect Dis* 143: 413, 1981.
106 Lambden PR et al: Biological properties of two distinct pilus types produced by isogenic variants of *Neisseria gonorrhoeae* P9. *J Bacteriol* 141: 393, 1980.
107 McChesney D et al: Genital antibody response to a parenteral gonococcal pilus vaccine. *Infect Immun* 36: 1006, 1982.
108 Schoolnik GK et al: A pilus peptide vaccine for the prevention of gonorrhea. *Prog Allergy* 33: 315, 1983.
109 Virji M, Heckels JE: The role of common and type-specific pilus antigenic domains in adhesion and virulence of gonococci for human epithelial cells. *J Gen Microbiol* 130: 1089, 1984.
110 Bessen D, Gotschlich EC: Interactions of gonococci with HeLa cells: Attachment, detachment, replication, penetration, and the role of protein II. *Infect Immun* 54: 154, 1986.
111 Rothbard JB et al: Antibodies to peptides corresponding to a conserved sequence of gonococcal pilins block bacterial adhesion. *Proc Natl Acad Sci USA* 82: 915, 1985.
112 Rothbard JB et al: Strain-specific and common epitopes of gonococcal pili. *J Exp Med* 160: 208, 1984.
113 Boslego J et al: Efficacy trial of a purified gonococcal pilus vaccine, in *Program and Abstracts of the 24th Interscience Conference on Antimicrobial Agents and Chemotherapy,* Washington, American Society for Microbiology, 1984.
114 Lindberg F et al: Gene products specifying adhesion of uropathogenic *Escherichia coli* are minor components of pili. *Proc Natl Acad Sci USA* 83: 1891, 1986.
115 Muir LL et al: Proteins that appear to be associated with pili in *Neisseria gonorrhoeae*. *Infect Immun* 56: 1743, 1988.
116 James JF, Swanson J: Color/opacity colonial variants of *Neisseria gonorrhoeae* and their relationship to the menstrual cycle, in *Immunobiology of Neisseria gonorrhoeae,* GF Brooks et al (eds). Washington, American Society for Microbiology, 1978, p 338.
117 Stromberg N et al: Identification of carbohydrate structures that are possible receptors for *Neisseria gonorrhoeae*. *Proc Natl Acad Sci USA* 85: 4902, 1988.
118 Densen P, Mandell GL: Gonococcal interactions with polymorphonuclear neutrophils: Importance of the phagosome for bactericidal activity. *J Clin Invest* 62: 1161, 1978.
119 Thongthai C, Sawyer WD: Studies in the virulence of *Neisseria gonorrhoeae:* I. Relation of colonial morphology and resistance to phagocytosis by polymorphonuclear leukocytes. *Infect Immun* 7: 373, 1973.
120 Siegel M et al: Gonococcal pili: Safety and immunogenicity in humans and antibody function in vitro. *J Infect Dis* 145: 300, 1982.
121 Virji M, Heckels JE: Role of anti-pilus antibodies in host defense against gonococcal infection studied with monoclonal anti-pilus antibodies. *Infect Immun* 49: 621, 1985.
122 Swanson J et al: Studies on gonococcus infection: X. Pili and leukocyte association factor as mediators of interactions between gonococci and eukaryotic cells *in vitro*. *Infect Immun* 11: 1352, 1975.
123 Casey SG et al: *Neisseria gonorrhoeae* survive intraleukocytic oxygen-independent antimicrobial capacities of anaerobic and aerobic granulocytes in the presence of pyocin lethal for extracellular gonococci. *Infect Immun* 52: 384, 1986.
124 Parsons NJ et al: A determinant of resistance of *Neisseria gonorrhoeae* to killing by human phagocytes: An outer membrane lipoprotein of about 20 kDa with a high content of glutamic acid. *J Gen Microbiol* 132: 3277, 1986.
125 Rest RF et al: Interactions of *Neisseria gonorrhoeae* with human neutrophils: Effect of serum and gonococcal opacity on phagocyte killing and chemiluminescence. *Infect Immun* 36: 737, 1982.
126 Shafer W et al: Antigonococcal activity of human neutrophil cathepsin G. *Infect Immun* 54: 184, 1986.
127 Shaw JH, Falkow S: Model for invasion of human tissue culture cells by *Neisseria gonorrhoeae*. *Infect Immun* 56: 1625, 1988.
128 McGee ZA et al: Mechanisms of mucosal invasion by pathogenic *Neisseria*. *Rev Infect Dis* 5 (suppl 4): S708, 1983.
129 Gregg CR et al: Toxic activity of purified lipopolysaccharide of *Neisseria gonorrhoeae* for human fallopian tube mucosa. *J Infect Dis* 143: 532, 1981.
130 Melly MA et al: Ability of monomeric peptidoglycan fragments from *Neisseria gonorrhoeae* to damage human fallopian-tube mucosa. *J Infect Dis* 149: 378, 1984.
131 Fleming TJ et al: Arthropathic properties of gonococcal peptidoglycan fragments: Implications for the pathogenesis of disseminated gonococcal disease. *Infect Immun* 52: 600, 1986.
132 Schwab JH et al: Association of experimental chronic arthritis with the persistence of group A streptococcal cell walls in the articular tissue. *J Bacteriol* 1728, 1967.
133 Rice PA, Kasper DL: Characterization of serum resistance of *Neisseria gonorrhoeae* that disseminate: Roles of blocking antibody and gonococcal outer membrane proteins. *J Clin Invest* 70: 157, 1982.
134 Harriman GR et al: Activation of complement by serum-resistant *Neisseria gonorrhoeae:* Assembly of the membrane attack complex without subsequent cell death. *J Exp Med* 156: 1235, 1982.
135 Joiner KA et al: Studies on the mechanism of bacterial resistance to complement-mediated killing: IV. C5b-9 forms high molecular weight complexes with bacterial outer membrane constituents on serum-resistant but not on serum-sensitive *Neisseria gonorrhoeae*. *J Immunol* 131: 1443, 1983.
136 Rice PA et al: Immunoglobulin G antibodies directed against protein III block killing of serum-resistant *Neisseria gonorrhoeae* by immune serum. *J Exp Med* 164: 1735, 1986.
137 Shafe WM et al: Identification of a new genetic site (*sac-3*$^{+}$) in

*Neisseria gonorrhoeae* that affects sensitivity to normal human serum. *Infect Immun* 35: 764, 1982.

138 McShan WM et al: A recombinant molecule from a disseminating strain of *Neisseria gonorrhoeae* that confers serum bactericidal resistance. *Infect Immun* 55: 3017, 1987.

139 Densen P et al: Specificity of antibodies against *Neisseria gonorrhoeae* that stimulate neutrophil chemotaxis: Role of antibodies directed against lipooligosaccharides. *J Clin Invest* 80: 78, 1987.

140 Rice PA et al: Natural serum bactericidal activity against *Neisseria gonorrhoeae* from disseminated, locally invasive, and uncomplicated disease. *J Immunol* 124: 2105, 1980.

141 Jaffe HW et al: Diagnosis of gonorrhea using a genetic transformation test on mailed clinical specimens. *J Infect Dis* 146: 275, 1982.

142 Spratt BG: Hybrid penicillin-binding proteins in penicillin-resistant strains of *Neisseria gonorrhoeae*. *Nature* 332: 173, 1988.

143 Phillips I: β-Lactamase-producing penicillin-resistant gonococcus. *Lancet* 2: 656, 1976.

144 Fayet O et al: β-Lactamase-specifying plasmids isolated from *Neisseria gonorrhoeae* have retained an intact right part of a Tn3-like transposon. *J Bacteriol* 149: 136, 1982.

145 Chen S-T, Clowes RC: Nucleotide sequence comparisons of plasmids pHD131, pJB1, pFA3, and pFA7 and β-lactamase expression in *Escherichia coli, Haemophilus influenzae,* and *Neisseria gonorrhoeae*. *J Bacteriol* 169: 3124, 1987.

146 Brunton J et al: Molecular nature of a plasmid specifying beta-lactamase production in *Haemophilus ducreyi*. *J Bacteriol* 148: 788, 1981.

147 Anderson B et al: Common β-lactamase-specifying plasmid in *Haemophilus ducreyi* and *Neisseria gonorrhoeae*. *Antimicrob Agents Chemother* 25: 296, 1984.

148 McNicol PJ et al: Transfer of plasmid-mediated ampicillin resistance from *Haemophilus* to *Neisseria gonorrhoeae* requires an intervening organism. *Sex Transm Dis* 13: 145, 1986.

149 Boslego JW et al: Effect of spectinomycin use on the prevalence of spectinomycin-resistant and of penicillinase-producing *Neisseria gonorrhoeae*. *N Engl J Med* 317: 272, 1987.

150 Lammel CJ et al: Antibody-antigen specificity in the immune response to infection with *Neisseria gonorrhoeae*. *J Infect Dis* 152: 990, 1985.

151 Hook EW III et al: Analysis of the antigen specificity of the human serum immunoglobulin G immune response to complicated gonococcal infection. *Infect Immun* 43: 706, 1984.

152 McMillan A et al: Antibodies to *Neisseria gonorrhoeae:* A study of the urethral exudates of 232 men. *J Infect Dis* 140: 89, 1979.

153 Tramont EC: Inhibition of adherence of *Neisseria gonorrhoeae* by human genital secretions. *J Clin Invest* 59: 117, 1977.

154 Brinton CC Jr et al: The development of a neisserial pilus vaccine for gonorrhea and meningococcal meningitis, in *Seminars in Infectious Disease,* L Weinstein, BN Fields (eds). New York, Thieme-Stratton, 1982, vol 4, p 140.

155 Plummer FA et al: Epidemiologic evidence for strain specific immunity to *Neisseria gonorrhoeae* in frequently infected women, in *Abstracts,* International Society STD Research, Atlanta, 1987, p 3.

156 Buchanan TM et al: Gonococcal salpingitis is less likely to recur with *Neisseria gonorrhoeae* of the same principal outer membrane protein antigenic type. *Am J Obstet Gynecol* 138: 978, 1980.

Chapter 14

# Gonococcal infections in the adult

Edward W. Hook III
H. Hunter Handsfield

## HISTORY

The major clinical manifestations of gonorrhea in men were described in ancient Chinese, Egyptian, Roman, and Greek literature as well as in the Old Testament.[1] The current term for the clinical syndromes referred to as gonorrhea (Greek, "flow of seed") is attributed to Galen (130 A.D.), who is said to have believed that the urethral exudate present in males with gonorrhea was semen. However, there is little recorded evidence of awareness that urethral discharge in men was linked with morbidity for women until relatively recently. In 1879, *Neisseria gonorrhoeae* was demonstrated by Neisser in stained smears of urethral, vaginal, and conjunctival exudates, making the gonococcus the second identified bacterial pathogen following the discovery of *Bacillus anthracis*.[2] *N. gonorrhoeae* was first cultured in vitro by Leistikow in 1882, and effective antimicrobial therapy in the form of sulfonamides was first applied in the 1930s.[3] In 1962 the availability of Thayer-Martin medium[4] greatly facilitated the diagnosis of gonorrhea and may have contributed to subsequent increases in numbers of cases of gonorrhea reported in women. Since the mid-1960s knowledge of the molecular basis of gonococcal–host interactions and gonococcal epidemiology have increased to the point where there are few other microbial pathogens which are as well described.

*N. gonorrhoeae* initially infects noncornified epithelium, most often of the urogenital tract and secondarily of the rectum, oropharynx, and conjunctivae. It is transmitted almost exclusively by sexual contact or perinatally, and infection most often remains localized to initial sites of inoculation. Ascending genital infections (salpingitis, epididymitis) and bacteremic dissemination, however, are relatively common and account for most of the serious morbidity due to gonorrhea. These complications are most common in populations that lack ready access to effective diagnosis and therapy.

## EPIDEMIOLOGY

### INCIDENCE

Relatively few countries have reporting systems that permit accurate estimation of the true incidence of gonorrhea. Figure 14-1 shows the reported annual incidence of gonorrhea in the United States and Sweden from 1955 through 1987.[5,6] Recent changes in gonorrhea incidence reflect the influence of multiple, sometimes opposing, trends for members of certain risk groups. At least part of the decline in gonorrhea in both countries has been attributed to the impact of behavioral changes made to reduce risks of infection with human immunodeficiency virus (HIV). However, these changes have not occurred uniformly within the population. Although national data are not available, studies from several North American and European cities[7,8] suggest that gonorrhea rates in homosexual or bisexual men have declined precipitously, while rates in other groups have changed less. Among white U.S. teenagers, gonorrhea rates may actually have increased slightly.[9]

The incidence of gonorrhea varies with age (Fig. 14-2). Eighty-two percent of reported cases in the United States in 1987 occurred in patients aged 15 to 29 years, with the highest rates occurring in the 20- to 24-year-old age group. The incidences in 15- to 19-year-old and 20- to 24-year-old women were 1455 and 1420 cases per 100,000 population, respectively. However, it is estimated that only about 50 percent of 15- to 19-year-old women in the United States were sexually experienced, compared with over 90 percent of the 20- to 24-year-old age group. Thus, despite similar overall rates, the reported incidence of gonorrhea was almost twice as high for sexually active adolescents as for sexually active women in the 20- to 24-year-old group.[5,9]

In the United States, reported cases of gonorrhea are about 10-fold higher in nonwhites than whites, a difference only partially explained by greater attendance of nonwhites at public clinics where reporting is more complete than in private health care settings.[10] Other demographic risk factors for gonorrhea include low socioeconomic status, urban residence, early onset of sexual activity, unmarried marital status, and a history of past gonorrhea.[10,12] Recent studies in Seattle documented that about 25

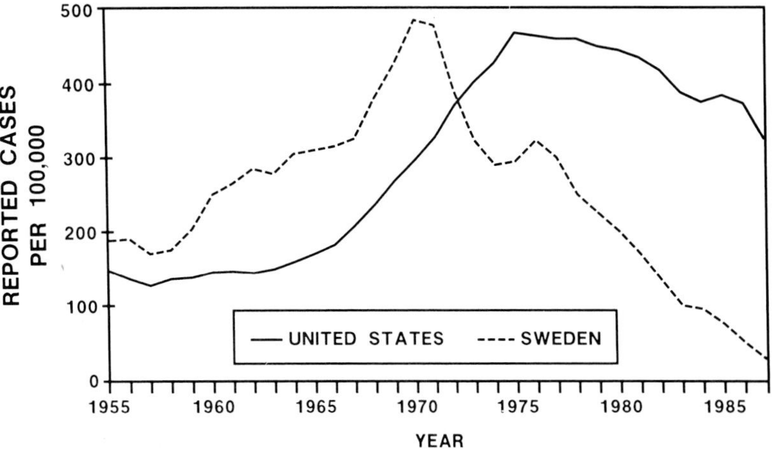


**Fig. 14-1.** Reported annual incidence of gonorrhea in the United States and Sweden from 1955 to 1987. *(From Centers for Disease Control,[5] D Danielsson, National Bacteriological Laboratory.[6])*

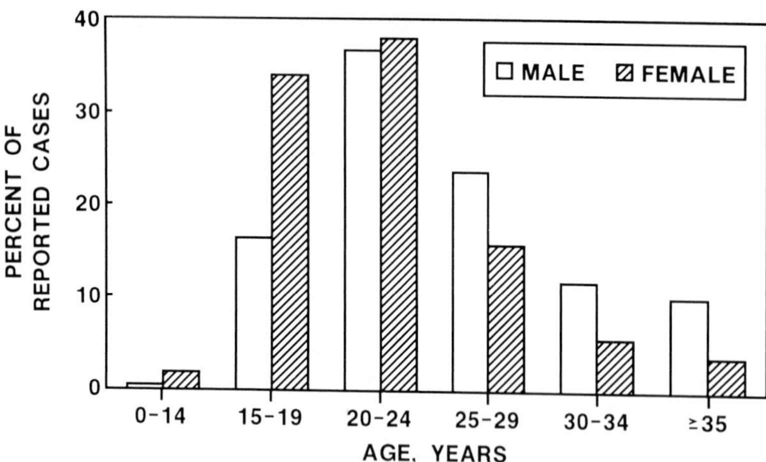


**Fig. 14-2.** Age and sex distribution of reported cases of gonorrhea in the United States, 1987. *(From Centers for Disease Control.[5])*

percent of sexually active 16- to 18-year-old black females living in low-socioeconomic-level, urban census tracts in 1986 to 1987 acquired gonorrhea each year.[11] In the 1980s, illicit drug use and prostitution also appear to have become increasingly associated with enhanced risk of gonorrhea, syphilis, and probably other sexually transmitted diseases (STDs) as well. Male homosexuality may no longer be strongly associated with gonorrhea because of changing sexual practices among many homosexual men as a consequence of concerns regarding AIDS.

The incidence of gonorrhea in the United States is seasonal: the highest rates occur in late summer while the lowest are in late winter and early spring, with nadirs tending to be about 20 percent lower than peaks.[10,13,14] The antimicrobial susceptibility of *N. gonorrhoeae* appears to fluctuate similarly.[14] The proportion of gonococcal isolates that are relatively resistant to penicillins and tetracyclines is slightly higher in late winter than in summer, possibly as a consequence of seasonal variation in antibiotic usage. Seasonal variations in sexual activity, access to health care, changing commitments in schedules of the young individuals at highest risk for gonorrhea, or other factors may also be involved in these seasonal fluctuations.

The efficiency of gonorrhea transmission is dependent on anatomic sites infected and exposed as well as number of exposures. The risk of acquiring urethral infection for a man following a single episode of vaginal intercourse with an infected woman is estimated to be 20 percent, rising to an estimated 60 to 80 percent following four exposures.[15] The prevalence of infection in women named as secondary sexual contacts of men with gonococcal urethritis has been reported to be 50 to 90 percent,[15,16] but no published studies have carefully controlled for number of exposures. It is likely that the single-exposure transmission rate from male to female is higher than that from female to male, in part because of retention of the infected ejaculate within the vagina. The risk of transmission by other types of sexual contact is less well defined. Gonorrhea transmission through insertive or receptive rectal intercourse presumably is relatively efficient. Transmission of pharyngeal infection during fellatio and cunnilingus has been documented and is thought to be rare, although conflicting data exist.[17,18] In women use of hormonal contraception may increase risk of acquiring gonorrhea[19,19a] and use of spermicides and/or the diaphragm clearly has a protective influence.[20,21] Transmission by fomites or through nonsexual contact is extremely rare but may account for rare cases of gonorrhea in infants.

Symptoms and the behavioral response to them also influence the transmission of gonorrhea. Previous reports that ≥80 percent of women with gonorrhea were asymptomatic were most often based on studies of women who were examined in screening surveys or who were referred to STD clinics because of sexual contact with infected men.[22] Symptomatic infected women who sought medical attention were thus often excluded from such surveys. However, as might be expected, >75 percent of women with gonorrhea attending acute care facilities such as hospital emergency room are symptomatic.[23] The true proportion of infected women who remain asymptomatic undoubtedly lies between these extremes. Appreciation of symptomatic infection in infected women is more difficult than in men because the clinical syndromes may be mistakenly attributed to other infectious processes, including urinary tract or vaginal infections.

Asymptomatically infected males and females contribute disproportionately to gonorrhea transmission because many symptomatic individuals cease sexual activity and seek medical care. However, the presence of urogenital symptoms does not assure that transmission will not occur. In a recent study of patients attending STD clinics in Baltimore, 38 percent of men and 46 percent of women presenting for symptom evaluation reported sexual exposure following the onset of the symptoms that brought them to the clinic.[24] The reasons for continued sexual activity despite the presence of symptoms may include the relative lack of severity of symptoms early in the course of disease, denial, and for women, the nonspecificity of urogenital symptoms. The observation that many transmitters of gonorrhea (and other STDs) do not spontaneously cease sexual activity and seek care emphasizes the importance of taking active steps to bring the partners of infected persons to treatment.

Asymptomatic infections occur in men as well as women, and the percentage of infected men who are asymptomatic probably varies with duration of infection. In a cohort of 81 men who acquired urethral infection at a defined time, the mean time to development of symptoms was 3.4 days, and only 2 (2.5 percent) remained asymptomatic for 14 days (Fig. 14-3).[25] Although this study was performed in a geographic area where the strains of *N. gonorrhoeae* most likely to cause asymptomatic urethral infections were uncommon, the incidence of asymptomatic urethral gonococcal infection in the general population also has been estimated at approximately 1 to 3 percent.[26]

## PREVALENCE

The prevalence of gonorrhea within communities tends to be dynamic, fluctuating over time and influenced by a number of interactive factors. Mathematical models for gonorrhea within

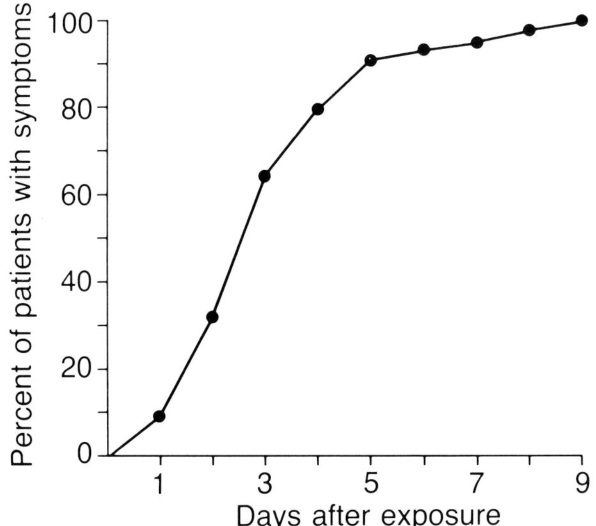


**Fig. 14-3.** Incubation period in 44 men with symptomatic gonococcal urethritis. *(From WO Harrison et al.*[25]*)*

communities suggest that gonorrhea prevalence is sustained not only by continued transmission by asymptomatically infected patients, but also by "core group" transmitters who are more likely than members of the general population to become infected and transmit gonorrhea to their sex partners.[27–29] Although members of the core group described in these mathematical models share a number of characteristics including geographic clustering (usually within inner cities) and low socioeconomic status, the core group probably actually comprises a number of heterogeneous subgroups. These include persons with repeated episodes of gonorrhea, those who fail to abstain from sex despite the presence of symptoms or knowledge of recent exposure, and patients who practice high-risk behaviors such as illegal drug use, prostitution, or prostitute patronage.[12,24,28] Finally, because the core group is defined primarily on behavioral grounds, membership in a core group is not a stable characteristic of an individual but may change over time. Several studies have provided empirical observations which support mathematical models of core-group transmission.[12,24,28]

While providing the focus for continued endemnicity of gonorrhea, core groups are not solely responsible for gonorrhea prevalence within communities. Disease prevalence is due to infections transmitted by both core-group and non-core-group members, the interaction between these two groups, and the movement of patients from one group to another. These factors in turn fluctuate with changes in normative social behavior, disease-control efforts, and other epidemiologic factors. At present, gonorrhea-control efforts are heavily invested in the concept of vigorous pursuit and treatment of infected core-group members and asymptomatically infected individiuals. Because about 40 percent of infected men and many women who are asymptomatic indeed have clinical findings compatible with gonorrhea,[23,26] patient education designed to modify the behavior or response to mild symptoms may also be an important yet unexplored part of gonorrhea control. In addition, however, control efforts to access the often-difficult-to-reach core-group transmitters are needed to assist in gonorrhea control. The mathematical models which suggest the role of core-group members in sustaining gonorrhea prevalence within communities also suggest that because gonorrhea transmission is not 100 percent efficient and because spontaneous cures occur, without hyperendemic transmission by core-group members, gonorrhea prevalence would decline, perhaps ultimately to zero.[27,29]

## EPIDEMIOLOGIC CORRELATES OF GONOCOCCAL TYPES

A variety of methods for gonococcal typing have been developed, as discussed in Chap. 13. Only auxotyping,[30] protein I serotyping,[31] or the two used in combination[32] have been widely used to study gonococcal epidemiology. Auxotyping classifies gonococci on the basis of stable nutritional requirements for a variety of amino acids and nucleosides, alone or in combination.[30] Examples of common auxotypes are strains requiring arginine (Arg), proline (Pro), uracil (U), methionine (M), or arginine, hypoxanthine, and uracil (AHU$^-$) for growth. Gonococci requiring none of the substrates are termed *prototrophic* (Proto) or are referred to by some authors as *wild type.* Protein I serotyping is based on the stable antigenic diversity of protein I, the protein present in largest quantity in the gonococcal outer membrane.[31] Protein I is divided into two mutually exclusive classes, protein IA and protein IB, each of which can be further subdivided into serovars in coagglutination assays using panels of protein IA- or protein IB-specific monoclonal antibody reagents. Each serovar is designated by its protein I type (IA or IB) and a numeral based on its coagglutination pattern (e.g., IA-4, IB-3). Using both auxotyping and serovar analysis, gonococci can be divided into a large number of auxotype/serovar (A/S) classes (e.g., AHU/IA-1, Pro/IB-3, Proto/IB-12), providing a highly discriminative tool for study of gonococcal epidemiology.[32]

Relatively large numbers (>50) of gonococcal A/S classes usually are present in communities simultaneously,[32,33] and new strains continue to be detected over time. The distribution of isolates within A/S classes tends to be uneven, with a few A/S classes contributing disproportionately to the total number of isolates. These predominant A/S classes generally persist within communities for months or years. In most studies using these methods, many more A/S classes are detectable only intermittently or even only once during a sampling interval and then are not detected again.

The factors that determine which A/S classes will become predominant and which will be seen only transiently may include biological characteristics of the strain or the host. Alternatively, epidemiologic factors such as prostitute transmission or importation by travelers may be important. During a 12-week study of consecutive patients with gonorrhea seen at a Seattle STD clinic,[32] 489 isolates were collected from 390 patients. These isolates could be divided into 57 different A/S classes. Some A/S classes were isolated only from heterosexual men and women (e.g., AHU/IA-1, AHU/IA-2), while for other A/S classes, isolates were obtained almost exclusively from homosexual or bisexual men (e.g., Arg/IB-2, Proto/IB-20). During the study, one strain (Proto/IB-3) was not detected until week 6 and over the next 2 weeks was isolated from one woman, one homosexual man, and 10 heterosexual men. During the next few weeks, isolates from heterosexual men continued to far outnumber those from women, and over the subsequent year, this strain became one of the predominant gonococcal A/S classes seen in the city. Interviews of the patients infected by the Proto/IB-3 strain early in the outbreak revealed that one infected female acknowledged over 100 different sexual partners over the preceding 2 months, suggesting that she may have played an important role in the introduction and establishment of this gonococcal strain in the community. Thus, the Proto/IB-3 strain may have become common in Seattle not because of specific biological factors, but because of its chance transmission to members of a core population by a high-frequency transmitter.

Some gonococcal strain types are associated with specific clinical manifestations of disease. In Seattle during the early 1970s, AHU/IA-1 and AHU/IA-2 strains caused >90 percent of asymptomatic urethral infections in men[34] and the majority of cases of disseminated gonococcal infections,[35] but were less common in symptomatic men and in women with gonococcal salpingitis.[36] These strains grow more slowly than other strains, are particularly susceptible to the penicillins and tetracyclines, and tend to be resistent to the complement-mediated bactericidal activity of normal human serum.[37] Since the 1970s, the prevalence of AHU/IA strains in Seattle has diminished, as have the numbers of patients with disseminated gonococcal infection and the numbers of men with asymptomatic urethral infections.[38] These changes occurred shortly after institution of contact tracing for gonorrhea and with routine treatment of asymptomatic male sexual partners of infected women.

## PATHOLOGY

In adults, only mucous membranes lined by columnar, cuboidal, noncornified squamous epithelial cells are susceptible to gonococcal infection. The initial event in gonococcal infection is the adherence of *N. gonorrhoeae* to mucosal cells in a process mediated by pili and other surface proteins.[39,40] The organism is then pinocytosed by the epithelial cells, which transport viable, sometimes dividing, gonococci from the mucosal surface to subepithelial spaces.[41] In fallopian tube organ culture models, simultaneous with attachment of gonococci to nonciliated epithelial cells, gonococcal lipooligosaccharide (endotoxin) impairs ciliary motility and contributes to destruction of surrounding ciliary cells.[42] This process may promote further attachment of additional organisms. Progressive mucosal cell damage and submucosal invasion are accompanied by a vigorous polymorphonuclear leukocytic response, submucosal microabscess formation, and exudation of purulent material into the lumen of the infected organ. In untreated infections, polymorphonuclear leukocytes are gradually replaced by mononuclear cells, and abnormal round cell infiltration has been reported to persist for several weeks or months after gonococci can no longer be isolated.[41] The molecular mechanisms of gonococcal invasion and infection are more fully discussed in Chap. 13.

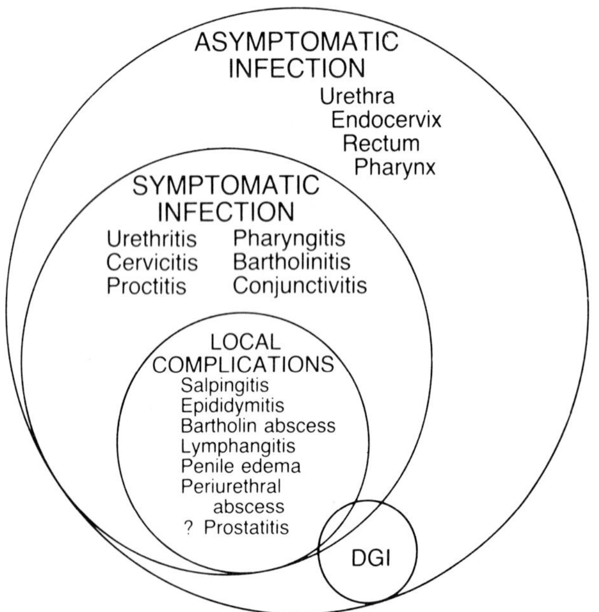


**Fig. 14-4.** Clinical spectrum of gonococcal infection. DGI = disseminated gonococcal infection.

## CLINICAL MANIFESTATIONS: UNCOMPLICATED GONOCOCCAL INFECTIONS

Despite the focus of many patients and even some clinicians on symptomatic local infections, clinical gonorrhea is manifested by a broad spectrum of clinical presentations including asymptomatic and symptomatic local infections, local complicated infections, and systemic dissemination. Figure 14-4 estimates the relative proportion of individuals with each of the major clinical syndromes and shows the interrelations between them in a somewhat simplified form.

### URETHRAL INFECTION IN MEN

Acute anterior urethritis is the most common manifestation of gonococcal infection in men. The incubation period ranges from 1 to 14 days or even longer; however, the majority of men develop symptoms within 2 to 5 days, as was the case in 36 (82 percent) of 44 men with uncomplicated gonorrhea in one of the few studies in which the time of exposure could be clearly defined (Fig. 14-3).[25] The predominant symptoms are dysuria or urethral discharge. Although initially scant and mucoid or mucopurulent in appearance, in most males the urethral exudate becomes frankly purulent and relatively profuse within 24 h of onset (Fig. 14-5).[41] Dysuria usually begins subsequent to development of discharge. Variable degrees of edema and erythema of the urethral meatus commonly accompany gonococcal urethritis. Approximately one-quarter of patients develop only a scant or minimally purulent exudate, grossly indistinguishable from that associated with nongonococcal urethritis,[43,44] and a minority never develop overt signs and symptoms of urethritis.[25,26] The severity of symptoms is partly determined by the infecting strain of *N. gonorrhoeae*, as discussed above. Without treatment, the usual course of gonococcal urethritis is spontaneous resolution over a period of several weeks, and ≥95 percent of untreated patients become asymptomatic within 6 months.[41] Subsequent asymptomatic carriage of *N. gonorrhoeae* may occur, but probably is exceptional.

Complications of gonococcal urethritis include epididymitis (Chap. 53), acute or chronic prostatitis (Chap. 54); so-called posterior urethritis, which may be associated with stranguria and urinary urgency; seminal vesiculitis; and infections of Cowper's and Tyson's glands. These have been infrequently documented using modern diagnostic techniques and are now rare in industrialized societies.

### UROGENITAL INFECTION IN WOMEN

The endocervical canal is the primary site of urogenital gonococcal infection in women. Urethral colonization is present in 70 to 90 percent of infected women,[45–47] but is uncommon in the

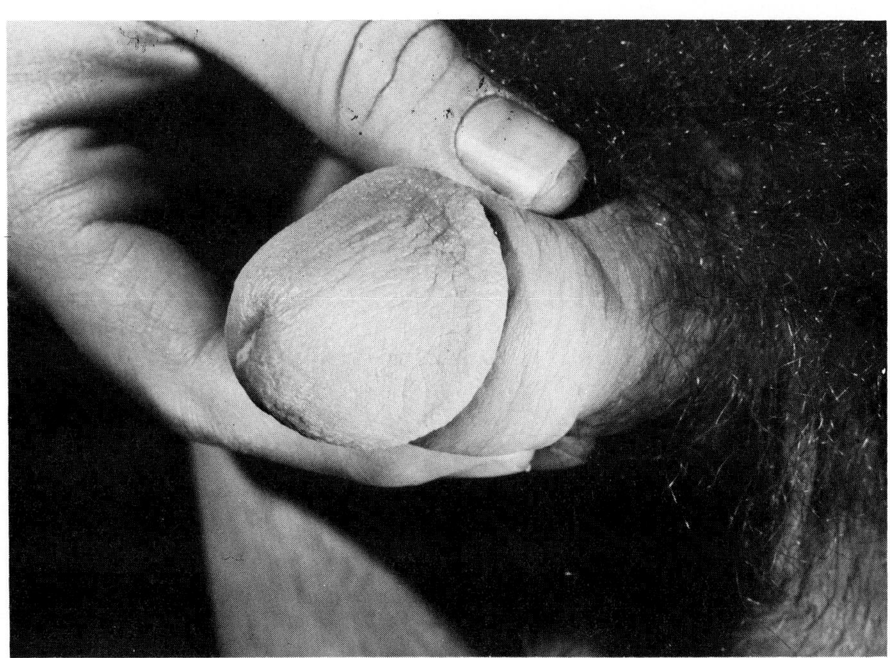

**Fig. 14-5.** Purulent urethral discharge and penile edema in a patient with gonococcal urethritis.

absence of endocervical infection, except in hysterectomized women, in whom the urethra is the usual site of infection.[48] Infection of the periurethral (Skene's) gland or Bartholin's gland ducts is also common, but probably is rare in the absence of endocervical or urethral infection.

The incubation period for urogenital gonorrhea in women is less certain and probably more variable than in men, but most who develop local symptoms apparently do so within 10 days of infection.[49,50] The most common symptoms are those of most lower genital tract infections in women (Chap. 46) and include increased vaginal discharge, dysuria, intermenstrual uterine bleeding, and menorrhagia, each of which may occur alone or in combination and may range in intensity from minimal to severe.[23,51] Although the physical examination may be normal, many infected women have cervical abnormalities that include purulent or mucopurulent cervical discharge, erythema and edema of the zone of ectopy, and mucosal bleeding that is easily induced by swabbing the endocervix.[51] Purulent or mucoid urethral exudate may occasionally be expressed from the urethra, periurethral glands, or the Bartholin's duct (Fig. 14-6). The clinical assessment of women for gonorrhea is often confounded, however, by the nonspecificity of these signs and symptoms and by the high prevalence of coexisting cervical or vaginal infections with *Chlamydia trachomatis, Trichomonas vaginalis, Candida albicans,* herpes simplex virus, and a variety of other organisms (Chap. 46).

The manifestations of gonorrhea during pregnancy are not significantly different from those in nonpregnant women except that pelvic inflammatory disease is probably less common and pharyngeal infection appears to be more prevalent than in nonpregnant women.[52] Reported complications of genital gonorrhea in pregnancy include spontaneous abortion, premature rupture of fetal membranes, premature delivery, and acute chorioamnionitis (Chap. 64), as well as ophthalmia neonatorum, pharyngeal infections, and other syndromes in the newborn (Chap. 65).

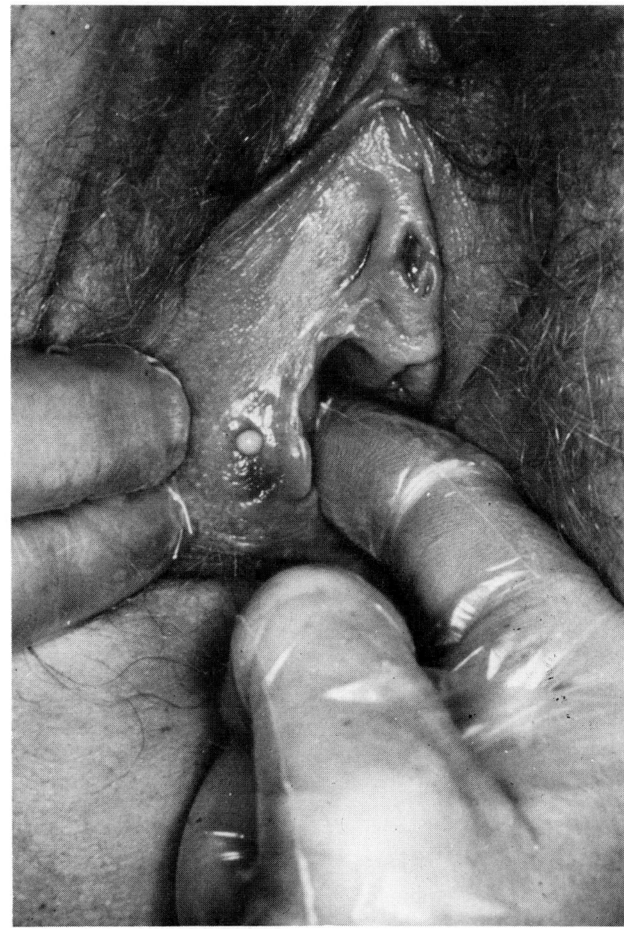

**Fig. 14-6.** Purulent exudate expressed from the Bartholin's gland duct of a woman with gonococcal Bartholin's gland abscess. *(From JA Davies et al., Br J Vener Dis 54:409, 1978.)*

## RECTAL INFECTION

The rectal mucosa is infected in 35 to 50 percent of women with gonococcal cervicitis and is a frequent site of infection in homosexual men; it is the only site of infection in approximately 5 percent of women with gonorrhea and 40 percent of homosexually active men.[45–47,53–56] In women, rectal gonorrhea is usually asymptomatic, whereas in homosexual men gonococcal infection is often demonstrated in patients with overt proctitis. Among homosexual men, rectal gonorrhea is due to direct inoculation through receptive rectal intercourse. In contrast, most rectal infections in women occur without acknowledged rectal sexual contact and are assumed to result from local spread of infected cervical secretions. The prevalence of rectal infection in women is positively correlated with the duration of endocervical infection,[54] further supporting the thesis that infection is usually due to perineal contamination by cervicovaginal exudate. Rectal infection in men occurs rarely, if ever, in strictly heterosexual men.

The symptoms of rectal gonococcal infection in men range from minimal anal pruritus, painless mucopurulent discharge (often manifested only by a coating of stools with exudate), or scant rectal bleeding, to symptoms of overt proctitis, including severe rectal pain, tenesmus, and constipation.[54,56] External inspection of the anus only occasionally shows erythema and abnormal discharge, but anoscopy commonly reveals mucoid or purulent exudate (often localized to the anal crypts), erythema, edema, friability, or other inflammatory mucosal changes.[55] Several studies have suggested that fewer than 10 percent of rectal gonococcal infections in men and women are symptomatic, but many of these studies may have ignored or failed to elicit more subtle or ill-defined symptoms. Moreover, most studies have been affected by sample bias, failing to distinguish among patients being screened for gonorrhea, those attending spontaneously because of symptoms, and those responding to epidemiologic investigation of infected partners. One study[55] found that among homosexual men examined because they were sexual contacts of men with gonorrhea, 87 (57 percent) of 152 infected men had rectal symptoms, compared with 66 (41 percent) of 162 men from whom *N. gonorrhoeae* was not isolated ($p = 0.01$). However, coinfection with other pathogens was not investigated. A prospective study that controlled for the reason for the visit showed that while a history of recent exposure to a sexual partner with gonorrhea was common in asymptomatically infected patients, in patients attending the clinic for other reasons, *N. gonorrhoeae* was isolated from 31 (27 percent) of 114 symptomatic men but from only 6 (9 percent) of 64 asymptomatic men ($p < 0.01$).

## PHARYNGEAL INFECTION

Among patients with gonorrhea, pharyngeal infection occurs in 3 to 7 percent of heterosexual men, 10 to 20 percent of heterosexual women, and 10 to 25 percent of homosexually active men. However, the pharynx is the sole site of infection in less than 5 percent of patients irrespective of gender or sexual orientation.[17,54,58–60] Gonococcal infection is transmitted to the pharynx by orogenital sexual contact and is more efficiently acquired by fellatio than by cunnilingus.[61] Occasional cases may be due to autoinoculation from anogenital infection. Ancedotal reports suggest that gonococcal infection may cause acute pharyngitis or tonsillitis and occasionally is associated with fever or cervical lymphadenopathy, but over 90 percent of pharyngeal infections are asymptomatic.[17,58,59] Evaluation of pharyngeal symptoms is confounded, however, by the intriguing observation that among clients of STD clinics, sore throat and perhaps overt pharyngitis are correlated with a history of fellatio, but not with isolation of *N. gonorrhoeae* or other sexually transmitted organisms.[17,61] Cunnilingus has not been associated with pharyngeal symptoms.

The clinical and epidemiologic significance of pharyngeal gonococcal infection is uncertain. The occasional occurrence of symptomatic pharyngitis and a possible increased risk of disseminated gonococcal infection in persons with pharyngeal gonorrhea[17] are countered by the usual absence of symptoms and a spontaneous cure rate that approaches 100 percent within 12 weeks of infection.[62,63] In addition, the transmission of pharyngeal gonorrhea to sex partners is inefficient and relatively rare, although some studies suggest that pharyngeal infection may be transmitted to the urethra by fellatio more readily than previously described.

## UNCOMPLICATED INFECTION OF OTHER SITES

Gonococcal conjunctivitis is rare in adults; it is most often seen in patients with concomittent anogenital gonorrhea, presumably due to autoinoculation.[64] Accidental conjunctival infection has been emphasized as a hazard for laboratory personnel working with *N. gonorrhoeae*.[65,66] An outbreak of 13 cases of gonococcal conjunctivitis was attributed to the cultural practice of ocular irrigation with urine.[67] Although usually described as a severe infection with a high risk of sequelae, at least in adults, mild or asymptomatic conjunctival gonorrhea infection occurs as well.

Primary cutaneous infection with *N. gonorrhoeae* has been reported[68–70] and usually presents as a localized ulcer of the genitals, perineum, proximal lower extremities, or finger. In many reports, simultaneous infection with other etiologic agents such as herpes simplex virus, *Haemophilus ducreyi*, and other pyogenic organisms was not excluded, and primary gonococcal infection was not differentiated from secondary colonization of a preexisting lesion. Gonococcal infection of a congenitally patent median graphe duct of the penis is an uncommon but well-documented occurrence.[69] Such infections usually occur in patients with anogenital gonorrhea, but exceptions have been reported.[70]

## DIFFERENTIAL DIAGNOSIS OF UNCOMPLICATED GONORRHEA

In males, gonococcal urethritis usually causes more florid signs and symptoms than nongonococcal urethritis and has a more abrupt onset, more prominent dysuria, and a urethral discharge that is more profuse and more purulent in appearance.[43,44] Additionally, the incubation period for gonorrhea usually is shorter than that of nongonococcal urethritis. Nonetheless, there is sufficient overlap in all these features that clinical differentiation often is unreliable and must be corroborated by laboratory tests.[43] For the diagnosis of urogenital infection in women and for anorectal pharyngeal infection, clinical differentiation of gonococcal from other causes is even less reliable than for urethritis in men, and laboratory diagnosis is mandatory. Nonetheless, a careful history and use of clinical predictors of infection for directing presumptive therapy in populations at increased risk is appropriate and desirable, because expeditious therapy is likely to reduce complications and reduce further transmission of infection. Differential diagnosis is discussed more completely in Chaps. 46, 52, and 55.

## COMPLICATED GONOCOCCAL INFECTIONS

### LOCAL COMPLICATIONS IN MEN

#### Epididymitis

In men the most common local complication of gonococcal urethritis is epididymitis (Chap. 53), a syndrome that occurred in up to 20 percent of infected patients prior to the availablity of modern antimicrobial therapy.[41] At present, the most common causes of acute epididymitis in patients under age 35 are *C. trachomatis, N. gonorrhoeae,* or both organisms.[71] Patients with acute epididymitis tend to present with unilateral testicular pain and swelling, and most patients with gonococcal epididymitis have overt urethritis when they present.

#### Lymphangitis and urethral stricture

Penile lymphangitis, sometimes associated with regional lymphadenitis, is an uncommon minor complication of gonococcal urethritis, as is generalized penile edema ("bull-headed clap"), a syndrome that also may accompany nongonococcal urethritis or genital herpes.[72] The pathogenesis of penile edema is unclear; most such patients lack palpable cords or other clear signs of penile thrombophlebitis or lymphangitis. Postinflammatory urethral strictures as complications of untreated gonococcal infection were common in the preantibiotic era but are now rare.[41] Many such strictures, however, probably were related to repeated infection or were due to the caustic urethral irrigations used for treatment, and stricture is rare today if effective systemic antimicrobial therapy is instituted promptly. Periurethral abscesses also are rare.

### LOCAL COMPLICATIONS IN WOMEN

#### Salpingitis

Acute salpingitis, or pelvic inflammatory disease, is the most common complication of gonorrhea in women, occurring in an estimated 10 to 20 percent of those with acute gonococcal infection.[73,74] Salpingitis is the most common of all complications of gonorrhea, as well as most important in terms of public health impact, both because of acute manifestations and because of the long-term sequelae (infertility and ectopic pregnancy) associated with this syndrome. Patients with gonococcal salpingitis usually present with various combinations of lower abdominal pain, dyspareunia, abnormal menses, intermenstrual bleeding, or other complaints compatible with intraabdominal infection.[75] On physical examination these patients are usually found to have lower abdominal, uterine, or adnexal tenderness, cervical motion pain, abnormal cervical discharge, and sometimes an adnexal mass or tuboovarian abscess.[75] Gram-stained smears of cervical secretions may show gram-negative intracellular diplococci. However, as in women with uncomplicated gonococcal cervicitis, the Gram stain is negative in 40 to 60 percent of women with gonococcal salpingitis. Other findings that may or may not be present include fever, leukocytosis, elevation of the erythrocyte sedimentation rate, and increased levels of C-reactive protein.[75] Women with gonococcal salpingitis often appear more acutely ill than women with nongonococcal salpingitis, are more often febrile (74 percent versus 22 percent), and are more likely to present during the first 3 days of symptoms (32 percent versus 15 percent).[75] Despite the apparently greater clinical severity of gonococcal salpingitis, laparoscopic studies show that the severity of tubal disease is similar in women with gonococcal or nongonococcal salpingitis.[75] The pathophysiology, differential diagnosis, and clinical spectrum of acute salpingitis are more fully discussed in Chap. 49.

Apart from salpingitis, Bartholin's gland abscess is the most common urogenital complication of gonorrhea in women. *N. gonorrhoeae* was isolated from the Bartholin's gland ducts of 52 (28 percent) of 183 women with urogenital gonorrhea, 10 of whom (6 percent) had enlargement and tenderness of the gland.[76] Other bacteria, including *C. trachomatis,* are responsible for many cases of bartholinitis, but tests for gonococcal infection are indicated for all women with this syndrome.

## SYSTEMIC COMPLICATIONS: DISSEMINATED GONOCOCCAL INFECTION

Disseminated gonococcal infection (DGI), usually manifested by the acute arthritis-dermatitis syndrome, is the most common systemic complication of acute gonorrhea and occurs in 0.5 to 3 percent of patients with untreated mucosal gonorrhea.[77–79] The clinical manifestations arise from gonococcal bacteremia and are most often clinically manifest as acute arthritis, tenosynovitis, dermatitis, or a combination of these findings. Patients with clinical manifestations of DGI are often stratified on the basis of culture results into proven, probable, and possible DGI.[80] Patients with positive cultures from blood, joint fluid, skin lesions, or otherwise sterile sources constitute less than 50 percent of DGI cases and are considered to have proven DGI.[77–80] In more than 80 percent of DGI patients, *N. gonorrhoeae* may be cultured from the primary mucosal site(s) of infection (anogenital or pharyngeal cultures) or from a sexual partner;[77–80] in the absence of positive blood or other sterile-site cultures, these patients are usually referred to as having probable DGI. Patients with an appropriate clinical syndrome and the expected response to therapy but with negative cultures for *N. gonorrhoeae* are referred to as having possible DGI. However, recognition of patients with DGI is sometimes delayed because of the wide variety of clinical findings associated with this syndrome and the mistaken assumption that patients with gonococcal bacteremia have high fever, marked leukocytosis, or other signs of clinical toxicity.

As suggested by the pseudonym arthritis-dermatitis syndrome, the most common clinical manifestations of DGI are joint pain and skin lesions. Although the "classic" skin lesion of gonococcal dermatitis is a tender, necrotic pustule on an erythematous base, in many patients, skin lesions may also evolve from, or present as, macules, papules, pustules, petechiae, bullae, or ecchymoses.[77–80] The skin lesions tend to be located on the distal portions of extremities and usually number fewer than 30.[78,80] Many patients with gonococcal dermatitis have arthralgia or tenosynovitis early in the disease, and frank arthritis with effusion tends to occur somewhat later. Approximately 30 to 40 percent of patients with DGI have overt arthritis.[77–80] Any joint may be involved, although DGI most often involves wrist, metacarpal-phalangeal, ankle, or knee joints. In patients with gonococcal arthritis, synovial fluid cultures are rarely positive in patients with synovial fluid leukocyte counts <20,000 per cubic millimeter, whereas cultures are often positive in patients with >40,000 white blood cells per cubic millimeter.[79–80] The manifestations of gonococcal arthritis and differentiation of this process from other acute arthritides are more fully discussed in Chap. 61.

Proving infection in patients with DGI is sometimes difficult. The bacteremia associated with DGI is not continuous, and positive blood cultures become less common as the duration of clinical signs and symptoms increases. Overall, only 20 to 30 percent of DGI patients have positive blood cultures.[77–80] In at least some cities AHU/IA-1 and AHU/IA-2 strains of *N. gonorrhoeae* most often cause DGI; these strains also tend to be associated with asymptomatic urogenital infection, increased susceptibility to penicillin G, and resistance to the complement-mediated bactericidal activity of normal human serum.[78,79] Although most gonococci isolated from patients with DGI are "serum resistant," strains isolated from patients with suppurative arthritis are less resistant than strains isolated from patients presenting with tenosynovitis or dermatitis.[79,81] These organisms also are more likely to be inhibited by the concentrations of vancomycin contained in selective media for gonococcal isolation from mucosal sites (e.g., modified Thayer-Martin medium) and by the sodium polyanetholsulfonate anticoagulant used in many blood culture media.[82–84] Each of these problems may be overcome through use of alternative media; however, use of alternative media is relatively uncommon because of lack of knowledge of their availability. In addition, DGI is often not included in the differential diagnosis of acute, asymmetric arthritis or dermatitis in young, sexually active patients because of the erroneous expectation that patients with DGI are likely to have signs and symptoms of urogenital infection. Mucosal infection in patients with disseminated gonococcal infection often is asymptomatic. All of these problems contribute to underdiagnosis of DGI.

Disseminated gonococcal infection is more common in women than in men.[77–80] In most cases bacteremia probably begins 7 to 30 days after infection; in about half of women with DGI, the onset of symptoms occurs within 7 days following menstruation.[77–80] Several studies have also cited pregnancy and pharyngeal gonorrhea as risk factors for DGI.[17,77–80] Deficiency of complement either due to inherited complement deficiency or due to episodic complement deficiency in association with other diseases such as lupus erythematosus may predispose individuals to gonococcal or meningococcal bacteremia.[78,79,85] Only a small percentage of patients with DGI, however, have complement deficiency syndromes, and routine screening of DGI patients for complement deficiency is probably not indicated. Such screening should be performed, however, in patients with second episodes of systemic gonococcal or meningococcal infection.[78,79,85]

The characteristic response to appropriate antimicrobial therapy with high doses of penicillin has been utilized as evidence of DGI in patients from whom *N. gonorrhoeae* could not be isolated.[80] Over 90 percent of patients are subjectively improved within 48 h of initiating therapy, and more than 90 percent of febrile patients become afebrile over the same period.[80] More recently, DGI due to PPNG[86] or gonococci with chromosomally mediated antibiotic resistance[87] has been heralded by failure to respond clinically to penicillin therapy; at the present time, only ceftriaxone or other antibiotics with proven activity against antibiotic-resistant gonococci should be used for therapeutic trials.

### Gonococcal Endocarditis and Meningitis

Gonococcal endocarditis is an uncommon complication of gonococcal bacteremia, occurring in an estimated 1 to 3 percent of patients with DGI.[77,78] Nonetheless, recognition of gonococcal endocarditis among patients with DGI is essential because of the possibility of rapidly progressive valvular damage with life-threatening consequences. The aortic valve appears to be most often infected in patients with gonococcal endocarditis.

Fewer than 25 cases of gonococcal meningitis have been reported. Case reports of this complication describe patients with typical presentations of acute bacterial meningitis, usually without typical findings of DGI.[88,89] *N. gonorrhoeae* is indistinguishable from *N. meningitidis* on Gram's stain of CSF.

## MENINGOCOCCAL INFECTIONS

Several reports have documented that infection or colonization with *N. meningitidis* may occur at all mucosal sites compatible with sexual transmission. There are data to suggest that, although rare in comparison to gonorrhea, meningococcal infections may mimic nearly all the clinical manifestations of gonorrhea. Pharyngeal colonization with *N. meningitidis* was documented in 17.2 percent of 2224 patients attending an STD clinic from 1970 to 1972,[17] a rate comparable to that in the general population.[90] However, subgroups of patients attending STD clinics have been found to have differing rates of carriage. Among 398 STD clinic patients with gonorrhea, *N. meningitidis* was isolated from the oropharynges of 44 (52 percent) of 85 homosexual men, compared with 58 (19 percent) of 313 heterosexual men and women ($p < 0.0001$). In addition, *N. meningitidis* was isolated significantly less frequently from heterosexual blacks than from heterosexual whites ($p < 0.0001$).[91] The relative prevalences parallel the relative frequencies with which these population groups acknowledge orogenital sexual practices (homosexual men > heterosexual whites > heterosexual blacks). Other investigators reported a similar prevalence (42.5 percent) of pharyngeal meningococcal colonization in 815 homosexual men attending an STD clinic and demonstrated an inverse relationship between meningococcal and gonococcal pharyngeal colonization.[60]

Genital and anorectal colonization with *N. meningitidis* also occurs. In the New York City gonorrhea screening program, the frequency of isolation of this organism from the urethra, endocervix, or anal canal tripled from 1975 to 1979.[92] Among clients of a municipal STD clinic, meningococci were isolated from the anal canal in 15 (2.1 percent) of 731 homosexual men and 2 (0.2 percent) of 1197 women, and from the urethra of 3 (0.4 percent) of 669 homosexual men.[93] In a similar study,[94] *N. meningitidis* was isolated from the urethra of 4 (0.2 percent) of 1728 presumptively heterosexual men, compared with 15 (1.1 percent) of 1363 homosexual men ($p < 0.01$), and from the anal canal in 36 (2.4 percent) of 1481 homosexual men. In the same study, 15 (13 percent) of 114 urethral isolates and 36 (21 percent) of 175 anal canal isolates of oxidase-positive gram-negative diplococci from homosexual men were confirmed as *N. meningitidis* rather than *N. gonorrhoeae*. In contrast, only four (1.1 percent) of 368 urethral isolates from heterosexual men were *N. meningitidis*.[94] Thus, all suspicious anorectal or urethral isolates from homosexual men, as well as pharyngeal isolates from all patients, should be tested to distinguish *N. gonorrhoeae* from *N. meningitidis*.

The pathogenicity of anogenital meningococcal infection and the frequency with which it produces clinical disease are unclear, and no systematic studies have been performed to determine its mode of acquisition or the prevalence of infection in the sex partners of colonized patients. However, >80 percent of meningococcal isolates in this setting are serogroupable and hence presumably pathogenic; in Seattle, New York, and Chicago, serogroups B and C accounted for 40 to 60 percent and 5 to 20 percent of isolates, respectively.[60,91,92] Several case reports have linked meninogococcal isolation to urethritis, epididymitis, vaginal discharge, acute salpingitis, and DGI-like syndromes.[38,90,92,93,95] Therapy has not been formally studied, but rectal or genital meningococcal infections have been eradicated in small numbers of patients receiving treatment with regimens recommended by the Centers for Disease Control for gonorrhea. Thus, the preponderance of evidence suggests that genital meningococcal infection often is sexually transmitted and, when detected, should be treated as gonorrhea is.

## LABORATORY DIAGNOSIS

The laboratory diagnosis of gonococcal infections depends primarily on identification of *N. gonorrhoeae* at infected sites by microscopic examination of stained smears or culture, or occasionally by immunochemical or genetic detection of the organism or its products. Details of several techniques, and particularly culture, are included in Chap. 73.

## IDENTIFICATION OF *Neisseria gonorrhoeae* IN SECRETIONS

### Culture

Isolation of *N. gonorrhoeae* is the diagnostic standard for gonococcal infections. Currently available antibiotic-containing selective media (e.g., modified Thayer-Martin medium) have diagnostic sensitivities of 80 to 95 percent for promptly incubated specimens, depending in part on the anatomic site being cultured (Table 14-1). For urethral specimens from symptomatic men, selective and nonselective media are equally sensitive because the concentration of gonococci in the urethra usually exceeds that of other flora. In contrast, selective media are preferred for culturing the endocervix, rectum, and pharynx, where other, less fastidious bacteria often outnumber *N. gonorrhoeae*.[83,84] The highest yield from all sites probably results when both selective and nonselective media are inoculated simultaneously with specimens obtained using separate swabs.[83,96,97] However, the incremental yield is small, and this procedure is probably not sufficiently cost-effective to be recommended for routine use.

**Table 14-1. Frequency of Isolation of *Neisseria gonorrhoeae* by Site from Patients with Uncomplicated Gonorrhea***

| | *N* | Total positive number (%) | Only site positive, number (%) |
|---|---|---|---|
| *Women*† | 162 | | |
| Endocervix | | 155 (96) | 75 (46) |
| Anal canal | | 62 (38) | 3 (2) |
| Pharynx | | 35 (22) | 4 (3) |
| *Heterosexual men* | 177 | | |
| Urethra | | 177 (100) | 166 (94) |
| Pharynx | | 11 (6) | 0 |
| *Homosexual men* | 355 | | |
| Urethra | | 205 (58) | 146 (41) |
| Anal canal | | 177 (50) | 109 (31) |
| Pharynx | | 62 (17) | 18 (5) |

* Analysis limited to patients for whom all indicated sites were cultured; single cultures on modified Thayer-Martin medium were used.
† Women who had undergone hysterectomy were excluded.
SOURCE: Data on women and heterosexual men are from Handsfield et al.;[57] data on homosexual men are combined from Handsfield et al.[57] and Tice and Rodriguez.[60]

For women, single cultures on most selective media detect 80 to 90 percent of cervical infections.[45,46,83,97] Although the urethra, Bartholin's ducts and Skene's glands are commonly infected, they are rarely the sole site of infection in women with intact cervices and therefore are not usually cultured. In women who have undergone hysterectomies, however, urethral culture gives highest yield.[48] *N. gonorrhoeae* may be isolated from the anal canal of 35 to 50 percent of women with gonorrhea, and this is the sole site of infection in up to 5 percent.[45,46,53] Similarly, the pharynx is infected in about 5 to 20 percent of women with gonorrhea but is the sole site of infection in fewer than 5 percent.[17,45,46] The proportion of women found to have a positive culture from the anal canal or pharynx alone probably would be still lower if duplicate endocervical specimens were routinely cultured.[97] Thus, for women, cultures of the urethra, accessory gland ducts, anal canal, and pharynx should be considered optional, depending on symptoms, sites exposed, culture methods employed, and available resources.

The sites to be cultured in men are also dependent on sexual orientation and the anatomic sites exposed. For heterosexual men, culture of urethral exudate alone is usually sufficient, but pharyngeal cultures may be useful for men with pharyngitis who practice cunnilingus or for men who have performed cunnilingus with a women known to have gonorrhea.[17] Among homosexually active men, the rectum is infected almost as frequently as the urethra.[57,60,98] Isolated pharyngeal infection occurs in about 5 percent of infected homosexual men.[17,57,60,98] Although gonococcal urethritis is common, asymptomatic urethral infection is rare in this population.[57,60] Thus, in screening asymptomatic homosexual men for whom all three sites are potentially exposed, anorectal culture gives the highest yield, and pharyngeal and urethral cultures are desirable but have lower yield. However, these issues have not been reexplored since the mid-1980's, when most urban homosexually active men made major changes in sexual behavior in response to the AIDS epidemic.

Several reports have documented failure of vancomycin-containing selective culture media to support growth of vancomycin-sensitive gonococci.[82,99] The prevalence of such strains is highly variable, but may account for up to 30 percent of gonococcal isolates in some geographic areas.[82,84,99] The ability to culture these organisms also is inoculation-dependent, with greater inhibition occurring with smaller inocula.[82,84,99] Most vancomycin-sensitive strains are of the more fastidious AHU auxotype.[82] Thus, use of vancomycin-containing media in some geographic areas may selectively impair gonorrhea diagnosis in heterosexuals, whites, and asymptomatically infected patients, who are more likely than others to be infected with these AHU strains and may harbor smaller numbers of organisms.[82]

### Stained smears

Gram's stain, methylene blue, acridine orange, and several other dyes have been used to prepare clinical material for microscopic examination for gonococci, but Gram's stain has been the most

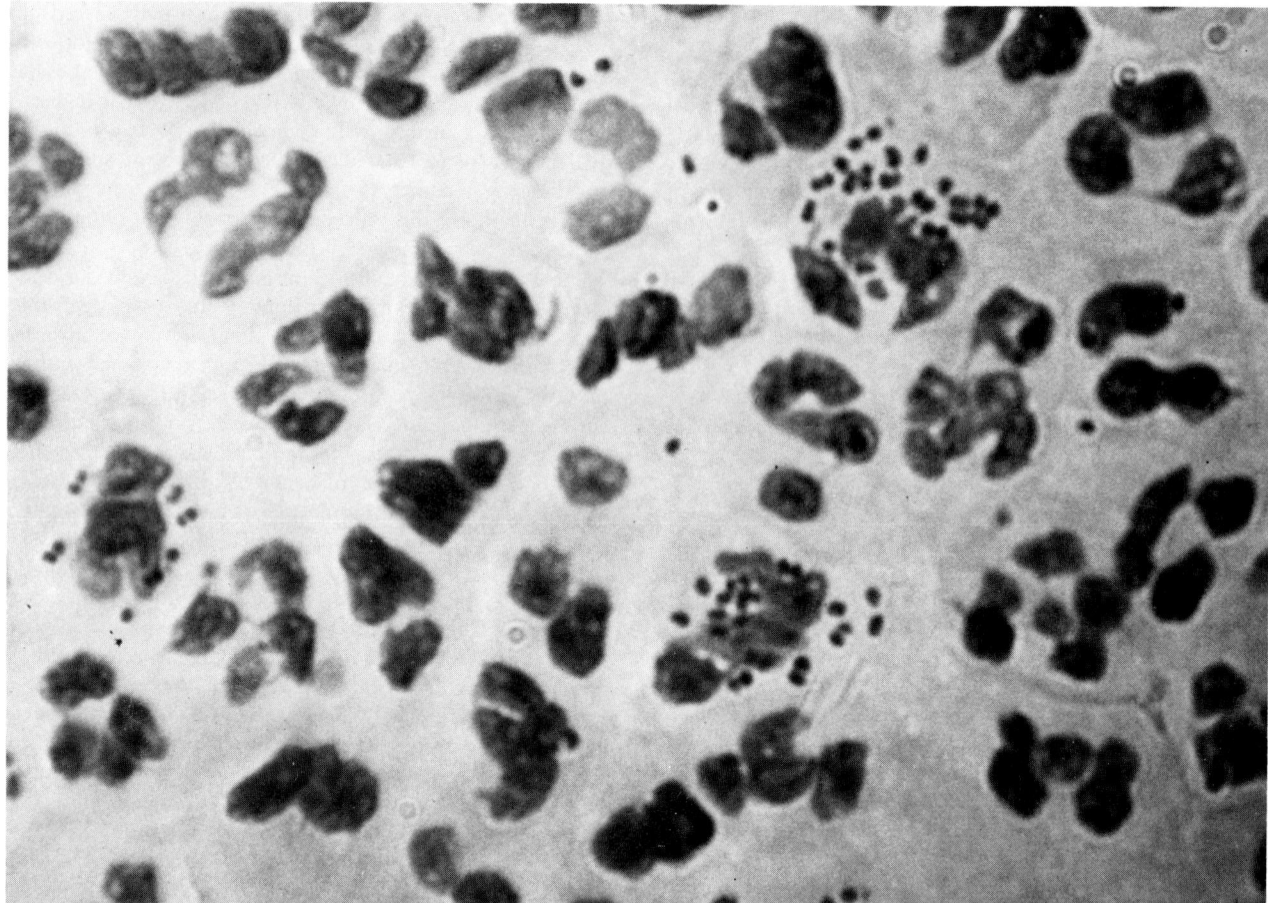

**Fig. 14-7.** Gram-stained smear showing polymorphonuclear leukocytes with intracellular gram-negative diplococci in urethral exudate from a man with gonococcal urethritis (×1000).

extensively studied. For examination of clinical material, a smear is considered positive for gonorrhea when gram-negative diplococci with typical morphology are identified within or closely associated with polymorphonuclear leukocytes (Fig. 14-7); it is considered equivocal if only extracellular organisms or morphologically atypical intracellular gram-negative diplococci are seen; and negative if no gram-negative diplococci are present. Nonpathogenic *Neisseriaceae* are generally not cell-associated; however, *N. meningitidis* may also be cell-associated and is morphologically indistinguishable from *N. gonorrhoeae*. *Acinetobacter* species are bipolar-staining gram-negative bacilli that, contrary to earlier reports, are easily distinguished from *N. gonorrhoeae* by experienced microscopists. Table 14-2 shows the sensitivity and specificity of gram-stained smears for various categories of genital and rectal infection relative to isolation of *N. gonorrhoeae*.

For evaluation of men with symptoms and signs of urethritis, the urethral smear is sufficiently sensitive and specific that culture may be considered optional for routine care.[100] This depends in part, however, on specimen collection technique and the experience of the microscopist. In addition, isolation of the organism is necessary to test for antimicrobial resistance. Accordingly, in most settings in industrialized nations, isolation of *N. gonorrhoeae* usually should be attempted.

Although smears from the endocervix or rectum are less sensitive than those from the urethra, positive smears of properly collected specimens are highly specific when examined by experienced personnel, and they facilitate expeditious therapy of infected patients.[73,100,101] It has often been incorrectly stated that stained smears are not diagnostically useful in women. However, positive endocervical smears have a high predictive value in women likely to have gonorrhea, making this test clinically useful in settings in which the index of suspicion is high.[73,100,101] For

**Table 14-2. Sensitivity and Specificity of Gram-Stained Smears for Detection of Genital or Anorectal Gonorrhea**

| Site and clinical setting | Sensitivity* | Specificity* |
|---|---|---|
| *Urethra:* | | |
| Men with symptomatic urethritis | 90–95 | 95–100 |
| Men with asymptomatic urethral infection | 50–70 | 95–100 |
| *Endocervix:* | | |
| Uncomplicated gonorrhea | 50–70 | 95–100 |
| Pelvic inflammatory disease | 60–70 | 95–100 |
| *Anorectum:* | | |
| Blind swabs | 40–60 | 95–100† |
| Anoscopically obtained specimens | 70–80 | 95–100† |

*Sensitivity = percent of patients with positive cultures who have positive Gram-stained smears. Specificity = percent of patients with negative cultures whose Gram-stained smears also are negative.

†The studies showing 95–100% specificity for anorectal smears did not report whether meningococcal infection was distinguished from gonorrhea. Until further data are available, a positive anorectal smear should be considered highly specific for either gonococcal or meningococcal infection.

SOURCE: Compiled from Handsfield et al,[26] Jacobs and Kraus,[43] Thin and Shaw,[46] Barlow and Phillips,[47] Wallin,[50] Rothenberg et al,[100] Wald,[101] William et al,[102] Deheragoda.[103]

example, for women with symptoms or signs of lower genital tract infection or salpingitis, an endocervical smear showing typical intracellular gram-negative diplococci supports the diagnosis of gonorrhea. On the other hand, smears have a lower predictive value and are less cost-effective for screening asymptomatic women with normal physical examinations. Thus, culture remains the standard for gonorrhea diagnosis in women, and stained smears should be utilized as an adjunct to, but not replacement for, culture. The sensitivity of anorectal smears for evaluation of symptomatic patients at risk for rectal gonorrhea is enhanced when the exudate is obtained by direct visualization using an anoscope rather than blindly,[102] even though anoscopy does not apparently improve the sensitivity of culture.[103] Smears are not commonly obtained from the urethra or accessory gland ducts of women, but should be performed if abnormal exudate is expressed or the patient has had a hysterectomy. As for endocervical smears, the predictive value of a positive anorectal, urethral, or accessory duct smear is higher in symptomatic patients than in asymptomatic individuals being screened for gonorrhea. The Gram's stain smear has not been systemically studied in pharyngeal gonococcal infection, but is generally believed to be both insensitive and nonspecific; it is not recommended.

### Other rapid diagnostic techniques

Fluorescein-conjugated antigonococcal antibodies have been employed to detect gonococci in secretions, but this method has not proved sufficiently sensitive or specific for routine use;[104] modifications using monoclonal antibodies are under investigation. Immunologic or biochemical detection of gonococcal antigens or metabolic products, including surface proteins, endotoxin, and oxidase or other enzymes, are also under investigation[105–108] as is detection of gonococcal DNA using hybridization technologies.[109,110] Endotoxin detection by *Limulus* amebocyte lysate assay has been studied extensively, but has not demonstrated sufficient sensitivity or specificity to warrant routine use, especially for endocervical or rectal infections.[105] There continues to be a need for accurate nonculture diagnostic methods for use in situations in which culture diagnosis is not readily available.

### Collection of clinical specimens

Urethral exudate from men may be obtained by passage of a small swab or bacteriologic loop 2 to 4 cm into the urethra[26] or by collecting the first 10 to 20 ml of voided urine.[111,112] Although the latter method obviates the discomfort of passing a urethral swab or loop, collection and culture of urine is time-consuming, depends in part on the ability of the patient to provide a proper specimen, and requires prompt processing because the urine from some individuals is rapidly bactericidal for *N. gonorrhoeae*.[113] For collection of endocervical specimens, the cervix should be cleansed of external exudate or vaginal secretions and a swab inserted 1 to 2 cm into the external os and rotated gently for up to 10 sec.[114] When personal or logistic contraints preclude speculum examination, a vaginal specimen may be obtained by a clinician or the patient using a swab or a tampon;[115] with this technique there is a modest reduction in culture sensitivity and a marked reduction in the sensitivity of gram-stained smears. Anorectal specimens from patients without symptoms of proctitis may be obtained by blindly passing a swab 2 to 3 cm into the anal canal, using lateral pressure to avoid entering any fecal mass.[102] If gross fecal contamination of the swab occurs, it should be discarded and another specimen obtained. For symptomatic patients, anorectal specimens should be obtained under direct vision using anoscopy, which increases the sensitivity of the smear.[102,103] Pharyngeal specimens are obtained by swabbing the posterior pharynx, including the tonsillar areas and faucial pillars.

## SEROLOGIC DIAGNOSIS

Serologic tests have been developed to detect antibodies to *N. gonorrhoeae* or its components using complement fixation, immunoprecipitation, bacterial lysis, immunofluorescence, hemagglutination, latex agglutination, enzyme-linked immunoabsorbance, and other techniques.[116] Many of these methods have proved useful for studies of the immune response and pathogenesis of gonorrhea. However, most reported serodiagnostic tests have sensitivities ≤70 percent and specificities ≤80 percent for patients with uncomplicated gonorrhea and thus are not useful for screening, case finding, or diagnosis.[117] For example, if an idealized test whose sensitivity and specificity were both 90 percent were used to screen a population with a gonorrhea prevalence of 2 percent, the predictive value of the positive test (the probability that the patient with the positive test had gonorrhea) would be only 16 percent, compared with a 100 percent predictive value for positive culture. Although attractive on theoretical grounds, available serologic techniques are not sufficiently sensitive or specific for routine use.[118]

## THERAPY OF GONOCOCCAL INFECTIONS

### ANTIMICROBIAL SUSCEPTIBILITY OF *N. gonorrhoeae* AND DEVELOPMENT OF RESISTANCE

Most gonococci are susceptible in vitro to a wide variety of antimicrobial agents, including the penicillins, cephalosporins, tetracyclines, macrolides, quinolones, rifampin, and most aminocyclitol antibiotics. Relative or absolute resistance to several antibiotics, however, is relatively easily selected for in the laboratory, and in vivo development of resistance continues to be the driving force for changes in recommended antimicrobial therapy of gonorrhea (Table 14-3). In the mid-1930s, sulfanilamide was introduced and quickly became the agent of choice for treatment of gonorrhea, supplanting the use of local irrigation with antiseptic solutions such as potassium permanganate.[3,41] By 1944, however, many gonococci had become resistant to sulfanilamide therapy, and treatment failure occurred in about one-third of patients.[3] Fortunately, in 1943 the first reports of the near 100 percent utility of penicillin for gonorrhea treatment were published,[119] and by the end of World War II, as penicillin became available to the general public, it quickly became the therapy of choice for gonorrhea. Unfortunately, relative resistance to the penicillins became apparent by the early 1950s.[120,121] Despite progressively increasing resistance since that time, the penicillins remained the drugs of choice for gonorrhea therapy for the next 25 years, because their excellent therapeutic/toxic ratio permitted increments in the dose to overcome gradually increasing penicillin resistance. By the early 1970s, 18 to 90 percent of gonococci from various parts of the world had developed chromosomally mediated "low-level" penicillin resistance, with minimal inhibitory concentrations (MICs) ≥0.12 μg/ml; in southeast Asia and in the Philippines, penicillin MICs exceeded 0.25 μg/ml in ≥45 percent of the strains.[120] Similar trends in antimicrobial susceptibility to tetracyclines and other antibiotics were seen at the same time.

Table 14-3. Antimicrobial Resistance Mechanisms of *Neisseria gonorrhoeae*

| | Plasmid-mediated | | |
|---|---|---|---|
| | β-Lactam resistance | Tetracycline resistance | Chromosomally mediated |
| Resistance factor | Single-step acquisition of one of multiple plasmids (4.4, 3.2, 7.2 Md) encoding for β-lactamase production | Single-step acquisition of a 25.2-Md *tet M*–containing plasmid | Cumulative effect of multiple chromosomal mutations producing a spectrum of antimicrobial sensitivities |
| Mechanism | β-Lactamase production | Unknown; increased protein synthesis noted in strains acquiring the plasmid | Multiple mechanisms including<br>Decreased cell wall permeability<br>Increased concentration or decreased affinity of penicillin-binding proteins<br>Ribosomal changes |
| Antimicrobials | β-Lactam antibiotics | Tetracyclines | β-Lactam, tetracyclines, erythromycin, spectinomycin, quinolones |
| Detection | Rapid single-step screening procedures | Disk sensitivity testing highly predictive | Agar dilution susceptibility testing (time-consuming); disk sensitivity testing imprecise and poorly standardized |
| Frequency | Geographic variation, but overall 3% of U.S. isolates tested by CDC Gonococcal Isolate Surveillance Project (GISP) | Geographic variation, but overall 3% of U.S. isolates (GISP) | Geographic variation; variation with different antimicrobials; in the GISP, rates in the U.S.A. were<br>Penicillin G 16%<br>Tetracycline 46%<br>Spectinomycin-ceftriaxone <0.1% |

In 1972, in an effort to deal with increasing penicillin resistance among gonococci, the recommended dose of procaine penicillin for gonorrhea therapy was doubled from 2.4 to 4.8 million units and the coadministration of 1 g of probenecid was recommended to augment penicillin's effect by delaying excretion of the drug.[122] It was hoped that this high-dose therapy would help circumvent further development of gonococcal penicillin resistance. Initially this strategy appeared to be successful; in the United States between 1972 and 1978, the proportion of gonococci with penicillin G MICs $> 0.5$ μg/ml fell from 22 to 3 percent, and relative tetracycline resistance (MIC $\geq 2.0$ μg/ml) fell from 19 percent to under 3 percent of strains.[14] By the late 1970s, however, progressive development of relative resistance to penicillin was noted. Subsequently, problems of treatment were aggravated by recognition of plasmid-mediated resistance to penicillin[123,124] and to the tetracyclines.[125]

## Penicillinase-producing *Neisseria gonorrhoeae* (PPNG)

In 1976, strains of *N. gonorrhoeae* with high-level penicillin resistance due to plasmid-mediated production of β-lactamase were reported for the first time.[123] Such strains were recognized at about the same time in west Africa, the far east, Europe, and North America.[124,126] The β-lactamase plasmids from strains that originated in west Africa typically had a molecular mass of 3.2 megadaltons, while plasmids from strains originating in the far east had a 4.4-megadalton β-lactamase plasmid.[126] These organisms rapidly became widespread, and in some geographic areas (parts of Africa and the far east) soon outnumbered penicillinase-negative strains.[126] In the United States, the incidence of PPNG infections (Fig. 14-8) gradually rose from the time of their introduction in 1976 through 1979; during this interval, most such patients or their sex partners had traveled overseas.[126] Endemic transmission increased gradually until 1985, when PPNG rates increased dramatically.[127] By 1988, PPNG accounted for over 40,000 gonorrhea cases in the United States, or >4 percent of reported gonorrhea.[128] Within the United States, as in the rest of the world, there is substantial geographic variation in PPNG prevalence. By early 1988, in south Florida and New York City, PPNG prevalence exceeded 33 and 10 percent, respectively, while in other regions of the country these infections remained uncommon.[127–129]

## Higher-level chromosomal resistance

In 1983, an outbreak of increased treatment failures in Durham, N.C., caused by gonococci that did not produce β-lactamase but were unusually resistant to penicillin G (MICs 2.0 to 4.0 μg/ml) served to refocus interest on the problem of chromosomally mediated antimicrobial resistance.[130] This outbreak occurred as the result of introduction of a single gonococcal strain containing several previously described chromosomal antibiotic resistance loci (*pen A, mtr, pen B*) as well as a possible new resistance locus.[131] This strain apparently was introduced into the community by a single high-frequency transmitter.[130] Subsequently, others reported problems due to gonococci with clinically significant penicillin resistance (MIC $\geq 1.0$ μg/ml) on the basis of chromosomal mutations.[132,133] These organisms, which also tend to be relatively resistant to tetracycline (MIC $\geq 2.0$ μg/ml), can be detected reliably only by agar-dilution MIC testing, a cumbersome technique which is not readily available in many locations. In 1987, institution of nationwide antimicrobial resistance surveillance by the Centers for Disease Control (CDC) demonstrated that this form of resistance has become quite common.[133]

## High-level tetracycline resistance

In 1985, reports from the CDC focused attention on another new problem: high-level, plasmid-mediated tetracycline-resistant *N. gonorrhoeae* (TRNG).[134] TRNG strains harbor a 25.2-megadalton plasmid derived from the 24.5-megadalton conjugative plasmid and owe their resistance to acquisition of a *tet M* gene coding for high-level tetracycline resistance.[134,135] Such gonococci have MICs to tetracycline hydrochloride of ≥16 μg/ml and are essentially impervious to clinically obtainable levels of the tetracyclines. The prevalence of TRNG strains appears to vary geographically, but they have been detected in all areas where they have been sought.[134] The highest levels have been reported

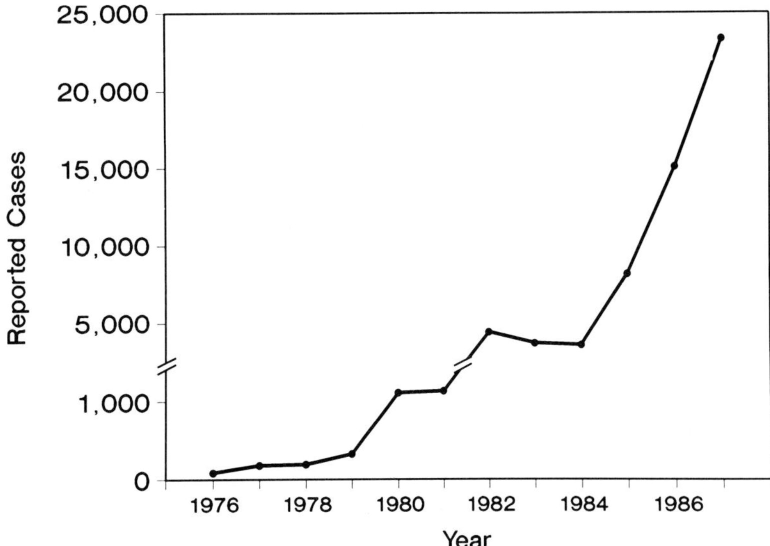


**Fig. 14-8.** Reported annual incidence of gonorrhea due to penicillinase-producing *Neisseria gonorrhoeae* in the United States from 1976 through 1987. *(From Centers for Disease Control.[5])*

in the northeastern United States and especially in the Baltimore area, where 15 to 20 percent of isolates in 1986 to 1988 were TRNG.[33,134]

## Spectinomycin resistance

In 1987, an outbreak of *N. gonorrhoeae* with high-level, presumably chromosomally mediated resistance to spectinomycin was reported in U.S. military personnel in Korea.[136] Investigation of this outbreak provided empirical evidence of the effect of selective antimicrobial pressure on the development of antimicrobial resistance. In Korea, because of the high prevalence of PPNG, in 1981 spectinomycin had been adopted as the drug of choice for gonorrhea therapy.[136] By 1983, however, reports of spectinomycin treatment failures were beginning to occur in patients with gonorrhea, and over the next 2 years the prevalence of spectinomycin-resistant *N. gonorrhoeae* was noted to increase. The prevalence of PPNG declined from a peak of nearly 45 percent to approximately 13 percent during the period that spectinomycin was the drug of choice for gonorrhea therapy. These data suggest that the antimicrobial use patterns within the community constitute a driving force for development of antimicrobial resistance. Following recognition of this outbreak, ceftriaxone became the drug of choice for treatment of gonorrhea in U.S. military personnel in Korea.[136] Sporadic cases of spectinomycin-resistant gonorrhea have been reported elsewhere, but such strains remain rare in the United States.[137,138]

In 1986, as the problems of antimicrobial resistance in *N. gonorrhoeae* in the United States were becoming apparent, the CDC reinstituted the process of sentinel gonococcal surveillance.[133] By early 1989, data from the systematic monthly testing of gonococcal isolates from 20 U.S. cities demonstrated that nearly 50 percent of isolates have one form of antimicrobial resistance or another.[128] In addition, the CDC sentinel surveillance system has confirmed the substantial geographic diversity of antimicrobial-resistant *N. gonorrhoeae*.[128,133]

## CHOICE OF TREATMENT REGIMENS FOR *N. gonorrhoeae*

The choice of antimicrobial agents for gonorrhea therapy is influenced by a variety of factors in addition to the antimicrobial activity of drugs for *N. gonorrhoeae*. Pharmacokinetic studies have demonstrated that serum levels of antimicrobial agents equal to or greater than three times the MIC of the infecting strain of *N. gonorrhoeae* for ≥8 h are needed to reliably cure uncomplicated infection.[139] In general, single-dose therapy is preferred for gonorrhea in order to overcome problems of patient compliance. In addition, the choice of antimicrobial agents for therapy should reflect local patterns of antimicrobial resistance and the probability that patients with acute gonococcal infection are coinfected or have recently been exposed to other STD agents. Among coinfecting agents for patients with gonorrhea in the United States, *Chlamydia trachomatis* is preeminent. Approximately 15 to 25 percent of men and 30 to 50 percent of women with acute urogenital gonorrhea are coinfected with *C. trachomatis*.[10,44,74,140] In addition, substantial numbers of women with acute gonococcal infection have simultaneous *Trichomonas vaginalis* infections, and a small percentage of patients have been exposed to infectious syphilis at the time of sexual contact as well. In Africa and other areas where chancroid is prevalent, patients may have been exposed to *Haemophilus ducreyi* at the time of acquisition of gonorrhea.

Since 1985, the treatment recommendations published by the CDC for the United States have recommended single-dose therapy with medications effective for eradication of *N. gonorrhoeae*, followed by 7 days of therapy expected to reliably eradicate *C. trachomatis* infections (either tetracycline or erythromycin).[141] This approach has been shown to be effective for therapy of both infections.[140] In the few regions where antimicrobial resistance of *N. gonorrhoeae* is not yet a problem, single-dose therapy with either 4.8 million units of procaine penicillin IM plus 1.0 g probenecid or a combination of 2.0 g ampicillin or 2.0 g amoxicillin orally plus 1.0 g probenecid remains acceptable, followed by a 7-day course of antichlamydial therapy. In areas where antimicrobial resistance is more common or where surveillance is incomplete, ceftriaxone (250 mg) or spectinomycin (2.0 g) IM probably should be used for routine initial therapy.[142] These drugs also should be used for all infections which persist following treatment using any of the other regimens.[142]

The dose of ceftriaxone currently recommended for therapy of uncomplicated gonorrhea by the CDC is a single injection of 250 mg IM,[141,142] although 125 mg IM has been successfully used in several high-volume STD clinics.[143] The smallest commercially available unit of ceftriaxone is 250 mg, so this dose is most convenient for most settings. Either dose is highly effective for rectal and pharyngeal, as well as genital, gonorrhea.[144] Although a small percentage (<1%) of patients treated with ceftriaxone fail antimicrobial therapy, clinically significant ceftriaxone resistance had not been reported through 1988. The major drawbacks of ceftriaxone therapy for gonorrhea are the requirement for parenteral administration and the potential (albeit low) for allergic reactions of patients allergic to β-lactam antibiotics.

In 1984, a report was published describing the utility of norfloxacin, a new quinolone antibiotic, for treating antibiotic-resistant gonococcal infections.[145] Enthusiasm for gonorrhea therapy with earlier quinolones (nalidixic acid and rosoxacin) was tempered by the tendency of gonococci to rapidly become resistant to the former and by the unacceptable neurotoxicity (primarily vestibular) of the latter.[146] Since that time, a number of other newer quinolones (ciprofloxacin, ofloxacin, enoxacin, fleroxicin, temafloxacin, and others) have been evaluated as single-dose regimens with promising results.[146] On the other hand, recent reports of quinolone resistance among gonococcal isolates from the Philippines,[147] where rosoxacin has been widely used to treat gonorrhea for several years, have raised important questions regarding the long-term utility of these otherwise relatively well tolerated, orally active antimicrobials for gonorrhea therapy.

Each of the currently recommended treatment regimens has specific advantages and disadvantages that should be utilized to individualize therapy for gonorrhea. For example, the ampicillin-probenecid or amoxicillin-probenecid regimens are the easiest treatment regimens to administer and are highly acceptable to most patients, but these regimens are associated with lower cure rates than other regimens even for urogenital infections caused by susceptible gonococci. Similarly, while efficacious for anogenital gonorrhea, spectinomycin hydrochloride is not efficacious for treatment of pharyngeal gonorrhea.[148] The long recommended procaine penicillin–probenecid regimen is cumbersome to administer, is poorly tolerated by some patients, carries the risk of acute procaine reactions, and is ineffective for many patients infected with antibiotic-resistant gonococci; there is little justification for its continued use. For treatment of homosexual men with gonorrhea, the ceftriaxone regimen is preferred over other regimens. The strains of gonococci that occur in homosexual men are more likely to harbor the antibiotic resistance mutation (*mtr*)[149] which makes these organisms somewhat more resistant to the penicillins and thus results in higher treatment failure rates when the ampicillin(amoxicillin)-probenecid and tetracycline regimens are utilized. Similarly, because spectinomycin may fail to cure up to 50 percent of pharyngeal infections,[148] it is not useful in homosexual men.

## FOLLOW-UP

Repeat cultures for test of cure are recommended for all patients with gonorrhea.[141,142] Test-of-cure cultures should not be performed until at least 4 to 5 days following the last dose of tetracycline, since detectable serum levels of this drug are present for 3 days following completion of therapy.[150] All known infected sites should be recultured. In addition, in women, follow-up anorectal cultures should be obtained, since 30 percent of treatment failures are detected only by anorectal culture, regardless of whether anorectal infection was sought or detected prior to treatment.[151]

## MANAGEMENT OF SEX PARTNERS

Most authorities recommend "epidemiologic" treatment of all recent sex partners of patients with gonorrhea, prior to the availability of culture results, in order to prevent complications and curtail the transmission.[152,153] The definition of *recent* depends on the clinical and epidemiologic settings; in most instances, all partners exposed within 2 weeks prior to the onset of symptoms or to diagnosis of the index case should be treated. For patients with asymptomatic gonococcal infection, however, extending contact tracing to 1 month may prove useful for control efforts.

## PREVENTION

Properly used condoms provide a high degree of protection against acquisition and transmission of genital infection.[24,154] The diaphragm and cervical cap may also reduce transmission and acquisition of endocervical infection.[19,155] Topical spermicidal and bactericidal agents have been shown recently to clearly reduce the probability of infection by both *N. gonorrhoeae* and *C. trachomatis* in patients using these gels.[20,21] Urinating, washing, and douching after intercourse are assumed by many to be beneficial in prevention of gonorrhea, but controlled data are lacking. In addition, certain practices such as douching are now increasingly being associated with harmful outcomes. Prophylactic administration of antibiotics immediately or soon after sexual exposure clearly reduces risk of infection.[25] However, this practice is likely to select and facilitate transmission of antibiotic-resistant strains of *N. gonorrhoeae*. In addition, except in very high-risk settings, routine antibiotic prophylaxis is unlikely to be cost-effective.

# References


1 Rosebury T: *Microbes and Morals.* New York, Viking, 1971.

2 Kampmeier RH: Identification of the gonococcus by Albert Neisser. *Sex Transm Dis* 5:71, 1978.

3 Kampmeier RH: Introduction of sulfonamide therapy for gonorrhea. *Sex Transm Dis* 10:81, 1983.

4 Thayer JD, Martin JE: Selective medium for the cultivation of *N. gonorrhoeae* and *N. meningitidis*. *Public Health Rep* 79:49, 1964.

5 Centers for Disease Control: *Sexually Transmitted Disease Statistics, Calendar Year 1987,* No. 136. Atlanta, US Public Health Service, 1988, pp 1–58.

6 Danielsson D, National Bacteriological Laboratory: Unpublished data. Ørebro and Stockholm, Sweden, 1988.

7 Judson FN: Fear of AIDS and gonorrhoea rates in homosexual men, letter. *Lancet* 2:159, 1983.

8 Handsfield HH: Decreasing incidence of gonorrhea in homosexually active men. *West J Med* 143:469, 1985.

9 Rice RJ et al: Gonorrhea in the United States 1975–84: Is the giant only sleeping? *Sex Transm Dis* 14:83, 1987.

10 Barnes RC, Holmes KK: Epidemiology of gonorrhea: Current perspectives. *Epidemiol Rev* 6:1, 1984.

11 Rice RJ et al: Unpublished data.

12 Brooks GF et al: Repeated gonorrhea: An analysis of importance and risk factors. *J Infect Dis* 137:161, 1978.

13 Wright PA, Judson FN: Relative and seasonal incidences of the sexually-transmitted diseases: A two-year statistical review. *Br J Vener Dis* 54:433, 1978.

14 Reynolds GH et al: The national gonorrhea therapy monitoring study: II. Trends and seasonality of antibiotic resistance of *Neisseria gonorrhoeae*. *Sex Transm Dis* 6 (suppl):103, 1979.

15 Holmes KK et al: An estimate of the risk of men acquiring gonorrhea by sexual contact with infected females. *Am J Epidemiol* 91:170, 1970.
16 Hooper RR et al: Cohort study of venereal disease: I. The risk of gonorrhea transmission from infected women to men. *Am J Epidemiol* 108:136, 1978.
17 Wiesner PJ et al: Clinical spectrum of pharyngeal gonococcal infections. *N Engl J Med* 288:181, 1973.
18 Tice RW, Rodriguez VL: Pharyngeal gonorrhea. *JAMA* 246:2717, 1981.
19 McCormack WM et al: Effect of menstrual cycle and method of contraception on recovery of *Neisseria gonorrhoeae. JAMA* 247: 1292, 1982.
19a Louv WC et al: Oral contraceptive use and the risk of chlamydial and gonococcal infections. *Am J Obstet Gynecol* 160:396, 1989.
20 Cates W Jr et al: Sex and spermicides: Preventing unintended pregnancy and infection. *JAMA* 248:1636, 1982.
21 Louv WC et al: A clinical trial of nonoxynol-9 for preventing gonococcal and chlamydial infections. *J Infect Dis* 158:518, 1988.
22 Pedersen AHB, Bonin P: Screening females for asymptomatic gonorrhea infection. *Northwest Med* 70:255, 1971.
23 McCormack WM et al: Clinical spectrum of gonococcal infection in women. *Lancet* 2:1182, 1977.
24 Upchurch DM et al: Behavioral contributions to acquisition and transmission of *Neisseria gonorrhoeae.* (Submitted.)
25 Harrison WO et al: A trial of minocycline given after exposure to prevent gonorrhea. *N Engl J Med* 300:1074, 1979.
26 Handsfield HH et al: Asymptomatic gonorrhea in men: Diagnosis, natural course, prevalence and significance. *N Engl J Med* 290:117, 1974.
27 Yorke JA et al: Dynamics and control of the transmission of gonorrhea. *Sex Transm Dis* 5:51, 1978.
28 Rothenberg RB: The geography of gonorrhea: Empirical demonstration of core group transmission. *Am J Epidemiol* 117:688, 1983.
29 May RM: The transmission and control of gonorrhea. *Nature* 291:376, 1981.
30 Carifo K, Catlin BW: *Neisseria gonorrhoeae* auxotyping: Differentiation of clinical isolates based on growth responses on chemically defined media. *Appl Microbiol* 26:223, 1973.
31 Knapp JS et al: Serological classification of *Neisseria gonorrhoeae* with use of monoclonal antibodies to gonococcal outer membrane protein I. *J Infect Dis* 150:44, 1984.
32 Knapp JS et al: Epidemiology of gonorrhea: Distribution and temporal changes in *Neisseria gonorrhoeae* auxotype/serovar class. *Sex Transm Dis* 14:26, 1987.
33 Hook EW III et al: Determinants of emergence of antibiotic-resistant *Neisseria gonorrhoeae. J Infect Dis* (in press).
34 Crawford G et al: Asymptomatic gonorrhea in men: Caused by gonococci with unique nutritional requirements. *Science* 196:1352, 1977.
35 Knapp JS, Holmes KK: Disseminated gonococcal infection caused by *Neisseria gonorrhoeae* with unique nutritional requirements. *J Infect Dis* 132:204, 1975.
36 Draper DL et al: Auxotypes and antibiotic susceptibilities of *Neisseria gonorrhoeae* from women with acute salpingitis: Comparison with gonococci causing uncomplicated genital tract infections in women. *Sex Transm Dis* 8:43, 1981.
37 Knapp JS et al: Phenotypic and epidemiologic correlates of auxotype in *Neisseria gonorrhoeae. J Infect Dis* 138:160, 1978.
38 Rompalo AM et al: The acute arthritis-dermatitis syndrome: The changing importance of *Neisseria gonorrhoeae* and *Neisseria meningitidis. Arch Intern Med* 147:281, 1987.
39 Pierce WA, Buchanan TM: Attachment role of gonococcal pili: Optimum conditions and quantitation of adherence of isolated pili to human cells *in vitro. J Clin Invest* 61:931, 1978.
40 King GL, Swanson J: Studies on gonococcus infection: XV. Identification of surface proteins of *Neisseria gonorrhoeae* correlated with leukocyte association. *Infect Immuno* 21:575, 1978.
41 Pelouze PS: *Gonorrhea in the Male and Female.* Philadelphia, Saunders, 1941.
42 Gregg CR et al: Toxic activity of purified lipopolysaccharide of *Neisseria gonorrhoeae* for human fallopian tube mucosa. *J Infect Dis* 143:432, 1981.
43 Jacobs NF, Kraus SJ: Gonococcal and nongonococcal urethritis in men: Clinical and laboratory differentiation. *Ann Intern Med* 82:7, 1975.
44 Handsfield HH: Gonorrhea and nongonococcal urethritis: Recent advances. *Med Clin North Am* 62:925, 1978.
45 Schmale JD et al: Observation on the culture diagnosis of gonorrhea in women. *JAMA* 210:312, 1969.
46 Thin RN, Shaw EJ: Diagnosis of gonorrhea in women. *Br J Vener Dis* 55:10, 1979.
47 Barlow D, Phillips I: Gonorrhea in women: Diagnostic, clinical, and laboratory aspects. *Lancet* 1:761, 1978.
48 Judson RN, Ruder MA: Effect of hysterectomy on genital infections. *Br J Vener Dis* 55:434, 1979.
49 Platt R et al: Risk of acquiring gonorrhea and prevalence of abnormal adnexal findings among women recently exposed to gonorrhea. *JAMA* 250:320, 1983.
50 Wallin J: Gonorrhea in 1972: A 1-year study of patients attending the VD unit in Uppsala. *Br J Vener Dis* 51:41, 1974.
51 Curran JW et al: Female gonorrhea: Its relation to abnormal uterine bleeding, urinary tract symptoms, and cervicitis. *Obstet Gynecol* 45:195, 1975.
52 Corman LC et al: The high frequency of pharyngeal gonococcal infection in a prenatal clinic population. *JAMA* 230:568, 1974.
53 Klein EJ et al: Anorectal gonococcal infection. *Ann Intern Med* 86:340, 1977.
54 Kinghorn GR, Rashid S: Prevalence of rectal and pharyngeal infection in women with gonorrhea in Sheffield. *Br J Vener Dis* 55:408, 1979.
55 Lebedeff DA, Hochman EB: Rectal gonorrhea in men: Diagnosis and treatment. *Ann Intern Med* 92:463, 1980.
56 Quinn TC et al: The polymicrobial origin of intestinal infections in homosexual men. *N Engl J Med* 309:576, 1983.
57 Handsfield HH et al: Correlation of auxotype and penicillin susceptibility of *Neisseria gonorrhoeae* with sexual preference and clinical manifestations of gonorrhea. *Sex Transm Dis* 7:1, 1980.
58 Tice AW, Rodriguez VL: Pharyngeal gonorrhea. *JAMA* 246:2717, 1981.
59 Bro-Jorgensen A, Jensen T: Gonococcal pharyngeal infections: Report of 110 cases. *Br J Vener Dis* 49:491, 1973.
60 Janda WM et al: Prevalence and site-pathogen studies of *Neisseria meningitidis* and *N. gonorrhoeae* in homosexual men. *JAMA* 244:2060, 1980.
61 Sackel SG et al: Orogenital contact and the isolation of *Neisseria gonorrhoeae, Mycoplasma hominis,* and *Ureaplasma urealyticum* from the pharynx. *Sex Transm Dis* 6:64, 1979.
62 Wallin J, Siegel MS: Pharyngeal *Neisseria gonorrhoeae*: Colonizer or pathogen? *Br Med J* 1:1462, 1979.
63 Hutt DM, Judson FN: Epidemiology and treatment of oropharyngeal gonorrhea. *Ann Intern Med* 104:655, 1986.
64 Thatcher RW, Pettit TH: Gonorrheal conjunctivitis. *JAMA* 215:1494, 1971.
65 Bruins SC, Tight RR: Laboratory-acquired gonococcal conjunctivitis. *JAMA* 241:274, 1979.
66 Podgore JK, Holmes KK: Ocular gonococcal infection with little or no inflammatory response. *JAMA* 246:242, 1981.
67 Valenton MJ, Abendanio R: Gonorrheal conjunctivitis. *Can J Ophthalmol* 8:421, 1973.
68 Chapel T et al: The microbiological flora of penile ulcerations. *J Infect Dis* 137:50, 1978.
69 Robinson L, Alergant CD: Gonococcal infection of the penis. *Br J Vener Dis* 49:364, 1973.
70 Scott MJ Jr, Scott MJ Sr: Primary cutaneous *Neisseria gonorrhoeae* infections. *Arch Dermatol* 118:351, 1982.

71 Berger RE et al: Etiology, manifestations and therapy of acute epididymitis: Prospective study of 50 cases. *J Urol* 121:750, 1979.

72 Wright RA, Judson FN: Penile venereal edema. *JAMA* 241:157, 1979.

73 Eschenbach DA et al: Polymicrobial etiology of acute pelvic inflammatory disease. *N Engl J Med* 293:166, 1975.

74 Holmes KK et al: Salpingitis: Overview of etiology and epidemiology. *Am J Obstet Gynecol* 138:893, 1980.

75 Svensson L et al: Differences in some clinical and laboratory parameters in acute salpingitis related to culture and serologic findings. *Am J Obstet Gynecol* 138:1017, 1980.

76 Rees E: Gonococcal bartholinitis. *Br J Vener Dis* 43:150, 1967.

77 Holmes KK et al: Disseminated gonococcal infection. *Ann Intern Med* 74:979, 1979.

78 Masi AT, Eisenstein BI: Disseminated gonococcal infection (DGI) and gonococcal arthritis (GCA): II. Clinical manifestations, diagnosis, complications, treatment and prevention. *Semin Arthritis Rheum* 10:173, 1981.

79 O'Brien JA et al: Disseminated gonococcal infection: A prospective analysis of 49 patients and a review of pathophysiology and immune mechanisms. *Medicine* 2:395, 1983.

80 Handsfield HH et al: Treatment of the gonococcal arthritis-dermatitis syndrome. *Ann Intern Med* 84:661, 1976.

81 Rice PA, Goldenberg DL: Clinical manifestations of disseminated infection caused by *Neisseria gonorrhoeae* are linked to differences in bactericidal reactivity of infecting strains. *Ann Intern Med* 95: 175, 1985.

82 Merrett S et al: *Neisseria gonorrhoeae* strains inhibited by vancomycin in selective media and correlation with auxotype. *J Clin Microbiol* 14:94, 1981.

83 Bonin P et al: Isolation of *Neisseria gonorrhoeae* on selective and nonselective media in a STD clinic. *J Clin Microbiol* 92:218, 1984.

84 Reichart CA et al: Comparison of GC-Lect and modified Thayer-Martin media for isolation of *Neisseria gonorrhoeae*. *J Clin Microbiol* (in press).

85 Petersen BH et al: *Neisseria meningitidis* and *Neisseria gonorrhoeae* bacteremia associated with C6, C7, or C8 deficiency. *Ann Intern Med* 90:917, 1979.

86 Rinaldi RZ et al: Penicillin-resistant gonococcal arthritis: A report of four cases. *Ann Intern Med* 97:43, 1982.

87 Strader KW et al: Disseminated gonococcal infection caused by chromosomally mediated penicillin-resistant organisms. *Ann Intern Med* 104:365, 1986.

88 Sazeed ZA et al: Gonococcal meningitis: A review. *JAMA* 219:1730, 1972.

89 Rice RJ et al: Phenotypic characterization of *Neisseria gonorrhoeae* isolated from three cases of meningitis. *J Infect Dis* 153:362, 1986.

90 Apicella MA: *Neisseria meningitidis,* in *Principles and Practices of Infectious Diseases,* GL Mandell et al (eds). New York, Wiley, 1979, p 1640.

91 Handsfield HH, Knapp JS, Holmes KK. Unpublished data.

92 Faur YC et al: Isolation of *N. meningitidis* from patients in a gonorrhea screening program: A four-year survey in New York City. *Am J Public Health* 71:53, 1981.

93 Judson FN et al: Anogenital infection with *Neisseria meningitidis* in homosexual men. *J Infect Dis* 137:458, 1978.

94 Carlson BL et al: Isolation of *Neisseria meningitidis* from anogenital specimens from homosexual men. *Sex Transm Dis* 7:71, 1980.

95 William DC et al: *Neisseria meningitidis:* Probable pathogen in two related cases of urethritis, epididymitis, and acute pelvic inflammatory disease. *JAMA* 242:1653, 1979.

96 Danielsson D, Johannisson G: Culture diagnosis of gonorrhea: A comparison of the yield with selective and non-selective gonococcal culture media inoculated in the clinic and after treatment of specimens. *Acta Derm Venereol* (Stockh) 53:75, 1973.

97 Judson FN, Werness BA: Combining cervical and anal-canal specimens for gonorrhea on a single culture plate. *J Clin Microbiol* 12: 216, 1980.

98 McMillan A, Young H: Gonorrhea in the homosexual man: Frequency of infection by culture site. *Sex Transm Dis* 5:146, 1978.

99 Windall JJ et al: Inhibitory effects of vancomycin on *Neisseria gonorrhoeae* in Thayer-Martin medium. *J Infect Dis* 142:775, 1980.

100 Rothenberg RB et al: Efficacy of selected diagnostic tests for sexually transmitted diseases. *JAMA* 235:49, 1976.

101 Wald ER: Diagnosis by Gram stain in the female adolescent. *Am J Dis Child* 131:1094, 1977.

102 William DC et al: The utility of anoscopy in the rapid diagnosis of symptomatic anorectal gonorrhea in men. *Sex Transm Dis* 8:16, 1981.

103 Deheragoda P: Diagnosis of rectal gonorrhea by blind anorectal swabs compared with direct vision swabs taken via a proctoscope. *Br J Vener Dis* 53:311, 1977.

104 Thin RNT et al: Direct and delayed methods of immunofluorescent diagnosis of gonorrhea in women. *Br J Vener Dis* 47:27, 1970.

105 Prior RB, Spagna VA: Application of *Limulus* test device in rapid evaluation of gonococcal and nongonococcal urethritis in males. *J Clin Microbiol* 14:256, 1981.

106 Takeguchi MW et al: Enzymatic detection of *Neisseria gonorrhoeae. Br J Vener Dis* 56:304, 1980.

107 Demetriou E et al: Evaluation of an enzyme immunoassay for detection of *Neisseria gonorrhoeae* in an adolescent population. *JAMA* 252:247, 1984.

108 Danielsson D et al: Diagnosis of urogenital gonorrhea by detecting gonococcal antigen with a solid phase enzyme immunoassay (Gonozyme). *J Clin Pathol* 36:674, 1983.

109 Janik A et al: Genetic transformation as a tool for detection of *Neisseria gonorrhoeae. J Clin Microbiol* 4:71, 1976.

110 Jaffe HW et al: Diagnosis of gonorrhea using a genetic transformation test on mailed clinical specimens. *J Infect Dis* 146:275, 1982.

111 Murray ES et al: New options for diagnosis and control of gonorrheal urethritis in males using uncentrifuged first voided urine (FVU) as a specimen for culture. *Am J Public Health* 69:596, 1979.

112 Luciano AA, Grubin L: Gonorrhea screening: Comparison of three techniques. *JAMA* 243:680, 1980.

113 McCutchan JA et al: Role of urinary solutes in natural immunity to gonorrhea. *Infect Immun* 15:149, 1977.

114 Ris HW, Dodge RW: Gonorrhea in adolescent girls in a closed population: Prevalence, diagnosis and treatment. *Am J Dis Child* 123: 185, 1972.

115 McCormack WM et al: Evaluation of the vaginal tampon as a means of obtaining cultures for *Neisseria gonorrhoeae. J Infect Dis* 128: 129, 1973.

116 Sandstrom E, Danielsson D: A survey of gonococcal serology, in *Genital Infections and Their Complications,* D Danielsson et al (eds). Stockholm, Almqvist and Wiksell, 1975, p 253.

117 Holmes KK et al: Is serology useful in gonorrhea? A critical analysis of factors influencing serodiagnosis, in *Immunobiology of Neisseria Gonorrhoeae,* GF Brooks et al (eds). Washington, American Society for Microbiology, 1978, p 370.

118 Dans PE et al: Gonococcal serology: How soon, how useful and how much? *J Infect Dis* 135:330, 1977.

119 Mahoney JF et al: The use of penicillin sodium in the treatment of sulfonamide-resistant gonorrhea in men. A preliminary report. *Am J Gonorr Vener Dis* 27:525, 1943.

120 Sparling PF: Antibiotic resistance in the gonococcus, in *The Gonococcus,* RB Roberts (ed). New York, Wiley, 1978, p. 111.

121 Martin JE et al: Comparative study of gonococcal susceptibility to penicillin in the United States, 1955–1969. *J Infect Dis* 122:459, 1970.

122 Centers for Disease Control. Recommended treatment schedules for gonorrhea—March 1972. *MMWR* 21:82, 1972.

123 Phillips I: Beta-lactamase producing, penicillin-resistant gonococcus. *Lancet* 2:656, 1976.

124 Roberts M et al: Molecular characterization of two beta-lactamase specifying plasmids from *Neisseria gonorrhoeae. J Bacteriol* 131: 557, 1977.

125 Centers for Disease Control: Tetracycline-resistant *Neisseria gonorrhoeae*—Georgia, Pennsylvania, New Hampshire. *MMWR* 34: 563, 1985.
126 Perine PL et al: Epidemiology and treatment of penicillinase-producing *Neisseria gonorrhoeae. Sex Transm Dis* 6(suppl):152, 1979.
127 Centers for Disease Control: Penicillinase-producing *Neisseria gonorrhoeae*—United States, 1986. *MMWR* 36:107, 1987.
128 Zenilman JM et al: Unpublished data, 1988.
129 Zenilman JM et al: Penicillinase-producing *Neisseria gonorrhoeae* in Dade County, Florida: Evidence of core-group transmitters and the impact of illicit antibiotics. *Sex Transm Dis* 15:45, 1988.
130 Faruki H et al: A community-based outbreak of infection with penicillin-resistant *Neisseria gonorrhoeae* not producing penicillinase (chromosomally mediated resistance). *N Engl J Med* 313:607, 1985.
131 Faruki H, Sparling PF: Genetics of resistance in a non-beta-lactamase-producing gonococcus with relatively high-level penicillin resistance. *Antimicrob Agents Chemother* 30:856, 1986.
132 Hook EW III et al: Auxotype/serovar diversity and antimicrobial resistance of *Neisseria gonorrhoeae* in two mid-sized American cities. *Sex Transm Dis* 14:141, 1987.
133 Centers for Disease Control: Sentinel surveillance system for antimicrobial resistance in clinical isolates of *Neisseria gonorrhoeae. MMWR* 36:585, 1987.
134 Centers for Disease Control: Tetracycline-resistant *Neisseria gonorrhoeae*—Georgia, Pennsylvania, New Hampshire. *MMWR* 34:563, 1985.
135 Morse SA et al: High-level tetracycline resistance in *Neisseria gonorrhoeae* is result of acquisition of streptococcal *tet-M* determinant. *Antibicrob Agents Chemother* 30:664, 1986.
136 Boslego JW et al: Effect of spectinomycin use on the prevalence of spectinomycin-resistant and of penicillinase-producing *Neisseria gonorrhoeae. N Engl J Med* 317:272, 1987.
137 Ison CA et al: Spectinomycin resistant gonococci. *Br Med J* 287:1827, 1983.
138 Ashford WA et al: Spectinomycin-resistant penicillinase producing *Neisseria gonorrhoeae. Lancet* 2:1035, 1981.
139 Jaffe HW et al: Pharmacokinetic determinants of penicillin cure of gonococcal urethritis. *Antimicrob Agents Chemother* 15:587, 1979.
140 Stamm WE et al: Effect of treatment regimens for *Neisseria gonorrhoeae* on simultaneous infections with *Chlamydia trachomatis. N Engl J Med* 310:545, 1984.
141 Centers for Disease Control. Sexually transmitted diseases guidelines, 1985. *MMWR* 31(suppl):335, 1985.
142 Centers for Disease Control: Antibiotic-resistant strains of *Neisseria gonorrhoeae.* Policy guidelines for detection, management, and control. *MMWR* 36(suppl):, 1987.
143 Handsfield HH, Hook EW III: Ceftriaxone for treatment of uncomplicated gonorrhea: Routine use of a single 125 mg dose in a sexually transmitted disease clinic. *Sex Transm Dis* 14:227, 1987.
144 Judson FN et al: Comparative study of ceftriaxone and spectinomycin for treatment of pharyngeal and anorectal gonorrhea. *JAMA* 253:1417, 1985.
145 Crider SR et al: Treatment of penicillin-resistant *Neisseria gonorrhoeae* with oral norfloxacin. *N Engl J Med* 311:137, 1984.
146 Dallabetta GA, Hook EW III: Treatment of sexually-transmitted diseases with quinolone antimicrobial agents, in *Quinolone Antimicrobial Agents,* JS Wolfson, DC Hooper (eds). Washington, DC, American Society for Microbiology, 1989, p. 125.
147 Joyce MP et al: *In vitro* sensitivity of *Neisseria gonorrhoeae* to quinolone antibiotics in the Republic of the Philippines, abstracted (no E19). *Abstracts of the Sixth International Pathogenic Neisseria Conference, Pine Mountain, Georgia,* 1988.
148 Kraus SJ: Incidence and therapy of gonococcal pharyngitis. *Sex Transm Dis* 6(suppl):143, 1979.
149 Morse SA et al: Gonococcal strains from homosexual men have outer membranes with reduced permeability to hydrophobic molecules. *Infect Immun* 37:432, 1982.
150 Judson FN, Rothenberg RR: Tetracycline treatment of uncomplicated male gonorrhea. *J Am Vener Dis* 125:499, 1972.
151 Schroeter AL, Reynolds G: The rectal culture as a test of cure of gonorrhea in the female. *J Infect Dis* 125:499, 1972.
152 Hart G: Epidemiologic treatment for syphilis and gonorrhea. *Sex Transm Dis* 7:149, 1980.
153 Judson FN, Maltz AB: A rational basis for the epidemiologic treatment of gonorrhea in a clinic for sexually transmitted diseases. *Sex Transm Dis* 5:89, 1978.
154 Barlow D: The condom and gonorrhea. *Lancet* 2:811, 1977.
155 Stone KM et al: Personal protection against sexually transmitted diseases. *Am J Obstet Gynecol* 155:180, 1986.

Chapter 15

# Biology of *Chlamydia trachomatis*

Julius Schachter

## TAXONOMY

*Chlamydia trachomatis* is one of the two species within the genus *Chlamydia* (Table 15-1).[1] *C. trachomatis* is an important cause of blindness and sexually transmitted diseases of humans. The other species, *Chlamydia psittaci*, is a common pathogen of avian species and domestic mammals but involves humans only as a zoonosis.[2] The newly described TWAR strains have no known animal reservoir and only infect humans.[3] They are currently considered as *C. psittaci* but are genetically different and may belong in a new species.[4] Some *C. psittaci* strains are sexually transmitted in their natural hosts and one—the guinea pig inclusion conjunctivitis (GPIC) agent—may offer a potentially useful animal model for the study of sexually transmitted chlamydial infections.[5,6]

The two species are identified on the basis of two relatively simple laboratory tests (Table 15-2). The simpler involves staining infected cells with iodine to determine whether the inclusions contain glycogen (*C. trachomatis* inclusions do, while *C. psittaci* inclusions don't). The second and less reliable test involves testing for susceptibility to sulfonamides: *C. trachomatis* strains are susceptible and *C. psittaci* strains are usually resistant. Each of these species contains many different strains possessing a variety of serologic and biologic properties. Unfortunately, technical restrictions dictated by their growth cycle have limited studies on the physiology of these organisms and thus markers for more sophisticated attempts at speciation have not been identified.

The need for better tools for speciation is particularly acute within *C. trachomatis*. This species contains three biovars that are probably different organisms.[1] The murine biovar is not known to infect humans. The biovar causing human lymphogranuloma venereum (LGV) contains three serovars. The trachoma biovar includes strains that cause common human genital tract diseases (urethritis, cervicitis, salpingitis, infant diseases, etc.) and trachoma. DNA homology within the LGV and trachoma biovars is almost complete. The mouse biovar is less related (30 to 60 percent homology), but there is essentially no (less than 10 percent) homology with *C. psittaci*.

**Table 15-1. Human Diseases Caused by Chlamydiae**

| Species | Serovar* | Disease |
|---|---|---|
| *C. psittaci* | Many unidentified serovars | Psittacosis |
| *C. psittaci* | TWAR | Respiratory disease |
| *C. trachomatis* | L1, L2, L3 | Lymphogranuloma venereum |
| *C. trachomatis* | A, B, Ba, C | Hyperendemic blinding trachoma |
| *C. trachomatis* | D, E, F, G, H, I, J, K | Inclusion conjunctivitis (adult and newborn), nongonococcal urethritis, cervicitis, salpingitis, proctitis, epididymitis, pneumonia of newborns |

*Predominant, but not exclusive association of serovar with disease.
SOURCE: J Schachter.[26]

**Table 15-2. Usual Properties of *Chlamydia* spp.**

| | *C. trachomatis* | *C. psittaci* |
|---|---|---|
| Sulfonamide susceptibility | + | − |
| Iodine staining inclusions | + | − |
| Natural host | Human | Avian, lower mammals |

The trachoma and LGV biovars are related serologically but differ not only in the diseases they produce but also in the type of cells they parasitize (in vivo and in vitro), in experimental host range and a variety of other biological properties related to the infectious process (Table 15-3). The trachoma biovar has a very limited host spectrum in terms of susceptible cell types. In the natural host it appears to infect only squamocolumnar cells; macrophages are not infected. LGV strains are more invasive and appear to be more efficient at replication in macrophages. Neither will grow in polymorphonuclear leukocytes.

The chlamydiae are distinguished from all other microorganisms on the basis of a unique growth cycle[1] (Fig. 15-1). It involves an alternation between two highly specialized morphologic forms that are adapted to either intracellular or extracellular environments. Because of this cycle chlamydiae have been placed in their own order and family (Chlamydiales, Chlamydiaceae). They are obligate intracellular parasites and cannot be cultured on artificial media. Chlamydiae are restricted to an intracellular lifestyle because they lack the ability to synthesize high-energy compounds. Thus they depend on the host cell to supply them with ATP (adenosine triphosphate) and necessary nutrients. Moulder has called them "energy parasites."[7] They lack a system for electron transport, have no cytochromes, and cannot synthesize ATP and GTP (guanine triphosphate). The growth cycle initially involves attachment and penetration into susceptible host

**Table 15-3. Properties of LGV and Other Trachoma Biovars of *C. trachomatis***

| Properties | LGV | Trachoma |
|---|---|---|
| I Sulfonamide susceptibility | + | + |
| II Iodine-staining inclusions | + | + |
| III Host spectrum | | |
| A Natural host: humans | + | + |
| 1. Mucosal surfaces | − | + |
| 2. Lymphoid | + | − |
| B Produce follicular conjunctivitis in subhuman primates | − | + |
| C Lethal to mice (intracerebral) | + | − |
| IV Growth in cell culture | | |
| A Form plaques | + | − |
| B Marked enhancement by centrifugation | − | + |
| C Infectivity enhanced by treating cells with DEAE | − | + |
| D Infectivity reduced by treating cells with neuraminidase | − | + |
| E Infectivity blocked by saturating cell surface with heat-killed homologous organism | − | + |

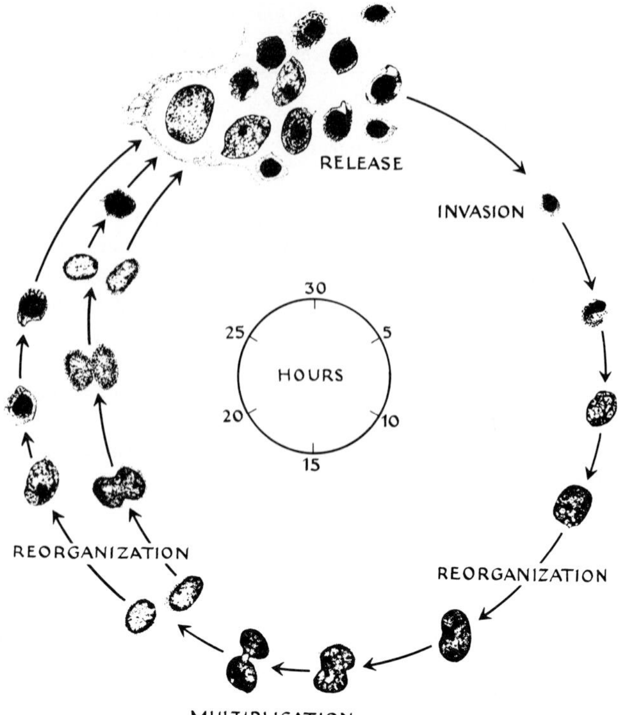


**Fig. 15-1.** Growth cycle of the *Chlamydia*. (*From JW Moulder.*[7])

cells.[8,9] The attachment process may involve specific receptor sites; presence of these sites could determine which cells are naturally susceptible.[10,11] Penetration of *Chlamydia* into the host cell involves an enhanced phagocytic process which is induced by the chlamydiae. Once they penetrate the cell they remain within a phagocytic vesicle throughout the growth cycle, but the chlamydiae specifically inhibit phagolysosomal fusion. Heat-killed or antibody-treated chlamydiae are not ingested at an enhanced rate and fail to inhibit phagolysosomal fusion. These two properties, induced phagocytosis and prevention of phagolysosomal fusion, are probably the major virulence factors of this organism.

## HISTORY

The human diseases caused by *Chlamydia trachomatis* have been recognized since antiquity.[12] Trachoma is described in Egyptian papyri. LGV was probably described by John Hunter in the eighteenth century. The genital tract infections, such as nongonococcal urethritis and neonatal ophthalmia caused by *C. trachomatis,* were not recognized until it was possible to categorize these conditions following the identification of the gonococcus. With the introduction of ocular (Credé) prophylaxis with silver nitrate drops to prevent ophthalmia neonatorum, and of cultural and smear methods of diagnosing gonococcal infections, it became apparent that conjunctivitis in infants and urethritis in adult males both had nongonococcal forms.

*C. trachomatis* was first visualized in 1907 by Halberstaedter and Prowazek in stained conjunctival scrapings taken from orangutans that had been inoculated with human trachomatous material. They quickly identified the typical intracytoplasmic inclusions, but initially they assumed that the organism was a protozoan. Shortly thereafter, similar inclusions were identified in human material from trachoma cases and then in conjunctival scrapings taken from infants with inclusion blennorrhea. Inclusions were then found in the genital tracts of mothers of the affected infants and in the urethras of the fathers. In the first decade of this century the presence of these inclusions was associated with nongonococcal urethritis.[13]

*C. trachomatis* was first isolated from patients with lymphogranuloma venereum. In the 1930s the growth cycle of the LGV organism (as seen following intracerebral inoculation in mice and then in eggs) was noted to be similar to that found for the psittacosis organism which had been isolated during the psittacosis pandemic of 1929–1930. The trachoma agent proved more difficult to recover, not being infective for mice. It was isolated by inoculation of embryonated hens' egg yolk sacs by T'ang and associates in the 1950s.[14] These results were soon confirmed by a number of research teams in different parts of the world. In retrospect it is likely that a previous isolation claim, by Macchiavello, was probably valid—but it was not confirmed and the isolate was lost. The first isolate of *Chlamydia* (other than LGV agents) from the genital tract was made in 1959 by Jones, Collier, and Smith, who recovered *C. trachomatis* from the cervix of the mother of an infant with ophthalmia neonatorum.[15] In 1964, chlamydiae were first recovered from the urethras of men epidemiologically associated with conjunctivitis cases.[16,17]

For a number of years there were very few groups actively pursuing the study of chlamydial genital tract infections. One of the reasons for this lack of interest was the lack of a technology which lent itself to screening large numbers of specimens. All of the early isolation studies (from 1960 to 1965) were performed using yolk-sac isolation procedures and thus were not clinically relevant because they could take up to 6 weeks to provide definitive answers. Dunlop and his colleagues at the Institute of Ophthalmology in London were the pioneering group that provided much of the impetus for continued research on chlamydial genital tract infections. In a series of studies they found a number of anatomic sites of the genitourinary system could be infected with *Chlamydia* and showed that approximately one-third of men with nongonococcal urethritis were carrying the organism in their urethras.[18–20] A major technical breakthrough by Gordon and his colleagues in developing a tissue culture isolation procedure for *C. trachomatis* made it possible to screen large numbers of specimens and to obtain the results of an isolation attempt in 48 to 72 h, which made the diagnosis clinically useful.[21] A number of other English research groups independently demonstrated that one-third to one-half of men with nongonococcal urethritis had chlamydial infections.[22–25] In recent years the clinical syndromes associated with these infections rapidly expanded[26] (Table 15-1) (see Chaps. 16, 17, and 66).

## EPIDEMIOLOGY

### SEXUALLY TRANSMITTED CHLAMYDIAL INFECTIONS

There are two major modes of transmission of *C. trachomatis:* sexual, and congenital. LGV is always transmitted sexually. In industrialized western society virtually all *C. trachomatis* infections are sexually transmitted, except those of neonates, who may acquire infection from their mother during birth. Men who acquire infection with non-LGV *C. trachomatis* strains usually develop nongonococcal urethritis 1 to 2 weeks postinfection. Because chlamydiae are obligate intracellular parasites and can only survive by a replicative cycle that results in death of the infected host cells, they must be considered to be pathogens at all times and are not part of the normal flora of the male or female genital tract. They, however, do not always produce clinically apparent infections. For specific discussions of the epidemiology of these sexually transmitted infections see Chaps. 16 and 17.

If infective genital tract discharges are inoculated into the eye either during sexual activity or by hand to eye contact, conjunctivitis may develop.[12,26,27] The disease caused by the trachoma biovar is called inclusion conjunctivitis, reflecting the diagnostic cytologic findings. In adults it is an acute follicular conjunctivitis which tends to follow a self-limited course. Keratitis and micropannus are common. Occasionally the disease persists beyond a few months and clinical features consistent with the diagnosis of trachoma may develop. Visual debility is rare. However, the regular appearance of corneal involvement (with the exception of Herbert's peripheral pits) similar to that found in classical trachoma, has led some workers to suggest that chlamydial infection of the eye represents a spectrum from mild, self-limited, acute, follicular conjunctivitis to chronic trachoma. The clinical picture is determined by the immunologic status of the host: previous exposure and hypersensitivity result in more severe disease, and reinfections or complicating bacterial infections interfere with spontaneous healing.[12,26,27]

Infants exposed to *Chlamydia* by passage through the infected birth canal may also acquire the infection and can develop a number of diseases, including conjunctivitis and pneumonia (see Chap. 66). At least 60 to 70 percent of exposed infants acquire chlamydial infection.[28] Thus both horizontal and vertical transmission of *C. trachomatis* occur in industrialized society.

## ENDEMIC TRACHOMA

Child to child transmission is the most common method of chlamydial transmission in trachoma endemic areas.[12,26,27,29] In many developing countries trachoma is endemic and in some it is hyper- or holoendemic. Several hundred million people are known to be afflicted with trachoma and millions have been blinded. In holoendemic areas children acquire the infection very early, either from persistently infected adults in their families or from exposure to other infected children. In some communities all are infected by 2 years of age. Poor hygiene and unsanitary conditions contribute to the spread of the organism. Flies act as mechanical vectors in spreading infective ocular discharges. The disease begins as an acute mucopurulent conjunctivitis (often complicated by secondary bacterial infections) that becomes a chronic follicular keratoconjunctivitis, sometimes accompanied by a significant pannus (corneal neovascularization) formation. In hyperendemic areas active disease usually wanes when the children are 6 to 10 years old. Most of the children will be left with minor sequelae when the disease becomes inactive and there will be no effect on vision. Some children with moderate to severe trachoma will develop badly scarred conjunctivae as a result of the necrosis of follicles. This scarring in the upper tarsal plate of the conjunctiva may, with time, result in distortion of the upper eyelid. The inturned upper lid margin causes the eyelashes to abrade and ultimately break down the corneal epithelium. It may take 25 or 30 years for this process to evolve fully, as the scars contract with age. The blindness seen in adults of greater than 40 years of age usually reflects early childhood trachoma. In a hyperendemic area age-specific blindness rates at age 60 may be 20 percent or more.

## SEROVAR DISTRIBUTION

There are few studies aimed at determining the distribution of serovars in a community. There appear to be no biological markers associated with the different serovars that would tend to make such typing relevant from either the clinical or the public health viewpoint. In trachoma endemic areas usually only one or two serovars are recovered in a community.[27,30] Most infections within a household appear to be of the same serovar.

The genital serovars are not evenly distributed. L2 appears to be the most common of the LGV serovars and the DE serovars are the most commonly recovered trachoma biovars.[31] The A serovar has never been recovered from the genital tract, but the B serovar, which is commonly associated with endemic trachoma, has also been shown to cause genital tract infection. Specific monoclonal antibodies are available which can distinguish among the different serovars, but until this identification becomes more meaningful it will remain a research procedure.[32]

# BIOLOGY

## DEVELOPMENTAL CYCLE

The developmental cycle of chlamydiae sets them apart from all other bacteria. There are some differences in inclusion morphology within the chlamydiae, but both species appear to have essentially identical developmental cycles. The cycle may be divided into several steps: (1) initial attachment of the elementary body to the host cell; (2) entry into the cell; (3) morphologic change to the reticulate body with intracellular growth and replication; (4) morphologic change to elementary body; and (5) release of infectious particles.

The infectious particle, the elementary body (EB), is relatively resistant to the extracellular environment but is not metabolically active. This particle changes to a metabolically active and dividing form called the reticulate particle (RB or initial body) at some time within the first 6 to 8 h after entering the host cell. This reorganization process is poorly understood. After the RB stage has been reached, *Chlamydia* use host-cell substrates to synthesize their own RNA, DNA, and protein.[33] Glycogen accumulates within the inclusions of *C. trachomatis,* reaching levels detectable by iodine stain at approximately 30 to 48 h postinfection.[34] The RBs divide by binary fission from approximately 8 h postentry into the cell to approximately 18 to 24 h. This is the stage of greatest metabolic activity when the organisms are most sensitive to inhibitors of cell-wall synthesis and of bacterial metabolic activity. At approximately 18 to 24 h some of the RBs reorganize into the smaller infectious EBs. RBs are approximately 1 μm in diameter and do not appear to be electron-dense; the EBs are approximately 350 nm in diameter and have an electron-dense center. Beyond 18 to 24 h the numbers of EBs increase and appear to predominate, although both EBs and RBs are found in the inclusion. This entire cycle takes place within the phagosome, which obviously undergoes a large increase in size. At some time between 48 to 72 h the cell ruptures, releasing the infectious EB.

Phagolysosomal fusion does not occur until the death of the cell is imminent. This inhibition has been attributed to a chlamydial surface antigen because antibody-treated EBs do not inhibit phagolysosomal fusion.

The RBs are not stable outside the host cell. Thus, as part of their unique growth cycle, the *Chlamydia* appear to have evolved two morphologic entities—the compact stable EB which successfully persists in the extracellular environment and is responsible for cell to cell and host to host transmission, and the highly labile RB which represents the metabolically active and vegetative form which is noninfective and does not survive outside the host cell.

The EB is toxic. If many particles are ingested (multiplicities on the order of 100 EBs per host cell) the host cell may die with no resultant progeny.[35] Large concentrations of *Chlamydia* inoculated intravenously into mice will also kill the animal by a toxic "death" which appears to be a result of damage to the vascular endothelium. *Chlamydia* do not produce an extracellular toxin.

### Attachment

The attachment of *C. psittaci* and the LGV biovar of *C. trachomatis* to cells is highly efficient, as is penetration. Saturation of the cultured cell's surface is not observed.[11] Heating prevents attachment; the host cells have a trypsin-sensitive attachment site that is quickly regenerated. In contrast, the trachoma biovar attaches inefficiently, saturation can be demonstrated, and heating the organism does not inhibit attachment, nor does trypsinization of host cells keep them from attaching.[11,37] The trachoma biovar may have a more specialized attachment site than the LGV biovar; this may explain its more limited host range.

The initial contact of the chlamydial EB with the susceptible host cell may involve a specific receptor-ligand interaction, but no such structures have clearly been identified. For some strains attachment may be charge-dependent. DEAE-dextran pretreatment of cells leads to marked enhancement of attachment and entry of the trachoma biovar but not for *C. psittaci* or the LGV biovar.[11] Treatment with negatively charged molecules such as heparin can inhibit chlamydial infectivity and elute EBs from the surface of host cells.[38] The attachment of *Chlamydia* to host cells and inhibition of phagolysosomal fusion are inhibited by specific antibody, by mild heat treatment (56°C for 30 min), or trypsinization.[36,39] However, Hackstadt and Caldwell found that surface proteolysis of EBs did not impair infectivity, although major outer membrane protein (MOMP) was dramatically cleaved and largely removed from the surface.[40] Polyclonal antibody to MOMP neutralized infectivity but did not inhibit attachment or penetration.[41] Similarly, monoclonal antibody to a species-specific *C. trachomatis* MOMP antigen neutralized infectivity of two serovars (L2 and I) but did not reduce attachment to susceptible cells.[42]

### Cell entry

Once attached the EB is rapidly internalized by the host cell. If a mixture of EBs and *Escherichia coli* or yeast are presented to susceptible host cells, the *Chlamydia* will be preferentially ingested.[36] Many of the cells that the *Chlamydia* infect are not considered phagocytes; *Chlamydia* induce phagocytosis by the nonprofessional phagocytes.[43]

The mechanism of chlamydial uptake is controversial. Ultrastructural studies on the entry of *Chlamydia* into susceptible cells suggest that they enter through clathrin-coated pits. This suggests that chlamydial entry is via a pathway similar to receptor-mediated endocytosis.[44] However, inhibitors of receptor-mediated endocytosis such as monodansylcadaverine or amantadine did not inhibit LGV biovar uptake in HeLa cells.[45]

### Intracellular growth

The chlamydial particle enters the cell within a phagosome and stays within that phagosome through its entire life cycle, but phagolysosomal fusion does not take place.[9] An inhibitor of phagolysosomal fusion appears to be an EB surface protein antigen.[46] The inhibitory signal is not present on the RB surface, since after RBs are ingested there is fusion.[47] Inhibition is specific to the chlamydial phagosome, as fusion can take place in other phagosomes in the same cell.[48]

Approximately 8 h after entry into the cell the EB (diameter approximately 350 nm) has changed into an RB which has a diameter of approximately 800 to 1000 nm. The rigid structure of the EB is lost and the RB is more permeable, allowing it to take up ATP and required nutrients. The inclusion (and the RB) acts essentially as a reverse mitochondria, with ATP and other nutrients entering the inclusion from the host cell.[49] The RBs divide by binary fission for approximately 20 to 24 h. About that time some of the RBs become EBs by a condensation process which is not clearly understood. Other RBs continue to divide. During replication of the RBs there is budding and blebbing of the outer membrane. Intermediate forms are also seen (Fig. 15-1). The mature inclusion contains hundreds to thousands of elementary bodies. The entire cytoplasm of the cell may be displaced by the inclusion. At the conclusion of the infectious cycle lysosomal enzyme activity is noted.[50]

## MORPHOLOGY AND COMPOSITION

The chlamydiae are structurally complex microorganisms which possess cell walls and membranes (Fig. 15-2) quite analogous in structure to the cell walls of gram-negative bacteria.[51]

Although *Chlamydia* do have a cell wall, it does not appear to contain muramic acid. It is likely that the chlamydial cell wall is unique among bacterial species and probably represents a specialized structure which is compatible with the requirements of the chlamydial growth cycle. Traces of muramic acid have been found, but in quantities inadequate to maintain structural integrity by a peptidoglycan layer.[52] The cell wall consists of subunits

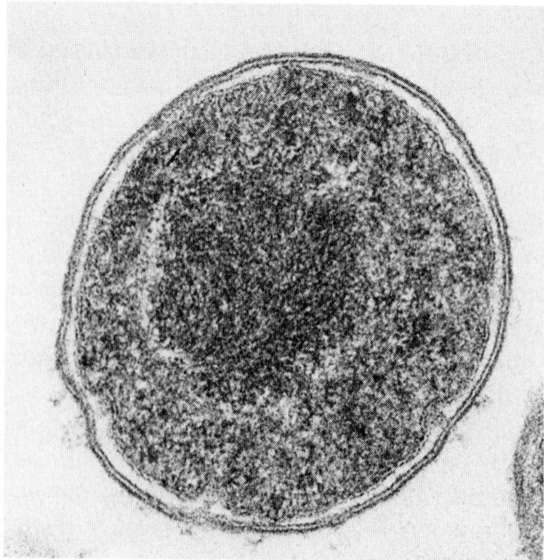

**Fig. 15-2.** Electron photomicrograph of a thin section of a *C. trachomatis* elementary body (strain L2/434). The trilaminar outer membrane and inner cytoplasmic membrane of the elementary body are illustrated. 118,000 magnification. (*From HD Caldwell.*[54])

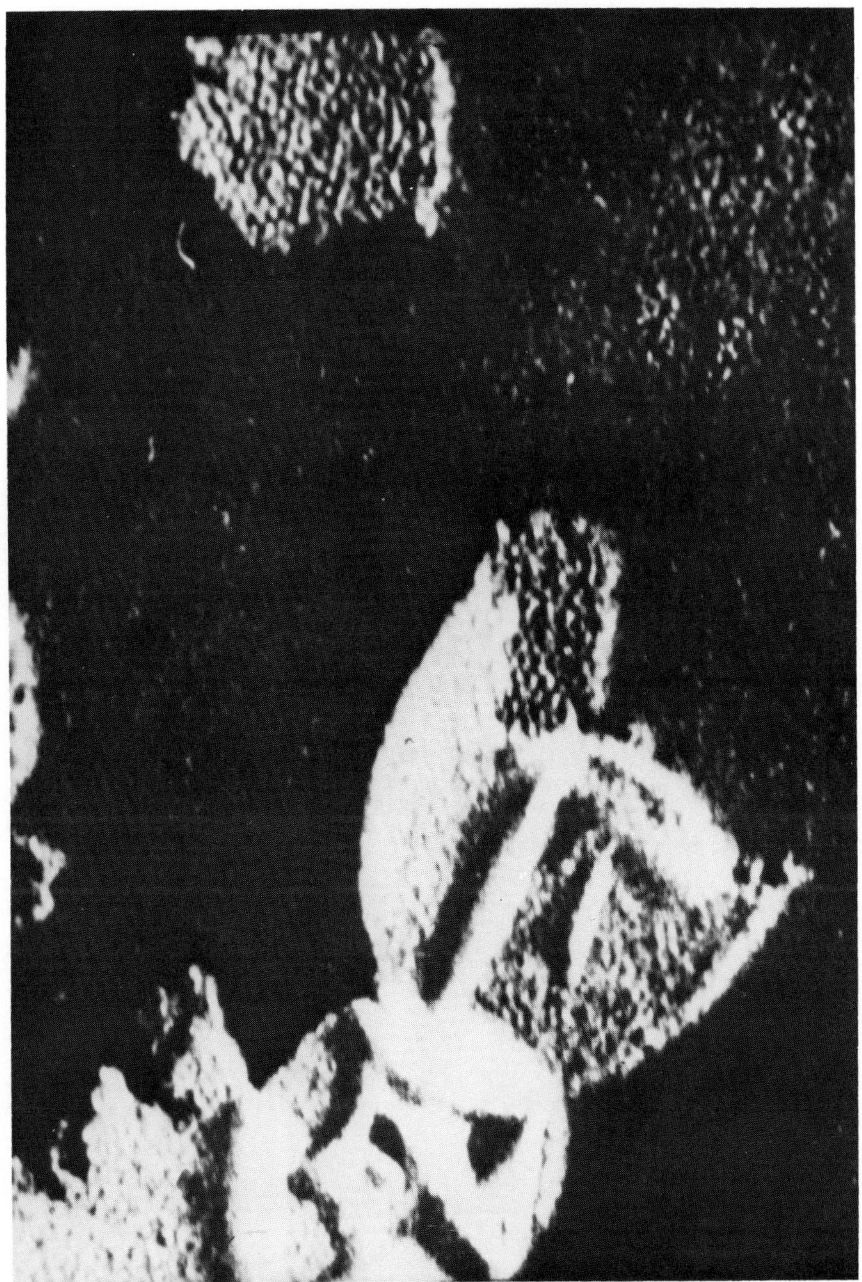

**Fig. 15-3.** Fine structure of cell wall of meningopneumonitis organism. Shadowed preparation showing regular geometric arrangement of subunits approximately 20 nm in diameter, × approximately 75,000 magnification. (*From A Matsumoto and GP Manire.*[51])

approximately 20 nm in diameter arranged in a regular geometric pattern (Fig. 15-3).[53] The outer membrane of *Chlamydia* contains a major outer membrane protein (MOMP) which is approximately 30 percent of the weight of the organism and approximately 60 percent of the weight of the outer membrane.[54] The size of this protein varies by serovar with a molecular weight range of 38 to 43 kilodaltons.[55] It appears to be the major structural protein and functions in maintaining the structural integrity of the cell wall.[54] It is a cysteine-rich protein which is linked by disulfide bonds to itself and to two other proteins of approximately 15 and 60 kilodaltons to maintain structural rigidity.[56,57] It is possible that the major structural changes that occur when the EB changes to an RB represent a reduction of the disulfide links within the EB outer membrane. RB outer membrane structure is in some respects similar to that of the EB, although there is less disulfide bridging between MOMP and the other cysteine-rich proteins.[56,58] In the beginning of the growth cycle MOMP is reduced to the monomeric form. MOMP is found in the outer membrane throughout the life cycle, whereas these other proteins are synthesized later in the cycle.[56,58,59] Synthesis of these other proteins probably is regulated so that they appear at the time the EBs form.

Supporting the concept that the EB-RB transformation is partly dependent on reduction of disulfide bonds is the observation that reduced and alkylated MOMP functions as a porin.[60] Reduction of EBs with dithiothreitol results in increased glutamine oxidation, reduced infectivity, decreased osmotic stability, and change to staining characteristics of the RB.[61] MOMP is apparently a transmembrane protein with surface antigenic components responsible, at least in part, for serovar complex reactivity. Other surface antigens, responsible solely for serovar specifically, appear to have a molecular weight of 25,000 to 30,000.[62] The common group antigen, which has a carbohydrate reactive moiety, may be released from the particles by treatment with detergents such as deoxycholate.[63]

The chemical composition of the organism appears to be approximately 35 percent protein and 40 to 50 percent lipid. Both RNA and DNA are found, although reticulate particles, being metabolically active, have more RNA. *Chlamydia* cannot utilize thymidine[64] and contain no detectable thymidine kinase.[65] It is likely that requirements for DNA synthesis are met through a uridine and thymidylic synthetase pathway. The host cell's thymidine kinase may play a role.

Electron micrographs show a regular arrangement of spikelike protuberances in a limited area of the EB surface (Fig. 15-4).[66] The function of these projections is not known, but from their arrangement it is likely that they are involved in attachment and possibly in transfer of molecules into or out of the EB particle.

*Chlamydia* appear to contain a number of penicillin-binding proteins.[67] The lack of muramic acid and peptidoglycan is diffi-

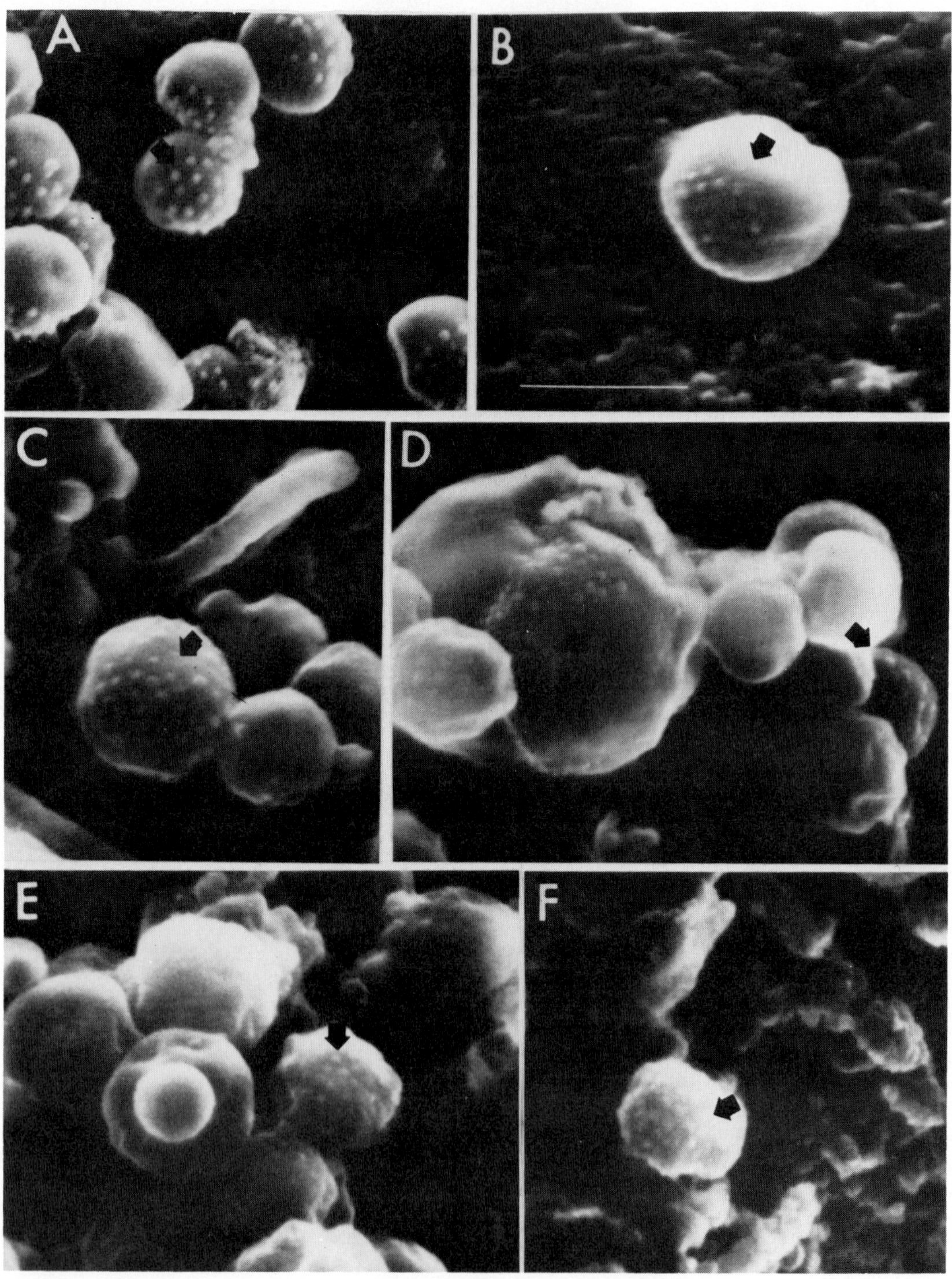


**Fig. 15-4.** Scanning electron micrograph of two strains of *C. psittaci* and four strains of *C. trachomatis* settled onto L cells. (*a*) *C. psittaci* (6BC). (*b*) *C. psittaci* (feline pneumonitis). (*c*) *C. trachomatis* (mouse pneumonitis). (*d*) *C. trachomatis* (440L). (*e*) *C. trachomatis* (G17). (*f*) *C. trachomatis* (UW57). Arrows point to prominent arrays of projections. The bar in (*b*) represents 0.5 μm × 50,000 magnification. (*From WM Gregory et al.*[66])

cult to reconcile with the known inhibitory effects of penicillins. The effect of penicillin in other bacteria is known to involve inhibition of cross-linking between tetrapeptide side chains of peptidoglycan, and *Chlamydia* therefore probably have similar cross-linked tetrapeptides. These presumably are linked to something other than peptidoglycan. Cycloserine, an inhibitor of tetrapeptide synthesis, is active against *Chlamydia* and its effect can be reversed by d-alanine, suggesting that this model is correct.[68]

## GROWTH AND CULTURE

Because *Chlamydia* are obligate intracellular parasites, it is necessary to supply a living host cell to support their growth. Tissue culture isolation procedures have made chlamydial isolation clinically relevant. The organism can be recovered from patients in 48 to 72 h—a time period consistent with other bacteriologic procedures. A number of cell lines have been used and a variety of treatments, physical or chemical, have been employed to increase the susceptibility of these cells to chlamydial infection.[12]

Modification of the cells' charge by pretreatment of the monolayers with DEAE-dextran enhances attachment by non-LGV *C. trachomatis* strains.[69] The single most important step in enhancing infection is centrifugation of the inoculum onto the tissue culture monolayer.[21,70] With the exception of LGV strains, the *C. trachomatis* strains are not efficient at attaching to and infecting cells in vitro. Indeed a convenient method of differentiating LGV from the trachoma biovar strains is to measure the enhancement of infectivity achieved with centrifugation, for it is minimal with the LGV strains and $>10^2$ for the non-LGV strains. The centrifugal forces used (ca. 2500 g) are probably inadequate to sediment the chlamydial particles, and the effects may be on the cultured cell membranes.

The most commonly used procedures involve either iododeoxyuridine (IUDR) pretreatment of cells or treatment of cells with cycloheximide after centrifugation of the inoculum[71,72] (see Chap. 74 for detailed discussion of these methods). The growth of chlamydiae within the cell basically requires that the cell receive its required nutrients. The growth of *Chlamydia* in cell culture can be regulated by the amino acid concentration in the medium. Deprivation of the essential amino acids can render productive chlamydial infections to a nonproductive state. Addition of the required amino acids will then trigger growth of the chlamydiae.[73] Synthetic abilities of the host cell are stopped by the action of cycloheximide and under these conditions, *C. psittaci* required isoleucine, valine, and phenylalanine.[74] *C. trachomatis* requires histidine, while *C. psittaci* does not.[75] Different *C. trachomatis* serovars show different nutritional requirements.[75] Cysteine is needed for the production of the cysteine-rich proteins that are important in EB rigidity. Cysteine deprivation prevents the final differentiation of EBs from RBs, but replication during the RB phase appears to be almost normal.[76]

RBs can use amino acids derived from either the host cell nutrient pool or from degradation of host protein. L cells and *C. psittaci* require L-isoleucine, as neither synthesizes it. If L-isoleucine is added to an infected L cell population carried in minimal medium, both *Chlamydia* and L cells will replicate.[74] Inhibition of L cell metabolism in a deficient medium will allow chlamydiae to grow; they are obviously using small amounts of the amino acid released by degradation of host protein.

RBs harvested at 20 h, but not EBs purified from *C. psittaci* and *C. trachomatis* infected cells, support ATP-dependent and antibiotic susceptible synthesis of proteins. MOMP and 12.5 and 60 kilodalton cysteine-rich protein are produced at a lesser rate than in infected cells.[77] Chlamydiae are capable of incorporating carbon from glucose-6-phosphate, pyruvate, and isoleucine into a trichloroacetic acid insoluble fraction.[78] Chlamydial inclusions and RBs function, in a sense, as reverse mitochondria, with ATP entering and ADP being excreted.[49]

Cyclic AMP (cAMP) inhibits chlamydial growth, and the action has been shown to be on the RB to EB transformation.[79] RBs appear to have a receptor protein for cAMP.[80] Hormone levels may affect chlamydial growth and metabolism, possibly by effects on cAMP concentrations. Estradiol enhances the growth of *C. psittaci* and *C. trachomatis* in HeLa cells.[81,82]

## GENETICS

Difficulties in preparing adequate quantities of purified organisms and lack of suitable markers have restricted genetic studies, and little is known concerning the biological aspects of chlamydial genetics. The DNA of *C. trachomatis* strains have a G plus C (guanine plus cytosine) content of 44 to 45 percent.[83] Chlamydiae have one of the smallest bacterial genomes (approximately one-half the size of neisserial or rickettsial DNA).[84] DNA homology within chlamydial species is virtually complete, but surprisingly (in view of their biologic similarities) there is little interspecies homology. Restriction endonuclease analysis may provide the basis for molecular fingerprinting of some chlamydial strains.[85]

Relatively few *C. psittaci* strains have been analyzed for the presence of plasmids. All *C. trachomatis* serovars contain a 4.4 megadalton plasmid.[86] It is present as a multimeric form. Restriction endonuclease cleavage patterns of the plasmid differed for the single LGV strain compared with the other *C. trachomatis* strains tested.[86] Functions of the plasmid genes are not known, although some of the gene products are expressed during *C. trachomatis* infection in cell culture. The gene products appear relatively late in the developmental cycle, during the multiplication of RBs and condensation from RB to EB.[85] Polypeptides encoded by these plasmids have been synthesized in an in vitro transcription translation system and the polypeptides were not immunoreactive with antiserum prepared against chlamydiae.[87]

The sequence of the 16S RNA genes of *Chlamydia psittaci* and *Chlamydia trachomatis* has been determined and there is only a 5 percent difference between the two species.[88] The sequence is similar to that of other eubacteria.

Wenman and Lovett were the first to succeed in cloning a chlamydial gene into *E. coli* and obtaining expression of an antigen.[89] Since then the MOMP genes of several serovars have been cloned. Chlamydial LPS has been successfully cloned into *E. coli* and is expressed in the outer membrane.[90] Because of its important structural and antigenic role the studies with the gene responsible for MOMP have been of particular interest. The amino acid sequence of MOMP is now known for serovars L1, L2, B, and C.[91,92] The L1 serovar MOMP contains 371 amino acids, whereas B and L2 contain 372 and C contains 375. The molecular weights fall between 39.5 and 40.5 kilodalton. MOMP genes encode a 22 amino acid leader (signal) peptide. There are five conserved and four variable domains within the structural genes; two of the variable sequences encode for hydrophilic segments. The most variable segments are approximately 11 amino acids long; one occurs in the amino terminal half, the other in the carboxyl terminal half of the MOMP. These variable domains may be responsible for subgroup or serovar-specific antigenic reactivity.

## PATHOGENESIS

The pathogenesis of any of the infections with *C. trachomatis* has not been elucidated. It is clear that lymphogranuloma venereum is a systemic infection involving lymphoid tissues. In vitro studies have shown the organisms are capable of replicating within macrophages.[93] To date all information suggests that non-LGV *C. trachomatis* strains have a very limited host range in vivo. They appear to be almost exclusively parasites of squamocolumnar-columnar epithelial cells. Because they are obligate intracellular parasites and kill host cells at the end stages of their growth cycle, these chlamydial strains must cause some cell damage where they persist. There is no in vivo evidence for latency in the sense of persistence of nonreplicating chlamydiae. The disease process and clinical manifestations of chlamydial infections probably represent the combined effects of tissue damage resulting from chlamydial replication as well as the inflammatory responses caused by the presence of chlamydiae and necrotic material from the destroyed host cells. There is an abundant immune response to chlamydial infection (in terms of circulating antibodies or cell-mediated responses) and there is now evidence that chlamydial diseases result in part from hypersensitivity or are diseases of immunopathology.[12,27,94] There must be some sort of protective immune response to the organisms, because chlamydial infections tend to follow a fairly self-limited acute course resolving into a low-grade persistent infection which may last for years. These infections may be activated by a variety of stimuli, of which steroids represent one class. Other reactivating agents also presumably exist.

LGV is a lymphoproliferative disease. Other chlamydiae appear to be capable of causing a localized lymphoproliferative response in the sense that they can induce follicle formation in the mucous membranes. Although such a response is most well known for the conjunctiva (trachoma and inclusion conjunctivitis), follicular cervicitis and probably follicular urethritis (cobblestone appearance of Waelsch urethritis) are recognized entities. Follicles induced by *C. trachomatis* are true lymphoid follicles with germinal centers.

Trachoma has long been considered a disease in which reinfection is important.[27] It has been speculated that hypersensitivity to chlamydial antigens contributed to disease severity. In vaccine trials, a deleterious outcome, followed inadequate vaccination, and more severe disease was seen after heterotypic infection.[12,27,95] Resistance to reinfection appears to be predominantly serovar-specific. Using nonhuman primates, Taylor and colleagues found that repeated (weekly) conjunctival instillation of *C. trachomatis* will result in a disease with many of the manifestations of trachoma, including conjunctival scarring.[96] Similarly, in an experimental salpingitis model, Patton and colleagues found that severe salpingitis in nonhuman primates was also in part dependent on previous exposure to chlamydiae.[97] A common pathologic end point of chlamydial infection is scarring of the affected mucous membranes. This is what ultimately leads to the blindness in trachoma and to the infertility and ectopic pregnancy after acute salpingitis.

In the guinea pig inclusion conjunctivitis (GPIC) model a triton-soluble extract of EBs induced an ocular hypersensitivity reaction if dropped onto the conjunctiva of previously infected, but not naive, animals.[98] The reactive material appears to be genus-specific as similar results were obtained when the same extract was dropped onto the eyes of nonhuman primates that had been infected with the trachoma agent.[99] The specific allergen for this ocular hypersensitivity reaction has not been identified. A clue has come from studies indicating that a sensitizing protein antigen of 57 kilodaltons is excreted into the supernate of GPIC-infected cells that have been treated with penicillin (Morrison and Caldwell, personal communication).

In animal models chlamydial infection induces lymphokines that may play a role in controlling the infection, and which could also contribute to pathologic consequences. Lymphokines can induce collagen deposition, collagenase production, and fibroblast proliferation. It is possible that they are involved in development of the scarring. Gamma interferon and interleukins can be found in the tears of children with trachoma (Rothermel and Schachter, unpublished).

There are no satisfactory animal models for genital *C. trachomatis* infection. Nonhuman primates are susceptible to ocular and genital infections with the trachoma biovar. Much has been learned about the pathogenesis and immunity in ocular infections. Data suggesting prior exposure are important in the poor outcome after oviduct infection has been obtained in this model.[97] Because of expense and difficulty in obtaining a large number of nonhuman primates, attempts have been made to develop models in smaller animals. The genital tract of female mice that have been treated with progesterone can be infected and ascending infections can result in salpingitis and infertility.[100] Some workers have attempted to exploit naturally occurring chlamydial infection in smaller animals. The *C. psittaci* guinea pig inclusion conjunctivitis agent and the mouse pneumonitis biovar of *C. trachomatis* are both capable of infecting genital tracts of their natural host.[5,6,101] They are sexually transmitted and can cause tubal factor infertility as a result of ascending infection in the female genital tract.[102,103]

## ANTIMICROBIAL SUSCEPTIBILITY

Growth of chlamydia in the laboratory is discussed fully in Chap. 74. There is no universally accepted protocol for testing antibiotic susceptibility of *C. trachomatis*. A number of different procedures have been used, and the data presented in Table 15-4 present the range of results obtained for inhibitory levels in tissue culture systems. The simplest procedures involve infection of cell culture with a standard inoculum followed by addition of an antibiotic-containing medium. After an appropriate incubation period inclusion counts are performed and the concentration of antibiotic resulting in 50 or 100 percent reduction in inclusion count is accepted as the minimum inhibitory concentration (MIC). This procedure tends to overestimate the activity of the drugs tested. A more rigorous test involves blind passage of inclusion negative monolayers in an effort to assure that the drugs in question actually killed the *Chlamydia*, and the minimum concentration where no inclusions are detected on passage is considered to be the minimal cidal level.[104] The most rigorous test of antimicrobial activity involves attempts to sterilize established infections in cell culture systems. In this system the tissue culture monolayers are infected with *C. trachomatis* for approximately 48 h and then different drug levels are added to the infected cell culture systems. After a subsequent 24 h incubation period, the cell cultures are washed and passed to determine whether chlamydiae have been eradicated. This procedure is likely to underestimate the effective levels of drugs in that the antibiotics are being added at a time after they would tend to be active [during active replication or metabolism (which peaks at less than 48 h)] and the technique

**Table 15-4. Minimum Inhibitory Concentration (MIC) of Antimicrobial Agents for *C. trachomatis***

| Drug | MIC, μg, or unit/ml |
|---|---|
| Rifampin | 0.005–0.25 |
| Rosaramycin | 0.025–0.25 |
| Tetracyclines | 0.03–1.0 |
| Erythromycin | 1–1.0 |
| Ofloxacin | 0.5–1.0 |
| Ampicillin | 0.5–10.0 |
| Penicillin | 1.0–10.0 |
| Sulfamethoxazole | 0.5–4.0 |
| Clindamycin | 2–16 |
| Spectinomycin | 32–100 |
| Gentamicin | 500 |
| Vancomycin | 1000 |

SOURCE: J Schachter.[26]

suffers from technical objections concerning potential carry-over of drugs into the second passage.

*Chlamydia trachomatis* is susceptible to sulfonamides.[1] The organisms produce their own folic acid and are susceptible to the action of the sulfonamides and to trimethoprim. Sulfonamides have been clinically effective in trachoma and lymphogranuloma venereum but are not used in treating most genital tract infections with *Chlamydia* because these drugs are not active against other organisms producing similar diseases.[26] Tetracyclines and erythromycin are generally considered the drugs of choice in managing chlamydial genital tract infections. The organisms are highly susceptible in vitro and in vivo to the action of the antibiotics.[26,104] Resistance to these drugs has never been shown to occur naturally. Although there are documented treatment failures where chlamydiae have been isolated from patients following treatment, the recovered agents have been found to be wholly susceptible to the antibiotics. There is a suggestion that relative resistance to erythromycin has been developing, but there are no data to suggest that this has reached clinically relevant levels.[105] Rifampin, which is highly active in vitro, has not been widely used to treat human chlamydial infections. Resistance to this drug can be readily developed by passage in the laboratory in the presence of low concentrations of the antibiotic.[106]

Aminoglycosides are not active against *Chlamydia,* and this has led to their widespread use in controlling bacterial contamination in clinical specimens being tested for the presence of *Chlamydia.* Common antifungal drugs such as amphotericin B and nystatin are also inactive against *Chlamydia,* as are the nitroimidazoles used to treat *Trichomonas* infections.

Penicillins are active against *Chlamydia* in vitro but they are not clinically useful. By analogy from animal studies it has been calculated that levels on the order of 20 to 30 million units of penicillin per day would be required for antichlamydial activity in vivo. Cephalosporins are not active. *Chlamydia* do have a bacterialike cell wall, and its synthesis can be inhibited by penicillins, but only in the early phases of the growth cycle. Addition of penicillins to infected cells in vitro cannot be expected to show marked activity after 16 to 20 h of infection, as at that stage active cell wall synthesis is minimal. It is likely that one of the cell wall inhibitors will be found to be clinically active against chlamydiae. Quinolones are active in vitro and some of them undoubtedly will be clinically useful.

## IMMUNOLOGY

There is little knowledge concerning the structure and chemistry of chlamydial antigens.[107] The biological role of antibodies or cell-mediated immunity, resulting from exposure to chlamydial antigens, in either enhancing or protecting against disease or infection is not yet clear. Much of the difficulty in studying chlamydial antigens is due to technical problems in obtaining adequate quantities of organisms required for the physicochemical fractionation procedures that are commonly used to study antigenic structure. Thus, these organisms are ideal candidates for study by modern techniques of molecular biology and genetics. What is clear is that *Chlamydia* are highly complex organisms which contain antigens of genus, species, subspecies, and serovar specificity.[107]

The most easily detected antigen is the chlamydial group antigen, shared by all members of the genus. This antigen is responsible for the complement-fixing reactions that have been commonly used to diagnose psittacosis or lymphogranuloma venereum. The group antigen is heat-stable and periodate-sensitive and can be extracted from infected tissues with ether or detergents such as sodium lauryl sulfate or sodium deoxycholate. Dhir and colleagues isolated a large water-soluble polysaccharide (ca. $10^6$ molecular weight) by alkaline hydrolysis of partially purified group antigen.[108] The reactive moiety was found to be a ketodeoxyoctanoic acid. Other, apparently protein, group antigens have been identified but have not been characterized. The major genus-specific antigen has been identified as lipopolysaccharide (LPS).[109]

Chlamydial EBs and RBs contain an LPS antigenically similar to that of other gram-negative bacteria. It demonstrates a positive limulus lysate test. It is structurally similar to the lipid A and KDO core of LPS from rough (Re) mutants of *Salmonella typhimurium.*[110] The chemical composition of the chlamydial LPS is also similar to that of *Salmonella typhimurium* LPS but appears to contain a unique constituent, 3-hydroxydocosanoic acid.[111]

Chlamydial LPS has two antigen sites. One is identical to that of the other bacteria, and the other is *Chlamydia*-specific.[112] *Acinetobacter calcoaceticus* LPS can be used as the CF antigen for antichlamydial antibodies, but not all sera positive against the chlamydial antigen will react to the *Acinetobacter* LPS.[110]

The antigens responsible for delayed hypersensitivity tests, such as the Frei test, which has been used in diagnosing lymphogranuloma venereum, have not been studied using modern techniques. The major antigen here is probably the LPS common group antigen because it is heat-stable and sensitive to periodate. *C. psittaci* strains have been used successfully to prepare Frei antigens. There also appear to be specific antigens involved in delayed hypersensitivity responses, as more specific antigenic preparations could be prepared by acid extraction from the crude group antigen.

Species-specific antigens appear to be shared by all members of a chlamydial species. They are probably membrane-associated. They have been demonstrated by indirect hemagglutination, immunodiffusion with sonicated organisms, and crossed immunoelectrophoresis with solubilized organisms. One of these species-specific antigens has been purified to homogeneity by immunoabsorption with monospecific antibody.[113] It is common to *C. trachomatis,* pronase, and heat-sensitive, and of large molecular weight ($1.55 \times 10^5$ daltons). Antibody to this antigen is found in convalescent human sera from patients with lymphogranuloma venereum or those with high levels of antibody following other *C. trachomatis* infections.

The subspecies or serovar-specific antigens are common only to selected strains within chlamydial species. These antigens have been the basis for a variety of serologic tests used for the classification of *C. trachomatis* isolates. They appear to be associated with the mortality observed following intravenous inoculation of mice with large quantities of viable chlamydiae. This death is termed a "toxic death" because it cannot be accounted for by multiplication of the organism; deaths occur within 24 h, before a single cycle of replication can occur. The "toxic" effect of chlamydiae can be prevented by preincubation of the inoculum with hyperimmune serum. This "toxin" neutralization is strain-specific and was first used to classify a variety of *C. psittaci* isolates.[114] A similar approach was used with *C. trachomatis* isolates, and it was found that immunization of mice could prevent lethality from homotypic toxic challenge. A mouse toxicity prevention test (MTPT) was developed which yielded a number of specific *C. trachomatis* serovars.[115,116] These serovars are identical to those shown by the microimmunofluorescence test (micro-IF).[117] The responsible antigens appear to be on the MOMP molecule.

To date 15 serovars of *C. trachomatis* have been identified.[32] A, B, and C serovars are usually associated with hyperendemic blinding trachoma in developing countries; D through K have been associated with oculogenital disease in industrialized societies, and L1, L2, and L3 are LGV serotypes. These serotypes fall into two broad complexes (B and C) by micro-IF. Each complex shows extensive cross reaction within the complex but little reaction with the other complex. Serovar-specific monoclonal antibodies are now available for typing purposes.

It is likely that immunity to infection, although relatively weak, is dependent upon the serovar-specific surface antigens. Although conflicting results have been obtained concerning the nature and properties of these antigens, it is likely that some disparate results reflect the use of crude chlamydial preparations in the assays. Sacks and MacDonald have identified a type-specific antigen from *C. trachomatis* serotype A and shown it to be a heat-labile, pronase-sensitive, surface antigen with an apparent subunit molecular weight of 27,000 daltons.[62]

MOMP appears to contain epitopes of serovar, serogroup, and species specificity.[118–120] Minor genus-specific reactivity has also been shown. MOMP and the other two proteins of 60 and 12 to 15 kilodaltons may be copurified by sarkosyl extraction of EBs. The 60- to 62-kilodalton proteins are important immunogens and are often found as a doublet.[121] While MOMP appears to be the immunodominant antigen, there may be a more selective response to 60- to 62-kilodalton proteins. The 60-kilodalton proteins are surface-exposed and have species-specific antigens. In contrast, the 15-kilodalton proteins are not on the EB surface. They contain antigens of species and biovar specificity.[122] Monoclonal antibodies directed against MOMP are neutralizing in cell culture and protective against toxic effects after intravenous inoculation of mice with live EBs. They can also neutralize infectivity for ocular infection in subhuman primates.[123] Monoclonal antibodies against nonsurface subspecies or species-specific epitopes or against the LPS neither protected mice nor neutralized infectivity for the eye. The neutralization reactions appear to be serovar- or serogroup-specific.[124]

The outer membrane of *Chlamydia* is a particularly interesting structure because in the EB it represents a target for immune attack. A number of functions have been identified with putative protective antigens in the outer membrane. Factors such as specific attachment, enhanced phagocytosis, and phagolysosomal fusion inhibition are all neutralized by specific antibody. Although a number of protein antigens have been identified and MOMP has been shown to induce a neutralizing antibody, no virulence antigen has been specifically identified.

## CONTROL OF CHLAMYDIAL INFECTION BY THE HOST

In the majority of chlamydial infections only a relatively small proportion of cells at affected sites are infected. Because each inclusion releases hundreds of viable EBs and relatively few nearby cells are infected, there must be control mechanisms that limit infectivity. The mechanisms are not clear. Lymphokines have been shown to have an inhibitory effect on chlamydiae.[125] *Chlamydia trachomatis* is sensitive to alpha, beta, and gamma interferons.[126] The lymphokine which inhibits *Chlamydia* in human macrophages and in mice has been identified as gamma interferon.[127,128] Interferon delays the developmental cycle so that the RBs persist longer.[129,130] This may result in persistent inapparent infection and may also play a role in immunopathogenesis. The mode of action appears to be the same as in other systems, involving depletion of tryptophan, making it unavailable to the chlamydiae.[131] The effect is reversible by addition of exogenous tryptophan. It is likely that mechanisms such as the apparent effect of gamma interferon represent control of infection rather than protection against new infection. They may be involved in clearance. It is possible that neutralizing antibody plays a role, but the mechanism by which neutralizing antibody would act is not known. Antibody against MOMP has been shown to neutralize infectivity, but surprisingly it did not interfere with chlamydial attachment, ingestion, or inhibition of phagolysosomal fusion.[41]

## IMMUNITY

Immunity induced by chlamydial infection is not well understood. It is clear that single infections will not result in solid immunity to reinfection. Multiple infections, homo- or heterotypic, are common. Unfortunately, the natural infection is not readily quantifiable in terms of inoculum size and thus relative degrees of immunity may exist which are overcome with a sufficiently large challenge. Some immunity probably develops following initial or serial infection. In screening studies, younger women have higher cervical infection rates than older women; older women also have higher antibody levels on average. Many culture-negative individuals attending STD clinics have IgM antibody to the organism.[132] This antibody could result from recent exposure and rapid resolution of the infection or its ablation by an immune response.

The only human chlamydial infection which has been subjected to extensive vaccine studies is trachoma. Unfortunately these studies were performed without a sophisticated knowledge of the chlamydial immune response. These results have been summarized elsewhere.[12,27] The results from field studies on vaccine trials and infection of human volunteers and subhuman primates indicate that there is a short-lived relative immunity by reinfection with homotypic challenge. More severe disease may result from heterotypic infection, which may also follow vaccination with a poor (i.e., nonprotective) immunogen.

Data from ocular infection with *C. psittaci* in guinea pigs and *C. trachomatis* in subhuman primates suggest an important role for antibody in host defense.[133–135] There are many possible modes of action. Antibody is capable of neutralizing chlamydial infectivity in cell culture. It may inhibit attachment of the organism to the surface of a nonprofessional phagocyte, or result in failure to inhibit phagolysosomal fusion. It may prevent a morphologic shift of the EBs and RBs by cross-linking surface proteins. Antibody that blocks attachment of *C. psittaci* to L cells will enhance attachment to macrophages.[136]

*Chlamydia* do not appear to survive well in polymorphonuclear leukocytes (PMN).[137] It is possible that antibody-enhanced phagocytosis plays an important role in clearance of infection and in resistance to reinfection. *Chlamydia* are rapidly internalized by human PMNs, and the majority are rendered noninfectious within 1 h. Most of the EBs are found in PMN phagosomes where lysosomal fusion has occurred.[138] The mechanism of killing by PMNs is not known, but it is likely that oxygen-dependent and -independent mechanisms are involved. Killing is still seen in the presence of inhibitors such as azide or cyanide.[137] Both species of chlamydiae act as polyclonal stimulators of B lymphocytes.[139] Stimulation can be effected in mice that are LPS nonresponders, suggesting that something other than the genus-specific antigen is responsible.

Lymphocytes clearly play an important role in resistance to infection and in clearance of primary infection. T-cell-deficient mice do not produce significant levels of antichlamydial antibody.[140] Lymphocyte transformation, in vitro, and delayed-type hypersensitivity reactions are also T-cell-dependent. They can be found in heterozygous mice and in mice who received thymus transplants but are not observed in the nude athymic mouse.[141,142]

Williams and colleagues have exploited the nude (athymic) mouse model of respiratory infection with the mouse pneumonitis biovar of *C. trachomatis* to dissect the immune response.[140,142–144] Results of these studies have suggested a defense role for both antibody and CMI responses.

## VACCINE AND VIRULENCE FACTORS

Because the responsible surface antigens would be likely vaccine candidates, efforts to identify the factors responsible for attachment, enhanced uptake, and inhibition of phagolysosomal fusion will continue to be stressed. All evidence to date suggests that MOMP must be an extremely important antigen in some of these activities. Inhibition of these virulence determinants appears to be serovar-specific. The only antigenic sites of that specificity that have been clearly identified are on MOMP. A likely alternative approach to vaccine development will be to use information obtained from sequence analysis of the MOMP genes to synthesize peptides reflecting the variable (presumed serovar-specific) sites on the protein.[91] Because these variable sequences are fairly short, approximately 11 amino acids long, their synthesis should be relatively easy. Incorporation of the synthetic peptides into appropriate carriers could allow development of experimental vaccines and tools for identifying virulence factors.

The importance of T cells in immunity appears to be a recurring theme. Both humoral and CMI responses are T-cell-dependent. Identification of specific T cell recognition sites on the EB surface (or on MOMP) may be crucial to understanding chlamydial immunity, particularly because they may not be the antigenic epitopes.

A real problem with vaccine development will be generating immune responses that appear to be better than those that occur after natural infection. While much progress is being made on the microbiologic front, particularly in cloning the MOMP genes and identifying the potential antigenic sites, it is clear that considerable input from immunologists will be required to generate optimal methods for antigen presentation to enhance mucous-membrane immunity.

## References


1 Moulder JW et al: Order II. Chlamydiales Storz and Page 1971, in *Bergey's Manual of Systematic Bacteriology,* NR Krieg, JG Holt (eds). Baltimore, Williams and Wilkins, 1984, vol 1, pp 729–739.

2 Meyer KF: The host spectrum of psittacosis-lymphogranuloma venereum (PL) agents. *Am J Ophthalmol* 63:1225, 1967.

3 Grayston JT et al: A new *Chlamydia psittaci* strain, TWAR, isolated in acute respiratory tract infections. *N Engl J Med* 315:161, 1986.

4 Campbell LA et al: Characterization of new *Chlamydia* agent, TWAR, as a unique organism by restriction endonuclease analysis and DNA-DNA hybridization. *J Clin Microbiol* 25:1911, 1987.

5 Murray ES: Guinea pig inclusion conjunctivitis virus. I. Isolation and identification as a member of the psittacosis-lymphogranuloma-trachoma group. *J Infect Dis* 114:1, 1964.

6 Mount DT et al: Experimental genital infection of male guinea pigs with the agent of guinea pig inclusion conjunctivitis and transmission to females. *Infect Immun* 8:925, 1973.

7 Moulder JW: Intracellular parasitism: Life in an extreme environment. *J Infect Dis* 130:300, 1974.

8 Byrne GI: Requirements of ingestion of *Chlamydia psittaci* by mouse fibroblasts (L cells). *Infect Immun* 14:645, 1976.

9 Friis RR: Interaction of L cells and *Chlamydia psittaci:* Entry of the parasite and host responses to its development. *J Bacteriol* 110:706, 1972.

10 Levy NJ: Wheat germ agglutinin blockage of chlamydial attachment sites: Antagonism by N-acetyl-D-glycosamine. *Infect Immun* 25: 946, 1979.

11 Kuo CC et al: Effect of polycations, polyanions and neuraminidase on the infectivity of trachoma-inclusion conjunctivitis and lymphogranuloma venereum organisms in HeLa cells: Sialic acid residues as possible receptors for trachoma-inclusion conjunctivitis. *Infect Immun* 8:74, 1973.

12 Schachter J, Dawson CR: *Human Chlamydial Infections.* Littleton, PSG Publishing Co, 1978, p 273.

13 Lindner K: Gonoblennorrhoe, einschlussblennorrhoe und trachoma. *Graefes Arch Clin Exp Ophthalmol* 78:380, 1911.

14 T'ang FF et al: Trachoma virus in chick embryo. *Natl Med J China* 43:81, 1957.

15 Jones BR et al: Isolation of virus from inclusion blennorrhoea. *Lancet* 1:902, 1959.

16 Jones BR: Ocular syndromes of TRIC virus infection and their possible genital significance. *Br J Vener Dis* 40:3, 1964.

17 Rose L, Schachter J: Genitourinary aspects of inclusion conjunctivitis. *Invest Ophthalmol* 3:680, 1964.

18 Dunlop EMC et al: Relation of TRIC agent to "non-specific" genital infection. *Br J Vener Dis* 42:77, 1966.

19 Dunlop EMC et al: Infections by TRIC agent and other members of the Bedsonia group with a note on Reiter's disease: III. Genital infection and diseases of the eye. *Trans Ophthalmol Soc UK* 86:321, 1966.

20 Dunlop EMC et al: Genital infection in association with TRIC virus infection of the eye. III. Clinical and other findings. Preliminary report. *Br J Vener Dis* 40:33, 1964.

21 Gordon FB, Quan AL: Isolation of the trachoma agent in cell culture. *Proc Soc Exp Biol Med* 118:354, 1965.

22 Darougar S et al: Chlamydial infection: Advances in the diagnostic isolation of *Chlamydia*, including TRIC agent, from the eye, genital tract and rectum. *Br J Vener Dis* 48:416, 1972.

23 Oriel JD et al: Chlamydial infection: Isolation of *Chlamydia* from patients with nonspecific genital infection. *Br J Vener Dis* 131:376, 1975.

24 Richmond SJ et al: Chlamydial infection: Role of *Chlamydia* subgroup A in nongonococcal and postgonococcal urethritis. *Br J Vener Dis* 48:437, 1972.
25 Dunlop EMC et al: Isolation of *Chlamydia* from the urethra of a woman. *Br Med J* 2:386, 1972.
26 Schachter J: Chlamydial infections. *N Engl J Med* 298:428, 490, 540, 1978.
27 Grayston JT, Wang SP: New knowledge of chlamydiae and the diseases they cause. *J Infect Dis* 132:87, 1975.
28 Schachter J et al: Prospective study of perinatal transmission of *Chlamydia trachomatis. JAMA* 255:3374, 1986.
29 Jones BR: The prevention of blindness from trachoma. *Trans Ophthalmol Soc UK* 95:16, 1975.
30 Treharne JD: The community of epidemiology of trachoma. *Rev Infect Dis* 7:760, 1985.
31 Kuo C-C et al: Immunotypes of *Chlamydia trachomatis* isolates in Seattle, Washington. *Infect Immun* 41:865, 1983.
32 Barnes RC et al: Rapid immunotyping of *Chlamydia trachomatis* with monoclonal antibodies in a solid-phase enzyme immunoassay. *J Clin Microbiol* 22:609, 1985.
33 Moulder JW: The relation of the psittacosis group (chlamydiae) to bacteria and viruses. *Annu Rev Microbiol* 20:107, 1966.
34 Weiss E: Comparative metabolism of rickettsia and other host dependent bacteria. *Zentralb Bakteriol* 206:292, 1968.
35 Kellog KR et al: Toxicity of low and moderate multiplicities of *Chlamydia psittaci* for mouse fibroblasts (L cells). *Infect Immun* 18:531, 1977.
36 Byrne GI, Moulder JW: Parasite-specified phagocytosis of *Chlamydia psittaci* and *Chlamydia trachomatis* by L and HeLa cells. *Infect Immun* 19:598, 1978.
37 Lee CK: Interaction between a trachoma strain of *Chlamydia trachomatis* and mouse fibroblasts (McCoy cells) in the absence of centrifugation. *Infect Immun* 31:584, 1981.
38 Becker Y: The Chlamydia: Molecular biology of procaryotic obligate parasites of eucaryocytes. *Microbiol Rev* 42:274, 1978.
39 Hatch TP et al: Attachment of *Chlamydia psittaci* to formaldehyde-fixed and unfixed L cells. *J Gen Microbiol* 125:273, 1981.
40 Hackstadt T, Caldwell HD: Effect of proteolytic cleavage of surface-exposed proteins on infectivity of *Chlamydia trachomatis. Infect Immun* 48:372, 1985.
41 Caldwell HD, Perry LJ: Neutralization of *Chlamydia trachomatis* infectivity with antibodies to the major outer membrane protein. *Infect Immun* 38:745, 1982.
42 Peeling R et al: In vitro neutralization of *Chlamydia trachomatis* with monoclonal antibody to an epitope on the major outer membrane protein. *Infect Immun* 46:484, 1984.
43 Moulder JW: Comparative biology of intracellular parasitism. *Microbiol Rev* 49:298, 1985.
44 Hodinka RL, Wyrick PB: Ultrastructural study of mode of entry of *Chlamydia psittaci* into L-929 cells. *Infect Immun* 54:855, 1986.
45 Ward ME, Murray A: Control mechanisms governing the infectivity of *Chlamydia trachomatis* for HeLa cells: Mechanisms of endocytosis. *J Gen Microbiol* 130:1765, 1984.
46 Eissenberg LG et al: *Chlamydia psittaci* elementary body envelopes: Ingestion and inhibition of phagolysosome fusion. *Infect Immun* 40:741, 1983.
47 Brownridge EA, Wyrick PB: Interaction of *Chlamydia psittaci* reticulate bodies with mouse peritoneal macrophages. *Infect Immun* 24:697, 1979.
48 Eissenberg LG, Wyrick PB: Inhibition of phagolysosome fusion is limited to *Chlamydia psittaci*-laden vacuoles. *Infect Immun* 32:889, 1981.
49 Hatch TP et al: Adenine nucleotide and lysine transport in *Chlamydia psittaci. J Bacteriol* 150:662, 1982.
50 Doughri AM et al: Mode of entry and release of chlamydiae in infections of intestinal epithelial cells. *J Infect Dis* 126:652, 1972.
51 Matsumoto A, Manire GP: Electron microscopic observations on the fine structure of cell walls of *Chlamydia psittaci. J Bacteriol* 104:1332, 1970.
52 Garrett AJ et al: A search for the bacterial mucopeptide component, muramic acid, in *Chlamydia. J Gen Microbiol* 80:315, 1974.
53 Matsumoto A, Manire GP: Electron microscopic observations on the effects of penicillin on the morphology of *Chlamydia psittaci. J Bacteriol* 101:278, 1970.
54 Caldwell HD et al: Purification and partial characterization of the major outer membrane protein of *Chlamydia trachomatis. Infect Immun* 31:1161, 1981.
55 Salari SH, Ward ME: Polypeptide composition of *Chlamydia trachomatis. J Gen Microbiol* 123:197, 1981.
56 Hatch TP et al: Structural and polypeptide differences between envelopes of infective and reproductive life cycle forms of *Chlamydia. J Bacteriol* 157:13, 1984.
57 Newhall WJ, Jones RB: Disulfide-linked oligomers of the major outer membrane protein of *Chlamydia. J Bacteriol* 154:998, 1983.
58 Newhall WJ: Biosynthesis and disulfide cross-linking of outer membrane components during the growth cycle of *Chlamydia trachomatis. Infect Immun* 55:162, 1987.
59 Hatch TP et al: Synthesis of disulfide-bonded outer membrane proteins during the developmental cycle of *Chlamydia psittaci* and *Chlamydia trachomatis. J Bacteriol* 165:379, 1986.
60 Bavoil P et al: Role of disulfide bonding in outer membrane structure and permeability in *Chlamydia trachomatis. Infect Immun* 44:479, 1984.
61 Hackstadt et al: Disulfide-mediated interaction of chlamydial major outer membrane protein: Role in the differentiation of chlamydiae? *J Bacteriol* 161:25, 1985.
62 Sacks DL, MacDonald AB: Isolation of a type-specific antigen from *Chlamydia trachomatis* by sodium dodecyl sulfate polyacrylamide gel electrophoresis. *J Immunol* 122:136, 1979.
63 Jenkin HM et al: Species-specific antigens from the cell walls of the agents of meningopneumonitis and felinepneumonitis. *J Immunol* 86:123, 1961.
64 Pelc SR, Crocker TT: Differences in utilization of labelled precursors for the synthesis of deoxyribonucleic acid in cell nuclei and psittacosis virus. *Biochem J* 78:1, 1961.
65 Lin H-S: Inhibition of thymidine kinase activity and deoxyribonucleic acid synthesis in L cells infected with the meningopneumonitis agent. *J Bacteriol* 96:2054, 1968.
66 Gregory WM et al: Arrays of hemispheric surface projections on *Chlamydia psittaci* and *Chlamydia trachomatis* observed by scanning electron microscopy. *J Bacteriol* 138:241, 1979.
67 Barbour AG et al: *Chlamydia trachomatis* has penicillin-binding proteins but not detectable muramic acid. *J Bacteriol* 151:420, 1982.
68 Moulder JW et al: Inhibition of the growth of agents of the psittacosis group by D-cycloserine and its specific reversal by D-alanine. *J Bacteriol* 85:707, 1963.
69 Kuo CC et al: Primary isolation of TRIC organisms in HeLa 229 cells treated with DEAE-dextran. *J Infect Dis* 125:665, 1972.
70 Weiss E, Dressler HR: Centrifugation of rickettsiae and viruses onto cells and its effect on infection. *Proc Soc Exp Biol Med* 103:691, 1960.
71 Wentworth BB, Alexander ER: Isolation of *Chlamydia trachomatis* by use of 5-iodo-2-deoxyuridine-treated cells. *Appl Microbiol* 27:912, 1974.
72 Ripa KT, Mardh PA: New simplified culture technique for *Chlamydia trachomatis,* in *Nongonococcal Urethritis and Related Infections,* KK Holmes, D Hobson (eds). Washington, DC, American Society for Microbiology, 1977, p 323.
73 Bader JP, Morgan HR: Latent viral infections of cells in culture. VI. Role of amino acids, glucose, and glutamine in psittacosis virus propagation in L cells. *J Exp Med* 106:617, 1958.
74 Hatch TP: Competition between *Chlamydia psittaci* and L cells for host isoleucine pools: A limiting factor in chlamydial multiplication. *Infect Immun* 12:211, 1975.
75 Allan I, Pearce JH: Amino acid requirements of strains of *C. trachomatis* and *C. psittaci* growing in McCoy cells: Relationship with clinical syndrome and host origin. *J Gen Microbiol* 129:2001, 1983.
76 Stirling P et al: Interference with transformation of chlamydiae from

productive to infective body forms by deprivation of cysteine. *FEMS Microbiol Lett* 19:133, 1983.

77 Hatch TP et al: Synthesis of protein in host-free reticulate bodies of *Chlamydia psittaci* and *Chlamydia trachomatis*. *J Bacteriol* 162:938, 1985.

78 Weiss E, Wilson NN: Role of exogeneous adenosine triphosphate in catabolic and synthetic activities of *Chlamydia psittaci*. *J Bacteriol* 97:719, 1969.

79 Ward ME, Salari H: Control mechanisms governing the infectivity of *Chlamydia trachomatis* for HeLA cells—Modulation of cyclic nucleotides, prostoglandins and calcium. *J Gen Microbiol* 128(part 3):639, 1982.

80 Kaul R, Wenman WM: Cyclic AMP inhibits developmental regulation of *Chlamydia trachomatis*. *J Bacteriol* 168:722, 1986.

81 Bose SK, Goswami PC: Enhancement of adherence and growth of *Chlamydia trachomatis* by estrogen treatment of HeLa cells. *Infect Immun* 53:646, 1986.

82 Moses EB et al: Enhancement of growth of the chlamydial agent of guinea pig inclusion conjunctivitis in HeLa cells by estradiol. *Curr Microbiol* 11:265, 1984.

83 Kingsbury DT, Weiss E: Lack of deoxyribonucleic acid homology between species of the genus *Chlamydia*. *J Bacteriol* 96:1421, 1968.

84 Kingsbury DT: Estimate of the genome size of various microorganisms. *J Bacteriol* 98:1400, 1979.

85 Peterson EM, de la Maza LM: Characterization of DNA by restriction of endonuclease cleavage. *Infect Immun* 41:604, 1983.

86 Palmer L, Falkow S: A common plasmid of *Chlamydia trachomatis*. *Plasmid* 16:52, 1986.

87 Joseph T et al: Molecular characterization of *Chlamydia trachomatis* and *Chlamydia psittaci* plasmids. *Infect Immun* 51:699, 1968.

88 Weisburg WG et al: Eubacterial origin of chlamydiae. *J Bacteriol* 167:570, 1986.

89 Wenman WM, Lovett MA: Expression in *E. coli* of *Chlamydia trachomatis* antigen recognized during human infection. *Nature* 296: 68, 1982.

90 Nano FE, Caldwell HD: Expression of chlamydial genus-specific lipopolysaccharide epitope in *Escherichia coli*. *Science* 228:742, 1985.

91 Stephens RS et al: Diversity of *Chlamydia trachomatis* major outer membrane protein genes. *J Bacteriol* 169:3879, 1987.

92 Pickett MA: Complete nucleotide sequence of the major outer membrane protein gene from *Chlamydia trachomatis* serovar L1. *FEMS Microbiol Lett* 42:185, 1987.

93 Kuo C-C: Cultures of *Chlamydia trachomatis* in mouse peritoneal macrophages: Factors affecting organism growth. *Infect Immun* 20:439, 1978.

94 Hanna L et al: Human cell-mediated immune response to chlamydial antigens. *Infect Immun* 23:412, 1979.

95 Grayston JT: Trachoma vaccine, in *International Conference on the Application of Vaccines against Viral, Rickettsial, and Bacterial Diseases of Man*. Washington, DC, Pan American Health Organization, 1971, p 311.

96 Taylor HR et al: An animal model of trachoma: II. The importance of repeated infection. *Invest Ophthalmol Vis Sci* 23:507, 1982.

97 Patton DL et al: Distal tubal obstruction induced by repeated *Chlamydia trachomatis* salpingeal infections in pig-tailed macaques. *J Infect Dis* 155:1292, 1987.

98 Watkins NG et al: Ocular delayed hypersensitivity: A pathogenic mechanism of chlamydial conjunctivitis in guinea pigs. *Proc Natl Acad Sci USA* 83:7480, 1986.

99 Taylor HR et al: Pathogenesis of trachoma: The stimulus for inflammation. *J Immunol* 138:3023, 1987.

100 Tuffrey M et al: Infertility in mice infected genitally with a human strain of *Chlamydia trachomatis*. *J Reprod Fertil* 78:251, 1986.

101 Barron AL et al: Immune response in mice infected in the genital tract with mouse pneumonitis agent (*Chlamydia trachomatis* biovar). *Infect Immun* 44:82, 1984.

102 Schachter J et al: Hydrosalpinx as a consequence of chlamydial salpingitis in the guinea pig, in *Chlamydial Infections*, P-A Mårdh, KK Holmes, JD Oriel, P Piot, J Schachter (eds). Amsterdam, Elsevier, 1982, p 371.

103 Swensen CE et al: *Chlamydia trachomatis* induced salpingitis in mice. *J Infect Dis* 148:1101, 1983.

104 Ridgway GL et al: A method for testing antibiotic susceptibility of *Chlamydia trachomatis* in a cell culture system. *J Antimicrob Chemother* 2:71, 1976.

105 Mourad A et al: Relative resistance to erythromycin in *Chlamydia trachomatis*. *Antimicrob Agents Chemother* 18:696, 1980.

106 Schachter J: Rifampin in Chlamydia infections. *Rev Infect Dis* 5(suppl 3):S562, 1983.

107 Schachter J, Caldwell HD: Chlamydiae. *Annu Rev Microbiol* 34: 285, 1980.

108 Dhir SP et al: Immunochemical studies on chlamydial group antigen (presence of a 2-keto-3-deoxycarbonate as immunodominant group). *J Immunol* 109:116, 1972.

109 Nurminen M et al: The genus-specific antigen of *Chlamydia:* Resemblance to the lipopolysaccharide of enteric bacteria. *Science* 220:1279, 1983.

110 Nurminen M et al: Immunologically related ketodeoxyoctonate-containing structures in *Chlamydia trachomatis*, Re mutants of *Salmonella* species, and *Acinetobacter calcoaceticus* var. *anitratus*. *Infect Immun* 44:609, 1984.

111 Nurminen M et al: Chemical characterization of *Chlamydia trachomatis* lipopolysaccharide. *Infect Immun* 48:573, 1985.

112 Brade L et al: Antigenic properties of *Chlamydia trachomatis* lipopolysaccharides. *Infect Immun* 48:569, 1985.

113 Caldwell HD et al: Antigen analysis of chlamydiae by two dimensional immunoelectrophoresis: II. A trachoma-LGV specific antigen. *J Immunol* 115:969, 1975.

114 Manire GP, Meyer KF: The toxins of the psittacosis-lymphogranuloma group of agents: III. Differentiation of strains by the toxin neutralization test. *J Infect Dis* 86:241, 1950.

115 Bell SD et al: Immunization of mice against toxic doses of homologous elementary bodies of trachoma. *Science* 130:626, 1959.

116 Alexander ER et al: Further classification of TRIC agents from ocular trachoma and other sources of the mouse toxicity prevention test. *Am J Ophthalmol* 63:1469, 1967.

117 Wang SP, Grayston JT: Immunologic relationship between genital TRIC, lymphogranuloma venereum and related organisms in a new microtiter indirect immunofluorescence test. *Am J Ophthalmol* 70:367, 1970.

118 Caldwell HD, Schachter J: Antigenic analysis of the major outer membrane protein of *Chlamydia* spp. *Infect Immun* 35:1024, 1982.

119 Stephens RS et al: Monoclonal antibodies to *Chlamydia trachomatis:* Antibody specificities and antigen characterization. *J Immunol* 128:1083, 1982.

120 Batteiger BE et al: Antigenic analysis of the major outer membrane protein of *Chlamydia trachomatis* with murine monoclonal antibodies. *Infect Immun* 53:530, 1986.

121 Newhall WJ et al: Analysis of the human serological response to protein of *Chlamydia trachomatis*. *Infect Immun* 38:1181, 1982.

122 Zhang X-Y et al: The low-molecular-mass, cystein-rich outer membrane protein of *Chlamydia trachomatis* possesses both biovar- and species-specific epitopes. *Infect Immun* 55:2570, 1987.

123 Zhang X-Y et al: Protective monoclonal antibodies recognize epitopes located on the outer membrane protein of *Chlamydia trachomatis*. *J Immunol* 138:575, 1987.

124 Lucero ME, Kuo C-C: Neutralization of *Chlamydia trachomatis* cell culture infection by serovar-specific monoclonal antibodies. *Infect Immun* 50:595, 1985.

125 Byrne GI, Faubion CL: Lymphokine-mediated microblastic mechanisms restrict *Chlamydia psittaci* growth in macrophages. *J Immunol* 128:469, 1982.

126 Czarniecki CW et al: Interferon-induced inhibition of *Chlamydia trachomatis:* Dissociation from other biological activities of interferons, in *Interferons as Cell Growth Inhibitors and Antitumor Factors*. New York, Alan R Liss, 1986, p 467.

127 Rothermel CD et al: Gamma interferon is the factor in lymphokine

that activates human macrophages to inhibit intracellular *Chlamydia psittaci* replication. *J Immunol* 131:2542, 1983.

128 Byrne GI, Kreuger DA: Lymphokine-mediated inhibition of Chlamydia replication in mouse fibroblasts is neutralized by anti-gamma interferon immunoglobulin. *Infect Immun* 42:1152, 1983.

129 Rothermel CD: *Chlamydia* and human monocytes: Relationship between parasite growth and host cell differentiation, in *Abstracts of the Annual Meeting of the American Society for Microbiology 1985*. Washington, DC, American Society for Microbiology, 1985, p 30 (abstract B75).

130 Shemer Y, Sarov I: Inhibition of growth of *Chlamydia trachomatis* by human gamma interferon. *Infect Immun* 48:592, 1985.

131 Byrne GI et al: Introduction of tryptophan catabolism is the mechanism for gamma-interferon-mediated inhibition of intracellular *Chlamydia psittaci* replication. *Infect Immun* 53:347, 1986.

132 Philip RN et al: Fluorescent antibody responses to chlamydial infection in patients with lymphogranuloma venereum and urethritis. *J Immunol* 112:2126, 1974.

133 Ahmad A et al: Resistance to reinfection with a chlamydial agent (guinea pig inclusion conjunctivitis agent). *Invest Ophthalmol Vis Sci* 16:549, 1977.

134 Barenfanger J, MacDonald AB: The role of immunoglobulin in the neutralization of trachoma infectivity. *J Immunol* 113:1607, 1974.

135 Rank RG, Barron AL: Humoral immune response in acquired immunity to chlamydial genital infection of female guinea pigs. *Infect Immun* 39:463, 1983.

136 Gardner M: Differences between the interaction of *Chlamydia psittaci* (6BC) with professional (mouse macrophages) and nonprofessional (mouse fibroblasts) phagocytes, in *Abstracts of the Annual Meeting of the American Society for Microbiology 1977*. Washington, DC, American Society for Microbiology, 1977, abstract D6.

137 Yong EC et al: Toxic effects of human polymorphonuclear leukocytes on *Chlamydia trachomatis*. *Infect Immun* 37:422, 1982.

138 Yong EC et al: Degradation of *Chlamydia trachomatis* in human polymorphonuclear leukocytes: An ultrastructural study of peroxidase-positive phagolysosomes. *Infect Immun* 53:427, 1986.

139 Levitt D et al: Both species of *Chlamydia* and two biovars of *Chlamydia trachomatis* stimulate mouse B lymphocytes. *J Immunol* 136:4249, 1986.

140 Williams DM et al: The role of antibody in host defense against the agent of mouse pneumonitis. *J Infect Dis* 145:200, 1982.

141 Rank RG et al: Chronic chlamydial genital infection in congenitally athymic nude mice. *Infect Immun* 48:847, 1985.

142 Williams DM et al: Cellular immunity to the mouse pneumonitis agent. *J Infect Dis* 149:630, 1984.

143 Williams DM et al: Primary murine *Chlamydia trachomatis* pneumonia in B-cell-deficient mice. *Infect Immun* 55:2387, 1987.

144 Williams DM et al: Role of natural killer cells in infection with the mouse pneumonitis agent (murine *Chlamydia trachomatis*). *Infect Immun* 55:223, 1987.

# Chapter 16

# *Chlamydia trachomatis* infections of the adult

Walter E. Stamm
King K. Holmes

Since the early 1970s, *Chlamydia trachomatis* has been recognized as a genital pathogen responsible for an increasing variety of clinical syndromes, many closely resembling infections caused by *Neisseria gonorrhoeae* (Table 16-1). Because few practitioners have access to facilities for isolation of *C. trachomatis*, these infections must usually be diagnosed and treated without benefit of microbiological confirmation. Newer, noncultural diagnostic tests utilizing antigen-detection methods have in part addressed this problem but are likewise not available to many clinicians. Unfortunately, many chlamydial infections, particularly in women, are difficult to diagnose clinically and elude detection because they produce few or no symptoms and because the symptoms and signs they do produce are nonspecific. The increased incidence of these infections has thus in large part resulted from inadequate laboratory facilities for their detection and eventual treatment, the nonspecific signs and symptoms chlamydial infections produce, the lack of familiarity clincians have with these infections, and the lack of resources so far directed toward screening of high-risk patients, contact tracing, and treatment of infected partners.

## EPIDEMIOLOGY

### INFECTIONS IN MEN

The prevalence of chlamydial urethral infection has been assessed in populations of men attending general medical clinics, STD clinics, adolescent medicine clinics, and student health centers and ranges from 3 to 5 percent of asymptomatic men seen in general medical settings to 15 to 20 percent of all men seen in STD clinics.[1–5] Among military personnel, Podgore et al. found an 11 percent prevalence of asymptomatic urethral chlamydial infection compared with a 2 percent prevalence of urethral gonococcal infection.[6] Rates of chlamydial urethral infection of 13 to 15 percent have also been reported among sexually active boys attending adolescent medicine clinics.[7,8] Prevalence and site of mucosal infection as judged by positive culture appear to be strongly correlated with both age and sexual preference. Of 1221 patients screened for urethral infection in an STD clinic, 5 percent of homosexual men and 14 percent of heterosexual men had positive urethral cultures for *C. trachomatis*,[5] and in both groups prevalence decreased in each 5-year period from age 19 to age 39 (Fig. 16-1). Serologic evidence of chlamydial infection increased with age in heterosexuals but appeared relatively constant with increasing age in homosexual and bisexual men.[5] In other studies, both nongonococcal urethritis (NGU) and postgonococcal urethritis (PGU) were due to *C. trachomatis* less frequently in homosexual men than in heterosexual men.[1,9] The prevalence of chlamydial infection has generally been higher in nonwhites than in whites. In one screening study, 19 percent of nonwhite and 9 percent of white heterosexual males had urethral chlamydial infection.[5] Evidence of chlamydial infection has been infrequent in sexually inexperienced populations.

Chlamydial infection is a cause of proctitis in homosexual men who practice receptive rectal intercourse without condom protection.[10–12] Thus, both urethral and rectal chlamydial infections contributed to the high prevalence of serum antibody to *C. trachomatis* in homosexual men in the pre-AIDS era.

Pharyngeal infection with *C. trachomatis* has been demonstrated in 3 to 6 percent of men and women attending STD clinics and correlates with a history of recent orogenital contact.[13] Most such infections are asymptomatic. Among adolescents attending a teen clinic, only 1 percent were culture-positive for *C. trachomatis* in the pharynx.[14] Earlier serologic studies suggesting an etiologic role for *C. trachomatis* in nonstreptococcal community-acquired pharyngitis have not been supported by more recent attempts to isolate *C. trachomatis* from patients with pharyngitis.[15–17] The earlier serologic studies may have been measuring antibodies against the TWAR strain of chlamydia.[18]

The incidence of *C. trachomatis* infection in men has not been well defined, since in most countries these infections are not officially reported, are not microbiologically confirmed, and may often be asymptomatic, thus escaping detection. It has been es-

**Table 16-1. Clinical Parallels Between Genital Infections Caused by *N. gonorrhoeae* and *C. trachomatis***

| | Resulting clinical syndrome | |
|---|---|---|
| Site of infection | *N. gonorrhoeae* | *C. trachomatis* |
| *Men:* | | |
| Urethra | Urethritis | NGU, PGU |
| Epididymis | Epididymitis | Epididymitis |
| Rectum | Proctitis | Proctitis |
| Conjunctiva | Conjunctivitis | Conjunctivitis |
| Systemic | Disseminated gonococcal infection | Reiter's syndrome |
| *Women:* | | |
| Urethra | Acute urethral syndrome | Acute urethral syndrome |
| Bartholin's gland | Bartholinitis | Bartholinitis |
| Cervix | Cervicitis | Cervicitis, cervical metaplasia |
| Fallopian tube | Salpingitis | Salpingitis |
| Conjunctiva | Conjunctivitis | Conjunctivitis |
| Liver capsule | Perihepatitis | Perihepatitis |
| Systemic | Disseminated gonococcal infection | Reactive arthritis |

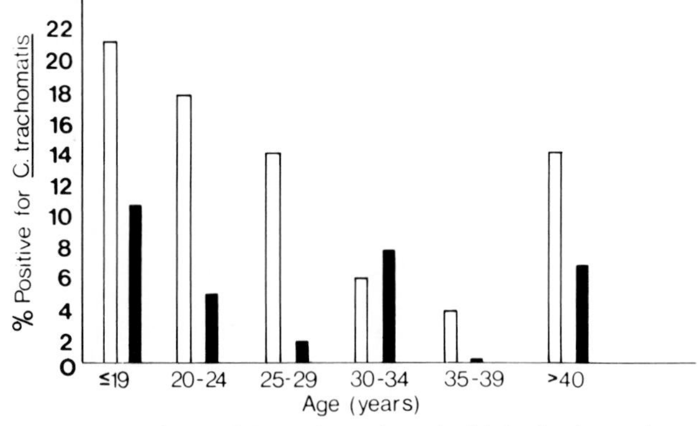


**Fig. 16-1.** Prevalence of *C. trachomatis* urethral infection by age in men attending an STD clinic. *Open bars* = heterosexual men; *solid bars* = homosexual or bisexual men.

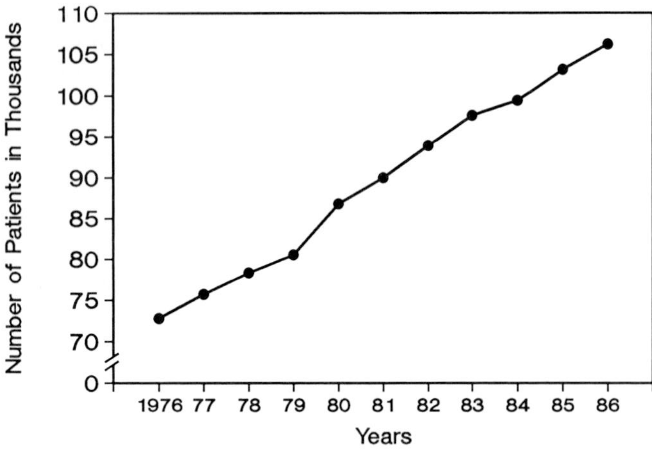


Fig. 16-2. Cases of NGU by year in England and Wales. *(Data from D Catteral.)*

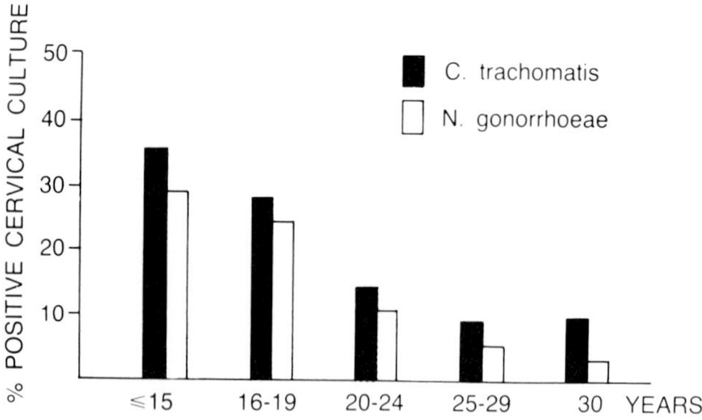


Fig. 16-3. Prevalence of *C. trachomatis* and *N. gonorrhoeae* cervical infection by age in women attending an STD clinic. *Open bars = N. gonorrhoeae; solid bars = C. trachomatis.*

timated, however, that more than 2 million cases of NGU occur annually in men in the United States.[19] If one assumes that 40 percent of NGU cases result from chlamydia, then over 800,000 cases of symptomatic chlamydial urethritis in men occur annually. The number of asymptomatic new cases which occur annually cannot be estimated with accuracy. Since the number of reported cases of NGU has increased dramatically since the early 1970s and 1980s in England and Wales, where this condition is reportable (Fig. 16-2), one can reasonably conclude that *C. trachomatis* infections in men have also increased dramatically in incidence over this period.

The transmissibility of genital chlamydial infections to males has not yet been extensively studied. In a recent study, male partners of women who had either chlamydial or gonococcal cervicitis were found to be infected with these agents 28 and 81 percent of the time, respectively.[20] Male partners of women with dual infections were also more often infected with gonorrhea than with chlamydia (77 and 28 percent, respectively)[20]. Although this study suggests that *N. gonorrhoeae* is more transmissible than *C. trachomatis*, the differing lengths of incubation period of these two agents and differing efficiency of isolation from the urethra could explain the results.

## INFECTIONS IN WOMEN

The prevalence of chlamydial infection has been studied in pregnant women, in women attending gynecology or family planning clinics, in women attending STD clinics, and in college students. Prevalence of infection in these studies has ranged from 3 to 5 percent in asymptomatic women to over 20 percent in women seen in STD clinics.[21–35] During pregnancy, 5 to 7 percent of women generally have been culture-positive,[36–42] though a 21 percent prevalence in a population of inner-city black women[39] and a 26 percent prevalence among Navaho women have been reported.[42] Demographic factors associated with an increased risk of chlamydial isolation in at least several studies include young age, nonwhite race, single marital status, and use of oral contraceptives.[21,25,34,35] The proportion of sexually active women with positive cervical cultures for *C. trachomatis* has been highest for women aged 15 to 21 and declines strikingly thereafter (Fig. 16-3), while the prevalence of serum antibody to *C. trachomatis* increases with age until about 30, when it plateaus at approximately 50 percent. Sexually inexperienced populations rarely exhibit chlamydial cervical infections. In a recent study evaluating a 50 percent sample of all sexually active Alaskan Inuit women living in remote villages, 114 (23 percent) of 493 had cervical infection with *C. trachomatis*.[43] In sexually active populations in which little diagnostic testing and/or specific treatment is being used, the prevalence of infection may thus reach surprisingly high levels.

The incidence of *C. trachomatis* genital infection has been even less well defined in women than in men. Because the infection produces no specific symptoms, is rarely confirmed microbiologically, and is not reported, virtually no incidence data are yet available. However, since many studies have shown that *C. trachomatis* can be isolated from the cervix of 60 to 70 percent of female sex partners of men with chlamydial NGU, it seems certain that the incidence of chlamydial infections in women has paralleled the increasing incidence in men. Transmissibility has also been poorly defined. A recent comparative study of partners of men with either chlamydial or gonococcal urethritis found that these women were infected 45 and 80 percent of the time, respectively.[20] Among female partners of men with both infections, 45 percent had chlamydial infection and 64 percent had gonorrhea.

## NATURAL HISTORY OF CHLAMYDIAL INFECTION

Several studies in the United States indicate that approximately 5 percent of neonates acquire chlamydial infection perinatally,[36,37] yet antibody prevalence in later childhood before onset of sexual activity may exceed 20 percent.[44] Acquisition of infection during childhood has not yet been well documented, but could occur from infected siblings or parents. Childhood upper respiratory, eye, or middle ear infections with *C. trachomatis* might explain this rise in antibody prevalence between the neonatal period and adolescence,[1] as could chlamydial genital infections acquired by children as a result of sexual abuse (see Chap. 72). Alternatively, cross-reacting antibody to TWAR chlamydial strains producing upper respiratory infections during childhood could account for some or all of this apparent increasing seroprevalence to *C. trachomatis* (see Chap. 15). The name *Chlamydia pneumoniae* has recently been proposed for the TWAR strain, which has a low degree of DNA homology with *C. trachomatis* or *C. psittaci*.

In adolescence, the incidence of culture-positive symptomatic genital chlamydial infections rises sharply, as does antibody prevalence. Asymptomatic infection also occurs commonly, and long-lived but unrecognized urethral, rectal, and cervical infections undoubtedly occur. Both rectal and urethral infections contribute to the high antibody prevalence found in homosexual men.

Much remains to be learned about the natural history of genital infections due to *C. trachomatis*, but on the basis of knowledge of the natural history of trachoma and of limited studies of untreated men and nonpregnant women,[22,45] subacute and chronic asymptomatic infection of genital mucosal surfaces undoubtedly occurs. The reported occurrence of chlamydial respiratory infection during immunosuppression suggests that impaired immunity may be followed by reemergence of symptomatic infection from a chronic latent focus.[46,47] Recrudescence of ocular trachoma years after leaving an endemic area has also been shown to occur during topical cortisone therapy.[48] It is not certain yet whether pregnancy, also a state associated with depressed cell-mediated immunity, may be associated with reactivation of genital chlamydial infection.[49] Current evidence indicates that chlamydial infection has not been a problem in AIDS patients.[50] Similarly, the interactions between ocular trachoma, lymphogranuloma venereum (LGV), and non-LGV genital and perinatal infection have not been extensively studied. It is not known, for example, whether the epidemiology or manifestations of genital chlamydial infections are altered in LGV or trachoma endemic areas, but such studies are in progress.[51]

## CLINICAL MANIFESTATIONS

Genital infections caused by *C. trachomatis* closely parallel those due to *N. gonorrhoeae* in terms of clinical manifestations (Table 16-1). Both organisms preferentially infect columnar or transitional epithelium of the urethra, with extension to the epididymis; the endocervix, with extension to the endometrium, salpinx, and peritoneum; and the rectum. Both organisms can produce extensive subepithelial inflammation, epithelial ulceration, and scarring. Rarely, both organisms can produce systemic manifestations, but the pathogenesis of the systemic manifestations of *C. trachomatis* infection is still poorly understood.

## INFECTIONS IN MEN

### Urethritis

Although Koch's postulates have not been specifically fulfilled, persuasive evidence suggests that *C. trachomatis* causes 35 to 50 percent of NGU in heterosexual men.[52–61] The frequency of chlamydial isolation in men with recent onset of NGU has been remarkably consistent from study to study, despite differences in patient population and methodology.[52–54] When female partners of *C. trachomatis*–positive and *C. trachomatis*–negative men with NGU were examined, 60 to 75 percent of the former and 0 to 10 percent of the latter had chlamydial cervicitis,[55–59] consistent with sexual transmission of *C. trachomatis* having resulted in NGU. Immunotyping of isolates from both partners has shown concordance of immunotypes in most couples.[52] Serum IgM antichlamydial antibody is frequently found in culture-positive men with NGU but rarely in culture-negative men with NGU.[60] Finally, placebo-controlled treatment trials of men with NGU or therapeutic trials utilizing drugs such as spectinomycin, which have little effect upon chlamydia, indicate that most men given placebo or ineffective therapy for *C. trachomatis* remain culture-positive and symptomatic until effective treatment is given.[61–64] Elimination of chlamydia thus coincides with resolution of symptoms. Although *C. trachomatis* has not been experimentally inoculated into the human urethra, baboons and chimpanzees develop chlamydial urethritis accompanied by serologic evidence of infection after urethral inoculation[65,66]

Clinically, chlamydia-positive and chlamydia-negative NGU cannot be differentiated on the basis of signs or symptoms. Both usually present after a 7- to 21-day incubation period with dysuria and mild to moderate whitish or clear urethral discharge. Examination reveals no abnormalities other than the discharge in most cases; associated adenopathy, focal urethral tenderness, and meatal or penile lesions should suggest herpetic urethritis. Abnormal prostatic examinations have not been convincingly linked to chlamydial urethritis.

*C. trachomatis* urethral infection is more often asymptomatic than gonococcal urethral infection, and when symptoms occur, they are milder with chlamydial urethritis.[5,67] However, many men with asymptomatic chlamydial urethral infection exhibit persistent urethral leukocytosis [$\geq$4 polymorphonuclear leukocytes (PMNs) per $\times 1000$ field] on Gram stains of urethral secretions or persistent pyuria in a first-void urine, indicating ongoing inflammation.[67]

Postgonococcal urethritis occurring in heterosexual men, like NGU, frequently results from infection with *C. trachomatis*. These patients probably acquire gonorrhea and chlamydial infection simultaneously but, due to the longer incubation period of *C. trachomatis*, develop a biphasic illness if their original gonorrhea is treated with an agent that does not eradicate chlamydia. It remains possible, however, that gonococcal infection causes reactivation of latent chlamydial infection. Coinfection with these two agents occurs in from 15 to 35 percent of heterosexual men with gonorrhea but rarely in homosexual men.[9] Of men infected with both chlamydia and *N. gonorrhoeae* who are treated with penicillin, ampicillin, gentamicin, or spectinomycin, 80 percent or more develop symptomatic PGU, or urethral leukocytosis without symptoms.[52,54,68]

### Epididymitis

Berger and coworkers have shown that *C. trachomatis* causes most cases of what was previously termed idiopathic epididymitis in young, heterosexually active males.[69] In this study, chlamydial and gonococcal epididymitis was usually associated with urethritis caused by *C. trachomatis* and *N. gonorrhoeae* in patients who were less than 35 years of age and sexually active, while patients with epididymitis who were older than 35 years generally had coliform infections and a history of urologic disease or instrumentation (see Chap. 53). Clinically, chlamydial epididymitis presents as unilateral scrotal pain, swelling, tenderness, and fever in a young male who often has associated chlamydial urethritis, though the urethritis may be asymptomatic. Men with chlamydial epididymitis improve rapidly with tetracycline treatment, supporting the causal role of *C. trachomatis*.[70]

*Chlamydia trachomatis* also produces mild epididymitis in monkeys after introduction of the organism into the vas deferens.[71] Antibody production, stimulation of cell-mediated immunity to chlamydial antigens, histologic findings, and subsequent recovery of *C. trachomatis* from the monkey's urethra support the causative role of *C. trachomatis* in this model.[71,72] However, the epididymitis is mild, organisms have not been recovered from the epididymis, and the effects of repeated inoculation have not been studied. Thus, animal experiments have not yet elucidated the pathogenesis of chlamydial epididymitis.

### Prostatitis

Despite continued study, the role of *C. trachomatis* in causing nonbacterial prostatitis remains controversial (see Chap. 54). Mårdh and coworkers reported that only 13 percent of patients with nonbacterial prostatitis had antibodies to *C. trachomatis* in serum or in expressed prostatic secretions,[73] and none had positive cultures from expressed prostatic secretions. They speculated that negative cultures could have resulted from the antichlamydial effects of spermine and zinc in prostatic secretions.[74] More recently, Nilsson reported recovery of *C. trachomatis* from the expressed prostatic secretions of 26 men with acute NGU, all of whom were considered to have cytologic evidence of prostatitis.[75] Bruce and colleagues also reported frequent isolation of chlamydia from urine, prostatic fluid, and prostatic expressate of men with nonbacterial prostatitis.[76] These studies have not convincingly demonstrated the presence of chlamydia in the prostate itself, and the definition of prostatitis used is disputed. However, Poletti and colleagues performed transrectal biopsies of the prostate in 30 men with known positive urethral cultures for *C. trachomatis* and a diagnosis of nonbacterial prostatitis based on prostatic tenderness or swelling upon digital palpation; the organism was recovered from 10 of 30 prostatic specimens.[77] These studies require confirmation. Taken together, these studies are inconclusive regarding the role of *C. trachomatis* in nonbacterial prostatitis. Further studies should utilize a careful case definition (including cell counts in expressed prostatic secretions), conventional histologic studies, immunohistochemical study of biopsied tissue, serologic studies, and evaluation of response to therapy.

### Proctitis

The chronic, indolent form of LGV which results from secondary spread of *C. trachomatis* of the LGV immunotypes from the genitalia to the rectum, usually in women, is discussed in Chap 17. *C. trachomatis* of non-LGV immunotypes also has been isolated from the rectal mucosa of infants, heterosexual women, and homosexual men. The clinical manifestations of rectal infection in infants and adult women have not been studied extensively.

Recent prospective evaluation of homosexual men indicates that *C. trachomatis* of either the genital immunotypes D to K or LGV immunotypes can produce proctitis.[10,12] LGV immunotypes usually produce a primary ulcerative proctitis and a histopathologic picture of giant cell formation and granulomas identical to those seen in acute Crohn's disease. Non-LGV immunotypes produce milder infections, ranging from asymptomatic infection to symptomatic proctitis resembling gonococcal proctitis with rectal pain and bleeding, mucous discharge, and diarrhea.[78] Most *C. trachomatis*–infected patients have abnormal numbers of PMNs in their rectal Gram stain, and on sigmoidoscopy, those with symptoms exhibit friable rectal mucosa. *C. trachomatis* appeared to be responsible for up to 15 percent of proctitis in our studies of homosexual males, and treatment with tetracycline promptly cured these patients.

### Reiter's syndrome

Both Reiter's syndrome (urethritis, conjunctivitis, arthritis, and characteristic mucocutaneous lesions) and reactive tenosynovitis or arthritis without the other components of Reiter's syndrome have been related to genital infection with *C. trachomatis*.[79] Recent studies of untreated men with characteristic Reiter's syndrome using the microimmunofluorescent (micro-IF) antibody assay also indicate that preceding or concurrent infection with *C. trachomatis* is present in more than 80 percent (Chap. 61).[79–81] Many men with Reiter's syndrome exhibit marked lymphocyte stimulation by chlamydial antigens in in vitro blastogenesis assays.[80] Fluorescein-conjugated monoclonal antibodies have been used to demonstrate what appear to be *C. trachomatis* elementary bodies in the joint fluid and synovial biopsies of patients with Reiter's syndrome, suggesting dissemination of infection beyond the mucosal site of entry in such patients.[82]

Like postenteric (salmonella, shigella, yersinia) arthritides, sacroilliitis, and spondylitis, Reiter's syndrome occurs with increased frequency in patients with the HLA-B27 haplotype.[82,83] The HLA-B27 haplotype appears to confer a 10-fold increased risk of developing Reiter's syndrome. However, among a large series of HLA-B27-positive men with chlamydial urethritis but with no other manifestations of Reiter's syndrome, none went on to develop Reiter's syndrome after onset of therapy with a tetracycline.[84]

## INFECTIONS IN WOMEN

### Cervicitis

While many women with chlamydia isolated from the cervix have no signs or symptoms of infection, at least a third generally have local signs of infection.[85] Most commonly found are mucopurulent discharge (37 percent of women) (Plates 15 and 16) and hypertrophic ectopy (19 percent). Hypertrophic ectopy refers to an area of ectopy that is edematous, congested, and bleeds easily (see Chap. 46). Cervical follicles can be visualized colposcopically in some women with chlamydial infection of the cervix,[86] but this finding has been uncommon in our experience and that of others.[31] Paavonen et al. recently reported that colposcopic features of immature squamous metaplasia of the zone of ectopy are associated with chlamydial infection.[86] The number of PMN leukocytes in cervical mucus is correlated with chlamydial infection of the cervix. Brunham et al. reported that $\geq$10 PMN leukocytes per $\times$1000 field was best correlated.[87] Attention to collection of the specimens, and to selective counting of PMNs in cervical mucus rather than in areas containing vaginal epithelial cells, is important. We currently use a cutoff of $\geq$30 PMN leukocytes per $\times$1000 field in Gram-stained smears of cervical mucus as best correlated with chlamydial (or gonococcal) cervicitis. There appears to be a wide range of normal leukocyte values in women without cervical infection, perhaps due to the influence of the menstrual cycle, contraceptive practices, sexual activity, and other infections. Women who exhibit signs of chlamydial cervicitis (mucopurulent discharge, hypertrophic ectopy) yield greater numbers of chlamydial inclusion-forming units on primary isolation in tissue culture than women who have chlamydial infection without cervicitis.[88] Whether infections associated with cervicitis have been more recently acquired has not been established.

The prevalence of *C. trachomatis* infection appears greater in women with ectopy than in those without ectopy.[85] Ectopy may predispose women to chlamydial infection by exposing a greater number of susceptible columnar epithelial cells, making infection more likely upon exposure. Alternatively, ectopy may increase the shedding of *C. trachomatis* from the cervix, or *C. trachomatis* infection of the cervix may cause ectopy. Cervical ectopy is normally present in 60 to 80 percent of sexually active adolescents

(Plate 13) and then declines in prevalence in the third and fourth decades. This may help explain the high prevalence of cervical chlamydial infections in adolescents. Oral contraceptives have also been associated with increased risk of cervical *C. trachomatis* infection, probably because their use promotes ectopy; the increased risk appears limited to oral contraceptive users with ectopy.[25,85]

Clinical recognition of chlamydial cervicitis depends upon a high index of suspicion and a careful cervical examination. As discussed above, findings suggestive of chlamydial infection include easily induced endocervical bleeding, mucopurulent endocervical discharge, and edema of an area of ectopy. The differential diagnosis of mucopurulent discharge from the endocervical canal in a young, sexually active woman includes gonococcal endocervicitis, salpingitis, endometritis, IUD-induced inflammation, or other causes (see Chap. 46). Gram stain of appropriately collected mucopurulent endocervical discharge from patients with chlamydial endocervicitis also usually shows >30 PMN leucocytes per $\times 1000$ field, absence of gonococci, and only occasional bacteria. Similarly, the observation of purulent (yellow or green) colored cervical discharge on a cervical swab collected from such patients (a positive "swab test"; see Chap. 46) correlates with the presence of chlamydial and/or gonococcal infection.[87] Unfortunately, the majority of women with chlamydial infection cannot be distinguished from uninfected women by clinical examination or by these simple tests.

Nearly all women with endocervical chlamydial infection have or develop antibodies to *C. trachomatis* in serum as assessed by the micro-IF assay. Only 20 to 30 percent exhibit IgM antibody at the time of diagnosis, however, suggesting that many newly diagnosed cervical infections in women are not recent but long-lived. Local cervical antibody has been reported in only 30 to 50 percent of cases,[89] but in our experience over 70 pecent of culture-positive women have local antibody.[49] Sequential culturing of untreated women has demonstrated that chlamydial infection may persist for weeks or months without development of symptoms, or may spontaneously resolve.[22,32]

The relation of chlamydial cervical infection to cytologic atypia, including reactive and metaplastic atypia and dysplasia, is discussed in Chap. 48. The cervical Pap smear frequently shows a characteristic pattern of inflammation in chlamydial infection, which can alert the cytopathologist and clinician to the need for further tests for chlamydia.

## Urethritis

Screening studies in STD clinics suggest that of women cultured for *C. trachomatis* at both the cervix and urethra, 50 percent of positive women yield chlamydia from both sites and 25 percent from either site alone.[25,58] Paavonen reported that women who had *C. trachomatis* in their cervix and urethra were more likely to complain of dysuria than women with cervical infection alone.[58] Isolated urethral infection, without cervical infection, appears to increase in prevalence with age.[25] Case reports have previously suggested that symptoms of dysuria and frequency occur in women with chlamydial urethritis, pyuria, and no bacteriuria or other urinary pathogens, and our prospective evaluation of young women with the acute urethral syndrome (dysuria and frequency without bacteriuria of $\geq 10^5$ conventional uropathogens per milliliter of urine) has implicated chlamydia as an important cause of dysuria in young, sexually active women.[26] Of 16 women with sterile pyuria, 10 had cultural and/or serologic evidence of infection with *C. trachomatis*, compared with less than 10 percent of women from the same population who lacked urinary symptoms or who had coliform cystitis. Women with chlamydial infection who were given placebo remained culture-positive and symptomatic until given active antimicrobial therapy, while those given doxycycline improved rapidly.[90]

Although urethral symptoms may develop in women with chlamydial infection, the majority of female STD clinic patients with urethral chlamydial infection do not have dysuria or frequency.[25] Even in women with chlamydial urethritis causing the acute urethral syndrome, signs of urethritis (urethral discharge, meatal redness, or swelling) are infrequent,[26] although the presence of mucopurulent cervicitis in a woman with dysuria and frequency should suggest the diagnosis. *C. trachomatis* urethritis should be suspected in young, sexually active women with dysuria, frequency, and pyuria, especially if they have had a new sex partner within the last month or a sex partner with NGU. Other correlates of chlamydial urethral syndrome include duration of dysuria of more than 7 to 10 days, lack of hematuria, lack of suprapubic tenderness, and use of birth control pills. An abnormal urethral Gram stain showing $\geq 10$ PMNs per oil immersion field in women with dysuria but without coliform bacteriuria supports the diagnosis of chlamydial urethritis but is also found in women with gonococcal or trichomonal infection of the urethra.[91]

## Bartholinitis

Like gonococci, *C. trachomatis* may produce an exudative infection of Bartholin's ducts. Davies et al. studied 30 women who had clinical evidence of bartholinitis, and isolated *N. gonorrhoeae* and *C. trachomatis* from the ductal exudate of 24 and 9 women, respectively.[92] Of the 9 chlamydia-positive women, 7 had concurrent gonorrhea, but 2 were sex partners of men with NGU and had no evidence of gonococcal infection. Purulent infections of Bartholin's ducts may thus be due to chlamydial infection, either alone or with concurrent gonococcal infection.

## Endometritis

Histologic evidence of endometritis, often with immunohistologic and/or cultural evidence of *C. trachomatis*, is present in nearly one-half of patients with chlamydial mucopurulent cervicitis[97–99] and can be demonstrated in nearly all patients with chlamydial salpingitis. The presence of endometritis in patients with chlamydial cervicitis correlates with a history of abnormal vaginal bleeding (Chap. 50).[99]

It is now clear that *C. trachomatis* infection is associated with endometritis.[93–97] Mårdh and coworkers first described two women from whom *C. trachomatis* was recovered by uterine aspiration, despite negative cervical cultures.[93] Both women exhibited signs of salpingitis and developed serologic evidence of chlamydial infection. Concomitant endometritis probably explains the menorrhagia and metrorrhagia often seen in women with salpingitis. These studies, like previous evidence gathered in monkeys infected with *C. trachomatis*,[96] indicate that chlamydia cervicitis probably spreads through the endometrial cavity to reach the fallopian tubes. Subsequent studies have shown that chlamydial endometritis is characterized by infiltration of the endometrial stroma by plasma cells, and infiltration of the endometrial superficial epithelium by PMN leukocytes.

Besides nonpuerperal endometritis, Wager and coworkers have shown an association of intrapartum fever and late postpartum endometritis with untreated antenatal *C. trachomatis* infection.[100] Others have confirmed this association (Chap. 64).[36]

### Salpingitis

The proportion of acute salpingitis cases due to *C. trachomatis* varies geographically and with the population studied. In Sweden, Mårdh and colleagues found that 19 of 53 women with salpingitis had chlamydial infections of the cervix and that of those with cervical infection who had laparoscopy, 6 of 7 grew *C. trachomatis* in a culture from the fallopian tube.[101] These authors found that 80 percent of 60 consecutive women with acute salpingitis had antibodies to *C. trachomatis,* with 37 percent exhibiting serologic evidence of acute chlamydial infection. Other serologic studies of women with salpingitis also suggest the etiologic role of chlamydia.[102–104] Our own studies, with P. Wølner-Hanssen and D. Eschenbach, of Seattle women with laparoscopically confirmed salpingitis and histologically confirmed endometritis indicate that 80 to 90 percent have proven chlamydial or gonococcal infection, usually confirmed in the upper genital tract, with the proportion having either chlamydial or gonococcal infection being approximately equal. An interesting treatment study by Rees and colleagues further supports the role of chlamydia in salpingitis.[105] Among 343 women randomly treated for gonorrhea with either penicillin or tetracycline, a significantly greater proportion of those who received penicillin went on to develop salpingitis; persistence of cervical *C. trachomatis* was associated with many but not all cases of salpingitis. As discussed in Chaps. 49 and 50, and elsewhere,[106–110] many cases of chlamydial salpingitis are associated with mild or absent symptoms or signs, despite progressive tubal scarring, resulting in ectopic pregnancy or infertility. Studies in animals (Chaps. 49 and 50) also support the causative role of chlamydia in salpingitis.[(111,112)]

### Perihepatitis (Fitz-Hugh–Curtis syndrome)

Since its description by Fitz-Hugh and Curtis, perihepatitis occurring after or with salpingitis has been considered a complication of gonococcal infection. Recent studies suggest that chlamydial infection may in fact be more commonly associated with perihepatitis than is *N. gonorrhoeae* (see Chap. 51).[113–115] Perihepatitis should be suspected in young, sexually active women who develop right-upper-quadrant pain, fever, nausea, or vomiting. Evidence of salpingitis may or may not be present.

## OTHER CHLAMYDIAL INFECTIONS IN ADULTS

Since *C. trachomatis* causes a distinctive pneumonia syndrome in neonates (Chap. 66), several studies have assessed the etiologic role of chlamydia in adults with pneumonia. Two case reports and small studies suggest that *C. trachomatis* is an occasional cause of pneumonitis in immunocompromised adults.[116–118] Tack and coworkers isolated *C. trachomatis* from the lower respiratory secretions of 5 immunosuppressed patients with pneumonia and from 1 patient with acute bronchitis.[46] *C. trachomatis* was also isolated from the eye and nasopharynx and from bronchial brushings in 3 of these patients. None of these 6 patients developed serologic evidence of *C. trachomatis* infection, and 3 had concomitant cytomegalovirus infection. On the other hand, Meyers and coworkers demonstrated sustained IgM and IgG antibody rises to *C. trachomatis* in 3 patients who developed interstitial pneumonia after marrow transplantation, but lung tissue examined by culture and fluorescent antibody techniques from these patients and from 63 other transplant patients with pneumonia provided no evidence of chlamydial infection.[116] Histologic or cultural evidence of *C. trachomatis* infection could not be demonstrated in 48 lung biopsies from AIDS patients with pneumonia.[50] Komaroff and coworkers found serologic evidence of recent chlamydial infections in 4 out of 19 adults with community-acquired pneumonia not due to common bacterial or viral pathogens.[119] However, in retrospect these may have been antibodies to *C. pneumoniae* rather than to *C. trachomatis.*[120] At this point, there is little evidence to suggest that *C. trachomatis* causes community-acquired pneumonia in adults.

*Chlamydia trachomatis* may on occasion produce culture-negative endocarditis,[121] and serologic studies in one patient suggested that meningoencephalitis resulted from chlamydial infection.[122] Other uncommon infections in adults, including peritonitis and postmenopausal vaginitis, have been attributed to chlamydia.[123,124]

## DIAGNOSIS

Chapter 74 discusses in detail the cytologic, tissue-culture, antigen-detection, and serologic methods for diagnosis of *C. trachomatis* infections. Aspects relevant to deciding whom to test, what test to use, the collection of specimens, and the interpretation of results in adult patients are presented below.

## SPECIMEN COLLECTION

Specimens must be appropriately collected and transported to maximize the chances of isolating *C. trachomatis* or demonstrating its presence by antigen detection in infected patients. Being obligate intracellular pathogens, chlamydiae are best isolated from cell scrapings rather than from purulent discharges, secretions, or urine. Hence it is imperative to ensure that specimens from the urethra, cervix, or rectum contain cells scraped from each of these respective sites. Swabs can be used for this purpose as effectively as and more easily than curettes. Small cytologic brushes can be effectively used to collect cervical specimens. Cervical specimens should be obtained only after mucus and debris have been removed from the os with a swab. For urethral specimens, a thin urethrogenital swab on an aluminum shaft is preferred, while for cervical or rectal specimens, a thicker plastic-shafted swab should be used. Wooden-shafted swabs reduce the number of inclusion-forming units in specimens stored in transport media for as short a period as 6 to 12 h, and thus should not be used for culture. Some lots of swabs with calcium alginate tips have been found to depress recovery of *C. trachomatis.* Thus, rayon- or cotton-tipped swabs may be preferable.

After a specimen is obtained for culture, it should be placed immediately into sucrose-phosphate transport medium containing antibiotics, usually gentamicin, vancomycin, and nystatin. The specimen should then be refrigerated, transported on ice, and inoculated as soon as possible, preferably within 24 h. Inclusion counts decline only 0 to 15 percent after 6 to 24 h of refrigeration, but counts decline rapidly after 24 h. Thus, if inoculation cannot be accomplished within 6 to 24 h, specimens are better frozen at −70°C until inoculation can take place. Swabs for antigen detection should be placed in the manufacturer's transport medium. Refrigeration is unnecessary.

## CULTURE AND ANTIGEN-DETECTION METHODS

Confirmation of chlamydial infection by culture involves (1) collecting a specimen containing as many epithelial cells as possible,

(2) preventing bacterial overgrowth of the specimen by the addition of antibiotics to the transport medium, (3) centrifuging the specimen to maximize contact between elementary bodies and the tissue culture monolayer, (4) using an antimetabolite to inhibit replication of the tissue culture cells, and (5) using iodine, Giemsa, or immunofluorescence staining to detect mature inclusions in infected cells.

The sensitivity and specificity of currently available isolation methods for *C. trachomatis* from genital specimens are unknown, as no standard for comparison exists. In untreated patients cultured repeatedly for *C. trachomatis,* 70 to 80 percent are repeatedly positive on serial cultures; negative patients usually remain negative on repetitive cultures.[1,61,90]

The expense and time required to perform *C. trachomatis* cultures have been a major hindrance to their more widespread availability for diagnostic purposes. Noncultural methods for detection of *C. trachomatis* antigen in infected secretions have been eagerly awaited and are not commercially available. Two general approaches to antigen detection have been taken: direct immunofluorescence staining of smears using monoclonal antibodies, and detection of chlamydial antigen eluted from swabs and measured by enzyme-linked immunosorbent assay (ELISA) methods.[125] Chapter 74 compares the sensitivity and specificity of these tests with culture methods.

## SEROLOGIC TECHNIQUES

Serologic tests have not been routinely used for diagnosis of chlamydial genital tract infections other than LGV. Two major problems have precluded the successful use of serologic studies for the diagnosis of an individual patient's genital infection. First, the baseline prevalence of antibody in populations which are sexually active and likely to be at risk for *C. trachomatis* infection is high, often ranging from 45 to 65 percent of persons tested. Seropositivity increases with age and sexual activity, and in most studies 95 to 100 percent of those who are culture-positive are seropositive. The high prevalence of seropositivity in culture-negative, asymptomatic patients presumably results from previous infection or from persisting, chronic asymptomatic infection not easily detected with current culture techniques.

The second major difficulty precluding effective use of serodiagnosis results from the asymptomatic or minimally symptomatic nature of many chlamydial infections. Lack of an abrupt onset of symptoms means that many patients are seen during periods when IgM antibody or rising or falling titers of IgG antibody cannot be demonstrated, and hence these serologic parameters of recently acquired infection are often absent. This particularly applies to women. Onset of symptoms is more abrupt in men with NGU, and seroconversion can be documented in most men who are still seronegative when first seen; IgM antichlamydia antibodies have been found in up to 80 percent of culture-positive men who have no previous history of NGU.[60]

Superficial genital tract infection (urethritis, cervicitis) generally produces micro-IF antibody titers in the range of 1:8 to 1:256, but rarely higher. Of men with NGU who were initially seronegative but later developed IgG antibody to chlamydia, 60 percent developed titers between 1:8 and 1:32 while 40 percent were between 1:64 and 1:256.[60] In adults, higher antibody titers (≥1:256) have more often been seen in women with salpingitis; even higher titers (often ≥1:1024) have been seen in adults with perihepatitis or LGV, but further data are needed to assess the diagnostic significance of high antibody titers in single specimens.

## WHEN TO USE DIAGNOSTIC TESTING

All women suspected of having *C. trachomatis* genital infections on the basis of symptoms, signs, or exposure history, including women with suspected mucopurulent cervicitis, endometritis, pelvic inflammatory disease, acute urethritis, or acute proctitis, as well as women whose male partners have gonorrhea or NGU, should have specific diagnostic testing. As described above, the diagnosis of many of these conditions is difficult to establish on clinical grounds alone, and the presence of a positive chlamydial test is thus of great value in confirming the suspected diagnosis. Although women in these categories should be empirically treated with tetracycline or doxycycline without awaiting test results, a specific confirmation of *C. trachomatis* infection clarifies the diagnosis, improves the patient's understanding of her illness, probably enhances mediation compliance, and facilitates management of sexual partners.

Second, unrecognized *C. trachomatis* infections should be identified by appropriate screening of women in high-risk groups. Such groups include all women attending STD clinics or other clinics (family planning clinics, juvenile detention centers, and abortion clinics, for example) where the prevalence of infection exceeds 10 to 12 percent. Physicians should screen women who have specific risk factors associated with chlamydial infections: adolescent age range, a new sexual partner, multiple sexual partners, racial/ethnic groups found to be at high risk in the local setting, and signs of cervicitis. Strong consideration should be given to screening all unmarried pregnant women and pregnant women with one or more of these risk characteristics.

In men, given both the relative paucity of serious complications that arise from *C. trachomatis* infections and the considerably greater proportion of infections that can be accurately diagnosed on clinical grounds alone, both specific diagnostic testing and screening for *C. trachomatis* infections should be given a lower priority than in women. Thus, when resources limit the numbers of tests that can be done (in public health clinics, for example), tests that are available should be used primarily for women. However, knowledge of the role of *C. trachomatis* in NGU has prognostic implications (>90 percent cure rate for patients positive for *C. trachomatis* compared with 50 percent for those who are negative), fosters more aggressive identification and treatment of female partners, and has educational benefits for both patient and physician. Specific diagnostic testing thus provides a number of benefits even though most infected men with symptoms or signs of urethritis can be treated empirically with tetracycline before the test results are known.

Up to one-third of heterosexual men with *C. trachomatis* urethral infection attending STD clinics lack symptoms of urethritis, and a case can be made for routine screening tests for *C. trachomatis* in such clinics to identify these persons. Alternatively, such men could be screened for increased numbers of PMN leukocytes in first-voided urine specimens by microscopy or leukocyte esterase testing, or for increased PMN leukocytes (e.g., ≥5 per × 1000 field) on Gram-stained urethral smear, and those with abnormal findings could be selected for specific testing for chlamydia. This approach warrants further evaluation. Asymptomatic partners of women with mucopurulent cervicitis, pelvic inflammatory disease, or asymptomatic chlamydial infection should also be screened and then given empirical therapy. The use of empirical therapy without specific testing foregoes an opportunity to identify still other sexual contacts who should be evaluated and treated and thus fosters continuation of the epidemic and reinfection of the patient. In homosexual men with

Table 16-2. Diagnosis of *C. trachomatis* Infections in Men*

| Associated findings | Clinical criteria | Laboratory criteria | |
|---|---|---|---|
| | | Presumptive | Diagnostic |
| NGU | Dysuria, urethral discharge | Urethral GS with 5 or more PMN/high-power (×1000) field; pyuria on FVU | Positive culture or direct antigen test (urethra) |
| Acute epididymitis | Fever, epididymal or testicular pain, evidence of NGU, epididymal tenderness or mass | As for NGU | As for NGU; positive culture on epididymal aspirate |
| Acute proctitis (non-LGV strain) | Rectal pain, discharge, bleeding; abnormal anoscopy (mucopurulent discharge, pain, spontaneous or induced bleeding) | Rectal GS with 1 or more PMN/high-power (×1000) field | Positive culture or direct FA (rectal) |
| Acute proctocolitis (LGV strain) | Severe rectal pain, discharge, hematochezia; markedly abnormal anoscopy (as above) with lesions extending into colon; fever lymphadenopathy | Rectal GS with 1 or more PMN/high-power (×1000) field | Positive culture or direct FA (rectal); complement fixation antibody titer |

*GS = Gram stain; PMN = polymorphonuclear leukocytes; NGU = nongonococcal urethritis; FA = fluorescent antibody; FVU = first-void urine; LGV = lymphogranuloma venereum. Reproduced with permission from the *Annals of Internal Medicine.*

suspected proctitis, *C. trachomatis* testing should be done to confirm the suspected diagnosis. Tables 16-2 and 16-3 summarize diagnostic criteria for various *C. trachomatis* infections in men and women, respectively.

## SELECTION OF THE APPROPRIATE TEST

Selection of the most appropriate laboratory test for detection of *C. trachomatis* depends on local availability and expertise, the prevalence of infection in the test population, and the purpose of the test. Isolation in cell culture remains the most sensitive and specific test and thus should be used when it is available and when transport conditions, cost, and other logistic factors permit its use.

Because of its high specificity, cell culture may be of greatest value in screening low-risk populations. Although they have not yet been extensively evaluated in this setting, the positive and negative predictive values of the antigen-detection test are likely to be lowest in low-risk groups. An alternative approach in such low-prevalence settings may be to screen patients with antigen tests, but to confirm positive antigen-detection tests by culture. In populations of women in which the prevalence of infection exceeds 10 percent, both the direct smear test and the ELISA test provide satisfactory sensitivity and specificity, rapid turnaround time, and simplified transport conditions.

## THERAPY

Although in vitro susceptibility testing for *C. trachomatis* has not been rigorously standardized, studies to date have found little strain-to-strain variation in minimum inhibitory concentrations of individual antimicrobials against chlamydia.[126–129] The most active drugs against *C. trachomatis* in tissue culture are rifampin and the tetracyclines, followed by macrolides, sulfonamides, some fluoroquinolones, and clindamycin.

The majority of clinical evidence regarding the effectiveness of various antimicrobials against *C. trachomatis* has been accumulated in men with NGU (Table 16-4). Two general principles have emerged from these studies: penicillin, ampicillin, cephalosporins, and spectinomycin in single-dose regimens given for treatment of gonorrhea usually do not eradicate concomitant chlamydial infection, and 7 or more days of treatment with tetracyclines or

Table 16-3. Diagnosis of *C. trachomatis* Infections in Women*

| Associated findings | Clinical criteria | Laboratory criteria | |
|---|---|---|---|
| | | Presumptive | Diagnostic |
| Mucopurulent cervicitis | Mucopurulent cervical discharge, cervical ectopy and edema, spontaneous or easily induced cervical bleeding | Cervical GS with greater than 30 PMN/high-power (×1000) field in nonmenstruating women | Positive culture or direct antigen test (cervix) |
| Acute urethral syndrome | Dysuria-frequency syndrome in young sexually active women; recent new sexual partner; often more than 7 days of symptoms | Pyuria, no bacteriuria | Positive culture or direct antigen test (cervix or urethra) |
| PID | Lower abdominal pain; adnexal tenderness on pelvic exam; evidence of MPC often present | As for MPC; cervical GS positive for gonorrhea; endometritis on endometrial biopsy | Positive culture or direct antigen test (cervix, endometrium, tubal) |
| Perihepatitis | Right upper quadrant pain, nausea, vomiting, fever; young sexually active women; evidence of PID | As for MPC and PID | High-titer IgM or IgG antibody to *C. trachomatis* |

*GS = Gram stain; PMN = polymorphonuclear leukocytes; PID = pelvic inflammatory disease; MPC = mucopurulent cervicitis. Reproduced with permission from the *Annals of Internal Medicine.*

**Table 16-4. Summary of Selected Studies Evaluating Oral Antimicrobial Treatment of *C. trachomatis* Urethritis in Men**

| Regimen | Efficacy* | Reference |
|---|---|---|
| Minocycline, 200 mg stat., then 100 mg q 12 h for 6 days | 11/12 (92%) | 133 |
| Tetracycline, 500 mg qid for 7 days | 35/35 (100%) | 63 |
| Erythromycin stearate, 500 mg q 12 h for 2 weeks | 30/31 (97%) | 134 |
| Doxycycline, 200 mg for 2 days, then 100 mg for 12 days | 50/52 (96%) | 135 |
| Deteclo, qd for 7 days | 11/12 (92%) | 131 |
| Deteclo, qd for 21 days | 16/16 (100%) | |
| Minocycline, 200 mg stat., then 100 mg bid for 6 days | 39/40 (98%) | 136 |
| Rifampin, 600 mg qd for 6 days | 52/53 (98%) | |
| Erythromycin stearate, 500 mg q 12 h for 15 days | 27/30 (90%) | 138 |
| Lymecycline, 300 mg q 12 h for 10 days | 21/24 (88%) | |
| Lymecycline, 300 mg q 12 h for 20 days | 18/21 (86%) | |
| Pivampicillin, 750 mg tid for 7 days | 19/22 (86%) | 130 |
| Doxycycline, 200 mg for 1 day, then 100 mg for 6 days | 56/57 (98%) | 143 |
| Trimethoprim-sulfamethoxazole, 160 and 800 mg bid, respectively, for 10 days | 18/20 (90%) | |
| Erythromycin, 500 mg bid for 10 days | 18/23 (78%) | |
| Trimethoprim-sulfadiazine, 160 and 500 mg, respectively, in 1 tablet bid for 14 days | 18/19 (95%) | 61 |
| Tetracycline, 250 mg qid for 7 days | 21/24 (88%) | 139 |
| Tetracycline, 500 mg qid for 7 days | 33/36 (92%) | |
| Rosaramicin, 250 mg qid for 7 days | 38/42 (90%) | |
| Amoxicillin, 750 mg tid for 10 days | 6/6 (100%) | 137 |
| Ciprofloxacin, 500 mg bid for 7 days | 5/13 (38%) | 140a |

*Studies cited here performed chlamydia cultures before, just after, and 2 to 3 weeks following completion of treatment; efficacy, as expressed in this table, equals the number of patients with negative chlamydia cultures on visit 2 or 3 divided by the number of patients returning for follow-up visits 2 and 3. Eradication of chlamydia was usually, but not always, associated with clinical resolution of signs and symptoms.

macrolides eradicates *C. trachomatis* from nearly all men, at least as determined by short-term follow-up.[130–139] However, chlamydial infection recurs 3 to 6 weeks after treatment in 5 to 10 percent of these men and cannot be clearly designated as reinfection or relapse. Most such recurrences are of the same immunotype as the original infecting strain,[52] and nearly all cause recurrent clinical evidence of urethritis. In addition, despite apparent elimination of *C. trachomatis,* 10 to 15 percent of men develop persisting or relapsing symptoms, perhaps due to simultaneous infection with another agent.

In men with NGU, trials using either placebos or agents, such as spectinomycin, which are ineffective against *C. trachomatis* have clearly established the greater effectiveness of specific antimicrobial treatment in eliminating both signs and symptoms of infection and in eradicating chlamydia.[61,64] Clinical trials indicate that tetracycline hydrochloride, doxycycline, minocycline, triple tetracycline, erythromycin, and trimethoprim-sulfamethoxazole all achieve comparable clinical cure rates of approximately 85 to 95 percent in men with chlamydial NGU (see Chap. 52). Of the newer fluoroquinolones, ofloxacin has reported cure rates in this range, while ciprofloxacin has been associated with more frequent failures.[140a] Although relatively ineffective against *C. trachomatis* in vitro and when administered as a single dose, amoxicillin, when given as 750 mg PO tid for 10 days, apparently eliminated chlamydia from six men with NGU followed for 24 to 48 days.[137] Pivampicillin in high dosage gave similar results.[130] Although symptoms usually subsided as cultures became negative in these studies, the possibility cannot be excluded that latent chlamydial infection persisted after amoxicillin or pivampicillin treatment. Because of its effectiveness and low cost, tetracycline hydrochloride has been the most widely used agent for treatment of NGU. The recommended length of therapy ranges from 7 to 21 days. However, in two studies in which 7 days of therapy were compared with 21 days of therapy with tetracycline or minocycline, no difference was found.[132,133] Thus, there is as yet no evidence that prolongation of tetracycline therapy beyond 1 week is necessary, provided that sex partners can be treated concurrently. In Reiter's syndrome, the value of tetracycline therapy has not been studied, either in terms of clinical response of NGU or in terms of improvement of other features of the syndrome. Men with either idiopathic epididymitis or proven chlamydial epididymitis should receive doxycycline, 100 mg PO bid for 10 days. In a small treatment trial, ampicillin, 3.5 g followed by 500 mg PO qid, appeared less effective than tetracycline in these patients.[70]

Fewer studies have assessed the effectiveness of antimicrobial treatment of uncomplicated cervical or urethral chlamydial infection in women (Table 16-5). Those data available suggest that tetracycline, 500 mg qid for 7 days, successfully eliminates *C. trachomatis* from the cervix through 3 weeks of follow-up.[140–146] Erythromycin, when given as 500 mg PO qid for 7 to 14 days, is also effective as is ofloxacin, 200 mg PO bid.[147] A small double-blind, placebo-controlled trial indicates that doxycycline, 100 mg PO bid for 10 days, successfully eliminated *C. trachomatis* from the cervix and urethra of women with the acute urethral syndrome.[90] Treatment of salpingitis is discussed in Chaps. 49 and 50.

## PREVENTION

A major hindrance to effective prevention of chlamydial genital tract infection is the absence of specific diagnostic testing in most STD clinics or physicians' offices. At least 40 percent of all chlamydial infections seen in STD clinics are asymptomatic, and an even greater proportion of chlamydial infections in sexually active populations not seeking health care are probably asymptomatic. Establishment of diagnostic screening procedures for *C.*

**Table 16-5. Summary of Selected Studies Evaluating Antimicrobial Treatment of *C. trachomatis* Cervicitis in Women**

| Regimen | Efficacy | Reference |
|---|---|---|
| Deteclo, 300 mg bid for 7 days | 20/20 (100%) | 141 |
| Oxytetracycline, 250 mg qid for 14 days | 49/50 (98%) | 134 |
| Oxytetracycline, 250 mg qid for 21 days | 145/161 (90%) | 140 |
| Erythromycin, 500 mg bid for 15 days | 13/17 (76%) | 138 |
| Lymecycline, 300 mg bid for 10 days | 18/20 (90%) | |
| Lymecycline, 300 mg bid for 20 days | 14/14 (100%) | |
| Doxycycline, 200 mg stat., then 100 mg bid for 8 days | 10/10 (100%) | 142 |
| Trimethoprim-sulfadiazine, 160 and 500 mg, respectively, in 1 tablet bid for 14 days | 15/15 (100%) | 61 |
| Doxycycline, 100 mg bid for 10 days | 15/15 (100%) | |
| Doxycycline, 200 mg stat., then 100 mg bid for 9 days | 55/58 (95%) | 143 |
| Erythromycin, 500 mg bid for 10 days | 36/39 (92%) | |
| Trimethoprim-sulfamethoxazole, 160 and 800 mg, respectively, in 1 tablet for 10 days | 37/40 (93%) | |
| Tetracycline, 500 mg qid for 7 days | 6/6 (100%) | 144 |
| Tetracycline, 250 mg qid for 7 days | 6/6 (100%) | |
| Rosaramicin, 250 mg qid for 7 days | 9/11 (82%) | |
| Erythromycin, 250 mg qid for 7 days | 10/10 (100%) | |
| Tetracycline, 500 mg qid for 7 days | 21/22 (95%) | 145 |
| Erythromycin, 250 mg qid for 7 days | 12/12 (100%) | |
| Sulfisoxazole, 500 mg qid for 10 days | 8/8 (100%) | |
| Ciprofloxacin, 500 mg bid for 7 days | 30/35 (86%) | 147 |
| Pivampicillin, 700 mg bid for 7 days | 26/26 (100%) | 148 |

*trachomatis* in high-risk populations seen in STD clinics, family planning clinics, prenatal clinics, juvenile detention centers, adolescent medicine clinics, and gynecology clinics seems critical to identify and treat asymptomatically infected individuals who constitute the major reservoir for *C. trachomatis*.

Empirical treatment of women who are sex partners of men with NGU is recommended even when specific diagnostic testing is performed. At least 30 percent of these women will be culture-positive if tested, and many will be asymptomatic and lack signs of infection. All women identified as recent partners of men with NGU should be carefully examined for mucopurulent cervicitis and salpingitis and then treated with tetracycline, 500 mg PO qid for 7 days or doxycycline, 100 mg bid for 7 days; or with erythromycin, 500 mg PO qid for 7 to 14 days, if pregnant or possibly pregnant.

The diagnosis of chlamydial mucopurulent cervicitis cannot be as easily and reliably established as the diagnosis of NGU. For this reason, specific diagnostic testing is strongly recommended in such patients. If testing is not done, however, women who have clear-cut mucopurulent cervicitis and a negative culture for gonorrhea should be assumed to have chlamydial infection. They should be treated with the tetracycline or erythromycin regimens outlined above, and their sex partners should be identified and examined for evidence of urethritis. Gram stains in men without symptoms may reveal asymptomatic urethral leukocytosis, which has been associated with chlamydial infection. Until further data are available, partners of women with mucopurulent cervicitis or salpingitis should probably also receive tetracycline, 500 mg PO qid for 7 days.

Since coinfection with chlamydia occurs in 15 to 25 percent of heterosexual men and 30 to 40 percent of women with gonorrhea, postgonococcal chlamydial morbidity (PGU, epididymitis, mucopurulent cervicitis, salpingitis) and chlamydial transmission can be prevented by increased use of treatment regimens for gonorrhea that are also effective against chlamydia. Combined therapy with a single-dose regimen effective against gonorrhea (ampicillin, spectinomycin, ceftriaxone, or other of the newer cephalosporins), followed by a regimen effective against chlamydia (doxycycline, 100 mg bid, or tetracycline hydrochloride, 500 mg qid for 7 days) is currently recommended.

With implementation of most of these recommendations in Seattle–King County in the late 1970s, facilitated by public funding for chlamydia cultures in 1979, the prevalence of *C. trachomatis* cervical infection among women attending the Harborview Medical Center STD Clinic has fallen significantly from 14 percent in 1980 to 1982 to 10 percent in 1983 to 1986. No accompanying decline was seen in males attending the clinic, perhaps due to the fact that a higher proportion of these infections are symptomatic. Although this decline in prevalence among women may be related to changes in sexual behavior as well, the decline in *C. trachomatis* infection has been more dramatic than for other STDs, such as gonorrhea and syphilis. We believe that prevention of genital *C. trachomatis* infection may be a readily achievable goal with appropriate use of the above measures, particularly screening to identify unrecognized cases.

## References


1 Schachter J: Chlamydial infections. *N Engl J Med* 298: 428, 1978.

2 Schachter J et al: Are chlamydial infections the most prevalent venereal disease? *JAMA* 231: 1252, 1975.

3 Thelin I et al: Contact tracing in patients with genital chlamydial infection. *Br J Vener Dis* 56: 259, 1980.

4 McMillan A et al: Chlamydial infection in homosexual men: Frequency of isolation of *Chlamydia trachomatis* from the urethra, ano-rectum, and pharynx. *Br J Vener Dis* 57: 47, 1981.

5 Stamm WE et al: *Chlamydia trachomatis* urethral infections in men. Prevalence, risk factors, and clinical manifestations. *Ann Intern Med* 100: 47, 1984.

6 Podgore JK et al: Asymptomatic urethral infections due to *Chlamydia trachomatis* in male military personnel. *J Infect Dis* 146: 828, 1982.

7 Sadof MD et al: Dipstick leukocyte esterase activity in first-catch urine specimens. A useful screening test for detecting sexually

transmitted diseases in the adolescent male. *JAMA* 258: 1932, 1987.

8 Adger H et al: Screening for *Chlamydia trachomatis* and *Neisseria gonorrhoeae* in adolescent males: Value of first catch urine examination. *Lancet* 2: 944, 1984.

9 Bowie WR et al: Etiologies of postgonococcal urethritis in homosexual and heterosexual men: Roles of *Chlamydia trachomatis* and *Ureaplasma urealyticum*. *Sex Transm Dis* 5: 151, 1978.

10 Stamm WE et al: *Chlamydia trachomatis* proctitis, in *Chlamydial Infections*, PA Mårdh et al (eds). Amsterdam, Elsevier, 1982, pp 111–115.

11 Goldmeier D, Darougar S: Isolation of *Chlamydia trachomatis* from the throat and rectum of homosexual men. *Br J Vener Dis* 53: 184, 1977.

12 Quinn TC et al: *Chlamydia trachomatis* proctitis. *N Engl J Med* 305: 195, 1981.

13 Jones RB et al: *Chlamydia trachomatis* in the pharynx and rectum of heterosexual patients at risk for genital infection. *Ann Intern Med* 102: 757, 1985.

14 Neinstein LS, Inderlied C: Low prevalence of *Chlamydia trachomatis* in the oropharynx of adolescents. *Pediatr Infect Dis* 5: 660, 1986.

15 Komaroff AL et al: Serological evidence of chlamydial and mycoplasmal pharyngitis in adults. *Science* 221: 927, 1983.

16 Gerber MA et al: Role of *Chlamydia trachomatis* in acute pharyngitis in young adults. *J Clin Microbiol* 20: 993, 1984.

17 Husseltein et al: Frequency of *Chlamydia trachomatis* as a cause of pharyngitis. *J Clin Microbiol* 22: 858, 1984.

18 Schachter J: *Chlamydia psittaci:* Reemergence of a forgotten pathogen. *N Engl J Med* 315: 189, 1986.

19 Evaluations and Statistical Services Section, Venereal Disease Control Division, Centers for Disease Control, Atlanta, Ga.

20 Lycke E et al: The risk of transmission of genital *Chlamydia trachomatis* infection is less than that of genital *Neisseria gonorrhoeae* infection. *Sex Transm Dis* 7: 6, 1980.

21 Richmond SJ et al: Value and feasibility of screening women attending STD clinics for cervical chlamydial infections. *Br J Vener Dis* 56: 92, 1980.

22 McCormack WM et al: Fifteen month follow-up study of women infected with *Chlamydia trachomatis*. *N Engl J Med* 300: 123, 1979.

23 Oriel JD et al: Chlamydial infections of the cervix. *Br J Vener Dis* 50: 11, 1974.

24 Hilton AL et al: Chlamydia A in the female genital tract. *Br J Vener Dis* 50: 1, 1974.

25 Brunham R et al: Epidemiological and clinical correlates of *C. trachomatis* and *N. gonorrhoeae* infection among women attending an STD clinic. *Clin Res* 29: 47A, 1981.

26 Stamm WE et al: Causes of the acute urethral syndrome in women. *N Engl J Med* 303: 409, 1980.

27 Paavonen J et al: Genital chlamydial infections in patients attending a gynecological outpatient clinic. *Br J Vener Dis* 54: 257, 1978.

28 Ripa KT et al: *Chlamydia trachomatis* cervicitis in gynecologic outpatients. *Obstet Gynecol* 52: 698, 1978.

29 Schachter J et al: Chlamydiae as agents of sexually transmitted diseases. *Bull WHO* 54: 245, 1976.

30 Persson K et al: Prevalence of nine different microorganisms in the female genital tract. *Br J Vener Dis* 55: 429, 1979.

31 Oriel JD et al: Infection of the uterine cervix with *Chlamydia trachomatis*. *J Infect Dis* 137: 443, 1978.

32 Johannisson G et al: Genital *C. trachomatis* infection in women. *Obstet Gynecol* 56: 671, 1980.

33 Robertson P, Schachter J: Failure to identify venereal disease in lesbian population. *Sex Transm Dis* 8:75, 1981.

34 Saltz GR et al: *Chlamydia trachomatis* cervical infections in female adolescents. *J Pediatr* 98: 981, 1981.

35 Bowie WR et al: Prevalence of *C. trachomatis* and *N. gonorrhoeae* in two populations of women. *Can Med Assoc J* 124: 1477, 1981.

36 Harrison HR et al: *Chlamydia trachomatis* infection in pregnancy: Epidemiology and outcomes, abstracted (no 516). Read at the Twenty-first Interscience Conference on Antimicrobial Agents and Chemotherapy. Washington, DC, American Society for Microbiology, 1981.

37 Hammerschlag MR et al: Prospective study of maternal and infantile infection with *Chlamydia trachomatis*. *Pediatrics* 64: 142, 1979.

38 Martin DH et al: Prematurity and perinatal mortality in pregnancies complicated by maternal *Chlamydia trachomatis* infection. *JAMA* 247: 1585, 1982.

39 Martin DH et al: High prevalence of chlamydial infections in an inner city obstetrical population, abstracted (no 515). Read at the Twenty-first Interscience Conference on Antimicrobial Agents and Chemotherapy. Washington, DC, American Society for Microbiology, 1981.

40 Chandler JW et al: Ophthalmia neonatorum associated with maternal chlamydial infections. *Trans Am Acad Ophthalmol Otolaryngol* 83: 302, 1977.

41 Frommell GT et al: Chlamydial infection of mothers and their infants. *J Pediatr* 95: 28, 1979.

42 Harrison HR et al: Cervical *Chlamydia trachomatis* and mycoplasmal infections in pregnancy. Epidemiology and outcomes. *JAMA* 250: 1721, 1983.

43 Toomey KE et al: Unrecognized high prevalence of *Chlamydia trachomatis* cervical infection in an isolated Alaskan population. *JAMA* 258: 53, 1987.

44 Black SB et al: Serologic evidence of chlamydial infection in children. *J Pediatr* 98: 65, 1981.

45 Stamm WE, Cole B. Asymptomatic *Chlamydia trachomatis* urethritis in men. *Sex Transm Dis* 13: 163, 1986.

46 Tack KJ et al: Isolation of *Chlamydia trachomatis* from the lower respiratory tract of adults. *Lancet* 1: 116, 1980.

47 Ormsby HL et al: Topical therapy in inclusion conjunctivitis. *Am J Ophthalmol* 35: 1811, 1952.

48 Ito JI et al: Pneumonia due to *Chlamydia trachomatis* in an immunocompromised adult. *N Engl J Med* 307: 95, 1982.

49 Brunham BC et al: Cellular immune response during uncomplicated genital infection with *Chlamydia trachomatis* in humans. *Infect Immun* 34: 98, 1981.

50 Moncada JV et al: Prevalence of *Chlamydia trachomatis* lung infection in patients with acquired immune deficiency syndrome. *J Clin Microbiol* 23: 986, 1986.

51 Ballard RC et al: The epidemiology of chlamydial infections of the eye and genital tract in South Africa. Third International Meeting on Sexually Transmitted Diseases, Antwerp, Belgium, 1980.

52 Holmes KK et al: Etiology of nongonococcal urethritis. *N Engl J Med* 292: 1199, 1975.

53 Oriel JD et al: Chlamydial infection: Isolation of *Chlamydia* from patients with non-specific genital infection. *Br J Vener Dis* 48: 429, 1972.

54 Richmond SJ et al: Chlamydial infection: Role of *Chlamydia* subgroup A in non-gonococcal and post-gonococcal urethritis. *Br J Vener Dis* 48: 437, 1972.

55 Dunlop EMC et al: Chlamydia and non-specific urethritis. *Br J Vener Dis* 2: 575, 1972.

56 Alani MD et al: Isolation of *Chlamydia trachomatis* from the male urethra. *Br J Vener Dis* 53: 88, 1977.

57 Terho P: *Chlamydia trachomatis* in NGU. *Br J Vener Dis* 54: 251, 1978.

58 Paavonen J: *Chlamydia trachomatis*-induced urethritis in female partners of men with nongonococcal urethritis. *Sex Transm Dis* 6: 69, 1979.

59 Lassus A et al: Erythromycin and lymecycline treatment of chlamydia-positive and chlamydia-negative NGU: A partner controlled study. *Acta Derm Venereol (Stockh)* 59: 278, 1979.

60 Bowie WR et al: Etiology of nongonococcal urethritis: Evidence of *Chlamydia trachomatis* and *Ureaplasma urealyticum*. *J Clin Invest* 59: 735, 1977.

61 Paavonen J et al: Treatment of NGU with trimethoprim-sulpha-

diazine and with placebo: A double-blind partner-controlled study. *Br J Vener Dis* 56: 101, 1980.

62 Bowie WR et al: Differential response of chlamydial and ureaplasma-associated urethritis to sulphafurazole (sulfisoxazole) and aminocyclitols. *Lancet* 2: 1276, 1976.

63 Handsfield HH et al: Differences in the therapeutic response of chlamydia-positive and chlamydia-negative forms of nongonococcal urethritis. *J Am Vener Dis Assoc* 2: 5, 1976.

64 Prentice MJ et al: NGU: A placebo controlled trial of minocycline in conjunction with laboratory investigations. *Br J Vener Dis* 52: 269, 1976.

65 Digiacomo RF et al: Chlamydial infection of the male baboon urethra. *Br J Vener Dis* 51: 310, 1975.

66 Taylor-Robinson D et al: Microbiological, serological and histopathological features of experimental *Chlamydia trachomatis* urethritis in chimpanzees. *Br J Vener Dis* 57: 36, 1981.

67 Schwartz SL, Kraus SJ: Persistent urethral leucocytosis and asymptomatic chlamydial urethritis. *J Infect Dis* 140: 614, 1979.

68 Oriel JD et al: Infection with *Chlamydia* group A in men with urethritis due to *Neisseria gonorrhoeae*. *J Infect Dis* 131: 376, 1975.

69 Berger RE et al: *Chlamydia trachomatis* as a cause of acute "idiopathic" epididymitis. *N Engl J Med* 298: 301, 1978.

70 Berger RE et al: Etiology, manifestations, and therapy of acute epididymitis: Prospective study of 50 cases. *J Urol* 121: 750, 1979.

71 Moller BR, Mårdh PA: Experimental epididymitis and urethritis in grivet monkeys provoked by *Chlamydia trachomatis*. *Fertil Steril* 34: 275, 1980.

72 Berger RE et al: Epididymitis induced in *Macaca nemestrina* with *Chlamydia trachomatis* (submitted for publication).

73 Mårdh PA et al: Role in *Chlamydia trachomatis* in non-acute prostatitis. *Br J Vener Dis* 54: 330, 1978.

74 Mårdh PA et al: Inhibiting effect on the formation of chlamydial inclusions in McCoy cells by seminal fluid and some of its components. *Invest Urol* 17: 510, 1980.

75 Nilsson S et al: Isolation of *Chlamydia trachomatis* from the urethra and from prostatic fluid in men with signs and symptoms of acute urethritis, in Studies on *C. trachomatis* as a cause of lower urogenital tract infections. *Thesis Acta Dermatovener* suppl 93, 1981.

76 Bruce AW et al: The role of chlamydiae in genitourinary disease. *J Urol* 126: 625, 1981.

77 Poletti F et al: Isolation of *Chlamydia trachomatis* from the prostatic cells in patients affected by nonacute abacterial prostatis. *J Urol* 134: 691, 1985.

78 Rompalo AM et al: Potential value of rectal-screening cultures for *Chlamydia trachomatis* in homosexual men. *J Infect Dis* 153: 888, 1986.

79 Kousa M et al: Frequent association of chlamydial infection with Reiter's syndrome. *Sex Transm Dis* 5: 57, 1978.

80 Martin DH et al: Urethral chlamydial infections in men with Reiter's syndrome, in *Chlamydial Infections*, PA Mårdh et al (eds). Amsterdam, Elsevier, 1982, pp 107–111.

81 Bowie WR: personal communication, 1981.

82 Keat AC et al. *Chlamydia trachomatis* and reactive arthritis: The missing link. *Lancet* i: 72, 1987.

83 Brewerton DA et al: Reiter's disease and HLA 27. *Lancet* 2: 996, 1973.

84 Keat AC et al: Role of *Chlamydia trachomatis* and HLA-B27 in sexually acquired reactive arthritis. *Br Med J* 1: 605, 1978.

85 Harrison HR et al: Cervical *Chlamydia trachomatis* infection in university women: Relationship to history, contraception, ectopy and cervicitis. *Am J Obstet Gynecol* 153: 244, 1985.

86 Paavonen J et al. Colposcopic manifestations of cervical and vaginal infections. *Obstet Gynecol Surv* 43: 373, 1988.

87 Brunham RC et al: Mucopurulent cervicitis—the ignored counterpart in women of urethritis in men. *N Engl J Med* 311: 1, 1984.

88 Hobson D et al: Quantitative aspects of chlamydial infection of the cervix. *Br J Vener Dis* 56: 156, 1980.

89 Richmond SJ et al: Antibodies to *Chlamydia trachomatis* in cervicovaginal secretions. *Sex Transm Dis* 7: 11, 1980.

90 Stamm WE et al: Treatment of the acute urethral syndrome. *N Engl J Med* 304: 956, 1981.

91 Wallin JE et al: Urethritis in women attending an STD clinic. *Br J Vener Dis* 57: 50, 1981.

92 Davies JA et al: Isolation of *Chlamydia trachomatis* from Bartholin's ducts. *Br J Vener Dis* 54: 409, 1978.

93 Mårdh PA et al: Endometritis caused by *Chlamydia trachomatis*. *Br J Vener Dis* 57: 191, 1981.

94 Gump DW et al: Endometritis related to *Chlamydia trachomatis* infection. *Ann Intern Med* 95: 61, 1981.

95 Hamark B et al: Bacteriological cultures from the endometrial cavity in patients with acute salpingitis. *Acta Obstet Gynecol Scand [Suppl]* 93: 55, 1981.

96 Moller BR et al: Salpingitis og endometritis forårsaget af *Chlamydia trachomatis*. *Ugeskr Laeger* 172: 3319, 1980.

97 Wasserheit JN et al: Microbial causes of proven pelvic inflammatory disease and efficacy of clindamycin and tobramycin. *Ann Intern Med* 104: 187, 1986.

98 Sweet RL et al: Failure of beta-lactam antibiotics to eradicate *Chlamydia trachomatis* in the endometrium despite apparent clinical cure of acute salpingitis. *JAMA* 250: 2641, 1983.

99 Paavonen J et al: Prevalence and manifestations of endometritis among women with cervicitis. *Am J Obstet Gynecol* 152: 280, 1985.

100 Wager GP et al: Puerperal infectious morbidity: Relationship to route of delivery and to antepartum *Chlamydia trachomatis* infection. *Am J Obstet Gynecol* 138: 1028, 1980.

101 Mårdh PA et al: *Chlamydia trachomatis* infection in patients with acute salpingitis. *N Engl J Med* 296: 1377, 1977.

102 Eschenbach DA et al: Polymicrobial etiology of acute pelvic inflammatory disease. *N Engl J Med* 293: 166, 1975.

103 Treharne JD et al: Antibodies to *Chlamydia trachomatis* in acute salpingitis. *Br J Vener Dis* 55: 26, 1979.

104 Simmons PD et al: Antichlamydial antibodies in pelvic inflammatory disease. *Br J Vener Dis* 55: 419, 1979.

105 Rees E: The treatment of pelvic inflammatory disease. *Am J Obstet Gynecol* 138: 1041, 1980.

106 Mårdh PA: Ascending chlamydial infection in the female tract, in: D Oriel et al (eds). *Chlamydial Infections*. London, Cambridge University Press, 1986, pp 173–185.

107 Svensson L et al: Differences in some clinical and laboratory parameters in acute salpingitis related to culture and clinical findings. *Am J Obstet Gynecol* 138: 1017, 1980.

108 Bowie WR et al: Acute pelvic inflammatory disease in outpatients. *Ann Intern Med* 95: 685, 1981.

109 Osser S et al: Epidemiologic and serodiagnostic aspects of chlamydial salpingitis. *Obstet Gynecol* 59: 206, 1982.

110 Brunham RC et al: Etiology and outcome of acute pelvic inflammatory disease. *J Infect Dis* 158: 510, 1988.

111 Moller BR et al: Experimental pelvic inflammatory disease provoked by *Chlamydia trachomatis* and *Mycoplasma hominis* in grivet monkeys. *Am J Obstet Gynecol* 138: 990, 1980.

112 Patton D et al: *Chlamydia trachomatis* salpingitis in the pig-tailed macaque, in *Chlamydial Infections*, PA Mårdh et al (eds). Amsterdam, Elsevier, 1982, pp 399–405.

113 Muller-Schoop JW et al: *Chlamydia trachomatis* as a possible cause of peritonitis and perihepatitis in young women. *Br J Vener Dis* 1: 1022, 1978.

114 Wolner-Hanssen P et al: Perihepatitis in chlamydial salpingitis. *Lancet* 1: 901, 1980.

115 Dalaker K et al: *Chlamydia trachomatis* as a cause of perihepatitis associated with pelvic inflammatory disease. *Br J Vener Dis* 57: 41, 1977.

116 Meyers JD et al: *Chlamydia trachomatis* infection as a cause of pneumonia after human marrow transplantation. *Transplantation* 36: 130, 1983.

117 Tack KJ et al: Isolation of *Chlamydia trachomatis* from the lower respiratory tract of adults. *Lancet* i: 116, 1980.
118 Cunningham D et al: T-cell lymphoblastic lymphoma of the uterus complicated by *Chlamydia trachomatis* pneumonia. *Postgrad Med J* 62: 55, 1986.
119 Komaroff AL et al: *Chlamydia trachomatis* infection in adults with community-acquired pneumonia. *JAMA* 245: 1319, 1981.
120 Schachter J: Human *Chlamydia psittaci* infection in chlamydial infections, in D Oriel et al (eds). *Proceedings of the Sixth International Symposium on Human Chlamydial Infections*. London, Cambridge University Press, 1986.
121 vander Bel-Kahn JM et al: *Chlamydia trachomatis* endocarditis. *Am Heart J* 95: 627, 1978.
122 Myhre EB, Mårdh PA: *Chlamydia trachomatis* infections in a patient with meningoencephalitis. *N Engl J Med* 304: 910, 1981.
123 Lannigan R et al: *Chlamydia trachomatis* peritonitis and ascites following appendectomy. *Can Med Assoc J* 123: 295, 1980.
124 Goldmeier D et al: Chlamydial vulvovaginitis in a post menopausal woman. *Lancet* 2: 476, 1981.
125 Stamm WE: Diagnosis of *Chlamydia trachomatis* genitourinary infections. *Ann Intern Med* 108: 710, 1988.
126 Ridgway GL et al: A method for testing the antibiotic susceptibility of *Chlamydia trachomatis* in a cell culture system. *J Antimicrob Chemother* 2: 71, 1976.
127 Treharne JD et al: Susceptibility of chlamydiae to chemotherapeutic agents, in *Nongonococcal Urethritis and Related Infections*, KK Holmes, D Hobson (eds). Washington, DC, American Society for Microbiology, 1977, pp 214–223.
128 Blackman HJ et al: Antibiotic susceptibility of *Chlamydia trachomatis*. *Antimicrob Agents Chemother* 12: 673, 1977.
129 Kuo C et al: Antimicrobial activity of several antibiotics and a sulfonamide against *Chlamydia trachomatis* organisms in organ culture. *Antimicrob Agents Chemother* 12: 80, 1977.
130 Johannison G et al: Susceptibility of *Chlamydia trachomatis* to antibiotics in vitro and in vivo. *Sex Transm Dis* 6: 50, 1979.
131 Thambar IV et al: Double-blind comparison of two regimens in the treatment of NGU. *Br J Vener Dis* 55: 284, 1979.
132 Bowie WR et al: Therapy for nongonococcal urethritis: Double-blind randomized comparison of two doses and two durations of minocycline. *Ann Intern Med* 95: 306, 1981.
133 Prentice MJ et al: Non-specific urethritis: A placebo-controlled trial of minocycline in conjunction with laboratory investigations. *Br J Vener Dis* 52: 269, 1976.
134 Oriel JD et al: Comparison of erythromycin stearate and oxytetracycline in the treatment of non-gonococcal urethritis. *Scott Med J* 22: 375, 1977.
135 Perroud HM, Vulliemin JF: L'hyclate de doxycycline dans le traitment des uretrites non-gonoccicques. *Schweiz Med Wochenschr* 108: 412, 1978.
136 Coufalik ED et al: Treatment of nongonococcal urethritis with rifampicin as a means of defining the role of *Ureaplasma urealyticum*. *Br J Vener Dis* 55: 36, 1979.
137 Bowie WR et al: Eradication of *Chlamydia trachomatis* from the urethras of men with NGU by treatment with amoxicillin. *Sex Transm Dis* 8: 79, 1981.
138 Lassus A et al: Erythromycin and lymecycline treatment in chlamydia-positive and chlamydia-negative nongonococcal urethritis: A partner-controlled study. *Acta Derm Venereol (Stockh)* 59: 278, 1979.
139 Stamm WE, Holmes KK: Comparison of rosaramicin and tetracycline for the treatment of NGU, in *Current Chemotherapy and Infectious Diseases*, JD Nelson, C Grassi (eds). Washington, DC, American Society for Microbiology, 1980, vol 1, pp 269–270.
140 Rees E et al: Chlamydia in relation to cervical infection and pelvic inflammatory disease, in *Nongonococcal Urethritis and Related Infections*, D Hobson, KK Holmes (eds). Washington, DC, American Society for Microbiology, 1977, pp 67–77.
140a Arya O et al: Evaluation of ciprofloxacin 500 mg twice daily for one week in treating uncomplicated gonococcal, chlamydial and nonspecific urethritis in men. *Genitourin Med* 62: 170, 1986.
141 Waugh MA, Nayyar KC: Triple tetracycline (Deteclo) in the treatment of chlamydial infection of the female genital tract. *Br J Vener Dis* 53: 96, 1977.
142 Ripa KT et al: *Chlamydia trachomatis* cervicitis in gynecologic patients. *Obstet Gynecol* 52: 698, 1978.
143 Johannison G: Studies on *Chlamydia trachomatis* as a cause of lower urogenital tract infection. *Acta Derm Venereol* 93 (suppl) 29, 1981.
144 Brunham RC et al: Rosaramicin, erythromycin and tetracycline in the treatment of urogenital infection with *Chlamydia trachomatis* in women, abstracted. Read at the Twelfth International Congress of Chemotherapy. Florence, Italy, 1981.
145 Bowie WR: Seven to ten day antimicrobial regimens for *Chlamydia trachomatis* cervical infection. *Clin Res* 28: 43A, 1980.
146 Hunter J et al: Response to treatment of chlamydial infection of uterine cervix. *Lancet* 2: 848, 1979.
147 Ahmed-Jushuf IH et al: Ciprofloxacin treatment of chlamydial infections of urogenital tracts of women. *Genitourin Med* 64: 14, 1988.
148 Cramers M et al: Pivampicillin compared with erythromycin for treating women with genital *Chlamydia trachomatis* infection. *Genitourin Med* 64: 247, 1988.

Chapter 17

# Lymphogranuloma venereum

Peter L. Perine
A. Olu Osoba

Lymphogranuloma venereum (LGV) is one of the sexually transmitted diseases caused by *Chlamydia trachomatis*. A sporadic disease in North America, Europe, and Oceania, LGV is highly prevalent in parts of Africa, Asia, and South America. It is also known variously as tropical or climatic bubo,[1] strumous bubo,[2] poradenitis inguinalis,[3] Durand-Nicolas-Favre disease,[3,4] lymphogranuloma inguinale, and the fourth, fifth, or sixth venereal disease.[5] LGV is preferred because it is less easily confused with granuloma inguinale.

LGV is a chronic disease that has a variety of acute and late manifestations. Three stages of infection, more or less analogous to those of venereal syphilis, are recognized.[6] The infrequent primary lesion is a small, inconspicuous genital papule or herpetiform ulcer of short duration and few symptoms. The secondary stage is characterized by acute lymphadenitis with bubo formation (the inguinal syndrome), and/or acute hemorrhagic proctitis (the anogenitorectal syndrome) together with fever and other symptoms caused by systemic spread of infection. The vast majority of patients recover from LGV after the secondary stage without sequela, but in a few patients the persistence of chlamydia in anogenital tissue incites a chronic inflammatory response and the development of genital ulcers, fistulas, rectal strictures, and genital elephantiasis. Antibiotic treatment during the secondary stage prevents these late complications, which otherwise may require surgical repair.

LGV is usually caused by one of three serovars of *C. trachomatis:* L1, L2, and L3 (see Chap. 15). As a general rule these serovars cannot be distinguished from those causing trachoma and other genital tract infections.[7] Other *C. trachomatis* strains have been isolated from infected tissue taken from patients who have symptoms compatible with genitoanorectal LGV.[8,9]

Throughout most of its history LGV has been confused with other diseases, particularly with the lymphadenopathy of syphilis and genital herpes and the buboes of chancroid. Confusion was caused in part by the failure to recognize the common etiology of the different manifestations of LGV, which were often described as distinct clinical or pathological entities. Durand, Nicolas, and Favre established the disease as a clinical and pathological entity in 1913,[4] and Phylactos deduced a common etiology of climatic bubo and LGV in 1922,[10] but the greatest advancement to the study of LGV was the development of a "specific" skin test by Frei in 1925.[11] This test established the etiology of LGV proctocolitis and rectal stricture.[12] In 1930 LGV chlamydia were isolated from buboes by intracerebral inoculation of monkeys,[10] and LGV chlamydia were grown in embryonated eggs in 1935.[13] The latter achievement made possible the commercial manufacture of large amounts of standardized antigen for Frei tests and serodiagnostic tests.

The first effective drugs for treatment of LGV were the sulfonamides, which were introduced in the late 1930s.[14] Although other drugs have since been developed for treatment of LGV[15] and serodiagnostic tests have been refined to give greater specificity, we still do not fully understand the pathogenesis of this disease.

A thorough review of the history of LGV is a study in itself and will not be attempted here. The monograph on LGV published by Stannus in 1933[5] lists 933 references and, together with the excellent reviews published by Koteen in 1945[16] and Favre and Hellerström in 1954,[10] describes the historical background of the disease.

## EPIDEMIOLOGY

LGV is a sporadic disease throughout North America, Europe, Australia, and most of Asia and South America. It is endemic in east[17] and west Africa,[18] India,[19] parts of southeastern Asia,[20] South America,[21] and the Caribbean.[22] Few countries require official notification of LGV cases, and the lack of standard diagnostic criteria renders reported cases somewhat suspect. Since 1950 no country in Europe reported more than a few dozen cases of LGV annually,[21] and the average for the United States was 595 cases per year, with slight increases during the wars in Korea and Vietnam.[23] By contrast, one municipal clinic in Ethiopia reports several thousand cases of acute LGV annually.[17] Most of the reported LGV cases in nonendemic areas occur in sailors, soldiers, and travelers who acquire the infection while visiting or living in an endemic area.[20] Like other sexually transmitted diseases, LGV is more common in urban than in rural areas, among the sexually promiscuous, and among the lower socioeconomic classes.[22] However, much of the reported epidemiology on LGV is based on the results of serologic tests and/or Frei skin tests that are not specific for the disease. When such tests are used in large prevalence studies (e.g., in venereal disease clinics and municipal hospitals), a large segment of the population is inevitably found to have positive test results but no history or physical evidence of the disease. Many such studies conducted in the United States in the 1930s claimed that 20 to 40 percent of blacks and 2 to 5 percent of whites were or had at one time been infected with LGV.[10,16,24] Such studies probably demonstrated the high prevalence of other *C. trachomatis* infections in these highly selected patient populations rather than a true racial difference. Of interest are early reports from Africa and South America which stated that climatic bubo was uncommon in all but white expatriates.[25]

Acute LGV occurs most frequently during the third decade, which corresponds to the age of peak sexual activity. Extragenital[10,16] and adolescent infections have also been reported,[10] and material from ruptured buboes and other infected tissue poses a risk to research and health care personnel.[26,27]

Acute LGV is reported much more frequently in men than in women, with the ratio often reaching 5:1 or greater.[28] This is because symptomatic infection is much less common in women, who usually are diagnosed during early infection only if they develop acute proctocolitis or, less commonly, inguinal buboes. Late complications such as hyperplasia, ulceration and hypertrophy of the genitalia (esthiomene), and rectal strictures are reported to be more frequent in women than in men.[16,24] Homosexual men who are recipients of anal intercourse may also present with acute proctocolitis rather than inguinal buboes[9] and may develop rectal strictures.[22]

The frequency of infection following exposure is unknown. LGV is probably not as contagious as gonorrhea. Primary herpetiform lesions, urethritis, cervicitis, proctocolitis, and chronic ulcerations are probably the most infectious forms of LGV. Although supporting evidence is limited, the endocervix is apparently the most common site of acute infection in women. The cervix may remain infected for periods of weeks or months, as has been demonstrated for other serovars of *C. trachomatis*.[29] Conjugal infections are said to be common.[10,30] Congenital transmission does not occur, but infection may be acquired during passage through an infected birth canal.

## PATHOGENESIS

Chlamydia cannot penetrate intact skin or mucous membrane; these organisms probably gain entry through minute lacerations and abrasions. Laboratory-acquired infections following inhalation of highly concentrated virulent cultures have been reported.[27]

LGV is predominantly a disease of lymphatic tissue.[31] The essential pathological process is thrombolymphangitis and perilymphangitis with spread of the inflammatory process from infected lymph nodes into the surrounding tissue. The lymphangitis is marked by proliferation of endothelial cells lining the lymph vessels and the lymph channels in lymph nodes. Lymph nodes draining the site of primary infection rapidly enlarge and form small, discrete areas of necrosis surrounded by densely packed endothelial cells.[32] The necrotic areas attract polymorphonuclear leukocytes and enlarge to form characteristic triangular- or quadrangular-shaped "stellate abscesses." Inflammation mats the adjacent lymph nodes together by periadenitis, and as the inflammation progresses, abscesses coalesce and rupture the node, forming loculated abscesses, fistulas, or sinus tracts.

The inflammatory process lasts several weeks or months before subsiding. Healing takes place by fibrosis, which destroys the normal structure of lymph nodes and obstructs subcutaneous and submucous lymph vessels. The resulting chronic edema and sclerosing fibrosis causes induration and enlargement of the affected parts. Fibrosis also compromises the blood supply to the overlying skin or mucous membrane, and ulceration occurs. In the rectum this results in destruction and ulceration of the mucosa, transmural inflammation of the bowel wall, obstruction of lymphatic drainage, and formation of a fibrotic, inflammatory stricture. Numerous adhesions form which fix the lower part of the sigmoid and rectum to the wall of the pelvis and neighboring organs.[32,33]

Although the primary pathological process in LGV may be localized to one or two groups of lymph nodes, the organisms spread systemically in the bloodstream and can enter the central nervous system.[34] Dissemination and local extension of disease is limited by host immunity. Delayed hypersensitivity (as evidenced by positive skin tests) and specific chlamydia antibody can be demonstrated 1 to 2 weeks after infection.[35] Chlamydial cytoplasmic inclusions can also be demonstrated within tissue phagocytes early in the course of infection.[13] Host immunity ultimately limits chlamydial multiplication but may not eliminate these organisms from the body, and a state of latency ensues.[15] Viable chlamydia have been isolated from late lesions as long as 20 years after initial infection.[36] Much of the tissue damage in LGV is probably caused by cell-mediated hypersensitivity to chlamydial antigens. Persistence of LGV in tissues or repeated infections by the same or related serovars of *C. trachomatis* may be important in developing systemic disease.[37] It is of interest that repeated subcutaneous or intravenous injections of Frei antigen were used to treat LGV in the 1930s with some success,[38] possibly by desensitizing the host to chlamydia.

## CLINICAL MANIFESTATIONS

### PRIMARY LESION

The primary lesion of LGV may take one of four forms: a papule, a shallow ulcer or erosion, a small herpetiform lesion, or nonspecific urethritis.[28] The most common is the herpetiform ulcer, which appears at the site of infection after an incubation period of 3 to 12 days or longer.[10,24,30,32] Asymptomatic and inconspicuous (although occasionally multiple and deeply erosive), it is found in 3 to 53 percent of patients,[39,40] heals rapidly, and leaves no scar.[28,32] The most common site of occurrence in men is the coronal sulcus, followed by the frenum, prepuce, penis, urethra, glans, and scrotum.[10] In women it appears most commonly on the posterior vaginal wall, the fourchette, the posterior lip of the cervix, and the vulva.[6,10,39] If located intraurethrally, the ulcer or erosion may cause nonspecific urethritis with a thin, mucopurulent discharge.[16,20] Other uncommon types of primary lesions are balanitis[30] and nodular ulcerations.[10,16,32]

Primary LGV lesions in men may be associated with a cordlike lymphangitis of the dorsal penis and formation of a large, tender lymphangial nodule, or "bubonulus".[10] Bubonuli may rupture and form draining sinuses and fistulas of the urethra as well as fibrotic, deforming scars at the base of the penis.[41] Lymphangitis is very often accompanied by local and regional edema, which may produce varying degrees of phimosis in men and genital swelling in women.[30] (See Table 17-1)

Cervicitis and urethritis are probably more common manifestations of primary LGV than reported statistics indicate.[30] The urethritis is usually asymptomatic and follows a mild course. Cervicitis may extend locally and could conceivably cause perimetritis or salpingitis, which are known to occur in other genital chlamydial infections.[15,29]

### INGUINAL SYNDROME

Inflammation and swelling of the inguinal lymph nodes is the most common manifestation of the secondary stage of LGV in men[20,24] and is the reason why most patients seek medical attention.[28] Other lymph nodes may be involved; the likelihood of such involvement depends on the location of the primary lesion (Table 17-2). The incubation period for this manifestation is 10

**Table 17-1. Lesions of Lymphogranuloma Venereum**

| Early | Late |
|---|---|
| *Inguinal syndrome:* | |
| Primary genital lesion(s)<br>Inguinal buboes<br>Bubonulus | Genital elephantiasis<br>Genital ulcers and fistulas |
| *Anorectal syndrome:* | |
| Proctitis | Rectal stricture<br>Lymphorrhoids<br>Perirectal abscesses<br>Anal fistula |
| *Other:* | |
| Urethritis<br>Cervicitis<br>Salpingitis<br>Parametritis | Frozen pelvis<br>Infertility |
| Conjunctivitis<br>Regional lymphadenitis<br>Meningitis | Scarring |

**Table 17-2. Site of Primary LGV Infection Determining Subsequent Lymphatic Involvement**

| Site of primary infection | Affected lymph nodes |
|---|---|
| Penis, anterior urethra | Superficial and deep inguinal |
| Posterior urethra | Deep iliac, perirectal |
| Vulva | Inguinal |
| Vagina, cervix | Deep iliac, perirectal, retrocrural, lumbosacral |
| Anus | Inguinal |
| Rectum | Perirectal, deep iliac |

to 30 days, but it may be delayed for as long as 4 to 6 months after infection.[36,39] It is important to note that LGV can occur as an acute symptomatic infection without apparent lymph node localization or tissue reaction at the point of infection.

The inguinal bubo is unilateral in two-thirds of cases[16,24] (Fig. 17-1). It begins as a firm, slightly painful mass which enlarges over 1 to 2 weeks. The inguinal bubo was described by William Wallace[42] in 1833:

> The skin becomes red; and is then found to be adherent to the surface of the tumour, over which it could be previously moved—the bubo then for the most part increases with rapidity; the pain becomes of a throbbing kind; some degree of fever sets in, marked by an acceleration of pulse, an increase of heat, loss of appetite, imperfect sleep, with a general feeling of indisposition.

The constitutional symptoms associated with inguinal buboes may be associated with systemic spread of chlamydia. During this stage of infection, LGV organisms have been recovered from the blood and the cerebrospinal fluid of patients both with and without symptoms of meningoencephalitis and abnormal cerebrospinal fluid.[34,43,44] Other manifestations of systemic spread are hepatitis,[45,46] pneumonitis,[28] and possibly arthritis.[47] Erythema nodosum, erythema multiforme, and eye ground changes (papillary edema) are also reported.[16,30,44]

As the bubo enlarges, the male patient complains of severe pain in the groin. He walks with a limp, bent at the waist in an attempt to limit pain. Within 1 to 2 weeks the bubo becomes fluctuant, and the skin overlying the bubo takes on a characteristically livid color ("blue balls") that predicts rupture of the bubo.[24] Rupture through the skin usually relieves pain and fever.[16,44] Numerous sinus tracts are formed which drain thick, tenacious, yellowish pus for several weeks or months with little or no discomfort.[48] Healing takes place slowly, leaving callous and contracted scars in the inguinal region. The disappearance of the inguinal bubo usually marks the end of the disease in men, and the majority suffer no serious sequela.[24,49] Bubonic relapse occurs in about 20 percent of untreated cases.[49]

Only about one-third of inguinal buboes become fluctuant and rupture; the others slowly involute and form firm inguinal masses without undergoing suppuration.[16,24] In about 20 percent of cases the femoral lymph nodes are also affected and may be separated from the enlarged inguinal lymph nodes by Poupart's ligament; this process creates a groove that is said to be pathognomonic for LGV[28] (Fig. 17-2). Simultaneous involvement of the deep iliac lymph nodes occurs in about 75 percent of cases and may cause formation of a large pelvic mass which, fortunately, seldom suppurates.[30,44] Extragenital primary lesions produce lymphadenitis and bubo formation in the lymph nodes draining the lesions; these extragenital buboes do not differ symptomatically or pathologically from inguinal buboes.[16]

In large-series studies of LGV in women, only 20 to 30 percent present with the inguinal syndrome.[24,50] About one-third of female cases without proctitis, however, complain of lower abdominal and back pain, especially when supine.[44] This symptom is characteristic of involvement of the deep pelvic and lumbar lymph nodes and may be mistaken for acute appendicitis[28] or a tuboovarian abscess.[16,44] Numerous adhesions may form, fixing the pelvic organs together.[44]

Other infectious diseases causing inguinal lymphadenitis and bubo formation are plague, tularemia, and tuberculosis. More common causes of inguinal lymphadenitis without suppuration, which are frequently misdiagnosed as LGV, are genital herpes, syphilis, chancroid, and Hodgkin's disease.[30] Small lesions on the feet or lower extremities may cause significant inguinal adenopathy. In nonendemic areas, however, the syndrome is most frequently mistaken for an incarcerated inguinal hernia[51] or lymphoma.[52]

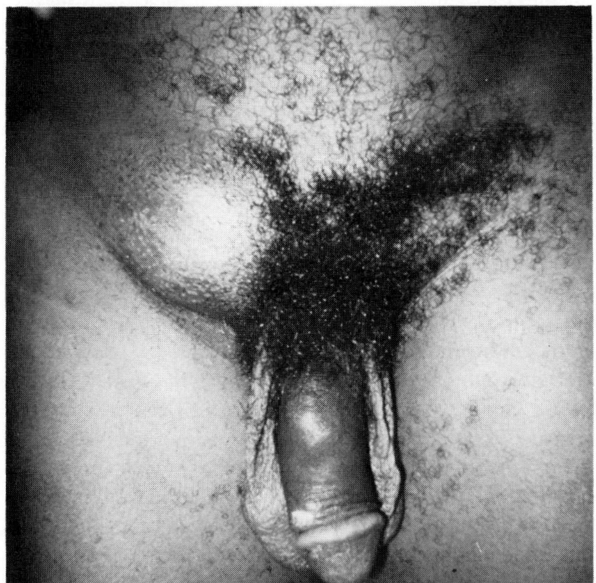

**Fig. 17-1.** Early inguinal syndrome of LGV showing superficial, primary preputial erosion, dorsal penile lymphangitis, and right inguinal bubo.

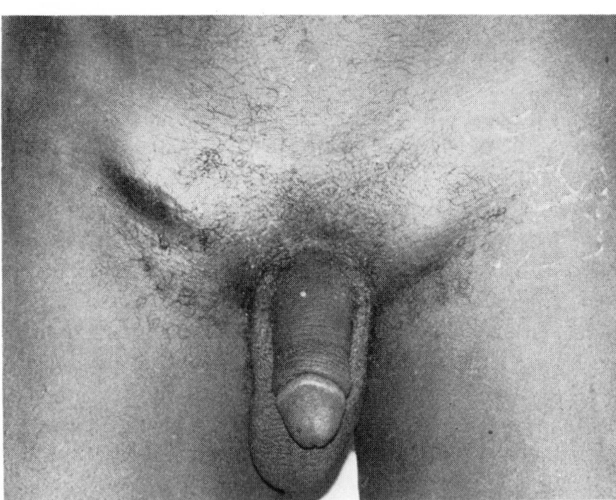

**Fig. 17-2.** Early inguinal syndrome of LGV showing a small vesicular primary lesion and bilateral inguinal lymphadenitis with cleavage of the enlarged right inguinal and femoral lymph nodes by the inguinal ligament, the characteristic "groove" sign.

## ANOGENITORECTAL SYNDROME

The subacute manifestations of this syndrome are proctocolitis and hyperplasia of intestinal and perirectal lymphatic tissue (lymphorrhoids). The chronic or late manifestations are perirectal abscesses, ischiorectal and rectovaginal fistulas, anal fistulas, and rectal stricture or stenosis.[22,30]

In men, the rectal mucosa can be directly inoculated with chlamydia during receptive anal intercourse or by lymphatic spread from the male posterior urethra. In women, the rectal mucosa can also be directly inoculated with chlamydia during anal intercourse, or it can be contaminated by migration of infectious vaginal secretions or by lymphatic spread from the cervix and posterior vaginal wall. The vast majority of patients with the anorectal syndrome are women or homosexual men.[50,53–57]

The early symptoms of rectal infection are anal pruritus and a mucous rectal discharge caused by local or diffuse edema of the anorectal mucosa. The mucosa becomes hyperemic and friable after a period of several weeks and bleeds easily when traumatized.[53,56,57] Multiple, discrete, superficial ulcerations with irregular borders appear on the mucosa, and are gradually replaced by granulation tissue. A chronic inflammatory process invades the bowel wall, and noncaseous granulomas and crypt abscesses form.[53,56] With secondary bacterial infection of the rectal mucosa, the discharge becomes mucopurulent. If left untreated, the granulomatous process progressively involves all layers of the bowel wall. The muscle layers are replaced by fibrous tissue;[33,53] in women the rectovaginal septum may be eroded and a rectovaginal fistula may be formed.[54] Contraction of the fibrous components of the granulation tissue over a period of months or years causes partial (stricture) or complete (stenosis) blockage of the rectum.[33,53,54]

Symptoms of proctocolitis include fever, rectal pain, and tenesmus.[16,22,54] The lower left quadrant of the abdomen is tender, and the pelvic colon may be palpably thickened. The rectal mucosa feels granular on digital examination, and movable, enlarged lymph nodes may be palpated immediately under the bowel wall.[54] There are no pathognomonic sigmoidoscopic findings. The inflammatory process may be localized to one segment of bowel or it may occur at several different levels concurrently, but it is usually limited to that portion below the peritoneal reflection.[22,33,54]

Additional symptoms that occur with rectal stricture are varying degrees of constipation, passage of "pencil" stools, attacks of ileus with colic and abdominal distension, and weight loss.[24,30,53,58] The stricture usually forms 2 to 5 cm above the anocutaneous margin, where the perirectal lymphatic tissue is the richest.[22,54] It is usually annular or tubular in shape,[58] and its proximal margins are granular (Fig. 17-3). If the palpating finger can be introduced through the aperture of the nondistensible and rigid stricture, the mucous membrane above it has a normal consistency.[54] By contrast, the mucous membrane below the stricture generally shows ulcerative and granulomatous proctitis, which makes the digital examination very painful.[24] Although the stricture often is very narrow, complete bowel obstruction (rectal stenosis) is rare but may cause bowel perforation and peritonitis, which is the usual cause of death in LGV.[30,59]

The rectal mucosa below the stricture and the skin around the anus are frequent sites for formation of perirectal abscesses and anal fissures.[55,58] These may also occur as the only manifestation of chronic anogenitorectal LGV. Obstruction of the lymphatic and venous drainage of the lower rectum produces perianal outgrowths of lymphatic tissue which grossly resemble hemorrhoids

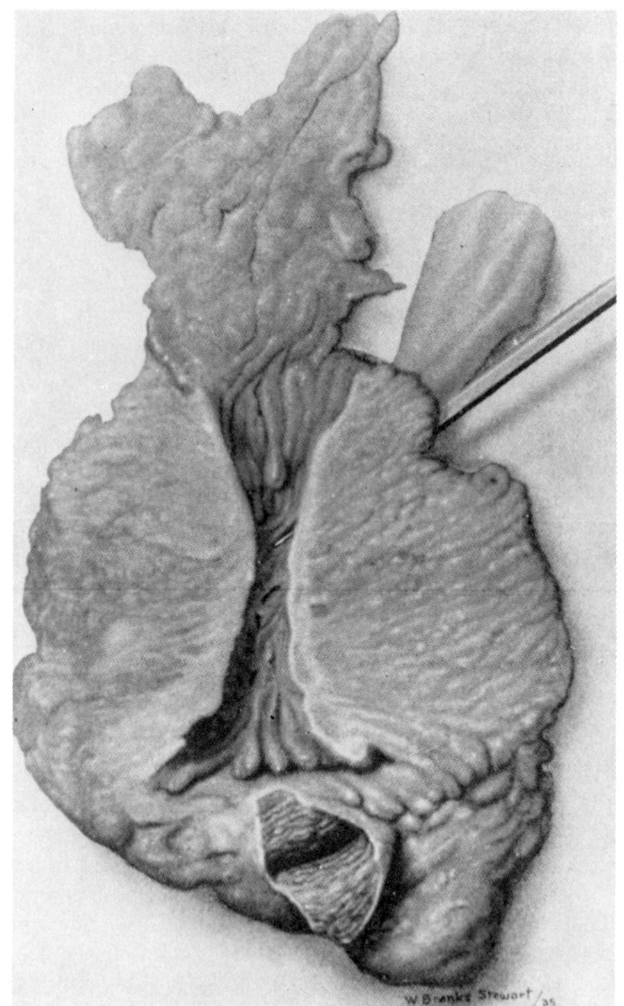

Fig. 17-3. Necropsy specimen of an LGV rectal stricture containing an ileosigmoidal fistula. (*From LL Lichtenstein.*[60])

but are called *lymphorrhoids*[60] or *perianal condylomas.*[58] Histologically these anal tags are composed of dilated lymph vessels with perilymphatic inflammation.[16,24]

The clinical and histological picture of early LGV proctocolitis is identical to that seen in inflammatory bowel disease,[61,62] and there has been considerable debate in the medical literature concerning a possible etiologic role for LGV in regional ileitis (Crohn's disease) and ulcerative colitis.[63] Schuller et al.[64] demonstrated specific LGV antibody in the serum of 38 out of 55 patients with Crohn's disease, but subsequent studies showed no serologic evidence of chlamydia infection in either Crohn's disease or ulcerative colitis.[65–67]

Several groups have isolated non-LGV *C. trachomatis* serovars from male homosexuals with proctocolitis.[9,56,57] The sigmoidoscopic and biopsy findings in these patients differ from those found in LGV infections; the inflammatory process is not as intense or as invasive as that caused by LGV serovars, and hypertrophic mucosal "follicles" predominate. Non-LGV proctocolitis may prove to be more common than that caused by LGV, but it is not known if non-LGV serovars will cause rectal stricture if left untreated.

The rectal stricture of LGV may resemble that caused by trauma, actinomycosis, tuberculosis, schistosomiasis, and malignancy.[22,30,58] It is most frequently mistaken for rectal cancer, and a biopsy should be taken to exclude this diagnosis. The incidence of rectal cancer in patients with LGV rectal stricture has ranged from 2 percent[68] to 5 percent.[69] In a study of 106 LGV patients who subsequently developed carcinoma, Rainey[69] proposed a causal relationship between LGV rectal stricture and the development of rectal cancer, hypothesizing that the chronic irritation of LGV predisposes the rectal stricture to malignant transformation.

## ESTHIOMENE

*Esthiomene* (Greek, "eating away"), a primary infection affecting the lymphatics of the scrotum, penis, or vulva, may cause chronic progressive lymphangitis, chronic edema, and sclerosing fibrosis of the subcutaneous tissues of these structures.[24,50] This results in induration and enlargement of the affected parts, and ultimately in ulceration. In the earliest stages the ulceration is superficial, but it gradually becomes more invasive and destructive. The vast majority of patients with esthiomene are women, and many authorities prefer to restrict the use of the term to this sex.

Chronic ulcerations are extremely painful. In women they are most common on the external surface of the labia majora, on the genitocrural folds, and on the lateral regions of the perineum[30] (Figs. 17-4, 17-5). The edema may extend from the clitoris to the anus and interfere with normal function. Urethral and vaginal stenosis and fistula formation have been reported.[16,24,50]

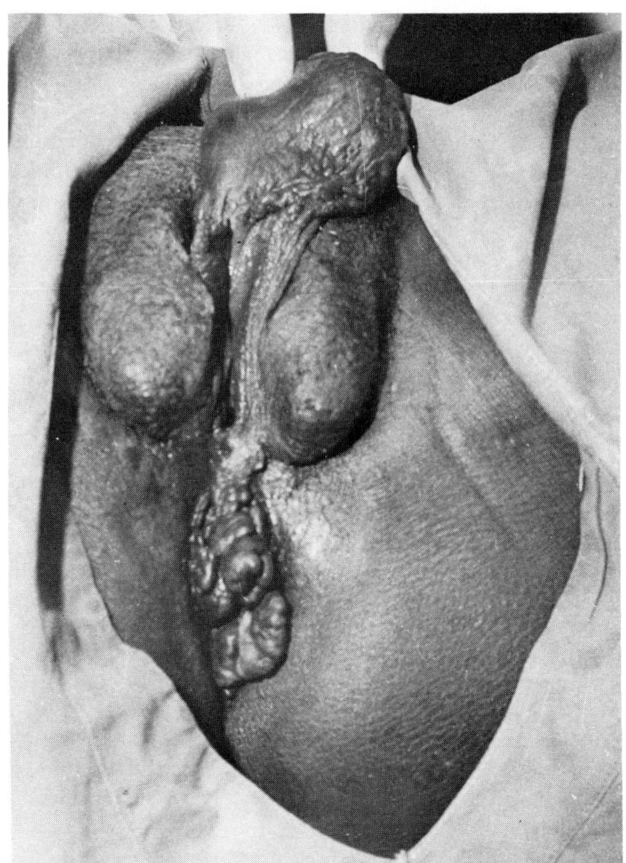

**Fig. 17-5.** Elephantiasis of the labia and clitoris in a woman with late lymphogranuloma venereum. (*Courtesy of M.I. unit, Ibadan University, Nigeria.*)

## OTHER MANIFESTATIONS

There is a tendency for women to develop papillary growths on the mucosa of the urethral meatus; these growths cause dysuria, frequency, and urinary incontinence with some perimeatal ulceration.[50] Penile, scrotal, or perineal sinuses may develop with or without urethral stenosis.[18,50] Coutts[30] refers to this symptom complex as the *urethrogenitoperineal syndrome.*

Penoscrotal elephantiasis appears from 1 to 20 years after infection.[30] It may affect only the prepuce, the prepuce and the penis, the scrotum alone, or all of the male external genitalia. The genital tissue is indurated and often deformed. The scrotum may reach monstrous size, but this is unusual.[24] Other conditions such as filariasis and mycosis must be considered in the differential diagnosis.

Follicular conjunctivitis, often accompanied by lymphadenitis of the maxillary and posterior auricular nodes,[16] can occur at any stage of LGV. The conjunctiva is infected by autoinoculation of infectious discharge. This condition may be analogous to Parinaud's oculoglandular syndrome.[30]

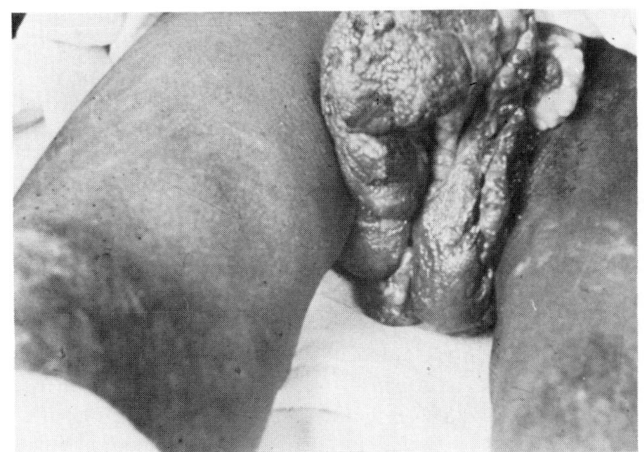

**Fig. 17-4.** Esthiomene of late lymphogranuloma venereum in a woman.

Primary LGV lesions of the mouth and pharynx can occur as the result of fellatio or cunnilingus. This results in lymphadenitis of the submaxillary or cervical lymph nodes.[26] Cases of supraclavicular lymphadenitis with mediastinal lymphadenopathy and pericarditis have also been reported.[70,71] Coutts[47] has recovered LGV from the gallbladder wall (in cases of chronic cholecystitis) and from fibrous perihepatic (in cases of Fitz-Hugh–Curtis syndrome), abdominal, and pelvic adhesions.

Erythema nodosum and other skin manifestations occur in about 10 percent of LGV cases during the early stages of infection.[10] Their appearance may be precipitated by surgical manipulation of infected lymph nodes.[16] The malnutrition associated with rectal stricture was a frequent cause of pellagra in the preantibiotic era.[24]

## DIAGNOSIS

Mild leukocytosis with an increase in monocytes and eosinophils frequently accompanies early bubonic and anogenitorectal LGV.[20,22,25] A more significant polymorphonuclear leukocytosis is found routinely in patients whose LGV buboes, abscesses, etc., are superinfected with pyogenic bacteria.[16] The only other clinical laboratory abnormality found with regularity is an elevated gamma-globulin concentration due to an increase of IgA, IgG, and IgM immunoglobulins.[17] Anticomplement activity is commonly associated with hypergammaglobulinemia.[72–74]

The diagnosis of LGV is usually based on (1) a positive Frei skin test, (2) a positive complement-fixation (CF) or other serological test for LGV, (3) isolation of LGV chlamydia from infected tissue and secretions in mice, embryonated eggs, or tissue culture, and (4) histological identification of chlamydia in infected tissue. Although histopathological changes in LGV are not unique, they are sufficiently distinct to differentiate LGV buboes, bubonuli, and rectal strictures from similar lesions caused by other sexually transmitted agents.[24,32,75]

## FREI TEST

The original Frei test antigen was pus obtained from unruptured buboes, diluted in saline, and sterilized by heating.[11] Not only was the risk of bacterial contamination of this antigen considerable, but it could easily be inactivated by too much heating and standardization of its potency was impossible.[76] Nevertheless a positive test in a patient with clinical findings compatible with LGV generally indicated present or past infection.[77] The successful culture of LGV in large amounts in the yolk sac of chick embryos led to the commercial manufacture of standardized antigen (Lygranum) in 1940.[78] The test consisted of intradermal injections of 0.1 ml of Lygranum into the skin of one forearm and a similar volume of control yolk sac material into the other forearm. The test was read at 48 h, and a positive result was the development of a papule at least 6 × 6 mm in the principal diameters, provided that the papule produced by the control was 5 × 5 mm or smaller. The same antigen was also used in complement-fixation serodiagnostic tests for LGV[79] after Melczer and Sipos[80] demonstrated the complement-fixing property of LGV in 1937.

The Frei skin test usually becomes positive after the appearance of buboes 2 to 8 weeks after infection.[10,16,77] In the older literature it was said that the Frei test was positive in about 95 percent of patients with bubonic LGV and in about 90 percent of those with ulcerative elephantiasis.[6] The lack of sensitivity in the early stages of LGV is a distinct disadvantage.[46]

Since the Frei antigen is common to all *Chlamydia*, the specificity of a positive reaction has limited its diagnostic usefulness, particularly in the past two decades when the prevalence of other chlamydial infections has risen considerably.[15] The Frei test tends to remain positive for several years and possibly for life despite treatment.[77,81] For these reasons, commercial manufacture of Frei antigen was discontinued in 1974.

## COMPLEMENT-FIXATION TEST

The CF test is more sensitive and is positive earlier than the Frei test.[16,30,43] There is no correlation between the CF antibody titer and the intensity of the Frei reaction,[16,82] although in a given patient there is often close agreement between the two.[77] Like the Frei test, the CF test gives cross reactions in infections caused by other chlamydial infections, and the antibody may persist in high or low titer for many years.[77,83] In general, active LGV infections have CF titers of 1:64 or greater,[28,77,82–84] but high CF titers are occasionally found in asymptomatic patients and those with other chlamydial infections.[82,83] Titers below 1:64 in a patient suspected of LGV on clinical grounds should be interpreted with caution.

Although a rise in CF titer of two or more dilutions may occur in early LGV,[82] most patients with documented LGV initially have high CF titers that show little difference between serum specimens obtained during acute infection and at 6 weeks into convalescence.[46,82] Variations in CF titer can also be caused by changes in both the concentration of test antigen and the test procedure.

## NEUTRALIZING ANTIBODY

LGV-neutralizing antibody is measured by mixing test serum with virulent mouse brain emulsion;[35] if the test serum contains LGV antibody, the mixture will not produce meningoencephalitis when inoculated into the brains of mice.[16]

## MICROIMMUNOFLUORESCENT (MICRO-IF) TEST

The micro-IF test is considerably more sensitive than the CF test;[35,85,86] although the micro-IF antibody reacts broadly with other *C. trachomatis* strains,[85] it is usually possible to demonstrate the antigenic type of the infecting strain by the pattern of reactivity.[9,17,35] In LGV, acute-phase serum usually contains very high titers of micro-IF antibody.[9,17,56] The major disadvantage of the micro-IF test is that it is used primarily in a few specialized laboratories and is not routinely available.

## OTHER SEROLOGICAL TESTS

A radioisotope precipitation (RIP) test was used by Philip et al.[35] to detect LGV antibody. In this procedure antiglobulin is used to precipitate otherwise nonsedimentable complexes of radiolabeled meningopneumonitis chlamydia and chlamydia antibody. The proportion of radioactivity removed from the system is a measure of the amount of antibody present. The test is more sensitive than the micro-IF, but unless specific LGV antigens are used, it suffers from the same lack of specificity as the CF test. It is also available in only a few specialized laboratories.

A trachoma-LGV-specific antigen extracted from LGV chlamydia grown in tissue culture has been used in a counterimmunoelectrophoresis test to detect antibodies in LGV patients.[87] It has about the same sensitivity and specificity as the micro-IF test.

The future potential of serovar-specific monoclonal chlamydial antibodies is being investigated. These antibodies will probably lead to the commercial manufacture of test reagents and different test systems (e.g., enzyme-linked immunosorbent assay, or ELISA) that will greatly increase the availability of specific serodiagnostic tests for LGV.

## ISOLATION OF LGV

Chlamydia can be isolated from infected tissue by inoculation of mouse brain, yolk sac, or tissue culture.[15,16,88] The recovery rate depends on the method used and the source of the inoculum. Bubo pus is the most practical clinical material.[28] Wall[82] compared the recovery rate from bubo biopsy or pus in mice and yolk sac; chlamydia were cultured from 85 percent of patients, with a higher recovery rate in mice (98 percent) than in yolk sac (78 percent). Other studies report much lower recovery rates.[46,89]

For the past 15 years, HeLa-229[90] and McCoy[91] tissue-culture cell lines have been used to isolate LGV chlamydia. The reported recovery rate from buboes, genital tissue, or rectal tissue ranges from 24 to 30 percent,[17,35,46] which is much lower than that reported for nongonococcal urethritis.[15,88]

## CYTOLOGY

The elementary and inclusion bodies of chlamydia can be visualized both outside and inside cells in secretions and infected tissues by using Giemsa's, iodine, and fluorescent antibody staining methods.[30,88,92] Cytology has not been very successful for diagnosis of LGV,[32] often because of the frequent contamination of specimens by bacteria and other artifacts.

## OTHER DIAGNOSTIC PROCEDURES

Various radiological procedures have been used in LGV. Lymphography demonstrates the extent of lymph node involvement but does not outline buboes or reveal specific changes.[93] Barium enema findings in rectal strictures caused by LGV are said to be characteristic and quite different from cancer: the LGV stricture is elongated, in contradistinction to the stricture produced by cancer; it produces little alteration in the mucosal pattern of the bowel; and it has a tendency to form fistulas which tend to reenter the lumen of the rectum.[94,95]

## TREATMENT

A variety of different drugs have been used to treat LGV, but there is no singularly effective drug that will assure bacteriologic cure. A major problem in evaluating a given drug is the relative lack of criteria by which efficacy can be measured.[96] The natural history of LGV is highly variable, and spontaneous remission is common.[44,49]

Sulfonamides were the first drugs to show efficacy in LGV by promoting reduction in the size of buboes, healing of fistulas, etc.[14,75,97] The lesions were not sterilized even after many months of therapy,[14] and CF titers may show little or no change.[98] In experimentally infected mice, 20 percent remained infected with LGV despite the most extensive sulfonamide therapy.[97]

A number of different antibiotics have been used to treat LGV. Penicillin and streptomycin were the first to be used but were found ineffective, although penicillin has some activity against chlamydia in vitro.[97] The next antibiotics used were the tetracyclines, which proved to be quite effective in the management of the primary and secondary stages of LGV.[49,83,99] Similar effectiveness was found with chloramphenicol,[96] erythromycin[100] and minocycline,[19] and rifampin.[101]

## BUBONIC LGV

Greaves et al.[49] attempted the only comparative treatment study of bubonic LGV. The relative effectiveness of oral chlortetracycline, oxytetracycline, chloramphenicol, or sulfadiazine was compared with patients treated symptomatically with aspirin. The tetracyclines and chloramphenicol were given in a dosage of 500 mg qid for 14 days following a loading dose of 1 g. Sulfadiazine was given in a dose of 2 g initially, followed by 4 g daily in divided doses for 10 to 28 days. The relative effectiveness of each drug was measured by the duration of inguinal adenopathy and the occurrence of bubonic relapse, sinus formation, or skin lesions after completion of therapy. Unfortunately, the average number of patients treated with each drug was 6.5, which limits the statistical validity of the results.

The duration of the bubo after treatment was the same in all the drug-treated groups and was not significantly shorter compared with the duration of the bubo in those given symptomatic therapy. Although specific chemotherapy had only a minimal effect in shortening the duration of the bubonic lesion (31 days versus 69 days), there was a more frequent occurrence of complications among the symptomatically treated control group. They observed a marked reduction in CF antibody titer in drug-treated cases, which suggests that the amount of LGV present in infected tissues was reduced, if not eliminated. Other workers have shown that lymph nodes that were proved to be infective before tetracycline were found to be negative after therapy.[102]

Minocycline, in a loading oral dose of 300 mg followed by 200 mg bid for 10 days, has been used with success to treat acute bubonic LGV and a limited number of cases of proctitis.[19] Only limited information is available on treatment of LGV with erythromycin.[100]

Fever abates and patients usually experience prompt relief of bubo pain and tenderness and feel much improved 1 to 2 days after starting antibiotics.[17,20] The bubo seldom suppurates after therapy begins, but fluctuant buboes may require frequent needle-and-syringe aspiration to prevent rupture.[17]

## ANOGENITORECTAL LGV

Banov[53] reported the immediate and long-term effects of chlortetracycline, oxytetracycline, chloramphenicol, and erythromycin in cases of rectal stricture. Criteria used to compare the different drugs were subjective, the patients were not randomly assigned treatments, and the dosage schedules were variable. With the exception of erythromycin (only three cases studied), all drugs were effective. Apparently these drugs reduced the inflammatory edema of the rectal stricture but had no effect on scar tissue. In contrast to bubonic LGV, antibiotics had no immediate effect on the titer of CF antibody. No case of anal or rectovaginal fistula was cured by drugs alone.

The response of proctocolitis to antibiotics is usually dramatic. Symptoms are completely relieved and the rectal mucosa heals within a few weeks after treatment.[22,56] Occasional tetracycline treatment failures in proctocolitis have been reported.[22,57]

The recommended antibiotic treatment for both bubonic and anogenitorectal LGV is tetracycline, 2 g daily in divided doses for 2 to 4 weeks.[36] Dual infections with other sexually transmitted diseases are common in LGV patients,[16,22,30] and these should be treated appropriately.

## SURGICAL TREATMENT

Surgical treatment of the acute inguinal syndrome should be limited to aspiration of fluctuant lymph nodes and occasional incision and drainage of abscesses.[22] Before the advent of sulfonamides, surgical extirpation of buboes was recommended,[22,25] although it was probably a prominent factor in the development of postoperative elephantiasis of the genitals by further blocking normal lymphatic drainage.[39] Under antibiotic coverage there is little risk that incision or aspiration of fluctuant buboes will lead to formation of sinuses.[20,51]

Spontaneous resolution of a fibrous LGV rectal stricture never occurs, but the inflammatory process and the diameter of the stricture may be dramatically improved by antibiotic treatment.[22,53] Dilation of the stricture using elastic bougies under direct vision may be necessary but poses a significant risk of bowel perforation. It should be limited to soft, short strictures not extending above the peritoneal reflection and should be abandoned if the stricture splits easily or if bleeding occurs.[22]

A variety of different surgical procedures may be required for advanced rectal stricture. The indications for operation are bowel obstruction, persistent rectovaginal fistula, and gross destruction of the anal canal, anal sphincter, and perineum.[22] Plastic operations on the vulva, penis, and scrotum may be required for esthiomene and genital elephantiasis.[30] None of these procedures should be attempted without antibiotic treatment, and, if possible, antibiotics should be given for several months before the decision to perform surgery is made.[103]

## PREVENTION

Prevention of LGV in nonendemic areas is predicated on identification and treatment of sexual contacts of proved or suspected cases. These contacts should receive prophylactic antibiotic treatment if recently exposed to infection, so as to prevent reinfection as well as to eliminate a potential reservoir. The increasing prevalence of anorectal LGV in male homosexuals in the United States should be kept in mind when a young male presents with symptoms of proctocolitis.

Control of LGV in endemic areas presents a formidable problem. Diagnostic and treatment facilities are very limited, and patients often do not seek medical attention until after late complications are well-established. The only hope appears to be that with the passage of time the standards of living and hygiene in endemic areas will improve to the point where health education and medical care are readily available.

# References


1 Godding CC: On non-venereal bubo. *Br Med J* 2:842, 1896.

2 Klotz HG: Uber die Entwickelung der sogenannten strumösen Bubonen und die indicationen fur die fruhzeitige Exstirpation derselben. *Berl Klin Wochenschr* 1:132, 1890.

3 Fiessinger N: Diagnostic des adenopathies chroniques. *J Des Practiciens* 39:162, 1925.

4 Durand M et al: Lymphogranulomatose inguinale subaiguë d'origine génitale probable; peut-être venerienne. *Province Med (Paris)* 24:55, 1913.

5 Stannus HS: *A Sixth Venereal Disease.* London, Bailliere, Tindall and Cox, 1933.

6 Sokes JH et al: Lymphogranuloma venereum. *Am J Med Sci* 197:575, 1939.

7 Grayston JT, Wang SP: New knowledge of chlamydiae and the diseases they cause. *J Infect Dis* 132:87, 1975.

8 Schachter J, Meyer KF: Lymphogranuloma venereum: II. Characterization of some recently isolated strains. *J Bacteriol* 99:636, 1969.

9 Schachter J: Confirmatory serodiagnosis of lymphogranuloma venereum proctitis may yield false-positive results due to other chlamydial infections of the rectum. *Sex Transm Dis* 8:26, 1981.

10 Favre M, Hellerström S: The epidemiology, aetiology and prophylaxis of lymphogranuloma inguinal. *Acta Derm Venereol [Suppl] (Stockh)* 34(30):1, 1954.

11 Frei W: Eione neue Hautreaktion bei Lymphogranuloma inguinale. *Klin Wochenschr* 4:2148, 1925.

12 Frei W, Koppel A: Ulcus vulvae chronicum elephantiasticum (esthiomène) und sogennates Syphilôme anorectal als Folgeerscheinungen der Lymphogranulomatosis inguinales. *Klin Wochenschr* 7:2331, 1928.

13 Miyagawa Y: Studies on the characteristics of Miyagawanella lymphogranulomatis. *Jpn J Exp Med* 26:157, 1956.

14 Jones H et al: Studies on lymphogranuloma venereum: III. The action of the sulfonamides on the agent of lymphohgranuloma venereum. *J Infect Dis* 76:55, 1945.

15 Schachter J: Chlamydial infections. *N Engl J Med* 298:428, 490, 540, 1978.

16 Koteen H: Lymphogranuloma venereum. *Medicine* 24:1, 1945.

17 Perine PL et al: Diagnosis and treatment of lymphogranuloma venereum in Ethiopia, in *Current Chemotherapy and Infectious Diseases.* Washington, American Society for Microbiology, 1980, pp. 1280–1282.

18 Osoba AO: Sero-epidemiological study of lymphogranuloma venereum in Western Nigeria. *Afr J Med Sci* 6:125, 1977.

19 Sowmini CN et al: Minocycline in the treatment of lymphogranuloma venereum. *J Am Vener Dis Assoc* 2:19, 1976.

20 Abrams AJ: Lymphogranuloma venereum. *JAMA* 205:199, 1968.

21 Willcox RR: Importance of the so-called "other" sexually-transmitted diseases. *Br J Vener Dis* 51:221, 1975.

22 Annamuthodo H: Rectal lymphogranuloma venereum in Jamaica. *Ann R Coll Surg Engl* 29:141, 1961.

23 Blount J: Personal communication, Venereal Disease Control Division, Centers for Disease Control, Atlanta.

24 D'Aunoy R, von Haam E: Venereal lymphogranuloma. *Arch Pathol* 27:1032, 1939.

25 Butler CS: Climatic bubo. *US Navy Med Bull* 20:1, 1924.

26 Thorsteinsson SB et al: Lymphogranuloma venereum: A cause of cervical lymphadenopathy. *JAMA* 235:1882, 1976.

27 Harrop GA et al: New clinical conceptions of lymphogranuloma venereum. *Trans Assoc Am Physicians* 56:101, 1941.

28 Schachter J: Lymphogranuloma venereum and other nonocular *Chlamydia trachomatis* infections, in *Nongonococcal Urethritis and Related Infections,* D Hobson, KK Holmes (eds). Washington, American Society for Microbiology, 1977, pp 91–97.

29 Johannisson G et al: Genital *Chlamydia trachomatis* infection in women. *Obstet Gynecol* 56:671, 1980.

30 Coutts WE: Lymphogranuloma venereum: A general review. *Bull WHO* 2:545, 1950.

31 Schachter J, Osoba AO: Lymphogranuloma venereum. *Br Med Bull* 39:151, 1983.

32 Smith EB, Custer RP: The histopathology of lymphogranuloma venereum. *J Urol* 63:546, 1950.

33 Ault GW: Venereal disease of the anus and rectum. *Am J Syph* 21:430, 1937.

34 Sabin AB, Aring CD: Meningoencephalitis in man caused by the virus of lymphogranuloma venereum. *JAMA* 120:1376, 1942.

35 Philip RN et al: Study of chlamydia in patients with lymphogranuloma venereum and urethritis attending a venereal disease clinic. *Br J Vener Dis* 47:114, 1971.

36 Dan M et al: A case of lymphogranuloma venereum of 20 years duration: Isolation of *Chlamydia trachomatis* from perianal lesions. *Br J Vener Dis* 56:344, 1980.

37 Quinn TC et al: Experimental proctitis due to rectal infection with *Chlamydia trachomatis* in nonhuman primates. *J Infect Dis* 154:833, 1986.

38 Kornblith BA: Lymphogranuloma venereum: Treatment of 300 cases with special reference to the use of Frei antigen intravenously. *Am J Med Sci* 198:231, 1939.

39 Rothchild TPE, Higgins GA: Acute lymphogranuloma venereum: A

short review with observations on the surgical implications and changing geographical distribution. *J Urol* 68:918, 1952.

40 Mehus A et al: Etiology of genital ulcers in Swaziland. *Sex Transm Dis* 10:33, 1983.

41 Hopsu-Havu VB, Sonck CE: Infiltrative, ulcerative, and fistular lesions of the penis due to lymphogranuloma venereum. *Br J Vener Dis* 49:193, 1973.

42 Wallace W: A treatise on the venereal diseases. London, Burgess, Hill, 1833, p 348.

43 Beeson PB et al: Isolation of virus of lymphogranuloma venereum from blood and spinal fluid of a human being. *Proc Soc Exp Biol Med* 63:306, 1946.

44 von Haam EV, D'Aunoy R: Is lymphogranuloma inguinale a systemic disease? *Am J Trop Med Hyg* 16:527, 1936.

45 Bjerke JR, Hovding G Jr: Lymphogranuloma venereum with hepatic involvement. *Acta Derm Venerol (Stockh)* 57:90, 1977.

46 Schachter J et al: Lymphogranuloma venereum: I. Comparison of the Frei test, complement fixation test, and isolation of the agent. *J Infect Dis* 120:372, 1969.

47 Coutts WE: Contribution to the knowledge of lymphogranulomatosis venereum as a general disease. *J Trop Med Hyg* 39:13, 1936.

48 Prehn DT: Lymphogranuloma venereum and associated diseases. *Arch Dermatol Syph* 35:231, 1937.

49 Greaves AB et al: Chemotherapy in bubonic lymphogranuloma venereum. *Bull WHO* 16:277, 1957.

50 Torpin et al: Lymphogranuloma venereum in the female: A clinical study of ninety-six consecutive cases. *Am J Surg* 43:688, 1939.

51 Najafi JA et al: Surgical aspects of inguinal lymphogranuloma venereum. *Milit Med* 144:697, 1979.

52 Mauff AC et al: Problems in the diagnosis of lymphogranuloma venereum. *S Afr Med J* 63:55, 1983.

53 Banov L: Rectal stricture of lymphogranuloma venereum: Some observations from a five-year study of treatment with the broad spectrum antibiotics. *Am J Surg* 88:761, 1954.

54 Mathewson C Jr: Inflammatory strictures of the rectum associated with venereal lymphogranuloma. *JAMA* 110:709, 1938.

55 Greaves AB: The frequency of lymphogranuloma venereum in persons with perirectal abscesses, fistulae in ano, or both. *Bull WHO* 29:797, 1963.

56 Quinn TC et al: *Chlamydia trachomatis* proctitis. *N Engl J Med* 305:195, 1981.

57 Levine JS et al: Chronic proctitis in male homosexuals due to lymphogranuloma venereum. *Gastroenterology* 79:563, 1980.

58 Saad EA et al: Ano-rectal-colonic lymphogranuloma venereum. *Gastroenterology* 97:89, 1962.

59 Jorgensen L: Lymphogranuloma venereum. *Acta Pathol Microbiol Scand* 47:113, 1959.

60 Lichtenstein LL: Rectal stricture: A clinical analysis of 58 cases with observations on 154 Frei-positive cases of lymphogranuloma inguinale. *Am J Surg* 31:111, 1936.

61 de la Monte SM et al: Follicular proctocolitis and neuromatous hyperplasia with lymphogranuloma venereum. *Hum Pathol* 16: 1025, 1985.

62 Munday PE, Taylor-Robinson D: Chlamydia infection in proctitis and Crohn's disease. *Br Med Bull* 39:155, 1983.

63 Crohn BR et al: Regional ileitis, a pathologic and clinical entity. *JAMA* 99:1323, 1932.

64 Schuller JL et al: Antibodies against chlamydia of lymphogranuloma venereum type in Crohn's disease. *Lancet* 1:19, 1979.

65 Swarbrick ET et al: Chlamydia, cytomegalovirus, and yersinia in inflammatory bowel disease. *Lancet* 2:11, 1979.

66 Taylor-Robinson D et al: Low frequency of chlamydial antibodies in patients with Crohn's disease and ulcerative colitis. *Lancet* 2: 1162, 1979.

67 Mårdh PA et al: Lack of evidence for an association between infection with *Chlamydia trachomatis* and Crohn's disease as indicated by micro-immunofluorescence antibody tests. *Acta Pathol Microbiol Scand* [B] 88:57, 1980.

68 Levin I et al: Lymphogranuloma venereum, rectal stricture and carcinoma. *Dis Colon Rectum* 7:129, 1964.

69 Rainey R: The association of lymphogranuloma inguinale and cancer. *Surgery* 35:221, 1954.

70 Sheldon WH et al: Lymphogranuloma venereum of supraclavicular lymph nodes with mediastinal lymphadenopathy and pericarditis. *Am J Med* 5:320, 1948.

71 Bernstein DI et al: Mediastinal and supraclavicular lymphadenitis and pneumonitis due to *Chlamydia trachomatis* serovars L, and $L_2$. *N Engl J Med* 311:1543, 1984.

72 Lassus A et al: Auto-immune serum factors and IgA elevation in lymphogranuloma venereum. *Ann Clin Res* 2:51, 1970.

73 Sonck CE et al: Autoimmune serum factors in active and inactive lymphogranuloma venereum. *Br J Vener Dis* 49:67, 1973.

74 Williams RD, Gutman AB: Hyperproteinemia with reversal of the albumin: Globulin ratio in lymphogranuloma inguinale. *Proc Soc Exp Biol Med* 34:91, 1936.

75 Tucker HA: Inguinal lymphogranuloma venereum in the male. *Am J Syph Gon Vener Dis* 29:619, 1945.

76 Frei W: On the skin test in lymphogranuloma inguinale. *J Invest Dermatol* 1:367, 1938.

77 King AJ et al: Intradermal tests in the diagnosis of lymphogranuloma venereum. *Br J Vener Dis* 32:209, 1956.

78 Grace AW et al: A new material (Lygranum) for performance of the Frei test for lymphogranuloma venereum. *Proc Soc Exp Biol Med* 45:259, 1940.

79 McKee CM et al: Complement fixation test in lymphogranuloma venereum. *Proc Soc Exp Biol Med* 44:410, 1940.

80 Melczer M, Sipos K: Komplementbindungsversuche bei lymphogranuloma inguinale. *Arch Dermatol Syph* 176:176, 1937.

81 Grace AW: Persistence of a positive Frei reaction after treatment of venereal lymphogranuloma with sulfonamide drugs. *Vener Dis Inform* 22:349, 1941.

82 Wall MJ et al: Studies on the complement fixation reaction in lymphogranuloma venereum. *Am J Syph Gon Vener Dis* 31:289, 1947.

83 Greaves AB, Taggart SR: Serology, Frei reaction, and epidemiology of lymphogranuloma venereum. *Am J Syph Gon Vener Dis* 37:273, 1953.

84 Goldberg J, Banov L Jr: Complement fixation titers in tertiary lymphogranuloma venereum. *Br J Vener Dis* 32:37, 1956.

85 Wang SP et al: A simplified method for immunological typing of trachoma-inclusion conjunctivitis-lymphogranuloma venereum organisms. *Infect Immun* 7:356, 1973.

86 Schachter J et al: Chlamydiae as agents of human and animal diseases. *Bull WHO* 49:443, 1973.

87 Caldwell HD, Kuo CC: Serologic diagnosis of lymphogranuloma venereum by counterimmunoelectrophoresis with a *Chlamydia trachomatis* protein antigen. *J Immunol* 118:442, 1977.

88 Paavonen J: Chlamydial infections: Microbiological, clinical and diagnostic aspects. *Med Biol* 57:152, 1979.

89 Shaffer MF et al: Use of the yolk sac of the developing chicken embryo in the isolation of the agent of lymphogranuloma venereum. *J Infect Dis* 75:109, 1944.

90 Kuo CC et al: Primary isolation of TRIC organisms in HeLa 229 cells treated with DEAE-dextran. *J Infect Dis* 125:665, 1972.

91 Gordon FB, Quan AL: Isolation of the trachoma agent in cell culture. *Proc Soc Exp Biol Med* 118:354, 1965.

92 Klotz SA et al: Hemorrhagic proctitis due to lymphogranuloma venereum serogroup L2. *N Engl J Med* 308:1563, 1983.

93 Osoba AO, Beetlestone CA: Lymphographic studies in acute lymphogranuloma venereum infection. *Br J Vener Dis* 52:399, 1976.

94 Annamunthodo H, Marryatt J: Barium studies in intestinal lymphogranuloma venereum. *Br J Radiol* 24:53, 1961.

95 Piersol GM et al: Lymphogranuloma venereum: A systemic disease. *Trans Assoc Am Physicians* 53:275, 1938.

96 Greenblatt RB: Antibiotics in treatment of lymphogranuloma venereum and granuloma inguinale. *Ann NY Acad Sci* 55:1082, 1952.

97 Rake G: Chemotherapy of lymphogranuloma venereum. *Am J Trop Med Hyg* 28:555, 1948.
98 Grace AW, Rake G: Complement fixation test for lymphogranuloma. *Arch Dermatol Syph* 48:619, 1943.
99 Wright LT et al: The treatment of lymphogranuloma venereum with Terramycin. *Antibiot Chemother* 1:193, 1951.
100 Banov L Jr, Goldberg J: Erythromycin treatment of lymphogranuloma venereum, in *Antibiotics Annual. 1953–1954,* H Welch, F Martín-Ibánẽz (eds). New York, Medical Encyclopedia, 1953, pp 475–479.
101 Menke HE et al: Treatment of lymphogranuloma venereum with rifampicin. *Br J Vener Dis* 55:379, 1979.
102 Wright LT et al: Aueromycin: A new antibiotic with virucidal properties: 1. A preliminary report on successful treatment in twenty-five cases of lymphogranuloma venereum. *JAMA* 138:408, 1948.
103 Osoba AO: Medical treatment of late complications of lymphogranuloma venereum. *West Afr J Pharmacol Drug Res* 3:71, 1976.

# Chapter 18

# Biology of *Treponema pallidum*

Daniel M. Musher

*Treponema pallidum,* the causative organism of syphilis, is one of a small group of treponemes, members of the order Spirochaetales, which are virulent for human beings. *T. pallidum* is indistinguishable by known morphological, chemical, or immunologic methods from treponemes which cause yaws, pinta, or endemic syphilis and which are currently designated as *T. pallidum* subsp. *pertenue, T. carateum,* or *T. pallidum* var. *Bosnia,* respectively.[1-3] Other pathogenic treponemes include *T. cuniculi,* which infects lagomorphs, and *T. hyodysenteriae,* which causes diarrheal disease in swine. The other members of the genus *Treponema* are free-living organisms widely distributed in nature and generally not known to cause disease. DNA hybridization[2] has shown that the treponemes which cause disease in humans are very closely related (perhaps identical) and as a group differ from the other treponemes; the one exception may be *T. cuniculi,* which has not been subjected to this kind of study. Except for *T. hyodysenteriae,* the virulent treponemes cannot be grown in bacteriologic liquid media (see below).

## STRUCTURE

*T. pallidum* has a length of 6 to 15 μm (usually 10 to 13 μm) and a width of only 0.15 μm, which renders it below the level of resolution and, therefore, not visible by light microscopy—hence, the reliance upon the dark field microscope in clinical practice or upon electron microscopy in special clinical and investigational situations.[4] This organism has regular, tight spirals; when fixed, it appears wavelike with a wavelength of 1.1 μm and an amplitude of 0.2 to 0.3 μm. Dark field microscopic examination of a wet preparation reveals a rotatory motion with flexion and back-and-forth motion that are said to be characteristic of the virulent treponemes.[5] *T. pallidum* in vivo may be surrounded by an amorphous outer layer,[6] perhaps resulting from production of mucopolysaccharides.[7] The outer membrane includes a number of different proteins which have been characterized by polyacrylamide gel electrophoresis[8] and many of which have been shown to participate in immunologic responses to infection.[9,10] An electron-dense (peptidoglycan) layer and a cytoplasmic membrane can be demonstrated by electron microscopy,[4,11] Between the outer membrane and the electron-dense layer are found flagella (axial fibrils); these are assumed to play a role in locomotion, although their location within the outer membrane and the failure of antiflagellar antibodies to immobilize certain cultivable spirochetes raises questions about this assumption. Figure 18-1 shows the appearance of *T. pallidum.*

## METABOLISM AND CULTIVATION

Studies of *T. pallidum* are severely restricted by the inability to readily grow this organism in vitro, which has hindered study of metabolism, toxin production, and antigenic composition and has also made it difficult to examine dose-response relationships or the induction of immunity. Limited replication has been observed in vitro in the presence of mammalian cells at 34 to 35°C.[12,13] Growth seems to be best in the presence of 3 to 5% $O_2$ and 5% $CO_2$ in $H_2$; thus, the traditional suggestions that

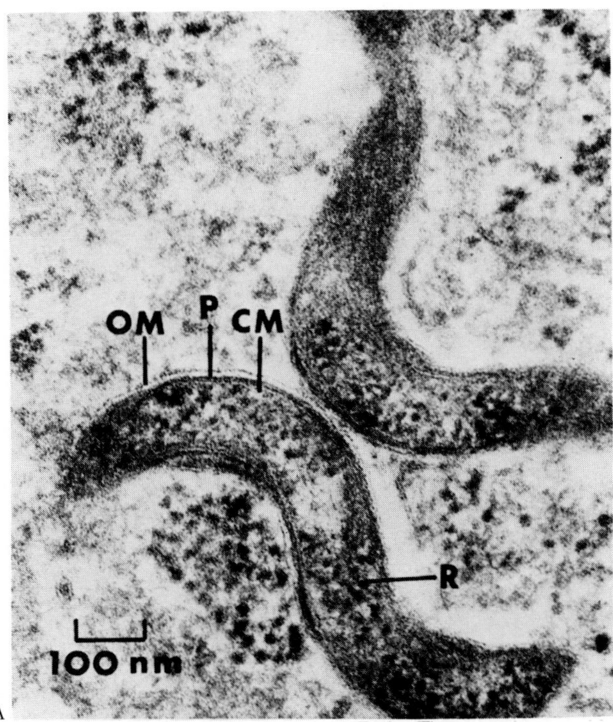


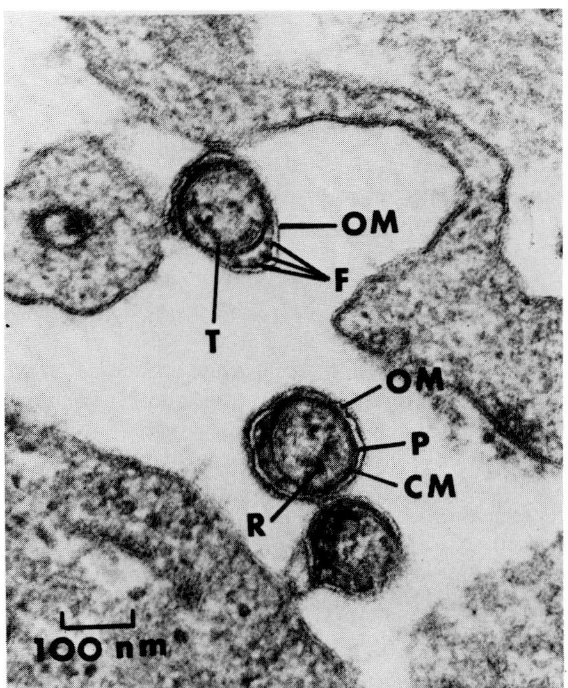


**Fig. 18-1.** (*a*) Longitudinal and (*b*) cross section of *T. pallidum* showing outer membrane (OM), flagella (F), peptidoglycan layer (P), cytoplasmic membrane (CM), cytoplasmic tubules (T), and ribosomes (R). (*Courtesy of K. Hovind-Hougen.*)

*T. pallidum* is an obligate anaerobe is incorrect. *T. pallidum* metabolizes glucose and pyruvate aerobically,[14] has a cytochrome system, and has superoxide dismutase and catalase activity.[15] Under optimal in vitro conditions, treponemal replication time is similar to that reported in vivo, namely, about 30 h.[16]

## PATHOGENESIS

### ANIMAL MODELS

Animal models to study syphilis have also been problematic.[1] Experimental primary infection can be produced in rabbits, and they also develop secondary lesions. Hamsters and guinea pigs develop atypical lesions at injection sites, and infection may also be produced in immunosuppressed mice, but only with the greatest difficulty. In discussing the pathogenesis of syphilis, it is generally assumed that there is no essential difference between experimentally induced infection in rabbits and naturally acquired infection in humans, at least in the early, active phase of infection. This assumption results from the close parallels between infection in rabbits and in humans and is necessary because of the paucity of available information derived from human studies. There is no known parallel in the rabbit, or in any other animal, including subhuman primates, for tertiary syphilis.

### EARLIEST STAGE OF INFECTION

The skin and mucous membranes provide the initial protective barrier against infection by *T. pallidum*. Implantation of treponemes subcutaneously (intradermally) probably occurs at sites of macroscopically invisible abrasions produced during sexual intercourse. The rotatory motion of the virulent treponeme has been said to enable it to penetrate cells or burrow between them, but there are no data to support this simplistic view. It is most unlikely that the treponeme penetrates an unbroken, keratinized epidermal layer.

Epidemiologic data show that about one-third of people who have sexual intercourse with an infected subject will become infected themselves. Although it is not possible to estimate the number of organisms needed to cause a naturally occurring infection in humans, the number of *T. pallidum* that will produce an infection following injection into rabbits is very small. This number is calculated from studies in which the concentration of treponemes in a suspension is determined by dark field microscopy; this suspension is then diluted serially, and aliquots are injected into rabbits. Injection of a large inoculum (e.g. $10^7$ organisms) may cause a chancre to appear in 5 to 7 days. With smaller inocula the incubation period becomes longer. Inoculation of 50 to 100 organisms is followed by an incubation period of about 3 weeks. Further dilution leads to less regular production of lesions with an incubation period that reaches but does not exceed 5 weeks.[1,17] An experimental study in previously uninfected human volunteers produced strikingly similar results.[18] Whereas one might have assumed that prior experience with *T. pallidum* might lead to a more prolonged incubation period,[1,19] one recent study[20] has suggested the opposite result, namely, that the incubation period is slightly shorter in rabbits that are acutely infected. This observation has been related to a proposed immunosuppressive state caused by the infection. The minimal infective dose by the intravenous route is much greater (around $10^5$ organisms), which is consistent with other models of infection. For example, intraperitoneal injection of one virulent pneumococcus into mice is lethal, but a much larger inoculum must be given intravenously in order to cause progressive infection.

Once treponemes find their way into dermal sites, normal serum constituents may have an antitreponemal effect,[21] perhaps resulting from cross-reactivity between *T. pallidum* and other gram-negative organisms and/or nonpathogenic treponemes that colonize the alimentary tract. Normal human serum has been shown to exert low-grade treponemicidal activity in vitro.[22] However, factors that govern natural species immunity to syphilis are unknown, as is the case with most other infections. Serum bactericidal activity does not appear to be an important contributing factor to the ability of mice or guinea pigs to resist infection, and a variety of other factors ranging from the role of killer-lymphocytes to the availability of receptor sites on host cells need to be considered.

#### Adherence

Viable *T. pallidum* attach by one or both ends to mammalian cells in vitro (Fig. 18-2), although they rarely, if ever, penetrate these cells;[23,24] adherence occurs only if the treponemes are viable and is inhibited by preincubating them with antitreponemal antibody. A specialized receptor site on the end of the treponeme has not been documented by electron microscopy.[11] Interaction between surface components and lectins has been used to suggest that the ligand is a mucopolysaccharide;[7] however, the ability to bind lectins may be nonspecific, and several lines of evidence, including the finding that the ligand is destroyed by trypsin, may indicate a protein composition.[25] Some studies have suggested that adherent *T. pallidum* damage tissues.[26] It should be noted that neither conventional toxins nor lipopolysaccharide A (endotoxin) have been detected in *T. pallidum*.

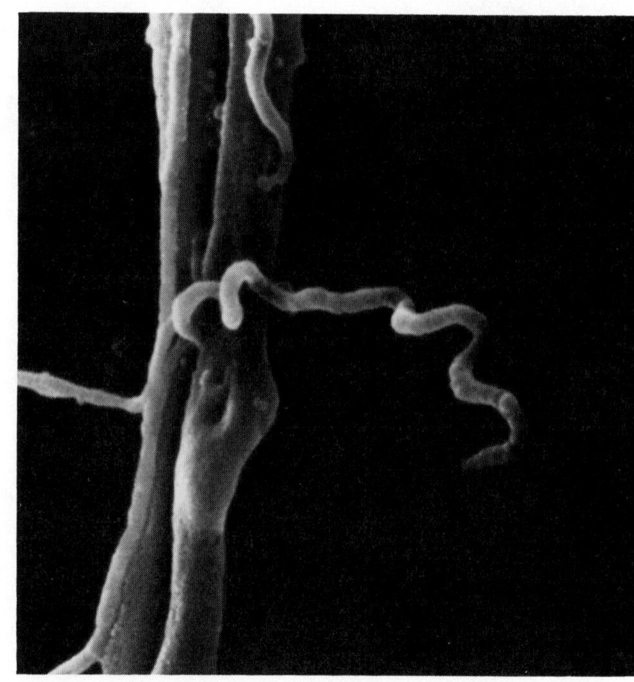

**Fig. 18-2.** *T. pallidum* adheres to cultured rabbit testicular cells by a specialized end structure. (*Courtesy of J. Baseman.*)

## Host response

**Neutrophils.** The initial cells attracted to an area of bacterial invasion are polymorphonuclear leukocytes (PMNs); the same is true of the response to invasion by *T. pallidum*.[27] Studies in our laboratory have shown that *T. pallidum* generates chemotactic substances (presumably the C5a component of the complement cascade) during in vitro incubation with normal human serum and have verified that PMNs are the first cells to accumulate at the site of intradermal treponemal injection.[28] We also found that incubating PMNs with *T. pallidum* stimulates a chemiluminescent response suggesting that a reaction takes place at the PMN membrane. We were surprised to find by electron-microscopic examination that phagocytosis occurs readily; soon after exposure to PMNs in vitro or in vivo, treponemes are seen within phagocytic vacuoles. The treponemes did not even need to be preincubated with serum or complement before this reaction took place. The fact that *T. pallidum* is readily phagocytized by PMNs in vitro or in vivo without additional opsonization is consistent with the finding that host IgG is present on the surface of the organism.[29,30] Presumably, complement is present as well, although this has not been demonstrated.

Our hypothesis, when we began these studies, had been that *T. pallidum* resists ingestion by phagocytic cells, perhaps because the external, amorphous layer functions as a capsule. It now appears more likely, although it is still speculative, that these organisms are ingested but not necessarily killed. Possible mechanisms include coating of treponemes with substances that make them nonsusceptible to lysosomal enzymes, failure of granules to fuse with phagocytic vacuoles, or persistence of treponemes outside of phagosomes but within the cytoplasm. Alternatively, only some treponemes may be ingested; others that are able to resist phagocytosis for whatever reason may then be responsible for disease. It remains a fascinating and enigmatic question how this slow-growing pathogenic treponeme with an estimated dividing time of 30 h is able to escape initial host defense and establish lesions.

**Lymphocytes.** Once *T. pallidum* have penetrated the epithelial layer, the organisms replicate locally; simultaneously, some organisms escape and may be trapped in draining lymph nodes. PMNs accumulate in the area, soon thereafter to be replaced by thymus-dependent lymphocytes.[31,32] B cells that contain surface antibody to *T. pallidum* may also be present.[33]

Studies showing large numbers of thymus-dependent lymphocytes within a few days of the initial infection have generally used large inocula; in the natural situation this tissue reaction occurs more slowly but presumably follows the same pattern. Lymphocytes predominate, with macrophages and occasional PMNs also noted. In addition, the primary chancre contains a large amount of mucoid material consisting mainly of hyaluronic acid and chondroitin sulfate; the exact origin and properties of this substance are not fully understood, but some authorities believe this material may modulate or alter immune responses. Thus the chancre, the initial lesion arising at a site of treponemal infection, contains a mucoid center and is surrounded by a cellular infiltrate that is chiefly lymphocytic, with infiltrating cells being found most prominently in a perivascular location.

**Macrophages.** During the incubation period, proliferation of treponemes is associated with stimulation of cell-mediated and humoral immunity. Evidence showing that a line of sensitized thymus-dependent lymphocytes appears in primary syphilitic lesions has already been cited.[31,32] Presumably an initial treponeme-macrophage interaction allows for processing of antigens, followed by proliferation of clones of thymus-dependent lymphocytes. Perhaps ingestion by PMNs is also involved in antigen processing. These cells, in the presence of treponemal antigen, presumably produce lymphokines which attract and/or activate macrophages. Activated macrophages have been shown to ingest *T. pallidum* in vitro in the presence of exogenous antibody.[34] Ingestion in vivo has also been said to occur, correlating with a decline in the number of detectable treponemal forms, and the presence of degenerating treponemes is demonstrable in phagocytic vacuoles;[31,35] it is not certain whether killing by macrophages or ingestion of damaged treponemal forms is responsible. The antigens involved in the sensitization reaction have not been identified, but splenic and lymph node lymphocytes obtained from rabbits 1 week after challenge with a large dose of treponemes have been shown to proliferate in vitro during exposure to sonicated treponemes.[36]

## Humoral-antibody responses

**Specific Treponemal Antibodies.** The fact that B-cell stimulation has taken place is inferred from the presence of a variety of antibodies that are present in the serum of most patients by the time they seek medical attention for a syphilitic chancre. Antibodies directed against treponemal antigens are detected in 80 percent or more of cases of primary syphilis by (1) the fluorescent treponemal antibody (FTA-ABS) test after absorption of serum with the nonvirulent *T. phagedenis* (formerly called *T. reiteri*)[37,38] or by (2) the newer *T. pallidum*-hemagglutinating antibody tests which can be done in an ordinary laboratory without using a fluorescent microscope.[38–40] The *T. pallidum* immobilization test (TPI), which detects immobilization and inactivation of *T. pallidum* by serum antibody in vitro in the presence of exogenous complement, is positive in a smaller proportion of cases of primary syphilis.[41] It is still not known if these antibodies are directed against the same or different antigens or, in the case of TPI antibody, whether IgG or IgM is chiefly involved. Recent studies have documented the sequential emergence of IgM and IgG reactive with individual outer-membrane proteins of *T. pallidum* during the course of syphilis.[9,42]

**Nontreponemal (Anticardiolipin) Antibodies.** Antibody against cardiolipin is also present in primary syphilis and is detected in about two-thirds of cases by the Venereal Disease Research Laboratory (VDRL) or the rapid plasma reagin (RPR) tests which are modifications of the initial Wassermann reaction.[37,43] Cardiolipin is a substance which constitutes about 10 percent of treponemal lipids and is also present in mammalian tissues. An interesting and unanswered question is whether the antibody is directed against altered mammalian tissue, which results from syphilitic infection and the host response to treponemal components, or against treponeme-incorporated mammalian lipids, whether they be normal or altered.

**Circulating Immune Complexes.** Circulating complexes may be detected in some patients with primary syphilis and in the majority of those with secondary syphilis.[44–46] These complexes contain immunoglobulin (mainly $IgG_1$ and $IgG_3$), complement, and identifiable outer membrane proteins of *T. pallidum*. The presence of human antigens including fibronectin, and antibody to fibronectin[46] suggests a possible link between VDRL-reactivity and autoimmune diseases.

Thus, by the time of the primary syphilitic lesion, both humoral and cell-mediated immune mechanisms have been activated. Treponeme-sensitized lymphocytes and activated macrophages are present in lesions, and antitreponemal humoral antibody is detectable in serum. The number of treponemes has begun to decrease, although treponemes (usually extracellular[47]) are still present. All these observations suggest that the infection is being controlled, especially in the case of a relatively slow-growing and non-toxin-producing organism. The proof of the effectiveness of this immune response at this point would be spontaneous resolution of infection.

## SECONDARY STAGE

The occurrence of secondary syphilis indicates that the host response to this unusual infection remains incompletely understood. For, as the local immune process appears to be bringing the primary infection under control, a remarkable phenomenon occurs: the manifestations of generalized infection appear. Widespread, small, individual lesions are seen in naturally infected human subjects 3 to 6 weeks after the primary chancre has appeared. Their characteristics and time of appearance reflect several processes: (1) the hematogenous spread of treponemes throughout the body; (2) the establishment of lesions in the skin, an area that may offer better growth conditions for *T. pallidum* because of reduced temperature; and (3) the development of some degree of systemic immunity which modifies the appearance of these disseminated lesions. If not for this last-named feature, these lesions would all look like primary chancres, which is exactly what happens when previously uninfected rabbits are infected intravenously with *T. pallidum.* In fact, on occasion, a human being has a florid form of infection (called malignant secondary syphilis by some authorities) which, for whatever reason, is reminiscent of the infection that follows intravenous challenge in rabbits.

Additional evidence for the generalized nature of secondary syphilis derives from the varied manifestations of this infection in human subjects, including malaise, fever, generalized lymph node enlargement, hepatitis, arthritis, glomerulonephritis, and central nervous system involvement. Some authorities believe that a more florid form of secondary syphilis occurs in patients who have the acquired immunodeficiency syndrome, but, at the time of this writing (1987), this is controversial.

The disseminated stage of naturally acquired syphilis, with its innumerable small lesions, persists for weeks or months. Patients with this stage of disease have high antibody titers by all measures, including specific treponemal and nontreponemal tests; most have a positive TPI as well. Perhaps an important clue to the persistence of the disease is the finding that delayed-type hypersensitivity to treponemal antigens is usually absent.[48,49] Nevertheless, animal studies suggest that intradermal challenge with *T. pallidum* is not likely to lead to new chancres. This situation is common in parasitic diseases and is called *premunition:* the host resists rechallenge but is unable to clear the initial infection. While at this stage lesions are more controlled (i.e., less exuberant) than disseminated lesions would be, and while the host is resistant to a new infection, persistence of organisms and activity of disease underscore the point that a state of true immunity has not been achieved. At a time when local immunity has brought the initial chancre under control and there is ample evidence for an active, systemic immune reaction, the host is unable to eradicate systemic infection. Circulating immune complexes may be deposited in the kidneys[50,51] and the skin[52] where they contribute, to a varying degree, to the observed histopathologic changes.

## DEVELOPMENT OF IMMUNITY: LATENCY

Eventually, the host suppresses the infection sufficiently so that no lesions are clinically apparent. This stage is called latency. Delayed-type hypersensitivity to *T. pallidum* is uniformly present at this time[48,49] and may be important, together with humoral antibody, in finally controlling infection. The acquisition of immunity in rabbits also appears to correlate with the appearance of inducible factors that inhibit macrophage migration.[53] In the pretreatment era, after the host's immune response had seemingly controlled the infection (as evidenced by onset of latency), relapse of disseminated, secondary lesions still occurred in up to one-fourth of cases.[54]

This unusual evolution of infection has led to a number of studies of cell-mediated and humoral immunity. Syphilitic infection in rabbits has been shown to stimulate acquired cellular resistance,[55] a reaction that is mediated by thymus-dependent lymphocytes.[56] Evidence for a biological role of activated macrophages has been mixed, with most results having been negative. Systemic treatment with agents that activate macrophages, such as *Mycobacterium bovis* (BCG) or *Propionibacterium parvum,* does not alter the rate of clearance of intravenously injected *T. pallidum* or the progression of syphilitic infection.[57,58] One set of investigators reported more rapid clearance of treponemes from a local site of injection if macrophages were first activated locally;[35] others disagree.[57,59] Transfusing lymphocytes from syphilis-immune rabbits into normal rabbits using inbred strains did not transfer immunity to syphilis;[60] however, immunity to *T. pallidum* var. *Bosnia* has been transferred in hamsters by using this same approach,[61] and there is a report that local infusion of immune lymphocytes at a site of treponemal infection provides protection.[62]

It also has been difficult to demonstrate a full protective role for humoral immunity despite the presence of TPI antibody, which immobilizes and inactivates *T. pallidum* in vitro.[41] Infusions of relatively large amounts of globulin at the time of treponemal inoculation delay the onset of infection and attenuate it, but surprisingly do not prevent it altogether.[63,64] Thus, lesions still appear at initial challenge sites after catabolism of the infused antibody. This contrasts with our general understanding of humoral immunity in other infections. For example, if a mouse is infused with a sufficient amount of immune serum prior to pneumococcal or streptococcal challenge to provide protection initially, infection certainly does not appear later on. In contrast, *T. pallidum* seems to persist at the site of inoculation despite the presence of infused antibody. Virulent treponemes display a remarkable capacity to resist the attempts of the host, both humoral and cellular, to eradicate them. On the basis of the evidence to date, it is reasonable to believe that an interaction between cellular and humoral immune mechanisms is probably necessary to terminate active syphilitic infection, but it is obvious that much remains unknown. One cannot even be certain that this general assertion will ultimately prove to be correct.

## TERTIARY STAGE

Even when syphilis finally appears to be arrested, we know that this often only reflects a latent period. *T. pallidum* can sometimes be isolated in latency from infected tissues both in humans and in experimentally injected animals.[1] From 1 to 20 years or more after disseminated infection has given way to latency, tertiary syphilis becomes clinically apparent. Gummas may appear in soft tissue or viscera. These large granulomatous lesions suggest an immunologic response, which is assumed to reflect a response to treponemal antigens. However, this has not been easy to demonstrate. Some investigators used a silver stain to show treponemes were always present in gummas; others suggested that in many cases this represented an artifact.[65] One report has used immunofluorescent techniques to demonstrate treponemes in a single, and somewhat atypical, case.[66] Gummas do not appear in areas where one would necessarily expect large numbers of treponemes to have persisted after active disease (for example, they have a predilection to appear at sites of trauma, such as elbows and knees), although the trauma might have facilitated their persistence through unknown mechanisms. They also appear in the testis and the liver, but not in lymph nodes. One might find an explanation for each of these observations individually; taken together, though, the picture is one of confusion. Neurosyphilis is even more difficult to understand because different syndromes occur, associated with different histologic appearances. Perhaps the immunologically privileged nature of the central nervous system contributes to this situation.

## EVIDENCE FOR ABERRANT IMMUNE RESPONSES

All these observations have stimulated interest in what might be considered aberrant aspects of the immune response to syphilitic infection. The problem with these studies is that varying results have been obtained, and even when perturbations in immunity are found, it is difficult to relate them directly to observed events in the evolution of syphilis. For example, some workers have shown that the response of peripheral blood lymphocytes to nontreponemal or treponemal antigens is depressed during syphilis; there have been different opinions as to whether serum factors or abnormalities in the lymphocytes themselves are responsible.[67–70] Others have found lymphocyte responses to be normal. The mechanism by which serum might suppress lymphoblastic responses in vitro, specifically whether mucopolysaccharides and/or immune complexes are responsible, is still uncertain; treponemal mucopolysaccharides (glycosaminoglycans) which are present in serum and tissue extracts of infected rabbits may bind mitogens, thereby preventing the interaction with lymphocytes.[71]

Other immunologic studies have focused on abnormal immunoglobulin response in syphilis, showing greatly suppressed IgG responses to a nontreponemal, T-lymphocyte-dependent antigen early in active infection.[72] IgM responses were found to be increased severalfold. Technical problems precluded this same kind of observation using treponemal antigen. Circulating immune complexes may be responsible for suppression of IgG responses;[73] failure to bring syphilitic infection under control could be due to the host's inability to make an appropriate bactericidal antibody directed against an essential antigen. These findings are analogous to those in some chronic parasitic infections. Abundant evidence for immunologic responsiveness does not, a priori, lead to rejection of this possibility since responses to some treponemal antigens could be normal or increased while other responses could be suppressed. At the present time, the biological importance of abnormal immunoglobulin responses in syphilis is not understood.

## IMMUNE RESPONSE: PROSPECTS FOR A VACCINE

Over the past several decades there has been much discussion about a vaccine to protect against syphilis. My view remains[74] that there are so many unusual features of the clinical progression of syphilis and there is so much unknown about the biology of the infecting organism that this discussion is still premature. Outer membrane proteins that are immunogenic might be used as vaccines and their efficacy studied in experimental infection. Since there is substantial question about the ability of humoral factors to bring infection under control, it is not known whether this approach will successfully identify biologically important antigens. Several investigators have succeeded in cloning *Escherichia coli* to produce antigens from *T. pallidum;* this method could be used to generate protein antigens for a treponemal vaccine if such a product were thought to be desirable. It seems safe to say that we are still many years away from development of an effective vaccine.

# References


1 Turner TB, Hollander DH: Biology of the treponematoses. *WHO Monogr Ser* 35:1, 1957.
2 Fieldsteel AH, Miao RH: Genetics of treponema, in *Pathogenesis and Immunology of Treponemal Infection,* RF Schell, DM Musher (eds). New York, Dekker, 1982.
3 Fohn MJ et al: Specificity of antibodies from patients with pinta for antigens of *Treponema pallidum* subspecies *pallidum. J Infect Dis* 156:000, 1987.
4 Hovind-Hougen K: Determination by means of electron microscopy of morphological criteria of value for classification of some spirochetes, in particular treponemes. *Acta Pathol Microbiol Scand [B]* 255 (suppl):1, 1976.
5 Clarkson KA: Technique of darkfield examination. *Med Tech Bull* 7:199, 1956.
6 Zeigler JA et al: Demonstration of extracellular material at the surface of pathogenic *T. pallidum* cells. *Br J Vener Dis* 52:1, 1976.
7 Fitzgerald TJ et al: Relationship of *Treponema pallidum* to acidic mucopolysaccharides. *Infect Immun* 24:252, 1979.
8 Norris SG et al: Identity of *Treponema pallidum* subsp. *pallidum* polypeptides: Correlation of sodium dodecyl sulfate-polyacrylamide gel electrophoresis results from different laboratories. *Electrophoresis* 8:77, 1987.
9 Hanff PF et al: Humoral immune response in human syphilis to polypeptides of *Treponema pallidum. J Immunol* 129:1287, 1982.
10 Baker-Zander SA et al: Antigens of *Treponema pallidum* recognized by IgG and IgM antibodies during syphilis in humans. *J Infect Dis* 151:264, 1985.
11 Hovind-Hougen K: Morphologic anatomy of *Treponema,* in *Pathogenesis and Immunology of Treponemal Infection,* RF Schell, DM Musher (eds). New York, Dekker, 1982.
12 Fieldsteel AH et al: Cultivation of virulent *Treponema pallidum* in tissue culture. *Infect Immun* 32:908, 1981.
13 Jenkin H: Cultivation of treponemes, in *Pathogenesis and Immunology of Treponemal Infection,* RF Schell, DM Musher (eds). New York, Dekker, 1982.
14 Baseman JB et al: Virulent *Treponema pallidum:* Aerobe or anaerobe? *Infect Immun* 13:704, 1976.
15 Austin FE et al: Distribution of superoxide dismutase, catalase, and peroxidase activities among *Treponema pallidum* and other spirochetes. *Infect Immun* 33:372, 1981.
16 Cumberland MC, Turner TB: The rate of multiplication of *Treponema pallidum* in normal and immune rabbits. *Am J Syph Gon Vener Dis* 33:201, 1949.
17 Magnuson HJ et al: The minimal infectious inoculum of *Spirochaeta*

*pallida* (Nichols strain) and a consideration of its rate of multiplication in vivo. *Am J Syph Gon Vener Dis* 32:1, 1948.

18 Magnuson HJ et al: Inoculation syphilis in human volunteers. *Medicine* 35:33, 1956.

19 Magnuson HJ et al: The rate of development and degree of acquired immunity in experimental syphilis. *Am J Syph Gon Vener Dis* 32:418, 1948.

20 Fitzgerald TJ: Accelerated lesion development in experimental syphilis. *Infect Immun* 34:478, 1981.

21 Hederstedt B: Studies on the *Treponema pallidum* immobilizing activity in normal human serum: 2. Serum factors participating in the normal serum immobilization reaction. *Acta Pathol Microbiol Scand* [C] 84:135, 1976.

22 Bishop NH, Miller JN: Humoral immune mechanisms in acquired syphilis, in *Pathogenesis and Immunology of Treponemal Infections*, RF Schell, DM Musher (eds). New York, Dekker, 1982.

23 Fitzgerald TJ et al: *Treponema pallidum* (Nichols strain) in tissue cultures: Cellular attachment, entry, and survival. *Infect Immun* 11:1133, 1975.

24 Hayes NS et al: Parasitism by virulent *Treponema pallidum* of host cell surfaces. *Infect Immun* 17:174, 1977.

25 Alderete JF, Baseman JB: Surface characterization of virulent *Treponema pallidum*. *Infect Immun* 30:814, 1980.

26 Fitzgerald TJ: Toxic activities of *Treponema pallidum*, in *Pathogenesis and Immunology of Treponemal Infection*, RF Schell, DM Musher (eds). New York, Dekker, 1982.

27 Rich AR et al: Experiments demonstrating that acquired immunity in syphilis is not dependent on allergic inflammation. *Bull Johns Hopkins Hosp* 52:179, 1933.

28 Musher DM et al: The interaction between *Treponema pallidum* and human polymorphonuclear leukocytes. *J Infect Dis* 147:77, 1983.

29 Hovind-Hougen K et al: Electron microscopy of treponemes subjected to the *Treponema pallidum* immobilization (TPI) test: II. Immunoelectron microscopy. *Acta Pathol Microbiol Scand* [C] 87:263, 1979.

30 Alderete JF, Baseman JB: Surface-associated host proteins on virulent *Treponema pallidum*. *Infect Immun* 26:1048, 1979.

31 Lukehart SA et al: Characterization of lymphocyte responsiveness in early experimental syphilis: II. Nature of cellular infiltration and *Treponema pallidum* distribution in testicular lesions. *J Immunol* 124:461, 1980.

32 Baker-Zander S, Sell S: A histopathologic and immunologic study of the course of syphilis in the experimentally infected rabbit: Demonstration of long-lasting cellular immunity. *Am J Pathol* 101:387, 1980.

33 Soltani K et al: Detection by direct immunofluorescence of antibodies to *Treponema pallidum* in the cutaneous infiltrates of rabbit syphilomas. *J Infect Dis* 138:222, 1978.

34 Lukehart SA, Miller JN: Demonstration of the in vitro phagocytosis of *Treponema pallidum* by rabbit peritoneal macrophages. *J Immunol* 121:2014, 1978.

35 Hardy PH et al: Macrophages in immunity to syphilis: Suppressive effect of concurrent infection with *Mycobacterium bovis* BCG on the development of syphilitic lesions and growth of *Treponema pallidum* in tuberculin-positive rabbits. *Infect Immun* 26:751, 1979.

36 Lukehart SA et al: Characterization of lymphocyte responsiveness in early experimental syphilis: I. In vitro response to mitogens and *Treponema pallidum* antigens. *J Immunol* 124:454, 1980.

37 Moore MB Jr, Knox JM: Sensitivity and specificity in syphilis serology: Clinical implications. *South Med J* 48:963, 1965.

38 Garner MF et al: *Treponema pallidum* haemagglutination test for syphilis: Comparison with the TPI and FTA-ABS tests. *Br J Vener Dis* 48:470, 1972.

39 Lesinski J et al: Specificity, sensitivity and diagnostic value of the TPHA test. *Br J Vener Dis* 50:334, 1974.

40 Rudolph AH: The microhemagglutination assay for *Treponema pallidum* antibodies (MHA-TP), a new treponemal test for syphilis: Where does it fit? *J Am Vener Dis Assoc* 3:3, 1976.

41 Turner TB et al: Protective antibodies in the serum of syphilitic patients. *Am J Hyg* 48:173, 1948.

42 Baker-Zander SA et al: Antigens of *Treponema pallidum* recognized by IgG and IgM antibodies during syphilis in humans. *J Infect Dis* 151:264, 1985.

43 Musher DM: A reactive VDRL in an asymptomatic patient, in *Current Clinical Topics in Infectious Diseases*: 9, JS Remington and MN Swartz (eds). New York, McGraw-Hill, 1988, pp 147–157.

44 Solling J et al: Circulating immune complexes in syphilis. *Acta Derm Venereol (Stockh)* 58:263, 1978.

45 Engel S, Diezel W: Persistent serum immune complexes in syphilis. *Br J Vener Dis* 56:221, 1980.

46 Baughn RE et al: Characterization of the antigenic determinants and host components in immune complexes from patients with secondary syphilis. *J Immunol* 136:1406, 1986.

47 Penn CW: Avoidance of host defenses by *Treponema pallidum* in situ and on extraction from infected rabbit testes. *J Gen Microbiol* 126:69, 1981.

48 Marshak LC, Rothman S: Skin testing with a purified suspension of *Treponema pallidum*. *Am J Syph Gon Vener Dis* 35:35, 1951.

49 Thivolet J et al: Étude de l'intradermoreaction aux suspensions de treponemes formolées (souche Nichols pathogène) chez les syphilitiques et les sujets normaux. *Ann Inst Pasteur Lille* 84:23, 1953.

50 Bhorade MS et al: Nephropathy of secondary syphilis: A clinical and pathological spectrum. *JAMA* 216:1159, 1971.

51 Gamble CN, Reardan JB: Immunopathogenesis of syphilitic glomerulonephritis: Elution of antitreponemal antibody from glomerular immune-complex deposits. *N Engl J Med* 292:449, 1975.

52 Jorizzo JL et al: Role of circulating immune complexes in human secondary syphilis. *J Infect Dis* 153:1014, 1986.

53 Metzger M et al: Cell-mediated immunity in experimental syphilis in rabbits. *Arch Immunol Ther Exp (Warsz)* 25:25, 1977.

54 Clark EG, Danbolt N: The Oslo study of the natural course of untreated syphilis: An epidemiologic investigation based on a re-study of the Boeck-Bruusgaard material. *Med Clin North Am* 48:613, 1964.

55 Schell RF, Musher DM: Detection of nonspecific resistance to *Listeria monocytogenes* in rabbits infected with *Treponema pallidum*. *Infect Immun* 9:658, 1974.

56 Schell R et al: Induction of acquired cellular resistance following transfer of thymus-dependent lymphocytes from syphilitic rabbits. *J Immunol* 114:550, 1975.

57 Graves SR, Johnson RC: Effect of pretreatment with *Mycobacterium bovis* (strain BCG) and immune syphilitic serum on rabbit resistance to *Treponema pallidum*. *Infect Immun* 12:1029, 1975.

58 Baughn RE et al: Effect of sensitization with *Propionibacterium acnes* on the growth of *Listeria monocytogenes* and *Treponema pallidum* in rabbits. *J Immunol* 118:108, 1977.

59 Graves S: Susceptibility of rabbits to *Treponema pallidum* after infection with *Mycobacterium bovis*. *Br J Vener Dis* 44:394, 1979.

60 Baughn RE et al: Inability of spleen cells from chancre-immune rabbits to confer immunity to challenge with *Treponema pallidum*. *Infect Immun* 17:535, 1977.

61 Schell RF et al: Endemic syphilis: Transfer of resistance to *Treponema pallidum* stain Bosnia A in hamsters with cell suspension enriched in thymus-derived cells. *J Infect Dis* 141:752, 1980.

62 Metzger M: The role of immunologic responses in protection against syphilis, in *The Biology of Parasitis Spirochetes*, RC Johnson (ed). New York, Academic Press, 1976, pp 327–337.

63 Turner TB et al: Effects of passive immunization on experimental syphilis in the rabbit. *Johns Hopkins Med J* 133:241, 1973.

64 Weiser RS et al: Immunity to syphilis: Passive transfer in rabbits using serial doses of immune serum. *Infect Immun* 13:1402, 1976.

65 Turner TB: Personal communication.

66 Handsfield HH et al: Demonstration of *Treponema pallidum* in a cutaneous gumma by indirect immunofluorescence. *Arch Derm* 719:677, 1983.

67 Musher DM et al: Lymphocyte transformation in syphilis: An in vitro correlate of immune suppression in vivo? *Infect Immun* 11:1261, 1975.

68 Pavia CS et al: Selective responses of lymphocytes from *Treponema*

*pallidum* infected rabbits to mitogens and *Treponema reiteri. Infect Immun* 15:417, 1977.

69 Wicher V, Wicher K: In vitro cell response of *Treponema pallidum*-infected rabbits: II. Inhibition of lymphocyte response to phytohaemagglutinin by serum of *T. pallidum*-infected rabbits. *Clin Exp Immunol* 24:487, 1977.

70 Ware JL et al: Serum of rabbits infected with *Treponema pallidum* (Nichols) inhibits in vitro transformation of normal rabbit lymphocytes. *Cell Immunol* 42:363, 1979.

71 Baughn RE, Musher DM: Reappraisal of lymphocyte responsiveness to concanavalin A during experimental syphilis: Evidence that glycosaminoglycans in the sera and tissues interfere with active binding sites on the lectin and not with the lymphocytes. *Infect Immun* 35:552, 1982.

72 Baughn RE, Musher DM: Altered immune responsiveness associated with experimental syphilis in the rabbit: Elevated IgG and depressed IgA response to sheep erythrocytes. *J Immunol* 120:1691, 1978.

73 Baughn RE et al: Detection of circulating immune complexes in the sera of rabbits with experimental syphilis: Possible role in immunoregulation. *Infect Immun* 29:575, 1980.

74 Musher DM et al: The role of a vaccine for syphilis. *Sex Transm Dis* 4:163, 1977.

# Chapter 19
# Natural history of syphilis

P. Frederick Sparling

*Know syphilis in all its manifestations and relations, and all other things clinical will be added unto you.*

Sir William Osler, 1897

Syphilis is one of the most fascinating diseases of humans. Its remarkably variable and long drawn-out course raises many unanswered questions about the nature of the host-parasite interaction. The disease has been of great historical importance not only for the practice of medicine, but also because of its effect on many persons who played important roles in the history of the western world. It was an extremely common infection only a few decades past, with prevalence in various autopsy series in the first half of the twentieth century of 5 to 10 percent.[1,2] In certain groups of low socioeconomic status studied in the prepenicillin era, syphilis affected 25 percent or more of the population.[3] Widespread use of antibiotics now has reduced the incidence of early syphilis to manageable proportions, and recognized new cases of late syphilis have decreased even more remarkably. Nevertheless, this classic disease is still very important from many points of view. In this chapter, the origins of the disease are discussed briefly, and the course of the untreated and treated disease is analyzed. More detailed coverage of the pathogenesis of syphilis is found in Chap. 18; the clinical manifestations, in Chaps. 20 to 23.

## ORIGINS

### COLUMBIAN THEORY

Syphilis was epidemic in late fifteenth century Europe and the early stages were apparently often unusually severe by contemporary standards. The rapid spread and considerable effects of the disease throughout Europe in the last decade of the fifteenth century caused it to be termed the Great Pox, in contrast to another scourge, smallpox. The disease received its present name from the poem by Fracastoro in 1530 about the afflicted shepherd, Syphilus. The late complications of syphilis were recognized early, and were frequently mentioned by many Elizabethan authors.

The late-fifteenth century European epidemic coincided with the return of Columbus from America in 1493, causing many to assume that the disease was acquired from natives in the West Indies, and carried back to a nonimmune (and therefore particularly susceptible) population in Europe. Certainly, if this did occur, conditions were ripe for rapid transmission, because Europe was engaged in wars at that time, and the movement of the troops and their camp followers created a perfect vehicle for rapid spread of a sexually transmitted disease. On the other hand, there are biblical and ancient Chinese writings which are consistent with descriptions of late cutaneous syphilis, although other illnesses such as tuberculosis or leprosy could have caused similar descriptions to be written. An illness suggestive of syphilis apparently was not described in early American natives. These and other considerations led some to speculate that venereal syphilis did not arise suddenly in Europe after 1493, but may have been endemic already, only to become more widespread and severe as a consequence of the wars which coincided with the return of Columbus and his men.

### THE ENVIRONMENTAL THEORY

Some scholars have suggested that venereal syphilis is merely a variant of other treponemal diseases which are common in other parts of the world. This idea, formerly championed by Hudson,[4] was recently raised again in a slightly altered form by Hollander.[5] The notion is that *Treponema pallidum,* the causative agent of venereal syphilis, is really the same species as *T. pallidum* subspecies *pertenue,* the causative agent of yaws (a disabling cutaneous and osseous disease of the tropics); *T. pallidum* spp. *carateum,* the causative agent of pinta (a less destructive cutaneous disease found in certain parts of rural Central and South America); and *T. pallidum* spp. *bosnia,* the causative agent of nonvenereal syphilis, which is found in arid parts of the near east and surrounding territory. According to this hypothesis, all treponematoses are merely variants of a single disease, the expression of which has been modified by environmental factors, especially temperature. Consistent with this idea is evidence by DNA-DNA hybridization of the close relationship between *T. pallidum* and *T. pallidum pertenue,*[6] and other studies which demonstrate their considerable antigenic similarities.[7,8] Although the various pathogenic treponemal species do exhibit some differences in host range in animals,[8] this probably reflects relatively minor genetic variations.

Current studies in several laboratories on the molecular genetics and immunology of *T. pallidum*[9–11] may help to resolve questions of the relatedness of the pathogenic treponemes of humans, which is important to future considerations of programs for eradication of syphilis and other treponematoses. It will remain for future historians to argue about the origins of syphilis; short of creation of an "Andromeda strain," it probably will never be possible to know for certain when and how any of the major infectious diseases arose. (The current human immunodeficiency syndrome epidemic may be just such an instance!)

## THE COURSE OF UNTREATED SYPHILIS

The natural history of the disease, already quite well known in the nineteenth century, became even more clear after the discovery of *T. pallidum* by Schaudinn and Hoffmann in 1905[12] and after introduction of serological tests shortly thereafter. In the following section an overview of the course of the disease is presented, followed by a more complete description of a few of the attempts at a definitive analysis of the natural course of the illness.

### TRANSMISSION

The disease is usually acquired by sexual contact, with the obvious and important exception of congenital syphilis, where the infant innocently acquires the infection by transplacental transmission of *T. pallidum.* Transmission by sexual contact requires exposure to moist mucosal or cutaneous lesions, and therefore a person ordinarily only is able to transmit syphilis during the first few years of infection, during the time of susceptibility to spontaneous mucocutaneous secondary relapses (see below).

The rate of acquisition of syphilis from an infected sexual partner has been estimated at about 30 percent, based on a placebo-controlled study of the efficacy of various antibiotics in aborting syphilis in known contacts within the previous 30 days of patients with primary or secondary syphilis.[13] The $ID_{50}$ of the rabbit-adapted Nichols strain of *T. pallidum* for human volunteers by intracutaneous inoculation was estimated to be 57 organisms, which was similar to the $ID_{50}$ for rabbits;[14] if the $ID_{50}$ for humans of native or "street strains" of *T. pallidum* on mucosal surfaces is similar, exposure to a relatively few organisms suffices to initiate infection.

Syphilis is a systemic disease shortly after its inception,[15] and women may transmit infection to their fetus in utero shortly after onset of infection. Transmission to the fetus in utero has been documented as early as the ninth week of pregnancy.[16] Women may remain potentially infectious for the fetus for many years, although the risk of infecting a fetus declines gradually during the course of untreated illness; after about 8 years there is little risk even in the untreated mother (see Chap. 67).

## THE STAGES OF SYPHILIS

### Primary

The untreated illness typically results in a primary lesion, the chancre, from 10 to 90 days (average 3 weeks) from exposure. The lesion is usually single but may be multiple, and although it is usually painless and associated with regional adenopathy, frequent exceptions occur (see Chap. 20). Primary lesions in nongenital sites may be particularly likely to have atypical appearance, especially in the anal area. Untreated, the primary lesion heals in a few weeks.

### Secondary

Within a few weeks or months (or less commonly, coincident with the primary lesion) a variable systemic illness develops, characterized by low-grade fever, malaise, sore throat, headache, adenopathy, and cutaneous or mucosal rash (see Chap. 20). This secondary stage of illness may be accompanied by alopecia, and up to 10 percent of patients have mild hepatitis.[17] Rarely, a form of nephrotic syndrome develops.[18] Evolution of secondary lesions is a manifestation of widespread hematogenous and lymphatic dissemination of *T. pallidum,* as evidenced by the infectious transfer of disease to susceptible animals with blood, lymph nodes, liver biopsy, and cerebrospinal fluid (reviewed in Ref. 15). A single sample of renal tissue was negative in an animal transfer test,[15] consistent with other evidence that the pathogenesis of secondary syphilitic nephropathy involve deposition of immune complexes[18] rather than infection of renal tissue by *T. pallidum.*

There is interest in this possible role of depression of the cellular immune response in the observed waxing and waning of the lesions of early (primary and secondary) syphilis. Many investigators have observed depression of specific and nonspecific lymphocyte responses in vitro coincident with the lesions of early syphilis in humans[19] and rabbits;[20,21] the hypothesis that depression of cellular immune responses to *T. pallidum* antigens is in some way involved in recrudescence of active lesions in secondary syphilis is attractive but still unproved. There is evidence for circulating immune complexes in early syphilis,[21] which could be responsible for some of the clinical manifestations and perhaps contributes to the depression of cellular immune responses. In this context, it is interesting to recall that old clinical and experimental observations established that there is temporary immunity to new infection during active early syphilis ("chancre immunity"),[22] although individuals previously treated for early syphilis were susceptible to experimental infection.[14] The role of the immune responses in the pathogenesis of early syphilis and in resistance to infection is discussed more completely in Chap. 18 and elsewhere.[23–25]

### Latency

By definition, persons with historical or serological evidence for syphilis but with no clinical manifestations have latent syphilis. This has been somewhat arbitrarily divided into early latency and late latency, on the basis of the time when untreated individuals are likely to have spontaneous mucocutaneous (infectious) relapses. In the Oslo study of untreated syphilis, secondary relapses occurred in 25 percent of patients, with most in the first year and a steadily decreasing incidence until 5 years had elapsed.[26] The U.S. Public Health Service therefore defines *early* (potentially infectious) *latency* as 1 year from onset of infection, whereas others prefer a longer interval before designating the infection as *late latent.* Since neurosyphilis may be asymptomatic or subtle, and cardiovascular syphilis also may be difficult to detect on physical examination, assignment of a diagnosis of latent syphilis requires both a careful physical examination and an examination of cerebrospinal fluid.

### Tertiary

The principal morbidity and mortality of syphilis in adults is due to the variable occurrence of later manifestation illness in the skin, bones, central nervous system, or viscera, particularly the heart and great vessels.

**Gumma.** Late cutaneous and osseous manifestations formerly were very common, but have become exceedingly rare in present practice. These lesions (*gummas*) have characteristic gross and microscopic appearance. Because gummas usually responded dramatically and rapidly to specific therapy, they were classified as benign late syphilis (Chap. 23), even though untreated they frequently led to destruction of soft tissues or bone. The pathogenesis of gummas was uncertain; spirochetes could be demonstrated in lesions,[15] but limited experiments in previously infected humans suggested that gummas might have been the result of a hypersensitivity response to endogenous or exogenous *T. pallidum* antigen.[14] Lesions of late benign syphilis sometimes occurred for an extended period from as few as 2 to over 40 years from onset of infection. Gummas of critical organs (heart, brain, liver) could be fatal.

**Cardiovascular.** Involvement of the heart and aorta by *T. pallidum* (Chap. 22) occurred roughly 10 to 30 years following onset of infection. Spirochetes could be demonstrated in large numbers in the infected aorta at postmortem,[15] but the critical effect was probably due to a vasculitis of the vasa vasorum. The most usual result was an aneurysm of the ascending aorta or other great vessels, and/or aortic valve insufficiency and heart failure due to dilatation of the aortic ring.

**Neurological.** Involvement of the central nervous system led to a number of different syndromes (Chap. 21), occurring over an extended period from 1 or 2 years to more than 30 years from onset of infection. The pathogenesis of late central nervous system syphilis is not understood completely. In syphilitic meningitis, *T. pallidum* could be demonstrated easily in cerebrospinal fluid, and in general paresis (syphilitic meningoencephalitis) spirochetes were also easily demonstrable (reviewed in Ref. 15). The common denominator of these illnesses also may be a small-vessel vasculitis (Chap. 21). In contrast, spirochetes could not be demonstrated in the spinal cord or other tissues in patients with tabes dorsalis, leading to the suggestion that loss of posterior column function in tabes dorsalis could have been the result of an immunologic attack on spinal cord tissue. Inability to create an animal model of neurosyphilis has greatly hindered further understanding of these devastating but interesting syndromes.

## THE OSLO STUDY

Probably all of the important clinical manifestations of syphilis were recognized by physicians of the nineteenth century, prior to introduction by Wassermann in 1906 of the first serological test for syphilis. It was not certain, however, what was the fate of the individual untreated patient, other than knowledge that some persons seemed to develop late destructive complications but others escaped unscathed. Our present understanding of this issue is based primarily on a large prospective study of patients conducted in Oslo from 1890 to 1910 by Professor Boeck, and subsequently followed up retrospectively by Bruusgaard[27] and later by Gjestland et al.[26]

Boeck was concerned that therapy available in 1890 (principally mercurials) might be more toxic than the disease itself, and therefore instigated a study of the fate of selected patients with untreated early primary or secondary syphilis. Diagnosis was based strictly on clinical criteria, since neither dark field microscopy nor serology was available for most of the initial phase of the study. Patients with lesions typical of early infectious syphilis were hospitalized until no longer infectious, but they were not treated. One-half of the males and three-fourths of the females were observed with lesions of secondary syphilis only. More females than males were admitted to the study because of the greater availability of hospital beds for females. This introduced a positive bias into the overall outcome since females fared better than males. A total of 2181 cases were entered, later shown to comprise only 1978 different patients. Patients were hospitalized approximately 3 months, although a few remained in hospital for 10 to 12 months, illustrating the long periods in which untreated patients were thought to be potentially infectious.

The most valuable data from the Oslo study came from a monumental follow-up and reappraisal conducted by Gjestland nearly 50 years after Boeck instigated the study. By limiting the original group of 1978 patients to the 1404 who were Norwegian residents of Oslo, some follow-up information was obtained from 1949 to 1951 on over 80 percent of the study group, a remarkable figure considering the number of years which had passed. Of the original group, 259 were still alive and 83 percent of these were examined intensively in hospital. Only one-sixth had received any therapy (and of these, almost all received it late in the course), usually too little to be of any clinical importance. Several important findings emerged and are discussed below.

### Frequency of secondary relapse

Prior to 1950, it was often stated that relapse of secondary syphilitis frequently was the result of inadequate therapy, which by interfering with the host immune response actually made it more likely that a patient would suffer later complications. Gjestland's observation that 23.6 percent of untreated patients suffered at least one secondary relapse clearly showed that waxing and waning was a normal part of the course of untreated syphilis. About one-quarter of patients with a relapse had more than one relapse. About 90 percent of secondary relapses occurred in the first year, and 94 percent within the first 2 years, but some occurred over 4 years later. Relapses affected the mouth, throat, or anogenital areas in 85 percent of patients, who were thus likely to be infectious during a relapse of secondary syphilis.

### Benign late syphilis (gumma)

This was the most frequent late (tertiary) manifestation, affecting 14.4 percent of males and 16.7 percent of females. The most frequently involved organs were skin (70 percent), bone (9.6 percent), and mucosa (10.3 percent). Only 10 percent of patients had gummas of more than a single type of tissue (e.g., bone and skin). Similar to secondary syphilis, gummas remitted only to recur later in the same or another site in about one-fourth of males and one-third of females, with up to seven discrete episodes. Gummas occurred anywhere from 1 to 46 years after onset of infection, usually within the first 15 years.

### Cardiovascular syphilis

No patients infected before age 15 developed late cardiovascular syphilis. Overall, 13.6 percent of males and 7.6 percent of females developed cardiovascular complications, usually within 30 to 40 years of onset. If persons under 15 were excluded, 14.9 percent of males and 8.0 percent of females developed cardiovascular syphilis (Table 19-1). These figures, although frequently quoted in reviews of the Oslo study, are almost certainly an underestimate, since only a minority of the Oslo patients were autopsied, and the prevalence of cardiovascular syphilis was much higher in the autopsied group (Table 19-2). Since the clinical diagnosis of gumma was more obvious than that of other late forms of syphilis, it is possible that the incidence of gummas actually was not greater than that of cardiovascular or neurological syphilis.

### Neurosyphilis

Late syphilis of the nervous system developed in 9.4 percent of males and 5.0 percent of females. Curiously, although neurosyphilis did develop in persons infected before age 15, it did so rarely in persons infected after age 40 (zero of 28 males, 2 of 45 females). Onset from time of infection varied depending on the

**Table 19-1. Prevalence of Cardiovascular Syphilis among Persons Acquiring Syphilis after Age 15 in the Oslo Study of Untreated Syphilis**

| | Males, % (N = 303) | Females, % (N = 584) |
|---|---|---|
| Aortic insufficiency | 7.3 | 3.3 |
| Aortic aneurysm | 3.6 | 1.5 |
| Uncomplicated aortitis | 2.6 | 2.9 |
| Coronary stenosis | 0.7 | 0.3 |
| Aortitis (found at death) | 0.7 | 0.0 |
| Total | 14.9 | 8.0 |

SOURCE: Gjestland.[26]

**Table 19-2. Cardiovascular Syphilis in the Oslo Study of Untreated Syphilis: Comparison of Known Study Group with Autopsied Patients**

| | Percent in known study group | Percent in autopsied group |
|---|---|---|
| Uncomplicated aortitis | | |
| Male | 2.6 | 9.3 |
| Females | 2.9 | 11.2 |
| Complicated aortitis (aortic insufficiency, aneurysms, coronary stenosis) | | |
| Males | 12.2 | 25.3 |
| Females | 5.1 | 10.4 |

SOURCE: Gjestland.[26]

type of neurosyphilis; meningovascular disease typically occurred in the first 15 to 18 years of infection, whereas paresis occurred after 20 to 25 years and tabes after about 30 years. The frequency distribution of different types of neurosyphilis is shown in Table 19-3. Although recognized neurosyphilis was somewhat less common than either gumma or cardiovascular syphilis, it may have been the most important clinically by virtue of its occurrence at an earlier age than cardiovascular disease and its significant morbidity and mortality.

### Other observations

The probability of dying directly as a result of untreated syphilis in the Oslo study was 17.1 percent in males and 8 percent in females after 40 years of infection. Syphilis was the second leading cause of death in males and fifth leading cause in females (tuberculosis was first in each group). Life expectancy seemed to be reduced to an extent greater than could be attributed to the recognized specific late manifestations. Among patients with benign late syphilis, 21 percent developed cardiovascular, neurological, or other more severe forms of late syphilis, as compared to 16 percent of patients who did not develop benign late syphilis; there was no evidence to confirm the previous clinical impression that development of benign late syphilis protected from other serious complications. Men fared less well than women, particularly regarding cardiovascular and neurosyphilis, where they ran a 2:1 risk compared to females of developing such complications. Overall, only 28 percent of patients developed recognized late complications; 72 percent survived to old age with no obvious ill effects. If autopsies had been performed more often, more mild forms of late syphilis surely would have been discovered, so the often-quoted figure of 72 percent surviving without late complications certainly is too generous.

**Table 19-3. Prevalence of Recognized Neurosyphilis in the Oslo Study of Untreated Syphilis**

| | Frequency, % | |
|---|---|---|
| Type | Males (N = 331) | Females (N = 622) |
| Diffuse meningovascular | 3.6 | 1.7 |
| General paresis | 3.0 | 1.7 |
| Tabes dorsalis | 2.5 | 1.4 |
| Gumma of brain | 0.3 | 0.2 |
| Total | 9.4 | 5.0 |

SOURCE: Gjestland.[26]

Despite flaws, particularly some uncertainty about the initial diagnosis in the absence of dark field examination or serological tests for syphilis, nonrandomized selection of patients, absence of a suitably selected control group, insufficient autopsies (24 percent), and irregular performance of lumbar punctures, the Oslo study is highly valuable because of the large sample size, nearly total absence of treatment, excellent long-term follow-up, and entry of a reasonably homogeneous group of patients each of whom was in the early stages of infectious syphilis.

## THE TUSKEGEE STUDY

In 1932, a second study of the natural history of ostensibly untreated syphilis was undertaken by the U.S. Public Health Service in Macon County, Alabama, home of the Tuskegee Institute. This study, generally known as the Tuskegee study, has been harshly criticized in recent years on ethical grounds[28,29] because written informed consent was never obtained from the involved patients. Some have suggested that the patients were duped into participating by giving them the impression that they were receiving treatment, when in fact considerable effort was made to prevent adequate treatment with either arsenicals or, when they later became available, penicillin and other antibiotics.[29] Because the study was limited to black males, some have chosen to view the study as essentially racist.[28,29]

It is not the purpose of this writer to undertake a thorough review of the ethics of the study, nor to try to defend it except to say that there is no evidence that there was conscious malintent on the part of those who organized and carried out the study. The rationale for the study apparently was the concept that the considerable toxicity of arsenicals, the principal antisyphilitic available at the time, might be worse than the disease, since the early results of the Oslo study[27] indicated that the majority of untreated syphilitics suffered no late effects of the disease. There was concern that the Oslo study was flawed by lack of proper controls, and by insufficient rate of autopsies. There also was a question in the minds of many clinicians of the time about differences in the natural history of syphilis in different racial groups (reviewed in Ref. 29).

In 1932 a serological survey of men of Macon County, Alabama, revealed that about one-fourth had a positive test for syphilis. Those with infectious lesions of early syphilis were treated with arsenicals. A total of 412 other men who had a history of previous lesions of early syphilis but who no longer were considered infectious were enrolled in the study. Many of those received a short, subcurative course of arsenical therapy.[30] A matched group of 204 seronegative controls also was selected. The composition of these groups changed slightly with time; when some controls were later found to have acquired syphilis, they were switched to the syphilis group. All patients and controls received an entry physical exam, lumbar puncture, and chest films. An attempt was made to reexamine these men at periodic intervals, and to obtain as many autopsies as possible. Results of follow-up were excellent, since after 20 years only about 10 percent of patients were totally lost, and approximately two-thirds of patients who died had been autopsied.[30]

Results were published at intervals by different teams who conducted the periodic reviews.[30–33] Unfortunately, a comprehensive report never has been published. The principal finding was an increased mortality rate in the syphilitic group, estimated to be 20 percent loss of life expectancy at the 12-year follow-up[33] and 17 percent at the 20-year follow-up.[31] Most of the excess mortality occurred in the first 20 years; little additional increment was noted in a report after 30 years.[32] As in the Oslo study, not all mortality could be directly attributed to specific lesions of late syphilis. Other significant differences between syphilitics and controls after 20 years included a higher frequency in the syphilitics of significant cardiac complaints and cardiac enlargement, a higher frequency of "arteriosclerosis," and a higher frequency of hypertension. After 30 years, remaining survivors had similar frequencies of hypertension, but a higher proportion of syphilitics had an abnormal electrocardiogram.[32]

Specific lesions of late syphilis were found in about 14 percent of syphilitics at the 20-year follow-up[31] and in 12 percent of examined syphilitic survivors at the thirtieth year of the study.[32] The findings are summarized in Table 19-4. Cardiovascular syphilis was the most frequent finding; there was a roughly similar frequency of benign late syphilis (usually of bone) and of neurosyphilis.

By the twentieth year of the study, about two-thirds of the syphilitic patients had received some therapy, but only 7 percent had received curative doses of penicillin.[30] Partial treatment had no obvious effect on development of late syphilis,[31] but was associated with increased frequency of seroreversal (reversion to a negative test for anticardiolipin antibodies). After 20 years of follow-up, cardiovascular or neurosyphilis was considered the primary cause of death in 30 percent of the infected men.[31]

The Tuskegee study did add to our knowledge of the course of the illness, but the findings were not dramatic and most were not unexpected. The increased frequency of hypertension and of deaths not due to specific lesions of late syphilis appear the most noteworthy findings. The study did not prove whether syphilis had a different course in whites and blacks, but comparisons to other studies suggest that there are few differences which can be attributed to race.

## THE ROSAHN STUDY

A third large study of the natural course of syphilis was conducted by Paul Rosahn, the results of which are available in a comprehensive monograph.[1] Unlike the Oslo or Tuskegee studies, this study was based entirely on a review of autopsy materials. Any study based on dead patients obviously has actual or potential bias toward poor outcomes, but the study nevertheless is of great value. A cross-sectional review was made of all autopsies conducted at Yale University School of Medicine from 1917 to 1941; among almost 4000 persons over age 20 at death, 9.7 percent had clinical, laboratory, or autopsy evidence of syphilis. (The hospital population was weighted toward lower socioeconomic groups, over 90 percent of whom were white.) About one-half of patients had received no therapy.

Overall, 51 percent of syphilitic patients had anatomic lesions attributable to syphilis at autopsy. Among untreated patients only, 39 percent had lesions attributable to syphilis. Among clinically diagnosed patients (diagnosis made during life), about 30 percent developed late anatomic lesions of syphilis (very similar to the Oslo study), and about 20 percent died because of syphilis. Most lesions were cardiovascular. Among 77 patients with untreated syphilis with late anatomic lesions at autopsy, 83 percent of lesions were cardiovascular, 7.6 percent were neurological, and 8.5 percent were gummas. Many patients had multiple lesions.

Patients with positive serological tests were more likely to have anatomic lesions and to have died because of them, than those with negative serological tests, suggested that persistence of positive VDRL-type tests was associated with disease activity. About one-fourth of patients with late lesions at autopsy had negative anticardiolipin serological tests before death, confirming once again the frequency of negative VDRL-type tests among patients with tertiary syphilis.

Syphilis was associated with reduced likelihood of living past 70 years of age. Part of the excess mortality may not have been due to morphologically recognized late complications.

In summary, the Rosahn study was similar in many respects to the other large studies (Oslo, Tuskegee). Each study demonstrated increased mortality due to syphilis, and indicated that 15 to 40 percent of untreated patients develop recognizable late (tertiary) complications. The Tuskegee and Rosahn studies, which had the highest autopsy rates, showed the highest frequencies of cardiovascular syphilis. At least 60 percent of untreated patients did not develop late recognizable anatomic complications, and about 80 percent did not die primarily because of syphilis.

## STUDIES IN THE ANTIBIOTIC ERA

No comprehensive study analogous to the studies cited above has been carried out in the past 30 years. There is clear evidence that penicillin treatment of acquired early syphilis almost always prevents late complications of the disease. There has been debate

**Table 19-4. Tertiary Syphilis in the Tuskegee Study**

| | Syphilitic study group | |
|---|---|---|
| Type | 20-Year follow-up[31] (N = 159) | 30-Year follow-up[32] (N = 90) |
| Benign late syphilis | 6 (4%) | 1 (1%) |
| Cardiovascular syphilis | 10 (6%) | 7* (8%) |
| Aneurysm | 3 | |
| Aortic insufficiency | 5 | |
| Aneurysm and aortic insufficiency | 2 | |
| Neurological syphilis | 7 (4%) | 3* (3%) |
| Paresis | 1 | |
| Tabes | 1 | |
| Optic atrophy | 2 | |
| Tabes and optic atrophy | 2 | |
| Tabes, optic atrophy, aneurysm | 1 | |
| Total | 23 (14%) | 11 (12%) |

*Specific types of illness not reported.

about the apparent persistence of *T. pallidum* in humans[34] and animals[35] after penicillin therapy, but there is little convincing evidence as to the importance of these observations.[15] Late manifest neurosyphilis may be an exception; high-dose intravenous penicillin is probably indicated in an attempt to assuredly kill *T. pallidum* in the central nervous system of these patients (see Chap. 21).

Statistical studies published by the U.S. Public Health Service[36] strongly suggest that intentional or unintentional antibiotic therapy of early syphilis is preventing some proportion of late syphilis. There was a sharp decline in rates of reported early syphilis in the 1950s, followed by a threefold rise in the 1960s, which rates have been maintained roughly to the present. In contrast, there was only a minor secondary rise in reported early latent syphilis in the 1960s and 1970s, and a steady, continuous decline in late (tertiary) and late latent syphilis rates in the same interval (Table 19-5). Antibiotics apparently are aborting some of the recognized late complications of syphilis.

Gumma seems to have disappeared from the contemporary scene, since few young or middle-aged clinicians have seen a proved case. There is also a suggestion that tabes dorsalis has become quite rare.[37] However, a survey of hospital records of patients with positive serologies in Denmark from the years 1961 to 1970 disclosed about equal numbers of patients with previously undiagnosed tabes, paresis, aortic insufficiency, and aortic aneurysm.[38] A variety of anecdotal experiences,[39] including the author's unpublished clinical observations indicate that all of the classic forms of late syphilis of the central nervous system continue to turn up intermittently in large tertiary care hospitals, although diagnostic confusion is not at all uncommon in such patients. Variant forms of neurosyphilis which are difficult to classify do occur,[39] but they also occurred in the preantibiotic era (see Chap. 21). Suggestions of the relatively common occurrence of subtle or highly atypical forms of neurosyphilis presenting primarily with seizures and/or peripheral neuropathies or pupillary abnormalities[40] are difficult to evaluate, since a study which makes this claim is based to a considerable degree on positive fluorescent treponemal antibody-absorption (FTA-ABS) tests on cerebrospinal fluid. This test is not standardized for this purpose, and its clinical meaning is suspect.

There have been few recent studies to evaluate the prevalence of newly diagnosed cardiovascular syphilis. An interesting paper published in 1970 by Prewitt[41] analyzed syphilitic patients seen at the Memphis-Shelby County (Tennessee) Venereal Disease Clinic for signs of aortic insufficiency. All were over 35 years old and had a history of treatment for syphilis and/or a reactive FTA-ABS test. Of 317 patients examined, 26 (8 percent) had the murmur of aortic insufficiency, including 14 of 97 (14 percent) apparently untreated patients. Among the untreated patients, 9 of 27 (33 percent) over age 70 but only 5 of 70 (7 percent) less than age 70 had aortic regurgitation. The murmur was faint in about one-half of patients, and about 80 percent had little or no functional disability. The implication was that syphilitic aortic insufficiency may be much more common today than usually appreciated, at least in sexually transmitted disease clinics. One wonders whether the apparent long delay in onset of signs and symptoms, and the relatively mild form of the disease was due to partial or complete but inadvertent antibiotic therapy.

**Table 19-5. Reported Rates of Syphilis in the United States of America, 1947–1977 (Representative Years)**

| | Case rates per 100,000 | | |
|---|---|---|---|
| Year | Primary, secondary | Early latent | Late, late latent |
| 1947 | 66.4 | 73.9 | 86.6 |
| 1952 | 6.9 | 24.0 | 69.1 |
| 1957 | 3.9 | 10.6 | 54.2 |
| 1962 | 11.5 | 10.7 | 43.3 |
| 1967 | 10.8 | 8.0 | 31.7 |
| 1972 | 11.8 | 10.1 | 21.0 |
| 1977 | 9.5 | 9.9 | 10.4 |

SOURCE: Centers for Disease Control.[36]

## CONCLUSION

Syphilis is still common, particularly in certain sectors of the population. Late complications may be relatively less of a problem than in the preantibiotic era, but alertness to the possibility of late syphilis and awareness of the pleiotropic clinical manifestations of late syphilis are crucial if these forms of the disease are to be diagnosed and treated properly. The principal concern must be vigilance in finding, treating, and preventing early syphilis. Because all forms of syphilis, particularly certain types of late syphilis, are less common than in the glory days of syphilis as a clinical specialty, it is important to teach others and to remind ourselves of the multiple faces of the great actor, *lues venerea*. These are covered in considerable detail in Chaps. 20 to 23 and 67.

Since syphilis is an independent risk factor for seropositivity to HIV,[42] and since early syphilis may be atypical and quite severe in HIV-infected persons (author's unpublished observations), vigilance in diagnosis, therapy, and prevention of syphilis is now more important than ever.

# References


1 Rosahn PD: Autopsy studies in syphilis. *Journal of Venereal Disease Information,* supplement no 21, U.S. Public Health Service, Venereal Disease Division, 1947.

2 Symmers D: Anatomic lesions in late acquired syphilis: A study of 314 cases based on the analysis of 4,880 necropsies at Bellevue Hospital. *JAMA* 66:1457, 1916.

3 Olansky S et al: Untreated syphilis in the male Negro: Environmental factors in the Tuskegee study. *Public Health Rep* 69:691, 1954.

4 Hudson ER: Treponematoses and African slavery. *Br J Vener Dis* 40: 43, 1963.

5 Hollander DH: Treponematosis from pinta to venereal syphilis revisited: Hypothesis for temperature determination of disease patterns. *Sex Transm Dis* 8:34, 1981.

6 Fieldsteel AH: Genetics of *Treponema,* in *Pathogenesis and Immunology of Treponemal Infection,* RF Schell, DF Musher (eds). New York, Marcel Dekker, 1983, p 39.

7 Schell RF et al: Acquired resistance of hamsters to challenge with homologous and heterologous virulent treponemes. *Infect Immun* 37:617, 1982.

8 Turner TB, Hollander DH: Biology of the treponematoses. *WHO Monograph Ser* 35:1, 1957.

9 Walfield AM et al: Expression of *Treponema pallidum* antigens in *Escherichia coli. Science* 216:522, 1982.

10 Stamm LV et al: Expression of *Treponema pallidum* antigens in *Escherichia coli* K-12. *Infect Immun* 36:1238, 1982.

11 Robertson SM et al: Murine monoclonal antibodies specific for virulent *Treponema pallidum* (Nichols). *Infect Immun* 36:1076, 1982.

12 Schaudinn FR, Hoffmann E: Vorläufiger Bericht über das Vorkommen von Spirochaeten in syphilitischen Krakheitsproducten und bei Papillomen. *Arbeiten aus dem K Gesundheitsamte* 22:527, 1905.
13 Schroeter AL et al: Therapy for incubating syphilis: Effectiveness of gonorrhea treatment. *JAMA* 218:711, 1971.
14 Magnuson HJ et al: Inoculation syphilis in human volunteers. *Medicine* 35:33, 1956.
15 Turner TB et al: Infectivity tests in syphilis. *Br J Vener Dis* 45:183, 1969.
16 Harter CA, Benirschke K: Fetal syphilis in the first trimester. *Am J Obstet Gynecol* 124:705, 1976.
17 Fehér J et al: Early syphilitic hepatitis. *Lancet* 2:896, 1975.
18 Gamble CN, Reardan JB: Immunopathogenesis of syphilitic glomerulonephritis: Elution of antitreponemal antibody from glomerular immune-complex deposits. *N Engl J Med* 292:449, 1975.
19 Levene GM et al: Reduced lymphocyte transformation due to a plasma factor in patients with active syphilis. *Lancet* 2:246, 1969.
20 Pavia CS et al: Selective in vitro response of thymus-derived lymphocytes from *Treponema pallidum*-infected rabbits. *Infect Immun* 18:603, 1977.
21 Baker-Zander SA et al: Serum regulation of in vitro lymphocyte responses in early experimental syphilis. *Infect Immun* 37:568, 1982.
22 Chesney AM: Immunity in syphilis. *Medicine* 5:463, 1926.
23 Wicher K, Wicher V: Immunopathology of syphilis, in *Pathogenesis and Immunology of Treponemal Infection,* RF Schell, DF Musher (eds). New York, Marcel Dekker, 1983, p 161.
24 Baughn RE: Immunoregulatory effects in experimental syphilis, in *Pathogenesis and Immunology of Treponemal Infection,* RF Schell, DF Musher (eds). New York, Marcel Dekker, 1983, p 271.
25 Folds JD: Cell mediated immunity, in *Pathogenesis and Immunology of Treponemal Infection,* RF Schell, DF Musher (eds). New York, Marcel Dekker, 1983, p 315.
26 Gjestland T: The Oslo study of untreated syphilis: An epidemiologic investigation of the natural course of syphilitic infection based on a restudy of the Boeck-Bruusgaard material. *Acta Derm Venereol* 35 ([*Suppl*] (*Stockh*) 34):1, 1955.
27 Bruusgaard E: Über das schicksal der nicht specifisch behandelten leuktiker. *Arch Dermatol Syph* (*Berlin*) 157:309, 1929.
28 Brandt AM: Racism and research: The case of the Tuskegee syphilis study. *Hastings Cent Rep* December 1978, p 21.
29 Jones JH: *Bad Blood.* New York, Free Press, 1981.
30 Schuman SH et al: Untreated syphilis in the male Negro: Background and current status of patients in the Tuskegee study. *J Chronic Dis* 2:543, 1955.
31 Olansky S et al: Untreated syphilis in the male Negro. X: Twenty years of clinical observation of untreated syphilitic and presumably nonsyphilitic groups. *J Chronic Dis* 4:177, 1956.
32 Rockwell DH et al: The Tuskegee study of untreated syphilis. *Arch Intern Med* 114:792, 1964.
33 Heller JR Jr, Bruyere PT: Untreated syphilis in the male Negro. II: Mortality during 12 years of observation. *J Vener Dis Inform* 27:34, 1946.
34 Yobs AR et al: Do treponemes survive adequate treatment of late syphilis? *Arch Dermatol* 91:379, 1965.
35 Yobs AR et al: Further observations on the persistence of *Treponema pallidum* after treatment in rabbits and humans. *Br J Vener Dis* 44: 116, 1968.
36 Centers for Disease Control: *Sexually Transmitted Disease Fact Sheet,* ed 34. US Department of Health, Education, and Welfare Publication 79-8195.
37 Kampmeier RH: Whatever has happened to locomotor ataxyl!, editorial. *J Am Vener Dis Assoc* 3:51, 1976.
38 Fischer A et al: Tertiary syphilis in Denmark 1961–1970: A description of 105 cases not previously diagnosed or specifically treated. *Acta Derm Venerol* (*Stockh*) 56:485, 1976.
39 Luxon L et al: Neurosyphilis today. *Lancet* 1:90, 1979.
40 Hooshmand H et al: Neurosyphilis: A study of 241 patients. *JAMA* 219:726, 1972.
41 Prewitt TA: Syphilitic aortic insufficiency: Its increased incidence in the elderly. *JAMA* 211:637, 1970.
42 Rabkin CS et al: Prevalence of antibody to HTLV-III/LAV in a population attending a sexually transmitted disease clinic. *Sex Transm Dis* 14:48, 1987.

# Chapter 20
# Early syphilis in the adult

R. N. Thin

## DEFINITIONS

Venereal syphilis was defined by Stokes[1] as an "infectious disease due to *Treponema pallidum*, of great chronicity, systemic from the outset, capable of involving practically every structure of the body in its course, distinguished by florid manifestations on the one hand and years of complete asymptomatic latency on the other, able to simulate many diseases in the fields of medicine and surgery, transmissible to offspring in man, transmissible to certain laboratory animals, and treatable to the point of presumptive cure." All this remains true. The sexually transmitted form is acquired syphilis, while infection in utero produces congenital syphilis.

Both congenital and acquired syphilis are divided into early and late stages. Early acquired syphilis is further subdivided into an incubation period, primary, secondary, and early latent stages. The division between early and late latent disease is taken as 1 year by the U.S. Public Health Service based on the higher rate of relapse of secondary syphilis in the Oslo study (see below) during the first year of the disease. In Britain the dividing line is usually taken as 2 years[2] based on infectivity. The early stage may be extended to 4 years or longer, for occasionally a mother has given birth to a congenital syphilitic infant more than 2 years after becoming infected.

## HISTORY

There are two hypotheses concerning the origin of syphilis. One, the unitarian theory, suggests that it first appeared in the tropics transmitted by casual contact, like yaws and endemic syphilis. When the disease spread to temperate climates where more clothing was worn, sexual intercourse provided the only opportunity for contact, so the disease became the sexually transmitted infection we now know.[3] The other, or Columbian theory, suggested that the disease arose in American Indians and was brought to Europe with the return of Columbus in 1493 from his discovery of America. Members of his crews subsequently took part in the siege of Naples by Charles VIII of France. Warfare in the fifteenth century allowed spread of sexually transmitted disease among soldiers and camp followers of both sides. At that time the disease became known as the "French disease" among Italians and the "Italian disease" among the French. The disease received its name from a poem written in 1530 by Fracastoro about an infected shepherd named Syphilis.

Though the late manifestations were well recognized by authors and artists in the Middle Ages in Europe, the long incubation period and prolonged course delayed recognition of the natural history of syphilis. By the eighteenth century syphilis and gonorrhea were understood to be sexually transmitted. The most important contributions to our understanding of syphilis were made from 1891 onward. In Oslo that year, Professor Boeck, who believed that therapy was ineffective and perhaps more toxic than the disease, set up a prospective study. Patients with early syphilis were entered over the ensuing 20 years; they were not treated but were followed until 1951.[4] Originally 1978 patients entered the study, but the main findings concerned 1404 Oslo residents and follow-up information was obtained on 80 percent—a remarkable achievement. Although the study can be criticized on various grounds such as the absence of dark field microscopy and selection of cases, it provides a fascinating account of the natural history of syphilis and gives the best information on this subject. Though most interest centers on late disease it does provide important information on secondary syphilis. For example, relapse in secondary syphilis occurred in 25 percent of cases affecting the mouth, throat, and anogenital region. Clinical relapse could be repeated but did not have any undue prognostic implication. The only other study which resembles the Oslo study is the Tuskegee study, which started in 1932 at Macon County, Alabama. This study was limited to black males who again did not receive curative therapy and who were followed for 30 years.[5] The study included a group of seronegative controls. No comprehensive report was published and findings largely confirmed existing understanding. Natural history is discussed in greater detail in Chap. 19.

The important laboratory advances started in 1905 when Schaudinn and Hoffman of Hamburg discovered the causative organism, which they originally called *Spirochaeta pallidum* but later changed to *Treponema pallidum*. The following year in Berlin, Wassermann described the serological reaction which still bears his name. In 1909, Erlich of Frankfurt produced an organic arsenical, 606 or Salvarsan, which had a therapeutic effect when given intravenously and led to the development of other more effective arsenicals. The most important advance in therapy came in 1943 when penicillin (which had been discovered by Fleming and developed by Florey in Oxford), was successfully used by Mahoney and his colleagues to treat syphilis. Moore[6] summarized the various trials of different penicillin regimens that were studied and set the foundation for modern therapy.

Although the early discoveries came from Europe, further advances were concentrated in the United States. Many flocculation tests for circulating antibodies were described, but they all had drawbacks. In 1946, Harris et al.[7] described the Harris or Venereal Disease Research Laboratory (VDRL) slide test, a flocculation reaction which has proved reliable, easy, cheap, and reproducible worldwide. This procedure has since been modified and simplified to give the Rapid Plasma Reagin (RPR) test and the Automated Reagin Test (ART). These techniques all detect nonspecific lipoidal antibodies, and nonspecific reactions occur. In 1949, Nelson and Mayer[8] described the first specific test, the *Treponema pallidum* immobilization (TPI) test. Since then the more widely used fluorescent treponemal antibody absorbed (FTA-ABS), the *Treponema pallidum* hemagglutination (TPHA), and the microhemagglutination (MHA-TP) tests have come into more general use. Though an enzyme-linked immunoassay (ELISA) was described in 1975,[9] this technique has not yet been widely adopted. Serological tests are discussed in detail in Chaps. 75 and 76.

## EPIDEMIOLOGY

Syphilis is a worldwide disease, and like all sexually transmitted diseases multiple factors affect its spread. There is evidence of a general decline in incidence in Western countries since 1860.[6] It is difficult in many countries to obtain comprehensive data. Britain has a national recording system which has various limitations but gives reasonably accurate trends. The overall figures for syphilis in Britain are shown in Fig. 20-1. The rise in the incidence of syphilis in World War II was mirrored in other countries including the United States. The smaller rise between 1971 and 1980 was due to primary and secondary syphilis in homosexual men, who contributed 45.9 percent of the total in 1971 and 58.0 percent in 1977.[10,11] In both studies homosexually acquired infections were concentrated in the West End of London, but in the second study increases were noted throughout England. The fall in recent years in the incidence of syphilis in men is attributed to the reduction in early disease in homosexuals, especially in London.[12] Age-related data show early syphilis to be concentrated in young adults with many more cases in males than in females.

In the United States, following the increase in World War II there was an abrupt fall in the incidence of syphilis like that seen in Britain. This was followed by a gradual decline, but from 1978 to 1982 there was an increase in primary and secondary syphilis. The incidence of these two forms fell after 1982. This is probably due to a decline in early syphilis among urban homosexuals related to reduced partner changing which, as in Britain, reflects the fear of HIV infection. In contrast there are also reports of local increases of early infectious syphilis in heterosexuals.[13]

It is difficult to obtain accurate data from other countries, but a few pointers are available. The situation in Amsterdam appears similar to that in London, with a decline in syphilis related to a change in behavior by homosexual men.[14] In contrast Singapore experienced an increase of early infectious syphilis from 1980 to 1984.[15] Among the factors suggested were prostitution, reduced prescription of procaine penicillin for gonorrhea because of penicillinase-producing strains of *Neisseria gonorrhoeae* (PPNG), loss of herd immunity following elimination of nonvenereal treponemal disease, and mobility of the at-risk population. Homosexual spread among men did not appear to be an important factor.

Sexually transmitted diseases are more prevalent in large cities than in small towns. Recent studies have shown clustering of cases within towns, and one study shows this applies to syphilis in Seville, indicating enhanced opportunity for spread.[16]

## PATHOGENESIS

*T. pallidum* probably requires a break in squamous or columnar epithelum to enter the body—macroscopic and microscopic trauma readily occurs during sexual contact. Some organisms lodge at the site of entry; others escape via the lymphatic system to the regional lymph nodes and disseminate throughout the body. Wherever they lodge they may proliferate and stimulate an immune response.

Small inocula of treponemas can lead to infection, and sexual exposure to a person with active mucocutaneous syphilis carries a risk of acquiring syphilis of up to 60 percent. A placebo controlled study of efficacy of antibiotics in aborting syphilis in contacts suggested 30 percent infectivity.[17] Studies of infection in pairs of partners in the United States and Britain before and after the introduction of penicillin indicated infection in 48 to 62 percent of secondary contacts.[18–21]

In general the incubation period has a mean of 21 days with extremes of 10 to 90 days.[2,22,23] Experimentally, large inocula are associated with short incubation periods and small inocula with longer periods, but reasons for incubation periods over 5 weeks are unclear.

The immunobiology and pathogenesis of syphilis in humans and the immune response still pose many problems (discussed in Chap. 18). Untreated disease runs a roughly predictable but variable course; reasons for the clinical variability are obscure. For example, though neurosyphilis usually takes about 10 years to develop it has long been known that clinical neurosyphilis may appear in the secondary stage.[1] In part, clinical variation in expression of disease reflects difference in the immune status of the host.

The most important condition affecting the immune system currently seen in the age group hitherto most at risk for acquired early syphilis is human immunodefiency virus (HIV) infection. HIV infection impairs the helper/inducer T lymphocytes which carry the glycoprotein molecule CD4 on their surface. This molecule acts as a receptor for HIV. CD4 receptors are also present on some monocytes and macrophages. CD4 T lymphocytes become steadily depleted during the course of the disease, impairing

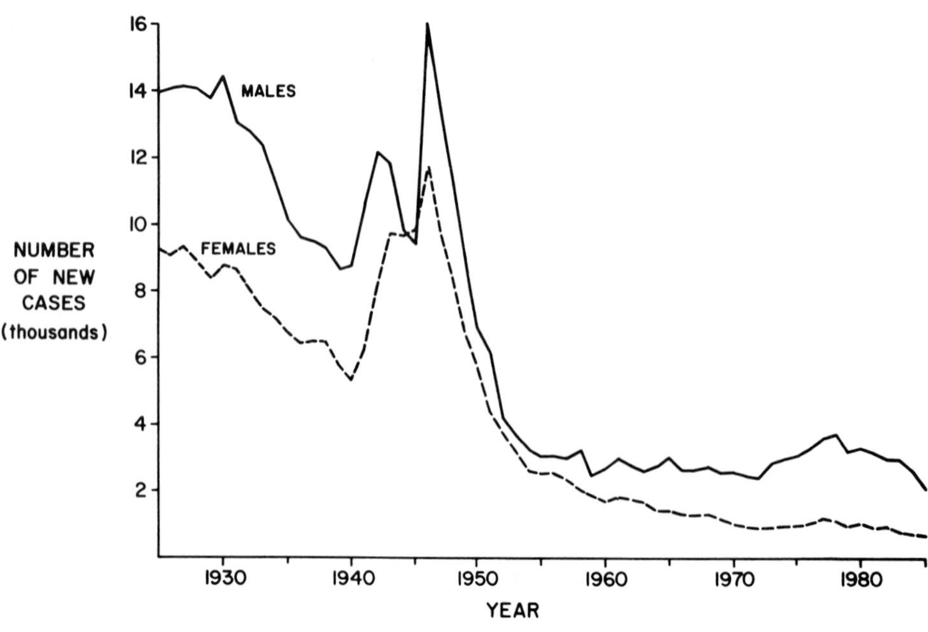


**Fig. 20-1.** Reported incidence of syphilis from specialist clinics in the United Kingdom from 1925 to 1985.

the immune response to infection (Chap. 29). Reports have recently appeared showing that early acquired syphilis, like other infections, may pursue a malignant course in patients with HIV infection.[24–27] Neurosyphilis may develop earlier after the onset of disease, and treatment with benzathine penicillin may be more likely to be followed by neurosyphilis than in immunocompetent patients. One patient with HIV infection and Kaposi sarcoma appeared to have secondary syphilis, diagnosed by biopsy with negative results to VDRL and FTA-ABS tests. The serological tests subsequently converted to positive.[28] It is prudent to screen all patients with HIV infection for syphilis and vice versa. Similar problems may arise occasionally in patients with immune depression due to disease such as T cell leukemia or antineoplastic chemotherapy.[29]

Some immunity to infection develops as indicated by the latent stage, and about 60 percent of infected patients remain in this stage without therapy.[4] Late clinical syphilis may be a response to endogenous or exogenous treponemal antigen.[30] Although immunity to syphilis develops slowly with chronic infection, it may be lost after curative therapy; a 22-year-old female treated for congenital syphilis presented 2 years later with primary acquired syphilis.[31]

## CLINICAL MANIFESTATIONS

### PRIMARY SYPHILIS

The first clinical manifestation is usually a local lesion at the site of entry. This is usually a site of genital trauma, such as the coronal sulcus, glans, frenum, prepuce, and shaft of the penis, and near the anus, in the anal canal or rectum in the homosexual or bisexual male. In the female the lesion is found on the fourchette or elsewhere on the vulva and on the cervix. Unilateral edema may accompany labial lesions, but rectal and cervical lesions may be asymptomatic (see Plates 37–41).

The lesion starts as a dull red macule which rapidly becomes papular and then ulcerates. The classical ulcer, the chancre, is rounded with a well-defined margin, and a rubbery, thickened, indurated base; it is painless and nontender and produces more serum and less blood than ulcers due to other causes (Figs. 20-2 and 20-3). The early chancre has a clear red base, but later this becomes covered with a gray slough.

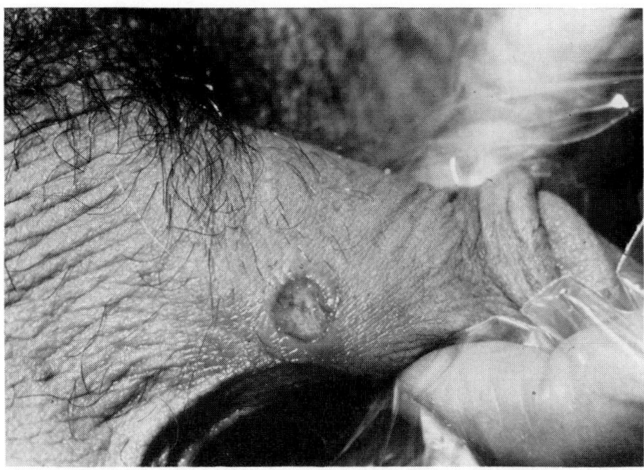

**Fig. 20-2.** Primary chancre of the shaft of the penis; typical clear-based lesion with indurated margin. (*Courtesy of E Stolz.*)

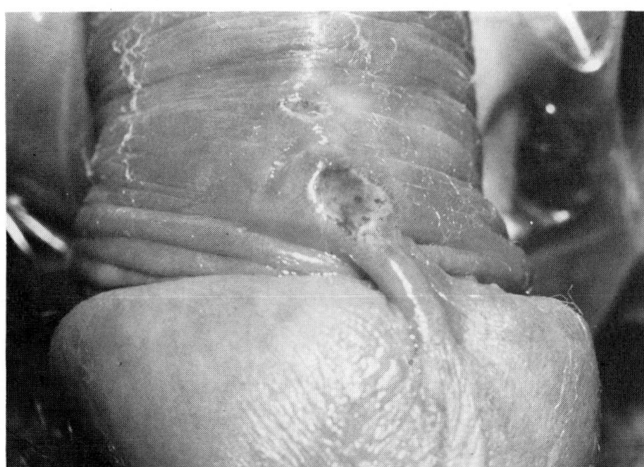

**Fig. 20-3.** Small primary chancre of the penis. (*Courtesy of E Stolz.*)

Classical chancres are becoming less common, at least in the Western parts of the world, and all genital and anorectal ulcers in at-risk persons should be regarded as suspect. Chancres have been reported at other sites including lips (Fig. 20-4), tongue, tonsils, breasts, and fingers. Lesions at extragenital sites may be atypical, and a high index of suspicion is necessary to make this diagnosis.

Untreated, a chancre will persist for 3 to 6 weeks and then heal. Relapse of the primary chancre is rare and is called monorecidive or chancre redux. Another rare phenomenon, a gumma at the site of the original chancre, is called pseudo-chancre redux.

In most cases regional lymphadenopathy develops within a week of the appearance of the chancre. Nodes are painless, nontender, small to moderate in size, rubbery in consistency, and nonsuppurative. With genital and anal chancres nodes are often bilateral, but with chancres elsewhere they are unilateral.

If an ulcer becomes secondarily infected with pyogenic bacteria, it may be painful and tender, and the nodes may develop the same features.

### SECONDARY SYPHILIS

*T. pallidum* disseminates widely throughout the body. Wherever organisms lodge they may multiply, and about 3 to 6 weeks after

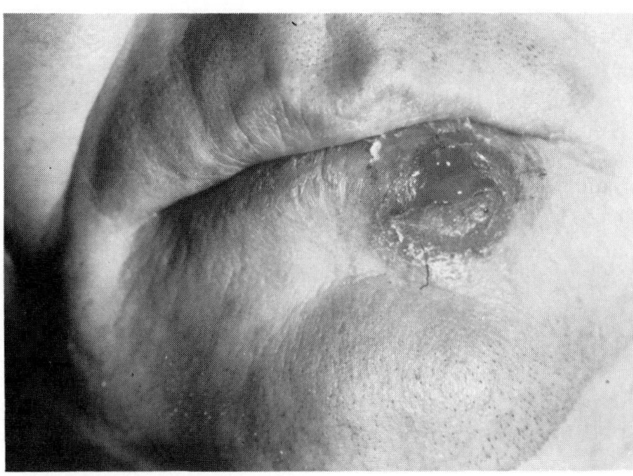

**Fig. 20-4.** Primary syphilitic chancre of the lip. (*Courtesy of E Stolz.*)

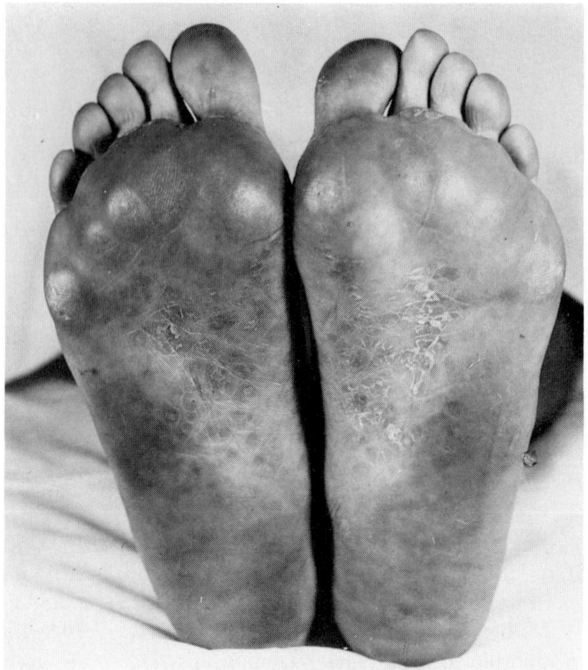

Fig. 20-5. Secondary syphilis: rash on soles of the feet.

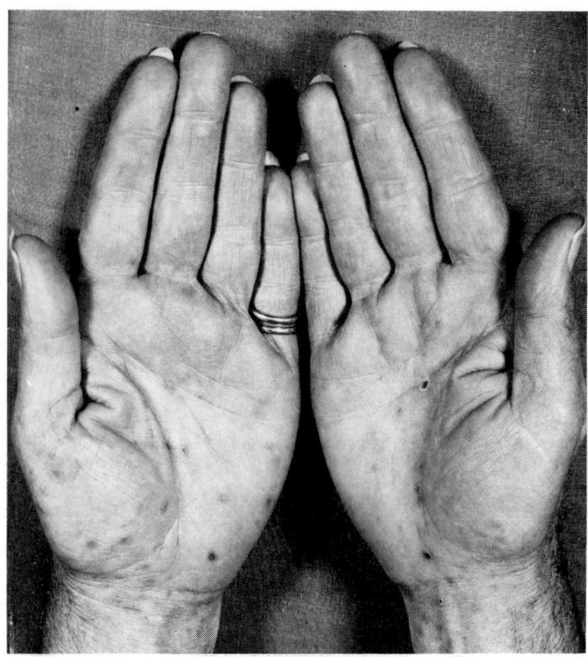

Fig. 20-6. Secondary syphilis: rash on palms.

the appearance of the chancre the symptoms and signs of secondary syphilis appear. It is at this stage that the disease is seen to be systemic. The more common symptoms include sore throat, malaise, headaches, weight loss, variable fever, and musculoskeletal pains.[1,32] The common signs include a rash in 75 to 100 percent, lymphadenopathy in 50 to 86 percent, and mucosal ulceration in 6 to 30 percent.[2,32] The chancre may, rarely, persist into the secondary stage.

The rash starts as a faint macular eruption of rose pink rounded lesions 0.5 to 1.0 cm in diameter on the trunk and flexor surfaces of the upper limbs. It gradually becomes dull red and papular and spreads to involve the whole body, characteristically including the palms and soles, where the papules gradually become squamous (Figs. 20-5 and 20-6; Plates 42–45). Once the papular stage is reached the rash is polymorphic and is usually nonirritant.

Variations of the rash include follicular lesions, annular lesions which are described as more common in blacks than whites, and so-called corymbose lesions with one central papule surrounded by a ring of smaller ones. Papules may be dense on the forehead, where they are described as corona veneris. Papules affecting intertriginous areas may become eroded and fissured when they are called split papules; such lesions are found at the angles of the mouth, nasolabial fold, and behind the ears (Fig. 20-7). In warm, moist areas papules may become large and raised and may resemble viral warts, but they are characteristically broad and flat—so-called condylomata lata. These may develop around the anus, on the scrotum, on the vulva, and in hot, humid climates have been reported in the nasolabial folds, under the chin, behind the ears, in the axillae, and in antecubital folds, between the toes, under the breasts, and in the umbilicus.[32]

Lesions resembling pustules may occur as a result of the impaired blood supply—endarteritis obliterans. The center of the papule necroses and is replaced by scaly dry keratin or squames, giving a pustular appearance. These lesions may also be called rupial but occur in less than 1 percent of cases.[1,32]

Patchy alopecia may be a late manifestation, often being present without other features (Fig. 20-8). Diffuse thinning of the hair on the scalp has also been described as well as on the outer half of the eyebrows, eyelashes, and beard.

With or without treatment all manifestations of secondary syphilis resolve. Pustules may heal with hypo- or hyperpigmentation. One characteristic area of skin where the rash may heal leaving hyperpigmentation is the neck, especially posteriorly. Here patchy depigmentation may be referred to as leukoderma colli or collar of Venus.

The adenopathy of secondary syphilis may be generalized. In addition to inguinal nodes the suboccipital, posterior cervical, axillary, and epitrochlear nodes become involved. Enlargement resembles that seen in primary syphilis, the nodes being only moderately enlarged, rubbery, discrete, and nontender.

Mucosal ulcers, or "mucous patches" as they are called in secondary syphilis, may affect any mucous membrane, the mouth

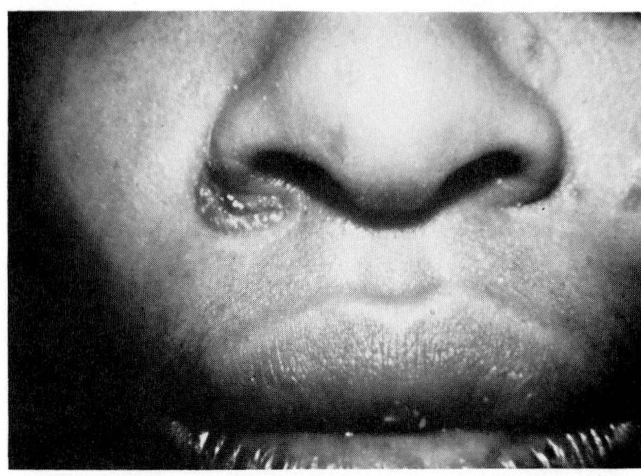

Fig. 20-7. Secondary syphilis: split papule of the nasal fold.

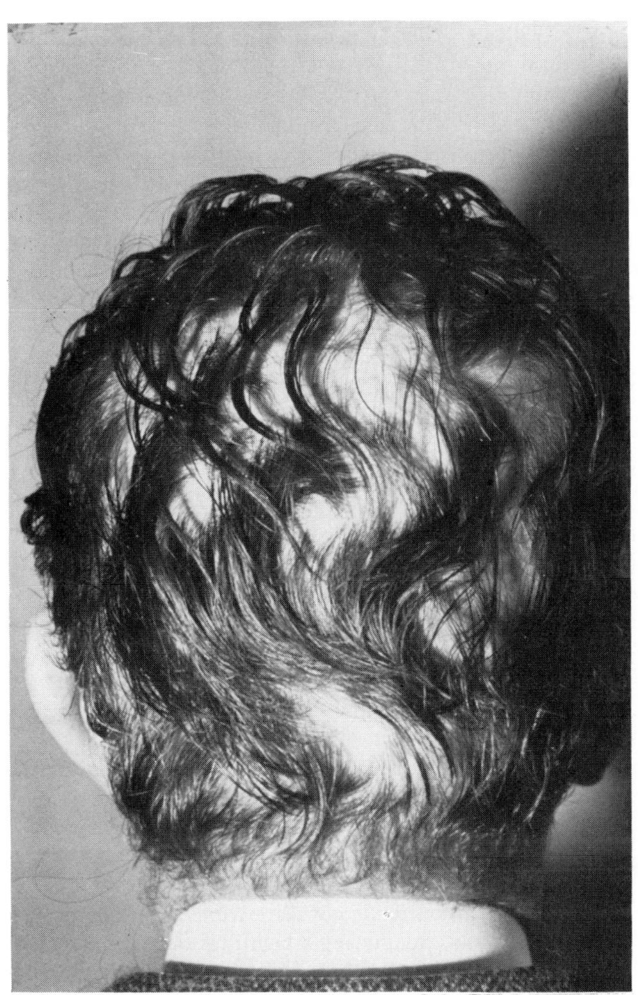

Fig. 20-8. Secondary syphilis: moth-eaten alopecia. (*Courtesy of E Stolz.*)

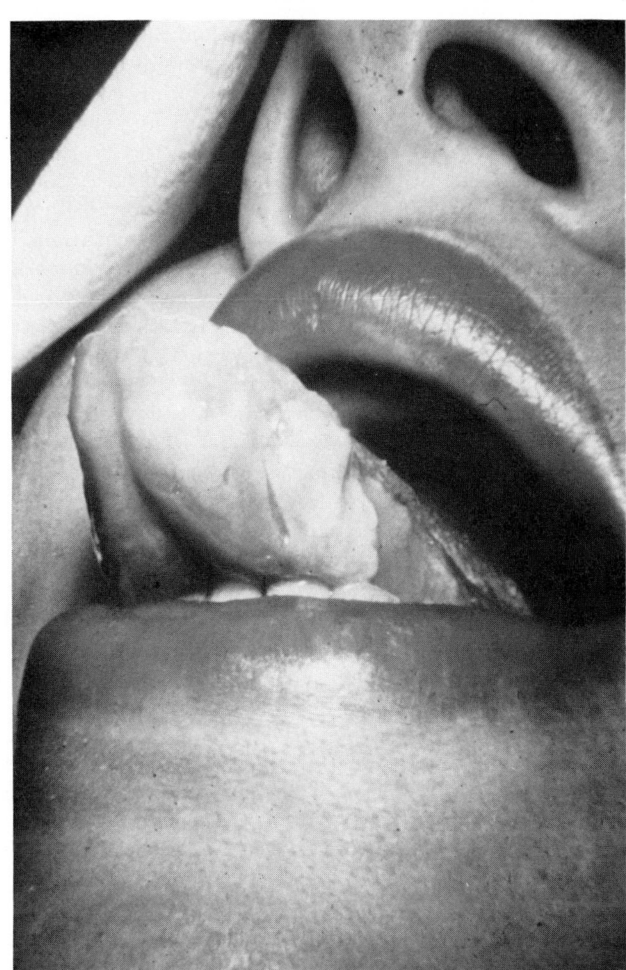

Fig. 20-9. Secondary syphilis: mucous patch of the tongue.

(Fig. 20-9), pharynx, larynx, and genitals being the most commonly affected. The ulcers are described as having a dull red base or a grayish slough. Careful examination will reveal very superficial lesions barely distinguishable from the surrounding epithelium. Involvement of other systems is described as occurring in 10 percent of cases or less.[2] Arthritis, bursitis, and osteitis have all been described. Bone pain is occasionally a prominent symptom, and destructive bone lesions may occur.[32] An enlarged liver may be palpable, and hepatitis is recognized as a feature of secondary syphilis; a disproportionally high alkaline phosphatase concentration used to be regarded as characteristic, but not all reports support this finding.[33–35] The nephrotic syndrome due to syphilitic glomerulonephritis, an immune complex deposit disease, is occasionally seen and more rarely hemorrhagic nephritis.[36–38] These conditions respond to penicillin therapy. Gastric ulceration and gastritis have been reported,[33] and an enlarged spleen may be palpable. Silent anterior iritis may be commoner than is generally recognized, occurring more often in relapse of secondary syphilis than in the first attack. Acute choroiditis is occasionally seen.[2]

Though not usual practice, examination of the cerebrospinal fluid shows abnormalities in a proportion of patients varying in different series; meningitis, cranial nerve palsies, transverse myelitis, thrombosis of cerebral arteries, and syphilitic nerve deafness have all been described.[39,40] (See Chap. 21.)

# DIAGNOSIS

## PRIMARY SYPHILIS

### Clinical suspicion

The prerequisite in diagnosis is clinical suspicion. The age, sexual behavior, and contact history are important factors in alerting the physician. A single painless, indurated, nontender ulcer gives a high probability of primary syphilis. Multiple painful lesions reduce the probability and suggest secondary syphilis. Syphilis must also be considered in the diagnosis of oral and anorectal ulcers and occasionally when ulcers are noted at other sites.

### Dark field microscopy

Dark field microscopy[41] is the investigation of first choice. It is widely regarded as sensitive and specific in the diagnosis of primary syphilis.[42] However, actual data are lacking; Hart[43] discussed predictive values of dark field microscopy, comparing it with the VDRL test. He concluded that expertise in this technique was important for accurate diagnosis. The technique of dark field microscopy is considered in detail in Chap. 75. Important practical points to remember are to clean lesions thoroughly with physiologic saline, to squeeze the lesion and scrape firmly, and to collect serum rather than blood. *T. pallidum* can be readily identified by an experienced microscopist from its characteristic spiral morphology and from its mobility, which is much greater than saprophytic treponemes. The latter will cause concern only when ulcers are found on or near mucosal surfaces.

If dark field microscopy is not immediately available, exudate may be sent to a laboratory in a capillary tube provided transit time is only a few hours. Alternatively, the specimen may be examined in the laboratory by staining with fluorescein-labeled *T. pallidum* globulin and using a fluorescent microscope. For this technique samples may be sent on a slide fixed in acetone. Unfortunately, these "mail in" tests are not widely available in the United States or in many other countries.

If the initial dark field examination is negative in a suspect case, the procedure should be repeated on at least two successive days. The patient should bathe the lesions with physiologic saline between examinations. A negative examination does not exclude the diagnosis—there may be too few organisms to be identified, the lesion may be healing, or topical or systemic and treatment may have been given. Secondary infection may obscure an otherwise positive dark field. A nontreponemicidal antimicrobial such as sulfisoxazole 1 g four times daily for 5 days or co-trimoxazole 2 × 480 mg tablets twice daily can be given and the lesion bathed in physiologic saline.

If it is known that antiseptics have been applied to a suspect chancre, a superficial enlarged regional lymph node may be aspirated and the aspirate examined by dark field microscopy (Fig. 20-10).

### Serological tests

Serological tests provide only indirect evidence of primary syphilis but can be a useful adjunct in diagnosis, especially when antimicrobials have been taken, negating dark field microscopy, or in situations where this technique is unavailable. The VDRL becomes reactive some 14 days after the appearance of the chancre and is reactive in 50 to 70 percent of patients at the time of diagnosis.[44] The more sensitive FTA-ABS test becomes reactive around the time of the appearance of the chancre and at the time of diagnosis is reactive in 70 to 90 percent of cases.[45] The MHA-TP gives results similar to the FTA-ABS. It is because of this delay in reactivity that dark field microscopy is the investigation of first choice in primary syphilis. Furthermore, dark field microscopy provides a diagnosis in minutes whereas at best serological tests take several hours.

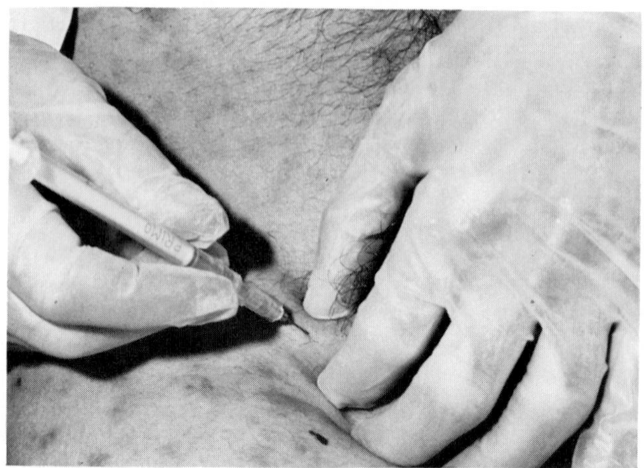

**Fig. 20-10.** Technique for node aspiration, for purpose of preparation of a dark field examination. (*Courtesy of E Stolz.*)

A presumptive diagnosis of primary syphilis can be made in patients where the dark field examination is negative, if they have suggestive clinical features supported by a history of contact and have reactive serological tests provided these include a reactive FTA-ABS or MHA-TP results. If there is doubt in the interpretation of the initial investigations, the serological tests should be repeated. A rising VDRL titer indicates a high probability of primary syphilis.

## SECONDARY SYPHILIS

### Clinical suspicion

As with primary syphilis, a high index of suspicion is important. Features which suggest a high probability of secondary syphilis include a papular rash affecting the palms and soles, condylomata lata and mucous patches, especially if there is lymphadenopathy and malaise.

### Dark field microscopy

Dark field examinations should be undertaken on papules, condylomata lata, or, in their absence, on a mucous patch; saprophytic treponemes on mucosal surfaces may cause confusion. The preferred lesion is a papule at a distance from an orifice.

### Serological tests

Serological tests are virtually always reactive in secondary syphilis, the VDRL test often having a high titer (reactive at a serum dilution of 1:16 or higher). Excessive amounts of antibody can interfere with the test, leading to a nonreactive, weakly reactive, or atypical reaction (the prozone phenomenon). This effect can be prevented by diluting the serum. Typical clinical features, repeated reactive results to the VDRL test in titer 1 in 16 or higher, and a reactive FTA-ABS or MHA-TP result lead to a presumptive diagnosis of secondary syphilis. Skin biopsy may be quite helpful (Figs. 20-11 and, 20-12).

## LATENT INFECTION

In latent infection there are, by definition, no positive clinical features. Diagnosis depends on positive results to serological tests which must include a VDRL or similar test and an FTA-ABS or MHA-TP test. At least two samples taken at an interval of a week must be examined. If there are conflicting results, further samples are necessary. The CSF should be examined to exclude CNS involvement (Chap. 21). A chest radiograph may be indicated on occasion to look for calcification in the ascending aorta. Further investigation such as CT or ultrasound scans may be considered if CSF or chest radiograph show suspicious abnormalities.

## DIFFERENTIAL DIAGNOSIS

### Primary syphilis

All genital ulcers, and all anorectal lesions in at-risk persons should be regarded as possible primary syphilis. Differential diagnosis of a primary chancre includes genital herpes simplex, sec-

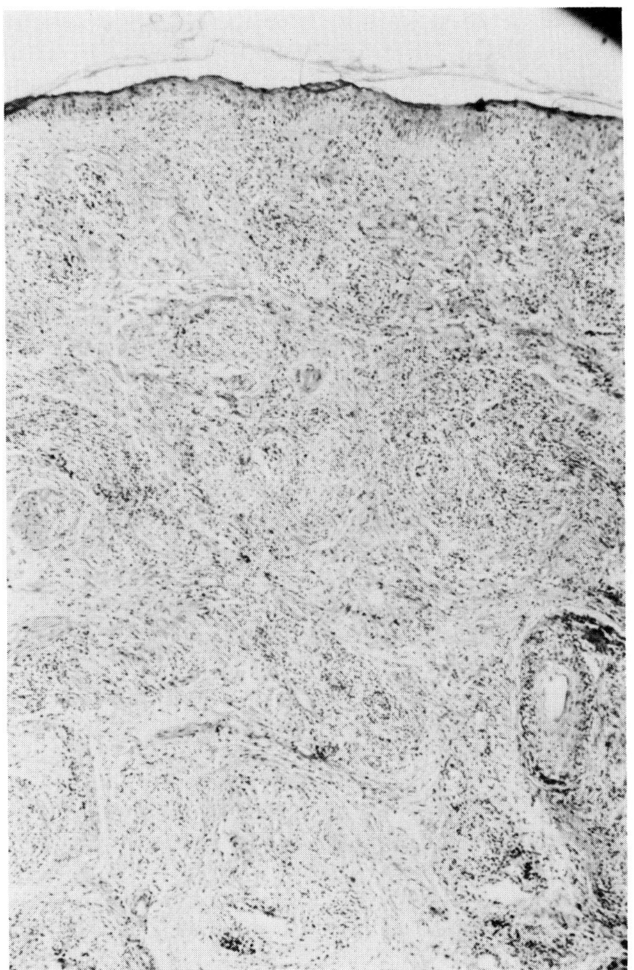

**Fig. 20-11.** Secondary syphilis: skin biopsy. H&E stain. Dense round cell infiltrate and vasculitis. (*Courtesy of E Stolz.*)

ondary syphilis, erosive balanitis, trauma with or without secondary pyogenic infection, scabies, furuncle, and less commonly herpes zoster, carcinoma, fixed drug eruption, Vincent's ulcers, and orogenital ulceration including Reiter's syndrome (or the sexually acquired reactive arthritis syndrome), Stevens-Johnson's syndrome, and Behçet's syndrome. If there has been exposure in a tropical climate or a contact has been in such a climate, one should consider chancroid, granuloma inguinale, lymphogranuloma venereum, tuberculosis, and amoebic ulceration.

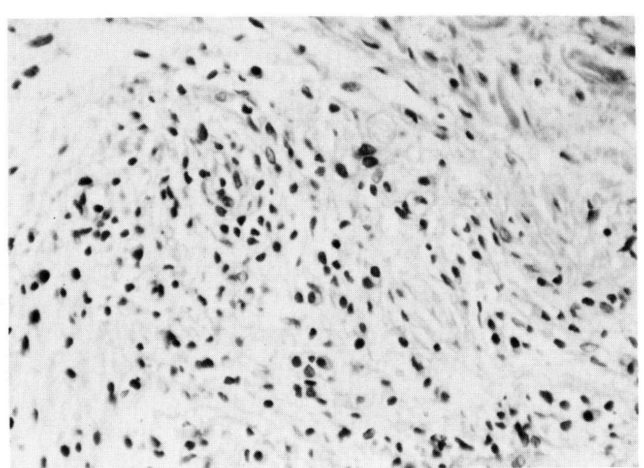

**Fig. 20-12.** Secondary syphilis: skin biopsy. H&E stain. Focal lymphocytic and plasma cell infiltrate. (*Courtesy of E Stolz.*)

### Secondary syphilis

An enormous range of conditions must be included in the differential diagnosis of secondary syphilis and can only be outlined here. An early manifestation is fever which may precede other features, sometimes for several weeks; so syphilis must be included in the (less common) causes of fever of obscure origin. The macular rash may resemble a drug eruption, measles, rubella, pityriasis rosea, pityriasis (tinea) versicolor, seborrheic dermatitis, erythema multiforme, rose spots of typhoid fever, and leprosy. The papular rash may resemble drug eruption, lichen planus, acne vulgaris, and scabies. Squamous eruption may be confused with psoriasis or seborrheic dermatitis. Annular lesions may resemble fungal infection, impetigo, erythema multiforme, and more rarely the annular form of lichen planus and granuloma annulare. Condylomata lata may be confused with human papilloma virus warts. The alopecia due to secondary syphilis must be distinguished from alopecia areata.

Though the macular eruption was described by Stokes[1] as the most common eruption, Chapel[32] found maculopapular eruptions more common and related this to earlier presentation. In contrast to classical descriptions, Chapel[32] did not find lesions denser on flexor than on extensor surfaces. Palms and soles are the most common sites, and he also noted that itch may occur. Harris[33] commented that in a series of 60 patients with secondary syphilis who underwent skin biopsies in a specialist dermatology hospital, the diagnosis was not suspected in 10 percent of cases and was not thought to be the most likely diagnosis in a further 15 percent. These findings emphasize the need for a high index of suspicion.

The lymphadenopathy of secondary syphilis resembles that of glandular fever (EBV and CMV mononucleosis), HIV infection, Hodgkin's disease, and lymphomas. Secondary syphilis, HIV disease, and glandular fever may be difficult to distinguish clinically, for they may all present with fever, malaise, sore throat, rashes, and lymphadenopathy in young men. When considering any one of these conditions, it is prudent to investigate for the others.

The mucosal ulceration of secondary syphilis may resemble that seen in herpes simplex and the orogenital ulceration syndromes mentioned above. The mucosal ulcers of secondary syphilis should be distinguished from primary latent syphilis.

## TREATMENT

Intramuscular penicillin remains the antimicrobial of choice for the treatment of all stages of syphilis in patients who are not hypersensitive.[2,46,47] There is no evidence of the development of *T. pallidum* resistant to penicillin. The aim is to maintain a prolonged low concentration of penicillin within the tissues, but this must be continuous.[47] There is evidence that penetration of long-acting benzathine penicillin into the central nervous system is poor[48] but, because of convenience, this is preferred in many centers. Furthermore Dunlop[49] has cast doubt on the concentration of penicillin in the central nervous system achieved by conventional doses of procaine penicillin used in Britain. As indicated above,[25,26] there is now grave doubt concerning the efficacy of benzathine penicillin in the presence of HIV disease.

## PRIMARY AND SECONDARY SYPHILIS

For primary and secondary syphilis the recommended therapy is benzathine penicillin G 2.4 million units (1.2 million units into each buttock) by intramuscular injection at a single session.[45] If it is certain the course will be completed, one may give aqueous procaine penicillin G 600,000 units daily by intramuscular injection for 8 to 12 days.[2] For patients hypersensitive to penicillin, tetracycline hydrochloride 500 mg may be given by mouth four times daily for 15 days.[46]

## LATENT INFECTION

Latent syphilis present for less than 1 year should be treated with the same regimens as primary or secondary syphilis. If latent infection has been present for more than 1 year, the recommended regimens are benzathine penicillin 2.4 million units by intramuscular injection once a week for 3 successive weeks, aqueous procaine penicillin G 600,000 units by intramuscular injection daily for 15 days, or tetracycline hydrochloride 500 mg by mouth four times daily for 30 days.[2,46] Care must be taken to ensure compliance when patients are taking oral therapy. For patients who cannot tolerate tetracycline and are hypersensitive to penicillin, preferred therapy is erythromycin stearate 500 mg four times daily by mouth for 15 to 30 days. Follow-up is important, for there are anecdotes of treatment failure after erythromycin.[50]

Other regimens such as doxycycline 100 mg two or three times daily and various cephalosporins such as cephalexin 500 mg four times daily for 15 days have been suggested, but experience with them is limited.[47] Dunlop,[49] usually a proponent of high-dose therapy, suggests ampicillin 500 mg four times daily by mouth with probenecid to increase penetration into the CSF and the eye, but warns that this produces satisfactory concentrations of penicillin only in the absence of diarrhea. He also suggests that amoxycillin may be more effective.[49] Faber et al.[51] suggest amoxycillin 6 g daily plus probenecid 2 g daily for 15 days to give adequate CSF concentrations. Alternative regimens for neurosyphilis also include 24 million units of aqueous penicillin G intravenously for 8 to 10 days[25,26,52] or doxycycline 200 mg twice daily for 21 days.[53] Neurosyphilis and therapy for neurosyphilis are discussed fully in Chap. 21.

## PREGNANT PATIENTS

The treatments of choice for the pregnant patient are the parenteral penicillin regimens outlined above. When the patient is hypersensitive to penicillin, the erythromycin regimens outlined should be prescribed. However, erythromycin may fail to cross the placental barrier;[50] so mother and child should be followed with great care.

## JARISCH HERXHEIMER REACTION

The Jarisch Herxheimer reaction commonly develops a few hours after the first dose of antimicrobial for the treatment of primary and secondary syphilis and subsides within 24 h. Systemic manifestations include fever, malaise, headache, musculoskeletal pain, nausea, and tachycardia. A primary lesion may swell and the lesions of secondary syphilis may appear for the first time. The reaction must be differentiated from penicillin hypersensitivity and procaine reactions. The patient should be warned about the reaction, and the only management required in early syphilis is reassurance, fluids, and aspirin or paracetamol. The Herxheimer reaction is more common in early syphilis but is more serious in late syphilis.

## FOLLOW-UP

Though treatment failure has been reported in up to 10 percent of cases of early infectious syphilis, it is rare in the writer's experience, which mainly concerns the use of procaine penicillin. In practice it is often difficult to distinguish treatment failure from reinfection. As recurrence either from treatment failure or reinfection is a possibility, all cases should be followed up if possible. One satisfactory routine is to see patients monthly for the first 3 months, then 6, 9, 12, and 24 months after the beginning of therapy.[54] Others advocate more frequent visits.[2,26] As the clinical features will resolve without therapy, serological tests must be undertaken as well as clinical examination. The response of the VDRL titer should be monitored. The other lipoidal antigen nontreponemal tests, namely, the RPR test or ART, serve equally well. As far as possible the same test should be used before and after therapy because the results otherwise are not strictly comparable. In a careful analysis of data from patients with primary and secondary syphilis treated with recommended therapy, the VDRL titer declined approximately fourfold 3 months after treatment and eightfold after 6 months.[55] In primary syphilis the VDRL test is usually nonreactive 1 year after treatment[56] and in secondary syphilis it is nonreactive 2 years after treatment.[57] The FTA-ABS and MHA-TP remain positive. Careful follow-up is especially important after oral therapy.

### Treatment failure

Treatment failure must be considered in early infectious syphilis if clinical signs persist or reappear, the VDRL titer remains high, the VDRL titer does not fall as indicated, or the VDRL titer rises. In such cases, retreatment is indicated.

## PREVENTION

### BEHAVIOR MODIFICATION

The decline in syphilis in some cities[12–14] is most probably due to reduction in partner change and safer sexual practices. This has been due partly to formal education programs and partly to the understanding homosexual and bisexual men have acquired informally or through their organizations. It is clear that education can have a considerable effect on sexual behavior. This has not been achieved in the heterosexual population in other areas,[13] maybe because of lack of education, lack of targeting, and lack of the stimulus generated by a fear of a fatal disease (AIDS).

### PARTNER MANAGEMENT

An essential part of the management of early infectious syphilis is ensuring examination, investigation, and if necessary treatment of all at-risk sexual partners. For primary syphilis these will be partners during the previous 3 months or, if the source of infection is determined, all partners following the last sexual contact with the source. For secondary syphilis, at-risk partners will be all those during the preceding 6 to 12 months depending again on whether the source can be identified.

## OTHER METHODS

Diagnostic and treatment facilities must be maintained. Serological testing for high- and low-risk groups must be continued including patients attending treatment clinics, at-risk individuals attending other facilities, blood donors, and pregnant women. Education programs remain important and must be targeted at those at risk. All prevention and control methods must be coordinated at local clinics to ensure maximum effect.

# References


1 Stokes JH et al: *Modern Clinical Syphilology*, 3d ed. Philadelphia, Saunders, 1945.
2 King A et al: *Venereal Diseases*, 4th ed. London, Bailliere Tindall, 1980.
3 Hudson EH: *Non-venereal Syphilis*. Edinburgh, Livingston, 1958.
4 Gjestland T: The Oslo study of untreated syphilis: An epidemiologic investigation of the natural course of the syphilitic infection based upon a re-study of the Boeck-Bruusgard material. *Acta Derm Venereol* 35, *suppl* 34 (*Stockh*): 1, 1955.
5 Rockwell DH et al: The Tuskegee study of untreated syphilis. *Arch Intern Med* 114:792, 1964.
6 Moore J Earle: *Penicillin in Syphilis*. Springfield, IL, Thomas, 1946.
7 Harris A et al: Microflocculation test for syphilis using cardiolipin antigen. *J Vener Dis Inf* 27:169, 1946.
8 Nelson RA, Mayer MM: Immobilisation of Treponema pallidum in vitro by antibody produced in syphilitic infection. *J Exp Med* 89: 369, 1949.
9 Veldkamp J, Visser AM: Application of the enzyme linked immunosorbent assay (ELISA) in the serodiagnosis of syphilis. *Br J Vener Dis* 51:227, 1975.
10 British Co-operative Clinical Group: Homosexuality and venereal disease in the United Kingdom. *Br J Vener Dis* 49:329, 1973.
11 British Co-operative Clinical Group: Homosexuality and venereal disease in the United Kingdom—A sexual study. *Br J Vener Dis* 56:6, 1980.
12 Communicable Diseases Surveillance Centre: Sexually transmitted disease in Britain 1985. *Communicable Disease Report* 87/45:3, 1987.
13 Wilder MH et al: Increases in primary and secondary syphilis—United States. *MMWR* 36:393, 1987.
14 Coutinho RA et al: Influence of special surveillance programmes and AIDS on declining incidence of syphilis in Amsterdam. *Genitourin Med* 63:210, 1987.
15 Thirumoorthy T et al: Epidemiology of infectious syphilis in Singapore. *Genitourin Med* 62:75, 1986.
16 Alvarez-Dardet C et al: Urban clusters of sexually transmitted diseases in the city of Seville. *Sex Transm Dis* 12:166, 1985.
17 Shroeter AL et al: Therapy for incubating syphilis: Effectiveness of gonorrhoea treatment. *JAMA* 218:711, 1971.
18 Klingbeil LJ, Clark EG: Studies in the epidemiology of syphilis. *J Vener Dis Inf* 22:1, 1941.
19 von Wersssouwetz JK: The incidence of infection in contacts of early syphilis. *J Vener Dis Inf* 28:132, 1948.
20 Alexander LJ, Schoch AG: Prevention of syphilis. *Arch Derm Syphilol* 59:1, 1949.
21 Schober P et al: How infectious is syphilis? *Br J Vener Dis* 59:217, 1983.
22 Robertson DHH et al: *Clinical Practise in Sexually Transmissable Diseases*. Tunbridge Wells, England, Pitman, p 94.
23 Sparling PF: Natural history of syphilis, in *Sexually Transmitted Diseases*, KK Holmes et al (eds). New York, McGraw-Hill, 1984, p 229.
24 Johns DR et al: Alteration in the natural history of neurosyphilis by concurrent infection with the human immunodeficiency virus. *N Engl J Med* 316:1569, 1987.
25 Berry CD et al: Neurologic relapse after benzathine penicillin therapy for secondary syphilis in a patient with HIV infection. *N Engl J Med* 316:1587, 1987.
26 Tramont EC: Syphilis in the AIDS era. *N Engl J Med* 316:1600, 1987.
27 Beck-Sague CM et al: Neurosyphilis and HIV infection. *N Engl J Med* 317:1473, 1987 (letter).
28 Hicks CB et al: Seronegative secondary syphilis in a patient infected with the human immunodeficiency virus (HIV) with Kaposi sarcoma. *Ann Intern Med* 107:492, 1987.
29 Gorsuch AN et al: Rapid development of syphilis in a long standing diabetic. *Postgrad Med J* 57:183, 1981.
30 Magnuson HJ et al: Inoculation syphilis in human volunteers. *Medicine* 35:33, 1956.
31 Pavithran K: Acquired syphilis in a patient with late congenital syphilis. *Sex Transm Dis* 14:120, 1987.
32 Chapel TA: The signs and symptoms of secondary syphilis. *Sex Transm Dis* 7:161, 1980.
33 Harris JRW: *Recent Advances in Sexually Transmitted Diseases,* 3d ed. Edinburgh, Churchill Livingston, 1981, p 73.
34 Campisi D, Whitcomb C: Liver disease in early syphilis. *Arch Intern Med* 139:365, 1978.
35 Feher J et al: Early syphilitic hepatitis. *Lancet* 2:896, 1975.
36 Bhorade MS et al: Nephropathy of secondary syphilis: A clinical and pathological spectrum. *JAMA* 216:1159, 1971.
37 Gamble CN, Reardon JB: Immunopathogenesis of syphilitic glomerulonephritis: Elution of antitreponemal antibody from glomerular immune-complex deposits. *N Engl J Med* 292:449, 1975.
38 O'Regan S et al: Treponemal antigen in congenital and acquired syphilitis nephritis? Demonstration by immunofluorescence studies. *Ann Intern Med* 85:325, 1976.
39 Wetherill JH et al: Syphilis presenting as an acute neurological illness. *Br Med J* 1:1157, 1965.
40 Willcox RR, Goodwin PG: Nerve deafness in early syphilis. *Br J Vener Dis* 47:401, 1971.
41 *Manual of Tests for Syphilis*. Atlanta, Venereal Disease Programme, US Communicable Disease Center, 1969 (USPHS publication 411).
42 *Criteria and Techniques for the Diagnosis of Early Syphilis*. Atlanta, Centers for Disease Control, 1979 (DHEW publication 98-376).
43 Hart G: Syphilis tests in diagnostic and therapeutic decision making. *Ann Intern Med* 104:368, 1986.
44 Wende RB et al: The VDRL slide test in 322 cases of dark field positive primary syphilis. *South Med J* 64:5, 1971.
45 Duncan WC et al: The FTA-ABS test in dark field positive primary syphilis. *JAMA* 228:859, 1974.
46 Centers for Disease Control: 1985 STD treatment guidelines *MMWR* 34:suppl 45, 1985.
47 Panconesi E et al: Treatment of syphilis: A short critical review. *Sex Transm Dis* 8:321, 1981.
48 Rein MF: Treatment of neurosyphilis. *JAMA* 246:2613, 1981.
49 Dunlop EMC: Survival of treponemas after treatment: Comments, clinical conclusions and recommendations. *Genitourin Med* 61:293, 1985.
50 Hashisaki P et al: Erythromycin failure in the treatment of syphilis in a pregnant woman. *Sex Transm Dis* 10:36, 1983.
51 Faber WR et al: Treponemicidal levels of Amoxicillin in cerebrospinal fluid after oral administration. *Sex Transm Dis* 10:148, 1983.
52 Yim CW et al: Neurosyphilis and HIV infections. *N Engl J Med* 317:1474, 1987 (letter).

53 Yim CW et al: Penetration of oral doxycycline into the cerebrospinal fluid of patients with latent or neurosyphilis. *Antimicrob Agents Chemother* 23:347, 1985.
54 Thin RN: *Lecture Notes on Sexually Transmitted Diseases*. Oxford, Blackwells, 1982, pp 37, 43.
55 Brown ST et al: Serological response to syphilis treatment: A new analysis of old data. *JAMA* 253:1296, 1985.
56 Fiumara NJ: Treatment of seropositive primary syphilis: An evaluation of 196 patients. *Sex Transm Dis* 4:92, 1977.
57 Fiumara NJ: Treatment of secondary syphilis: an evaluation of 204 patients. *Sex Transm Dis* 4:96, 1977.

# Chapter 21
# Neurosyphilis

Morton N. Swartz

The manifestations of central nervous system syphilis, readily recognized by physicians practicing three or four decades ago, are unfamiliar to many physicians today as a result of the relative rarity of this condition. A rise has not occurred in the number of cases of neurosyphilis stemming from untreated early syphilis acquired either during World War II or during the period of increased sexual permissiveness that began in the 1960s. It is as yet unknown whether the increase in atypical manifestations of venereal diseases in the male homosexual population is masking cases of early syphilis. By escaping detection and treatment, such early syphilis may become responsible for a future reemergence of neurosyphilis. There has been a slight increase in recent years in the incidence of acute syphilitic meningitis, an early form of neurosyphilis.

## PATHOGENESIS

The very early and frequent invasion of the meninges by *Treponema pallidum* during systemic dissemination of syphilitic infection is indicated by several lines of evidence. First, *T. pallidum* has been demonstrated, by animal inoculation, in the cerebrospinal fluid of patients with untreated primary and secondary syphilis.[1–3] It has been reported that the spirochete may be recovered from 15 to 40 percent of "normal" spinal fluids in early syphilis.[2] More recently, *T. pallidum* has been isolated by animal inoculation from the CSF of the one patient with primary syphilis studied, 8 of 16 patients with secondary syphilis, and none of 11 patients with latent syphilis.[4] Second, abnormalities in the CSF have been noted in 13 percent of patients with untreated primary syphilis,[5] 25 to 40 percent of patients with untreated secondary syphilis,[5,6] and 13.9 percent of untreated patients with primary and secondary syphilis.[7]

## CLASSIFICATION AND CHRONOLOGY

The multitude of histopathologic reactions induced, anatomic sites involved, and clinical syndromes produced by neurosyphilis make classification complex. A helpful schema is that utilized by Merritt et al. in their classic monograph on neurosyphilis[8] (Table 21-1). Although this classification indicates the existence of distinctive individual forms of neurosyphilis, features of several of the entities commonly coexist, producing, for example, combinations of meningitis and vasculitis or tabes and paresis. This is not surprising when one considers that neurosyphilis fundamentally is a very chronic meningitis capable of producing vascular and parenchymatous sequelae in the cerebrum and spinal cord. Although neurosyphilis is almost always a consequence of acquired syphilis, involvement of the central nervous system (CNS) can also be a feature of congenital syphilis. Indeed, the major categories of acquired neurosyphilis (asymptomatic neurosyphilis, acute syphilitic meningitis, cerebral meningovascular syphilis, paresis, tabes) also occur in congenital syphilis (Chap. 67).

**Table 21-1. Classification of Neurosyphilis**

*Asymptomatic neurosyphilis*
Early
Late

*Meningeal neurosyphilis*
Acute syphilitic meningitis
Spinal syphilitic pachymeningitis

*Meningovascular neurosyphilis*
Cerebral form
Spinal form

*Parenchymatous neurosyphilis*
General paresis
Tabes dorsalis
Optic atrophy

*Gummatous neurosyphilis*
Cerebral form
Spinal form

SOURCE: After HH Merritt et al.[8]

As noted earlier (Chap. 19), the frequent clinical involvement of the central nervous system in the natural history of untreated syphilis has been documented in long-term longitudinal studies performed earlier in this century. In the Oslo study of 953 persons with primary or secondary syphilis, 6.5 percent subsequently developed CNS involvement.[9,10] In the Tuskegee follow-up study in 1963, of 90 survivors of a group of black males with latent syphilis, 3.3 percent had CNS involvement.[11]

In the prepenicillin era (1932–1942) clinical neurosyphilis was an important element in the overall spectrum of syphilitic manifestations; for example, clinical neurosyphilis was found in 29 percent of 2263 cases of syphilis examined at the Boston City Hospital.[12] The most common forms of nervous system involvement were asymptomatic neurosyphilis (31 percent) and tabes (30 percent) (Table 21-2.) The incidence of paresis was probably underestimated since such patients were more likely to have been treated in psychiatric rather than general hospitals. In the antibiotic era the successful treatment of early syphilis (and perhaps the unwitting treatment of latent syphilis with penicillin administered in the treatment of other illnesses) has made neurosyphilis an uncommon disorder in many parts of the world. In the United States, neurosyphilis declined as the cause of initial admissions

**Table 21-2. Relative Frequencies of Different Types of Neurosyphilis***

| | Percentage of neurosyphilis cases |
|---|---|
| Asymptomatic neurosyphilis | 31 |
| Tabes | 30 |
| Paresis | 12 |
| Taboparesis | 3 |
| Vascular neurosyphilis | 10 |
| Syphilitic meningitis | 6 |
| Deafness | 1 |
| Optic neuritis | 3 |
| Meningomyelitis and other forms of spinal cord involvement | 3 |
| Other | 1 |

*Data on 676 patients with neurosyphilis examined at Boston City Hospital (1932–1942).
SOURCE: HH Merritt et al.[12]

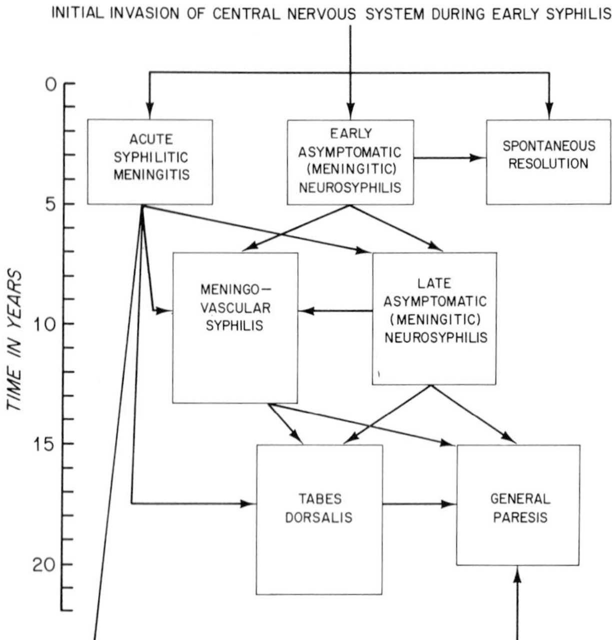


**Fig. 21-1.** Chronology of neurosyphilis. *(After HH Merritt et al.*[12]*)*

to mental hospitals from a rate of 4.3 cases per 100,000 population (in 1946) to 0.4 cases per 100,000 population (in 1960). In Great Britain deaths from general paresis fell from an annual figure of about 600 in 1941 to 24 in 1968; this decrease reflects both decreased incidence and increased efficacy of treatment.[13] In the United States in 1976, the last year in which the Centers for Disease Control recorded separately the number of cases of neurosyphilis, there were 2903 reported cases of neurosyphilis out of a total of 71,761 cases of syphilis.[14]

After the initial spirochetal invasion of the CNS has occurred, untreated or inadequately treated infection may take one of several courses: spontaneous resolution, asymptomatic syphilitic meningitis, or symptomatic acute syphilitic meningitis (Fig. 21-1). Progression of early asymptomatic or symptomatic meningeal infection eventuates either in continuing asymptomatic neurosyphilis or meningovascular syphilis (usually during the period from 5 to 12 years after primary infection) or in tabes or paresis. The progression often represents a continuum of changes rather than a series of discrete steps. It is unclear why some patients never develop neurosyphilis in the course of untreated syphilis or why some patients who do develop CNS syphilis manifest tabes and others paresis or meningovascular disease.

## CLINICAL MANIFESTATIONS

### ASYMPTOMATIC NEUROSYPHILIS

#### Symptoms and signs

Asymptomatic neurosyphilis is defined by the presence of abnormalities in the cerebrospinal fluid (CSF) in the absence of neurologic symptoms or findings. Thus, examination of the CSF is essential for diagnosis. Although the pathology of this phase of neurosyphilis is undefined, it is presumed that the changes are almost always confined to the meninges, at least in early asymptomatic neurosyphilis (Fig. 21-1). Slight chronic meningitis and ependymitis (but no evidence of endarteritis or encephalitis) were observed at autopsy of an untreated patient with late asymptomatic neurosyphilis (positive blood serology for 9 years); this patient died of an intercurrent acute pneumococcal pneumonia.[12]

Asymptomatic neurosyphilis has in the past been divided into an early stage (from 0 to 5 years after initial infection) and a late stage (over 5 years after initial infection). The maximum incidence of CSF abnormalities is observed between 12 and 18 months after initial infection; in the prepenicillin era a completely normal CSF examination after 2 years of latent untreated syphilitic infection afforded reasonable assurance that neurosyphilis would not develop.[12] Knowledge of the evolution of early asymptomatic neurosyphilis is based on earlier studies in patients who either had received no treatment or had been treated prior to the introduction of penicillin. The frequency of asymptomatic neurosyphilis tended to decrease with the passage of time; one cooperative study reported that at 3, 10, and 20 years following onset, the frequency was 20, 12.9, and 6.3 percent, respectively.[15] A reciprocal increase in the incidence of symptomatic neurosyphilis was noted in the same study.

Late asymptomatic neurosyphilis may occasionally be accompanied by evidence of syphilitic involvement of other organs, such as the aorta. Data on the prognosis of untreated late asymptomatic neurosyphilis in the prepenicillin era indicate progression of the infection to clinical neurosyphilis in 23 to 87 percent of the syphilis cases studied.[5] Since asymptomatic neurosyphilis has been found in elderly patients who have had syphilis for many years, it is clear that asymptomatic neurosyphilis does not invariably progress to clinical neurosyphilis.

#### Laboratory findings

Blood serology is positive in almost every case of asymptomatic neurosyphilis. The CSF shows in most instances a cell count of less than 100 lymphocytes per cubic millimeter, a normal or slightly elevated (<100 mg/dl) protein concentration, and a nontreponemal serologic test that is positive (in over 90 percent of patients).[12] When the colloidal gold test (a reflection of the globulin concentration) was routinely determined in the past, it most commonly showed a mid-zone curve, but it sometimes showed a first-zone curve or occasionally was normal. The first-zone, or *paretic,* curve was at one time thought to be pathognomonic of paresis, but it was frequently found in other forms of neurosyphilis and in a variety of nonsyphilitic diseases of the central nervous system. The mid-zone, or *leutic,* curve is common in all forms of neurosyphilis and can be observed in many other abnormal spinal fluids.

Prognosis during the arsenical era appeared to be related to the intensity of the CSF changes. In one study 6 percent of 73 patients with moderately positive CSF tests subsequently developed clinical neurosyphilis, whereas 33 percent of 36 patients with markedly positive CSF tests showed similar progression.[16]

### MENINGEAL SYPHILIS

#### Acute syphilitic meningitis

Even prior to the antibiotic era, acute syphilitic meningitis was relatively rare. In a 15-year (1920–1935) survey[17] of records of three Boston hospitals, only 80 definite cases were found. This study provides the most thorough and comprehensive description of the clinical and pathologic features of this disease. Acute syphilitic meningitis accounted for 6 percent of the cases of neurosyphilis (Table 21-2) and 1.4 percent of a total of 2263 syphilitic patients examined at the Boston City Hospital in the same 15-year period.

**Symptoms and Signs.** The incubation period in the majority of patients with syphilitic meningitis is less than 1 year. Fewer than 10 percent of patients have a secondary rash at the time of the meningitis; in about one-quarter of patients, meningitis is the first clinical manifestation of syphilis. Syphilitic meningitis is most common in young adults; rarely, it is a feature of early congenital syphilis.

The clinical presentations of acute syphilitic meningitis may be divided into several patterns for convenience, but these categories overlap extensively. The clinical constellation of headache, fever, photophobia, and stiff neck combined with CSF findings of a mild lymphocytic pleocytosis and a normal glucose concentration commonly suggests a viral aseptic meningitis. However, the identical picture, even in the absence of a secondary rash or a history of a chancre, may be caused by syphilitic meningitis.[18] A positive nontreponemal serology [the Venereal Disease Research Laboratory (VDRL) test] provides the important clue to diagnosis. In patients who have a positive VDRL test, the CSF serology is positive in over 90 percent at the first lumbar puncture; those patients with a negative CSF VDRL test are found to have positive test results on subsequent examinations. The response to penicillin is prompt, and fever and other clinical findings clear within several days. Relapse or progression to meningovascular or parenchymatous neurosyphilis probably does not occur when recommended therapy with penicillin has been administered (see Management, below).

*Acute syphilitic hydrocephalus* was the picture presented by one-third of the cases of syphilitic meningitis reported by Merritt and Moore.[17] Symptoms usually develop 3 to 7 months after primary infection, but they can appear as many as 6 years later. The principal symptoms (headache, nausea, and vomiting), are those of increased intracranial pressure. Fever is only low-grade or may be absent. Neck stiffness, Kernig's sign, and papilledema are the principal findings. The last is associated with only minor degrees of visual loss; this association indicates that the appearance of the optic disk is secondary to increased intracranial pressure rather than to primary optic neuritis. Cranial nerve palsies are not a feature; reflex changes are usually absent.

*Syphilitic meningitis with cerebral changes* accounted for one-quarter of the cases in the study of Merritt and Moore.[17] The symptoms (seizures, aphasia, and hemiplegia) are a combination of those of increased intracranial pressure and those of focal cerebral involvement. Clinical findings usually include stiff neck, confusion or delirium, and papilledema. Occasionally, cranial nerve palsies are present and most commonly involve the third and sixth cranial nerves.

*Syphilitic meningitis with prominent cranial nerve palsies* was found in about 40 percent of the cases of syphilitic meningitis reviewed by Merritt and Moore.[17] The principal neurologic manifestations are cranial nerve palsies and increased intracranial pressure (less marked and less frequent than in the preceding two forms of meningitis). The involvement of multiple cranial nerves, particularly the third, sixth, seventh, and eighth, is consistent with an extensive basilar meningitis.

Occasionally, a patient may be seen by a physician because of acute sensorineural hearing loss that subsequently is attributed to early syphilis. Such nerve deafness, commonly bilateral, is associated with syphilitic meningitis, which may be a minor element in the clinical picture and initially may be overlooked.[19] Deafness is commonly preceded by tinnitus and may develop over 1 or 2 weeks. The hearing loss primarily involves higher frequencies; vestibular involvement is uncommon. Usually there are no other clinical findings to suggest syphilis. Sensorineural deafness may occur in about 20 percent of patients with overt acute syphilitic meningitis; such deafness is common with other cranial nerve palsies. The serum VDRL test is positive, and mild abnormalities (pleocytosis of up to several hundred mononuclear cells and minimally increased protein) are present in the CSF. The CSF nontreponemal serology is usually positive but sometimes may not have converted by the time of treatment. Early acquired syphilis is a cause of potentially reversible sudden sensorineural deafness in a young adult that must be considered in diagnosis, even in the absence of clinical findings of secondary syphilis or of overt lymphocytic meningitis. The response to penicillin therapy is usually good, with return to normal hearing.[20,21] However, the dosage of penicillin should be the same as that employed for late neurosyphilis and not the same as that for secondary syphilis (see Management, below). Suboptimal therapy may be associated with recurrence of hearing loss several months later.

**Laboratory Findings.** In the extensive series reported by Merritt and Moore[17] in 1935, the blood Wassermann reaction was positive in only 64 percent of patients. However, these cases were studied before the introduction of more sensitive tests. The current serum reagin [VDRL and rapid plasma reagin (RPR)] and treponemal [fluorescent treponemal antibody-absorption (FTA-ABS)] tests are regularly positive in acute syphilitic meningitis. The CSF changes include elevated pressure, mononuclear pleocytosis of 10 to 500 cells per cubic millimeter (occasionally as high as 1000 to 2000 cells per cubic millimeter), elevated protein concentration (45 to 200 mg/dl), elevated globulin level, hypoglycorrhachia ($\leq$40 mg/dl) in 45 percent of cases, and first- or mid-zone colloidal gold curve in 90 percent of cases. Modern CSF reagin tests are almost uniformly positive.

Correlation between pathologic findings on auditory brainstem responses (suggesting occult brainstem involvement or cochlear nerve dysfunction) and cerebrospinal fluid abnormalities has been noted in 27 percent of 26 consecutive patients with secondary or early latent syphilis, all with normal neurological examinations.[22] Whether these preliminary findings indicate a subset of patients, who if untreated (or inadequately treated) would go on to develop sensorineural hearing loss associated with subsequent late syphilis, is not known.[23]

**Pathologic Changes.** The inflammatory process involves not only the meninges but also the ependyma (granular ependymitis). The meningeal infiltrate consists of lymphocytes and plasma cells located particularly in perivascular spaces. If the process becomes prolonged, fibroblastic organization ensues. Progressive inflammatory changes produce an endarteritis, which may result in thrombosis, vascular occlusion, and cerebral infarction. This process underlies the focal cerebral signs (aphasia, hemiplegia) and seizures that occur in some patients with acute syphilitic meningitis.

Acute syphilitic hydrocephalus develops as a result of obstruction, by organizing exudate, of CSF flow either from the posterior to middle crania fossa (communicating hydrocephalus) or from the fourth ventricle (obstructive hydrocephalus). Compression of cranial nerves by basilar exudate and fibrous organization most often accounts for the multiple cranial nerve palsies often observed during the course of syphilitic meningitis. Third cranial nerve involvement may also be a consequence of increased intracranial pressure.

**Diagnosis and Differential Diagnosis.** Diagnosis of acute syphilitic meningitis is based on the clinical picture of aseptic meningitis, lymphocytic response in the CSF (with or without mild hypoglycorrhachia), and positive reagin-type blood and CSF serology. A history of a recent chancre or secondary rash or the presence of generalized lymphadenopathy may suggest the diagnosis, but in many patients meningitis is the first clinical manifestation of syphilitic infection.

Differential diagnosis includes the various causes of a lymphocytic meningitis, including enteroviruses, leptospirosis, tuberculous meningitis, cryptococcal meningitis, and the meningitis of Lyme disease. The presence of rash with many echovirus infections may suggest early syphilis, but the serologic test for syphilis should be positive only in the latter. Tuberculous meningitis may closely mimic syphilitic meningitis by virtue of frequent cranial nerve involvement (particularly of the sixth cranial nerve) and hypoglycorrhachia. The demonstration of acid-fast organisms in the CSF or the presence of a positive VDRL test provides the basis for distinguishing between these conditions. The response to parenteral penicillin is evident within a few days in syphilitic meningitis. In patients with cryptococcal meningitis, CSF examination will usually demonstrate the presence of cryptococci or cryptococcal antigen. Leptospirosis, presenting as aseptic meningitis, may be suggested by a history of exposure to rodents or dogs and by a lack of cranial nerve or focal cerebral signs. However, diagnosis is established definitively only by a serologic (agglutination) test or by isolation of *Leptospira interrogans* from blood, spinal fluid, or urine. Acute syphilitic hydrocephalus may suggest the diagnosis of brain tumor because of prominent headache, vomiting, and papilledema. The presence of low-grade fever and signs of increased intracranial pressure might raise the question of brain abscess. CT scan and a serologic test for syphilis are of value in distinguishing between these diagnoses.

The clinical features, particularly the distinctive skin lesion, and epidemiology of Lyme disease serve to distinguish it from secondary syphilis when both present with the picture of lymphocytic meningitis. When Lyme disease occurs in the absence of extrameningeal findings (Bannwarth's syndrome), the distinction between the two processes becomes more difficult. The sera and CSF of patients with the neurologic involvement of Lyme disease are nonreactive in nontreponemal tests.[24,25] However, the sera of 11 percent of patients with Lyme disease have been reported to show reactivity on the FTA-ABS test.[26] Patients with syphilis show serologic reactivity with *Borrella burgdorferi:* 27 percent of 18 patients with various stages (primary, secondary, latent, late) of syphilis had positive ELISA tests for Lyme disease, and 61 percent had positive IFA tests.[25] Utilizing the clinical and epidemiologic features of the two diseases as well as VDRL reactivity and *B. burgdorferi* antibody testing of serum and CSF, distinction between the meningeal syndromes of the two spirochetal diseases can be readily made.

### Spinal pachymeningitis

Syphilitic spinal pachymeningitis is a very rare subacute inflammation in the meninges and dura produced by either a gumma or an unusually thick inflammatory reaction (hypertrophic pachymeningitis), which encases the spinal cord in a tough fibrous sheath.[12] Clinically, the process begins insidiously and progresses steadily over several months to a year, suggesting an enlarging tumor or possibly cervical spondylosis or a protruded intervertebral disk. Hypertrophic spinal pachymeningitis characteristically involves the cervical area and affects the posterior aspect of the dura. The principal manifestations include radicular pains and paresthesias in the arms and hands, followed by loss of tendon reflexes and wasting of muscles, segmental sensory loss below the involved area, and spastic paraparesis (extensor plantar responses, absent abdominal reflexes).[27] The neck is stiff. Long-tract signs are due to both cord compression and partial infarction of the cord. Fever is absent or low-grade.

CSF examination usually reveals yellow fluid with a high protein content (Froin's syndrome), a mild lymphocytic pleocytosis (up to 100 to 200 cells per cubic millimeter), and block to pressure elevation on jugular compression. Reagin-type serologic tests on blood and CSF are positive. Myelography shows a partial or complete extradural block.

Owing to the rarity of the condition, experience with treatment in the penicillin era is limited. In the arsenical era, antisyphilitic treatment was usually ineffective and neurosurgical intervention was employed to establish the diagnosis and remove the meningeal-dural mass. Treatment with procaine penicillin for 3 weeks has resulted in complete resolution of neurologic findings and clearing of partial myelographic block in one patient who was treated after 6 weeks of symptoms.[28]

## MENINGOVASCULAR SYPHILIS

### Cerebrovascular syphilis

Vascular neurosyphilis involves all parts (cerebrum, brainstem, and spinal cord) of the central nervous system. The common denominator is the production of areas of infarction secondary to syphilitic endarteritis. Although it is called vascular neurosyphilis, the process is almost invariably a meningovascular one, stemming from the chronic meningitis underlying all forms of central nervous system syphilis. Since lesions in the spinal cord produce a distinctive picture, they are considered separately (see Meningovascular Syphilis of the Spinal Cord, below). In the series from the Boston City Hospital[12] in the pre-penicillin era, 3 percent of patients with syphilis and 10 percent of patients with neurosyphilis had cerebrovascular syphilis (Table 21-2). Most patients with cerebrovascular syphilis are 30 to 50 years of age. Most cases occur 5 to 12 years after initial infection, which is earlier than the occurrence of paresis or tabes (Fig. 21-1), but cases have occurred after a latent period of less than 2 years (rarely, of only a few months).[12] The chronology of neurosyphilis is such that, if untreated, a patient with cerebrovascular syphilis may ultimately develop either tabes or paresis (Fig. 21-1). Also, the combination of active cerebrovascular neurosyphilis with general paresis or tabes may occur in the same patient. In the study of Merritt et al.,[12] 10 percent of the patients with cerebrovascular neurosyphilis had pupils that constricted on accommodation but not to light (Argyll Robertson pupils) but no other manifestations, at the time, of tabes or paresis.

**Symptoms and Signs.** The possibility of meningovascular syphilis should be considered when cerebrovascular accidents occur in a young adult. The onset of the symptoms is often abrupt. However, about half the cases described by Merritt et al.[12] had premonitory symptoms of headache, dizziness, insomnia, memory loss, or mood disturbances lasting for weeks or months. Psychiatric manifestations (personality and behavioral changes, slowing of mentation and speech) may be so prominent as to suggest the diagnosis of general paresis initially, until the onset of a stroke syndrome.[12,29] Among the most common manifestations are hemiparesis or hemiplegia (83 percent of cases), aphasia

(31 percent), and seizures (14 percent).[12] Among 241 patients with neurosyphilis studied at the Medical College of Virginia, adult-onset seizure disorders were prominent symptoms in 24 percent; of those with seizures, 40 percent had cerebrovascular syphilis.[30] Twelve percent of cases studied by Merritt et al.[12] had clinical evidence of more than one cerebral arterial occlusion. The most common sites of involvement, by far, were in the territory of the middle cerebral artery, but most other arteries (anterior cerebral, posterior cerebral, basilar, posterior inferior cerebellar) were occasionally occluded. The neurologic syndromes produced were comparable to those caused by arteriosclerotic thrombotic lesions, but in neurosyphilis the site of thrombosis more often involved smaller branches and produced less extensive infarcts.

Occlusion of the middle cerebral artery on the dominant side of the brain produces aphasia, contralateral hemiplegia, hemianesthesia, and homonymous hemianopia. With involvement of more distal branches, the hemiplegia and hemianesthesia affect the arm and the face more than the leg.

Occlusion of branches of the anterior cerebral artery causes contralateral hemiplegia and hemianesthesia that chiefly affect the leg. Abulia, contralateral grasp and suck reflexes, and transient mutism may also be clinical features.

Occlusion of the posterior cerebral artery results in *thalamic* (Déjérine-Roussy) *syndrome:* transient contralateral hemiparesis, contralateral severe impairment of superficial and deep sensation followed by severe spontaneous burning pain in the same area, choreoathetoid movements, and ataxia of the hand. A contralateral homonymous hemianopia is frequently observed along with thalamic syndrome.

Occlusion of the posterior inferior cerebellar or vertebral artery results in lateral medullary syndrome: contralateral loss of pain and temperature sense; ipsilateral Horner's syndrome, hoarseness, and dysphagia; ipsilateral palatal paralysis and diminished gag reflex; vestibular abnormalities (vomiting, vertigo, nystagmus); hiccup; ipsilateral ataxia of limbs; and ipsilateral impaired sense of pain over the face. Occlusion of other smaller branches of the vertebral and basilar arteries may produce a variety of brainstem syndromes.

Although distinctive occlusive cerebrovascular syndromes have been features of cerebrovascular syphilis in the past when syphilis was more likely to run its course untreated or inadequately treated, nowadays the clinical picture may be atypical. An example is that of a 64-year-old woman with a history of "drop attacks" suggesting vertebrobasilar artery disease, who was found to have positive blood and CSF serology and elevated CSF protein concentration (165 mg/dl) and cell count (40 cells per cubic millimeter). The drop attacks ceased after penicillin therapy.[31]

**Laboratory Findings.** Serum reagin and antitreponemal antibody tests are positive in meningovascular syphilis. The CSF cell count is usually between 10 and 100 cells per cubic millimeter (virtually all lymphocytes), which is in keeping with a smoldering low-grade syphilitic meningitis in patients whose clinical picture reflects primarily occlusive vascular disease. The CSF protein concentration is elevated (40 to 250 mg/dl), the colloidal gold test (if done) is usually mid-zone in type, and the CSF VDRL test is usually positive.

Angiographic changes have been reported in cerebrovascular syphilis. These include diffuse irregularity and "beading" of anterior and middle cerebral arteries and segmental (sausagelike) dilatation of the pericallosal artery.[32] In contrast to the short, irregular sites of atherosclerotic disease, the areas of arterial narrowing in cerebrovascular syphilis tend to be longer and smoother. Vascular neurosyphilis, rather than atherosclerosis, is also suggested when angiographic changes occur in the supraclinoid portion of the internal carotid artery and the proximal portions of the anterior or middle cerebral arteries, in the absence of stenotic changes at the carotid bifurcation (a common site of atherosclerosis).[33]

Computed tomography shows low-density areas with variable degrees of contrast enhancement, consistent with multifocal infarctions. Magnetic resonance imaging shows focal regions of high signal intensity on T2-weighted sequences, compatible with foci of ischemia.[34]

**Pathologic Changes.** The characteristic histologic changes of the arteritis of cerebrovascular neurosyphilis (Heubner's endarteritis) consist of infiltration by lymphocytes and plasma cells of the vasa vasorum and the adventitia (and ultimately the media) of large- and medium-sized arteries. Occlusion of the vasa vasorum results in destruction of the smooth muscle and elastic tissue of the media. Concentric proliferation of subintimal fibroblasts narrows the lumen progressively until it is occluded by thrombus formation. Infarction, subsequent scar formation, and cavitation (if the infarcted area is sizable) occur as in atherosclerotic cerebrovascular disease.

**Diagnosis and Differential Diagnosis.** The diagnosis is suggested when an acute cerebrovascular accident occurs in a young adult without a history of hypertension or findings suggestive of embolic cardiac disease (infective endocarditis, atrial thrombus, or myxoma) and when there is a positive serum VDRL test or a history of previously untreated or inadequately treated early syphilis. Since cerebrovascular syphilis is essentially always accompanied by some degree of meningitis, a lymphocytic pleocytosis in the CSF at the time of the thrombosis supports this diagnosis. A positive CSF serology is important in establishing the diagnosis. In the older age group, the problem is compounded by the greater likelihood of coexisting cerebral atherosclerosis, which may also be responsible for a stroke even though the patient has meningeal (asymptomatic) neurosyphilis.

Differential diagnosis includes other causes of stroke syndromes such as hypertension (lacunar strokes), atherosclerotic vascular disease, cerebral emboli, or various types of cerebral vasculitis. Angiographic changes in cerebral vessels in systemic lupus erythematosus may be indistinguishable from those of syphilitic arteritis, and those in polyarteritis nodosa may also be somewhat similar to those of syphilitic arteritis.[33] Spinal fluid findings will direct attention to the diagnosis of cerebrovascular syphilis.

## Meningovascular syphilis of the spinal cord

Meningovascular syphilis of the spinal cord consists principally of *syphilitic meningomyelitis* (the most common form) and *spinal vascular syphilis (acute syphilitic transverse myelitis).* Spinal syphilis has always been very rare, representing only about 3 percent of cases of neurosyphilis. It is almost always associated with cerebral involvement, but the disease of the cord may be preeminent. The basic underlying process is chronic spinal meningitis, which may result in parenchymatous degeneration of the cord directly or through the mediacy of vascular thrombosis. Thus, the picture in some cases is predominantly that of chronic meningitis with cord damage (degeneration and atrophy of peripheral myelinated fibers); in other cases the picture is that of cord infarction or myelomalacia.[35]

**Symptoms and Signs.** The onset of *syphilitic meningomyelitis* is usually gradual. It occurs after a prolonged latent period (commonly 20 to 25 years), at the same time as parenchymatous neurosyphilis might be expected. The earliest symptoms are frequently weakness or paresthesias of the legs.[12] Fever is not a feature. The weakness progresses to paraparesis or paraplegia, which is often asymmetric. The other principal symptoms are urinary and fecal incontinence and variable sensory disorders (pain, paresthesias) in the legs. Although the process may occasionally appear stationary, complete remissions (such as those that characterize multiple sclerosis) do not occur in the untreated patients. On examination the legs are weak and spastic, and deep tendon reflexes are hyperactive; ankle clonus is present. Abdominal reflexes are absent, and extensor plantar responses can be elicited. A sensory level is present in about one-third of patients. The most frequent sensory abnormalities are loss of position and vibratory sense in the lower extremities. The clinical picture may be more complex when meningomyelitis develops in the course of tabes or general paresis, or when spinal artery thrombosis supervenes, changing the spastic paraparesis to a flaccid paraplegia. Nowadays, the full-blown picture may not present itself, since antibiotic therapy can arrest progression of the process.[36]

The classic manifestations of *spinal vascular syphilis* are those of a transection of the spinal cord, usually at a thoracic level: abrupt onset of flaccid paraplegia, sensory level on the trunk, and urinary retention.[12] The patient is not febrile. Most cases occur at about the same time after initial infection as does cerebrovascular syphilis. In some patients, transection of the cord is incomplete. After the state of "spinal shock" abates, the clinical picture becomes one of spastic paraplegia with extensor plantar responses and automatic emptying of the bladder. Arterial occlusion does not always produce a spinal transection syndrome. Occasionally only a portion of the cord is infarcted, as in Brown-Séquard hemisection syndrome (ipsilateral paralysis and loss of position and vibratory sense below the level of the lesion, and contralateral loss of pain and temperature sense below the level of the lesion).

**Laboratory Findings.** Blood serologic (nontreponemal antibody) tests are regularly positive except in burned-out or old, treated cases. CSF examination discloses mild pleocytosis (10 to 300 lymphocytes per cubic millimeter), mildly elevated protein concentration (45 to 250 mg/dl), normal dynamics, and a positive VDRL test or similar serologic test for syphilis, except in burned-out or old, treated cases.[12] If a myelogram is performed, no abnormalities are disclosed.[37]

**Diagnosis and Differential Diagnosis.** The diagnosis of syphilitic spinal thrombosis is made on the clinical picture of an abrupt flaccid paraplegia developing in a patient with a consistent spinal fluid formula and positive blood and CSF serologies. Other causes of a picture of acute transverse myelitis must be distinguished. These include anterior spinal artery occlusion (secondary to dissecting aortic aneurysm or vasculitis), spinal epidural abscess or infective granuloma, epidural hemorrhage, and cord compression by metastatic tumor or by vertebral destruction due to osteomyelitis. Myelography or CT scanning with the newer third-generation instruments are necessary to evaluate the presence of epidural block by external masses. Roentgenograms of the spine, radionuclide scans, and CT scans can reveal vertebral body osteomyelitis and vertebral displacement. Infectious polyneuritis may resemble this clinical picture as well; the absence of early bladder involvement, the absence of cells in the CSF, and a negative serologic test for syphilis would be expected with this process.

Syphilitic meningomyelitis is of more gradual onset. Differential diagnosis may include multiple sclerosis and subacute combined degeneration. The latter is usually distinguished by associated achlorhydria, macrocytic anemia, and lack of CSF pleocytosis. Positive serologic tests of blood and CSF are essential in making the diagnosis of syphilitic meningomyelitis.

## PARENCHYMATOUS NEUROSYPHILIS

### General paresis

General paresis (also known as paretic neurosyphilis, dementia paralytica, and general paralysis of the insane) is a meningoencephalitis associated with direct invasion of the cerebrum by *T. pallidum.* The clinical illness is a chronic process that evolves over many years and declares itself in middle to late adult life. Untreated, the course is progressively downhill, terminating in death. This form of late syphilis develops 15 to 20 years after initial infection. Prior to World War II, patients with this disease made up 5 to 10 percent of all first admissions of psychotic patients to psychiatric hospitals.[38,39] Although this disease is now rare,[40] it appears to account for about the same percentage of the cases of neurosyphilis as formerly: 12 percent in the Boston City Hospital series in the 1930s[12] and 10 percent in the series from Medical College of Virginia Hospitals from 1965 to 1970.[30]

**Symptoms and Signs.** The clinical picture is that of a combination of psychiatric manifestations and neurologic findings. It may mimic almost any type of psychiatric or neurological disorder. The illness is commonly insidious in onset but may occasionally become suddenly evident. The early features are usually of a psychiatric nature, and the course of illness is that of a dementing process. Early symptoms include gradual memory loss, impairment of intellectual function, and personality changes (Table 21-3). As the disease progresses, these symptoms are magnified and others appear: defects in judgment, emotional lability, delusions, and inappropriate social or moral behavior. Grandiose delusions and megalomania, although dramatic manifestations traditionally considered classic features of general paresis, occur in only 10 to 20 percent of cases.[41] These delusions, often accompanied by hypomania, may take many forms, including those of great wealth or political power, extraordinary physical or intellectual prowess, or inappropriate social or political importance. Depression has been reported in some studies as the predominant presenting feature and the most common initial diagnosis in patients with paresis.[40]

**Table 21-3. Symptoms of General Paresis**

| Early | Late |
|---|---|
| Irritability | Defective judgment |
| Memory loss | Emotional lability (depression, agitation, euphoria) |
| Personality changes | Lack of insight |
| Impaired capacity to concentrate and learn | Confusion and disorientation |
| Carelessness in appearance | Delusions of grandeur |
| Headache | Paranoia |
| Insomnia | Seizures |

Adult-onset seizures, noted in 15 to 20 percent of patients,[41] may be the initial manifestation of paresis and may bring to medical attention a patient who has shown minimal or no evidence of mental aberrations to his or her family. In patients with paresis of apparently sudden clinical onset, the earliest indication of the disease may be seizures, transient ischemic attacks, or an apparent stroke with loss of consciousness (*apoplectiform attacks*), followed by hemiparesis, monoplegia, or aphasia. After such episodes, persisting confusion or psychotic behavior characteristic of paresis becomes apparent.

The most common neurologic findings in general paresis are pupillary abnormalities; lack of facial expression (a characteristic flattening of the facial lines, or *paralytic facies*); tremors of the lips, tongue ("trombone tongue"), facial muscles, and fingers; and impaired handwriting and speech (Table 21-4). The earliest speech disorder is faulty enunciation and slurring of consonants, often best elicited with the use of test phrases such as "Methodist Episcopal" and "Around the rugged rock the ragged rascal ran." Speech becomes progressively thicker, and the problem may be compounded by the development of dysnomia or global aphasia. Pupillary abnormalities are common in paresis and may be present in other forms of neurosyphilis. A true Argyll Robertson pupil is not frequent in early paresis; at this stage the pupils may be large (rather than miotic), unequal, and sluggishly reactive to light and accommodation. Over the course of months, normal pupils may change to the Argyll Robertson type defined by the following characteristics: (1) the retina is sensitive (i.e., eye is not blind); (2) pupils are small, fixed, and do not react to strong light; (3) pupils react normally to convergence-accommodation; (4) mydriatics (atropine) fail to dilate pupil fully; and (5) pupils do not dilate on painful stimuli. Argyll Robertson pupils are observed more frequently in tabes than in paresis.

As the untreated paretic process advances, apathy, hypotonia, unsteadiness, dementia, and physical deterioration become the major elements in the clinical picture. Frequent focal or generalized seizures accompany progressive deterioration and eventuate in a bedridden, paralyzed, incontinent state. The term *Lissauer's dementia paralytica* has been used to describe a small group of atypical cases of paresis which showed focal neurological signs and at autopsy exhibited striking atrophy of certain cerebral convolutions,[12] particularly in the frontal and temporal lobes. Such patients initially had focal seizures followed by hemiparesis, hemianopia, or aphasia which subsequently cleared. With repetition of the seizures, the postictal neurologic changes gradually became permanent.

**Table 21-4. Neurological Signs of General Paresis***

| Sign | Percent |
|---|---|
| *Common* | |
| Pupillary abnormalities | 57 |
| Argyll Robertson pupils | 26 |
| Slurred speech | 28 |
| Expressionless facies | — |
| Tremors (tongue, face, hands) | 18 |
| Impaired handwriting | — |
| Reflex abnormalities (↑ or ↓) | 52 |
| *Uncommon* | |
| Focal signs | 1–2 |
| Eye muscle palsies | — |
| Optic atrophy | 2 |
| Extensor plantar responses | — |

*Where percentages are noted they are derived from compilation of 134 cases from two series studies dealing with patients observed in the period 1950–1969[40,41]

SOURCE: After K Dewhurst;[40] K Dawson-Butterworth and PEM Heathcote[41]

As noted earlier, the various forms of neurosyphilis do not necessarily exist as pure entities. Thus, in occasional patients with paresis, neurologic examination might reveal absent deep tendon reflexes in the lower extremities and loss of position and vibratory senses.

The duration of untreated paresis, fron the onset of detectable mental symptoms till death, has ranged from a few months, in cases of sudden onset, to 4 or 5 years.[12] Uncommonly, spontaneous but transitory remissions in mental symptomatology have occurred but have not altered the ultimate evolution of the disorder. In the pre-penicillin era, treatment of paresis with malaria plus arsenicals benefited 33 to 50 percent of cases by arresting progression of the disease and allowing some type of occupational activity. The shorter the duration and the milder the symptoms at the institution of therapy, the better the prognosis. The introduction of penicillin therapy dramatically improved the capability to halt progression of paresis (see Management, below).

Communicating hydrocephalus has complicated a few cases of general paresis and, despite clearing of CSF abnormalities after treatment with large doses of penicillin, has accounted for either lack of clinical improvement or progressive deterioration. The patients showed gait apraxia, akinetic mutism, incontinence, and pyramidal tract signs along with severe dementia.[42] Isotope cisternograms showed early ventricular entry of the radionuclide and absence of parasagittal radioactivity. CSF shunting produced immediate improvement in several cases. Impairment of CSF absorption by chronic meningitis and meningeal fibrosis in general paresis appears to be the pathogenesis of this process.

**Laboratory Findings.** The blood nontreponemal serology has been reported positive in 95 to 100 percent of cases of paresis.[12,41,43] In a study emphasizing the current atypical presentation of neurosyphilis, only 48.5 percent of 241 patients with a diagnosis of neurosyphilis had a positive nontreponemal serology.[30] However, 56.3 percent of the patients had a history of earlier treatment for syphilis, and only 12 of the 241 patients had the clear-cut clinical picture of paresis. Thus, this series may not be as discordant with other studies as it appears, since prior treatment may have been sufficient to induce seroconversion (without preventing the subsequent development of neurosyphilis) and the majority of cases of atypical neurosyphilis may not have represented formes frustes of paresis. The serum FTA-ABS test is uniformly positive in patients with paresis.

Abnormalities of the CSF are found in essentially all cases of untreated paresis.[12] The characteristic CSF findings, the so-called paretic formula, consist of (1) normal or, occasionally, slightly increased pressure; (2) lymphocytic pleocytosis (usually 8 to 100 lymphocytes per cubic millimeter); (3) increased protein concentration (usually 50 to 100 mg/dl); (4) increased globulin concentration; (5) positive colloidal gold reaction, when performed (80 percent first-zone type, e.g., 5555432100; 20 percent mid-zone type); (6) normal or, occasionally, mildly reduced glucose; and (7) reactive nontreponemal test. The CSF nontreponemal tests show a very high specificity, and false-positive VDRL test is extremely unusual. Thus, a positive CSF VDRL test is very strong evidence for a diagnosis of neurosyphilis. However, CSF nontreponemal tests may have a sensitivity of less than 100 percent. CSF Wassermann reactions have been reported negative in some patients with clinically diagnosed neurosyphilis (occasionally general paresis, but more often tabes).[2,41,44] It is unclear whether subsequent repetition of the tests or use of the current, more sensitive nontreponemal tests would have shown positive results in those patients with paresis and a negative CSF Wassermann reaction. A patient with a clinical diagnosis of meningovascular syphilis, evidence of dementia, and a negative CSF VDRL test result was found at autopsy to have evidence of neurosyphilis.[45] From the brief description given, it is not clear whether general paresis was either the clinical or the postmortem diagnosis. Another patient with a clinical diagnosis of general paresis and an initially negative (but subsequently positive) serum VDRL test had nonreactive CSF VDRL tests on three CSF specimens. Brain biopsy revealed a meningoencephalitis with neuronal degeneration and increased numbers of astrocytes and microglial cells in the cortex. A spirochete, stained with indirect fluorescent antibody, was demonstrated in the biopsy.[46] Paresis with a negative CSF examination may occur in a patient whose neurosyphilitic process has been arrested by treatment, leaving persistent mental changes.

To enhance the sensitivity of serologic tests of the CSF in suspected cases of neurosyphilis, the CSF FTA test has been studied recently.[47–49] Although results indicated that the FTA tests were more frequently positive than other CSF tests in all stages of syphilis, there are problems with the specificity of this test. False-positive reactions occur in 0.5 to 4.5 percent.[50] In addition, a reactive CSF FTA-ABS result may not indicate active neurosyphilis, since the reactivity may be produced by diffusion of serum immunoglobulins into the CSF.[51] Also, contamination of a CSF specimen with very small amounts of FTA-positive blood can produce a false-positive CSF FTA test.[52] For these reasons the interpretation of a positive CSF FTA test is unclear.[53] At present, a positive CSF FTA test alone in a patient with neurologic findings of uncertain nature does not establish a diagnosis of neurosyphilis.

Nontreponemal and treponemal test results have a major role in diagnosis of neurosyphilis. However, certain considerations may make interpretation of test results difficult in an individual case:

1. VDRL seroreactivity is present in only about 70 percent of patients with late (cardiovascular and nervous system) syphilis; in a study of neurosyphilis, including many cases with atypical presentations reported in 1972,[30] only about 50 percent of patients had a positive nontreponemal serology.
2. CSF VDRL may be negative in occasional clinically characteristic cases of neurosyphilis,[45,46,54] and the entire CSF analysis (VDRL, cell count, protein concentration) may be normal in some patients with reactive FTA-ABS (serum and CSF) thought to have clinical neurosyphilis.[54]
3. Although abnormalities occur in the CSF of 25 to 40 percent of patients with untreated secondary syphilis,[5,6] indicating early involvement of the nervous system, treatment with penicillin usually prevents any progression to symptomatic neurosyphilis. Such treatment would cause reversion of the serum VDRL to negative, but the serum FTA-ABS would remain positive. Would the transient initial (asymptomatic) invasion of the meninges prior to penicillin therapy for secondary syphilis induce antitreponemal antibody synthesis locally in the central nervous system? Further, would such CSF FTA-ABS antibodies persist thereafter despite eradication of nervous system infection, much as serum FTA-ABS reactivity persists after successful treatment of early syphilis?
4. CSF FTA-ABS may be reactive as a result of diffusion of serum immunoglobulins into the CSF, or as a result of contamination of the CSF by a small amount of FTA-ABS positive blood, rather than because of local antibody synthesis in the central nervous system. What should the physician conclude concerning an older adult with (or without) a history of prior treated early syphilis who years later has a reactive serum FTA-ABS (or TPHA), atypical neurologic or psychiatric findings, and CSF abnormalities (minimal pleocytosis and slightly elevated protein) that include reactive FTA-ABS or TPHA? Is this a patient whose serum (and CSF) treponemal test reactivity merely represents prior infection and whose current neurologic syndrome has a nonsyphilitic etiology, or is this a patient with active neurosyphilis lacking serum and CSF VDRL reactivity? The matter is controversial and opposing views have been stated.[54–57] Evaluation depends largely on interpretation of the CSF treponemal test results.

New approaches, not yet widely applied clinically, may help resolve the dilemma. Intrathecal antibody synthesis, exhibiting oligoclonal characteristics, would be consonant with the diagnosis of neurosyphilis. Although a CSF-IgG index (CSF IgG:serum IgG/CSF albumin:serum albumin) of >0.7 is indicative of IgG synthesis within the central nervous system,[58,59] it would be consistent not only with neurosyphilis but also with a variety of other infectious or inflammatory processes. Specificity would be provided by demonstration that intrathecal IgG (and IgM) production consisted of antitreponemal antibodies. An intrathecal *Treponema pallidum* antibody (ITPA) index

$$\frac{\text{TPHA-IgG titer in CSF}}{\text{total IgG in mg in CSF}} \Big/ \frac{\text{TPHA-IgG titer in serum}}{\text{total IgG in mg in serum}}$$

can provide such specificity.[60] A TPHA index

$$\text{CSF-TPHA titer} \Big/ \frac{\text{CSF albumin (mg/dl)} \times 10^3}{\text{serum albumin (mg/dl)}}$$

has been applied to the same end.[61] Evidence for intrathecal antitreponemal antibody synthesis can also be provided when the serum/CSF ratio of TPHA is at least four times lower than the corresponding ratio for adenovirus hemagglutinating antibody. A CSF *T. pallidum*–specific IgM ELISA has been shown to have a sensitivity of 100 percent (on a small number of patients with symptomatic neurosyphilis) and a specificity of 98 percent.[62] However, patients with asymptomatic neurosyphilis are nonreactive in the test. In another study, local synthesis within the central nervous system of antitreponemal IgM antibodies was indicated in 19 patients with untreated neurosyphilis by CSF IgM ELISA antibody levels/mg total IgM in CSF that were 3- to 75-fold higher than corresponding serum levels.[63]

The EEG is abnormal in 80 percent of patients with paresis. The CT scan has recently been used to evaluate cerebral syphilis including paresis.[64,65] In one patient with clinical paresis, a CT scan showed extensive regions of decreased attenuation of the cerebral white matter, particularly in the frontal lobes and paraventricular areas of the parietal lobes. Enlargement of cortical sulci and associated ventricular dilation were also present.[64] From these preliminary findings it would seem that neurosyphilis can show the CT-scan pattern observed in demyelinating disorders. In another patient exhibiting clinical features, particularly of meningovascular syphilis but also of tabes and possibly of paresis, a CT scan showed cortical atrophy and multiple areas of hypodensity in both cerebellar hemispheres and in the brainstem (these findings are consistent with infarctions).[64] Multiple nodular enhancing lesions on CT at the base of the brain in another patient with meningovascular syphilis showed complete clearing 3 months after a 10-day course of intravenous penicillin.[66] Godt et al.[65] found both enhancing lesions (gummas) and generalized cortical and subcortical atrophy in several patients with neurosyphilis.

Chest roentgenograms may show widening of the aorta, consistent with syphilitic aortitis, which occasionally coexists with parenchymatous neurosyphilis.

**Pathologic Changes.** Grossly, the brain in general paresis shows varying degrees of thickening of the meninges, consistent with chronic meningitis and fibrosis. Cerebral atrophy is prominent. The frontal pole and the tips of the temporal lobes are particularly involved. Demyelinization of cerebral white matter is often present and usually correlates with the extent of cortical neuron loss.[67] A characteristic finding is that of granular ependymitis, formed of whorls of subependymal astrocytes. Microscopically, the changes consist of (1) meningeal and perivascular infiltration with lymphocytes and plasma cells, (2) degeneration and loss of nerve cells, (3) proliferation of microglia and astrocytes, (4) iron deposition in vessel walls and in microglia, and (5) the presence of spirochetes in brain tissue (demonstrated by Dieterle silver stain, animal inoculation, or indirect FTA test).

**Diagnosis and Differential Diagnosis.** The diagnosis is based on the clinical picture, which is readily recognizable in its full-blown form but is more difficult to define when atypical or incomplete, plus characteristic spinal fluid abnormalities. Although the CSF is reputedly abnormal in all untreated cases of general paresis, the same changes may occur during the course of other types of neurosyphilis. Thus, the combination of preexisting CSF changes of asymptomatic syphilitic meningitis with a variety of organic brain syndromes may be misdiagnosed as general paresis. These syndromes include cerebral tumor, subdural hematoma, cerebral arteriosclerosis, Alzheimer's disease, multiple sclerosis, senile dementia, and chronic alcoholism. The findings on CT scan, the presence of pupillary changes, and a history of drug or alcohol abuse are helpful in correct diagnosis. Hallucinations are prominent in delirium tremens but are rare in general paresis. However, alcoholic deterioration and Korsakoff's psychosis may present a picture of memory loss, inappropriate behavior, mood swings, and poor judgment that is difficult to distinguish from paresis.

An adult-onset seizure disorder may be a manifestation of paresis or of an atypical form of neurosyphilis. Paresis can be excluded when CSF abnormalities are absent. When CSF changes of neurosyphilis are present, the question becomes one of whether the seizures represent epilepsy in a patient with asymptomatic neurosyphilis or whether they are the manifestations of syphilitic brain injury. The presence of focal neurologic findings in patients with neurosyphilis-produced seizures helps to resolve the question. The combination of seizures and focal findings may be found in both general paresis and meningovascular syphilis. Distinguishing between the two is probably not very important, since both are treated with penicillin.

## Tabes dorsalis

Tabes dorsalis has become uncommon, reflecting the overall decline in neurosyphilis of all types. In the prepenicillin era it accounted for about one-third of patients with neurosyphilis.[12] Among several hundred patients with neurosyphilis treated in neurologic clinics in Poland from 1956 to 1965, tabes dorsalis was the most frequent diagnosis (43.6 percent). However, in 60 percent of the tabetic patients the process appeared to have "burned out" (i.e., there was an absence of CSF abnormalities) either spontaneously or as a result of the previous use of antibiotics in the treatment of intercurrent illnesses.[68] In a study of late complications of syphilis involving about one-third of the population of Finland between 1963 and 1968, 66 cases of neurosyphilis were identified; of these, two-thirds involved tabes dorsalis.[69] In the 1960s, 30 cases of neurosyphilis (10 of tabes) were seen in one regional neurological center in England over a 3½-year period (1964 to 1968); over the next 8½ years only 16 cases (4 of tabes) were encountered.[43] At present, a patient with far-advanced tabes dorsalis is a rarity in most developed countries.

The onset of symptoms of tabes occurs in the majority of untreated patients in the fifth and sixth decades of life after an average latent period of 20 to 25 years.

**Symptoms and Signs.** The early clinical features of tabes are lightning pains, paresthesias, diminished deep tendon reflexes (manifestations of posterior root and posterior column dysfunction), and poor pupillary responses to light. In more advanced stages of the disease, other symptoms and signs become prominent (Table 21-5). *Lightning pains* are sudden paroxysms of severe stabbing pains lasting for a few minutes at a time. They usually occur in the lower extremities but may be felt anywhere on the body. They may occur at long intervals or may persist in attacks lasting for several days at a time. Relief of such pains may be provided by treatment with carbamazepine (200 mg orally, two to four times daily).[70] Paresthesias are frequently felt on the legs or trunk. Hyperesthesia may be present in the areas involved by lightning pains; such areas may serve as trigger zones that precipitate bouts of pain when touched.

*Visceral crises* are related to lightning pains, tending to recur in attacks of marked severity that may mimic acute surgical emergencies. The most common form is a gastric crisis consisting of intense epigastric pain, nausea, and vomiting. Intestinal crises (abdominal pain and diarrhea), rectal crises (painful tenesmus), and laryngeal crises (pain in larynx, hoarseness, stridor) are rare.

**Table 21-5. Symptoms and Signs of Tabes Dorsalis***

| | Percent |
|---|---|
| *Symptoms* | |
| Lightning pains | 75 |
| Ataxia | 42 |
| Bladder disturbances | 33 |
| Paresthesias | 24 |
| Visceral crises | 18 |
| Visual loss (optic atrophy) | 16 |
| Rectal incontinence | 14 |
| *Signs* | |
| Pupillary abnormalities | 94 |
| Argyll Robertson pupils | 48 |
| Absent ankle jerks | 94 |
| Absent knee jerks | 81 |
| Romberg's sign | 55 |
| Impaired vibratory sense | 52 |
| Impaired position sense | 45 |
| Impaired touch and pain sense | 13 |
| Ocular palsies | 10 |
| Charcot's joints | 7 |

*Data from 150 cases.
SOURCE: After HH Merritt et al.[12]

In some patients, impotence and urinary retention or dribbling, resulting from an insensitive, hypotonic bladder, may be early symptoms of sacral root dysfunction.

Other symptoms become evident with more advanced tabes: broad-based, stamping gait, which becomes worse in the dark; diminished vision due to optic atrophy; Charcot's joint (unstable, painless, uninflamed, markedly enlarged joint with overproduction of bone due to repeated trauma to this anesthetic structure); and mal perforant (a painless penetrating trophic ulcer on the plantar surface at the base of a toe).

Sluggish pupillary reactivity to light is an early finding in tabes; true Argyll Robertson pupil is a later feature of the disease. Loss of vibration sense and inability to feel passive movement in joints are among the first detectable signs of this disease. Other sensory abnormalities include loss of deep pain perception (e.g., on forceful pinching of the Achilles tendon) and development of patchy areas of hypalgesia and hypesthesia over the trunk and extremities (Hitzig's zones).

Diminished or absent knee and ankle reflexes are almost essential diagnostic findings in tabes (Table 21-5). Muscular power is usually well maintained until the late stages. Plantar responses are flexor; if a Babinski sign is present, it indicates the coexistence of meningovascular syphilis, general paresis, or some unrelated disorder of the central nervous system. Ataxia is evident on heel-to-shin and finger-to-nose testing.

Involvement of cranial nerves (particularly the second, third, and sixth) is often overlooked in tabes. Primary optic atrophy appears as sharply defined, grayish white optic disks with conspicuous physiologic cupping, visible lamina cribrosa, and narrowed retinal arteries. If untreated, visual loss progresses to blindness over months to years. The changes of syphilitic optic atrophy are irreversible. Oculomotor nerve palsy was observed in 10 percent of cases of tabes reported by Merritt et al.[12] The ptosis and flabbiness of facial muscles probably contributes in a large measure to the so-called tabetic facies. Ptosis is due to third cranial nerve weakness and is likely to be bilateral. The presence of ptosis may suggest the possibility of myasthenia, but it is not aggravated by fatigue or ameliorated by edrophonium chloride (Tensilon).[30] Divergent strabismus may also result from third cranial nerve palsy. Oculomotor weakness is thought to be due to an associated basilar meningitis. This would account for its occasional improvement after penicillin therapy. Eighth cranial nerve involvement (hearing loss with or without accompanying vestibular symptomatology) is not uncommon.

The clinical course of untreated tabes usually evolves over a period of years. Early manifestations are lightning pains and paresthesias, decreased or absent reflexes, oculomotor palsies, visceral crises, urinary incontinence, and sluggish or nonreactive pupils. Ataxia occurs in the moderately advanced stage of tabes. In the untreated patient the time from the onset of tabes to the development of ataxia may be 6 months to 25 years; the longer the duration of the preataxic phase, the slower the subsequent course. In the prepenicillin era, far-advanced tabes was observed with complete incapacitation due to blindness, ataxia, deafness, and loss of bladder control. In some late cases, Charcot's joints present problems because of joint deformity, instability, and susceptibility to fractures. The spine (particularly the lumbar spine) may be the site of a Charcot joint (Charcot's spine, tabetic spinal arthropathy). The osseous changes include dense irregular sclerosis, large parrot-beak osteophytes, scoliosis, and disk-space narrowing.[71] Although the lesion itself is painless, distressing pain may be produced by impingement of the hypertrophic bone or by a disk protruding on posterior nerve roots.[72]

Tabes may burn out with time, even without treatment. Lightning pains may persist even when early treatment has been successful; their presence, therefore, does not indicate continued syphilitic infection. Antibiotic treatment cannot reverse the extensive changes of advanced disease.

**Laboratory Findings.** The laboratory findings in tabetic neurosyphilis may be quite variable, depending on the stage of tabes, whether partial or full treatment has been administered in the past, and whether the process has spontaneously burned out. In the prepenicillin era, negative blood Wassermann reactions were reported in 40 percent of cases in one series studied;[2] another study reported negative Wassermann or Hinton test reactions in 12 percent of cases.[12] In a more recent study (conducted from 1963 to 1968) of 40 patients with tabes, 10 percent had negative blood VDRL titers.[69] In a 1972 study of seven patients with long-standing tabes, the blood Wassermann reaction was negative in six patients. All but one patient had been treated repeatedly in previous years but continued to have lightning pains and other manifestations of tabes. The one patient with the positive serology was the one untreated individual.[70] The treponemal serologic tests remain positive.

The CSF findings among 100 patients with tabes in the prepenicillin era, including a large number of patients with old, arrested cases, were reported by Merritt et al.:[12] (1) cell count was normal in 50 percent, and lymphocytic pleocytosis (5 to 160 lymphocytes per cubic millimeter) was found in 50 percent (practically all untreated cases); (2) globulin concentration was increased; (3) protein concentration was elevated (45 to 100 mg/dl) in 50 percent; (4) colloidal gold test curve of mid-zone type was found in 55 percent; and (5) the Wassermann or the Hinton test was positive in 72 percent. Normal CSF can be found in the late stages of treated or burned out tabes in a patient who continues to have lightning pains and Charcot's joints; this finding reflects the irreversible damage already produced in the spinal cord and dorsal roots.

**Diagnosis and Differential Diagnosis.** A clinical diagnosis of tabes is most likely in a patient with lightning pains and ataxia who exhibits findings of absent deep tendon reflexes, Argyll Robertson pupils, and a positive Romberg sign. Early and atypical cases present greater problems in diagnosis, and only the results of serologic testing and spinal fluid examination may lead to the correct diagnosis.[43] A mixed clinical picture of taboparesis may also be a source of diagnostic confusion. As noted earlier, blood and CSF serologic changes may revert to normal in treated and burned-out cases with continuing symptoms.

Differential diagnosis includes a variety of neurologic disorders. Although knee and ankle jerks may be lost in meningovascular syphilis of the spinal cord, lightning pains and pupillary changes are not usually present; ultimately, hyperactive reflexes and extensor plantar responses develop. Adie's syndrome (absent deep tendon reflexes and myotonic pupil) can be distinguished from tabes by the fact that the pupil is not miotic. This syndrome also lacks the lightning pains and ataxia of tabes, and serologic tests are negative and CSF examination is normal. Diabetic neuropathy may mimic tabes (diabetic pseudotabes) by producing sluggish pupillary reactivity, ptosis, pains, and ataxia and by absent deep tendon reflexes. However, in diabetic and other types of peripheral neuropathy, the pain is burning in character rather than shooting, as is typical of tabes and the serologic findings are negative. Combined system disease is similar to tabes in producing ataxia and bladder disturbances, but lightning pains are not a feature. Extensor plantar responses are found in combined system disease but not in tabes.

### Optic atrophy

Syphilitic optic atrophy, with the same ocular manifestations as occur in tabes dorsalis, may appear as an isolated manifestation of neurosyphilis.[73] The usual symptoms are those of progressive visual loss involving first one eye and then the other. As in cases of tabes, CSF abnormalities are usually present in the untreated patient. In addition to occurring as an isolated manifestation of neurosyphilis without clinical evidence of prior ocular inflammation, optic atrophy may result from prior syphilitic optic neuritis (see Current Atypical Presentations of Neurosyphilis). The visual evoked response (VER) may make it possible to distinguish primary from postneuritic optic atrophy on the basis of a normal latency in the former.[74] Penicillin treatment can usually prevent further progression of visual loss.

## GUMMAS OF THE NERVOUS SYSTEM

### Cerebral gummas

Intracerebral gummas are extremely rare; only one was encountered among 676 cases of neurosyphilis at the Boston City Hospital over a 15-year period in the prepenicillin era.[12] The features are those of a cerebral neoplasm, brain abscess, or tuberculoma; the diagnosis is usually made when the patient is operated on for a suspected intracranial mass lesion. A gumma has been described in a patient with the clinical picture of syphilitic meningitis.[75] A low-density nonenhancing area was observed by CT scan in the right frontal region, and on biopsy this showed coagulation necrosis with a surrounding infiltrate of round cells and giant cells; these observations are consistent with a gumma. The gumma was clinically asymptomatic in this patient. The clinical course is subacute. CSF findings include mild lymphocytic pleocytosis (30 to 150 cells per cubic millimeter), increased pressure, increased protein, and positive nontreponemal serology. Angiographic findings are similar to those of other cerebral inflammatory processes; there is a hypervascular blush zone surrounding the focal area of gummatous necrosis.[76]

### Gumma of the spinal cord

Gumma of the spinal cord is fundamentally a granuloma of the meninges compressing the cord. The clinical picture is that of a cord tumor: root pains, spastic paraplegia, urinary and fecal incontinence, and loss of sensation below the lesion. The progression is subacute. The CSF findings consist of dynamic block, markedly elevated protein (over 350 mg/dl), and a positive nontreponemal serologic test.

## CONGENITAL NEUROSYPHILIS

### Classification and chronology

Symptomatic congenital neurosyphilis is very rare now because of early treatment of the infected pregnant mother or of the congenitally infected infant diagnosed at birth before overt central nervous system disease has become evident. Invasion of the CNS probably occurs during the first few months or years; it is the same meningovascular process observed in acquired syphilis. Asymptomatic involvement of the nervous system may occur in up to 60 percent of cases of untreated congenital syphilis.[77] The same syndromes described in acquired syphilis also occur in the congenital form of infection; as in the acquired form, overlap is frequent. The chronology is also roughly comparable: (1) *meningitis* between the third and twelfth months of infancy, (2) *meningovascular neurosyphilis* during the first 2 years of life, (3) *paresis or tabes* usually in adolescence but at any time from 6 to 21 years of age. One or more of the features of congenital syphilis are evident in most patients with congenital neurosyphilis.

### Congenital syphilitic meningitis

The clinical manifestations of congenital syphilitic meningitis are similar to those of pyogenic meningitis in infants. The onset may be insidious, and attention is not drawn to the illness until a seizure occurs. The neck may or may not be stiff, enlargement of the head and bulging fontanelles may become evident, and palsies of the third, sixth, and seventh cranial nerves may develop. Complications include communicating hydrocephalus, severe mental retardation, and blindness, particularly if the infant is not treated promptly. The CSF findings include lymphocytic pleocytosis (250 to 500 cells per cubic millimeter), elevated protein concentration (50 to 200 mg/dl), and a positive serologic test for syphilis.

### Congenital meningovascular syphilis

Congenital meningovascular syphilis represents a continuing smoldering meningitis with accompanying chronic arteritis and occlusion of cerebral arteries. The arteritis is the main element in the clinical syndrome resulting in hemiplegia, hemianopia, and seizures. The CSF findings are mild lymphocytic pleocytosis, mild protein elevation, and positive serology.

### Congenital paresis (juvenile paresis)

Congenital paresis often develops in children with defective mental or physical growth since infancy, but 60 percent of the cases studied by Menninger[78] showed normal mental development until the onset of symptoms at puberty. The earliest changes are in personality, behavior, and intelligence; the changes may develop insidiously or appear suddenly. Forgetfulness, indifference, stubbornness, and irritability become prominent as behavior becomes erratic and schoolwork deteriorates. Progressive dementia becomes the major feature. If the child was mentally retarded from infancy, the mental deficiency becomes more profound. Neurologic symptoms accompany these mental changes. Seizures occur in half of the cases. As in the adult form, tremors, choreiform movements, dysarthria, and incoordination appear. Sucking and grasp reflexes may be present. Pupils are usually irregular and dilated, and they fail to respond to light (and sometimes to accommodation). Optic atrophy and chorioretinitis are frequent. Hyperactive tendon reflexes and extensor plantar responses become evident as the disease advances.[12,79] The CSF changes are the same as those in adult paresis.

The clinical picture and course may mimic that of subacute sclerosing panencephalitis (SSPE). The positive blood and CSF serology in paresis and the high level of measles antibody in the CSF in SSPE serve to distinguish between these diagnoses. Treatment, even with penicillin, often produces no changes in the clinical picture, even though the CSF pleocytosis may be eliminated and the protein level reduced. Occasionally, a patient may exhibit some limited clinical improvement after antibiotic treatment.[80]

### Congenital tabes

Congenital tabes is less frequent than paresis. The early symptoms are loss of vision and incontinence. Lightning pains, which are so common in adult tabes, are much rarer in the congenital form. Gross ataxia is unusual. Fixed dilated pupils, as in congenital paresis, are almost always present; optic atrophy and cranial nerve palsies (particularly involving extraocular muscles) are also frequent. Absent deep tendon reflexes and impaired position and vibration sense are usually found on examination. The CSF changes are similar to those in acquired tabes. The clinical course is usually slowly progressive and more benign than in adult tabes.

## CURRENT ATYPICAL PRESENTATIONS OF NEUROSYPHILIS

During the past two decades, as the incidence of neurosyphilis has continued to decline, attention has been drawn to unusual patterns and atypical presentations of this disease.[30,31,81,82] One reason for this may be decreased familiarity among physicians with early and less frequent manifestations of neurosyphilis than was formerly the case. It also is possible that the clinical features and the course of neurosyphilis have been modified by the use of inadequate doses of penicillin administered for the treatment of early or late syphilis or for the treatment of intercurrent illnesses during the latent stage of syphilis. Patients have been described (1) whose only clinical features were blurring of vision, CSF changes (slight lymphocytic pleocytosis and a positive nontreponemal serologic test), and Argyll Robertson pupils (which disappeared after antisyphilitic therapy);[83] or (2) whose findings consisted of isolated bilateral oculomotor nerve paresis, positive serologic findings in blood and CSF, and minimal CSF pleocytosis;[84] or (3) whose only findings consisted of sudden tinnitus, deafness, dizziness, and positive VDRL and FTA reactions in both blood and CSF.[36]

Hooshmand et al. emphasized the frequency with which atypical symptoms or findings occurred among 241 cases of neurosyphilis diagnosed in one medical center between 1965 and 1970.[30] Since the cases described often did not have the full constellation of features characteristic of classical neurosyphilis (Argyll Robertson pupils, lightning pains, Charcot's joints), the diagnostic standards employed in this study are of paramount importance. They included one or another of the following sets of criteria: (1) positive blood FTA-ABS serology along with neurologic or ophthalmologic findings suggestive of neurosyphilis, (2) unexplained neurological illness with positive blood and CSF FTA-ABS tests and CSF showing more than five white blood cells per cubic millimeter, or (3) positive FTA-ABS results in blood and CSF in patients with progressive neurologic diseases in whom other etiologic considerations had been excluded. Thus, the diagnosis of neurosyphilis depended on the clinical evaluation of symptoms and signs, which individually are not pathognomonic, and the results of serologic tests and CSF examination. The most prominent symptoms, which occurred in about one-quarter of the patients in this group, were those of an adult-onset seizure disorder. The seizure disorder was accompanied by a few manifestations of meningovascular syphilis somewhat more often than by incomplete pictures of tabes or general paresis. Another atypical presentation was with mild symmetrical ptosis and a partial picture of tabes. Cerebrovascular accidents, confusional syndromes, and dementing illnesses (possible formes frustes of general paresis) were other presenting clinical manifestations.

In patients with partial or atypical clinical features of neurosyphilis, the serologic findings and CSF changes assume a major role in diagnosis. In the series of Hooshmand et al.,[30] the blood nontreponemal serology was reactive in 48.5 percent; the CSF nontreponemal serology was positive in 100 (55.7 percent) of the 176 patients on whom it had been performed. In almost 90 percent of the patients, the CSF cell counts were 10 or less per cubic millimeter, and in about 60 percent the protein level was in the normal range. CSF FTA-ABS tests were performed in 156 of the 241 patients and were positive in all. From the data given, it is not clear in how many patients the serologic and CSF diagnosis of neurosyphilis was based primarily on the positive CSF FTA-ABS test. However, as noted earlier (see General Paresis), a positive blood FTA-ABS test (with a negative nontreponemal reaction) may be an indication of a previous, but now inactive, syphilitic infection. A reactive CSF FTA test may occur in patients with no other CSF changes or clinical findings of neurosyphilis.[49] Thus, at this point, caution clearly is warranted in making a diagnosis of neurosyphilis based only on the finding of a reactive CSF FTA test in a patient with unexplained neurologic abnormalities. Otherwise, one might be in the position of attributing to a syphilitic etiology a variety of neurologic findings that are in fact due to an atherosclerotic, hypertensive, infectious, degenerative, or other process; this can be particularly problematic when treating older adults. Also, patients with moderately advanced, but cured, parenchymatous neurosyphilis may exhibit further clinical findings that suggest progression of the syphilitic infection but actually are due to other intercurrent diseases.

The presence of other CSF findings, such as a positive VDRL test and pleocytosis, provides a much stronger basis for attributing an atypical neurological picture to neurosyphilis, or at the very least provides a basis for the diagnosis of asymptomatic neurosyphilis accompanied by some other central nervous system process. However, in many of the atypical cases of neurosyphilis described in recent years,[30] CSF pleocytosis was minimal or absent and the protein level was normal. Such findings emphasize the previous considerations about the significance of a positive CSF FTA test as the sole laboratory finding pointing to a diagnosis of active or inactive syphilis of the nervous system. Among a group of 11 patients with progressive neurologic symptoms diagnosed as neurosyphilis, the CSF VDRL test was nonreactive in six patients (the CSF FTA test was positive in all five of these patients in whom it was determined), the cell count was increased ($>$ 5 cells per cubic millimeter) in five patients, and the protein level was abnormal in seven patients.[85] In one patient the CSF VDRL test was negative, the CSF FTA test was positive, the cell count and the protein level were normal, and the CSF gamma globulin (normally $<$ 12 percent) was increased to 25 percent of the CSF protein. In another patient the only CSF abnormalities were a positive CSF FTA test, a protein level of 75 mg/dl, and a gamma globulin level of 19 percent. If the clinical picture in these cases had been atypical and the serum VDRL test nonreactive (only the serum FTA-ABS test was positive), would they have represented examples of atypical active neurosyphilis or of some other neurologic disorder in a patient with latent or previously treated inactive syphilis? Hopefully, the utility of the determination of local immunoglobulin synthesis in the central nervous system in the diagnosis of neurosyphilis (see General Paresis, Laboratory Findings) will be validated by further study and will resolve the problem. If this type of determination cannot be performed in the available laboratory, the therapeutic approach should be to treat the possibility of neurosyphilis with penicillin and observe the clinical response while continuing to investigate other possible causes of the neurologic picture.

## Acute syphilitic optic neuritis and chorioretinitis

Acute optic neuritis and perineuritis, characterized by acute marked visual loss and swelling of the optic disks, may occur during early syphilitic meningitis or may accompany secondary syphilis without overt meningitis.[86,87] Occasionally, inflammatory cells can be observed in the vitreous or aqueous. Syphilitic optic neuritis can be distinguished from the papilledema of syphilitic meningitis by the prominent visual loss of the former. In the case of retrobulbar syphilitic optic neuritis, funduscopic examination is normal. Diffuse syphilitic neuroretinitis describes the uncommon patient with secondary syphilis who has optic papillitis, opaque retinal edema, prominent vitreous inflammation, and retinal vasculitis.[88] Treatment consists of intravenous penicillin G as for syphilitic meningitis.

# MANAGEMENT

## ANTIBIOTIC THERAPY

The introduction of penicillin in the treatment of neurosyphilis strikingly simplified and improved the therapy and outcome in this disease. At first, repeated intramuscular injections of aqueous penicillin were administered every 3 to 4 hours for a total dosage of 2 to 3 million units over a period of 8 to 16 days.[12] By the early 1950s it was established that the administration of 6 to 10 million units of penicillin (as either procaine penicillin G or procaine penicillin in oil with aluminum monostearate) over a period of 18 to 21 days produced a good therapeutic response in over 90 percent of treated cases as indicated by CSF examination. In the occasional patient who did not respond to such a program, repeated courses of increased dosage of penicillin were usually successful in arresting the infection. In one series, spinal fluid findings indicated that the disease was arrested in each of 462 patients with various forms of neurosyphilis treated in this fashion.[89] In a multicenter study involving treatment of over 1000 patients with paresis, a total penicillin dosage of 6 million units was judged to be adequate.[90] Patients who required re-treatment to arrest the infection had received less than 6 million units of penicillin initially. For about the past decade it has been generally accepted that treatment with 7.2 million units of benzathine penicillin G (2.4 million units intramuscularly weekly for 3 doses) is adequate treatment for all forms of neurosyphilis, but there have been some disconcerting observations about patients who have received this treatment (see below). The most recent recommendations of the Centers for Disease Control[91] involve the use of either intravenous aqueous penicillin G for 10 days, intramuscular procaine penicillin G for 10 days, or weekly injections of benzathine penicillin G for 3 doses (Table 21-6). Intravenous penicillin G for 10 to 15 days is the most reasonable therapy to employ for symptomatic neurosyphilis. This assures penicillin concentrations in the CSF which are continuously at least severalfold above the minimally treponemicidal concentration of 0.018 μg/ml during therapy.[92] Intravenous penicillin G is similarly advocated for treatment of asymptomatic neurosyphilis;[93] alternatively, daily aqueous procaine penicillin G (plus probenecid) for 10 to 14 days would be preferable to benzathine penicillin G, which is no longer advocated by the World Health Organization, although it remains among the drug regimens listed by the Centers for Disease Control.

**Table 21-6. Drug Regimens for Treatment of Neurosyphilis**

1. *Aqueous crystalline penicillin G:* 12 to 24 million units intravenously daily (2 to 4 million units every 4 h) for 10 days, followed by *benzathine penicillin G* 2.4 million units intramuscularly weekly for 3 doses
2. *Aqueous procaine penicillin G:* 2.4 million units intramuscularly daily plus *probenecid* 500 mg orally 4 times daily, both for 10 days, followed by *benzathine penicillin G* 2.4 million units intramuscularly weekly for 3 doses
3. *Benzathine penicillin G:* 2.4 million units by intramuscular injection weekly for 3 doses
4. *Tetracycline hydrochloride:** 500 mg orally 4 times daily for 30 days

*For patients who are allergic to penicillin.
SOURCE: After Centers for Disease Control.[91]

## ADEQUACY OF RECOMMENDED DOSAGES

Questions have arisen about the appropriateness of the previously recommended intramuscular penicillin treatment schedules for neurosyphilis. The recommended dosages for the treatment of all forms of late syphilis have been gauged to maintain serum spirochetocidal levels of 0.031 unit or more per milliliter.[94] Spirochetocidal levels are not achieved in the CSF of patients receiving intramuscular benzathine penicillin G therapy for neurosyphilis. No detectable penicillin was found in the CSF of 12 of 13 patients receiving benzathine penicillin G intramuscularly in high dosage (3.6 million units per week for 4 weeks).[95] In another patient treated with 600,000 units of aqueous procaine penicillin G intramuscularly daily, the peak CSF penicillin level 3 h after injection was less than 0.017 unit per milliliter.[95] Consistent with these observations is the reported isolation by rabbit inoculation of *T. pallidum* from the CSF of a patient who had been treated with 1.2 million units of benzathine penicillin G intramuscularly three times weekly for 3 weeks.[96]

It is now apparent that therapeutic failures and late clinical progression of neurosyphilis can sometimes occur with previously recommended intramuscular penicillin treatment programs.[97] In 1966 Short et al.[98] described two treatment failures (8 percent) among 26 patients who received 4.8 million units of benzathine penicillin G (two injections of 2.4 million units each spaced 7 to 10 days apart). More recently a patient was described in whom atypical syphilitic basilar meningitis developed 1 year after treatment for latent syphilis with 2.4 million units of benzathine penicillin G, injected intramuscularly once weekly for 3 weeks.[99] Prior to treatment the only abnormality in the CSF had been an elevated protein level. One year later the patient was admitted to the hospital with complete right oculomotor nerve paresis; CSF findings included 16 mononuclear cells per cubic millimeter, an elevated protein level, and a positive VDRL test. Three months following intravenous treatment with penicillin (20 million units daily for 21 days), the third cranial nerve palsy had almost completely disappeared, and the CSF showed clearing of the pleocytosis and a fourfold reduction in the VDRL titer.

Studies of larger groups of patients have reinforced doubts raised about the adequacy of prior recommended doses of penicillin in the treatment of neurosyphilis. The long-term follow-up (average 17 years) of a group of 64 patients with general paresis treated with penicillin (3 to 30 million units, cumulative) indicated that 39 percent developed new neurological signs during that interval.[100] The new findings observed were major ones such as seizures, hemiparesis, paraplegia, tabes dorsalis, and their frequency was many times in excess of the prevalence rates for cerebrovascular disease or epilepsy in adults without syphilis but of comparable age. Hooshmand et al. reported 10 patients with tabes or meningovascular syphilis who continued to show clinical evidence of active neurosyphilis and continued CSF pleocytosis after what generally had been considered an adequate course of treatment (9 million units of penicillin G administered over 3 weeks).[30] Symptomatic improvement and clearing of the CSF pleocytosis followed intramuscular treatment with 20 million units of procaine penicillin G administered over a period of 3 weeks. In the same study of 89 patients with neurosyphilis followed up for at least 2 years after completion of a 3-week course of treatment (20 to 24 million units of procaine penicillin G) five clinical failures were observed (four with general paresis and one with the picture of an "organic brain syndrome"). In the latter cases, CSF cell counts and protein values remained normal. Whether these "failures" represented further progression of the infection despite treatment or the consequences of already established structural changes is unclear from the report.

The information cited above strongly suggests that intramuscular dosages of penicillin that were previously considered adequate are sometimes insufficient to eradicate syphilitic infection of the central nervous system. More intensive treatment of neurosyphilis seems warranted, particularly if the patient is symptomatic and has not responded to initial antibiotic therapy. Two such intensive treatment regimens are the 3-week program (intramuscular administration of 20 to 24 million units of penicillin) of Hooshmand et al.[30] and the preferable high-dose intravenous penicillin G program (Table 21-6). These regimens produce peak CSF spirochetocidal levels of over 0.3 μg/ml.

Cellular immunity is known to play an important role in syphilis.[101] Since cellular immunity may be severely depressed in patients with human immunodeficiency virus (HIV) infection, neurosyphilis might be expected to take different clinical forms and/or be more difficult to treat successfully in patients with HIV infection. Two recent reports suggest that this is the case.[102,103] Therapy for neurosyphilis in HIV-infected persons should be undertaken with high-dose intravenous penicillin G, and careful follow-up observation is necessary.

## FOLLOW-UP AND RE-TREATMENT

The CSF findings are usually a dependable index of the activity of neurosyphilis and provide a measure of the effectiveness of antibiotic therapy. However, occasional patients with active neurosyphilis (19 percent in one series)[30] exhibit no CSF pleocytosis.[31,36,85] In some of these patients with no cells in the CSF prior to treatment, mild pleocytosis (6 to 20 cells per cubic millimeter) occurs briefly 1 to 3 weeks after the start of penicillin therapy. In patients in whom adequate initial penicillin therapy has arrested the infection, repeat CSF examination at 3 to 6 months shows a normal cell count and, if originally increased, a decrease in the concentration of protein.[104] Further CSF examination 1 year after treatment shows a continued fall in the protein level and a decrease in the titer of the nontreponemal serologic test. However, the latter may not become completely negative for several years or longer and is not per se an indication of active neurosyphilis under these circumstances. If the CSF cell count does not return to normal in 3 to 6 months or if, having returned to normal, the count rises again in relapse, then re-treatment is indicated. If relapse, as judged by the CSF formula, has not occurred during a period of 2 years after adequate penicillin therapy, it is unlikely to occur.

Clinical and CSF examinations should be performed 3 months after antibiotic treatment of patients with neurosyphilis and then at 6-month intervals, until the CSF findings return to normal. Thereafter, reevaluation should be performed annually for several years. This is particularly important in the cases of patients who have been treated with alternative antibiotics, because limited data are available on the long-term efficacy of such therapeutic programs. Blood serologic testing should be performed at 6 and 12 months and thereafter at yearly intervals for at least 3 years.[97]

## PROGNOSIS

In the prepenicillin era, untreated or inadequately treated asymptomatic neurosyphilis progressed over a 5- to 18-year period to clinical neurosyphilis in 23 to 87 percent of cases;[5] the percentage depended to some extent on the duration of the asymptomatic neurosyphilis when first diagnosed. Although the optimal dosage, preparation, or duration of penicillin administration in the treatment of asymptomatic neurosyphilis has not been established, penicillin clearly is effective therapy. Among 765 patients treated with varying dosages of penicillin (2.4 to more than 9 million units) for asymptomatic neurosyphilis, only one subsequently went on to develop symptomatic disease and was considered an unequivocal treatment failure.[105]

The clinical course of untreated acute syphilitic meningitis cannot be determined from the literature for lack of a sizable series of cases. However, its unfavorable course can be surmised from the available data on patients who had received poor treatment by the standards of the prepenicillin era. In one compilation of 31 such patients, the process progressed in 20 (65 percent) to the development of paresis, tabes, or other types of neurosyphilis.[12] The results of penicillin therapy of acute syphilitic meningitis have been very good, with clearing of the CSF changes and lack of progression to parenchymatous neurosyphilis.

The immediate prognosis for a patient with cerebral arterial occlusion due to meningovascular syphilis is usually better than that for a patient with a similar thrombosis on an atherosclerotic basis because of the younger age of the former and the greater likelihood that the arteries involved are smaller. Treatment, even in the prepenicillin days, was effective, and most patients had no further cerebrovascular accidents. In the series of Merritt et al.,[12] only 10 percent of patients had further cerebral thromboses, and those who did were in an older age group in which atherosclerotic disease may have played a role. Penicillin therapy in effective dosage has usually been effective in clearing the CSF changes and in preventing progressive clinical disease. Obviously, it cannot reverse structural damage that has already occurred. The report of Hooshmand et al. cited earlier, however, is disconcerting and runs counter to this encouraging outlook.[30] In that report there were 10 apparent failures among patients with meningovascular syphilis who received 9 million units of procaine penicillin G over a period of 3 weeks or more.

The course of untreated general paresis is progressive, and the outcome is eventually fatal. The duration of life from the onset of identifiable mental symptoms to death usually ranges from a few months to 4 or 5 years,[12] but an occasional untreated patient with so-called stationary paresis has survived for 10 years. The earlier reports of results of penicillin treatment of paresis indicated a relatively low rate (6 to less than 20 percent) of failure of response in the CSF, of clinical progression, or of late complications.[106,107] More recent studies involving longer-term follow-up indicate the development of new neurological signs in 39 percent of patients treated with penicillin.[100] Progression of the disease may occur even in the absence of reactive CSF tests.

Among a group of 58 hospitalized patients with paresis treated with one or more courses of penicillin, 26 (45 percent) improved and were discharged from the hospital; this result clearly indicates that this form of neurosyphilis is not hopeless, particularly when treatment is instituted as soon as clinical symptoms become evident.[40] It is unclear whether the development of new signs in patients with paresis treated with what has been considered adequate penicillin dosage is due to persistence of treponemes in the CSF,[96,108] to the need for spirochetocidal concentrations of penicillin in the CSF, or to an increased susceptibility to other neurologic processes. Further study of these treatment failures is needed.

The prognosis of tabes dorsalis is variable, and the disease can be compatible with long life. About 4 to 10 percent of untreated cases become spontaneously arrested at an early stage. In the prepenicillin era, treatment improved or arrested the clinical course in over 80 percent of cases. However, in view of the nature of the underlying pathology, disappearance of many of the clinical findings would not be expected. Similarly, many of the residual signs and symptoms may persist after penicillin therapy. The most satisfactory therapeutic results are achieved in early cases of tabes in which the CSF findings are markedly abnormal.

## References


1 Chesney AM, Kemp JE: Incidence of *Spirochaeta pallida* in cerebrospinal fluid during early stage of syphilis. *JAMA* 83:1725, 1924.

2 Stokes JH et al: *Modern Clinical Syphilology*, 3d ed. Philadelphia, Saunders, 1944, p 8.

3 Merritt HH et al: *Neurosyphilis*. New York, Oxford, 1946, p 7.

4 Lukehart SA et al: Isolation of virulent *Treponema pallidum* from cerebrospinal fluid of patients with early syphilis. *Clin Res* 32 (2):374A, 1984.

5 Hahn RD, Clerk EG: Asymptomatic neurosyphilis: A review of the literature. *Am J Syph Gon Vener Dis* 30:305, 1946.

6 Merritt HH: Early clinical and laboratory manifestations of syphilis of the central nervous system. *N Engl J Med* 223:446, 1940.

7 Dattner B: *The Management of Neurosyphilis*. New York, Grune & Stratton, 1944.

8 Merritt HH et al: *Neurosyphilis*. New York, Oxford, 1946, p 21.

9 Gjestland T: The Oslo study of untreated syphilis: An epidemiologic investigation of the natural course of the syphilitic infection based upon a re-study of the Boeck-Bruusgaard material. *Acta Derm Venereol [Suppl] (Stockh)* 35(34):11, 1955.

10 Clark EG, Danbolt N: The Oslo study of the natural course of untreated syphilis: An epidemiologic investigation based on a restudy of the Boeck-Bruusgaard material. *Med Clin North Am* 48: 613, 1964.

11 Rockwell DH et al: The Tuskegee study of untreated syphilis: The 30th year of observation. *Arch Intern Med* 114:792, 1964.

12 Merritt HH et al: *Neurosyphilis*. New York, Oxford, 1946.

13 Martin JP: Conquest of general paresis. *Br Med J* 2:159, 1972.

14 Personal communication with Centers for Disease Control, Atlanta, GA.

15 O'Leary PA et al: Cooperative clinical studies in the treatment of syphilis: Asymptomatic neurosyphilis. *Vener Dis Inf* 18:45, 1937.

16 Moore JE, Hopkins HH: Asymptomatic neurosyphilis: VI. The prognosis of early and late neurosyphilis. *JAMA* 95:1637, 1930.

17 Merritt HH, Moore M: Acute syphilitic meningitis. *Medicine* 14: 119, 1935.

18 Melvin ET, Mildvan D: Acute syphilitic meningitis: A case report. *Mt Sinai J Med NY* 46:201, 1979.

19 Willcox RR, Goodwin PG: Nerve deafness in early syphilis. *Br J Vener Dis* 47:401, 1971.

20 Alergant CD: Eighth nerve deafness in early syphilis: Report of a case. *Br J Vener Dis* 41:300, 1965.

21 Balkany TJ, Dans PE: Reversible sudden deafness in early acquired syphilis. *Arch Otolaryngol* 104:66, 1978.

22 Löwhagen G-B et al: Central nervous system involvement in early syphilis. Part II. Correlation between auditory brainstem responses (ABR) and cerebrospinal fluid abnormalities. *Acta Derm Venereol (Stockh)* 63:530, 1983.

23 Steckelberg JM, McDonald TJ: Otologic involvement in late syphilis. *Laryngoscope* 94:753, 1984.

24 Pachner AR, Steere AC: The triad of neurologic manifestations of Lyme disease: Meningitis, cranial neuritis, and radiculoneuritis. *Neurology* 35:47, 1985.

25 Russell H et al: Enzyme-linked immunosorbent assay and indirect immunofluorescence assay for Lyme disease. *J Infect Dis* 149:465, 1984.

26 Magnarelli LA et al: Cross-reactivity in serological tests for Lyme disease and other spirochetal infections. *J Infect Dis* 156:183, 1987.

27 Agdal N et al: Pachymeningitis cervicalis hypertrophica syphilitica. *Acta Derm Venereol (Stockh)* 60:184, 1980.

28 Gribble LD: Syphilitic spinal pachymeningitis. *S Afr Med J* 2:1326, 1972.

29 Holmes MD et al: Clinical features of meningovascular syphilis. *Neurology* 34:553, 1984.

30 Hooshmand H et al: Neurosyphilis: A study of 241 patients. *JAMA* 219:726, 1972.

31 Joffe R et al: Changing clinical picture of neurosyphilis: Report of seven unusual cases. *Br Med J* 1:211, 1968.

32 Liebeskind A et al: Unusual segmental cerebrovascular changes. *Radiology* 106:119, 1973.

33 Vatz KA et al: Neurosyphilis and diffuse cerebral angiopathy: A case report. *Neurology* 24:472, 1974.

34 Holland BA et al: Meningovascular syphilis: CT and MR findings. *Radiology* 158:439, 1986.

35 Adams RA, Merritt HH: Meningeal and vascular syphilis of the spinal cord. *Medicine* 23:181, 1944.

36 Luxon L et al: Neurosyphilis today. *Lancet* 1:90, 1979.

37 Fisher M, Poser CM: Syphilitic meningomyelitis. *Arch Neurol* 34: 785, 1977.

38 Catterall RD: Neurosyphilis. *Br J Hosp Med* 17:585, 1977.

39 Moore M, Merritt HH: Role of syphilis of the nervous system in the production of mental disease. *JAMA* 107:1292, 1936.

40 Dewhurst K: The neurosyphilitic psychoses today: A survey of 91 cases. *Br J Psychiatry* 115:31, 1969.

41 Dawson-Butterworth K, Heathcote PEM: Review of hospitalized cases of general paralysis of the insane. *Br J Vener Dis* 46:295, 1970.

42 Gimenez-Roldan S et al: Dementia paralytica: Deterioration from communicating hydrocephalus. *J Neurol Neurosurg Psychiatry* 42: 501, 1979.

43 Heathfield KWG: The decline of neurolues. *Practitioner* 217:753, 1976.

44 Dewhurst K: The composition of the cerebrospinal fluid in the neurosyphilitic psychoses. *Acta Neurol Scand* 45:119, 1969.

45 Burke AW: Syphilis in a Jamaican psychiatric hospital: A review of 52 cases including 17 of neurosyphilis. *Br J Vener Dis* 48:249, 1972.

46 Ch'ien L et al: Seronegative dementia paralytica: Report of a case. *J Neurol Neurosurg Psychiatry* 33:376, 1970.

47 Escobar MR et al: Fluorescent antibody tests for syphilis using cerebrospinal fluid: Clinical correlation in 150 cases. *Am J Clin Pathol* 53:886, 1970.

48 Mahony JDH et al: Evaluation of the CSF-FTA-ABS test in latent and tertiary treated syphilis. *Acta Derm Venereol (Stockh)* 52:71, 1972.

49 Jaffe HW et al: Tests for treponemal antibody in CSF. *Arch Intern Med* 138:252, 1978.

50 Madiedo G et al: False positive VDRL and FTA in cerebrospinal fluid. *JAMA* 244:688, 1980.

51 McGeeney T et al: Utility of the FTA-ABS test of CSF in the diagnosis of neurosyphilis. *Sex Transm Dis* 6:195, 1979.

52 Davis LE, Sperry S: The CSF-FTA test and the significance of blood contamination. *Arch Neurol* 6:68, 1979.

53 Jaffe HW: The laboratory diagnosis of syphilis: New concepts. *Ann Intern Med* 83:846, 1975.
54 Musher DM et al: Evaluation and management of an asymptomatic patient with a positive VDRL reaction in *Current Clinical Topics in Infectious Disease-9*, JS Remington, MN Swartz (eds). New York, McGraw-Hill, 1988, p 147.
55 Burke JN, Schaberg DR: Neurosyphilis in the antibiotic era. *Neurology* 35:1368, 1985.
56 Jordan KG: Diagnostic criteria for neurosyphilis. *Neurology* 36: 1273, 1986.
57 Jaffe HW, Kabins SA: Examination of cerebrospinal fluid in patients with syphilis. *Rev Infect Dis* 4:S842, 1982.
58 Pedersen NS et al: Specificity of immunoglobulins synthesized within the central nervous system in neurosyphilis. *Acta Pathol Microbiol Immunol* 90:97, 1982.
59 Vartdal F et al: Neurosyphilis: Intrathecal synthesis of oligoclonal antibodies to *Treponema pallidum*. *Ann Neurol* 11:35, 1981.
60 Prange HW et al: Relationship between neurological features and intrathecal synthesis of IgG antibodies to *Treponema pallidum* in untreated and treated human neurosyphilis. *J Neurol* 230:241, 1983.
61 Gschnait F et al: Cerebrospinal fluid immunoglobulins in neurosyphilis. *Br J Vener Dis* 57:238, 1981.
62 Lee JB et al: Detection of immunoglobulin M in cerebrospinal fluid from syphilis patients by enzyme-linked immunosorbent assay. *J Clin Microbiol* 24:736, 1986.
63 Müller F et al: Demonstration of locally synthesized immunoglobulin M antibodies to *Treponema pallidum* in the central nervous system of patients with untreated neurosyphilis. *J Neuroimmunol* 7:43, 1984/85.
64 Ganti SR et al: Computed tomography of cerebral syphilis. *J Comput Assist Tomogr* 5:345, 1981.
65 Godt P et al: The value of CT in cerebral syphilis. *Neuroradiology* 18:197, 1979.
66 Moskovitz BL et al: Meningovascular syphilis after "appropriate" treatment of primary syphilis. *Arch Intern Med* 142:139, 1982.
67 Escobar A, Nieto D: in *Neuro-Syphilis in Pathology of Central Nervous System*, J Minkler (ed). New York, McGraw-Hill, 1968, vol 3, p 2448.
68 Towpik J, Nowakowska E: Changing patterns of late syphilis. *Br J Vener Dis* 46:132, 1970.
69 Aho K et al: Late complications of syphilis: A comparative epidemiological and serological study of cardiovascular syphilis and various forms of neurosyphilis. *Acta Derm Venereol (Stockh)* 49:336, 1969.
70 Ekbom K: Carbamazepine in the treatment of tabetic lightning pains. *Arch Neurol* 26:374, 1972.
71 McNeel DP, Ehne G: Charcot joint of the lumbar spine. *J Neurosurg* 30:55, 1969.
72 Ramani PS, Sengupta RP: Cauda equina compression due to tabetic arthropathy of the spine. *J Neurol Neurosurg Psychiatry* 36:260, 1973.
73 Hahn RD: Tabes dorsalis with special reference to primary optic atrophy. *Br J Vener Dis* 33:139, 1957.
74 Kerty E et al: Visual evoked response in syphilitic optic atrophy. *Acta Ophthalmol* 64:553, 1986.
75 Kaplan JG et al: Luetic meningitis with gumma: Clinical, radiographic, and neuropathologic features. *Neurology* 31:464, 1981.
76 Tsai FY et al: Angiographic findings with an intracranial gumma. *Neuroradiology* 13:1, 1977.
77 Ingall D, Norins L: Syphilis, in *Infectious Diseases of the Fetus and Newborn Infant*, JS Remington, JO Klein (eds). Philadelphia, Saunders, 1976, p 433.
78 Menninger WC: *Juvenile Paresis*. Baltimore, Williams & Wilkins, 1936.
79 Carruthers MM et al: A case of congenital paresis in 1966. *Ann Intern Med* 66:1204, 1967.
80 Platou RV: Treatment of congenital syphilis with penicillin. *Adv Pediatr* 4:37, 1949.
81 Koffman O: The changing pattern of neurosyphilis. *Can Med Assoc J* 74:807, 1956.
82 Modified neurosyphilis, editorial. *Br Med J* 2:647, 1978.
83 Lanigan-O'Keefe LM: Return to normal of Argyll-Robertson pupils after treatment. *Br Med J* 2:1191, 1977.
84 Jordan K et al: Bilateral oculomotor paralysis due to neurosyphilis. *Ann Neurol* 3:90, 1978.
85 Kolar OJ, Burkhart JE: Neurosyphilis. *Br J Vener Dis* 53:221, 1977.
86 Weinstein JM et al: Acute syphilitic optic neuritis. *Arch Ophthalmol* 99:1392, 1981.
87 Hotson JR: Modern neurosyphilis: A partially treated chronic meningitis. *West J Med* 135:191, 1981.
88 Folk JC et al: Syphilitic neuroretinitis. *Am J Ophthalmol* 95:480, 1983.
89 Dattner B: Late results of penicillin therapy in neurosyphilis. *Trans Am Neurol Assoc* 77:127, 1952.
90 Hahn RD et al: The results of treatment in 1,086 general paralytics the majority of whom were followed for more than five years. *J Chronic Dis* 7:209, 1958.
91 Centers for Disease Control: 1985 STD treatment guidelines. *MMWR* 34(4S):suppl Oct 18, 1985.
92 Schoch PE, Wolters EC: Penicillin concentrations in serum and CSF during high-dose intravenous treatment for neurosyphilis. *Neurology* 37:1214, 1987.
93 Simon RP: Neurosyphilis. *Arch Neurol* 42:606, 1985.
94 Mohr JA et al: Neurosyphilis and penicillin levels in cerebrospinal fluid. *JAMA* 236:2208, 1976.
95 Yoder FW: Penicillin treatment of neurosyphilis: Are recommended dosages sufficient? *JAMA* 232:270, 1975.
96 Tramont EC: Persistence of *Treponema pallidum* following penicillin G therapy: Report of two cases. *JAMA* 236:2206, 1976.
97 Centers for Disease Control: Syphilis: Recommended treatment schedules, 1976. *Ann Intern Med* 85:94, 1976.
98 Short DH et al: Neurosyphilis: The search for adequate treatment. *Arch Dermatol* 93:87, 1966.
99 Greene BM et al: Failure of penicillin G benzathine in the treatment of neurosyphilis. *Arch Intern Med* 140:1117, 1980.
100 Wilner E, Brody JA: Prognosis of general paresis after treatment. *Lancet* 2:1370, 1968.
101 Pavia et al: Cell-mediated immunity during syphilis: A review. *Br J Vener Dis* 54:144, 1978.
102 Johns DR et al: Alteration in the natural history of neurosyphilis by concurrent infection with the human immunodeficiency virus. *N Engl J Med* 316:1569, 1987.
103 Berry CD et al: Neurologic relapse after benzathine penicillin therapy for secondary syphilis in a patient with HIV infection. *N Engl J Med* 316:1587, 1987.
104 Dattner B et al: Criteria for the management of neurosyphilis. *Am J Med* 10:463, 1951.
105 Hahn RD et al: Penicillin treatment of asymptomatic central nervous system syphilis: I. Probability of progression to symptomatic neurosyphilis. *Arch Dermatol* 74:355, 1956.
106 Hahn RD et al: Penicillin treatment of general paresis (dementia paralytica). *Arch Neurol Psychiatry* 81:557, 1959.
107 Weickhardt G: Penicillin therapy in general paresis. *Am J Psychiatry* 105:63, 1948.
108 Collart P et al: Significance of spiral organisms found, after treatment, in late human and experimental syphilis. *Br J Vener Dis* 40:81, 1964.

# Chapter 22
# Cardiovascular syphilis*

Bernadine P. Healy

At the turn of this century, syphilis was a major cause of cardiovascular disease. In 1894 William Osler devoted considerable attention in his textbook of medicine to syphilitic arteriosclerosis and aneurysms.[1] Thirty years later Richard Cabot in his book *Facts on the Heart*[2] devoted nearly 100 pages to this condition. Cabot considered it one of the leading causes of "harmful cases"; syphilitic heart disease was one-fifth as common as rheumatic valvular disease and one-ninth as prevalent as hypertensive heart disease. At the present time, syphilitic heart disease is relatively uncommon. However, there is evidence that syphilis, along with other venereal diseases, is on the rise, particularly among the homosexual population.[3] Whether the increase in venereal disease that has been witnessed in recent years will result in an increase in cardiovascular syphilis as this century closes remains to be seen. Regardless of its incidence, syphilitic heart disease may present unpredictably after a long latent period and needs to be considered in the evaluation of diseases of the aorta and aortic valve. Since adequate therapy of early syphilis will prevent the development of cardiovascular syphilis, this should be one of the goals of every venereal disease control program.

## PATHOLOGY AND PATHOPHYSIOLOGY

The cardiovascular system is not clinically affected in the early stages of syphilis, but it is involved morphologically in up to 80 percent of occurrences of the tertiary stage of the disease,[4] although clinical manifestations of cardiovascular syphilis may occur in only about 10 percent of such occurrences. In the tertiary stage, aortic, coronary ostial, valvular, and myocardial lesions of syphilis have been described, but aortitis is the most common lesion, accounting for the majority of clinical manifestations[5–13] (Figs. 22-1 and 22-2).

*Treponema pallidum* presumably spreads to the heart during the early stages of syphilis, possibly via the lymphatics, and the organisms lodge in the aortic wall, where they remain dormant for years. The spirochetes appear to have a predilection for the vasa vasorum of the aorta, particularly the proximal aorta, producing transmural inflammatory lesions resulting in endarteritis of these vessels. The proximal portions of the coronary arteries near the ostia sometimes are involved by the obliterative endarteritis. This inflammatory process, which is rich in perivascular lymphocytes and plasma cells, continues for years, long after evidence of early syphilis has passed. This suggests that the lesions of late cardiovascular syphilis have an immunologic basis, as has been proposed for other forms of tertiary syphilis.

Although the initial insult is primarily to the small nutrient vessels of the aorta, all three layers of aortic wall are affected by the process. Probably because of obliteration of the lumen of the vasa vasorum, the aortic media develops patchy necrosis with subsequent focal scarring. The medial destruction is also associated with the destruction of the important elastic tissue of the media, which sets the stage for subsequent aortic dilatation and aneurysm formation. The adventitia, which contains the prominently inflamed vasa vasorum, undergoes fibrous thickening. The overlying aortic intima becomes diffusely diseased, with atherosclerotic changes involving virtually the entire intimal surface of the affected aorta. The extensive plaque formation has been described as "tree barking," and the calcification accompanying these complicated atherosclerotic plaques accounts for the eggshell calcification of the proximal aorta that is often evident radiographically (Fig. 22-3).

Although rarely present in the tertiary stage of syphilis, syphilitic gummas may infiltrate the aortic wall or myocardium. Gummas, which are focal, circumscribed zones of necrosis containing inflammatory cells and often giant cells enclosed by fibrous tissue, are morphologically similar to the granulomatous lesions of tuberculosis or sarcoidosis. The end stage of the gumma is a fibrous scar. Little is known of the clinical manifestations of gummas in the heart because of their rarity and the difficulty of clinical recognition, but it is likely that the same complications of ventricular arrhythmias and the same valve dysfunctions that may occur in other granulomatous conditions affecting the heart, such as sarcoid, may also occur with syphilis.

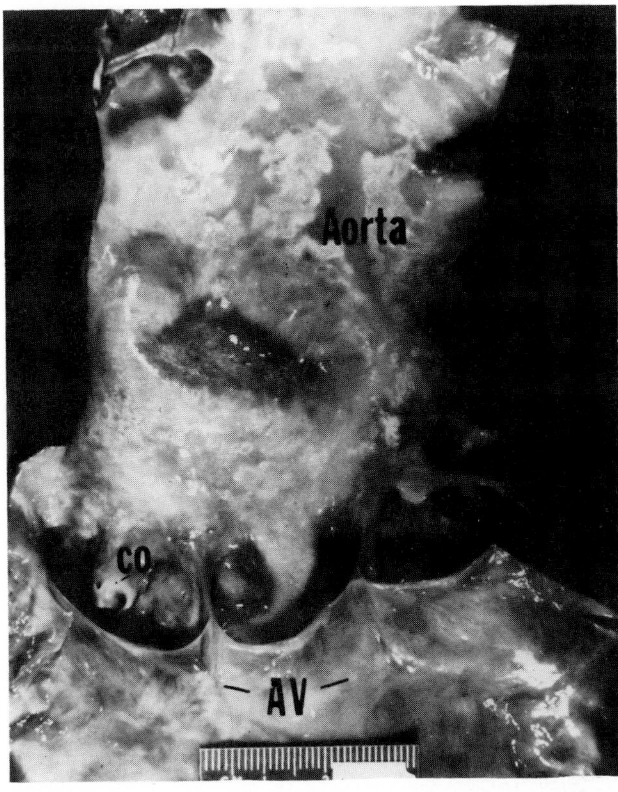


**Fig. 22-1.** Proximal aorta and aortic valve from a patient with syphilitic aortitis. The atherosclerotic process extensively involved the aortic root area and was less prominent in the distal aorta, which is the reverse of the atherosclerotic pattern ordinarily seen. The cusps of the aortic valve (AV) are thickened because of mild aortic insufficiency, and some intimal plaque is evident around the coronary ostia (CO), which may be critically narrowed in syphilis.

*Supported by grant P50-HL-17655 from the National Institutes of Health, Public Health Service, Department of Health and Human Services and by the Peter Belfer Laboratory for Myocardial Research.

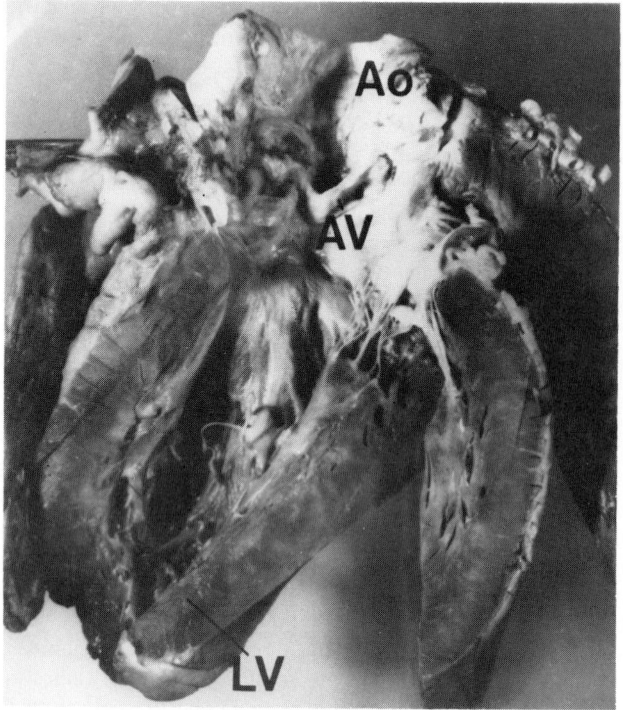


Fig. 22-2. Heart of a patient who died with syphilitic aortic insufficiency. The aortic valve leaflets are thickened and rolled. The proximal aorta (Ao) is involved by atherosclerotic plaques which demarcate the area of syphilitic aortitis. The left ventricle (LV) is hypertrophied and moderately dilated as a result of the long-standing aortic insufficiency.

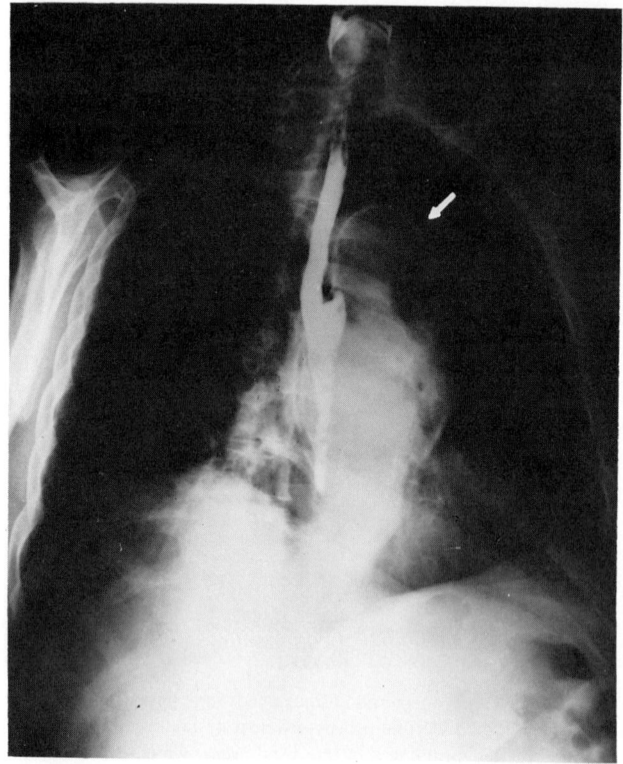

Fig. 22-3. Chest radiograph, after barium swallow, of a 56-year-old man with a history of incompletely treated syphilis. Marked calcification can be seen within the aneurysm of the ascending aorta (*arrow*). (*Courtesy BW Gayler.*)

## CONGENITAL SYPHILIS

Prenatal, or congenital, syphilis may involve the heart, but cardiovascular lesions similar to those of acquired syphilis are exceedingly rare in this form of syphilis. When prenatal death occurs due to spirochetemia, focal inflammatory lesions with scarring may be seen in most of the body organs, including the heart, and live organisms may be identified in the affected tissues. After birth, in addition to the characteristic mucocutaneous and skeletal abnormalities of early congenital lues, secondary and tertiary syphilis may develop. However, for unclear reasons, aortitis and aortic insufficiency do not seem to occur. This subject is discussed more fully in Chap. 67.

## CLINICAL MANIFESTATIONS OF ACQUIRED CARDIOVASCULAR SYPHILIS

Since syphilis of the cardiovascular system becomes clinically manifest only in the tertiary stage of the disease, which is preceded by a latent period of 15 to 30 years, most patients with clinical evidence of cardiovascular lues are between 40 and 55 years of age; men are affected three times as often as women. The described pathological changes account for the three major clinical cardiac problems posed by lues: thoracic aneurysm formation, aortic valve incompetence, and coronary ostial stenosis. As it is not active infection but already present degenerative changes which cause dysfunction at this late stage, antibiotic therapy is not helpful for cardiovascular syphilis.

## AORTIC ANEURYSM

The luetic aneurysm, the most common manifestation of tertiary syphilis, virtually always involves the thoracic aorta and particularly involves the proximal ascending aorta immediately at and above the sinuses of Valsalva. Over 60 percent of syphilitic aneurysms involve the ascending portion of the thoracic aorta and 25 percent involve the transverse arch.[14] Rarely, syphilitic aneurysms can occur, mainly in the innominate artery, where they may present with cerebral emboli.[14] These aneurysms are typically fusiform or saccular in type. Dissecting aneurysms do not occur, probably because of the medial scarring and wall thickening of the chronic inflammatory process.[13]

Isolated luetic aneurysms frequently are undetected and asymptomatic for years. Symptoms eventually develop because the aneurysm had encroached on surrounding structures or has ruptured. In some cases a luetic aneurysm has been known to erode through the chest wall and present as a chest wall mass. More typically the patient presents with persistent chest pain or with symptoms of a mass lesion compressing adjacent structures, such as hoarseness from recurrent laryngeal nerve pressure. A rare presentation may be with the superior vena cava syndrome, and in association with cough, dyspnea, dysphagia, and hemoptysis, may be misdiagnosed as lung cancer.[15] Another dramatic presentation may be erosion of the chest wall. Physical findings of luetic aneurysms, however, are minor most of the time. Indeed if aortic insufficiency is not present, there may be no detectable abnormalities on cardiac examination. The heart sounds have been described, however, as tambouric in quality, in part because of the dilated and noncompliant aorta. The chest radiograph may be normal or show a mediastinal mass with typical egg-shell calcification outlining the aneurysm (Fig. 22-3). This finding, however, may also be seen in severely atherosclerotic aortas or aortas from patients of advanced age and is not specific for syphilis. The precise definition of the aneurysm is achieved by aortic root angiography, which would ordinarily be performed in a patient who presents with a complex of symptoms such as persistent chest pain and mediastinal mass compatible with an aneurysm.

Management of luetic aneurysms is largely dictated by symptoms. If a patient presents with evidence of an expanding aneurysm or with chest pain or symptoms of encroachment on adjacent tissue, surgical resection would be appropriate therapy.

## CORONARY ARTERY DISEASE

The coronary arteries may be primarily involved in syphilis, but almost always only the ostia or the most proximal few millimeters of the coronary arteries are affected. The cause of the coronary arterial disease is an obliterative endarteritis of the type that involves the aorta. When the luetic process significantly narrows the coronary ostia, it may lead to ischemic heart disease, including angina pectoris or sudden death. Probably because of the proximal nature of the coronary lesions, patients with syphilitic coronary disease typically die suddenly or develop chest pain rather than develop an acute occlusion of the left main coronary artery. Ordinarily, the acute coronary occlusion would involve such an extensive mass of left ventricular myocardium that the patient would not likely survive long enough to evolve a clinically apparent myocardial infarct. The diagnosis of syphilitic coronary disease should be considered in a patient who has been shown, by coronary angiography, to have isolated right or left main coronary ostial narrowing without atherosclerosis in the rest of the coronary tree and who has a history of syphilis or other signs of cardiovascular syphilis. At the present time, management of symptomatic coronary ostial disease, particularly when the left coronary is involved, should be coronary artery bypass surgery; there is sufficient evidence now that patients with left main coronary narrowing have improved survival with surgery.[16]

Coronary artery bypass surgery may be more complicated when severe luetic aortitis is also present, as a severely calcified ascending aorta may make aortic cross-clamping more risky and grafting of the vein graft into the aorta difficult. An innominate artery–coronary artery bypass graft has been reported in one patient because of the latter problem.[17] Alternatively, an internal mammary artery graft can be used, which does not require an aortic anastomosis.[18]

## AORTIC VALVE DISEASE

Pure aortic regurgitation without stenosis is a common cardiovascular manifestation of syphilis, occurring in roughly 30 percent of patients with tertiary syphilis of the cardiovascular system. The aortic regurgitation appears to be due to aortic root dilatation with stretching of the aortic valve, leading in many cases to widening of the aortic valve commissures, thickening of the aortic valve leaflets, and a variable amount of aortic valve incompetence. Aortic insufficiency typically presents in patients who are 50 years of age or older, in whom the etiology often may be unclear. The severity of aortic insufficiency may range from mild to severe and largely determines both the clinical course and its management.

Physical findings of luetic aortic insufficiency include diastolic blowing along the lower left sternal border, increased aortic second sound, and if the aortic insufficiency has been severe enough, a prominent left ventricle which is both hypertrophied and dilated. A tambourlike quality of the second heart sound has been commonly described in syphilitic aortic valve disease, probably due to the aortic root dilatation. This is not a specific finding, since other conditions may also lead to a tambouric second sound. If aortic stenosis also is present, the cause is highly unlikely to be syphilis. The differential diagnosis of chronic pure aortic insufficiency (i.e., without a component of stenosis) includes only a few major conditions.[19] Other causes of chronic pure aortic insufficiency include healed infective endocarditis, congenitally malformed valves, Marfan's syndrome, ankylosing spondylitis, Reiter's syndrome, trauma with cusp dehiscence, or an aneurysm in a sinus of Valsalva (Table 22-1). In old age, ectasia of the aorta may lead to some stretching of the aortic valve and mild aortic insufficiency. Cardiovascular syphilis can usually be distinguished from these other conditions by a complex of findings including aortic root disease, a tricuspid aortic valve with normality of the other cardiac valves, and the absence of stigmata of metabolic and connective tissue diseases. Distinguishing among these entities has implications for management. For example, if a patient with Marfan's syndrome requires aortic valve replacement, the proximal aortic root dilatation and thinning that extend to the sinuses of Valsalva, where the coronary ostia reside, are usually so extensive that repair of the entire proximal aortic root (with coronary artery bypass) is required. In contrast, in syphilis the region of the sinuses of Valsalva is thickened and scarred and only mildly dilated, and surgical repair can usually be accomplished well above the sinuses of Valsalva.

**Table 22-1. Causes of Aortic Regurgitation**

| | Syphilis | Ankylosing spondylitis | Marfan's syndrome | Rheumatic |
|---|---|---|---|---|
| Average age | 50 | 45 | 30 | 45 |
| Usual sex | Men | Men | Men | Men |
| Aortic regurgitation | + + + + | + + + + | + + + + | + + + |
| Mitral regurgitation | 0 | + | + + + | + + + + |
| Conduction disturbances | + | + + + + | 0 | 0 |
| Aorta | | | | |
| Adventitial scarring | + + + | + + + | 0 | 0 |
| Medial degeneration | + + + | + + + | + + + + | 0 |
| Intimal proliferation | + + | + + | 0 | 0 |
| Limited to sinuses of Valsalva | 0 | + | 0 | 0 |
| Aortic cusp thickening | Focal | Diffuse | Focal | Diffuse |
| Anterior mitral leaflet thickening | 0 | + + | + | + + + + |

SOURCE: After Bulkley and Roberts.[19]

Management of syphilitic aortic insufficiency is dictated by the symptoms and hemodynamic status of the patient. Congestive heart failure and chest pain are indications for valve replacement. Unfortunately, symptoms often develop at a time when the heart has already been destructively restructured, hypertrophied, and dilated, and despite valve replacement, a secondary valvular myocardiopathy remains. Technical aspects of surgery for syphilitic aortic insufficiency are generally no more difficult than for rheumatic valvular disease; the area of the sinuses of Valsalva and the most proximal aortic root tend to be scarred and thickened and therefore provide a good foundation for valve implantation. It should be stressed that the state of the aorta should be carefully assessed both before and after valve replacement. Progressive thoracic aortic dilatation can occur after aortic valve replacement for syphilitic aortic valve disease and may require surgical repair, as well.[20]

## SUMMARY

Cardiovascular syphilis in its tertiary phase may lead to aortic aneurysms, aortic insufficiency, coronary stenosis, and rarely myocarditis. Its clinical presentation is characterized by the functional disorder resulting from cardiac involvement and at times may be difficult to distinguish from other more common varieties of cardiac disease. Although cardiovascular syphilis may be prevented by appropriate therapy of early syphilis, this is a disease which most likely will continue to be seen. Understanding of its pathology and pathophysiology is important to its recognition and subsequent management.

## References

1 Osler W: *The Principles and Practice of Medicine*. 1894. Reprint. AM Harvey et al (eds). New York, Appleton-Century-Crofts, 1919.

2 Cabot RC: *Facts on the Heart*. Philadelphia, Saunders, 1926.

3 Adler MW: Syphilis: Clinical features. *Br Med J* 288:468, 1984.

4 Robbins SL, Cotran RS: *Pathologic Basis of Disease*. Philadelphia, Saunders, 1979, p 408.

5 Gould SE: *Pathology of the Heart*. Springfield, IL, Charles C Thomas, 1960, pp 906–908.

6 Martland HS: Syphilis of the aorta and heart. *Am Heart J* 6:1, 1930.

7 Carr JG: The gross pathology of the heart in cardiovascular syphilis. *Am Heart J* 6:30, 1930.

8 Saphir O: Syphilitic myocarditis. *Arch Pathol* 13:266, 1932.

9 Bruenn HG: Syphilitic disease of the coronary arteries. *Am Heart J* 9:421, 1934.

10 Steel D: The roentgenological diagnosis of syphilitic aortitis: A review of forty proved cases. *Am Heart J* 6:59, 1930.

11 Webster B et al: Studies in cardiovascular syphilis: III. The natural history of syphilitic aortic insufficiency. *Am Heart J* 46:117, 1953.

12 Heggtveit HA: Syphilitic aortitis: A clinicopathologic autopsy study of 100 cases, 1950 to 1960. *Circulation* 29:346, 1964.

13 Roberts WC et al: Nonrheumatic valvular cardiac disease: A clinicopathologic survey of 27 different conditions causing valvular dysfunction. *Cardiovasc Clin* 5:333, 1973.

14 Tadavarthy SM et al: Syphilitic aneurysms of the innominate artery. *Radiology* 139:31, 1981.

15 Phillips PL et al: Syphilitic aortic aneurysm presenting with the superior vena cava syndrome. *Am J Med* 71:171, 1981.

16 Bulkley BH, Roberts WC: Atherosclerotic narrowing of the left main coronary artery: A necropsy analysis of 152 patients with fatal coronary heart disease and varying degrees of left main narrowing. *Circulation* 53:823, 1976.

17 Weinstein G, Killen DA: Innominate artery–coronary artery bypass graft in a patient with calcific aortitis. *J Thorac Cardiovasc Surg* 79:312, 1980.

18 Loop FD et al: Influence of the internal-mammary-artery graft on 10-year survival and other cardiac events. *N Engl J Med* 314:1, 1986.

19 Bulkley BH, Roberts WC: Ankylosing spondylitis and aortic regurgitation. Description of the characteristic cardiovascular lesion from study of eight necropsy patients. *Circulation* 48:1014, 1973.

20 Nancarrow PA, Higgins CB: Progressive thoracic aortic dilatation after valve replacement. *AJR* 142:669, 1984.

Chapter 23

# Late benign syphilis

Rudolph H. Kampmeier

*Late benign syphilis* represents an inflammatory process [either proliferative or destructive (gummatous)] that involves structures generally not essential to the maintenance of life and that occurs in both acquired and prenatal infection. The overwhelming majority of these manifestations occur in the skin and the bones, with a lesser frequency in the mucosae and certain of the viscera, muscles, and ocular structures. Resulting scar tissue may impair functions of the structures involved. (Gumma of the myocardium, brain, spinal cord or of the trachea with stenosis may be anything but benign!)

Tumors or swellings, ulcers, and destructive lesions of the nasopharynx were associated with syphilis, either implicitly or explicitly, as early as the sixteenth century. Syphilis of bone was described by a Polish physician, Jan Knolle, in 1763. The first systematic studies of late benign lesions were made by Rudolf Virchow, the "father of pathology," in 1858 and by S. Wilkes in 1863. The former not only described the gross lesions but provided the basic description of the histopathologic hallmarks of the late benign disease.[1]

## INCIDENCE

The reduction within the professional life of the author of a formerly common form of disease to one which most readers may never see is nothing short of remarkable. The most acceptable data concerning the frequency of late benign syphilis in an untreated population of syphilitic patients are those provided by the Boeck-Bruusgaard study. A critical review of this clinical material in 1955 showed that 15.8 percent of the 1147 patients in the study "sooner or later" developed late benign lesions of the skin, mucous membranes, or bones and joints. These manifestations occurred more frequently among women (17.3 percent) than men (13.7 percent). Among those observed to have late benign disease, 25 percent of the men and 34.7 percent of the women had from two to seven episodes of this manifestation.[2]

**Table 23-1. Distribution of Late Benign Lesions as to Site and Race**

| Site | Black | White |
|---|---|---|
| Skeletal (all types) | 123 | 55 |
| Skin | 124 | 47 |
| Upper respiratory tract (nose, throat, larynx) | 50 | 19 |
| Mucous membrane (mouth) | 41 | 19 |
| Eye (all types) | 43 | 11 |
| Visceral (liver, stomach, etc.) | 23 | 14 |
| Lower respiratory tract | 2 | 2 |
| Mediastinum | 3 | 1 |
| Lymph nodes | 7 | — |
| Genital tract (female) | 4 | — |
| Penis | 3 | 2 |
| Testes | 3 | 1 |
| Skeletal muscle | 3 | 1 |
| Totals | 429 | 172 |

Table 23-1 shows the frequency with which late benign syphilis was encountered in the Vanderbilt syphilis clinic from 1925 to 1943. It must be emphasized that patients commonly had more than one tissue involved simultaneously. The decreased incidence of late disease with the passage of years (Fig. 23-1) was the result of intensive case finding followed by treatment of early and latent syphilis with arsenicals and, after 1946, with penicillin.[3,4]

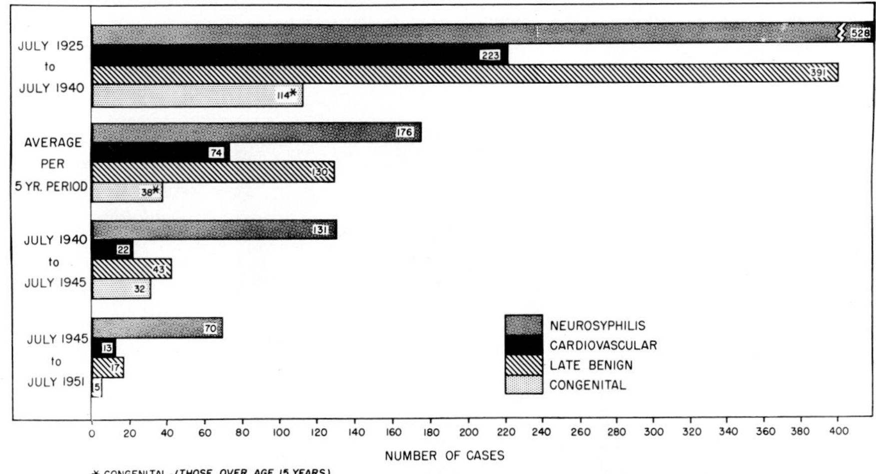


**Fig. 23-1.** The decrease in the incidence of late syphilis in the Vanderbilt University Hospital Syphilis Clinic. *Congenital = those over age 15. The experience of the first 15 years could not be broken down by 5-year periods; therefore, a 5-year average for this period is used for purposes of comparison. The figures marked by an asterisk represent the incidence of disease in which the diagnosis was made on ambulant clinic patients and does not include diagnoses made on ward patients. Unfortunately, figures subsequent to 1951 cannot be included; with the discontinuance of the syphilis clinic that year, the syphilitic patients were absorbed into the general medical and/or specialty clinics. Therefore, syphilitic disease was often not diagnosed and recorded. The diagnoses of syphilis that were made did not represent the critical diagnoses made in the syphilis clinic, which utilized history meetings and which included the consensus of three or four clinicians experienced in the disease. (*From RH Kampmeier.*[4])

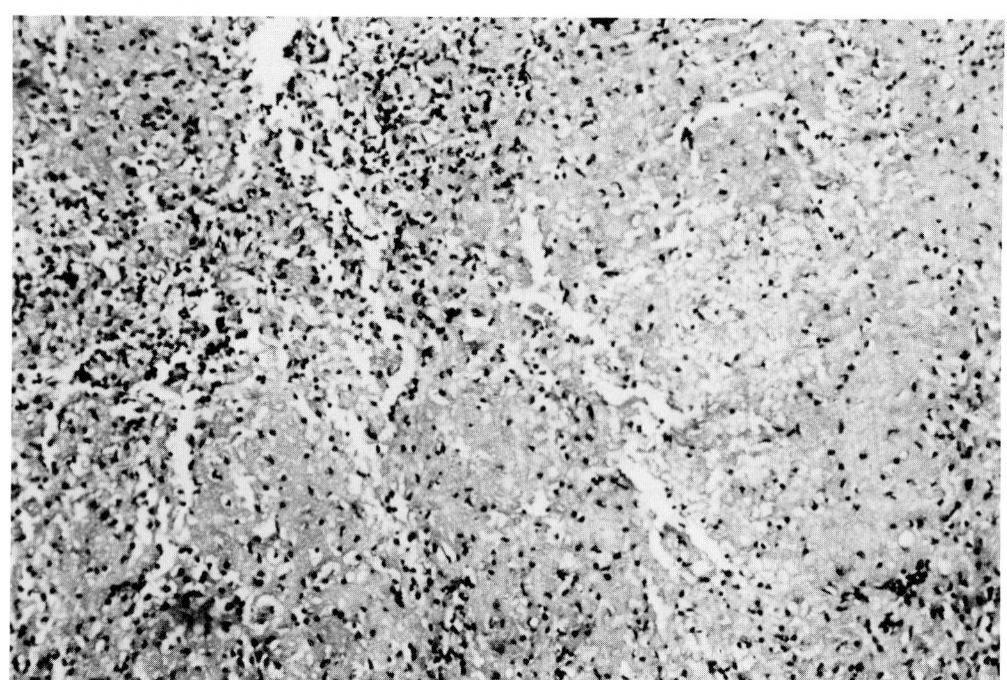

**Fig. 23-2.** Photomicrograph of a gummatous lesion in the testis of a 50-year-old black man.[14] An ill-defined area of necrosis with architectural distortion is surrounded by scar and lymphocytic infiltrate. Giant cells are not detected in this lesion (H & E). (*Courtesy of Dr. Robert Collins.*)

## PATHOGENESIS

It is generally accepted that the gumma represents a maximal inflammatory (allergic) response to a few organisms. The demonstration of *Treponema pallidum* in this lesion is difficult; animal inoculation is rarely successful, silver stains usually are unrewarding; an instance of success with indirect immunofluorescence has been reported. From extensive experience in endemic syphilis, Grin of Yugoslavia proposed two explanations for gumma formation: (1) reactivation of treponemes in a sensitized patient with untreated or inadequately treated venereal or endemic syphilis and (2) superinfection in a host already in an allergic state from a previous infection.[5] The best evidence in support of an allergic, or hypersensitivity, basis for the gumma was provided by Magnuson et al., who inoculated volunteers in Sing Sing Prison with the Nichols strain of *T. pallidum*. In the Sing Sing study, gummas developed only in persons with a history of previous syphilis. Among 26 inoculated prisoners who had been adequately treated earlier, 10 developed lesions (including one gumma) at the site of inoculation; of 5 who had been treated adequately for congenital syphilis, 1 developed a gumma at the site of inoculation.[6] Magnuson et al. concluded that superinfection in a sensitized patient may explain gumma formation. However, Gjestland believed superinfection had a minor role in the Oslo patients who developed gummas.[7] Olansky quoted experimental studies in rabbits by Collart et al., in which the administration of cortisone

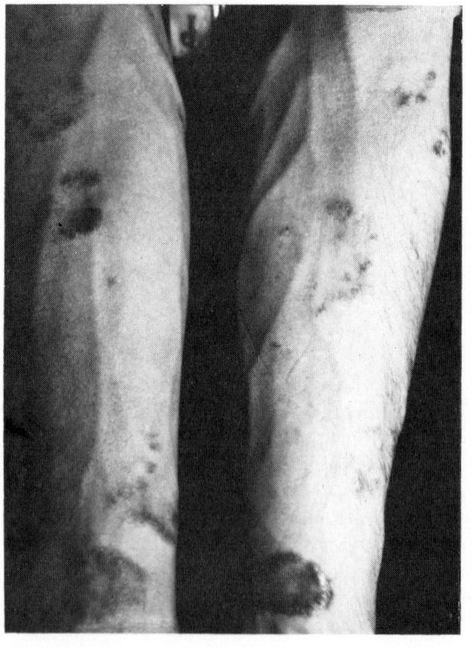

A

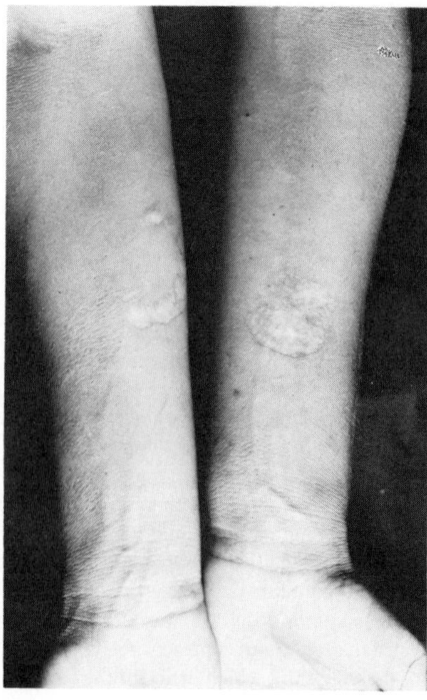

B

**Fig. 23-3.** (*a*) Nodular syphilid. (*b*) Characteristic residual scars from noduloulcerative syphilis. (*From RH Kampmeier, Essentials of Syphilology, Philadelphia, Lippincott, 1943.*)

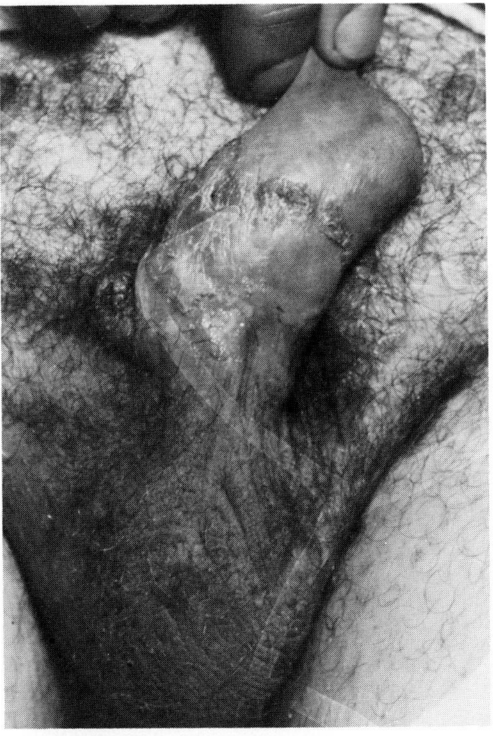

A

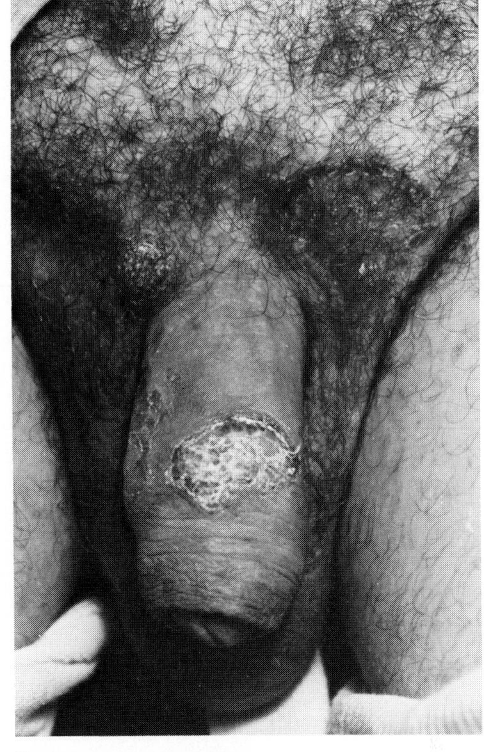

B

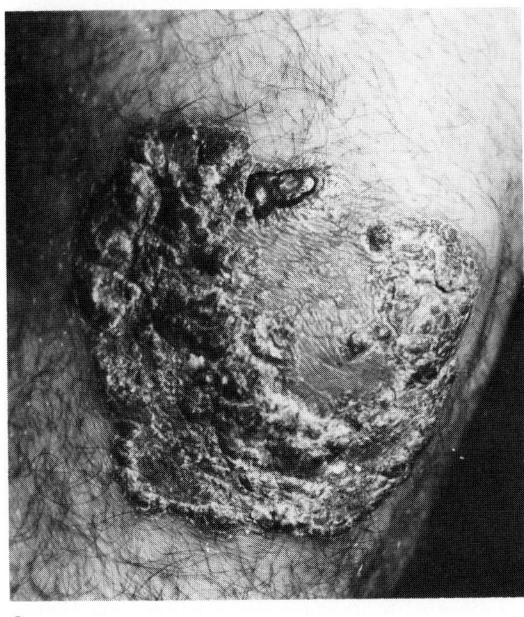

C

**Fig. 23-4.** (*a*) Nodular syphilid on inferior side of the penis. (*b*) Nodular syphilid of the pubic area and solitary gumma on dorsum of the penis. (*c*) Nodular syphilid of the knee. There were signs of aortic incompetency. (*From RH Kampmeier, Essentials of Syphilology, Philadelphia, Lippincott, 1943.*)

seemed to have altered the animals' immunity and thus permitted the development of a lesion of late syphilis.[8] That there may be other factors at times is suggested by the observations by members of the faculty at Vanderbilt University School of Medicine that osseous syphilis upon occasion has followed local trauma in a person in a late latent stage.

## PATHOLOGY

Syphilitic inflammation is generally relatively mild but chronic, and slow destruction of tissue leads to eventual fibrosis. The early inflammatory nodule has a granulomatous character closely resembling the lesion of tuberculosis. Grossly, gummas are nodules which may be found in any tissue or organ and may vary from microscopic size to many centimeters in diameter. The necrotic material in the larger nodules is of a gummy consistency, hence the term gumma. The histologic picture shows coagulative necrosis surrounded by lymphocytes and mononuclear cells; multinucleated giant cells appear only rarely. Ghosts of preexisting structures may be detected. The lesion is encapsulated by proliferating connective tissue with vascularized connective tissue extending outward from the necrotic area (Fig. 23-2). When the skin or mucous membrane is involved, an ulcer develops. Deep scarring accompanies the healing of gummas.

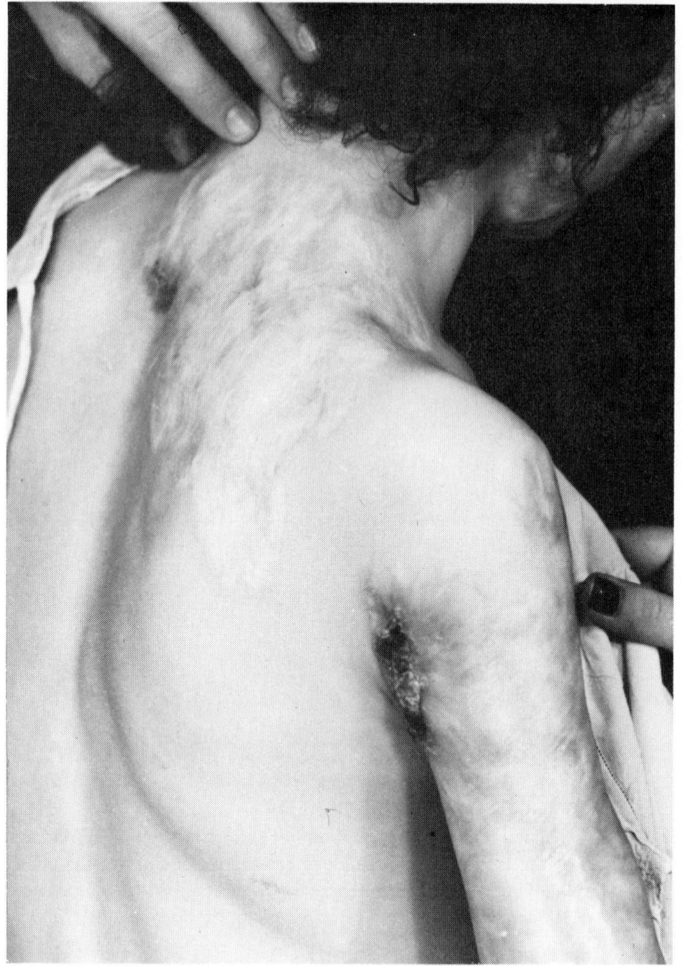

A

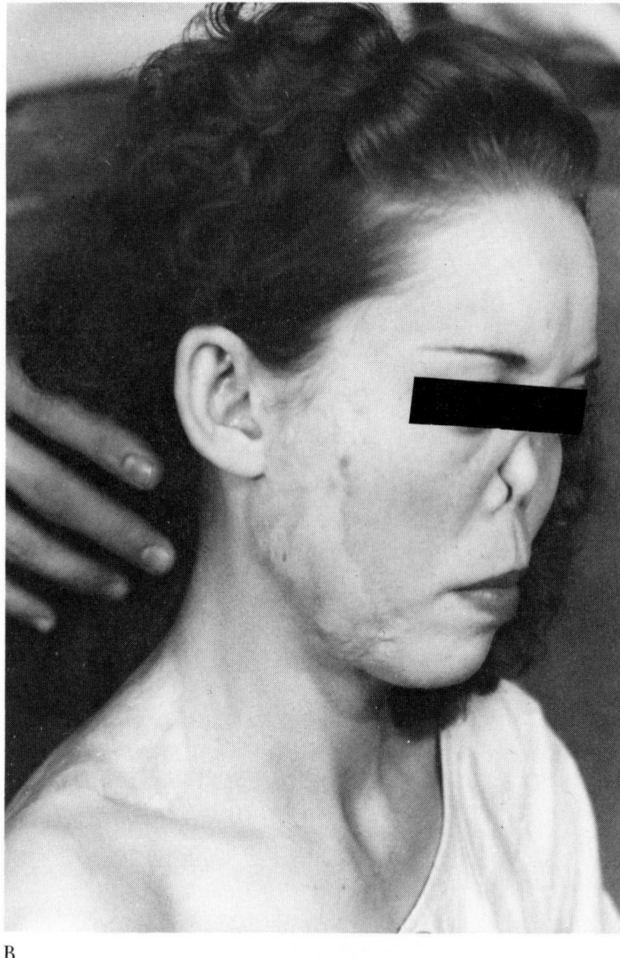

B

Fig. 23-5. (*a*) Atrophic scars on shoulder, arm, and (*b*) face following years of progressing noduloulcerative syphilids from congenital syphilis in a 14-year-old girl. An active area is visible at posterior axillary fold. Note the saddle-shaped nose. (*From RH Kampmeier, Physical Examination in Health and Disease, Philadelphia, Davis, 1970.*)

## CLINICAL MANIFESTATIONS

It is well to recall Osler's words:

> Syphilis simulates every other disease. It is the only disease necessary to know. One then becomes an expert dermatologist, an expert laryngologist, an expert alienist, an expert oculist, an expert internist, and an expert diagnostician.[9]

This aphorism may be put into other words as follows: The presence of any chronic inflammation, tumefaction or tumor, or destructive lesion of any tissue or organ of the body requires that syphilis be considered in the differential diagnosis.*

## SKIN

The late syphilid is considered first because of its frequency (see Table 23-1) and visualization as a prototype lesion involving tumefaction with or without softening (ulceration) and healing with scar formation. Two forms may appear: nodular or noduloulcerative, and a solitary lesion.

### Nodular and noduloulcerative lesions

Basically the *nodular lesion* is a deep indurated nodule that varies from pinhead to pea size and is brownish red in color. The multiple nodules are distributed usually in an arciform pattern with predilection for the face, the scapular and interscapular areas, and the extremities. They may remain for weeks or months and may heal without breaking down but still may show scarring. If nodular lesions break down to the noduloulcerative form, they heal leaving an atrophic noncontractile scar (Figs. 23-3 to 23-5). If untreated, they will heal, but over time (up to years) new nodules appear at the margins of the previous site with serpiginous progress and may eventually cover by scar an area as large as the whole back. Resolution of this syphilid is prompt under treatment. (A nonhealing area requires biopsy because of probable epithelioma.) A variant of this lesion on the palms or soles is a squamous or psoriasiform lesion without ulceration or scarring.

*A few, very rare examples of late syphilis are included to emphasize that no tissue or organ is immune to gummatous disease and that there is therefore a need for the consideration of syphilis in differential diagnosis.

## The solitary gumma

The solitary gumma is a subcutaneous process that involves the skin secondarily. It is more common on the thighs, buttocks, shoulders, forehead, and scalp. As it becomes necrotic, it has the characteristics of a "cold abscess," as in other granulomatous diseases. It may drain through one or more areas (Fig. 23-6).

# SKELETON

Tertiary syphilis of bones is about as common as gumma of the skin (Table 23-1). Although the gumma is a destructive process, it may be hidden by the osseous or periosteal reaction. A detailed radiologic study was made of 115 bones involved in 67 patients[10]: tibia, 34; clavicle, 17; skull, 15 (Fig. 23-7); fibula, 15; humerus, 5; rib, 4; ulna, 3; scapula, 3; malar, 2; mandible, 2; and 1 each for facial, sternum, spine, radius, metacarpal, metatarsal, phalanx, patella, and ischium. Although the basic lesion is the gumma, the radiographic manifestations (see Fig. 23-8) were classified as follows:

1. Periostitis, periosteal thickening with increased density in laminated layers (27 bones).
2. Gummatous osteitis, destructive or osteomyelitic lesions, usually with periosteal or endosteal changes and sclerosis of the surrounding bone (72 bones).
3. Sclerosing osteitis, in which the increased density and periosteal change hide the gummatous lesion (16 bones).

The clinical characteristics include pain (especially nocturnal), tenderness, swelling, bony tumor, stiffness, and limited motion. Less common symptoms are heat, redness, and draining sinuses. Gumma of skeletal muscle is recognized by biopsy or by resolution of the tumor under therapy.

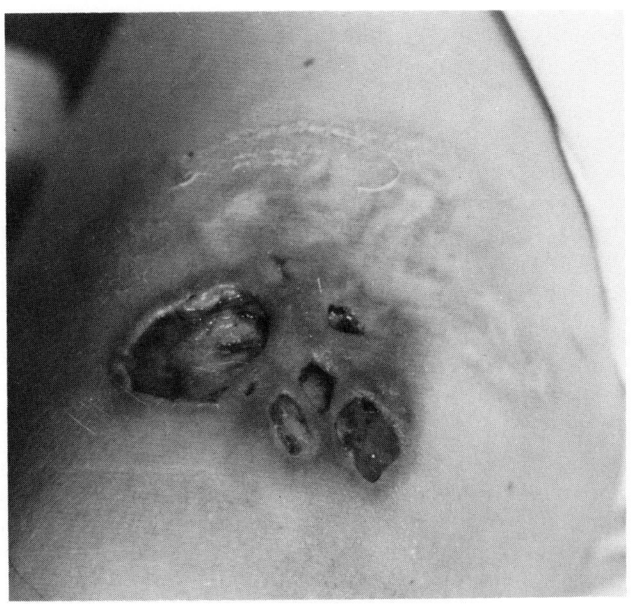

**Fig. 23-6.** Ulcerating solitary gumma of skin of 12 months' duration. Note scarring from spontaneous healing. Accompanying solitary ulcers on each shoulder and on the leg, 4 to 8 cm in diameter, began as pimples 7 months previously. (*From RH Kampmeier, Essentials of Syphilology, Philadelphia, Lippincott, 1943.*)

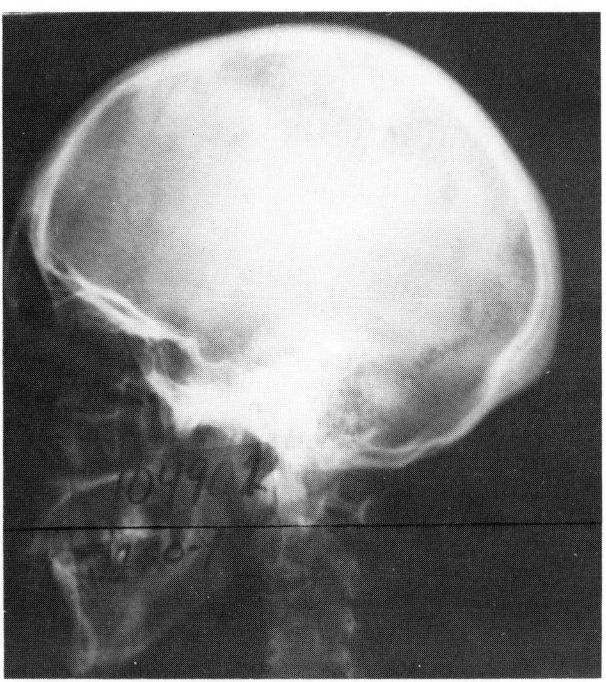

**Fig. 23-7.** Multiple areas of gummatous osteitis in patient shown in Fig. 23-15. (*From RH Kampmeier.*[3])

# UPPER RESPIRATORY TRACT, MOUTH, AND TONGUE

Gummatous osteitis of the nasal bones, hard palate, and nasal septum, as well as perichondritis of the latter used to be relatively common (Table 23-1 and Figs. 23-9 and 23-10). Labial involvement may occur in the noduloulcerative lesion of the face, as well as in a solitary gumma. Gumma of the tongue presents as a tumor (Fig. 23-11). Gumma of the soft palate leads to chronic ulceration, almost always with perforation. A history of chronic "sore throat" (actually difficulty in deglutition) lasting for weeks or months and the presence of an indolent ulcer are characteristic of tertiary involvement of the fauces and oropharynx. Deforming scars here provide the hallmark of such a process years before. Chronic hoarseness may suggest tumefaction or ulceration and/or destruction of the epiglottis or laryngeal structures (typical of gummatous involvement of the larynx), which are easily seen with a laryngeal mirror. (This lesion is not to be confused with the laryngitis not uncommonly associated with secondary syphilis, which is easily recognized by the experienced laryngologist.)

# LOWER RESPIRATORY TRACT

Late syphilitic disease of these structures is rare and usually difficult to prove etiologically. One patient who died from asphyxia was proved at postmortem examination to have a gumma at the bifurcation of the trachea. In several of our patients symptoms led to bronchoscopy, which revealed narrowed bronchi, and a biopsy diagnosis of "chronic inflammation." Resolution in response to *bismuth* and *iodides*, verified by follow-up bronchoscopy, certainly suggested a syphilitic etiology. Pulmonary syphilitic disease is very rare, and although a solitary tumor, nodule, or localized infiltrate is the more usual, a major diffuse infiltration has been observed (Fig. 23-12). Successful treatment by *iodides*

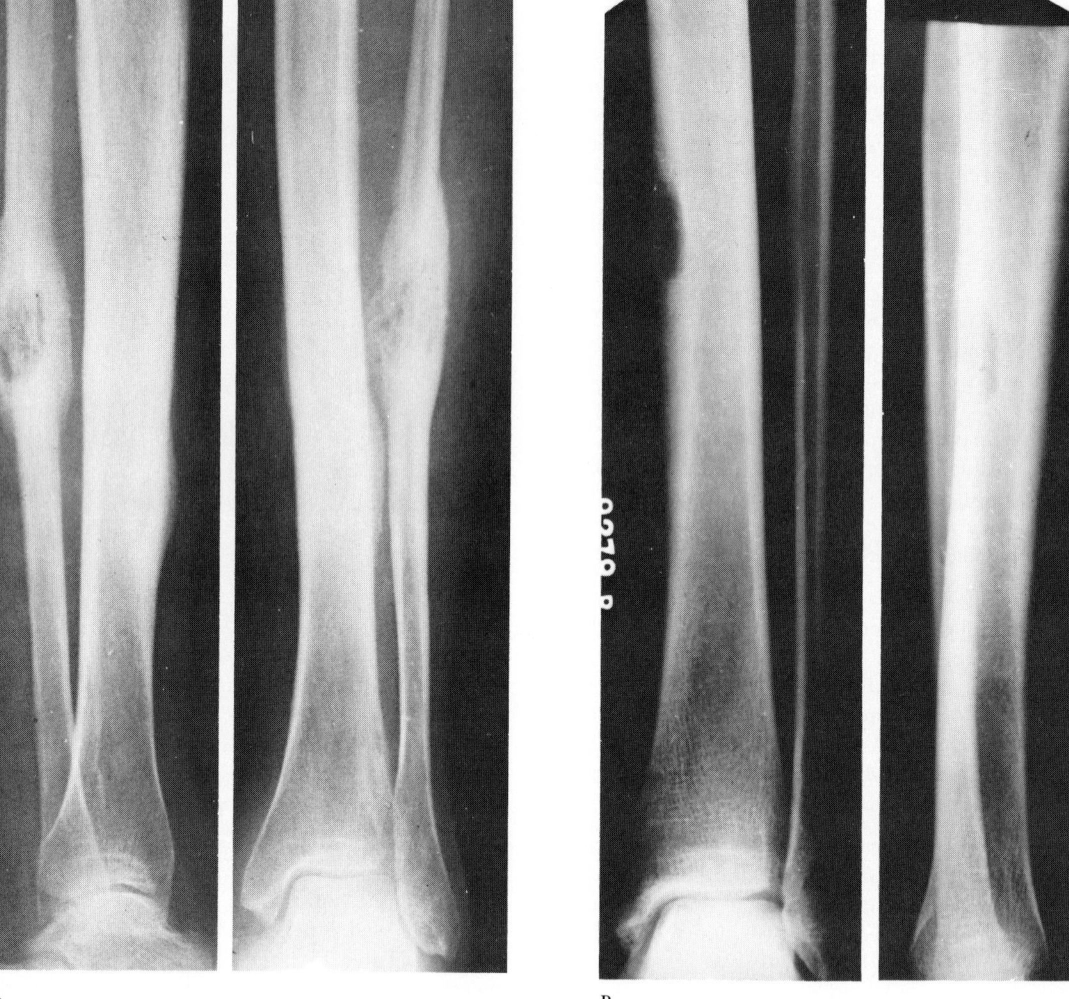


**Fig. 23-8.** (*a*) Periostitis of tibia without destruction; gummatous destruction of fibula. (*From RH Kampmeier, Essentials of Syphilology, Philadelphia, Lippincott, 1943.*) (*b*) Destructive cystlike lesion (gumma) of cortex with periosteal elevation and thickening. (*From HC Francis and RH Kampmeier, South Med J 36:556, 1953.*)

and *bismuth* adds certainty to the etiologic diagnosis of syphilis of the lung.

## DIGESTIVE SYSTEM

The clinical picture of the rare gumma of the esophagus suggests carcinoma.[11] Esophagoscopy may reveal an ulcer, tumor, or stricture. If biopsy does not show malignant cells, only a therapeutic trial may hold the answer (Fig. 23-13). Gumma of the diaphragm with esophageal obstruction occurs.[11] Gastric syphilis may mimic either a malignant or a benign gastric ulcer clinically and radiologically (Fig. 23-14). Seven instances of syphilis of the stomach were reported from Vanderbilt University Hospital,[12] and 93 cases were evaluated at the Mayo Clinic.[13] Commonly, such patients have been operated upon because of a mistaken diagnosis; others have required operation after antisyphilitic treatment resulted in obstructive scarring ("hourglass stomach").

Gumma of the liver (Fig. 23-15) is the most frequent type of gastrointestinal tertiary syphilis. Some patients remain asymptomatic but feel an abdominal mass merely by chance. However, there may be symptoms of low-grade fever, weight loss, and epigastric pain and tenderness. Splenomegaly often accompanies the disease. (For hepatomegaly accompanied by fever, common practice in the south early in this century was first to treat with quinine and, if unsuccessful, then to administer mercury and iodides. This regimen indicates that syphilitic hepatitis was frequently encountered.) Healing of gumma of the liver leaves a characteristic scar and, if multiple, gross deformity of the liver (*hepar lobatum*). Gumma of the pancreas has been reported but is rare.

## GENITOURINARY TRACT

Gumma of the bladder and kidney has been reported, but many experienced syphilologists have never seen a proven example. Gummatous involvement of the testes and of the female genital organs has been encountered.[14]

## ENDOCRINE SYSTEM

Gumma of the thyroid gland has been reported. Two instances of gumma of the adrenal glands accompanied by Addison's dis-

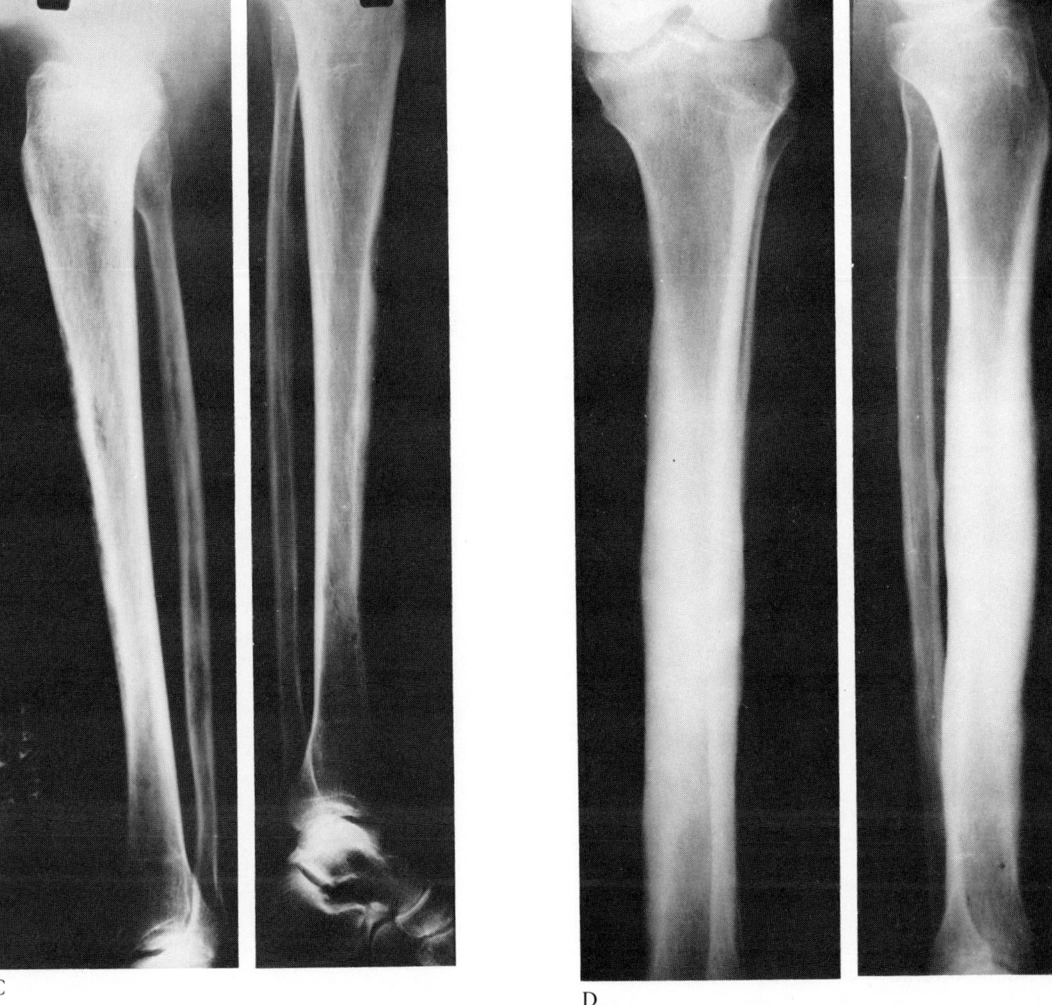


**Fig. 23-8** *(continued)* (*c*) Extensive, superficial destructive lesions in both tibias with almost complete absence of periosteal reaction; gummas with periosteal changes in the fibulas. (*From HC Francis and RH Kampmeier, South Med J 36:556, 1953.*) (*d*) Sclerosing osteitis; the roentgenograph shows wavy outlines of dense sclerotic bone without destruction. (*From HC Francis and RH Kampmeier, South Med J 36:556, 1953.*)

ease have been proved at autopsy in patients hospitalized at Vanderbilt University Hospital.

## BREAST

Gumma may appear as a tumor of the breast and then be diagnosed as syphilis by the surgical pathologist, or it may present as an ulcer which responds to antisyphilitic treatment (Fig. 23-16).

## OCULAR DISEASE

There is nothing specific about the iritis of late syphilis. Keratoiritis was common in congenital syphilis in the past. Disease of the choroid (syphilitic chorioretinitis) is a serious manifestation of late syphilis. The retinal exudate of the active phase upon resolution leaves characteristic scars in the choroidal pigment.

## MYOCARDIUM

The postmortem finding of myocardial gummas, especially of the left ventricle and commonly asymptomatic, has been reported upon occasion. Although complete heart block from gummatous involvement of the atrioventricular bundle has been documented rarely, we have encountered two instances[16] (Fig. 23-17).

## DIAGNOSIS, PROGNOSIS, AND TREATMENT

To consider syphilis and include it in the differential diagnosis is one-half of the diagnosis. Screening serologic tests are helpful because they are usually reactive, especially where there is extensive involvement of soft tissue (e.g., gumma of skin or liver). The serologic test results may be of high titer. The prozone phenomenon has been encountered in some cases, resulting in a falsely negative qualitative (VDRL) which has been shown to be positive upon retesting in appropriate dilutions of serum. On the other hand a negative reaction may accompany a localized lesion, e.g., as of bone.

The prognosis in untreated disease is dependent upon the site

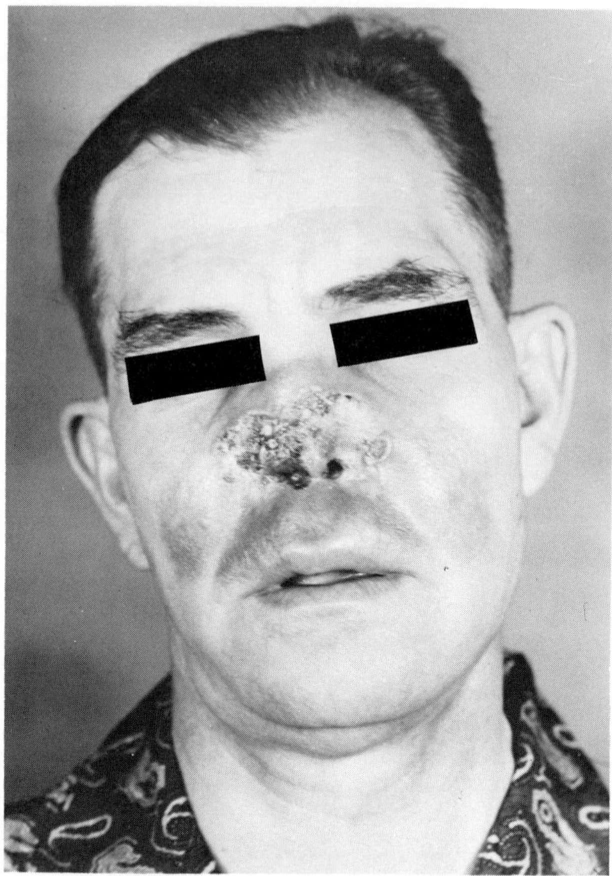

Fig. 23-9. Disease of the cartilagenous nasal septum.

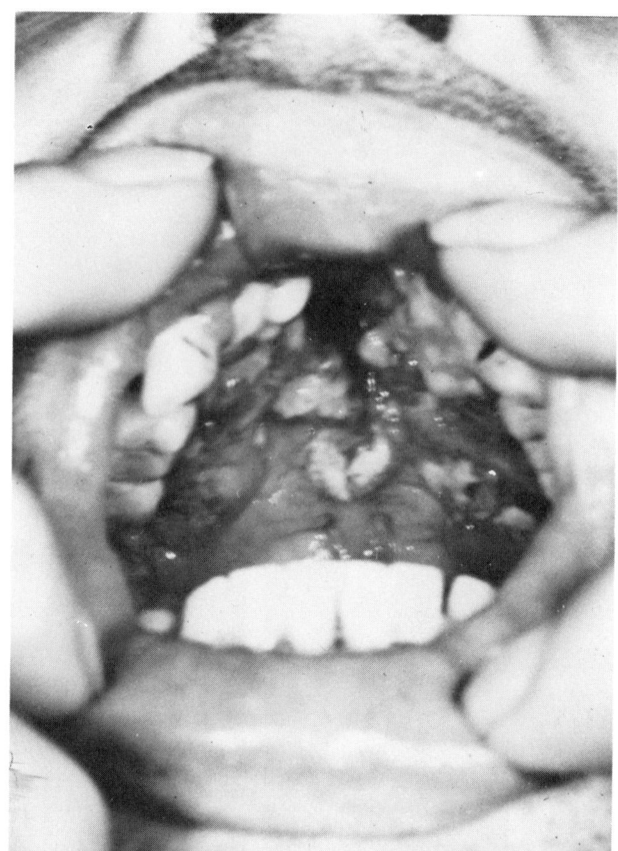

Fig. 23-10. Osteitis of hard palate with perforation. (*From RH Kampmeier, Physical Examination in Health and Disease, Philadelphia, Davis, 1970.*)

of involvement. Noduloulcerative cutaneous syphilis may alternately progress and heal for years. Bone lesions may heal spontaneously or end in draining sinuses from a chronic osteomyelitic process. Lesions of viscera tend to heal or lead to functional disability from scarring. (Numerous instances of hepar lobatum appeared in routine autopsies at Charity Hospital, New Orleans.) Untreated chronic retinitis causes impaired vision and even blindness.

## HEAVY METAL

The response of late benign disease to antisyphilitic treatment was prompt and dramatic with few exceptions. Syphilids usually healed quickly following the administration of iodides and a heavy metal. It should be recalled that healing might occur following the use of iodides only, as was noted 150 years ago. St. John[17] in his review of the literature stated that the response to chemotherapy was reported to be excellent, with resolution in over 90 percent of cases if four or more courses of arsenic and heavy metal were given; even with less than four courses, the "cure" rate was high. Incidentally, antibiotics have deprived the clinician of the certainty of a diagnosis by therapy. A clinical response of a late benign lesion to bismuth is specific for syphilis and offers proof of its etiology. Unfortunately, bismuth is not generally available for this purpose today, and the effective spectrum of antibiotic therapy is too broad to offer this certainty.

A Jarisch-Herxheimer reaction may be especially hazardous in late benign syphilis. An instance of chorioretinitis was observed in which an injection of arsenic produced an exacerbation of disease which led to almost complete destruction of the retina. One patient required tracheostomy following arsenotherapy for late latent syphilis with unknown laryngeal disease. Formerly, it was customary to initiate treatment for late latent syphilis and late benign disease with a course of bismuth and iodides. Penicillin also may induce a Jarisch-Herxheimer reaction. No one advises the caution we used in chemotherapy, however, because the rarity of gummatous disease has reduced the statistical likelihood of a serious Jarisch-Herxheimer reaction to near zero.

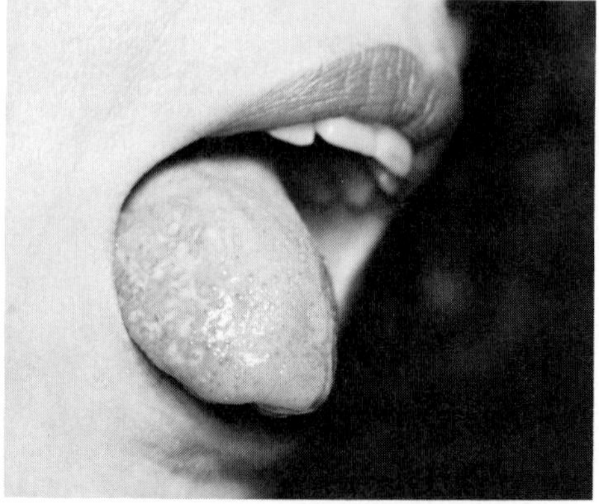

Fig. 23-11. Gumma of the tongue. (*From RH Kampmeier, Physical Examination in Health and Disease, Philadelphia, Davis, 1970.*)

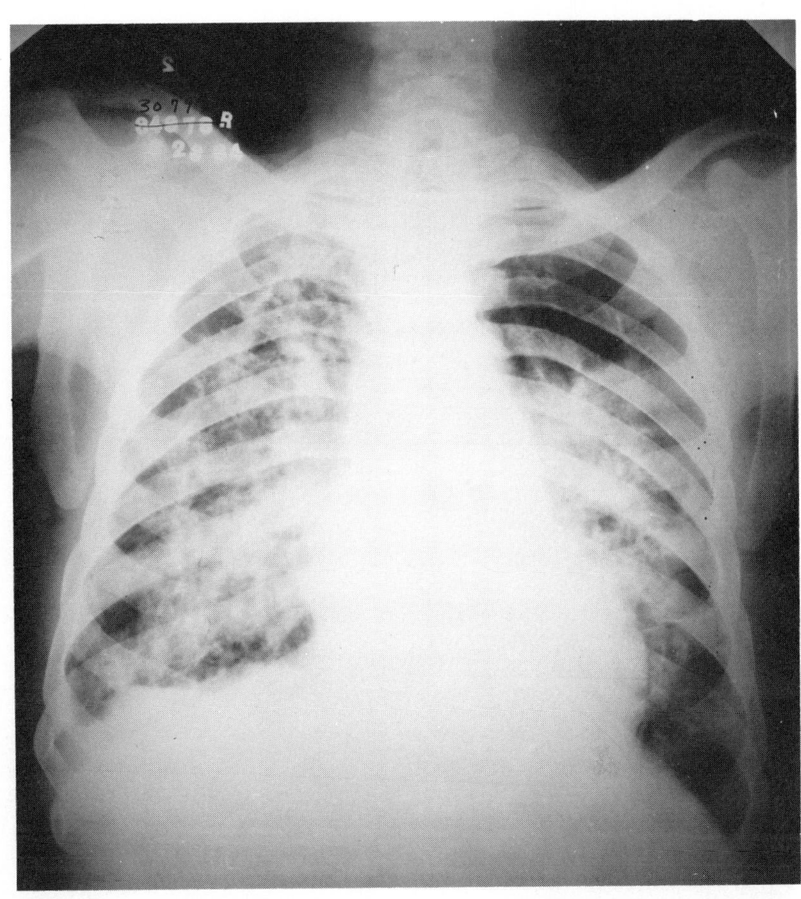

**Fig. 23-12.** Postmortem findings of gummatous infiltrates, syphilitic arteritis, and pulmonary fibrosis. There was accompanying aortitis in this patient.

## PENICILLIN

As shown in Fig. 23-1, late benign disease was approaching the vanishing point in the era before penicillin and this trend was enhanced by the efficacy of penicillin therapy for early syphilis. (For contrast to Table 23-1, a search in the medical records department for the past 15 years of the Vanderbilt University Hospital and the Metropolitan Nashville General Hospital revealed only one instance of gummatous disease.[14] The evaluation of treatment in a rare disease is difficult. St. John stated that "there are no controlled studies of penicillin in any large series of patients," and he referred to the writings of Tucker.[18] In 1948, after citing the first reported case of a syphilid treated with penicillin at the Mayo Clinic in 1944, Tucker reviewed the results of penicillin therapy in some detail in 34 patients having cutaneous lesions and in 16 with bone disease treated at the Johns Hopkins Hospital clinics. (These included the cases of a previous report.[19]) Of the first 18 patients treated for a syphilid, two had relapses and were re-treated. Sixteen patients who were followed for a mean of 911 days remained well after having received 1.7 million units of amorphous penicillin. Another 16 similar patients who received from 0.32 to 7.0 million units (10 received crystalline penicillin G) were well at the end of a mean of 364 days. The 16 patients who had syphilitic osteitis, osteomyelitis, and/or periostitis were treated with 0.6 to 7.0 million units of penicillin and were followed for a mean of 706 days. In one, although the bone lesion was under control, a syphilid developed 8 months later.

### Penicillin treatment in 12 cases of late benign syphilis

Because of the paucity of data on the treatment of late benign syphilis with penicillin, I will briefly review the cases of 12 patients who were treated between 1946, after penicillin became generally available, and 1951, when the Vanderbilt syphilis clinic was closed. Syphilitic patients were thereafter admitted to the general medical outpatient service.

Three patients had nodular syphilids and were treated respectively as follows: 2.4 million units of amorphous penicillin (40,000 units every 3 h); 7.2 million units of penicillin in beeswax and peanut oil (POB) in 15 days; 9.0 million units of procaine penicillin in 15 days. The lesions remained healed at 3 years, 1 year, and 1 year, respectively. (The second of these patients also had sclerosing osteitis of both tibias and findings of type III spinal fluid; when this patient was last seen 1 year after treatment, the osteitis remained unchanged radiologically but the spinal fluid showed a reduction in the number of cells to normal.) In one of these patients, treatment with 9.0 million units of POB was followed by disappearance of multiple subcutaneous masses in less than 60 days.

A patient with gummatous osteitis of the nasal septum and nasal bones was treated with 3.0 million units of amorphous penicillin (40,000 units every 3 h); the bridge of the nose collapsed, and findings of type II spinal fluid remained unchanged after 5 years. In another patient syphilitic osteitis of a rib with a

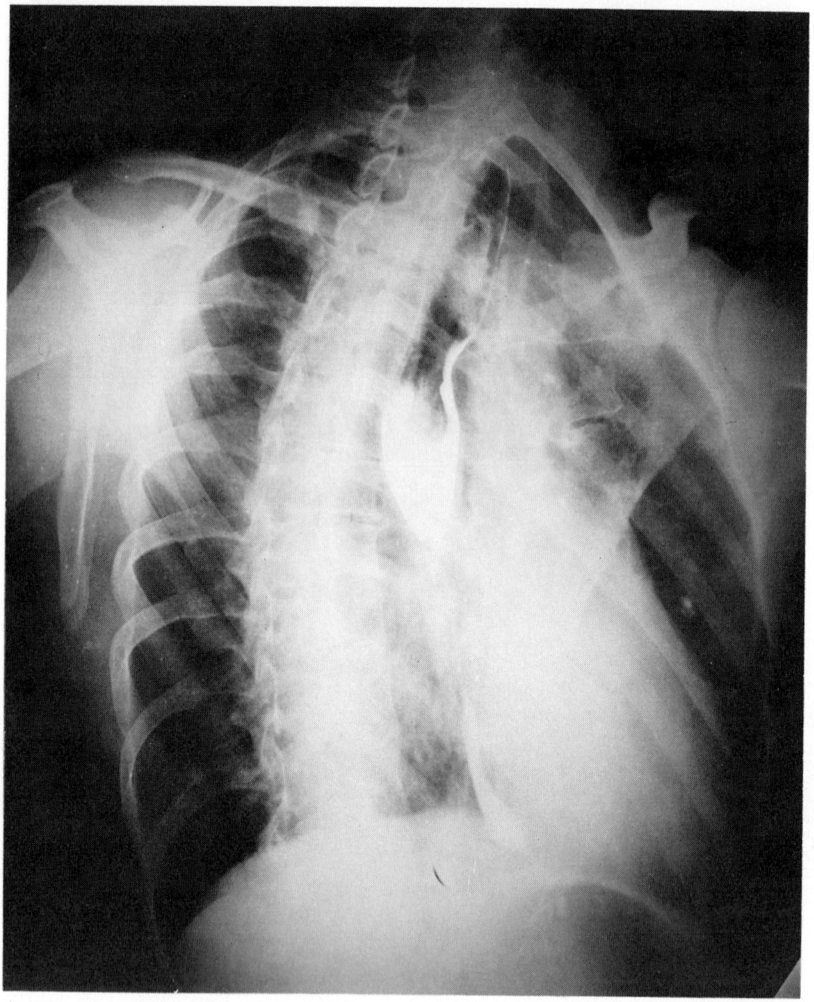
A

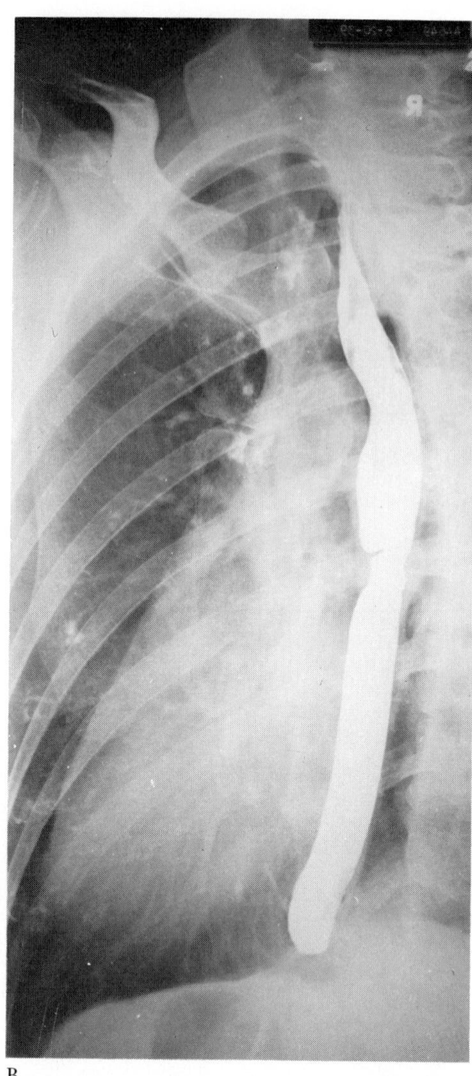
B

**Fig. 23-13.** (*a*) Obstructive lesion of the esophagus. (*b*) Residual slight constriction following administration of iodides, bismuth, and arsenic. (*From RH Kampmeier and E Jones.*[11])

draining sinus healed under treatment with five injections of 6.0 million units of POB and 60 mg arsenoxide and with three injections of bismuth; follow-up was only for 3 months.

Two women presented with painful swelling over the medial one-third of the clavicle and the sternoclavicular joint. X-rays of the first woman revealed enlargement of the medial end of the clavicle with irregular overgrowth of bone on the clavicular border and on the sternal border which crosses the joint space, and slight rarefaction and some sclerotic changes. For the second woman, the x-rays revealed destruction of bone and a thickened periosteum. The first of these patients had completed treatment with 47 injections of neoarsphenamine and 35 injections of bismuth for tabes dorsalis 15 months previously. The patients were treated with 7.8 million units and 9.0 million units of POB in 13 and 15 days, respectively. The pain, tenderness, and soft-tissue swelling responded to treatment. The radiologic changes in the first of these cases remained unchanged over 5 years. In the second case, although there was some filling-in of bone and thickening of the cortex, areas of rarefaction continued to be noted at 6 months.

A patient with gummatous hepatitis (Fig. 23-15) had accompanying osteitis of the parietal and occipital bones (Fig. 23-7) and the ilium. Treatment with 9.0 million unts of POB resulted in restitution of bone in the skull to normal by 15 months; the liver edge receded to the costal margin within 6 months.

A patient with a gumma of the tongue and periostitis of the sternum was treated with 9.0 million units of POB (Fig. 23-11). There was prompt response of both lesions, but the gumma left a residual notch at the border of the tongue and blood tests were negative 1 year after treatment. Three years later a draining ulcer developed on a thigh and was accompanied by serorelapse. Cultures for fungi proved negative; biopsy revealed only chronic inflammation. The ulcer was cured by three injections of water-soluble bismuth, followed by treatment with 6.0 million units of aluminum monostearate penicillin. The patient was well when seen last a year later.

A patient with tabes dorsalis who developed gastric symptoms was found to have a very large ulcer on the posterior surface of the fundus, which was interpreted by the radiologist as probably malignant. (Spinal fluid was of type II.) A surgical consultant advised against gastric resection in this 67-year-old man, who was considered a poor risk. He was treated with 9.0 million units of POB, which provided symptomatic relief. X-ray studies were negative some months later and again 1 year later.

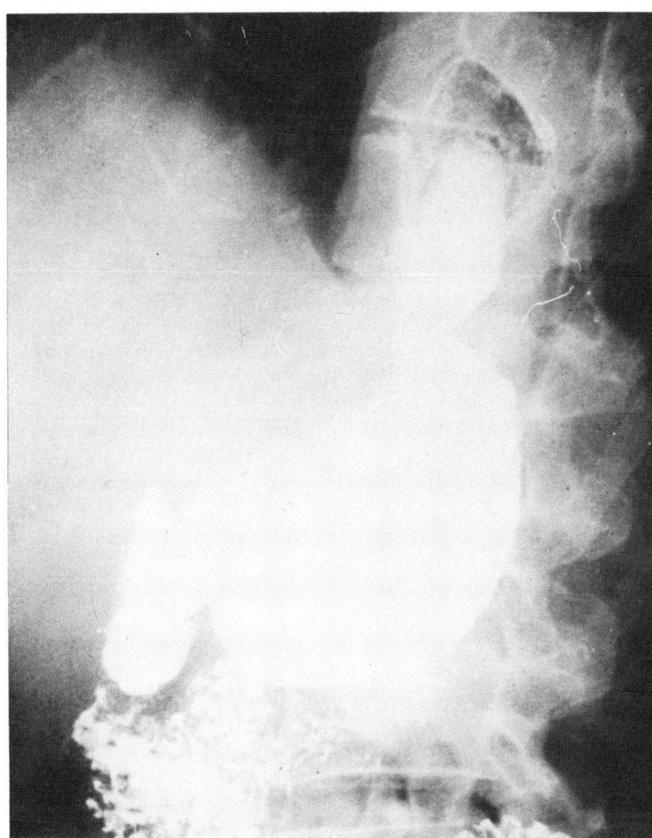

**Fig. 23-14.** Gummatous gastric ulcer. Radiological diagnosis of inoperable carcinoma. Resolution under bismuth and arsenic. (*From RH Kampmeier, Essentials of Syphilology, Philadelphia, Lippincott, 1943.*)

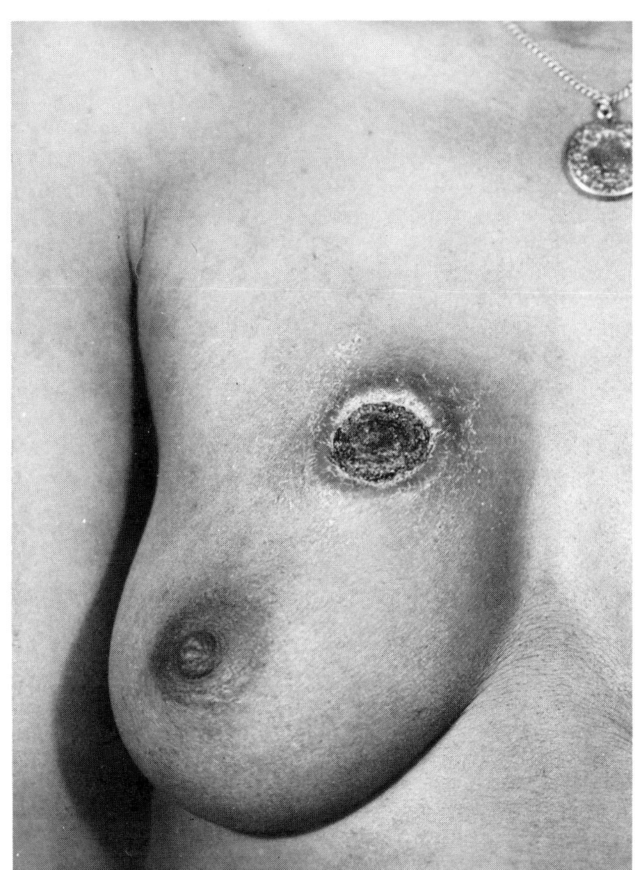

**Fig. 23-16.** Gumma of the breast. (*From RH Kampmeier.*[15])

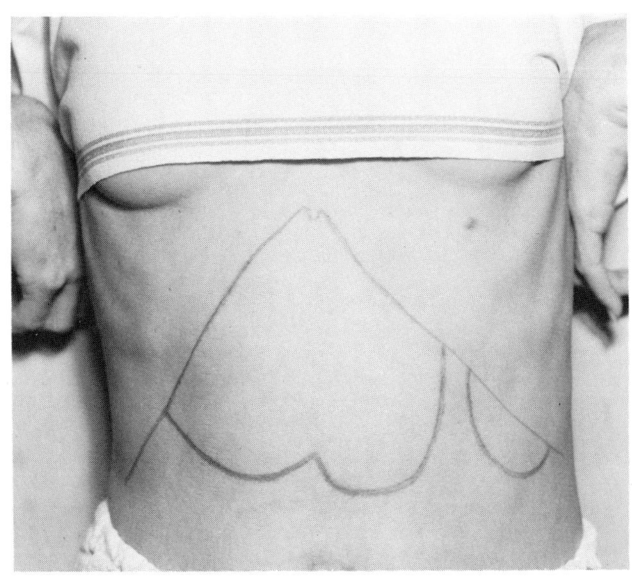

**Fig. 23-15.** Gummatous hepatitis with splenomegaly of the same patient as in Fig. 23-7. (*From RH Kampmeier.*[3])

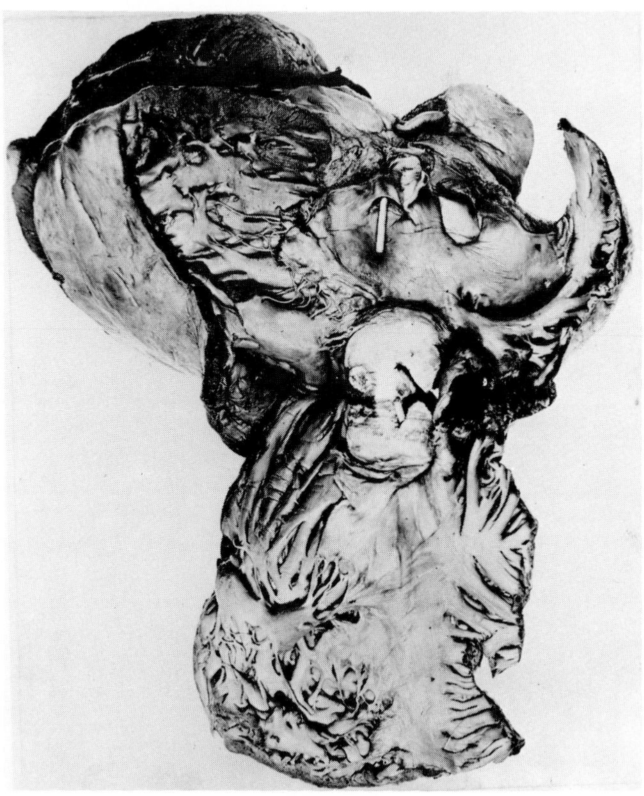

**Fig. 23-17.** Gumma involving the atrioventricular bundle and the right coronary artery. (*From A Weinstein, RH Kampmeier, RH Harwood. Courtesy AMA Arch Intern Med 100:90, Copyright 1957, AMA.*)

A 46-year-old man was admitted to the neurosurgical service with symptoms leading to diagnosis of a focal lesion (a tumor or gumma) of the frontoparietal area. The spinal fluid findings were those of type III. Treatment consisted of 4.0 million units of aqueous penicillin G and 14.0 million units of aluminum monostearate penicillin in 24 injections given 3 times weekly. The patient became asymptomatic, and 6 months later his spinal fluid showed improvement.

After Tucker had reviewed the experience at Johns Hopkins in the treatment of 34 patients having late benign syphilis, he concluded, "On the basis of reported data and an analysis of our own material, satisfactory results may be obtained in approximately 90% of such cases by the administration of a single course of penicillin alone."[18] The experience with treatment provided at the Vanderbilt syphilis clinic is in agreement with this statement. St. John, in his 1976 review of the literature on the treatment of late benign syphilis, found no subsequent therapeutic trials and accepted Tucker's recommendation of treatment with "at least two million units of penicillin if not more." A computer search for the past decade provides no further experience in the treatment of late benign syphilis other than in case reports.

## References


1 Kampmeier RH: Historical article: Clarification of the systemic manifestations of syphilis, especially in the tertiary stage. *Sex Transm Dis* 8:82, 1981.

2 Clark EG, Danbolt N: The Oslo study of the natural course of untreated syphilis. *J Chronic Dis* 2:311, 1955.

3 Kampmeier RH: The late manifestations of syphilis: Skeletal, visceral and cardiovascular. *Med Clin North Am* 48:667, 1964.

4 Kampmeier RH: Comments on the present day management of syphilis. *South Med J* 46:226, 1953.

5 Grin EI: *Epidemiology and Control of Endemic Syphilis: Report on a Mass Treatment Campaign in Bosnia.* WHO Monograph Series. Geneva, WHO, 1953.

6 Magnuson HJ et al: Inoculation syphilis in human volunteers. *Medicine (Baltimore)* 35:33, 1956.

7 Gjestland T: The Oslo study of untreated syphilis. *Acta Derm Venereol* [suppl] (Stockh) 35:34, 1955.

8 Collart P et al, quoted in Olansky S: Late benign syphilis (gumma). *Med Clin North Am* 48:653, 1964.

9 Bean RB, Bean WB: *Sir William Osler Aphorisms from His Bedside Teachings and Writings.* Springfield, IL, Charles C Thomas, 1961.

10 Francis HC, Kampmeier RH: The bone lesions in acquired tertiary syphilis. *South Med J* 36:556, 1943.

11 Kampmeier RH, Jones E: Esophageal obstruction due to gummata of esophagus and diaphragm. *Am J Med Sci* 201:539, 1941.

12 Harris S, Youmans JB: Syphilis of the stomach: A report of seven cases. *South Med J* 24:877, 1931.

13 Eusterman GB: Gastric syphilis: Observations based on 93 cases. *JAMA* 96:173, 1931.

14 Dao AH, Adkins RB: Bilateral gummatous orchitis. *South Med J* 73:954, 1980.

15 Kampmeier RH: Syphilis of the breast: Chancre and gumma. *Am Pract* 1:395, 1947.

16 Weinstein A et al: Complete heart block due to syphilis. *AMA Arch Intern Med* 100:90, 1957.

17 St John RK: Treatment of late benign syphilis: Review of the literature. *J Am Vener Dis Assoc* 3 (pt 2): 146, 1976.

18 Tucker HA: Penicillin in benign late and visceral syphilis. *Am J Med* 5:702, 1948.

19 Dexter DD, Tucker HA: Penicillin treatment of benign late gummatous syphilis: A report of twenty-one cases. *Am J Syph Gonor Vener Dis* 30:211, 1945.

# Chapter 24

# Chancroid and *Haemophilus ducreyi*

Allan R. Ronald
William Albritton

## DEFINITION

Chancroid is an acutely ulcerative disease, usually of the genitals, often associated with an inguinal bubo, due to infection with *Haemophilus ducreyi*, a gram-negative, facultative anaerobic bacillus that requires hemin (X factor) for growth.

## HISTORY

Chancroid, or soft chancre (ulcus molle), was first differentiated from syphilis, or hard chancre, by Ricord in France in 1838. At the University of Naples in 1889, Ducrey inoculated the skin of the forearm of three patients with purulent material from their own genital ulcer.[1] At weekly intervals he inoculated a new site with material from the most recent ulcer and was able to maintain serial ulcers through as many as 15 generations. He described it as a short, compact streptobacillary rod ($1.5 \times 0.5$ μm) that is nicely rounded at the ends and has an indentation at the sides. It was found both within and without neutrophils. He concluded that it was responsible for the soft chancre and further stated that others were incorrect in their attribution of a major role to the "common microorganisms of suppuration" in the pathogenicity of the ulcer or the bubo. Within 3 years this work was confirmed by Krefting,[2] and Unna subsequently described the histology of the chancroidal ulcer and visualized the clumps and chains of gram-negative rods in the lesion.[3]

Sullivan[4] in his review of chancroid in 1940 credited Lenglet in 1898 and Bezancon, Griffin, and LeSourd in 1900 with the first successful cultures of *H. ducreyi*, although Himmel[5] cited the successes of earlier investigators. Teague and Deibert reported the isolation of *H. ducreyi* from up to 80 percent of patients with suspected clinical chancroid.[6] In subsequent studies Teague and Deibert demonstrated that serum (rabbit or sheep), a red blood cell extract (rabbit), and casein digest or peptone were necessary to obtain good growth of *H. ducreyi* on agar media.[7] In 1944 Beeson also noted that both serum and red cells were necessary to support the growth of the organism, but neither X nor V factor appeared to be essential.[8]

In 1913 Ito carried out intradermal tests both with *H. ducreyi* from culture and with pus from a chancroidal bubo.[9] A papule, 8 mm or more in diameter, appearing between the third and seventh days was interpreted as a positive test. In 1923 Reenstierna at the Pasteur Institute confirmed Ito's work.[10] The test became positive in over 90 percent of patients 2 or more weeks after the appearance of the genital ulcer. The value of the Ito-Reenstierna intradermal test was confirmed by Greenblatt and Sanderson,[11] and a commercial antigen was marketed by Lederle Laboratories for intradermal testing; it is no longer commercially available.

Despite considerable clinical investigation into chancroid and its etiology during the first four decades of this century, controversy as to the etiologic agent still existed. In 1935 the U.S. Public Health Service stated that "this is a local disease of the external generative organs in which a sore develops. The cause of this sore is believed to be an infection with a germ, although some physicians question the part which this germ plays."[12] Other historically relevant information can be found in the review of Sullivan in 1940[4] and the series of articles from the VDRL chancroid studies.[13–15]

## EPIDEMIOLOGY

Chancroid is a sexually transmitted disease more prevalent in individuals from lower socioeconomic groups who frequent prostitutes.[16] The presence of a foreskin makes males more susceptible to *H. ducreyi*.[17] Also, men have a markedly higher incidence of the disease than women do. Chancroid has not been well characterized in male homosexuals. *H. ducreyi* appears to be spread from person to person only by sexual contact with no known alternate routes. Autoinoculation of fingers or other sites is reported occasionally. Fomites have not been shown to play any role in transmission.

Several studies have characterized epidemic chancroid in the military. In Korea, 32 percent of venereal disease among American military was considered to be chancroid. In Korea, the ratio of gonorrhea to chancroid to syphilis was 14:8:1 in white troops and 21:11:1 in black troops.[18] Among Australian troops during the Vietnamese conflict, 23 percent of men with chancroid were circumcised, compared with 60 percent of men with other venereal diseases.[17]

Until recently, few epidemiologic studies have been carried out in civilian populations in Western societies. During the past decade, epidemics of chancroid have occurred similar to the 1975 to 1977 experience in Winnipeg.[16,19–22] Prostitutes appear to be the reservoir of disease in each of these epidemics. The ratio of males to females with chancroid in most nonmilitary epidemics has been 10:1.

There is no evidence for a continuing reservoir of *H. ducreyi* in the absence of clinical cases of chancroid. Although studies from Sheffield, England, suggested that *H. ducreyi* commonly coinfects herpetic ulcers and can be frequently isolated from genital secretions and the oropharynx of otherwise healthy individuals, attempts to repeat these studies in other communities have failed to show any asymptomatic reservoir in the absence of ulcers.[23,24]

The annual incidence of chancroid decreased markedly in the United States between 1950 and 1978.[21] In 1947, the incidence was 6.4 cases per 100,000 population. It fell to between 0.3 and 0.6 cases per 100,000 with fewer than 1000 cases reported annually. Clusters of chancroid continued to be seen at seaports with microepidemics introduced from time to time by individuals, many of whom had returned from tropical countries. However, in 1985, the number of reported cases rose above 2000 for the first time since 1956 and further increased to 3418 cases in 1986.[21] This rapid increase in reported cases of chancroid has continued through 1987 and 1988, with the majority of cases occurring in New York City, Dallas, Boston, and several communities in Florida. In the absence of well-organized eradication programs, infected individuals will presumably travel to nonendemic areas and establish new foci of disease.

Genital ulcer disease due to *H. ducreyi* is a major public health and medical problem in many third world countries.[25] In Nairobi, Kenya, over 5000 patients with chancroid are seen annually in the one major clinic for sexually transmitted disease. Among prostitutes, the prevalence of genital ulcers ranges from 5 to 35 percent. *H. ducreyi* can be cultured from approximately 50 percent of these ulcers.[26] The risk of chancroid following coitus with a sexual partner with active genital ulcer disease has been investigated in Nairobi.[27] The source contacts of 10 men with chancroid were all women with genital ulcers. None of these men had contracted their infection from a female without visible lesions. Among 29 secondary contacts of men with culture proven chancroid, 17 had ulcers. Although *H. ducreyi* can cause urethritis, the urethra has not been shown to be a reservoir for this organism.[28] It is presumed that individuals capable of transmitting the infection to others have ulcers. In women, ulcers may often be subclinical, and sexual activity continues.[26,27] Thus, promiscuous women with ulcers and few if any symptoms become an efficient reservoir for continued dissemination of *H. ducreyi* to their sexually promiscuous clients and subsequently to their spouses.

Proper epidemiologic studies of *H. ducreyi* require techniques to type or fingerprint strains and follow them within the population of patients with chancroid. Recent published studies have had some success using plasmids,[29] outer membrane proteins,[30,31] enzyme profiles,[32] and indirect immunofluorescence[33] as epidemiologic markers. However, additional studies are needed to define the extended population genetics of *H. ducreyi.*

## ETIOLOGY

### TAXONOMY AND BIOCHEMISTRY

*H. ducreyi* is a gram-negative, facultative anaerobic bacillus that requires hemin (X factor) for growth, reduces nitrate to nitrite, and has a DNA guanosine-plus-cytosine content of 0.38 mole fraction. The organism is small, nonmotile and non-spore-forming, and shows typical streptobacillary chaining on Gram stain. The ultrastructural characteristics of the *H. ducreyi* cell wall were well described by Kilian and Theilade,[34] Lwoff and Pirosky,[35] and Killian,[36] and Hammond et al.[37] demonstrated the organism's need for hemin for growth. The latter two studies demonstrated the absence of enzymatic activity in the hemin biosynthetic pathway by use of the porphyrin test described by Biberstein et al.[38] and subsequently by Kilian.[39] *H. ducreyi* also lacks the ferrochelatase or heme synthetase which catalyzes the insertion of iron into the protoporphyrin nucleus and is found in some strains of *H. influenzae*. All strains reduce nitrate to nitrite when tested as described by Cowan and Steel.[40] These features, in addition to the guanosine-plus-cytosine content of less than 0.39 mole fraction, are sufficient to include the organism among the hemin-requiring species of *Haemophilus*. Although no unique colonial or biochemical characteristics have been demonstrated, *H. ducreyi* can be differentiated from other hemin-requiring strains of *Haemophilus* by its lack of requirement for nicotinamide adenine dinucleotide (NAD, V factor), its failure to produce $H_2S$, catalase, or indole, and its production of alkaline phosphatase. The Pasteur Institute strain CIP542 has been designated the type strain for the species.

*H. ducreyi* has few distinguishing biochemical features. Nitrate reduction is characteristic of the genus, and all strains reported are oxidase-positive and catalase-negative. Other than a positive Voges-Proskauer reaction and weak acid production with glucose and arabinose, most strains are biochemically inert when tested for a variety of chemical reactions. Although deficient in carbohydrate hydrolytic activity, *H. ducreyi* has a wide variety of peptide hydrolytic activities.[32,41,42]

Biochemical characteristics of differential value are given in Table 24-1.

Recent studies have demonstrated a rough type of lipopolysaccharide without O-antigenic side chains, but with a highly substituted 2-keto-3-deoxyoctulosonic acid (KDO) core for both virulent and avirulent strains of *H. ducreyi,* although some differences in electrophoretic mobilities were noted.[43,44]

## GROWTH AND NUTRITIONAL CHARACTERISTICS

*H. ducreyi* grows well on nutritionally enriched media such as chocolatized blood agar or hemoglobin agar with complex supplements such as IsoVitaleX (BBL) or CVA supplement (Gibco). Excellent growth is also obtained on a more defined agar medium containing peptone, glucose, glutamine, and hemin,[45] although some strains require cysteine and starch or albumin as well. Growth in heart infusion broth with 10% fetal calf serum has been reported.[46] Growth is best at 30 to 33°C in a water-saturated atmosphere, and some strains show improved growth with $CO_2$.[46] All isolates will grow anaerobically.[47] Hemin requirements of *H. ducreyi* are higher than those of other hemin-requiring species, with most strains requiring 25 to 50 μg/ml for growth compared with 1 to 10 μg/ml for *H. haemoglobinophilus* or *H. influenzae*. The added requirement for albumin for some strains could explain the earlier findings of a serum requirement for this species.[8] Primary isolation growth conditions appear to be more pH-, moisture-, $CO_2$-, temperature-, and media-dependent than that required for working with laboratory-adapted strains.[47]

**Table 24-1. Differential Biochemical and Nutritional Characteristics of *Haemophilus* spp. and Other Fastidious Gram-Negative Rods**

| | X factor required | V factor required | Lysine decarboxylase | Glucose, acid | Sucrose, acid | Lactose, acid | Catalase | Oxidase | Nitrate reductase | Alkaline phosphatase |
|---|---|---|---|---|---|---|---|---|---|---|
| *H. ducreyi* | + | − | − | V† | − | − | − | + | + | + |
| *H. haemoglobinophilus* | + | − | − | + | + | − | + | + | + | − |
| *H. aphrophilus* | −* | − | − | + | + | + | − | − | + | + |
| *Actinobacillus actinomycetemcomitans* | − | − | − | + | − | − | + | + | + | + |
| *Eichenella corrodens* | − | − | + | − | − | − | − | + | + | − |
| *Cardibacterium hominis* | − | − | − | + | + | − | − | + | − | − |

*X factor is usually required on primary isolation but may not be needed after repeated passage. The porphyrin test, however, is positive.
†Variable.

## IMMUNOCHEMISTRY

Very little is known regarding the immunochemistry of *H. ducreyi*. Previous studies have shown both a delayed hypersensitivity response[12] and an antibody response in patients with chancroid and in experimental animals. Antibodies have been detected by complement fixation,[48] agglutination,[49] precipitation,[50] and indirect fluorescent antibody tests.[51] In most studies intact cells or whole-cell antigen preparations were used. Autoagglutination of *H. ducreyi* in saline suspensions has given confusing results, and its growth in entangled chains makes it difficult to obtain a homogeneous suspension.

Cross-reactivity of antisera produced against crude *H. ducreyi* antigens with antigen extracts from other *Haemophilus* species is readily demonstrated. However, such cross-reactivity is not surprising; cross-reactivity of capsular and noncapsular antigens with antisera produced against other *Haemophilus* species has been previously reported.[52] Hansen and Loftus described monoclonal antibodies reactive with all strains of *H. ducreyi*.[53]

## GENETICS

Little is known regarding the genetics of *H. ducreyi*. Except for minor variations, strains of *H. ducreyi* appear to be a serologically and biochemically homogeneous group. The guanosine-plus-cytosine content of the chromosomal DNA of *H. ducreyi* is similar to that of other species of hemin-requiring *Haemophilus*, but DNA hybridization studies have shown a lack of relatedness between *H. ducreyi* and other *Haemophilus* species.[54]

Strains of *H. ducreyi* have been shown to carry 5.7- or 7.0-megadalton ampicillin-resistance plasmids which contain the complete, functional Tn2-like ampicillin-resistance transposon and are highly homogenous with a 4.4-megadalton *H. influenzae* plasmid, a 4.1-megadalton *H. parainfluenzae* plasmid, and the 3.2- and 4.1-megadalton plasmids from *Neisseria gonorrhoeae*[55] Strains have also been shown to carry a plasmid identical to the gonococcal 3.2-megadalton plasmid[56] and a unique 2.6-megadalton plasmid which confer resistance to penicillin.[57] This suggests that the ampicillin transposon, although possibly of enteric origin, has been transposed into a group of related, small non-self-transmissible plasmids shared by several genera.[55,58]

Self-transfer of antibiotic-resistance plasmids and mobilization of non-self-transferable plasmids have been demonstrated in conjugative matings between *H. ducreyi* and other species.[59,60] The ability of *H. ducreyi* to accept and donate plasmids during conjugation suggests that widespread dissemination of antibiotic-resistance determinants and other genes is possible in this species despite its lack of genome relatedness to other members of the genus *Haemophilus*.

## PATHOGENESIS

The histologic features of chancroid have been well described, and ulcer biopsy has been used as a diagnostic tool. Sheldon and Heyman noted three discrete zones of chancroid.[61] The superficial layer consists of necrotic tissue, fibrin, neutrophils, and many gram-negative coccobacilli. The middle zone shows edema and newly formed blood vessels perpendicular to the surface of the ulcer. The deep layer manifests a dense infiltrate of neutrophils, plasma cells, and leukocytes with fibroblastic proliferation. Older lesions may have distinct lymphoid follicle formation in the deep layer.

The pathogenesis of genital ulcers due to *H. ducreyi* has not been extensively investigated. Trauma or abrasion is thought to be necessary for organisms to penetrate the epidermis, and the skin must be scarified in order to induce experimental chancroid lesions on the forearm. The inoculum size required for infection is not known, and no toxins or extracellular enzymes of *H. ducreyi* have been described. In lesions the organism is usually present within both macrophages and neutrophils and is also free in clumps in the interstitium.

In the rabbit model as well as in human studies, some strains of *H. ducreyi* have been shown to be virulent, whereas others are apparently avirulent.[37,62] Several investigators have shown that virulence can be lost with serial cultivation, and strains lose the capacity to produce skin lesions.[63] Avirulent organisms have been reported to be more susceptible to antimicrobial agents, particularly polymyxin.[37,62]

Recent studies demonstrated that virulent strains of *H. ducreyi* are relatively resistant to phagocytosis and killing by human polymorphonuclear leukocytes and are resistant to complement-mediated killing by normal human and rabbit sera.[64,65] Minor differences in lipopolysaccharide (LPS) profiles were also observed, suggesting involvement of the classic pathway of complement activation in serum killing to avirulent strains.[43] These studies and the subsequent work initiated by Abeck and Johnson[66] should lead to a clear understanding of the virulence factors of *H. ducreyi*.

The lymphadenitis associated with genital ulcer disease due to *H. ducreyi* is associated with pyogenic inflammatory response. Suppuration is associated with vast numbers of neutrophils and a paucity of bacilli. Presumably, some unknown and unique characteristics of *H. ducreyi* enable it to produce the suppurating bubo. The nature of the factors responsible has not been explored, and the almost complete absence of microorganisms in the bubo pus is also unexplained.

The role of the immune response as related to either disease susceptibility or pathogenesis is unknown.

## CLINICAL MANIFESTATIONS

The incubation period is usually between 4 and 7 days and is rarely less than 3 days or more than 10 days. No prodromal symptoms are recognized.

Males usually present with a complaint referable directly to the ulcer or to inguinal tenderness. Depending on the site of the ulcer, women often present with less obvious symptoms including pain on voiding, pain on defecation, rectal bleeding, dyspareunia, or vaginal discharge. On occasion, patients of both sexes have been admitted with the diagnosis of acute nonreducible inguinal hernia.

The chancre begins as a tender papule surrounded by erythema. Over the course of 24 to 48 h it becomes pustular, eroded, and ulcerated. Vesicles are not seen at any stage of the disease. The ulcer is usually quite painful in males, but it frequently is not painful in females. Most females with ulcers are unaware of their infection. The ulcer has ragged undermined edges, is sharply demarcated, and is without induration. The base of the ulcer may be covered by a gray or yellow necrotic purulent exudate, and its friable granulomatous base may bleed on scraping (Plates 31 and 32). There is little inflammation of the surrounding skin. Several ulcers may merge to form giant ulcers (greater than 2 cm) or serpiginous ulcers. Occasionally, lesions may remain pustular, the so-called dwarf chancroid, and resemble a folliculitis or py-

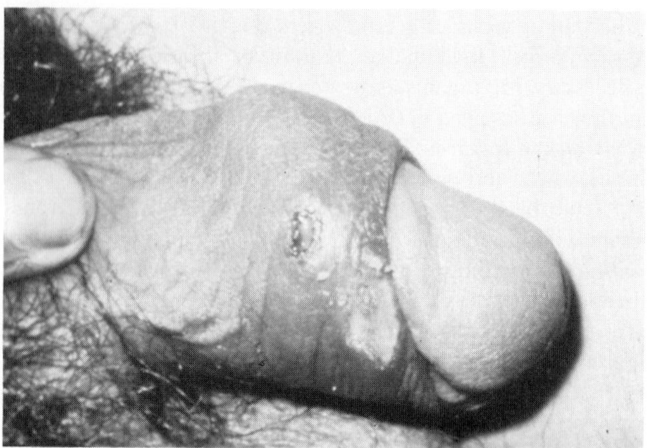

**Fig. 24-1.** Typical chancroidal ulcer in a male.

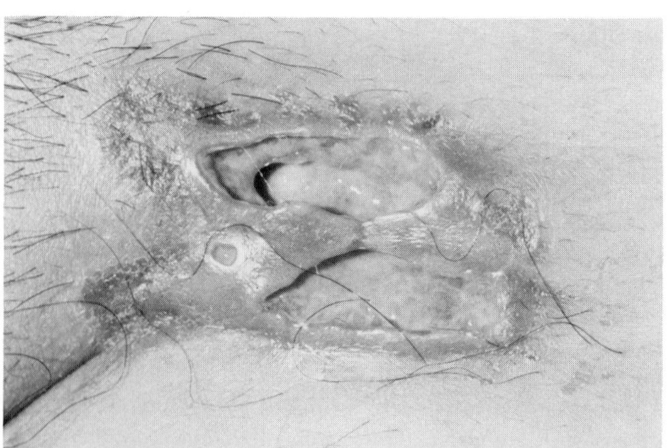

**Fig. 24-3.** Ruptured inguinal bubo in a patient with chancroid; extensive destruction of soft tissues and skin is evident.

ogenic infection.[67] One-half of men have a single ulcer.[19] The mean number of discrete ulcers in women in one study was 4.5.[26]

Most lesions in males are on either the external or internal surface of the prepuce, on the frenulum, or in the coronal sulcus (Fig. 24-1, Plate 31). The glans meatus and the shaft of the penis can also be involved but are involved less frequently. Edema of the prepuce is common. *H. ducreyi* can cause purulent urethritis. In an STD clinic in Nairobi, 1 to 2 percent of men who present with acute purulent urethritis are infected with *H. ducreyi.*[28]

In females the majority of lesions are at the entrance to the vagina and include lesions on the fourchette, labia, vestibule, and clitoris (Plate 32). Longitudinal ulcers are often present at the posterior fourchette. Large periurethral ulcers are not uncommon. Vaginal wall ulcers can occur, usually by extension from the introitus, and are often painless. In a study of 34 women with chancroid, five had perianal ulcers and three had ulcerative lesions of the cervix.[19] Rectovaginal fistulas have been reported as a complication of chancroid. Extragenital lesions are less common but have been described on the breasts, the fingers, and the thighs, and within the mouth. It is assumed that trauma and abrasions are important in the pathogenesis of the chancroidal ulcer and account for the distribution of lesions.

Chancroid may be confused with other forms of genital ulcers, including syphilis, genital herpes, and donovanosis. The differential diagnosis of genital ulcers is discussed in Chap. 59.

Painful inguinal adenitis is a characteristic feature of chancroid and may be present in up to 50 percent of patients. The adenitis is unilateral in most patients and erythema of the overlying skin is usually present (Fig. 24-2). Buboes can progress to become fluctuant with spontaneous rupture. Recalcitrant serpiginous spreading ulceration can occur with destruction of both skin and soft tissue (Fig. 24-3). In our study, 22 of 30 patients with buboes greater than or equal to 5 cm in diameter on presentation either had spontaneous drainage or required drainage by either aspiration or incision for improvement of symptoms and more rapid cure.[19] Bubo pus is usually thick, creamy, and viscous. Both lymphadenitis and bubo formation are less common in females.

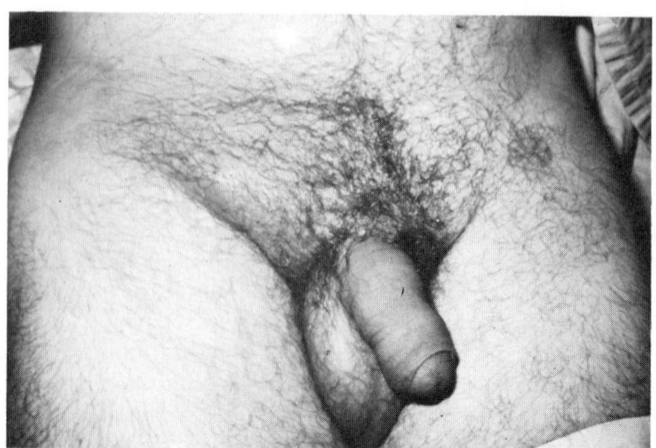

**Fig. 24-2.** Typical unilateral inguinal bubo in a patient with chancroid.

Mild constitutional symptoms can accompany the illness. However, *H. ducreyi* has not been shown to cause systemic infection or to spread to distant sites. Occasionally, superinfection with anaerobes including *Fusobacterium* spp. or *Bacteroides* spp. leads to gangrenous phagedenic ulceration and extensive destruction of genital tissue. Cicatrix formation with phimosis is a late complication of chancroid that may require circumcision.

*H. ducreyi* has not been noted to cause opportunistic infection or to become more invasive in immunocompromised hosts. It has not been reported to cause disease in infants born to women with active chancroid at delivery.

## NATURAL HISTORY

Before the era of antimicrobial therapy, genital ulcer disease due to *H. ducreyi* was a protracted illness with slow and often incomplete resolution. In one study the mean duration of ulcer disease prior to hospitalization was 34 days, and for 479 men the average duration of hospitalization was 30 days.[68] During World War I, the average time lost from duty with chancroid was 25 days.[69]

Improved hygiene and the use of saline soaks seem to promote granulation of tissue and gradual reepithelialization of the ulcer. However, recurrence was common. In one study, following healing but on early return to prostitution, 26 percent of women were noted to have recurrent ulcers within 2 months and almost always at the site of the previous lesion.[70] In this study, reinfection could not be differentiated from relapse, although biopsies showed a thin epithelium over healed ulcers, suggesting a predisposition for recurrence at these sites.

Occasionally, without treatment genital ulcers and inguinal abscesses have been reported to persist for years.

## LABORATORY DIAGNOSIS

The laboratory diagnosis of chancroid depends on the isolation of *H. ducreyi* from a genital ulcer or bubo and the exclusion of other diseases associated with similar clinical findings, especially ulcers due to herpes simplex, syphilis, and lymphogranuloma venereum.

Either cotton or calcium alginate swabs are suitable for a specimen collection. Swabs should be taken from the purulent ulcer base. The organism will only survive for 2 to 4 h on a swab unless refrigerated. No satisfactory transport system has been developed. The numbers of *H. ducreyi* in ulcer exudates are substantial and probably in the range of $10^7$ to $10^8$/ml of pus. On the other hand, no organisms are seen in bubo pus, and culture from the bubo is always sterile unless it has ruptured and an inguinal abscess is present. Ducrey made this observation in his classic paper describing the etiologic agent in 1889.[1]

Direct examination of clinical material by a Gram's stain[71] or electron microscopy[72] has been suggested but may be misleading because of the polymicrobial flora of most genital ulcers.[73] Specific immunochemical staining with fluorescent antibody may be of help in preliminary identification of the organism,[51] but every attempt should be made to confirm the diagnosis by cultural procedures.

Primary isolation of *H. ducreyi* from genital lesions has been reported with varying success. Hammond et al.[74] reported an isolation rate of 56 percent when a selective medium of chocolate agar enriched with 1% IsoVitaleX (BBL) containing 3 μg/ml vancomycin was used during a period of a localized epidemic of chancroid. Sottnek et al.[46] reported success on primary isolation utilizing heart infusion agar with 5% defibrinated rabbit blood or 10% fetal bovine serum plus vancomycin. A starch aggregation medium has been reported to be useful in primary isolation,[47,75] but most field studies have demonstrated a need for at least two primary isolation media to maintain culture sensitivity above 80 percent, and the best single media have been prepared from a nutritionally rich agar base supplemented with hemoglobin and serum, such as gonococcal agar supplemented with hemoglobin and fetal calf serum.[76,77]

Small, nonmucoid, yellow-gray, semiopaque or translucent colonies that can be pushed intact across the agar surface usually appear in 2 to 4 days but may appear as late as 7 days after inoculation. A zone of α hemolysis is seen on plates containing rabbit blood. A water-saturated atmosphere containing 5 to 10% $CO_2$ and a reduced incubation temperature of 33 to 35°C are important for primary cultivation of this organism.[47]

Presumptive identification can be made by demonstrating short, gram-negative bacilli with occasional streptobacillary chaining from solid media and the inability of isolates to produce porphyrin from δ-aminolevulinic acid by the porphyrin test. Confirmatory identification requires the demonstration of a hemin (X factor) requirement for growth and the absence of a requirement for NAD (V factor) on media otherwise nutritionally enriched and with the growth conditions previously described (see Table 24-1). The porphyrin test[39] is the preferred method of demonstrating hemin requirement, and the oxidase test requires tetramethyl-*p*-phenylenediamine, as demonstrated by Nobre[78] and others. Organisms resembling *H. ducreyi* have been isolated from genital ulcers.[79]

Alternatives to culture diagnosis have not been well described. Monoclonal antibodies which are specific for *H. ducreyi* have been produced[53,80] and have been used to detect antigen in lesion material from experimentally infected animals and patients with chancroid. The lack of DNA homology of strains of *H. ducreyi* with other organisms should also allow the development of specific DNA probes for the nonculture diagnosis of chancroid.

Attempts have been made to develop a serological test for chancroid. Complement fixation, precipitin, and agglutination tests are positive in some patients with genital ulcer disease due to *H. ducreyi*. Museyi et al. have recently described an enzyme-linked immunosorbent assay (ELISA) using whole lysed *H. ducreyi* as the antigen source; the test appears to have considerable specificity and sensitivity.[81] The nature and duration of the antibody response and its significance in altering susceptibility to information with *H. ducreyi* are unknown.

## ANTIMICROBIAL SUSCEPTIBILITY

In studies reported between 1940 and 1960, *H. ducreyi* was shown to be susceptible in vitro to tetracycline, streptomycin, chloramphenicol, sulfonamides, and penicillin.[62,82–84] Recent studies from diverse regions show that clinically significant antimicrobial resistance has become common.[85–89] Plasmid-mediated antibiotic resistance in *H. ducreyi* has been described for ampicillin,[90] sulfonamides,[91] chloramphenicol,[92] tetracycline,[93] streptomycin, and kanamycin.[94]

Newer macrolide antibiotics, quinolones, and some second- and third-generation parenteral cephalosporins also have enhanced in vitro activity against *H. ducreyi* (Table 24-2).[94a]

## TREATMENT

Prior to the advent of the sulfonamides, a variety of poorly studied therapeutic approaches to chancroid were used. Circumcision was standard therapy. Apparently buboes rarely developed after circumcision.[67]

Sulfonamides were discovered to be effective therapy for chancroid in 1938.[95] Sulfanilamide was prescribed for 7 to 14 days. Cultures became negative for *H. ducreyi* within 48 h. The average time to healing was less than 10 days.[96,97] Five days of therapy was shown to be comparable to longer regimens.[96] The average duration of hospitalization during World War II was reduced from 25 to 11 days, and the average duration for healing was reduced from 32 to 15.7 days.[98,99] Prior to the emergence of β-lactamase-producing strains of *H. ducreyi*, oral ampicillin appeared to be an effective regimen.[19] Streptomycin in a dosage of 1 g daily for 5 days was adequate therapy for 93 percent of patients with chancroid in U.S. troops in Korea.[18] However, buboes more often developed and progressed to suppuration during treatment compared with treatment with either chloramphenicol or oxytetracycline.[18]

**Table 24-2. Antimicrobial Susceptibility of Clinical Isolates of *H. ducreyi***

| | Range, mg/l | $MIC_{50}$, mg/l | $MIC_{90}$, mg/l |
|---|---|---|---|
| Sulfonamides* | 0.25–128 | 64 | 128 |
| Ampicillin* | 0.03–128 | 16 | 128 |
| Vancomycin | 4–128 | 8 | 64 |
| Tetracycline* | 0.125–64 | 16 | 32 |
| Trimethoprim | 0.125–32 | 4 | 16 |
| Kanamycin* | 0.5–8 | 2 | 8 |
| Chloramphenicol* | 0.25–16 | 0.25 | 8 |
| Rifampin | 0.004–1 | 0.008 | 0.016 |
| Erythromycin | 0.0005–0.032 | 0.008 | 0.030 |
| Ciprofloxacin | 0.003–0.03 | 0.003 | 0.007 |
| Ceftriaxone | 0.001–0.004 | 0.002 | 0.002 |

*Antimicrobials currently associated with plasmid-mediated resistance in *H. ducreyi*.

SOURCE: After Hammond et al,[37] Sanson-Le Pors et al,[85] Slootmans et al,[86] Bilgeri et al,[87] Sturm,[88] and Bowmer et al.[108]

The genital ulcer may follow a course different from that of the bubo. Prior to the advent of antimicrobial agents, repeated aspiration was often required. With therapy, a single aspiration is usually sufficient, even in patients with large buboes.[19] Patients with inguinal lymphadenitis without suppuration usually respond without developing a bubo.

During the 1970s, resistant strains of *H. ducreyi* emerged and treatment failures were common. During the Vietnam conflict, tetracycline and chloramphenicol were found to be ineffective regimens.[100] However, kanamycin in a dosage of 500 mg twice daily for 6 to 14 days and intravenous cephalothin 3 g daily for 7 days were successfully used to treat chancroid.[101,102]

In 1983, Fast et al. correlated clinical treatment response with in vitro resistance in Nairobi and showed that clinical failure could be anticipated if *H. ducreyi* were not eradicated from the ulcer within 72 h of initiation of therapy.[89] Subsequent studies in Nairobi and elsewhere have shown that treatment does not need to be continued until the ulcer has reepithelized. Studies in Rotterdam, Korea, and Kenya confirmed the effectiveness of trimethoprim-sulfamethoxazole for chancroid with very few failures.[89,103,104] In a subsequent study, Plummer et al. showed that a single dose of a trimethoprim-sulfonamide regimen was as effective as more prolonged courses of therapy.[82] However, in Thailand, emergence of resistance to trimethoprim and sulfonamides has reduced the effectiveness of this regimen.[105] Several studies have found erythromycin to be very effective with clinical resolution of ulcers within 1 to 2 weeks.[106,107] The Centers for Disease Control at present recommends 500 mg erythromycin four times per day or trimethoprim-sulfamethaxazole one double-strength tablet (160 mg trimethoprim and 800 mg sulfamethoxazole) for 7 days.

A long-acting third-generation cephalosporin, ceftriaxone, has been shown in two separate studies to cure chancroid if given as an intramuscular dose of 250 mg.[105,108] Other regimens shown to be effective include amoxicillin in combination with clavulanic acid.[109,110] A three-day regimen given in a dose of 375 mg three times daily has been shown to be as effective as a longer course of therapy. Clavulanic acid effectively blocks the β-lactamase and permits amoxicillin to eradicate *H. ducreyi*. Spectinomycin has also been successful, although the cure rate is slightly less than 90 percent.[111]

The quinolones may prove to be very useful agents for the treatment of chancroid. In preliminary studies, both rosoxacin and enoxacin were satisfactory alternatives to standard regimens.[112,113] Ciprofloxacin in a dose of 500 mg twice daily for 3 days cured all 40 men treated in Kenya.[114] Fleroxacin given as a single dose of 200 mg also was found to cure over 95 percent of HIV-seronegative men with chancroid.[115] Further studies are required to determine both the dose and the duration of quinolone regimens.

Relapse after complete healing occurs at the site of the original ulcer in about 5 percent of patients. Treatment with the original regimen is usually successful. If the sexual partner is not treated, reinfection can be anticipated following sexual reexposure. We recommend that all sexual partners of patients with clinical chancroid be treated with the regimen used to cure the index patient.

## EPIDEMIOLOGIC ASSOCIATION WITH HUMAN IMMUNODEFICIENCY VIRUS–1

Recent studies in Africa provide substantial evidence that chancroid is a risk factor for the heterosexual spread of HIV-1.[116–118] Among 115 men presenting with genital ulcers, 63 percent of the HIV-1-seropositive men reported a prior episode of genital ulcers compared with 31 percent of the HIV-1-seronegative men.[117] Among 340 men in the same Nairobi clinic with a sexually transmitted disease, 63 percent of HIV-1-positive men had a past history of ulcers compared with only 19 percent of HIV-negative men.[118] Among prostitutes who have a very high seroincidence of HIV-1, 60 percent of seroconverting women experienced one or more episodes of genital ulcers prior to conversion compared with 45 percent of HIV-1-seronegative women.[119] This relation became stronger with a dose response when the number of ulcer episodes per month was determined. Among seroconverting prostitutes, the number of ulcer episodes per month was 0.11 compared with 0.04 among prostitutes who remained seronegative.[119]

In a seroincidence study, of 429 seronegative men presenting with sexually transmitted disease acquired from an HIV-1-infected prostitute cohort, acquisition of HIV-1 was strongly correlated with both genital ulcer disease and the presence of a foreskin.[120] Both were independent risk factors that increased the risk of seroconversion from less than 1 percent in 118 circumcised men with urethritis to 6 percent in 93 circumcised men with ulcers to 29 percent in 55 uncircumcised men with genital ulcers.[120]

Similar associations between genital ulcers and HIV-1 infection have been reported from Zambia.[121]

Genital ulcers apparently render women more susceptible to infection with HIV-1 following heterosexual contact with infected men. The presence of genital ulcers in HIV-1-infected women dramatically increases the probability that their sexual partners will become infected. Presumably, genital ulcers facilitate the passage of HIV-1 into vaginal secretions. In Africa and probably in many other developing countries, most genital ulcers are due to chancroid.

Recently, we observed that both men and women with chancroid and asymptomatic HIV-1 infection are much more likely to fail treatment.[122] This observation has major implications for treatment protocols in countries in which HIV-1 is prevalent. In Kenya, over 30 percent of men and women with chancroid are HIV-1 seropositive. If both pathogens are present, chancroid and HIV-1 presumably act synergistically with increased infectivity, susceptibility, and, for *H. ducreyi,* failure to respond to treatment. It may be that chancroid is one of the major reasons for the rapid heterosexual spread of HIV-1 in eastern and southern Africa. In Nairobi, Kenya, it appears that perhaps one-third of HIV-1 infections in prostitutes and at least one-half of HIV-1 infections in their clients are related to concomitant infection with *H. ducreyi.*[117–119]

## PREVENTION AND CONTROL

Intervention and strategies to control *H. ducreyi* become an urgent priority if its association with HIV-1 is established. Among military populations, measures to prevent chancroid were only moderately effective.[69] In Winnipeg on two occasions, and in southern California, widespread treatment of prostitutes with ulcers and prostitutes named as sexual contacts of men with ulcers effectively eradicated the disease in both populations.[16,19,123] The absence of symptoms in many female source contacts, despite the presence of ulcers, made eradication difficult without programs to carry out contact tracing. Most women do not seek treatment despite numerous ulcers, and most prostitutes continue to be sexually active.[124]

If other studies confirm the lack of any important reservoir for

*H. ducreyi* other than promiscuous women with ulcers, control programs should be possible. The use of condoms by clients dramatically reduces the acquisition of ulcers by prostitutes.[125]

Eradication of *H. ducreyi* from sexually promiscuous individuals may be an achievable goal. The known epidemiology of chancroid suggests that effective control measures targeted to select populations should halt the spread of this disease. The use of condoms, regular pelvic examination of prostitutes, early effective intervention of infectious lesions, contact tracing, and other strategies all need urgent critical evaluation in order to control or eradicate chancroid and thereby perhaps reduce the rate of heterosexual spread of HIV-1.

## References


1 Ducrey A: Experimentelle Untersuchungen über den Ansteckungsstoff des weichen Schankers und über die Bubonen. *Monatshr Prakt Dermatol* 9: 387, 1889.

2 Krefting R: Ueber die für Ulcus Molle specifische Mikrobe. *Arch Dermat Syphilis Erganzungshefte* 24: 14, 1892.

3 Unna PG: Der Streptobacillus des weichen Schankers. *Monatshr Prakt Dermatol* 14: 485, 1892.

4 Sullivan M: Chancroid. *Am J Syph* 24: 482, 1940.

5 Himmel J: Contribution à l'étude de l'immunité des animaux vis-à-vis du bacille du chancre mou. *Ann Inst Pasteur* 15: 928, 1901.

6 Teague O, Deibert O: The value of the cultural method in the diagnosis of chancroid. *J Urol* 4: 543, 1920.

7 Teague O, Deibert O: Some observations on the bacillus of unna-ducrey. *J Med Res* 43: 61, 1922.

8 Beeson PB: Studies on Chancroid: IV. The Ducrey bacillus: Growth requirements and inhibition by antibiotic agents. *Proc Soc Exp Biol Med* 61: 81, 1946.

9 Ito T: Klinische und bacteriologische Studien über Ulcus Molle und Ducreysche Streptobazillen. *Arch Dermatol Syph* 116: 341, 1913.

10 Reenstierna J: Chancre mou experimental chez le singe et le lapin. *Acta Dermatol Venereol* 2: 1, 1921.

11 Greenblatt RB, Sanderson ES: The diagnostic value of the intradermal chancroidal skin test. *Arch Dermatol Syph* 36: 486, 1937.

12 Greenblatt RB, Sanderson ES: The intradermal chancroid bacillary antigen test as an aid in the differential diagnosis of the venereal bubo. *Am J Surg* 41: 384, 1938.

13 Deacon WE et al: VDRL chancroid studies: I. A simplified procedure for the isolation and identification of *Haemophilus ducreyi*. *J Invest Dermatol* 26: 399, 1956.

14 Kaplan W et al: VDRL chancroid studies: III. Use of Ducrey skin test vaccines on rabbits. *J Invest Dermatol* 26: 415, 1956.

15 Ajello GW et al: Nutritional studies of a virulent strain of *Haemophilus ducreyi*. *J Bacteriol* 72: 802, 1956.

16 Blackmore CA et al: An outbreak of chancroid in Orange County, California: Descriptive epidemiology and disease-control measures. *J Infect Dis* 151: 840, 1985.

17 Hart G: Venereal disease in a war environment: Incidence and management. *Med J Aust* 1: 808, 1975.

18 Asin J: Chancroid: A report of 1402 cases. *Am J Syph Gon Vener Dis* 36: 483, 1952.

19 Hammond GW et al: Clinical, epidemiological, laboratory and therapeutic features of an urban outbreak of chancroid in North America. *Rev Infect Dis* 2: 867, 1980.

20 Lykke-Olesen L et al: Epidemic of chancroid in Greenland, 1977–78. *Lancet* i: 654, 1979.

21 Schmid GP et al: Chancroid in the United States, reestablishment of an old disease. *J Am Med Assoc* 258: 3265, 1987.

22 Becker TM et al: *Haemophilus ducreyi* infection in South Florida: A race disease on the rise? *South Med J* 80: 182, 1987.

23 Kinghorn GR et al: Genital colonization with *Haemophilus ducreyi* in the absence of ulceration. *Eur J Sex Transm Dis* 1: 89, 1983.

24 Diaz-Mitoma F et al: Etiology of non-vesicular genital ulcers in Winnipeg. *Sex Transm Dis* 14: 33, 1987.

25 Kibukamusoke JW: Venereal disease in East Africa. *Trans R Soc Trop Med Hyg* 59: 642, 1965.

26 Plummer FA et al: Clinical and microbiologic studies of genital ulcers in Kenyan women. *Sex Transm Dis* 12: 193, 1985.

27 Plummer FA et al: Epidemiology of chancroid and *Haemophilus ducreyi* in Nairobi. *Lancet* 2: 1293, 1983.

28 Kunimoto DY et al: Urethral infection with *Haemophilus ducreyi* in men. *Sex Transm Dis* 15: 37, 1988.

29 Handsfield H et al: Molecular epidemiology of *Haemophilus ducreyi* infections. *Ann Intern Med* 95: 315, 1981.

30 Odumeru JA et al: Characterization of cell proteins of *Haemophilus ducreyi* by polyacrylamide gel electrophoresis. *J Infect Dis* 148: 710, 1983.

31 Taylor DN et al: Antimicrobial susceptibility and characterization of outer membrane proteins of *Haemophilus ducreyi* isolated in Thailand. *J Clin Microbiol* 21: 442, 1985.

32 van Dyck E, Piot P: Enzyme profile of *Haemophilus ducreyi* strains isolated on different continents. *Eur J Clin Microbiol* 6:40, 1987.

33 Slootmans L et al: Typing *Haemophilus ducreyi* by indirect immunofluorescence assay. *Genitourin Med* 61: 123, 1985.

34 Kilian M., Theilade J: Cell wall ultrastructure of strains of *Haemophilus ducreyi* and *Haemophilus piscium*. *Int J Systematic Bacteriol* 25: 351, 1975.

35 Lwoff A, Pirosky I: Determination du facteur de croissance pour *Haemophilus ducreyi*. *CR Seances Soc Biol (Paris)* 124: 1169, 1937.

36 Killian M: A taxonomic study of the genus *Haemophilus* with the proposal of a new species. *J Gen Microbiol* 93: 9, 1976.

37 Hammond GW et al: Antimicrobial susceptibility of *Haemophilus ducreyi*. *Antimicrob Agents Chemother* 13: 608, 1978.

38 Biberstein EL et al: Action of *Haemophilus* cultures on δ-aminolevulinic acid. *J Bacteriol* 86: 814, 1963.

39 Kilian M: A rapid method for the differentiation of *Haemophilus* strains. *Acta Pathol Microbiol Scand [B]* 82: 835, 1974.

40 Cowan ST, Steel KJ: *Manual for the Identification of Medical Bacteria*. Cambridge University Press, 1965, chap. 8

41 Sturm AW, Zanen HC: Enzymic activity of *Haemophilus ducreyi*. *J Med Microbiol* 18: 181, 1984.

42 Casin IM et al: The enzymatic profile of *Haemophilus ducreyi*. *Ann Microbiol (Inst Pasteur)* 133B: 379, 1982.

43 Odumeru JA et al: Relationship between lipopolysaccharide composition and virulence of *Haemophilus ducreyi*. *J Med Microbiol* 23: 155, 1987.

44 Abeck D et al: *Haemophilus ducreyi* produces rough lipopolysaccharide. *FEBS Microbiol Lett* 42: 159, 1987.

45 Hammond GW et al: Determination of the hemin requirement of *Haemophilus ducreyi*: Evaluation of the porphyrin test and media used in the satellite growth test. *J Clin Microbiol* 7: 243, 1978.

46 Sottnek FO et al: Isolation and identification of *Haemophilus ducreyi* in a clinical study. *J Clin Microbiol* 12: 170, 1980.

47 Sturm AW, Zanen HC: Characteristics of *Haemophilus ducreyi* in culture. *J Clin Microbiol* 19: 672, 1984.

48 Saelhof CC: Complement fixation in chancroidal infection. *Urol Cutaneous Rev* 30: 224, 1926.

49 Saelhof CC: Observations on chancroidal infection. *J Infect Dis* 35: 591, 1924.

50 Reymann F: Type differentiation of *Haemophilus ducreyi*. *Acta Pathol Microbiol Scand* 27: 364, 1950.

51 Denys GA et al: An indirect fluorescent antibody technique for *Haemophilus ducreyi*. *Health Lab Sci* 15: 128, 1937.

52 Branefors P: A serologic study of somatic antigens from *Haemophilus influenzae* and two related species. *Int Arch Allergy Appl Immunol* 59: 143, 1979.

53 Hansen EJ, Loftus TA: Monoclonal antibodies reactive with all strains of *Haemophilus ducreyi*. *Infect Immunol* 44: 196, 1984.

54 Casin I et al: Lack of deoxyribonucleic acid relatedness between *Haemophilus ducreyi* and other *Haemophilus* species. *Int J Syst Bacteriol* 35: 23, 1985.

55 McNicol PJ, Ronald AR: The plasmids of *Haemophilus ducreyi. J Antimicrob Chemother* 14: 561, 1984.
56 Anderson B et al: Common β-lactamase-specifying plasmid in *Haemophilus ducreyi* and *Neisseria gonorrhoeae. Antimicrob Agents Chemother* 25: 296, 1984.
57 Ronald AR: Unpublished observations.
58 Brunton J et al: Origin of small β-lactamase-specifying plasmids in *Haemophilus* species and *Neisseria gonorrhoeae. J Bacteriol* 168: 374, 1986.
59 Deneer HG et al: Mobilization of nonconjugative antibiotic resistance plasmids in *Haemophilus ducreyi. J Bacteriol* 149: 726, 1982.
60 McNicol PJ et al: Characterization of a *Haemphilus ducreyi* mobilizing plasmid. *J Bacteriol* 165: 657, 1986.
61 Sheldon WH, Heyman A: Studies on chancroid: I. Observations on the histology with an evaluation of biopsy as a diagnostic procedure. *Am J Pathol* 22: 415, 1946.
62 Thayer JD et al: In vitro sensitivity of *Haemophilus ducreyi* to several antibiotics. *Antibiot Chemother* 5: 132, 1955.
63 Dienst RB: Virulence and antigenicity of *Hemophilus ducreyi. Am J Syph Gon Vener Dis* 32: 289, 1948.
64 Odumeru JA et al: Role of lipopolysaccharide and complement in susceptibility of *Haemophilus ducreyi* to human serum. *Infect Immunol* 50: 495, 1985.
65 Odumeru JA et al: Virulence factors of *Haemophilus ducreyi. Infect Immunol* 43: 607, 1984.
66 Abeck D, Johnson AP: Identification of surface-exposed proteins *Haemophilus ducreyi. FEMS Microbiol Lett* 44: 49, 1987.
67 Gaisin A, Heaton CL: Chancroid: Alias the soft chancre. *Int J Dermatol* 3: 188, 1975.
68 Rauschkolb JE: Circumcision in treatment of chancroidal lesions of male genitalia. *Arch Dermatol Syph* 39: 319, 1939.
69 Moore JE: The diagnosis of chancroid and the effect of prophylaxis upon its incidence in the American expeditionary forces. *J Urol* 4: 169, 1920.
70 Lao DG, Trussell RE: Chancroid in women in Manila. *Am J Syph* 31: 277, 1947.
71 Borchardt KA, Hoke AW: Simplified laboratory technique for diagnosis of chancroid. *Arch Dermatol* 102: 190, 1970.
72 Marsch WC et al: Ultrastructural detection of *Haemophilus ducreyi* in biopsies of chancroid. *Arch Dermatol Res* 263: 153, 1978.
73 Chapel T et al: The microbiological flora of penile ulcerations. *J Infect Dis* 137: 50, 1978.
74 Hammond W et al: Comparison of specimen collection and laboratory techniques for isolation of *Haemophilus ducreyi. J Clin Microbiol* 7: 39, 1978.
75 Hafiz S et al: Sheffield medium for cultivation of *Haemophilus ducreyi. Br J Vener Dis* 60: 196, 1984.
76 Dylewski J et al: Laboratory diagnosis of *Haemophilus ducreyi*: Sensitivity of culture media. *Diagn Microbiol Infect Dis* 4: 241, 1986.
77 Kunimoto DY et al: Field testing of modified Bieling media for the isolation of *Haemophilus ducreyi* in Kenya. *Eur J Clin Microbiol* 5: 673, 1986.
78 Nobre GN: Identification of *Haemophilus ducreyi* in the clinical laboratory. *J Med Microbiol* 15: 243, 1982.
79 Ursi JP et al: Characterisation of an unusual bacterium isolated from genital ulcers. *J Med Microbiol* 15: 97, 1982.
80 Schalla WO et al: Use of dot-immunobinding and immunofluorescence assays to investigate clinically suspected cases of chancroid. *J Infect Dis* 153: 879, 1986.
81 Museyi K et al: Use of an enzyme immunoassay to detect serum IgG antibodies to *Haemophilus ducreyi. J Infect Dis* 157: 1039, 1988.
82 Plummer FA et al: Single-dose therapy of chancroid with trimethoprim-sulfametrole. *N Engl J Med* 309: 67, 1983.
83 Wetherbee DG et al: In vitro antibiotic effects on *Haemophilus ducreyi. J Vener Dis Inform* 33: 462, 1949.
84 Reymann F: Sensitivity of *Haemophilus ducreyi* to penicillin, streptomycin and sulfathiazole. *Acta Pathol Microbiol Scand* 26: 309, 1949.
85 Sanson-Le Pors MJ et al: *In-vitro* susceptibility of thirty strains of *Haemophilus ducreyi* to several antibiotics including six cephalosporins. *J Antimicrob Chemother* 11: 271, 1983.
86 Slootmans L et al: Susceptibility of 40 *Haemophilus ducreyi* strains to 34 antimicrobial products. *Antimicrob Agents Chemother* 24: 564, 1983.
87 Bilgeri YR et al: Antimicrobial susceptibility of 103 strains of *Haemophilus ducreyi* isolated in Johannesburg. *Antimicrob Agents Chemother* 22: 686, 1982.
88 Sturm AW: Comparison of antimicrobial susceptibility patterns of fifty-seven strains of *Haemophilus ducreyi* isolated in Amsterdam from 1978 to 1985. *J Antimicrob Chemother* 19: 187, 1987.
89 Fast MW et al: Antimicrobial therapy of chancroid: An evaluation of five treatment regimens correlated with in vitro sensitivity. *Sex Transm Dis* 10: 1, 1983.
90 Brunton JL et al: Plasmid-mediated ampicillin resistance in *Haemophilus ducreyi. Antimicrob Agents Chemother* 15: 294, 1979.
91 Albritton WL et al: Plasmid-mediated sulfonamide resistance in *Haemophilus ducreyi. Antimicrob Agents Chemother* 21: 159, 1982.
92 Roberts MC et al: Molecular characterization of chloramphenicol-resistant *Haemophilus parainfluenzae* and *Haemophilus ducreyi. Antimicrob Agents Chemother* 28: 176, 1985.
93 Albritton WL et al: Plasmid-mediated tetracycline resistance in *Haemophilus ducreyi. Antimicrob Agents Chemother* 25: 187, 1984.
94 Sanson-LePors MJ et al: Plasmid-mediated aminoglycoside phosphotransferases in *Haemophilus ducreyi. Antimicrob Agents Chemother* 28: 315, 1985.
94a LeSaux N et al: In vitro activity of ceftriaxone, cefetamet (Ro 15-8074), ceftetrame (Ro 19-5247; T-2588), and fleroxacin (Ro 23-6240; Am-833) versus *Neisseria gonorrhoeae* and *Haemophilus ducreyi. Antimicrob Agents Chemother* 31: 1153, 1987.
95 Hanschell HM: Sulfanilamide in the treatment of chancroid. *Lancet* 1: 886, 1938.
96 Combes FC et al: Treatment of chancroid with sulfathiazole: Investigation of the minimal effective dose. *Am J Syph* 27: 700, 1943.
97 Culp OS: Treatment of chancroid with sulfanilamide. *Am J Syph* 24: 622, 1940.
98 Satulsky EM: Management of chancroid in a tropical theater: Report of 1,555 cases. *JAMA* 127: 259, 1943.
99 Harp VC: Observations of chancroid therapy with and without sulfathiazole. *Am J Syph Gon Vener Dis* 30: 361, 1946.
100 Kerber RE et al: Treatment of chancroid: A comparison of tetracycline and sulfisoxazole. *Arch Dermatol* 100: 604, 1969.
101 Marmar JL: The management of resistant chancroid in Vietnam. *J Urol* 107: 807, 1972.
102 Storey G: Clinical manifestations of chancroid. *Br J Urol* 42: 738, 1970.
103 Nayyar KC et al: Rising incidence of chancroid in Rotterdam. Epidemiological, clinical, diagnostic and therapeutic aspects. *Br J Vener Dis* 55: 439, 1979.
104 Fitzpatrick JE et al: Treatment of chancroid: Comparison of sulfamethoxazole trimethoprim with recommended therapies. *JAMA* 246: 1804, 1981.
105 Taylor DN et al: Comparative study of ceftriaxone and trimethoprim-sulfamethoxazole for the treatment of chancroid in Thailand. *J Infect Dis* 152: 1002, 1985.
106 Carpenter JL et al: Erythromycin therapy of chancroid. *Sex Transm Dis* 8: 192, 1981.
107 Plummer FA et al: Antimicrobial therapy of chancroid: Effectiveness of erythromycin. *J Infect Dis* 148: 726, 1983.
108 Bowmer MI et al: Single-dose ceftriaxone for chancroid. *Antimicrob Agents Chemother* 31: 67, 1987.
109 Fast MV et al: Treatment of chancroid by clavulanic acid with amoxycillin in patients with β-lactamase-positive *Haemophilus ducreyi* infection. *Lancet* 2: 509, 1982.
110 Ndinya-Achola JO et al: Augmentin in the treatment of chancroid: Three day oral course. *Genitourin Med* 62: 202, 1986.

111 Fransen L et al: A comparison of single-dose spectinomycin with five days of trimethoprim/sulfamethoxazole for the treatment of chancroid. *Sex Transm Dis* 14: 98, 1987.
112 Haase DA et al: Clinical evaluation of rosoxacin for the treatment of chancroid. *Antimicrob Agents Chemother* 30: 39, 1986.
113 Naamara W et al: Therapy of chancroid with enoxacin. *Genitourin Med* (in press).
114 Namaara W et al: Therapy of chancroid with enoxacin. *Genitourin Med* 164: 189, 1988.
115 MacDonald K et al: 27th Interscience Conference on Antimicrobial Agents and Chemotherapy, Oct 4–7, 1987. Sheraton Center Hotel, The New York Hilton, New York. Abstract 821, p 240.
116 Piot P et al: Retrospective seroepidemiology of AIDS virus infection in Nairobi populations. *J Infect Dis* 155: 1108, 1987.
117 Greenblatt RM et al: Genital ulceration as a risk factor for human immunodeficiency virus infection. *AIDS* 2: 47, 1988.
118 Simonsen JN et al: Human immunodeficiency virus infection in men with sexually transmitted diseases. *N Engl J Med* 319: 274, 1988.
119 Plummer FA et al: IV International Conference on AIDS, June 12–16, 1988. Stockholm International Fairs, Stockholm, Sweden. Abstract 4554, p 200, book 2.
120 Melbye M et al: Evidence of heterosexual transmission and clinical manifestation of human immunodeficiency virus infection and related conditions in Lusaka, Zambia. *Lancet* 2: 1113, 1986.
121 Cameron DW et al: IV International Conference on AIDS, June 12–16, 1988. Stockholm International Fairs, Stockholm, Sweden. Abstract 4061, p 275, book 1.
122 Cameron DW et al: IV International Conference on AIDS, June 12–16, 1988. Stockholm International Fairs, Stockholm, Sweden. Abstract 7637, p 334, book 2.
123 Jessamine P et al: Clinical and Investigative Medicine, Annual Meeting for the Canadian Society for Clinical Investigation, Royal College of Physicians and Surgeons of Canada, September 23–26, 1988, Ottawa, Ontario. Abstract R-432, p C66.
124 D'Costa LJ et al: Prostitutes are a major reservoir of sexually transmitted diseases in Nairobi, Kenya. *Sex Transm Dis* 12: 64, 1985.
125 Cameron DW et al: IV International Conference on AIDS, June 12–16, 1988. Stockholm International Fairs, Stockholm, Sweden. Abstract 6517, p 276, book 2.

# Chapter 25
# Donovanosis

Gavin Hart

## HISTORY

Donovanosis is a chronic, progressively destructive bacterial infection of the genital region, generally regarded to be sexually transmitted. The disease has been known by many names, including granuloma contagiosa, granuloma Donovani, granuloma inguinale tropicum, granuloma pudendi tropicum, sclerosing granuloma, and ulcerating granuloma of the pudenda; but the most common synonyms are granuloma inguinale and granuloma venereum.

Donovanosis was probably first described by McLeod in 1882. The causative organism was discovered by Donovan in 1905 and until recently was known as *Donovania granulomatis*. Because of the characteristics of the organism, particularly a prominent capsule, a relationship with *Klebsiella* has often been suggested. However, possibly due to the difficulty in growing *Calymmatobacterium granulomatis* on artificial media, its biochemical and bacteriologic characteristics have not been defined sufficiently to support this classification, and it must currently be regarded as an organism of uncertain affiliation.

## BIOLOGY OF ORGANISM

The infectious agent is *C. granulomatis*, a gram-negative bacterium measuring 1.5 by 0.7 μm. In tissue smears the bacteria appear enclosed in vacuolar compartments in large histiocytic cells or occasionally in polymorphonuclear leukocytes or plasma cells.[1] The bacteria reproduce in multiple foci within these cells until the vacuole contains 20 to 30 organisms, which mature and are then liberated when the infected cell ruptures (Figs. 25-1 and 25-2; Plate 96).

The organisms have a surrounding cell membrane and overlying cell wall and possess a sharply defined capsule when mature.

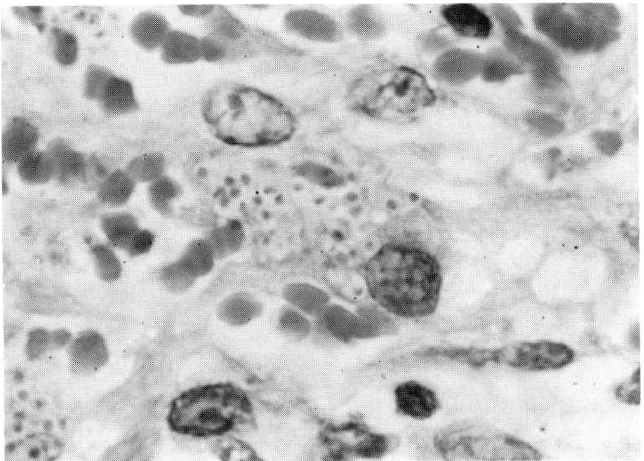

Fig. 25-1. Donovanosis. H&E stain of biopsy specimen, showing intracytoplasmic Donovan bodies.

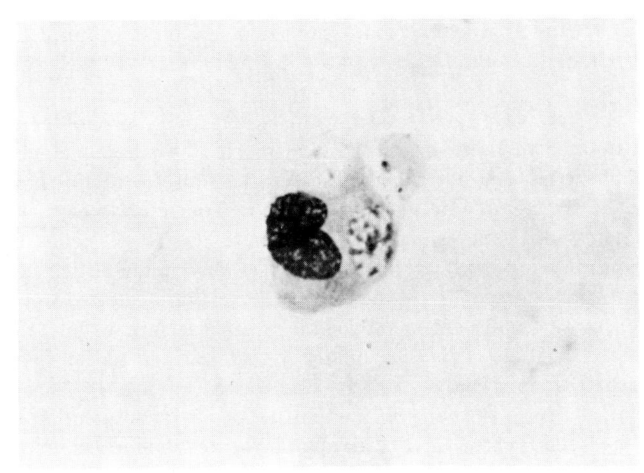

Fig. 25-2. Donovanosis. Giemsa's stain of a crust preparation from a biopsy specimen, showing a single cell with many intra-cytoplasmic Donovan bodies.

Small filamentous projections, of the size of bacterial fimbriae or pili, extend from the cell wall. Electron microscopy reveals electron-dense granules measuring 35 to 45 μm in diameter in the periphery of the cell.[2] Culture in the chick embryonic yolk sac has been reported.[3]

## IMMUNOLOGY AND PATHOGENESIS

The primary lesion begins as an indurated nodule which erodes to form a beefy, exuberant, granulomatous heaped ulcer. This usually progresses slowly, often coalescing with adjacent lesions or forming new lesions by autoinoculation, particularly in the perineal region. Extensive acanthosis and dense dermal infiltrate, mainly plasma cells and histiocytes, occur. Some polymorphonuclear lymphocytes are present in focal collections or scattered throughout the infiltrate, but lymphocytes are rare. The pronounced marginal epithelial proliferation may simulate early epitheliomatous change.[4] The infecting organisms invade mononuclear endothelial cells, and when mature feature metachromatic bars that stain blue or black with Wright's stain (Plate 96). The pathognomonic feature of donovanosis is the large infected mononuclear cell, 25 to 90 μm in diameter, containing many intracytoplasmic cysts filled with deeply staining Donovan bodies (Figs. 25-1 and 25-2).

Metastatic hematogenous spread to bones, joints, and liver occasionally occurs. Occasionally, the lymphatics are involved, but the frequently seen so-called suppurating bubo of the groin is in fact a subcutaneous granuloma (Plate 34). Secondary infection may occur, aggravating tissue destruction and residual scarring.

## EPIDEMIOLOGY

Although rarely reported in the United States, United Kingdom, and other developed countries, donovanosis is among the most prevalent sexually transmitted diseases in some developing communities. In West New Guinea, up to 25 percent of some populations were infected in the 1920s, and 23.5 percent of male patients attending one urban venereal disease clinic in 1972 had donovanosis.[5] The disease is endemic among aborigines living in the central deserts of Australia,[6] and is common in India, the

Caribbean, Africa,[7] and many other tropical or subtropical environments. A recent epidemic of 20 cases was reported from Texas.[8]

The role of sexual transmission is controversial. Goldberg[9] postulated that the vagina is often infected by autoinoculation from the rectum, but clinical disease occurs after sexual or nonsexual trauma of infected sites. Anal intercourse is closely associated with rectal lesions of homosexual patients and penile lesions in their partners.[10] In most cases, lesions cannot be detected in sexual contacts, but a number of studies have detected infection in 12 to 52 percent of marital or other steady sexual partners.[11] The disease is only mildly contagious, and repeated exposure is apparently necessary for the development of most clinical cases. The long incubation period or inconspicuous lesions (such as rectal or vaginal) favor low detection rates in sexual partners.

Zigas[12] screened a New Guinea population and detected lesions in 4.4 percent of the children 1 to 4 years of age and in 4.9 percent of persons over age 15, whereas no disease was detected in the other age groups. He suggested that the young children were probably infected by sitting on the laps of diseased parents or relatives, whereas adult infection was associated with sexual intercourse.

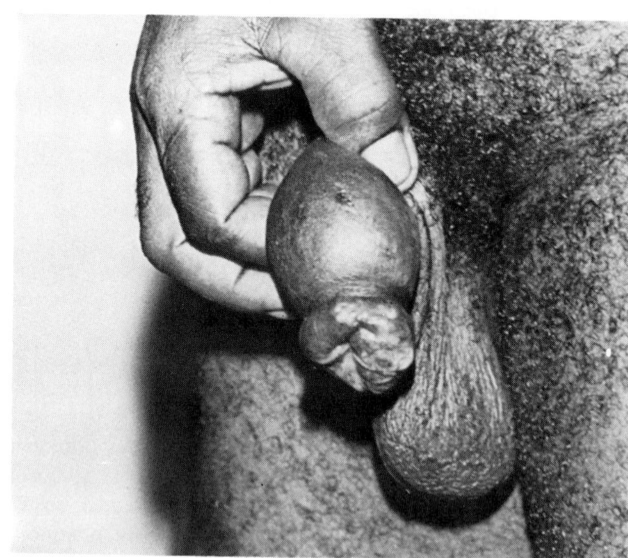

**Fig 25-4.** Donovanosis. Ulceration of the preputial margin may lead to severe phimosis and preputial distention with urine or urethral discharge.

## CLINICAL MANIFESTATIONS AND SEQUELAE

The incubation period has been ill-defined but is probably 8 to 80 days. The disease begins as single or multiple subcutaneous nodules which erode through the skin to produce clean, granulomatous, sharply defined lesions which are usually painless. (Plate 33, Fig. 25-3) These lesions, which bleed readily on contact, slowly enlarge; there may be abundant, beefy-red granulation tissue. Secondary infection may contribute to necrotic debris on an ulcer or at its margin, but surrounding cellulitis rarely occurs. Fibrosis occurs concurrently with extension of the primary lesion and phimosis or lymphedema of distal tissues is common in the active phase of the disease (Plate 35; Fig. 25-4). Inguinal involvement may mimic the buboes of other genital infections (pseudobuboes).

The genitalia are involved in 90 percent of the cases, the inguinal region in 10 percent, the anal region in 5 to 10 percent, and distant sites in 1 to 5 percent.[12] A verrucous form of disease is particularly likely to occur in the perianal area (Plate 36; Fig. 25-5). Lesions are limited to the genitalia in approximately 80 percent of cases and to the inguinal region in less than 5 percent. Cervical or intravaginal lesions may be an uncommon cause of vaginal bleeding[13] but may account for the predominance of females among patients who suffer hematogenous spread of the organism.[14]

In the male, lesions most commonly occur on the prepuce or glans; in the female, lesions on the labia are the most common (Fig. 25-6). The most common distant sites infected are on the head (mouth, lips, throat, face), but involvement of the liver, thorax, and bones[15,16] has also been reported. These distant sites are usually associated with primary lesions of the genitals, but primary lesions of the mouth[17] and axilla[18] have been reported.

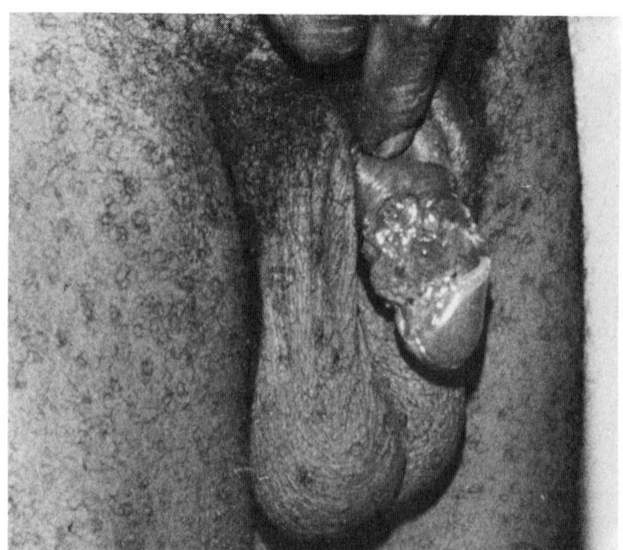

**Fig. 25-3.** Donovanosis. Typical beefy granuloma of the penis.

## DIAGNOSIS

The clinical manifestation is highly suggestive of the diagnosis in most cases. However, the diagnosis is readily confirmed by a

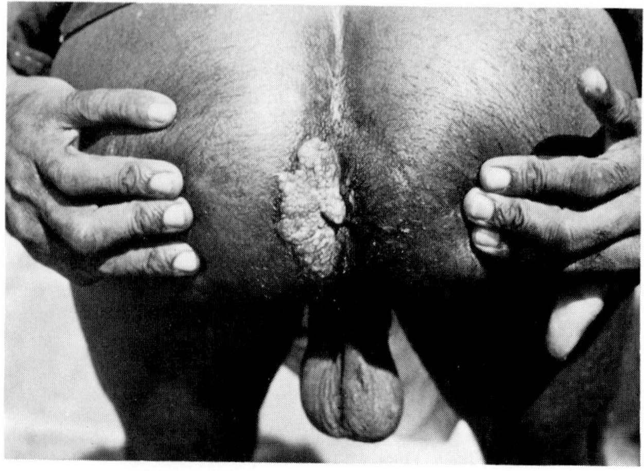

**Fig. 25-5.** Perianal donovanosis. (*Courtesy of CN Sowmini.*)

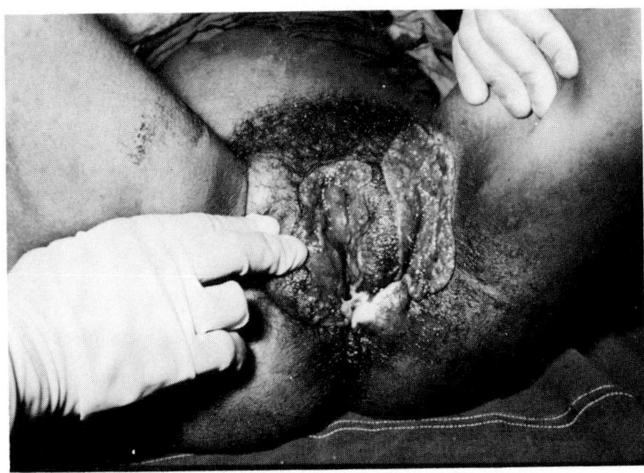

**Fig. 25-6.** Vulvar donovanosis. (*Courtesy of CN Sowmini.*)

stained crush preparation from the lesion. A piece of clean granulation tissue from a lesion is spread against the slide to be examined. The impression obtained is air dried and stained with Wright's or Giemsa's stain.

Donovan bodies appear as clusters of blue- or black-staining organisms with a safety pin appearance (from bipolar chromatin condensation) in the cytoplasm of large mononuclear cells (Figs. 25-1 and 25-2; Plate 96).

The crush preparation is designed to facilitate interpretation by minimizing the amount of debris and other organisms which may occur on superficial smears. However, identification of Donovan bodies in Papanicolaou smears has been reported.[19,20] The features on smear from cervical lesions include intact capillaries indicative of epithelial and stromal ulceration, marked inflammatory cell infiltrate consisting predominantly of neutrophils, epithelioid histiocytes representing granuloma formation, and Donovan bodies located in characteristic single or multiple intracytoplasmic vacuoles within large histiocytes.[20] No multinucleated giant cells and very few lymphocytes were observed, providing an important distinction from some chronic granulomatous conditions.

Light microscopic examination of biopsy specimens which have been formalin-fixed and wax embedded is a less reliable diagnostic procedure since the pathognomonic Donovan bodies are infrequently seen. However, the organisms may be identified by electron microscopy or by light microscopy of sections prepared for electron microscopy by glutaraldehyde fixation and plastic embedding.[1]

Investigation for other sexually transmitted disease is often warranted in patients in whom donovanosis is suspected. Coexisting syphilis and gonorrhea have been reported.[14]

## DIFFERENTIAL DIAGNOSIS

Unusual presentations of donovanosis may cause confusion with a wide variety of diseases. However more common manifestations of the disease also lead to frequent misdiagnosis. Some cases of chancroid simulate donovanosis.[21]

## CARCINOMA

Carcinoma is a frequent misdiagnosis of penile donovanosis, particularly by inexperienced clinicians, and the correct diagnosis is often revealed only by preoperative biopsy or postoperative histological examination of tissue excised as carcinoma. This confusion may occur relatively early in the disease process (Fig. 25-7). In advanced cases of donovanosis or when unusual sites are affected, the simulation of carcinoma may be even more convincing.[22] With external lesions diagnostic confusion is resolved definitively by histologic examination, but where this is not readily available therapeutic trial with chloramphenicol or other appropriate antibiotics solves the problem within a few weeks.

## SECONDARY SYPHILIS

Perianal donovanosis lesions (Fig. 25-5) are frequently diagnosed as condylomata lata. This situation usually presents to the consultant as persisting condylomata lata following penicillin therapy—a story that is virtually diagnostic of donovanosis in areas where the disease is common. Syphilis serology may add to the confusion because it may be positive due to past or concomitant treponemal infection, although the reagin titer is usually low, which makes secondary syphilis unlikely.

## AMEBIASIS

The distinction between amebiasis and donovanosis may be very difficult because both may produce necrotic ulceration of the penis following anal intercourse, and the two diseases may coexist. If the diagnosis cannot be resolved by histologic examination (which may show Donovan bodies and/or trophozoites of *E. histolytica*), therapeutic trial with chloramphenicol is warranted if all findings are consistent with a diagnosis of donovanosis.

## CONCURRENT INFECTIONS

Because patients with donovanosis often delay for many months before seeking treatment,[5,7,23] they frequently have more than one infection at the time of presentation. Often a second infection (such as gonorrhea) may be more distressing than donovanosis and is the reason for seeking treatment, but asymptomatic disease

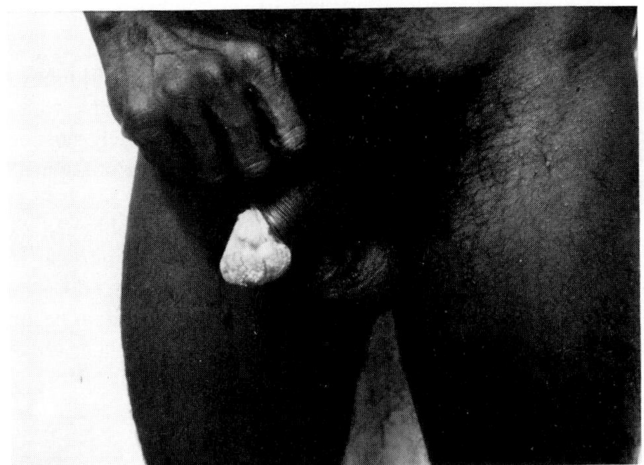

**Fig. 25-7.** Penile donovanosis mimicking carcinoma. (*Courtesy of CN Sowmini.*)

(e.g., syphilis) commonly coexists with the donovanosis. Consequently, the diagnosis of one disease does not exclude others and patients with donovanosis should be screened for other diseases which are common in the subgroup of the population from which they come.

## MANAGEMENT

Many antibiotics have been used for treatment but some are potentially toxic and others have proved to be of variable effectiveness. Chloramphenicol (0.5 g every 8 h orally) and gentamicin (1 mg/kg twice a day) are probably the most effective drugs and cure most lesions within 3 weeks.[24] However, many clinicians are reluctant to use these drugs as first choice because of toxicity. Streptomycin (1 g twice a day intramuscularly) has remained highly effective in some areas[25] but in others has only maintained its usefulness for a limited time.[24]

Ampicillin is sometimes effective[26] but may require prolonged administration (0.5 g four times a day orally for 12 weeks).[27] Penicillin is not effective.[28]

Erythromycin (0.5 g every 6 h orally) has proved to be effective[29] and may be considered in pregnancy, but the results are often disappointing unless it is combined with another antibiotic.[30] Co-trimoxazole (two tablets every 12 h for 10 days) has also proved to be effective.[31] Lincomycin (0.5 g four times a day orally) has also been used successfully in a small number of patients.[26,30]

Tetracycline (0.5 g every 6 h orally) is probably the most widely used drug[29,30] for treating donovanosis and, although resistance has been encountered, is recommended as first-line therapy in developed communities where there are high compliance and follow-up rates, with chloramphenicol or gentamicin reserved for resistant cases. Lincomycin, or possibly erythromycin, could be used for pregnant patients. Chloramphenicol, which is cheap and highly effective and is associated with higher compliance rates than tetracycline (possibly because of gastrointestinal side effects of the latter drug), may be the most appropriate drug in developing communities.

Medication should be continued until lesions have completely healed. If drugs are stopped before this time (after a minimum of 3 weeks of therapy) healing usually continues but the recurrence rate is greater.

If an antibiotic is effective, clinical response should be evident in 7 days. Within a few days of the start of treatment, the lesions become paler, less exuberant, and less friable. Shrinking of the lesions by peripheral epithelization is evident after 7 days, and total healing, except in severe cases, usually occurs within 3 to 5 weeks. Relapse occurs frequently, especially if an antibiotic is discontinued before the primary lesion has completely subsided. An area of depigmentation may occur at the border of the healed lesion (Fig. 25-8).

Donovan bodies are usually not found in smears obtained after 5 to 10 days of treatment. If treatment is discontinued at this stage, the lesion often continues to heal, but Donovan bodies may reappear within 7 to 10 days, and the lesion may again become active.

## PREVENTION AND CONTROL

No method of prophylaxis has been assessed. The disastrous sequelae such as complete genital erosion or urethral occlusion are caused solely by delay in seeking treatment. If treated at the time of appearance of the initial subcutaneous nodule, donovanosis is a benign disease. The primary aim of the control campaign, therefore, should be to encourage the population to seek treatment as soon as they are aware of genital or inguinal lesions.

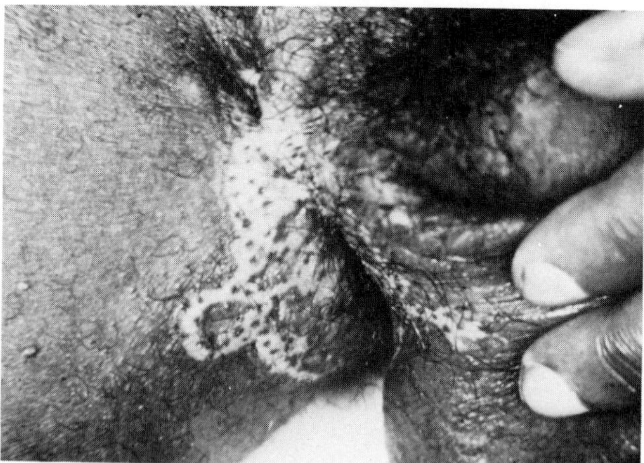

Fig. 25-8. Donovanosis. Depigmented irregular scar at borders of healed lesion.

Control measures have never been evaluated, but yearly screening of the total male population aged 15 to 40 years reduced the prevalence to below 1 percent in one community.[32]

## References


1 Dodson RF et al: Donovanosis: A morphologic study. *J Invest Dermatol* 62:611, 1974.
2 Kuberski T et al: Ultrastructure of Calymmatobacterium granulomatis in lesions of granuloma inguinale. *J Infect Dis* 142:744, 1980.
3 Anderson K et al: Etiologic consideration of *Donovania granulomatis* cultured in three cases in embryonic yolks. *J Exp Med* 8:451, 1945.
4 Nayar M et al: Donovanosis—A histopathological study. *Indian J Pathol Microbiol* 24:71, 1981.
5 Hart G: Psychological and social aspects of venereal disease in Papua New Guinea. *Br J Vener Dis* 50:453, 1974.
6 Mitchell KM et al: Donovanosis in Western Australia. *Genitourin Med* 62:191, 1986.
7 Bhagwandeen BS, Naik KG: Granuloma venereum (granuloma inguinale) in Zambia. *East Afr Med J* 54:638, 1977.
8 Rosen T et al: Granuloma inguinale. *J Am Acad Dermatol* 11:433, 1984.
9 Goldberg J: Studies on granuloma inguinale: VII. Some epidemiological considerations of the disease. *Br J Vener Dis* 40:140, 1964.
10 Marmell M: Donovanosis of the anus in the male: An epidemiologic consideration. *Br J Vener Dis* 34:213, 1958.
11 Hart G: *Chancroid, Donovanosis, Lymphogranuloma Venereum.* US Department of Health, Education, and Welfare Publication no (CDC) 75-8302, 1975.
12 Zigas V: Medicine from the past: Donovanosis project in Goilala (1951–1954). *Papua New Guinea Med J* 14:148, 1971.
13 Murugan S et al: Vaginal bleeding in granuloma inguinale. *Br J Vener Dis* 58:200, 1982.
14 Brigden MB, Guard R: Extragenital granuloma inguinale in North Queensland. *Med J Aust* 2:565, 1980.
15 Kirkpatrick DJ: Donovanosis (granuloma inguinale): A rare cause of osteolytic bone lesions. *Clin Radiol* 21:101, 1970.
16 Schneider J et al: Extragenital donovanosis: Three cases from Western Australia. *Genitourin Med* 62:196, 1986.

17 Garg BR et al: Donovanosis (granuloma inguinale) of the oral cavity. *Br J Vener Dis* 51:136, 1975.

18 Spagnolo DV et al: Extragenital granuloma inguinale (Donovanosis) diagnosed in the United Kingdom: A clinical, histological and electron microscopical study. *J Clin Pathol* 37:945, 1984.

19 De Boer A et al: Cytologic identification of Donovan bodies in Granuloma inguinale. *Acta Cytol* 28:126, 1984.

20 Leiman G et al: Cytologic detection of cervical granuloma inguinale. *Diagn Cytopathol* 2:138, 1986.

21 Kraus SJ et al: Pseudogranuloma inguinale caused by *Haemophilus ducreyi*. *Arch Dermatol* 118:494, 1982.

22 Jofre ME et al: Granuloma inguinale simulating advanced pelvic cancer. *Med J Aust* 2:869, 1976.

23 Lal S, Nicholas C: Epidemiological and clinical features in 165 cases of granuloma inguinale. *Br J Vener Dis* 46:461, 1970.

24 Maddocks I et al: Donovanosis in Papua New Guinea. *Br J Vener Dis* 52:190, 1976.

25 Lal S: Continued efficacy of streptomycin in the treatment of granuloma inguinale. *Br J Vener Dis* 47:454, 1971.

26 Breschi LC et al: Granuloma inguinale in Vietnam: Successful therapy with ampicillin and lincomycin. *Am Vener Dis Assoc* 1:118, 1975.

27 Thew MA et al: Ampicillin in the treatment of granuloma inguinale. *JAMA* 210:866, 1969.

28 Robinson HM: The treatment of granuloma inguinale, lymphogranuloma venereum, chancroid and gonorrhea. *Arch Dermatol Syph* 64: 284, 1951.

29 Robinson HM, Cohen MM: Treatment of granuloma inguinale with erythromycin. *J Invest Dermatol* 20:407, 1953.

30 Ashdown LR, Kilvert GT: Granuloma inguinale in northern Queensland. *Med J Aust* 1:146, 1979.

31 Garg BR et al: Efficacy of co-trimoxazole in donovanosis. *Br J Vener Dis* 54:348, 1978.

32 Vogel LC: Een granuloma-venereum (donovanosis): Epidemic in Suid Niew Guinea (1920). *Ned Tijdschr Geneeskd* 109:2425, 1965.

# Chapter 26

# Genital mycoplasmas

Aaron Eli Glatt
William M. McCormack
David Taylor-Robinson

In 1937 Dienes and Edsall[1] first reported the isolation of a mycoplasma from a human—from an abscess of Bartholin's gland. Since then, 12 mycoplasmas have been isolated from human sources, mainly oropharyngeal and genital mucous membranes. Three species commonly cause disease in humans. *Mycoplasma pneumoniae* causes atypical pneumonia. *Mycoplasma hominis* and *Ureaplasma urealyticum* (T mycoplasmas, T strains, ureaplasmas) can frequently be isolated from the human genital tract. A fourth species, *Mycoplasma genitalium,* has been isolated from men with nongonococcal urethritis.[2–5] It has been shown to be a urogenital tract pathogen in higher primates[6,7,8] and has been implicated in human disease as well.[4,9] This chapter will attempt to outline current concepts of the role of *M. hominis, U. urealyticum,* and *M. genitalium* in human disease. For a more detailed consideration of the biology and immunology of mycoplasmas, the reader is referred to several recent reviews.[3,10–14]

## EPIDEMIOLOGY

### COLONIZATION OF INFANTS AND CHILDREN

Infants presumably become colonized with genital mycoplasmas during passage through the birth canal; infants who are delivered by cesarean section are colonized less often than those delivered vaginally.[15,16] Ureaplasmas have been isolated from the genitalia of up to one-third of infant girls, and *M. hominis* from a smaller proportion.[15,17,18] The mucosa of the male genital tract is probably less exposed, and this is reflected in the less frequent recovery of mycoplasmas from the genital tract of infant boys.[18] Mycoplasmas, mainly ureaplasmas, have been isolated from the nose and throat of about 15 percent of infants of both sexes.[15] Other studies have demonstrated higher rates,[19] especially in babies in special care units.[16] Sanchez and Regan[20] found that 59 (45 percent) of 132 infants born to mothers colonized with *U. urealyticum* had at least one site culture positive for *U. urealyticum.* It is likely that infant-colonization figures vary from one population to another, depending upon the proportion of pregnant women who are colonized.

Neonatal colonization tends not to persist. With age there is a progressive decrease in the proportion of infants who are colonized. Genital mycoplasmas are seldom recovered from urine or genital specimens from prepubertal boys,[21,22] whereas 5 to 22 percent of prepubertal girls have been found to be colonized with *U. urealyticum* and 8 to 17 percent with *M. hominis.*[19,21,23,24] In sexually abused children, these figures rise to 30 to 48 percent and 12 to 34 percent, respectively.[24,25]

**Table 26-1. Sexual Experience and Colonization with Genital Mycoplasmas in Normal Men**

| Number of partners | Number studied | Percent with ureaplasmas | Percent with *M. hominis* |
|---|---|---|---|
| 0 | 36 | 3 | 0 |
| 1 | 32 | 19 | 0 |
| 2 | 23 | 26 | 4 |
| 3–5 | 42 | 41 | 14 |
| 6–14 | 29 | 45 | 14 |
| >14 | 16 | 56 | 13 |

SOURCE: McCormack et al.[26]

### COLONIZATION OF ADULTS

Following puberty, colonization occurs primarily as a result of sexual contact.[19,26–29] Sexually mature individuals who have no history of sexual contact are infrequently colonized with genital mycoplasmas. Colonization increases in relation to the number of different sexual partners (Tables 26-1 and 26-2). With increasing sexual experience, colonization increases more rapidly in women than in men, which suggests that women are more susceptible to colonization with these organisms.

Genital mycoplasmas have been isolated more often from black than from white men[30] and from black than from white women.[17,28,31–34] Some feel that these findings are related to various socioeconomic variables and/or sexual activity.[28,35] However, in a study which was carefully controlled for sexual experience, black women were colonized significantly more often with *M. hominis* and *U. urealyticum* than other women were.[36] This study also demonstrated that barrier contraceptives are associated with lower ureaplasmal colonization rates.

Socioeconomic status is also related to genital mycoplasmal colonization. In Boston, *M. hominis* was isolated from 53.6 percent and ureaplasmas from 76.3 percent of clinic patients at a municipal hospital, compared with 21.3 percent and 52.9 percent, respectively, of patients visiting private obstetricians and gynecologists in the same area.[33] Whether these statistically significant results are a reflection of a difference in sexual experience or whether other environmental factors are involved is unknown.

Genital mycoplasmas can be isolated with considerable frequency from the genital tract of men and women. It is against this background that studies of the role of these microorganisms in human disease must be viewed.

**Table 26-2. Sexual Experience and Vaginal Colonization with Mycoplasmas**

| Number of partners | Number studied | Percent with ureaplasmas | Percent with *M. hominis* |
|---|---|---|---|
| None | | | |
| No genital contact | 47 | 8.5 | 0 |
| Genital contact | 38 | 39.5 | 2.6 |
| 1 | 190 | 34.7 | 4.2 |
| 2 | 90 | 72.2 | 12.2 |
| 3–5 | 135 | 68.1 | 18.5 |
| >6 | 71 | 77.5 | 31.0 |

SOURCE: McCormack et al.[27]

## CLINICAL MANIFESTATIONS AND SEQUELAE

### ROLE OF GENITAL MYCOPLASMAS IN DISEASES OF THE GENITAL TRACT IN MEN

#### Nongonococcal urethritis

Although mycoplasmas were first associated with nongonococcal urethritis almost 40 years ago, confusion persists as to their role in this condition. The results of more recent studies support earlier data[10] indicating that *M. hominis* is not a cause of nongonococcal urethritis.[37–40] Indeed, some workers have isolated *M. hominis* less frequently from urethritis patients than from controls.[41] The response to various antimicrobial agents has also not supported the association of this mycoplasma with nongonococcal urethritis.[10,41,42]

Inoculation of primates with *M. genitalium* isolated from a patient with nongonococcal urethritis has resulted in urethritis and persistent recovery of the organism.[6,8] Antibody to *M. genitalium* was not present prior to inoculation nor in the first 4 to 6 weeks after inoculation.[8] Thereafter, at least eightfold increases in serum antibody were observed associated with an increased number of organisms in the urethra. Likewise *M. genitalium* was isolated from the blood of two male chimpanzees when large numbers of organisms were present in the urethra.[6] The late antibody response in chimpanzees suggests that similar late responses in humans could easily be missed unless widely separated paired sera are tested. In 22 men with nongonococcal urethritis, 19 with gonorrhea and 22 controls, *M. genitalium* was isolated putatively from 32, 12, and 10 percent respectively and from 42 percent of the first group when chlamydiae were not present.[4] Fourfold or greater antibody rises were present in 4 (29 percent) of the nongonococcal urethritis patients, versus only 2 (12 percent) of those without urethritis. Hooton et al.[43] have used a DNA probe to determine the prevalence of urethral infection with *M. genitalium*. It was found most frequently (27 percent) in men with persistent or recurrent nongonococcal urethritis, suggesting that it may account for some of these cases, and more frequently in homosexual or bisexual men than in heterosexual men. Further studies are necessary to establish fully what role *M. genitalium* plays in human urethritis.

It is now well established that *Chlamydia trachomatis* causes 34 to 50 percent of cases of nongonococcal urethritis.[37,39,40] There are two prerequisites to assessing the role of *U. urealyticum* in nongonococcal urethritis. First, *C. trachomatis* must be sought; second, the groups of men must be of comparable sexual experience because sexual experience is a major determinant of colonization with ureaplasmas.[26] In six studies,[40,44–48] ureaplasmas were isolated significantly more often from patients with chlamydia-negative nongonococcal urethritis than from patients who were chlamydia-positive or from control groups of men or from both. In contrast, other studies[37,49] did not find this to be the case. If ureaplasmas are involved in the pathogenic process, it would be reasonable to expect them to be present in larger numbers than if they had only a commensal role. Several investigators[40,44,47,48] have reported quantitative data to support the latter hypothesis. They isolated *U. urealyticum* in larger numbers from men with nonchlamydial, nongonococcal urethritis than from men who had chlamydial urethritis or from comparable men who did not have urethritis.

Shepard[50] used suboptimal doses of doxycycline to treat patients with nongonococcal urethritis. There was a temporary disappearance of both symptoms and ureaplasmas from the urine, and return of symptoms was associated with reappearance of the organisms. A similar phenomenon was also noted in a man who was given a short course of tetracycline therapy for nongonococcal urethritis.[51] A causative role cannot be inferred from these data, however, because other tetracycline-sensitive organisms were not sought.

Another approach to understanding the role of ureaplasmas in this disease is to treat patients with antibiotics that have differential activity against *U. urealyticum* and *C. trachomatis*. Bowie et al.[52] treated men with aminocyclitols, which are active against ureaplasmas but not against chlamydiae, or with sulfisoxazole, which is active against chlamydiae but not against ureaplasmas. When correlated with the results of pretreatment cultures, the clinical results suggested that both chlamydiae and ureaplasmas could cause urethritis. When patients who had nongonococcal urethritis were treated with rifampicin, which is active against chlamydiae but not against ureaplasmas, chlamydiae were isolated from only 1 of 53 men who were initially chlamydiae-positive, whereas ureaplasmas were isolated from 55 of 68 men who were initially ureaplasma-positive. Furthermore, 44 percent of men whose ureaplasmas persisted failed to recover symptomatically, whereas only about 8 percent of men whose ureaplasmas disappeared were not cured clinically.[42]

Another approach is to relate the development of postgonococcal urethritis to the presence of putative causes of nongonococcal urethritis in pretreatment urethral specimens. After treatment of gonococcal urethritis with penicillin, postgonococcal urethritis developed in virtually all men whose pretreatment urethral specimens contained *C. trachomatis* as well as *Neisseria gonorrhoeae*. Among men who were not colonized by *U. urealyticum*, postgonococcal urethritis was significantly associated with *C. trachomatis* infection ($p < 0.02$). Among men without *C. trachomatis* infection, postgonococcal urethritis developed in 11 of 18 men (61 percent) who had *U. urealyticum* infection and in 5 of 18 men (28 percent) who did not ($p = 0.09$).[53] Regardless of whether *C. trachomatis* was present, postgonococcal urethritis developed in 13 (87 percent) of 15 men with $10^3$ or more *U. urealyticum* organisms in pretreatment urine cultures.[53]

Serologic studies of the role of *U. urealyticum* in nongonococcal urethritis have been disappointing. The standard mycoplasmacidal test is a sensitive measure of antibody to *M. hominis*, but antibody responses to ureaplasmas are difficult to demonstrate.[54] However, using a new enzyme-linked immunosorbent assay (ELISA), an antibody response to *U. urealyticum* was demonstrated in 12 (67 percent) of 18 patients with nongonococcal urethritis.[55] Ten (83 percent) of 12 had IgM increases consistent with acute infection. On the other hand, of 40 subjects with negative cultures for ureaplasmas, only 4 (10 percent) and 3 (7.5 percent) were IgG and IgM seropositive, respectively. Further work is necessary to refine the ELISA, but it offers promise as a useful research tool.

Perhaps the most convincing evidence linking *U. urealyticum* to nongonococcal urethritis comes from a study in which two of the authors inoculated themselves intraurethrally with strains of *U. urealyticum* that had been isolated from different patients who had nongonococcal urethritis.[56] The strains had been cloned during nine passages on mycoplasmal media. Both subjects had negative urethral cultures for potentially pathogenic microorganisms before inoculation. Both subjects developed urethritis and a transient metabolism-inhibition antibody response. Similarly, persistent large numbers of *U. urealyticum* organisms were noted in the urethra of a hypogammaglobulinemic man with recurrent urethritis.[57] Repeated antibiotic treatments correlated with symptomatic and microbiological cure. These results indicate that some ureaplasmas are likely to be pathogenic under natural conditions.

Shepard and Lunceford[58] have associated serovar 4 of Black[59] with nongonococcal urethritis. Over 50 percent of 122 men with nongonococcal urethritis from whom ureaplasmas were isolated had this serovar, compared with 24 percent of 125 colonized individuals who were symptom-free. However, the specimens from some of the controls had been collected from 1 to 3 years earlier, and this means that temporal changes in the distribution of serovars cannot be excluded. Studies of small groups of patients have shown no particular serovar to be associated with nongonococcal urethritis.[59] Furthermore, approximately 10 to 40 percent of genital cultures contain more than one serovar.[54] Serotyping procedures can easily mistype isolates unless various precautions are taken. Monospecific sera improve accuracy, but the data reported so far do not suggest that specific serovars are regularly associated with specific clinical syndromes.[54]

Thus, it would appear that *U. urealyticum* is responsible for some cases of nongonococcal urethritis, although it is unclear what proportion of the cases of nongonococcal urethritis from which ureaplasmas can be recovered are actually due to ureaplasmas. The recovery of *U. urealyticum* from the urethra of a man who has nongonococcal urethritis does not necessarily mean that ureaplasmas are the cause of his urethritis.

## Prostatitis

Hofstetter et al.[60] studied men with what was described as urethroprostatitis. Mycoplasmas, mainly ureaplasmas, were isolated significantly more often and in greater numbers from patients with disease than from normal men who served as controls. Since it is difficult to determine whether organisms in prostatic secretions actually come from the prostate, it is interesting that Hofstetter et al.[60] isolated mycoplasmas from tissues obtained by use of a perineal biopsy. Meares[61] and Vinje et al.[62] failed to recover ureaplasmas from men with chronic nonbacterial prostatitis.

Peeters and associates evaluated 85 men with prostatitis of unknown origin.[63] Ureaplasma organisms were isolated from 40 (47.1 percent) of patients and from 13 (25.9 percent) of 51 healthy men who served as controls ($p = 0.02$). *Mycoplasma hominis* was recovered from 10 (11.8 percent) of the men who had prostatitis and from 2 (3.9 percent) of the healthy men ($p = 0.26$). Mårdh and Colleen[64] recovered *M. hominis* from 10 percent of 79 patients with chronic prostatitis and from none of the 20 normal age-matched controls. One colonized patient had mycoplasmacidal serum antibodies to *M. hominis*.[65]

In recent studies by Brunner[66] and Weidner,[67] the isolation of ureaplasmas in relatively large numbers ($>10^3$ organisms per milliliter) from semen or prostatic secretions (as opposed to urine or urethral secretions) was associated with a favorable response to treatment with tetracycline and with the presence of leukocytes in the semen. Using these criteria Brunner associated ureaplasmas with prostatitis in 82 (13.3 percent) of 597 patients who had prostatitis, and Weidner implicated ureaplasmas in 46 (11.2 percent) of 412 men who had urethroprostatitis. Thus, while it may appear that *U. urealyticum* plays a role in a small proportion (10 to 15 percent) of cases of "nonspecific" nonbacterial prostatitis, the extent to which these cases represent "acute or chronic" infections is not clear. Biopsies taken under transrectal ultrasound control from the prostates of 50 men with chronic prostatitis, defined by the Stamey technique, were found to contain chronic inflammatory cells but no microorganisms (A. Doble and D. Taylor-Robinson, unpublished data). It seems that a role for the genital mycoplasmas in the truly chronic condition has not been established.

## Epididymitis

Studies[68–70] have shown that in heterosexual men under 35 years of age, most cases of epididymitis are due to *N. gonorrhoeae* or *C. trachomatis*, whereas in older men and homosexuals, gram-negative rods are usually responsible. Genital mycoplasmas were sought in these studies; although ureaplasmas were recovered from urethral specimens from many of the men who had epididymitis, $>10^3$ organisms were isolated from only one man, and no ureaplasmas were recovered from percutaneous aspirates of the inflamed epididymis. Although the investigators concluded that ureaplasmas do not play an etiologic role in epididymitis, ureaplasmas may do so occasionally because recently the organisms have been isolated from the epididymal aspirate of a patient with nonchlamydial epididymitis in association with a greater than fourfold serologic antibody response.[70a]

## Reiter's disease

Sexually acquired reactive arthritis (SARA) occurring in men who have or have recently had nongonococcal urethritis, and the less common Reiter's disease, in which conjunctivitis occurs, also are seen primarily in men who are genetically predisposed, i.e., who have the HLA-B27 histocompatibility antigen. When exposed to infectious and, possibly, other stimuli, these individuals develop the disease. *Chlamydia trachomatis* is apparently capable of initiating this pathophysiologic process. In two studies *C. trachomatis* was recovered from the urethra of upward of half of men with untreated SARA or Reiter's disease, and serologic investigations implicated the microorganism in these cases.[71,72] When a fluorescein-labeled monoclonal antibody to *C. trachomatis* was used, chlamydial elementary bodies were found in joint material of five of eight patients with SARA (and in one synovial biopsy) but in none of eight controls.[73] All five chlamydia-positive patients also had a serum antibody response to *C. trachomatis*.

The role, if any, of *U. urealyticum* and *M. hominis* in SARA or Reiter's disease is unclear. These organisms have been isolated from the genital tract of patients with SARA or Reiter's disease as frequently as from patients with nongonococcal urethritis.[10] Keat et al.[74] found that HLA-B27-positive men who had chlamydia-negative nongonococcal urethritis were just as likely to develop arthritis as men who were chlamydia-positive were. These data suggest that agents associated with nongonococcal urethritis other than *C. trachomatis* may play a role in SARA and Reiter's disease. Attempts to isolate mycoplasmas from diseased joints have not been very fruitful. Early reports of recovery have not been consistently confirmed, probably because most of these were spurious as a result of contamination by mycoplasmas in cell cultures. Serologic studies have been of limited utility.[10,75] The ureaplasmal stimulation of peripheral lymphocytes and synovial fluid round cells from patients with Reiter's disease[76] is of interest, although it may reflect no more than prior exposure to the microorganisms.

## ROLE OF GENITAL MYCOPLASMAS IN DISEASE OF THE GENITAL TRACT IN WOMEN

### Bartholin's abscess

Genital mycoplasmas have been isolated from Bartholin's gland abscesses,[1,10] although many of these abscesses had ruptured or been opened surgically before the specimens were obtained. Thus, it is not clear to what extent the results represented superficial colonization of these abscesses by mycoplasmas present in the vagina. Lee et al.[77] obtained percutaneous aspirates from 34 intact Bartholin's gland abscesses, which were examined for genital mycoplasmas and other organisms. Eight abscesses contained gram-negative bacilli and four contained *N. gonorrhoeae*. Twelve abscesses contained one or more vaginal microorganisms, including anaerobes and facultative organisms. Genital mycoplasmas were isolated from vaginal specimens from most of the patients. *Mycoplasma hominis*, however, was isolated from only one (along with other vaginal organisms) and *U. urealyticum* from none of the aspirates. Thus, it would appear that genital mycoplasmas are not an important cause of Bartholin's gland abscesses.

### Vaginitis

Women who have bacterial vaginosis (nonspecific vaginitis) are more likely to have positive cultures for *M. hominis* and to have larger numbers of the organisms than are women who do not have vaginitis.[10,29,78] Bacterial vaginosis is characterized by a homogeneous malodorous vaginal discharge and is thought to result from the replacement of the normal vaginal microflora by a more complex flora that includes *Gardnerella vaginalis* and various anaerobic bacteria.[79–81] *Mycoplasma hominis* could conceivably play a role in bacterial vaginosis, as a primary pathogen or more likely in a symbiotic relationship with other microorganisms. In a study in which women with nonspecific vaginitis were compared with controls who did not have vaginitis, both *G. vaginalis* and *M. hominis* were recovered significantly more often from the women with vaginitis.[81] While mycoplasmas are resistent in vitro to metronidazole, such treatment eliminated *G. vaginalis* and *M. hominis* from many of the subjects. Eradication of *G. vaginalis* was correlated with a clinical response, but eradication of *M. hominis* but not *G. vaginalis* with doxycycline did not cure women of their vaginitis.[81] Thus, the contribution of *M. hominis* to the pathologic changes in bacterial vaginosis is not clear. *Ureaplasma urealyticum* has been less consistently associated with vaginitis, several investigators reporting its recovery about as often from controls as from patients with vaginitis.[10,29] However, Gravett and Eschenbach noted that the number of *U. urealyticum* organisms is increased considerably in women with bacterial vaginosis.[82]

### Pelvic inflammatory disease

Pelvic inflammatory disease is an ascending infection in which organisms present in the vagina and cervix invade the endometrium, fallopian tubes, and surrounding structures.[83] *Chlamydia trachomatis* and *N. gonorrhoeae* are the organisms that are isolated most frequently from patients with pelvic inflammatory disease.[83–87] A mixture of aerobic and anaerobic bacteria has been implicated as a cause of this condition by some investigators.[88–91] It is against this background that we will consider the role of the genital mycoplasmas.

The studies which first convincingly suggested a role for genital mycoplasmas in pelvic inflammatory disease were conducted by Mardh and Westrom.[92] *Mycoplasma hominis* was isolated from the tubes of 4 of 50 women (8 percent) with salpingitis. In no case did tubal specimens from women without salpingitis yield *M. hominis*. More recently, Wasserheit et al. performed laparoscopy and did endometrial biopsies on 36 women with suspected pelvic inflammatory disease.[86] *Chlamydia trachomatis* or *N. gonorrhoeae* were identified in 11 of 14 women with both salpingitis and endometritis, in 2 of 9 with salpingitis or endometritis, and in none of 13 patients who had neither ($p < 0.0001$). *Mycoplasma hominis* organisms were not isolated from any of the patients, whereas two patients with salpingitis and endometritis did have positive cultures for ureaplasmas. On the other hand, in another recent laparoscopy study, *M. hominis* was isolated directly from the fallopian tubes of 11 percent of women with salpingitis but from only 3 percent of those without disease (C. M. Stacey, P. E. Munday, and D. Taylor-Robinson, unpublished data).

Investigators have recovered *M. hominis* more frequently from vaginal and cervical specimens from women who have pelvic inflammatory disease than from normal women.[84,88,91,93] However, *M. hominis* is often recovered from patients who have bacterial vaginosis (see above). Since the aforementioned studies linking the isolation of *M. hominis* from lower genital tract specimens in patients with pelvic inflammatory disease did not include evaluation for bacterial vaginosis, the data are difficult to interpret. *Ureaplasma urealyticum* has been less extensively studied but has been isolated from the fallopian tubes of patients with pelvic inflammatory disease[92,94] as well as from pelvic fluid obtained by culdocentesis from such patients.[94–96]

In several studies, antibody to *M. hominis*[91] and fourfold rises in antibody titer to *M. hominis*[88,97] were found more often among women who had pelvic inflammatory disease than among controls. In several such studies the antibody titer rises were associated with the isolation of *M. hominis* from the lower genital tract[98,99] or from the inflamed fallopian tubes[97] (C. M. Stacey et al., unpublished data). Mårdh also found an increased level of IgM in 34 percent of patients with acute salpingitis. This was associated with the isolation of *M. hominis* and with the presence of indirect hemagglutinating antibody to the mycoplasma.[100] Mårdh and colleagues have shown high coinfection rates in endometrial cultures in pelvic inflammatory disease.[101] This has led to the theory that epithelial damage caused by other microorganisms allows contact between *M. hominis* and the immune system and thus an antibody elevation.[102]

*Mycoplasma genitalium* has also been implicated in pelvic inflammatory disease. Twelve (38.7 percent) of 31 women with pelvic inflammatory disease and no antibody to *M. hominis* or *C. trachomatis* had a fourfold or greater elevation in *M. genitalium* antibody titer.[9] In another study,[103] antibody responses to *M. genitalium* were not detected in patients with pelvic inflammatory disease. Others have shown that approximately one-quarter of infertile women have antibody to *M. genitalium*, although there is no correlation with abnormal hysterosalpingograms as there is when antibody to *C. trachomatis* is associated with infertility.[104]

In fallopian tube organ cultures, *N. gonorrhoeae* produced profound damage to the epithelium.[105] In contrast, *M. hominis* multiplied and persisted but did not cause damage.[106] However, scanning electron microscope examination showed that the organisms induced pathologic changes in the form of ciliary swelling.[107] This may be due to the effect of ammonia produced by mycoplasmal metabolism. Ureaplasmas of human origin have been inoculated into fallopian tube organ cultures without obvious damage ensuing.[106] Studies in intact animals may be more relevant than studies in organ cultures. Female grivet monkeys infected with *M. hominis* developed a self-limited acute salpingitis and parametritis.[108] Further studies in grivet monkeys have shown that ascending *M. hominis* infection of the genital tract must be preceded by mechanical injury of the epithelial barrier and that subsequent spread occurs via blood and lymph vessels rather than by the canalicular route.[109] *Mycoplasma genitalium* also has been shown to produce severe endosalpingitis and/or persistent shedding of organisms in monkeys.[6,7]

These data suggest that genital mycoplasmas can cause pelvic inflammatory disease. Additional studies are needed to determine the relative contribution of *M. hominis*, *M. genitalium*, and *U. urealyticum* to the etiology of contemporary pelvic inflammatory disease.

## Fever following abortion

Dramatic changes in the incidence and severity of infected abortions have occurred since the legalization of pregnancy termination in the 1970s. Life-threatening endomyometritis is much rarer today.

In 1970, Harwick et al. reported the isolation of *M. hominis* from the blood of 4 of 51 women who had febrile abortions but not from 53 women who had afebrile abortions.[110] Furthermore, antibody responses to *M. hominis* were detected in 50 percent of women who had febrile abortions but in only 2 of 14 women (14 percent) who had afebrile abortions. More recently, Plummer and colleagues isolated *M. hominis* from two infected febrile women within 24 h after spontaneous abortion.[111] Thus, *M. hominis* appears to cause some cases of fever following abortion. Since patients with this infection have recovered with or without appropriate antimicrobial treatment, mycoplasmas do not appear to be particularly virulent in this setting.

## Postpartum fever

Endometritis is the most common cause of postpartum fever. Cesarian section is the major risk factor. Endometritis is much less common after vaginal delivery, and such infections also tend to be less severe and often remit spontaneously. Postpartum fever is also classified as early (first 24 to 48 h) or late.

Genital mycoplasmas as well as other vaginal microorganisms can be found transiently in the bloodstream following vaginal delivery. Mycoplasmas were recovered from the blood of 26 of 327 women (8 percent) a few minutes after delivery; *M. hominis* was recovered from 10 women, *U. urealyticum* from 15 women, and both species from 1 woman. This transient bloodstream invasion was not associated with postpartum fever.[112]

As detailed elsewhere,[10,113] there have been many reports describing individual patients with postpartum fever from the blood of whom *M. hominis* has been isolated a day or more after delivery. An antibody response was seen in nearly all cases.[114,115] Lamey isolated *M. hominis* from the bloodstream of 9 of 125 febrile postpartum women, compared with none of 60 afebrile postpartum patients ($p < 0.005$).[116] Thus, *M. hominis* causes postpartum fever, presumably by causing endometritis. The patients develop a low-grade fever a day or two after delivery, are not severely ill, and recover uneventfully even without antibiotic therapy.[111,114]

Platt et al. sought to determine how often *M. hominis* endometritis occurs without bloodstream invasion.[117] They evaluated 535 women who had been delivered vaginally and found that 23 women had unexplained postpartum fever and that *M. hominis* was the only agent significantly associated with it. Occurrence of fever was most strongly associated with a low or absent titer of mycoplasmacidal antibody to *M. hominis* at delivery. However, Gravett et al. found no difference between the recovery of genital mycoplasmas from women with intrapartum fever and from controls.[118]

Verinder reported three women who developed septic arthritis due to *M. hominis* a few days after a normal vaginal delivery.[119] In these cases, the organisms presumably entered the bloodstream during or after delivery and were deposited in the joints.

The relation between vaginal colonization with *M. hominis* and postpartum fever is unclear. In a study of over 300 women who were delivered consecutively at Boston City Hospital, however, no such association was seen.[115] Harrison et al. evaluated 1365 pregnant women and showed that *M. hominis* (but not *U. urealyticum*) was associated with fever and/or endometritis after vaginal delivery (relative risk 7.3).[35] Further studies by the group supported the lack of association of ureaplasma colonization and postpartum fever.[120]

Employing protected transcervical catheters, Eschenbach obtained endometrial cultures from 51 febrile postpartum women, 87 percent of whom underwent cesarian section.[121] Seven (14 percent) had ureaplasmas as the sole isolate, two (4 percent) had *M. hominis* and *U. urealyticum*, and 30 others (59 percent) had both mycoplasmas (22 ureaplasma, 8 *M. hominis*) and bacteria. Eschenbach et al. found that *G. vaginalis* was the most common endometrial isolate in early febrile postpartum women, but that nearly 20 percent had ureaplasmas as a sole isolate.[122] From 3 of 18 such patients, ureaplasmas were also isolated from the blood. Antibiotic therapy with agents ineffective in vitro against mycoplasmas resulted in improvement in most of these patients[122,123] and in others like them.[116]

Williams and associates took intraoperative transabdominal specimens from 77 women undergoing cesarian sections.[124] Lower-uterine-segment cultures yielded ureaplasmas in 6 (42 percent) of 15 women with endometritis compared with 4 (10 percent) of 40 uninfected controls. *Mycoplasma hominis* was not isolated. There was a high degree of coisolation of virulent bacteria with the ureaplasmas, suggesting that ureaplasmas may play a symbiotic role in the pathogenesis of endometritis following cesarian section or could possibly just be a marker of the disease.

Berman et al. studied more than 1200 Navajo women and found that women undergoing cesarian section had a higher rate of postpartum endometritis if *M. hominis* was present on predelivery endocervical culture.[125] The association between vaginal colonization and postpartum fever is likely to be best seen when there is prolonged labor and prolonged rupture of the membranes.[126] In a study in which the amniotic surface of placentas obtained at cesarean section was tested, Jones and Tobin found that patients who had placental cultures positive for *M. hominis* or ureaplasmas were more likely to be febrile after delivery than those who had negative cultures.[127]

Late postpartum fever is often due to extragenital causes, althought pelvic infection is also a factor. Hoyme et al. isolated ureaplasmas from the endometrium of 6 of 18 patients with late endometritis; in 4 it was the sole isolate.[128] Others have implicated *C. trachomatis*.[122] Further work is necessary to define the role of mycoplasmas in the etiology of late postpartum endometritis.

In summary, *M. hominis* is capable of causing postpartum fever, but further studies are needed to define more fully its contribution in relation to that of other microorganisms. *Ureaplasma urealyticum* appears to be important in post–cesarian section fever and may be important in late postpartum fever along with other organisms.

## ROLE OF GENITAL MYCOPLASMAS IN DISORDERS OF THE URINARY TRACT

### Urinary calculi

When ureaplasmas were inoculated directly into the bladder or renal pelvis, magnesium ammonium phosphate (struvite) calculi developed in the bladders of male (but not female) rats.[129] Since treating the animals with an inhibitor of urease prevented stone formation, the production of calculi was presumably related to the urease activity of the ureaplasmas.[130] Other workers[67] isolated ureaplasmas not only from urine collected from the ureter and renal pelvis, but also from the renal cortex and medulla of two patients who came to surgery with calculi in the ureter or renal pelvis. These interesting findings remain to be evaluated in larger groups of patients.

### Pyelonephritis and urinary tract infection

*Mycoplasma hominis* does not appear to play a role in acute cystitis.[131,132] Similar isolation rates for the organism have been demonstrated in symptomatic women and in controls,[131] and the organism was not found in suprapubic aspirates. However, ureaplasmas were cultured from 4 of 15 suprapubic aspirates from women with acute urethral syndrome of unclear etiology.[133] McDonald et al.[134] recovered ureaplasmas from suprapubic aspirates of urine from 20 of 101 patients with urinary tract infections; in 7 they were the sole isolate. Further studies are necessary to establish the role of *U. urealyticum* in lower urinary tract infection.

Thomsen[135] isolated *M. hominis* from the upper urinary tract of 3 women and ureaplasmas from the renal pelvis of 2 women in a group of 40 patients with chronic pyelonephritis; however, *M. hominis* was not isolated from the upper urinary tract of 40 patients with noninfectious urinary tract diseases. Only 1 of the 3 patients who harbored *M. hominis* had associated bacteriuria, but all 3 patients had an acute exacerbation of pyelonephritis; 2 of them developed antibody to *M. hominis*. In addition, Thomsen isolated *M. hominis* from the upper urinary tract of 7 of 80 patients with acute pyelonephritis; in 4 of these cases, the microorganism was isolated in pure culture.[136] Antibodies to *M. hominis*, measured by indirect hemagglutination, were found in serum and in urine from some of these patients.[137] *Ureaplasma urealyticum* was isolated from the upper urinary tract of five patients, one of whom was also infected by *M. hominis*. The ureaplasmal isolation rate, however, was not statistically different from that in the control group.[136] Thomsen and Lindskov[138] examined urine samples from 702 patients with pyuria. Nine patients who had pyelonephritis had *M. hominis* isolated from their urine and had antibodies to *M. hominis* in the urine. Only two of the nine had bacteriuria.

Thus, *M. hominis* appears to cause a small proportion of cases of acute pyelonephritis. *Ureaplasma urealyticum* causes pyelonephritis less often if it causes the disease at all.

## ROLE OF GENITAL MYCOPLASMAS IN BLOODSTREAM INVASION

The occurrence of *M. hominis* in the blood is not entirely confined to women. This mycoplasma was isolated from the blood of five febrile men who had had obstruction, manipulation, or surgery of the genitourinary tract.[139] Blood cultures from which *M. hominis* was isolated have also been reported in two patients following trauma[140] and in a patient with chronic lymphocytic leukemia and prostatic obstruction.[141]

## ROLE OF GENITAL MYCOPLASMAS IN WOUND INFECTIONS

Steffenson and colleagues recently described four patients with sternal wound infections and mediastinitis associated with *M. hominis*. Three of the patients had heart or heart-lung transplants.[142] Mandibular fracture complicated by *M. hominis* infection has also been described.[143]

## ROLE OF GENITAL MYCOPLASMAS IN DISORDERS OF REPRODUCTION

### Involuntary infertility

Mycoplasmas could conceivably reduce fertility in men by inhibiting spermatogenesis, causing the formation of abnormal spermatozoa, reducing the motility of sperm, or impairing the passage of spermatozoa as a consequence of damaging the genital tract. In women, mycoplasmas might interfere directly with the transmission of spermatozoa and with the fertilization of ova. Inflammation and its attendant scarring, caused by mycoplasmas, could also interfere with the movement and implantation of ova and so reduce fertility. Each of these mechanisms has been proposed at one time or another, and they have been reviewed in detail elsewhere.[144]

Ureaplasmas may decrease sperm motility and number[146–149] and are associated with an abnormal appearance of spermatozoa.[146–149] Elimination of *U. urealyticum* correlated with improvement in sperm motility, quantity, and appearance.[150–152] Yet, in 33 men with ureaplasmas in their semen, none had *U. urealyticum* isolated from their vas deferens,[153] supporting the concept that sperm are "infected" with ureaplasmas at the time of ejaculation.

*Ureaplasma urealyticum* has been isolated more often from genital specimens from infertile than from fertile couples by some investigators[144,154–155] but not by others.[156–159] However, Cassell and colleagues found ureaplasmas twice as commonly in a subpopulation of women whose infertility was associated with a "male factor" than in other women.[34] In several studies,[160–162] *U. urealyticum* was recovered more often from endometrial specimens from infertile women than from fertile women. This is consistent with the finding of granulomatous endometrial lesions in patients with abnormal reproductive histories who were colonized with ureaplasmas.[163] However, in one of these studies,[162] although ureaplasmas were recovered more often from endometrial aspirates from infertile (26 percent) than from fertile (8 percent) women, endometrial isolation was about the same for women with unexplained infertility as it was for women whose cause of infertility was known.

As reviewed elsewhere,[10] conception rates ranging from 23 to 84 percent have been recorded among ureaplasma-colonized infertile couples who were treated with tetracyclines. In one study, however, the conception rate among untreated ureaplasma-positive infertile women was the same after 1 year (28 percent) as it was among untreated women who were not colonized by *U. urealyticum* (27 percent).[159] In contrast, Busolo et al. reported that conception had occurred in 5 (26.3 percent) of 19 doxycycline-treated patients in whom high concentrations ($10^5$ or greater) of ureaplasmas were eradicated; there were no conceptions among 29 couples in whom ureaplasmas persisted after treatment with doxycycline.[152] Similarly, Toth et al. successfully eradicated ureaplasmas from 129 infertile couples; the 3-year conception rate was 60 percent compared with only 5 percent for 32 infertile couples in whom ureaplasmas could not be eliminated ($p < 0.001$).[164] In contrast, Upadhyaya and colleagues were able to eradicate ureaplasmas from 91 percent of infertile couples; subsequent pregnancy rates were the same whether or not the ureaplasmas were eradicated.[155]

The most logical approach to understanding the role, if any, of *U. urealyticum* in infertility is to conduct large, properly controlled, double-blind studies in which couples with well-defined, unexplained infertility are randomly assigned to receive antimicrobial agents or placebo. Harrison et al.[165] treated couples who had primary infertility of unknown cause with doxycycline or placebo (Table 26-3). Although a 28-day course of the antibiotic eradicated *M. hominis* and ureaplasmas, the rate of conception (17 percent) was no higher in those treated with the drug than in those given placebo. Three other studies also failed to show an association between administration of tetracycline to ureaplasma-colonized couples and conception.[162,166,167]

Thus, although *U. urealyticum* is associated with altered motility of sperm, its role in infertility remains unclear.

## Habitual spontaneous abortion and stillbirth

Although Foulon et al.[168] found ureaplasmas more often in endocervical specimens from women with a history of spontaneous abortion (especially recurrent spontaneous abortion) than in a control group of women, most investigators have found no relation between lower genital tract colonization with ureaplasmas and fetal loss.[10,32,35,169–171] However, none of these studies could exclude the possibility that a smaller subgroup was indeed at higher risk. Normal amniotic fluid (intact membranes, transabdominal amniocentesis) does not contain mycoplasmas (*M. hominis* or *U. urealyticum*)[171] except very late in pregnancy.[118,172] Ureaplasmas have been isolated in pure cultures from chorion, amnion, and decidua of a spontaneous abortus[173] and from discolored amniotic fluid of two women with severe chorioamnionitis who subsequently had preterm labor.[174] *Ureaplasma urealyticum* has also been isolated more frequently from spontaneously aborted fetuses, stillborns, or premature infants than from induced abortions or normal full-term infants.[175–179] Clearly, there is an association between infection of the products of conception

**Table 26-3. Treatment of Infertility: Controlled Double-Blind Study**

| Treatment group | Number studied | Conceptions | |
|---|---|---|---|
| | | Number | Percent |
| Doxycycline | 30 | 5 | 17 |
| Placebo | 28 | 4 | 14 |
| Nothing | 30 | 5 | 17 |

SOURCE: Harrison et al.[165]

by ureaplasmas and spontaneous abortion. However, the association is difficult to evaluate since the comparability of the various groups of women remains unsure and because the role of other microorganisms often was not assessed.

The ability to isolate mycoplasmas from aborted fetuses and stillborn infants is not due entirely to superficial contamination; the organisms have been isolated from the lungs[178,180] and from the brain, heart, and viscera.[10,178] Isolation from the respiratory tract presumably indicates aspiration of infected amniotic fluid (fetuses with pneumonia almost always have chorioamnionitis[181]), whereas isolation from the heart and viscera may be indicative of hematogenous spread. Isolation of *M. hominis* and *U. urealyticum* from the central nervous system of preterm infants,[182] and meningitis[183] and chronic lung disease or pneumonia[184] secondary to ureaplasma infection have also been reported recently. In relation to bloodstream invasion, 2 of 10 women who had *M. hominis* in the blood immediately after delivery had stillborn infants, whereas only 1 of 301 women from whom the mycoplasma was not isolated had a stillbirth.[112] Unfortunately, none of these observations answers the major question of whether abortion of the fetus occurs because mycoplasmas invade it and cause its death or whether the fetus dies for some other reason and is then invaded by the organisms.

Jones[185] found complement-fixing antibody to *M. hominis* in 29 percent of sera from 70 women after abortion but in only 15 percent of sera from 100 normal pregnant women before delivery; however, the occurrence of this mycoplasma in the cervix of the women in the two groups was about the same. Recently, Quinn noted highly significant differences between the prevalence of ureaplasmal antibody in normal pregnancies compared with pregnancies with poor outcomes.[186] In normal cases, elevated antibody was present in 6.5 percent of neonates. In contrast, 77.3 percent of stillbirths and 69.3 percent of neonatal deaths had antibody elevations ($p < 0.001$). Chorioamnionitis was present in most and also correlated with ureaplasmas being grown from the placenta.[187] These serologic data support the concept that ureaplasmal infections occur more commonly in women who have poor pregnancy outcomes than in those who have normal pregnancies. It is, however, noteworthy that others have recorded entry of mycoplasmas into the circulation[112] and stimulation of an antibody response quite frequently during or after a normal pregnancy,[112,188] so that an increased frequency of antibody in itself is not supportive evidence for mycoplasmas causing the abortions.

Mycoplasmas are sensitive to several broad-spectrum antibiotics. Fetal loss, if due to these organisms, could conceivably be prevented by appropriate antimicrobial therapy. In one study,[189] six women who had had a total of 29 unsuccessful pregnancies were given demeclocycline beginning before or shortly after conception and continuing for 28 weeks. Before treatment, five of the women were tested for genital mycoplasmas, and four were found to be colonized. Although one woman had an early abortion and another a stillbirth, three of the other women carried to term and the fourth had a premature infant. Other reports by the same group of workers are similar,[190] describing successful pregnancies after antibiotic treatment of women who were colonized by ureaplasmas and who had had frequent abortions previously. These investigators have postulated that mycoplasmal infection is a cause of reproductive failure.[191] However, to conclude that this is so seems inadvisable because specimens were not examined for other microorganisms, such as *C. trachomatis*.[192] Stray-Pedersen et al. used doxycycline to treat women who had previously experienced spontaneous abortions.[160] A large proportion of these women subsequently had normal pregnancies. Quinn et al. reported that the few habitual aborters to whom they gave erythromycin delivered normal babies more frequently than those given a placebo.[193]

Despite these studies, the role of antimicrobial agents in preventing spontaneous abortion remains unsettled because either the antibiotic-treatment trials have been uncontrolled or the numbers of persons studied have been too few. There is a need for further placebo-controlled trials, especially since many women who have previously experienced abortions deliver normally when brought into hospital.[194]

## Chorioamnionitis

Shurin et al.[195] isolated *U. urealyticum* from newborn infants (but not mothers) twice as frequently when there was an associated histologically severe chorioamnionitis (Table 26-4). Many workers have suggested that chorioamnionitis might be due to mycoplasmal infection.[174,179,180,187,196–198] Gibbs also found *M. hominis* more often in amniotic fluid of patients with clinical evidence of intrauterine infection (35 percent) in late pregnancy than in amniotic fluid of asymptomatic patients (8 percent) ($p < 0.001$);[199] identical isolation rates, however, were found for *U. urealyticum* in both groups. In contrast, women whose amniotic fluid contained genital mycoplasmas did not develop intrapartum fever more frequently than control women without mycoplasmal isolation.[118] Others have found that length of labor correlated with mycoplasmal recovery from the chorion[200] and that infection appeared to be the result rather than the cause of ruptured membranes.[201] Thus, the association between chorioamnionitis and colonization of the infant could be spurious. However, several studies[195,197,199] have taken into account the duration of rupture of the membranes in their analysis and still found a significant association between chorioamnionitis and mycoplasmal infection.

## Low birth weight

Unexpected observation in the early 1960s indicated that the rates of low-birth-weight deliveries were unexpectedly low in pregnant women who had received tetracycline. Administration of tetracycline was not associated with any measurable demographic variable,[202,203] and the most likely possibility that emerged was that the genital mycoplasmas were involved.

Klein et al.[15] then showed that the rates of isolation of genital mycoplasmas from the noses and throats of newborn infants were roughly inversely proportional to birth weight (Table 26-5). The presumed colonization of the mucous membranes of the infant during the birth process may have represented either greater susceptibility of the newborn infant to such colonization or passage through a more heavily infected field. Direct transmission in utero seemed unlikely because of the low frequency of colonization of infants delivered by cesarean section.[15] A prospective study was then conducted in which specimens were taken from 484 prenatal patients at the time of the first prenatal visit, and the culture results were tabulated in terms of birth weight. The data show that there was a distinct relation between the presence of both species of genital mycoplasmas and low birth weight (Table 26-6).[17]

Other groups of workers have been unable to associate ureaplasmal colonization with birth weight.[120,204–206] Embree et al. studied placentas from 446 high-risk pregnancies and 108 normal pregnancies and found that isolation of ureaplasmas was associated with prematurity, low birth weight, and intrauterine growth retardation.[198] Similar findings were described by others.[179,196] Although Foy,[204] Embree,[198] Ross,[206] and Zlatnick and colleagues[200] did not find a relation between the isolation of *M. hominis* and birth weight, di Musto et al.[207] and Romano et al.[208] noted that *M. hominis*–colonized mothers gave birth to infants with lower mean weight then mothers who were not colonized.

Additional evidence supports the association of ureaplasmas with low birth weight. In one study, 246 women who were colonized with *U. urealyticum* at the first prenatal visit were examined for rises in serum mycoplasmacidal antibody titer to any serotype of *U. urealyticum*.[209] The mean birth weight was 3006 ± 565 g for those with a fourfold rise in titer, and 3239 ± 488 g for those without a significant rise in titer ($p < 0.01$).

In a double-blind study,[172] 250 mg of erythromycin or a placebo was given four times daily for 6 weeks (Table 26-7). Those treated with erythromycin during the third trimester had a higher mean birth weight (3331 g) than did the placebo group (3187 g) ($p < 0.05$). Although treatment with erythromycin failed to eradicate vaginal colonization with ureaplasmas, it may have prevented ascending infection.

**Table 26-4. Relation of Chorioamnionitis to Colonization of Infants with *Ureaplasma urealyticum****

| Chorioamnionitis | Number studied | *U. urealyticum* Number | *U. urealyticum* Percent |
|---|---|---|---|
| Present | 48 | 18 | 37.5 |
| Absent | 116 | 22 | 19.0 |

*$p < 0.05$
SOURCE: Shurin et al.[195]

**Table 26-5. Mycoplasmal Colonization of Neonates**

| Birth weight, g | Number studied | Percent colonized with mycoplasmas* |
|---|---|---|
| ≤1500 | 3 | 100 |
| 1500–2000 | 16 | 31 |
| 2001–2500 | 49 | 14 |
| 2501–3000 | 47 | 15 |
| 3001–3500 | 69 | 12 |
| >3500 | 37 | 8 |

**M. hominis* and/or *U. urealyticum* isolated from nose and/or throat.
SOURCE: Klein et al.[15]

**Table 26-6. Mycoplasmal Colonization during Pregnancy: Relation to Birth Weight**

| | Number | Mean birth weight, g |
|---|---|---|
| *U. urealyticum* isolated* | 384 | 3099† |
| *U. urealyticum* not isolated | 100 | 3297† |
| *M. hominis* isolated* | 229 | 3084‡ |
| *M. hominis* not isolated | 255 | 3187‡ |

*Isolated from cervical cultures and/or from urine at first prenatal clinic visit.
†$p < 0.003$.
‡$p = 0.054$.
SOURCE: Braun et al.[17]

Table 26-7. Mean Birth Weights of Infants Born to Participants Who Took Erythromycin or Placebo

| Length of treatment, trimester of enrollment | Treatment group | No. studied | Birth weight: Mean, g | Birth weight: Standard deviation | $p$* |
|---|---|---|---|---|---|
| Six weeks | | | | | |
| Second | Placebo | 98 | 3249.5 | 474.2 | NS |
| | Erythromycin | 101 | 3238.9 | 512.1 | |
| Third | Placebo | 84 | 3187.4 | 500.5 | 0.042 by equal variance 2-sample t-test (one-tailed) |
| | Erythromycin | 64 | 3330.7 | 490.5 | |
| Less than 6 weeks | | | | | |
| Second | Placebo | 138 | 3118.5 | 572.4 | NS |
| | Erythromycin | 128 | 3224.9 | 569.7 | |
| Third | Placebo | 107 | 3138.6 | 540.9 | NS |
| | Erythromycin | 105 | 3082.6 | 580.8 | |

*NS = not statistically significant.
SOURCE: McCormack et al.[172]

## DIAGNOSIS

### COLLECTION OF SPECIMENS

In men, the genital mycoplasmas colonize the urethral mucosa and can be found under the foreskin of uncircumcised men. Tarr et al. found that intraurethral specimens were somewhat more productive than meatal specimens (86 percent vs. 76 percent sensitivity) for the recovery of *U. urealyticum*.[210] In their study all men who were colonized with *U. urealyticum* were identified by one of these two specimens. They also found that *M. hominis* was recovered most often from the urethra of circumcised men (79 percent sensitivity), whereas the coronal sulcus was more likely to be colonized in uncircumcised men (83 percent sensitivity). In women, vaginal specimens are more likely to contain mycoplasmas than are specimens obtained from the endocervical canal, posterior fornix, and periurethral area.[211] Urine specimens provide an indirect means of sampling the genital mucosa. Urine samples are easier to obtain than genital specimens but are somewhat less frequently positive.

### HANDLING OF SPECIMENS

Specimens should be inoculated immediately into medium. They should not be allowed to dry. Once in medium, the specimens should be transported to the laboratory as soon as possible, preferably within 24 h, and in the meantime the medium should be kept at 4°C. This is particularly important if an estimation of the number of organisms in a specimen is to be made. Urine samples should also be kept cool and, for greater isolation sensitivity, centrifuged at 600 g.

### ISOLATION AND IDENTIFICATION

Mycoplasmas are gram-negative but do not take up counterstain sufficiently well for the small individual organisms to be recognized on microscopic examination of Gram-stained clinical specimens. Diagnosis depends on culturing specimens on appropriate media with identification of isolates. The basic medium is a beef heart infusion broth, available commercially as PPLO (pleuropneumonia-like organism) broth, supplemented with fresh yeast extract (10% vol/vol; 25% wt/vol) and horse serum (20% vol/vol). The latter supplies cholesterol or related sterols which are required by all mycoplasmas.[10] Higher yields may be achieved using SP-4 medium, which is usually used for spiroplasmas and fastidious mycoplasmas.[212] Further modifications (addition of $CO_2$, pH changes, addition of *M. hominis* antiserum, etc.) may be necessary for *M. genitalium*, which is a slow-replicating, fastidious, and difficult-to-isolate glucose-fermenting obligate aerobe.[212–214] Genital mycoplasmas grow well in broth medium under atmospheric conditions, but on agar, colonies develop best in an atmosphere of 95% $N_2$ and 5% $CO_2$.

Clinical material is added to separate vials of broth containing phenol red (0.002%) and arginine, urea, or glucose. Knowledge of the metabolic activity of mycoplasmas is utilized in order to detect their growth in broth medium. *M. hominis* metabolizes arginine to ammonia, thus raising the pH of medium from an initial 7.0. Ureaplasmas grow best at pH 6.0 or less, and they possess a urease which breaks down urea to ammonia so that a similar color change is produced. Glucose-fermenting mycoplasmas cause a decrease in the pH of the medium which initially is set usually at 7.8. Aliquots of medium from cultures showing these color changes are subcultured onto agar medium. The addition of manganous sulfate to agar medium results in brown-colored ureaplasmal colonies, so aiding their detection. However, manganese may inhibit certain strains,[215] and calcium chloride may be a useful alternative.[216] Use of this liquid-to-agar technique provides the most sensitive method for the isolation both of ureaplasmas[217,218] and of *M. hominis*.[217] Culturing ureaplasmas takes no more than 1 to 2 days, and culturing *M. hominis* takes up to about 1 week. However, 2 to 3 months may be required for some glucose-fermenting mycoplasmas (bovine plasma albumin may extend the duration of viability and numbers of some mycoplasmas[219]).

Colonies of *M. hominis* are about 200 to 300 μm in diameter and have a characteristic "fried egg" appearance because their growth is in the agar at the center of the colony and only on the surface of the agar at the periphery. Ureaplasmas were originally termed T strains or T mycoplasmas (*T* for "tiny") because they produce very small colonies (15 to 60 μm in diameter). These colonies usually lack surface peripheral growth. Colonial morphology is, however, an unreliable means of identification. Increasing the volume of agar[220] and buffering the medium[221] have been shown to increase ureaplasmal colony size. Furthermore, if colonies of *M. hominis* are crowded together, they may be small and lack peripheral surface growth.

*Mycoplasma hominis* produces nonhemolytic pinpoint colonies on blood agar, but the organisms cannot be visualized in Gram-stained smears of these colonies. *Mycoplasma hominis* also grows in most routine blood culture media without changing their appearance; blind subculture onto blood agar can be used in a diagnostic bacteriology laboratory to diagnose bloodstream invasion with *M. hominis*.[114]

Antibacterials such as penicillin are usually added to mycoplasmal media to inhibit bacterial growth. Thallium acetate has also been used for this purpose. Since ureaplasmas and some glucose-fermenting mycoplasmas are sensitive to thallium acetate,[3,222] it probably ought to be omitted from the media when these organisms are being sought. Erythromycin and lincomycin have a differential effect on genital mycoplasmas in vitro.[223] Erythromycin is more active against *U. urealyticum* than against *M. hominis*, whereas lincomycin inhibits *M. hominis* but not ureaplasmas. These differences in susceptibility have been used to separate the genital mycoplasmas in culture.[217,224]

## SEROTYPING

Both *M. hominis* and *U. urealyticum* have been shown to have multiple serovars. Lin et al.[225] have shown that there are at least seven serovars of *M. hominis*. Repeat infections are not uncommon, and the original strain may not persist in the genital tract.[54] Two different serotyping systems have been proposed for *U. urealyticum*. Black[59] described eight serovars, and Lin et al.[226] described 11 serovars. Recent work in which the prototype organisms for each of the two typing systems have been compared has shown that some serovars are unique to each system. Thus, the actual number of serovars of *U. urealyticum* may be 16 or more, falling into 2 large serogroups.[54,227,228] More than one ureaplasmal serovar is present at the same time in 10 to 40 percent of genital cultures.[54] Although the data are scanty, none of the work to date has suggested that any particular serovar is convincingly associated with any particular disease process.[54] More work is needed in this area.

## NONCULTURE IDENTIFICATION

Immunoassays have been used to detect antigens of various mycoplasmal species.[68,229,230] Diagnosis can be obtained quickly (often on the same day), and the test is relatively inexpensive. However, improvements in sensitivity are necessary before these tests can replace culture, and none is available currently except in a research setting. Mycoplasma-specific enzyme not present in mammalian tissue can be detected by monoclonal antibody,[54] but further data are necessary to judge its diagnostic value. Likewise, DNA/RNA probes hold promise[228] but are currently available only in research settings.

## MANAGEMENT

Since mycoplasmal culture facilities are still not generally available to clinicians, management depends upon recognizing clinical syndromes for which mycoplasmas could be responsible and providing therapy which will be adequate to eliminate mycoplasmas.

*Mycoplasma hominis* causes some cases of pelvic inflammatory disease. Tetracyclines are active against many strains of *M. hominis* as well as against *C. trachomatis*, which is a more important cause of pelvic inflammatory disease. Initial treatment for pelvic inflammatory disease should include antibiotics active against *N. gonorrhoeae*, *C. trachomatis*, *M. hominis*, and anaerobes; the Centers for Disease Control currently recommend either cefoxitin and doxycycline, or clindamycin and gentamicin. With emergence of tetracycline-resistant *M. hominis*,[231] clindamycin is the only obvious alternative, pending more data on the quinolones.

Similarly, *M. hominis* can cause fever following abortion and appears to be a major cause of fever following vaginal delivery. Treatment of fever in these situations with an antibiotic that is effective against *M. hominis*, such as clindamycin, appears to be warranted. *Mycoplasma hominis* is resistant to erythromycin.

The weight of accumulated evidence suggests that *C. trachomatis*, *U. urealyticum*, and possibly *M. genitalium* are causes of nongonococcal urethritis. The usual treatment of nongonococcal urethritis with tetracycline is effective against *C. trachomatis* and against most isolates of *M. genitalium* and *U. urealyticum*. However, about 10 percent of ureaplasmas are resistant to tetracycline,[47,232–234] with about 40 percent of tetracycline-resistant strains exhibiting cross-resistance to erythromycin.[233] This is partially due to the presence of the *tetM* DNA sequence described previously as a cause of *M. hominis* resistance.[231,234] Of the quinolones, ofloxacin shows the most activity against *U. urealyticum*; other quinolones are less active,[235] and spectinomycin has some activity. Few data are available regarding other choices. Patients with nongonococcal urethritis due to tetracycline-resistant organisms usually have no clinical response to the administration of tetracycline.[236] This pattern is different from that seen in most treatment failures in which the symptoms of urethritis resolve while the patient is receiving tetracycline and then recur 1 or 2 weeks after cessation of therapy. Thus, patients with nongonococcal urethritis who show no response at all to treatment with tetracycline should be examined if possible for resistant ureaplasmas and should be treated with an alternative antibiotic active against these organisms—possibly erythromycin or a quinolone.

For conditions in which a mycoplasmal cause has not been proved, it is difficult to justify either examination for the organisms or treatment directed against them. These ubiquitous organisms can be isolated from genital specimens taken from approximately one-half of normal, sexually experienced adults. Thus, culture of genital specimens from adults with an idiopathic disorder will result in isolation of either *M. hominis* or *U. urealyticum* (or both) from about one-half of such patients. To consider the organisms a cause of the disorder on the basis of such a predictable microbiological finding is not warranted, and to routinely provide antimycoplasmal therapy in such instances is not defensible.

## PREVENTION

Regular use of barrier contraceptives retards genital colonization with mycoplasmas,[26,36] but the organisms are so widespread that it is difficult to visualize any approach that would prevent a significant proportion of sexually experienced adults from eventually becoming colonized.

Women who are at risk of developing postpartum fever due to *M. hominis* can be identified prior to delivery on the basis of a low mycoplasmacidal antibody titer to *M. hominis* and its isolation from the vagina. In patients so identified, it may be possible after delivery to intervene with an antibiotic that is active against *M. hominis* and thus prevent postpartum fever. This area is worthy of study.

The data on erythromycin treatment of pregnant women who were colonized with ureaplasmas suggest that the examination of pregnant women for ureaplasmas and treatment of ureaplasma-positive women with erythromycin during the third trimester could prevent chorioamnionitis and low birth weight in some populations. These data need to be confirmed in other studies before such a prophylactic approach can be advocated. Recommending the administration of any medication to large numbers of pregnant women cannot be taken lightly.

There are no immunizing preparations available for the genital mycoplasmas. A much better understanding of the immunology of genital mycoplasmal infections is required before work directed toward the development of a vaccine can begin.

## REFERENCES


1 Dienes L, Edsall G: Observations on the L-organism of Klieneberger. *Proc Soc Exp Biol Med* 36:740, 1937.

2 Tully JG et al: A newly discovered mycoplasma in the human urogenital tract. *Lancet* 1:1288, 1981.

3 Taylor-Robinson D et al: Urogenital mycoplasma infections of man: A review with observations on a recently discovered mycoplasma. *Isr J Med Sci* 17:524, 1981.

4 Taylor-Robinson D et al: Microbiological and serological study of non-gonococcal urethritis with special reference to *Mycoplasma genitalium*. *Genitourin Med* 61:319, 1985.

5 Tully JG et al: *Mycoplasma genitalium*, a new species from the human urogenital tract. *Int J Syst Bacteriol* 33:387, 1983.

6 Tully JG et al: Urogenital challenge of primate species with *Mycoplasma genitalium* and characteristics of infection induced in chimpanzees. *J Infect Dis* 153:1046, 1986.

7 Moller BR et al: Acute upper genital tract disease in female monkeys provoked experimentally by *Mycoplasma genitalium*. *Br J Exp Pathol* 66:417, 1985.

8 Taylor-Robinson D et al: Urethral infection in male chimpanzees produced experimentally by *Mycoplasma genitalium*. *Br J Exp Pathol* 66:95, 1985.

9 Moller BR et al: Serological evidence implicating *Mycoplasma genitalium* in pelvic inflammatory disease. *Lancet* 1:1102, 1984.

10 Taylor-Robinson D, McCormack WM: Mycoplasmas in human genitourinary infections, in *The Mycoplasmas*, JG Tully, RF Whitcomb (eds). New York, Academic, 1979, vol 3, chap X.

11 Current insights in mycoplasmology. *Yale J Biol Med* 56:357, 695, 1983.

12 Biology and pathogenicity of mycoplasmas. *Isr J Med Sci* 20:750, 800, 866, 1984.

13 International symposium on *Mycoplasma hominis*—a human pathogen. *Sex Transm Dis* 10(4 suppl):226, 1983.

14 Ureaplasmas of humans. *Pediatr Infect Dis* 5(6 suppl):S292, 1986.

15 Klein JO et al: Colonization of newborn infants by mycoplasmas. *N Engl J Med* 280:1025, 1969.

16 Taylor-Robinson D et al: The occurrence of genital mycoplasmas in babies with and without respiratory distress. *Acta Pediatr Scand* 73:383, 1984.

17 Braun P et al: Birth weight and genital mycoplasmas in pregnancy. *N Engl J Med* 284:167, 1971.

18 Foy HM et al: Acquisition of mycoplasmata and T-strains during infancy. *J Infect Dis* 121:579, 1970.

19 Iwasaka T et al: Hormonal status and mycoplasma colonization in the female genital tract. *Obstet Gynecol* 68:263, 1986.

20 Sanchez PJ, Regan JA: Vertical transmission of *Ureaplasma urealyticum* in full term infants. *Pediatr Infect Dis* 6:825, 1987.

21 Lee Y-H et al: The genital mycoplasmas: Their role in disorders of reproduction and in pediatric infections. *Pediatr Clin North Am* 21:457, 1974.

22 Foy H et al: Prevalence of *Mycoplasma hominis* and *Ureaplasma urealyticum* (T-strains) in urine of adolescents. *J Clin Microbiol* 2:226, 1975.

23 Hammerschlag MR et al: Microbiology of the vagina in children: Normal and potentially pathogenic organisms. *Pediatrics* 62:57, 1978.

24 Hammerschlag MR et al: Colonization of sexually abused children with genital mycoplasmas. *Sex Transm Dis* 14:23, 1987.

25 Coury DL et al: *Ureaplasma urealyticum* and *Mycoplasma hominis* colonization among sexually abused children. *Pediatr Infect Dis* 5(6 suppl):S351, 1986.

26 McCormack WM et al: Sexual experience and urethral colonization with genital mycoplasmas: A study in normal men. *Ann Intern Med* 78:696, 1973.

27 McCormack WM et al: Sexual activity and vaginal colonization with genital mycoplasmas. *JAMA* 221:1375, 1972.

28 Shafer MA et al: Microbiology of the lower genital tract in post-menarchal adolescent girls: Difference by sexual activity, contraception and presence of non-specific vaginitis. *J Pediatr* 107:974, 1985.

29 Hill GB et al: Bacteriology of the vagina. *Scand J Urol Nephrol* 86(suppl):23, 1984.

30 Lee Y-H et al: Reevaluation of the role of T-mycoplasmas in non-gonococcal urethritis. *J Am Vener Dis Assoc* 3:25, 1976.

31 Cassell GH et al: Incidence of genital mycoplasmas in women at the time of diagnostic laparoscopy. *Yale J Med Biol* 56:557, 1983.

32 Harrison HR: Prospective studies of *Mycoplasma hominis* in pregnancy. *Sex Transm Dis* 10(4 suppl):311, 1983.

33 McCormack WM et al: Colonization with genital mycoplasmas in women. *Am J Epidemiol* 97:240, 1973.

34 Cassell GH et al: Microbiologic study of infertile women at the time of diagnostic laparoscopy. Association of ureaplasmas with a defined subpopulation. *N Engl J Med* 308:502, 1983.

35 Harrison HR et al: Cervical *Chlamydia trachomatis* and mycoplasmal infections in pregnancy. Epidemiology and outcomes. *JAMA* 250:1721, 1983.

36 McCormack WM et al: Vaginal colonization with *Mycoplasma hominis* and *Ureaplasma urealyticum*. *Sex Transm Dis* 13:67, 1986.

37 Holmes KK et al: Etiology of nongonococcal urethritis. *N Engl J Med* 292:1199, 1975.

38 Bowie WR et al: Bacteriology of the urethra in normal men and men with nongonococcal urethritis. *J Clin Microbiol* 6:482, 1977.

39 Oriel JD: Role of genital mycoplasmas in nongonococcal urethritis and prostatitis. *Sex Transm Dis* 10(4 suppl):263, 1983.

40 Brunner H et al: Quantitative studies on the role of *Ureaplasma urealyticum* in non-gonococcal urethritis and chronic prostatitis. *Yale J Med Biol* 56:545, 1983.

41 Taylor-Robinson D: The role of mycoplasmas in non-gonococcal urethritis: A review. *Yale J Med Biol* 56:537, 1983.

42 Coufalik ED et al: Treatment of nongonoccal urethritis with rifampicin as a means of defining the role of *Ureaplasma urealyticum*. *Br J Vener Dis* 55:36, 1979.

43 Hooton TM et al: Prevalence of *Mycoplasma genitalium* determined by DNA probe in men with urethritis. *Lancet* 1:266, 1988.

44 Bowie WR et al: Etiology of nongonococcal urethritis: Evidence for *Chlamydia trachomatis* and *Ureaplasma urealyticum*. *J Clin Invest* 59:735, 1977.

45 Wong JL et al: The etiology of nongonococcal urethritis in men attending a venereal disease clinic. *Sex Transm Dis* 4:4, 1977.

46 Prentice MJ et al: Non-specific urethritis: A placebo-controlled tiral of minocycline in conjunction with laboratory investigations. *Br J Vener Dis* 52:269, 1976.

47 Hawkins DA et al: Unsuccessful treatment of non-gonococcal urethritis with rosoxacin provides information on the aetiology of the disease. *Genitourin Med* 61:51, 1985.

48 Hunter JM et al: *Chlamydia trachomatis* and *Ureaplasma urealyticum* in men attending a sexually transmitted diseases clinic. *Br J Vener Dis* 57:130, 1981.

49 Taylor-Robinson D et al: *Ureaplasma urealyticum* and *Mycoplasma hominis* in chlamydial and non-chlamydial nongonococcal urethritis. *Br J Vener Dis* 55:30, 1979.
50 Shepard MC: Quantitative relationship of *Ureaplasma urealyticum* to the clinical course of nongonococcal urethritis in the human male, in *Mycoplasmas of Man, Animals, Plants, and Insects,* JM Bove, JF Duplan (eds). Paris, Institut National de la Santé et de la Recherche Médicale, 1974, vol 33, chap **X**.
51 MacLeod AD et al: Prolonged eradication of urogenital mycoplasmas after administration of tetracycline to men in the Antarctic. *Br J Vener Dis* 52:337, 1976.
52 Bowie WR et al: Differential response of chlamydial and ureaplasma-associated urethritis to sulphafurazole (sulfisoxazole) and aminocyclitols. *Lancet* 2:1276, 1976.
53 Bowie WR et al: Etiologies of postgonococcal urethritis in homosexual and heterosexual men: Roles of *Chlamydia trachomatis* and *Ureaplasma urealyticum*. *Sex Transm Dis* 5:151, 1978.
54 Lin JS: Human mycoplasmal infections: Serologic observations. *Rev Infect Dis* 7:216, 1985.
55 Brown MB et al: Measurement of antibody to *Ureaplasma urealyticum* by an enzyme-linked immunosorbent assay and detection of antibody responses in patients with nongonococcal urethritis. *J Clin Microbiol* 17:288, 1983.
56 Taylor-Robinson D et al: Human intra-urethral inoculation of ureaplasmas. *Q J Med* 46:309, 1977.
57 Taylor-Robinson D et al: *Ureaplasma urealyticum* causing persistent urethritis in a patient with hypogammaglobulinaemia. *Genitourin Med* 61:404, 1985.
58 Shepard MC, Lunceford CD: Serological typing of *Ureaplasma urealyticum* isolates from urethritis patients by an agar growth inhibition method. *J Clin Microbiol* 8:566, 1978.
59 Black FT: Modifications of the growth inhibition test and its application to human T-mycoplasmas. *Appl Microbiol* 25:528, 1973.
60 Hofstetter A: Mykoplasmeninfektionen des Urogenitaltraktes. *Hautarzt* 28:295, 1977.
61 Meareş EM Jr: Bacterial prostatitis vs "prostatosis": A clinical and bacteriological study. *JAMA* 224:1372, 1973.
62 Vinje O et al: Laboratory findings in chronic prostatitis—with special reference to immunological and microbiological aspects. *Scand J Urol Nephrol* 17:291, 1983.
63 Peeters MF et al: Role of mycoplasmas in chronic prostatitis. *Yale J Med Biol* 56:551, 1983.
64 Mårdh P-A, Colleen S: Search for uro-genital tract infections in patients with symptoms of prostatitis: Studies on aerobic and strictly anaerobic bacteria, mycoplasma, fungi, trichomonads and viruses. *Scand J Urol Nephrol* 9:8, 1975.
65 Mårdh P-A et al: Infections of the genital and urinary tracts with mycoplasmas and ureaplasmas, in *Genital Infections and Their Complications,* D Danielsson et al (eds). Stockholm, Amqvist and Wiksell, 1975, chap **X**.
66 Brunner M et al: Studies on the role of *Ureaplasma urealyticum* and *Mycoplasma hominis* in prostatitis. 147:807, 1983.
67 Weidner W et al: Ureaplasmal infections of the male urogenital tract, in particular prostatitis, and semen quality. *Urol Int* 4:5, 1985.
68 Harnisch JP et al: Aetiology of acute epididymitis. *Lancet* 1:819, 1977.
69 Berger RE et al: Chlamydia trachomatis as a cause of acute "idiopathic" epididymitis. *N Engl J Med* 298:301, 1978.
70 Hawkins DA et al: Microbiological survey of acute epididymitis. *Genitourin Med* 62:342, 1986.
70a Jalil N et al: Infection of the epididymis by *Ureaplasma urealyticum*. *Genitourin Med* 64:367, 1988.
71 Kousa M et al: Frequent association of chlamydial infection with Reiter's syndrome. *Sex Transm Dis* 5:57, 1978.
72 Keat AC et al: Evidence of *Chlamydia trachomatis* infection in sexually acquired reactive arthritis. *Ann Rheum Dis* 39:431, 1980.
73 Keat A et al: *Chlamydia trachomatis* and reactive arthritis: The missing link. *Lancet* 1:72, 1987.
74 Keat AC et al: Role of *Chlamydia trachomatis* and HLA-B27 in sexually acquired reactive arthritis. *Br Med J* 1:605, 1978.
75 Taylor-Robinson D et al: The association of *Mycoplasma hominis* with arthritis. *Sex Transm Dis* 10(4 suppl):341, 1983.
76 Ford DK et al: Cell-mediated immune responses of synovial mononuclear cells in Reiter's syndrome against ureaplasmal and chlamydial antigens. *J Rheum* 7:751, 1980.
77 Lee Y-H et al: Microbiological investigation of Bartholin's gland abscesses and cysts. *Am J Obstet Gynecol* 129:150, 1977.
78 Paavonen J et al: *Mycoplasma hominis* in nonspecific vaginitis. *Sex Transm Dis* 10(4 suppl):271, 1983.
79 Spiegel CA et al: Anaerobic bacteria in nonspecific vaginitis. *N Engl J Med* 303:601, 1980.
80 Blackwell AL et al: Anaerobic vaginosis (nonspecific vaginitis): Clinical, microbiological and therapeutic findings. *Lancet* 2:1379, 1983.
81 Pheifer TA et al: Nonspecific vaginitis: Role of *Haemophilus vaginalis* and treatment with metronidazole. *N Engl J Med* 298:1429, 1978.
82 Gravett MG, Eschenbach DA: Possible role of *Ureaplasma urealyticum* in preterm premature rupture of the fetal membrane. *Pediatr Infect Dis* 5(6 suppl):S253, 1986.
83 Sweet RL: Colonization of the endometrium and fallopian tubes with *Ureaplasma urealyticum*. *Pediatr Infect Dis* 5(6 suppl):S244, 1986.
84 Kinghorn GR et al: Clinical and microbiological investigation of women with acute salpingitis and their consorts. *Br J Obstet Gynaecol* 93:869, 1986.
85 Mårdh P: Introductory address: Clinical and microbiol etiology of pelvic inflammatory disease. *Sex Transm Dis* 11(4 suppl):428, 1984.
86 Wasserheit JN et al: Microbial causes of proven pelvic inflammatory disease and efficacy of clindamycin and tobramycin. *Ann Intern Med* 104:187, 1986.
87 Moller BR: The role of mycoplasmas in the upper genital tract of women. *Sex Transm Dis* 10(4 suppl):281, 1983.
88 Eschenbach DA et al: Polymicrobial etiology of acute pelvic inflammatory disease. *N Engl J Med* 293:166, 1975.
89 Mårdh P-A et al: *Chlamydia trachomatis* infection in patients with acute salpingitis. *N Engl J Med* 296:1377, 1977.
90 Dodson MG, Faro S: The polymicrobial etiology of acute pelvic inflammatory disease and treatment regimens. *Rev Infect Dis* 7(suppl 4):S696, 1985.
91 Mårdh P: Mycoplasmal PID: A review of natural and experimental infections. *Yale J Med Biol* 56:529, 1983.
92 Mårdh P-A, Westrom L: Tubal and cervical cultures in acute salpingitis with special reference to *Mycoplasma hominis* and T-strain mycoplasmas. *Br J Vener Dis* 46:179, 1970.
93 Moller BR et al: Chlamydia, mycoplasmas, ureaplasmas and yeasts in the lower genital tract of females. Comparison between a group attending a venereal disease clinic and a control group. *Acta Obstet Gynecol Scand* 64:145, 1985.
94 Sweet RL et al: Use of laparoscopy to determine the microbial etiology of acute salpingitis. *Am J Obstet Gynecol* 134:68, 1980.
95 Solomon F et al: Infections associated with genital mycoplasma. *Am J Obstet Gynecol* 116:785, 1973.
96 Sweet RL: Colonization of the endometrium and fallopian tubes with *Ureaplasma urealyticum*. *Pediatr Infect Dis* 5(6 suppl):S244, 1986.
97 Mårdh P-A, Westrom L: Antibodies to *Mycoplasma hominis* in patients with genital infections and in healthy controls. *Br J Vener Dis* 46:390, 1970.
98 Moller BR et al: *Chlamydia trachomatis, Mycoplasma hominis* and *Neisseria gonorrhoeae* infection in patients with signs of pelvic inflammatory disease. *Sex Transm Dis* 8:198, 1981.
99 Miettinen A et al: Enzyme immunoassay for serum antibody to *Mycoplasma hominis* in women with acute pelvic inflammatory disease. *Sex Transm Dis* 10(4 suppl):289, 1983.
100 Mårdh P-A: Increased serum levels of IgM in acute salpingitis related to the occurrence of *Mycoplasma hominis*. *Acta Pathol Microbiol Scand [B]* 78:726, 1970.
101 Mårdh P-A et al: Endometritis caused by *Chlamydia trachomatis*. *Br J Vener Dis* 57:191, 1981.

102 Lind K et al: Importance of *Mycoplasma hominis* in acute salpingitis assessed by culture and serological tests. *Genitourin Med* 61:185, 1985.
103 Lind K, Kristensen GB: Significance of antibodies to *Mycoplasma genitalium* in salpingitis. *Eur J Clin Microbiol* 6:205, 1987.
104 Moller BR et al: Serologic evidence that chlamydia and mycoplasmas are involved in infertility of women. *J Reprod Fertil* 73:237, 1985.
105 Carney FE Jr, Taylor-Robinson D: Growth and effect of *Neisseria gonorrhoeae* in organ cultures. *Br J Vener Dis* 49:435, 1973.
106 Taylor-Robinson D, Carney FE Jr: Growth and effect of mycoplasmas in fallopian tube organ cultures. *Br J Vener Dis* 50:212, 1974.
107 Mårdh P-A et al: Studies on ciliated epithelia of the human genital tract: I. Swelling of the cilia of fallopian tube epithelium in organ cultures infected with *Mycoplasma hominis*. *Br J Vener Dis* 52:52, 1976.
108 Moller BR et al: Experimental infection of the genital tract of female grivet monkeys by *Mycoplasma hominis*. *Infect Immun* 20:248, 1978.
109 Moller BR, Freundt EA: Experimental infection of the genital tract of female grivet monkeys by *Mycoplasma hominis*: Effects of different routes of infection. *Infect Immun* 26:1123, 1979.
110 Harwick HJ et al: *Mycoplasma hominis* and abortion. *J Infect Dis* 121:260, 1970.
111 Plummer DC et al: Bacteraemia and pelvic infection in women due to *Ureaplasma urealyticum* and *Mycoplasma hominis*. *Med J Aust* 146:135, 1987.
112 McCormack WM et al: Isolation of genital mycoplasmas from blood obtained shortly after vaginal delivery. *Lancet* 1:596, 1975.
113 Eschenbach DA: *Ureaplasma urealyticum* as a cause of post partum fever. *Pediatr Infect Dis* 5(6 suppl):S258, 1986.
114 Wallace RJ Jr et al: Isolation of *Mycoplasma hominis* from blood cultures in patients with postpartum fever. *Obstet Gynecol* 51:181, 1978.
115 McCormack WM et al: Genital mycoplasmas in postpartum fever. *J Infect Dis* 127:193, 1973.
116 Lamey JR et al: Isolation of mycoplasmas and bacteria from the blood of postpartum women. *Am J Obstet Gynecol* 143:104, 1982.
117 Platt R et al: Infection with *Mycoplasma hominis* in post-partum fever. *Lancet* 2:1217, 1980.
118 Gravett MG et al: Preterm labor associated with subclinical amniotic fluid infection and with bacterial vaginosis. *Obstet Gynecol* 67:229, 1986.
119 Verinder DGR: Septic arthritis due to *Mycoplasma hominis*: A case report and review of the literature. *J Bone Joint Surg* [Br] 60:224, 1978.
120 Harrison HR: Cervical colonization with *Ureaplasma urealyticum* and pregnancy outcome: Prospective studies. *Pediatr Infect Dis* 5(6 suppl):S266, 1986.
121 Eschenbach DA et al: Endometrial cultures obtained by a triple-lumen method from afebrile and febrile post partum women. *J Infect Dis* 153:1038, 1986.
122 Eschenbach DA et al: Bacterial vaginosis during pregnancy: An association with prematurity and postpartum complications. *Scand J Urol Nephrol* 86(suppl):213, 1984.
123 Rosene K et al: Polymicrobial early post partum endometritis with facultative and anaerobic bacteria, genital mycoplasmas and *Chlamydia trachomatis*: Treatment with piperacillin or cefoxitin. *J Infect Dis* 153:1028, 1986.
124 Williams CM et al: Clinical and microbiological risk evaluation for post-Cesarian section endometritis by multivariate discriminant analysis: Role of intraoperative mycoplasma, aerobes, and anaerobes. *Am J Obstet Gynecol* 156:967, 1987.
125 Berman SM et al: Low birth weight prematurity, and post-partum endometritis. Association with prenatal cervical *Mycoplasma hominis* and *Chlamydia trachomatis* infections. *JAMA* 257:1189, 1987.
126 Caspi E et al: Isolation of *Mycoplasma* from the placenta after cesarean section. *Obstet Gynecol* 48:682, 1976.
127 Jones DM, Tobin BM: Isolation of mycoplasmas and other organisms from the placenta after caesarean section. *J Med Microbiol* 2:347, 1969.
128 Hoyme UB et al: Microbiology and treatment of late postpartum endometritis. *Obstet Gynecol* 68:226, 1986.
129 Friedlander AM, Braude AI: Production of bladder stones by human T mycoplasmas. *Nature* 247:67, 1974.
130 Lamm DL et al: Medical therapy of experimental infection stones. *Urology* 10:418, 1977.
131 Stamm WE et al: Etiologic role of *Mycoplasma hominis* and *Ureaplasma urealyticum* in women with the acute urethral syndrome. *Sex Transm Dis* 10(4 suppl):318, 1983.
132 Thomsen AC: Occurrence and pathogenicity of *Mycoplasma hominis* in the upper urinary tract: A review. *Sex Transm Dis* 10:(4 suppl):323, 1983.
133 Gilbert GL et al: Bacteriuria due to ureaplasmas and other fastidious organisms during pregnancy: Prevalence and significance. *Pediatr Infect Dis* 5(6 suppl):S239, 1986.
134 McDonald MI et al: *Ureaplasma urealyticum* in patients with acute symptoms of urinary tract infection. *J Urol* 128:517, 1982.
135 Thomsen AC: The occurrence of mycoplasmas in the urinary tract of patients with chronic pyelonephritis. *Acta Pathol Microbiol Scand [B]* 83:10, 1975.
136 Thomsen AC: Occurrence of mycoplasmas in urinary tracts of patients with acute pyelonephritis. *J Clin Microbiol* 8:84, 1978.
137 Thomsen AC: Mycoplasmas in human pyelonephritis: Demonstration of antibodies in serum and urine. *J Clin Microbiol* 8:197, 1978.
138 Thomsen AC, Lindskov HO: Diagnosis of *Mycoplasma hominis* pyelonephritis by demonstration of antibodies in urine. *J Clin Microbiol* 9:681, 1979.
139 Simberkoff MS, Toharsky B: Mycoplasmemia in adult male patients. *JAMA* 236:2522, 1976.
140 Ti TY et al: Isolation of *Mycoplasma hominis* from the blood of men with multiple trauma and fever. *JAMA* 247:60, 1982.
141 DeGirolami PC, Madoff S: *Mycoplasma hominis* septicemia. *J Clin Microbiol* 16:566, 1982.
142 Steffenson DO et al: Sternotomy infections with *Mycoplasma hominis*. *Ann Intern Med* 106:204, 1987.
143 Lee YH et al: Wound infections with *Mycoplasma hominis*. *JAMA* 218:252, 1971.
144 Styler M, Shapiro SS: Mollicutes (mycoplasma) in infertility. *Fertil Steril* 44:1, 1985.
145 Naessens A et al: Recovery of microorganisms in semen and relationship to sperm sample. *Fertil Steril* 45:101, 1986.
146 Fowlkes DM et al: T-mycoplasmas and human infertility: Correlation of infection with alterations in seminal parameters. *Fertil Steril* 26:1212, 1975.
147 Busolo F et al: Mycoplasmic localization patterns on spermatozoa of infertile men. *Fertil Steril* 42:412, 1984.
148 Toth A et al: Light microscopy as an aid in predicting ureaplasma infection in human semen. *Fertil Steril* 30:586, 1978.
149 Hofstetter A et al: Genitale Mykoplasmenstämme als Ursache der männlichen Infertilität. *Helv Chir Acta* 45:329, 1978.
150 Swenson CE et al: *Ureaplasma urealyticum* and human infertility: The effect of antibiotic therapy on semen quality. *Fertil Steril* 31:660, 1979.
151 Toth A, Lesser ML: *Ureaplasma urealyticum* and infertility: The effect of different antibiotic regimens on the semen quality. *J Urol* 128:705, 1982.
152 Busolo F et al: Microbial flora in semen of asymptomatic infertile men. *Andrologia* 16:269, 1984.
153 Taylor-Robinson D: Evaluation of the role of *Ureaplasma urealyticum* in infertility. *Pediatr Infect Dis* 5(6 suppl):S262, 1986.
154 Gnarpe H, Friberg J: Mycoplasma and human reproductive failure: I. The occurrence of different mycoplasmas in couples with reproductive failure. *Am J Obstet Gynecol* 114:727, 1972.
155 Upadhyaya M et al: The role of mycoplasmas in reproduction. *Fertil Steril* 39:814, 1983.
156 de Louvois J et al: Frequency of mycoplasma in fertile and infertile couples. *Lancet* 1:1073, 1974.
157 André D et al: Rôle des mycoplasmes dans la stérilité. Étude de 150 femmes stériles. *J Gynecol Obstet Biol Reprod (Paris)* 7:51, 1978.

158 Matthews CD et al: The frequency of genital mycoplasma infection in human fertility. *Fertil Steril* 26:988, 1975.
159 Nagata Y et al: Mycoplasma infection and infertility. *Fertil Steril* 31:392, 1979.
160 Stray-Pedersen B et al: Uterine T-mycoplasma colonization in reproductive failure. *Am J Obstet Gynecol* 130:307, 1978.
161 Koren Z, Spigland I: Irrigation technique for detection of *Mycoplasma* intrauterine infection in infertile patients. *Obstet Gynecol* 52:588, 1978.
162 Stray-Pedersen B et al: Infertility and uterine colonization with *Ureaplasma urealyticum. Acta Obstet Gynecol Scand* 61:21, 1982.
163 Horne HW et al: Sub-clinical endometrial inflammation and T-mycoplasma: A possible cause of human reproductive failure. *Int J Fertil* 18:226, 1973.
164 Toth A et al: Subsequent pregnancies among 161 couples treated for *T-mycoplasma* genital tract infection. *N Engl J Med* 308:505, 1983.
165 Harrison RF et al: Doxycycline treatment and human infertility. *Lancet* 1:605, 1975.
166 Matthews CD et al: T-mycoplasma genital infection: The effect of doxycycline therapy on human unexplained infertility. *Fertil Steril* 30:98, 1978.
167 Idriss WM et al: On the etiologic role of *Ureaplasma urealyticum* (T-mycoplasma) infection in infertility. *Fertil Steril* 30:293, 1978.
168 Foulon W et al: Epidemiology and pathogenesis of *Ureaplasma urealyticum* in spontaneous abortion and early premature labor. *Pediatr Infect Dis* 5(6 suppl):S353, 1986.
169 Harrison HR: Cervical colonization with *Ureaplasma urealyticum* and pregnancy outcome: Prospective studies. *Pediatr Infect Dis* 5(6 suppl):S266, 1986.
170 Munday PE et al: Spontaneous abortion—an infectious etiology? *Br J Obstet Gynecol* 91:1177, 1984.
171 Thomsen AC et al: The infrequent occurrence of mycoplasmas in amniotic fluid from women with intact fetal membranes. *Acta Obstet Gynecol Scand* 63:425, 1984.
172 McCormack WM et al: Effect on birth weight of erythromycin treatment of pregnant women. *Obstet Gynecol* 69:202, 1987.
173 Kundsin RB et al: Strain of mycoplasma associated with human reproductive failure. *Science* 157:1573, 1967.
174 Cassell GM et al: Isolation of *Mycoplasma hominis* and *Ureaplasma urealyticum* from amniotic fluid at 16–20 weeks of gestation: Potential effect on outcome of pregnancy. *Sex Transm Dis* 10(4 suppl):294, 1983.
175 Kundsin RB, Driscoll SG: The role of mycoplasmas in human reproductive failure. *Ann NY Acad Sci* 174:794, 1970.
176 Robertson JA et al: Serotypes of *Ureaplasma urealyticum* in spontaneous abortion. *Pediatr Infect Dis* 5(6 suppl):S270, 1986.
177 Caspi E et al: Early abortion and *Mycoplasma* infection. *Isr J Med Sci* 8:122, 1972.
178 Sompolinsky D et al: Infections with mycoplasma and bacteria in induced midtrimester abortion and fetal loss. *Am J Obstet Gynecol* 121:610, 1975.
179 Kundsin RB et al: *Ureaplasma urealyticum* incriminated in perinatal morbidity and mortality. *Science* 213:474, 1981.
180 Tafari N et al: Mycoplasma T strains and perinatal death. *Lancet* 1:108, 1976.
181 Driscoll SG: Chorioamnionitis: Perinatal morbidity and mortality. *Pediatr Infect Dis* 5(6 suppl):S273, 1986.
182 Waites KB et al: Chronic *Ureaplasma urealyticum* and *Mycoplasma hominis* infections of central nervous system in preterm infants. *Lancet* 2:17, 1988.
183 Garland SM, Murton LJ: Neonatal meningitis caused by *Ureaplasma urealyticum. Pediatr Infect Dis* 6:868, 1987.
184 Cassell GH et al: Association of *Ureaplasma urealyticum* infection of the lower respiratory tract with chronic lung disease and death in very-low-birth-weight infants. *Lancet* 2:240, 1988.
185 Jones DM: *Mycoplasma hominis* in abortion. *Br Med J* 1:138, 1967.
186 Quinn PA: Evidence of an immune response to *Ureaplasma urealyticum* in perinatal morbidity and mortality. *Pediatr Infect Dis* 5(6 suppl)S282, 1986.
187 Quinn PA et al: Chorioamnionitis: Its association with pregnancy outcome and microbial infection. *Am J Obstet Gynecol* 156:379, 1987.
188 Lin J-SL et al: Serologic studies of human genital mycoplasmas: Distribution of titers of mycoplasmacidal antibody to *Ureaplasma urealyticum* and *Mycoplasma hominis* in pregnant women. *J Infect Dis* 137:266, 1978.
189 Driscoll SG et al: Infections and first trimester losses: Possible role of mycoplasmas. *Fertil Steril* 20:1017, 1969.
190 Kundsin RB: Mycoplasma in genitourinary tract infection and reproductive failure. *Prog Gynecol* 5:275, 1970.
191 Horne HW Jr et al: The role of mycoplasma infection in human reproductive failure. *Fertil Steril* 25:380, 1974.
192 Mårdh P-A et al: Endometritis caused by *Chlamydia trachomatis. Br J Vener Dis* 57:191, 1981.
193 Quinn PA et al: Evidence supporting the role of genital mycoplasma infections in habitual spontaneous abortions, in *Proceedings of the Third Meeting of the International Organization for Mycoplasmology*, Custer, SD, September 1980.
194 Hawkins DF: Sex hormones in pregnancy, in *Obstetric Therapeutics*, DF Hawkins (ed). London, Bailliere Tindall, 1974, Chap **X**.
195 Shurin PA et al: Chorioamnionitis and colonization of the newborn infant with genital mycoplasmas. *N Engl J Med* 293:5, 1975.
196 Kundsin RB et al: Association of *Ureaplasma urealyticum* in the placenta with perinatal morbidity and mortality. *N Engl J Med* 310:941, 1984.
197 Hillier SL et al: The association of *Ureaplasma urealyticum* with preterm birth, chorioamnionitis, post partum fever, intrapartum fever and bacterial vaginosis. *Pediatr Infect Dis* 5(6 suppl):S349, 1986.
198 Embree JE et al: Placental infection with *Mycoplasma hominis* and *Ureaplasma urealyticum*: Clinical correlation. *Obstet Gynecol* 56:475, 1980.
199 Gibbs RS et al: *Mycoplasma hominis* and intrauterine infection in late pregnancy. *Sex Transm Dis* 10(4 suppl):303, 1983.
200 Zlatnick FJ et al: Chorionic mycoplasmas and prematurity. *J Reprod Med* 31:1106, 1986.
201 Lamont RF et al: Spontaneous early preterm labour associated with abnormal genital bacterial colonization. *Br J Obstet Gynaecol* 93:804, 1986.
202 Elder HA et al: The natural history of asymptomatic bacteriuria during pregnancy: The effect of tetracycline on the clinical course and the outcome of pregnancy. *Am J Obstet Gynecol* 111:441, 1971.
203 Elder HA et al: Effect of tetracycline on outcome of pregnancy in non-bacteriuric patients. Presented at the Eighth Interscience Conference on Antimicrobial Agents and Chemotherapy, New York, October 21–23, 1968.
204 Foy HM et al: Isolation of *Mycoplasma hominis*, T-strains, and cytomegalovirus from the cervix of pregnant women. *Am J Obstet Gynecol* 106:635, 1970.
205 Harrison RF et al: Genital mycoplasmas and birth weight in offspring of primigravid women. *Am J Obstet Gynecol* 133:201, 1979.
206 Ross JM et al: The effect of genital mycoplasmas on human fetal growth. *Br J Obstet Gynecol* 88:749, 1981.
207 di Musto JC et al: *Mycoplasma hominis* type I infection and pregnancy. *Obstet Gynecol* 41:33, 1973.
208 Romano N et al: Mycoplasmas in pregnant women and in newborn infants. *Boll Ist Sieroter Milan* 55:568, 1976.
209 Kass EH et al: Genital mycoplasmas as a cause of excess premature delivery. *Trans Assoc Am Physicians* 94:261, 1981.
210 Tarr PI et al: Comparison of methods for the isolation of genital mycoplasmas from men. *J Infect Dis* 133:419, 1976.
211 McCormack WM et al: Localization of genital mycoplasmas in women. *Am J Obstet Gynecol* 112:920, 1972.
212 Tully JG et al: Evaluation of culture media for the recovery of *My-*

*coplasma hominis* from the human genital tract. *Sex Transm Dis* 10(4 suppl):256, 1983.

213 Taylor-Robinson D: Mycoplasma infection of the human genital tract with particular reference to non-gonococcal urethritis. *Ann Microbiol (Paris)* 135A:129, 1984.

214 Furr PM, Taylor-Robinson D: Microimmunofluorescence technique for detection of antibody to *Mycoplasma genitalium*. *J Clin Pathol* 37:1072, 1984.

215 Robertson JA, Chen MH: Effects of manganese on the growth and morphology of *Ureaplasma urealyticum*. *J Clin Microbiol* 19:857, 1984.

216 Shepard MC, Robertson JA: Calcium chloride as an indicator for colonies of *Ureaplasma urealyticum*. *Pediatr Infect Dis* 5(6 suppl):S349, 1986.

217 Braun P et al: Methodologic investigations and prevalence of genital mycoplasmas in pregnancy. *J Infect Dis* 121:391, 1970.

218 Taylor-Robinson D et al: Comparison of techniques for the isolation of T-strain mycoplasmas. *Nature* 222:274, 1969.

219 Taylor-Robinson D, Behnke J: The prolonged persistence of mycoplasmas in culture. *J Med Microbiol* 23:89, 1987.

220 Lee Y-H et al: Effect of agar volume, inoculum size, and Hepes buffer on the size of T-mycoplasmal colonies. *J Lab Clin Med* 84:766, 1974.

221 Manchee RJ, Taylor-Robinson D: Enhanced growth of T-strain mycoplasmas with *N*-2-hydroxyethylpiperazine-$N^1$-2-ethanesulfonic acid buffer. *J Bacteriol* 100:78, 1969.

222 Lee Y-H et al: T-mycoplasmas from urine and vaginal specimens: Decreased rates of isolation and growth in the presence of thallium acetate. *J Infect Dis* 125:318, 1972.

223 Braun P et al: Susceptibility of genital mycoplasmas to antimicrobial agents. *Appl Microbiol* 19:62, 1970.

224 Robertson JA: Bromothymol blue broth: Improved medium for detection of *Ureaplasma urealyticum* (T-strain mycoplasma). *J Clin Microbiol* 7:127, 1978.

225 Lin J-S, Kass EH: Serological reactions of *Mycoplasma hominis*: Differences among mycoplasmacidal, metabolic inhibition, and growth agglutination tests. *Infect Immun* 10:535, 1974.

226 Lin J-SL et al: Serologic typing of human genital T-mycoplasmas by a complement-dependent mycoplasmacidal test. *J Infect Dis* 126:658, 1972.

227 Horowitz SA et al: Can group- and serovar-specific proteins be detected in *Ureaplasma urealyticum*. *Pediatr Infect Dis* 5(6 suppl): S325, 1986.

228 Razin S, Yogev D: Genetic relatedness among *Ureaplasma urealyticum* serotypes (serovars). *Pediatr Infect Dis* 5(6 suppl):S300, 1986.

229 Miettinen A et al: Detection of *Mycoplasma hominis* antigen in clinical specimens by using a 4 layer modification of enzyme immunoassay. *J Immunol Methods* 69:267, 1984.

230 Kotani H et al: New method of identification and serodiagnosis for genital mycoplasmas by immunobinding assay. *Pediatr Infect Dis* 5(6 suppl):S349, 1986.

231 Roberts MC et al: Tetracycline-resistant *Mycoplasma hominis* strains contain streptococcal tetM sequences. *Antimicrob Agents Chemother* 28:141, 1985.

232 Evans RT, Taylor-Robinson D: The incidence of tetracycline-resistant strains of *Ureaplasma urealyticum*. *J Antimicrob Chemother* 4:57, 1978.

233 Taylor-Robinson D, Furr PM: Clinical antibiotic resistance of *Ureaplasma urealyticum*. *Pediatr Infect Dis* 5(6 suppl):S335, 1986.

234 Roberts MC, Kenny GE: Dissemination of the tetM tetracycline resistance determinant to *Ureaplasma urealyticum*. *Antimicrob Agents Chemother* 29:350, 1986.

235 Aznar J et al: Activities of new quinolone derivatives against genital pathogens. *Antimicrob Agents Chemother* 27:76, 1985.

236 Stimson JB et al: Tetracycline-resistant *Ureaplasma urealyticum*: A cause of persistent nongonococcal urethritis. *Ann Intern Med* 94:192, 1981.

## Chapter 27

# Enteric bacterial pathogens: *Shigella, Salmonella, Campylobacter*

Gerald T. Keusch

In recent years, the recognized spectrum of sexually transmitted diseases has been broadened considerably. Perhaps most notable among the "new" sexually transmitted diseases are the organisms which cause enteritis or proctitis, especially in gay males (the "gay bowel syndrome"). The clinical aspects of these syndromes are discussed in Chap. 55; this chapter reviews the microbiology and epidemiology of the bacteria most commonly associated with sexually transmitted enteritis.

## HISTORY, EPIDEMIOLOGY, AND CLINICAL MANIFESTATIONS

### HISTORY

The recorded history of the enteric bacterial pathogens is surely as long as the history of the human race. Numerous descriptions of diarrhea and dysentery appear in the Bible, and their common occurrence undoubtedly accounts for their failure to make the list of the top 10 plagues. Throughout history, the course of military campaigns has often been decided as much by the call to stool as by the call to battle. Beginning about a century ago and continuing to the present, specific etiologic agents have been discovered by careful microbiological and epidemiological study. Recent work has been particularly fruitful in uncovering many of the features and mechanisms of pathogenesis in a virtual renaissance in the study of diarrhea. Entirely new concepts of shigellosis and salmonellosis have been developed, and previously unrecognized etiologic agents, such as *Campylobacter*, have emerged as important causes of diarrheal disease. In the last decade, these agents have been recognized as common causes of enteritis in homosexual men.

### EPIDEMIOLOGY

From the time of Moses, in one of the earliest published epidemiological studies,[1] it was recognized that to control diarrheal disease one must control the spread of feces in the environment. The circle of transmission from oral ingestion to anal excretion to oral ingestion has led some authorities to categorize the enteric bacterial diseases as filth diseases; the role of feces, fingers, flies, fomites, food, fluids, and more recently, various forms of fornication is well known. However, it must be remembered that the epidemiology of the individual agents is as much a consequence of their specific biological properties as it is the result of environmental (or host) factors.

#### *Shigella*

*Shigella* are highly host-adapted bacteria; they are natural pathogens only of humans and certain species of higher primates. As a consequence, one human infection is almost invariably traceable to another human, although the route may deviate through food or fluids.[2] Another feature of importance is the capacity of small inocula to cause symptomatic infection. Experimental infections of human volunteers with a few hundred to a few thousand viable shigellae is easily accomplished.[3] Hence, the principal route of infection for these organisms is by contact spread. Since convalescent or asymptomatic carriers may have $10^2$ to $10^3$ bacteria per gram of stool, while active cases excrete $10^5$ to $10^8$ shigellae per gram of stool, it is easy to see how anal-oral spread can readily occur among household contacts.

First noted in 1974, homosexually transmitted shigellosis has been documented in such large U.S. cities as San Francisco, Seattle, and New York.[4–7] In contrast to trends in prevalence of *Shigella* species in the general U.S. population, where *S. sonnei* has predominated over the past two decades,[2] *S. flexneri* has accounted for the majority of cases among homosexuals.[8] The magnitude of this association is reflected in a greater than five-fold increase in *S. flexneri* isolates in adult males over this time period, in comparison with no change or a decrease in women and children, respectively. In addition, the median age of the patient with *S. flexneri* had increased from 5 to 26 years.[8] By 1985, one-fourth of all *S. flexneri* isolates in the United States were from men 20 to 59 years of age. Although it cannot be unequivocally shown that this increase is solely accounted for by transmission among homosexuals, all evidence is consistent with this view.[9] Shigellosis is known to be a colonic disease and the organism is able to invade this organ.[2,3] In orally acquired infection, colonic lesions are most prominent in the rectum and become progressively less severe as the ileocecal junction is approached, indicating a tropism for the most distal portion of the bowel.[10] Thus, it is possible that direct inoculation of *Shigella* during anal intercourse could result in infection of the susceptible rectal mucosa. Alternatively, the practice of fellatio after anal intercourse could also lead to transmission of an oral infectious inoculum. In San Francisco, where concern for HIV infection has altered sexual practices among male homosexuals, the incidence of shigellosis has decreased by 30 percent among the target group in the past few years.[11]

#### *Salmonella*

There are three species of *Salmonella, S. typhi, S. choleraesuis*, and *S. enteritidis*, the last of which contains almost 2000 distinct serotypes. Non-host-adapted serotypes of *S. enteritidis* are the cause of most *Salmonella* gastroenteritis. The infections may be traced to another human host, but food—especially poultry, eggs, milk, or water—is most often implicated.[12] Hence, *salmonellosis* is usually a food-borne gastroenteritis (commonly classified as *food poisoning with fever*). Outbreaks of common-source salmonellosis have been documented for a number of vehicles, including dried and whole milk, milk chocolate, poultry, pork, shellfish, and powdered eggs.[12] The surface of hen's eggs and the interior of cracked or even grade A uncracked eggs[13] may also be culture-positive.

While such vehicles account for most outbreaks, person-to-person spread certainly occurs, particularly among male homosexuals. Like shigellosis, spread of salmonella between male sexual partners is promoted by the practice of anilingus and of fellatio after anal intercourse. The minimal infectious dose in normal adult volunteers is around $10^5$ organisms, but influencing this are such host factors as gastric acidity, composition of the normal bacterial flora, and age of the host.[12] Because acid pH rapidly and significantly reduces viability of the salmonellae, the intermediate infectious dose and the efficacy of the normal gastric acid barrier may protect most individuals from direct transmission of salmonella gastroenteritis during sexual activity. Hypochlorhydric subjects or postgastrectomy patients are clearly at greater risk to salmonella infections. Inoculum size is reduced by 100-fold if protected in food or in other vehicles.

*Salmonella typhi* and other causes of enteric fever are highly host-adapted to humans. The epidemiological route is always traceable to another human, whether case or carrier. Many interesting, intricate, and ingenious routings, however, may be involved in carrying the organism to a susceptible new human host. Usually a food or water vehicle is the direct carrier of the infecting dose. Volunteer studies using the virulent Quailes strain have demonstrated that at least $10^5$ organisms are required to produce disease under these conditions.

### *Campylobacter*

The classification of *Campylobacter* is both confusing and evolving at the present time (Table 27-1). The genus can be conveniently divided into two big groups on the basis of the catalase reaction, since human pathogens are found only among the catalase-positive species. The latter can be further divided according to temperature tolerance. One subgroup, typified by the prototypic *Campylobacter*, originally called *Vibrio fetus* but now renamed *C. fetus* ssp. *fetus* (usually more simply called *C. fetus*), grow well at temperatures ranging from 25 to 37°C. The existence of thermophilic species, defined as the ability to grow at 42°C but not at 25°C, was first reported by King in 1957[14] who described a group of "related *Vibrios*" exhibiting this property. Current use of better selective media have allowed the culture and identification of several separate species among thermophilic *Campylobacters*, including the most common species causing human illness, the hippurate-positive *C. jejuni*.[15] Two hippurate-negative thermophilic strains also cause human infection, *C. coli* and *C. laridis*, the latter distinguished in part because of its naladixic acid and cephalothin resistance.[16] Human infections typically result from ingestion of contaminated food or liquids. *C. jejuni* is rapidly killed by gastric acid, but it can survive for weeks in chilled milk or water.[17] The most common sources of infection are unpasteurized milk, undercooked poultry, and contaminated water sources. In common source outbreaks, usually around 25 percent of those exposed develop clinical illness. Although solid data are not yet available concerning the infective dose, it appears that some subjects will become ill after ingestion of as few as 500 organisms.[17]

More recently, a group of similar bacteria designated "*Campylobacter*-like organisms" (CLOs) has been found to cause diarrhea, especially in male homosexuals.[18] The CLOs resemble the typical *Campylobacter* in being catalase- and oxidase-positive, microaerophilic, motile, curved gram-negative rods, but they differ in colonial morphology, in some biochemical reactions, and in growth temperature requirements.[19] The group includes three species biochemically resembling *C. jejuni*, except that they are not thermophilic, are cephalothin-sensitive, and are also distinct by DNA hybridization techniques.[20] A fourth CLO, *C. pyloris*, is unique in its habitat and microbiological characteristics. This organism colonizes the stomach, is very strongly urease-positive, and has been epidemiologically associated with acute and chronic gastritis and possibly with gastric and/or duodenal ulcer disease,[21] although showing no special predilection for the homosexual population. Two *C. jejuni*-like CLOs are now sufficiently characterized to propose new species names, *C. cinaedi* (formerly CLO type 1) and *C. fennelliae* (formerly CLO type 2).[20] These CLOs are, in some clinical series, the most common isolate from patients with "gay bowel syndrome"; however, because of their antibiotic sensitivity pattern they will not be isolated if cephalothin containing *Campylobacter* selective media are used.[18]

In a recent study in San Francisco, pathogens were recovered from nearly 50 percent of adults with diarrhea and *C. jejuni* was identified in three-fifths of these.[22] *C. jejuni* and *Shigella* together accounted for 53 percent of diarrhea among homosexual men, and in contrast to the rest of the population, *Shigella* sp. outnumbered *C. jejuni* by 2:1. In Seattle, the two pathogens accounted for 10 percent of the total symptomatic infections in homosexuals, with a 2:1 edge for *C. jejuni*.[23] Pathogens were also found in two-fifths of asymptomatic homosexual subjects, which together with the frequent finding of nonpathogenic protozoa, indicates the intensity of exposure to infected feces among this group. The most common presentation was that of proctocolitis, defined as diarrhea with lower abdominal cramps and mucosal abnormalities extending above 15 cm from the rectum, as detected by sigmoidoscopy.[9]

## CLINICAL MANIFESTATIONS

Clinical manifestations of infection due to the three groups of organisms are similar but still distinctive.

### *Shigella*

Shigellae are the classic cause of bacillary dysentery, a clinical syndrome characterized by frequent passage of small volumes of frankly bloody, mucoid stools, accompanied by abdominal

**Table 27-1. Classification of the Genus *Campylobacter***

| | Selected characteristics | | | | | Growth temperature | |
|---|---|---|---|---|---|---|---|
| | Drug sensitivity | | | | | | |
| Species | Naladixic | Cephalothin | Hippurate | $H_2S$ | Nitrate | 25°C | 42°C |
| *C. fetus* | R | S | – | – | + | + | – |
| *C. jejuni* | S | R | + | – | + | – | + |
| *C. coli* | S | R | – | – | + | – | + |
| *C. laridis* | R | R | – | – | + | – | + |
| *C. cinaedi* | S | S | – | – | + | – | – |
| *C. fennelliae* | S | S | – | – | – | – | – |
| *C. hyointestinalis* | R | S | – | + | + | ± | + |

*Note:* R = resistant; S = susceptible.

**Table 27-2. Relative Severity of Infections Due to the Genus *Shigella***

| Species | Frequency of isolation in U.S. | Clinical manifestations: Dysentery | Diarrhea | Hemolytic uremic syndrome | Other extraintestinal |
|---|---|---|---|---|---|
| *S. dysenteriae* type 1 | Nil* | + + + + | + + | + | + |
| *S. flexneri* | 20–30% | + + | + + + | ± | + |
| *S. boydii* | Nil | + + | + + + | 0 | + |
| *S. sonnei* | 70–80% | + | + + + + | 0 | + |

*Isolation of *S. dysenteriae* type 1 in the United States occurred in the early 1970s as the result of the epidemic in Mexico and Central America at that time.

cramps, tenesmus, and fever.[24] However, most cases of clinical shigellosis begin with watery diarrhea which may or may not progress to the dysentery syndrome. This is somewhat dependent on the species involved (Table 27-2). *Shigella dysenteriae* type 1 causes the most severe illness, often progressing so rapidly from diarrhea to dysentery that the former is not even noticed, whereas *S. sonnei* generally causes only a self-limited diarrhea.

In the United States, *S. dysenteriae* 1 infection is distinctly unusual and is invariably imported. *S. sonnei* accounts for over three-fourths of the isolates in the general population and usually causes a mild to moderate watery diarrhea. *S. flexneri*, the predominant isolate in the homosexual population, results in more intensive disease, with much more inflammatory component. New manifestations are also being seen in these patients. For example, cutaneous shigellosis has been reported in a 22-year-old male homosexual who presented with a tender penile furuncle from which a pure culture of *S. flexneri* was isolated.[25]

## *Salmonella*

Salmonellae cause four clinical types of infection: acute gastroenteritis, enteric (typhoid) fever, septicemia with or without focal systemic lesions, and an asymptomatic carrier state[26] (Table 27-3). Enteric fever has become uncommon in the United States (and will not be discussed here) as the number of human host reservoirs has diminished with improved sanitation. The number of cases of salmonella gastroenteritis, however, has increased due to increasing use of potentially contaminated processed foods, as well as to poor food-storage practices which favor the multiplication of microorganisms. Clinical manifestations of salmonella gastroenteritis, including fever, headache, vomiting, abdominal pain, and diarrhea, usually begin 24 to 36 h after the inoculum is consumed.[12,26] Respiratory symptoms such as cough can occur, producing a symptom complex that patients may describe as *intestinal flu*. Sporadic cases that are not investigated microbiologically thus go undiagnosed in contrast to the larger common-source outbreaks which are generally well studied. Bacteremia is frequently detected if blood cultures are obtained early in the infection, and this may become clinically significant in a few patients; generally, bacteremia is transient and self-limited without therapy.[26] The diarrhea is watery, and it often contains mucus and, on occasion, blood.[12] Microscopic examination of the stool reveals a few erythrocytes but usually shows large numbers of leukocytes. In a few patients dysenteric symptoms appear, including frankly bloody stools, tenderness over the sigmoid colon, and tenesmus. The resemblance of this phase of disease to shigellosis is supported by endoscopic demonstration of colonic mucosal edema, hyperemia, friability, petechial hemorrhages, and histologic evidence of mucosal inflammation, crypt abscess, and focal epithelial necrosis.[27,28]

## *Campylobacter*

*Campylobacter jejuni* causes shigella-like illness, ranging from self-limiting watery diarrhea to febrile bloody diarrhea with abdominal pain.[29–31] Diarrhea is often preceded by a prodromal febrile period accompanied by nausea, malaise, headache, myalgia, backache, and abdominal pain. After a day or so, the pain becomes colicky and diarrhea begins. Fresh blood and/or mucus is seen in some instances, but microscopic examination demonstrates the presence of erythrocytes in most patients, along with many inflammatory cells. The fever is often short-lived, and the

**Table 27-3. Clinical Manifestations of Different *Salmonella* Serovars**

| Species | Host range (preference) | Clinical syndrome: Acute gastroenteritis | Enteric fever | Septicemia | Focal invasive infections |
|---|---|---|---|---|---|
| *S choleraesuis* | Narrow (swine) | 0 | 0 | + + + + | + + |
| *S. typhi* | Narrow (humans) | 0 | + + + + | + + + +* | + +† |
| *S. enteritidis* serovar: | | | | | |
| *typhimurium* | Broad‡ | + + + | ± | + | + |
| *enteritidis* | Broad | + + + + | 0 | 0 | 0 |
| *pullorum* | Narrow (chickens) | 0 | 0 | 0 | 0 |
| *paratyphi* A | Narrow (humans) | 0 | + + | + + + +* | +† |
| *paratyphi* B | Narrow (humans) | 0 | + + | + + + +* | +† |
| *paratyphi* C | Narrow (humans) | 0 | + + | + + + +* | +† |

*Bacteremia occurs as part of the enteric fever syndrome.
†Invasion of gallbladder and Peyer's patches occur as part of the enteric fever syndrome.
‡Most gastroenteritis strains are typically non-host-adapted with a broad range of host preference.

acute diarrhea usually subsides in 2 to 3 days. In perhaps 10 percent of patients, the abdominal pain and tenderness may persist, or recurrent fever or diarrhea may occur. In some patients the intensity of the abdominal pain and tenderness, accompanied by bloody diarrhea, leukocytosis with a left shift, and an elevated erythrocyte sedimentation rate, may lead to the diagnosis of an acute surgical abdomen. While appendicitis may indeed be found at laparotomy, more often only diffuse bowel inflammation and mesenteric adenitis are found. Sigmoidoscopy in some patients has revealed erythema, edema, granularity, exudation, and focal contact bleeding of colonic mucosa. Histologic examination is consistent with an acute colitis,[32] and toxic dilation has been reported in such patients.[33]

Clinical disease due to CLOs is similar to *C. jejuni*, including diarrhea, abdominal cramps, bloody stool, and even tenesmus. Proctocolitis is present when patients are examined by endoscopy, with anal discharge, pain, and fever as clinical features, and inflammation present by proctosigmoidoscopy and by histological examination of rectal biopsies. Mucosal friability, ulcers, crypt abscesses, and inflammation of the lamina propria are all present, and are similar to findings in other bacterial inflammatory bowel diseases, such as shigellosis. It is now also known that these organisms can be systemically invasive in homosexual men, and they may be isolated from blood and be associated with systemic symptoms including fever, chills, and arthralgias.[34] Presumptive diagnosis can be made by dark field examination of stool for organisms with a characteristic darting spiral-like motility typical of the Campylobacters. A recent report describes recovery of another thermophilic species, *C. hyointestinalis*, previously believed to be a swine pathogen, from a male homosexual with proctitis.[35] This organism is otherwise quite similar to *C. fetus*, except that it produces $H_2S$ in triple sugar iron agar (TSI), is often pigmented, and does not grow well at 25°C. Identification is confirmed by other, more complex, laboratory tests.

### Systemic Invasion

All three of these pathogens can cause clinically severe bacteremia[36–39] or persistent enteric infection[38,40,41] in patients with acquired immunodeficiency syndrome (AIDS). Five patients with *Shigella* sepsis have been reported in AIDS patients, and as might be expected, all were due to *S. flexneri*.[36] Eight AIDS patients were seen in one institution over 28 months with recurrent *Salmonella typhimurium* septicemia, and in 5 patients, the infection occurred prior to the confirmed diagnosis of AIDS.[37] *S. typhimurium* sepsis occurred in two-thirds of patients with salmonellosis among 71 AIDS patients in another series.[38] Recurrent salmonellosis developed in 2 patients, even though appropriate antibiotics were given. In San Francisco, 14 percent of *Salmonella* infections occurring in men during the period of January 1982 to June 1986 were in AIDS patients.[42] An incidence of 384/100,000 male AIDS patients was calculated. Using data in the literature, a similar rate of 46/100,000 AIDS patients in the United States has been derived.[43] These rates of *Salmonella* sepsis in AIDS are to be compared with an estimated 0.3/100,000 in the general population. However, gastrointestinal symptoms are present in less than half of AIDS patients with Salmonellosis compared with over 90 percent of the general population. A multiply resistant *C. jejuni* caused a 7-month chronic diarrhea in another AIDS patient,[41] and 4 patients in another series[40] had recurrent infection with the same strain of *C. jejuni*, as determined by the identical biochemical and serological characteristics of the isolates.

## GROWTH, PHYSIOLOGY, AND CULTURE

### *SHIGELLA*

The genus *Shigella* belongs to the tribe Eschericheae in the family Enterobacteriaceae and is closely related to *Escherichia coli*. Unlike *E. coli*, they do not ferment lactose, although *S. sonnei* is able to do so slowly, and the organisms are nonmotile. Surprisingly for the potent illness they cause, shigellae are not the most hardy of bacteria; they do not survive well in high atmospheric temperatures, are subject to desiccation, may be overgrown by the acid-producing fecal flora, and quickly and quietly die in acidic stools.

Routine isolation and identification of *Shigella* in feces involves first using selective media and then using biochemical and serological agglutination reactions to confirm identity. Selective media are employed with two purposes in mind: (1) to suppress the growth of components of the normal fecal flora that might otherwise overgrow the pathogen, and (2) to detect fermentation of lactose by a color reaction. A variety of media have been developed for this purpose, such as MacConkey's bile salt, xylose-lysine-deoxycholate (XLD), Hektoen enteric (HE), and tergitol-7-triphenyltetrazolium chloride (T7T) agars. The yield of positives is enhanced by using several selective media and by preliminary enrichment incubation in broth inhibitory to nonpathogens, such as Hajna's gram-negative (GN) broth. Stool samples that cannot be rapidly processed should be inoculated to holding medium, such as buffered glycerol-saline transport medium.

Lactose-negative colonies are screened for their ability to ferment glucose (shigellae are positive) and produce gas (nearly all shigellae are negative). Triple sugar iron (TSI) agar slants are frequently used for this purpose. Glucose fermentation in the butt produces acid which turns the indicator yellow, while the slant remains red (alkaline) because the organism cannot aerobically metabolize lactose or sucrose. The medium also detects $H_2S$ production as a black reaction product (ferrous sulfide), usually positive in the salmonellae (which also produce an acid butt-alkaline slant) but negative in the shigellae. The presumptive diagnosis is supported by negative motility and using antisera to the group antigens of *S. dysenteriae* (A), *S. flexneri* (B), *S. boydii* (C), or *S. sonnei* (D). Further biochemical identification is unnecessary for routine purposes.

### *SALMONELLA*

The genus *Salmonella* is classified in the tribe Salmonelleae, as part of the family Enterobacteriaceae. Like shigellae, salmonellae ferment glucose but not lactose or sucrose, and they are facultatively anaerobic. Unlike shigellae, salmonellae are invariably motile and almost always $H_2S$-positive. The strategy to isolate *Salmonella* is similar to that adopted for *Shigella;* indeed the salmonellae grow well on minimally selective media (such as MacConkey's), moderately selective media (including XLD, HE, and SS), and even on highly selective media (such as bismuth sulfite). The latter is therefore the most effective selective medium for the isolation of *Salmonella,* including *S. typhi.* Tetrathionate and selenite-F broth enrichment media are also satisfactory for salmonellae but are inhibitory to many shigellae.

Classification of a *Salmonella* isolate into the three species is simple. *Salmonella typhi* is readily identified because it gives a characteristic alkaline slant-acid butt TSI pattern with no gas produced and just a trace of $H_2S$. Confirmation is obtained by negative citrate (Simmons' citrate agar) and ornithine decarboxylase reactions, and by serological means. All of the nearly 2000 members of the species *S. enteritidis* are distinguished by a combination of biochemical reactions and serological tests for capsular (K), somatic (O), and flagellar (H) antigens. For convenience, these serovars will subsequently be referred to by the serotype designation alone. Individual salmonellae possess multiple O and H antigens which result in agglutination reactions with specific antisera. Serogroups (designated by capital letters A, B, C, etc.) are established on the basis of the presence of certain major O antigens. Of the salmonellae, *S. typhi* and *S. paratyphi* C alone possess an important capsular or envelope antigen named *Vi*. Because of shared group antigens, many organisms will be classified together in each major O serogroup. These can be distinguished by the pattern of H antigens present. To accomplish this, organisms are grown in broth culture to increase motility and develop flagellar antigens. A panel of H-specific antibodies is used to determine which immobilize the isolate because it posesses that H antigen.

It is not a simple task to identify the majority of the individual members of the species *S. enteritidis;* a large battery of typing sera must be maintained for this purpose. Fortunately, the majority of infections are caused by only a few serotypes, and procedures using a small number of individual and pooled typing sera can be tailored to these possibilities. Identification of rare isolates is of particular value for surveillance and epidemiological studies; reference public health laboratories can be used for this purpose. Isolation of rare or exotic serotypes is thus of epidemiological importance, but the diseases they cause are undistinguishable on clinical grounds.

## *CAMPYLOBACTER*

The genus *Campylobacter* (from the Greek *campylo,* "curved," and *bacter,* "rod") is composed of highly motile, oxidase-positive, curved gram-negative rods. Originally classified as *Vibrio* because of these properties, *Campylobacter* are microaerophilic and nonfermentative and have a distinctive DNA composition. *Campylobacter* grow optimally in 5 to 6% $O_2$, grow poorly in air or under anaerobic conditions, and require $CO_2$. Use of antibiotic selective media is critical for isolation of Campylobacters, whereas the growth of CLOs depends on the use of cephalothin-free media since these organisms are quite sensitive to this antibiotic. However, screening all stool samples sent to the routine clinical microbiology laboratory for invasive enteric pathogens is not very cost-effective. At the University of Virginia, the cost per positive culture (including 40 percent with *Shigella* or *Salmonella,* and 60 percent with *Campylobacter*) was over \$250.[44] When cultures were performed only on stools with fecal leukocytes, the cost per positive was reduced to \$30, and 75 percent of the samples yielded a pathogen. Addition of patient-selection criteria should also be useful. Thus, male homosexuals who present with proctitis should have stool cultures looking for *Campylobacter* species, especially CLOs. A wet mount of fresh stool examined by phase contrast microscopy may also reveal to the trained eye the characteristic darting, corkscrew motility of the organism.

Once isolated, the classification of the different *Campylobacter* species in the clinical laboratory relies on a few simple procedures, including growth characteristics at 25, 37, and 42°C, hippurate hydrolysis, nitrate reduction, $H_2S$ production, and susceptibility to naladixic acid and cephalothin (Table 27-1). However, there may be some confusion because test results can be variable, as they may depend on consistency of performance; for example, steady incubator temperature for temperature tolerance tests or use of fresh reagents for $H_2S$ production. Unusual or uncertain isolates, including CLOs and in particular *C. hyointestinalis,* should be sent to a reference laboratory for confirmation.

## PATHOGENESIS

All of the organisms under consideration here share a basic virulence trait that influences the kind of disease they produce, namely, the ability to penetrate intestinal epithelial cells and cause tissue pathology.[45] In no instance, however, is this invasion mechanism fully understood. Differences in the site of and response to invasion among the pathogens also point out the likelihood of major biological differences among them. Invasion properties are clearly related to the small infectious dose of these organisms that is required in humans, and they are therefore a crucial factor in the direct sexual transmission of infection. In addition, various types of enterotoxins have been described in the three organisms.

## *SHIGELLA*

Invasion mechanisms are best understood for *Shigella.*[46,47] It is of obvious benefit for the survival of the organism to reach an intracellular locus where they are protected from various host defenses such as antibody, complement, or phagocytic cells. It is also this property which presumably permits establishment of infection with as few as 10 viable *S. dysenteriae* 1 by mouth.[48] This tiny dose is the most important factor favoring contact spread from host to host without the need for enrichment in food or water.

Invasion of cells and survival of shigellae within the cytoplasm is controlled by both chromosomal and plasmid genes.[46,47] At least three regions of the chromosome are involved, the rhamnose, histidine, and purine E loci. If *E. coli–Shigella* hybrids are created by insertion of *E. coli* DNA from these regions into *Shigella,* the hybrids are found to invade intestinal epithelial cells but neither multiply nor survive, and they cause no symptoms. Transfer of the same loci in the other direction from virulent *Shigella* to avirulent *E. coli* K12 does not result in invasive or virulent transconjugants either. Additional factors are needed, and these have now been found to be controlled by genes present on large (120 to 140 megadaltons) plasmids.[46,47] Several of the critical genes are present within a cloned 22-megadalton fragment of the large *S. flexneri* invasion plasmid. One, the *ipa* gene (for invasion plasmid antigen), controls several outer membrane polypeptides expressed on the bacterial surface in a strategic location to serve in recognition of attachment sites on gut cells. The other gene is called *inv* (for the invasion gene), which may function in the insertion of ipa gene products into the cell membrane, allowing the internalization process to proceed.

There are also other putative virulence-associated genes on the same large plasmid, including vir F (known to control binding of the dye Congo red dye, which is a marker of surface charge) and vir G (which codes for a hemolysin that probably functions in escape of the organism from endocytic vesicles to the cytoplasm).

A second virulence trait is the protein Shiga toxin, so named because it was first described in *S. dysenteriae* 1 (Shiga's bacillus). Identical or very similar toxins are produced by other *Shigella* species as well. This toxin binds to a specific intestinal cell membrane glycolipid,[49] as demonstrated in the rabbit intestine where it is present specifically on the villus cell.[50] Its action to inhibit cellular protein synthesis results in functional impairment of the villus cell and a decrease in the absorptive capacity for sodium and chloride without change in anion secretion by the crypt cell. The decrease in NaCl absorption and unopposed anion secretion is sufficient to result in net accumulation of fluid in the bowel lumen. The role of the toxin in the dysentery phase of shigellosis is uncertain but may explain intestinal epithelial cell pathology in dysentery, since it is cytotoxic to the colonic cell.[51,52] The mechanism of action, inhibition of protein synthesis, is identical to that of the toxic plant lectin, ricin. Both molecules are N-glycosidases, specifically hydrolyzing adenine residue 4324 in the 28S rRNA of the 60S ribosomal subunit.[53] This action irreversibly inactivates the ribosome and inhibits protein synthesis.

## *SALMONELLA*

*Salmonella* are systemically invasive, resulting in positive blood cultures early in the course of gastroenteritis.[12,26] The minimum oral infectious dose of gastroenteritis strains of *Salmonella* in normal adult volunteers is around $10^5$ organisms. Studies in experimental animals, summarized by Turnbull,[12] indicate that the ileum is the major site of infection; cecal and colonic lesions occur as well, but less commonly. The invasion process has been studied by Takeuchi, using *S. typhimurium* in a guinea pig model.[54] When the organisms closely approach the epithelial cell brush border (<35 nm), microvilli appear to melt away and the organism enters the cell in a membrane-bound vesicle. Turnbull and Richmond[55] have also shown invasion by *S. enteritidis* into cecal epithelial cells in the 1-day-old chick, also within vesicles. In both models organisms penetrate into the lamina propria, from which they presumably enter the bloodstream to produce early bacteremia. Giannella et al. have shown that, whereas invasion is necessary for virulence, it is not sufficient to evoke a secretory process; the organism must also induce a local polymorphonuclear leukocyte inflammatory response.[56] Pretreatment with nitrogen mustard to deplete leukocytes blunts the secretory response.[57] In spite of the inflammation, the permeability barrier function of the gut is maintained; neither $^{51}$Cr-tagged albumin nor $^{14}$C-tagged mannitol appear in the gut lumen in infected rhesus monkeys or in the rabbit ileal loop model.[58] Not all inflammation-provoking strains cause secretion, however. This observation suggests the possibility of enterotoxin activity as well,[59] but this remains an unproven hypothesis in spite of considerable investigation. Both cholera-like secretory toxins and Shiga-like cytotoxins have been described.[60,61]

## *CAMPYLOBACTER*

The oral infectious dose of *Campylobacter* for humans is variable, and in some individuals as few as 500 organisms will suffice.[17] Evidence that the organism is invasive includes the pathology of the gut, the bloody inflammatory exudate present in stool, and the frequency of positive blood cultures.[29,62] Experimental studies in primary 10-day-old chicken embryo cell cultures, and in 3- to 8-day-old chicks have provided direct evidence of this.[29,63] Chick embryo cells are heavily invaded within 24 h after exposure to $10^8$ bacteria. Organisms are present within vesicles in the cytoplasm, and as the bacteria multiply, the host cells show degenerative changes and die by 36 h. In the intact chicks, *Campylobacter* are recovered from small bowel and cecum, are present within epithelial cells, and are found in blood and liver in one-fourth to one-third of the animals. The younger birds also develop bloody diarrhea.[63]

Increasing evidence shows that *Campylobacter* strains causing watery diarrhea produce enterotoxins resembling cholera toxin.[17] These toxins are reported to be similar to cholera toxin in molecular weight (60 to 70 kilodaltons), in binding to Gml ganglioside and causing elongation of CHO cells, in being neutralized by anticholera toxin antibody, in possessing a similar B subunit and resulting in fluid secretion in appropriate animal models. Guerrant et al. have recently described a different kind of toxin in polymyxin-B extracts of bacterial suspensions from 5/12 strains of *C. jejuni*.[64] They found a Shiga-like toxin *Campylobacter* cytotoxin, which, similar to the *Salmonella* toxin, was not neutralized by Shiga toxin antibody. Whether or not these toxins exert similar actions on gut epithelial cell function as Shiga toxin when released intracellularly by invading organisms is not known at this time.

## IMMUNE RESPONSE

Shigella infections lead to production of serum antibodies against somatic O antigens of the organism and to production of neutralizing antibody to the cytotoxin.[24] The relationship of these antibodies to protection against disease is not clear. Parenteral immunization with killed bacteria or formalin toxoid preparations in humans or simian hosts, respectively, which stimulate serum antibodies, do not protect against oral bacterial challenge.[45–47]

The efficacy of oral live vaccines prepared from noninvasive *Shigella* strains, nonmultiplying streptomycin-dependent mutants, or *Shigella–E. coli* hybrids indicates the presence of important immune host defenses at the mucosal surface.[65] The protection induced is strain-specific;[65] however, neither the antigens involved nor the nature of the immune response is known. Insertion of *Shigella* somatic antigens by genetic manipulation onto the surface of colonizing *E. coli* does not lead to a protective response.

Little is known of the immune response to salmonella gastroenteritis.[66] Perhaps investigative enthusiasm has been diminished by the realization that there are so many diverse antigenic determinants among the large number of potential pathogens; little hope exists for finding a simple polyvalent vaccine. Nevertheless, a live attenuated mutant *S. typhimurium*, which synthesizes an incomplete O antigen because it lacks the enzyme uridine diphosphogalactose-4-epimerase, has produced excellent protection in 1-day-old chicks challenged 2 weeks later.[67]

There also is a paucity of information on the immune response to *C. jejuni* because the organism is so new to the list of significant enteric pathogens. Patients with *Campylobacter* gastroenteritis do develop serum antibodies detectable by either a serum bactericidal assay or an indirect immunofluorescence technique employing autologous isolates as the antigen.[29,30] Low titers have been found in control sera, suggesting either prior infection with *C. jejuni* or cross-reaction with other bacterial antigens, and the specificity is not yet known. Antitoxin antibodies have also been reported.[68]

## GENETICS AND ANTIMICROBIAL SUSCEPTIBILITY

### *SHIGELLA*

Observations in Japan during the 1950s on antibiotic susceptibility of clinical isolates of *Shigella* have had a major impact on our understanding of the biology of microorganisms in the environment. Whereas *Shigella* were highly susceptible to sulfonamides (Su) in the mid-1940s in Japan, by 1952 over 80 percent had become resistant. As newer antibiotics were introduced into clinical use, strains resistant to tetracycline (TC), chloramphenicol (CM), or streptomycin (SM) also emerged. In 1956 and 1957 an explosive increase in strains resistant to all four drugs was noted. It was also observed that such multiply resistant strains might occur during therapy of an initially sensitive isolate during the course of treatment with one drug alone. Since this is clearly unlikely on a mutation-selection basis, it was suggested that drug resistance might be transferred from a resident *E. coli* strain to the invading pathogen. When this was independently demonstrated in 1959 by Akiba et al. and by Ochiai et al.,[69,70] the field of plasmid biology was born, for the genetic information was found to be contained on a transferable extrachromosomal circular DNA called an *R factor*. Spread of R factors among the Enterobacteriaceae, aided by the selective pressures of antibiotic usage, has occurred since that time. This spread accounts for the increasing difficulty in selecting antimicrobial therapy for many of these organisms. Genetic information for virulence factors may also be on plasmid DNA, often in transposons that can jump from plasmid to plasmid or from plasmid to chromosome.[71] Spread of R factors containing such transposons can simultaneously transfer virulence and antibiotic resistance.

Within the genus *Shigella*, the majority of strains of *S. sonnei*, the epidemic strains of *S. dysenteriae* type 1 from Mexico, Central America, and Bangladesh, and many isolates of *S. flexneri* are resistant to one or more antibiotics, usually including TC, CM, SM, and Su.[72] Ampicillin (AM) and trimethoprin-sulfamethoxazole (TMP-SMX) resistance has been variable, increasing in many geographic areas as the drugs have been extensively used, but also for unknown reasons diminishing in prevalence in some places as well. This makes it mandatory to continuously monitor antimicrobial susceptibility of *Shigella* in each locale so that appropriate therapy can be selected. The Mexico–Central America pandemic strain of the period 1969–1971 had R factors that mediated resistance to CM, TC, SM, and Su. These R factors were 80 megadaltons in size, were of the O compatibility group, were $fi^-$ phenotype, and transferred identical levels of antibiotic resistance to *E. coli* K12. The R factor from the epidemic of *S. dysenteriae* type 1 in Bangladesh was identical in resistance markers but associated with either a 62- or 52-megadalton band on gels. Current strains in Africa, India, and Bangladesh are also AM and TMP-SMX resistant, and it has been necessary to resort to naladixic acid as the drug of choice in this setting.[72] Naladixic acid resistance has been found, however, leaving few choices.[73,74] The new 4-quinolones are a good choice at this time, although their safety in children less than 17 years of age is not certain.[75,76]

### *SALMONELLA*

Salmonella gastroenteritis is self-limiting and, because antimicrobials previously available do not shorten the clinical illness[77,78] and actually prolong the period of convalescent carriage, most experts have considered their use to be contraindicated except in patients with systemic invasion and focal infections. The advent of quinolones has once again raised the possibility of effective therapy for this group of organisms.[79,80]

The resistance patterns of *S. typhimurium* are more complex than those of *S. typhi*, but the former can harbor the same plasmids found in *S. typhi*, including a 135-megadalton R factor mediating resistance to CM, TC, SM, and Su, and the TnA transposon.[81] *Salmonella typhimurium*, the most common salmonella isolated from infected humans, thus could serve as a reservoir for R plasmids in the genus. Other multiply resistant serotypes have emerged from time to time as the cause of miniepidemics.[82,83] Continued surveillance for salmonellae is thus mandatory in order to guide initial antibiotic choices in each locale.

### *CAMPYLOBACTER*

Little is known about plasmid-mediated antimicrobial resistance in *C. jejuni*. TC-resistant strains occur in which both intraspecies and interspecies transfer (to *C. fetus* ssp. *fetus*) has been documented, but not to *E. coli*.[84] *Campylobacter jejuni* is not very susceptible to penicillins, trimethoprim, or trimethoprim-sulfamethoxazole.[85,86] Over 90 percent of strains are highly sensitive to erythromycin or clindamycin, while nearly all strains are susceptible to low concentrations of chloramphenicol, gentamicin, or furazolidone.

## PREVENTION

In principle, it seems rather straightforward to supply clean water, to preclude bacterial contamination and growth of microorganisms in food by employing appropriate food-handling techniques from farm to kitchen, to encourage personal hygiene to minimize person-to-vehicle or person-to-person spread (including direct transmission related to sexual activity), and to dispose of feces and sewage in a sanitary fashion. In practice, none of these measures is simple to institute. Were this the case, surveillance and containment of cases and carriers due to highly host-adapted species theoretically could lead to eradication of the agent in the population.

In the case of *Shigella*, killed vaccines administered parenterally do not work.[48] Nor has there been any remarkable success with presentation of killed antigens to the gut surface. Rather, live oral vaccines thus far appear to be the best approach. Several principles have been employed in constructing vaccine strains, largely through the work of Formal and colleagues. Because invasion is of paramount importance to the pathogenesis of disease[45] noninvasive bacterial variants have been selected for use. Should penetration occur, a second level of attenuation has been added by constructing *Shigella–E. coli* hybrids to impair the ability of shigellae to survive.[46] These hybrid organisms penetrate the gut cell but they are rapidly cleared, and the hybrid organism is avirulent. A third level of attenuation can be included by employing SM-dependent mutants that fail to grow in the absence of added antibiotic. A noninvasive variant of an SM-dependent *Shigella–E. coli* hybrid would then represent a triple attenuation. Various attenuated strains have in fact been proved to induce protective immunity in humans,[87] although in no instance has an effective, stable, nonreverting strain free of side effects become available.[88]

A recent approach has been to move the genes for important *Shigella* surface antigens into an avirulent *E. coli* which will colonize the intestine; however, the initial studies have demonstrated a failure to induce protective immunity.[45,46] Attempts are now being made to employ the gal-E mutant of *S. typhi* as a carrier cell for the plasmid-determined form I antigen of *S. sonnei*. For the *S. typhimurium*, use of gal-E mutant live oral vaccines appears promising in experimental animals.[67]

A second concept is to employ ecological approaches to prevent colonization by the invading pathogen. The normal flora is protective against both *Shigella* and *Salmonella enteritidis*, particularly the exclusive *Bifidobacterium* flora of the breast-fed infant, and components of the flora of the older individual that produce low pH, high Eh (oxidation-reduction potential), and volatile fatty acids in the colon.[89,90] Successful colonization of hosts with a stable, interfering flora has not been achieved, however.

Several modes for interruption of pathogenesis appear feasible from a theoretical point of view.[91] By inhibiting the receptor-mediated cell-cell or cell-toxin contacts that initiate the disease process, symptoms might be prevented even though infection per se is not. Receptor competition therapy, blockade, or modulation or reversal of binding interactions using soluble carbohydrate haptens or hydrophobic affinity gels has been proposed.[91] Pharmacologic agents have also been proposed as a means of inhibiting the biochemical mechanisms or inflammatory response involved in disease production.[92] However, it will be necessary to ensure that such treatment will do no harm on a long-term basis, regardless of short-term effectiveness.

Although there are no solutions at present, we have at least begun to develop new approaches to the invasive diarrheas.

## References


1 Deuteronomy 23:12–13.

2 Keusch GT: Shigellosis, in *Bacterial Infections of Humans: Epidemiology and Control*, AS Evans, H Feldman (eds). New York, Plenum, 1982, p 487.

3 Levine MM et al: Pathogenesis of *Shigella dysenteriae* 1 (Shiga) dysentery. *J Infect Dis* 127:261, 1973.

4 Dritz SK, Back AF: *Shigella* enteritis venereally transmitted. *N Engl J Med* 291:1194, 1974.

5 Dritz SK et al: Patterns of sexually transmitted enteric diseases in a city. *Lancet* 2:3, 1977.

6 Bader M et al: Venereal transmission of shigellosis in Seattle-King County. *Sex Transm Dis* 4:89, 1977.

7 Drusin LM et al: Shigellosis: Another sexually transmitted disease? *Br J Vener Dis* 52:348, 1976.

8 Tauxe RV: The persistence of *Shigella flexneri* in the United States: The increased role of the adult male. *Am J Public Health* (In press).

9 Quinn TC: Clinical approach to intestinal infections in homosexual men. *Med Clin North Am* 70:611, 1986.

10 Speelman P et al: Distribution and spread of colonic lesions in shigellosis: A colonoscopic study. *J Infect Dis* 150:899, 1984.

11 Department of Public Health, City and County of San Francisco: Shigellosis in San Francisco, 1977–1985. *San Francisco Epidemiological Bull* 2:1, 1986.

12 Turnbull PCB: Food poisoning with special reference to salmonella: Its epidemiology, pathogenesis and control. *Clin Gastroenterol* 8:663, 1979.

13 St Louis ME et al: The emergence of grade A eggs as a major source of *Salmonella enteritidis* infections. New implications for the control of salmonellosis. *JAMA* 259:2103, 1988.

14 King EO: Human infections with *Vibrio fetus* and a closely related vibrio. *J Infect Dis* 101:119, 1957.

15 Blaser MJ et al: *Campylobacter* enteritis in the United States. *Ann Intern Med* 98:360, 1983.

16 Tauxe RV et al: Illness associated with *Campylobacter laridis*, a newly recognized *Campylobacter* species. *J Clin Microbiol* 21:222, 1985.

17 Walker RI et al: Pathophysiology of *Campylobacter* enteritis. *Microbiol Rev* 50:81, 1986.

18 Quinn TC et al: Infections with *Campylobacter jejuni* and *Campylobacter*-like organisms in homosexual men. *Ann Intern Med* 101:187, 1984.

19 Fennell CL et al: Characterization of *Campylobacter*-like organisms isolated from homosexual men. *J Infect Dis* 149:58, 1985.

20 Totten PA et al: *Campylobacter cinaedi* (sp. nov.) and *Campylobacter fenneliae* (sp. nov.): Two new *Campylobacter* species associated with enteric disease in homosexual men. *J Infect Dis* 151:131, 1985.

21 Warren JR, Marshall BJL: Unidentified curved bacilli on gastric epithelium in active chronic gastritis. *Lancet* i:1273, 1983.

22 Siegel D et al: Predictive value of stool examination in acute diarrhea. *Arch Pathol Lab Med* 111:715, 1987.

23 Quinn TC et al: The polymicrobial origin of intestinal infections in homosexual men. *N Engl J Med* 309:576, 1983.

24 Keusch GT: Shigella infections. *Clin Gastroenterol* 8:645, 1979.

25 Stoll DM: Cutaneous shigellosis. *Arch Dermatol* 122:22, 1986.

26 Rubin RH, Weinstein L: *Salmonellosis: Microbiologic, Pathologic, and Clinical Features*. New York, Stratton Intercontinental Medical Book Corp, 1977.

27 Mandal BK, Mani V: Colonic involvement in salmonellosis. *Lancet* 1:884, 1976.

28 Schofield PF et al: Toxic dilation of the colon in salmonella colitis and inflammatory bowel disease. *Br J Surg* 66:5, 1979.

29 Butzler JP, Skirrow MB: *Campylobacter* enteritis. *Clin Gastroenterol* 8:737, 1979.

30 Blazer MJ et al: *Campylobacter* enteritis: Clinical and epidemiologic features. *Ann Intern Med* 91:179, 1979.

31 Karmali MA, Fleming PC: *Campylobacter* enteritis in children. *J Pediatr* 94:527, 1979.

32 Lambert ME et al: *Campylobacter* colitis. *Br J Med* 1:857, 1979.

33 Pockros PJ et al: Toxic megacolon complicating *Campylobacter* enterocolitis. *J Clin Gastroenterol* 3:318, 1986.

34 Quinn TC et al: New developments in infectious diarrhea. *Disease-A-Month* 32:174, 1986.

35 Fennell CL et al: Isolation of "*Campylobacter hyointestinalis*" from a human. *J Clin Microbiol* 24:146, 1986.

36 Baskin DH et al: *Shigella* bacteremia in patients with the acquired immune deficiency syndrome. *Am J Gastoenterol* 82:338, 1987.

37 Glaser JB et al: Recurrent *Salmonella typhimurium* bacteremia associated with the acquired immunodeficiency syndrome. *Ann Intern Med* 102:189, 1985.

38 Smith PD et al: *Salmonella typhimurium* enteritis and bacteremia in the acquired immunodeficiency syndrome. *Ann Intern Med* 102:207, 1985.

39 Pasternak J et al: Bacteremia caused by *Campylobacter*-like organism in two male homosexuals. *Ann Intern Med* 101:339, 1984.

40 Perlman D et al: Persistent *Campylobacter jejuni* infections in patients infected with the human immunodeficiency virus (HIV). *Ann Intern Med* 108:540, 1988.

41 Dworkin B et al: Persistence of multiply antibiotic-resistant *Campylobacter jejuni* in a patient with acquired immune deficiency syndrome. *Am J Med* 80:965, 1986.

42 Celum CL et al: Incidence of salmonellosis in patients with AIDS. *J Infect Dis* 156:998, 1987.

43 Sperber SJ, Schleupner CJ: Salmonellosis during infection with human immunodeficiency virus. *Rev Infect Dis* 9:925, 1987.

44 Guerrant RL et al: Evaluation and diagnosis of acute infectious diarrhea. *Am J Med* 78 (suppl 6B):91, 1985.

45 Formal SB et al: Invasive enteric pathogens. *Rev Infect Dis* 5:S702, 1983.

46 Kopecko DJ et al: Genetic determinants of virulence in *Shigella* and dysenteric strains of *Escherichia coli:* Their involvement in the pathogenesis of dysentery. *Curr Top Microbiol Immunol* 118:71, 1985.

47 Hale TL, Formal SB: Pathogenesis of *Shigella* infections. *Pathol Immunopathol Res* 6:117, 1987.

48 Levine MM et al: Pathogenesis of *Shigella dysenteriae* (Shiga) dysentery. *J Infect Dis* 127:261, 1973.

49 Jacewicz M et al: Isolation of a shigella toxin binding glycolipid from rabbit jejunum and HeLa cells and its identification as globotriaosylceramide. *J Exp Med* 163:1391, 1986.

50 Kandel G et al: Shigella toxin selectively targets villus but not crypt cells in rabbit jejunum, providing an explanation for its enterotoxic activity. *Gastroenterology* 92:1459, 1987.

51 Keenan KP et al: Morphologic evaluation of the effects of Shiga toxin and *E. coli* Shiga-like toxin on the rabbit intestine. *Am J Pathol* 125:69, 1986.

52 Moyer MP et al: Cytotoxicity of Shiga toxin for primary cultures of human colonic and ileal epithelial cells. *Infect Immun* 55:1533, 1987.

53 Endo Y et al: Site of action of a Vero toxin (VT2) from *Escherichia coli* 0157:H7 and of Shiga toxin on eukaryotic ribosomes. RNA N-glycosidase activity of the toxins. *Eur J Biochem* 171:45, 1988.

54 Takeuchi A: Electron microscope studies of experimental salmonella infection: I. Penetration into the intestinal epithelium by *Salmonella typhimurium. Am J Pathol* 50:109, 1967.

55 Turnbull PCB, Richmond JE: A model of salmonella enteritis: The behavior of *Salmonella enteritidis* in chick intestine studied by light and electron microscopy. *Br J Exp Pathol* 59:64, 1978.

56 Giannella RA et al: Pathogenesis of salmonellosis: Studies of fluid secretion, mucosal invasion, and morphologic reaction in the rabbit ileum. *J Clin Invest* 52:441, 1973.

57 Giannella RA: Importance of the intestinal inflammatory reaction in salmonella mediated intestinal secretion. *Infect Immun* 23:140, 1979.

58 Giannella RA et al: Role of plasma filtration in the intestinal fluid secretion mediated by infection with *Salmonella typhimurium. Infect Immun* 13:470, 1976.

59 Peterson JW: *Salmonella* toxins, in *Pharmacology of Bacterial Toxins,* F Dorner, J Drews (eds). Oxford, Pergamon, 1986, pp 227–234.

60 Wallis TS et al: Enterotoxin production by *Salmonella typhimurium* strains of different virulence. *J Med Microbiol* 21:19, 1986.

61 Panigrahi D et al: Evaluation of immuno-dot-blot assay for detection of cholera-related enterotoxin antigen in *Salmonella typhimurium. J Clin Microbiol* 25:702, 1987.

62 Blaser MJ et al: Acute colitis caused by *Campylobacter fetus* ss *jejuni. Gastroenterology* 78:448, 1980.

63 Ruiz-Palacios GM et al: Experimental *Campylobacter* diarrhea in chickens. *Infect Immun* 34:250, 1981.

64 Guerrant RL et al: Production of a unique cytotoxin by *Campylobacter jejuni. Infect Immun* 55:2526, 1987.

65 Levine MM et al: New knowledge on pathogenesis of bacterial enteric infection as applied to vaccine development. *Microbiol Rev* 47:510, 1983.

66 Stephen J et al: Salmonellosis: In retrospect and prospect. *CIBA Found Symp* 112:175, 1985.

67 Pritchard DG et al: Effects of Gal-E-mutant of *Salmonella typhimurium* on experimental salmonellosis in chickens. *Avian Dis* 22:562, 1978.

68 Ruiz-Palacios GM et al: Serum antibodies to heat-labile enterotoxin of *Campylobacter jejuni. J Infect Dis* 152:413, 1985.

69 Akiba T et al: On the mechanism of development of multiple drug resistant clones of *Shigella. Jpn J Microbiol* 4:219, 1960.

70 Ochiai K et al: Inheritance of drug resistance (and its transfer) between *Shigella* strains and between *Shigella* and *E. coli* strains. *Nihon Iji Shimpo* 34:1861, 1959.

71 So M et al: The *E. coli* gene encoding heat stable toxin is a bacterial transposon flanked by inverted repeats of IS 1. *Nature* 277:453, 1979.

72 Salam MA, Bennish M: Therapy of shigellosis. 1. Randomized, double blind trial of naladixic acid in childhood shigellosis. *J Pediatr* (in press).

73 Keusch GT, Bennish M: Shigellosis, in *Bacterial Infections of Humans, Epidemiology and Control,* 2nd Ed, AS Evans, P Brachman (eds). New York, Plenum, in press.

74 Panhotra BR: Naladixic-acid-resistant *Shigella dysenteriae* 1. *Lancet* 1:763, 1985.

75 Rogerie F et al: Comparison of norfloxacin and naladixic acid for treatment of dysentery caused by *Shigella dysenteriae* 1 in adults. *Antimicrobial Agents Chemother* 29:883, 1986.

76 Keusch GT: Antimicrobial therapy for enteric infections and typhoid fever: State of the art. *Rev Infect Dis* 10:S199, 1988.

77 Dixon JMS: Effect of antibiotic treatment on duration of excretion of *S. typhimurium* by children. *Br Med J* 2:1343, 1965.

78 Nelson JD et al: Treatment of *Salmonella* gastroenteritis with ampicillin, amoxicillin, or placebo. *Pediatrics* 65:1125, 1980.

79 Pilcher H et al: Ciprofloxacin in the treatment of acute bacterial diarrhea: A double blind study. *Eur J Clin Microbiol* 5:241, 1986.

80 Jewes LA: Antimicrobial therapy of non-typhi salmonella and shigella infection. *J Antimicrobial Chemother* 19:557, 1987.

81 Alfaro G: Genetic stability and transfer inhibition of plasmids in strains of *Salmonella typhi. Rev Lat Am Microbiol* 20:223, 1978.

82 Lintz D et al: Nosocomial salmonella epidemic. *Arch Intern Med* 136:968, 1976.

83 McConnell MM et al: The value of plasmid studies in the epidemiology of infections due to drug-resistant *Salmonella wien. J Infect Dis* 139:178, 1979.

84 Taylor DE et al: Transmissible tetracycline resistance in *Campylobacter jejuni. Lancet* 2:797, 1980.

85 Vanhoof R et al: Susceptibility of *Campylobacter fetus* subsp *jejuni* to twenty nine antimicrobial agents. *Antimicrob Agents Chemother* 14:553, 1978.

86 Walder M: Susceptibility of *Campylobacter fetus* subsp *jejuni* to twenty antimicrobial agents. *Antimicrob Agents Chemother* 16:37, 1979.

87 Levine MM et al: Shigellosis in custodial institutions: V. Effect of intervention with streptomycin-dependent *Shigella sonnei* vaccine in an institution with endemic disease. *Am J Epidemiol* 104:88, 1976.

88 Levine MM et al: Shigellosis in custodial institutions: IV. *In vivo* stability and transmissibility of oral attenuated streptomycin-dependent shigella vaccines. *J Infect Dis* 131:704, 1975.

89 Bohnhoff M, Miller CP: Enhanced susceptibility to salmonella infection in streptomycin-treated mice. *J Infect Dis* 111:117, 1962.

90 Maier BR et al: *Shigella:* Indigenous flora interactions in mice. *Am J Clin Nutr* 25:1433, 1972.

91 Keusch GT: Specific membrane receptors: Pathogenetic and therapeutic implications in infectious diseases. *Rev Infect Dis* 1:517, 1979.

92 Field M: New strategies for treating watery diarrhea. *N Engl J Med* 297:1121, 1977.

Chapter 28

# Biology of human immunodeficiency virus and related viruses

Ashley T. Haase

*In the memories of those who lived through them, the grim days of the plague do not stand out like vivid flames, ravenous and inextinguishable, but like the slow deliberate progress of some monstrous thing crushing out all upon its path.*

Albert Camus, *The Plague,* 1947

## INTRODUCTION

This opening chapter on AIDS begins with a quotation from Camus's novel *The Plague,* which captures the somber sense of the magnitude of this plague of our times. The chapter is intended as an overview and introduction to the more detailed treatments of the epidemiology, clinical picture, and immunobiology of AIDS (Chaps. 29–32), and as a primer on the molecular biology of retroviruses, the family of viruses to which the human immunodeficiency virus (HIV) belongs.

## DEFINITIONS: VIRAL TAXONOMY AND ORIGINS

The etiologic agent of AIDS is a member of a subfamily of retroviruses called *lentiviruses* because they characteristically cause slow (Latin *lentus* = "slow") infections in which months or years separate invasion of the host from the appearance of symptoms.[1,2] By contrast, the other subfamilies of retroviruses (Table 28-1) either transform cells in culture and induce tumors in a variety of species (oncogenic retroviruses) or establish persistent and inapparent infections which in tissue culture are manifest by vacuole formation in cells (the *spuma* [Latin] of the spumavirinae refers to the "foamy" appearance of the infected cell). Lentiviruses also cause cytotoxic effects in culture, typically fusing and killing the host cell, and differ in many other respects from retroviruses in the other subfamilies. All retroviruses, however, have in common RNA genomes which are replicated via a DNA intermediate in the cell. The name *retro*virus refers to this reversed flow of genetic information catalyzed by an RNA-directed DNA polymerase, or reverse transcriptase, of the virus.

Table 28-1. Retroviridae

| Subfamily | Prototypic members |
|---|---|
| Oncovirinae | |
| *Genera:* | |
| Oncovirus C | Rous sarcoma virus |
| Oncovirus B | Mouse mammary tumor virus |
| Oncovirus D | Mason-Pfizer monkey virus |
| Lentivirinae | Visna virus |
| Spumavirinae | Foamy virus |

Table 28-2. Lentivirinae

| Virus | Host species | Disease |
|---|---|---|
| Visna | Sheep | Wasting, paralysis |
| Maedi | Sheep | Pneumonia |
| Progressive pneumonia virus | Sheep | Pneumonia |
| Zwoegerziekte | Sheep | Pneumonia |
| Caprine arthritis encephalitis virus (CAEV) | Sheep, goats | Arthritis, encephalitis |
| Equine infectious anemia virus (EIAV) | Horses | Fever, anemia |
| Bovine lentivirus | Cows | Lymphadenopathy |
| Feline lentivirus | Cats | Immunodeficiency |
| Simian immunodeficiency virus (SIV) | Monkeys | Immunodeficiency |
| Human immunodeficiency virus (HIV) | Man | Neurologic disease, immunodeficiency, wasting |

The lentiviruses are responsible for slowly evolving infections of animals (sheep, goats) which eventually result in wasting and paralytic disease (visna), pneumonia (maedi), or arthritis (caprine arthritis and encephalitis) (Table 28-2). These viruses and progressive pneumonia virus and Zwoegerziekte constituted the initial members of the subfamily of lentiviruses.[3] With the discovery of HIV as the first human lentivirus,[4,5] renewed interest has greatly expanded the subfamily to include retroviruses that cause relapsing fever and anemia in horses (equine infectious anemia virus, or EIAV[6]) and retroviruses associated with immunosuppressive diseases in cows,[7] cats,[8] and old world monkeys.[9] HIV is related by similarities in genome organization, nucleotide and amino acid sequences, and immunologic cross-reactivity to the simian viruses (Fig. 28-1), but the divergence of sequences is too extensive to support the theory that HIV arose by horizontal transmission from a primate reservoir to humans.[10,11] It is now clear that HIV is not closely related as initially thought[12] to the human T-lymphotropic viruses HTLV-I and HTLV-II (see Chap. 33), except in host range (T cells) and in properties such as transactivation.[13]

The origins of HIV and other lentiviruses are obscure, but they do not appear to have arisen from endogenous sequences embedded in the genomes of some species, probably because these viruses do not infect germ line cells. Lentiviruses are, therefore, referred to as exogenous viruses. All lentiviruses are genetically heterogeneous, with the greatest diversity in the region of the genome encoding a major glycosylated protein of the viral envelope. By three-dimensional mapping of sequence similarities, HIV isolates can be divided into two major groups, HIV-1 and HIV-2, the latter of which is most closely related to simian immunodeficiency virus (SIV).[14] HIV-1 and HIV-2 are antigenically distinct and have been reported to differ in pathogenicity as well, but it now appears that the "nonpathogenic" HIV-2 (designated HTLV-4) may have been a simian virus contaminant.[15–18]

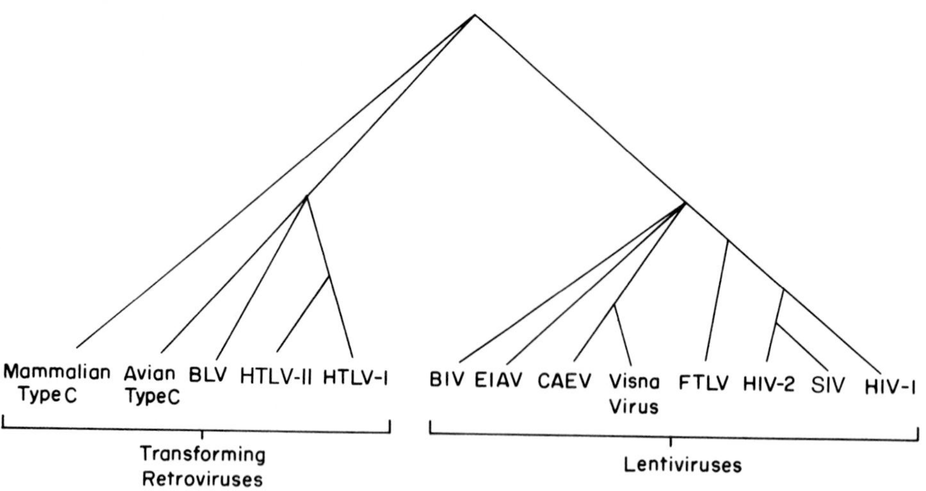


**Fig. 28-1.** Taxonomic relationships of retroviruses. Although a good approximation, these relationships remain controversial (see also Fig. 33-1). Abbreviations: BLV, bovine leukemia virus; BIV, bovine immunodeficiency virus; EIAV, equine infectious anemia virus; CAEV, caprine arthritis encephalitis virus; FTLV, feline T lymphotropic virus; SIV, simian immunodeficiency virus. (*Modified from D Ho, N Engl J Med 317:278, 1987, with permission.*)

## HISTORY

Retroviruses in general, and the lentiviruses in particular, were amongst the first viruses linked to specific diseases.[2] At the turn of the century, Valle and Carre (1904) demonstrated the transmissibility of equine infectious anemia by bacteria-free filtrates, and a few years later Ellerman and Bang (1908) and Rous (1911) showed that leukemias and fibrosarcomas in chickens are similarly transmissible. During the 1950s, as animal virology became firmly established with methods for cultivation of viruses in tissue culture, the viruses responsible for Rous sarcoma and many other kinds of cancer in a variety of species were visualized by electron microscopy. The spherical particles associated with these viruses were classified into three morphologically distinct types. Type A particles exist only within cells, whereas types B and C generally are first visible in sections of infected cells as crescentic structures which mature by budding. The extracellular particles have an electron-dense core and an envelope covered by knobs or spike-like structures. The B-type particles have long and prominent spikes and an eccentric core; type C particles have less prominent knobs protruding from the envelope and a central core; the more recently described type D particle is found both intracellularly and extracellularly and has an eccentric nucleoid and shorter spikes than B particles.

In the ensuing two decades, biochemical characterization of the retroviruses provided a detailed picture of the structure, composition, and novel mode of replication of these viruses. Certainly the highlight of this period was the provirus hypothesis[19] advanced by Howard Temin in 1963–1964 to explain the block in the replication of RNA-containing tumor viruses by drugs which act on DNA. The independent discovery by Temin and Mizutani[20] and by Baltimore[21] of an RNA-dependent DNA polymerase (reverse transcriptase) which could synthesize a DNA intermediate from RNA, overcame the widespread skepticism in the scientific community of the validity of the hypothesis and led quickly to the convincing proof by Hill and Hillova[22] that DNA from infected cells contains all the information necessary to confer on uninfected cells the ability to produce new retroviruses.

The confluence and maturation of technologies for the analysis of viruses and the cultivation of cells in culture led to the discovery of human retroviruses. In 1976, Gallo and his coworkers found that addition of conditioned medium from human embryonic cells would sustain the growth of human T lymphocytes.[23] This growth factor, interleukin-2 (IL-2), made it possible to establish long-term cultures of T cells from leukemic patients and thus provided the basis for the isolation of retroviruses[24,25] from relatively uncommon T-cell leukemias, designated human T-lymphotropic virus types I and II (HTLV-I, HTLV-II) by Gallo and coworkers, and adult T-cell leukemia (ATL) viruses by Japanese scientists.[26]

These discoveries, and increasing evidence that the newly described acquired immunodeficiency syndrome might be the result of infection of T helper cells, led Gallo to propose that a variant of HTLV-I might be the cause of AIDS.[27] In 1983, Essex et al. reported that 25 to 30 percent of AIDS patients had antibodies which cross reacted with an HTLV-I membrane antigen.[28] In retrospect, this may well have represented coinfection of individuals with both HTLV-I and HIV. The story of the actual etiologic agent of AIDS begins in 1983 with Montagnier's isolation of a nontransforming retrovirus from a patient with the AIDS-related lymphadenopathy syndrome.[29] The French isolate, called lymphadenopathy virus (LAV), was soon shown to selectively infect $CD4^+$ lymphocytes and to resemble EIAV far more closely than HTLV-I or HTLV-II. At the same time (1984), Gallo described a tissue culture system for isolation and production of retroviruses from AIDS patients; the system was used to obtain the necessary reagents for serologic assays.[30] With this solid experimental foundation, progress was rapid, and by the summer of 1984 investigators had shown that HTLV-III (the designation of the retrovirus Gallo et al. isolated from AIDS patients) could be isolated from large numbers of individuals with AIDS or with various syndromes preceding AIDS, and that antibodies to viral proteins were detectable in virtually every case.[31,32] After considerable debate, the causative agent of AIDS was renamed the human immunodeficiency virus,[33] replacing the designations LAV/HTLV-III and ARV, after an AIDS-related retrovirus isolated by Levy.[34]

The story of the AIDS retrovirus now merges with that of the lentiviruses. By 1985, a comparison of the morphology, genome structure, and nucleotide sequence of HIV with other retroviruses established its classification as the first human lentivirus,[4,5] knowledge which immediately predicted many of the unusual host–virus interactions and the formidable and unprecedented difficulties which must be overcome to control a slow infection.[35] The contemporary scene is one of enormous activity directed to the problems of control of HIV infection and to other issues taken up in the remainder of this chapter. To conclude this section on an optimistic note, the striking compression in the history of retrovirology, from decades to months, is testimony to the progress and commitment of the scientific community to meeting the challenges of this great scourge.

## EPIDEMIOLOGY

The epidemiology of HIV is discussed more fully in Chaps. 31 and 32. HIV-infected cells, and probably to a much lesser extent HIV viral particles, circulate in the bloodstream and are present in a variety of tissue fluids, but only blood, semen, vaginal secretions, and possibly milk have been implicated in the spread of HIV. Transmission occurs from these sources by sexual contact, exposure to blood or blood components, or perinatally (mother to neonate). The high-risk groups are therefore homosexual and bisexual males, IV drug users, certain transfusion recipients, hemophiliac patients and others exposed to blood or blood products, and children born to mothers with AIDS or in high-risk groups.[36] Heterosexual transmission, often from sexual intercourse with infected prostitutes, IV drug users, or bisexual men, while less frequent in the United States and Europe, contributes significantly to AIDS in Africa.[37]

HIV can also enter the body through cuts, scratches, and abrasions in the skin, or by direct contact with mucosal surfaces. Percutaneous exposures have resulted in rare but well-documented instances of infection in health care or laboratory workers.[38] However, there is no evidence for transmission by casual contact, by prolonged nonsexual contact in households with infected individuals, by ingestion, by inhalation, or by insect bites.[39] The incidence of infection in health care workers, even with documented exposures, is extremely low (< 1 percent). HIV is readily inactivated by alcohols, chlorine bleach, aldehydes, and other commonly used disinfectants.[40]

## THE BIOLOGY OF HIV

### STRUCTURE OF THE VIRUS

The salient properties which distinguish retroviruses, briefly alluded to in the section on taxonomy, are summarized in more detail in Table 28-3. The distinctive features of HIV are presented in a structural model of the virus in Fig. 28-2.[41] Mature virions are roughly spherical and about 100 nm in diameter (Fig. 28-3), but the range in sizes and shapes is extensive. In addition to typical spherical particles, there are comet-shaped virions and virions with blebs or tails varying in diameter from 70 to 160

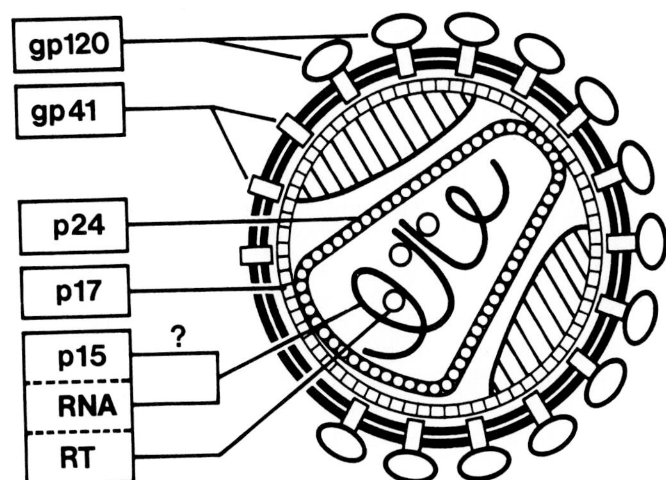


Fig. 28-2. Structural model of the organization of HIV. (*From HR Gelderblom et al,*[41] *with permission.*)

**Table 28-3. Taxonomic Features of Retroviridae**

| | |
|---|---|
| Nucleic acid | Linear positive-sense single-stranded RNA (60–70 S) composed of two identical subunits (30–35 S); 5′ cap structure ($m^7G^5ppp^5NmpNp$); polyadenylated 3′ end; repeated sequences at 3′ and 5′ ends; tRNA base-paired to genome complex |
| Protein | About 60% by weight; gag, internal structural proteins; pol, reverse transcriptase, protease, integrase; env, envelope proteins (1-2) |
| Lipid | About 35% by weight; derived from cell membrane |
| Carbohydrate | About 4% by weight; associated with env proteins |
| Physicochemical properties | Density 1.16–1.18 g/ml in sucrose, 1.16–1.21 g/ml in cesium chloride; sensitive to lipid solvents, detergents, and heat inactivation (56°C, 30 min); highly resistant to UV- and X-irradiation |
| Morphology | Spherical enveloped virions (80–120 nm in diameter), variable surface projections (8 nm in diameter), icosahedral capsid containing a ribonucleoprotein complex with a core shell (nucleoid) |

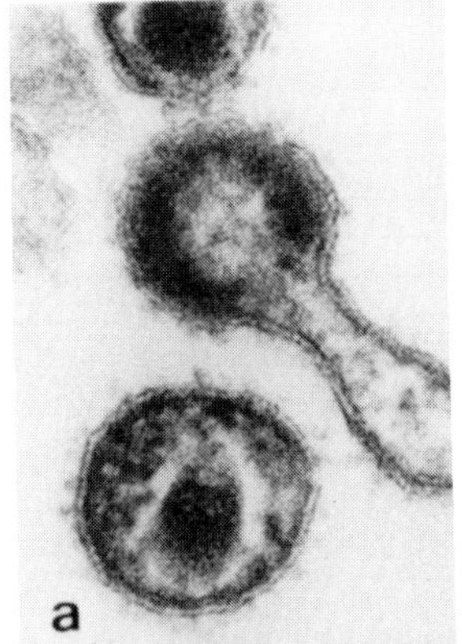


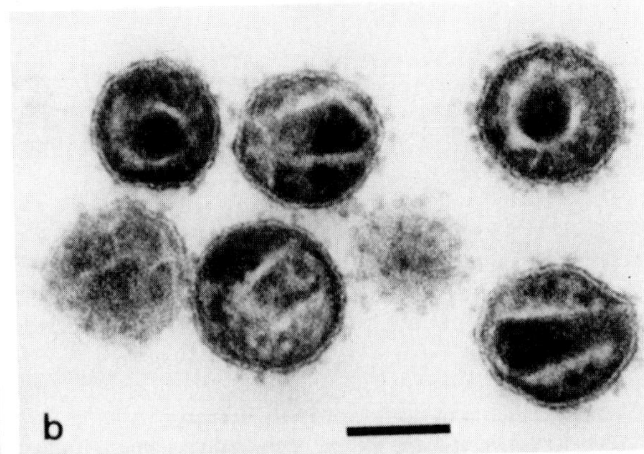


Fig. 28-3. Electron micrographs of thin sections of HIV. (*a*) The most completely budded particle contains an open, electron-dense RNP shell apposed to the viral membrane. Virus surface projections are visible on the left half of the bud. (*b*) "Mature" particles showing different core orientations, lateral-bodies, and a continuous dense layer adjacent to the inner membrane. Bar represents 100 nm. (*From HR Gelderblom et al,*[41] *with permission.*)

nm.[42] Some 70 to 80 knoblike projections protrude above the surface of the virion, and these envelope structures have two component glycoproteins,[43,44] gp120 and gp41.* The conical virion core is typical of all lentiviruses, but there are two lateral bodies of unknown composition that may be unique to HIV.[41] The major structural polypeptide of the virus and the core is p24; other polypeptides derived from a common precursor form a shell around the core (p17), or complex with virion RNA (p15).[41]

Viral RNA has not been characterized extensively, but, by analogy to other retroviruses,[2] is presumed to be a dimer with two identical linear molecules of about 9000 nucleotides which resemble mRNAs in having plus-stranded polarity, a methylated cap structure at the 5′ end, and polyadenylated 3′ termini. A tRNA base paired near the 5′ end of the viral RNA serves as the primer for the minus strand during DNA synthesis (see the section on replication).

## STRUCTURE AND FUNCTIONS OF THE PROVIRUS AND ITS mRNAs

The organization of the HIV proviral DNA genome and details of each region are illustrated in Fig. 28-4. The size of the genome varies from about 9200 (HIV-1) to 9600 (HIV-2) nucleotides.[45,46] Genes for the structural proteins (*gag*, *env*), reverse transcriptase, a protease and integrase (*pol*), and long terminal repeats (LTRs) are common to all retroviruses. However, HIV also has five or six additional genes—designated *vif* (previously known as *sor*), *vpr* (previously *R*), *tat*, *rev* (previously *art/trs*), and *nef* (previously *3′orf*)—which regulate viral gene expression. The transactivator (*tat*)[47,48] gene product p14[49] acts in *trans* in the nucleus[50] of infected cells to increase production of viral structural proteins. It may do this in part by preventing termination of viral RNA synthesis in the responding region downstream from the start site for transcription (TAR element).[51,52] The gene product p19[53] of *rev* (regulator of expression of virion proteins, previously known as *art*, antirepression transactivator) enhances synthesis of *gag* and *env* by relieving the repressive effects of inhibitory sequences in the mRNAs[54] and by ensuring correct splicing (hence, the alternative previous designation of the gene as *trs* for *trans regulator of splicing*). These genes act in concert to modulate levels of gene expression through positive (*tat* and *rev*) or negative (*rev*) effects.[55] A third regulatory gene, *nef* (negative regulatory factor) is encoded by the open reading frame at the 3′ end of the genome, and down regulates viral gene expression. It may be responsible in part for the ability of the virus to lie completely dormant.[55–57]

The structural and replicative genes are transcribed either as full-length (9.2 kb) genomic mRNAs (*gag*, *pol*) or subgenomic species of about 4 to 5 kb (*env*), formed by splicing 5′ leader sequences to the body of the mRNA.[58] Subsequently, the mRNAs are translated into polyprotein precursors, and these precursors

*The convention in retrovirology is to use a prefix for the protein followed by the molecular weight $\times 10^{-3}$. Thus, gp120 is a glycosylated protein with a molecular weight of 120,000.

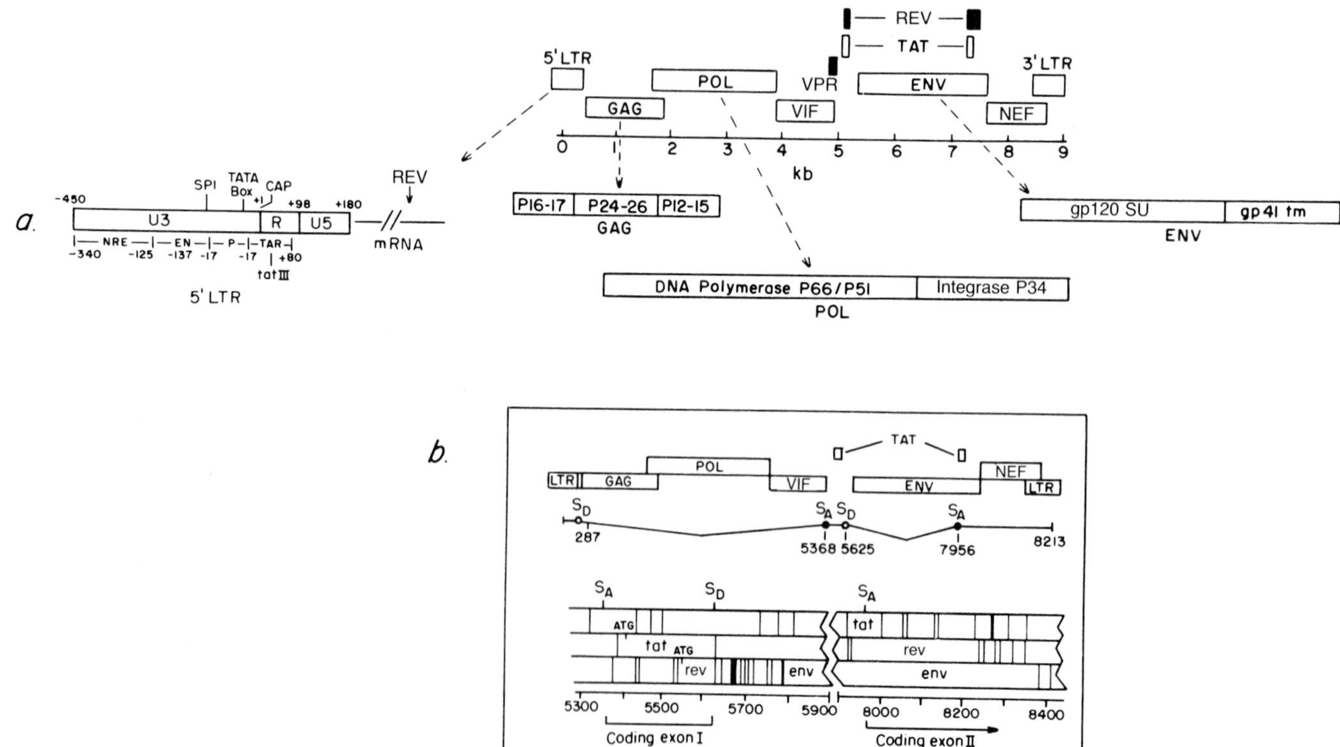


**Fig. 28-4.** HIV provirus. (*a*) See text for explanation. (*b*) Complex splicing of *tat* and *rev*. $S_D$ = slice donor sequences. $S_A$ = splice acceptor sequences. Numbers indicate nucleotide number. Vertical bars in the exploded view represent stop codons in the three reading frames. ATG indicates initiator codons; *tat*, *rev*, and *env* are the open reading frames for the respective coding exons.

are cleaved by proteases into the mature gene products. The *gag* precursor protein (pr55$^{gag}$), the initial translational product of the 9.2 kb mRNA, is processed in order from the amino terminus into p17, p24, and p15.[45] The reverse transcriptase is the product of the *pol* gene. Proteolytic cleavages generate two species, p66/p51 and p34 (p51 and p66 share amino termini, implying an additional cleavage site in the smaller species).

The primary translational product of the *env* gene is a glycosylated precursor (gp160) which is processed into an extracellular (su) portion gp120, and a smaller transmembrane (tm) anchor (gp41). N-terminal signal sequences in the precursor ultimately direct the protein to the cell surface, and sequences in the first half of the amino end of the molecule provide sites for glycosylation which increase the apparent molecular weight of the external glycoprotein from 65,000 to 120,000.

The proviral DNA is flanked by LTRs formed by copying sequences repeated at both ends of the viral RNA genome (*R*) and sequences unique to the 5′ end (*U5*) and 3′ end (*U3*). The LTRs contain sequences which play critical roles in regulating gene expression.[59] The region (Fig. 28-4*a*) designated NRE, for *negative regulatory element*, down regulates gene expression; the region designated EN, for *enhancer*, increases gene expression. *P* signifies the *promoter* region for transcription with its TATA box located upstream of the start site (the positive or negative numbers in Fig. 28-4 refer to the number of nucleotides to the right or left of the start site). Finally, there are regions which affect levels of mRNAs by interactions with cellular transcriptional factors (e.g., sp1) or the products of the *tat* and *rev* genes. These interactions occur in regions close to the 5′ capped end of the mRNA (CAP) in the transactivation responsive region in *R* (TAR), or downstream in the body of the mRNA (indicated by the arrow from *rev*).

The small mRNAs (about 2 kb) for these regulatory genes are generated by complex splicing mechanisms. The *tat* transcript, for example, comprises untranslated leader sequences in the *gag* gene joined to a short middle exon derived from sequences following *vif*, and a longer exon from *env* and 3′ sequences (Fig. 28-4*b*).

The roles of *vif* and *vpr* in the life cycle of HIV are not fully understood, but they serve essential functions. Viral particles, for example, are made without the *vif* gene product p23, but they are not infectious.[60–62]

## REPLICATION

The life cycle of HIV (see Fig. 28-5) begins with the attachment of virus to T helper lymphocytes and other cells with the CD4 cell surface antigen.[63] This specific interaction, mediated by a glycosylated domain near the carboxy terminus of gp120,[64,65] is followed by fusion of the viral envelope,[66] and entry of virions. The reverse transcriptase then synthesizes a double-stranded DNA copy of the RNA genome by a complex mechanism which involves a series of transcriptional jumps generating a linear molecule flanked by two LTRs.[2] Viral DNA subsequently becomes stably associated with the infected cell through integration into the chromosomal DNA of its host (proviral genome).[67] Integration into host DNA is facilitated by the viral integrase and appears to be at random sites. Although integration is generally assumed to be an obligatory event in the life cycle of retroviruses, this may not necessarily be the case. In cells infected by HIV and other lentiviruses there are often several hundred copies of extrachromosomal DNA that could serve as templates for synthesis of viral RNA, and in fact do so in the case of animal lentiviruses (visna).[68,69]

Viral DNA is transcribed by host cell RNA polymerase II, and the resulting viral mRNAs are translated into the structural proteins. After glycosylation and proteolytic processing, the viral subcomponents are either inserted into the membrane of the infected cell or complex with genomic RNAs to form the ribonucleoprotein (RNP) cores. Virions are assembled in a budding process which begins at the cell surface with the appearance of a crescentic density (the cores) beneath regions of the cell membrane containing the viral envelope components. Completion of the budding process releases a viral particle in which the core briefly retains its crescentic appearance before condensing into the dense nucleoid characteristic of the mature virion. Although Fig. 28-5 depicts only extracellular virus, virions also form intracellularly in cytoplasmic vacuoles of lymphocytes and monocytes.[70]

The rate and extent of virus production in tissue culture systems is governed by the products of the previously described regulatory genes *tat*, *rev*, and *nef*, and by the products of a number of cellular genes. These include Sp1 and other as yet undefined cellular transcriptional activators;[71] NF κB, a nuclear protein which induces kappa-chain antibody synthesis in B cells;[72] cytokines;[73] and perhaps other products made by T cells activated by mitogens, antigens, or allogenic stimulation.[74] Coinfection by viruses in the herpes and papovavirus families may also reactivate transcription of latent HIV.[75,76]

## PATHOGENESIS

There are still many questions about the postinfection events that eventually lead to AIDS. For this reason, the reconstruction of pathogenesis that follows supplements current knowledge about HIV with experience drawn from the analysis of animal lentivirus infections.[35]

## INITIAL PHASES OF INFECTION: ENTRY, MULTIPLICATION, DISSEMINATION

In the first step of infection, invasion of the host, HIV is introduced (probably mainly inside cells) into the bloodstream, either directly or from other sites through intimate contact with infected secretions. Virus attaches and penetrates T helper lymphocytes, monocytes, and macrophages,[77] and possibly epithelial cells,[78] to initiate the multiplication stage of infection. Within the first week or two, individuals become viremic, and circulation of cell-free virus spreads the infection to secondary sites where a variety of cell types may participate in replication, including dendritic cells,[79] promyelocytes,[80] microglia,[81] endothelium,[82] astrocytes, and oligodendrocytes.[83,84] The broader host cell range of HIV (beyond T-lymphotropism), which has recently been recognized, may reflect the presence of low-density CD4 receptors or possibly other viral receptors in other cell types.

## IMMUNE RESPONSE

During the period of viral dissemination, the infected individual mounts both a humoral and a cell-mediated response (Fig. 28-6). IgM antibodies to HIV have been detected as early as 5 days postinfection, and seroconversion is often complete by the second

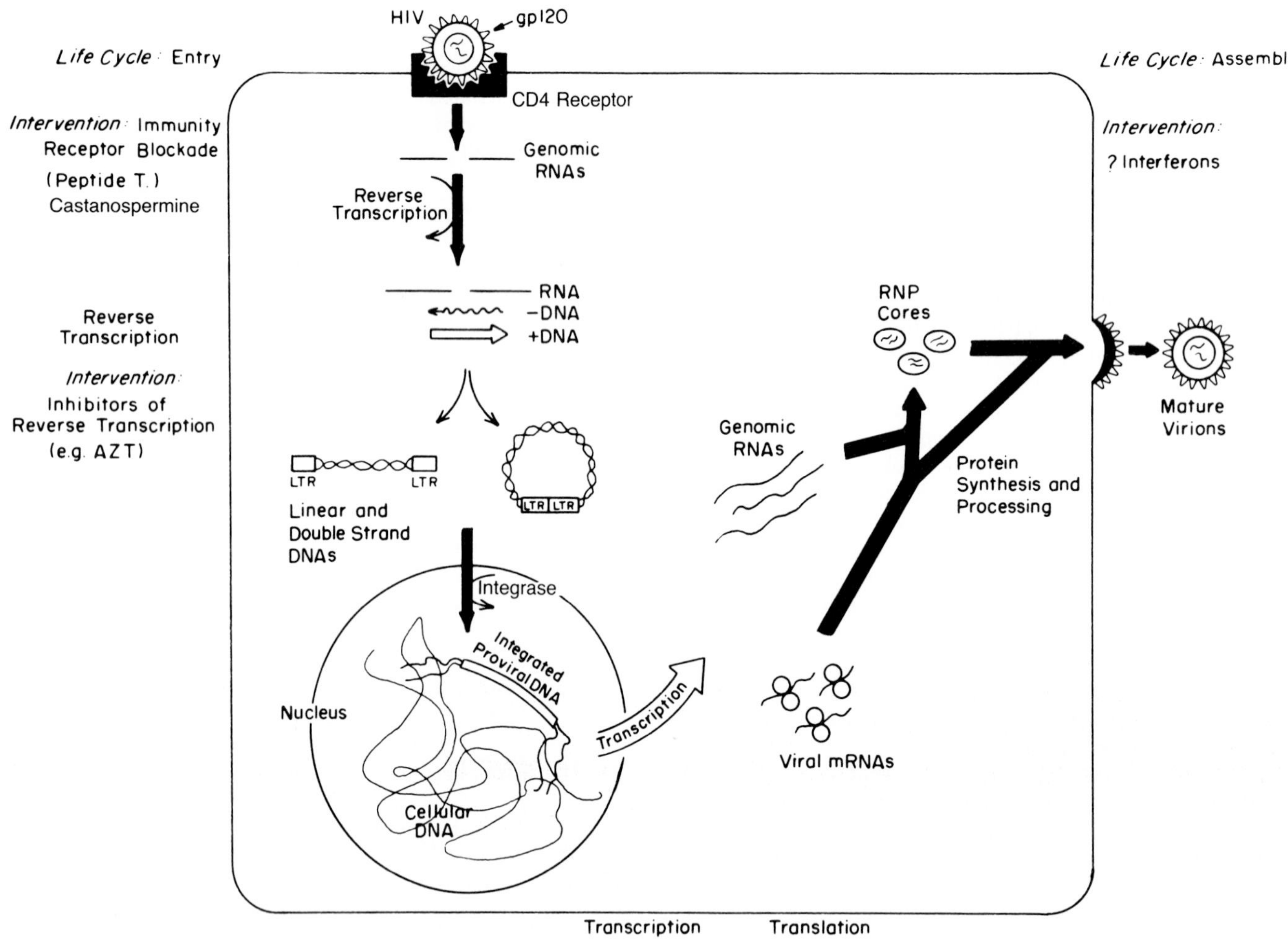


**Fig. 28-5.** HIV life cycle with points of potential intervention. HIV binds to the CD4 cell surface antigen and enters the cell, where the released viral RNA genomes are copied into DNA. Synthesis is initiated at the 5′ end of the viral RNA using the bound tRNA as primer. Ribonuclease H activity of the reverse transcriptase degrades the RNA in the RNA-DNA hybrid to free sequences complementary to the repeated sequences at the 5′ and 3′ end of the RNA. Base pairing of the (−) strand DNA to the 3′ end of a second viral RNA accomplishes the first transcriptional jump and provides one of the LTRs. As the (−) strand DNA is elongated, ribonuclease H cleavage of RNA at a polypurine tract provides the primer for (+) strand DNA synthesis. In a second transcriptional jump this species is transferred to the end of (−) strand DNA to form the second LTR. A viral integrase facilitates the integration of viral DNA into the host genome. In a productive life cycle viral DNA is transcribed and translated to generate the RNA cores and viral subcomponents which are assembled into viral particles at the cell surface.

to seventh weeks (occasionally much longer). These first antibodies are directed against gp160 and p24 but, in time, antibodies to all other structural proteins and nonstructural proteins are demonstrable,[85–87] and IgM is replaced by other immunoglobulin classes (IgG, and IgA in saliva[88]). Functionally, antibodies to HIV mediate antibody-dependent cytotoxicity and neutralize virus in vitro.[89–92] However, neutralizing antibodies elicited by the viral glycoproteins are generally present only in low titer.[92] Although soluble p24 antigen is cleared from plasma in association with the humoral immune response, only to reappear late in the course of infection coincident with declining antibody titers,[93–95] the relation between these events is not clear. A correlation with clinical status has been taken as evidence that humoral immunity is capable of containing infection, but this relation does not hold in all studies or populations,[95] and the presence of neutralizing antibody is a poor predictor of the $CD4^+/CD8^+$ cell ratio and/or clinical status.[92] Furthermore, passive administration of immune globulin containing high titers of anti-HIV neutralizing antibody has failed to protect chimpanzees from subsequent virus challenge.[96]

Although antibody may inhibit HIV infectivity, even for a brief period after attachment of virus to cells, some antibodies may have an opposite, enhancing effect. Thus, immune enhancement of HIV infectivity, mediated by attachment of antibody-virus complexes to cellular Fc and C receptors, has been recently described. The role such antibodies play in the pathogenesis of AIDS is uncertain, however.

The cellular immune response to HIV is mediated by class I restricted virus-specific cytotoxic lymphocytes (CTLs) bearing the cell surface marker CD8[97,98]; and $CD8^+$ cells that suppress viral replication apparently independent of direct cytotoxicity.[99] CTLs recognize both *gag* and *env* gene products irrespective of the

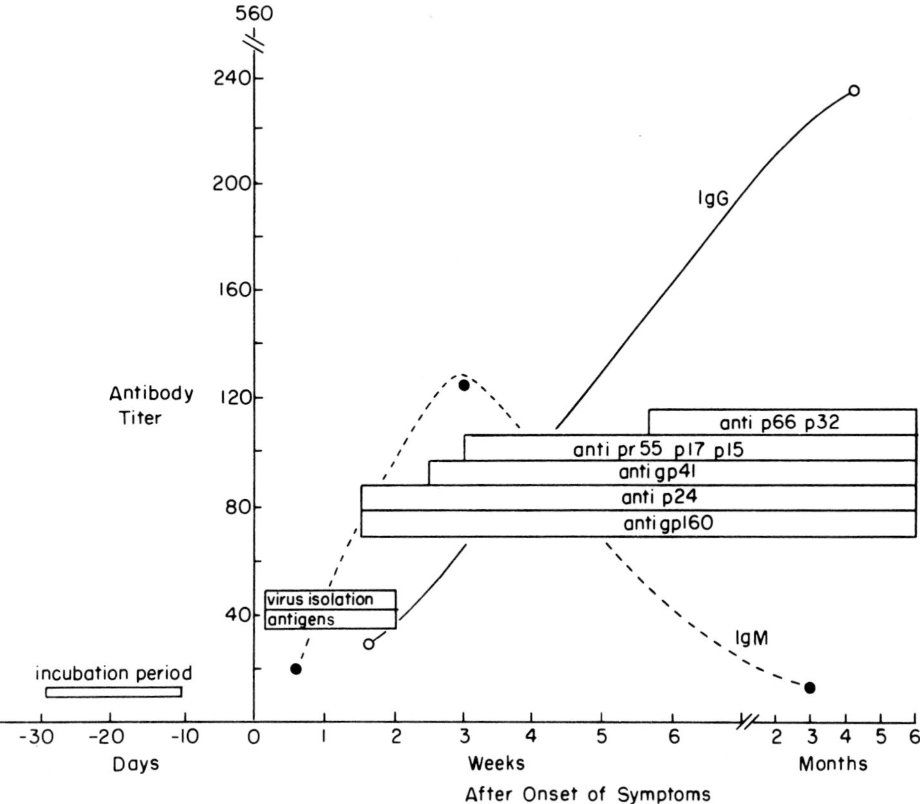


Fig. 28-6. Hypothetical time course of relation of viral isolation and antigenemia to the humoral immune response. Virus may be isolated from peripheral blood lymphocytes throughout the course of the infection, while cell-free viremia again becomes common late in disease.

intracellular location of intact *gag* products and the polymorphic nature of the viral glycoproteins.

## PERSISTENCE, LATENCY, AND THE TROJAN HORSE MECHANISM OF DISSEMINATION

Despite the immune response, all lentiviruses typically persist in their hosts.[35] HIV establishes latent and persistent infections in tissue culture,[100] and infected cells and viral antigens have been detected in a few individuals as long as 6 to 14 months before overt seroconversion.[101] The perplexing and vexing ability of lentiviruses to elude immune surveillence has been attributed to restricted gene expression in the majority of infected cells.[35] Most infected cells harbor the viral genome in an immunologically silent state in which viral antigens are not produced or are not presented in sufficient quantities for efficient detection and destruction by host defenses. This explanation holds not only for perpetuation of infection in tissues, but also for dissemination of virus, which likely occurs in monocytes/macrophages. This insidious mode of spread of lentiviruses in and between individuals has been referred to as the *Trojan Horse* mechanism of spread.[35]

## DAMAGE TO CELLS AND TISSUES

Lentiviruses fuse infected and uninfected cells to form giant cells and syncytia which degenerate as the characteristic cytopathic effect (CPE) of infections in vitro.[35] For HIV, fusion is mediated by interactions between CD4 on the cell's surface and the amino terminus of gp41.[102] Cell fusion, however, is not the only mechanism of cell death in culture, as HIV kills T cells without fusion and there are viral mutants which fuse without killing.[103] A toxic effect of accumulated extrachromosomal viral DNA has also been invoked as an alternative mechanism of retroviral CPE, but this seems unlikely to operate in lentivirus infections as the number of copies of viral DNA can be dissociated from cytotoxicity.[35]

In moving from the pathogenesis of cell injury in vitro to pathology at the organismal level, the mechanisms may be expected to be more complex. In the first place, although the dysfunction and depletion of $CD4^+$ helper cells is central to the immunocompromised state in AIDS (see Chap. 29), only a minor fraction of the lymphocyte population contains viral RNA (1 in 10,000 to 100,000 cells[104]). This discrepancy between the profound general effects of infection and the limited number of infected cells implies an amplification mechanism set in motion by viral replication. Current speculations include (1) destruction of progenitor cells or other immune cell subsets which affect T-cell proliferation and function, (2) elimination of uninfected cells through syncytium formation with infected cells, (3) shedding of the viral glycoprotein which is directly[105] or indirectly immunosuppressive [by inducing prostaglandin ($PGE_2$) release from monocytes or inciting an immune attack against gp120 bound to the CD4 receptor of uninfected cells[106]], (4) an autoimmune state with a target antigen of cellular origin induced by HIV which stimulates production of antilymphocyte antibodies.[107]

## THE NEUROLOGIC MANIFESTATIONS OF AIDS

Some neurologic abnormality eventually occurs in the majority of symptomatic HIV-infected individuals, and neurologic disease may be the presenting or predominant manifestation of infection[108] (see Chap. 30). The most common pathologic alteration, pallor and rarefaction of white matter, is associated with inflammatory foci of mononuclear cells around blood vessels and in the neuroparenchyma. This subacute encephalitis, which resembles the histopathologic changes in visna,[35] primarily affects subcortical areas and most frequently causes a characteristic dementia with motor deficits. There is also a vacuolar myelopathy associated with AIDS which has no known counterpart in the lentivirus infections of animals.[109]

The pathogenesis of the neurologic disorder, like the immunosuppressive state, is not well understood. HIV clearly invades the CNS, but the infected cells for the most part are not neurons or glial cells but endothelium, monocytes, and macrophages from the CNS (microglia) and periphery.[81–84] Again, of necessity, indirect mechanisms have been advanced to account for the damage to nerve cells: (1) release of cytotoxins and proteases from macrophages, leading to innocent-bystander damage; (2) alteration in the blood–brain barrier adversely affecting neurologic function; (3) immunopathologic effects analogous to visna, from accumulation of inflammatory cells; (4) competitive interactions between gp120 and neuroleukin, a nerve growth factor required for survival of neurons.[110]

## THE ROLE OF SOLUBLE FACTORS IN PATHOGENESIS

Several facets of AIDS may be the result of shedding or secretion of soluble factors from the virus or from host cells, particularly monocytes. The monokine IL-1, induced by infection with HIV, is pyrogenic and thus may play a role in the persistent fevers seen in some infected individuals. IL-1 is also part of a feedback loop of immunoregulation in which excessive levels of $PGE_2$ may contribute to immunosuppression. There has been speculation that another monokine, tumor necrosis factor (TNF), or cachectin, might be involved in the striking cachexia of AIDS and in "slim disease," a clinical variant of African AIDS (see Chap. 32). HIV infection may cause polyclonal B cell activation, an effect perhaps mediated by the similarities between gp120 and neuroleukin which is a lymphokine for B cells as well as growth factor for neurons. Finally, the increased incidence of Kaposi's sarcoma may be the result in part of the release of endothelial growth factors from infected cells.

## PROSPECTS FOR CONTROL

### THE PROBLEMS: INTRACELLULAR AND ORGAN HAVENS; ANTIGENIC VARIATION

This concluding section on HIV addresses general principles of prevention, eradication, and treatment of infection. To begin with, HIV must be considered a problem of unprecedented difficulty because of the mechanisms which allow the virus to persist, spread, and cause disease in the face of natural immunity. These mechanisms include covert infection of cells in tissues, blood, and secretions, and refuge in the CNS (beyond the blood–brain barrier). In addition, lentiviruses spawn antigenic variants which in principle may be freed temporarily from immune restraints. The unique problems of lentiviruses as intracellular pathogens provide a compelling rationale to seek a means to maintain dormancy and prevent progression to disease, in addition to programs devoted to prevention and eradication.

Measures to control HIV can be considered within the framework of the viral life cycle (Fig. 28-5) as blocks to entry of the virus or subsequent steps of viral DNA synthesis and gene expression. Collectively the goals of these strategies are (1) to diminish the aggregate burden of infected cells, (2) to attenuate the deleterious effects of viral infection in the individual who already harbors the virus by mitigating the destructive effects of replication, and (3) to interdict the spread of virus in and between individuals. With this framework in mind, the various approaches will be considered under the traditional headings of vaccines and antiviral agents.

## VACCINES, ANTIGENIC VARIATION, AND IMMUNOPROPHYLAXIS

To date, the largest efforts to control the spread of HIV have been directed toward the production of a subunit vaccine composed of antigens which elicit neutralizing antibody (gp160, gp120, gp41, p17). These gene products have been synthesized by recombinant DNA technology in *E. coli,* mammalian cells, or insect (baculovirus) vectors[111–113] and combined with an adjuvant (muramyl dipeptides, or immune-stimulating complexes, iscoms) to enhance immunogenicity. The adjuvant function can be provided by the vector when the recombinant genes are incorporated into viral vectors (vaccinia, adenovirus, or *Ty,* the yeast retrotransposon).[114,115] Immunogenic regions of gp120 or p17 which elicit a T-cell response and/or neutralizing antibody have also been identified as potential peptide vaccine candidates.[116,117] Underlying all these efforts is the tacit assumption, yet unproven, that specific neutralizing antibody, proper T-cell responses, or a combination of both may provide protection against exogenous infection with HIV.

The variability in the *env* gene of HIV[118,119] found between isolates from different individuals or from the same individual has been a source of considerable concern, because of parallels to antigenic variation in animal lentivirus infections, particularly EIAV.[35] In the latter case, the rapid emergence of mutated viruses which are no longer neutralized by antibodies to preexisting antigenic variants provides a mechanism for persistence and dissemination between infected animals and accounts for the episodic character of disease. However, while it may be necessary to develop a multivalent vaccine with components of HIV-1 and the distantly related HIV-2, there is little solid evidence to suggest that antigenic variation is a major mechanism for the persistence of lentiviruses, with the exception of EIAV.[35]

Thus far, subunit viral products have been shown to elicit neutralizing antibodies and a cellular immune response in goats, primates, and man, and one of the recombinant viral vaccines (gp120) is currently in phase I (toxicity) testing in human volunteers. However, the initial results in animal models have proved disappointing. Chimpanzees immunized with vaccinia HIV gp120 developed virus-specific antibody and activated T cells but were not protected on challenge with HIV.[120]

Although passive immunoprophylaxis has been successful with other viruses, such as hepatitis B virus, recent attempts to protect chimpanzees with passively administered neutralizing antibody resulted in failure.[96] Although the dose of challenge virus was large in these studies (approximately 100 chimpanzees 50 percent infective doses), the failure of antibody to protect against infection suggests that it will not be easy to develop effective means of active or passive immunoprophylaxis.

## ANTIVIRALS

In addition to vaccine development, there is a large-scale search underway for agents which interfere at different stages in the life cycle of HIV (see Fig. 28-5). Dextran sulfate and soluble recombinant CD4 may work by preventing attachment of HIV to cells.[121] The plant alkaloid castanospermine inhibits viral entry by altering glycosylation of the viral glycoprotein.[122] Reverse transcription can be preferentially blocked (compared with cellular DNA polymerases) by dideoxynucleotide terminators.[123] One of these, 3-azido-3′-dideoxythymidine (AZT), is currently in clinical use (see Chap. 30). Foscarnet, an inhibitor of the DNA polymerase of herpes simplex, also blocks replication of HIV at the step of reverse transcription.[124] A number of other agents to which HIV shows susceptibility in vitro interfere with the capping or splicing of mRNA (ribavirin, antisense oligonucleotides[125,126]) or later steps in synthesis and assembly of virion subcomponents. Interferon inducers, interferons per se, and possibly tumor necrosis factor (TNF) all inhibit HIV in vitro, possibly at the stage of viral maturation.[127,128]

Despite the efficacy of those agents in vitro, and to some extent clinically (AZT), there is currently no drug or combination of drugs which has the desired characteristics of low toxicity for prolonged administration, good penetration into the CNS, and high viral inhibitory activity. Thus, the urgent quest for anti-HIV therapy continues along traditional and novel lines. In the latter class, antisense oligonucleotides, perhaps in viral vectors,[35] and novel drugs targeted against the viral regulatory gene products (*tat*, etc.) or viral protease hold special promise for the future.[121,129] Certainly, it is too early to predict efficacy of these agents in humans, but, again, the unique aspects of lentivirus interactions with their hosts may make it more realistic to expect a spectrum of agents with effects ranging from total prevention to moderation of disease.

## References


1 Haase AT: The slow infection caused by visna virus. *Curr Top Microbiol Immunol* 72:101, 1975.

2 Teich N, Varmus HE (eds): *RNA Tumor Viruses*, 2d ed. New York, Cold Spring Harbor Laboratory, 1982.

3 Stowring L et al: Serological definition of the lentivirus group of retroviruses. *J Virol* 29:523, 1979.

4 Gonda MA et al: Sequence homology and morphologic similarity of HTLV-III and visna virus, a pathogenic lentivirus. *Science* 227:173, 1985.

5 Sonigo P et al: Nucleotide sequence of the visna lentivirus: Relationship to the AIDS virus. *Cell* 42:369, 1985.

6 Chiu IM et al: Nucleotide sequence evidence for relationship of AIDS retrovirus to lentiviruses. *Nature* 317:366, 1985.

7 Gonda MA et al: Characterization and molecular cloning of a bovine lentivirus related to human immunodeficiency virus. *Nature* 330: 388, 1987.

8 Pedersen NC et al: Isolation of a T-lymphotropic virus from domestic cats with an immunodeficiency-like syndrome. *Science* 235: 790, 1987.

9 Daniel MD et al: Isolation of T-cell tropic HTLV-III-like retrovirus from macaques. *Science* 228:1201, 1985.

10 Franchini G et al: Sequence of simian immunodeficiency virus and its relationship to the human immunodeficiency viruses. *Nature* 328:539, 1987.

11 Chakrabarti L et al: Sequence of simian immunodeficiency virus from macaque and its relationship to other human and simian retroviruses. *Nature* 328:543, 1987.

12 Arya SK et al: Homology of genome of AIDS-associated virus with genomes of human T-cell leukemia viruses. *Science* 225:927, 1984.

13 Wong-Staal F et al: Human T-lymphotropic retroviruses. *Nature* 317:395, 1985.

14 Lott TJ et al: Three-dimensional similarity mapping reveals nucleotide sequence relationships among human immunodeficiency virus (HIV) isolates. *Gene* 57:247, 1987.

15 Clavel F et al: Isolation of a new human retrovirus from West African patients with AIDS. *Science* 233:343, 1986.

16 Kanki PJ et al: Human T-lymphotropic virus type 4 and the human immunodeficiency virus in West Africa. *Science* 236:827, 1987.

17 Clavel F et al: Molecular cloning and polymorphism of the human immune deficiency virus type 2. *Nature* 324:691, 1986.

18 Hahn BH et al: Relation of HTLV-4 to simian and human immunodeficiency-associated viruses. *Nature* 330:184, 1987.

19 Temin HM: Mechanism of cell transformation by RNA tumor viruses. *Ann Rev Microbiol* 25:609, 1971.

20 Temin HM et al: RNA-dependent DNA polymerase in virions of Rous sarcoma virus. *Nature* 226:1211, 1970.

21 Baltimore D: RNA-dependent DNA polymerase in virions of RNA tumor viruses. *Nature* 226:1209, 1970.

22 Hill M et al: Virus recovery in chicken cells treated with Rous sarcoma cell DNA. *Nature New Biol* 237:30, 1972.

23 Gallagher RE et al: Growth and differentiation in culture of leukemic leukocytes from a patient with acute myelogenous leukemia and re-identification of type-C virus. *Proc Natl Acad Sci USA* 72: 4137, 1975.

24 Poiesz BJ et al: Detection and isolation of type C retrovirus particles from fresh and cultured lymphocytes of a patient with cutaneous T-cell lymphoma. *Proc Natl Acad Sci USA* 77:7415, 1980.

25 Poiesz BJ et al: Isolation of a new type C retrovirus (HTLV) in primary uncultured cells of a patient with Sezary T-cell leukaemia. *Nature* 294:268, 1981.

26 Yoshida M et al: Isolation and characterization of retrovirus from cell lines of human adult T-cell leukemia and its implication in the disease. *Proc Natl Acad Sci USA* 79:2031, 1982.

27 The chronology of AIDS research. *Nature* 326:435, 1987.

28 Essex M et al: Antibodies to cell membrane antigens associated with human T-cell leukemia virus in patients with AIDS. *Science* 220:859, 1983.

29 Barré-Sinoussi F et al: Isolation of a T-lymphotropic retrovirus from a patient at risk for acquired immune deficiency syndrome (AIDS). *Science* 220:868, 1983.

30 Popovic M et al: Detection, isolation, and continuous production of cytopathic retroviruses (HTLV-III) from patients with AIDS and pre-AIDS. *Science* 224:497, 1984.

31 Gallo RC et al: Frequent detection and isolation of cytopathic retroviruses (HTLV-III) from patients with AIDS and at risk for AIDS. *Science* 224:500, 1984.

32 Schüpbach J et al: Serological analysis of a subgroup of human T-lymphotropic retroviruses (HTLV-III) associated with AIDS. *Science* 224:503, 1984.

33 Coffin J et al: Human immunodeficiency viruses. *Science* 232:697, 1986.

34 Levy JA et al: Isolation of lymphocytopathic retroviruses from San Francisco patients with AIDS. *Science* 225:840, 1984.

35 Haase T: Pathogenesis of lentivirus infections. *Nature* 322:130, 1986.

36 Curran JW et al: The epidemiology of AIDS: Current status and future prospects. *Science* 229:1352, 1985.

37 Piot P et al: Retrospective seroepidemiology of AIDS virus infection in Nairobi populations. *J Infect Dis* 155:1108, 1987.

38 CDC: Update: Human immunodeficiency virus infections in health-care workers exposed to blood of infected patients. *MMWR* 36:285, 1987.

39 Friedland GH et al: Lack of transmission of HTLV-III/LAV infection

to household contacts of patients with AIDS or AIDS-related complex with oral candidiasis. *N Engl J Med* 314:344, 1986.
40 Martin LS et al: Disinfection and inactivation of the human T lymphotropic virus type III/lymphadenopathy-associated virus. *J Infect Dis* 152:400, 1985.
41 Gelderblom HR et al: Fine structure of human immunodeficiency virus (HIV) and immunolocalization of structural proteins. *Virology* 156:171, 1987.
42 Stannard LM et al: The morphology of human immunodeficiency virus particles by negative staining electron microscopy. *J Gen Virol* 68:919, 1987.
43 Schüpbach J et al: Serological analysis of a subgroup of human T-lymphotropic retroviruses (HTLV-III) associated with AIDS. *Science* 224:503, 1984.
44 Sarngadharan M et al: Antibodies reactive with human T-lymphotropic retroviruses (HTLV-III) in the serum of patients with AIDS. *Science* 224:506, 1984.
45 Ratner L et al: Complete nucleotide sequence of the AIDS virus, HTLV-III. *Nature* 313:277, 1985.
46 Guyader M et al: Genome organization and transactivation of the human immunodeficiency virus type 2. *Nature* 326:662, 1987.
47 Sodroski J et al: Trans-acting transcriptional regulation of human T-cell leukemia virus type III long terminal repeat. *Science* 227:171, 1985.
48 Arya SK et al: Trans-activator gene of human T-lymphotropic virus type III(HTLV-III). *Science* 229:69, 1985.
49 Goh WC et al: Identification of a protein encoded by the trans activator gene tatIII of human T-cell lymphotropic retrovirus type III. *J Virol* 59:181, 1986.
50 Hauber J et al: Trans-activation of human immunodeficiency virus gene expression is mediated by nuclear events. *Proc Natl Acad Sci USA* 84:6364, 1987.
51 Rosen CA et al: The location of cis-acting regulatory sequences in the human T cell lymphotropic virus type III (HTLV-III/LAV) long terminal repeat. *Cell* 41:813, 1985.
52 Kao SY et al: Anti-termination of transcription within the long terminal repeat of HIV-1 by *tat* gene product. *Nature* 330:489, 1987.
53 Knight DM et al: Expression of the *art/trs* protein of HIV and study of its role in viral envelope synthesis. *Science* 236:837, 1987.
54 Sodroski J et al: A second post-transcriptional trans-activator gene required for HTLV-III replication. *Nature* 321:412, 1986.
55 Haseltine WA, Wong-Stahl F: The molecular biology of the AIDS virus. *Sci Am* 259:52, 1988.
56 Luciw PA et al: Mutational analysis of the human immunodeficiency virus: The orf-B region down-regulates virus replication. *Proc Natl Acad Sci USA* 84:1434, 1987.
57 Franchini G et al: Cytoplasmic localization of the HTLV-III 3′orf protein in cultured T cells. *Virology* 155:593, 1986.
58 Muesing MA et al: Nucleic acid structure and expression of the human AIDS/lymphadenopathy retrovirus. *Nature* 313:450, 1985.
59 Chen ISY et al: Regulation of AIDS virus expression. *Cell* 47:1, 1986.
60 Kan NC et al: Identification of HTLV-III/LAV *sor* gene product and detection of antibodies in human sera. *Science* 231:1553, 1986.
61 Fisher AG et al: The *sor* gene of HIV-1 is required for efficient virus transmission in vitro. *Science* 237:888, 1987.
62 Strebel K et al: The HIV *"A"* (*sor*) gene product is essential for virus infectivity. *Nature* 328:728, 1987.
63 Dalgleish AG et al: The CD4 (T4) antigen is an essential component of the receptor for the AIDS retrovirus. *Nature* 312:763, 1984.
64 Lasky LA et al: Delineation of a region of the human immunodeficiency virus type 1 gp20 glycoprotein critical for interaction with the CD4 receptor. *Cell* 50:975, 1987.
65 Matthews TJ et al: Interaction between the human T-cell lymphotropic virus type $III_B$ envelope glycoprotein gp120 and the surface antigen CD4: Role of carbohydrate in binding and cell fusion. *Proc Natl Acad Sci USA* 84:5424, 1987.
66 Stein BS et al: pH-Independent HIV entry into CD4-positive T cells via virus envelope fusion to the plasma membrane. *Cell* 49:659, 1987.
67 Panganiban AT: Retroviral DNA integration. *Cell* 42:5, 1985.
68 Shaw GM et al: Molecular characterization of human T-cell leukemia (lymphotropic) virus type III in the acquired immune deficiency syndrome. *Science* 226:1165, 1984.
69 Harris JD et al: Slow virus visna: Reproduction in vitro of virus from extrachromosomal DNA. *Proc Natl Acad Sci USA* 81:7212, 1984.
70 Meyenhofer MF et al: Ultrastructural morphology and intracellular production of human immunodeficiency virus (HIV) in brain. *J Neuropathol Exp Neurol* 46:474, 1987.
71 Okamoto T et al: Demonstration of virus-specific transcriptional activator(s) in cells infected with HTLV-III by an in vitro cell-free system. *Cell* 47:29, 1986.
72 Nabel G et al: An inducible transcription factor activates expression of human immunodeficiency virus in T cells. *Nature* 326:711, 1987.
73 Folks TM et al: Cytokine-induced expression of HIV-1 in a chronically infected promonocyte cell line. *Science* 238:800, 1987.
74 Tong-Starksen SE et al: Human immunodeficiency virus long terminal repeat responds to T-cell activation signals. *Proc Natl Acad Sci USA* 84:6845, 1987.
75 Mosca JD et al: Herpes simplex virus type-1 can reactivate transcription of latent human immunodeficiency virus. *Nature* 325:67, 1987.
76 Gendelman HE et al: Trans-activation of the human immunodeficiency virus long terminal repeat sequence by DNA viruses. *Proc Natl Acad Sci USA* 83:9759, 1986.
77 Gartner S et al: The role of mononuclear phagocytes in HTLV-III/LAV infection. *Science* 233:215, 1986.
78 Adachi A et al: Productive, persistent infection of human colorectal cell lines with human immunodeficiency virus. *J Virol* 61:209, 1987.
79 Patterson S et al: Susceptibility of human peripheral blood dendritic cells to infection by human immunodeficiency virus. *J Gen Virol* 68: 1177, 1987.
80 Levy JA et al: AIDS-associated retroviruses (ARV) can productively infect other cells besides human T helper cells. *Virology* 147:441, 1985.
81 Vazeux R et al: AIDS subacute encephalitis. *Am J Path* 126:403, 1987.
82 Wiley CA et al: Cellular localization of human immunodeficiency virus infection within the brains of acquired immune deficiency syndrome patients. *Proc Natl Acad Sci USA* 83:7089, 1986.
83 Gyorkey F et al: Human immunodeficiency virus in brain biopsies of patients with AIDS and progressive encephalopathy. *J Infect Dis* 155:870, 1987.
84 Stoler MH et al: Human T-cell lymphotropic virus type III infection of the central nervous system. *JAMA* 256:2360, 1986.
85 Gaines H et al: Antibody response in primary human immunodeficiency virus infection. *Lancet* ii:1249, 1987.
86 Cooper DA et al: Antibody response to human immunodeficiency virus after primary infection. *J Infect Dis* 155:1113, 1987.
87 Arya SK et al: Three novel genes of human T-lymphotropic virus type III: Immune reactivity of their products with sera from acquired immune deficiency syndrome patients. *Proc Natl Acad Sci USA* 83: 2209, 1986.
88 Archibald DW et al: Secretory IgA antibodies to human immunodeficiency virus in the parotid saliva of patients with AIDS and AIDS-related complex. *J Infect Dis* 155:793, 1987.
89 Weiss RA et al: Neutralization of human T-lymphotropic virus type III by sera of AIDS and AIDS-risk patients. *Nature* 316:69, 1985.
90 Robert-Guroff M et al: HTLV-III-neutralizing antibodies in patients with AIDS and AIDS-related complex. *Nature* 316:72, 1985.
91 Rook AH et al: Sera from HTLV-II/LAV antibody-positive individuals mediate antibody-dependent cellular cytotoxicity against HTLV-III/LAV-infected T cells. *J Immunol* 138:1064, 1987.
92 Prince AM et al: Prevalence, clinical significance, and strain specificity of neutralizing antibody to the human immunodeficiency virus. *J Infect Dis* 156:268, 1987.
93 Goudsmit J et al: Expression of human immunodeficiency virus antigen (HIV-Ag) in serum and cerebrospinal fluid during acute and chronic infection. *Lancet* ii:177, 1986.

94 Groopman JE et al: Serological Characterization of HTLV-III Infection in AIDS and related disorders. *J Infect Dis* 153:736, 1986.

95 Barin F et al: Human immunodeficiency virus antigenemia in patients with AIDS and AIDS-related disorders: A comparison between european and central African populations. *J Infect Dis* 156:830, 1987.

96 Prince AM et al: Failure of a human immunodeficiency virus (HIV) immune globulin to protect chimpanzees against experimental challenge with HIV. *Proc Natl Acad Sci USA* 85:6944, 1988.

97 Walker BD et al: HIV-specific cytotoxic T lymphocytes in seropositive individuals. *Nature* 328:345, 1987.

98 Plata F et al: AIDS virus-specific cytotoxic T lymphocytes in lung disorders. *Nature* 328:348, 1987.

99 Walker CM et al: $CD8^+$ lymphocytes can control HIV infection in vitro by suppressing virus replication. *Science* 234:1563, 1986.

100 Folks T et al: Induction of HTLV-III/LAV from a nonvirus-producing T-cell line: Implications for latency. *Science* 231:600, 1986.

101 Ranki A et al: Long latency precedes overt seroconversion in sexually transmitted human-immunodeficiency-virus infection. *Lancet* ii:589, 1987.

102 Lifson JD et al: AIDS retrovirus induced cytopathology: Giant cell formation and involvement of CD4 antigen. *Science* 232:1123, 1986.

103 Somasundaran M et al: A major mechanism of human immunodeficiency virus-induced cell killing does not involve cell fusion. *J Virol* 61:3114, 1987.

104 Harper ME: Detection of lymphocytes expressing human T-lymphotropic virus type III in lymph nodes and peripheral blood from infected individuals by in situ hybridization. *Proc Natl Acad Sci USA* 83:772, 1986.

105 Mann DL et al: HTLV-III large envelope protein (gp120) suppresses PHA-induced lymphocyte blastogenesis. *J Immunol* 138:2640, 1987.

106 Lyerly HK et al: Human T-cell lymphotropic virus $III_B$ glycoprotein (gp120) bound to CD4 determinants on normal lymphocytes and expressed by infected cells serves as target for immune attack. *Proc Natl Acad Sci USA* 84:4601, 1987.

107 Stricker RB et al: An AIDS-related cytotoxic autoantibody reacts with a specific antigen on stimulated $CD4^+$ T cells. *Nature* 327:710, 1987.

108 Price RW et al: AIDS encephalopathy. *Neurol Clin* 4:285, 1986.

109 Petito CK et al: Vacuolar myelopathy pathologically resembling subacute combined degeneration in patients with the acquired immunodeficiency syndrome. *N Engl J Med* 312:874, 1985.

110 Lee MR et al: Functional interaction and partial homology between human immunodeficiency virus and neuroleukin. *Science* 237:1047, 1987.

111 Putney SD et al: HTLV-III/LAV-neutralizing antibodies to an *E. coli*-produced fragment of the virus envelope. *Science* 234:1392, 1986.

112 Rusche JR et al: Humoral immune response to the entire human immunodeficiency virus envelope glycoprotein made in insect cells. *Proc Natl Acad Sci USA* 84:6924, 1987.

113 Lasky LA et al: Neutralization of the AIDS retrovirus by antibodies to a recombinant envelope glycoprotein. *Science* 233:209, 1986.

114 Hu SL et al: Expression of AIDS virus envelope gene in recombinant vaccinia viruses. *Nature* 320:537, 1986.

115 Adams SE et al: The expression of hybrid HIV:Ty virus-like particles in yeast. *Nature* 329:68, 1987.

116 Cease KB et al: Helper T-cell antigenic site identification in the acquired immunodeficiency syndrome virus gp120 envelope protein and induction of immunity in mice to the native protein using a 16-residue synthetic peptide. *Proc Natl Acad Sci USA* 84:4249, 1987.

117 Palker TJ et al: A conserved region at the COOH terminus of human immunodeficiency virus gp120 envelope protein contains an immunodominant epitope. *Proc Natl Acad Sci USA* 84:2479, 1987.

118 Wong-Staal F et al: Genomic diversity of human T-lymphotropic virus type III (HTLV-III). *Science* 229:759, 1985.

119 Hahn BH et al: Genetic variation in HTLV-III/LAV over time in patients with AIDS or at risk for AIDS. *Science* 232:1548, 1986.

120 Hu SL et al: Effect of immunization with a vaccinia-HIV *env* recombinant on HIV infection of chimpanzees. *Nature* 328:721, 1987.

121 Yarchoan R et al: AIDS therapies. *Sci Am* 259:110, 1988.

122 Walker BD et al: Inhibition of human immunodeficiency virus syncytium formation and virus replication by castanospermine. *Proc Natl Acad Sci USA* 84:8120, 1987.

123 Mitsuya H et al: Long-term inhibition of human T-lymphotropic virus type III/lymphadenopathy-associated virus (human immunodeficiency virus) DNA synthesis and RNA expression T cells protected by 2′,3′-dideoxynucleosides in vitro. *Proc Natl Acad Sci USA* 84:2033, 1987.

124 Sarin PS et al: Inhibition of HTLV-III/LAV replication by foscarnet. *Biochem Pharmacol* 34:4075, 1985.

125 Vogt MW et al: Ribavirin antagonizes the effect of azidothymidine on HIV replication. *Science* 235:1376, 1987.

126 Zamecnik PC et al: Inhibition of replication and expression of human T-cell lymphotropic virus type III in cultured cells by exogenous synthetic oligonucleotides complementary to viral RNA. *Proc Natl Acad Sci USA* 83:4143, 1986.

127 Montefiori DC et al: Antiviral activity of mismatched double-stranded RNA against human immunodeficiency virus in vitro. *Proc Natl Acad Sci USA* 84:2985, 1987.

128 Hammer SM et al: In vitro modification of human immunodeficiency virus infection by granulocyte-macrophage colony-stimulating factor and γ interferon. *Proc Natl Acad Sci USA* 83:8734, 1986.

129 Mitsuya H et al: Strategies for antiviral therapy in AIDS. *Nature* 325:773, 1987.

# Chapter 29

# Immunology of HIV infection

Scott Koenig
Anthony S. Fauci

## INTRODUCTION

The acquired immunodeficiency syndrome (AIDS) is caused by two distinct but related human retroviruses which have been named human immunodeficiency viruses I and II (HIV-1 and HIV-2). The vast majority of recognized cases of AIDS throughout the world are caused by HIV-1. HIV-1, originally called human T-cell lymphotropic (leukemia) virus type III (HTLV-III), lymphadenopathy-associated virus (LAV), and AIDS-related retrovirus (ARV), was first isolated from the peripheral blood and lymph nodes of patients with AIDS and AIDS-related complex (ARC) in the United States, Europe, and Central Africa.[1–5] It has become one of the most extensively studied viruses and within the class of retroviruses appears to be one of the most complex. HIV-1 contains an approximately 10-kilobase (kb) single-stranded RNA genome with at least nine known genes (see Chap. 28).[6,7] Three structural genes (*env, gag,* and *pol*) are complemented by six other genes (*tat, rev, vif, nef, vpr, vpu*), some of which have important regulatory functions. The envelope protein is a ligand for the CD4 molecule, the receptor for HIV, which is expressed most notably on a major population of lymphocytes that is critical for normal immune function. The regulatory proteins produced control viral replication and may affect expression of host cellular genes to alter normal cellular physiology and function.

Isolates of HIV-1 are typified by their marked heterogeneity, particularly within segments of the envelope region.[8] Yet despite these differences, all forms of HIV-1 appear to cause immunologic dysfunction and devastating clinical sequelae. Current projections are that approximately 30 percent of seropositive individuals will develop AIDS within 5 years of infection, with some predictions that all HIV-infected patients will eventually succumb to AIDS in the absence of effective antiretroviral therapy.[9] There are, however, HIV isolates that differ in their biological properties in vitro, particularly with respect to virulence, cytopathicity, and cellular tropism. It seems plausible that these differences might alter virulence in vivo and influence the resultant clinical outcome. The isolation of more cytopathic variants from individual patients with clinical progression over time supports this contention.[10] The emergence of new variants may occur as the result of point mutations in particular isolates or through recombination of different isolates to generate virions with different biological properties. With further molecular analysis and serologic classification of new variants, it may ultimately be possible to assign certain genotypes and serotypes to HIV-1 isolates and catalogue them in terms of their potential pathogenicity.

HIV-2[11,12] is another human retrovirus, originally called lymphadenopathy-associated virus 2, that was initially isolated from AIDS patients and healthy individuals in western Africa, and more recently from patients in Europe and the western hemisphere. Sera from these individuals showed only minimal reactivity against *gag*-associated proteins of HIV-1 and virtually no reactivity against the envelope proteins of HIV-1 in Western blots and radioimmunoprecipitation (RIP) assays. In contrast, serologic patterns against simian immunodeficiency virus (SIV) proteins were similar to those of sera from animals infected with the African green monkey and macaque isolates of SIV. These observations subsequently prompted the cloning and sequencing of this new AIDS-associated virus.[13] As expected, it was found to be distinct from SIV but structurally more related to it than to HIV-1. However, the HIV-2 isolates that have been characterized appear to be similar to HIV-1 in their biological and clinical properties.

Infection with HIV has been shown to occur by homosexual and heterosexual contact, through blood or blood components, or by maternal-fetal transmission (see Chap. 31). Although rare individuals have been shown to develop a severe, acute illness following infection, the majority of patients either develop a mild mononucleosis-like disorder or are asymptomatic upon initial infection. As a result of this acute infection, an individual usually mounts a detectable immune response to HIV within several weeks manifested by the development of antibodies to the various protein components of HIV; this production of antibody serves as the principal means of detecting infection in a patient. For some, a period of over a year may elapse before an HIV-specific humoral immune response can be detected by currently available technology. While different serologic patterns may emerge in a given individual, the most frequent course of a serologic response is the development of antibodies to the core or *gag* proteins followed by a response to the *env* components (see Chap. 79). A transient antibody response to the *nef* gene product may appear before the responses to the *gag* and *env* proteins (A. Ranki, unpublished observation). Following serologic conversion, the clinical syndrome of AIDS may develop after a long variable time course. In advanced disease, humoral responses may wane and loss of responses to *gag* or other HIV proteins may occur.

While a complete understanding of the pathogenesis of AIDS has not emerged, certain observations in the clinic and laboratory have been documented that provide a framework for elucidating pathogenic mechanisms. A central feature to the development of AIDS is the loss of competency of the immune system as the result of infection with HIV. Immune impairment may be derived from depletion of cellular components or through their altered function. Although all components of the immune system are at least indirectly affected by infection with HIV, the loss of a competent inducer T-cell compartment results in the most devastating clinical consequences in adults. These individuals may succumb to a panoply of opportunistic infectious agents requiring T-cell immunity for their containment (see Chap. 30). The most notable include certain viruses, fungi, mycobacteria, and protozoa.[14,15] *Pneumocystis carinii* pneumonia (PCP) is caused by the pathogen most frequently associated with mortality in AIDS patients, a complex organism which was originally thought to be a protozoon, but which has been shown recently to be related to fungi.[16] The reasons for the predominance of this organism above all others in causing morbidity for HIV-infected patients in this country are elusive. Similarly, while there is a general assumption that the immune system plays an important role against neoplastic transformation, the reason why particular tumors such as Kaposi's sarcoma and B-cell lymphoma occur is unclear. The development of these tumors is certainly influenced by factors other than a breakdown in immune surveillance and may include mechanisms such as the induction of particular growth factors by HIV, expression or induction of an oncogene, or coinfection with other oncogenic pathogens. A recent study has described the development of vascular dermal sarcomas in transgenic mice expressing the HIV-1 *tat* gene, suggesting a role for this single HIV gene in the etiology of Kaposi's sarcoma.[17]

The initial competency or stage of development of a patient's immune system at the time of infection with HIV may influence subsequent clinical manifestations. Newborn populations infected with HIV are at particular risk of developing bacterial infections since they do not have the advantage of having developed preformed humoral immunity to common bacterial pathogens. Therapeutic intervention with prophylactic systemic immunoglobulin has resulted in a more favorable clinical outcome in these pediatric AIDS patients.

The goal of this chapter is to provide an understanding of the manner in which HIV can affect immune function and how disruption of the immune system may contribute to the development of AIDS.

## LYMPHOCYTE TROPISM OF HIV

The first major advance in AIDS research was the ability to isolate the etiologic agent of this disorder. This was achieved by coculturing peripheral blood mononuclear cells (PBMCs) and lymph node cells from patients with phytohemagglutinin (PHA)-stimulated PBMCs from healthy individuals. Lymphoblasts that expressed the CD4 molecule on their surface were identified as the subpopulation that could support viral growth.[18–20] Similarly, human tumor cell lines bearing the CD4 molecule also could be infected with the virus, while T cell lines that did not express CD4 were not susceptible to infection.

The selectivity of HIV for CD4-bearing cells is the result of the binding of the viral envelope protein to the CD4 molecule, which serves as the receptor for the virus (Fig. 29-1).[21] The importance of this molecule was originally suggested by the observation that antibodies to some, but not all, of the determinants of CD4 can block infection with HIV.[22] Antibodies to CD4 which recognize epitopes that are not within the binding site (e.g., OKT4) can be used to coprecipitate the CD4 molecule and HIV envelope.[21] Human cell lines which normally do not express CD4 and cannot be infected with HIV can be rendered susceptible to the virus by transfecting the gene for CD4 and inducing CD4 expression.[23] Other cell surface receptors besides CD4 may need to be concomitantly expressed. This is suggested by the observation that expression of human CD4 in a murine cell line did not generate a permissive cell line for HIV, even though this cell line could support HIV replication through the transfection of an infectious DNA clone of HIV. One such protein may facilitate the fusion between HIV envelope and cell membrane proteins. The critical role of CD4 expression with respect to the permissiveness of T cells for HIV infection is further substantiated by the ability of soluble forms of the CD4 molecule to prevent infection of cells with HIV.[24] Consequently, the soluble form of the CD4 molecule is currently being examined for its efficacy in inhibiting infection in patients. Several recent reports have identified the particular regions within the amino-terminal portion of the CD4 molecule that bind to gp120.[25,26] Of interest is the observation that while many of the known monoclonal antibodies to CD4 can prevent binding of HIV, none exclusively recognizes the specific epitope to which the envelope protein binds (Q. Satentau, unpublished observations).

At least one site near the carboxy end of the gp120 envelope molecule has been determined to be involved in binding to CD4,[27] although other regions within the gp120 and gp41 proteins may participate in binding as well. Frame-shift mutations generated in both amino- and carboxy-terminal regions of the gp120 envelope protein have impaired envelope binding to the CD4 molecule.[28] Similarly, defects in processing of the precursor envelope molecule gp160 to gp120 and gp41 interfere with amino-terminal envelope binding. A block in envelope processing may prevent some critical regions involved in viral fusion from gaining access to the cell membrane. Fusion proteins have been shown to be important in the infectivity of paramyxoviruses, and conserved amino acid sequences from the fusion regions of measles and respiratory syncytial virus are found within the transmembrane portions of HIV-1 and HIV-2. In addition, antibodies that block fusion of visna, a lentivirus which infects sheep, can prevent in vitro infection of ovine monocytes (O. Narayan, unpublished observation).

Infection of cells with HIV is accompanied by the loss of CD4 expression and is not associated with significant losses of other cell membrane–associated proteins. With HIV binding there may be transient initial modulation of CD4 which does not appear to be associated with phosphorylation and endocytosis of the CD4 molecule. Phosphorylation and endocytosis of CD4 are observed when cells are treated with either phorbol esters (TPA) or antigen. In one experimental system, mutation of the CD4 gene that re-

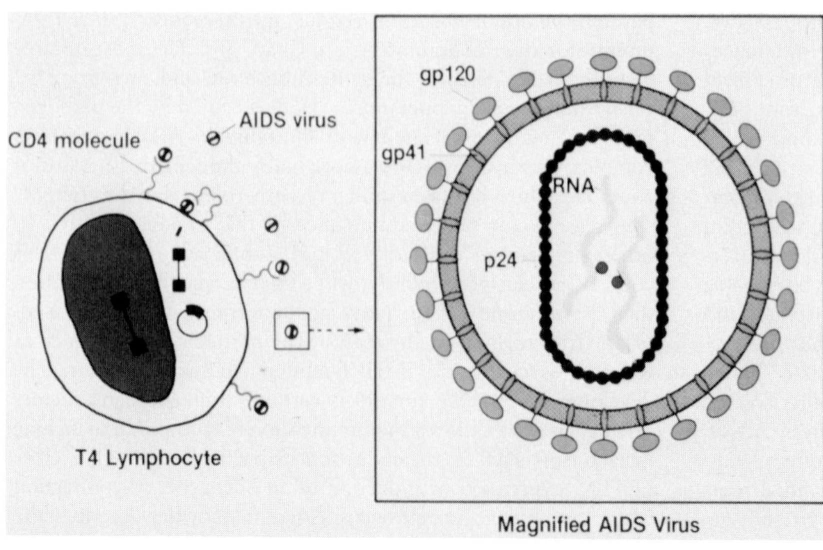


**Fig. 29-1.** Interaction between HIV envelope proteins and the CD4 molecule on T lymphocytes.

sulted in the expression of CD4 which lacked its cytoplasmic tail and thus prevented TPA-induced endocytosis did not impair HIV infection.[29] It is therefore likely that viral entry is dependent on membrane fusion without endocytosis of CD4. The persistent loss of CD4 expression with active HIV replication may be due to a decrease in CD4 mRNA expression and protein production, or to the formation of intracytoplasmic complexes between CD4 and HIV envelope protein that prevent transport of CD4 to the membrane surface.[30]

HIV is cytopathic for CD4-bearing cells although susceptibility may vary among CD4-bearing tumor lines. In vitro cytopathic effects may be manifested by the formation of syncytia, fragile multinucleated forms with engorged cytoplasm, that erupt and release viral and cellular contents. Under experimental conditions, these syncytia develop through fusion of infected cells expressing the HIV envelope and uninfected cells displaying the CD4 molecule (Fig. 29-2).[31–34] Multinucleated giant cells containing HIV have been seen in vivo in brain tissue[35] and lymph nodes,[36] but it is unclear if these multinucleated cells form in a manner analogous to the formation of syncytia observed in vitro or contribute to CD4-cell losses in vivo. Not all the cellular losses observed in vitro are attributable to syncytia formation, since HIV infection of some cell lines can result in marked cellular senescence in the absence of significant syncytia formation. MT-4, an HTLV-I-transformed cell line, is an example of one such line that is particularly susceptible to the cytopathic effects of HIV but forms few syncytia. This implies that several mechanisms may be responsible for the cytopathic properties of HIV (see below). In one study, in vitro cytopathic properties of HIV-1 correlated with the density of CD4 expression on tumor cell lines, with more substantial cell loss observed in those lines with the highest expression.[30] However, others have seen marked cytopathicity of HIV-1 in some cell lines even in the presence of modest CD4 expression. This suggests that the magnitude of infection and cytopathic properties may be influenced by a number of factors including CD4 membrane density, the activation state of the cell, and the level of expression of certain factors[37] (e.g., NFkB) which can influence viral transcription or translation.

The in vitro cytopathic effects of HIV on $CD4^+$ lymphocytes may parallel laboratory observations made on the circulating peripheral blood lymphocytes in AIDS patients. The hallmark of the syndrome and the immunologic defect is the depletion of circulating $CD4^+$ lymphocytes. This population defines the subset of T cells that serves as the functional helper and inducer cells in an immune response. A subset of $CD4^+$ lymphocytes can function also as specific cytotoxic cells, particularly in response to infection with certain viruses.

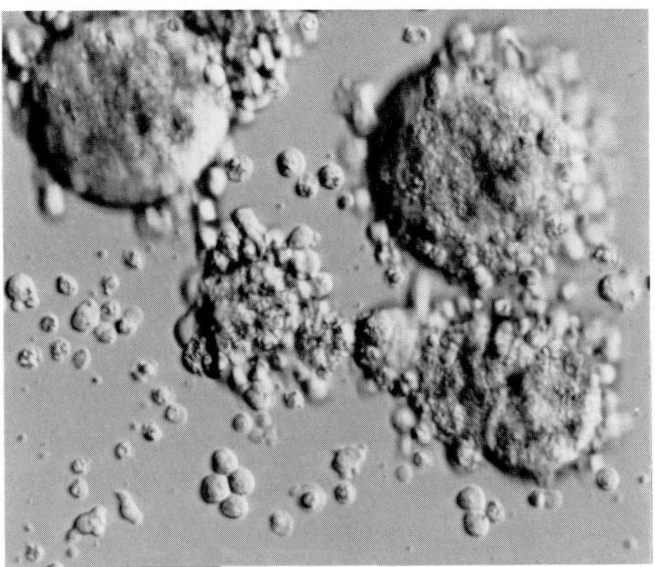

**Fig. 29-2.** Syncytia formation by HIV-envelope-expressing lymphocytes and CD4-bearing tumor cells. (*Photograph by C. Fox.*)

Normally, $CD4^+$ cells recognize and respond to antigen in association with a major histocompatibility protein on "presenting" cells such as monocytes and dendritic cells, and recruit and stimulate other T cells and B cells in the production of a cellular or humoral response, respectively. The initial step in the stimulation of the antigen-specific $CD4^+$ lymphocyte is the binding of a "processed" form of the antigen in association with the class II histocompatibility molecule by the antigen-specific receptor (TCR). The TCR is structurally and functionally associated with another group of proteins called the CD3 complex. In the presence of interleukin-1 (IL-1) produced by macrophages, these $CD4^+$ cells elaborate IL-2, express a high-affinity form of the IL-2 receptor on their surface, and proliferate. Part of the inductive capacity of the $CD4^+$ population for other cell types is due to this production of IL-2, a stimulant for T cells, B cells, and natural killer (NK) cells. Other lymphokines produced by $CD4^+$ lymphocytes, such as gamma interferon (γ-IFN), IL-4, and tumor necrosis factor (TNF-β), have stimulatory properties on other cell types as well. Thus, with the multiple functions performed and regulated by the CD4 cell, loss of the CD4 population can have dire functional consequences on the immune system.

The severity of $CD4^+$-lymphocyte depletion somewhat correlates with the clinical disorder in HIV-seropositive individuals (see Chap. 30). Patients with a history of opportunistic infection (OI), usually PCP, characteristically have the lowest number of $CD4^+$ cells.[38–41] In fact, individuals without a clinical history of OI and extremely low $CD4^+$-lymphocyte counts (0–200/mm$^3$) are at imminent risk for developing AIDS with OI. The rate of $CD4^+$ lymphocyte loss varies greatly among patients. Initial losses during the primary infection may be partially reconstituted, and many years of clinical latency may evolve into periods of gradual and progressive attrition of $CD4^+$ lymphocytes or episodes of precipitous decline in these cell counts. HIV antigenemia may be present prior to seroconversion and during periods of marked $CD4^+$-cell loss (see Chap. 79).

Early clinical studies suggested that some $CD4^+$ subsets may be preferentially depleted in some HIV-infected groups. Certain subsets of $CD4^+$ cells have been defined by the presence of other coexpressed cell surface antigens. For example, one group reported preferential loss of $CD4^+Leu8^+$ cells in lymphadenopathy patients,[42] an observation which was not universally made.[43] The CD4 subset which may function as an "inducer" of T helper cells, and has been defined by the monoclonal antibody 4B4, may be the population that is especially susceptible to HIV infection and depletion, since it is one of the first T cells to be activated in the generation of the specific immune response. However, selective loss of $4B4^+$ T cells in AIDS patients was not observed in one report. In an experimental model of simian immunodeficiency involving a lentivirus that induces an AIDS-like disorder in macaques this $4B4^+$ $CD4^+$ T-cell population was found to be preferentially lost during infection (R. Desrosiers, unpublished observation). Future prospective examinations of the phenotypes of circulating lymphocytes in high-risk HIV-seronegative individuals and T-cell subpopulation changes that develop after seroconversion should help to clarify this issue.

In addition to the direct cytopathic effects of HIV on $CD4^+$

lymphocytes observed in the in vitro models of infection, other mechanisms may contribute to the CD4⁺-lymphocyte depletion observed in vivo. It has been found that at any given point in time, one cell in $10^4$ to $10^6$ PBMCs in the circulation is expressing HIV RNA.[44] While this figure may slightly underestimate the total number of infected cells due to technical limitations in virion detection in the reported studies, it would seem that the bone marrow reserves should be able to compensate for this degree of $CD4^+$-cell loss. Impairment of normal marrow differentiation could result from HIV infection of lymphocyte precursors or other critical cell populations that regulate lymphoid differentiation. In one study, in vitro T-cell colony formation of bone marrow from AIDS patients has been found to be depressed.[45] Others have reported that the growth of colony-forming units of granulocytes/monocytes (CFU-GM) and erythroid burst-forming units (BFU-E) in bone marrow from AIDS patients was impaired when cultured in the presence of sera from HIV-infected individuals. HIV could be isolated from some of these bone marrow specimens as well.[46] A recent study has demonstrated that $CD34^+$ cells, progenitor cells for the monocytic series, can be infected in vitro with HIV.[47] Therefore, direct infection of precursor cells and immune responses to HIV-infected bone marrow cells may thwart normal marrow function.

Several autoimmune mechanisms have been proposed to cause CD4-lymphocyte depletion.[48,49] Since the CD4 molecule serves as a receptor for both HIV and class II molecules, it has been hypothesized that during the course of the normal immune response to HIV, both a cross-reactive and cytopathic response against class II–bearing cells and an anti-idiotypic humoral response against CD4-bearing cells might occur. While autoantibodies are present in infected individuals, these cytopathic effects have not been demonstrated. A small percentage of HIV-seropositive individuals have been found to generate anti-CD4 antibodies; however, the vast majority of these antibodies are not anti-idiotypic and in one study appeared to be directed against the carboxy terminus of the CD4 molecule (J. Sodrowski et al., unpublished report). Experimentally, anti-idiotypic antibodies generated against monoclonal antibodies that recognize the T4a epitope (which blocks HIV infection) can bind to HIV, albeit weakly, since the monoclonal antibodies recognizing the T4a epitope are situated close to, but not directly at, the site of HIV-envelope binding (Q. Sattentau, unpublished observations).

Autoimmune responses may be generated against neoantigens or activation antigens in chronically infected patients. In one study, an activation antigen with a molecular weight of 18,000 has been identified on PHA-activated $CD4^+$ lymphocytes, and sera from the majority of HIV-seropositive individuals contained antibody which could recognize these cells.[50] Further investigations are necessary to define this antigen and correlate its appearance with CD4 depletion. An interesting observation reported recently is that HIV envelope-specific $CD4^+$ cytotoxic T cells from HIV-seronegative individuals could lyse uninfected activated $CD4^+$ cells that process recombinant gp120 envelope protein.[51,52] $CD8^+$ cells could not process the recombinant protein. This suggests an alternative mechanism for CD4-cell depletion that is not directly dependent on an active HIV infection of the susceptible cells. For this mechanism to significantly contribute to $CD4^+$-cell loss in vivo, either large numbers of $CD4^+$ envelope-specific cytotoxic T lymphocytes (CTLs) would need to be generated in patients, or already processed soluble envelope antigen would need to be presented in association with class I histocompatibility proteins for recognition by $CD8^+$ HIV envelope-specific CTLs.

On the other hand, either processed or nonprocessed secreted envelope proteins bound to $CD4^+$ HIV-infected cells could be recognized by circulating envelope-specific antibodies in the sera of infected patients. $CD16^+$ NK cells could bind to the Fc region of these antibodies and lyse uninfected $CD4^+$ cells in a manner irrespective of major histocompatibility complex (MHC) proteins. The latter process is called antibody-dependent cellular cytotoxicity (ADCC). $CD16^+$ cells with lytic activity against target cells binding gp120 in vitro have been characterized in a majority of healthy seropositive individuals and may mediate cytolysis by this mechanism.[53]

## INFECTION OF MACROPHAGES WITH HIV

While early in vitro studies of the cytopathic effects of HIV on T cells appeared to correlate with the in vivo findings of $CD4^+$-cell depletion, there were some concurrent observations that indicated that infection of other cell types may occur. Armstrong et al.[54] first demonstrated infection of follicular dendritic cells by electron microscopy in a patient with lymphadenopathy, and Belsito and colleagues[55] noted reduced numbers of Langerhans cells in the skin of AIDS patients. Both these cell types function in antigen presentation in their respective organ systems, and, at least in the case of Langerhans cells, CD4 antigen can be detected on the surface of these cells. Macrophages, which can express the CD4 protein and serve to process antigen in the circulation and tissues, thus seemed to be a likely candidate for infection with HIV. Initially, it was found that tumor cell lines of the monocyte lineage could support the growth of HIV.[56] It was then reported that purified populations of PBMCs from HIV-seronegative patients could be infected with a T-cell-derived HIV isolate and, furthermore, that HIV could be detected in similar adherent non-T-cell populations from HIV-seropositive individuals.[57–59] The importance of infection of monocytes and macrophages in vivo was highlighted by the observation that this is the predominant cell type found in brain tissue in HIV-infected individuals with encephalopathy. This has been demonstrated through viral isolation and by in situ hybridization, immunohistochemical, and electron microscopic techniques.[60–63] HIV isolates derived from brain tissue have been successfully passaged in peripheral blood macrophages, and it appears that such viral isolates preferentially, but not exclusively, replicate in macrophages. Likewise, it was reported in one of the studies that HIV isolates passaged successively through T cells would not propagate in macrophages derived from the peripheral blood.[59]

HIV-1 isolates with different cellular affinities and growth patterns may be derived from individual patients. For example, one group of investigators reported that an HIV isolate obtained from a brain biopsy differed from an isolate obtained from the same patient's cerebrospinal fluid (CSF) in biological and structural properties.[64] The CSF-derived isolate could be passaged in monocytes while the brain-biopsy-derived HIV isolate could not. Restriction-enzyme analysis of these two isolates demonstrated unique patterns. Recent observations of HIV infection of monocytes using monocyte-colony-stimulating factor (M-CSF) in vitro support the concept that particular isolates may have a proclivity to infect certain types of cells and replicate in a manner different from what has been described for T cells. For instance, in one study, the replication of isolates derived from the PBMCs of AIDS patients repeatedly passaged in macrophages showed a pattern of membrane-associated virions budding within vesicles in the cytoplasm.[65] These cells showed few particles budding from the cell surface. Similar observations were made following the in vitro infection of bone marrow precursor cells committed to differentiation into cells of the monocyte/macrophage lineage[47] (Fig. 29-3). Whether or not this growth pattern is peculiar to these in vitro conditions is unclear. If similar patterns of replication occur in vivo, an explosive release of virions may occur by the activation of HIV-infected macrophages. Cells that predominantly or exclusively replicate HIV within the cytoplasm may be partially sequestered from host immune defenses, and this may be a means by which viral persistence is achieved.

## HIV INFECTION OF OTHER CELLS

There have been isolated reports that other cells may support the growth of HIV. The evidence has included the use of tumor cell lines propagated in vitro with some of the characteristics of normal tissue as well the in situ detection of HIV in biopsy and autopsy specimens from seropositive individuals. The role of HIV infection in these tissue types in the pathogenesis of AIDS or in dysfunction of particular organ systems is unclear. Cell types reported to be subject to infection with HIV include endothelial cells,[61] cervical cells,[66] colorectal cells,[67] argentaffin cells,[68] retinal cells,[69] transformed B cells,[70] and bone-marrow-derived circulating dendritic cells.[71] Some, but not all, of these cell types have been shown to express either CD4 mRNA or CD4 protein.

## ACTIVATION OF LATENT HIV INFECTION

Productive infection of T cells with HIV in vitro or viral isolation from PBMCs of HIV-infected patients requires cell activation. Some experiments indicated that HIV replication could be induced in latently infected cells following exposure of the cells in vitro to PHA.[2,18,72] For individuals infected with HIV, antigenic stimulation experienced in their normal environment might induce a similar response. In one group of experiments, it was demonstrated that when PBMCs derived from HIV-uninfected individuals had been activated by antigen (such as the soluble antigens tetanus toxoid and keyhole limpet hemocyanin) prior to

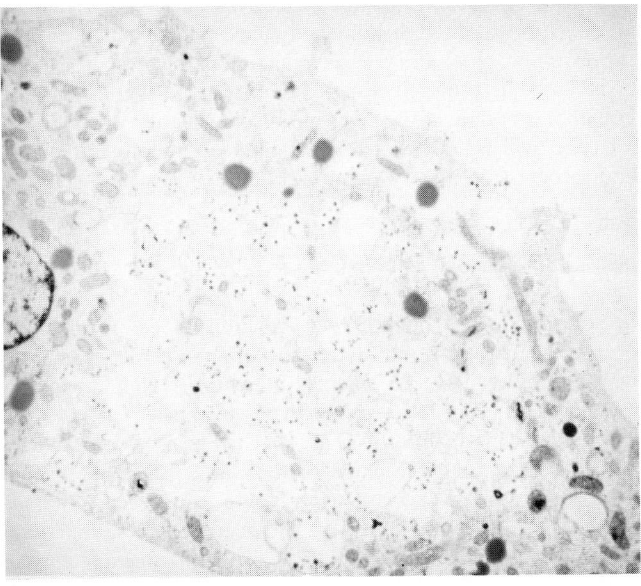

A

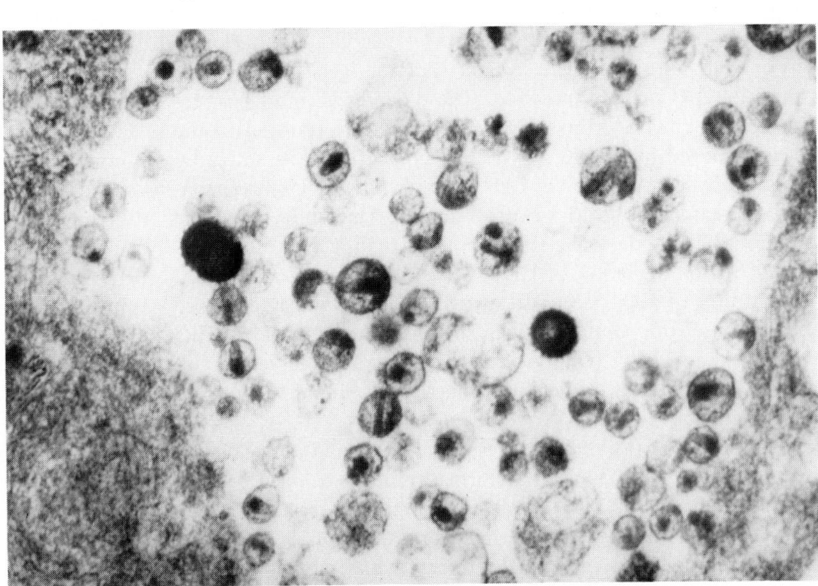

B

**Fig. 29-3.** Infection of bone marrow cells with HIV. (*A*) Low- and (*B*) high-power magnification of HIV particles within intracytoplasmic vesicles. (*Electron micrograph by J. Orenstein.*)

exposure to HIV, they were 10 to 100 times more susceptible to viral replication than PBMCs that had been preincubated without antigen.[73]

Concurrent infections with viral pathogens such as cytomegalovirus (CMV), Epstein-Barr virus (EBV), hepatitis B, and herpes simplex virus may activate latent HIV and induce viral expression in those individuals infected with HIV. This may occur through the activation of cells involved in specific immune response to these viruses or through the production of non-HIV viral-specific products that may influence HIV replication. It has been shown in vitro that HIV expression can be upregulated in cells following transfection of HIV-infected cells with DNA from heterologous viruses or by cotransfection of full-length infectious HIV clones with heterologous genes from DNA viruses[74–77] (see Chap. 36).

In addition to mitogens, antigens, and viruses, cytokines that are elaborated in the normal immune response appear to play a role in the induction of productive HIV infection from a latent or low-level chronic infection. Studies using chronically infected cell lines indicated that a variety of cytokines, including granulocyte/macrophage-colony-stimulating factor (GM-CSF) and tumor necrosis factor (TNF)-α, can produce cellular inductive signals with consequent upregulation of HIV infection.[78,79] Further investigation of this phenomenon suggests that enhanced HIV expression by cytokines reflects induction of the promotor region of HIV by the transactivating effect of a DNA-binding protein. Full understanding of the mechanisms of activation of latent HIV infection will be essential for attempts to develop strategies to limit progression of HIV-induced disease.

## IMMUNE DEFECTS IN T CELLS

In addition to the quantitative depletion of T4 lymphocytes, prominent qualitative or functional immunologic abnormalities may be observed in HIV-infected individuals. This impairment may be detected in HIV-seropositive individuals even at a stage when significant quantitative losses of CD4-bearing cells have not been observed. Unfractionated PBMCs from AIDS patients may manifest profound decreases in response to mitogens, alloantigens, and soluble antigens.[80–82] The degree of these functional changes is variable, but depression of T-cell function appears more pronounced in AIDS patients with opportunistic infections than in individuals with other HIV-related conditions.

PBMCs from AIDS patients frequently exhibit a diminution in response to mitogens such as pokeweed mitogen (PWM), concanavalin A (Con A), and PHA. These depressed mitogenic responses by PBMCs from AIDS patients can be restored to the levels achieved by PBMC cultures of control subjects solely by using equivalent numbers of $CD4^+$ lymphocytes in cultures from AIDS patients and healthy control donors. This implies that the functional T-cell defect in the response to mitogen is intimately related to the depletion of $CD4^+$ T cells. However, similar reconstitution of $CD4^+$ cells from AIDS patients did not restore the response to a soluble antigen such as tetanus toxoid.[80] This suggests that $CD4^+$ lymphocytes responsive to soluble antigen are either selectively depleted or functionally impaired in these AIDS patients.

This defect in proliferation response to soluble antigen does not appear to be due to an abnormality in the antigen presentation required for such responses. Studies performed with PBMCs of identical twins, in which one sibling had AIDS and the other was healthy and HIV-seronegative, demonstrated that monocytes from the seronegative twin were incapable of reconstituting a defective tetanus toxoid response of $CD4^+$ lymphocytes from the twin with AIDS. This defect could not be explained by the presence of suppressor cells in the AIDS patient, since no depression in responsiveness was seen when PBMCs from the AIDS patient were mixed with PBMCs from the healthy twin (S. Koenig, unpublished observations).

In support of this qualitative defect in proliferative responses to soluble antigen, a large proportion of a cohort of asymptomatic, HIV-seropositive homosexual men exhibited an absence of a response to tetanus toxoid, including individuals with normal numbers of circulating $CD4^+$ cells.[83] A similar defect has also been seen with other test antigens[84] and most likely reflects abnormalities across the spectrum of the antigen-specific T-cell repertoire. In a prospective study of the proliferative responses of individual healthy HIV-seropositive individuals to soluble antigens, mitogens, and alloantigens, loss of response to the soluble protein of influenza was invariably one of the first immune defects observed (G. Shearer, unpublished observation). If the lack of responsiveness to soluble proteins reflects the selective depletion of antigen-responsive cells, one would expect a more global quantitative loss of the $CD4^+$ cells accompanying this functional abnormality, and this is not observed. Because the decreased response to soluble antigen appears early in the course of HIV infection, and even in those individuals with circulating $CD4^+$ lymphocyte counts in the normal range, a functional impairment of T4 cells may represent a critical initial step in the progressive immune defects seen with HIV infection.

There is some in vitro evidence of functional abnormalities of T4 cells caused by exposure to HIV or viral products in the absence of a productive or cytopathic infection. In one study,[73] exposure of PBMCs stimulated in vitro with a soluble antigen in the presence of noncytopathic concentrations of HIV resulted in a marked inhibition of proliferation responses to soluble antigens and, to a lesser extent, to mitogens. Other studies[85] have shown that certain purified subunits of HIV, particularly gp120 envelope protein, could inhibit antigen-specific responses when exposed to lymphocytes, even though they would be incapable of producing infection. In the setting of an active HIV infection, discrete cell-activation pathways have been shown to be selectively inhibited.[86]

Several potential mechanisms could explain the impairment of T4-cell function with exposure to HIV in the absence of a productive HIV infection. Antigen-specific responses of T4 cells require the interaction of the CD4 molecule expressed on the surface of the T4 cells with the class II MHC molecule situated on the antigen-presenting cell. In addition, antigen, in conjunction with class II molecules, binds to the CD3-Ti antigen receptor complex on T lymphocytes. It is conceivable that HIV envelope binds avidly to the CD4 molecule on the T4 cell and could interfere with the normal interaction of the CD4 molecule with the class II MHC molecule on the antigen-presenting cell.[87,88] As responses of T4 cells to mitogens are probably not dependent on interaction of the CD4 and class II MHC molecules, the cellular activation pathway of mitogen stimulation could bypass this step and induce an essentially normal proliferative response in cells rendered refractory to antigenic stimulation. This would be consistent with the observations noted earlier of normal mitogen responses under certain circumstances in which a selective defect in antigen responses is seen.

Another possibility is that exposure of T cells to HIV or its products might cause a postreceptor signal transduction defect that mitogen, but not antigen, can at least partially override. Since the triggering of cells by soluble antigens and mitogens occurs through different pathways,[89] it is possible that envelope binding to the CD4 molecule may preferentially impair the antigen-specific pathway. It has recently been observed that HIV-infected T cells have a defect in the calcium mobilization necessary for activation when they are stimulated through the CD3-Ti complex but not through the CD2-dependent pathway.[86]

IL-2 has an important role in the generation of T-cell activation and response. In the absence of adequate IL-2 or the expression of its receptor, T cells will not divide. A functional defect in IL-2 or IL-2 receptor gene expression may contribute to functional abnormalities observed in AIDS patients.[90] Some, but not all, reports have demonstrated decreased IL-2 production by PBMCs from AIDS patients.

In addition to the deficiencies noted in proliferative responses to antigen, AIDS patients demonstrate impaired cytotoxic responses.[91–93] For instance, depressed HLA class I restricted CTL responses against CMV and influenza have been observed in patients early in the course of their disease. This depressed function involves responses mediated by CD8$^+$ cells, which typically are not infected with HIV, suggesting that another component of the immune system must be involved in the response. Although directly mediated by CD8$^+$ cells, MHC class I restricted CTL activity is characteristically dependent on an intact CD4$^+$ cell inducer function. The observed impairment of this response no doubt reflects CD4$^+$ cell dysfunction. This implies that the reconstitution of appropriate CD4$^+$ cell function should ameliorate this cytotoxic defect if the effector function of CD8$^+$ cells is intact. Supporting this notion, in vitro T-cell-mediated cytotoxicity to CMV was restored with the addition of IL-2,[94] possibly by bypassing the required CD4$^+$ inductive signals. In addition, CD8$^+$ cytotoxic responses against alloantigens appear to be relatively preserved early in the course of HIV infection, although they may be impaired in more progressive disease. In this regard, CD4$^+$ cells are thought not to be necessary for induction of alloreactive responses.

## IMMUNE DEFECTS IN MACROPHAGES

It is now well established that monocytes and macrophages can be infected with HIV and play an important role in the pathogenesis of HIV infection. The virus can infect cells of the monocyte/macrophage lineage through attachment to the CD4 molecule expressed on the surface of certain subsets of the cells, or via phagocytosis. Recently, antibody-mediated enhancement of HIV infection has been demonstrated in vitro in the U937 cell line,[95] probably by an Fc-receptor-dependent pathway. Virus can be isolated from monocytes and macrophages in the blood and various organs of HIV-infected individuals. An important difference between HIV infection of monocytes and T lymphocytes is that monocytes are relatively refractory to the cytopathic effects of the virus. Persistence of HIV infection in monocytes thus may help to explain the inability of an HIV-specific immune response to clear the body of virus. Furthermore, because HIV-infected monocytes are found in the circulation, these cells may be responsible for disseminating the virus to various parts of the body including the brain, the lung, and perhaps the bone marrow.

Although many monocyte activities appear to be preserved in AIDS patients, a number of functional abnormalities of these cells have also been reported, including defective chemotaxis and killing of particular microorganisms. Certain of these abnormalities may reflect direct infection of monocytes by HIV. However, given the relatively low number of infected circulating monocytes, it is more likely that epiphenomena, as a consequence of HIV infection, contribute to these measured abnormalities. Some of the functional defects observed in monocyte function may reflect deficient inductive signals from CD4$^+$ cells. For example, γ-IFN produced by normal CD4$^+$ cells is capable of reconstituting certain defective functions of monocytes, although following prolonged courses of intravenous γ-IFN, impaired monocyte respiratory burst activity persists in these AIDS patients.

Chemotaxis is the monocyte function most frequently observed to be impaired in HIV-infected patients.[96,97] Yet, this defect is not necessarily specific to HIV infection, since many patients chronically ill from other viral and malignant disorders also have depressed chemotactic responses. Reports from many studies indicate that a range of functions appear to remain intact in monocytes derived from HIV-infected patients. These include phagocytic activity,[98] ADCC,[97] tumoricidal activity,[99] cytotoxicity against *Toxoplasma gondii* and *Chlamydia psittaci* in response to γ-IFN,[100] and fungicidal activity against *Aspergillus fumigatus*, *Cryptococcus neoformans*, and *Thermoascus crustaceus*,[98] as well as *Candida*.[101] Slight impairment of C3-receptor-mediated clearance of autologous red cells has been reported in AIDS patients, although this was seen in other infected patients without AIDS.[102]

Macrophages from AIDS patients also appear to function normally in soluble-antigen presentation, in both syngeneic and MHC-class-II-compatible systems. Minimal differences have been observed in soluble-antigen presentation by circulating monocytes using highly enriched cell populations derived from AIDS patients and their healthy identical twins. Similar results have been found by others using MHC-class-II-compatible presenting cells.[103] In one report, decreased expression of class II antigens was observed on monocytes of patients with AIDS.[104] In another study, a higher proportion of HIV-infected lymphadenopathy patients, compared with normal individuals, demonstrated a low proliferative response to anti-T3 antibody. This impairment was corrected by the addition of normal allogeneic macrophages, suggesting that accessory-cell function in this T-cell-dependent response was defective.[105] In the experimental setting exposing macrophages to supernatants containing HIV, impaired antigen presentation has been observed in vitro (H. Mitsuya, unpublished observations). This defect may be due to infection of the macrophages with HIV, may be caused by a particular HIV protein, or a factor induced by HIV in the cell lines used. In vivo, in a focus of active viral replication (e.g., lymph node), defective antigen presentation by infected macrophages may contribute to impairment of a local immune response.

HIV infection may directly and/or indirectly influence secretion of monokines such as IL-1[106] and TNF. Although it has generally been felt that IL-1 production and secretion by monocytes are relatively preserved, some findings suggest that inhibitors of IL-1 may be present in the circulation of AIDS patients. These issues, and their clinical significance, need further clarification.

HIV infection of monocytes and macrophages in the brain is associated with neuropsychiatric abnormalities ranging from the asymptomatic state to meningoencephalitis and dementia, and occurs in about 60 percent of HIV-infected individuals (see Chap. 30). Several mechanisms involving monocytes and macrophages have been proposed that may contribute to the pathology of dementia in AIDS patients.[107] Infected monocytes and macrophages may release chemotactic factors that lead to the infiltration of the brain with inflammatory cells. Alternatively, activated and infected macrophages may release factors that are toxic for the growth of neurons or can stimulate glial cells. Reactive glial cells have been found in intimate contact with macrophages in the brains of AIDS patients.

It has been observed in vitro that the HIV envelope protein can inhibit neuronal growth.[108] A putative nerve growth factor, neuroleukin, has been implicated in this process. One proposed pathogenic mechanism involves a partial sequence homology between HIV gp120 and neuroleukin, and suggests that HIV envelope could compete for binding to the growth factor receptor on neurons and inhibit neuroleukin-induced neuronal growth. Recently, peptide sequences derived from other regions of HIV have been reported to inhibit developing neurons from murine spinal cord in vitro.[109] Whether infected macrophages or other cells in the central nervous system release concentrations of viral envelope sufficient to inhibit the growth of human neurons in vivo needs further assessment.

## IMMUNE DEFECTS IN B CELLS

B-cell function and humoral immunity are markedly abnormal in patients with AIDS. Beyond the consequences of deficient numbers of CD4$^+$ T helper cells in initiating specific antibody production, intrinsic B-cell physiology and activity are altered in HIV-infected individuals. AIDS patients characteristically develop polyclonal B-cell activation, manifested by hypergammaglobulinemia, spontaneous B-cell proliferation, and increased spontaneous secretion of immunoglobulin in vitro.[13,14,110–115] In symptomatic individuals, serum levels of IgG, IgA, and IgD are elevated,[110–112,115] with more variable changes noted in IgM. Generally IgM levels appear to be relatively normal in adults with AIDS; either IgM hypergammaglobulinemia or IgM hypogammaglobulinemia may be found in pediatric AIDS patients.[114]

In contrast to the increased spontaneous activity noted in B cells from AIDS patients, antigen-specific and -nonspecific B-cell responses are impaired.[110] In vitro proliferative responses to antigens and mitogens are decreased, as is PWM-induced immunoglobulin synthesis.[113] In vivo responses of AIDS patients to primary and secondary immunizations are poor with reduced specific antibody production to both protein and polysaccharide antigens.[110,116] An inability to mount an adequate IgM response to antigenic challenge is an obvious and clinically significant humoral defect. The consequences are most debilitating in HIV-infected infants and children who have not previously been exposed to a variety of pathogenic bacterial organisms and must rely on a primary initial IgM response for immune protection. Certain adult AIDS patients also appear to have an increased susceptibility to certain pyogenic bacteria, which in part reflects defective humoral responses.[117]

The polyclonal hyperactivity of the B-cell limb of the immune response in AIDS patients may be induced by multiple factors. Several well-established polyclonal B-cell activators such as EBV and CMV frequently are found to coinfect this patient population and may contribute to this observed phenomenon.[115,118] Despite the apparent inability of HIV to directly infect normal, untransformed B cells, the effects of viral proteins on B-cell activity may account for some of the observed in vivo changes. Both intact infectious HIV and disrupted viral particles induce polyclonal activation of normal B cells with proliferative responses and immunoglobulin synthesis comparable to that of other B-cell mitogens.[115,118,119] Recently, peptides synthesized from HIV published sequences caused comparable responses.[120] Whether these responses reflect direct effects solely on B cells, or require T cells to secrete soluble factors or to "present" concentrated peptides from HIV to induce this polyclonal response, remains to be resolved.

Increased spontaneous transformation of B cells of AIDS patients by EBV in vitro has been reported and is thought to reflect impaired T-cell and NK-cell surveillance, not necessarily related to intrinsic B-cell dysfunction. This phenomenon may be associated with the increased incidence of B-cell lymphomas observed in AIDS patients. It is important to note, however, that despite the ability of HIV to infect EBV-transformed B cells in vitro, there is no evidence of HIV integration in the B-cell lymphomas of AIDS patients.[121] The high incidence of these lymphomas in AIDS patients may be associated with increased transformation by EBV and simply reflect the high incidence of coinfection with EBV in these individuals. There is no current indication that nontransformed B cells can be infected with HIV, nor have HIV-infected B cells been identified in HIV-seropositive individuals.

In addition to the stimulatory effects of viral particles on B cells, HIV has been found to suppress EBV-induced immunoglobulin production by purified B cells.[122] The mechanism of this suppressive effect is unclear.

## IMMUNE DEFECTS IN NATURAL KILLER CELLS

The majority of NK cell activity is attributed to a circulating population of large granular lymphocytes (LGL), which constitute approximately 10 percent of lymphocytes and bear CD16 on their surface. A smaller circulating population of CD16$^-$ cells expressing the product of the T-cell receptor $\gamma$-$\delta$ gene also have been shown to have NK-cell activity.[123] NK cells are capable of killing virally infected cells, tumor cells, and allogeneic cells. They are thought to have a central role in immunosurveillance against viral infections and spontaneously developing tumors.

The number of circulating NK cells does not appear to be significantly decreased with HIV infection, even in those patients who have developed AIDS. These cells bind normally to their target cells;[124,125] however, compared with cells from uninfected individuals, these cells have diminished cytotoxic capability.[124–130] Using lysis of tumor cell lines as a standard of NK activity, NK-cell function measured in unfractionated PBMCs from AIDS patients has been found to be depressed when compared with healthy seronegative controls. NK function can be enhanced or restored to normal levels when activated by IL-2, Con A, or TPA and calcium ionophore.[124,130,131] Thus, NK cells from AIDS patients appear to be intrinsically intact and able to perform their cytolytic function once activated. However, postbinding or "triggering" defects interfere with their ability to be activated and to function normally.

## OTHER IMMUNOLOGIC ABNORMALITIES

A number of other factors have been proposed to account for some of the immune defects seen in AIDS patients. In addition to hypergammaglobulinemia, circulating autoantibodies[131–135] and circulating immune complexes[136,137] have been detected in AIDS patients. The clinical consequences of an elevation in circulating immune complexes are unclear, but may have relevance to certain symptoms such as arthritis, nephritis, and thrombocytopenia, which are sometimes seen in HIV-infected individuals.

Elevated levels of acid-labile alpha interferon,[138,139] alpha 1 thymosin,[140] and beta 2 microglobulin[141] have been reported in patients with AIDS, but these observations are of unknown clinical significance. Antibodies to alpha 1 thymosin[142] appear to cross-react with p17 and may be effective in viral neutralization.

## IMMUNE RESPONSE TO HIV

There are many components of the immune system which may respond to infection with HIV. Some of these responses may limit viral replication while others may inadvertently enhance the spread and replication of the virus. In order to design a successful vaccine against HIV or devise immune-mediated therapeutic modalities to inhibit viral spread, it is critical to delineate which arms of the immune system can participate in generating a successful immune response to HIV and to identify the structural elements of the virus which are recognized by this system. The effectiveness of specific elements of the immune response to eliminate HIV may be dictated by conditions peculiar to lentiviral infection or HIV per se. In this regard, the route of infection by HIV is primarily through blood or mucosal surfaces, and the humoral and cell-mediated responses generated in these body compartments differ. Secretory antibody may be vital for protection against sexually transmitted HIV but should not have a major role in transfusion-acquired or needle-associated infection. There may be regional differences in the type of T-cell immunity as well, especially in epithelial-associated responses.[143] In addition, the induction of a successful response in the peripheral blood may not confer immunity in a more immunologically privileged region such as the central nervous system, which also sequesters HIV.

There appear to be strong selective pressures for inducing changes within the envelope regions of HIV, creating a greater diversity than has been seen in the case of influenza. Hypothetically, point mutations in the HIV strain in a given patient could result in single amino acid substitutions in immunodominant regions resulting in altered antigenicity and enhanced virulence of the variants. Thus, an initially successful immune response to a given isolate may be rendered impotent. Recent studies using the polymerase chain reaction (PCR) to analyze envelope sequence changes in isolates from individual patients support this notion (S. Wain-Hobson, unpublished observations). In the case of equine infectious anemia virus, another lentivirus, induction of neutralizing antibody in an infected pony results in the selection of variants that escape antibody recognition.[144]

The immunosuppressive nature of this virus diminishes the prospects for protective immunity. While the primary cause of immunosuppression in humans relates to the loss of the $CD4^+$ cells, immunologic abnormalities precede substantial circulating $CD4^+$ cell loss. The causes of these defects are unclear, but some possible mechanisms have been discussed above. A relatively intact immune system may be required for novel vaccination schemes to bolster specific immunity in individuals already infected with HIV.

Induction of an immune response to HIV in HIV-seronegative individuals could potentially enhance HIV propagation after exposure. Antibody with inadequate neutralizing capacity may recognize live cell-free virus, associate with macrophages through the Fc receptor, and facilitate viral entry and replication in these cells.[95] Even if a vaccine demonstrates efficacy, appropriate personal and public health precautions will need to be observed in vaccinated individuals at high risk for infection.

Many different responses may contribute to the development of protective immunity (Table 29-1). These may include neutralizing and cytolytic antibodies, ADCC responses, MHC-restricted T-cell cytotoxic responses, and NK-cell-mediated lysis.

Neutralizing antibodies remove free virions from the circulation and prevent spread of the viral infection. Precise mechanisms of viral neutralization are unclear since both free and cell-associated virions are involved in the propagation of HIV infection. For some viruses, such as respiratory syncytial virus and hepatitis A virus, production of antibody with in vitro neutralizing capacity correlates with protection in individuals exposed to these viruses. Passive transfer of antibody from individuals immunized to these viruses confers protection to unimmunized recipients. For HIV, several different in vitro neutralizing assays have been devised, but it is unclear if the presence of these antibodies in vivo can confer to the HIV-infected individual protection from further disease progression. Furthermore, there is no evidence to support the notion that the presence of neutralizing antibody to HIV would be protective for the uninfected individual exposed to HIV. A recent study indicated that passive transfer of antibody from individuals with high titers of neutralizing activity to chimpanzees could not prevent infection of these animals when challenged with HIV.[145]

In addition to recognizing free or newly bound virions, antibodies may be directed against cell-associated viral proteins. The antibody may associate with the virion as it buds through the cell membrane. Alternatively, some unassembled viral proteins may be expressed on the cell membrane apart from the virion and may be subject to recognition by antibody. *Nef* may be one of these proteins as it has been shown to be myristilated and thought to serve as a G-binding protein.[146] The attachment of free gp120 envelope protein from whole or disrupted virions to the CD4 molecule of uninfected cells may contribute to the attrition of the CD4 compartment via inopportune recognition by envelope-specific antibody or cytotoxic cells.

The specificity for neutralizing antibody either may be broad, as in the case of the group-specific response, which may recognize heterogeneous isolates of HIV, or may be restricted, as in the case of the type-specific responses that recognize closely related strains.[147] The potential specificity differences of the neutralizing antibodies are the result of the marked diversity within the HIV envelope, where regions of less than 50 percent amino acid homology among HIV-1 strains are interposed with sequences that are more highly conserved.

The specificity of neutralizing antibody has been examined in animal systems as well as in patients infected with HIV-1. Overlapping the sequences which Lasky et al.[27] defined as participating in the binding of the envelope protein to CD4 is a sequence determined by Cease et al.[148] that stimulates T-helper-cell responses in mice immunized with HIV-1 envelope proteins. These sequences are found within a conserved region of gp120. This site was defined as potentially immunogenic based on a computer model which predicted the α-helical and amphipathic regions of the envelope protein. In contrast to this T-cell-helper site in this conserved area is the region within the second hypervariable domain of gp120 which contains three overlapping peptides that

**Table 29-1. Immune Response to HIV**

1. Neutralizing antibodies
2. Cytolytic antibodies
3. Antibody-dependent cellular cytotoxicity
4. T-cell-mediated cytotoxicity
5. Natural killer cell cytotoxicity

have been defined as being important in cell fusion,[149] the induction of MHC-class-I-restricted cytotoxic T lymphocytes in mice,[150] and type-specific neutralization.[151] In the latter study, antibody resulting from immunization with envelope from the HIV-$1_{III-B}$ strain could not neutralize the HIV-$1_{RF}$, and vice versa. Human sera from HIV-infected individuals appear also to recognize this epitope in a type-specific manner. However, this may be one of many immunogenic domains, and identifying conserved regions that elicit group-specific neutralizing antibodies or cell-mediated responses is still feasible. For example, Ho et al. have found a peptide within a conserved portion of the envelope regions that could generate a group-specific neutralizing response in rabbits against both HIV-$1_{IIIB}$ and HIV-$1_{RF}$ isolates.[152]

Sera obtained from patients representing the full clinical spectrum of HIV infection have been shown to have neutralizing capabilities.[153–155] One study demonstrated group specificity of the neutralizing antibodies derived from patients; preferential neutralization can be seen against matched serum and a viral isolate from a given patient. The ability of neutralizing antibody to confer protection is questionable, however; some studies demonstrated a correlation of the presence of neutralizing antibody with an earlier clinical stage and loss of titers with disease progression, while other studies showed no correlation at all.

Antibody-dependent cytotoxic processes may participate in surveillance against HIV.[156,157] Any cytotoxic cell bearing Fc receptors such as NK cells or macrophages can participate in this process. However, the incorporation of HIV by endocytosis into a macrophage, a cell that is a reservoir for infection in vivo, may actually facilitate viral propagation if the virions are not destroyed by phagolysosomal contents. Sera derived from HIV-seropositive individuals has been shown to mediate ADCC in vitro, and some groups have reported a decrease in ADCC activity in sera derived from individuals with AIDS compared with healthy HIV-seropositive donors. However, this decrease in ADCC activity may merely reflect a global defect in immune function in clinically advanced individuals. ADCC activity appears to best correlate with the presence of antibodies to the envelope protein, although antibodies directed against other viral proteins may be involved as well.

NK cells may participate in eliminating HIV-infected cells.[158] Cells with different phenotypes may be involved in this response and may include those which express both CD16 and Leu19. In addition, T cells, particularly those with $\gamma$-$\delta$ T-cell receptor rearrangement, theoretically may be involved in lysing HIV-infected cells in an MHC-unrestricted manner. Enriched populations of LGLs from seronegative individuals, which contain the majority of NK activity, have been shown to mediate a small cytolytic response against HIV-infected targets. This response can be augmented with IL-2. Weinhold et al.[53] have reported that the majority of HIV envelope-specific cytotoxicity found in the peripheral blood of seropositive individuals is MHC-unrestricted and is mediated by CD16-positive cells by an ADCC-dependent mechanism.

Cytotoxic T cells appear in unusually high frequency and may be demonstrated by direct assay in fresh unfractionated PBMCs obtained from HIV-seropositive individuals.[159–161] Cells with similar cytotoxic activity can be cultured from bronchoalveolar lavage fluids[162] and CSF of HIV-infected patients.[163] Both MHC-restricted and -unrestricted responses have been reported. CTLs have been demonstrated against *env, gag, pol, nef,* and *vif* gene products, and efforts are now focused on identifying the particular epitopes recognized by clonal lines of CTLs. Some of those clonal lines have demonstrated group specificity by virtue of their ability to lyse target cells from different HIV-1 isolates.[161] Thus, conserved epitopes of HIV-1 are immunogenic in seropositive individuals.

It has yet to be established whether or not CTLs to HIV are beneficial or harmful to HIV-infected individuals. Certainly the presence of CTLs has correlated with protection against disseminated herpesvirus infections, and they appear to be important in animal models of retrovirus-induced leukemia. Some have argued that incomplete elimination of virally infected cells may enhance dissemination. The presence of $CD8^+$ cells from HIV-seropositive individuals appears to inhibit the ability to isolate HIV from $CD4^+$ cells in vitro, and this may involve HIV-specific cytolytic mechanisms.[164] Further efforts to define this process in in vitro and in vivo models are necessary.

## THERAPY FOR THE IMMUNE DEFECTS

In the setting of the profound depression in immune function seen in patients with AIDS, clinical investigators have attempted to replace, restore, or enhance immunologic function by various approaches. Limited clinical trials have included (1) single and sequential transfer of lymphocytes or PBMCs from HIV-seronegative HLA-matched siblings or identical twins;[165,166] (2) infusion of bone marrow from these same donors;[165] (3) intermittent or continuous infusion of IL-2;[167] (4) parenteral administration of $\gamma$-IFN; and (5) administration of various antigen nonspecific immunomodulators (e.g., Ampligen). Most of the clinical trials are still in progress. Some of these studies were conducted before any effective therapy was available to inhibit viral replication. In many of the investigations, the prospects for any sustained restoration of immune function were poor considering the advanced clinical stage of the participants. As most of these clinical investigations were performed in single patients or as phase I trials, efficacy of treatment could not be fully evaluated.

Limited laboratory data from these early studies have demonstrated transient increases in circulating $CD4^+$ cells and sporadic improvement in some in vitro immune parameters in some of the patients, particularly those receiving cell transfers. In no case has sustained laboratory or clinical improvement been reported. While these initial efforts have not been especially encouraging, in the absence of chemotherapeutic agents to prevent replication of HIV, it is not surprising that adaptively transferred mature $CD4^+$ lymphocytes or stem cells would eventually succumb to infection with HIV.

The success of some of the immunomodulators in restoring immune competency will be dependent on several factors. Intervention will need to be attempted early in a patient's clinical course before profound lymphocyte depletion occurs. A correlation between efficacy and number of circulating lymphocytes has been shown recently in a study of AIDS patients with Kaposi's sarcoma treated with a combination of $\alpha$-IFN and azidothymidine.[168] Also, cytokines with stimulatory properties on the immune system, including those that may be cytotoxic for HIV-infected cells (e.g., TNF), may under certain conditions enhance HIV expression and inadvertently result in further immune compromise or disease progression.[79] In this regard, in a phase I study of patients with Kaposi's sarcoma treated with $\gamma$-IFN, clinical progression was seen particularly in patients treated with the highest doses of this agent (H. C. Lane, unpublished observation). Finally, active replication of HIV would have to be suppressed by an effective antiretroviral agent in order to prevent infection of the reconstituted immune system (see Chap. 30).

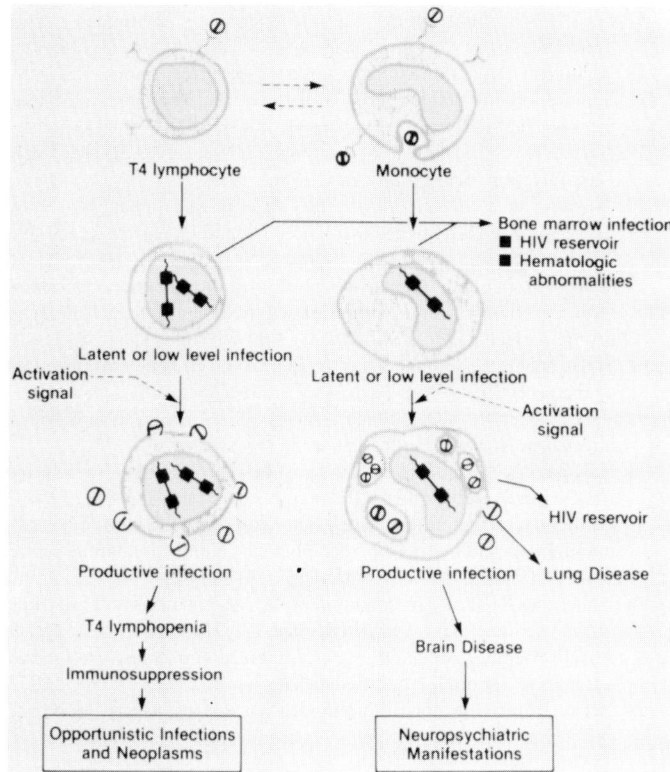


**Fig. 29-4.** Mechanisms of pathogenesis of HIV.

## CONCLUDING REMARKS

Over the past several years, we have developed an understanding of the structural and biological properties of HIV and its relation to the development of AIDS. Using various laboratory parameters and in vitro model systems, we have achieved an appreciation for many of the potential mechanisms that may contribute to the pathogenesis of this disorder (Fig. 29-4). Both quantitative and qualitative lymphocyte defects are pervasive in HIV-infected individuals and promote the development of AIDS. Macrophages are an important reservoir for infection and may be implicated in the neurologic disorders that develop in these patients. However, there are still major voids in our understanding of the precise mechanisms by which HIV causes $CD4^+$ lymphocyte depletion and functional abnormalities in vivo, and the role of the immune response to HIV in either protecting individuals from or contributing to the pathogenesis of AIDS. These questions need to be pursued in order to facilitate attempts to develop effective vaccines and therapeutic modalities.

### ACKNOWLEDGMENT

The authors would like to acknowledge the assistance of Dr. M. Hamburg and M. Rust.

## References


1 Barré-Sinoussi F et al: Isolation of a T lymphotropic retrovirus from a patient at risk for acquired immune deficiency syndrome (AIDS). *Science* 220:868, 1983.
2 Gallo RC et al: Frequent detection and isolation of cytopathic retrovirus (HTLV-III) from patients with AIDS and at risk for AIDS. *Science* 224:500, 1984.
3 Levy JA et al: Isolation of lymphocytopathic retroviruses from San Francisco patients with AIDS. *Science* 225:840, 1984.
4 Coffin J et al: Human immunodeficiency viruses. *Science* 232:697, 1986
5 Popovic M et al: Detection, isolation, and continuous production of cytopathic retroviruses (HTLV-III) from patients with AIDS and pre-AIDS. *Science* 224:497, 1984.
6 Rabson AB, Martin MA: Molecular organization of the AIDS retrovirus. *Cell* 40:477, 1985.
7 Gallo R et al: HIV/HTLV gene nomenclature. *Nature* 333:504, 1988.
8 Benn S et al: Genomic heterogeneity of AIDS retroviral isolates from North America and Zaire. *Science* 230:949, 1985.
9 Public Health Service, DHHS: *Quarterly Report to the Domestic Policy Council on the Prevalence and Rate of Spread of HIV in the United States, July, 1988.* Atlanta, Centers for Disease Control, 1988.
10 Cheng-Mayer C et al: Biologic features of HIV-1 that correlate with virulence in the host. *Science* 240:80, 1988.
11 Brun-Vezinet F et al: Lymphadenopathy-associated virus type 2 in AIDS and AIDS-related complex. *Lancet* 1:128, 1987.
12 Clavel F et al: Human immunodeficiency virus type 2 infection associated with AIDS in West Africa. *N Engl J Med* 316:1180, 1987.
13 Clavel F et al: Molecular cloning and polymorphism of the human immune deficiency virus type 2. *Nature* 324:691, 1986.
14 Masur H et al: An outbreak of community-acquired *Pneumocystis carinii* pneumonia: Initial manifestation of cellular immune dysfunction. *N Engl J Med* 305:1431, 1981.
15 Siegel FP et al: Severe acquired immunodeficiency in male homosexuals, manifested by chronic perianal ulcerative herpes simplex lesions. *N Engl J Med* 305:1439, 1981.
16 Edman JC et al: Ribosomal RNA sequence shows *Pneumocystis carinii* to be a member of the fungi. *Nature* 334:519, 1988.
17 Vogel J et al: The HIV *tat* gene induces dermal lesions resembling Kaposi's sarcoma in transgenic mice. *Nature* 335:606, 1988.
18 Klatzmann D et al: Selective tropism of lymphadenopathy associated virus (LAV) for helper-inducer T lymphocytes. *Science* 225:59, 1984.
19 Dalgleish AG et al: The CD4 (T4) antigen is an essential component of the receptor for the AIDS retrovirus. *Nature* 312:763, 1984.
20 Klatzmann D et al: T-lymphocyte T4 molecule behaves as the receptor for human retrovirus LAV. *Nature* 312:767, 1984.
21 McDougal JS et al: Binding of HTLV-III/LAV to $T4^+$ T cells by a complex of the 110 K viral protein and the T4 molecule. *Science* 231:382, 1985.
22 Sattentau QJ et al: Epitopes of the CD4 antigen and HIV infection. *Science* 234:1120, 1986.
23 Maddon PJ et al: The T4 gene encodes the AIDS virus receptor and is expressed in the immune system and the brain. *Cell* 47:333, 1986.
24 Lifson JD et al: Synthetic CD4 peptide derivatives that inhibit HIV infection and cytopathicity. *Science* 241:712, 1988.
25 Clayton LK et al: Substitution of murine for human CD4 residues identifies amino acids critical for HIV-gp120 binding. *Nature* 335: 363, 1988.
26 Berger EA et al: A soluble recombinant polypeptide comprising the amino-terminal half of the extracellular region of the CD4 molecule contains an active binding site for human immunodeficiency virus. *Proc Natl Acad Sci USA* 85:2357, 1988.
27 Lasky LA et al: Delineation of a region of the human immunodeficiency virus type 1 gp120 glycoprotein critical for interaction with the CD4 receptor. *Cell* 50:975, 1987.
28 Kowalski M et al: Functional regions of the envelope glycoprotein of human immunodeficiency virus type 1. *Science* 237:1351, 1987.
29 Maddon P et al: HIV infection does not require endocytosis of its receptor, CD4. *Cell* 54:865, 1988.
30 Hoxie JA et al: Alterations in T4 (CD4) protein and mRNA synthesis in cells infected with HIV. *Science* 234:1123, 1986.
31 Sodrowski J et al: Role of the HTLV-III/LAV envelope in syncytium formation and cytopathicity. *Nature* 322:470, 1986.

32 Lifson JD et al: AIDS retrovirus induced cytopathology: Giant cell formation and involvement of CD4 antigen. *Science* 232:1123, 1986.
33 Lifson JD et al: Induction of CD4-dependent cell fusion by the HTLV-III/LAV envelope glycoprotein. *Nature* 323:725, 1986.
34 Yoffe B et al: Fusion as a mediator of cytolysis in mixtures of uninfected CD4$^+$ lymphocytes and cells infected by human immunodeficiency virus. *Proc Natl Acad Sci USA* 84:1429, 1987.
35 Epstein LG et al: Progressive encephalopathy in children with acquired immune deficiency syndrome. *Ann Neurol* 17:488, 1988.
36 Ewing EP et al: Primary lymph node pathology in AIDS and AIDS-related lymphadenopathy. *Arch Pathol Lab Med* 109:977, 1985.
37 Nabel G, Baltimore D: An inducible transcription factor activates expression of human immunodeficiency virus in T cells. *Nature* 326: 711, 1987.
38 Lane HC et al: Correlation between immunologic function and clinical subpopulations of patients with the acquired immune deficiency syndrome. *Am J Med* 78:417, 1985.
39 Mittelman et al: Analysis of T cell subsets in different clinical subgroups of patients with the acquired immune deficiency syndrome. *Am J Med* 78:951, 1985.
40 Polk BF et al: Predictors of the acquired immunodeficiency syndrome developing in a cohort of seropositive homosexual men. *N Engl J Med* 316:61, 1987.
41 Goedert JJ et al: Effect of T4 count and cofactors on the incidence of AIDS in homosexual men infected with human immunodeficiency virus. *JAMA* 257:331, 1987.
42 Giorgi JV et al: Selective alterations in immunoregulatory lymphocyte subsets in early HIV (human T-lymphotropic virus type III/ lymphadenopathy-associated virus) infection. *J Clin Immunol* 7: 140, 1987.
43 Nicholson JKA et al: Alterations of functional subsets of T helper and T suppressor cell populations in acquired immunodeficiency syndrome (AIDS) and chronic unexplained lymphadenopathy. *J Clin Immunol* 5:269, 1985.
44 Harper ME et al: Detection of lymphocytes expressing human T-lymphotropic virus type III in lymph nodes and peripheral blood from infected individual by *in situ* hybridization. *Proc Natl Acad Sci USA* 83:772, 1986.
45 Winkelstein A et al: Defective in vitro T cell colony formation in the acquired immunodeficiency syndrome. *J Immunol* 134:151, 1985.
46 Donahue RE et al: Suppression of in vitro haematopoiesis following human immunodeficiency virus infection. *Nature* 326:200, 1987.
47 Folks TM et al: Infection and replication of HIV-1 in purified progenitor cells of normal human bone marrow. *Science* 242:919, 1988.
48 Klatzmann D, Gluckman JC: HIV infection: Facts and hypotheses. *Immunol Today* 7:291, 1986.
49 Ziegler JL, Stites DP: Hypothesis: AIDS is an autoimmune disease directed at the immune system and triggered by a lymphotropic retrovirus. *Clin Immunol Immunopathol* 41:305, 1986.
50 Stricker RB et al: An AIDS related cytotoxic autoantibody reacts with a specific antigen on stimulated CD4+ T cells. *Nature* 327: 170, 1987.
51 Siliciano RF et al: Analysis of host-viral interactions in AIDS with anti-gp120 T cell clones: Effect of HIV sequence variation and a mechanism for CD4+ cell depletion. *Cell* 54:561, 1988.
52 Lanzavecchia A et al: T cells can represent antigens such as HIV gp120 targeted to their own surface molecules. *Nature* 334:530, 1988.
53 Weinhold KJ et al: Cellular anti-gp120 cytolytic reactivities in HIV-1 seropositive individuals. *Lancet* I:902, 1988.
54 Armstrong GA et al: Follicular dendritic cells and virus-like particles in AIDS-related lymphadenopathy. *Lancet* 2:230, 1984.
55 Belsito DV et al: Reduced Langerhans' cell Ia antigen and ATPase activity in patients with the acquired immunodeficiency syndrome. *N Engl J Med* 310:1279, 1984.
56 Levy JA et al: AIDS-associated retrovirus (ARV) can productively infect other cells besides human T helper cells. *Virology* 147:441, 1985.
57 Ho DD et al: Infection of monocyte/macrophages by human T lymphotropic virus type III. *J Clin Invest* 77:1712, 1986.
58 Nicholson JKA et al: In vitro infection of human monocytes with human T-lymphotropic virus type III/lymphadenopathy-associated virus (HTLV-III/LAV). *J Immunol* 137:323, 1986.
59 Gartner S et al: The role of mononuclear phagocytes in HTLV-III/ LAV infection. *Science* 233:215, 1986.
60 Koenig S et al: Detection of AIDS virus in macrophages in brain tissue from AIDS patients with encephalopathy. *Science* 233:1089, 1986.
61 Wiley CA et al: Cellular localization of human immunodeficiency virus infection within the brains of acquired immune deficiency syndrome patients. *Proc Natl Acad Sci USA* 83:7089, 1986.
62 Stoler MH et al: Human T cell lymphotropic virus type III infection of the central nervous system. *JAMA* 256:2360, 1986.
63 Vazeux R et al: AIDS subacute encephalitis: Identification of HIV-infected cells. *Am J Pathol* 126:403, 1987.
64 Koyanagi Y et al: Dual infection of the central nervous system by AIDS viruses and distinct cellular tropisms. *Science* 64:819, 1987.
65 Gendelman HE et al: Efficient isolation and propagation of human immunodeficiency virus on recombinant colony-stimulating factor 1–treated monocytes. *J Exp Med* 167:1428, 1988.
66 Pomerantz RJ et al: Human immunodeficiency virus (HIV) infection of the uterine cervix. *Ann Intern Med* 108:321, 1988.
67 Adachi A et al: Productive, persistent infection of human colorectal cell lines with human immunodeficiency virus. *J Virol* 61:209, 1987.
68 Nelson JA et al: Human immunodeficiency virus detected in bowel epithelium from patients with gastrointestinal symptoms. *Lancet* I:8580, 1988.
69 Pomerantz RJ et al: Infection of the retina by human immunodeficiency virus type 1. *N Engl J Med* 317:1643, 1987.
70 Montagnier L et al: Adaption of lymphadenopathy associated virus (LAV) to replication in EBV-transformed B lymphoblastoid cell lines. *Science* 225:63, 1984.
71 Patterson S, Knight SC: Susceptibility of human peripheral blood dendritic cells to infection by human immunodeficiency virus. *J Gen Virol* 68:1177, 1987.
72 Zagury D et al: Long-term cultures of HTLV-III-infected T cells: A model of cytopathology of T cell depletion in AIDS. *Science* 2:850, 1985.
73 Margolick JB et al: Amplification of HTLV-III/LAV infection by antigen-induced activation of T cells and direct suppression by virus of lymphocyte blastogenic responses. *J Immunol* 138:1719, 1987.
74 Gendelman HE et al: Transactivation of the human immunodeficiency virus terminal repeat sequence by DNA viruses. *Proc Natl Acad Sci USA* 83:9759, 1986.
75 Mosca JD et al: Herpes simplex virus type-1 can reactivate transcription of latent human immunodeficiency virus. *Nature* 325:67, 1987.
76 Davis MG et al: Immediate-early gene region of human cytomegalovirus transactivates the promoter of human immunodeficiency virus. *Proc Natl Acad Sci USA* 84:8642, 1987.
77 Ostrove JM et al: Activation of the human immunodeficiency virus by herpes simplex virus type 1. *J Virol* 61:3726, 1987.
78 Folks TM et al: Cytokine-induced expression of HIV-1 in a chronically infected promonocyte cell line. *Science* 238:800, 1987.
79 Clouse KA et al: Monokine regulation of human immunodeficiency virus-1 expression in a chronically infected human T cell clone. *J Immunol* 142:431, 1989.
80 Lane HC et al: Qualitative analysis of immune function in patients with the acquired immunodeficiency syndrome. *N Engl J Med* 313:79, 1985.
81 Smolen JS et al: Deficiency of the autologous mixed lymphocyte reaction in patients with classic hemophilia treated with commercial factor VIII concentrate. *J Clin Invest* 75:1828, 1985.
82 Gupta S et al: Autologous mixed lymphocyte reaction in man: XIV. Deficiency of the autologous mixed lymphocyte reaction in acquired immune deficiency syndrome (AIDS) and AIDS related complex (ARC). In vitro effect of purified interleukin-1 and interleukin-2. *Clin Exp Immunol* 58:395, 1984.

83 Fauci AS: AIDS: Immunopathogenic mechanisms and research strategies. *Clin Res* 35:503, 1987.

84 Shearer GM et al: Prospective study of cytotoxic T lymphocyte responses to influenza and antibodies to human T lymphotropic virus-III in homosexual men. *J Clin Invest* 76:1699, 1985.

85 Shalaby MR et al: The effects of human immunodeficiency virus recombinant envelope glycoprotein on immune cell functions *in vitro*. *Cell Immunol* 110:140, 1987.

86 Linette GP et al: HIV-1 infected T cells show a selective signaling defect after perturbation of CD3/antigen receptor. *Science* 241:573, 1988.

87 Gay D et al: Functional interaction between human T-cell protein CD4 and the major histocompatibility complex HLA-DR antigen. *Nature* 626, 1987.

88 Doyle C, Strominger JL: Interaction between CD4 and class II MHC molecules mediates cell adhesion. *Nature* 330:256, 1987.

89 Alcover A et al: Functional and molecular aspects of human T lymphocyte activation via T3-T1 and T11 pathways. *Immunol Rev* 95:5, 1987.

90 Fauci AS: The human immunodeficiency virus: Infectivity and mechanisms of pathogenesis. *Science* 239:617, 1988.

91 Shearer GM et al: Functional T lymphocyte immune deficiency in a population of homosexual men who do not exhibit symptoms of acquired immune deficiency syndrome. *J Clin Invest* 74:496, 1984.

92 Sheridan JF: Cell-mediated immunity of cytomegalovirus (CMV) and herpes simplex virus (HSV) antigens in the acquired immune deficiency syndrome: Interleukin-1 and interleukin-2 modify in vitro responses. *J Clin Immunol* 4:304, 1984.

93 Rook AH et al: Deficient, HLA-restricted, cytomegalovirus-specific cytotoxic T cells and natural killer cells in patients with the acquired immunodeficiency syndrome. *J Infect Dis* 152:627, 1985.

94 Rook AH et al: Interleukin-2 enhances the depressed natural killer and cytomegalovirus-specific cytotoxic activities of lymphocytes from patients with the acquired immune deficiency syndrome. *J Clin Invest* 72:398, 1983.

95 Takeda A et al: Antibody-enhanced infection by HIV-1 via Fc-receptor mediated entry. *Science* 242:580, 1988.

96 Smith PD et al: Monocyte function in the acquired immune deficiency syndrome. *J Clin Invest* 74:2121, 1984.

97 Poli G et al: Monocyte function in intravenous drug abusers with lymphadenopathy syndrome and in patients with acquired immunodeficiency syndrome: Selective impairment of chemotaxis. *Clin Exp Immunol* 62:136, 1985.

98 Washburn RG et al: Phagocytic and fungicidal activity of monocytes from patients with acquired immunodeficiency syndrome. *J Infect Dis* 151, 1985.

99 Kleinerman ES et al: Activation of monocyte-mediated tumoricidal activity in patients with acquired immunodeficiency syndrome. *J Clin Oncol* 3:1005, 1985.

100 Murray HW et al: Impaired production of lymphokines and immune (gamma) interferon in the acquired immunodeficiency syndrome. *N Engl J Med* 310:883, 1984.

101 Estevez ME et al: Early defect of phagocytic cell function in subjects at risk for acquired immunodeficiency syndrome. *Scand J Immunol* 24:215, 1986.

102 Bender BS et al: Demonstration of defective C3-receptor-mediated clearance by the reticuloendothelial system in patients with acquired immunodeficiency syndrome. *J Clin Invest* 79:715, 1987.

103 Hofmann B et al: Immunological studies in the acquired immunodeficiency syndrome. *Scand J Immunol* 23:669, 1986.

104 Heagy W et al: Decreased expression of human class II antigens on monocytes from patients with acquired immune deficiency syndrome. *J Clin Invest* 74:2089, 1984.

105 Prince HE et al: Defective monocyte function in acquired immune deficiency syndrome (AIDS): Evidence from a monocyte-dependent T-cell proliferative system. *J Clin Immunol* 5:21, 1985.

106 Enk C et al: Interleukin 1 activity in the acquired immunodeficiency syndrome. *Scand J Immunol* 23:491, 1986.

107 Price RW et al: The brain in AIDS: Central nervous system HIV-1 infection and AIDS dementia complex. *Science* 239:586, 1988.

108 Lee MR et al: Functional interaction and partial homology between human immunodeficiency virus and neuroleukin. *Science* 237:1047, 1987.

109 Brenneman DE: Neuronal cell killing by the envelope protein of HIV and its prevention by vasoactive intestinal peptide. *Nature* 335:639, 1988.

110 Lane HC et al: Abnormalities of B-cell activation and immunoregulation in patients with the acquired immunodeficiency syndrome. *N Engl J Med* 309:453, 1983.

111 Chess Q et al: Serum immunoglobulin elevations in the acquired immunodeficiency syndrome (AIDS): IgG, IgA, IgM, and IgD. *Diagn Immunol* 2:148, 1984.

112 Papadopoulos NM, Frieri M: The presence of immunoglobulin D in endocrine disorders and diseases of immunoregulation, including the acquired immunodeficiency syndrome. *Clin Immunol Immunopathol* 32:248, 1984.

113 Anderson KC et al: Isolation and functional analysis of human B cell populations. *J Immunol* 134:820, 1985.

114 Pahwa SG et al: Defective B-lymphocyte function in homosexual men in relation to the acquired immunodeficiency syndrome. *Ann Intern Med* 101:757, 1984.

115 Amann AJ et al: Acquired immune dysfunction in homosexual men: Immunologic profiles. *Clin Immunol Immunopathol* 27:315, 1983.

116 Amann AJ et al: B-cell immunodeficiency in acquired immune deficiency syndrome. *JAMA* 251:1447, 1984.

117 Polsky B et al: Bacterial pneumonia in patients with the acquired immunodeficiency syndrome. *Ann Intern Med* 104:38, 1986.

118 Yarchoan R et al: Mechanisms of JB cell activation in patients with acquired immunodeficiency syndrome and related disorders. *J Clin Invest* 78:439, 1985.

119 Schnittman SM et al: Direct polyclonal activation of human B lymphocytes by the acquired immune deficiency syndrome virus. *Science* 233:1084, 1986.

120 Nair MPN et al: Immunoregulatory activities of human immunodeficiency virus (HIV) protein: Effect of HIV recombinant and synthetic peptides on immunoglobulin synthesis and proliferative responses by normal lymphocytes. *Proc Natl Acad Sci USA* 85:6498, 1988.

121 Pelicci PG et al: Multiple monoclonal B-cell expansions and *c-myc* oncogene rearrangements in AIDS-related lymphoproliferative disorders: Implications for lymphomagenesis. *J Exp Med* 164:2049, 1986.

122 Pahwa S et al: Stimulatory and inhibitory influences of human immunodeficiency virus on normal B lymphocytes. *Proc Natl Acad Sci USA* 83:9124, 1986.

123 Borst J et al: A T-cell receptor γ/CD3 complex found on cloned functional lymphocytes. *Nature* 325:683, 1987.

124 Bonavida B et al: Mechanisms of defective NK cell activity in patients with acquired immunodeficiency syndrome (AIDS) and AIDS-related complex. *J Immunol* 137:1157, 1986.

125 Katzman M, Lederman MM: Defective postbinding lysis underlies the impaired natural killer activity in factor VIII-treated, human T lymphotropic virus type III seropositive hemophiliacs. *J Clin Invest* 77:1057, 1986.

126 Rook AH et al: Deficient, HLA-restricted, cytomegalovirus-specific cytotoxic T cells and natural killer cells in patients with the acquired immunodeficiency syndrome. *J Infect Dis* 152:627, 1985.

127 Pollack MS et al: Lymphocytotoxic antibodies to non-HLA antigens in the sera of patients with acquired immunodeficiency syndrome (AIDS), in *Non-HLA Antigens in Health, Aging, and Malignancy.* New York, Liss, 1983, pp 209–213.

128 Lew F et al: Natural killer cell function and modulation of α-IFN and IL-2 in AIDS patients and prodromal subjects. *Clin Lab Immunol* 14:115, 1984.

129 Creemers PC et al: Evaluation of natural killer cell activity in patients with persistent generalized lymphadenopathy and acquired immunodeficiency syndrome. *Clin Immunol Immunopathol* 36:141, 1985.

130 Rook AH et al: Interleukin 2 enhances the natural killer cell activity of acquired immunodeficiency syndrome patients through a γ-interferon-independent mechanism. *J Immunol* 134:1503, 1985.

131 Reddy MM et al: Differential effects of interferon-a2a and interleukin-2 on natural killer cell activity in patients with acquired immune deficiency syndrome. *J Biol Response Mod* 3:379, 1984.
132 Kloster BE et al: Lymphocytoxic antibodies in the acquired immune deficiency syndrome (AIDS). *Clin Immunol Immunopathol* 30:330, 1984.
133 Williams RC Jr et al: Lymphocyte-reactive antibodies in acquired immune deficiency syndrome. *J Clin Immunol* 4:118, 1984.
134 Dorsett B et al: Anti-lymphocyte antibodies in patients with the acquired immune deficiency syndrome. *Am J Med* 78:621, 1985.
135 Tomar RH et al: Cellular targets of antilymphocyte antibodies in AIDS and LAS. *Clin Immunol Immunopathol* 37:37, 1985.
136 McDougal JS et al: Immune complexes in the acquired immunodeficiency syndrome (AIDS). *J Clin Immunol* 5:130, 1985.
137 Gupta S, Licorish K: Circulating immune complexes in AIDS. *N Engl J Med* 310:1530, 1984.
138 DeStefano E et al: Acid-labile human leukocyte interferon in homosexual men with Kaposi's sarcoma and lymphadenopathy. *J Infect Dis* 146:451, 1982.
139 Buimovici-Klein E et al: Long-term follow-up of serum-interferon and its acid-stability in a group of homosexual men. *AIDS Research* 2:99, 1986.
140 Hersh EM et al: Elevated serum thymosin $alpha_1$ levels associated with evidence of immune dysregulation in male homosexuals with a history of infectious diseases or Kaposi's sarcoma. *N Engl J Med* 308:45, 1983.
141 Bhalla RB: Abnormally high concentrations of beta 2 microglobulin in acquired immunodeficiency syndrome (AIDS) patients. *Clin Chem* 29:1560, 1983.
142 Sarin PS: Neutralization of HTLV-III/LAV replication by anti-serum to thymosin $\alpha_1$. *Science* 232:1135, 1986.
143 Goodman T, Lefrancois L: Expression of the γ-delta T-cell receptor on intestinal CD8+ intraepithelial lymphocytes. *Nature* 333:855, 1988.
144 Montelaro et al: Antigenic variation during persistent infection by equine infectious anemia virus, a retrovirus. *J Biol Chem* 259:10539, 1984.
145 Prince AM et al: Failure of HIV immune globulin to protect chimpanzees against experimental challenge with HIV. *Proc Natl Acad Sci USA* 85:6944, 1988.
146 Guy B et al: HIV F/3′ *orf* encodes a phosphorylated GTP-binding protein resembling an oncogene product. *Nature* 330:266, 1987.
147 Willey RL et al: Identification of conserved and divergent domains within the envelope gene of the acquired immunodeficiency syndrome retrovirus. *Proc Natl Acad Sci USA* 83:5038, 1986.
148 Cease KB et al: Helper T-cell antigenic site identification in the acquired immunodeficiency syndrome virus gp120 envelope protein and induction of immunity in mice to the native protein using a 16-residue synthetic peptide. *Proc Natl Acad Sci USA* 84:4249, 1987.
149 Rusche JR et al: Antibodies that inhibit fusion of human immunodeficiency virus-infected cells bind a 24-amino acid sequence of the viral envelope, gp120. *Proc Natl Acad Sci USA* 85:3198, 1988.
150 Takahashi H et al: An immunodominant epitope of the human immunodeficiency virus envelope glycoprotein gp160 recognized by class I major histocompatibility complex molecule-restricted murine cytotoxic T lymphocytes. *Proc Natl Acad Sci USA* 85:3105, 1988.
151 Palker TJ et al: Type-specific neutralization of the human immunodeficiency virus with antibodies to *env*-encoded synthetic peptides. *Proc Natl Acad Sci USA* 85:1932, 1988.
152 Ho DD et al: Second conserved domain of gp120 is important for HIV infectivity and antibody neutralization. *Science* 239:1021, 1988.
153 Robert-Guroff M: HTLV-III neutralizing antibodies in patients with AIDS and AIDS-related complex. *Nature* 316:72, 1985.
154 Weiss RL et al: Neutralization of human T-lymphotropic virus type III by sera from AIDS and AIDS-risk patients. *Nature* 316:69, 1985.
155 Weiss RA et al: Variable and conserved neutralization antigens of human immunodeficiency virus. *Nature* 324:572, 1986.
156 Rook AH et al: Sera from HTLV-III/LAV antibody-positive individuals mediate antibody-dependent cellular cytotoxicity against HTLV-III/LAV infected T cells. *J Immunol* 139:2263, 1987.
157 Ojo-Amaize EA et al: Antibodies to human immunodeficiency virus in human sera induce cell-mediated lysis of human immunodeficiency virus-infected cells. *J Immunol* 139:2263, 1987.
158 Ruscetti FW et al: Analysis of effector mechanism against HLTV-1 and HTLV-III/LAV infected lymphoid cells. *J Immunol* 136:3619, 1986.
159 Walker BD et al: HIV-specific cytotoxic T lymphocytes in seropositive individuals. *Nature* 328:345, 1987.
160 Walker BD et al: HIV-1 reverse transcriptase is a target for cytotoxic T lymphocytes in infected individuals. *Science* 240:64, 1988.
161 Koenig S: Group specific, major histocompatibility complex class I restricted cytotoxic responses to human immunodeficiency virus-1 envelope proteins by cloned peripheral blood T cells from an HIV infected individual. *Proc Natl Acad Sci USA* 85:8638, 1988.
162 Plata F et al: AIDS virus-specific cytotoxic T lymphocytes in lung disorders. *Nature* 328:348, 1987.
163 Sethi KK et al: Phenotypic heterogeneity of cerebrospinal fluid-derived HIV-specific and HLA-restricted cytotoxic T-cell clones. *Nature* 335:178, 1988.
164 Walker CM et al: CD8+ lymphocytes can control HIV infection in vitro by suppressing virus replication. *Virology* 234:1563, 1986.
165 Lane et al: Partial immune reconstitution in a patient with the acquired immunodeficiency syndrome. *N Engl J Med* 311:1099, 1984.
166 Vilmer E: Clinical and immunological restoration in patients with AIDS after marrow transplantation, using lymphocyte transfusions from the marrow donor. *Transplantation* 44:25, 1987.
167 Lane HC et al: Use of interleukin-2 in patients with acquired immunodeficiency syndrome. *J Biol Response Mod* 3:512, 1984.
168 Lane HC et al: Anti-retroviral effects of interferon-α in AIDS-associated Kaposi's sarcoma. *Lancet* II:1218, 1988.

# Chapter 30

# Clinical manifestations of HIV infection in adults in industrialized countries

Martin S. Hirsch

## HISTORY

The clinical spectrum of infections associated with the human immunodeficiency viruses (HIV) continues to evolve. Although individual cases of unexplained immunosuppression accompanied by opportunistic infection were recognized in industrialized societies during the 1960s and 1970s,[1] 1981 proved to be a turning point in the recognition of a new syndrome. In June of that year, a short report in the *Morbidity and Mortality Weekly Report (MMWR)* of the United States Centers for Disease Control described five cases of *Pneumocystis carinii* pneumonia occurring in previously healthy men in the Los Angeles area.[2] Over the next several months, similar cases were described elsewhere, as were apparent outbreaks of other immunodeficiency-associated conditions, including Kaposi's sarcoma, mucosal candidiasis, disseminated cytomegalovirus infection, and chronic perianal herpes simplex virus ulcers.[3–6] The common features of the patients were that they had evidence of T lymphocyte dysfunction manifested by hyporesponsiveness to mitogens and antigens, and that they were either homosexual men or intravenous drug abusers.

By the end of 1982, it was clear that the outbreak of a new acquired immunodeficiency syndrome (AIDS) was not limited to a few cities or to two defined populations. Over 800 cases had been reported from over 30 states and the afflicted populations included Haitian immigrants, hemophiliacs, transfusion recipients, sex partners of bisexual males and intravenous drug abusers, and children born to mothers at risk. All these observations pointed to a transmissible agent spread through genital secretions and blood, and efforts at isolating and identifying an etiologic agent intensified.

Several infectious agents were suggested as possible etiologic agents for this newly described immunodeficiency syndrome, including human retroviruses. The first isolation of a retrovirus, initially called lymphadenopathy-associated virus (LAV), from a patient in Paris[7] was largely ignored until April 1984, when scientists at the National Cancer Institute in Bethesda confirmed the isolation and greatly expanded the evidence linking this retrovirus, called human T-lymphotropic virus III by the U.S. group, to the immunodeficiency syndrome.[8–10] Identification of the etiologic virus, since renamed human immunodeficiency virus type I (HIV-1), has permitted further characterization of the natural history of infection and the spectrum of disease associated with the agent. Moreover, first steps toward control of HIV-1 infection have been taken through development of public health measures to limit the spread of infection and antiviral chemotherapy to prolong lives of infected individuals.

In 1986, a second human immunodeficiency virus (HIV-2) was isolated in West Africa.[11] Subsequent isolates have been reported from Europe and North America.[12,13] Although there is controversy regarding the relative pathogenicity of HIV-2, it appears clear that HIV-2, like HIV-1, is capable of causing both AIDS and neurologic disease.[11–13]

## STAGES OF HIV INFECTION

With each passing year, the spectrum of illness associated with HIV infection has broadened. Whether this broad spectrum reflects differences in virus tropism, host response, or cofactors is uncertain. Several classification systems for HIV-related illnesses have been proposed. The two most widely utilized have been the CDC[14] and the Walter Reed[15] classification systems (Tables 30-1 and 30-2). The CDC classification offers the advantage of simplicity, whereas the Walter Reed system utilizes laboratory abnormalities, e.g., T helper cell numbers and cutaneous delayed hypersensitivity reactivity to help with staging. Although categorization is somewhat artificial and often misleading to patients, it is useful for surveillance, epidemiologic studies, and studies of therapeutic intervention. For the purposes of this chapter, the most recent CDC classification system[14] will be utilized.

## ACUTE PRIMARY INFECTION SYNDROMES (GROUP I)

Many HIV seroconversions are asymptomatic or subclinical. However, some seroconverters will develop a self-limited mononucleosis or influenza-like syndrome characterized by fever, rigors, arthralgias, myalgias, malaise, lethargy, anorexia, nausea, diarrhea, sore throat, and a truncal maculopapular, urticarial, or vesicular rash.[16,17] Neurological signs and symptoms may predominate, including headaches, stiff neck, retro-orbital pain, neuritis, myelopathy, photophobia, irritability, depression, or frank encephalopathy.[16–18] The illness may last 2 to 3 weeks but usually results in clinical recovery.

Laboratory abnormalities may include transient leukopenia, lymphopenia, relative monocytosis, thrombocytopenia, and elevated erythrocyte sedimentation rate. T4/T8 ratios in peripheral blood may become inverted, largely as a result of increased T8 cells, and atypical lymphocytes may be seen on blood smears.

**Table 30-1. CDC Classification for HIV Infections**

| | |
|---|---|
| Group I | Acute infection |
| Group II | Asymptomatic infection* |
| Group III | Persistent generalized lymphadenopathy* |
| Group IV | Other disease: |
| Subgroup A | Constitutional disease |
| Subgroup B | Neurologic disease |
| Subgroup C | Secondary infectious diseases |
| Category C-1 | Specified secondary infectious diseases listed in the CDC surveillance definition for AIDS+ |
| Category C-2 | Other specified secondary infectious diseases |
| Subgroup D | Secondary cancers+ |
| Subgroup E | Other conditions |

*Patients in Groups II and III may be subclassified on the basis of a laboratory evaluation.

+Includes those patients whose clinical presentation fulfills the definition of AIDS used by CDC for national reporting.

Table 30-2. The Walter Reed Staging Classification for HIV Infection

| WR stage | HIV antibody or virus detection | Chronic lymphadenopathy | T helper cells/mm³ | Delayed hypersensitivity | Thrush | Opportunistic infections |
|---|---|---|---|---|---|---|
| 0 | – | – | >400 | + | – | – |
| 1 | + | – | >400 | + | – | – |
| 2 | + | + | >400 | + | – | – |
| 3 | + | ± | <400 | + | – | – |
| 4 | + | ± | <400 | Partial anergy | – | – |
| 5 | + | ± | <400 | Complete and/or | + | – |
| 6 | + | ± | <400 | Partial or complete anergy | ± | + |

Incubation periods ranging from a few days up to 3 months have been described,[19] and seroconversion has occurred from 1 to 10 weeks after onset of acute illness. HIV can be isolated from blood (mononuclear cells or plasma) and HIV p24 antigen can often be detected in plasma during the acute illness.[16,20] HIV has been isolated from CSF during episodes of acute meningitis.[17] Antibodies to HIV in serum were detected by IgM IFA as early as 5 ± 3 days after onset of illness by one group.[19] These peaked at 24 ± 17 days and disappeared by 81 ± 27 days. IgG IFA titers were detectable somewhat later (11 ± 3 days), peaked at 133 ± 63 days, and persisted. Other investigators have found radioimmunoprecipitation (RIPA) and Western blot assays to be positive within 2 weeks of clinical illness, whereas enzyme-linked immunosorbent assays (ELISA) became positive later.[21] Positivity by ELISA varied in time from day 31 ± 14 to 58 ± 32 depending on the kit used.

## ASYMPTOMATIC INFECTION (GROUP II) AND PERSISTENT GENERALIZED LYMPHADENOPATHY (GROUP III)

Although still classified separately, there is increasing evidence that the prognosis of asymptomatic infection with or without lymphadenopathy is similar. Diagnosis of asymptomatic infection is usually made on the basis of a repeatedly positive HIV antibody screening test (e.g., ELISA) confirmed by a supplemental antibody assay such as Western blotting, immunofluorescence, or RIPA. (See Chap. 79.) Isolation of HIV from peripheral blood or detection of a surrogate marker such as HIV p24 antigen in serum may also be utilized to detect infection, particularly in those individuals who have not yet seroconverted.[22]

The duration of an asymptomatic carrier state is unpredictable but may be prolonged. In adults, mean asymptomatic incubation periods before development of AIDS have been estimated at 7 to 9 years.[23] The longest studied group is the San Francisco City Clinic Cohort Study, in which 6700 homosexual and bisexual men who enrolled in hepatitis B studies between 1978 and 1980 have been followed.[24] After 88 months of infection, 36 percent of the orginally asymptomatic HIV carriers had developed AIDS and another 40 percent had other signs or symptoms of infection; only 20 percent remained asymptomatic.[22] Studies in other high-risk groups (e.g., hemophiliacs, transfusion recipients) indicate a 25 to 30 percent incidence of AIDS over a 5- to 6-year period.[25]

Within the population of HIV-infected asymptomatic individuals, laboratory testing is useful to predict risk of progression to AIDS. Commonly employed blood tests include a complete blood count, including differential white blood cell count and platelet determination. The most useful and available single measurement of prognosis appears to be the number of CD4 positive cells in peripheral blood. Although the ratio of CD4 to CD8 cells (T4/T8 ratio) may give similar information, it reflects changes not only in the critically important T helper cell but also in T cytotoxic-suppressor cells which may be increased during other infections (e.g., cytomegalovirus, hepatitis B, or Epstein-Barr virus). In one study of homosexual men with persistent generalized lymphadenopathy (PGL), progression to AIDS over 20 months was 60 percent in those with fewer than 200 CD4 cells/mm³, compared with 10 percent in those with greater than 350 CD4 cells/mm³;[26] other studies have given similar results. Additional laboratory assays that may predict progression to AIDS are diminished lymphocyte proliferative responses to antigens, diminished natural killer cell activity, production of circulating levels of acid labile interferon or detection of circulating B-2 microglobulin.[27–30] See Chapter 29 for a summary of immunologic abnormalities described in patients infected with HIV.

It is not clear what viral, host, or environmental factors are responsible for the variable disease progression among HIV-infected individuals. Certain other infectious agents (e.g., cytomegalovirus), genetic factors, and lifestyles have all been postulated as cofactors in pathogenesis, but none has been clearly established. In a Multicenter AIDS Cohort Study (MACS) of homosexual and bisexual HIV seropositive men, decreased numbers of CD4 cells, increased numbers of CD8 cells, high titers of CMV antibodies, low levels of HIV antibodies, and history of sex with someone in whom AIDS developed were independently associated with subsequent progression to AIDS.[31] It is not clear whether these are determinants or merely markers of disease progression.

Asymptomatic HIV carriers often have persistent generalized lymphadenopathy (PGL), defined as palpable lymphadenopathy (nodes ≥ 1 cm) at two or more extrainguinal sites for more than 3 months in the absence of an identifiable cause other than HIV infection. Nodal histology demonstrates pronounced follicular hyperplasia with prominent capillary endothelial cell proliferation. HIV particles are sometimes observed within follicular dendritic cells. As patients develop clinical symptoms (i.e., progress to CDC category IV), lymph node histology changes to reflect atrophy of germinal centers progressing to lymphocyte depletion and fibrosis. Thus, lymph node regression may, paradoxically, herald disease progression. Although lymph node biopsy was once performed frequently, its major utility now is to rule out Kaposi's sarcoma or lymphoma in individual nodes that are disproportionately enlarged.

Lymphadenopathy, itself, does not appear to be a good predictor of disease progression. Several studies have shown a similar progression in asymptomatic individuals with or without lymphadenopathy.[32] Thus, differentiation between CDC categories II and III appears more artificial than real.

## Table 30-3. CDC Case Definition of AIDS (1987)

I. *Without laboratory evidence regarding HIV infection.* If laboratory tests for HIV were not performed or gave inconclusive results and the patient had no other cause of immunodeficiency listed in section I.A below, then any disease listed in section I.B indicates AIDS if it was diagnosed by a definitive method.
   A. Causes of immunodeficiency that disqualify diseases as indicators of AIDS in the absence of laboratory evidence for HIV infection.
      1. High-dose or long term systemic corticosteroid therapy or other immunosuppressive/cytotoxic therapy ≤ 3 months before the onset of the indicator disease
      2. Any of the following diseases diagnosed ≤ 3 months after diagnosis of the indicator disease: Hodgkin's disease, non-Hodgkin's lymphoma (other than primary brain lymphoma), lymphocytic leukemia, multiple myeloma, any other cancer of lymphoreticular or histiocytic tissue, or angioimmunoblastic lymphadenopathy
      3. A genetic (congenital) immunodeficiency syndrome or an acquired immunodeficiency syndrome atypical of HIV infection, such as one involving hypogammaglobulinemia
   B. Indicator diseases diagnosed definitively
      1. Candidiasis of the esophagus, trachea, bronchi, or lungs
      2. Cryptococcosis, extrapulmonary
      3. Cryptosporidiosis with diarrhea persisting > 1 month
      4. Cytomegalovirus disease of an organ other than liver, spleen, or lymph nodes in a patient > 1 month of age
      5. Herpes simplex virus infection causing a mucocutaneous ulcer that persists longer than 1 month; or bronchitis, pneumonitis, or esophagitis for any duration affecting a patient > 1 month of age
      6. Kaposi's sarcoma affecting a patient < 60 years of age
      7. Lymphoma of the brain (primary) affecting a patient <60 years of age
      8. Lymphoid interstitial pneumonia and/or pulmonary lymphoid hyperplasia (LIP/PLH complex) affecting a child <13 years of age
      9. *Mycobacterium avium* complex or *M. kansasii* disease, disseminated (at a site other than or in addition to lungs, skin, or cervical or hilar lymph nodes)
      10. *Pneumocystis carinii* pneumonia
      11. Progressive multifocal leukoencephalopathy
      12. Toxoplasmosis of the brain affecting a patient >1 month of age

II. *With laboratory evidence for HIV infection.* Regardless of the presence of other causes of immunodeficiency (I.A), in the presence of laboratory evidence for HIV infection, any disease listed above (I.B) or below (II.A or II.B) indicates a diagnosis of AIDS.
   A. Indicator diseases diagnosed definitively
      1. Bacterial infections, multiple or recurrent (any combination of at least two within a 2-year period), of the following types affecting a child <13 years of age: septicemia, pneumonia, meningitis, bone or joint infection, or abscess of an internal organ or body cavity (excluding otitis media or superficial skin or mucosal abscesses), caused by *Haemophilus, Streptococcus* (including pneumococcus), or other pyogenic bacteria.
      2. Coccidioidomycosis, disseminated (at a site other than or in addition to lungs or cervical or hilar lymph nodes)
      3. HIV encephalopathy (also called "HIV dementia," "AIDS dementia," or "subacute encephalitis due to HIV")
      4. Histoplasmosis, disseminated (at a site other than or in addition to lungs or cervical or hilar lymph nodes)
      5. Isosporiasis with diarrhea persisting >1 month
      6. Kaposi's sarcoma at any age
      7. Lymphoma of the brain (primary) at any age
      8. Other non-Hodgkin's lymphoma of B-cell or unknown immunologic phenotype and the following histologic types:
         *a.* Small noncleaved lymphoma (either Burkitt or non-Burkitt type)
         *b.* Immunoblastic sarcoma (equivalent to any of the following, although not necessarily all in combination: immunoblastic lymphoma, large-cell lymphoma, diffuse histiocytic lymphoma, diffuse undifferentiated lymphoma, or high-grade lymphoma)
         *Note:* Lymphomas are not included here if they are of T-cell immunologic phenotype or their histologic type is not described or is described as "lymphocytic," "lymphoblastic," "small cleaved," or "plasmacytoid lymphocytic"
      9. Any mycobacterial disease caused by mycobacteria other than *M. tuberculosis*, disseminated (at a site other than or in addition to lungs, skin, or cervical or hilar lymph nodes)
      10. Disease caused by *M. tuberculosis*, extrapulmonary (involving at least one site outside the lungs, regardless of whether there is concurrent pulmonary involvement)
      11. *Salmonella* (nontyphoid) septicemia, recurrent
      12. HIV wasting syndrome (emaciation, "slim disease")
   B. Indicator diseases diagnosed presumptively
      *Note:* Given the seriousness of diseases indicative of AIDS, it is generally important to diagnose them definitively, especially when therapy that would be used may have serious side effects or when definitive diagnosis is needed for eligibility for antiretroviral therapy. Nonetheless, in some situations, a patient's condition will not permit the performance of definitive tests. In other situations, accepted clinical practice may be to diagnose presumptively based on the presence of characteristic clinical and laboratory abnormalities.
      1. Candidiasis of the esophagus
      2. Cytomegalovirus retinitis with loss of vision
      3. Kaposi's sarcoma
      4. Lymphoid interstitial pneumonia and/or pulmonary lymphoid hyperplasia (LIP/PLH complex) affecting a child <13 years of age
      5. Mycobacterial disease (acid-fast bacilli with species not identified by culture), disseminated (involving at least one site other than or in addition to lungs, skin, or cervical or hilar lymph nodes)
      6. *Pneumocystis carinii* pneumonia
      7. Toxoplasmosis of the brain affecting a patient >1 month of age

III. *With laboratory evidence against HIV infection.* With laboratory test results negative for HIV infection, a diagnosis of AIDS for surveillance purposes is ruled out unless:
   A. All the other causes of immunodeficiency listed above in section I.A are excluded; *and*
   B. The patient has had either:
      1. *Pneumocystis carinii* pneumonia diagnosed by a definitive method; *or*
      2. *a.* Any of the other diseases indicative of AIDS listed above in section I.B diagnosed by a definitive method; *and*
         *b.* A T-helper/inducer (CD4) lymphocyte count $<400/mm^3$

## SYMPTOMATIC HIV INFECTION (GROUP IV)

After a variable period of asymptomatic HIV seropositivity, a variety of signs or symptoms may herald clinical deterioration. Chronic fevers, night sweats, diarrhea, weight loss, herpes zoster, oral thrush, or hairy leukoplakia may occur individually, simultaneously, or sequentially. The term AIDS-related complex (ARC) is often used to characterize the presence of two or more symptoms and two or more laboratory findings indicative of immune dysfunction. Unfortunately, definitions of ARC have varied, and this term is not used in the CDC classification system.

To be categorized in CDC group IVA, one or more of the following must be present: fever persisting more than 1 month, involuntary weight loss of greater than 10 percent of baseline or diarrhea for more than 1 month, in the absence of a concurrent illness or condition other than HIV infection to explain the findings. It is becoming clear, however, that this definition of HIV-constitutional disease is too narrow to reflect the increasing spectrum of HIV-associated systemic disease. HIV may directly or indirectly involve multiple organ systems, leading to a variety of clinical syndromes.

Similarly, definitions of AIDS have changed over time, reflecting a greater understanding of the relationships among HIV, wasting syndromes, the nervous system, opportunistic infections, and neoplasms.[33] The revised CDC definition of AIDS is shown in Table 30-3. Once the diagnosis of AIDS has been made, the 1-year survival is often less than 1 year, although considerable variability exists, depending on factors such as age, sex, risk group, and tissue diagnosis.[34] For example, black women who acquire AIDS through IV drug abuse have a particularly poor prognosis, whereas white homosexual men 30 to 34 years old who present with only Kaposi's sarcoma have a 1-year survival probability of over 80 percent.

## MANIFESTATIONS OF HIV INFECTION BY BODY SYSTEM

### SKIN AND MUCOUS MEMBRANES

Cutaneous manifestations of the acute primary infection (Group I) have consisted of a truncal maculopapular eruption in approximately 50 percent of patients. Occasional patients will have more diffuse eruptions that may involve the oropharynx. Sometimes these may be urticarial or vesicular.[16,17] These are self-limited and resolve within 1 to 3 weeks.

As immune deficiency develops later in the course of HIV infection, a variety of mucocutaneous manifestations develop. These may be of infectious, neoplastic, allergic, or undefined etiology. It is unclear which, if any, of the mucocutaneous manifestations are caused by HIV directly, although infection of skin Langerhans cells and cervical monocytes, lymphocytes, and endothelial cells has been reported.[35,36] Table 30-4 lists some of the conditions observed in HIV-infected patients.

**Table 30-4. Mucocutaneous Manifestations of HIV Infection**

Infections
- Viruses:
  - Herpes simplex
  - Varicella zoster
  - Molluscum contagiosum
  - Human papilloma virus
  - Hairy leukoplakia (? EBV)
- Bacteria:
  - *Myocobacterium avium* or *M. marinum*
  - *Treponema pallidum* (syphilis)
  - *Staphylococcus aureus*
- Fungi:
  - *Candida albicans*
  - *Cryptococcus neoformans*
  - *Histoplasma capsulatum*
- Mites:
  - Scabies

Neoplasms
- Kaposi's sarcoma
- Squamous cell carcinomas
- Basal cell carcinomas
- Cutaneous lymphomas (?)

Miscellaneous
- Seborrheic dermatitis
- Telangiectasis
- Ichthyosis
- Erythroderma
- Papules
- Drug reactions

Infections with herpes simplex types 1 and 2 are often quite severe and chronic. If untreated, they can become erosive and secondarily infected. Herpes zoster can disseminate or become chronic. We have seen zoster ulcers from which varicella zoster virus could be isolated persist for over 6 months in an HIV-infected patient. Moreover, the appearance of herpes zoster in a previously asymptomatic HIV carrier may herald progression to AIDS.[37] Molluscum contagiosum, induced by a poorly defined pox virus, occurs commonly in genital or facial areas and may require surgery or cryosurgery for eradication. A number of other opportunistic pathogens, including *Candida albicans, Myobacterium avium* complex, *Cryptococcus neoformans, Histoplasma capsulatum,* and papilloma viruses may also cause skin lesions in HIV-infected patients. Some of these opportunistic infections are covered in Chap. 57.

Of particular note is the seborrheic dermatitis that develops in up to 83 percent of patients with AIDS.[38,39] It is frequently severe and may resemble psoriasis in its appearance, with papular and scaling lesions involving scalp (sometimes with alopecia), face, trunk, groin, and extremities. Diffuse erythroderma may be seen as well. Although the pathogenesis of HIV-associated hyperkeratotic disorders is unclear, both ketoconazole and topical steroids have been reported to be useful in their management.[40]

Papular eruptions with noncoalescing 2- to 5-mm skin-colored papules, often pruritic in nature, have been described in over 20 percent of patients with AIDS.[41] These papules, histologically characterized by a nonspecific perivascular mononuclear cell infiltration, often persist for prolonged periods.

Allergic skin reactions occur in over 50 percent of AIDS patients treated with trimethoprim-sulfamethoxazole.[42] An erythematous, maculopapular rash is often associated with fever, neutropenia, thrombocytopenia, and transaminase elevation. The mechanisms underlying HIV-associated drug hypersensivity are unclear.

The principal mucocutaneous neoplasm observed in HIV-infected individuals is Kaposi's sarcoma. This and other neoplastic complications of HIV infection will be discussed later in this chapter as well as in Chap. 56. In addition to Kaposi's sarcoma of the mouth, a number of other oral manifestations of HIV infection are common. Oral candidiasis, observed in over 80 percent of patients with ARC or AIDS, often predicts the imminent development of more serious opportunistic infections.[43] Oral candidiasis can often be controlled by topical therapy with nystatin or clotrimazole. Extension into the esophagus, sometimes presenting with dysphagia, requires the use of oral ketoconazole or low-dose intravenous amphotericin B. It must be remembered, however, that esophageal candidiasis may be present without any symptoms.

Hairy leukoplakia is a newly described disorder observed commonly in HIV-infected individuals.[44,45] Like oral candidiasis, it may be predictive of AIDS development. Raised white areas on the tongue or buccal mucosa appear, often with a corrugated or "hairy" surface. Histologically, excessive keratinization without inflammatory response is observed; intraepithelial Langerhans cells are depleted, perhaps as a result of previous HIV infection. Both papilloma-like viruses and Epstein-Barr virus (EBV) have been detected in lesions, although HIV itself has not been found. Satisfactory clinical response to oral acyclovir has been reported.[46]

Infection of the genital tract by HIV appears common, as the virus is readily excreted in both semen[47] and cervical secretions.[48] It is not clear whether local genital infection necessarily results in tissue damage, although there is an association between genital ulcerative lesions and HIV infection, in both men and women.[36,49] Whether HIV actually causes such lesions is unknown currently.

## GASTROINTESTINAL TRACT

The gastrointestinal tract is a major target organ in HIV infection, particularly among homesexual men.[50–52] Rectal tissue may be a major portal of entry and certain colonic cells can be infected with HIV.[53] In situ hybridization of biopsy specimens from rectum and duodenum has demonstrated HIV-infected cells in bowel crypts and lamina propria.[54]

Gastrointestinal symptoms including anorexia, nausea, vomiting, and diarrhea are described by the majority of symptomatic HIV-infected patients.[52] Significant weight loss occurs in nearly all patients with AIDS, and in HIV carriers is highly predictive of AIDS development. The role of HIV, itself, as a pathogen in these observed gastrointestinal disorders is unclear. Multiple other pathogens may be involved (Table 30-5), including viruses (cytomegalovirus, herpes simplex), chlamydiae, bacteria (*Shigella, Salmonella, Campylobacter,* mycobacteria), and parasites (*Giardia,* cryptosporidia, isospora, amoeba, *Strongyloides*). In one study, thorough diagnostic evaluations conducted on patients with AIDS and diarrhea (including esophagogastroduodenoscopy and colonoscopy) revealed one or more enteric pathogens in 85 percent, 69 percent of which were improved on treatment.[55]

Gastrointestinal infection with cytomegalovirus (CMV) is extremely common,[56] and it is possible that HIV and CMV may interact in the pathogenesis of tissue damage in the bowel and elsewhere.[57] CMV infection of the bowel most often presents as a diffuse colitis associated with watery or bloody diarrhea and abdominal pain.[56] CMV esophagitis, gastritis, or cholangitis may also be present. Localized ulcers of the colon may lead to toxic dilation and rarely perforation. CMV gastrointestinal infections appear to respond to the acyclovir derivative ganciclovir, although controlled trials have not yet been reported.[58] Chronic herpes simplex anal and perianal infections are common in homosexual men with HIV infection and may require prolonged suppressive therapy with oral acyclovir.[59]

**Table 30-5. Gastrointestinal Manifestations of HIV Infections**

Opportunistic infections
Viruses:
- *Herpes simplex* (proctitis, esophagitis, oral, perianal)
- Cytomegalovirus (esophagitis, enteritis, cholangitis, colitis)
- Papilloma (condyloma accuminata)

Chlamydiae: *Chlamydia trachomatis* (proctitis)
Fungi: *Candida albicans* (esophagitis, thrush)
Bacteria:
- *Salmonella* (colitis)
- *Shigella* (colitis)
- *Campylobacter* (colitis)
- *C. difficile* (colitis)
- *Neisseria gonorrhoeae* (proctitis)
- *Treponema pallidum* (proctitis, perianal)

Parasites:
- *Giardia lamblia* (enteritis)
- Cryptosporidia (enteritis)
- Microsporidia (enteritis)
- *Isospora belli* (enteritis)
- *Strongyloides stercoralis* (enteritis)
- *Entamoeba histolytica* (colitis)

Infections with *Entamoeba histolytica, Giardia lamblia, Isospora belli,* cryptosporidia species, and microsporidia species of protozoa are particulary common in homosexual men with HIV infection.[52] Cryptosporidia and isospora may both cause severe protracted diarrhea with brush border maldigestion and malabsorption, resulting in profound weight loss.[60] Cryptosporidia may in addition cause biliary tract disease, often in conjunction with CMV, presenting as cholecystitis or cholangitis.[61] Diagnosis of cryptosporidia or *I. belli* infections depends on identification of the oocyst form in stained specimens. Treatment of cryptosporidial infections has generally been unsatisfactory, although spiramycin is currently undergoing placebo-controlled trials. In contrast, *I. belli* infections respond promptly to trimethoprim-sulfamethoxazole, and possibly metronidazole, although prolonged suppression may be required.[60]

*Mycobacterium avium* complex infection may present with intestinal involvement characterized by diarrhea, malabsorption, weight loss, and fever. Small-bowel biopsy may resemble Whipple's disease. Diagnosis is based on identification of *M. avium* on biopsy and/or in stool or blood cultures. No uniformly successful treatment has been described, although a variety of regimens are under investigation.

The clinical courses of salmonella and campylobacter gastrointestinal infections in HIV-infected patients often differ from that seen in noninfected, immunologically intact individuals. They may be protracted and relapsing with recurrent bacteremias, thus necessitating chronic suppresive antibiotic regimens for adequate control.[52]

Several malignancies of the gastrointestinal tract must be differentiated from other causes of bowel dysfunction. These include Kaposi's sarcoma which occurs throughout the bowel, small-bowel lymphomas of various types (undifferentiated, Burkitt-like), and squamous cell carcinoma of the rectum and anus. These are discussed in Chap. 56.

## ENDOCRINE SYSTEM

There is currently no evidence that HIV directly infects cells of the endocrine system. However, a number of endocrine disorders may develop in the course of HIV infection.

Hypogonadism is common in men with HIV infection and may be the first endocrine abnormality detected.[62] It appears to reflect progression of disease with cachexia and weight loss. Among men with ARC or AIDS, decreased libido, impotence, and decreased serum testosterone are frequent. Serum gonadotropin levels are reduced and responses to gonadotropin-releasing hormone administration are normal.[62]

Adrenal insufficiency may be observed as a result of disseminated cytomegalovirus or *M. avium* infection involving the adrenal gland,[63] but most HIV-infected individuals appear to have intact adrenal cortisol reserve.[62] Similarly, thyroid function appears intact in most HIV-infected men.[62] Thus, at present there is no evidence that the commonly observed wasting syndrome of HIV infection has an endocrine basis.

## KIDNEYS

HIV-infected individuals are subject to several forms of renal injury. AIDS-associated nephropathy (or AIDS-related glomerulopathy) is characterized by proteinuria (> 3.5 g per day) and focal segmental glomerulosclerosis.[64,65] This syndrome results in renal failure within a few weeks and is minimally responsive to hemodialysis. It appears disproportionately common in black male intravenous drug abusers and to a lesser extent in Haitians, but the mechanisms of its development are unclear.

A second renal abnormality observed in patients with AIDS is characterized by diffuse mesangial hyperplasia.[65] This does not appear to be frequently associated with clinically overt renal disease but is detected at autopsy. Glomerular mesangial deposits of IgM and C3 suggest immune complex deposition, although the antigen is undefined.

Kidney damage may also result from ischemia or nephrotoxic factors, particularly drugs including pentamidine, aminoglycosides, trimethoprim-sulfamethoxazole, meclofenamate, and radiocontrast agents.[64] This form of injury may lead to acute renal failure that is responsive to hemodialysis.

## HEART AND LUNGS

Rare patients with AIDS may develop a congestive cardiomyopathy with four-chamber dilatation, myofibrillar loss, and focal myocarditis.[66] The pathogenetic mechanisms involved in this late AIDS complication are unclear.

Lymphocytic interstitial pneumonitis (LIP) is a common manifestation of pediatric AIDS but is also seen in adults.[67] It is not clear whether this condition is the same as that called nonspecific interstitial pnemonitis (NIP) by others.[68] In one series of adult patients with AIDS, the latter disorder was diagnosed in 38 percent of all patients (41 of 110) and accounted for 32 percent (48 of 152) of all episodes of clinical pneumonitis.[68] The etiology of LIP or NIP is unknown, though in children both EBV and HIV have been implicated in LIP. Histological studies demonstrate interstitial inflammation with lymphocytes, plasma cells, moderate edema, and fibrin deposition. The clinical features of patients with NIP or LIP are similar to those seen in patients with *Pneumocystis carinii* pneumonia (PCP), but in contrast to PCP, the course often resolves or stabilizes without specific therapy. The role for corticosteroid therapy is unclear.

Multiple opportunistic infections may present with pulmonary manifestations (Table 30-6). Pneumocystis pneumonia remains the most common presenting opportunistic infection in AIDS; it will be discussed in detail in Chap. 57.

**Table 30-6. Pulmonary Complications of HIV Infections**

Opportunistic infections
- *Pneumocystis carinii*
- Cytomegalovirus
- *Cryptococcus neoformans*
- *Mycobacterium avium* complex
- *M. tuberculosis*
- *M. kansasii*
- *Histoplasma capsulatum*
- *Neisseria asteroides*
- Other (pyogenic bacteria, herpes simplex, *Toxoplasma gondii, Staphylococcus stercoralis, Candida albicans, Legionella pneumophila*)

Neoplasms
- Kaposi's sarcoma
- Lymphoma

Miscellaneous
- Lymphoid interstitial pneumonitis (LIP)
- Nonspecific interstitial pneumonitis (NIP)

## HEMATOLOGIC SYSTEM

As discussed earlier, the major hematologic abnormalities observed during progressive HIV infections are decreases in the numbers and functional capabilities of CD4 positive helper T lymphocytes. However, hematologic abnormalities are not limited to lymphocytes. Anemia, thrombocytopenia, and granulocytopenia may all be seen in individual patients. Peripheral cytopenias are often associated with bone marrow hyperplasia rather than hypoplasia.[70] Although the pathogenesis of these abnormalities is probably multifactorial, antibodies in patient sera directed against the envelope glycoprotein of HIV (gp120) appear capable of suppressing the growth of hematopoietic progenitors from HIV seropositive but not seronegative controls,[71] suggesting that such antigens are expressed on the bone marrow precursor cells. The progenitors, themselves, appear capable of responding to both erythropoietin and granulocyte-macrophage colony stimulating factor (GMCSF) in vitro[71] and to GMCSF in vivo.[72] Alterations of regulatory T lymphocytes within bone marrow may also be involved in the pathogenesis of the observed hematopoietic abnormalities.[73]

Immune thrombocytopenic purpura occurs in up to 10 percent of HIV-infected individuals and may, at times, be the only clinical evidence of infection.[74] Manifestations include easy bruisability, epistaxis, gingival or rectal bleeding, and petechiae. In approximately 15 percent, the thrombocytopenia is asymptomatic. Several mechanisms have been proposed for the thrombocytopenia including direct infection of platelets or megakaryocytes by HIV, immune complex formation, and novel antibodies directed against a platelet membrane antigen of 25,000 daltons.[75] The therapy of thrombocytopenia in HIV-infected patients has included splenectomy, azidothymidine, corticosteroids, and intravenous immune globulin.[76,94]

Anemia is observed in the vast majority of patients with AIDS. Reticulocyte counts are generally depressed and red cell morphology is normal.[70,77] Although positive Coombs tests and erythrophagocytosis have been described, these appear to be rare events. The mechanisms of the anemia seen in advanced disease are varied and may include infection of bone marrow cells by HIV or opportunists (eg., *M. avium* complex), immune mechanisms, administered drugs, (eg., azidothymidine), or nutritional deficiencies.

Circulating lupuslike anticoagulants are frequently observed in patients with AIDS.[78] These inhibitors prolong the activated partial thromboplastin time (PTT) and are typically directed against phospholipid components of the prothrombin activator complex involved in coagulation. Thrombotic complications are rare and the PTT is usually only moderately prolonged.

## NERVOUS SYSTEM

A number of opportunistic infections (toxoplasmosis, cryptococcosis, mycobacterial infection, progressive multifocal leukoencephalopathy) can present with neurologic manifestations. Lymphomas of the central nervous system also are being recognized with increasing frequency. These opportunistic infections and neoplasms are reviewed in Chaps. 56 and 57. In this chapter, we summarize the effects of HIV, itself, on the nervous system.

HIV enters the nervous system early in infection, perhaps carried by monocyte-macrophages from the peripheral blood.[79,80] Clinical and pathological features of neurological disorders associated with HIV are shown in Table 30-7. Several mechanisms have been proposed to explain the neurological manifestations of HIV infection. HIV infections of brain macrophages, endothelial cells, and glial cells have been described. However, the pathogenesis of the abnormalities observed remains poorly defined.[81]

HIV subacute encephalitis has also been called AIDS encephalopathy or the AIDS dementia complex. The characteristic syndrome of progressive cognitive impairment accompanied by motor and behavioral abnormalities may occur in 25 to 65 percent of patients with AIDS.[82,83] HIV neurologic disease can occur in the absence of clinical immunodeficiency, suggesting the possibility of neurotropic HIV strains.

Early in the course of HIV subacute encephalitis, symptoms relate to cognitive impairment, particularly forgetfulness, loss of concentration, and slowness of thought. Nearly 50 percent of patients report symptoms of motor dysfunction, such as loss of balance or leg weakness.[82] Behavioral symptoms such as apathy, social withdrawal, depression, and personality changes are present in about 40 percent. Behavioral changes are the only initial abnormalities in about 20 percent. Psychomotor slowing associated with a blunted affect may be the only abnormal finding. Organic psychosis develops occasionally as a prominent early manifestation.

The course of HIV encephalopathy is usually progressive, evolving slowing over a period of several months to a year.[83] The mean survival time from the onset of severe dementia is usually less than 6 months. As the disease progresses, there is gradual deterioration in cognitive function as well as evidence of progressive motor and behavioral abnormalities. Late in the course, psychomotor slowing is a prominent manifestation in about 80 percent of affected patients.[82] Other common late signs and symptoms include ataxia, hypertonia, weakness, tremor, incontinence, and psychiatric disturbances including organic psychosis, frontal release signs, myoclonus, and seizures. Severe dementia with global cognitive impairment is frequently associated with akinetic mutism, incontinence, paraparesis, and myoclonus or seizures. Patients usually remain alert even late in the course. Lethargy and coma most often occur in the setting of systemic illness.

Routine diagnostic studies including cerebrospinal fluid analysis, computed tomographic (CT) scans, and electroencephalography usually show nonspecific abnormalities in patients with subacute encephalitis. Cerebrospinal fluid abnormalities are present in 85 percent.[82] A mild mononuclear pleocytosis with a range of 5 to 50 leukocytes/mm$^3$ is found in about 20 percent. About 60 percent have an elevated cerebrospinal fluid protein level ranging from 0.5 to 1 g/liter.[82] Hypoglycorrhachia is rare. The CT scan shows differing degrees of diffuse cerebral atrophy in 80 to 90 percent of affected patients with occasional low-density lesions in white matter.[82,83] Magnetic resonance imaging is more sensitive than the CT scan and frequently shows white matter abnormalities in addition to cerebral atrophy.[82,83] Electroencephalography may demonstrate differing degrees of generalized slowing in a nonspecific pattern.[83]

Histopathologic findings include cerebral atrophy, gliosis of cortex and white matter, small foci of tissue necrosis, microglial nodules, foci of demyelination, perivascular inflammation, and multinucleated giant cells.[84] Lesions are most frequent in white

**Table 30-7. Major Neurologic Disorders Associated with HIV Infection**

| Disorder | Prevalence, % | Clinical features |
|---|---|---|
| **Opportunistic infections** | | |
| *Toxoplasma gondii* | 10 | Focal seizures, altered consciouness, CT-ring enhancing lesions |
| *Cryptococcus neoformans* | 4–8 | Headache, confusion, seizures, CSF cryptococcal antigen |
| Progressive mutifocal leukoencephalopathy | 1–4 | Limb weakness, gait abnormalities, visual loss, altered mental state, CT + MRI-white matter lesions |
| Lymphoma | 5–10 | Diplopia, weakness, encephalopathy; CT contrast-enhancing lesions |
| **HIV-related** | | |
| Subacute encephalitis | 25–65 | Cognitive deficits, memory loss, psychomotor slowing, pyramidal tract signs, ataxia, weakness, depression, organic psychosis, incontinence, myoclonus, seizures |
| Peripheral neuropathies: Chronic distal symmetric polyneuropathy | 10–50 | Painful dysesthesias, numbness paresthesias, weakness, autonomic dysfunction |
| Chronic inflammatory demyelinating polyneuropathy | | Weakness, sensory deficits, mononeuropathy multiplex, cranial nerve palsies, hyporeflexia or areflexia, cerebrospinal fluid pleocytosis |
| Vacuolar myelopathy | 11–22 | Gait ataxia, progressive spastic paraparesis, posterior column deficits, incontinence |
| Aseptic meningitis | 5–10 | Headache, fever, meningeal signs, cranial nerve palsies, cerebrospinal fluid pleocytosis |

matter, cerebral cortex, amygdala, basal ganglia, and hippocampus.

A vacuolar myelopathy affecting posterior and lateral columns occurs in 11 to 22 percent of patients with AIDS.[84,85] A syndrome of progressive spastic paraparesis evolves over a period of months, with gait ataxia, leg weakness, upper motor neuron signs, incontinence, and posterior column deficits;[85] 90 percent of these patients also have some dementia. Pathologic findings include vacuolar degeneration affecting white matter, most commonly at the thoracic level of the lateral columns.

Distal symmetric polyneuropathy, inflammatory demyelinating polyneuropathies, and other peripheral nerve disorders are also seen in HIV-infected patients.[86] As many as 95 percent of patients with AIDS have histopathologic evidence of peripheral nerve disease.[79] Symptoms of peripheral neuropathy are reported by about 50 percent of affected patients.

The most common type of neuropathy is a chronic, distal, symmetric, predominantly sensory, polyneuropathy.[87,88] This disorder occurs most frequently in patients with AIDS but also occurs in patients with other HIV-related conditions. Painful dysesthesias or paresthesias are the most common symptoms (48 percent); weakness is reported by 33 percent, and evidence of autonomic dysfunction occurs in at least 10 percent.[79] Findings on neurologic examination include distal small and large fiber sensory deficits, weakness, diminished distal deep tendon reflexes, and orthostatic hypotension. Nerve conduction studies have shown evidence of a distal axonal or mixed axonal and demyelinating polyneuropathy.[88] Clinical features include weakness, relatively mild sensory deficits, areflexia, and electrophysiologic evidence of a predominantly demyelinating neuropathy. Occasionally a multifocal pattern with cranial nerve involvement and mononeuropathy multiplex is seen.[88] This disorder is distinguished from Guillain-Barré syndrome by a cerebrospinal fluid pleocytosis ranging from about 10 to 50 cells/mm$^3$.[86] The course often evolves during a period of weeks to months, but patients may have spontaneous alleviation of symptoms or may respond to steroids or plasmapheresis.[86] Histologic findings include demyelination, axonopathy, and mononuclear cell infiltration.[79]

Other neurologic disorders have been associated rarely with HIV infection. Polymyositis responding to treatment with steroids has been described in patients with the AIDS-related complex or otherwise asymptomatic serologic evidence of HIV infection.[89] An autonomic neuropathy presenting with syncopal episodes associated with bradycardia and postural hypotension may lead to cardiorespiratory arrest after invasive procedures, e.g., needle aspiration of the lung.[90] Acute leukoencephalitis and cerebral granulomatous angiitis associated with isolation of HIV from cerebrospinal fluid and brain in patients without immunodeficiency have been described, as has a severe progressive diffuse leukoencephalopathy associated with AIDS.[79]

## OCULAR MANIFESTATIONS

A variety of ocular manifestations are seen in patients infected with HIV. Cotton-wool spots, representing focal areas of retinal ischemia, are present in the majority of patients with AIDS or ARC.[91,92] The pathogenesis of these lesions is not clear, although occlusion of retinal arterioles and capillaries secondary to immune complex deposition or perivasculitis has been proposed. HIV has been isolated from retinas, and immunohistochemical staining demonstrated HIV antigens within retinal endothelial and neuroretinal cells,[92] suggesting that the virus itself may be responsible for cotton-wool spots in some patients.

Ocular infections secondary to a variety of opportunists including CMV, cryptococcus, toxoplasma, mycobacteria, candida, herpes simplex, and varicella zoster have been reported in patients with AIDS. Orbital and conjunctival Kaposi's sarcoma has been noted as well.[91] Of these, the most common and severe infection is CMV retinitis, occurring in 25 to 35 percent of patients with AIDS.[93] Characteristic features include a "brush fire" appearance of hemorrhages and exudates, vasculitis with perivascular sheathing, and unrelenting contiguous progression to retinal necrosis and opacification, often resulting in visual loss. Stabilization or improvement has been noted in the majority of patients treated with intravenous ganciclovir, although prolonged maintenance therapy is required.[93]

## TREATMENT

Treatment of individual opportunistic infections and neoplasms is covered in Chaps. 56 and 57. This chapter will review developments in the treatment of the underlying HIV infection. Progress in the development of antivirals to treat HIV infections has moved rapidly. Within 3 years from the time AIDS was associated definitively with HIV, 3′azido-3′-deoxythymidine (AZT, zidovudine, Retrovir) was licensed for use in this disorder.[94]

In 1985, Mitsuya et al.[95] demonstrated that AZT inhibited HIV-1 replication in vitro at concentrations of $>0.1\ \mu M$ ($>0.37\ \mu g/ml$), whereas inhibition of the multiplication of infected lymphocytes was observed only at concentrations $>1$ m$M$. Some cells are more sensitive than lymphocytes to the cytotoxic effects of AZT; in particular, hematopoietic progenitor cells are inhibited by concentrations of $0.9 \pm 0.1\ \mu M$. In addition, in some cells (e.g., primary human monocyte-macrophages) AZT may be less active against HIV, possibly because of diminished phosphorylation.[96] The apparent retroviral selectivity of AZT is a result of a preferential interaction of the 5′-triphosphate of AZT (AZTTP) with reverse transcriptase. AZT is converted by cellular thymidine kinase to a monophosphate form (AZTMP). The monophosphate is subsequently converted by a cellular thymidylate kinase into a diphosphate and by other cellular enzymes to its active triphosphate form. AZTTP inhibits HIV-1 reverse transcriptase approximately 100 times more effectively than it does cellular polymerase alpha. AZTTP binds preferentially to HIV-1 reverse transcriptase, and the incorporation of azidothymidylate into the growing DNA strand leads to chain termination. Furthermore, AZTMP competitively inhibits thymidylate kinase, an action resulting in reduced levels of thymidine-5′-triphosphate (dTTP).

After oral dosing, AZT is rapidly absorbed, with peak serum concentrations occurring at 30 to 90 min. The mean AZT half-life is about 1 h. Chronic dosing of 250 mg every 4 h results in peak and trough concentrations of 0.62 and 0.16 μg/ml, respectively. The average bioavailability of the oral AZT capsule is 65 percent, and total urinary recovery is 90 percent. Because AZT is metabolized primarily by glucuronidation, drugs that inhibit this step (e.g., probenicid) can increase the half-life of AZT. AZT penetrates the blood-brain barrier effectively, and this penetration results in antiviral concentrations within the CSF.

From February 1986 to the end of June 1986, 282 patients with AIDS or ARC were enrolled in a clinical trial conducted at

12 different centers in the United States.[97,98] Patients with AIDS were within 4 months of their first attack of *P. carinii* pneumonia, and patients with ARC had severe clinical signs (e.g., significant weight loss or oral thrush).

By September 1986, the study was terminated by an independent data safety monitoring board. Nineteen patients (12 with AIDS, 7 with ARC) in the placebo group had died, compared with only one who received AZT. Furthermore, there was a significant difference in opportunistic infections (OI) in patients who received placebo (45 OI) compared with AZT recipients (24 OI). Patients who received AZT generally gained weight, whereas placebo recipients lost weight. Karnofsky scores of functional capability also improved in AZT recipients but did not improve in the placebo groups. Individuals who received AZT generally showed an increase in CD4 cells, although this effect was lost after 5 months in patients with AIDS and over 12 months in patients with ARC. Of patients who received AZT, 29 percent developed skin test reactivity to at least one antigen, while only 9 percent of placebo recipients lost skin anergy. The exact mechanisms by which these effects occurred are not fully elucidated, but preliminary data from several centers suggest that HIV-1 p24 antigenemia is reduced in AZT recipients, a finding probably reflecting diminished virus replication in vivo.

The decreased mortality rates observed in patients treated with AZT were also seen during extended follow-up of the originally enrolled patients. After 36 weeks of observation, 9 (6.2 percent) of the original 145 patients randomized to AZT had died, compared with 29 (39.3 percent) of the original 137 patients who were randomized to placebo and received less than three total weeks of AZT therapy (Burroughs Wellcome, unpublished observation). AZT treatment was, thus, associated with a sixfold decrease in mortality after 36 weeks of study. The estimated mortality of the AZT group, followed for 1 year, was 10.3 percent.

AZT treatment did produce some side effects during the placebo-controlled study. Macrocytic anemia occurred frequently in the AZT group and made transfusions necessary in 40 patients (compared with 11 in the placebo group). Another side effect that also made AZT dose reduction necessary was neutropenia in 16 percent.[98] Headache was the most common adverse symptom observed. Nausea, myalgia, and insomnia were also reported more frequently in recipients of AZT. These adverse effects were reversible and generally tolerable for patients with AIDS or severe ARC.

Rare instances of pancytopenia with hypocellular marrow have been described.[94] Patients who enter therapy with poor bone marrow reserve secondary to opportunistic infection (e.g., *M. avium* complex) or with vitamin $B_{12}$ deficiency have more toxicity than patients with sufficient marrow reserve. In addition, other adverse effects such as fever, rash, and nail pigmentation have been observed. Rarely, patients have developed apparent CNS toxicity, usually manifested by reversible confusion. AZT has, however, also been reported to lead to neurological improvement in three patients with the HIV dementia complex,[99] an observation making interpretation of neurological changes difficult. Anecdotal case reports also suggest that AZT may benefit certain patients with HIV-associated thrombocytopenia, psoriasis, or lymphocytic interstitial pneumonia, but such reports will require confirmation in larger studies.[94]

Although it is tempting to extrapolate from the one completed placebo-controlled trial and several anecdotal case reports to other HIV-associated conditions, such extrapolations are dangerous and unwise. Except in carefully controlled trials, it is recommended that AZT be limited to those patients with symptomatic HIV infection and a history of pneumocystis pneumonia or less than 200/mm$^3$ CD4 cells. Controlled trials are currently underway in asymptomatic HIV carriers, as well as in patients with early ARC, and localized Kaposi's sarcoma. Until results from such trials are available, it is impossible to predict accurately whether the potential benefits of AZT in such situations outweigh the considerable risks.

The currently recommended dosage of AZT for adults is 200 mg every 4 h, although the dose administered in the placebo-controlled trial was 250 mg every 4 h. Trials sponsored by the NIH AIDS Clinical Trials Group are comparing maintenance doses of 200 and 100 mg every 4 h in an attempt to determine whether toxicity can be reduced without sacrificing clinical benefit.

Frequent monitoring of complete blood counts (hemoglobin, hematocrit, leukocytes, differential, platelets) is necessary in patients receiving AZT.[94] Changes in mean corpuscular volume generally occur before other alterations but do not necessarily predict subsequent toxicity. Renal and liver function tests should be monitored as well. Measurement of CD4 lymphocytes or p24 antigen in blood may reflect drug effect but are not necessary for monitoring a patient's clinical improvement.

The proper management of AZT toxicity has not been resolved. For moderate granulocytopenia (750 to 1300/mm$^3$), dose reduction to 100 mg every 4 h is recommended. If toxicity returns at the lower dose schedule, further reductions in dose may be necessary. For more severe granulocytopenia, temporary dose discontinuation should be considered.

For hemoglobin/erythrocyte toxicity, patients may be transfused for severe reductions (6.5 to 7.9 g/dl). If transfusion requirements are greater than four units every 21 days, dose reduction or discontinuation is indicated. Others may attempt dose reduction before transfusion for hemoglobin reductions betwen 8 and 10 g/dl.

Several other drugs have shown anti-HIV activity in vitro and are in various stages of clinical investigation. Many of these are reverse transcriptase inhibitors. Some, such as suramin, have proved too toxic for widespread use. Others, including dideoxycytidine, foscarnet, and dideoxyinosine are in phase I trials.[100]

Agents have also been developed which may act at other sites of HIV replication including attachment (soluble CD4, dextran sulfate, AL721, and peptide T) and posttranscriptional processing, assembly, or release (ribavirin, interferons, glycosylation inhibitors). Some of these compounds are in clinical trial, while others are in earlier stages of development.[94,100]

Combination therapy of HIV infection is also under active investigation. Several drug combinations are synergistic against HIV replication in vitro (AZT plus interferon alpha, AZT plus acyclovir) and are in clinical trials.[100] Others (ribavirin and AZT) are antagonistic.[101] Although in vitro interactions may not necessarily reflect conditions in the patient, combinations showing antagonism in the laboratory should be used clinically only under carefully controlled conditions.

It may also be possible to stimulate immune responses by the use of biological response modifiers such as interleukin-2, interferon gamma, leukocyte-derived immunomodulators (IMREG-1), or granulocyte-macrophage colony stimulating factor.[72] Use of these agents alone may be a double-edge sword, however, since stimulation of macrophages or lymphocytes may actually activate latent HIV, at least in vitro.[102] An immunodulator-antiviral combination approach is worthy of study, and clinical trials of AZT plus either interleukin-2 or granulocyte-macrophage colony stimulating factor are underway.

## PREVENTION OF HIV INFECTION

The ultimate goal of development of a safe and effective HIV vaccine is probably years away. Approaches toward that goal are discussed in Chap. 28. Current efforts at prevention must be aimed at limiting the spread of HIV from individual to individual. Understanding the primary modes of transmission (blood and genital secretions) has allowed the development of blood screening techniques that have improved the safety of our blood and organ supplies for transfusion and transplantation.

Recommendations for behavior modification among risk groups (sexually active men and women, intravenous drug users) are now familiar to the informed public, i.e., maintenance of mutually monogamous relationships, avoiding contact of genital secretions with mucous membranes through utilization of a latex condom, abstaining from drugs or utilization of sterile needles without sharing.[103] Avoidance of pregnancy in HIV-seropositive women and use of universal precautions by health care workers are also recommended.

Acceptance of these guidelines by populations at risk is variable and depends on complex social factors. Sexual and drug practices are not always amenable to radical change. Moreover, the message given may depend on the moral or ethical views of the messenger. In addition, the degree of risk to large segments of the population remains poorly defined.

Nevertheless, among certain high-risk populations, there is evidence of dramatic behavioral change over the past several years. For example, in San Francisco cohort studies of homosexual men, numbers of sexual partners declined dramatically between 1978 and 1985.[104] Similar observations have been made elsewhere.[103] Approaches to prevention of spread in drug abuser populations have included expanded methadone and residential treatment programs, various outreach efforts, and experimental needle exchange programs. However, behavior change among drug abusers has been less widely adopted than among homosexual men.[103]

## References


1 Huminer D et al: AIDS in the pre-AIDS era. *Rev Infect Dis* 9:1102, 1987.
2 Pneumocystis pneumonia—Los Angeles. *MMWR* 30:250, 1981.
3 Kaposi's sarcoma and pneumocystis pneumonia among homosexual men—New York City and California. *MMWR* 30:305, 1981.
4 Gottlieb MS et al: Pneumocystis carinii pneumonia and mucosal candidiasis in previously healthy homosexual men. *N Engl J Med* 305:1425, 1981.
5 Masur H et al: An outbreak of community-acquired pneumocystis carinii pneumonia. Initial manifestations of cellular immune dysfunction. *N Engl J Med* 305:1431, 1981.
6 Siegal FP et al: Severe acquired immunodeficiency in male homosexuals, manifested by chronic perianal ulcerative herpes simplex lesions. *N Engl J Med* 305:1439, 1981.
7 Barre-Sinoussi F et al: Isolation of a T-lymphotropic retrovirus from a patient at risk for AIDS. *Science* 220:868, 1983.
8 Popovic M et al: Detection, isolation, and continuous production of cytopathic retroviruses (HTLV-III) from patients with AIDS and pre-AIDS. *Science* 224:497, 1984.
9 Gallo RC et al: Frequent detection and isolation of cytopathic retroviruses (HTLV-III) from patients with AIDS and at risk for AIDS. *Science* 224:500, 1984.
10 Sarngadharan M et al: Antibodies reactive with human T-lymphotropic retroviruses (HTLV-III) in the serum of patients with AIDS. *Science* 224:506, 1984.
11 Clavel F et al: Isolation of a new human retrovirus from West African patients with AIDS. *Science* 233:343, 1986.
12 Clavel F et al: Human immunodeficiency virus type 2 infection associated with AIDS in West Africa. *N Engl J Med* 316:1180, 1987.
13 AIDS due to HIV-2 infection. *MMWR* 37:33, 1988.
14 Classification system for human T-lymphotropic virus type III/lymphadenopathy-associated virus infections. *MMWR* 35:334, 1986.
15 Redfield RR et al: The Walter Reed staging classification for HTLV III/LAV infection. *N Engl J Med* 314:131, 1986.
16 Cooper DA et al: Acute AIDS retrovirus infection. Definition of a clinical illness associated with seroconversion. *Lancet* 1:537, 1985.
17 Ho DD et al: Primary human T-lymphotropic virus type III infection. *Ann Intern Med* 103:880, 1985.
18 Calabrese LH et al: Acute infection with the human immunodeficiency virus (HIV) associated with brachial neuritis and exanthematous rash. *Ann Intern Med* 107:849, 1987.
19 Tindall B et al: Characterization of the acute clinical illness associated with human immunodeficiency virus infection. *Arch Intern Med* 148:945, 1988.
20 Cooper DA et al: Antibody response to human immunodeficiency virus after primary infection. *J Infect Dis* 155:1113, 1987.
21 Gaines H et al: Antibody responses in primary human immunodeficiency virus infection. *Lancet* 1:1249, 1987.
22 Kessler HA et al: Diagnosis of human immunodeficiency virus infection in seronegative homosexuals presenting with an acute viral syndrome. *JAMA* 258:1196, 1987.
23 Curran JW et al: Epidemiology of HIV infection and AIDS in the United States. *Science* 239:610, 1988.
24 Jaffe HW et al: The Acquired Immunodeficiency Syndrome in a cohort of homosexual men. *Ann Intern Med* 103:210, 1985.
25 Eyster ME et al: Natural history of human immunodeficiency virus infections in hemophiliacs: Effects of T-cell subsets, platelet counts, and age. *Ann Intern Med* 107:1, 1987.
26 Gottlieb MS et al: T cell phenotyping in the diagnosis and management of AIDS and AIDS-related diseases. *Curr Top AIDS* 1:225, 1987.
27 Bonavida B et al: Mechanism of defective NK cell activity in patients with acquired immunodeficiency syndrome (AIDS) and AIDS-related complex. *J Immunol* 137:1157, 1986.
28 Lane HC et al: Qualitative analysis of immune function in patients with the acquired immunodeficiency syndrome–evidence for a selective defect in soluble antigen recognition. *N Engl J Med* 313:79, 1985.
29 Kreiss JK et al: Antibody to human T cell leukemia virus membrane antigens, beta-microglobulin levels, and thymosin alpha levels in hemophiliacs and their spouses. *Ann Intern Med* 100:178, 1984.
30 Seligman M et al: Immunology of human immunodeficiency virus infection and the acquired immunodeficiency syndrome—An update. *Ann Intern Med* 107:234, 1987.
31 Polk BF et al: Predictors of the Acquired Immunodeficiency Syndrome developing in a cohort of seropositive homosexual men. *N Engl J Med* 316:61, 1987.
32 Melbye M et al: The natural history of human immunodeficiency virus infection. *Current Topics in AIDS* 1:57, 1987.
33 Revision of the CDC surveillance case definition for acquired immunodeficiency syndrome. *MMWR* 36:35, 1987.
34 Rothenberg R et al: Survival with the acquired immunodeficiency syndrome. Experience with 5833 cases in New York City. *N Engl J Med* 317:1297, 1987.
35 Tschachler E et al: Epidermal Langerhans cells—A target for HTLV III/LAV infection. *J Invest Dermatol* 88:233, 1987.
36 Pomerantz RJ et al: Human immunodeficiency virus infection of the uterine cervix. *Ann Intern Med* 108:321, 1987.
37 Friedman-Kien AE et al: Herpes zoster: A possible early clinical sign for the development of acquired immunodeficiency syndrome in high risk individuals. *J Am Acad Dermatol* 14:1023, 1986.
38 Eisenstat BA et al: Seborrheic dermatitis and butterfly rash in AIDS. *N Engl J Med* 311:189, 1984.
39 Mathes BM et al: Seborrheic dermatitis in patients with acquired

immunodeficiency syndrome. *J Am Acad Dermatol* 13:947, 1985.

40 Kaplan MH et al: Dermatologic findings and manifestations of acquired immunodeficiency syndrome (AIDS). *J Am Acad Dermatol* 16:485, 1987.

41 James WD et al: A papular eruption associated with human T cell lymphotropic virus type III disease. *J Am Acad Dermatol* 13:563, 1985.

42 Gordin F et al: Adverse reactions to timethoprim-sulfamethoxazole in patients with the acquired immunodeficiency syndrome. *Ann Intern Med* 100:495, 1984.

43 Klein RS et al: Oral candidiasis in high-risk patients as the initial manifestations of the acquired immunodeficiency syndrome. *N Engl J Med* 311:354, 1984.

44 Greenspan JS et al: Replication of Epstein-Barr virus within the epithelial cells of oral "hairy" leukoplakia, an AIDS-associated lesion. *N Engl J Med* 313:1564, 1985.

45 Greenspan D et al: Relationships of oral hairy leukoplakia to infection with the human immunodeficiency virus and the risk of developing AIDS. *J Infect Dis* 155:475, 1987.

46 Resnick L et al: Regression of oral hairy leukoplakia after orally administered acyclovir therapy. *JAMA* 259:384, 1988.

47 Ho D et al: Isolation of human T-lymphotropic virus-III from semen and blood of a healthy homosexual man. *Science* 226:451, 1984.

48 Vogt MW et al: Isolation of HTLV-III/LAV from cervical secretions of women at risk for AIDS. *Lancet* 1:525, 1986.

49 Simonsen JN et al: Human immunodeficiency virus infection among men with sexually transmitted diseases–experiences from a center in Africa. *N Engl J Med* 319:274, 1988.

50 Kotler DP et al: Enteropathy associated with the acquired immunodeficiency syndrome. *Ann Intern Med* 101:421, 1984.

51 Gillin JS et al: Malabsorption and mucosal abnormalities of the small intestine in the acquired immunodeficiency syndrome. *Ann Intern Med* 102:619, 1985.

52 Quinn TC: Gastrointestinal manifestations of human immunodeficiency virus. *Curr Top AIDS* 1:155, 1987.

53 Adachi A et al: Productive, persistent infection of human colorectal cell lines with human immunodeficiency virus. *J Virol* 61:209, 1987.

54 Nelson JA et al: Human immunodeficiency virus detected in bowel epithelium from patients with gastrointestinal symptoms. *Lancet* 1:259, 1988.

55 Smith PD et al: Intestinal infections in patients with the acquired immunodeficiency syndrome (AIDS). *Ann Intern Med* 108:328, 1988.

56 Levinson W et al: Cytomegalovirus colitis in acquired immunodeficiency—A chronic disease with varying manifestations. *Am J Gastroenterol* 80:445, 1985.

57 Skolnik PR et al: Bidirectional interactions between human immunodeficiency virus and cytomegalovirus. *J Infect Dis* 157:508, 1988.

58 Masur H et al: Effect of 9-(1,3-dihydroxy-2-propoxymethyl) guanine for cytomegalovirus infection in patients with the acquired immunodeficiency syndrome. *Ann Intern Med* 104:41, 1986.

59 Straus SE et al: Oral acyclovir to suppress recurring herpes simplex virus infections in immunodeficient patients. *Ann Intern Med* 100:522, 1984.

60 Soave R et al: AIDS commentary—Cryptosporidium and Isospora belli infections. *J Infect Dis* 157:225, 1988.

61 Blumberg RS et al: Cytomegalovirus and cryptosporidium associated acalculous gangrenous cholecystitis. *Am J Med* 76:1118, 1984.

62 Dobs AS et al: Endocrine disorders in men infected with human immunodeficiency virus. *Am J Med* 84:611, 1988.

63 Green LW et al: Adrenal insufficiency as a complication of the acquired immunodeficiency syndrome. *Ann Intern Med* 101:497, 1984.

64 Rao TKS et al: The types of renal disease in the acquired immunodeficiency syndrome. *N Engl J Med* 316:1062, 1987.

65 Pardo V et al: AIDS-related glomerulopathy: Occurrence in specific risk groups. *Kidney Int* 31:1167, 1987.

66 Cohen IS et al: Congestive cardiomyopathy in association with the Acquired Immunodeficiency Syndrome. *N Engl J Med* 315:628, 1986.

67 Solal-Celigny P et al: Lymphoid interstitial pneumonitis in acquired immunodeficiency syndrome-related complex. *Am Rev Respir Dis* 131:956, 1985.

68 Suffredini AF et al: Nonspecific interstitial pneumonitis: A common cause of pulmonary disease in the Acquired Immunodeficiency Syndrome. *Ann Intern Med* 107:7, 1987.

69 Murray JF et al: Pulmonary complications of the Acquired Immunodeficiency Syndrome: An update. *Am Rev Respir Dis* 133:504, 1987.

70 Frontiera M et al: Peripheral blood and bone marrow abnormalities in the acquired immunodeficiency syndrome. *West J Med* 147:157, 1987.

71 Donahue RE et al: Suppression of in vitro haematopoiesis following human immunodeficiency virus infection. *Nature* 326:200, 1987.

72 Groopman JE et al: Effect of recombinant human granulocyte-macrophage colony stimulating factor on myelopoiesis in the acquired immunodeficiency syndrome. *N Engl J Med* 317:593, 1987.

73 Stella CC et al: Defective in vitro growth of the hemopoietic progenitor cells in the Acquired Immunodeficiency Syndrome. *J Clin Invest* 80:286, 1987.

74 Morris L et al: Autoimmune thrombocytopenic purpura in homosexual men. *Ann Intern Med* 96:714, 1982.

75 Stricker RB et al: Target platelet antigen in homosexual men with immune thrombocytopenia. *N Engl J Med* 313:1375, 1985.

76 Pollak AN et al: Successful intravenous immune globulin therapy for human immunodeficiency virus-associated thrombocytopenia. *Arch Intern Med* 148:695, 1988.

77 Spivak JL et al: Hematologic abnormalities in the acquired immune deficiency syndrome. *Am J Med* 77:224, 1984.

78 Cohen AJ et al: Circulating coagulation inhibitors in the acquired immunodeficiency syndrome. *Ann Intern Med* 104:175, 1986.

79 Gabuzda DH et al: Immunohistochemical identification of HTLV-III antigen in brains of patients with AIDS. *Ann Neurol* 20:289, 1986.

80 Price RW et al: The brain in AIDS: Central nervous system HIV-1 infection and AIDS dementia complex. *Science* 239:586, 1988.

81 Ho DD et al: Pathogenesis of infection with human immunodeficiency virus. *N Engl J Med* 317:278, 1987.

82 Navia BA et al: The AIDS dementia complex. I. Clinical features. *Ann Neurol* 19:517, 1986.

83 Navia BA et al: The acquired immunodeficiency dementia complex as the presenting or sole manifestation of human immunodeficiency virus infection. *Arch Neurol* 44:65, 1987.

84 de la Monte SM et al: Subacute encephalomyelitis of AIDS and its relation to HTLV-III infection. *Neurology* 37:562, 1987.

85 Petito CK et al: Vacuolar myelopathy pathologically resembling subacute combined degeneration in patients with the acquired immunodeficiency syndrome. *N Engl J Med* 312:874, 1985.

86 Cornblath DR et al: Inflammatory demyelinating peripheral neuropathies associated with human T-cell lymphotropic virus type III infection. *Ann Neurol* 21:32, 1987.

87 Snider WD et al: Neurological complications of acquired immunodeficiency syndrome: Analysis of 50 patients. *Ann Neurol* 14:403, 1983.

88 Levy RM et al: Neurological manifestations of the acquired immunodeficiency syndrome (AIDS): Experience at UCSF and review of the literature. *J Neurosurg* 62:475, 1985.

89 Dalakas MC et al: Polymyositis associated with AIDS retrovirus. *JAMA* 256:2381, 1986.

90 Craddock C et al: Cardiorespiratory arrest and autonomic neuropathy in AIDS. *Lancet* ii:16, 1987.

91 Schuman JS et al: Acquired immunodeficiency syndrome (AIDS). *Surv Ophthalmol* 31:384, 1987.

92 Pomerantz RJ et al: Infection of the retina by human immunodeficiency virus type 1. *N Engl J Med* 317:1643, 1987.

93 D'Amico DJ et al: Ophthalmoscopic and histologic findings in cytomegalovirus retinitis treated with BW-B759U. *Arch Ophthalmol* 109:1788, 1986.

94 Hirsch MS: AIDS Commentary—Azidothymidine. *J Infect Dis* 157:427, 1988.

95 Mitsuya HK et al: 3′azido-3′-deoxythymidine (BWA509U): an antiviral agent that inhibits the infectivity and cytopathic effect of human T lymphotropic virus type III/lymphadenopathy-associated virus in vitro. *Proc Natl Acad Sci USA* 82:7096, 1985.

96 Richman DD et al: Failure of dideoxynucleosides to inhibit human immunodeficiency virus replication in cultured human macrophages. *J Exp Med* 166:1144, 1987.

97 Fischl MA et al: The efficacy of azidothymidine (AZT) in the treatment of patients with AIDS and AIDS-related complex—A double-blind placebo-controlled trial. *N Engl J Med* 317:185, 1987.

98 Richman DD et al: The toxicity of azidothymidine (AZT) in the treatment of patients with AIDS and AIDS-related complex—A double-blind, placebo-controlled trial. *N Engl J Med* 317:192, 1987.

99 Yarchoan R et al: Response of human-immunodeficiency virus associated neurological disease to 3′-azido-3′-deoxythymidine. *Lancet* 1:132, 1987.

100 Vogt MW et al: Treatment of Human Immunodeficiency Virus infection. *Infect Dis Clin North Am* 1:323, 1987.

101 Vogt MW et al: Ribavirin antagonizes the effect of azidothymidine on HIV replication. *Science* 235:1376, 1987.

102 Folks TM et al: Cytokine-induced expression of HIV-1 in a chronically infected promonocyte cell line. *Science* 238:800, 1987.

103 Fineberg HV: Education to prevent AIDS: Prospects and obstacles. *Science* 239:592, 1988.

104 Winkelstein W et al: Diagnosis of human immunodeficiency virus infection in seronegative homosexuals presenting with an acute viral syndrome. *Am J Public Health* 76:685, 1987.

Chapter 31

# The epidemiology of HIV infection in industrialized countries

Scott D. Holmberg
James W. Curran

## HISTORICAL PERSPECTIVE

Sporadic, unrecognized cases of the acquired immunodeficiency syndrome (AIDS) may have occurred in the United States and Europe as early as 1952.[1] However, the AIDS epidemic is usually demarcated by the report in mid-1981 of *Pneumocystis carinii* pneumonia (PCP), an unusual infection previously reported only in immunosuppressed patients, in five young homosexual men in Los Angeles.[2] At about the same time, Kaposi's sarcoma (KS), previously known as a rare tumor of elderly men of Mediterranean origin, was observed in young homosexual men in New York City. By early July 1981, 26 cases of KS were identified in homosexual men, four of whom also had PCP.[3] Aggressive KS had been noted in Africans in Europe in the late 1970s,[4] and in 1982, some European researchers realized that AIDS cases were occurring in citizens of their own countries as well.

AIDS was thought from the beginning to possibly be the result of infection with a transmissible agent, and a number of studies of homosexual men supported this hypothesis before human immunodeficiency virus (HIV) was identified.[5,6] Compared with homosexual men without AIDS, those with AIDS had substantially more sexual partners, were more likely to have had a history of sexually transmitted diseases (STDs), and had more (anonymous) partners from gay bathhouses.[5] The suspicion that AIDS resulted from a sexually transmissible agent was further reinforced in early 1982 when public health officials in southern California became aware that several men with AIDS had had sexual contact with one another; 40 of the first 216 AIDS cases in homosexual men in the United States could be linked sexually to one another.[7,8]

Herpes group viruses, nitrate inhalants, or some other infectious or toxic agent(s), alone or in concert, were originally considered in the etiology of AIDS; however, attention shifted in 1982 to retroviruses because one of the few known retroviruses at that time, feline leukemia virus, caused immunodeficiency in cats, and the only known human retrovirus, human T-cell leukemia virus type 1 (HTLV-I), had a predilection for T-lymphocytes. Before the recognition of lymphadenopathy virus (LAV) in France[9] in 1983 and human T-lymphotropic virus type III (HTLV-III) in the United States[10] in 1984—both now termed HIV—epidemiologic attention had shifted to behavioral risk factors for infection in homosexual men.

Between 1978 and 1980, about 6700 homosexual men in San Francisco gave serum and were interviewed as part of studies of hepatitis B prevalence, incidence, and vaccine efficacy. About 1600 men have been reexamined subsequently in studies of AIDS and HIV infection. HIV-antibody positivity increased in these men from 4.5 percent in 1978 to over 70 percent in 1986 (Fig. 31-1). However, because AIDS was recognized as an STD before the actual agent was identified, and because many men changed their behavior accordingly, actual rates of HIV-seroconversion peaked in 1982 (Fig. 31-1).

Despite the changed behavior of homosexual men, this group accounts for over 70 percent of AIDS cases in developed countries. Because of the long incubation period between HIV infection and disease, reported AIDS cases have continued to increase dramatically in North America (Fig. 31-2) and in Europe.[12] By early 1988, over 66,000 cases had been reported from industrialized nations to the World Health Organization (WHO) (Table 31-1).[13]

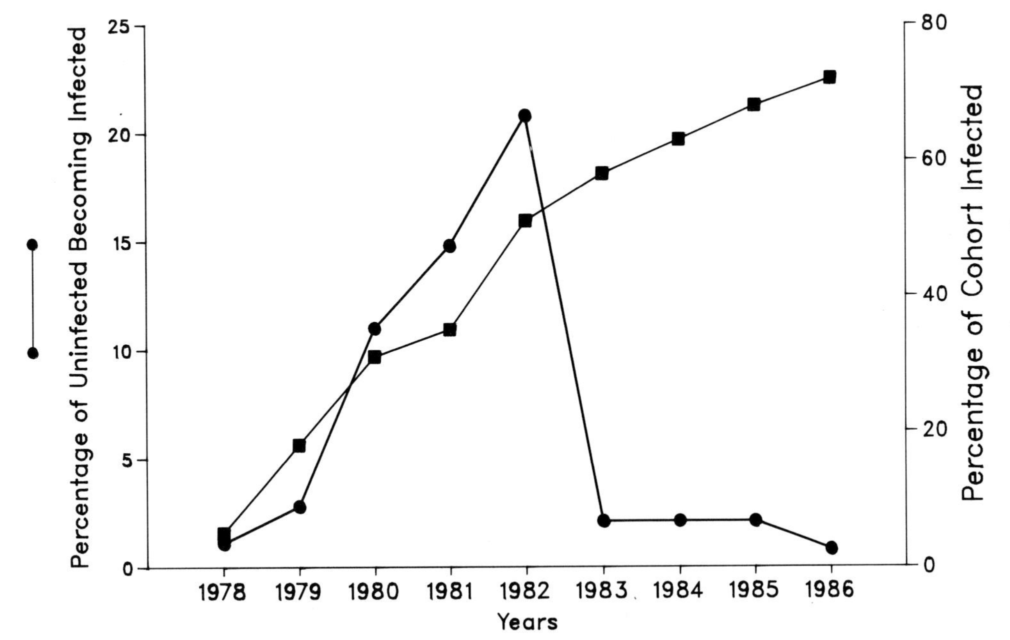


**Fig. 31-1.** Incidence and prevalence of HIV infection in the San Francisco City Clinic/CDC study of homosexual and bisexual men. Incidence of HIV is calculated from serum samples collected regularly and frequently from 283 men who took part in studies of hepatitis B between 1978 and 1986. (*From Ref. 11.*)

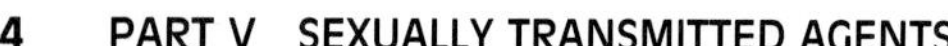


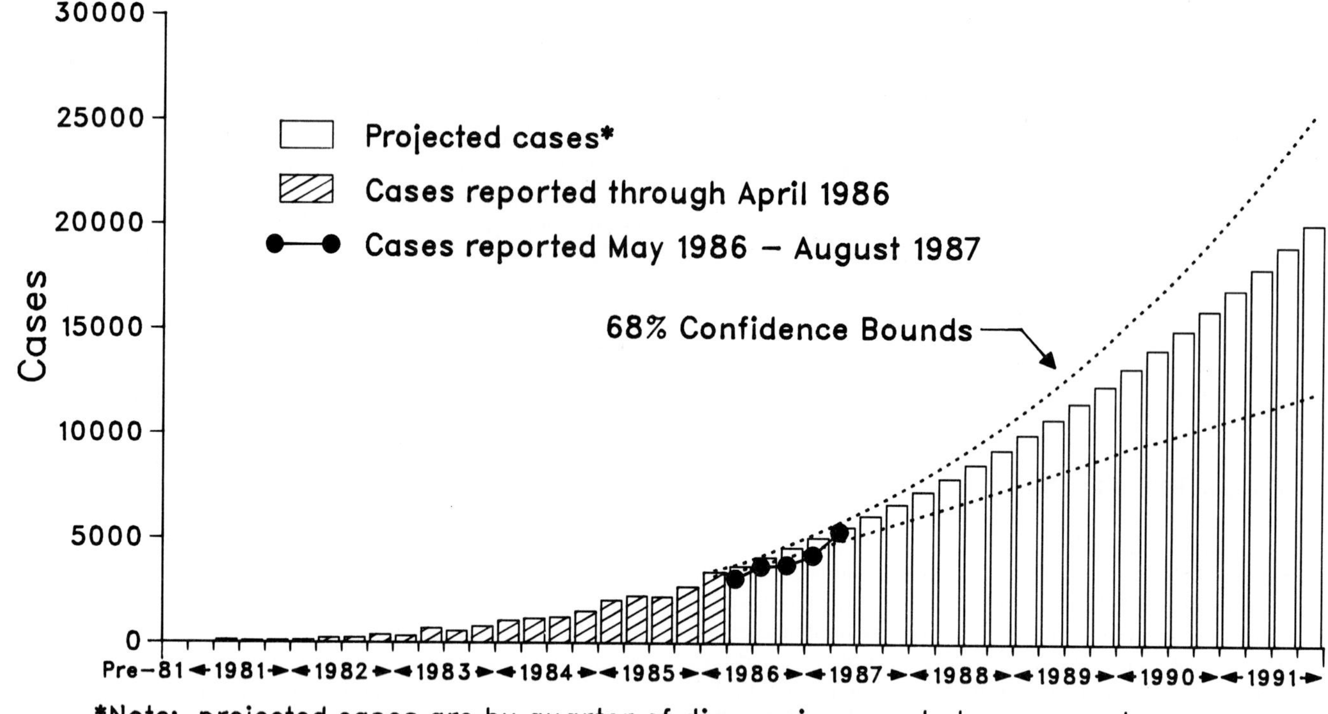


**Fig. 31-2.** Incidence of AIDS in the United States, by quarter of diagnosis as projected from cases reported to CDC as of April 30, 1986 (shaded bars), projected through 1991 (open bars), and reported to CDC between May 1, 1986, and August 31, 1987 (black circles). (*From Ref. 22.*)

**Table 31-1. Approximate Distribution of Adult AIDS Cases by Risk Activity in Industrialized Nations, March 1988**

| Country of report (reported cases*) | Approximate percentage of cases belonging to groups at risk for AIDS | | | | | | |
|---|---|---|---|---|---|---|---|
| | Homosexual and bisexual men | Intravenous-drug abusers | Homo-bisexual drug abusers | Heterosexuals (immigrants†) | Transfusion recipients | Persons with hemophilia | Unknown and other |
| North America | | | | | | | |
| USA (53,069) | 66 | 16 | 8 | 4 (2) | 2 | 1 | 3 |
| Canada (1488) | 78 | <1 | 4 | 11 (9) | 2 | 1 | 3 |
| Total (54,557) | 66 | 16 | 8 | 4 (2) | 2 | 1 | 3 |
| Europe | | | | | | | |
| France (3073) | 66 | 9 | 3 | 17 (15) | 1 | 2 | 2 |
| FRG (1760) | 79 | 6 | 1 | 3 | 7 | 4 | <1 |
| UK (1227) | 87 | 1 | 2 | 2 | 1 | 4 | 3 |
| Italy (1411) | 28 | 59 | 5 | 1 | 3 | 2 | 2 |
| Spain (718) | 22 | 54 | 9 | 1 | <1 | 11 | 4 |
| Switzerland (355) | 69 | 10 | 5 | 9 (6) | 2 | 2 | 3 |
| Netherlands (420) | 91 | 3 | 0 | 2 | 1 | 1 | 2 |
| Belgium (297) | 23 | 2 | 0 | 62 (55) | 8 | 1 | 4 |
| Other European countries‡ (905) | — | — | — | — | — | — | — |
| Total (10,166) | 67 | 14 | 3 | 5 | 3 | 4 | 4 |
| Pacific | | | | | | | |
| Australia (758) | 88 | <1 | 2 | 1 | 7 | 1 | 1 |
| New Zealand (66) | 88 | <1 | 0 | <1 | <1 | 4 | 2 |
| Japan (59) | 41 | <1 | 0 | 4 | 1 | 53 | <1 |
| Total (883) | 85 | <1 | 2 | 1 | 6 | 5 | 1 |

As compiled from Ref. 11–21.

*Representing 65,606 (80.5%) of the 81,433 AIDS cases reported to the World Health Organization as of February 29, 1988.

†Immigrants from countries of west and central Africa and from Haiti, where heterosexual spread is believed to be the dominant mode of transmission.

‡Includes Denmark (228 cases), Sweden (165), Austria (139), Portugal (90), Greece (88), Norway (70), Ireland (33), Yugoslavia (26), Finland (24), Luxembourg (9), Czechoslovakia (8), Hungary (8), GDR (4), USSR (4), Bulgaria (3), Poland (3), and Romania (3).

—indicates risk activity data not available.

## INCIDENCE AND PREVALENCE OF HIV INFECTION AND AIDS

Surveillance for HIV infection began in the United States shortly after the first cases were recognized.[22] The first surveillance case definition included the presence of certain reliably diagnosed diseases, such as KS and PCP, occurring in persons without a known cause for their immune impairment.[23] After HIV was identified and as a clearer picture of the protean manifestations of HIV infection has emerged, the case definition has been modified to include persons with many unusual or aggressive infections or tumors in whom HIV infection has been indicated by a positive HIV-antibody test (see Chap. 30).[24] Patients in the United States who have fulfilled these case definitions have been reported to the Centers for Disease Control (CDC) in Atlanta since 1981[22] and, worldwide, to the World Health Organization (WHO) Collaborating Centre on AIDS in Paris since 1984.[12,13] Because the surveillance system for AIDS cases relies on the ability and willingness of persons to diagnose and report AIDS cases through local, regional, and national health agencies, there is concern that AIDS cases may be considerably underreported. In the United States, attempts to assess the reliability of case reports have included matching death registry data with AIDS case reports. One such study showed in late 1985 that 83 to 100 percent of persons dying of AIDS in four major urban centers in the United States were being appropriately reported to CDC,[25] indicating that the reporting system yielded reliable data on actual AIDS incidence in those areas at that time.

It is very difficult, however, to extrapolate reports of AIDS to the actual incidence and prevalence of HIV infection. For example, in the San Francisco cohort of homosexual men described above, the estimated ratio of HIV-seropositive men to men with AIDS was 825:1 in 1980; in 1984, the estimated ratio had declined to 28:1.[22] The relative prevalence of seropositivity and AIDS in most areas of the United States probably lies between these ratios. To project the magnitude of the AIDS epidemic in the United States and develop strategies for control, public health, scientific, and government leaders convened at the Coolfont Conference Center in West Virginia in June 1986. They estimated that by the end of 1991, 270,000 AIDS cases will have occurred and that 179,000 of these persons will have died.[26] The conferees estimated that 1.0 to 1.5 million Americans had been infected by HIV by 1986.

To better define the prevalence of HIV infection, a review of current knowledge was undertaken from September through November 1987. Data obtained from 50 studies of homosexual and bisexual men indicated an HIV seroprevalence in them of 20 to 50 percent in most major cities; in 88 studies of intravenous-drug abusers (IVDAs), HIV-antibody prevalence was as high as 50 to 65 percent in New York City and environs and below 5 percent in areas other than the East Coast.[11] In a few limited studies, HIV infection generally ranged from 0 to 1.2 percent for persons without identified risks. About 1 percent of heterosexual men and women attending an STD clinic in a borough of New York City, who denied risk behavior for HIV infection or known sexual contact with persons in AIDS risk groups, were found to be infected.[11] While estimates resulting from current data vary widely, they are consistent with the earlier estimate from the Coolfont Conference of 1.0 to 1.5 million HIV-infected Americans.[11] A so-called family of surveys, now in progress at hospitals, college campuses, STD and other clinics, prisons, alternate testing centers (for HIV), and other sites, is expected to yield useful and more accurate incidence and trend data regarding HIV infections.

The proportion of AIDS cases occurring in known high-risk groups in Europe loosely conforms with patterns seen in the United States and Canada,[27] but some differences may be observed even between contiguous countries (Table 31-1). For example, proportionately many more AIDS cases are seen in IVDAs in southern than in northern European cities.[27] Other countries have disproportionately more AIDS cases in certain other groups, such as central Africans living in France or persons with hemophilia in Japan. While the 53,000 reported AIDS cases in the United States may represent about 20 to 30 HIV infections per case, this ratio may be much higher or lower in other countries. Changing HIV infection incidence in homosexual men and different incidence and prevalence of HIV infection in IVDAs in different cultures and countries further confound such comparisons.[12]

## MODES OF TRANSMISSION AND MAJOR GROUPS AT RISK OF HIV INFECTION

HIV, the causative agent of AIDS, can be transmitted in three ways: sexually, through exposure to contaminated blood or needles, and perinatally. In developed countries, these three modes of transmission occur under a wide variety of circumstances, and many factors may influence the spread of HIV from one person to another.

### SEXUAL TRANSMISSION: HOMOSEXUAL MEN

Homosexual men have remained the most affected group in almost all developed countries (Table 31-1). Of the 50,000 U.S. AIDS patients reported to CDC as of January 1, 1988, over 36,000 (72 percent) are homosexual or bisexual men [including homosexual and bisexual men who also use intravenous (IV) drugs]. However, HIV infection rates in selected cohorts of homosexual men in major U.S. cities have clearly declined (Fig. 31-1). This has been attributed to changed sex practices in response to the AIDS epidemic, such as having fewer or only one sex partner, using condoms, and other practices to avoid the exchange of semen.[28,29] Objective evidence of such changes can also be found in the declining incidence of other STDs, such as gonorrhea, in homosexual men since 1982.[30] Declines in HIV infection and other STDs in homosexual men have also been noted in Europe, where heterosexual IVDAs account for an ever-increasing proportion of AIDS cases.[31]

However, decreases in HIV infection rates in homosexual and bisexual men obscure the fact that in cities such as San Francisco, where half or more of homosexual men have HIV infection, relatively few exposures may lead to infection. Also, it is expected that the number of AIDS cases in homosexual men will continue to increase as persons infected years ago become ill. It will probably be several more years before the incidence of AIDS in homosexual men substantially decreases.

### SEXUAL TRANSMISSION: HETEROSEXUAL PERSONS

Heterosexual citizens of most industrialized countries who deny risk activities for HIV infection, such as homosexual activity or IV-drug abuse, comprise about 2 percent of all reported AIDS cases (Table 31-1). Early in the AIDS epidemic, some women who had AIDS denied drug abuse but said they had had sexual contact with men who were IVDAs, bisexual, or hemophilic.[32,33]

Thus, it became apparent early in the epidemic that heterosexual male-to-female transmission of HIV could occur. Although scientists had recovered HIV from cervical secretions and although menstruating women bleed per vagina, some researchers were originally skeptical that female-to-male transmission could occur frequently or at all. However, it was soon clearly established that female-to-male transmission does occur. Men who deny risks for exposure other than frequent prostitute contact in the United States[34] or Africa[35] may acquire HIV infection and develop AIDS.

How easily is HIV transmitted from woman to man? A recent study of heterosexual partners (usually spouses) of persons infected by transfusion showed that 2 (8 percent) of 25 husbands of transfusion-infected women had HIV antibodies after 2 years. Intensive interviews by experienced personnel failed to establish any risk other than contact with the HIV-infected wife.[36] Rates of heterosexual spread are much lower than would be observed with other STDs, such as gonorrhea or syphilis (Table 31-2). Most HIV-infected spouses of HIV-infected hemophilic men or transfusion recipients had had hundreds of unprotected sexual contacts by the time they were discovered to be HIV-seropositive and were interviewed. This suggests that the average risk of HIV infection from a single heterosexual contact may be less than 0.1 percent.[36,39] However, such a statistic obscures reports of persons becoming infected after only one or a few sexual contacts with an HIV-infected partner.[36] Thus, it appears that host or viral factors influence the transmissibility of and susceptibility to HIV and that low rates of heterosexual transmission on a population basis cannot accurately predict a person's risk of infection from a single contact.

Although European countries such as France and Belgium report high percentages of AIDS cases among heterosexuals, these cases are mainly among Africans residing in those countries (Table 31-1). The penetrance of HIV into the non-drug-abusing heterosexual communities of industrialized nations does not now appear to be extensive[11,31] and may not be in the future.[44] For example, military recruits and blood donors in the United States have seroprevalences of HIV-antibody of 0.15 and 0.02 percent, respectively,[11] and most of these infected persons have been found to be homosexual or bisexual men or IVDAs.

Although the ability of HIV to infect the general populations of industrialized nations apparently has been low to date, rates of HIV infection in specific groups, especially inner-city minorities, may be high. A study of sexually active heterosexuals attending an STD clinic in New York City indicates that about 1 percent (2/248) of those with no known risk are HIV-seropositive from frequent and frequently anonymous heterosexual contacts in an area highly endemic for AIDS. Of 47 women who reported sexual contact with members of groups at risk for AIDS (usually IVDAs), seven (15 percent) were HIV-seropositive (M.A. Chiasson and A.R. Lifson, personal communications). Likewise, 6.3 percent of men and 3.0 percent of women attending an STD clinic in Baltimore were found to be HIV-seropositive;[45] many of the women had been infected by heterosexual contact with IVDAs or bisexual men.

## NEEDLE-BORNE TRANSMISSION: INTRAVENOUS-DRUG ABUSERS (IVDAs)

After homosexual and bisexual men, IVDAs are the next largest category of AIDS patients in the Western world. Heterosexual IVDAs comprise 16 percent of AIDS cases reported in the United States and over 50 percent of AIDS cases reported in Italy and Spain (Table 31-1). The extent of drug use since 1978, needle-sharing frequency, and time spent in "shooting galleries" all increase one's risk of HIV infection.[46,47] In some shooting galleries, needles may be shared up to 50 times. Conversely, use of sterile needles and length of time in treatment (methadone) programs are associated with lower rates of infection. Geography also seems to play a role: in the United States, about 80 percent of all IVDA AIDS cases occur in New York City and northern New Jersey, and actual zones of decreasing HIV-seropositivity have been described with increasing distance from downtown Manhattan.[47,48]

There are an estimated 200,000 to 400,000 IVDAs in New York City and 750,000 to 1.1 million in the entire United States. Current seropositivity in New York City is 60 percent.[48] Even in those attending methadone maintenance clinics in one study, about one-third are HIV-seropositive.[46] In Europe, seroprevalence of HIV among IVDAs is estimated to be about 40 to 50 percent in West Germany; 70 percent in Milan, Italy; and 17 percent in Denmark.[28] Furthermore, unlike homosexual men whose self-reported changes in sexual behavior are reflected in actual decreases in HIV seroconversion rates, IVDAs continue to seroconvert at a high rate. In one study, about 8 to 10 percent of those attending methadone maintenance clinics in the Bronx, New York City, were still seroconverting for HIV every year (P.A. Selwynn and E.E. Schoenbaum, personal communication). It is difficult to study IVDAs outside methadone treatment programs. Thus, although it is likely, it is not known whether IVDAs in the community are becoming infected at higher rates than are IVDAs in programs to stop their IV-drug habit.

**Table 31-2. Rates of Heterosexual Transmission of Human Immunodeficiency Virus (HIV) Reported from Various Studies**

| Partners of persons with AIDS | Male-to-female spread: fraction of exposed persons infected, % | Female-to-male spread: fraction of exposed persons infected, % |
|---|---|---|
| Partners of IVDAs*[37] | 41/88 (47) | 7/12 (58) |
| Partners of IVDAs[38] | 3/6 (50) | 1/3 (33) |
| Partners of IVDAs[39] | 5/12 (42) | |
| Partners of Haitian immigrants[40] | 6/11 (55) | 5/5 (100) |
| Partners of hemophilic men[40] | 2/21 (10) | — |
| Partners of hemophilic men[39] | 4/19 (21) | — |
| Partners of hemophilic men[41] | 4/25 (16) | — |
| Partners of hemophilic men[42,43] | 77/772 (10) | — |
| Partners of bisexual men[39] | 12/55 (22) | — |
| Partners of transfusion-infected persons[36] | 10/55 (18) | 2/25 (8) |
| Partners of transfusion-infected men[39] | 1/4 (25) | |

*Intravenous-drug abusers.

IVDAs are an important link between the reservoir of the HIV-infected population and the uninfected heterosexual population. Women who acquire HIV infection from sexual contact with men in high-risk groups for AIDS more frequently report sexual contact with IVDAs than with bisexual men, transfusion-infected men, or hemophilic men.[49] Conversely, female-to-male spread of HIV may result from contact with prostitutes, who are often IVDAs or sex partners of IVDAs.[50] Finally, about 80 percent of U.S. pediatric AIDS cases occur in infants born to HIV-infected mothers (see below); most of these infected mothers are IVDAs or their sex partners. Thus, the current high prevalence and continued incidence of HIV infection in IVDAs is not a problem limited to themselves.

## BLOOD-BORNE TRANSMISSION: BLOOD AND ORGAN RECIPIENTS

With the availability and widespread use of an enzyme immunoassay for screening blood for HIV antibodies, HIV infections from blood transfusion have been almost completely eliminated. Such screening began by April 1985 in almost all U.S. blood collection centers and shortly thereafter in most European countries. However, before the widespread screening, an estimated 12,000 U.S. residents may have been infected by transfused blood and survived the illness or procedure for which they received blood.[51] One epidemiologic study of recipients of blood from donors who subsequently developed AIDS or were found to have HIV infection showed that the likelihood of being infected from a presumably HIV-infective unit is virtually 100 percent, and that the type of blood component received does not apparently influence that risk.[52]

Because a recently infected donor may not have yet developed antibody to HIV, blood donations during this "window period"—estimated to be about 3 months after infection—will not test positive on HIV-antibody screening. It is rare for blood to slip through donor self-deferral and HIV-antibody screening, but it does occur.[53] Estimates of the number of such infective units being transfused range from 72 to 460 per year, i.e., about 1/40,000 to 1/250,000 transfused units in the United States yearly.[51,54] About 60 percent of blood components are transfused to persons who do not survive the condition for which they were hospitalized. Thus, a worst-case estimate of the current chances of acquiring HIV infection from receiving a single unit of blood is probably less than 1 in 100,000 and should not deter someone who needs blood from receiving it.

Since screening of blood cannot detect every infectious unit, self-deferral from donating by donors who think they have been at risk of HIV infection continues to be very important in protecting the blood supply.[55] Epidemiologic studies have shown that HIV-infected persons who gave infective but test-negative blood did so for various reasons: they did not perceive themselves to have been at risk of HIV infection; they felt pressured by employers or colleagues to donate; or they wished to be screened for HIV antibody.[51,54] Seropositive donors who are detected by screening for HIV antibody tend to be members of minority groups living in urban, economically depressed settings,[49] to whom it is difficult to deliver preventive health messages.

## HEMOPHILIC PERSONS

AIDS in hemophilic persons was first reported in 1982,[56] providing strong support for the theory of a transmissible (infectious) agent as the cause of AIDS. Persons with hemophilia—virtually all men—receive clotting factors harvested from plasma of thousands of blood donors, typically receiving about 70,000 units of clotting factor concentrates each year. (One unit is defined as the amount of factor VIII or IX present in 1 ml of normal fresh frozen plasma.) Thus, hemophilic men are exposed to many blood-borne infections, usually viral. Given their particular exposure, it is not surprising that men with hemophilia in the United States, Europe, South America, and Japan were quickly and extensively infected with HIV.

Several investigations in different areas of the United States indicate a rise in HIV-antibody seroprevalence in hemophilic men from about 10 percent in 1980 to as high as 80 percent in 1984.[57] A similar rise in HIV seroprevalence in French hemophilic men was also observed.[58] In Japan, testing of serum from 252 men with hemophilia in 1985 showed that 91 (38.4 percent) were HIV-seropositive.[59] As with homosexual men, greatest incidence of HIV infection—as measured by HIV seroconversion—appears to have occurred in 1982 and 1983. Frequent users of factor VIII concentrates from those years are virtually all infected. Hemophilia B patients are somewhat less likely than hemophilia A patients to have become infected, probably because hemophilic B patients often receive fresh frozen plasma or cryoprecipitate rather than factor concentrate and use less factor concentate in general. Also, the process employed to produce factor IX may differ slightly from that used to produce factor VIII concentrate. Still, a study conducted in 1983 showed that 39 percent of hemophilia B patients are also HIV-infected.[60] Hemophilic persons comprise 1 percent of adult and 5 percent of pediatric AIDS cases reported in the United States. However, given the rarity of hemophilia and the long incubation between HIV infection and AIDS, these data imply widespread infection among the estimated 10,000 hemophilia A and 5000 hemophilia B patients in the United States. Indeed, direct studies show high HIV seroprevalence in both types of hemophilic men.

A method for heat treatment of factor concentrates was found effective in 1984 in eliminating HIV that had been spiked into these concentrates. Heat treatment has since been widely adopted, making infection of previously uninfected persons with hemophilia exceedingly rare in developed nations.[61] However, a few infections, described in Canada and France, have occurred after use of inadequately heat-treated products, i.e., products treated 30 h or less and treated with "dry" rather than "wet" heat (R. Remis, personal communication).

## NEEDLE-BORNE AND BLOOD-BORNE TRANSMISSIONS: HEALTH CARE WORKERS

Early reports in England and the United States indicated that HIV infections were occurring in a few health care workers with needle-stick exposures.[62,63] To evaluate the risk to health care workers, a number of studies have prospectively followed health care workers who have had accidental sticks with needles used on AIDS patients or HIV-infected persons. An ongoing CDC study has so far found that, of 917 health care workers with such exposures, only 4 (0.4 percent) have seroconverted to the virus (R. Marcus, personal communication). Previous studies, and reviews of collections of such studies, indicate that the risk of HIV infection from accidental needle stick is low, apparently about 1 percent or less per stick.[64–66] This rate can be compared with risk for hepatitis B infection from accidental needle stick, usually estimated at 12 percent per stick. Furthermore, some of the needle-stick exposures resulting in HIV infection have been unusual, involving deep sticks with large amounts of infected blood injected.[62,63] Nonetheless, even such low risk of infection with a potentially fatal virus causes great concern among health care professionals.

Studies of seroconversion in health care workers after mucosal exposure to infectious blood have been undertaken by various centers, but none of 292 health care workers with such exposures have been found to be HIV-antibody-positive.[64–66] In a prospective study of health care workers at the National Institutes of Health, more than 2000 skin and mucous membrane exposures to blood or body fluids of AIDS patients did not result in HIV infection.[67] The first report of HIV transmission from mucosal exposure to infectious blood was of a mother who developed HIV antibody while tending her chronically ill child.[68] In 1987, CDC reported the results of investigations of three incidents involving young female health professionals who apparently acquired HIV infection through contact with infected blood.[69] These cases indicated that blood-to-mucosa transmission of HIV, although very rare, may occur. Because of this possibility, CDC guidelines for health-care workers have been reevaluated and continue to reinforce the importance of "universal precautions" in preventing exposure to potentially infectious clinical material.[70]

## PERINATAL TRANSMISSION

Children may acquire HIV infection through any of the mechanisms listed above, such as by transfusion of blood or antihemophilic clotting factors and, rarely, through sexual exposures. However, in most countries, most HIV transmission to children is perinatal; in the United States, 78 percent of children under 13 years old who have AIDS have a parent with or at risk for AIDS.[71–74] Because most pediatric AIDS cases result from perinatal transmission (in developed countries, usually from IV-drug-abusing mothers), the demographic characteristics of pediatric AIDS cases reflect those of their parents. Eighty percent are black or Hispanic;[75] 75 percent reside in New York, New Jersey, Florida, and California. As many as 30,000 births to infected drug-abusing women may have occurred already in greater New York City alone,[47] and the New York State Department of Health estimates that 1 of 61 births in New York City is to an HIV-infected woman. These numbers underscore the fact that perinatal transmission is closely linked to HIV infection in IVDAs and their sex partners.

The actual risk of HIV infection in the perinatal period has varied widely from report to report—from 0 to 100 percent—although pooled data and larger studies suggest that infants born to infected mothers have a 40 to 60 percent risk of acquiring infection from their infected mothers.[74] Assessment of infection in newborn infants is complicated by the initial presence of HIV antibody acquired passively from their mothers. Thus, HIV-antibody tests do not reflect the infection status of infants until they have been able to clear maternal antibodies and elicit antibodies on their own if truly infected (usually not until 9 months of age). Also, seroreversion has been reported in HIV-infected infants; so a negative HIV-antibody test in the first year of life may not ensure lack of perinatal infection.[76]

## TRANSMISSION IN OTHER AT-RISK POPULATIONS: PROSTITUTES, PRISONERS

HIV infection in female prostitutes in the United States is primarily associated with IV-drug abuse.[77] In Europe, none of 505 non-drug abusing prostitutes in London, Paris, and Nuremberg, West Germany, were found to be infected, whereas 24 (75 percent) of 32 prostitutes in Pordenone, Italy, and Zurich, Switzerland, who abused IV drugs were HIV-seropositive.[77] U.S. prostitutes had rates of HIV infection ranging from 0 percent in Las Vegas (where prostitutes were previously screened for HIV) to 57 percent in cities of northern New Jersey. Overall, about 20 to 30 percent of prostitutes in major U.S. cities may be infected, but rates vary depending on their use of IV drugs and numbers and types of sex partners.[77] Risk of transmission from these prostitutes to their male customers is hard to estimate. In a few instances in which numbers of sexual contacts resulting in female-to-male spread of HIV could be specified,[36,39] it seems that the average risk of such transmission from any single sexual contact is less than 0.1 percent (see above under Sexual Transmission: Heterosexual Persons). However, sexual transmission of HIV has been observed after only one or a few contacts with an HIV-infected person.[36]

As early as 1983, AIDS was identified as a special problem among inmates of U.S. correctional facilities, especially in mid-Atlantic states.[78] Although there has been concern that needle sharing and homosexual behavior in prisons might result in high rates of transmission in U.S. prisons, some preliminary data suggest that this may not be the case. Testing of over 1300 inmates of the Maryland Division of Corrections has shown a steady seroprevalence of 6.5 to 7.0 percent in 36 months of testing from 1985 through 1987. Also, men who had been incarcerated for many years, i.e., from before the start of the AIDS epidemic, were infrequently found to be HIV-infected (Ref. 78 and D. Vlahov, personal communication). Most HIV infections in U.S. prisoners can be related to IV-drug use before incarceration.

## UNPROVED MODES OF HIV TRANSMISSION

Considerable epidemiologic and laboratory investigation has been devoted to the putative transmission of HIV by unproved routes, such as by casual contact, human or insect bites, or fomites, food, or water. To date, there is no proof that HIV infection can be contracted from such sources.[79]

When data from several studies are combined[36,80] over 442 family members and household (nonsexual) contacts of AIDS patients have been tested for HIV antibody. Although some of these persons shared eating utensils, toothbrushes, razors, or toilets with AIDS patients and kissed AIDS patients on the lips,[36] none have been found HIV-seropositive. Transmission in more casual circumstances—such as in schools or workplaces—must be even less likely than in family settings; no such instance of transmission inside or outside the family has been documented.

To date, reports of 31 persons bitten by AIDS patients have been published; none of these bitten persons have been found HIV-seropositive on testing many months later.[81,82] HIV is rarely recovered from the saliva of HIV-infected persons,[83] and it survives poorly in saliva.[84]

There has been concern over mosquitoes as possible vectors of HIV, but this seems very unlikely. HIV-infected children in Africa have other identifiable risks for their infection, usually birth to an infected mother or transfusion with HIV-infected blood.[33,85] Purported transmission of HIV by mosquitoes in an indigent area of Florida was found on closer examination to be the result of heterosexual spread and IV-needle sharing.[86] HIV does not replicate in mosquitoes infected under artificial laboratory conditions.[87]

Finally, there are no reports of HIV transmission by food, water, or fomites. HIV survival in the environment is limited; it is rapidly inactivated by heat, sunlight, and many other environmental conditions.[88]

## RISK FACTORS FOR SUSCEPTIBILITY TO AND TRANSMISSIBILITY OF HIV

Large cohort studies of homosexual men in developed countries have yielded important data about behavioral risk factors for HIV infection. These studies have uniformly shown that large numbers of sexual partners and high percentage of sexual acts involving receptive anal intercourse, unprotected by condoms, both substantially increase a homosexual man's likelihood of becoming infected by HIV.[89–94] The data regarding risk of HIV infection from insertive anal intercourse and from receptive or insertive oral intercourse have been much less clear, mainly because it is almost impossible to find a sufficient number of persons who engage in just one of these activities to the exclusion of other sexual activities. However, because these types of sexual relations involve the exchange of semen or mucosal-mucosal (and perhaps blood-to-blood) contact, they should not generally be regarded as safe sex practices in regard to HIV transmission.

Another risk factor that has emerged from several recent studies is a previous history of genital ulcer disease, such as chancroid, syphilis, or herpes simplex virus type 2 (HSV-2). Genital ulcer disease is more common in HIV-infected than in noninfected African female prostitutes;[95,96] and in a recent study of homosexual men in Seattle, HIV-antibody-positive men more frequently than uninfected men had demonstrable antibodies to HSV-2 (77 vs. 37 percent).[97] This and similar studies of already HIV-infected persons cannot exclude the possibility that HIV and HSV-2 infections result independently from a primary risk factor (sexual activity). However, in a recent study of serum samples collected from homosexual men in San Francisco, HSV-2 infection preceded, and apparently predisposed, to HIV seroconversion in homosexual men. Sixty-eight percent of 62 HIV-infected homosexual men had antibody to HSV-2 before or at HIV seroconversion compared with 47 percent of 61 HIV-uninfected men who had had serum samples drawn from them in the same years as the HIV seroconverters.[98] It seems biologically plausible that HSV-2 might predispose to HIV infection because inapparent and unrecognized lesions of penile, vaginal, and rectal mucosa might allow the easier passage of HIV to the bloodstream. In regard to this, recently observed increases in chancroid and syphilis in U.S. cities may facilitate the spread of HIV.

Biologic host factors that might enhance transmissibility from an HIV-infected to an uninfected person are hard to evaluate unless one can identify probable or definite transmitters of HIV. One group of investigators has closely followed the wives of 25 hemophilic men for several years. Four (16 percent) of these wives became infected, and their seroconversion occurred after their husbands had been HIV-infected for many years and had had substantial decrements in helper T cells (T4 cells, CD4-positive cells).[41] Preliminary data from a study of homosexual partner-pairs in Boston also indicate that men who had probably transmitted HIV to their partners had higher suppressor T cells (T8 cells, CD8-positive cells) and lower helper:suppressor T-cell ratios than did men who had not transmitted HIV to their (still uninfected) partners (C.R. Horsburgh, Jr., and G.R. Seage III, personal communication). These interesting, but preliminary, findings indicate that there may be periods of greater infectivity early and/or late in HIV infection, periods associated with viremia and antigenemia and with the absence of HIV antibody.[99]

## FUTURE SPREAD OF HIV AND FUTURE CASES OF AIDS IN INDUSTRIALIZED COUNTRIES

The future of the AIDS epidemic is hard to predict because of the lack of critical answers about the natural history of infection with the virus (see Chap. 30).[100] Specifically, the incubation period between HIV infection and AIDS and the proportion of HIV-infected persons who will ultimately develop AIDS are both unknown; these issues will remain difficult to specify until the AIDS epidemic "peaks." However, mathematical models of the epidemic can be constructed. Depending on assumptions used, these indicate that the mean incubation period is 8 years or longer and that probably at least 50 percent of, and perhaps all, HIV-infected persons who survive long enough will ultimately develop AIDS.[101]

Given these and other assumptions, it appears that there will continue to be geometric increases in AIDS cases in North America and Europe for the immediate future. Figure 31-2 shows the incidence of AIDS in the Unites States by quarter of diagnosis projected from cases reported as of April 1986.[102] A polynomial model was fitted to the adjusted case counts as transformed by the Box-Cox method.[22] Reported cases in the past 2 years neatly fit the model and are close to the estimates made by public health, academic, and scientific officials at the Coolfont Conference in West Virginia in 1986.[26] Similar projections for AIDS cases in Europe have been equally grim and indicate geometric increases in AIDS cases for the immediate future.[12]

In the United States and Europe, spread of HIV has declined substantially in some populations of homosexual men, and spread by transfused blood and blood products (clotting factors) has been virtually eliminated. Cases in heterosexuals are expected to increase in number and percentage of reported AIDS cases; however, most heterosexual spread of HIV has thus far been to sex partners of persons in risk groups for AIDS. Because of the long incubation period between infection and disease, reported AIDS cases in all groups will continue to increase in the immediate future. In the long term, because of continued seroconversions in IVDAs and transmission from them to sex partners and neonates, drug abusers will account directly and indirectly for an ever-increasing percentage of AIDS cases in North America[11] and Europe.[31]

## EPIDEMIOLOGIC APPROACHES TO CONTROL OF HIV TRANSMISSION

As for other STDs, control of HIV transmission first requires education about and modification of unsafe sex practices.[103] Several simple precautions can completely or almost completely reduce a person's risk for HIV infection.

Many persons in the industrialized world have not been members of risk groups for HIV infection and have been either celibate or monogamous with someone who has not been infected. These persons are not at risk of sexual acquisition of HIV if their and their partners' behavior does not change. In situations in which it is uncertain whether one or both partners have been exposed sexually or otherwise to HIV, these persons should be encouraged to have antibody testing to determine their infection status.[104] Patients attending STD clinics should be especially targeted for screening and counseling.[45] Some persons who think they may have been infected in the past, and those who want to avoid infection, should practice sex that eliminates the exchange of potentially infectious body fluids, e.g., semen. Condoms, although not 100 percent effective in all circumstances, may still reduce seminal transmission of HIV.[105]

Needle-borne transmission of HIV will continue as long as infected needles are shared by IVDAs. One important preventive measure is to increase the availability of methadone and other drug-cessation clinics. In New York City and many other U.S. cities, thousands of addicts await placement in such programs because there are still not enough programs to accommodate them. Another measure that has been considered in the United States and the United Kingdom and implemented in some European countries is to make clean needles widely available. In the Netherlands, Ireland, and Switzerland, there are programs to exchange used for sterile injection equipment; in Copenhagen, free syringes and needles are distributed to IVDAs in health centers.[31] This intervention requires further evaluation, but it may be most effective when coupled with strong counseling and readily available drug-treatment programs.

The risk for HIV infection from blood transfusion has been practically but not completely eliminated by donor deferral and blood screening. Because the risk of HIV infection from receipt of blood and blood products is so low, autologous predonation of blood is not necessary to assure a low risk for HIV infection, although it may reduce one's risk of non-A, non-B hepatitis and may help the general blood supply.[106] Because blood donors are screened and factor concentrates are heat-treated, there should be no transmission by such concentrates unless heat-treatment procedures are inadequate.

Perinatal transmission is mainly a problem of HIV-infected pregnant IVDAs and their partners in industrialized countries; programs to reduce such transmission must concentrate mainly on this group. Pregnant women, especially in cities such as New York where an estimated 1 in 61 births are to HIV-infected women, are being increasingly encouraged to have HIV-antibody testing before or early in their pregnancies. However, it is difficult to get educational and preventive messages to inner-city minority women, the group most likely to be HIV-infected through their own or their parent's drug use, and to encourage them to have early prenatal care when they might be tested for HIV. Also, as discussed above, drug-treatment programs need to be made readily available to women who are IVDAs.

Health care workers may minimize their low risk of occupational HIV infection by wearing gloves and handling potentially infectious material such as blood with great care. Although transmission has rarely occurred through other exposures, most health care workers virtually eliminate their risk of infection by cautious handling and wearing gloves while working with HIV-infected patients and their clinical material.

One special issue that has arisen in the control of AIDS epidemic is the role of antibody testing. A convocation of health, academic, medical, scientific, and the ethical leaders in the United States was almost unanimous in rejecting mandatory HIV antibody testing for most segments of the population. However, these experts were equally convinced that such testing and counseling should be widely available and strongly promoted for those who may have been exposed to HIV.[104]

Contact tracing, as is done for other STDs, may be appropriate in certain circumstances, such as for the heterosexual contacts of persons infected by blood or blood product transfusions. However, contact tracing is often not practical for other groups, such as homosexual men who may have had numerous (often anonymous) contacts during the AIDS epidemic. For such groups, widespread voluntary testing and counseling is probably more effective in identifying HIV-infected persons.

## ECONOMIC AND SOCIAL CONSEQUENCES OF THE AIDS EPIDEMIC

The U.S. Public Health Service estimates that 270,000 reported cases and 179,000 deaths from AIDS will have occurred in the United States by the end of 1991.[26] Assuming that no highly effective therapy for AIDS will have been developed by then, the implications for health-care delivery are enormous. The direct economic cost for hospitalization of AIDS patients has been estimated to be $50,380 in Boston[107] and $41,499 in San Francisco.[108] (An earlier estimate of $147,000 per patient nationwide[109] was based on the increased length and frequency of hospitalizations for AIDS patients at that time.) In the absence of vaccines or cures, the Public Health Service estimates that there will be 74,000 new AIDS cases in 1991 in addition to the 71,000 AIDS patients alive at the beginning of that year.[26] The estimated direct cost for hospitalization of these persons is 8 to 16 billion dollars, about 1.2 to 2.4 percent of total projected health care expenditures in 1991.[110] The burden on already strained resources in many city hospitals, the incremental need for hospital beds in some communities, the possible need to build special separate facilities, and the planning for hospital and health care worker needs will be tremendous.[111,112] The cost to the economy in terms of lost output, e.g., time lost from work owing to AIDS morbidity and mortality—estimated at about $600,000 per patient—may be higher than total direct treatment costs for AIDS patients.[113]

The economic implications are much broader than just these direct costs of hospitalization, costs that are markers of much wider demands on the health and social service sectors of the economy. As many as 40 to 50 percent of HIV-infected persons may have manifestations of infection other than AIDS or other conditions requiring hospitalization. Some of these conditions may require extensive workup and treatment. The costs of antibody testing and counseling at blood banks and alternate test sites add to the economic impact of the AIDS epidemic. About 18 million units of blood are collected in the United States each year and require HIV-antibody (and perhaps in the future other) testing. Research and prevention efforts by federal and local governments and by pharmaceutical companies trying to develop new therapeutic or preventive modalities add yet other costs of the AIDS epidemic. The cost of a year's supply of azidothymidine (AZT), about $10,000 when this drug became commercially available in 1987, reflects ever-increasing drug-development costs. This figure does not include physician fees, transfusions, and other treatments and tests associated with receiving AZT.

Finally, persons who are HIV-positive (and many of those who are HIV-seronegative) require counseling and support, even when they may have no symptoms requiring treatment.

For all these direct and indirect costs, there are perhaps as many unmeasurable and incalculable costs in terms of other "resources" that developed nations consider precious. One measure of these is "years of potential life lost" before 65 years of age (YPLLs), which serve as an index of the loss to society of persons in their economic and creative prime. Since AIDS is predominantly a fatal disease of the young, YPLLs more truly indicate the real loss to industrialized societies from this epidemic. In the United States, there will be an estimated 1.1 million YPLLs in 1990 alone.[110] The hysteria surrounding the AIDS epidemic has resulted in considerable, often inappropriate, responses by industries, schools, prisons, social services (such as police and fire departments), hospitals, and the community. Ignorance and hysteria about AIDS have endangered basic civil and human liberties and, in some cases, diminished services for persons most in need. One of the saddest aspects of the AIDS epidemic has been its indirect cost to societies that value open and free social exchange.

## References


1 Huminer D et al: AIDS in the pre-AIDS era. *Rev Infect Dis* 9:1102, 1987.

2 Centers for Disease Control: *Pneumocystis* pneumonia—Los Angeles. *MMWR* 30:250, 1981.

3 Centers for Disease Control: Kaposi's sarcoma and *Pneumocystis* pneumonia among homosexual men—New York City and California. *MMWR* 30:305, 1981.

4 Clumeck N et al: Acquired immune deficiency syndrome in black Africans (letter). *Lancet* 1:642, 1983.

5 Jaffe HW et al: National case-control study of Kaposi's sarcoma and *Pneumocystis carinii* pneumonia in homosexual men. Part I. Epidemiologic results. *Ann Intern Med* 99:145, 1983.

6 Marmor M et al: Risk factors for Kaposi's sarcoma in homosexual men. *Lancet* 1:1083, 1982.

7 Centers for Disease Control: A cluster of Kaposi's sarcoma and *Pneumocystis carinii* pneumonia among homosexual male residents of Los Angeles and Orange Counties, California. *MMWR* 31:305, 1982.

8 Auerbach DM et al: Cluster of cases of the acquired immune deficiency syndrome: Patients linked by sexual contact. *Am J Med* 76: 487, 1984.

9 Barré-Sinnousi F et al: Isolation of a T-lymphotropic retrovirus from a patient at risk for acquired immune deficiency syndrome (AIDS). *Science* 220:868, 1983.

10 Gallo RC et al: Frequent detection and isolation of cytopathic retroviruses (HTLV-III) from patients with AIDS and at risk of AIDS. *Science* 224:500, 1984.

11 Centers for Disease Control: Human immunodeficiency virus infection in the United States. *MMWR* 36 (suppl): 6S, 1987.

12 Downs AM et al: AIDS in Europe: Current trends and short term predictions estimated from surveillance data, January 1981–June 1986. *AIDS* 1:53, 1987.

13 World Health Organization: Acquired immunodeficiency syndrome (AIDS)—Data as of 29 February 1988. *Weekly Epidemiol Rec* 63: 69, 1988.

14 Anonymous: Latest UK figures for AIDS. *Lancet* 1:934, 1987.

15 Anonymous: AIDS today. *NZ Med J* 100:89, 1987.

16 Brunet JB, Ancelle RA: The international occurrence of the acquired immunodeficiency syndrome. *Ann Intern Med* 103:670, 1985.

17 Elmslie K, Nault P: AIDS surveillance in Canada. *Can Med Assoc J* 135:780, 1986.

18 Swinbanks D: Woman's AIDS death in Japan produces shock waves. *Nature* 325:387, 1987.

19 Whyte BM et al: Epidemiology of the acquired immunodeficiency syndrome in Australia. *Med J Aust* 146:65, 1987.

20 World Health Organization: Acquired immunodeficiency syndrome (AIDS): Situation in the WHO European region as of 31 December 1986. *Weekly Epidemiol Rec* 62:117, 1987.

21 World Health Organization: Acquired immunodeficiency syndrome (AIDS): Situation in the WHO European region as of March 31, 1987. *Weekly Epidemiol Rec* 2:229, 1987.

22 Curran JW et al: Epidemiology of HIV infection and AIDS in the United States. *Science* 239:610, 1988.

23 Centers for Disease Control: Update on acquired immune deficiency syndrome (AIDS)—United States. *MMWR* 31:507, 1982.

24 Centers for Disease Control: Revision of the CDC surveillance case definition for acquired immunodeficiency syndrome. *MMWR* 36 (suppl): 3S, 1987.

25 Hardy AM et al: Review of death certificates to assess completeness of AIDS case reporting. *Public Health Rep* 102:286, 1987.

26 Public Health Service: Coolfont report: A PHS plan for prevention and control of AIDS and the AIDS virus. *Public Health Rep* 101:341, 1986.

27 Brunet J-B et al: Report on the European Community Workshop on Epidemiology of HIV Infections: Spread among intravenous drug abusers and the heterosexual population. *AIDS* 1:59, 1987.

28 McKusick L et al: Reported changes in the sexual behavior of men at risk for AIDS, San Francisco, 1982–1984—The AIDS Behavior Research Project. *Public Health Rep* 100:622, 1985.

29 Centers for Disease Control: Self-reported changes in sexual behavior among homosexual and bisexual men from the San Francisco City Clinic Cohort. *MMWR* 36:187, 1987.

30 Centers for Disease Control: Declining rates of rectal and pharyngeal gonorrhea among males—New York City. *MMWR* 33:295, 1984.

31 Ancelle-Park R et al: AIDS and drug addicts in Europe (letter). *Lancet* 2:626, 1987.

32 Centers for Disease Control: Immunodeficiency among female sexual partners of males with acquired immune deficiency syndrome (AIDS)—New York. *MMWR* 31:697, 1983.

33 Harris C et al: Immunodeficiency in female sexual partners of men with the acquired immunodeficiency syndrome. *N Engl J Med* 308: 1181, 1983.

34 Chamberland ME et al: Acquired immunodeficiency syndrome in the United States: An analysis of cases outside high-incidence groups. *Ann Intern Med* 101:617, 1984.

35 Quinn TC et al: AIDS in Africa: An epidemiologic paradigm. *Science* 234:977, 1986.

36 Peterman TA et al: Risk of human immunodeficiency virus transmission from heterosexual adults with transfusion-associated infections. *JAMA* 259:55, 1988.

37 Steigbigel NH et al: Heterosexual transmission of infection and disease by the human immunodeficiency virus (HIV) (abstract), in *III International Conference on AIDS. Abstracts volume.* Washington, DC, US Department of Health and Human Services, 1987, p 106.

38 Fischl MA et al: Evaluation of heterosexual partners, children, and household contacts of adults with AIDS. *JAMA* 257:640, 1987.

39 Padian N et al: Male-to-female transmission of human immunodeficiency virus. *JAMA* 258:788, 1987.

40 Kreiss JK et al: Antibody to human T-lymphotropic virus type III in wives of hemophiliacs: Evidence for heterosexual transmission. *Ann Intern Med* 102:623, 1985.

41 Goedert JJ et al: Heterosexual transmission of human immunodeficiency virus: Association with severe depletion of T-helper lymphocytes in men with hemophilia. *AIDS Res Hum Retroviruses* 3:355, 1988.

42 Jason JM et al: HTLV-III/LAV antibody and immune status of household contacts and sexual partners of persons with hemophilia. *JAMA* 255:212, 1986.

43 Centers for Disease Control: HIV infection and pregnancies in sex-

ual partners of HIV-seropositive hemophilic men. *MMWR* 36:593, 1987.

44 May RM, Anderson M: Transmission dynamics of HIV infection. *Nature* 326:137, 1987.

45 Quinn TC et al: Human immunodeficiency virus infection among patients attending clinics for sexually transmitted diseases. *N Engl J Med* 318:197, 1988.

46 Selwyn PA et al: Natural history of HIV infection in intravenous drug abusers (IVDAs) (abstract), in *III International Conference on AIDS. Abstracts volume.* Washington, DC, US Department of Health and Human Services, 1987, p 2.

47 Selwyn PA: AIDS: What is now known. II. Epidemiology. *Hosp Pract* 21:127, 1986.

48 Lange WR et al: The geographic distribution of human immunodeficiency virus (HIV) antibodies in parenteral drug abusers (PDAs) (abstract), in *III Internation Conference on AIDS. Abstracts volume.* Washington, DC, US Department of Health and Human Services, 1987, p 71.

49 Ward JW et al: Epidemiologic characteristics of blood donors with antibody to human immunodeficiency virus. *Transfusion* 28:298, 1988.

50 Centers for Disease Control: Antibody to human immunodeficiency virus in female prostitutes. *MMWR* 36:157, 1987.

51 Peterman TA et al: Estimating the risks of transfusion-associated immune deficiency syndrome and human immunodeficiency virus infection. *Transfusion* 27:371, 1987.

52 Ward JW et al: Risk of human immunodeficiency virus infection from blood donors who later developed the acquired immunodeficiency syndrome. *Ann Intern Med* 106:61, 1987.

53 Centers for Disease Control: Transfusion-associated human T-lymphotropic virus type III/lymphadenopathy-associated virus infection from a seronegative donor—Colorado. *MMWR* 24:389, 1986.

54 Ward JW et al: Human immunodeficiency virus transmission by blood transfusions screened negative for HIV antibody. *N Engl J Med* 318:473, 1988.

55 Centers for Disease Control: Update: Revised Public Health Service definition of persons who should refrain from donating blood and plasma—United States. *MMWR* 34:547, 1985.

56 Centers for Disease Control: *Pneumocystis carinii* pneumonia among persons with hemophilia A. *MMWR* 31:365, 1982.

57 Johnson RE et al: Acquired immunodeficiency syndrome among patients attending hemophilia treatment centers (1978 to June 1984) and mortality experience of US hemophiliacs (1968 to 1978). *Am J Epidemiol* 121:797, 1985.

58 Mathez D et al: LAV/HTLV-III seroconversion and disease in hemophiliacs treated in France (letter). *N Engl J Med* 314:118, 1986.

59 Ikegami N and the Collaborative Study Group of National Hospitals: Prevalence of antibodies to AIDS-associated retrovirus in in- and out-patients in Japan. *AIDS Res* 2 (suppl): S29, 1986.

60 Eyster ME et al: Prospective study of AIDS in hemophiliacs with elevated interferon alpha levels (abstract), in *III International Conference on AIDS. Abstracts volume.* Washington, DC, US Department of Health and Human Services, 1987, p 21.

61 Centers for Disease Control: Survey of non-US hemophilia treatment centers for HIV seroconversion following therapy with heat-treated factor concentrates. *MMWR* 36:121, 1987.

62 Anonymous: Needlestick transmission of HTLV-III from a patient infected in Africa. *Lancet* 2:1376, 1984.

63 Weiss SH et al: HTLV-III infection among health care workers: Association with needle-stick injuries. *JAMA* 254:2089, 1985.

64 Henderson DK et al: Risk of nosocomial infection with human T-cell lymphotropic virus type III/lymphadenopathy-associated virus in a large cohort of intensively exposed health care workers. *Ann Intern Med* 104:644, 1986.

65 McCray E: The Cooperative Needlestick Surveillance Group: Occupational risk of the acquired immunodeficiency syndrome among health care workers. *N Engl J Med* 314:1127, 1986.

66 Gerberding JL et al: Risk of transmitting the human immunodeficiency virus, cytomegalovirus, and hepatitis B virus to health care workers exposed to patients with AIDS and AIDS-related condition. *J Infect Dis* 156:1, 1987.

67 Curran JW et al: Epidemiology of HIV infection and AIDS in the United States. *Science* 239:610, 1988.

68 Centers for Disease Control: Apparent transmission of human T-lymphotropic virus type III/lymphadenopathy-associated virus infection from a child to a mother providing health care. *MMWR* 35: 76, 1986.

69 Centers for Disease Control: Update: human immunodeficiency virus infections in health care workers exposed to blood of infected patients. *MMWR* 36:285, 1987.

70 Centers for Disease Control: Recommendations for prevention of HIV transmission in health-care settings. *MMWR* (suppl) 36:1S, 1987.

71 Ammann AJ: The acquired immunodeficiency syndrome in infants and children. *Ann Intern Med* 103:734, 1985.

72 Scott GB et al: Mothers of infants with the acquired immunodeficiency syndrome. Evidence for both symptomatic and asymptomatic carriers. *JAMA* 253:363, 1985.

73 Cowan MJ et al: Maternal transmission of acquired immunodeficiency syndrome. *Pediatrics* 73:382, 1984.

74 Oxtoby MJ et al: National trends in perinatally acquired AIDS, United States (abstract), in *III International Conferences on AIDS. Abstracts volume.* Washington, DC, US Department of Health and Human Services, 1987, p 157.

75 Centers for Disease Control: Acquired immunodeficiency syndrome among blacks and Hispanics—United States. *MMWR* 35:663, 1986.

76 Borkowsky W et al: Human-immunodeficiency-virus infections in infants negative for anti-HIV by enzyme-linked immunoassay. *Lancet* 1:1168, 1987.

77 Centers for Disease Control: Antibody to human immunodeficiency virus in female prostitutes. *MMWR* 36:157, 1987.

78 Centers for Disease Control: Acquired immunodeficiency syndrome in correctional facilities: A report of the National Institute of Justice and the American Correctional Association. *MMWR* 35:195, 1986.

79 Lifson AR: Do alternate modes for transmission of human immunodeficiency virus exist (review)? *JAMA* 259:1353, 1988.

80 Friedland GH et al: Lack of transmission of HTLV-III/LAV infection to household contacts of patients with AIDS or AIDS-related complex with oral candidiasis. *N Engl J Med* 314:344, 1986.

81 Tsoukas C et al: Risk of transmission of HTLV-III/LAV from human bites (poster), in: *Program and Abstracts of the II International Conference on AIDS.* Paris, France, L'Association pour la Recherche sur les Deficits Immunitaires Viro-Induits, 1986, p 125.

82 Drummond J: Seronegative 18 months after being bitten by a patient with AIDS (letter). *JAMA* 256:2342, 1986.

83 Ho DD et al: Infrequency of isolation of HTLV-III virus from saliva in AIDS (letter). *N Engl J Med* 313:1606, 1985.

84 Fultz PN: Components of saliva inactivate human immunodeficiency virus (letter). *Lancet* 2:1215, 1986.

85 Mann JM et al: Risk factors for human immunodeficiency virus seropositivity among children 1-24 months old in Kinshasa, Zaire. *Lancet* 2:654, 1986.

86 Centers for Disease Control: Acquired immunodeficiency syndrome in Western Palm Beach County, Florida. *MMWR* 35:609, 1986.

87 Jupp, PG, Lyons SF: Experimental assessment of bedbugs (*Cimex lectularius* and *Cimex hemipterus*) and mosquitoes (*Aedes aegypti formosus*) as vectors of human immunodeficiency virus. *AIDS* 1: 171, 1987.

88 Quinnan JV et al: Inactivation of human T-cell lymphotropic virus, type III by heat, chemicals, and irradiation. *Transfusion* 26:481, 1986.

89 Darrow WW et al: Risk factors for human immunodeficiency virus (HIV) infections in homosexual men. *Am J Public Health* 77:479, 1987.

90 Goedert JJ et al: Determinants of retrovirus (HTLV-III) antibody and immunodeficiency conditions in homosexual men. *Lancet* 2: 711, 1984.

91 Jaffe HW et al: The acquired immunodeficiency syndrome in a co-

hort of homosexual men. A six-year follow-up study. *Ann Intern Med* 103:210, 1985.
92 Polk BF et al: Predictors of the acquired immunodeficiency syndrome developing in a cohort of seropositive homosexual men. *N Engl J Med* 316:61, 1987.
93 Winkelstein W Jr et al: Sexual practices and risk of infection by the human immunodeficiency virus. The San Francisco Men's Health Study. *JAMA* 257:321, 1987.
94 Goedert JJ et al: Three-year incidence of AIDS in five cohorts of HTLV-III-infected risk group members. *Science* 231:992, 1986.
95 Kreiss JK et al: AIDS virus infection in Nairobi prostitutes. Spread of the epidemic to East Africa. *N Engl J Med* 314:414, 1986.
96 Plummer FA et al: Incidence of human immunodeficiency virus (HIV) infection and related disease in a cohort of Nairobi prostitutes (abstract), in *III International Conference on AIDS. Abstracts volume.* Washington, DC, US Department of Health and Human Services, 1987, p 6.
97 Handsfield HH et al: Association of anogenital ulcer disease with human immunodeficiency virus infection in homosexual men (abstract), in *III International Conference on AIDS. Abstracts volume.* Washington, DC, US Department of Health and Human Services, 1987, p 206.
98 Holmberg SD et al: Prior herpes simplex virus type 2 infection as a risk factor for HIV infection. *JAMA* 259:1048, 1988.
99 Goudsmit J et al: IgG response to human immunodeficiency virus in experimentally infected chimpanzees mimics the IgG response in humans. *J Infect Dis* 155:327, 1987.
100 Hopkins DR: Key epidemiologic questions about AIDS and infection with HTLV-III/LAV. *Public Health Rep* 101:234, 1986.
101 Holmberg SD, Curran JW: The natural history of human immunodeficiency virus (HIV) infection, in *The Immunobiology and Pathogenesis of Persistent Virus Infections,* C Lopez, HS Margolis (eds). Washington, DC, American Society for Microbiology, 1988; 180–201.
102 Morgan WM, Curran JW: Acquired immunodeficiency syndrome: Current and future trends. *Public Health Rep* 101:459, 1986.
103 Koop CE: *Surgeon General's Report on the Acquired Immune Deficiency Syndrome.* Washington, DC, US Department of Health and Human Services, 1986.
104 Centers for Disease Control: Public Health Service guidelines for counseling and antibody testing to prevent HIV infection and AIDS. *MMWR* 36:509, 1987.
105 Feldenblum PJ, Fortney JA: Condoms, spermicides, and the transmission of human immunodeficiency virus: A review of the literature. *Am J Public Health* 78:52, 1988.
106 Surgenor DM: The patient's blood is the safest blood. *N Engl J Med* 316:542, 1987.
107 Seage GR III et al: Medical care costs of AIDS in Massachusetts. *JAMA* 256:3107, 1986.
108 Scitovsky AA et al: Medical care costs of patients with AIDS in San Francisco. *JAMA* 256:3103, 1986.
109 Hardy AM et al: The economic impact of the first 10,000 cases of acquired immunodeficiency syndrome in the United States. *JAMA* 255:209, 1986.
110 Scitovsky AA et al: *Final Report: Estimating the Direct and Indirect Economic Costs of Acquired Immunodeficiency Syndrome,* 1985, 1986, and 1990. Atlanta, GA, Centers for Disease Control, 1986.
111 Hardy AM: Planning for the health care needs of patients with AIDS (editorial). *JAMA* 256:3140, 1986.
112 Weinberg DS, Murray HW: Coping with AIDS: The special problems of New York City. *N Engl J Med* 317:1469, 1987.
113 Bloom DE, Carliner G: The economic impact of AIDS in the United States. *Science* 239:604, 1988.

Chapter 32

# Unique aspects of human immunodeficiency virus and related viruses in developing countries

Thomas C. Quinn

## INTRODUCTION

Over the past several years, the acquired immunodeficiency syndrome (AIDS) has become a global pandemic. By August 1988, over 100,000 cases of AIDS had been reported to the World Health Organization from 144 countries. Since many other cases remain unrecognized and unreported, particularly in developing countries which lack the infrastructure necessary for diagnosis and accurate surveillance, it is estimated that over 250,000 cases of AIDS have probably occurred worldwide.[1,2] An additional 500,000 individuals are estimated to be infected with the etiologic agent of AIDS, the human immunodeficiency virus (HIV), and to have symptoms associated with this viral infection referred to as AIDS-related complex (ARC). Furthermore, an estimated 5 to 10 million individuals may already be infected with HIV.[1–3] It is this latter pool of asymptomatic infected individuals which represents the major human reservoir of HIV infection. Thousands of additional AIDS cases will eventually develop and millions of other individuals may become infected following sexual or parenteral contact with these asymptomatic carriers of the virus.

Unfortunately, the vast majority of both asymptomatic and symptomatic infected people reside in developing countries where the economic and social effects of this disease will have their greatest impact. Because of the limited financial resources of these countries, the challenge to control this epidemic will be greatest within those areas where traditional efforts to control other infectious diseases through vaccines or other measures have always lagged behind more technologically advanced countries. Because of the present lack of an effective vaccine or curative therapy it is evident that HIV infection and AIDS will continue to escalate throughout all areas of the world. However, the greatest increase will be in developing countries, particularly in Africa where the means to control this disease may be more limited.[4]

## HISTORICAL PERSPECTIVE

### HIV-1

AIDS was first recognized as a clinical entity in 1981 with reports of life-threatening opportunistic infections and Kaposi's sarcoma occurring among homosexual men residing in the United States.[5,6] Following the recognition of AIDS in the United States, similar cases were identified among Haitian patients residing in the United States and among Africans residing in Europe.[7–12] Pape et al., in a systematic survey, identified 229 patients with AIDS in Haiti between 1979 and 1984.[13] There is substantial evidence that HIV was present in Africa prior to this period. Serologic analysis of sera from Africa which had been stored since 1959 demonstrated evidence of HIV infection in an individual residing in Kinshasa, Zaire.[14] By 1970, one of 500 (0.2 percent) pregnant women residing in Kinshasa, Zaire, was found to be seropositive for HIV.[15] A retrospective review of clinical records for suspected AIDS cases among Africans or other individuals who visited Africa included a Danish surgeon who was apparently exposed to HIV in Zaire between 1972 and 1975, and subsequently developed AIDS in 1976.[16] In a retrospective analysis of sera collected in 1976 from 659 residents of the remote Equateur Province of Zaire, 5 (0.8 percent) individuals were positive for antibody to HIV.[17] Following culture of these sera, one isolate of HIV was recovered from an antibody-positive individual who subsequently died of AIDS in 1978.[18]

Clinically, AIDS appears to have been uncommon in Africa prior to the late 1970s. Hospital chart reviews in Europe identified only a few cases suggestive of AIDS among Africans or others who traveled to and from Africa prior to 1978.[7,19] The absence of aggressive Kaposi's sarcoma or changes in Kaposi's sarcoma epidemiology in Uganda (1951–1976), northeastern Zaire (1971–1983), Zambia (pre-1973), and Kinshasa (pre-1980) provides further indirect evidence against widespread HIV-associated disease during this period.[20]

These findings prompted a series of investigations to determine the presence of AIDS within central Africa.[21–29] By the early 1980s, epidemics of atypical aggressive Kaposi's sarcoma associated with HIV seropositivity were documented in Zaire, Zambia, and Uganda.[23–25] Epidemic increases in a chronic life-threatening enteropathic illness referred to as "slim disease" were identified during this same time period in Zaire, Uganda, and Tanzania.[26,27] In Rwanda, an epidemic of esophageal candidiasis was detected in 1983 in a hospital where approximately 300 esophagoscopies had been performed annually since 1979.[28] In addition, a careful surveillance of cryptococcal meningitis in Kinshasa, Zaire starting prior to 1960 showed a rapid increase in the annual number of cases starting in 1978, with an over sevenfold increase in 1978–1984 compared with the period 1959–1977.[21,29] By October 1983, two separate studies in Kinshasa, Zaire, and Kigali, Rwanda, confirmed the presence of 38 and 26 cases of AIDS, respectively, in these areas.[21,22] As in Haiti, these cases were equally distributed among men and women and were not associated with traditional risk factors for HIV infection such as homosexuality or IV drug use.

Longitudinal studies, particularly in urban centers of central Africa, have demonstrated increasing numbers of AIDS cases among both men and women, particularly those with promiscuous sexual lifestyles. For example, among female prostitutes in Nairobi, Kenya, HIV seroprevalence rose from 4 percent in 1980 to 88 percent in 1987 (Fig. 32-1).[4,30] For men attending a sexually transmitted disease clinic in Nairobi, Kenya, the rate of HIV infection rose from 1 percent in 1980 to 22 percent in 1988. Similarly, even among the general population, rates of HIV infection have risen from 0 percent in 1980 to 3 percent in 1988 in Nairobi and from 0.2 percent in 1970 to 8 percent in 1986 among pregnant women in Kinshasa, Zaire.

Unlike the urban centers of Africa, HIV infection in rural Africa has remained relatively stable (Table 32-1). For example, HIV seroprevalence has remained low among the residents of the Equateur Province of Zaire at 0.8 percent between 1976 and 1986, whereas HIV seroprevalence has increased tenfold among pregnant women in Kinshasa, Zaire, during the same time period.[17] It is likely, therefore, that social changes with disruption

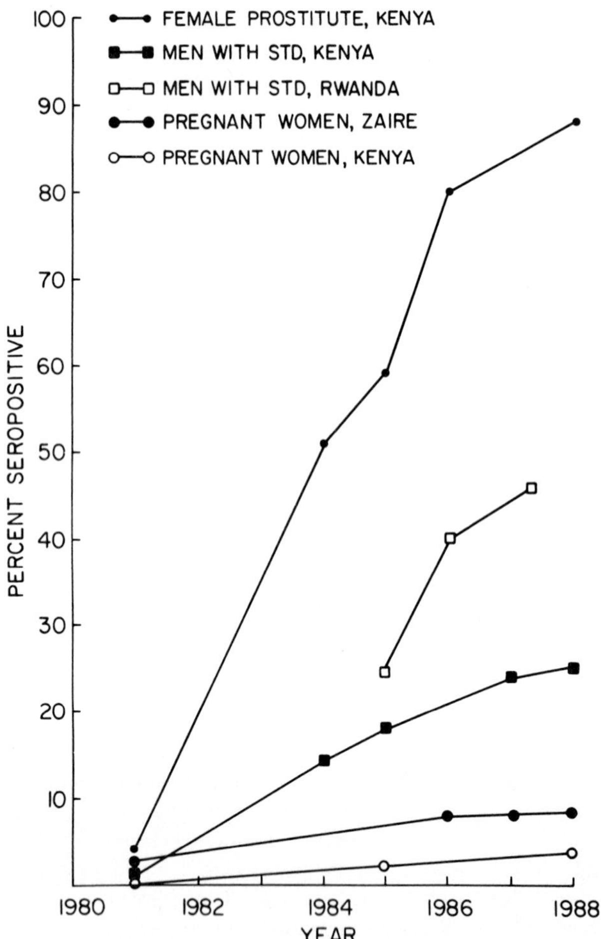


Fig. 32-1. Longitudinal seroprevalence of HIV infection in selected populations in Kenya, Zaire, and Rwanda. (Data from Piot et al.)

**Table 32-1. Comparison of HIV Prevalence Rates in Healthy Adults Residing in Major Cities versus Rural Areas for Selected African Countries**

| Country | Area | HIV prevalence (%) |
|---|---|---|
| Cameroon | Yaounde (1987) | 0.5 |
| | Maroua, semirural (1986) | 0.5 |
| | Mora, rural (1985) | 0.0 |
| Central African Republic | Bangui (1987) | 7.8 |
| | Bambari, semirural (1987) | 3.7 |
| Gabon | Libreville (1986) | 1.8 |
| | Franceville (Western province) (1986) | 0.3 |
| | Hout Ogone Province (1986) | 0.0 |
| Kenya | Nairobi (1985–86) | 2.4 |
| | 15K outside Nairobi (1985) | 0.9 |
| | NE Kenya Sololo (1986) | 0.9 |
| Rwanda | Kigali (1985) | 18.0 |
| | 2 remote rural areas (1985) | 4.5 |
| Tanzania | Dar es Salaam (1986) | 3.6 |
| | Bukoba, rural towns (1986) | 16.0 |
| | Arusha, rural towns (1986) | 0.7 |
| Congo | Brazzaville (1986) | 5.0 |
| | Pointe Noire, semirural (1985) | 0.0 |
| Zaire | Kinshasa (1987) | 5.6 |
| | Yambuku, remote village (1986) | 1.0 |

of traditional lifestyles may be partly responsible for the rapid spread of HIV infection in some areas of Africa.

Introduced at a later time, HIV infection appears to have become established in the countries of Latin America in the late 1970s. Importation of HIV-infected blood units and coagulation factor VIII and factor IX concentrates from the United States and Europe, as well as visitors from these and other industrialized countries, may have been responsible for the introduction of HIV to Latin America. While Brazil had less than 25 reported cases of AIDS in 1982, over 2000 had been reported by the end of 1987.[2] Similarly, HIV infection appears to have been introduced to Asia sometime in the early 1980s, although the number of AIDS cases remains relatively small in these areas. Seroprevalence rates among prostitutes in India, the Philippines, and Indonesia confirm the presence of HIV infection at relatively low levels (1 to 5 percent).[1,31–33] It can be anticipated, given the right conditions of sexual promiscuity, unscreened blood transfusions, or use of unsterilized needles, that HIV infection will become rapidly established within high-risk members of these populations.

## HIV-2

In 1985, during studies in West Africa, Kanki and others found atypical anti-HIV antibody patterns in prostitutes residing in Dakar, Senegal, an area where AIDS had not been previously reported.[34,35] By radioimmunoprecipitation, these Senegalese sera reacted more strongly with a retrovirus that had been previously isolated from African green monkeys and captive macaques and which was referred to as the simian immunodeficiency virus (SIV).[36] Serologic surveys using SIV antigens identified seropositive individuals among female prostitutes, patients with tuberculosis, and patients attending STD clinics.[37] Clavel and colleagues then isolated a virus from HIV-1 seronegative AIDS patients in Guinea-Bissau and the Cape Verde Islands in West Africa which he initially named LAV-2, but which was later renamed HIV-2.[38] Genetic and serologic studies have demonstrated remarkable cross-reactivity between HIV-2 and SIV. Thus both scientific groups had independently identified human infection with a retrovirus distinct from HIV-1.[39–42] With the subsequent development of a serologic test for HIV-2, evidence for infection with this virus has been found in most countries of West Africa, and to a lesser extent in Europe and South America, with one case reported in the United States.[43–45] Since this virus behaves like HIV-1 in terms of transmission patterns, it is probable that epidemic spread of HIV-2 may resemble that of HIV-1 over the foreseeable future.

## EPIDEMIOLOGY

The true extent of HIV and related retroviral infections in developing countries can only be estimated roughly from limited serologic and surveillance reports. In many of these countries, infectious disease surveillance capabilities are limited because of weaknesses in the health care infrastructure and inadequate resources. In addition, the CDC/WHO definition of AIDS typically requires sophisticated laboratory support for the diagnosis of opportunistic infections and malignancies and exclusion of other known causes of immunodeficiency, and is therefore not applicable or practical for developing countries.[46,46a] Nevertheless, in an attempt to measure the extent of HIV infection in their people, many countries have instituted limited forms of AIDS surveillance and have performed serologic studies for HIV in selected populations.

## AIDS SURVEILLANCE

Of the 80,994 AIDS patients reported from the Americas by August 1988, 90 percent were from the United States.[1,2] Outside of the United States, Brazil has reported 2956 cases, with cases increasing from 801 at the end of June 1986 to 1695 at the end of June 1987. Canada has reported a total of 1809 cases with only slight increases over the last 2 years. Other countries in the Americas with over 100 cases include Haiti, Mexico, Dominican Republic, Trinidad and Tobago, Bahamas, Colombia, Argentina, and Venezuela. In Africa, a total of 14,939 cases were reported by August 1988, with 44 countries reporting at least one or more cases (Fig. 32-2). Uganda, Tanzania, Kenya, Rwanda, Burundi, and Zambia have each reported more than 500 cases, while Zimbabwe and Zaire have each reported more than 300 cases. The highest number of cases has been reported from urban areas in central, eastern, and southern Africa. Although cases were first officially reported from Africa in the second half of 1982, nearly 70 percent of all cases were reported in 1987, illustrating both increased recognition of cases and increased government cooperation and reporting.

AIDS surveillance in Africa was initially established in Kinshasa, Zaire, between July 1984 and February 1985, when 332 cases were identified for an adjusted annual incidence of approximately 176 cases per million population.[47] The incidence in adult Kinshasa residents was approximately 380 cases per million since nearly all the reported cases occurred among persons 20 years of age or older. Peak age-specific incidence rates of 786 per million and 601 per million were present among 30- to 39-year-old men and women, respectively. By the end of 1986, the annual incidence was approximately 200 cases per 100,000 adults, and preliminary data from 1987 suggest that these rates may actually exceed 300 cases per 100,000.[48] However, these are probably minimal estimates since the data reflect only recognized or reported cases of AIDS in several hospitals within one city.

In Asia, 277 cases have been reported from 22 countries with more than 5 cases reported from Thailand, India, the Philippines, and Hong Kong. The low number of reported AIDS cases and the documented low seroprevalence rates even among female prostitutes in Asia suggest that HIV infection has only recently been introduced within this area of the world.[33]

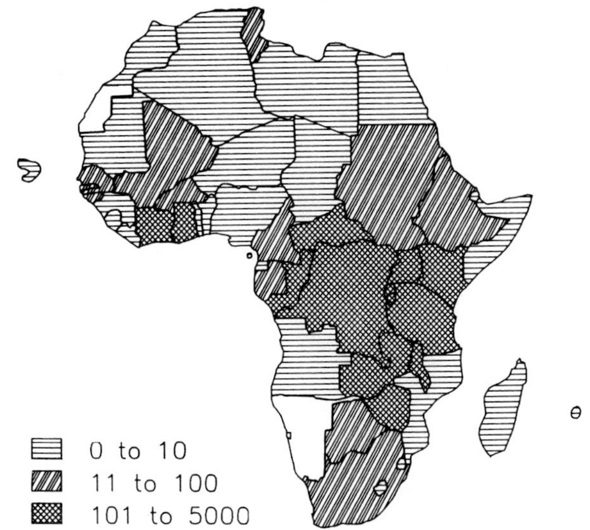


**Fig. 32-2.** Countries of Africa that have reported cases of AIDS to the World Health Organization as of April 1988.

Common to all areas of the world, the major modes of transmission of HIV are sexual, parenteral, and perinatal. The relative frequency of these three types of transmission, and the interval since HIV introduction and subsequent dissemination result in three distinct epidemiologic patterns (Fig. 32-3).[1] Pattern 1 of HIV infection is characteristic of that observed in developed countries such as western Europe, North America, some areas of South America, Australia, and New Zealand. Homosexual and bisexual men and IV drug users are the major affected groups. The virus was probably initially introduced into homosexual men in the mid-1970s or early 1980s, and up to 50 percent of the homosexual men in urban areas are infected. IV drug abuse accounts for the next largest proportion of HIV infections and in some areas, such as southern Europe, IV drug users are responsible for the majority of HIV infections. Heterosexual and subsequently perinatal transmission are not presently a major problem, but both modes of transmission are expected to increase

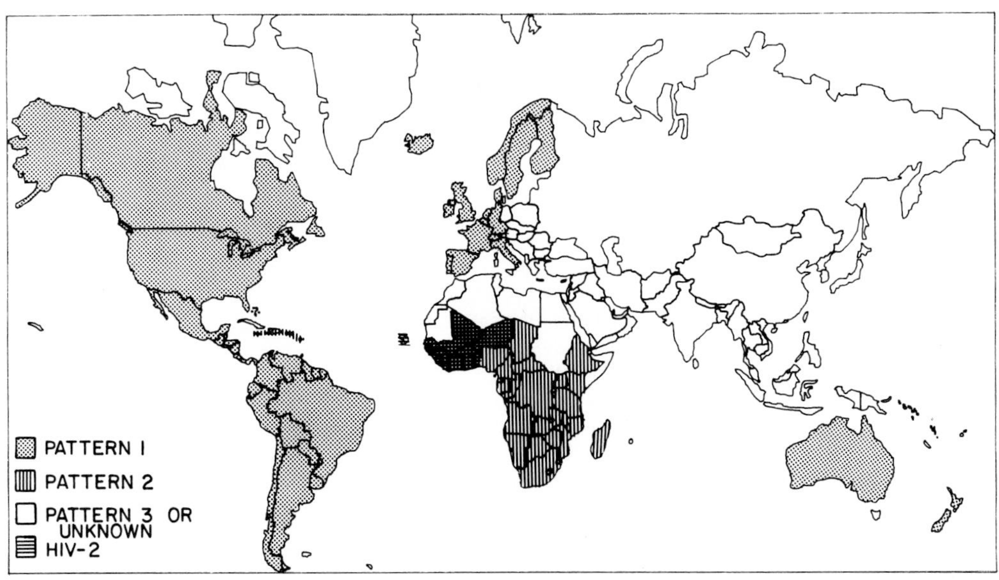


**Fig. 32-3.** Patterns of HIV-1 and HIV-2 infection in the world. Pattern 1 consists primarily of homosexual and bisexual men and IV drug users. Pattern 2 consists of heterosexual cases, and pattern 3 represents those areas with recent introduction of HIV among persons with multiple sex partners. (Adapted from Piot et al.)

within the near future, particularly among inner-city minority populations. Transmission via contaminated blood or blood products no longer continues to be a major problem, although thousands of individuals were infected by this route prior to 1985.

In pattern 2, characteristic of countries in Africa, the Caribbean, and some areas of South America, heterosexuals appear to be the major population group infected. The virus may have been introduced into these populations in the early to late 1970s, but serologic surveys within the past year demonstrate infection in up to 25 percent of 20- to 40-year-old individuals in some urban areas of Africa (Tables 32-1 and 32-2). As a sexually transmitted disease, seroprevalence rates appear to be extremely high (up to 80 percent) among female prostitutes (Table 32-2). Homosexual transmission does not appear to be an important factor in the spread of HIV in these areas, although it may exist to a lesser degree. Because of the equal sexual distribution, perinatal transmission has become a major problem as 5 to 15 percent of women are HIV seropositive. Unlike pattern 1 countries, transfusion of HIV infected blood continues to be a major public health problem in these areas. Nonsterilized needles and syringes may also account for an undetermined proportion of HIV infections.

Pattern 3 is found in the countries of Asia, the Pacific region, the Middle East, eastern Europe, and some rural areas of South America where the virus may have been introduced only within the last several years. Because of this recent introduction, limited spread has occurred among persons with multiple sexual partners, including both homosexual and heterosexual individuals. HIV infection rates among prostitutes remain less than 5 percent in contrast to that observed in pattern 2. Since few women have evidence of HIV infection, perinatal transmission has not become a major problem. Transfusion of HIV-infected blood has also not become a significant problem except for recipients of imported blood or blood products from other countries where the blood is not routinely screened.

**Table 32-2. Comparisons of HIV Prevalence among Various Population Subgroups for Selected African Countries**

| Country and year | Risk group | HIV prevalence (%) |
|---|---|---|
| Ghana (1987) | Blood donors and patients | 4.7 |
| | Prostitutes | 25.2 |
| Ivory Coast (1987) | Pregnant women | 2.6 |
| | Prostitutes | 17.0 |
| Kenya (1985) | Pregnant women | 2.0 |
| | STD clinic patients | 7.5 |
| | Prostitutes | 51 |
| Rwanda (1987) | Married blood donors | 6.5 |
| | Single blood donors | 20.2 |
| Tanzania (1986) | Pregnant women | 3.6 |
| | Bar maids | 28.8 |
| Uganda (1986) | Blood donors | 10.8 |
| | Pregnant women | 13.0 |
| | Prostitutes | 80.0 |
| Zambia (1985) | Male blood donors and hospital workers | 17.2 |
| | Male STD clinic patients | 45.5 |
| Congo (1985) | Pregnant women | 11.0 |
| | Sterility problems patients | 16.6 |
| Zaire (1986) | Pregnant women | 5.6 |
| | Prostitutes | 27.0 |

## HIV-2

Preliminary serologic surveys have demonstrated a high prevalence of HIV-2 in the countries of West Africa, specifically Guinea-Bissau, the Cape Verde Islands, Senegal, Burkina Faso, Ivory Coast, Guinea, Mauritania, and the Gambia.[43,44] Countries of central and eastern African where infection by HIV-1 has reached epidemic proportions have shown little evidence of HIV-2 infection. In West Africa, infection rates may range from 0.3 to 17 percent in the general population, based on studies in blood donors, to as high as 64 percent in some high-risk populations such as female prostitutes (Table 32-3).[34,35,43,44,49,50] Available data, although limited, suggest that HIV-2 infected persons come from the same risk groups as those infected by HIV-1, with heterosexual activity being the predominant mode of transmission. Unfortunately, little epidemiologic information is available regarding HIV-2 infection because of difficulty in serologic diagnosis due to serologic cross-reaction with HIV-1.[51]

HIV-2 is now being reported outside of West Africa, predominantly in Europe, in South America, and the United States.[43–45] It is likely that HIV-2 will spread to other geographic areas and that active surveillance for HIV-2 infection will be necessary in all parts of the world. The simultaneous occurrence of HIV-1 and HIV-2 will have implications for diagnostic services, blood donor screening programs, and vaccine development.

## TRANSMISSION PATTERNS

### SEXUAL TRANSMISSION

The predominant mode of HIV transmission throughout the world is sexual, with homosexual transmission being more common in developed countries and bisexual and heterosexual transmission being more common in developing countries. For example, in 1984 bisexuality was the most common risk factor for HIV infection (36 percent) in Haitian men, and the male-to-female sex ratio among Haitian AIDS patients was 3:1.[13] Since then, the male-to-female ratio has approached 1:1, and homosexuality or bisexuality is far less frequent a risk factor than heterosexual activity.[52] Heterosexual transmission and vertical transmission from mother to infant have now become the pre-

**Table 32-3. Seroprevalence of HIV-2 in Selected Populations of West Africa**

| Population | Number tested | Prevalence (%) |
|---|---|---|
| **Pregnant women:** | | |
| Senegal | 72 | 4.2 |
| Guinea | 119 | 1.7 |
| Burkina Faso | 58 | 1.7 |
| Ivory Coast | 365 | 0.3 |
| **Hospitalized patients:** | | |
| Senegal | 178 | 2.2 |
| Guinea-Bissau | 123 | 15.4 |
| Ivory Coast | 40 | 5.0 |
| **Prostitutes:** | | |
| Senegal | 403 | 15.0 |
| Guinea-Bissau | 39 | 64.0 |
| Burkina Faso | 308 | 20.4 |
| Ivory Coast | 232 | 20.0 |

Data adapted from Kanki et al.[44,49]

dominant modes of transmission in Haiti.[53] When first studied in 1985, HIV infection in Trinidad was predominantly found among homosexual men, especially those in contact with homosexual men in the United States,[54] but more recent data indicate that heterosexual transmission is increasing.[55] Similar patterns of sexual transmission are emerging in other developing countries of Latin America such as Brazil, Mexico, and the Dominican Republic.[1,56–58]

In Africa heterosexual transmission has been the predominant mode of transmission for many years.[1,4] Even among the first imported AIDS cases diagnosed in Europe, the vast majority of patients from Africa or the Caribbean failed to acknowledge the traditional risk behaviors of homosexuality or IV drug use. In 1987, 80 percent of patients from Africa and the Caribbean who were diagnosed in Europe continued to deny these risk factors, and AIDS cases were equally distributed among both men and women.[59] Among these cases, a high level of sexual activity with multiple partners was the apparent risk factor, rather than any specific sexual orientation.

As in developed countries, AIDS in developing countries primarily affects young and middle-aged persons. The sex and age distribution of AIDS cases reflects patterns seen with other sexually transmitted diseases, in which the incidence and morbidity rates are higher among younger women and slightly older men.[4] In a study of 500 AIDS cases in Kinshasa, Zaire, in 1986, the mean age of male cases was 37.4 vs. 30.0 years for women. Women with AIDS were more likely than men to be unmarried (61 vs. 36 percent), and nearly one-third of the married AIDS patients had at least one previous marriage or "union libre" (persistent cohabitation without formal marriage). One-third of the AIDS patients reported having had at least one sexually transmitted disease during the 3 years preceding their illness.[4]

Serologic studies of HIV infection in Africa also confirm an overall equal HIV infection rate among the sexes, but with rates peaking among women at a slightly earlier age than men. Data concerning HIV seroprevalence among 5099 healthy people (2982 men and 2117 women) in Kinshasa, Zaire show a bimodal distribution of antibody, with prevalence peaks under 1 year of age and among young adults age 16 to 19 years (Fig. 32-4).[4] While other factors may influence the distribution of HIV infection, this pattern is strongly suggestive of a sexually transmitted disease with higher prevalence rates among younger sexually active women.[60] The combination of passive antibody transfer and transmission of virus from mother to infant is probably responsible for the high seroprevalence rate in young children.

While bidirectional heterosexual transmission of HIV infection appears to be limited in the United States and Europe, there is biological and clinical evidence of bidirectional transmission in Africa. First, HIV theoretically can be transmitted bidirectionally among heterosexuals since the virus can be isolated from semen as well as cervicovaginal secretions.[61–63] Second, African male AIDS patients as well as expatriate males with AIDS who previously lived in Africa frequently report a history of sex with prostitutes, and the presence of HIV in male heterosexuals attending clinics for sexually transmitted diseases is increasing, suggesting female-to-male transmission.[64,65] Further evidence of such transmission comes from household studies with AIDS patients in Zaire and Uganda in which HIV antibody was significantly higher among spouses (61 to 68 percent) and in infants of infected mothers than in other household members or controls.[66,67] In both studies, there was no significant difference in HIV seropositivity rates among either the male or female sexual partner of the index case. While these household studies document high rates of infection among spouses of the infected persons, they do not permit assessment of directionality of HIV transmission. This needs to be addressed in prospective cohort studies of sexual partners of newly seroconverted HIV-infected individuals. Finally, several clusters of African AIDS cases have been identified, and the chronology of events suggests both female-to-male and male-to-female transmission of HIV.

Risk factors associated with HIV infection among heterosexuals include the number of sexual partners, sex with a prostitute, being a prostitute, and being a sexual partner of an infected person.[68–72] Specific sexual activity, including anal intercourse, which was reported by only 4 to 8 percent of female AIDS patients and female prostitutes, was not associated with HIV infec-

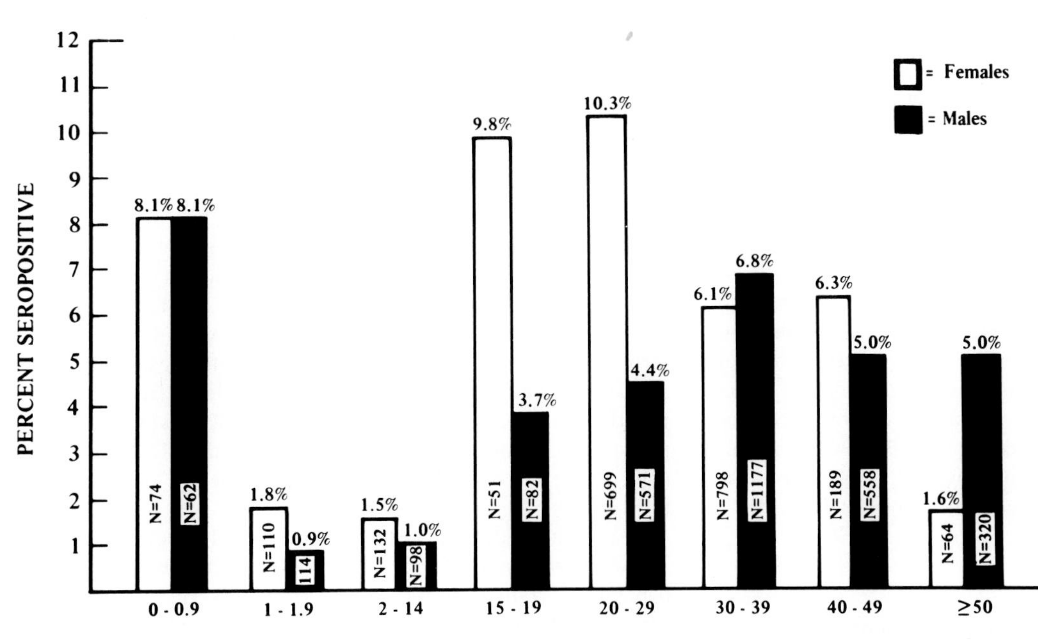


**Fig. 32-4.** HIV seroprevalence rates among 5099 healthy persons by age in Kinshasa, Zaire, 1984–1985. Sample population consisted of 2982 men and 2117 women. Positive patients had sera that were repeatedly reactive on a commercially available ELISA and were Western blot-positive. In age groups 16 to 19 years and 20 to 29 years, seroprevalence rates were significantly higher in women (10.3 percent) than in men (4.3 percent). For 50 to 59 years of age, seroprevalence rates were significantly higher in men (5.0 percent) than in women (1.6 percent). (From TC Quinn, et al.[4])

tion in surveys in Kenya, Zaire, Rwanda, and Zambia.[71–73] Thus, receptive anal intercourse, which is a major risk factor for HIV infection in male homosexuals, may not be a requirement for heterosexual transmission.

Genital ulcers and other sexually transmitted diseases appear to facilitate sexual transmission of HIV, as is evident from several studies in Africa. Among Nairobi prostitutes, HIV seropositivity was significantly associated with a history of sexually transmitted diseases such as gonorrhea, genital ulcers, and syphilis.[71] In a prospective study of 116 initially seronegative prostitutes followed for 2 years in Nairobi, 54 (76 percent) of 71 women with one or more episodes of genital ulcer disease seroconverted compared with 20 (44 percent) of 45 women lacking such disease.[74,75] In studies in Zambia and Kenya, seropositivity in men was correlated with the presence of genital ulcers.[72,76] In another prospective study of men with a STD and a history of recent prostitute exposure, 13 (14 percent) of 91 men with genital ulcer disease seroconverted during a 3-month follow-up period compared with 3 (3 percent) of 108 men with urethritis.[77] Since the men did not have genital ulcers at the time of intercourse with a prostitute, it is probable that the acquisition of HIV infection by men with genital ulcers is an index of infectivity of the female sex partner rather than related to the susceptibility of the male partner.[1] In this study, a single sexual exposure was apparently associated with a female-to-male transmission rate of 5 to 10 percent provided particular cofactors were present. This is considerably higher than previously estimated in other population groups. Genital ulcers and other STDs such as *Chlamydia trachomatis* may allow penetration of HIV into the bloodstream by causing epithelial disruption or may increase susceptibility by increasing the population of T-helper lymphocytes, the target cells for HIV, at the site of infection within the genital tract.[1]

In a case control study from Nairobi, uncircumcised men were found to have an increased risk of HIV infection compared with circumcised men.[78] Although genital ulcers were associated with HIV infection and uncircumcised men were known to have an increased risk of chancroid, uncircumcised men had a higher HIV seroprevalence independent of genital ulcers or sexual activity. Thus, the occurrence of balanitis or enhanced viral survival under the foreskin could possibly increase susceptibility to HIV infection.

Oral contraception is another factor that may increase susceptibility of women to heterosexual HIV infection. In a prospective study of Nairobi prostitutes, the incidence of HIV infection was significantly greater in oral contraceptive users [29 (80 percent) of 35] than in nonusers [46 (57 percent) of 81].[75] This association persisted after controlling for such covariates as the number of sexual partners, history of STDs, and condom use. A similar finding was evident among female prostitutes in Zaire in whom HIV seropositivity was significantly correlated with the taking of oral medications to prevent pregnancy or sexually transmitted diseases.[73] Possible mechanisms for increased susceptibility to HIV among oral contraceptive users include an increased area of cervical ectropion, increased concomitant *C. trachomatis* infection, direct immunosuppressive effects of oral contraceptives, or less frequent use of barrier contraceptives by those on oral contraceptives. The role of oral contraceptives as a potential factor for increasing HIV susceptibility requires further study.

## PERINATAL TRANSMISSION

With increasing prevalence of HIV infection among young sexually active women, an increasing rate of infection is being documented among their children. Perinatal transmission of HIV may occur in utero through transplacental passage of HIV, at the time of delivery when there is a maternal-fetal blood exchange, or postnatally through breast feeding or other possible routes. The efficiency of and risk factors associated with perinatal infection remain unknown, and prospective studies are currently underway in high-risk areas. In North America and Europe, HIV infection has been documented to occur in 30 to 65 percent of infants born to HIV-seropositive mothers.[79–82]

Preliminary data from Kinshasa, Zaire and Nairobi, Kenya suggest that approximately 40 to 50 percent of children born to HIV antibody positive mothers have IgM antibody to HIV either in cord blood or at the 3-month follow-up visit.[83,84] In Kinshasa, Zaire, 22 percent of 351 children born to HIV-positive mothers died within 3 months after birth compared with only 1 percent of 351 children born to seronegative mothers. Immunologic studies performed in concert with testing for IgM antibodies in cord blood demonstrated a marked association between low number of T4 cells in the mother and the probability of HIV transmission to the child.[85]

The contribution of breast feeding in perinatal transmission of HIV is unclear at present, although HIV has been isolated from breast milk and anecdotal cases of probable postnatal transmission through breast milk have been reported.[81,86,87] It is likely, however, that breast feeding represents only a small incremental risk of mother-to-infant transmission compared with in utero or peripartum transmission, and further studies are warranted before recommendations regarding breast feeding by HIV-infected women are made.

With increased evidence of perinatal transmission, a major concern has been raised regarding the safety and immunogenicity of immunizations given to HIV-infected children.[88–90] Because the morbidity and mortality of childhood diseases is so high in unvaccinated children regardless of HIV status, the World Health Organization has recommended that measles, poliomyelitis, diphtheria, tetanus, and pertussis immunizations be given to all children regardless of the HIV serologic status.[91] BCG should be given to all children in tuberculous endemic areas except for HIV-infected children with AIDS-related symptoms.

## TRANSFUSIONS

The importance of blood transfusions and HIV transmission in developing countries is exemplified by the 2 to 18 percent seroprevalence rate of HIV infection rate among blood donors in central Africa and some Caribbean countries.[28,92–94] Among African AIDS patients diagnosed either in Africa or in Europe, approximately 5 to 10 percent report having received at least one blood transfusion during the previous 5 years.[47] In one large case control study of seropositive healthy persons in Kinshasa, Zaire, 9.3 percent of HIV seropositives compared with 4.8 percent of seronegatives reported receiving blood transfusions.[95] Similarly, 31 percent of hospitalized seropositive children aged 2 to 24 months, born to seronegative mothers, had a history of blood transfusions prior to their present hospitalization. Only 7 percent of seronegative control children of the same age had a similar history.[96]

In a recent study which examined the role of blood transfusions in the transmission of HIV among African children, 147 (14.1 percent) of 1046 pediatric patients at Mama Yemo Hospital in Kinshasa, Zaire, had a history of previous blood transfusion.[97] Forty (3.8 percent) of these 1046 pediatric patients were HIV seropositive, and there was a strong dose response association between blood transfusion and HIV seropositivity. The odds ratio of being HIV seropositive increased to 43 in children who had received 3 or more blood transfusions. In a follow-up study of 167 hospitalized children with acute malaria, 21 (12.6 percent) were HIV seropositive.[98] Ten of the 11 HIV seropositive acute malaria patients had received blood transfusions during the index hospitalization and at least 4 of these children were documented to have been seronegative prior to the transfusion. Follow-up of these 4 children demonstrated the development of IgM antibodies and the persistence of IgG antibodies to HIV 6 months after receiving these blood transfusions. These studies document the high risk of HIV infection from transfusions in these regions.

The impact of HIV transmission via blood transfusion may be substantial in some developing countries where blood donations are not routinely screened for HIV. Presently, efforts to exclude high-risk donors in developing countries on epidemiologic or clinical grounds have thus far been unsuccessful, and blood screening for HIV has been limited by the lack of financial resources necessary for routine testing and for adequate facilities for blood banking. With the development and introduction of rapid diagnostic tests, transmission via blood transfusions can theoretically be limited if screening becomes a routine practice.

## INJECTIONS

While intravenous drug abuse is exceedingly rare in poorly developed and impoverished areas, injections with unsterilized needles administered for medical purposes may play an analogous role in terms of exposure to HIV. In an HIV seroprevalence study of 2384 hospital workers in Kinshasa, significantly more seropositive than seronegative workers reported receiving medical injections during the previous three years. Among those reporting injections, seroprevalence was nearly twice as high in those with 5 or more injections then in those who had received fewer than 5 injections.[95] In a study of hospitalized seropositive children aged 1 to 24 months in Kinshasa, Zaire, 16 seropositive children who had been born to seronegative mothers had received more injections than seronegative children born to seronegative mothers.[96] These data suggest that injections and scarifications may be associated with HIV infection. However, it is difficult to distinguish whether that association is truly causal or simply reflects treatment for early symptoms of HIV infection or other illnesses such as sexually transmitted diseases.

## TRANSMISSION VIA OTHER ROUTES

As in Europe and the United States, there is no evidence to support casual or household transmission of HIV in developing countries. In household studies, performed in Kinshasa, Uganda, and Haiti, the rate of HIV seropositivity did not differ significantly between the nonspousal household contacts of AIDS cases and household contacts of uninfected controls.[53,66,67] Similarly, no association has been observed among hospital workers with any measure of patient or blood contact and HIV seroprevalence.[95] In addition, the absence of HIV infection among expatriates who lack recognized risk factors for HIV infection, despite living in close proximity to possibly infected individuals, reaffirms the apparent lack of casual transmission of HIV infection.[4]

Epidemiologic data from tropical areas as well as in the United States also argue against arthropod transmission.[1,4,99] In Africa, the sex and age-specific distribution of HIV seroprevalence are inconsistent with vector-borne transmission. The low seroprevalence rate among children 1 to 14 years of age and among persons over 50 years of age, and the significantly higher rate among adults 20 to 49 years of age, argues against vector-borne transmission, which is traditionally higher in young children.[4] Virtually all seropositive children studied in most countries have identifiable risk factors for HIV infection such as maternal infection, history of blood transfusion, and/or multiple injections.[79,96,100] The lack of evidence for household clustering of HIV, except as explained by heterosexual or perinatal routes, also argues against mechanical vector transmission over short distances such as might occur with bedbugs or mosquitoes following interrupted feedings. The geographic distribution of HIV infection and other arthropod-borne diseases such as malaria also appears to be discordant in some areas.[101] The low titer of HIV in the blood of infected persons and the small amount of blood on insects' mouth parts reinforce the improbability of mechanical transmission of HIV by insect vectors.[102]

## NATURAL HISTORY OF HIV INFECTION

Studies on the natural history of HIV-1 and HIV-2 infection in individuals residing in tropical areas are limited, since these studies have only recently been instituted. In central Africa, disease progression in HIV-1 infected heterosexuals appears similar to that observed for homosexual men.[1,103,104] In Zaire, 6.3 percent of 56 individuals who had seroconverted between 1984 and 1986 had developed AIDS-related conditions (ARC) by the end of 1986 and 5 percent had developed AIDS.[105] Among 91 men and women who were already seropositive at enrollment in the cohort in 1984, 16.3 percent had ARC in 1986, 3.3 percent had AIDS, and 11.9 percent had died from suspected AIDS over this 2-year period. In Nairobi, Kenya, 6 percent of HIV seropositive female prostitutes developed severe illness during the 12 months of follow-up.[1] Among African men and women with lymphadenopathy syndrome or AIDS-related complex followed in Europe, the annual progression rates to AIDS were 1.1 and 20.7 percent, respectively.[106]

While prognostic factors have been identified for disease progression among European and American HIV infected individuals, little is known about factors that may affect disease progression in people residing in developing countries. It has been hypothesized that endemic infectious agents widely prevalent throughout Africa may serve as cofactors in increasing HIV susceptibility and/or disease progression.[107] Immunologic studies have also demonstrated a significant elevation of activated lymphocytes and immune complexes among African heterosexual and U.S. homosexual populations compared with the U.S. heterosexual population.[107] These data demonstrated that the immune systems of African heterosexuals, similar to those of U.S. homosexual men, are in a chronically activated state associated with chronic viral or parasitic antigenic exposure which may cause them to be particularly susceptible to HIV infection or disease progression. Prospective studies are warranted in different populations to examine the specific impact of these viral, bacterial, and parasitic infections and other antigenic stimuli on the susceptibility to and development of HIV disease.

## ETIOLOGY

As discussed in Chap. 30, AIDS is characterized by the occurrence of life-threatening opportunistic infections and malignancies occurring in individuals who have severe depression of the cell-mediated immune system due primarily to the loss of T-helper lymphocytes. Clinical, epidemiologic, immunologic, and virologic investigations in both developed and developing countries have firmly established that the causative agent of AIDS is a retrovirus which selectively infects the T-helper lymphocyte and eventually causes death of the cell. The predominant human retrovirus isolated from these patients is referred to as HIV-1, whereas the human retrovirus found to cause AIDS predominantly among residents of West Africa is referred to as HIV-2 (see Chap. 28).

The virulence of HIV-1 and HIV-2 lies in their unique ability to progressively weaken the immune system that provides protection against opportunistic pathogens (see Chap. 29). HIV is capable of replicating within a limited number of cells in the human body including lymphocytes, macrophages, and cells of the central nervous system. It has been shown that both HIV-1 and HIV-2 have a specific tropism for the CD4 receptor of the T-helper lymphocyte based on interaction of this receptor with the viral envelope protein, gp120.[108,109] After specific binding to the CD4 lymphocyte, HIV enters the cytoplasm of the cell by an unknown mechanism. Within the cytoplasm of the cell the uncoated single-stranded viral RNA is transcribed into double-stranded DNA via the enzyme reverse transcriptase. The double-stranded circular DNA enters the nucleus where it integrates into the host cell DNA. These viral genes may remain integrated for the lifetime of the cell, and consequently the infection of the individual is lifelong. Stimulation of the infected lymphocyte activates viral replication resulting in viral budding from the lymphocyte, cytolysis of the infected cell, and subsequent infection of other T4 lymphocytes. In vitro activation can be achieved via mitogenic, antigenic, or allogenic stimulation.[110,111] In vivo, potential activators include other pathogens such as cytomegalovirus, hepatitis B virus, and herpes simplex virus, as well as allogenic stimulation from exposure to semen or blood components.[112]

## VIRAL HETEROGENEITY

HIV isolates have been recovered from patients residing in tropical areas and compared with viral isolates from North America and Europe by restriction enzyme analysis and Southern blot analysis.[113–115] In most cases, North American and European viral isolates are slightly different from one another but exhibit little geographic specificity. African and Haitian isolates are also different from one another, but as a group are more diverse and heterogeneous than the isolates from North America and Europe, having more unique restriction sites and 40 percent fewer conserved sites.[113–115] The genomic variability is greatest within the envelope (*env*) gene.

Although retroviral genomes have not been extensively characterized, antigenic variation involving the viral envelope is a characteristic feature of lentiviruses. Neutralization studies show that different antigenic strains of equine infectious anemia virus (EIAV) can be identified in individual diseased horses.[116] Similar changes have been mapped to the *env* gene of visna virus.[117] It has also been reported, primarily from central Africa, that HIV can be isolated from antibody-negative adults with clinical AIDS symptoms.[118] Hybridization studies with HIV probes under stringent conditions indicate an overall high degree of homology between these and prototype HIV viruses, suggesting that some African HIV-infected patients fail to make detectable antibodies to HIV or their antibodies may be bound in immune complexes not detectable by current techniques.[43]

This diversity of antibody response to HIV-1 and the recovery of retroviral isolates from antibody-negative AIDS patients led to the recent discovery of HIV-2 from patients with AIDS-like symptoms in West Africa.[37,38] These individuals were suffering from opportunistic infections usually associated with HIV-1 infection, but their antibody responses against HIV-1 were atypical. These isolates, referred to as HIV-2, were related to HIV-1 in terms of morphology, cell tropism, and in vitro cytopathic effect on CD4+ cells.[39–41] Following the molecular cloning of HIV-2 isolates, genomic analysis indicated that HIV-1 and HIV-2 shared a similar genomic organization, suggesting a common evolutionary origin, but differed significantly in terms of nucleotide sequences. The more conserved *gag* and *pol* gene displayed a 56 and 66 percent nucleotide sequence homology, respectively, and less than 60 percent amino acid identity.[40–42] The sequence homology for other viral genes, particularly *env,* was even lower, making HIV-1 and HIV-2 only 42 percent homologous overall. Although HIV-2 is serologically cross-reactive with simian immunodeficiency virus (SIV), similar genomic studies demonstrate only 70 percent homology between the two viruses.[41,42] In summary, HIV-2 appears to be evolutionarily more closely related to SIV than to HIV-1. It is likely that the time of divergence of HIV-1 and HIV-2 was earlier than the beginning of the current epidemics, and that a virus ancestor with similar properties and pathogenic potential probably existed a long time ago in the human population. The emergence of the AIDS epidemic was likely the result of simultaneous modifications of epidemiologic parameters in west and central Africa, such as rapid urbanization, leading to the infection of larger populations.[40]

## CLINICAL MANIFESTATIONS

Clinical features of HIV infection are diverse and range from asymptomatic infection to involvement with a wide variety of opportunistic infections, HIV-induced encephalopathy, and/or malignancies. Clinical manifestations may vary in different populations according to the relative frequency of other endemic opportunistic infections. In contrast to what is observed in developed countries, patients in tropical areas present with gastrointestinal and dermatologic features more frequently than the pulmonary symptoms commonly seen in the AIDS patients in the United States.[13,26,47,119,120] However, any of the spectrum of opportunistic infections and malignancies that has been described in American and European patients with HIV infection may also occur in patients residing in tropical areas, but with different frequencies.

Following exposure to HIV, seroconversion occurs within 6 to 12 weeks, frequently in association with a nonspecific viral illness. Symptoms may include fever, arthralgia, headache, nausea, generalized lymphadenopathy, a macular skin eruption, or neurologic manifestations.[121,122] Although seroconversion frequently may go unnoticed, in occasional cases a severe life-threatening encephalopathy may develop.[123] In one study in Kinshasa, Zaire, most patients who seroconverted after receiving HIV seropositive blood transfusions developed fever within several weeks of the transfusion and subsequently developed persistent generalized lymphadenopathy.[124]

It is well recognized that the vast majority of HIV-infected individuals remain asymptomatic for many years. However, as HIV infection progresses, nonspecific signs and symptoms of illness appear which are referred to as ARC. These symptoms include unintentional weight loss, malaise, fatigue, lethargy, anorexia, abdominal discomfort, diarrhea, fever, night sweats, headache, pruritic skin lesions, amenorrhea, lymphadenopathy, and splenomegaly. These symptoms and signs are frequently intermittent and may disappear spontaneously during certain periods.

Several detailed clinical studies among African and Haitian patients help provide some information regarding the clinical presentation of AIDS in these areas.[13,47,125–127] In a recent review of 196 AIDS patients diagnosed in Kinshasa, Zaire, the mean duration of symptoms prior to diagnosis was 11.8 months (range 1 to 78 months, medium 8 months).[47] Symptoms consisted of profound weight loss (mean 29 percent of body weight; 99 percent of patients), fever (81 percent of patients), diarrhea (68 percent), cough (37 percent), dysphagia (35 percent), pruritis (30 percent), and dyspnea (23 percent). The most commonly observed opportunistic infections among these and other patients included oral esophageal candidiasis, central nervous system cryptococcosis, toxoplasmosis, tuberculosis, and cryptosporidiosis in approximately equal frequency (14 to 25 percent). In contrast to American and European AIDS patients, of which approximately 63 percent eventually develop *Pneumocystis carinii* pneumonia, pneumocystis was found in only 14 percent of African patients diagnosed in Europe.[8]

Weight loss is found in nearly all symptomatic HIV-infected patients residing in tropical areas, and it is generally progressive. It is frequently the first sign of HIV infection and in some patients may be the only one throughout their disease. It is frequently accompanied with diarrhea, and in studies in tropical areas such as central Africa and Haiti, diarrhea and weight loss are present in over 80 percent of patients who progress to AIDS. This may reflect a greater susceptibility to gastrointestinal pathogens common to a specific geographic location.[128] Malebranche and colleagues[120] demonstrated that the primary clinical features at presentation of 29 AIDS patients residing in Haiti were unexplained chronic diarrhea, fever, extreme weight loss, anorexia, and multiple opportunistic infections. Chronic diarrhea was by far the most common clinical presentation in these patients, being present in all but 2 patients. At the time of diagnosis 24 patients had had diarrhea for over 6 months. The diarrhea was described as constant, intermittent, watery, and unresponsive to therapy. Infections included oral esophageal candidiasis in 27 of 29 patients, *Mycobacterium tuberculosis* in 7, cryptosporidiosis in 11, and cytomegalovirus and herpes simplex virus infection of the gastrointestinal tract in 4 and 3 patients, respectively.

Similar clinical presentations of HIV infection have been described among African AIDS patients.[4,19,27,127,128] Multiple studies have described the clinical presentation of HIV infection in Africans as consisting of fever, weight loss of more than 10 percent body weight, and diarrhea.[8,21,47] Serwadda et al. reported the association of a diarrheal illness, referred to as "slim disease," in rural Uganda and Tanzania, with HIV infection.[26] The clinical presentation of "slim disease" was essentially identical to enteropathic AIDS, with the major symptoms of weight loss and unexplained diarrhea present in over 80 percent of cases. Of patients with clinical diarrhea and weight loss of 10 kg or more, all were found to be seropositive for HIV and all were anergic to skin test antigens, reflecting underlying immunosuppression. In limited studies, oral esophageal candidiasis was evident in 80 percent of cases, *Cryptosporidia* in 20 to 30 percent, *Isopora* in 10 percent, and *Entamoeba histolytica, Strongyloides stercoralis, Giardia lamblia, Salmonella,* and *Mycobacterium* infection each in approximately 5 to 10 percent of patients.[8] Overall, specific pathogens were not identified in 25 to 50 percent of the patients with chronic diarrhea and HIV infection.[129] Some of these patients may have histologic evidence of cytomegalovirus infection at autopsy, whereas others have nonspecific inflammation and evidence of chronic malabsorption such as partial villus atrophy with crypthyperplasia.[126] These findings strongly suggest that malabsorption in association with chronic diarrheal illness may contribute to significant weight loss in these HIV-infected patients. While individual opportunistic infectious agents may differ from patient to patient, the underlying pathologic process involving the gastrointestinal tract is similar among most HIV-infected patients.[128]

Many HIV-infected patients in the tropics develop mucocutaneous lesions. In one study, a generalized papular pruritic eruption referred to as "prurigo" was found in approximately 20 percent of African patients with HIV infection.[130] Lesions are symmetrically distributed over the body but are frequently found on the extremities. Clinically, these papules are pruritic and patients may scratch their lesions, resulting in superinfection, scarring, and hyperpigmentation. Histologically, the lesions are nonspecific and include perivascular infiltration of the skin and subcutaneous tissues with mononuclear cells and a variable number of eosinophils. The etiology of this eruption is presently unknown. In HIV endemic areas, the diagnostic accuracy of this papular pruritic eruption is relatively high. In one study in Kinshasa, Zaire, 87 percent of consecutive adult outpatients with prurigo were HIV antibody positive.[130]

Another common infection seen early in HIV-infected patients is varicella zoster infection. Approximately 10 percent of HIV-infected patients may develop recurrent zoster infection during the course of their illness.[131] The clinical features of zoster are very similar to classical zoster in nonimmunocompromised patients, except that zoster in HIV-infected patients tends to be more recurrent, with a 22 percent recurrence rate in one study. The occurrence of zoster may precede the appearance of opportunistic infection by several months or years, but its predictive value is relatively high in an endemic area for HIV infection.[131,132]

Localized oral candidiasis occurring in an adult who is not on antibiotics or steroids, and who does not have a hematologic malignancy or diabetes mellitus or other immunosuppressive disease, is highly predictive for the diagnosis of HIV infection in both developing and developed countries.[133,134] In addition, the development of oral candidiasis in an ARC patient is a poor prognostic sign, as many of these patients will develop opportunistic infections within the ensuing months. Among African and Haitian patients with HIV infection approximately 45 to 55 percent of patients may present with oral candidiasis as one of their more prominent clinical features.[13,120,126,129] Since endoscopy is not routinely performed in many developing areas, it is uncertain how frequent esophageal candidiasis may occur, although 61 percent of African patients with oral candidiasis in one study[129] complained of dysphagia, suggesting the presence of esophageal candidiasis.

Among African and Haitian AIDS patients, tuberculosis appears to be one of the earliest opportunistic infections among HIV-infected individuals.[135–137] In Zaire, 53 (33 percent) of 159 confirmed pulmonary patients hospitalized at a tuberculosis sanitarium were HIV-positive, including 10 (67 percent) of 15 patients with extrapulmonary tuberculosis.[135] Seropositivity in these cases was significantly associated with anergy to intradermal tuberculin, and history of blood transfusion during the previous 5 years. Among patients with tuberculosis, there was no significant association between HIV infection and extent of radiographic lesions, duration of disease, or initial response to treatment. However, HIV infection was more commonly present in patients with extrapulmonary tuberculosis lesions. HIV infection may substantially complicate both the management of individual patients with tuberculosis and strategies for tuberculosis control in countries where HIV infection occurs.

Another clinical characteristic of AIDS in Africa is the appearance of aggressive disseminated Kaposi's sarcoma. Kaposi's sarcoma of a chronic variety has been present in some areas of central Africa for at least the last 30 years.[23–25] The aggressive form of Kaposi's sarcoma associated with HIV infection has now been reported predominantly in the same areas where classic endemic Kaposi's sarcoma is prevalent such as Uganda, Zambia, Tanzania, Rwanda, and Zaire.[23,25,47] This aggressive form is histologically similar to but clinically different from classic Kaposi's sarcoma. The aggressive form of Kaposi's sarcoma occurs as multiple black plaques, macules, or nodules on black skin, or as purple lesions on white skin. Lesions may appear on all parts of the body and disseminate to lymph nodes and internal organs, predominantly pulmonary and gastrointestinal organs. Within the mouth, the lesions are frequently found on the hard palate. Diagnosis is by biopsy, which reveals spindle-shaped endothelial cells with intracellular clefts and extravasated erythrocytes.

The origin of this sarcoma in relationship to AIDS remains unclear. Comparative studies of the chronic endemic form of Kaposi's sarcoma and the new aggressive variety have failed to isolate any clear causative agents. Within developed countries it is primarily found only among homosexual men,[138] and in developing countries it has been primarily identified in areas where the endemic form was known to exist previously.[25] Initial data implicated human cytomegalovirus in both chronic and aggressive forms, since CMV is highly endemic in many areas of Africa where this tumor appears, and disseminated cytomegalovirus is very common in homosexual men with HIV disease. However, molecular hybridization studies have failed to identify this virus in the chronic African form, suggesting a different etiology for this tumor.[139]

## PEDIATRIC AIDS

Clinical features of HIV infection among children in developing countries are even less specific than those described for adults. In one study among 368 hospitalized children in Kinshasa, Zaire, aged 2 to 14 years, seropositivity in 40 (11 percent) children was associated with the diagnosis of malnutrition, pneumonia, and anemia.[100] Of hospitalized patients with both malnutrition and pneumonia, 31 percent were seropositive and the mortality rate of seropositive children was over three times greater than that for seronegative children. In Bangui, Central African Republic, 21 (12.3 percent) of 175 children with malnutrition, and 25 (24.8 percent) of 101 mothers were HIV-seropositive, whereas only 3 (3.1 percent) of 96 healthy children were seropositive.[140] Pneumonitis, diarrhea, lymphadenopathy, oral thrush, and dermatitis were each more frequently seen in the seropositive children than in seronegative malnourished children. Thus, pediatric HIV disease in Africa resembles HIV disease in children in the United States.[79] However, it is difficult to distinguish HIV-associated disease in Africa on the clinical grounds of failure to thrive, malnutrition, and pulmonary disease, as these are common pediatric problems in the tropics.

## HIV-2

Little is known regarding the clinical spectrum of HIV-2 infection among West Africans where the virus appears to be endemic. It is evident from some clinical reports, however, that HIV-2 is associated with an immunologic deficiency and a clinical illness similar to AIDS. Clavel et al.[141] recently described the clinical features of 30 patients with HIV-2 of whom 17 had AIDS, 4 had AIDS-related complex, 1 had diffuse lymphadenopathy, 2 had other clinical problems, and 6 were asymptomatic. The most common clinical presentation of HIV-2 was chronic diarrhea in 14 patients, and severe weight loss in 13 patients, similar to that described for HIV-1 disease among Africans, or patients with "slim disease."[26,27] Infections frequently diagnosed in these HIV-2 patients included *Isospora belli, Cryptosporidium, Mycobacterium tuberculosis,* aspergillosis, and *Pneumocystis carinii* pneumonia. Four HIV-2 infected patients had Kaposi's sarcoma, 4 had diffuse lymphadenopathy, 1 had cerebral lymphoma, and 1 had acute encephalitis. Thus, even though HIV-2 infection is frequently seen among healthy individuals, as is HIV-1,[43,44,49] the clinical spectrum of HIV-2 infection appears to be similar to that observed for HIV-1 in the tropics.[141]

## DIAGNOSIS AND MANAGEMENT

The diagnosis of HIV-1 and HIV-2 infections is based on serology by ELISA with confirmatory tests such as Western blot or immunofluorescent antibody assays. Highly sensitive and specific assays for HIV-1 were developed following the initial isolation of HIV-1[8,142,143] and have been widely available since 1985. While these assays may have a low predictive value in low-prevalence populations,[144] they are highly reliable in detecting HIV infection in high-risk patients. Serologic diagnosis for HIV-1 is discussed in more detail in Chapter 79.

The diagnosis of HIV-2 infection in clinically suspect patients remains problematic. As discussed earlier, the viral proteins of HIV-2, even though divergent from HIV-1, are 50 percent conserved with respect to the *gag* and *pol* gene products.[40–42] Thus, HIV-2 antibody-positive sera recognize the core proteins of HIV-1 but not the envelope proteins, owing to the greater than 70 percent divergence for amino acids encoded by *env*. Similarly, HIV-1 antibody-positive sera may react with the *gag* and *pol* proteins of HIV-2 but not with HIV-2 envelope glycoproteins. Thus, sera from individuals with antibody to HIV-2 may cross-react or be totally missed by the current serologic assays for HIV-1 depending upon the titer of antibody to *gag* and *pol*, or *env* proteins. Currently, the HIV-1 ELISA test used for screening U.S. blood donors may detect 42 to 92 percent of HIV-2 infections depending upon the stage of infection, due to this cross-reactivity.[51] Several HIV-2 ELISAs have been commercially developed and are being utilized in conjunction with HIV-1 ELISA to detect the presence of either virus. As recombinant antigens for these two viruses are utilized in diagnostic assays, increased specificity may be achieved and accurate diagnosis of HIV-1 or HIV-2 infection may be possible.[145] Presently, however, there are reports of serologic profiles in some individuals suggesting double infection with HIV-1 and HIV-2.[146–149] Most of these cases originate from the Ivory Coast where 20 percent of the AIDS patients have an HIV-1 specific serum reactivity, 32 percent are HIV-2 reactive, and 50 percent have dual reactivity.[149] These data suggest either that the patients with dual reactivity are infected with both viruses or that there is considerable serologic cross-reactivity. Additional laboratory studies are warranted to discriminate between the two viral infections.

For the diagnosis of AIDS, documentation of opportunistic infections, malignancies, or selected systemic diseases in association with HIV seropositivity are required to fulfill the WHO/CDC case definition for AIDS[46a] (Chapter 30). However, in many developing countries, diagnostic and laboratory facilities may be insufficient to reliably diagnose the diseases required by the WHO/CDC definition. Thus, for surveillance purposes and to enable clinicians to diagnose AIDS in the absence of sophisticated diagnostic facilities, a clinical case definition of AIDS was developed in 1985 for use in developing countries (Table 32-4).[150]

In an attempt to validate this case definition in Africa, 174 inpatients at one hospital in Kinshasa, Zaire, were examined, of whom 34 percent had antibody to HIV.[151] For detection of HIV seropositivity, the WHO clinical case definition had a sensitivity of 59 percent, specificity of 90 percent, and a positive predictive value of 74 percent. Sensitivity could be improved to 75 percent by including moderate to severe asthenia as a major clinical sign. The sensitivity for the diagnosis of "full-blown" AIDS is probably higher, since all patients with HIV antibody were considered when evaluating the validity of the case definition, including patients with coincidental HIV seropositivity, ARC, and AIDS. The major problem in the differential diagnosis of AIDS was tuberculosis, which has many of the same signs and symptoms commonly seen in HIV infection. Of 12 HIV seronegative patients in Kinshasa meeting the criteria of the clinical AIDS case definition, 9 (75 percent) had tuberculosis.

A simplified clinical case definition for pediatric AIDS has also been proposed by WHO (Table 32-4). In a survey to examine this case definition, 21 (13 percent) of 159 hospitalized children in Kinshasa were found to be seropositive for HIV.[152] The WHO clinical case definition for pediatric AIDS was found to be fairly specific (87 percent), but it lacked sensitivity (35 percent). As a consequence, the predictive value for HIV seropositivity was only 25 percent. The low predictive value of the case definition for pediatric AIDS is most likely due to the frequent occurrence of malnutrition and diarrheal and respiratory diseases that are highly endemic within this population, and which mimic the symptoms of HIV infection. As more clinical data become available, the development of clinical definitions that maximize both sensitivity and specificity for HIV disease should be encouraged for surveillance and epidemiologic purposes.

To improve the sensitivity and the positive predictive value of the clinical case definitions, it is advisable to confirm clinical suspicion with HIV serology. Other elements of the patient's history and physical examination not mentioned in the clinical definition may be helpful in the differential diagnosis. Diagnosis of HIV infection should be suspected in symptomatic patients with a high number of sexual partners, those who have had sexual contact with prostitutes, prostitutes themselves, and among those who have had sexual contact with a known HIV-infected person or a person who presents with symptoms or signs of HIV. Recent history of blood transfusions or frequent exposure to unsterilized needle injections should also increase suspicion for HIV infection.

A diagnosis of HIV infection may also become apparent during follow-up of the patient. Most symptoms and signs of HIV disease are persistent and frequently resistant to therapy. If the patient initially does not meet criteria of the clinical case definition and serologic diagnosis is not available, the patient should be followed until resolution of this disease, or progression of disease when the diagnosis of HIV infection becomes evident.

In many developing countries tuberculosis is widely endemic, and most immunocompetent individuals will respond to an intradermal tuberculin skin test. A simple diagnostic method in suspect AIDS patients is the presence of cutaneous anergy to tuberculin. Such cutaneous anergy, even in the presence of tuberculosis, is significantly associated with HIV seropositivity. This test is particularly practical for young adults who are not severely ill, but cutaneous anergy may occur in elderly individuals or those with severe illnesses even in the absence of HIV infection.

Laboratory data which are suggestive of HIV infection include an elevated sedimentation rate, neutropenia, lymphopenia (less than 1500 $mm^3$), and anemia. In many cases the platelet count may be normal, but thrombocytopenia has been documented as a prognostic indicator for progression to AIDS in HIV-infected individuals.[153] With respect to lymphocyte phenotyping, the finding of depressed T-helper lymphocytes (<400) had a sensitivity of 97 percent and specificity of 88 percent for HIV infection in one study in Africa.[154] These tests are costly and time-consuming and are not routinely available in many developing countries. Other diagnostic assays which are not widely available include HIV culture and HIV antigen detection which remain research procedures limited to selected laboratories.

**Table 32-4. Provisional WHO Clinical Case Definition for AIDS Where Diagnostic Resources Are Limited**

**Adults**

AIDS in an adult is defined by the existence of at least two of the major signs associated with at least one minor sign, in the absence of known causes of immunosuppression such as cancer or severe malnutrition or other recognized etiologies.

**Major signs**
(a) Weight loss > 10% of body weight
(b) Chronic diarrhea > 1 month
(c) Prolonged fever > 1 month (intermittent or constant)

**Minor signs**
(a) Persistent cough for > 1 month
(b) Generalized pruritic dermatitis
(c) Recurrent herpes zoster
(d) Oropharyngeal candidiasis
(e) Chronic progressive and disseminated herpes simplex infection
(f) Generalized lymphadenopathy

The presence of generalized Kaposi's sarcoma or cryptococcal meningitis is sufficient for the diagnosis of AIDS.

**Children**

Pediatric AIDS is suspected in an infant or child presenting with at least two major signs associated with at least two minor signs in the absence of known causes of immunosuppression.

**Major signs**
(a) Weight loss or abnormally slow growth
(b) Chronic diarrhea > 1 month
(c) Prolonged fever > 1 month

**Minor signs**
(a) Generalized lymphadenopathy
(b) Oropharyngeal candidiasis
(c) Repeated common infections (otitis, pharyngitis, and so forth)
(d) Persistent cough > 1 month
(e) Generalized dermatitis
(f) Confirmed maternal HIV infection

## PREVENTION AND CONTROL

With estimates of several million HIV-infected people worldwide, it is evident that HIV has created a major global health problem. While some countries have relatively high rates of infection among selected populations, other areas of the world are just now beginning to identify infected individuals and the impact of this disease will continue to increase. Control of HIV infection must become a public health priority in all countries of the world. With the lack of an effective vaccine and no promise of curative therapy within the near future, primary prevention is the only effective means to control HIV infection and AIDS. Virologic and epidemiologic studies have confirmed that HIV is predominantly spread via intimate sexual contact, primarily among homosexual men in the United States and Europe and among heterosexuals in tropical regions such as central Africa and Haiti.[1,103] Other modes of transmission include unscreened blood transfusions, the sharing of needles and syringes by intravenous drug users, and transmission from mother to infant either in utero or perinatally. Repeated use of unsterilized blood-contaminated needles and syringes may also play a role in the spread of HIV in developing countries. Each of these modes of transmission must be dealt with effectively in the development of a comprehensive control program.

The prevention of HIV infection in developing countries will be exceedingly complex given the social, political, and economic context of the third world, and for reasons related to many of the factors which have already facilitated HIV transmission. Rapid urbanization in many parts of Africa and South America has resulted in economic and sociologic changes that have influenced behavior and have affected the health infrastructure. The lack of financial resources severely limits rapid expansion of a control program which is both vertically and horizontally oriented. For example, public health officials cannot immediately upgrade blood transfusion services to prevent HIV infection, if the per person cost of the proposed intervention is likely to be approximately 10 to 30 times the annual per capita public health budget.[4] Implementation of blood bank screening for HIV may not be practical in areas where blood banking does not even exist.

In order to meet these challenges, the World Health Organization and other international health agencies are providing assistance to developing countries in the development of AIDS control programs.[155] Basic tenents of the program include the following stepwise strategy:

1. Initial assessment of the national HIV situation by seroepidemiologic studies along with evaluation of existing resources
2. Strengthening of the health infrastructure in order to support AIDS-related epidemiologic laboratory, clinical, and prevention activities
3. Education and information programs regarding AIDS and its prevention directed to the general public, risk groups in the population, and health care workers at all levels
4. Exchange of information including the reporting of AIDS cases

The principal goal of these programs remains the prevention of HIV transmission to uninfected persons. Prevention of sexual transmission through reduction in the number of sexual partners or use of condoms will necessarily be educational, and creative approaches to this activity will be required. The most important target group are individuals exhibiting high-risk behavior, and their sexual partners. Depending on the area, this may mean all sexually active men and women, and particularly persons with sexually transmitted diseases such as prostitutes and other promiscuous individuals. Community-based approaches to STD control for prostitutes and promiscuous individuals, with the establishment of area health committees selected by target group members, is usually more effective and acceptable to the group at risk.[155] Reduction of the risk of sexual transmission is primarily based on limiting the number of sexual partners, avoidance of unsafe sexual practices, and consistent use of condoms. A mutually monogamous relationship between seronegative individuals, and the use of condoms between partners of unknown serologic status, should help prevent the further spread of sexual transmission of HIV.

Changes in medical practices, including traditional practices, may be required to reduce the transmission risk associated with injections, scarifications, and blood transfusions. In Africa, blood transfusions are probably the second most important route of HIV transmission accounting for up to 10 percent of infection in adults and up to 30 percent in children. Screening of donated blood for HIV is an absolute necessity and can have an immediate impact on the spread of AIDS. Education programs aimed at physicians regarding the risk of HIV transmission through transfusion and the development of stringent criteria for the need for transfusion, linked with the increased availability of rapid diagnostic assays which may not require traditional blood banks, should be effective in preventing HIV transmission through blood transfusions.[156,157]

Prevention of HIV transmission through injections is theoretically feasible by using disposable needles and syringes. However, this may be too costly in many countries, and health care workers should be intensively trained to reduce the number of injections to a minimum and to systematically and properly sterilize reusable needles and syringes. Health education programs should inform the population about the risk of HIV transmission through contaminated needles and other skin-piercing instruments without eroding confidence in the immunization and medical programs.

Preventing perinatal transmission of HIV infection requires prevention of HIV infection in women of childbearing age, and counseling on contraception for HIV-seropositive women. These issues are extremely complex as they relate to fundamental social and psychological concerns such as sexual behavior and procreation. Prevention may require repeated campaigns to recruit both men and women who are considering becoming parents into voluntary testing and counseling programs.

The challenges for AIDS prevention in developing and developed countries are similar. The major difference is that the national resources required to build and sustain the epidemiologic, laboratory, clinical, and prevention activities outlined above are not sufficient in many developing areas. International health agencies will be required to provide a coordinated international effort, providing financial, scientific, educational, and technical support to those countries requesting assistance. Integration of these control programs into existing health and educational programs will require the full support by appropriate governmental agencies. Without immediate action in these areas, it is likely that the AIDS epidemic will continue to spread throughout all countries with alarming speed.

## References

1 Piot P et al: AIDS: An international perspective. *Science* 239:573, 1988.

2 World Health Organization: Acquired immunodeficiency syndrome (AIDS)—Data as of December 9, 1987. *Weekly Epidemiol Rec.*

3 Institute of Medicine: *Confronting AIDS; Direction for Public Health, Health Care and Research.* Washington, DC, National Academy Press, 1986.

4 Quinn TC et al: AIDS in Africa: An epidemiologic paradigm. *Science* 234:955, 1986.

5 Centers for Disease Control: *Pneumocystis pneumonia*—Los Angeles. *MMWR* 30:250, 1981.

6 Centers for Disease Control: Kaposi's sarcoma and *Pneumocystis* pneumonia among homosexual men—New York City and California. *MMWR* 30:305, 1981.

7 Clumeck N et al: Acquired immune deficiency syndrome in black Africans. *Lancet* i: 642, 1983.

8 Clumeck N et al: Acquired immune deficiency syndrome in African patients. *N Engl J Med* 310:492, 1984.

9 Pitchenik AE et al: Opportunistic infections and Kaposi's sarcoma among Haitians. *Ann Intern Med* 98:277, 1983.

10 Taelman H et al: Syndrome d'immunodeficience acquise chez trois patients du Zaire. *Ann Soc Belge Med Trop* 63:73, 1983.

11 Pitchenik AE et al: Tuberculosis, atypical mycobacterium, and the acquired immunodeficiency syndrome among Haitian and non-Haitian patients in South Florida. *Ann Intern Med* 101:641, 1985.

12 Brunet JB et al: Acquired immunodeficiency syndrome in France. *Lancet* i: 700, 1983.

13 Pape JW et al: The acquired immunodeficiency syndrome in Haiti. *Ann Intern Med* 103:674, 1985.

14 Nahmias AJ et al: Evidence for human infection with an HTLV-III/LAV-like virus in Central Africa, 1959. *Lancet* 1:1279, 1986.

15 Brun-Vezinet F et al: Prevalence of antibodies to lymphadenopathy associated retrovirus in African patients with AIDS. *Science* 226: 453, 1985.

16 Bygbjerg IC: AIDS in a Danish surgeon. *Lancet* i:925, 1983.

17 Nzilambi N et al: The prevalence of infection with human immunodeficiency virus over a 10-year period in rural Zaire. *N Engl J Med* 318:276, 1988.

18 Getchell JP et al: Human immunodeficiency virus isolated from a serum sample collected in 1976 in Central Africa. *J Infect Dis* 156: 833, 1987.

19 Biggar RJ et al: ELISA HTLV retrovirus antibody reactivity associated with malaria and immune complexes in healthy Africans. *Lancet* ii:520, 1985.

20 Safai B, Good RA: Kaposi's sarcoma: A review and recent developments. *Clin Bull* 10:52, 1980.

21 Piot P et al: Acquired immunodeficiency syndrome in a heterosexual population in Zaire. *Lancet* ii:65, 1984.

22 Van de Perre P et al: Acquired immunodeficiency syndrome in Rwanda. *Lancet* ii:62, 1984.

23 Bayley AC: Aggressive Kaposi's sarcoma in Zambia, 1983. *Lancet* i:1318, 1983.

24 Bayley AC et al: HTLV-III distinguishes atypical and endemic Kaposi's sarcoma in Africa. *Lancet* i:359, 1985.

25 Downing RG et al: African Kaposi's sarcoma and AIDS. *Lancet* i:475, 1984.

26 Serwadda D et al: Slim disease: A new disease in Uganda and its association with HTLV-III infection. *Lancet* ii:849, 1985.

27 Marquart K-H et al: Slim disease (AIDS). *Lancet* ii:186, 1985.

28 Van de Perre P et al: Antibody to HTLV-III in blood donors in Central Africa. *Lancet* i:336, 1985.

29 Vandepitte J et al: AIDS and cryptococcosis (Zaire, 1977). *Lancet* i:925, 1983.

30 Piot P et al: Retrospective seroepidemiology of HIV infection in Nairobi populations. *J Infect Dis* 155:1108, 1987.

31 Simoes EA et al: Evidence for HTLV-III infection in prostitutes in Tamil Nadu (India). *Indian J Med Res* 1987, p 335.

32 Kunhl P et al: Human immunodeficiency virus antibody screening in blood donors from India, Nigeria and Thailand. *Vox Sang* 52: 203, 1987.

33 Monzon OT: AIDS and infection due to HIV (AIDS virus) basic information. *Philipp J Nurs* 57:43, 1987.

34 Barin F et al: Serological evidence for virus related to simian T-lymphotropic retrovirus III in residents of West Africa. *Lancet* 2: 1387, 1985.

35 Kanki PJ et al: Antibodies to simian T-lymphotropic retrovirus type III in African green monkeys and recognition of STLV-III viral proteins by AIDS and related sera. *Lancet* i: 1330, 1985.

36 Daniel MD et al: Isolation of T-cell tropic HTLV-III-like retrovirus from macaques. *Science* 228:1201, 1985.

37 Kanki PJ et al: New human-T-lymphotrophic retrovirus related to simian T-lymphotrophic virus type III (STLV-III AGM). *Science* 232:238, 1986.

38 Clavel F et al: Isolation of a new human retrovirus from West African patients with AIDS. *Science* 233:343, 1986.

39 Clavel F et al: Molecular cloning and polymorphism of the human immune virus type 2. *Nature* 324:691, 1986.

40 Guyader M et al: Genome organization and transactivation of the human immunodeficiency virus type 2. *Nature* 326:662, 1987.

41 Hahn BH et al: Relation of HTLV-IV to simian and human immunodeficiency-associated viruses. *Nature* 330:184, 1987.

42 Kornfeld H et al: Cloning of HTLV-IV and its relation to simian and human immunodeficiency virus. *Nature* 326:610, 1987.

43 Clavel F: HIV, the West African AIDS virus. *AIDS* 1:135, 1987.

44 Kanki PJ: West African human retroviruses related to STLV-III. *AIDS* 1:141, 1987.

45 Centers for Disease Control: AIDS due to HIV infection—New Jersey. *MMWR* 37, 1988.

46 Centers for Disease Control: Revision of the CDC case definition for AIDS. *MMWR* 36:1S, 1987.

46a Report on a WHO Collaborative Meeting on AIDS. *Bull WHO* 64:37, 1986.

47 Mann JM et al: Surveillance for AIDS in a Central African city. *JAMA* 255:3255, 1986.

48 Ryder R et al: Community surveillance for HIV infection in Zaire. Third International Conference on AIDS, Washington, DC, 1987, p 57.

49 Kanki PJ et al: Human T-lymphotropic virus type 4 and the human immunodeficiency virus in West Africa. *Science* 827, 1987.

50 Desrosiers RC, Letvin NL: Animal models for acquired immunodeficiency syndrome. *Rev Infect Dis* 9:438, 1987.

51 Denis F et al: Efficacy of five enzyme immunoassays for antibody to HIV in detecting antibody to HTLV-IV. *Lancet* 1:324, 1987.

52 Pape JW et al: Risk factors associated with AIDS in Haiti. *Am J Med Sci* 291:4, 1986.

53 Collaborative Study Group of AIDS in Haitian-Americans: Risk factors for AIDS among Haitians residing in the United States. Evidence of heterosexual transmission. *JAMA* 257:635, 1987.

54 Bartholomew C et al: Racial and other characteristics of human T cell leukemia/lymphoma (HTLV-I) and AIDS (HTLV-III) in Trinidad. *Br Med J* 290:1243, 1985.

55 Biggar RJ: AIDS and HIV infection: Estimates of the magnitude of the problem worldwide in 1985/1986. *Clin Immunol Immunopathol* 45:297, 1987.

56 Padian NS: Heterosexual transmission of acquired immunodeficiency syndrome: International perspectives and national projections. *Rev Infect Dis* 9:947, 1987.

57 Koenig RE et al: Prevalence of antibodies to the human immunodeficiency virus in Dominicans and Haitians in the Dominican Republic. *JAMA* 257:631, 1987.

58 Castro BG et al: Human immunodeficiency virus infection in Brazil (Letter). *JAMA* 257:2592, 1987.

59 Mann JM: The global AIDS situation. *World Health Stat Q* 40:185, 1987.

60 Aral SO, Holmes KK: Epidemiology of sexually transmitted diseases, in *Sexually Transmitted Diseases,* KK Holmes, Mårdh PA, Sparling PF, et al (eds). New York, McGraw-Hill, pp 127–141.

61 Vogt MW et al: Isolation patterns of the human immunodeficiency virus from cervical secretions during the menstrual cycle of women at risk for the acquired immunodeficiency syndrome. *Ann Intern Med* 106:380, 1987.

62 Wofsy CB et al: Isolation of AIDS-associated retroviruses from gen-

ital secretions of women with antibodies to the virus. *Lancet* i:527, 1986.

63 Zagury D et al: HTLV-III in cells cultured from semen of two patients with AIDS. *Science* 226:449, 1984.

64 Van de Perre P et al: Seroepidemiological study on sexually transmitted diseases and hepatitis B in African promiscuous heterosexuals in relation to HTLV-III infection. *Eur J Epidemiol* 3:14, 1987.

65 Vittecoq D et al: Acquired immunodeficiency syndrome after travelling in Africa: An epidemiological study in seventeen Caucasian patients. *Lancet* 1:612, 1987.

66 Mann JM et al: Prevalence of HTLV-III/LAV in household contacts of patients with confirmed AIDS and controls in Kinshasa, Zaire. *JAMA* 256:721, 1986.

67 Sewankambo NK et al: HIV infection through normal heterosexual contact in Uganda. *AIDS* 1:113, 1987.

68 Clumeck N et al: Heterosexual promiscuity among African patients with AIDS. *N Engl J Med* 311:182, 1985.

69 Clumeck N et al: Seroepidemiological studies of HTLV-III antibody prevalence among selected groups of heterosexual Africans. *JAMA* 254:2599, 1985.

70 Van de Perre P et al: Female prostitutes: A risk group for infection with human T-cell lymphotropic virus type III. *Lancet* ii: 524, 1985.

71 Kreiss JK et al: AIDS virus infection in Nairobi prostitutes: Spread of the epidemic to East Africa. *N Engl J Med* 314:414, 1986.

72 Melbeye M et al: Evidence for heterosexual transmission and clinical manifestations of human immunodeficiency virus infection and related conditions in Lusaka, Zambia. *Lancet* 2:1113, 1986.

73 Mann JM et al: Sexual practices associated with LAV/HTLV-III seropositivity among female prostitutes in Kinshasa, Zaire. Second International Conference on AIDS, Paris, France, 1986, p 105.

74 Piot P et al: Heterosexual transmission of HIV. *AIDS* 2:1, 1988.

75 Plummer FA et al: Incidence of human immunodeficiency virus (HIV) infection and related disease in a cohort of Nairobi prostitutes. Third International Conference on AIDS, Washington, DC, 1987, p 6.

76 Greenblatt RM et al: Genital ulceration as a risk factor for human immunodeficiency virus infection in Kenya. *AIDS* 2:47, 1988.

77 Cameron DW et al: Female-to-male heterosexual transmission of HIV infection in Nairobi. Third International Conference on AIDS, Washington, DC, 1985, p 25.

78 Cameron DW et al: International Conference on Antimicrobial Agents and Chemotherapy. Washington, DC, 1987.

79 Rogers MF: AIDS in children: A review of the clinical, epidemiologic and public health aspects. *Pediatr Infect Dis* 4:230, 1985.

80 Lapointe N et al: Transplacental transmission of HTLV-III virus. *N Engl J Med* 312:1325, 1985.

81 Ziegler JB et al: Postnatal transmission of AIDS-associated retrovirus from mother to infant. *Lancet* 896, 1985.

82 Mok JQ et al: Infants born to mothers seropositive for human immunodeficiency virus. Preliminary findings from a multicenter European study. *Lancet* 1:1164, 1987.

83 Nzila N et al: Perinatal HIV transmission in two African hospitals. Third International Conference on AIDS, Washington, DC, 1987, p 158.

84 Braddick M et al: Congenital transmission of HIV in Nairobi, Kenya. Third International Conference on AIDS, Washington, DC, 1987, p 158.

85 Francis H et al: Immunologic profile of mothers in perinatal transmission of HIV infection. Third International Conference on AIDS, Washington DC, 1987, p 214.

86 Thiry L et al: Isolation of AIDS virus from cell free breast milk of three healthy virus carriers. *Lancet* 2:891, 1985.

87 Lepage P et al: Postnatal transmission of HIV from mother to child. *Lancet* 2:400, 1987.

88 Von Reyn CF et al: Human immunodeficiency virus infection and routine childhood immunization. *Lancet* 2:689, 1987.

89 Halsey NA, Henderson DA: HIV infection and immunization against other agents. *N Engl J Med* 316:683, 1987.

90 Redfield RR et al: Disseminated vaccinia in a military recruit with human immunodeficiency virus (HIV) disease. *N Engl J Med* 316: 673, 1987.

91 World Health Organization: Special programme on AIDS and expanded programme on immunization. *Weekly Epidemiol Rec* 62:297, 1987.

92 Brun-Vezinet F: Seroepidemiological studies of LAV in Central Africa. International Symposium on African AIDS, Brussels, Belgium.

93 Mhalu F et al: Prevalence of HIV antibodies in healthy subjects and groups of patients in some parts of Tanzania. Third International Conference on AIDS, Washington, DC, TP86, 1987, p 76.

94 Liskin L et al: AIDS a public health crisis. *Popul Rep* 14:L193, 1986.

95 Mann JM et al: HTLV-III/LAV seroprevalence among hospital workers in Kinshasa, Zaire: Lack of association with occupational exposure. *JAMA* 256:3099, 1986.

96 Mann JM et al: Risk factors for human immunodeficiency virus seropositivity among children 1–24 months old in Kinshasa, Zaire. *Lancet* 2:654, 1986.

97 Greenberg AE et al: Malaria and the transmission of HIV via blood transfusions in a pediatric population in Kinshasa, Zaire. *JAMA* 259:545, 1988.

98 Nguyen-Dinh P et al: Malaria and human immunodeficiency virus infection in children in Kinshasa, Zaire. *Bull WHO* 65:607, 1987.

99 Castro KG et al: Transmission of HIV in Belle Glade, Florida: Lessons for other communities in the United States. *Science* 239:193, 1988.

100 Mann JM et al: HTLV-III/LAV seroprevalence in pediatric inpatients 2–14 years old in Kinshasa, Zaire. *J Pediatrics* 78:673, 1986.

101 Greenberg AE et al: Evaluation of serological cross-reactivity between antibodies to plasmodium and HTLV-III/LAV. *Lancet* ii:247, 1986.

102 Zuckerman AJ: AIDS and insects. *Br Med J* 292:1094, 1986.

103 Curran JW et al: Epidemiology of HIV infection and AIDS in the United States. *Science* 239:610, 1988.

104 Mann JM et al: Natural history of HIV infection in Zaire. *Lancet* 2:707, 1986.

105 Ngaly B et al: Continuing studies on the natural history of HIV infection in Zaire. Third International Conference on AIDS, Washington, DC, 1987, p 2.

106 DeWitt S et al: Disease outcome among heterosexual Africans with HIV infection. Third International Conference on AIDS, Washington, DC, 1987, p 120.

107 Quinn TC et al: Serologic and immunologic studies in patients with AIDS in North America and Africa: The potential role of infectious agents as cofactors in human immunodeficiency virus infection. *JAMA* 257:2617, 1987.

108 Klatzmann D et al: Selective tropism of lymphadenopathy associated virus (LAV) for helper-inducer T lymphocytes. *Science* 225:59, 1984.

109 McDougal JS et al: Binding of HTLV/III/LAV to T4+ T-cells by a complex of the 110K viral protein and the T4 molecule. *Science* 231:382, 1986.

110 McDougal JS et al: Cellular tropism of the human retrovirus HTLV-III/LAV: I. Role of T-cell activation and depression of the T4 antigen. *J Immunol* 135:3151, 1985.

111 Zagury D et al: Long-term cultures of HTLV-III infected T-cells: A model of cytopathology of T-cell depletion in AIDS. *Science* 231:850, 1986.

112 Fauci AS: The human immunodeficiency virus: Infectivity and mechanisms of pathogenesis. *Science* 239:617, 1988.

113 Benn S et al: Genomic heterogeneity of AIDS retroviral isolates from North America and Zaire. *Science* 230:949, 1985.

114 Wong-Staal F et al: Genomic diversity of human T-lymphotropic virus type III (HTLV-III). *Science* 229:759, 1985.

115 Ferns RB et al: Characterization of monoclonal antibodies against the human immunodeficiency virus (HIV) gag products and their use in monitoring HIV isolate variation. *J Gen Virol* 68:1543, 1987.

116 Salinovich O et al: Rapid emergence of novel antigenic and genetic variants of equine infectious anemia virus during persistent infection. *J Virol* 57:71, 1986
117 Narayan O et al: Virus mutation during slow infection: Temporal development and characterization of mutants of visna virus recovered from sheep. *J Gen Virol* 41:343, 1978.
118 McCormick VB et al: Isolation of LAV/HTLV-III virus from African AIDS patients and from persons without AIDS or IgG antibody to LAV/HTLV-III. *Am J Trop Med Hyg* 36:102, 1987.
119 DeHovitz JA et al: Clinical manifestations and therapy of *Isospora belli* infection in patients with the acquired immunodeficiency syndrome. *N Engl J Med* 315:87, 1986.
120 Malebranche R et al: Acquired immunodeficiency syndrome with severe gastrointestinal manifestations in Haiti. *Lancet* ii:873, 1983.
121 Cooper DA et al: Acute AIDS retrovirus infection. Definition of a clinical illness associated with seroconversion. *Lancet* i:537, 1985.
122 Tindall B et al: Characterization of the acute clinical illness associated with human immunodeficiency virus infection. *Arch Intern Med* 148:945, 1987.
123 Carne CA et al: Acute encephalopathy coincident with seroconversion for anti-HTLV-III. *Lancet* ii:1206, 1985.
124 Colebunders R et al: Transmission of HIV following blood transfusion in Africans. Fourth International Conference on AIDS, 1988.
125 Clumeck N et al: Some epidemiological and clinical characteristics of African AIDS. *Antibiot Chemother* 38:41, 1987.
126 Vieira J et al: Acquired immune deficiency in Haitians: Opportunistic infections in previously healthy Haitian immigrants. *N Engl J Med* 308:125, 1983.
127 Biggar RJ et al: Clinical features of AIDS in Europe. *Eur J Cancer Clin Oncol* 20:165, 1984.
128 Quinn TC: Gastrointestinal manifestations of human immunodeficiency virus, in *Current Topics in AIDS*, MS Gottlieb et al (eds). New York, Wiley, 1987.
129 Colebunders R et al: Persistent diarrhea in Zairian AIDS patients: An etiologic study. *Am J Gastroenterol* 82:859, 1987.
130 Colebunders R et al: Generalized papular pruritic eruption: A manifestation of HIV infection in African patients. *AIDS* 1:117, 1987.
131 Colebunders R et al: Herpes zoster in African patients: A clinical predictor of human immunodeficiency virus infection. *J Infect Dis* 157:314, 1988.
132 Melbye M et al: Risk of AIDS after herpes zoster. *Lancet* 1:728, 1987.
133 Klein RS et al: Oral candidiasis in high-risk patients as the initial manifestation of the acquired immunodeficiency syndrome (AIDS). *N Engl J Med* 311:354, 1984.
134 Quinn TC: Early symptoms and signs of AIDS and the AIDS-related complex, in *AIDS: A Basic Guide for Clinicians*, P Ebbesen et al (eds). Copenhagen, Munksgaard, 1984, pp 69–83.
135 Mann J et al: Association between HTLV-III/LAV infection and tuberculosis in Zaire (Letter). *JAMA* 256:346, 1986.
136 Pitchenik AE et al: Tuberculosis, atypical mycobacteriosis, and the acquired immunodeficiency syndrome among Haitian and non-Haitian patients in south Florida. *Ann Intern Med* 101:641, 1984.
137 Guerin JM et al: Acquired immune deficiency syndrome: Specific aspects of the disease in Haiti. *Ann NY Acad Sci* 437:254, 1984.
138 Safai B et al: The natural history of Kaposi's sarcoma in the acquired immunodeficiency syndrome. *Ann Intern Med* 103:744, 1985.
139 Ambinder RF et al: Lack of cytomegalovirus association with endemic African Kaposi's sarcoma. *J Infect Dis* 156:193, 1987.
140 Lesbordes JL et al: Malnutrition and HIV infection in children in the Central African Republic. *Lancet* 2:337, 1986.
141 Clavel F et al: Human immunodeficiency virus type 2 infection associated with AIDS in West Africa. *N Engl J Med* 316:1180, 1987.
142 Brun-Vezinet F et al: Detection of IgG antibodies to lymphadenopathy-associated virus in patients with AIDS or lymphadenopathy syndrome. *Lancet* i:1253, 1984.
143 Sarngadharan MG et al: Antibodies reactive with human T lymphotropic retrovirus (HTLV-III) in the serum of patients with AIDS. *Science* 224:506, 1984.
144 Mortimer PP, Clewley JP: Serological tests for human immunodeficiency virus, in *Current Topics in AIDS*, MS Gottlieb et al (eds). Chichester, England, Wiley, 1987, vol 1, pp 133–154.
145 Gnann JW Jr et al: Synthetic peptide immunoassay distinguishes HIV type 1 and HIV type 2 infections. *Science* 237:1346, 1987.
146 Foucault C et al: Double HIV-1 and HIV-2 seropositivity among blood donors (Letter). *Lancet* ii:165, 1987.
147 Rey MA et al: HIV-1 and HIV-2 double infection in French homosexual male with AIDS-related complex (Letter). *Lancet* 1:388, 1987.
148 Rey F et al: HIV-1 and HIV-2 double infection in Central African Republic. *Lancet* 2:1391, 1986.
149 Denis F et al: Prevalence of human T-lymphotropic retroviruses type III (HIV) and type IV in Ivory Coast. *Lancet* ii:408, 1987.
150 World Health Organization: Acquired immunodeficiency syndrome (AIDS). WHO/CDC case definition for AIDS. *Weekly Epidemiol Rec* 61:69, 1986.
151 Colebunders R et al: Evaluation of a clinical case definition of acquired immunodeficiency syndrome in Africa. *Lancet* 1:492, 1987.
152 Colebunders RL et al: Evaluation of a clinical case definition of AIDS in African children. *AIDS* 1:151, 1987.
153 Kaslow RA et al: Infection with the human immunodeficiency virus: Clinical manifestations and their relationship to immune deficiency. *Ann Intern Med* 107:474, 1987.
154 Francis H et al: Diagnosis of HIV infection in Africa: Comparison of ELISA and immunologic assays. *Am J Trop Med Hyg* 38:641, 1988.
155 Ngugi EN et al: Effect of an AIDS education program on increasing condom use in a cohort of Nairobi prostitutes. Third International Conference on AIDS, Washington, DC, 1987, p 157.
156 Carlson JR et al: Rapid, easy, and economical screening test for antibodies to human immunodeficiency virus. *Lancet* i:361, 1987.
157 Quinn TC et al: Rapid latex agglutination assay using recombinant envelope polypeptide for the detection of antibody to the human immunodeficiency virus. *JAMA* 260:510, 1988.

# Chapter 33
# Clinical pathobiology of HTLV-I infection

Richard Marlink
M. Essex

## INTRODUCTION

The first naturally occurring human retrovirus to be discovered is now termed human T-lymphotropic virus type I (HTLV-I).[1] This virus has been shown to be a prototype for numerous isolates of a type of retrovirus found to be endemic in certain regions of the world.[2] The role of retroviruses in the development of cancer or other diseases has long been suspected, but it was not until this discovery that a distinct retroviral agent was identified and associated with human disease.[3]

From epidemiologic studies it appears that HTLV-I has primarily blood-borne and sexual transmission routes and usually only results in a "carrier state" in chronically infected individuals.[4] Most individuals infected with HTLV-I remain healthy but reveal the presence of antibodies to the virus. However, the regular presence of the viral agent in patients suffering from a particular rare T-cell malignancy, adult T-cell leukemia/lymphoma (ATL), the clustering of ATL cases in areas where HTLV-I is endemic and the integration of HTLV-I provirus in ATL tumor cells all point to an important role for HTLV-I in the pathogenesis of this human neoplasm. Within endemic areas HTLV-I has also been implicated in the pathogenesis of certain other lymphatomatous malignancies, in the propensity for immune suppression, and in the development of a chronic progressive myelopathy. Further information on mechanisms of oncogenesis and immune dysfunction will certainly be obtained from the study of this "first" human retrovirus.

## RETROVIRUSES

### MECHANISMS OF REPLICATION

HTLV-I is a member of the large group of RNA viruses known as *retroviruses.* These viral agents are distinct in the molecular genetics of their replication, as this group of viruses has been shown to require reverse transcription for replication, hence their name *retro*virus (see also Chap. 28). The reverse transcriptase enzyme, described by Temin[5] and Baltimore,[6] has the ability to transcribe DNA from RNA, the reverse direction of normal eukaryotic transcription. This enzyme, present by definition in all retroviruses, allows the transcription of a DNA template from the RNA viral genome after cellular attachment and penetration has occurred (see Fig. 28-5). The DNA template of the viral genome can then integrate into the host cell's genome in what is called a *proviral* form. Once integrated, the provirus can undergo varying degrees of transcription and translation to produce the complete RNA virus, or the proviral DNA can remain latent in the host genome and be transmitted to progeny cells at the time of cell division. When the RNA viral genome is made, it is protected by central *core* proteins and packaged with its reverse transcriptase and other polymerases. An *envelope* then buds from the surface of the cytoplasmic membrane, and the core particle with enzymes are assembled inside the envelope to form a mature virion.

### MECHANISMS OF TRANSMISSION AND TRANSFORMATION

Retroviruses are also distinct in their modes of transmission. They are the only known group of viruses which can be transmitted from generation to generation in an inherited, or *vertical,* fashion, as well as in a *horizontal* fashion as an infectious agent.[7] Those retroviruses which are vertically transmitted only are known as *endogenous* retroviruses and normally are not expressed or activated, except perhaps during embryonic development.[8] To date, these endogenous retroviruses constitute a large group of animal retroviruses and have not been shown to be definitively involved in any pathologic process in humans.

The horizontally acquired, or *exogenous,* retroviruses, on the other hand, can be involved in oncogenic transformation in both animals and humans.[8,9] At least two basic mechanisms may be involved in retroviral transformation. One is through a transforming cellular *onc* gene, which usually but not always represents a protein kinase, that the virus acquires through recombination. This cellular *onc* gene, or oncogene, is reinserted into the cellular genome by the integration of the proviral form of the retrovirus within an area of the genome where the gene will not be under its usual cellular control. These transforming *onc* genes, therefore, are naturally occurring genes derived from the cellular genome which have become incorporated in an aberrant fashion. When retroviruses acquire such genes they can transform a variety of cell types and are, therefore, useful in studying oncogenesis. These "altered" retroviruses, however, usually do not survive in nature since they may be replication-defective.[10]

Transformation involving "chronic leukemia viruses," such as HTLV-I, is most likely due to a different mechanism of retrovirus-related oncogenesis, the regulatory reprogramming of an infected cell and its progeny at the genetic level. In the case of HTLV-I and related viruses, this is done through a transactivation of transcription (TAT), and it involves a long induction period. The TAT mechanism is mediated by a specific gene in the viral genome. The altered transcription that results from this integrated viral message may then lead to transformation or immortalization of the infected cell.[11,12] A "family tree" of certain transactivating retroviruses is shown in Fig. 33-1, showing the evolutionary relationship of HTLV-I to other mammalian exogenous retroviruses with this type of transcriptional regulation.

## HTLV-I

### IDENTIFICATION

In the later half of the 1970s, Takatsuki and colleagues[13] described an unusual clustering of T-cell leukemia/lymphoma patients in certain southern islands of Japan. The abnormally large percentage of an unusual T-cell phenotype among the lymphoid malignancies on these islands led to the search for a transmissible agent by investigators in Japan and the United States. The even-

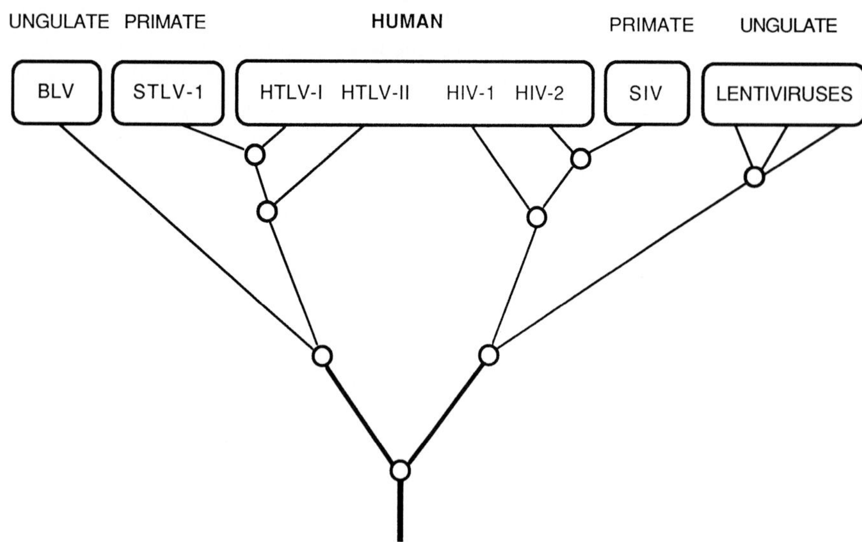


**Fig. 33-1.** Evolutionary relationship of certain mammalian retroviruses which may display *tat* transacting transcriptional regulation (TAT). Natural hosts are noted at top of figure. BLV = bovine leukemia virus; STLV-I = simian T-lymphotropic virus type I; HTLV-I, -II = human T-lymphotropic virus type I, type II; HIV-1, -2 = human immunodeficiency virus type 1, type 2; SIV = simian immunodeficiency virus. See also Figure 28-1. (*After F Wong-Staal and RC Gallo.*[9])

tual discovery of HTLV-I was made feasible by the previous development of the ability to sustain the growth of T lymphocytes with a T-cell growth factor, interleukin-2 (IL-2).[14] Lymphocytes from a patient in the United States with a diagnosis of cutaneous T-cell lymphoma (CTCL) were cultured, and a continuous cell line was established which was transformed and expressed the virus HTLV-I.[1]

## DESCRIPTION OF THE VIRUS

HTLV-I is similar to other C-type retroviruses in that the envelope glycoproteins bud from the cytoplasmic membrane of an infected cell and assembly of the core components of the virus is not seen by electron microscopy until the components are assembled at the site of budding.[1,15,16] HTLV-I is different from many animal type C retroviruses in that its reverse transcriptase utilizes $Mg^{2+}$ as its divalent cation, rather than $Mn^{2+}$, for optimal enzymatic activity. The complete viral particle is about 100 nm in diameter, and its core is morphologically distinct from HIV-1 and HIV-2, the two known types of human immunodeficiency retroviruses (see Chap. 28).

Like other retroviruses, HTLV-I has *gag*, *pol*, and *env* genes which code for core proteins, polymerase and endonuclease proteins, and envelope proteins respectively. *Long terminal repeat* sequences (LTRs) are located at each end of the provirus and help regulate the transcription of the other viral genes. A unique region of the genome is located next to the 3′ LTR. Encoded from within this region is the protein responsible for TAT activity, essential in the transforming capabilities of the virus in culture.[17,18] This TAT protein, with the proposed name $tax_1$ for HTLV-I,[19] may induce the host cell to proliferate by binding to cellular regulatory sequences which may control the production of IL-2 receptor (IL-2R),[20–22] thereby inducing leukemic growth through an increase in the number of cellular receptors and/or independent regulation of this T-cell growth factor. Several of the basic biological characteristics of this virus are listed in Table 33-1.

**Table 33-1. Biological Characteristics of HTLV-I**

1. HTLV-I integrates into host cell DNA at random sites.
2. Integration may then lead to immortalization of cells in a monoclonal or oligoclonal pattern.
3. Immortalization is via a *transacting transcription*, or TAT, mechanism.
4. HTLV-I-transformed cells in vitro are remarkably similar to primary HTLV-I leukemia cells.
5. Malignancies associated with HTLV-I infection do not show consistent chromosomal alterations.

The virus contains several protein antigens that induce antibodies in infected people. The major *gag* gene product is p24. This antigen induces antibodies in most infected people and is present in large amounts in both infected cells and virus particles. The amino-terminal *gag* gene phosphoprotein, p19, is also immunogenic in most people. When sources of antigen are taken from infected cells, larger precursor forms that contain both p24 and p19, such as p55, p38, and p28, are also found. Nonspecific antibodies that cross react with p19 are sometimes found since this antigen apparently contains epitopes that are related to certain normal cellular antigens.

The *env* gene encodes a polyprotein that is 61,000 to 65,000 daltons in its glycosylated form. It is subsequently cleaved to give rise to an amino-terminal, external glycoprotein designated gp45 and to a carboxy-terminal, transmembrane protein, p21E. The gp61 and gp45 are regularly immunogenic, inducing antibodies in virtually all infected seropositive individuals.

## CLOSELY RELATED HUMAN RETROVIRUS: HTLV-II

Most of the viruses isolated from HTLV-I endemic regions are highly related in nucleic acid sequence and in their protein products and are, therefore, collectively termed HTLV-I. A second member of the human T-lymphotropic virus family was first isolated from a patient with a T-cell variant of hairy cell leukemia[23] and given a separate type distinction, HTLV-II. HTLV-II is less related by nucleic acid homology than the different isolates of HTLV-I and differs slightly both in the ultrastructural appearance of its mature viral particles[24] and in the size of its immunogenic protein products.[25] The role of HTLV-II in disease pathogenesis is less clear than that of HTLV-I, but seroepidemiologic studies are confounded by a considerable serologic cross-reactivity between HTLV-I and HTLV-II, especially with respect to conserved regions in the deduced amino acid sequences of the major *gag* and *env* gene products.[26,27] Indirect in vitro evidence has suggested that HTLV-I antibody reactivity detected in certain cohorts of intravenous drug users in New York City may be directed against HTLV-II, rather than against HTLV-I.[28] Overall, the actual geographic distribution of HTLV-II is unclear due to this extensive serologic cross-reactivity between HTLV-I and HTLV-II.

## EPIDEMIOLOGY

Once HTLV-I was isolated and propagated in the laboratory, serologic assays for detection of antibodies to HTLV-I could be developed and utilized to study the distribution, transmission, and natural history of infection. After the initial identification of ATL clustering in Japan, a second focus of an aggressive T-cell malignancy, then called T-cell lymphosarcoma cell leukemia (TLCL), was described as a clinical entity among Caribbeans living in the United Kingdom[29] and shown to be associated with a high degree of seropositivity to HTLV-I. Increased seroprevalence to HTLV-I was subsequently shown in Africa,[30,31] in the southeastern United States,[32] in the northern regions of South America,[33] and in southern Italy.[34] Evidence of HTLV-I exposure has even been shown in certain areas of Alaska and northern Sweden.[35] When extensively studied, such as in Japan and the Caribbean, endemic foci of HTLV-I are characterized by an increased prevalence of healthy HTLV-I carriers and an elevated incidence of T-cell-related malignancies (see Table 33-2).

## TRANSMISSION

Similar to the human immunodeficiency viruses (HIVs), HTLV-I, and HTLV-II are horizontally acquired exogenous retroviruses, capable of blood-borne or sexual transmission. Early seroepidemiologic studies in Japan have implicated blood transfusions as a significant mode of HTLV-I transmission in certain populations.[36,37] Partially because of HTLV-I's sporadic geographic distribution, its long latency period, and its wide disease/infection ratio, widespread blood bank screening for HTLV-I has not yet taken place outside Japan. This situation will change, however, in the near future.

Antibodies to HTLV-I (and/or HTLV-II) have been noted in certain groups of intravenous drug addicts in the United States,[28] in the United Kingdom,[38] and in Italy.[39] The implications for future disease pathogenesis, especially in relation to concomitant exposure to HIV-I in this population, have yet to be determined.

Sexual transmission of HTLV-I has been documented, but the relative efficiency of this mode of transmission is unknown. Several surveys have shown a marked increase in seropositivity as certain populations reach sexually active ages[40] and have demonstrated transmission among sexual partners.[41,42] The persistence of high prevalence rates in geographic areas and the seropositive carrier rates among certain families suggest that HTLV-I infection, like HIV infections, is not likely to be casually acquired.

Studies in Japan indicate that there may be a differential propensity for transmission between the sexes. The prevalence of HTLV-I infection in Japan increases with age for both sexes,[43,44] but in older seropositive carriers, a larger proportion may be women.[44,45] Whether this seroprevalence difference between males and females represents relative infectiousness or susceptibility is presently unknown.

Transplacental transmission of this virus has not been conclusively documented, but acquisition of viral infection can occur early in childhood, perhaps related to close mother–child contact or transmission via breast milk.[46] In fact, utilizing an animal model for HTLV-I transmission, Miyoshi and colleagues have shown that transmission via milk can occur in laboratory-infected rabbits.[47]

**Table 33-2. Epidemiologic Features of HTLV-I**

1. HTLV-I is an exogenous, horizontally transmitted retrovirus.
2. Transmission can occur by sexual or intimate contact, by exposure to blood or blood products, or by breast feeding.
3. Infection with HTLV-I is characterized by a long latency period prior to disease development and a low risk for development of disease.
4. Geographic and familial clustering of seropositivity to HTLV-I is seen, which may be very sporadic within countries or regions.
5. Increased incidence of ATL and other HTLV-I-associated sequelae may occur in HTLV-I endemic regions.

## CLINICAL MANIFESTATIONS

### ATL

Adult T-cell leukemia/lymphoma (ATL) is an aggressive non-Hodgkins' lymphoma (NHL), frequently associated with hypercalcemia, that is closely linked to previous exposure to HTLV-I. Several of the clinical and pathologic features of this disease are outlined in Table 33-3 (also see Fig. 33-2).

The usual presence of skin involvement in HTLV-I-related malignancies and the evidence for a smoldering clinical state sometimes preceding the leukemic or aggressive lymphomatous stage of ATL have led to the use of the term *cutaneous T-cell lymphoma* (CTCL) in other regions, especially in the Western Hemisphere. The terminology is in keeping with the existence of a separate clinical state without hypercalcemia and possessing a much better prognosis than frank ATL. Most cases of CTCL,

**Table 33-3. Adult T-Cell Leukemia/Lymphoma**

A. *Clinical Manifestations*
   1. T-cell leukemia and/or stage IV lymphoma commonly with
      - Bone marrow infiltration
      - Lymphadenopathy
      - Infiltrating skin involvement
      - Hepatomegaly
      - Splenomegaly
   2. Hypercalcemia and possible lytic bone lesions
   3. Propensity for pyogenic infections and/or opportunistic infections
B. *Pathologic Features*
   1. Histologic
      - A skin, lymph node, or bone marrow biopsy usually shows large cell, mixed, or unclassifiable NHL with anti-Tac+ (IL-2 receptor) and usually T4 phenotype
      - Lymphocytes with convoluted nuclei seen by light and electron microscopy
      - Acid phosphatase activity, partially tartrate-resistant, in neoplastic cells
   2. Laboratory
      - Positive HTLV-I serologic studies
      - Anemia and thrombocytopenia, common
      - Degree of hypercalcemia and leukocytosis correlated with prognosis

however, are not associated with positive HTLV-I serologic studies[50] and probably warrant a separate clinical classification. Antibodies to HTLV-I are usually also absent in classic cases of mycosis fungoides and Sézary syndrome, although since their clinical and histologic features may also overlap or be confused with smoldering ATL, caution must be used when interpreting data concerning HTLV-I exposure and these syndromes.

A typical case of ATL occurs later in life, with the typical age at presentation being in the fifth or sixth decade. The prognosis is grim. The neoplastic process is aggressive and usually not responsive to chemotherapy once "full-blown" leukemia or lymphoma develops. The patient's age, gender, or degree of skin, bone marrow or liver involvement do not seem to significantly alter the prognosis of ATL. A high number of circulating white blood cells may predict a poorer prognosis, as may the degree of hypercalcemia.[51–55,61]

The hypercalcemia seen with ATL has been postulated to be related to the production of a lymphokine or other factor secreted by the neoplastic cells which stimulates osteoclastic activity. Increased osteoclastic activity is seen in ATL-positive bone marrow biopsies, even in areas of bone which are not involved with leukemic infiltration.[55] Certain HTLV-I-transformed lymphocyte cell lines may be able to uniquely metabolize the physiologically inactive 25-hydroxyvitamin $D_3$ to the active 1,25-dihydroxyvitamin $D_3$.[56] If this in vitro observation applies to transformed HTLV-I infected cells in vivo, it may play a future role in explaining and, perhaps, in treating the abnormal calcium regulation seen in ATL.

## B-CELL CLL

Less clear than the relationship between ATL and HTLV-I exposure, an association between other malignancies and HTLV-I may exist. There are numerous reports of other forms of leukemia or lymphoma associated with a "relatively" high degree of seropositivity to HTLV-I. In the Caribbean[57] and perhaps in Africa,[58] reports of a higher than expected seroprevalence to HTLV-I have been made involving patients with chronic lymphocytic leukemia (CLL) with B-cell phenotype. The clinical features of these B-cell CLL cases are similar to those of CLL seen in regions not endemic for HTLV-I. In one patient from Jamaica, cultured B cells from a CLL case did not show viral components, yet a T-cell line established from the patient displayed the HTLV-I provirus.[59]

## HTLV-I and IMMUNOSUPPRESSION

The apparently indirect role HTLV-I plays in the pathogenesis of the previously mentioned B-cell CLL could be due in part to a certain degree of immunosuppression that has been associated with HTLV-I infection.[43] The profound depletion of T4 helper lymphocytes seen with HIV infection (see Chaps. 29 and 30) is not a hallmark of the pathogensis of HTLV-I disease, yet death in a significant number of ATL patients is due to infections. These infections may not be treatment-related and many times involve pyogenic organisms, manifesting as septicemias, pneumonias, or urinary tract infections. Especially in Japan and the United States, perhaps related to available diagnostic capabilities, both minor and systemic opportunistic infections are also seen in ATL patients.[49,60,61]

Since many types of leukemia or lymphoma may be associated with a relative degree of immunosuppression, it is of greater significance that increased susceptibility to common infections appears to be related to HTLV-I seropositivity alone. When infectious disease wards were surveyed on the southern Japanese island of Kyushu, 42 percent of hospitalized patients were HTLV-I seropositive, a threefold increase from the background seropositivity among healthy adults from the same region.[43] The infectious diseases for which these patients were hospitalized were varied and included bacterial pneumonia, hepatitis, and pyelonephritis. Of further interest, an extremely high percentage of patients with strongyloides infections in one study in Okinawa were also seropositive for HTLV-I, with many showing monoclonal integration of proviral DNA, increased numbers of abnormal lymphocytes, and other indicators of smoldering ATL.[62] Again, it could be postulated that perhaps an immunodeficiency caused by HTLV-I exposure could be predisposing this population to other endemic infections.

This apparent susceptibility to various infectious diseases requires further study, as does a more specific observation by Miyoshi and collegues in Kochi, Japan.[63,64] These investigators have reported three cases of AIDS-like diseases (*Pneumocystis carinii* pneumonia in two cases and cryptococcal meningitis in a third case) which occurred in young patients seropositive for HTLV-I and seronegative for HIV, with no other reasons for immunosuppression. Absent responses to delayed-type hypersensitivity (DTH) skin testing and reduced numbers of T-helper lymphocytes were also seen in these patients. These cases differ from the previous reports of opportunistic infections indicative of a depressed cellular immunity in ATL patients, in that severe opportunistic infections occurred in HTLV-I seropositive patients not yet afflicted with ATL.

Specific in vitro and in vivo definitions of the immune defects present in HTLV-I infection are scarce. Certain T-cell functions in HTLV-I-infected cell lines are altered,[65] and functionally the primary leukemic cells from HTLV-I patients may act more as suppressor cells, even though they may carry the T4 phenotype.[66] HTLV-I carriers may show a reduced Epstein-Barr virus (EBV)-specific memory T-cell response in an in vitro system.[67] The relationships of these laboratory observations to the previously described clinical observations have yet to be elucidated.

Concurrent infections with both HIV and HTLV-I have been reported, and the potential for either an acceleration of the cytopathic effects of HIV[68] or an increase in the neoplastic potential of HTLV-I[69] has been suggested in these situations. In vitro observations that HIV expression is facilitated in lymphocyte cultures also infected with HTLV-I[70] may be related to the fact that the TAT protein of HTLV-I ($tax_1$) may also transactivate the LTR of HIV-1.[71] This facilitated expression of HIV could possibly occur in vivo and may then portend a worse prognosis for individuals exposed to both HIV and HTLV-I.

## HTLV-I AND NEUROTROPISM

Since 1985, groups of patients have been reported in the Caribbean[72] and in Japan[73] who have presented with a chronic progressive myelopathy in association with high titers of HTLV-I antibodies, with ATL-like cells in their serum or CSF, and with intra blood–brain-barrier synthesis of HTLV-I antibodies.[74,75] Just as there is clustering of ATL cases in HTLV-I endemic regions and an extremely high percentage of ATL cases show evidence of exposure to HTLV-I, this chronic progressive myelopathy appears to be a distinct disease entity associated with HTLV-I.

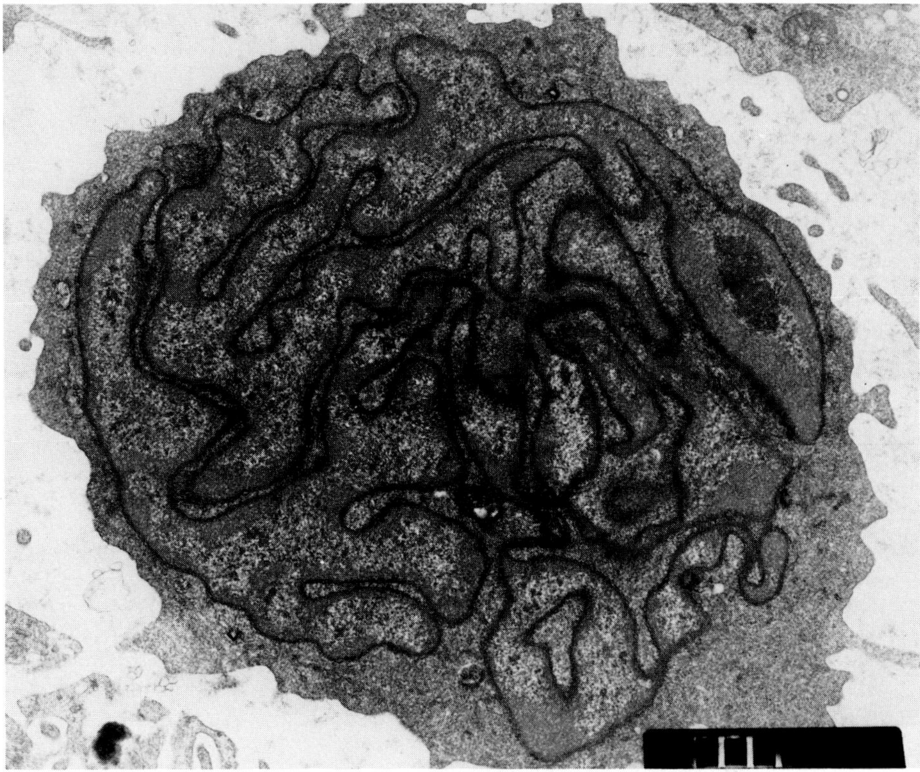

**Fig. 33-2.** Electron micrograph of a T-lymphocyte infected with HTLV-I from a patient with ATL, showing lobulated and convoluted nucleus. (*Courtesy of S Hawari, Mallory Institute of Pathology, Boston.*)

The reports from the Caribbean have grouped this myelopathy with tropical spastic paraparesis (TSP), since TSP has already been described in both an epidemic form, perhaps related to toxins or nutritional factors, and an endemic form, which has been seen in certain tropical countries.[76] The cases reported from Japan have been referred to as HTLV-I-associated myelopathy (HAM) and share many of the clinical and laboratory abnormalities seen with HTLV-I-seropositive TSP cohorts, leading to the conclusion that TSP and HAM represent a single disease entity.[77] This entity is characterized by spastic paraparesis with a propensity for weakness and variable sensory abnormalities in the lower extremities. Bladder dysfunction is common. The clinical course may be prolonged or, on occasion, rapidly progressive.

In addition to the presence of anti-HTLV-I antibodies in these patients, an increase in OKT4-, OKDR-, and IL-2R-positive lymphocytes and a decrease in OKT8-positive lymphocyte subsets may be present.[78] These laboratory alterations are similar to what may be demonstrated in ATL patients.[79]

Myelopathies and numerous other central nervous system abnormalities have been described in AIDS and HIV-infected individuals (reviewed in Ref. 80; see also Chap. 30). Thus, it is not surprising that a specific myelopathy has been recognized which is either directly or indirectly related to HTLV-I infection.

## DIAGNOSIS OF HTLV-I INFECTION

With the discovery of additional clinical entities associated with HTLV-I infection and with the recognition that there are large numbers of asymptomatic "carriers" of HTLV-I in endemic areas who may be blood donors, the development of laboratory techniques for the determination of HTLV-I infection is of increasing importance.[81–83] Serologic assays, similar to those used for detection of antibodies to the AIDS virus (see Chap. 79), are available for determination of HTLV-I exposure. The performance characteristics of screening assays, such as the enzyme-linked immunosorbent assay (ELISA or EIA) or the particle agglutination assay, have not been as extensively studied as those of the widely used HIV screening tests. Confirmatory serologic tests for HTLV-I exposure include infected-cell membrane fluorescence, fixed-cell fluorescence, Western blotting (WB), and radioimmunoprecipitation (RIPA), but their interpretation is also not widely standardized and requires various degrees of technical experience. Also, since HTLV-I produces less antigen in continuous cell lines compared with HIV, and since nonspecific reactivities to nonviral antigens are common in HTLV-I confirmatory assays, the sensitivity and specificity of various HTLV-I serologic assays have yet to be fully determined.

In large-scale survey of serum from almost 40,000 blood donors throughout the United States, 0.025 percent were confirmed to be reactive for HTLV-I antibodies.[84,85] The confirmation of the initial screening EIAs used to detect the reactive samples necessitated both WB and RIPA. This latter procedure, however, is presently suited only for research laboratories due to the high cost and technical labor required for its performance. One can see, therefore, that after a repeatedly reactive EIA is found by screening in a blood bank setting, a straightforward confirmatory assay for HTLV-I antibodies may not be readily available.

In the future, the determination of HTLV-I exposure may be improved by DNA amplification techniques, especially in cases where an antibody response may be undetectable.[86,87]

## TREATMENT OF HTLV-I INFECTION

Inhibition of the in vitro infectivity of HTLV-I has been shown with the antiretroviral drug azidothymidine.[88] Since the vast majority of individuals infected with HTLV-I will not develop pathologic complications secondary to their exposure, antiviral treatment of individuals seropositive to HTLV-I has not yet been evaluated. Also, since the disease ATL is due to a proliferation of a single HTLV-I-altered cell, rather than to continuous virus replication, it seems unlikely that antiviral drugs will be as effective in this setting as they are for HIV infection and AIDS. Humoral immunity against HTLV-I infection may be elicited in primates with HTLV-I envelope proteins,[89] and this lends encouragement for the possible development of a vaccine against HTLV-I in the future.

## REFERENCES


1 Poiesz BJ et al: Detection and isolation of type C retrovirus particles from fresh and cultured lymphocytes of a patient with cutaneous T-cell lymphoma. *Proc Natl Acad Sci USA* 77:7415, 1980.
2 Watanabe et al: HTLV-I (US isolate) and ATLV (Japanese isolate) are the same species of human retrovirus. *Virology* 133:238, 1984.
3 Shaw GM et al: Human T-cell leukemia virus: Its discovery and role in leukemogenesis and immunosuppression. *Adv Intern Med* 30:1, 1984.
4 The T- and B-cell Malignancy Study Group: Statistical analyses of clinico-pathological, virological and epidemiological data on lymphoid malignancies with special reference to adult T-cell leukemia/lymphoma: A report of second nationwide study of Japan. *Jpn J Clin Oncol* 15:517, 1985.
5 Temin HJ, Mijtzutani Y: RNA-dependent DNA polymerase in virions of Rous sarcoma virus. *Nature* 226:1211, 1970.
6 Baltimore D et al: Viral RNA-dependent DNA polymerase virus of RNA tumor viruses. *Nature* 226:1209, 1970.
7 Varmus HE et al: The origin and structure of endogenous retroviral DNA. *Ann Ny Acad Sci* 354:379, 1980.
8 Essex M: Horizontal and vertical transmission of retroviruses, in *Viruses Associated with Human Cancer,* LA Phillips (ed). New York and Basel, Dekker, 553, 1983.
9 Wong-Staal F, Gallo RC: Human T-lymphotropic retroviruses. *Nature* 317:395, 1985.
10 Cooper GM: Cellular transforming genes. *Science* 217:801, 1982.
11 Lobach DF et al: Retroviruses and human cancer: Evaluation of T-lymphocyte transformation by human T-cell leukemia virus. *Cancer Invest* 3(2):145, 1985.
12 Yoshida M, Seiki M: Recent advances in the molecular biology of HTLV-I: Trans-activation of viral and cellular genes. *Ann Rev Immunol* 5:541, 1987.
13 Takatsuki K et al: Adult T cell leukemia in Japan, in *Topics in Hematology,* S Sero et al (eds). Amsterdam, Excerpta Medica, pp. 73–77, 1977.
14 Morgan DA et al: Selective *in vitro* growth of T-lymphocytes from normal human bone marrows. *Science* 193:1007, 1976.
15 Miyoshi I et al: A novel T-cell line derived from adult T-cell leukemia. *Gann* 71:155, 1980.
16 Reitz MS Jr et al: Characterization and distribution of nucleic acid sequence of a novel type-C retrovirus isolated from neoplastic human T-lymphocytes. *Proc Nat Acad Sci USA* 78:1887, 1981.
17 Lee TH et al: Antigens encoded by the 3′ terminal region of human T-cell leukemia virus. *Science* 226:57, 1984.
18 Sodroski et al: The human T-cell leukemia virus x-*lor* region encodes a transcriptional activator protein. *Science* 228:1430, 1985.
19 Gallo R et al: HIV/HTLV gene nomenclature. *Nature* 333:504, 1988.
20 Tsudo et al: Failure of regulation of Tac antigen/TCGF receptor on adult T-cell leukemia cells by anti-Tac monoclonal antibody. *Blood* 61(5):1014, 1983.
21 Sugamura K et al: Human retrovirus-induced IL-2 receptors and their possible role in transduction of continuous cell growth signal. *Int Symp Princess Takamatsu Cancer Res Fund* 15:269, 1984.
22. Teshigawara K et al: Adult T leukemia cells produce a lymphokine that augments interleukin 2 receptor expression. *J Mol Cell Immunol* 2:17, 1985.
23 Kalyanaraman VS et al: A new subtype of human T-cell leukemia virus (HTLV-II) associated with a T-cell variant of hairy cell leukemia. *Science* 218:571, 1982.
24 Gelmann EP et al: Molecular cloning of a new unique human T-leukemia virus (HTLV-$II_{mo}$). *Proc Natl Acad Sci USA* 81:933, 1984.
25 Lee TH et al: Human T-cell leukemia virus specific antigens. *Int Symp Princess Takamatsu Cancer Res Fund* 15:197, 1985.
26 Lee TH et al: Serologic cross-reactivity between envelope gene products of type I and type II human T-cell leukemia virus. *Proc Natl Acad Sci USA* 81:7579, 1984.
27 Sodroski J et al: Sequence of the envelope glycoprotein gene of type II human T lymphotropic virus. *Science* 225:421, 1984.
28 Robert-Guroff M et al: Prevalence of antibodies to HTLV-I, -II, and -III in intravenous drug abusers from an AIDS endemic region. *JAMA* 225(22):3133, 1986.
29 Catovsky D et al: Adult T-cell lymphoma-leukemia in blacks from the West Indies. *Lancet I*:639,1982.
30 Hunsmann G et al: Antibodies to ATLV/HTLV-1 in Africa. *Med Microbiol Immunol* 173:167, 1984.
31 Saxinger et al: Human T-cell leukemia virus (HTLV-1) antibodies in Africa. *Science* 225:1473, 1984.
32 Blayney DW et al: The human T-cell leukemia-lymphoma virus in the southeastern United States. *JAMA* 250:1048, 1983.
33 Robert-Guroff M et al: Seroepidemiologic studies on human T-cell leukemia/lymphoma virus, type I, in *Human T-Cell Leukemia/Lymphoma Virus*, RC Gallo et al (eds). Cold Spring Harbor, Cold Spring Harbor Press, p 285, 1984.
34 Mansari V et al: Human T-cell leukemia/lymphoma virus (HTLV-I) DNA: Detection in Italy in a lymphoma and in a Kaposi sarcoma patient. *Int J Cancer* 34:891, 1984.
35 Robert-Guroff M et al: Prevalence of HTLV-I in arctic regions. *Int J Cancer* 36:651, 1985.
36 Hinuma Y et al: Adult T-cell leukemia: Antigen in an ATL cell line and detection of antibodies to the antigen in human sera. *Proc Natl Acad Sci USA* 78:6476, 1981.
37 Okochi K, Sato H: A retrospective study on transmission of adult T-cell leukemia virus by blood transfusion: Seroconversion in recipient. *Vox Sang* 46:245, 1984.
38 Teddler RS et al: Low prevalence in the UK of HTLV-I and HTLV-II infection in subjects with AIDS, with extended lymphadenopathy, and at risk of AIDS. *Lancet II*:125, 1984.
39 Gradilone A et al: HTLV-I and HIV infection in drug addicts in Italy. *Lancet* II:753, 1986.
40 Blattner WA et al: HTLV: Epidemiology and relationship to disease. *Int Symp Princess Takamatsu Cancer Res Fund* 15:93, 1985.
41 Nakano S et al: Search for possible routes of vertical and horizontal transmission of adult T-cell leukemia virus. *Gann* 75:1044, 1984.
42 Kajiyama W et al: Intrafamilial transmission of adult T-cell leukemia virus. *J Infect Dis* 154:851, 1986.
43 Essex M et al: Seroepidemiology of human T-cell leukemia virus in relation to immunosuppression and the acquired immunodeficiency syndrome, in *Human T-cell Leukemia/Lymphoma Viruses*, RG Gallo et al (eds). Cold Spring Harbor, Cold Spring Harbor Press, 335, 1984.
44 Tajima K et al: Epidemiological analysis of the distribution of antibody to adult T-cell leukemia-virus-associated antigen: Possible horizontal transmission of adult T-cell leukemia virus. *Gann* 73:893, 1982.
45 Kondo T et al: Risk of adult T-cell leukemia/lymphoma in HTLV-I carriers. *Lancet II*:159, 1987.
46 Komuro A et al: Vertical transmission of adult T-cell leukemia virus. *Lancet I*:240, 1983.
47 Hirose S et al: Milk-borne transmission of human T-cell leukemia virus type I in rabbits. *Virology* 162(2):487, 1988.
48 Tajima K, Kuroishi T: Estimation of rate of incidence of ATL among ATLV (HTLV-I) carriers in Kyushu. *Jpn J Clin Oncol* 15(2):423, 1985.
49 Yamaguchi K et al: Proposal for smoldering adult T-cell leukemia (smoldering ATL): A clinicopathologic study of 5 cases. *Blood* 62: 758, 1983.

50 Winckler LA, Bunn PA: Cutaneous T-cell lymphoma: a review. *Hematology* I:49, 1983.
51 Hanaoka M: Progress in adult T-cell leukemia research. *Acta Pathol Jpn* 32(suppl 1):171, 1982.
52 Takasuki K et al: Clinical aspects of adult T-cell leukemia/lymphoma (ATL). *Int Symp Princess Takamatsu Cancer Res Fund* 15:51, 1985.
53 Gibbs WN et al: Adult T-cell leukemial lymphoma in Jamaica and its relationship to human T-cell leukemia/lymphoma virus type I associated lymphoproliferative disease, in *Retroviruses in Human Lymphoma/Leukemia*, M Miwa et al (eds). Utrecht, Tokyo/VNU Science Press, p 77, 1985.
54 Tamura K et al: Clinical analysis of 33 patients with adult T-cell leukemia (ATL)-diagnostic criteria and significance of high-and-low-risk ATL. *Int J Cancer* 37:335, 1986.
55 Jaffe ES et al: The pathologic spectrum of adult T-cell leukemia/lymphoma in the United States. *Am J Surg Pathol* 8(4):263, 1984.
56 Reichel H et al: 25-Hydroxyvitamin D3 metabolism by human T-lymphotropic virus-transformed lymphocytes. *J Clin Endocrinol Metabol* 65(3):519, 1987.
57 Blattner WA et al: Human T-cell leukemia/lymphoma virus associated lymphoreticular neoplasia in Jamaica. *Lancet II*:61, 1983.
58 Fleming AF: The epidemiology of lymphomas and leukaemias in Africa. An overview. *Leukemia Res* 9:735, 1985.
59 Clark JW et al: Molecular and immunologic analysis of a chronic lymphocytic leukemia virus. *Cancer* 56(3):495, 1985.
60 Blayney DW et al: The human T-cell leukemia/lymphoma virus associated with American adult T-cell leukemia/lymphoma. *Blood* 62(2):401, 1983.
61 Bunn PA et al: Clinical course of retrovirus-associated adult T-cell lymphoma in the United States. *N Engl J Med* 309:257, 1983.
62 Nakada K et al: Monoclonal integration of HTLV-I proviral DNA in patients with stronglyoidiasis. *Int J Cancer* 40:145, 1987.
63 Miyoshi I: AIDS-like opportunistic infections in HTLV-I carriers. Presented at ARC International Symposium on Viruses and Cancer, Martinique, Jan 8–10, 1986.
64 Kobayashi M et al: HTLV-positive T-cell lymphoma/leukemia in an AIDS patient. *Lancet I*:1361, 1984.
65 Popovic M et al: Alteration of T-cell functions by infection with HTLV-I or HTLV-II. *Science* 226:459, 1984.
66 Yamada Y et al: Phenotypic and functional analysis of leukemic cells from 16 patients with adult T-cell leukemia/lymphoma. *Blood* 61: 192, 1983.
67 Katusuki T et al: Immune suppression in healthy carriers of adult T-cell leukemia retrovirus (HTLV-I): Impairment of T-cell control of Epstein-Barr virus-infected B-cells. *Jpn J Cancer Res* 78(7):639, 1987.
68 Bartholomew C et al: Progression to AIDS in homosexual men coinfected with HIV and HTLV-I in Trinidad. *Lancet* II: 1469, 1987.
69 Harper M et al: Concomitant infection with HTLV-I and HTLV-III in a patient with T8 lymphoproliferative disease. *N Engl J Med* 315:1073, 1986.
70 De Rossi A et al: Differential response to cytopathic effects of human T-lymphotropic virus type-III (HTLV-III) superinfection in T4 (helper) and T8 (suppressor) T-cell clones transformed by HTLV-I. *Proc Natl Acad Sci USA* 83:4927, 1986.
71 Siekevitz M et al: Activation of the HIV-I LTR by T cell mitogens and the trans-activator protein of HTLV-I. *Science* 238:1575, 1987.
72 Gessain A et al: Antibodies to human T-lymphotropic virus type-I in patients with tropical spastic paraparesis. *Lancet II*:407, 1985.
73 Osame M et al: HTLV-I-associated myelopathy, a new clinical entity. *Lancet I*:1031, 1986.
74 Osame M et al: Chronic progressive myelopathy associated with elevated antibodies to human T-lymphotropic virus type I and adult T-cell leukemialike cells. *Ann Neurol* 22(2):117, 1987.
75 Vernant JC et al: Endemic tropical spastic paraparesis associated with human T-lymphotropic virus type I: A clinical and seroepidemiological study of 25 cases. *Ann Neurol* 21:123, 1987.
76 Román GC: The neuroepidemiology of tropical spastic paraparesis. *Ann Neurol* 23(suppl):S113, 1988.
77 Román GC, Osame M: Identity of HTLV-I-associated tropical spastic paraparesis and HTLV-I-associated myelopathy. *Lancet I*:651, 1988.
78 Itoyama Y et al: Altered subsets of peripheral blood lymphocytes in patients with HTLV-I associated myelopathy (HAM). *Neurology* 38:816, 1988.
79 Hatlori T et al: Surface phenotype of Japanese adult T-cell leukemia cells characterized by monoclonal antibodies. *Blood* 58:645, 1981.
80 McArthur JC: Neurologic manifestations of AIDS. *Medicine* 66(6):407, 1987.
81 Lee TH et al: Antigens expressed by human T-cell leukemia virus-transformed cells, in *Human T-Cell Leukemia Virus*, RC Gallo et al (eds). Cold Spring Harbor, Cold Spring Harbor Press, p 111, 1984.
82 Chosa T et al: Analysis of anti-HTLV-I antibody by strip radioimmunoassay, immunosorbent assay and membrane immunofluorescence assay. *Leuk Res* 10:605, 1986.
83 Weiss SH: Laboratory detection of human immunodeficiency viruses, in *AIDS and Other Manifestations of HIV Infection*, GP Wormer et al (eds). Park Ridge, NJ, Noyes Publications, p 270, 1987.
84 Fang CT et al: Detection of antibodies to human T-lymphotropic virus type I (HTLV-1). *Transfusion* 28(2):179, 1988.
85 Williams AE et al: Seroprevalence and epidemiological correlates of HTLV-I infection in US blood donors. *Science* 240:643, 1988.
86 Duggan D et al: HTLV-I-induced lymphoma mimicking Hodgkin's disease. Diagnosis by polymerase chain reaction amplification of specific HTLV-I sequences in tumor DNA. *Blood* 71(4):1027, 1988.
87 Abbott M et al: Enzymatic gene amplification: Qualitative and quantitative methods for detecting proviral DNA amplified in vitro. *J Inf Dis* 158(6):1158, 1988.
88 Matsushita S et al: Pharmacological inhibition of in vitro infectivity of human T lymphotropic virus type-I. *J Clin Invest* 80(2):394, 1987.
89 Nakamura H et al: Protection of cynomologus monkeys against infection by human T-cell leukemia virus type-I by immunization with viral *env* gene products produced in *Escherichia coli. Int J Cancer* 40(3):403, 1987.

# Chapter 34
# Biology of the herpesviruses

Patricia G. Spear

A few key characteristics differentiate the herpesviruses from other viruses. The genome is a linear, double-stranded DNA ranging in size from 125,000 to 250,000 base pairs. The virion is composed of the DNA-containing core; an icosahedral capsid, which is about 100 nm in diameter and exhibits in the electron microscope exactly 162 morphological units, or capsomeres, on its surface; and an outer lipid-containing membrane or envelope. Herpesviruses use both the nucleus and the cytoplasm of the host cell for their replication.

Six different human herpesviruses have been recognized to date, including herpes simplex viruses types 1 and 2 (HSV-1 and HSV-2), varicella-zoster virus (VZV), Epstein-Barr virus (EBV), cytomegalovirus (CMV) (see Chap. 36), and the recently discovered[1–3] human herpesvirus 6 (HHV-6). All are marvelously well adapted to their natural host, being endemic in all human populations and carried by a significant number of individuals in each population. Each of the human herpesviruses appears to be more closely related to biologically similar herpesviruses of animals than to each other (excepting the close relationship between HSV-1 and HSV-2).

The pathology and epidemiology of herpesvirus infections depend not only on viral replication and associated cytotoxicity but also on the capacity of herpesviruses to establish latent infections, and subsequently to be activated from the latent state. The term *productive infection* will be used here to describe, at the cell level, an infection in which the invading virus replicates to yield progeny virus and the cell is killed. *Latent infection* or *latency* means that the genome of the invading virus is stably maintained by the cell (in the cell nucleus) with only limited expression of viral genes, no production of progeny virus, and no evident virus-induced cytotoxicity. Latent infections can be converted to productive infections by factors and stimuli that have not yet been clearly defined, resulting in reactivation of virus replication, possibly at levels sufficient to cause clinical symptoms. An important feature of disease caused by HSV in particular, and VZV to a lesser extent, is recurrence of lesions due to periodic or sporadic reactivation of latent virus.

Although this chapter will focus primarily on HSV, other human and animal herpesviruses will be mentioned when comparisons are informative. The power of comparative studies has been enhanced by the availability of complete genomic nucleotide sequences,[4–6] which permit identification of many conserved genes and also of apparently unrelated genes encoded by different herpesviruses.

## HISTORY AND TAXONOMY

Cutaneous lesions resulting from herpesvirus infections were known to be caused by transmissible agents (see Chap. 35) before viruses were recognized or defined in present-day terms. When it was established that nucleic acid is the genetic material and with development of the electron microscope, both events occurring in the 1940s, it became possible to develop reliable criteria for the classification of viruses.[7,8] The classification of viruses depends principally on structural features of the virion (extracellular infectious particle) and on properties of the viral genome.

HSV was one of the first viruses to be examined in the electron microscope by the then newly developed technique of negative staining. Wildy et al.[9] deduced from their photographs that the virion consists of a core, capsid, and envelope and that the capsid has icosahedral symmetry and 162 capsomers on its surface. Russell[10] first demonstrated unequivocally that the genome of HSV is DNA. Estimates of genome size changed over the years (from smaller to larger values) as methods for isolation of the DNA improved. We now know from nucleotide sequence analysis[6] that the size of the HSV-1 genome is of the order of 152,260 base pairs.

The genomes of the various herpesviruses are clearly evolutionarily related but differ in size, in organization of unique and repeated sequences, and in gene content and order. To illustrate these points, Fig. 34-1 shows maps of three herpesvirus genomes with the locations of repeated sequences and of a subset of viral genes (those encoding glycoproteins).

Available information indicates that a single map suffices for HSV-1 and HSV-2, although some homologous open reading frames or noncoding regions may differ in length because of insertions or deletions of genetic information. The order of homologous genes on the HSV and VZV genomes is for the most part colinear; moreover, very few genes are found in one genome and not the other, and vice versa.[6,11] On the other hand, comparison of the HSV or VZV genome with the EBV genome (or the CMV genome not shown) reveals only small blocks of colinear homologous genes, due in part to differences in gene order.[6,12,13] Divergence of the herpesviruses has been accompanied by rearrangements of the genomes (inversions, translocations, etc.), as well as by divergence of individual genes and distinctive additions or deletions of genetic information.

A classification of the herpesviruses made primarily on the basis of biological properties[14] is concordant with evolutionary inferences that can be drawn from nucleotide sequence analyses. Both HSV and VZV were assigned to the subfamily Alphaherpesvirinae, CMV to the subfamily Betaherpesvirinae, and EBV to the subfamily Gammaherpesvirinae.

In the 1950s, with the development of methods to propagate cells and viruses in culture and to quantitate viruses by plaque assay, it became possible to study the biochemistry and molecular biology of viral replication in cell culture. The first plaque assay for HSV was described in 1957,[15] and studies of HSV replication and gene expression in cultured cells have proceeded at an accelerating pace since then. Armed with information about the interactions of HSV with cultured cells, investigators are beginning to use the powerful tools now available (including in situ hybridization and immunocytochemistry) to probe the interactions of HSV with the cells of organized tissues obtained from infected animals and humans. We can expect a wealth of new findings relevant to pathogenesis and immune responses in the near future.

## MOLECULAR EPIDEMIOLOGY

The diseases caused by herpesviruses are endemic. Transmission of infection usually requires intimate contact between individuals. Often, the transmitting party is an asymptomatic shedder of in-

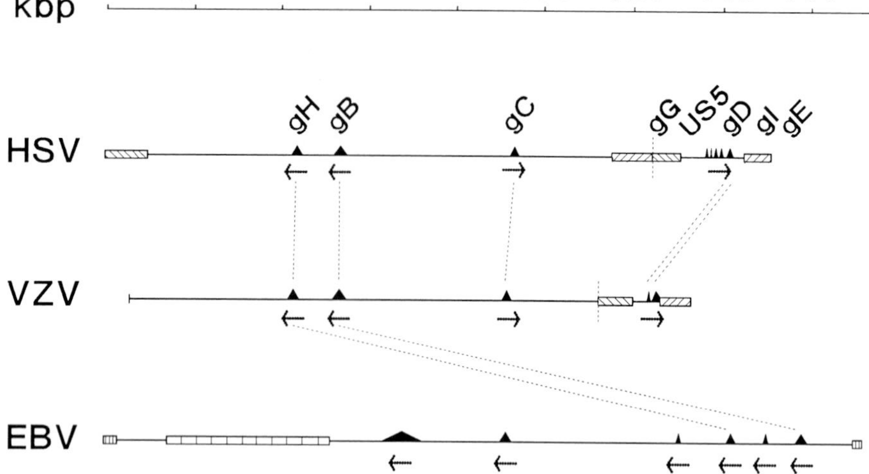


**Fig. 34-1.** The genomes of three human herpesviruses, HSV, VZV, and EBV, showing the positions of repeated sequences and of selected genes. The scale of these maps is in thousands of base pairs (kbp). The hatched boxes on the HSV and VZV maps represent repeated sequences present in two copies with inverted orientation. The open boxes on the EBV genome represent multiple repeated sequences all in the same orientation. The filled pyramids mark the locations of genes encoding membrane glycoproteins. Both VZV and EBV encode glycoproteins homologous to HSV gB and gH, as indicated by the dashed lines. In addition, VZV encodes glycoproteins homologous to HSV gC, gI, and gE. Any other evolutionary relationships that may exist among the glycoproteins encoded by these three viruses are not readily evident from primary sequence analysis. The HSV genes are for the most part colinear with related VZV genes, whereas related EBV genes have a different order. The VZV glycoproteins are designated, in order from left to right, gpIII, gpII, gpV, gpIV, and gpI. The EBV glycoproteins (two of which have not yet been detected or characterized and are therefore called by the names of open reading frames) are designated BPLF1, gp350/220, gp35, gp85, BILF2, and gp110. These maps are based largely on the nucleotide sequence analyses of Baer et al.,[4] Davison and Scott,[5] and McGeoch et al.[6]

fectious virus. Sexually transmitted forms of disease are important but are not the only forms of disease caused by HSV. CMV can also be sexually transmitted (see Chap. 36).

It was recognized in the 1960s that there are two distinct serovars of HSV.[16,17] Moreover, it was noted that type 1 (HSV-1) strains were usually isolated from labial, facial, and ocular lesions and from brain lesions in encephalitis, whereas type 2 (HSV-2) strains were usually isolated from genital lesions and from tissues of newborn infants who became infected during delivery through an infected birth canal.[18]

It is clear that HSV-1 and HSV-2 are closely related to one another. Although a complete sequence of the HSV-2 genome has not yet been reported, it is likely that every HSV-1 gene has a homologue encoded by HSV-2, and vice versa, and that all homologous genes occupy identical positions on each genome. Genetic recombination between HSV-1 and HSV-2 readily occurs, and the recombinants are viable, although they may be less virulent in animals than either parental strain. It is also clear that HSV-1 and HSV-2 have evolved separately and diverged somewhat during the recent past (recent in relation to the time scale for divergence of the other human herpesviruses). Certain of the HSV-1 genes, for example, encode larger or smaller proteins than the homologous HSV-2 genes, because of type-specific insertions or deletions of genetic information within the coding sequences.[19]

Strains belonging to a single HSV serotype also exhibit genetic variation, although of a lower order than that found between strains of different serotype (see Chap. 77). The biology of the herpesviruses favors the generation and maintenance of a certain amount of genetic diversity, consistent with maintenance of function, among the viruses circulating within a human population at any given time. Every infected individual is a long-term carrier of virus and may produce and shed virus periodically or continuously over a period of years in the face of pressures applied by protective immune responses. Moreover, the virus strain transmitted among members of a particular family may have a totally different lineage, traceable through generations of humans, than the virus strain transmitted among members of the family next door, assuming only a nodding acquaintance between members of the two families.

It is not surprising, therefore, that restriction endonuclease polymorphisms are easily detectable among epidemiologically unrelated strains of HSV.[20] Use of as few as four or five endonucleases that cut the genome at 10 to 20 sites is usually sufficient to differentiate between two HSV strains, of the same or different serotype, isolated from any two individuals who are unacquainted. Conversely, virus isolates obtained sequentially from a single individual or from known contacts exhibit no easily detectable restriction endonuclease polymorphisms. This has made it possible to trace the sources of infections occurring in clusters, such as in a nosocomial outbreak.[21] It remains to be determined whether or how these genetic differences observed among HSV strains influence biological activity or virulence of the strains.

## MOLECULAR BIOLOGY OF VIRAL REPLICATION AND LATENCY

Despite the fact that HSV infections outside the laboratory are, for the most part, limited to humans, the virus has an extremely broad host range. Just as many animal species can be experimentally infected with HSV, many types and species of cultured cells will support HSV replication. On the other hand, the other human herpesviruses have a much more limited host range, are fastidious about the cell types in which they will replicate, and, in general, are much more difficult to propagate in cell culture. Consequently, the molecular details of viral replication are more completely understood for HSV than for the other human herpesviruses.

## VIRAL REPLICATION

### Entry of virus into the cell

Viral replication starts with adsorption of virus to a susceptible cell. Viral glycoproteins in the virion envelope bind to components of the cell surface in a cascade of interactions that culminates in penetration of the nucleocapsid into the cell cytoplasm. At least for HSV, this penetration can be effected by fusion of the virion envelope with the plasma membrane of the cell;[22,23] endocytosis of the virion is not required.

There are at least seven virus-encoded glycoproteins in the virion envelope of HSV and perhaps eight (an eighth open reading frame that could encode a membrane glycoprotein has been identified).[19,24] At least three of these glycoproteins, designated gB, gD, and gH, are essential for infectivity because appropriate mutations in any one can render the virion noninfectious.[25–28] The other four glycoproteins (gC, gE, gG, and gI) may not be essential under all conditions for infectivity. Deletions of the genes encoding these glycoproteins do not eliminate infectivity,[29–31] at least in cell culture, although adsorption or penetration could be somewhat less efficient than with wild-type virus.

It is important to know how all these glycoproteins are organized in the virion envelope in order to understand how they function in infectivity. Only limited information is available at present. Studies of the solubilized glycoproteins have failed to reveal any multimeric units except homodimers of gB.[32,33] Electron microscopy of virions labeled with gold-tagged antibodies (Fig. 34-2) has permitted the demonstration that three of the glycoproteins (gB, gC, and gD) constitute three morphologically distinct spikes projecting from the virion envelope.[34]

Recent evidence demonstrates that the initial cell surface receptor for HSV-1 and HSV-2 is heparan sulfate,[35] which is related in structure to heparin and is a major glycosaminoglycan moiety of ubiquitous cell surface proteoglycans. Both gB and gC are heparin-binding proteins (gC probably makes the first contact with the cell surface), and either glycoprotein, acting independently, can mediate the initial adsorption of virus to cells (D. WuDunn et al., unpublished studies). Following this initial adsorption, gB, gD, and gH must interact with other, as yet unidentified, cell surface components so as to induce membrane fusion. This hypothesis is based on a number of observations, including the following: (1) Virions devoid of gB or gD can bind to cells but cannot penetrate;[26,27] (2) monoclonal antibodies specific for gB, gD, or gH can neutralize infectivity by blocking penetration without having any effect on adsorption;[23,36,37,37a] (3) transformed cells that express gD are resistant to HSV infection; virus can adsorb to the cells but penetration does not occur.[38,39] This latter observation suggests that gD expressed by the cell may somehow tie up a cell surface component normally required for interaction with gD in virions during penetration.

It is evident from the foregoing that the molecular events required for HSV entry into a cell are complex and involve multiple virion components and probably also multiple cell surface components, including heparan sulfate. It seems likely that entry of other herpesviruses is also a complex process, involving different sets of cell surface components for each virus.

In only one other instance has a cell surface receptor for a herpesvirus been identified. Adsorption of EBV to B lymphocytes is mediated at least in part by binding of the virion glycoprotein gp350/220 to CR2,[40,41] a receptor for the C3d component of complement. It is of interest that EBV gp350/220 binds to a complement receptor and that HSV gC mimics a complement receptor. HSV gC binds to the C3b component of complement and can accelerate decay of C3b.[42,43] These two viral glycoproteins could be evolutionarily related although the degree of primary sequence homology is weak and limited.

Suggestive results pertaining to interactions of CMV with cells have been reported. First, one of the CMV glycoproteins has surprising similarity in sequence to human class I major histocompatibility complex (MHC) antigens.[44] Second, $\beta_2$-microglob-

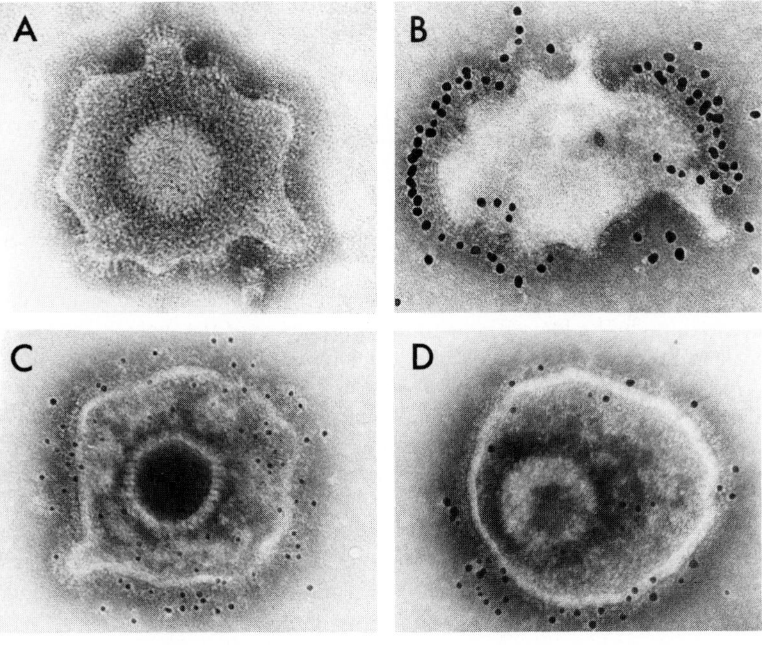


**Fig. 34-2.** Electron micrographs of negatively stained HSV, showing different kinds of spikes projecting from the virion envelope. The most prominent spikes are composed of gB, as shown by the decoration of these spikes with gold-labeled anti-gB (*B*). Similarly, long slender structures, difficult to resolve, are gC (*C*), and some of the short fuzzlike structures are gD (*D*). Similar figures were published by Stannard et al.[34] (*Courtesy of LM Stannard.*)

ulin, the invariant chain of class I MHC antigens, binds to virions and enhances infectivity of the virions, leading the authors to suggest that adsorption of virus to cells is mediated by the $\beta_2$-microglobulin.[45]

## Intracellular synthesis of viral components

Once the nucleocapsid enters the cytoplasm of the cell, the genome is released and delivered to the nucleus. There the viral genes are transcribed by cell polymerase II under control of viral regulatory components, some of which are brought into the cell along with the genome.[46] Only a limited subset of the viral genes can be transcribed at first—the immediate-early, or $\alpha$, genes, which encode mostly regulatory proteins. Optimal transcription of the $\alpha$ genes requires the activity of a viral regulatory protein called $\alpha$-TIF or VP16.[47–49] This viral regulatory protein is a virion constituent localized between the capsid and the envelope and is one of the important viral proteins that is delivered to the cell along with the viral genome.

Once the $\alpha$ genes have been transcribed and translated into the $\alpha$-proteins, one or more of these proteins enables the next wave of transcription for expression of the early, or $\beta$, genes. The $\beta$ genes encode enzymes and other proteins required for viral DNA replication, including thymidine kinase and DNA polymerase (both important targets of currently used antiviral drugs). Following $\alpha$- and $\beta$-gene expression and DNA replication, the late, or $\gamma$, genes can be expressed to produce most of the virion proteins and glycoproteins.

Herpesviruses and certain other DNA viruses have provided excellent experimental systems for the study of eukaryotic gene expression and its regulation, in part because these viruses use the cell machinery for transcription and processing of transcripts to yield functional mRNAs. The virus superimposes on this cell machinery its own regulatory factors which aid in targeting cell transcription factors to virus-specific nucleotide sequences. Interestingly, herpesviruses differ from other DNA viruses and from the cell in that most herpesvirus genes expressed during productive infection are free of introns (intervening sequences that are removed from RNA transcripts by splicing to yield the functional mRNAs).[50] The significance of this is not yet understood.

After synthesis of the HSV proteins in the cytoplasm, most of the proteins are transported to the nucleus, where they serve as regulatory factors, enzymes involved in DNA replication, or structural components of the nucleocapsid. Viral glycoproteins are made on membrane-bound ribosomes and become distributed to all the membranes of the cell except the mitochondrial membranes.

## Assembly and egress of virions

Nucleocapsids are assembled in the nucleus of the cell and acquire an envelope by budding through modified patches of the inner nuclear membrane that presumably contain viral glycoproteins. Virions can be observed in the perinuclear space and in cytoplasmic vesicles. Evidence has been presented that egress of HSV virions is by way of the Golgi apparatus and transport vesicles normally involved in secretion.[51] The finding that expression of gD in transformed cells renders the cells resistant to penetration by HSV[38,39] suggests a role for gD in egress of virions from cells (in addition to its role in virion infectivity). Specifically, expression of gD in membranes of the infected cell may permit progeny virions to exit the cell without penetrating into the cytoplasm from cytoplasmic vesicles or the cell surface.

There is some uncertainty whether the process of envelopment and egress described above applies to all herpesviruses. With herpesviruses such as VZV, with which production of cell-free virus is not nearly so efficient as with HSV, progeny nucleocapsids can be detected in the cytoplasm and may appear to be budding through a cytoplasmic membrane. It has been proposed that nucleocapsids may somehow get to the cytoplasm and then be enveloped by budding through a cytoplasmic membrane into a vesicle.[52] Alternatively, what appears to be envelopment at a cytoplasmic membrane may actually be deenvelopment resulting from fusion of progeny virions with a cytoplasmic membrane. Because of absence of a mechanism to prevent such fusion, there would be significant loss of progeny from the infectious yield of the infected cell.

## Fate of the cell that produces virus

Herpesviruses kill the cells in which they replicate. For HSV at least, inhibition of cell functions starts with entry of the nucleocapsid into the cell. A viral gene product introduced into the cell along with the nucleocapsid somehow causes degradation of preexisting cytoplasmic mRNAs such that cell protein synthesis is immediately inhibited.[53] Other viral factors produced after infection inhibit or alter various host functions, including DNA replication and RNA processing. For the most part, the viral inhibitory factors have not been identified or characterized.

# THE LATENT STATE

The ability of herpesviruses to persist for life in their natural hosts depends in large part on their ability to establish latent infections. As mentioned above, the latent state is one in which the viral genome is stably maintained in the cell nucleus with expression of only a limited subset of viral genes. The latently infected cell is not killed by the virus; viral gene products expressed may even stimulate cell division. Virions or infectious virus cannot be recovered from latently infected tissue immediately after its removal from an experimental animal or human cadaver, but reactivation of latent virus to the replicating state, yielding infectious virus, can often be achieved by in vitro cultivation of the explanted tissue.

Limited information about the state and expression of herpesvirus genomes in latency is available, principally for HSV in neurons and for EBV in B lymphocytes. In both cases the target cell is ordinarily in a nondividing state. EBV induces proliferation of the latently infected B cells, causing cell division even in the absence of antigenic stimulation. HSV is not known to induce the proliferation of latently infected cells. This apparent difference between cells latently infected with EBV and those latently infected with HSV may in part account for the observed differences in viral gene expression during latency, as described below.

Available information about HSV latency has come principally from in vivo studies, in part because it is not certain that the authentic latent state has yet been established or maintained in cultured cells. Evidence has been presented that the HSV genomes present in sensory ganglia of latently infected mice and humans are probably episomal and circular,[54–56] in contrast to virion-associated genomes, which are linear. Analyses of both animal and human tissues revealed the presence in latently infected cells of transcripts from one specific region of the viral genome[57–67] (Figs. 34-3 and 34-4). The transcripts detected, called the latency-associated transcripts (LATs), have some unusual properties. They are transcribed from the DNA strand opposite that encoding one of the immediate-early or α proteins, the one designated ICP0 or IE110. The transcripts contain relatively little poly(A) and appear to be retained in the nucleus of the cell. Two different spliced forms of the same transcription product have been detected.[68,69] There are open reading frames that could be translated, but no evidence has yet been obtained that the RNA serves as mRNA. Small amounts of this RNA are made during productive infection of cultured cells, but apparently only one form which may not be spliced. This RNA product made during productive infection cannot be classified as an α-, β-, or γ-gene product; it belongs to a unique kinetic class.[70]

Studies with a viral mutant unable to produce LATs have revealed that the LATs are not absolutely essential for the establishment of latency in experimental animals, or for the reactivation of latent virus.[71] This is very puzzling inasmuch as LAT expression is clearly a good marker for the latent state induced by wild-type virus. Intense efforts are currently directed at investigating the role of LAT in HSV latency and in identifying any other viral genes that may be expressed. Results obtained by in situ hybridization suggest that a region of the viral genome just downstream of that encoding the LAT may also be expressed in latently infected cells,[60,61,67]

This work may be facilitated by experimental systems being developed for the investigation of HSV latency in cultured cells. Infection of neurons with HSV in vitro usually results in productive infection and death of the cells. Recently, however, it was shown that infection of cultured neurons in the presence of nerve growth factor resulted in a nonproductive interaction of virus with a fraction of the cells. Removal of nerve growth factor then activated viral replication.[72,73] This system shows great promise for characterization of the state and expression of the HSV genomes associated with the cells. Other experimental systems have been developed in which nonneuronal cells are nonproductively infected with virus by use of inhibitors and supraoptimal temperatures.[74–76] For all these experimental systems, it remains to be seen whether the state of latency obtained is similar to that which occurs in vivo.

Viral genome maintenance and expression in the latent state are better understood for EBV[77] than for any other herpesvirus, in large part because latently infected B lymphocytes can be isolated from humans and propagated in vitro without induction of virus production. The EBV genome in latently infected cells exists as covalently closed circular episomes. A specific mechanism may exist to join the ends through direct repeat sequences found at

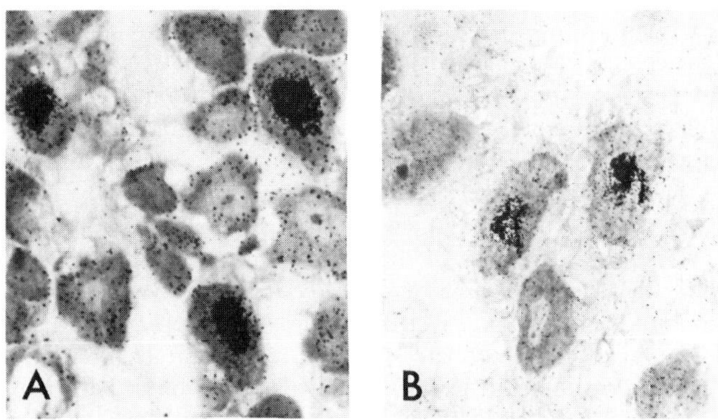


**Fig. 34-3.** Detection of HSV-1 latency-associated transcripts (LATs) in neurons of peripheral ganglia by in situ hybridization and autoradiography. The black autoradiographic grains are localized over nuclei of some of the neurons in mouse tissue (*A*) and human tissue (*B*) taken from latently infected subjects. Experimental details are given in publications by Stevens et al.[57,65] (*Courtesy of JG Stevens.*)

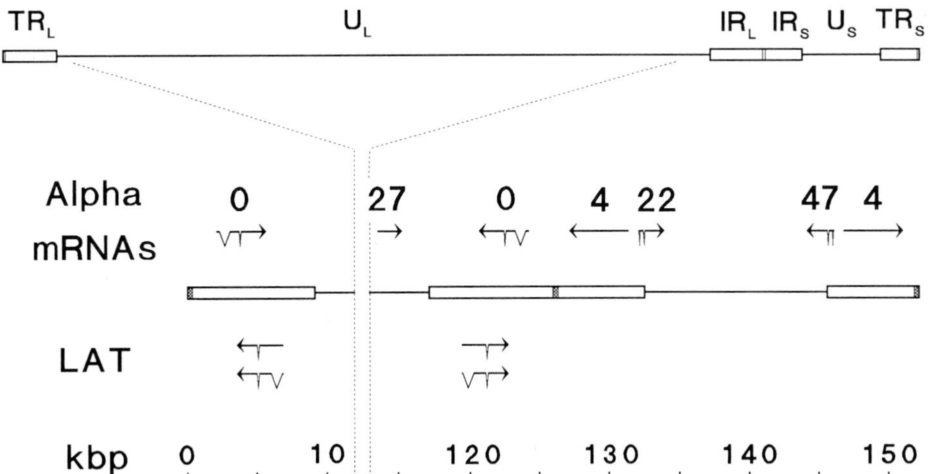


**Fig. 34-4.** RNAs transcribed from selected regions of the HSV genome. At top is a representation of the entire HSV genome, showing the positions of unique ($U_L$, $U_S$) and repeated sequences ($TR_L$ and $IR_L$ are inverted repeats, as are $IR_S$ and $TR_S$). In the middle is shown an expanded representation of the repeated sequences and adjacent unique sequences. The immediate-early or α, genes are transcribed first during virus replication, followed by the transcription of all other viral genes. The products encoded by α-mRNAs are designated ICP0 (or IE110), ICP27 (or IE63), ICP4 (or IE175), ICP22 (or IE68), and ICP47 (or IE12). In latently infected cells, only the latency-associated transcripts (LATs) have been detected to date. It is not known whether these transcripts serve as mRNAs. Direction of transcription is indicated for each RNA as well as the positions of introns spliced out. The scale is in thousands of base pairs (kbp). (*Drawn from information published by McGeoch et al.*[6] *and Wechsler et al.*[68])

each end. The EBV genome persists in multiple copies per cell nucleus and is replicated in concert with cell DNA. Cell polymerase catalyzes the replication of the viral genomes in latently infected cells whereas viral polymerase does so during productive infection.

The only EBV gene products expressed in the latent state include several nuclear proteins and a couple of membrane-associated proteins.[77] One of the nuclear proteins interacts with a viral origin of DNA replication, directing cell polymerase where to initiate replication.[78] The other nuclear proteins and the membrane proteins are probably required for immortalization of the lymphocytes. Latently infected B lymphocytes differ phenotypically from uninfected B lymphocytes in that the former can replicate indefinitely without antigenic stimulus.

## PATHOGENESIS

### SEROTYPE-SPECIFIC ASPECTS OF DISEASE

It is difficult to define HSV-1-specific and HSV-2-specific aspects of pathogenicity in human disease, except perhaps for differences in the frequency of recurrent lesions (Chap. 35). Many features of infections caused by HSV-1 and HSV-2 are indistinguishable. Despite the fact that HSV-1 and HSV-2 strains are usually isolated from different anatomic sites, it is clear that strains of either serotype can initiate and establish infection at whatever site they are inoculated. Although encephalitis in adults is almost invariably caused by HSV-1 and meningitis is more frequently associated with genital infections (where HSV-2 isolations are more frequent than HSV-1 isolations) (Chap. 35), it cannot be assumed that intrinsic properties of each serotype solely determine whether encephalitis or meningitis can occur. The anatomic site at which inoculation occurs or the age of the host at the time of exposure at different sites may also be important factors in determining the nature of systemic disease.

The fact remains, however, that HSV-1 and HSV-2 strains differ in a number of ways that can be assessed by analyses of nucleotide and amino acid sequences, by serologic tests, and by tests of pathogenicity in various experimental systems. One way to account for these differences, even if their physiologic significance is not yet evident, is to postulate that HSV-1 and HSV-2 evolved from a common ancestor after establishment of this ancestor in separate ecologic niches (facial/ocular tissues and genital tissues) defined by anatomic site and source of virus for inoculation. If genital infections usually resulted from inoculation with virus shed from genital tissues, and facial infections from facial tissues, then conditions would be right for emergence of the two serotypes with subtle differences in properties dictated by subtle differences in requirements for optimal maintenance within and transmission from the two anatomic sites.

An interesting discussion of HSV-1–HSV-2 divergence relative to changes in primate mating habits has recently been published in the context of analyzing the divergence of several herpesvirus-encoded enzymes.[79] The authors argue that the ancestral virus from which HSV-1 and HSV-2 evolved may have depended in part on oral-genital modes of transmission, as occurs with the B virus of old world monkeys due to self oral-genital contact as well as male-female oral-genital contact. They argue further that adoption by our ancestors of bipedal stance and face-to-face mating posture permitted oral and genital sites to "become microbiologically somewhat isolated from each other," thereby permitting the separate evolution of oral and genital strains of HSV.

### DETERMINANTS OF HSV PATHOGENICITY

#### Cell and tissue tropism

The pattern of tissue and organ damage caused by primary HSV infection and by reactivation of latent virus is in part determined by the types of cells in which the virus can replicate and in which latent infections can occur. Judging from studies of cultured cells and from the nature of disseminated disease in infants and immunocompromised adults, it appears that many human cell types are susceptible to HSV infection and can support viral replication. This is consistent with the finding that heparan sulfate, a ubiquitous cell surface glycosaminoglycan, is the initial receptor for HSV. Conversely, EBV infects few human cell types (B lymphocytes and some epithelial cells) and uses CR2 (a receptor for the complement component C3d) as its initial receptor. The limited distribution of CR2 appears to be a major determinant in the limited host range of EBV.

Despite the ability of HSV to infect many cell types, HSV disease is often localized to the body surface at the site of inoculation and to the sensory ganglia of nerves communicating with this site. Undoubtedly, an effective immune response is in part responsible for limiting the spread of infection. The possibility exists, however, that there are nonimmunologic barriers to the spread of infection in the normal adult. For example, certain cell types in fully differentiated tissues may not be able to support HSV replication, either because of inaccessibility or lack of required cell surface receptors or because of lack of other factors needed for biosynthesis of viral components. With the discovery that cell surface heparan sulfate can be the initial receptor for HSV, it will be important to determine whether precise patterns of sulfation on the repeating disaccharide units are required for HSV adsorption (as is required for the interactions of some heparin-binding proteins with heparan sulfate or heparin). If so, probes for heparan sulfate and for particular sulfation patterns in heparan sulfate can be developed in order to examine human tissues from individuals of different ages for presence or absence of these patterns. In addition, the other cell surface receptors for HSV, and key intracellular components required for HSV replication or latency, must be identified in order that their distribution in fully differentiated and developing tissues can be assessed.

As indicated above, neurons of the peripheral nervous system can harbor latent HSV genomes. Virus presumably gains access to these neurons via the nerve endings located near the site of inoculation where viral replication takes place. The sites at which recurrent mucocutaneous lesions occur are apparently determined by the locations of nerve endings of the neurons from which virus has been reactivated. Although the presence of HSV DNA in human brain tissue has been reported[80] and latent HSV genomes and LATs can be detected regularly in the central nervous system of experimentally infected mice,[54,55,60] it remains to be determined whether presence of HSV genomes in the central nervous system is a regular feature of latent infections in humans. In a recent study,[55] HSV DNA was detected in both the peripheral and central nervous systems of latently infected mice but only in trigeminal ganglia, not brain stems, of HSV-seropositive humans who died of causes unrelated to herpesvirus infection. Clearly, HSV can penetrate to the human central nervous system, as evidenced by the sporadic cases of HSV-induced encephalitis. It is unclear how the virus gets to the brain in these cases and whether there are factors predisposing to encephalitis in addition to HSV infection.

Although attention has focused on the neuron as the cell type harboring latent HSV genomes, recent results obtained with experimental animals indicate that latent virus can also be found, long after recovery from the primary infection, in nonneuronal tissue at the site of inoculation. Specifically, the production of infectious virus was induced by cultivation in vitro of tissues explanted from the footpads[81,82] or corneas[83,84] of latently infected mice, whereas no infectious virus could be detected in these tissues immediately on explant. This has been the accepted operational definition for latency in the past, for example, in earlier studies that identified sensory ganglia as sites of latency. A better operational definition, for the present, may be expression of LATs in the absence of most other viral transcripts (LAT appears to be a good marker for cells latently infected with wild-type virus even if LAT-negative viral mutants retain the ability to establish latency). The possibility that latent HSV genomes could persist in nonneuronal human tissues, particularly in corneas, has important implications. Therefore, additional analyses of animal and human tissues are awaited with great interest, particularly studies designed to identify cell types in addition to neurons that can harbor HSV genomes expressing the LATs.

Latent infections with HSV and with other herpesviruses are problematic because the latent state is relatively unstable. There can be frequent activation of viral replication with or without recurrence of disease, depending on the immune status of the individual as well as on other poorly defined factors.[85] Unfortunately, little is known, in molecular terms, about the mechanism of reactivation of viral replication.

### Immune responses

HSV rarely causes severe disseminated disease in adults, except when cell-mediated immunity is compromised. Among infected (seropositive) individuals who have no known immunologic defects, the responses to infection typically range from no clinical signs and symptoms to localized lesions, sometimes with mild to moderate systemic symptoms, and perhaps followed by periodic recurrences of localized lesions. Virus reactivation and replication probably occur periodically even in asymptomatic individuals, judging from virus isolations and from sustained antibody levels.

Several questions about protective immunity, all of which remain to be adequately answered, are raised by these observations. What accounts for absence of clinical disease in some infected individuals (relative avirulence of the infecting HSV strain, innate resistance of certain cell types, better or different kinds of immune responses to certain antigens, other antiviral mechanisms)? Which antigens induce the immune responses that prevent localized or disseminated disease? What kinds of immune responses are most protective against localized or disseminated disease? Are the protective mechanisms effective against localized disease qualitatively different than those that protect against disseminated disease, or only quantitatively different?

Because deficiencies of cell-mediated immunity, rather than antibody synthesis, are associated with increased incidence of disseminated disease caused by HSV,[86] it seems likely that cell-mediated effector mechanisms are most important for preventing spread of infection. Moreover, recurrent localized herpetic lesions can occur in the face of high antiviral antibody titers. It would probably be a mistake to assume that antibodies are of no importance, however, given the interrelatedness of the various arms of the immune system and the possibilities that antibodies can regulate certain aspects of the immune response as well as act as immediate antimicrobial effectors.

In attempts to identify HSV antigens that can induce protective immunity in experimental animal systems, attention has been focused mostly on the virion envelope glycoproteins. The rationale has been that because these glycoproteins are exposed on the surfaces both of virions and of infected cells, they are most likely to be the targets recognized by antibodies as well as cytotoxic T cells. As it happens, this rationale may be misguided with respect to the requirements for T-cell recognition. For HSV,[87] cytomegalovirus,[88] and other viruses, cytotoxic T cells can recognize and kill cells that express viral proteins not normally displayed on the cell surface, because the T cells actually "see" only peptide fragments of antigen produced by catabolic processes and presented on cell surfaces in association with MHC antigens.[89]

It is therefore difficult to predict which antigens are most important in inducing protective cell-mediated responses. Possibly many of the 70-odd proteins encoded by HSV contribute to the induction of protective immunity, making it difficult to identify a few key immunogens. In experimental animal systems, at least three of the HSV glycoproteins have been isolated and tested as vaccines by a variety of protocols. All were shown to induce protective immunity, and even in some instances to induce protection against establishment of latency.[90–95] Ideally, many isolated viral antigens would be tested by a single protocol, and degree of protection against disease or establishment of latency would be compared with that obtained by immunization with killed or attentuated whole virus. Although this is unlikely to be done on the scale that might be desired, it is hoped that systematic tests of viral glycoproteins and early viral proteins as immunogens will be carried out.

Some of the viral glycoproteins expressed by HSV may not only induce immune responses but also modulate immune effector mechanisms in ways that have not yet been precisely defined. The viral glycoprotein designated gE binds to the Fc region of IgG and is responsible (perhaps along with gI) for the expression of Fc receptors on the surfaces of infected cells.[96–98] The viral glycoprotein gC (mentioned above in the context of its heparin-binding activity and role in viral adsorption) binds to the complement component C3b and is responsible for the expression of C3b receptors on infected cells.[42,99] In the presence of normal aggregated IgG, infected cells are protected somewhat from immune cytolysis.[100] Moreover, interaction of gC with C3b can accelerate decay of this pivotal component in the complement cascade,[43] and virions containing gC appear to be somewhat protected against complement-mediated neutralization.[101] These observations suggest that gE and gC may protect infected cells or virions from damage due to immune effector mechanisms. It remains to be determined, however, whether these activities observed in vitro have relevance in vivo and whether the binding activities of gE and gC might not serve other functions as well. As discussed above, gC participates in the adsorption of virus to cells, at least in part through its heparin-binding activity.

Immune responses to viral antigens can, in some instances, cause as much or more damage in affected tissues as the cytopathology associated with viral replication. This kind of immunopathology appears to be important in some cases of herpetic keratitis, where there is deep stromal damage, but probably does not figure as importantly in other kinds of herpetic lesions or disseminated disease.

## TRANSFORMATION OF CELLS BY HSV

Most, if not all, DNA viruses encode proteins that can stimulate certain cell activities. For example, papillomaviruses and certain of the herpesviruses, such as EBV, induce the proliferation of latently infected cells, overriding normal controls on cell division. The epidermal hyperplasias or warts induced by papillomaviruses and the lymphoproliferation caused by EBV are usually benign proliferations unless immune responses are inadequate or unless secondary factors contribute to the viral-induced transformation to cause malignant transformation of the infected cells.

There is no evidence that HSV induces the proliferation of latently infected cells or that infection with HSV is causally associated with any human malignancy. Early suspicions that HSV might be an etiologic agent of cervical carcinoma were based mostly on seroepidemiologic studies.[102] These suspicions have been lessened, if not laid to rest, by recent findings that papillomavirus DNA, not HSV DNA, can regularly be detected in cervical carcinomas.

Although it has not been ruled out that HSV could be a cofactor in the causation of cervical carcinoma and other tumors, evidence for or against such a role will be difficult to obtain. The reason is that experimental models of HSV transformation have not yielded clues about reliable viral markers in cells putatively transformed by HSV. The introduction of certain fragments of the HSV genome into cells in vitro has been associated with malignant transformation of the cells. In contrast to cells transformed by other DNA viruses, however, it has not been possible to demonstrate that the transformed phenotype required retention of any of the viral DNA or expression of any particular HSV protein.[103]

## ANTIVIRAL AGENTS

Most of the drugs now in use for therapy of herpesvirus infections (Chap. 35) are nucleoside analogues or other agents that interfere with viral DNA replication.

The most successful drug in this class is acyclovir (ACV), which is highly selective against cells infected with HSV and other herpesviruses (e.g., VZV) that encode thymidine kinases.[104] This selectivity is based on properties of two of the viral enzymes involved in DNA replication. First, viral thymidine kinase can phosphorylate and thus activate ACV whereas human thymidine kinases tend not to use this analogue as a substrate. Second, viral DNA polymerase is more sensitive to inhibition by phosphorylated ACV than cell DNA polymerases are. Unfortunately, mutations in either of these viral enzymes can render the viral mutant resistant to ACV.[105] ACV-resistant mutants have been isolated (but not frequently) from drug-treated patients[106] and are almost always deficient in thymidine kinase. ACV is less effective against CMV, apparently because this virus does not encode a thymidine kinase. Ganciclovir, an analogue of ACV that does not require viral thymidine kinase for initial phosphorylation, is being evaluated for efficacy against CMV disease[107] (see Chap. 36).

As more is learned about the molecular interactions essential for HSV replication and for the establishment of latency, attention is likely to be focused on developing new drugs or agents that can block interactions specifically required by the virus. Known inhibitory agents, even if themselves not therapeutically useful, can provide structural information needed to design drugs with antiviral activity. For example, analogues of heparin might bind selectively to virus and block its adsorption to cells without possessing all the other pharmacologic activities of heparin. Also, antiviral activity might be a property of small molecules designed to mimic the antigen-combining sites of neutralizing antibodies that efficiently block viral penetration.

Clues about essential and potentially inhibitable molecular interactions also come from recent findings that cells expressing certain HSV gene products are resistant to infection by, or replication of, HSV. As mentioned above, HSV cannot penetrate cells expressing HSV gD.[38,39] In addition, viral gene expression is aborted in cells expressing a mutant form of the HSV regulatory protein VP16.[108] In both instances, it is likely that the viral protein expressed by the cell saturates sites on cell components required for interaction with proteins of the infecting virus. When the cell components have been identified and the nature of the virus–cell interactions defined, it may be possible to design drugs that can block the required interactions without toxicity to uninfected cells.

## PROSPECTS FOR AN EFFECTIVE HSV VACCINE

Most of the viral vaccines in use protect against systemic diseases such as poliomyelitis, measles, etc. For these diseases, the goal in vaccination is to induce immunity as good as that induced during recovery from natural disease, which often confers long-lasting protection against another episode of the disease.

Severe disseminated disease is a rare feature of HSV infection, except for infants or immunocompromised individuals. Immunity developing during the course of natural infection is probably sufficient to prevent such disseminated disease. On the other hand, recovery from localized disease caused by HSV is often not associated with sufficient immunity to prevent recurrent mucocutaneous lesions or to prevent reinfection with the formation of new lesions and the establishment of new reservoirs of latent virus.

Vaccination is not likely to be an effective approach to preventing severe disease in infants or immunocompromised individuals except, indirectly, by reducing the overall incidence of latent infections and the frequency of virus shedding due to reactivation. The greatest demand for a vaccine comes from other groups, principally from individuals who suffer the periodic recurrences of facial, ocular, or genital lesions.

Criteria for success of an HSV vaccine would therefore include ability to reduce the frequency of latent infections established during primary encounter with the virus or to reduce the frequency of lesions resulting from reactivation of latent virus or, preferably, both. Given that better protection would be demanded from a vaccine than results during recovery from natural infection, it might be necessary to accept a higher frequency of incomplete protection among vaccinated individuals than has been considered acceptable for other vaccines. Moreover, safety of any potential vaccine is an overriding consideration inasmuch as the vaccine would probably be targeted principally at ameliorating non-life-threatening disease.

Live attenuated, as well as subunit, HSV vaccines have been proposed. The major advantages of a live vaccine (lower input doses, exposure of the immune system to all viral antigens) are offset by the likelihood that even attenuated HSV can establish latent infections. The difficulties in developing effective subunit vaccines stem from our ignorance as to which of the 70-odd viral proteins are the best immunogens for protective immunity and ignorance as to how to present these antigens so as to stimulate protective immunity.

A trial to induce protection in human subjects (at risk for acquiring sexually transmitted herpetic disease) by immunization with a mixed glycoprotein vaccine did not yield satisfactory results despite the induction of antiglycoprotein antibodies and T-cell responses.[109,110] These disappointing results could be due to correctable inadequacies in the nature and composition of the vaccine and should not discourage further efforts, particularly because promising results have been obtained in experimental animal systems. As mentioned above, immunization of experimental animals with isolated viral proteins (for the most part, only glycoproteins have been tested to date) or mixtures of viral antigens has proved to reduce the severity of localized lesions and systemic disease and, in some instances, has reduced the incidence of latency.

## SUMMARY

Despite the remarkable diversity of the human herpesviruses with respect to the diseases they cause, latent infection and subsequent reactivation of viral replication are key aspects of the biology and pathology of them all. The prevalence and epidemiology of herpesvirus-induced diseases are determined in large part by the fact that latently infected individuals experience periodic reactivation and production of transmissible virus, whether or not clinical symptoms accompany the virus production. The management of immunocompromised patients is complicated by the facts that most of us carry one or more latent herpesviruses and that reactivation of these viruses can be devastating in the absence of normal immune responses. In immunocompetent individuals, however, it is principally HSV, and to a lesser extent VZV, that causes recurrent disease through reactivation of latent virus. This kind of disease poses difficult, but interesting, challenges for prevention and treatment.

### ACKNOWLEDGMENTS

I thank my colleagues, Drs. René Santos, Betsy Herold, and Nico van der Walt, for critical reviews of this chapter. Some of the work described here was supported by the Marietta Klinman Memorial Grant for Cancer Research from the American Cancer Society and by grants CA19264 and CA21776 from the National Institutes of Health.

# References

1 Salahuddin SZ et al: Isolation of a new virus, HBLV, in patients with lymphoproliferative disorders. *Science* 234:596, 1986.

2 Josephs SF et al: Genomic analysis of the human B-lymphotropic virus (HBLV). *Science* 234:601, 1986.

3 Lopez C et al: Characteristics of human herpesvirus-6. *J Infect Dis* 157:1271, 1988.

4 Baer R et al: DNA sequence and expression of the B95-8 Epstein-Barr virus genome. *Nature* 310:207, 1984.

5 Davison AJ, Scott JE: The complete DNA sequence of varicella-zoster virus. *J Gen Virol* 67:1759, 1986.

6 McGeoch DJ et al: The complete DNA sequence of the long unique region in the genome of herpes simplex virus type 1. *J Gen Virol* 69:1531, 1988.

7 Lwoff A et al: A system of viruses. *Cold Spring Harbor Symp Quant Biol* 27:51, 1962.

8 Wildy P: Classification and nomenclature of viruses (First Report of the ICNV). *Monogr Virol* 5:181, 1971.

9 Wildy P et al: The morphology of herpes virus. *Virology* 12:204, 1960.

10 Russell WC: Herpesvirus nucleic acid. *Virology* 16:355, 1962.

11 Davison AJ, McGeoch DJ: Evolutionary comparisons of the S segments in the genomes of herpes simplex virus type 1 and varicella-zoster virus. *J Gen Virol* 67:597, 1986.

12 Davison AJ, Taylor P: Genetic relations between varicella-zoster virus and Epstein-Barr virus. *J Gen Virol* 68:1067, 1987.

13 Kouzarides T et al: Large-scale rearrangement of homologous regions in the genomes of HCMV and EBV. *Virology* 157:397, 1987.

14 Roizman B: The family Herpesviridae: General description, taxonomy, and classification, in *The Herpesviruses,* Roizman B (ed). New York and London, Plenum, 1982, vol 1, p 1.

15 Kaplan AS: A study of the herpes simplex virus–rabbit kidney cell system by the plaque technique. *Virology* 4:435, 1957.

16 Schneweis KE: Serologische Untersuchungen zur Typendifferenzierung des *Herpesvirus hominis. Z Immunitaetsforsch Exp Ther* 124:24, 1962.

17 Plummer G: Serological comparison of the herpesviruses. *Br J Exp Pathol* 45:135, 964.

18 Nahmias AJ, Dowdle WR: Antigenic and biologic differences in *Herpesvirus hominis. Prog Med Virol* 10:110, 1968.

19 McGeoch DJ et al: DNA sequence and genetic content of the *Hin*dIII *l* region in the short unique component of the herpes simplex virus type 2 genome: identification of the gene encoding glycoprotein G, and evolutionary comparisons. *J Gen Virol* 68:19, 1987.

20 Hayward GS et al: Anatomy of herpes simplex virus DNA: Strain differences and heterogeneity in the locations of restriction endonuclease cleavage sites. *Proc Nat Acad Sci USA* 72:1768, 1975.

21 Buchman TG et al: Restriction endonuclease fingerprinting of herpes simplex virus DNA: A novel epidemiological tool applied to a nosocomial outbreak. *J Infect Dis* 138:488, 1978.

22 Morgan C et al: Electron microscopy of herpes simplex virus: I. Entry. *J Virol* 2:507, 1968.

23 Fuller AO, Spear PG: Anti-gD antibodies that permit adsorption but block infection by herpes simplex virus prevent virion-cell fusion at the cell surface. *Proc Nat Acad Sci USA* 84:5454, 1987.

24 McGeoch DJ et al: Sequence determination and genetic content of the short unique region of the genome of herpes simplex virus type 1. *J Mol Biol* 181:1, 1985.

25 Sarmiento M et al: Membrane proteins specified by herpes simplex viruses: III. Role of glycoprotein VP7($B_2$) in virion infectivity. *J Virol* 29:1149, 1979.

26 Cai W et al: Role of glycoprotein B of herpes simplex virus type 1 in viral entry and cell fusion. *J Virol* 62:2596, 1988.

27 Ligas MW, Johnson DC: A herpes simplex virus mutant in which glycoprotein D sequences are replaced by β-galactosidase sequences binds to but is unable to penetrate into cells. *J Virol* 62:1486, 1988.

28 Desai PJ et al: Excretion of non-infectious virus particles lacking glycoprotein H by a temperature-sensitive mutant of herpes simplex virus type 1: Evidence that gH is essential for virion infectivity. *J Gen Virol* 69:1147, 1988.

29 Homa FL et al: Molecular basis of the glycoprotein C-negative phenotypes of herpes simplex virus type 1 mutants selected with a virus-neutralizing monoclonal antibody. *J Virol* 58:281, 1986.

30 Longnecker R, Roizman B: Generation of an inverting herpes simplex virus 1 mutant lacking the L-S junction *a* sequences, an origin of DNA synthesis, and several genes including those specifying glycoprotein E and the α47 gene. *J Virol* 58:583, 1986.

31 Neidhardt H et al: Herpes simplex virus type 1 glycoprotein E is not indispensable for viral infectivity. *J Virol* 61:600, 1987.

32 Sarmiento M, Spear PG: Membrane proteins specified by herpes simplex viruses: IV. Conformation of the virion glycoprotein designated VP7($B_2$). *J Virol* 29:1159, 1979.

33 Claesson-Welsh L, Spear PG: Oligomerization of herpes simplex virus gB. *J Virol* 60:803, 1986.

34 Stannard LM et al: Herpes simplex virus glycoproteins associated with different morphological entities projecting from the virion envelope. *J Gen Virol* 68:715, 1987.

35 WuDunn D, Spear PG: Initial interaction of herpes simplex virus with cells is binding to heparan sulfate. *J Virol* 63:52, 1989.

36 Highlander SH et al: Neutralizing monoclonal antibodies specific for herpes simplex virus glycoprotein D inhibit virus penetration. *J Virol* 61:3356, 1987.

37 Highlander SL et al: Monoclonal antibodies define a domain on herpes simplex virus glycoprotein B involved in virus penetration. *J Virol* 62:1881, 1988.

37a Fuller AO et al: Neutralizing antibodies specific for glycoprotein H of herpes simplex virus permit viral attachment to cells but prevent virion-cell fusion required for penetration. *J Virol* (in press).

38 Campadelli-Fiume G et al: Entry of herpes simplex virus 1 in BJ cells that constitutively express viral glycoprotein D is by endocytosis and results in the degradation of the virus. *J Virol* 62:159, 1988.

39 Johnson RM, Spear PG: Herpes simplex virus glycoprotein D mediates interference with herpes simplex virus infection. *J Virol* 63:819, 1989.

40 Nemerow GR et al: Identification of gp350 as the viral glycoprotein mediating attachment of Epstein-Barr virus (EBV) to the EBV/C3d receptor of B cells: Sequence homology of gp350 and C3 complement fragment C3d. *J Virol* 61:1416, 1987.

41 Tanner J et al: Epstein-Barr virus gp350/220 binding to the B lymphocyte C3d receptor mediates adsorption, capping and endocytosis. *Cell* 50:203, 1987.

42 Friedman HM et al: Glycoprotein C of HSV-1 functions as a C3b receptor on infected endothelial cells. *Nature* 309:633, 1984.

43 Fries LF et al: Glycoprotein C of herpes simplex virus type 1 is an inhibitor of the complement cascade. *J Immunol* 137:1636, 1986.

44 Beck S, Barrell BG: Human cytomegalovirus encodes a glycoprotein homologous to MHC class-I antigens. *Nature* 331:269, 1988.

45 Grundy JE et al: $\beta_2$-microglobulin enhances the infectivity of cytomegalovirus and, when bound to the virus, enables class I HLA molecules to be used as a virus receptor. *J Gen Virol* 68:793, 1987.

46 Roizman B, Batterson B: Herpesviruses and their replication, in *Virology,* Fields BN (ed). New York, Raven, 1985, p 497.

47 Post LE et al: The regulation of alpha genes of herpes simplex virus: Expression of chimeric genes produced by fusion of thymidine kinase with alpha gene promoters. *Cell* 24:555, 1981.

48 Campbell MEM et al: Identification of herpes simplex virus DNA sequences which encode a *trans*-acting polypeptide responsible for stimulation of immediate early transcription. *J Mol Biol* 180:1, 1984.

49 Pellet PE et al: Nucleotide sequence and predicted amino acid sequence of a protein encoded in a small herpes simplex virus DNA fragment capable of *trans*-inducing alpha genes. *Proc Natl Acad Sci USA* 82:5870, 1985.

50 Wagner EK: Individual HSV transcripts, in *The Herpesviruses,* Roizman B (ed). New York and London, Plenum, 1985, vol 3, p 45.

51 Johnson DC, Spear PG: Monensin inhibits the processing of herpes simplex virus glycoproteins, their transport to the cell surface and the egress of virions from infected cells. *J Virol* 43:1102, 1982.

52 Jones F, Grose C: Role of cytoplasmic vacuoles in varicella-zoster virus glycoprotein trafficking and virion envelopment. *J Virol* 62: 2701, 1988.

53 Fenwick ML: The effects of herpesviruses on cellular macromolecular synthesis, in *Comprehensive Virology,* Fraenkel-Conrat H, Wagner RR (eds). New York and London, Plenum, 1984, vol 19, p 359.

54 Rock DL, Fraser NW: Detection of HSV-1 genome in central nervous system of latently infected mice. *Nature* 302:523, 1983.

55 Efstathiou S et al: Detection of herpes simplex virus–specific DNA sequences in latently infected mice and in humans. *J Virol* 57:446, 1986.

56 Mellerick DM, Fraser NW: Physical state of the latent herpes simplex virus genome in a mouse model system: evidence suggesting an episomal state. *Virology* 158:265, 1987.

57 Stevens JG et al: RNA complementary to a herpesvirus alpha gene mRNA is prominent in latently infected neurons. *Science* 235:1056, 1987.

58 Puga A, Notkins AL: Continued expression of a poly $(A)^+$ transcript of herpes simplex virus type 1 in trigeminal ganglia of latently infected mice. *J Virol* 61:1700, 1987.

59 Spivack JG, Fraser NW: Detection of herpes simplex virus type 1 transcripts during latent infection in mice. *J Virol* 61:3841, 1987.

60 Deatly AM et al: Latent herpes simplex virus type 1 transcripts in peripheral and central nervous system tissues of mice map to similar regions of the viral genome. *J Virol* 62:749, 1988.

61 Wagner EK et al: Physical characterization of the herpes simplex virus latency-associated transcript in neurons. *J Virol* 62:1194, 1988.

62 Rock DL et al: Detection of latency-related viral RNAs in trigeminal ganglia of rabbits latently infected with herpes simplex virus type 1. *J Virol* 61:3820, 1987.

63 Croen KD et al: Latent herpes simplex virus in human trigeminal ganglia. Detection of an immediate early gene "anti-sense" transcript by in situ hybridization. *N Engl J Med* 317:1427, 1987.

64 Steiner I et al: Latent herpes simplex virus type 1 transcription in human trigeminal ganglia. *J Virol* 62:3493, 1988.

65 Stevens JG et al: Prominence of the herpes simplex virus latency-associated transcript in trigeminal ganglia from seropositive humans. *J Infect Dis* 158:117, 1988.

66 Gordon YJ et al: RNA complementary to herpes simplex virus type 1 ICPO gene demonstrated in neurons of human trigeminal ganglia. *J Virol* 62:1832, 1988.

67 Krause PR et al: Detection and preliminary characterization of herpes simplex virus type 1 transcripts in latently infected human trigeminal ganglia. *J Virol* 62:4819, 1988.

68 Wechsler SL et al: Fine mapping of the latency-related gene of herpes simplex virus type 1: Alternative splicing produces distinct latency-related RNAs containing open reading frames. *J Virol* 62:4051, 1988.

69 Wagner EK et al: The herpes simplex virus latency-associated transcript is spliced during the latent phase of infection. *J Virol* 62:4577, 1988.

70 Spivack JG, Fraser NW: Expression of herpes simplex virus type 1 (HSV-1) latency-associated transcripts and transcripts affected by the deletion in avirulent mutant HFEM: Evidence for a new class of HSV-1 genes. *J Virol* 62:3281, 1988.

71 Javier RT et al: A herpes simplex virus transcript abundant in latently infected neurons is dispensable for establishment of the latent state. *Virology* 166:254, 1988.

72 Wilcox, CL, Johnson EM: Nerve growth factor deprivation results in the reactivation of latent herpes simplex virus in vitro. *J Virol* 61:2311, 1987.

73 Wilcox CL, Johnson EM: Characterization of nerve growth factor–dependent herpes simplex virus latency in neurons in vitro. *J Virol* 62:393, 1988.

74 Shiraki K, Rapp F: Establishment of herpes simplex virus latency in vitro with cycloheximide. *J Gen Virol* 67:2497, 1986.

75 Scheck AC et al: Prolonged herpes simplex virus latency in vitro after treatment of infected cells with acyclovir and human leukocyte interferon. *Antimicrob Agents Chemother* 28:589, 1986.

76 Russell J, Preston CM: An in vitro latency system for herpes simplex virus type 2. *J Gen Virol* 67:397, 1986.

77 Dambaugh T et al: The virus genome and its expression in latent infection, in *The Epstein-Barr Virus: Recent Advances,* Epstein MA, Achong BG (eds). London, William Heineman Medical, 1986, p 13.

78 Yates JL et al: Stable replication of plasmids derived from Epstein-Barr virus in various mammallian cells. *Nature* 313:812, 1985.

79 Gentry GA et al: Sequence analyses of herpesviral enzymes suggest an ancient origin for human sexual behavior. *Proc Natl Acad Sci USA* 85:2658, 1988.

80 Fraser NW et al: Herpes simplex type 1 DNA in human brain tissue. *Proc Natl Acad Sci USA* 78:6461, 1981.

81 Clements GB, Subak-Sharpe JH: Herpes simplex virus type 2 establishes latency in the mouse footpad. *J Gen Virol* 69:375, 1988.

82 Al-Saadi SA et al: Herpes simplex virus type 2 latency in the footpad of mice: Effect of acycloguanosine on the recovery of virus. *J Gen Virol* 69:433, 1988.

83 Claoue CM et al: Does herpes simplex virus establish latency in the eye of the mouse? *Eye* 1:525, 1987.

84 Abghari SZ, Stulting RD: Recovery of herpes simplex virus from ocular tissues of latently infected inbred mice. *Invest Ophthalmol Vis Sci* 29:239, 1988.

85 Hill TJ: Herpes simplex virus latency, in *The Herpesviruses,* Roizman B (ed). New York and London, Plenum, 1985, vol 3, p. 175.

86 Rouse BT: Role of adaptive immune defense mechanisms in herpes simplex resistance, in *Immunobiology of Herpes Simplex Virus Infection,* Rouse BT, Lopez C (eds). Boca Raton, Fla, CRC Press, 1984, p 107.

87 Martin S et al: Herpes simplex virus type 1-specific cytotoxic T lymphocytes recognize virus nonstructural proteins. *J Virol* 62:2265, 1988.

88 Reddehase MJ, Koszinowski UH: Significance of herpesvirus immediate early gene expression in cellular immunity to cytomegalovirus infection. *Nature* 312:369, 1984.

89 Klein J: The major histocompatibility complex and protein recognition by T lymphocytes. *Adv Exp Med Biol* 225:1, 1987.

90 Schrier RD et al: Type-specific delayed hypersensitivity and protective immunity induced by isolated herpes simplex virus–infected target cells. *J Immunol* 130:1413, 1983.

91 Long D et al: Glycoprotein D protects mice against lethal challenge with herpes simplex virus types 1 and 2. *Infect Immun* 37:761, 1984.

92 Cremer KJ et al: Vaccinia virus recombinant expressing herpes simplex virus type 1 glycoprotein D prevents latent herpes in mice. *Science* 228:737, 1985.

93 Dix RD, Mills J: Acute and latent herpes simplex virus neurological disease in mice immunized with purified virus-specific glycoproteins gB or gD. *J Med Virol* 17:9, 1985.

94 Rooney JF et al: Immunization with a vaccinia virus recombinant expressing herpes simplex virus type 1 glycoprotein D: Long-term protection and effect of revaccination. *J Virol* 62:1530, 1988.

95 Berman PW et al: Efficacy of recombinant glycoprotein D subunit vaccines on the development of primary, recurrent, and latent genital infections with herpes simplex virus type 2 in guinea pigs. *J Infect Dis* 157:897, 1988.

96 Baucke RB, Spear PG: Membrane proteins specified by herpes simplex viruses: V. Identification of an Fc-binding glycoprotein. *J Virol* 32:779, 1979.

97 Para MF et al: Similarities and differences in the Fc-binding glycoprotein (gE) of herpes simplex virus types 1 and 2 and tentative mapping of the viral gene for this glycoprotein. *J Virol* 41:137, 1982.

98 Johnson DC et al: Herpes simplex virus immunoglobulin G Fc receptor activity depends on a complex of two viral glycoproteins, gE and gI. *J Virol* 62:1347, 1988.

99 Seidel-Dugan C et al: C3b receptor activity on transfected cells expressing glycoprotein C of herpes simplex virus types 1 and 2. *J Virol* 62:4027, 1988.

100 Adler R et al: Possible role of Fc receptors on cells infected and transformed by herpesvirus: Escape from immune cytolysis. *Infect Immun* 21:442, 1978.

101 McNearney TA et al: Herpes simplex virus glycoproteins gC-1 and gC-2 bind to the third component of complement and provide protection against complement-mediated neutralization of viral infectivity. *J Exp Med* 166:1525, 1987.

102 Rawls WE: Herpes simplex viruses and their roles in human cancer, in *The Herpesviruses,* Roizman B (ed). New York and London, Plenum, 1985, vol 3, p 241.

103 Galloway DA, McDougall JK: The oncogenic potential of herpes simplex virus: Evidence for a 'hit-and-run' mechanism. *Nature* 302: 21, 1983.

104 Elion GB et al: Selectivity of action of an antiherpetic agent, 9-(2-hydroxyethoxymethyl) guanine. *Proc Natl Acad Sci USA* 74:5716, 1977.

105 Schnipper LE, Crumpacker CS: Resistance of herpes simplex virus to acycloguanosine: Role of viral thymidine kinase and DNA polymerase loci. *Proc Natl Acad Sci USA* 77:2270, 1980.

106 Crumpacker CS: Significance of resistance of herpes simplex virus to acyclovir. *J Am Acad Dermatol* 18:190, 1988.

107 Whitley RJ: Ganciclovir—have we established clinical value in the treatment of cytomegalovirus infections? *Ann Intern Med* 108:452, 1988.

108 Friedman AD et al: Expression of a truncated viral *trans*-activator selectively impedes lytic infection by its cognate virus. *Nature* 335:452, 1988.

109 Mertz GJ et al: Herpes simplex virus type-2 glycoprotein subunit vaccine: tolerance and humoral and cellular immune responses in humans. *J Infect Dis* 150:242, 1984.

110 Zarling JM et al: Herpes simplex virus (HSV)-specific proliferative and cytotoxic T-cell responses in humans immunized with an HSV type 2 glycoprotein subunit vaccine. *J Virol* 62:4481, 1988.

# Chapter 35

# Genital herpes

Lawrence Corey

Genital herpes simplex virus (HSV) infection has emerged as a disease of public health importance. The disease has been clinically recognized since the 1700s, and major advances in the understanding of its natural history and epidemiology have emerged in the last three decades. The morbidity of the illness, its frequent recurrence rates, and its complications such as aseptic meningitis and neonatal transmission have made this entity of great concern to patients and health care providers.

## HISTORY

The word *herpes* (from the Greek "to creep") has been used in medicine for at least 25 centuries. Cold sores (herpes febrilis) were described by the Roman physician Herodotus in 100 A.D.[1] Genital herpes was first described by the French physician Jean Astruc in 1736,[2] and the first English translation appeared in his treatise on venereal disease in 1754. The disease was well recognized by nineteenth century venereologists. In 1893 Unna diagnosed genital herpes in 9.1 percent of 846 prostitutes visiting his infirmary.[3] In 1886, Diday and Doyon published the monograph *Les Herpes génitaux,* in which they observed that genital herpes often appeared after a venereal infection such as syphilis, chancroid, or gonorrhea. They also described cases of recurrent genital herpes.[4]

In the late nineteenth century, fluid from oral-labial infection was shown to be infectious to other humans. The disease was successfully transferred to rabbits in the early twentieth century, and HSV was grown in vitro in 1925.[5–7] In 1921, Lipshutz inoculated material from genital herpetic lesions into the skin of humans, eliciting clinical infection within 48 to 72 h in six persons and within 24 days in one person. In other experiments, he observed that rabbits developed corneal infection more readily with strains originating from genital sites than with those from oral-labial sites. While he surmised that there were epidemiologic and clinical differences between oral and genital herpes,[8] most workers felt that the viruses of genital and labial herpes were identical. In the early 1960s, Schneeweiss in Germany and Dowdle and Nahmias in the United States reported that HSV could be divided by neutralization tests into two antigenic types and that there was an association between the antigenic type and the site of viral recovery.[9–12] These observations led to the benchmark studies on the epidemiology of genital herpes in the late 1960s.

## EPIDEMIOLOGY

### PREVALENCE OF GENITAL HSV INFECTIONS

The reported prevalence of genital herpes depends upon the demographic and clinical characteristics of the patient population studied and whether clinical or laboratory techniques, or both, are used for diagnoses. Seroepidemiologic studies have shown a wide disparity between antibody prevalence and clinical infection, indicating that many persons acquire asymptomatic infection.[12,13] In addition, many persons with clinically symptomatic HSV infection do not attend physicians' offices. Thus there are great differences between the prevalence of type 1 (HSV-1) and type 2 (HSV-2) infection and the frequency of symptomatic genital and oral-labial HSV infection seen by medical practitioners. In the United Kingdom in 1985, genital HSV infections accounted for approximately 3 percent of all visits to sexually transmitted disease (STD) clinics.[14] Nationwide statistics for genital herpes are not available in the United States. Genital HSV infection was diagnosed in 8.1 percent of all persons attending the STD clinics in King County, Washington, in 1984 (Fig. 35-1) with new problems. Some decrease in clinically diagnosed genital HSV infection has occurred in King County since 1985, with figures for total and new patient visits of 3.9 and 6.5 percent, respectively, in 1986. HSV has been isolated from 0.3 to 5.4 percent of males and 1.6 to 10 percent of females attending STD clinics in Western countries.[15–17] In non-STD-clinic patient populations, HSV has been isolated from the genital tract in from 0.25 to 5.0 percent of patients. Many of these patients are asymptomatic.[18–21] In STD clinics seeing a high proportion of non-Caucasians, genital herpes is reported only one-eighth to one-twelfth as frequently as *Neisseria gonorrhoeae* infection.[22] Student health centers seeing middle- and upper-class young adults, in whom the prevalence of gonococcal infection is very low, report that genital HSV infections are 7 to 10 times more common than gonorrhea.[23]

Many studies have shown that the prevalence of genital HSV increased markedly between the early 1960s and 1980s. For example, between 1968 and 1973, the reported incidence of genital HSV infection nearly doubled each year in Auckland, New Zealand.[24] In the years 1970 to 1976, the incidence of HSV infections, as detected by the routine cytologic screening of Papanicolaou smears obtained from cervical scrapings from women attending a gynecology clinic in Bangkok, Thailand, increased from 0.2 cases per 1000 patients to 6.9 cases per 1000 patients.[25] Similarly, visits to practitioners in the United States for first-episode genital HSV increased substantially between 1966 and 1981.[26] Concomitant with this increase in genital HSV infection has been an increase in neonatal HSV infection in the United States. In King County, Washington, the incidence of neonatal HSV infection has risen from 3.6 cases per 100,000 live births

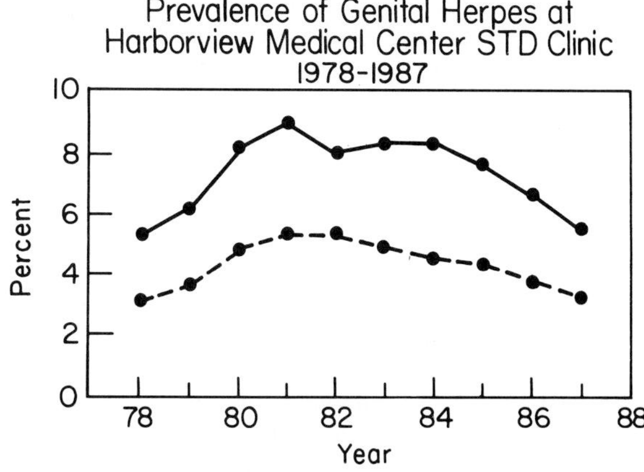


Fig. 35-1. Prevalance of diagnosed genital HSV infection in patients attending the King County STD Clinic between 1978 and 1987. The solid line reflects the percentage of new patient visits in which genital HSV was diagnosed, while the dashed line represents all patient visits in which genital HSV was diagnosed.

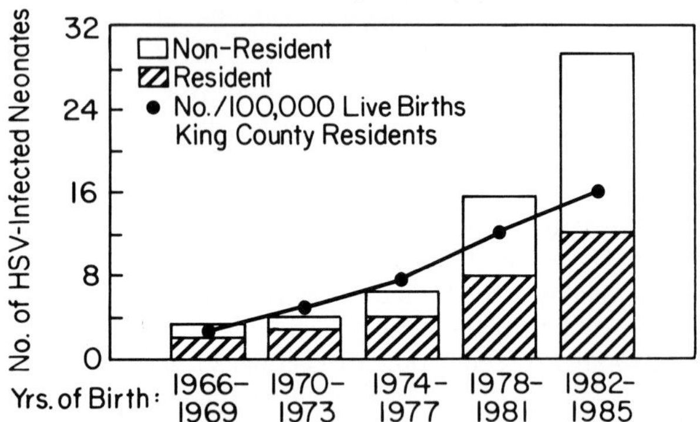


Fig. 35-2. Incidence of neonatal HSV infection in King County, Washington, from 1966 to 1985.

in the years 1966 to 1969 to 5.3 in 1970 to 1973, 7.8 in 1974 to 1977, 11.8 in 1978 to 1981, and 15.4 in 1982 to 1985 (Fig. 35-2).[27] While some persons have suggested that these figures may represent an increased recognition of the disease, the concomitant rise in reported neonatal HSV infection seen throughout the United States suggests that in many population groups there has been a marked increase in HSV-2 infections during this time period.[27,28]

## DEMOGRAPHIC CHARACTERISTICS OF PATIENTS WITH GENITAL HERPES

Genital HSV infections occur in all population groups. HSV-2 antibody prevalence rates are higher in nonwhite than in white populations.[27] However, symptomatic infection is relatively more common in whites.[29] Recent evidence suggests that the presence of HSV-1 antibody increases the frequency with which HSV-2 infection is asymptomatic.[19] This observation and other health care behavioral issues may explain the difference in seroprevalence and clinically symptomatic HSV infection.

While other STDs are identified in patients with genital HSV, HSV may often be the first STD acquired by many individuals. Genital herpes was the first STD acquired by 60 percent of the genital HSV patients seen in one series in Seattle. Past *N. gonorrhoeae* infection was present in less than 1 percent of these patients.[30] However, in other population groups, an association between *N. gonorrhoeae* and genital herpes has been demonstrated,[15,16] and patients recruited from STD clinics often have concomitant genitourinary infections.[19]

## PREVALENCE OF HSV ANTIBODY

Prevalence of antibody to HSV increases with age and correlates with socioeconomic status.[12,28,31–35] Some serologic tests such as the standard complement fixation antibody assay do not distinguish between HSV-1 and HSV-2 (see Chap. 77). Other serologic tests—neutralization, indirect immunofluorescence, passive hemagglutination, indirect hemagglutination, enzyme-linked immunosorbent assay (ELISA), and radioimmunoassay (RIA)—which partially distinguish antibodies to HSV-2 from antibodies to HSV-1 have been developed[34–37] (see Chap. 77). However, serologic cross-reactions between the two HSV types are common in these assays, as the predominant antibody responses appear to be directed as type-common rather than type-specific antigenic determinants.[38–40] It is difficult, therefore, to detect the presence of HSV-2-specific antibody in the presence of high titers of HSV-1 antibody. Because of this, serologic assays using whole-virus antigens underestimate the true prevalance of HSV-2 infection. Recently, this problem has been overcome by the development of newer type-specific serologic assays which accurately allow the detection of HSV-2 in the presence of HSV-1 antibodies and vice versa.[41,42] For a fuller discussion of these serologic assays, see Chap. 77.

Serosurveys of western populations in the post-World War II era found that 80 to 100 percent of middle-aged adults of lower socioeconomic status possessed antibodies to HSV, compared with 30 to 50 percent of adults of higher socioeconomic groups.[43–45] In the United States in the 1970s, HSV-1 antibodies were detected in about 50 percent of high and 80 percent of lower socioeconomic class persons by age 30.[43] In STD clinics, about 60 percent of attendees had HSV-1 antibody. In western Europe HSV-1 infection in young adults appears 10 to 20 percent more frequently than in the United States.[46]

Antibodies to HSV-2 are not routinely detected in sera until puberty, and antibody prevalence rates correlate with past sexual activity. HSV-2 antibodies were detected in 80 to 90 percent of female prostitutes, up to 75 percent of adults of lower socioeconomic status, 50 percent of randomly selected heterosexual men and women attending STD clinics, and 70 to 80 percent of randomly selected homosexual men attending STD clinics.[12,19,43,47] Recent studies have shown HSV-2 antibody prevalence rates to be about 5 to 10 percent higher in women than in men.[41,42] In the general U.S. population, HSV-2 antibody prevalence rates range from 20 to 40 percent in Caucasian to 30 to 60 percent in non-Caucasian populations.[46a] Most obstetric populations have a 30 percent HSV-2 seroprevalence rate when new serologic techniques are used.[46] HSV-2 seroprevalence rates in the general population in Europe and other areas of the world are not available.[48,49] In Australia, HSV-2 seroprevalence rates appear 10 to 15 percent lower than in the United States.[50]

## PATHOGENESIS

Transmission of HSV infection most frequently occurs through close contact with a person who is shedding virus at a peripheral site, mucosal surface, or secretion. Since HSV is readily inactivated at room temperature and by drying, aerosol and fomite spread are unusual means of transmission.[51–53]

Infection occurs via inoculation of virus onto susceptible mucosal surfaces (e.g., the oropharynx, cervix, conjunctivae) or through small cracks in the skin. HSV infection is associated with focal necrosis and ballooning degeneration of cells, production of mononucleated giant cells, and eosinophilic intranuclear inclusions (Cowdry type A bodies).[54] The initial cellular response is predominantly polymorphonuclear, followed by a lymphocytic response. When viral replication is restricted, lesions reepithelialize.

Concomitant with initial infection, HSV ascends peripheral sensory nerves and enters sensory or autonomic nerve root ganglia where latency is established (see Chap. 34).[55–58] When cocultivation techniques are used, HSV-2 (and rarely HSV-1) has been isolated from S3 and S4 sacral nerve root ganglia.[57] The biological mechanism by which latency is established and the nature of the virus–cell interaction that results in latency is incompletely understood (see Chap. 34). Latency can be established after both symptomatic and asymptomatic initial infection. Similarly, recrudescenct productive infection may be clinically symptomatic or asymptomatic. Reinfection with different strains of virus has also been demonstrated; however, this appears to be an infrequent event, and recurrences are almost always due to reactivation of the initial strain of virus from latently infected ganglia.[59,60]

The mechanism by which HSV establishes latency is unknown. Recent work has established that only partial transcripts of genes for HSV proteins are present in latently infected ganglionic neurons.[61] A segment of RNA that was transcribed in the complementary sense (*antisense*) and which overlaps the gene for the immediate-early protein ICP0 has been found in the nuclei of 0.1 to 5 percent of latently infected neurons (see Chap. 34). This latency-associated transcript is not found in high abundance in acutely infected cells.[61,62] Mutants with deletion of this segment of the genome can, however, establish latency, suggesting that this part of the HSV genome is not necessary to establish latency, but may be important in maintaining it. The mechanism of HSV reactivation is, at present, also not known. What is, however, clear is that the state of the HSV genome in the latently infected cell differs from that in the productively infected cell.[63]

Several hypotheses have been promulgated to account for intermittent recrudescences of disease.[64] The so-called ganglion-trigger hypothesis suggests that a stimulus (hormonal, immunologic, physical) affects the interaction between the host ganglion cell and the virus such that partial expression of genes for viral proteins no longer occurs, productive infection ensues, and virions move down the peripheral nerve, infect epidermal cells, and produce the characteristic skin lesions. The travel time for the virus in the nerve often appears too long to account for the rapidity of recurrences following ganglionic stimulation, however. In addition, antibody titers against HSV remain constant for long periods of time and are unaffected by recurrences, suggesting frequent antigenic stimulation. The "skin trigger theory" postulates that small amounts of infectious virus are made by the ganglion cells and frequently reach the skin cells via nerves. The body's defense mechanism normally eliminates these "microfoci" of infection, but temporary local suppression of immunity allows visible lesions to form. One argument against this hypothesis is that virus has not been demonstrated in epidermal cells between episodes of productive infection. Nonetheless, in guinea pigs and rabbits persistence of virus in the genital tract and cornea has been documented.[65] As local skin trauma such as sunburn, epilation, and surgery may precipitate recurrent lesions, the skin trigger theory would account for these observations better than the ganglion trigger theory.[65a] Further understanding of the factors involved in establishing and maintaining latency or in reactivating latent virus are needed before one can resolve or interpret these theories.

## CLINICAL MANIFESTATIONS OF GENITAL HERPES

The clinical manifestations and recurrence rate of genital herpes are influenced by viral type and host factors such as past exposure to HSV-1, previous episodes of genital herpes, and gender. The effects of host factors such as age, race, site of inoculation, or genetic background on the acquisition of infection or expression of disease are poorly understood. Many HSV infections (both HSV-1 and HSV-2) are asymptomatic. Retrospective studies suggest that as many as 50 to 70 percent of HSV-2 infections are asymptomatic. Recent prospective studies suggest, however, that most first infections are clinically symptomatic, albeit mild. Many are not likely to result in the patient's attendance at the physician's office[66] Thus, the frequency of truly asymptomatic infection may not be as high as previously thought.

## FIRST EPISODE OF GENITAL HERPES

The clinical manifestations of genital herpes vary greatly, depending in part on whether the patient is experiencing the first episode of infection or has recurrent disease. First episodes of genital herpes often are associated with systemic symptoms, involve multiple genital and extragenital sites, and have a prolonged duration of viral shedding and lesions.[30] Patients with first episodes of genital herpes who have clinical or serologic evidence of prior HSV infection have a milder illness than those experiencing true primary infection (i.e., the first infection with either HSV-1 or HSV-2).[67–69] About 50 percent of persons who presented to the Seattle STD clinic with their first episode of symptomatic genital herpes had primary infection with either HSV-1 or HSV-2.[19] Most persons with nonprimary first episodes of genital HSV infection have serologic evidence of past HSV-1 infection.[70] However, in some series about 25 percent of persons who state they are experiencing their first episodes of symptomatic genital herpes have serologic evidence of past HSV-2 in their sera, indicative of past asymptomatic acquisition of HSV-2.[71]

Genital HSV-1 infections have been reported with increasing frequency in some populations, especially in persons experiencing first episodes of infection.[72–74] Most genital HSV-1 infections are true primary infections, as several studies have shown genital HSV-1 infection recurs much less frequently than genital HSV-2 infection.[30,206,208] About 25 percent of all first episodes of true primary genital HSV are due to HSV-1.[30] Overall 5 to 15 percent of all first episodes of genital herpes are caused by HSV-1.

Prior oral-labial HSV-1 infection appears to protect against the acquisition of genital HSV-1 disease.[70] In addition, prior HSV-1 infection ameliorates the severity of first episodes of genital (HSV-2) herpes.[19,30] Persons with first-episode nonprimary genital HSV-2 infection are less likely to have systemic symptoms and more likely to have a shorter duration of symptoms and signs than persons with primary genital herpes due to either HSV-1 or HSV-2 (Table 35-1). The severity of local symptoms, duration of viral shedding from lesions, and duration of lesions appear similar in patients with primary HSV-1 and those with primary HSV-2 disease.

## PRIMARY GENITAL HERPES

Primary genital HSV-2 infection is characterized by a high frequency and prolonged duration of systemic and local symptoms. Fever, headache, malaise, and myalgias are reported in nearly 40 percent of men and 70 percent of women with primary HSV-2 disease ($p < 0.05$) (Table 35-2). Systemic symptoms appear early in the course of the disease, usually reach a peak within the first 3 to 4 days after onset of lesions, and gradually recede over the subsequent 3 to 4 days (Fig. 35-3).

Pain, itching, dysuria, vaginal or urethral discharge, and tender inguinal adenopathy are the predominant local symptoms of disease. Painful lesions are reported in 95 percent of men (mean duration 10.9 days) and 99 percent of women (mean duration 12.2 days) with primary HSV infection. Dysuria, both external and internal, appears more frequently in women (83 percent)

**Table 35-1. Relation between Viral Type, Presence of HSV Antibody in Acute Sera, and Severity of Disease in Patients with First-Episode Genital Herpes***

| | Primary HSV-1 infection | Primary HSV-2 infection | Nonprimary HSV-2 infection† |
|---|---|---|---|
| Number in study | 20 | 189 | 76 |
| Percent with systemic symptoms | 58 | 62 | 16 |
| Mean duration local pain, days | 12.5 | 11.8 | 8.7 |
| Mean number of lesions | 24.3 | 15.5 | 9.5 |
| Percent with bilateral lesions | 100 | 82 | 55 |
| Percent forming new lesions during course of disease | 68 | 75 | 45 |
| Mean duration viral shedding from genital lesions, days | 11.1 | 11.4 | 6.8 |
| Mean duration lesions, days | 22.7 | 18.6 | 15.5 |

*Only one patient with complement fixation and/or neutralizing antibody in acute-phase sera had HSV-1 isolated from the genital lesions.
†$p < 0.05$ for each comparison between nonprimary and primary HSV-2 infection (chi square or student's t-test).

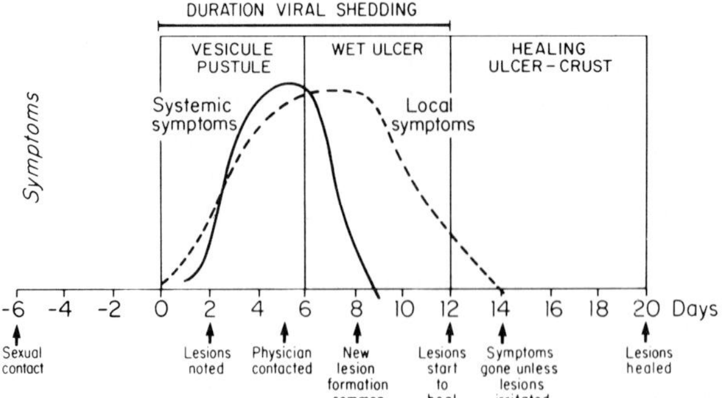


Fig. 35-3. Clinical course of primary genital herpes.

than in men (44 percent). The isolation of HSV from the urethra and urine of both men and women with primary genital herpes suggests that in addition to external dysuria resulting from urine touching active genital HSV lesions, HSV urethritis and/or cystitis may account for the higher frequency and longer duration of dysuria in women.

Urethral discharge and dysuria is noted in about one-third of men with primary HSV-2 infection of the external genitalia. HSV can be isolated from a urethral swab or from first-voided urine of these men. The urethral discharge is usually clear and mucoid, and the severity of dysuria is often out of proportion to the amount of urethral discharge elicited on genital examinations. Gram's stain of the urethral discharge usually reveals between 5 and 15 polymorphonuclear leukocytes per oil-immersion field. Occasionally a mononuclear cell response is seen.

The clinical symptoms of pain and irritation from lesions gradually increase over the first 6 to 7 days of illness, reach their maximum intensity between days 7 and 11 of disease, and gradually recede over the second week of illness (Fig. 35-3). Tender inguinal adenopathy usually appears during the second and third week of disease and often is the last symptom to resolve. Inguinal and femoral lymph nodes when palpated are generally found to be firm, nonfluctuant, and tender. Suppurative lymphadenopathy is a very uncommon manifestation of genital herpes.

**Table 35-2. Clinical Symptoms and Signs of Primary Genital HSV-2 Infection in Men and Women Followed at the University of Washington Genital HSV Clinic**

| | Men | Women |
|---|---|---|
| Percent with constitutional symptoms | 39* | 68 |
| Percent with meningitis symptoms | 11* | 36 |
| Percent with local pain | 95 | 99 |
| Mean duration of local pain, days (range) | 10.9 (1–40) | 11.9 (1–37) |
| Percent with dysuria | 44* | 83 |
| Mean duration of dysuria, days (range) | 7.2 (2–20)** | 11.9 (1–26) |
| Percent with urethral/vaginal discharge | 27** | 85 |
| Mean duration discharge, days | 5.6** | 12.9 |
| Percent with tender adenopathy | 80 | 81 |
| Mean duration adenopathy, days | 8.6** | 14.2 |
| Mean area of lesions, $mm^2$ (range) | 427 (6–1671) | 550 (8–3908) |
| Mean duration viral shedding from lesions, days | 10.5 | 11.8 |
| Percent with HSV isolated from urethra | 28* | 76 |
| Percent with HSV isolated from cervix | — | 88 |
| Mean duration viral shedding from cervix, days | — | 11.4 |
| Mean duration lesions, days | 16.5 | 19.7 |

* $p < 0.05$ by chi square.
**$p < 0.05$ by student's t-test.

## Clinical signs and duration of viral shedding in primary genital herpes

In both men and women with primary genital HSV infection, widely spaced bilateral pustular or ulcerative lesions on the external genitalia are the most frequent presenting sign. Lesions are characteristically described as starting as papules or vesicles which rapidly spread over the genital area. At the time of the first clinic visit, multiple small pustular lesions which coalesce into large areas of ulcerations are usually present (Plates 25, 26, and 28). The size and shape of the ulcerative lesions vary greatly between patients. These ulcerative lesions persist from 4 to 15 days until crusting and/or reepithelialization occurs. In general, lesions in the penile and mons areas crust over before complete reepithelialization ensues. Crusting does not occur on mucosal surfaces. Residual scarring from lesions is uncommon. New lesion formation (the development of new areas of vesiculation or ulceration during the course of infection) occurs in over 75 percent of patients with primary genital herpes. New lesions usually form between days 4 and 10 of disease.

The median duration of viral shedding as defined from the onset of lesions to the last positive culture is about 12 days (Table 35-2). The mean time (about 10.5 days) from the onset of vesicles to the appearance of the crust stage correlates well with the duration of viral shedding. However, since there is considerable overlap between the duration of viral shedding and the duration of crusting and since mucosal lesions don't crust, patients should be advised not to resume sexual activity until lesions have completely reepithelialized. The mean time from the onset of lesions to complete reepithelialization of all lesions appears slightly longer in women (19.5 days) than in men (16.5 days).

## Frequency and appearance of HSV cervicitis in first episodes of genital herpes

Ninety percent of women with primary genital HSV-2 infection, 70 percent of women with primary genital HSV-1 infection, and 70 percent of women with first-episode nonprimary genital HSV-2 infection have concomitant HSV cervicitis.[30,74] The high rate of isolation of HSV from the cervix in initial episodes contrasts sharply with the 12 to 20 percent isolation rate in women who present with recurrent external genital lesions (Table 35-5).[30,75] Primary genital HSV cervicitis may be symptomatic (purulent vaginal discharge) or asymptomatic.[19,76] In most cases of primary HSV cervicitis, the cervix appears abnormal to inspection. The appearance may include areas of diffuse or focal friability and redness, extensive ulcerative lesions of the exocervix, or severe necrotic cervicitis (Plate 14). HSV infection of the cervix usually involves the squamous epithelium of the exocervix in contrast to the mucopurulent cervicitis of *Chlamydia trachomatis* and *N. gonorrhoeae* infection. Clinical differentiation may be difficult, although cervical necrosis and ulceration are highly correlated with HSV cervicitis.

In women with primary genital herpes, the mean duration of viral shedding from the cervix (11.4 days) is similar to that from lesions of the external genitalia.

## Pharyngeal infection

HSV infection of the pharynx is commonly seen in association with primary genital herpes and may be the presenting complaint in about 20 percent of patients with either primary HSV-1 or primary HSV-2 infections. Both HSV-1 and HSV-2 may cause pharyngitis. Both HSV types may be associated with oral-genital exposure to the source contact.[77,78] In children, autoinoculation of the genital area during the course of primary HSV-1 gingivostomatitis occasionally may be seen. HSV pharyngitis is much less frequently seen in patients with concomitant nonprimary first-episode genital herpes or patients with recurrent genital herpes (1 percent). In the author's experience, HSV was isolated from the pharynx in 70 percent of persons with primary genital herpes who complained of sore throat during the acute episode of the disease. Viral cultures of the pharynx were obtained from 20 patients with primary HSV-2 who did not complain of sore throat; HSV was not isolated from the pharynx in any of these patients, which indicates that HSV pharyngitis is usually symptomatic. Clinical signs of HSV pharyngitis may vary from mild erythema to a diffuse ulcerative pharyngitis.[77–80] The inflammatory response to these large areas of ulceration may produce a whitish exudate; when the exudate is wiped away the extensive ulceration may be visualized. In rare cases severe swelling of the posterior pharynx resulting in obstruction of the airway may occur.[81] Extension of the ulcerative posterior pharyngeal lesions into the anterior gingival area may occur. Most patients with HSV pharyngitis have tender cervical nodes, and constitutional symptoms such as fever, malaise, myalgia, and headache are common. Many are misdiagnosed as having streptococcal pharyngitis and/or infectious mononucleosis.

Previous studies of HSV pharyngitis have shown the entity to be a common form of infection in college-age students and almost invariably to be due to primary infection with HSV-1.[80] Reactivation of HSV pharyngeal lesions rarely leads to symptomatic pharyngitis. Instead, recurrent oral-labial lesions or asymptomatic salivary gland shedding are seen. Reactivation of HSV-2 in the trigeminal ganglia occurs much less frequently than reactivation of latent HSV-1 in the trigeminal nerve root.[78] A recent study in Seattle showed HSV to be the most common cause of pharyngitis in STD clinic attendees, streptococcus the second most common, and *Mycoplasma pneumoniae* the third (W. Lafferty and L. Corey, personal observations).

Table 35-3. Complications of Primary Genital HSV-2 Infection

| | Approximate frequency, percent |
|---|---|
| Central nervous system complications | |
| Stiff neck, headache, and photophobia | 28 |
| Hospitalized with aseptic meningitis | 5 |
| Sacral autonomic nervous system radiculopathy* | 1 |
| Transverse myelitis | rare |
| HSV pharyngitis | 10 |
| Development of extragenital lesions | |
| Lip | 3 |
| Buttock, groin | 9 |
| Breast | 2 |
| Finger | 6 |
| Eye | 1 |
| Disseminated cutaneous infection | <0.5 |
| Direct extension of disease | |
| Pelvic inflammatory disease syndrome (including endometritis) | 1.8 |
| Pelvic cellulitis | rare |
| Suppurative lymphadenitis | <0.5 |
| Fungal superinfection | |
| Yeast vaginitis | 14 |

*Constipation, urinary retention, and sacral anesthesias.
SOURCE: After references 43–79, 99.

## COMPLICATIONS OF GENITAL HERPES

The complications of genital herpes are related both to local extension and to spread of virus to extragenital sites. Development of lesions at extragenital cutaneous sites (Table 35-3) and central nervous system involvement and fungal superinfection are the most frequently encountered complication. Complications of primary genital herpes occur more frequently in women than in men.

### Central nervous system complications

**Aseptic Meningitis.** Central nervous system involvement may occur in several forms, including aseptic meningitis, transverse myelitis, or what has been called the sacral radiculopathy syndrome.[82–84] In one series of patients with primary genital HSV-2 infection, stiff neck, headache, and photophobia on two consecutive examinations were reported in 36 percent of women and 13 percent of men ($p < 0.001$). Hospitalization was required for clinically overt aseptic meningitis in 6.4 percent of women and 1.6 percent of men with primary HSV-2 infections.[30] A study of genital herpes in the early 1900s reported a high frequency of CSF pleocytosis in patients without overt clinical evidence of meningeal irritation, suggesting that meningeal involvement may be a frequent occurrence with genital herpes.[85]

Both HSV-1 and HSV-2 have been isolated from CSF,[86,87] although isolations of HSV-2 are much more common. HSV has been isolated from 0.5 to 3.0 percent of patients presenting to the hospital with aseptic meningitis[87,88] HSV aseptic meningitis appears to be more frequently associated with genital than with oral-labial infection.[89,90] In contrast, HSV encephalitis in older children or adults is rarely due to HSV-2 infection.[91] Fever, headache, vomiting, photophobia, and nuchal rigidity are the predominant symptoms of HSV aseptic meningitis. Meningeal symptoms usually start from 3 to 12 days after onset of genital lesions. Symptoms generally reach a maximum 2 to 4 days into the illness and gradually recede over 36 to 72 h. The CSF in HSV aseptic meningitis is usually clear, and the opening pressures may be elevated. White blood cell counts in the CSF may range from 10 to over 1000 cells per cubic millimeter (mean 550). The pleocytosis is predominantly lymphocytic in adults, although early in the course of disease and in neonates a predominantly polymorphonuclear response may be seen. The CSF glucose level is usually more than 50 percent of the blood glucose level, although hypoglycorrhachia has been reported; the CSF protein level is slightly elevated.[92] If cultures are obtained within 24 h of onset of headache and photophobia, HSV may be grown from the CSF. The differential diagnosis of HSV aseptic meningitis includes diseases which result in neurologic involvement and genital ulcerations: sacral herpes zoster, Behçet's syndrome, collagen vascular disease, inflammatory bowel disease, porphyria, and benign recurrent aseptic meningitis (Mollaret's syndrome). In STD populations, a primary seroconversion illness due to human immunodeficiency virus (HIV-1) should also be considered (see Chap. 30).

Aseptic meningitis associated with genital herpes appears to be a benign albeit uncomfortable disease in immunocompetent persons. Signs and symptoms of encephalitis are unusual, and neurologic sequelae are rare. Use of systemic antiviral chemotherapy for primary genital herpes decreases the subsequent development of aseptic meningitis.[93] Controlled trials of intravenous acyclovir for established HSV meningitis have not been conducted. However, it is the author's recommendation that intravenous acyclovir 5 mg/kg q 8 h be given for hospitalized symptomatic patients. Once symptoms are resolved, oral therapy can be continued. Higher doses of intravenous acyclovir should be utilized for patients with HSV-1 encephalitis, and oral therapy should not be attempted.

**Other Neurologic Complications.** Both transverse myelitis and autonomic nervous sytem dysfunction have been described in association with genital HSV infection.[83–85] Symptoms of autonomic nervous system dysfunction include hyperesthesia or anesthesia of the perineal, lower back, and sacral regions; difficulty urinating; and constipation. Physical examination reveals a large bladder, decreased sacral sensation, and poor rectal and perineal sphincter tone. In men, a history of impotence and absent bulbocavernous reflexes may be present. CSF pleocytosis may be present. Electromyography usually reveals slowed nerve conduction velocities and the presence of fibrillation potentials in the affected area, and urinary cystometric examination shows a large atonic bladder. Most cases gradually resolve over 4 to 8 weeks.[94–97]

Transverse myelitis occasionally occurs in association with primary genital HSV infection.[97–99] Decreased deep-tendon reflexes and muscle strength in the lower extremities, as well as the above-described autonomic nervous system signs and symptoms, are present. In one reported case, significant residual dysfunction was present years later.[99] Whether autonomic nervous system dysfunction results from viral invasion of the central nervous system or an unusual immunologic response to infection is unknown. Controlled clinical trials of antivirals or anti-inflammatory medications have not been performed.

## Extragenital lesions

The development of extragenital lesions during the course of infection is a common complication of first-episode primary genital herpes but is uncommon in nonprimary or recurrent genital herpes. Extragenital lesions are also more common in women than in men with primary genital herpes, 26 percent vs. 8 percent ($p < 0.05$). Extragenital lesions are most frequently located in the buttock, groin, or thigh area, although finger and eye sites are also involved. Characteristically, the extragenital lesions develop after the onset of genital lesions, often during the second week of disease. The distribution of lesions on the extremities and/or areas near the genital lesions, and their occurrence well into the course of disease, suggest that the majority of extragenital lesions develop by autoinoculation of virus rather than viremic spread.[100] Anatomic differences, especially contact with infected cervical-vaginal secretions, are the most likely explanation for the apparent increased risk of extragenital lesions in women. One recent survey of herpetic infections of the hand found HSV-2 to be much more common than HSV-1.[101]

## Disseminated infection

Blood-borne dissemination evidenced by the appearance of multiple vesicles over widespread areas of the thorax and extremities occurs rarely in persons with primary mucocutaneous herpes.[102,103] Cutaneous dissemination usually occurs early in the disease and is often associated with aseptic meningitis, hepatitis, pneumonitis, or arthritis.[104,105] Other complications of primary genital HSV-2 infection include monoarticular arthritis,[106,107] hepatitis,[108,109] thrombocytopenia,[110] and myoglobinuria.[111] Pregnancy may predispose to severe visceral dissemination of primary genital HSV disease.[112–114] Severe mucocutaneous and occasionally visceral dissemination of disease may occur in patients with atopic eczema.[115–118] In immunosuppressed patients, especially those with impaired cellular immune responses, reactivation of genital HSV infection can be associated with viremic spread of virus to multiple organs.[119–123] These patients may develop interstitial pneumonia, hepatitis, and pneumonitis, similar to the manifestations of disseminated infection of the neonate. Disseminated visceral infection in the immunosuppressed and pregnant patient is a disease of high mortality. Systemic antiviral chemotherapy should be given.

## Local extention of disease

Both HSV-1 and HSV-2 have been shown to be rare causes of pelvic inflammatory disease.[124,125] Some patients with primary cervical HSV infection may manifest lower abdominal pain and adnexal uterine tenderness. Occasionally, this represents dual infection with other sexually transmitted pathogens such as *N. gonorrhoeae* and *C. trachomatis*. However, extension of HSV infection into the uterine cavity has been reported, as has laparascopic evidence of vesicular fallopian tube lesions from which HSV has been isolated.[124]

## Superinfection

Bacterial superinfection of genital herpes in nonimmunosuppressed patients is uncommon. In rare cases, pelvic cellulitis presenting as an advancing erythema and swelling of the perineal area is encountered. In this instance systemic antimicrobial therapy should be administered.

Fungal superinfection is, however, frequently encountered during the course of initial genital herpes. In one series, monilial vaginitis was reported in 14 percent of women with first episodes of genital disease.[30] In another study of women attending an STD clinic, concomitant *Candida* infection was reported significantly more frequently in women with HSV than in those without.[19] Characteristically, vaginal fungal infection develops during the second week of disease and is associated with a change in character of the vaginal discharge, and reemergence of local symptoms such as vulvar itching and irritation. Typical hyphal forms can be demonstrated on potassium hydroxide examination of vaginal secretions. If the condition is symptomatic, treatment with clotrimazole and/or nystatin is recommended (see Chap. 45).

## SUMMARY OF THE CLINICAL COURSE OF INITIAL GENITAL HERPES

First-episode genital HSV infection is a disease of both systemic and local manifestations. Over one-half of the patients with primary genital herpes suffer from constitutional complaints, and one-third complain of headache, stiff neck, and mild photophobia during the first week of disease. Herpes progenitalis is clearly a misnomer in initial genital HSV infection.

Patients with serologic evidence of prior HSV-1 infection are less apt to have constitutional symptoms and have a lower rate of complications and a shorter duration of disease than persons with true primary genital herpes. Neutralizing antibody to HSV has been shown to inactivate extracellular virus and interrupt the spread of HSV infection.[126] In addition, a cellular immune response to HSV antigens appears earlier in persons with nonprimary genital HSV than in persons with true primary infection.[128] It is likely that both these immune mechanisms account for the clinical differences between primary and nonprimary first episodes of genital infection.

Although the duration of viral shedding from external genital lesions is similar in men and women with primary genital herpes, the duration of symptoms and the frequency of complications are greater in women. One potential explanation may be the high frequency of cervical and urethral involvement in women; the greater surface area of involvement may account for the increased severity of clinical disease in women.

## RECURRENT GENITAL HERPES: CLINICAL SIGNS AND SYMPTOMS

In contrast to first episodes of genital infection, recurrent genital herpes is characterized by symptoms, signs, and anatomic sites of infection localized to the genital region.[30,75,127,129] Local symptoms such as pain and itching are mild compared with the symptoms in initial genital infection, and the duration of the episode usually ranges from 8 to 12 days or less (Tables 35-4 and 35-5). Approximately 50 percent of persons with recurrent genital herpes develop symptoms in the prodromal phase of illness (i.e., prior to the appearance of lesions) (Table 35-4). Prodromal symptoms vary from a mild tingling sensation, occurring 30 min to 48 h prior to the eruption, to shooting pains in the buttocks, legs, or hips 1 to 5 days prior to the episode. In many patients these symptoms of sacral neuralgia are the most bothersome part of the episode.

**Table 35-4. Prevalence and Duration of Clinical Symptoms of Recurrent Genital Herpes in Patients Followed at the University of Washington Genital HSV Clinic**

| | Males | Females |
|---|---|---|
| Number in Study | 218 | 144 |
| Percent experiencing prodromal symptoms | 53 | 43 |
| Percent with pain | 67* | 88 |
| Mean duration pain, days (range) | 3.9 (1–14)** | 5.9 (1–13) |
| Percent with itching | 85 | 87 |
| Mean duration itching, days (range) | 4.6 (1–16) | 5.2 (1–15) |
| Percent with dysuria | 9 | 27 |
| Percent with urethral/vaginal discharge | 4 | 45 |
| Mean duration discharge, days (range) | 1.7 (1–5)** | 5.3 (1–14) |
| Percent with tender lymph nodes | 23 | 31 |
| Mean duration tender nodes, days (range) | 9.2 (1–25)** | 5.9 (1–15) |

* $p < 0.01$ by chi square.
**$p < 0.01$ by student's t-test.

As with initial genital disease, symptoms of recurrent genital herpes tend to be more severe in women (Table 35-4). In several series of studies, painful genital lesions were reported more frequently (60 to 90 percent) in women (mean duration 5.9 days) than in men (30 to 70 percent, 3.9 days, respectively). In addition, pain is reported to be more severe in women. Two-thirds of male patients report minimal local pain during the course of infection. Dysuria was reported in only 17 percent of women with recurrent disease. Most reported only external dysuria, and isolation of HSV from the urethra was uncommon in both sexes (3 to 9 percent).

Lesions of recurrent genital HSV are usually confined to one side, with an area of involvement approximately one-tenth that of primary genital infection (Plate 27). The average duration of viral shedding from the onset of lesions is about 4 days, and the

**Table 35-5. Clinical Signs of Recurrent Genital Herpes in Patients Followed at the University of Washington Genital HSV Clinic**

| | Males | Females |
|---|---|---|
| Number in study | 218 | 144 |
| Mean number of lesions at onset of episode, days (range) | 7.5 (1–25) | 4.8 (1–15) |
| Mean lesion area, mm$^2$ (range) | 62.7 (2–270) | 53.5 (4–208) |
| Percent with bilateral lesions | 15* | 4 |
| Percent forming new lesions during episode | 43* | 28 |
| Mean duration of new lesion formation, days (range) | 5.2 (1–15) | 5.4 (1–15) |
| Percent with extragenital lesions | 3 | 5 |
| Mean time to crusting, days (range) | 4.1 (1–15) | 4.7 (2–13) |
| Mean time to healing, days (range) | 10.6 (5–25) | 9.3 (4–29) |
| Mean duration viral shedding from lesions, days (range) | 4.4 (1–20) | 4.1 (2–14) |
| Percent shedding virus from cervix | — | 12 |
| Duration viral shedding from cervix days (range) | — | 3.2 (1–16) |

*$p < 0.05$ by chi square.

mean time from the onset of lesions to crusting of lesions averages between 4 and 5 days for both men and women (Table 35-5). The mean time from onset of vesicles to complete reepithelialization of lesions is about 10 days. Although symptoms of recurrent genital disease are more severe in females, objective signs of disease are relatively similar in the two sexes.

Only about 10 to 30 percent of women who present with recurrent genital lesions experience concomitant cervical infection. When cervical infection is present, the duration of cervical viral shedding is short, the shedding occurs early in the episode, and the infection is often without visible cervical lesions, unless routine colposcopy is performed (see the section on HSV cervicitis below).

In summary, the symptoms of recurrent genital herpes are often mild, and external genital lesions are usually unilateral. However, considerable variation in the severity and duration of disease exists among patients. In addition, the severity of individual recurrent episodes of disease in any one patient may vary greatly during the course of disease. Some recurrences have only one to two lesions lasting 6 to 7 days, while others may be associated with 15 to 20 lesions lasting 12 to 16 days.

### "Atypical" genital HSV infection

Recent studies showing the widespread seroprevalence of HSV-2 infection have provoked reevaluations of the overall clinical spectrum of genital HSV in various population groups. Whereas the classic clinical findings of genital HSV are described above, more-recent studies have illustrated the diverse clinical spectrum of genital HSV. For example, in a recent survey in which randomly selected women attending an STD clinic were intensively sampled for HSV, HSV was isolated from 30 percent of women with genital lesions not clinically felt to be herpetic; many of these lesions were small linear ulcerations, felt to be due to trauma. Women with serologic evidence of HSV-2 have been shown to have more "atypical" genital fissures and cracks than women without HSV antibodies; suggesting that HSV-2 is often the cause of these lesions.[130] These observations indicate that all genital ulcerations and fissures should be examined and evaluated for herpes. Laboratory diagnostic tests such as viral cultures and the use of type-specific serologic studies should be employed by clinicians (see Chap. 77).

## OTHER CLINICAL SYNDROMES ASSOCIATED WITH GENITAL HSV INFECTION

### HSV cervicitis

HSV may involve the cervix alone, without involvement of the external genitalia. Cervical HSV infection may be asymptomatic or may present as a mucopurulent cervicitis. In a recent survey of women attending an STD clinic, HSV was isolated from the cervix of 4 percent of randomly selected women attendees.[19] Of these women with HSV cervicitis, half had concomitant first-episode genital lesions, 15 percent had both cervical HSV and recurrent genital lesions, and 35 percent had only HSV cervicitis. Evidence of cervical lesions on routine speculum examination was present in 50 percent of these women; almost all with first-episode infections. An additional 15 percent of women were found to have HSV lesions when examined with colposcopy. In total, colposcopy detected lesions in 65 percent of women with HSV cervicitis. Papanicolaou smear revealed evidence of HSV cervicitis in 60 percent of women from whom HSV was isolated. Thus, even the most detailed clinical examination and cytologic testing will pick up only 65 to 70 percent of cervical HSV infection.

### Herpes simplex proctitis

HSV has been isolated from rectal mucosa and rectal biopsies in men and women with symptoms of rectal pain and discharge.[131–135] In a prospective study of 100 consecutive homosexual men who presented to an STD clinic with symptoms of rectal discharge and pain, HSV was isolated from rectal swabs and/or rectal biopsies in 23 percent.[131] In men with nongonococcal proctitis, HSV was the most frequent pathogen isolated.

HSV proctitis differs from gonococcal proctitis in that fever, systemic symptoms, severe rectal pain, discharge, tenesmus, and evidence of sacral autonomic nervous system dysfunction may be seen.[132–140] Patients usually present with acute onset of rectal pain, discharge, tenesmus, constipation, and blood and/or mucoid rectal discharge. Fever, malaise, and myalgia are common, and urinary retention, dysesthesia of the perineal region, and impotence may be reported. External perianal lesions are seen in about one-half of the patients. Anoscopy and/or sigmoidoscopy generally reveals a diffuse, friable rectal mucosa, although occasionally discrete ulcerations of the rectal mucosa may be present (Plates 73 and 74). In most cases the pathologic condition is limited to the lower 10 cm of the rectum. Rectal biopsies of involved mucosa generally reveal diffuse ulcerations and lymphocytic infiltration. If multiple histologic sections are obtained, intranuclear inclusions may be demonstrated in rectal biopsies in about 40 percent of cases.[135] Both HSV-1 and HSV-2 have been isolated from patients with HSV proctitis.[133,135] Recurrences of this disease have been described and may be mild and/or asymptomatic. Controlled clinical evaluation of the use of systemic acyclovir suggests some clinical benefit.[140] With decreasing frequency of unprotected anorectal intercourse among homosexual men, HSV proctitis is being seen less frequently.

Rectal HSV infection may also be seen in women. Over 75 percent of anorectal HSV infections in women are asymptomatic.[19,130] In women there appears to be little association between anorectal HSV infection and rectal intercourse (recent or past). Serologic studies suggest that reactivation of latent sacral ganglionic HSV infection may result in asymptomatic rectal shedding of HSV in the anorectal canal. The importance of rectal HSV infection of women in transmission of HSV-2 remains to be assessed.

### Genital ulcerations

HSV infection causes 40 to 60 percent of genital ulcerations in patients presenting to gynecologic practices or STD clinics in the United States.[141,142] The varied size, symptoms, and appearance of genital HSV lesions may make clinical diagnosis of genital ulcerations, especially single genital ulcerations, difficult. HSV may be isolated from many lesions attributed by patients to trauma or irritation. In addition, clinical differentiation of genital ulcerations due to HSV, *Treponema pallidum*, and *Haemophilus ducreyi* is often uncertain (Plates 31, 32, 37–41) (see Chaps. 20 and 24). As discussed in Chap. 77, the sensitivity of a viral culture for detecting HSV in a lesion is only 50 percent, because the ulcer persists beyond the time virus is readily recovered from the lesion. Thus, lack of isolation of HSV from a genital lesion does not rule out HSV as the initiating course; repeated samplings earlier in the course of lesions may be necessary.

## Asymptomatic HSV infection

One of the least understood aspects of the natural history of genital herpes is asymptomatic viral shedding. HSV has been cultured from the lower genitourinary tract of asymptomatic women and men. In women the anatomic sites of asymptomatic shedding include the cervix, vulva, rectum, and urethra. In men, asymptomatic shedding may be documented by swab cultures of the penile skin and/or urethra. The frequency of detecting asymptomatic HSV infection is, in part, a function of the frequency of sampling.

Transmission of genital herpes can occur by sexual contact with an asymptomatic excreter of virus. This appears to be an important source of infection, especially in the seronegative sexual contact.[143–145] Asymptomatic excretion has been demonstrated in saliva and in cervical and seminal secretions. Douglas and Spruance have demonstrated asymptomatic excretion of HSV in saliva in 2 percent of adults,[146,147] and there are reports of transmission of genital HSV-1 infection from oral-genital sex during a period of asymptomatic salivary excretion of virus.[144] Asymptomatic cervical viral shedding has been shown to result in both horizontal and vertical transmission of disease.[143–145,148] Centifanto isolated HSV from seminal secretions from nearly 20 percent of men undergoing routine vasectomy,[149] but a subsequent study failed to isolate HSV in over 600 semen samples taken from men with recurrent genital HSV infection. HSV has been isolated infrequently from prostatic secretion or biopsies.[150]

The frequency of asymptomatic cervical HSV infection and risk factors associated with it are not well studied. Rattray et al. followed six women with twice-weekly viral cultures of the cervical and vulvar area.[151] In this small group of women with recurrent genital herpes, asymptomatic HSV infection of the cervix accounted for 1 of 23 clinical and virologic recurrences of genital herpes. Adam et al. also demonstrated transient asymptomatic excretion of HSV from the cervix of three women who were sampled regularly over 3 months.[152] HSV antigen has been demonstrated in cervical-vaginal secretions when HSV culture was negative.[153,154] While false-positive immunofluorescent assays can be seen, these data may also reflect short but frequent periods of viral shedding in which infectious virus is quickly inactivated by local immune mechanisms, or episodes of defective viral replication. These studies indicate that the pattern of viral shedding from the cervix is intermittent, similar to the intermittent appearance of external genital lesions.

Frequency of sampling is a major factor affecting studies of symptomatic HSV shedding. In a recent review of 27 women who performed home cultures, asymptomatic vulvar or cervical shedding occurred in more than 80 percent of women who submitted more than 50 daily home cultures.[154] The asymptomatic shedding rate varied from 0.5 to 2 percent of the days these HSV-2 seropositive women were sampled. Thus, asymptomatic shedding is an infrequent but not negligible problem in patients with HSV-2. Asymptomatic shedding from the vulva is as frequent as that from the cervix. Vulvar shedding probably reflects small lesions not noticeable to either patient or clinician.

The anatomic site of asymptomatic shedding in men is less well understood. Most asymptomatic shedding in men appears to be from small penile lesions not identifiable by examination, analogous to asymptomatic vulvar shedding in women. Asymptomatic shedding of HSV in semen appears uncommon and when present is usually associated with first-episode primary infection.[150,155]

## Genital herpes virus infection in the immunocompromised patient

Although much of the literature of HSV infections in the immunosuppressed patient has concentrated on oral-labial disease, the increasing prevalence of genital herpes has resulted in an increasing awareness of the consequences of genital herpes in immunosuppressed patients. Immunocompromised patients have both more frequent and more prolonged mucocutaneous HSV infections.[156–158] Mucocutaneous HSV infections in the immunocompromised host are usually associated with systemic complaints, prolonged local symptoms, and durations of viral shedding greater than 30 days.

Over 70 percent of renal and bone marrow transplant recipients who have serologic evidence of past HSV infection reactivate latent HSV infection within the first month after transplantation.[159,160] Recurrent genital herpes in immunosuppressed patients often results in the development of large numbers of vesicles which coalesce into deep, often necrotic, ulcerative lesions.[161] Dissemination of virus may occur. Ramsey et al. reported the isolation of HSV-2 from lung parenchyma of 1 of 15 adult bone marrow transplant recipients who developed herpes simplex virus pneumonitis.[162] The administration of prophylactic acyclovir prior to bone marrow transplantation has decreased the incidence of reactivated HSV disease.[163,166] Several studies have demonstrated the utility of topical, oral, or intravenous acyclovir in shortening the course and accelerating the healing of mucocutaneous HSV infection in the immunocompromised patient.[167] In general most episodes of mucocutaneous herpes in the immunosuppressed patient should be treated, usually with oral or intravenous acyclovir.

## HSV infection in the HIV-infected patient

Severe HSV infections are among the most common clinical presentations and manifestations of HIV infection. Almost all homosexual men with HIV infection possess antibodies to HSV; 80 to 90 percent to HSV-1 and 80 to 95 percent to HSV-2.[47,168] In those with both HSV-1 and HSV-2 antibodies, reactivation of genital lesions appears to be more frequent than reactivation of oral-labial lesions.[78] Characteristically, HIV-infected patients with HSV present with persistent chronic mucocutaneous ulcerations often involving large areas of perianal, scrotal, or penile areas.[169] Pain and lesions may be present for months, and secondary infections with *Candida* are extremely common. Lesions respond to oral acyclovir therapy (400 mg five times per day), and many patients benefit from chronic suppressive therapy.[166] Recently, TK-negative mutants which are resistant to acyclovir have been isolated with increasing frequency from HIV-infected patients with persistent HSV infection nonresponsive to systemic acyclovir (see below). Treatment with alternative drugs such as Foscarnate may produce healing, although recurrences often occur.

As with most aspects of HIV infection, the severity and frequency of reactivation of HSV increase over the course of HIV infection, i.e., as the patient develops progressive immunodeficiency.[169] In vitro, HSV-1 and HSV-2 gene products transactivate gene regulatory elements, of HIV and may increase the amount of HIV replication.[170] Similar interactions may be seen with cytomegalovirus (CMV) or Epstein-Barr virus (EBV) (see Chap. 36). The role of herpesvirus infections in the progression of HIV disease remains to be determined, although little evidence currently exists to suggest that the in vitro observations of the effect of HSV on HIV replication have any in vivo correlates.

### Role of HSV in acquisition of HIV

Several studies have shown that genital ulcerations and, in particular, the presence of HSV-2 antibodies are risk factors in the acquisition of HIV.[47,171,172] Chancroid infection appears to be the major cause of genital ulceration in Africa. Several studies in the United States have demonstrated that the seroprevalence of HSV-2 is higher in HIV-infected than in HIV-noninfected homosexual men. Although difficult to control well, retrospective and prospective studies of homosexual men in Seattle and San Francisco have shown that the risk of HIV acquisition increases after seroconversion to HSV-2.[47,168,172] As most persons with HSV antibodies develop genital ulcerations in which activated T cells are present, it appears that easier access of HIV to its cellular target may be one potential explanation for this phenomenon. Whether control of genital ulcerations or treatment of HSV infection will decrease the acquisition rate of HIV remains to be determined. These data, however, indicate that more attention should be paid to identifying and counseling the chronic carrier of HSV-2 in high-risk populations.

## RECURRENCE RATE OF GENITAL HSV INFECTION

There are still many gaps in our knowledge concerning the natural history of genital herpes, especially its chronicity. Long-term prospective studies of its rate of recurrence in persons who acquire symptomatic primary infection are unavailable. Many basic questions remain unanswered. Does the frequency of disease change over time? What trigger factors influence recurrences of infection?

Limited prospective studies of patients with primary genital herpes infection have shown that about 60 percent of patients with HSV-1 genital infections develop recurrences within the first 12 months of infection. This is much less than the 90 percent recurrence rate after primary HSV-2 infection (Fig. 35-4). Vaginal inoculation of mice with HSV-1 strains is also much less likely to establish latency in sacral nerve root ganglia than HSV-2 infection.[173] A biological difference between the two viruses may account for their difference in recurrence rates and for the well-known anatomic predilection for HSV-2 infections to be "below the waist" (see Chap. 34).

Both the severity of the initial episode and the host immune response to disease appear to influence the subsequent recurrence rate of disease. Patients with primary genital HSV-2 infection who develop high titers of HSV-2 complement-independent neutralizing antibody in convalescent sera are more likely to develop recurrences than those who do not develop anti-HSV neutralizing antibody.[70] More severe disease as measured by prolonged viral shedding and lesions was also associated with the development of higher titers of neutralizing antibodies as well as antibodies to HSV-specified glycoproteins.[174] Development of high titers of complement-independent neutralizing antibody in convalescent-phase sera after primary infection may reflect a high degree of antigenic exposure and/or a large number of latently infected cells in sacral nerve root ganglia. In the mouse model of mucocutaneous HSV infection, high levels of neutralizing antibody in convalescent sera have been associated with increased numbers of latently infected ganglionic cells.[175]

Recurrence rates of genital herpes vary greatly between individuals. Over the first 2 years of follow-up after primary HSV-2 infection, the median rate of recurrence is five episodes per year. Men tend to have slightly higher recurrence rates than women. Prior HSV-1 infection does not appear to influence the percentage of persons who subsequently have recurrences. However, persons with prior HSV-1 infection who acquire symptomatic HSV-2 infection appear to have lower recurrence rates during the second and third years of follow-up than those followed after primary HSV-2 infection.[175a] Genetic factors related to host immune response may also play a role in the frequency of reactivation.[175b]

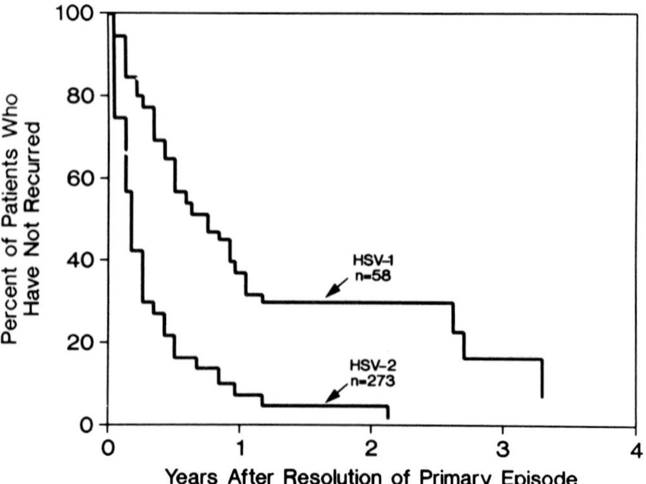


Fig. 35-4. Recurrence rates after primary HSV-1 and HSV-2 infection.

## GENITAL HSV INFECTIONS IN PREGNANCY

A major concern of pregnant patients with genital herpes is the possibility of transmission of the infection to the neonate. Neonatal herpes is a disease of high mortality and morbidity[176–178] (see Chap. 70). Transmitting this STD to a newborn can have devastating effects on the parents as well. Both intrauterine and intrapartum transmission of HSV infection have been described.[179,180] When evaluating the pregnant woman with genital herpes, it should be remembered that the severity of the clinical disease, incidence of cervicitis, duration and titer of viral shedding, and potential of developing viremia differ among patients. In addition, these variables are quite different in primary compared with recurrent HSV infection. The relative risk of transmission to the neonate and the subsequent management of the infection vary accordingly.

## EPIDEMIOLOGY OF HERPES IN PREGNANCY

The prevalence of genital HSV infection during pregnancy as well as the relative incidence of neonatal HSV infection is influenced by the socioeconomic status, age, and past sexual activity of the patient population studied. In the United States, serologic evidence of past HSV-2 infection is present in about 30 percent of middle class women attending prenatal clinics; the percentage is 50 to 70 percent in nonwhite lower socioeconomic obstetric populations. Despite this high serologic prevalence, clinical evidence of HSV is much less. In Seattle, in an obstetric population with a 30 percent prevalence of antibodies to HSV-2, a past or current history of genital HSV was present in only 8 percent of women.

Estimates of the incidence of neonatal herpes have varied from 1 in 3000 to 1 in 20,000 live births.[177] Neonatal HSV infection is not a reportable disease in the United States, but the overall frequency of neonatal HSV infection in the United States has been estimated to be approximately 1 in 7500 live births, or about 700 cases nationally each year. In many areas neonatal herpes has increased in frequency over the last decade. In King County, Washington, the rate was 16 per 100,000 live births in 1982 to 1985 (Fig. 35-2).[27]

## CLINICAL COURSE OF GENITAL HERPES IN PREGNANCY

While it is stated that pregnancy adversely affects the severity and recurrence rate of genital HSV infection, studies comparing the clinical signs and symptoms of disease in matched nonpregnant and pregnant populations are unavailable. Recent studies have indicated that most of the clinical manifestations of recurrent genital herpes, including the frequency of HSV cervicitis, duration of lesions, pain, and constitutional symptoms, are similar in pregnant and nonpregnant women.[181,182] However, the frequency and severity of recurrences do appear to increase over the course of pregnancy.[182] Visceral dissemination of HSV in pregnant women acquiring primary genital disease has been described,[112–114] especially if infection is acquired in the third trimester, but it is rare. Systemic antiviral chemotherapy with intravenous acyclovir should be initiated in pregnant women who have evidence of disseminated infection, especially hepatitis, pneumonitis, or coagulopathy, even though the potential effects of the drug on the fetus are uncertain (see below).

## EFFECTS OF HSV ON PREGNANCY OUTCOME

Studies in the 1960s in lower socioeconomic class populations suggested that genital HSV infection is associated with an increased frequency of spontaneous abortion and premature delivery.[183,184] These studies also suggested that primary HSV cervicitis has a higher risk of complications than other types of disease. Recently, Brown et al. accumulated 28 cases of women who acquired first-episode genital HSV in pregnancy.[185] Pregnancy morbidity was seen only in the 15 women with clinical primary infection, that is, those with fever, constitutional symptoms, and severe lesions. Women with serologic and clinical nonprimary infection had no pregnancy morbidity. Neonatal HSV and prematurity were most frequently seen in women who acquired primary genital infection during the third trimester.[185]

Several explanations for the difference in neonatal morbidity in women with primary versus recurrent genital HSV infection are possible. With primary disease, both hematogenous spread of HSV and ascending chorioamnionitis may produce neonatal infection and disease.[186] Recurrent vulvar genital herpes is usually not associated with concomitant cervicitis. In fact, there is currently little evidence to suggest that women with recurrent genital herpes have increased rates of neonatal morbidity. Several clinical series and a recent population-based study of women with recurrent genital HSV infection in pregnancy suggested no effect of clinical recurrent infection on neonatal outcome including birth weight and gestational age.[181,182,187]

## MATERNAL–INFANT TRANSMISSION OF DISEASE

The major source of HSV infection to the newborn is through contact with the infected maternal genital tract at the time of delivery.[148,176,177] Transmission of HSV from mother to infant occurs mainly during asymptomatic episodes of maternal infection.[148] In recent studies, over 70 percent of infants with neonatal HSV infection were born to mothers without symptoms or signs of infection at delivery. Studies defining the relative risk of transmission of clinically significant infection during vaginal delivery through an HSV-infected birth canal are just beginning to emerge. Primary genital herpes appears to result in a much greater frequency of transmission of herpes to the infant than recurrent genital infection does.[182,184] In several small series, the risk of transmission of disease to the infant from a woman with primary HSV infection was found to be as high as 50 percent (20 to 50 percent).[177,182] The risk of neonatal transmission through vaginal delivery in women with recurrent HSV cervicitis appears to range from 0 to 8 percent, and most studies estimate it at 3 to 5 percent.[187–190] Factors determining whether an exposed infant becomes infected are not completely defined, but include virus titer, local environmental and immune factors, use of fetal monitoring devices, cellular immune responses of the neonate, and titer of maternal antibody in serum and/or amniotic fluid.[191,192] Studies by Yeager et al. have indicated that those infants who are exposed to infectious maternal secretions but who do not develop neonatal herpes have higher maternal neutralizing antibody titers than those exposed infants who go on to develop neonatal herpes.[190]

## MANAGEMENT OF PREGNANT WOMEN WITH GENITAL HERPES

The management of the pregnant woman with genital HSV infection must be individualized and based on the clinical course of disease in the mother as well as the availability of virologic and laboratory support. While critical information still needs to be gathered before optimal management of women with genital herpes can be developed, some guidelines concerning the use of diagnostic virologic services as well as the use of cesarean section can be made.

The acquisition of primary disease during pregnancy carries the risk of potential transplacental transmission of virus to the neonate. In some women, primary infection results in spontaneous abortion. One common question raised by patients with first episodes of genital herpes during pregnancy who do not abort is the use of amniocentesis to determine if intrauterine infection, and hence a congenitally infected child, is present. Recent evidence suggests that false-positive as well as false-negative information may result from this procedure.[193] Uninfected infants have been delivered despite the antepartum isolation of HSV from amniotic fluid. In addition, antiviral substances in amniotic fluid may make isolation of virus from the infant difficult. Thus, amniocentesis at present does not appear to be a reliable test for predicting the presence or absence of a congenitally infected infant.

The vast majority of pregnant women with recurrent genital herpes deliver normal infants, and routine amniocentesis is not recommended in these women or in those who have experienced recurrent episodes of genital herpes in the early stages of pregnancy.

Criteria for laboratory screening and surveillance procedures, as well as delivery procedures, for women with recurrent genital HSV infections are the most frequently encountered problems of obstetricians managing pregnant women with genital herpes. It is obvious from the high prevalence rate of HSV-2 infection in pregnancy (antibody prevalence 30 to 60 percent depending on the population studied) and the low incidence of neonatal disease (1:3000 to 1:20,000 live births) that only a few infants are at risk of acquiring disease. Cesarean section is therefore not routinely warranted for all women with recurrent genital disease. As intrapartum transmission of infection accounts for the vast majority of cases, only those women who shed HSV at the time of delivery need be considered for abdominal delivery. In the past, the American College of Obstetrics and Gynecology and other authorities recommended that patients with genital herpes have weekly cultures of the cervix and/or vulva to determine the presence of asymptomatic viral shedding at or near term.[187,194] However, several studies have shown no correlation between recurrences prior to delivery, even recurrences in the third trimester, and the presence of viral shedding at term.[181,182,187] As such, weekly cytologic and virologic monitoring is no longer advocated. Unfortunately, a rapid, reliable diagnostic method for detection of asymptomatic cervical shedding of HSV is not available. While rapid assays such as ELISA, FA, and routine DNA-hybridization methods have sensitivity equal to that of viral cultures from specimens from genital lesions, when compared with viral isolation they have reduced sensitivity for asymptomatic shedding (see Chap. 77). Because of the low prevalence of shedding HSV at delivery in the general population (<1 percent), these assays also have low positive predictive value for detecting genitourinary HSV infection at the time of delivery.

Patients with recurrent genital herpes should be encouraged to come to the delivery room early at the time of delivery. At this time, careful examination of the external genitalia and the cervix should be performed. In addition, a swab of the cervix and/or vulvar area for viral isolation should be taken. Women who have no clinical evidence of lesions should be delivered vaginally. The presence of active lesions of the cervix or external genitalia, i.e., clinical evidence of herpesvirus infection of the lower genital tract, is an indication for abdominal delivery. This policy will result in the exposure of some infants to episodes of cervical and/or vulvar shedding. As discussed earlier, recent data suggest that only 1 to 6 percent of infants exposed to maternal genital excretions containing HSV develop neonatal herpes.[188] Identification of such infants and communication of an HSV exposure to the attending pediatrician is necessary.[195,196] Currently, it is the policy of most authorities to take samples from these infants (throat, nasopharynx, eyes, and rectal area) for culture for HSV shedding immediately and then at 5- to 10-day intervals. Any clinical evidence of lethargy, skin lesions, or other symptoms of neonatal HSV should be evaluated promptly. All infants from whom HSV is isolated after 24 h of delivery should be treated with systemic antiviral chemotherapy. For a fuller discussion of the presentation of neonatal HSV and its therapy see Chap. 70.

The relation between the duration of ruptured membranes in women with clinically apparent lesions and the potential for transmission of HSV to the infant has also been an area of indecision. Delivery of infants by cesarean section, even from women with intact membranes, occasionally results in neonatal herpes.[195] Prolonged contact with infected secretions may increase the relative risk of acquisition of disease. Many authorities recommend that if membranes have been ruptured for over 4 to 6 h, cesarean section no longer be considered for infant HSV prophylaxis. However, as noted earlier, only 15 to 25 percent of women with recurrent external genital lesions have concomitant HSV cervicitis. Thus, the majority of infants born of mothers with recurrent external genital herpes do not come in prolonged contact with infected genital secretions until the late stages of labor, that is, until exposure to the lower genital canal. Thus in women with recurrent genital herpes who have active external genital lesions at the time of labor, this author still recommends abdominal delivery, providing that no evidence of cervical involvement has been demonstrated by prior virologic monitoring techniques and/or cervical cytologic techniques.

## HOSPITAL ISOLATION OF INFANTS BORN TO WOMEN WITH GENITAL HSV INFECTION

Infants born by cesarean section to women prior to the rupture of membranes or by vaginal delivery to women with no evidence of recent HSV infection are at minimal risk of developing HSV infection, and most hospitals do not recommend segregating the infant from the rest of the newborn nursery. If a more cautionary approach is desired, the infant can be put into an Isolette to make hospital personnel aware of the necessity to use wound and skin precautions and proper hand-washing techniques.

Infants born of women at risk of transmitting disease to the neonate (i.e., women with active lesions) should be placed in isolation.[194] Viral cultures, liver-function studies, and CSF examinations should be obtained, and the infant should be observed closely for the first month of life. Any symptoms of neonatal disease (e.g., poor feeding, fever, hypothermia, skin lesions, or central nervous system signs such as seizures) should be investigated expeditiously for evidence of neonatal HSV infection.[196,197] Management of contact between infant and mother should also be handled on an individual basis. In women who acquire primary genital herpes late in pregnancy, the high incidence of extragenital lesions and the potential of viremia suggest that separation of mother and infant is warranted. As recurrent genital herpes is rarely associated with frequent dissemination of disease or the development of extragenital lesions on exposed extremities, protection of the infant from exposure to infected genital secretions is adequate. When handling the infant in the hospital, the mother should wear a gown and observe proper hand-washing techniques. We allow rooming in with the mother once she has been taught protective measures and is cognizant of the importance of washing her hands between touching her genitalia and touching the infant. There is a greater risk that the newborn will acquire HSV infection from oral-labial herpes than from genital HSV.[198] Thus, nursery personnel and other adults with external labial lesions caused by HSV should also be excluded from intimate contact with the newborn infant.[199]

## DIAGNOSIS OF GENITAL HERPES

### CLINICAL DIAGNOSIS

The differentiation between genital HSV infection and other infectious or noninfectious causes of genital ulceration may be difficult. If multiple grouped vesicles are present or if there is a history of prior lesions of similar size, duration, and character at or near the site of observed attack, HSV infection is the most likely cause of the ulceration. Lesions of genital herpes are painful when touched, and this clinical sign may be useful in differentiating coalesced genital herpetic ulcers from other causes such as *T. pallidum*. It should, however, be remembered that occasionally both organisms may coexist in the same lesion.[200] A persistent, tender, large ulcerative lesion in a patient at risk of *T. pallidum* infection, especially one in whom nontender, rubbery bilateral inguinal adenopathy is present, should raise the suspicion that both pathogens may be present.

Both primary and recurrent HSV infection are accompanied by tender lymphadenopathy. The inguinal nodes upon palpation are usually mildly tender, nonfixed, and only slightly firm. Suppuration, commonly seen with *H. ducreyi* and/or lymphogranuloma venereum, is only rarely seen in genital HSV infection. Nontender, rubbery, firm lymph nodes are more commonly seen with *T. pallidum* infection. Because of the diversity of the signs and symptoms of HSV infections, laboratory confirmation of the cause of genital ulcers should be sought whenever possible.[201]

Noninfectious causes of genital ulcerations, such as inflammatory bowel disease (Crohn's disease) or mucosal ulcerations associated with Behçet's syndrome, may also be confused with genital herpes. These noninfectious causes are usually associated with ulcers that persist for much longer periods of time than those associated with recurrent genital herpes. In addition, the lesions themselves appear larger and deeper than those typically seen in genital HSV infection. A history of persistent lesions waxing and waning with the symptoms of bowel disease is usually elicited in those who have genital ulcerations and a mucocutaneous manifestation of Crohn's disease. Persistent oral lesions, conjunctivitis, and/or central nervous system disease may help differentiate Behçet's syndrome from recurrent genital herpes. The overlap between primary genital HSV infection with conjunctivitis and aseptic meningitis and Behçet's syndrome may, however, cause diagnostic confusion. Persistent lack of laboratory evidence of HSV infection is often useful in establishing the clinical diagnosis of these noninfectious entities.

Despite these descriptions, the clinical manifestations of genital herpes vary considerably; many patients have atypical genital lesions, linear ulcerations with little pain and no erythema, or atypical furuncles. In the United States, most genital ulcerations in heterosexual persons are caused by HSV. However, in other populations *H. ducreyi* and *T. pallidum* may be more prevalent.

## LABORATORY DIAGNOSIS

A detailed discussion of the laboratory diagnosis of genital herpes is presented in Chap. 77. Laboratory confirmation of genital herpes should be performed on all persons in whom a definitive clinical diagnosis cannot be made. Knowledge of the diagnosis is useful in (1) explaining the potential infectivity during episodes of lesions, (2) persuading women to have annual Papanicolaou smears, (3) selecting women at future risk for transmitting the infection to the neonate, and (4) confirming the diagnosis in those for whom antiviral chemotherapy is prescribed. Viral isolation is the most sensitive and specific method of confirming a diagnosis of genital herpes. In most clinical situations, the rapid appearance of HSV in tissue culture (1 to 4 days) makes viral isolation the preferred method for laboratory confirmation when genital herpes is suspected. Alternatively, rapid detection methods such as cytologic examination or immunofluorescence may be used.

Demonstration of a rise in anti-HSV antibody titer in sera drawn early in the course of and after an episode of disease has limited utility in the diagnosis of genital herpes. Serodiagnosis is useful in documenting primary infection, because nearly all patients with primary genital herpes seroconvert. A diagnostic rise in specific antibodies may also be seen in those with nonprimary first episodes of genital herpes.[70] The sensitivity of these serologic procedures is not, however, as high as that of viral isolation. Less than 10 percent of patients with recurrent episodes of disease experience a serologic rise in antibody titer between acute and convalescent sera.[70]

The development of new type-specific serologic methods (see Chap. 77) provides the opportunity to determine if a person is an asymptomatic carrier of HSV-2. As most HSV-2 appears to be transmitted from persons who have undiagnosed disease or asymptomatic infection, more active identification of HSV-2 carriers has been advocated. Past infection with HSV-2 can be identified by the presence of HSV-2 antibodies in serum. If one has HSV-2 antibodies and a genital lesion, it is likely the genital ulceration is caused by HSV, although, as discussed above, other causes are possible.

## THERAPY OF GENITAL HERPES

The therapy of genital herpes includes the following goals: (1) preventing infection and/or (2) shortening the clinical course of disease and reducing the frequency of complications of primary infection such as aseptic meningitis and urinary retention, (3) preventing the development of latency and subsequent clinical recurrences after initial genital infection, (4) preventing subsequent recurrences of disease in those with established latency, (5) decreasing the transmission of disease, and (6) eradicating established latent infection. Major advances in the therapy of genital herpes have been made in the last 7 years, although not all the goals described above have been achieved.

## ACYCLOVIR

The mainstay of the therapy of genital HSV infection is the antiviral acyclovir (ACV). ACV is an acyclic nucleoside analogue that is a substrate for HSV-specified thymidine kinase (TK).[202,203] Acyclovir is selectively phosphorylated by HSV-infected cells to ACV-monophosphate (ACV-MP). Cellular enzymes then phosphorylate ACV-MP to ACV-triphosphate (ACV-TP), a competitive inhibitor of viral DNA polymerase[204,205,205a] (see Fig. 35-5). ACV-TP is incorporated into the growing DNA chain of the virus and causes chain termination.

ACV has potent in vitro activity against both HSV-1 and HSV-2.[204] In animal models, topical or systemic ACV markedly reduces the severity of mucocutaneous HSV infections and, if administered within 96 h after inoculation of virus, prevents ganglionic latency.[205] Numerous trials of ACV in primary and recurrent genital herpes have been conducted. In primary genital HSV infection, intravenous ACV (5 mg/kg q 8 h for 5 days), oral ACV (200 mg five times a day for 10 to 14 days), and topical

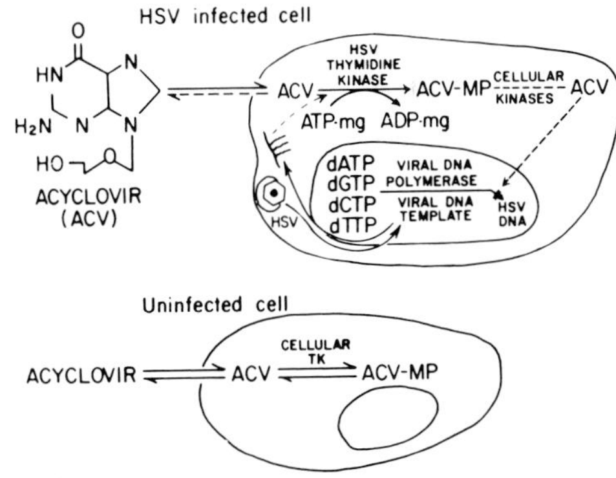


Fig. 35-5. Mechanism of action of acyclovir.

ACV (5% in polyethylene glycol ointment) all reduce the duration of symptoms and viral shedding, and speed healing.[206–209] Table 35-6 shows the relative effectiveness of these therapies in these studies. Systemic therapy prevents new lesion formation, and because of the high incidence of urethral, cervical, and oral infections, systemic therapy (oral ACV) is preferable in first-episode infections. The clinical effect of ACV on first-episode infection is considerable, reducing fever and constitutional symptoms within 48 h of initiating therapy and rapidly relieving symptoms. Thus all patients with first-episode genital HSV infection who present with active lesions should be treated, and because the natural history of disease is for symptoms to progressively increase during the first week, early initiation of therapy is recommended. The author's personal recommendation is to initiate therapy with 200 mg orally five times per day (1 g total daily dose) in persons with presumptive first episodes while awaiting the result of cultures. If an alternative diagnosis is present and cultures are negative, then therapy is discontinued. While treatment of first-episode infection markedly shortens the course of the first episode, it has no discernible effect on the long-term natural history of recurrences at currently utilized dosages.[208,210] Thus patients still need to be counseled about the clinical manifestations and high rate of recurrence, especially among those with HSV-2 infection.

## Treatment of recurrent genital herpes

As discussed earlier, the duration of lesions and symptoms of recurrent genital herpes are considerably less than in first-episode infection. In addition, the number of lesions and their duration may vary greatly among individuals and among episodes in a single individual. In general, persons enrolled in antiviral trials for evaluation of therapies for genital herpes have had from 5 to 15 lesions per episode. Thus, when one is deciding whether to initiate antiviral chemotherapy for recurrent genital herpes, one should consider the severity of infection and relative benefit to the patient.

Oral ACV has given the most consistent therapeutic benefit in reducing the duration of recurrent attacks of genital herpes.[211,212]

**Table 35-6. Treatment of Primary Genital Herpes with Acyclovir: Comparison of Intravenous, Oral, and Topical Preparation** (Percent Reduction Compared with Control Group)

| | Intravenous acyclovir | Oral acyclovir | Topical acyclovir |
|---|---|---|---|
| Number in Study | 27 | 59 | 51 |
| Duration of viral shedding from genital lesions | 85% | 80% | 55% |
| Duration of viral shedding from cervix | 89% | 92% | 65% |
| Reduction in new lesion formation | Yes | Yes | No |
| Time to complete crusting of lesions | 54% | 46% | 34% |
| Time to complete healing of lesions | 57% | 35% | 29% |
| Local itching | 75% | 33% | 55% |
| Local pain | 57% | 44% | 26% |
| Dysuria | 43% | 50% | 12%* |
| Vaginal discharge | 64% | 25% | 16%* |
| Systemic symptoms | Yes | ±* | No |

*Not statistically significant from placebo-treated control group.

A series of studies have demonstrated that both physician- and patient-initiated therapy reduces the duration of lesions and shortens the time virus can be isolated from lesions. However, the effect on symptoms such as local pain and itching is less than the effect on viral shedding and lesion healing. While in most studies oral-ACV recipients tend to have a shorter period of painful genital lesions than placebo recipients, these differences are not statistically significant. Patient-initiated therapy tends to offer greater benefit than physician-initiated therapy because it tends to be initiated earlier.[211] The currently recommended dose is 200 mg orally five times daily. At these dosages and duration, oral ACV has few side effects. Occasional nausea has been reported. Idiosyncratic reactions such as fever and rash have been reported.

The effectiveness of topical ACV on recurrent genital HSV is controversial. In the United States, a 5% topical preparation in polyethlene glycol produced an antiviral effect but little clinical benefit.[206] In Europe, where the preparation is 5% ACV in an aqueous cream, more consistent therapeutic benefit has been achieved.[213] No enhanced benefit is seen if both the oral and topical preparations are utilized simultaneously.[214]

Table 35-7 summarizes current recommendations for the use of ACV in treating genital herpes episodes.

**Table 35-7. Current Status of Antiviral Chemotherapy of Mucocutaneous HSV Infections**

| Type of infection | Treatment and benefits |
|---|---|
| *Mucocutaneous HSV infections* | |
| Immunosuppressed patients | |
| Acute symptomatic first or recurrent episodes | IV or oral ACV relieves pain and speeds healing; with localized external lesions, topical ACV may be beneficial. |
| Suppression of reactivation | IV or oral ACV taken daily prevents recurrences during high-risk periods (e.g., immediately after transplant); lesions will recur when therapy is discontinued. |
| Immunocompetent patients | |
| First episodes of genital herpes | Oral ACV is the treatment of choice. IV ACV may be used if severe disease or neurologic complications are present; topical ACV may be beneficial in patients without cervical, urethral, or pharyngeal involvement. |
| Symptomatic recurrent genital herpes | Oral ACV has some benefit in shortening lesions and viral excretion time; routine use for all episodes not recommended. |
| Suppression of recurrences | Daily oral ACV prevents reactivation of symptomatic recurrences. While licensure is at present limited to 6 months, recent studies suggest courses of up to 18 months are safe. |
| First episodes of oral-labial HSV | Oral ACV has not yet been formally studied but is likely to be effective. |
| Recurrent episodes of oral-labial HSV | Topical ACV is of no clinical benefit; oral ACV has minimal benefit. |

**Table 35-7. Cont.**

| Type of infection | Treatment and benefits |
|---|---|
| Oral-labial UV-provoked HSV | One study indicates oral ACV will prevent UV-provoked lesions when started 24 h prior to exposure and continued through exposure period, usually 7–21 days. |
| Herpetic whitlow | Anecdotal reports suggest oral ACV is beneficial. |
| HSV proctitis | Oral ACV will shorten the course of disease. |
| Herpetic eye infections | Topical trifluorothymidine, vidarabine, idoxuridine, acyclovir, and interferon are all beneficial; debridement may be required; topical steroids may worsen disease. |
| **Antiviral Dosages** | |
| Immunosuppressed patients | IV ACV 5 mg/kg q 8 h for 7–14 days, depending on response. Oral ACV 200–400 mg p.o. 5 times a day for 7–14 days. Topical ACV 4–6 times a day for 7–10 days. |
| Immunocompetent patients | IV ACV 5 mg/kg q 8 h for 5 days. |
| First-episode genital herpes | Oral ACV 200 mg p.o. 5 times a day for 10 days. |
| Recurrent genital herpes | Oral ACV 200 mg p.o. 5 times a day for 5 days. |
| CNS HSV infections | IV ACV 10 mg/kg q 8 h for 10 days. Oral ACV not recommended. |
| **Suppression of HSV Infection** | |
| Immunosuppressed patients | 400 mg p.o. tid (higher dosages can be utilized if clinically necessary). |
| Immunocompetent patients | ACV 200 mg tid or 400 mg p.o. bid (higher or lower dosages can be utilized depending on clinical response). |

## Suppressive acyclovir

Recurrence rates of genital herpes vary in individuals over time. Most patients who seek medical attention for recurrent genital HSV infection report from five to eight recurrences per year.

Several studies have shown that oral ACV given daily to patients with frequently recurring genital HSV (4 to 12 episodes per year) is effective in preventing clinical recurrences of genital herpes.[215–218] Acyclovir in does of 200 mg two to five times daily for up to 2 years will prevent recurrences in 65 to 85 percent of patients as long as therapy is continued. Suppressive therapy in persons with frequently recurring disease produces considerable relief of symptoms and has been of major medical and psychosocial benefit to these patients.

The dosage of oral ACV for suppressive therapy of genital herpes has varied. Early studies suggested that therapies consisting of 200-mg capsules taken two, three, four, or five times a day were of relatively similar efficacy.[215] Recent studies have shown that 400 mg bid or 200 mg qid are the best initial starting dosages in immunocompetent patients.[218] After 2 to 3 months of therapy, it is often possible to reduce the dosage over time to 200 mg three times a day or even 400 mg once daily. More than 90 percent of persons with frequently recurring genital herpes who are immunocompetent have a significant reduction in the number of clinical recurrences on suppressive therapy, although breakthrough recurrences still occur. Up to 25 percent of persons on suppressive therapy develop a breakthrough recurrence each 3-month period.[218] Thus, it is likely that most patients on chronic suppressive therapy will at some time develop a breakthrough. Compared with untreated recurrences, breakthrough recurrences are associated with milder symptoms, shorter duration of viral shedding, and shorter duration of lesions.[215,219] Studies are not available on the effect of chronic suppressive ACV on the frequency of asymptomatic genital tract shedding of HSV and how this may impact on subsequent risk of transmission of disease. Published reports and the author's own experience indicate that occasional cases of transmission may occur during therapy, usually due to sexual activity at the time of a mild breakthrough recurrence.[143]

## Toxicity of suppressive acyclovir

Because frequently recurring genital herpes may plague a patient for years, many patients desire to take oral ACV for prolonged periods. Preclinical animal studies of ACV showed no drug-related carcinogenicity, effect on fertility, or abnormal fetal development.[220] Although acyclovir has been shown to have mutagenic potential in 2 of 22 in vitro systems, the implications of the results for humans treated with chronic suppressive therapy for long periods are unknown. Chronic suppressive ACV taken at dosages of 200 mg five times a day or 200 mg two times a day has had no effect on spermatic function in males.[150] Side effects of daily suppressive oral ACV are uncommon. In fact, data from a multicenter trial of over 1000 patients taking suppressive therapy for 1 year showed no significant clinical or laboratory toxicity.[219] In general, it is the author's policy to do serum creatinine and liver function studies at 6-month intervals on patients on chronic suppressive therapy, but many practitioners do not feel that this is necessary.

One of the major issues facing the clinician managing a patient with genital herpes is the use of intermittent versus chronic suppressive ACV. The most common criteria on which to base this decision are the number of outbreaks, the severity of the outbreaks, and the impact of the disease on the patient's overall sense of well-being. Patients with frequently recurring genital herpes who have considerable physical discomfort, emotional upset, and potential for transmission of infection to sexual partners are candidates for chronic suppressive therapy.[221] Persons who have three to four genital recurrences per year are probably best managed with supportive care and acute intermittent oral therapy. Similarly, persons with frequent recurrences who are minimally symptomatic and not at risk of transmitting infection to an uninfected partner may also be best served by supportive or intermittent therapy. The cost of chronic therapy ($1.50 to $2.50 per day) may also affect this decision. Studies indicate that it takes from 5 to 7 days of therapy before clinical effect can be seen.[215] Intermittent use, for example weekend therapy, has been associated with subsequent clinical recurrences and transmission of disease, indicating that ACV must be administered on a daily basis.[222]

## Acyclovir in pregnancy

Although ACV is not teratogenic in animals, until studies defining its role and safety in pregnancy are available, the use of oral ACV in pregnancy generally cannot be advocated. Recent studies have indicated that first-episode primary genital herpes at or near term is of high morbidity to the patient and infant,[188] and anecdotal observations have suggested the utility of intravenous ACV therapy in this setting.[223] Currently, no data are available to indicate if ACV will prevent the morbidity of primary genital HSV infection at or near term. This situation, fortunately rare, must be handled on an individual basis.

One theoretical use for short-term suppressive ACV therapy is in pregnant women with recurrent genital herpes; ACV administration late in the third trimester might prevent outbreaks near the time of delivery and thereby avoid the need for cesarean section. The incidence of HSV infection in neonates born to women with HSV-2 antibody is low (about 1 in 2000 births), so routine use of ACV in seropositive women to prevent neonatal HSV infection is not cost-effective. Among women with frequently recurring genital HSV infection who have a high rate of cesarean section, effective prophylaxis would be desirable. However, no studies are available showing the safety or utility of suppressive oral ACV therapy in pregnancy, especially its effect on asymptomatic viral shedding. Similarly, no data are available to suggest that short-term ACV therapy is useful as a "morning-after pill" to protect seronegative individuals from primary infection after contact with a sexual partner who has active lesions. If ACV increased the frequency of asymptomatic primary infection, this strategy might even be harmful.

## Emergence of resistance

In vitro resistance to ACV can result from TK-deficient, TK-altered, or DNA polymerase–resistant strains of HSV. TK deficiency is the most common mechanism of HSV resistance to ACV.[224–227] Animal studies have suggested that TK-deficient mutants are less virulent and less able to establish neural latency.[228] However, some of these strains have been shown to be able to establish ganglionic latency, albeit less often than wild-type TK-positive strains. Acyclovir-resistant strains of HSV have been recovered from patients who have never been treated with ACV.[226,227] The clinical significance of ACV resistance is further confounded by the observation that TK-deficient mutants have been isolated from lesions of patients who have responded to treatment with ACV. No clear relation has been established between response to prophylactic therapy and in vitro susceptibility testing of specific clinical isolates. Similarly, the relation between in vitro resistance to ACV and the subsequent development of breakthrough recurrences while on suppressive ACV is unclear. Some studies have found breakthrough isolates resistant in vitro to ACV whereas in other patients, HSV isolates were susceptible.[216,226] Most of the resistant isolates of ACV have been from immunocompromised patients undergoing multiple courses of therapy for established infection. Recently it appears that increasing ACV resistance has been seen in HIV-infected patients who have received long courses of intermittent and/or suppressive therapy.[229] This has been associated with persistent cutaneous lesions which have cleared with the use of alternative antiviral chemotherapy, especially intravenous Foscarnate. These observations indicate that ACV-resistant mutants can be associated with severe clinical disease and may be eradicated with an alternative chemotherapy. Thus, continued surveillance of HSV strains associated with breakthrough recurrences and/or persistent mucocutaneous infection is needed. At present, routine in vitro testing of HSV isolates for ACV sensitivity is not recommended. However, patients who report clinically documented persistent HSV infections while on chronic suppressive therapy and/or have persistent mucocutaneous infections, especially those who have HIV infection, should have their isolates tested for ACV resistance. If the current increase in ACV resistance that is being noted in HIV-infected patients continues, alternative antiviral chemotherapy may become an important aspect of the primary care physicians' treatment of HSV infections.

# OTHER ANTIVIRALS

The role of other antiviral agents in the therapy of genital herpes has remained controversial. In the United States, no other antivirals for the therapy of genital herpes are available. However, in other areas of the world other agents such as vidarabine monophosphate, isoprinosine, various interferon preparations, and foscarnate are available. A brief review of these compounds follows.

## Foscarnate

Foscarnate, an investigational drug in the United States, is a viral DNA polymerase inhibitor similar in structure to phosphonoacetic acid. In vitro it has potent antiviral activity and has been quite effective in speeding the healing of lesions in animal models.[230] It is an insoluble compound and can be effectively administered only intravenously or topically. Systemically it has caused some renal toxicity and causes changes in calcium and phosphorous balance, and as such has been reserved for therapy of serious herpes virus infection, especially cytomegalovirus infection in immunosuppressed patients. Foscarnate appears to be the preferred drug for treatment of disease due to ACV-resistant strains of HSV. In men one study demonstrated a reduction in healing time with 0.3% topical foscarnet cream compared with placebo.[231] However, a collaborative Canadian trial by Sacks et al. of 0.3% foscarnate cream in men and 1% in women demonstrated little overall effect on reducing symptoms or lesions, although some effect of foscarnate cream in reducing viral shedding from lesions, especially in men, was present. Thus, the medication appears to afford little clinical benefit in this setting.[232]

## Vidarabine

Vidarabine (adenine arabinoside, ara-A) is an antiviral compound which selectively inhibits HSV DNA polymerase. Intravenous ara-A is effective in decreasing the mortality of HSV encephalitis and neonatal herpes.[232–234] In comparative trials, ACV has been shown to be more effective for HSV encephalitis in adults.[235,236] For neonatal herpes, the drugs appear to be of nearly equivalent efficacy when given intravenously at comparable dosages. Topically applied 3% ara-A cream and a 10% cream made from the more soluble monophosphate derivative, ara-AMP, are ineffective in shortening the course of initial or recurrent genital and oral-labial infections.[237] Intramuscular ara-AMP has given inconsistent results in genital HSV infections, and because of the greater innate mutagenicity of vidarabine compared with ACV, it is not a drug that can be recommended for routine therapy.

### Idoxuridine, 2-deoxy-D-glucose, Lysine

Topical application of idoxuridine (IDU) (Stoxil) has also been investigated in therapy of oral and genital herpes. Topical preparations of IDU cream are ineffective in genital HSV infection. Several studies comparing IDU in dimethyl sulfoxide (DMSO) have been conducted.[238–240] A 30% IDU-DMSO mixture shortened viral shedding in both initial and recurrent genital herpes; however, no effect was noted on the duration of symptoms, rate of healing, or subsequent recurrence rate of disease.[240] In addition, toxicity associated with prolonged ulceration of genital lesions was seen with a 40% IDU-DMSO mixture. DMSO is not approved for use in the United States. Routine treatment of genital HSV infections with topical IDU in DMSO is not currently recommended. Neither topical 2-deoxy-D-glucose nor oral lysine have been effective in treating genital herpes.[241–243]

## TOPICAL SURFACTANTS AND ANTISEPTICS

HSV is a lipid-enveloped virus, and dissolution of the envelope reduces infectivity. Double-blind placebo-controlled investigations of topical surfactants such as ether and chloroform have shown these medications to be ineffective in shortening the course or duration of initial or recurrent genital or oral-labial HSV infection.[244,245] Similarly well-controlled double-blind investigations of povidone iodine, silver, and zinc compounds on human genital HSV infection have not been conducted.[243] A recent trial of a topical surfactant Intervir-A (*p*-disobutyl phenyl poly ethoxyethanol and polyoxyethylene-10-oleyl ether) claimed to show efficacy in alleviating pain and speeding healing of genital HSV infection.[246] Details of the stage of illness and viral type were not reported, and confirmation of the efficacy of this preparation is needed before recommendations regarding its use can be made.[247]

## PHOTODYNAMIC INACTIVATION

Double-blind placebo-controlled trials of photodynamic inactivation using neutral red and/or proflavine dyes showed them to be ineffective in shortening the course of recurrent genital or oral infection.[248,249] In vitro, this approach to treatment was shown to render HSV capable of causing cell transformation. These agents should not be used for therapy of HSV infection.

## INTERFERONS

The advent of recombinant-DNA-derived interferon has produced renewed interest in the treatment of genital herpes with interferons. A study of 9 million units daily of recombinant-DNA-derived alpha interferon given intramuscularly with and without topical ACV for first-episode genital herpes failed to show any benefit on the disease course either in speeding healing of lesions or in preventing future recurrences of disease.[250,251] In another study, intravenous leukocyte interferon had little effect in reducing the duration of viral shedding in patients with genital HSV-2 infection and had no effect on shortening the duration of lesions of either viral type.[252] Thus, it appears that systemic interferon preparations have little clinical benefit in first-episode infections.

A topical interferon preparation in nonoxynol-9 gel has been utilized to treat acute episodes of recurrent genital HSV infection.[253,254] In these studies, some clinical benefit in relieving pain and speeding healing has been achieved. Continued exploration of these findings is underway. In general, treatment of recurrent genital herpes with systemic interferons has shown this approach to be ineffective and toxic (fever, malaise, myalgias, and neuralgias). Similarly, prophylaxis of recurrences with injectable recombinant-DNA-produced interferons has shown no efficacy of these preparations.[255]

## ISOPRINOSINE

While isoprinosine probinex has been advocated for the therapy of recurrent genital HSV infections, little data exist regarding its therapeutic efficacy. Recent trials have shown the ineffectiveness of this medication for the treatment of genital herpes. Isoprinosine probinex with and without ACV had no benefit compared with ACV alone in the treatment or prophylaxis of genital HSV infection.[256,257]

## IMMUNE MODULATORS

Immune modulators such as levamisole and transfer factors have received some attention for the therapy of genital HSV infection. Controlled clinical trials of levamisole have shown no effect in recurrent mucocutaneous infection.[258,259]

Few studies of transfer factor in mucocutaneous HSV infection have been reported. In a small study conducted at Emory University in Atlanta, Georgia, transfer factor offered no clinical benefit in preventing recurrences of genital herpes.[260] The fluctuations in in vitro cellular immune responses to HSV antigens appear more marked and more frequent than those to varicella-zoster antigens and may make preparation of an effective transfer factor more difficult. No studies have been performed of transfer factor in prevention of primary genital herpes.

## HETEROLOGOUS AND HOMOLOGOUS VACCINES

Many heterologous vaccines such as smallpox, bacillus Calmette-Guérin (BCG), influenza, and polio vaccines have been used as therapies for genital HSV infection.[261] Controlled studies of smallpox vaccine in recurrent oral-labial herpes and BCG vaccine in recurrent genital herpes indicated that the vaccines are ineffective in reducing the recurrence rate of disease.[262] Two recent deaths from disseminated vaccinia infection indicate that use of smallpox vaccine is a potentially dangerous form of therapy which should be actively discouraged.[263]

Inactivated-HSV vaccines are available in Europe (Lupidon G and Lupidon H). Well-controlled evaluations of these vaccines have not been performed, and these preparations are currently unavailable in the United States. Both purified-subunit HSV vaccines and live-virus vaccines are currently under development.[264–267]

## PROPHYLAXIS OF INFECTION

Currently, no proven effective means of prophylaxis of HSV has been established. Barrier forms of contraception, especially condoms, may decrease transmission of disease, especially from episodes of asymptomatic infection. Transmission of disease when lesions are present may still occur despite the use of condoms. Spermicides contain the topical surfactant nonoxynol-9, which inactivates HSV in vitro. Nonoxynol-9 has been shown to be ineffective in the treatment of established genital HSV infection.[69] No data are available, however, to determine if it would be effective in decreasing transmission of disease. With the high incidence of asymptomatic infection and atypical infection, development of an effective HSV vaccine appears to afford the best approach to the prevention of HSV. It is hoped that the vaccines under development will enter clinical trials rapidly.[268,269]

## SUMMARY

Genital HSV infection is a disease of major public health importance. In the last 2 decades genital herpes infection has increased in prevalence in many population groups, especially white middle-class men and women between the ages of 15 and 35 years. First-episode genital HSV infection is a disease of multiple anatomic sites, lasts 3 to 4 weeks, and has a high rate of complications. In contrast, episodes of recurrent genital disease are of much milder intensity and duration. The major morbidity of recurrent genital herpes is its frequency of recurrence, its chronicity, and its effects on the patient's personal relationships and sexuality. The transmission of disease to the neonate is a major concern to women. Studies in the last few years have shown effectiveness of the antiviral compound acyclovir in reducing many of the clinical manifestations of genital herpes. However, HSV-2 infection is still epidemic in most parts of the world. Greater attention to the diagnosis of the asymptomatic carrier and greater emphasis on the recognition of HSV as a cause of genital ulceration is also needed. This is especially relevant with recent data showing that HSV-2 is a risk factor in the acquisition of HIV. Further investigations on the mechanism of recurrence and risk factors associated with recurrence will hopefully provide the tools to attempt to control this disease. In the meantime, knowledge of the natural history of the disease will aid the physician in providing the patient with the information necessary to understand this complex entity, including its long-term complications, and attempt to decrease the transmission to sexual partners and neonates. In this way the physician may do much toward allowing the patient to cope with the psychological and physical components of this illness.

## References


1 Wildy P: Herpes history and classification, in *The Herpes Viruses*, Kaplan AS (ed). New York, Academic, 1973, pp 1–25.
2 Astruc J: *De Morbis Venereis Libri Sex*. Paris, 1736.
3 Hutfield DC: History of herpes genitalis. *Br J Vener Dis* 42:263, 1966.
4 Diday P, Doyon A: *Les Herpes Génitaux*. Paris, Masson et Cie, 1886.
5 Baum O: Über die Ubentragbarkeit des Herpes Simplex auf die kaninchen Hourhaut. *Derm Wochenschr* 70:105, 1920.
6 Cruter W: Das Herpesvirus sein aetiologische und klinische Bedeutung. *Münch Med Wochenschr* 71:1058, 1924.
7 Parker F, Nye RW: Studies on filterable viruses: II. Cultivation of herpes virus. *Am J Pathol* 1:337, 1925.
8 Lipschutz B: Untersuchungen über die Aetiologie der Krankheiten der Herpesgruppe (Herpes zoster, Herpes genitalis, Herpes febrilis). *Arch Dermatol Symp (Berlin)* 136:428, 1921.
9 Dowdle WR et al: Association of antigenic type of *Herpesvirus hominis* with site of viral recovery. *J Immunol* 99:974, 1967.
10 Nahmias AJ, Dowdle WR: Antigenic and biologic differences in *Herpesvirus hominis*. *Prog Med Virol* 10:110, 1968.
11 Nahmias AJ et al: Relation of pock size on chorioallantoic membrane to antigenic type of *Herpesvirus hominis*. *Proc Soc Exp Bio Med* 174:1022, 1968.
12 Nahmias AJ et al: Antibodies to *Herpesvirus hominis* types 1 and 2 in humans. *Am J Epidemiol* 91:539, 1970.
13 Stavraky KM et al: Sexual and socioeconomic factors affecting the risk of past infections with herpes simplex virus type 2. *Am J Epidemiol* 118:109–21, 1983.
14 Medical Office.
15 Wentworth BB et al: Isolation of viruses, bacteria and other organisms from venereal disease clinic patients: Methodology and problems associated with multiple isolations. *Health Lab Sci* 10:75, 1973.
16 Jeansson S, Molin L: On the occurrence of genital herpes simplex virus infection. *Acta Derm Venereol* 54:479, 1974.
17 Jeansson S, Molin L: Genital *Herpesvirus hominis* infection: A venereal disease. *Lancet* 1:1064, 1970.
18 Rauh JL et al: Genital surveillance among sexually active adolescent girls. *J Pediatr* 90:844, 1977.
19 Koutsky LA et al: Spectrum of symptomatic and sozyiliunt genital herpes in women attending an STD clinic. Int. Faculty STD Research. 7th meeting Atl. Georgia Aug 2–5 1987.
20 Knox GE et al: Comparative prevalence of subclinical cytomegalovirus and herpes simplex virus in the genital and urinary tracts of low-income urban women. *J Infect Dis* 140:419, 1979.
21 Vesterinen E et al: clinical and virological findings in patients with cytologically diagnosed gynecologic herpes simplex infection. *Acta Cytol (Baltimore)* 21:199, 1977.
22 *STD Fact Sheet,* 35th ed. US Department of Health and Human Services, Public Health Service, Centers for Disease Control, Atlanta, 1981, pp 5–12.
23 Sumaya CV et al: Genital infections with herpes simplex virus in university student populations. *Sex Transm Dis* 7:16, 1980.
24 MacDougall ML: Genital herpes simplex in the female, 1968 to 1973. *NZ Med J* 82:33, 1975.
25 Srinannoboon S: Cytologic study of herpes simplex infection and dysplasia in the female genital tract. *J Med Assoc Thai* 62:201, 1979.
26 Becker TM et al: Genital herpes infections in private practice in the United States, 1966–1981. *J Am Med Assoc* 253:1601, 1985.
27 Sullivan-Bolyai J et al: Neonatal herpes simplex virus infection in King County, Washington: Increasing incidence and epidemiological correlates. *J Am Med Assoc* 250:3059, 1983.
28 Rawls WE et al: Genital herpes in 2 social groups. *Am J Obstet Gynecol* 110:682, 1971.
29 Corey L, Spear PG. Infections with herpes simplex viruses. *N Engl J Med* 314:686, 749, 1986.
30 Corey L et al: Clinical course of genital herpes simplex virus infections in men and women. *Ann Inter Med* 48:973, 1983.
31 Nahmias AJ, Roizman D: Infection with herpes simplex virus 1 and 2. *N Engl J Med* 19:667, 1973.
32 Josey W et al: The epidemiology of type 2 (genital) herpes simplex virus infection. *Obstet Gynecol Surv* 27:295, 1972.
33 Wentworth BB, Alexander ER: Seroepidemiology of infections due to members of the herpesvirus group. *Am J Epidemiol* 94:496, 1971.
34 Nahmias AJ et al: Antibodies to *Herpesvirus hominis* types 1 and

2 in humans: Patients with genital infections. *Am J Epidemiol* 92:539, 1970.
35 Rawls WE et al: Measurement of antibodies to herpesvirus types 1 and 2 in human sera. *J Immunol* 104:599, 1970.
36 Plummer G et al: Type 1 and 2 herpes simplex viruses: Serological and biological differences. *J Virol* 5:51, 1970.
37 Prakash SS, Seth P: Evaluation of indirect hemagglutination and its inhibition in the differentiation between antibodies to herpes simplex virus types 1 and 2 for seroepidemiologic studies: Use of a II/I index threshold of 85 and an assay of type-specific antibodies. *J Infect Dis* 139:524, 1979.
38 Yeo J et al: Studies on cross reactive antigens in herpes viruses. *Virology* 108:256, 1981.
39 McClung H et al: Relative concentration in human sera of antibodies to cross reacting and specific antigens of HSV virus types 1 and 2. *Am J Epidemiol* 194:192, 1976.
40 Eberle R, Courtney RJ: Assay of type-specific and type-common antibodies to herpes simplex virus types 1 and 2 in human sera. *Infect Immun* 31:1062, 1981.
41 Ashley RL et al: Comparison of Western blot and gG-specific immunodot enzyme assay for detecting HSV-1 and HSV-2 antibodies in human sera. *J Clin Microbiol* 26:662, 1988.
42 Lee FK et al: Detection of herpes simplex virus type 2 specific antibody with glycoprotein G. *J Clin Microbiol* 22:642, 1985.
43 Guinan ME et al: Genital herpes simplex virus infection. *Epidemiol Rev* 7:127, 1988.
44 Porter DD et al: Prevalence of antibodies to EB virus and other herpesviruses. *JAMA* 208:1675, 1979.
45 Duenas A et al: Herpesvirus type 2 in a prostitute population. *Am J Epidemiol* 95:483, 1972.
46a Daling J et al: Sexual practices, sexually transmitted diseases, and the incidence of anal cancer. *N Engl J Med* 317:973, 1987.
47 Stamm WE et al: Association between genital ulcer disease and acquisition of HIV infection in homosexual men. *JAMA* 260:1429, 1988.
48 Vestergaard BF, Rune SJ: Type-specific herpes simplex virus antibodies in patients with recurrent duodenal ulcer. *Lancet* 1:1273, 1980.
49 Smith IW, Peutherer JF: The incidence of *Herpesvirus hominis* antibody in the population. *J Hyg (Lond)* 65:395, 1967.
50 Cunningham T, Corey L: Personal observations.
51 Cesario TC et al: Six years' experience with herpes simplex virus in a children's home. *Am J Epidemiol* 90:416, 1969.
52 Selling B, Kibrick S: An outbreak of herpes simplex among wrestlers (*Herpes Gladiatorum*). *N Engl J Med* 170:979, 1964.
53 Stern H et al: Herpetic whitlow, a form of cross-infection in hospitals. *Lancet* 2:871, 1959.
54 Naib ZM: Exfoliative cytology of viral cervico-vaginitis. *Acta cytol (Baltimore)* 10:126, 1966.
55 Cook ML, Stevens JG: Pathogenesis of herpetic neuritis and ganglionitis in mice: Evidence for intra-axonal transport of infection. *Infect Immun* 7:272, 1973.
56 Barringer JR, Swoveland P: Recovery of herpes simplex virus from human trigeminal ganglions. *N Engl J Med* 188:648, 1973.
57 Barringer JR: Recovery of herpes simplex virus from human sacral ganglions. *N Engl J Med* 291:828, 1974.
58 Warren KG et al: Isolation of latent herpes simplex virus from the superior cervical and vagus ganglions of human beings. *N Engl J Med* 198:1068, 1978.
59 Buchman TG et al: Demonstration of exogenous genital reinfection with herpes simplex virus type 2 by restriction endonuclease fingerprinting of viral DNA. *J Infect Dis* 140:295, 1979.
60 Schmidt O et al: Exogenous reinfection is an uncommon occurrence in patients with symptomatic genital herpes. *J Infect Dis* 149, 1984.
61 Stevens JG et al: RNA complementary to a herpesvirus alpha gene mRNA is prominent in latently infected neurons. *Science,* 235: 1056, 1987.
62 Croen KD et al: Latent herpes simplex virus in human trigeminal ganglia: Detection of an immediate early gene "anti-sense" transcript by in situ hybridization. *N Engl J Med* 317:1427, 1987.
63 Rock DL, Fraser NW. Latent herpes simplex virus type 1 DNA contains 2 copies of the virion DNA joint region. *J Virol* 55:849, 1985.
64 Hill TJ. Herpes simplex virus latency, In *The Herpesviruses,* Roizman B (ed). New York, Plenum, 1985, vol 3, pp 175–240.
65 Stanbury LR et al: Genital herpes in guinea pigs: Pathogenesis of primary infection and description of recurrent disease. *J Infect Dis* 146:397, 1983.
65a Haverkos HW et al: Reactivation of type 1 herpes simplex virus by thoracolumbar neurosurgery. *Ann Int Med* 101:503, 1984.
66 Double-blind placebo-controlled trial of a herpes simplex virus type-2 glycoprotein vaccine in persons at high risk for genital herpes infection. *J Infect Dis,* in press.
67 Kaufman RH et al: Clinical features of herpes genitalis. *Cancer Res* 33:1446, 1973.
68 Adams HG et al: Genital herpetic infection in men and women: Clincal course and effect of topical application of adenine arabinoside. *J Infect Dis* 133:A151, 1976.
69 Vontver AL et al: Clinical course and diagnosis of genital herpes simplex virus infection and evaluation of topical surfactant therapy. *Am J Obstet Gynecol* 133:548, 1979.
70 Reeves WC et al: Risk of recurrence after first episodes of genital herpes: Relation to HSV type and antibody response. *N Engl J Med* 305:315, 1981.
71 Bernstein D et al: Serologic analysis of first episode nonprimary genital herpes simplex virus infection. *Am J Med* 77:1055, 1984.
72 Kalinyak JE et al: Incidence and distribution of herpes simplex virus types 1 and 2 from genital lesions in college women. *J Med Virol* 1:175, 1977.
73 Smith EW et al: Virological studies in genital herpes. *Lancet* 2:1089, 1976.
74 Barton IG et al: Association of HSV-1 with cervical infection. *Lancet* 2:1108, 1981.
75 Guinan ME et al: The course of untreated recurrent genital herpes simplex infection in 27 women. *N Engl J Med* 304:759, 1981.
76 Josey WE et al: Genital herpes simplex infection in the female. *Am J Obstet Gynecol* 96:493, 1966.
77 Embil JA et al: Concurrent oral and genital infection with an identical strain of herpes simplex virus type 1. *Sex Transm Dis* 8:70, 1981.
78 Lafferty WE et al. Recurrences after oral and genital herpes simplex virus infection: Influence of anatomic site and viral type. *N Engl J Med* 316:1444, 1987.
79 Evans AS, Dick EC: Acute pharyngitis and tonsilitis in University of Wisconsin student. *JAMA* 190:699, 1964.
80 Glezen WP et al: Acute respiratory disease of university students with special reference to the etiologic role of *Herpesvirus hominin. Am J Epidemiol* 101:111, 1975.
81 Tustin AW, Kaiser AB: Life threatening pharyngitis caused by herpes simplex virus type 2. *Sex Transm Dis* 6:23, 1979.
82 Ross CAC, Stevenson J: Herpes simplex meningoencephalitis. *Lancet* 2:682, 1961.
83 Klastersky J et al: Ascending myelitis in association with herpes simplex virus. *N Engl J Med* 187:182, 1972.
84 Caplan LR et al: Urinary retention probably secondary to herpes genitalis. *N Engl J Med* 197:920, 1977.
85 Ravaut P, Darre M: Les reactions nerveuses au cours de herpes genitaux. *Ann Dermatol Syph (Paris)* 5:481, 1904.
86 Olson LC et al: Herpesvirus infections of the human central nervous system. *N Engl J Med* 272:1271, 1967.
87 Skoldenberg B et al: Herpes simplex virus 2 and acute aseptic meningitis. *Scand J Infect Dis* 7:227, 1975.
88 Meyer HM et al: Central nervous system syndromes of "viral" etiology. *Am J Med* 29:334, 1960.
89 Morison RE et al: Adult meningoencephalitis caused by *Herpesvirus hominis* type 2. *Am J Med* 56:540, 1974.

90 Craig C, Nahmias A: Different patterns of neurologic involvement with herpes simplex virus types 1 and 2: Isolation of herpes simplex virus from the buffy coat of two adults with meningitis. *J Infect Dis* 127:365, 1973.

91 Whitley RJ et al: Adenine arabinoside therapy of biopsy proven herpes simplex virus encephalitis: National Institute of Allergy and Infectious Diseases Collaborative Antiviral Study. *N Engl J Med* 197:289, 1977.

92 Brenton DW: Hypoglycorrhachia in herpes simplex type 2 meningitis. *Arch Neurol* 37:317, 1980.

93 Corey L et al: Intravenous acyclovir for the treatment of primary genital herpes. *Ann Intern Med* 98:914, 1983.

94 Riehle RA, Williams JJ: Transient neuropathic bladder following herpes simplex genitalis. *J Urol* 122:263, 1979.

95 Oates JK, Greenhouse PR: Retention of urine in anogenital herpetic infection. *Lancet* 1:691, 1978.

96 Jacome DE, Yanez GF: Herpes genitalis and neurogenic bladder and bowel. *J Urol* 124:752, 1980.

97 Goldmeier D et al: Urinary retention and intestinal obstruction associated with anorectal herpes simplex virus infection. *Br Med J* 1:425, 1975.

98 Samarasinghe P et al: Herpetic proctitis and sacral radiomyelopathy: a hazard for homosexual men. *Br Med J* 2:365, 1979.

99 Shturman-Ellstein R et al: Myelitis associated with genital herpes in a child. *J Pediatr* 88:523, 1976.

100 Crane LR, Lerner AM: Herpetic whitlow: a manifestation of primary infection with herpes simplex virus type 1 and 2. *J Infect Dis* 137:855, 1978.

101 Gill JM et al: Herpes simplex virus infections of the hand. A profile of 79 cases. *Am J Med* 84:89, 1988.

102 Nahmias AJ: Disseminated herpes simplex virus infections. *N Engl J Med* 282:684, 1979.

103 Kipping R, Downie A: Generalized infection with herpes simplex. *Br Med J* 10:247, 1948.

104 Ruchman I, Dodd K: Recovery of herpes simplex virus from the blood of a patient with herpetic rhinitis. *J Lab Clin Med* 35:434, 1950.

105 Auch Moedy JL et al: Fatal disseminated herpes simplex virus infection in a healthy child. *Am J Dis Child* 135:45, 1981.

106 Friedman HM et al: Acute monarticular arthritis caused by herpes simplex virus and cytomegalovirus. *Am J Med* 69:241, 1980.

107 Shelley WB: Herpetic arthritis associated with disseminated herpes simplex virus and cytomegalovirus. *Am J Med* 69:241, 1980.

108 Joseph TJ, Vogt PJ: Disseminated herpes with hepatoadrenal necrosis in an adult. *Am J Med* 56:735, 1974.

109 Flewett TH et al: Acute hepatitis due to herpes simplex in an adult. *J Clin Pathol* 22:60, 1969.

110 Whittaker JA, Hardson MD: Severe thrombocytopenia after generalized HSV-2 infection. *South Med J* 72:864, 1978.

111 Schlesinger JJ et al: Myoglobinuria associated with herpes group viral infections. *Arch Intern Med* 138:422, 1978.

112 Koberman T et al: Maternal death secondary to disseminated *Herpesvirus hominis*. *Am J Obstet Gynecol* 137:742, 1980.

113 Goyette RE et al: Fulminant hepatitis during pregnancy. *Obstet Gynecol* 43:191, 1974.

114 Young EJ et al: Disseminated herpesvirus infection associated with primary genital herpes in pregnancy. *JAMA* 235:2731, 1976.

115 Wenner HA: Complications of infantile eczema caused by virus of herpes simplex: (a) Description of the clinical characteristics of an unusual eruption and (b) identification of an associated filterable virus. *Am J Dis Child* 67:247, 1944.

116 Mailman CJ et al: Recurrent eczema herpeticum. *Arch Dermatol* 89:815, 1964.

118 Wheeler CE Jr, Abele DC: Eczema herpeticum, primary and recurrent. *Arch Dermatol* 93:162, 1966.

119 Keane JT et al: *Herpesvirus hominis* hepatitis and disseminated intravascular coagulation: Occurrence in an adult with pemphigus vulgaris. *Arch Intern Med* 126:1312, 1976.

120 Sutton AL et al: Fatal disseminated *Herpesvirus hominis* type 2 infection in an adult with associated thymic dysplasia. *Am J Med* 56:545, 1974.

121 Schneidman DW et al: Chronic cutaneous herpes simplex. *JAMA* 241:592, 1979.

122 St. Geme JW et al: Impaired cellular resistance to herpes simplex virus in Wiskott-Aldrich syndrome. *N Engl J Med* 173:229, 1965.

123 Linnemann CC et al: *Herpesvirus hominis* type 2 meningoencephalitis following renal transplantation. *Am J Med* 61:703, 1976.

124 Lehtinen M et al: Detection of herpes simplex virus in women with acute pelvic inflammatory disease. *J Infect Dis* 152:78, 81, 1985.

125 Abraham AA: *Herpesvirus hominis* endometritis in a young woman wearing an intrauterine device. *Am J Obstet Gynecol* 131: 340, 1978.

126 Notkins AL: Immune mechanisms by which the spread of viral infections is stopped. *Cell Immunol* 11:478, 1974.

127 Guinan ME et al: Course of an untreated episode of recurrent genital herpes simplex infection in 27 women. *N Engl J Med* 304: 759, 1981.

128 Corey L et al: Cellular immune response in genital herpes simplex virus infection. *N Engl J Med* 199:986, 1978.

129 Parker JD, Bantalval JE: Herpes genitalis: Clinical and virological studies. *Br J Vener Dis* 43:212, 1967.

130 Koutsky LA et al. Clinical spectrum of urogenital and anorectal HSV infection in women: Diagnostic strategies for a high risk population. Unpublished data.

131 Quinn TC et al: The etiology of anorectal infection in homosexual men. *Am J Med* 71:395, 1981.

132 Waugh MA: Anorectal *Herpesvirus hominis* infection in men. *J Am Vener Dis Assoc* 3:68, 1976.

133 Goldmeier D: Proctitis and herpes simplex virus in homosexual men. *Br J Vener Dis* 56:111, 1980.

134 Levine JB, Saeed M: *Herpesvirus hominis* (type 1) proctitis. *J Clin Gastroenterol* 1:225, 1979.

135 Goodell SE et al: Herpes simplex virus: Proctitis. *N Engl J Med* 309:868, 1983.

136 Curry JP et al: Proctitis associated with *Herpesvirus hominis* type 2 infection. *Can Med Assoc J* 119:485, 1978.

137 Goldmeier D: Herpetic proctitis and sacral radiculomyelopathy in homosexual men. *Br Med J* 2:549, 1979.

138 Samarasinghe PL et al: Herpetic proctitis and sacral radiomyelopathy: A hazard for homosexual men. *Br Med J* 2:365, 1979.

139 Jacobs SC et al: Acute motor paralytic bladder in renal transplant patients with anogenital herpes infection. *J Urol* 123:426, 1980.

140 Rompalo AM et al: Oral acyclovir for treatment of first-episode herpes simplex virus proctitis. *JAMA* 259:2879, 1988.

141 Chapel T et al: Microbiological flora of penile ulcerations. *J Infect Dis* 137:50, 1978.

142 Kinghorn GR et al: Pathogenic microbial flora of genital ulcers in Sheffield with particular reference to herpes simplex virus and *Haemophilus ducreyi*. *Br J Vener Dis* 58:377, 1982.

143 Rooney JJ et al: Acquisition of genital herpes from an asymptomatic sexual partner. *N Engl J Med* 314:1561, 1986.

144 Mertz GJ et al: Transmission of genital herpes in couples with one symptomatic and one asymptomatic partner: A prospective study. *J Infect Dis* 157:1169, 1988.

145 Mertz GJ et al: Frequency of acquisition of first episode genital infection with herpes simplex virus from symptomatic and asymptomatic source contacts. *Sex Transm Dis* 12:33, 1985.

146 Douglas RG Jr, Couch RB: A prospective study of chronic herpes simplex virus infection and recurrent herpes labialis in humans. *J Immunol* 104:289, 1970.

147 Spruance SL. Pathogenesis of herpes simplex labialis: Excretion of virus in the oral cavity. *J Clin Microbiol* 19:675, 1984.

148 Whitley RJ et al: The natural history of genital herpes simplex virus infection of mother and newborn. *Pediatrics* 66:489, 1980.

149 Centifano YM et al: Herpesvirus type 2 in the male genitourinary tract. *Science* 318:1972, 1978.

150 Douglas JM et al: A double-blind placebo-controlled trial of the effect of chronic oral acyclovir on sperm production in men with frequently recurrent genital herpes. *J Infect Dis* 157:588, 1988.
151 Rattray MC et al: Recurrent genital herpes among women: Symptomatic versus asymptomatic viral shedding. *Br J Vener Dis* 54: 262, 1978.
152 Adam E et al: Persistence of virus shedding in asymptomatic women after recovery from herpes genitalis. *Obstet Gynecol* 564: 171, 1979.
153 Moseley R et al: Comparison of the indirect immunoperoxidase and direct immunofluorescence techniques with viral isolation for the diagnosis of genital herpes simplex virus infection. *J Clin Microbiol* 13:93, 1981.
154 Stenzel Poore M et al: Herpex simplex in genital secretions. *Sex Transm Dis* 14:17, 1987.
154a Brock BV et al: Frequency of asymptomatic shedding of HSV in women. *Sex Transm Dis* (in press).
155 Deture FA et al: Herpes virus type 2 study of semen in male subjects with recurrent infections. *J Urol* 120:449, 1978.
156 Montgomerie JZ et al: Herpex simplex virus infection after renal transplantation. *Lancet* 2:867, 1969.
157 Whitley RJ et al: Infections caused by the herpes simplex virus in the immunocompromised host: natural history and topical acyclovir therapy. *J Infect Dis* 150:323, 1984.
158 Wade JC et al: Intravenous acyclovir to treat mucocutaneous herpes simplex virus infection after marrow transplantation: a double-blind trial. *Ann Intern Med* 96:265, 1982.
159 Meyers JD et al: Infection with herpes simplex virus and cell-mediated immunity after marrow transplant. *J Infect Dis* 142:338, 1980.
160 Pass RF et al: Identification of patients with increased risk of infection with herpes simplex virus after renal transplantation. *J Infect Dis* 140:487, 1979.
161 Whitley RJ: Mucocutaneous herpes simplex virus infections in immunocompromised patients. *Am J Med* 73:236, 1982.
162 Ramsey PG et al: Herpes simplex virus pneumonia: Clinical presentation and pathogenesis. *Ann Intern Med* 97:813, 1982.
163 Saral R et al: Acyclovir prophylaxis of herpes-simplex-virus infections: A randomized double-blind controlled trial in bone marrow-transplant recipients. *N Engl J Med* 305:63, 1981.
164 Shepp DH, et al: Oral acyclovir therapy for mucocutaneous herpes simplex virus infections in immunocompromised marrow transplant recipients. *Ann Intern Med* 102:723, 1985.
165 Mitchell CD et al: Acyclovir therapy for mucocutaneous herpes simplex infections in immunocompromised patients. *Lancet* 1: 1389, 1981.
166 Gold D, Corey L: Acyclovir prophylaxis of herpes simplex virus infection. *Antimicrob Agents Chemother* 31:361, 1987.
167 Straus SE et al: Oral acyclovir to suppress recurring herpes simplex virus infection in immunodeficient patients. *Ann Int Med* 100:522, 1984.
168 Holmberg SB et al: Prior HSV type 2 infection as a risk factor for HIV infection. *JAMA* 259:1048, 1988.
169 Siegel FP et al: Acquired immunodeficiency in male homosexuals manifested by chronic perianal ulcerative herpes simplex lesions. *N Engl J Med* 305:1439, 1988.
170 Mosca JD et al: Herpes simplex virus type 1 can reactivate transcription of latent human immunodeficiency virus. *Nature* 325:67, 1987.
171 Kreiss JK et al: AIDS virus infection in Nairobi prostitutes: Spread of the epidemic to East Africa. *N Engl J Med* 314:414, 1986.
172 Holmberg SB et al: Prior HSV-2 type 2 infection as a risk factor for HIV infection. *JAMA* 259:1048, 1988.
173 Richards JT et al: Differences in neurovirulence of herpes simplex virus type 1 and type 2 isolates in four experimental infections of mice. *J Infect Dis* 144:464, 1981.
174 Zweerink HJ, Corey L: Virus specific antibodies for HSV-2 in sera from patients with genital herpes virus infection. *Infect Immun* 37:413, 1982.
175 Klein RJ et al: Orofacial herpes simplex virus infection in hairless mice: Latent virus in trigeminal ganglia after topical antiviral treatment. *Infect Immun* 20:130, 1978.
175a Corey L et al: Effect of prior HSV-1 infection on the natural history of genital herpes. Abstract 821, 20th ICAAC, October 23–26, 1988, Los Angeles.
175b Kapadia A et al: Familial herpes simplex infection associated with activation of the complement system. *Am J Med* 67:122, 1979.
176 Nahmias AJ et al: Newborn infection with *Herpesvirus hominis* types 1 and 2. *J Pediatr* 75:1194, 1969.
177 Nahmias AJ et al: Herpes simplex, in *Infectious Diseases of the Fetus and Newborn Infant,* Remington JS, Klein JO (eds). Philadelphia, Saunders, pp 636–78, 1983.
178 Stagno S and Whitley RJ: Herpes virus infections of pregnancy: Part II: Herpex simplex virus and varicella zoster infection. *N Engl J Med* 313:1327, 1985.
179 Florman A et al: Intrauterine infection with herpes simplex virus: Resultant congenital malformations. *JAMA* 225:129, 1973.
180 Chalub EG et al: Congenital herpes simplex type II infection with extensive hepatic calcification, bone lesions and cataracts: Complete postmortem examination. *Dev Med Child Neurol* 19:527, 1977.
181 Vontver LA et al: Recurrent genital herpes simplex virus infection in pregnancy: Infant outcome and frequency as asymptomatic recurrences. *Am J Obstet Gynecol* 143:75, 1982.
182 Brown ZA et al: Genital herpes in pregnancy: Risk Factors associated with recurrences and asymptomatic shedding. *Am J Obstet Gynecol* 153:24, 1985.
183 Naib ZM et al: Association of maternal genital herpetic infection with spontaneous abortion. *Obstet Gynecol* 35:260, 1970.
184 Nahmias AJ et al: Perinatal risk associated with maternal genital herpes simplex virus infection. *Am J Obstet Gynecol* 110:825, 1971.
185 Brown ZA et al: Effects on infants of first episode genital herpes during pregnancy. *N Engl J Med* 317:1247, 1987.
186 Hain J et al: Ascending transcervical herpes simplex infection with intact fetal membranes. *Obstet Gynecol* 56:106, 1980.
187 Wolf ME: Women with genital herpes and risk of postpartum endometritis. Abstract, Society for Epidemiologic Research, June 15–17, 1988, Vancouver, BC.
187 Arvin AM et al: Failure of antepartum maternal cultures to predict the infant's risk of exposure to herpes simplex virus at delivery. *N Engl J Med* 315:796, 1986.
188 Prober CG et al: Low risk of herpes simplex virus infections in neonates exposed to the virus at the time of vaginal delivery to mothers with recurrent genital HSV infections. *N Engl J Med* 316: 240, 1987.
189 Tejani N et al: Subclinical herpes simplex genitalis infections in the perinatal period. *Am J Obstet Gynecol* 135:547, 1979.
190 Yeager AS: Genital herpes simplex infections: Effect of asymptomatic shedding and latency on management of infections in pregnant women and neonates. *J Invest Dermatol* 83:053s, 1984.
191 Yeager AS et al: Relationship of antibody to outcome in neonatal herpes simplex virus infections. *Infect Immun* 29:532, 1980.
192 Parvey LS, Ch'ien LT: Neonatal herpes simplex virus infection introduced by fetal monitor scalp electrodes. *Pediatrics* 65:1140, 1980.
193 Zervoudakis IA et al: Herpes simplex in the amniotic fluid of an unaffected fetus. *Obstet Gynecol* 55:16s, 1980.
194 Committee on Fetus and Newborn and Committee on Infectious Diseases: Perinatal herpes simplex virus infections. *Pediatrics* 66: 147, 1980.
195 Light IJ, Linnemann CC: Neonatal herpes simplex infection following delivery by cesarean section. *Obstet Gynecol* 44:496, 1974.
196 Whitley RJ et al. Changing presentation of herpes simplex virus infection in neonates. *J Infect Dis* 158:109, 1988.

197 Sullivan-Bolyai J et al: Presentation of neonatal HSV infections: Implications for a change in therapeutic strategy. *Pediatr Infect Dis* 5:309, 1986.
198 Light IJ: Postnatal acquisition of herpes simplex virus by the newborn infant: A review of the literature. *Pediatrics* 63:480, 1979.
199 Linnemann CC et al: Transmission of herpes-simplex virus type 1 in a nursery for the newborn: Identification of viral isolates by DNA "fingerprinting." *Lancet* 1:964, 1978.
200 Chapel TA et al: Simultaneous infection with *Treponema pallidum* and herpes simplex virus. *Cutis* 24:191, 1979.
201 Corey L et al: Genital herpes simplex virus infection: Current concepts in diagnosis, therapy and prevention. *Ann Intern Med* 98: 973, 1983.
202 Schaeffer HJ et al: 9-(2-Hydroxyethoxymethyl) guanine activity against viruses of herpes group. *Nature* 272:583, 1978.
203 Elion GB et al: Selectivity of action of an antiherpetic agent, 9-(2-hydroxyethoxymethyl) guanine. *Proc Natl Acad Sci* USA 74:5716, 1977.
204 Crumpacker CS et al: Growth inhibition by acycloguanosine of herpesvirus isolated from human infections. *Antimicrob Agents Chemother* 15:642, 1979.
205 Dorsky DI, Crumpacker CS. Acyclovir: Drugs 5 years later. *Ann Intern Med* 207:859, 1987.
205a Brigden D, Whitman P. The clinical pharmacology of acyclovir and its prodrug. *Scand J Infect Dis (Suppl)* 47:33, 1985.
206 Corey L et al: Double blind placebo controlled trial of topical acyclovir in first and recurrent episodes of genital herpes simplex virus infection. *N Engl J Med* 106:1313, 1982.
207 Bryson YJ et al: Treatment of first episodes of genital herpes simplex virus infections with oral acyclovir: a randomized double blind controlled trial in normal subjects. *N Engl J Med* 308:916, 1983.
208 Mertz GJ et al: Double-blind placebo-controlled trial of oral acyclovir in the first episode genital herpes simplex virus infection. *JAMA* 252:1147, 1984.
209 Corey L et al: Intravenous acyclovir for the treatment of primary genital herpes. *Ann Int Med* 98:914, 1983.
210 Corey L et al: Risk of recurrence after treatment of first episode genital herpes with intravenous acyclovir. *Sex Transm Dis* 12:215, 1985.
211 Reichman RC et al: Treatment of recurrent genital herpes simplex infections with oral acyclovir: a controlled trial. *JAMA* 251:2103, 1984.
212 Nilsen AE et al: Efficacy of oral acyclovir in treatment of initial and recurrent genital herpes. *Lancet* 2:572, 1982.
213 Fiddian AP et al: Topical acyclovir in the treatment of genital herpes: a comparison with systemic therapy. *J Antimicrob Chemother* 12(suppl B):67, 1983.
214 Kinghorn GR et al: Efficacy of combined treatment with oral and topical acyclovir in first episode genital herpes. *Genitourin Med* 62:186, 1986.
215 Douglas JM et al: A double blind study of oral acyclovir for suppression of recurrences of genital herpes simplex virus infection. *N Engl J Med* 310:1551, 1984.
216 Straus SE et al: Suppressing of frequently recurring genital herpes: a placebo-controlled double blind trial of oral acyclovir. *N Engl J Med* 310:1545, 1984.
217 Halsos AM et al: Oral acyclovir suppression of recurrent genital herpes: a double-blind, placebo-controlled crossover study. *Acta Derm Venereol (Stockh)* 65:59, 1985.
218 Mindel A et al: Dosage and safety of long term suppressive therapy for recurrent genital herpes. *Lancet* 1:926, 1988.
219 Mertz GJ et al: Long term acyclovir suppression of frequently recurring genital herpes simplex virus infection: a multi-center double blind trial. *JAMA* 260(2):201, 1988.
220 Tucker WE: Preclinical toxicology of acyclovir: an overview. *Am J Med* 73:(1A):27–30, 1982.
221 Gold D, Corey L: Acyclovir prophylaxis for herpes simplex virus infection. *Antimicrob Agents Chemother* 31:361, 1987.
222 Straus SE et al: Double blind comparison of weekend and daily regimens of oral acyclovir for suppression of recurrent genital herpes. *Antiviral Res* 6:151, 1986.
223 Lagrew DC et al: Disseminated herpes simplex virus infection in pregnancy: successful treatment with acyclovir. *JAMA* 252:2038, 1984.
224 Coen DM, Schaffer PA: Two distinct loci confer resistance to acycloguanosine in herpes simplex virus type 1. *Proc Natl Acad Sci USA* 77:2265, 1980.
225 Barry DW et al: Clinical and laboratory experience with acyclovir-resistant herpes viruses. *J Antimicrob Chemother* 18(suppl B):75, 1986.
226 Nusinoff-Lehrman S et al: Recurrent genital herpes and suppressive oral acyclovir therapy: relationship between clinical outcome and in vitro drug sensitivity. *Ann Int Med* 204:686, 1986.
227 McLaren C et al: In vitro sensitivity to acyclovir in genital herpes simplex viruses from acyclovir treated patients. *J Infect Dis* 148: 868, 1983.
228 Field HJ, Darby G. Pathogenicity in mice of strains of herpes simplex virus which are resistant to acyclovir in vitro and in vivo. *Antimicrob Agents Chemother* 17:209, 1980.
229 Crumpacker CL et al: Acyclovir resistant HSV-2 isolates in patients with HIV infection. *N Engl J Med* (in press).
230 Alenius S et al: Therapeutic effects of foscarnet sodium and acyclovir on cutaneous infection due to herpes simplex virus type 1 in guinea pigs. *J Infect Dis* 145:569, 1982.
231 Wallin J et al: Topical treatment of recurrent genital herpes infection with foscarnate. *Scand J Infect Dis* 17:165, 1985.
232 Sacks SL et al: Clinical course of recurrent genital herpes and treatment with foscarnet cream. Results of a Canadian multicenter trial. *J Infect Dis* 155:178, 1987.
233 Whitley RJ et al: Adenine arabinoside therapy of biopsy-proved herpes simplex encephalitis: National Institute of Allergy and Infectious Diseases Collaborative Antiviral Study. *N Engl J Med* 297: 389, 1977.
234 Whitley RJ et al: Vidarabine therapy of neonatal herpes simplex virus infection. *Pediatrics* 66:495, 1980.
235 Whitley R et al: Vidarabine versus acyclovir therapy in herpes simplex encephalitis. *N Engl J Med* 314:144, 1986.
236 Skoldenberg B et al: Acyclovir versus vidarabine in HSV encephalitis: randomized multicenter study in conservative Swedish patients. *Lancet* 2:707, 1984.
237 Spruance SL et al: Ineffectiveness of topical adenine arabinoside 5′-monophosphate in the treatment of recurrent herpes simplex labialis. *N Engl J Med* 300:1180, 1979.
238 MacCallum FO, Juel-Jensen BE: Treatment of herpes simplex virus skin infection with IDU in dimethylsulfoxide: Results of double-blind controlled trial. *Br Med J* 2:805, 1966.
239 Davidson-Parker JD: A double blind trial of idoxuridine in recurrent genital herpes. *J Antimicrob Chemother* 3(suppl):131, 1977.
240 Silvestri DL et al: Ineffectiveness of topical idoxuridine in dimethylsulfoxide for genital herpes. *JAMA* 248:953, 1982.
241 Kern ER et al: Failure of 2-deoxy-D-glucose in treatment of experimental cutaneous and genital herpes simplex virus (HSV) infections. *J Infect Dis* 146:159, 1982.
242 Milman N et al: Failure of lysine treatment in recurrent herpes simplex labialis. *Lancet* 2:942, 1978.
243 Scheibel M, Jessen O: Lysine prophylaxis in recurrent herpes simplex labialis: A double-blind controlled crossover study. *Acta Derm Venereol (Stockh)* 60:85, 1979.
244 Friedrich EG Jr, Masukawa T: Effect of povidone-iodine on herpes genitalis. *Obstet Gynecol* 45:337, 1975.
245 Corey L et al: Ineffectiveness of topical ether for the treatment of genital herpes simplex virus infection. *N Engl J Med* 199:237, 1978.
246 Goldberg CB: Controlled trial of 'Intervir-A' in herpes simplex virus infection. *Lancet,* March:703, 1986.
247 Gold D et al: Topical surfactant therapy for recurrent HSV infection. *Lancet* 2:283, 1986.
248 Myers MG et al: Failure of neutral-red photo-dynamic inactivation

in recurrent herpes simplex virus infections. *N Engl J Med* 292:945, 1975.

249 Felbee TD et al: Photodynamic inactivation of herpes simplex. *JAMA* 223:289, 1973.

250 Levin MJ et al: Comparison of recombinant leukocyte interferon-alpha (rIFN-2A) with topical acyclovir for the treatment of first episode herpes genitalis and prevention of subsequent recurrences. *Antimicrob Agents Chemother* Unpublished data.

251 Mendelson J et al: Effect of recombinant interferon alpha c 2 on clinical course of first episode genital herpes infection and subsequent recurrences. *Genitourin Med* 62:97, 1986.

252 Pazin GJ et al: Leukocyte interferon for treating first episodes of genital herpes in women. *J Infect Dis* 156:891, 1987.

253 Rapp F, Wrzos H: Synergistic effect of human leukocyte interferon and nonoxynol 9 against herpes simplex virus type 1. *Antimicrob Agents Chemother* 28:449, 1985.

254 Lassus A et al: Efficacy of interferon and placebo in the treatment of recurrent genital herpes: A double-blind trial. *Sex Transm Dis* 14:185, 1987.

255 Kuhls TL et al: Suppression of recurrent genital herpes simplex virus infection with recombinant $a_2$ interferon. *J Infect Dis* 154: 437, 1986.

256 Mindel A et al: Treatment of first attack genital herpes, acyclovir versus inosine pranobex. *Lancet* 1:1171, 1987.

257 Mindel A, Carney O: Suppression of frequently recurring genital herpes. Acyclovir versus inosine pranobex. Abstract 89, International Congress and Symposium Services. 1988.

258 Spruance SL et al: Treatment of recurrent herpes simplex labialis with levamisole. *Antimicrob Agents Chemother* 15:662, 1979.

259 Bierman SM: Double-blind crossover study of levamisole as immunoprophylaxis for recurrent herpes progenitalis. *Cutis* 21:352, 1978.

260 Starr SE: Immunotherapy for recurrent herpetic infections. *Cutis* 20:596, 1977.

261 Kern AB, Schiff BL: Smallpox vaccinations in the management of recurrent herpes simplex: A controlled evaluation. *J Invest Dermatol* 33:99, 1959.

262 Douglas JM et al: Ineffectiveness and toxicity of BCG vaccine for the prevention of recurrent genital herpes. *Antimicrob Agents Chemother* 27:203, 1985.

263 Centers for Disease Control: Adverse reactions to smallpox vaccinations—1978. *MMWR* 28:265, 1979.

264 Mertz GJ et al: Herpes simplex virus type-2 glycoprotein-subunit vaccine: tolerance and humoral and cellular responses in humans. *J Infect Dis* 150:242, 1984.

265 Meignier B: Vaccination against herpes simplex virus infection, in *The Herpesviruses,* Roizman B and Lopez C (eds). New York, Plenum, 1985, vol 4, pp 265–269.

266 Allen WP, Rapp F. Concept review of genital herpes vaccines. *J Infect Dis* 145:413, 1982.

267 Pescador-Sanchez L et al: The effect of adjuvants on the efficacy of a recombinant HSV glycoprotein vaccine. *J Immunol* 141:1720, 1988.

268 Lasky LA et al: Protection of mice from lethal herpes simplex virus infection by vaccination with a secreted form of cloned glycoprotein D. *Biotechnology* 2:527, 1984.

269 Meigneir B et al: In vivo behavior of genetically engineered herpes simplex viruses R7017 and R7020: Contruction and evaluation in rodents. *J Infect Dis* 158:602, 1988.

# Chapter 36

# Cytomegalovirus as a sexually transmitted infection

Lynn Smiley
Eng-Shang Huang

## DEFINITION AND HISTORY

Cytomegaloviruses (CMV) are a group of viruses within the betaherpesvirinae subfamily of the herpesviridae family.[1] They are widely distributed and have been isolated from human, green monkey, squirrel monkey, chimpanzee, horse, mouse, guinea pig, and many low mammalian species. Infection with this group of viruses typically results in a characteristic enlargement of cells with the appearance of distinctive intranuclear and cytoplasmic inclusion bodies which has led to the common name of cytomegalovirus. Although the cytomegaloviruses share many structural and biologic similarities, there is a lack of genetic relatedness among human CMV, mouse CMV, and simian CMV as determined by nucleic acid hybridization.[2] In general, these viruses show a high degree of species specificity. In humans, cytomegaloviruses cause asymptomatic as well as severe infections which may be followed by either persistent or latent infections.

In vivo and in vitro infection of cells with human CMV produces cell enlargement with typical Cowdry's type A intranuclear inclusions resembling those associated with herpes simplex virus (HSV) infection. These types of histologically distinct cells are commonly found in the tissues of patients with fatal infections.[3] Cytomegalic cells were first described by Jesionek and Kiolemenoglou in 1904,[4] who observed these protozoan-like cells in the kidneys, lung, and liver of a premature infant. In the same year, Ribbert[5] demonstrated similar cytomegalic cells in the kidneys of a neonate and the parotid glands of two older infants studied at autopsy. In 1921, Goodpasture and Talbot found cytomegalic cells in the kidneys, lung, and liver of a 6-week-old infant dying from pneumonia. They thought that these giant cells resulted from chronic inflammation and suggested the term "cytomegalia" to emphasize their unusual size.[6] These investigators, like their predecessors, concluded that the inclusions originated from infection with a protozoa or the agent of syphilis. In 1921, Lipschutz recognized the similarity between these cytomegalic inclusion bodies and those seen in herpetic lesions, and postulated a viral etiology for cytomegalic inclusion disease. This groundwork led to the demonstration of a viral etiology by Cole and Kuttner,[7] who found that filtered extracts from submaxillary glands of adult guinea pigs were able to induce cytomegalic inclusion-bearing cells in young animals. Wyatt et al.[8] and Fetterman[9] reported typical inclusion-bearing cells in urine sediments from patients and introduced exfoliative cytology as a diagnostic tool for detecting cytomegalic inclusion disease. Finally, in 1956, using tissue culture methods, Smith isolated "human salivary gland virus" from infants dying of cytomegalic inclusion disease.[10] The unifying term "cytomegalovirus" was suggested by Weller[11] to reflect the morphological change in virus-infected cells.

The isolation of CMV from cervical secretions[12] and semen[13] and the demonstration of an association between CMV infection and chronic cervicitis[14] provided early evidence that CMV might be a sexually transmitted disease. Identical virus strains have since been isolated from asymptomatic homosexual men living in the same geographic area.[15,16] This virus is often isolated from the body fluids of homosexual men with the acquired immunodeficiency syndrome (AIDS).

## MOLECULAR VIROLOGY

**Virion Structure.** Human CMV is a double-stranded DNA virus with a genome of 150 million daltons, about 240 kb. Its genome is the most complex of all the DNA viruses, and approximately 50 percent larger than the genome of HSV. The density of viral DNA is about 1.716 $g/cm^3$, which is slightly higher than that of human host-cell DNA; this corresponds to a G+C content of 56 to 58 percent.[17] Intact viral DNA is composed of covalently bonded long (L) and short (S) segments, each of which contains L and S unique sequences flanked by homologous repetitive sequences, respectively (Fig. 36-1). Because of an inverted rightward or leftward orientation of the L and S segments, DNA isomers with four symmetrical arrangements similar to that of HSV DNA may be found in purified CMV DNA.[18] DNA-DNA reassociation kinetics studies indicate that individual human CMV isolates share at least 80 percent sequence homology with the prototype strain AD-169.[19] As a group, however, the degree of homology existing among CMV strains is greater than that between HSV type 1 and type 2, which is about 50 percent (see Chap. 35), making it impossible to classify cytomegaloviruses into subgroups or subtypes. The genomic polymorphism of CMV is vividly demonstrated by digestion of purified viral DNA with restriction endonucleases and analysis of the digestion products by agarose gel electrophoresis.[19,20] As shown in Fig. 36-2, each CMV isolate has its own distinct DNA restriction pattern. No epidemiologically unrelated strains share identical DNA restriction patterns. Identical patterns have been demonstrated, however, in viruses obtained sequentially from a patient with recurrent infections, and in viruses isolated from sexual partners or from pregnant women and their offspring.[16,21] Antigenic variation among CMV strains can be demonstrated by neutralization tests,[22] complement fixation,[19] or electroimmunodiffusion.[23]

Morphologically, CMV resembles other herpesviruses. Electron microscope observations show that the enveloped virion is approximately 200 nm in diameter. It consists of a naked virus containing a spherical DNA-protein-complex core, about 60 nm in diameter, surrounded by a 110-nm icosahedral capsid with 162 capsomeres.[24] The naked virion is surrounded by an envelope with a single or double membrane structure which is acquired during budding from the nuclear or cytoplasmic membrane of the infected cell. CMV is sensitive to lipid solvents or detergents which destroy the integrity of the viral envelope. Frequently, some membrane-bound particles ("dense bodies") are found associated with the virus in cytoplasmic inclusions, as well as in the extracellular fluid of infected cultures. The dense body has a size of 300 nm and consists of spherical particles surrounded by a membrane similar to that of the viral envelope. It does not contain viral DNA but shares most of the polypeptides contained in the purified virion.[25,26]

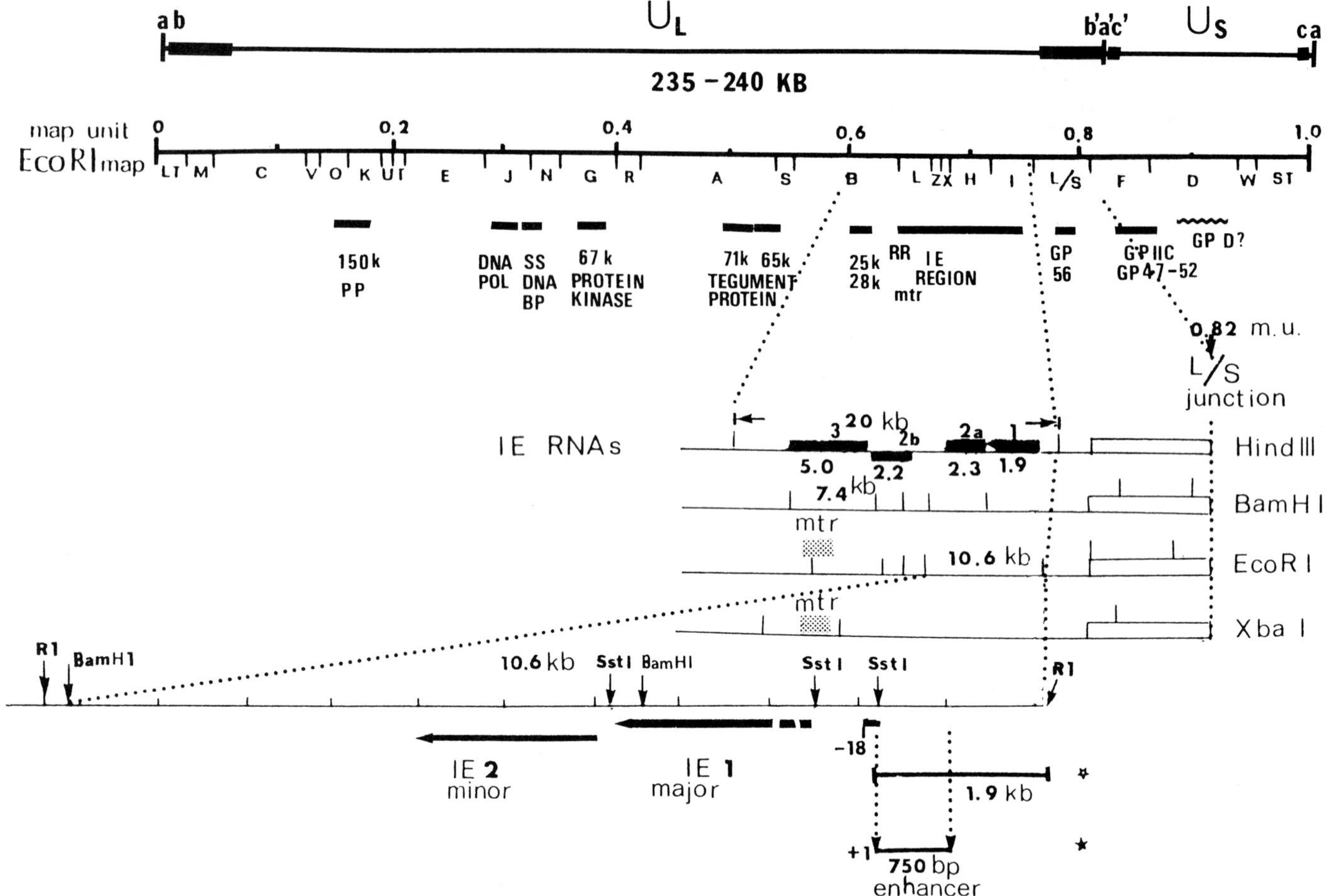


Fig. 36-1. Diagram of the CMV DNA restriction map (EcoR1) showing relative locations of CMV IE genes: tegument proteins, 67K phosphorylated protein, and DNA polymerase.

SDS-polyacrylamide gel electrophoresis reveals that purified CMV virions contain at least 33 polypeptides with molecular weights ranging from 11,000 to 290,000 daltons.[26–28] At least eight glycoproteins are associated with the virion, and antisera to these glycoproteins can neutralize virus infectivity in vitro.[26] Two major capsid proteins with molecular weights of 150 and 34 kilodaltons constitute the virion capsid. Between the capsid and viral envelope are two tegument proteins of 68 and 72 kilodaltons, which form a bridge between the capsid and virion.[26,28] These tegument proteins may play a role in the regulation of CMV gene expression as they are able to regulate the activity of the CMV immediate-early promoter (see below). A DNA polymerase and a protein kinase have been found associated with CMV virions purified from the extracellular fluid of infected cultures.[29] A 67 kilodalton CMV-specific phosphorylated protein encoded by a CMV gene at 0.37 to 0.39 map units contributes to this protein kinase activity.[30,31]

**Viral Gene Regulation.** In permissive human fibroblasts, CMV gene expression is regulated by a cascade of regulatory elements sequentially acting at both transcriptional and translational levels.[32] Three main stages of gene expression resembling those of HSV have been defined: immediate-early (IE), early, and late.[33] Following adsorption, penetration, and uncoating of the virus, a group of viral RNAs referred to as IE RNAs are synthesized within 1 to 4 h from regions of the long unique sequence of CMV DNA. This group of RNAs is transcribed from IE genes even in the presence of the protein synthesis inhibitor, cyclohexamide. The translation products of IE RNAs are called the IE antigens or alpha proteins. One of the IE genes (gene 3) has been designated as a morphological transforming region, because it encompasses a region which is able to morphologically transform mammalian cells in vitro. The resulting transformed cells are tumorigenic in experimental animals.[16,34] IE protein synthesis is essential for subsequent transcription and translation of the early genes, also called the beta genes. Early antigens (beta proteins) are defined as those proteins synthesized before viral DNA replication. These comprise the enzymes involved in nucleoside metabolism, viral DNA replication (such as virus-specific DNA polymerase, ribonucleotide reductase, etc.), and other factors which are required for the switch to late gene (gamma gene) expression. Late genes are those genes expressed after viral DNA synthesis; these genes primarily encode viral structural polypeptides. The beta group of proteins are essential for full-scale late gene expression.

CMV has a strong IE promoter-enhancer region located upstream of the coding sequences of the IE gene 1. This promoter-enhancer seems to have little cell or species preference and is active in bacteria and many mammalian cells.[35,36] Recombinant plasmids containing this DNA can be used to promote the expression of foreign proteins in many cells. The observed activity of the CMV promoter-enhancer is more than 100-fold higher than

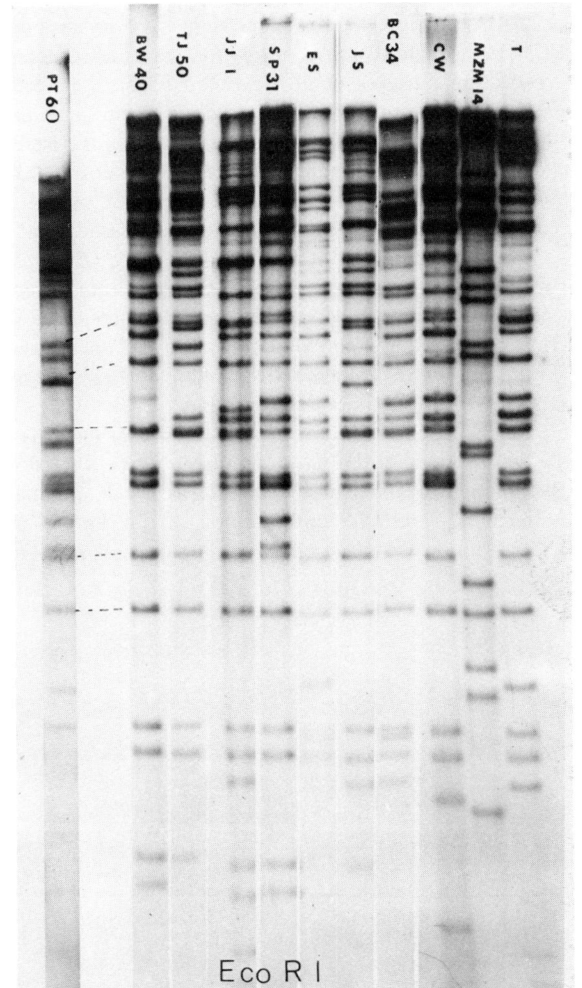


**Fig. 36-2.** Restriction enzyme analysis of virus DNAs from various CMV isolates. Purified $^{32}$P-labeled CMV DNAs were digested with EcoR1 and then subjected to 1 percent agarose gel electrophoresis. Strain MZM 14 is a chimpanzee CMV shown for comparison. Others are human clinical isolates. Viral DNA polymorphism is evident.[16]

the activity of the early promoter of SV40 virus.[35,36] The CMV IE gene 1 product has been found to be able to autoregulate its own promoter.[37]

In view of the fact that almost all homosexual men with AIDS are actively infected with human CMV, it has been hypothesized that an interaction between CMV and human immunodeficiency virus (HIV) may contribute to the pathogenic effects of HIV infection. A potential molecular interaction between the CMV IE gene and the HIV promoter has been demonstrated in experiments involving DNA transfection and transient gene expression.[38] A gene product derived from the IE region of human CMV, in particular IE region 2, can transactivate the expression of the bacterial chloramphenicol acetyltransferase (CAT) gene when it is linked to the promoter of HIV, the long terminal repeat (LTR). The CMV IE transactivator increases the level of mRNA transcribed from the plasmid carrying the CAT gene under HIV LTR control. This transcriptional activation appears to be additive, not synergistic, with that of the *tat* gene product which is encoded by HIV and known to activate its LTR (see Chap. 28). In addition, the CMV IE gene product activates a promoter construct in which the *cis*-acting *tat* responsive region has been deleted, suggesting that the mode of action of these two transactivators may be different. These in vitro results indicate that the human CMV IE gene product might stimulate HIV gene expression, thereby potentiating the consequences of HIV infection in persons with concurrent CMV infection.[38] The possibility of such an interaction is strengthened by the recent observation that CMV and HIV may coinfect the same cell types.[39]

**Antiviral Drugs and CMV.** Infection of human fibroblasts with CMV leads not only to the stimulation of host cell DNA polymerase synthesis but also to the induction of a novel, virus-specific DNA polymerase. This virus-encoded DNA polymerase is a beta protein which is expressed at the early stage of virus infection.[40] It exhibits unique chromatographic behavior, template specificity, and salt and drug sensitivities distinct from that of host cell enzymes. In contrast to the host cell enzyme, this virus-specific DNA polymerase is extremely sensitive to phosphonoacetate and the triphosphate derivatives of 9-(1,3-dihydroxy-2-propoxymethyl)guanine (gancyclovir, or DHPG), 1-(2′-deoxy-2′-fluoro-beta-D-arabinofuranosyl)-5-iodocytosine (FIAC), and -5-iodouracil (FIAU).[41–43] Therefore, phosphonoacetate, FIAC, and gancyclovir are considered potent anti-CMV compounds capable of differentially inhibiting CMV DNA replication in vitro. In contrast, acyclovir has relatively little activity against this virus.

CMV late gene expression occurs 36 to 48 h after virus infection. At this stage, viral structural proteins are synthesized, cellular DNA synthesis is shut off, and infectious virus is released. The production of late proteins is fully dependent on viral DNA replication. Inhibition of CMV DNA replication by phosphonoacetate or gancyclovir prevents the synthesis of late viral structural proteins.[44]

## EPIDEMIOLOGY

CMV infections are ubiquitous and usually asymptomatic.[11] CMV infection is endemic rather than epidemic; there is no seasonal variation. Viral transmission occurs by intimate person-to-person contact. Potential sources of virus include saliva, urine, semen, breast milk, blood, transplanted donor organs, and cervical and vaginal secretions. The prevalence of CMV infection in the adult population ranges from 40 percent in Europe to almost 100 percent in Africa and the Far East.[45,46] In general, the prevalence of CMV infection is related to the socioeconomic status of a population and, to a certain extent, to the geographic location. The age-specific prevalence in general is lower in Europe, Australia, and certain regions of America, and significantly higher in underdeveloped countries. In Africa and some regions of the Far East, almost every adult has acquired CMV infection before age 35. Approximately 15 to 20 percent of third trimester pregnant women and 15 to 20 percent of children under 1 year of age in the Far East shed virus in cervical secretions or urine, respectively.[12,47] In the United States, this rate is 1.5 to 13.5 percent.[48]

**Maternofetal Transmission.** Maternal infections play an important role in transmission of CMV to neonates, whereas sexual transmission becomes a predominant mode of transmission in adult life. CMV can be reactivated during gestation, and the virus may be transmitted to the fetus in utero despite circulating maternal antibody. Approximately 1 percent of infants (0.4 percent in higher socioeconomic groups to 2.2 percent in lower socioeconomic groups) are found to be congenitally infected at birth.[48–50] Congenital infections may follow primary, reactivated, or recurrent maternal infections. Following primary maternal infection, CMV is transmitted to 40 to 50 percent of the offspring, and 5 to 10 percent of these congenitally infected infants will become symptomatic.[51] An adverse outcome is more likely when infection occurs during the first trimester.[52] Although maternal immunity to CMV does not protect the fetus from intrauterine infection, some evidence suggests that maternal immunity reduces the severity of infection in the infant.[52,53] In different populations, primary infection occurs in 0.7 to 4 percent of susceptible seronegative women.[53–57] An additional 8 to 60 percent of infants become infected during the first 6 months of life, probably as the result of acquiring infection during passage through the birth canal or as the result of breast-feeding.[53,58,59] The next wave of CMV infection occurs in day care centers or nursery schools.[60] Viral transmission among preschool children in day care centers is extremely high. CMV infection rates subsequently increase rapidly at the age of entry into school. By puberty, approximately 40 to 80 percent of youths have been infected with CMV.[54] In some lower socioeconomic areas, 90 to 100 percent of the population may be infected during childhood.[54]

**Sexual Transmission.** Sexual transmission is a significant mode of spread for CMV. Virus may be isolated from the uterine cervix, semen, and saliva,[13] although the relative roles played by each of these potential sources of virus is not clear. Approximately 8 to 10 percent of women, either pregnant or nonpregnant, shed CMV from the cervix,[54] and approximately 30 percent of asymptomatic homosexual men have CMV in their semen.[16,61] Jordan et al.[62] reported that 16 of 120 (13.3 percent) women at risk for STD had cervical CMV infection. Willmott[63] studied 531 females visiting a British STD clinic and found that 6.6 percent were positive for CMV. The level of sexual activity is a stronger predictor of CMV infection than race, age, or socioeconomic status.[64,65] Handsfield et al.[64] reported that viruses with identical DNA restriction patterns could be isolated from heterosexual partners. In another study, CMV was isolated from the semen of 13 of 40 (30 percent) homosexual males studied in the Research Triangle area of North Carolina.[16] Virus particles could be demonstrated inside the sperm as well as in the extracellular seminal fluids (see Fig. 36-3). DNA restriction analysis revealed that four isolates from different individuals shared the same DNA restriction pattern, while an additional pair shared another uniquely identical pattern (Fig. 36-4).[16] This sharing of identical DNA restriction patterns indicates the epidemiological relatedness of virus strains among these men and strongly implies sexual transmission of CMV.

Compared with heterosexual men, homosexual men are significantly more likely to be CMV culture positive. Infection in homosexual men is associated with increased age, number of sexual partners, and the practice of anal-receptive intercourse.[61,66] Among CMV seropositive homosexual men, those

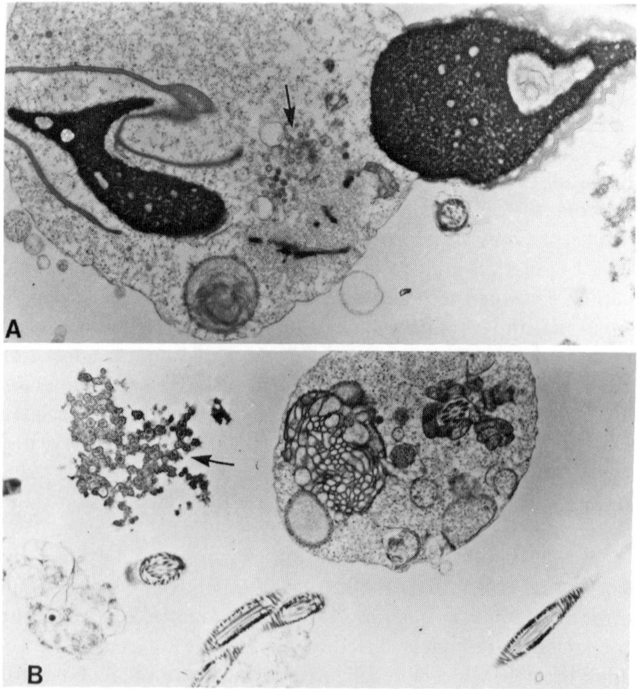


Fig. 36-3. Electron micrographs of semen samples from asymptomatic homosexual men with active CMV infection. (A) Intracellular location of viral particles (arrow); (B) extracellular viral particles (arrow).[15,16]

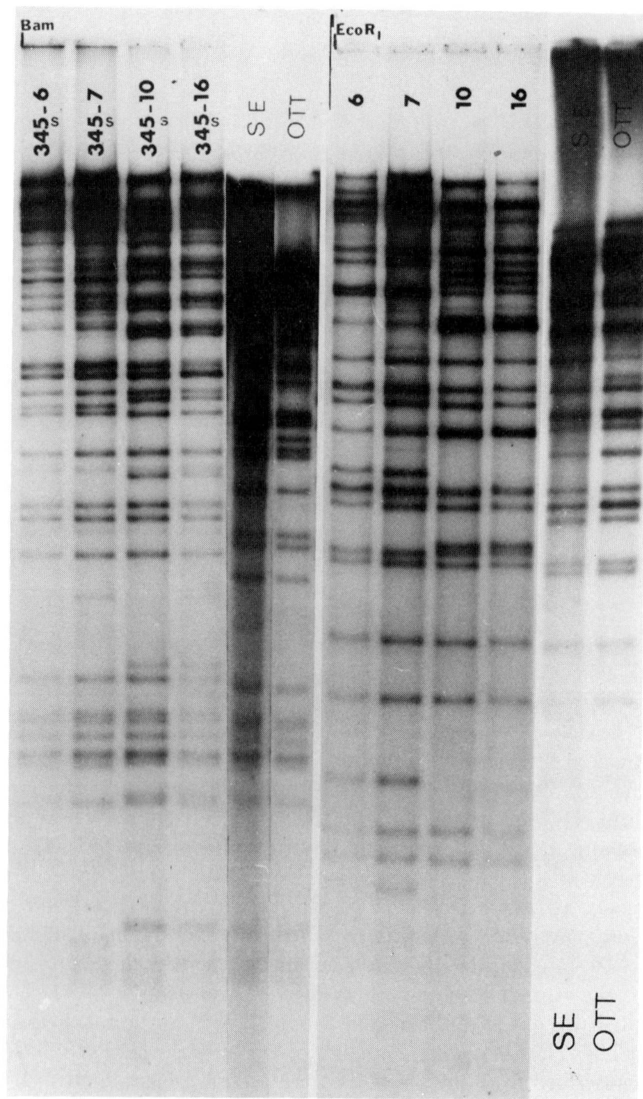


Fig. 36-4. Restriction enzyme analysis of viral DNA from various CMV isolates from semen of asymptomatic homosexual men. $^{32}$P-labeled viral DNAs were subjected to BamH1 (left) and EcoR1 (right) restriction enzyme digestion. Viral strains 345-6, 345-7, SE, and OTT share identical restriction patterns, while strains 345-10 and 345-16 are identical.[16]

cultured for virus excreted CMV more frequently and for a longer duration in the semen than in urine.[66] Excretion of CMV in semen is significantly associated with HIV seropositivity in asymptomatic homosexual men.[67] These results suggest that HIV infection could also promote localized reactivation of cervical CMV, which is seen in otherwise healthy pregnant women.[68] Independent of infection with HIV, CMV seropositivity and CMV excretion are associated with increased T-suppressor lymphocyte counts and reduced T-helper/T-suppressor ratios.[66,69] In both situations, shedding of virus is intermittent and occurs in the absence of significant alterations in humoral immunity.

**Transfusion-Transmitted CMV.** In addition to sexual and maternofetal transmission, primary or recurrent CMV infection occasionally follows blood transfusions or organ transplantation. Several studies provide conclusive data to indicate that blood transfusions are an important source of CMV infection.[46] Transfusion of leukocyte-enriched blood products increases the risk of CMV infection. Conversely, it has been demonstrated that the use of leukocyte-depleted or cryopreserved red blood cells reduces the risk of CMV infection.[70] Ho[46] has summarized data from 12 studies on a total of 1550 transfusion recipients. Of these patients, 14 percent developed primary infection with CMV. In an additional 10 percent, reactivation or recurrent infection occurred. Symptomatic illness associated with transfusion-acquired primary CMV infections is more common in premature infants than in older persons. Between 50 and 90 percent of infants who acquire primary infection develop various forms of CMV-induced disease, including interstitial pneumonitis and severe jaundice. The mortality can approach 40 percent.[46]

**CMV Infection in Immunosuppressed Populations.** CMV infection is very common in immunosuppressed populations and in patients with AIDS. In renal allograft recipients, an average of 53 percent of seronegative patients acquire primary CMV infection, and 85 percent of seropositive subjects develop CMV recurrences. Similar rates occur in cardiac and bone marrow transplant recipients. About 70 to 85 percent of the transplant recipients become symptomatic with primary infection, while only 20 to 40 percent develop symptoms with recurrent infections.[46] The mortality rate of CMV interstitial pneumonitis in transplant patients with primary CMV infection is higher than in patients with recurrent infection.[46] Male homosexuals or bisexuals with AIDS have extremely high rates of CMV infection, as almost 100 percent of them excrete CMV in body fluids. This phenomenon does not exist in other populations at high risk for AIDS, such as drug abusers or hemophiliacs. The rate of CMV infection among these other groups is less than that in homosexual men with AIDS, and is close to that of similar populations without AIDS. In hemophiliacs tested at the University of North Carolina, 60 percent were CMV seropositive regardless of HIV status or type and amount of clotting factor usage. HIV infection status correlated with clotting factor usage, whereas CMV was significantly associated only with age (Smiley et al., in preparation).

## CLINICAL MANIFESTATIONS

**Neonatal Infection.** Although many CMV infections are asymptomatic, the wide spectrum of CMV-associated diseases in newborns and immunocompromised hosts clearly establishes this virus as a significant pathogen. Clinical manifestations of congenital CMV infection range from minimal involvement to severe CMV disease with neurological abnormalities, hepatosplenomegaly, jaundice, chorioretinitis, and petechiae.[71] Most congenitally infected infants (≥90 percent) are asymptomatic at birth, however. Nonetheless, 5 to 20 percent of these infants may develop late manifestations of CMV infection such as hearing loss and poor intellectual performance.[50,51,70–73] Congenital or perinatal CMV infections are usually persistent with chronic viral excretion over months or years.[74]

**Infection in Normal Hosts.** Primary CMV infections in normal children and adults are also usually asymptomatic but may be associated with a mononucleosis-like illness involving fever, lethargy, myalgias, headache, and mild hepatitis.[75] A similar illness, the postperfusion syndrome, may develop after transfusion of large amounts of blood. CMV causes 8 percent of all infectious mononucleosis syndromes.[76] CMV mononucleosis often resembles mononucleosis due to Epstein-Barr virus (EBV), another member of the herpesviridae family, but certain clinical features differ. CMV infected patients are older with a mean age of 28 years, compared with EBV infected patients, who have a mean age of 19 years.[77] With CMV mononucleosis, the duration of fever is longer (mean duration 18 days) than in patients with EBV (mean duration 10 days).[78] Pharyngitis, tonsillitis, lymphadenopathy, and lymphocytosis with atypical lymphocytes are more commonly associated with EBV than with CMV.[77] Parenthetically, EBV has been recovered from the uterine cervix, suggesting the possibility that it also may be sexually transmitted like CMV and HSV. Another cause of a mononucleosis-like syndrome that must be considered in sexually active adults is HIV (see Chap. 30). Other complications of CMV infections in normal hosts are rare and include rash, granulomatous hepatitis, Guillain-Barré syndrome, meningoencephalitis, myocarditis, pneumonitis, hemolytic anemia, and thrombocytopenia.

**Infection in Immunocompromised Persons.** In immunocompromised patients, CMV infection may be asymptomatic or may act as an opportunist causing serious illness with high morbidity and mortality. Adverse effects of CMV infection following organ transplantation include syndromes directly related to the virus, including severe mononucleosis-like syndromes, leukopenia, pneumonitis, retinitis, and gastrointestinal ulcerations.[46] In addition, there may be indirect effects including superinfection and a possibly increased risk of graft rejection. The high incidence of CMV infection following transplantation may be attributed to reactivation of latent virus by immunosuppressive drugs, as well as transmission of virus by latently infected donor tissues.[79] It is important whether infection occurring after transplantation is primary or reactivated, as primary infections result in more serious disease.[80,81]

In AIDS, CMV causes variable clinical manifestations similar to those described following transplantation.[82] Patients with AIDS more commonly develop erosive CMV esophagitis, pneumonitis, adrenalitis, retinitis, or meningoencephalitis.

## LABORATORY DIAGNOSIS

A laboratory diagnosis of suspected CMV infection may be confirmed by several methods, including viral isolation, serology, electron microscopy, histologic evaluation, immunohistochemical staining of tissues, and/or nucleic acid hybridization techniques.

CMV infection may be demonstrated histopathologically by detection of characteristic large cells with intranuclear and occasional cytoplasmic inclusions in biopsy or autopsy materials. The presence of these cytomegalic cells suggests CMV infection, but virological or serological confirmation is still desirable.

**Serologic Diagnosis.** A serologic diagnosis may be made by comparing antibody titers present in acute-phase sera with those in convalescent phase specimens obtained 2 to 3 weeks later. A seroconversion or fourfold or greater rise in titer is diagnostic of recent (but not necessarily primary) infection. Single serum samples are useful for seroepidemiologic studies but are of little value for diagnosis of CMV infections. If congenital infection is suspected, both maternal and infant sera should be examined. The presence of only IgG class antibodies to CMV in the infant's serum indicates passive acquisition of maternal antibodies. Detection of IgM CMV antibodies usually indicates congenital infection. Because IgM antibodies may persist for months, detection of IgM in a single sample generally has limited usefulness in adults.[83]

Common serologic methods include the complement fixation (CF) test, indirect immunofluorescent antibody (IFA) test, indirect hemagglutinin (IHA) test, anticomplement immunofluorescence (ACIF), latex agglutination, and the enzyme-linked immunosorbent assay (ELISA). Presently, the ELISA is the most extensively used because of its sensitivity and ease of performance. In contrast, the sensitivity and specificity of the CF test is poor. Screening sera by CF at a 1:8 dilution may miss some low-titer but positive sera, whereas screening at less than 1:8 is impractical because of nonspecific reactions and the anticomplementary nature of many samples. Antigenic variation among CMV strains may result in false-negative results if the strain causing infection is significantly different from the antigen source used in the CF assay. Significant antibody titer rises are detected earlier using IFA than CF, but false positives occur in the IFA test in patients who have rheumatoid factor. IFA tests are also time-consuming and must be interpreted cautiously because of the CMV-induced IgG-Fc receptor expressed by some infected cells.[84] The ACIF test avoids the false-positive problem with IFA since complement is fixed only by antigen-antibody complexes.

**Virus Isolation.** CMV may be cultured from throat washings, urine, cervical swab, blood (buffy coat), or biopsy specimens. In the evaluation of immunocompromised patients, buffy coat cultures are a better indicator of symptomatic infection than positive CMV cultures from urine or throat washings.[85] Positive isolates from urine should be interpreted cautiously, because shedding may persist up to 2 years after initial infection. Human fibroblast cells best support the growth of CMV and are therefore routinely used for diagnostic purposes. False-negative cultures may result if specimens are mishandled. Optimally, blood should be obtained in EDTA or citrated tubes, while throat and cervical washings should be placed in appropriate culture media before transport. All specimens should be placed on wet ice and transported promptly to the laboratory. The time required for isolation of virus depends somewhat on the quantity of virus present. If titers are high, cultures may become positive within 2 to 10 days. Other cultures may take up to 6 weeks to exhibit cytopathic effects consistent with CMV infection. Because of this, specific approaches permitting more rapid diagnosis are important, especially in the management of immunosuppressed patients with a potentially rapidly progressive CMV disease such as retinitis. In such settings the centrifugation-culture technique is presently the diagnostic method of choice.[86–88] This involves centrifugation of the specimen onto monolayer cell cultures and the subsequent assay for early CMV antigens by either immunofluorescence, immunoperoxidase staining, or ELISA using monoclonal antibodies.

**Other Diagnostic Approaches.** Immunofluorescent microscopy of tissue sections with monoclonal antibodies has also been successfully used by some laboratories.[89,90] At the present time, nucleic acid hybridization techniques[91,92] are not practical for the routine diagnostic laboratory because these methods are technically complex and probes are not commercially available. We have, however, designed a rapid method to detect CMV DNA in urine of infected subjects. Viral particles in urine or exfoliated cells are first precipitated with polyethylene glycol (PEG) at a final concentration of 12 percent. DNA is extracted and subjected to dot-blot hybridization using either biotinylated or P-32-labeled CMV DNA probes. Hybridization time may be shortened to 2 h. If a biotinylated DNA probe is used, results can be obtained in one afternoon. More recently, the sensitive polymerase chain reaction (PCR) method using CMV-specific synthetic oligonucleotide primers has been used successfully to detect viral DNA in various clinical samples in the authors' laboratory.

## TREATMENT

Interferon (IFN), transfer factor, adenine arabinoside, acyclovir, and combinations of these agents have been tried without success for treatment of congenital CMV infection or severe CMV disease in transplant patients.[93–99] However, human IFN-alpha and recombinant IFN have been shown to be efficacious in preventing serious CMV disease in seropositive renal transplant patients.[100,101] Combination therapy with newer antiviral drugs and biologic response modifiers such as IFN should continue to be tested in patients with severe CMV disease.

Based on preclinical and clinical data, the most promising drugs currently available for the treatment of CMV disease include phosphonoformate (foscarnet sodium, PFA) and gancyclovir (DHPG, 9-[1,3-dihydroxy-2-propoxymethyl] guanine). Phosphonoformate selectively inhibits CMV DNA polymerase and consequently reduces viral replication.[102–105] Following preliminary trials demonstrating that phosphonoformate was well tolerated,[106,107] controlled studies were initiated to evaluate its efficacy in immunosuppressed patients. At present, these studies remain in progress. Recently, phosphonoformate has been reported to have resulted in resolution of CMV retinitis in five patients with AIDS.[108] Gancyclovir, also known as DHPG,[109] is structurally related to acyclovir and has good in vitro activity against CMV[44,110] (see above). In herpes simplex virus infection, gancyclovir is phosphorylated by the virus-specific thymidine kinase and then by cellular enzymes to the triphosphate form which inhibits the herpes DNA polymerase. CMV appears to lack a thymidine kinase, however, so it is not yet clear how this drug precisely inhibits CMV replication. The lack of viral thymidine kinase accounts for the poor sensitivity of CMV to acyclovir; gancyclovir may be more active because of greater phosphorylation by cellular enzymes. Data on the treatment of some forms of CMV disease with gancyclovir are encouraging but largely uncontrolled. The drug is generally well tolerated, but reversible neutropenia is a frequent adverse reaction. Patients with CMV retinitis or colitis usually stabilize or improve on therapy but patients with CMV pneumonia often respond poorly.[111–114] Also, if treatment is terminated, most AIDS patients relapse; therefore, maintenance therapy is necessary. Treatment of CMV disease with phosphonoformate or gancyclovir may be beneficial, but more effective and less toxic therapeutic regimens must be developed for both acute and chronic use. The development of a new series of gancyclovir derivatives (7-deazadenosine nucleosides) which inhibit CMV replication offers promise.[115,116]

## PREVENTION

There is a need for methods to prevent CMV disease following intrauterine transmission of virus, after transplantation procedures or during the development of AIDS. Approaches to prevention that have been studied thus far include both passive and active immunization. It is worthwhile noting that no prevention strategies have yet been tested in controlled studies involving patients with AIDS. To assess the potential impact of prevention strategies, it is relevant to examine the level of protection offered by natural immunity. Although it does not totally prevent reactivation or recurrent infection, natural immunity can prevent severe disease. In comparison with CMV seropositive renal transplant recipients, CMV seronegative recipients of kidneys from seropositive donors are at significantly higher risk for serious CMV disease.[81,117] The use of these prevention strategies is therefore based on the premise that passive immunization will result in protection similar to naturally acquired immunity, even if disease is not totally prevented.

Although cell-mediated immunity is important, circulating antibody has some value in preventing CMV disease.[118–122] Studies in bone marrow and renal transplant patients[119,120,123,124] reveal that passive immunization with intravenous hyperimmune globulin results in a modification of clinical disease. This is especially important in situations where an organ donor is known to be seropositive or the use of seronegative blood products cannot be guaranteed.

Two live attenuated CMV vaccines (AD169 and Towne strain passage 125) have been shown to be safe and immunogenic in young adults[125] and renal transplant patients.[126,127] However, immunity wanes rapidly following immunization. Two double-blind, placebo-controlled Towne vaccine trials, carried out in seronegative recipients of seropositive donor kidneys, revealed that vaccine afforded only partial protection from severe CMV disease.[128] Analysis of viruses shed after transplantation in these patients provided evidence against vaccine strain latency, since restriction endonuclease studies revealed these isolates to be wild-type and not vaccine-related.[129] However, owing to the unstable nature of CMV, it is possible that the attenuated live vaccine may have lost infectivity during preparation and storage. It is not surprising, therefore, that vaccine virus was not isolated from vaccinees. Several laboratories are developing inactivated subunit vaccines, in part because of the theoretical possibility that live CMV might be oncogenic.[16,34] Combinations of various prevention strategies might be most useful in the future.

## References


1 Roizman B et al: Herpesviridae. Definition, provisional nomenclature and taxonomy. *Intervirology* 16: 201, 1982.
2 Huang ES, Pagano JS: Cytomegalovirus. II. Lack of relatedness to herpes simplex type I and II, Epstein-Barr virus and non-human cytomegalovirus. *J Virol* 13: 642, 1974.
3 Hanshaw JB: Cytomegalovirus, in *Virology Monographs,* S Gard et al (eds). New York, Springer-Verlag, 1968, p 2.
4 Jesionek A, Kiolemenoglou B: Über einen befund von protozoenartigen gebilden in den organen eines heriditarluetischen fotus. *Munch Med Wochenschr* 15: 1905, 1904.
5 Ribbert H: Über protozoenartige zelien in der niere eines syphilitischen neugeborenen und in der parotis von kindern. *Zentralbl Allg Pathol* 15: 945, 1904.
6 Wright HT Jr: Cytomegalovirus, in *The Herpesviruses,* AS Kaplan (ed). New York, Academic, 1973, p 354.
7 Cole R, Kuttner AG: A filtrable virus present in the submaxillary glands of guinea pigs. *J Exp Med* 44: 855, 1926.
8 Wyatt JP et al: Generalized cytomegalic inclusion disease. *J Pediatr* 36: 271, 1950.
9 Fetterman GH: A new laboratory aid in the clinical diagnosis of inclusion disease of infancy. *Am J Clin Pathol* 22: 424, 1952.
10 Smith MG: Propagation in tissue cultures of a cytopathogenic virus from human salivary gland virus disease. *Proc Soc Exp Biol Med* 92: 424, 1956.
11 Weller TH: The cytomegalovirus: Ubiquitous agents with protean clinical manifestations. *N Engl J Med* 285: 203, 1971.
12 Alexander ER: Maternal and neonatal infection with cytomegalovirus in Taiwan. *Pediatr Res* 1: 210, 1967.
13 Lang DJ, Kummer JF: Demonstration of cytomegalovirus in semen. *N Engl J Med* 287: 756, 1972.
14 Alexander ER: Possible etiologies of cancer of the cervix other than herpesviruses. *Cancer Res* 33: 1486, 1973.
15 Huang ES: The role of cytomegalovirus infection in Kaposi's sarcoma, in *AIDS: The Epidemic of Kaposi's Sarcoma and Opportunistic Infection,* AE Friedman-Kien (ed). New York, Masson, 1984, p 111.
16 Huang ES et al: Molecular epidemiology and oncogenicity of human cytomegalovirus, in *Biochemical and Molecular Biology of Cancer,* CC Harris (ed). UCLA Symposium on Molecular Biopsy. New Series 40: 323, 1986.
17 Huang ES et al: Human cytomegalovirus. I. Purification and characterization of viral deoxyribonucleic acid. *J Virol* 12: 1473, 1973.
18 Kilpatrick BA, Huang ES: Human cytomegalovirus genome: Partial denaturation map and organization of genome sequences. *J Virol* 24: 261, 1977.
19 Huang ES et al: Detection of human cytomegalovirus and analysis of strain variation. *Yale J Biol Med* 49: 29, 1976.
20 Kilpatrick BA et al: Analysis of cytomegalovirus genomes with restriction endonuclease HindIII and EcoR1. *J Virol* 18: 1095, 1976.
21 Huang ES et al: Molecular epidemiology of cytomegalovirus infection in women and their infants. *N Engl J Med* 303: 958, 1980.
22 Weller TH et al: Seriologic differentiation of viruses responsible for cytomegalic inclusion disease. *Virology* 12: 130, 1960.
23 Sweet GH et al: Antigens of human cytomegalovirus: Electroimmunodiffusion assays and comparison among strains. *J Gen Virol* 43: 707, 1979.
24 Montplaisir S et al: Electron microscopy in the rapid diagnosis of cytomegalovirus: Ultrastructural observation and comparison of methods of diagnosis. *J Infect Dis* 125: 533, 1972.
25 Sarov I, Ahady I: The morphogenesis of human cytomegalovirus: Isolation and polypeptide characterization of cytomegalovirus and dense bodies. *Virology* 66: 474, 1975.
26 Stinski MF: Human cytomegalovirus: Glycoproteins associated with virions and dense bodies. *J Virol* 19: 594, 1976.
27 Kim KS et al: Analysis of structural polypeptides of purified human cytomegalovirus. *J Virol* 20: 604, 1976.
28 Stinski MF: Synthesis of proteins and glycoproteins in cells infected with human cytomegalovirus. *J Virol* 23: 751, 1977.
29 Mar EC et al: Human cytomegalovirus-associated DNA polymerase and protein kinase activities. *J Gen Virol* 57: 149, 1981.
30 Davis MG et al: Mapping and expression of a human cytomegalovirus major viral protein. *J Virol* 52: 129, 1984.
31 Davis MG, Huang ES: Nucleotide sequence of a human cytomegalovirus DNA fragment encoding a 67-kilodalton phosphorylated viral protein. *J Virol* 56: 7, 1985.
32 Stinski MF: Organization and expression of the immediate early genes of human cytomegalovirus. *J Virol* 46: 1, 1983.

33 Wathen MW, Stinski MF: Temporal patterns of human cytomegalovirus transcription: Mapping the viral DNAs synthesized at immediate early, early and late times after infection. *J Virol* 41: 462, 1982.
34 Nelson JA et al: Structure of the transforming regions of human cytomegalovirus AD-169. *J Virol* 49: 109, 1984.
35 Boshart MF et al: A very strong enhancer is located upstream of an immediate early gene of human cytomegalovirus. *Cell* 41: 521, 1985.
36 Davis MG, Huang ES: Transfer and expression of plasmids containing human cytomegalovirus immediate-early gene promoter-enhancer sequences in eukaryotic and prokaryotic cells. *Biotechnol Appl Biochem* 10: 6, 1988.
37 Stinski MF, Roehr TJ: Activation of the major immediate-early gene of human cytomegalovirus by cis-acting elements in the promoter-regulatory sequence and by virus-specific trans-acting components. *J Virol* 55: 431, 1985.
38 Davis MG et al: Immediate-early gene region of human cytomegalovirus trans-activates the promoter of human immunodeficiency virus. *Proc Natl Acad Sci USA* 84: 8642, 1987.
39 Nelson JA et al: HIV and HCMV coinfect brain cells in patients with AIDS. *Virology* 165: 286, 1988.
40 Huang ES: Human cytomegalovirus III. Virus-induced DNA polymerase. *J Virol* 16: 298, 1975.
41 Huang ES: Human cytomegalovirus IV. Specific inhibition of virus-induced DNA polymerase activity and viral DNA replication by phosphonoacetic acid. *J Virol* 16: 1560, 1975.
42 Mar EC et al: Inhibition of cellular DNA polymerase alpha and human cytomegalovirus-induced DNA polymerase by the triphosphates of 9-(2-hydroxyethoxymethyl) guanine and 9-(1,3-dihydroxy-2-propoxymethyl)guanine. *J Virol* 53: 776, 1985.
43 Mar EC et al: Human cytomegalovirus-induced DNA polymerase and its interaction with the triphosphate of 1-(2′-deoxy-2′-fluoro-B-D-arabinofuranosyl)-5-methyluracil, -5-iodocytosine, and -5-methylcytosine. *J Virol* 56: 846, 1985.
44 Mar EC et al: Effect of 9-(1,3,-dihydroxy-2-propoxymethyl)guanine on human cytomegalovirus replication *in vitro*. *Antimicrob Agents Chemother* 24: 518, 1983.
45 Krech U: Complement-fixing antibodies against cytomegaloviruses in different parts of the world. *Bull WHO* 49: 103, 1973.
46 Ho M: *Cytomegalovirus, Biology and Infection*. New York, Plenum, 1982.
47 Numazaki Y et al: Primary infection with human cytomegalovirus: Virus isolation from healthy and pregnant women. *Am J Epidemiol* 91: 410, 1970.
48 Stagno S et al: Congenital cytomegalovirus infection: Occurrence in an immune population. *N Engl J Med* 296: 1254, 1977.
49 Hanshaw JB: Congenital cytomegalovirus infection: A fifteen year perspective. *J Infect Dis* 123: 555, 1971.
50 Starr JE et al: Inapparent congenital cytomegalovirus infection: Clinical and epidemiologic characteristics in early infancy. *N Engl J Med* 282: 1075, 1970.
51 Stagno S et al: Congenital cytomegalovirus infection: The relative importance of primary and recurrent maternal infection. *N Engl J Med* 306: 945, 1982.
52 Stagno S et al: Primary cytomegalovirus infection in pregnancy: Incidence, transmission to fetus, and clinical outcome. *JAMA* 256: 1904, 1986.
53 Stagno S et al: Maternal cytomegalovirus infection and perinatal transmission, in *Clinical Obstetrics and Gynecology*, GE Knox (ed). Philadelphia, Lippincott, 1982, p 563.
54 Alford CA et al: Epidemiology of cytomegalovirus, in *The Human Herpesviruses: An Interdisciplinary Perspective*, A Nahmias et al (eds). New York, Elsevier, 1981, p 159.
55 Ahlfors K et al: Congenital cytomegalovirus infection: On the relation between type and time of maternal infection and infant's symptoms. *Scand J Infect Dis* 15: 129, 1983.
56 Grant S et al: A prospective study of cytomegalovirus infection in pregnancy. I. Laboratory evidence of congenital infection following maternal primary and reactivated infection. *J Infect Dis* 143: 24, 1981.
57 Griffiths PD et al: A prospective study of primary cytomegalovirus infection in pregnant women. *Br J Obstet Gynaecol* 87: 308, 1980.
58 Hayes K et al: Cytomegalovirus in human milk. *N Engl J Med* 287: 177, 1972.
59 Stagno S et al: Breast milk and the risk of cytomegalovirus infection. *N Engl J Med* 302: 1073, 1980.
60 Pass RF et al: Cytomegalovirus infection in a day-care center. *N Engl J Med* 307: 477, 1982.
61 Mintz L et al: Cytomegalovirus infections in homosexual men: An epidemiology study. *Ann Intern Med* 99: 326, 1983.
62 Jordan MC et al: Association of cervical cytomegaloviruses with venereal disease. *N Engl J Med* 288: 932, 1973.
63 Willmott FE: Cytomegalovirus in female patients attending a VD clinic. *Br J Vener Dis* 51: 278, 1975.
64 Handsfield HH et al: Cytomegalovirus infection in sexual partners: Evidence for sexual transmission. *J Infect Dis* 151: 344, 1985.
65 Embil JA et al: Association of cytomegalovirus and herpes simplex virus infections of the cervix in four clinic populations. *Sex Transm Dis* 12: 224, 1985.
66 Collier AC et al: Cytomegalovirus infection in homosexual men: Relationship to sexual practices, antibody to HIV and cell-mediated immunity. *Am J Med* 82: 593, 1987.
67 Rinaldo CR et al: Excretion of cytomegalovirus in semen associated with HTLV-III seropositivity in asymptomatic homosexual men. *J Med Virol* 20: 17, 1986.
68 Montgomery R et al: Recovery of cytomegalovirus from the cervix in pregnancy. *Pediatrics* 49: 524, 1972.
69 Greenberg SB et al: Lymphocyte subsets and urinary excretion of cytomegalovirus among homosexual men attending a clinic for sexually transmitted diseases. *J Infect Dis* 150: 330, 1984.
70 Tolkoff-Rubin NE et al: Cytomegalovirus infection in dialysis patients and personnel. *Ann Intern Med* 89: 625, 1978.
71 Weller TH, Hanshaw JB: Virologic and clinical observations on cytomegalic inclusion disease. *N Engl J Med* 266: 1233, 1962.
72 Reynolds DW et al: Inapparent congenital cytomegalovirus infection with elevated cord IgM levels. Causal relationship with auditory and mental deficiency. *N Engl J Med* 290: 291, 1974.
73 Hanshaw JB et al: School failure and deafness after "silent" congenital cytomegalovirus infection. *N Engl J Med* 295: 468, 1976.
74 Gold E et al: Cytomegalovirus, in *Viral Infections of Humans*, 2d ed, AS Evans (ed). New York, Plenum, 1982, p 167.
75 Kumar ML et al: Congenital and postnatally acquired cytomegalovirus infections: Long-term follow-up. *J Pediatr* 104: 674, 1984.
76 Klemola E et al: Infectious mononucleosis like disease with negative heterophile agglutination test. Clinical features in relation to Epstein-Barr virus and cytomegalovirus antibodies. *J Infect Dis* 121: 608, 1970.
77 Evans AS: Infectious mononucleosis and related syndromes. *Am J Med Sci* 276: 325, 1978.
78 Hoagland RJ: *Infectious Mononucleosis*. New York, Grune & Stratton, 1976, p 52.
79 Chou S: Acquisition of donor strains of cytomegalovirus by renal transplant recipients. *N Engl J Med* 314: 1418, 1986.
80 Chatterjee SN, Jordan GW: Prospective study of the prevalence and symptomatology of cytomegalovirus infection in renal transplant recipients. *Transplantation* 28: 457, 1979.
81 Smiley ML et al: The role of pretransplant immunity in protection from cytomegalovirus disease following renal transplantation. *Transplantation* 40: 157, 1985.
82 Macher AM et al: Death in the AIDS patient: Role of cytomegalovirus (letter). *N Engl J Med* 309: 1454, 1983.
83 Horwitz CA et al: Heterophil-negative infectious mononucleosis and mononucleosis-like illnesses. *Am J Med* 63: 947, 1977.
84 Keller R et al: An IgG-Fc receptor induced in cytomegalovirus-infected human fibroblasts. *J Immunol* 116: 772, 1976.
85 Klemola E et al: Cytomegalovirus mononucleosis in previously healthy individuals. *Ann Intern Med* 71: 11, 1969.

86 Gleaves CA et al: Rapid detection of cytomegalovirus in MRC-5 cells inoculated with urine specimens by using low-speed centrifugation and monoclonal antibody to early antigen. *J Clin Microbiol* 19: 917, 1984.

87 Gleaves CA et al: Comparison of standard tube and shell vial cell culture techniques for the detection of cytomegalovirus in clinical specimens. *J Clin Microbiol* 21: 217, 1985.

88 Swenson PD, Kaplan MH: Rapid detection of cytomegalovirus in cell culture by indirect immunoperoxidase staining with monoclonal antibody to an early nuclear antigen. *J Clin Microbiol* 21: 669, 1985.

89 Goldstein LC et al: Monoclonal antibodies to cytomegalovirus: Rapid identification of clinical isolates and preliminary use in diagnosis of cytomegalovirus pneumonia. *Infect Immun* 38: 273, 1982.

90 Volpi A et al: Rapid diagnosis of pneumonia due to cytomegalovirus with specific monoclonal antibodies. *J Infect Dis* 147: 1119, 1983.

91 Myerson D et al: Diagnosis of cytomegaloviral pneumonia by *in situ* hybridization. *J Infect Dis* 150: 272, 1984.

92 Spector SA et al: Detection of human cytomegalovirus in clinical specimens by DNA-DNA hybridization. *J Infect Dis* 150: 121, 1984.

93 Thomas IT et al: Transfer-factor treatment in congenital cytomegalovirus infection. *Lancet* 2: 1056, 1977.

94 Balfour HH et al: Acyclovir in immunocompromised patients with cytomegalovirus disease. A controlled trial at one institution. *Am J Med* 73 (1A): 241, 1982.

95 Meyers JD et al: Treatment of cytomegalovirus pneumonia after marrow transplant with combined vidarabine and human leukocyte interferon. *J Infect Dis* 146: 80, 1982.

96 Meyers JD et al: The use of acyclovir for cytomegalovirus infections in the immunocompromised host. *J Antimicrob Chemother* 12 (suppl B): 181, 1983.

97 Meyers JD et al: Recombinant leukocyte A interferon for the treatment of serious viral infections after marrow transplant: A phase 1 study. *J Infect Dis* 148: 551, 1983.

98 Wade JC et al: Treatment of cytomegalovirus pneumonia with high-dose acyclovir. *Am J Med* 73 (1A): 249, 1982.

99 Wade JC et al: Treatment of cytomegalovirus pneumonia with high-dose acyclovir and human leukocyte interferon. *J Infect Dis* 148: 557, 1983.

100 Hirsch MS et al: Effects of interferon-alpha on cytomegalovirus reactivation syndromes in renal transplant recipients. *N Engl J Med* 308: 1489, 1983.

101 Weimar W et al: The incidence of cytomegalo- and herpes simplex virus infections in renal allograft recipients treated with high dose recombinant leukocyte interferon: A controlled study. *Scand J Urol Nephrol Suppl* 92: 37, 1985.

102 Oberg B: Antiviral effects of phosphonoformate (PFA, Foscarnet sodium). *Pharmacol Ther* 19: 387, 1983.

103 Prusoff WH et al: Overview of the possible targets for viral chemotherapy, in *Targets for the Design of Antiviral Agents,* RJ Walker, E Declerg (eds). New York, Plenum, 1984, p 1.

104 Prusoff WH et al: Basic biochemical and pharmacological aspects of antiviral agents. *Antiviral Res* 1 (suppl): 1, 1985.

105 Erikson B, Oberg B: Phosphonoformate and phosphonoacetate, in *Antiviral Drugs and Interferon. The Molecular Basis of Their Activity,* Y Becker (ed). Boston, Martinus Nijhoff Publishing, 1984, p 127.

106 Ringden O et al: Foscarnet for cytomegalovirus infections. *Lancet* 1: 1503, 1985.

107 Ringden O et al: Pharmacokinetics, safety and preliminary experiences using foscarnet in the treatment of cytomegalovirus infections in bone marrow and renal transplant recipients. *J Antimicrob Chemother* 17: 373, 1986.

108 Walmsley S et al: Treatment of cytomegalovirus retinitis with trisodium phosphonoformate (abstr 568), in Abstracts of the 26th Interscience Conference on Antimicrobial Agents and Chemotherapy. Washington, American Society for Microbiology, 1986.

109 Swallow DL, Kampfer GL: The laboratory selection of antiviral agents. *Br Med Bull* 41: 322, 1985.

110 Ashton WT et al: Activation by thymidine kinase and potent antiherpetic activity of 2′-nor-2′deoxy-guanosine (2′ NDG). *Biochem Biophys Res Commun* 108: 1716, 1982.

111 Shepp DH et al: Activity of 9-[hydroxy-1-(hydroxymethyl) ethoxymethyl] guanine in the treatment of cytomegalovirus pneumonia. *Ann Intern Med* 103: 368, 1985.

112 Rosecan LR et al: Antiviral therapy for cytomegalovirus retinitis in AIDS with dihydroxypropoxymethylguanine. *Am J Ophthalmol* 101: 405, 1986.

113 Laskin OL et al: Use of gancyclovir to treat serious cytomegalovirus infections in patients with AIDS. *J Infect Dis* 155: 323, 1987.

114 Collaborative DHPG Treatment Study Group: Treatment of serious cytomegalovirus infections with 9-(1,3-dihydroxy-2-propoxymethyl) guanine in patients with AIDS and other immunodeficiencies. *N Engl J Med* 314:801, 1986.

115 Duke AE et al: In vitro and in vivo activities of phosphate derivatives of 9-(1,3-dihydroxy-2-propoxymethyl) guanine against cytomegalovirus. *Antiviral Res* 6: 299, 1986.

116 Turk SR et al: Pyrrolo [2,3,-d]pyrimidine nucleosides as inhibitors of human cytomegalovirus. *Antimicrob Agents Chemother* 31: 544, 1987.

117 Betts RF: The relationship of epidemiology and treatment factors to infection and allograft survival in renal transplantation, in *CMV Pathogenesis and Prevention of Human Infection,* SA Plotkin et al (eds). New York, Alan R Liss, 1984, p 87.

118 Yeager AS et al: Prevention of transfusion-acquired cytomegalovirus infections in newborn infants. *J Pediatr* 98: 281, 1981.

119 Meyers JD et al: Prevention of cytomegalovirus infection by cytomegalovirus immune globulin after marrow transplantation. *Ann Intern Med* 98: 442, 1983.

120 Winston DJ et al: Cytomegalovirus immune plasma in bone marrow transplant recipients. *Ann Intern Med* 97: 11, 1982.

121 O'Reilly RJ et al: A randomized trial of intravenous hyperimmune globulin for the prevention of cytomegalovirus infection following marrow transplantation: Preliminary results. *Transplant Proc* 15: 1405, 1983.

122 Bowden RA et al: Cytomegalovirus immune globulin and seronegative blood products prevent primary cytomegalovirus infection after marrow transplantation. *N Engl J Med* 314: 1006, 1986.

123 Winston DJ et al: Intravenous immune globulin for prevention of cytomegalovirus infection and interstitial pneumonia after bone marrow transplantation. *Ann Intern Med* 106: 12, 1987.

124 Snydman DR et al: Use of cytomegalovirus immune globulin to prevent cytomegalovirus diseases in renal-transplant recipients. *N Engl J Med* 317:1049, 1987.

125 Fleisher GR et al: Vaccination of pediatric nurses with live attenuated cytomegalovirus. *Am J Dis Child* 136: 294, 1982.

126 Plotkin SA et al: Clinical trials of immunization with the Towne 125 strain of human cytomegalovirus. *J Infect Dis* 134: 470, 1976.

127 Gehrz RC et al: Cytomegalovirus vaccine: Specific humoral and cellular immune responses in human volunteers. *Arch Intern Med* 140: 936, 1980.

128 Plotkin SA et al: Towne-vaccine-induced prevention of cytomegalovirus disease after renal transplants. *Lancet* 1: 528, 1984.

129 Plotkin SA, Huang E-S: Cytomegalovirus vaccine virus (Towne strain) does not induce latency. *J Infect Dis* 152: 395, 1985.

Chapter 37

# Biology of human genital tract papillomaviruses*

Keerti V. Shah

about 14 from mucosal sites and the remaining from cutaneous sites.[7] The genital tract is the reservoir for all but two of the mucosal HPVs. As with many other sexually transmitted pathogens, HPV infections produce varied effects. These are described in different sections of this book. Acute infections may be asymptomatic or produce exophytic or flat condylomas (Chap. 38); chronic, persistent infections may result in intraepithelial neoplasia and squamous cell carcinoma (Chap. 48); and children infected at birth may develop juvenile-onset respiratory papillomatosis (Chap. 71). The diagnostic methods for HPVs are described in Chap. 78.

## HISTORY

The viral etiology of warts (papillomas) was established early in the twentieth century by experimental transmission of the disease with cell-free filtrates of wart extracts.[1] In the mid-1930s, the papilloma of the cottontail rabbit provided the first model for mammalian tumor viruses.[2] Papillomavirus particles were visualized soon after electron microscopy came into general use. However, little progress was made in the understanding of the biology of these infections because the viruses could not be propagated in cell cultures. In the late 1970s, this difficulty was bypassed to some extent when it became possible to clone the viral genomes directly from infected tissues into bacterial plasmid vectors. The availability of the cloned viral genomes provided the means to compare viruses isolated from different sites and to examine suspect tissues for the presence of viral genomic sequences by nucleic acid hybridization.[3,4] In the mid-1970s it was recognized that the cervix was frequently infected with human papillomaviruses (HPVs) and that low-grade intraepithelial neoplasia of the cervix, a precursor lesion of carcinoma of the cervix, was essentially indistinguishable from HPV infection at that site.[5,6] To date, more than 50 HPV types have been characterized,

*This work was supported in part by NIH grant #AI16959.

## GENERAL PROPERTIES

Papillomaviruses are small naked viruses with an icosahedral symmetry (Fig. 37-1) and a double-stranded circular DNA genome. The viral capsid is made up of at least two proteins: a 53- to 59-kilodalton polypeptide which accounts for more than 80 percent of the viral protein, and a minor 70-kilodalton polypeptide. In addition, the viral genome is complexed with low-molecular-weight histones of cellular origin.

## THE VIRAL GENOME

Excellent detailed reviews of the organization and functions of the viral genome are available.[7–10] Here, the information is summarized briefly. The genome contains about 8000 base pairs and has a molecular weight of $5 \times 10^6$. A number of human and animal HPVs have been completely sequenced. An analysis of these sequences shows that all of the open reading frames (ORFs; potential coding regions) of HPVs are located on one strand. The experimental data on viral transcripts and viral proteins confirm that only one DNA strand is transcribed. All human and animal papillomaviruses display a broadly similar genomic organization as indicated by the locations and sizes of the ORFs (Fig. 37-2).

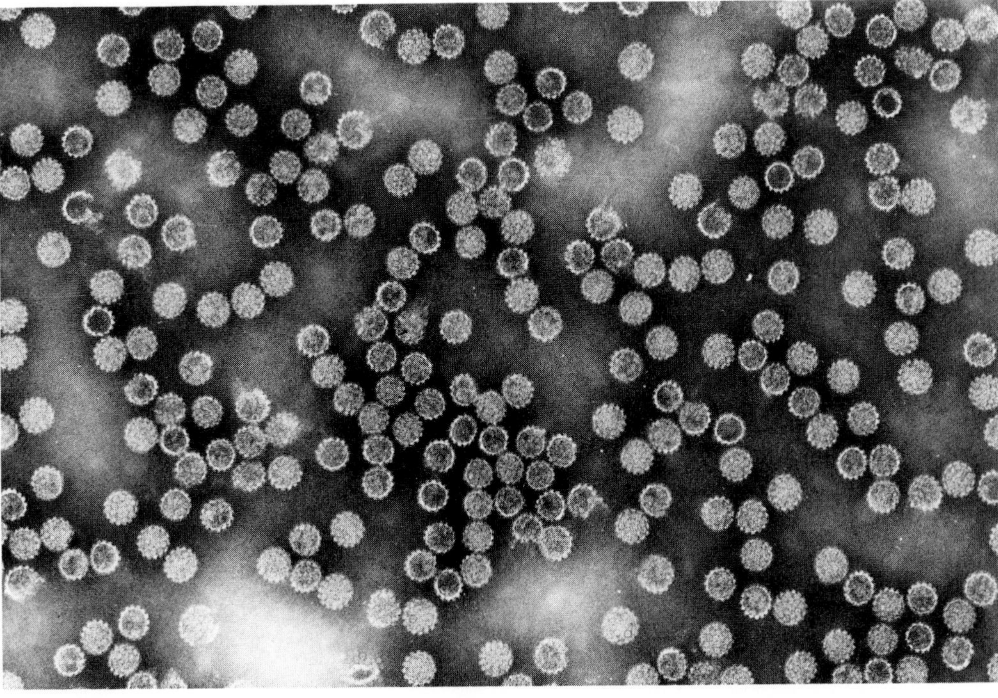

Fig. 37-1. Electron micrograph of purified virus from a human plantar wart negatively stained with potassium phosphotungstate; ×140,000.

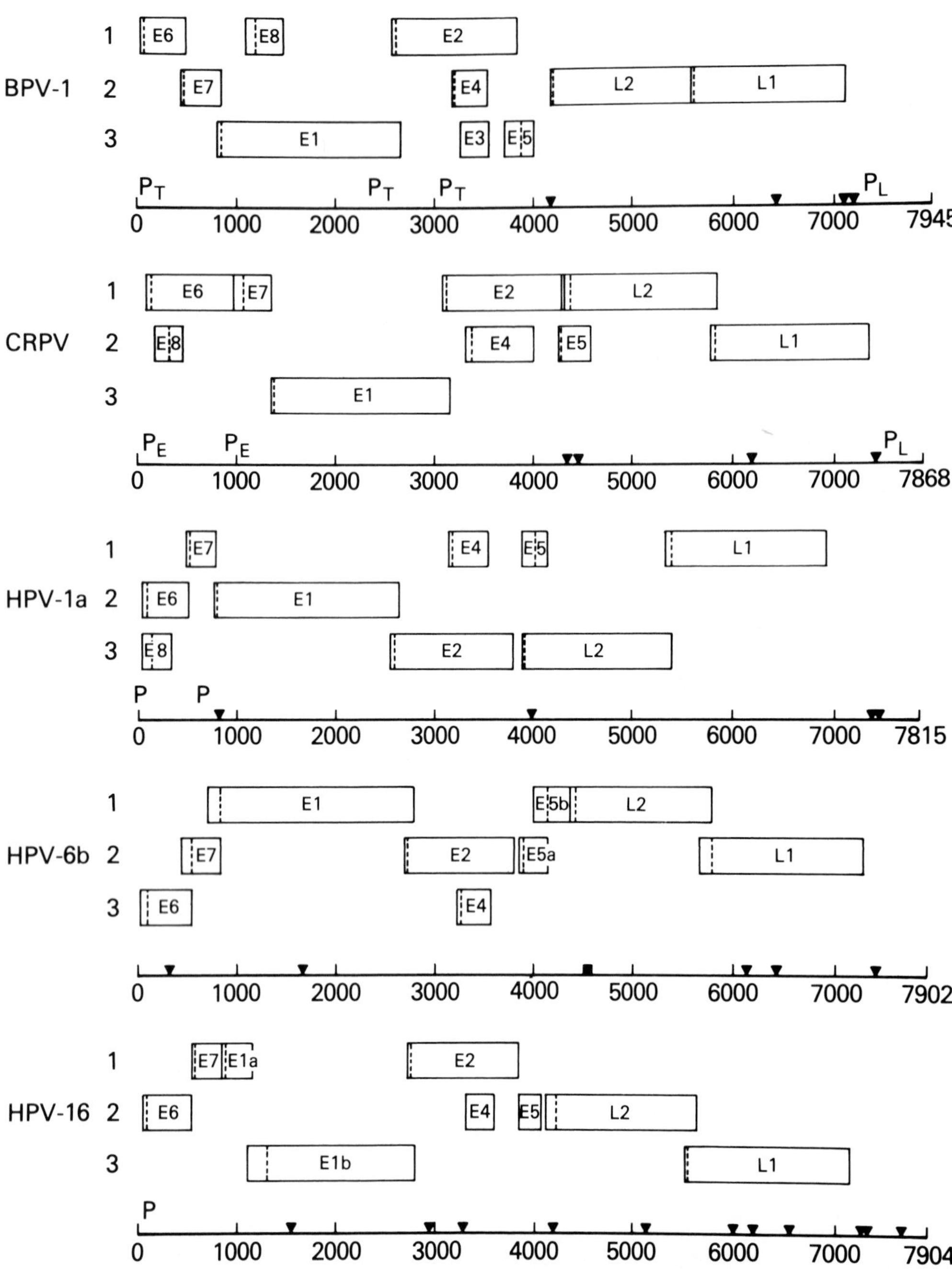


**Fig. 37-2.** Genomic organization of papillomaviruses. The genomes of bovine papillomavirus type 1 (BPV-1), cottontail rabbit papillomavirus (CRPV), and HPV types 1a, 6b, and 16 are compared. ORFs are shown as open boxes. Dashed vertical lines in ORFs indicate the position of the first methionine codon. Putative transcriptional promoters are indicated by *P*. $P_T$ represents start sites for BPV-1 transformed cell mRNA, $P_L$ start site for late region mRNA, and $P_E$ start sites for CRPV mRNA in a carcinoma cell line. Polyadenylation signals are indicated by solid triangles (▼) or solid squares (■). (*Reprinted with permission from Baker.*[13])

The functions of the papillomavirus ORFs are assigned mostly on the basis of cellular transformation assays with bovine papillomavirus (BPV) genomes; at present, there are few biologic assays available for HPVs. The viral genome is divided into an "early" region (about 4.5 kb) which is necessary for transformation, a "late" region (about 2.5 kb) which codes for capsid proteins, and a regulatory region (about 1 kb) which contains the origin of replication and control elements for transcription and replication. The transcription and protein products of the ORFs are poorly understood, so the designations "early" and "late" for the location on the genome are only for convenience. There are eight ORFs in the early region (E1 to E8) and two ORFs in the late region (L1, L2) (Table 37-1). Some viral messages are made with contribution from more than one ORF. ORFs E3 and E8 are not found consistently in all papillomavirus genomes and they probably do not represent coding sequences. ORF E1 is required for episomal replication of BPV in mouse fibroblasts. It contains sequences homologous to T antigens of simian virus 40. ORF E2 of BPV has been shown to have transactivating and transrepressing functions.[11] E4 protein of HPV-1 is expressed abundantly in plantar warts,[12] but high expression of E4 does not occur in lesions associated with other HPVs. E5 and E6 code for transforming proteins of BPV. E6 and E7 may code for the transforming proteins of HPVs. No specific functions have been identified for E5 of HPVs. L1 codes for the major capsid protein which contains group-specific epitopes. L2 codes for a minor capsid protein which may be important in the determination of host range.[13]

Table 37-1. Characteristics and Functions of Papillomavirus ORFs

| ORF | Characteristics | Function |
|---|---|---|
| E1 | In the middle of early region; largest of all ORFs for all HPVs; portions homologous to polyomavirus T antigens | Episomal replication |
| E2 | At 3′ end of early region; beginning of E2 overlaps with end of E1; middle portion most variable among HPVs | Full-length E2 product activates transcription by binding to specific sequences in regulatory region; truncated E2 product represses transcription |
| E3 | Present only in some papillomavirus genomes; contained within E2 ORF; has no initiation codon | Unknown |
| E4 | Contained within E2 ORF; very variable among HPVs | E4-related protein abundantly synthesized in HPV-1 induced warts |
| E5 | At 3′ end of early region; codes for a short very hydrophobic polypeptide | Major transforming protein of BPV |
| E6 | At 5′ end of early region; carboxy terminus has basic amino acids | Transforming protein of BPV and possibly of HPVs |
| E7 | At 5′ end of early region | High copy number in BPV; possible transforming protein of HPVs |
| E8 | At 5′ end of early region; present in only some papillomaviruses | Unknown |
| L1 | In 3′ half of late region; well conserved | Codes for major 55-kDa capsid protein; has genus-specific epitopes |
| L2 | In 5′ half of late region; overlaps slightly with L1; middle portion variable | Codes for minor capsid protein; may be involved in host range determination |

## TAXONOMY AND CLASSIFICATION

All human and animal papillomaviruses belong to the genus *Papillomavirus* which constitutes one of the two genera of the family Papovaviridae. The other genus, *Polyomavirus,* contains viruses related to simian virus 40 of Asian macaques, polyoma virus of mice, and BK and JC viruses of humans.[14] Papillomaviruses and polyomaviruses were grouped together in 1962 because they share the properties of small size, nonenveloped virion, icosahedral capsid, superhelical double-stranded DNA genome, and the nucleus as the site of multiplication.[15] Subsequent research has revealed that despite these similarities, papillomaviruses and polyomaviruses are not evolutionarily related. As described earlier, papillomaviruses carry all of their genetic information in one DNA strand. In contrast, polyomaviruses contain about one-half of the information in each strand. Members of each genus share nucleotide sequences and antigenic determinants; such relationships are not seen between members of the two genera. Papillomaviruses infect suface epithelia, producing warts or related pathology at the site of entry on the skin or mucous membranes. Polyomaviruses reach internal organs by the process of viremia. In nature, papillomaviruses stimulate cell growth and are associated with benign or malignant tumors. Polyomaviruses produce their pathogenic effect by lytic infection.

Papillomaviruses are highly species-specific. With the exception of bovine papillomaviruses which may infect horses,[16] naturally occurring interspecies transmission is not described. Papillomaviruses are classified first by their natural hosts (human, bovine, canine, etc.) and then by the degree of genetic relatedness among viruses infecting that host species. Papillomaviruses may produce pure epithelial proliferation (papillomas: e.g., all human types, some bovine types, canine and rabbit papillomaviruses) or a combined epithelial and fibroblastic proliferation (fibropapillomas: e.g., some bovine types, viruses of sheep and elk). In deer, the fibroblastic element in the tumor is so predominant that the tumors are referred to as fibromas. In some instances, viruses causing similar lesions in different species (e.g., fibropapillomas in cattle and deer) show greater nucleotide sequence homology than viruses causing different lesions in the same species (e.g., papillomas and fibropapillomas of cattle).[17]

All papillomaviruses share some nucleotide sequences. Among the viral genomes, the most conserved areas include the carboxy-terminal half of E1, the N- and C-terminal ends of E2, and L1. The least conserved areas include the regulatory region, and E4, E5, and L2. By convention, if two papillomavirus DNAs hybridize less than 50 percent in a liquid reassociation kinetics reaction, they are regarded as different types.[18] In terms of relating this value to nucleotide sequence homology, the closely related genital tract viruses HPV-6 and HPV-11 show an overall nucleotide sequence homology of 82 percent and give a value of 25 percent hybridization in liquid reassociation kinetics reactions.[19] Viral DNAs of any one type which display polymorphisms in their restriction enzyme sites are designated subtypes (a,b,c, etc.).

Diagnostic tests take advantage of the genetic interrelatedness of papillomaviruses (Chap. 78). For example, DNA hybridization is carried out under "nonstringent" conditions (low effective temperature) when the objective is to screen a specimen for any HPV. Under these conditions, an HPV probe is able to detect not only homologous sequences but also weakly hybridizing heterologous sequences of related HPVs.

## PATHOGENESIS

Warts are generally benign, self-limiting tumors which regress after a time. All the layers of the normal epithelium are represented in the wart and the basement membrane is not breached. The initial event in wart formation is very probably trauma to the epithelium and the entry of the virus into one or a few cells of the basal germinal layer. Basal cells are the only cells in the epithelium which are capable of dividing. Papillomaviruses multiply exclusively in the nucleus. Infection with the virus stimulates cell growth, leading to an irregularly thickened prickle cell layer and a granular layer which contains foci of vacuolated "koilocytic" cells with nuclear changes. Warts show abnormal mitoses in suprabasal layers of the tumor. On the skin and in some genital lesions, the cornified layer of nonnucleated dead cells may display hyperkeratosis. Viral replication is closely tied in with differentiation of the epithelium. Only the early functions of the virus are expressed in the deeper layers of the epithelium whereas both early and late functions are expressed in the superficial differentiated layers of the epithelium. Therefore, viral particles and viral capsid proteins are absent in basal cells but are found in the more superficial layers of the epithelium. Cells which produce virus particles do not divide and are destined to die. Productive infection is associated with a variety of nuclear changes which include enlargement, hyperchromasia, degeneration, and pyknosis. The affected cells also display perinuclear cavitation (koilocytosis). The presence of infectious virus particles in the most superficial layers of the epithelium provides opportunities for transmission to a susceptible contact. As a rule, virus particles are abundant in plantar and common warts, but relatively scarce in genital and respiratory papillomas.

Papillomaviruses have not yet been propagated in tissue culture. In human keratinocyte cultures infected with HPV-1, viral DNA is replicated and some viral transcripts are made but viral capsid protein and viral particles are not synthesized, and the viral DNA is lost after a few passages.[20,21] It is possible that the precise requirements of cellular differentiation required for productive infection are not fulfilled by the cells grown in vitro. Kreider et al.[22] have devised a system in which the natural conditions are apparently reproduced and complete virus particles are made. Fragments of susceptible tissue (cervical epithelium, foreskin) are exposed to virus-positive condyloma extract and transplanted beneath the renal capsule of athymic nude mice. The cells of the tissue fragment multiply and form cysts. After a period of 3 to 6 months, the cells display viral cytopathic effects similar to those in naturally occurring condylomas and also synthesize capsid proteins and viral particles. This system has been used to demonstrate the varying susceptibility of different tissues to an HPV-11 isolate.[23] It has not yet been possible to propagate other HPVs in this system. Studies of G6PD phenotypes in heterozygous women suggest that warts are of clonal origin, arising from infection of a single cell or a small group of cells.[24,25] Normal tissues of these women contain both phenotypes of the enzyme, but wart tissues exhibit one or the other phenotype. This implies that all the cells of a wart should contain the viral genome and that the infection does not spread from cell to cell.

## RELATIONSHIP TO CANCER

Some human and animal papillomaviruses are associated with naturally occurring cancers (Table 37-2). Progression of papillomavirus-associated lesions to invasive cancer displays several common characteristics. First, only some of the virus types that infect a species have oncogenic potential. For example, in the rare human dermatological disorder epidermodysplasia verruciformis (EV), which occurs on a background of a genetically inherited immunodeficiency, more than 20 different HPV types are recovered from pigmented macular lesions of the skin.[26] However, only two types, HPV-5 and HPV-8, predominate in the squamus cell carcinomas which arise from some of these lesions.[27] Similarly, the human genital tract is infected with over a dozen HPVs. However, a majority of the squamous cell cancers of the lower genital tract are associated with only two of these viruses, HPV-16 and HPV-18. The distinction between oncogenic and nononcogenic viruses is not absolute, however. HPV-6 and HPV-11, which are commonly found in exophytic condylomas, are associated occasionally with severe dysplasia and malignant tumors in both genital and respiratory tracts.[28–30] Five types of BPV are recognized in cattle. One of them, BPV-4, which produces alimentary tract papillomas is associated with malignant progression of the lesion.[31] The molecular basis for the difference in the oncogenic potential of these papillomaviruses has not yet been elucidated. Second, there is a long time period between the initial infection and the development of invasive cancer. This period may be between 5 and 40 years in humans (Table 37-2). Third, cofactors are often involved in malignant conversion. Carcinomas in EV patients arise preferentially in lesions which are exposed to sunlight.[26,27] Respiratory papillomas generally run a benign course but progression to malignancy is not uncommon in individuals who received radiation therapy for the treatment of the disease.[32] The importance of cofactors is most clearly demonstrated in the occurrence of alimentary tract carcinomas in cattle in Scotland.[31] In geographic locations where bracken fern forms a part of the natural diet of the cattle, BPV-4 induced papillomas are increased in number, occupy more sites in the alimentary tract, and progress to carcinoma. Sunlight plays a role in the development of papillomavirus-associated carcinomas in the eye and skin of cattle and in the skin of sheep.[33] The rodent *Mastomys natalensis* papillomavirus (MnPV)-associated skin carcinomas represent an unusual situation.[34] In virus-infected *Mastomys* colonies, the animal at birth contains the viral genome in every cell. Keratoacanthomas and skin carcinomas which occur frequently in these animals are correlated with increased transcriptional activity of the viral genome.[35]

The long latent period and the need for cofactors for progression of papillomas to malignancy are consistent with a multistep mechanism of carcinogenesis. It is hypothesized, for instance, that

**Table 37-2. Naturally Occurring Malignant Tumors Associated with Papillomaviruses**

| Virus type | Host | Characteristics of tumor | Cofactors |
|---|---|---|---|
| HPV-5, HPV-8 | Man | Squamous cell carcinoma in EV lesions; many years after initial lesions | Sunlight; immunologic defect |
| HPV-16, HPV-18 | Man | Cervical and vulvar cancer; 5–30 years after infection | Not known. Suspected cofactors include oncogene expression, cellular mutation, tobacco metabolites, etc. |
| Not known; probably HPV-6 and HPV-11 | Man | Laryngeal carcinoma; 5–40 years after radiation therapy | X-irradiation |
| BPV-4 | Cattle | Alimentary tract carcinomas | Bracken fern |
| Not known | Cattle | Eye and skin carcinomas | Sunlight |
| Not known | Sheep | Skin carcinomas | Sunlight |
| Cottontail rabbit papillomavirus | Rabbit | Skin carcinomas | |
| *Mastomys* papillomavirus | Multimammate mouse | Skin carcinomas in infected laboratory colonies | Not known |

papillomavirus infection may lead to "immortalization" of the cells, but that a second event (ultraviolet light, x-irradiation, cellular mutations, etc.) is required for the development of the invasive tumor.

## VIRAL GENOMES IN CANCERS

There are marked differences in the state and functional activity of papillomavirus genomes in cancers of different species. For example, in cattle, the BPV-4 genome is readily detected in alimentary tract papillomas but is apparently lost in the carcinomas.[36] In cottontail rabbit carcinomas, the genome is present in an unintegrated episomal form.[37] In contrast, in human genital tract cancers, the HPV genomes are present and integrated into the cellular DNA. Viral integration has been found in all cervical cell lines which contain HPV-16 and HPV-18, as well as in many high-grade and invasive lesions associated with these viruses.[38–40] Integration is not site-specific with respect to the cellular DNA but may occur in the proximity of cellular proto-oncogenes, or at a fragile site on the chromosome.[41,42] It is not known if the integration event is related to amplification of some of the cellular proto-oncogenes,[41,43] which has been described to occur in late stages of cervical carcinomas.

There is some specificity with respect to the site on the circular viral genome where the break occurs for integration. In cell lines derived from cervical carcinoma, viral genomes of HPV-16 and HPV-18 are found to be almost always interrupted in the E1/E2 region.[39,44,45] This break would disrupt the function of the E2 ORF. In the bovine papillomavirus model the E2 ORF codes for two opposing trans-acting regulatory functions. The product of the full-length E2 increases transcription of the early genes whereas the product of the C-terminal portion of the E2 represses the transcription of these genes.[11,46,47] The E2 ORF of HPV-16 probably codes for similar functions.[48] However, it is not yet clear how a break in the E1/E2 region would promote malignant transformation in an HPV-16 or HPV-18-associated lesion.

These is accumulating evidence that the regions of the HPV genome which are necessary for the initiation and maintenance of transformation are the E6 and E7 ORFs. After the break in the E1/E2 region which accompanies integration, E6, E7, and part of the E1 ORF can still be transcribed from the early viral promoter. E6 and E7 proteins are consistently detected in HPV-associated cervical carcinoma cells lines and in cells transformed in vitro by HPVs.[38,39,44,45,49–51] Mapping of HPV-16 specific transcripts in genital tract lesions has shown that E6 and E7 transcripts are consistently found in preinvasive as well as invasive cancers.[52]

Experimental studies also support the role of E6/E7 as transforming proteins. The E7 ORF of HPV-16 transforms a continuous rat cell line.[53] The E6/E7 region of HPV-16 cooperates with the *ras* proto-oncogene in tumorigenic transformation of primary rat kidney cells.[54] Recently, tissue-specific constitutive enhancers have been identified in the regulatory regions of HPV-16 and HPV-18 and it has been suggested that they may have an important role in the expression of E6/E7 ORFs in cervical carcinogenesis.[55]

It is widely believed that the progression of HPV-associated lesions to malignancy requires additional cellular events. The possibility of oncogene activation has already been mentioned. Studies of somatic hybrids of HeLa cells and normal human cells have suggested that cellular genes exercise "surveillance" over HPV replication in infected cells and that mutations of these cellular genes are required for the development of the fully transformed phenotype.[56] Cellular mutation has been proposed as the mechanism for the emergence of a fully transformed phenotype among murine NIH 3T3 cells which carry integrated HPV-16 genome.[57]

## TRANSMISSION AND EPIDEMIOLOGY

Papillomavirus infections are transmitted through abrasions of the skin (cutaneous HPVs), by sexual contact (genital tract HPVs), and during passage through an infected birth canal (some genital tract HPVs). The epidemiology of sexually transmitted HPVs is discussed in Chap. 38 and 48 and details of intrapartum transmission are given in Chap. 71. Therefore, the discussion here will be confined to some virologic aspects of transmission of genital tract HPVs.

Except for HPV-13 and HPV-32 which exclusively infect the oral cavity, the genital tract serves as a reservoir for all mucosal viruses. Each genital HPV type infects certain sites preferentially and produces a defined spectrum of pathological effects. The patterns of infection with HPV-6, HPV-11, and HPV-16, three of the most prevalent genital tract HPVs, are compared in Table 37-3. All three types cause asymptomatic infections and are also found in exophytic and flat condylomas. HPV-6 and HPV-11 predominate in the exophytic lesions. In high-grade intraepithelial neoplasias and invasive cancers, HPV-6 and HPV-11 are virtually absent whereas HPV-16 is associated with 50 percent or more of these lesions. HPV-6 and HPV-11 are especially effective at infecting extragenital mucosal sites and are responsible for nearly all respiratory tract and conjunctival papillomas. HPV lesions of the oral cavity may be caused by several genital tract HPVs, by other HPVs which exclusively infect this site, and rarely by cutaneous HPVs.[58]

Like other sexually transmitted infections, HPV may be transmitted from an infected maternal genital tract to the offspring. Such transmission is responsible for juvenile-onset respiratory papillomatosis (Chap. 71). It is estimated that only a small proportion of children at risk (born to infected mothers) develop respiratory papillomatosis.[59] Transmission most likely occurs intrapartum as the fetus passes through an infected birth canal. Disease in the child may be manifest as early as a few months or as late as 10 or more years after birth. As already mentioned, HPV-6 and HPV-11 account for nearly all respiratory papillomas. Other HPV types present in the maternal genital tract are either not transmitted to the offspring, or if transmitted are producing effects which are not yet recognized.

**Table 37-3. Characteristics of Three Genital Tract HPVs**

| | HPV type | | |
|---|---|---|---|
| | 6 | 11 | 16 |
| *Genital tract* | | | |
| Asymptomatic | + | + | + |
| Exophytic condyloma | + + + + | + + + | + |
| Flat condyloma | + + | + + | + + |
| Low-grade intraepithelial neoplasia | + | + | + |
| High-grade intraepithelial neoplasia | ± | ± | + + + |
| Invasive cancer | | | + + + |
| *Extragenital sites* | | | |
| Respiratory papilloma | + + | + + + | |
| Conjunctival papilloma | + + | + + | |
| Oral cavity papilloma | + | + | + |

## IMMUNOLOGIC RESPONSE

There are as yet no suitable reagents for the measurement of type-specific humoral or cellular responses to HPVs. Nonetheless, many early observations have underscored the importance of immune functions in the biology of papillomaviruses. Warts increase in number and size in conditions that depress T cell functions (e.g., pregnancy, organ transplantation). Histologic examination of regressing warts shows evidence of cellular immune response. Warts are not as prevalent in adults as they are in children. It has been suggested that the lower prevalence in adults is a result of immunity acquired following infections in childhood. Using viral particles obtained from clinical lesions as antigen, attempts have been made to demonstrate humoral and cell-mediated responses to cutaneous HPVs by a variety of techniques.[60,61] It is difficult to evaluate the results of some of these early studies because they were performed with material pooled from clinical lesions (which may have contained more than one HPV type) and because the protocols applied in different laboratories were not uniform. More recently, proteins coded by the different ORFs of several HPV types have been generated from bacterial expression vectors and synthetic peptides corresponding to presumed antigenic sites have been prepared. However, the use of these reagents in immunologic tests has not yet provided firm data on the nature, magnitude, and type specificity of the humoral and cellular immune responses to HPV infections.[62]

## PREVENTION

The prospects for the development of an effective immunization against HPVs are not bright. It is not known if natural infection with an HPV type confers protection against subsequent reinfection with the same type. Recurrence of genital warts is common but it is not clear whether this is a result of an incomplete cure of a previous infection, reactivation of a latent infection, new infection with a different HPV type, or reinfection by the same HPV type. If natural infection does not protect against subsequent infection with the same HPV type, effective immunization may be difficult to achieve. Moreover, attempts to develop vaccines against infections which are strictly mucosal and do not have a systemic phase generally have been unsuccessful. There are no suitable animal models of the disease, making it difficult to investigate which antigenic determinants of the virus might mediate protective immunity. Despite the above, immunization of cattle by subcutaneous injection of formalin-inactivated extracts of bovine papillomas, or with capsid proteins expressed in bacterial vectors, is believed to be effective against infection with BPV.[63,64] In the past, immunization with inactivated autologous condyloma extracts has been tried to treat recalcitrant condylomas in man, with conflicting results.[65] At present, avoidance of high-risk behavior appears to be the only feasible way to prevent HPV infections of the genital tract.

## References


1 Ciuffo G: Innesto positivo con filtrato di verrucae volgare. *Giorn Ital Mal Venereol* 48:12, 1907.

2 Shope R: Infectious papillomatosis of rabbits. *J Exp Med* 58:607, 1933.

3 Orth G et al: Characterization of a new type of human papillomavirus that causes skin warts. *J Virol* 24:108, 1977.

4 Gissmann L et al: Human papillomaviruses: Characterization of four different isolates. *Virology* 76:569, 1977.

5 Meisels A et al: Condylomatous lesions of the cervix. II. Cytologic, colposcopic and histopathologic study. *Acta Cytol* 21:379, 1977.

6 Purola E, Savia E: Cytology of gynecologic condyloma acuminatum. *Acta Cytol* 21:26, 1977.

7 Pfister H, Fuchs PG: Papillomaviruses: Particles, genome organisation and proteins, in *Papillomaviruses and Human Disease*, K Syrjanen et al (eds). Berlin, Springer-Verlag, 1987, p 1.

8 Broker T: Structure and genetic expression of papillomaviruses. *Obstet Gynecol Clin North Am* 14:329, 1987.

9 Howley PM et al: Molecular aspects of papillomavirus-host cell interactions. *Banbury Rpt* 21:261, 1986.

10 Pettersson U et al: Organization and expression of papillomavirus genomes, in *The Papovaviridae, Vol. 2, the Papillomaviruses*, NP Salzman, PM Howley (eds). New York, Plenum, 1987, p 67.

11 Lambert PF et al: A transcriptional repressor encoded by BPV-1 shares a common carboxy-terminal domain with the E2 transactivator. *Cell* 50:69, 1987.

12 Doorbar J et al: Identification of the human papilloma virus-la E4 gene products. *EMBO J* 5:355, 1986.

13 Baker CC: Sequence analysis of papillomavirus genomes, in *The Papovaviridae, Vol. 2, The Papillomaviruses*, NP Salzman, PM Howley (eds). New York, Plenum, 1987, p 321.

14 Shah KV: Papovaviruses, in *Virology*, BN Fields et al (eds). New York, Raven, 1985, p 371.

15 Melnick J: Papova virus group. *Science* 135:1128, 1962.

16 Lancaster W, Olson C: Animal papillomaviruses. *Microbiol Rev* 46:191, 1982.

17 Lancaster WD, Sundberg JP: Characterization of papillomaviruses isolated from cutaneous fibromas of white-tailed deer and mule deer. *Virology* 123:212, 1982.

18 Coggin JR, zur Hausen H: Workshop on papillomaviruses and cancer. *Cancer Res* 39:545, 1979.

19 Dartman K et al: The nucleotide sequence and genome organization of human papilloma virus type 11. *Virology* 151:124, 1986.

20 LaPorta RF, Taichman LB: Human papilloma viral DNA replicates as a stable episome in cultured human epidermal keratinocytes. *Proc Natl Acad Sci USA* 79:3393, 1982.

21 Christian CB et al: Infection of cultured human cells of respiratory tract origin with human papillomavirus type 1, in *Cancer Cells 5/Papillomaviruses*, BM Steinberg et al (eds). New York, Cold Spring Harbor Laboratory, 1987, p 165.

22 Kreider JW et al: In vivo transformation of human skin with human papillomavirus type 11 from condylomata acuminata. *J Virol* 59:369, 1986.

23 Kreider JW et al: Susceptibility of various human tissues to transformation in vivo with human papillomavirus type 11. *Int J Cancer* 39:459, 1987.

24 Murray R et al: Possible clonal origin of common warts (verruca vulgaris). *Nature* 232:51, 1971.

25 Buscema J et al: Genetic investigation of the cellular origin of vulvovaginal condylomata acuminata, in *Cancer Cells 5/Papillomaviruses*, BM Steinberg et al (eds). New York, Cold Spring Harbor Laboratory, 1987, p 245.

26 Orth G: Epidermodysplasia verruciformis: A model for understanding the oncogenicity of human papillomaviruses. *Ciba Found Symp* 120:157, 1986.

27 Orth G: Epidermodysplasia verruciformis, in *The Papovaviridae, Vol. 2, The Papillomaviruses*, NP Salzman, PM Howley (eds). New York, Plenum, 1987, p 199.

28 Rando RF et al: The noncoding region of HPV-6vc contains two distinct transcriptional enhancing elements. *Virology* 155:545, 1986.

29 Byrne JC et al: Human papillomavirus-11 DNA in a patient with chronic laryngotracheobronchial papillomatosis and metastatic squamous-cell carcinoma of the lung. *N Engl J Med* 317:873, 1987.

30 Crissmann JD et al: Squamous papillary neoplasia of the adult upper aerodigestive tract. *Human Pathol* (in press).

31 Jarrett WFH et al: High incidence area of cattle cancer with a possible

interaction between an environmental carcinogen and a papillomavirus. *Nature* 274:215, 1978.

32 Rabbett WF: Juvenile laryngeal papillomatosis: The relation of irradiation to malignant degeneration in this disease. *Ann Otol Rhinol Laryngol* 74:1149, 1965.

33 Sundberg JP: Papillomavirus infections in animals, in *Papillomaviruses and Human Disease*, K Syrjanen et al (eds). Berlin, Springer-Verlag, 1987, p 240.

34 Amtmann E et al: Tumor induction in the rodent *Mastomys natalensis* by activation of endogenous papilloma virus genomes. *Nature* 308:291, 1984.

35 Amtmann E, Wayss K: Papillomaviruses and carcinogenic progression II. The *Mastomys natalensis* papillomavirus, in *Papillomaviruses and Human Disease*, K Syrjanen et al (eds). Berlin, Springer-Verlag, 1987, p 187.

36 Campo MS, Jarrett WFH: Papillomavirus infection in cattle: Viral and chemical cofactors in naturally occurring and experimentally induced tumours. *Ciba Found Symp* 120:117, 1986.

37 Wettstein FO: Papillomaviruses and carcinogenic progression I. Cottontail rabbit (Shope) papillomavirus, in K Syrjanen et al (eds): *Papillomaviruses and Human Disease*, Berlin, Springer-Verlag, 1987, p 167.

38 Durst M et al: The physical state of human papillomavirus type 16 DNA in benign and malignant tumors. *J Gen Virol* 66:1515, 1985.

39 Schwarz E et al: Structure and transcription of human papillomavirus sequences in cervical carcinoma cells. *Nature* 314:111, 1985.

40 Yee C et al: Presence and expression of human papillomavirus sequences in human cervical carcinoma cell lines. *Am J Pathol* 119:361, 1985.

41 Durst M et al: Papillomavirus sequences integrate near cellular oncogenes in some cervical carcinomas. *Proc Natl Acad Sci USA* 84:1070, 1987.

42 Popescu N et al: Human papillomavirus type 18 DNA is integrated at a single chromosome site in cervical carcinoma cell line SW756. *J Virol* 51:1682, 1987.

43 Riou G et al: C-myc proto-oncogene expression and prognosis in early carcinoma of the uterine cervix. *Lancet* 1:761, 1987.

44 Baker CC et al: Structural and transcriptional analysis of human papilloma-virus 16 sequences in cervical carcinoma cell lines. *J Virol* 61:962, 1987.

45 Schneider-Gadicke A, Schwarz E: Different human cervical carcinoma cell lines show similar transcription patterns of human papillomavirus type 18 early genes. *EMBO J* 5:2285, 1986.

46 Haugen TH et al: *Trans*-activation of an upstream early gene promoter of bovine papilloma virus-1 by the product of the viral E2 gene. *EMBO J* 6:145, 1987.

47 Spalholz BA et al: Transactivation of the BPV transcriptional regulatory element by the E2 gene product. *J Virol* 61:2128, 1987.

48 Phelps WC, Howley PM: Transcriptional *trans*-activation by the human papillomavirus type 16 E2 gene product. *J Virol* 61:626, 1987.

49 Androphy EJ et al: Identification of the HPV-16 E6 protein from transformed mouse cells and human cervical carcinoma cell lines. *EMBO J* 6:989, 1987.

50 Banks L et al: Identification of human papillomavirus type 18 E6 polypeptide in cells derived from human cervical carcinomas. *J Gen Virol* 68:1351, 1987.

51 Seedorf K et al: Identification of early proteins of the human papilloma viruses types 16 (HPV 16) and type 18 (HPV 18) in cervical carcinoma cells. *EMBO J* 6:139, 1987.

52 Shirasawa H et al: Transcriptional differences of the human papillomavirus type 16 genome between precancerous lesions and invasive carcinomas. *J Virol* 62:1022, 1988.

53 Kanda T et al: Human papillomavirus type 16 open reading frame E7 encodes a transforming gene for rat 3Y1 cells. *J Virol* 62:610, 1988.

54 Matlashewski G et al: Human papillomavirus type 16 DNA cooperates with activated *ras* in transforming primary cells. *EMBO J* 6:1741, 1987.

55 Gius D et al: Inducible and constitutive enhancer domains in the noncoding region of human papillomavirus type 18. *J Virol* 62:665, 1988.

56 zur Hausen H: Human genital cancer results from deficient cellular control of papillomavirus gene expression. *Lancet* II:489, 1986.

57 Noda T et al: Progression of the phenotype of transformed cells after growth stimulation of cells by a human papillomavirus type 16 gene function. *J Virol* 62:313, 1988.

58 Syrjanen SM: Human papillomavirus infections in the oral cavity, in *Papillomaviruses and Human Diseases*, K Syrjanen et al (eds). Berlin, Springer-Verlag, 1987, p 104.

59 Shah K et al: Rarity of cesarean delivery in cases of juvenile-onset respiratory papillomatosis. *Obstet Gynecol* 68:795, 1986.

60 Chardonnet Y et al: Cell-mediated immunity to human papillomavirus. *Clin Dermatol* 3:156, 1985.

61 Kienzler J-L: Humoral immunity to human papillomaviruses. *Clin Dermatol* 3:144, 1985.

62 Li C-CL et al: Identification of the human papillomavirus-6b L1 open reading frame protein in condylomas and corresponding antibodies in human sera. *J Virol* 61:2684, 1987.

63 Pilacinski WP et al: Immunization against bovine papillomavirus infection. *Ciba Found Symp* 120:136, 1986.

64 Spadbrow PB: Immune response to papillomavirus infection, in *Papillomaviruses and Human Disease*, K Syrjanen et al (eds). Berlin, Springer-Verlag, 1987, p 333.

65 Pass F, Shah KV: Immunology of human papovaviruses, in *Comprehensive Immunology: Immunology of Infections,* AJ Nahmias, RJ O'Reilly (eds). New York, Plenum, 1982, p 225.

# Chapter 38

# Genital human papillomavirus infection

David Oriel

## DEFINITIONS

A *wart* is an epidermal tumor caused by a papillomavirus. *Condylomata acuminata,* "pointed condylomas," are warts with a particular clinical appearance (see below), and the term should not be used as a synonym for anogenital warts.

## HISTORY

Anogenital warts were evidently quite common in the ancient world.[1] For many years after syphilis appeared in Europe in the late fifteenth century, they were thought to be a part of this disease. When this belief was discarded, they were attributed to gonorrhea instead. After the discovery of the gonococcus in 1879, it became clear that many patients with warts did not have gonorrhea, and they were then attributed to genital irritation by secretions "disordered through venery." This led to the term *venereal warts,* which is still sometimes used. Eventually, however, a series of studies beginning in the late nineteenth century and continuing for 50 years showed that this theory also was wrong, and that anogenital warts were caused by a human papillomavirus (HPV).[2] Until the 1970s it was believed that all types of wart were caused by the same virus, but it is now known that there are multiple types of HPV with predilections for particular tissues (see Chap. 37).[3]

Although some early workers believed that genital warts were infectious, this was confirmed only in 1954, when an outbreak of vulvar warts among the wives of soldiers returning from the Korean war was described.[4] The incubation period was estimated as 4 to 6 weeks. The idea that genital warts were a venereal disease was violently attacked at the time but has since been confirmed many times.

Recognition that HPV infection of the cervix could cause inconspicuous flat lesions requiring colposcopy for identification is quite recent. It began with the suggestion that some cervical abnormalities previously regarded as a form of cervical intraepithelial neoplasia (CIN) closely resembled warts both cytologically and histologically.[5] This idea was soon confirmed, and it was also observed that subclinical warty lesions were common throughout the genital tract. Associations between cervical "flat condylomas" and CIN were first reported in 1977.[5,6] Virological studies subsequently showed that DNA sequences of several types of HPV could be identified not only in anogenital warts but in many varieties of genital neoplasia. The earlier view that anogenital warts were a harmless, if troublesome, condition has now been abandoned.

## EPIDEMIOLOGY

### PREVALENCE

Data on the prevalence of genital warts in the general population are scanty. A group of 771 married women in King County, Washington, was asked if they had ever had genital warts; 6 percent said that they had, and this figure was fairly consistent among 5-year age groups from ages 20 to 34 years.[7] Subclinical HPV infection is common. Studies of unselected cervical smears have shown the presence of koilocytotic atypia, indicative of HPV infection (see Chap. 37), in 1 percent of women in Quebec and in 1.3 percent in Sydney.[5,8] Furthermore, HPV sequences have been identified in many individuals with no clinical signs of infection. In Germany, sequences of HPV 6, 11, 16, or 18 have been identified in 31 (5.8 percent) of 530 smears from the glans penis of healthy men aged 16 to 79 years.[9] In another study, 10 percent of women aged 15 to 50 years with normal cervical smears were positive for HPV DNA.[10]

### INCIDENCE

Anogenital warts are often diagnosed in people who attend clinics for sexually transmitted diseases (STD). In the United Kingdom the disease is reportable from clinics. In 1985, 58,960 new cases of warts were reported, constituting 14.8 percent of all infections treated. This is an increase of 85 percent over 1980, when 31,780 new cases of warts were seen, 10.0 percent of all infections treated.[11] The total national incidence must be much higher than these figures suggest, because the disease is not reportable from other specialities or from general practice. In the United States there has also been a substantial increase in new cases of genital warts during the last decade, and the incidence rates are now approximately double those reported from the United Kingdom.[12,13] Today, genital warts are the commonest viral STD, three times as common as genital herpes, and their incidence is exceeded only by gonorrhea and chlamydial infection.

### AGE OF ONSET

Most genital warts are seen in young adults. The age of onset in men has been reported as between 16 and 25 years (maximal at age 22 years), and in women between 16 and 25 years (maximal at age 19 years). Gonorrhea shows a similar age distribution.[2]

### INFECTIVITY

As a rule, genital HPV infections are transmitted by direct sexual contact. In an early study[2] it was shown that nearly two-thirds of sex partners of individuals with genital warts developed the disease after an average incubation period of 2 to 3 months. Similar results have been reported in a recent investigation;[14] 90 male partners of women with genital warts were examined, and 62 (69 percent) were found to have histologically confirmed warts themselves. Genital lesions in sex partners identified through contact tracing are often inconspicuous, and careful examination may be needed to identify them.[14,15] The transfer of HPV by fomites plays a part in the epidemiology of skin warts;[16] whether this occurs with genital strains of HPV is not known.

## ASSOCIATED INFECTIONS

Many people with genital warts have other sexually transmitted infections. In a study from an STD clinic in the United Kingdom[17] 10 percent of men with penile warts had gonorrhea, and 17 percent nongonococcal urethritis; 12 percent of women with vulvar warts had gonorrhea, and 12 percent trichomoniasis. Concomitant infections are also present in patients with genital warts seen in dermatologic practice.[18]

## INVOLVEMENT OF NONGENITAL AREAS

Genital strains of HPV can infect nongenital sites. Of these, the commonest is the anus. Approximately 8 percent of men with penile warts, and 20 percent of women with vulvar warts have anal warts,[2] exemplifying the multicentric nature of genital HPV infections. Anal warts occurring alone are strongly associated with anoreceptive intercourse.[19,20] Therefore, although they are sometimes found in women, they are much commoner in homosexual or bisexual men; it has been reported in a study from New York City that 22 percent of a group of such men either had anal warts at the time of examination or had had them in the past.[20] Noncondylomatous wart virus infection of the anal canal has recently been demonstrated.[21] Anal smears from 102 homosexual men were stained by Papanicolaou's method, and 45 (44 percent) showed features of papillomavirus infection. Many of the patients had had anal warts in the past, but only 5 had warts at the time of the examination. The average age of onset of anal warts is similar to that of genital warts, and associated infections are common. Anal warts contain predominantly HPV 6 DNA sequences,[22] and it seems likely that the virus is transmitted by sexual contact with a partner with a penile HPV infection. In homosexual men anal warts are much commoner than penile warts;[19,20] the reason for this is uncertain, but may relate to lowered local immunity to HPV (see below).

In the past, condylomata acuminata in the mouth were regarded as rare, but they are diagnosed more frequently today.[23,24] Some patients with condylomas of the lips, tongue, or palate have concomitant genital or anal warts, and some give a history of oral sex with an infected partner. Transmission of HPV by orogenital contact is clearly possible, but the genotypes involved have not yet been identified.

## INVOLVEMENT OF CHILDREN

Anogenital warts are not uncommon in prepubertal children; they can occur at any age, and affect girls more often than boys.[25] They can arise in several ways. (1) They can appear in infants born to mothers with genital warts.[26] In such cases, warts do not appear for several weeks, which suggests that infection occurs during delivery, but a case has been described in which they were present at birth, indicating that antenatal infection can occur.[27] The risk to an infant exposed to HPV infection from the mother during delivery is not known. (2) It is also believed that anogenital warts in children can follow close nonsexual contact within a family.[25,28] (3) Anogenital warts may follow sexual abuse; this has been variously estimated as being responsible for 30 to 80 percent of cases.[29] The long incubation period of the warts, and the existence of several possible routes of infection, cause problems in interpreting their significance.[30,31] Limited studies of genital wart material from children have shown HPV 6, 11, and 16 DNA sequences.[28] This indicates infection from a genital site but provides no information concerning how this has occurred. A case has been described recently in which a 5-year-old boy's perianal warts appeared to be due to autoinoculation from a finger wart, as sequences of HPV 2 were found in biopsies from both sites.[32] Further studies of the epidemiology and virology of this disease are clearly required.

Laryngeal papillomatosis in children is also closely associated with maternal genital warts, and is discussed in Chap. 71.

## ETIOLOGY

Genital warts are caused by infection of the epidermis by specific HPV types. The subject is described in detail in Chap. 37. In the majority of lesions sequences of HPV 6 and 11 are found, but sometimes HPV 16 or other types are present. The relationship between genital warts and common skin warts was much discussed in the past, but there is no clinical or virological evidence of any close association between the two. Nevertheless, a small number of patients with common skin warts develop similar warts on the genitals. Autoinoculation with HPV 1, 2, or 4 seems a likely explanation; as these types have been identified in some genital wart material.[33]

## PATHOGENESIS

### HISTOPATHOLOGY AND CYTOLOGY

Papillomaviruses are epitheliotropic, and their replication depends on the presence of a differentiating squamous epithelium. Viral DNA, but not viral structural protein, can be detected in the lower layers of the epithelium. Capsid antigen and infective virus are present in only the superficial differentiated cell layers.[34]

Anogenital warts show the general histologic features of viral warts. The basal cell layer is intact, and the border with the dermis clear-cut (Fig. 38-1). The prickle cell layer is hyperplastic (acanthosis). The dermal papillae are elongated. Hyperkeratosis is not usually a feature unless the warts have been present for a long time or unsuccessfully treated; as a rule, the stratum corneum consists of only one or two layers of parakeratotic cells. Koilocytes are scattered throughout the outer cell layers of genital warts. They are mature squamous cells in which a large clear perinuclear zone is sharply demarcated from the peripheral cytoplasm. Their nuclei may be enlarged and hyperchromasic, and double or multiple nuclei are often seen.[35] Ultrastructural studies show virus particles in some of the cell nuclei. Koilocytosis appears to represent a specific cytopathic effect of HPV.[36] The histopathology of flat cervical condylomas resembles that of condylomata acuminata. Papanicolaou-stained smears show koilocytosis, and in many specimens cytologic features of CIN are also seen (see below).

Immunochemical methods can be used to demonstrate HPV capsid proteins in both smears and biopsies. On the whole, there is a good correlation between this technique and the demonstration of virus particles by electron microscopy; approximately 50 percent of condylomata acuminata give positive results by both methods.[34]

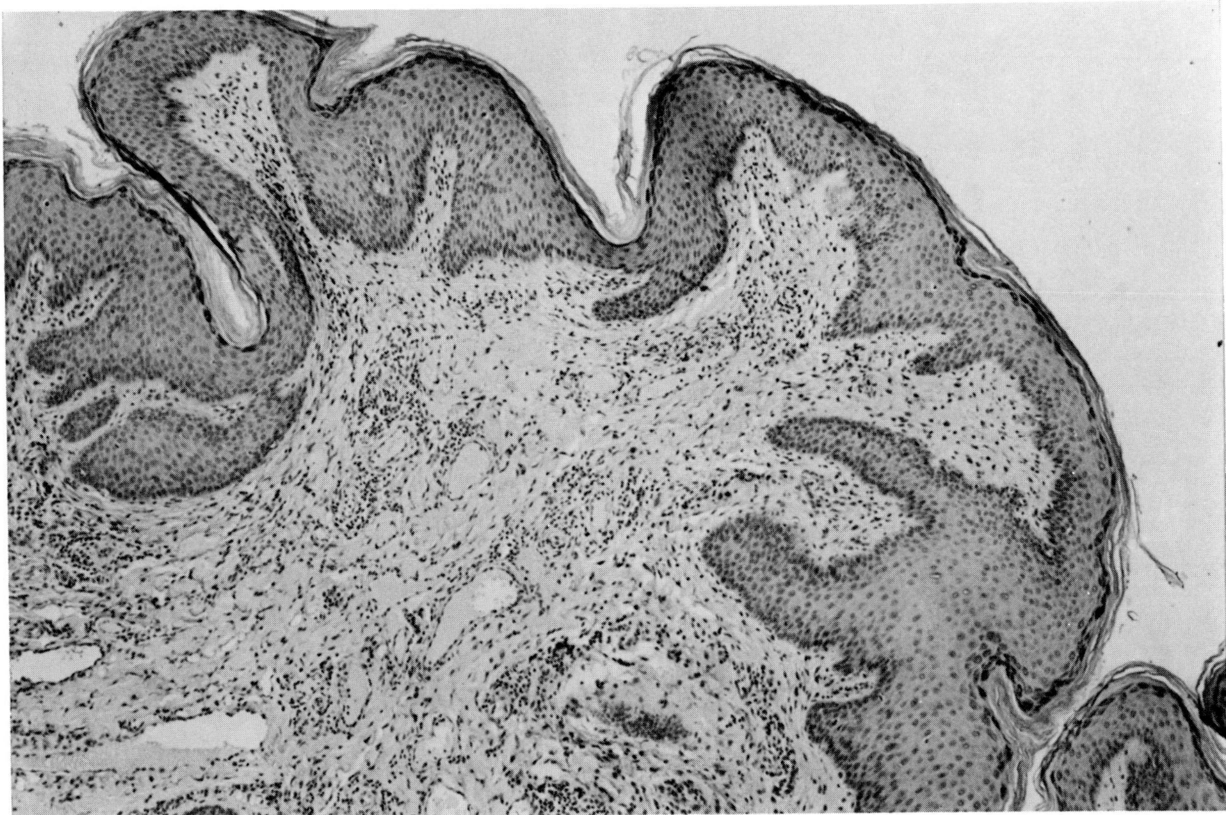

**Fig. 38-1.** Biopsy of condyloma acuminatum, showing acanthosis, elongated dermal papillae, and sharp border with the dermis. H&E stain. (*Courtesy of E. Stolz.*)

## RISK FACTORS

In adults, exposure to the causal agent of genital warts is usually by sex contact with a partner with a clinical or subclinical infection. It would be expected that increasing numbers of sex partners would increase the risk of infection, and this has been demonstrated in women in a recent study.[37] The presence of warts on other parts of the body is a conceivable, although weak, risk factor. In babies, exposure to HPV in the birth canal is strongly associated with the development of both anogenital and laryngeal warts.

The risk of developing genital warts for women who have ever smoked has been reported as 3.7 times that of lifetime nonsmokers, and the long-term use of oral contraceptives may also increase the risk of HPV infection.[37] A possible explanation for these associations is their effect on immune responses, which are known to be affected by both cigarette smoking and high circulating levels of estrogenic and progestagenic steroids. There have been reports of an increased risk of condylomata acuminata, and of CIN, in women who are immunosuppressed.[38]

## IMMUNOLOGY

Little is known about host defenses to HPVs.[39] There is no in vitro system which supports growth of these viruses, so that information about the immune response to viral antigens is scanty. Antibodies to a bovine type common papillomavirus antigen have been detected by ELISA more often in patients with genital warts than in controls,[40] but the nature of these antibodies is uncertain. Molecular cloning and DNA sequencing techniques are being used to characterize genital papillomavirus proteins, and serological studies of responses to recombinant antigens should provide useful information.

Since there are no suitable in vitro infected target cells, it has been difficult to investigate cell-mediated immune responses (CMI) to HPV. At present, techniques which rely on the recognition of specific antigen by primed lymphocytes are used, but studies of patients with skin warts have shown only small and transitory responses in these tests, and data from patients with genital warts are not available. It has been reported that nonspecific CMI responses are to some extent defective in patients with a long history of genital warts.[41] In the future, it may prove possible to create a suitable target cell for T-cell studies by introducing viral genes into cells; the use of such molecular techniques should greatly facilitate the study of HPV-host interactions.

## CLINICAL MANIFESTATIONS

### GENITAL WARTS IN MEN

Genital warts in men are pleomorphic. Condylomata acuminata (exophytic condylomas) are the most frequent (Fig. 38-2). They are soft, fleshy, and vascular. They often appear first on the frenum, coronal sulcus, glans penis, and the lining of the prepuce, areas which are liable to trauma during intercourse, allowing entry of an infecting agent. They can also present on the shaft of the penis and the scrotum. Papular warts appear on relatively dry areas, particularly the shaft of the penis (Fig 38-3); they are

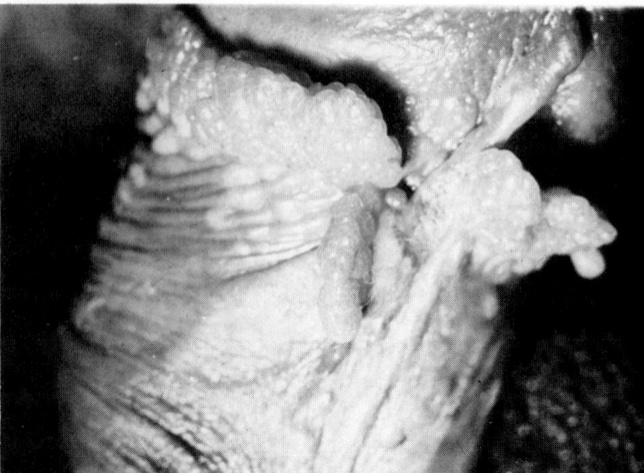

Fig. 38-2. Penile condylomata acuminata.

usually multiple, and vary between 1 and 5 mm in diameter. Common warts occasionally appear on the shaft of the penis (Fig. 38-4), usually in association with similar lesions on nongenital skin. The urethra is often affected by exophytic condylomas, either alone or in association with other lesions; 80 percent are in the terminal urethra, but they can spread and involve the proximal urethra.[42] Men with urethral condylomas may complain of urethral bleeding or discharge, or of a reduction in urinary stream, but many are symptomless. Examination reveals characteristic condyloma tissue in the terminal urethra. It is often difficult to determine the extent of the disease in men with a narrow meatus. Because they are inconspicuous, it has been suggested that urethral condylomas may be an important source of infection to others.[15] Condylomata acuminata of the bladder are rare, and nearly always associated with urethral condylomas.[42]

Flat condylomas affect the same areas as exophytic warts; they are usually multiple, and may be confluent. (Fig. 38-5) As a rule they are subclinical, and the affected areas cannot be clearly iden-

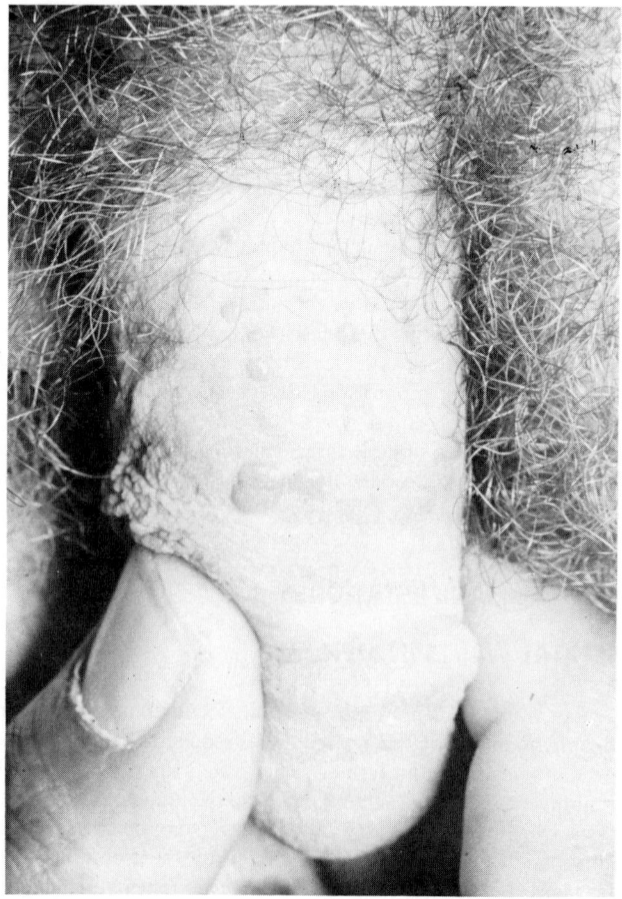

Fig. 38-3. Multiple papular warts of shaft of penis.

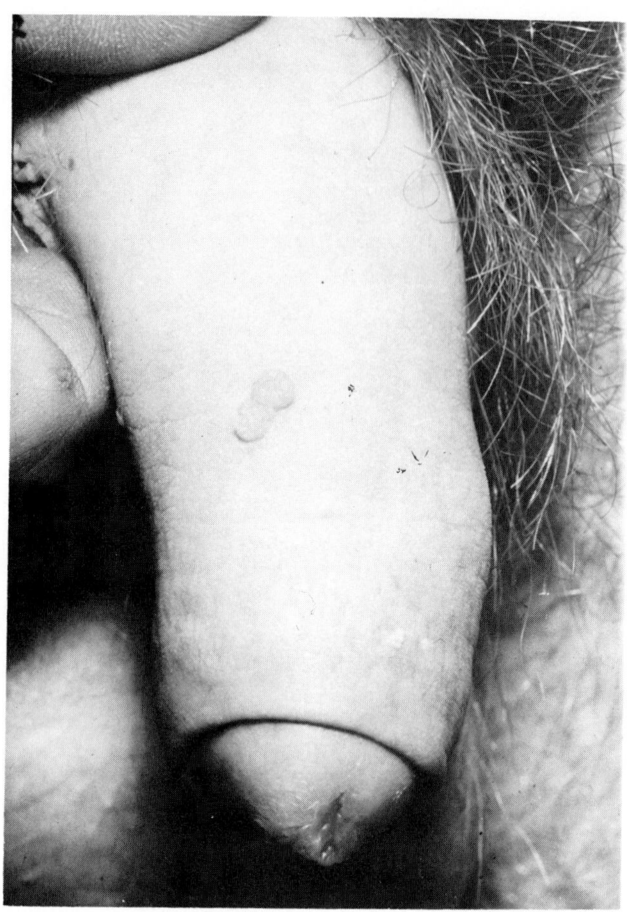

Fig. 38-4. Penile common wart (verruca vulgaris). This lesion is unlikely to respond to podophyllin.

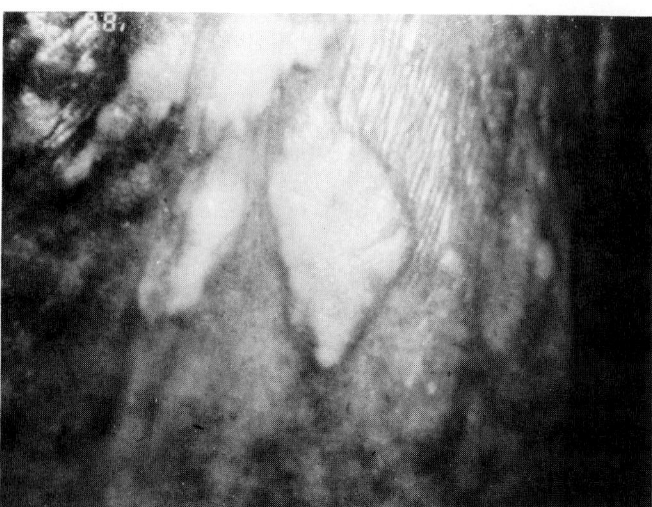

Fig. 38-5. Subclinical wart virus infection of the penis. These lesions become apparent after the application of 5 percent acetic acid.

tified unless acetic acid solution is applied and a colposcope or other source of magnification used.

## GENITAL WARTS IN WOMEN

Exophytic condylomas usually appear first at the fourchette and adjacent labia, and may spread quite rapidly to other parts of the vulva (Fig. 38-6); in 20 percent of cases condylomas also appear on the perineum and perianal area. Any part of the vagina may be affected, and in a few women the vagina may be entirely occupied by condylomatous tissue. Papular warts affect the outer parts of the genitals, such as the labia majora and perineum.

Subclinical HPV infection of the vulva has been identified only recently. It takes the form of "microwarts" (Fig. 38-7) or of flat lesions of the vulva visible by colposcopy after the application of acetic acid. Fissuring of these areas can be a cause of vulvodynia and dyspareunia.[43]

For many years exophytic condylomas were regarded as the only manifestation of infection of the cervix by HPV. They are present in about 6 percent of women with vulvar warts, and occasionally occur alone.[2] During the last decade it has become clear that subclinical infection of the cervix is common, however, and the colposcope has proved invaluable in its recognition. The term "flat condyloma" has been used to describe noncondylomatous wart virus infection of the cervix. The colposcopic changes are well recognized.[45] After the cervix has been treated with 5 percent acetic acid the transformation zone shows areas which are white, often with a raised and roughened surface. (Fig. 38-8) Punctation indicates the presence of small intraepithelial vascular loops. If the cervix is now treated with iodine solution, the acetowhite epithelium fails to stain, while the fully differentiated squamous epithelium stains deeply. It has been shown that about 50 percent of women with vulvar warts show evidence of cervical HPV infection.[46]

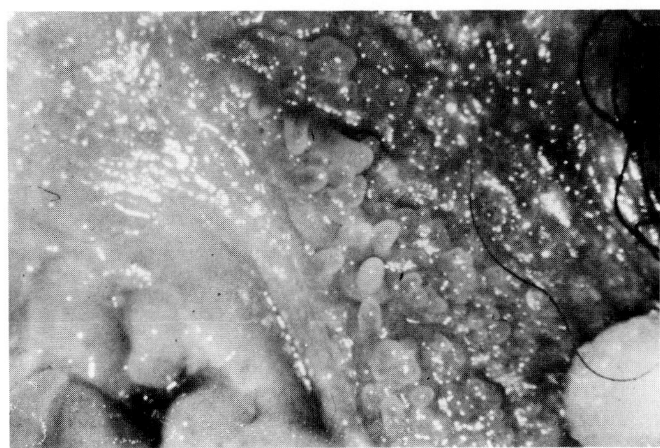

Fig. 38-7. Vulvar "microwarts."

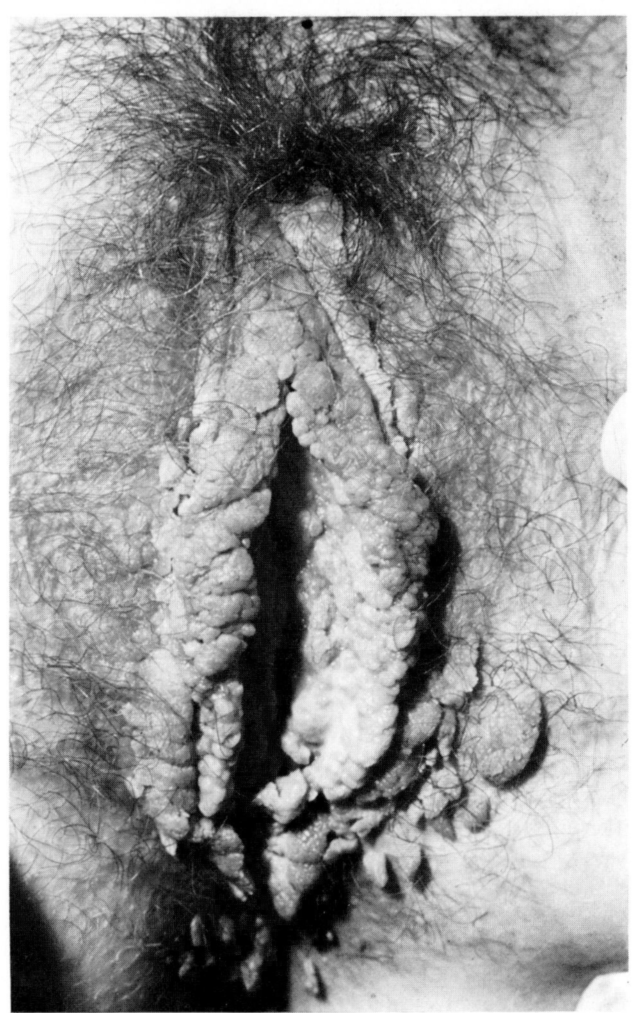

Fig. 38-6. Extensive condylomata acuminata of the labia and immediately adjacent sites. (*Courtesy of E. Stolz.*)

Studies by colposcopy, cytology, and histology have shown an association between HPV infection and CIN; this association has been reported by different authors as between 25 and nearly 100 percent of women with CIN.[36,47] Its significance in the etiology of cervical cancer is discussed in Chap. 48.

## ANAL WARTS

Perianal warts are usually condylomata acuminata (Fig. 38-9). They are multifocal, and may reach a substantial size. Internal

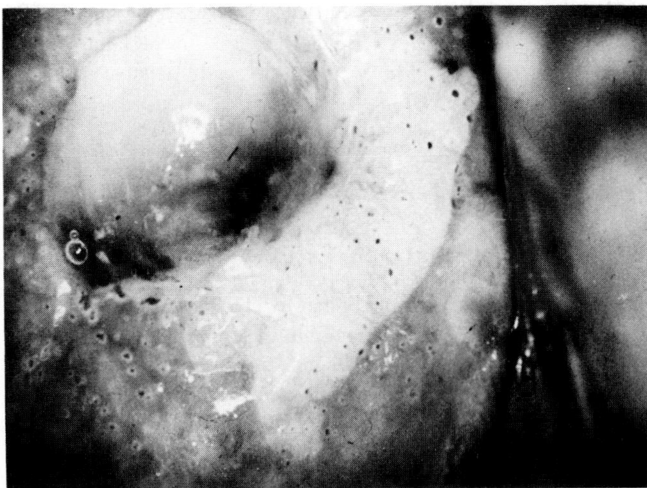

Fig. 38-8. Flat condyloma of the cervix after treatment with 5 percent acetic acid. The epithelium is white and slightly raised, and punctuation is visible.

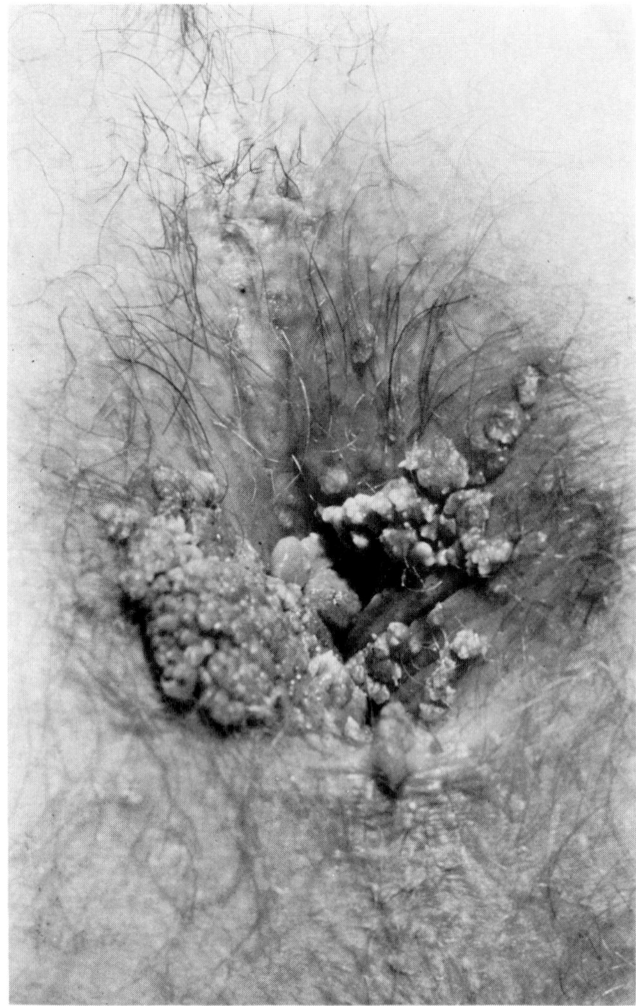

**Fig. 38-9.** Anal condylomata acuminata. (*Courtesy of E. Stolz.*)

condylomas affect over 50 percent of men with external warts;[48] most of these are in the anal canal, but they can occur above the pectinate line. Noncondylomatous HPV infection of anorectal mucosa also occurs in homosexual men. In one study,[49] 45 (44 percent) of 102 rectal smears from such men showed koilocytosis. Many of the men had previously been treated for perianal warts, but only two of those who were cytologically positive still had warts at the time of examination. The association between anorectal dysplasia and HPV is discussed below.

## GIANT CONDYLOMA

Genital and anal condylomata acuminata may reach a substantial size. Large vulvar condylomas may occur in women with conditions in which cell mediated immunity is reduced, such as pregnancy and Hodgkin's disease, or who are receiving immunosuppressive therapy. The giant condyloma (Buschke-Loewenstein tumor) is an uncommon tumor. In most of the recorded cases the penis has been affected,[50] but it has been described on the vulva and perianal area.[51] An initial wartlike lesion enlarges relentlessly to form a locally invasive, destructive but nonmetastasizing tumor. Despite its formidable clinical behavior, histologically it appears to be benign, consisting of condyloma acuminatum tissue.[50] There has been much discussion about its nature.

Transformation into a metastasizing squamous carcinoma has been reported,[52] and it has been suggested that a giant condyloma may be a well-differentiated carcinoma from the beginning.[53] Its histological identity with condyloma acuminatum suggests a possible viral etiology, and HPV 6 or 11 DNA has been identified in some giant condylomas.[54] Whether other factors are also involved is not known.

## HPV AND GENITAL NEOPLASIA

For several years evidence has been accumulating which implicates specific HPV types in the pathogenesis of genital epithelial neoplasia. These data may be summarized (see also Chap. 37):

1. Genital warts are an STD. Carcinoma of the cervix behaves like an STD, major risk factors being multiple sex partners and an early age at first intercourse. It should be noted that these risk factors have not been shown to apply to cancer of the penis or vulva.[55]
2. HPV DNA, particularly HPV 16 and 18, has been repeatedly found in squamous cervical cancers, the higher grades of CIN and cervical cancer cell lines.[56,57] This association is also present, although less consistently, with neoplasia of the vulva and penis.[58]
3. HPV DNA is integrated into the genome of the host cell in invasive cancers but is episomal in lower grades of intraepithelial neoplasia.[59]
4. Associations have been found between CIN and vulvar warts, cervical HPV infection, and HPV infection in sex partners.[46,60,61]
5. The outcome of cervical HPV infection appears to depend in part on the viral type, infection with HPV 16 being more likely to progress than infection with HPV 6 or 11.[62]

This evidence is persuasive but not totally convincing. HPV DNA is frequently present in normal genital epithelia.[9,10] Series of patients with neoplasia in whom various HPV types have been identified are mostly small, and control patients are not always well matched for demographic variables and sexual behavior. Comparison between groups may be partly invalidated by different methods of specimen collection and different hybridization procedures. Although carcinoma in situ is a more sinister lesion than superficial dyskaryosis in prospective studies, it is not a malignant neoplasm and the causes of progression to invasive cancer are not known. It is possible that current high levels of intraepithelial neoplasia of the cervix, vulva, penis, and anus are the result of infection by HPVs which produce lesions which mimic "genuine" intraepithelial neoplasia but which are inherently harmless.[63] It is not certain whether viral DNA is an active participant in promoting tumor growth, or simply evidence of an old infection.[64] The virus may initiate early cell change, but not participate in subsequent events which culminate in invasive cancer.

HPV infection may indeed be a major factor in the pathogenesis of genital epithelial cancer, but carcinogenesis may be a complex multistep process involving several different factors at each stage of development.[35] Much further work, including well-controlled, prospective clinical studies, will be needed to clarify these issues.

## DIAGNOSIS

Anogenital warts must be differentiated from other papillomatous lesions of the area, which include anatomical variants, infective conditions, and neoplasms. In men, parallel rows of sebaceous glands on the corona of the penis and grouped yellow ectopic sebaceous glands (Fordyce's spots) which occur on the inner and outer side of the prepuce are anatomical variants which are easily recognized. In women, epithelial papillae and small sebaceous glands are common on the vulva, and perianal fibroepithelial polyps affect both sexes.

The most important infective lesions to be distinguished from anogenital warts are the condylomata lata of secondary syphilis, which appear on moist areas such as the vulva and anus. They are more rounded than warts. Other signs of secondary syphilis are also present, and dark field microscopy of serum from the condylomas shows motile treponemes, while serological tests for syphilis are strongly positive. In the tropics, the granulating lesions of donovanosis may be confused with anogenital condylomata acuminata (see Chap. 25). The umbilicated tumors of molluscum contagiosum are usually easily distinguished from warts (see Chap. 39).

Distinguishing warts from neoplastic conditions is obviously important but may not be easy. Vulvar and penile intraepithelial neoplasia lesions may be single or multiple, and pigmented or nonpigmented. These may resemble genital warts, and indeed the two diseases may occur together.[65–67] There is no easy solution to this diagnostic problem, but it is clearly important to biopsy any lesions which appear atypical or which respond poorly to treatment. The laboratory detection of HPV infection is described in Chap. 78. The colposcopic, cytologic, and histopathologic features which differentiate noncondylomatous wart virus infection of the cervix from CIN have been mentioned above, and are discussed in detail in Chap. 48.

## TREATMENT

It is often said that most warts will disappear sooner or later without treatment. While there are data to support such a statement for skin warts, the evidence for spontaneous regression of anogenital warts is only anecdotal. This disease is worrying for the patient, and in some cases anogenital HPV infection may contribute to the development of neoplasia. It is not yet possible to predict the future behavior of any particular anogenital wart, and thus there is no alternative to aiming for the complete elimination of all lesions, difficult though this may be. Sex partners should always be examined, for they may have not only warts but penile, vulvar, or cervical intraepithelial neoplasia. For this reason, examination of a female partner should always include cervical cytology. Before anogenital warts are treated, diagnostic tests for possible associated infections should be performed. In the case of children, the diagnosis of another infection may be of medicolegal importance.

Over the years many treatment modalities for this disease have been tried, and no one method has emerged as superior to all others. The procedures in use today include cytotoxic agents, surgery, and immune modulating methods. Antiviral therapy has had only a limited success.[68] Topical idoxuridine and acyclovir are ineffective. Treatment with interferons, whose action is in part antiviral, appears more promising and is discussed below.

## CYTOTOXIC AGENTS

Podophyllin resin is extracted from the rhizome of *Podophyllum peltatum* and *P. emodi,* which grow respectively in North America and the Himalayas. It contains cytotoxic lignans, of which podophyllotoxin is the most active. Podophyllin is applied to warts as a 20 percent solution in ethanol or tincture of benzoin and allowed to dry. It is washed off after 3 to 4 h, but with subsequent applications this interval can be lengthened to 12 h. Treatment is repeated once or twice a week. Because of the risk of irritation of the skin adjacent to the warts, it should be applied by a doctor or paramedical worker.

The major objection to podophyllin is that treatment failures are common. It has been reported[69] that only 22 percent of penile warts were cured by one, and a further 16 percent by two, applications. If there has been no real improvement after a month's treatment, an alternative should be used. Podophyllin is potentially toxic. There have been several reports of severe systemic side effects following generous applications to large condylomas. These toxic effects include blood dyscrasias, hepatotoxicity, and neuropathy[70] and may be particularly severe in pregnancy.[71] Not more than 0.5 ml of 20 percent podophyllin should be applied at any one time, and it should not be used at all during pregnancy. Podophyllin may have oncogenic and teratogenic potential,[72,73] so it should not be applied to the cervix, and prolonged treatment (which in any case is unlikely to be successful) should be avoided.

A 0.5 percent solution of podophyllotoxin in ethanol has recently been used for the self-treatment of penile warts. Good results have been claimed,[74] but it is too soon to decide the place of this approach in the treatment of anogenital warts.

5-Fluorouracil (5-FU) is a cytotoxic agent which has been used for the treatment of genital warts. Its effect is variable, and it is liable to cause unacceptable soreness. Intraurethral condylomata acuminata have been successfully treated by the application of 5 percent 5-FU cream after each voiding for up to 8 days.[75]

Trichloracetic acid is applied undiluted and washed off after 4 h. It is weakly destructive and rather painful, and numerous treatments may be required. It is sometimes effective against small warts but has no advantages over other treatment modalities.

## SURGERY

Cryotherapy is effective against both genital and anal warts provided that they are not too large or extensive. A cryoprobe operated by nitrous oxide is a useful piece of equipment. Freezing is continued until there is an iceball 1 to 2 mm larger than the diameter of the wart.[76] Cryotherapy is painful, and a local anesthetic is recommended unless only one or two small lesions are being treated.

Electrocautery under local anesthesia is effective but only practicable at certain sites, such as the shaft of the penis, the labia majora, and the perianal area. For other genital areas, and for patients with extensive disease or with lesions affecting the urethra or cervix, cautery or diathermy under general anesthesia may be preferable. $CO_2$ laser treatment is now increasingly used. Under colposcopic control the extent and depth of tissue destruction can be carefully controlled, and the treatment of warts and the destruction of premalignant lesions, if present, can be combined. Healing is more rapid after laser vaporization than after cautery or diathermy. Laser therapy can be used against warts in any site, but it should be emphasized that special training and experience, and skill in colposcopy, are needed.

A scissor excision technique for the treatment of perianal and intraanal warts has given good results, with low recurrence rates and avoidance of scarring and anal stenosis.[77] If the disease is not extensive, this procedure can be used for outpatients.[78]

## IMMUNE MODULATING METHODS

Interferons (IFN) show some antiviral activity, but their action against anogenital warts is believed to be due to their effect on cell-mediated immunity. Intramuscular IFN-alpha and -beta have been used on a small scale for the treatment of recalcitrant genital warts.[79,80] There has been a definite, if variable, therapeutic effect but side effects are troublesome. With the object of achieving high local IFN concentrations without causing systemic reactions, several studies have examined the effect of intralesional therapy. In a placebo-controlled trial, repeated injections of IFN-alpha directly into genital warts have been shown to be effective and reasonably well tolerated.[81] However, the treatment is laborious and still not altogether free from side effects. In the future, intralesional or perilesional IFN therapy may have a place as an adjunct to surgical treatment, but more studies are needed to establish its value. Hitherto, topical IFN therapy for anogenital warts has given disappointing results.

## PREVENTION

Efforts to prevent an STD may be justified by how many people are affected, the severity of its effects, and the probability that preventive action will influence either of these. Anogenital warts are undoubtedly common, and their incidence appears to be increasing. Adverse effects include enlargement in pregnancy, laryngeal papillomatosis in children, and a possible risk of intraepithelial neoplasia and squamous cancer. At present there are not enough data from prospective studies to quantify the likelihood of these events. Nevertheless, the continuous escalation in the number of new cases of these infections must cause concern and preventive measures should be considered, although at present it is not possible to decide the priority which these should receive.

The most important strategy for the prevention of anogenital warts is the examination of sex partners, and the treatment of those found to be affected. Unfortunately, epidemiologic treatment, which is of particular value in STDs with a long incubation period, is impossible and surveillance of exposed individuals for several months presents obvious problems. Some asymptomatic women with cervical condylomas may be identified by routine cervical cytology; their treatment, and examination of their partners, is a useful preventive measure. Screening of other groups for warts is hardly practicable. It would be expected, although evidence is lacking, that the use of condoms would give protection from HPV infection. Otherwise, measures for prevention are based on health education and behavior modification as described in Chap. 88. Control strategies for cervical cancer through cytology and colposcopy are described in Chap. 48. Until the natural history of this disease, and the role of HPV in its pathogenesis, are more clearly understood the routine identification of these viruses, or of individual HPV types, cannot be regarded as a useful preventive measure.

## References


1 Bafverstedt B: Condylomata acuminata—Past and present. *Acta Derm Venereol (Stockh)* 47:476, 1967.
2 Oriel JD: Natural history of genital warts. *Br J Vener Dis* 47:1, 1971.
3 McCance DJ: Human papillomaviruses and cancer. *Biochim Biophys Acta* 823:195, 1986.
4 Barrett TJ et al: Genital warts—A venereal disease. *JAMA* 154:333, 1954.
5 Meisels A et al: Condylomatous lesions of the cervix II: Cytologic, colposcopic and histopathologic study. *Acta Cytol* 21:379, 1977.
6 Purola E, Savia E: Cytology of gynecologic condyloma acuminatum. *Acta Cytol* 21:26, 1977.
7 Daling JR et al: History of genital warts in a selected population. *Lancet* i:157, 1984.
8 Reid R et al: Noncondylomatous cervical wart virus infection. *Obstet Gynecol* 55:476, 1980.
9 Grussendorf-Conen et al: Human papillomavirus genomes in penile smears of healthy men. *Lancet* ii:92, 1986.
10 de Villiers EM et al: Human papillomavirus infections in women with and without abnormal cytology. *Lancet* ii:703, 1987.
11 Report 1987:Sexually transmitted diseases in Britain: 1985. *Communicable Disease Reports* 87/45, 1987.
12 Editorial note: Condylomata acuminata—United States 1966–1981. *JAMA* 250:336, 1983.
13 Chuang T-Y et al: Condylomata acuminata in Rochester, Minnesota 1950–1978. 1:Epidemiology and clinical features. *Arch Dermatol* 120:469, 1984.
14 Sand PK et al: Evaluation of male consorts of women with genital human papillomavirus infection. *Obstet Gynecol* 68:679, 1986.
15 Levine RU et al: Cervical papillomavirus infection and intraepithelial neoplasia: A study of male sex partners. *Obstet Gynecol* 64:16, 1984.
16 Bunney MH: *Viral Warts: Their Biology and Treatment.* New York, Oxford University Press, 1982, p 10.
17 Kinghorn G: Genital warts: Incidence of associated genital infections. *Br J Dermatol* 99:405, 1978.
18 Farris GM et al: The investigation of patients with genital warts. *Br J Dermatol* 111:736, 1984.
19 Oriel JD: Anal warts and anal coitus. *Br J Vener Dis* 47:373, 1971.
20 Carr G, William DC: Anal warts in a population of gay men in New York City. *Sex Transm Dis* 4:56,1977.
21 Frazer IH et al: Association between anorectal dysplasia, human papillomavirus and human immunodeficiency virus in homosexual men. *Lancet* ii:657, 1986.
22 McCance DJ et al: Human papillomavirus in condylomata acuminata of the anus. *J Clin Pathol* 39:927, 1986.
23 Judson FN: Condyloma acuminatum of the oral cavity: A case report. *Sex Transm Dis* 8:218, 1981.
24 Lutzner MA et al: Different papillomaviruses as the causes of oral warts. *Arch Dermatol* 118:393, 1982.
25 Stumpf PG: Increasing occurrence of condylomata acuminata in premenarchal children. *Obstet Gynecol* 56:262, 1980.
26 Zamora S et al: Condyloma acuminatum in a 2½ year old girl. *J Urol* 129:145, 1983.
27 Tang CK: Congenital condylomata acuminata. *Am J Obstet Gynecol* 131:912, 1978.
28 Rock B et al: Genital tract papillomavirus infection in children. *Arch Dermatol* 122:1129, 1986.
29 de Jong AR et al: Condylomata acuminata in children. *Am J Dis Child* 136:704, 1982.
30 Bender ME: New concepts of condylomata acuminata in children. *Arch Dermatol* 122:1121, 1986.
31 Schachner L, Hankin DE: Assessing child abuse in childhood condyloma acuminatum. *J Am Acad Dermatol* 12:157, 1985.
32 Fleming KA et al: DNA typing of genital warts and a diagnosis of sexual abuse of children. *Lancet* ii:454, 1987.
33 Krzyzek RA et al: Anogenital warts contain several distinct species of human papillomavirus. *J Virol* 36:236, 1980.

34 McCance DJ: Genital papillomavirus infection: Virology, in *Recent Advances in Sexually Transmitted Diseases No 3,* JD Oriel et al (eds). Edinburgh, Churchill Livingstone, 1986, p 109.
35 Koss JG: Carcinogenesis in the uterine cervix and human papillomavirus infection, in *Papillomaviruses and Human Disease,* K Syrjanen et al (eds). Berlin, Springer-Verlag, 1987, p 235.
36 Meisels A et al: Lesions of the uterine cervix associated with papillomavirus and their clinical consequences, in *Advances in Clinical Ctyology,* LG Koss et al (eds). New York, 1984, vol 2, p 1.
37 Daling JR et al: Risk factors for condyloma acuminatum in women. *Sex Transm Dis* 13:16, 1986.
38 Schneider V et al: Immunosuppression as a high-risk factor in the development of condyloma acuminatum and squamous neoplasia of the cervix. *Acta Cytol* 27:220, 1983.
39 Kirchner H: Immunobiology of human papillomavirus infection. *Progr Med Virol* 33:1, 1986.
40 Baird PJ: Serological evidence for the association of papillomavirus and cervical neoplasia. *Lancet* ii:17, 1983.
41 Avgerinou G et al: Reduction of cell mediated immunity in patients with genital warts of long duration. *Genitourin Med* 62:396, 1986.
42 de Benedictis TJ: Intraurethral condylomata acuminata: Management and a review of the literature. *J Urol* 118:767, 1977.
43 von Krogh G: Treatment of human papillomavirus-induced lesions, in *Papillomaviruses and Human Disease,* K Syrjanen et al (eds). Berlin, Springer-Verlag, 1987, p 296.
44 Meisels A et al: Human papillomavirus infection of the cervix. *Int J Gynecol Pathol* 1:75, 1982.
45 Reid R et al: Non-condylomatous cervical wart virus infection. *Obstet Gynecol* 55:476, 1980.
46 Walker PG et al: Abnormalities of the uterine cervix in women with vulval warts. *Br J Vener Dis* 59:120, 1983.
47 Reid R et al: Genital warts and cervical cancer III: Subclinical papillomavirus infection and cervical neoplasia are linked by a spectrum of continuous morphologic and biologic change. *Cancer* 53:943, 1984.
48 Schlappner OLA, Shaffer EA: Anorectal condylomata acuminata: A missed part of the condyloma spectrum. *Can Med Assoc J* 118:172, 1978.
49 Medley G: Anal smear test to diagnose occult anorectal infection with human papillomavirus in men. *Br J Vener Dis* 60:205, 1984.
50 Ananthakrishnan N et al: Loewenstein-Buschke tumour of penis—A carcinomimic. Report of 124 cases with review of the literature. *Br J Urol* 53:460, 1981.
51 Judge JR: Giant condyloma acuminatum involving vulva and rectum. *Arch Pathol* 88:46, 1969.
52 South LM et al: Giant condyloma of Buschke and Loewenstein. *Clin Oncol* 3:107, 1977.
53 Tessler AN, Applebaum SM: The Buschke-Loewenstein tumor. *Urology* 20:36, 1982.
54 Gissmann L et al: Analysis of human genital warts (condylomata acuminata) and other genital tumours for human papillomavirus type 6 DNA. *Int J Cancer* 29:143, 1982.
55 Hellberg D: Penile cancer: Is there an epidemiological role for smoking and sexual behaviour? *Br Med J* 295:1306, 1987.
56 Gissmann L, Schwartz E: Persistence and expression of human papillomavirus DNA in genital cancer, in *Papillomaviruses*, D Evered et al (eds). Chichester, Wiley, 1986, p 190.
57 Macnab et al: Human papillomavirus in clinically and histologically normal tissue of patients with genital cancer. *N Engl J Med* 315:1052, 1986.
58 McCance DJ et al: Human papillomavirus types 16 and 18 in carcinomas of the penis in Brazil. *Int J Cancer* 37:55, 1986.
59 Durst M et al: The physical state of human papillomavirus type 16 DNA in benign and malignant genital tumors. *J Gen Virol* 66:1515, 1985.
60 Syrjanen KJ: Human papillomavirus lesions in association with cervical dysplasias and neoplasias. *Obstet Gynecol* 62:617, 1983.
61 Campion MJ: Increased risk of cervical neoplasia in the consorts of men with penile condylomata. *Lancet* i:943, 1985.
62 Campion MJ et al: Progressive potential of mild cervical atypia: Prospective cytological, colposcopic and virological study. *Lancet* ii:237, 1986.
63 Leading article: Cervical intraepithelial neoplasia. *Lancet* ii:365, 1982.
64 Yee C et al: Presence and expression of human papillomavirus sequences in human cervical carcinoma cells. *Am J Pathol* 119:361, 1985.
65 Wade TR et al: Bowenoid papulosis of the genitalia. *Arch Dermatol* 115:306, 1979.
66 Laohadtanaphorn S et al: Multicentric pigmented carcinoma in situ of the vulva in association with vulvar condylomata acuminata. *Aust NZ J Obstet Gynecol* 19:249, 1979.
67 Campion MJ, Singer A: Vulval intraepithelial neoplasia: Clinical review. *Genitourin Med* 63:147, 1987.
68 Kinghorn GR: Genital papillomavirus infections: Treatment, in *Recent Advances in Sexually Transmitted Diseases 3,* JD Oriel et al (eds). Edinburgh, Churchill Livingstone, 1986, p 147.
69 von Krogh G: Topical treatment of penile condylomata acuminata with podophyllin, podophyllotoxin and colchicine. *Acta Derm Venereol* 58:163, 1978.
70 Slater GE et al: Podophyllin poisoning: Systemic toxicity following cutaneous application. *Obstet Gynecol* 52:94, 1978.
71 Chamberlain MJ et al: Toxic effect of podophyllin in pregnancy. *Br Med J* 3:391, 1972.
72 Gueson EJ et al: Dysplasia following podophyllin treatment of vulvar condylomata acuminata. *J Reprod Med* 6:159, 1971.
73 Karol MD et al: Podophyllum: Suspected teratogenicity from topical application. *Clin Toxicol* 16:283, 1980.
74 von Krogh G: Topical self-treatment of penile warts with 0.5% podophylotoxin in ethanol for four or five days. *Sex Transm Dis* 14:135, 1987.
75 Dretler SP, Klein LA: The eradication of intraurethral condylomata acuminata with 5 per cent 5-fluorouracil cream. *J Urol* 113:195, 1975.
76 Simmons PD et al: Cryotherapy versus electrocautery in the treatment of genital warts. *Br J Vener Dis* 57:273, 1981.
77 Thomson JFS, Grace RH: Treatment of perianal and anal condylomata acuminata. A new operative technique. *J R Soc Med* 71:181, 1978.
78 McMillan A et al: Outpatient treatment of perianal warts by scissor excision. *Genitourin Med* 63:114, 1987.
79 Schonfeld A et al: Intramuscular human interferon-beta injections in the treatment of condylomata acuminata. *Lancet* i:1038, 1984.
80 Gall SA et al: Interferon for the therapy of condyloma acuminatum. *Am J Obstet Gynecol* 153:157, 1985.
81 Eron LJ et al: Interferon therapy for condylomata acuminata. *N Engl J Med* 315:1059, 1986.

# Chapter 39
# Molluscum contagiosum

John Munroe Douglas, Jr.

## DEFINITION AND HISTORY

Molluscum contagiosum is a benign papular condition of the skin and mucous membranes which is often sexually transmitted in adults. It is caused by the molluscum contagiosum virus (MCV), a member of the poxvirus family. The characteristic appearance of molluscum contagiosum was first described in 1817 by Bateman, who called the disorder "molluscum," a common term then for pedunculated lesions. Additionally, he described this condition as "contagiosum" to signify its apparent transmissibility, which he felt was due to the "milky fluid" which could be expressed from lesions.[1–3] In 1841, Henderson and Paterson each described in this fluid cellular elements with large intracytoplasmic inclusion bodies, subsequently termed Henderson-Paterson or molluscum bodies, which they felt were responsible for causation and transmission of the disease.[1–3] Subsequent reports of successful transmission of infection to humans by direct inoculation of lesion material supported an infectious etiology. Suspicion initially focused on a parasitic or bacterial agent, but the report by Lipschutz in 1911 of tiny "elementary bodies" within the molluscum bodies and the documentation of disease transmission by a "filterable agent" by Juliusberg in 1905 and Wile and Kingery in 1919 pointed to a virus as the etiologic agent.[1–3] In the early 1930s, Goodpasture demonstrated a marked similarity between the cellular inclusions and elementary bodies of molluscum contagiosum, fowl pox, and vaccinia and concluded that all were members of the same family of viruses.[3,4]

## EPIDEMIOLOGY

Characterization of the epidemiology of infection with MCV has been limited by several factors. In most patients, the lesions cause few problems and are self-limited.[1,2,5–8] It is likely that many infected patients do not seek medical attention, and there are few population-based data on those patients who do since molluscum contagiosum is usually not a reportable disease. Furthermore, there is currently no in vitro system for cultivation of MCV,[2,3,9,10] which has restricted studies of virus transmission, asymptomatic infection, and seroprevalence and forced epidemiologic studies to rely on detection of characteristic clinical lesions by physical examination.[2]

Molluscum contagiosum appears to be spread by both sexual and nonsexual routes of transmission.[1–3,5–8,11–13] In adults, lower abdominal, thigh, and genital lesions are more common than those in extragenital locations.[2,5,6] The suspicion that genital molluscum contagiosum is sexually transmitted is indirect but is supported by a frequent history of contact with multiple sexual partners and prostitutes, the history and presence of other STD, the presence of genital lesions in sexual partners, and peak ages of occurrence (20 to 29 years) which are similar to those of other STD.[2,5,6–8,13–15] There is no information about the efficiency of sexual transmission of MCV. The nonvenereal form of disease occurs primarily in children on the face, trunk, and extremities and appears to be transmitted by direct contact with the skin of infected individuals and/or fomites.[1–3,8,11,12] Involvement of multiple members of a household occurs in 25 percent of families studied,[2,8] although whether this represents skin-to-skin or fomite-to-skin transmission is not clear. Several studies have associated molluscum contagiosum with baths and swimming.[1,2,8,12] Nonsexual transmission has also been reported in the patients of a surgeon with hand lesions and in association with wrestling, tatooing, and the use of gymnastic equipment and towels.[1–3]

The most consistent information on rates of genital molluscum contagiosum comes from the STD clinic system of England which has reported cases since 1971.[15] The absolute and relative numbers of cases have increased dramatically since the early 1970s. In 1982, there were 1378 new cases of molluscum contagiosum, a fourfold increase from 1971.[13,15] These cases comprised 0.27 percent of new cases attending STD clinics and represented 2.94 new cases of molluscum contagiosum/100,000 population of all ages, an increase of 40 percent since 1978.[13] In the United States, data from STD clinics are based on samples of representative facilities and are thus more limited. From 1977 to 1981, the proportion of clinic visits for molluscum contagiosum was stable and ranged from 0.3 percent in Columbus, Ohio to 1.0 percent in Denver, Colorado.[14] Five times as many cases were noted in men as in women, and the rates in whites were 2 to 4 times higher than those in nonwhites.[14] Data from a longitudinal survey of private physicians demonstrated a different trend, with an 11-fold increase in visits by adults for molluscum contagiosum from 1966 to 1983.[14]

Rates of nonvenereal molluscum contagiosum have been estimated from patients identified in dermatology clinics and in population-based surveys, mostly based on children with extragenital lesions.[1,2,8,11,12,16] This form of disease appears to be uncommon in North America and Europe, accounting for only 0.1 to 1.2 percent of patients attending dermatology clinics.[1,8] In other areas community surveys indicate that the disease is much more common. Among villagers in Fiji and New Guinea, visible lesions were detected in 4.5 and 7 percent of the population respectively.[8,11] Most cases were in children, and in surveys restricted to children in Fiji, New Guinea, and Japan, prevalence rates have been reported to range from 6 to 22 percent.[8,11,12] During an outbreak of molluscum contagiosum in East Africa, 17 percent of the village population and 52 percent of children more than 2 years old developed lesions.[16]

Seroepidemiologic studies of MCV are limited in number and difficult to compare because of varying techniques and sources of antigen and lack of adequate controls.[2,3,11,17,18] Studies using an indirect immunofluorescent technique with fixed sections of molluscum contagiosum lesions appear most promising and have found low titers of antibody in 69 to 89 percent of patients with visible lesions.[11,17,18]

## ETIOLOGY

Although never convincingly replicated in vitro, MCV has been purified from skin lesions and is considered to be a poxvirus on the basis of size, structure, chemical composition, physical characteristics, and behavior.[2,3,19] Like the vaccinia virus, with which it has been most extensively compared, ultrastructural studies of MCV reveal a brick-shaped particle, approximately 300 × 220 × 100 nm in dimension, consisting of a biconcave viral core

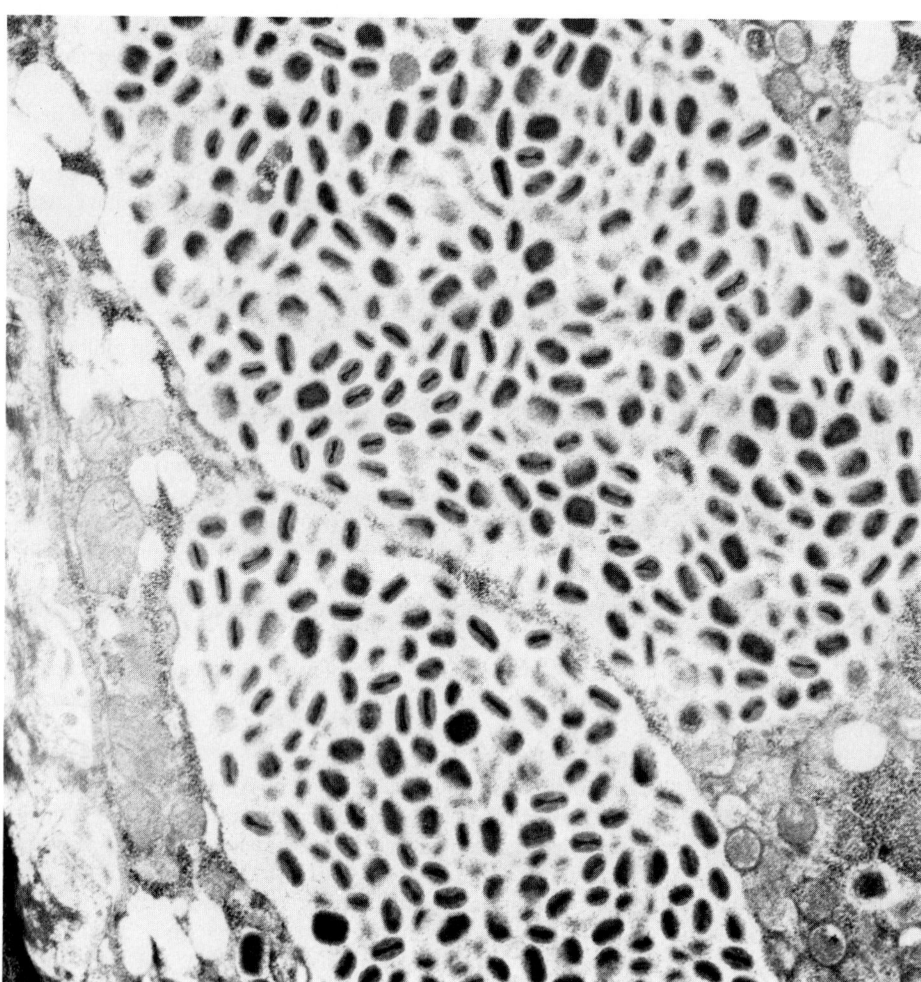

**Fig. 39-1.** Transmission electron micrograph of a molluscum body filled with molluscum contagiosum virus. A biconcave core is visible within many of the virions. Original magnification × 30,000. (*Courtesy of BA Werness.*)

enclosed by an inner membrane and an outer envelope[2,3,19] (Fig. 39-1). The viral genome consists of a single molecule of linear double-stranded DNA with terminal or near-terminal intrastrand covalent links; its molecular weight is 118 megadaltons, corresponding to 178 kilobase pairs.[2,10] Characteristic of the poxvirus family, MCV replicates in the cytoplasm in discrete electron-dense areas known as "viral factories."[2,3,19,20] In contrast, however, MCV lacks serologic cross-reactivity with other family members[2,3,18] and is unable to rescue other types of heat-inactivated poxviruses in mixed infection by the process known as nongenetic reactivation.[2,3] Because of these distinctions, MCV is designated as an unclassified poxvirus.

Attempts at experimental cultivation of MCV have been frustrating. The disease has not been transmitted to animals, and even human transmission experiments are variably successful.[2,3] The virus cannot be replicated in cell culture; while one report described propagation of MCV in WI-38 and human amnion cells,[21] no successful reproduction of this work has been reported.[2,9] Virions derived from molluscum contagiosum lesions will, however, cause functional changes in a variety of cell lines, inducing interferon production and producing a characteristic cytopathic effect (CPE).[2,3,9] Electron microscopic studies indicate that virus particles penetrate the cell by phagocytosis, undergo envelope uncoating, and progress to the stage of free virus cores within 8 to 12 h.[3,9] However, it is the subsequent step, "second-stage uncoating" of the inner membrane to release viral DNA into the cytoplasm, which fails to occur in vitro, blocking completion of the replication cycle.[2,3,9] The cytopathic changes of cell swelling, rounding, and clumping appear within 24 h and seem to require early viral gene function since they can be blocked by inhibitors of RNA and protein synthesis. The CPE is transitory, however, regressing within 4 days and disappearing during serial propagation of cell lines after three to four passages.[2,3,9]

Characterization of viral strains has been limited by difficulties with in vitro cultivation. A recent evaluation of virions from skin lesions by SDS-polyacrylamide gel electrophoresis identified seven major polypeptides and showed variability between patients, suggesting a potential for use in strain evaluation.[22] The evaluation of viral DNA may be a more powerful tool for molecular analysis. Limited studies indicate a similar restriction endonuclease pattern among epidemiologically related lesions,[23] and the cloning of MCV DNA and its use in restriction enzyme analysis was recently reported.[10]

## PATHOGENESIS

The pathologic changes induced by MCV infection are very characteristic and generally limited to the epidermis[1-3,19] (Fig. 39-2). Molluscum contagiosum lesions consist of focal areas of hyperplastic epidermis surrounding cyst-shaped lobules filled with keratinized debris and degenerating molluscum bodies. In the basal layer, the nuclei and cytoplasm of the keratinocytes are enlarged; this is the only layer in which mitotic figures are seen. By the spindle layer, cells begin to display cytoplasmic vacuolization and enlargement and then replacement by eosinophilic compart-

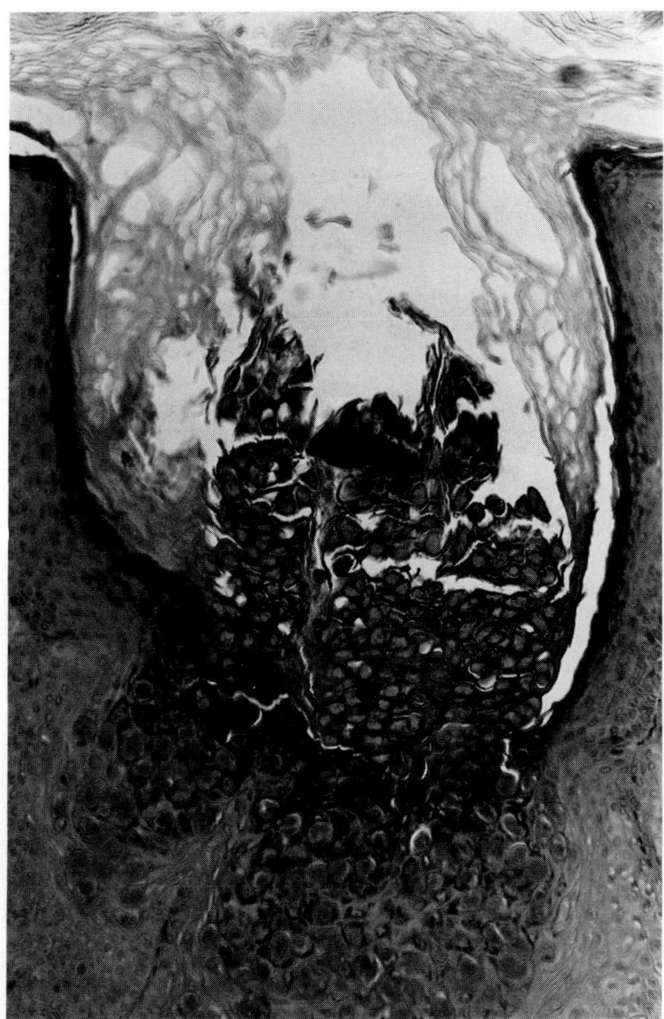

**Fig. 39-2.** Biopsy of a molluscum contagiosum lesion showing an area of epidermal hyperplasia surrounding a cystic lobule. Keratinocytes in the upper epidermis as well as those desquamated into the lobule demonstrate large round intracytoplasmic molluscum bodies. Hemotoxylin and eosin stain. (*Courtesy of BA Werness.*)

mentalized globules, the molluscum bodies, which compress the nuclei to the cell periphery. In the granular layer, the molluscum bodies become more homogeneous with loss of their internal structural markings and are finally desquamated into the cystic lobules.[1–3,19] Dermal changes are usually limited to stromal proliferation, although inflammation occurs in up to 20 percent of clinical lesions, with edema, vascular proliferation and thrombosis, and infiltration of the necrotic epithelium by lymphocytes, histiocytes, neutrophils, and occasionally multinucleated giant cells.[2,3,19,24]

Ultrastructural studies of molluscum contagiosum lesions demonstrate free virus cores in all layers of the epidermis, even in mitotic cells of the basal layer.[19,20] Second-stage uncoating of the cores, replication of viral DNA, and the formation of viral factories do not occur, however, until the spindle and granular layers. The molluscum bodies which develop in these layers are composed of large masses of maturing virions[19,20] (Fig. 39-1). The presence of the virus from the basal layer outward in a progressively maturing form suggests that infection of the epidermis with MCV involves infection of basal keratinocytes initially, perhaps by trauma, with a "latent phase" lasting until the spindle layer when second-stage uncoating occurs.[19,20]

The role of host immunity in the control of MCV infection has been poorly defined, although the greater prevalence of lesions in children than in adults[8,11,16] suggests the acquisition of host resistance with age. The inflammatory reaction noted above may indicate evidence of a cell-mediated immune response to MCV antigens, as the appearance of inflammation often precedes the resolution of lesions.[24,25] Case reports of widespread lesions in patients with impaired T-cell function, especially those with AIDS, also argue for the importance of cell-mediated immunity.[26–28] The role of humoral immunity remains unclear, although the presence of low levels of antibody in most patients regardless of disease duration suggests that it must be minor.[2,17,18]

## CLINICAL MANIFESTATIONS

The incubation period of molluscum contagiosum averages 2 to 3 months and may range from 1 week to 6 months.[1,2,6] Most patients are asymptomatic, the diagnosis being made incidental to another problem; a minority complain of itching or tenderness.[1,2,5–8] Lesions begin as tiny pinpoint papules which grow over several weeks to a diameter of 3 to 5 mm, occasionally enlarging to 10 to 15 mm, producing the "giant molluscum."[1,2,6] The papules are smooth, firm, and dome-shaped, with a highly characteristic central umbilication from which caseous material can be expressed (Fig. 39-3). They are usually flesh-colored but can appear gray-white, yellow, or pink. In adults, lesions most often occur on the thighs, inguinal region, buttocks, and lower abdominal wall and less commonly on the external genitalia and perianal region, especially mucosal surfaces, a pattern contrasting with the distribution of genital warts.[2,5–7] Children more typically develop lesions on the face, trunk, and extremities; lesions on the palms, soles, and mucous membrane are rare.[1,2,5,6,8,12] A linear distribution of lesions often occurs, suggesting autoinoculation by scratching.[1,2,6] Lesions are usually more widespread in children than they are in adults, and while adults with genital molluscum contagiosum rarely develop extragenital lesions, 10 to 50 percent of children with molluscum contagiosum have lesions in the genital region.[8]

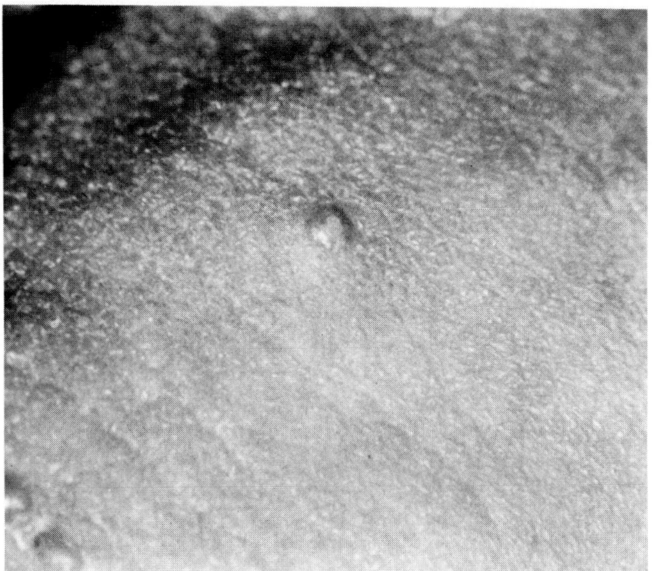

**Fig. 39-3.** Solitary molluscum contagiosum lesion with typical dome shape and central umbilication. (*Courtesy of AC Cardozo.*)

In normal hosts, the number of lesions usually varies between 10 and 20, ranging from 1 to 100; patients with impaired host defenses, however, may develop hundreds of lesions.[2,5–8,26–28] Widespread involvement of eczematous areas has been described in patients with atopic dermatitis and attributed to skin disruption, use of topical steroids, and/or an underlying immunological disorder.[2,26,29] Patients with frankly abnormal cell-mediated immunity are also at risk of developing extensive outbreaks of lesions; cases have been described in patients with sarcoidosis, Hodgkin's disease, and AIDS, and in those receiving immunosuppressive therapy.[2,26–28] Of interest, the distribution of lesions in these patients, including homosexual men with AIDS, is usually over the face and trunk rather than the genital region.[27,28]

The most frequent complication of molluscum contagiosum, bacterial superinfection, occurs in up to 40 percent of cases.[2,6,8] Another common problem is "molluscum dermatitis," appearing 1 to 15 months after the onset of skin lesions in approximately 10 percent of patients.[2,6,25] The dermatitis consists of a sharply bordered eczematoid reaction 3 to 10 cm in diameter around an individual lesion, may involve only a portion of an individual's lesions, and usually disappears as the lesion resolves.[2,25] Lesions of the eyelid may induce a unilateral conjunctivitis; the pattern is usually that of a chronic follicular or papillary conjunctivitis, but corneal changes with a punctate epithelial keratitis similar to that of trachoma can also occur.[2] Other inflammatory conditions seen in association with molluscum contagiosum include folliculitis, sycosis barbae, erythema annulare centrifugum, and pseudoleukemia cutis.[2] Although it has been suggested that the lesions of molluscum contagiosum, like genital warts, may increase during pregnancy, there is little information on this issue. Infection does not appear to affect the outcome of pregnancy, and while lesions have been reported in a child as young as 1 week old, no documented case of maternal-fetal transmission of infection has been reported.[7]

The average duration of untreated molluscum contagiosum is reported to be approximately 2 years, ranging from 2 weeks to 4 years.[2,6,8,11,30] Individual lesions usually resolve within 2 months.[30] Recurrences of lesions after clearance have been noted in 15 to 35 percent of patients;[8,30] whether these represent new infections or exacerbation of subclinical or latent infection is not clear. The East African outbreak which occurred suddenly in 17 percent of villagers during refeeding after a famine[16] raises the question of reactivation of a chronic infection.

## DIAGNOSIS

The clinical diagnosis of molluscum contagiosum is usually made easily on the basis of the characteristic, pearly, umbilicated papule with the caseous center found on the face, trunk, extremities, or genital region.[2,6] Lesions are most frequently misdiagnosed as common or genital warts or keratoacanthomas.[2,6,8] Other considerations in the differential diagnosis include syringomas, plane warts, lichen planus, epithelial and intradermal nevi, seborrheic dermatitis, basal cell epithelioma, infection with herpes simplex and varicella zoster virus, and atopic dermatitis.[2,6,31] In atypical cases the diagnosis can be confirmed by demonstrating the pathognomonic enlarged epithelial cells with intracytoplasmic molluscum bodies on cytologic or histologic studies.[2,6] Thinly spread smears of material expressed from lesion cores stained by Wright, Giemsa, or Gram's stain will demonstrate sheets of infected cells, and hematoxylin- and eosin-stained sections of punch biopsies will reveal the characteristic epidermal histopathologic changes[2,6,19] (Fig. 39-2). Other diagnostic techniques include detection of MCV antigen with fluorescent antibody studies and visualization of the abundant viral particles by electron microscopy.[2] Although not used for diagnostic purposes, the CPE induced in cell culture by MCV may be confused with that of herpes simplex virus; one clinical laboratory reported that up to 10 percent of specimens from genital lesions producing a CPE were caused by MCV.[31] Additional considerations in a patient with molluscum contagiosum include diagnostic studies for other STD in those with genital lesions[2,6] and the possibility of an immunodeficiency, such as HIV infection[27,28] in those with widespread lesions. The question of whether genital lesions in children should prompt an investigation of sexual abuse is unresolved, although the presence of additional extragenital lesions supports a nonsexual route of transmission.[32]

## TREATMENT AND PREVENTION

Treatment of molluscum contagiosum is generally simple and accomplished by eradicating lesions with mechanical destruction or techniques to induce local epidermal inflammation.[2,6] While treatment hastens resolution of individual lesions and may thereby reduce autoinoculation and transmission to others, the high frequency of recurrences and the benign and self-limited nature of the infection must be weighed against the pain and potential for scarring induced by destructive therapies, especially in children.[2,6,33] Controlled studies evaluating different therapeutic approaches have not been performed. The simplest and most widely used methods are excisional curettage or expression of the core of the lesion by direct pressure;[2,6,33] these procedures are often followed by cauterization of the lesion base with electrodesiccation or a chemical agent such as phenol, silver nitrate, trichloroacetic acid, or iodine.[2,6,8] Cryotherapy with liquid nitrogen is an alternative mode of direct destruction.[2,6,33] For tiny lesions which may be difficult to curette or express, topical application of irritating agents such as podophyllin, cantharadin, tretinoin, silver nitrate, phenol, or trichloroacetic acid have been recommended;[2,6,33] these often require more than a single treatment. No therapy is very effective in immunocompromised patients, presumably because of the increased occurrence of new lesions.[26–29] Bacterial superinfection and molluscum dermatitis may require systemic antibiotics or topical corticosteroids, respectively.[33] Because of the difficulties with in vitro cultivation of MCV, nothing is known of its sensitivity to antiviral agents. Case reports describing the use of methisazone,[29] an antipoxviral agent, and interferon[34] in the therapy of refractory lesions suggest little clinical benefit. A small uncontrolled trial of systemic isoprinosine, a broad-spectrum antiviral agent with immunomodulating properties, showed clearance of lesions in 77 percent of patients within 4 weeks, although the authors speculated that the drug would not be likely to benefit immunocompromised hosts.[35]

# References


1 Low RC: Molluscum contagiosum. *Edinburgh Med J* 53:657, 1946.

2 Brown ST et al: Molluscum contagiosum. *Sex Transm Dis* 8:227, 1981.

3 Postlethwaite R: Molluscum contagiosum: A review. *Arch Environ Health* 21:432, 1970.

4 Goodpasture EW: Borreliotoses: Fowl-pox, molluscum contagiosum, variola-vaccinia. *Science* 77:119, 1933.

5 Cobbold RJC, MacDonald A: Molluscum contagiosum as a sexually transmitted disease. *Practitioner* 204:416, 1970.
6 Felman YM, Nikitas JA: Sexually transmitted molluscum contagiosum. *Dermatol Clin* 1:103, 1983.
7 Wilkin JK: Molluscum contagiosum venereum in a women's outpatient clinic: A venereally transmitted disease. *Am J Obstet Gynecol* 128:531, 1977.
8 Postlethwaite R et al: Features of molluscum contagiosum in the north-east of Scotland and in Fijiian village settlements. *J Hyg (Lond)* 65:281, 1967.
9 McFadden G et al: Biogenesis of pox-viruses: Transitory expression of molluscum contagiosum early functions. *Virology* 94:297, 1979.
10 Darai G et al: Analysis of the genome of molluscum contagiosum virus by restriction endonuclease analysis and molecular cloning. *J Med Virol* 18:29, 1986.
11 Sturt RJ et al: Molluscum contagiosum in villages of the West Sepik district of New Guinea. *Med J Aust* 2:751, 1971.
12 Niizeki K et al: An epidemic study of molluscum contagiosum: Relationship to swimming. *Dermatologica* 169:197, 1984.
13 Chief Medical Officer of the Department of Health and Social Security: Sexually transmitted diseases: Extract from the annual report. *Genitourin Med* 61:204, 1985.
14 Becker TM et al: Trends in molluscum contagiosum in the United States, 1966–1983. *Sex Trans Dis* 13:18, 1986.
15 Oriel JD: The increase in molluscum contagiosum. *Br Med J* 294:74, 1987.
16 Murray MJ et al: Molluscum contagiosum and herpes simplex in Maasai pastoralists; Refeeding activation of virus infection following famine? *Trans R Soc Trop Med Hyg* 74:371, 1980.
17 Epstein WL et al: Viral antigens in human epidermal tumors: Localization of an antigen to molluscum contagiosum. *J Invest Dermatol* 40:51, 1963.
18 Shirodaria PV, Matthews RS: Observations on the antibody responses in molluscum contagiosum. *Br J Dermatol* 96:29, 1977.
19 Reed RJ, Parkinson RP: The histogenesis of molluscum contagiosum. *Am J Surg Pathol* 1:161, 1977.
20 Epstein WL, Fukuyama K: Maturation of molluscum contagiosum virus (MCV) in vivo: Quantitative electron microscopic autoradiography. *J Invest Dermatol* 60:73, 1973.
21 Francis RD, Bradford HB: Some biological and physical properties of molluscum contagiosum virus propagated in cell culture. *J Virol* 19:382, 1976.
22 Oda H et al: Structural polypeptides of molluscum contagiosum virus: Their variability in various isolates and location within the virion. *J Med Virology* 9:19, 1982.
23 Parr RP et al: Structural characterization of the molluscum contagiosum virus genome. *Virology* 11:247, 1977.
24 Henao M, Freeman RG: Inflammatory molluscum contagiosum. *Arch Dermatol* 90:479, 1964.
25 Kipping HF: Molluscum dermatitis. *Arch Dermatol* 103:106, 1971.
26 Pauly CR et al: Atopic dermatitis, impaired cellular immunity and molluscum contagiosum. *Arch Dermatol* 114:391, 1978.
27 Redfield RR et al: Severe molluscum contagiosum infection in a patient with human T cell lymphotrophic (HTLV-III) disease. *J Am Acad Dermatol* 13:821, 1985.
28 Katzman M et al: Molluscum contagiosum and the acquired immunodeficiency syndrome: Clinical and immunological details of two cases. *Br J Dermatol* 116:131, 1987.
29 Solomon LM, Telner P: Eruptive molluscum contagiosum in atopic dermatitis. *Can Med Assoc J* 95:978, 1966.
30 Hawley TG: The natural history of molluscum contagiosum in Fijiian children. *J Hyg (Camb)* 68:631, 1970.
31 Dennis J et al: Molluscum contagiosum, another sexually transmitted disease: Its impact on the clinical virology laboratory. *J Infect Dis* 151:376, 1985.
32 Schactner L, Hankin D: Reply to, Is genital molluscum contagiosum a cutaneous manifestation of sexual abuse in children? *J Am Acad Dermatol* 14:848, 1986.
33 Ginsburg CM: Management of selected skin and soft tissue infections. *Pediatr Infect Dis* 5:735, 1986.
34 Mayumi M et al: Selective immunoglobulin M deficiency associated with disseminated molluscum contagiosum. *Eur J Pediatr* 145:99, 1986.
35 Gross G: Systemic treatment of mollusca contagiosa with inosiplex. *Acta Derm Venereol (Stockh)* 66:76, 1986.

Chapter 40

# Viral hepatitis

Stanley M. Lemon
John E. Newbold

## HISTORY AND DEFINITIONS

Although viral hepatitis is unquestionably an ancient disease, only in recent years has an appreciation emerged of the diversity of infectious agents capable of causing hepatic inflammation and the clinical syndrome of acute jaundice associated with malaise, nausea, vomiting, and occasionally fever. Over one hundred years ago, the occurrence of hepatitis (probably type B) following vaccination for smallpox with materials containing human lymph clearly demonstrated the infectious nature of this disease, as well as the potential infectivity of human body fluids. Clinical descriptions of what was almost certainly type A hepatitis date from the mid-nineteenth century, although the infectious nature of this syndrome, then termed "catarrhal jaundice," was not clearly recognized until human transmission studies were carried out in the early twentieth century. Extensive epidemics of both "short-incubation, infectious hepatitis" and "long-incubation, homologous serum hepatitis" during the Second World War spurred intensive epidemiologic and clinical investigations which led to the recognition of the two different forms of viral hepatitis now known as types A and B. The distinctions between these entities were confirmed and extended by the landmark studies of Krugman and associates at the Willowbrook Institution during the 1950s and 1960s, studies which included the development of a crude vaccine for type B hepatitis derived by heat treatment of human serum. The era of modern hepatitis virology, however, began with the discovery of Australia antigen (now known to be the envelope antigen of the hepatitis B virus) by Blumberg and associates in 1965, and its subsequent association with hepatitis B. Knowledge in this area has since continued to expand rapidly, and at least five distinctly different human viruses are now recognized as causative agents of acute viral hepatitis (see Table 40-1).

Hepatitis A virus (HAV), hepatitis B virus (HBV), hepatitis delta virus (HDV), and at least two agents of non-A, non-B hepatitis (NANB) (so called because of the absence of associated serologic markers of hepatitis A and B) share a remarkable predilection for involvement of the liver despite profound differences in physical structure, pathobiology, and epidemiology. HAV is an RNA-containing picornavirus, similar in many respects to poliovirus, and known to cause only acute and not chronic hepatic disease. HBV, on the other hand, is a DNA-containing hepadnavirus, associated with both acute and chronic forms of hepatitis as well as hepatocellular carcinoma. HDV is a unique, defective RNA virus that is dependent on coinfection with HBV for replication and expression of disease. Two distinctly different NANB viruses are recognized to cause enterically transmitted disease (NANB-E virus) or posttransfusion hepatitis (NANB-P). Although relatively little is known about the epidemiology and biology of these two viruses, recent advances in the recognition of particles or antigens associated with these infections hold significant promise for improving our understanding of NANB hepatitis in the near future. In addition to these "classical" hepatitis viruses, yellow fever virus may cause extensive hepatic inflammation and remains an important cause of morbidity and mortality in some regions of the world. Lesser degrees of hepatic inflammation often accompany primary infection with cytomegalovirus and Epstein-Barr virus, and other commonplace viruses (herpes simplex, varicella zoster, rubeola, coxsackievirus, and adenovirus) have on occasion caused significant hepatic disease.

It is appropriate to focus attention on the hepatitis viruses in a textbook concerned with sexually transmitted diseases. Sexual activity may profoundly influence the transmission of both HAV and HBV, even though both viruses are also commonly transmitted by other means. Vaccines are available for prevention of hepatitis B (and may soon be available for hepatitis A), providing a unique means of prevention among sexually transmitted diseases. Their use must be considered in populations at risk for STD. The role played by sexual transmission in the spread of HDV and the NANB viruses is much less certain, and requires further investigation.

**Table 40-1. Human Hepatitis Viruses**

| Designation | Virus type | Nucleic acid | Particle size, nm | Known antigens | Modes of transmission* | Acute disease | Chronic disease |
|---|---|---|---|---|---|---|---|
| Hepatitis A virus (HAV) | Picornavirus | ssRNA | 27 | HAV | ET<br>ST<br>PT (rare) | Yes | No |
| Hepatitis B virus (HBV) | Hepadnavirus | dsDNA | 42 | HBsAg<br>HBcAg<br>HBeAg | HT<br>ST<br>PT<br>NT | Yes | Yes |
| Hepatitis delta virus (HDV) | Unclassified | ssRNA | 36 | HBsAg<br>HDAg | PT<br>ST(?) | Yes | Yes |
| Enteric non-A, non-B virus (NANB-E) | Unclassified | ssRNA(?) | 30 | NANB-E | ET | Yes | No |
| Posttransfusion non-A, non-B virus (NANB-P) | Unclassified | ssRNA(?) | 40(?) | NANB-P | PT | Yes | Yes |

*Documented modes of transmission: ET, enterically transmitted; HT, horizontally transmitted (see text); NT, perinatal transmission; PT, parenterally transmitted; ST, sexually transmitted.

# HEPATITIS A

## HEPATITIS A VIRUS (HAV)

**Physical Characteristics and Replication Cycle.** HAV was first visualized by Feinstone and associates[1] in fecal suspensions from human volunteers. It is a small 27-nm, spherical, nonenveloped particle, with a buoyant density in CsCl of 1.33 g/cm$^3$.[2] The RNA genome of HAV has been molecularly cloned and the complete nucleotide sequences of several strains have been determined.[3] Virion RNA is single-stranded and nonsegmented, 7478 bases in length, and organized into a 5′ noncoding region 734 bases long, followed by a single long open reading frame capable of encoding a polyprotein of 2227 amino acids, and a short 3′ noncoding region which terminates in a 3′ polyadenylic acid tract (Fig. 40-1). A small, genome-linked protein (VPg) is covalently attached to the 5′ end of virion RNA.[4] Purified virion RNA may serve as messenger for the synthesis of viral antigens, indicating that the viral genome is positive-stranded, and full-length cloned complementary DNA is also infectious in cell cultures.[5]

Current concepts of the replication of HAV[6] are largely derived from knowledge of the replication of other picornaviruses (such as poliovirus) which closely resemble HAV in particle structure and genomic organization. Virion RNA acts as messenger for synthesis of a large polyprotein which is thought to be cotranslationally processed by virus-specified proteases into both structural and nonstructural proteins. The genomic sequence suggests the presence of four viral capsid proteins, only three of which (VP1, VP2, and VP3, ranging from 222 to 300 amino acid residues in length) have been unequivocally demonstrated in purified virus preparations. Virion RNA also serves as template for negative-strand RNA synthesis. As with other picornaviruses, replication occurs in the cytoplasm of the infected cell and RNA transcription proceeds asymmetrically, with an excess of positive-strand molecules synthesized under direction of a virus-specified RNA polymerase. Although the many similarities evident between HAV and poliovirus have prompted the classification of HAV as enterovirus type 72, HAV shows only very limited identity with other enteroviruses at the nucleotide level, and this classification may be premature. HAV probably would be classified better within a unique genus of picornaviruses.

Alone among the human hepatitis viruses, HAV may be propagated in cell cultures. In most in vitro systems, HAV does not produce a cytopathic effect;[7] there is no shutdown in host cell protein synthesis such as occurs with poliovirus infection. A variety of primate cell lines are permissive for HAV, but primary isolation of wild-type virus is difficult and frequently entails a period of several weeks (or longer) between inoculation of cell cultures and the first detection of viral antigen. Thus, virus isolation is not a viable approach to diagnosis. Furthermore, virus yields from cell culture are relatively low, complicating conventional approaches to vaccine development.[8] Recently, several cell culture-adapted HAV variants have been reported to induce cytopathic effects in vitro.

Only a single antigenic specificity has been associated with HAV, and no significant antigenic differences have been found among strains collected from widely separated geographic regions.[9] Substantial evidence suggests that the critical antigen(s) of HAV are conformationally determined and are thus "assembled" rather than "linear" structures determined solely by the primary amino acid sequences of the capsid protein.[8] Analysis of HAV using neutralizing murine monoclonal antibodies indicates the presence of an immunodominant antigenic site on the virus capsid that is involved in antibody-mediated neutralization. Recent studies have demonstrated that one of the amino acid residues of VP3 contributes to this site.[10] However, the conformational nature of the HAV antigen has thus far prevented development of a vaccine based on expression of recombinant cDNA.

**Pathobiology.** Chimpanzees, several species of marmosets, and New World owl monkeys are susceptible to HAV and may be infected by either oral or parenteral administration of virus.[11] Although disease in these primates is usually mild compared with symptomatic infections in adult humans, the course of the infection is otherwise very similar. Infection of the hepatocyte is central to the pathogenesis of hepatitis A. Studies with animal models have provided conflicting evidence for the replication of virus within the gastrointestinal epithelium,[8] even though relatively large amounts of virus are present in feces from 1 to 4 weeks after exposure[12] (Fig. 40-2). The bulk of fecal virus shedding thus occurs prior to the onset of hepatocellular disease. HAV, presumably replicated within hepatocytes, is found in the bile,[13] and it is thought that this is the source of most virus shed in the feces. Viral antigen is present within the cytoplasm of the hepatocyte, as well as within germinal centers of the spleen and lymph nodes and along the glomerular basement membrane in some primates.[14] There is a viremia which roughly parallels the shedding of virus in the feces, but which is of lower magnitude.[15] At the onset of hepatic inflammation, the titer of infectious virus is greatest in liver, followed by feces, and then serum. Viral antigen may be detected in the feces as late as 2 weeks after the onset of symptoms,[16] but chronic fecal shedding of virus has not been observed. Epidemiologic studies noting the disappearance of HAV from closed populations with the passage of time argue against its existence.[17]

The mechanisms responsible for hepatocellular damage are not known.[8] At present, however, most authorities consider type A hepatitis to be due to an immunopathologic response to infection of the hepatocyte, rather than to a direct cytopathic effect of the virus.

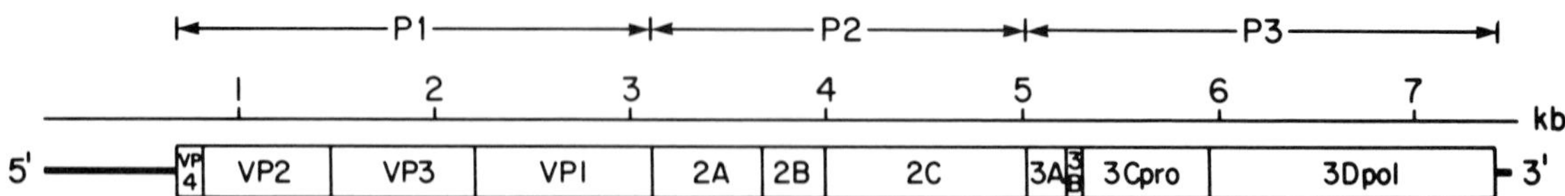


**Fig. 40-1.** Genomic organization of hepatitis A virus. The single-stranded (+)-sense RNA genome has a 5′ untranslated region approximately 750 bases in length, followed by a long open reading frame (boxed region). The open reading frame can be divided into P1 (capsid proteins VP1, VP2, VP3, and possibly VP4), P2 (nonstructural proteins of uncertain function), and P3 [protease (3Cpro), 5′ genome-linked protein VPg (3B), and RNA polymerase (3Dpol)] regions. There is a short 3′ untranslated region, followed by a polyadenylic acid tail. Translation of the RNA is cap-independent and leads to synthesis of a large polyprotein which is cotranslationally processed with some (all?) cleavages mediated by the viral-encoded protease.

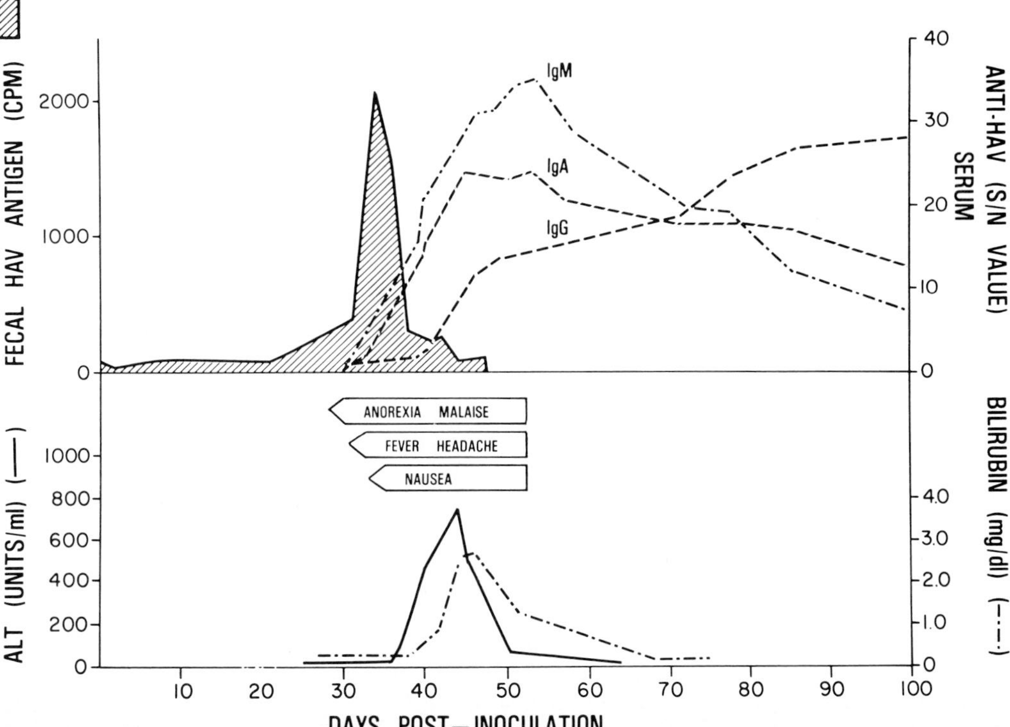


Fig. 40-2. Experimental hepatitis A virus infection in a 21-year-old male volunteer. Fecal HAV and immunoglobulin-specific anti-HAV were measured by solid-phase radioimmunoassay. Feces from days 33 and 35 were shown to contain infectious HAV by passage to primates. (*Reprinted by permission from N Engl J Med.*[8])

**Immunity.** Antibody to the virus (anti-HAV) generally appears in the serum concurrent with the earliest evidence of hepatocellular disease (Fig. 40-2). Early antibody is comprised largely of IgM, although IgG may also be present shortly after the onset of symptoms.[18] Both IgG and IgM antibody have viral neutralizing actvity.[19] IgG anti-HAV persists for life and confers protection against reinfection.[20] Reexposure of seropositive individuals may lead to increases in anti-HAV titer but is not associated with liver disease. Both fecal and serum IgA anti-HAV have been described,[21] but their role in protection against HAV infection is uncertain. Only limited information is available concerning cellular immune mechanisms, although both NK cell and HLA-restricted cytotoxic T-cell activities have been described.[22,23] Along with interferon induction, such cellular effector mechanisms may play a role in clearing virus from the infected liver.

**Transmission.** Spread of HAV between individuals is almost uniformly due to fecal-oral transmission. Virus transmission is facilitated by conditions which favor fecal-oral spread, including sexual practices involving oral-anal contact. Saliva may contain very small amounts of infectious HAV,[24] but it is likely that virus in saliva represents a trivial source for transmission in comparison with the much greater titers of virus present in the feces. The potential for household transmission and even common-source outbreaks is enhanced by the extraordinary physical stability of the virus.[25] Virus is concentrated from contaminated waters by filter-feeding shellfish; hepatitis A may result if such shellfish are ingested uncooked. Although parenteral transmission has occurred with transfused blood, such instances are rare because the viremia is relatively brief in duration.

## EPIDEMIOLOGY

**Population Studies.** Overall, evidence suggests that hepatitis A has become less prevalent in developed nations during the past several decades, possibly as a result of continuing improvements in sanitation.[26] Because of this trend, the percentage of the adult population susceptible to the virus has undoubtedly increased and will probably continue to do so. The prevalence of antibody is currently only 15 to 25 percent in American military populations (S.M. Lemon, unpublished data). In the United States, the prevalence of anti-HAV is clearly related to age as well as socioeconomic factors.[27,28] The age-related nature of antibody prevalence in some Western countries appears to be due largely to a cohort effect created by the decreasing incidence of hepatitis A infection. In some developed countries the median age of infection has been shown to be increasing.[26] Significant international differences exist in the age-related prevalence of anti-HAV, however. In contrast to the United States and northern Europe, infection usually occurs during early childhood in many developing nations,[29] often at an age at which symptoms of hepatitis A are minimal or absent (see below). This situation may be changing, however, as sanitary conditions improve in these countries, leading to increased susceptibility to the virus among young adults. The potential impact of this effect is typified by an epidemic of hepatitis A in Shanghai which reportedly involved over 600,000 persons in early 1988.

**Endemic Hepatitis A.** The vast majority of hepatitis A infections occur sporadically, presumably as a result of person-to-person spread of virus, and in many cases may not be recognized as hepatitis. In a recent study conducted in five "sentinel" counties within the United States, 41 percent of reported cases of sporadic viral hepatitis were due to HAV.[30] In these counties, the annual incidence of HAV ranged from 3.8 (Jefferson County, Alabama) to 32.6 (San Diego County, California) per 100,000 persons.

Preschool day care facilities, especially those enrolling children under the age of 2 years, play a significant role in the spread of HAV. It has been estimated that up to 40 percent of all cases of hepatitis A within one American community were related to either attendance at a day care center or exposure to a child enrolled in such a facility.[31] The majority of infected children under the age of 2 years do not become icteric and are not recognized as having hepatitis. Nevertheless, such children appear to efficiently shed virus, and transmission of virus from them is facilitated by their lack of toilet training. Subsequent infection of older siblings, parents, and baby-sitters (all of whom are more likely to develop classic signs of hepatitis) is therefore common. In recent years, there also has been increasing recognition of hepatitis A among drug addicts.[32] This association probably reflects the general level of hygiene among such persons but may also be due at least in part to occasional needle-borne transmission of virus.

**Sexual Transmission.** Hepatitis A, like other predominantly enteric infections, may be transmitted during sexual activity. However, the importance of sexual transmission of HAV varies widely among different populations. Sexual transmission probably plays a greater role in the spread of HAV in industrialized nations which have good public health sysytems than in developing nations with inadequate sanitary and water systems. Sexual behavior may influence antibody prevalence rates (Table 40-2), but this is not invariably the case. In Halifax, Nova Scotia, anti-HAV was found over three times more frequently among patients from an STD clinic than among normal blood donors, but these populations may not have been socioeconomically comparable.[33] Homosexual STD clinic patients in New York City and Copenhagen did not possess serologic evidence of past infection more often than matched controls.[28,34] Nevertheless, of 102 homosexual males recruited from an STD clinic in Seattle, 30 percent had anti-HAV, compared with only 12 percent of age and socioeconomically matched heterosexual males.[35] The risk of previous infection was related to age, number of sex partners, and duration of homosexuality. Furthermore, an annual infection rate of 22 percent was observed when seronegative homosexual men were followed prospectively. Men reporting frequent oral-anal exposure were found to be at significantly increased risk of becoming infected with HAV. In retrospect, it is apparent that an epidemic of hepatitis A had probably occurred within this group of homosexual men during the study period. In general, these men had been homosexual for many years (mean = 12.4 years for those without anti-HAV), and if the annual risk of acquiring hepatitis A were constant at 22 percent, the expected antibody prevalence would have been far greater than the observed 30 percent. An epidemic of hepatitis A has been described among male homosexuals in Copenhagen,[36] suggesting that similar hepatitis A outbreaks may not be uncommon among urban homosexual males. In addition, many acute HAV infections were noted among male homosexual participants in a hepatitis B vaccine trial in New York City.[37] One in five men were anti-HAV-positive at the start of this study, and an annual attack rate of about 4.5 percent was noted during the 2 years of follow-up. These cases were evenly distributed among the population at risk and did not appear to occur in identifiable groups or clusters.

A survey of Danish men who were reactive in various serologic tests for syphilis revealed a higher anti-HAV prevalence among homosexuals (36 percent) than among heterosexuals (20 percent).[38] Moreover, the prevalence of anti-HAV correlated with the number of episodes of syphilis in younger homosexual males. Yet another study involving STD patients suggests that the presence of anti-HAV may be related to the number of lifetime sexual partners.[39] Within the United States, the Sentinel County study of viral hepatitis carried out by the Centers for Disease Control beginning in 1979 demonstrated a marked male predominance among cases of hepatitis A (65 percent).[30] Furthermore, 15 percent of hepatitis A cases occurred in persons who reported a homosexual preference. All of these data suggest that HAV may be commonly transmitted among male homosexuals.

Despite these studies, hepatitis A differs from most other sexually transmitted pathogens, including other predominantly enteric organisms such as shigella, in at least two important ways. First, infection with the virus produces solid immunity so that symptomatic reinfection occurs infrequently if ever.[8,20] Second, the infected individual is infectious for a relatively brief period of time. There is no prolonged carrier state. Thus, to maintain sexual transmission of HAV within a population, several host conditions appear to be required. These include: (1) a high degree of susceptibility among the population at risk, as defined by negative tests for anti-HAV, (2) sexual promiscuity, so that multiple partners may be exposed during the relatively brief period when virus is shed, and (3) sexual practices facilitating fecal-oral spread of virus. The outbreaks of hepatitis A observed among homosexual men in Seattle and Copenhagen included all these elements, and further suggest that the introduction of virus into the sexually active population is an additional requirement.[35,36]

**Common Source Outbreaks.** Although common source outbreaks due to food or water contaminated with hepatitis A virus may be highly dramatic and involve large numbers of patients, such outbreaks account for only a small proportion of all hepatitis A infections. Infection of a food handler is commonly incriminated in such outbreaks.

**Table 40-2. Prevalence of Anti-HAV in Patients Attending STD Clinics**

| Sexual preference / sex | Location | % with anti-HAV | Reference |
|---|---|---|---|
| Heterosexual / males | Halifax, NS | 39 | 33 |
| Heterosexual / females | Halifax, NS | 39 | 33 |
| Heterosexual / males | Seattle | 12 | 35 |
| Heterosexual / both | Copenhagen | 16 | 34 |
| Heterosexual / males | Denmark | 20 | 38 |
| Homosexual / males* | New York City | 23 | 37 |
| Homosexual / males | Halifax, NS | 42 | 33 |
| Homosexual / males | Seattle | 30 | 35 |
| Homosexual / males | Copenhagen | 28 | 34 |
| Homosexual / males | Denmark | 36 | 38 |

*HBV vaccine study participants.

## CLINICAL MANIFESTATIONS OF HEPATITIS A

In the individual patient, acute illness due to hepatitis A virus is indistinguishable from that due to hepatitis B or non-A, non-B viruses.[8] The incubation period of hepatitis A is relatively short, averaging about 4 weeks (Fig. 40-2). Under the age of 3 years, less than 1 in 10 infected children develop symptoms of hepatitis, whereas most infected adults are symptomatic.[40] Symptoms are often abrupt in appearance, although there may be a prodromal period of low-grade fever, malaise, headaches, and myalgias. Anorexia, nausea, and vomiting occur early in the illness, and diarrhea is not uncommon, especially among children.[8] The specific diagnosis of viral hepatitis, however, is often not suggested until the occurrence of dark urine or jaundice. Serum aminotransferase elevations are similar in magnitude to those seen in acute hepatitis B, although they generally do not persist as long. Most infected individuals will have normal aminotransferase levels by 6 weeks after the onset of symptoms, although 10 to 20 percent of cases may have minor enzyme abnormalities persisting for up to 3 months.[41] Chronic hepatitis has yet to be documented following hepatitis A. Although jaundice may occasionally be prolonged for several weeks or more ("cholestatic hepatitis"), it is not indicative of severe hepatocellular disease and uniformly resolves with time. In recent years, attention has focused on occasional cases of "relapsing hepatitis A" with symptomatic and chemical evidence of recurrent hepatitis in the year following acute type A hepatitis. The pathobiology of this condition is uncertain, but it always resolves without progression to chronic hepatitis. Hepatitis A accounts for less than 10 percent of all cases of fulminant hepatitis,[42] and the mortality in acute symptomatic hepatitis A is probably less than 0.1 to 0.2 percent.

## DIAGNOSIS OF HAV INFECTION

Diagnosis of hepatitis A rests entirely on serologic methods. Although anti-HAV may be detected by a variety of techniques, antibody is usually measured by solid-phase radioimmunoassay or enzyme-linked immunosorbent assay. Absence of anti-HAV is strong evidence against current infection with HAV. However, the detection of anti-HAV in a patient with hepatitis does not prove that infection is recent or responsible for current symptoms. A specific serodiagnosis requires the demonstration of IgM anti-HAV, which is present in virtually all patients with acute hepatitis A and may be detected by sensitive antibody-capture immunoassays for as long as 6 months after the onset of symptoms.[8]

## PREVENTION OF HEPATITIS A

**Passive Immunization.** Immune globulin (IG), if administered within 2 weeks of exposure, is 80 to 90 percent effective in protecting against illness associated with HAV infection.[43] Infection is also probably prevented if IG is given soon enough after exposure. Postexposure prophylaxis (0.02 ml/kg intramuscularly) is recommended for all household and sexual contacts of patients with hepatitis A, as well as for individuals with exposure to day care centers or other institutional facilities within which significant transmission of HAV has been documented.[44] Postexposure prophylaxis is generally not recommended in the setting of a common source outbreak, because such outbreaks are usually recognized only well into their course when IG may no longer be effective in prevention of disease. However, it is difficult to exclude the possibility of a beneficial effect in individual cases.[40] Preexposure IG prophylaxis (0.06 ml/kg body weight every 5 months) has been recommended for travelers to endemic areas in developing countries, especially when such travel is off the major tourist routes and into the local economy.[44] Lesser doses of IG provide protection for shorter time periods. Adverse reactions to IG are minimal and are generally limited to local and allergic manifestations which occur in about 1 percent of all recipients. There is good evidence that immune globulin distributed commercially within the United States is not capable of transmitting the human immunodeficiency virus (HIV) or other bloodborne agents such as HBV.

**Active Immunization.** Phase 1 clinical trials have been conducted with both formalin-inactivated, whole virus vaccines and candidate live, attenuated virus vaccines. Formalin-inactivated virus vaccines are very immunogenic and have been shown to be effective in preventing disease following live-virus challenge of primates.[45] Although the costs of producing such a vaccine for general use may prove to be prohibitive because of the relatively low yield of virus in cell culture, it is probable that such vaccines will become available for limited clinical use within the next several years. With respect to attenuated vaccines, HAV variants which have been serially passed in cell culture have been shown to be attenuated for man and capable of eliciting neutralizing, presumably protective, antibodies.[46] Such vaccines offer potential economic and biologic advantages over inactivated vaccines,[8] but a good balance between attenuation and immunogenicity has not yet been reached. In addition, significant questions remain to be answered regarding the genetic stability of attenuated virus and the risk posed by fecal shedding of such virus variants. Although the genomes of several HAV strains have been molecularly cloned and virion capsid proteins have been expressed from cDNA, efforts to develop a recombinant, subunit vaccine have thus far been stymied by the conformational nature of the critical HAV antigens.

## HEPATITIS B

## HEPATITIS B VIRUS (HBV)

**Physical and Chemical Characteristics.** HBV is a hepadnavirus and thus one of a family of related DNA viruses infecting the livers of a variety of avian and mammalian species. The HBV virion (also known as the Dane particle) is a complex, double-shelled 42-nm spherical particle with an outer surface envelope surrounding a core structure containing a small DNA genome. This genome is unique among human viruses in that it is a circular DNA molecule which is double-stranded for 50 to 85 percent of its length, with a total genome length equivalent to double-stranded DNA of approximately 3200 base pairs.[47] The genomes of several HBV strains have been molecularly cloned and fully sequenced. The partially double-stranded DNA consists of a long strand which is (−)-sense (i.e., antimessenger sense) and a shorter (+)-sense strand which overlap at their 5′ ends (see Fig. 40-3).[48] Within the (+)-strand, there are four overlapping, open reading frames utilizing all three translation frames (i.e., encoding different amino acids from the same nucleotide sequences). Given the small size of the genome, this parsimonious use of the genomic

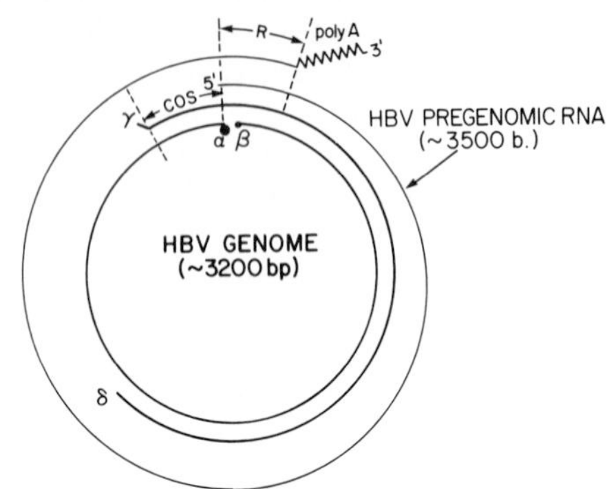


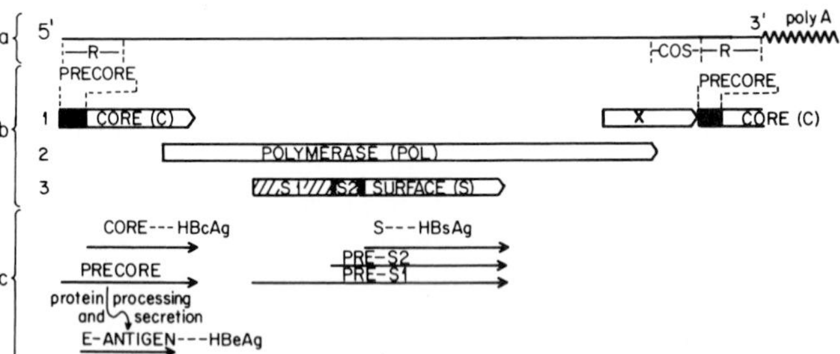


**Fig. 40-3.** Organization of the hepatitis B virus genome. Panel A depicts the relationship between the Dane particle DNA and the RNA pregenome. α and β identify the unique 5′ and 3′ ends of the long or (−)-sense DNA strand. γ is the unique 5′ end, while δ represents the variable 3′ end of the short or (+)-sense strand. The 5′ and 3′ ends of the pregenomic RNA are marked. The region "R" represents a terminally redundant sequence that is present in the RNA pregenome. It is approximately 10 percent of the genome size; thus the pregenomic RNA is 1.1 genome equivalents. The cohesive overlap region between the 5′ ends of the (+) and (−)-sense DNA strands is designated "cos." Panel B depicts the relationship between the pregenome RNA (a), the open reading frames encoded therein (b), and presently characterized protein products (c). Three distinct translation frames are present (marked 1, 2, and 3). The nature of the products of the *pol* and "X" genes remains uncertain.

DNA provides for a relatively large amount of genetic information. There are no regions of the DNA that are nontranslated. The four open reading frames are thought to encode a viral DNA polymerase, two core proteins (core and precore), a family of three surface envelope proteins (see below), and the "X" protein. There is tentative evidence that the latter protein may be a trans-activator of HBV gene expression, and thus possibly analogous to the *tat* gene of HIV (see Chap. 28). Studies carried out in recent years indicate that the DNA genome of HBV replicates via reverse transcription of an intermediate RNA molecule (the "pregenome").[49] The replication cycle of HBV thus resembles in gross detail that of the RNA-containing retroviruses, including HIV. Indeed the genomic organizations of these viruses bear some superficial similarities (Fig. 40-3).

In addition to the genomic DNA, the HBV core contains a DNA polymerase which is thought to have reverse transcriptase activity, and possibly a protein kinase as well.[50] DNA polymerase present within the HBV core is active in situ in the presence of appropriate deoxynucleoside triphosphates, using as a template the single-stranded portion of the circular genome.[51] This endogenous polymerase reaction is the basis of an assay for detection and quantitation of virus particles which has been used for research purposes. The major core protein is a 21-kilodalton molecule with specific antigenic activity (hepatitis B core antigen, or HBcAg). HBcAg is released from the intact virion by detergent treatment which removes the surface envelope and leaves an intact 27-nm core particle. More vigorous disruption of the virus core results in the release of an antigenically distinct, soluble viral antigen (HBeAg).[52] Although antigenically distinct and used for a number of years as a serum marker for HBV infectivity, it has been recognized only recently that the HBeAg molecule is closely related to HBcAg, being derived by protease processing and secretion from the precore molecule (see Fig. 40-3).[53] The DNA sequences unique to the precore region specify a signal peptide which directs the precore protein into a secretory pathway; in this process both the amino terminal signal peptide and a carboxy terminal peptide are cleaved from the precore protein to generate HBeAg.

The surface envelope surrounding the virus core is a complex structure containing as its major antigen a 24-kilodalton glycoprotein (hepatitis B surface antigen, or HBsAg, also called the S protein, and previously known as "hepatitis-associated antigen" or "Australia antigen"). An antigenic determinant common to all strains of hepatitis B ("a") is associated with HBsAg. In addition, two pairs of mutually exclusive allelic antigens ("y" and "d", "w" and "r") have been defined.[54] Of the four possible major subtype combinations, only three ("ayw," "adw," and "adr") have been found with any degree of frequency, and these occur in distinct, but possibly changing, geographic and demographic distributions. Also present in the Dane particle envelope are two related proteins, pre-S1 (42 kilodaltons) and pre-S2 (36 kilodaltons). The pre-S1, pre-S2, and S molecules all share the 226 amino acids of the S protein at their carboxy terminus: they are coterminal translation products of the open reading frame encoding the S-protein, but represent products of translation from different AUG initiation codons and are derived from distinct mRNAs[48] (Fig. 40-3). The roles of pre-S1 and pre-S2 in the biology of HBV remain controversial, although pre-S2 has been proposed to contain the virion receptor binding site. The inclusion of these antigens in future vaccines may result in improved immunogenicity (see below). HBsAg is usually produced in excess by infected hepatocytes and, in most carriers of HBV, incomplete 22-nm spherical or tubular HBsAg particles greatly outnumber intact Dane particles in the blood. These particles, as well as the surface envelope of the Dane particle, also contain host cell derived materials, including human albumin.

**Replication Cycle of HBV.** Attempts to propagate the virus in conventional cell cultures have not been successful, although several continuous cell lines have been derived from human hepatoma tissue which contain integrated HBV DNA and continuously synthesize HBsAg in vitro. More recently, transfection of human hepatoma-derived cells with tandem copies of cloned HBV genomic DNA has led to the selection of cell lines with stably integrated viral DNA which produce Dane particles detectable by electron microscopy and which are infectious for chimpanzees.[55,56]

Early studies with the duck hepadnavirus (duck hepatitis B virus, or DHBV) and subsequent work with HBV led to the novel conclusion that replication of this DNA virus proceeds via an RNA genomic intermediate.[49] This conclusion was based on the identification of immature intracellular core particles containing full-length RNA genomic intermediates and reverse transcriptase activity, and the observation that synthesis of (−)-strand viral DNA is not inhibited by actinomycin-D (which typically blocks DNA-directed but not RNA-directed DNA synthesis). Current

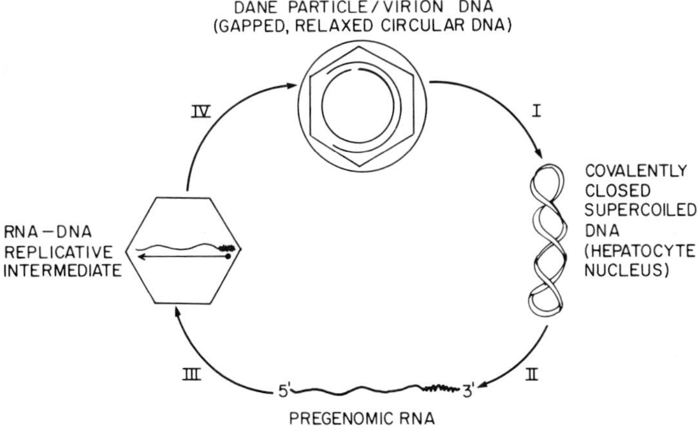


**Fig. 40-4.** Replication cycle of hepatitis B virus. (*Adapted from D Ganem and H Varmus.*[48])

concepts concerning the replication of HBV may be summarized briefly as follows (Fig. 40-4). After attachment and penetration of the hepatocyte, synthesis of the incomplete (+)-strand of the gapped virion DNA is accomplished, presumably under direction of the viral DNA polymerase, and upon ligation by cellular enzyme(s) forms a fully double-stranded circular DNA molecule (covalently closed circular DNA). This supercoiled episomal DNA does not replicate by a DNA-dependent DNA synthesis mechanism and serves only a transcriptional role;[57] nonetheless, its amplification and persistence in the cell is central to the replication cycle of the virus. The covalently closed circular DNA serves in the nucleus as template for subgenomic (+)-strand RNA transcripts for the envelope proteins (S, pre-S1, and pre-S2) as well as a somewhat greater than full-length (+)-sense RNA genomic intermediate (the viral "pregenome"). There is only a single polyadenylic acid addition site located within the core gene, and all the messengers therefore are 3′ coterminal; no splicing of RNA transcripts has yet been detected. Subgenomic messengers have not been identified for the core protein, the "X" protein, or the DNA polymerase, which are currently presumed to be derived from pregenomic RNA acting as messenger. The pregenomic RNA serves a dual role, however, as it is also encapsulated within immature cytoplasmic core particles along with the DNA polymerase (reverse transcriptase). Within the immature core particle, the long (−)-sense DNA strand is synthesized by reverse transcription from pregenomic RNA, probably with concomitant degradation of the RNA. Subsequently, (+)-sense DNA is replicated from the full-length (−)-strand, but this process is prematurely interrupted by the completion of viral assembly and release of virus from the cell. The result is a partially double-stranded DNA molecule encapsulated within the Dane particle.

The mechanism by which the cellular pool of supercoiled HBV DNA is expanded is uncertain. It has been suggested that amplification might be the result of intracellular nuclear reinfection with immature Dane particles;[57] alternatively, it might result from exogenous reinfection of the hepatocyte by additional virions. During viral replication, double-stranded HBV DNA may be integrated at a low frequency into host chromosomal DNA. Unlike conventional retroviruses, however, this process is not obligatory for viral replication. Furthermore, integration appears to be a random event.

Several features of the replication cycle require further investigation. However, the involvement of a unique reverse transcriptase in a complex replication cycle suggests that effective antiviral drugs may eventually be developed.

**Pathobiology.** Following exposure, virus presumably gains access to the liver via the bloodstream. HBsAg is found within the cytoplasm of hepatocytes, whereas HBcAg is usually restricted to the hepatocyte nucleus.[58] There is evidence that HBV may also replicate within certain mononuclear cells of the bone marrow or blood,[59] but the liver is the primary site of HBV replication. This tropism may result in part from the involvement of tissue-specific virus enhancer regions and promoters regulating HBV gene expression, the presence of virus-specific receptors on only certain cell types, or both. There is no evidence for replication of the virus at mucosal surfaces.

The majority of infections are self-limited[60] (Fig. 40-5). HBsAg may appear in the blood as early as 6 days after parenteral exposure, although this interval is usually from 1 to 2 months after mucosal exposures.[61] Shortly afterward, circulating Dane

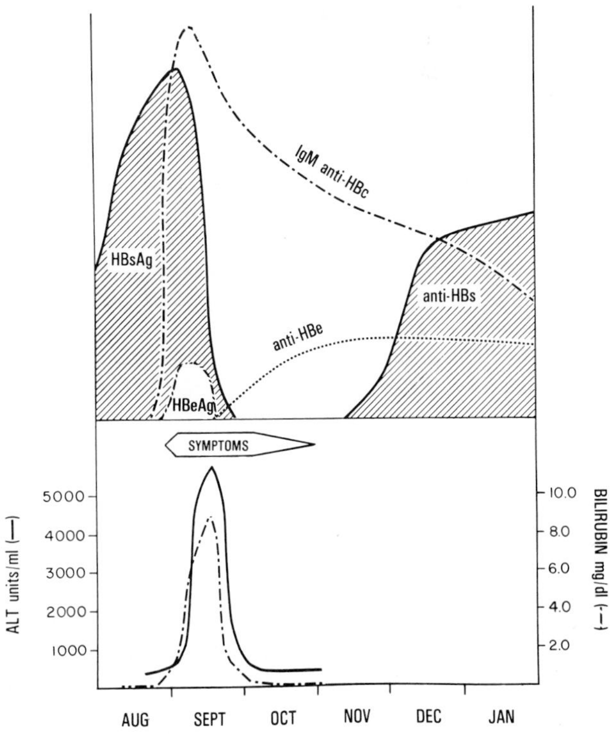


**Fig. 40-5.** Acute, self-limited hepatitis B infection occurring in a 49-year-old laboratory technician. HBV-related antigens and antibodies were measured by solid-phase immunoassays.

particles, HBeAg, and DNA polymerase may be detected. This stage of detectable viremia is often brief. HBsAg synthesis is more abundant and typically more persistent, however, and it may be detected for up to 5 months or in some cases even longer.[60,61] The first humoral immune response to the virus, consisting of IgM antibody to HBcAg (IgM anti-HBc), develops shortly after the appearance of HBsAg.[60,62] Following the disappearance of circulating DNA polymerase and HBeAg, antibody to HBeAg (anti-HBe) may also be detected. Over 95 percent of infected normal adults will eventually clear HBsAg from the circulation, and most, but not all, of these individuals develop antibody to HBsAg (anti-HBs). There may, however, be a delay of weeks to months prior to the first appearance of anti-HBs, even after the disappearance of HBsAg. During this so-called window period, anti-HBc and anti-HBe are the only serum markers of HBV infection. Symptoms of hepatitis usually develop after HBsAg has been circulating in the blood for 3 to 6 weeks,[60] and usually occur while HBsAg is still present (approximately 90 percent of patients). Symptoms may develop during the "window period," however, or even after the appearance of anti-HBs.[60,62] The appearance of anti-HBs signals the resolution of the infection. This antibody is protective against reinfection[37] and represents responses against the S, pre-S1, and pre-S2 proteins. Anti-HBc and anti-HBs usually persist for years following infection.

A small proportion (probably <5 percent) of infected adults are not able to clear HBsAg from their blood and become chronic HBsAg carriers (Fig. 40-6). Such individuals frequently have little or no evidence of acute liver disease when initially infected. Development of the chronic carrier state is more frequently seen in individuals who are immunocompromised (e.g., previous HIV infection). Almost all infants who are infected neonatally become carriers. HBsAg may persist in the blood of these individuals for years in large and relatively constant amounts, and may be associated with the presence of either HBeAg or anti-HBe. Carriers with HBeAg usually have circulating Dane particles and detectable DNA polymerase activity;[63] such carriers should be considered to be especially infectious.[64,65] Chronic HBsAg carriers typically have very high titers of anti-HBc and usually do not have anti-HBs. Atypical individuals, however, may have both HBsAg as well as anti-HBs directed against a different HBsAg subtype. While most persistent HBsAg carriers are asymptomatic and do not have evidence of significant liver disease, a minority have elevated serum aminotransferases and the histologic picture of chronic active hepatitis. This lesion may in some cases progress to cirrhosis and death. The delta virus (HDV) plays an important role in promoting severe liver disease associated with HBV infection (see below). The presence of HBeAg correlates with significant liver disease, and seroconversion from HBeAg to anti-HBe in carriers with chronic hepatitis is frequently followed by resolution of liver function abnormalities.[66] The carrier state itself may spontaneously resolve in some cases.

The mechanism responsible for hepatocellular damage in either acute or chronic HBV infection is not known. Because immunosuppressed patients are less likely to develop overt signs of hepatitis and because replication of large quantities of virus occurs in many totally healthy carriers, it seems likely that the host immune response is intimately involved in the expression of liver disease. Cytotoxic effector cells capable of killing HBsAg-bearing target cells have been found by some but not all investigators. Of perhaps greater importance are reports of virus-specific, histocompatibility-restricted, cytotoxic T cells with activity directed against HBcAg-bearing hepatocytes.[67]

There is a strong association between persistent HBV infection and primary carcinoma of the liver.[68] Infection with HBV usually precedes the development of hepatocellular carcinoma by years, although the tumor occasionally develops during childhood. Cell lines initiated from hepatoma tissues synthesize 22-nm HBsAg particles and contain integrated HBV DNA. HBV DNA has also been detected directly within tumor tissue.[69] Nevertheless, it remains uncertain whether HBV by itself is directly oncogenic, or only one of several important factors involved in tumorigenesis. The related woodchuck hepadnavirus (WHV), however, is capable of inducing hepatocellular carcinoma in experimental infections under controlled conditions. The association of HBV with hepatocellular carcinoma is found worldwide, but hepatocellular carcinoma is a significant problem mainly in those countries where the HBsAg carrier rate is high and neonatal transmission of virus frequent.

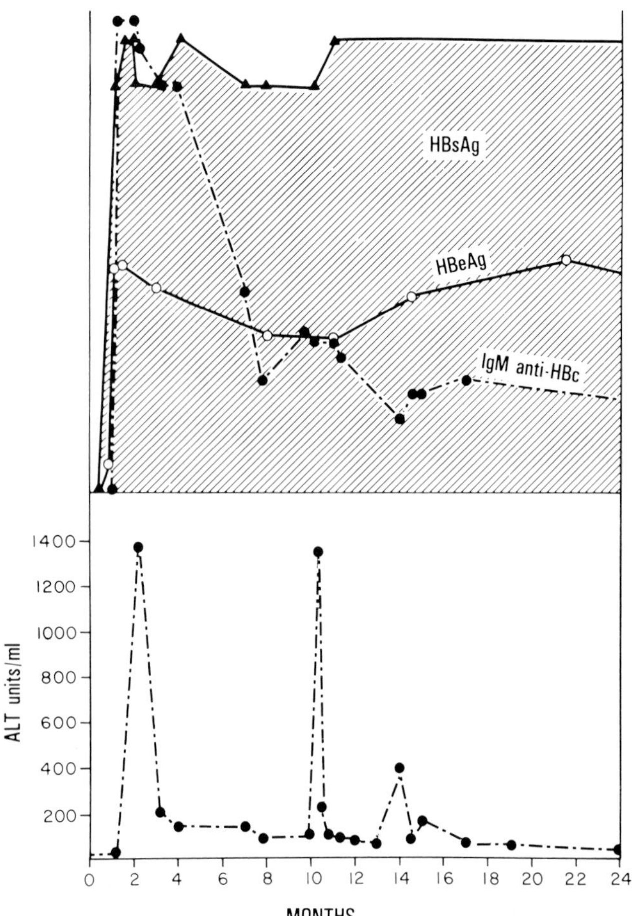


**Fig. 40-6.** Acute hepatitis B infection progressing to the chronic HBsAg carrier state and chronic active hepatitis. HBsAg was measured by reverse passive hemagglutination, other HBV markers by solid-phase radioimmunoassay. (*Sera and HBsAg results courtesy of S Krugman.*)

**Immunity.** Infection with HBV is marked by the development of antibody directed against each of the individual viral antigens: anti-HBs, anti-HBc, and anti-HBe (Fig. 40-5). Of these, the antibody most clearly associated with a protective effect against reinfection is anti-HBs.[37,60] This protection extends to all HBV subtypes. Anti-HBc at best plays an uncertain role in protection. While the presence of anti-HBe in the blood of a HBsAg carrier suggests a relative lack of infectivity, there is no evidence that anti-HBe by itself has any protective effect. The role cell-mediated immunity plays in protection against reinfection is not known.

**Transmission.** The transmission of HBV may be categorized into four general modes: parenteral, sexual, perinatal, and "horizontal" (defined as occurring in the absence of recognized parenteral, sexual, or perinatal exposure). Blood is obviously a major source of virus for transmission, as it may contain very high titers of virus. Transfusion has, however, become an infrequent cause of hepatitis B since the introduction of sensitive methods for detecting HBsAg in donor units.[70] While parenterally acquired HBV remains common among drug addicts and needle-stick accidents are a source of infection for health care workers, HBV is much more commonly transmitted by nonparenteral means. HBsAg has been found in the saliva, vaginal secretions, and semen of infected individuals,[71–73] and the presence of Dane particles has been confirmed in saliva by electron microscopy.[74] Of greater relevance, HBV DNA may be detected by molecular hybridization in both saliva and semen of some HBeAg-positive carriers.[75,76] Quantitative Southern blot analysis has shown that the quantity of virus in saliva and semen is usually one thousandfold less than that present simultaneously in the blood but still may be as high as $10^6$ viral particles per milliliter.[75] Most of the virus appears to be extracellular, but there may also be cell-associated virus in these secretions. The presence of virus in saliva and semen presumably reflects leakage from the circulation, and not the replication of virus at oropharyngeal or genital sites. Carriers with very high serum titers of virus (determined by hybridization) are more likely to have virus detectable in these secretions. There may also be a positive correlation with the serum HBeAg titer.[75] Although studies directly examining the infectivity of various body fluids are limited, it is probably correct to state that any body fluid or secretion may be infectious.

Transmission of HBV to members of the families of HBsAg carriers is well documented, and multiple epidemiologic surveys suggest that "horizontal" transmission to young children is probably the most common means of transmission of this virus worldwide. The exact mechanism by which this occurs is not known, however. It is uncertain whether virus is commonly transmitted by oral exposure to infected secretions such as saliva. Early experiments demonstrated that HBV-containing serum was infectious when given orally to susceptible individuals,[77] but the virus inoculum used in these studies included large amounts of exogenous protein which may have protected the virus from inactivation by mucosal enzymes, gastric acid, or bile. More recent attempts to transmit HBV to susceptible nonhuman primates by oral administration of infectious saliva were unsuccessful, even though the saliva transmitted infection when administered parenterally.[78] Such evidence suggests that the oropharynx is a relatively hostile portal of entry for HBV but is compatible with reports that bites by infected individuals may transmit infection. It is probable that most "horizontal" transmission within families and among young children is due to inapparent parenteral exposures to saliva or blood. Such exposures may be relatively infrequent but are apt to occur over an extended period of household (or perhaps classroom) contact with a persistently infected virus carrier.

Numerous studies indicate that both heterosexual and homosexual intercourse may be associated with transmission of HBV. The evidence for sexual transmission among male homosexuals is overwhelming and points to participation in rectal intercourse and exposure to large numbers of sexual partners as primary risk factors.[79,80] In addition to epidemiologic evidence supporting heterosexual spread of HBV, human semen has been shown to transmit infection when instilled into the vagina of susceptible gibbons.[78]

HBV is commonly transmitted from HBsAg carrier mothers to their infants.[65,81] As infected infants usually become chronic carriers, perinatal transmission of virus is largely responsible for maintenance of the carrier pool in areas of high HBV endemicity such as Taiwan. Perinatal transmission is also frequent following acute maternal HBV infection in the third trimester. The presence of maternal HBeAg is associated with an increased risk of transmission of virus to the newborn.[65,81] While intrauterine infection has been noted, most infections probably occur at the time of birth or shortly thereafter. Transmission may be due to direct contamination of the infant's circulation with maternal blood at the time of delivery. The presence of HBsAg and anti-HBc in cord blood does not necessarily indicate that infection has occurred, however, as both may disappear with time. Cord blood IgM anti-HBc is not helpful in identifying infection in newborns. If the infant has no evidence of infection by the fourth month of life, he or she has a high probability of remaining free of infection subsequently. While HBsAg may be found in breast milk, there is no epidemiologic evidence to incriminate breast-feeding as a major factor in transmission of the virus.

## EPIDEMIOLOGY

**Population Studies.** Dramatic differences exist between various regions of the world in terms of the prevalence of HBV.[65,82] In regions of Southeast Asia and Africa, >90 percent of the population may have serologic evidence of past or current HBV infection, and 10 to 20 percent of adults may be HBsAg-positive. In contrast, among a total of 2163 New York City volunteer blood donors, only 7.2 percent had past exposure to HBV, and only 0.4 percent were HBsAg-positive.[82] Striking differences in HBsAg carrier rates have also been noted between ethnically disparate groups living within the same geographic area.[83] Within the United States, the seroprevalence generally increases with age and lower socioeconomic status, and is higher among blacks and persons of oriental ancestry.[79,82] In addition, health care workers are at increased risk of HBV infection, largely acquired through inapparent means but correlating with exposure to blood.[84]

**Sexually Transmitted HBV.** Sexual transmission of HBV was first suggested by the occurrence of acute hepatitis B among sexual contacts of HBsAg carriers.[85] An increased prevalence of HBsAg and anti-HBs has since been noted among prostitutes and individuals attending venereal disease clinics, but such studies are difficult to control for possibly important socioeconomic variables.[34,79,86] Overall, however, the most striking serologic evidence relating HBV transmission to sexual practices has been found among male homosexuals (Table 40-3).

Of over 600 male homosexuals in New York City, solicited for study through recognized homosexual organizations and health clinics in the mid-1970s, 4.6 percent were found to be HBsAg carriers and 51.1 percent were found to have had past infection to the virus as evidenced by HBsAg or anti-HBs positivity.[79] These men were predominantly Caucasian, under 40 years of age, and highly educated. Female homosexuals did not seem to be at increased risk as only 6.3 percent had anti-HBs and none were carriers. Of the males studied, 23 percent gave a past history of viral hepatitis, and in these individuals the total seroprevalence rate was 65 percent. There was a high degree of correlation between promiscuity and serologic evidence of past HBV infection. Of those with less than 10 sex partners during the previous 6 months, only 30.9 percent had been infected with

Table 40-3. Serum HBV Markers in Male Homosexuals

| | All individuals, % | | | HBsAg-positive only, % | | |
|---|---|---|---|---|---|---|
| Location | HBsAg | Anti-HBs | Anti-HBc* | HBeAg | Anti-HBe | Reference |
| New York City | 5.2 | 54 | 10 | 61 | 28 | 87,96 |
| USA (multicenter) | 6.1 | 52 | 3 | 65 | 16 | 80 |
| London | 5.2 | 38 | Not done | Not done | Not done | 142 |
| Denmark† | 5.6 | 61 | Not done | Not done | Not done | 38 |

*Percentage shown is for those with only anti-HBc.
†All men had positive syphilis serologies.

HBV, compared with 60.5 percent of those with more than 10 sex partners. The highest rates for HBsAg (7.5 percent) were found among men reporting predominant or exclusive involvement in rectal intercourse, while those reporting oral-genital sex had significantly lower rates for both HBsAg (2.3 percent), and anti-HBs (39 vs. 51 percent). The duration of homosexuality was also related to past HBV infection, and was more important than age at the time of screening. Illicit drug use did not appear to be an important variable. A similarly high overall prevalence of HBV markers has been documented among male homosexuals in several additional studies (Table 40-3).[34,80,87–89] Based on previous estimates that approximately 4 percent of North American white males are exclusively homosexual, Dietzman et al.[88] estimated that approximately 27 percent of adult males with serologic evidence of HBV infection acquired it through a homosexual exposure. This figure may well be an underestimate, especially when applied to certain urban populations. In this regard it is interesting that there is an excess of unmarried, usually never married, males among HBsAg-positive volunteer blood donors.[82]

There appear to be several reasons why male homosexuals have been at such dramatically increased risk of acquiring hepatitis B infection. One of the most important factors is the number of sexual partners. The typical homosexual male frequenting Denver's steam baths in the late 1970s had eight different male sexual contacts per month.[90] These contacts were largely anonymous. Such an individual may have had contact with over 1000 different sexual partners during his homosexual lifetime. In addition, the high HBsAg carrier rate found among homosexual males resulted in frequent sexual exposure to HBsAg-positive partners. Schreeder et al.[80] estimated that the average openly homosexual male had 4.2 sexual contacts with HBsAg-positive men annually. However, these studies were conducted in the years immediately preceding the recognition of the acquired immunodeficiency syndrome, and the subsequent adoption of safe sex practices by many homosexual men appears to have altered the epidemiology of HBV in this high-risk group. Although the overall incidence of hepatitis B increased within the United States from 1982 to 1987, the proportion of hepatitis B cases associated with homosexual activity fell from 20 to 9 percent in four sentinel counties studied by the Centers for Disease Control.[91] In contrast, the proportion attributed to heterosexual contact (i.e., sexual contact with a patient with hepatitis, an HBV carrier, or with multiple partners) increased from 15 to 22 percent during this same period.

In general, female homosexuals are less promiscuous than male homosexuals. Szmuness et al.[79] found the mean number of sex partners for male homosexuals over a 6-month interval was 20, compared with 1.6 for female homosexuals. This may in part explain their lesser risk of HBV infection. Another factor may be that males may be more likely to become chronic virus carriers than females following acute HBV infection.

Involvement in either receptive or insertive anal intercourse is a second important factor influencing the risk of acquisition of HBV among homosexually active males.[79,80] Nonspecific proctitis is not uncommon among homosexual men practicing anal intercourse, and breakdown of normal mucosal barriers may facilitate transmission of virus. In one study, over a quarter of homosexual men had experienced rectal bleeding during a 4-month period of time, and this was found to be related both to the number of sex partners as well as to involvement in receptive anal intercourse.[80] In this same study, insertive oral-anal contact was also associated with HBV infection, although the reason for this association was less certain. Of note, oral-genital or oral-oral contact between homosexual men had little apparent influence on the risk of becoming infected with HBV. In another survey, approximately one-fifth of male homosexuals reported rectal bleeding after intercourse and 9 to 16 percent had fissures, cracks, or tears in the rectum or anal skin over a 12-month period.[92] In yet another study, 13 of 22 homosexual, HBsAg-positive men were found to have rectal mucosal lesions, usually consisting of multiple, punctate bleeding points within 6 cm of the anal verge.[93] HBsAg was identified in swab specimens from such lesions, as well as in swabs taken from apparently normal rectal mucosa and anal sphincters. HBsAg was identified in feces from these homosexual men, a finding which may in part explain the risk of infection associated with insertive oral-anal contact.

Another important factor is that HBsAg-positive male homosexuals are very likely to be HBeAg-positive, possibly reflecting their relatively recent acquisition of HBV as adults (Table 40-3). HBeAg is associated with an increased risk of transmission of virus following heterosexual[94] and needle-stick[64] exposures as well as with an increased risk of perinatal transmission,[72] and its presence implies a high risk of infectivity for homosexual men. The titer of HBeAg may correlate with the amount of virus present in semen and saliva.[75] Approximately 65 percent of HBsAg-positive homosexual men are positive for HBeAg while anti-HBe may be detected in 25 percent.[95–97] In contrast, only about 10 percent of asymptomatic HBsAg-positive blood donors are HBeAg-positive.

Many homosexual men who are HBsAg-positive have at least chemical evidence of chronic liver disease. In New York City, 62 percent of male homosexual carriers had total serum alanine aminotransferase levels of greater than 40 Karmen units, and 48 percent had levels greater than 60 Karmen units.[79] These rates are roughly twice those seen in other groups of asymptomatic carriers. Looked at in another way, Hentzer et al.[34] found elevated serum alanine aminotransferase levels in 9 out of 95 asymptomatic homosexual males. Eight of these individuals were HBsAg-positive. The histologic lesion responsible for these changes is uncertain, as is its implication for the long-term health of these carriers. The risk of eventual development of primary liver carcinoma among HBsAg-positive homosexuals is not well established but may be appreciable. However, hepatocellular carcinoma has not emerged as a major problem in homosexual men with the acquired immunodeficiency syndrome, and thus this risk does not appear to be substantially increased by immunosuppression due to HIV infection.

There is considerable evidence to support the transmission of hepatitis B by heterosexual contact as well. Sexual partners of HBsAg-positive carriers frequently have serologic evidence of HBV infection.[85,94,98] In one study, either HBsAg or anti-HBs was found in 27 percent of spouses of HBsAg carriers, but in only 11 percent of spouses of noncarrier controls.[79] However, nonsexual family contacts of HBsAg carriers also frequently have serologic evidence of past HBV infection. On the other hand, sexual partners of individuals with acute hepatitis B are clearly at increased risk of acquiring infection when compared with other members of the household. Mosley[99] reported that 18 percent of susceptible cohabiting spouses eventually became infected with HBV whereas other family members generally did not. Similarly, Koff et al.[100] found intrafamilial spread of HBV to be confined to susceptible sexual partners in this setting. The risk of heterosexual transmission appears to be higher when the HBsAg-positive partner has detectable serum HBV DNA.[101] This is not surprising, since the amount of virus in saliva and semen is related to the magnitude of the viremia.[75] While virus may actually be transmitted by vaginal intercourse among cohabiting sexual partners, it is also possible that it may be transmitted by inapparent parenteral exposures resulting from the sharing of razors, toothbrushes, or other personal articles.[99] As described above, transmission of virus through exchange of saliva plays an uncertain role.

The prevalence of hepatitis B virus infection among white heterosexuals attending a clinic for sexually transmitted diseases in Arizona, who were without other risk factors such as intravenous drug abuse, has been shown to be related to numbers of previous sex partners.[102] Serum markers of HBV infection were present in 21 percent of those with five or more sex partners during the preceding 4 months, but in only 6 percent of those with fewer than five partners. A similar correlation existed for total numbers of lifetime sex partners, among both male and female clinic patients. In addition, a similar survey of heterosexual college students without other risk factors for HBV acquisition also demonstrated a positive correlation between numbers of previous sex partners and risk of HBV infection.[102] At present, it is estimated that approximately one in five reported cases of acute hepatitis B in the United States may have been contracted through heterosexual exposure.[91]

**Hepatitis in Military Populations.** The reported rates for hepatitis B in American soldiers have been considerably higher than those for comparable civilian populations, although it must be realized that most civilian cases go unreported. Hepatitis B has been responsible for the majority of cases of acute viral hepatitis occurring among U.S. soldiers, both at home and abroad. In a study conducted during 1978–1979, 69 percent of hepatitis cases occurring among American troops in Europe were due to HBV, as were 74 percent of hepatitis cases among American troops stationed in Korea.[103] The relative importance of parenteral and nonparenteral transmission of virus among soldiers is not known. Both circumstantial and direct evidence, however, suggests a major role for sexually acquired hepatitis B, especially among soldiers assigned overseas to areas where local populations have high HBsAg carrier rates.[103,104]

## CLINICAL MANIFESTATIONS OF HBV INFECTION

Many adults infected with HBV probably have silent infections which result in permanent and solid immunity. Only one-third of seropositive male homosexuals relate a past history of viral hepatitis.[79] However, in a placebo-controlled trial of an HBV vaccine conducted among homosexual men in New York City, 64 percent of infections in placebo recipients were associated with clinical evidence of disease.[37] Compared with hepatitis A, however, acute hepatitis B is a more serious disease. The onset of illness is generally more insidious than that due to HAV, and evidence of hepatocellular disease resolves more slowly. The incubation period is usually from 40 to 110 days but may be shorter with large-inoculum parenteral exposures and may be prolonged by administration of globulin preparations.[61] A small proportion (1 percent or less) of icteric adults develop acute hepatic failure, and about three out of four of these unfortunate patients will die as a result of their infection. Hepatitis B virus is present in about one-half of all patients with fulminant hepatitis, although infection with HDV may be responsible for disease in many of these patients (see below). As a rule, elderly patients tolerate acute hepatitis more poorly than younger individuals.

Approximately 15 to 20 percent of patients develop a transient serum sickness–like illness during the prodromal or early acute stage of hepatitis B.[105] This syndrome is characterized by an erythematous macular or maculopapular, occasionally urticarial skin rash, polyarthralgias, and frequently frank arthritis. The arthritis may be migratory, is frequently symmetrical, and may involve both large joints of the extremities as well as the proximal interphalangeal joints of the hands. Synovial fluid findings are variable, but leukocyte counts as high as 90,000 per cubic millimeter (often with a predominance of neutrophils) have been reported. Serum aminotransferases are usually elevated and may be the best clue to the proper diagnosis.

A striking feature of hepatitis B is the development of persistent infection. Out of 429 hospitalized patients with acute icteric hepatitis B, 43 became persistent carriers of HBsAg in one study.[106] The overall frequency with which acute infection in normal adults leads to the chronic carrier state is probably much lower, however, as these hospitalized patients represented a selected population. A long-term follow-up study of American soldiers infected with HBV present in contaminated yellow fever vaccine administered during 1941–1942 failed to show a detectable number of HBsAg carriers.[107] Up to a third of chronic HBsAg carriers develop histologic evidence of chronic active hepatitis, while the remainder may have only a benign form of liver disease characterized by minimal inflammatory changes on liver biopsy.[106] While chronic active hepatitis may progress to cirrhosis and death, it more frequently remits spontaneously even in moderately advanced cases.[108] Although most persistent HBV infections are well tolerated by the host, a wide variety of immunopathological conditions are associated with persistent circulating HBsAg, including generalized necrotizing vasculitis (polyarteritis nodosa), chronic membranous and membranoproliferative glomerulonephritis, essential mixed cryoglobulinemia, and perhaps polymyalgia rheumatica.

## DIAGNOSIS OF HBV INFECTION

Approximately 90 percent of patients with acute hepatitis B have HBsAg detectable in their serum when they first present for medical care.[60,62] This antigen may be detected by any of a variety of sensitive assay methods, including radioimmunoassay, enzyme-linked immunosorbent assay, and reverse passive hemagglutination. Approximately 10 percent of patients with acute HBV infection are HBsAg-negative, however, and these cases are more difficult to document. In such patients, anti-HBc is uniformly present while anti-HBs may be found in some. Anti-HBs and anti-HBc generally are detected by solid-phase immunoassay and both persist for many years after acute infection; their presence is not diagnostic of acute hepatitis B. Specific tests for IgM anti-HBc, however, have proved very useful in the diagnosis of acute infection.[62] IgM anti-HBc may be detected by antibody-capture immunoassay in almost all cases of acute hepatitis B, and persists after acute infection for 6 to 24 months. While many chronic HBsAg carriers have persistent IgM anti-HBc, the titer is usually substantially lower than that found in acute infection and it is usually not detected in commercial assays (thus preserving IgM anti-HBc as a specific marker for acute infection). The IgM antibody is often 7S rather than 19S IgM in chronic carriers.[109]

A useful approach capable of detecting the greatest possible number of hepatitis B infections is to test first for anti-HBc (Table 40-4). If absent, HBV infection is effectively ruled out. If anti-HBc is present, tests for HBsAg and IgM anti-HBc will establish whether or not the infection is active and recent. If HBsAg is not detectable, testing for anti-HBs will determine the immune status. Although in practice these tests are often carried out concurrently as part of a "hepatitis panel," such a staged approach to testing makes biologic sense and ultimately may prove more economical. The presence of HBeAg in an HBsAg-positive individual should suggest a high degree of infectivity,[64,65] and conversion of HBeAg to anti-HBe in a patient with chronic hepatitis B may signal a resolution of hepatocellular disease, and in some cases even herald an end to the HBsAg carrier state.[66] Overall, however, the clinical value of HBeAg/anti-HBe testing is questionable.

**Table 40-4. Serologic Diagnosis of Hepatitis Virus Infections**

*Step 1 (patient has acute hepatitis):*

| | | IgM anti-HAV Positive | IgM anti-HAV Negative |
|---|---|---|---|
| Anti-HBc | Positive | Acute hepatitis A ? hepatitis B, obtain HBsAg and IgM anti-HBc (step 2) | ? hepatitis B, obtain HBsAg and IgM anti-HBc (step 2) |
| | Negative | Acute hepatitis A | Non-A, non-B, rule out EBV and CMV |

*Step 2 (anti-HBc is positive):*

| | | IgM anti-HBc Positive | IgM anti-HBc Negative |
|---|---|---|---|
| HBsAg | Positive | Acute hepatitis B, follow HBsAg to rule out development of carrier state | HBV carrier; get anti-HD to exclude delta superinfection |
| | Negative | Acute hepatitis B, obtain anti-HBs to confirm resolution of infection | Previous HBV; probable acute non-A, non-B; rule out EBV and CMV |

IgM anti-HAV: IgM-specific antibody to HAV
Anti-HBc: Antibody to HBV core antigen
IgM anti-HBc: IgM-specific antibody to HBV core antigen
HBsAg: HBV surface (envelope) antigen
Anti-HBs: Antibody to HBV surface antigen (immunity)
Anti-HD: Antibody to hepatitis delta antigen
Anti-HAV: Antibody to HAV (useful to determine immunity)

## PREVENTION

**Active Immunization: Preexposure Prophylaxis.** The plasma-derived vaccine licensed within the United States (Heptavax-B, Merck, Sharp & Dohme) contains 22-nm HBsAg particles which have been extensively purified, with any residual infectivity destroyed by formalin treatment.[110,111] There is no evidence that this vaccine harbors any adventitous viral agents, including HIV.[111,112] Its safety and efficacy were conclusively demonstrated in two large, placebo-controlled, randomized, double-blind trials carried out among homosexual males in the United States.[37,92,113] Subjects in these studies received three doses (either 40 or 20 μg each) intramuscularly in the deltoid region at 0, 1, and 6 months. The most common side effect was soreness at the injection site, which occurred after approximately 16 percent of all vaccine administrations. In the New York trial,[37,92] 77 percent of recipients were anti-HBs-positive 1 month after the second injection (which was given 4 weeks after the first), and over 95 percent of vaccine recipients possessed anti-HBs after the third dose. Administration of the third injection resulted in higher titers of anti-HBs in those individuals who were already anti-HBs-positive, and presumably extended the period until booster doses might be necessary. Immunity appears to last 5 years or longer.[114]

In the New York study, the incidence of acute hepatitis B was reduced by 92.1 percent in vaccine recipients compared with placebo recipients over a 2-year follow-up period, and the incidence of all HBsAg-positive infections was reduced 88.9 percent.[92] Protection was highly correlated with the development of detectable anti-HBs. Over half of the identifiable HBV events occurring in the immunized population consisted of seroconversion to anti-HBc, in the absence of either detectable HBsAg or chemical evidence of liver damage. In contrast, such events accounted for only a quarter of HBV infections among placebo recipients. Protection against hepatitis B was evident within a few weeks of the first administration of the vaccine, despite the fact that the typical incubation period is 6 to 8 weeks for this disease. This suggests that postexposure administration of the vaccine may be at least partially effective. Other studies indicate that concurrent administration of up to 3 ml of hyperimmune globulin (see below) and vaccine (at separate body sites) does not significantly lessen the antibody response to the vaccine and results in both an immediate and prolonged anti-HBs response.[115] The vaccine must not be frozen prior to administration (this reduces immunogenicity) and should not be administered by buttocks injection.[111,116] For optimal immunogenicity, the vaccine must be deposited in the deltoid muscle. HIV infection is known to blunt the immune response to this vaccine.[117]

Although over 4,400,000 doses of this vaccine were distributed between 1982 and 1987 in the United States, its overall impact on hepatitis B rates has been negligible. Over the period from 1981 to 1985, the incidence of hepatitis B actually increased from 9.2 to 11.5 per 100,000 in the U.S. population.[111] Several factors are responsible for this lack of impact on disease incidence, including the cost of the vaccine (still approximately $100 for a three-dose immunization series) and a lack of programs targeting this vaccine to truly high-risk groups (intravenous drug users, homosexual men, and promiscuous heterosexuals).

In 1986, a recombinant vaccine for hepatitis B (Recombivax HB, Merck, Sharp & Dohme) was licensed for use within the United States. This product contains highly purified HBsAg expressed from a yeast vector containing recombinant HBV DNA.[118] The recombinant HBsAg is nonglycosylated, but the vaccine is similar in most other respects to the plasma-derived vaccine, including cost. The recombinant vaccine is formulated at 10 μg per dose rather than the 20 μg per dose used for plasma-derived vaccine, and it might therefore be somewhat less immunogenic.[111] There are no recognized differences in the safety of these two vaccines. The plasma-derived and recombinant vaccines do not contain appreciable quantities of pre-S1 and pre-S2 proteins. Experimental recombinant vaccines containing these additional proteins are under evaluation and may ultimately prove to have superior immunogenicity. Hopefully, as additional vaccines join the marketplace, the cost of hepatitis B immunization will come down.

Preexposure vaccination should be the mainstay of any program to prevent hepatitis B. Vaccine is recommended for sexual and household contacts of hepatitis B carriers as well as homosexually active males, health care workers with exposure to blood, clients and staffs of institutions for the developmentally disabled, hemodialysis patients, users of illicit injectable drugs, and recipients of some blood products (Table 40-5).[111] Vaccine should also be considered for heterosexually active persons with multiple partners (including prostitutes), inmates of correctional facilities, and some travelers to HBV endemic regions.

Either vaccine should be given as three 1-ml intramuscular injections in the deltoid region, at months 0, 1, and 6. Hemodialysis patients should receive twice the normal dose of plasma-derived vaccine (40-μg doses) because the antibody response is frequently poor in such patients. It might be reasonable to extend this recommendation to persons known to be HIV-infected as well.[117] Whether or not vaccine recipients should first be screened for HBV serologic markers is a decision which should be based on the cost of testing, the cost of vaccine, and the probability of prior HBV infection. The presence of any HBV marker would obviate the need for the vaccine. In general, it makes sense to screen homosexual males and other very high-risk individuals prior to immunization, both to learn their HBV status (many will be HBsAg carriers, see Table 40-3) and because many will not require the vaccine. There is, however, no harm done to the HBsAg-positive patient by inadvertent administration of the vaccine. Generally, postimmunization anti-HBs testing is not recommended, but this may be useful for individuals at especially high risk of exposure, or who are at risk of not responding well to the vaccine (i.e., immunocompromised persons, persons with preexisting HIV infection, and older men). In some individuals

**Table 40-5. Persons for Whom Hepatitis B Vaccination Is Recommended or Should Be Considered[44,111]**

Preexposure
- Persons for whom vaccine is recommended:
  - Health care workers having blood or needle-stick exposures
  - Clients and staff of institutions for the developmentally disabled
  - Hemodialysis patients
  - Homosexually active men
  - Users of illicit injectable drugs
  - Recipients of certain blood products
  - Household members and sexual contacts of HBV carriers
  - Special high-risk populations
- Persons for whom vaccine should be considered:
  - Inmates of long-term correctional facilities
  - Heterosexually active persons with multiple sexual partners
  - International travelers to HBV endemic areas

Postexposure
- Infants born to HBV-positive mothers
- Health care workers having needle-stick exposures to human blood

failing to mount a detectable anti-HBs response after three doses of vaccine, a fourth dose may result in seroconversion. There are no recommendations for routine booster immunizations at present.[117]

Over the next several decades, the impact of HBV immunization will be most dramatic in its prevention of perinatal infection in regions where HBV infection is highly endemic and contributes significantly to morbidity and mortality due to cirrhosis and hepatoma. Immunization of the newborn is essentially postexposure prophylaxis and is enhanced by the simultaneous administration of both hyperimmune globulin and vaccine. This topic is addressed in the next section.

**Passive Immunoprophylaxis: Postexposure Prophylaxis.** Passive immunization with globulin preparations, unlike vaccine, provides immediate but only temporary protection, and its use should be reserved for postexposure prophylaxis. There is little doubt that hepatitis B immune globulin (HBIG) is effective in preventing hepatitis B when given following percutaneous or mucosal exposure to HBV, while the efficacy of regular IG is less certain.[43,119] Relatively little information is available which directly addresses the efficacy of globulin preparations in preventing sexual transmission of HBV, however. One study has compared the efficacy of HBIG (anti-HBs 1:200,000) and IG (an older preparation, devoid of anti-HBs) in preventing hepatitis B infection among spouses of patients with icteric acute hepatitis B.[120] During the 6 months following administration of the globulin, only 1 of 25 spouses receiving HBIG but 9 of 33 spouses receiving IG developed acute symptomatic hepatitis B. Furthermore, asymptomatic seroconversion to anti-HBs was noted in 22 percent of IG recipients, but only 4 percent of HBIG recipients.

Current recommendations call for postexposure prophylaxis following significant percutaneous or mucosal exposure to blood or other body fluids with a high probability of containing HBV.[44] HBIG (0.06 ml/kg) is preferred over IG (0.06 ml/kg) and must be given as soon as possible after exposure (preferably within 24 to 48 h). A second dose is recommended 1 month after the first unless concomitant immunization with hepatitis B vaccine is begun. HBIG and vaccine may be given concurrently, but at different sites.[115] The decision to proceed with active immunization depends on the likelihood of continuing exposure to HBV-containing material.

Similar measures are recommended for sexual contacts of patients who are HBsAg-positive.[44] Exposures to acute hepatitis B and chronic hepatitis B infections are managed somewhat differently, however. For heterosexual partners of patients with acute hepatitis B, a single dose of HBIG is recommended, with a second dose given if there is continuing sexual exposure and the index patient remains HBsAg-positive. It is wise to test contacts for HBsAg, anti-HBs, and anti-HBc before administering HBIG, as the presence of any of these markers would obviate the need for prophylaxis.[120] Once a need for prophylaxis is established clinically, however, administration of HBIG should not be delayed more than 48 h by any testing. Prophylaxis of nonsexual household contacts of patients with acute hepatitis B is not warranted unless there is overt exposure to blood. Heterosexual partners of chronic HBsAg carriers should be given vaccine in addition to a single dose of HBIG. The first dose of vaccine should be given concurrent with the HBIG, but at a second site. Homosexual men or promiscuous heterosexuals with multiple sex partners who present with a history of hepatitis B exposure should be similarly managed. Concurrent administration of vaccine is justified in these cases by the likelihood of continued exposure to the virus.

Simultaneous administration of vaccine and HBIG to neonates born to HBsAg-positive mothers is highly effective in preventing perinatally transmitted HBV infection.[121] HBIG (0.5 ml IM) should be given to such infants within 12 h of birth, with concomitant initiation of a three-dose (10-μg) vaccine series at an alternate site.[44] It is now recommended that all pregnant women be screened in advance for HBsAg, as strategies restricting screening to high-risk groups have been shown to miss a large proportion of carrier mothers.[122] Prophylaxis of the newborn is an especially important aspect of the control of HBV infections, as prevention of perinatal transmission is likely to prevent development of a lifelong carrier state. Widespread prophylaxis of the newborn should lead to a dramatic reduction of the adult HBV carrier pool in subsequent generations.

## TREATMENT

There are few reliable data which suggest that any antiviral agent is effective in the treatment of acute hepatitis B. However, human interferon has shown promise in the treatment of chronic hepatitis due to HBV, particularly when combined with pulse/withdrawal courses of corticosteroids.[123] Some antivirals (e.g., adenine arabinoside or even acyclovir) may interfere with hepadnavirus replication, but there are no good data suggesting that such therapies lead to clinical benefits. Corticosteroids alone may be detrimental, in both severe acute hepatitis B and also HBsAg-positive chronic active hepatitis.[108,124]

## HEPATITIS DELTA VIRUS (HDV)

Understanding of this unique pathogen and its substantial contribution to HBV-associated liver disease has emerged rapidly over the past few years. Because it is a defective virus, the replication of HDV is absolutely dependent upon simultaneous HBV infection for essential helper functions. Thus HDV infects only patients with active HBV infection. The HDV virion is a 35-nm particle found in the blood.[125,126] It has an outer envelope consisting of HBsAg and an amorphous core containing delta antigen (HDAg) complexed with a small, circular, single-stranded RNA molecule 1689 bases in length.[127] This genomic RNA has a very high G + C content and extensive intramolecular complementarity resulting in its assuming a rodlike, predominantly double-stranded secondary structure. Both genomic- and antigenomic-sense RNA is present in the liver of infected individuals. Replication of the viral RNA is thought to occur by a "rolling circle" mechanism, with the RNA molecule capable of autocatalytic cleavage. The delta antigen is a highly basic phosphoprotein with RNA-binding capabilities.[128] It is encoded by one of three open reading frames in the antigenomic-sense RNA, making HDV a negative-stranded RNA virus. It is not known whether other open reading frames in the antigenomic- and genomic-sense RNA are expressed. Although HBsAg, encoded by the HBV genome, is an integral part of the HDV virion, it seems unlikely that HBV provides additional helper functions facilitating HDV replication.

HDV infection may occur as a "coinfection" with acute hepatitis B in an individual who was previously susceptible to HBV, or as a "superinfection" in an HBV carrier.[129] Either type of infection may result in severe hepatitis with fulminant disease and death. Coinfections are often marked by a biphasic serum aminotransferase response, while superinfections may be associated with transient (at times permanent) suppression of HBV replication markers. Those who survive acute coinfections usually go on to complete recovery and do not seem to be at an increased risk of becoming chronic HBV carriers. On the other hand, HBV carriers surviving HDV superinfections frequently become carriers of HDV as well, and often subsequently show evidence of significant chronic liver disease.[129]

The diagnosis of HDV infection is generally dependent upon demonstration of antibody to HDAg (anti-HD) as this is the only widely available test. However, the anti-HD response in coinfections is often transient and of low magnitude, and thus probably frequently missed. In superinfections, anti-HD typically rises to and persists at high levels, signifying persistent HDV infection. Another marker of use in detection of both acute and chronic HDV infection is IgM anti-HD, but this test is not generally available to clinicians. Detection of HDV RNA in serum, either by hybridization using RNA probes[130] or by enzymatic amplification of cDNA (viz., polymerase chain reaction) reverse transcribed from virion RNA (P. Becherer and S. M. Lemon, unpublished data), shows promise and this approach may ultimately prove to be the diagnostic method of choice. One of the most useful means of distinguishing acute HDV/HBV coinfections from HDV superinfection of a chronic HBsAg carrier is by measurement of IgM anti-HBc (Table 40-4). Indeed, persons presenting with what appears to be acute type B hepatitis who lack this serum marker should be suspected of having HDV superinfection.

HDV is found in the blood of anti-HD positive HBsAg carriers, and the prevalence of anti-HD among American carriers is strongly associated with parenteral drug abuse, hemophilia, or a history of multiple transfusions.[131] Geographic differences in the distribution of HDV are striking, however, and anti-HD is significantly more prevalent among HBsAg carriers from Middle Eastern and Mediterranean countries. In South America, outbreaks of fulminant delta hepatitis with high mortality rates have been reported among native Americans, possibly representing widespread superinfection of HBsAg carriers.

It is not clear whether HDV is sexually transmitted, but this is likely to be the case. Homosexually active males who are HBsAg-positive generally have a low prevalence of anti-HD compared with other carrier groups.[131,132] Accordingly, compared with drug addicts, a smaller percentage of homosexual men presenting with acute HBsAg-positive hepatitis in Los Angeles have anti-HD.[129] These men also have a lower overall mortality than drug addicts, reflecting their lower frequency of HDV infection. Nonetheless, HDV coinfection has been found in 14 percent of homosexually active men from Los Angeles presenting with acute HBsAg-positive hepatitis,[129] and delta hepatitis occurs in such men in the absence of a history of transfusions or parenteral drug abuse. A recent survey found anti-HD antibodies in 9 to 15 percent of HBsAg-positive homosexual men living in Los Angeles and San Francisco, but only 0 to 1 percent of HBsAg-positive homosexual men in Chicago and Pittsburgh.[132] In the West Coast groups, the presence of anti-HD was correlated with sexual activity as measured by numbers of previous sex partners, as well as intravenous drug abuse. Because of the severity of liver disease accompanying acute and chronic HDV infections and the large existing pool of anti-HD-negative, HBsAg-positive homosexual men, the potential for sexual transmission of HDV is a concern worthy of continuing attention.

Although there is no specific means for prevention of HDV infection (particularly in the person who is already HBsAg-positive), immunization with hepatitis B vaccine provides protection against HDV by preventing the necessary helper virus infection.

## POSTTRANSFUSION NON-A, NON-B HEPATITIS (NANB-P)

Very little is known about the nature of the infectious agents responsible for NANB-P hepatitis, despite intensive research efforts. Chimpanzees are susceptible to NANB infection and will develop evidence of hepatocellular injury 2 to 13 weeks after the inoculation of infectious serum,[133,134] but multiple reports of antigen/antibody systems or virus particles associated with NANB infection have not gained general acceptance. As this book goes to press, however, there are reports in the press (not yet formal publications) describing the molecular cloning of a (+)-sense viral RNA genome (~10 kb) and the expression of an antigen reactive with antisera from many patients with NANB-P hepatitis.[135] If true, this development represents a breakthrough in what has been a very difficult biologic problem and should herald the acquisition of significant new information about this important disease.

The frequency with which NANB-P infection occurs in the absence of liver disease is of course not known. The incubation period of posttransfusion NANB hepatitis ranges from 2 to 15 weeks with a mean of about 7 weeks.[136] Recognized cases of posttransfusion hepatitis are usually milder than hepatitis associated with HAV or HBV, and most cases are anicteric. Viremia may be present as early as 12 days prior to the onset of acute hepatitis, may persist for years, and has been documented by chimpanzee challenge even in the absence of abnormal serum aminotransferases. The most striking feature of NANB infection to emerge thus far, however, is a strong association of these agents with chronic liver disease. Chronic active hepatitis develops in as many as 30 percent of posttransfusion NANB infections.[137,138] Patients with this form of chronic active hepatitis appear to follow a relatively benign course, with most cases entering spontaneous biochemical remissions. However, cirrhosis may develop more frequently than previously thought.

The epidemiology of NANB hepatitis is that of a blood-borne virus and is in many respects probably very similar to that of HBV. Currently, NANB hepatitis is responsible for over 80 percent of cases of posttransfusion hepatitis. NANB hepatitis also frequently occurs in the absence of transfusion, however, accounting for approximately 25 percent of sporadic cases of acute viral hepatitis in this country.[30] Fewer than one in five sporadic NANB cases appear to be related to illicit self-injection. Little is known about specific mechanisms of nonparenteral transmission of these agents, including the possibility of sexual transmission. An attack rate of 1.13 to 2.8 percent was observed among homosexual men during the 15-month course of the hepatitis B vaccine trial, roughly one-fifth to one-tenth the rate of hepatitis B observed among placebo recipients in the trial.[37] In the Sentinel County study carried out by the Centers for Disease Control,[30] homosexual preference was an acknowledged risk factor in only 4 percent of NANB cases, compared with 12 percent of HBV cases and 15 percent of HAV cases. Unlike hepatitis A and B, cases of NANB hepatitis did not show male predominance and were equally distributed among males and females. In another study, only one in nine asymptomatic homosexual men with elevated aminotransferase levels lacked evidence of HBV infection, suggesting that NANB agents are a relatively minor cause of chronic liver disease in these men.[34]

The diagnosis of NANB hepatitis requires the exclusion of infection with HAV, HBV, cytomegalovirus, and Epstein-Barr virus. Because of its potential for sexual transmission, infection with cytomegalovirus particularly should be considered in cases of mild hepatitis occurring in homosexual men (see Chap. 36). Although not every study has shown a beneficial effect, IG (10 ml) may be effective in the prevention of at least icteric posttransfusion hepatitis following multiple transfusions.

## ENTERICALLY TRANSMITTED NON-A, NON-B HEPATITIS (NANB-E)

In the late 1970s, several large, apparently water-borne outbreaks of hepatitis occurred in India.[139] These epidemics were shown to be due to neither HAV nor HBV, indicating the existence of a form of NANB hepatitis capable of water-borne transmission. In the past several years, studies have associated this infection with a 30-nm virus particle found in the feces of infected individuals,[140] leading to use of the term "enterically transmitted non-A, non-B hepatitis" or NANB-E. Assays for antibody have been developed, but these are technically very difficult and not yet widely applied. In its clinical characteristics, the disease appears to resemble hepatitis A, but it has been associated with a strikingly high incidence of death in infected pregnant women.[139] The epidemiology is poorly understood, but outbreaks have been recently identified in Mexico, suggesting that the virus may have a worldwide distribution, particularly in developing and semiequatorial regions. There is no information concerning the possibility that this virus might be sexually transmitted.

## MANAGEMENT OF ACUTE VIRAL HEPATITIS

Most patients with acute hepatitis follow an uneventful course leading to complete recovery. Restrictions on diet and activity are not required beyond that which patients desire for their own comfort. Hospitalization is best avoided because of the risk of nosocomial spread but should be considered for patients over 40 years old, with underlying disease, or with severe illness (bilirubin greater than 15 mg/dl or significant prolongation of the prothrombin time). Containment within the hospital should be directed at feces in patients with hepatitis A, and at prevention of blood exposures in other types of hepatitis.[141] No specific therapy is clearly beneficial, and the primary purpose of hospitalization is to ensure adequate supportive care and monitoring. Corticosteroids should not be used.[124] Hospitalized patients should be watched closely for early signs of hepatic failure. If encephalopathy develops, aggressive medical management should include reduction in dietary protein, cleansing of the bowel, oral nonabsorbable antibiotics, discontinuation of all sedative-hypnotics, and correction of coagulation deficiencies with fresh frozen plasma. Mortality remains high despite the best medical care.

A careful attempt at virus-specific diagnosis should be made using available serologic techniques (Table 40-4). It is advisable to test sexual partners of patients with acute HBV infection for HBsAg, anti-HBs, and anti-HBc. Prior infection will be frequently documented, and this may reduce the anxieties of both the patient and the partner. Specific recommendations for prophylaxis have been reviewed above. Loss of sexual desire frequently accompanies acute viral hepatitis, and sexual abstinence may be practical while patients are ill. Although intercourse is best avoided while the patient is HBsAg- (and especially HBeAg-) positive, such a recommendation should only be made in acute and not chronic infections and should be modified as circumstances require. The use of condoms may reduce the risk of sexual transmission of

HBV and provide protection in addition to that afforded by HBIG and immunization, but the efficacy of condoms in this setting has not been studied.

## References


1 Feinstone SM et al: Hepatitis A: detection by immune electron microscopy of a viruslike antigen associated with acute illness. *Science* 182: 1028, 1973.
2 Lemon SM et al: Infectious hepatitis A virus particles produced in cell culture consist of three distinct types with different buoyant densities in CsCl. *J Virol* 54: 78, 1985.
3 Cohen JI et al: Complete nucleotide sequence of wild-type hepatitis A virus: Comparison with different strains of hepatitis A virus and other picornaviruses. *J Virol* 61: 50, 1987.
4 Weitz M et al: Detection of a genome-linked protein (VPg) of hepatitis A virus and its comparison with other picornaviral VPgs. *J Virol* 60: 124, 1986.
5 Cohen JI et al: Hepatitis A virus cDNA and its RNA transcripts are infectious in cell culture. *J Virol* 61: 3035, 1987.
6 Ticehurst JR et al: Replication of hepatitis A virus: New ideas from studies with cloned cDNA, in *Molecular Aspects of Picornaviral Infection and Detection,* B Semler, E Ehrenfeld (eds). Washington, ASM Press, 1988, in press.
7 Provost PJ, Hilleman MR: Propagation of human hepatitis A virus in cell culture in vitro. *Proc Soc Exp Biol Med* 160: 213, 1979.
8 Lemon SM: Type A viral hepatitis: New developments in an old disease. *N Engl J Med* 313: 1059, 1985.
9 Lemon SM, Binn LN: Antigenic relatedness of two strains of hepatitis A virus determined by cross-neutralization. *Infect Immun* 42: 418, 1983.
10 Lemon SM, Ping L-H: Antigenic structure of hepatitis A virus, in *Molecular Aspects of Picornavirus Infection and Detection,* B Semler, E Ehrenfeld (eds). Washington, ASM Press, 1988. in press.
11 Lemon SM: Animal models in hepatitis research, in *Clinical Hepatology,* G Csomos, H Thaler (eds). Berlin, Springer-Verlag, 1983, p 244.
12 Dienstag JL et al. Faecal shedding of hepatitis A antigen. *Lancet* i: 765, 1975.
13 Schulman AN et al: Hepatitis A antigen particles in liver, bile, and stool of chimpanzees. *J Infect Dis* 134: 80, 1976.
14 Mathiesen LR et al: Localization of hepatitis A antigen in marmoset organs during acute infection with hepatitis A virus. *J Infect Dis* 138: 369, 1978.
15 Lemon SM et al: Cell-culture adapted variant of hepatitis A virus selected for resistance to neutralizing monoclonal antibody retains virulence in owl monkeys, in *Viral Hepatitis and Liver Disease,* AJ Zuckerman (ed). New York, Alan R Liss, 1988, p 70.
16 Coulepis AG et al: Detection of hepatitis A virus in the feces of patients with naturally acquired infections. *J Infect Dis* 141: 151, 1980.
17 Skinhøj P et al: Hepatitis A in Greenland: Importance of specific antibody testing in epidemiologic surveillance. *Am J Epidemiol* 105: 140, 1977.
18 Locarnini SA et al: The antibody response following hepatitis A infection. *Intervirology* 8: 309, 1977.
19 Lemon SM, Binn LN: Serum neutralizing antibody response to hepatitis A virus. *J Infect Dis* 148: 1033, 1983.
20 Decker RH et al: Serologic studies of transmission of hepatitis A in humans. *J Infect Dis* 139: 74, 1979.
21 Yoshizawa H et al: Diagnosis of type A hepatitis by fecal IgA antibody against hepatitis A antigen. *Gastroenterology* 78: 114, 1980.
22 Kurane I et al: Human lymphocyte responses to hepatitis A virus-infected cells: Interferon production and lysis of infected cells. *J Immunol* 135: 2140, 1985.
23 Vallbracht A et al: Cell-mediated cytotoxicity in hepatitis A virus infection. *Hepatology* 6: 1308, 1986.
24 Purcell RH et al: Hepatitis A virus, in *Viral Hepatitis and Liver Disease,* GN Vyas et al (eds). New York, Grune & Stratton, 1984, p 9.
25 Siegl G et al: Stability of hepatitis A virus. *Intervirology* 22: 218, 1984.
26 Frösner GG et al: Decrease in incidence of hepatitis A infections in Germany. *Infection* 6: 259, 1978.
27 Szmuness W et al: The prevalence of antibody to hepatitis A antigen in various parts of the world: A pilot study. *Am J Epidemiol* 106: 392, 1977.
28 Szmuness W et al: Distribution of antibody to hepatitis A antigen in urban adult populations. *N Engl J Med* 295: 755, 1976.
29 Burke DS et al: Age-specific prevalence of hepatitis A virus antibody in Thailand. *Am J Epidemiol* 113: 245, 1981.
30 Francis DP et al: Occurrence of hepatitis A, B, and non-A/non-B in the United States: CDC Sentinel County hepatitis study. *Am J Med* 76: 69, 1984.
31 Hadler SC et al: Hepatitis A in day-care centers: A community-wide assessment. *N Engl J Med* 302: 1222, 1980.
32 Centers for Disease Control: Hepatitis A among drug abusers. *MMWR* 37: 297, 1988.
33 McFarlane ES: Prevalence of antibodies to hepatitis A antigen in patients attending a clinic for treatment of sexually transmitted diseases. *Sex Transm Dis* 7: 87, 1980.
34 Hentzer B et al: Viral hepatitis in a venereal clinic population. *Scand J Infect Dis* 12: 245, 1980.
35 Corey L, Holmes KK: Sexual transmission of hepatitis A in homosexual men: Incidence and mechanism. *N Engl J Med* 302: 435, 1980.
36 Høybye G et al: An epidemic of acute viral hepatitis in male homosexuals: Etiology and clinical characteristics. *Scand J Infect Dis* 12: 241, 1980.
37 Szmuness W et al: Hepatitis B vaccine: Demonstration of efficacy in a controlled clinical trial in a high-risk population in the United States. *N Engl J Med* 303: 833, 1980.
38 Kryger P et al: Increased risk of infection with hepatitis A and B viruses in men with a history of syphilis: Relation to sexual contacts. *J Infect Dis* 145: 23, 1982.
39 McFarlane ES et al: Antibodies to hepatitis A antigen in relation to the number of lifetime sexual partners in patients attending an STD clinic. *Br J Vener Dis* 57: 58, 1981.
40 Lednar WM et al: Frequency of illness associated with epidemic hepatitis A virus infections in adults. *Am J Epidemiol* 122: 226, 1985.
41 Dienstag JL: Hepatitis A virus, in *Progress in Liver Diseases* IV, H Popper, F Schaffner (eds). New York, Grune & Stratton, 1979, p 343.
42 Rakela J et al: Hepatitis A virus infection in fulminant hepatitis and chronic active hepatitis. *Gastroenterology* 74: 879, 1978.
43 Seeff LB, Hoofnagle JH: Immunoprophylaxis of viral hepatitis. *Gastroenterology* 77: 161, 1979.
44 Advisory Committee on Immunization Practices: Recommendations for protection against viral hepatitis. *MMWR* 34: 313, 1985.
45 Binn LN et al: Preparation of a prototype inactivated hepatitis A virus vaccine from infected cell cultures. *J Infect Dis* 153: 749, 1986.
46 Provost PJ et al: New findings in live, attenuated hepatitis A vaccine development. *J Med Virol* 20: 165, 1986.
47 Robinson WS: The genome of hepatitis B virus. *Annu Rev Microbiol* 31: 357, 1977.
48 Ganem D, Varmus H: The molecular biology of the hepatitis B viruses. *Annu Rev Biochem* 56: 651, 1987.
49 Summers J, Mason WS: Replication of the genome of a hepatitis B-like virus by reverse transcription of an RNA intermediate. *Cell* 29: 403, 1982.
50 Albin C, Robinson WS: Protein kinase activity in hepatitis B virus. *J Virol* 34: 297, 1980.
51 Robinson WS: DNA and DNA polymerase in the core of the Dane particle of hepatitis B. *Am J Med Sci* 270: 151, 1975.
52 Takahashi K et al: Demonstration of hepatitis B e antigen in the core of Dane particles. *J Immunol* 122: 275, 1979.

53 Ou J et al: Hepatitis B gene function: The precore region targets the core antigen to cellular membranes and causes secretion of the e antigen. *Proc Natl Acad Sci USA* 83: 1578, 1986.

54 Bancroft WH et al: Detection of additional antigenic determinants of hepatitis B antigen. *J Immunol* 109: 842, 1972.

55 Sureau C et al: Production of hepatitis B virus by a differentiated human hepatoma cell line after transfection with cloned circular HBV DNA. *Cell* 47: 37, 1986.

56 Acs G et al: Hepatitis B virus produced by transfected HepG2 cells causes hepatitis in chimpanzees. *Proc Natl Acad Sci USA* 84: 4641, 1987.

57 Tuttleman J et al: Formation of the pool of covalently closed circular viral DNA in hepadnavirus-infected cells. *Cell* 47: 451, 1986.

58 Ray MB et al: Differential distribution of hepatitis B surface antigen and hepatitis B core antigen in the liver of hepatitis B patients. *Gastroenterology* 71: 462, 1976.

59 Korba BE et al: Hepadnavirus infection of peripheral blood lymphocytes *in vivo*: Woodchuck and chimpanzee models of viral hepatitis. *J Virol* 58: 1, 1986.

60 Hoofnagle JH et al: Serologic responses in hepatitis, in *Viral Hepatitis*, GN Vyas et al (eds). Philadelphia, Franklin Institute Press, 1978, p. 219.

61 Krugman S et al: Viral hepatitis, type B: Studies on natural history and prevention re-examined. *N Engl J Med* 300: 101, 1979.

62 Lemon SM et al: IgM antibody to hepatitis B core antigen as a diagnostic parameter of acute infection with hepatitis B virus. *J Infect Dis* 143: 803, 1981.

63 Hindman SH et al: "e" antigen, Dane particles, and serum DNA polymerase activity in HBsAg carriers. *Ann Intern Med* 85: 458, 1976.

64 Alter HJ et al: Type B hepatitis: The infectivity of blood positive for e antigen and DNA polymerase after accidental needlestick exposure. *N Engl J Med* 295: 909, 1976.

65 Okada K et al: e antigen and anti-e in the serum of asymptomatic carrier mothers as indicators of positive and negative transmission of hepatitis B virus to their infants. *N Engl J Med* 294: 746, 1976.

66 Hoofnagle JH et al: Seroconversion from hepatitis B e antigen to antibody in chronic type B hepatitis. *Ann Intern Med* 94: 744, 1981.

67 Eddleston ALWF et al: Lymphocyte cytotoxicity to autologous hepatocytes in chronic hepatitis B virus infection. *Hepatology* 2: 122S, 1982.

68 Beasley RP et al: Hepatocellular carcinoma and hepatitis B virus: A prospective study of 22,707 men in Taiwan. *Lancet* ii: 1129, 1981.

69 Summers J et al: Hepatitis B virus DNA in primary hepatocellular cancer tissue. *J Med Virol* 2: 207, 1978.

70 Aach RD, Kahn RA: Post-transfusion hepatitis: Current perspectives. *Ann Intern Med* 92: 539, 1980.

71 Heathcote J et al: Hepatitis B antigen in saliva and semen. *Lancet* i: 71, 1974.

72 Villarejos V et al: Role of saliva, urine and feces in transmission of type B hepatitis. *N Engl J Med* 291: 1375, 1974.

73 Darani M, Gerber M: Hepatitis B antigen in vaginal secretions. *Lancet* ii: 1008, 1974.

74 Macaya G et al: Dane particles and associated DNA-polymerase activity in the saliva of chronic hepatitis B carriers. *J Med Virol* 4: 291, 1979.

75 Jenison S et al: Quantitative analysis of hepatitis B virus DNA in saliva and semen of chronically infected homosexual men. *J Infect Dis* 156: 299, 1987.

76 Davison F et al: Detection of hepatitis B virus DNA in spermatozoa, urine, saliva, and leucocytes of chronic HBsAg carriers. A lack of relationship with serum markers of replication. *J Hepatol* 4: 37, 1987.

77 Krugman S, Giles JP: Viral hepatitis: New light on an old disease. *JAMA* 212: 1019, 1970.

78 Scott RM et al: Experimental transmission of hepatitis B virus by semen and saliva. *J Infect Dis* 142: 67, 1980.

79 Szmuness W et al: On the role of sexual behavior in the spread of hepatitis B infection. *Ann Intern Med* 83: 489, 1975.

80 Schreeder MT et al: Hepatitis B in homosexual males: Prevalence of HBV infection and factors related to transmission. *J Infect Dis* 146: 7, 1982.

81 Stevens CE et al: Vertical transmission of hepatitis B antigen in Taiwan. *N Engl J Med* 292: 771, 1975.

82 Szmuness W et al: Socio-economic aspects of the epidemiology of hepatitis B, in *Viral Hepatitis*, GN Vyas et al (eds). Philadelphia, Franklin Institute Press, 1978, p 297.

83 Gust ID et al: A seroepidemiologic study of infection with HAV and HBV in five Pacific islands. *Am J Epidemiol* 110: 237, 1979.

84 Dienstag JL, Ryan DM: Occupational exposure to hepatitis B virus in hospital personnel: Infection or immunization? *Am J Epidemiol* 115: 26, 1982.

85 Hersh T et al: Nonparenteral transmission of viral hepatitis type B (Australia antigen-associated hepatitis). *N Engl J Med* 285: 1363, 1971.

86 Frosner GG et al: Prevalence of hepatitis B antibody in prostitutes. *Am J Epidemiol* 102: 241, 1975.

87 Szmuness W: Large-scale efficacy trials of hepatitis B vaccines in the USA: Baseline data and protocols. *J Med Virol* 4: 327, 1979.

88 Dietzman DE et al: Hepatitis B surface antigen (HBsAg) and antibody to HBsAg: Prevalence in homosexual and heterosexual men. *JAMA* 238: 2625, 1977.

89 Lim KS et al: Role of sexual and non-sexual practices in the transmission of hepatitis B. *Br J Vener Dis* 53: 190, 1977.

90 Judson FN et al: Screening for gonorrhea and syphilis in the gay baths—Denver, Colorado. *Am J Public Health* 67: 740, 1977.

91 Centers for Disease Control: Changing patterns of groups at high risk for hepatitis B in the United States. *MMWR* 37: 429, 1988.

92 Szmuness W et al: A controlled clinical trial of the efficacy of the hepatitis B vaccine (Heptavax B): A final report. *Hepatology* 1: 377, 1981.

93 Reiner NE et al: Asymptomatic rectal mucosal lesions and hepatitis B surface antigen at sites of sexual contact in homosexual men with persistent hepatitis B virus infections. *Ann Intern Med* 96: 170, 1982.

94 Perrillo RP et al: Hepatitis B e antigen, DNA polymerase activity, and infection of household contacts with hepatitis B virus. *Gastroenterology* 76: 1319, 1979.

95 Murphy BL et al: Serological testing for hepatitis B in male homosexuals: Special emphasis on hepatitis B e antigen and antibody by radioimmunoassay. *J. Clin Microbiol* 11: 301, 1980.

96 Szmuness W et al: Prevalence of hepatitis B "e" antigen and its antibody in various HBsAg carrier populations. *Am J Epidemiol* 113: 113, 1981.

97 Tedder RS et al: Contrasting patterns and frequency of antibodies to the surface, core, and e antigens of hepatitis B virus in blood donors and in homosexual patients. *J Med Virol* 6: 323, 1980.

98 Heathcote J et al: Role of hepatitis B antigen carriers in nonparenteral transmission of the hepatitis B virus. *Lancet* ii: 370, 1974.

99 Mosley JW: The epidemiology of viral hepatitis: An overview. *Am J Med Sci* 270: 253, 1975.

100 Koff RS et al: Contagiousness of acute hepatitis B: Secondary attack rates in household contacts. *Gastroenterology* 72: 297, 1977.

101 Tassopoulas NC et al: Detection of hepatitis B virus DNA in asymptomatic hepatitis B surface antigen carriers: Relation to sexual transmission. *Am J Epidemiol* 126: 587, 1987.

102 Alter MJ et al: Hepatitis B virus transmission between heterosexuals. *JAMA* 256: 1307, 1986.

103 Lemon SM et al: Etiology of viral hepatitis in American soldiers. *Am J Epidemiol* 116: 438, 1982.

104 Scott RMcN et al: Factors relating to transmission of viral hepatitis in a United States military population stationed in Thailand. *Am J Epidemiol* 113: 520, 1981.

105 Sergent JS: Extrahepatic manifestations of hepatitis B infection. *Bull Rheum Dis* 33: 1, 1983.

106 Redeker AG: Viral hepatitis: Clinical aspects. *Am J Med Sci* 270: 9, 1975.

107 Seeff LB et al: A serological follow-up of the 1942 epidemic of

postvaccination hepatitis in the United States Army. *N Engl J Med* 316: 965, 1987.

108 Lam KC et al: Deleterious effect of prednisolone in HBsAg-positive chronic active hepatitis. *N Engl J Med* 304: 380, 1981.

109 Sjogren MH et al: Clinical significance of low molecular weight (7-8S) immunoglobulin M antibody to hepatitis B core antigen in chronic hepatitis B virus infections. *Gastroenterology* 91: 168, 1986.

110 Buynak EB et al: Development and chimpanzee testing of a vaccine against human hepatitis B. *Proc Soc Exp Biol Med* 151: 694, 1976.

111 Advisory Committee on Immunization Practices CDC: Update on hepatitis B prevention. *MMWR* 36: 353, 1987.

112 Francis DP et al: The safety of hepatitis B vaccine: Inactivation of the AIDS virus during routine vaccine manufacture. *JAMA* 256: 869, 1986.

113 Francis DP et al: The prevention of hepatitis B with vaccine: Report of the Centers for Disease Control multi-center efficacy trial among homosexual men. *Ann Intern Med* 97: 362, 1982.

114 Hadler SC et al: Longterm immunogenicity and efficacy of hepatitis B vaccine in homosexual men. *N Engl J Med* 315: 209, 1986.

115 Szmuness W et al: Passive-active immunisation against hepatitis B: Immunogenicity studies in adult Americans. *Lancet* i: 575, 1981.

116 Weber DJ et al: Obesity as a predictor of poor antibody response to hepatitis B plasma vaccine. *JAMA* 254: 3187, 1985.

117 Collier A et al: Antibody to human immunodeficiency virus (HIV) and suboptimal response to hepatitis B vaccination. *Ann Intern Med* 109: 101, 1988.

118 Emini EA et al: Production and immunological analysis of recombinant hepatitis B vaccine. *J Infection* 13 (suppl A): 3, 1986.

119 Lemon SM: Viral hepatitis, in *Sexually Transmitted Diseases*, 1st ed, K Holmes et al (eds). New York, McGraw-Hill, 1984, p 479.

120 Redeker AG et al: Hepatitis B immune globulin as a prophylactic measure for spouses exposed to acute type B hepatitis. *N Engl J Med* 293:1055, 1975.

121 Stevens CE et al: Yeast-recombinant hepatitis B vaccine: Efficacy with hepatitis B immune globulin in prevention of perinatal hepatitis B virus transmission. *JAMA* 257: 2612, 1987.

122 Advisory Committee for Immunization Practices: Prevention of perinatal transmission of hepatitis B virus: Prenatal screening of all pregnant women for hepatitis B surface antigen. *MMWR* 37: 342, 1988.

123 Aach RD: The treatment of chronic type B viral hepatitis. *Ann Intern Med* 109: 89, 1988.

124 Gregory PB: The demise of corticosteroid therapy for acute viral hepatitis. *Gastroenterology* 80: 404, 1981.

125 Rizetto M et al: The hepatitis B virus-associated δ antigen: Isolation from liver, development of solid-phase radioimmunoassays for δ antigen and anti-δ, partial characterization of δ antigen. *J Immunol* 125: 318, 1980.

126 Rizetto M et al: δ-agent: Association of δ-antigen with hepatitis B surface antigen and RNA in serum of δ-infected chimpanzees. *Proc Natl Acad Sci USA* 77: 6124, 1980.

127 Wang K-S et al: Structure, sequence and expression of the hepatitis delta (δ) viral genome. *Nature* 323: 508, 1986.

128 Chang M-F et al: Human hepatitis delta antigen is a nuclear phosphoprotein with RNA-binding activity. *J Virol* 62: 2403, 1988

129 DeCock KM et al: HDV infection in the Los Angeles area, in *The Hepatitis Delta Virus and Its Infection*, M Rizetto et al (eds). New York, Alan R Liss, 1987.

130 Negro F et al: Chronic hepatitis D virus (HDV) infection in hepatitis B virus carrier chimpanzees experimentally infected with HDV. *J Infect Dis* 158: 151, 1988.

131 Rizetto M et al: Epidemiology of HBV-associated delta agent: Geographical distribution of anti-delta and prevalence in polytransfused HBsAg carriers. *Lancet* i: 1215, 1980.

132 Solomon RE et al: Human immunodeficiency virus and hepatitis delta virus in homosexual men: A study of four cohorts. *Ann Intern Med* 108: 51, 1988.

133 Alter HJ et al: Transmissible agent in non-A, non-B hepatitis. *Lancet* i: 459, 1978.

134 Tabor E et al: Transmission of non-A, non-B hepatitis from man to chimpanzee. *Lancet* i: 463, 1978.

135 Ezzell C: Candidate cause identified of non-A, non-B hepatitis. *Nature* 333: 195, 1988.

136 Feinstone SM et al: Transfusion-associated hepatitis not due to viral hepatitis type A or B. *N Engl J Med* 292: 767, 1975.

137 Berman M et al: The chronic sequelae of non-A, non-B hepatitis. *Ann Intern Med* 91: 1, 1979.

138 Rakela J, Redeker AG: Chronic liver disease after acute non-A, non-B viral hepatitis. *Gastroenterology* 77: 1200, 1979.

139 Khuroo MS: Study of an epidemic of non-A, non-B hepatitis. Possibility of another human hepatitis virus distinct from post-transfusion non-A, non-B type. *Am J Med* 80: 818, 1980.

140 Arankalle VA et al: Aetiological association of a virus-like particle with enterically-transmitted non-A, non-B hepatitis. *Lancet* i: 550, 1988.

141 Favero MS et al: Guidelines for the care of patients hospitalized with viral hepatitis. *Ann Intern Med* 91: 872, 1979.

142 Coleman JC et al: Hepatitis B antigen and antibody in a male homosexual population. *Br J Vener Dis* 53: 132, 1977.

# Section 3
# Ectoparasites

## Chapter 41
# Human lice

Stephan A. Billstein

The order *Anaplura* includes over 400 species of sucking lice, which are ectoparasites of mammals. Sucking lice are dorsoventrally compressed, wingless, and small, with retractable piercing-sucking mouthparts. One species is the cause of a common sexually transmitted disease: pubic lice, or "crabs."

Three species of lice infest human beings: *Phthirus pubis,* the crab louse; *Pediculus humanus humanus,* the body louse; and *Pediculus humanus capitis,* the head louse. This chapter focuses principally on pubic lice, but head and body lice will be briefly considered for purposes of comparison.

### LIFE CYCLE AND REPRODUCTION

Lice have five stages in their life cycle: egg (or nit), three nymphal stages, and the adult stage. All stages occur on the host. Sucking lice undergo a simple metamorphosis in which immature lice are morphological miniatures of adults, but have no reproductive ability.

The egg of the crab louse is smaller than the eggs of either the head or body louse, which measure approximately 0.8 mm long and 0.3 mm wide.[1] The nit is oval in shape and opalescent in color; it contains a cap (operculum) which comes off intact when the egg hatches (Fig. 41-1). An egg will hatch within 5 to 10 days after being incubated in the heat of the host's body. Interestingly, the young nymph emerges through the cap by sucking air into its body, and expelling it from its anus until a cushion of compressed air is formed, which then pops the cap open and allows the nymph to escape.[2] Over a period of 8 to 9 days, the nymph produces three molts. The louse remains on the body, and requires frequent blood meals after having hatched. When lice reach adulthood, mating occurs after approximately 10 h and continues until the lice die. The female louse lays approximately four eggs per day.

In the case of the body louse, the egg case is attached to hair or clothing by a cementlike material secreted by the female louse. After hatching, the empty shell may stick to hair or clothing for some time. It is often difficult to remove by washing or shampooing, or by vinegar or organic solvents. If all else fails, the empty egg cases eventually are moved away either by growth of the hair, by the use of a fine-tooth comb, or by cutting the hair.

Little is known about the actual life span of the adult louse. Under artificial conditions, lice have survived for about 1 month. Ambient temperature, humidity, and availability of human blood are thought to influence the life span of all types of human lice. Off the host, all stages of the louse can be expected to die within 30 days, regardless of temperature. Unfed adult head and body lice can survive for up to 10 days, whereas adult pubic lice rarely survive more than 24 h off the host.[3] Lice leave the host voluntarily only when the host has died or becomes febrile, or when there is close personal contact with another host.

The life of a louse is dependent on human blood. When ready to feed, the louse anchors its mouth to the skin, stabs an opening through the skin, pours saliva into the wound to prevent clotting, and pumps blood from the wound into its digestive system. During feeding, dark-red feces may be deposited on the skin.

The pubic louse has greatly enlarged middle and hind legs and claws; the abdomen is wider than it is long, giving it the appearance of a crab (Fig. 41-2). Pubic lice are about 1 mm in length. Adult head and body lice have a longer body (approximately 3 mm in females and 2 mm in males), and relatively

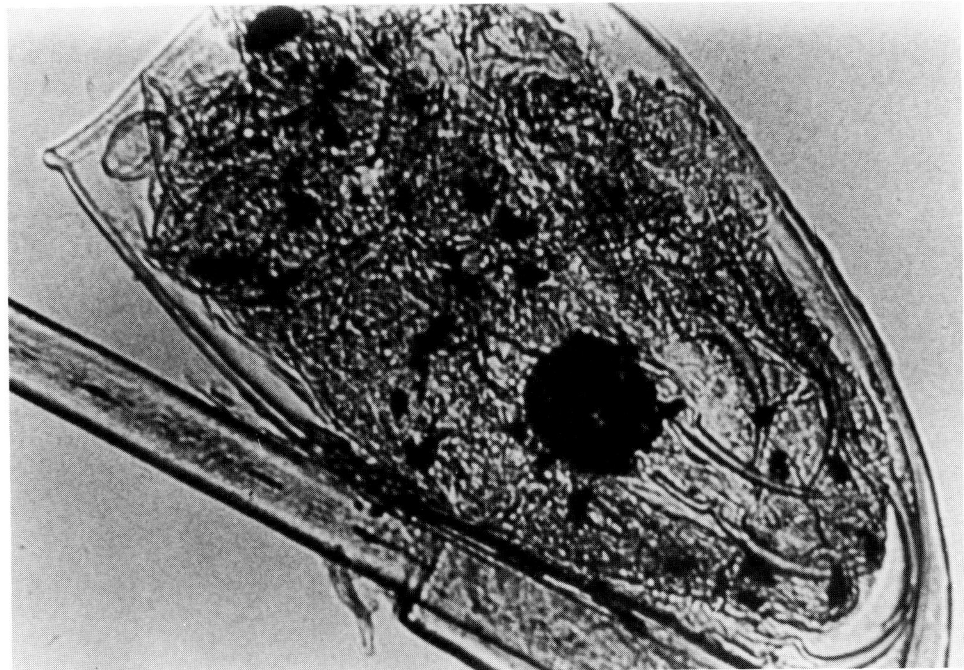

**Fig. 41-1.** Close-up micrograph of a louse nit (egg).

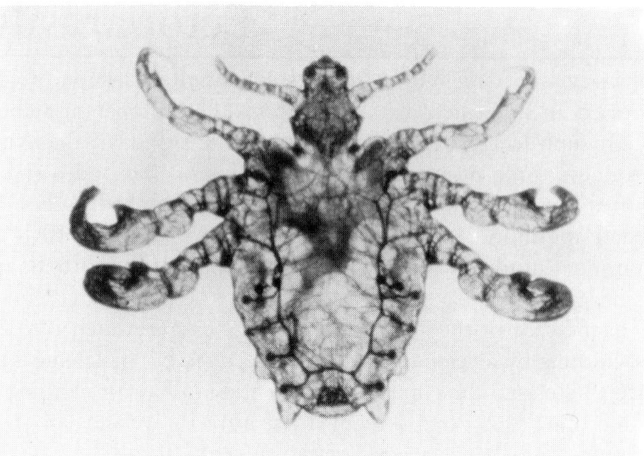

**Fig. 41-2.** Pubic louse after recent blood meal. *(Courtesy of V. D. Newcomer.)*

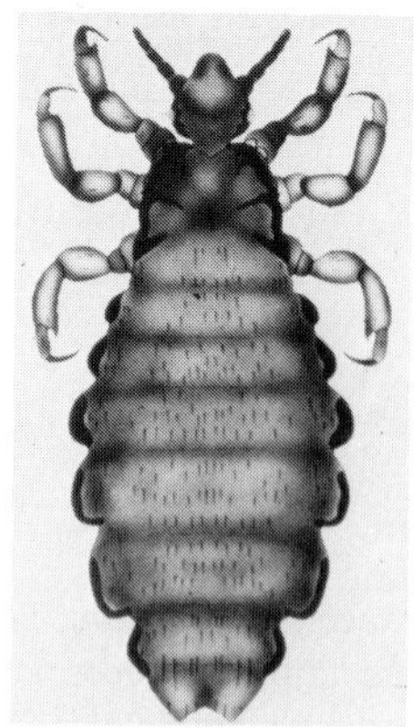

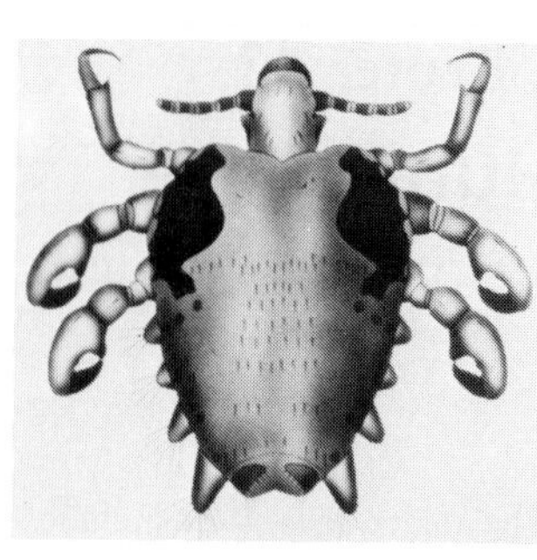

**Fig. 41-3.** Comparison of the gross structure of *(left)* the head louse and *(right)* the pubic louse.

shorter middle and hind legs (Fig. 41-3). The pubic louse has three parts: a head (with a pair of eyes), a thorax (with three pairs of legs), and a segregated abdomen. At the end of each leg, there is a hooklike claw and opposing thumb, which enable the louse to maintain its hold on hair (Fig. 41-4).

A difference between the body and head louse and the pubic louse involves their grasping ability. The grasp of the pubic louse's claw matches the diameter of pubic and axillary hairs; hence, it is not only found in the pubic area (Fig. 41-5, Plate 79), but also has been recovered from the axillae, beard areas of the face, eyelashes (Fig. 41-6), and eyebrows. The diameter of the head louse's claw's grasp seems to be uniquely adapted to the diameter of the scalp hair. Therefore, it is very difficult to transplant head lice to other areas of the body.

Another difference between the species is that of egg laying. Adult female pubic lice and head lice glue their eggs to hairs, while the female body louse usually ovoposits on the fiber or in the seams of clothing.

A third difference is the rate of movement. Pubic lice seem to be the most sedentary. Nuttal and Payot recorded public lice moving at a maximum of 10 cm in a day.[4] Body lice can wander as much as 35 mm in a 2-hour period. Temperature, ambient humidity, and availability of a blood meal also influence the rate of movement. Lice do not like light, and will move frantically to escape light.

## EPIDEMIOLOGY

It is estimated by sales figures on pediculocides that more than 3 million cases of pediculosis are treated each year in the United States. Most cases are due to head and pubic lice infestations. Infestation by body lice seems to be less common in this country. Epidemics of louse-borne relapsing fever and epidemic typhus are now rare, since the body louse is the only species implicated as their vector. Mass epidemics of these diseases have resulted when

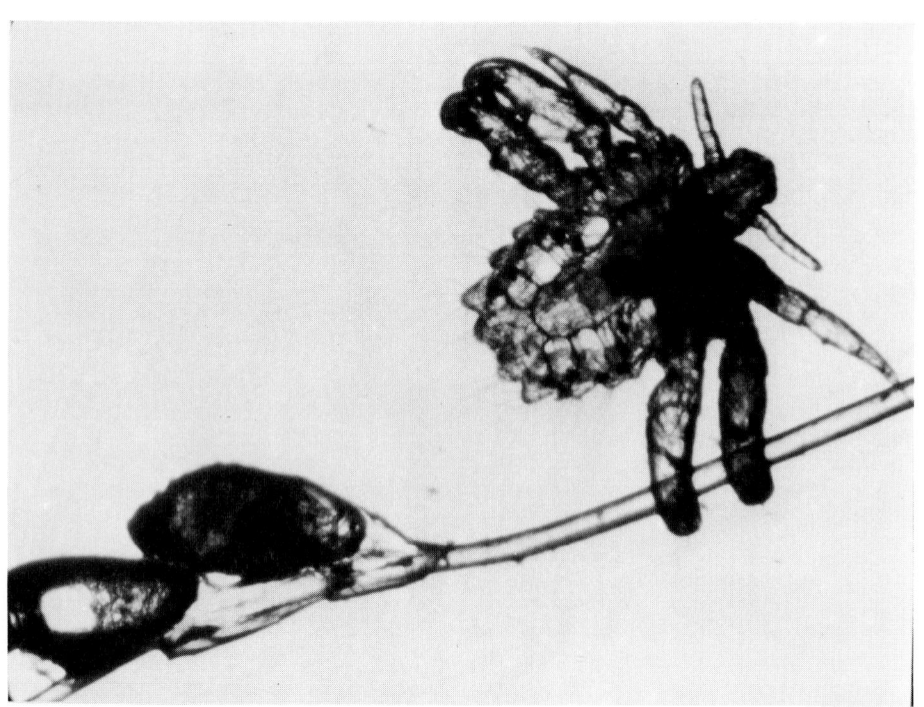

**Fig. 41-4.** Pubic louse and nits on a hair follicle. *(Courtesy of V. D. Newcomer.)*

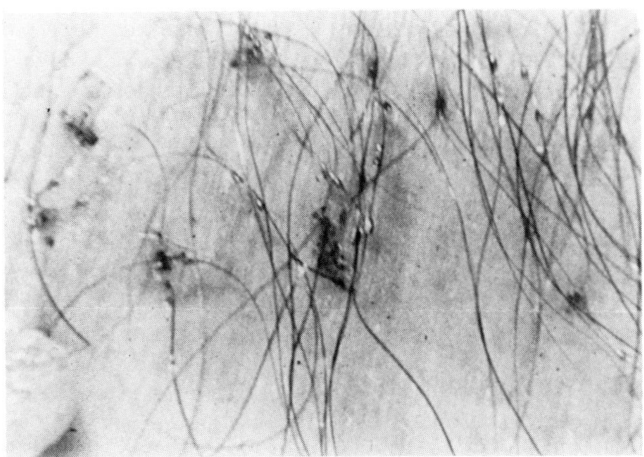

Fig. 41-5. Adult pubic lice and nits.

large populations have lived in unsanitary conditions as in times of famine, disaster, and war.

"Vagabond's disease" is a diagnosis made in persons who continually harbor these lice, and whose skin becomes hardened and darkly pigmented as a result of frequent louse bites and patient response.

## TRANSMISSION

Human lice are transmitted from one person to another primarily by intimate contact. Although all types of human lice are relatively host-specific, crab lice occasionally have been reported to infest dogs. Both head and body lice are transmitted by sharing personal articles such as hairbrushes, combs, towels, or clothing. Pubic lice do not seem to spread as rapidly as other human lice when off the host. They have a shorter life span (24 h compared to several days for other lice), and their movements are more lethargic. Sexual transmission is considered to be the most important means of pubic lice transmission. However, there are documented cases of transmission from toilet seats, beds, and egg-infested loose hairs dropped by infested persons on shared objects.

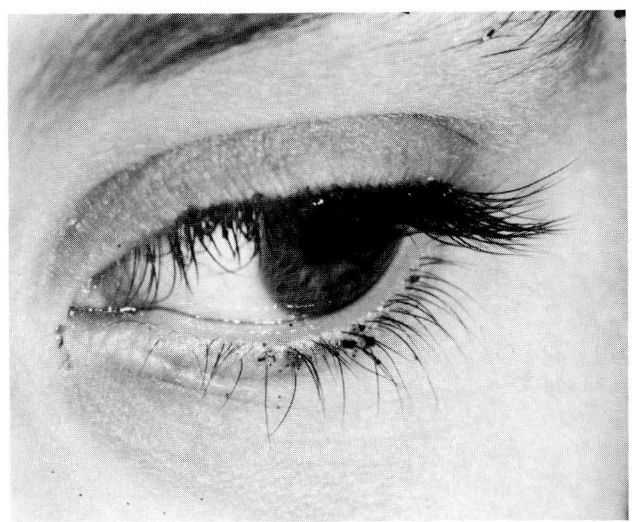

Fig. 41-6. Adult pubic lice and nits on eyelashes. *(Courtesy of E. Stolz.)*

The population with the highest incidence of pubic lice is similar to that of gonorrhea and syphilis: single persons, ages 15 to 25. Prevalence of pubic lice infestation declines gradually to age 35 and is rare in persons older than 35. Head lice are most common in children up to 6 years of age.

## CLINICAL MANIFESTATIONS

Sensitivity to the effect of louse bites varies with the individual. When previously unexposed persons are bitten, there may either be no signs or symptoms or a slight sting with little or no itching or redness. At least 5 days must pass before allergic sensitization can occur. At that point, the main symptom is itching, which leads to scratching, erythema, irritation, and inflammation. An individual who has been bitten by a large number of lice over a short period of time may have mild fever, malaise, and increased irritability.

Apparently, many persons eventually develop some degree of immunity to the bite of the louse. Persons infested for a long time may even become oblivious to the lice on their bodies. The opposite may also occur. Excessive scratching may lead to superinfection. Characteristic small "blue spots" may appear in the skin, as the result of the crab louse bites; these persist for several days.

## DIAGNOSIS

Diagnosis of lice infestation is made by (1) taking a careful history from the patient, (2) considering lice infestation as a possible or probable cause of the patient's signs and symptoms, and (3) careful examination of the patient. Both adult lice and their eggs (nits) are easily seen by the naked eye (Figs. 41-5, 41-6, Plate 79).

Head lice characteristically are found on the scalp surface with the nits attached to the hair. Since scalp hair grows at a rate of about 0.4 mm per day, and nits of the head louse usually hatch within 9 days, most of the unhatched nits are within 5 mm of the scalp surface. Nits on scalp hair are usually cemented at an oblique angle which helps to distinguish them from foreign material which slides up and down and frequently surrounds the hair.

Upon examination of the groin or pudendal area, pubic lice may be perceived as scabs over what first were thought to be "scratch papules." When taking a closer look, if nits appear on the hairs, the proper diagnosis becomes obvious. If the "crust" is removed and placed on a glass slide for microscopic examination, the crust often walks away before the cover glass is in place. When no adult lice are available, the demonstration of nits under the microscope will also confirm the diagnosis.

When one sees with the naked eye white flakes on the hair, other possible considerations are seborrheic dermatitis (dandruff flakes), hair casts, solidified globules of hair spray, and certain accretions on hair shafts.

## MANAGEMENT

Treatment and disinfection regimens should be individualized. Ideally the regimen should employ a pediculocide which effectively will kill both the adults and the eggs. Also, examination of partners and other household contacts of the patient should be made so that both source and spread cases can be treated.

Both nonprescription and prescription medications are currently available. For these medications to be ovocidal, the pediculocide should remain in contact with the eggs for at least 1 h. In the experience of the author, the most effective nonprescription products contain pyrethrins and piperonyl butoxide.[5] Two products, Rid (liquid and shampoo) and Triple X (liquid and shampoo) contain 0.3 percent pyrethrins and 3.0 percent piperonyl butoxide. A single application of either of these compounds usually is effective on both adult lice, and eggs. Recent studies[6,7] have indicated that a small percentage of patients will require reapplication 7 to 10 days after the first treatment. Rid has a fine-tooth comb in the package to help dislodge the dead nits upon treatment completion. The oldest marketed product in this group is an A-200 Pyrinate (shampoo). It contains 0.165 percent pyrethrins and 2.0 percent piperonyl butoxide. This medication requires two applications 7 days apart, as the initial one is often not lethal for the nits. Other over-the-counter pediculocides currently available in the United States include Cuprex (31 percent tetrahydronaphthalene, 0.03 percent copper oleate), and Barc (0.18 percent pyrethrins, 2.2 percent piperonyl butoxide). They are allegedly less effective than the former drugs in treatment of lice infestations in a public health clinic setting.

Kwell, a 1.0 percent gamma benzene hexachloride preparation (lotion, shampoo, and cream), is the most commonly used prescription medication currently available. Scabene, marketed in late 1981, is the same formulation but is available only as a lotion. In the United States, it has also been available at times as a commercial insecticide, Lindane. In using this drug, the patient should be advised to divide the day into three 8-h segments. A shower is taken before each of two 1 percent gamma benzene hexachloride applications. Each application must remain on the affected area for the 8-h period, after which another shower is advised. After the third shower, no further application is required. Other prescription medications available include emulsions of 20 percent or greater of benzyl benzoate, 10 percent sulfur ointment, and Eurax (10 percent crotamiton). All three are effective but have disadvantages in that they require several days' applications and/or impart an unpleasant odor to the patient.

The use of 1 percent gamma benzene hexachloride has several disadvantages. It can be percutaneously absorbed when applied to a severely excoriated skin. Case reports have alluded to mild signs and symptoms of neurotoxicity when it has been ingested, applied too frequently, not washed off as directed, or used on massively excoriated skin. In one study,[8] 9 percent of a single dose was found in the urine in a badly excoriated patient in the 5 days following the treatment. No other studies, however, have shown blood, tissue, and urine levels.[9,10] Gamma benzene hexachloride use should be avoided on small children, pregnant women, and individuals with massive excoriations or multiple lesions over the scrotum.

Itching is an important feature of all lice infestations. The initial treatment with a pediculocide may be effective for killing both the adult lice and the eggs, but the itching may continue because of allergic reaction and/or irritation. The possibility of posttreatment pruritis should be discussed with the patient; a mild topical antipruritic/anti-inflammatory cream or ointment may also be prescribed. The patient should be reevaluated 4 to 7 days after initial treatment. Attention to these considerations is crucial, as it often prevents excessive pediculocide use and may prevent parasitophobia and feelings of "being unclean."

Additional prescription medications include: 6 percent sulfur in petrolatum which may be useful for infants who cannot tolerate other therapies; a 5 to 10 percent thiobendazole cream; DDT (currently not available in the United States and known to have resistant strains); and malathion (currently not available in the United States).

The most recent entry into the United States pediculocide market is 1 percent primethrin (Nix). Primethrin is a synthetic pyrethroid related chemically to the pyrethrins. It is photostable and thermostable and has a low mammalian toxic effect and a broad spectrum of insecticidal activity. Compared with pyrethrins, its marked stability in the presence of light is believed to give it residual activity. It has been shown to persist on the hair shaft for more than 10 days. As complete ovocidal activity is lacking, this residual property is believed to be the mechanism for overcoming this drawback. This prescription medication was introduced in the United States in 1986. The current package insert indication is for the treatment of head lice. Studies[6,7] have compared 1 percent primethrin marketed as a creme rinse with a shampoo (Kwell). Statistical significance was achieved in studies showing a success rate of 97 to 99 percent eradication of the infestation using Nix versus a 43 to 85 percent success rate with the shampoo mixture. One study[11] compared these two products for treatment of pubic lice. That study showed, at 10 days post-initial application, a 43 percent failure rate with primethrin and a 40 percent failure rate with the Kwell shampoo.

The current recommended administration of primethrin creme rinse is applying it for 10 min after thoroughly washing the area first, then gently rinsing off the area. If signs and symptoms persist, another application may be warranted 7 to 10 days later.

All pediculocides interfere with function of the louse nerve ganglion, leading to respiratory paralysis and death. An exception is the use of vaseline on pubic lice attached to the eyelids or eyelashes; its action smothers lice by mechanical obstruction of the respiratory apparatus.

Ridding the patient's clothing and fomites of adult lice and nits is an important part of the treatment regimen. Laundering these items in hot water (125°F) or dry cleaning kills the adults, nymphs, or nits. Nonwashable items may be treated with any of a variety of pyrethrin-piperonyl butoxide containing disinfectants (such as R and C spray, Li-Ban Spray, Black Flag, and Raid). It is important to inform the patient that these products should be used on inanimate or nonwashable items only.

## CONTROL ASPECTS

In discussion of epidemic control of lice infestations with administrators of schools or institutions, or control measures with and for an individual, the following set of guidelines can be recommended:

1. Document that lice are truly the cause of the problem.
2. Diagnose which louse species is involved.
3. Establish an effective therapeutic regimen including: (a) treatment of the individual with a pediculocide which kills adults and nits; (b) environmental disinfection; (c) treatment of household and intimate contacts; and (d) reassurance to the infested that they are not "unclean" and that they will get better.[8]

Lice infestation may cause anxiety and embarrassment, but it is totally curable with no long-term effects.

## References


1 Barnes AM, Keh B: The biology and control of lice on man. *California Vector Views* 6:7, 1959.
2 Slonka GF: Life cycle and biology of lice. *J School Health* 47:349, 1977.
3 Keh B, Poorbaugh JH: Understanding and treating infestations of lice on humans. *California Vector Views* 18:23, 1971.
4. Nuttall GHF: Combating lousiness among soldiers and civilians. *Parasitology* 10:411, 1918.
5. Billstein S, Laone P: Demographic study of head lice infestations in Sacramento County children. *Int J Dermatol* 18:301, 1979.
6 Brandenburg K et al: 1% permethrin cream rinse vs. 1% lindane shampoo in treating pediculosis capitis. *AJDC* 140:894, 1986.
7 Taplin D et al: Permethrin 1% creme rinse for the treatment of pediculus humanus var capitis infestation. *Ped Dermatol* 3:344, 1986.
8 Jaranek D: Personal communication.
9 Rasmussen JE: The problem of lindane. *J Am Acad Dermatol* 5:507, 1981.
10 Shacter B: Treatment of scabies and pediculosis with lindane preparations: An evaluation. *J Am Acad Dermatol* 5:517, 1981.
11 Kalter DC et al: Treatment of pediculosis pubis. *Arch Dermatol* 123:1315, 1987.

# Chapter 42
# Scabies

Milton Orkin
Howard Maibach

## HISTORY

Bonomo's discovery in 1687 of the itch mite (*Sarcoptes scabiei*) marked scabies as the first disease in humans with known cause; unfortunately, two centuries passed before this was generally accepted. Von Hebra (1816–1880), the father of modern dermatology, delineated much of our basic knowledge about scabies. He noted the relative unimportance of fomites in its transmission; however, this concept was not generally accepted until a century later, when reintroduced by Mellanby[1] as a result of studies of experimentally induced scabies in volunteers during World War II. At the same time, Heilesen[2] wrote a monograph on scabies, which remains another rich source. Mellanby and Heilesen's incisive studies form the scientific foundation for contemporary knowledge of this infestation.

## BIOLOGY OF THE ORGANISM

The adult female itch mite has a rounded body and four pairs of legs and measures 400 μm in length. It walks rapidly on human skin, covering 2.5 cm per min.[3] Finding a suitable location, it burrows into the horny layer to the boundary of the stratum granulosum. The burrow provides its home for life, approximately 30 days (Plate 80). Within hours of burrowing, it begins laying enormous eggs (two or three a day), which progress through larval and nymphal stages to form adult mites in 10 days. The average number of adult female mites on an infested patient is 11.

The mites concentrate in special sites; two-thirds of these sites are on the hands and wrists. Since the eruption may be caused in part by immature stages of the mite and by sensitization, the distribution of adult female mites does not parallel that of the typical scabietic lesions. In primary infestation, itching or eruption does not occur for several weeks, the time required for sensitization.

## IMMUNOLOGY AND PATHOGENESIS

Epidemics of scabies occur in 30-year cycles with a 15-year gap between the end of one epidemic and the beginning of the next; the epidemics usually last about 15 years.[4] The cause of the current pandemic is not clear. Although a number of factors (poverty, poor hygiene, sexual promiscuity, misdiagnosis, increased travel, and demographic and ecological considerations) promote development of scabies, the causes are probably multifactorial.

Increasing information suggests that immunologic factors (humoral and cell-mediated) are important. This topic was recently reviewed,[5] and the following findings were found to be of additional pertinence:

1. Frentz and associates[6] demonstrated IgE deposits, by direct immunofluorescence, in the vessel walls of the upper dermis of some patients with scabies; indirect immunofluorescence was negative. Hoefling and Schroeter[7] found a cutaneous vasculitis-like pattern on direct immunofluorescence of dermal vessels, with the presence of IgM and C3 conjugates (IgE not available); granular deposits of IgM and IgG in the dermal-epidermal junction had a pattern similar to lupus erythematosus.
2. Van Neste and Salmon[8] noted that circulating immune complexes increased in the serum of patients with treated scabies; subsequent study suggested that antigens or substances derived from the scabies mite were not involved in the immune complexes.[9]
3. Falk,[10] studying serum immunoglobulins in patients with scabies, noted that 40 percent of patients had significantly lower IgA, higher IgG, higher IgM, and higher IgE than did uninfected persons.

   Falk and Bolle[11] studied IgE antibodies to housedust mite, *Dermatophagoides pteronyssinus,* in patients with scabies and observed elevation of IgE levels, even in nonatopic individuals, suggesting that IgE against human scabies mite cross reacts with *D. pteronyssinus;* they believe that scabies infestation is often associated with atopic disease. Follow-up of these patients showed a distinct decrease in total serum IgE concentrations and of circulating IgE antibodies to *D. pteronyssinus* in nonatopic patients after treatment, but only slight decrease in the atopic group.[12]
4. Falk and Bolle,[13] utilizing an extract from adult female scabietic mites, reported positive intracutaneous (immediate type) reactions in individuals who had scabies less than a year prior to testing, but negative reactions in patients with scabies more than a year previously. Passive transfer (Prausnitz-Küstner) was positive. These findings indicated that immediate type hypersensitivity (type I) occurs with scabies infestation. Activation of the cellular arm of the immune system in scabies remains largely unexplored.[14]
5. An increased frequency of HLA-A11 was demonstrated in nonatopic patients with scabies.[15] This suggests a potential genetic susceptibility to scabies, but this must be confirmed in other populations.

Orkin has noted an interrelationship in some patients between scabies and atopic dermatitis: difficulty in differentiating scabies from variations of atopic dermatitis (especially papular urticaria); a significant number of patients in whom scabies seems combined with atopic dermatitis, with the latter persisting after the scabies is cleared; and a high incidence of scabietic hypersensitivity sequelae (nodular scabies, dyshidrosiform syndrome[16]) in patients with an atopic background.

## EPIDEMIOLOGY

The socioeconomic characteristics of patients with this infestation are representative of those of the general population. The frequency of scabies in black Americans appears to be significantly lower than in white Americans and in some other racial group.[17]

Although it is unwise to be dogmatic about the way in which a particular patient contracted scabies, close personal contact is usually involved.[18] The long incubation period, usual in individuals infested for the first time, may make it difficult to trace the source. If one member of the household becomes infested, multiple members or the entire family may eventually be affected unless specific treatment is instituted. When several members of a family or group complain of a pruritic eruption, scabies is a likely diagnosis.[19]

In sexually active young adults (ages 15 to 40), sexual transmission is likely. Although syphilis and gonorrhea are frequently transmitted by brief sexual contact, scabies is more likely to be transmitted when the partners spend the night together. Scabies is one of the few sexually transmitted diseases which is also commonly nonsexually transmitted in households to individuals of all ages.

The greater the parasite load in an individual, the greater the likelihood of transmission; the importance of those few individuals with high parasite rates, such as patients with crusted scabies, in transmitting scabies is obvious. Immature mites are capable of causing infestation, although the usual cause is probably the newly fertilized adult female.

Scabies is frequent in school-age children but is unlikely to be transmitted in schools.[20] Outbreaks are not uncommon in nursing homes, hospitals, and other institutions. Nosocomial outbreaks of scabies occur; presumably many instances are not reported.[21]

## CLINICAL MANIFESTATIONS

### CLASSIC SCABIES

In the current cycle, classic scabies (Table 42-1) is seen less frequently. Itching is characteristically nocturnal. Lesions are roughly symmetrical. The hands are often the first areas involved; lesions (frequently eczematous) occur mainly on the finger webs and the sides of the digits (Figs. 42-1, 42-2). The flexor surfaces of the wrist are commonly involved, as are the extensor surfaces of the elbows (lesions may be nodular, but more commonly are dry and eczematous) and the anterior axillary folds.[19] The female breasts may have eczematous lesions resembling those of Paget's disease. Papular lesions are usually present on the abdomen, particularly around the umbilicus in a spokelike arrangement. The disease may affect the lower portion of the buttocks in the crease where they join the upper part of the thighs (Plate 82); impetiginous crusting on the buttocks should make one suspicious of scabies. Penile involvement is characteristic: nodules may dominate or chancriform changes or pyoderma (Plate 83) may be present. In adults, the upper back, neck, face, scalp, palms, and soles are seldom involved.

**Table 42-1 Diagnosis of Scabies**

1. Suggestive
   *a.* Distribution: Hands, wrists, elbows, anterior axillary folds, areolae of female breasts, abdomen, genitals, buttocks
   *b.* Morphology: Typically polymorphic. Burrows are pathognomonic
   *c.* Nocturnal pruritus
   *d.* Contact cases (highly suggestive)
   *e.* Response to "specific" therapy
   *f.* Skin biopsy in inflammatory or nodular lesions
2. Diagnostic: Identification of the mite (success rate varies with experience and persistence)
   *a.* Microscopic study: Skin scrapings or other techniques
   *b.* Skin biopsy (performed in difficult cases): Sections may reveal mites or fecal pellets

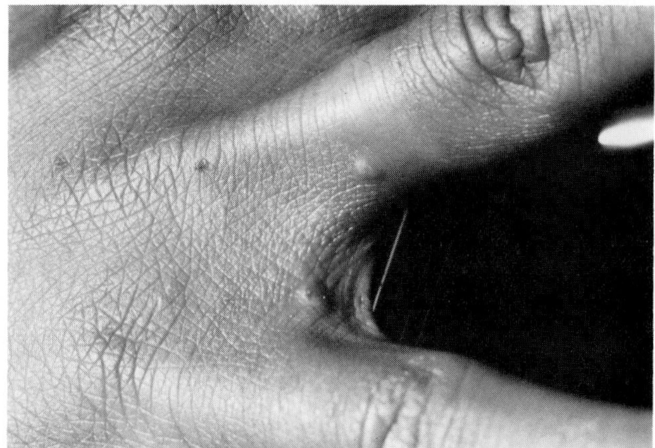

**Fig. 42-1** Papules in the interdigital area, highly suggestive of scabies. (*Courtesy of E. Stolz.*)

The pathognomonic burrow is a short, wavy, dirty-appearing line which often crosses skin lines; it is most common on the fingerwebs (Fig. 42-2), volar wrists, elbows, and penis. At most sites, small, erythematous, often excoriated papules are encountered; many of these may be "larval papules",[22] an important morphological component of the current cycle. Secondary eczematization and infection may overshadow other features, making diagnosis more difficult. Many dermatoses present with monomorphous lesions; scabies is usually a polymorphous disease. An exception is the occasional patient with scabies in whom urticaria is the only cutaneous manifestation.

### SPECIAL FORMS OF SCABIES

These are seen much more commonly in the current cycle.

#### Scabies in the clean

There is a definite increase in the incidence of scabies in clean persons. The disease is easily misdiagnosed in these cases because lesions may be barely observable and burrows may be difficult to find.[23] The person presumably removes many mites with frequent bathing (soap destroys many life forms). In these cases,

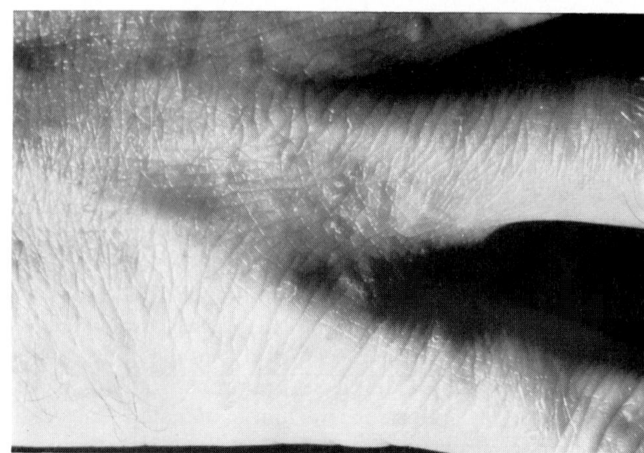

**Fig. 42-2.** Multiple scabietic burrows and papules are present on the fingerwebs. (*Courtesy of A. Hoke.*)

larval papules may be significant. Meticulous physical examination will suggest the diagnosis, which is confirmed by identification of the mite.

## Scabies incognito[23]

Corticosteroid administration (topical or systemic) may ameliorate symptoms and signs of scabies while the infestations and transmissibility persist. This frequently results in unusual clinical presentations, atypical distribution, and an unusual extent of involvement, which in some instances closely simulates a variety of other entities. It will be of interest to see if scabies incognito occurs after use of hydrocortisone (0.5%) over-the-counter preparations.

## Nodular scabies

The ratio of nodular to other forms of scabies is 1:15 or greater. The nodules are reddish brown and pruritic and occur on covered parts, most frequently male genitalia, groin, and axillary regions. Mites are seldom identified in nodules present for more than a month. The disease frequently remains misdiagnosed for long periods; histiocytosis X and lymphoma are considered clinically. The histologic features are similar to those of lymphoma (especially Hodgkin's disease) and arthropod bites.

Diagnosis is facilitated by the overlapping occurrence or recent history of more typical scabies (usually responding to scabicides). The nodules probably develop as a hypersensitivity reaction.

Although the nodular form of scabies clears spontaneously, the nodules may persist for months to more than a year despite antiscabietic therapy. The nodules frequently subside with nightly application of tar gel for 2 to 3 weeks. They also may improve or clear with intralesional injections of corticosteroid (triamcinolone acetonide, 5 mg/ml).

## Scabies in infants and young children

Misdiagnosis is frequent in such cases because of low index of suspicion, secondary eczematous changes (possibly widespread) suggesting other conditions, and atypical distribution to include head, neck, palms, and soles.[24] Vesicles are common. Secondary bacterial infection, manifest as pustules, bullous impetigo, severe crusting or ecthyma, is frequent. Poor feeding and failure to gain weight appropriately are characteristic features in scabies contracted during the neonatal period.[25]

Children recently adopted from foreign countries, especially Korea and Vietnam, have a high frequency of scabies, which often appears after the children arrive at their destination.[23]

## Animal-transmitted scabies

This condition is not uncommon in the United States. Although persons may be infested with mites from various animals, dogs (usually puppies) are the major source. Animal mites do not differ morphologically from human mites but differ biologically. Humans are infested inadvertently by direct or indirect contact. The condition often goes undiagnosed.

The frequency of scabies in dogs has increased since 1963 throughout the United States. The external surface of the ears is the most frequent site of predilection, corresponding to the high frequency of hand involvement in human scabies. In the United States and Canada in the past decade, a number of regional outbreaks of canine scabies transmitted to humans have been reported. Canine-transmitted scabies in humans differs from human scabies in that the former has greater ease of transmission, different distribution patterns, absence of burrows, and shorter incubation period.

Animal-transmitted scabies is self-limited (several weeks). The animal should be treated by a veterinarian skilled in veterinary dermatology. Symptomatic family members may be treated with supportive measures. It is unnecessary to treat asymptomatic members of the household or sexual contacts outside the household, since the condition usually is not contagious between humans.

## Crusted (Norwegian) scabies

This rare condition is highly contagious, even on casual contact, because of the myriad of mites in the exfoliating scales. Local or regional epidemics of more typical forms of scabies frequently result, usually in hospitals or other institutions. Crusted scabies is a psoriasiform dermatosis of the hands and feet, with dystrophy of the nails and a variable erythematous, scaling eruption that may become generalized; it usually takes a number of months for this morphology to become fixed. Pruritus is minimal. The disease shows a predilection for the mentally retarded, physically debilitated, or immunologically deficient (from congenital or iatrogenic cause). Crusted scabies is a rare complication in renal transplant patients receiving immunosuppressive therapy.

An abortive papular form of scabies, probably due to infestation with immature forms (without adult females), has been noted in fellow patients and particularly in medical, nursing, and supportive staff exposed to patients with crusted scabies. This eruption consists of erythematous papules, similar to papular urticaria, on the arms and legs.

Therapy for crusted scabies is similar to that for the more common types, although this type responds more slowly and may require repeated applications of scabicides. Use of a keratolytic agent before application of the scabicide may facilitate resolution.

## Scabies with other sexually transmitted diseases

Sexual transmission of scabies, particularly in sexually active young adults, is common. This infestation is frequently seen at venereal disease clinics and may coexist with gonorrhea, syphilis, pediculosis pubis, and other sexually transmissible conditions. A diagnosis of scabies, particularly when penile lesions are present, should prompt search for coexisting sexually transmitted disease, beginning with culture for gonorrhea and serologic test for syphilis. The frequency of asymptomatic gonorrhea is high in female patients with scabies, particularly in the 15- to 29-year age group.[26] The chancre of syphilis (the so-called chancre galeuse) is sometimes seen in a cutaneous lesion of scabies.[27]

## Atypical scabies with HIV infection

Atypical (crusted or "exaggerated") scabies may occur in patients with HIV infection.[28] It is one of the many types of opportunistic infections and cutaneous manifestations seen in patients with AIDS.

## Secondary infections and their complications

Secondary bacterial infections may complicate scabies. Nephritogenic streptococcal strains may colonize scabietic lesions and lead to acute glomerulonephritis. This has been reported mainly in tropical areas, but recently has been reported in Canada and France; its potential is universal.

## DIFFERENTIAL DIAGNOSIS

Scabies is a great imitator. Differential diagnosis includes nearly all pruritic dermatoses,[29] including atopic dermatitis, contact dermatitis, prurigo, papular urticaria, pyoderma, pruritus due to systemic disease, pruritic dermatoses of pregnancy, infectious eczematoid dermatitis, insect bites, cheyletiella dermatitis, excoriations, lichen planus, dermatitis herpetiformis, mastocytosis, urticaria, and pediculosis, as well as syphilis, keratosis follicularis, and vasculitis.

## DIAGNOSIS (Table 42-2)

Table 42-2. Laboratory Techniques for Microscopic Study

1. Skin scrapings
2. Needle extraction of mite
3. Epidermal shave biopsy
4. Burrow ink test (BIT)
5. Curettage of burrows
6. Swab technique with clear cellophane adhesive
7. Topical tetracycline, then Wood's light
8. Punch biopsy

## LABORATORY TECHNIQUES FOR MICROSCOPIC STUDY

1. *Skin scrapings* Recently developed, unexcoriated papules or burrows are located with the help of a hand lens or head loupe. Mineral oil is placed on a sterile scalpel blade and allowed to flow into the lesions.[30] Vigorous scraping with the blade about six or seven times removes the top of burrows or papules. The oil and scraped material are transferred to a glass slide, and a cover slip is applied. Diagnosis is confirmed by the presence of any stage of the mite or the typical fecal pellets, which outnumber the living organisms. (Fig. 42-3, Plate 80).
2. *Sewing needle or pin to prick out mite from undamaged burrows*[1,2,31] The needle is used to perforate the burrow at the site of the mite (the "dark point" in white patients and the "white point" in black patients); the needle is moved tangential to the skin from side to side; the mite will grip the end of the needle, then transfer the mite to the slide.
3. *Epidermal shave biopsy*[32] Locate a suspicious papule or burrow, elevate the papule between the thumb and forefinger (or use curved forceps for elevation), and gently "saw" off the top of the lesion with a 15 scalpel blade held parallel to the skin surface. The biopsy is so superficial that bleeding should not occur nor should local anesthesia be necessary. The biopsy material is placed on a glass slide and examined with a light microscope. Care should be taken if dealing with a small child. Martin and Wheeler[32] reported 90 to 95 percent positive findings in patients in whom scabies was the leading diagnosis.
4. *Burrow ink test (BIT)*[33] Gently rub the scabietic papule with the underside of an inexpensive fountain pen, covering the papule with ink; immediately wipe off the surface ink from the lesion with an alcohol pad. In the BIT-positive lesion the ink will track down the mite burrow by forming a characteristic dark zigzag line running across and away from the papule. The BIT has the advantage over the superficial shave

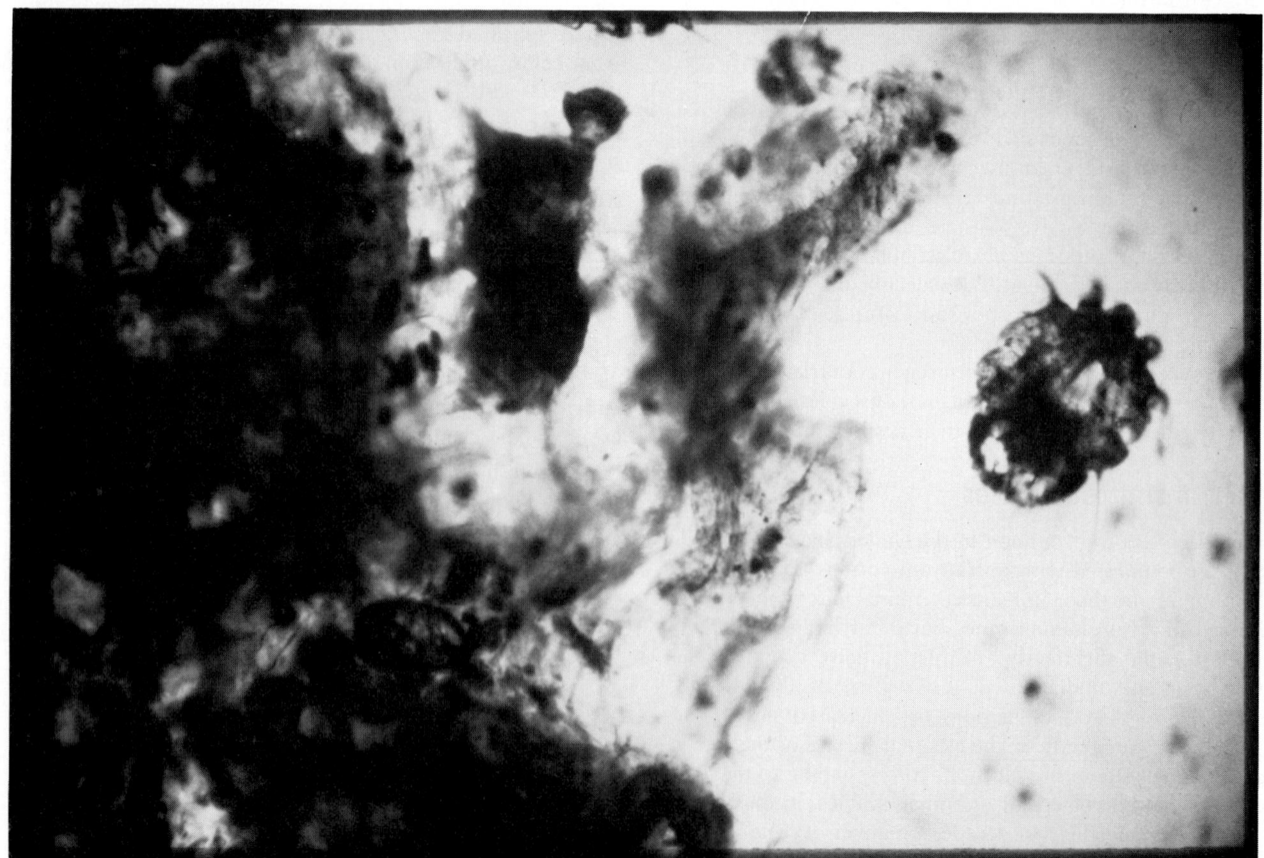

Fig. 42-3. Skin scrapings of unexcoriated papules fortuitously disclose adults, larva, eggs, and fecal pellets, any of which would be diagnostic.

biopsy of being painless and more useful in the child or uncooperative patient; however, there may be false-negative tests with the BIT. Some prefer use of the BIT to identify suspicious lesions, followed by a superficial shave biopsy (Plate 81).

5. *Curettage of burrows*[34] Superficially curette the long axis of a burrow, or across the summit of a papule, and deposit the curetting on a clean slide with the aid of a scalpel, then place one to two drops of mineral oil on the curetting and cover with a cover slip. This technique is particularly valuable in infants, small children, and uncooperative patients.
6. *Skin-swab technique with clear cellophane adhesive tape*[35] Clean the skin with ether, then apply cellophane tape to the lesion and remove with brisk movement; strips of adhesive tape are stuck on the slide (six strips of the same lesion on one slide) and the slide is examined microscopically.
7. *Topical tetracycline to area of suspected burrows* Apply topical tetracycline, wipe off, and examine area with Wood's light.
8. Punch biopsies can also be used to demonstrate mites or products.

## THERAPY

Specific measures for nodular scabies, animal-transmitted scabies, and crusted scabies are discussed in the sections describing these forms.

## PRINCIPLES[36]

The choice of a drug for treatment of scabies must take into account efficacy and potential toxicity. There has been limited interest in comparative, controlled efficacy trials of scabicides.

Patients tend to apply the drugs more frequently and over longer periods than prescribed. Limiting the quantity prescribed prevents overtreatment dermatitis, which the patient may mistake for persistence of the scabies, and minimizes percutaneous penetration. Approximately 30 mg (1 oz) of a topical preparation is required to cover adequately the trunk and extremities of an average adult; proportionately less is needed for children and infants. The scabicide should be applied thinly but thoroughly from the neck downward to all areas, with special attention to the hands, feet, and intertriginous areas.

Selective treatment of asymptomatic family members at high risk for acquiring the infestation from a confirmed case may be appropriate.[37] If the patient routinely shares a bed with another person, the probability is high that transmission to that person has already occurred, and therefore treatment of the asymptomatic bed partner is justified. Sexual contacts should also be treated simultaneously. It is less significant to treat those with minimal skin-to-skin contact with an infested family member.

Twenty-four hours after effective therapy, the patient can no longer transmit the disease. However, symptoms and signs may not clear for weeks, since the hypersensitivity state does not cease immediately on mite destruction. The patient should be alerted to this possibility so that he or she will know what to expect. Intimate apparel should be washed and dried by machine (hot cycle in each), washed and ironed, or boiled.

Treatment can fail if the patient does not follow instructions. Reinfestation from an outside source does not occur commonly except with sexual transmission. Dermatitis, generally from too frequent use of a scabicide, is usually irritant in nature. Resistance can be proved only by again demonstrating the mites in patients in whom there is reasonable assurance that the medication has been properly applied. Acarophobia (delusions of parasitosis) is not uncommon with or without scabies; diagnosis should not be made until examination fails to show infestation.

## SPECIFIC AGENTS

Commonly used scabicides and instructions for their use are presented in Table 42-3.[38]

### Lindane cream or lotion

Lindane cream or lotion is easy to use and effective. Allergic contact dermatitis from this agent has not been documented; irritant contact dermatitis from too frequent use is not uncommon. Of a single dose of lindane in acetone applied to the forearm, 9 percent can be accounted for in the urine;[39] cutaneous absorption has been verified in scabietic and normal children by Ginsburg and associates.[40] Studies of acute toxicity have shown central nervous system (CNS) toxicity. Careful studies to determine the presence or absence of subclinical CNS toxicity have not been performed, nor has CNS toxicity from appropriately used topical therapy been proved.[41] Clinical CNS toxicity has been limited to misuse situations.

Until appropriate toxicological data become available, we prefer not to use lindane in infants, young children, or pregnant women, nor should it be used in patients with seizure disorders or in patients with other neurologic disease. In older children and nonpregnant adults, an application of the lotion is left on for 8 to 12 h and washed off thoroughly; the lotion should be kept away from the eyes and mucous membranes. A second application is appropriate only when there is evidence of failure of compliance (the family should be instructed again), reinfestation, or resistance.

Kramer et al.[42] reviewed the reports of adverse drug reactions to lindane cream or lotion and concluded that this scabicide was safe to use in infants and small children, as long as the manufacturer's instructions were followed. However, Kramer and as-

**Table 42-3. Therapy of Scabies**

| Lindane* | Crotamiton* | Sulfur |
|---|---|---|
| Cream or lotion, 1% (Gammexane, Kwell, Quellada, Scabene) | Cream, 10% (*N*-ethyl-*o*-crotonotoluidide; Eurax) | Precipitated sulfur, 6% |
| 1. Apply one thin layer to entire trunk and extremities and leave on for 8–12 h. | 1. Massage medication into skin from neck downward nightly for two nights. | 1. Apply preparation to trunk and extremities nightly for three nights. |
| 2. At end of 8–12 h, shower or bathe to thoroughly remove medication; change intimate apparel and bed linen. | 2. Twenty-four hours after second application, wash off medication thoroughly; change intimate apparel and bed linen. | 2. Twenty-four hours after last application, bathe to thoroughly remove medication; change intimate apparel and bed linen. |

**Nonrefillable* prescription should be made for only amount needed.

sociates suggested additional precautions: (1) hot bath or shower should be avoided before the application; (2) each application should be limited to 6 h; (3) repeat treatments should be limited to a maximum of two applications separated by at least 1 week; (4) to prevent licking or mouthing the drug during the application period, the infant or young child should be fully clothed or under the direct observation of a responsible adult.

### Sulfur

Used for centuries, sulfur is generally prescribed as precipitated sulfur (5 to 10%) in petrolatum. The ointment is applied nightly for three successive nights. Patients find it less acceptable than modern scabicides because of odor, messiness and staining. We prefer precipitated sulfur in infants, in small children, in pregnant and lactating women, as well as in patients with seizure disorders or other neurologic diseases.

### Crotamiton

Crotamiton has not been a highly effective scabicide in our experience and that of others. Sensitization occurs rarely but not in scabies therapy. Crotamiton cream should be thoroughly massaged into the skin from the neck downward, with particular attention to the hands, feet, and intertriginous areas; a second application should be administered 24 h later.

The clinical experience of crotamiton in the treatment of infants and young children with scabies was addressed. Cubela and Yawalkar[43] found five daily applications of crotamiton cream necessary for adequate (cure rate of 70 percent) treatment of scabies; the crotamiton cream was far better than the crotamiton lotion. Konstantinov et al.[44] reported 100 percent cure rate with five applications of either crotamiton cream or lotion in 50 hospitalized scabietic infants and small children. In both studies the crotamiton was well tolerated and no side effects were noted. Future studies may confirm that five consecutive daily applications of crotamiton are better than the two currently recommended.

## ACCOMPANYING MEDICATIONS

An oral antipruritic medication, such as an antihistamine or salicylate, may be used simultaneously with the scabicide. For the pruritus that characteristically lingers after adequate antiscabietic therapy, a hydrocortisone preparation may provide symptomatic relief in adults, and a lubricating agent or emollient may be helpful in infants and small children.

Most patients with secondarily infected scabies do not require systemic antibacterial therapy; the bacterial aspect clears with scabicidal therapy. When bacterial infection is extensive, some physicians prefer to also utilize oral antibacterial agents. The organism probably will be either *Staphylococcus aureus* or betahemolytic streptococci group A. The agents employed should depend on knowledge of the sensitivity of bacteria in that geographic location: it is rarely necessary to perform culture and sensitivity studies except for epidemiologic purposes. The use or avoidance of systemic antimicrobials does not alter the likelihood of developing poststreptococcal glomerulonephritis.

In a rare instance of incapacitating posttreatment itching in an adult, a short course of systemic corticosteroid therapy, such as a 7- to 10-day course of prednisone at initial dosage of 40 mg per day, gives prompt, dramatic relief.

## PREVENTION

Early diagnosis and treatment with an effective scabicide for the patient as well as appropriate household and sexual contacts of infested persons is the key to prevention. A high index of suspicion on the part of the clinician is important. Attempting to prove the diagnosis by demonstrating the organism will help to prevent overdiagnosis.

# References


1 Mellanby K: *Scabies,* 2d ed. London, Classey, 1972.
2 Heilesen B: Studies on *Acarus scabiei* and scabies. *Acta Derm Venereol [Suppl] (Stockh)* 26(14):1, 1946.
3 Mellanby K: Biology of the parasite, in *Scabies and Pediculosis,* M Orkin et al (eds). Philadelphia, Lippincott, 1977, pp 8–16.
4 Orkin M: Resurgence of scabies. *JAMA* 217:593, 1971.
5 Orkin M, Maibach HI: Scabies, a current pandemic. *Postgrad Med* 66:52, 1979.
6 Frentz G et al: Immunofluorescence studies in scabies. *J Cutan Pathol* 4:191, 1977.
7 Hoefling KK, Schroeter AL: Dermatoimmunopathology of scabies. *J Am Acad Dermatol* 3:237, 1980.
8 Van Neste D, Salmon J: Circulating antigen-antibody complexes in scabies. *Dermatologica* 157:221, 1978.
9 Van Neste D, Salmon J: Immune complexes in scabies. *Dermatologica* 160:131, 1980.
10 Falk ES: Serum immunoglobulin values in patients with scabies. *Br J Dermatol* 102:57, 1980.
11 Falk ES, Bolle R: IgE antibodies to house dust mite in patients with scabies. *Br J Dermatol* 102:283, 1980.
12 Falk ES: Serum IgE before and after treatment for scabies. *Allergy* 36:167, 1981.
13 Falk ES, Bolle R: In vitro demonstration of specific immunological hypersensitivity to scabies mite. *Br J Dermatol* 103:367, 1980.
14 Van Neste D: Immunologic studies in scabies. *Int J Dermatol* 20:264, 1981.
15 Falk ES, Thorsby E: HLA antigens in patients with scabies. *Br J Dermatol* 104:317, 1981.
16 Bjornberg A, Friis B: Persistent pustulosis in children adopted from Asia: A sequela of scabies? *Int J Dermatol* 17:69, 1978.
17 Alexander AM: Role of race in scabies infestation. *Arch Dermatol* 114:627, 1978.
18 Mellanby K: Epidemiology of scabies, in *Scabies and Pediculosis*, M Orkin et al (eds). Philadelphia, Lippincott, 1977, pp 60–63.
19 Epstein E Sr, Orkin M: Scabies: Clinical aspects, in *Scabies and Pediculosis*, M Orkin et al (eds). Philadelphia, Lippincott, 1977, pp 17–22.
20 Juranek D, Schultz MG: Epidemiologic investigations of scabies in the United States, in *Scabies and Pediculosis*, M Orkin et al (eds). Philadelphia, Lippincott, 1977, pp. 64–72.
21 Gooch JJ et al: Nosocomial outbreak of scabies. *Arch Dermatol* 114:897, 1978.
22 Shelley WB, Wood MG: Larval papule as a sign of scabies. *JAMA* 236:1144, 1976.
23 Orkin M: Today's scabies. *JAMA* 233:882, 1975.
24 Hurwitz S: Scabies in babies. *Am J Dis Child* 126:226, 1973.
25 Burns BR et al: Neonatal scabies. *Am J Dis Child* 133:1031, 1979.
26 Nielsen AO et al: Gonorrhea in patients with scabies. *Br J Vener Dis* 52:394, 1976.
27 Beek CH, Mellanby K: Scabies, in *Handbook of Tropical Dermatology and Medical Mycology*, RDGP Simon (ed). Amsterdam, Elsevier, 1953, pp 875–888.
28 Sadick N et al: Unusual features complicating human T-lymphotropic virus type III infection. *J Am Acad Dermatol* 15:482, 1986.
29 Orkin M, Maibach HI: Current concepts in parasitology: This scabies pandemic. *N Engl J Med* 298:496, 1978.

30 Muller G et al: Scraping for human scabies: A better method for positive preparations. *Arch Dermatol* 107:70, 1973.

31 Lomholt G: Demonstration of sarcoptes scabiei. *Arch Dermatol* 114:1096, 1978.

32 Martin WE, Wheeler CE Jr: Diagnosis of human scabies by epidermal shave biopsy. *J Am Acad Dermatol* 1:335, 1979.

33 Woodley D, Saurat JH: The Burrow Ink Test and the scabies mite. *J Am Acad Dermatol* 4:715, 1981.

34 Howell JB: Office diagnosis of scabies. *Arch Dermatol Syph* 62:144, 1950.

35 Proenca N: Skin-swab technique with adhesive tape. *Cutis* 17:802, 1976.

36 Orkin M et al: Treatment of today's scabies and pediculosis. *JAMA* 236:1136, 1976.

37 Orkin M et al: Treatment of household and sexual contacts of patients with scabies, in *Controversies in Dermatology*, E Epstein Sr (ed). Philadelphia, Saunders, 1983.

38 Orkin M et al: Scabies: A practical protocol for managing the pandemic. *Mod Med* 46:66, 1978.

39 Feldman RH, Maibach HI: Percutaneous penetration of some pesticides and herbicides in man. *Toxicol Appl Pharmacol* 28:126, 1974.

40 Ginsburg CM et al: Absorption of lindane (gamma benzene hexachloride) in infants and children. *J Pediatr* 91:998, 1977.

41 Maibach HI, Orkin M: Adverse reaction to treatment in *Cutaneous Infestations and Insect Bites*, M Orkin and HI Maibach (eds). New York, Marcel Dekker, 1985.

42 Kramer MS et al: Operational criteria for adverse drug reactions in evaluating suspected toxicity of a popular scabicide. *Clin Pharmacol Therap* 27:149, 1980.

43 Cubela V, Yawalkar SJ: Clinical experience with crotamiton cream and lotion in treatment of infants with scabies. *Br J Clin Pract* 32:229, 1978.

44 Konstantinov D et al: Crotamiton cream and lotion in the treatment of infants and young children with scabies. *J Int Med Res* 7:443, 1979.

# Chapter 43
# *Trichomonas vaginalis* and trichomoniasis

Michael F. Rein
Miklós Müller

Trichomoniasis, an infection with a flagellated protozoon, *Trichomonas vaginalis*, is a common sexually transmitted infection. *T. vaginalis* was described by Donné as early as 1836[1] but was for a long time regarded as a commensal. Its role as a primary pathogen of the human urogenital tract is now undisputed. The pathogenicity of the organism was established in the first half of this century by inoculating volunteer women[2] and men[3] with axenically cultured *T. vaginalis*. A significant percentage of these persons developed clinically apparent trichomoniasis. Although in *T. vaginalis* infections other pathogens are often present, contributing to the clinical picture, recent evaluation of symptoms and signs in trichomoniasis,[4] controlled for other known pathogens, permitted the description of the disease entity trichomoniasis. Therapy of human trichomoniasis was inadequate until the 1960s when metronidazole and subsequently other 5-nitroimidazole derivatives were found to be highly effective systemic drugs.[5]

Two other distinct species of trichomonads that inhabit humans have been recently reviewed.[6] *Trichomonas tenax* is found in the mouth, often in association with gingivitis. It is unclear whether *T. tenax* actually contributes to the inflammatory process or whether it merely colonizes the anaerobic periodontal crevices. Similarly, *Pentatrichomonas hominis* is found in the large intestine, often in association with acute diarrheal syndromes, but its role as a pathogen is also undefined. The three species have a pronounced site specificity, and association of vaginal trichomoniasis with infestation of the mouth or the rectum has never been convincingly established. Indeed, experimental inoculation of the other trichomonad species into the vagina does not produce infection, and *T. vaginalis* cannot establish infection in the mouth or colon.[6]

Current knowledge of trichomonads of humans and the diseases they cause is discussed in detail in a recent monograph.[7]

## THE ORGANISM

*T. vaginalis* is generally ovoid, but in specimens obtained directly from patients its shape may be less regular, with ameboid properties.[8,9] The organism is 10 to 20 μm wide, although trichomonads freshly isolated from patients with more severe disease may be smaller than those from asymptomatic cases or from cultures.[10] In fresh preparations, the organism is recognized by its jerky, swaying motion. At higher magnification (×400) one can observe the beating flagella and the undulating membrane.

Locomotion is provided by four free anterior flagella and a recurrent flagellum attached to an undulating membrane which extends for about two-thirds of the length of the cell (Fig. 43-1). There is a large nucleus with the scattered chromatin characteristic of eukaryotic cells. A highly developed Golgi complex is referred to as the parabasal apparatus. Skeletal organelles include an axostyle, which consists of microtubules running more or less axially through the body and projecting at the posterior end to form a slender spike.[8,9] The cross-striated costa is situated just below the undulating membrane. The cytoplasm is rich in glycogen granules and contains free and membrane-bound ribosomes. Large vacuoles, possibly of endocytic origin, are often present. Relatively large, dense granules are located along the axostyle and costa. These membrane-limited chromatic granules, called hydrogenosomes,[11,12] stain intensely with basic dyes and occur only in certain other anaerobic protozoa and fungi. *T. vaginalis* contains no mitochondria. The structure of *T. vaginalis* is described in detail in Ref. 8.

*T. vaginalis* attaches to mucous membranes. An adhesin has been described.[13] In attached cells, an organelle-free dense zone develops in the area of contact.[14] The membranes of the parasite and mucosal cells interdigitate in the zone of contact. Blocking

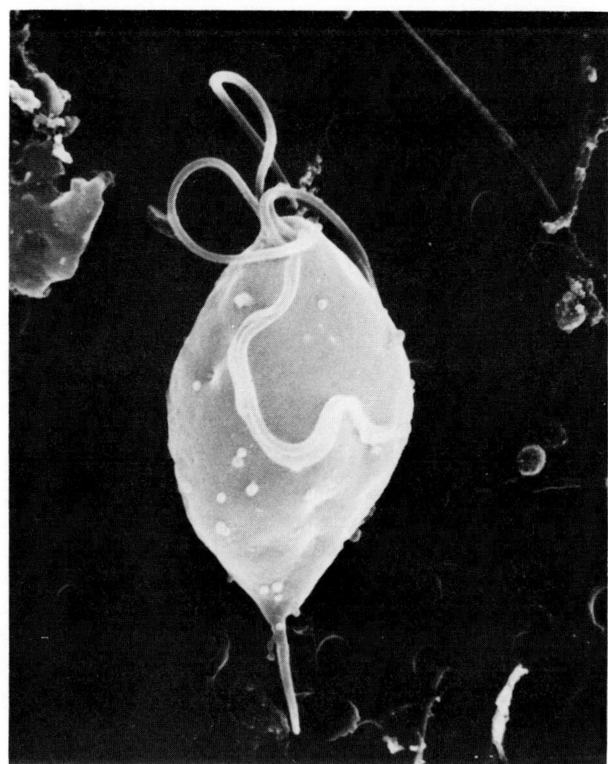

Fig. 43-1. Scanning electron micrograph of *Trichomonas vaginalis*. Three of the four anterior flagella (and the origin of the fourth), the undulating membrane with its trailing flagellum, and the axostyle protruding at the end of the body are clearly seen. ×6000 magnification. (*From A Warton, BM Honigberg, J Protozool 26:56, 1979.*)

of this process by the microfilament inhibitor cytochalasin B inhibits attachment.[15,16]

Most soluble nutrients are transported through the cell membrane, but *T. vaginalis* ingests bacteria and other particulate matter by phagocytosis.[9,17] Food vacuoles formed in this way fuse with lysosomes, and their contents are digested. The overall contribution of endocytosis to the nutrition of *T. vaginalis* is not known.

*T. vaginalis* is usually described as anaerobic; optimal in vitro growth occurs under moderately anaerobic conditions. The organism has a fermentative energy metabolism.[11,18] Its major metabolic end products are glycerol, lactate, acetate, carbon dioxide, and, under anaerobic conditions, molecular hydrogen. The first two are formed by cytosolic glycolysis whereas the latter are produced from pyruvate in the hydrogenosomes by an enzyme system similar to those present in obligately anaerobic bacteria, which differs markedly from the pyruvate metabolizing systems of aerobes and facultative anaerobes. The biosynthetic capabilities of the organism are limited. It requires a number of nutrients including a carbohydrate, preformed purines, pyrimidines, fatty acids, and sterols.

*T. vaginalis* reproduces by binary fission and exists only as a vegetative cell. Cysts and other forms resistant to the environment have never been documented convincingly.[8,9]

Differences among strains and isolates of *T. vaginalis* have been clearly defined. Serotypes with unique and common antigens have been identified by a variety of immunological techniques.[9,19] The surface expression of various antigens is subject to regulation and might be correlated with changes in virulence.[20] Isoenzyme patterns of various isolates also differ.[21,22] Certain isolates contain double-stranded RNA viruses.[23] Strains of different sizes[10] and rates of growth[9] have been identified, and these characteristics might be related to virulence. Isolates differ in their ability to produce inflammation in a variety of experimental systems (see below).

## EPIDEMIOLOGY

The predominant role of sexual contact in the transmission of human genitourinary trichomoniasis is well established. The epidemiology of this disease has been reviewed recently.[24,25]

## PREVALENCE IN WOMEN

Because in most countries trichomoniasis is not reportable, incidence figures are sketchy, and those existing are often outdated. The National Drug and Therapeutic Index suggests that about 2 million cases of trichomoniasis were treated by office-based physicians in the United States during a 12-month period ending in June 1974;[26] 2.5 to 3 million American women were then thought to contract trichomoniasis annually.[26] In the seventies the World Health Organization estimated 180 million cases of trichomonal infection were acquired annually worldwide.[26]

The prevalence of trichomoniasis in specific groups correlates with the general level of sexual activity. Trichomoniasis has been diagnosed in about 5 percent of women in family planning clinics or among married female employees, compared with 13 to 25 percent of women attending gynecology clinics, and 50 to 75 percent of prostitutes. The prevalence of trichomoniasis among women in STD clinics has ranged from 7 to 32 percent.[4,26] In a series of consecutive cases seen in a primary health care unit attending because of vaginal discharge, 9 percent presented with trichomoniasis.[27]

In many countries, trichomoniasis has, during the last decade, become less and less commonly seen in women attending gynecological clinics. A Swedish STD clinic reported a prevalence of trichomoniasis of 5.4 percent in 1980 while in 1987 it was only 0.7 percent.[28]

The method of contraception used affects the prevalence of trichomoniasis. Trichomoniasis was significantly associated with nonuse of barrier methods (4 vs. 20 percent) and nonuse of oral contraceptives (20 vs. 34 percent).[4] The rate of oral contraceptive use is somewhat lower among women with trichomoniasis than among women with other sexually transmitted diseases.[29,30] Estrogens have no direct effect on trichomonad growth but may act by changing the vaginal environment.[30] Although contraceptive foam is highly active against trichomonads in vitro,[31] a clinical protective effect has not been documented.

## PREVALENCE IN MEN

Information on the prevalence of trichomoniasis in men is even more sketchy because of the large fraction of asymptomatic cases, the frequently self-limited nature of the infection, and the difficulty in diagnosis. The infection was diagnosed in the late seventies in up to 4 percent of men attending STD clinics.[32] In the sixties a prevalence of 5 to 20 percent was reported among men with nongonococcal urethritis.[33–37] More recent studies indicate much lower prevalence figures of trichomoniasis in men.

## SEXUAL TRANSMISSION

Several lines of evidence support the importance of the venereal acquisition of trichomoniasis. Trichomoniasis is most prevalent among the sexual partners of patients with documented infection. The organism is usually demonstrated in 30 to 40 percent of the male sexual partners of infected women.[9,28,34,37] A prevalence of 70 percent was observed among men who had sexual contact with infected women within the previous 48 h; only 33 percent of men were infected if their last contact was 2 weeks previously.[38] Trichomoniasis is generally documented in at least 85 percent of the female partners of infected men.[9] Asymptomatically infected men are probably an important vector and perhaps a reservoir of disease, and eventual control of trichomoniasis depends on effective treatment of men as well as women. Several studies have suggested an increased cure rate in women following treatment of their regular sexual partners.[39–42]

Detection of trichomonads in young, premenarchal girls can indicate sexual abuse.[43]

A decade ago trichomoniasis could be diagnosed in 8 to 62 percent of women with gonorrhea.[44–46] Of clinical significance is the high prevalence of gonorrhea in women with trichomoniasis.[29,30,32,33,44–46] The prevalence of gonorrhea is 1.4 to 3 times higher among women with trichomoniasis than among women without this infection.[4,46] Trichomonads have been isolated from 16 to 20 percent of men with gonococcal urethritis.[28,46] These associations make it imperative that patients with trichomoniasis be evaluated for the presence of other sexually transmitted diseases.

An inoculum of less than $10^4$ trichomonads will initiate experimental infection in women[2] and of $4 \times 10^6$ cells will initiate infection in men.[3]

## NONVENEREAL TRANSMISSION

Perinatal acquisition of disease represents the most frequent form of nonvenereal transmission. Such infection has been reported in about 5 percent of female babies born of infected mothers.[47–49]

Nonvenereal acquisition of *T. vaginalis* by adults must be relatively infrequent. The site specificity of the organism means that infection can follow only intravaginal or intraurethral inoculation.

The organism is very sensitive to desiccation, but if not desiccated it can survive for several hours in various body fluids (urine, semen, vaginal exudates). It also can survive in or on moist objects (sponges, towels, toilet seats, etc.).[24] In spite of the possibility of transmission via objects contaminated with body fluids, no well-documented cases have been reported.

## PATHOGENESIS

The mechanisms by which *T. vaginalis* causes disease remain to be elucidated. Clinical and experimental observations suggest that the virulence of the organism, susceptibility and reactivity of the host, and features of epidemiology, such as combined infections, all contribute to clinical severity.

## OBSERVATIONS IN HUMAN INFECTIONS

### Urogenital infection

Trichomoniasis due to *T. vaginalis* is an infection almost exclusively of the urogenital tract.

In adult women with trichomoniasis, the organisms are isolated from the vagina in over 95 percent of infections and from the urinary tract only in less than 5 percent.[50] Only areas covered by squamous but not by columnar epithelium are involved.[14] Although the exterior of the cervix shares in the vaginal inflammatory response, trichomonads are isolated from the endocervix in no more than 13 percent of women.[50] Endocervical specimens should not be used in an attempt to diagnose trichomoniasis.

The urethra and Skene's glands are infected in 90 percent of cases.[28,50,51] Dysuria and discharge from the urethra or Skene's ducts may result, and a wet mount examination of material recovered from the urethra yields organisms in more than half of infected women.[51] Organisms have been isolated from bladder urine.[40] In prepubescent girls, the vagina does not support growth of trichomonads, and the urinary tract may be the only site of infection.

The greatest significance of these extravaginal genitourinary sites of infection is that organisms may persist there even after they have been eliminated from the vagina by local therapy as advocated presently in pregnant women.

Involvement proximal to the cervix is extremely rare, possibly because of the relative resistance of columnar epithelium.[14]

The urethra is the most common site of infection in men. Involvement of other parts of the urogenital tract is much less frequently documented. Trichomonads have been identified in epididymal aspirates,[52] and prostatic involvement has been suggested.[34,53] Although trichomonads are frequently identified in the urine of infected men, infestation of the bladder is not well documented. Trichomonads have been isolated from the subpreputial sac[34] and from lesions of the penis.[45,54]

Trichomonads, probably *T. vaginalis*, have been occasionally isolated from the kidney and once from a perinephric abscess.[55]

### Extraurogenital infection

Infestation by *T. vaginalis* outside the urogenital tract is extremely rare.[6] Disseminated infection with *T. vaginalis* has never been described even in severely immunocompromised patients, suggesting that the site specificity of infection depends on factors other than traditionally recognized host defenses. Whether *T. vaginalis* is particularly fastidious with respect to microenvironment or whether only a very select range of host cells is susceptible for attachment is unclear.

Trichomonads were repeatedly detected at extraurogenital sites, e.g., lungs and pleural cavity[56–58] and cerebrospinal fluid,[59] usually in cases with severe underlying disease. The organisms were rarely identified as *T. vaginalis* but in most cases were probably *Trichomonas tenax* or *Pentatrichomonas hominis*.[6]

### Host-parasite relationships

Trichomonal infection of women ranges from an asymptomatic carrier state to profound, acute, inflammatory disease. About one-third of asymptomatically infected women become symptomatic within 6 months, suggesting that changes in the host may contribute to pathogenetic expression. Some observers have noted the frequency with which symptoms of trichomoniasis either appear or exacerbate during or immediately following the menstrual period.[60] This observation also suggests that the vaginal microenvironment affects the pathogenicity of trichomonads and may vary from time to time in the same patient. Other factors in the vaginal microenvironment, including menstrual blood, pH, oxidation-reduction potential, hormonal levels, or other microbes, may contribute to the expression of pathogenicity (see Chap. 12). The frequency with which asymptomatic trichomoniasis eventually becomes symptomatic supports the contention that asymptomatic infection should be treated when it is diagnosed.

Infected male sexual partners of women with florid disease are usually asymptomatic.[33,34] The absence of an inflammatory response in the male urethra to infection with the same strain of trichomonads producing severe disease in the vagina further supports the argument that the pathogenicity of trichomonads is dependent on features of the site of infection.

### Pathologic observations

Trichomonal infection in women usually elicits an acute inflammatory response resulting in a vaginal discharge containing large numbers of polymorphonuclear neutrophils (PMN). Trichomonads are found in the vaginal cavity, or adhering to the epithelial surfaces; there is no invasion of the mucosa.[14] Colposcopy reveals proliferation and a characteristic double cresting of mucosal capillaries[61] and microhemorrhages.[4] Only squamous epithelium is involved.[14]

Large numbers of PMN are observed in the vaginal cavity. Biopsies show migration of PMN into the deeper epithelial layers. The number of PMN in discharge correlates roughly with the degree of the patient's symptoms.

Cytopathologic and histopathologic changes associated with

urogenital trichomoniasis in women[62] and men[63] have been reviewed recently.

## EXPERIMENTAL INFECTIONS

The pathogenicity of *T. vaginalis* has been studied in animal models and in tissue cultures.[9,64–66] In common laboratory animals (e.g., rodents) persistent, symptomatic vaginal infections have not been obtained yet; thus most models employ ectopic, intraperitoneal, and subcutaneous infections. Squirrel monkeys have been developed recently as promising models for vaginal infections.[67] Additional information has come from studies of infected organ and tissue cultures. Although sometimes contradictory, experimental work generally supports the concepts that trichomonads vary in their pathogenicity and that host factors also contribute to the clinical expression of disease. It is generally held that *T. vaginalis* destroys the epithelial cells it contacts, although the mechanism(s) of cytotoxicity are unknown.[15,68]

## IMMUNITY AND IMMUNE RESPONSE

Repeated trichomonal infections are common, and clinically significant protective immunity does not appear to occur in trichomoniasis. There are no data suggesting that trichomoniasis is more severe or becomes disseminated in neutropenic or immunocompromised patients. Some degree of systemic immunity can be demonstrated in experimental subcutaneous infections of mice. Immune reactions to *T. vaginalis* in humans and experimental animals have recently been reviewed.[69]

### HUMORAL IMMUNE RESPONSE

Serum antibody, usually at low titers, has been detected in human infections by a variety of techniques including complement fixation, agglutination, passive hemagglutination, and indirect fluorescence.[9,70–73] This antibody response is usually considered insufficiently reliable for diagnostic purposes.

Antitrichomonal IgA has been detected in three-quarters of women with acute trichomoniasis but also in almost half of women without current infection.[73] Lower levels of antitrichomonal antibody were seen in patients with a larger parasite load,[73] suggesting that local antibody may have some role in host defense. Local antibody has not been detected in male urogenital trichomoniasis.[74] Trichomonads activate serum complement via the alternative pathway, and they are susceptible to complement-mediated lysis to a variable degree, dependent on the isolate.[75]

### CELL-MEDIATED IMMUNITY

#### Delayed hypersensitivity

Delayed hypersensitivity develops in natural human infection and has been demonstrated by intradermal injection of killed protozoa or fragments in 27 to 82 percent of women and 37 to 75 percent of men with acute infection,[9] but the reaction is not useful diagnostically. Trichomonads contain and release substances which activate T lymphocytes.[76]

#### Phagocytic cells and lymphocytes

The predominant cell type responding to natural infection is the PMN as shown by the high numbers of these cells in the vaginal exudate. Trichomonads contain and release substances chemoattractive to PMN.[77] PMN may be observed to attach to trichomonads in fresh preparations from acute infections. Phagocytosis of trichomonads by PMN has been observed in subcutaneous abscesses in mice.[78] In vitro, PMN are capable of rapidly killing *T. vaginalis* using oxidative bactericidal systems.[79] Groups of PMN have also been observed to disrupt trichomonads and phagocytize the pieces.[79] Phagocytosis of trichomonads by macrophages is occasionally observed in human infections,[80] and macrophages have been shown to kill trichomonads in vitro.[81] The actual contribution of phagocytic cells to host defenses in natural infection remains to be defined.

## CLINICAL FEATURES

### DISEASE IN WOMEN

The percentage of women harboring trichomonads who have symptoms varies with the manner in which cases are selected and ranges from 50 to 90 percent.[4,9,29,33,82] Women attend vaginitis clinics primarily because of symptoms. The percentage of trichomonal infections which are asymptomatic is obviously correspondingly low in that population. Infected women often have insufficiently severe symptoms to prompt them to seek medical attention but on questioning indicate some mild urogenital complaints. Trichomonad infection, as mentioned above, is often accompanied by infections with other organisms; thus often it is difficult to attribute the symptoms and signs observed to *T. vaginalis* alone.[4] Many women attend STD clinics as the sexual partners of men infected with other pathogens, and in this population the percentage of asymptomatic cases is higher. Clinical aspects of trichomoniasis in women have been reviewed in detail[82] and are summarized in Table 43-1.

#### History

Vaginal discharge is noted by about 50 to 75 percent of women diagnosed in STD clinics as having trichomoniasis.[4,9,29,33,82,83] The discharge is described as malodorous by only about 10 percent of patients.[33] Malodorous discharge, particularly when associated with little vulvovaginal irritation, may be more suggestive of bacterial vaginosis (see Chaps. 46 and 47). Vaginal pruritus is described by one-quarter to one-half of patients and is often severe. Up to one-half of infected patients note some degree of dyspareunia. Dysuria and, more rarely, urinary frequency are mild and resemble the discomfort of cystitis.

Lower abdominal pain is not a common complaint but has been described by 5 to 12 percent of women.[9,33,82] It is possible that this discomfort results from pelvic lymphadenitis. The clinician must, however, always be suspicious that lower abdominal pain actually represents coincident salpingitis due to other sexually transmitted organisms.

Tender inguinal adenopathy is described by small numbers of affected women.[9,60]

Many women note that the symptoms of trichomoniasis begin or exacerbate during or immediately following the menstrual period.[60] The cyclical nature of symptoms makes determination of

**Table 43-1. Prevalence of Clinical Features among Women with Trichomoniasis (from Ref. 82 with data added from Ref. 4)**

| Symptoms, signs, and laboratory findings | Prevalence, % |
|---|---|
| Symptoms: | |
| None | 9–56 |
| Discharge | 50–75 |
| Malodorous | 10–67 |
| Irritating, pruritic | 23–82 |
| Dyspareunia | 10–50 |
| Dysuria | 30–50 |
| Lower abdominal discomfort | 5–12 |
| Signs: | |
| None | ~15 |
| Diffuse vulvar erythema | 10–37 |
| Excessive discharge | 50–75 |
| Yellow, green | 5–42 |
| Frothy | 8–50 |
| Vaginal wall inflammation | 20–75 |
| Strawberry cervix | |
| Naked eye | 1–2 |
| Colposcopy | ~45 |
| Laboratory findings: | |
| pH > 4.5 | 66–91 |
| Positive whiff test | ~75 |
| Wet mount | |
| Excess PMN | ~75 |
| Motile trichomonads | 40–80 |
| Fluorescent antibody | 80–90 |
| Gram stain | <1 |
| Acridine orange | ~60 |
| Giemsa stain | ~50 |
| Papanicolaou smear | 56–70 |

an incubation period particularly difficult, but most workers have found incubation periods varying from 3 to about 28 days in experimental and natural infections.[60]

### Physical examination

The vulva is diffusely erythematous or excoriated in less than one-tenth to one-third of patients.[4,33] Vaginal discharge may be sufficient to run out onto the vulva even before a speculum is introduced. The labia range from pallid in mild disease to markedly erythematous and even edematous with more severe infection, although edema is more likely to be seen in candidiasis.[4] On insertion of the speculum, excessive discharge is observed in one-half to three-quarters of infected women[29,33,39,42,82,83] (Plate 21). The typical discharge of trichomoniasis is often described as being yellow-green and frothy, and the presence of a yellow vaginal discharge suggests trichomoniasis;[4] such typical discharge is seen in a minority of patients. The discharge is gray in about three-quarters and yellow or green in less than half of the cases.[4,36,82,83] It is visibly frothy in 8 to 50 percent of infected women,[4,40,82] and a frothy discharge is also seen in bacterial vaginosis (see Chap. 46).

The vaginal walls are erythematous in 20 to 75 percent of patients, and in more severe cases, they may have a granular appearance. The external surface of the cervix is usually involved in the same process. Punctate hemorrhages (colpitis macularis) of the cervix may result in a strawberry appearance (Plate 20) which is observed by the naked eye in only about 1 to 2 percent of cases,[29] but in 45 percent by colposcopy.[4] Its presence strongly suggests trichomoniasis.

Some patients with trichomoniasis, the proportion dependent on the population studied, show no evidence of vaginal inflammation on physical examination.

## DISEASE IN MEN

The majority of men with trichomonal infection remain asymptomatic. Many come to treatment because they are the sexual partners of women with symptomatic disease. The percentage of men with symptoms depends strongly on the method by which the cases are collected. If the population observed includes many men referred because they are the sexual partners of women with symptomatic disease, the proportion of asymptomatic male cases will increase. If the population contains many men presenting with nongonococcal urethritis, the series will be biased in favor of symptomatic cases. Thus symptomatic men accounted for about 10 to 50 percent of cases in various series.[33–35] In unselected populations fewer patients will be symptomatic. Urogenital trichomoniasis in men is reviewed in Refs. 25 and 34.

### Urethritis

It is reasonably well established that *T. vaginalis* is one cause of nongonococcal urethritis (NGU). Trichomonads are isolated from about 5 percent[33,35,37,84] to 15 to 20 percent of men with NGU.[34] This strong association does not prove an etiologic role for the trichomonad, however, because these series were not controlled for other causes of NGU such as *Chlamydia trachomatis* or *Ureaplasma urealyticum*. Trichomonal infection is more closely associated with NGU that fails to respond to treatments active against the latter agents.[34,71,72] Subsequent response to metronidazole supports the diagnosis.

An etiologic role of *T. vaginalis* in male urethritis was strongly supported by volunteer studies. Three out of five men inoculated intraurethrally with axenically cultured trichomonads developed urethral symptoms.[3] In addition, rising titers of antitrichomonal antibody were detected in men with urethritis from whom trichomonads were isolated.[25,34,71]

The incubation period compares with those of other forms of NGU,[72] as does the spectrum of symptoms. Discharge is described by 50 to 60 percent of symptomatic men.[33,35,38] In about one-third of cases it is frankly purulent, in another third mucopurulent, and the remainder have a mucoid discharge.[25,33,34,37] The discharge is usually present in very small amounts and may be apparent only as an opalescent bead visible at the meatus upon arising which disappears after micturition.[35,38,45] As in other forms of nongonococcal urethritis, the discharge may be intermittent.[72] Dysuria is experienced by less than one-quarter of men and mild pruritus by another quarter.[33,35,38] Mild urethral irritation is noted upon questioning by up to 50 percent of men,[33] and some describe a characteristic burning immediately after coitus.[39] Frank urinary frequency is relatively uncommon, being described by about 5 percent of infected men.[33,72]

Trichomonal urethritis is apparently self-limited for the majority of men. The organism can be recovered from 70 percent of men who have had sex with infected women within 48 h, but the prevalence drops to 33 percent by 2 weeks after the last sexual exposure.[38] It is possible that antitrichomonal properties of prostatic fluid contribute to the rate of spontaneous resolution.[84]

Urethral stricture of any etiology may make it difficult to cure trichomonal urethritis. About 10 percent of men exhibiting relapsing or persistent infection had some degree of stricture, and urologic evaluation is recommended for patients with relapsing trichomonal urethritis.[33–35,38,85]

### Other conditions

A few cases of acute, nongonococcal epididymitis have been attributed to trichomonal infection.[34,35,52,86] In some cases, trichomonads were observed in epididymal aspirates. The association was strongest for patients whose epididymitis did not respond to treatment with tetracyclines.[86] Coincident studies for *C. trachomatis* infection were not done in these studies, which were performed before that agent was known to be a cause of genital infection.

The prostate is said to be involved in up to 40 percent of infected patients,[34,53,71,72] but such involvement is usually asymptomatic. Two of five experimentally inoculated men developed clinical signs of prostatic inflammation.[3] The diagnosis has been entertained in men whose prostatitis did not respond to treatment with tetracyclines or some other standard antibacterial agents.[34]

It is not clear whether *T. vaginalis* actually causes genital ulcers or, more likely, merely colonizes ulcers caused by other agents.

## PEDIATRIC DISEASE

Babies born of infected mothers may contract trichomoniasis during the birth process. This risk is generally estimated as up to 5 percent.[47–49] Trichomoniasis is diagnosed in 4 to 17 percent of babies examined because of vaginal discharge.[47,87] Occasionally infected children have fever and appear fussy. Children should be treated when the diagnosis is made. In children, trichomonads can infect the urinary tract as well as the vagina.

## COMPLICATIONS

Compared with other sexually transmitted diseases, no late complications of trichomoniasis are known. Its medical significance derives primarily from its high incidence, the physical and emotional discomfort it causes, the economic consequences of time lost from work, and the cost of therapy itself. Some complications have been suggested, but these are not as well documented as those due to other sexually transmitted diseases. Thus it seems unlikely that trichomoniasis is a reversible cause of infertility, although trichomonads have been isolated from about 10 percent of some series of infertile men.[34] Such association does not, of course, imply causality. Some in vitro interactions between spermatozoa and trichomonads have been reported,[34] but their significance is not known.

## TRICHOMONIASIS IN PREGNANCY

Trichomoniasis seems to have little if any effect on pregnancy. Older studies reporting increased incidence of premature rupture of the membranes or a postpartum syndrome of fever, sometimes associated with a foul-smelling excretion or frank endometritis, were inadequately controlled for coincident infections or other factors.

## MALIGNANCY

Cancer of the cervix behaves epidemiologically as if it were a sexually transmitted disease. It is therefore not surprising that trichomoniasis has been linked in several series to carcinoma of the cervix (reviewed in Ref. 62). These series share the weakness that they were not controlled for other sexually transmitted pathogens, such as papillomavirus, which are strongly correlated with cervical malignancy. The true oncogenic potential of trichomoniasis is undefined but probably not significant.

## DIAGNOSIS

## CLINICAL DIAGNOSIS

Although certain signs and symptoms are predictive for female and male trichomoniasis, these are insufficient to establish the diagnosis, which requires the detection of the parasite either by direct microscopic examination or by culture (reviewed in Ref. 88).

Male urogenital trichomoniasis is impossible to differentiate clinically from nongonococcal urethritis (NGU) of other etiologies. Response to treatment, however, may provide useful diagnostic information. NGU that fails to respond to standard therapy active against chlamydiae and ureaplasmas may indicate trichomoniasis.

## MICROSCOPIC EXAMINATION

### In women

Definitive diagnosis of trichomoniasis depends on demonstration of the organism. With the speculum in place, material can be recovered for examination by sweeping the anterior and posterior fornices with a cotton swab or platinum loop. The cotton swab can be agitated in 1 ml of saline in a test tube and a drop of the resulting suspension transferred to a microscope slide. Alternatively, a drop of saline can be put on the microscope slide and a loop of vaginal material mixed in the drop directly on the slide. In either case, the preparation is covered with a cover slip and then briefly and gently warmed in order to increase trichomonad motility prior to examination. The slide should be examined at low (×100) and then medium (×400) magnification. If a standard bright field microscope is used, the substage condenser should be racked down or the substage diaphragm closed to increase contrast. Phase contrast microscopy is becoming more generally available and makes evaluation of the wet mount easier. Trichomonads are also readily identified by dark field examination of the suspension. *T. vaginalis* is destroyed on a potassium hydroxide preparation.

In the typical wet mount from a patient with trichomoniasis (Fig. 43-2), the epithelial cells are relatively clean with their edges sharply defined, and the nucleus is easily identified. In florid infection, epithelial cell turnover may be rapid, and one observes increased numbers of parabasilar cells.[9] These are ovoid and about two-thirds the size of typical squamous cells.

In trichomoniasis one usually sees increased numbers of PMN. There normally are a few PMN in vaginal discharge, probably of cervical origin, and PMN may be present in a ratio of about 1:1 with epithelial cells in the wet mount from normal women. About half the patients with trichomoniasis, however, have numbers of PMN far in excess of one per epithelial cell. Small num-

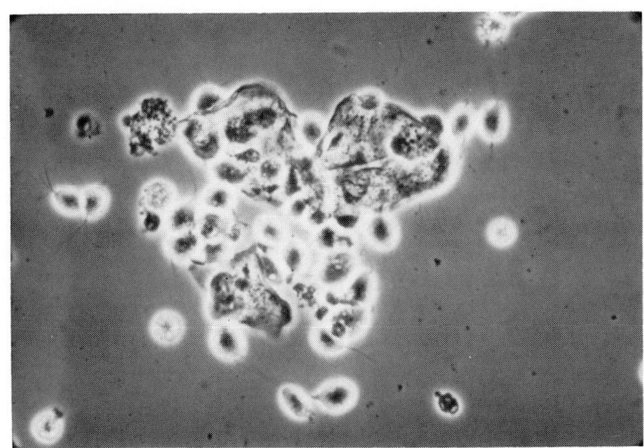

**Fig. 43-2.** Phase photomicrograph of vaginal wet mount showing epithelial cells, polymorphonuclear neutrophils, and trichomonads. (*Courtesy of Centers for Disease Control, Atlanta.*)

bers of PMN do not rule out infection. It must be remembered that PMN in the vaginal pool may be of cervical origin, and excess PMN are seen in vaginal fluid of women with mucopurulent cervicitis.

Bacteria are easily recognized in the wet mount and are either rods or, frequently, coccobacilli. Concurrent infection with *Candida albicans* or *Gardnerella vaginalis* is common, and these organisms should be sought on the wet mount.

The diagnosis of trichomoniasis is made by observing the parasites. They are ovoid and slightly larger than PMN (Fig. 43-2); they are best recognized by their motility. By phase or dark field microscopy, the individual flagella and undulating membrane are easily recognized. Observation of a single trichomonad establishes the diagnosis. Unfortunately, the wet mount reveals trichomonads in only approximately 40 to 80 percent of cases.[4,28,89–91] Thus at least one-quarter of women with trichomoniasis will not be diagnosed correctly if the wet mount is used alone.

Various stained smears (with Giemsa, acridine orange,[90] and other methods) have been proposed to diagnose trichomoniasis. They have the advantage of allowing microscopy to be deferred to a more suitable time or place. However, they have no apparent diagnostic advantage over the wet mount, and recognition of trichomonads in stained preparations requires more experience than noticing the motile organisms in fresh mounts. Gram stain is not recommended because PMN and trichomonads appear similar by this method.

Trichomonads are often reported on Papanicolaou (Pap) smears from the cervix. Pap smears have a sensitivity of about 60 to 70 percent,[4,82,89] equivalent to the wet mount. Trichomonads may be difficult to identify on Pap smear, leading to false positives as well.

Identification of trichomonads by immunofluorescent antibody[91] or by an ELISA[92,93] or latex agglutination[94] are promising[91] but still experimental techniques.[95] Each has a sensitivity of over 90 percent.

### In men

It is quite difficult to demonstrate *T. vaginalis* directly in male urine or genital secretions. Indeed only 50 percent of men with documented trichomoniasis had trichomonads identified on their first examination in one series.[38] Because small numbers of trichomonads may be present in male infection and these may be reduced by micturation, it is best to examine men prior to first voiding.[35] Trichomonads may be revealed by gently scraping the urethral mucosa with a small platinum loop and transferring the material to a drop of saline on a microscope slide for direct observation by wet mount or for staining.[60] Neither method will reveal infection in more than 30 percent of cases.[96,97] Examination of the sediment of a first morning urine, particularly after prostatic massage, will reveal trichomonads in about 15 percent of cases not diagnosed by direct examination of urethral material.[34,72]

## CULTURE

A variety of media for the diagnosis of trichomoniasis have been studied and are roughly comparable. Formulas are given in several publications.[76,88,98] Trichosel broth medium (Baltimore Biological Laboratory) is quite suitable for routine diagnostic work. Some strains of this protozoon or cultures inoculated with only a few cells might fail to grow. Cultures should preferably be incubated anaerobically. Most isolates show growth within 48 h, but negative cultures should be held for 7 days. Details of culture methods and progress toward development of defined media have been reviewed in Ref. 98.

Most studies suggest that in excess of 95 percent of cases in women can be diagnosed by culture.[4,91,95]

In view of the difficulty of finding trichomonads by direct microscopy in men, culture plays an important role in the diagnostic work. In material recovered from the urethra *T. vaginalis* will grow in approximately 60 percent of cases.[38,96] Additional cases will be detected by culturing the urine sediment, especially after prostatic massage.

## SERODIAGNOSIS

Although serum antibodies can be detected at low titers in many patients with trichomoniasis, serodiagnosis is currently experimental and appears to add little to direct microbiological techniques in the diagnosis of trichomoniasis.

## THERAPY

The treatment of trichomoniasis was revolutionized by the development of the 5-nitroimidazoles, first metronidazole and subsequently a number of related drugs (tinidazole, ornidazole, etc.) of similar efficacy.[2] *T. vaginalis* is not susceptible to a wide variety of other antimicrobial agents.[99] In vitro activity by an anthelminthic benzimidazole, mebendazole, was observed,[99] but this compound has as yet received no clinical testing. Therapy of trichomoniasis has been reviewed in detail.[5,100]

## METRONIDAZOLE AND OTHER 5-NITROIMIDAZOLES

### Susceptibility of *T. vaginalis*

Most strains of *T. vaginalis* are highly susceptible to metronidazole and related drugs with minimal inhibitory concentrations of 1 μg/ml or less when tested under anaerobic conditions.[101–104] Minimum trichomonacidal concentrations have ranged from 0.25 to 16 μg/ml.[101,102,104] Effective concentrations measured under aerobic conditions are higher.[102,104,105] Large samples of

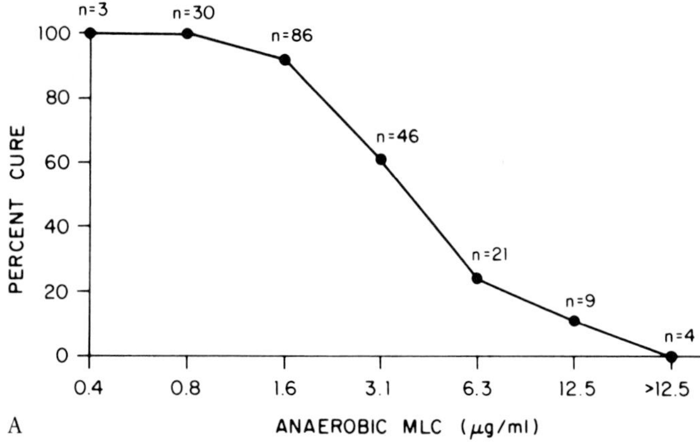


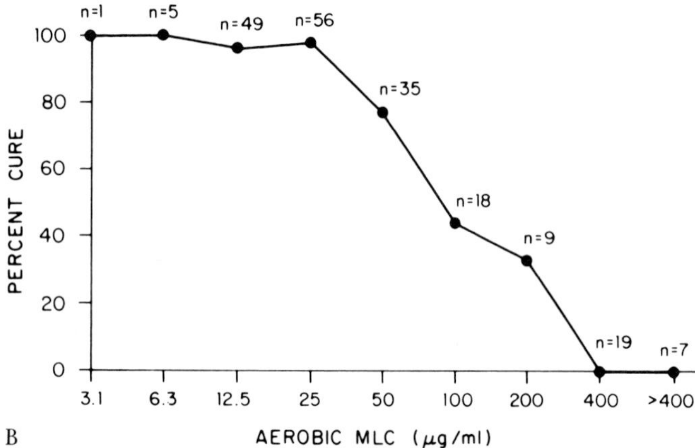


**Fig. 43-3.** Relationship of treatment outcome and minimal lethal concentration of metronidazole for *Trichomonas vaginalis* isolates determined under anaerobic (*a*) and aerobic (*b*) conditions. Total number of isolates tested was 199, which included 53 isolates from treatment-refractory patients. (*From Ref. 104.*)

isolates manifest a continuum of susceptibility. Treatment results show a definite but not absolute correlation with in vitro results[104] (Fig. 43-3). Susceptibility levels to other 5-nitroimidazoles are similar.[101]

Recently, isolates of *T. vaginalis* with relatively high levels of resistance to metronidazole were obtained from patients who were not cured by repeated courses of the drug.[103,105–107] Testing under aerobic conditions enhances the differences between susceptible and resistant organisms in their minimal trichomonacidal concentrations.[105–107] High aerobic values (>50 μg/ml) provide a good indication of clinically significant resistance. They are, however, determined under conditions different from those prevailing in natural infection. Thus they are unrealistically high and should not be regarded as representing blood levels needed to eliminate the infection.[106]

## Pharmacology

Peak serum levels following the oral administration of 500 mg of metronidazole are approximately 10 μg/ml. Peak serum levels following a single 2-g dose are about 40 μg/ml. The serum half-life of the drug is of the order of 6 to 8 h.[108] Pharmacokinetic problems are not responsible for treatment failures.[109] Other 5-nitroimidazoles differ somewhat from metronidazole in their pharmacological behavior.[108]

## Mode of action of 5-nitroimidazoles

Metronidazole and other 5-nitroimidazole drugs are selectively active not only against *T. vaginalis* but also against other anaerobic microorganisms, protozoa (*Entamoeba histolytica, Giardia lamblia*) as well as bacteria (e.g., *Bacteroides* and *Clostridium* species). This selectivity is correlated with metabolic differences between anaerobes and aerobes.[110–112] Ferredoxins, low-redox potential proteins, play a major role in the energy metabolism of anaerobes but not of aerobes. The 5-nitroimidazoles are not microbicidal by themselves, but the low-redox potential proteins effectively reduce the nitro group, which leads to the formation of highly cytotoxic products within the microbial cells.[112] These products have not yet been identified, but they are known to be short-lived and quickly decomposed into nontoxic end products. Aerobiosis interferes with the reduction process and diminishes the antianaerobic activity of the 5-nitroimidazoles.[104]

## Treatment of trichomoniasis

The frequency of infection of the urethra and periurethral glands in women dictates that systemic chemotherapy be given to effect a permanent cure. Therapy eradicating only vaginal trichomonads may leave organisms behind in the urinary tract, resulting in subsequent endogenous reinfection.

The recommended treatment of trichomoniasis in women consists of 2.0 g of metronidazole administered as a single oral dose (or of another 5-nitroimidazole preparation in a comparable dose). This regimen is highly effective, with reported cure rates in the range of 82 to 88 percent of women.[41,42,104,113,114] When sexual partners are treated simultaneously the cure rate is often in excess of 95 percent.[41,42,113,114] When metronidazole was first introduced, the recommended treatment schedule was 250 mg orally three times daily for 7 days, which has cured about 95 percent of the patients. The single-dose regimen was first recommended for tinidazole. Extensive testing demonstrated that this regimen is applicable to metronidazole treatment as well. Its advantages include better patient compliance, a lower total dose (38 percent of multidose regimens), a shorter time during which the patient's anaerobic bacterial flora is subject to alteration by the drug, and a shorter period during which the patient should abstain from consumption of alcohol. On the other hand, simultaneous treatment of sexual partners appears to be more important with the single-dose than with the multidose regimens.[41,42]

The 7-day multidose regimen is highly effective in curing men,[33,37] but single-dose regimens have not been extensively or systematically evaluated. One recent report indicates a 40 percent failure rate with the single-dose regimen in men.[37]

## Treatment of asymptomatic male sexual partners

When women are treated with a 1-week course of metronidazole, the relapse rate is very low, even if sexual partners are not treated.[42] Asymptomatic male sexual partners of infected women should, however, be treated simultaneously on an epidemiologic basis. Such epidemiologic treatment is generally accepted in the case of most other sexually transmitted diseases.

When women are treated with the single-dose regimens, simultaneous treatment of sexual partners is necessary to achieve maximal cure rates.[41,42]

### 5-Nitroimidazole resistance

As discussed above, treatment with metronidazole or other 5-nitroimidazoles results in a cure rate close to but definitively less than 100 percent. Patients who were not cured with the first regimen often respond favorably to repeating the standard treatment.[5,104,106] Some patients, however, prove to be refractory to repeated standard treatments. If reinfection also can be excluded, the cause of treatment failure can be a genuine resistance of the given *T. vaginalis* strain to 5-nitroimidazoles.[105,106] Increased doses of drug and longer treatment can be necessary to cure patients refractory to standard treatment,[5,105–107] if properly conducted testing demonstrates decreased drug susceptibility of the pathogen. Some authors have used intravenous metronidazole.[115]

### Pregnancy

Treatment of trichomonal infection in pregnant women is unsatisfactory.[116] Metronidazole readily crosses the placenta, and maternal and fetal levels of the drug are equal. Although studies on women who received standard multiple doses of metronidazole during the first trimester of pregnancy indicate that the drug produced no harmful effects, it is prudent not to use this drug in the first trimester.[116] Among treated women neither the incidence of perinatal death (2.5 percent) nor the incidence of spontaneous abortion (11 percent) was higher than expected in the population studied. In this group 3.8 percent of pregnancies resulted in babies with developmental anomalies, which was slightly higher than expected.[40] Thus there has been some concern about the possible teratogenicity of metronidazole. An evaluation of 61 women treated during pregnancy found no congenital malformations, and concluded that the drug could be administered safely during the second or third trimester.[117]

In general, it seems prudent to avoid all drugs during pregnancy if possible, and one might therefore approach symptomatic trichomoniasis in pregnancy with local therapies. Local application of various vaginal creams (see below) has cured some women, or one might initially attempt gentle douching with a solution of 2 tablespoons of vinegar in a quart of water daily and then twice weekly. Such treatment may reduce symptoms to tolerable levels. After the patient is beyond the first trimester, treatment with a single dose of metronidazole can be employed.

Povidone-iodine douches should probably be avoided in pregnancy because increased serum levels of iodine may suppress fetal thyroid development.[118]

### Adverse reactions

**Acute Toxicities.** Many patients taking metronidazole complain of a disagreeable or metallic taste. Nausea was described by about 10 percent of patients taking a single 2-g dose.[42] Transient neutropenia with peripheral white blood counts of 1000 to 1400 was observed in 7.5 percent of patients treated with multiple doses of metronidazole.[119] This reaction was never associated with significant infectious complications.

**Interaction with Alcohol.** In certain individuals, metronidazole has a disulfiram-like effect; thus it can produce a variety of systemic symptoms including nausea and flushing. Patients should be cautioned concerning consumption of alcohol while on treatment.

**Interaction with Other Drugs.** Metronidazole has been observed to prolong the prothrombin time in patients taking warfarin,[120] presumably by competing for binding sites on serum proteins. Patients on oral anticoagulants should be carefully monitored during therapy with metronidazole.

**Superinfection.** Metronidazole is active against many anaerobic bacteria and therefore significantly affects the normal anaerobic flora of the gastrointestinal and urogenital tracts. Pseudomembranous colitis has been occasionally observed following the treatment of trichomonal vaginitis with metronidazole.[121] Vaginal candidiasis has been described in up to 16 percent of patients treated with 1 week of metronidazole,[42,122] but the incidence of candidial superinfection is much lower in other series.[123] It is our practice to admininster topical antifungal agents to women whose vaginal wet mount reveals large numbers of yeasts and who are being treated with a 1-week course of metronidazole. It is reasonable to assume that the risk of superinfection is reduced with the single-dose regimen because of the shorter duration of its effect on normal bacterial flora.

**Carcinogenicity.** When high doses of metronidazole were administered on a long-term basis, recipient mice manifested an excess of lung tumors,[124] but other species, such as hamsters, did not show a similar effect.[125] Metronidazole is mutagenic for certain bacteria which are good predictors of carcinogenic potential in animals.[126]

A cohort of 771 women treated with metronidazole during the period 1960 through 1969 was followed for 15 to 25 years and showed no statistically significant increase of cancer morbidity and mortality over the expected rate.[127] Bronchogenic cancer was observed at a higher than expected rate for the overall population, but when adjusted for smoking habits this again did not exceed the expected rate. These data confirm a shorter-term evaluation of the same cohort.[128] The risk to humans of short-term low-dose metronidazole treatment is extremely small. The drug should not be administered indiscriminately, however, but only when clinically or epidemiologically warranted. The lowest effective total therapeutic dose should be employed.

## IMMUNIZATION

A vaccine for active immunization against trichomoniasis has been introduced in several European countries. This vaccine (Solco Trichovac, Solco Co., Switzerland) consists of killed cells of "aberrant lactobacilli" isolated from the vagina of women with trichomoniasis.[129] The bacteria in the vaccine were claimed to share antigens with *T. vaginalis,* but this observation could not be confirmed.[130,131] Although a number of papers suggest a beneficial effect for this vaccine, its efficacy remains to be evaluated in well-controlled double-blind prospective studies. In view of this consideration and of the lack of immunological basis for efficacy, the use of the vaccine cannot be recommended until results of controlled tests become available. More details on this topic are provided in Ref. 132.

## LOCAL THERAPIES

Because they have been associated with unacceptably high failure rates, the wide variety of topical therapies proposed over the years has fallen into disuse. Topical therapy should be reserved for clinical situations in which systemic nitroimidazole therapy is contraindicated.

An imidazole antifungal, clotrimazole, kills *T. vaginalis* after 48 h of exposure to 100 μg/ml in vitro. No effect was observed at levels less than 25 μg/ml, and its level of activity against protozoa was at least 50-fold lower than against fungi.[133] One hundred milligrams applied intravaginally for 6 days has been reported to cure 48 to 66 percent of patients by culture.[134] When cure was defined as relief of symptoms and elimination of the organism from wet mount, the same course cured 61 to 81 percent of women.[135,136] Recent unpublished experience (MFR) suggests a cure rate of only about 25 percent, which may be no better than the rate of spontaneous resolution. Such treatment may have a role, particularly during the first trimester of pregnancy, in relieving symptoms.

Aminocrine-allantoin-sulfonamide topical preparations are no longer available in the United States. Topical preparations containing sulfonamide alone are not indicated for the treatment of trichomoniasis.

## References


1 Kampmeier RH: Description of *Trichomonas vaginalis* by MA Donné. *Sex Transm Dis* 5:119, 1978.
2 Hesseltine HC et al: Experimental human vaginal trichomoniasis. *J Infect Dis* 71:127, 1942.
3 Lancely F, MacEntegart MC: *Trichomonas vaginalis* in the male: The experimental infection of a few volunteers. *Lancet* 4:668, 1953.
4 Wølner-Hanssen P et al: Clinical manifestations of vaginal trichomoniasis. *JAMA* 264:571, 1989.
5 Lossick JG: Treatment of *Trichomonas vaginalis* infections. *Rev Infect Dis* 4:801, 1982.
6 Honigberg BM: Trichomonads found outside the urogenital tract of humans, in *Trichomonads Parasitic in Humans,* BM Honigberg (ed). New York, Springer, 1989, p 344.
7 Honigberg BM (ed): *Trichomonads Parasitic in Humans,* New York, Springer, 1989.
8 Honigberg BM, Brugerolle G: Structure, in *Trichomonads Parasitic in Humans,* BM Honigberg (ed). New York, Springer, 1989. p 5.
9 Honigberg B: Trichomonads of importance in human medicine, in *Parasitic Protozoa,* JP Kreier (ed). New York, Academic, 1978, vol 2, p 275.
10 Winston RML: The relation between size and pathogenicity of *Trichomonas vaginalis. J Obstet Gynecol Br Comm* 81:399, 1974.
11 Müller M: The hydrogenosome. *Symp Soc Gen Microbiol* 30:127, 1980.
12 Müller M: Energy metabolism of protozoa without mitochondria. *Annu Rev Microbiol* 42:465, 1988.
13 Alderete JF, Garza GE: Identification and properties of *Trichomonas vaginalis* proteins involved in cytadherence. *Infect Immun* 56:28, 1988.
14 Nielsen MH, Nielsen R: Electron microscopy of *Trichomonas vaginalis* Donné. Interaction with vaginal epithelium in human trichomoniasis. *Acta Pathol Microbiol Scand* (B) 83:305, 1975.
15 Alderete JF, Garza GE: Specific nature of *Trichomonas vaginalis* parasitism of host cell surfaces. *Infect Immun* 50:701, 1985.
16 Cappuccinelli P, Varesio L: The effect of cytochalasin B, colchicine and vinblastine on the adhesion of *Trichomonas vaginalis* to glass surfaces. *Int J Parasitol* 5:57, 1975.
17 Francioli P et al: Phagocytosis and killing of *Neisseria gonorrhoeae* by *Trichomonas vaginalis. J Infect Dis* 147:87, 1983.
18 Müller M: Biochemistry of *Trichomonas vaginalis,* in *Trichomonads Parasitic in Humans,* BM Honigberg (ed). New York, Springer, 1989, p 53.
19 Krieger JN et al: Geographic variation among isolates of *Trichomonas vaginalis.* Demonstration of antigenic heterogeneity by using monoclonal antibodies and the indirect immunofluorescence technique. *J Infect Dis* 152:979, 1985.
20 Alderete JF: Alternating phenotypic expression of two classes of *Trichomonas vaginalis* surface markers. *Rev Infect Dis* 10(suppl 2): S408, 1988.
21 Proctor EM et al: Isoenzyme patterns of isolates of *Trichomonas vaginalis* from Vancouver. *Sex Transm Dis.* 15:181, 1988.
22 Nadler SA, Honigberg BM: Genetic differentiation and biochemical polymorphism among trichomonads. *J Parasitol* 74:797, 1988.
23 Wang AL, Wang CC: The double-stranded RNA in *Trichomonas vaginalis* may originate from virus-like particles. *Proc Natl Acad Sci USA* 83:7956, 1986.
24 Lossick JS: Epidemiology of urogenital trichomoniasis, in *Trichomonads Parasitic in Humans,* BM Honigberg (ed). New York, Springer, 1989. p 313.
25 Krieger JN: Epidemiology and clinical manifestations of urogenital trichomoniasis in men, in *Trichomonads Parasitic in Humans,* BM Honigberg (ed). New York, Springer, 1989, p 237.
26 Rein MF, Chapel TA: Trichomoniasis, candidiasis, and the minor venereal diseases. *Clin Obstet Gynecol* 18:73, 1975.
27 Holst et al: Bacterial vaginosis. Microbiology and clinical findings. *Eur J Clin Bacteriol* 6:536, 1987.
28 Schou M et al: *Trichomonas vaginalis* is now a very rare disease in Sweden. Scandinavian Society for Genitourinary Medicine, Vth meeting, 1988, p 37.
29 Fouts AC, Kraus SJ: *Trichomonas vaginalis:* Reevaluation of its clinical presentation and laboratory diagnosis. *J Infect Dis* 141:137, 1980.
30 Bramley M, Kinghorn G: Do oral contraceptives inhibit *Trichomonas vaginalis*? *Sex Transm Dis* 6:261, 1979.
31 Bolch OH, Warren JC: In vitro effects of Emko on *Neisseria gonorrhoeae* and *Trichomonas vaginalis. Am J Obstet Gynecol* 115: 1145, 1973.
32 Wright RA, Judson FN: Relative and seasonal incidences of the sexually transmitted diseases: A two year statistical review. *Br J Vener Dis* 54:433, 1978.
33 Wisdom AR, Dunlop EMC: Trichomoniasis: Study of the disease and its treatment in women and men. *Br J Vener Dis* 41:90, 1965.
34 Krieger JN: Urologic aspects of trichomoniasis. *Invest Urol* 18:411, 1981.
35 Catterall RD: Diagnosis and treatment of trichomonal urethritis in men. *Br Med J* 2:113, 1960.
36 Ronnike F: Discharge symptomatology in 1000 gynaecological cases examined with a view to *Trichomonas vaginalis:* Results of metronidazole (Flagyl) treatment. *Acta Obstet Gynecol Scand* 42(suppl 6):63, 1963.
37 Latif AS et al: Urethral trichomoniasis in men. *Sex Transm Dis* 14:9, 1987.
38 Weston TET, Nicol CS: Natural history of trichomonal infection in males. *Br J Vener Dis* 39:251, 1963.
39 Burch TA et al: Epidemiological studies on human trichomoniasis. *Am J Trop Med Hyg* 8:312, 1959.
40 Peterson WF et al: Metronidazole in pregnancy. *Am J Obstet Gynecol* 94:343, 1966.
41 Underhill RA, Peck JE: Causes of therapeutic failure after treatment of trichomonal vaginitis with metronidazole: Comparison of single dose treatment with a standard regimen. *Br J Clin Pract* 28:134, 1974.
42 Hager WD et al: Metronidazole for vaginal trichomoniasis: Seven day vs single dose regimens. *JAMA* 244:1219, 1980.
43 Jones JG et al: *Trichomonas vaginalis* infestation in sexually abused girls. *Am J Dis Child* 139:846, 1985.
44 Judson FN: The importance of coexisting syphilitic, chlamydial, mycoplasmal, and trichomonal infections in the treatment of gonorrhea. *Sex Transm Dis* 6:112, 1979.
45 Morton RS: Trichomoniasis: Clinical aspects, in *Recent Advances in Sexually Transmitted Diseases,* RS Morton, JRW Harris (eds). London, Churchill-Livingstone, 1975, p 210.

46 Rein MF: Epidemiology of gonococcal infection, in *The Gonococcus,* RB Roberts (ed). New York, Wiley, 1977, p 1.

47 Al-Salihi FL et al: Neonatal *Trichomonas vaginalis:* Report of 3 cases and review of the literature. *Pediatrics* 53:196, 1974.

48 Bramley M: Study of female babies of women entering confinement with vaginal trichomoniasis. *Br J Vener Dis* 52:58, 1976.

49 Robinson SC, Halifax NS: Observations on vaginal trichomoniasis. I. In pregnancy. *Can Med Assoc J* 84:948, 1961.

50 Grys E: Topography of trichomoniasis in the reproductive organ of the woman. *Wiad Parazytol* 10:122, 1964.

51 Wallin JE et al: Urethritis in women attending an STD clinic. *Br J Vener Dis* 57:50, 1981.

52 Fisher I, Morton RS: Epididymitis due to *Trichomonas vaginalis. Br J Vener Dis* 45:252, 1969.

53 Gardner WA et al: *Trichomonas vaginalis* in the prostate gland. *Arch Pathol Lab Med* 110:430, 1986.

54 Sowmini CN et al: Infections of the median raphe of the penis: Report of 3 cases. *Br J Vener Dis* 49:469, 1972.

55 Suriyanon V et al: *Trichomonas vaginalis* in a perinephric abscess: A case report. *Am J Trop Med Hyg* 24:776, 1975.

56 Walton BC, Bacharach T: Occurrence of trichomonads in the respiratory tract. Report of three cases. *J Parasitol* 49:35, 1963.

57 Hersh SM: Pulmonary trichomoniasis and *Trichomonas tenax. J Med Microbiol* 20:1, 1985.

58 Walzer PD et al: Empyema with *Trichomonas* species. *Am Rev Respir Dis* 118:415, 1978.

59 Masur H et al: A trichomonas species in a mixed microbial meningitis. *JAMA* 236:1978, 1976.

60 Catterall RD: Trichomonal infection of the genital tract. *Med Clin North Am* 56:1203, 1972.

61 Kolstad P: The colposcopical picture of *Trichomonas vaginalis. Acta Obstet Gynecol Scand* 43:388, 1965.

62 Gupta PK, Frost JK: Cytopathology and histopathology of female genital tract in *Trichomonas vaginalis* infection, in *Trichomonads Parasitic in Humans,* BM Honigberg (ed). New York, Springer, 1989, p 276.

63 Gardner WA, Culberson DE: Pathology of urogenital trichomoniasis in men, in *Trichomonads Parasitic in Humans,* BM Honigberg (ed). New York, Springer, 1989, p 293.

64 Honigberg BM: Biological and physiological factors affecting pathogenicity of trichomonads, in *Biochemistry and Physiology of Protozoa,* 2d ed, M Levandowsky, SH Hunter (eds). New York, Academic, 1979, vol 2, p 409.

65 Kulda J: Employment of experimental animals in studies of *Trichomonas vaginalis* infection, in *Trichomonads Parasitic in Humans,* BM Honigberg (ed). New York, Springer, 1989, p 112.

66 Honigberg BM: Host cell–trichomonad interactions and virulence assays using *in vitro* systems, in *Trichomonads Parasitic in Humans,* BM Honigberg (ed). New York, Springer, 1989, p 155.

67 Gardner WA: Experimental genital trichomoniasis in the squirrel monkey (*Saimiri sciureus*). *Genitourin Med* 63:188, 1987.

68 Krieger JN et al: Contact-dependent cytopathogenic mechanisms of *Trichomonas vaginalis. Infect Immun* 50:778, 1985.

69 Ackers JP: Immunologic aspects of human trichomoniasis, in *Trichomonads Parasitic in Humans,* BM Honigberg (ed). New York, Springer, 1989, p 36.

70 Matthews HM, Healy GR: Evaluation of two serologic tests for *Trichomonas vaginalis* infection. *J Clin Microbiol* 17:840, 1983.

71 Kuberski T: *Trichomonas vaginalis* associated with nongonococcal urethritis and prostatitis. *Sex Transm Dis* 7:135, 1980.

72 Kuberski T: Evaluation of the indirect hemagglutination technique for the study of *Trichomonas vaginalis* infections, particularly in men. *Sex Transm Dis* 5:97, 1978.

73 Ackers JP et al: Antitrichomonal antibody in the vaginal secretions of women infected with *T. vaginalis. Br J Vener Dis* 51:319, 1975.

74 Ackers JP et al: Absence of detectable local antibody in genitourinary tract secretions of male contacts of women infected with *Trichomonas vaginalis. Br J Vener Dis* 54:168, 1978.

75 Demeš P et al: Differential susceptibility of fresh *Trichomonas vaginalis* isolates to complement in menstrual blood and cervical mucus. *Genitourin Med* 64:176, 1988.

76 Mason PR, Patterson BA: Proliferative response of human lymphocytes to secretory and cellular antigens of *Trichomonas vaginalis. J Parasitol* 71:265, 1985.

77 Mason PR, Forman L: Polymorphonuclear cell chemotaxis to secretions of pathogenic and nonpathogenic *Trichomonas vaginalis. J Parasitol* 68:457, 1982.

78 Frost JK, Honigberg BM: Comparative pathogenicity of *Trichomonas vaginalis* and *Trichomonas gallinae* to mice. II. Histopathology of subcutaneous lesions. *J Parasitol* 48:898, 1962.

79 Rein MF et al: Trichomonacidal activity of human polymorphonuclear neutrophils: Killing by disruption and fragmentation. *J Infect Dis* 142:575, 1980.

80 Mantovanic A et al: Cytotoxicity of human peripheral blood monocytes against *Trichomonas vaginalis. Clin Exp Immunol* 46:391, 1981.

81 Landolfo S et al: Natural cell-mediated cytotoxicity against *Trichomonas vaginalis* in the mouse. *J Immunol* 124:508, 1980.

82 Rein MF: Clinical manifestations of urogenital trichomoniasis in women, in *Trichomonads Parasitic in Humans,* BM Honigberg (ed). New York, Springer, 1989, p 227.

83 Hughes HE et al: A clinical and laboratory study of trichomoniasis of the female genital tract. *J Obstet Gynecol Br Comm* 73:821, 1966.

84 Langley JG et al: Venereal trichomoniasis: Role of men. *Genitourin Med* 63:264, 1987.

85 Krieger JN et al: Evaluation of chronic urethritis. Defining the role of endoscopic procedures. *Arch Intern Med* 148:703, 1988.

86 Amar AD: Probable *Trichomonas vaginalis* epididymitis. *JAMA* 200:417, 1967.

87 Lang WR: Premenarchal vaginitis. *Obstet Gynecol* 13:723, 1959.

88 McMillan A: Laboratory diagnostic methods and cryopreservation of trichomonads, in *Trichomonads Parasitic in Humans,* BM Honigberg (ed). New York, Springer, 1989, p 299.

89 Spence MR et al: The clinical and laboratory diagnosis of *Trichomonas vaginalis* infection. *Sex Transm Dis* 7:168, 1980.

90 Hipp SS et al: Screening for *Trichomonas vaginalis* infection by use of acridine orange fluorescent microscopy. *Sex Transm Dis* 6:235, 1979.

91 Krieger et al: Diagnosis of trichomoniasis. Comparison of conventional wet-mount preparation with cytologic studies, cultures, and monoclonal antibody staining of direct specimens. *JAMA* 259:1223, 1988.

92 Yule A et al: Detection of *Trichomonas vaginalis* antigen in women by enzyme immunoassay. *J Clin Pathol* 40:566, 1987.

93 Watt RM et al: Rapid assay for immunological detection of *Trichomonas vaginalis. J Clin Microbiol* 24:551, 1986.

94 Carney JA et al: A new rapid agglutination test for the diagnosis of *Trichomonas vaginalis* infection. *J Clin Pathol.* 41:806, 1988.

95 Lossick JG: The diagnosis of vaginal trichomoniasis. (Editorial.) *JAMA* 259:1230, 1988.

96 Morton RS: Trichomoniasis: Laboratory aspects, in *Recent Advances in Sexually Transmitted Diseases,* RS Morton, JRW Harris (eds). London, Churchill-Livingstone, 1975, p 214.

97 Hess J: Review of current methods of the detection of *Trichomonas* in clinical material. *J Clin Pathol* 22:269, 1969.

98 Linstead DJ: Cultivation of trichomonads parasitic in humans, in *Trichomonads Parasitic in Humans,* BM Honigberg (ed). New York, Springer, 1989, p 91.

99 Sears SD, O'Hare J: In vitro susceptibility of *Trichomonas vaginalis* to 50 antimicrobial agents. *Antimicrob Agents Chemother* 32:144, 1988.

100 Lossick JG: Therapy of urogenital trichomoniasis, in *Trichomonads Parasitic in Humans,* BM Honigberg (ed). New York, Springer, 1989, p 326.

101 Korner B, Jensen HK: Sensitivity of *Trichomonas vaginalis* to metronidazole, tinidazole, and nifuratel in vitro. *Br J Vener Dis* 52:404, 1976.

102 Meingasser L et al: Studies on strain sensitivity of *Trichomonas vaginalis* to metronidazole. *Br J Vener Dis* 54:72, 1978.

103 Smith RF, DiDomenico A: Measuring the in vitro susceptibility of *Trichomonas vaginalis* to metronidazole. *Sex Transm Dis* 7:120, 1980.

104 Müller M et al: In-vitro susceptibility of *Trichomonas vaginalis* to metronidazole and treatment outcome in vaginal trichomoniasis. *Sex Transm Dis* 15:51, 1988.

105 Meingassner JG, Thurner J: Strain of *Trichomonas vaginalis* resistant to metronidazole and other 5-nitroimidazoles. *Antimicrob Agents Chemother* 15:254, 1979.

106 Lossick JG et al: In vitro drug susceptibility and doses of metronidazole required for cure in cases of refractory vaginal trichomoniasis. *J Infect Dis* 153:948, 1986.

107 Krajden S et al: Persistent *Trichomonas vaginalis* infection due to a metronidazole-resistant strain. *Can Med Assoc J* 134:1373, 1986.

108 Wood BA, Monro AM: Pharmacokinetics of tinidazole and metronidazole in women after single large oral doses. *Br J Vener Dis* 49:475, 1975.

109 Robertson DHH et al: Treatment failure in *Trichomonas vaginalis* infections in females. I. Concentrations of metronidazole in plasma and vaginal content during normal and high dosage. *J Antimicrob Chemother* 21:373, 1988.

110 Edwards DI: Mechanism of antimicrobial action of metronidazole. *J Antimicrob Chemother* 5:499, 1979.

111 Müller M: Action of clinically utilized 5-nitroimidazoles on microorganisms. *Scand J Infect Dis* 26:S31, 1981.

112 Müller M: Reductive activation of nitroimidazoles in anaerobic microorganisms. *Biochem Pharmacol* 35:37, 1986.

113 Dykers JR: Single dose metronidazole for trichomonal vaginitis. *N Engl J Med* 293:23, 1975.

114 Fleury FS: A single dose of two grams of metronidazole for *Trichomonas vaginalis* vaginitis. *Am J Obstet Gynecol* 128:320, 1977.

115 Dombrowski MP et al: Intravenous therapy of metronidazole-resistant *Trichomonas vaginalis*. *Obstet Gynecol* 69:524, 1987.

116 Robbie MD, Sweet RL: Metronidazole use in obstetrics and gynecology: a review. *Am J Obstet Gynecol* 145:865, 1983.

117 Rodin P, Hass G: Metronidazole and pregnancy. *Br J Vener Dis* 42:210, 1966.

118 Vorherr H et al: Vaginal absorption of povidone-iodine. *JAMA* 244:2628, 1980.

119 Rodin P et al: Flagyl in the treatment of trichomoniasis. *Br J Vener Dis* 36:147, 1960.

120 Kazmier FJ: A significant interaction between metronidazole and warfarin. *Mayo Clin Proc* 51:782, 1976.

121 Saginur R et al: Colitis associated with metronidazole therapy. *J Infect Dis* 141:772, 1980.

122 Clark JFJ, George T Jr: Control of concomitant vaginal moniliasis during metronidazole therapy for *Trichomonas vaginalis*. *J Natl Med Assoc* 58:464, 1966.

123 Beveridge MM: Vaginal moniliasis after treatment of trichomonal infection with Flagyl. *Br J Vener Dis* 38:220, 1962.

124 Rustia M, Shubik P: Induction of lung tumors and malignant lymphomas in mice by metronidazole. *J Natl Cancer Inst* 48:421, 1972.

125 Anonymous: Metronidazole (Flagyl) box warning. *FDA Drug Bull* April–May 1976.

126 Goldman P: Metronidazole. *N Engl J Med* 303:1212, 1980.

127 Beard CM et al: Cancer after exposure to metronidazole. *Mayo Clin Proc* 63:147, 1988.

128 Beard CM et al: Lack of evidence for cancer due to use of metronidazole. *N Engl J Med* 301:519, 1979.

129 Pavic R, Stojkovic L: Vaccination with Solco Trichovac. Immunological aspects of a new approach for therapy and prophylaxis of trichomoniasis in women. *Gynaecol Rundsch* 23(suppl):27, 1983.

130 Gombošová A et al: Immunotherapeutic effect of the lactobacillus vaccine, Solco Trichovac, in trichomoniasis is not mediated by antibodies cross reacting with *Trichomonas vaginalis*. *Genitourin Med* 62:107, 1986.

131 Alderete JF: Does lactobacillus vaccine for trichomoniasis, Solco Trichovac, induce antibody reactive with *Trichomonas vaginalis*? *Genitourin Med* 64:118, 1988.

132 Spiegel CA: Microflora associated with *Trichomonas vaginalis* infections and vaccination against vaginal trichomoniasis, in *Trichomonads Parasitic in Humans*, BM Honigberg (ed). New York, Springer, 1989, p 215.

133 Waitz JA et al: Chemotherapeutic evaluation of clotrimazole. *Appl Microbiol* 22:891, 1971.

134 Schnell JD: The incidence of vaginal candida and trichomonas infections and treatment of trichomonas vaginitis with clotrimazole. *Postgrad Med J* 50:S79, 1974.

135 Legal H-P: The treatment of trichomonas and candida vaginitis with clotrimazole vaginal tablets. *Postgrad Med J* 50:S81, 1974.

136 Lohmeyer H: Treatment of candidiasis and trichomoniasis of the female genital tract. *Postgrad Med J* 50:S78, 1974.

# Chapter 44

# Intestinal protozoa: *Giardia lamblia, Entamoeba histolytica,* and *Cryptosporidium*

Richard L. Guerrant
Cynthia S. Weikel
Jonathan I. Ravdin

Enteric protozoan pathogens are increasingly recognized causes of diarrhea. This chapter reviews the biology of the major protozoan causes of diarrhea: *Giardia lamblia, Entamoeba histolytica,* and *Cryptosporidium*. These protozoa may sometimes be transmitted by sexual practices that enable fecal-oral spread; *Cryptosporidium* infections present particularly severe problems in patients with the acquired immunodeficiency syndrome (AIDS).

## *GIARDIA LAMBLIA*

## HISTORY, EPIDEMIOLOGY, AND CLINICAL MANIFESTATIONS

### History

*Giardia lamblia* was probably first discovered by the inventor of the microscope, Anton van Leeuwenhoek, when he examined his own diarrheal stool. In a letter to the Royal Society on November 4, 1681, he described a number of "animalcules . . . approximately the size of a blood cell, with flattish bodies and several legs, moving much like a wood louse running up against a wall."[1] In 1859 Vilem D. F. Lambl described the parasite and called it *Cercomonas intestinalis*. However, since this organism was found in a number of asymptomatic individuals,[2] it was not considered to be a pathogen until it was repeatedly observed to be associated with diarrhea,[3–5] malabsorption,[6] and occasional tissue invasion.[7] Even the demonstration of experimental human infection in 36 percent of volunteers ingesting 10 to 25 *Giardia* cysts in water and the presence of moderate to marked diarrheal symptoms in 60 percent of 15 infected individuals left some question about the pathogenicity of this parasite.[8] There have since been numerous studies of the different strains of *Giardia,* the animal-host-species specificities, the morphological and functional characteristics of this flagellated protozoan, its in vitro cultivation, and the possible mechanisms by which it may cause enteric disease. As with *Entamoeba histolytica,* the in vitro cultivation of *Giardia lamblia* has enabled the study of different strains at the molecular level.

### Epidemiology

Several epidemiologic surveys have revealed that 2 to 9 percent of the population in many parts of the world excrete *Giardia* cysts[9,10] with increasing prevalence rates in tropical areas or for travelers; exposed infants and children have the highest prevalence rates.[11,12] This skewed distribution of giardiasis toward children is in distinct contrast to amebiasis, where gain and loss of infections (with a median duration of 2 years) appears to be independent of age.[13] The geographic and age distribution, as well as increased frequencies of giardiasis in institutions where hygienic standards are difficult to maintain, indicate that spread occurs by the fecal-oral route.[3,14] The human volunteer studies by Rendtorff[8] suggest that ingestion of relatively small numbers of cysts in food or water or by person-to-person contact results in infection. A food-borne outbreak was reported in which contamination of canned salmon apparently occurred after careful diaper changing of an infected infant.[15]

Waterborne giardiasis has been widely recognized in the last 15 years and is now the commonest reported parasitic infection in England and the United States.[16] Although first suggested by an outbreak of amebiasis and giardiasis in 1946 in a Tokyo apartment building where sewage-contaminated water was implicated (*Giardia* cysts were demonstrated in 80 percent of symptomatic individuals who did not have amebiasis),[4] attention was drawn to waterborne giardiasis by an outbreak in Aspen, Colorado, in 1965 when 11 percent of skiers and 5 percent of residents were infected and *Giardia* cysts were demonstrated in sewage that had contaminated the drinking water. A total of 23 additional outbreaks of giardiasis involving over 7000 individuals in the United States subsequently implicated water which was inadequately sedimented and filtered often despite bacteriologically adequate chemical disinfection.[16] These include a number of citywide outbreaks in Portland, Oregon, Aspen, Colorado, Rome, New York,[17] Camus, Washington, and Berlin, New Hampshire. From the Rome outbreak, cysts were found in city water which was shown to be infectious for beagle pups[17] (an experimental animal infection that had been described by Padchenko in the Russian literature in 1969). The greatest frequency of *Giardia* infections appeared to correlate with the season of greatest fecal contamination in a Colorado study.[18]

Studies of travelers from the United States and other countries to Leningrad and Moscow have noted impressive attack rates of giardiasis ranging from 22 to 41 percent.[19] In one study the mean incubation period was 14½ days and 69 percent of those infected were symptomatic.[19]

Besides humans, potential reservoirs include small animals such as beavers, which may be found contaminating even the remotest streams. As had been shown by Rendtorff in 1954,[20] *Giardia lamblia* cysts remain infectious for humans after holding in water for over 2 weeks. Furthermore, chemical disinfection of contaminated surface water, especially when cold, is inadequate, and appropriate flocculation, sedimentation, and filtration are necessary to remove infectious cysts. Cysts may also be killed by 2 to 5% phenol or lysol. Transmission may also occur with contaminated, uncooked foods[15] or by person-to-person contact in families, nurseries, institutions, and day-care centers.[3,9,14] Recently, primarily among sexually active male homosexuals, fecal-oral and rectal-genital spread of *Giardia* has been implicated.[21,22]

### Clinical manifestations

In endemic areas the majority of *Giardia* infections are asymptomatic; however, a significant portion of residents[18] and most previously uninfected travelers are symptomatic. The most characteristic symptoms include diarrhea of greater than 10 days' duration, cramping upper abdominal pain, bloating, flatulence, and weight loss.[17,19] Less commonly, nausea, vomiting, and fever may be seen.

Although the incubation period ranges from 1 to 8 weeks,

symptoms often precede the first detectable fecal shedding of the parasites; the median prepatency period in one study (14 days) was 6 days longer than the median incubation period (8 days).[23] Thus, it may be necessary to examine upper small bowel aspirates or repeated fecal specimens to document a diagnosis of giardiasis. While the infection is usually self-limited,[8] symptoms may intermittently recur or persist for prolonged periods up to months or even years.[24] The illness may last up to 6 or 7 weeks.[19]

Signs and symptoms of malabsorption, ranging from mild noninflammatory diarrhea, steatorrhea, or weight loss to a more severe celiac syndrome, especially in children,[6] are well documented with malabsorption of D-xylose, fat, carotene, vitamin A, folate, and vitamin $B_{12}$.[5,25,26] Malabsorption may be especially severe in patients with achlorhydria,[25] immunodeficiency,[25,27] protein-calorie malnutrition,[28] or bacterial overgrowth[29] complicating their illnesses. In patients with hypogammaglobulinemia, giardiasis can be associated with mucosal inflammation, villus flattening, and with lactase, maltase, or sucrase deficiency.[24,26,30] Likewise, giardiasis may mimic or accentuate the malabsorption seen in chronic pancreatitis.[31]

While *Giardia*-induced diarrhea is usually noninflammatory with only rare tissue invasion,[7] inflammatory proctitis and vaginitis have been reported.[32]

For poorly understood reasons, patients with giardiasis may rarely develop eosinophilia, urticaria, or other symptoms such as arthritis[33] that are suggestive of an immune response to an antigen exposed during acute diarrhea. These symptoms respond to specific antigiardial therapy.[34]

## STRUCTURE AND BIOLOGY OF THE ORGANISM

Named *Giardia* by Kunstler, who observed this genus in tadpole intestinal tracts in 1882, the genus was considered by Alexeieff and Dobell to be the same as the human flagellated protozoan. The genus and disease are called *Lamblia* and lambliasis in eastern Europe; however, most agree on the genus named *Giardia,* of which at least three species are recognized on the basis of morphology and host-species specificities.[35] Although species specificity is debated and size can be changed with host diet,[36] *Giardia* trophozoites usually measure 12 to 15 μm long by 5 to 15 μm wide and 1 to 4 μm thick. Cysts are usually 8 to 12 μm by 7 to 10μm.[37] Shaped like a horseshoe crab with a rounded dorsal surface and concave ventral surface, *Giardia* trophozoites have four pairs of posteriorly directed flagella from the lateral and ventral surfaces.

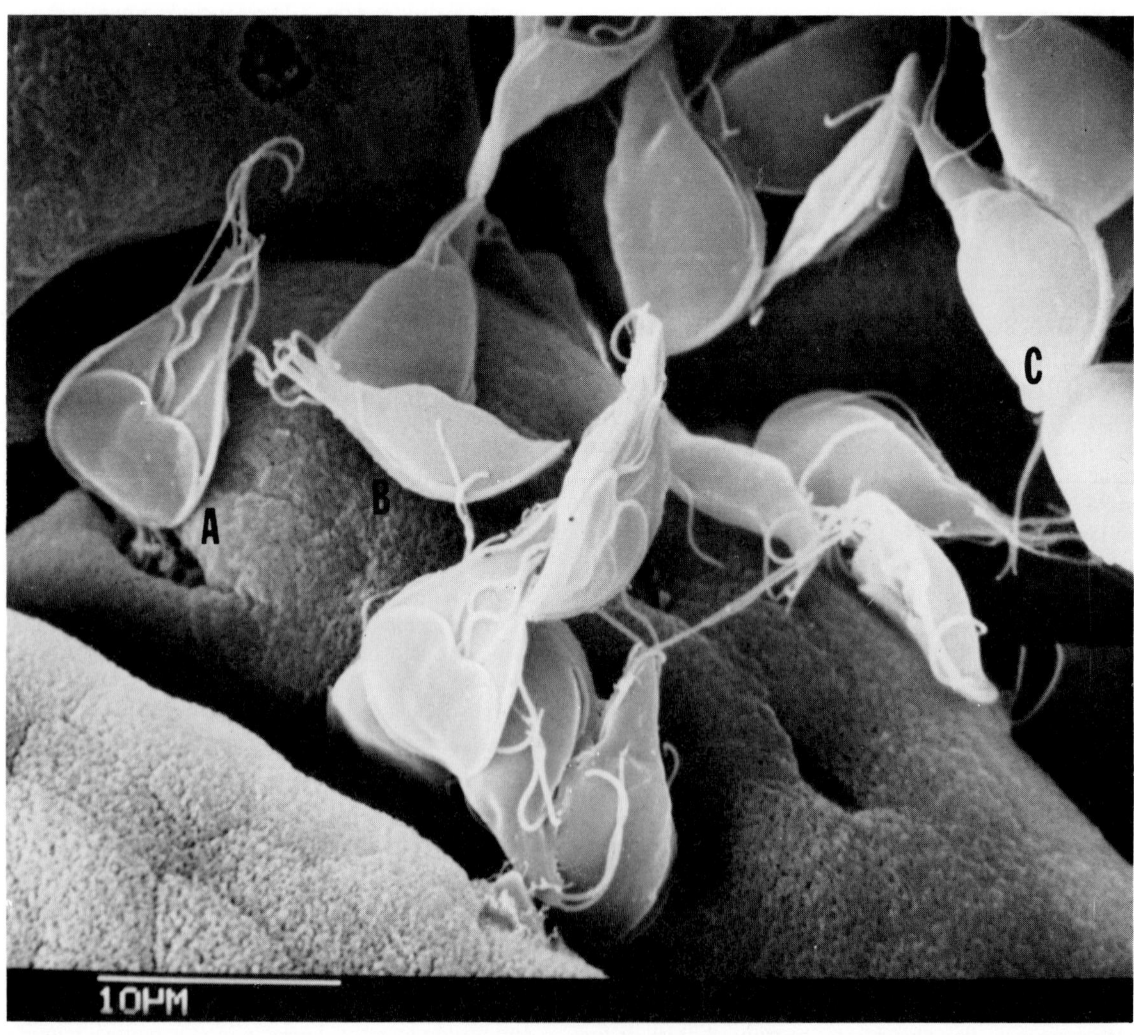


**Fig. 44-1.** Scanning electron micrograph of *Giardia lamblia* trophozoites from a jejunal biopsy of a patient with symptomatic giardiasis. (*a*) In the ventral view, flagella lead from the adhesive disk to the tapered posterior end. (*b*) In the lateral view, anterior flagella can be seen. (*c*) The dorsal view. (*Courtesy of R. L. Owen.*)

The trophozoite has a unique, anterior, ventral adhesive disk to which are attached a clockwise spiral of microtubules and contractile elements (Fig. 44-1). There is also a posterior vent in this disk where beating, ventral flagella appear to expel fluid that may help establish a mechanical suction for adherence of the parasite to mucosal or other surfaces.[38,39] Alternate suggestions include contractile or grasping actions by the disk. This adhesive disk is divided into two lobes, the medial surfaces of which are the median groove. Two nuclei lie dorsal to the adhesive disk lobes and the eight flagella appear to arise from basal bodies located anterior to the nuclei. Endocytic or exocytic vacuoles that have been shown to concentrate ferritin or even bacteria are also found adjacent to the disk and elsewhere.[40] There is recent evidence that *G. lamblia* have surface receptors for such lectins as wheat germ agglutinin that can be blocked by specific carbohydrates.[41] In addition, a 56-kilodalton protease-activated *Giardia* lectin has been isolated by SDS-PAGE from a lipopolysaccharide (LPS)-sepharose column.[42] The median body appears to be a tight packet of microtubules that lies between the posterior poles of the nuclei and appears to be unique to *Giardia* species.[39] The median bodies of *G. duodenalis (G. lamblia)* that infect humans, dogs, rabbits, and other mammals are characteristically claw-shaped and lie transversely across the trophozoite. *G. muris* from rodents or birds have small, central, round median bodies, and *G. agilia* from amphibians are long and narrow and have long, tear-shaped median bodies.[35–37] As with *E. histolytica*, differences among *G. lamblia* strains as to isoenzyme patterns,[43] antigens and surface proteins,[44,45] and restriction endonuclease patterns,[46] have been described. A double-stranded RNA virus has been described in the Portland I strain of *G. lamblia* that could infect another (WB) *G. lamblia* strain.[47] Recent evidence on the antigenic variation of a cysteine-rich 170-kilodalton protein expressed on the surface of certain *G. lamblia* suggest frequent rearrangements at the gene locus as well as long tandem repeats in the DNA.[48]

Trophozoites may encyst in response to a reduced pH, detachment, immunologic attack, or other hostile environments in vivo,[39] and encystment has been accomplished in vitro using primary bile salts.[49] Apparently, after a single division in the cyst and a period of maturation, two daughter trophozoites can be induced to excyst in vitro by special conditions and reduced pH.[50]

## GROWTH, PHYSIOLOGY, AND CULTURE

Although not successful with other *Giardia* strains, the human strain *G. duodenalis (G. lamblia)* has been cultured in vitro, first symbiotically with *Candida guillermandii* and then axenically (without other bacteria or parasites) by Meyer.[51] In 1978 Bingham and Meyer successfully cultured trophozoites that were obtained in vitro from cysts shed by humans and monkeys.[50] As shown by Visvesvara, the conditions for culture of *G. lamblia* in vitro are similar to those for culture of *E. histolytica; Giardia* may be more oxygen tolerant, but both parasites require serum and cysteine.[52,53] Bile salts have been shown to support growth of *G. lamblia.*[53,54] *Giardia* trophozoites can be preserved at low temperatures in glycerol or dimethyl sulfoxide.

The in vitro cultivation of *Giardia* trophozoites has enabled definition of their growth curves with doubling times of 7 to 40 h noted by different investigators.[52,53] *Giardia* appear to facultatively metabolize glucose to ethanol acetate and carbon dioxide via a flavin- rather than cytochrome-mediated electron-transport system or a Krebs cycle.[55]

## IMMUNOLOGY AND PATHOGENESIS

### Immunology and host response

A substantial number of studies of humoral and cellular immune responses to *Giardia* infection reveal a complexity ranging from partial, relative protection to possible roles in pathogenesis. Evidence for acquired resistance includes the skewed age distribution toward children (in contrast to amebiasis);[13] the observation that long-term residents of endemic areas appear to have a lower infection rate than short-term residents,[56] and the tendency for individuals in endemic areas to be infected asymptomatically. In addition, prior infection appears to result in acquired resistance to *G. muris* infection in the mouse model.[57]

The nature of acquired resistance appears to be related in part to local antibody production. Although initial humoral responses to *Giardia* infection are predominantly IgM, there follows an IgA and IgG response[58] that correlates with the severity of the histologic jejunal lesion.[59] Although debated by others,[60] the findings of Zinneman suggested that patients with giardiasis had lower secretory IgA levels.[27] Of seven patients with type 2 IgA and IgM deficiency and nodular small bowel lymphoid hyperplasia described by Hermans et al., six had giardiasis that improved with therapy.[61] Ament et al. have shown that hypogammaglobulinemic patients who acquired giardiasis develop enteric symptoms and malabsorption.[62] However, the frequent occurrence of selective IgA deficiency without recognized problems with giardiasis suggests that other Ig classes or possibly still other factors are also involved in protection against symptomatic *Giardia* infections. Human serum kills *G. lamblia* trophozoites via activation of the classical complement pathway.[63] IgM-supported complement-dependent lysis of *G. lamblia* has been demonstrated.[64] Anti-IgM treated mice develop heavy, prolonged infections (without any serum or local antibody responses) with *G. muris.*[65] Peyer's patch B cells show an early increase in surface IgM bearing cells followed by a switch to surface IgA-bearing cells with *G. muris* infection in mice.[66] The absence of severe disease with *Giardia* infections in AIDS patients (in contrast to, for example, cryptosporidial and mycobacterial infections) militates against a major primary role for cellular immunity in preventing symptomatic disease with *Giardia* infection.

In the mouse model, transient protective immunity can be transferred by milk to suckling offspring, possibly at the cost of loss of effective intestinal immunity by the nursing mother.[67] Whether this immunity is related to passive transfer of cellular or documented humoral immunity[68] or both remains to be determined. Murine and human biopsy studies have suggested roles for microfolded epithelial (M) cells overlying Peyer's patches in processing giardial antigens, for intralumenal migration of small lymphocytes that directly attack the parasite, or for intraepithelial large T lymphocytes or macrophages in the pathogenesis and resistance in *Giardia* infection.[37,39,69]

Evidence for a role for cell-mediated immunity in protection against *Giardia* infection again comes from the *G. muris* mouse model[70] in which athymic mice develop a prolonged *G. muris* infection.[71] Subsequent study has shown that the helper/inducer T lymphocytes (L3T4+), rather than the cytotoxic/suppressor (Ly − 2+) subset are responsible for clearance of murine *G. muris* infections.[72] Resistance to giardiasis may also be provided by toxic free fatty acids produced from breast milk by a bile salt stimulated lipase.[73,74]

The resistance to *Giardia* infection, however, is far from absolute. Normal human adults are usually susceptible to this widespread parasite; Rendtorff infected all 13 adults challenged with greater than 100 cysts.[8] Despite the evidence for increased susceptibility when specific humoral or cellular responses are impaired or absent, the relative infrequency of giardiasis in most patients with IgA deficiency and the acquisition of incomplete resistance by athymic nude mice[70] show that resistance to *Giardia* infection is complex and may involve both local humoral and cellular immune responses.

## Pathogenesis

The apparent increased frequency of giardiasis in patients with blood group A[75] may reflect less recognition of a shared parasite antigen with blood group A antigen[76] or the association of other traits with blood group A such as achlorhydria or differences in cell surface or mucus glycoproteins.

The initial stages in the pathogenesis of *G. lamblia* infection follow ingestion of a relatively small number of cysts (usually in water or by contact), and excystation of trophozoites in the upper small bowel where multiplication apparently occurs. Larger inocula probably cause more severe infection.[8] Although gastric acidity may contribute to excystation,[50] several investigators have noted increased symptoms with giardiasis in hypochlorhydric or postgastrectomy patients.

There are several tantalizing hypotheses regarding the mechanism by which *Giardia* alters small bowel function or histology to cause disease. Some have suggested that the close adherence of many trophozoites mechanically impede normal absorptive processes.[77] Holberton has shown evidence for a physical suction and some microvillus brush border damage under the ventral disk of *Giardia* trophozoites that resulted in deformation of the gut cell cortex.[38] Imprints of the ventral disks have also been demonstrated in the microvillous brush border in the mouse model with *G. muris* infection.[78] However, this has not been shown in humans, nor do symptoms correlate with density or intensity of infection.[79] Instead, symptoms have been correlated with lymphocytic infiltration in the jejunal epithelium[79] suggesting possible immunologic damage. Increased crypt cell production with lymphocytic infiltration has been noted in mice infected with *G. muris*.[80] Furthermore, Roberts-Thompson and Mitchell showed villus injury when T-lymphocytes were added to nude, athymic mice before infection with *Giardia*.[71] Inflammatory responses with plasma cell infiltrates are also seen in segmentally damaged mucosa, especially in immunoglobulin deficiency states.[81] Others have described direct invasion of the mucosa by trophozoites in vivo.[82] Whether this tissue damage relates to cytotoxic or enterotoxic products of *G. lamblia* is unclear at present. Malabsorption and specific brush border enzyme deficiencies are well recognized in giardiasis.[26] These findings might be explained in part by increased epithelial cell turnover with increased villus tip cell extrusion.[26,71] Others suggest that the parasite may compete with the host for nutrients.[77] Possible strain differences in pathogenicity have been suggested by studies in a gerbil model based on differences in surface antigens, patterns of infection, and homologous immune responses.[83,84]

Finally, the interaction of *Giardia* with other microorganisms appears to be important in certain instances. Whether by host-tissue damage or by actual carriage of other microorganisms by *Giardia*,[40] severe malabsorption and steatorrhea with giardiasis has been associated with small bowel bacterial overgrowth.[28,20] Concentrations of $10^3$ to $10^7$ bacteria (mostly enteric coliforms) have been described with giardiasis and malabsorption or steatorrhea that in some instances had to be eradicated before the symptoms resolved. Symptomatic responses to tetracycline without eradication of the *Giardia* have also been noted.[85] Bile salt deconjugation by bacterial overgrowth or by *Giardia* themselves has been postulated but has not been proved.[29] Smith and coworker failed to confirm direct bile salt deconjugation by *G. lamblia;*[86] however, direct uptake of bile salts by the parasite may be significant and clearly enhances its growth.[87] There is considerable promise of improved understanding of the pathogenesis of giardiasis with the development of the in vitro culture techniques as well as animal models of *Giardia muris* in mice and with recent studies of *G. lamblia* in gerbils, rats, and mice.

# DIAGNOSIS

## Examination of fresh and concentrated stool specimens

The diagnosis of *Giardia lamblia* infection can often be made by examining fresh or concentrated fecal specimens in cases of diarrhea that persist beyond the prepatency period of 5 to 7 days. As summarized in Table 44-1, the prompt examination of a fresh diarrheal stool specimen may reveal the striking motile trophozoites of *G. lamblia* on an unstained, direct, wet-slide preparation or a trichrome stained specimen for cysts or trophozoites before or after concentration (Fig. 44-2).

**Table 44-1. Diagnosis of *Giardia lamblia* Infection**

| Test | Sensitivity | Specificity |
|---|---|---|
| Fresh fecal exam for motile trophozoites | Better with active diarrhea | Specific in experienced hands, but finding *Giardia* does not prove disease causation |
| Stained, concentrated fecal exam | Approximately 34–98% | |
| Duodenal aspirate or string test | May be more sensitive than stool exam early in illness and in children (83–86%) | |
| Jejunal biopsy/imprint | Approaches 100% | |
| Serological tests: | | |
| IFA using patient's cysts or trophozoites | 89% of symptomatic patients | 71–100% |
| Immunodiffusion (with sonicated cysts) | 91% | Approaches 100% |
| IFA (with cultured trophozoites) | 97% ≥ 1:16 | 85–100% |
| ELISA (with cultured trophozoites) | 81% | 88% |

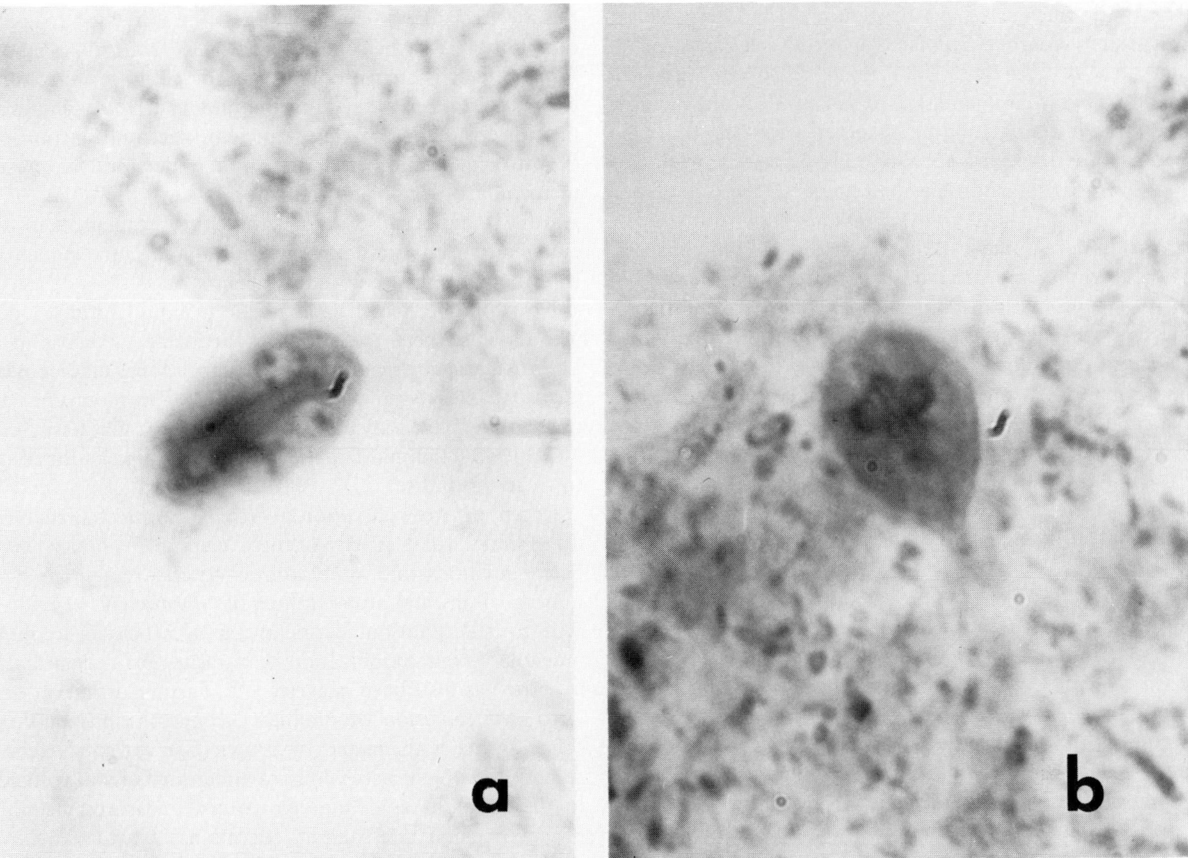


**Fig. 44-2.** *Giardia lamblia* (*a*) cyst and trophozoite (*b*) from fecal specimens of a patient with active giardiasis. Gomori-Wheatley trichrome stain, oil immersion ×640 magnification. (*Courtesy of G. R. Healy.*)

The diagnosis of *Giardia* infection is usually made by examining one to three stool specimens after concentration using such methods as flotation in 33% zinc sulfate (after clarification by centrifugation in water) or formalin-ether sedimentation in approximately 10 ml of 10% formalin suspension with 3 ml ether. The concentrate is then stained with 1% potassium iodide saturated with iodine. While some report that three concentrated fecal specimens are adequate to diagnose the vast majority of cases, others have shown that as few as 34 percent of stool specimens from patients with the parasite in the upper small bowel were positive. Barium, kaolin products, oily laxatives, antibiotics, antacids, paregoric, enemas, and cotton swabs will greatly reduce the value of the microscopic examination.

## Examination of small bowel contents or tissue

Although debated by some, from studies in adult volunteers,[88] several observers have reported an improved yield with examining duodenal aspirates or even small bowel biopsies in patients whose fecal examinations are negative for *Giardia*. Although this is more difficult and requires intubation, effective sampling of small bowel contents can also be accomplished with the string test (Entero-Test, Hedeco, Palo Alto, Calif.), which involves swallowing a gelatin capsule with one end of the 140-cm (or 90-cm for children) nylon line taped to the side of the mouth. Removal of the string after 4 to 6 h and examining the bile-stained mucus has been helpful in demonstrating *Giardia lamblia* trophozoites, particularly in young children and in adults early in their illness.

When jejunal biopsy is performed, one should examine a Giemsa-stained sample of the "imprint" of the tissue as well as the tissue itself for the purple-stained trophozoites.

## Serologic tests

Primarily because of limitations on antigen supply prior to in vitro cultivation of *Giardia*, little was known until very recently about serological responses to *Giardia* infections.

In 1976 Ridley and Ridley, using an indirect fluorescent antibody (IFA) test and patient isolates of cysts and trophozoites as antigen, found that 32 of 36 cases (89 percent) of giardiasis with malabsorption gave positive results, whereas none of two cases of giardiasis without malabsorption and none of 17 controls were positive. There was a crude correlation of severity of jejunal histopathology with antibody titer.[55] IFA titers fell in 11 of 19 cases (58 percent) 1 month or longer after therapy. Of 34 patients with malabsorption (mostly after travel to tropical areas) but negative stool and biopsy studies for *Giardia*, 10 (29 percent) had significant IFA antigiardial titers, which suggests that available diagnostic tests by direct examination may miss clinically significant giardiasis. These investigators also noted that use of mature cysts gave less reproducible results.

Washed, concentrated, sonicated *Giardia* cysts from fecal specimens were also used by Vinayak et al.[89] to develop an immunodiffusion test for giardiasis that was said to be 91 percent sensitive and negative in all 31 healthy or other parasite-infected controls.

Visvesvara and colleagues have developed an IFA test using axenically cultured *Giardia lamblia* trophozoites as antigen.[90] They found titers of 1:16 to 1:1024 among 29 of 30 patients with symptomatic giardiasis and 1:2 to 1:4 in 19 healthy controls. These positive titers could be absorbed with *Giardia* trophozoites in vitro. Fifteen patients with other parasitic infections for bacterial overgrowth syndromes had titers ≤ 1:16.

Smith et al. reported use of *Giardia lamblia* trophozoites cultivated in vitro in development of an enzyme-linked immunosorbent assay (ELISA) that appeared to be specific and sensitive with 81 percent of symptomatically infected patients developing antibody titer rises at 2 weeks to 15 months.[91] The sensitivity of an enzyme-linked immunosorbent (ELISA) assay for detection of *Giardia* antigen in feces has been 92 to 98 percent (probably more sensitive than fecal microscopy); the specificity is also high.[92–94]

## GENETICS, ANTIMICROBIAL SUSCEPTIBILITY, AND THERAPY

Axenic cultivation of *G. lamblia* has enabled studies of the genetics of strain variation[46–48] as well as in vitro sensitivity testing to antiparasitic agents.[95] Because the natural history of giardiasis is usually self-limited but occasionally recurrent over long periods of time, studies of the clinical efficacy of antigiardial therapy are difficult at best. As summarized in Table 44-2, quinacrine (Atabrine) 100 mg tid for 7 days is the recommended drug of choice in the United States and results in 80 to 100 percent cure rates.[9,25,96] Because of the occasional side effects of toxic psychosis, yellow staining of sclerae and skin, vomiting, and rare exfoliative dermatitis seen with quinacrine, a number of regimens of nitroimidazole derivatives have been used and are preferred by some. Metronidazole (Flagyl) 250 to 750 mg tid for 10 days effects 70 to 95 percent cure rates, respectively.[25] Single daily doses of metronidazole of 1.6 to 2.0 g for 2 to 3 days also appear to be effective, but may cause more gastrointestinal side effects. Other nitroimidazole derivatives, including tinidazole, nimorazole, and ornidazole (Ro 7-0207), have also been effective with possibly fewer side effects when given for 1 to 7 days.[97] Whether the mechanism of action of quinacrine is related to its relative distribution and then intercalation into DNA or to other membrane effects is currently unclear. The ability of nitroimidazoles to kill *Giardia* may relate to inhibition of DNA synthesis, competition for reducing equivalents with electron transport proteins or other mechanisms that are not understood at present. As metronidazole is not officially approved in the United States for giardiasis and because of concern about its mutagenicity and carcinogenicity in some experimental animals, the potential risks should be weighed before this agent is used.

Furazolidone, which is available in liquid form for pediatric use, has also been suggested.[96] Tartrazine, which is in certain Latin American preparations of furazolidone, may be related to serum sickness seen with this agent.[98] Paromomycin has been used in pregnant patients with symptomatic giardiasis.[99]

Table 44-2 summarizes the pertinent features of the drugs used to treat giardiasis.

Recent in vitro cultivation of *Giardia lamblia* has enabled studies of antigiardial activity of these agents.[95] Although the appropriate methods and standardized criteria remain to be determined, "4-day end point" killing of *Giardia* has been noted with 0.05 to 0.1 μg/ml quinacrine and with 5.0 to 6.4 μg/ml metronidazole.[35,51] Immobilization of parasites by antigiardial agents in vitro has also been suggested.[100] Further definition of the in vitro determination of inhibitory concentrations of these and other agents with axenically grown *Giardia* and amebas have recently become feasible and are under further study. In addition to the need for epidemiologic control measures including improved hygienic and sanitary conditions and water treatment to include flocculation, sedimentation, and filtration, the potential for exploring means for biological control of *Giardia* infections is now being opened by recent developments in in vitro culture technique and animal model. The roles of external and in vivo environments, pH, mucus, specific parasite and intestinal surface receptors, gut motility, and interaction with bacterial or other flora in causing or controlling disease are among the current frontiers in giardiasis research. Likewise, despite tantalizing suggestions of a protective role for cellular or humoral immunity, it remains unclear at present whether a vaccine might actually worsen the disease process in giardiasis.

**Table 44-2. Agents Used in the Treatment of Giardiasis**

| Agent | Dosage | Cure rate | Side effects |
|---|---|---|---|
| *Acridine derivative* | | | |
| Quinacrine (Atabrine) | 100 mg tid for 5–7 days | 63–100% | Occasional toxic psychosis; insomnia; headache; yellow sclerae, skin and urine; nausea; vomiting; rare exfoliative dermatitis. Contraindicated in patients with psoriasis. |
| | Pediatric: 6–8 mg/kg per day (or 2 mg/kg tid) for 5–7 days | 84–93% | |
| *Nitroimidazoles** | | | |
| Metronidazole (Flagyl) | 250 mg tid for 5–10 days | 56–70% | Nausea, headache, metallic taste, occasional insomnia, diarrhea, vertigo, paresthesia, rash, rare mild disulfiram-like reaction with alcohol, ataxia, urethral burning, reversible neutropenia (single daily dose metronidazole causes more gastrointestinal side effects; tinidazole reportedly causes fewer gastrointestinal side effects). |
| | 750 mg tid for 3–10 days | 95% | |
| | 1.6–2 g qd for 1–5 days | 91% | |
| | Pediatric: 15–25 mg/kg per day (or 5 mg/kg tid) for 5–7 days | 61–90% | |
| Tinidazole and others (nimorazole, ornidazole) | 2 g PO for 1 dose | 93–97% | |
| | 125 mg bid for 7 days | | |
| *Nitrofurantoin* | | | |
| Furazolidone (Furoxone) | 100 mg tid for 7 days | 72–92% | Occasional nausea, vomiting, headache, rare disulfiram-like reaction with alcohol, arthralgia, rash, urticaria, hemolysis, other blood dyscrasias. |
| | Pediatric: 1.5 mg/kg suspension qid for 7 days. | | |

*Not approved in the United States for giardiasis.

## *ENTAMOEBA HISTOLYTICA*

## HISTORY, EPIDEMIOLOGY, AND CLINICAL MANIFESTATIONS

### History

For over a century, amebiasis has been recognized as an invasive enteric illness in humans. The clinical syndrome of amebiasis and effective therapy are well known. In recent years there has been a renewed interest in pathogenesis of *E. histolytica* infections.

The early history of amebiasis has been reviewed extensively.[101] Although a British surgeon, Timothy Richard Lewis, first described amebas in human stool in 1869, Löesch is credited with the first description of amebic dysentery, in a patient from St. Petersburg, Russia, in 1875. Löesch also reproduced colitis in dogs by introducing the patient's stool orally or rectally. Koch first noted amebas in tissue specimens in 1887, and in 1893 Quincke and Roos first described amebic cysts. In 1903 Fritz Schaudinn named the parasite *E. histolytica* from its apparent capacity to destroy tissue. In 1912 Bernard Rogers found that emetine extracts from the ipecac root effectively cured amebic dysentery and liver abscesses. *E. histolytica* was definitively shown to be a human pathogen (as distinguished from the commensal *E. coli*) in human volunteer studies by Walker and Sellards in the Philippines in 1913.[102]

### Epidemiology

*Entamoeba histolytica* infects 10 percent of the world's population; although the vast majority are asymptomatic, invasive amebiasis is the third leading parasitic cause of death worldwide.[103] Epidemic outbreaks of amebiasis have been reported with food or water contamination from many areas.[4] However, endemic amebiasis as currently seen in the United States is acquired by the fecal-oral route, usually by person-to-person spread.[104] High-risk groups include residents of mental institutions (with stool cyst excretion rates up to 70 percent),[105] lower socioeconomic groups and recently emigrated Mexican-Americans in the southern United States,[105] and sexually promiscuous male homosexuals (with cyst excretion rates in San Francisco and New York as high as 20 percent).[106,107] However, the prevalence of *E. histolytica* infection in male homosexuals has declined in the last few years, probably along with the alteration in sexual practices within this group.[108] Overall prevalence rates in the United States are approximately 4 percent.[103] Foreign travel to highly endemic areas such as Mexico, India, the Middle East, and South America also increases the risk of amebic infection.[109]

Sexual transmission of *E. histolytica* results in enteric infection with possible dissemination or venereal infection in males and females. Amebic colitis occurs primarily in sexually active male homosexuals between 20 and 40 years of age with analingus being a significant risk factor for acquisition of ameba and *Giardia* infections. Penile and cervical amebiasis in conjugal partners is rare but reported.

### Clinical manifestations

Clinical syndromes with *E. histolytica* infection range from asymptomatic cyst excretion to acute rectocolitis, chronic nondysenteric intestinal disease (which can be confused with inflammatory bowel disease), typhloappendicitis, ameboma, or toxic megacolon. Extraintestinal amebiasis usually results from hepatic abscesses which may extend to pleuropulmonary disease, pericarditis, or peritonitis. Unusual extraintestinal manifestations include venereal genital lesions, cutaneous lesions, and brain abscess.

## STRUCTURE OF THE ORGANISM

*E. histolytica* trophozoites range in size from 10 to 60 μm, with an average size of 25 μm. Trophozoites contain a single 3- to 5-μm nucleus with fine peripheral chromatin and a central nucleolus (Fig. 44-3). The cytoplasm consists of a clear ectoplasm and a granular endoplasm that contains numerous vacuoles (Fig. 44-4). Cysts of *E. histolytica* average 12 μm in diameter (range 5 to 20 μm) and, depending on their maturity, contain one to four nuclei that have the same morphology as trophozoite nuclei. As in other members of the order Amoebidae, young *E. histolytica* cysts contain chromatoid bodies with smooth, rounded edges. Immature cysts may contain clumps of glycogen which stain with iodine.

Other members of the Entamoebidae family found in humans include *Entamoeba polecki, E. coli, E. gingavalis, Endolimax nana, Iodamoeba butschlii,* and *Dientamoeba fragilis. E. histolytica* and *E. hartmani* are recognized as two distinct species.[111] *E. hartmani* differs from *E. histolytica* in being smaller, having distinct antigenic differences, and being noninvasive.[111] Most experts agree that another nonpathogenic species of *Entamoeba* is the Laredo-like strain which grows in culture at lower temperatures (25 to 30°C) and does not cause clinical disease.[112]

Extensive electron-microscopic studies of *E. histolytica* reveal no mitochondria; ribonucleoprotein exists in helical arrays in the cytoplasm.[113–115] Endoplasmic and ectoplasmic vesicles are bound by a 120-Å double-layered membrane, much like the outer limiting membrane.[114]

Amebae also contain a uroid area where vesicles are noted external to the cell membrane.[116] An external fuzzy glycocalyx can be measured 20 to 30 nm on bacteria-associated trophozoites from tissue and 5 nm on axenic amebas.[117] Microfilament-like structures and actin have been identified in amebic trophozoites[118,119] and the actin gene has recently been cloned.[120] Microtubules have not been demonstrated. Apparent roles for microfilament, but not microtubule, function have been described in studies of the cytopathogenic capacity of *E. histolytica.*[121–123]

The surface membrane of *E. histolytica* has been well characterized biochemically. Amebae are agglutinated by the lectin concanavalin A,[124] which may be a marker for degree of pathogenicity of different strains.[124,125] Using concanavalin A binding to stiffen the external surface membrane, Aley et al. isolated relatively pure membrane preparations of *E. histolytica.*[126] Petri et al. have recently isolated the 170-kilodalton galactose/*N*-acetyl-*D*-galactosamine (Gal/GalNAc) inhibitable surface adherence lectin of *E. histolytica.*[125] Microfilament-depending capping, or aggregation of receptors, for concanavalin A or fluorescent-tagged antiameba antibody has been shown on *E. histolytica* and the capped membrane material characterized biochemically; but this capping capacity does not appear to correlate with virulence.[128,129] However, this process may help amebae avoid attack by host defenses.

In studies of surface-charge properties of *E. histolytica* trophozoites, Trissl has demonstrated a greater negative surface charge on axenic amebas than on monocontaminated or monoaxenic amebas and has suggested that virulence may be associated with

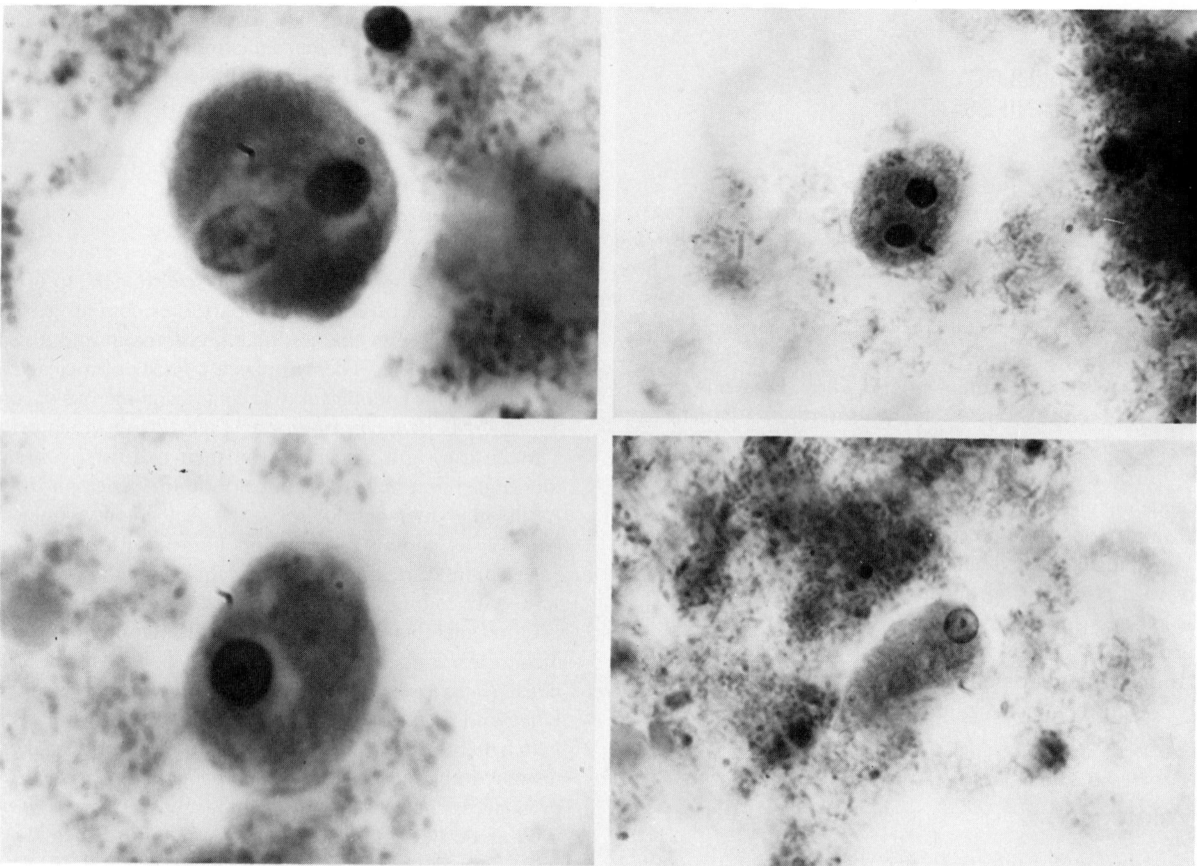

**Fig. 44-3.** *Entamoeba histolytica* trophozoites from fecal specimens of a patient with amebic colitis. Gomori-Wheatley trichrome stain, oil immersion. (*Right panel*) ×320 magnification. (*Left panel*) ×640 magnification. Note single nuclei with central, punctate karyosome, with delicate peripheral nuclear chromatin. The top two trophozoites also have an ingested red blood cell. (*Courtesy of G. R. Healy.*)

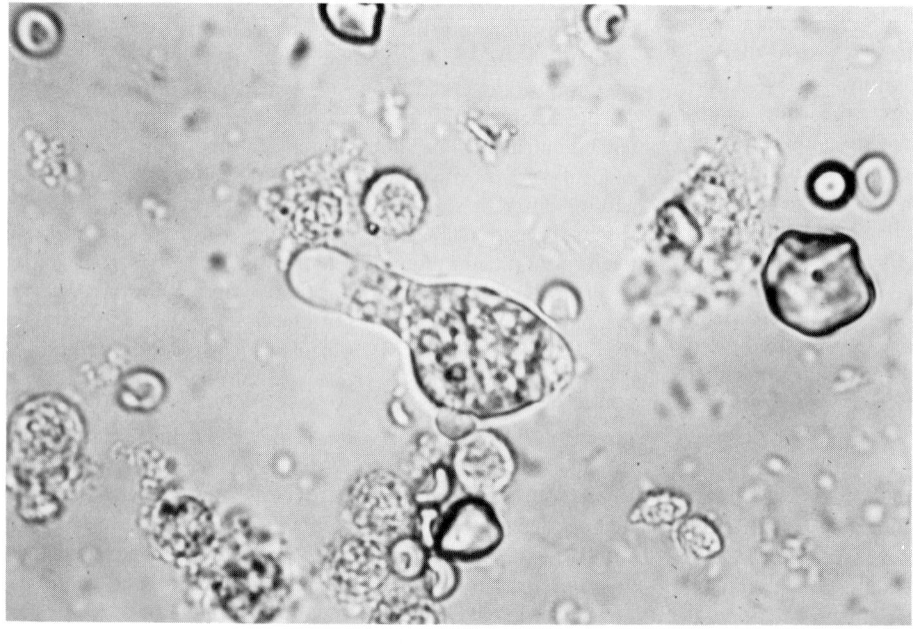

**Fig. 44-4.** *Entamoeba histolytica* trophozoites from a saline suspension of a vaginal specimen from a patient whose partner also had amebic colitis. A single typically motile trophozoite is seen.

reduced surface charges on the amebas.[125] Ravdin and coworkers found that an increased parasite surface membrane impedance was associated with decreased cytopathogenic activity.[129] Differences in surface charge warrant further study with regard to lectin agglutination and possibly pathogenicity.

## GROWTH, PHYSIOLOGY, AND CULTURE

### Life cycle

The life cycle of *E. histolytica* has been well characterized.[130,131] Cysts are the infective form of *E. histolytica* because they can survive outside the host for weeks to months in a moist environment. Infected individuals excrete up to 45 million cysts per day.[130] Ingestion of cysts from fecally contaminated sources is followed by excystation in either small or large bowel. The nuclei then divide to form eight nuclei (transient metacystic stage), cytoplasmic division occurs, and eight amebic trophozoites emerge.[102] The trophozoite population then resides in the large bowel, where tissue invasion may occur. *E. histolytica* cyst walls contain chitin, an oligosaccharide of *N*-acetyl-*D*-glucosamine, sialic acid, and other cyst-specific antigens.[132,133] Encystation is an active process; anaerobic glycolytic respiration, and DNA synthesis occur.[124] The conditions that induce encystation, excystation, and tissue invasion by amebas remain unclear and are the subject of current investigation.

Axenic cultivation of *E. histolytica* in medium without other organisms was first reported in 1961 by Diamond.[134] This was accomplished by microisolation of amebic cysts which were then introduced into a monophasic medium seeded with crithidial trypanosomes. A liquid medium was reported in 1968 and the current medium in use (TYI-S-33: trypticase, yeast extract, iron, serum) was developed in 1978.[135] These culture techniques have made it possible to grow amebas in large numbers and to maintain cultures for prolonged periods. Clonal growth of *E. histolytica* in semisolid medium was recently developed which allows quantitative cultures for drug susceptibility testing and other laboratory studies.[136] Studies of axenic culture in vitro have clarified nutritional and other requirements for amebic growth. These include requirements for cysteine, riboflavin ($B_2$), vitamin $B_{12}$, iron, serum, optimal pH, and low oxygen tension.[135]

## IMMUNOLOGY AND PATHOGENESIS

### Immunology and host response

There is no evidence that intestinal colonization by *E. histolytica* elicits a protective host immune response.[137] However, extensive but anecdotal evidence indicates that cure of amebic colitis or liver abscess is followed by resistance to subsequent invasive amebiasis.[138,139] The mechanisms of immune defense against *E. histolytica* infection have not been fully characterized. Serum from both healthy controls and infected patients (with high antibody titers to *E. histolytica*) are amebicidal to trophozoites through activation of the alternate complement pathway.[140,141] However, trophozoites that cause invasive disease are resistant to complement-mediated lysis and complement-resistant amebae can be selected in vitro by culture in normal human serum.[142,143] Serum antibodies and coproantibodies have been demonstrated to increase during invasive disease.[142,143] A protective role for humoral immunity is suggested by the presence of antibody to the parasite's galactose/*N*-acetyl-*D*-galactosamine (Gal/GalNAc) inhibitable adherence lectin.[144] Human immune sera can prevent amebic in vitro adherence,[144,145] despite the parasite's ability to aggregate and shed attached antibodies.[127] In addition to the Gal/GalNAc lectin, the parasite antigens most frequently recognized by human immune sera have been characterized,[146] which may be useful for development of diagnostic tests and vaccines. Production of mucosal antiamebic IgA antibodies has not been studied.

Cell-mediated immune (CMI) defense mechanisms appear to have a role in limiting invasive disease and possibly resistance to recurrent invasion following pharmacologic cure.[137] Following invasive amebiasis, the CMI response consists of antigen-specific lymphocyte blastogenesis with production of lymphokines (including gamma interferon) which activate monocyte-derived macrophages to kill *E. histolytica* trophozoites in vitro.[147–149] In addition, cured patients develop effective antigen-specific cytotoxic T lymphocyte activity for *E. histolytica* trophozoites.[148] However, in acute disease, CMI to *E. histolytica* is specifically depressed by a serum factor.[150] The high prevalence of *E. histolytica* intestinal infection in male homosexuals with AIDS or certain other clinical manifestations of HIV infection without an increased incidence of invasive amebiasis[108] suggests that host resistance to the initial amebic invasion of the colonic mucosa does not involve CMI mechanisms.

Nonimmune host defenses may be most important in prevention of parasite attachment to and disruption of the colonic mucosa. In animal models, mucus trapping of *E. histolytica* trophozoites occurs[151] and depletion of the colonic mucus blanket is always seen before parasite invasion.[152] Chadee and coworkers recently demonstrated that purified rat and human colonic mucins, which are rich in Gal/GalNAc residues, are high-affinity receptors for the ameba's Gal/GalNAc lectin, and mucin inhibits amebic adherence to and lysis of colonic epithelial cells in vitro.[153] Therefore, colonic mucin glycoproteins act as an important host defense by binding to the *E. histolytica* Gal/GalNAc adherence lectin; however, this interaction may facilitate intestinal colonization by amebae and thus promote parasitism by *E. histolytica.*

### Pathology

The pathology of human amebiasis provides clues to its pathogenesis. *E. histolytica* appears to exert a tissue lytic effect, for which the organism is named, whether in colon, liver, lung, or brain; this lytic effect leaves an amorphous, granular, eosinophilic material surrounding trophozoites in tissue[154] and can be studied in vitro. Consistent with the capacity to destroy leukocytes, inflammatory cells are found only at the periphery of amebic lesions and not adjacent to the trophozoites.[123,125,154,155]

The typical flask-shaped colonic ulcers are usually superficial, reaching only the muscularis mucosa level and separated by normal mucosa. Amebic trophozoites are seen in clusters in the periphery of necrotic areas. Light- and electron-microscopic studies have been alternatively interpreted as showing contact lysis of mucosal cells or diffuse mucosal damage prior to amebic invasion.[116,156] Current in vitro studies favor direct invasion and contact-dependent cytolysis by amebic trophozoites.

Liver pathology consists of the necrotic abscess and periportal fibrosis; however, the so-called abscess contains acellular, proteinaceous debris rather than white cells and is surrounded by a rim of amebic trophozoites.[154] Triangular areas of hepatic necrosis have been observed, possibly due to ischemia from amebic obstruction of portal vessels.[154] Periportal fibrosis alone, without trophozoites present, has been reported in patients with amebic colitis.[157] Whether this reflects past trophozoite invasion or host reaction to amebic antigens or toxins is currently unclear. "Amebic hepatitis" is a debated entity; liver function abnormalities commonly present with amebiasis are associated with periportal inflammation without demonstrable trophozoites.

## Pathogenesis

Pathogenesis of invasive amebiasis can be divided into four steps: (1) colonization of the intestine with a virulent *E. histolytica* trophozoite, (2) disruption of mucosal barriers with adherence to colonic epithelial cells, (3) lysis of adherent epithelial cells and host inflammatory cells, and (4) resistance to host humoral and cellular defense mechanisms with deep tissue invasion. Recent in vitro studies have markedly increased our understanding of the biochemical and molecular mechanisms of the pathogenesis of invasive amebiasis.

## Virulence

It is debated whether there exist distinct pathogenic and nonpathogenic strains of *E. histolytica.* Alternatively, all *E. histolytica* isolates may have the genetic capacity for pathogenicity, but expression of the necessary parasite proteins is modified by local intestinal factors. Sargeaunt and coworkers (reviewed in Ref. 158) demonstrated that starch gel electrophoresis of *E. histolytica* clinical isolates reveal patterns for the enzymes hexokinase, phosphoglucomutase, and glucosephosphate iomerase which are characteristic for invasive or noninvasive amebic infection at the time the sample was collected. The isoenzyme patterns are referred to as zymodemes; Sargeaunt[158] and others[159] propose that zymodeme studies reflect stable strain differences and that there is no need to treat individuals infected with *E. histolytica* expressing a "nonpathogenic" zymodeme. However, recent work by Mirelman and coworkers[160,161] conflicts with the assumption that an ameba's zymodeme pattern is a constant genetically determined trait. A single *E. histolytica* clone expressing a "nonpathogenic" zymodeme was induced by in vitro coculture with irradiated viable bacteria to express a "pathogenic" zymodeme pattern, lyse tissue culture cells, and cause liver abscess in hamsters.[161] Coculture with the original patients' bacterial flora resulted in the ameba reverting to a "nonpathogenic" zymodeme phenotype. As risks to the host or others of intestinal infection with "nonpathogenic" zymodemes has not been adequately studied, and considering the aforementioned in vitro experiments, we think it is best to assume that all *E. histolytica* isolates have the capacity to become pathogenic.

The previous studies and in vivo experiments have drawn attention to the association of *E. histolytica* with bacteria (reviewed in Ref. 162). Associated bacteria facilitated early culture of *E. histolytica* in vitro and Phillips et al. showed that bacteria were required for the establishment of invasive disease in germfree guinea pigs infected with amebae grown with *T. cruzii.*[163] They interpreted the role of bacteria to be one of providing an environment which enables amebae to grow in the colon.[164] Wittner and Rosenbaum subsequently demonstrated that amebae required direct association with viable bacteria for virulence and that a soluble virulence factor could not be demonstrated.[165] Recent axenic culture methods have allowed strains of amebae to retain virulence after prolonged periods (up to 9 years) of in vitro culture.[166] However, in vitro destruction of tissue culture cells by axenic trophozoites is stimulated by parasite ingestion of viable bacteria.[167] Associated bacteria are apparently useful by either accelerating the ameba's electron transport system or increasing its reducing capacity.[167] Viral particles have also been demonstrated in axenic amebae and can result in lysis of the amebae.[168] Viral passage from amebic strains of higher virulence to less virulent strains, however, does not consistently alter amebic virulence.[169]

Host nutritional factors appear to relate to the invasiveness of amebic infections. Weanling rats given protein-deficient diets are more susceptible to amebic infection; those already infected can eliminate the parasite when subsequently given high-protein diets.[169] High-carbohydrate, low-protein diets resulted in colonization but reduced tissue invasion.[170] Faust and Read have noted an association of a poor nutritional state with more invasive amebic disease in humans.[171] Wanke and Butler recently reported a very high mortality for amebic colitis in malnourished patients in Bangladesh.[172] Although iron feeding of experimental animals appears to increase the severity of experimental amebiasis, studies in humans do not reveal any correlation of invasive amebiasis with the serum iron or saturation of iron-binding proteins.[173] Finally, several investigators have noted an interesting association of ameba virulence and exposure of the parasite to cholesterol or liver passage.[174,175] The increased virulence apparently persists for weeks after cholesterol exposure and is therefore not a temporary membrane or nutritional effect; it remains to be further elucidated.

## Adherence mechanisms

*E. histolytica* trophozoites maintained in axenic culture must establish adherence in order to lyse target cells.[121,122] Ravdin and coworkers have demonstrated that in vitro adherence of *E. histolytica* trophozoites to Chinese hamster ovary (CHO) cells and human colonic mucins is exclusively mediated by the parasite's Gal/GalNAc inhibitable surface lectin.[122,153,176] The Gal/GalNAc lectin also participates in amebic in vitro adherence to human leukocytes,[147,176] rat and human colonic mucosa and submucosa,[145] human erythrocytes,[122,177] Chang liver cells,[178] opsonized bacteria or bacteria with Gal/GalNAc containing lipopolysaccharide,[179] and rat colonic epithelial cells.[153] Ravdin and coworkers[180] produced monoclonal antibodies which inhibited amebic adherence to CHO cells. Utilizing the lectin's carbohydrate binding activity and lectin specific monoclonal antibodies, Petri and coworkers recently isolated the *E. histolytica* Gal/GalNAc adherence lectin.[181] The galactose terminal glycoprotein, asialoorosomucoid (ASO) was more effective than asialofetuin and 1000-fold more effective than galactose in inhibiting amebic adherence to CHO cells. $^{35}$S methionine metabolically labeled amebic proteins from a culture filtrate or detergent solubilized amebae were applied to an ASO affinity column. After washing, a peak of $^{35}$S activity was eluted with galactose; SDS-PAGE under reducing conditions with autoradiography demonstrated a 170-kilodalton metabolically labeled amebic protein (Fig. 44-5). Petri et al. confirmed that the 170-kilodalton amebic protein purified is the Gal/GalNAc adherence lectin in three ways: (1) application of $^{35}$S methionine metabolically labeled amebic proteins to an adherence inhibitory H8-5 antibody-Affigel 10 column resulted in elution of the same 170-kilodalton protein, (2) the most adherence inhibitory monoclonal antibody, F-14,[152] exclusively rec-

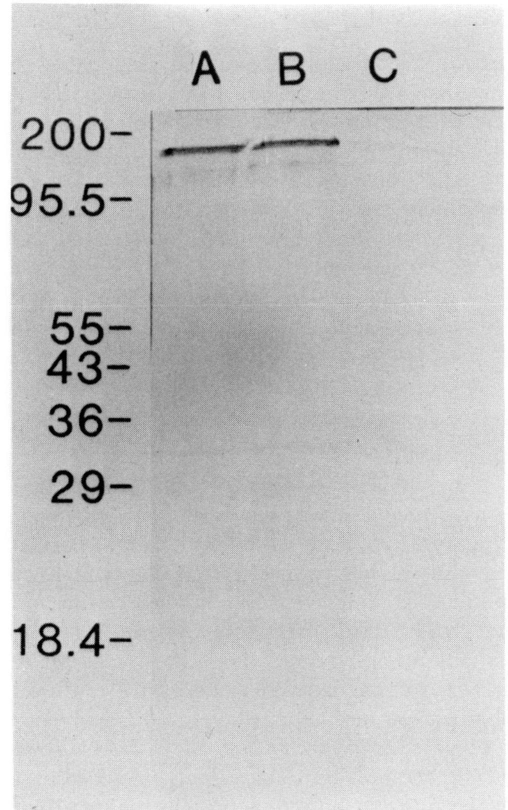


**Fig. 44-5.** Galactose inhibition of binding of the amebic adherence lectin to the asialoorosomucoid (ASOR) affinity column. Autoradiograph of SDS-PAGE of [$^{35}$S]methionine-labeled proteins eluted with galactose from an ASOR column to which conditioned medium (A), conditioned medium plus 0.5*M* dextrose (B), or conditioned medium plus 0.5*M* galactose (C) has been applied. The columns were extensively washed in 50 mM Tris, 200 mM NaCl, 10 mM $CaCl_2$, pH 7.35, and then eluted with 0.5*M* galactose in the above buffer. Galactose-eluted fractions were electrophoresed on 10% polyacrylamide gels and analyzed by autoradiography. (*From J Clin Invest 80:1238, 1987.*)

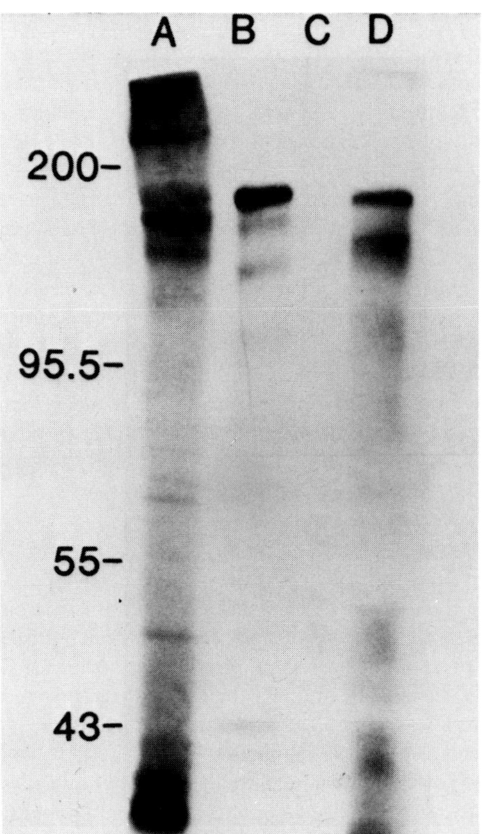


**Fig. 44-6.** Immunoprecipitation of [$^{35}$S]methionine-metabolically-labeled amebic protein with H8-5 and pooled human immune sera (PHIS). Autoradiograph of SDS-PAGE (10% acrylamide separating gel) of [$^{35}$S]methionine-labeled amebic proteins (A) immunoprecipitated with monoclonal antibody H8-5 (B), normal human serum (C), or PHIS (D). A 170-kilodalton metabolically labeled amebic protein was immunoprecipitated by lectin-specific H8-5 and PHIS and is the most intensively labeled antigen recognized by PHIS. (*From Infect Immun 55:2327, 1987.*)

ognized by immunoblotting the 170-kilodalton protein, purified by ASO affinity chromatography and lastly, (3) the Gal/GalNAc lectin purified by H8-5 immunoaffinity chromatography bound to CHO cells in a galactose-specific manner and competitively inhibited adherence of viable amebae. The *E. histolytica* Gal/GalNAc adherence lectin is the most prominent antigen immunoprecipitated by a pool of human immune sera (Fig. 44-6); immune sera from diverse geographic regions such as Mexico, India, United States, South Africa, and Zaire all recognize this adherence protein on immunoblotting.[127,182,183]

A chitotriose inhibitable lectin in *E. histolytica* homogenate which agglutinated erythrocytes was described by Kobiler and Mirelman.[184] In a high-ionic-strength buffer, amebic adherence to Henle cells was inhibitable by 40 percent with chitin.[185] The chitotriose inhibitable lectin may have a role in encystation.[133] Arroyo and Orozco[186] recently produced monoclonal antibodies which inhibit parasite adherence and ingestion of fixed human erythrocytes by up to 60 percent and on immunoblotting recognized a 112-kilodalton *E. histolytica* surface protein. Carbohydrate specificity of this putative amebic adhesin is not described; apparently more than one amebic adhesin mediates adherence to erythrocytes.[129]

## Cytolytic mechanisms

The pathology of invasive human amebiasis has a characteristic appearance: amebae are surrounded by amorphous granular debris, presumably due to tissue lysis.[154] Axenic *E. histolytica* trophozoites only kill target cells upon direct contact rather than via secreted cytotoxins.[121,122] Gal/GalNAc lectin-mediated adherence is required for lysis of target CHO cells, Chang liver cells, rat colonic epithelial cells, and human PMN or mononuclear cells.[122,173,176–178] Purified Gal/GalNAc lectin is a cytotoxin which induces rapid increases in target cell $[Ca^{++}]_i$.[187] Amebic cytolytic activity is dependent on parasite microfilament function,[121,122] $[Ca^{++}]_i$,[187,188] $Ca^{++}$-dependent parasite phospholipase A (PLA) activity,[188,189] and maintenance of an acid pH in amebic endocytic vesicles.[190] Establishment of adherence by *E. histolytica* trophozoites is followed by a marked sustained elevation of target cell $[Ca^{++}]_i$ which contributes to but may not be totally sufficient for target cell death.[187] Phorbol esters specifically augment amebic cytolytic activity.[191] An *E. histolytica* ionophore-like protein of 13 to 15 kilodaltons by SDS-PAGE induces lipid bilayers or vesicles to leak $Na^+$, $K^+$, and to a lesser extent $Ca^{++}$.[192–196] The amebic ionophore is packaged in dense intracellular aggregates and can depolarize erythrocytes;[194,195] although suggested, there is as yet no evidence that this ionophore directly participates in parasite cytolytic mechanisms. *E. histolytica* contains numerous proteolytic enzymes, including a cathepsin B protease,[196] an acidic protease,[197] a collagenase,[198] and a recently purified major neutral protease.[199] Proteases appear to be involved in dissolution of the extracellular matrix anchoring cells and tissue structure.[199] *E. histolytica* enterotoxigenic activity[200,201] may induce a secretory diarrheal component.

In vivo models of amebic liver abscess[202,203] and recent in vitro studies[178] demonstrate that parasite adherence to and lysis of host polymorphonuclear leukocytes enhances tissue destruction by release of toxic neutrophil oxidative products. A further understanding of the biochemical and molecular basis for the pathogenicity of *E. histolytica* should aid in the development of a vaccine or pharmacologic strategies to combat this disease.

## DIAGNOSIS

### Stool and proctoscopic examination

The key to laboratory diagnosis of colonic amebiasis is the stool examination. Three stool specimens or one purged specimen should be examined for maximum yield prior to use of barium, antacids, enemas, or antimicrobial or antiparasitic agents which will interfere with the microscopic examination.[204,205] If fecal specimens cannot be examined immediately, they should be refrigerated or fixed. Trophozoites in stool will rapidly lyse at room temperature or at 37°C. A saline wet mount should first be examined to establish the presence of amebic trophozoites or cysts. Differentiation of *Entamoeba* species requires permanent stains (trichrome or iron-hematoxylin) following fixation in 10% formalin or polyvinyl alcohol to reveal characteristic nuclear morphology, as described above (Figs. 44-3 and 44-4; Plate 67). The most common error in diagnosis is mistaking fecal leukocytes or macrophages for amebic trophozoites.[104] Of note, fecal leukocytes are usually pyknotic or absent in patients with amebic colitis, in contrast to bacterial dysentery, possibly because of the direct toxic effect of amebas on leukocytes.[123,125,154]

The stool examination is positive in approximately 90 percent of patients with invasive amebic colitis;[206] however, if the stool examination is negative in a suspected case of amebic colitis, proctoscopy or colonoscopy is indicated.[207,208] The margin of a colonic ulcer should be scraped (not swabbed, as amebic trophozoites may adhere to cotton swabs), and appropriate stains made of the scraping material, which often shows the parasite. If tissue is obtained, a careful search for invading trophozoites should be made on routine hematoxylin and eosin (H&E) and periodic acid-Schiff (PAS) stained material.

### In vitro cultivation

*E. histolytica* can be cultured from clinical specimens. Numerous culture media have been used, including liver extract (Cleveland and Collier), egg infusion media (Balamuth), and alcohol-egg extract of Nelson.[209] However, none is selective for *E. histolytica*. Both cyst and trophozoites can be cultured, a technique which can help differentiate *E. histolytica* from *E. coli*, *E. hartmani*, and the Laredo strain of *E. histolytica*. Cleveland and Collier's medium can be made more selective by adding rice powder and antibiotics (penicillin and streptomycin).[112] Failure of the culture to grow at low temperatures excludes the Laredo-like strain, which grows well at 23°C.[112] These methods can be used to document amebiasis in patients.

### Serology

Numerous techniques have been developed for study of the serological response to *E. histolytica* infection (Table 44-3). All methods are highly specific; patients with no exposure to amebas are rarely positive. These tests are usually quite sensitive for detection of patients with amebic liver abscess or invasive colitis, but are quite variable in asymptomatic cyst passers (Table 44-3). The indirect hemagglutination test (IHA) is the most widely used method at present in the United States.[142,210,211] The IHA uses antigen prepared from axenic cultures of *E. histolytica* (usually strain HK9). Serum is heat inactivated and added in serial dilutions to sheep or human red blood cells sensitized with amebic antigens. Hemagglutination is evaluated in comparison with known positive and negative controls.[212] IHA titers are usually elevated at the time of initial presentation with invasive amebiasis, often to titers of greater than or equal to 1:1024,[210] and then fall to lower levels at 2 to 11 years after therapy.[142,210,211] When repeated exposure or persistent infection renders the IHA less useful,[211] the gel diffusion precipitan test, which remains positive for shorter periods following acute illness (6 months), may be helpful.[211] Serological testing for amebiasis should be considered and may be quite helpful in differentiating inflammatory bowel disease from amebic colitis. Fewer than 2 percent of patients with inflammatory bowel disease and negative stool examinations for amebas have positive IHA titers.[210–212] Because of the widespread occurrence of amebiasis, patients in whom the diagnosis of inflammatory bowel disease is considered should have sera tested and stools examined for amebic infection, especially before steroid therapy is considered.

A rapid ELISA has been developed to detect amebic antigen in stool,[213–215] although its clinical usefulness has not yet been fully determined.

**Table 44-3. Systems in Use to Evaluate Serologic Response to Infection with *E. histolytica***

| Serological test | Percent positive in | | | |
|---|---|---|---|---|
| | Controls | Cyst passers | Rectocolitis | Liver abscess |
| Indirect hemagglutination | 0–7 | 8–15 | 81–98 | 83–100 |
| Indirect immunofluorescence | | | 57 | 57 |
| Countercurrent immunoelectrophoresis | 0–1.7 | | 87 | 95–100 |
| Agar gel diffusion | 0–18 | 1–52 | 55–95 | 80–100 |
| Enzyme-linked immunosorbent assay (ELISA) | | 50 | | 100 |
| Complement fixation | 0–16 | 28 | 85–90 | 83–100 |
| Cellulose acetate membrane precipitation | 0 | | 100 | |
| Immunoelectrophoresis | | | 87 | 93 |
| Latex agglutination | 0 | | 75 | 100 |
| Thin layer immunoassay | | | | 79 |

## TREATMENT

At present, drug susceptibility of *E. histolytica* is based on clinical activity and nonquantitative observations. Recent work with quantitative, clonal growth of *E. histolytica* provides a method for drug evaluation that can be standardized for static and amebicidal activities.[216,217] Appropriate drug therapy of amebiasis must take into account drug distribution (absorption, penetration, excretion in the intestinal tract) and sites of amebicidal activity. For example, antibiotics are usually active only in colonic and not in hepatic disease. Drugs that are active in all tissues include metronidazole, tiberal, tinidazole, dehydroemetine, and emetine hydrochloride.[206,218–220] Agents which may help eradicate gut luminal infection include diloxanide furoate, paromycin, bismuth iodide, and diiodohydroxyquin.[207,220,221] Tetracycline and erythromycin have some activity in colonic disease and chloroquine may be active in hepatic disease.[206] Recommended drug regimens, including dosages and possible adverse reactions, are outlined in Table 44-4.

## PREVENTION AND BIOLOGICAL CONTROL

At present, prevention of amebiasis rests on interference with fecal-oral transmission by improved hygiene, sanitation, water treatment, by abstaining from oral-anal-genital contact and by proper isolation of index cases.[222] Numerous tantalizing but unexplored possibilities for biological control also exist. One approach would be to prevent commensal carriage in the human host; and another, disregarding carriage, would be aimed at altering the parasite or host to avoid tissue invasion. Systemic and, especially, local intestinal immunity for alterations in microbial flora might well alter the parasite's carriage and shedding or its invasiveness. Recent isolation of the *E. histolytica* Gal/GalNAc adherence lectin and characterization of *E. histolytica* antigens further suggest the feasibility of vaccine development.

Certainly giardiasis and amebiasis rank among the widespread, often devastating human diseases for which the current renaissance of immunobiologic research holds great promise for many exciting developments. The groundwork that has been laid has already resulted in improved understanding of the biology of *Giardia* and amebas through in vitro culture and animal models. We now stand at the threshold of greatly improved understanding of the pathogenesis and, hopefully, eventual control of these two protozoan enteric parasitic infections.

# *CRYPTOSPORIDIUM*

## INTRODUCTION AND HISTORY

Organisms of the genus of *Cryptosporidium* are small (2 to 6 μm) coccidian protozoans that may inhabit the gastrointestinal, respiratory, and biliary tracts of a variety of animals including man. In 1907, Tyzzer first described this parasite as a cause of asymptomatic infection in the gastric glands of the common laboratory mouse.[223] In 1955, Slavin reported the first case of symptomatic diarrheal disease in poultry due to *Cryptosporidium*.[224] The parasite was subsequently demonstrated to be a pathogen of many animals and to cause epidemics of diarrheal disease. How-

**Table 44-4. Treatment of *E. histolytica* Infections**

| Drug | Dose and duration | Cure rate | Adverse reactions |
|---|---|---|---|
| | | **Cyst passage** | |
| Diloxanide furoate (obtain from CDC) | 500 mg tid for 10 days | 87–96% | Mild gastrointestinal upset (uncommon). |
| Diiodohydroxyquin (followed by tetracycline) | 650 mg tid for 20 days | 95% | Subacute optic neuropathy, dermatitis, diarrhea, headache. Avoid if hepatic disease or iodine intolerance. |
| Paromomycin | 300 mg/kg per day for 5–10 days | 80–90% | Gastrointestinal upset. |
| | | **Invasive colitis** | |
| Metronidazole* | 750 mg tid for 10 days<br>750 mg tid for 5 days†<br>2.4 g qd for 2–3 days†<br>50 mg/kg for 1 dose† | >90%<br>>90%<br>>90% | 10–20% Gastrointestinal upset (less with divided dosage), disulfiram effect, bitter taste, seizures, possible carcinogenesis. |
| Tetracycline | 250 mg qd for 14 days† | 90% | Gastrointestinal upset, hepatotoxicity, fungal suprainfection, teeth discoloration. |
| Dehydroemetine | 1–1.5 mg/kg per day IM for 5 days† | 80–90% | 25–50% cardiotoxicity (tachycardia, hypotension, angina, electrocardiograph changes, neuromuscular (tremor, muscle tenderness, and weakness), gastrointestinal. |
| | | **Liver abscess‡** | |
| Metronidazole | 750 mg tid for 5–10 days† or 2.4 g qd for 1–2 days† | 99% | See above. |
| Dehydroemetine (followed by chloroquine) | 1–1.5 mg/kg per day for 5 days† (600 mg qd for 2 days) | 90% (60% Alone) | See above. Gastrointestinal upset, headache, pruritus. |

*Alternate therapies to metronidazole with possibly less toxicity, but which are unavailable in the United States, include the following drugs: tinidazole, 50 mg/kg per day for 3 days (plus lumenal agent from the therapy for cyst passage), and tiberal, 15–30 mg/kg per day for 5 days (plus lumenal agent from the therapy for cyst passage).

†Plus lumenal agent from the therapy for cyst passage.

‡Aspiration of abscess not necessary for cure, but in experienced hands it may decrease symptoms and recovery time. The only absolute indication is a lack of response or worsening while the patient is on medical therapy for 3–5 days.

ever, the first instance of symptomatic human disease was first recorded in 1976 in a young immunocompetent child.[225] Human infection with *Cryptosporidium* was considered rare prior to 1982 and the result of opportunistic infection with a pathogen outside its normal host range. With the recognition of AIDS in the early 1980s, an increasing number of cases of severe cryptosporidiosis were reported.[226] In 1983, an outbreak of symptomatic cryptosporidiosis among animal handlers stimulated clinical interest leading to the recognition of this parasite as an important diarrheal pathogen in the immunocompetent host.[227]

## PATHOGENESIS

Historically, *Cryptosporidium* was assumed to be host-specific, similar to another coccidian parasite, *Eimeria.* Although the exact number of distinct species of *Cryptosporidium* is debated, recent studies indicate a limited number of valid species that can be distinguished by size, life-cycle characteristics, ability to transmit infection between animals (e.g., mammal to mammal vs. mammal to poultry), and chromosome pattern[228–233] (personal communication, W.L. Current). The primary mammalian species causing diarrheal disease is *Cryptosporidium parvum.*[229] A second species infecting the stomach of mammals is named *Cryptosporidium muris.*[223] Other apparent species include *Cryptosporidium baileyi* and *meleagridis* infecting poultry, as well as unnamed species infecting quail, guinea pigs, and possibly fish and reptiles.

Disease among animal hosts includes diarrhea in large mammals such as calves, piglets, lambs, foals, and goats, intestinal and respiratory disease in poultry or asymptomatic carriage in most rodents.[232] Persistent infection associated with diarrhea has been reported in nude (nu/nu) BALB/c mice when infected at 6 days of age; when inoculated at 42 days of age, only asymptomatic infection developed.[234] These observations and the fact that AIDS patients manifest severe symptomatic disease suggest that T lymphocytes, particularly the T helper subset, are important in recovery from infection and the development of protective immunity. In general, young animals are more susceptible to infection possibly due to innate resistance developing as the animal matures or the development of specific acquired protective immunity.[235] Experimentally, diarrheal disease develops in gnotobiotic animals monoinfected with *Cryptosporidium,* indicating that this parasite is a primary enteric pathogen.[236,237]

The life cycle of *Cryptosporidium* is similar to other coccidia (Fig. 44-7).[230,238] Infection is initiated when the host accidentally ingests oocysts. Although the infectious dose for many animal species is not clear, inoculation of 100 to 500 oocysts causes infection in 50 percent of Swiss-Webster mice.[239] A report of a researcher who acquired infection after a rabbit inoculated with *Cryptosporidium* coughed on him suggest that the infectious dose is also low in humans.[240] The asexual cycle of *Cryptosporidium* infection is initiated when gastric acid and proteolytic enzymes in the upper small bowel cause the oocyst wall to dissolve at its single suture resulting in a slitlike opening from which the four sporozoites can exit the oocyst.[241] The sporozoites are able to penetrate and parasitize the intestinal epithelial cells or potentially other epithelial surfaces contiguous to the gastrointestinal tract (i.e., respiratory or biliary tract epithelium). Within the host cells, sporozoites develop into trophozoites and, subsequently, type I meronts. The type I meront releases six to eight merozoites

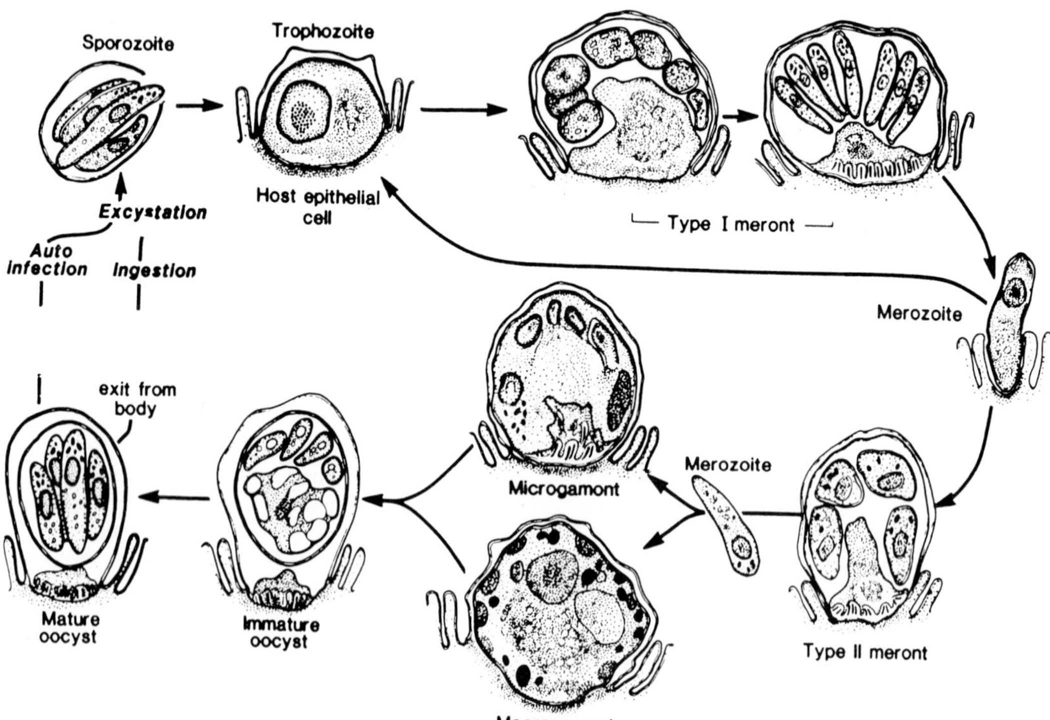


Fig. 44-7. Diagrammatic representation of the life cycle of *Cryptosporidium*. Sporozoites excyst from an oocyst and enter the microvillus of an epithelial cell, where they differentiate into trophozoites. Trophozoites undergo nuclear proliferation to form type 1 meronts. A merozoite leaves the type 1 meront to form either a type 1 or 2 meront. A merozoite leaves the type 2 meront to form microgamonts or a macrogamont. The microgamont fertilizes the macrogamont, which then develops into an oocyst. Oocysts sporulate in situ and either release sporozoites for autoinfection or pass from the body in the feces. (*From R Fayer, BLP Ungar, Microbiol Rev 50:458, 1986.*)

capable of reinfecting the host epithelial cell. Some of these merozoites develop into type II meronts containing four merozoites. These type II meronts release merozoites which initiate the sexual cycle of *Cryptosporidium* with the development of macrogamonts and microgamonts. Microgamonts are aflagellar but motile and fertilize macrogamonts, resulting in immature oocysts developing within the intestinal epithelial cell. Oocysts released from the host epithelial cell are either thin- or thick-walled and immediately able to initiate infection (i.e., fully sporulated). Thin-walled oocysts may excyst within the bowel, releasing sporozoites which reinfect the host epithelial cells. Thick-walled oocysts are excreted by the host and known to be extremely hardy. Thus, autoinfection of the host can occur due to either type I meronts or thin-walled oocysts, which may account for the ability of this parasite to cause sustained symptomatic infections in the immunocompromised host potentially lasting for the life of the individual.[238]

In general, the pathogenesis of *Cryptosporidium* infections is poorly understood. In humans, detailed studies of intestinal histopathology and function are provided only by case reports of immunocompromised patients, primarily with the acquired immunodeficiency syndrome. The intestinal mucosa usually appears intact and the enterocytes are generally well preserved by ultrastructural studies.[243,244] At the sites of parasite attachment to the enterocyte surface, microvilli are displaced and may be elongated next to the parasitic form. In addition, "peaking" of the host cell cytoplasm may occur at the point of attachment of the cryptosporidia.[242,243] In some infections, villous architecture by light microscopy is moderately to severely abnormal revealing crypt elongation and villous atrophy.[245,246] However, significant diarrhea ($\geq$ 1 liter per day) may occur with minimal histopathological change in the gut.[244] The degree and cell content of the inflammatory infiltrate in the lamina propria of gut infected with *Cryptosporidium* in clinically affected patients has ranged from minimal[247] to substantial[244–246] and may include plasma cells, lymphocytes, macrophages, and/or polymorphonuclear leukocytes. One limitation of these human case reports is that it is often not clear how extensively the patients were evaluated for additional enteropathogens. In animal studies, the degree of pathological abnormality has tended to correlate with the extent of infection and, in some species, such as calves, lambs, and piglets, with the severity of clinical illness.[235,237,248,249] In animals such as mice, rats, and guinea pigs, no obvious clinical illness occurs and pathologic findings range from inapparent to moderate.[249,250] In studies of spontaneously infested guinea pigs, cryptosporidial organisms have been observed deep in the cytoplasm of M cells overlying Peyer's patches, as well as associated with macrophages subjacent to the M cells suggesting antigenic sampling by the intestinal immune system.[251]

The mechanisms by which this parasite causes diarrhea in either the immunocompetent or immunocompromised host have not yet been elucidated. Both secretory (unaffected by fasting) and malabsorptive diarrhea have been reported in AIDS patients infected with *Cryptosporidium.*[244,252,253] D-xylose and B12 malabsorption, steatorrhea, and increased fecal alpha-1 antitrypsin clearance have been reported.[244,246,252,253] Radiographic studies have also showed results consistent with malabsorption such as flocculation of the barium, mucosal thickening, and dilation in the small bowel.[254] Animal studies have confirmed lactase deficiency and xylose malabsorption in calves infected with *Cryptosporidium.*[235,248] Detailed electron micrograph studies indicate that the parasite develops intracellularly in the host epithelial cell but is extracytoplasmic.[230,242] A striking electron-dense zone described as a "feeder organelle" forms at the interface between the parasite and the host cell.[230,242] It may be through this zone that the parasite receives nutrition as well as delivers parasite products capable of stimulating intestinal secretion. The observation that voluminous, watery diarrhea may occur in the immunocompromised host might suggest production of an enterotoxin or neurohumoral products by the parasite. Experimental results to date are mixed.[255–257] Similarly, the pathogenetic role of metabolic products from the inflammatory infiltrate in the lamina propria which may stimulate intestinal secretion[258] or the effect of other enteric infections on the clinical course of cryptosporidiosis have not been investigated.

## CLINICAL MANIFESTATIONS

Infection with *Cryptosporidium* has been documented in both immunocompetent and immunocompromised patient populations.[227,232,247,248,256,259,260] The clinical manifestations of cryptosporidiosis depend on the immune status of the host. In immunocompetent hosts, the majority of cases are sporadic, involving children or adults in both the developed and developing world.[259] Infection has also been reported in animal handlers,[227,232] homosexual men,[246] travelers,[261,262] and contacts of infected individuals (e.g. household contacts or hospital personnel).[232,260,263,264] In the immunocompetent host, infection results in a flulike, noninflammatory gastrointestinal illness characterized by malaise, anorexia, vomiting, fever, abdominal pain, and cramps. Blood and pus are not present in the stools and the fecal leukocyte examination is negative. Diarrhea lasts on average 6 to 14 days although some patients will have a more prolonged illness with diarrhea lasting a month, and rarely, 4 months.[247,260,265–267] Diarrhea may be much more severe (e.g., such as 17 liters of daily stool output) in immunocompromised hosts with defects in either humoral or cell-mediated immunity.[226,232,268] In this host, infection is frequently persistent and the resulting morbidity, for instance, in AIDS patients, may contribute to earlier mortality.[269] AIDS patients have been reported to develop extraintestinal infection involving the respiratory or biliary epithelium.[247,270–275] Although the contribution of respiratory cryptosporidiosis to clinical disease is unclear, individuals with biliary infection may present with the clinical picture of cholecystitis and may also be coinfected with cytomegalovirus.[247,275]

The incubation period of the infection is unclear but appears to be between 3 and 14 days.[232] In experimental data, the parasite can complete its developmental cycle in 3 days.[238] Until recently, asymptomatic carriage of the oocysts in clinically unaffected populations has been thought to be infrequent. For instance, in three studies examining predominantly asymptomatic homosexual men attending sexually transmitted diseases clinics, none of 375 individuals were found to have *Cryptosporidium* oocysts in their stools[276–278] In contrast, in these studies, *Giardia lamblia* was found in 3.3 to 6.5 percent and *Entamoeba histolytica* in 5.4 to 23.5 percent of the men. In studies examining the prevalence of infection with *Cryptosporidium* in developed countries such as the United States, Australia, or Europe, rates of infection in non-outbreak situations most often ranged from approximately $< 1$ to 5 percent. Among controls, only 0.6 percent of stools were positive.[232] In contrast, infection rates have been highest in developing countries with a range of 3 to 16.7 percent in individuals with symptoms and 3.2 percent in controls.[232,279–281] Recent data on the duration of oocyst excretion following clinical illness indicate that persistent asymptomatic oocyst excretion may occur.[265,266,282–284] Oocyst excretion lasts an average of 7 days postillness but may, on occasion, extend for several weeks.[265,266]

Several potential modes of transmission for *Cryptosporidium* have been identified. Earlier studies documented the potential for animal-to-human spread and *Cryptosporidium* is clearly a zoonotic infection.[227,232,248,259,268] Both domestic animals, e.g., calves, and companion animals such as puppies and kittens serve as potential sources of human infection. Increasing evidence indicates that person-to-person spread of this infection is important and is probably the major mode of transmission.[232,247,259,260,264] Human-to-human transmission is particularly well illustrated by the reports of outbreaks of diarrhea associated with *Cryptosporidium* infection in day care centers[266,285] and reports of intrafamilial spread of infection. In addition, water-borne outbreaks traced to surface water[286] or sewage contamination of chlorinated well water have been reported.[287] *Cryptosporidium* oocysts have been identified in treated sewage effluents and surface waters.[288,289] Unpasteurized milk has been postulated to be a potential source of *Cryptosporidium* infection, but there are, as yet, no definitive data.

Because the clinical syndrome associated with cryptosporidiosis is not unique, the differential diagnosis includes the extensive list of enteric pathogens which cause noninflammatory diarrhea. Rotaviruses and enterotoxigenic *E. coli* are the leading causes of noninflammatory diarrhea worldwide, especially among young children; Norwalk-like viruses must also be considered. In immunocompromised individuals (e.g., AIDS and bone marrow transplant patients), adenoviruses and coxsackieviruses may cause diarrhea.[290] *Giardia lamblia, Strongyloides stercoralis,* and *Isospora belli* are other potential parasitic causes of noninflammatory diarrhea. Epidemiologic data such as travel history, food ingestion (e.g., raw seafood), and recent antibiotic usage may be helpful in prioritizing the diagnostic possibilities.[291]

## DIAGNOSIS

The diagnosis of cryptosporidiosis is established by staining the stool with a modified acidfast technique specific for the oocyst stage of *Cryptosporidium* where the characteristic oocyst morphology is observed (Fig. 44–8). Examination of at least two fecal smears may be necessary for diagnosis,[265] and concentrating the stool may improve detection of the parasite particularly in nonacute illness or in evaluation of contacts of infected individuals.[232] Oocyst excretion may be intermittent; positive and negative smears from the same patient on the same day have been reported. In addition, a minority of the oocysts may not readily take up the acidfast stain and may appear as empty holes in a fecal smear.[292] This variability in the staining characteristics of the oocysts does not hinder diagnosis in experienced hands. Recently, a specific immunoglobulin M monoclonal antibody to the oocyst wall has been developed and marketed as a direct immunofluorescent antibody stain which is sensitive and specific.[293,294]

Although not available yet for clinical diagnosis, an enzyme-linked immunosorbent assay (ELISA) for detection of serum immunoglobulin M and G antibodies to *Cryptosporidium* has been developed.[295] Using both the IgG and IgM ELISA tests, 95 percent of the patients with cryptosporidiosis, including patients with AIDS, had detectable antibodies at the time of medical presentation. The ELISA should prove to be particularly helpful in epidemiologic studies of cryptosporidiosis.

## PREVENTION OF INFECTION AND THERAPY

The primary therapy for all forms of diarrheal illness including cryptosporidiosis is fluid and electrolyte replacement. Rehydration may be oral or intravenous depending on the clinical status and age of the patient. In studies to date, from 0 to 30 percent

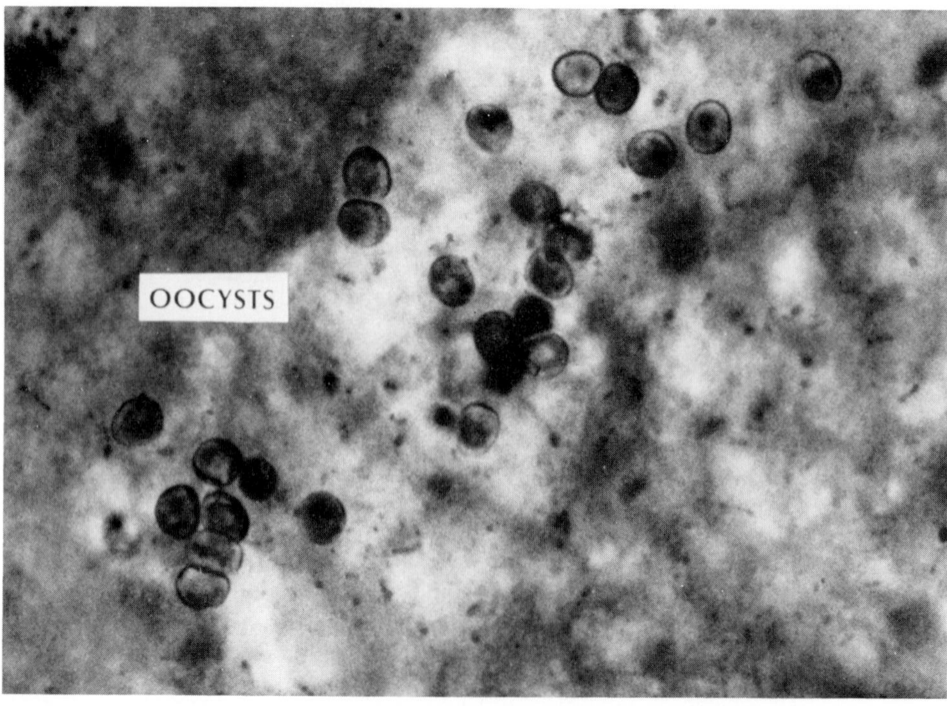


**Fig. 44-8.** *Cryptosporidium* oocysts stained with a modified acidfast stain. Oocysts are approximately 4 to 6 μm in diameter.

of immunocompetent patients have required hospital admission for intravenous rehydration during *Cryptosporidium* infections.[232,260,296–298] Although many drugs have been evaluated in animals or humans, no clearly effective pharmacologic therapy for cryptosporidiosis has emerged.[232,247,268,299] Uncontrolled data have suggested that spiramycin may inhibit infection and lead to clinical improvement.[300–302] A controlled clinical trial is presently underway.[247] Spiramycin is a macrolide antibiotic similar to erythromycin which is presently not commercially available in the United States but may be dispensed with permission from the U.S. Food and Drug Administration.[247] Development of an effective specific therapy for cryptosporidiosis has been hindered by the lack of a simple model for testing of drug sensitivity. Although nonspecific antidiarrheal therapies such as kaolin plus pectin (Kaopectate), antimotility agents (e.g., loperamide and paregoric) or bismuth subsalicylate (Pepto-Bismol) may be helpful in controlling symptoms, efficacy and safety in cryptosporidiosis have not been evaluated.

The thick-walled oocysts of *Cryptosporidium* are known to be very hardy and resistant to numerous tested disinfectants.[232] Only heat, and prolonged treatment (18 h) with 10% formalin or 5% ammonia, have been shown experimentally to reduce the infectivity of the oocysts.[248,303,304] Therefore, careful handwashing and enteric precautions in the hospital setting are important to interrupt person-to-person spread of infection.

Future research to better understand the ecologic niches of this parasite will be important in the development of measures to control the spread of infection.

## References


1 Leeuwenhoek AV: Letter no. 66 to the Royal Society, in *Tropical Medicine and Parasitology, Classic Investigations,* BH Kean et al (eds). Ithaca, Cornell University Press, 1978, vol 1, pp 4–5.

2 Monat HA, McKinney WL: Giardiasis: Question of pathogenicity. *US Naval Med Bull* 46:1204, 1946.

3 Ormiston G et al: Enteritis in a nursery home associated with *Giardia lamblia. Br Med J* 2:151, 1942.

4 Davis C, Ritdrie LS: Clinical manifestations and treament of epidemic amebiasis occurring in occupants of Mantetsu apartment building, Tokyo, Japan. *Am J Trop Med Hyg* 28:803, 1948.

5 Antia FP et al: Giardiasis in adults: Incidence, symptomatology and absorption studies. *Indian J Med Sci* 20:471, 1966.

6 Cortner JA: Giardiasis: A cause of celiac syndrome. *Am J Dis Child* 98:311, 1959.

7 Brandborg LL et al: Histological demonstration of mucosal invasion by *Giardia lamblia* in man. *Gastroenterology* 52:143, 1967.

8 Rendtorff R: The experimental transmission of human intestinal protosoan parasites: II. *Giardia lamblia* cysts given in capsules. *Am J Hyg* 59:209, 1954.

9 Petersen H: Giardiasis (lambliasis). *Scand J Gastroenterol* 7 (suppl 14):1, 1972.

10 Centers for Disease Control: Intestinal parasite surveillance; United States, 1976. *MMWR* 27:167, 1978.

11 Meuwissen JHETh et al: Giardiasis. *Lancet* 2:32, 1977.

12 Court JM, Stanton C: The incidence of *Giardia lamblia* infestation of children in Victoria. *Med J Aust* 2:438, 1959.

13 Knight R: Epidemiology and transmission of giardiasis. *Trans R Soc Trop Med Hyg* 74:433, 1980.

14 Black RE et al: Giardiasis in day-care centers: Evidence of person-to-person transmission. *Pediatrics* 60:486, 1977.

15 Osterholm MT et al: An outbreak of food-borne giardiasis. *N Engl J Med* 304:24, 1981.

16 Craun GF: Waterborne giardiasis in the United States: A review. *Am J Public Health* 69:817, 1979.

17 Shaw PK et al: A communitywide outbreak of giardiasis with evidence of transmission by a municipal water supply. *Ann Intern Med* 87:426, 1977.

18 Wright RA et al: Giardiasis in Colorado: An epidemiologic study. *Am J Epidemiol* 105:330, 1977.

19 Brodsky RE et al: Giardiasis in American travelers to the Soviet Union. *J Infect Dis* 130:319, 1974.

20 Rendtorff RC, Holt CJ: The experimental transmission of human intestinal protosoan parasites: IV. Attempts to transmit *Entamoeba coli* and *Giardia lamblia* cysts by water. *Am J Hyg* 60:327, 1954.

21 Meyers JD et al: *Giardia lamblia* infection in homosexual men. *Br J Vener Dis* 53:54, 1977.

22 Schmerin MJ et al: Giardiasis: Association with homosexuality. *Ann Intern Med* 88:801, 1978.

23 Jokipii AMM, Jokipii L: Prepatency of giardiasis. *Lancet* 1:1095, 1977.

24 Cain GD et al: Malabsorption associated with *Giardia lamblia* infestation. *South Med J* 61:532, 1968.

25 Wolfe MS: Giardiasis. *JAMA* 233:1362, 1975.

26 Hartong WA et al: Giardiasis: Clinical spectrum and functional-structural abnormalities of the small intestinal mucosa. *Gastroenterology* 77:61, 1979.

27 Zinneman HH, Kaplan AP: The association of giardiasis with reduced intestinal secretory immunoglobulin. *Am J Dig Dis* 17:793, 1972.

28 Mayoral LG et al: Intestinal malabsorption and parasitic disease: The role of protein malnutrition. *Gastroenterology* 50:856, 1966.

29 Tandon BN et al: Mechanism of malabsorption of giardiasis: A study of bacterial flora and bile salt deconjugation in upper jejunum. *Gut* 18:176, 1977.

30 Tompkins AM et al: Bacterial colonization of jejunal mucosa in giardiasis. *Trans R Soc Trop Med Hyg* 72:32, 1978.

31 Sheehy TW, Holley P: *Giardia*-induced malabsorption in pancreatitis. *JAMA* 233:1373, 1975.

32 Kacker PP: A case of *Giardia lamblia* proctitis presenting in a VD clinic. *Br J Vener Dis* 49:318, 1973.

33 Goobar JP: Joint symptoms in giardiasis. *Lancet* 1:1010, 1977.

34 Harris RH, Mitchell JH: Chronic urticaria due to *Giardia lamblia. Arch Dermatol Syphilol* 59:587, 1949.

35 Meyer EA, Radulescu S: *Giardia* and giardiasis. *Adv Parasitol* 17:1, 1979.

36 Tsuchiya H: Changes in morphology of *Giardia canis* as affected by diet. *Proc Soc Exp Biol Med* 28:708, 1931.

37 Owen RL: The ultrastructural basis of *Giardia* function. *Trans R Soc Trop Med Hyg* 74:429, 1980.

38 Holberton DV: Attachment of *Giardia:* A hydrodynamic model. *J Exp Biol* 60:207, 1974.

39 Owen RL: The immune response in clinical and experimental giardiasis. *Trans R Soc Trop Med Hyg* 74:443, 1980.

40 Nemanic PC et al: Ultrastructural observations on giardiasis in a mouse model: II. Endosymbiosis and organelle distribution in *Giardia muris* and comparison with *Giardia lamblia. J Infect Dis* 140: 222, 1979.

41 Hill DR et al: Lectin binding by *Giardia lamblia. Infect Immun* 34:733, 1981.

42 Lev B et al: Lectin activation in *Giardia lamblia* by host protease: A novel host-parasite interaction. *Science* 232:71, 1986.

43 Bertram MA et al: A comparison of isozymes of five axenic *Giardia* isolates. *J Parasitol* 69:793, 1983.

44 Smith PD et al: Antigenic analysis of *Giardia lamblia* from Afghanistan, Puerto Rico, Ecuador, and Oregon. *Infect Immun* 36:714, 1982.

45 Nash TE, Keister DB: Differences in excretory-secretory products and surface antigens among 19 isolates of *Giardia. J Infect Dis* 152: 1166, 1985.

46 Nash TE et al: Restriction-endonuclease analysis of DNA from 15

*Giardia* isolates obtained from humans and animals. *J Infect Dis* 152:62, 1985.

47 Wang AL, Wang CC: Discovery of a specific double-stranded RNA virus in *Giardia lamblia*. *Mol Biochem Parasitol* 21:269, 1986.

48 Adam RD et al: Antigenic variation of a cysteine-rich protein in *Giardia lamblia*. *J Exp Med* 167:109, 1988.

49 Gillin FD et al: Encystation and expression of cyst antigens by *Giardia lamblia* in vitro. *Science* 135:1040, 1987.

50 Bingham AK, Myer EA: *Giardia* excystation can be induced in vitro in acidic solutions. *Nature* 277:301, 1979.

51 Meyer EA: *Giardia lamblia:* Isolation and axenic cultivation. *Exp Parisitol* 39:101, 1976.

52 Visvesvara GS: Axenic growth of *Giardia lamblia* in Diamond's TPS-1 medium. *Trans R Soc Trop Med Hyg* 74:213, 1980.

53 Keister DB: Axenic culture of *Giardia lamblia* in TYI-S-33 medium supplemented with bile. *Trop Med Hyg* 487:77, 1983.

54 Gillin FD et al: Biliary lipids support serum-free growth of *Giardia lamblia*. *Am Soc Microbiol* 641:53, 1986.

55 Lindmark DG: Energy metabolism of the anaerobic protozoon *Giardia lamblia*. *Mol Biochem Parasitol* 1:1, 1980.

56 Wright RA, Vernon TM: Epidemic giardiasis at a resort lodge. *Rocky Mountains Med J* 73:208, 1976.

57 Roberts-Thomson IC et al: Acquired resistance to infection in an animal model of giardiasis. *J Immunol* 117:2036, 1976.

58 Thompson A et al: Immunoglobulin-bearing cells in giardiasis. *J Clin Pathol* 30:292, 1977.

59 Ridley MJ, Ridley DS: Serum antibodies and jejunal histology in giardiasis associated with malabsorption. *J Clin Pathol* 29:30, 1976.

60 Jones EG, Brown WR: Serum and intestinal fluid immunoglobulins in patients with giardiasis. *Am J Dig Dis* 19:791, 1974.

61 Hermans PE et al: Dysgammaglobulinemia associated with nodular lymphoid hyperplasia of the small intestine. *Am J Med* 40:78, 1966.

62 Ament ME et al: Structure and function of the gastrointestinal tract in primary immunodeficiency syndromes: A study of 39 patients. *Medicine* 52:227, 1973.

63 Hill DR et al: Susceptibility of *Giardia lamblia* trophozoites to the lethal effect of human serum. *J Immunol* 2046:132, 1984.

64 Deguchi M et al: Mechanism of killing of *Giardia lamblia* trophozoites by complement. *J Clin Invest* 1296:79, 1987.

65 Snider DP et al: Chronic *Giardia muris* infection in anti-IgM-treated mice. *J Immunol* 4153:134, 1985.

66 Carlson JR et al: Response of Peyer's patch lymphocyte subsets to *Giardia muris* infection in BALB/c mice. *Cell Immunol* 51:97, 1986.

67 Stevens DP, Frank DM: Local immunity in murine giardiasis: Is milk protective at the expense of maternal gut? *Trans Assoc Am Physicians* 91:268, 1978.

68 Andrews JS Jr, Hewlett EL: Protection against infection with *Giardia muris* by milk containing antibody to *Giardia*. *J Infect Dis* 143:242, 1981.

69 Kraft SC: The intestinal immune response in giardiasis. *Gastroenterology* 76:877, 1979.

70 Stevens DP et al: Thymus dependency of host resistance to *Giardia muris* infection: Studies in nude mice. *J Immunol* 120:680, 1978.

71 Roberts-Thomson IC, Mitchell GF: Giardiasis in mice: I. Prolonged infections in certain mouse strains and hypothymic (nude) mice. *Gastroenterology* 75:42, 1978.

72 Heyworth MF et al: Clearance of *Giardia muris* infection requires helper inducer T lymphocytes. *J Exp Med* 1743:165, 1987.

73 Gillin FD, Reiner DS: Human milk lipase kills parasitic intestinal protozoa. *Science* 221:1290, 1983.

74 Reiner DS et al: Human milk kills *Giardia lamblia* by generating toxic lipolytic products. *J Infect Dis* 825:154, 1986.

75 Zisman M: Blood-group A and giardiasis. *Lancet* 2:1285, 1977.

76 Ogilvie BM, Wilson RJ: Evasion of the immune response by parasites. *Br Med Bull* 32:177, 1976.

77 Barbieri D et al: Giardiasis in childhood: Absorption tests and biochemistry, histochemistry, light and electron microscopy of jejunal mucosa. *Arch Dis Child* 45:466, 1970.

78 Owen RL et al: Ultrastructural observations on giardiasis in a murine model: I. Intestinal distribution, attachment, and relationship to the immune system of *Giardia muris*. *Gastroenterology* 76:757, 1979.

79 Wright SG, Tomkins AM: Quantification of the lymphocytic infiltrate in jejunal epithelium in giardiasis. *Clin Exp Immunol* 29:408, 1977.

80 McDonald TT et al: Small intestinal epithelial cell kinetics and protozoal infection in mice. *Am Gastroenterol Assoc* 496:74, 1978.

81 Ament ME, Rubin CE: Relation of giardiasis to abnormal intestinal structure and function in gastrointestinal immunodeficiency syndromes. *Gastroenterology* 62:216, 1972.

82 Saha TK, Ghosh TK: Invasion of small intestinal mucosa by *Giardia lamblia* in man. *Gastroenterology* 72:402, 1977.

83 Blasevic M et al: *Giardia lamblia* infections in mongolian gerbils: An animal model. *J Infect Dis* 222:147, 1983.

84 Aggawal A, Nash TE: Comparison of two antigenically distinct *Giardia lamblia* isolates in gerbils. *Am J Med Hyg* 325:36, 1987.

85 Leon-Barua R: The possible role of intestinal bacterial flora in the genesis of diarrhea and malabsorption associated with parasitosis. *Gastroenterology* 55:559, 1968.

86 Smith PD et al: In vitro studies on bile acid deconjugation and lipolysis inhibition by *Giardia lamblia*. *Dig Dis Sci* 700:26, 1981.

87 Farthing MJG et al: Effects of bile and bile salts on growth and membrane lipid uptake by *Giardia lablia*. *Am Soc Clin Invest* 1727:76, 1985.

88 Nash TE et al: Experimental human infections with *Giardia lamblia*. *J Inf Dis* 156:974, 1987.

89 Vinayak VK et al: Demonstration of antibodies in giardiasis using the immunodiffusion technique with *Giardia* cysts as antigen. *Ann Trop Med Parasitol* 72:581, 1978.

90 Visvesvara GS et al: An immunofluorescence test to detect serum antibodies to *Giardia lamblia*. *Ann Intern Med* 93:802, 1980.

91 Smith PD et al: IgG antibody to *Giardia lamblia* detected by enzyme linked immunosorbent assay. *Gastroenterology* 80:1476, 1981.

92 Ungar BL et al: Enzyme-linked immunosorbent assay for the detection of *Giardia lamblia* in fecal specimens. *J Infect Dis* 90:149, 1984.

93 Green EL et al: Immunodiagnostic detection of *Giardia* antigen in feces by a rapid visual enzyme-linked immunosorbent assay. *Lancet* 691:2, 1985.

94 Nash TE et al: Usefulness of an enzyme-linked imunosorbent assay for detection of *Giardia* antigen in feces. *J Clin Microbiol* 1169:25, 1987.

95 Gillin FD, Diamond LS: Inhibition of clonal growth of *Giardia lamblia* and *Entamoeba histolytica* by metronidazole, quinacrine and other antimicrobial agents. *J Antimicrob Chemother* 8:305, 1981.

96 Bassily S et al: The treatment of *Giardia lamblia* infection with mepacrine, metronidazole and furazolidone. *J Trop Med Hyg* 73:15, 1970.

97 El-Masry NA et al: Treatment of giardiasis with tinidazole. *Am J Trop Med Hyg* 27:201, 1978.

98 Wolfe MS, Moede AL: Serum sickness with furazolidone. *Am J Trop Med Hyg* 27:762, 1978.

99 Davidson RA: Issues in clinical parasitology: The treatment of giardiasis. *Am J Gastroenterol* 79:256, 1984.

100 Jokipii L, Jokipii AMM: In vitro susceptibility of *Giardia lamblia* trophozoites to metronidazole and tinidazole. *J Infect Dis* 141:317, 1980.

101 Stilwell GG: Amebiasis: Its early history. *Gastroenterology* 28:606, 1955.

102 Walker EL, Sellards AW: Experimental entamoebic dysentery. *The Philippine J Sci B Trop Med* 8:253, 1913.

103 Walsh, JA: Prevalence of *Entamoeba histolytica* infection, in *Amebiasis: Human Infection by Entamoeba histolytica,* JI Ravdin (ed). New York, Wiley, 1988, pp 93–105.

104 Krogstad DJ et al: Amebiasis: Epidemiologic studies in the United States, 1971–1974. *Ann Intern Med* 88:89, 1978.

105 Thompson JE et al: Amebic liver abscess: A therapeutic approach. *Rev Infect Dis* 7:171, 1985.

106 Markell EK et al: Intestinal protozoa in homosexual men of the San

Francisco Bay area: Prevalence and correlates of infection. *Am J Trop Med Hyg* 33:239, 1984.

107 Ortega HB et al: Enteric pathogenic protozoa in homosexual men from San Francisco. *Sex Transm Dis* 11:59, 1983.

108 Druckman DA, Quinn TC: *Entamoeba histolytica* infection in homosexual men, in *Amebiasis: Human Infection by Entamoeba histolytica,* JI Ravdin (ed). New York, Wiley, 1988, pp 563–575.

109 Pearson RD, Hewlett EL: Amebiasis in travelers, in *Amebiasis: Human Infection by Entamoeba histolytica,* JI Ravdin (ed). New York, Wiley, 1988, pp 556–562.

110 Thomas JA, Antony AJ: Amebiasis of the penis. *Br J Urol* 48:269, 1976.

111 Goldman M et al: Antigenic analysis of *Entamoeba histolytica* by means of fluorescent antibody: II. *E. histolytica* and *E. hartmani. Exp Parasitol* 10:366, 1960.

112 Edelman MH, Spingarn CL: Cultivation of *Entamoeba histolytica* as a diagnostic procedure: A brief review. *Mt Sinai J Med (NY)* 43:27, 1976.

113 Miller JH et al: An electron microscopic study of *Entamoeba histolytica. J Parasitol* 47:577, 1961.

114 El-Hashimi W, Pittman F: Ultrastructure of *Entamoeba histolytica* trophozoites obtained from the colon and from *in vitro* cultures. *Am J Trop Med Hyg* 19:215, 1970.

115 Lushbaugh WB: Proteinases of *Entamoeba histolytica,* in *Amebiasis: Human Infection by Entamoeba histolytica,* JI Ravdin (ed). New York, Wiley, 1988, pp 219–231.

116 Pittman FE et al: Studies in human amebiasis: II. Light and electron-microscopic observations of colonic mucosa and exudate in acute amebic colitis. *Gastroenterology* 65:588, 1973.

117 Lushbaugh WB, Miller JH: Fine structural topochemistry of *Entamoeba histolytica* Schaudinn, 1903. *J Parasitol* 60:421, 1974.

118 Michel R, Schupp E: Cytoplasmic fibrils and their relation to ameboid movement of *Entamoeba histolytica,* in *Memorias de la Conferencia Internacional Sobre Amibiasis,* B Sepulveda, LS Diamond (eds). Mexico City, Instituto Mexicano del Seguro Social, 1976, pp 300–310.

119 Meza I et al: Isolation and characterization of actin from *Entamoeba histolytica. J Biol Chem* 258:3936, 1983.

120 Edman E et al: Genomic and cDNA actin sequences from a virulent strain of *Entamoeba histolytica. Proc Natl Acad Sci USA* 84:3024, 1987.

121 Ravdin JI, et al: Cytopathogenic mechanisms of *Entamoeba histolytica. J Exp Med* 152:377, 1980.

122 Ravdin JI, Guerrant RL: The role of adherence in cytopathogenic mechanisms of *Entamoeba histolytica.* Study with mammalian tissue culture cells and human erythrocytes. *J Clin Invest* 68:1305, 1981.

123 Guerrant RL et al: The interaction between *Entamoeba histolytica* and human polymorphonuclear leukocytes. *J Infect Dis* 143:83, 1981.

124 Martinez-Palomo A et al: Selective agglutination of pathogenic strains of *Entamoeba histolytica* induced Con A. *Nature* 245:186, 1973.

125 Trissl D et al: Surface properties related to concanavalin A-induced agglutination. *J Exp Med* 145:652, 1977.

126 Aley SB, Scott WA: Plasma cohn ZA membrane of *Entamoeba histolytica. J Exp Med* 152:391, 1980.

127 Petri WA et al: Recognition of the galactose- or N-acetylgalactosamine-binding lectin of *Entamoeba histolytica* by human immune sera. *Infect Immun* 55:2327, 1987.

128 Calderon J, Avila EE: Antibody-induced caps in *Entamoeba histolytica:* Isolation and electrophoretic analysis. *J Infect Dis* 153:927, 1986.

129 Ravdin JI et al: Impedance measurements and cytotoxicity in the presence of bepridil, verapamil, and cytochalasin D. *Exp Parasitol* 60:63, 1985.

130 Barker DC, Swales LS: Characteristics of ribosomes during differentiation from trophozoite to cyst in axenic *Entamoeba* species. *Cell Differ* 1:297, 1972.

131 Neal RA: Phylogeny: The relationship of *Entamoeba histolytica* to morphologically similar amebae of the four-nucleate cyst group, in *Amebiasis: Human Infection by Entamoeba histolytica,* JI Ravdin (ed). New York, Wiley, 1988, pp 13–26.

132 Chayen A, Avron B: *Entamoeba histolytica,* antigens and amoebiasis, in *Parasite Antigens in Protection, Diagnosis and Escape, Current Topics in Microbiology and Immunology,* M Parkhouse (ed). New York, Springer-Verlag, 1985, vol 120.

133 Mirelman D, Avron B: Cyst formation in *Entamoeba,* in *Amebiasis: Human Infection by Entamoeba histolytica,* JI Ravdin (ed). New York, Wiley, 1988, pp 768–781.

134 Diamond LS: Axenic cultivation of *Entamoeba histolytica. Science* 134:336, 1961.

135 Diamond LS et al: A new medium for the axenic cultivation of *Entamoeba histolytica* and other *Entamoeba. Trans R Soc Trop Med Hyg* 72:431, 1978.

136 Gillin FD, Diamond LS: Clonal growth of *Entamoeba histolytica* and other species of *Entamoeba* in agar. *J Protozool* 25:539, 1978.

137 Salata RA, Ravdin JI: Review of the human immune mechanisms directed against *Entamoeba histolytica. Rev Infect Dis* 8:261, 1986.

138 DeLeon A: Prognostico tardio en el absceso hepatico amibiano. *Arch Invest Med (Mex)* 1 (suppl 1):205, 1970.

139 Sepulveda B, Martinez-Palomo A: Immunology of amoebiasis by *Entamoeba histolytica,* in *Immunology of Parasitic Infections.* S Cohen and KS Warren (eds). Oxford, Blackwell Scientific Publications, 1982, p 170–191.

140 Ortiz-Ortiz L et al: Activation of the alternative pathway of complement by *Entamoeba histolytica. Clin Exp Immunol* 34:10, 1978.

141 Huldt G et al: Interactions between *Entamoeba histolytica* and complement. *Nature* 277:214, 1979.

142 Reed SL et al: Resistance to lysis by immune serum of pathogenic *Entamoeba histolytica. Trans R Soc Trop Med Hyg* 77:248, 1983.

143 Calderon J, Tovar R: Loss of susceptibility to complement lysis in *Entamoeba histolytica* HM1 by treatment with human serum. *Immunology* 58:467, 1986.

144 Petri WA, Ravdin JI: Cytopathogenicity of *Entamoeba histolytica. Eur J Epidemiol* 3:123, 1987.

145 Petri WA et al: Recognition of the galactose- or N-acetyl-galactosamine-binding lectin of *Entamoeba histolytica* by human immune sera. *Infect Immun* 55:2327, 1987.

146 Joyce MP, Ravdin JI: Antigens of *Entamoeba histolytica* are recognized by immune sera from liver abscess patients. *Am J Trop Med Hyg* 38:74, 1988.

147 Salata RA et al: Interaction of human leukocytes with *Entamoeba histolytica:* Killing of virulent amebae by the activated macrophage. *J Clin Invest* 76:491, 1985.

148 Salata RA et al: Patients treated for amebic liver abscess develop a cell mediated immune response effective *in vitro* against *Entamoeba histolytica. J Immunol* 136:2633, 1986.

149 Salata RA et al: The role of gamma interferon in the generation of human macrophages and T lymphocytes cytotoxic for *Entamoeba histolytica. Am J Trop Med Hyg* 37:72, 1987.

150 Salata RA et al: Immune sera suppresses the antigen specific proliferative response in T lymphocytes from patients cured of amebic liver abscess. 34th Annual Meeting of the American Society of Tropical Medicine and Hygiene, Miami, Florida, November 5, 1985.

151 Leitch GJ et al: *Entamoeba histolytica* trophozoites in the lumen and mucus blanket of rat colons studied *in vivo. Infect Immun* 47:68, 1985.

152 Chadee K, Meerovitch E: *Entamoeba histolytica:* Early progressive pathology in the cecum of the gerbil *(Meriones unguiculatus). Am J Trop Med Hyg* 34:283, 1985c.

153 Chadee K et al: Rat and human colonic mucins bind to and inhibit the adherence lectin of *Entamoeba histolytica. J Clin Invest* 80:1245, 1987.

154 Brandt H, Perez-Tamyo R: The pathology of human amebiasis. *Hum Pathol* 1:351, 1979.

155 Jarumilinta R, Kradolfer F: The toxic effect of *Entamoeba histolytica* on leukocytes. *Ann Trop Med Parasitol* 58:375, 1964.

156 Proctor EM, Gregory MA: The observation of a surface active ly-

sosome in the trophozoites of *Entamoeba histolytica* from the lower colon. *Ann Trop Med Parasitol* 66:339, 1972.

157 Chanduri RN, Saba TK: Liver biopsy study in intestinal amoebiasis. *Calcutta Med J* 53:39, 1956.

158 Sargeaunt PG: Zymodemes of *Entamoeba histolytica,* in *Amebiasis: Human Infection by Entamoeba histolytica,* JI Ravdin (ed). New York, Wiley, 1988, pp 370–387.

159 Allason-Jones E et al: *Entamoeba histolytica* as a commensal intestinal parasite in homosexual men. *N Engl J Med* 315:353, 1986.

160 Mirelman D et al: *Entamoeba histolytica:* Virulence enhancement of isoenzyme-stable parasites. *Exp Parasitol* 57:172, 1984.

161 Mirelman D et al: Changes in isoenzyme patterns of a cloned culture of nonpathogenic *Entamoeba histolytica* during axenization. *Infect Immun* 54:827, 1986.

162 Mirelman D: Ameba-bacterial relationship in amebiasis, in *Amebiasis: Human Infection by Entamoeba histolytica,* JI Ravdin (ed). New York, Wiley, 1988, pp 351–369.

163 Phillips BP et al: Studies on the ameba-bacterial relationship in amebiasis: Comparative results of the intracecal inoculation of germ free, monocontaminated, and conventional guinea pigs with *Entamoeba histolytica. Am J Trop Med Hyg* 4:675, 1955.

164 Phillips BP et al: Studies on the ameba-bacterial relationship in amebiasis: II. Some concepts on the etiology of the disease. *Am J Trop Med Hyg* 7:392, 1958.

165 Wittner M, Rosenbaum RM: Role of bacteria in modifying virulence of *Entamoeba histolytica. Am J Trop Med Hyg* 19:755, 1970.

166 Diamond LS et al: A comparison of the virulence of nine strains of axenically cultivated *E. histolytica* in hamster liver. *Arch Invest Med (Mex)* 5 (suppl 2):423, 1974.

167 Bracha R, Mirelman D: Virulence of *Entamoeba histolytica* trophozoites. Effects of bacteria, microaerobic conditions and metronidazole. *J Exp Med* 160:353, 1984.

168 Diamond LS et al: Viruses of *Entamoeba histolytica:* I. Identification of transmissible virus-like agents. *J Virol* 9:326, 1972.

169 Mattern CFT et al: Experimental amebiasis: IV. Amebal viruses and the virulence of *Entamoeba histolytica. Am J Trop Med Hyg* 28:653, 1979.

170 Ross GW, Knight R: Dietary factors affecting the pathogenicity of *Entamoeba histolytica* in rats. *Trans R Soc Trop Med Hyg* 6:560, 1973.

171 Faust EC, Read TR: Parasitologic surveys in Cali, Departmento del Valle, Columbia: V. Capacity of *Entamoeba histolytica* of human origin to utilize different types of starches in its metabolism. *Am J Trop Med Hyg* 8:293, 1959.

172 Wanke C, Butler T: Intestinal amebiasis in a hospital population in Bangladesh. Paper 1566, 25th ICAAC Conference, Minneapolis, Minnesota, 1985.

173 Diamond LS et al: *Entamoeba histolytica:* Iron and nutritional immunity. *Arch Invest Med (Mex)* 9 (suppl 1):329, 1978.

174 Lushbaugh WB et al: Effect of hamster liver passage on the virulence of axenically cultivated *Entamoeba histolytica. Am J Trop Med Hyg* 27:248, 1978.

175 Das SR, Ghoshal S: Restoration of virulence to rat of axenically grown *Entamoeba histolytica* by cholesterol and hamster liver passage. *Ann Trop Med Parasitol* 70:439, 1976.

176 Ravdin JI et al: The N-acetyl-D-galactosamine-inhibitable adherence lectin of *Entamoeba histolytica:* I. Partial purification and relation to amebic virulence *in vitro. J Infect Dis* 151:804, 1985.

177 Orozco ME et al: *Entamoeba histolytica:* Cytopathogenicity and lectin activity of avirulent mutants. *Exp Parasitol* 63:157, 1987.

178 Salata RA, Ravdin JI: The interaction of human neutrophils and *Entamoeba histolytica* increases cytopathogenicity for liver cell monolayers. *J Infect Dis* 154:19, 1986.

179 Bracha R, Mirelman D: Adherence and ingestion of *Escherichia coli* serotype 055 by trophozoites of *Entamoeba histolytica. Infect Immun* 40:882, 1983.

180 Ravdin JI et al: Production of mouse monoclonal antibodies which inhibit *in vitro* adherence of *Entamoeba histolytica* trophozoites. *Infect Immun* 53:1, 1986.

181 Petri WA et al: Isolation of the galactose-binding lectin which mediates the *in vitro* adherence of *Entamoeba histolytica. J Clin Invest* 80:1238, 1987.

182 Petri WA et al: Antigenic stability and immunodominance of the Gal/GalNAc adherence lectins of *Entamoeba histolytica. Am J Med Sci,* in press, 1988.

183 Ravdin JI et al: Correlation of clinical status and zymodeme analysis with serum Western blot recognition of *Entamoeba histolytica* antigens. Abstract 176, 36th Annual Meeting of the American Society of Tropical Medicine and Hygiene, Los Angeles, CA, December 1, 1987.

184 Kobiler D, Mirelman D: Lectin activity in *Entamoeba histolytica* trophozoites. *Infect Immun* 29:221, 1980.

185 Kobiler D, Mirelman D: Adhesion of *Entamoeba histolytica* trophozoites to monolayers of human cells. *J Infect Dis* 144:539, 1981.

186 Arroyo R, Orozco E: Localizacion e identification de adhemiba I., una proteina que participa en la adhesion de *Entamoeba histolytica* a eritrocitos humanos y celulas epiteliales. Abstract. X Seminario Sobre Amibiasis, Mexico, DF, October 6–8, 1986.

187 Ravdin JI et al: The relationship of free intracellular calcium ions to the cytolyte activity of *Entamoeba histolytica. Infect Immun* 56: 1505, 1988.

188 Ravdin JI et al: Effect of calcium and phospholipase A antagonists on the cytopathogenicity of *Entamoeba histolytica. J Infect Dis* 152: 542, 1985.

189 Long-Krug SA et al: The phospholipase A enzymes of *Entamoeba histolytica:* Description and subcellular localization. *J Infect Dis* 152: 536, 1985.

190 Ravdin JI et al: Acid intracellular vesicles and the cytolysis of mammalian target cells by *Entamoeba histolytica* trophozoites. *J Protozool* 33:478, 1986.

191 Weikel CS et al: Phorbol esters specifically enhance the cytolytic activity of *Entamoeba histolytica. Infect Immun* 56:1485, 1988.

192 Lynch EC et al: An ion channel forming protein produced by *Entamoeba histolytica. EMBO J* 1:801, 1982.

193 Young JD-E et al: Characterization of a membrane pore-forming protein from *Entamoeba histolytica. J Exp Med* 156:1677, 1982.

194 Rosenberg I, Gitler C: Subcellular fractionation of amoebapore and plasma membrane components of *Entamoeba histolytica* using self-generating percoll gradients. *Mol Biochem Parasitol* 14:231, 1985.

195 Young JD-E, Cohn ZA: Molecular mechanisms of cytotoxicity mediated by *Entamoeba histolytica:* Characterization of a pore-forming protein (PFP). *J Cell Biochem* 29:299, 1985.

196 Lushbaugh WB et al: Purification of cathepsin B activity of *Entamoeba histolytica* toxin. *Exp Parasitol* 59:328, 1985.

197 Scholze H, Werries E: A weakly acidic protease has a powerful proteolytic activity in *Entamoeba histolytica. Mol Biochem Parasitol* 11:293, 1984.

198 Muñoz MDL et al: The collagenase of *Entamoeba histolytica. J Exp Med* 155:42, 1982.

199 Keene WE et al: The major neutral proteinase of *Entamoeba histolytica. J Exp Med* 163:536, 1986.

200 McGowan K et al: *Entamoeba histolytica* causes intestinal secretion: Role of serotonin. *Science* 221:762, 1983.

201 Feingold C et al: Isolation, purification, and partial characterization of enterotoxin from extracts of *Entamoeba histolytica* trophozoites. *Infect Immun* 48:211, 1985.

202 Tsutsumi V et al: Cellular basis of experimental amebic liver abscess formation. *Am J Pathol* 117:81, 1984.

203 Chadee K, Meerovitch E: The pathogenesis of experimentally induced amebic liver abscess in the gerbil (*Meriones unguiculatus*). *Am J Pathol* 117:71, 1984.

204 Juniper K: Acute amebic colitis. *Am J Med* 33:377, 1962.

205 Ravdin JI, Guerrant RL: Current problems in diagnosis and treatment of amoebic infections, in *Current Clinical Topics in Infectious Diseases,* vol. 7, JS Remington, MN Swartz (eds). New York, McGraw-Hill, 1986, pp 82–111.

206 Adams EB, MacLeod IN: Invasive amebiasis: I. Amebic dysentery and its complications. *Medicine* 56:315, 1977.

207 Ravdin JI: Intestinal disease caused by *Entamoeba histolytica,* in *Amebiasis: Human Infection by Entamoeba histolytica,* JI Ravdin (ed). New York, Wiley, 1988, pp 495–510.

208 Blumencranz H et al: The role of endoscopy in suspected amebiasis. *Am J Gastroenterology* 78:15, 1983.

209 Healy GR: Diagnostic techniques for stool samples, in *Amebiasis: Human Infection by Entamoeba histolytica,* JI Ravdin (ed). New York, Wiley, 1988, pp 635–649.

210 Healy GR: Serology, in *Amebiasis: Human Infection by Entamoeba histolytica,* JI Ravdin (ed). New York, Wiley, 1988, pp 650–663.

211 Patterson M et al: Serologic testing for amoebiasis. *Gastroenterology* 78:1185, 1980.

212 Kessel JF et al: Indirect hemagglutination and complement fixation tests in amebiasis. *Am J Trop Med Hyg* 14:540, 1965.

213 Ungar BL et al: Use of a monoclonal antibody in an enzyme immunoassay for the detection of *Entamoeba histolytica* in fecal specimens. *Am J Trop Med Hyg* 34:465, 1985.

214 Palacios O et al: Determinacion del antigeno amibiano in heces por el matado elisa para la identificacion de *Entamoeba histolytica. Arch Invest Med (Mex)* 9 (suppl 1):339, 1978.

215 Randall GR et al: Use of the enzyme-linked immunosorbent assay (ELISA) for detection of *Entamoeba histolytica* antigen in faecal samples. *Trans R Soc Trop Med Hyg* 78:593, 1984.

216 Cedeño JR, Krogstad DJ: Susceptibility testing of *Entamoeba histolytica. J Infect Dis* 148:1090, 1983.

217 Cedeño JR, Krogstad DJ: *In vitro* antiamebic drug activity, in *Amebiasis: Human Infection by Entamoeba histolytica,* JI Ravdin (ed). New York, Wiley, 1988, pp 723–733.

218 Powell SJ: Therapy of amebiasis. *Bull NY Acad Sci* 47:469, 1971.

219 Sunoto SH et al: Tiberal (Ro 7-0207-Roche) in the treatment of intestinal amoebiasis—Part II. *Paediatr Indones* 16:403, 1976.

220 Norris SM, Ravdin JI: The pharmacology of antiamebic drugs, in *Amebiasis: Human Infection by Entamoeba histolytica,* JI Ravdin (ed). New York, Wiley, 1988, pp 734–740.

221 Wolfe MS: Nondysenteric intestinal amebiasis: Treatment with diloxanide furoate. *JAMA* 224:1601, 1973.

222 Walsh JA: Transmission of *Entamoeba histolytica* infection, in *Amebiasis: Human Infection by Entamoeba histolytica,* JI Ravdin (ed). New York, Wiley, 1988, pp 106–119.

223 Tyzzer EE: A sporozoan found in the peptic glands of the common mouse. *Proc Soc Exp Biol* 5:12, 1907.

224 Slavin D: *Cryptosporidium meleagridis* (sp. nor.). *J Comp Pathol* 65:262, 1955.

225 Nime FA et al: Acute enterocolitis in a human being infected with the protozoan *Cryptosporidium. Gastroenterology* 70:592, 1976.

226 Centers for Disease Control: Cryptosporidiosis: Assessment of chemotherapy of males with acquired immune deficiency syndrome (AIDS). *MMWR* 31:589, 1982.

227 Current WL, et al: Human cryptosporidiosis in immunocompetent and immunodeficient persons. *N Engl J Med* 308:1252, 1983.

228 Levine ND: Taxonomy and review of the coccidian genus *Cryptosporidium* (Protozoa, Apicomplexa). *J Protozool* 31:94, 1984.

229 Upton SJ, Current WL: The species of *Cryptosporidium* (Apicomplexa: Cryptosporidiidae) infecting mammals. *J Parasitol* 71:625, 1985.

230 Current WL, Reese NC: A comparison of endogenous development of three isolates of *Cryptosporidium* in suckling mice. *J Protozool* 33:98, 1986.

231 Current WL et al: The life cycle of *Cryptosporidium baileyi* n. sp. (Apicomplexa, Cryptosporidiidae) infecting chickens. *J Protozool* 33:289, 1986.

232 Fayer R, Ungar BLP: *Cryptosporidium* spp. and cryptosporidiosis. *Microbiol Rev* 50:458, 1986.

233 Mead JR et al: *Cryptosporidium* isolate comparison using field inversion gel electrophoresis. *Am Soc Trop Med Hyg,* in press.

234 Heine J et al: Persistent *Cryptosporidium* infection in congenitally athymic (nude) mice. *Infect Immun* 43:856, 1984.

235 Moon HW et al: Intestinal cryptosporidiosis: Pathogenesis and immunity. *Microecol Therap* 15:103, 1985.

236 Tzipori S et al: Enterocolitis in pigs caused by *Cryptosporidium* sp. purified from calf faeces. *Vet Parasitol* 11:121, 1982.

237 Heine J et al: Enteric lesions and diarrhea in gnotobiotic calves monoinfected with *Cryptosporidium* species. *J Infect Dic* 150:768, 1984.

238 Current WL, Haynes TB: Complete development of *Cryptosporidium* in cell culture. *Science* 224:603, 1984.

239 Ernest JA et al: Infection dynamics of *Cryptosporidium parvum* (Apicomplexa: Cryptosporiidae) in neonatal mice (Mus musculus). *J Parasitol* 72:796, 1986.

240 Blagburn BL, Current WL: Accidental infection of a researcher with human *Cryptosporidium. J Infect Dis* 148:772, 1983.

241 Reduker DW et al: Ultrastructure of *Cryptosporidium parvum* oocysts and excysting sporozoites as revealed by high resolution scanning electron microscopy. *J Protozool* 32:708, 1985.

242 Vetterling JM et al: Ultrastructure of *Cryptosporidium wrairi* from the guinea pig. *J Protozool* 18:218, 1971.

243 Lefkowitch JH et al: Cryptosporidiosis of the human small intestine: a light and electron microscopic study. *Hum Pathol* 15:746, 1984.

244 Modigliani R et al: Diarrhoea and malabsorption in acquired immune deficiency syndrome: A study of four cases with special emphasis on opportunistic protozoan infestations. *Gut* 26:179, 1985.

245 Meisel JL et al: Overwhelming watery diarrhea associated with a *Cryptosporidium* in an immunosuppressed patient. *Gastroenterol* 70:1156, 1976.

246 Soave R et al: Cryptosporidiosis in homosexual men. *Ann Intern Med* 100:504, 1984.

247 Soave R, Armstrong D. *Cryptosporidium* and cryptosporidiosis. *Rev Infect Dis* 8:1012, 1986.

248 Tzipori S: Cryptosporidiosis in animals and humans. *Microbiol Rev* 47:84, 1983.

249 Tzipori S et al: *Cryptosporidium*: Evidence for a single-species genus. *Infect Immun* 30:884, 1980.

250 Hampton JC, Rosario B: The attachment of protozoan parasites to intestinal epithelial cells of the mouse. *J Parasitol* 52:939, 1966.

251 Marcial MA, Madara JL: *Cryptosporidium*: Cellular localization, structural analysis of absorptive cell-parasite membrane-membrane interactions in guinea pigs, and suggestion of protzoan transport by M cells. *Gastroenterol* 90:583, 1986.

252 Koch KL et al: Cryptosporidiosis in a patient with hemophilia, common variable hypogammaglobulinemia, and the acquired immunodeficiency syndrome. *Ann Intern Med* 99:337, 1983.

253 Petras RE et al: Cryptosporidial enteritis in a homosexual male with an acquired immunodeficiency syndrome. *Cleve Clin Q* 50:41, 1983.

254 Berk RN et al: Cryptosporidiosis of the stomach and small intestine in patients with AIDS. *Am J Radiol* 143:549, 1984.

255 Garza DH et al: Enterotoxin-like activity in cultured cryptosporidia: Role in diarrhea. *Gastroenterology* 90:1424, 1986.

256 Casemore DP et al: *Cryptosporidium* species a "new" human pathogen. *J Clin Pathol* 38:1321, 1985.

257 Guerrant RL et al: Parasitic causes of diarrhea: An overview, in *Pathophysiology of Secretory Diarrhea*, E Lebenthal, M Duffey (eds). in press, 1988.

258 Musch MW et al: Stimulation of colonic secretion by lipoxygenase metabolites of archidonic acid. *Science* 217:1255, 1982.

259 Navin TR: Cryptosporidiosis in humans: Review of recent epidemiologic studies. *Eur J Epidemiol* 1:77, 1985.

260 Wolfson JS et al: Cryptosporidiosis in immunocompetent patients. *N Engl J Med* 312:1278, 1985.

261 Jokipii L et al: Cryptosporidiosis associated with traveling and giardiasis. *Gastroenterology* 89:838, 1985.

262 Soave R, Ma P: Cryptosporidiosis: Traveler's diarrhea in two families. *Arch Intern Med* 145:70, 1985.

263 Koch KL et al: Cryptosporidiosis in hospital personnel. *Ann Intern Med* 102:593, 1985.

264 Ribeiro CD, Plamer SR: Family outbreak of cryptosporidiosis. *Br Med J* 292:377, 1986.

265 Jokipii L, Jokipii AMM: Timing of symptoms and oocyst excretion in human cryptosporidiosis. *N Engl J Med* 315:1643, 1986.

266 Stehr-Green JK et al: Shedding of oocysts in immunocompetent individuals infected with *Cryptosporidium. Am J Trop Med Hyg* 36: 338, 1987.

267 Isaacs D et al: Cryptosporidiosis in immunocompetent children. *J Clin Pathol* 38:76, 1985.

268 Navin TR, Juranek DD: Cryptosporidiosis: Clinical, epidemiologic, and parasitologic review. *Rev Infect Dis* 6:313, 1984.

269 Navin TR, Hardy AM: Cryptosporidiosis in patients with AIDS. *J Infect Dis* 155:150, 1987.

270 Forgacs P et al: Intestinal and bronchial cryptosporidiosis in an immunodeficient homosexual man. *Ann Intern Med* 99:793, 1983.

271 Ma P et al: Respiratory cryptosporidiosis in the acquired immune deficiency syndrome. *JAMA* 252:1298, 1984.

272 Brady EM et al: Pulmonary cryptosporidiosis in acquired immune deficiency syndrome. *JAMA* 252:89, 1984.

273 Guarda LA et al: Human cryptosporidiosis in the acquired immune deficiency syndrome. *Arch Pathol Lab Med* 107:562, 1983.

274 Pitlik SD et al: Cryptosporidial cholecystitis. *N Engl J Med* 308:967, 1983.

275 Blumberg RS et al: Cytomegalovirus- and *Cryptosporidium*-associated acalculous gangrenous cholecystitis. *Am J Med* 76:1118, 1984.

276 McMillan A, McNeillage GJC: Comparison of the sensitivity of microscopy and culture in the laboratory diagnosis of intestinal protozoal infection. *J Clin Pathol* 37:809, 1984.

277 Jokipii L et al: Frequency, multiplicity and repertoire of intestinal protozoa in healthy homosexual men and in patients with gastrointestinal symptoms. *Ann Clin Res* 17:57, 1985.

278 Chaiszon MA et al: A prevalence survey for *Cryptosporidum* and other parasites in healthy homosexual men in New York City. Abstract 203. 34th Annual Meeting of the American Society of Tropical Medicine and Hygiene, November, 1985.

279 Addy PAK, Aikins-Bekoe P: Cryptosporidiosis in diarrhoeal children in Kumasi, Ghana. *Lancet* 1:735, 1986.

280 Smith G, Ende J: Cryptosporidiosis among black children in hospital in South Africa. *J Infect* 13:25, 1986.

281 Pape JW et al: Cryptosporidiosis in Haitian children. *Am J Trop Med Hyg* 36:333, 1987.

282 Hart CA et al: Gastro-enteritis due to *Cryptosporidium*: A prospective survey in a children's hospital. *J Infect* 9:264, 1984.

283 Baxby D et al: Shedding of oocysts by immunocompetent individuals with cryptosporidiosis. *J Hyg Camb* 95:703, 1985.

284 Ratnam S et al: Occurrence of *Cryptosporidium* oocysts in fecal samples submitted for routine microbiological examination. *J Clin Microbiol* 22:402, 1985.

285 Centers for Disease Control: Cryptosporidiosis among children attending day care centers. *MMWR* 33:599, 1984.

286 Centers for Disease Control: Cryptosporidiosis—New Mexico. *MMWR* 36:561, 1987.

287 D'Antonio RG et al: A waterborne outbreak of cryptosporidiosis in normal hosts. *Ann Intern Med* 103:886, 1985.

288 Musial CE et al: Detection of *Cryptosporidium* in water by using polyypropylene cartridge filters. *Applied Environ Microbiol* 53:687, 1987.

289 Madore MS et al: Occurrence of *Cryptosporidium* oocysts in sewage effluents and select surface waters. *J Parasitol* 73:702, 1987.

290 Yolken RH et al: Infectious enteriitis in bone-marrow transplant recipients. *N Engl J Med* 306:1009, 1982.

291 Symposium on Emerging Perspectives in Management and Prevention of Infectious Diseases. Ed by Neil HC. *Diarrheal Disease. Am J Med* 78 (suppl 6B):63, 1985.

292 Weikel CS et al: Cryptosporidiosis in Northeastern Brazil: Association with sporadic diarrhea. *J Infect Dis* 151:963, 1985.

293 Sterling CR, Arrowood MJ: Detection of *Cryptosporidium* sp. infections using a direct immunofluorescent assay. *Pediatr Infect Dis* 5:139, 1986.

294 Garcia LS et al: Fluorescence detection of *Cryptosporidium* oocysts in human fecal specimens by using monoclonal antibodies. *J Clin Microbiol* 25:119, 1987.

295 Ungar BLP et al: Enzyme immunoassay detection of immunoglobulin M and G antibodies to *Cryptosporidium* in immunocompetent and immunocompromised persons. *J Infect Dis* 153:570, 1986.

296 Holten-Andersen W et al: Prevalence of *Cryptosporidium* among patients with acute enteric infection. *J Infect* 9:277, 1984.

297 Montessori GA, Bischoff L: Cryptosporidiosis: A cause of summer diarrhea in children. *Can Med Assoc J* 132:1285, 1985.

298 Marshall AR et al: Cryptosporidiosis in patients at a large teaching hospital. *J Clin Microbiol* 25:172, 1987.

299 Weikel CS: Cryptosporidiosis: Diagnostic advances, treatment hurdles. *Hosp Ther* 13:109, 1988.

300 Centers for Disease Control: Update: Treatment of cryptosporidiosis in patients with acquired immunodeficiency syndrome (AIDS). *MMWR* 33:117, 1984.

301 Portnoy D et al: Treatment of intestinal cryptosporidiosis with spiramycin. *Ann Intern Med* 101:202, 1984.

302 Collier AC et al: Cryptosporidiosis after marrow transplantation: Person-to-person transmission and treatment with spiramycin. *Ann Intern Med* 101:205, 1984.

303 Campbell I et al: Effect of disinfectants on survival of *Cryptosporidium* oocysts. *Vet Rec* 111:414, 1982.

304 Anderson BC: Moist heat inactivation of *Cryptosporidium sp. Am J Public Health* 75:1433, 1985.

# Chapter 45
# Vulvovaginal candidiasis

Jack D. Sobel

## EPIDEMIOLOGY

Vulvovaginal candidiasis (VVC), also called candidal vaginitis, is found throughout the world. In many countries, candidal vaginitis remains the commonest cause of vaginal infection. This is particularly so in the hotter tropical and subtropical climates. In the United States candidal vaginitis is second only to bacterial vaginosis and is three times more frequent than trichomonas vaginitis.[1] Although candidal vaginitis is not a reportable disease, most authors feel that it is increasing in frequency, the most likely explanation being the widespread use of systemic and topical vaginal antimicrobial agents.

Point-prevalence studies indicate that *Candida* spp. may be isolated from the genital tract of 5 to 55 percent of asymptomatic, healthy women in the childbearing age;[2] the sensitivity of the culture technique influences the demonstrated prevalence. Most authors, however, feel the figure is closer to 20 percent.[3,4] The natural history of asymptomatic colonization is unknown, although both animal and limited human studies suggest that vaginal carriage may continue for several months and perhaps years. Several factors are associated with increased rates of asymptomatic vaginal colonization with *Candida*. These include pregnancy (30 to 40 percent), use of high-estrogen-content oral contraceptives, uncontrolled diabetes mellitus, and women frequenting *sexually transmitted disease* (STD) clinics.[4,5] The rarity of *Candida* isolation in premenarchal females and the lower prevalence of candida vaginitis after menopause emphasize the hormonal dependence of the infection.

Three subpopulations of women may be identified. Some women never develop symptomatic VVC throughout their lives; a second group suffers from infrequent isolated episodes; a third population suffers from repeated, recurrent, and often chronic infection. It has been estimated that approximately 75 percent of all women will experience at least one episode of VVC during their lifetime.[6] According to Hurley, approximately 40 to 50 percent of these will experience a further episode.[7] There are no accurate figures with regard to the size of the group with recurrent infection, although no busy practitioner will deny having several such patients.[8] Similarly, because *Candida* infection is not reportable, definitive statistical information on the incidence of VVC is difficult to obtain. If one relies on information obtained from microbiological laboratories, the information fails to distinguish between VVC and vaginal colonization with *Candida*. Furthermore, mixed infections commonly occur in symptomatic women in whom isolation of *Candida* does not confirm a causal relationship.

## MICROBIOLOGY

### The pathogen

Between 85 and 90 percent of yeasts isolated from the vagina are *Candida albicans* strains.[4,5,9,10] The remainder are other *Candida* spp., and *Torulopsi glabrata*,[5] the latter being the commonest next to *C. albicans*. Nonalbicans *Candida* spp. are capable of inducing vaginitis and are often more resistant to conventional therapy.[11] The recently described method of typing *C. albicans* established by Warnock and associates and by Odds and Abbott[13] has provided a useful method.[12,13] There was no evidence of selected strains having tropism for the vagina or being uniquely able to cause vaginitis.[14] Uniquely virulent strains have not been identified.[15]

*Candida* organisms are dimorphic, in that they may be found in humans in different phenotypic phases. In general, blastospores (blastoconidia) represent the phenotypic form responsible for transmission or spread, including the bloodstream phase, as well as the form associated with asymptomatic colonization of the vagina. In contrast, germinated yeast with the production of mycelia most commonly constitute the tissue-invasive form and are usually identified in the presence of symptomatic disease.

### Candida virulence factors

In order for *Candida* spp. to colonize the vaginal epithelium they must first adhere to the vaginal epithelial cells. *C. albicans* adheres in significantly higher numbers to such cells than do *C. tropicalis, C. krusei,* and *C. pseudotropicalis.*[16] This may explain the relative infrequency of the latter species causing vaginitis. All *C. albicans* strains appear to adhere equally well to both exfoliated vaginal and buccal epithelial cells. In contrast, there is considerable person-to-person variation in terms of vaginal epithelial cell receptivity to *Candida* organisms in adherence assays.[17] Nevertheless, *Candida* does not show increased cell affinity for vaginal cells from women with recurrent vulvovaginal candidiasis (VVC).[18] The significance of adherence in the pathogenesis of candidal vaginitis is suggested by the failure of a cerulenin-resistant mutant of *C. albicans,* which adhered poorly, to induce vaginitis in an experimental murine model of candidiasis.[19] Currently no epithelial cell receptor for *Candida* has been identified and the yeast adhesin appears to reside with the surface mannoprotein.

Germination of *Candida* enhances colonization[16,17] and facilitates tissue invasion. Using a mutant strain of *C. albicans* which failed to germinate at 37°C, Sobel and coworkers[20] demonstrated in vivo that the nongerminating mutant was incapable of inducing experimental candidal vaginitis.[20] The implications of this observation are that factors that enhance or facilitate germination tend to promote symptomatic vaginitis, whereas measures that inhibit germination may prevent vaginitis in women who are asymptomatic carriers of yeast.[21]

Little is known regarding the role of candidal proteolytic enzymes, toxins, and phospholipases in determining the virulence of the organisms. Recently, Soll and his team observed high-frequency heritable switching of colony morphology of *Candida* grown on amino-acid-rich agar at 24°C. The variant phenotypes represent, among other things, a varying capacity to spontaneously form mycelia. Although there is as yet no evidence that genetic switching occurs in vivo at 37°C, it provides an attractive hypothesis for the possibility of spontaneous in vivo transformation from asymptomatic colonization to symptomatic vaginitis, due to genetic selection of more virulent clones of *Candida* capable of causing acute invasive disease.[22]

## PATHOGENESIS

*Candida* organisms gain access to the vaginal lumen and secretions predominantly from the adjacent perianal area.[2,23,24] Candidal vaginitis is seen predominantly in women of childbearing age, and in the majority of cases a precipitating factor can be identified to explain the transformation from asymptomatic carriage to symptomatic vaginitis. A higher prevalence of VVC has been observed among women of low socioeconomic status and during pregnancy. VVC affects women of all socioeconomic strata.

Two fundamental questions are critical in understanding the pathogenesis of VVC. The first relates to the mechanism whereby asymptomatic colonization of the vagina changes to symptomatic VVC. The second concerns the mechanism whereby some women suffer from repeated and chronic vulvovaginal candidal infections.

Hurley and associates[7,9] have fostered the view that *C. albicans* is never a commensal in the vagina, in that clinicians could almost always detect vaginal pathology, even in asymptomatic patients from whom *Candida* was isolated. Subsequent investigations, however, have not corroborated this view and have demonstrated that many women carry *C. albicans* in the vagina without symptoms or signs of vaginitis, often with a low concentration of *Candida*.[25] These observations are compatible with the view that *C. albicans* may be a commensal or a pathogen in the vagina, and that changes in the host vaginal environment are usually necessary before the organism induces pathological effects.

### Predisposing factors

**Pregnancy.** The vagina during pregnancy shows an increased susceptibility to vaginal infection by *Candida* spp., resulting in both a higher prevalence of vaginal colonization as well as a higher rate of symptomatic vaginitis.[26] The rate of symptomatic vaginitis is maximally increased in the third trimester, and symptomatic recurrences are also common during pregnancy.[10,26] It is generally thought that the high levels of reproductive hormones—by providing a higher glycogen content in the vaginal environment—provide an excellent carbon source for *Candida*.[27] A more complex mechanism is probably likely, in that estrogens enhance adherence of *Candida* to vaginal epithelial cells (personal communication). Recently, a cytosol receptor or binding system for female reproductive hormones has been documented in *Candida albicans*.[28] These and other investigators demonstrated in vitro binding of female sex hormones to *Candida* as well as the capacity of certain hormones to enhance yeast mycelial formation and hence virulence.[28,29] Accordingly, it is postulated that the high levels of reproductive hormones encountered in pregnancy directly enhance yeast virulence. Not surprisingly, therefore, rates of cure of candidal vaginitis are significantly lower during pregnancy.[4]

**Oral Contraceptives.** Several studies have shown increased vaginal colonization with *Candida* following high-estrogen-content oral contraceptive use.[4] Almost certainly, the same mechanism operative in pregnancy applies to these subjects. Recent studies utilizing low-estrogen-content oral contraceptives have not found an increase in candidal vaginitis.[30,31]

**Diabetes Mellitus.** Vaginal colonization with *Candida* is more frequent in diabetic women. Although uncontrolled diabetes predisposes to symptomatic vaginitis, most diabetics are not afflicted by repeated infection.[3,4] It has become traditional to perform glucose tolerance tests in all women with recurrent VVC. The yield of these expensive studies is extremely low; testing, therefore, is not justified in premenopausal women. Occasionally women with recurrent VVC describe an association between "candy binges" and exacerbation of symptomatic vaginitis. For the most part, however, dietary restrictions have no place in the routine managment of yeast vaginitis.

**Antibiotics.** Onset of symptomatic VVC is frequently observed during courses of oral systemic antibiotics. Broad-spectrum antibiotics, such as tetracyclines, ampicillin, and oral cephalosporins, are mainly responsible for exacerbation of symptoms. Not only is symptomatic vaginitis frequently precipitated, but vaginal colonization rates increase from approximately 10 to 30 percent.[32,33] Antibiotics, both systemic and topical agents, are thought to act by eliminating the protective vaginal bacterial flora.[34] Thus the natural flora is thought to provide colonization resistance as well as preventing germination and hence superficial mucosal invasion by *Candida*. In particular, aerobic and anaerobic resident lactobacilli have been singled out as providing such a protective function. Auger and Joly found low numbers of lactobacilli in vaginal cultures obtained from women with symptomatic vaginitis.[35] Current concepts of the *Lactobacillus–Candida* interaction include competition for nutrients, as well as stearic interference by lactobacilli of receptor sites on vaginal epithelial cells for candida.[17] Other mechanisms include the elaboration of bacteriocins by lactobacilli which inhibit yeast proliferation and germination, as well as a direct antibiotic-induced stimulatory effect on growth of *Candida*.[36]

**Miscellaneous.** Among the factors that may have contributed to the increased incidence of VVC in Western societies has been the use of tight, restricting, poorly ventilated clothing and nylon underclothing with increased local, perineal moisture and temperature.[3,7] The use of well-ventilated clothing and cotton underwear may be of value in preventing infection.[37] There is no evidence confirming that iron deficiency predisposes to infection.[38] Anecdotal evidence suggests that the use of commercial douches, perfumed toilet paper, chlorinated swimming pools, or feminine hygiene sprays contributes to symptomatic vaginitis. Chemical contact, local allergy, or hypersensitivity reactions may alter the vaginal milieu and permit the transformation from asymptomatic colonization to symptomatic vaginitis.

### Source of infection

**Intestinal Reservoir.** Although the gastrointestinal tract may well be the initial source of *Candida* colonization of the vagina, there is considerable controversy regarding the role of the intestinal tract as a focus of reinfection in women with recurrent VVC.[39]

*Candida* were recovered on rectal culture from 100 percent of women with recurrent VVC.[40] This observation has been the basis of the concept of a persistent intestinal reservoir, and that reinoculation of the vagina occurs from the persistent rectal focus following apparent eradication of vaginal yeast by topical therapy. This hypothesis has been criticized, as several authors have found much lower concordance between rectal and vaginal cultures in patients with recurrent VVC.[14,23,24] Thus VVC recurred frequently in the absence of simultaneously positive rectal cultures. Two controlled studies using oral nystatin treatment, which reduces intestinal yeast carriage, failed to prevent symptomatic recurrence of vaginal candidiasis.[41,42] Furthermore, some women had persistent intestinal yeast carriage and failed to develop vaginal colonization. Nevertheless, in spite of mounting skepticism, the possibility that persistent gastrointestinal tract carriage is a source of vaginal reinfection cannot be entirely dismissed, especially since the majority of *Candida* strains isolated from the rectum and the vagina are identical.[24,43]

**Sexual Transmission.** Penile colonization with *Candida* is present in approximately 20 percent of male partners of women with recurrent vaginal candidiasis.[44,45,46] *Candida* are most commonly found in uncircumcised, usually asymptomatic, males in the vicinity of the coronal sulcus. Asymptomatic male genital colonization with *Candida* is four times more common in male sexual partners of infected women than in partners of uninfected women.[44] Infected partners usually carry identical strains.[24]

In spite of the aforementioned circumstantial evidence, direct confirmation that sexual transmission does occur is still lacking, and the contribution of sexual transmission to the pathogenesis of infection remains unknown. Based upon the prevalence of positive penile cultures, the role of sexual spread appears limited. Hence routine therapy of male partners, even those of women with recurrent VVC, is unlikely to substantially reduce recurrence rates. No single controlled study has shown that treatment of males prevents recurrence in females. Anecdotal evidence is available that anogenital and particularly orogenital contact may transmit infection, but adequate documentation is lacking.

**Vaginal Relapse.** After systemic and topical antibiotic therapy, negative vaginal cultures once more turn positive for *Candida* within 30 days in 20 to 25 percent of women, strongly supporting the hypothesis that vaginal relapse is responsible for recurrent vaginal infections.[4] Strains isolated before and after therapy are of the identical type in more than two-thirds of recurrences.[24] Symptomatic relief after clinically successful topical therapy of symptomatic vaginitis is accompanied by a drastic reduction in the number of viable yeasts in the vagina. Small numbers of the microorganisms persist, however, within the vaginal lumen, generally in numbers too small to be detected by conventional vaginal cultures.[14] It is also conceivable that small numbers of *Candida* might sojourn temporarily within superficial cervical or vaginal epithelial cells only to reemerge some weeks or months later.[47]

## Natural vaginal defense mechanisms

**Humoral System.** Patients with profound immunoglobulin deficiencies are not susceptible to vaginal yeast infections. Following acute vaginal candidal infection, systemic (IgM and IgG) and local (S-IgA) responses are elicited.[48,49] The protective role of local antibodies is unknown. Patients with recurrent infection do not lack antibody.[50] Lower local antibodies titers have been described during active vaginal infections, which may reflect an adsorption effect.

Elevated serum and vaginal *Candida*-specific IgE antibodies have been detected in some women with recurrent VVC[51,52] even though total IgE levels are normal.[52]

**Phagocytic System.** Although both polymorphonuclear leukocytes and monocytes play an important role in limiting systemic candidal infection and deep-tissue invasion,[53] these phagocytic cells are characteristically absent from vaginal fluid during candidal vaginitis. Accordingly, these phagocytic cells are not thought to play a role in influencing mucosal colonization or even preventing superficial invasion of the vaginal epithelium by *Candida*. In the rat model of experimental vaginal candidiasis, as in humans, histology of the vagina fails to demonstrate leukocytes in the vaginal fluid or stratified squamous epithelium, which remains intact. Polymorphonuclear cells can be seen concentrating within the underlying lamina propria but appear not to be presented with a chemotactic signal to induce migration into more superficial layers or vaginal fluid.

**Cell Mediated Immunity.** Oral thrush correlates well with depressed cell-mediated immunity seen in debilitated or immunosuppressed patients. This is particularly evident in patients with chronic mucocutaneous candidiasis or with AIDS. In this context, *Candida* are typically opportunistic pathogens. Accordingly, one might anticipate that lymphocytes similarly contribute to normal vaginal defense mechanisms preventing mucosal invasion by *Candida*.

Virtually all adult women with recurrent VVC have normal cutaneous delayed hypersensitivity reactions to multiple antigens, including those of *Candida*. Similarly, in vitro lymphocytic proliferation responses to mitogens in such women appear intact, although several authors have reported depressed lymphoblastic response to *Candida* antigens.[54–58] The possibility of a subpopulation of lymphocytes or serum factors inducing suppression of local genital tract lymphocytes or effector cells has been postulated.[57]

Recent studies by Witkin provide an attractive hypothesis of selective acquired immunodeficiency in women with recurrent VVC.[56] The observation is that of impaired in vitro T-lymphocyte response only to *Candida* antigen, while there is a normal proliferative response to mitogens and other non-*Candida* antigens. According to Witkin, reduced T-lymphocyte reactivity to *Candida* antigen is the result of the elaboration by the patient's macrophages of prostaglandin $E_2$, which blocks lymphocyte proliferation possibly by inhibiting interleukin-2 production. He further postulated that abnormal macrophage function could be the result of local IgE *Candida* antibodies present in the vagina of women with recurrent VVC, or the result of a serum factor in such patients.[52,59,60] Although this hypothesis requires confirmation, numerous investigators have observed decreased *Candida*-specific lymphocyte reactivity in vitro.[54–58] How T lymphocytes protect the vagina against symptomatic candidal vaginitis is unknown.

**Vaginal Flora.** Probably the most important defense against both candidal colonization and symptomatic inflammation is the normal natural bacterial flora. Any newly arrived *Candida* organism, in order to survive and persist, must initially adhere to epithelial cells and then grow, proliferate, and germinate in order to colonize the vaginal mucosa successfully. Although microbial competition for nutrients has long been considered the most important source of competition, animal studies suggest that lactobacilli and *Candida* frequently survive side by side.[61] The role of bacteriocins in inhibiting yeast growth and germination requires additional investigation[36] (see section on Antibiotics).

**Miscellaneous.** Although not studied in the vagina, various natural secretions have been shown to possess considerable antifungal activity. Pollock et al.[62] reported fungistatic and fungicidal activity against *C. albicans* of human parotid salivary histidine-rich polypeptides.

### Mechanisms involved in invasion and inflammatory response

During the symptomatic episode there is the conspicuous appearance of the germinated or filamentous forms of *Candida*. Germinated organisms not only enhance colonization but represent the dominant invasive phase capable of penetrating intact epithelial cells and invading the vaginal epithelium, although only the very superficial layers are involved.[63] Although symptoms are not strictly related to the yeast load, nevertheless clinical vaginitis does tend to be associated with greater numbers of organisms and with the germinated yeast phase.[5] Approximately $10^3$ to $10^4$ *Candida* per ml of vaginal fluid may be recovered in both symptomatic and asymptomatic states.[5]

The mechanism whereby *Candida* induces inflammation is not yet established. Yeast cells are capable of producing several extracellular proteases as well as phospholipases. The paucity of phagocytic cells in the inflammatory exudate possibly reflects the lack of chemotactic substances elaborated. Both blastoconidia and pseudohyphae are capable of destroying superficial cells by direct invasion.

Based on the clinical spectrum which varies from an acute florid exudative form with thick white vaginal discharge and large numbers of germinated yeast cells to the other extreme of absent or minimal discharge, fewer organisms, and yet severe pruritis, it is suggested that more than one pathogenic mechanism may exist. In the presence of pruritis alone, hypersensitivity or immune mechanisms are likely to be involved.[64,65] Thus it is of interest that not infrequently male partners of asymptomatic female carriers of *Candida* develop postcoital penile erythema and pruritis which usually lasts several hours only.

## CLINICAL MANIFESTATIONS

Acute pruritis and vaginal discharge are the usual presenting complaints, but neither symptom is specific to VVC and neither is invariably associated with disease. The most frequent symptom is that of vulvar pruritis, which is present in virtually all symptomatic patients. Vaginal discharge is not invariably present and is frequently minimal. Although described as typically cottage-cheese-like in character, the discharge may vary from watery to homogeneously thick. Vaginal soreness, irritation, vulvar burning, dyspareunia, and external dysuria are commonly present. Odor, if present, is minimal and nonoffensive. Examination frequently reveals erythema and swelling of the labia and vulva, often with discrete pustulopapular peripheral lesions. The cervix is normal, and vaginal mucosal erythema is present together with adherent whitish discharge. Characteristically, symptoms are exacerbated in the week preceding the onset of menses with some relief with the onset of menstrual flow.

It is apparent that a clinical spectrum of candidal vaginitis exists. In some patients a more exudative picture is apparent with copious discharge and white vaginal plaques satisfying the traditional description of vaginal thrush (see Plate 19). At the other end of the spectrum are those with minimal discharge and severe erythema particularly with extensive vulvar involvement often extending into the inguinal and perianal regions. In general, a quantitative relationship exists between the classic signs and symptoms of VVC, notably pruritis and vulvitis, and the extent of genital yeast colonization. Likewise surveys indicate a relative unreliability of the patient's own symptomatic assessment except in the case of pruritis.

Although *Candida* spp. occasionally cause extensive balanoposthitis in male partners of women with vaginal candidiasis, a more frequent event is a transient rash, erythema, and pruritis or a burning sensation of the penis which develops minutes or hours after unprotected intercourse. The symptoms are self-limiting and frequently disappear after showering. A history of postcoital penile rash was found in 20 percent of the partners of women with recurrent VVC (personal observation—unpublished).

## DIAGNOSIS

The relative lack of specificity of symptoms and signs precludes a diagnosis that is based on history and physical examination only. Neither clinical signs and symptoms alone nor culture confirmation of the presence of *Candida* should be regarded as a satisfactory basis for diagnosis. Regrettably both approaches are common in practice. In the Detroit Medical Center Candida Vaginitis Clinic, over 80 percent of physician-referred patients with a putative diagnosis of recalcitrant or recurrent VVC were found to have another cause of vaginitis and did not have VVC (personal observation). Bergsman and Berg emphasized that a patient's subjective symptoms are of no practical and consistent value in predicting VVC.[25] The most *Candida*-specific symptom is pruritis without discharge, and even this criterion correctly predicted VVC in only 38 percent of patients.[25]

Most patients with symptomatic vaginitis may be readily diagnosed on the basis of simple microscopic examination of vaginal secretions (Fig. 45-1). Accordingly, a wet-mount or saline preparation should routinely be done, not only to identify the presence of yeast cells and mycelia but also to exclude the presence of "clue cells" and motile trichomonads. Large numbers of white cells are also invariably absent and when present should suggest a mixed infection. The 10% potassium hydroxide preparation is extremely valuable and even more sensitive in diagnosing the presence of germinated yeast. Similarly, vaginal pH estimations reveal a normal pH (4.0 to 4.5) in candidal vaginitis, and the finding of a vaginal pH in excess of 5.0 should strongly alert clinicians to the possibility of bacterial vaginosis, trichomoniasis, or a mixed infection.

In spite of the value of direct microscopy, several studies have consistently revealed that up to 50 percent of patients with culture-positive symptomatic candidal vaginitis (responding to antimycotic therapy) will have negative microscopy.[23] Thus, although cultures are unnecessary if the wet-mount or KOH preparations show yeast and mycelia, vaginal culture should be performed in the presence of negative microscopy if VVC is suspected on the basis of symptoms or signs. Reliable clinical cultures can also be obtained by practitioners using Nickerson's medium or semiquantitative "slide-stix" cultures. The Pap smear is unreliable as a diagnostic modality, being positive in only about 25 percent.[66] Although vaginal culture is the most sensitive

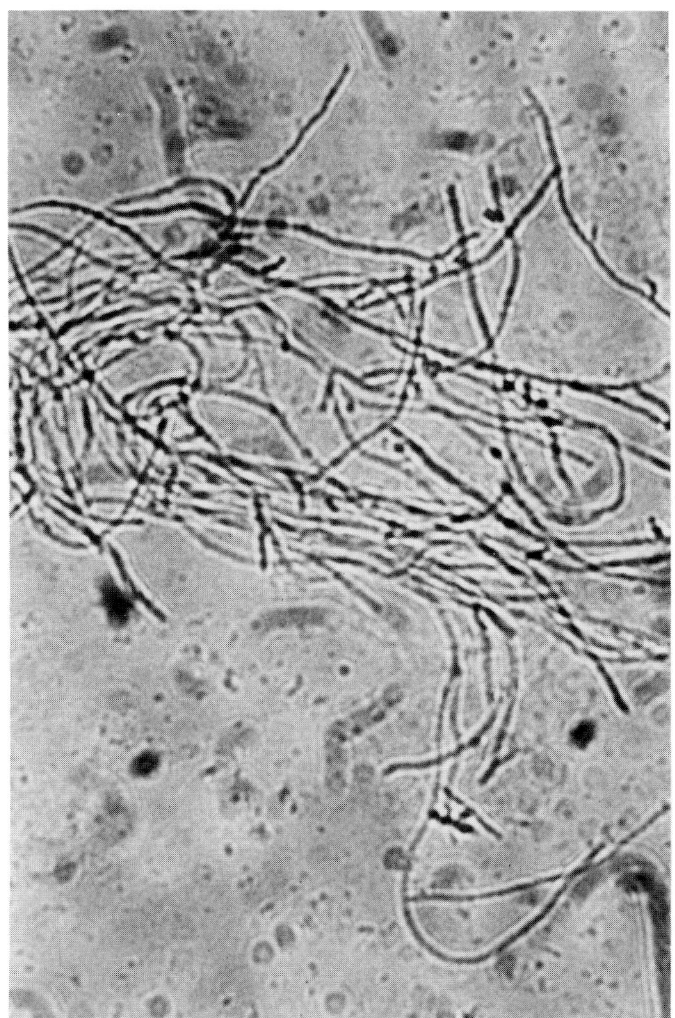

Fig. 45-1. Wet-mount examination of vaginal discharge from a woman with vulvovaginal candidiasis, showing mycelia. 1000× magnification.

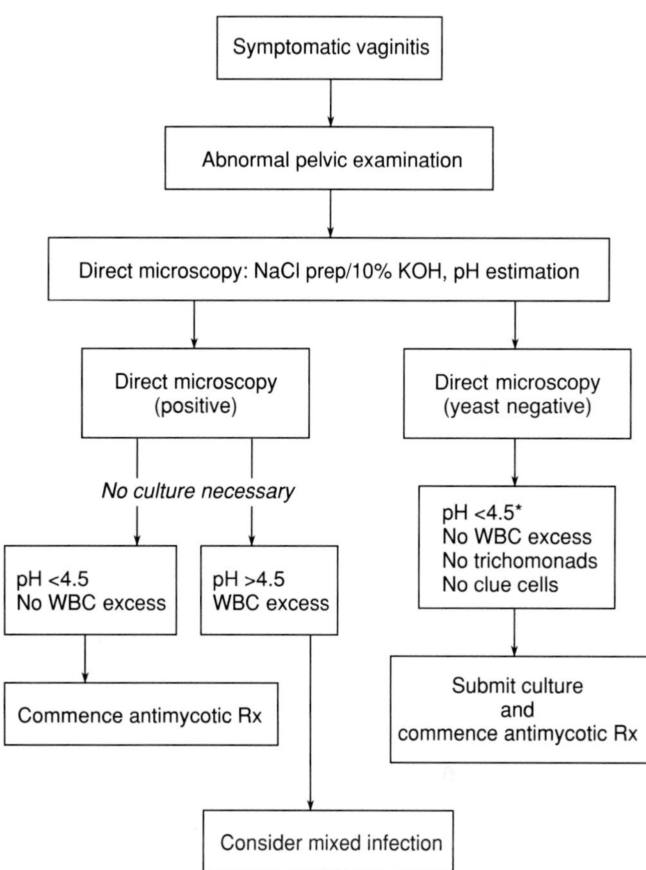


Fig. 45-2. Algorithm for diagnosis and treatment of vulvovaginal candidiasis.

method currently available for detecting *Candida*, a positive culture does not necessarily indicate that *Candida* is responsible for the vaginal symptoms. Odds et al.[4] have shown that direct microscopy positives usually correlate with relatively high yeast concentrations in vaginal secretions as confirmed by quantitative vaginal cultures. Their studies also suggested that in most women, the yeast cell numbers correlate with severity of clinical signs and symptoms, and finally that commensal yeast vaginal carriage tends to be associated with lower numbers of vaginal yeast. Diagnosis requires a correlation between clinical findings, microscopic examination, and finally, vaginal culture (Fig. 45-2). Although some prefer to use a selective medium, from a technical point of view there appears to be no significant difference or advantage in using Sabouraud agar, Nickerson's medium, or Microstix-Candida media, or in adding antibiotics such as chloramphenicol to the isolation medium. There is no reliable serological technique for the diagnosis of symptomatic candidal vaginitis.

Recently several commercial companies have reported success in achieving rapid and reliable diagnosis of candidal vaginitis, utilizing a latex agglutination slide technique employing polyclonal antibodies reactive with multiple *Candida* species and directed against yeast mannan.[67] One reported study revealed a sensitivity of 81 percent with a specificity of 98.5 percent.[67] The high specificity is a function of establishing a threshold for diagnosis based upon the higher antigen load present in symptomatic vaginitis, as compared with asymptomatic colonization. Quantitative cultures have revealed that commensal carriers of *Candida* tend to have less than 10 colonies per plate.

## TREATMENT

### Acute vaginitis

At the outset, clinicians should attempt to differentiate those women with infrequent episodes from those with chronic, recurrent, or recalcitrant VVC. This differentiation influences not so much the selection of the agent but rather the duration of therapy. In general, most physicians advise against treatment of asymptomatic vaginal carriage or colonization with *Candida*.

Numerous products are available for the treatment of symptomatic VVC (Table 45-1). In addition to the imidazoles listed in Table 45-1, and nystatin (a polyene), a number of other polyenes, ie., amphotericin B, candicidin, hamycin, meparticin, natamycin, trichomycin, have also been used in the therapy of candidal vaginitis. Among other miscellaneous agents used for the same purpose are boric acid, chlordantoin, cyclopiroxolamine, hydrogaphen, nifurtal, potassium sorbate, povidone iodine, and propionic acid. Antimycotic agents are available for topical or local administration (creams, lotions, aerosol sprays, vaginal tablets, suppositories, coated tampons) as well as for systemic use, which is administered orally. Currently, only ketoconazole has been widely used as an oral agent, although the newer triazoles

**Table 45-1. Therapy of Vulvovaginal Candidiasis**

| Drug | Formulation | Dosage |
|---|---|---|
| Butoconazole (Femstat) | 2% cream | 5 g at bedtime × 3 days |
| Clotrimazole (Gynelotrimin, Mycelex) | 1% cream | 5 g at bedtime × 7–14 days |
| | 10% cream | 5 g single application |
| | 100 mg vaginal tablet | 1 tablet at bedtime × 7 days<br>2 tablets at bedtime × 3 days |
| | 500 mg vaginal tablet | 1 tablet once |
| Miconazole (Monistat) | 2% cream | 5 g at bedtime × 7 days |
| | 100 mg vaginal suppository | 1 suppository at bedtime × 7 days |
| | 200 mg vaginal suppository | 1 suppository at bedtime × 3 days |
| | 1200 vaginal suppository | 1 suppository once |
| Econazole | 150 mg vaginal tablet | 1 tablet at bedtime × 3 days |
| Fenticonazole | 2% cream | 5 g at bedtime × 7 days |
| Tioconazole | 2% cream | 5 g at bedtime × 3 days |
| | 6.5% cream | 5 g at bedtime single dose |
| Terconazole | 2% cream | 5 g at bedtime × 3 days |
| Fluconazole | Oral tablet | 150 mg single dose |
| Ketoconazole (Nizoral) | 200 mg tablet | 400 mg orally daily × 5 days |
| Itraconazole | 100 mg tablet | 200 mg orally daily × 3 days |
| Nystatin (Micostatin, Nilstat) | 100,000-unit tablet | 1 tablet at bedtime × 14 days |

(itraconazole and fluconazole) appear to have an equivalent success rate with reduced toxicity and can be administered in shorter-duration regimens. Until these new azoles become available, the decision whether to use an oral or topical agent for acute candidal vaginitis is moot. Ketoconazole is not currently approved in the United States for use in acute candidal vaginitis. Nevertheless, Tooley in the United Kingdom, who evaluated 1710 patients' subjective preferences for different routes of administration in the treatment of candidal vaginitis, concluded that approximately half the study women preferred oral formulations, the remainder expressing a preference for different therapeutic modalities [topical creams (25 percent), hard pessaries (14 percent), and soft pessary (10 percent)].[68] In countries where both oral and topical modalities are available, patients should be given the opportunity of expressing their preference after the benefits and disadvantages of the different therapeutic options are explained.

Multiple studies have indicated both a clinical and mycological response of between 70 and 80 percent with topical nystatin.[69,70] Slightly higher response rates, i.e., 80 to 90 percent, can be expected with topical imidazoles administered over a 5- to 7-day period.[4] Several studies suggest that a marginally higher clinical and mycological response exceeding 90 percent is found with oral ketoconazole therapy. Nevertheless, the toxicity profile of ketoconazole is such that many practitioners have been reluctant to recommend oral therapy for a non-life-threatening disease, especially when so many topical alternatives are available. Rare side effects of ketoconazole include rash, nausea, gastrointestinal upset, anaphylaxis, and toxic hepatitis, which is thought to be idiosyncratic in nature and not dose-dependent. Hepatitis has been estimated to occur in 1 in 15,000 women, and rare fatal cases have been reported.[71] Ketoconazole also interferes in a dose-dependent manner with testicular synthesis of androgens and adrenal cortical synthesis of cortisol. Itraconazole has already been shown to be highly effective in treating acute VVC.[72,73] A single oral 150 mg dose of fluconazole, with a half-life over 20 h, was promising for VVC in a non-comparative trial.[73a] The phenylmorpholine derivative Ro 14-4767 is a novel antimycotic which has in preliminary studies been shown to be effective in topical therapy of experimental VVC. Chlordantoin and nifuratel are significantly less effective in eradicating *Candida* from the vagina than any of the polyene or azole antimycotics.

Tooley's study also revealed that women also generally preferred single-dose or short-course therapy to the more conventional 7- to 14-day therapy.[68] Accordingly, over the last few years because of patient preference and poor compliance, regimens have been developed in which the total dose of topical nystatin or the various imidazoles have remained the same or slightly reduced but the topical medications have been increased in size of each dose, so as to offer single-dose (single-day) or abbreviated courses of therapy. These new regimens are outlined in the table. In general, the shortened courses of therapy have in controlled studies been shown to be as effective as conventional topical therapy in relieving both symptoms and signs of infection, as well as achieving short-term negative cultures.[74–79] For the usual case of vulvovaginal candidiasis, these short-course regimens can now be considered efficacious. However, for severe cases the longer conventional 1-week or longer regimens are still advised. One reason for the efficacy of short courses is that the active compound persists at fungal inhibitory levels in vaginal secretions for up to 2 to 3 days after a single application of dosage formulations.[80] Plasma imidazole levels after vaginal treatment are very low, although the level of penetration of the active agents is undetermined. Short courses of therapy should not be prescribed in recalcitrant cases.

Another issue is the long-term follow-up of women with acute candidal vaginitis. Odds (1977), in analyzing multiple published reports of therapy with particular reference to mycological status of the vagina 30 days after conventional vaginal therapy, concluded that at least 20 percent of women who initially responded to conventional therapy and who were culture-negative and asymptomatic at the end of 1 week of therapy were culture-positive after 30 days.[69] He confirmed that antifungal formulations appeared not to influence mycological cure rates but that longer treatment duration was superior to shorter courses in terms of immediate mycological efficacy and prevention of mycological recurrence of vaginal yeasts. The clinical significance of this observation is unclear, but it supports the use of long duration of treatment in women prone to recurrent bouts of vulvovaginal candidiasis.

For the most part, topical vaginal antimycotic therapy is free of undesirable side effects. Occasionally local discomfort and burning are reported. This author has been made aware of several women who develop a contact hypersensitivity reaction to topical antimycotics, which may be a function of the chemical base or vehicle in the formulation rather than the specific imidazole component. These patients present with a persistent burning sensation particularly localized to the vaginal vestibule usually interpreted by the physician as a relapse or candidal reinfection, and additional antimycotic medication is empirically prescribed which aggravates the symptoms.

Gentian violet was the treatment of choice for vaginal yeast infections prior to the availability of polyenes and azole agents but has virtually no place today in the treatment of VVC. Similarly yogurt douches or topical live preparations of lactobacilli have no proved therapeutic efficacy.

## Acute vaginitis in pregnancy

As mentioned previously, management of VVC during pregnancy is more difficult, since clinical response tends to be slower and recurrences more frequent.[70,81,82] In general, most topical antifungal agents are effective, especially when prescribed for longer periods, i.e., 1 to 2 weeks. Although absorption of topical antifungals is minimal, the potential risk of vaginal antimycotic therapy to the developing fetus during the first trimester of pregnancy must be seriously considered and weighed against the benefit derived by the patient. Longer duration of therapy may be necessary to eradicate yeast infection. However, recently single high-dosage therapy with clotrimazole has been shown to be effective in pregnancy and may be considered for the initial therapeutic attempt.[83]

## Treatment of recurrent and chronic VVC

The management of women with recurrent and chronic VVC remains problematic. There has been considerable confusion primarily because of a lack of a clear, concise definition of what constitutes recurrent disease. A definition which appears reasonable is that of at least four mycologically proved symptomatic episodes in the previous 12 months, with exclusion of other common vaginal pathogens. The first step the clinician should take is to identify and eliminate possible underlying or predisposing causes. Uncontrolled diabetes must be controlled. Corticosteroids, other immunosuppresive agents, and hormones such as estrogens should be stopped where possible. Although most women with recurrent and chronic VVC have long since abandoned the use of oral contraceptives, this step should be considered by those still using them. In the author's experience[84] it was not found to be either beneficial or even necessary to discontinue low-dose estrogen oral contraceptive use when long-term antimycotic agents were prescribed. Similarly the yield of performing a glucose tolerance test in otherwise asymptomatic healthy premenopausal women to diagnose latent or chemical diabetes mellitus is extremely low and is not worthwhile.[85] Most women with recurrent VVC already avoid tight-fitting clothing and synthetic underwear. Douching with commercial preparations and vinegar is of no value and should be discouraged. Unfortunately, in the majority of women with recurrent or chronic VVC, no underlying or predisposing factor can be identified.[85]

In the past, physicians faced with women with recurrent VVC usually resorted to a method based on patient self-diagnosis and early initiation of self-treatment with topical therapy. The patient is given a repeat prescription and institutes therapy with the first recurrence of symptoms. In some women with two or three attacks per year this approach may be successful, using short courses of topical therapy, e.g. clotrimazole 500 mg, as single-dose therapy. The success of this method is primarily based on the patient's ability to make an accurate diagnosis. The availability of a slide agglutination test may facilitate self-diagnosis. The majority of this recalcitrant group of women, however, require a long-term maintenance suppressive prophylaxis regimen. Several studies have confirmed the success of long-term prophylactic therapy to significantly reduce the frequency of symptomatic episodes of VVC.[84,86,87] Because of the chronicity of therapy, the convenience of oral treatment is apparent, and the best suppressive prophylaxis has been achieved with a daily low-dose of oral ketoconazole, 100 mg daily over 6 months.[84] Once more the benefits of successful suppressive therapy must be weighed against the potential toxicity of long-term oral therapy. Low-dosage ketoconazole is remarkably free of dose-dependent side effects but is not free from idiosyncratic toxic reactions such as hepatitis. In all three reports of successful maintenance prophylaxis, cessation of antifungal prophylaxis was associated with resurgence of symptomatic infection in approximately half the studied women. The mechanism of the successful prophylaxis, particularly with low-dosage ketoconazole which results in subinhibitory vaginal concentrations only, is by no means clear. Possible explanations include a direct fungistatic effect, inhibition of germ tube formation, a direct effect of ketoconazole on vaginal epithelium,[88] and effects on the bacterial flora and immune system.

Dennerstein reported a reduced rate of recurrence in chronic VVC in 15 patients during a 3-month period of depo-medroxy progesterone acetate therapy.[89]

Chronic and recurrent VVC does not appear to be the result of resistant vaginal yeast.[24] Furthermore, long-term ketoconazole therapy was not associated with the development of increased candidal resistance to the drug or with a change in the species of *Candida* cultured from recurrent breakthrough episodes during maintenance therapy.[24] Rarely, however, in women who fail to respond to conventional therapy, one encounters unusual organisms which are resistant to standard therapy, such as *Saccharomyces cerevisiae*. Susceptibility testing should be reserved for these infrequent cases only. Three double-blind placebo-controlled trials evaluated topical antifungal treatment of male sex partners of women with recurrent VVC. None of the studies showed any significant reduction in the rate of recurrence in the female subjects. Accordingly routine topical therapy for male sexual partners of women with recurrent VVC is not currently recommended.

Another widely utilized measure to prevent recurrence is adding oral nystatin to the concomitant vaginal therapy. This method is aimed at reducing the risk of vaginal reinfection from a persistent intestinal reservoir. The merits of this theory have already been discussed under Pathogenesis. Short-term studies of simultaneous vaginal and oral therapy with nystatin have produced conflicting results regarding rates of recurrent VVC. Thus Milne and Warnock failed to show any benefit of concomitant nystatin therapy,[41] whereas a multicenter study[90] showed a modest reduction of vaginal reinfection. However, the latter study[90] did not extend further than 2 months following initial therapy. Accordingly there is a paucity of evidence supporting the widespread use of oral nystatin in both short- and long-term regimens.

An alternative approach to long-term maintenance anti-*Candida* therapy for recurrent VVC is the use of hyposensitization with a commercially available antigen. In a small study Rosedale and Braue achieved encouraging results,[91] but this study was uncontrolled.

Prophylactic antifungal medication is not routinely recommended to accompany antibiotic therapy in most women. However, in women with recurrent VVC and in whom antimicrobial agents have been identified as a frequent and inevitable precipitating factor, it may be prudent to simultaneously administer topical antimycotic therapy (not oral nystatin) together with antibiotics.

Finally in dealing with patients with chronic or recurrent VVC it is necessary to emphasize the importance of reassurance, support, and counseling. Chronic vaginitis results in chronic dyspareunia, and inevitably sexual and marital relations suffer, often irreversibly. Women should be reassured that today virtually all chronic victims can be adequately controlled if not cured.

## References


1 Center for Disease Control: Non-reported sexually transmitted diseases. *MMWR* 28: 61, 1979.
2 Drake TE, Maibach HI: Candida and candidiasis: Cultural conditions, epidemiology, and pathogenesis. *Postgrad Med* 53: 83, 1973.
3 Fleury FJ: Adult vaginitis. *Clin Obstet Gynecol* 24: 407, 1981.
4 Odds FC: *Candida and Candidosis.* Baltimore, University Park Press, 1979.
5 Oriel JD et al: Genital yeast infections. *Br Med J* 4: 761, 1972.
6 Berg AO et al: Establishing the cause of symptoms in women in a family practice. *JAMA* 251: 620, 1984.
7 Hurley R, De Louvois J: Candida vaginitis. *Postgrad Med J* 55: 645, 1979.
8 Fleury FJ: Recurrent candida vulvovaginitis. *Chemotherapy* 28 (suppl 1): 48, 1982.
9 Hurley R: Trends in candidal vaginitis. *Proc R Soc Med* 70 (suppl 4): 1, 1977.
10 Morton RS, Rashid S: Candidal vaginitis: Natural history, predisposing factors and prevention. *Proc R Soc Med* 70 (suppl 4): 3, 1977.
11 Horowitz BJ et al: *Candida tropicalis* vulvovaginitis. *Obstet Gynecol* 66: 229, 1985.
12 Warnock D et al: Epidemiological investigations of patients with vulvovaginal candidosis. *Br J Vener Dis* 55: 357, 1979.
13 Odds FC, Abbott AB: A simple system for the presumptive identification of *Candida albicans* and differentiation of strains with the species. *Sabouraudia* 18: 301, 1980.
14 Odds FC: Genital candidosis. *Clin Exp Dermatol* 7: 345, 1982.
15 Odds FC et al: Analysis of *Candida albicans* phenotypes from different geographical and anatomical sources. *J Clin Microbiol* 18: 849, 1983.
16 King RD et al: Adherence of *Candida albicans* and other candida species to mucosal epithelial cells. *Infect Immun* 27: 667, 1980.
17 Sobel JD et al: *C albicans* adherence to vaginal epithelial cells. *J Infect Dis* 143: 76, 1981.
18 Trumbore DJ, Sobel JD: Recurrent vulvovaginal candidiasis: Vaginal epithelial cell susceptibility to *Candida albicans* adherence. *Obstet Gynecol* 67: 810, 1986.
19 Lehner N et al: Pathogenesis of vaginal candidiasis: Studies with a mutant which has reduced ability to adhere in vitro. *Sabouraudia* 24: 127, 1986.
20 Sobel JD et al: Critical role of germination in the pathogenesis of experimental candidal vaginitis. *Infect Immun* 44: 576, 1984.
21 Sobel JD, Muller G: Ketoconazole prophylaxis in experimental vaginal candidiasis. *Antimicrob Agents Chemother* 25: 281, 1984.
22 Slutsky B et al: High frequency switching colony morphology in *Candida albicans. Science* 230: 666, 1985.
23 Bertholf ME, Stafford MJ: Colonization of *Candida albicans* in vagina, rectum, and mouth. *J Family Pract* 16: 919, 1983.
24 O'Conner MI, Sobel JD: Epidemiology of recurrent vulvovaginal candidiasis: Identification and strain differentiation of *Candida albicans. J Infect Dis* 154: 358, 1986.
25 Bergman JJ et al: Clinical comparison of microscopic and culture techniques in the diagnosis of Candida vaginitis. *J Family Pract* 18: 549, 1984.
26 Bland PB et al: Experimental vaginal and cutaneous moniliasis. Clinical and laboratory studies of certain monilias associated with vaginal oral and cutaneous thrush. *Arch Dermatol Syphilol* 36: 760, 1937.
27 McCourtie J, LG Douglas: Relationship between cell surface composition of *Candida albicans* and adherence to acrylic after-growth on different carbon sources. *Infect Immun* 32: 1234, 1981.
28 Powell BL et al: Estrogen receptor in *Candida albicans.* A possible explanation for hormonal influences in vaginal candidiasis. 23rd Interscience Conference on Antimicrobial Agents and Chemotherapy, Abstract 751, 1983, p 222.
29 Kinsman OS: Effect of mammalian steroid hormones and luteinizing hormone on germination of *C albicans.* American Society of Microbiology Conference on *Candida albicans,* Palm Springs, Abstract 27, May 16, 1987, p 13.
30 Apisarnthanarax P et al: Oral contraceptives and candidiasis. *Cutis* July 1974, p 77.
31 Davidson F, Oates JK: The pill does not cause "thrush." *Br J Obstet Gynecol* 92: 1265, 1985.
32 Caruso LJ: Vaginal moniliasis after tetracycline therapy. *Am J Obstet Gynecol* 90: 374, 1964.
33 Oriel JD, Waterworth PM: Effect of minocycline and tetracycline on the vaginal yeast flora. *J Clin Pathol* 28: 403, 1975.
34 Liljemark WF, Gibbons RJ: Suppression of *Candida albicans* by human oral streptococci in gnotobiotic mice. *Infect Immun* 8: 846, 1973.
35 Auger P, Joly J: Microbial flora associated with *Candida albicans* vulvovaginitis. *Obstet Gynecol* 55: 397, 1980.
36 Narayanan TK, Rao GR: Beta-indole-ethanol and beta-indolelactic acid production by candida species: Their antibacterial and autoantibiotic action. *Antimicrob Agents Chemother* 9: 375, 1976.
37 Hurley R: Recurrent candida infection. *Clin Obstet Gynecol* 8: 209, 1981.
38 Davidson F et al: Recurrent genital candidosis and iron metabolism. *Br J Vener Dis* 53: 123, 1977.
39 De Sousa HM, Van Uden N: The mode of infection in yeast vulvovaginitis. *Am J Obstet Gynecol* 80: 1096, 1960.
40 Miles MR et al: Recurrent vaginal candidiasis. Importance of an intestinal reservoir. *JAMA* 238: 1836, 1977.
41 Milne JD, Warnock DW: Effect of simultaneous oral and vaginal treatment on the rate of cure and relapse in vaginal candidosis. *Br J Vener Dis* 55: 362, 1979.
42 Vellupillai S, Thin RN: Treatment of vulvovaginal yeast infection with nystatin. *Practitioner* 219: 897, 1977.
43 Meinhof WL: Demonstration of typical features of individual *Candida albicans* strains as a means of studying sources of infection. *Chemotherapy* 28 (suppl 1): 51, 1982.
44 Rodin P, Kolator B: Carriage of yeasts on the penis. *Br Med J* 1: 1123, 1976.
45 Thin RN et al: How often is genital yeast infection sexually transmitted? *Br Med J* 2: 93, 1977.
46 Davison F: Yeasts and circumcision in the male. *Br J Vener Dis* 53: 121, 1977.
47 Garcia-Tamayo J et al: Human genital candidosis. Histochemistry, scanning and transmission electron microscopy. *Acta Cytol (Baltimore)* 26: 7, 1982.
48 Waldman RH et al: Immunoglobulin levels and antibody to *Candida albicans* in human cervicovaginal secretions. *Clin Exp Immunol* 10: 427, 1972.
49 Mathur S et al: Humoral immunity in vaginal candidiasis. *Infect Immun* 15: 287, 1977.
50 Gough PM et al: IgA and IgG antibodies to *Candida albicans* in the genital tract secretions of women with or without vaginal candidosis. *Sabouraudia* 22: 265, 1984.
51 Mathur S et al: Immunoglobulin E anti-Candida antibodies and candidiasis. *Infect Immun* 18: 257, 1977.

52 Witkin SS: IgE antibodies to *Candida albicans* in vaginal fluids of women with recurrent vaginitis. *Abstract Am Soc Micr Meeting*, Palm Springs, Abstract 9, May 16, 1987, p 10.
53 Diamond RD et al: Damage to pseudohyphae of *Candida albicans* by neutrophils in the absence of serum in vitro. *J Clin Invest* 61: 349, 1978.
54 Hobbs JR et al: Immunological aspects of candidal vaginitis. *Proc R Soc Med* 70(suppl 4): 11, 1977.
55 Syverson RE et al: Cellular and humoral immune status in women with chronic candida vaginitis. *Am J Obstet Gynecol* 123: 624, 1979.
56 Witkin SS et al: Inhibition of *Candida albicans*—Induced lymphocyte proliferation by lymphocytes and sera from women with recurrent vaginitis. *Am J Obstet Gynecol* 147: 809, 1983.
57 Mathur S et al: Antiovaria and anti-lymphocyte antibodies in patients with chronic vaginal candidiasis. *J Reprod Immunol* 2: 247, 1980.
58 Agarunowa JS et al: Risk of candidosis in patients with endocrinological disorders. *Mykosen* 29: 474, 1986.
59 Witkin SS: Inhibition of *Candida* induced lymphocyte proliferation by antibody to *Candida albicans*. *Obstet Gynecol* 68: 696, 1986.
60 Witkin SS et al: A macrophage defect in women with recurrent candida vaginitis and its reversal in vitro by prostaglandin inhibitors. *Am J Obstet Gynecol* 155: 790, 1986.
61 Savage DC: Microbial interference between indigenous yeast and lactobacilli in the rodent stomach. *J Bacteriol* 98: 1278, 1969.
62 Pollack JJ et al: Fungistatic and fungicidal activity of human parotid salivary histidine-rich polypeptides on *Candida albicans*. *Infect Immun* 44: 702, 1984.
63 Sobel JD, Muller G: Experimental vaginal candidiasis in rats. *Sabouraudia* 23: 199, 1985.
64 Kudelka NM: Allergy in chronic monilial vaginitis. *Ann Allergy* 29: 266, 1971.
65 Palacios HJ: Hypersensitivity as a cause of dermatologic and vaginal moniliasis resistant to topical therapy. *Ann Allergy* 37: 110, 1976.
66 Rosenberg M: Vaginal candidiasis: Its diagnosis and relation to urinary tract infection. *South Med J* 69: 1347, 1976.
67 Evans EGV et al: Criteria for the diagnosis of vaginal candidosis: Evaluation of a new latex agglutination test. *Eur J Obstet Gynecol Reprod Biol* 22: 365, 1986.
68 Tooley PJ: Patients and doctor preferences in the treatment of vaginal candidiasis. *Practitioner* 229: 655, 1985.
69 Odds FC: Cure and relapse with antifungal therapy. *Proc R Soc Med* 70 (suppl 4): 24, 1977.
70 Lang WE et al: Nystatin vaginal tablets in treatment of candidal vulvovaginitis. *Obstet Gynec* 8: 364, 1956.
71 Lewis JH et al: Hepatic injury associated with ketoconazole therapy: Analysis of 33 cases. *Gastroenterol* 86: 503, 1984.
72 Sanz FS, Palacia-Hernanz A: Randomized comparative trial of three regimens of Itraconazole for treatment of vaginal mycoses. *Rev Infect Dis* 9 (suppl 1): 139, 1987.
73 Calderon-Marquez JJ: Itraconazole in the treatment of vaginal candidiasis and the effect of treatment of the sexual partner. *Rev Infect Dis* 9 (suppl 1): 143, 1987.
73a Multicenter Study Group: Treatment of vaginal candidiasis with a single oral dose of fluconazole. *Eur J Clin Microbiol Infect Dis* 7:364, 1988.
74 Stein GE et al: Single dose tioconazole compared with three day treatment with clotrimazole in vulvovaginal candidiasis. *Antimicrob Agents Chemother* 29: 969, 1986.
75 Van der Meijdes WI et al: Double-blind comparison of 200 mg ketoconazole oral tablets and 1200 mg miconazole vaginal capsule in the treatment of vaginal candidosis. *Eur J Obstet Gynecol Reprod Biol* 22: 133, 1986.
76 Brown D et al: Butaconazole vaginal cream in the treatment of vulvovaginal candidiasis. Comparison with miconazole nitrate and placebo. *J Reprod Med* 31: 1045, 1986.
77 Loendersloot EW et al: Efficacy and tolerability of single-dose versus six-day treatment of candidal vulvovaginitis with vaginal tablets of clotrimazole. *Am J Obstet Gynecol* 152: 953, 1985.
78 Brewster E et al: Effect of Fenticonazole in vaginal candidiasis: A double-blind clinical trial versus clotrimazole. *J Intern Med Res* 14: 306, 1986.
79 Breuker G et al: Single-dose therapy of vaginal mycoses with clotrimazole vaginal cream 10%. *Mykosen* 29: 427, 1986.
80 Ritter W: Pharmacokinetic fundamentals of vaginal treatment with clotrimazole. *Am J Obstet Gynecol* 152: 945, 1985.
81 Wallenburg HCS, Wladimiroff JW: Recurrence of vaginal candidiasis during pregnancy: Comparison of miconazole and nystatin treatments. *Obstet Gynecol* 48: 491, 1976.
82 McNellis D et al: Treatment of vulvovaginal candidiasis in pregnancy. A comparative study. *Obstet Gynecol* 50: 674, 1977.
83 Lindeque BG, Van Niekerk WA: Treatment of vaginal candidiasis in pregnancy with a single clotrimazole 500 mg vaginal pessary. *South Am Med J* 65: 123, 1984.
84 Sobel JD: Recurrent vulvovaginal candidiasis. A prospective study of the efficacy of maintenance ketoconazole therapy. *N Engl J Med* 315: 1455, 1986.
85 Sobel JD: Recurrent vulvovaginal candidiasis. What we know and what we don't (editorial). *Ann Intern Med* 101: 390, 1984.
86 Sobel JD: Management of recurrent vulvovaginal candidiasis with intermittent Ketoconazole prophylaxis. *Obstet Gynecol* 65: 435, 1985.
87 Davidson F, Mould RF: Recurrent genital candidosis in women and the effect of intermittent prophylactic treatment. *Br J Vener Dis* 54: 176, 1978.
88 Kinsman OS et al: Hormonal factors in vaginal candidiasis in rats. *Infect Immun* 53: 498, 1986.
89 Dennerstein GJ: DepoProvera in the treatment of recurrent vulvovaginal candidiasis. *J Reprod Med* 31: 801, 1986.
90 Nystatin Multicenter Study Group: Therapy of candidal vaginitis: The effect of eliminated intestinal *Candida*. *Am J Obstet Gynecol* 155: 651, 1986.
91 Rosedale N, Browne K: Hyposensitisation in the management of recurring vaginal candidiasis. *Ann Allergy* 43: 250, 1979.

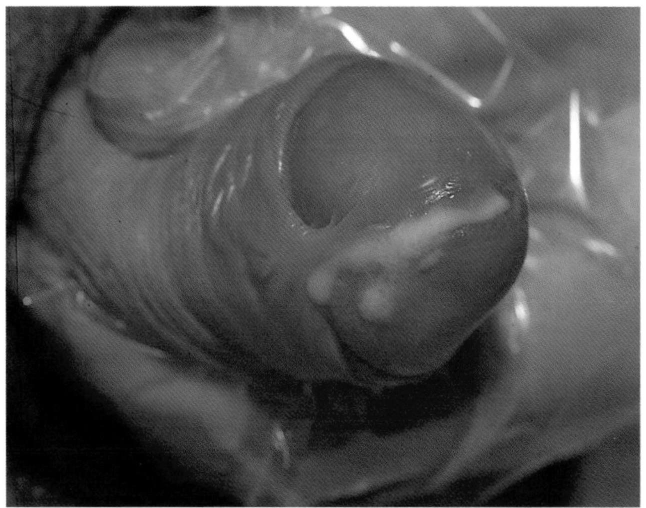

**Plate 1.** Gonococcal urethritis. Note profuse purulent urethral discharge and meatal erythema.

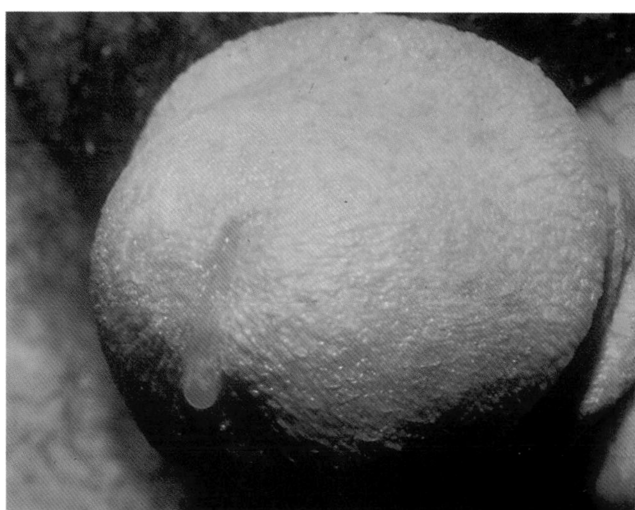

**Plate 2.** Chlamydial urethritis. Note the scant minimally purulent urethral discharge.

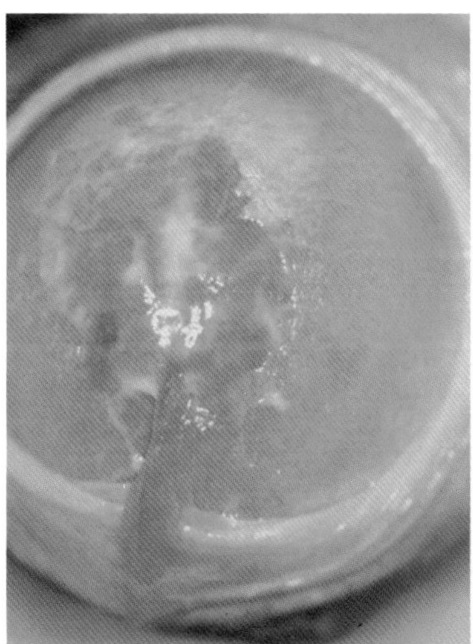

**Plate 3.** Nongonococcal urethritis and meatitis associated with Stevens-Johnson syndrome due to *Mycoplasma pneumoniae* pneumonitis. NGU also occurs as a manifestation of other systemic diseases, such as Reiter's syndrome.

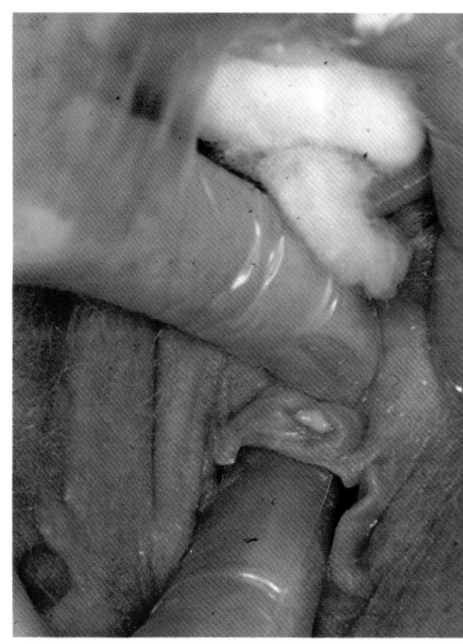

**Plate 4.** Urethritis in a female caused by *Neisseria gonorrhoeae*. Pus can be expressed from the urethral orifice by compressing the urethra against the pubic symphysis.

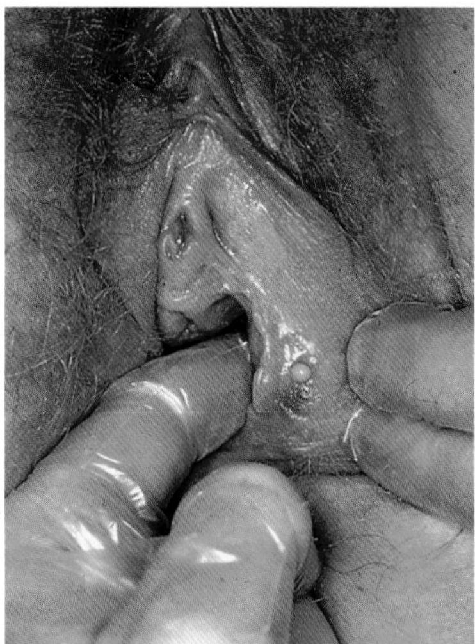

**Plate 5.** Acute bartholinitis caused by *Neisseria gonorrhoeae*. Pus is expressed from the orifice of Bartholin's duct, which opens in the posterior portion of the labia minor and runs posteriorly toward the rectum.

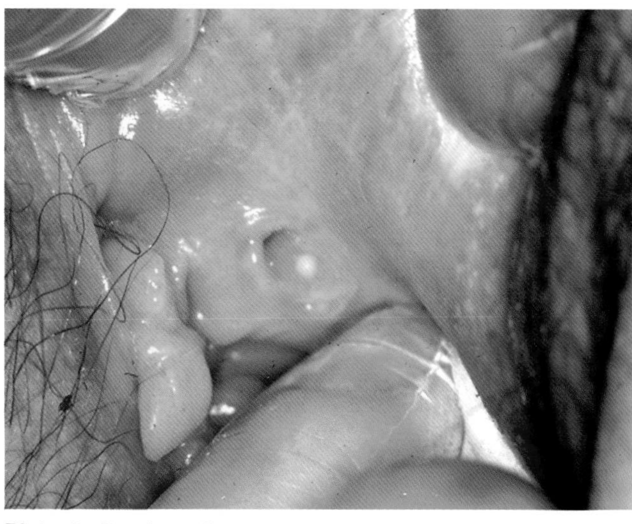

**Plate 6.** .Purulent discharge from Skene's gland. This can be caused by *Neisseria gonorrhoeae* or *Chlamydia trachomatis*.

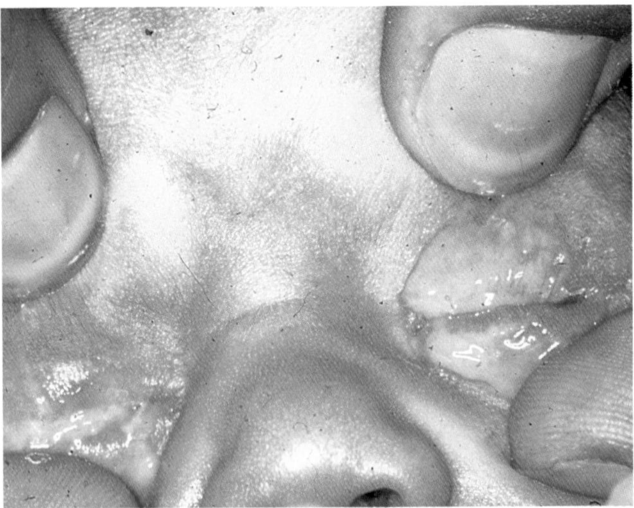

**Plate 7.** Neonatal gonococcal conjunctivitis. Note profuse purulent exudate.

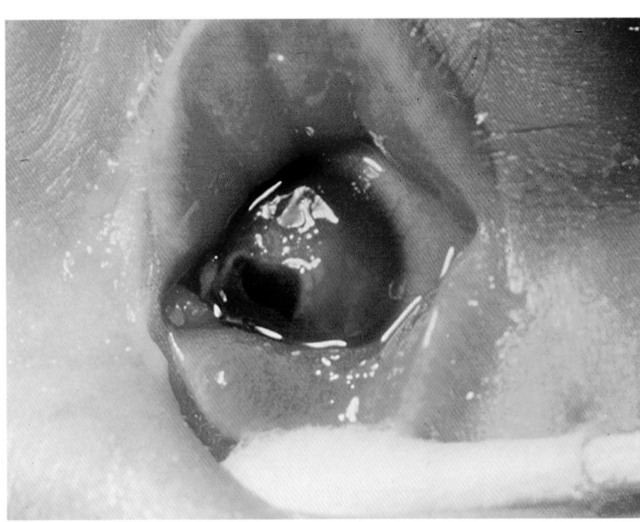

**Plate 8.** Neonatal conjunctivitis and keratitis. Both *Chlamydia trachomatis* and herpes simplex virus type 2 were isolated from the eye of this infant.

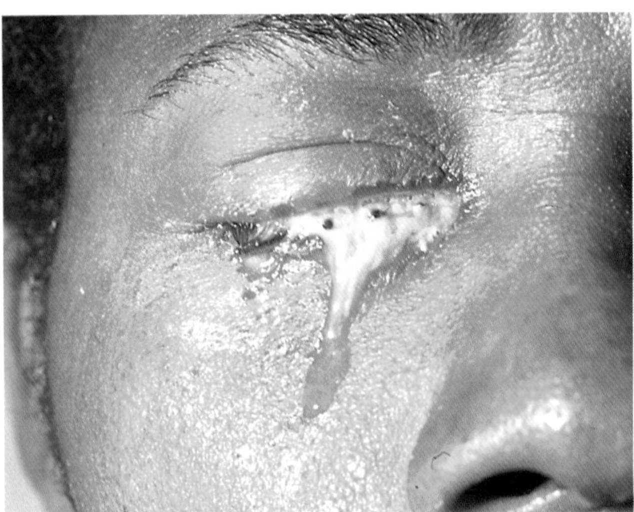

**Plate 9.** Acute gonococcal conjunctivitis in an adult.

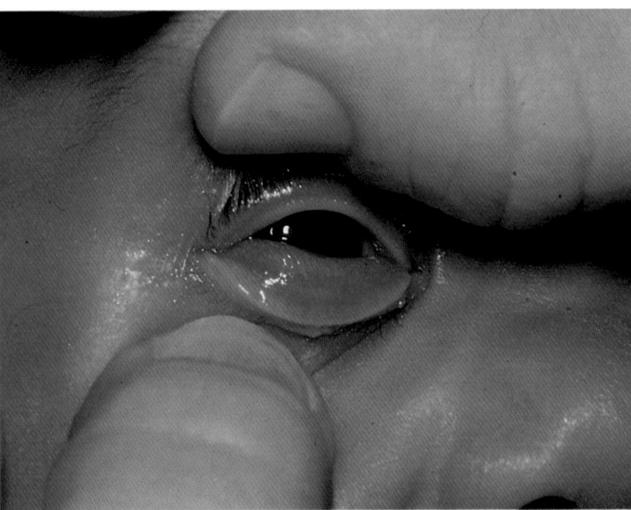

**Plate 10.** Acute recurrent chlamydial conjunctivitis in a two-month old infant. The follicular hyperplasia of the lower palpebral conjunctiva, seen in this recurrent infection, is usually not seen in the first episode of neonatal chlamydial conjunctivitis.

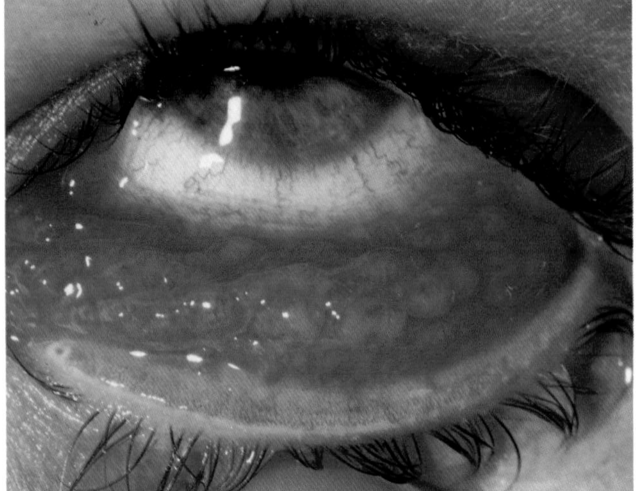

**Plate 11.** Paratrachoma in an adult, caused by a genital immunotype of *C. trachomatis*. Note the marked follicular appearance.

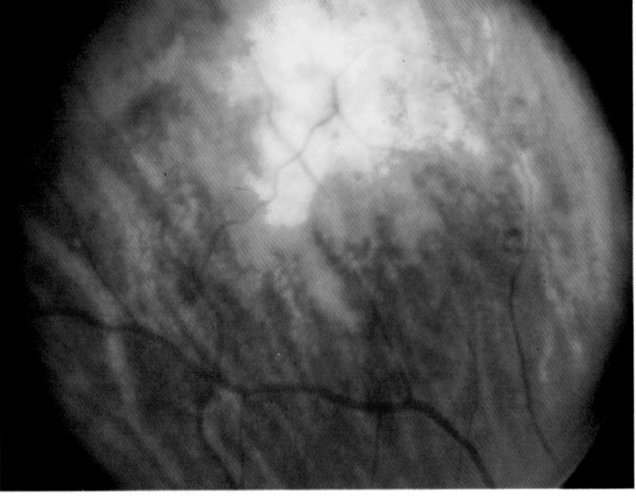

**Plate 12.** CMV chorioretinitis in a patient with AIDS.

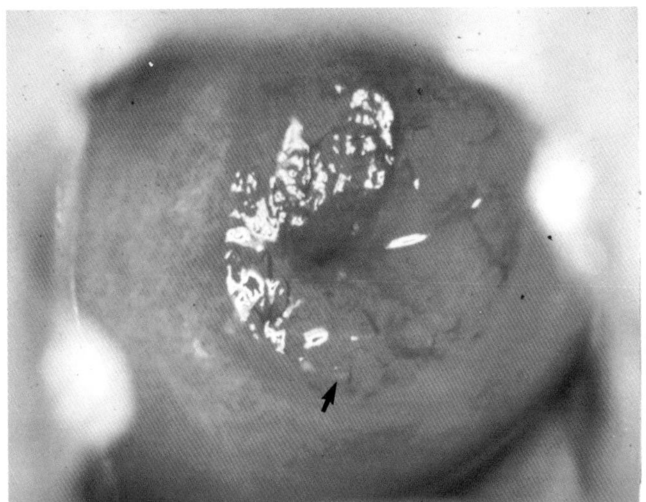

**Plate 13.** Cervical ectopy. Endocervical columnar epithelium is present in an ectopic position on the exocervix, giving a bright-red circumoral appearance. Note that the cervical mucus is clear, not purulent. However, also note the small vesicle (arrow) indicative of a very early primary HSV lesion, within the zone of ectopy.

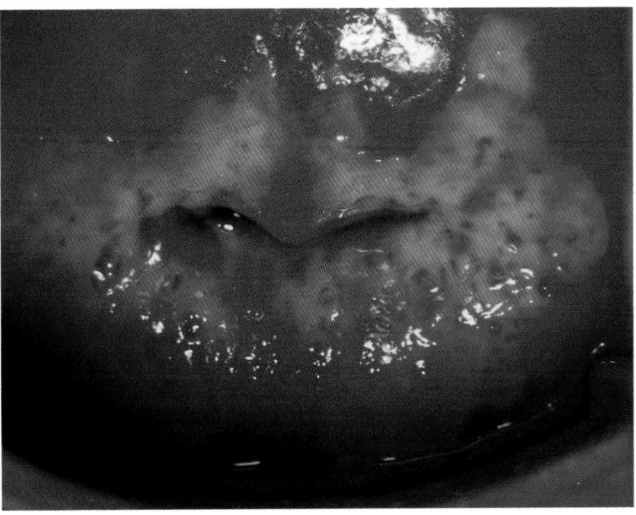

**Plate 14.** Severe primary HSV-2 cervicitis. HSV-2 produces both endocervicitis and ectocervicitis.

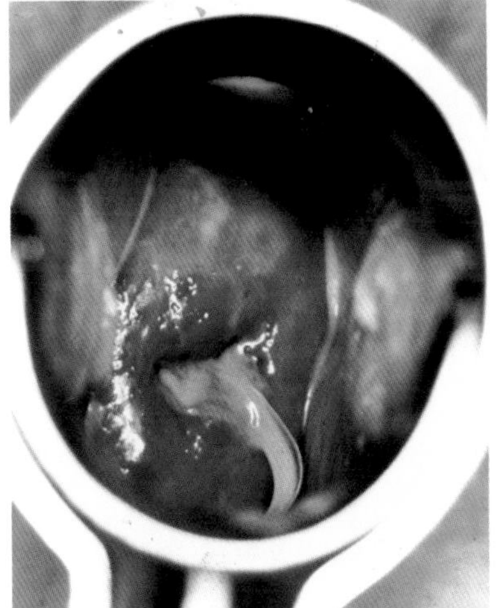

**Plate 15.** Mucopurulent cervicitis caused by *C. trachomatis.* Note pus mixed with mucus (indicating source from the endocervix); also note ectopy, edema, and bleeding.

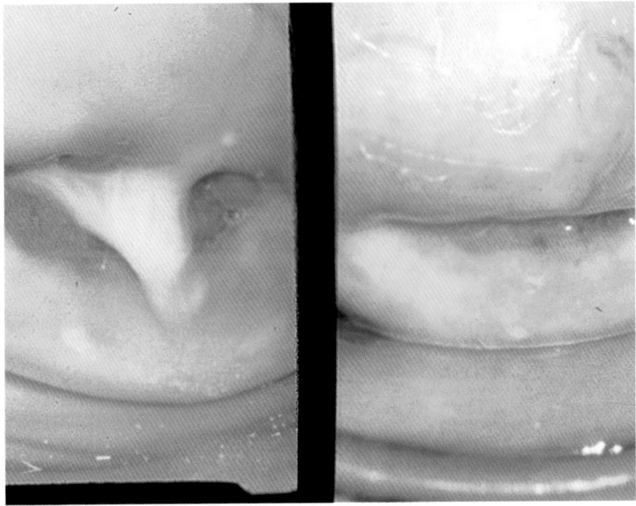

**Plate 16.** Mucopurulent cervicitis caused by *C. trachomatis,* before and after treatment with doxycycline.

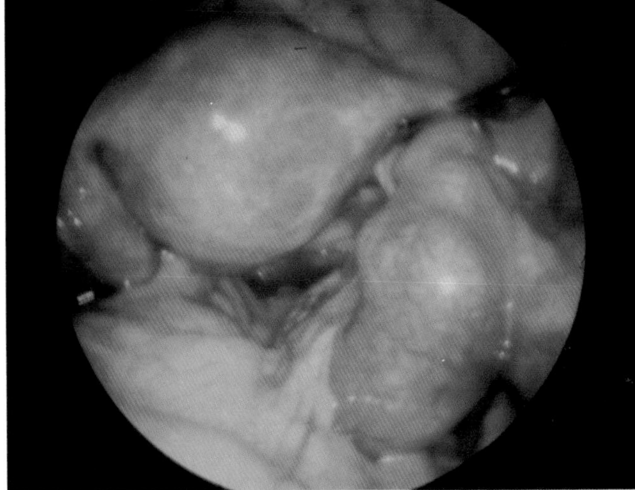

**Plate 17.** Proven chlamydial pyosalpinx. The right tube is swollen, tortuous, reddened, and filled with pus. The yellow omentum is adherent to the abdominal orifice of the tube.

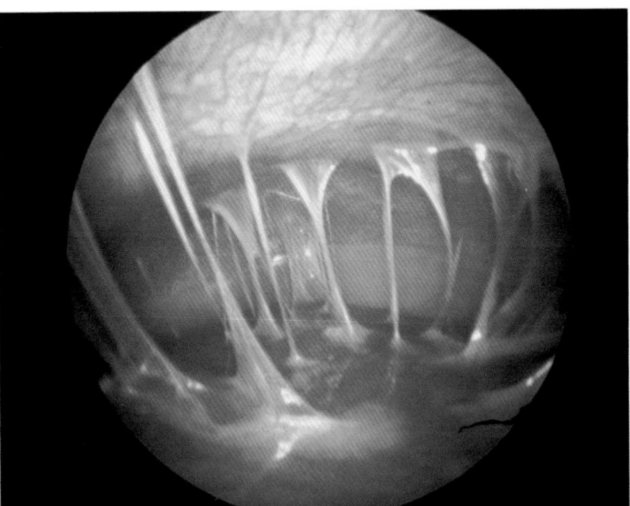

**Plate 18.** Laparoscopic view of perihepatic adhesions in a patient with Fitz-Hugh–Curtis syndrome of approximately six weeks duration.

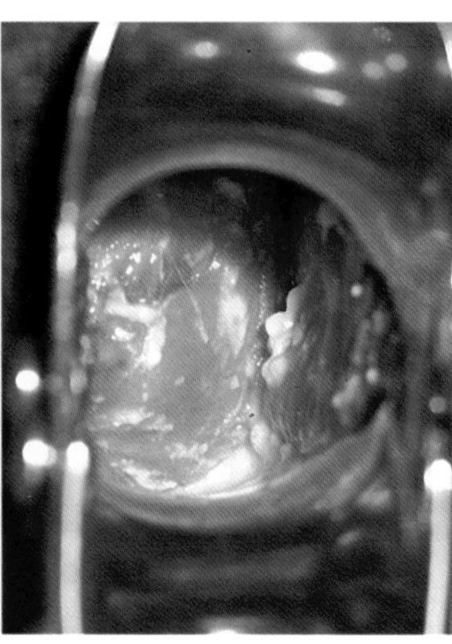

**Plate 19.** Cervical-vaginal candidiasis. Note the white nonhomogeneous curd-like, clumped exudate characteristic of candida infection.

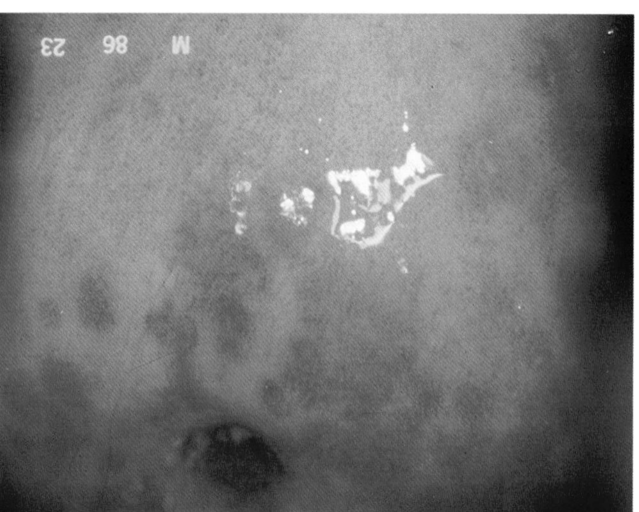

**Plate 20.** Colpophotograph of "strawberry cervix" showing petechiae on the ectocervix in a patient with trichomonal vaginitis and ectocervicitis.

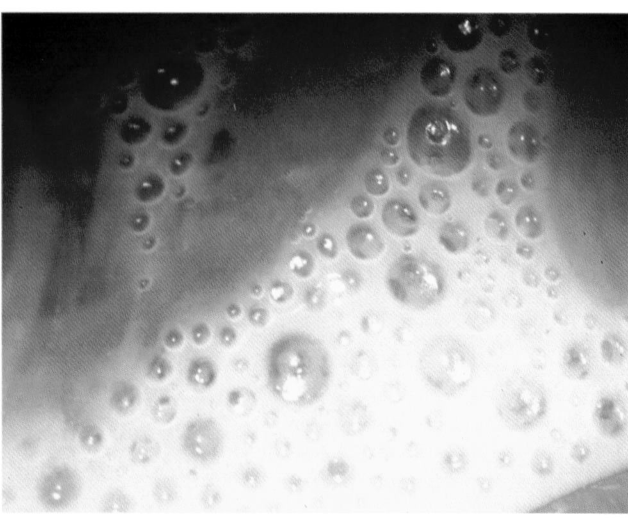

**Plate 21.** Profuse purulent vaginal discharge due to trichomoniasis. Color is yellow when viewed on a white swab. Appearance is occasionally frothy, as seen here.

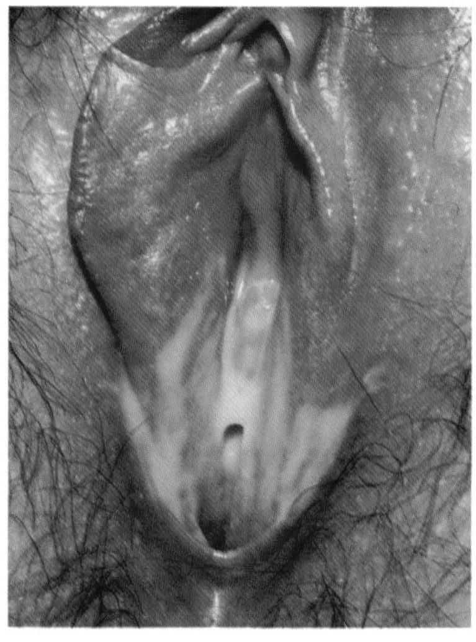

**Plate 22.** Bacterial vaginosis. Note white homogeneous discharge is uniformly adherent to the vaginal walls and flowing out onto the fourchette.

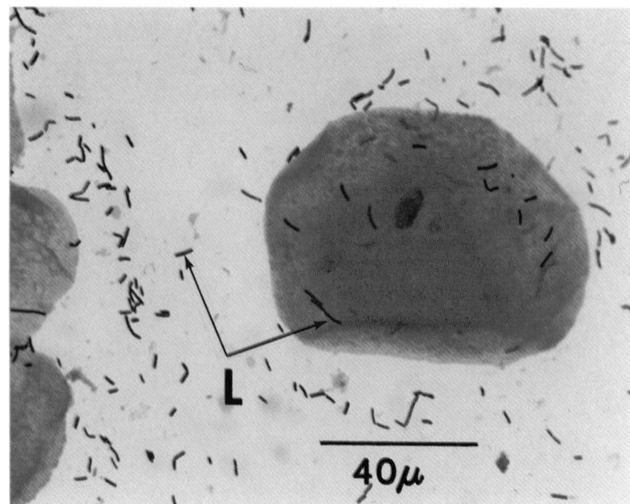


**Plate 23.** Gram's stain of normal vaginal flora. Note moderate number of lactobacilli (L) and normal epithelial cells.

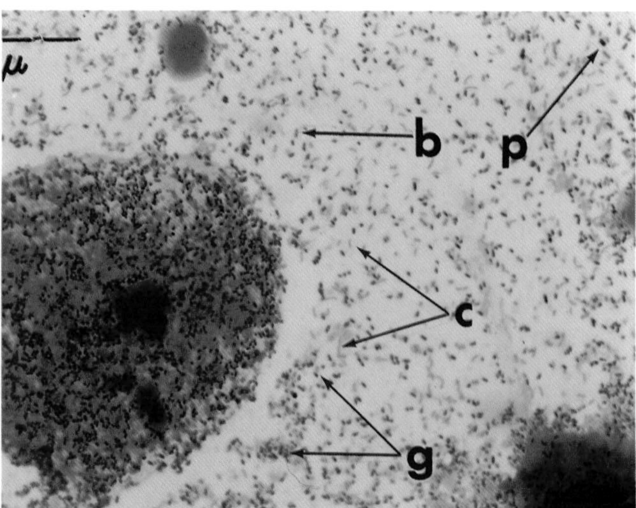


**Plate 24.** Gram's stain of vaginal fluid in bacterial vaginosis. Note gram-variable coccobacilli resembling *Gardnerella* (g), curved rods (c) representing *Mobiluncus*, gram-negative rods resembling *Bacteroides* (b), and gram-positive cocci resembling peptococci (p).

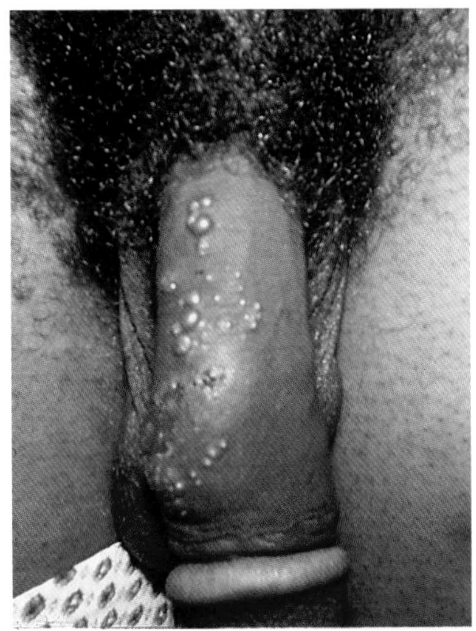

**Plate 25.** Severe primary HSV infection with extensive vesicles, ulcerations, and penile edema.

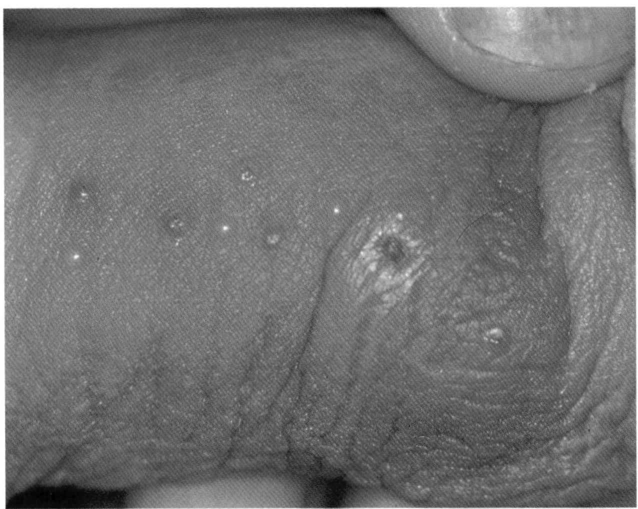

**Plate 26.** Less severe primary genital HSV infection showing intact vesicles and pustules with surrounding erythema together with an earlier lesion, which is crusted and healing.

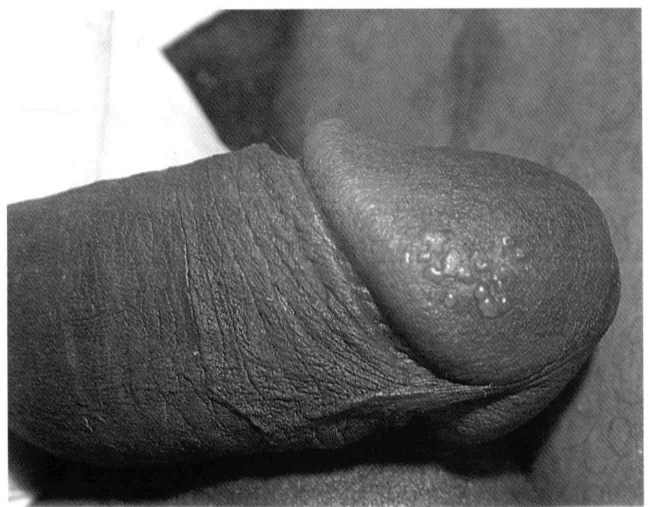

**Plate 27.** Recurrent HSV infection, showing grouped vesicles of the glans penis.

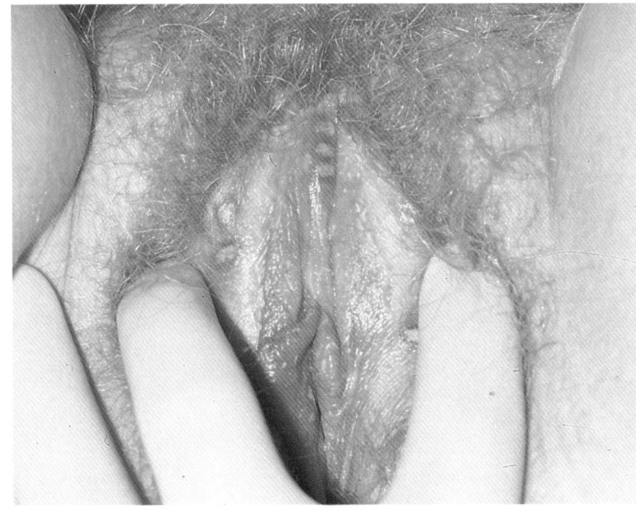

**Plate 28.** Primary genital herpes of the vulva.

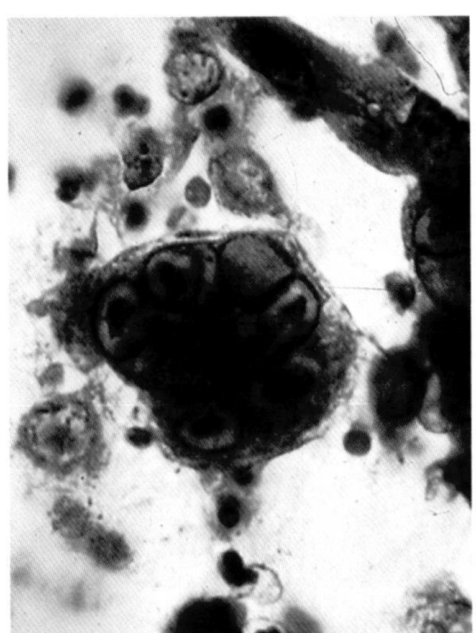

**Plate 29.** Wright-Giemsa stain of scrapings from a herpetic lesion (Tzanck smear) showing multinuclear giant cell and ground-glass appearance of nuclei with nuclear inclusions.

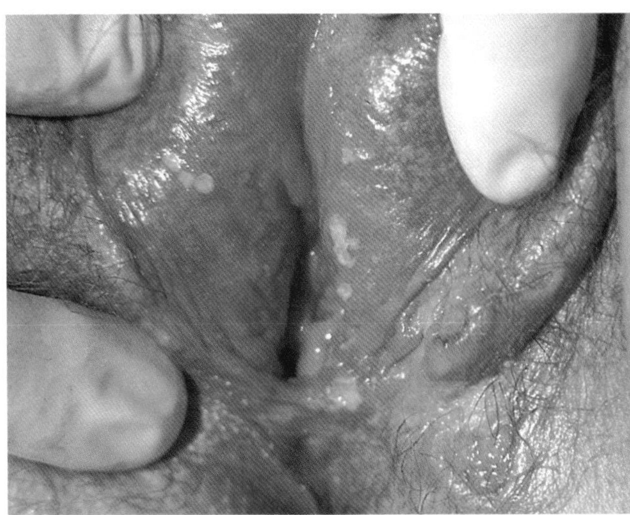

**Plate 30.** Behçet's syndrome. Ulcerations on inner and outer labia and perineum. In males, the ulcers usually involve the scrotum.

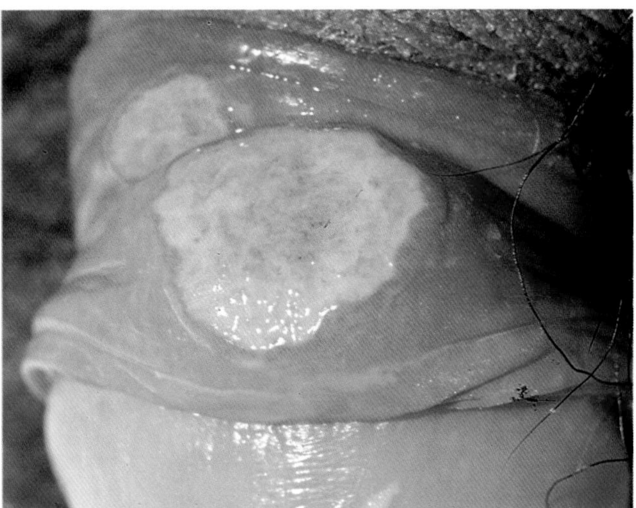

**Plate 31.** Chancroid ulcer involving the foreskin with "kissing" lesion of the penile shaft. Note serpiginous border of the ulcer, which is superficial and covered with a purulent exudate.

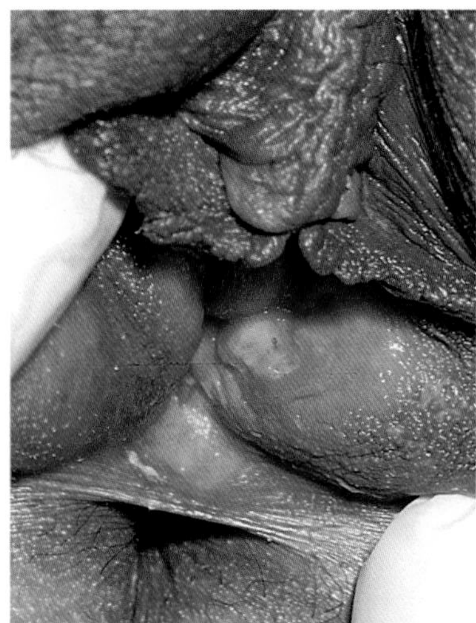

**Plate 32.** Chancroid ulcer of the fourchette in a female.

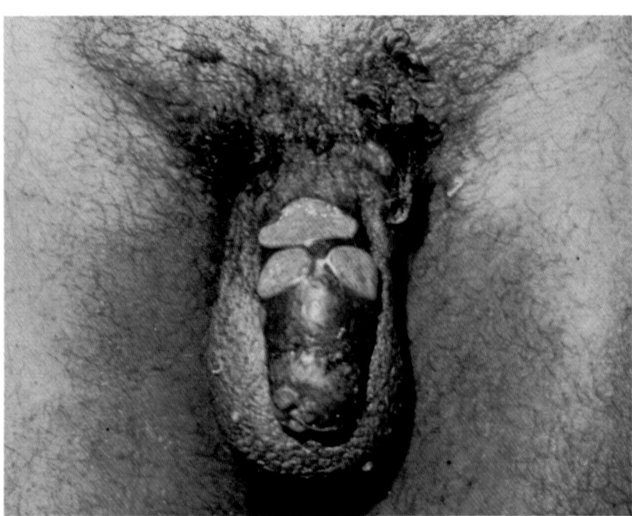

**Plate 33.** Diskoid form of donovanosis.

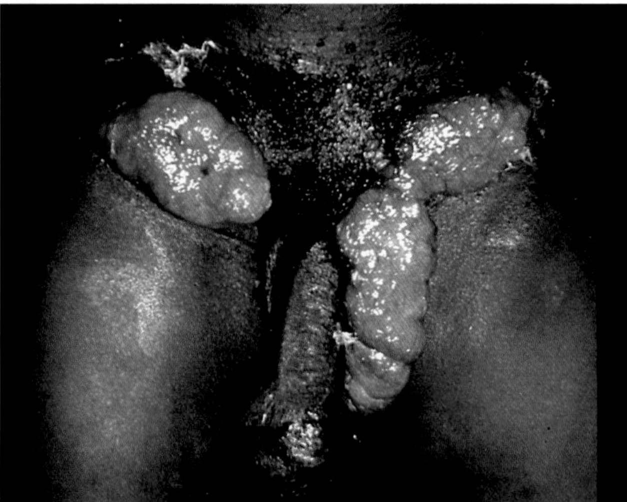

**Plate 34.** Donovanosis. Exuberant granulation tissue with lesions spreading from the penis and scrotum by continuity to one inguinal area, and also to the opposite inguinal area with an intervening skip area, producing pseudobuboes of both inguinal regions.

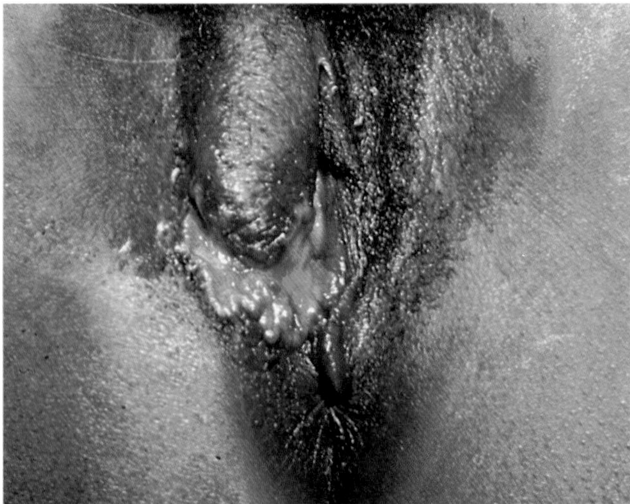

**Plate 35.** Donovanosis in the female with vulvar lymphedema.

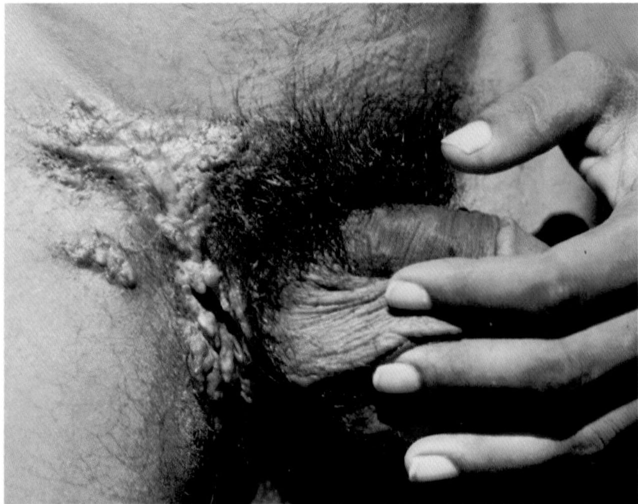

**Plate 36.** Verrucous form of donovanosis, with lesions spreading from the crural area to the inguinal area by continuity. Verrucous donovanosis is most often perianal.

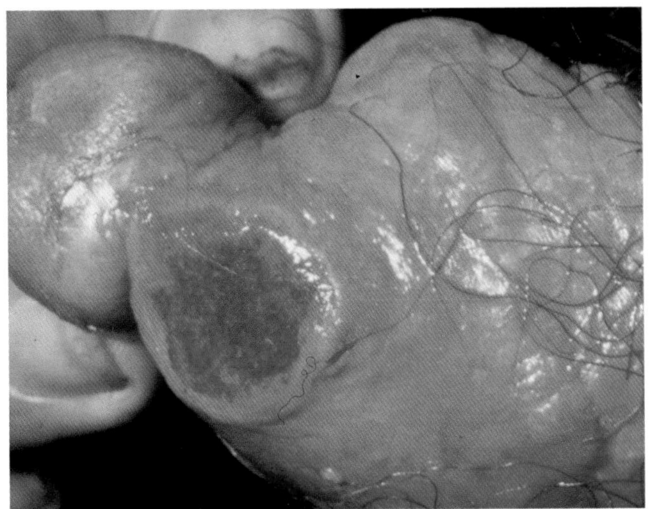

**Plate 37.** Primary syphilitic chancre of the penis. Note the rolled edges of the ulcer, the indurated button-like appearance, and the clean ulcer base.

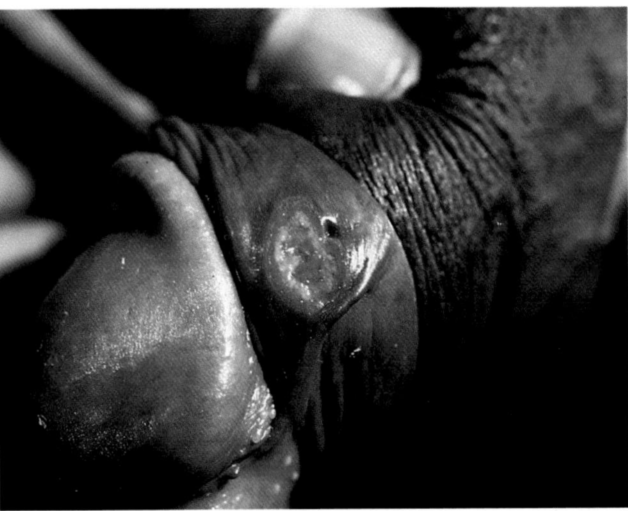

**Plate 38.** Penile chancre in primary syphilis. Classic lesions showing rolled indurated edges with clean ulcer base.

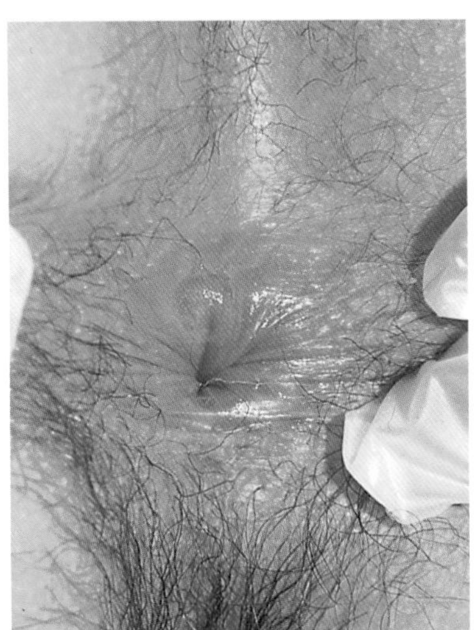

**Plate 39.** Primary perianal chancre in a homosexual man.

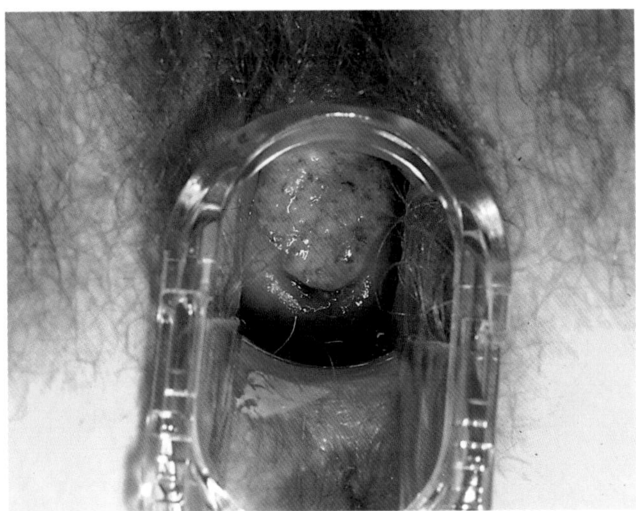

**Plate 40.** Primary syphilitic chancre of the cervix.

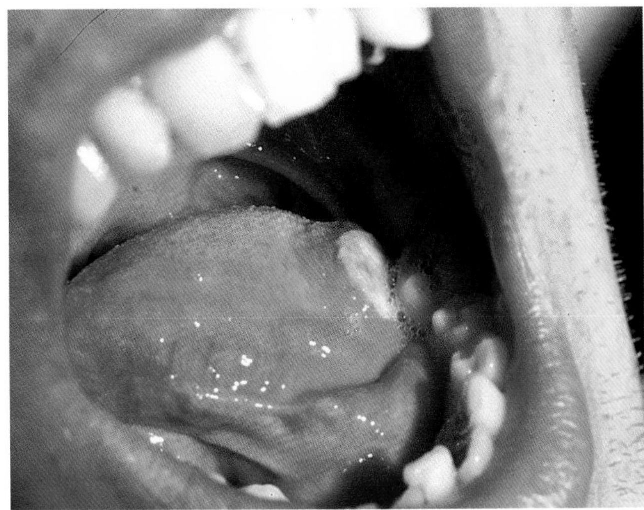

**Plate 41.** Primary chancre of the tongue.

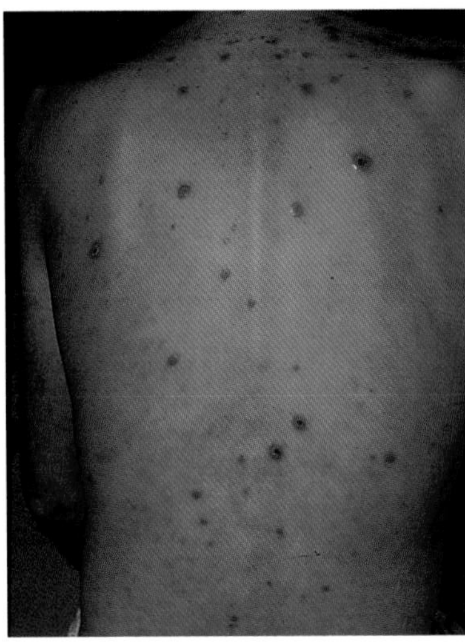

**Plate 42.** Pustular and macular lesions in secondary syphilis.

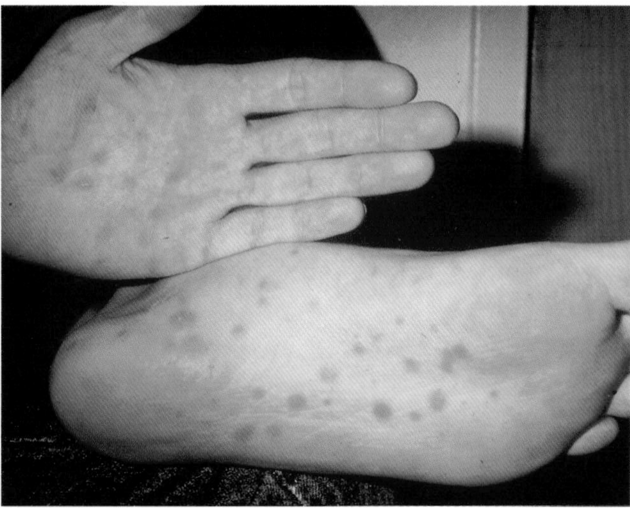

**Plate 43.** Secondary syphilitic rash of the palm and sole.

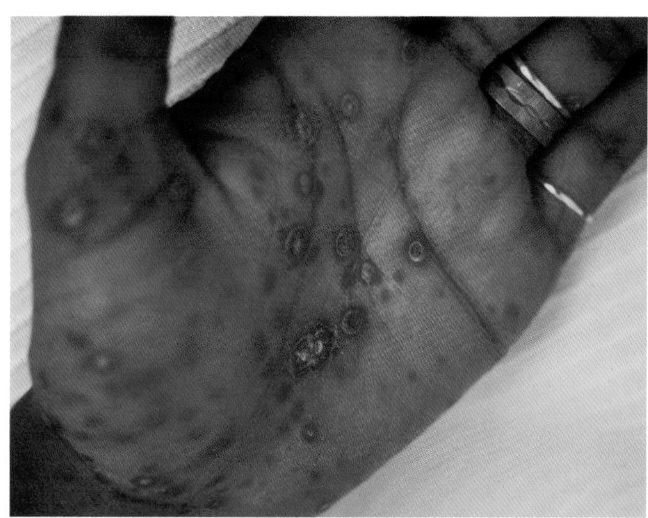

**Plate 44.** Secondary syphilitic rash of palm.

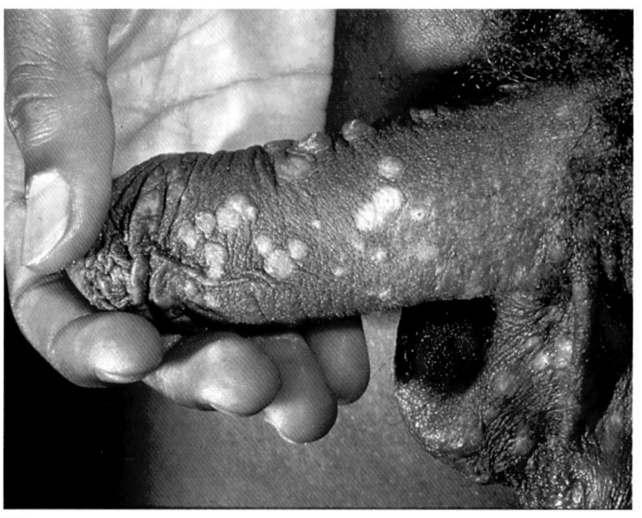

**Plate 45.** Secondary syphilitic lesions on the penis.

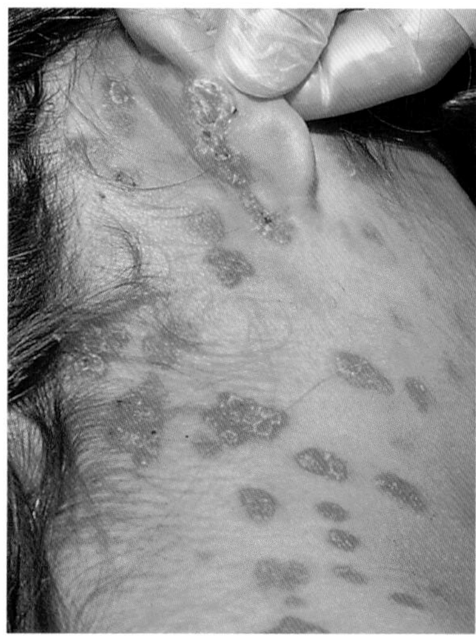

**Plate 46.** Psoriasiform secondary syphilis.

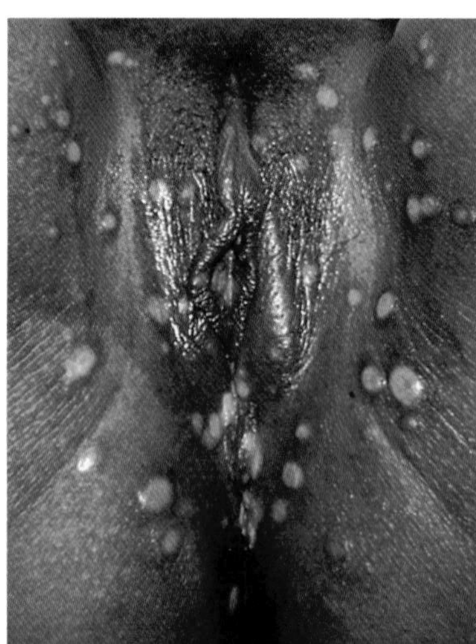

**Plate 47.** Perivulvar and perianal condyloma latum, in secondary syphilis.

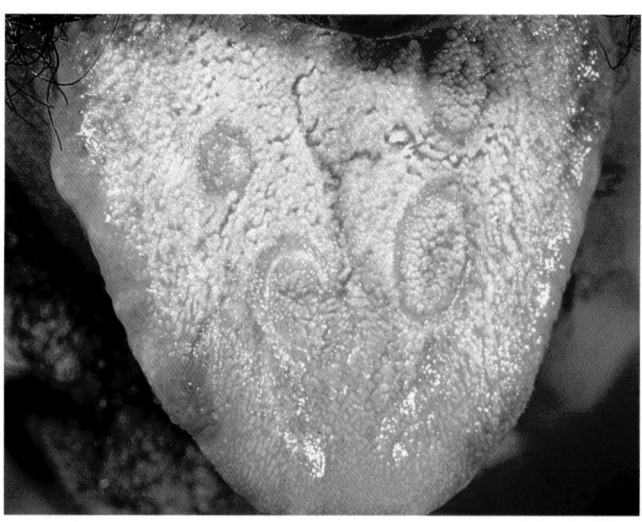

**Plate 48.** Mucus patches involving the tongue in secondary syphilis.

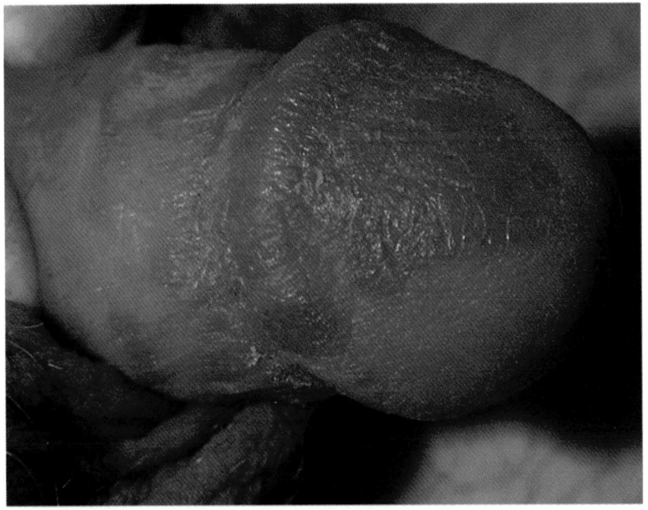

**Plate 49.** Seborrheic dermatitis of the glans and preputium of the penis. Red erythematous lesions, covered with yellowish-white scales. On the genitalia, seborrheic lesions are characteristically sharply defined.

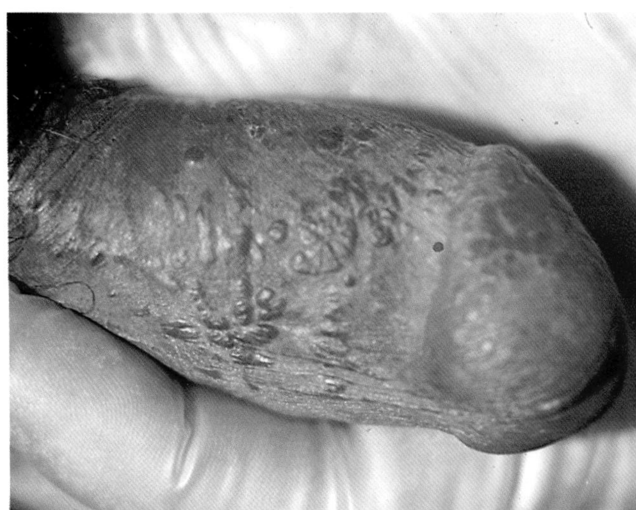

**Plate 50.** Lichen ruber planus of the penis. Brown, hyperpigmented papules on the penis. Reticulated white pattern on glans penis. Lichen ruber planus lesions may be flat, angular, and white linear striae (Wickham's striae) or atrophic variants can be seen.

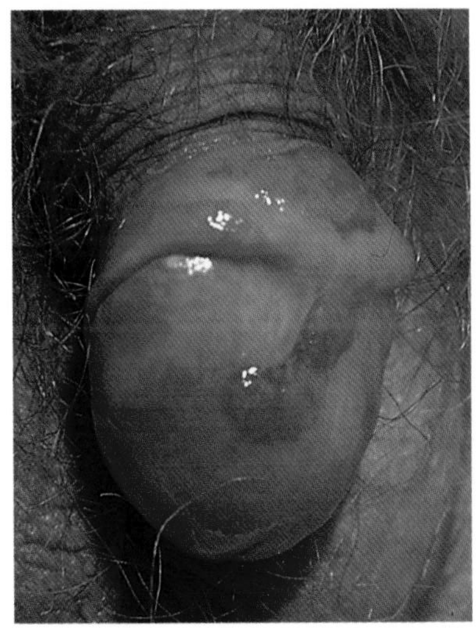

**Plate 51.** Plasmocellular balanitis. Patches of erythema with a shiny, smooth, and moist surface of glans and foreskin of the penis.

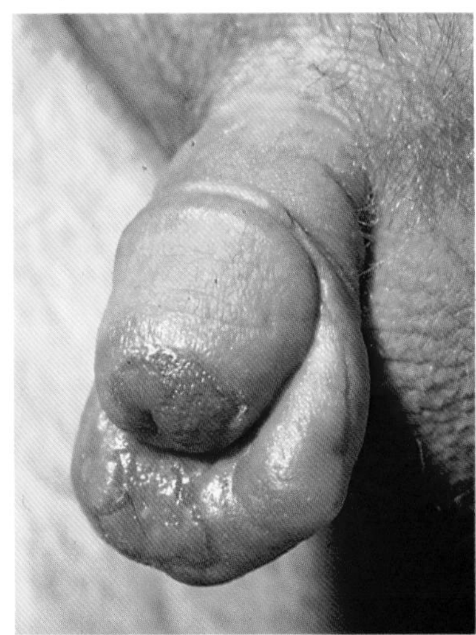

**Plate 52.** Erythroplasia of Queyrat. Red-colored, glazed, barely raised irregularly shaped plaques on glans and foreskin of the penis. These lesions also occur on the inner aspect of the vulva. Ulceration and crusting may occur.

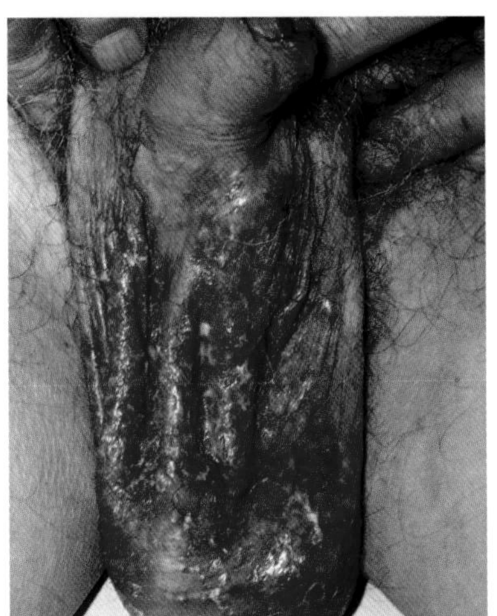

**Plate 53.** Scrotal candidiasis.

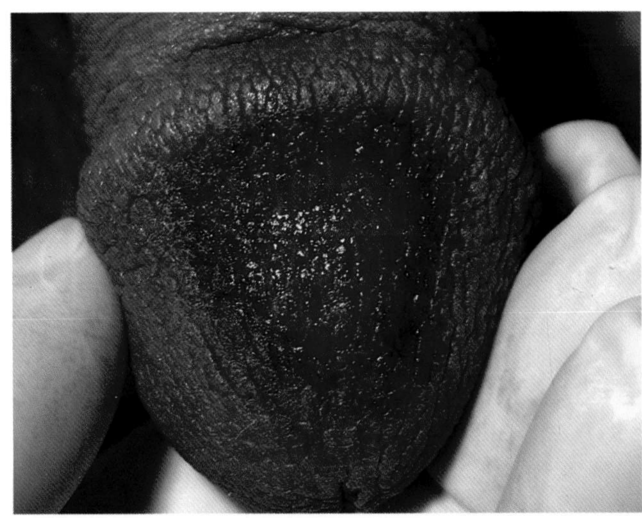

**Plate 54.** Fixed drug eruption of the glans penis due to tetracycline, showing an eroded surface and peripheral hyperpigmentation.

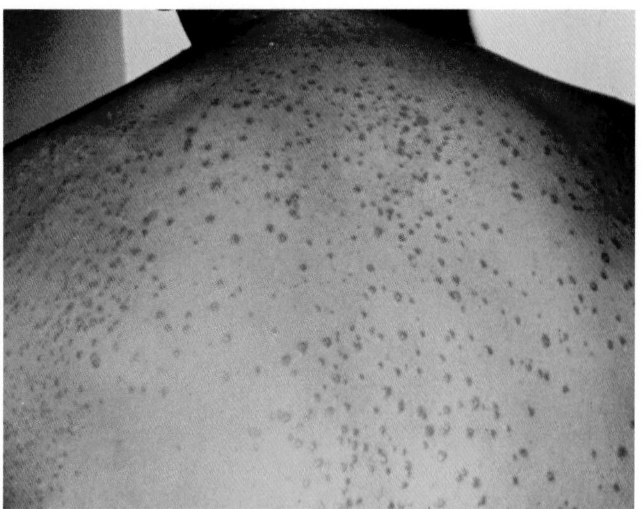

**Plate 55.** Droplike, or guttate, lesions of psoriasis. Such lesions are often seen with acute flares of the disease, often following streptococcal infection.

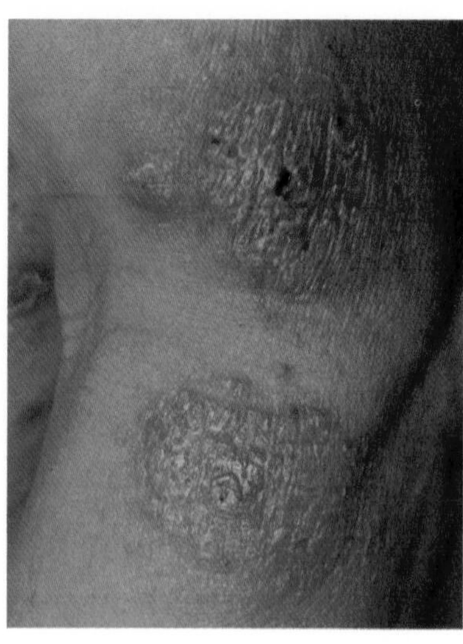

**Plate 56.** Morphologically these lesions look like psoriasis. In fact, they are psoriasiform lesions of secondary syphilis.

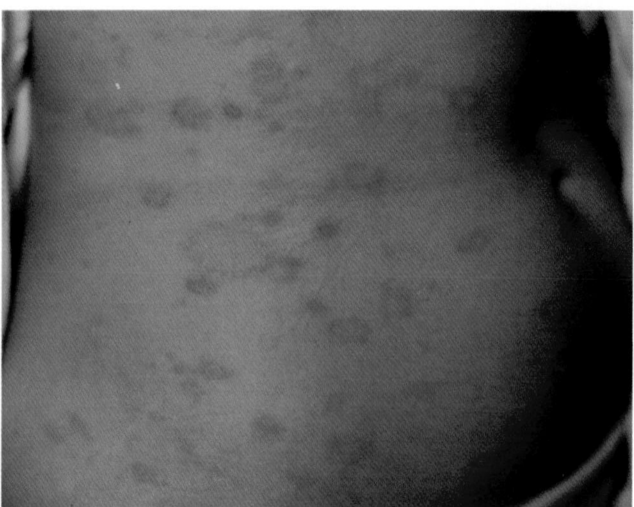

**Plate 57.** Characteristic lesions of pityriasis rosea.

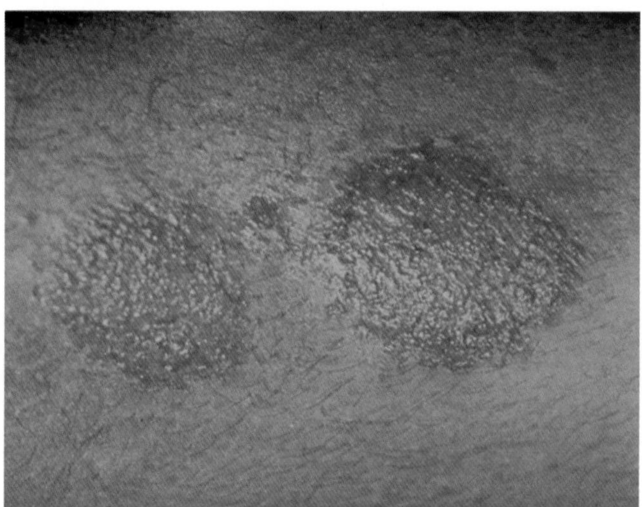

**Plate 58.** Scaling macules of nummular eczema.

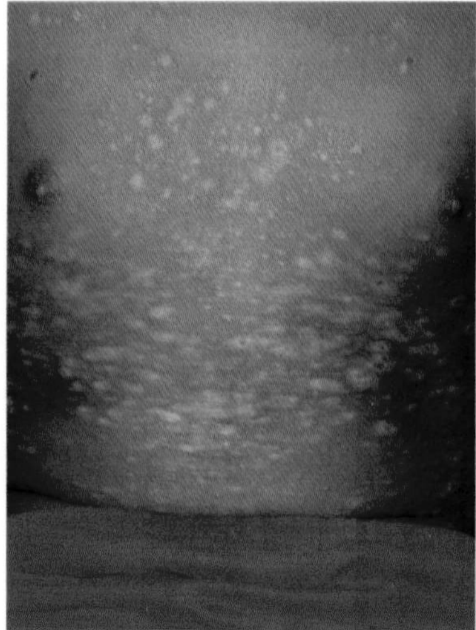

**Plate 59.** Lichen planus.

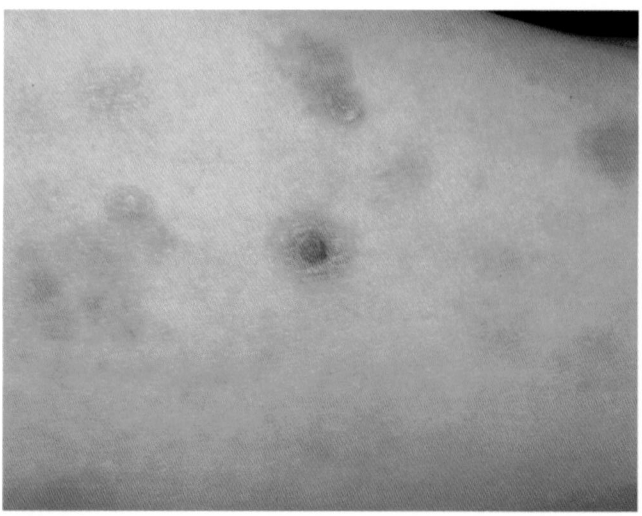

**Plate 60.** Pityriasis lichenoides et varioliformis acuta (PLEVA).

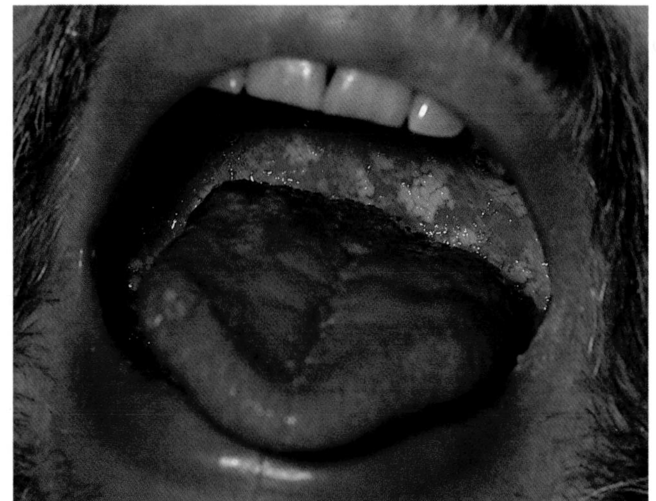

**Plate 61.** Oral thrush in a patient with HIV infection.

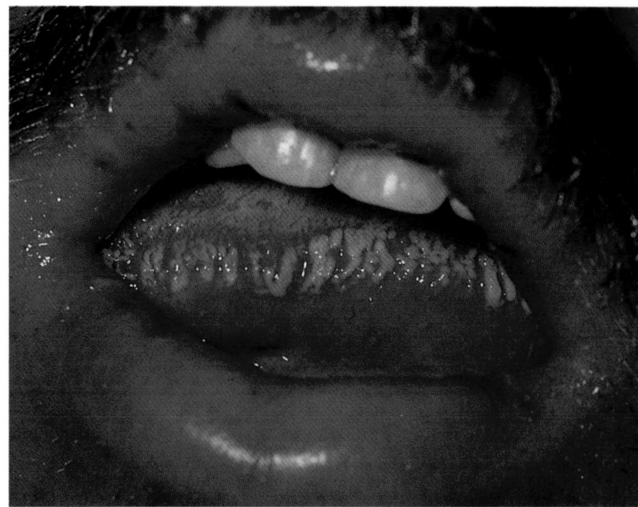

**Plate 62.** Oral hairy leukoplakia in a patient with HIV infection.

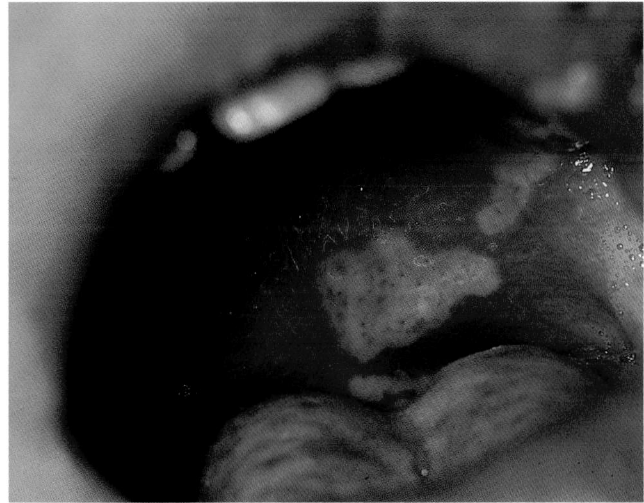

**Plate 63.** Oral herpes zoster (with cutaneous dissemination) in Group IVa HIV infection.

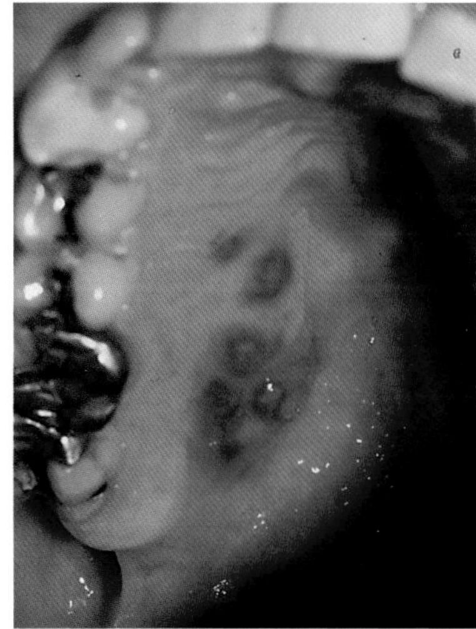

**Plate 64.** Kaposi's sarcoma in the palate as a manifestation of AIDS.

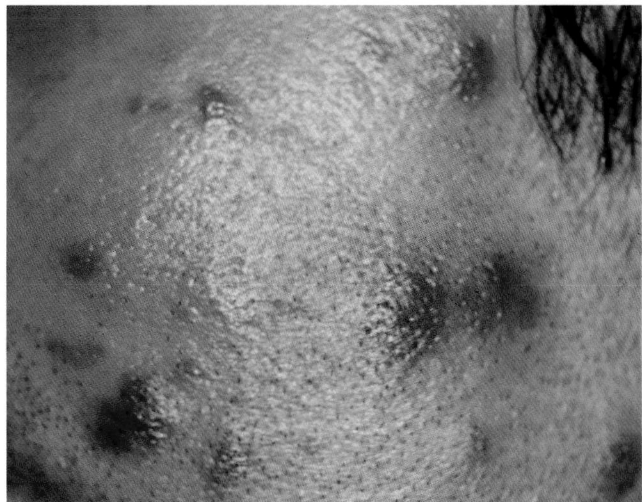

**Plate 65.** Kaposi's sarcoma on the face of a homosexually active man with AIDS.

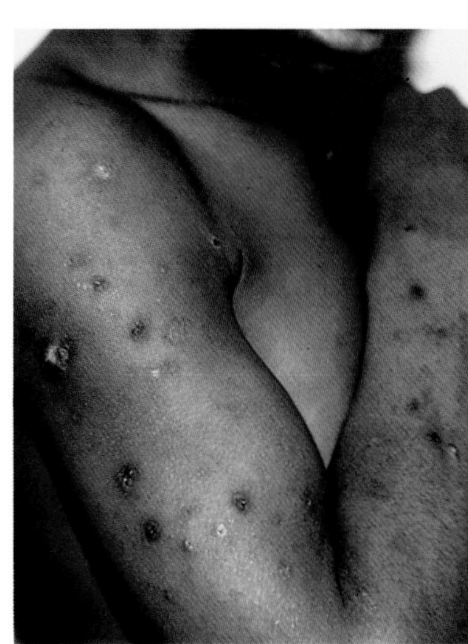

**Plate 66.** Pruritic excoriated rash on an African man with AIDS.

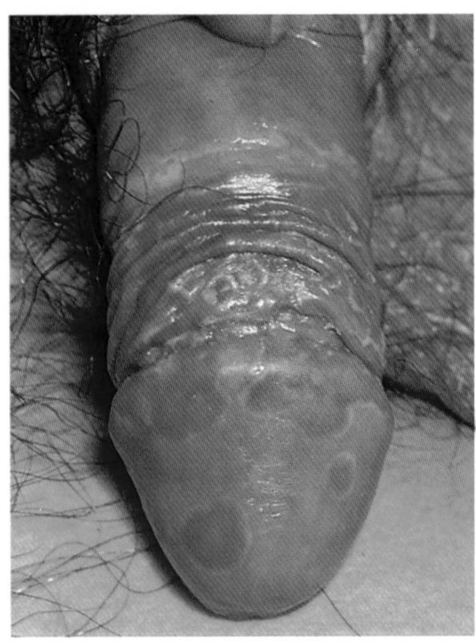

**Plate 67.** Circinate balanitis in Reiter's syndrome.

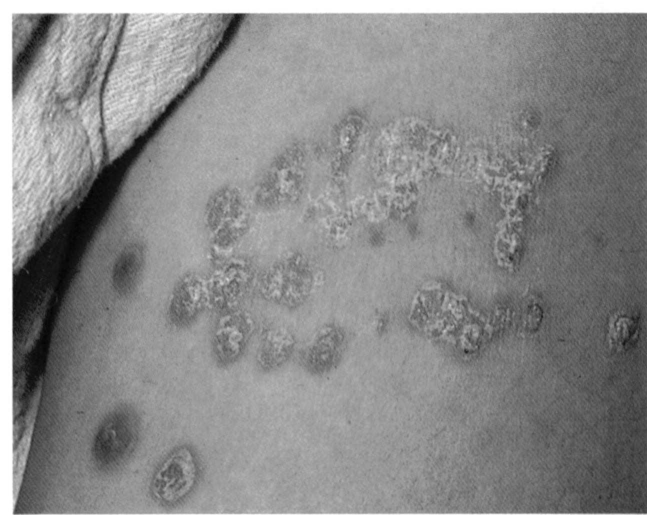

**Plate 68.** Keratodermia blenorrhagica in Reiter's syndrome.

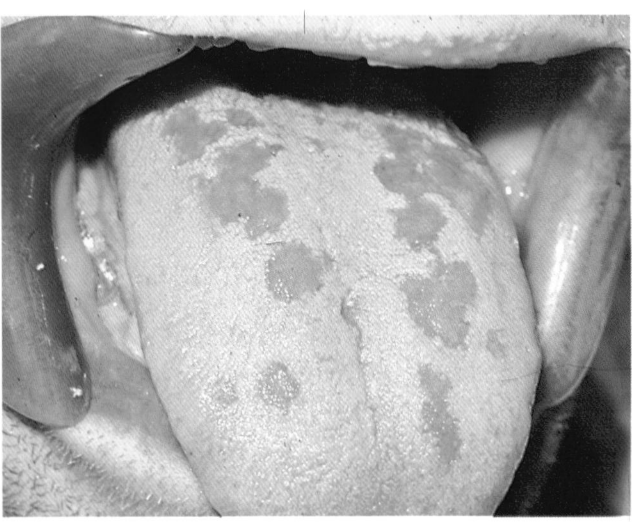

**Plate 69.** Superficial ulcerations of the tongue in Reiter's syndrome.

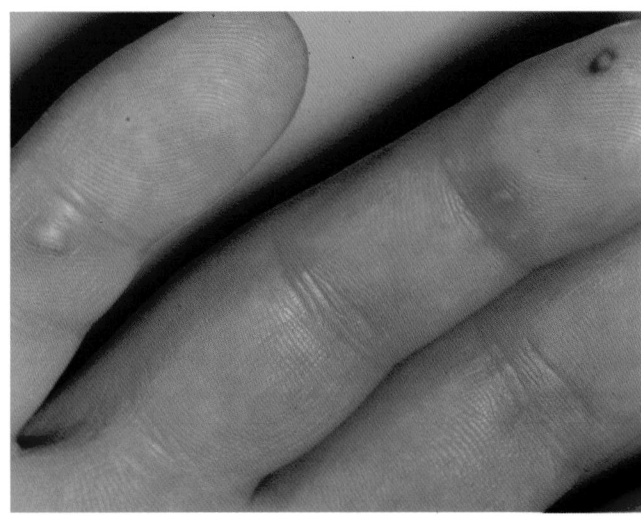

**Plate 70.** Typical distribution of skin lesions in disseminated gonococcal infection. Usually 5 to 20 such lesions are apparent on the extremities, generally sparing the face and trunk.

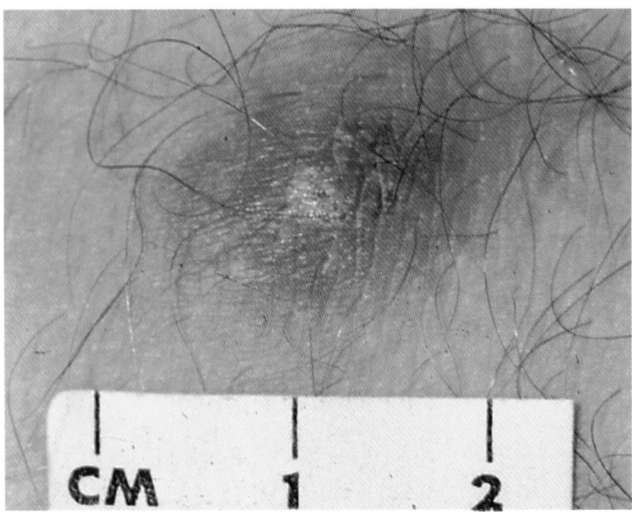


**Plate 71.** Hemorrhagic pustular lesion of disseminated gonococcal infection.

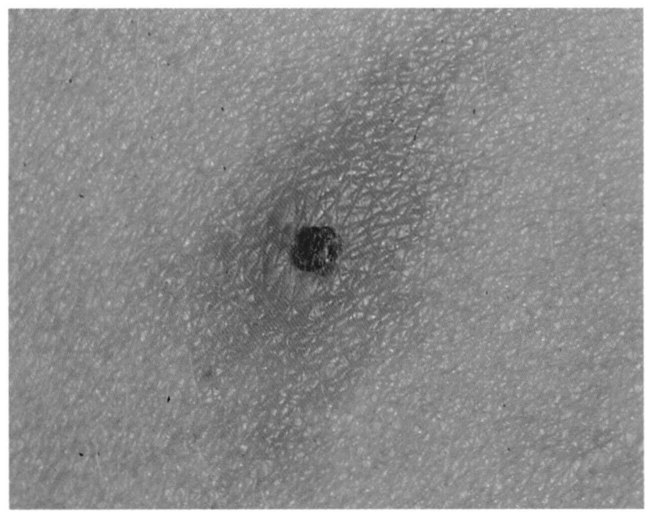

**Plate 72.** Crusted petechial lesion of disseminated gonococcal infection.

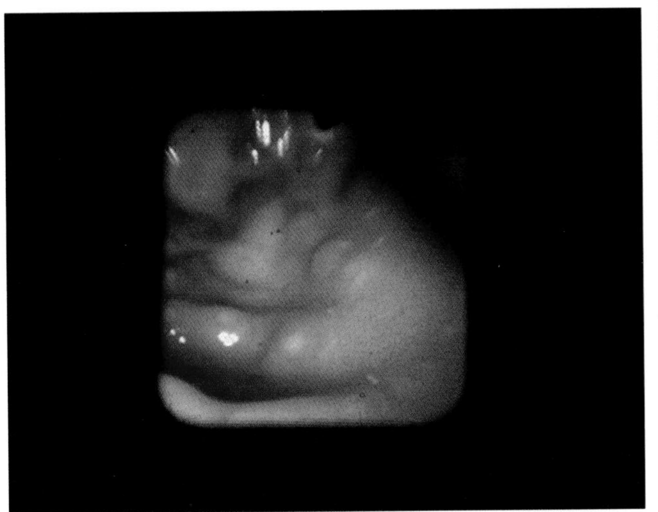

**Plate 73.** Short-bundle sigmoidoscopic view of the distal rectum in a patient with early primary anorectal herpes, showing intact vesiculopustules.

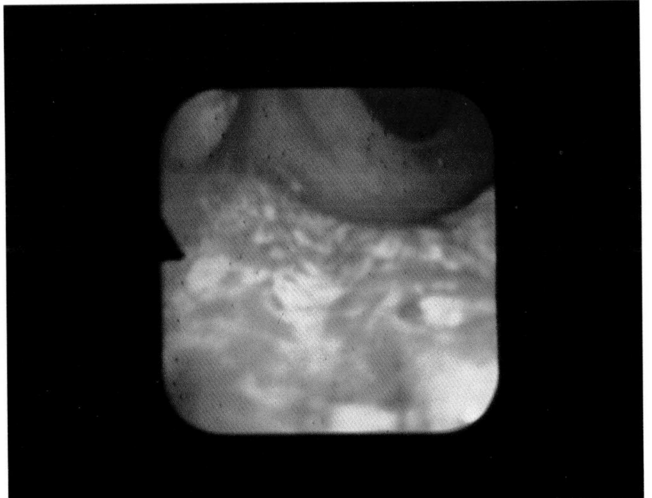

**Plate 74.** Short-bundle sigmoidoscopic view of primary anorectal herpes showing patchy bleeding and exudate extending up to 8 cm, with normal rectal mucosa above.

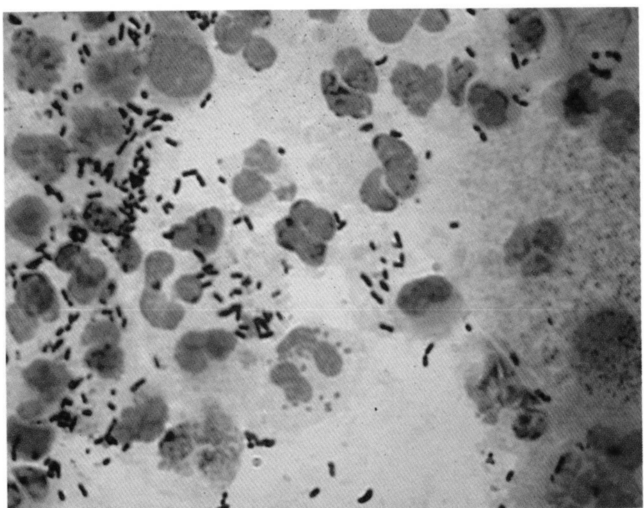

**Plate 75.** Gram-stained smear of exudate obtained at anoscopy showing one polymorphonuclear leukocyte containing gram-negative diplococci.



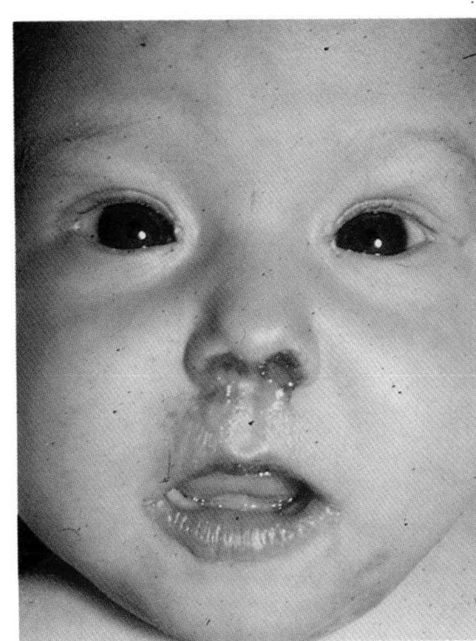

**Plate 76.** "Snuffles" associated with crusting and purulent nasal discharge in an infant with congenital syphilis.

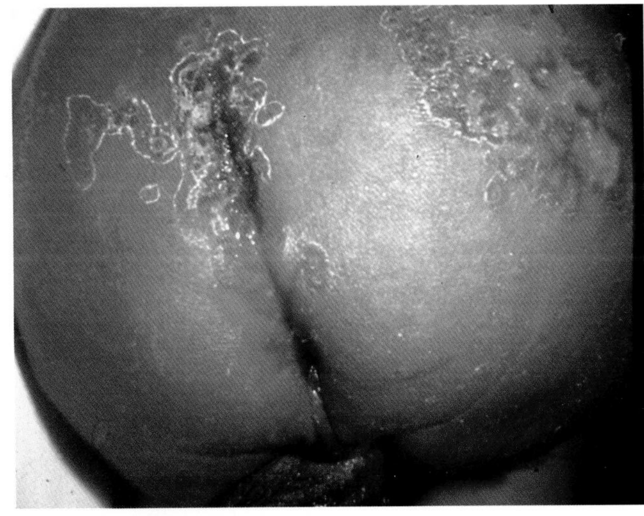

**Plate 77.** Neonatal HSV infection. Ulcers and crusted lesions on the buttocks.

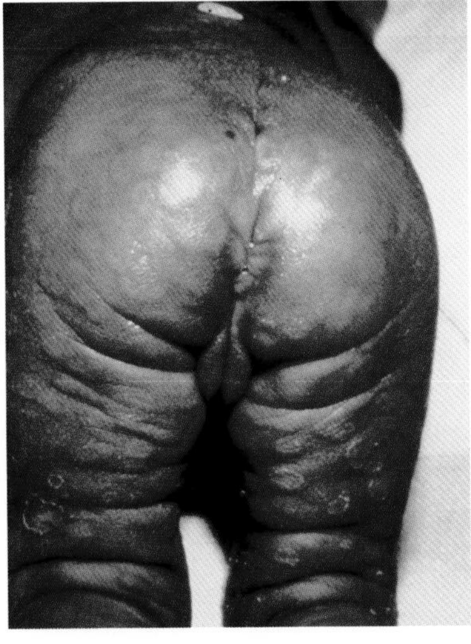

**Plate 78.** Congenital syphilis. Diffuse diskoid lesions associated with perianal lesions cover the entire body of this infant.

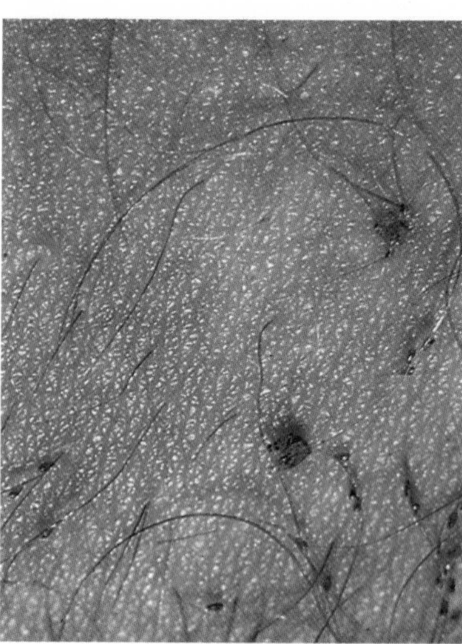

**Plate 79.** Heavy infestation with *Phthirus pubis,* showing nits (eggs) on pubic hair and adult crab lice holding onto pubic hairs.

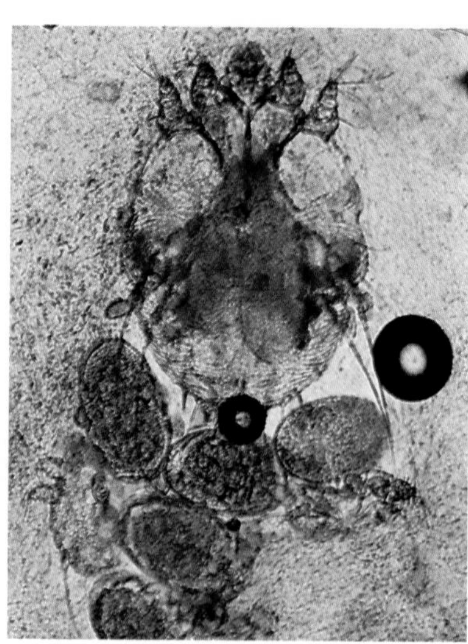

**Plate 80.** *Sarcoptes scabiei* mite with eggs in feces scraped from scabetic burrow.

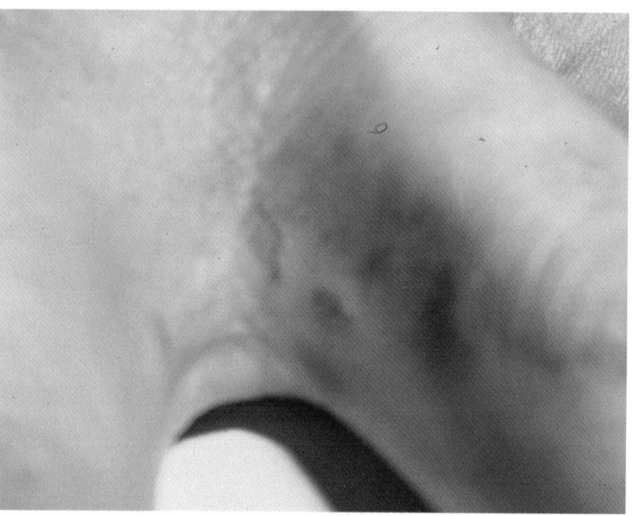

**Plate 81.** Intradermal burrow of scabies demonstrated by coating the skin with ink, then wiping away surface ink, leaving the intradermal burrow filled with ink.

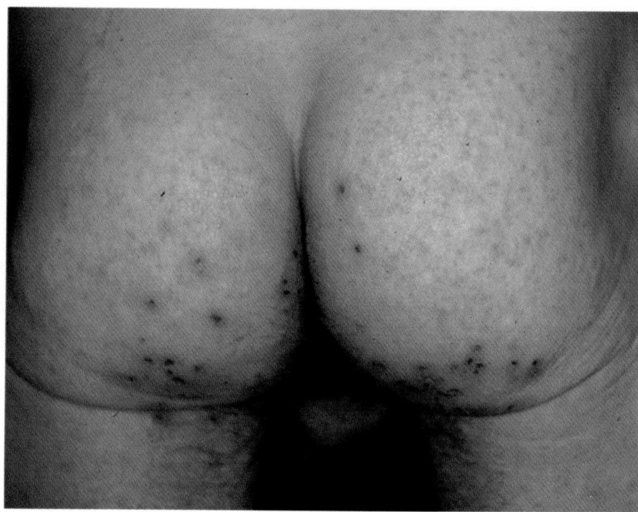

**Plate 82.** Grouped excoriations due to scabies on the lower buttocks, simulating dermatitis herpetiformis.

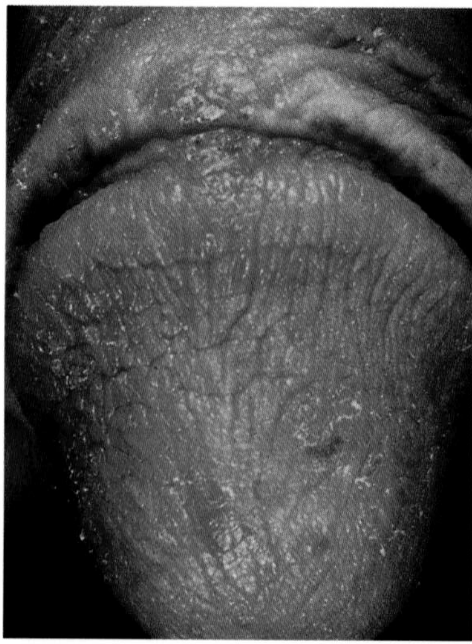

**Plate 83.** Scabies of the penis. Pyoderma of the penis is highly suggestive of scabies.

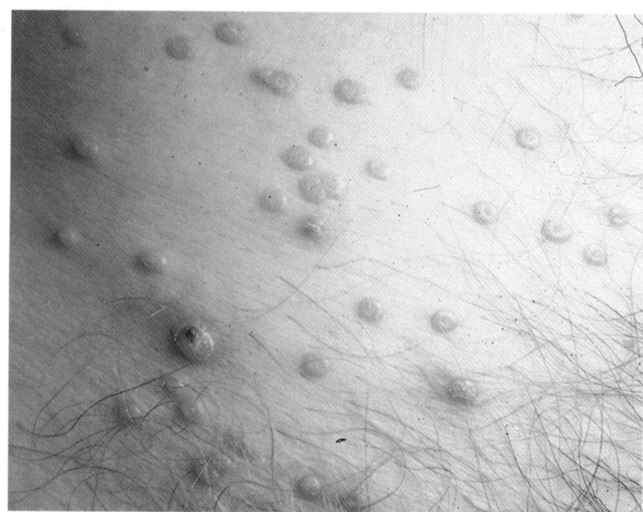

**Plate 84.** Molluscum contagiosum of the lower abdomen and suprapubic area in a patient with co-existing genital molluscum lesions. Note central umbilication and pale salmon color.

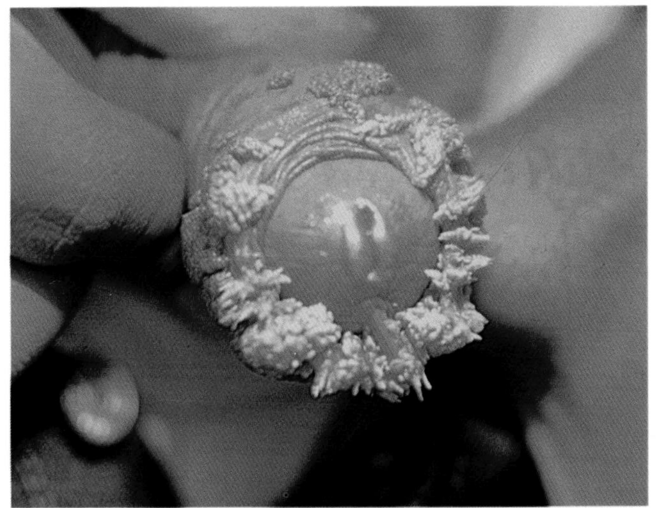

**Plate 85.** Extensive penile condylomata acuminata. Typically, exophytic visible condylomata of the external genitalia in the male and female are associated with HPV types 6 or 11.

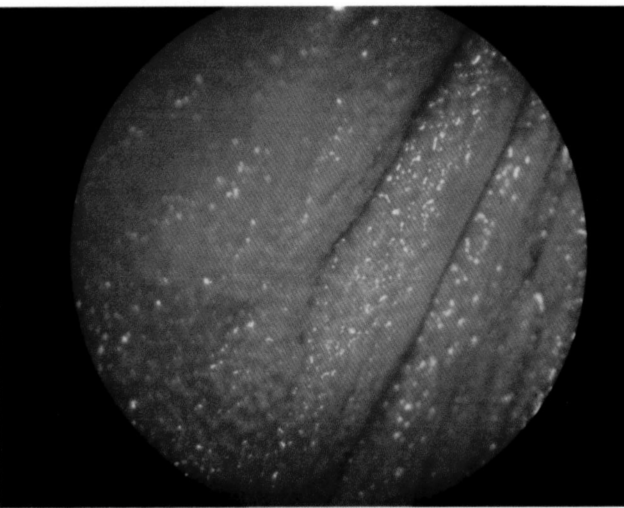

**Plate 86.** Vaginal asperities. Small somewhat-raised white dots diffusely scattered over the pink vaginal epithelium, following acetic acid treatment. Magnification 16×. It is suspected but not yet proven that these are associated with HPV infection of the vaginal epithelium.

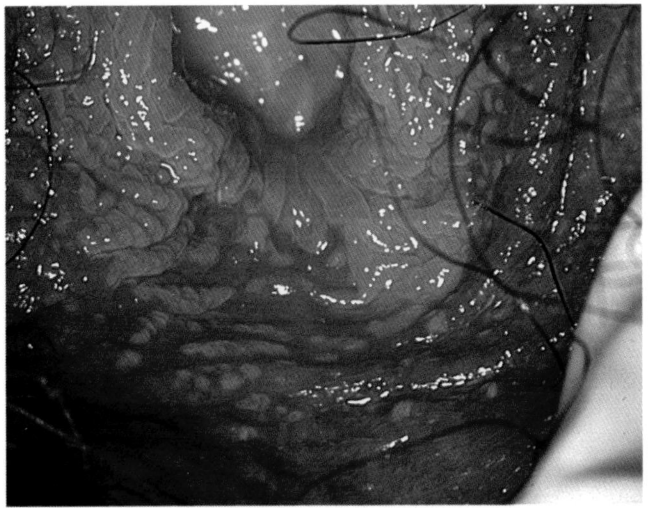

**Plate 87.** Appearance of "white epithelium" after application of acetic acid to the vulva. It is suspected that these lesions are associated with HPV infection.

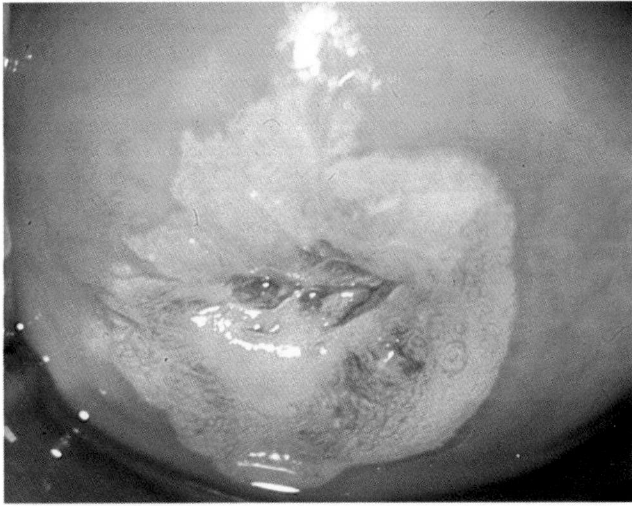

**Plate 88.** Appearance of "white epithelium" visualized with a colposcope through a green filter after application of acetic acid to the cervix. Opaque, white epithelium with sharp borders, as shown here, is associated with HPV infection.

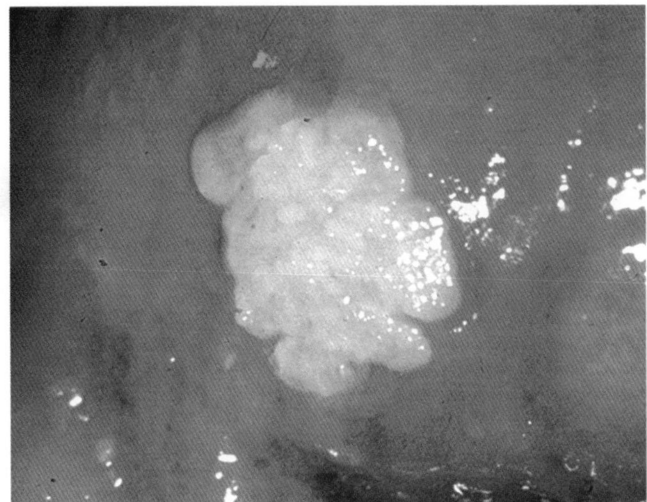

**Plate 89.** Cervical leukoplakia which is associated with dysplasia and cervical HPV infection.

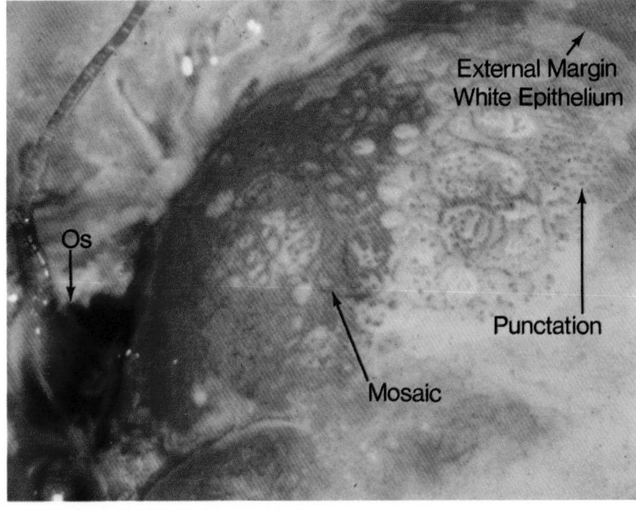


**Plate 90.** Severe dysplasia of the cervix as seen by colposcopy. This cervix displays features of punctation, mosaicism, and white epithelium.

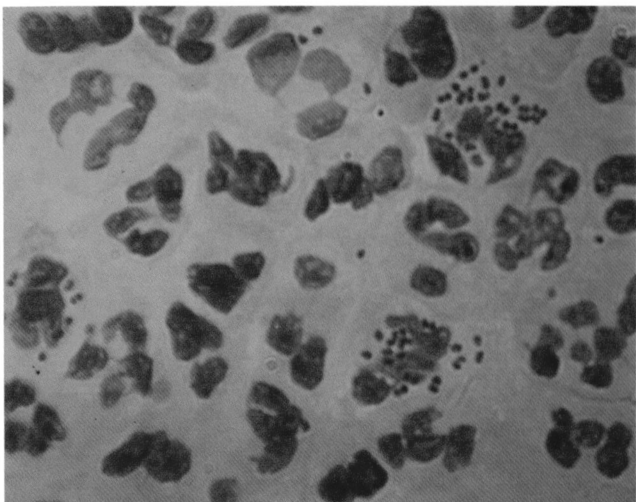

**Plate 91.** Gram stain of gonococcal urethritis, showing large number of Gram-negative intracellular diplococci.

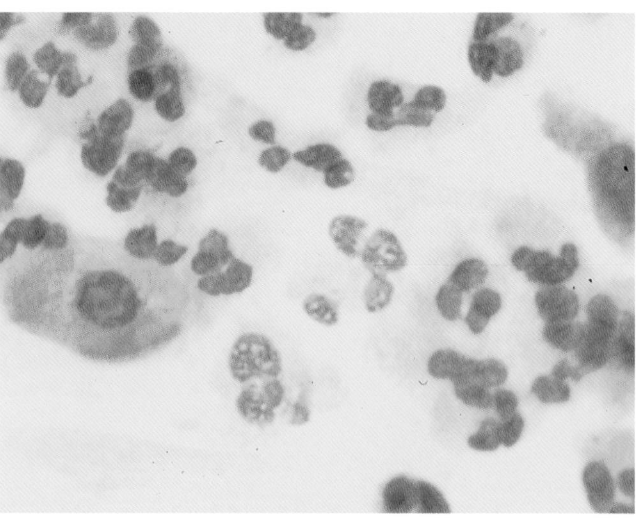

**Plate 92.** Smear from non-gonococcal urethritis. Note the presence of both polymorphonuclear leukocytes and occasional mononuclear leukocytes in the absence of Gram-negative diplococci.

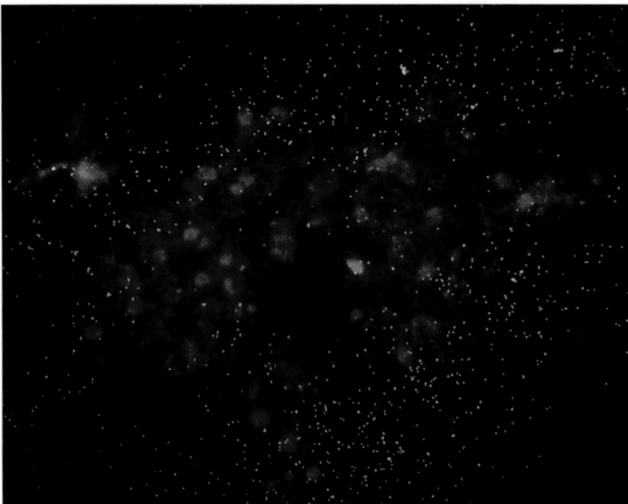

**Plate 93.** *C. trachomatic* elementary bodies visualized in endocervical exudate using fluorescein-conjugated species-specific monoclonal antibodies against *C. trachomatis*.

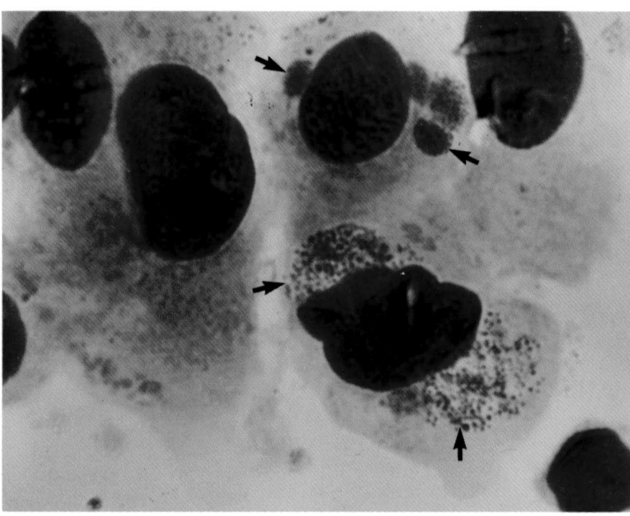

**Plate 94.** Giemsa-stained conjunctival scraping from neonatal inclusion conjunctivitis caused by *C. trachomatis* (arrows indicate chlamydial inclusions).

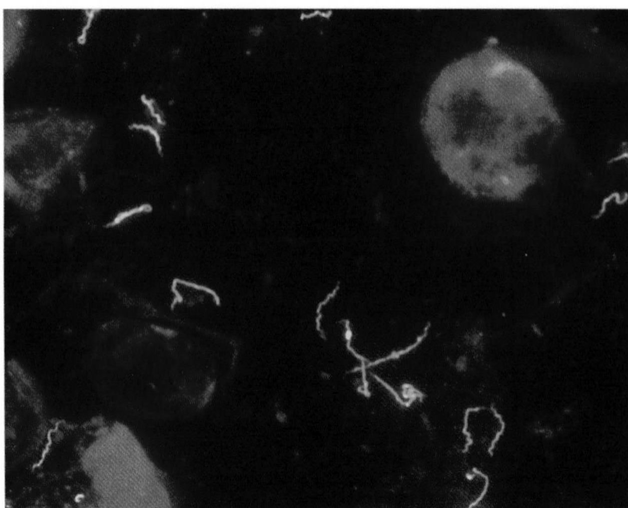

**Plate 95.** *Treponema pallidum* identified on direct smear from primary human chancre using species-specific fluoroscein-conjugated monoclonal antibody to *T. pallidum*.

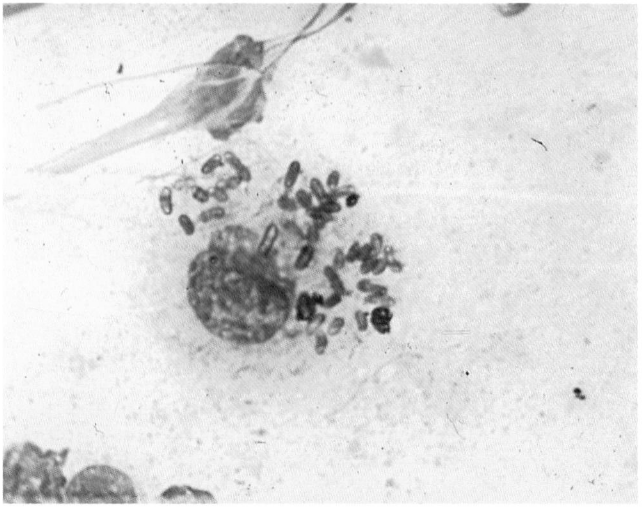

**Plate 96.** Impression smear from a punch biopsy obtained from the margin of a lesion of donovanosis and stained with Wright-Giemsa stain, showing typical donovan bodies.

# PART VI APPROACH TO COMMON CLINICAL SYNDROMES

## Chapter 46

# Lower genital tract infections in women: Cystitis, urethritis, vulvovaginitis, and cervicitis

King K. Holmes

Differences in male and female anatomy and reproductive physiology account for the greater risk of complications of certain STDs in women and also for the greater difficulty in differential diagnosis of urogenital infections in women. In fact, the difficulty in diagnosing sexually transmitted urogenital infections in women undoubtedly results in delay of proper therapy, which further contributes to the higher risk of complications in women and to the further spread of infection in the community.

In heterosexual men, gonococcal and chlamydial infections appear to be limited to the anterior urethra in most cases, though the frequency of extention of infection to the posterior urethra and genital adnexae has not been well studied. Symptoms and signs of urethral discharge are readily recognizable by both the patient and the clinician, and have come to represent the most monotonous aspect of venereology; knowledge of variations on this theme is limited.

On the other hand, in women several STD pathogens, including *Neisseria gonorrhoeae, Chlamydia trachomatis,* and herpes simplex virus (HSV), have predilection for infection of the urethra, cervix, and rectum simultaneously, producing more variable symptom patterns, each with a wide range of differential diagnostic possibilities. Furthermore, infections at any one site can produce symptoms that are poorly localized and are easy to erroneously ascribe to involvement of a contiguous site. For example, infections of the bladder, urethra, or vulva can produce similar symptoms, such as dysuria or dyspareunia, and infections of either the cervix or the vagina can produce abnormal vaginal discharge. Finally, lack of appreciation of the differing clinical signs of specific genital infections in women can often be attributed to inadequate inspection of the genitalia because of poor clinical skills, lack of speculums in many developing countries, or simple reluctance to perform the examination (see Fig. 46-1.) These factors preclude accurate clinical diagnosis, forcing the clinician to rely solely on microbiological diagnosis or history of exposure to STD.

Thus, an extraordinary sense of mystery prevails about urogenital infections in women. The vague terms still used to describe some of them, such as "nonspecific genital infection" and "lower genital tract infection," pose a barrier to accurate clinical diagnosis and therapy and should be abandoned. One of the major thrusts in venereology during the past 25 years has been toward improved detection of gonococcal infection in women. However, there is almost total reliance on contact tracing and "culture screening" to detect and reduce the "female reservoir" of gonorrhea. Because of the expense and limited availability of facilities for isolation of *C. trachomatis* in the past, there has been an unwarranted sense of futility about the prospects for diagnosis of chlamydial infection in women. Uncertainty about the usual etiologies of inflammatory conditions of the urinary tract, vulva, vagina, and cervix in women, the lack of consistent application of available laboratory testing where needed, and the failure to exclude coinfections when analyzing the clinical manifestations of any one particular infection add to the confusion and vagueness concerning classification of urogenital inflammation in women. Clinicians experience further difficulty in differentiating true inflammatory conditions from noninflammatory conditions, including functional, psychosomatic genitourinary complaints.

Although the etiology of certain genitourinary and anorectal inflammatory conditions in women is still not well understood, it is becoming increasingly possible to presumptively identify many common and potentially serious STDs in women on the basis of clinical observations of symptoms and signs, supplemented with selective use of relatively simple screening and confirmatory laboratory tests. More precise diagnosis of urogenital infection in women could make a major contribution to improved control of several important STDs in the community, and should lead to improved management strategies for genital infection in the individual patient. An etiologic classification of urogenital inflammatory syndromes in women is presented in Table 46-1 and each syndrome is further discussed below. Chapter 11 introduces an approach to the anatomy and physical examination of the female genital tract and is a useful background for this chapter. Chapters 43, 45, and 47 discuss the three most common nonviral vaginal infections (trichomoniasis, vulvovaginal candidiasis, and bacterial vaginosis, respectively), which are therefore not covered in detail here.

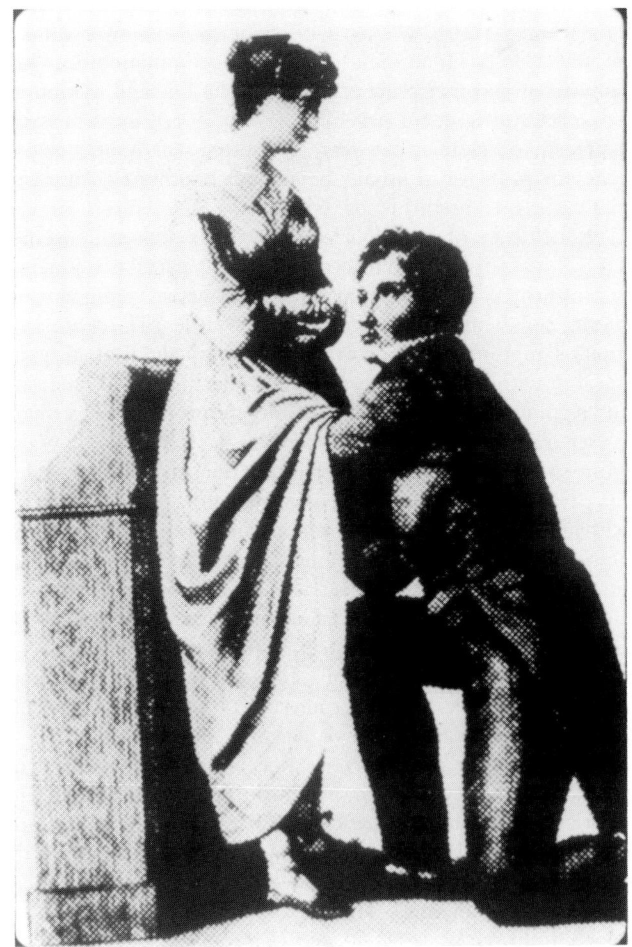

**Fig. 46-1.** Pelvic examination performed by a clinician not trained in sexually transmitted diseases.

**Table 46-1. Etiologic Classification of Lower Urogenital Inflammatory or "Pseudoinflammatory" Conditions in Adult, Premenopausal Women**

| Site involved | Usual microbial etiology | Idiopathic |
|---|---|---|
| Cystitis | Coliform bacteria<br>*Staph. saprophyticus* | Interstitial cystitis |
| Urethritis | *N. gonorrhoeae*<br>*C. trachomatis*<br>HSV | |
| Vulvitis | HSV, ?HPV<br>*C. albicans* | Vulvar papillomatosis<br>Vulvar vestibulitis<br>Essential vulvodynia |
| Vaginitis/ vaginosis | *T. vaginalis*<br>*C. albicans*<br>*G. vaginalis,* mycoplasmas, and anaerobic bacteria | Desquamative inflammatory vaginitis |
| Endocervicitis | *C. trachomatis*<br>*N. gonorrhoeae*<br>HSV | |
| Ectocervicitis | HSV<br>*T. vaginalis*<br>*C. albicans* | |

## CYSTITIS AND URETHRITIS

### EPIDEMIOLOGY AND ETIOLOGY

In the United States, women with symptoms of lower urinary tract infection (UTI) account for more than 5 million office visits to physicians in office practice each year.[1] In England, symptoms of dysuria and frequent urination have occurred in as many as 20 percent of women per year.[2] Symptoms of dysuria or frequency in women can usually be attributed either to acute bacterial cystitis, to urethritis, or to vulvitis.

The incidence of *acute bacterial cystitis* is highest in women 20 to 25 years of age, and this condition is a particularly common cause of urinary symptoms among sexually active young women. Among 263 women presenting to the Seattle STD clinic with urinary symptoms alone, or with both urinary and vaginal symptoms, but without clear signs of vaginal infection, 69 (26 percent) had "significant" bacteriuria ($\geq 10^5$ organisms per ml of urine).[3]

A separate study of female students at the University of Washington showed that the traditional criterion of $\geq 10^5$ uropathogens per ml of urine is insensitive for diagnosis of acute bacterial cystitis in women who present with dysuria and frequency.[4] This criterion was originally established in studies of women with acute pyelonephritis and in surveys of asymptomatic women, who have a low prevalence of bladder infection. However, among students with symptoms of dysuria specimens obtained by suprapubic aspiration or urethral catheterization frequently confirmed the presence of bladder infection, even when urines contained lower concentrations of bacteria, ranging from $10^2$ to $<10^5$ bacteria per ml. It is now accepted that in women with dysuria and frequency, from one-third to one-half of those with bacterial cystitis have "low-count" bacteriuria, with cultures yielding between $10^2$ and $10^5$ organisms per ml of urine.[5] In the two Seattle studies mentioned above, *Escherichia coli* has been the most common cause of symptomatic bacteriuria in young women, followed by *Staphylococcus saprophyticus, Proteus mirabilis, Klebsiella pneumoniae,* and *Enterobacter* sp. *Staph. saprophyticus* accounted for 11 percent of urinary tract infections in college women, and 17 percent in female STD clinic patients. Symptoms and signs of *E. coli* and *Staph. saprophyticus* infections were similar.[6]

The syndrome of dysuria and frequency in women whose urine does not contain $\geq 10^2$ of the above uropathogens has been called the "urethral syndrome" or, in the presence of pyuria, the "dysuria–sterile pyuria syndrome."[7]

Among university women with the urethral syndrome who had sterile bladder urines, the etiology was found to be related to the presence or absence of pyuria. Infection with *C. trachomatis* was demonstrated in 10 of 16 women with pyuria and 1 of 16 women without pyuria ($p = 0.002$).[8] *Pyuria* was defined as less than eight leukocytes per milliliter of uncentrifuged midstream urine, which is approximately equivalent to 10 leukocytes per 400 × microscopic field when 10 ml of urine have been centrifuged and the sediment resuspended in 1 ml of urine for microscopic examination under a cover slip. *N. gonorrhoeae* was not found to be associated with the urethral syndrome in this population of university students.

However, among indigent women attending a hospital emergency room, gonococcal infection was found to be significantly correlated with dysuria, accounting for 8 (61 percent) of 13 cases whose urine samples contained $<10^5$ uropathogens per milliliter.[9] Cultures for *C. trachomatis* were not obtained in that study. *C. trachomatis* is probably the major cause of the urethral syndrome among college students without bladder infection by uropathogens and among female contacts of men with nongonococcal urethritis,[10] whereas both *N. gonorrhoeae* and *C. trachomatis* may be important causes of the urethral syndrome among women who are at higher risk of gonorrhea.[11] HSV infections (especially primary infection), though not commonly found among women with the urethral syndrome, clearly produce urethritis, dysuria, and pyuria in young sexually active women, and can be mistaken for bacterial cystitis if vulvar lesions are not prominent or carefully sought. Dysuria in women who do not have bacteriuria or urethral infection with STD pathogens is often attributable to *vulvar inflammation* caused by genital herpes or by vulvovaginitis. For example, Komaroff et al. reported that in young women, dysuria was attributable to vaginitis more often than to UTI because vaginitis was so much more common than UTI.[12] However, when women were able to localize the dysuria as "internal" (i.e., felt inside the body) or "external" (felt on the vaginal labia as the stream of urine passed), only internal dysuria was correlated with UTI. As noted above, genital herpes can produce urethritis with internal dysuria, as well as vulvar lesions and external dysuria.

### DIAGNOSIS AND THERAPY

The characteristic features which help to differentiate the three major conditions that can result in dysuria in women are summarized in Table 46-2. The medical history, physical examination, and simple laboratory tests are all helpful in the differential diagnosis of dysuria.

An approach to the diagnosis of dysuria in young women is summarized in Fig. 46-2. The first step is to try to determine whether dysuria is internal or external, and to evaluate for vulvovaginitis or endocervicitis. Internal dysuria suggests cystitis or urethritis, while external dysuria suggests periurethral or vulvar inflammation caused by HSV or by *Candida albicans.* Even among those with internal dysuria, speculum examination is indicated to rule out vaginitis or mucopurulent cervicitis. The latter can be caused by the same organisms that cause urethritis and

Table 46-2. Characteristic Features Which Differ in the Three Major Causes of Dysuria in Women

| | Acute bacterial cystitis | Urethritis | Vulvitis |
|---|---|---|---|
| Predisposing factors | Previous cystitis<br>Diaphragm use<br>Onset of symptoms within 24 h after intercourse | New sex partner | History of genital herpes<br>Partner with genital herpes<br>Antibiotic use<br>History of recurrent vulvovaginal candidiasis |
| Symptoms | Internal dysuria<br>Duration of symptoms ≤4 days<br>Frequency and urgency<br>Gross hematuria | Internal dysuria<br>Duration of symptoms often ≥7 days with chlamydial urethritis | External dysuria<br>Vaginal discharge<br>Vulvar irritation, burning, pruritis, or lesions |
| Signs | Suprapubic tenderness | Mucopurulent cervicitis<br>Vulvar lesions | Vulvar lesions<br>Vulvitis<br>Curdlike vaginal exudate |
| Laboratory | Pyuria<br>Microscopic hematuria<br>Rapid nitrite test<br>Urine Gram stain<br>Urine culture | Pyuria<br>Urethral discharge or bartholinitis<br>Endocervical exudate<br>Cervical and urethral tests for *C. trachomatis* and *N. gonorrhoeae*<br>Test lesion for HSV | No pyuria<br>Test lesion for HSV<br>Test vaginal discharge for *C. albicans* |

can thus result in internal dysuria. Urinalysis should be performed in all cases to detect pyuria. For detection of pyuria, as well as for culture, the urine should be a midstream specimen collected by the clean-catch technique. Microscopic examination of unspun urine using a hemocytometer or calibrated chamber is the most sensitive and specific test for the presence or absence of pyuria.[13] Alternatively, leukocytes can be counted after centrifugation of the urine followed by resuspension of the sediment in 1 ml of urine and enumeration of white cells in 1 to 2 drops of urine placed on a microscope slide under a coverslip. This method is slightly less accurate than the first method. Another simple test for pyuria involves the use of a "dipstick" for detection of leukocyte esterase in urine. These dipsticks also often contain a screening test for production of nitrite from nitrate by coliform bacteria. While the sensitivity of the leukocyte esterase test appears to be lower than that of the chamber microscopy method for detection of pyuria, the simplicity and low cost of the test make it useful for screening women with dysuria, and for identifying those whose urine cultures should be carefully examined for "low-count" bacteriuria (i.e., $\geq 10^2$ organisms per ml).[13] Among women with dysuria, pyuria usually is indicative of acute bacterial cystitis in women at low risk for STD and may indicate either cystitis or urethritis in women at high risk for STD. In the STD clinic study discussed above,[3] 40 percent had pyuria. With respect to detecting $\geq 10^5$ organisms per ml of urine in these symptomatic women, pyuria had a sensitivity of 88 percent, specificity of 76 percent, positive predictive value of 61 percent, and negative predictive value of 93 percent. If pyuria is found microscopically or by leukocyte esterase test, urine can be examined microscopically for bacteriuria. Bacteria can be detected microscopically in urine by (1) preparation of a Gram stain of a fresh, midstream, clean-catch, uncentrifuged urine specimen and examination with an oil immersion lens (the presence of one bacterial organism per field is correlated with quantitative isolation of $\geq 10^5$ bacteria per milliliter of urine), or (2) examination of unstained, centrifuged urinary sediment of fresh urine under the high dry objective (detection of 100 organisms per field also correlates well with isolation of $\geq 10^5$ bacteria per milliliter of urine). These procedures are simple and should be available in any clinic or physicians' office. However, bacteria present in concentrations of $<10^5$ per ml of urine are not likely to be seen on Gram stain; hence this is not a sensitive test for bacteriuria. Urine culture is especially indicated for diagnosis in patients with pyuria who have no microscopic evidence of bacteriuria and for identification and susceptibility testing of uropathogens from women with recurrent bacterial cystitis. If the patient has pyuria without bacteriuria and is considered to be at risk for STD, or has signs of mucopurulent endocervicitis, specimens from the endocervix and urethra should be cultured for *N. gonorrhoeae* and, when possible, tested for *C. trachomatis*.

The diagnosis of urethritis due to *C. trachomatis, N. gonorrhoeae*, or HSV rather than the diagnosis of bacterial cystitis is favored by a recent history of acquiring a new sex partner. Genital herpes could be suggested by history of genital herpes, of exposure to a partner with genital herpes, or the presence of genital lesions (which can also result in external dysuria). Symptoms of abnormal vaginal discharge in the woman with internal dysuria suggest gonorrhea, chlamydial infection, or genital herpes. Infection with *N. gonorrhoeae* or *C. trachomatis* is suggested by the presence of expressible urethral discharge (Plate 4), inflammation of Skene's glands (Plate 6), bartholinitis (Plate 5), mucopurulent cervicitis (Plates 15 and 16), or proctitis. Findings which favor cystitis rather than urethritis include a history of previous cystitis, history of onset of symptoms within 24 h after sexual intercourse,[15] prominent frequency or urgency, and history of gross hematuria. Cystitis is also suggested by a history of current diaphragm use, which appears to increase the risk of cystitis in young women, either by obstruction to urine flow or, more likely, by altering the vaginal bacterial flora.[14] Acute onset of severe dysuria leading to consultation within 4 days after onset favors a diagnosis of bacterial cystitis (or perhaps gonococcal urethritis), whereas a history of gradual onset of milder symptoms and long duration of symptoms before seeking therapy (≥7 days) suggests chlamydial urethritis.[8] Suprapubic tenderness and microscopic hematuria are also highly suggestive of cystitis in the acutely dysuric patient.[8]

External dysuria due to vulvitis can be produced by genital herpes or by vulvovaginal candidiasis. Perhaps less common conditions discussed in Chapters 59 and 60 can also produce this symptom. In a recent study of trichomoniasis, no significant cor-

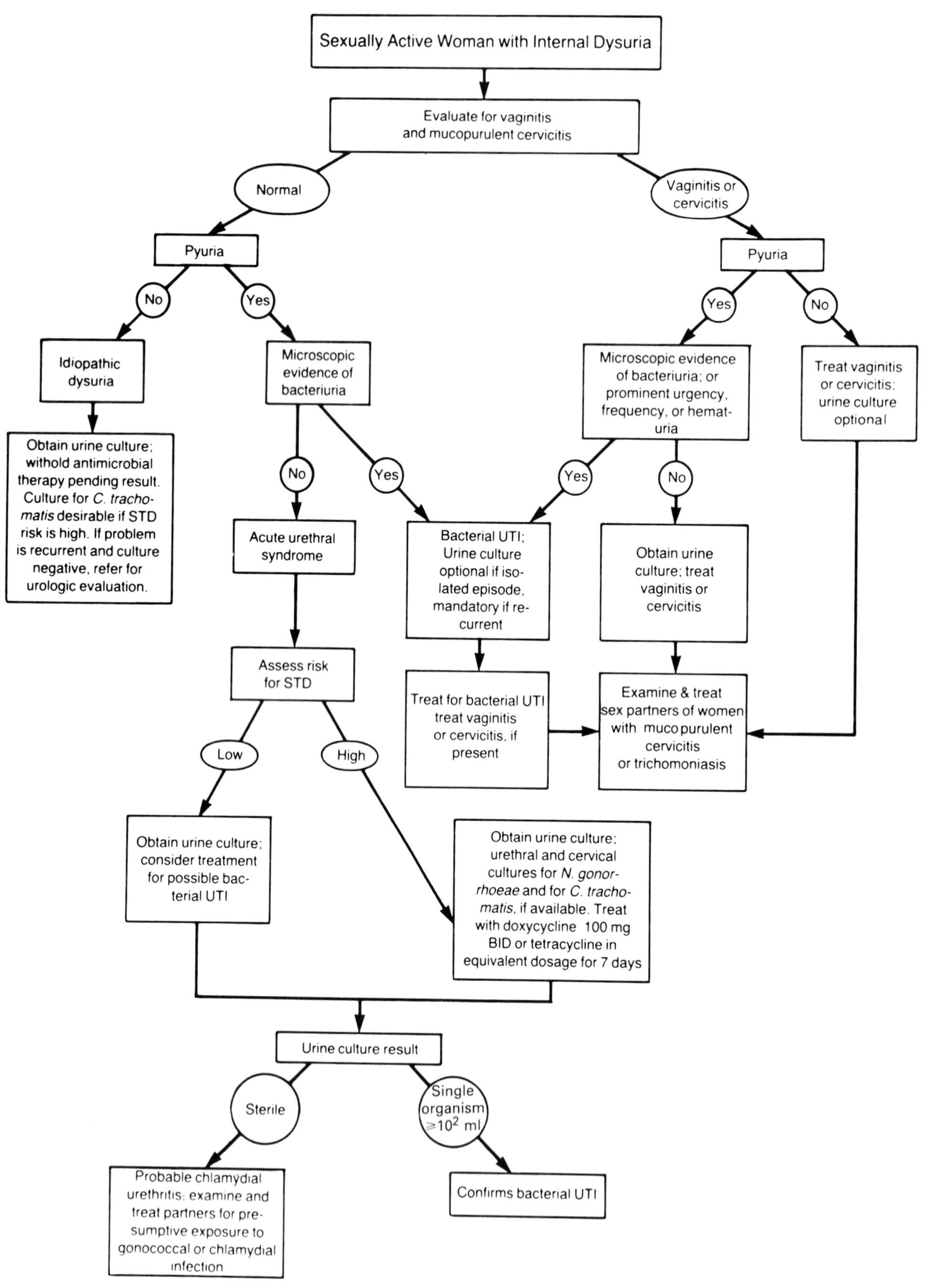


**Fig. 46-2.** Algorithm for management of sexually active woman with dysuria. For definition of pyuria, microscopic bacteriuria, and assessment of risk of STD, see text.

relation was found with dysuria or frequency, after adjustment for coinfections.[16] The patient with external dysuria should be questioned about history of genital herpes or exposure to herpes, or about risk factors for vulvovaginal candidiasis, such as recent antibiotic use.

Women with microscopic evidence of bacteriuria or with clinical findings suggestive of uncomplicated bacterial cystitis should be treated with short courses (preferably 3 days) of antimicrobial therapy, unless the temperature exceeds 101°F, symptoms have been present for longer than 1 week, or there is costovertebral angle pain or tenderness, which suggest the presence of pyelonephritis. A high proportion of coliform isolates from urine are resistant to sulfonamides, ampicillin, tetracyclines, and first-generation cephalosporins. These organisms, as well as *Staph. saprophyticus,* are generally susceptible to sulfamethoxazole-trimethoprim, trimethoprim alone, nitrofurantoin, the new quinolones, or amoxicillin-clavulanic acid. Fihn and colleagues[17] recently compared a single dose of trimethoprim (320 mg) plus sulfamethoxazole (1600 mg) with a 10-day course of trimethoprim (160 mg) plus sulfamethoxazole (800 mg) twice daily, for treatment of acute dysuria in 255 college women. Of these women, 216 (85 percent) had bacteriuria with $\geq 10^2$ organisms per ml of urine; 12 (5 percent) had *C. trachomatis* infection (of whom half also had bacteriuria); and 52 were considered to have vulvovaginal candidiasis (most of whom also had bacteriuria); 2 had genital herpes; one had gonorrhea; and none had trichomoniasis. There was no significant difference in the rate of resolution of symptoms with these two treatments. Thirteen days after the start of treatment, cure rates for those with acute bacterial cystitis were 76 percent in the single-dose group compared with 95 percent in the 10-day group ($p < 0.001$). However, at 6 weeks follow-up, cure rates were more similar (68 percent vs. 79 percent $p = 0.07$). Clinically important side effects were significantly more common with 10-day treatment (25 percent) than with single-dose treatment (12 percent). The authors suggested the need for evaluation of treatments of intermediate duration (e.g., 3 days) which might prove optimal. Women suspected of having urethritis due to chlamydia (because of pyuria without microscopic evidence of bacteriuria, together with other compatible clinical or epidemiological findings) should be treated with a tetracycline regimen such as 100 mg doxycycline twice daily for 1 week, while urine cultures are pending. This regimen was significantly more effective than placebo in curing symptoms of the urethral syndrome in women with pyuria[18] and would also be adequate in many bladder infections caused by common uropathogens. Male sex partners of women with suspected or confirmed gonococcal or chlamydial urethritis should be examined, and tested to exclude urethral infection, or should be treated for exposure to these agents (see Chaps. 14 and 16).

## VAGINAL INFECTIONS

### AGE-DEPENDENT DIFFERENCES IN VAGINAL ANATOMY, PHYSIOLOGY, AND FLORA

The normal anatomy, physiology, and microbial ecology of the vagina are age-dependent,[19] and there are also obvious age-dependent differences in the source of vaginal infections. These factors account for very different etiologies of vaginitis in neonates, infants and toddlers, prepubertal girls, and pre- and postmenopausal adults.

During the first month of life, the neonatal vagina, still under the influence of maternal estrogen, is lined by stratified squamous epithelium. From about 1 month of age until puberty, the vagina is lined by cuboidal cells, and the pH of vaginal fluid is normally about 7.0. After puberty, under the influence of estrogen, the vagina is lined by stratified squamous epithelium containing glycogen (Fig. 46-3). With growth of facultative $H_2O_2$-producing species of lactobacillus, such as *Lactobacillus acidophilus* and *Lactobacillus jenseni* to concentrations of approximately $10^9$ per ml of vaginal fluid, lactic acid is produced from glycogen, and the pH falls to 4.5, usually between 4.0 and 4.5, in normal adult women. The fall in pH, as well as the $H_2O_2$, are considered important in regulating the vaginal flora.[20] The oxidation-reduction potential (Eh) at the surface of the vaginal epithelium is approximately $0 \pm 50$ mV[21] in the absence of bacterial vaginosis, but is much lower in bacterial vaginosis.

The relative concentration of vaginal microbes has not been extensively characterized in neonates, infants, or prepubertal girls, but the facultative flora most often includes diphtheroids, *Staph. epidermidis*, γ-hemolytic streptococci, lactobacilli, and coliforms.[22,23] Coliforms are more common in the vagina before puberty (especially among toddlers still in diapers) than after puberty, whereas the reverse is true for lactobacilli which dominate the vaginal flora of normal postpubertal women.[20]

## VAGINITIS IN PREMENARCHAL GIRLS

The neonatal vaginal squamous epithelium is resistant to perinatally transmitted *N. gonorrhoeae* and *C. trachomatis* but is susceptible to perinatally transmitted vaginal candidiasis. Among older infants, the cuboidal vaginal epithelium is susceptible to *N. gonorrhoeae* and *C. trachomatis* but is resistant to candidiasis. Vaginal shedding of *C. trachomatis* does indeed sometimes appear after about 1 month of age in infants who were exposed perinatally but is not generally associated with overt signs of vaginitis in young infants. Vaginal infection by *N. gonorrhoeae* is rare among infants, and with few exceptions[24] it is thought to represent postnatal acquisition.

Among older premenarcheal girls, the etiology of vaginal symptoms is correlated with puberty status and with the presence or absence of objective signs of abnormal vaginal discharge. For example, in a study of 54 premenarcheal patients with suspected vaginitis and 52 age-matched controls,[25] a microbial pathogen was isolated from the vagina from 14 of 26 with abnormal vaginal discharge, zero of 26 with suspected vaginitis who had no vaginal discharge, and zero of 52 control subjects (Table 46-3). *N. gonorrhoeae* accounted for one-third of abnormal discharges in prepubertal girls, while *C. albicans* or "yeast" was isolated only from those premenarcheal girls who were considered to be pubertal (Tanner stages II, III, or IV) on the basis of breast growth.

*Streptococcus pyogenes* (group A β-hemolytic streptococci) and *Shigella sp.* are also recognized as causes of purulent or bloody vaginal discharge in prepubertal girls.[26–29] Any species of *Shigella* may cause vaginitis in children, but *Shigella flexneri* has been most often implicated and represented a significantly higher proportion of isolates from the vagina than from all other sites in one retrospective study.[28] Shigella vaginitis is often chronic, causes a bloody vaginal discharge in about 50 percent of recognized cases, and is associated with diarrhea in only about one-quarter of cases. The predilection of shigella for prepubertal

**Table 46-3. Pathogens Isolated from Vaginal Cultures from 52 Premenarcheal Girls with Suspected Vaginitis and 52 Age-Matched Controls**

| | Prepubertal | | Pubertal | | |
|---|---|---|---|---|---|
| Pathogens isolated | Discharge present (N = 12) | Discharge absent (N = 24) | Discharge present (N = 14) | Discharge absent (N = 2) | Control subjects (N = 52) |
| *Strep. pyogenes* | 0 | 0 | 1 | 0 | 0 |
| *N. gonorrhoeae* | 4 | 0 | 0 | 0 | 0 |
| *Shigella sonnei* | 1 | 0 | 0 | 0 | 0 |
| *C. albicans* or "yeast" | 0 | 0 | 8 | 0 | 0 |
| *C. trachomatis** | 0 | 0 | 0 | 0 | 0 |

*Specimens from 27 of 36 prepubertal girls with suspected vaginitis were cultured for *C. trachomatis.*
SOURCE: Paradise et al.[25]

rather than adult vaginitis may be partly attributable to poor survival of this organism below a pH of 5.5.

The etiologic roles of group B *Haemophilus influenzae* and coagulase-positive staphylococci in prepubertal vaginitis are controversial. As indicated in Table 46-3, no specific bacterial pathogen is found in a large proportion of prepubertal girls with abnormal vaginal discharge. However, intravaginal foreign body and poor perineal hygiene are among the leading predisposing factors in young girls, and *Enterobius vermicularis* (pinworm) is an acknowledged cause of vulvovaginitis. Although *C. trachomatis* has not been implicated as a common cause of prepubertal vaginitis, this agent was isolated from the vagina from about one-quarter of girls with gonococcal vaginitis and appeared to be responsible for postgonococcal vaginitis following penicillin treatment in such cases.[30] The occurrence of *C. trachomatis* infection in prepubertal sexually abused girls has been documented in several studies and is reviewed elsewhere.[31]

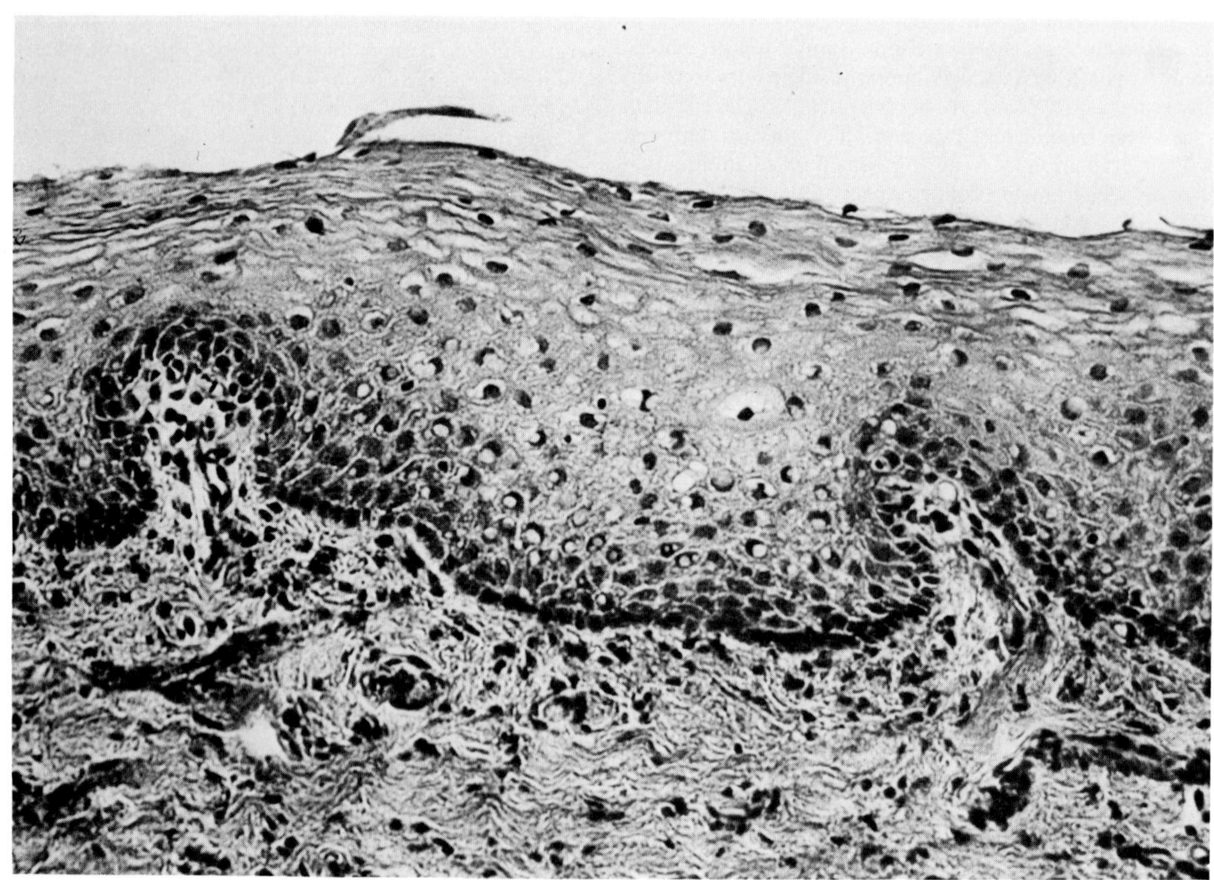

**Fig. 46-3.** Normal adult vaginal epithelium, showing the basal cell layer with overlying stratum spinosum. Note the absence of an overlying stratum corneum. The transit time for cells moving from the basal layer to the superficial surface of the vaginal epithelium has been estimated to be about 4 days, perhaps one-third that of normal epidermis.

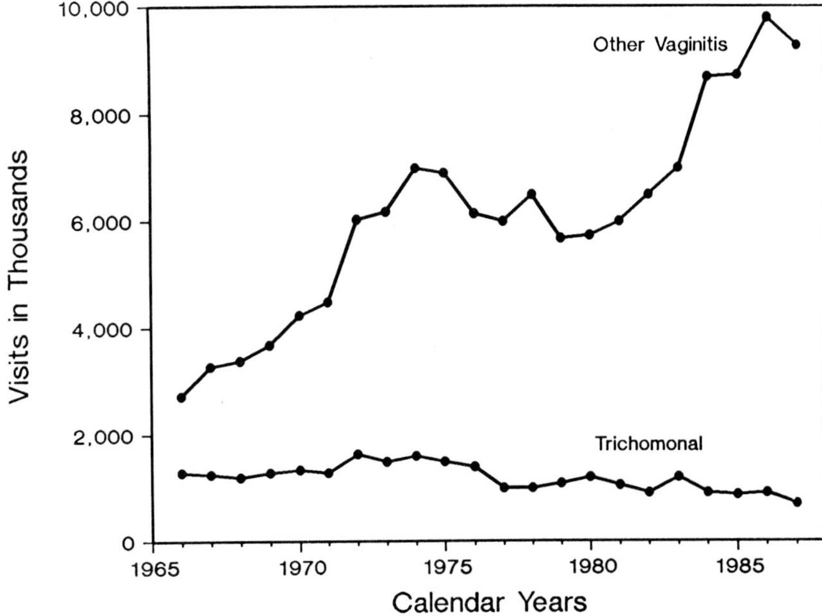


**Fig. 46-4.** Trends in number of office visits to physicians in private practices for trichomonal vaginitis and for "other vaginitis" (presumably including bacterial vaginosis), United States, 1966–1987. *(IMS, America.)*

## VAGINAL INFECTIONS IN ADULT WOMEN

Vaginal infections in adult women are among the most common problems in clinical medicine, being found in 28 percent of women attending STD clinics in one survey[32] and in an even higher percentage of women who were systematically examined for such infections in our own STD clinics (discussed below). Vaginal discharge is among the 25 most common reasons for consulting physicians in private office practice in the United States.[33] The three most common types of vaginal infections in adult women are vulvovaginal candidiasis, trichomoniasis, and bacterial vaginosis. These are discussed in Chaps. 43, 45, and 47. A possibly related syndrome, puerperal vaginal atrophy with dyspareunia, occurs postpartum in relation to the duration of breast-feeding, and is sometimes treated with topical estrogen.

In the United States, the number of visits to private physicians' offices for trichomonal vaginitis declined slowly from 1966 to 1987, but visits for other conditions classified as "vaginitis" (presumably including bacterial vaginosis, which does not appear to be associated with true vaginitis) increased from less than 3 million per year to nearly 10 million per year during the same period (Fig. 46-4). Vulvovaginal papilloma virus infections are discussed in Chapters 37 and 38.

Other types of vaginitis in adults include a destructive type of *ulcerative vaginitis* currently attributed to a toxin produced by *Staph. aureus* in women with toxic shock syndrome,[34,35] vaginal ulceration associated with use of vaginal tampons[36,37] or cervical caps, infections associated with other intravaginal foreign bodies, and miscellaneous uncommon vaginal infections.

In postmenopausal women, vaginal symptoms are very prevalent, and the usual forms of vaginal infection need to be considered and differentiated from vaginal atrophy.[38,39] The vaginal epithelium becomes thin with estrogen withdrawal, lubrication occurs less often with sexual arousal, the introitus narrows, and the depth of the vagina decreases. These atrophic changes have been found to be negatively correlated with frequency of intercourse and with circulating concentrations of gonadotrophins and androgens in postmenopausal women.[40]

A number of other perplexing, chronic vulvovaginal syndromes tend to involve women older than those most often affected by STD. These have been termed desquamative inflammatory vaginitis (also known as "erosive vaginal lichen planus"); vulvar vestibulitis; purulent vaginitis (not attributable to trichomoniasis or candidiasis); recurrent bacterial vaginitis; and essential vulvodynia. Since the etiology of these syndromes remains unknown, treatment is empiric, and should be as conservative as possible.

## CERVICITIS

Two types of cervicitis can be distinguished—*endocervicitis* (also known as *mucopurulent cervicitis*) and *ectocervicitis*. Causes of endocervicitis include *C. trachomatis*, *N. gonorrhoeae*, and herpes simplex virus. HSV infection can also be associated with ectocervicitis, and will be discussed separately below.

**Endocervicitis.** Urethritis in men represents the tip of the iceberg of infections caused by *C. trachomatis* and *N. gonorrhoeae*. Endocervicitis, together with subclinical urethral infections in both sexes, represents the portion of the iceberg which is largely unrecognized today. At present, control of these infections unfortunately is based largely on the clinical diagnosis of urethritis in the male and on treatment of the female sex partners of men with urethritis. This is particularly so in developing countries, where specific laboratory tests for *N. gonorrhoeae* and *C. trachomatis* are not widely available. Because endocervicitis produces symptoms less often than male urethritis, and symptoms of endocervicitis (e.g., vaginal discharge) are less distinctive than symptoms of urethritis, the careful assessment of clinical signs of mucopurulent cervicitis, and the appropriate use of laboratory tests for detection of subclinical infection of the female, are of paramount importance in the control of gonococcal and chlamydial infections.

Infection of the cervix represents a reservoir for sexual or perinatal transmission of pathogenic microorganisms, and might

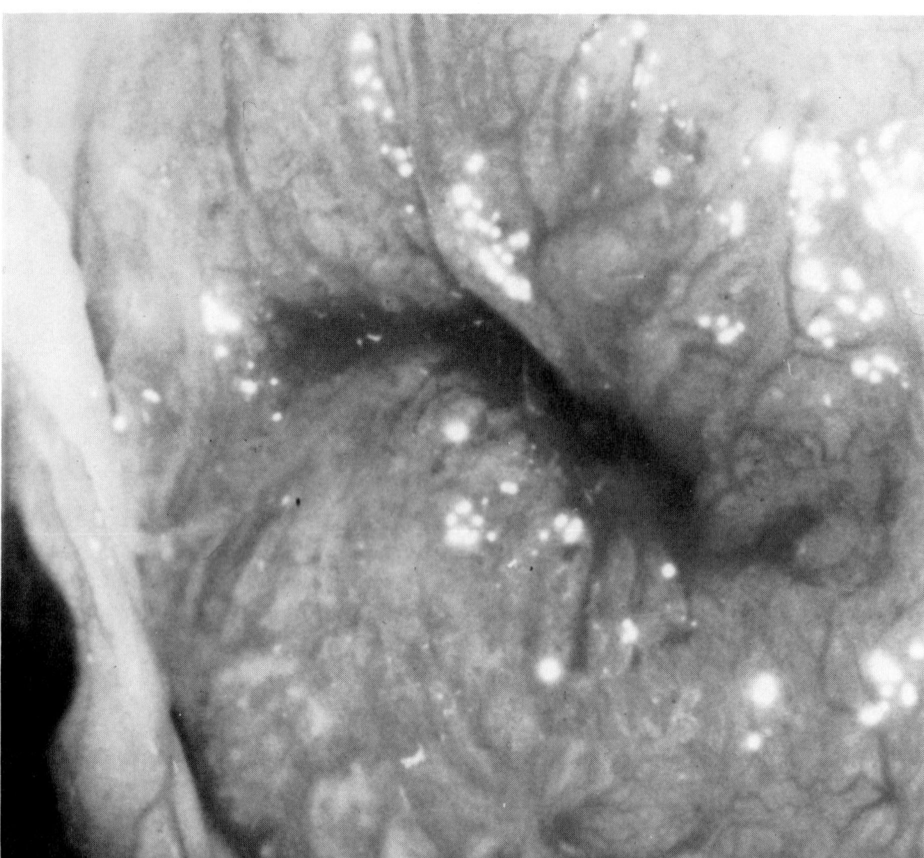

**Fig. 46-5.** Colpophotograph of the cervix infected with *C. trachomatis,* showing proliferation and dilation of subepithelial capillaries in the zone of ectopy.

lead to at least two possible types of complications in the female: (1) ascending intralumenal spread of pathogenic organisms from the cervix, producing endometritis and salpingitis; (2) ascending infection during pregnancy, resulting in chorioamnionitis, premature rupture of membranes, premature delivery, amniotic fluid infection, and puerperal infection.

The lack of widely recognized objective signs of cervical inflammation is illustrated by the confusing nomenclature for endocervicitis. Terms such as acute and chronic cervicitis, cervical erosion, cervical discontinuity, mucopurulent cervicitis, papillary cervicitis, follicular cervicitis, and hypertrophic cervicitis have all been used. This confusion results in part from the changes which occur in the cervix over the reproductive period and during the menstrual cycle[41–43] and in part from difficulty in differentiating normal ectopic columnar epithelium from endocervicitis. The latter differentiation is complicated by the fact that cervical ectopy (Plate 13) appears to be correlated with cervical infection by *C. trachomatis.*[44–46] Ectopy is present in the majority of younger teenage girls, and decreases steadily in prevalence with increasing age. Further, ectopy is significantly positively correlated with oral contraceptive use, independent of age (P Wolner-Hanssen, KK Holmes, unpublished data).

In this chapter, the term *mucopurulent endocervical discharge* (or *endocervical mucopus*)will be used to refer to yellow endocervical exudate or ≥30 neutrophils per 400 × microscopic field in endocervical mucus as demonstrated by Gram's stain (see below); *mucopurulent cervicitis* will refer to the appearance of the inflamed endocervix on physical examination—optimally by colposcopy—with manifestations such as yellow endocervical discharge, edema, and erythema of the zone of ectopy, and easily induced endocervical bleeding; and *endocervicitis* will refer to histopathologic features of endocervical inflammation.

**Definition and Etiology of Mucopurulent Cervicitis.** Rees et al. were particularly instrumental in establishing the relationship of *C. trachomatis* to cervicitis.[47] To further evaluate objective criteria for the clinical diagnosis of mucopurulent cervicitis, we studied 100 randomly selected women attending an STD clinic in Seattle for the correlation of selected cervical abnormalities with isolation of *C. trachomatis*, *N. gonorrhoeae*, and HSV.[48] The presence of yellow endocervical exudate, confirmed by the simple identification of yellow exudate on a white cotton-tipped swab specimen of endocervical secretions, correlated only with isolation of *C. trachomatis.* Mucopurulent secretions were present in 62 percent of women with cervical chlamydial infection and 12 percent of women with no cervical pathogen. Bleeding produced by collection of culture specimens from the endocervix, erythema (due to increased vascularity—see Fig. 46-5), and edema of the area of ectopy were also more common among women with *C. trachomatis* infection. Examples of some of these findings are shown in Plates 15 and 16. Microscopic detection of increased numbers of neutrophils demonstrated by Gram stain within strands of endocervical mucus, collected after first removing ectocervical vaginal cells with a large swab, and examined as described below, was also correlated with isolation of *C. trachomatis* (see Fig. 46-6 and 46-7).

In a more recent study of a larger series of women attending an STD clinic, we have found that the presence of yellow mucopus collected from the endocervix and visualized on a white

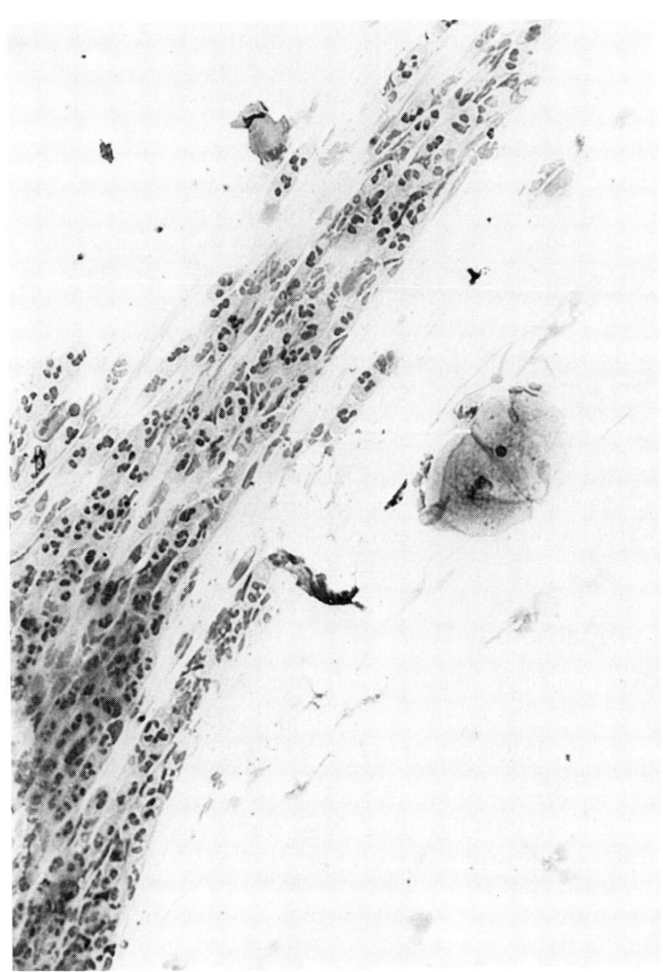

**Fig. 46-6.** Satisfactory smear of endocervical mucus from chlamydial mucopurulent cervicitis, showing many neutrophils in strands of mucus, with few contaminating vaginal squamous cells or bacteria.

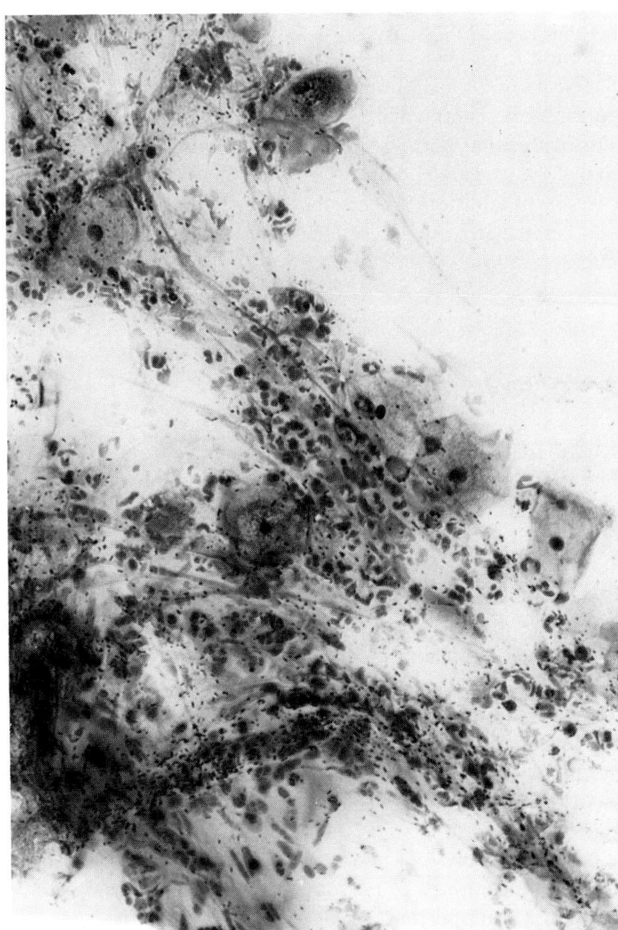

**Fig. 46-7.** Unsatisfactory smear of cervical mucus. Although moderate numbers of neutrophils are seen, the presence of many vaginal squamous cells and bacteria makes it difficult to tell whether the neutrophils originate in the cervix or the vagina.

swab was independently correlated both with chlamydial and with gonococcal infection of the endocervix (KK Holmes, unpublished data). In our initial study, chlamydial infection was best correlated with ≥10 neutrophils per 1000× microscopic field in endocervical mucus. In the more recent study, a cutoff of ≥30 neutrophils per 1000× field was better correlated with gonococcal or chlamydial infection. In a separate study of women attending family planning clinics, Handsfield et al. found that cervical chlamydial infection was correlated both with mucopurulent discharge and with easily induced cervical bleeding.[49] Histopathologic manifestations of endocervicitis are discussed below.

During 1987, the diagnosis of mucopurulent cervicitis was made by various clinicians in only 691 (18 percent) of 3825 women visiting the Seattle STD clinic, while during the same period, nongonococcal urethritis was identified in 1974 (30 percent) of 6608 heterosexual men visiting the clinic. Among a random sample of 773 women from the Seattle STD clinic who were carefully examined during 1984–1986 by a single clinician, the prevalence of mucopurulent cervical discharge, defined by the presence of yellow endocervical exudate, was 26 percent. *N. gonorrhoeae* or *C. trachomatis* was isolated from 45 percent of those with mucopurulent cervical discharge vs. 14 percent of those without it. Thus, with respect to isolation of *C. trachomatis* or *N. gonorrhoeae* in this population, the sensitivity of detecting mucopurulent cervical discharge was 54 percent, specificity 82 percent, positive predictive value 45 percent, and negative predictive value 86 percent. Among those without mucopurulent cervical discharge, additional findings of easily induced bleeding, edema or erythema of the zone of ectopy, or ≥30 neutrophils per 1000× field did not correlate well with chlamydial or gonococcal infection. Although mucopurulent cervicitis has been significantly correlated with endocervical infection in most if not all studies, the sensitivity, specificity, and predictive value have varied in different settings.[50–52] It is difficult to assess to what extent the variability is attributable to differences in patients, to differences in assessing mucopurulent cervicitis, or to differences in detection of *C. trachomatis*. Our experience suggest that correlation of isolation of *C. trachomatis* or *N. gonorrhoeae* from the cervix with detection of purulent (yellow) endocervical discharge by an inexperienced clinician is initially low (in which case identification of increased numbers of neutrophils in cervical mucus by an experienced laboratory technician is more reliable); but with training and experience, the correlation improves. It is likely that as experience with chlamydia diagnosis grows, skill in diagnosis of mucopurulent cervicitis will also increase. Nonetheless, we have also found that among university women undergoing routine annual examination, detection of purulent (yellow) endocervical exudate is not sensitive for screening for chlamydial infection.

The cause of mucopurulent cervicitis in the absence of proved gonococcal, chlamydial, or HSV infection remains uncertain. Various genital pathogens have been implicated, and it is likely that false negative cultures for chlamydia account for some cases.[53] In addition, it seems possible that oral contraceptive use and cervical ectopy per se may be associated with endocervical inflammation.[53]

## ECTOCERVICITIS

Routine colposcopic examination of female STD clinic patients has shown that cervical HSV infection is highly correlated with cervical ulcers or necrotic lesions, while trichomoniasis is correlated with colpitis macularis ("strawberry cervix"), and both *C. trachomatis* and cytomegalovirus infection of the cervix are correlated with colposcopic features of immature metaplasia.[54] Immature metaplasia was defined as faint acetowhite epithelium (white after application of acetic acid) with diffuse distal borders, occurring as fingerlike projections within the transformation zone, at the central margin of a squamocolumnar junction advancing centrally into the zone of ectopy. In a further analysis, colpitis macularis (Plate 20) was identified without magnification in only 2 (2 percent) of 108 women with trichomoniasis but was seen by colposcopy in 49 (45 percent) of the 108 with trichomoniasis vs. only 6 (1 percent) of 509 without trichomoniasis.[16] Cervical ulcerations or necrotic lesions were detected by colposcopy in 22 (65 percent) of 34 women with positive cervical cultures for HSV, and 11 (1.5 percent) of 745 with negative cultures for HSV (L Koutsky, unpublished data). *C. albicans*, like *T. vaginalis*, also can produce ectocervicitis, but both are associated with other manifestations of inflammation of the contiguous stratified squamous vaginal epithelium (Plates 19, 21).

## SPECIAL DIAGNOSTIC PROCEDURES

The presence of cervicitis can be confirmed by a variety of supplementary diagnostic procedures, most of which should be available to clinicians specializing in treatment of genital infections of women. These include Gram's stain of endocervical mucus, cervical cytology, colposcopy, and cervical biopsy. The microbial etiology of cervicitis can be presumptively established by Gram's stain of endocervical mucus and further substantiated by isolation of *C. trachomatis*, *N. gonorrhoeae*, or HSV or by detection of specific microbial antigens, for example, by direct immunofluorescence.

### Endocervical Gram's stain

Just as sputum is difficult to evaluate microscopically when contaminated by oropharyngeal cells and flora, the endocervical mucus is difficult to evaluate microscopically when contaminated by vaginal cells and flora. The ectocervix should therefore be wiped clean with a large swab before endocervical mucus is obtained for microscopy. Mucus is then obtained from the endocervical canal, rolled in a thin film over a slide, heat-fixed, and stained with Gram's stain. The slide is screened at low magnification ($\times$ 100) to identify strands of cervical mucus, to evaluate the extent of contamination by vaginal squamous cells, and to select representative areas of cervical mucus for examination with the oil immersion lens. The number of neutrophils per $\times$ 1000 field should then be counted in several representative fields. The presence of $\geq$ 30 per $\times$ 1000 field in mucus supports the diagnosis of cervicitis, unless heavy contamination by vaginal squamous cells (e.g., $>$ 100 squamous cells per slide) and vaginal flora (e.g., $>$100 bacteria per $\times$ 1000 field overlying cervical mucus) suggest that the neutrophils may have originated in the vagina rather than in the endocervix. Contamination of the specimen with vaginal flora can also obfuscate the detection of gonococci in endocervical mucus by Gram's stain. As discussed elsewhere, detection of gram-negative diplococci within neutrophils in properly collected endocervical mucus is highly specific, but gonococci can be identified by Gram's stain in only about 50 to 60 percent of women with cervical gonococcal infection.

### Cytopathology

Over 25 million cervical Pap smears are performed by physicians in private office practices in the United States each year for detection of cervical neoplasia. There is growing interest in the use of cervical cytological screening to identify women with cervicitis who require further microbiological studies.

The correlation of cervical intraepithelial neoplasia with human papilloma virus infection is described in Chap. 48. Cytological studies in STD clinic patients and in pregnant women have shown that *C. trachomatis* infection is significantly correlated with certain other epithelial cell changes and inflammatory cell patterns.[55] The epithelial cell changes include so-called reactive changes of metaplastic cells and endocervical cells. Inflammatory changes which are significantly correlated with *C. trachomatis* infection include the presence of transformed lymphocytes and of increased numbers of histiocytes and plasma cells, as well as increased numbers of neutrophils. Large, inclusion-containing vacuoles in endocervical and metaplastic cells also are correlated with *C. trachomatis* infection, but they are relatively nonspecific and are not present in the majority of women with chlamydial infection. Pap smears showing inflammation could be further tested by direct immunofluoroscence with fluorescein-conjugated monoclonal antibodies to identify specific cervical pathogens, as discussed below.[56] Use of cytopathology to identify cervical inflammation in addition to cervical neoplasia, represents an important approach to control of *C. trachomatis* infections in the future.

### Colposcopy and cervicography

Colposcopy has been increasingly used to evaluate women who have cervical cytological smears consistent with cervical intraepithelial neoplasia, and to obtain directed biopsies of colposcopically visible lesions. Cervicography (photographing the cervix with greater depth of field than seen with colposcopy) provides a permanent photographic record of cervical lesions.[57] Colposcopy and cervicography have potential utility for use in high-risk patients (e.g., in STD clinics), for screening examinations for cervical dysplasia,[58] and for cervical infection.[54] Colposcopic features of papillomavirus infection and of dysplasia are described in Chap. 48. Colposcopic features of mucopurulent cervicitis are described above and are illustrated in Plates 14 to 16, 19, and 20 and in Fig. 46-5. The sensitivity, specificity, and predictive value of colposcopy and cervicography as screening tests for dysplasia and cervical infection require further study in various clinical settings.

## Histopathology

In patients with endocervicitis due to *C. trachomatis*, cervical biopsy may show intraepithelial inclusions, which are located in columnar or metaplastic cells. Such inclusions are best demonstrated by immunofluorescence or immunoperoxidase staining (Fig. 46-8). By electron microscopy with special stains (Figs. 46-9 and 46-10), these can be shown to contain typical elementary and reticulate bodies of *C. trachomatis*. Inflammation surrounds endocervical glands in a patchy distribution, and lymphoid follicles, containing germinal center cells (transformed lymphocytes) can be identified in about two-thirds of patients (Fig. 46-11). The majority of cervical biopsy specimens from patients with chlamydia-positive endocervicitis show superficial focal endocervical microulcerations, reactive endocervical cellular changes, stromal and epithelial cellular edema, dilatation and proliferation of subepithelial capillaries, and stromal inflammatory infiltration, predominantly by plasma cells. These changes resemble those described in ocular trachoma.

There is surprisingly little recent information on the histopathology of cervical infection with *N. gonorrhoeae* or of initial and recurrent episodes of HSV cervicitis. We have observed that HSV infections differ from chlamydial and gonococcal infections in showing deep, necrotic ulceration with stromal infiltration predominantly by lymphocytes; whereas chlamydial cervicitis differs from gonococcal or HSV cervicitis in showing germinal centers and stromal infiltration predominantly by plasma cells (N Kiviat, unpublished data).

## Confirmatory microbiological studies

To provide a guide to therapy, patient counseling, and management of sex partners, a specific microbiological diagnosis is desirable in patients with cervicitis. This can be accomplished by isolation of *N. gonorrhoeae*, *C. trachomatis*, or HSV, or by immunologic detection of microbial antigens. A Gram stain of endocervical mucus should be performed in all patients with suspected cervicitis, for detection of gram-negative diplococci associated with neutrophils, as well as for quantitation of neutrophils. However, even if gonococci are identified by Gram stain, a culture for *N. gonorrhoeae* should also be performed in most settings to permit testing for beta-lactamase production. A confirmatory test for *C. trachomatis* is also desirable in women with mucopurulent cervicitis, even if gonococcal infection is found, since about one-third of women with gonorrhea had coexisting *C. trachomatis* infection, and the proportion is highest in the presence of endocervicitis. Handsfield et al.[49] found that in family planning clinics, where 9 percent of women had chlamydial infection, 90 percent of infections could be identified by obtaining cervical cultures from women with any two of the following five findings: age $\leq$24 years, new sex partner within 2 months, mucopurulent endocervical discharge, easily induced endocervi-

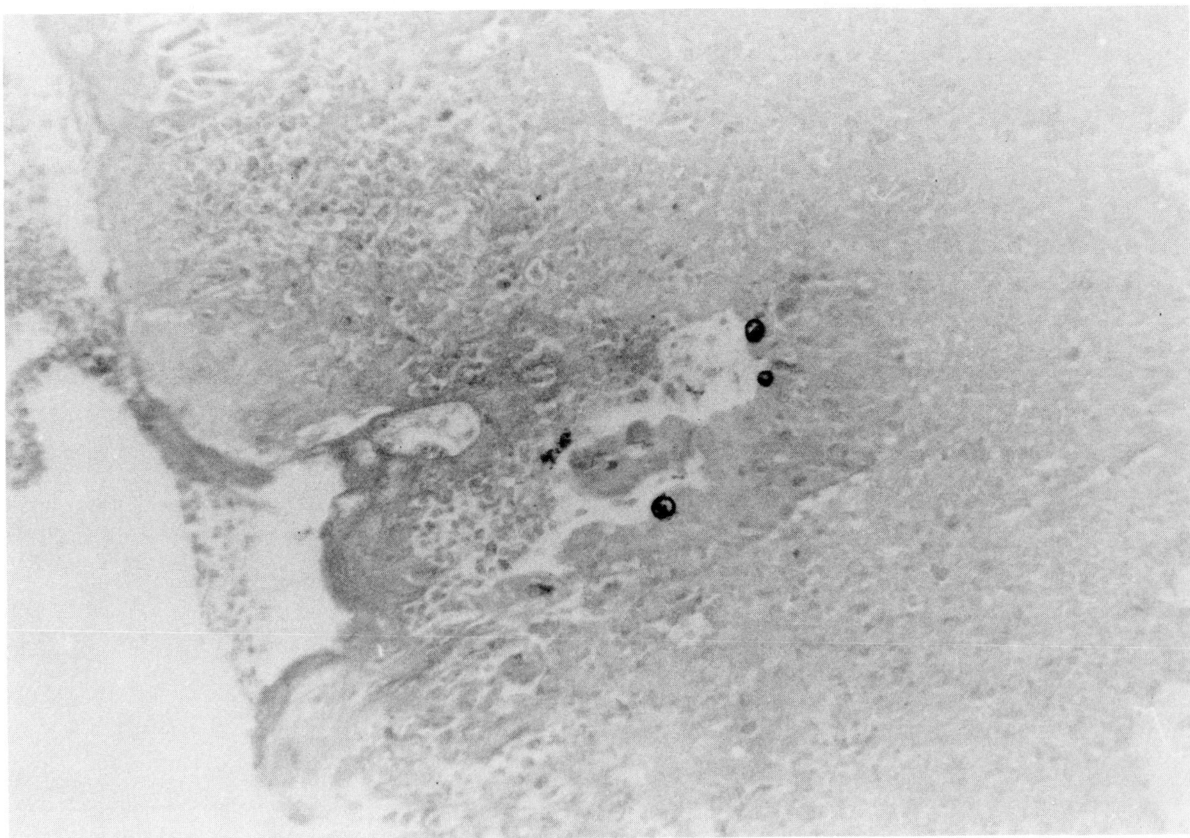

**Fig. 46-8.** Immunoperoxidase stain of a cervical biopsy specimen using monoclonal antibodies to *C. trachomatis* showing cervical intraepithelial chlamydial inclusions. *(Courtesy of N Kiviat.)*

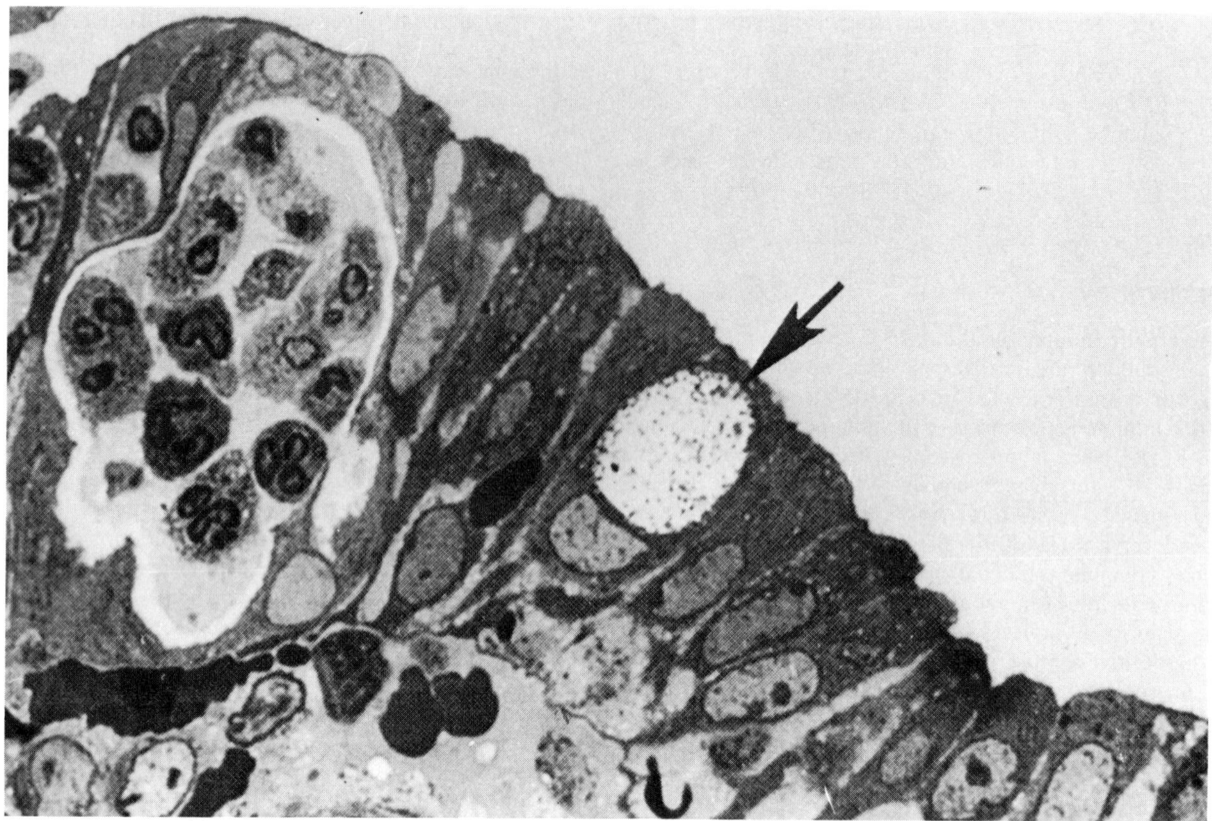

**Fig. 46-9.** Thin section of cervical biopsy showing a chlamydial inclusion in a columnar epithelial cell, compressing the nucleus to the base of the cell. Toluidine blue O stain, phase contrast, ×1000 magnification. *(Courtesy of J Swanson.)*

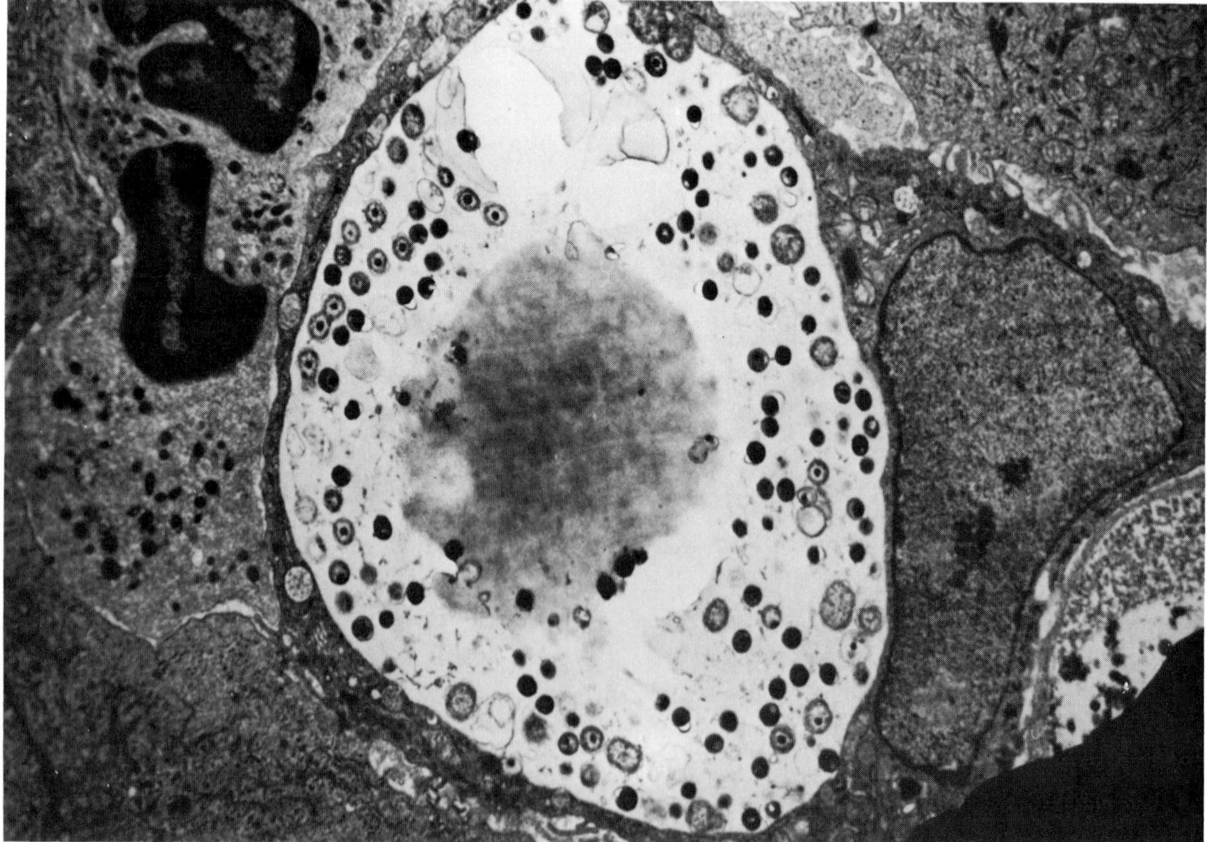

**Fig. 46-10.** Electron micrograph of a chlamydial inclusion in cervical biopsy tissue, showing compact elementary bodies, larger reticulate bodies, and intermediate forms which resemble bull's eyes. Uranyl acetate, lead citrate, ×12,000 magnification. *(Courtesy of J Swanson.)*

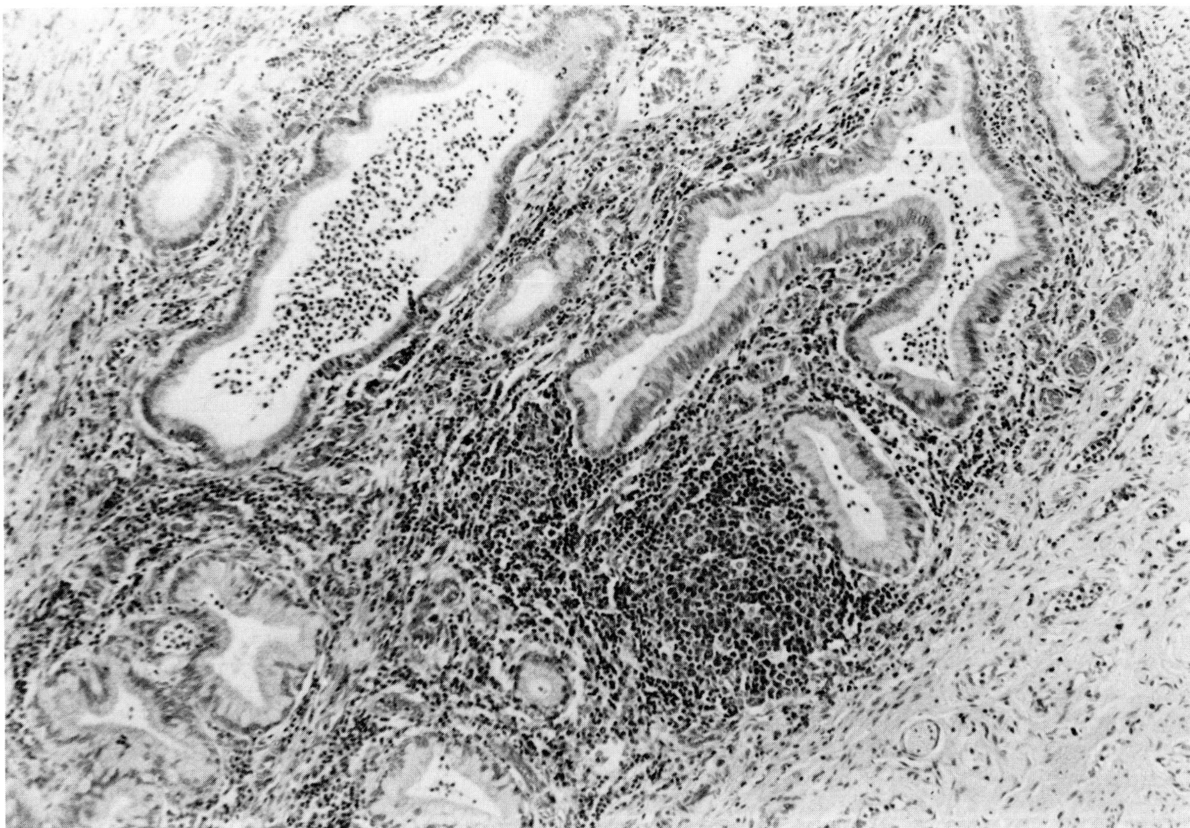

**Fig. 46-11.** Endocervical biopsy showing patchy periglandular inflammation associated with chlamydial infection. Several gland lumena are filled with neutrophils, with intraepithelial infiltration by neutrophils, and are surrounded by mononuclear cells, predominantly plasma cells. A rounded germinal center containing transformed lymphocytes is present.

cal bleeding, and no use of barrier contraception. If confirmatory tests are not available or affordable, empirical therapy can be given to women with mucopurulent cervicitis. However, the recent development of methods for immunological detection of *C. trachomatis* in endocervical specimens (Chap. 74) has made diagnostic testing for *C. trachomatis* more widely available. The presence of cervical lesions suggestive of HSV infection warrants confirmatory testing for HSV (Chap. 77). Viral isolation will permit differentation of HSV-1 from HSV-2, which has prognostic importance, since HSV-1 is less likely than HSV-2 to cause recurrent genital herpes. If colpitis macularis is seen, wet mount examination for motile trichomonads is usually positive.

## TREATMENT FOR MUCOPURULENT CERVICITIS

The 1985 Centers for Disease Control guidelines for treatment of STD[59] recommend treatment of mucopurulent cervicitis as recommended for uncomplicated gonorrhea if *N. gonorrhoeae* is found, and treatment as recommended for chlamydial infection if gonorrhea is not found. However, chlamydial infection should always be suspected in women with mucopurulent cervicitis, whether or not gonorrhea is found. Furthermore, a negative endocervical Gram stain for *N. gonorrhoeae* does not exclude gonorrhea. Among women with coexistent gonococcal and chlamydial infection of the cervix, persistence of *C. trachomatis* was more common after single-dose ampicillin therapy than after therapy with trimethoprim-sulfamethoxazole; and persistence or development of cervicitis after therapy was correlated with persistence of *C. trachomatis*.[60] Treatment of women with gonococcal infection with 4.8 million units of procaine penicillin G plus probenecid was associated with a significantly higher rate of posttreatment cervicitis and pelvic inflammatory disease than was treatment with drugs effective against *C. trachomatis* (tetracycline or trimethoprim-sulfamethoxazole.)[61] Treatment of cervical *C. trachomatis* infection with 500 mg of tetracycline hydrochloride 4 times daily for 7 days appears to be effective in eradicating *C. trachomatis* from the cervix (Chap. 16) and has been shown to eliminate mucopurulent endocervical discharge in nearly all women within 3 weeks after completion of therapy.[62] Thus, therapy for mucopurulent cervicitis should include a regimen active against *C. trachomatis*, such as the 7-day course of tetracycline described above. Alternatives include 100 mg doxycycline twice daily for 7 days or 500 mg erythromycin 4 times daily for 7 days. If coexisting gonococcal infection is found or suspected, additional therapy for gonorrhea should be provided, since tetracyclines are not reliable as sole therapy for gonorrhea in most areas of the world.

## PREVENTION

When used correctly, the condom can probably be regarded as highly effective in preventing sexual transmission of pathogens which infect the columnar epithelium of the urethra and endocervix (e.g., *N. gonorrhoeae*, *C. trachomatis*, and HSV); moderately effective in reducing sexual transmission of pathogens which can infect the squamous epithelium of the vulva and penis (e.g., HSV, *Treponema pallidum*, *H. ducreyi*, human papilloma virus); and ineffective in reducing sexual transmission of pathogens which infest the cornified skin or the cutaneous appendages (e.g., *Sarcoptes scabiei*, *Phthirus pubis*). Other intravaginal barrier contraceptives, such as the diaphragm, especially when used with antiseptic spermicides, might also be expected to reduce transmission of *N. gonorrhoeae* and *C. trachomatis*.[63]

## RELATIVE FREQUENCY OF LOWER GENITOURINARY INFECTIONS IN WOMEN

The relative frequency of the common forms of lower genitourinary infections in adult women discussed above depends upon the criteria used for diagnosis and upon the population studied. Table 46-4 summarizes the clinical diagnoses and microbiological diagnoses among women examined by generally similar techniques in three clinical settings.

Among 167 women with urinary or genital symptoms who were examined at the University of Washington Family Medicine Clinic, which serves a population demographically representative of the population of King county, 52 percent complained of urinary symptoms and 79 percent complained of vaginal symptoms.[64] Bacteriuria with $\geq 10^2$ uropathogens per milliliter of urine was documented in 18 of 87 women with urinary symptoms. Bacterial vaginosis was by far the commonest form of vaginal infection detected by the clinical examination, although *C. albicans* was detected five times more often by culture than by wet mount examination in 10% KOH in this study. Genital herpes, and infection with *T. vaginalis, N. gonorrhoeae,* and/or *C. trachomatis,* conditions which are clearly sexually transmitted, were each relatively uncommon in this population. Komaroff et al. also found that vaginal infection was more common than urinary infection among consecutive women with urogenital symptoms seen in a primary care clinic setting.[12] Fleury has also reported that in a private practice setting, bacterial vaginosis (NSV) was the most common form of vaginal infection, followed by candidal vaginitis, with trichomonal vaginitis being least common.[65]

Female college students attending the University of Washington Student Health Women's Clinic have been studied in two separate surveys. Among 397 consecutive women attending the clinic for any reason (series A), objective clinical evidence of vaginal infection was found in 39 percent.[66] Bacterial vaginosis and vaginal candidiasis were again much commoner than the sexually transmitted causes of cervicitis, although our criteria for the diagnosis of mucopurulent cervicitis had not yet been developed for use in this study.

In a second study of university students (series B), 823 women undergoing routine examination were more comprehensively evaluated and were compared with a group of 779 randomly selected women attending our STD clinic who were evaluated by exactly the same methods. Nearly all diagnoses, and the sexually transmitted pathogens such as *T. vaginalis, C. trachomatis, N. gonorrhoeae,* and HSV were much more common in the STD population (KK Holmes, unpublished data). Only one case of trichomoniasis and one of gonorrhea were found in the students. The rates of bacterial vaginosis and vulvovaginal candidiasis probably were higher in students in series A than in series B because the latter were seen for routine exam, the former for any reason, including genital symptoms. The addition of the sexually transmitted infections to those infections which might be re-

**Table 46-4. Percent Prevalence of Clinical and Microbiological Evidence of Lower Genital Tract Infections in Three Clinical Settings in Seattle**

| | University of Washington Family Medicine Clinic* (N = 167) | University of Washington Student Health Clinic Series A† (N = 397) | University of Washington Student Health Clinic Series B‡ (N = 823) | Seattle–King County Harborview Medical Center STD Clinic§ (N = 779) |
|---|---|---|---|---|
| **Clinical diagnoses** | | | | |
| Bacterial vaginosis | 19 | 21 | 6 | 38 |
| Vaginal candidiasis | 5 | 16 | 4 | 15 |
| Trichomonal vaginitis | 2 | 2 | 0 | 9 |
| Mucopurulent cervicitis | 4 | ND | 1 | 26 |
| Genital herpes | 0 | 0 | 0.5 | 11 |
| **Microbiologic diagnoses** | | | | |
| *Gardnerella vaginalis* isolated | 66 | 51 | 49 | 74 |
| *Candida albicans* isolated | 25 | 22¶ | 20 | 26 |
| *Trichomonas vaginalis* isolated | 7 | ND | 0.1 | 15 |
| *Chlamydia trachomatis* isolated | 5 | ND | 6 | 15 |
| *Neisseria gonorrhoeae* isolated | 2 | ND | 0 | 14 |
| HSV isolated | ND | ND | 0.1 | 8 |

ND = no data.

NOTE: Trichomonal vaginitis and mucopurulent cervicitis are much more common in STD clinic patients than in Student Health Clinic or Family Medicine Clinic patients. Similarly, sexually transmitted pathogens (*T. vaginalis, C. trachomatis, N. gonorrhoeae*) are much more common in the STD clinic patients.

*All 167 women had genitourinary symptoms, 64, 1980–1981.

†Consecutive women attending the Women's Clinic at the University of Washington Student Health Clinic,[66] 1979–1980.

‡Consecutive women attending the Women's Clinic for routine annual examination, 1984–1988.

§Randomly selected women attending the Seattle STD Clinic, 1984–1986.

¶225 of 397 women underwent culture of vaginal fluid on Sabouraud's agar for isolation of yeast.

garded as more often of endogenous origin (e.g., vulvovaginal candidiasis, urinary tract infection, and perhaps bacterial vaginosis) makes the differential diagnosis of urogenital symptoms more complex in the STD clinic setting than in other settings. Thus, careful clinical and microbiological studies are particularly necessary in the individual patient who is considered to be at high risk for STD.

## DIFFERENTIAL DIAGNOSIS AND MANAGEMENT OF VAGINAL DISCHARGE

Symptoms or signs of abnormal vaginal discharge may be attributable to vaginal infection or to cervicitis. Therefore the most important initial step in evaluation of vaginal discharge is exclusion of cervicitis, the more serious condition.

Mucopurulent cervicitis caused by *C. trachomatis* or *N. gonorrhoeae* must be differentiated from cervicitis caused by HSV, from vaginitis, and from simple cervical ectopy without inflammation, a common condition (Plate 13). Columnar epithelium lies in an exposed position on the ectocervix in the majority of adolescent girls at the onset of menarche. The prevalence of ectopy gradually declines through young adulthood. The term *ectropion,* sometimes used interchangeably with the term *ectopy,* has also been used to describe the patulous parous cervix, which opens as the blades of a vaginal speculum are spread, to expose the endocervix. Ectopy or ectropion, when not associated with visible or microscopic evidence of mucopurulent exudate, or with colposcopic epithelial abnormalities, is a normal finding and requires no therapy. Recurrent genital herpes involving the cervix alone produces lesions of the endocervix and the ectocervical squamous epithelium. Ectocervicitis due to trichomoniasis and vulvovaginal candidiasis are generally associated with vaginitis, as discussed above.

After the presence or absence of cervicitis is established, the next step involves establishing the presence or absence of vaginal infection. Not infrequently, cervicitis coexists with vaginal infection, particularly with bacterial vaginosis or trichomonal vaginitis; and bacterial vaginosis is common among women with trichomonal vaginitis.

The amount, consistency, and location of the discharge within the vagina should be noted. A sample of discharge should then be removed with a swab from the vaginal wall, avoiding contamination with cervical mucus. The color of vaginal discharge should be noted in comparison with the white color of the swab. The pH should be determined directly by rolling the swab containing the specimen on the pH indicator paper. An additional specimen should be removed with a swab and mixed first with a drop of saline, then with a drop of 10% KOH, on a microscope slide. The odor released after mixing the specimen with KOH is noted, and separate coverslips are placed on the saline and KOH wet mounts for microscopic examination to detect the presence and quantity of normal epithelial cells, clue cells, neutrophils, motile trichomonads, or fungal forms.

Although the sensitivity and specificity of symptoms and signs as outlined above and in Table 46-5 are not high, in many patients, symptoms and signs and microscopic wet mount findings correspond to a consistent pattern, and further studies are unnecessary. However, when symptoms or signs suggest a vaginal infection which cannot be confirmed by microscopic wet mount examination, further microbiological studies are indicated. Depending upon the clinical findings, these further studies may include culture for *C. albicans,* culture for *T. vaginalis,* or Gram stain of vaginal fluid to differentiate between normal flora and the flora characteristic of bacterial vaginosis. In women with prominent vaginal complaints but no abnormal findings, all three of these additional microbiological tests may be indicated to differentiate vaginal infection from other causes of vaginal symptoms, including functional complaints.[67]

We have recently assessed the symptoms and signs of bacterial vaginosis and vaginal trichomoniasis among randomly selected female STD clinic patients, by adjusting for coinfections and other potential confounders. Bacterial vaginosis (as independently defined by objective Gram stain criteria) was significantly correlated with symptoms of vaginal discharge (present, however, in only 17 percent of patients) or malodor (49 percent); and with signs of homogeneous discharge (69 percent), yellow discharge (32 percent), fishy odor of vaginal fluid in potassium hydroxide (43 percent), and vaginal fluid pH $\geq$4.7 (97 percent). Bacterial vaginosis was correlated with the presence of vaginal clue cells (81 percent), but not with the presence of increased numbers of neutrophils in cervical secretion or with increased numbers of white blood cells in vaginal fluid.[68] In contrast, in the same group of patients, trichomoniasis was significantly correlated with symptoms of yellow vaginal discharge (42 percent) and vulvar itching (60 percent); with colposcopic signs of colpitis macularis (44 percent); and with signs of purulent (yellow) vaginal discharge (59 percent), vulvar erythema (37 percent), and vaginal erythema (20 percent), as well as with an increased concentration of white blood cells in vaginal fluid.[69]

In a recent study from France[70] the clinical manifestations of cervicitis and vulvovaginitis were assessed by univariate analyses in relation to the presence of specific microbial pathogens. Findings were generally consistent with the above, and isolation of *C. albicans* was significantly associated with the symptom of vulvar pruritis and with signs of vulvitis and vaginitis.

Usual courses of treatment for vaginal infection are also summarized in Table 46-5. It is still common practice to prescribe metronidazole for bacterial vaginosis only for those who have complaints related to this condition. However, as discussed below, this could change if data implicating bacterial vaginosis as predisposing to upper genital infection and premature delivery are confirmed elsewhere.

Perhaps the most important aspect of the differential diagnosis of mucopurulent cervicitis is careful evaluation for complicating endometritis or salpingitis. As discussed below and in Chap. 50, endometritis, manifested by midline abdominal tenderness or menorrhagia, often with elevation of the erythrocyte sedimentation rate or peripheral white count, and with characteristic histopathological evidence of endometritis, is often present among women with mucopurulent cervicitis.

## GYNECOLOGICAL COMPLICATIONS OF LOWER GENITAL TRACT INFECTIONS IN WOMEN

Among STD clinic patients with mucopurulent cervicitis studied at the University of Washington, at least 40 percent have had histopathological evidence of plasma cell endometritis.[71] Jacobsen and Westrom have required the presence of purulent discharge in the vagina (leukocytes must outnumber other cell types) for the diagnosis of salpingitis.[72,73] It seems likely that such discharge is probably attributable to mucopurulent cervicitis in most if not all cases. Jacobsen and Weström state they have never seen

Table 46-5. Diagnostic Features and Management of Vaginal Infection in Premenopausal Adults

| | Normal vaginal exam | Yeast vaginitis | Trichomonal vaginitis | Bacterial vaginosis (NSV) |
|---|---|---|---|---|
| Etiology | Uninfected; *Lactobacillus* predominant | *Candida albicans* and other yeasts | *Trichomonas vaginalis* | Associated with *G. vaginalis,* various anaerobic bacteria, and mycoplasma |
| Typical symptoms | None | Vulvar itching and/or irritation, increased discharge | Profuse purulent discharge, vulvar itching | Malodorous, slightly increased discharge |
| Discharge: | | | | |
| Amount | Variable; usually scant | Scant to moderate | Profuse | Moderate |
| Color* | Clear or white | White | Yellow | Usually white or gray |
| Consistency | Nonhomogeneous, floccular | Clumped; adherent plaques | Homogeneous | Homogeneous, low viscosity; uniformly coating vaginal walls |
| Inflammation of vulvar or vaginal epithelium | None | Erythema of vaginal epithelium, introitus; vulvar dermatitis common | Erythema of vaginal and vulvar epithelium; colpitis macularis | None |
| pH of vaginal fluid† | Usually ≤4.5 | Usually ≤4.5 | Usually ≥5.0 | Usually ≥4.7 |
| Amine ("fishy") odor with 10% KOH | None | None | May be present | Present |
| Microscopy‡ | Normal epithelial cells; lactobacilli predominate | Leukocytes, epithelial cells; yeast, mycelia, or pseudomycelia in up to 80% | Leukocytes; motile trichomonads seen in 80–90% of symptomatic patients, less often in the absence of symptoms | Clue cells; few leukocytes; lactobacilli outnumbered by profuse mixed flora, nearly always including *G. vaginalis* plus anaerobic species, on Gram stain |
| Usual treatment | None | Miconazole or clotrimazole intravaginally each 100 mg daily for 7 days | Metronidazole or tinidazole 2.0 g orally (single dose) | Metronidazole 500 mg orally twice daily for 7 days |
| | | Nystatin, 100,000 units intravaginally twice daily for 7–14 days | Metronidazole 500 mg orally twice daily for 7 days | |
| Usual management of sex partners | None | None; topical treatment if candidal dermatitis of penis is present | Examine for STD; treat with metronidazole, 2 gm p.o. | Examine for STD; no treatment if normal |

*Color of discharge is determined by examining vaginal discharge against the white background of a swab.

†pH determination is not useful if blood is present.

‡To detect fungal elements, vaginal fluid is digested with 10% KOH prior to microscopic examination; to examine for other features, fluid is mixed (1:1) with physiologic saline. Gram's stain also is excellent for detecting yeasts and pseudomycelia and for distinguishing normal flora from the mixed flora seen in bacterial vaginosis but is less sensitive than the saline preparation for detection of *T. vaginalis.*

salpingitis laparoscopically in a patient who did not have a purulent vaginal discharge.[74] In contrast, U.S. gynecologists have not required the presence of mucopurulent cervicitis as a criterion for salpingitis, and in fact guidelines developed for diagnosis of salpingitis by a group of U.S. gynecologists and approved by the Obstetrics and Gynecology Infectious Disease Society did not include this criterion.[75]

It is important to note that the Scandinavians have encountered salpingitis caused by anaerobes much less frequently in recent years than has been the case in the United States. It can be hypothesized that mucopurulent cervicitis may be a predisposing factor for gonococcal and/or chlamydial salpingitis; whereas bacterial vaginosis may be the predisposing cause among women with salpingitis caused by those pathogens characteristically found in the vagina in bacterial vaginosis (e.g., *Bacteroides* sp., peptococci, *M. hominis, G. vaginalis*). This perspective is illustrated in Fig. 46-12. Among the set of randomly selected Seattle STD clinic patients described above, bacterial vaginosis was significantly associated with a clinical diagnosis of PID; and even after adjusting for coinfections and other potential confounders, bacterial vaginosis was significantly associated with moderate to severe adnexal tenderness.[68] Simultaneous mucopurulent cervicitis and bacterial vaginosis may be responsible for mixed tubal infections caused by the cervical pathogens *(N. gonorrhoeae, C. trachomatis)*, together with the bacterial vaginosis-associated organisms. Evaluation of these and other possible models for the interrelationship between upper and lower genital tract infection could lead to clearer understanding of the pathogenesis of salpingitis. A clearer understanding of pathogenesis and etiology of PID, and confirmation of the role of specific cervical and vaginal infections in leading to PID, might reduce the need for invasive diagnostic procedures and permit a more rational basis for selecting antimicrobial therapy in the individual patient. For example, it should be determined whether the presence of mucopurulent cervicitis increases the predictive value of a clinical diagnosis of PID, and the probability of upper genital infection with *C. trachomatis* or *N. gonorrhoeae*. Finally, as discussed in Chap. 64, there is also a great deal of current interest in defining the importance of cervical infection and bacterial vaginosis in causing complications of pregnancy. If the reported role of these conditions in predisposing to chorioamnionitis and premature delivery[76,77] is confirmed, an increased emphasis on proper management of these lower genital tract infections in pregnant women can be anticipated.

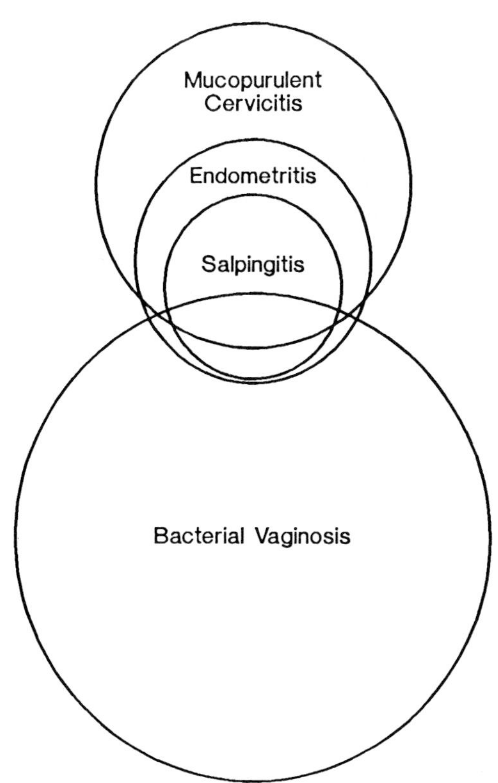


**Fig. 46-12.** Hypothetical relationship of upper genital tract infections to lower genital tract infections. In this model, among women with mucopurulent cervicitis, upper tract infections are attributable to *C. trachomatis* and *N. gonorrhoeae,* while among women with bacterial vaginosis, upper tract infections are attributable to bacterial vaginosis-associated vaginal organisms (e.g., *Mycoplasma hominis, Bacteroides* spp., and *Peptostreptococcus* spp). Upper tract infections in women with both bacterial vaginosis and mucopurulent cervicitis may be due to either or both sets of organisms. A second hypothesis advanced here is that salpingitis complicating mucopurulent cervicitis or bacterial vaginosis is associated with endometritis.

## References


1 Cypress BK: Patients' reasons for visiting physicians. National Ambulatory Medical Care Survey. United States, 1977–78, in *Vital and Health Statistics.* Data from the National Health Survey, Series 13; No. 56, DHHS Publication (PHS)82-1717. National Center for Health Statistics. Hyattsville, 1981.

2 Waters WE et al: Clinical significance of dysuria in women. *Br Med J* 2:754, 1970.

3 Wong ES et al: Urinary tract infection among women attending a clinic for sexually transmitted diseases. *Sex Transm Dis* 11:18, 1984.

4 Stamm WE et al: Diagnosis of coliform infection in acutely dysuric women. *N Engl J Med* 307:463, 1982.

5 Stamm WE: Quantitative urine cultures revisited. *Eur J Clin Microbiol* 3:279, 1984.

6 Latham RH et al: Urinary tract infections in young adult women caused by *Staphylococcus saprophyticus. JAMA* 250:3063, 1983.

7 Komaroff AL, Friedland G: The dysuria-sterile pyuria syndrome, editorial. *N Engl J Med* 3038:452, 1980.

8 Stamm WE et al: Causes of the acute urethral syndrome in women. *N Engl J Med* 303:409, 1980.

9 Curran JW: Gonorrhea and the urethral syndrome. *Sex Transm Dis* 4:119, 1977.

10 Paavonen J: *Chlamydia trachomatis*-induced urethritis in female partners of men with nongonococcal urethritis. *Sex Transm Dis* 6:69, 1979.

11 Panja SK: Urethral syndrome in women attending a clinic for sexually transmitted diseases. *Br J Vener Dis* 59:179, 1984.

12 Komaroff AL et al: Management strategies for urinary and vaginal infections. *Arch Intern Med* 138:1069, 1978.

13 Pfaller M et al: The usefulness of screening tests for pyuria in combination with culture in the diagnosis of urinary tract infection. *Diagn Microbiol Infect Dis* 6:207, 1987.

14 Fihn SD et al: Association between diaphragm use and urinary tract infection. *JAMA* 253:240, 1985.

15 Nicolle LE et al: The association of urinary tract infection with sexual intercourse. *J Infect Dis* 146:579, 1982.

16 Wølner-Hanssen P et al: Clinical manifestations of vaginal trichomoniasis. *JAMA* 261:571, 1989.
17 Fihn SD et al: Trimethoprim-sulfamethoxazole for acute dysuria in women: A single-dose or 10 day course. A double blind, randomized trial. *Ann Intern Med* 108:350, 1988.
18 Stamm WE et al: Treatment of the acute urethral syndrome. *N Engl J Med* 304:956, 1981.
19 Cruickshank R, Shaiman A: The biology of the vagina in the human subject. II: The bacterial flora and secretion of the vagina at various age-periods, and their relation to glycogen in the vaginal epithelium. *J Obstet Gynaecol Br Emp* 41:208, 1934.
20 Eschenbach DA et al: Prevalence of hydrogen peroxide-producing *Lactobacillus* species in normal women and women with bacterial vaginosis. *J Clin Microbiol* 27:251, 1989.
21 Holmes KK et al: Vaginal redox potential in bacterial vaginosis (nonspecific vaginitis). *J Infect Dis* 152:379, 1985.
22 Hardy GC: Vaginal flora in children. *Am J Dis Child* 62:939, 1941.
23 Hammerschlag MR et al: Microbiology of the vagina in children: normal and potentially pathogenic organisms. *Pediatrics* 62:57, 1978.
24 Gutman LT, Holmes KK: Gonococcal infection, in *Infectious Diseases of the Fetus and Newborn Infant,* 3d ed, JS Remington, JO Klein (eds). Philadelphia, Saunders, 1989.
25 Paradise JE et al: Vulvovaginitis in premenarcheal girls: Clinical features and diagnostic evaluation. *Pediatrics* 70:193, 1982.
26 Heller RH et al: Vulvovaginitis in the premenarcheal child. *J Pediatr* 74:370, 1969.
27 Singleton AF: Vaginal discharge in children and adolescents. *Clin Pediatr (Phila)* 19:799, 1980.
28 Murphy TV, Nelson JD: Shigella vaginitis: Report of 28 patients and review of the literature. *Pediatrics* 63:511, 1979.
29 Schwartz RH et al: Vulvovaginitis in prepubertal girls: The importance of group A streptococcus. *South Med J* 75:446, 1982.
30 Rettig PJ, Nelson JD: Genital tract infection with *Chlamydia trachomatis* in prepubertal children. *J Pediatr* 99:206, 1981.
31 Fuster CD, Neinstein LS: Vaginal *Chlamydia trachomatis* prevalence in sexually abused prepubertal girls. *Pediatrics* 79:234, 1987.
32 Centers for Disease Control: Nonreported sexually transmitted diseases. *MMWR* 28:61, 1979.
33 *1976 Summary: National Ambulatory Medical Care Survey, Advance Data from Vital and Health Statistics of the National Center for Health Statistics,* US Department of Health, Education, and Welfare no 30, July 13, 1978.
34 Larkin SM et al: Toxic shock syndrome: Clinical, laboratory, and pathologic findings in nine fatal cases. *Ann Intern Med* 96:858, 1982.
35 Paris AL et al: Pathologic findings in twelve fetal cases of toxic shock syndrome. *Ann Intern Med* 96:852, 1982.
36 Friedrich EG, Siegesmund KA: Tampon-associated vaginal ulcerations. *Obstet Gynecol* 55:149, 1980.
37 Barrett KF et al: Tampon-induced vaginal or cervical ulceration. *Am J Obstet Gynecol* 127:332, 1977.
38 Galask RP, Larsen B: Identifying and treating genital tract infections in postmenopausal women. *Geriatrics* 36:69, 1981.
39 Osborne NG et al: Genital bacteriology: A comparative study of premenopausal women with postmenopausal women. *Am J Obstet Gynecol* 135:195, 1979.
40 Leiblum S et al: Vaginal atrophy in the postmenopausal women. *JAMA* 249:2195, 1983.
41 Goldacre MJ et al: Epidemiology and clinical significance of cervical erosion in women attending a family planning clinic. *Br Med J* 1:748, 1978.
42 Singer A: The uterine cervix from adolescence to the menopause. *Br J Obstet Gynaecol* 82:81, 1975.
43 Pixley E: Basic morphology of the prepubertal and youthful cervix: Topographic and histologic features. *J Reprod Med* 16:221, 1976.
44 Arya OP et al: Epidemiological and clinical correlates of chlamydial infection of the cervix. *Br J Vener Dis* 56:37, 1980.
45 Tait IA et al: Chlamydial infection of the cervix in contacts of men with nongonococcal urethritis. *Br J Vener Dis* 56:37, 1980.
46 Harrison HR et al: Cervical *Chlamydia trachomatis* infection in university women: Relationship to history, contraception, ectopy, and cervicitis. *Am J Obstet Gynecol* 153:244, 1985.
47 Rees E et al: Chlamydia in relation to cervical infection and pelvic inflammatory disease, in *Nongonococcal Urethritis and Related Infections,* D Hobson, KK Holmes (eds). Washington, American Society of Microbiology, 1977, p 67.
48 Brunham RC et al: Mucopurulent cervicitis: The ignored counterpart of urethritis in the male. *N Engl J Med* 311:1, 1984.
49 Handsfield HH et al: Criteria for selective screening for *Chlamydia trachomatis* infection on women attending family planning clinics. *JAMA* 255:1730, 1986.
50 Schafer M-A et al: *Chlamydia trachomatis:* Important relationships to race, contraception, lower genital tract infection, and Papanicolaou smear. *J Pediatr* 104:141, 1984.
51 Kent GP et al: Screening for *Chlamydia trachomatis* infection in a sexually transmitted disease clinic: Comparison of diagnostic tests with clinical and historical risk factors. *Sex Transm Dis* 15:51, 1988.
52 Swinker ML et al: Prevalence of *Chlamydia trachomatis* cervical infection in a college gynecology clinic: Relationship to other infections and clinical features. *Sex Transm Dis* 15:133, 1988.
53 Paavonen J et al: Etiology of cervical inflammation. *Am J Obstet Gynecol* 154:556, 1986.
54 Paavonen J et al: Colposcopic manifestations of cervical and vaginal infections. *Obstet Gynecol Survey* 43:373, 1988.
55 Kiviat N et al: Cytologic manifestations of cervical and vaginal infections. I. Epithelial and cellular inflammatory changes. *JAMA* 253:989, 1985.
56 Kiviat NB et al: Cytologic manifestations of cervical and vaginal infections. II. Confirmation of *Chlamydia trachomatis* infection by direct immunofluorescence using monoclonal antibodies. *JAMA* 253:997, 1985.
57 Tawa K et al: A comparison of the Papanicolaou smear and the cervigram: Sensitivity, specificity, and cost analysis. *Obstet Gynecol* 71:229, 1988.
58 Wilson JD: Value of colposcopy in genitourinary departments. *Genitourin Med* 64:100, 1988.
59 1985 STD Treatment Guidelines. *MMWR* 43(suppl 4S), 1985.
60 Brunham RC et al: Treatment of concomitant *Neisseria gonorrhoeae* and *Chlamydia trachomatis* infections in women: Comparison of trimethoprim-sulfamethoxazole with ampicillin-probenecid. *Rev Infect Dis* 4:91, 1983.
61 Stamm WE et al: Effect of *Neisseria gonorrhoeae* treatment regimens on simultaneous infection with *Chlamydia trachomatis. N Engl J Med* 310:545, 1984.
62 Brunham RC et al: Therapy of cervical chlamydial infection. *Ann Intern Med* 97:216, 1982.
63 Rosenberg MJ et al: The contraceptive sponge's protection against *Chlamydia trachomatis* and *Neisseria gonorrhoeae. Sex Transm Dis* 14:147, 1987.
64 Berg AO et al: Establishing the cause of genitourinary symptoms in women in a family practice: Comparison of clinical examination and comprehensive microbiology. *JAMA* 251:620, 1984.
65 Fleury FJ: Adult vaginitis. *Clin Obstet Gynaecol* 24:407, 1981.
66 Amsel R et al: Nonspecific vaginitis: Diagnostic criteria and microbial and epidemiological associations. *Am J Med* 74:14, 1983.
67 McGuire LS et al: Psychosexual functioning in symptomatic and asymptomatic women with and without signs of vaginitis. *Am J Obstet Gynecol* 137:600, 1980.
68 Eschenbach DA et al: Diagnosis and clinical manifestations of bacterial vaginosis. *Am J Obstet Gynecol* 158:819, 1988.
69 Wølner-Hanssen P et al: Clinical manifestations of vaginal trichomoniasis. *JAMA* 261:571, 1989.
70 Lefevre JC et al: Lower genital tract infections in women: Comparison of clinical and epidemiological findings with microbiology. *Sex Transm Dis* 15:110, 1988.
71 Paavonen J: Prevalence and manifestations of endometritis among women with cervicitis. *Am J Obstet Gynecol* 152:280, 1985.
72 Weström L: Diagnosis, etiology and prognosis of acute salpingitis. Thesis. Student littatur, Lund, Sweden, 1976.

73 Weström L: Incidence, prevalence and trends of acute pelvic inflammatory disease and its consequences in industrialized countries. *Am J Obstet Gynecol* 138:880, 1980.
74 Jacobsen L: Differential diagnosis of acute pelvic inflammatory disease. *Am J Obstet Gynecol* 138:1006, 1980.
75 Hager DW et al: Criteria for diagnosis and grading of salpingitis. *Obstet Gynecol* 61:113, 1983.
76 Hillier SL et al: A case-control study of chorioamnionic infection and histologic chorioamnionitis in prematurity. *N Engl J Med* 319:972, 1988.
77 Martius J et al: Relationships of vaginal *Lactobacillus* sp., cervical *Chlamydia trachomatis*, and bacterial vaginosis to preterm birth. *Obstet Gynecol* 7:89, 1988.

# Chapter 47
# Bacterial vaginosis

Sharon Hillier
King K. Holmes

*Our knowledge of leukorrhea is unsatisfactory and incomplete. The majority of physicians neither appreciate the gross aspects of the condition nor discover the locality from which discharges arise, practically none of us possesses an adequate knowledge of the bacteria involved, and most clinicians admit that their curative efforts yield poor results.*

Arthur H. Curtis, M.D. (December 19, 1913[1])

## DEFINITION

Bacterial vaginosis (BV) is the most prevalent cause of vaginal symptoms among women of childbearing age. BV is often perceived by primary care physicians as a trivial and ill-defined syndrome of uncertain etiology which is a problem primarily for aesthetic reasons. These perceptions may account for the fact that ineffective treatments are still commonly prescribed for BV.

Bacterial vaginosis (nonspecific vaginitis) is a clinical entity characterized by symptoms of slightly increased quantities of malodorous vaginal discharge. Although it is conventional practice to make a diagnosis of bacterial vaginosis only after excluding other conditions that can be associated with vaginal discharge, such as trichomoniasis, vulvovaginal candidiasis, or cervicitis, these conditions can undoubtedly coexist with bacterial vaginosis. Physical examination and analysis of vaginal fluid reveal the following: a thin homogeneous, white, uniformly adherent vaginal discharge; elevation of the pH of vaginal fluid above 4.5; development of a fishy odor when vaginal fluid is mixed with 10% (wt/vol) KOH; and "clue cells" on microscopic examination of vaginal fluid. Gram stain of normal vaginal fluid shows a predominance of lactobacilli. In contrast, the Gram stain of vaginal fluid from a woman with bacterial vaginosis shows a decrease or absence of lactobacilli, and a predominance of gram-variable coccobacilli consistent with *Gardnerella vaginalis* or *Bacteroides* species. Culture of vaginal fluid reveals mixed flora that typically includes genital mycoplasmas, *Gardnerella vaginalis*, and anaerobic bacteria such as peptostreptococci, *Bacteroides* spp., and *Mobiluncus* spp. Biochemical analysis of vaginal fluid from women with bacterial vaginosis usually shows characteristic changes thought to be due to bacterial metabolism. The vaginal fluid contains an altered pattern of organic acids (e.g., increased succinate, decreased lactate). There are abnormal amounts of putrescine, cadaverine, and trimethylamine which probably contribute to the malodor. The pathogenesis of bacterial vaginosis has yet to be fully elucidated. Since there usually is little or no inflammation of the vaginal epithelium per se, the syndrome apparently represents a disturbance of the vaginal microbial ecosystem rather than a true tissue or epithelial infection. However, recent work has demonstrated an increased risk for prematurity and chorioamnionitis among pregnant women with BV, and suggests that BV may be a risk factor for pelvic inflammatory disease.

## HISTORY

Nearly a century ago, Doderlein described a nonmotile bacillus which he considered to be the normal flora of the vagina of pregnant women.[2] The Doderlein bacillus, as it became known, was later identified as being *Lactobacillus*. In 1899, Menge and Kronig reported that both facultative and strictly anaerobic microorganisms, as well as the Doderlein bacillus, could be isolated from the vagina of most women.[3] These early studies established that normal vaginal flora is comprised of a mixture of microorganisms, and that *Lactobacillus* spp. are the predominant species.

"Leukorrhea," or white discharge from the vagina, was the focus of much research in the first quarter of the century. It was thought that vaginal discharge resulted from infection of the uterus and was treated by curettage of the endometrium. In 1913, Curtis demonstrated that the endometria of women with leukorrhea lacked a white discharge, thus demonstrating that the discharge was of vaginal, not endometrial, origin. He observed that the vaginal flora of clinically normal married women consisted of Doderlein's bacilli, and that the greater the deviation of vaginal flora from the normal state, the greater the likelihood of vaginal discharge. Curtis was the first to link high concentrations of black-pigmented *Bacteroides*, curved anaerobic motile rods, and anaerobic cocci with discharge. He also recovered gram-variable diphtheroidal rods which probably represented *Gardnerella*. Thus, in 1913 many of the microorganisms which have been associated with bacterial vaginosis in more recent studies were found to be associated with this syndrome. Curtis's 1913 paper established three central themes; (1) that the vagina, and not the uterus, was the source of discharge, (2) that women having white discharge did not have large numbers of Doderlein bacilli, and (3) that the presence of anaerobic bacteria in the vagina, especially anaerobic rods, was correlated with vaginal discharge.

Research on vaginal flora continued in the early 1920s when Schroder reported that there were three different types of vaginal flora which corresponded to the "rheinheitgrad" (grade of cleanliness) of the vagina.[4] The flora of the first group, which was dominated by acid-producing rods (Doderlein's bacillus), was described as being least pathogenic. A second group had a mixed flora with Doderlein bacillus in the minority, while a third group had mixed flora with no Doderlein bacillus present. This third type of vaginal flora was designated as being the most pathogenic.

Despite Curtis's and Schroder's observation that vaginal discharge was associated with a shift in vaginal flora from predominant *Lactobacillus* to one dominated by anaerobes, other workers attempted to attribute the symptoms of nonspecific vaginitis to a single microorganism. In 1950, Weaver reported a link between lack of lactobacilli, presence of *Bacteroides* spp., and nonspecific vaginitis.[5] However, the lack of association of other aerobic and facultative bacteria with discharge led him to conclude that no particular organisms were associated with this syndrome. The recognition of the association of *Gardnerella vaginalis* with nonspecific vaginitis by Gardner and Dukes in 1955[6] (discussed below) provided the first clear evidence that *Gardnerella vaginalis* was associated with nonspecific vaginitis. However, because they failed (erroneously) to find an association between anaerobic bacteria and bacterial vaginosis, workers over the next 25 years tended to ignore the potential role of microorganisms other than *Gardnerella vaginalis*.

Because of the confusion surrounding the etiology of this syndrome, various names have been used to describe bacterial vaginosis. Prior to 1955, leukorrhea or nonspecific vaginitis were the terms most frequently used. Gardner and Dukes first applied the name *Haemophilus vaginalis* vaginitis to this syndrome in 1955, and today some clinicians use the term *Gardnerella vaginalis* vaginitis or vaginosis to describe this syndrome, while others have used the term anaerobic vaginosis.[7] Bacterial vaginosis is considered to be the name which best describes this syndrome, since BV is associated with vaginal overgrowth by several species of facultative and anaerobic bacteria,[8] and genital mycoplasmas. Since vaginal inflammation is not a feature of this infection, the term "vaginosis" has replaced the more familiar term "vaginitis."

## EPIDEMIOLOGY

How common is BV? The answer depends on the population studied. BV was diagnosed in 17 percent of the women seeking gynecologic care or having genitourinary symptoms in a family practice clinic,[9] and in 19 percent of consecutive women visiting the University of Washington Student Health Women's Clinic for any reason,[10] but in only 5 percent of those visiting the same clinic for routine annual examination (K. Holmes, unpublished data). By comparison, the prevalence of BV is higher among women attending sexually transmitted disease clinics: BV was diagnosed in 24 to 37 percent of women attending STD clinics in Uppsala, Sweden,[11] Seattle, Washington,[12] and Halifax, Nova Scotia.[13] Among pregnant women, Hill reported the prevalence of BV to be 16 percent among women visiting private physicians, 26 percent among those attending a prenatal teaching clinic, and 29 percent among those visiting a pregnancy-termination clinic.[14] Thus, the prevalence of BV has been lowest among women undergoing routine annual examinations and highest among those attending STD clinics. Among pregnant women the prevalence has been lowest in private patients and highest in those visiting a teaching clinic or requesting termination of pregnancy. We have found no difference in the prevalence of bacterial vaginosis in women tested in the second and third trimesters of pregnancy (S. Hillier, D. Eschenbach, unpublished data).

*Gardnerella vaginalis* is found significantly more often among sexually active women than among sexually inexperienced women,[10] but has nonetheless been recovered from 10 percent to 31 percent of sexually inexperienced adolescent girls.[15,16] While these studies demonstrate that *G. vaginalis* can be present in the absence of sexual activity, there is some evidence to support sexual transmission. Gardner[6] and Pheifer[17] detected *G. vaginalis* in the urethras of 79 and 86 percent of the male sex partners of women with BV, but not in the male controls. Ison and Easmon reported that 16 percent of 58 men attending a subfertility clinic had both *G. vaginalis* and anaerobes at concentrations of $10^3$ to $10^7$ organisms per milliliters of semen; however, the vaginal flora of the female sex partners was not examined.[18] In another recent study, the urethral, rectal, and oral flora of 23 male consorts of 22 women with BV were studied. *G. vaginalis* was recovered from two (9 percent) of the urethral samples, from one rectal sample, and from none of the throat specimens. *Mobiluncus* spp. was not recovered from the throat or urethral cultures of any of the men, but one rectal specimen yielded *M. curtisii.*[19] *Bacteroides* spp. were recovered from 4 (17 percent) and peptostreptococci from 12 (52 percent) of the urethral samples. The authors concluded that there was no evidence to support sexual transmission of these bacteria. However, a control group of men whose partners were normal was not studied. In our ongoing study, 25 male partners of women with BV were more likely than 16 males whose partners did not have BV to have urethral colonization with *G. vaginalis* (40 vs. 0 percent) (S. Hillier, B. Leite, K. K. Holmes, unpublished data). Taken together these studies suggest that some, but not all, male sex partners of women with BV are colonized with *Gardnerella, Mycoplasma*, and/or anaerobic bacteria, and that there may be an exchange of these microorganisms between partners during sexual intercourse. This concept is supported by the work of Piot et al. who showed that the *G. vaginalis* isolates from women with BV and from the urethra of their male sex partners belonged to identical biotypes more often than could be expected by chance ($p < 0.005$).[20] Larger controlled studies of the genital flora of women with BV and their partners are needed to clarify the role of the male partner as a reservoir for reinfection.

Is bacterial vaginosis sexually transmitted? The published literature contains conflicting evidence on the sexual transmissibility of BV, and few studies have examined the epidemiology of bacterial vaginosis as a clinical entity. There are two lines of evidence which suggest that bacterial vaginosis can be sexually transmitted: the recovery of BV-associated microorganisms from the male consorts of women with BV as discussed above, and the higher prevalence of BV among very sexually active women than among sexually inexperienced women. Amsel et al., in a study of female university students, found BV in 69 of 293 women who were sexually experienced and in none of 18 who were virgins ($p = 0.03$).[10] However, Bump and Bueschling have reported BV in 6 (12 percent) of 52 virgins.[21] Neither Amsel[10] nor Holst[19] found an association between age at first intercourse and BV, and Holst reported that women with BV did not have more sexual partners than normal women.[19]

Other epidemiological factors may also be important. Use of an intrauterine device was more common among women with BV in both Amsel's[10] (18.8 vs. 5.4 percent, $p < 0.001$) and Holst's[19] study (35 vs. 16 percent, $p < 0.25$). However, age, smoking status, history of abnormal Pap smears, days of menstrual flow, days since last menstrual period, form of menstrual protection, age at menarche, and years since menarche have not been associated with BV.[10,19]

## ETIOLOGY

### *Gardnerella vaginalis*

Leopold first reported the isolation of a small nonmotile nonencapsulated pleomorphic gram-negative rod from the genitourinary tract of women with cervicitis in 1953.[22] Two years later, Gardner and Dukes isolated this organism, which they named *Haemophilus vaginalis*, from 92 percent of 141 women with "bacterial vaginitis," from 20 percent of women with *Trichomonas vaginalis* infestation, from 4 percent of women with clinical moniliasis, and from none of 78 controls.[6] *H. vaginalis* was stated to be the sole bacterial isolate from the vagina from women with "vaginitis," despite the use of a variety of culture media under anaerobic as well as aerobic conditions. In an attempt to fulfill Koch's postulates, Gardner inoculated 15 women who were not infected by *H. vaginalis* with material from the vaginas of infected patients, and was able to reproduce the infection in 11 of 15 women. However, inoculation of pure *H. vaginalis* resulted in infection in only 1 of 13 women, even though *H. vaginalis* was isolated from the vagina of all of these women one or more weeks after they had been inoculated. Both Brewer[23] and Heltai[24] confirmed the association between nonspecific vaginitis and *H. vaginalis*. However, they did not find this organism to be the sole isolate from the vagina and concluded that *H. vaginalis* was not the sole etiologic agent of nonspecific vaginitis.

Adding to the uncertainty surrounding *H. vaginalis* was the lack of consensus on the taxonomic status of the microorganism. In 1963, Zinneman and Turner recommended the reclassification of the organism to the genus *Corynebacterium*, because under optimal growth conditions, it was gram-positive and formed polar granules.[25] Electron microscopy studies by Reyn et al. showed that the organism's cell wall resembled that of a gram-positive bacterium[26] while Criswell's electron microscopic studies of the same strain indicated that the organism was more probably gram-negative.[27] In 1980, Greenwood and Pickett resolved the issue by proposing a new genus, *Gardnerella*, "to include catalase and oxidase negative, gram negative to gram variable bacteria with laminated cell walls, which produce acetic acid as the major end product of fermentation."[28]

The body of literature over the past 30 years has substantiated Gardner and Dukes' observation that *Gardnerella vaginalis* is highly associated with bacterial vaginosis. However, with use of more sensitive culture media[29] *G. vaginalis* can be isolated, often in high concentrations, from women with no signs of vaginal infection. It is now thought that *G. vaginalis* somehow interacts with anaerobic bacteria and genital mycoplasmas (discussed below) to cause bacterial vaginosis.

## Anaerobic bacteria

Anaerobic rods and cocci were first isolated from the vagina in 1897[3] and were found to be associated with vaginal discharge by Curtis in the early part of this century.[1] Black-pigmented *Bacteroides* (the *Bacteroides melaninogenicus* group) and other *Bacteroides* spp. were linked with vaginitis by Hite in 1947,[30] Weaver in 1950,[5] and Hunter in 1958.[31] These investigators also noted a decrease in the proportion of women with lactobacilli among those with vaginal discharge. In 1979, Goldacre reported that gram-negative anaerobic bacilli were significantly more common among women with "troublesome vaginal discharge" than among normal women, and concluded that the association between genitourinary symptoms and anaerobes warranted further study.[32] In 1980, Spiegel analyzed the vaginal fluid from 53 women with bacterial vaginosis using quantitative anaerobic cultures and gas-liquid chromatography to detect the short-chain organic acid metabolites of the vaginal flora. *Bacteroides* spp. were isolated from 76 percent and *Peptococcus* (now called *Peptostreptococcus*) were recovered from 36 percent of the women with bacterial vaginosis; both types of anaerobes were isolated significantly less often from normal women.[8] The recovery of anaerobic species was directly correlated with a decrease in lactate and an increase in succinate and acetate in the vaginal fluid. After metronidazole therapy, the *Bacteroides* and peptostreptococci were not recovered from the women, and lactate again became the predominant organic acid in the vaginal fluid. Spiegel concluded that anaerobes interacted with *G. vaginalis* to cause bacterial vaginosis. Others have confirmed the association between anaerobes and BV.[11,33,34]

In our experience the *Bacteroides* spp. most commonly associated with BV are the black-pigmented species (*B. asaccharolyticus, B. intermedius, B. melaninogenicus, B. corporis,* and others), *B. bivius* and *B. ureolyticus*. Members of the *Bacteroides fragilis* group (*B. fragilis, B. ovatus, B. vulgatus, B. thetaiotaomicron*), which are common in the intestinal tract, are less commonly isolated from the vagina and are not associated with BV. Several species of fusobacteria have been isolated from women with BV, but much less frequently than the *Bacteroides* spp. Anaerobic gram-positive rods including anaerobic *Lactobacillus* spp., *Bifidobacterium* spp., and *Eubacterium* spp., may also be isolated from 10 to 30 percent of women with BV. Anaerobic gram-positive cocci (primarily peptostreptococci) are also usually recovered. Anaerobic gram-negative cocci (*Veillonella* spp.) are less frequently isolated. All these species are isolated less often from the normal vagina.

As research continued into the etiology of BV during the early 1980s another anaerobic microorganism, *Mobiluncus*, was implicated in the syndrome. A curved anaerobic rod was first observed by Gram stain of uterine discharge in 1895[35] by Kronig, was first isolated from the uterine discharge of women with postpartum fever by Curtis,[36] and was given the name "*Vibrio mulieris*" by Prevot in 1940.[37] Because this microorganism is nutritionally fastidious and strictly anaerobic, it was not detected by culture during the early studies of BV. However, in 1980, Durieux and Dublanchet characterized 18 strains of succinate-producing anaerobic curved rods which were isolated from women with vaginal discharge.[38] A number of researchers noted the association of this organism either with abnormal vaginal discharge or with clinical features of bacterial vaginosis.[39–42] Spiegel reported detection of this organism by direct Gram stain of the vaginal fluid from 31 (51 percent) of 62 women with BV and from none of 42 normal controls.[43] In 1984, Spiegel and Roberts proposed the genus name *Mobiluncus* for this motile rod. Two species were described: *M. curtisii* and *M. mulieris*.[44] *Mobiluncus* has been detected by DNA probe, culture, and/or Gram stain in 68 percent of women with BV in one study[45] and has recently been detected by fluorescent monoclonal antibodies in 50 percent of 107 women with and 17 (6 percent) of 291 women without clinical signs of BV.[11] The highest isolation rate for *Mobiluncus* spp. has been reported by Holst, who recovered *Mobiluncus* from the vagina and/or rectum of 29 (85 percent) of 34 women with BV. The isolation of *Mobiluncus* spp., from only the rectum of 7 of these women suggests that the gut may be a reservoir for this organism. *Mobiluncus* is always isolated from the vagina together with other organisms associated with BV.[46]

## Genital mycoplasmas

The association of genital mycoplasmas with vaginitis was noted in 1958 by Hunter and Long[31] who recovered pleuropneumonia-like microorganisms from 48 percent of 39 women with vaginitis and 14 percent of 48 control women ($p < 0.05$). Women harboring pleuropneumonia-like microorganisms, later recognized as mycoplasmas, were more likely to harbor other "abnormal" vaginal flora including anaerobic gram-negative rods and trichomonads. In 1970, Mendel reported that mycoplasmas were isolated from nearly half of patients with trichomoniasis or *Gardnerella vaginalis*, but that they were not linked to any specific disease.[47] Taylor-Robinson and McCormack first suggested that *Mycoplasma hominis* could have a role in nonspecific vaginitis, either in symbiosis with *Gardnerella vaginalis* and other organisms or as a sole pathogen.[48] This was supported by Pheifer et al. who reported that *M. hominis* was more prevalent among women with BV than among normal controls (63 vs. 10 percent).[17] In 1982, Paavonen et al. reported that *M. hominis* and *G. vaginalis* in vaginal fluid were each associated with bacterial vaginosis, as was the presence of succinate and other short-chain organic acids.[49] These authors concluded that the genital mycoplasmas should also be considered as potential etiologic agents of bacterial vaginosis, together with *G. vaginalis* and anerobic bacteria.

## Other microorganisms

*Escherichia coli* and other gram-negative bacteria, group B streptococci, enterococci, and most species of viridans streptococci are not associated with BV. However, two species of viridans group streptococci, *Streptococcus acidominimus* and *Streptococcus morbillorum*, each have been isolated significantly more often from the vaginas of women having bacterial vaginosis than from normal women.[50] There is no increase in colonization with coagulase-negative staphylococci or diphtheroids among those with BV.

It is apparent that no single organism is the etiologic agent of bacterial vaginosis. One multivariate analysis of vaginal flora data has shown that four categories of vaginal bacteria are independently associated with BV: *Mobiluncus* spp., *Bacteroides* spp., *Gardnerella vaginalis*, and *Mycoplasma hominis*.[51] The prevalence of each of these microorganisms is increased among women with BV. In addition, these organisms are present at 100- to 1000-fold greater concentrations among women with BV than among normal women. (See Figs. 47-1 through 47-4.)

## PATHOGENESIS

Bacterial vaginosis results from the replacement of the normal vaginal flora (*Lactobacillus*) with a mixed flora consisting of *Gardnerella vaginalis*, anaerobes, and *Mycoplasma hominis*.

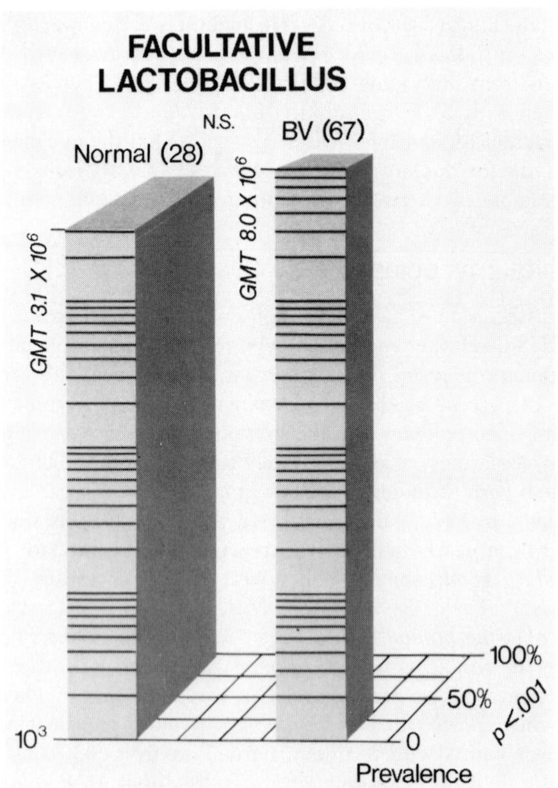


**Fig. 47-1.** While the prevalence of lactobacilli is decreased among women with BV, the geometric mean concentration (GMT) of lactobacilli among those who are colonized is about the same for women with or without BV. (*Courtesy of D. A. Eschenbach, unpublished data.*)

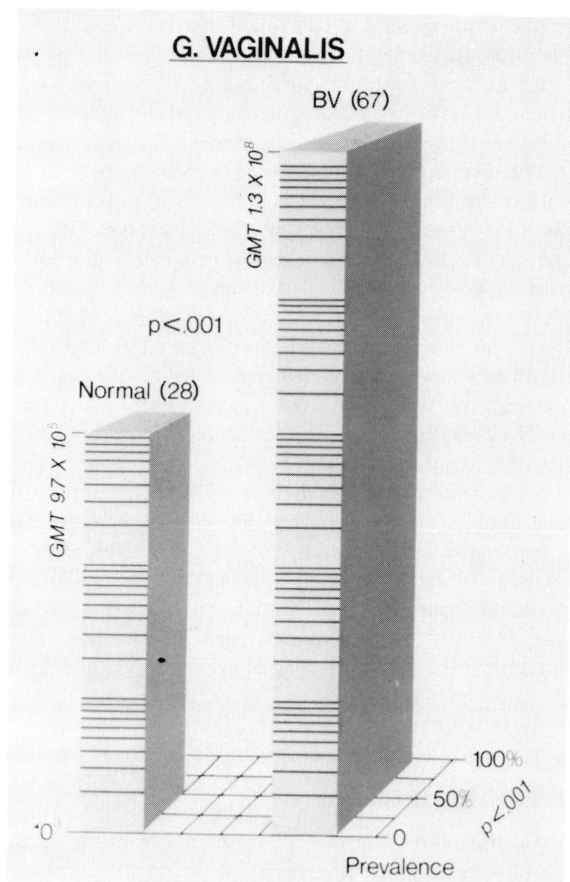


**Fig. 47-2.** The prevalence of *G. vaginalis* is nearly twice as high among women with bacterial vaginosis as among normal women. Among those who are colonized by *G. vaginalis*, the geometric mean concentration (GMT) of *G. vaginalis* for women with bacterial vaginosis is over 100 times higher than among normal women. (*Courtesy of D. A. Eschenbach, unpublished data.*)

Thus, most studies on the pathogenesis of BV have focused on how the microbial ecosystem of the vagina is altered. In an effort to experimentally reproduce the signs and symptoms of bacterial vaginosis, Criswell inoculated 29 normal pregnant women with 2 ml of suspension containing $2 \times 10^{10}$ *G. vaginalis*. Seven (24 percent) of the 29 women developed clinical signs of infection over the 3 weeks postinoculation.[52] However, no attempt was made to determine whether anaerobic bacteria or genital mycoplasmas were also present among those who acquired the clinical syndrome. In the grivet monkey model system, *Gardnerella vaginalis* or *Mobiluncus* sp. applied alone intravaginally did not cause signs of vaginitis. However, when two monkeys were inoculated with both *G. vaginalis* and *Mobiluncus*, vaginal discharge developed in both monkeys after 5 days.[53] These studies, together with epidemiologic data described above, are consistent with the notion that introduction of a particular set of organisms, perhaps via sexual intercourse, initiates the change in vaginal flora characteristic of BV.

*Lactobacillus* spp. may play a role in the ability of normal women to resist infection. Skarin has reported that vaginal lactobacilli inhibit *G. vaginalis, Mobiluncus,* and *Bacteroides* species in vitro.[54] While it has long been known that some strains of *Lactobacillus* produce $H_2O_2$,[55] recent studies have demonstrated that normal women are usually colonized by $H_2O_2$-producing

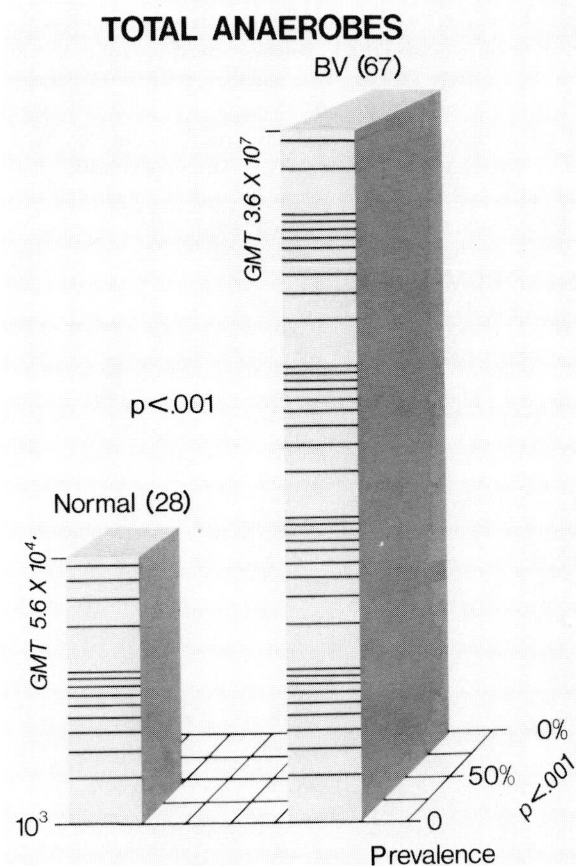


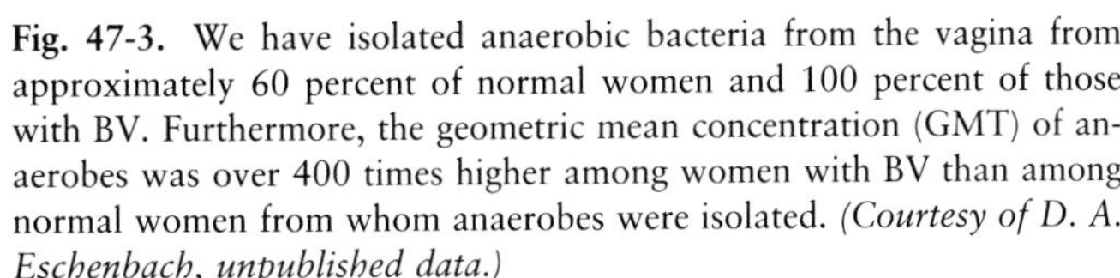

**Fig. 47-3.** We have isolated anaerobic bacteria from the vagina from approximately 60 percent of normal women and 100 percent of those with BV. Furthermore, the geometric mean concentration (GMT) of anaerobes was over 400 times higher among women with BV than among normal women from whom anaerobes were isolated. *(Courtesy of D. A. Eschenbach, unpublished data.)*

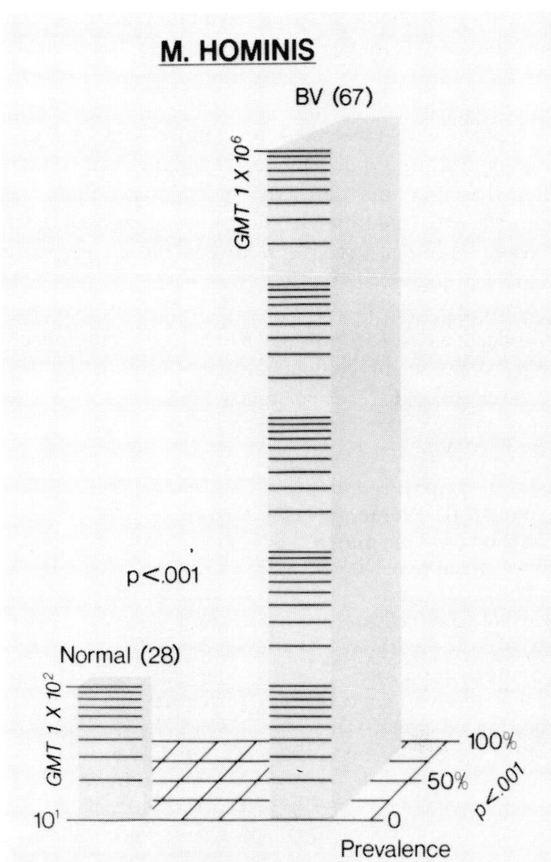


**Fig. 47-4.** We have isolated *Mycoplasma hominis* from 60 to 70 percent of women with BV and 20 percent of normal women. As with anaerobic bacteria and *Gardnerella vaginalis,* those women with BV have geometric mean concentrations (GMT) several logs higher than normal women colonized by *M. hominis*. *(Courtesy of D. A. Eschenbach, unpublished data.)*

strains of lactobacilli, while women with BV lack $H_2O_2$-producing strains. Further, during a prospective study, women colonized with $H_2O_2$-positive lactobacilli were less likely to develop bacterial vaginosis than were those women colonized with $H_2O_2$-negative lactobacilli.[56] The $H_2O_2$ produced by the vaginal lactobacilli may inhibit the growth of the *Bacteroides, Gardnerella, Mobiluncus,* and *Mycoplasma* in the vagina either directly via the toxic activity of $H_2O_2$ or by reacting with a halide ion in the presence of cervical peroxidase as part of the $H_2O_2$-halide-peroxidase antibacterial system. Further research is needed to clarify the role of $H_2O_2$-producing lactobacilli in modulating vaginal flora.

So far, no host factor has been identified that increases susceptibility to BV. A possible exception is IUD use, but the mechanisms by which IUD use may increase the risk of BV are not understood. The redox potential of the vaginal epithelial surface of women with BV is lower than that in normal women. After the women with BV were treated with metronidazole, the redox potential of the vaginal epithelium returned to the normal range, a result suggesting that the low vaginal Eh was not a persistent underlying host factor.[57]

It is thought that amines produced by the microbial flora, perhaps by microbial decarboxylases, account for the characteristic abnormal fishy odor which is produced when vaginal fluid is mixed with 10 percent KOH. This so-called "whiff test" is thought to be due to volatilization of aromatic amines including putrescine, cadaverine,[58] and trimethylamine[59] at alkaline pH. However, it is still unknown which, if any, organisms produce these amines. The microbial sources of the organic acids found in the vagina of normal women and women with BV is better defined.[8]

The effects of altered patterns of organic acids and of increased concentrations of certain amines are unknown, though it has been shown that certain organic acids found in the vagina with BV can be cytotoxic in sufficient concentration.[60] The effects of BV on the vaginal epithelium and on epithelial cell turnover have not yet been well studied. Nonetheless, there is evidence that the increased vaginal concentrations of anaerobic pathogens in BV may increase the risk of ascending upper genital tract infections discussed below.

## CLINICAL MANIFESTATIONS

In a recent case-control study involving sexually transmitted disease clinic patients with or without objective signs of BV by Gram stain criteria, bacterial vaginosis was significantly associated with symptoms of vaginal malodor (49 percent of patients with BV vs. 20 percent without BV) and vaginal discharge (50 percent of patients with BV vs. 37 percent without BV), although many women with this condition were asymptomatic.[12] Abdominal pain, pruritis, or dysuria were not associated with a clinical diagnosis of BV (Table 47-1). Examination revealed a nonviscous homogeneous, white, uniformly adherent vaginal discharge (69 percent women with vs. 3 percent of those without BV). This discharge is uniformly adherent to the vaginal walls and often visible on the labia and fourchette before insertion of a vaginal speculum (Plate 22). Although vaginal discharge was described as yellow by a third of women with BV, the number of polymorphonuclear leukocytes in vaginal discharge was not increased in this syndrome. Nearly all women with BV have a vaginal pH of ≥4.7 when measured with pH paper having an appropriate pH range, although this finding is by no means specific for BV. A fishy odor was noted when vaginal fluid was mixed with 10 percent KOH (the "whiff test") in 43 percent of those with vs. 1 percent of those without BV. Microscopic evaluation of vaginal fluid at high power (400×) revealed clue cells in 81 percent of those with vs. 6 percent of those without BV. Clue cells are epithelial cells whose margins are obscured by adherent bacteria (Fig. 47-5). Recent studies have demonstrated that clue cells are covered with *Gardnerella vaginalis*, as well as anaerobic species such as *Mobiluncus* (Plates 23 and 24).

## POSSIBLE COMPLICATIONS OF BACTERIAL VAGINOSIS

The morbidity of bacterial vaginosis has generally been measured in terms of the high prevalence of the condition and the associated

**Table 47-1. Symptoms and Signs among 661 Randomly Selected Women Attending a Sexually Transmitted Disease Clinic. Univariate and Multivariate Comparison of Patients with and without Gram Stain Criteria for Bacterial Vaginosis (See text for definition of Gram stain criteria)**

| | Bacterial vaginosis ($n$ = 311) % | No bacterial vaginosis ($n$ = 350) % | Univariate Odds ratio | Univariate $p$ | Multivariate* Odds ratio | Multivariate* $p$ |
|---|---|---|---|---|---|---|
| Symptoms | | | | | | |
| Chief complaint | | | | | | |
| None | 47 | 36 | 1.5 | 0.01 | 2.6 | 0.2 |
| Abdominal pain | 7 | 3 | 3.0 | 0.05 | 2.6 | 0.2 |
| Vaginal bleeding | 0.6 | 0.3 | 2.3 | 0.5 | 2.1 | 0.3 |
| Vaginal discharge | 17 | 7 | 2.9 | <0.0001 | 2.6 | 0.01 |
| Vulvar pruritus | 8 | 18 | 0.4 | <0.001 | 0.9 | 0.9 |
| Other (dysuria, ulcers) | 20 | 36 | 0.5 | <0.01 | 0.7 | 0.3 |
| Odor | 49 | 20 | 3.9 | <0.001 | 3.4 | <0.001 |
| Increased discharge | 50 | 37 | 1.7 | 0.001 | 1.3 | 0.005 |
| Yellow discharge | 24 | 17 | 1.6 | 0.01 | 1.2 | 0.08 |
| Abdominal pain | 45 | 35 | 1.5 | 0.01 | 1.2 | 0.4 |
| Increased amount of menstrual bleeding | 14 | 9 | 1.6 | 0.04 | 1.4 | 0.2 |
| Prolonged menses | 11 | 6 | 2.1 | 0.01 | 1.2 | 0.4 |
| Intermenstrual bleeding | 16 | 13 | 1.2 | 0.4 | 1.2 | 0.5 |
| Signs | | | | | | |
| Homogeneous discharge | 69 | 3 | 77 | <0.001 | 103 | <0.001 |
| Frothy discharge | 2 | 0 | | 0.007 | | |
| Increased discharge | 9 | 4 | 2.3 | 0.02 | 1.5 | 0.001 |
| Yellow vaginal discharge | 32 | 18 | 2.2 | 0.001 | 2.3 | 0.001 |
| Ectopy (any) | 51 | 52 | 1.0 | 0.8 | 1.1 | 0.8 |
| Ectopy (≥50%) | 7 | 8 | 0.8 | 0.4 | 1.2 | 0.8 |
| Mucopus | 28 | 21 | 1.5 | 0.03 | 1.2 | 0.4 |
| Adnexal tenderness⁺ | 4 | 0.3 | 12.9 | 0.002 | 9.2 | 0.04 |
| Uterine tenderness | 4 | 1 | 2.5 | 0.08 | 1.7 | 0.4 |
| Cervical motion tenderness | 3 | 0.6 | 4.6 | 0.04 | 2.8 | 0.2 |
| Clinical diagnosis of PID | 3 | 0 | | 0.003 | | |
| Macroscopic warts | 7 | 14 | 0.5 | 0.009 | 0.5 | 0.004 |
| Amine-like odor of vaginal fluid in potassium hydroxide | 43 | 1 | 88 | <0.001 | 113 | <0.001 |
| pH ≥ 4.7 | 97 | 47 | 30 | <0.001 | 23 | <0.001 |
| Mean pH ± SD | 5.0 ± 0.3 | 4.6 ± 0.3 | | | | |
| Microscopic result | | | | | | |
| Any clue cells | 81 | 6 | 69 | <0.001 | 75 | <0.001 |
| Clue cells ≥ 20% of epithelial cells | 78 | 5 | 72 | <0.001 | 88 | <0.001 |
| Cervical Gram stain ≥30 PMN/HPF | 28 | 22 | 1.4 | 0.08 | 1.1 | 0.7 |
| Vaginal wet mount ≥30 WBCs/HPF | 40 | 34 | 1.3 | 0.2 | 1.4 | 0.1 |
| Vaginal wet mount showing predominance of lactobacilli | 2 | 59 | 0.02 | <0.001 | 0.02 | <0.001 |

PID = pelvic inflammatory disease; PMNs = polymorphonuclear leukocytes; HPF = high power field; WBCs = white blood cells.

*Each sign was adjusted for age, race, parity, education, occupation, current smoking, age at first intercourse, lifetime sexual partners, *C. trachomatis*, *N. gonorrhoeae*, yeast, and herpes simplex virus in the analysis. Women with *Trichomonas vaginalis* were excluded from the analysis.

⁺Adnexal tenderness scored as moderate to severe.

SOURCE: Reference 12.

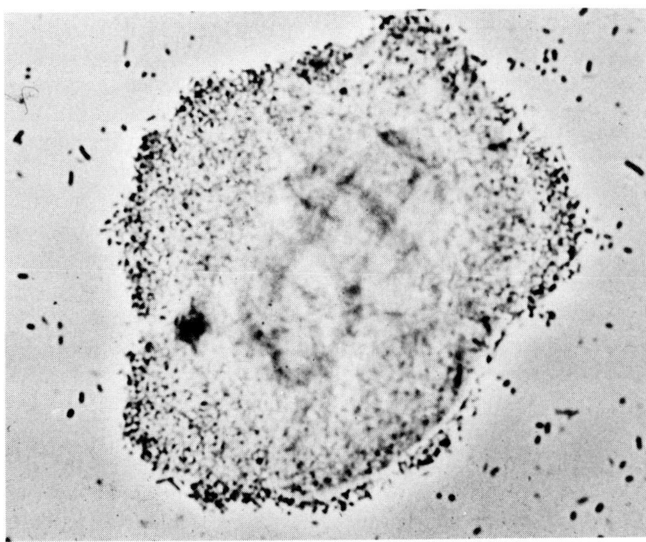

**Fig. 47-5.** Wet mount of vaginal fluid showing a typical clue cell from a woman with bacterial vaginosis. Note that the cell margins are obscured, ×1000 magnification.

psychological distress rather than in terms of the physical morbidity. However, the increased intravaginal concentrations of bacteria in bacterial vaginosis, together with the shift to a more virulent flora, may predispose to certain infectious obstetric complications, such as chorioamnionitis, amniotic fluid infection, and puerperal infectious morbidity, as well as to gynecologic complications such as pelvic inflammatory disease. Berman et al. recently reported that isolation of *Mycoplasma hominis* at the first prenatal visit was predictive of post-cesarean-section endometritis.[61] Our own data directly implicate bacterial vaginosis-associated organisms in amniotic fluid infection,[62] chorioamnionitis,[63] and postpartum endometritis and bacteremia.[64] Gravett demonstrated that BV, as diagnosed presumptively by gas chromatographic analysis of vaginal fluid, was significantly associated with preterm premature rupture of the membranes (odds ratio 2.0, 95 percent confidence interval 1.1 to 3.7), preterm labor (odds ratio 2.0, 95 percent confidence interval 1.1 to 3.5), and amniotic fluid infection (odds ratio 2.7, 95 percent confidence interval 1.1 to 6.1).[65] Martius showed that BV, as diagnosed by vaginal Gram smear, was associated with delivery before 37 weeks' gestation (odds ratio 2.3, 95 percent confidence interval 1.1 to 5.0).[51] We have recently found in a case-control study that BV is significantly associated with histologic evidence of chorioamnionitis, with recovery of BV-associated organisms from the space between the chorion and amnion, and preterm delivery.[63]

The concept that bacterial vaginosis may predispose nonpregnant women to polymicrobial upper genital tract infections, including endometritis and salpingitis, remains speculative. However, among randomly selected women attending an STD clinic, moderate to severe adnexal tenderness was detected in 11 (4 percent) of 293 women with BV vs. 1 (0.3 percent) of 333 women without BV (OR = 12.9, $p$ = 0.002).[12]

## DIAGNOSIS

Symptoms alone are not reliable for the diagnosis of bacterial vaginosis. Amsel et al. recommended basing the clinical diagnosis of bacterial vaginosis on the presence of three or four of the following signs:[10] (1) characteristic homogeneous white adherent discharge, (2) vaginal fluid pH> 4.5, (3) release of a fishy amine odor from vaginal fluid mixed with 10 percent KOH, and (4) presence of clue cells (usually representing at least 20 percent of vaginal epithelial cells). These simple clinical tests are inexpensive and available in most office settings. We agree with the original observation of Gardner and Dukes that detection of clue cells is the most useful single procedure for diagnosis of BV, but demonstration of the other features serves to support the microscopic interpretation of presence of clue cells.

### Discharge

The evaluation of the discharge can be difficult, especially when women have douched or have had recent intercourse. The discharge associated with bacterial vaginosis is white, nonfloccular, and adherent to the walls of the vagina and is not markedly increased over that normally seen. Some women with the other clinical signs of BV may have slight or no homogeneous discharge (Table 47-1), but BV should not be ruled out if the other, more objective signs are present.

### Vaginal fluid pH

The vaginal fluid pH should be measured using pH paper having appropriate range (pH 4.0 to 6.0). Commercially available pH paper which is suitable for this purpose includes colopHast® pH 4.0 to 7.0 (MCB Reagents, 480 Democrat Rd., Gibbstown, NJ 98027) or pHydrion paper® pH 3.0 to 5.5 (Micro Essential Laboratory, Brooklyn, NY 11210). Vaginal pH is best determined by swabbing the lateral and posterior fornices of the vagina, and then placing the sample directly on the pH paper. Alternatively, the pH paper can be placed on the surface of the speculum after it has removed from the vagina. The cervical mucus must be avoided since it has a higher pH (pH 7.0) than the vaginal fluid. Eschenbach has reported that none of 178 women with pH ≤ 4.4 had clue cells, while all of 257 women who had ≥ 20 percent clue cells had vaginal pH ≥ 4.7. Of these 257 women, 89 percent had a homogeneous discharge, an amine odor, or both.[12] Vaginal fluid pH has the greatest sensitivity of the four clinical signs, but the lowest specificity.

### Odor

Vaginal malodor is the most common symptom of women with BV, and release of the "fishy" amines from vaginal fluid after addition of 10 percent KOH greatly increases the detection of malodor. A drop of vaginal fluid should be placed on a glass slide and a drop of 10 percent KOH added. The amines are released immediately and the odor dissipates quickly. A coverslip may be placed over this preparation for microscopic exam for the hyphal forms associated with candidiasis. Although Bump has reported the KOH odor test to be the most powerful single predictor for diagnosis of BV,[66] we find this test is the least sensitive of the four clinical tests for diagnosis of BV. Eschenbach et al. reported a positive predictive value of only 76 percent[12] for this test compared with Gram stain diagnosis of BV.

### Wet mount exam for clue cells

Clue cells are squamous vaginal epithelial cells which are covered with many vaginal bacteria, giving them a stippled or granular appearance. The borders are obscured or fuzzy owing to adherence of small rods or cocci (Fig. 47-5). Recent studies have shown that *Gardnerella, Mobiluncus,* and other bacteria may adhere to the vaginal epithelial cells. Lactobacilli may also bind to exfoliated vaginal epithelial cells, although they are seldom present in high enough concentrations to completely obscure the edges of the epithelial cell and with experience should not be confused with true clue cells. We recommend that at least 20 percent of vaginal epithelial cells present be noted as clue cells to establish the diagnosis of BV. However, in our experience, even if only 1 to 20 percent of vaginal epithelial cells are noted to be clue cells by an experienced microscopist, this is highly correlated with Gram stain features of BV.

Clue cells are found by obtaining a sample of vaginal fluid with a swab and mixing this on a glass slide with a drop of normal saline. A coverslip should be placed over the suspension and 10 fields examined under high power (400×). This suspension can also be used for detection of motile trichomonads. The presence of clue cells is the finding most closely associated with the diagnosis of BV by Gram stain.[12]

## LABORATORY TESTS FOR DIAGNOSIS OF BACTERIAL VAGINOSIS

### VAGINAL CULTURE

Cultures for *Gardnerella vaginalis* are often obtained, but their usefulness for the diagnosis of BV is doubtful. While *G. vaginalis* can be recovered from nearly all women with BV, it has been recovered from up to 58 percent of those without composite clinical criteria for BV.[12] In one study, the presence of ≥3+ *G. vaginalis* by culture had a positive predictive value of only 49 percent with respect to composite clinical signs for the diagnosis of BV (Fig. 47-6).[12] Vaginal Gram stains had comparable levels of sensitivity, but a much greater specificity and predictive value than vaginal cultures for *G. vaginalis*. A positive vaginal culture for *G. vaginalis* in the absence of the clinical signs of BV should not be used as a basis for therapy. Likewise, *G. vaginalis* cultures are of little benefit for "test of cure" since many women without clinical signs of BV will be culture-positive for this organism following effective treatment.

### GRAM STAINED SMEARS OF VAGINAL FLUID

Diagnosis of BV by direct evaluation of vaginal Gram smears was first suggested by Dunkelberg,[67] and specific guidelines were later published by Spiegel.[68] This method is based upon the shift in flora associated with BV from predominance of lactobacilli (Fig. 47-7) to predominance of *Gardnerella* and anaerobic bacterial morphotypes (Fig. 47-8). Spiegel defined BV as the presence of *Gardnerella* plus some other bacterial morphotype, together with no more than five lactobacilli morphotypes per oil immersion field. This method has been reported to have 93 percent sensitivity and 79 percent specificity for diagnosis of BV as defined by clinical criteria.[12] The vaginal smear for Gram stain evaluation can be prepared at the same time that the wet mount is prepared by rolling (not streaking) the swab across the surface of a glass slide. The slide should be air-dried and can be stored for months or years prior to staining with no appreciable loss in quality. The slide should be heat-fixed and stained as usual in the clinical lab. The advantages of Gram stain for diagnosis are: the smear can be interpreted by standardized criteria by a microbiologist, it is suitable for quick screening, and it can be stored for batch reading or later confirmation if desired. We do not recommend treatment of women without symptoms or signs of BV, regardless of the presence of Gram stain features of BV. This view may change in the future if the role of BV as a risk factor for upper genital tract infection is confirmed.

### DIAGNOSTIC TESTS FOR BV BASED UPON METABOLIC PRODUCTS

Several methods have been published which are based on the detection of metabolic products of the microorganisms in the vaginal fluid of women with BV. We regard all of these to be tools for research on BV at the present time.

#### Gas chromatographic analysis of vaginal fluid

Gas chromatographic analysis of vaginal fluid can detect metabolic by-products of the bacteria living in the vagina. When lactobacilli are predominant, the lactic acid produced from glucose via the glycolytic pathway is the primary short-chain fatty acid

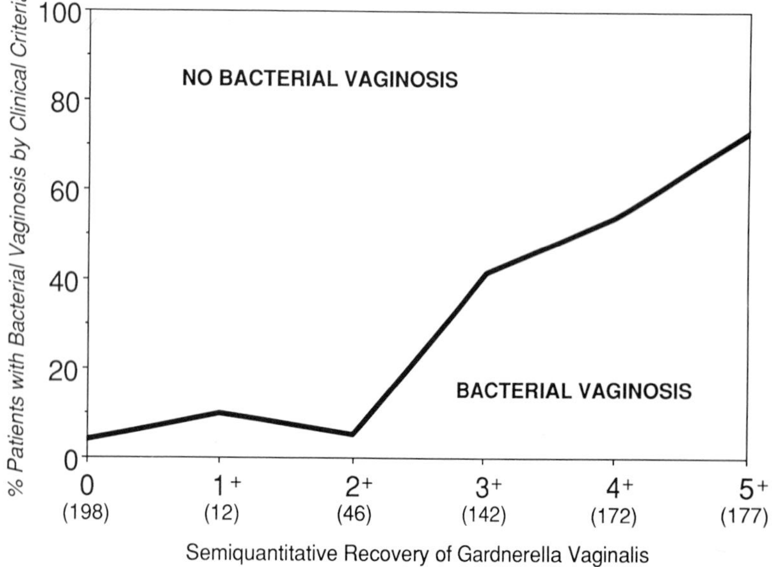


**Fig. 47-6.** Semiquantitative recovery of *Gardnerella vaginalis* from women with or without clinical signs of bacterial vaginosis. Of those women whose cultures yielded 3+ *G. vaginalis*, only half had BV. Even among women yielding 5+ *G. vaginalis*, 25 percent did not have clinical signs of BV. Because *G. vaginalis* can be isolated in high quantities from many women without clinical signs of BV, vaginal cultures for *Gardnerella* are not useful for diagnosis of BV.

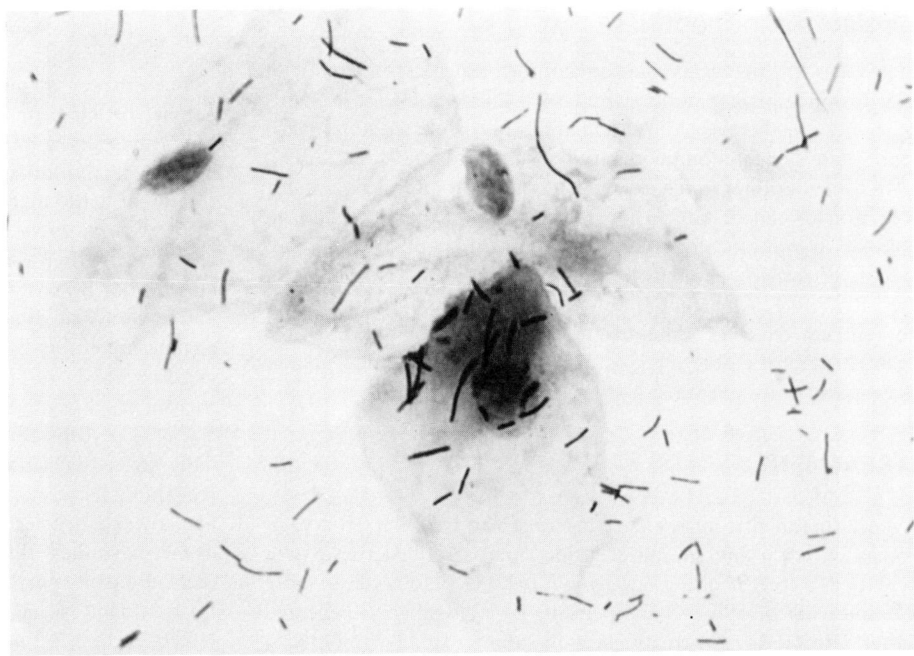

**Fig. 47-7.** Gram stain of normal vaginal fluid, showing gram-positive rods with blunt ends consistent with lactobacilli, ×1000 magnification.

present. Among women with BV, succinate, acetate, and less often other short-chain fatty acids including proprionate, butyrate, isobutyrate, or valeric acids can be detected. Since many of these bacteria also produce lactic acid during metabolism, lactic acid will usually be present as well. Spiegel[8] first described the gas chromatographic analysis of short-chain fatty acids of the vaginal fluid of women with BV and suggested that a succinate:lactate ratio of ≥0.4 was consistent with BV.

As described by Spiegel, this test had a 90 percent sensitivity and 97 percent specificity for the diagnosis of BV. However, in our studies up to 30 percent of vaginal wash specimens are not interpretable because there are no detectable peaks in the gas chromatographic analysis of the vaginal fluid specimens (Hillier, unpublished observation). In a study of 500 women attending a gynecology clinic, Thomason reported a sensitivity of 54 percent and a specificity of 94 percent for GLC[69] compared with clinical signs of BV.

## Thin-layer chromatography for determination of diamines in vaginal fluid

This test is based on the finding by Chen et al.[70] that women with clinical signs of BV have putrescine and cadaverine in the vaginal fluid. The sensitivity of this test was found to be 87 percent with a specificity of 86 percent. This test is suitable for screening large numbers of patient samples. With the appropriate equipment, about 60 to 100 vaginal washings can be analyzed by one person in 8 h.

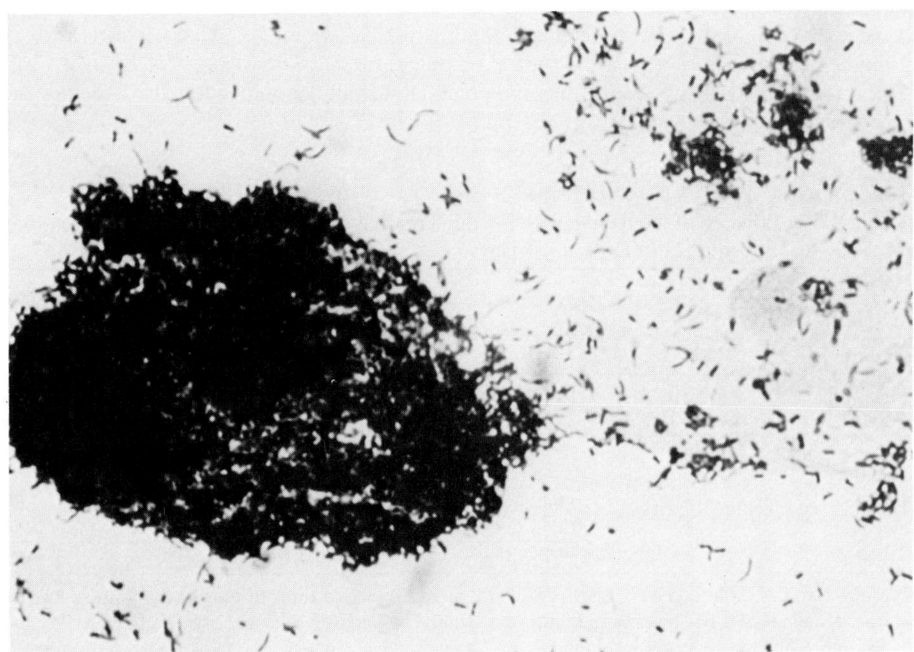

**Fig. 47-8.** Gram stain of vaginal fluid from a woman with bacterial vaginosis showing absence of lactobacilli and large numbers of gram-negative or gram-variable coccobacilli. Curved gram-variable rods are consistent with *Mobiluncus*. Note that epithelial cell on the left is a clue cell, while the epithelial cell to the right has clear margins, ×1000 magnification.

### Proline aminopeptidase test

The basis for this test is that some of the bacteria associated with BV produce proline aminopeptidase, while lactobacilli lack this enzyme. For this procedure vaginal fluid is incubated in a microtiter plate system along with enzyme substrate for 4 h at 35.5°C. After incubation, rapid garnet green is added to produce the color reaction. A red or pink color indicates a positive test, while an orange or yellow color is a negative test. In a study of 500 consecutive women, Thomason found that this test was 81 percent sensitive and 96 percent specific for diagnosis of BV as defined by clinical criteria.[69] The advantages claimed for this test over gas chromatographic analysis of vaginal fluid included greater sensitivity and lower cost and time required.

## TREATMENT

Many therapeutic agents have been used to treat bacterial vaginosis with varying success. Gardner first described triple sulfa cream as a treatment for *G. vaginalis* in 1955.[6] However, in more recent studies, only 27 (52 percent) of 52 women were cured after 7 to 10 days of treatment with sulfa cream.[17,71,72] Both *G. vaginalis* and *Bacteroides* are resistant to sulfonamides at the concentration usually considered clinically relevant. Although these organisms are inhibited by the concentrations found in the cream itself,[73,74] the clinical relevance of this is dubious. Sulfa creams have a low clinical efficacy rate and are inappropriate for treatment of BV.

There are many published studies on the efficacy of oral metronidazole given in doses of 800 to 1200 mg/day for 7 days. A number of investigators have proposed a single 2-g dose of metronidazole for treatment of BV. However, in studies comparing a single 2-g dose vs. 800 to 1200 mg of metronidazole per day for 7 days, 5 of 6 comparative studies of women followed 4 or more weeks after onset of therapy showed lower cure rates with the single-dose regimen.[7,74–78] When results from the 6 studies are combined, cure rates at least 4 weeks after therapy were 73 percent with this single dose vs. 82 percent with the 1-week dose ($p = 0.03$), Table 47-2.

A few women have been treated with 500-mg metronidazole tablets intravaginally for 7 days with 71 percent efficacy at 1 week.[79] Vaginal sponges containing 250 mg[80] to 1000 mg metronidazole have also been used as topical treatment for BV. The efficacy of this approach, which has the potential advantage of higher vaginal levels of drug with lower systemic side effects, is not yet known.

The efficacy of metronidazole is probably attributable to the activity of this drug against anaerobic bacteria[74] and the activity of its hydroxymetabolite against *G. vaginalis*.[81] Metronidazole and its metabolites are not active in vitro against *M. hominis*, yet treatment with metronidazole apparently eradicates this organism.[82] *Mobiluncus curtisii* is resistant to metronidazole,[43] but it is not yet known whether this plays a role in persistence or recurrence of BV after metronidazole treatment.

Clindamycin, another antibiotic which is particularly active against anaerobic bacteria and moderately active against *G. vaginalis* and *M. hominis* has been used in a topical cream for the treatment of bacterial vaginosis.[83] In a dose evaluation study, 5 g of 2 percent clindamycin cream applied intravaginally once daily for 7 days had an efficacy of 93 percent in 18 women reevaluated 4 weeks after onset of therapy. Lower concentrations had lower efficacies. If these preliminary findings are confirmed in larger studies, this compound may provide an alternative to metronidazole, particularly for the treatment of recurrent BV and for treatment of BV during pregnancy.

Beta lactam antibiotics, including ampicillin, amoxicillin, and pivampicillin, are less effective against BV than metronidazole. Cure rates for ampicillin have varied from 33 to 100 percent, with a mean of 66 percent.[17,72,85–86] A small trial of amoxicillin yielded a similar efficacy.[76] One possible explanation for the poor efficacy of beta lactam antibiotics is the production of beta lactamases by many of the *Bacteroides* spp. which can be isolated from the vagina. In a small study by Symonds, six women were treated with amoxicillin plus clavulanic acid, an inhibitor of beta lactamase, and all were cured.[87] In a larger open study (R. Barnes, K. Holmes, S. Hillier, C. Lipinski, unpublished), 14 of 18 women were cured using this regimen. Still, the relative inefficiency of penicillins compared with metronidazole may result not from beta lactamase production but from the nonselective activity of penicillin against normal lactobacilli, as well as against BV-associated flora. Accordingly, lactobacilli may repopulate the vagina more readily during metronidazole therapy than during ampicillin therapy,[84] which might contribute to the higher cure rate with metronidazole.

Erythromycin is not effective,[88] nor is tetracycline or doxycycline, which have reported efficacy of only 13 to 50 percent against BV.[17,72,89] Other alternative therapies which have been described include acetic acid gel,[90] and Dienoestrol cream,[91]

**Table 47-2. Efficacy of Metronidazole for the Treatment of BV. A Comparison of 2-g Single Dose vs. 800- to 1200-mg Daily Dose for 7 Days**

| | | Cure* 1–2 weeks after onset of therapy | | Cure ≥4 weeks after onset of therapy | |
|---|---|---|---|---|---|
| Author | Ref | 2 g | 7 g | 2 g | 7 g |
| Blackwell | 7 | 16/20 (80%) | 20/20 (100%) | 10/20 (50%) | 12/20 (60%) |
| Eschenbach | 75 | 27/33 (85%) | 39/52 (93%) | 24/35 (69%) | 29/38 (82%) |
| Hovik | 76 | — | — | 18/20 (90%) | 17/19 (89%) |
| Jerve | 77 | — | — | 70/83 (84%) | 83/97 (87%) |
| Jones | 74 | 41/47 (87%) | 30/33 (91%) | 24/34 (71%) | 22/28 (79%) |
| Swedberg | 78 | 39/46 (85%) | 35/36 (97%) | 20/34 (47%) | 26/30 (87%) |
| Total | | 124/148 (84%) | 125/131 (95%) $p^{\dagger} = 0.003$ | 166/226 (73%) | 191/232 (82%) $p^{\dagger} = 0.03$ |

*In most studies, failure is defined by persistence or recurrence of three of four of the following: clue cells, amine odor, homogeneous discharge, and elevated vaginal pH. For Swedberg, failure was defined by persistence or recurrence of clue cells.
†Chi square test for comparison of efficacy of 2-g vs. 7-g regimen.

which have been found to be unsatisfactory, with cure rates of only 7 and 6 percent. Povidone-iodine vaginal tablets, 200 mg twice daily for 2 weeks, were completely ineffective.[92]

## UNRESOLVED ISSUES IN PATIENT MANAGEMENT

### How common is late recurrence and why does it happen?

In 1955, Gardner noted that "before the advent of antibiotics and sulfonamides, the treatment of bacterial vaginitis was discouraging because eradication of the causative organism was difficult and recurrences were common."[6] Unfortunately, 35 years after Gardner made his initial observation, the treatment of BV can still be discouraging because of the high rate of recurrent infection. In our studies, up to 80 percent of women develop recurrent BV within 9 months after metronidazole therapy (unpublished data). The reasons for recurrence are not understood. Four possible explanations include (1) reinfection by a male partner who is colonized with BV-associated microorganisms, (2) recurrence due to the persistence of BV-associated microorganisms which are inhibited, but not killed, during therapy, (3) the failure to reestablish the normal, and perhaps protective, *Lactobacillus*-predominant flora following therapy, and (4) persistence of another, yet-unidentified host factor in the patient making her susceptible to recurrence. Until these questions are resolved, it is difficult to devise effective strategies for prevention of recurrence.

### Should male partners be treated?

While many women believe that they have contracted the infection from a male partner, no study to date has convincingly shown that treatment of the male partner decreases the rate of recurrence,[78] although randomized placebo-controlled trials with long-term follow-up in monogamous couples are lacking. For this reason, we do not recommend routine treatment of the male partner at present, but do believe better data on this approach are needed.

### Are over-the-counter preparations of lactobacilli useful?

A number of women have used over-the-counter lactobacilli products to attempt to reconstitute the vaginal flora. These include acidophilus milk, yogurt or various *Lactobacillus*-containing capsules, and powders available from health food stores. Some of the earliest treatments for bacterial vaginosis involved attempts to restore the vaginal flora by application of *Lactobacillus* preparations.[93,94] Butler reported that 18 of 19 patients were cured after receiving 1 to 8 applications of pure culture of human-derived strain of Doderlein bacillus at weekly intervals.[95] However, in a more recent study only 1 of 14 women were cured after applying yogurt intravaginally twice daily for 7 days.[91]

While the idea of inoculating the vagina with exogenous lactobacilli to restore the normal flora may be rational, there are a number of arguments against this course. Bacteria found in an ecologic niche are uniquely adapted to that particular environment. Therefore, the lactobacilli found in dairy products are commercial strains which have been adapted to the dairy food industry. A study by Wood showed that these commercial strains adhered more poorly to vaginal epithelial strains, when compared with human-derived strains of *Lactobacillus*.[96] Strains of lactobacilli which do not adhere well to vaginal epithelial cells are probably less likely to successfully colonize the vagina. We have recently reported that 9 of 16 *Lactobacillus* preparations commercially available in the United States were contaminated with other bacteria, and 5 of 16 did not contain $H_2O_2$-producing strains known to be protective in the vagina.[97] It is unlikely that available products are of therapeutic value for the treatment or prevention of BV.

### Should women with signs of BV be treated if they are asymptomatic?

In our experience, some women are aware of their discharge or odor but discount it because it has been present for months or even years. Thus, many women who do not present with symptoms will acknowledge symptoms of odor and/or discharge on questioning. Women with BV should be informed of their diagnosis, and treatment should be offered if requested. However, a recommendation for routine treatment of all women with BV awaits further studies defining risks of upper tract infection among women with BV.

### Should pregnant women with BV be treated?

Several studies have shown an association between bacterial vaginosis and pregnancy complications including preterm labor, preterm delivery, chorioamnionitis, and amniotic fluid infection. Although the studies suggest that BV may be a risk factor for pregnancy complications, the effect of treatment of BV during pregnancy to decrease the incidence of these complications has not been studied. Carefully controlled trials of treatment of BV among pregnant women must be conducted and must show benefit exceeding cost and risk of treatment before screening and treatment of all pregnant women with BV can be recommended.

Whether to treat pregnant women with symptomatic BV is dependent on the discretion of the clinician. While metronidazole, 500 mg twice daily for 7 days, is sometimes given after the first trimester, some clinicians have concerns about the possibility of a teratogenic effect of metronidazole in humans. Topical therapy with intravaginal metronidazole or clindamycin may be more acceptable for use during pregnancy; however, these therapies are not yet commercially available.

## PREVENTION

Since the microbiologic and host risk factors for acquisition of BV are poorly understood, it is difficult to define useful approaches for the prevention of this condition. Since BV is associated with sexual activity, abstinence or condom use may provide the best means of prevention. Since the prevalence of sexual transmission in BV is not well defined, and since concurrent treatment of male partners has not yet been shown to prevent recurrent BV, it cannot be recommended that the male sex partners of women with BV be treated. Recolonization of the vagina with lactobacilli may provide a host defense to infection by BV-associated organisms. However, deliberate vaginal recolonization has not yet been adequately evaluated as a method for prevention of BV. Similarly, treatment of BV has not yet been adequately evaluated as a method for preventing pregnancy and puerperal morbidity or postgynecological surgery morbidity.

## References

1 Curtis AH: On the etiology and bacteriology of leucorrhoea. *Surg Gynecol Obstet* 18: 229, 1914.

2 Doderlein A: *Das Scheidensekret und seine Bedeutung für das Puerperalfieber*. Leipzig, O. Durr. 1892.

3 Menge C, Kronig B: Bakteriologie des weiblichen Genitalkanales. *Monatschr Geburtsh* 9: 703, 1899.

4 Schroder R: Zur pathogenese und Klinik des vaginalen Fluors. *Zentralb Gynakol* 38: 1350, 1921.

5 Weaver JD et al: The bacterial flora found in nonspecific vaginitis vaginal discharge. *Am J Obstet Gynecol* 60: 880, 1950.

6 Gardner HL, Dukes CD: *Haemophilus vaginalis* vaginitis. A newly defined specific infection previously classified "nonspecific vaginitis." *Am J Obstet Gynecol* 69: 962, 1955.

7 Blackwell et al: Anaerobic vaginosis (nonspecific vaginitis): Clinical, microbiological and therapeutic findings. *Lancet* ii: 1379, 1983.

8 Spiegel CA et al: Anaerobic bacteria in nonspecific vaginitis. *N Engl J Med* 303: 601, 1980.

9 Berg AO et al: Establishing the cause of genitourinary symptoms in women in a family practice. *JAMA* 251: 620, 1984.

10 Amsel R et al: Nonspecific vaginitis: Diagnostic criteria and microbial and epidemiologic associations. *Am J Med* 74: 14, 1983.

11 Hallen A et al: Bacterial vaginosis in women attending STD clinic: Diagnostic criteria and prevalence of *Mobiluncus* spp. *Genitourin Med* 63: 386, 1987.

12 Eschenbach DA et al: Diagnosis and clinical manifestation of bacterial vaginosis. *Am J Obstet Gynecol* 158: 819, 1988.

13 Hill LH et al: Nonspecific vaginitis and other genital infections in three clinic populations. *Sex Transm Dis* 10: 114, 1983.

14 Hill LVH et al: Prevalence of lower genital tract infections in pregnancy. *Sex Transm Dis* 15: 5, 1988.

15 Shafer MA et al: Microbiology of the lower genital tract in postmenarchal adolescent girls: Differences by sexual activity, contraception, and presence of nonspecific vaginitis. *J Pediatr* 107: 974, 1985.

16 Bump RC et al: Sexually transmissable infections agents in sexually active and virginal asymptomatic adolescent girls. *Pediatrics* 77: 488, 1986.

17 Pheifer TA et al: Nonspecific vaginitis. Role of *Haemophilus vaginalis* and treatment with metronidazole. *N Engl J Med* 298: 1429, 1978.

18 Ison CA, Easmon CSF: Carriage of *Gardnerella vaginalis* and anaerobes in semen. *Genitourin Med* 60: 120, 1985.

19 Holst E et al: Bacterial vaginosis: Microbiological and clinical findings. *Eur J Clin Microbiol* 6: 536, 1987.

20 Piot P et al: Biotypes of *Gardnerella vaginalis*. *J Clin Microbiol* 22: 677, 1984.

21 Bump RC, Bueschling WJ: Bacterial vaginosis in virginal and sexually active adolescent females: Evidence against exclusive sexual transmission. *Am J Obstet Gynecol* 159: 935, 1988.

22 Leopold S: Heretofore undescribed organisms isolated from the genitourinary system. *US Armed Forces Med J* 4: 263, 1953.

23 Brewer JL et al: *Haemophilus vaginalis* vaginitis. *Am J Obstet Gynecol* 74: 834, 1957.

24 Heltai A, Taleghany P: Nonspecific vaginal infections: A critical evaluation of *Haemophilus vaginalis. Am J Obstet Gynecol* 77: 144, 1959.

25 Zinneman K, Turner GC: The taxonomic position of *"Haemophilus vaginalis" (Corynebacterium vaginale)*. *J Pathol Bacteriol* 85: 213, 1963.

26 Reyn A et al: An electron microscope study of this sections of *Haemophilus vaginalis* (Gardner and Dukes) and some possibly related species. *Can J Microbiol* 12: 1125, 1966.

27 Criswell BS et al: *Haemophilus vaginalis* 594, a gram-negative organism? *Can J Microbiol* 17: 865, 1972.

28 Greenwood JR, Pickett MJ: Transfer of *Haemophilus vaginalis* Gardner and Dukes to a new genus, *Gardnerella: G. vaginalis* (Gardner and Dukes) comb. nov. *Int J Syst Bacteriol* 30: 170, 1980.

29 Totten PA et al: Selective differential human blood bilayer media for isolation of *Gardnerella (Haemophilus) vaginalis*. *J Clin Microbiol* 15: 141, 1982.

30 Hite KE et al: A study of the bacterial flora of the normal and pathologic vagina and uterus. *Am J Obstet Gynecol* 53: 233, 1947.

31 Hunter CA, Long KR: A study of the microbiological flora of the vagina. *Am J Obstet Gynecol* 75: 865, 1958.

32 Goldacre MJ et al: Vaginal microbial flora in normal young women. *Br Med J* 1: 1450, 1979.

33 Piot P et al: The vaginal microbial flora in nonspecific vaginitis. *Eur J Clin Microbiol* 1: 301, 1982.

34 Fredricsson B et al: *Gardnerella*-associated vaginitis and anaerobic bacteria. *Gynecol Obstet Invest* 17: 236, 1984.

35 Kronig I: Über die Natur der Scheidenkeime, speciell über das Vorkommen anaerober Streptokokken im Scheidensekret Schwangerer. *Zentralb Gynakol* 19: 409, 1895.

36 Curtis AH: A motile curved anaerobic bacillus in uterine discharges. *J Infect Dis* 12: 165, 1913.

37 Prevot AR: *Manuel de Classification et de Determination des Bacteries Anaerobies*. Paris, Masson et Cie, 1940.

38 Durieux R, Dublanchet A: Les "vibrions" anaerobies des leucorrhees. I. Technique d'isolemont et sensibilité aux antibiotiques. *Med Mal Infect* 10: 109, 1980.

39 Hjelm E et al: Anerobic curved rods in vaginitis. *Lancet* ii: 1353, 1981.

40 Holst E et al: Characteristics of anaerobic comma-shaped bacteria recovered from the female genital tract. *Eur J Clin Microbiol* 1: 310, 1982.

41 Phillips I, Taylor E: Anaerobic curved rods in vaginitis. *Lancet* i: 221, 1982.

42 Sprott MS et al: Characteristics of motile curved rods in vaginal secretions. *J Med Microbiol* 16: 175, 1983.

43 Spiegel CA et al: Curved anaerobic bacteria in bacterial (nonspecific) vaginosis and their response to antimicrobial therapy. *J Infect Dis* 148: 817, 1983.

44 Spiegel CA, Roberts MC: *Mobiluncus* gen nov, *Mobiluncus curtisii* subsp. curtisii sp. nov., *Mobiluncus curtisii* subsp. *holmesii* subsp. nov., and *Mobiluncus mulieris* sp. nov., curved rods from the human vagina. *Int J Syst Bacteriol* 34: 177, 1984.

45 Roberts MC et al: Comparison of Gram stain, DNA probe, and culture for the identification of species of *Mobiluncus* in female genital specimens. *J Infect Dis* 152: 74, 1985.

46 Thomason JL et al: Clinical and microbiological characterization of patients with nonspecific vaginosis associated with motile, curved anaerobic rods. *J Infect Dis* 149: 801, 1984.

47 Mendel EB et al: *Mycoplasma* species in the vagina and their relation to vaginitis. *Obstet Gynecol* 35: 104, 1970.

48 Taylor-Robinson D, McCormack WM: The genital mycoplasmas. *N Engl J Med* 302: 1003, 1980.

49 Paavonen J et al: *Mycoplasma hominis* in nonspecific vaginitis. *Sex Transm Dis* 10: 271, 1983.

50 Rabe LK et al: Association of viridans group streptococci from pregnant women with bacterial vaginosis and upper genital tract infection. *J Clin Microbiol* 26: 1156, 1988.

51 Martius J et al: Relationships of vaginal *Lactobacillus* species, cervical *Chlamydia trachomatis* and bacterial vaginosis to preterm birth. *Obstet Gynecol* 71: 89, 1988.

52 Criswell BS et al: *Haemophilus vaginalis:* Vaginitis by inoculation from culture. *Obstet Gynecol* 33: 195, 1969.

53 Mardh P-A et al: The grivet monkey as a model for study of vaginitis. Challenge with anaerobic curved rods and *Gardnerella vaginalis*, in *Bacterial Vaginosis*, P-A Mardh, D Taylor-Robinson (eds). Stockholm, Almqvist and Wiksell, 1984, p 117.

54 Skarin A, Sylwan J: Vginal lactobacilli inhibiting growth of *Gardnerella vaginalis, Mobiluncus* and other bacterial species cultured from vaginal content of women with bacterial vaginosis. *Acta Pathol Microbiol Immunol Scand Sect B* 94: 399, 1986.

55 Whittenbury R: Hydrogen peroxide formation and catalase activity in the lactic acid bacteria. *J Gen Microbiol* 35: 13, 1964.

56 Hillier SL et al: $H_2O_2$-producing lactobacilli and *Bacteroides* species as predictors of acquisition of bacterial vaginosis during pregnancy: A prospective study. Abstracts Annual Meeting International Society for STD Research, 1987.

57 Holmes KK et al: Vaginal redox potential in bacterial vaginosis (nonspecific vaginitis). *J Infect Dis* 152: 379, 1985.
58 Chen KCS et al: Amine content of vaginal fluid from untreated and treated patients with nonspecific vaginitis. *J Clin Invest* 63: 828, 1979.
59 Brand JM, Galask, RP: Trimethylamine: The substance mainly responsible for the fishy odor often associated with bacterial vaginosis. *Obstet Gynecol* 63: 682, 1986.
60 Singer RE, Buchner BA: Butyrate and propionate: Important components of toxic dental placque extracts. *Infect Immun* 32: 458, 1981.
61 Berman SM et al: Low birth weight, prematurity, and postpartum endometritis. Association with prenatal cervical *Mycoplasma hominis* and *Chlamydia trachomatis* infection. *JAMA* 257: 1189, 1987.
62 Gravett MG et al: Preterm labor associated with subclinical amniotic fluid infection and with bacterial vaginosis. *Obstet Gynecol* 67: 229, 1986.
63 Hillier SL et al: Case-control study of chorioamnionic infection and chorioamnionitis in prematurity. *N Engl J Med* 319: 972, 1988.
64 Rosene K et al: Polymicrobiol early postpartum endometritis with facultative and anaerobic bacteria, genital mycoplasma, and chlamydia trachomatis: Treatment with pipericillin or celoxitin. *J Infect Dis* 153: 1028, 1986.
65 Gravett MG et al: Independent association of bacterial vaginosis and *Chlamydia trachomatis* infection with adverse pregnancy outcome. *JAMA* 256: 1899, 1986.
66 Bump RC et al: The prevalence, six-month persistence, and predictive values of laboratory indicators of bacterial vaginosis (nonspecific vaginitis) in asymptomatic women. *Am J Obstet Gynecol* 150: 917, 1984.
67 Dunkelberg WE: Diagnosis of *Haemophilus vaginalis* vaginitis by gram-stained smears. *Am J Obstet Gynecol* 91: 998, 1965.
68 Spiegel CA et al: Diagnosis of bacterial vaginosis by direct Gram stain of vaginal fluid. *J Clin Microbiol* 18: 170, 1983.
69 Thomason JL et al: Proline aminopeptidase as a rapid diagnostic test to confirm bacterial vaginosis. *Obstet Gynecol* 71: 607, 1988.
70 Chen KCS et al: Biochemical diagnosis of vaginosis: Determination of diamines in vaginal fluid. *J Infect Dis* 145: 337, 1982.
71 Pito P et al: A placebo-controlled, double-blind comparison of tinidazole and triple sulfonamide cream for the treatment of nonspecific vaginitis. *Am J Obstet Gynecol* 147: 85, 1983.
72 Malouf M et al: Treatment of *Haemophilus vaginalis* vaginitis. *Obstet Gynecol* 57: 711, 1981.
73 McCarthy LR et al: Antibiotic susceptibility of *Haemophilus vaginalis (Corynebacterium vaginale)* to 21 antibiotics. *Antimicrob Agents Chemother* 16: 186, 1977.
74 Jones BM et al: *In vitro* and *in vivo* activity of metronidazole against *Gardnerella vaginalis, Bacteroides* spp. and *Mobiluncus* spp. in bacterial vaginosis. *J Antimicrob Chemother* 16: 189, 1985.
75 Eschenbach DA et al: A dose-duration study of metronidazole for the treatment of nonspecific vaginosis. *Scand J Infect Dis Suppl* 40: 73, 1983.
76 Hovik P: Nonspecific vaginitis in an outpatient clinic. *Scand J Infect Dis* (Suppl) 40:107, 1983.
77 Jerve F et al: Metronidazole in the treatment of nonspecific vaginitis (NSV). *Br J Vener Dis* 60: 171, 1984.
78 Swedberg J et al: Comparison of single-dose vs. one-week course of metronidazole for symptomatic bacterial vaginosis. *JAMA* 254: 1046, 1985.
79 Bistoletti P et al: Comparison of oral and vaginal metronidazole therapy for nonspecific bacterial vaginosis. *Gynecol Obstet Invest* 21: 144, 1986.
80 Brenner WE, Dingfelder JR: Metronidazole-containing vaginal sponges for the treatment of bacterial vaginosis. *Adv Contracept* 2: 363, 1986.
81 Ralph ED, Amatnicks YE: Relative susceptibilities of *Gardnerella vaginalis (Haemophilus vaginalis), Neisseria gonorrhoeae,* and *Bacteroides fragilis* to metronidazole and its two major metabolites. *Sex Transm Dis* 7: 157, 1980.
82 Koutsky LA et al: Persistence of *Mycoplasma hominis* after therapy: Importance of tetracycline resistance and of coexisting vaginal flora. *Sex Transm Dis* 11: 374, 1983.
83 Hillier SL et al: Microbiologic efficacy of topical clincamycin for the treatment of bacterial vaginosis. Abstract Annual Meeting American Society for Microbiology, p 10, No A54, 1988.
84 Amsel R et al: Comparison of metronidazole, ampicillin, and amoxicillin for treatment of bacterial vaginosis (nonspecific vaginitis): Possible explanation for the greater efficacy of metronidazole, in *First United States Metronidazole Conference,* SM Finegold (ed). Biomedia Information Corp, New York, 1982.
85 Lee L, Schmale JD: Ampicillin therapy for *Corynebacterium vaginale (Haemophilus vaginalis)* vaginitis. *Am J Obstet Gynecol* 115: 786, 1973.
86 Rodgers HA et al: *Haemophilus vaginalis (Corynebacterium vaginale)* vaginitis in women attending public health clinics: Response to treatment with ampicillin. *Sex Transm Dis* 5: 18, 1978.
87 Symonds J, Biswas AK: Amoxicillin, augmentin, and metronidazole in bacterial vaginosis associated with *Gardnerella vaginalis. Genitourin Med* 62: 136, 1986.
88 Durfee MA et al: Ineffectiveness of erythromycin for treatment of *Haemophilus vaginalis*-associated vaginitis. *Antimicrob Agents Chemother* 16: 635, 1979.
89 Balsdon MJ et al: *Corynebacterium vaginale* and vaginitis: A controlled trial of treatment. *Lancet* i: 501, 1980.
90 Andersch B et al: Treatment of bacterial vaginosis with an acid cream: A comparison between the effect of lactate-gel and metronidazole. *Gynecol Obstet Invest* 21: 9, 1986.
91 Fredriccson B et al: Ecological treatment of bacterial vaginosis. *Lancet* i: 176, 1987.
92 Duttan IM et al: Aetiology and management of nonspecific vaginitis. *Br J Vener Dis* 58: 32, 1982.
93 Loser A: Des Fluor, seine Entste Lung und eine neue kausale Therapie Mittels des Baketerienproparates, Bazillosan. *Zentrabl Gynakol* 44: 417, 1920.
94 Mohler RW, Brown CP: Doderlein's bacillus in the treatment of vaginitis. *Am J Obstet Gynecol* 25: 718, 1933.
95 Butler BC, Beakley JW: Bacterial flora in vaginitis. A study before and after treatment with pure cultures of Doderlein bacillus. *Am J Obstet Gynecol* 79: 432, 1960.
96 Wood JR et al: *In vitro* and adherence *Lactobacillus* species to vaginal epithelial cells. *Am J Obstet Gynecol* 153: 740, 1985.
97 Hughes VL, Hillier SL: Lactobacilli from non-prescription products used for the treatment of vaginitis. Abstracts Annual Meetings American Society for Microbiology, p 368, No C218, 1988.

# Chapter 48

# Cervical neoplasia and other STD-related genital and anal neoplasias

Jorma Paavonen
Laura A. Koutsky
Nancy Kiviat

## INTRODUCTION

Among women, carcinoma of the uterine cervix is the second most common cancer in the world, and the most common cancer in many developing countries of Africa, South and Central America, Asia, and the Pacific.[1] For 1980, it was estimated that there were 465,600 new cases of cervical cancer detected worldwide, making it the fifth most common cancer among both sexes, preceded only by cancers of the stomach, lung, breast, and colon or rectum.

Cancer of the cervix virtually always starts in the area of the transformation zone at the squamocolumnar junction and usually begins as a focus of cells that are abnormal or dysplastic but not malignant. As shown in Fig. 48-1, the squamocolumnar junction is dynamic and changes location on the cervix throughout a women's lifetime. Because the epithelium defined by the squamocolumnar junction undergoes considerable change during a woman's reproductive years and because dysplasia as well as sexually transmitted infections of the cervix are most common during these same years, it has been hypothesized that the interaction of squamocolumnar change, STD, and dysplasia largely determines a woman's risk for developing invasive cervical cancer. Although carcinomas of the penis, vagina, vulva, and anus each are detected 5 to 50 times less often than carcinoma of the cervix, current evidence suggests that they are morphologically similar and that they share a common sexually transmitted etiology.[2–4]

Over the last decade, evidence implicating sexually transmitted human papillomavirus (HPV) in the etiology of these tumors has become compelling (see Chap. 37). Evidence implicating other sexually transmitted infections including *Treponema pallidum, Neisseria gonorrhoeae, Trichomonas vaginalis,* herpes simplex virus (HSV), and *Chlamydia trachomatis* is now much weaker than the evidence implicating HPV.

Unlike most other carcinomas, genital tract and anal carcinomas are easily preventable because the cervix, vagina, vulva, anus, and penis are readily accessible to cytologic, colposcopic, and histopathologic examination and because simple surgical excision or destruction of intraepithelial neoplastic or dysplastic lesions has proved to be highly effective in preventing progression to malignancy. However, until Pap smear screening becomes more widely available in developing countries and all women with cytologic evidence of cervical intraepithelial neoplasia (CIN) are referred for colposcopy, histologic confirmation, and treatment when indicated, the global incidence of invasive cervical cancer is likely to remain high.

This chapter reviews the evidence that links genital and anal cancers with sexually transmitted diseases (STDs), offers practical guidelines for the prevention, diagnosis, and early treatment of precancerous lesions, and briefly discusses emerging technologies that will be applied to the diagnosis and management of these lesions in the future.

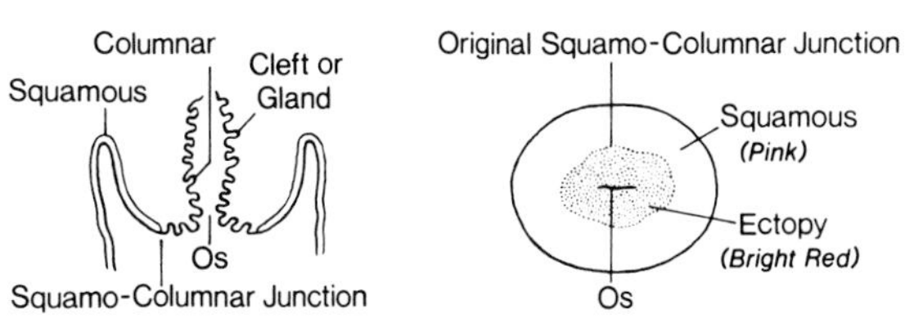


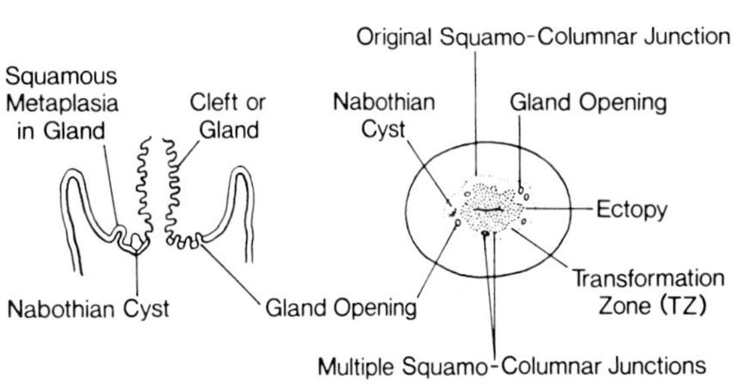


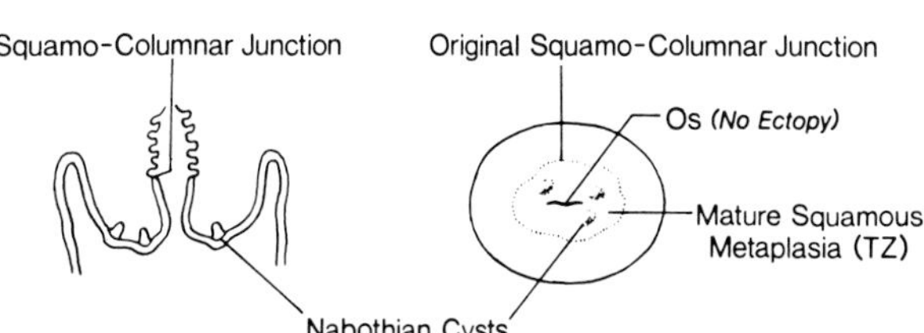


**Fig. 48-1.** These diagrams show the change in location of the squamocolumnar junction on the uterine cervix from menarche (12 years) through initiation of sexual activity (21 years) and menopause (45 years).

## HISTORICAL OVERVIEW

As early as 1842, Rigoni-Stern[5] reported that cancer of the uterus (site unspecified) occurred less frequently among cloistered nuns than among married women. Since this initial report, other studies have confirmed the association between various measures of sexual exposure and development and squamous cell neoplasms of the cervix,[6] anus,[7] and vulva.[8]

Papanicolaou's observation, reported in 1943, that exfoliated cervical cells from the area of the squamocolumnar junction that pooled in the vaginal fornices could be used for early detection of even a small cervical lesion was a major breakthrough. This discovery permitted development of cytologic cervical screening programs which have contributed to the decline by 78 percent in the incidence and mortality rates of cervical cancer in the United States over the last 35 years.[9,10] Although the concept that premalignant intraepithelial lesions are stages in a continuum provided the basis for implementing population-based cytologic screening programs in the early 1950s, it was not until Richart and Barron reported their observations on the natural history of dysplasia in 1969 that the progressive potential of early precancerous lesions became widely accepted.[11]

During the 1930s and 1940s work with the Shope papillomavirus, i.e., cottontail rabbit papillomavirus (CRPV), was providing important clues to the role of viruses in tumor production. Despite the fact that CRPV was the first DNA virus known to be oncogenic in mammals and was also the first tumor-inducing agent studied in conjunction with chemical agents acting as cocarcinogens,[12,13] the relation of this group of viruses to human tumors, particularly those of the genital tract, was not recognized for at least another 40 years.

In 1956, Koss and Durfee[14] described the cytologic and histologic features now known to be characteristic of genital wart virus infection of the cervix. Initially, these features were thought to be a variant of dysplasia and not manifestations of warts. It was not until the 1970s that Meisels and Fortin[15] and Purola and Savia[16] linked these characteristic cellular changes, often seen in association with dysplasia, with genital papillomavirus infection. The inability to cultivate papillomavirus in cells was (and is) a barrier to research on these viruses. The advent of recombinant DNA technology led to the cloning of HPV DNA and to the recognition of heterogeneity among this group of viruses based upon studies of DNA homology and restriction enzyme analysis.[17–20] Of the 60 types identified between 1976 and 1989, 20 are thought to infect primarily genital tract and anal epithelium, and two of these (HPV 16 and 18) have been most strongly linked with the development of genital tract and anal cancers.

## DEFINITIONS

As seen in Table 48-1, a variety of different types of malignancies occur at all genital and anal sites, and the majority of tumors are of the squamous cell type. Squamous cell lesions of the anus and genital tract, which are felt to be neoplastic in nature, are generally divided into (1) invasive cancer, and (2) noninvasive lesions. The latter lesions, called dysplasias or intraepithelial neoplasias, were first described on the cervix and are felt to vary in malignant potential. Similar squamous cell pathology has subsequently been described in other areas of the genital tract or anus of males and females.

## INVASIVE SQUAMOUS CELL CANCER

The term "invasive" is applied to tumors in which the malignant cells have penetrated the underlying basement membrane and have infiltrated the stroma. The morphology of invasive squamous cell cancer of the cervix, vagina and vulva, penis, and anus is similar. Cancers are graded as well, moderately, or poorly differentiated (grades I to III). Grade I, or well-differentiated carcinoma, most resembles normal squamous epithelium with many keratinizing cells and keratin pearls present. Grade II, or moderately differentiated cancer, shows less keratin formation with greater nuclear polymorphism and more mitoses present. Grade III, or poorly differentiated squamous cell cancer, is composed of cells with a high nuclear/cytoplasmic ratio and many mitotic figures, but no keratin formation.[21]

It is a common practice in the case of cervical and vulvar lesions (and in some laboratories for cancers at other genital sites) to further classify invasive cancers as being either frankly invasive or microinvasive. There is not yet a consensus as to the exact criteria necessary for a diagnosis of cervical microinvasive cancer, but the definition proposed by the Society of Gynecologic Oncologists (SGO) states that malignant cells should not penetrate more than 2 mm below the basement membrane and that lymphatic or vascular invasion should be absent. More recently, some pathologists and gynecologists have proposed that lesions in which the malignant cells have penetrated to a depth of 5 mm without vascular and/or lymphatic invasion, or lesions in which malignant cells penetrate to a depth of 3 mm but where vascular and/or lymphatic invasion is present, be classified separately as "occult carcinoma."[22]

## NONINVASIVE SQUAMOUS CELL EPITHELIAL LESIONS

Genital tract lesions known as dysplasias or intraepithelial neoplasias comprise a spectrum of lesions of varying malignant potential and are far more common than invasive squamous cancers. To understand the current classification systems for these lesions and the controversies surrounding them, it is important to understand how these systems have evolved.

Early in this century, pathologists observed that the normal cervical epithelium adjacent to areas of invasive cancer was frequently completely replaced by cells which were morphologically identical to tumor cells, but which were confined to the area

**Table 48-1. Distribution (Percent) of Genital and Anal Cancers by Histologic Type [Surveillance, Epidemiology, and End Results (SEER) Program, United States, 1973–1977[10]]**

| Total *N*: | Cervix 6549 | Vagina 353 | Vulva 876 | Female anus 394 | Male anus 230 | Penis 370 |
|---|---|---|---|---|---|---|
| Histologic types:* | | | | | | |
| Carcinoma, NOS | 11.0 | 7.2 | 3.8 | 3.3 | 2.2 | 3.5 |
| Papillary carcinoma, NOS | 0.4 | 2.2 | 3.1 | 0.3 | 0.9 | 5.4 |
| Squamous cell carcinoma | 75.6 | 67.0 | 74.4 | 49.2 | 44.3 | 85.4 |
| Transitional cell carcinoma, NOS | 0.1 | 0.7 | 0.1 | 30.2 | 22.2 | 0.5 |
| Adenocarcinoma, NOS | 7.2 | 6.1 | 1.3 | 10.4 | 22.2 | — |
| Melanomas | — | 3.6 | 6.4 | 1.9 | — | 1.6 |
| Other tumors | 5.7 | 13.2 | 10.9 | 4.7 | 8.2 | 3.6 |

*NOS = not otherwise specified.

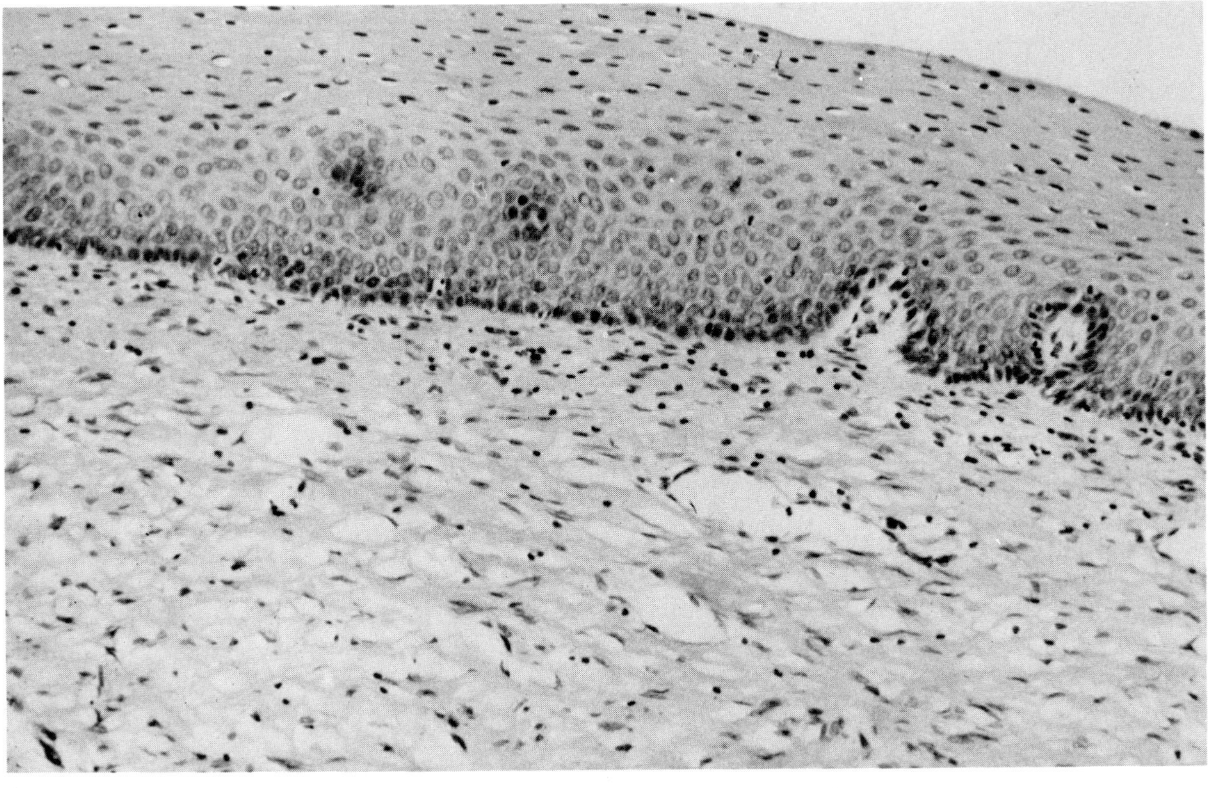

A

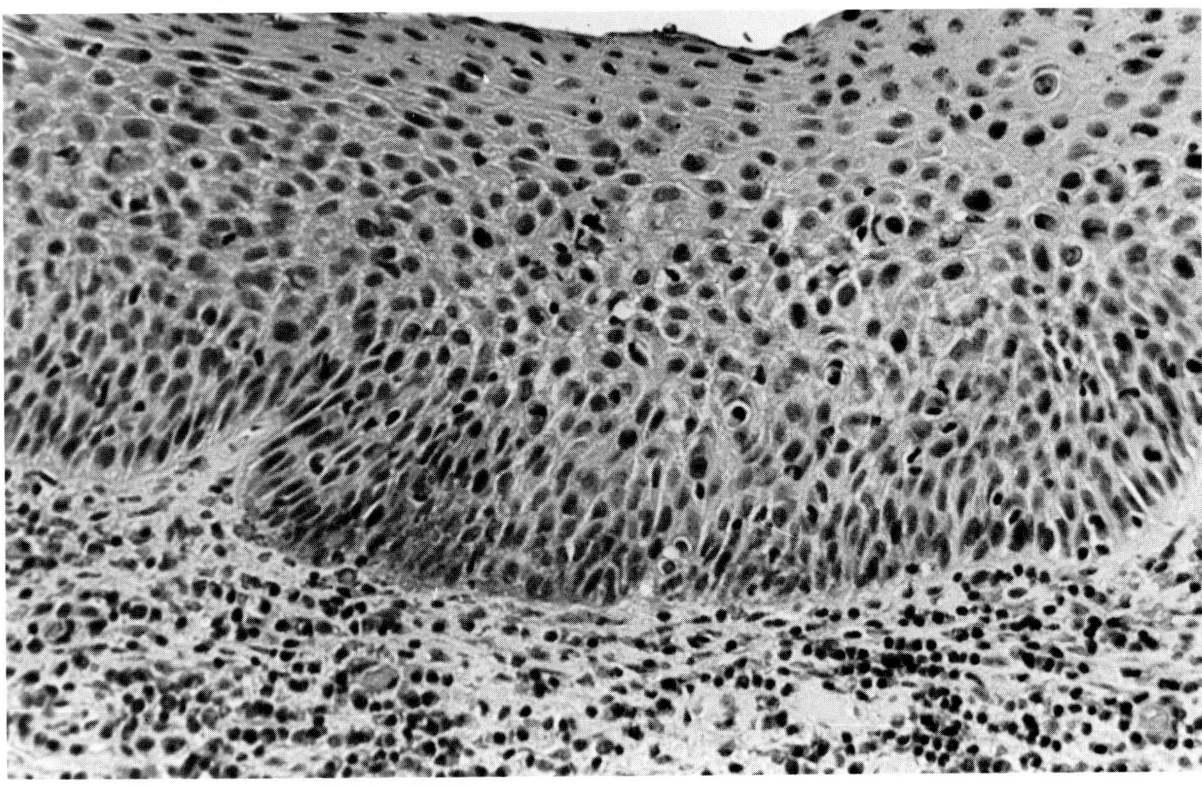

B

**Fig. 48-2.** Cervical biopsies (H&E stain) demonstrating histopathological characteristics of cervical intraepithelial neoplasia (CIN). (*a*) Normal stratified squamous epithelium, showing normal maturation and differentiation, with progression from the narrow basal cell layer through the intermediate cell layer to horizontally oriented superficial squamous cells. ×125 magnification. (*b*) CIN grade I: Abnormal maturation and loss of differentiation is shown involving lower one-third of the epithelium where there is crowding of cells, nuclear hyperchromasia, and vertically oriented cells. ×300 magnification.

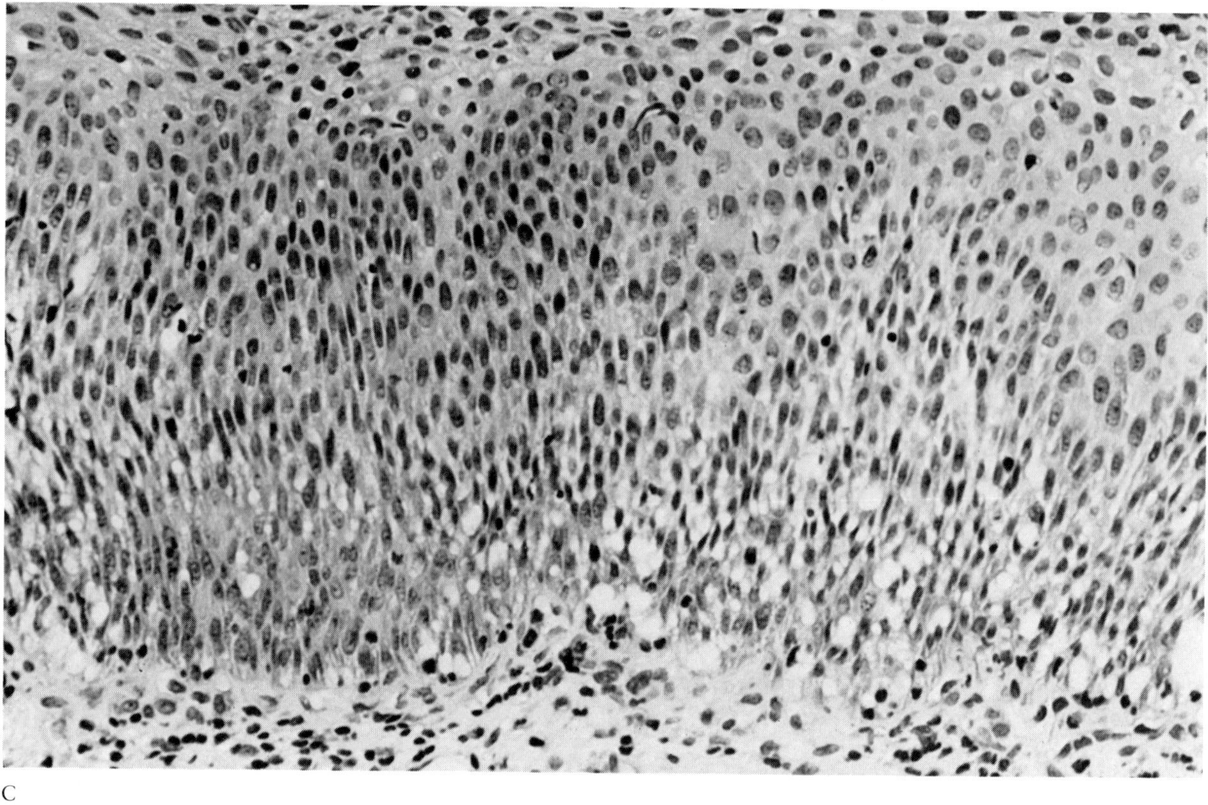

C

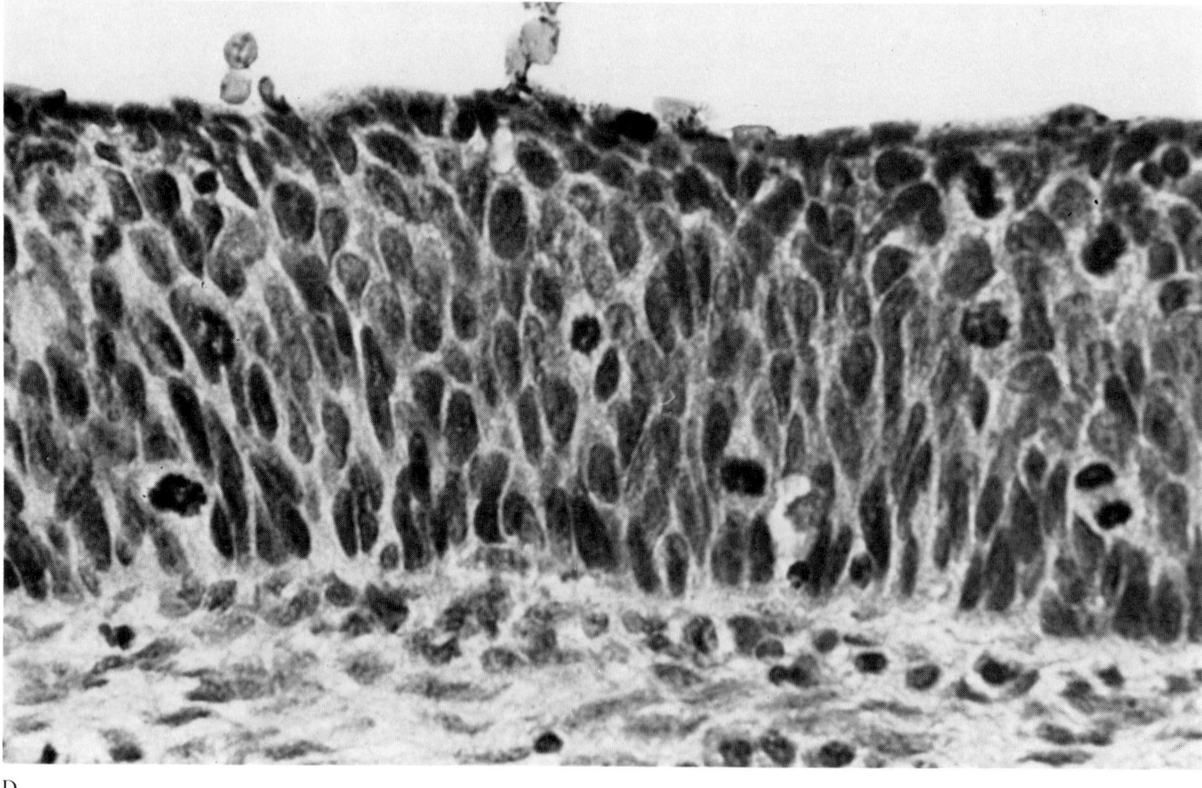

D

Fig. 48-2. (*continued*) (*c*) CIN grade II: Abnormal maturation and loss of differentiation and polarity is shown as it involves at least the lower two-thirds of the epithelium. ×300 magnification. (*d*) CIN grade III: Abnormal maturation and loss of differentiation that shows involvement of the full thickness of the epithelium. (Some, but not all, pathologists attempt to differentiate severe dysplasia from CIS within the CIN grade III category; as bases for differentiation they use preservation of a single layer of flattened epithelium at the surface in CIN grade III but not CIS, and greater nuclear crowding in CIS.) ×500 magnification.

normally occupied by epithelial cells. Such lesions were designated as carcinoma in situ (CIS) of the cervix. It was soon appreciated that a wide spectrum of abnormal lesions of the cervix existed, ranging from those of carcinoma in situ to lesions partially composed of cells with features similar to those of CIS, but also containing less worrisome cells which shared certain features with normal cervical epithelial cells. Pathologists felt that the latter lesions (called dysplasias or CINs today) represented the very earliest morphologic changes associated with cervical cancer, and many attempted to develop hierarchical systems for classification for these lesions which reflected their potential biological behavior. The belief was that the greater the percentage of the thickness of the epithelium occupied by undifferentiated cells, the more likely was the development of CIS and later invasive cancer.

The many classification systems that were developed to describe these early lesions of cervical cancer became confusing for clinicians concerned with patient treatment. In 1961, the First International Congress of Exfoliative Cytology, and the Committee on Histologic Terminology for Lesions of the Uterine Cervix were convened, and an agreement was reached on nomenclature for classification of noninvasive cervical epithelial lesions.[23] Lesions were classified by both histology and cytology as either "carcinoma in situ" or "dysplasia." Carcinoma in situ was defined as a lesion in which the entire thickness of the surface epithelium showed no differentiation, but in which no invasion had yet occurred. The term dysplasia was reserved for all other disturbances of differentiation of the squamous epithelium for which the malignant potential was unclear. Pathologists, however, were encouraged to categorize these dysplasias as mild, moderate, or severe, as they increasingly resembled carcinoma in situ, as reflected by the increasing percentage of the thickness of the lesion occupied by undifferentiated cells. It was soon apparent that this classification system presented a practical problem: pathologists were unable to reproducibly distinguish between severe dysplasia and carcinoma in situ.[24–26] Attempting to alleviate this problem, Richart[27] proposed that these lesions of the cervix all be viewed as a continuum of premalignant changes which he divided into three grades: cervical intraepithelial neoplasia grade I (CIN I), grade II (CIN II), and grade III (CIN III), corresponding to mild, moderate, and severe dysplasia or carcinoma in situ. The grouping of severe dysplasia and CIS in the category CIN III recognizes the fact that pathologists have difficulty in distinguishing between severe dysplasia and CIS. Histologically, in CIN I lesions the lower one-third of the epithelium is composed of abnormal immature cells, with differentiation occurring in the upper two-thirds of the epithelium. In CIN II, differentiation does not occur until the upper third of the epithelium. In CIN III there is a full thickness of undifferentiated cells[28,29] (Fig. 48-2). Clearly, however, as discussed below under Cytology, since surface scrapes (Pap smears) of the cervix are able to detect abnormal cells from lesions consistent with CIN I or CIN II by histology, the differentiating epithelium in the upper portion of all lesions also contains characteristic abnormal cells (Fig. 48-3). The histologic and cytologic classification of these abnormal cells is discussed in detail below.

Recent developments concerning the probable role of HPV in cervical cancer and precancer, as discussed below, have reoriented the conceptualization of classifying cervical epithelial pathology. Some pathologists have suggested that specific histologic findings could successfully segregate "low-risk lesions" containing HPV 6 or 11 from "high-risk" lesions containing HPV 16, 18, or 31[30,31] and have proposed that lesions be classified as either condyloma, presumably containing only primarily low-risk types of HPV (6 or 11); or as CIN with or without koilocytosis (frequently containing high-risk HPV types 16, 18). However, for several reasons, we currently do not recommend attempting to divide lesions into condyloma on the one hand or dysplasia with or without koilocytosis on the other. Although CIN III lesions most often do contain HPV 16, 18, or 31, morphology is unable to reliably predict the type of HPV found in CIN I and II.[32] Furthermore, much of what was previously diagnosed as mild dysplasia or CIN I is currently recognized as having the morphologic changes associated with productive HPV infection and is frequently called "condyloma." The inter- and intraobserver reproducibility for segregation of lesions as condyloma vs. CIN I vs. CIN II vs. CIN III by either cytology or histology has been shown by a number of studies to be less than satisfactory, and some lesions classified as condyloma have been shown to progress to CIS.[4] Thus, it would seem prudent to avoid attempting to divide low-grade lesions into "condyloma" (implying a purely infectious lesion having no malignant potential) or "CIN I" (implying a lesion which may have malignant potential). At present, as discussed below in the Cytology section, lesions should be classified morphologically according to traditional histologic criteria for CIN regardless of whether changes consistent with HPV are present or not and regardless of the HPV type

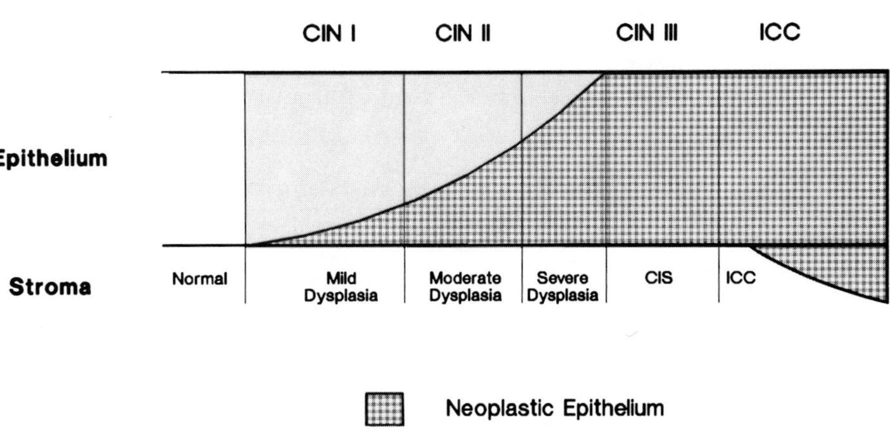


Fig. 48-3. Diagram showing the increase in atypical and neoplastic epithelium, relative to normal epithelium, detected within sections showing increasing severity of dysplasia, CIS, and invasive cervical carcinoma.

present. Further, treatment still is based on morphology, not on the type of HPV DNA present.

The nomenclature for the precancerous states of vaginal, vulvar, anal, and penile squamous epithelium is similar to that of the cervix,[33] being termed vaginal intraepithelial neoplasia (VAIN I, II, III), vulvar intraepithelial neoplasia (VIN I, II, III), anal intraepithelial neoplasia (AIN I, II, III), and penile intraepithelial neoplasia (PIN I, II, III). It is currently preferred to avoid using terms such as "Bowen's disease" or "Bowenoid papulosis" unless used in conjunction with the intraepithelial neoplasia nomenclature system. As in the case of cervical dysplasia, cytologic or histologic features suggestive of HPV infection at these other genital and anal sites should be reported in addition to, but not in place of, reported neoplastic features. There appears to be a remarkable morphologic similarity between CIN and VIN, although the risk for progression of VIN to invasive carcinoma is thought to be much lower than for CIN.[34]

Table 48-3. Age-Adjusted Genital and Anal Cancer Incidence for 1969–1971, 1973–1977, and 1981–1985, All Races, SEER Programs, United States[9,10]

| | 1969–1971 incidence per 100,000 | | 1973–1977 incidence per 100,000 | | 1981–1985 incidence per 100,000 | |
|---|---|---|---|---|---|---|
| | Females | Males | Females | Males | Females | Males |
| Cervix | 16.7 | | 12.4 | | 8.0 | |
| Vagina | 0.6 | | 0.7 | | 0.7 | |
| Vulva | 1.8 | | 1.6 | | 1.5 | |
| Penis | | 1.0 | | 0.9 | | 0.8 |
| Anus | 0.6 | 0.4 | 0.7 | 0.5 | 0.9 | 0.7 |

## INCIDENCE AND PREVALENCE

In the United States, as in other countries, the incidence of carcinoma of the cervix is at least 5 times higher than the incidence of carcinoma of the vagina, vulva, anus, and penis (Table 48-2). Overall, 69 percent of women in the United States who are 18 years of age or older had a Pap smear as part of a screening examination during the 3 years preceding 1987, and an additional 8 percent had one for a health problem during the same period.[9] Screening programs have never been implemented for the detection of precancerous lesions of the vulva, vagina, anus, or penis, and the incidence of invasive tumors of these sites has remained low and relatively constant over the last two decades (Table 48-3).

For all genital tract and anal cancers, except cancer of the vulva, the incidence is higher among blacks than among whites, and 5-year relative survival is generally better for whites than for blacks. Among all races, the median age of diagnosis for carcinoma of the cervix is 53 years, which is at least 10 years younger than the median age of diagnosis of carcinoma of the vagina (67 years), vulva (70 years), anus (females, 66 years; males, 63 years), and penis (66 years). As shown in Fig. 48-4, the incidence of all genital tract and anal cancers increases with age, with cervical cancer showing a sharp early rise between the ages of 20 and 40 with a slow steady rise thereafter. The incidence for the other tumors remains low until about age 45, and then increases exponentially (vulvar) or relatively linearly (vaginal, anal, and penile). Although the incidence of vulvar carcinoma is 60 percent higher among whites than among blacks, the 5-year relative survival is 36 percent higher for whites than for blacks, a difference that can be explained in part by the fact that tumors are detected at an earlier stage in whites than in blacks. Among whites, 62 percent of vulvar cancers compared with only 46 percent among blacks were detected while still locally invasive, showing no regional or distant metastases.[9]

## INTERNATIONAL TRENDS

Figure 48-5 shows the incidence of cervical and penile cancer estimated from data collected from tumor registries that were maintained in several countries between 1968–1971 and 1977–1982.[35,36] The incidence of cervical cancer declined in all of the areas shown, except Recife, Brazil; whereas the incidence of penile cancer increased slightly in most areas between the two periods studied. The incidence of both cervical and penile cancer appears to be very high in Latin America, a finding which may be in part due to the difficulty in collecting accurate denominator data. Also, there is a statistically significant positive correlation between the country-specific rates of cervical and penile carcinoma for these data.

## AGE-SPECIFIC TIME TRENDS IN THE INCIDENCE OF INVASIVE GENITAL TRACT AND ANAL CANCERS

As shown in Fig. 48-6, the incidence of invasive cervical cancer (ICC) within each 5-year age category has declined in the United States for both blacks and whites over the last 15 years, with black women showing relatively greater rates of decline.

In several countries where Pap smears have been used at less

Table 48-2. Age-Adjusted Incidence, Mortality, and 5-year Relative Survival Rates for Genital Tract and Anal Cancer, SEER Program, United States[9]

| | Incidence/$10^5$ (1981–1985) | | Mortality/$10^5$ (1981–1985) | | % survival (1979–1984) | | Median age of diagnosis in years (1981–1985) | |
|---|---|---|---|---|---|---|---|---|
| | Blacks | Whites | Blacks | Whites | Blacks | Whites | Blacks | Whites |
| Cervix | 16.5 | 7.9 | 6.3 | 2.5 | 58.6 | 66.7 | 53 | 53 |
| Vagina | 1.4 | 0.7 | 0.5 | 0.2 | 61.9 | 56.2 | 64 | 67 |
| Vulva | 1.0 | 1.6 | 0.3 | 0.3 | 53.9 | 73.7 | 59 | 71 |
| Anus: | | | | | | | | |
| Female | 1.2 | 0.9 | 0.3 | 0.1 | 51.2 | 57.0 | 62 | 67 |
| Males | 0.8 | 0.7 | 0.2 | 0.1 | 48.6 | 60.7 | 57 | 63 |
| Penis | 1.0 | 0.8 | 0.2 | 0.2 | 64.5 | 68.6 | 62 | 62 |

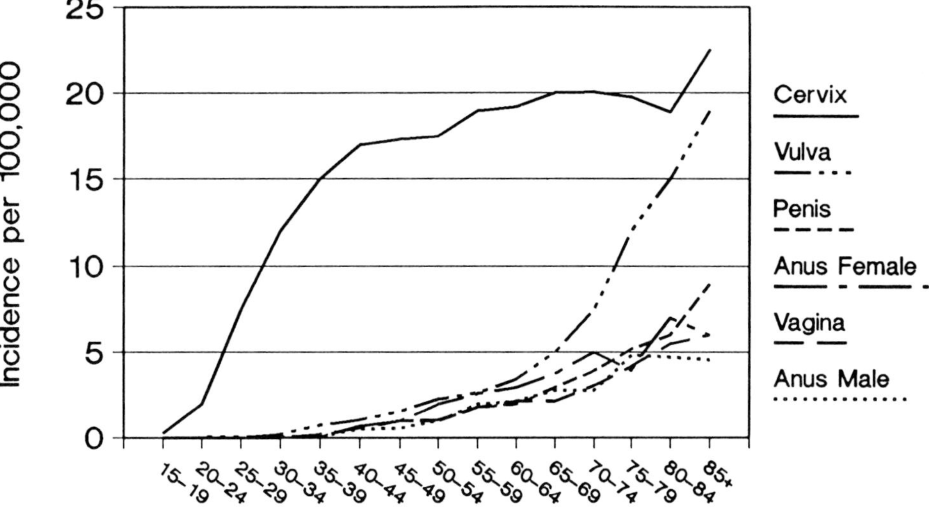


Fig. 48-4. Age- and sex-specific incidence of invasive cancers of the cervix, vulva, penis, anus, and vagina in the United States: Data from the SEER Program, 1981–1985.[9]

frequent intervals or where screening has focused on older women than in the United States, incidence and death rates for ICC have increased among young women in recent years. For example, the death rates among women less than 35 years of age doubled between 1970 and 1979 in England and Wales, suggesting the start of an ominous trend. However, the number of deaths among women under 35 years of age still represents less than 5 percent of all deaths from cervical cancer.[37–39] In Canada, the incidence of ICC for women 34 years of age and younger increased slightly from 1960 to 1983.[40] In Australia, between 1972 and 1976, both the incidence of and mortality from ICC increased in women of less than 40 years of age,[41–43] with approximately 15 to 20 percent of all ICC occurring in this age group. Similarly, in New Zealand, the incidence and mortality rates of cervical cancer declined among women over 35 years of age but rose in those age 35 or less.[44] As noted above, and reported by Chow et al.[45] and Chu et al.[46], data from the United States do not show an increase in incidence of ICC at younger ages when comparing the rates for the time intervals presented in Fig. 48-6. However, slight increases in incidence of carcinoma in situ of the cervix for women less than 26 years of age and in mortality rates from invasive cervical cancer have been observed, particularly among white women during the period 1981 to 1985. For example, among whites, age-specific mortality per 100,000 increased between 1969–1971 and 1981–1985 from 0.1 to 0.2 for women 20 to 24 years of age, from 0.5 to 0.8 for women 25 to 29 years of age, from 1.2 to 1.7 for women 30 to 35 years of age, and from 2.1 to 2.8 for women 35 to 39 years of age.[9]

## PREVALENCE OF PRECURSOR LESIONS

The reported prevalence of cytologic changes consistent with CIN has varied from 0.43 to 24 percent, with the highest prevalence reported for an STD clinic in Wales (Table 48-4). Despite the fact that Pap smear screening has been widespread in industrialized countries including the United States for the last two decades,

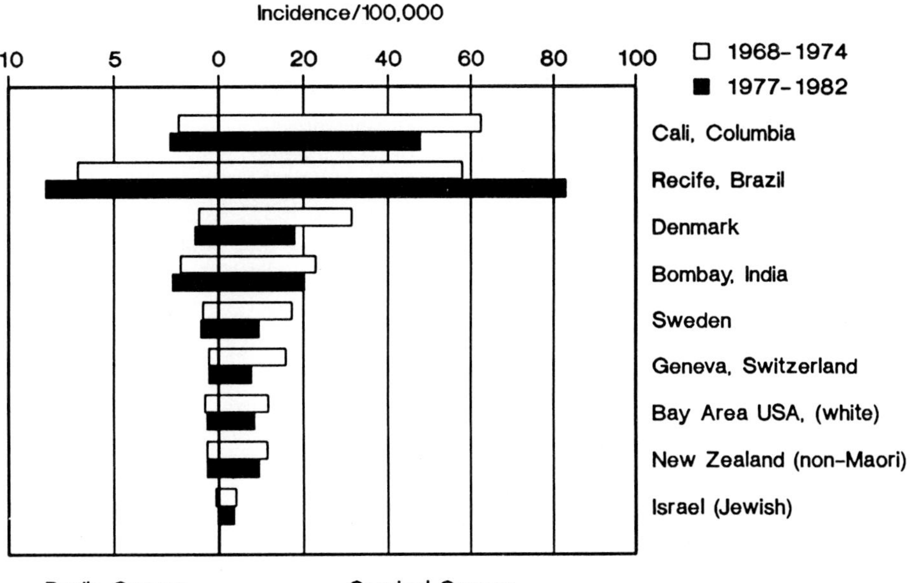


Fig. 48-5. Age-adjusted sex-specific incidence of invasive cancer of the cervix and penis in countries with established tumor registries during the years 1968–1974 and 1977–1982.[35,36]

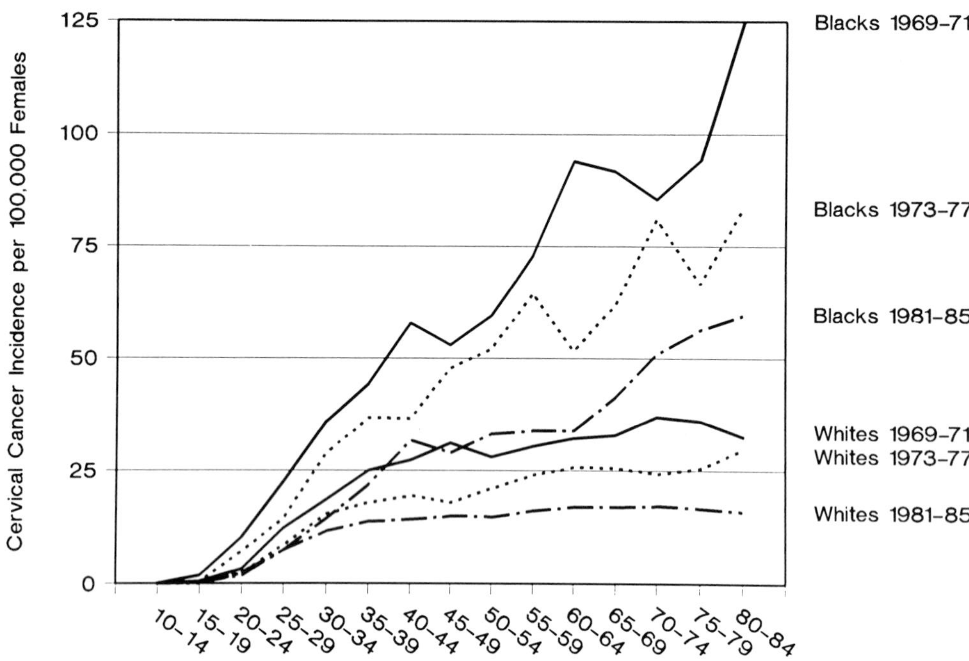


**Fig. 48-6.** Age-specific incidence of invasive cervical cancer among black and white women in the United States: Data from the SEER Program, 1969–1971, 1973–1977, and 1981–1985.[9,10]

methods of obtaining exfoliated cells and interpreting and reporting microscopic findings have never been well standardized, making it nearly impossible to compare results from different laboratories and different time periods. This becomes readily apparent when examining the data in Table 48-4. For example, during the early to mid-1980s, the prevalence of dysplasia in two similar STD clinics (Denver and Seattle) was 1.72 and 13.66 percent, respectively.

There are no good data on the prevalence of intraepithelial neoplasia or CIS of the vagina, vulva, anus, or penis, but it is thought that the prevalence of these lesions is much lower than for cervical neoplasia. VAIN in the upper vagina usually represents a distal extension of CIN. Ferguson and MacLure in 1963[73] published 27 cases of vaginal CIS or dysplasia that were found among 151 patients who had "false-positive" Pap smears. Timonen et al.[74] identified 23 primary vaginal dysplasias among 12,000 patients screened during one year, giving a prevalence of 2 per 1000. Woodruff in 1981[75] reported that less than 300 cases of CIS of the vagina had been recorded in the literature. Since vaginal cancer is so uncommon, screening for vaginal cancer has not received the same degree of emphasis as screening for cervical neoplasms.

During the 1970s, concomitantly with the increasing prevalence of vulvar HPV infections, the prevalence of VIN lesions reportedly increased[75–77] and the mean age of patients with VIN appeared to be declining from approximately 50 years to less than 30 years.[76,77]

## ETIOLOGY

Since 1950, at least three studies have documented low incidence and mortality of cervical cancer among nuns.[78–80] In contrast, subsequent wives of husbands whose previous wife had cervical cancer have been shown to be at increased risk.[81] In most studies, total number of sexual partners has been a strong predictor for cervical neoplasia.[82,83] In 1982, Buckley et al.[84] reported that among women reporting only one lifetime sexual partner, those whose husbands reported six or more sexual partners appeared to have approximately a fourfold higher risk for cervical neoplasia than women whose husbands reported having had fewer than six partners. Recently, Zunzunegui[85] showed that among South American women residing in California, the total number of sexual partners of the husband was highly associated with occurrence of ICC in the wife, whereas the woman's sexual partner history was not. Martinez, Graham, and Smith et al.[86–88] have reported an increased occurrence of cervical cancer in partners of men with penile carcinoma. Increased numbers of sexual partners has also been associated with carcinoma of the anus.[7]

The epidemiologic evidence correlating sexual behavior with CIN and ICC has led to an extensive search for specific STD agents acting as carcinogens in genital and anal cancers. History of venereal infections has been linked with cancers of the cervix, penis, and anus.[7,83,89] During the last 50 years, attention has shifted from one organism to another about every 10 years, from syphilis in the 1940s, to gonorrhea, trichomoniasis, and herpes simplex virus-2 in the 1970s, and currently to papillomavirus in the 1980s. Other pathogens that have been implicated in one or more studies during this period include mycoplasmas, *Gardnerella vaginalis,* cytomegalovirus, Epstein-Barr virus, and *C. trachomatis.*

Several case control studies have linked current cigarette smoking with cancers of the cervix,[82,90–92] vulva,[8] anus,[7] and penis.[93] A problem with interpreting results from these studies is the possibility that the reported associations reflect confounding sexual exposures not measured by number of sexual partners. Also, laboratory evidence of HPV infection was not sought in these studies. Nonetheless, there is evidence that cervical mucus from cigarette smokers is more likely than mucus from nonsmokers to be mutagenic,[94] and that cigarette smokers have a reduced Langerhans' cell population in the cervix, suggesting a local immunologic effect of smoking on cervical epithelium.[95] These data raise the question as to whether smoking may act as a risk factor in the development of some cervical cancers.

Although results from studies of oral contraceptive use and cervical cancer are not conclusive, there appears to be a slightly increased risk for cervical cancer associated with use, particularly long-term use, of hormonal contraceptives.[96] Alternative theories

Table 48-4. Detection of Cervical Dysplasia by Pap Smear in Different Clinical Settings around the World

| Reference | Area, years | Clinic setting | Number screened | Patients with suspected: Dysplasia, % | Carcinoma in situ (CIS), % | Cervical cancer,[†] % | Total % |
|---|---|---|---|---|---|---|---|
| | | North America—ob-gyn or family planning clinics | | | | | |
| 47 | Los Angeles (1952–1959) | Ob-gyn | 19,192 | 0.54 | 0.51 | 0.25 | 1.30 |
| 48 | Canada (1961–1967) | Ob-gyn | 75,000* | 1.07 | 0.36 | 0.20 | 1.56 |
| 49 | N.Y. City (1965–1968) | Planned Parent. | 39,954 | 1.20 | 0.50 | 0.45 | 2.15 |
| 50 | United States (1975–1978) | Ob-gyn | 34,318 | 1.41 | 0.12 | 0.06 | 2.17 |
| 51 | Seattle (1977–1978) | Planned Parent. | 8,504 | 5.75 | 0.15 | 0 | 5.90 |
| 52 | United States (1981) | Ob-gyn | 796,337 | 2.03 | 0.28 | 0.01 | 2.33 |
| 53 | U.S. (23 states) (1981–1983) | Planned Parent. | 1,045,059 | 2.15 | 0.18 | 0.001 | 2.33 |
| Unpub. | Seattle (1985) | Ob-gyn-HMO | 77,209* | 1.42 | 0.28 | 0.18 | 1.89 |
| Unpub. | Seattle (1985) | Ob-gyn | 127,800* | 1.24 | 0.16 | N.S. | 1.40 |
| | | Europe, Australia, and New Zealand—ob-gyn or family planning clinic | | | | | |
| 54 | Finland (1963–1971) | Ob-gyn | 406,348* | 0.55 | 0.16 | 0.05 | 0.76 |
| 55 | Sweden (1967–1975) | Ob-gyn | 930,127 | 0.99 | 0.30 | 0.14 | 1.37 |
| 56 | Germany (1971–1976) | Ob-gyn | 503,870* | 0.60 | 0.32 | 0.05 | 0.97 |
| 57 | Yorkshire, U.K. (1976–1977) | Ob-gyn | 97,250* | 2.45 | 2.28 | 1.12 | 2.93 |
| 58 | Netherlands (1979) | Ob-gyn | 116,090* | 2.21 | 0.36 | N.S. | 2.57 |
| 59 | Christchurch, New Zealand (1982–1985) | Family plan. | 28,858* | 2.88 | 0.42 | 0 | 3.29 |
| 60 | New Zealand (1985) | Ob-gyn | 2,782 | 4.60 | 0.68 | N.S. | 5.28 |
| 61 | West. Austral. (1983) | Ob-gyn | 8,970 | 1.60 | 0.29 | 0.02 | 1.91 |
| | | International, agrarian—ob-gyn or family planning clinics | | | | | |
| 62 | Trinidad (pre-1969) | Family plan. | 2,633 | 4.50 | 0.80 | 0 | 5.24 |
| 62 | Barbados (pre-1969) | Ob-gyn | 5,000 | 4.16 | 0.88 | 0.50 | 5.54 |
| 63 | New Delhi (1976–1970) | Not stated | 16,815 | 1.74 | 0.11[‡] | N.S. | 1.85 |
| 63 | Agra (1967–1970) | Not stated | 26,094 | 6.27 | 0.59[‡] | N.S. | 6.86 |
| 63 | Haiti (1976–1979) | Ob-gyn | 2,695* | 3.41 | 0.07 | 2.15 | 5.64 |
| 63 | Cameroon (1977) | University women's | 300 | 7.8 | 0.70 | 0 | 8.33 |
| 64 | New Delhi (1976–1982) | Ob-gyn | 68,436 | 1.33 | 0.08 | 0.07 | 1.47 |
| 65 | Egypt (1981–1985) | Ob-gyn | 4,458 | 0.59 | 0.12 | 0.11 | 0.99 |
| | | Adolescents—ob-gyn or family planning clinics | | | | | |
| 66 | Houston (1962–1968) | Ob-gyn | 10,246 | 2.82 | 0.07 | 0 | 2.89 |
| 67 | So. Calif. (1976) | Ob-gyn | 2,655 | 7.02 | 0.04 | 0 | 7.06 |
| 68 | Milan, Italy (1978–1984) | Ob-gyn | 2,097 | 5.91 | 0.10 | 0 | 6.01 |
| 52 | United States (1981) | Ob-gyn | 199,154 | 1.77 | 0.09 | 0 | 1.86 |
| 53 | U.S. (23 states) (1981–1983) | Planned Parent. | 372,498 | 1.59 | 0.05 | 0 | 1.64 |
| 61 | West. Austral. (1983) | Ob-gyn | 703 | 0.43 | 0.14 | 0 | 0.99 |
| | | High risk | | | | | |
| 69 | Taipei, Taiwan (1977) | Prostitute | 750 | 0.93 | 0.13 | 0 | 1.06 |
| 51 | Seattle (1977–1978) | STD | 764 | 11.39 | 0.13 | 0 | 11.52 |
| 70 | Perth, Australia (1978–1982) | STD | 2,992 | 2.0 | 0.2 | 0 | 2.21 |
| 71 | Denver (1981–1983) | STD | 697 | 1.72 | 0 | 0 | 0.44 |
| 72 | England (1982) | STD | 15,730 | 6.18 | 0.60[‡] | N.S. | 6.76 |
| 72 | Wales (1982) | STD | 620 | 24.19 | 2.70[‡] | N.S. | 26.94 |
| 32 | Seattle (1984–1986) | STD | 454 | 12.8 | 0.90 | 0 | 13.66 |

*Number screened based on number of Pap smears, not on number of women.
[†]N.S. = not stated.
[‡]Includes women with cytologic findings suggestive of invasive carcinoma.

that have so far received little support from experimental or epidemiologic data are that cervical cancer may be caused by exposure to spermatozoa[97] or uncircumcized sex partners.[98]

The epidemiology of cervical cancer, as with other cancers, suggests that progression to malignancy is a multistage process. Thus, regardless of evidence linking HPV infection to cervical cancer, the role of heredity, infections, and other acquired factors must be further assessed.

In the following review of the evidence associating specific sexually transmitted agents with the development of genital and anal neoplasia, results from molecular, biochemical, seroepidemiologic, and clinical studies are presented, unless such studies have been described in another chapter (e.g., the evidence linking HPV with genital cancer is discussed in Chaps. 37 and 38).

## VIRAL AGENTS IN THE ETIOLOGY OF GENITAL NEOPLASIA

### HPV

Of the 60 human papillomavirus types detected, at least 20 are specifically associated with anal or genital lesions. HPV types 6 and 11 are primarily associated with condylomatous lesions, whereas HPV types 16, 18, 31, 33, 35, and 39 are primarily associated with papular or subclinical premalignant and malignant lesions. Some of the newer HPV types, namely, HPV types 41 to 45, and 51 to 56, and 59 have also been detected in tissue from genital lesions.

As discussed in Chaps. 37 and 38, the molecular and biochemical evidence supporting a link between HPV and cancers of the genital tract and anus is quite strong. The epidemiologic evidence is less well developed, in part because current methods of detecting the virus in clinical specimens are less than optimally sensitive, specific, and reliable. The considerable variability between the findings of different research groups with respect to the types of HPV associated with specific clinical entities is probably due to differences in laboratory technique, methods of obtaining samples, choice of study populations, and perhaps differences in the geographical distribution of specific HPV types.

**Detection of HPV DNA in Genital Tract and Anal Cancers.** Figure 48-7 shows a comparison of results obtained from studies of cervical, vulvar, penile, and anal neoplasia that used molecular hybridization techniques to detect HPV 6 or 11 and HPV 16 or 18.[99–128] As shown in this figure, the relationships between specific types of human papillomavirus and tumors of the cervix, vulva, penis, and anus are similar for each site. HPV 16 or 18 DNA has been detected in less than 25 percent of specimens obtained from the cervix, vulva, penis, or anus classified as condyloma or intraepithelial neoplasia grade 1, and in 40 to 80 percent of specimens from these sites showing higher grades of neoplasia. As shown in Table 48-5, HPV 16, 18, or 31 DNA has been detected in only 1 to 18 percent of cervical specimens obtained from women with normal Pap smears. The evidence implicating HPV 16 or 18 in the etiology of most genital tract and anal tumors is consistent with reports of an increased risk for a second primary genital tract tumor among women with an earlier genital tract tumor.[129,130] Also, the HPV 16 link with cervical cancer does not appear to be a recent phenomenon, as Collins et al.[131] showed that HPV 16 DNA could be detected from a similar proportion of cervical cancer specimens sampled in each decade beginning in 1932, the first year that stored specimens were available.

Also shown in Fig. 48-7, HPV 16 or 18 DNA was detected in 68 percent of 28 adenocarcinomas of the cervix, a proportion comparable with that obtained for squamous cell carcinomas of the cervix. HPV 16 or 18 DNA has been detected in vaginal carcinomas[100,104,115] and was detected in vaginal specimens of all five women who developed vaginal intraepithelial neoplasia among a group of 959 women exposed to diethylstilbestrol in utero (four with HPV 6 and one with HPV 16).[132]

The relation between HPV 16 or 18 and adenocarcinoma of the cervix requires further study because recent evidence[110,111,116,133] suggests that compared with HPV 16, HPV 18 is detected more frequently in adenocarcinomas and in more aggressively invasive squamous cell cancers. It will be important to distinguish between HPV 18 and HPV 16 in future studies of cervical carcinomas.

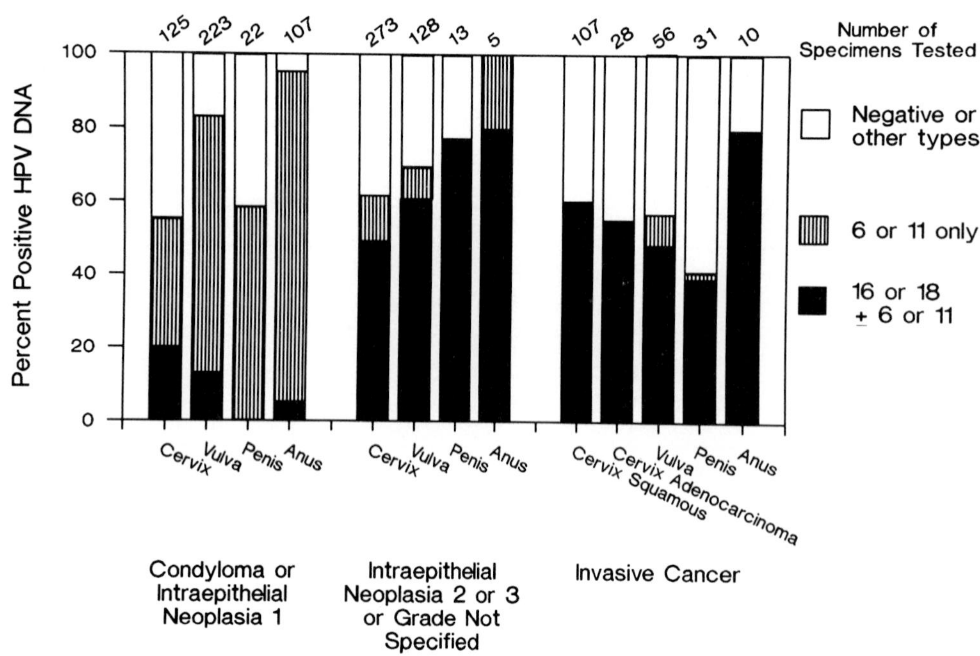


Fig. 48-7. Detection of HPV DNA in neoplastic specimens obtained from the cervix,[99,102–107,109–111,116] from the vulva,[99–101,108,112–115,118–122] from the penis,[102,113,114,117,123,124] and from the anus.[113,115,118,125–128]

Table 48-5. Prevalence of HPV DNA Detected in Cervical Specimens Obtained from Women with and without Cytologic Evidence of CIN and Who Attended Gynecology Clinics between 1984 and 1988

| Country, year | Reasons for attending clinic | Hybridization method (probes) | Detection of HPV DNA among: Women without cytologic evidence of cervical intraepithelial neoplasia | | Women with cytologic evidence of cervical intraepithelial neoplasia | |
|---|---|---|---|---|---|---|
| | | | Any HPV | HPV 16, 18, 31 | Any HPV | HPV 16, 18, 31 |
| France, 1986[134] | Cancer screening or treatment | Dot (6,11,16,18) | 4/311(1%) | 4/311(1%) | 14/47(30%) | 12/47(26%) |
| U.S., 1986[135] | Routine gyn. examination | Southern (6,11,16,18,31) | 21/188(11%) | 2/188(1%) | 10/11(91%) | 3/11(27%) |
| England, 1986[136] | Referred for inflammatory smears | Southern (6,11,16,18) | 12/79(15%) | 8/79(10%) | 12/27(44%) | 8/27(30%) |
| | Treatment for conditions unrelated to cervical neoplasia | | 12/104(12%) | 9/64(9%) | Not done | Not done |
| Germany, 1987[137] | Routine screening | Filter in situ (6,11,16,18) | 806/8755(9%) | Not typed | 97/282(34%) | Not typed |
| Germany, 1987[138] | Not stated but not pregnant | Southern (11,16,18) | 12/96(13%) | 7/96(7%) | Not done | Not done |
| | Pregnancy (88% in second trimester) | | 26/92(28%) | 17/92(18%) | Not done | Not done |
| U.S., 1987[139] | Pregnancy (tested in first trimester) | Southern and reverse (6,11,16,16,18,31) | 14/215(7%) | 5/215(2%) | 12/19(63%) | 10/19(53%) |
| U.S., 1988[32] | Routine annual examination university students | Dot blot and Southern (6,11,16,18,31) | 30/466(6%) | 24/466(5%) | 18/54(33%) | 16/54(30%) |
| | Random sample of women attending an STD clinic | | 22/358(6%) | 18/358(5%) | 24/62(39%) | 13/62(21%) |

**HPV DNA in Normals and in Cervical Intraepithelial Neoplasia.** Results from seven studies[32,134–139] of the prevalence of detecting HPV DNA in cervical samples are shown in Table 48-5. In all seven studies, exfoliated cell samples were obtained from the cervix and tested by Southern, dot, or filter in situ hybridization for evidence of HPV 6 or 11 and HPV 16 or 18 infection and, in a few studies, for the presence of other human papillomavirus types. Among nonpregnant women with negative, noninflammatory smears, HPV DNA was detected in from 1 to 13 percent of women tested, with five of six studies showing a prevalence of at least 6 percent. The prevalence of HPV types 16, 18, or 31 ranged from 1 to 9 percent, and overall, these types were detected in about half (range of 10 to 100 percent) of the HPV DNA positive specimens obtained in these studies. Also shown in Table 48-5 is the detection of HPV DNA in 30 to 91 percent of cervical specimens obtained from nonpregnant women with cytologic evidence of CIN. HPV 16, 18, or 31 DNA was msot commonly detected in specimens showing cytologic evidence of CIN but also was detected frequently from specimens that were cytologically negative. De Villiers et al.[137] found that detection of HPV DNA was inversely related to age, with the highest prevalence found among women less than 25 years of age (14 percent of 994) and the lowest prevalence among those who were at least 56 years of age (4 percent of 2027). These data are presented in Fig. 48-8, which compares the age-specific prevalences of cervical HPV DNA, CIN 1 or 2 CIN 3, and invasive

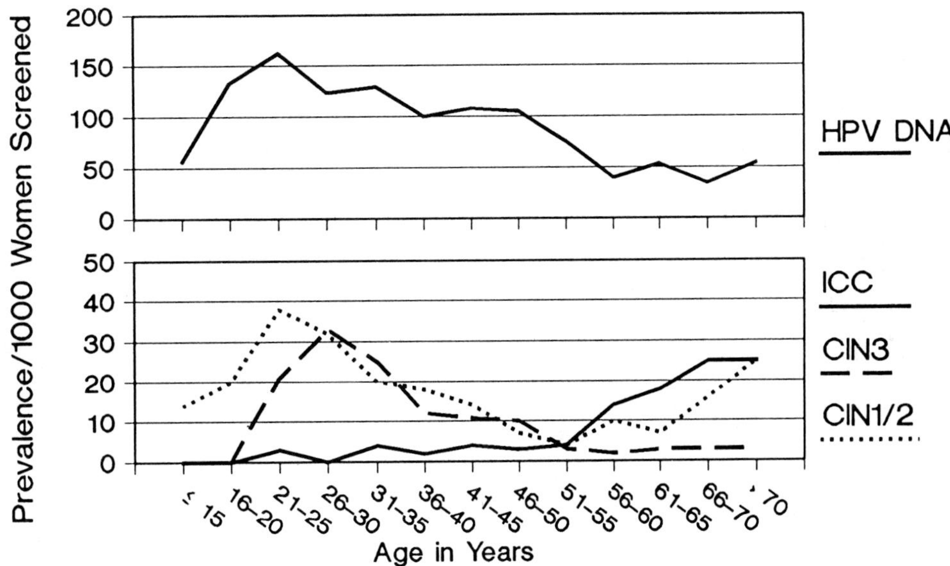


Fig. 48-8. Age-specific prevalence of HPV DNA, CIN 1–2, CIS, and invasive cervical cancer among 9295 women attending gynecology clinics in 1984. *(Data from de Villiers et al.*[137]*)*

cervical carcinoma. HPV DNA was found most commonly in women in their early twenties, that is, during the years when cytologic evidence of CIN and clinical evidence of genital warts were also most common.[140–142] The peak prevalence of CIN 3 was found in the late twenties, while the rate of invasive cervical cancer began to rise approximately two to three decades later.

Wickenden et al.[143] showed that the prevalence of HPV DNA was also high in women who had been successfully treated for CIS by laser therapy. They found that 48 percent of such women with cytologically and colposcopically normal cervices were positive for HPV DNA without any evidence of recurrent CIN. In order to explain the discrepancy between the high prevalence of HPV in normal women and the low rate of genital squamous cell carcinomas in the population, zur Hausen[144] suggested a mechanism of failing intracellular control of persisting viral genomes in proliferating cells, leading to development of neoplasia in some individuals. Such a model also could explain the long interval between the primary infection and the appearance of neoplasia.

## HSV

Soon after Rawls et al.[145] first isolated herpes simplex virus type 2 (HSV-2) from specimens of smegma from male STD clinic patients, Naib et al.[146] observed that cervical carcinoma or dysplasia was present in approximately 25 percent of cervical biopsy specimens from patients with cytological evidence of HSV infection. Several seroepidemiologic studies carried out in the 1970s indicated that women with CIN, CIS, and/or ICC were two to ten times more likely than controls to have antibody titers to HSV-2.[83] However, recent studies have not confirmed earlier results.[147] The major problem in most seroepidemiologic studies has been lack of careful matching of cases and controls for potential confounding factors, most importantly sexual behavior. Another problem with previous seroepidemiologic studies of the relationship between HSV and cervical neoplasia has been the difficulty in discriminating between serum antibody responses to HSV-1 and HSV-2. Seroepidemiologic studies of cervical neoplasia that have been reported to date have not used newer assays, which are better at differentiating antibody to HSV-2 from antibody to HSV-1.[148]

Frenkel et al.[149] were the first to report HSV-2 DNA in cervical cancer tissue. More recently, using Southern blot hybridization and defined fragments to viral DNA as probes, Galloway and McDougall[150] detected viral DNA sequences in 3 of 9 cervical tumors. Park et al.[151] detected viral DNA in 1 of 8 such tumors, and Prakash et al.[152] in 2 of 13 ICC specimens. HSV-specific RNA has been found in premalignant and malignant cervical tissue by in situ hybridization techniques.[153] Rodent cells transformed in vitro by HSV-2 have been reported to express a number of HSV-specific antigens including VP 143,[154] ICP 10,[155] and thymidine kinase.[156] Galloway et al.[157] identified a 737 base-pair fragment of HSV-2 DNA that transforms rodent cells in vitro. They found no evidence that this insertion sequence–like fragment encodes a polypeptide, suggesting that it can initiate transformation without involvement of a viral protein ("hit and run" hypothesis). However, there have been no reproducible reports on transformation of primate cells by HSV.

MacNab et al.[104] studied the association of HSV and HPV with cervical, vulvar, endometrial, and vaginal cancer by obtaining tumor specimens and specimens from histologically normal tissue of the same patients (internal controls). Hybridization to the HindIIIa clone of HSV-2 was detected in only 1 cervical tumor and 1 vulvar tumor (9 percent) among the 22 genital cancers studied. HPV 16 DNA was detected in 21 (84 percent) of the 25 tumors.

Di Luca and colleagues[158] also studied the simultaneous presence of HSV and HPV sequences in tumors of the female lower genital tract, by probing DNA from 13 cervical and vulvar intraepithelial neoplasias and 30 invasive carcinomas with cloned fragments of HSV-2 DNA and HPV 16 and 18 DNA. Four (31 percent) intraepithelial neoplasias and 4 (13 percent) invasive carcinomas hybridized to BglII N sequences of HSV-2. On the other hand, HPV 16 or HPV 18 DNA was detected in 92 percent of the intraepithelial neoplasias and in 53 percent of the invasive carcinomas. All 8 samples that hybridized to HSV-2 BglII N were also positive for HPV 16 or 18.

These results are in agreement with others showing that HSV DNA sequences are not often detected in genital tumors as tested by Southern blot hybridization, whereas DNA sequences hybridizing to HPV 16 or HPV 18 have been detected in over 50 percent of genital neoplasias (Fig. 48-7). Taken together, these observations suggest that HSV-2 is not a major etiologic agent in cervical neoplasia, but they do not rule out its involvement in some of the cases.[159] HSV DNA does not appear to be consistently retained or to code for a transforming protein. It remains possible that HSV and HPV might cooperate in oncogenesis, each playing a different role. More definitive seroepidemiologic studies of possible interactions between HSV and HPV in cervical cancer are needed.

## Cytomegalovirus, Epstein-Barr virus, and adenovirus

Human cytomegalovirus (CMV), a member of the human herpesvirus group, is capable of producing a latent infection in the human host. CMV can be sexually transmitted and has been isolated from the cervix of STD clinic patients.[160] Although CMV readily causes typical morphological alterations in endocervical epithelial cells in vitro, specific cytologic features in cervical specimens obtained from women have been difficult to demonstrate.[161] Melnick et al.[162] isolated CMV from 2 of 10 cervical cancer biopsies from patients with an advanced stage of the disease. Seroepidemiological studies of the association between CMV infection and cervical neoplasia have given inconclusive results.[163–165]

Albrecht and Rapp[166] transformed hamster embryo fibroblasts with ultraviolet-irradiated CMV. These transformed cells were tumorigenic in Syrian hamsters. Nelson et al.[167] demonstrated transformation of NIH 3T3 cells and primary rat embryo cells transfected with cloned restriction endonuclease DNA fragments of CMV strain AD169. Subsequently, Nelson et al.[168] determined the nucleotide sequence of the viral insert and open reading frames that might code for a gene product involved in transformation. The longest open reading frame in the fragment of the transforming region could code for a polypeptide with 41 amino acids. However, the CMV strains may vary considerably in their nucleotide sequence, and transformation studies with recent clinical isolates have not been performed.

Epstein-Barr virus (EBV), like CMV, belongs to the herpesvirus group. Infectious mononucleosis, the best-known syndrome associated with EBV, is associated with a variety of cutaneous and mucosal manifestations, including genital lesions.[169–171]

Although EBV is primarily a lymphotrophic virus, Sixbey et al.[172] demonstrated replication of EBV in human epithelial cells infected in vitro. Primary explant cultures of human ectocervix obtained from hysterectomy specimens were used in their experiments. EBV receptor was expressed in the human epithelial cells.[173] More recently, Sixbey et al.[174] reported detection of EBV genome in cervical epithelial cells from 5 (18 percent) of 28 women (2 with acute infectious mononucleosis and 3 seropositive women who were attending an STD clinic).

EBV is best known for its predilection for infecting and transforming B cells and for its association with endemic Burkitt's lymphoma. In addition, convincing evidence links this virus with the development of another epithelial cell carcinoma, undifferentiated nasopharyngeal carcinoma (NPC). EBV DNA is consistently detected in NPC biopsy material, and recently Young et al.[175] showed that an EBV latent protein, EBNA1, could be detected in 24 (83 percent) of 29 NPC biopsy specimens. Other latent proteins, including EBNA 2 and 3, were not detected, suggesting a pattern of EBV epithelial cell interaction in NPC which differed from that seen in EBV–lymphoid cell interactions in Burkitt's lymphoma. This result was subsequently confirmed by another group.[176] In addition, experimental molecular virologic studies have identified latent-infection viral genes and their products which caused transfected rat-1 cell clones to grow more densely, to lose contact inhibition, to lose anchorage dependence, and to be tumorigenic in nude mice.[177,178]

In summary, (1) EBV is associated with nasopharyngeal epithelial cell malignancy, (2) EBV infection of cervical epithelial cells occurs naturally, and (3) mechanisms for EBV-related tumorigenesis are unfolding from recent investigations. The association of this virus with chronic infection and tumors of the genital tract should be examined.

Adenovirus has occasionally been isolated from the cervix, and cytological alterations suspected to be caused by adenoviruses have been reported.[179] The effects of adenoviruses on monolayer cultures of human ectocervical and endocervical epithelial cells in vitro consist of hypertrophy of the cytoplasm and nucleus, development of pathological mitotic figures, fragmentation and aggregation of chromatin, and the appearance of intranuclear inclusion bodies.[180] However, the role of adenovirus infection in the development of cervical disease and abnormal cytologic atypias remains to be elucidated.

## HIV

Immunosuppression, whether inherited, as in epidermodysplasia verruciformis (EV), or acquired as a result of immunosuppressive therapy, increases the risk of genital tract and anal cancers. Invasive genital tract cancers are more common among immunosuppressed renal transplant patients as compared with controls,[181–184] and, as discussed in Chap. 37, skin cancers develop more often among individuals with EV than among individuals in the general population. An increase in invasive cancers of the anus, penis, cervix, vulva, or vagina among individuals infected with HIV has yet to be reported. However, because several investigators[185–192] have reported that genital or anal intraepithelial neoplasia is more common than expected among individuals with HIV infection, it is possible that invasive tumors will develop more frequently among HIV-infected vs. uninfected individuals. On the other hand, even if this is the case, the shortened life span of these individuals could mean that their lifetime risk for *invasive* genital or anal cancer is no greater than observed for the general population. Individuals infected with HIV should be closely monitored prospectively to define the risk of developing genital and anal neoplasia.

## Other STDs

Although sexually transmitted bacterial, chlamydial, protozoan, and fungal infections are probably not independent causes of genital and anal cancers, their capacity to induce chronic inflammation or irritation or to produce mutagenic metabolites[193] may increase risk of genital and/or anal carcinogenesis.

Several studies carried out in the 1930s to 1950s indicated that women with cervical cancer were more likely than those without to have serologic evidence of syphilis.[98] Rojel in 1953[194] explored this association among prostitutes and found that syphilis was equally common in prostitutes with or without cervical cancer, suggesting the existence of another carcinogen that was associated with acquisiton of *T. pallidum*.

Beral[195] compared mortality patterns for ICC with trends in incidence of gonorrhea in Great Britain, and found striking similarities. In cohorts of women, mortality rates from cervical cancer rose and fell consistently with the rise and fall in incidence of gonorrhea and syphilis some 20 years earlier. Additional studies have shown similar correlations between rates of gonorrhea and cervical neoplasia.[196–198]

Papanicolaou and Wolinska[199] described cellular changes including nuclear enlargement, irregularity, and hyperchromasia in cytological smears associated with the presence of *T. vaginalis*. Some investigators have demonstrated a higher rate of *T. vaginalis* infection in women with dysplasia or CIS than in the general population,[200] while others have not.[48,201] Experimentally, Patten[202] demonstrated that the cervix in mice inoculated vaginally with *T. vaginalis* underwent dysplastic changes, but that in each case cytology returned to normal after inoculations were discontinued.

In bacterial vaginosis (BV), which is the most common cause of abnormal vaginal discharge in many clinical settings (see Chaps. 46 and 47), the normal lactobacillus-dominated vaginal flora is replaced by one that includes *G. vaginalis*, *Mobiluncus* sp., *Bacteroides* sp., anaerobic gram-positive cocci, and mycoplasmas. Vaginal fluid of women with BV contains a characteristic pattern of organic acid microbial metabolites and amines.[203]

In a case control study, Guijon et al.[204] reported that cytologic or histopathologic evidence of HPV infection (koilocytosis) and altered vaginal flora consistent with BV were associated with CIN, and that these associations were independent of sexual behavior. One hypothesis is that nitrosamines (which are carcinogenic) are produced as metabolic microbial products under the anaerobic conditions of trichomoniasis or BV. However, this hypothesis has never been formally tested.[205]

Several studies have demonstrated an association between *C. trachomatis*, an inflammatory pattern and benign cytologic atypias seen on Pap smears;[206] however, the interpretation of many of these reports is heavily clouded by the lack of uniform criteria used to describe the cellular abnormalities. Cytologic changes consistent with CIN have been found more often in *C. trachomatis* culture-positive women than in culture-negative control women.[207–209] At least three seroepidemiologic studies have demonstrated an association between serum antichlamydial antibodies and CIN.[164,210]

Syrjänen et al.[211] evaluated the role of *C. trachomatis* in the development of CIN and the synergism between *C. trachomatis* and HPV among 418 women prospectively followed by cytology, colposcopy, and biopsy and found no correlation between *C. trachomatis* and cytologic atypia, and no evidence that *C. trachomatis* altered the natural history of HPV lesions.

*C. albicans* can adhere to genital tract epithelium, causes vulvovaginitis, often with ectocervicitis, and has been associated with the appearance of atypical superficial cells[161] but not with cervical neoplasia.

In summary, studies of the association of cervical neoplasia with sexually transmitted viruses, bacteria, and chlamydial infections are still few and none have included comprehensive microbiological and serological testing for putative infectious risk factors, with appropriate adjustment for coinfections and other relevant exposures in analyses. Only HPV has been consistently found to be associated with cervical dysplasias and invasive cervical cancer. Nonetheless, pathogens like *C. trachomatis* that cause cervical inflammation and epithelial damage resulting in metaplasia may increase the number of cells susceptible to neoplastic transformation by other oncogenic agents. In one study which controlled for age, residence, and number of sexual partners (<5,5 +), Daling et al.[7] found that among women but not among heterosexual men, antibodies to HSV-2 or to *C. trachomatis* were associated with anal cancer.

## NATURAL HISTORY

Most of our knowledge of the natural history of genital neoplasia is based on studies of cervical lesions showing dysplasia progressing to CIS. A few early studies examined progression from lesions showing CIS to those showing invasion, and a few recent studies have examined progression from cervical HPV infection to CIS. Results from these studies are discussed below.

### DEVELOPMENT OF INVASIVE CARCINOMA OF THE CERVIX AMONG WOMEN WITH CIS

During the 1940s through the 1960s, women with CIS diagnosed on histology were prospectively followed to ascertain the proportion which eventually become invasive. A wide variation in the proportion of cases progressing to ICC was observed (range of eight studies was 0 to 71 percent, with a median of 34 percent).[212] Because biopsies (which may have removed small lesions) were performed for the initial diagnosis, and because length of observation varied, results from these studies must be interpreted with caution. In addition to prospective studies of patients with CIS, retrospective reviews of biopsy specimens taken from patients known to have subsequently developed ICC have been performed.[213] For instance, Jones et al.[214] reviewed 1024 cases of ICC seen over a 16-year period and found 24 cases who had cervical biopsies taken at least 1 year prior. Seventeen patients (71 percent) had CIS lesions, 4 had no abnormality, and 3 had mild atypia.

### DEVELOPMENT OF CIS AMONG WOMEN WITH DYSPLASIA

Results from four studies of women with cytologic evidence of dysplasia who were followed with repeat Pap smears and without biopsy until a lesion showed CIS or until study termination are presented in Table 48-6. In these studies, cohorts were defined on the basis of cytologic findings rather than histology, thereby eliminating concern that a biopsy may have altered the natural course of the lesion. However, cytologic classification systems, enrollment criteria, length and frequency of follow-up, and statistical determination of progression were different for each study. For example, Richart and Barron[11] enrolled a woman who had had three dysplastic Pap smears, thereby ensuring the stability of the lesion. In contrast, Jordan et al.[217] enrolled only women who had had two negative Pap smears prior to the Pap smear that showed dysplasia, thereby perhaps reducing the problem of smears falsely negative for CIS on enrollment.

Within each cytologic category, progression to CIS was observed more frequently in the Richart and Barron study than in any of the other three studies. Based on life table analysis of 10 years of data, Richart and Barron[11] projected that 50 percent of mild dysplasias would progress to CIS in 5 years if left untreated.

**Table 48-6. Development of Carcinoma in situ among Women with Cytologic Evidence of Dysplasia: Summary of Four Studies**

| Principal author, year | Cytologic system* | Cytologic entry criterion | Cohort definition | Number in cohort | Months of follow-up | % progressing to ≥carcinoma in situ |
|---|---|---|---|---|---|---|
| Richart, 1969[11] | O[215] | 3 dysplastic smears | Mild dysplasia | NS† | Projected progression at 60 months (life table analysis) | 50 |
| | | | Mod. dysplasia | NS | | 70 |
| | | | Severe dysplasia | NS | | 95 |
| | | | Any dysplasia | | | 48 |
| Patten, 1978[216] | P[216] | 1 dysplastic smear | Mild dysplasia | 3299 | 60 months | 0.5 |
| | | | Mod. dysplasia | 661 | | 2.4 |
| | | | Severe dysplasia | 125 | | 10.4 |
| Jordan, 1981[217] | W[218] | 2 negative smears | Mild dysplasia | 708 | 60 months | 1.1 |
| | | | Mod. dysplasia | 164 | | 1.8 |
| | | | Severe dysplasia | 52 | | 7.7 |
| | | 3 dysplastic smears | Any dysplasia | 65 | | 19.0 |
| Nasiell, 1983, 1986‡[219,220] | W[218] | 1 dysplastic smear | Mild dysplasia | 555 | Projected progression at 60 months (life table analysis) | 15.0 |
| | | | Mod. dysplasia (no biopsy) | 410 | | 26.0 |
| | | | Mod. dysplasia (biopsy) | 484 | | 21.0 |

*Organization of cytologic classification scheme used to classify cytologic findings: O = Okagaki, P = Patten, W = World Health Organization.
†Numbers of subjects followed not specified.
‡No difference in biopsied vs. nonbiopsied group for the mild dysplasia group.

Progression of mild dysplasia to CIS during a similar interval was shown in less than 20 percent of women followed in each of the other three studies.[216,217,219,220]

The discrepancy between results obtained by Richart and Barron and in the other studies listed in Table 48-6 has been attributed to the fact that all women enrolled in Richart and Barron had had at least three abnormal cytology smears. However, analysis of the data from Jordan et al.[217] on the subset of women who had at least three dysplastic Pap smears suggests that this cannot be the only explanation. Progression to CIS within 5 years was estimated at 48 percent in the Richart and Barron study, and at only 19 percent of women enrolled with three dysplastic smears in the study of Jordan et al. It is also likely that a large portion of what was classified as mild, moderate, or severe dysplasia in the Richart and Barron study would have been classified, in other studies that used different cytologic classification systems, as evidence of early carcinoma in situ because Richart and Barron classified the severity of dysplasia on the basis of the relative proportion of abnormal cells that were of basal cell type. We consider the presence of any dysplastic cells that have morphologic features similar to basal cells to be most consistent with severe dysplasia or CIS. In addition, the criteria used by Richart and Barron may have reflected the size of the lesion more closely than it reflected different stages of CIN. Further, as discussed earlier, the fact that mild dysplasia tends to be associated with multiple HPV types, while severe dysplasia tends to be associated with HPV 16 or 18[4] calls into question whether these lesions should in fact be viewed as stages in a continuum. Also, it must be emphasized that cytology is basically a technique for screening for dysplasia, not a technique for staging severity of dysplasia—which is dependent on histologic studies of colposcopically directed biopsies.

In summary, since the diagnosis of cervical precancer by cytology is not based on universally standardized and objective criteria, studies of the natural history of cytologic abnormalities are not strictly comparable. The weight of evidence indicates that women with CIN 3 or CIS are more likely to develop invasive cervical carcinoma than are women with CIN 1 or 2. The weight of evidence also suggests that progression from mild or moderate dysplasia to CIS occurs in less than 50 percent of women over a 5-year period. It also appears that the risk of progression is dictated not only by initial severity of cytologic evidence of dysplasia, but also the size and appearance of the lesion by colposcopy or cervicography,[221,222] and perhaps by the presence of infection with high-risk HPV types, as discussed below.

## DEVELOPMENT OF CIS OR ICC AMONG WOMEN WITH CERVICAL HPV INFECTION

Mitchell et al.[223] followed 846 women with cytological evidence of HPV infection for the development of cervical neoplasia. CIS developed in 30 women (3.6 percent) during the next 6 years (compared with 1.9 expected cases of CIS), giving a relative risk of 15.6. The risk was greater in young (<25) women than in older (>29) women (38.7 vs. 8.1).

In a prospective study, Campion et al.[224] followed (without biopsy) 100 women with CIN 1 lesions detected at least three times by Pap smear during the 10 months prior to the start of follow-up. Over a period of 1 to 12 months, 26 percent progressed to CIN 3; the overall prevalence of HPV 16 was 39 percent, but it was 85 percent for those who progressed to CIN 3. Since all 26 cases of CIS were detected within 12 months of satisfying enrollment criteria, it is possible that a portion of these women were misclassified as CIN 1 (despite three repeated smears) at the beginning of the follow-up period and therefore were not true cases of progressive disease.

## DEVELOPMENT OF CIN AMONG WOMEN WITH PAP SMEARS SHOWING ATYPIA

Melamed and Flehinger[225] followed cohorts of women with negative Pap smears (28,791 women) or with Pap smears that were atypical but not abnormal enough to be classified as dysplasia (1223 women). Within 72 months, less than 5 percent of women with an initially negative smear compared with 20 percent of those with an atypical smear showed progression to dysplasia. Progression to a lesion showing at least CIS was observed in 1.2 percent of the negative group and 6.7 percent of the group with atypical smears.

In a recent study, Paavonen et al.[226] followed 124 STD clinic patients referred because of a single smear showing benign atypia. The mean follow-up time was 22 months, ranging from 1 to 59 months. After 30 months of follow-up the cumulative rate of progression to biopsy-confirmed CIN 2 to 3 was 14 percent for all women with benign atypias on referral cytology. Metaplastic cell atypia had a significantly higher rate of progression than superficial cell atypia (Fig. 48-9). This study provides evidence of the potential significance of metaplastic atypia as a precursor of CIN.

## NATURAL HISTORY OF SQUAMOUS CELL NEOPLASIAS OF OTHER SITES

Although vulvar intraepithelial neoplasia (VIN) lesions carry a potential for developing into invasive cancer, this rarely occurs. The term microinvasive vulvar cancer has also been introduced, and microinvasive lesions should always be regarded as invasive cancer. Approximately one-half of invasive vulvar carcinomas occur multifocally, and one-half develop as isolated ulcerative lesions. Although VIN lesions have been rare, an increasing incidence and prevalence has been reported from many countries, particularly in young women. Atypia consistent with VIN grade 1 to 2 has been reported in approximately 20 percent of patients with evidence of subclinical vulvar HPV infection.[77]

The natural history of VIN lesions in young women still remains largely unknown, although occasional malignant progression has been reported.[227] Buscema et al.[76] followed 102 patients with CIS of the vulva for 1 to 15 years. The average age of the patients was 47 years, with 40 percent under age 41; 28 percent had associated cervical dysplasia. Only 4 (4 percent) of the 102 patients with vulvar CIS developed invasive cancer during the follow-up; of these, 2 were postmenopausal and 2 were immunosuppressed because of underlying systemic disease. Friedrich et al.[228] reported 50 cases of CIS of the vulva, 9 of whom received no treatment. Five of the 9 patients experienced spontaneous regression, and only one case progressed to invasive vulvar carcinoma. This occurred in a 21-year-old severely immunosuppressed patient.

Crum et al.[229] reported 41 cases of VIN, of whom 4 (10 percent) developed carcinoma within 3 years of follow-up. The mean age of patients with progressive disease was 55 years. They concluded that young patients with VIN have a low risk of progression, whereas older patients have a higher risk of progression.

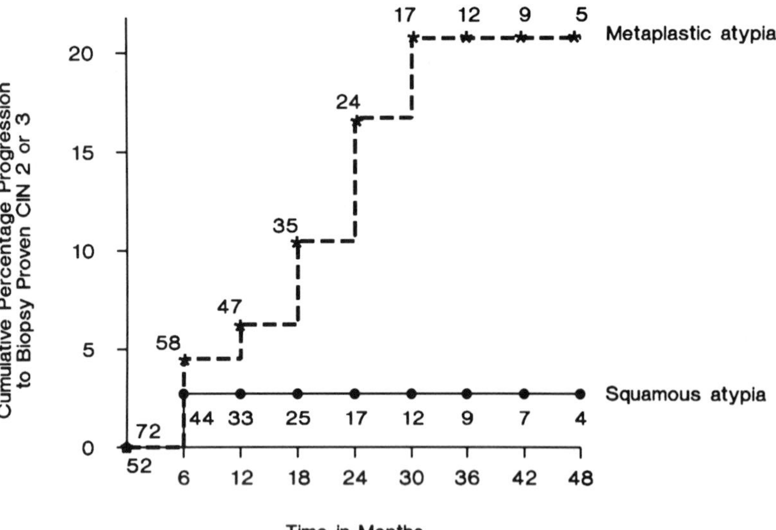


Fig. 48-9. Progression of metaplastic cell atypia and superficial cell atypia to biopsy-confirmed CIN 2 to 3 among women attending an STD clinic.[226]

Bonnekoh[230] also reported 2 young women aged 30 and 33 with Bowenoid papulosis of the vulva who developed invasive squamous cell carcinoma of the perineal and vulvar region.

Clearly more studies are needed of the natural history of VIN, the progressive potential of different grades of VIN lesions, and the risk factors associated with progression. Until they are done, the management of such patients should probably be as conservative as possible, and a period of observation seems justified.

There are even fewer data concerning the natural history of early vaginal squamous cell neoplasias, although the natural history of invasive vaginal carcinoma is thought to be similar to that of ICC. Rutledge[231] has shown a progression from VAIN to invasive carcinoma in several patients. Lenechan et al.[232] reviewed 59 cases of VAIN seen in a colposcopy clinic in Toronto between 1971 and 1984. Three patients (5 percent) developed invasive carcinoma of the vagina after local ablative techniques ($CO_2$ laser or electrocautery).

Although recent data show that HPV DNA can be detected in over 50 percent of anal and penile lesions showing intraepithelial neoplasia (see Fig. 48-7), these lesions, like those of the vulva, appear to be less likely than their counterparts in the cervix to progress to invasion.

## CYTOLOGY

Gynecologic cytology as we know it today dates from the early part of this century, when George Papanicolaou attempted to examine vaginal aspirates to detect clinically asymptomatic cervical cancer. He found that in addition to being able to detect cells from clinically inapparent invasive cancer, he could also detect cells from lesions of carcinoma in situ, and less worrisome cells from lesions which today are classified as dysplasias.[233] Since that time, "Pap" screening has been widely adopted and is credited, at least in part, for the dramatic decrease in the incidence of cervical cancer.[54,234]

The basis for classification of cervical abnormalities detected on Pap smears is, by necessity, different from that used on biopsy material since cytology examines only surface cells of a lesion. In invasive cancer and CIS, the surface cells are similar to those deep in the lesion, and so it is easy to see how cytology can detect such conditions. However, as explained above, histologically, lesions are classified as mild dysplasia (CIN I) or moderate dysplasia (CIN II) based on the percentage of the deep epithelium occupied by undifferentiated cells. Cytologic diagnosis is possible in such lesions because the differentiation that occurs in the upper portion of the epithelium of CIN I and II lesions is abnormal and these lesions shed surface cells with characteristic morphologic changes.

The criteria necessary for a cytologic diagnosis of invasive squamous cancer are well established, and the reader is referred to textbooks of cytology for an in-depth discussion of the subject.[235] Briefly, the diagnosis requires the presence of cells with nuclear and cytoplasmic changes associated with malignancies, as well as a characteristic background on which one typically sees necrotic debris, old blood, and inflammation.

## CYTOLOGIC CLASSIFICATION OF ABNORMAL BUT NOT INVASIVE CELLS

Generally, cells without the features of frankly invasive tumors are classified as dyskaryotic or suggestive of CIN or, if they show less severe changes, as atypical. Cells from lesions histologically consistent with CIN show abnormal nuclear and cytoplasmic changes including an increase in the nuclear/cytoplasmic ratio, increased and abnormally distributed nuclear chromatin, and abnormal nuclear and cytoplasmic conformation.[235]

Papanicolaou termed such individual abnormal cells as dyskaryotic to distinguish them from cells from obviously invasive tumors, and classified them as showing "superficial cell dyskaryosis," "intermediate cell dyskaryosis," "parabasal cell dyskaryosis," or "endocervical cell dyskaryosis" according to the normal cervical epithelial cells to which these abnormal cells bore the most resemblance.[233] Cytopathologists continue to classify individual abnormal cells in a somewhat similar fashion. Abnormal cells have been classified as showning (1) mild or superficial dyskaryosis or changes suggestive of CIN I, (2) moderate or intermediate cell dyskaryosis or changes consistent with CIN II, or (3) severe or parabasal cell dyskaryosis or changes consistent with CIN III. Cells are assigned an increasing grade of CIN or dysplasia as their nuclear to cytoplasmic ratio increases. In summary, the higher the grade of dysplasia, the less the cell resembles a normal superficial cell and the more it resembles the undifferentiated cells seen in CIS. A new classification scheme proposed by a 1988 National Cancer Institute Workshop on Classification of Cervical and Vaginal Cytology (personal communication, Diane Solomon, 1989) recommends that squamous cell intraepithelial lesions showing changes consistent with intraepithelial neoplasia be classified simply as either "low-grade" or "high-grade" (Table 48-7).

Many different grades of abnormal cells may be present on a smear, since CIN is frequently a multifocal disease, and while pathologists have generally agreed on how to classify individual abnormal cells, many systems for cytologic classification of the smear as a whole have been developed since Papanicolaou's time. In the system most widely used today (the World Health Organization classification system), the overall diagnosis of a smear is determined by the grade of the most abnormal cell present, regardless of the number of such cells present.[218] Thus, if a smear contains many abnormal cells showing changes suggestive of a mild dysplasia, but also cells with changes consistent with severe dysplasia, the overall diagnosis would be "changes suggestive of severe dysplasia."

Depending on the population screened, from 5 up to 25 percent (e.g., in patients from an STD clinic) have cellular changes on their smears which are abnormal but which fail to meet the criteria for a diagnosis of dysplasia. Cellular changes that are frequently placed in such a category include cells showing parakeratosis, hyperkeratosis, mild nuclear enlargement, abnormalities in cytoplasmic configuration, and binucleation. The significance of these changes is poorly understood. However, as mentioned above, several studies have suggested that at least a certain percentage of these atypias progress and thus repeat cytology is suggested. Furthermore, repeat cytology within a short period of time may show more severely dysplastic cells that were presumably absent or overlooked in the original cytologic sample.[225,226] We analyzed the microbiological and clinical correlates of minor changes in squamous, metaplastic, and endocervical cells in a study of 165 STD clinic patients using the classification system presented in Table 48-8. Minimal squamous atypia was significantly associated with yeast infection, moderate squamous atypia and koilocytosis were significantly associated with cervical condylomata visualized by colposcopy, while reactive or mildly atypical metaplastic changes were associated with *C. trachomatis* infection.[161] Similar studies are needed in which DNA probes for HPV are also used to further assess the cause of minor cytologic atypias.

**Table 48-7. Suggested Classification of Squamous Epithelial Cell Cytologic Changes***

Atypical squamous cells of undetermined significance (specify recommended follow-up and/or type of further investigation)
Squamous intraepithelial lesions [comment on presence or absence of cellular changes consistent with human papillomavirus (HPV) infection]
- Low-grade squamous intraepithelial lesion, encompassing:
  - Cellular changes consistent with HPV infection
  - Mild dysplasia/CIN 1
- High-grade squamous intraepithelial lesion, encompassing:
  - Moderate dysplasia/CIN 2
  - Severe dysplasia/CIN 3
  - Carcinoma in situ/CIN 3

Squamous carcinoma

*Summarized from abstract presented at the Workshop on Terminology and Classification of Vaginal Cytology, National Cancer Institute, December 1988.

## CYTOLOGIC CLASSIFICATION OF HPV-ASSOCIATED LESIONS

The classification of abnormal cervical cells by cytology has been reexamined in light of recent recognition of the role of HPV in cervical precancer and cancer and has presented the cytopathologist with a new set of problems in terms of diagnosis of HPV and classification of smears containing HPV-associated changes. Koilocytes or cells with distinct perinuclear halos (see Fig. 48-10) can be frequently identified in abnormal Pap smears and have been associated with clinical and colposcopic evidence of HPV infection and with the presence of HPV DNA in the cervix. Although many laboratories make the diagnosis of HPV based on the presence of such cells, studies have shown poor intra- and interobserver reproducibility for identification of such cellular changes.[32,236] Some pathologists also feel that cervical dyskeratosis, including hyperkeratosis (squamous cells without nuclei) and parakeratosis (abnormally small, rounded squamous cells with pyknotic nuclei), is indicative of HPV infection.[15,237] However, the sensitivity and specificity of this finding for the diagnosis of HPV infection is unknown. Fortunately, DNA probe technology which offers high specificity for a diagnosis of HPV will become increasingly available over the next few years.

**Table 48-8. Cytological Classification of "Benign" Atypias Not Sufficient to Be Termed Consistent with CIN**

| | Cell type | Cell arrangement | Nucleo-cytoplasmic ratio | Nuclear chromatin | Nuclear contour | Cytoplasm |
|---|---|---|---|---|---|---|
| Squamous reactive atypia | Superficial intermediate | Single cells | Normal to slightly increased | Chromocenters present | Regular | Small perinuclear halo |
| Squamous nonkoilocytotic atypia | Superficial intermediate | Single cells and thick groups | Variable | Slightly increased | Regular; binuclear | Dense; eosinophilic to orangiophilic (dyskaratosis) |
| Koilocytotic atypia | Superficial intermediate | Single cells and thick groups | Variable | Slightly increased or opaque | Irregular; bi- or multinucleation | Distinct "halo" around nucleus with dense outer rim of cytoplasm |
| Metaplastic atypia | Metaplastic | Single cells and thick groups | Slightly increased | Slightly increased; nucleoli can be present | Irregular | Dense to lacy cytoplasm |

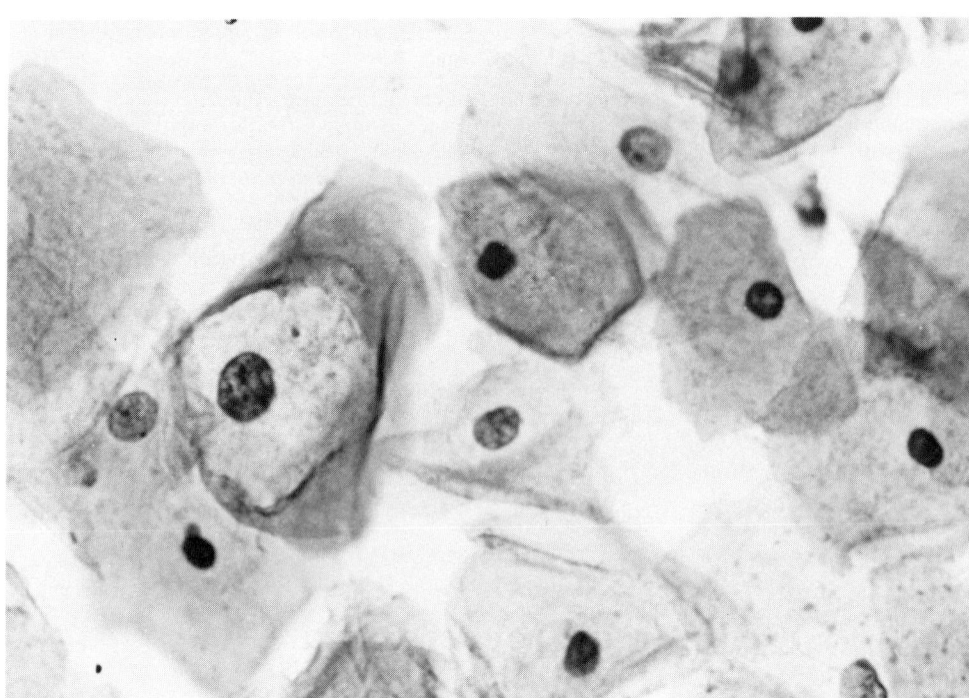

**Fig. 48-10.** Papanicolaou smear showing cytologic findings suggestive of infection by HPV. Note the koilocyte with a distinct perinuclear halo.

As noted above with regard to cervical biopsies, and discussed further below, a U.S. National Cancer Institute workshop has proposed that cytologic smears showing cellular changes suggestive of HPV infection without features of dysplasia should be classified together with smears showing changes consistent with mild dysplasia, under the category "low-grade intraepithelial squamous cell lesions."

## REPORTING OF CYTOLOGIC FINDINGS

Despite the fact that most cytology laboratories use the same systems for classification of individual atypical cells as well as for diagnosis of the overall smear, there is almost no agreement as to how these findings should be reported to clinicians.

In his *Atlas of Exfoliative Cytology*[238] Papanicolaou proposed that the results of cervical smear cytologies be reported by using a five-class system: class I: absence of atypical or abnormal cells; class II: atypical cells (reactive) but no malignant or premalignant cell changes; class III: atypical cells suggestive of but not diagnostic of malignancy; class IV: cells strongly suggestive of malignancy; and class V: cytology consistent with malignancy. This system predated the development of the dysplasia and CIN systems for histologic classification of cervical epithelial pathology (discussed above). Therefore, it is not clear how one should classify smears containing mild vs. moderate vs. severely dysplastic cells within the Papanicolaou class system. By the time the dysplasia and CIN systems were developed, many cytology laboratories had already been using the Papanicolaou classification system. Some laboratories abandoned this system and began to use descriptive diagnoses (cells consistent with mild moderate or severe dysplasia), other laboratories continued to use only the traditional Papanicolaou class system, but most have attempted to continue to use the Papanicolaou class system while including information about the "grade" of dysplasia or CIN present. This has resulted in further confusion. One survey[239] of 121 cytotechnologists, pathologists, and clinicians reported that 58 percent were using a combination of a descriptive diagnosis and the Papanicolaou class system, while 38 percent used a descriptive diagnosis alone and 5 percent used the Papanicolaou class alone to report cytologic findings. Considerable lack of agreement occurred as to assignment of a class to smears containing mildly and moderately dysplastic cells. In a questionnaire as to how various changes would be classified, mild dysplasias were put into class I, II, and III by 1, 59, and 36 percent of respondents, respectively, while moderate dysplasias were placed in class I, II, and III by 4, 76, and 12 percent of respondents.

Even greater disagreement occurred for lesions considered to be less than CIN (discussed below) such as inflammatory atypia, squamous atypia, hyperkeratosis, parakeratosis, and atypical endocervical cells. To some extent the confusion as to how to classify such changes reflects uncertainty about the natural history of these lesions. Given this confusion as well as the fact that it is important to be able to compare cytologic and histologic findings, it is probably best to avoid the use of any "class" system and to use descriptive diagnoses employing accepted terminology that will allow for comparison of cytologic and histologic findings. The 1988 NCI workshop concluded that "the Papanicolaou Class System is not acceptable in the modern practice of diagnostic pathology." It recommended that cervical cytology laboratory reports include (1) a statement of the adequacy of the specimen for diagnostic evaluation; (2) a general categorization of the smear as normal or abnormal; (3) a descriptive diagnosis, including evidence of infection, inflammation and reactive changes, and epithelial cell abnormalities involving squamous cells, glandular cells, or other epithelial neoplasias. Squamous cell abnormalities should be classified as outlined in Table 48-7. As discussed above, it is proposed that changes consistent with intraepithelial neoplasia are graded as either "high-" or "low-" grade squamous intraepithelial neoplasia, with an accompanying comment about cellular changes consistent with HPV infection, if applicable. Cellular changes consistent with HPV infection (without features of "dysplasia" or "CIN") may be used as a separate diagnostic term, although it is recommended that it be included under the designation of low-grade squamous intraepithelial lesion.

## SENSITIVITY AND SPECIFICITY OF CYTOLOGIC SCREENING

Whether or not Pap smears are effective for screening for cervical cancer and precancer is hotly debated. False-negative smears have been said to range from 1.1 to 62.5 percent.[240,241] However, it is clear that in countries where systematic Pap screening and appropriate follow-up has been instituted mortality from cervical cancer has dramatically decreased.[234] The effectiveness of cytology for prevention of cervical cancer depends on a number of factors including selection of those to be screened, frequency of screening, success in implementing screening programs, obtaining adequate smears and reading them appropriately, and finally instituting therapy.

## APPROPRIATE COLLECTION OF SPECIMENS

Despite the fact that many studies have shown that false-negative cytologies are frequently the result of inadequate sampling in collection of specimens,[242,243] there is no agreement as to how smears should be collected and what constitutes an adequate smear. Papanicolaou first proposed using vaginal pool aspirates for screening for cervical cancer, but it was quickly appreciated that since most dysplasia occurs at the area of the squamocolumnar junction, an adequate collection technique should involve sampling this area. In 1947, Ayres proposed using a wooden spatula to scrape the cervix itself to obtain a "surface biopsy" of the area most often involved with pathology. Samples obtained in this fashion often contain a greater number of dysplastic cells than the vaginal pool aspirate.[240] However, when the cervix is sampled with the Ayres spatula, the "false-negative" rate of cytology, based on comparison with biopsy, rereading of smears, and obtaining two or more cervical cytology samples, has been reported to be from 2 to 62 percent. The addition of an endocervical sample has been shown to lower false-negative rates for cytology.[240,244] Furthermore, since it is known that cervical squamous epithelial pathology most often occurs at the squamocolumnar junction, it has been proposed that the presence of endocervical cells on a smear would be an indication of adequacy of sampling of this area. This concept is supported by several studies such as that of Elias et al.,[245] who found that the odds of finding dysplastic cells consistent with mild to moderate or severe dysplasia and with carcinoma in situ or microinvasive carcinoma was 2.2 and 4.4 greater among women with endocervical cells present on their smear than among those without endocervical cells present. Although collection of endocervical material can be accomplished using a cotton-tipped applicator, brush, or aspirator (see Fig. 48-11), some data suggest that a cytology brush is superior to a cotton-tipped applicator for collection of endocervical cells in all age groups including pregnant women.[246] Others, however, claim that the presence of endocervical mucus alone is indicative of an adequate smear.[235] Several studies have shown that in addition to collection of endocervical samples, immediate repeated sampling of the cervix can significantly increase the number of dysplastic cells present on the smear.[243]

The question as to whether smears should be collected on one slide or two slides has not been adequately addressed. Our own experience in screening women from an STD clinic who have dense inflammation in their endocervical canal, and women attending an outpatient gynecology department clinic for routine examination, suggests that separation of the endocervical and ectocervical samples as shown in Fig. 48-11 is particularly useful in a population with a high rate of endocervical infection. Further studies should be done assessing this question, in terms of cost and sensitivity for detection of atypical cells, as well as for assessing the presence of endocervicitis.

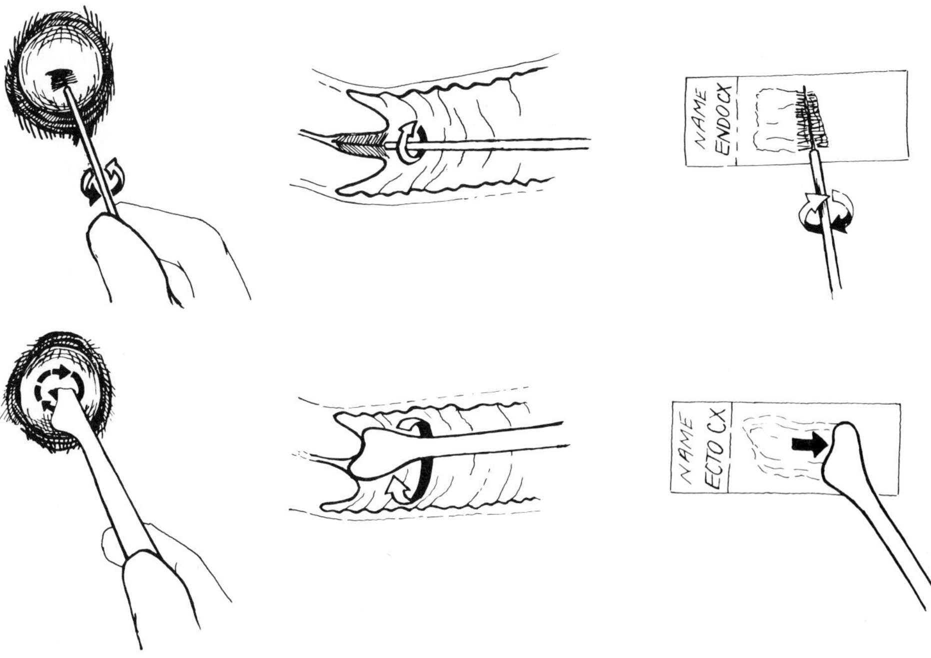


**Fig. 48-11.** Diagram demonstrating the recommended sampling technique for obtaining a Papanicolaou smear.

## INTERPRETATION OF CYTOLOGIC SMEAR

Correct interpretation of cytologic smears depends on a number of factors including (1) the availability of properly trained cytotechnologists and pathologists, (2) a working environment that rewards accurate screening, (3) adequate quality assurance programs, and (4) continuing education. In the past 10 years, most cytotechnology schools have had difficulty in recruiting students because the field is demanding and pay is fairly low. Unfortunately, in many laboratories cytotechnologists are paid by the number of slides they screen, a practice that does not reward careful, accurate screening. It is encouraging that recently several states in the United States have limited the number of slides cytotechnologists can screen per day. In addition, it appears that many states will follow the example of New York and mandate specific quality assurance programs and periodic reaccreditation of cytotechnologists.[247]

## CYTOLOGY AT OTHER GENITAL TRACT SITES

Sampling of exfoliating cells has also occasionally been used for other sites including vagina, vulva,[248] and anus.[249,250] Anal smears may prove to be of considerable importance in screening for anal cancer and precancer in homosexual men, a population known to be at high risk for this disease. However, the sensitivity and specificity of exfoliative cytology at these sites for diagnoses of epithelial pathology has not been established.

## NEW DEVELOPMENTS IN THE DETECTION OF CERVICAL PATHOLOGY

Over the next few years, sensitive and specific tests for diagnosis of HPV will become available (see Chap. 78). Although up to 30 percent of women with normal cytology have been found to harbor cervical HPV 16 or 18, over 50 percent of those with HPV DNA detected at the cervix have been found concurrently to have dyslastic cells present on their cervical smears. Detection of cervical HPV DNA may be useful in identifying a group of women who are at high risk for false-negative cytology.

## COLPOSCOPY

The colposcope is a magnifying optical instrument that provides a magnified view of the living tissue. Colposcopy is a noninvasive outpatient procedure; it is relatively simple, can be done quickly, and is generally not painful. One of the most important advantages of colposcopy is that it offers the opportunity to examine large anatomic areas of surface epithelium (cervix, vagina, vulva, anus) and to carefully map the lesions found.

During the last 50 years colposcopy has been used to evaluate women with atypical cervical cytology to determine the most significant lesion sites for obtaining targeted biopsies for histopathologic examination.[251,252] Only recently, colposcopy has been used as a routine diagnostic test to detect specific cervicovaginal infections.[226,226a] For the technical details of the colposcopic examination the reader is referred to standard textbooks of colposcopy.[224,225]

## NORMAL COLPOSCOPIC FINDINGS

Normal colposcopic findings include stratified glycogen-containing squamous epithelium covering the vagina and ectocervix, single-layered mucus-secreting glandular epithelium covering the endocervix, the squamocolumnar junction, and the typical transformation zone (T zone) where squamous metaplasia takes place when subcolumnar reserve cells multiply and become stratified during the process called squamous metaplasia. The origin of the subcolumnar reserve cells is not well understood, but they are believed to be pluripotential cells from the endocervical mucosa or stroma. Gland openings and Nabothian cysts are simple landmarks to identify the location and extent of the T zone.

## ABNORMAL COLPOSCOPIC FINDINGS

Atypical transformation zone refers to colposcopic changes produced either by crowding of the epithelial layer with excessive proliferation of cells, thus changing the optical density of the epithelium, or by changes in the vascularization of the epithelium which has acquired neoplastic potential. Atypical T zone findings include leukoplakia (white lesion visible before the application of 5% acetic acid, also known as keratosis), acetowhite epithelium (white lesion visible only after application of acetic acid), vascular atypia including patterns referred to as mosaicism, punctation, and abnormal vessels. The more marked the color change to white that takes place after the application of acetic acid and the sharper the lesion borders are, the higher is the likelihood of intraepithelial neoplasia. Mosaicism and punctation appear (Plate 90) when rete peg formation, i.e., elongated stromal papilli, occurs during metaplasia. In vascular atypia, the intercapillary distance has a positive association with the histopathologic severity of the lesion. The vascular appearance is enhanced with the use of a green filter. Normal blood vessels show regular treelike branching whereas abnormal vessels show corkscrew appearance, caliber changes, and abrupt changes in direction. The presence of abnormal vessels predicts a severe lesion and is suggestive of microinvasive carcinoma at least.

Colposcopically, it is relatively easy to distinguish between typical and atypical T zone findings. Atypical T zone findings are called either nonsignificant, i.e., not suggestive of CIN, or significant, i.e., suggestive of CIN 1 to 2, or highly significant, i.e., suggestive of at least CIN 3. This interpretation is based on the color tone of the lesion after the application of 5% acetic acid, sharpness of the demaraction borders between the lesion and the surrounding epithelium, surface contour, and vascular atypia. The extent of the lesion is important, although the size alone should not be considered as a diagnostic criterion. The graphic documentation of colposcopic findings is based on the use of commonly accepted abbreviations and sketch drawings. Colpophotographs can provide additional information although they cannot completely replace a quality graphic documentation.

Deriving a colposcopic index, or score, is helpful in quantitating the atypical T zone findings and shows a relatively good correlation with the histopathologic findings.[253]

## COLPOSCOPY IN THE MANAGEMENT OF CERVICAL NEOPLASIA

Colposcopy has proved to be a useful adjunct to cytology for the detection and localization of cervical, vaginal, and vulvar intraepithelial neoplasias. The colposcopist attempts to visualize the lesion and to determine (1) whether the colposcopic examination is adequate, (2) the histopathologic severity of the lesions, and (3) the location of the worst lesion(s) to obtain colposcopically directed biopsies. If the entire squamocolumnar junction cannot be seen (because a portion or all of the junction lies within the endocervical canal), the colposcopic examination is termed inadequate, or unsatisfactory. This problem occurs in approximately 15 to 20 percent of women, less often in young women.[254] In patients with inadequate colposcopy, an endocervical curettage, conization, or both are required for diagnosis.

The accuracy of diagnosis made by colposcopically directed biopsy has been compared with that determined by subsequent conization or hysterectomy.[255–257] These studies report concordance rates between 67 and 95 percent. Accuracy improves with the expertise of the colposcopist and should approach 100 percent with experience.

There is some controversy on the use of routine endocervical curettage (ECC). Some colposcopists recommend that an ECC should be performed whenever colposcopically directed biopsy is obtained,[258,259] whereas some colposcopists feel that an ECC is needed only in situations when the total squamocolumnar junction cannot be adequately visualized (inadequate colposcopy).[257,260,261]

## COLPOSCOPIC MANIFESTATIONS OF SPECIFIC CERVICAL AND VAGINAL INFECTIONS

Changes in the cervix or vagina caused by specific infectious agents can also be defined by colposcopy. For instance, *T. vaginalis* causes vascular changes comprising patchy areas of fine punctation also called strawberry cervix, or colpitis macularis. Vulvovaginal candidiasis shows characteristic cottage cheese–like discharge, increased erythema, and capillary dilatation with hairpin or comma-shaped capillaries. Mucopurulent cervicitis caused by *C. trachomatis* is often associated with edema and erythema of the area of ectopy and the transformation zone. Cervical ulcerations visible by colposcopy are associated with genital HSV infection. Small ectocervical ulcerations or ulcerations occurring in the transformation zone are often difficult to diagnose without the colposcope.

Other causes of cervical ulceration besides advanced ICC and genital herpes include primary syphilis, lymphogranuloma venereum, chancroid, tuberculosis, toxic shock syndrome, and trauma. Colposcopic diagnosis of classical condyloma acuminata is relatively easy. With the recognition of subclinical papillomavirus infections (SPI, flat condyloma) many colposcopists have attempted to develop criteria that would allow specific diagnosis of HPV infection and discrimination of HPV infection from true CIN,[262–266] but this has rapidly led to very confusing nomenclature with questionable reproducibility. The sensitivity, specificity, and predictive value of colposcopy in comparison with cytology, immunoperoxidase staining of HPV antigen, detection of HPV DNA, or histopathologic diagnosis of HPV infection has not been adequately tested.

Paavonen et al.[226] recently used colposcopic screening to define the colposcopic manifestations of several specific vaginal and cervical infections, adjusting for coinfections, in randomly selected STD clinic patients. Particularly noteworthy were the associations of endocervical mucopus with *C. trachomatis*, *N. gonorrhoeae*, and HSV; the strong association of "strawberry cervix" with *T. vaginalis;* the correlation of hypertrophic ("follicular") cervicitis with *C. trachomatis;* the association of immature metaplasia with CMV and *C. trachomatis;* and the association of cervical ulcers with HSV. The presence of an atypical T zone was associated only with koilocytosis, but not with any of the other specific pathogens studied, thus supporting other studies linking HPV and cervical neoplasia. In addition to atypical T zone, other colposcopic features significantly positively associated with koilocytosis were leukoplakia, satellite lesions, and ectocervical asperities (Plate 86), suggesting that these features are indicative of HPV infection.

## COLPOSCOPIC EXAMINATION OF THE PENIS AND ANUS

Magnified penile surface scanning (MPSS) is the name given to colposcopic examination of the penis.[117,123,267–269] Application of 5% acetic acid and colposcopy augments the detection and diagnosis of subclinical HPV infections and penile intraepithelial neoplasias (PIN). Macules and papules are the most common manifestations of SPI in the male.[117] Colposcopic examination of anal epithelium may also be used to locate and evaluate anal and perianal lesions, but at this time, less is known about the value of anal colposcopy than about penile or cervical colposcopy for the diagnosis of intraepithelial neoplasia or HPV infection.

## CERVICOGRAPHY

Cervicography is a relatively new method for cervical cancer detection developed by Stafl.[270] A cervicogram provides a photographic documentation of normal or abnormal cervical patterns and is obtained by using a cerviscope, which is a 35-mm camera equipped with a special lens system and light source to provide considerable depth of field, and which provides a 16× magnified colposcopic image of the cervix (Cerviscope, National Testing Laboratories, St. Louis, MO). Cervicograms can be obtained by a technician and sent to an expert for evaluation. Cervicography has not yet been used extensively, but it may prove complementary to cytologic screening.

Spitzer et al.[271] evaluated 97 patients with atypical Pap smears with repeat smear, cervicography, and colposcopy, and found that in the detection of CIN lesions cervicography was more sensitive than a repeat smear, but less so than colposcopy. Forty-two percent of the colposcopically detected lesions would have gone undetected by repeat Pap smears, compared with 11 percent by cervicography. Jones et al.[272] evaluated 236 women referred because of atypical, but not dysplastic Pap smears, by colposcopy, repeat Pap smears, and cervicography. Overall, 58 (25 percent) patients had biopsy-proved CIN. Repeat Pap smears identified only 17 percent of these patients, colposcopy 97 percent, and cervicography 81 percent. However, among women who are not selected on the basis of abnormal cytologic smears, cervicography appears less specific than cytology in screening for CIN. Unsatisfactory and defective cervigrams have been a frequent problem,[273] and cervicography has not been proved cost-effective. The rate of uninterpretable cervicograms is higher in older women than in younger women because the squamocolumnar junction is high in the endocervical canal, and therefore, cervicography is probably not useful in patients over 45.[271]

## MANAGEMENT OF THE PATIENT WITH ATYPICAL CERVICAL CYTOLOGY

Figure 48-12 illustrates a clinical algorithm used in our clinic for the management of patients with an atypical cervical cytology. More or less identical clinical algorithms have been proposed by several investigators.[274–277] As demonstrated in the algorithm, abnormal cervical cytologic findings can be divided into those which appear benign and those which suggest dysplasia. While the clinical management of patients with cytologic smears showing dyskaryotic changes consistent with CIN is well established (i.e., referral for colposcopy and colposcopically directed biopsy), the management of patients with so-called nondyskaryotic or benign atypias is controversial. The most frequent benign atypias are inflammatory changes associated with cervicovaginal infections. However, as discussed above, a proportion of benign atypia is associated with an underlying intraepithelial neoplasia. Thus, a repeat examination for definitive diagnosis is required. In noncompliant patients likely to be lost to further long-term follow-up, this should be scheduled as soon as possible. If inflammatory changes are noted, specific diagnostic tests for causes of endocervicitis and ectocervicitis should be performed (see Chap. 46), and any infections found should be treated. The once-common practice of prescribing vaginal sulfonamide creams for women with inflammatory changes in cervical smear, prior to repeating the smear, has no rational basis and should be discouraged.

Many clinicians recommend that patients with benign atypias should have smears repeated at 2 to 6 months[274,278] or at 12 months,[275] whereas others recommend immediate referral for colposcopy and colposcopically directed biopsy.[279–281] The difficulty with the latter recommendation is that the referral of all women with smears showing benign atypia would place an extraordinarily heavy burden on colposcoy and histopathology services, and the cost-effectiveness of this approach has not been established. At the present time, resources are not available in most settings to offer colposcopy to all women whose smears are reported as showing benign atypia. In a recent editorial, Fox[278] argued for increased referrals for colposcopic examination of women with any cytologic atypia, on the grounds that cervical cytologic screening is an unreliable method of detecting cervical neoplasia. Although no comprehensive national records are available to indicate how many women would then require colposcopy service, it can be estimated that at least 10 such cases are identified for every case of CIN 3.

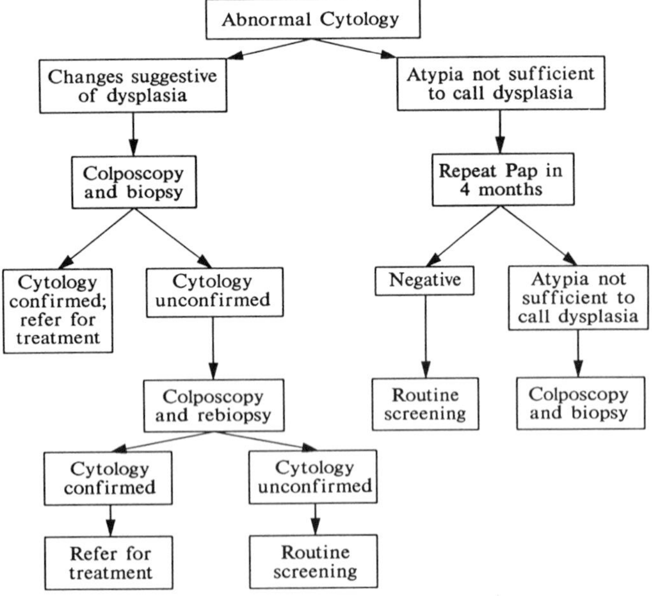


Fig. 48-12. Algorithm for management of women with abnormal Pap smears.

## TREATMENT OF GENITAL SQUAMOUS CELL NEOPLASIAS

This section will discuss treatment modalities of various genital squamous cell neoplasias in a broad sense, and the reader should refer to standard textbooks of gynecologic oncology for specific details of treatment.

## CERVICAL CARCINOMA

Treatment for early microinvasive carcinoma ranges from cervical conization to radical hysterectomy with pelvic node dissection and radiotherapy. The overall recurrence rate is only approximately 1 percent regardless of the criteria used for case definition and the method of treatment. It is generally thought that lesions with no stromal vascular involvement and lesions that are not confluent and are less than 3 mm in depth may be treated conservatively by hysterectomy with excision of the vaginal cuff. Treatment of other forms of ICC is based on the stage of disease as defined by the International Federation of Gynecologists and Obstetricians (FIGO) classification.[22] Radical surgery, radiotherapy, chemotherapy, or combinations of these are used. The selection of treatment should be individualized, and the best results can be obtained when there is a good teamwork between gynecologists, radiotherapists, and oncologists with a particular interest and experience. Surgical treatment with radical hysterectomy and lymphadenectomy (Wertheim operation) can be offered to patients with stage Ib or IIa disease according to the FIGO classification.[22] Preoperative and/or postoperative radiotherapy (intracavitary or external irradiation) is used in most cases. It is not within the scope of this chapter to describe the entire operative procedure or details of the radiotherapy or other treatment regimens such as chemotherapy used for more advanced disease.

## VAGINAL AND VULVAR CARCINOMA

For every carcinoma of the vagina, an estimated 45 cervical carcinomas and 3 vulvar carcinomas occur. Criteria for the diagnosis of carcinoma of the vagina include the following: the primary growth must arise from the vagina, the cervix must be intact and free of tumor, and there must be no evidence of primary tumor arising in other sites. Treatment requires individualization and is more difficult than the treatment of the cervix because of the thin walls and intermediate position between bladder and rectum. The selection of treatment is based on the stage of the disease, the tumor volume, the site of origin in the vagina, and its potential to spread. Surgery by vaginectomy is designed for superficial lesions at any level of the vagina. Surgical treatment can rarely be conservative because of the close proximity of the rectum and the bladder. Hence, ultraradical surgery with pelvic exenterization is often necessary. Small tumors arising from the upper vagina can be treated by radical hysterectomy with lymph node dissection. Cure rates are generally poor except in stage I disease.

## PENILE AND ANAL CARCINOMA

Squamous cell carcinoma of the anus is usually treated by a radical opreation, i.e., a combination excision of the rectum and anus and formation of a permanent colostomy. Radiotherapy can, in some cases, be used for patients with tumors unsuitable for local excision. Anal cancer and its metastases in lymph nodes are particularly radiosensitive. Small tumors under 2 cm and in situ tumors arising at the anal margin can be excised locally. However, most anal cancers are not suitable for local excision. Treatment of carcinoma of the penis includes excision of localized lesions with excision 2 cm proximal to the most proximal area of induration when localized lesions are extensive. Radiotherapy is equally effective in the treatment of small localized lesions. With clinical and pathologic evidence of inguinal metastases, inguinal node dissection is carried out after treatment of the primary tumor. There is no evidence that penectomy is superior. Definitive surgery is rarely possible in patients with inoperable nodal metastases or evidence of spread beyond the inguinal lymph nodes.[282]

## CERVICAL INTRAEPITHELIAL NEOPLASIA

In part because of its accessibility, the treatment of CIN has been rewarded with cure rates approaching 100 percent. This success rate is unparalleled in most areas of oncology but demands critical selection of patients and of modalities of treatment, and careful attention to posttreatment follow-up. The ideal management of a CIN lesion is the simplest method of destroying or removing the lesion. Once the extent of the lesion has been accurately localized, the severity of the lesion suspected by cytology has been histopathologically confirmed, and the possibility of invasion has been eliminated, the method of tissue destruction is probably not very critical. Ideally, treatment should be individualized.

Local biopsy excision of small single focus of early CIN is certainly a valid mode of therapy when accomplished in conjunction with colposcopy. Local excision, however, has no place in the treatment of multifocal or extensive disease or when disease is suspected in the endocervical canal. Hysterectomy still remains a treatment alternative for CIS in some cases when fertility is not an important issue. However, there is little place for hysterectomy in the treatment of other CIN lesions except when there are other concomitant gynecologic indications for hysterectomy or hysterectomy is chosen as a method of sterilization.

Conization of the cervix uteri was first described in 1815 in France, and it was described in the American literature in 1861. Since the 1950s several techniques have been described for inpatient or outpatient cervical conization. In addition to qualifying as a major tool for the diagnosis of CIN, cold-knife conization is widely employed as a definitive therapy for CIN. Cold-knife conization is mandatory when colposcopic expertise is not available. Further indications for cold-knife conization include inadequate colposcopy (squamocolumnar junction not fully visualized), positive ECC, or discrepancy between cytology and histopathology findings.

In Norway, Kolstad and Klem[283] treated a series of 1121 patients who had CIS by performing therapeutic conizations in 795 cases and hysterectomy in 238 cases. In the conization group 2.3 percent had recurrent CIS and 0.9 percent later developed ICC, and the corresponding figures in the hysterectomy group were 1.2 and 2.1 percent, respectively. These recurrent lesions developed from 5 to 25 years after initial therapy in both groups. Ahlgren et al.[284] reported on 343 women with CIS treated by conization; in 93 percent cervical cytology remained normal over 1 to 5 years of follow-up. In a much larger series from Sweden, Bjerre et al.[285] evaluated 2099 women treated by cold-knife conization of whom 1500 had CIS. No recurrence was reported in 87 percent, but 200 (13 percent) had subsequent positive cytology, of whom 117 were retreated by conization. However, even the most well-designed cone biopsy may not remove 100 percent of the lesion. Rubio et al.[286] in a detailed pathologic review of 354 cone biopsies found an interesting correlation between the size of the cone specimen and finding of residual disease. If the margins were positive, the recurrence rate was 39 percent, compared with 3 percent if the margins were negative, i.e., the lesion had been removed completely.

One of the problems with cold-knife conization is the relatively high complication rate, including postoperative hemorrhage, cervical stenosis and scarring, increased risk for subsequent preterm deliveries, and infertility. For instance, Luesley et al.[287] studied the complication rate among 915 women who underwent cone biopsy: 13 percent developed postoperative hemorrhage, 17 percent developed cervical stenosis, and 4 percent had infertility or pregnancy complications. These complications make cold-knife conization a less attractive treatment modality in very young women. Therefore, more simple outpatient treatment modalities such as cryotherapy and carbon dioxide laser treatment have been rapidly gaining popularity over cold-knife conization.

The local destruction of cervical tissue by electrocautery (hot cautery) is a procedure that has been used for the treatment of cervical lesions for several decades. Younge et al.[288] treated patients with CIS by electrocautery, and cured 26 of 27 of those who had surface lesions, but only 37 percent of those with crypt involvement. In Richart and Sciarra's series of 170 patients,[289] 2 patients later developed cervicovaginal scarring, 7 patients developed severe cervical canal stenosis, 3 patients had postoperative hemorrhage, and one patient developed PID.

A recent report[290] concerned 776 cases with CIN treated with outpatient electrocautery without anesthesia. The initial cure rate of 89 percent was surprisingly high; no difference in the cure rates was seen for different degrees of CIN, including CIS, and no complications were reported. The follow-up rate was 75 percent for one year and 46 percent for 5 years. There were few late recurrences, and most were retreated with electrocautery. Nevertheless, electrocautery is no longer recommended for the treatment of CIN because of fear of frequent complications and its failure to eradicate deep lesions.

Tissue destruction can also be accomplished by freezing of the cells. Cryocautery was introduced by Townsend and Ostergard[291] almost 20 years ago. It involves freezing of the lesion by passing liquid nitrogen for a period of 3 min through a specially designed metal probe pressed against the cervix. This produces a "freeze ball" which extends 3 mm out from the sides and down from the end of the cryoprobe. A "thaw" phase of 3 min is then followed by refreeze (so-called double freeze technique). Tissue necrosis results from this procedure, and most patients experience a profuse watery discharge for 2 to 3 weeks. Total reepithelialization is complete in 7 to 10 weeks.[292]

Cryocautery has the distinct advantage over electrocautery that it is virtually painless, bloodless, and has low risk for scarring. One disadvantage is that reepithelialization with squamous metaplastic activity usually moves the squamocolumnar junction high up in the endocervical canal. Thus, the value of cytology and colposcopy in particular in the postcryocautery follow-up evaluation is markedly reduced.

Several literature reviews of failure rates (i.e., persistence of disease) after initial cryotherapy for CIN have been published.[293–295] The overall failure rate approximates 8 percent for CIN 1 and 2, and 17 percent for CIN 3. However, much lower failure rates have been reported. For instance, Richart et al.[222] analyzed long-term results involving 2839 patients treated by cryotherapy for CIN in nine different institutions. The cumulative risk of developing CIN after successful cryotherapy (after three negative Pap smears) was 0.4 percent at 5 years, 0.4 percent at 10 years, and 0.4 percent at 14 years.

Major causes of failure include a positive ECC, inadequate colposcopic examination (squamocolumnar junction not fully visible), inadequate depth of freezing, very extensive lesions, and glandular involvement. Thus, cryotherapy is now considered contraindicated in patients with CIN who have inadequate colposcopy, or positive ECC, or exceptionally extensive lesions. Furthermore, because of the higher rate of treatment failures cryotherapy is no longer considered the treatment of choice for CIN 3 lesions, even if the ECC is negative.

Laser (light amplified by stimulated emission of radiation) treatment was introduced in gynecology approximately 10 years ago and has provided another outpatient treatment modality. The advantages of laser treatment include precise tissue destruction under colposcopic guidance, minimal damage to surrounding tissue, low risk for postoperative hemorrhage, rapid healing with practically no scarring, and decreased risk for postoperative infections. A new squamocolumnar junction is formed at the external os and is usually easily visible colposcopically. This greatly facilitates the cytologic and colposcopic evaluation during the follow-up. Furthermore, concomitant multifocal lesions in the vagina and vulva can easily be treated simultaneously. Three different techniques can be used for laser destruction of the transformation zone in the treatment of CIN: dome-shaped laser vaporization of the cervical tissue to a depth of 0.7 cm, cylindrical laser conization, usually to a depth of 1.5 to 2 cm, and the combination of both (i.e., a cowboy-hat shaped destruction of the cervical tissue). For specific details of the laser technique the reader is referred to standard textbooks.

In a recent literature review[294] the failure rates after initial laser treatment were 7 percent for CIN 1, 11 percent for CIN 2, and 19 percent for CIN 3, giving an overall failure rate of 14 percent. Other studies have generally given much lower failure rates, usually in the range of 6 percent,[296,297] which can be in part attributed to important improvements in the laser technique, such as the use of high power densities, destruction of the entire transformation zone, and treatment to a depth of at least 0.7 cm.

Carbon dioxide laser treatment seems better than cryotherapy for lesions larger than 3 cm in diameter and those with up to 5 mm extension into the endocervical canal.[298] Similarly, CIN 3 lesions respond better to laser than to cryotherapy, which is not surprising because the depth control with cryotherapy certainly is much less precise than with laser therapy.

The technique of laser excisional conization has been rapidly gaining popularity after several studies have demonstrated that it can be safely performed in outpatient clinics without general anesthesia. The major advantage of laser conization over vaporization is that the whole lesion is available for histopathologic investigation. Baggish[299] compared laser excisional conization and laser vaporization for the treatment of CIN. The cure rate for CIN 3 was 97 percent for conization compared with 91 percent for vaporization.

Topical chemotherapy, mainly with bleomycin or 5-fluorouracil (5-FU) has been used in the treatment of CIN by some authors[300,301] with a relatively poor success rate. The lack of enthusiasm for topical chemotherapy is due to the fact that CIN often involves glandular crypts which are not accessible to topical medication, and secondly because CIN is relatively easily treated by destructive methods such as laser. Meyskens et al.[302] conducted a phase I trial of the 0.05% vitamin A derivative, beta-all-trans-retinoic acid (TRA), delivered via a collagen sponge and cervical cap for CIN 1 and 2 in 35 patients, but complete resolution of CIN was not seen, and the toxicity was unacceptably high. Surwit et al.[303] used TRA for CIN 2 and 3 in 18 patients, and also observed vaginal toxicity and poor success rate. Similarly, interferons have not been very successful in the treatment of CIN.[304–306]

## VAGINAL INTRAEPITHELIAL NEOPLASIA

The most common site of VAIN is the upper third of the vagina, and the majority of patients have multifocal lesions. The treatment of choice for VAIN through the 1960s was partial or total vaginectomy with or without radiation, and was associated with considerable morbidity and loss of sexual function. In the 1970s less traumatic treatment modalities emerged, including colposcopically directed excisional biopsies, cryotherapy, laser therapy, and topical 5-FU. Laser therapy[232,307,308] and 5-FU[309] proved to be most successful with 85 to 90 percent cure rates. However, in some studies the recurrence rate of VAIN after 5-FU treatment has been unacceptably high.[310] 5-FU has been used in a variety of ways. Concentrations of 5-FU in vaginal creams have varied from 1 to 20 percent (usually 5 percent), and the total amount applied per treatment has varied from 1 to 5 g of cream, with daily (or nightly) or twice daily applications. The disadvantages of 5-FU include local toxicity frequently leading to the development of gential ulcerations, and long treatment courses. Application of a petroleum-based jelly to the vulva and perineum prior to intravaginal insertion of 5-FU cream may reduce the frequency of vulvar or perineal irritation and ulceration.

## VULVAR INTRAEPITHELIAL NEOPLASIA

Through the 1960s vulvectomy was the standard treatment for vulvar carcinoma in situ (VIS). However, in recent years, the trend has been toward using less aggressive treatment modalities, the reason being the relatively high rate of spontaneous regression of VIN lesions. The risk for invasion has been reported to vary from 0 to 6 percent.[76,228,311,312] In general, vulvectomy is not needed to rule out invasion in VIN. The preferred treatment of VIS is "skinning excision," ranging from excisional biopsy to skinning vulvectomy.[228,312–315] Laser has now replaced skinning vulvectomy in the treatment of VIN including VIS.[316–319] Reid[320] has been particularly instrumental in describing in detail the surgical technique and efficacy of extended laser ablation of all colposcopically recognizable lesions of the vulva. The rationale of using $CO_2$ laser to treat VIN is to destroy the entire area of multifocal abnormal epithelium to a shallow depth, so that rapid healing takes place. If the destruction does not extend below middermis, superficial laser vulvectomy gives a cosmetically good result. In a recent literature review of the use of topical 5-FU for VIS[309] the overall failure rate was 59 percent, which is clearly higher than after destructive treatment modalities.

## PENILE AND ANAL INTRAEPITHELIAL NEOPLASIA

Subclinical penile lesions associated with intraepithelial neoplasia (PIN or Bowenoid papulosis) are becoming increasingly recognized with increasing use of magnified penile surface scanning and application of acetic acid.[267–269,321] Although the potential of progression of such lesions is very low, female sexual partners are at increased risk for cervical neoplasia. Treatment of men with penile intraepithelial neoplasia may be important in the prevention of cervical neoplasia in women. The spontaneous regression rate of subclinical (papular) penile papillomavirus infections is not known. Lesions suggestive of PIN should be biopsied, and preferably treated with the local ablation using carbon dioxide laser surgery under colposcopic guidance. Cryotherapy, using a double freezing technique with a very small cryoprobe tip, is an alternative treatment. The freezing produces a local necrosis; the lesion usually disappears and the skin heals nicely. An advantage of laser therapy over cryotherapy is that it is easier with the former to treat the skin or mucosa adjacent to the lesion. Perhaps this partly accounts for the higher success rate with laser therapy than with cryotherapy.

Perianal and anal condylomas are most difficult to treat; the anal area is very sensitive to pain, bleeding is a problem, and the lesions are easy to miss. Anal condylomas occur occasionally in men with penile condylomas and frequently in women with genital condylomas. Therefore, performing proctoscopy during the colposcopic examination is recommended. Atypical subclinical lesions consistent with anal intraepithelial neoplasia (AIN) are often seen in homosexual men[322] and in heterosexual men and women with multifocal genital squamous cell neoplasia. HPV 16 is found in 8 percent of visible anal warts,[127] but penile and anal infections with HPV 16 probably are subclinical in most cases. Identification of HPV 16 DNA has been related to the grade of intraepithelial neoplasia of the lesion (see Fig. 48-7). Diagnosis of AIN can be difficult, since many conditions including condyloma acuminatum, hemorrhoids, lichen sclerosus, chronic fistula-in-ano, and Crohn's disease can coexist. Topical treatment modalities, for instance, 5-fluorouracil, have been used with poor success. Perianal and intra-anal laser therapy is the most effective treatment for AIN, although the natural history of such lesions is unknown and comparative treatment studies have not been performed.

## PREVENTION AND CONTROL

Only a few years ago genital warts were regarded as a trivial disease. Recent evidence linking HPV with genital and anal neoplasia heralds a new era of scientific investigation into the pathogenesis of HPV which must be matched by continuous training and education of medical and paramedical professionals. The current uncertainty as to the role of papillomaviruses in genital and anal pathology presents major problems for clinicians who must decide whether and how to treat patients who may be infected by an oncogenic virus. Clinicians feel frustrated repeatedly treating genital warts which usually are due to infection by low-risk HPV types 6 or 11; while at the same time they worry how to manage patients with subclinical HPV infections, some of which are associated with the high-risk HPV 16 or 18 types.

It is of utmost importance to develop valid and well-standardized methods for the diagnosis of type-specific HPV infections. At present, HPV typing is still too complicated and too expensive for routine laboratory service. However, as simpler HPV screening techniques become commercially available and the cost becomes affordable, it will be possible to assess individual lesions more precisely. This will then undoubtedly guide development of more effective patient management strategies and therapeutic procedures.

Will routine Pap smear still remain the most cost-effective way to identify all women who are at risk of developing invasive cancer? Certainly the track record for Pap smear screening programs is good, particularly in Nordic countries. On the other hand, many studies have shown shortcomings of the Pap smear and suggest that more standardization and quality control are needed in specimen collection and in the interpretation of the test. The need for quality control also applies to HPV DNA testing, particularly as these techniques move from research laboratories to large-scale screening studies and to clinical use.

Should all women who undergo routine gynecologic examination and Pap smear also receive testing for HPV DNA? Are all HPV-positive women at increased risk for cervical neoplasia or only those infected with certain HPV types, and how should such women be followed? Data from several recent and ongoing studies show that a large proportion (up to 50 percent) of women with cervical HPV 16 to 18 infection are cytologically negative. How should we manage such cases? Should they all be called back for repeat Pap smear, or should they be referred for colposcopy? Colposcoping cytologically negative women found to be positive for HPV DNA probably would present a major challenge in clinical practice. Colposcopy is generally used to evaluate women referred for cytologic atypia consistent with dysplasia, and has really not been adequately evaluated as a screening procedure. Should all atypical (multifocal) colposcopically detected lesions be biopsied? The high frequency of HPV DNA in the normal cervix, together with the much lower incidence of cervical cancer, suggests that if HPV infection is an essential step in the causal pathway of genital and anal neoplasias, the actual risk of invasive cancer to the individual with HPV infection is low. Other events may be needed to initiate malignant transformation. Thus, clearer definitions of other specific risk factors involved are needed to help formulate cost-effective prevention and control programs.

Counseling of patients found to have HPV infections follows the general principles for the control of other STDs. Counseling should include guidelines on safe sex practices to help change behaviors that increase risk for STDs and the consequences of STDs, such as genital neoplasia. Health education should include counseling to promote avoiding multiple partners and casual sex, to encourage compliance with treatment and follow-up, to promote and facilitate examination of sex partners, and to encourage the use of barrier contraception. Proper condom use with new partners should be strongly encouraged to prevent sexual transmission of HPV.

More data are needed on the benefits of systematic examination for evidence of HPV infection of male partners of women with CIN. The yield of magnified penile surface scanning with a colposcope, distal urethroscopy (using a nasal speculum, for instance), and anoscopy should be further analyzed. Papular lesions should be biopsied under local anesthesia to define the prevalence of PIN in such men. Female sex partners of men with PIN should undergo cervical Pap smear (and testing for HPV DNA if available).

As with cytological screening, it appears that there should be an expansion of colposcopy services in clinics serving high-risk populations, such as STD clinics. The questions that still require answering include who should be colposcoped, when, and by whom? With the limited resources available, most centers will only be able to offer colposcopy to women with cytologic evidence of CIN, or those with repeated cytology reports suggesting less significant benign atypia. We feel it is not appropriate to consider colposcopy as a special procedure performed only by gynecologists. General practitioners, venereologists, and physicians specializing in infectious diseases should receive training in colposcopy. After all, the colposcope is a relatively simple magnifying optical instrument that should be relatively easy to master by anybody who is adequately aware of the physiology and anatomy of the female (and male) genital tract. However, supervision by an acknowledged consultant gynecologic colposcopist should be available, and colposcopically directed local destructive therapy should be performed only by well-trained experts. Lastly, any increase in colposcopy services must be accompanied with increased governmental support and funding for the associated cytology, histopathology, nursing, and other services.

The strong association of HPV with malignant and premalignant genital squamous cell neoplasias certainly makes it tempting to speculate whether HPV-specific vaccination or specific antiviral therapy could be used to prevent and control such tumors. A decrease in the incidence of cervical cancer following vaccination would provide persuasive evidence of an etiologic role for HPV in tumor development. A WHO expert committee[3] has outlined general strategies for vaccination against papillomaviruses. Assuming that HPV infection is an essential step in the cause of genital and anal cancers, it has been estimated that prevention and control of genital HPV infections related to the development of such cancers would decrease the overall incidence of human cancer by approximately 20 percent. Thus, basic research on the immunology and therapy of HPV infections should be given a high priority.

## References


1 Parkin DM et al: Estimates of the worldwide frequency of sixteen major cancers in 1980. *Int J Cancer* 41:184, 1988.

2 Zur Hanssen H: Papillomaviruses in human cancer. *Cancer* 59: 1692, 1987.

3 World Health Organization. Genital human papillomavirus infections and cancer: Memorandum from a WHO meeting. *Bull WHO* 65:817, 1987.

4 Koutsky LA et al: Epidemiology of genital human papillomavirus infection. *Epidemiol Rev* 10:122, 1988.

5 Rigoni-Stern D: Fatti statistici relativi alle malattie cancerose. *Gior Serv Progr Pathol Terap* 2:507, 1842.

6 Cramer DW: Uterine cervix, in *Cancer Epidemiology and Prevention*, D Schottenfeld, JF Fraumeni (eds). Philadelphia, Saunders, 1982, p 881.

7 Daling JR et al: Sexual practices, sexually transmitted diseases, and the incidence of anal cancer. *N Engl J Med* 317:973, 1987.

8 Newcomb PA et al: Incidence of vulvar carcinoma in relation to menstrual, reproductive, and medical factors. *J Natl Cancer Inst* 73: 391, 1984.

9 National Cancer Institute. Division of Cancer Prevention and Control: 1987 Annual Cancer Statistics Review. NIH Publ 88-2789, US Department of Health and Human Services, 1988.

10 Young JL Jr et al (eds): Surveillance, Epidemiology and End Results: Incidence and Mortality Data: 1973–77. NCI Monograph 47, Bethesda, MD, NIH Publ 81-2330, 1981.

11 Richart RM et al: A follow-up study of patients with cervical dysplasia. *Am J Obstet Gynecol* 105:386, 1969.

12 Rous P et al: Carcinomatous changes in virus-induced papillomas of the skin of the rabbit. *Proc Soc Exp Biol Med* 32:578, 1935.

13 Rous P et al: The carcinogenic effect of papilloma virus on the tarred skin of rabbits. I. Description of the phenomenon. *J Exp Med* 67: 399, 1938.

14 Koss LG, Durfee GR: Unusual patterns of squamous epithelium of the uterine cervix: Cytologic and pathologic study of koilocytotic atypia. *Ann NY Acad Sci* 63:1245, 1956.

15 Meisels A et al: Condylomatous lesions of the cervix and vagina. I. Cytologic patterns. *Acta Cytol* 20:505, 1976.

16 Purola E et al: Cytology of gynecologic condyloma acuminatum. *Acta Cytol* 21:26, 1977.

17 Gissmann L et al: Human papilloma viruses: Physical mapping and genetic heterogeneity. *Proc Natl Acad Sci USA* 73:1310, 1976.

18 Gissmann L et al: Human papilloma viruses (HPV): Characterization of four different isolates. *Virology* 76:569, 1977.

19 Gissmann L et al: Partial characterization of viral DNA from human genital warts (condylomata acuminata). *Int J Cancer* 25:605, 1980.

20 Orth G: Characterization of a new type of human papillomavirus that causes skin warts. *J Virol* 24:108, 1977.

21 Reagan JW, Fu YS: The uterine cervix, in *Principles and Practice of Surgical Pathology*, SG Silverberg (ed). New York, Wiley, 1983, vol 2, p 1247.

22 Ferenczy A, Winkler B: Carcinoma and metastatic tumors of the cervix, in *Blaustein's Pathology of the Female Genital Tract*, 3d ed, RS Kurman (ed). New York, Springer-Verlag, 1987, p 219.

23 Weid GL: *Proceedings of the First International Congress on Exfoliative Cytology*. Philadelphia, Lippincott, 1961.

24 Cocker J et al: Consistency in the histological diagnosis of epithelial abnormalities of the cervix uteri. *J Clin Pathol* 21:67, 1968.

25 Siegler EE: Microdiagnosis of carcinoma in situ of the uterine cervix. A comparative study of pathologists' diagnoses. *Cancer* 9:463, 1956.

26 Kirkland JA: Atypical epithelial changes in the uterine cervix. *J Clin Pathol* 16:150, 1963.

27 Richart RM: Natural history of cervical intraepithelial neo plasia. *Clin Obstet Gynecol* 10:748, 1968.

28 Barron BA, Richart RM: A statistical model of the natural history of cervical carcinoma based on a prospective study of 557 cases. *J Natl Cancer Inst* 41:1343, 1968.

29 Richart RM: Cervical intraepithelial neoplasia, in *Pathology Annual*, SC Summers (ed). New York, Appleton Century Crofts, 1973, p 301.

30 Crum CP et al: Human papillomavirus type 16 and early cervical neoplasia. *N Engl J Med* 310:880, 1984.

31 Crum CP et al: Cervical papillomaviruses separate within morphologically distinct precancerous lesions. *J Virol* 54:675, 1985.

32 Kiviat NB et al: Prevalence of genital papillomavirus infection among women attending a college student health clinic in an STD clinic. *J Infect Dis* 159:293, 1989.

33 Report of the ISSVD Terminology Committee. Proceedings of the VIII World Congress, Stockholm Sweden. *J Reprod Med* 31:973, 1986.

34 Jeffcoate N: *Principles of Gynecology*, 5th ed. Butterworths, London, 1987.

35 Muir CS et al: *Cancer Incidence in Five Continents*, vol V. Scientific Publications 88, IARC, Lyon, 1988.

36 Waterhouse J et al: *Cancer Incidence of Five Continents*, vol III. Scientific Publication 15, IARC, Lyon, 1976.

37 Draper GJ et al: Changing patterns of cervical cancer rates. *Br Med J* 287:510, 1983.

38 McGregor JE: Mortality from carcinoma of cervix uteri in Britain. *Lancet* 2:774, 1978.
39 Cook GA et al: Trends in cervical cancer and carcinoma in situ in Great Britain. *Br J Cancer* 50:367, 1984.
40 Carmichael JA et al: Cervical carcinoma in women aged 34 and younger. *Am J Obstet Gynecol* 154:264, 1986.
41 Armstrong B et al: Increasing mortality from cancer of the cervix in young Australian women. *Med J Aust* 1:460, 1981.
42 Bourne RG et al: Invasive carcinoma of the cervix in Queensland. *Med J Aust* 1:156, 1983.
43 Roberts AW et al: Invasive carcinoma of the cervix in young women. *Med J Aust* 2:333, 1985.
44 Green GH: Rising cervical cancer mortality in young New Zealand women. *NZ Med J* 89:89, 1979.
45 Chow W-H et al: Decline in the incidence of carcinoma in situ of the cervix. *Am J Public Health* 76:1322, 1986.
46 Chu J et al: Decreasing incidence of invasive cervical cancer in young women. *Am J Obstet Gynecol* 157:1105, 1987.
47 Stern E: Epidemiology of dysplasia. *Obstet Gynecol Surv* 24:711, 1969.
48 Meisels A: Dysplasia and carcinoma of the uterine cervix. IV. A correlated cytologic and histologic study with special emphasis on vaginal microbiology. *Acta Cytol* 13:224, 1969.
49 Dubrow H et al: A stuyd of factors affecting choice of contraceptives. *Obstet Gynecol Surv* 24:1012, 1969.
50 Fasal E et al: Factors associated with high and low risk of cervical neoplasia. *J Natl Cancer Inst* 66:631, 1981.
51 Briggs RM et al: High prevalence of cervical dysplasia in STD clinic patients warrants routine cytologic screening. *Am J Public Health* 70:1212, 1980.
52 Sadeghi SB et al: Prevalence of cervical intraepithelial neoplasia in sexually active teenagers and young adults. Results in data analysis of mass Papanicolaou screening of 796,337 women in the United States in 1981. *Am J Obstet Gynecol* 148:726, 1984.
53 Sadeghi SB et al: Prevalence of dysplasia and cancer of the cervix in a nationwide, Planned Parenthood population. *Cancer* 61:2359, 1988.
54 Hakama M et al: Mass screenings for cervical cancer in Finland 1963–71. *Ann Clin Res* 7:101, 1975.
55 Pettersson F et al: Evaluation of screening for cervical cancer in Sweden: Trends in incidence and mortality 1958–1980. *Int J Epidemiol* 14:521, 1985.
56 Soost H-J et al: Results of cytologic mass screening in the Federal Republic of Germany. *Acta Cytol* 26:445, 1982.
57 Parkin DM et al: Cervical cytology screening in two Yorkshire areas: Results of testing. *Public Health* 96:3, 1982.
58 Boon ME et al: Simultaneous condyloma acuminatum and dysplasia in the uterine cervix. *Acta Cytol* 25:393, 1981.
59 Hicks SJ et al: Increased incidence of cervical intraepithelial neoplasia grade 3 and human papillomavirus infection at a family planning clinic. *NZ Med J* 100:647, 1987.
60 Jones RW et al: Cervical cytology in the Auckland region. *NZ Med J* March 23, 1988, p 132.
61 Armstrong BK et al: Cervical cytology in western Australia 1983. Reports to the Cancer Foundation of Western Australia. NH & MRC Research Unit in Epidemiology and Preventative Medicine, University of Western Australia, 1984.
62 Valiant HW: Family planning programs and detection of cervical neoplasia: Appropriate partners. *Obstet Gynecol Surv* 24:1023, 1969.
63 Lunt R: Worldwide early detection of cervical cancer. *Obstet Gynecol* 63:708, 1984.
64 Luthra UK et al: Natural history of precancerous and early cancerous lesions of the uterine cervix. *Acta Cytol* 31:226, 1987.
65 Hammad MMA et al: Low prevalence of cervical intraepithelial neoplasia among Egyptian females. *Gynecol Oncol* 28:300, 1987.
66 Kaufman RH et al: Cervical cytology in the teen-age patient. *Am J Obstet Gynecol* 108:515, 1970.
67 Feldman MJ et al: Abnormal cervical cytology in the teen-ager: a continuing problem. *Am J Obstet Gynecol* 126:418, 1976.
68 Zaninetti P et al: Characteristics of women under 20 with cervical intraepithelial neoplasia. *Int J Epidemiol* 15:477, 1986.
69 Sebastian JA: Cancer of the cervix—a sexually transmitted disease. Cytologic screening in a prostitute population. *Am J Obstet Gynecol* 131:620, 1987.
70 Armstrong BK et al: Time trends in prevalence of cervical cytological abnormality in women attending a sexually transmitted disease clinic and their relationship to trends in sexual activity and specific infections. *Br J Cancer* 54:669, 1986.
71 Tavelli BG et al: Cost-yield of routine Papanicolaou screening in a clinic for sexually transmitted diseases. *Sex Transm Dis* 12:110, 1985.
72 British Co-operative Clinical Group: Cervical cytology screening in sexually transmitted diseases clinics in the United Kingdom. *Genitourin Med* 63:40, 1987.
73 Ferguson JH et al: Intraepithelial carcinoma, dysplasia, and exfoliation of cancer cells in the vaginal mucosa. *Am J Obstet Gynecol* 87:326, 1963.
74 Timonen S et al: Dysplasia of the vaginal epithelium. *Gynaecologia* 162:125, 1966.
75 Woodruff JD: Carcinoma in situ of the vagina. *Clin Obstet Gynecol* 24:485, 1981.
76 Buscema J et al: Carcinoma in situ of the vulva. *Obstet Gynecol* 55:225, 1980.
77 Campion MJ: Clinical manifestations and natural history of genital human papillomavirus infection. *Obstet Gynecol Clin North Am* 14:363, 1987.
78 Gagnon F: Contribution to the study of the etiology and prevention of cancer of the cervix of the uterus. *Am J Obstet Gynecol* 60:516, 1950.
79 Kinlen LJ et al: Meat and fat consumption and cancer mortality: a study of strict religious orders in Britain. *Lancet* 1:946, 1982.
80 Fraumeni JF et al: Cancer mortality among nuns: Role of marital status in etiology of neoplastic disease in women. *J Am Cancer Inst* 42:455, 1969.
81 Kessler I: Venereal factors in human cervical cancer: Evidence from marital clusters. *Cancer* 39:1912, 1977.
82 Harris RWC et al: Characteristics of women with dysplasia or carcinoma in situ of the cervix uteri. *Br J Cancer* 42:359, 1980.
83 Hulka BS. Risk factors for cervical cancer. *J Chronic Dis* 35:3–11, 1982.
84 Buckley JD et al: Case-control study of the husbands of women with dysplasia or carcinoma of the cervix uteri. *Lancet* i:1010, 1981.
85 Zunzunegui MV et al: Male influences on cervical cancer risk. *Am J Epidemiol* 123:302, 1986.
86 Martinez I: Relationship of squamous cell carcinoma of the cervix uteri to squamous cell carcinoma of the penis among Puerto Rican women married to men with penile carcinoma. *Cancer* 24:777, 1969.
87 Graham S et al: Genital cancer in wives of penile cancer patients. *Cancer* 44:1870, 1979.
88 Smith PG et al: Mortality of wives of men dying with cancer of the penis. *Br J Cancer* 41:422, 1980.
89 Hall NEL et al: Penis, in *Cancer Epidemiology and Prevention*, D Schottenfeld, JF Fraumeni (eds). Philadelphia, Saunders, 1982, p 958.
90 Brinton LA et al: Cigarette smoking and invasive cervical cancer. *JAMA* 255:3265, 1986.
91 Clarke EA et al: Smoking as a risk factor in cancer of the cervix: Additional evidence from a case-control study. *Am J Epidemiol* 115: 59, 1982.
92 La Vecchia C et al: Cigarette smoking and the risk of cervical neoplasia. *Am J Epidemiol* 123:22, 1986.
93 Hellberg D et al: Penile cancer: Is there an epidemiologic role for smoking and sexual behavior: *Br Med J* 295:1306, 1987.

94 Holly EA et al: Mutagenic mucus in the cervix of smokers. *J Natl Cancer Inst* 76:983, 1986.
95 Barton SE et al: Effect of cigarette smoking on cervical epithelial immunity: A mechanism for neoplastic change? *Lancet* Sept 17, 1988:652.
96 Beral et al: Oral contraceptive use and malignancies of the genital tract. *Lancet* 2:1331, 1988.
97 Reid BL et al: Sperm basic proteins in cervical carcinogenesis: Correlation with socioeconomic class. *Lancet* 2:60, 1978.
98 Kessler I: Etiological concepts in cervical carcinogenesis. *Gynecol Oncol* 12:S7, 1981.
99 Reid R, et al: Sexually transmitted papillomaviral infections I The anatomic distribution and pathologic grade of neoplastic lesions associated with different viral types. *Am J Obstet Gynecol* 156:212, 1987.
100 Ikenberg H: Lack of c-myc gene amplification in genital tumours with different HPV status. *Lancet* 2:77, 1987.
101 Lehn H et al: Transcription of episomal papillomaviris DNA in human condylomata acuminata and Buschke-Löwenstein tumours. *J Gen Virol* 65:2003, 1984.
102 de Villiers E-M et al: Analysis of benign and malignant urogenital tumors for human papillomavirus infection by labelling cellular DNA. *Med Microbiol Immunol* 174:281, 1986.
103 McCance DJ et al: Prevalence of human papillomavirus type 16 DNA sequences in cervical intraepithelial neoplasia and invasive carcinoma of the cervix. *Br J Obstet Gynecol* 92:1101, 1985.
104 MacNab JCM et al: Human papillomavirus in clinically and histologically normal tissue of patients with genital cancer. *N Engl J Med* 315:1052, 1986.
105 Fuchs PG et al: Papillomavirus infections in cervical tumors of Austrian patients, in *Papillomaviruses: Cancer Cells*, BV Steinberg, JL Brandsma, LB Taichman (eds). Cold Spring Harbor, NY, Cold Spring Harbor Laboratory 1987, vol 5, p 297.
106 Tsunokawa Y et al: Presence of human papillomavirus type-16 and type-18 DNA sequences and their expression in cervical cancers and cell lines from Japanese patients *Int J Cancer* 37:499, 1986.
107 Yoshikawa H et al: Occurrence of human papillomavirus types 16 and 18 DNA in cervical carcinomas from Japan: Age of patients and histological type of carcinomas. *Jpn J Cancer Res* 76:667, 1985.
108 Kulski JK et al: DNA sequences of human papillomavirus types 11, 16 or 18 in invasive cervical carcinoma of Western Australian women. *Immunol Cell Biol* 65:77, 1987.
109 Lörincz AT et al: Characterization of human papillomavirus in cervical neoplasias and their detection in routine clinical screening, in *Viral Etiology of Cervical Cancer*, R Peto, H zur Hansen (eds). Banbury Report 21, Cold Spring Harbor, NY, Cold Spring Harbor Laboratory 1986, p 225.
110 Kurman RJ et al: Analysis of individual human papillomavirus types in cervical neoplasia: a possible role for type 18 in rapid progression. *Am J Obstet Gynecol* 159:293, 1988.
111 Tase T: Human papillomaviris types and localization of adenocarcinoma and adenosquamous carcinoma of the uterine cervix: a study by in situ DNA hybridization. *Cancer Res* 48:993, 1988.
112 Sutton GP et al: Human papillomavirus deoxyribonucleic acid in lesions of the female genital tract: Evidence for type 6/11 in squamous carcinoma of the vulva. *Obstet Gynecol* 70:564, 1987.
113 Henderson BR et al: Detection of specific types of human papillomavirus in cervical scrapes, and scrapes, and anogenital biopsies by DNA hybridization. *J Med Virol* 21:381, 1987.
114 Gross G, et al: Bowenoid papulosis: A venereally transmissible disease as reservoir for HPV 16. in *Viral Etiology of Cervical Cancer*, R Peto, H zur Hausen, (eds). Cold Spring Harbor, NY, Cold Spring Harbor Laboratory, 1986, p 149.
115 Gupta J et al: Association of human papillomavirus type 16 with neoplastic lesions of the vulva and other genital sites by in situ hybridization. *Am J Pathol* 127:206, 1987.
116 Barnes W et al: Possible prognostic significance of human papillomavirus type in cervical cancer. *Gynecol Oncol* 29:267, 1988.
117 Barrasso R et al: High prevalence of papillomavirus-associated penile intraepithelial neoplasia in sexual partners of women with cervical intraepithelial neoplasia. *N Engl J Med* 317:916, 1987.
118 Bergeron C et al: Multicentric human papillomavirus infections of the female genital tract: correlation of viral types with abnormal mitotic figures, colposcopic presentation, and location. *Obstet Gynecol* 69:736, 1987.
119 Tomita Y et al: Detection of human papillomavirus DNA in genital warts, cervical dysplasias and neoplasias. *Intervirology* 25:151, 1986.
120 Wells M et al: Demonstrations of human papillomavirus types in paraffin processed tissue from human anogenital lesions by in-situ DNA hybridization. *J Pathol* 152:77, 1987.
121 Buscema J et al: The predominance of human papillomavirus type 16 in vulvar neoplasia. *Obstet Gynecol* 71:603, 1988.
122 Kaufman RH et al: The cryosurgical therapy of cervical intraepithelial neoplasia. III. Continuing follow-up. *Am J Obstet Gynecol* 131:381, 1978.
123 Rosemberg SK et al: Sexually transmitted papillomaviral infection in men. *Obstet Gynecol Clin N Am* 14:495, 1987.
124 Villa LL et al: Human papillomavirus DNA sequences in penile carcinomas in Brazil. *Int J Cancer* 37:853, 1986.
125 Beckmann AM et al: Detection and localization of human papillomavirus DNA in human genital condylomas by in situ hybridization with biotinylated probes. *J Med Virol* 16:265, 1985.
126 Parker BJ et al: The clinical management and laboratory assessment of anal warts. *Med J Aust* 147:59, 1987.
127 McCance DJ et al: Human papillomavirus in condylomata acuminata of the anus. *J Clin Pathol* 39:927, 1986.
128 Hill SA, Coghill SB: Human papillomavirus in squamous carcinoma of anus. *Lancet* 2:1333, 1986.
129 Sherman KJ et al: Multiple primary tumors in women with vulvar neoplasms: a case-control study. *Br J Cancer* 57:423, 1988.
130 Schneider A et al: Multifocal squamous neoplasia of the female genital tract: significance of human papillomavirus infection of the vagina after hysterectomy. *Obstet Gynecol* 70:294, 1987.
131 Collins JE et al: Detection of human papillomavirus DNA sequences by in situ DNA-DNA hybridisation in cervical intraepithelial neoplasia and invasive carcinoma: a retrospective study. *J Clin Pathol* 41:289, 1988.
132 Bornstein J et al: Human papillomavirus associated with vaginal intraepithelial neoplasia in women exposed to diethylstilbestrol in utero. *Obstet Gynecol* 70:75, 1987.
133 Wilczynski SP et al: Human papillomaviruses and cervical cancer: analysis of histopathologic features associated with different viral types. *Human Pathol* 19:697, 1988.
134 Pratili MA et al: Recherche de papillomavirus humains dans des cellules épithéliales du col utérin: fréquence des types 16 et 18. Résultats préliminaires d'une étude clinique, cytologique et virologique. *J Gynecol Obstet Biol Reprod (Paris)* 15:45, 1986.
135 Lörincz AT et al: Correlation of cellular atypia and human papillomavirus deoxyribonucleic acid sequences in exfoliated cells of the uterine cervix. *Obstet Gynecol* 68:508, 1986.
136 Toon PG et al: Human papillomavirus infection of the uterine cervix of women with and without cytological signs of neoplasia. *Br Med J* 293:1261, 1986.
137 De Villiers E-M et al: Human papillomavirus infections in women with and without abnormal cervical cytology. *Lancet* 2:703, 1987.
138 Schneider A et al: Increased prevalence of human papillomaviruses in the lower genital tract of pregnant women. *Int J Cancer* 40:198, 1987.
139 Fife KH et al: Symptomatic and asymptomatic cervical infections with human papillomavirus during pregnancy. *J Infect Dis* 156:904, 1987.
140 Chuang T-Y et al: Condyloma acuminatum in Rochester, Minnesota, 1950–1978. Parts I and II. *Arch Dermatol* 120:469, 1984.
141 Oriel JD: Natural history of genital warts. *Br J Vener Dis* 47:1, 1971.
142 Becker TM et al: Genital human papillomavirus infection: a growing concern. *Obstet Gynecol Clin N Am* 14:389, 1987.

143 Wickenden C et al: Screening for human papillomaviruses in the female genital tract by DNA hybridization of cervical scrapes. Meeting of the Pathological Society of Great Britain and Ireland, University of Oxford, January 7–9, 1987. Abstract 252.
144 Zur Hausen H: Intracellular surveillance of persisting viral infections: Human genital cancer resulting from a failing cellular control of papillomavirus gene expression. *Lancet* 2:489, 1986.
145 Rawls WE et al: A search for viruses in smegma, premalignant and early malignant cervical tissues: The isolation of herpesviruses with distinct antigenic properties. *Am J Epidemiol* 87:647, 1968.
146 Naib ZM et al: Genital herpetic infection. Association with cervical dysplasia and carcinoma. *Cancer* 23:940, 1969.
147 Vonka V et al: Prospective study on the relationship between cervical neoplasia and herpes simplex type 2 virus. I. Epidemiological characteristics. *Int J Cancer* 33:49, 1984.
148 Sherlock CH et al: Type specificity of complement-fixing antibody against herpes simplex virus type 2 AG-4 early antigen in patients with asymptomatic infection. *J Clin Microbiol* 24:1093, 1986.
149 Frenkel N et al: A DNA fragment of herpes simplex virus type 2 and its transcription in human cervical cancer tissue: *Proc Natl Acad Sci USA* 69:3784, 1972.
150 Galloway DA et al: The oncogenic potential of herpes simplex viruses: Evidence for a 'hit and run' mechanism. *Nature* 302:21, 1983.
151 Park M et al: Detection of herpes simplex virus type 2 DNA restriction fragments in human cervical carcinoma tissue. *EMBO J* 2:1029, 1983.
152 Prakash SS et al: Herpes virus type 2 and human papillomavirus type 16 in cervicitis, dysplasia and invasive cervical carcinoma. *Int J Cancer* 35:51, 1985.
153 McDougall JK et al: Herpesvirus-specific RNA and protein in carcinoma of the uterine cervix. *Proc Natl Acad Sci USA* 79:3853, 1982.
154 Flannery VL et al: Expression of an early nonstructural antigen of herpes simplex virus in cells transformed in vitro by herpes simplex virus. *J Virol* 21:284, 1977.
155 Jarriwalla RJ et al: Tumorigenic transformation induced by a specific fragment of DNA from herpes simplex virus type 2. *Proc Natl Acad Sci USA* 77:2279, 1980.
156 Rapp F: The challenge of herpesviruses. *Cancer Res* 44:1309, 1984.
157 Galloway DA et al: Small fragments of herpesvirus DNA with transforming activity contain insertion sequence-like structures. *Proc Natl Acad Sci USA* 81:4736, 1984.
158 Di Luca D et al: Simultaneous presence of herpes simplex virus and human papillomavirus sequences in human genital tumors. *Int J Cancer* 40:763, 1987.
159 Zur Hausen H: Human genital cancer: synergism between two virus infections or synergism between a virus infection and initiative agents? *Lancet* 2:489, 1982.
160 Chandler SH et al: The epidemiology of cytomegaloviral infection in women attending a sexually transmitted disease clinic. *J Infect Dis* 152:597, 1985.
161 Kiviat NB et al: Cytologic manifestations of cervical and vaginal infections. I. Epithelial and inflammatory cellular changes. *JAMA* 253:989, 1985.
162 Melnick JL et al: Association of cytomegalovirus (CMV) infection with cervical cancer: Isolation of CMV from cell culture derived from cervical biopsy. *Intervirology* 10:115, 1978.
163 Pacsa A et al: Herpesvirus antibodies and antigens in patients with cervical anaplasia and in controls. *J Natl Cancer Inst* 55:775, 1975.
164 Paavonen J et al: Genital Chlamydia trachomatis infection in patients with cervical atypia. *Obstet Gynecol* 54:289, 1979.
165 Hart H et al: Lack of association of cytomegalovirus antibody level with carcinoma of the uterine cervix. *Gynecol Obstet Invest* 14:300, 1982.
166 Albrecht T et al: Malignant transformation of hamster embryo fibroblasts following exposure to ultraviolet-irradiated human cytomegalovirus. *Virology* 55:53, 1973.
167 Nelson JA et al: Transformation of NIH 3T3 cells with cloned fragments of human cytomegalovirus strain AD169. *J Virol* 43:83, 1982.
168 Nelson JA et al: Structure of the transforming region of human cytomagalovirus AD169. *J Virol* 49:109, 1984.
169 Brown ZA et al: Genital ulceration and infectious mononucleosis: report of a case. *Am J Obstet Gynecol* 127:673, 1977.
170 Lawee D et al: Solitary penile ulcer associated with infectious mononucleosis. *Can Med Assoc J* 129:146, 1983.
171 Portnoy J et al: Recovery of Epstein-Barr virus for genital ulcers. *N Engl J Med* 311:966, 1984.
172 Sixbey JW et al: Replication of Epstein-Barr virus in human epithelial cells infected in vitro. *Nature* 306:480, 1983.
173 Sixbey JW et al: A second site for Epstein-Barr virus shedding: The uterine cervix. *Lancet* 2:1122, 1986.
174 Sixbey JW et al: Human epithelial cell expression of an Epstein-Barr virus receptor. *Clin Res* 34:533A, 1986.
175 Young LS et al: Epstein-Barr virus gene expression in nasopharyngeal carcinoma. *J Gen Virol* 69:1051, 1988.
176 Fähraeus R et al: Expression of Epstein-Barr virus encoded proteins in nasopharyngeal carcinoma. *Int J Cancer* 42:329, 1988.
177 Henderson EE: Physiochemical-viral synergism during Epstein-Barr virus infection: A review. *J Nat Cancer Inst* 80:476, 1988.
178 Richtsmeier WJ: Epstein-Barr virus-associated malignancies. *CRC Crit Rev Clin Lab Sc* 25:105, 1987.
179 Laverty CR et al: Adenovirus infection of the cervix. *Acta Cytol* 21:114, 1977.
180 Vesterinen E et al: Cytopathogenecity of cytomegalovirus to human ecto- and endocervical epithelial cells in vitro. *Acta Cytol* 19:473, 1975.
181 Halpert R et al: Human papillomavirus and lower genital neoplasia in renal transplant patients. *Obstet Gynecol* 68:251, 1986.
182 Rudlinger R et al: Human papillomavirus infections in a group of renal transplant recipients. *Br J Dermatol* 115:681, 1986.
183 Sillman FH, Sedlis A: Anogenital papillomavirus infection and neoplasia in immunodeficient women. *Obstet Gynecol Clin N Am* 14:537, 1987.
184 Schneider V et al: Immunosuppression as a high-risk factor in the development of condyloma acuminatum and squamous neoplasia of the cervix. *Acta Cytol* 27:220, 1983.
185 Frazer IH et al: Association between anorectal dysplasia, human papillomavirus, and human immunodeficiency virus infection in homosexual men. *Lancet* 2:657, 1986.
186 Eron LJ et al: Interferon therapy for condylomata acuminata. *N Engl J Med* 315:1059, 1986.
187 Douglas JM Jr et al: The effect of asymptomatic infection with HTLV-III on the response of anogenital warts to intralesional treatment with recombinant alpha2 interferon. *J Infect Dis* 154:331, 1986.
188 Bradbeer C: Is infection with HIV a risk factor for cervical intraepithelial neoplasia? (Letter to the editor). *Lancet* 2:1277, 1987.
189 Spurrett B et al: Cervical dysplasia and HIV infection (Letter to the editor). *Lancet* 1:237, 1988.
190 Crocchiolo P et al: Cervical dysplasia and HIV infection (Letter to the editor). *Lancet* 1:238, 1988.
191 Byrne M et al: Cervical dysplasia and HIV infection (Letter to the editor). *Lancet* 1:239, 1988.
192 Kent C et al: The role of anal/genital warts in HIV infection (Letters). *JAMA* 258:85, 1987.
193 Mackowiak PA: Microbial oncogenesis. *Am J Med* 82:79, 1987.
194 Rojel J: The interrelation between uterine cancer and syphilis: A pathodemographic study. *Acta Pathol Microbiol Scand* 97:13, 1953.
195 Beral V: Cancer of the cervix: A sexually transmitted infection. *Lancet* 1:1037, 1974.
196 Lynge E et al: Cohort trends in incidence of cervical cancer in Denmark in relation to gonorrheal infection. *Acta Obstet Gynecol Scand* 64:291, 1985.
197 Starreveld AA et al: The latency period of carcinoma in situ of the cervix. *Obstet Gynecol* 62:348, 1983.
198 Furgyik S et al: Gonorrheal infection followed by an increased frequency of cervical carcinoma. *Acta Obstet Gynecol Scand* 59:521, 1980.

199 Papanicolaou GN et al: Vaginal cytology in trichomonas infestation. *Int Rec Med Gen Pract Clin* 168:551, 1955.

200 Thomas DB: An epidemiologic study of carcinoma in situ and squamous dysplasia of the uterine cervix. *Am J Epidemiol* 98:10, 1973.

201 Koss LG et al: Trichomonas vaginalis cervicitis and its relationship to cervical cancer. A histological study. *Cancer* 12:1171, 1959.

202 Patten SF Jr et al: An experimental study of the relationship between Trichomonas vaginalis and dysplasia in the uterine cervix. *Acta Cytol* 7:187, 1963.

203 Chen KCS et al: Biochemical diagnosis of vaginitis by determination of diamines in the vaginal fluid. *J Infect Dis* 145:337, 1982.

204 Guijon FB: The association of sexually transmitted diseases with cervical intraepithelial neoplasia: a case-control study. *Am J Obstet Gynecol* 151:185, 1985.

205 Pavic N: Is there a local production of nitrosamines by the vaginal microflora in anaerobic vaginosis/trichomoniasis? *Med Hypotheses* 15:433, 1984.

206 Mårdh P-A et al: *Chlamydia.* New York, Plenum Press, 1989 (in press).

207 Paavonen J et al: Cytologic findings in cervical chlamydial infection. *Med Biol* 58:174, 1980.

208 Cevenini R et al: Cytological and histopathological abnormalities of the cervix in genital Chlamydia trachomatis infections. *Br J Vener Dis* 57:334, 1981.

209 Carr MC et al: Chlamydia, cervicitis and abnormal Papanicolaou smears. *Obstet Gynecol* 23:27, 1979.

210 Schachter J et al: Chlamydia trachomatis and cervical neoplasia. *JAMA* 248:2134, 1982.

211 Syrjänen K et al: Coexistent chlamydial infections related to natural history of human papillomavirus lesions in uterine cervix. *Genitourin Med* 62:345, 1986.

212 Spriggs AI et al: Progression and regression of cervical lesions. *J Clin Pathol* 33:517, 1980.

213 Lange P: Clinical and histological studies on cervical carcinoma. *Acta Pathol Microbiol Scand* 50(suppl 143):13, 1960.

214 Jones HW Jr et al: Re-examination of biopsies taken prior to the development of invasive carcinoma of the cervix, in *Proceedings of the Third National Cancer Conference,* Philadelphia, Lippincott, 1956, p 678.

215 Okagaki T et al: Diagnosis of anaplasia and carcinoma in situ by differential cell counts. *Acta Cytol* 6:343, 1962.

216 Patten SF: Diagnostic cytology of the uterine cervix. *Monographs in Clinical Cytology: Diagnostic Cytopathology of the Uterine Cervix.* New York, S Karger, 1978, p 141.

217 Jordan SW et al: The significance of cervical cytologic dysplasia. *Acta Cytol* 25:237, 1981.

218 Roitton G, Chrostopherson WM: Cytology of the female genital tract, in *Histological Classification of Tumors,* no 8. Geneva, World Health Organization 1973.

219 Nasiell K et al: Behavior of mild cervical dysplasia during long-term follow-up. *Obstet Gynecol* 67:665, 1986.

220 Nasiell K et al: Behavior of moderate cervical dysplasia during long-term follow-up. *Obstet Gynecol* 61:609, 1983.

221 Richart RM et al: An analysis of "long-term" follow-up results in patients with cervical intraepithelial neoplasia treated by cryotherapy. *Am J Obstet Gynecol* 137:823, 1980.

222 Richart RM: The patient with an abnormal Pap smear-screening techniques and management. *N Engl J Med* 302:332, 1980.

223 Mitchell H et al: Prospective evaluation of risk of cervical cancer after cytological evidence of human papillomavirus infection. *Lancet* 1:573, 1986.

224 Campion MJ et al: Progressive potential of mild cervical atypia: prospective cytological, colposcopic and virological study. *Lancet* 2:237, 1986.

225 Melamed MR et al: Non-diagnostic squamous atypia in cervicovaginal cytology as a risk factor for early neoplasia. *Acta Cytol* 20:108, 1976.

226 Paavonen J et al: Natural history of benign cytologic atypias in an STD clinic population. *Acta Cytologica* 1989 (in press).

226a Paavonen J et al: Colposcopic manifestations of cervical and vaginal infections. *Obstet Gynecol Surv* 43:323, 1988.

227 Jones RW et al: Carcinoma in situ of the vulva: A review of 31 treated and 5 untreated cases. *Obstet Gynecol* 68:499, 1986.

228 Friedrich EG et al: Carcinoma in situ of the vulva: A continuing challenge. *Am J Obstet Gynecol* 136:830, 1980.

229 Crum CP et al: Vulvar intraepithelial neoplasia (severe atypia and carcinoma in situ). A clinicopathologic analysis of 41 cases. *Cancer* 54:1429, 1984.

230 Bonnekoh B et al: Transition to cutaneous squamous cell carcinoma in 2 patients with Bowenoid papulomatosis. *Z Hautkr* 62:773, 1987.

231 Rutledge F: Cancer of the vagina. *Am J Obstet Gynecol* 102:806, 1968.

232 Lenehan PM et al: Vaginal intraepithelial neoplasia: Biologic aspects and management. *Obstet Gynecol* 68:333, 1986.

233 Papanicolaou GN: A survey of the actualities and potentialities of exfoliative cytology in cancer diagnosis. *Ann Med* 30:661, 1948.

234 Cramer DW: The role of cervical cytology in the declining morbidity and morality of cervical cancer. *Cancer* 34:2018, 1974.

235 Koss LG: *Diagnostic Cytopathology,* 3d ed. Philadelphia, Lippincott, 1979, p 337.

236 Horn PL et al: Reproducibility of the cytologic diagnosis of human papillomavirus infection. *Acta Cytol* 29:692, 1985.

237 Schneider A et al: Sensitivity of the cytologic diagnosis of cervical condyloma in comparison with HPV DNA hybridization studies. *Diagn Cytopathol* 3:250, 1987.

238 Papanicolaou G: *Atlas of Exfoliative Cytology.* Massachusetts, Commonwealth Fund by University Press, 1954.

239 Maguire NG: Current use of the Papanicolaou class system in gynecologic cytology. *Diagn Cytopathol* 4:169, 1988.

240 Richart RM, Vailant HW: Influence of cell collection techniques upon cytological diagnosis. *Cancer* 18:1474, 1965.

241 Rylander E: Negative smears in women developing invasive cancer. *Acta Obstet Gynecol Scand* 56:115, 1977.

242 Gay JD et al: False-negative results in cervical cytologic studies. *Acta Cytol* 29:1043, 1985.

243 Sedlis A et al: Evaluation of two simultaneous obtained cervical smear: a comparison study. *Acta Cytol* 18:291, 1974.

244 Vooijs GP et al: Relationship between diagnoses of epithelial abnormalities and the composition of cervical smears. *Acta Cytol* 29: 323, 1985.

245 Elias A et al: The significance of endocervical cells in the diagnosis of cervical epithelial changes. *Acta Cytol* 27:225, 1983.

246 Kawaguchi K et al: The value of the cytolbrush for obtaining cells from the uterine cervix. *Diagn Cytopathol* 3:262, 1987.

247 Koss LG: The Papanicolaou test for cervical cancer—a triumph and a tragedy. *JAMA* 261:737, 1989.

248 Nauth H: Cytology of the exfoliative layer in normal and diseased vulvar skin. *Acta Cytol* 26:269, 1982.

249 Webb AJ: Cytologic diagnosis of anorectal and rectosigmoid lesions by a simple smear technique. *Acta Cytol* 23:524, 1979.

250 Medley Y: Anal smear test to diagnose occult anorectal infection with human papillomaviruses in men. *Br J Vener Dis* 60:205, 1984.

251 Kolstad P et al: *Atlas of Colposcopy,* 2d ed. Baltimore, University Park Press, 1977.

252 Coppleson M et al: *Colposcopy. A Scientific and Practical Approach to the Cervix and Vagina in Health and Disease,* 2d ed. Springfield, IL, Charles C Thomas, 1978.

253 Reid R et al: Genital warts and cervical cancer. VII. An improved colposcopic index for differentiating benign papillomaviral infections from high-grade cervical intraepithelial neoplasia. *Am J Obstet Gynecol* 153:611, 1985.

254 Singer A: The uterine cervix from adolescence to the menopause. *Br J Obstet Gynecol* 63:613, 1984.

255 Townsend DE et al: Abnormal Papanicolaou smears: Evaluation by colposcopy, biopsies, and endocervical curettage. *Am J Obstet Gynecol* 108:429, 1970.

256 Stafl A et al: Colposcopic diagnosis of cervical neoplasia. *Obstet Gynecol* 41:168, 1973.

257 Jawaheri G et al: Diagnostic value of colposcopy in the investigation of cervical neoplasia. *Am J Obstet Gynecol* 137:588, 1980.
258 Hatch KD et al: Role of endocervical curettage in colposcopy. *Obstet Gynecol* 65:403, 1985.
259 Kaufman RH et al: The cryosurgical therapy of cervical intraepithelial neoplasia. III. Continuing follow-up. *Am J Obstet Gynecol* 131:381, 1978.
260 Wetrich DW: An analysis of the factors involved in the colposcopic evaluation of 2194 patients with abnormal Papanicolaou smears. *Am J Obstet Gynecol* 154:1339, 1986.
261 Moseley KR et al: Necessity of endocervical curettage in colposcopy. *Am J Obstet Gynecol* 154:992, 1986.
262 Walker PG et al: Colposcopy in the diagnosis of papillomavirus infection of the uterine cervix. *Br J Obstet Gynecol* 90:1082, 1983.
263 Kirkup W et al: Cervical intraepithelial neoplasia and "warty" atypia: a study of colposcopic, histological and cytological characteristics. *Br J Obstet Gynecol* 89:571, 1982.
264 Väyrynen M et al: Colposcopy in women with papillomavirus lesions of the uterine cervix. *Obstet Gynecol* 65:409, 1985.
265 Follen MM et al: Colposcopic correlates of cervical papillomavirus infection. *Am J Obstet Gynecol* 157:809, 1987.
266 Schneider A et al: Colposcopy is superior to cytology for the detection of early genital human papillomavirus infection. *Obstet Gynecol* 71:236, 1988.
267 Levine RU et al: Cervical papillomavirus infection and intraepithelial neoplasia: a study of male sexual partners. *Obstet Gynecol* 64:16, 1984.
268 Sand PK et al: Evaluation of male consorts of women with human papillomavirus infection. *Obstet Gynecol* 68:679, 1986.
269 Krebs H-B et al: Human papillomavirus-associated lesions of the penis: colposcopy, cytology, and histology. *Obstet Gynecol* 70:299, 1987.
270 Stafl A: Cervicography: A new method for cervical cancer detection. *Am J Obstet Gynecol* 139:815, 1981.
271 Spitzer M et al: Comparative utility of repeat Papanicolaou smears, cervicography, and colposcopy in the evaluation of atypical Papanicolaou smears. *Obstet Gynecol* 69:731, 1987.
272 Jones DE et al: Evaluation of the atypical Pap smear. *Am J Obstet Gynecol* 157:544, 1987.
273 Blythe JG: Cervicography: A preliminary report. *Am J Obstet Gynecol* 152:192, 1985.
274 Singer A: The abnormal cervical smear. *Br Med J* 293:1551, 1986.
275 Berget A et al: Cervical intraepithelial neoplasia. Examination, treatment and follow-up. *Obstet Gynecol Surv* 40:545, 1985.
276 Noumoff JS: Atypia in cervical cytology as a risk factor for intraepithelial neoplasia. *Am J Obstet Gynecol* 156:628, 1987.
277 Briggs RM et al: Cervical intraepithelial neoplasia, in *Sexually Transmitted Diseases,* KK Holmes, P-A Mårdh, PF Sparling, PJ Wiesner (eds). New York, McGraw-Hill, 1984, p 589.
278 Fox H: Cervical smears: new terminology and new demands. *Br Med J* 294:1307, 1987.
279 Campion MJ et al: Complacency in diagnosis of cervical cancer. *Br Med J* 294:1337, 1987.
280 Kohan S et al: Colposcopic screening of women with atypical Papanicolaou smears. *J Reprod Med* 30:383, 1985.
281 Walker EM et al: Does mild atypia on a cervical smear warrant further investigation? *Lancet* 2:672, 1986.
282 Prout Garnick MB: Carcinoma of the penis, in Holland JF, Frei E (eds). *Cancer Medicine,* 2d ed. Philadelphia, Lea & Febiger, 1982, p 1934.
283 Kolstad P et al: Long-term follow-up of 1121 cases of carcinoma in situ. *Obstet Gynecol* 48:125, 1976.
284 Ahlgren M et al: Conization as treatment of carcinoma in situ of the uterine cervix. *Obstet Gynecol* 46:135, 1975.
285 Bjerre B et al: Conization as only treatment of carcinoma in situ of the uterine cervix. *Am J Obstet Gynecol* 125:143, 1976.
286 Rubio CA et al: Big cones and little cones. *Histopathology* 2:133, 1978.
287 Luesley DM et al: Complications of cone biopsy related to the dimensions of the cone and the influence of prior colposcopic assessment. *Br J Obstet Gynecol* 92:158, 1985.
288 Younge PA et al: A study of 135 cases of carcinoma in situ of the cervix at the Free Hospital for Women. *Am J Obstet Gynecol* 58: 867, 1949.
289 Richart RM et al: Treatment of cervical dysplasia by outpatient electracauterization. *Am J Obstet Gynecol* 101:200, 1968.
290 Deigan EA et al: Treatment of cervical intraepithelial neoplasia with electrocautery: A report of 776 cases. *Am J Obstet Gynecol* 154:255, 1986.
291 Townsend DE et al: Cryocauterization for pre-invasive cervical neoplasia. *J Reprod Med* 6:171, 1971.
292 Underwood PB Jr et al: Cryosurgery: Its use for the abnormal Pap smear. *Cancer* 38:546, 1976.
293 Charles EH et al: Cryosurgical treatment of cervical intraepithelial neoplasia. *Obstet Gynecol Surv* 35:539, 1980.
294 Stein DS et al: Laser vaporization in the treatment of cervical intraepithelial neoplasia. *J Reprod Med* 30:179, 1985.
295 Figge DC et al: Cryotherapy in the treatment of cervical intraepithelial neoplasia. *Obstet Gynecol* 62:353, 1983.
296 Bellina JH et al: Carbon dioxide laser management of cervical intraepithelial neoplasia. *Am J Obstet Gynecol* 141:828, 1981.
297 Jordan JA et al: The treatment of cervical intraepithelial neoplasia by laser vaporization. *Br J Obstet Gynecol* 92:394, 1985.
298 Ferenczy A: Comparison of cryo- and carbon dioxide laser therapy for cervical intraepithelial neoplasia. *Obstet Gynecol* 66:793, 1985.
299 Baggish MS: A comparison between laser excisional conization and laser vaporization for the treatment of cervical intraepithelial neoplasia. *Am J Obstet Gynecol* 155:39, 1986.
300 Masuda H et al: Loval therapy of carcinoma of the uterine cervix. *Cancer* 48:1899, 1981.
301 Price GL, Chuprevich TW: Topical f-fluorouracil treatment of transformation zone intraepithelial neoplasia of cervix and vagina. *Obstet Gynecol* 60:467, 1982.
302 Meyskens FL et al: A phase I trial of beta-all-trans-retinoic acid delivered via a collagen sponge and a cervical cap for mild or moderate intraepithelial cervical neoplasia. *J Natl Cancer Inst* 71:921, 1983.
303 Surwit EA et al: Evaluation of topically applied trans-retinoic acid in the treatment of cervical intraepithelial neoplasia. *Am J Obstet Gynecol* 143:821, 1982.
304 Choo YC et al: Intravaginal application of leukocyte interferon gel in the treatment of cervical intraepithelial neoplasia (CIN). *Arch Gynecol* 237:51, 1985.
305 Möller BR et al: Treatment of dysplasia of the cervical epithelium with an interferon gel. *Obstet Gynecol* 62:625, 1983.
306 De Palo G et al: Human fibroblast interferon in cervical and vulvar intraepithelial neoplasia associated with viral cytopathic effects. A pilot study. *J Reprod Med* 30;404, 1985.
307 Stafl A et al: Laser treatment of cervical and vaginal neoplasia. *Am J Obstet Gynecol* 128:128, 1977.
308 Townsend DE et al: Treatment of vaginal carcinoma in situ with the carbon dioxide laser. *Am J Obstet Gynecol* 143:565, 1982.
309 Sillman FH et al: A review of lower genital intraepithelial neoplasia and the use of topical 5-fluorouracil. *Obstet Gynecol Surv* 40:190, 1985.
310 Ballon SC et al: Topical 5-fluorouracil in the treatment of intraepithelial neoplasia of the vagina. *Obstet Gynecol* 54:163, 1979.
311 Forney JF et al: Management of carcinoma in situ of the vulva. *Am J Obstet Gynecol* 127:801, 1977.
312 DiSaia PJ et al: Surgical approach to multifocal carcinoma in situ of the vulva. *Am J Obstet Gynecol* 140:136, 1981.
313 Rutledge F et al: Treatment of intraepithelial carcinoma of the vulva by skin excision and graft. *Am J Obstet Gynecol* 102:806, 1968.
314 Caglar H et al: Vulvar intraepithelial neoplasia. *Obstet Gynecol* 60: 346, 1982.
315 Iversen T et al: Squamous cell carcinoma in situ of the vulva. A clinical and histopathological study. *Gynecol Oncol* 11:224, 1981.

316 Baggish MS, Dorsey JH: $CO_2$ laser for the treatment of vulvar carcinoma in situ. *Gynecol Oncol* 57:371, 1981.
317 Townsend DE et al: Management of vulvar intraepithelial neoplasia by carbon dioxide laser. *Obstet Gynecol* 60:49, 1982.
318 Bernstein SG et al: Vulvar carcinoma in situ. *Obstet Gynecol* 61: 304, 1983.
319 Leuchter RS et al: Treatment of vulvar carcinoma in situ with the $CO_2$ laser. *Gynecol Oncol* 19:314, 1984.
320 Reid R: Superficial laser vulvectomy. I. The efficacy of extended superficial ablation for refractory and very extensive condyloma. *Am J Obstet Gynecol* 151:1047, 1985.
321 Campion MJ et al: Subclinical penile human papillomavirus infection and dysplasia in consorts of women with cervical neoplasia. *Genitourin Med* 64:90, 1988.
322 Nash G et al: Atypical lesions of the anal mucosa in homosexual men. *JAMA* 256:873, 1986.

# Chapter 49

# Acute pelvic inflammatory disease (PID)

Lars Weström
Per-Anders Mårdh

## TERMINOLOGY AND DEFINITIONS

Pelvic inflammatory disease (PID) is defined as the acute clinical syndrome associated with ascending spread of microorganisms (unrelated to pregnancy or surgery) from the vagina or cervix to the endometrium, fallopian tubes, and/or contiguous structures.[1]

PID might include endometritis, parametritis, salpingitis, oophoritis, pelvic peritonitis, and pelvic (tubal, tubo-ovarian) abscess. In the literature, the diagnoses PID and acute salpingitis are often used synonymously for ascending genital infection involving the fallopian tubes. An ascending genital infection might also involve the appendix (periappendicitis)[2] and liver capsule (perihepatitis)[3] (see Chap. 51), as well as the splenic capsule (perisplenitis).[4]

In this chapter, PID caused by sexually transmitted pathogens such as *Neisseria gonorrhoeae* or *Chlamydia trachomatis* is termed *STD-associated PID*. Other cases of PID are termed *endogenous PID*, although some of the pathogens implicated in such cases also may be sexually transmitted.

## HISTORY

In 1683, Mauriceau was the first to describe inflammatory tumors of the uterine adnexa in puerperal infections.[5] Around 1870, autopsy reports were given on such "adnexitis." Between 1879 and 1911, four important milestones were set in the history of PID. One of these had immediate consequences, but the relevance of the other three to PID became apparent only a half century later. The first milestone was Neisser's discovery of the gonococcus in 1879. Bacteriologists and clinicians soon documented the strong correlation between "adnexitis" (PID) and gonococcal infection. The concept of PID as a disease mainly associated with gonorrhea dominated clinical thinking until modern times. The second discovery occurred in 1898, when Nocard and Roux[6] isolated the agent causing pleuropneumonia in cattle. In 1937, pleuropneumonia-like organisms (PPLO)—later mycoplasmas—were isolated from the human genital tract,[7] and in 1970, *Mycoplasma hominis* was reported as an etiological agent in acute salpingitis.[8,9]

The third discovery was the linking to one another of neonatal inclusion conjunctivitis, female inclusion cervicitis, and male urethritis by Halberstaedter and von Prowazek in 1907[10] and Lindner in 1911.[11] Successive improvements in methods of isolating the causative organism—*Chlamydia trachomatis*—came later.[12–14] In 1977, *C. trachomatis* was isolated from the fallopian tubes in cases of salpingitis.[15,16] Many studies have now documented *C. trachomatis* as one of the major etiological agents in PID.

The fourth milestone from this dynamic period at the turn of the century was laparoscopy, at first from a methodological point of view described by Kelling in 1902, and later applied in clinical medicine by Jacobaeus in 1910.[17] In PID, laparoscopy was applied for diagnosis and collection of specimens in 1969.[18] Laparoscopy soon proved to be an invaluable tool in clinical research on PID.

In 1946, Falk[19] contributed to the concept of PID as an ascending infection by showing that interruption of the canalicular route of spread from the lower to the upper female genital tract prevented PID.

Starting a century ago and for many decades thereafter, surgery was the undisputed therapy for PID. In 1919, Ahlström[20] introduced conservative treatment. He showed that such treatment resulted in a 90 percent clinical recovery. After the advent of antimicrobial chemotherapy in the thirties and antibiotic treatment in the forties, nonsurgical treatment of PID has become the rule and surgery the exception. In prospective studies on women given a laparoscopic diagnosis of PID, the earlier well-known long-term consequences of PID in terms of infertility and ectopic pregnancy were quantitatively defined.[21]

## EPIDEMIOLOGY AND ETIOLOGY

### General remarks

Acute PID is caused by two major groups of microorganisms: *STD agents* and organisms belonging to the *endogenous flora of the lower genital tract.*

During the past three decades, the majority of cases of PID (up to 80 percent) in the industrialized countries seem to have been caused by—or at least associated with—sexually transmitted microorganisms, especially in young persons.[22–31] The proportion of cases of PID caused by sexually transmitted organisms is related to factors that influence the overall incidence of STDs in the community, such as sexual and religious attitudes and traditions, economic and demographic factors, as well as other vaguely defined and unpredictable behavioral and environmental influences (see Chap. 2). Likewise, the proportions of women who are exposed to risk factors for PID, such as legal abortions or use of IUDs, or protective factors such as use of condoms or oral contraceptives, differ from population to population.

When studying reports on the epidemiology of PID, and on the role of different STD agents in PID, it is important to keep in mind the above factors as well as the following considerations:

- There are no generally accepted criteria for the clinical diagnosis of PID.
- In most regions, the disease is not reportable.
- Most studies of microbial etiology are based on rates of isolation from the cervix and not from the upper genital tract.
- Most studies have concerned only one or a limited number of PID-causing microorganisms. This is important, because double infections are common in the lower genital tract (see below).

Furthermore, there is growing evidence of an epidemic of asymptomatic "silent" PID running parallel to the clinically overt cases (see Chap. 50).

The epidemiology of PID in general is discussed below. The influence of the different causative organisms will be discussed under Etiology and that of other risk or protective factors under Pathophysiology.

## EPIDEMIOLOGY

### Prevalence and incidence

In the United States, an estimated 857,000 episodes of acute PID occurred each year around 1980.[32] In some industrialized countries (e.g., the United States, England, Sweden), estimates of the incidence of PID based on regional studies,[33–36] national surveys,[32,36–38] or extrapolations based on the prevalence of gonorrhea,[39,40] range from 9.5 to 14.0 cases of PID per 100 women per year in the fertile years, with a peak incidence of 18 to 20 per 1000 per year for ages 15 to 24 years. Adjustment for sexual activity reveals the highest annual incidence per 1000 *sexually active* women to be in the teenage group (see below).

From the developing countries, available data are meager but suggest that both STD and PID are common in parts of Africa, whereas in India acute PID seems to be of comparatively little importance.[41] It has been suggested that the high proportion of infertile women in some geographical areas might be a consequence of a high incidence of PID.[41,42]

### Trends

Age-specific incidence rates show a marked increase of PID over the years up to the early 1980s,[34,36–39,43] the increase running roughly parallel to that of STD in general.[37,38,43–44] The rates have been highest and have shown the greatest increases in women under the age of 25.[38,43]

In Sweden, it was estimated that women in the birth cohort of 1945 had a cumulative rate of first episodes of PID by their 25th birthday of 110/1000, whereas the corresponding figure for women in the 1950 birth cohort was 125/1000.[44]

In the United States, Washington et al.[45] noted that the ratio of nonwhite to white women hospitalized for acute PID decreased from 3.3 during 1970–1974 to 2.5 during 1975–1981, indicating that the overall rise in hospitalization rates (4.9 per 1000 to 5.3 per 1000) was almost entirely due to an increase in PID among young white women during the period.

On the other hand, in Sweden, a significant (40 percent) *decrease* of hospital discharge rates for salpingitis has been noted since 1978.[44] Available information indicates that the decrease in hospital discharge rates mirrors a decrease also of the total incidence of clinically diagnosed PID. The decrease of PID was coincident with a nationwide decrease in gonorrhea (see Chap. 2) and a decrease in chlamydial infections regionally.[35] A shift toward clinically and laparoscopically milder disease was also documented during the same period.[44]

### Age distribution and parity

The age distribution of women with PID is the same as that of those afflicted by STD in general (Fig. 49-1).[43,46] In most series, three out of four women afflicted with PID have been below the age of 25 (Fig. 49-2), an equally large proportion have been nulliparous, and half have never been pregnant (Fig 49-3).

### Ratio of STD-associated PID to "endogenous" PID

This ratio must depend on the incidence of PID-causing sexually transmitted pathogens among women. In general, the ratio of STD-associated PID to "endogenous" PID decreases with increasing age of the women.[34] In one study,[35] the total annual incidence of PID was 11.9 per 1000 sexually active women aged 20 to 24 and 79 percent of PID cases were associated with chlamydia and/or gonorrhea. In the 30- to 34-year age group, the corresponding figures were 4.0 per 1000 women and 55 percent. However, "endogenous" PID tends to run a clinically more severe course,[34,35,47] and in regions and age groups where women consult at hospitals only for severe PID, this might give an impression of a falsely low ratio of STD-associated to "endogenous" PID. The comparatively low sensitivity of clinical and laboratory diagnosis of genital chlamydial infections also may give a falsely low ratio of STD-associated to endogenous PID.

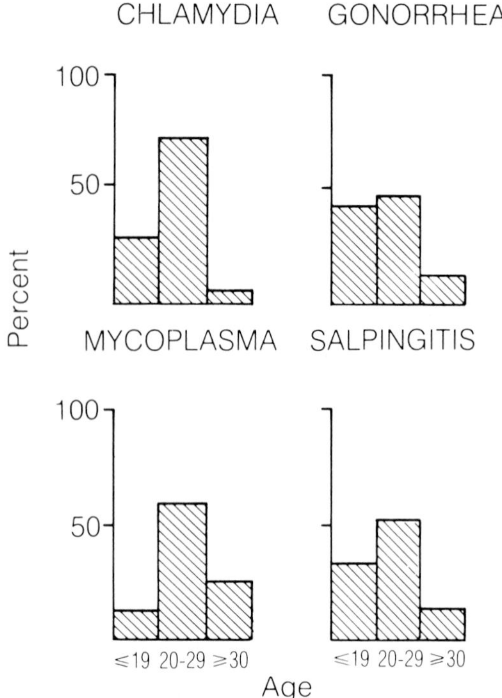


**Fig. 49-1.** Age distribution of women with lower genital tract infection from whom cervical specimens yielded growth of *N. gonorrhoeae*, *C. trachomatis*, or *M. hominis;* compared with age distribution of all women with laparoscopically verified acute PID. (From Refs. 8, 9, 34, 35, 46, 47.)

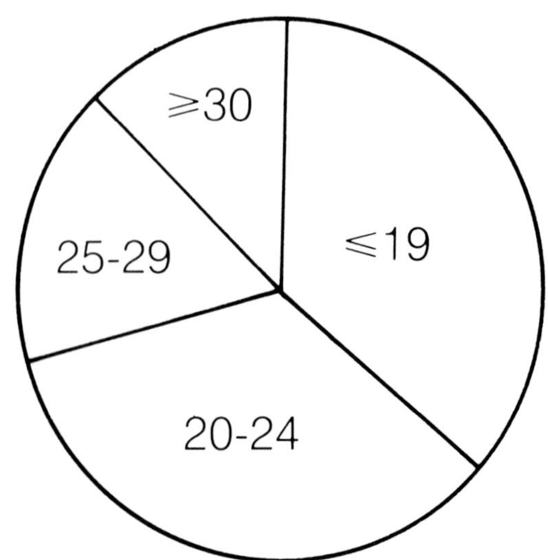


**Fig. 49-2.** Age distribution of 2400 women treated for laparoscopically verified acute PID. (From Refs. 34, 46.)

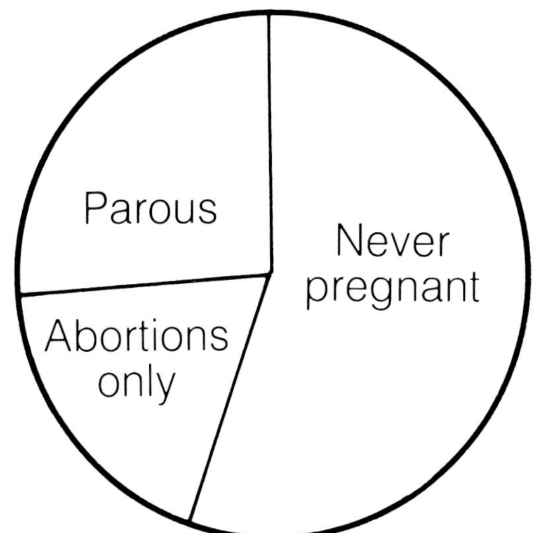


**Fig. 49-3.** Parity of 2400 women treated for laparoscopically verified acute PID. (From Refs. 34, 46.)

In assessing the relative importance of sexually transmitted "exogenous" pathogens vs. that of "endogenous" organisms in causing PID, it should be noted that some investigators believe that "exogenous" pathogens such as *N. gonorrhoeae* and *C. trachomatis* actually may initiate some cases of PID that are ultimately caused by endogenous organisms.[48] On the other hand, some investigators believe that some of the "endogenous" organisms which cause PID are, in general, also sexually transmitted (e.g., see Chaps. 46, 47).

## MICROBIAL ETIOLOGY

### General aspects

The multitude of species in the lower genital tract of all women as well as the inaccessibility of the fallopian tubes for sampling have long been major obstacles in studies of the etiology of PID. Modern studies, using culdocentesis or intra-abdominal sampling during laparoscopy, as well as studies of endometrial specimens, have shed new light on the etiology and pathophysiology of PID (see below). Still, discrepancies between microbial isolates from the lower and upper genital tract are common in cases of PID. Furthermore, isolates made from cul-de-sac specimens do not always correlate with findings in samples from the fallopian tubes in the same patient.[24,49]

A major limitation of the use of serology in studies of the etiology of PID is that genital infections not involving the upper genital tract might also provoke a serological response. Furthermore the patient with PID is from a serologic point of view often in the convalescence phase of the antibody response. Another limitation is the frequent inability of these techniques to distinguish between past and current infection.

### *Neisseria gonorrhoeae*

*N. gonorrhoeae* is the "classic" PID-causing agent, accepted as such for over one hundred years. In cases of PID, the organism has been recovered from the cervix, the endometrium,[50] and the fallopian tubes and pelvic cavity.[46,50] A cytotoxic effect of gonococci[51] and a ciliostatic effect of gonococcal endotoxin[52] have been demonstrated in organ cultures of human fallopian tube. The organism has not been isolated from macroscopically normal tubes.

Of women with cervical gonorrhea, it has been estimated that 10 to 19 percent develop symptoms of acute PID.[37] Certain characteristics of the gonococci may be related to their propensity to cause tubal infections, e.g., auxotype, penicillin resistance,[26,53] the forming of transparent colonies on agar,[26,54] and serovar.[55] The rates of isolation of gonococci from fallopian tubes or from cul-de-sac specimens from patients with PID and cervical gonorrhea have been low—usually between 10 and 20 percent.[24,47,56] The rate of recovery of gonococci from the upper genital tract in cases of gonorrhea-associated PID has been inversely related to the duration of symptoms, the organism being more often isolated from the fallopian tubes early in the clinical course of PID.[24,46,57,58,59] This could be attributable to gradual disappearance of gonococci from the fallopian tubes as the duration of tubal gonococcal infection increases. Alternatively, it is possible that true tubal gonococcal infection causes severe symptoms and early presentation; whereas patients who present after a longer duration of symptoms actually have milder, more tolerable symptoms because they do not really have salpingitis, or they have salpingitis caused by other organisms.

*N. gonorrhoeae* has been isolated from the lower genital tract in as many as 85 percent of women with acute PID.[24,50,60] Generally, reports from Europe have given much lower rates (5 to 27 percent) than reports from the United States and Canada (44 to 70 percent).[24] Coincident with the epidemic curve of gonorrhea, the proportions of women with PID who have gonorrhea have increased, leveled out, and decreased in proportion to the incidence of gonorrhea.[24,37,38,44] *In Sweden, the annual incidence of gonorrhea per 100,000 population decreased from an all-time high of 484 in 1970 to 68 in 1985.*[44] *During the same period, the proportion of women with PID who had gonorrhea decreased from 50 to 5 percent.*[44]

### *Chlamydia trachomatis*

*C. trachomatis* is now established as an important etiological agent in acute and chronic PID.

The organism has been demonstrated in the cervix, the endometrium,[61–64] and the fallopian tubes.[15,16,22,24,30,46,65–69] In experimental infections in grivet monkeys[70] and rabbits,[71] Koch's postulates have been fulfilled. IgM and IgG antibodies to the organism increase significantly during the course of naturally occurring infections in women.[22–24,72,73] In contrast to *N. gonorrhoeae, C. trachomatis* has been isolated from the upper genital tract from women with "chronic" PID.[67,74] In acute PID, the proportion of women with cervical infection who have demonstrable tubal infection with the same organism is higher for chlamydial infection than for gonorrhea.[22,24] The organism has rarely been isolated from cul-de-sac specimens.[24,49]

In European studies of PID, *C. trachomatis* was isolated from the lower genital tract in 31.4 percent (range 5 to 46 percent) of 1946 studied cases, and from the upper genital tract in 10.5 percent of studied cases. The highest yield from the upper genital tract was from 6 out of 7 chlamydia cervix-positive patients with PID.[22] IgG antibody to *C. trachomatis* at a titer of 1:64 or higher has been detected in 61 percent of laparoscopically verified cases of PID.[22,23,25,27,28,30,31,68,72–75] A fourfold or greater change in the titer of serum antibody to *C. trachomatis* was found in 25 percent of the cases.[30,68,72,73,75] The combined results from these European studies suggest that *C. trachomatis* was the causative agent in at least 60 percent of the cases—four times more often than *N. gonorrhoeae*. In Europe, the ratio of chlamydia- to gonorrhea-associated PID continues to increase.

The incidence of chlamydia-associated PID has been strikingly age-dependent.[29,30,31,35] From 1977 through 1980, the annual incidences of chlamydia-associated PID was 6.2 per 1000 women 15 to 19 years of age and 2.8 per 1000 women 25 to 29 years of age.[35]

In the United States, the number of cases of uncomplicated genital chlamydial infection was estimated as 3 to 5 million cases per year in the early eighties.[76] Recent studies[27,65,66,77] have given cultural and serological evidence of *C. trachomatis* as an etiological agent in up to 38 percent[65] of hospitalized cases, and up to 52 percent[27,78] of women treated as outpatients for PID.

## *Mycoplasma hominis*

*M. hominis* was incriminated as a possible cause of PID in the late sixties.[8,9] In later, mainly Scandinavian, studies, *M. hominis* has been demonstrated in the cervix, the endometrium,[78,79,80] and the fallopian tubes[8,78,81] in cases of PID. The organism can frequently be isolated from the vagina and cervix of women without cervicitis or PID, but has not been isolated from macroscopically normal tubes. Significant changes in antibodies to the organism have been demonstrated in patients with PID during the course of the disease.[9,78,79,81,82] In grivet monkeys, direct inoculation of *M. hominis* into the fallopian tubes provoked salpingitis.[78,83] In organ cultures of human fallopian tubes, a cytopathogenic effect has been demonstrated after inoculation infection with *M. hominis*.[84]

*M. hominis* has been recovered from the cervix from 243 (61 percent) of 399 women with PID, and from the upper genital tract from 12 (7.3 percent) of 165 women with PID who had positive cervical cultures.[8,78,79,81] During the course of acute PID, a significant change of antibody to *M. hominis* has been seen by enzyme immunoassay in 23 percent of followed cases,[82] and by indirect hemagglutination assay in 43 percent of cervix-culture-positive and 15 percent of cervix-culture-negative patients.[9,78,79,82] Thus, although *M. hominis* is infrequently isolated from fallopian tubes, serologic findings suggest a role of *M. hominis* in up to 30 percent of patients with PID. *M. hominis*–associated PID was evenly distributed in the different age groups, and differed in this respect from PID associated with *C. trachomatis* or *N. gonorrhoeae*.[80]

## *Mycoplasma genitalium*

Antibody to *M. genitalium* is also common in women with PID,[85] although the specificity of serologic tests for this agent remains uncertain. This mycoplasma species has also been found to produce salpingitis in experimental infections in grivet monkeys. Clinical studies of *M. genitalium* have been hampered by difficulties in recovering the organism; microbiological recovery takes 3 months. The recent introduction of a DNA probe for *M. genitalium* might soon increase our knowledge on the role of this organism in PID.

## *Ureaplasma urealyticum*

*U. urealyticum* has been isolated from the fallopian tubes in occasional cases of PID.[8,78,86] A significant increase of serum metabolism-inhibiting antibody to the organism has been demonstrated in one case.[9] Attempts at producing salpingitis in grivet monkeys using *U. urealyticum* have failed. Ureaplasmas are common isolates from the lower genital tract of patients with PID, but also from carefully selected nonpregnant sexually active control women.[87] The role, if any, of *U. urealyticum* in PID must be minimal.

## "Mixed" infections with STD agents

Isolation from the lower genital tract of more than one species of sexually transmitted pathogens is common in patients with acute PID.[24,28,31,75,86] Thus, in patients with "gonorrhea-associated" PID, a cervical infection with *C. trachomatis* was found in 28 percent of the cases.[75] Among patients with "mycoplasma-associated PID," strong correlations were found with concomitant isolations of *C. trachomatis, N. gonorrhoeae*, or both.[79,81]

These results illustrate the need for cultures of the upper genital tract in studies of the role of different STD agents in PID.

## "Endogenous" microbial agents

In women with bacterial vaginosis, the microbial flora of the lower genital tract contains a variety of aerobic, facultative, and strictly anaerobic bacterial species[88] (see also Chap. 47). In women with PID, the same spectrum of species has by and large been demonstrated in the upper genital tract, pelvic cavity, and cul-de-sac fluid.[39,49,56,58,59,69,86,89–96] Among species thus encountered in the upper genital tract have been facultative and anaerobic streptococci, including group B streptococci and peptostreptococci, *Escherichia coli, Gardnerella vaginalis, Bacteroides* species (especially *B. melaninogenicus* and *B. bivius* in recent studies) as well as clostridial and actinomyces species. In many patients with PID, more than one such species have been isolated from the upper genital tract or cul-de-sac fluid.[24,26,56,86,91,93,94] This has given rise to the concept of PID having a "polymicrobial" etiology.[56] While polymicrobial infection has been repeatedly demonstrated by cultures obtained at laparoscopy, results of cultures obtained by culdocentesis or transcervical endometrial aspiration should be interpreted with caution because of possible contamination with vaginal bacteria.

Isolation of these "endogenous" microorganisms from the upper genital tract in PID has been proportionally more common in clinically severe—often suppurative—infection than in cases with clinically benign disease.[24,46,47] In cases of PID with a clinically and laparoscopically early and mild appearance, anaerobic cultural techniques generally have revealed no growth of anaerobic bacteria.[29,47]

A "polymicrobial" flora of endogenous species have also been common findings in long-standing cases, in somewhat older women,[34] in women with repeated PID,[56,57,89,96] as well as in women with PID who are using an IUD.[97,98]

## Virus

Few attempts have been made at isolating virus from the upper genital tract in cases of PID. In a series of 15 patients,[8] virus was isolated from the fallopian tubes in two instances (Coxsackie B5, and ECHO 6, respectively). In one case, HSV type 2 was isolated from the endometrium and fallopian tube in chlamydia-associated salpingitis.[99]

Although in these few cases laboratory contamination cannot be excluded, further studies are warranted on the possible role of viral infections in the upper genital tract.

### Miscellaneous agents

Primary respiratory tract pathogens such as group A streptococci, pneumococci, *Haemophilus influenzae*, and *M. pneumoniae* have been isolated from the fallopian tubes in a few patients with salpingitis.[24,90] *Campylobacter fetus* is another rare cause of PID, as evidenced by a case in which septicemia also occurred.[100] Invasion of the tubes by *Enterobius vermicularis*[101] as well as *Trichomonas vaginalis*[8] has been repeatedly documented.

Among tropical diseases which might be associated with infections of the upper female genital tract are filariasis and schistosomiasis. Few data are, however, available on the prevalence, epidemiology, and pathophysiology of genital infections caused by those agents.

### Unknown etiology

In some 20 percent of cases of clinical acute PID with laparoscopically verified inflammatory reactions of the fallopian tubes, hitherto applied cultural techniques on tubal speciments have given no growth of any organism.[24] In many such cases, serologic examinations for the commonly accepted pathogens have also been negative. The patients in this category are characterized by being comparatively older (28 percent over 30 years), having longer duration of pelvic pain (38 percent over 3 days), having a normal ESR (53 percent), and presenting mild inflammatory changes at laparoscopy (53 percent).[102]

## PATHOPHYSIOLOGY AND RISK FACTORS

### Genital tract microbiology in normal women

In healthy women in the fertile ages, the vaginal microbial flora contains a multitude of species but is usually dominated by lactobacilli.[88] Some studies have shown quantitative and qualitative variations with the menstrual cycle, sexual intercourse, pregnancy, and use of contraceptives, as well as with the age of the woman.[88,103]

It has long been taken for granted that the upper genital tract in normal women should be sterile. However, recent studies suggest that microorganisms might (temporarily?) colonize or infect the endometrial cavity[104,105] as well as the fallopian tubes and pelvic cavity[69,106,107] in a proportion of women with no signs of a genital infection.

## PATHOPHYSIOLOGY

### General aspects

By definition, PID is caused by microorganisms which ascend from the lower genital tract.[1] Many studies have suggested a continuum of infection of the cervix, endometrium, and fallopian tubes with *N. gonorrhoeae*,[50] *C. trachomatis*,[61,62,64–66,109,110] and *M. hominis*,[78,79] as well as a histopathologic continuum including cervicitis, cervicitis/endometritis, and cervicitis/endometritis/salpingitis.[63–66,69,108] As noted above, sexually transmitted pathogens (e.g., *N. gonorrhoeae*, and perhaps *C. trachomatis*) are proportionally more often isolated from the upper genital tract in short-standing and comparatively mild disease, whereas "endogenous" organisms are proportionally more often isolated in clinically more advanced disease.[22,26,29,47,56–59,89–96] In clinically severe cases with abscess formation, strictly anaerobic species (e.g., *Bacteroides* sp.) are common isolates.[56,90,93–96] These observations have led to the speculation that in many cases of PID, STD organisms initiate the tubal inflammatory reaction (monomicrobial phase). It has been hypothesized by some investigators that the tubal mucosa thus "primed" is thereafter invaded by opportunists from the endogenous flora of the lower genital tract (polymicrobial phase), and that as in all soft tissue mixed infections, tissue destruction and lowered redox potential favor anaerobes, which gradually become dominating. In general, the clinical appearance of PID follows this hypothetical sequence of tubal isolates in that "monomicrobial" early disease associated with sexually transmitted pathogens is usually clinically mild or even asymptomatic, whereas the patient with "polymicrobial" PID is more severely ill.

### Route of spread

The concept of a canalicular spread of the microbial agents through the endometrium and endosalpinx was founded by the observations by Falk in 1946, cited above.[19] Since then, much support has been published for this concept. The simultaneous presence of cervicitis, endometritis, and salpingitis has been documented in many patients with PID. Falk's original observations have later been confirmed by Hajj,[109] who found no case of PID after tubal sterilization in 3500 women, and by Vessey et al.,[110] who found no case of PID in a prospective cohort study of 2243 sterilized women.

On the other hand, in the preantibiotic era, a noncanalicular spread of cervical infections was reported.[90] Lymphatic drainage of the cervix parametrially as well as along the surface of the uterus was documented early[111] and later reconfirmed.[112] In one recent study, the finding of acute salpingitis (proximal stump abscess) was reported in women who were sterilized.[113] In animal experiments it has been found that genital infections with *M. hominis* spread mainly to the parametria.[70] In women with clinically suspected PID but normal fallopian tubes at laparoscopy, it has been postulated that the pelvic pain could be explained by a parametrial lymphatic spread of the infection.[114] More studies of this concept are necessary.

Intra-abdominally, pelvic infection can spread to the appendix and cause periappendicitis[2] and paracolically to the liver surface causing perihepatitis.[3] Perisplenitis has also been reported in cases of PID.[4]

### Mechanisms of spread

**Cervix.** It is widely believed that the cervix offers a functional barrier for the ascent of microorganisms, although direct proof for this is incomplete. A functional barrier may be attributable to the rheological properties of the cervical mucus plug,[115] as well as to antibodies, enzymes, and other components of the cervical secretions. The protective effect of the functional barrier against the ascent of spermatozoa (and perhaps microorganisms) is at its lowest during ovulation[115] and when the mucus plug is absent[90] (i.e., during menstruation), and at its highest under the influence of progesterone.[115]

**Ectopy.** It has been suggested that extension of the cervical cylindrical epithelium out on the surface of the portio (ectopy) should facilitate infection by chlamydia.[116] The presence and surface area of cervical ectopy have been correlated with cervical infection with *C. trachomatis*.[116,117]

**Uterus.** The muscular activity of the myometrium might be important for the mechanical transport of particles through the genital tract. Coital (orgasmic) contractions of the myometrium have been demonstrated,[118] as has an increased myometrial activity in IUD-using women. Such activity is decreased in women administered progesterone.[119] These observations are in accordance with the findings that acute PID is seen only in sexually active women, is proportionally more common in IUD-using women, and is less often seen in women administered progesterone (see below).

**Menstruation.** Retrograde menstrual blood flow from the uterine cavity through the fallopian tubes has been demonstrated in the majority (90 percent) of women with patent tubes.[120] Microorganisms might spread with such blood, contributing to the development of PID. Clinical studies show that symptoms of PID caused by *N. gonorrhoeae* or *C. trachomatis*[39,46,77] begin more often during or immediately after menstruation than in midcycle or premenstrually.

**Spermatozoa.** Microorganisms that can adhere to human spermatozoa include *N. gonorrhoeae*,[121] *C. trachomatis*,[122] *M. hominis*,[123] and other bacteria.[124] In vitro, spermatozoa with such adherent bacteria can propagate through cervical ovulatory secretion[124] and egg albumin.[122] In a recent study, Friberg et al.[125] recovered spermatozoa with adherent chlamydia from the pelvic cavity of two women with acute PID.

Although the collected results from several clinical and epidemiological studies[98,110,126,129] suggest indirectly that sperm migration through the female genital tract might play a role in the pathophysiology of PID, there are very plausible alternative explanations for the results of each of these studies.

## RISK FACTORS FOR PID

### Age

The risk of acquiring PID seems to decrease with increasing age among sexually experienced women. The relative risks of PID in women who were culture-positive from the cervix for *N. gonorrhoeae*, *C. trachomatis*, or both, assigning a relative risk of 1.0 in the 15- to 19-year age group were 0.7 for women 20 to 24; 0.4 for women 25 to 29, and 0.2 for women 30 to 34.[35]

In sexually active teenage girls living in a region with an annual incidence of gonorrhea of 2255 per 100,000 per year, the risk of acquiring PID was calculated to be 1:8 in girls aged 15, 1:10 in 16-year-olds, and 1:80 in women 24 years of age.[34]

So far, there is no proved explanation for this age-dependent risk of PID, although age-related changes in immunological factors, in ectopy, and in the functional cervical barrier against ascending infection might be important.

### Sexual activity

Many authors[60,127,128] have emphasized the nonvirginity of patients with acute PID. PID is a rarity in celibatory nuns, for instance.[127] The risk of acquiring an STD and, hence, an STD-associated PID, is correlated to the numbers of sexual partners.[39] In women with only one sexual partner, the risk of PID has been found to correlate also with coital frequency.[98] The relationship of sexual activity to risk of PID is valid even for PID which is not associated with *N. gonorrhoeae* or *C. trachomatis*.

### Contraceptives

During the past twenty years, many studies have concerned the influence on the risk of PID of use of different methods of contraception.[129–136] Although few studies in this field can avoid criticism, most—but not all[135]—agree on the following four points:

1. Use of combined (i.e., estrogen/progesterone) contraceptive pills decreases the risk that a lower tract genital infection will ascend to the upper genital tract. Among the many possible explanations are progesterone-induced changes in the cervical mucus and decreased myometrial activity, and direct effect of estrogen or progestin on growth of chlamydia in the upper genital tract. Recent studies have provided evidence for protection against ascending chlamydia infection[137] but not against gonococcal infection (P. Wölner-Hanssen, D. Eschenbach, K.K. Holmes, unpublished data).
2. Use of oral contraceptives modifies the clinical course and the laparoscopic findings in patients who have PID,[137] in that OC-using women generally have a clinically and laparoscopically milder infection[130] and lower GMT (1:25) of antichlamydial IgG antibody than nonusers (1:109).[137]
3. Use of an IUD increases the risk of PID.[98,136] However, the first estimates of a 3- to 9-fold risk increase of PID in IUD users were falsely high because pill users were included among the controls. The risk of PID is higher during the weeks after insertion or change of an IUD[98] than during continuous use of the device. The use of a Dalkon shield device carried a significantly higher risk of PID than the use of copper-medicated devices.[129] Women using progesterone medicated devices have been reported to have a decreased risk of PID as compared with users of other types of IUD.[132,133] In IUD-using women who had only one sexual partner, the risk of PID was not significantly different from that of noncontraceptors but was found to be correlated more with coital frequency.[98]
4. Use of condoms, or of pessaries or sponges containing the spermicidal surfactant nonoxynol-9, prevents to a certain extent infection with sexually transmitted organisms such as *N. gonorrhoeae* and *C. trachomatis* and hence decreases the risk of PID caused by these organisms.[138–140]

Computing recent risk estimates from the literature as well as results from epidemiological studies in Lund, Sweden, we arrive at the relative risks of PID given in Table 49-1 in women using different contraceptive methods as compared with sexually active noncontraceptors.[141]

### "Iatrogenic" PID

Operative procedures such as cervical dilatation, curettage, tubal insufflation, hysterosalpingography, IUD insertion, and legal

**Table 49-1. Relative Risk of PID Related to Use of Contraceptives in Women 20 to 29 Years of Age in Lund, Sweden 1970–1974[141]**

| Contraceptive method | Relative risk of PID |
|---|---|
| Noncontraceptors | 1.0 |
| IUD | 1.5 |
| Oral contraceptives | 0.3 |
| Barrier methods | 0.6 |

abortion carry a small risk of infectious complications if professionally performed. In series of PID cases, such iatrogenic procedures have preceded the onset of PID by less than 4 weeks in 10 to 12 percent of the cases.[18,37,47]

PID has been reported as a postoperative complication in 0 to 13 percent of women undergoing first trimester legal abortion by vacuum curettage[142–144] as well as after hysterosalpingography.[145] The rate of postoperative PID after legal abortion[144,146] or HSG[147] was decreased significantly by prophylactic treatment with doxycycline but not with metronidazole or tinidazole.

In women applying for legal abortion and examined for preabortion levels of serum antibody to *C. trachomatis,* it was found that the risk of postabortion PID was inversely correlated to presence of antibody to certain chlamydial antigens (implying that antibody to such antigens might prevent postabortion chlamydial PID).[148]

### Repeated infections

Up to one-third of women who have had one episode of PID suffer from repeated bouts.[44,46] A high rate of recurrence is common even after a first episode of non-STD-associated PID.[46] In young women, the second and following episodes of PID are less often associated with gonococcal and chlamydial infection than is the first episode.[46,57] A second infection usually (56 percent) appears within 1 year of the first episode.[37,46,47]

The high rate of repeated bouts of PID has been explained by the following:

1. Failure to examine and treat sex partners of women with gonorrhea or chlamydia-associated PID results in reinfection. In Lund, Sweden, a significant decrease (from 16 to 4 percent) of second episodes of PID was seen in prospectively followed cases of PID coincident with initiation of partner examination and treatment in cases of chlamydia-associated PID.[44]
2. Inadequate treatment may cause a relapse of the first infection as opposed to reinfection.[34,37,48] From France[67,74] have come reports (not yet confirmed elsewhere) of the isolation of *C. trachomatis* from the fallopian tubes many years after the initial episode.
3. Postinfection tubal damage may render the fallopian tubes more vulnerable for infection by opportunistic species of the lower genital tract flora. This is supported by the observation of a lower rate of gonococcal or chlamydial infection in second bouts of PID, even in populations at high risks for these infections.[57]
4. Factors such as young age, sexual promiscuity, and low socioeconomic status which place the woman at high risk for STD in general continue to place her at risk for reinfection after the first episode of PID.

## PATHOLOGY

It is noteworthy that current understanding of the pathologic manifestations of PID is largely limited to descriptive analyses of gross pathology and histopathology. The specific mechanisms responsible for initiation of inflammation, tissue injury, and scarring in PID have been less extensively studied than in infections of many other organ systems.

## ENDOMETRITIS

Histopathologically, some pathologists consider endometritis difficult to separate from the physiological, cycle-related infiltration of the endometrium with leukocytes. However, in cases where *N. gonorrhoeae* has been recovered from the endometrial cavity, diffuse infiltration of the endometrium by polymorphonuclear leukocytes and areas of epithelial necrosis have been reported.[50,90] Infiltration of the endometrium with plasma cells seems to be the hallmark of endometrial infection by *C. trachomatis* but can also be seen in endometrial gonococcal infection (N. Kiviat, unpublished data).[61–63,108] Germinal centers containing transformed lymphocytes are also characteristic of chlamydial endometritis. Plasma-cell endometritis may be patchy, which means that the diagnosis might be missed. Endometritis is usually present in cases with salpingitis, but can also be found in women with suspected PID who have normal tubes at laparoscopy.[99]

## SALPINGITIS

*Microscopically* the inflammatory process starts in the mucosal surface epithelium and extends to the subepithelial tissue.[90] The mucosal cells show cloudy swelling, patchy necrosis, and deciliation.[90] In the subepithelial tissue a marked infiltration of inflammatory cells appears. Initially this consists of polymorphonuclear leucocytes, but later mononuclear cells and plasma cells predominate.[65,66] A marked edema causes swelling of the mucosal folds, which tend to adhere to one another, causing an impression of sealed luminal pockets (follicular salpingitis). The tubal lumen is filled with an exudate containing inflammatory and epithelial cells and cell debris. Later the inflammatory process involves the muscularis and extends through all layers to the serosa, on which fibrin deposits appear.

*Macroscopically* in early mild cases of salpingitis, the fallopian tubes are swollen and their serosal surface slightly reddened. The tubal mucosa, as seen at the open fimbriated ends, is congested and fiercely red. A purulent or seropurulent exudate is seen at or in the abdominal ostia of the tubes. The tubes are freely movable.[21,46]

In moderately severe disease, inflammatory changes are more advanced. The tubes are not freely movable, often covered by patchy fibrin deposits, and tend to adhere to nearby pelvic structures such as the ovaries and the broad ligament.

In severe salpingitis and pelvic peritonitis, the infectious process has spread to the pelvic peritoneum. The pelvic structures show intense congestion and the organs adhere to one another. Laparoscopy at this stage of the disease reveals the entire pelvic cavity to be occluded by an inflammatory mass in which the anatomical structures are difficult to define. The infectious process can lead to tissue destruction with tubal or tubo-ovarian abscess formation. Most often the omentum adheres to the pelvic structures and the infectious process remains confined to the pelvic cavity. Generalized peritonitis is uncommon.[90]

## HEALING AND REPAIR

In the vast majority of cases, endometritis heals without scarring. Aschermann's syndrome is rarely seen after endometritis that is not associated with curettage or abortion.

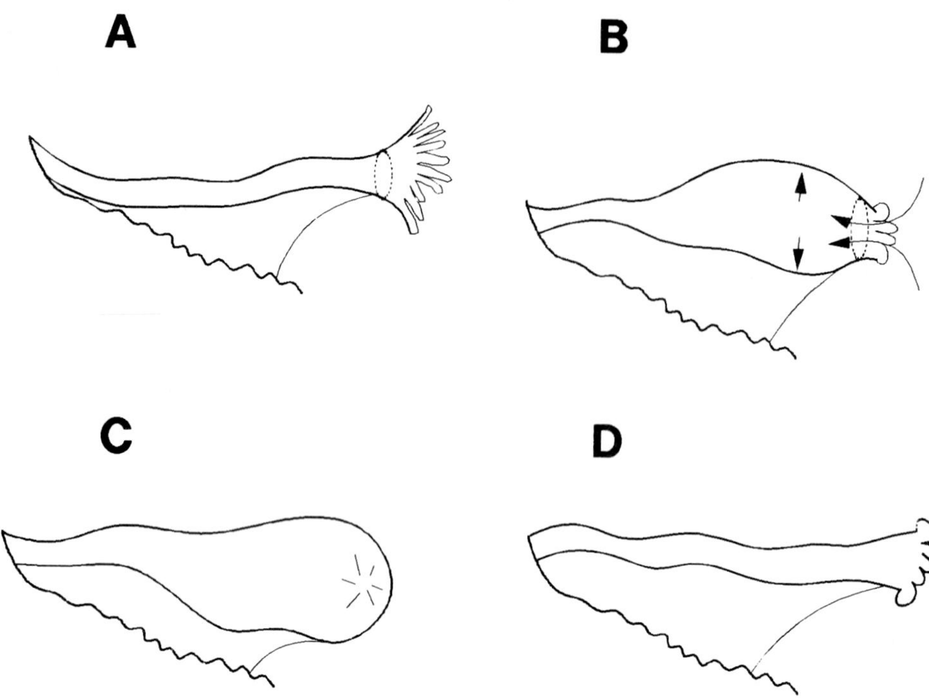


**Fig. 49-4.** Pathophysiology of postinflammatory damage to the fallopian tubes. (*a*) Normal fallopian tube. (*b*) Acutely inflamed tube. (*c*) Postinflammatory sactosalpinx. (*d*) Postinflammatory rigid but patent tube with "paraphimotic" abdominal ostium.

In the fallopian tubes, the inflammatory edema of the subserosal layers causes an increase in volume and pressure. This causes the serosa to give away along the margin of the mesosalpinx. The result will be a swelling of the entire organ as well as a shortening of the mesosalpinx. In most women, the part of the fallopian tube close to its fimbriated end lacks mesosalpinx. Here, the serosa cannot yield to the volume increase. The result will be a functional fibrous ring through which is drawn the tube's outermost part including the fimbriae (Fig. 49-4). This postulated process brings the fimbriae in close proximity to one another. During the combined processes of inflammation and repair, the fimbriae "heal" together, thereby sealing off the infectious process in the tubes from the pelvic cavity (Fig. 49-4).

In the pelvic cavity, the inflammatory reaction causes serosal cell death and damage to the pelvic peritoneal surfaces. Inflammatory exudate and fibrin deposits tend to "glue" adjacent surfaces to one another. Organization of such adhesions with ingrowing fibroblasts results in intrapelvic adhesions.

The process of repair goes on simultaneously with the infectious process. When the infection has been overcome, the inflammatory reaction gradually subsides as repair continues, resulting in either complete restitution or varying degrees of scarring or functional impairment.

The persisting morphological damage seen in some cases after a pelvic infection can be divided into three types—each appearing alone or in various combinations with one another on one or both sides in the pelvic cavity:

1. Endosalpingeal mucosal damage and damage to the tubal wall
2. Tubal occlusion
   *a*. Distal
   *b*. Proximal
3. Peritubal damage
   *a*. Restricted mobility
   *b*. Adhesions

In the mucosal epithelium, the process of repair often leaves little persisting damage, although intraluminal mucosa to mucosa adhesions may be formed.[149] The deciliation of the initial phase often is temporary.[150] The subserosal interstitial tissue of the tubes might become infiltrated by fibrocytes, resulting in a macroscopically normal but rigid tube, often with a "paraphimotic" abdominal ostium (Fig. 49-4). The functional capacity of such tubes has been little studied. Although often patent, it is logical to assume that restricted mobility, tubal rigidity, paraphimotic ostium, and intraluminal adhesions result in an impaired ovum pickup mechanism as well as a decreased ability of ovum and blastocyst transport. Decreased fecundity as well as a proportionally increased risk of a tubal pregnancy should follow.

The best documented end result of PID with respect to fertility is occlusion of the distal end of the fallopian tube.[90] The end result is a club- or retort-shaped tube, closed in its distal end (sactosalpinx) and often distended by serous fluid (hydrosalpinx). In many cases, the glued-together fimbriae can be identified as a star-shaped scar on the serosal surface (Fig. 49-4).

In a proportion of cases of tubal infertility, the tube is occluded proximally, i.e., close to its uterine portion. In the majority of such cases, the remaining part of the tube seems completely normal. The etiology of proximal occlusion has been disputed. Endometriosis is probably a more common cause than infection, except in cases presenting with other stigmata of postinfection damage.

Pelvic adhesions may form between inflamed areas of the tubes, the uterus, the ovaries, the broad ligaments, the bowel, and the pelvic walls. Such adhesions are most often seen between the tubes and adjacent surfaces of the uterus and the broad ligament as well as the ovaries. Adhesions interfere with the normal mobility of the organs as well as with ovum pickup.

## CLINICAL MANIFESTATIONS AND DIAGNOSIS

### General aspects

Clinically, acute PID can vary from asymptomatic to a life-threatening condition. In gonococcal and chlamydial PID, the patient is generally not seriously ill. The lower genital tract infection

**Table 49-2. Correlation of Clinical and Laboratory Abnormalities with Laparoscopic Findings in 2220 Cases Given a Clinical Diagnosis of Acute Salpingitis[36]**

| Clinical and laboratory abnormalities | Laparoscopic diagnosis | | Percent of women with salpingitis presenting the symptoms or signs |
|---|---|---|---|
| | Salpingitis, % | Normal or other, % | |
| Low abdominal pain *plus* signs of an LGTI* *plus* motion tenderness | 61.2 | 38.8 | 16.1 |
| As above *plus* one or more of the following: ESR ≥ 15 mm/h; temperature > 38.0°C; palpable adnexal mass: | | | |
| + one of the above abnormalities | 78.3 | 21.7 | 28.3 |
| + two of the above abnormalities | 89.6 | 10.4 | 38.7 |
| + all three abnormalities | 95.6 | 4.4 | 16.9 |

*LGTI = lower genital tract infection, as defined by the presence of inflammatory cells outnumbering other cellular elements on wet mount examination of vaginal fluid.

preceding PID may pass unnoticed or cause only slight and transient symptoms from the lower genital and/or urinary tracts. Cervicitis associated with chlamydia and/or gonorrhea is asymptomatic in the majority of cases. The lower genital tract infection may have been present for months before being complicated by PID. The onset of pelvic or low abdominal pain is usually regarded as the first symptom of ascending infection.

The diagnosis of acute PID is usually made on the basis of clinical criteria and the results of laboratory procedures. However, the clinical criteria used vary between doctors and institutions. Routine laparoscopy for the diagnosis of salpingitis has revealed that commonly used clinical criteria for acute salpingitis are correct in only about 65 percent of cases. In general, the positive predictive value of a clinical diagnosis of PID is lowest in patients presenting with few symptoms and signs of the disease (Table 49-2). Because the laparoscopic diagnosis of *salpingitis* should be highly specific when performed by an experienced laparoscopist and also because differential diagnostic mistakes could be avoided, liberal use of laparoscopy has been proposed.[18,49] However, laparoscopic findings may occasionally be normal in patients with symptoms of PID who have objective evidence of endometritis and/or endosalpingitis. For obvious reasons, laparoscopy cannot be routinely applied in all clinical situations.

Thus, for the diagnosis and management of acute PID, two dilemmas are met with. First the low accuracy of (varying) clinical criteria, weighed against the expenses and risks of laparoscopy, and second the difficulties in agreeing upon clinical criteria that are not too strict (and exclude patients with mild disease) or too liberal (and include patients with other or no disease). Uniform clinical criteria have been proposed for the diagnosis of acute salpingitis.[151,152] Likewise, clinical and laboratory findings have been analyzed, to identify patients who most need laparoscopy.[153] So far, however, none of those approaches has been clinically evaluated or generally agreed upon.

Below is presented the experience in Lund of clinical manifestations and diagnosis of acute PID as based on laparoscopically verified cases. In general, the minimum clinical criteria for performing laparoscopy on a case of assumed PID were: acute low abdominal or pelvic pain, objective signs of an infection of the lower genital tract (LGTI), plus increased (motion) tenderness at a pelvic examination.[18,46,102] Using these minimum criteria, laparoscopy revealed acute salpingitis in 65 percent, other pelvic pathology in 12 percent, and normal intrapelvic findings in 23 percent. The last mentioned group thus comprised women with a genital infection and pelvic pain but no laparoscopically demonstrable inflammation of the fallopian tubes or pelvic cavity.

## SYMPTOMS

The general condition of the average patient afflicted with acute PID is not much affected. Using the minimum criteria mentioned above, only about 3 percent of patients with PID were considered seriously ill at admission.[18,46]

The pain associated with PID was usually subacute in onset, bilateral low abdominal or pelvic, and dull in character. In an American study, onset of pain was seen within 1 week of the first menstrual day in 55 percent of cases with gonorrhea-associated PID and 57 percent of cases with chlamydia-associated PID.[77] Of patients who fell ill within 7 days of the first menstrual day, 81 percent had either gonorrhea or chlamydial infection or both. Of patients falling ill premenstrually, 66% had a non-STD-associated PID.[77] In the Lund study, brief duration of abdominal pain (less than 3 days) was significantly correlated with gonorrhea-associated disease and with age older than 30 years.[46] Abdominal pain exceeded 1 week significantly more often among women with chlamydia-associated PID than among those with non-chlamydial disease[102] (Table 49-3).

Irregular bleeding was commonly reported in PID (Table 49-4) and was significantly more common with chlamydia-associated PID than with other cases of PID (Table 49-3). In young women, reports of irregular uterine bleeding of recent onset should always arouse suspicion of a genital infection (endometritis), especially if she is not taking hormonal contraceptives.

Dysuria was reported by about one-fifth of patients with PID (Table 49-4). This symptom relates to the common (5 to 20 per-

**Table 49-3. Clinical and Laboratory Abnormalities in Women with Laparoscopically Verified Acute Salpingitis Associated with Cervical Infection with *Neisseria gonorrhoeae* ($n$ = 19) or *Chlamydia trachomatis* ($n$ = 68) or Neither Organism ($n$ = 64)[102]**

| Clinical or laboratory abnormality | Percent of women presenting with symptoms or signs of PID associated with | | |
|---|---|---|---|
| | Gonorrhea | Chlamydia | Neither |
| Pelvic pain: | | | |
| ≤ 3 days | 32 | 15 | 38 |
| > 10 days | 21 | 41 | 27 |
| Temperature > 38.0°C | 52 | 22 | 30 |
| Palpable adnexal mass | 52 | 25 | 20 |
| ESR ≥ 30 mm/h | 32 | 65 | 19 |
| Irregular bleeding | 25 | 40 | 30 |

**Table 49-4. Percent Prevalence of Symptoms, Signs, and Laboratory Abnormalities Among 807 Women Subjected to Laparoscopy Because of Clinically Suspected Salpingitis.[18,46,102] All Women Had (as Inclusion Criteria) Abdominal Pain, Adnexal Tenderness, and Objective Evidence of Purulent Vaginal Discharge**

| | Laparoscopic diagnosis | | | Laparoscopic diagnosis | |
|---|---|---|---|---|---|
| Symptoms | Salpingitis, % | No salpingitis,* % | Signs and laboratory abnormalities | Salpingitis, % | No salpingitis,† % |
| Abnormal discharge | 55 | 51 | Temperature > 38.0°C | 41 | 20 |
| Irregular bleeding | 36 | 43 | Palpable mass | 49 | 25 |
| Dysuria | 19 | 20 | ESR ≥ 15 mm/h | 76 | 53 |
| Vomiting | 10 | 9 | WBC > 10,000/ml blood† | 59 | 33 |
| Anorectal symptoms | 7 | 3 | Acute phase reactants‡ | 79 | 24 |
| | | | Decreased isoamylases§ | 90 | 20 |

*Normal intraperitoneal findings; assumed to have lower genital tract infection or endometritis (see text).
†WBC was determined in 240 cases.
‡Antichymotrypsin, orosomucoid, or acute-phase reactants including CRP, determined in 95 cases (see text).
§Determined in peritoneal fluid in 95 cases (see text).

cent) isolation of chlamydia, gonococci, and mycoplasmas from the urethra in cases with PID.[24,46,78,79]

Only about half of the patients with PID reported an increased or changed vaginal discharge (Table 49-4). This illustrates that the lower genital infection preceding the PID often may pass unnoticed, and also that the patient's report of the presence or absence of a vaginal discharge should not be relied upon for the diagnosis of genital infections in general.

In the Swedish studies, nausea and vomiting were infrequent symptoms in PID (Table 49-4), perhaps reflecting the small proportion in those studies who had developed peritonitis. In acute cases, the presence of vomiting points more to a disease of the gastrointestinal tract (e.g., appendicitis) than to a genital infection (see below). About 7 percent of patients with PID reported symptoms of proctitis (i.e., frequent stools and/or passage of mucus) (Table 49-4). Chills were infrequent, whereas dyspareunia was a common complaint.[46]

Pain or discomfort in the right upper abdominal quadrant as symptoms of a possible concomitant perihepatitis were spontaneously reported by 5 percent in series of patients with PID.[3,29,30] This is important, because in some cases of PID, this is the dominating symptom and might mislead the examining clinician to direct examination toward cholecystitis or pleuritis instead of the correct diagnosis of a genital infection (see Chap. 51).

It is noteworthy that the symptoms given in Table 49-4 were equally often reported by patients who had normal laparoscopic findings and were thus considered to have lower genital infection only. In view of recent data, some of them might have had an endometritis. As a consequence, the symptoms given by the patients give little information as to the presence or absence of salpingitis.

## OBJECTIVE FINDINGS

### Clinical

A rectal temperature of more than 38°C was recorded in one-third of the laparoscopically verified cases of salpingitis in Lund.[46] Another 8 percent reported a transient febrile episode before consulting. Febrile illness (i.e., rectal temperature > 38.0°C) was more common in patients with gonorrhea-associated salpingitis and in severe polymicrobial disease than in the generally more benign chlamydial infections (Table 49-3). Of women with no salpingitis at laparoscopy, 20 percent had fever at admittance (Table 49-4).

Palpable adnexal swellings were found in half (Table 49-4) of the patients with acute salpingitis. The frequency of this sign was correlated with the severity of laparoscopic signs of inflammation. However, adnexal swelling was reported by experienced examiners before laparoscopy in one-fourth of the cases with normal findings at laparoscopy, indicating the low predictive value of this finding on pelvic examination in patients with pelvic pain.

Women who have an ascending infection in the genital tract should have objective signs of an infection in the lower genital tract. In all laparoscopically verified cases of salpingitis in the Swedish studies,[46,102,116] microscopic examination of a wet mount of the vaginal contents revealed a marked increase in the number of inflammatory cells; i.e., inflammatory cells outnumbered all other cellular elements in the smear. In no instance of PID was the smear similar to that of healthy women (i.e., few or no leukocytes, dominance of gram-positive rod flora, "clean" vaginal epithelial cells, and a pH below 4.5). The presence of increased numbers of inflammatory cells in vaginal fluid was used as an inclusion criterion in many of these studies. Subsequent experience has confirmed that a normal wet mount examination of vaginal contents in women with acute pelvic pain provides strong evidence against PID, although exceptions occur.

### Laboratory tests

The results of commonly used laboratory tests in PID, as found in laparoscopically verified cases of salpingitis, are summarized in Table 49-4.

The number of white blood cells (WBC) in peripheral blood exceeded 10,000/ml blood in just under two-thirds of patients with salpingitis, but also in one-third of women with no signs of salpingitis at laparoscopy (Table 49-4).[46] An erythrocyte sedimentation rate (ESR) of ≥ 15 mm/h at admission was seen in 75 percent of patients with salpingitis, but also in half of those with no evidence of salpingitis at laparoscopy (Table 49-4). In patients with salpingitis the presence and degree of an elevated ESR, and elevation of the WBC count, correlated with the severity of the inflammatory reactions as seen at laparoscopy.[46]

Antichymotrypsin, orosomucoid, and/or C-reactive protein were increased in serum in 80 percent of the cases of salpingitis, but also in one out of four women with no laparoscopic evidence of salpingitis.[46] With salpingitis, the concentration of orosomucoid was increased more often than that of antichymotrypsin, but orosomucoid was elevated also in 12 percent of women without laparoscopic evidence of salpingitis. The concentration of antichymotrypsin was normal in such cases, but also in half of the patients with salpingitis.[46]

All the laboratory tests described above are nonspecific and were found to discriminate poorly between cases with laparoscopically mild salpingitis and those with genital infection not involving the tubes.[46] In some patients of the latter category, elevated WBC, ESR, and/or acute-phase reactant proteins might have been caused by endometritis or parametritis (which were not studied).

Isoamylases specific for the genital tract are produced by epithelial cells in the cervix and the fallopian tubes.[154] They are also demonstrable in peritoneal fluid collected from the cul-de-sac. During electrophoresis, the specific genital isoamylases move faster toward the anode than pancreatic and salivary isoamylases. The activities of the genital isoamylases in the peritoneal fluid are high in healthy women but are diminished or absent in tubal infections (and in pregnancy).[154] Specific genital isoamylases were absent or decreased in peritoneal fluid in 90 percent of cases of acute salpingitis, 7 percent of women with no genital infection, and 22 percent of women judged as having lower genital infection only.[154] Of all the laboratory tests used, this was found to be the most specific for salpingitis.[46]

Weström[46] analyzed the presence of inflammatory cells in peritoneal fluid obtained at laparoscopy. In 12 patients with acute salpingitis, the range of WBC per ml of peritoneal fluid was 3.1 to $3.7 \times 10^3$, and in 36 women with no genital infection the range was 0.3 to $1.3 \times 10^2$. Paavonen et al.[155] found "an inflammatory cell pattern" in peritoneal fluid in 10 out of 15 patients with PID. Peritoneal fluid was successfully obtained by cul-de-sac puncture in 80 percent of the cases. However, admixture of peripheral blood might be a problem, and the presence of WBC in peritoneal fluid does not discriminate between PID and inflammatory reactions of other organs in the peritoneal cavity.

As discussed below, attempts have been made at correlating the presence of histological evidence of endometritis with laparoscopic evidence of salpingitis.[65,69,155,156] An endometrial biopsy can be obtained as an office procedure. However, in patients with suspected PID, antibiotic treatment should be instituted after such a procedure.

## DIAGNOSIS

### Clinical and common laboratory tests

No symptom or sign is pathognomonic for PID. Because a lower genital infection precedes most, if not all, cases of PID, recognition of such an infection in a woman with pelvic pain should increase the predictive value of a clinical diagnosis of PID. This is most easily done using direct microscopy of a wet mount of the vaginal contents (see above). Examination of cervical mucus for the presence of an increased number of polymorphonuclear leucocytes (e.g., $\geq$ 30 per oil immersion field) also has been advocated as a method for establishing the presence of mucopurulent cervicitis caused by *N. gonorrhoeae* or *C. trachomatis*.[78] (See also Chap. 46.) If low abdominal pain, objective signs of a lower genital infection, and increased (motion) tenderness at a pelvic examination were used as minimum criteria of a provisional clinical diagnosis of PID, laparoscopy revealed salpingitis in 6 out of 10 such patients (Table 49-2).[36] The probability of salpingitis thereafter increased with additional symptoms and signs of disease (Table 49-2). The clinical picture of "classic" PID (low abdominal pain, pelvic tenderness, adnexal mass, fever, and elevated ESR) was found in only 16 percent of women with salpingitis. In cases with few symptoms and signs of disease, the extent to which the different levels of the genital tract were involved in the infectious process was virtually impossible to determine using only clinical criteria. In this respect, the commonly used nonspecific laboratory tests (ESR, WBC, acute-phase reactants) also gave little guidance.[46] It is possible that some of the women in this series[46] who lacked laparoscopic evidence of salpingitis actually had endometritis and may therefore have had PID. However, from the prognostic standpoint, infections of the fallopian tubes are more important than endometritis, and none of the symptoms and signs listed in Table 49-4 were useful in differentiating patients with mild or moderately severe salpingitis from those without salpingitis.

"Mixed models" of different symptoms, signs, and laboratory abnormalities have been proposed for the diagnosis of salpingitis.[153] Theoretically, with such models, the proportion of women who would need laparoscopy for verification of a diagnosis of salpingitis might be reduced by half.[153]

### Invasive techniques

**Cul-de-sac Puncture.** For the diagnosis of acute salpingitis, analyses of the genital isoamylases had a sensitivity of 85 percent and a specificity of 70 percent.[154] Corresponding figures for detecting elevated concentrations of WBC in peritoneal fluid, as presented above, suggest higher specificity. However, only small numbers of patients were studied, and specimens could not be obtained from at least 20 percent.

**Endometrial Biopsies.** Among women with clinically suspected PID, histopathological evidence of endometritis has been identified in approximately 90 percent of those with, and in from 10 to 33 percent of those without laparoscopic signs of salpingitis.[155,156]

**Laparoscopy.** This method has become "the gold standard" for diagnosis of acute salpingitis.[18] In clinical research on PID it is indispensable. For routine clinical diagnostic work, the expenses and risks of the procedure must be considered.[157] The risk of making differential diagnostic errors, of missing a correct diagnosis of salpingitis in cases presenting with few symptoms or signs, or of making an erroneous diagnosis of salpingitis in cases with only a lower genital infection and hence causing unnecessary alarm in the patient—all argue for liberal use of laparoscopy. In women in whom the differential diagnostic problems include salpingitis, appendicitis, or ectopic pregnancy, we feel laparoscopy is mandatory.

In the series of diagnostic laparoscopies from Lund, Sweden, laparoscopy has been used in over 3000 instances, with no mortality. Serious perioperative complication necessitated a laparotomy in three patients, all of whom had uneventful recoveries with no sequela. Minor complications such as bleeding from the laparoscopy wound and transient fall in blood pressure were seen in about 2 percent of the cases (Weström, unpublished data). In 1 percent, laparoscopy failed to provide a diagnosis because intra-abdominal adhesions were too extensive (Weström, op. cit.). Use of laparoscopy did not aggravate the infectious process.[18,46]

The differentiation between slight inflammatory changes in the tubes and normal conditions may be difficult for less experienced laparoscopists. Reddening and slight edema of the tubes can be seen at menstruation and in early pregnancy, but an inflammatory exudate is never seen under normal conditions and should always be sought and identified (eventually using pressure on the tubes) in doubtful cases. It has been argued that a fallopian tube with an early endosalpingitis might appear normal during laparoscopy. This is, however, uncommon, as evidenced by the fact that only 1 of 184 women who underwent laparoscopy because of assumed salpingitis, but were found to have normal tubes subsequently, developed acute salpingitis as revealed at a repeat laparoscopy.[46] Of these 184 women, 100 were followed to determine their fertility (see control group, below). None of the 100 became infertile because of tubal factors. It should be observed, however, that about half of these women were treated with antibiotics after laparoscopy.

The laparoscopic findings at different stages of salpingitis have been described above.

## Etiological diagnosis

**Culture.** To establish the microbial etiology of a tubal infection, specimens for microbiological studies should ideally be obtained from the tubal mucosa. This can be done during laparoscopy or laparotomy. At laparoscopy, various techniques have been used for safely obtaining specimens. These include swabbing the tubal mucosa with cotton-tipped sticks or brushes, aspiration of tubal contents into thin plastic catheters, puncture and aspiration of closed cavities and abscesses, as well as biopsy of the fimbriated ends of the fallopian tubes.[49,158] However, the sensitivities of such methods for obtaining specimens from the upper genital tract have not been compared.

Analyses of specimens obtained by culdocentesis or endometrial aspiration are less conclusive.[24,49,61–66,104,105] Culdocentesis carries a risk of contamination from the vagina and bowel, and is not reliable for the diagnosis of a tubal chlamydial infection.[24] Similarly, endometrial aspiration may be contaminated by organisms from the vagina or cervix.

Cultures from cervical specimens do not give conclusive information on the etiology of the *tubal* infection. Cervical cultures for STD agents should nevertheless be performed because the results of such cultures do help predict the etiology of endometrial and tubal infection, and should be used as guidance for contact tracing and treatment. Furthermore, isolation of *N. gonorrhoeae* or *C. trachomatis* from the cervix may increase the predictive value of a clinical diagnosis of PID (P. Wolner-Hanssen, unpublished data). Negative chlamydial cultures from the cervix have been reported in women with chlamydial PID as evidenced by positive endometrial and/or tubal cultures in some studies,[61,69] but this has been very uncommon in other studies.[65,78]

For the detection of etiological agents in endometrial, tubal, and cul-de-sac specimens, direct antigen detection[65,66,108] or DNA probes[159] might be used along with culture. In this respect, direct antigen detection in endometrial specimens obtained as an outpatient procedure seems most promising. Thus, Kiviat et al.[65] found the use of fluorescein-conjugated antibody stain to be more sensitive than culture for the detection of *C. trachomatis* in endometrial and tubal specimens in PID. Extended studies in this field will probably clarify many obscurities concerning the etiology of upper genital tract infections in PID.

**Serology.** Antibody determinations on single serum specimens give little information on the etiology of an upper genital tract infection.[24,160] As in other infectious diseases, analyses of serial serum samples are most useful. However, even significant change in the titers of serum IgM and/or IgG antibodies may not be indicative of the etiology of PID per se, because cervicitis can also elicit an antibody response. In both chlamydial and gonococcal salpingitis, stationary or undetectable antibody titers might be found in PID patients with a positive tubal or endometrial culture for the organism in question.[24,73] The results of serial antibody determinations often come too late to be of any guidance for therapy.

## Ultrasonography

Ultrasonography has been of no use in mild or moderately severe cases of PID but can aid in the diagnosis of abscesses and provides an objective means of following abscess healing during conservative antibiotic treatment.

These limitations of ultrasonography so far also apply to computed x-ray tomography and nuclear magnetic resonance imaging. Further research is needed in the use of intravaginal ultrasonography for diagnosis of PID.

# CLINICAL SYNDROMES IN RELATION TO ETIOLOGICAL DIAGNOSIS

In a given case of PID, the clinical picture gives no definite etiological diagnosis, but certain observations might give a clue of the microbial etiology. In gonorrhea-associated PID, the typical patient is young and from the lower socioeconomic strata of society. She has a short duration of abdominal pain before consulting. More often than in chlamydia-associated cases, she is febrile and has palpable adnexal swelling. Although the clinical picture may be rather florid, her general condition is surprisingly good (Table 49-3).

Chlamydial salpingitis also is seen most often in young patients but may be clinically milder. Svensson et al.[102] found that these patients often consulted after a longer (7 to 9 days) period of abdominal pain, less often were febrile, but more often had an elevated ESR—often to 30 to 50 mm/h (Table 49-3). Clinical findings were not impressive. Laparoscopy often reveals more pronounced inflammation of the fallopian tubes than could be expected from the clinical picture (see Plate 17). Onset of abdominal pain during or immediately after menstrual bleeding points to gonococcal or chlamydial infection.

The patient with a mixed infection is generally somewhat older. Often it is not her first infection. In countries where IUDs are readily available she is often an IUD user. The clinical course is variable, but the onset may be acute, and some patients with polymicrobial or monomicrobial "endogenous" PID (especially those with tubo-ovarian abscess) are more prostrate than patients with gonococcal or chlamydial infection. Palpable adnexal swellings, febrile illness, and peripheral blood leucocytosis are common.

# DIFFERENTIAL DIAGNOSIS

In women with low abdominal or pelvic pain and tenderness and objective signs of lower genital infection, the most common and difficult diagnostic problem is to determine whether infection involves the fallopian tubes. Among such patients, as mentioned above, symptoms, signs, and the laboratory tests discriminate poorly between those with and without salpingitis. From the point of view of treatment, differentiation between endometritis and salpingitis might be regarded as irrelevant, but from the point of view of fertility prognosis, it seems vital to distinguish between infections that involve the tubes and those which do not. Only laparoscopy seems to be reliable for this purpose.

**Table 49-5. Differential Diagnosis of Acute Salpingitis: Erroneous Clinical and Laparoscopic Diagnoses[18]**

| Clinical diagnosis salpingitis before laparoscopy | | Laparoscopic diagnosis salpingitis | |
|---|---|---|---|
| Laparoscopic diagnosis, % | | Clinical diagnosis before laparoscopy, % | |
| Acute salpingitis | 65.4 | Ovarian tumor | 22.0 |
| Normal findings | 22.6 | Acute appendicitis | 19.8 |
| Acute appendicitis | 2.9 | Ectopic pregnancy* | 17.6 |
| Pelvic endometriosis | 2.0 | "Chronic PID" | 11.0 |
| Corpus luteum bleeding | 1.5 | Acute peritonitis | 6.6 |
| Ectopic pregnancy* | 1.4 | Pelvic endometriosis | 5.5 |
| "Chronic PID" | 0.7 | Fibroids | 5.5 |
| Ovarian tumor | 0.9 | Unclear pelvic pain | 5.5 |
| Mesenteric lymphadenitis | 0.7 | Miscellaneous | 6.5 |
| Miscellaneous | 1.9 | | |
| | $N = 814$ | | $N = 91$ |

*Study performed 1960–1967 (see text).

In one large series,[18] 12 percent of women subjected to laparoscopy because of suspected salpingitis had other intrapelvic pathology. In laparoscopies performed because of a preoperative diagnosis other than PID, an infection of the fallopian tubes was sometimes found. The diagnostic findings from that study are summarized in Table 49-5.

For the immediate management of a case of suspected PID, two important differential diagnoses must be considered, acute appendicitis and ectopic pregnancy. Failures in these considerations might seriously endanger the patient. In acute appendicitis, the period of abdominal pain is generally shorter, symptoms from the gastrointestinal tract more prominent, and the patient more prostrate than in acute PID. A shift from initially diffuse abdominal pain to right lower quadrant pain is typical of appendicitis. The ESR is most often normal in acute appendicitis. Surgeons and gynecologists removing "typically inflamed" appendixes should be careful to visualize the adnexa and to cut open the removed appendix in order to differentiate between primary appendicitis and appendicitis secondary to a tubal infection (see Chap. 51). Diagnostic laparoscopy should be used liberally when the clinical differentiation between salpingitis and appendicitis is ambiguous.

During the past decade, the incidence of ectopic pregnancy has more than doubled in many countries.[40,161,162] It is now becoming a most important and common differential diagnostic problem in women in the fertile ages who have acute abdominal pain. In an early ectopic pregnancy, no menstrual period has been missed, and the commonly applied laboratory tests are normal. In an ectopic pregnancy, the woman who formerly menstruated regularly now often has metrorrhagia. However, metrorrhagia can also occur in PID, due to endometritis. In many instances, it is impossible to differentiate between an early ectopic pregnancy and early mild PID using only clinical criteria. *Before giving the patient a diagnosis of PID, it is in such instances mandatory to exclude pregnancy by using a sensitive pregnancy test (detecting at least 40 IU of chorionic gonadotropin per ml of urine or blood).* During the past few years at the Department of Gynecology in Lund, Sweden, ectopic pregnancy has been found more often than PID in young women presenting with acute abdominal pain and metrorrhagia (Weström L, unpublished data).

## TREATMENT

In women in the fertile ages, the ultimate objective of therapy should be to preserve fertility. Therefore, conservative treatment with rest and antibiotics should be the rule, surgery the exception.

## CONSERVATIVE TREATMENT

### General aspects

Women with severe infections and/or unclear diagnosis should be observed and treated in hospital until the diagnosis is established and the patient is afebrile. Although no significant difference with regard to future fertility has been proved between women treated in hospital and women treated as outpatients, it seems wise to limit outpatient treatment regimens to parous women with mild or moderately severe disease in whom good compliance with treatment at home can be expected. If treated with antibiotics as an outpatient, the woman should rest at home, avoid coitus, and obtain and record body temperature twice daily. Follow-up pelvic examinations and ESR determinations can be limited to once a week. We monitor the wet smears of the vaginal contents, and seek to eliminate evidence of lower genital inspection as well as signs of upper genital infection. With correct antibiotic treatment this usually takes at least 14 days.

*In all cases of PID, the patient's sexual partner(s) should be examined (including cultures for N. gonorrhoeae and tests for C. trachomatis) and treated if he or the patient was infected with either of these pathogens.*

If the woman is using an IUD, the device should be removed and appropriate contraceptive counseling given.

### Choice of antibiotics

In most cases, antimicrobial treatment has to be instituted before the microbial etiology has been established. In severely ill patients and those subjected to operative diagnosis and therapy, antibiotic treatment should be started intravenously. As to the initial choice of antibiotic regimen, two main lines of therapy can be outlined:

1. In young women with a *clinically mild or moderately severe* infection, the disease is most often associated with a sexually transmitted infection. Accordingly, the initial treatment should be selected to eradicate *N. gonorrhoeae, C. trachomatis,* and *M. hominis.* If these women are treated as outpatients, the following antibiotics are recommended: Cefoxitin 2.0 g IM along with probenecid 1.0 g by mouth *or* ceftriaxone 250 mg IM, *followed by* doxycycline 100 mg by mouth twice daily for 14 days.[1] In areas where penicillin-resistant strains are uncommon (e.g., $< 1$ percent of all isolates), amoxicillin 3.0 g by mouth plus probenecid 1.0 g by mouth could be substituted for cefoxitin-probenecid or ceftriaxone. Ceftriaxone could be continued on a once daily parenteral basis, either at home or in the office, although the benefits of repeated

doses of ceftriaxone over single dose treatment for ambulatory treatment of PID have yet to be compared. Doxycycline (or another tetracycline) should not be used as the sole drug for treatment of PID. In febrile cases with palpable adnexal swellings, hospitalization for parenteral therapy is clearly preferable. The sensitivity pattern of any gonococci isolated should be determined and the treatment changed if found not optimal.

2. *Clinically severe infections* (prostrate, febrile, palpable adnexal swelling), especially those necessitating surgery, are often caused by mixed anaerobic/facultative bacteria. In such cases intravenous treatment should be started immediately using one of the following regimens:[1] (a) Doxycycline 100 mg IV twice a day *plus* cefoxitin 2.0 g IV four times a day. IV treatment should be continued for at least 4 days followed by oral doxycycline 100 mg twice daily for a total course of 14 days of therapy. (b) Clindamycin 900 mg IV 3 times a day *plus* gentamicin or tobramycin 2.0 mg/kg body weight IV followed by 1.5 mg/kg IV 3 times a day in patients with normal renal function. IV treatment should be continued for at least 4 days, and if the patient improves, followed by clindamycin 450 mg by mouth 4 times daily to complete at least 14 days of therapy. This treatment regimen is probably not optimal with regard to *C. trachomatis* or *N. gonorrhoeae.*

If an IUD is present, it should be removed. In women with adnexal abscesses it might be wise to consider drainage if the patient does not respond to therapy within 24 h.

The results of cultures obtained from the lower and/or upper genital tract before start of treatment must be considered and might eventually guide a revision of the therapy.

## SURGERY

Operative procedures are indicated in life-threatening disease, in failure of conservative treatment, and in abscesses. They may also be considered in the somewhat older woman who does not want to maintain her fertility.

When operating, the surgeon should be as conservative as possible. Total pelvic "clean-outs" are rarely indicated. Even after severe disease treated with abscess drainage, pregnancy might follow.[163,164]

Diagnostic laparoscopy is contraindicated in patients for whom a laparotomy is clearly indicated.

## TREATMENT RESULTS

(See also Prognosis.) In the majority of cases, acute PID is clinically a self-limited disease with apparent recovery even if untreated.[60] However, before the advent of chemotherapy, repeated flare-ups of symptoms and signs of disease were common, indicating a chronic infection.[89,90] With correctly chosen antibiotic therapy of the patient and her partner, the current treatment results are good with respect to eradication of sexually transmitted pathogens from the cervix and clinical recovery. It has been shown that correct treatment together with evaluation and treatment of partner(s) significantly decreases the proportion of women who get repeated infections within 1 year after treatment.[44]

The only unequivocal proof of preserved reproductive *function* after PID is an intrauterine pregnancy. In women who had been treated between 1960 and 1974 with different antibiotic regimens, who had had only one bout of laparoscopically verified salpingitis, and who later exposed themselves to a chance of pregnancy, follow-up studies revealed postinfection tubal infertility in 10 to 13 percent, regardless of therapy.[165] However, note that the regimens used would not be chosen today in view of our current knowledge of the microbial etiology of PID.

The reasons why different antibiotic regimens gave roughly the same fertility prognosis might be not only that the antibiotics used were not optimal but also that the process of repair might cause later functional disturbances of the fallopian tubes. If so, this certainly emphasizes early institution of treatment, preferably before the infection has reached the fallopian tubes. In experimental infections in mice, it has been shown that the proportion of animals with postinfection tubal pathology was related to the delay until onset of therapy.[166]

## PROGNOSIS

## MORTALITY

The prognosis of acute PID *quo ad vitam* is good. In the preantibiotic era, Holtz in 1930[167] reported a mortality of 1.3 percent in a series of 1262 patients with PID. After the advent of chemotherapy, death from acute PID has been rare. In Sweden, six fatalities were reported in just over 100,000 episodes of PID in women under the age of 40 from 1970 through 1980. In the United States, the mortality rate for PID was 0.29 per 100,000 female population 15 to 44 years of age in 1979.[168] The most common cause of death in PID is rupture of a tubo-ovarian abscess with generalized peritonitis. In such instances, the mortality is still 6 to 8 percent.[169]

## LATE SEQUELAE

### General aspects

From the clinical point of view, the vast majority of women with acute PID recover completely, but some are left with postinfection damage to different structures of the reproductive system as described above. Such damage comprises the morphological basis for the late sequelae of acute PID, which include chronic pain due to adhesions, infertility, and increased risk of a tubal pregnancy due to tubal scarring. To this might be added an increased risk of repeated episodes of PID as discussed above.

Because many women postpone pregnancy and childbirth until long after the acute PID episode, impairment of their reproductive capability will not be revealed until years after the acute episode. In our series, over half of the women protected themselves against pregnancy for more than 3 years after acute PID.[21] A consequence of this is that follow-up studies on fertility after PID must be extended to 5 years—preferably more. In order to obtain information more rapidly on an eventual post-PID tubal damage, different methods have been applied for evaluating tubal patency. Thus, Bret and Legros in 1959[170] used tubal insufflation to demonstrate patent fallopian tubes in 20 out of 50 women treated for PID. Fifteen of those women eventually became pregnant. Hysterosalpingography has been used by a number of authors.[60,171,172] Patent fallopian tubes after PID were found in 38

Table 49-6. Pregnancy Rates after Acute Pelvic Inflammatory Disease

| Author(s) | Ref. | Year | No. of patients | Diagnosis | Antibiotic treatment | Follow-up time, years | Pregnancy rate, % Total | Pregnancy rate, % Corrected* |
|---|---|---|---|---|---|---|---|---|
| Holtz | 167 | 1930 | 804 | Clinical | No | Over 4 | 17 | 25 |
| Haffner | 176 | 1939 | 164 | Clinical | No | Over 4 | — | 42.2 |
| Bret and Legros | 170 | 1959 | 50 | Clinical | Yes | NG† | 30 | — |
| Hedberg and Spetz | 175 | 1958 | 324 | Clinical | Only in GC‡ | 2 | 30 | 70 |
| Sundén | 177 | 1959 | 52 | Visual | Yes | 3 | 58 | — |
| Viberg | 128 | 1964 | 108 | Clinical | Yes | NG† | — | 24 |
| | | | | | No | NG† | — | 16 |
| Falk | 60 | 1965 | 283 | Visual | Yes | 2.5 | — | 81 |
| Weström | 21 | 1975 | 415 | Visual | Yes | 9 | 64 | 79 |

*Patients who were voluntarily infertile or lost at follow-up are excluded.
†NG = not given.
‡Only women with gonorrhea-associated PID received antibiotic treatment.

to 87 percent of cases. In two small series, a second-look laparoscopy was used to evaluate tubal morphology after PID.[173,174] The results showed bilateral tubal occlusion in 2/13 and 2/64 women, respectively. In a few of the above series, these findings were correlated with later infertility/fertility.

Results of follow-up with respect to infertility/fertility in a number of studies are summarized in Table 49-6. In these studies diagnostic criteria for PID, proportion of women followed, treatment, and follow-up time varied.

The most extensive long-term follow-up after PID is the still ongoing study from Lund, Sweden.[21,37,165,178,179] A review of the results so far obtained is given below. The population analyzed comprised 1204 women between 15 and 34 years of age who were treated for one or more episodes of laparoscopically verified acute salpingitis between 1960 and 1979. None of the women had any known abnormality capable of impairing infertility at the time of their infection. In another 150 women, comparable with the patients in age, parity, and socioeconomic status, a laparoscopy for clinically suspected PID revealed entirely normal intrapelvic conditions. These women served as controls. All salpingitis cases and controls were followed until their first pregnancy. Those not becoming pregnant were followed until December 1984. Pregnancies were subdivided into intrauterine or ectopic. The women who did not become pregnant were divided into voluntarily infertile and involuntarily infertile. The latter category was further subdivided into women with proved post-salpingitis tubal occlusion, and women (couples) with other causes for infertility or incompletely examined couples.

The detailed results are given in Table 49-7 and in Fig. 49-5 and are discussed below.

## Chronic abdominal pain

Abdominal pain lasting longer than 6 months and causing the woman to seek medical advice was reported by 18.1 percent of women who had had salpingitis and by 5 percent of the controls. Similar figures were reported by Falk[60] in 1965. Chronic pelvic pain was more common in women who were infertile and was also correlated with the number of episodes of PID.[21,34] The most common pathologic finding in women with chronic pelvic pain was pelvic adhesions—a finding which has been documented also by others.[180,181] The pain in many of those women responded well to continuous treatment with progesterone or danazole, i.e., similar to the treatment of endometriosis.[34,46]

## Infertility

In the preantibiotic era, the rates of pregnancy after acute PID in women who were followed and who exposed themselves to a chance of pregnancy were 25 to 45 percent (Table 49-6). After the advent of chemotherapy, the corresponding figures have been 24 to 80 percent (Table 49-6).

In the series from Lund, 17.2 percent of the women with salpingitis and none of the controls who exposed themselves to a possible pregnancy were infertile because of tubal occlusion after one or more infections. After only one episode of salpingitis, 11.4 percent became infertile from post-salpingitis damage. The latter figure remained constant through the years of study and was irrespective of treatment given.[165,179]

The postinfection infertility rate was significantly lower (13.9 percent) in the age group 15 to 24 years than in women 24 to 34 years (25.7 percent) (Table 49-7).

Table 49-7. Infertility Due to Tubal Occlusion after Laparoscopically Verified Acute Salpingitis in 708 Patients and after Laparoscopy in 150 Control Subjects. All Patients and Controls Exposed Themselves to a Chance of Pregnancy and Either Conceived or Had a Diagnosis of Infertility and Tubal Occlusion[178]

| No. of episodes of PID | No. of women | Percent infertile due to tubal occlusion by age group: 15–24 years* | 25–34 years* | Total 15–34 years* |
|---|---|---|---|---|
| None (control subjects) | 150 | 0 | 0 | 0 |
| One, total | 484 | 9.4 | 19.2 | 11.4 |
| Mild disease | | 3.5† | 7.8† | 6.1† |
| Moderately severe disease | | 10.8† | 22.0† | 13.4† |
| Severe disease | | 27.3† | 40.0† | 30.0† |
| Two | 163 | 20.9 | 31.0 | 23.1 |
| Three or more | 61 | 51.6 | 60.0 | 54.3 |

*Age at time of first episode of PID.
†Percent of those in subgroup.

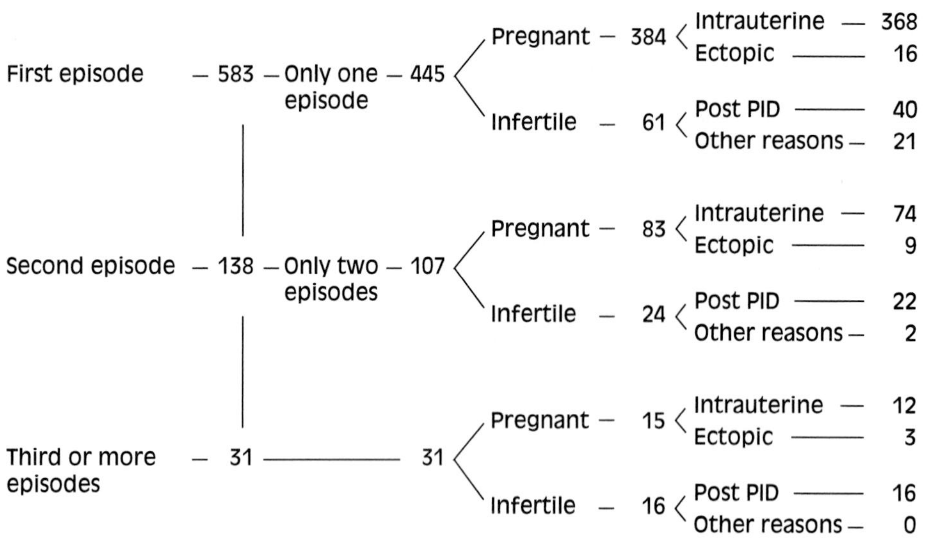


Fig. 49-5. Reproductive events after acute PID in 583 women, 15 to 24 years of age, with laparoscopically verified disease, who all exposed themselves to a chance of pregnancy (only first pregnancy after PID is included; voluntarily infertile women excluded).[178]

The infertility rate increased significantly with the number of episodes of salpingitis in one and the same woman (Table 49-7). With each new bout of PID the infertility rate roughly doubled. In women who had had only one episode of salpingitis, the infertility rate increased with the severity of the inflammatory changes seen at laparoscopy (Table 49-7). Among the 150 controls included in the study, none had infertility because of a tubal occlusion.

In women younger than 25 years of age, those who had had gonorrhea-associated salpingitis had significantly better fertility prognosis than those who had had nongonococcal salpingitis.[21,178] On the other hand, in a later study, Svensson et al.[182] found that for women who experienced a single episode of salpingitis, there was no difference in infertility rates following gonorrhea-associated salpingitis, chlamydia-associated salpingitis, both gonorrhea- and chlamydia-associated salpingitis, and neither gonorrhea- nor chlamydia-associated salpingitis. Follow-ups of larger numbers of patients are clearly needed to confirm these impressions.

In seroepidemiological studies of infertile and fertile women attempts have been made to correlate tubal infertility with the presence of serum antibody to *C. trachomatis*,[67,105,182–192] *N. gonorrhoeae*,[42,190] *M. hominis*,[78,190,193,194] and *M. genitalium*.[193] The combined results suggest a significant role of chlamydia and gonococci,[42,67,105,183–193] a possible role of *M. hominis*,[190,193] and no significant role of *M. genitalium*[193] in tubal infertility.

As mentioned, in the Lund series pill users more often had a laparoscopically mild salpingitis than noncontraceptors and users of other methods. A logical conclusion should be that the risk of infertility should be less in women who used contraceptive pills at the time of their disease episode. In an ongoing comprehensive computer analysis of the material from Sweden,[179] preliminary estimates of the relative risks of infertility related to use of contraceptives in a ⅛ random sample of women who had had only one infection were: noncontraceptors 1.0, barrier users 0.79, pill users 0.53, and IUD users 0.99. However, in this analysis, age was not accounted for.

In women who experienced one episode of severe PID, we found fertility preserved in 60 percent. Similarly, fertility was preserved in 37 (62.7 percent) of 59 women treated by colpotomy for pelvic abscess as reported by Rivlin.[163] Thus, even in severe disease, fertility is preserved in over half of the women. This definitely argues against radical surgery in such cases.

## Ectopic (tubal) pregnancy

In any population the number of ectopic pregnancies is related to the prevalence of fertile women exposed to the chance of pregnancy and to the distribution of risk factors for ectopic pregnancy among such women. Commonly accepted risk factors include increased age, postinfection and postoperative tubal damage, other tubal pathology, and use of an IUD.

From 1937 through the mid-fifties, the ratios of ectopic to intrauterine pregnancies have been rather constant.[40] After that, significant increases have been reported from almost all countries in the industrial Western Hemisphere.[40,161,162,195] The reasons for this increase have been disputed. Increased use of IUDs, increased age of women at time of pregnancy, increasingly conservative surgical treatment of ectopic pregnancy—leaving the tube intact and thus permitting a recurrence, and impact of the PID epidemic have all been discussed as possible reasons. However, because of the use of improved diagnostic methods (sensitive pregnancy tests, ultrasonography, laparoscopy) it is likely that a large proportion of otherwise self-limiting or self-healing ectopic pregnancies are revealed today as compared with earlier periods. This must be remembered when analyzing the increase.

In prospective studies of the ratio of ectopic to intrauterine pregnancies after PID, Holtz in 1930 found 1:200[167]; Haffner in 1939, 1:169[176]; and Krohn et al. in 1952, 1:129.[196] In our follow-up studies, the ratio for the *first* pregnancy after salpingitis was 1:16, in *all* pregnancies after salpingitis 1:24, and in the control women 1:147.[21]

Based on a comprehensive survey of large series of retrospective studies on the ratios of ectopic to intrauterine pregnancies, Urquhart[40] calculated an index of 0.27 ectopic pregnancies per 100 woman-years of noncontraception among women who had never had PID and an index of 2.0 for women in the post-PID state. In a recent study, the corresponding risks for 20- to 29-year-old women was calculated to be 0.3 and 2.0, respectively.[195] Thus, women in the post-PID state have a seven- to tenfold increased risk for ectopic pregnancy as compared with women who have never had the disease.

In two studies[197,198] serum antibody to *C. trachomatis* was found to be significantly more prevalent and to have significantly higher GMT in women operated because of ectopic pregnancy than in age-matched women with intrauterine pregnancy.

## IMPACT OF THE POST-PID STATE ON FEMALE FECUNDITY

### Clinically overt disease

Estimates of the current "crude infertility rate" in Europe and the United States have shown that by the end of 1 year unprotected sexual intercourse, 10 to 15 percent of married or cohabitating couples will fail to conceive.[199]

In our follow-up of infertility after salpingitis,[178] we found a rate of infertility *not* attributable to salpingitis of about 4 percent in both patients and controls.

If infertility and ectopic pregnancy as sequelae to the PID epidemic were of significance, increases in both these events should be demonstrable during the past decades. As mentioned, ectopic pregnancy has increased both numerically and in proportion to intrauterine pregnancy during the past 20 years. In the United States, several surveys have shown an increase in nonsurgical female sterility since 1965.[200–202] By and large, such infertility has doubled (see also Chap. 63). Using a multivariate analysis, Mosher and Aral in 1985[202] reported that "available evidence shows a strong association between STD, PID, and infertility trends." They calculated that STD, operating through PID, accounted for one-half to one-third of the infertility increase.

A flowchart is given in Fig. 49–5 of the reproductive events after acute PID in a cohort of 583 women, 15 to 24 years of age, who were seeking pregnancy after their first episode of laparoscopically verified PID.[178] Among women seeking pregnancy who had experienced one episode of acute PID, 12.6 percent in the age group 15 to 24 years, and 25 percent in the age group 25 to 34 years, were either infertile from their infection or had had an ectopic pregnancy.

### "Silent" PID

The figures given above were based on clinically proved cases of PID. During the past few years, we have increasing evidence of an epidemic of silent, asymptomatic tubal infections running parallel to the clinically overt cases (see Chap. 50).

Although such evidence strongly indicates the existence of an epidemic of "silent" infertility-producing PID, we have so far little information of the magnitude of this problem or of the etiology and pathophysiology of such infections. Further studies are certainly indicated in this field.

## PROPHYLAXIS AND FUTURE ASPECTS

As is evident from the above, acute PID is most often a complication of a sexually transmitted infection. Apart from exposure to STDs, other risk factors as well as protective factors have been identified. If an infection has been established in the upper genital tract, infertility and subfertility seem to be inevitable in a proportion of cases, even with the currently used treatment regimens.[165]

The strategy for preventing the late sequelae of PID therefore must follow two main lines: (1) control of PID-producing sexually transmitted infections, and (2) prevention of lower genital infection from ascending to the upper genital tract.

Public and professional education are prerequisites for achievement of both these goals. Education must be given to persons of all categories in medicine as well as to paramedical and social professions (including politicians). Public education should be concentrated on risk-exposed persons, started early in life, and repeated.

Strategies for the control of STD in general are given in the final section (X) of this book. As to PID specifically, these strategies must focus mainly on chlamydia and gonorrhea—especially the former. Examinations for chlamydial infection should be performed frequently in all high-risk persons of both sexes regardless of symptoms or findings.[203] The use of condoms should be encouraged. Sexual partners of women with PID should be examined and treated; partners of young women with PID should be considered for treatment with a tetracycline, even if the woman is not found to have gonococcal or chlamydial infection.

Women at risk for gonococcal or chlamydial infection should be screened for cervical infection before operative or diagnostic procedures involving penetration of the cervical mucus barrier, in order to prevent introduction of these organisms into the endometrium. Hormonal contraception should be recommended to young nulliparous women who may be at risk for chlamydial infection if there is no contraindication for oral contraceptives.

### Future aspects

During the past decade in Sweden, "classical" PID has decreased, and clinically and laparoscopically mild cases represent a higher proportion of those cases that are now recognized.[44] These changes may reflect an overall decrease of upper genital tract infections in women, but also perhaps a decline in clinically overt gonococcal PID, thus permitting a proportional increase of clinically more silent chlamydial PID. It remains to be seen whether those changes in Sweden predict changes that will also occur in other settings.

In the first edition of this book, the need was noted for development of simple, safe, and specific methods both for diagnosis of PID per se, and for establishing the etiology of PID. In these respects, the recently published studies on use of endometrial biopsy for diagnosis of PID as well as of use of antigen detection for diagnosis of chlamydial infection, and DNA probes for *M. genitalium* are promising. During the past few years, a number of practical animal models have been utilized for the studies on the pathophysiology,[204–207] immunology,[207] and sequelae[166,208–209] of PID in experimental systems. However, despite an ever-increasing armamentarium of antibiotics, we do not yet know the optimal treatment of PID with respect to preservation of fertility. Research using second-look laparoscopy might expedite collection of information, complementing the only functional test currently available—an intrauterine pregnancy.

## References


1 Centers for Disease Control: Antibiotic-resistant strains of *Neisseria gonorrhoeae*. Policy guidelines for detection, management, and control. *MMWR* 36:55, 1987.

2 Mårdh P-A, Wölner-Hanssen P: Periappendicitis and chlamydial salpingitis. *Surg Gynecol Obstet* 160:304, 1985.

3 Wölner-Hanssen P, Mårdh P-A: Perihepatitis and chlamydial salpingitis. *Lancet* i:901, 1980.

4 Gatt D, Jantet G: Perisplenitis and perinephritis in the Fitz-Hugh-Curtis syndrome. *Br J Surg* 74:110, 1987.
5 Diepgen P: Die Frauenheilkunde der Alten Welt, in *Handbuch der Gynäkologie*, W Stoeckel (ed). München, Verlag von JF Bergman, 1937, vol XII, part 1, p 97.
6 Nocard E, Roux ER: Le microbe de la péripneumonie. *Ann Inst Pasteur* 12:240, 1898.
7 Dienes L, Edsall G: Observations on the L-organism of Klineberger. *Proc Soc Exp Biol Med* 36:740, 1937.
8 Mårdh P-A, Weström L: Tubal and cervical cultures in acute salpingitis with special reference to *Mycoplasma hominis* and T-strain mycoplasmas. *Br J Vener Dis* 46:179, 1970.
9 Mårdh P-A, Weström L: Antibodies to *Mycoplasma hominis* in patients with genital infections and in healthy controls. *Br J Vener Dis* 46:390, 1970.
10 Halberstaedter L, von Prowazek S: Zur Ätiologie des Trachoms. *Dtsch Med Wochenschr* 33:1285, 1907.
11 Lindner K: Gonoblenorrhöe, Einschlussblenorrhöe, und Trachom. *Graefes Arch Ophthalmol* 78:345, 1911.
12 Tang FF et al: Studies on the etiology of trachoma with special reference to isolation of the virus in chick embryo. *Chin Med* 75: 429, 1957.
13 Gordon FB, Quan AL: Isolation of the trachoma agent in cell culture. *Proc Soc Exp Biol Med* 118:354, 1965.
14 Ripa KT, Mårdh P-A: Cultivation of *Chlamydia trachomatis* in cyclo-heximide-treated McCoy cells. *J Clin Microbiol* 6:388, 1977.
15 Eilard T et al: Isolation of Chlamydia in acute salpingitis. *Scand J Infect Dis* (suppl) 9:82, 1976.
16 Mårdh P-A et al: *Chlamydia trachomatis* as an etiological agent in acute salpingitis, in *Nongonococcal Urethritis and Related Infections*, D Hobson, KK Holmes (eds). Washington, DC, American Society for Microbiology, 1977, p 77.
17 Wittman I: The history of peritoneoscopy, in *Peritoneoscopy*, I Wittman (ed). Budapest, Akadémiai Kiadó. Hungarian Academy of Sciences, 1966, vol I, p 3.
18 Jacobson L, Weström L: Objectivized diagnosis of acute pelvic inflammatory disease. *Am J Obstet Gynecol* 105:1088, 1969.
19 Falk HC: Interpretation of the pathogenesis of pelvic infections as determined by cornual resection. *Am J Obstet Gynecol* 52:66, 1946.
20 Ahlström E: Die Behandlung nicht tuberkulöser Adnexentzündungen. *Acta Obstet Gynecol Scand* 5:765, 1919.
21 Weström L: Effect of acute pelvic inflammatory disease on fertility. *Am J Obstet Gynecol* 121:707, 1975.
22 Mårdh P-A et al: *Chlamydia trachomatis* infection in patients with acute salpingitis. *N Engl J Med* 296:1377, 1977.
23 Treharne J et al: Antibodies to *Chlamydia trachomatis* in acute salpingitis. *Br J Vener Dis* 55:26, 1979.
24 Mårdh P-A: An overview of infectious agents in salpingitis, their biology, and recent advances in methods of detection. *Am J Obstet Gynecol* 138:933, 1980.
25 Paavonen J: *Chlamydia trachomatis* in acute salpingitis. *Am J Obstet Gynecol* 138:957, 1980.
26 Holmes KK et al: Salpingitis; Overview of etiology and epidemiology. *Am J Obstet Gynecol* 138:893, 1980.
27 Bowie WR, Jones H: Acute PID in outpatients: Association with *Chlamydia trachomatis* and *Neisseria gonorrhoeae*. *Ann Intern Med* 95:685, 1981.
28 Möller BR et al: Infection with *Chlamydia trachomatis*, *Mycoplasma hominis*, and *Neisseria gonorrhoeae* in patients with acute pelvic inflammatory disease. *Sex Transm Dis* 8:198, 1981.
29 Gjönnaess H et al: Pelvic inflammatory disease; Etiologic studies with emphasis on chlamydial infection. *Obstet Gynecol* 59:550, 1982.
30 Weström L, Mårdh P-A: Chlamydial salpingitis. *Br Med Bull* 39:145, 1983.
31 Magnússon SS et al: Lower genital tract infection with *Chlamydia trachomatis* and *Neisseria gonorrhoeae* in Icelandic women with salpingitis. *Am J Obstet Gynecol* 155:602, 1986.
32 Curran JW: Economic consequences of pelvic inflammatory disease in the United States. *Am J Obstet Gynecol* 138:484, 1980.
33 Wright NH, Laemmle P: Acute pelvic inflammatory disease in an indigent population. *Am J Obstet Gynecol* 101:779, 1968.
34 Weström L, Mårdh P-A: Pelvic inflammatory disease; Epidemiology, diagnosis, clinical manifestations, and sequela, in *International Perspectives on Neglected Sexually Transmitted Disease: Impact on Venerology, Infertility, and Maternal and Child Health*, KK Holmes, P-A Mårdh (eds). New York, McGraw-Hill, 1983, p 235.
35 Weström L et al: Chlamydial and gonococcal infection in a defined population of women. *Scand J Infect Dis* 32:157, 1982.
36 WHO Scientific Group: Nongonococcal urethritis and other selected sexually transmitted diseases of public health importance. *WHO Tech Rep Ser* 660:95, 1981.
37 Weström L: Incidence, prevalence, and trends of acute pelvic inflammatory disease and its consequences in industrialized countries. *Am J Obstet Gynecol* 138:880, 1980.
38 Adler MW: Trends for gonorrhea and pelvic inflammatory disease in England and Wales and for gonorrhea in a defined population. *Am J Obstet Gynecol* 138:901, 1980.
39 Eschenbach D et al: Pathogenesis of acute pelvic inflammatory disease: Role of contraception and other risk factors. *Am J Obstet Gynecol* 128:838, 1977.
40 Urquhart J: Effect of the venereal disease epidemic on the incidence of ectopic pregnancy—Implications for the evaluation of contraceptives. *Contraception* 19:151, 1979.
41 Muir DG, Belsy MA: Pelvic inflammatory disease and its consequences in the developing world. *Am J Obstet Gynecol* 138:913, 1980.
42 Mabey DC et al: Tubal infertility in the Gambia, chlamydial and gonococcal serology in women with tubal obstruction compared with pregnant controls. *Bull WHO* 63:1107, 1985.
43 Gray R, Campbell O: Epidemiological trends of pelvic inflammatory disease in contraceptive use, in *Intrauterine Contraception. Advances and Future Prospects*, GI Zatuchni et al (eds). Philadelphia, Harper & Row, 1985, p 398.
44 Weström L: Decrease in incidence of women treated in hospital for acute salpingitis in Sweden. *Genitourin Med* 64:59, 1987.
45 Washington AE et al: Hospitalization for PID. Epidemiology and trends in the U.S. 1975–81. *JAMA* 251:25, 1984.
46 Weström L: *Diagnosis, Aetiology, and Prognosis of Acute Salpingitis* (Thesis). Lund, Sweden, Studentlitteratur, 1976.
47 Weström L, Mårdh P-A: Acute salpingitis—Aspects on aetiology, diagnosis and prognosis, in *Genital Infections and Their Complications*, D Danielsson et al (eds). Stockholm, Almqvist & Wiksell, 1975, p 157.
48 Sweet RL et al: Failure of beta-lactam antibiotics to eradicate *Chlamydia trachomatis* in the endometrium despite apparent clinical cure of acute salpingitis. *JAMA* 250:2641, 1983.
49 Sweet RL et al: Microbiology and pathogenesis of acute salpingitis as determined by laparoscopy. What is the appropriate site to sample? *Am J Obstet Gynecol* 138:985, 1980.
50 Runge H: Gonorrhoe der Weiblichen Geschlechtsorgane, in *Biologie und Pathologie des Weibes*, L Seitz, A Amreich (eds). Berlin, Urban & Schwartzenberg, 1953, vol V, p 413.
51 McGee Z et al: Pathogenic mechanisms of *Neisseria gonorrhoeae*: Observations on damage to human fallopian tubes in organ culture by gonococci of colony type 1 or 4. *J Infect Dis* 143:413, 1981.
52 Mårdh P-A et al: Studies on ciliated epithelia of the human genital tract. III. Mucociliary wave pattern in organ cultures of human Fallopian tubes challenged with *Neisseria gonorrhoeae* and gonococcal endotoxin. *Br J Vener Dis* 55:256, 1979.
53 Draper DL et al: Auxotypes and antibiotic susceptibilities of *Neisseria gonorrhoeae* from women with acute salpingitis. *Sex Transm Dis* 8:43, 1981.
54 Draper DL et al: Comparison of virulence markers of peritoneal and fallopian tube isolates with cervical *Neisseria gonorrhoeae* isolates from women with acute salpingitis. *Infect Immunol* 27:882, 1980.

55 Buchanan TM et al: Gonococcal salpingitis less likely to recur with *Neisseria gonorrhoeae* of the same principal outer membrane protein antigenic type. *Am J Obstet Gynecol* 138:978, 1980.
56 Eschenbach D et al: Polymicrobial etiology of acute pelvic inflammatory disease. *N Engl J Med* 293:166, 1975.
57 Sweet RL et al: Etiology of acute salpingitis: Influence of episode number and duration of symptoms. *Obstet Gynecol* 58:62, 1981.
58 Curtis AH: Bacteriology and pathology of fallopian tubes removed at operation. *Surg Gynecol Obstet* 36:621, 1921.
59 Hundley JM et al: Bacteriological studies in salpingitis with special reference to gonococcal viability. *Am J Obstet Gynecol* 60:977, 1950.
60 Falk V: Treatment of acute non-tuberculous salpingitis with antibiotics alone and in combination with glucocorticoids. *Acta Obstet Gynecol Scand* 44(suppl 6), 1965.
61 Mårdh P-A et al: Endometritis caused by *Chlamydia trachomatis*. *Br J Vener Dis* 57:191, 1981.
62 Winkler B et al: Chlamydial endometritis. A histological and immunohistochemical analysis. *Am J Surg Pathol* 8:771, 1984.
63 Paavonen J et al: Prevalence and manifestations of endometritis among women with cervicitis. *Am J Obstet Gynecol* 152:275, 1986.
64 Jones RB et al: Recovery of *Chlamydia trachomatis* from the endometrium of women at risk for chlamydial infection. *Am J Obstet Gynecol* 155:35, 1986.
65 Kiviat NB et al: Localization of *Chlamydia trachomatis* infection by direct immunofluorescence and culture. *Am J Obstet Gynecol* 154: 865, 1986.
66 Wasserheit JN et al: Microbial causes of proven PID and efficacy of Clindamycin and Tobramycin. *Ann Intern Med* 104:187, 1986.
67 Henry-Suchet J et al: Microbiology specimens obtained by laparoscopy from controls and from patients with pelvic inflammatory disease infertility with tubal obstruction. *Am J Obstet Gynecol* 138: 1022, 1980.
68 Ripa KT et al: *Chlamydia trachomatis* infection in patients with laparoscopically verified acute salpingitis. Results of isolation and antibody determinations. *Am J Obstet Gynecol* 138:960, 1980.
69 Paavonen J et al: Microbiological and histological findings in acute pelvic inflammatory disease. *Br J Obstet Gynaecol* 94:454, 1987.
70 Möller RB et al: Experimental infection of the genital tract provoked by *Chlamydia trachomatis* and *Mycoplasma hominis* in grivet monkeys. *Am J Obstet Gynecol* 138:990, 1980.
71 Patton D et al: Experimental salpingitis in rabbits provoked by *Chlamydia trachomatis*. *Fertil Steril* 37:691, 1982.
72 Skaug K et al: Chlamydial serum IgG antibodies in patients with acute salpingitis by an enzyme linked immunoassay. *Acta Pathol Microbiol Scand* (Sec C) 90:67, 1982.
73 Mårdh P-A et al: Antibodies to *Chlamydia trachomatis, Mycoplasma hominis,* and *Neisseria gonorrhoeae* in sera from patients with acute salpingitis. *Br J Vener Dis* 57:125, 1981.
74 Henry-Suchet J et al: Microbiologic study of chronic inflammation associated with tubal factor sterility: Role of *Chlamydia trachomatis*. *Fertil Steril* 47:274, 1987.
75 Kristensen GB et al: Infection with *Neisseria gonorrhoeae* and *Chlamydia trachomatis* in women with acute salpingitis. *Genitourin Med* 61:179, 1985.
76 Judson FN: Assessing the number of genital chlamydial infections in the U.S. *J Reprod Med* 30:269, 1985.
77 Sweet R et al: The occurrence of chlamydial and gonococcal salpingitis during the menstrual cycle. *JAMA* 255:2062, 1986.
78 Wølner-Hanssen P, et al: Outpatient treatment of pelvic inflammatory disease with cefoxitin and doxycycline. *Obstet Gynecol* 71:595, 1988.
79 Möller RB: *Chlamydia and Mycoplasmas in Pelvic Inflammatory Disease* (Thesis), Odense, Denmark, FADL's Forlag, 1985.
80 Miettinen A et al: Epidemiologic and clinical characteristics of pelvic inflammatory disease associated with *Mycoplasma hominis, Chlamydia trachomatis,* and *Neisseria gonorrhoeae*. *Sex Transm Dis* 13: 24, 1986.
81 Lind K et al: Importance of *Mycoplasma hominis* in acute salpingitis assessed by culture and serologic tests. *Genitourin Med* 61:185, 1985.
82 Miettinen A et al: Enzyme immunoassay for serum antibody to *Mycoplasma hominis* in women with acute PID. *Sex Transm Dis* 10: 276, 1983.
83 Möller BR et al: Experimental infection of the genital tract of female grivet monkeys by *Mycoplasma hominis*. *Infect Immunol* 20:248, 1978.
84 Mårdh P-A et al: Studies on ciliated epithelia of the human genital tract. I. Swelling of the cilia of fallopian tube epithelium in organ cultures infected with *Mycoplasma hominis*. *Br J Vener Dis* 52:52, 1976.
85 Möller BR et al: Serological evidence implicating *Mycoplasma genitalium* in pelvic inflammatory disease. *Lancet* i:1102, 1984.
86 Brihmer C et al: Salpingitis; aspects on diagnosis and etiology: A 4 year study from a Swedish hospital. *Eur J Obstet Gynecol Reprod Biol* 3:211, 1987.
87 Mårdh P-A, Weström L: T-mycoplasmas in the genital tract of the female. *Acta Pathol Microbiol Scand* (Sec B) 78:367, 1970.
88 Bartlett JC et al: Quantitative bacteriology of the vaginal flora. *J Infect Dis* 136:271, 1977.
89 Molnàr G, Geder L: Über Bakterienzüchtung and Antibiotikaempfindlichkeit bei chronischen Entzündungen der Adnexe und Parametrien. *Wien Klin Wochenschr* 70:226, 1958.
90 Heynemann T: Entzündungen der Adnexe, in *Biologie und Pathologie des Weibes,* L Seitz, A Amreich (eds). Berlin, Urban & Schwarzenberg, 1953, vol V, p 19.
91 Lukasik J: A comparative evaluation of the bacteriological flora of the uterine cervix and fallopian tubes in cases of salpingitis. *Am J Obstet Gynecol* 87:1028, 1963.
92 Widholm O, Kallio H: Suppurative adnexal infections. Report on 830 patients treated in 1947–61. *Gynecologia (Basel)* 160:321, 1965.
93 Lip J, Burgoyne X: Cervical and peritoneal flora associated with salpingitis. *Obstet Gynecol* 28:561, 1966.
94 Chow AW et al: The bacteriology of acute pelvic inflammatory disease. Value of cul-de-sac cultures and relative importance of gonococci and other aerobic and anaerobic bacteria. *Am J Obstet Gynecol* 122:876, 1975.
95 Mendling W, Krasemann C: Bakteriologische Befunde und therapeutische Konsequenzen bei Adnexitis. *Geburtsh Frauenheilk* 46: 462, 1986.
96 Thompson SE et al: The microbiology and therapy of acute pelvic inflammatory disease in hospitalized patients. *Am J Obstet Gynecol* 136:179, 1980.
97 Persson E et al: *Actinomyces israelii* in the genital tract of women with and without intrauterine contraceptive devices. *Acta Obstet Gynecol Scand* 62:563, 1983.
98 WHO Scientific Group: The mechanism of action, safety, and efficacy of intrauterine devices. *WHO Tech Rep Ser* 753, 1987.
99 Paavonen J et al: Endometritis and acute salpingitis associated with *Chlamydia trachomatis* and herpes simplex virus type 2. *Obstet Gynecol* 65:288, 1985.
100 Brown WJ, Sutter R: *Campylobacter fetus* septicemia with concurrent salpingitis. *J Clin Microbiol* 6:72, 1977.
101 Saffos RM, Rhatigan RM: Unilateral salpingitis due to *Enterobius vermicularis*. *Am J Clin Pathol* 67:296, 1977.
102 Svensson L et al: Differences in some clinical and laboratory parameters in acute salpingitis related to culture and serological findings. *Am J Obstet Gynecol* 138:1017, 1980.
103 Kivijärvi A et al: Microbiology of vaginitis associated with the intrauterine contraceptive device. *Br J Obstet Gynecol* 91:917, 1981.
104 Heinonen PK et al: Anatomic sites of upper genital infection. *Obstet Gynecol* 66:384, 1985.
105 Cleary RE, Jones RB: Recovery of *Chlamydia trachomatis* from the endometrium in infertile women with serum antichlamydial antibodies. *Fertil Steril* 44:233, 1985.

106 Weisner D et al: Bakteriologische Untersuchungen von Douglas-flüssigkeit. *Geburtsh Frauenheilk* 40:233, 1985.
107 Spence MR et al: A comparative evaluation of vaginal, cervical, and peritoneal flora in normal healthy females. *Sex Transm Dis* 9:762, 1981.
108 Winkler B et al: Immunoperoxidase localization of chlamydial antigens in acute salpingitis. *Am J Obstet Gynecol* 152:275, 1985.
109 Hajj SN: Does sterilization prevent pelvic infection? *J Reprod Med* 20:289, 1978.
110 Vessey M et al: Tubal sterilization: Findings in a large prospective study. *Br J Obstet Gynaecol* 90:203, 1983.
111 Iwanow NS: Über die Verbreitungswege der Entzündungsprozesse in den inneren weiblichen Geschlechtsorganen. *Arch Gynäkol* 149: 124, 1932.
112 Eicher E et al: In vivo studies with direct sky blue of the lymphatic drainage of the internal genitals in women. *Am J Obstet Gynecol* 67:1277, 1954.
113 Vermesh M et al: Acute salpingitis in sterilized women. *Obstet Gynecol* 69:265, 1987.
114 Wölner-Hanssen P et al: Laparoscopy in women with chlamydial infection and pelvic pain: A comparison of patients with and without salpingitis. *Obstet Gynecol* 61:299, 1983.
115 Odeblad E: The functional structure of human cervical mucus. *Acta Obstet Gynecol Scand* 47 (suppl 1):39, 1968.
116 Svensson L et al: *Chlamydia trachomatis* in women attending a gynaecological outpatient clinic with lower genital tract infection. *Br J Vener Dis* 57:259, 1981.
117 Harrison HR: Cervical *Chlamydia trachomatis* infection in university women: Relationship to history of contraception, ectopy, and cervicitis. *Am J Obstet Gynecol* 153:244, 1985.
118 Masters W, Johnson V: *Human Sexual Response.* Boston, Little Brown, 1966, p 116.
119 Bengtsson LP: Hormonal effects on human myometrial activity. *Vitam Horm* 31:257, 1973.
120 Halme J et al: Retrograde menstruation in healthy women and in patients with endometriosis. *Obstet Gynecol* 64:151, 1984.
121 James-Holmquest G et al: Differential attachment by piliated and non-piliated *Neisseria gonorrhoeae* to human sperm. *Inf Immunol* 9:897, 1974.
122 Wölner-Hanssen P, Mårdh P-A: In vitro tests of the adherence of *Chlamydia trachomatis* to human spermatozoa. *Fertil Steril* 42:102, 1984.
123 McCormack W et al: The genital mycoplasmas. *N Engl J Med* 288:78, 1973.
124 Toth A et al: Evidence for microbial transfer by spermatozoa. *Obstet Gynecol* 59:556, 1982.
125 Friberg J et al: *Chlamydia trachomatis* attached to spermatozoa recovered from the peritoneal cavity in patients with salpingitis. *J Reprod Med* 32:120, 1987.
126 Toth A et al: Development of infections of the genitourinary tract in wives of infertile males and possible role of spermatozoa in development of salpingitis. *Surg Gynecol Obstet* 159:565, 1984.
127 Stemmer U: Über die Ursachen von Eileiterentzündungen. *Zentralbl Gynakol* 63:1062, 1941.
128 Viberg L: Acute inflammatory conditions of the adnexa. *Acta Obstet Gynecol Scand* 43 (suppl 4), 1964.
129 Lee NC et al: Type of IUD and the risk of PID. *Obstet Gynecol* 62:1, 1983.
130 Svensson L et al: Contraceptives and acute salpingitis. *JAMA* 251:2553, 1984.
131 Rubin G et al: Oral contraceptives and pelvic inflammatory disease. *Am J Obstet Gynecol* 144:630, 1982.
132 Lukkainen T et al: Five year experience with levonorgestrel releasing IUD's. *Contraception* 33:139, 1986.
133 Soderstrom RM: Will progesterone save the IUD? *J Reprod Med* 28:305, 1983.
134 Wölner-Hanssen P et al: Laparoscopic findings and contraceptive use in women with signs and symptoms suggestive of acute salpingitis. *Obstet Gynecol* 66:233, 1985.
135 Washington AE et al: Oral contraceptives, *Chlamydia trachomatis* infections and pelvic inflammatory disease. *JAMA* 253:2246, 1985.
136 Senanayake P, Kramer DG: Contraception and the etiology of PID: New perspectives. *Am J Obstet Gynecol* 138:852, 1980.
137 Wölner-Hanssen P: Oral contraceptive use modifies the manifestations of pelvic inflammatory disease. *Br J Obstet Gynaecol* 93:619, 1986.
138 Cramer DW et al: The relationship of tubal infertility to barrier method and oral contraceptive use. *JAMA* 257:2446, 1987.
139 Rosenberg MJ et al: Effect of the contraceptive sponge on chlamydial infection, gonorrhea and candidiasis. A comparative clinical trial. *JAMA* 257:2308, 1987.
140 Kelly JP et al: In vitro activity of the spermicide nonoxynol-9 against *Chlamydia trachomatis. Antimicrob Agents Chemother* 27:760, 1985.
141 Weström L: Pelvic inflammatory disease (PID) and the intrauterine device: A causal relationship? in *International Forum,* D Edelmann (ed). *Int J Gynecol Obstet* 17:509, 1980.
142 Avonts D, Piot P: Genital infections in women undergoing therapeutic abortion. *Eur J Obstet Gynaecol* 20:53, 1985.
143 Qvigstad E et al: Pelvic inflammatory disease associated with *Chlamydia trachomatis* infection after therapeutic abortion. *Br J Vener Dis* 59:189, 1983.
144 Schiötz H, Csángó PA: A prospective study of *Chlamydia trachomatis* in first trimester legal abortion. *Ann Clin Res* 17:60, 1985.
145 Möller BR et al: Pelvic inflammatory disease after hysterosalpingography with *Chlamydia trachomatis* and Mycoplasma hominis. *Br J Obstet Gynaecol* 91:1181, 1984.
146 Heisterberg L: Prophylactic antibiotics in women with a history of pelvic inflammatory disease undergoing first trimester abortion. *Acta Obstet Gynecol Scand* 66:15, 1987.
147 Pittaway DE et al: Prevention of acute pelvic inflammatory disease after hysterosalpingography: Efficacy of doxycycline prophylaxis. *Am J Obstet Gynecol* 147:623, 1983.
148 Brunham RC et al: Postabortal *Chlamydia trachomatis* salpingitis: Correlating risk with antigen-specific serological responses and with neutralization. *J Infect Dis* 155:749, 1987.
149 Nordenskjöld F, Ahlgren M: Laparoscopy in female infertility. *Acta Obstet Gynecol Scand* 62:609, 1983.
150 Donnez J et al: Fimbrial ciliated cells percentage and epithelial height during and after salpingitis. *Eur J Obstet Reprod Biol* 17:293, 1984.
151 Monif G: Clinical staging of acute bacterial salpingitis and its therapeutic ramifications. *Obstet Gynecol* 143:489, 1982.
152 Hager WD et al: Criteria for diagnosis and grading of salpingitis. *Obstet Gynecol* 61:113, 1983.
153 Hadgu A et al: Predicting acute PID: A multivariate analysis. *Am J Obstet Gyneol* 155:954, 1986.
154 Skude G et al: Isoamylases in the female genital tract, in *Progress in Clinical Enzymology,* DM Goldberg et al (eds). New York, Masson, 1983, vol 12, p 277.
155 Paavonen J et al: Comparison of endometrial biopsy and peritoneal fluid testing with laparoscopy in diagnosis of acute PID. *Am J Obstet Gynecol* 151:645, 1985.
156 Kiviat N et al: Histopathologic manifestations of endometritic. (Unpublished data.)
157 Ledger WJ: Laparoscopy in the diagnosis and management of patients with suspected salpingo-oophoritis. *Am J Obstet Gynecol* 138:1012, 1980.
158 Mårdh P-A et al: Sampling, specimen obtaining, and isolation techniques in the diagnosis of chlamydial and other genital infections. *Sex Transm Dis* 8:280, 1981.
159 Pao CC et al: Deoxyribonucleic acid hybridization analysis for the detection of urogenital *Chlamydia trachomatis* infection in women. *Am J Obstet Gynecol* 156:195, 1987.
160 Puolakkainen M et al: Persistence of chlamydial antibodies after pelvic inflammatory disease. *J Clin Microbiol* 23:924, 1986.
161 Dorfman SF et al: Ectopic pregnancy mortality, United States, 1979 to 1980: Clinical aspects. *Obstet Gynecol* 64:386, 1984.

162 Centers for Disease Control: Ectopic pregnancy—United States 1981–1983. *MMWR* 35:289, 1986.

163 Rivlin ME: Clinical outcome following vaginal drainage of pelvic abscess. *Obstet Gynecol* 61:169, 1983.

164 Hager WD: Follow-up of patients with tubo-ovarian abscess(es) in association with salpingitis. *Obstet Gynecol* 61:680, 1983.

165 Weström L et al: Infertility after acute salpingitis: Results of treatment with different antibiotics. *Curr Ther Res* 26:752, 1979.

166 Swensen CE et al: The effect of tetracycline treatment on chlamydial salpingitis and subsequent fertility in the mouse. *Sex Transm Dis* 13:40, 1986.

167 Holtz F: Klinische Studien über die nicht-tuberkulöse Salpingo-oophoritis. *Acta Obstet Gynecol Scand* 10 (suppl 1), 1930.

168 Grimes DA: Deaths due to STD. *JAMA* 255:1727, 1986.

169 Mickal A et al: Ruptured ovarian abscess. *Am J Obstet Gynecol* 100:432, 1968.

170 Bret AJ, Legros R: Corticothérapie générale et locale et récupération fonctionelle tubaire. *Gynecol Obstet (Paris)* 58:522, 1959.

171 Hüter KE, Hartmann P: Antiphlogistiche Kortikosteroide in Kombination mit Tetracyklin in der Behandlung entzündlicher Genitalerkrankungen der Frau. *Geburth Frauenheilk* 18:1221, 1959.

172 Hedberg E, Ånberg A: Gonorrheal salpingitis: Views on treatment and prognosis. *Fertil Steril* 16:125, 1965.

173 Wölner-Hanssen P, Weström L: Second look laparoscopy after acute salpingitis. *Obstet Gynecol* 61:702, 1983.

174 Brihmer C, Brundin J: Second look laparoscopy after treatment of acute salpingitis with doxycycline/benzyl penicillin procaine or trimethoprim-sulfamethoxazole. *Scand J Inf Dis Suppl* 53:65, 1988.

175 Hedberg E, Spetz S: Acute salpingitis. View on prognosis and treatment. *Acta Obstet Gynecol Scand* 37:131, 1958.

176 Haffner J: Resultatene av den konservative og operative salpingittbehandling. *Nord Med* 111:2255, 1939.

177 Sundén B: The results of conservative treatment of salpingitis diagnosed at laparotomy and laparoscopy. *Acta Obstet Gynecol Scand* 38:286, 1959.

178 Weström L: Impact of sexually transmitted diseases on human reproduction: Swedish studies of infertility and ectopic pregnancy, in *Sexually Transmitted Diseases Status Report, NIAID Study Group.* Washington, DC, NIH Publications 1980, No 81-2213, p 43.

179 Weström L et al: Preliminary data: CDC/Lund joint multivariate computer analysis of pelvic inflammatory disease in Lund, Sweden 1960–1984.

180 Grossman MJ et al: Perihepatic adhesions in infertility patients with prior pelvic inflammatory disease. *J Reprod Med* 26:625, 1981.

181 Kresch AJ et al: Laparoscopy in 100 women with pelvic pain. *Obstet Gynecol* 64:672, 1984.

182 Svensson L et al: Infertility after acute salpingitis with special reference to *Chlamydia trachomatis* associated infections. *Fertil Steril* 40:322, 1983.

183 Punnonen R et al: Chlamydial serology in infertile women by immunofluorescence. *Fertil Steril* 31:656, 1979.

184 Moore DE et al: Association of *Chlamydia trachomatis* with tubal infertility. *Fertil Steril* 34:303, 1980.

185 Jones RB et al: Correlation between serum antichlamydial antibodies and tubal factors as a cause of infertility. *Fertil Steril* 38:553, 1982.

186 Gump DW et al: Infertile women and *Chlamydia trachomatis* infection, in *Chlamydial Infections,* P-A Mårdh et al (eds). Amsterdam, Elsevier, 1982, p 193.

187 Kane JL et al: Evidence of chlamydial infection in infertile women with and without fallopian tube obstruction. *Fertil Steril* 42:843, 1984.

188 Conway D et al: Chlamydial serology in infertile and fertile women. *Lancet* i:191, 1984.

189 Brunham RC et al: *Chlamydia trachomatis:* Its role in tubal infertility. *J Infect Dis* 152:127, 1985.

190 Tjiam KH et al: Prevalence of antibodies to *Chlamydia trachomatis, Neisseria gonorrhoeae,* and *Mycoplasma hominis* in infertile women. *Genitourin Med* 61:175, 1985.

191 Kosseim M, Brunham RC: Fallopian tube obstruction as a sequela to *Chlamydia trachomatis* infection. *Eur J Clin Microbiol* 5:584, 1986.

192 Robertson JN et al: Chlamydial and gonococcal antibodies in sera of infertile women with tubal obstruction. *J Clin Pathol* 40:377, 1987.

193 Möller RB et al: Serological evidence that chlamydiae and mycoplasmas are involved in infertility of women. *J Reprod Fertil* 73:237, 1985.

194 Gump DW et al: Lack of association between genital mycoplasmas and infertility. *N Engl J Med* 310:937, 1984.

195 Weström L et al: Incidence, trends, and risks of ectopic pregnancy in a defined population of women. *Br Med J* 282:15, 1981.

196 Krohn L: New etiological factor in ectopic pregnancy. *JAMA* 150:1291, 1952.

197 Svensson L et al: Ectopic pregnancy and antibodies to *Chlamydia trachomatis. Fertil Steril* 44:313, 1985.

198 Brunham RC et al: *Chlamydia trachomatis* infection in women with ectopic pregnancy. *Obstet Gynecol* 67:722, 1986.

199 Lenton EA et al: Long-term follow-up of the apparently normal couple with a complaint of infertility. *Fertil Steril* 28:913, 1977.

200 Mosher WD: Infertility trends among US couples 1965–1976. *Fam Plann Perspect* 14:22, 1982.

201 Mosher WD, Pratt WF: Reproductive impairments among married couples. United States Center for Health Statistics. *Vital Health Stat* 1982.

202 Mosher DW, Aral SO: Factors related to infertility in the United States 1965–1976. *Sex Transm Dis* 12:117, 1985.

203 Stamm WE, Holmes KK: Measures to control *Chlamydia trachomatis* infections: An assessment of new national policy guidelines. *JAMA* 256:1178, 1986.

204 Tuffrey M et al: Salpingitis in mice induced by human strains of *Chlamydia trachomatis. J Reprod Fertil* 78:251, 1986.

205 Kane JL et al: Chlamydial pelvic infection in cats: A model for the study of human pelvic inflammatory disease. *Genitourin Med* 61: 311, 1987.

206 Patton DL et al: Chlamydial infection of subcutaneous fimbrial transplants in cynomologus and rhesus monkeys. *J Infect Dis* 155: 299; 1987.

207 Patton DL: Immunopathology and histopathology of experimental chlamydial salpingitis. *Rev Infect Dis* 7:746, 1985.

208 Tuffrey M et al: Infertility in mice infected genitally with a human strain of *Chlamydia trachomatis. J Reprod Fertil* 78:251, 1986.

209 Patton DL et al: Distal tubal obstruction induced by repeated *Chlamydia trachomatis* salpingitis infections in pig-tailed macaques. *J Infect Dis* 155:1292, 1987.

# Chapter 50

# Atypical pelvic inflammatory disease: subacute, chronic, or subclinical upper genital tract infection in women

Pål Wølner-Hanssen
Nancy B. Kiviat
King K. Holmes

**Definition.** Pelvic inflammatory disease is a clinical syndrome caused by ascending spread of microorganisms from the lower to the upper genital tract. The syndrome is usually associated with abdominal pain of recent onset, but also with other symptoms from various organ systems, including the genital tract (recent onset of dyspareunia, menorrhagia, dysmenorrhea, and vaginal discharge); the gastrointestinal tract (nausea, vomiting, and perhaps symptoms of proctitis); and the urinary tract (dysuria, and perhaps urgency and frequency). In most cases of acute pelvic inflammatory disease, however, abdominal pain is the primary reason for consulting a clinician. For the clinician then, abdominal pain is usually a *conditio sine qua non* for a clinical diagnosis of pelvic inflammatory disease, or for considering laparoscopy to verify suspected acute salpingitis.[1] Even when salpingitis is an unexpected finding during laparoscopy or laparotomy performed for reasons other than acute pelvic inflammatory disease, abdominal pain has usually been a part of the symptomatology (see Table 49-5). Thus, in almost every case of acute pelvic inflammatory disease described in the literature, abdominal pain has been present. However, a growing body of evidence suggests that acute pelvic inflammatory disease with lower abdominal pain as the chief complaint may represent the "tip of the iceberg," and that there may be large numbers of women with relatively or completely painless upper genital tract infection. In this chapter the term "atypical pelvic inflammatory disease" is suggested for pelvic inflammatory disease not causing abdominal pain. Atypical pelvic inflammatory disease can be inferred when tubal occlusion or adhesions are found in women with no history of pelvic inflammatory disease; and confirmation of atypical pelvic inflammatory disease can be based on demonstration of inflammation of the fallopian tubes or endometrium in the absence of abdominal pain. Isolation of usual pathogens from inflamed fallopian tubes in the absence of lower abdominal pain would constitute the best evidence that pelvic inflammatory disease caused by these pathogens can be atypical in clinical presentation.

## HISTORY

Much of the knowledge of atypical pelvic inflammatory disease is based on indirect evidence or on direct evidence which is unconfirmed. Therefore, the history of such evidence will be critically reviewed in this chapter.

### Direct evidence for ongoing atypical pelvic inflammatory disease and for subclinical upper genital tract infection

**Endometritis and Endometrial Infection.** Recently, Paavonen et al.[2] demonstrated histopathologic evidence of endometritis (ten or more plasma cells in any of six tissue sections) in 47 percent of women who had mucopurulent cervicitis without symptoms of pelvic inflammatory disease (i.e., neither moderate to severe adnexal tenderness nor an oral temperature of ≥38°C). After reviewing the raw data, we have found that 65 percent of those culture-positive for *Chlamydia trachomatis* in the cervix had endometritis. Histopathologic features of endometritis were not significantly associated with isolation of *C. trachomatis* from the endometrium, but no attempts were made to detect chlamydial antigens in the endometrial tissue. In contrast, plasma cell endometritis was seen in only one (3 percent) of 35 endometrial biopsy specimens obtained from asymptomatic women who underwent evaluation for infertility. Sweet et al.[3] have reported persistence of *C. trachomatis* in the endometrium of women treated for pelvic inflammatory disease. Among 13 women with *C. trachomatis* infection before treatment, endometrial aspirates following cephalosporin treatment yielded *C. trachomatis* in 12 cases, despite disappearance of abdominal pain. The endometrial cultures were not verified with in situ detection of *C. trachomatis* antigens to exclude contamination from the cervix, and endometrial biopsies were not done to determine the presence or absence of endometritis. Nonetheless, these findings suggest that *C. trachomatis* may persist in the endometrium without causing pain.

*C. trachomatis* has also been recovered from the endometrium of infertile women. Thus, Cleary and Jones[4] isolated *C. trachomatis* from the endometrium of five (26 percent) of 19 infertile women who had serum antibodies to *C. trachomatis.* These women had no clinical evidence of acute pelvic inflammatory disease at the time of examination. By history, it seemed unlikely that the chlamydial infection was of recent onset. The endometrial cultures were not verified by in situ detection of *C. trachomatis* to rule out contamination from the cervix. In contrast to this study, Gump et al.[5] were unable to recover *C. trachomatis* from the cervix of any of 203 infertile women. Endometrial specimens were obtained from 185 of the women, only one of which was culture-positive for *C. trachomatis.* Similarly, Brunham et al.[6] failed to isolate *C. trachomatis* from the cervix of any of 17, and Guderian and Trobough[7] recovered the organism from the cervix of no more than 4 percent of 151 infertile women. Sellors et al.[8] failed to isolate *C. trachomatis* from the cervix and the fallopian tubes of 52 women with tubal factor infertility. We conclude that in the future, studies of the relationship of chlamydial infection of the endometrium to endometritis in women without abdominal pain should include not only cultures, but also histopathologic studies of the endometrium and in situ immunoperoxidase or immunofluorescent staining for *C. trachomatis.*

**Salpingitis and Tubal Infection.** Henry-Suchet et al.[9] reported isolation of *C. trachomatis* from the fallopian tubes of 6 (15 percent) of 39 infertile women who had no clinical or laparoscopic evidence of acute salpingitis, and from 7 (23 percent) of 30 women with so-called viscous pelvis (yellowish, viscous effusion in the cul-de-sac, redness of the peritoneum, and adnexal pseudocysts) (Table 50-1). *C. trachomatis* has also been isolated from the fallopian tubes of 2 of 20 women undergoing tubal ligation in the immediate postpartum period.[10] Neither patient reported a history of either pelvic inflammatory disease or sexually transmitted diseases, and neither exhibited any symptoms suggestive of salpingitis. Other researchers have so far not confirmed these remarkable findings. For example, Patton et al.[11] failed to isolate *C. trachomatis* from the tubes of 60 infertile women with distal tubal scarring, 47 percent of whom had serum antibodies to the organism. However, the majority of these women had been treated with different antibiotics prior to the laparoscopy (Patton DL, personal communication). None of the 67 infertile women with tubal adhesions or occlusions reported by Ånestad et al.[12] had systematically been treated with antibiotics during the previous 12 months, but the authors failed to recover *C. trachomatis* from the cervix or fallopian tubes of any of them. We believe that these studies are inconclusive and that future research should involve laparoscopic examination of infertile patients who had risk factors for chlamydial infection, but with no history of pelvic inflammatory disease, who have not been given antimicrobial therapy before the procedure. Specimens from the fallopian tubes should be cultured in reputable laboratories, and isolates should be saved and sent to reference laboratories for confirmation.

## Evidence of past atypical pelvic inflammatory disease among infertile women

As summarized in Table 50-2, several studies have demonstrated that a large proportion of infertile women with tubal adhesions or occlusion have no history of past pelvic inflammatory disease[(5–8,12–18)] even among those with serum antibodies to *C. trachomatis*. Patton and coworkers[19] examined tubal biopsies from women with scarred tubes using light microscopy and electron microscopy, and found no difference between women with or without a history of pelvic inflammatory disease with respect to tubal morphology and histopathology.

The relationship of tubal infertility to serum antibody to *N. gonorrhoeae* has been less well studied. Among 57 infertile women, however, Tjiam et al.[18] identified gonococcal pili antibodies in 61 percent of those with and in 25 percent of those without scarred fallopian tubes. Less than a third of women with gonococcal pili antibodies had chlamydial antibodies, and half of them lacked a history of pelvic inflammatory disease. These data suggest that *N. gonorrhoeae* may also cause atypical pelvic inflammatory disease. The weakness of this type of data is, of course, that the lack of remembered history of acute pelvic inflammatory disease does not exclude the possibility that these women may have experienced previous episodes of chlamydial or gonococcal salpingitis with abdominal pain that was never diagnosed by a clinician as a salpingitis and that was subsequently forgotten by the patient.

## Evidence of atypical pelvic inflammatory disease among women with ectopic pregnancy

Ectopic pregnancy is an important sequela of salpingitis. The yearly number of ectopic pregnancies in the United States increased from 17,800 in 1970 to 69,600 in 1983.[20] It has been estimated that at least half of all ectopic pregnancies can be attributed to previous pelvic inflammatory disease.[21] Recently, it has been reported that many women with ectopic pregnancy have no past history of pelvic inflammatory disease, despite the presence of serum antibodies to *C. trachomatis*. Svensson et al.[22] studied 112 women with ectopic pregnancy, of whom 73 (65 percent) had serum antibodies to *C. trachomatis*. Of those with such antibodies 20 (31 percent) had no past history of pelvic inflammatory disease. Brunham et al.[23] reported that of 50 women with tubal pregnancy, only 5 had a past history of pelvic inflammatory disease. Of 32 women who lacked other risk factors for ectopic pregnancy such as history of IUD use or tubal ligation, 18 (56 percent) had serum antibody to *C. trachomatis*. Of these 18, no more than 5 had a history of pelvic inflammatory disease. In summary, these studies suggest that a significant proportion of women with ectopic pregnancy, particularly those who have no other risk factors, may have had chlamydial infection, and that many of these had atypical rather than typical pelvic inflammatory disease. The proportion of ectopic pregnancies attributable to previous salpingitis may therefore exceed 50 percent.

## Evidence of atypical pelvic inflammatory disease among IUD users

Intrauterine devices (IUD) have been implicated in severe acute pelvic inflammatory disease such as tuboovarian abscesses,[24] but there is some evidence that IUD use also may be associated with atypical pelvic inflammatory disease. Of 69 infertile, past IUD users studied by Guderian and Trobough,[7] 49 (71 percent) had tubal occlusion or adnexal adhesions or both. Of these 49, the cause of tubal scarring was unexplained in 30 (61 percent). Of 25 women in this study who had an IgG antibody titer to *C. trachomatis* of 512 or higher, only 6 (24 percent) reported a past history of pelvic inflammatory disease. Smith et al.[25] studied tubal segments obtained from healthy women undergoing laparoscopic sterilization. Cultures were performed for anaerobic and

**Table 50-1. Infection with *C. trachomatis* among Infertile Women without Clinical Evidence of Acute Infection**

| Author | Number of patients | Culture site | Findings at surgery | *C. trachomatis* isolated, % |
|---|---|---|---|---|
| Henry-Suchet et al.[9] | 30 | Tubes | "Viscous pelvis"* | 23 |
| | 39 | Tubes | Old adhesions | 15 |
| | 49 | Tubes | Normal tubes | 2 |
| Patton et al.[11] | 60 | Tubes | Old adhesions | 0 |
| Ånestad et al.[12] | 67 | Cervix, tubes | Adhesions, occlusion | 0 |
| | 38 | Cervix, tubes | Normal tubes | 3 |
| Cleary and Jones[4] | 19 | Endometrium | No surgery | 26 |
| Gump et al.[5] | 185 | Endometrium | No surgery | 1 |
| Brunham et al.[6] | 17 | Cervix | Not specified | 0 |
| Guderian and Trobough[7] | 151 | Cervix | Not specified | 4 |
| Sellors et al.[8] | 52 | Cervix, tubes | Not specified | 0 |

*Viscous pelvis: yellow, viscous cul-de-sac fluid, adnexal pseudocysts, peritoneal redness.

**Table 50-2. History of Pelvic Inflammatory Disease and Presence of Chlamydial Antibodies among Infertile Women**

| Author | Findings at surgery | Chlamydial antibodies, %* | No history of PID, % | No history of PID among those with antibody to *C. trachomatis*, % |
|---|---|---|---|---|
| Punnonen et al.[13] | Sactosalpinx | 91 | 39 | 39 |
| Moore et al.[14] | Distal occlusion | 73 | 45 | 62 |
| | Adnexal adhesions | 21 | 58 | — |
| Jones et al.[15] | Tubal abnormality | 60 | 81 | 84 |
| Gump et al.[5] | Adnexal adhesions | 36 | — | 53 |
| Kane et al.[16] | Hydrosalpinx | 36 | 63 | 72 |
| Conway et al.[17] | Hydrosalpinx/adhesions | 75 | 75 | — |
| Brunham et al.[6] | Hydrosalpinx/adhesions | 72 | 61 | — |
| Tjiam et al.[18] | Adhesions or occlusion | 21 | 30 | 17 |
| Sellors et al.[8] | Tubal occlusion | 80 | 69 | 65† |
| Guderian and Trobough[7] | Residues of PID | 83 | 58 | 70 |
| Ånestad et al.[12] | Tubal occlusion | 91 | 66 | — |
| | Adnexal adhesions | 84 | 92 | — |

*Serum IgG and IgM.
†Personal communication.

aerobic bacteria, and were sterile in all cases. Cultures for *C. trachomatis* were not performed. Plasma cell infiltrates were found in the tubal submucosa in 47 percent of IUD users and in only 1 percent of non-IUD users. In addition, endometrial plasma cell infiltrates were seen in 50 percent of the IUD users. Gusberg[26] examined 40 IUD users by endometrial biopsy and found focal endometritis in 55 percent. Mishell et al.[27] examined 75 hysterectomy specimens from women between 25 and 35 years of age; all contained a Lippes loop. Culture specimens were transfundally collected to prevent contamination from the cervical flora. All five specimens containing a device inserted less than 24 h prior to surgery, and 5 (9 percent) of 54 containing a device put in more than 24 h prior to surgery were culture-positive. Plasma cell endometritis was diagnosed in 45 percent of the hysterectomy specimens. This study shows that introduction of an IUD contaminates the uterine cavity and that these microorganisms disappear rapidly from most but not all women, at least when the IUD has a monofilament string.[28] Chlamydial cultures were not performed at the time of this study. Retrospective studies by Daling et al.[29] and Cramer et al.[30] showed that infertile women with damaged fallopian tubes were more likely to have used certain IUDs in the past than were fertile women. Among 56 infertile patients with primary tubal infertility (diagnosis based either on an abnormal hysterosalpingogram or on findings during surgery), who had ever used an IUD, 17 (30 percent) had a history of IUD-related pelvic inflammatory disease.[29] The remaining 39 past IUD users may or may not have had IUD-related atypical pelvic inflammatory disease. In the Cramer study, only 12 percent of 89 infertile women who had ever used an IUD had a history of pelvic inflammatory disease.

In summary, these data strongly suggest that many IUD users have chronic endometritis and endosalpingitis, but do not indicate what the role of infection may be in causing these changes. The evidence also suggests that IUD-related salpingitis is a risk factor for tubal infertility and may be atypical.

### Evidence of postpartum atypical pelvic inflammatory disease

Secondary infertility is the predominant type of infertility in certain developing countries. For example, in some African countries 52 percent of infertility is secondary.[31] In these countries, 85 percent of female infertility can be attributed to past infection. The rate of tubal occlusion among infertile women from these countries is two to three times higher than it is among infertile women from developing Latin American, Asian, and East Mediterranean countries, or from developed countries. Up to a third of gynecologic admissions to African hospitals are caused by pelvic infections, about half of which are puerperal. Plummer et al.[32] recovered *C. trachomatis* from 21 percent and *N. gonorrhoeae* from 7 percent of 1013 pregnant women in Nairobi. Overall, 20 percent of the women in the study developed clinical evidence of postpartum endometritis or salpingitis or both. Among women with postpartum endometritis who were infected with *N. gonorrhoeae* or *C. trachomatis* or both, 68 percent of endometritis was attributable to either organism. Of 32 women in Seattle with antepartum chlamydial infection, 7 (32 percent) developed late postpartum endometritis.[33] The diagnosis of the upper genital tract infection was based on the presence of signs such as fever, uterine tenderness, or purulent lochia. However, in a smaller study by Hoyme et al.[34] only 3 of 19 women referred because of suspected late postpartum endometritis (symptoms developed 7 or more days after delivery) had fever. Twelve of the 19 women were infected with *C. trachomatis*. The clinical manifestations of endometritis were felt to be mild in this study, raising the possibility that the clinical spectrum of late postpartum endometritis includes even milder, subclinical cases. To what degree the tubes are involved in late postpartum endometritis is not known and requires study. The mild clinical manifestations of late postpartum endometritis are no guarantee that tubes are not infected. Moore et al.[14] found that two-thirds of infertile women with chlamydial antibodies and obstructed tubes had been previously pregnant. As mentioned, half of the women in the study had no history of pelvic inflammatory disease. Thus, the high secondary infertility rate in certain populations may, in part, be a result of a high rate of postpartum infections that produce atypical pelvic inflammatory disease.

## EPIDEMIOLOGY

The incidence of atypical pelvic inflammatory disease is unknown. The condition, as we have defined it, is subclinical or at least not associated with pain. Most of the time atypical pelvic inflammatory disease is recognized retrospectively, among infertile women or among those with ectopic pregnancy. The disease is not reportable, and no surveillance studies have been performed. The frequency of occurrence of atypical pelvic inflammatory disease can therefore only be indirectly inferred, for example, by studies of the prevalence of upper genital tract infection and inflammation in women with no symptoms or with symptoms other than abdominal pain.

To assess the possible contribution of endometritis to abnormal menstrual bleeding in women with no clinical evidence of acute pelvic inflammatory disease, all endometrial biopsies obtained at Harborview Medical Center between 1981 and 1985 from nonpregnant women, 40 years old or younger, were reviewed. No standardized criteria had been used for the diagnosis of endometritis at the time of biopsy. For the review of the slides, one or more plasma cells per 120× field of endometrial stroma was used as the minimal criterion for endometritis. During studies of women who had clinical evidence of acute, typical, pelvic inflammatory disease, and who had undergone laparoscopy and endometrial biopsy, endometritis as defined above was associated with acute salpingitis (Kiviat N, unpublished data). Initially, endometritis had been identified in only 15 (15 percent) of the 102 cases of abnormal bleeding. On reviewing the specimens, 49 (48 percent) of the 102 cases met the criterion for endometritis. Cultures for microbial pathogens were not performed in these patients. One of 17 specimens with endometritis stained with monoclonal antibodies to *C. trachomatis,* however, showed chlamydial inclusions.

The possible relationship of menorrhagia (here defined as perceived abnormally heavy bleeding during the last menstrual period compared with previous periods) and metrorrhagia to certain cervical microorganisms was next studied in 463 randomly selected Seattle STD-clinic patients with no abdominal pain. *N. gonorrhoeae, C. trachomatis,* and *Mycoplasma hominis* each was significantly more often isolated from the lower genital tract of women with menorrhagia than from those with no abnormal bleeding. As shown in Table 50-3, the associations between menorrhagia and these STD infections were limited to nonusers of oral contraceptives, suggesting that menorrhagia in oral contraceptive users could have been related to effects of the ingested hormones rather than to effects of infection. Bacterial vaginosis was also significantly associated with menorrhagia in nonusers of oral contraceptives.

Among nonusers of oral contraceptives, infections with *C. trachomatis* and *N. gonorrhoeae* were also more common among those with metrorrhagia, although none of these associations were significant. In this study, endometrial biopsies and cultures were not obtained to confirm the hypothesis that these infections produced abnormal menstrual bleedings by causing endometritis.

From these data, one can attempt to estimate the prevalence of atypical pelvic inflammatory disease, relative to that of typical pelvic inflammatory disease in this study population. Among 777 randomly selected women attending the STD clinic at Harborview Medical Center, nine were considered to have acute pelvic inflammatory disease of whom five were infected with *N. gonorrhoeae* or *C. trachomatis* or both, and 461 had no abdominal pain. Of these 461 women, 55 had menorrhagia, and 16 of those with menorrhagia were infected with *C. trachomatis* or *N. gonorrhoeae* or both. Thus, if those with menorrhagia plus chlamydial or gonococcal infection had endometritis, admittedly a tenuous assumption, and one assumes that all five with clinical evidence of chlamydial or gonococcal pelvic inflammatory disease actually had the condition, then the ratio of atypical to typical pelvic inflammatory disease would be 16 to 5. Similarly, of the 461 women, 55 had mucopurulent cervicitis (purulent cervical discharge or 30 or more polymorphonuclear leukocytes per 1200× field in cervical Gram stains) associated with infection by *C. trachomatis* or *N. gonorrhoeae,* as did all five of those with symptomatic pelvic inflammatory disease who had chlamydial or gonococcal infection. If one assumes that at least half of the 55 had endometritis (based upon the above-mentioned results of endometrial biopsies from women with mucopurulent cervicitis or menorrhagia), then the ratio of atypical to typical pelvic inflammatory disease would be 27 to 5. This ratio seems improbably high, and we believe it is necessary to determine the prevalence of histopathologic evidence of endometritis, and to obtain direct evidence by immunopathologic techniques for endometrial infection with *C. trachomatis* or *N. gonorrhoeae* among women who have mucopurulent cervicitis, or who have menorrhagia. The relationship of bacterial vaginosis to endometritis among those with menorrhagia also needs further study. Further studies are also required to see how frequently endometritis is accompanied by subclinical salpingitis, and whether endometritis per se may cause infertility.

## PATHOGENESIS

The clinical spectrum of pelvic inflammatory disease probably ranges from lack of symptoms to severe illness. It is possible that patients with endometritis may have symptoms only of vaginal discharge (due to mucopurulent cervicitis) or abnormal menstrual bleeding. The question is, why is pelvic inflammatory disease painless in some patients and painful in others? Is the pain of

**Table 50-3. Presence of Various Genital Infections among Women with and without Menorrhagia, Stratified by Oral Contraceptive (OC) Use. Patients Randomly Selected from Women Attending an STD Clinic**

| | Non OC users menorrhagia, % | | | | OC users menorrhagia, % | | | |
|---|---|---|---|---|---|---|---|---|
| Microorganisms | Present $n = 42$ | Absent $n = 258$ | $P$ | Odds ratio | Present $n = 13$ | Absent $n = 148$ | $P$ | Odds ratio |
| *C. trachomatis* | 21 | 10 | 0.03 | 2.4 | 0 | 21 | 0.066 | — |
| *N. gonorrhoeae* | 26 | 12 | 0.01 | 2.6 | 8 | 9 | 0.89 | 0.9 |
| *C. trachomatis* and/or *N. gonorrhoeae* | 36 | 19 | 0.014 | 2.4 | 8 | 26 | 0.15 | 0.2 |
| *M. hominis* | 75 | 49 | 0.003 | 3.4 | 23 | 40 | 0.23 | 0.5 |
| *U. urealyticum* | 90 | 85 | 0.41 | 1.7 | 77 | 86 | 0.39 | 0.6 |
| *G. vaginalis* | 86 | 73 | 0.09 | 2.2 | 69 | 64 | 0.69 | 1.3 |
| Bacterial vaginosis | 68 | 37 | <0.001 | 3.8 | 15 | 30 | 0.27 | 0.4 |

acute pelvic inflammatory disease attributable to peritonitis? Symptomatic pelvic inflammatory disease is usually associated with some degree of peritonitis, i.e., with leukocytic exudate in pelvic peritoneal fluid, with or without associated erythema of the peritoneum. In fact, tubal erythema and exudate are parts of the laparoscopic definition of salpingitis. Thus, lack of peritonitis may explain atypical pelvic inflammatory disease. The occurrence of peritonitis may be related to the size of the inoculum at the time of infection, the virulence of the infective pathogen, the effectiveness of the host immune response, and patency of the fallopian tubes.

A possible role of oral contraceptive use in the development of silent chlamydial pelvic inflammatory disease deserves special attention. Several studies have pointed out that use of oral contraceptives is associated with a higher rate of cervical infection with *C. trachomatis.*[35–38] Many other studies have suggested that oral contraceptives protect against typical, symptomatic pelvic inflammatory disease.[39–42] Washington et al.[43] attempted to explain this apparent paradox by suggesting that oral contraceptive use could promote chlamydial infection of the cervix and then cause atypical pelvic inflammatory disease. Further studies are needed to see whether oral contraceptive use promotes atypical pelvic inflammatory disease among women infected with *C. trachomatis.*

## DIAGNOSIS

The diagnosis of atypical pelvic inflammatory disease has usually been retrospective. That is, old adnexal adhesions and hydrosalpinx have been detected in infertile women who had no past history of pelvic inflammatory disease. The diagnosis of atypical pelvic inflammatory disease in the absence of symptoms of abdominal pain is obviously problematic, and recommendations here await confirmation in future studies. Nevertheless, it seems prudent at present to consider the diagnosis of endometritis in women who have mucopurulent cervicitis, menorrhagia, or both, particularly in those not using oral contraceptives. Sometimes cervicitis is easily recognizable due to yellow endocervical mucopus, erythema, and friability (see Chap. 46 and Plates 15 and 16). At other times cervicitis may be inapparent. In conjunction with obtaining a routine endocervical cytology smear, it probably would be good practice to take a brief look at the color of the endocervical specimen before it is streaked onto the microscope slide. Yellow mucus would warn of a possible infection, and further evaluation should follow. Subtle signs of uterine tenderness should not be dismissed, since it has been shown that uterine tenderness and peripheral leukocytosis are associated with histopathologic features of endometritis in such patients.

Diagnostic tests for gonococcal and chlamydial infection of the cervix should be performed, and those found to have mucopurulent cervicitis should be treated promptly, for example, with ceftriaxone followed by doxycycline (see Chap. 46). Endometrial biopsy might be a helpful aid in distinguishing those with anovulatory bleeding from those who have an infection. Presently, at least in the United States, most cases of menometrorrhagia in young women are first considered dysfunctional and treated with hormones. Endometrial biopsies are reserved for older women to rule out endometrial neoplasia. However, endometrial biopsy might also be indicated in sexually active young women to rule out endometritis. Although the status of the fallopian tubes has not been studied via laparoscopy in women with mucopurulent cervicitis, or menorrhagia alone, because it has been hard to justify laparoscopy in such patients, it will be of interest in the future to attempt to assess tubal findings in women with mucopurulent cervicitis or menorrhagia who need laparoscopy for other reasons, such as for infertility evaluation or for tubal sterilization.

## PREVENTION AND THERAPY

Prevention of silent chlamydial pelvic inflammatory disease requires prevention of *C. trachomatis* infection per se. In addition, early recognition and treatment of cervical chlamydial infections and atypical pelvic inflammatory disease should be pursued. Prevention and therapy of cervical chlamydial infections are discussed in Chaps. 16 and 46 and will not be repeated in detail here.

While it is generally believed that a 7- to 10-day course of tetracycline is sufficient to eradicate *C. trachomatis,* the evidence for this is based upon relatively short-term follow-up. Jones and Batteiger[44] recently reported late recurrence of *C. trachomatis* infection in 28 percent of patients in a retrospective study of STD clinic patients who underwent repeated cultures for the agent. Of these, 14 of 38 recurred with a serovar identical to the originally infecting strain. In a recent study, we treated 57 women with cervical *C. trachomatis* with tetracycline for 7 days, and prospectively followed them at 3-month intervals. The cumulative rate of recurrence was 31 percent after one year and 46 percent after 2 years of follow-up. These studies do not distinguish treatment failures from reinfection from untreated or new partners. Henry-Suchet and Douyel[45] reported persistence or recurrence of fallopian tube chlamydial infection in 46 percent of patients after a 1- to 2-month course of tetracycline therapy. These patients were presumably monogamous, and their partners had been treated. The conception rate was significantly lower among women with persisent *C. trachomatis* than among women successfully treated. We view these results with skepticism, since strains of *C. trachomatis* resistant to tetracyclines have not been reported from other areas of the world. Nevertheless, further studies should include long-term follow-up after the presently recommended 2-week course of treatment for pelvic inflammatory disease and 1-week treatment for uncomplicated mucopurulent cervicitis with doxycycline, to exclude possible persistence of the original infecting serovar of *C. trachomatis* after therapy.

# References


1 Jacobson L, Weström L: Objectivized diagnosis of pelvic inflammatory disease. *Am J Obstet Gynecol* 105:1088, 1969.

2 Paavonen J et al: Prevalence and manifestations of endometritis among women with cervicitis. *Am J Obstet Gynecol* 152:280, 1985.

3 Sweet RL et al: Failure of beta-lactam antibiotics to eradicate *Chlamydia trachomatis* in the endometrium despite apparent clinical cure of acute salpingitis. *JAMA* 250:2641, 1983.

4 Cleary RE, Jones RB: Recovery of *Chlamydia trachomatis* from the endometrium in infertile women with serum antichlamydial antibodies. *Fertil Steril* 44:233, 1985.

5 Gump DW et al: Evidence of prior pelvic inflammatory disease and its relationship to *Chlamydia trachomatis* antibody and intrauterine contraceptive device use in infertile women. *Am J Obstet Gynecol* 146:153, 1983.

6 Brunham RC et al: *Chlamydia trachomatis*: Its role in tubal infertility. *J Inf Dis* 152:1275, 1985.

7 Guderian AM, Trobough GE: Residues of pelvic inflammatory disease in intrauterine device users: A result of the intrauterine device or *Chlamydia trachomatis* infection? *Am J Obstet Gynecol* 154:497, 1986.

8 Sellors JW et al: Tubal factor infertility: An association with prior chlamydial infection and asymptomatic salpingitis. *Fertil Steril* 49:451, 1988.

9 Henry-Suchet J et al: *Chlamydia trachomatis* associated with chronic inflammation in abdominal specimens from women selected for tuboplasty. *Fertil Steril* 36:599, 1981.

10 Menchaca A et al: Incidence of *Chlamydia trachomatis* in peripartum fallopian tubes. *J Reprod Med* 33:199, 1988.

11 Patton DL et al: Silent pelvic inflammatory disease: Morphological, physiological, and serological findings. *Am J Obstet Gynecol* 73:622, 1989.

12 Ånestad G et al: Infertility and chlamydial infection. *Fertil Steril* 48: 787, 1987.

13 Punnonen R et al: Chlamydial serology in infertile women by immunofluorescence. *Fertil Steril* 31:656, 1979.

14 Moore DE et al: Increased frequency of serum antibodies to *Chlamydia trachomatis* in infertility due to distal tubal disease. *Lancet* ii: 574, 1982.

15 Jones RB et al: Correlation between serum antichlamydial antibodies and tubal factor as a cause of infertility. *Fertil Steril* 38:553, 1982.

16 Kane JL et al: Evidence for chlamydial infection in infertile women with and without fallopian tube obstruction. *Fertil Steril* 42:843, 1984.

17 Conway D et al: Chlamydial serology in fertile and infertile women. *Lancet* i:191, 1984.

18 Tjiam KH et al: Prevalence of antibodies to *Chlamydia trachomatis, Neisseria gonorrhoeae*, and *Mycoplasma hominis* in infertile women. *Genitourin Med* 61:175, 1985.

19 Patton DL et al: A morphological and physiological analysis of the tubal epithelium, *Abstracts of the International Society for STD Research*, 7th International Meeting, Atlanta, GA, August 2–5, 1987.

20 Centers for Disease Control: Ectopic pregnancy—United States, 1981–83. *MMWR* 35:289, 1986.

21 Weström L et al: Incidence, trends, and risks of ectopic pregnancy in a population of women. *Br Med J* 282:15, 1981.

22 Svensson L et al: Ectopic pregnancy and antibodies to *Chlamydia trachomatis*. *Fertil Steril* 44:313, 1985.

23 Brunham RC et al: *Chlamydia trachomatis* infection in women with ectopic pregnancy. *Obstet Gynecol* 67:722, 1986.

24 Scott WC: Pelvic abscess in association with intrauterine contraceptive device. *Am J Obstet Gynecol* 131:149, 1978.

25 Smith MR et al: A frequent response to intrauterine contraception. *J Reprod Med* 16:159, 1976.

26 Gusberg SB: Comments on Willson et al. *Am J Obstet Gynecol* 114: 134, 1972.

27 Mishell DR et al: The intrauterine device: A bacteriologic study of the endometrial cavity. *Am J Obstet Gynecol* 96:119, 1966.

28 Skangalis M et al: Microbial presence in the uterine cavity as affected by varieties of intrauterine contraceptive devices. *Fertil Steril* 37:263, 1982.

29 Daling JR et al: Primary tubal infertility in relation to the use of an intrauterine device. *N Engl J Med* 312:937, 1985.

30 Cramer DW et al: Tubal infertility and the intrauterine device. *N Engl J Med* 312:941, 1985.

31 Cates WJ et al: Worldwide patterns of infertility: Is Africa different? *Lancet* 2:596, 1985.

32 Plummer FA et al: Postpartum upper genital tract infections in Nairobi, Kenya: Epidemiology, etiology, and risk factors *J Inf Dis* 156: 92, 1987.

33 Wager GP et al: Puerperal morbidity: Relationship to route of delivery and to antepartum *Chlamydia trachomatis* infection. *Am J Obstet Gynecol* 138:1028, 1980.

34 Hoyme U et al: The microbiology and treatment of late postpartum endometritis. *Obstet Gynecol* 67:229, 1986.

35 Hilton AL et al; *Chlamydia* A in the female genital tract. *Br J Vener Dis* 50:1, 1974.

36 Kinghorn GR, Waugh MA: Oral contraceptive use and prevalence of infection with *Chlamydia trachomatis* in women. *Br J Vener Dis* 57:187, 1981.

37 Svensson L et al: *Chlamydia trachomatis* in women attending a gynecological outpatient clinic with lower genital tract infection. *Br J Vener Dis* 57:259, 1981.

38 Tait IA et al: Chlamydia infection of the cervix in contacts of men with nongonococcal urethritis. *Br J Vener Dis* 56:37, 1980.

39 Weström L et al: The risk of pelvic inflammatory disease in women using intrauterine contraceptive device as compared to nonusers. *Lancet* 2:221, 1976.

40 Eschenbach DA et al: Pathogenesis of acute pelvic inflammatory disease: Role of contraception and other risk factors. *Am J Obstet Gynecol* 128:838, 1977.

41 Faulkner WL, Ory HW: Intrauterine devices and acute pelvic inflammatory disease. *JAMA* 235:1851, 1976.

42 Senanayake P, Kramer DG: Contraception and the etiology of pelvic inflammatory disease: New perspectives. *Am J Obstet Gynecol* 138:852, 1980.

43 Washington AE et al: Oral contraceptives, *Chlamydia trachomatis* infection, and pelvic inflammatory disease. A word of caution about protection. *JAMA* 253:2246, 1985.

44 Jones RB, Batteiger BE: Human immune response to *Chlamydia trachomatis* infections, in *Chlamydial Infections*, D Oriel et al (eds). Cambridge, Cambridge University Press, 1986, p 423.

45 Henry-Suchet J, Douyel P: Treatment of culture documented intrapelvic *Chlamydia trachomatis* infection in women selected for tuboplasties: Preliminary results, in *Chlamydial Infections,* D Oriel et al (eds). Cambridge, Cambridge University Press, 1986, p 201.

# Chapter 51

# Fitz-Hugh–Curtis syndrome

David A. Eschenbach
Pål Wølner-Hanssen

## HISTORY

A syndrome caused by salpingitis and perihepatitis was first reported in 1920 by Stajano, a Uruguayan physician.[1] However, the syndrome was named after two Americans, Fitz-Hugh and Curtis, who reported their findings without knowledge of Stajano's report. In 1930, Curtis[2] described the presence of "violin string" adhesions between the liver and the anterior abdominal wall among women who also had gross pathological evidence of previous tubal infection. These adhesions were discovered during laparotomies performed for reasons other than acute salpingitis, and he deduced that they were the cause of acute pleuritic upper abdominal pain in other patients he had treated for acute salpingitis.[3] He further reasoned that the chronic tubal and liver abnormalities probably resulted from a prior gonococcal infection.

In 1934, Fitz-Hugh, an internist,[4] described a localized peritonitis of the anterior liver surface, the diaphragm, and the anterior abdominal wall in a patient with upper abdominal pain and tenderness who was undergoing a laparotomy for suspected acute cholecystitis. The gallbladder and the genital organs were normal, and a drainage tube was left in the subhepatic region. Fitz-Hugh reported:

> After cogitating overnight, we decided that what we had seen was probably the acute stage of the process which had been reported in its chronic form by Curtis. Accordingly, smears were made from the drainage tract, and we were promptly rewarded by the finding of a beautiful spread of typical gram negative intracellular biscuit-shaped diplococci.

A biopsy from this patient established the presence of perihepatitis. Inflammation was found confined to the liver capsule with minimal parenchymal involvement. The clinical features, pathophysiology, and differential diagnosis were thoroughly described by Fitz-Hugh, who called the syndrome *acute gonococcal perihepatitis*.[5] A comprehensive review of the early literature on perihepatitis was published by Stanley in 1946.[6] More recent studies suggesting that *Chlamydia trachomatis* may, in fact, be responsible for most cases of perihepatitis are reviewed below.

## ETIOLOGY

It was previously believed that *Neisseria gonorrhoeae* was the only organism responsible for perihepatitis. However, *N. gonorrhoeae* has been isolated from the liver in this syndrome in only a few instances,[7,8] and gram-negative diplococci were demonstrable in perihepatic exudate in only a few additional cases. In reported series of patients only one-third to one-half of patients with clinical Fitz-Hugh–Curtis (FHC) syndrome have had cervical gonococcal infection.[9–11] By modern methods, a single cervical culture is at least 80 percent sensitive in the recovery of *N. gonorrhoeae* among women with acute salpingitis.[12,13] Thus, it is unlikely that *N. gonorrhoeae* was present in the majority of women with salpingitis and perihepatitis who had negative cultures for the organism. The relative absence of data concerning isolation of *N. gonorrhoeae* directly from the surface of the liver may reflect the infrequent number of laparoscopies or laparotomies attempted when this disease is present.

Very little new information of the bacteriology or pathogenesis of the syndrome has been added from the 1930s until recently, when it became apparent that *Chlamydia trachomatis*[9,14–16] can also cause perihepatitis (Table 51-1). Müller-Schoop et al.[14] first reported serological evidence of chlamydial infection among 11 women with peritonitis, including 7 with perihepatitis. Changes in titer of microimmunofluorescent (micro-IF) antibody to *C. trachomatis* consistent with acute *C. trachomatis* infection were observed in 6 of 7 young women with perihepatitis. The relationship between these findings and perihepatitis remained uncertain, because none of the 7 women with perihepatitis had visual evidence of salpingitis. Subsequently, Wølner-Hanssen et al.[15] reported 4 cases of laparoscopically verified salpingitis with perihepatitis; 3 had perihepatitis confirmed during laparoscopy and the fourth had typical right upper quadrant pain without findings of perihepatic inflammation at laparoscopy. Serology was consistent with acute chlamydial infection in all 4 patients, and 3 had *C. trachomatis* recovered from the cervix. *N. gonorrhoeae* was not

**Table 51-1. Microbiological and Serological Evidence of *C. trachomatis* Infection and Microbiologic Evidence of *N. gonorrhoeae* Infection in Women with Acute Perihepatitis**

| | | | | Serodiagnosis of acute chlamydial infection | | | |
|---|---|---|---|---|---|---|---|
| Study | No. of cases | *N. gonorrhoeae* isolated | *C. trachomatis* isolated | IgM titer ≥ 16 | IgG titer ≥ 1024 | IgM or IgG seroconversion or fourfold change in titer | Total with serodiagnosis of acute chlamydial infection |
| Müller-Schoop et al.[14] | 7 | 2 | ND | 5 | 4 | 3/5 | 6 |
| Wølner-Hanssen et al.[15] | 4 | 0/3 | 3/3 | 1 | 2 | 3/4 | 4 |
| Wang et al.[9] | 23 | 7 | 3/10 | 10 | 13 | 14/18 | 20 |
| Paavonen et al.[16] | 15 | 0 | 6/11 | 4 | 7 | 4/11 | 10 |
| Gjønnaess[18] | 18 | 0 | 7 | — | — | — | — |
| Wølner-Hanssen[20] | 13 | 0 | 11/13 | 6/10 | 9* | 10/12* | 10 |
| Darougar[21] | 10 | 0/7 | 1/6 | 9/10 | — | — | — |
| Total | 90 | 9/86(10%) | 31/61(51%) | 26/59(44%) | 44/72(61%) | 34/50(68%) | 50/62(81%) |

*From original data.

isolated from any of the three patients tested. Among 23 consecutive women with acute salpingitis and clinical manifestations of perihepatitis studied in Seattle, *N. gonorrhoeae* was isolated from 7 (30 percent) of 23 and *C. trachomatis* from 3 of 10.[9] Serological evidence of acute *C. trachomatis* infection was found in 20 (87 percent) of the women, including all 12 from whom paired sera were collected at least 6 weeks apart. Only 47 percent of comparison women with clinical salpingitis but without symptoms of perihepatitis had serologic results consistent with acute chlamydial infection. Paavonen et al.[16] recovered *C. trachomatis* from the cervix or urethra of 6 patients but did not recover *N. gonorrhoeae* from the cervix of any of 15 patients with FHC syndrome. Twelve of these 15 had evidence of *C. trachomatis* infection, by either culture or serology (IgM antibody, fourfold change, or a high antibody titer).[16]

In many recent reports, attempts were made to recover *C. trachomatis* and other organisms from the tubes and/or liver surfaces. Dalaker et al.[17] recovered *C. trachomatis* from the cervix and fallopian tubes in 2 of 4 women with salpingitis and perihepatitis. Gjønnaess et al.[18] recovered *C. trachomatis* from the cervix in 7 of 18 women and from the fallopian tubes in 3 of 17 women with perihepatitis. Specimens for bacterial culture were obtained from the liver surface of 9 women, but no organisms were identified in these specimens. None of the 18 women had *N. gonorrhoeae* recovered from the genital tract. Henry-Suchet and coworkers[19] reported recovery of *C. trachomatis* from the liver surface of 5 of 9 of women with perihepatitis. Wølner-Hanssen et al.[20] reported a series of 13 women with laparoscopic evidence of both acute salpingitis and perihepatitis. All women had evidence of *C. trachomatis* infection, but none had positive cultures for *N. gonorrhoeae*. *C. trachomatis* was recovered from the liver surface in 2 of 8 women.

The geometric mean titer of antibody to *C. trachomatis* among seropositive patients is exceptionally high in the FHC syndrome; it is comparable with titers seen in cases of lymphogranuloma venereum. In the Seattle studies, the geometric mean titer was 1:724 in women with FHC syndrome vs. 1:138 in matched comparison women who had pelvic inflammatory disease without FHC syndrome ($p < 0.05$).[9] Similarly, in a Swedish study[19] the geometric mean titer of antibodies to *C. trachomatis* was significantly higher (1:1021) among the women with perihepatitis than among those women with chlamydial salpingitis but without perihepatitis (1:69). Moreover, patients with FHC syndrome more often have IgM antibodies to *C. trachomatis* than those with salpingitis alone. In the Swedish study,[20] IgM antibodies to *C. trachomatis* were detected in 60 percent of patients with perihepatitis and in 9 percent of those who had only salpingitis without perihepatitis. In the Seattle study,[9] 11 (48 percent) of 23 patients with FHC had IgM antibodies to *C. trachomatis*.

In summary, both *N. gonorrhoeae* and *C. trachomatis* have reportedly been isolated from the hepatic area of patients with perihepatitis. There is no evidence that other organisms commonly cause perihepatitis among women with salpingitis. In a tabulation of recently published reports, *N. gonorrhoeae* was isolated from about 10 percent and *C. trachomatis* from about 50 percent of women with perihepatitis (Table 51-1). Serologic evidence of acute *C. trachomatis* infection was present in 81 percent.

## PATHOLOGY

Unfortunately, only a few liver biopsy samples are available for review from humans with perihepatitis. In the first case described by Fitz-Hugh,[4] an acute inflammatory reaction was present on the liver capsule and in the connective tissue adjacent to the capsule. Some regenerating liver cells were also observed in the area.[5] In a case described by Wølner-Hanssen et al., the liver capsule was thickened and had a white blood cell infiltrate and capillary proliferation.[22] In two other reports,[11,23] including the only report in which *N. gonorrhoeae* was recovered from the liver,[11] the liver histology was normal in the area sampled by a needle biopsy. The main histologic changes appear to be confined to the liver capsule.

The gross pathology observed during the early phase of the disease includes areas of purulent and fibrinous peritonitis on the liver capsule and hemorrhagic areas of adjacent parietal peritoneum.[24] Approximated adhesions between the liver surface and the abdominal wall may also be present in acute cases (Fig. 51-1). These adhesions may break during laparoscopy, probably because of abdominal expansion during gas insufflation. Therefore, the liver may sometimes appear normal, but on close inspection, small areas of capillary bleeding on the abdominal peritoneum, and a fibrinous ridge or ring on the liver surface may be found.[8] The characteristic thin, usually avascular, violin string adhesions that have been observed between the liver capsule and the anterior abdominal wall in at least half of the reported cases undoubtedly represent a late stage of perihepatitis[4] (Fig. 51-2 and Plate 18). These adhesions probably persist indefinitely. Subdiaphragmatic abscess has been reported,[25] but it is a rare complication. Liver abscesses have not been associated with *N. gonorrhoeae* or *C. trachomatis* and when present are usually caused by coliform, streptococcal, and mixed aerobic-anaerobic infections, in association with pelvic abscesses or other intraabdominal infections.

## PATHOGENESIS

Experimental *C. trachomatis* perihepatitis has been produced in a grivet monkey[26] by performing a tubal ligation and injecting *C. trachomatis* into the endometrial cavity after curettage. One

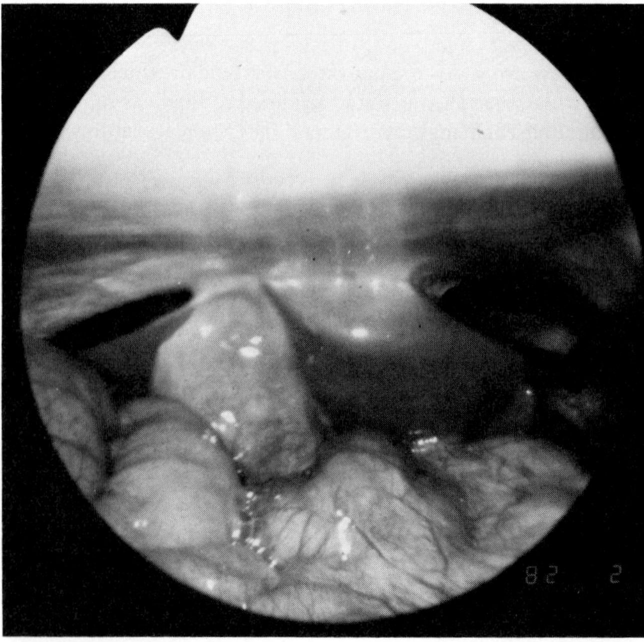

**Fig. 51-1.** Laparoscopic view of an early stage Fitz-Hugh–Curtis syndrome with the liver surface closely adherent to the anterior abdominal wall.

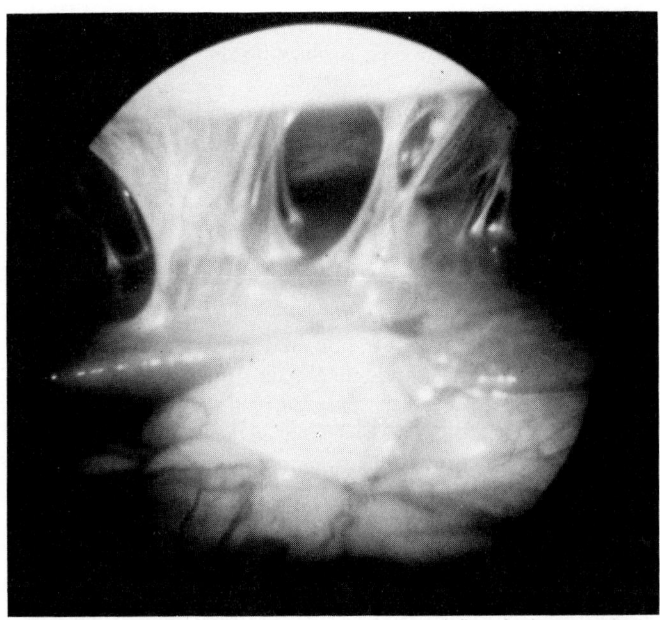

**Fig. 51-2.** Laparoscopic view of a later stage of Fitz-Hugh–Curtis syndrome demonstrating fibrous adhesions, including "violin string adhesions," between the liver surface and the anterior abdominal wall.

of the two monkeys inoculated developed peritonitis and perihepatitis. *C. trachomatis* was recovered from the endometrium but not from the surface of the spleen or intestine of that monkey. The liver was not cultured. Because the fallopian tubes had been ligated, peritonitis could not have been produced by direct tubal spread. However, adnexal blood vessels were surrounded by inflammation, and the liver infection most likely occurred as a result of the spread of endometrial infection through either blood vessels or lymphatics.

Only a minority of women with salpingitis develop perihepatitis. Host factors or microbial virulence factors that predispose to perihepatitis are not well defined. Circumstantial evidence suggests that prior genital infection may predispose to perihepatitis. Many women with gonococcal perihepatitis have previously had gonorrhea and/or salpingitis.[4,6,23] In our studies, women with chlamydia-associated perihepatitis frequently had serologic evidence of a previous infection with a heterologous chlamydial immunotype.[9] Of the 11 patients with clinical perihepatitis associated with IgM antibody to *C. trachomatis*, 7 had serum IgM antibody directed against a serovar of *C. trachomatis* different from the serovar against which the predominant IgG antibody was directed. These data suggest that reinfection with a heterologous immunotype may predispose women to perihepatitis. Recent evidence suggests that repetitive chlamydial infection is associated with an increasingly severe inflammatory reaction in the conjunctiva[27] and in the fallopian tubes.[28] These data support the possibility that FHC results, in part, from an immunopathologic response to repeated chlamydial infections. Oral contraceptive use seems to protect women with *C. trachomatis* or salpingitis from developing perihepatitis.[20] It is possible that sex steroids protect against perihepatitis by reducing the immunologic response to infection.

A further unsettled aspect of the pathogenesis of perihepatitis is the mode of spread of organisms from the pelvis to the liver. Three mechanisms have been proposed: (1) direct intraperitoneal spread, (2) lymphatic spread, and (3) hematogeneous spread. There is evidence that each of these mechanisms could account for transport of organisms from the pelvis to the liver.

Certainly, purulent material from the end of the fallopian tube can collect in the pelvis or among loops of bowel, and purulent material has been observed on the liver surface. In fact, when a woman is supine, the "subhepatic space" represents the most dependent portion of the abdominal cavity above the pelvis, and material from the pelvis would be expected to collect in this space. Mechanisms of peritoneal fluid movement have been thoroughly reviewed.[30] The thin film of peritoneal fluid is drawn by capillary action, peristalsis, and body motion toward the diaphragm. The fluid is drawn into diaphragmatic lacunae, both by a differential pressure gradient between the thoracic and peritoneal cavities and by the action of the diaphragm. From the lacunae the fluid is propelled into and along the thoracic duct by the thoracic movements. Approximately one-quarter of tagged erythrocytes introduced into the pelvis reach the systemic circulation within 48 h through these routes.[30] The possibility of spread of bacteria from the pelvis to the liver surface is suggested by the rapid recovery from the liver surface of particulate matter placed in the pelvis.[31]

The direct transabdominal spread from the fallopian tube to the liver is the most widely recognized route. However, it is clear that alternative hematogenous and lymphatic pathways exist for spread of genital infection to the liver. Perihepatitis has been reported among males with gonococcal urethritis who had tenderness localized to the upper abdomen.[11,32] We have seen perihepatitis develop in women with tubal obstruction from tubal ligation or prior infection, and vascular or lymphatic spread seems more likely than direct peritoneal spread in these cases. Vascular or lymphatic spread is also suggested in the experimental grivet monkey infection model described above.[26] Most lymphatic drainage from the lower abdomen that passes through the liver enters the right portion of the liver, which could explain why the majority of patients with perihepatitis develop only right-sided upper abdominal pain. In fact, evidence for gonococcal lymphatic spread exists, although it seldom is recognized clinically. *N. gonorrhoeae* has been recovered from an inguinal lymph node,[33] and lymphadenopathy has been reported in 102 (36 percent) of 285 males with gonococcal urethritis.[34]

The occurrence of gonococcal bacteremia is, of course, well documented in the gonococcal arthritis-dermatitis syndrome, and tenosynovitis has been reported in patients with clinical manifestations of salpingitis and perihepatitis.[6,31,35,36] *N. gonorrhoeae* was isolated from the blood of one patient with salpingitis, tenosynovitis, typical pustular skin lesions, and right upper abdominal pain and tenderness.[35] These authors considered the concurrence of gonococcemia and perihepatitis to be coincidental. However, the presence of abnormal liver function tests in up to 30 percent of patients with gonococcemia[37,38] suggests hepatitis is common with gonococcemia. Isolation of *C. trachomatis* from blood of patients with perihepatitis has not been attempted, but the high IgG titer to *C. trachomatis* and the high erythrocyte sedimentation rate in these women with perihepatitis[9,10,18,29] may reflect an unusually large amount of chlamydial antigen in the lymphatic and/or blood.

Animal models of gonococcal salpingitis or perihepatitis have not been developed. It has, however, been observed that experimental gonococcal endocarditis in rabbits causes hepatitis with hepatic abscesses,[39] scattered microabscesses containing gonococci, and focal liver cell necrosis.

The vast majority of women who develop perihepatitis have clinical or visual evidence of salpingitis. Even most patients who have "normal" pelvic findings on a physical exam have overt salpingitis when the fallopian tubes are visualized at laparoscopy. However, in some patients who have been explored, no abnormality of the fallopian tubes was observed.[4] In such patients endosalpingitis or endometritis may have been the original source of infection. Alternatively, there is a small proportion of patients who develop FHC syndrome from pelvic infections other than salpingitis. Patients with appendicitis[3] or other abdominal infections occasionally develop perihepatitis.

In summary, at least two organisms, *N. gonorrhoeae* and *C. trachomatis*, have been associated with perihepatitis. The relative importance of the two organisms is uncertain, and the role of other agents, such as mycoplasma, coliforms, and anaerobes, requires further study. Chlamydial reinfection with a new immunotype may especially predispose to perihepatitis. Perihepatitis probably arises from salpingitis through a direct peritoneal spread from the tubes, or by lymphatic and hematogenous routes.

## INCIDENCE

The reported rate of perihepatitis depends upon the criteria used for diagnosis. Jacobsen and Weström have observed pleuritic upper quadrant pain and tenderness among 7 (4 percent) of 190 salpingitis patients with cervical *N. gonorrhoeae* and among 10 (4 percent) of 252 salpingitis patients without cervical *N. gonorrhoeae*.[40] Upper quadrant abdominal pain has been reported among 12 percent of patients with acute salpingitis,[13] but it is not clear how many of these patients had the severe pleuritic pain traditionally associated with FHC syndrome. In a subset of our patients, upper quadrant liver edge tenderness was present in 33 percent of 91 salpingitis patients with and 19 percent of 113 without cervical *N. gonorrhoeae*. Among 137 adolescents with salpingitis,[14] right upper quadrant tenderness or hepatic enlargement was noted among 27 (20 percent) and serum glutamine phosphotransferase was abnormally elevated in 19 (32 percent) of 50.

Applying more stringent criteria for the diagnosis of perihepatitis, Onsrud observed perihepatitis in 38 (14 percent) of 274 patients with laparoscopically verified salpingitis.[24] Of these 38 patients with visualized perihepatitis, 24 had right upper quadrant pain and tenderness. Patients without upper quadrant pain tended to have less pronounced perihepatitis at laparoscopy than the patients with such symptoms. Thus, symptomatic perihepatitis occurred in 9 percent and asymptomatic perihepatitis occurred in 5 percent of the 274 patients with visualized salpingitis.[24] A somewhat lower prevalence was present in another study where 17 (5 percent) of 339 women with laparoscopically confirmed salpingitis also had perihepatitis.[29]

In summary, the diagnosis of perihepatitis has been made on the basis of typical symptoms in up to 20 percent[14] and on the basis of laparoscopic findings in 5 to 15 percent of women with salpingitis[18,29] while liver tenderness and abnormal liver function tests have been found in a larger percentage. Approximately 1 percent of sexually active women are estimated to acquire salpingitis annually. With the high rate of salpingitis occurring in sexually active females between the ages of 15 and 35, perihepatitis undoubtedly becomes one of the common causes, if not the most common cause, of upper quadrant pain in women of this age group.

## CLINICAL MANIFESTATIONS

A clinical diagnosis of perihepatitis should be suspected whenever a sexually active female presents with pleuritic upper quadrant pain. The syndrome occurs almost exclusively among women, although there are reports of men thought to have this syndrome.[11,32] In men, however, perihepatitis has been secondary to gonococcemia.

Usually, the onset of upper quadrant pain is relatively sudden and dramatic. The upper abdominal pain has been most frequently described on the right side. Pain occasionally radiates to the top of the shoulder and, rarely, to the back. The pain is exacerbated by breathing, coughing, or movement of the torso. Most frequently symptoms of lower abdominal pain are present, sometimes with fever, nausea, vomiting, increased vaginal discharge, menorrhagia, dysmenorrhea, or dyspareunia. In 60 percent of patients the onset of upper abdominal pain occurs at the same time as the lower abdominal pain from the salpingitis, but in 30 percent of patients the onset of pain occurs up to 14 days after the lower abdominal pain and in the remainder the pain starts up to 6 days before the lower abdominal pain (Eschenbach, personal observations). However, the upper abdominal pain is commonly so severe that a history of lower abdominal pain caused by salpingitis may not be volunteered by the patient. Symptoms of salpingitis may be so mild that lower abdominal symptoms and signs either are difficult to elicit or are absent. It should be noted that chlamydial salpingitis may be more indolent than gonococcal salpingitis. When the upper abdominal pain is severe, the physician's attention may focus entirely on the possibility of upper abdominal pathology and the diagnosis of salpingitis may be overlooked unless a careful pelvic examination is performed. Infrequently, the initial salpingitis will have been inadequately treated, and the patient will suddenly develop upper abdominal symptoms while receiving antibiotics.

## DIAGNOSIS

As with most patients with overt salpingitis, the pelvic exam usually reveals obvious manifestations of salpingitis, such as cervical, uterine, and adnexal tenderness, but these findings are, in some cases, more subtle. An adnexal mass may be present as the only abnormality of the pelvic examination. Manifestations of gonococcemia, including skin lesions, tenosynovitis, and arthritis occasionally occur.[35] The temperature was elevated above 38°C in 40 percent of patients in one study.[14] This is similar to the rate of fever in patients with salpingitis but no perihepatitis.

Signs of generalized peritonitis may be present. The upper abdominal tenderness and rigidity can be so marked that distinct liver tenderness is impossible to differentiate from generalized peritoneal signs. Liver tenderness is usually demonstrable in patients without generalized peritonitis. A classic friction rub[4] on auscultation over the liver surface is unusual. Scleral icterus should suggest other causes of hepatic disease.

As in uncomplicated salpingitis, the white blood cell count is elevated in only about 30 percent and the sedimentation rate is initially elevated in 30 to 45 percent[13,14] of patients, although in one series 82 percent of women with perihepatitis had an ESR ≥ 30 mm/h.[29] These laboratory abnormalities tend to be found in patients with the most severe and obvious clinical disease. Liver enzyme determinations should be made to exclude the possibility of viral hepatitis. Slight elevations of bilirubin and serum enzymes occur in 25 to 50 percent of patients with perihepatitis.[13,14] The chest x-ray occasionally demonstrates a small amount of pleural fluid. Although the gallbladder is usually visualized during an oral cholecystogram, perihepatitis can occasionally cause nonfilling of the gallbladder. Thus, this test cannot differentiate women with perihepatitis from those with cholecystitis. However, the ultrasound examination of the gallbladder and common bile duct is normal in patients with FHC syndrome. Thus, a normal ultrasound examination of the upper quadrant in the context of right upper quadrant pain in a young woman with abnormal pelvic examination findings is useful to differentiate FHC syndrome from acute cholecystitis.

Endocervical *N. gonorrhoeae* can be demonstrated by Gram stain in about one-half of patients with gonorrhea; a gonorrhea culture is mandatory because it is more sensitive. The presence of intracellular diplococci on Gram stain in a woman with signs and symptoms of perihepatitis is very helpful in supporting the diagnosis. However, *N. gonorrhoeae* has been isolated from the cervix of only 10 percent of women with perihepatitis in recent European studies (Table 51-1), and a failure to recover *N. gonorrhoeae* certainly does not exclude perihepatitis. Cervical and urethral *C. trachomatis* cultures are also necessary. Serologic evidence of acute chlamydial infection can also be obtained by demonstrating the presence of IgM antibody, a rise in antibody titer in serial sera, or a very high (e.g. ≥ 1:1024) titer of IgG antibody in the micro-IF test. In adults, tests for serum antibody to *C. trachomatis* have generally been useful for the diagnosis of lymphogranuloma venereum and Fitz-Hugh–Curtis syndrome, although experience with the latter is limited.

Direct observation of the liver and pelvis through the laparoscope is the most definitive method of diagnosing salpingitis and perihepatitis. Typical findings are described above. Similar findings may also occur on the splenic surface, suggesting that perisplenitis is another manifestation of salpingitis.[41]

## DIFFERENTIAL DIAGNOSIS

It is important to establish a diagnosis accurately and rapidly when severe upper abdominal pain is present because of the wide variety of therapies that are used to treat the diverse causes of upper abdominal pain. Perihepatitis most commonly simulates acute cholecystitis. However, most women with cholecystitis are older in contrast to patients with salpingitis, who are usually between the ages of 15 and 25.

Viral hepatitis is a common disease among young women. Among women with mild liver tenderness and liver enzyme elevations, serologic tests for hepatitis A and B should be performed, in addition to tests for infectious mononucleosis. Other diseases with potentially similar clinical manifestations include hepatitis non-A, non-B, alcoholic hepatitis, drug-induced hepatitis, secondary syphilis, toxic shock syndrome, and hepatitis caused by various types of bacteremia.

Because of the pleuritic component and occasional referral of the pain to the right shoulder or subcapsular area, pneumonia, pleuritis, or pleurodynia must also be considered. If posterior back pain is present, acute pyelonephritis or a perinephric abscess must be excluded. Other diagnoses which have been mistaken for the disease include perforated gastric or duodenal ulcer, acute pancreatitis, and liver or subdiaphragmatic abscess. Primary intra-abdominal infections other than salpingitis (e.g., appendicitis) also need to be excluded in the patient with perihepatitis.

Clues that favor a diagnosis of perihepatitis in a woman with right upper quadrant pain include young age, acute or subacute onset of severe pain, pleuritic pain, right upper quadrant localization of pain (as opposed to biliary colic with midepigastric localization), negative hepatitis A and B serologic studies, demonstration of mucopurulent cervicitis, uterine and adnexal tenderness on pelvic examination, and a normal ultrasound examination of the gallbladder. However, some of the diseases which can masquerade as perihepatitis cannot be excluded without surgical exploration, and occasionally a surgical disease such as appendicitis can produce perihepatitis.[3] Thus, visual confirmation of perihepatitis is desirable. A therapeutic trial of antimicrobials can support the diagnosis but should be preceded by laparoscopy whenever possible.

## THERAPY

Standard treatment regimens recommended for salpingitis (see Chap. 49) are adequate also for treatment of perihepatitis. For perihepatitis, we recommend use of doxycycline, 100 mg bid together with cefoxitin 2 g qid, both given intravenously for at least 4 days. After a definite clinical response occurs, doxycycline should be given orally to complete a total of 14 days of therapy. It is likely that most of the upper abdominal pain results from the acute liver capsule inflammation, because the pain usually resolves rapidly following antibiotic therapy. The acute pain also resolves rapidly when therapy is started even in patients who have already formed firm liver adhesions. These liver adhesions usually persist indefinitely, and as Curtis discovered, they frequently are incidentally discovered in asymptomatic patients years after the perihepatitis has occurred. However, some patients will continue to have upper quadrant pain following adequate antibiotic therapy. This pain may be pleuritic and tends to be exacerbated by motion which stretches the adhesions. Occasionally, patients with chronic right upper quadrant pain require laparoscopic lysis of the adhesions.[42]

# References


1 Stajano C: La reacción frénica en ginecologia. *Sem Med* 27:243, 1920.
2 Curtis AH: A cause of adhesions in the right upper quadrant. *JAMA* 94:1221, 1930.
3 Curtis AH: Adhesions of the anterior surface of the liver. *JAMA* 99: 2010, 1932.
4 Fitz-Hugh T Jr: Acute gonococcic peritonitis of the right upper quadrant in women. *JAMA* 102:2094, 1934.
5 Fitz-Hugh T Jr: Acute gonococcic perihepatitis: A new syndrome of right upper quadrant abdominal pain in young women. *Rev Gastroenterol* 3:125, 1936.
6 Stanley MM: Gonococcic peritonitis of the upper part of the abdomen in young women. *Arch Intern Med* 78:1, 1946.
7 Kimball LW, Knee S: Gonococcal perihepatitis in a male. *N Engl J Med* 282:1082, 1970.
8 Mauro E: Le syndrome abdominal droit supérieur au cours des annexites gonococciques (syndrome de Fitz-Hugh). *Presse Med* 46: 1919, 1938.
9 Wang SP et al: *Chlamydia trachomatis* infection in Fitz-Hugh–Curtis syndrome. *Am J Obstet Gynecol* 139:1034, 1980.
10 Semchyshyn S: Fitz-Hugh and Curtis syndrome. *J Reprod Med* 22: 45, 1979.
11 Litt IF, Cohen MI: Perihepatitis associated with salpingitis in adolescents. *JAMA* 240:1253, 1978.
12 Eschenbach DA et al: Polymicrobial etiology of acute pelvic inflammatory disease. *N Engl J Med* 293:166, 1975.
13 Sweet RL et al: Etiology of acute salpingitis: Influence of episode number and duration of symptoms. *Obstet Gynecol* 58:62, 1981.
14 Müller-Schoop JW et al: *Chlamydia trachomatis* as possible cause of peritonitis and perihepatitis in young women. *Br Med J* 1:1022, 1978.
15 Wølner-Hanssen P et al: Perihepatitis and chlamydial salpingitis. *Lancet* 1:901, 1980.
16 Paavonen J et al: Association of *Chlamydia trachomatis* infection with Fitz-Hugh–Curtis syndrome. *J Infect Dis* 144:176, 1981.

17 Dalaker K et al: *Chlamydia trachomatis* as a cause of acute perihepatitis associated with pelvic inflammatory disease. *Br J Vener Dis* 57:41, 1981.

18 Gjønnaess H et al: Pelvic inflammatory disease. Etiological studies with emphasis on chlamydial infection. *Obstet Gynecol* 59:550, 1982.

19 Henry-Suchet J et al: Peri-hepatites (syndrome de Fitz-Hugh Curtis) infra-clinques au cours de salpingites ou de sterilites tubaires. Cultures positives pour *Chlamydia trachomatis* dans les adherences perihepatiques. *Presse Med* 12:1725, 1983.

20 Wølner-Hanssen P: Oral contraceptive use modifies the manifestations of pelvic inflammatory disease. *Br J Obstet Gynecol* 93:619, 1986.

21 Darougar S et al.: Chlamydia and the Curtis–Fitz-Hugh syndrome. *Br J Vener Dis* 57:391, 1981.

22 Wølner-Hanssen P et al: Chlamydial perihepatitis. *Scand J Infect Dis* 32 (suppl):77, 1982.

23 Vickers FN, Maloney PJ: Gonococcal perihepatitis. *Arch Intern Med* 114:120, 1964.

24 Onsrud M: Perihepatitis in pelvic inflammatory disease associated with intrauterine contraception. *Acta Obstet Gynecol Scand* 59:69, 1980.

25 Scott GD: Subdiaphragmatic gonorrheal abscess. *JAMA* 96:1681, 1931.

26 Møller BR, Mårdh P-A: Experimental salpingitis in grivet monkeys by *Chlamydia trachomatis. Acta Pathol Microbiol Scand* [B] 88: 107, 1980.

27 Wang SP, Grayston JT: Local and systemic antibody response to trachoma eye infections in monkeys, in *Trachoma and Related Disorders Caused by Chlamydial Agents*, RE Nichols (ed). Amsterdam, Excerpta Medica, 1971, p 217.

28 Wølner-Hanssen P et al: Severe salpingitis in pig-tailed macaques after repeated cervical infections followed by a single tubal inoculation with *Chlamydia trachomatis,* in *Chlamydial Infections,* D Oriel, G Ridgway, J Schachter, D Taylor-Robinson, M Ward (eds). Proceedings of the Sixth International Symposium on Human Chlamydial Infections. Cambridge, Cambridge University Press, 1986, p 371.

29 Wølner-Hanssen P: Pathogenesis and manifestations of chlamydial pelvic inflammatory disease. Thesis, University of Lund, Lund, 1985.

30 Schildt BE, Eiseman B: Peritoneal absorption of $Cr_{51}$ tagged erythrocytes: Its influence by pneumoperitoneum and Fowlers position. *Acta Chir Scand* 119:397, 1960.

31 Courtice FC, Simonds WJ: Physiological significance of lymph drainage of the serous cavities and lungs. *Physiol Rev* 34:419, 1954.

32 Francis TI, Osoba AO: Gonococcal perihepatitis (Fitz-Hugh–Curtis syndrome) in a male patient. *Br J Vener Dis* 48:187, 1972.

33 Dahl R, Dans PE: Gonococcal lymphadenitis. *Arch Intern Med* 134: 1116, 1974.

34 Akers WA: Tender inguinal lymph nodes and gonococcal urethritis. *Milit Med* 137:107, 1972.

35 Lassus A, Kousa M: Gonococcal perihepatitis and gonococcaemia: Presentation of a case with cutaneous manifestations. *Br J Vener Dis* 49:48, 1973.

36 von Knorring J, Nieminen J: Gonococcal perihepatitis in a surgical ward. *Ann Clin Res* 11:66, 1979.

37 Holmes KK et al: Disseminated gonococcal infection. *Ann Intern Med* 74:979, 1971.

38 Williams RH: Gonococcal endocarditis: A study of 12 cases with 10 postmortem examinations. *Arch Intern Med* 61:26, 1938.

39 Kaspar RL, Drutz DJ: Perihepatitis and hepatitis as complications of experimental endocarditis due to *Neisseria gonorrhoeae* in the rabbit. *J Infect Dis* 136:37, 1977.

40 Jacobsen L, Weström L: Objectivized diagnosis of acute pelvic inflammatory disease. *Am J Obstet Gynecol* 105:1088, 1969.

41 Gatt D, Jantet G: Perisplenitis and perinephritis in the Curtis–Fitz-Hugh syndrome. *Br J Surg* 74:110, 1987.

42 Reichert JA, Valle RF: Fitz-Hugh–Curtis syndrome, a laparoscopic approach. *JAMA* 236:266, 1976.

# Chapter 52
# Urethritis in males

William R. Bowie

## DEFINITIONS

Urethritis, manifested by urethral discharge, dysuria, or itching at the end of the urethra, is the response of the urethra to inflammation of any etiology. The characteristic physical finding is urethral discharge, and the pathognomonic confirmatory laboratory finding is an increased number of polymorphonuclear leukocytes (PMN) on Gram stain of a urethral smear or in the sediment of the first-voided urine. Urethritis is called gonococcal, or gonorrhea, when *Neisseria gonorrhoeae* is detected, and nongonococcal if *N. gonorrhoeae* cannot be detected. The term nongonococcal urethritis (NGU) is preferable to the term nonspecific urethritis, because NGU has specific causes and some of these have been elucidated. Of these, *Chlamydia trachomatis* and *Ureaplasma urealyticum* are the most frequent. NGU occurring soon after curative therapy for urethral gonorrhea is called postgonococcal urethritis (PGU).

## HISTORY

In the 1800s, even prior to the discovery of *N. gonorrhoeae,* the existence of several types of urethritis was already suspected. By the 1880s, after isolation of *N. gonorrhoeae* and introduction of the Gram stain, differentiation of gonococcal from nongonococcal urethritis became possible. In the early 1900s, intracytoplasmic inclusions which today are considered characteristic of chlamydiae were seen in urethral smears of some men with urethritis. The development which had the greatest impact on clinical differentiation of gonococcal and nongonococcal urethritis, however, was the introduction of the sulfonamides and penicillins for treatment of urethritis. With penicillin in particular, gonococcal urethritis was curable, but NGU usually was not. Progress in therapy of NGU came with introduction of tetracyclines and macrolides. Further insight into the etiology of NGU came with the discovery of *Ureaplasma urealyticum* in 1954[1] and the development of cell culture isolation techniques for *Chlamydia trachomatis* in 1965.[2] Treatment recommendations for gonorrhea are now undergoing significant revisions because of dramatic increases in gonococcal resistance to penicillins and tetracyclines.[3,4]

## ETIOLOGY

Organisms that are proved or possible causes of sexually transmitted urethritis are listed in Table 52-1.

### *Neisseria gonorrhoeae*

The causal role of *N. gonorrhoeae* in male urethritis is well established and is reviewed in Chap. 14. Several aspects which are important for management of urethritis deserve reemphasis here. These include the frequency of asymptomatic infection, the increasing resistance of isolates of *N. gonorrhoeae* to traditional treatments, and the high frequency of concurrent *C. trachomatis* infection. Although most new cases of gonococcal urethritis are symptomatic, many studies have emphasized that gonococcal urethritis can be asymptomatic or minimally symptomatic.[5] As many as two-thirds of men in the community who are found to have urethral gonorrhea by routine screening or by contact tracing have no symptoms at all, or they have such mild symptoms that they are able to ignore them. These are the men who are most likely to remain sexually active and to spread gonorrhea. Asymptomatic men appear especially likely to have the arginine, hypoxanthine, and uracil requiring auxotrophs of *N. gonorrhoeae* that are often associated with disseminated gonococcal infection.[6]

Gradually increasing resistance of *N. gonorrhoeae* to penicillins in the 1950s, 1960s, and 1970s resulted in the need for progressively higher doses of penicillins in conjunction with probenecid to obtain a cure. In 1976, penicillinase-producing *N. gonorrhoeae* (PPNG), which were totally resistant to penicillin on the basis of plasmid-mediated β-lactamase production were recognized. These isolates were initially most prevalent in Southeast Asia and Africa but have now spread worldwide. More recently, chromosomally mediated resistance to penicillin has reached a level in some strains (chromosomally mediated resistant *N. gonorrhoeae,* CMRNG) where even the large doses of penicillin currently used do not reliably eradicate *N. gonorrhoeae.*[7] Finally, high-level resistance to tetracycline is being seen with increasing frequency in gonococci (tetracycline-resistant *N. gonorrhoeae,* TRNG).[8] These isolates are usually penicillin-sensitive. Antimicrobial resistance in gonococci is discussed further in Chaps. 13 and 14

### *Chlamydia trachomatis*

Multiple types of evidence indicate that *C. trachomatis* is a major cause of NGU and PGU (Ref. 9 and Chap. 16). Key evidence is summarized below.

#### Isolation

Studies have repeatedly shown that *C. trachomatis* can be isolated from the urethras of 25 to 60 percent (usually 30 to 40 percent)

**Table 52-1. Etiology of Sexually Transmitted Urethritis in Males**

- Gonococcal:
  - *Neisseria gonorrhoeae*
- Nongonococcal:
  - *Chlamydia trachomatis,* 30–50%
  - *Ureaplasma urealyticum,* 10–40%
  - Neither, 20–30%
    - *Trichomonas vaginalis,* rare
    - Yeasts, rare
    - Herpes simplex virus, rare
    - Adenoviruses, rare
    - *Haemophilus* sp., rare
    - *Bacteroides ureolyticus* ?
    - *Mycoplasma genitalium* ?
    - Other bacterial ?
    - Other ???

**Table 52-2. Recovery of *C. trachomatis* from Males with Nongonococcal Urethritis (NGU), Gonococcal Urethritis (GU), Postgonococcal Urethritis (PGU), and Symptomless Controls**

| Country | Investigator | Year | NGU* | GU* | PGU* | Controls* | References |
|---|---|---|---|---|---|---|---|
| U.K. | Dunlop et al. | 1972 | 44/99 (44) | | | | 10 |
| U.K. | Oriel et al. | 1972 | 49/135 (36) | | | 0/31 (0) | 11 |
| U.K. | Richmond et al. | 1972 | 40/103 (39) | 32/99 (32) | 17/21 (81) | 5/92 (5) | 12 |
| U.K. | Oriel et al. | 1975 | | 15/44 (34) | 11/23 (48) | | 13 |
| U.K. | Oriel et al. | 1975 | 33/133 (25) | | | | 14 |
| U.S.A. | Schacter et al. | 1975 | 27/76 (36) | 2/18 (11) | | 0/57 (0) | 15 |
| U.S.A. | Smith et al. | 1975 | 34/131 (26) | | | | 16 |
| U.S.A. | Holmes et al. | 1975 | 48/113 (42) | 13/69 (19) | 12/20 (60) | 4/58 (7) | 17 |
| U.K. | Oriel et al. | 1976 | 125/262 (48) | 35/141 (25) | | 3/74 (4) | 18 |
| U.K. | Prentice et al. | 1976 | 43/136 (32) | | | | 19 |
| U.S.A. | Bowie et al. | 1976 | 36/91 (40) | | | | 20 |
| Sweden | Johannisson et al. | 1977 | 44/103 (43) | | 11/15 (73) | | 21 |
| U.K. | Alani et al. | 1977 | 116/385 (30) | 13/118 (11) | 9/59 (15) | | 22 |
| U.K. | Vaughan-Jackson et al. | 1977 | | 30/95 (32) | 26/49 (53) | | 23 |
| U.S.A. | Bowie et al. | 1977 | 23/69 (33) | | | 1/39 (3) | 24 |
| U.S.A. | Segura et al. | 1977 | 71/180 (39) | | | | 25 |
| U.S.A. | Wong et al. | 1977 | 21/67 (31) | 4/99 (4) | | 3/85 (4) | 26 |
| Finland | Paavonen et al. | 1978 | 39/75 (52) | | | | 27 |
| Finland | Terho | 1978 | 93/159 (58) | | | 0/64 (0) | 28 |
| Finland | Terho | 1978 | | 38/133 (29) | 30/50 (60) | | 29 |
| Norway | Csango | 1978 | 36/81 (44) | | | | 30 |
| Sweden | Ripa et al. | 1978 | 74/284 (26) | 15/88 (17) | | | 31 |
| Switzerland | Perroud et al. | 1978 | 124/238 (52) | 32/139 (23) | 15/19 (79) | 1/40 (3) | 32 |
| U.S.A. | Bowie et al. | 1978 | | 23/121 (18) | 10/26 (38) | | 33 |
| U.S.A. | Bowie et al. | 1978 | 78/211 (37) | | | | 34 |
| U.S.A. | Smith et al. | 1978 | | 31/143 (22) | | | 35 |
| U.S.A. | Swartz et al. | 1978 | 35/107 (33) | 12/61 (20) | | 6/112 (5) | 36 |
| Finland | Lassus et al. | 1979 | 75/181 (45) | | | | 37 |
| U.K. | Coufalik et al. | 1979 | 93/217 (43) | | | | 38 |
| U.K. | Taylor-Robinson et al. | 1979 | 263/726 (36) | | | | 39 |
| Canada | Bowie et al. | 1980 | 80/200 (40) | | | | 40 |
| U.S.A. | Root et al. | 1980 | 19/96 (20) | | | | 41 |

*Number culture-positive/number examined (percent culture-positive).

of men who have NGU, 4 to 35 percent (usually 15 to 25 percent) of men with urethral gonorrhea, and 0 to 7 percent of men without obvious urethritis (Table 52-2). When asymptomatic men are screened to exclude the presence of pyuria, the rate of isolation is only 0 to 3 percent.[24] However, in one study of 97 asymptomatic United States military men, *C. trachomatis* was isolated from 11 men, whereas *N. gonorrhoeae* was isolated from only two.[42] *C. trachomatis* is less frequently isolated from homosexual men with NGU.[34]

## Serologic studies

Most patients with NGU who are seen in sexually transmitted disease (STD) clinics have existing antibody to *C. trachomatis* demonstrable in acute-phase sera by microimmunofluorescence (micro-IF), and it is unusual to document seroconversion or a fourfold increase in micro-IF antibody in such patients.[17] However, in a highly selected group of men with NGU who had relatively few sex partners and no previous history of urethritis, 9 of 10 men who were culture-positive for *C. trachomatis* and who were symptomatic for less than 10 days seroconverted.[24] IgM micro-IF antibody, a transiently detectable antibody that allows diagnosis of recent infection despite preexisting antibody, was detected in specimens from 16 of 20 men whose cultures were *C. trachomatis*-positive, compared with 3 of 39 patients with NGU whose cultures were negative ($p < 0.0001$).[24] These results indicated that recent acquisition of chlamydia, rather than reactivation of latent infection, was associated with urethritis.

## Postgonococcal urethritis

PGU provides an opportunity for prospective assessment of the ability of *C. trachomatis* to produce urethritis. Gonorrhea has a shorter incubation period than chlamydial urethritis, so that men with both infections can present with gonorrhea while the chlamydial urethritis is still incubating. When gonorrhea is treated with antimicrobials—such as penicillin, ampicillin, ceftriaxone, single-dose fluoroquinolones, or spectinomycin—that do not eradicate *C. trachomatis*, PGU develops in most men who have concurrent *C. trachomatis* infections (Table 52-2), and the rate of development of PGU is much greater in patients infected with *C. trachomatis* than in men with gonorrhea without *C. trachomatis* infection. The rate of development of PGU is lower if an antimicrobial such as tetracycline that is active against *C. trachomatis* is used.

## Studies of various treatments

Other evidence supporting the role of *C. trachomatis* as a urethral pathogen is that its selective eradication results in alleviation of urethritis in men infected with *C. trachomatis*.[20,24,38] Use of sulfonamides or rifampin, which are active against *C. trachomatis* but overall have a poor record in the treatment of NGU, resulted in clinical responses in most men infected with *C. trachomatis*, but in a significantly smaller proportion of men without *C. trachomatis*.[20,24,38] However, a better response in *C. trachomatis*-positive NGU patients than in chlamydia-negative NGU is also observed with a broader-spectrum antimicrobial, tetracycline.[43]

Persistence or recurrence of NGU within 6 weeks of initiation of a 7-day course of tetracycline, 2 g per day, was seen in 17 percent of men whose cultures were *C. trachomatis*-positive, compared with 47 percent of those whose cultures were *C. trachomatis*-negative ($p = 0.01$). In a subsequent study with minocycline, persistent or recurrent NGU developed within 6 weeks of initiation of therapy in 17 percent of 78 *C. trachomatis*-positive men compared with 35 percent of 133 men without *C. trachomatis* infection ($p < 0.005$).[34]

### Urethral inoculation of primates

When the urethra of a nonhuman primate is infected experimentally,[44] discharge and pyuria are not usually detected. However, urethral follicles develop, and urethral cultures may remain positive for *C. trachomatis* for as long as 3 months.

## ETIOLOGY OF *C. trachomatis*-NEGATIVE NGU

Several types of data indicate that *C. trachomatis* is usually not the cause of urethritis when *C. trachomatis* is not isolated. If men had false-negative cultures, further culture attempts might eventually demonstrate the organism. However, when initial urethral specimens are negative for *C. trachomatis,* they usually remain negative when the patients are followed without treatment.[43] Cervical cultures from female sex partners of men with *C. trachomatis*-negative NGU are likely to be *C. trachomatis*-negative.[11,17,22,27,37] In most cases of *C. trachomatis* culture-negative NGU there is no serological evidence of recent *C. trachomatis* infection.[24] *C. trachomatis*-negative NGU responds poorly to certain antimicrobials which are active against *C. trachomatis.* Sulfonamides, rifampin, and tetracyclines produce much poorer responses in *C. trachomatis*-negative than in *C. trachomatis*-positive NGU.[20,24,34,38,40,43]

### *Ureaplasma urealyticum*

#### Isolation

The most likely cause of many *C. trachomatis*-negative cases of NGU is *U. urealyticum.* Case-control studies of the association of *U. urealyticum* with NGU must account for the fact that urethral colonization is common in men without urethritis, and is strongly correlated with the total number of female sex partners.[45] In general, *U. urealyticum* has been isolated more often from patients with NGU than from control groups when the control group was less sexually active than the NGU group, but not when the sexual activity of the two groups was comparable (reviewed by McCormack et al.[46]). The serum antibody response to *U. urealyticum* in NGU has not been as impressive as the antibody response to *C. trachomatis.*[24]

However, other evidence is consistent with a pathogenic role for *U. urealyticum.* When men with relatively few sex partners and no previous episodes of urethritis were studied, the rate of isolation and concentration of *U. urealyticum* in first-voided urine were significantly greater in men with *C. trachomatis*-negative NGU than in those with *C. trachomatis*-positive NGU, or in a comparison group without urethritis.[24] In that study the comparison group without urethritis had actually had more sex partners than the other groups.[24] Results in other studies are shown in Table 52-3. Although cases were not stratified by history of urethritis or number of sex partners in some studies, *U. urealyticum* was isolated more often from *C. trachomatis*-negative than from *C. trachomatis*-positive NGU patients in many of these studies. Data compiled from three Seattle studies[20,24,34] showed that *U. urealyticum* was isolated significantly more often from men with a first episode of urethritis than from those who had had previous episodes or from men without urethritis; and among men with NGU, *U. urealyticum* was isolated more often from men with five or fewer sex partners than from those with six or more partners.

#### Studies of various treatments

The results of selective eradication of *U. urealyticum* also support a pathogenic role in NGU. Sulfonamides and rifampin are active against *C. trachomatis,* but not against *U. urealyticum,* whereas spectinomycin and streptomycin are active against *U. urealyticum,* but not against *C. trachomatis.* In men whose cultures were *C. trachomatis*-negative but *U. urealyticum*-positive, the urethritis responded poorly to sulfonamides and rifampin.[20,24,38] Urethritis responded well to streptomycin or spectinomycin when *U. urealyticum* was eradicated, but not when *U. urealyticum* persisted.[20] In other studies, Shepard, using suboptimal doses of doxycycline to treat patients with NGU, showed that with the disappearance of *U. urealyticum,* symptoms disappeared and with the reappearance of *U. urealyticum,* symptoms recurred.[47] Cultures for *C. trachomatis* were not performed in this study, however. In another study, NGU persisted 6 to 12 days after onset of minocycline therapy significantly more often in men infected with tetracycline-resistant *U. urealyticum* than in those infected with tetracycline-sensitive *U. urealyticum,* and persistent NGU correlated with persistence of the tetracycline-resistant strains.[48] Root et al. also demonstrated that there was a strong correlation between the tetracycline resistance of *U. urea-*

**Table 52-3. Recovery of *C. trachomatis* (C) and *U. urealyticum* (U) from Men with NGU**

| Country | Investigator | Year | C+U+ | C+U− | C−U+ | C−U− | Number | Reference |
|---|---|---|---|---|---|---|---|---|
| U.S.A. | Holmes et al. | 1975 | 29 (26)* | 19 (17) | 41 (36) | 24 (21) | 113 | 17 |
| U.K. | Prentice et al. | 1976 | 9 (11) | 16 (20) | 38 (47) | 18 (22) | 81 | 19 |
| U.S.A. | Bowie et al. | 1976 | 21 (23) | 15 (16) | 42 (46) | 13 (14) | 91 | 20 |
| U.S.A. | Bowie et al. | 1977 | 11 (16) | 15 (22) | 35 (51) | 8 (12) | 69 | 24 |
| U.S.A. | Wong et al. | 1977 | 4 (13) | 8 (27) | 12 (40) | 6 (20) | 30 | 26 |
| Finland | Paavonen et al. | 1978 | 11 (15) | 28 (37) | 10 (13) | 26 (35) | 75 | 27 |
| U.S.A. | Bowie et al. | 1978 | 38 (18) | 40 (19) | 87 (41) | 46 (22) | 211 | 34 |
| U.K. | Coufalik et al. | 1979 | 58 (27) | 35 (16) | 70 (32) | 54 (25) | 217 | 38 |
| U.K. | Taylor-Robinson et al. | 1979 | 138 (19) | 125 (17) | 246 (34) | 217 (30) | 726 | 39 |
| Canada | Bowie et al. | 1980 | 22 (11) | 58 (29) | 73 (37) | 47 (24) | 200 | 40 |
| U.S.A. | Root et al. | 1980 | 8 (8) | 11 (11) | 50 (52) | 27 (28) | 96 | 41 |

*Number in subgroup (percent of total study).

*lyticum* and the persistence of *U. urealyticum* after tetracycline treatment.[41]

## Urethral inoculation of primates

Intraurethral inoculation of *U. urealyticum* has been performed in two men and several nonhuman primates. The first man developed dysuria and frequency of urination, associated with pyuria and positive cultures for *U. urealyticum.*[49] Symptoms and signs disappeared with eradication of the *U. urealyticum* by minocycline. The second man developed urine containing mucus threads containing PMN which persisted after minocycline treatment despite the eradication of *U. urealyticum.*[49] Intraurethral inoculation of *U. urealyticum* into nonhuman primates has resulted in colonization of the urethra for various periods of time and was associated with increased numbers of PMN leukocytes on endourethral smear in some animals.[50,51]

## Serotyping

There are at least 14 serovars of *U. urealyticum.*[52] It is possible that only one or several of the serovars produce urethritis. Shepard found serovar 4 in 52 percent of 122 isolates from men with NGU, compared with 25 percent of 125 isolates from asymptomatic, but not necessarily normal, men.[53] Other data also indicated that *U. urealyticum* serovar 4 was frequently associated with asymptomatic pyuria as well.[53] However, while some groups have also demonstrated an association of urethritis with serovar 4,[54] others have not.[55,56]

## Postgonococcal urethritis

In contrast to the strong association between PGU and *C. trachomatis,* the association between PGU and *U. urealyticum* is weak. Among *C. trachomatis*-negative men with gonorrhea who received treatment with penicillins, which are not active against *U. urealyticum,* PGU developed in 11 (61 percent) of 18 who had *U. urealyticum* compared with 5 (28 percent) of 18 without *U. urealyticum* infection ($p = 0.09$).[33] In two other studies involving cultures for *C. trachomatis* and *U. urealyticum, U. urealyticum* was not shown to be associated with PGU.[17,23]

The accumulated evidence cited above is consistent with a role for *U. urealyticum* as a urethral pathogen, but it does not prove that *U. urealyticum* is a cause of urethritis, it does not establish what proportion of urethritis cases can be attributed to this agent, and it does not resolve the question as to why colonization with *U. urealyticum* so often occurs without apparent urethritis. It is possible that only certain serovars produce urethritis, that urethritis occurs predominantly on first exposure to *U. urealyticum,* that only a proportion of men colonized by *U. urealyticum* are susceptible to development of urethritis, or that urethritis produced by *U. urealyticum* is frequently subclinical and self-limited.

# OTHER CAUSES OF NGU

## Bacteria

Even if both *C. trachomatis* and *U. urealyticum* are etiologic agents in NGU, 20 to 30 percent of heterosexual men with NGU have neither organism initially isolated (Table 52-3). Most homosexual men with NGU actually have neither organism isolated.[34] The observation that *C. trachomatis*-negative, *U. urealyticum*-negative men responded least well to therapy with a tetracycline is consistent with a different etiology in these men. Of 46 such men, NGU persisted or recurred within 6 weeks after initiation of minocycline therapy in 24, or 52 percent.[34] All but one of these 24 men actually improved during minocycline therapy but subsequently had recurrent NGU soon after stopping therapy. This failure rate was significantly greater than that for men from whom *C. trachomatis* or *U. urealyticum* was initially isolated. Prentice et al. also found that men from whom neither organism was initially isolated showed good responses to treatment on short-term follow-up.[19] This initial response to therapy is consistent with but does not prove a bacterial or mycoplasmal etiology of *C. trachomatis*-negative *U. urealyticum*-negative NGU.

Most studies of the aerobic and anaerobic urethral flora have not yet revealed significant differences between *C. trachomatis*-positive and *C. trachomatis*-negative patients with NGU.[36,57] Because organisms were classified in broad taxonomic categories, it is possible that some subgroups of pathogenic organisms were not identified. However, seeking specific organisms, there are preliminary data supporting a possible role for *Bacteroides ureolyticus*[58,59] and another genital mycoplasma, *M. genitalium.*[60] These can be recovered from men with urethritis and can produce urethritis in some animal models, but their role and frequency as putative causes of urethritis are uncertain. *Haemophilus influenzae* and *Haemophilus parainfluenzae* are likely real but infrequent causes of urethritis.[61] Similarly, coliforms may cause a few cases of urethritis in homosexual men.[62] Other organisms have been proposed as potential causes of NGU, but their role has either not been assessed by others (*Haemophilus equigenitalis,* the agent of contagious equine metritis[63]) or has not been confirmed by other groups (*Staphylococcus saprophyticus*[57,64,65] and *Corynebacterium genitalium* type 1[65,66]).

## Viruses

Urethritis occurs in approximately 30 percent of men with primary genital herpes simplex virus (HSV) infection, and in a much lower percentage of men with recurrent genital HSV infection.[67] Most such patients have penile lesions, but some cases of NGU are due to HSV not associated with genital lesions. However, in comparative studies, HSV was not isolated at higher frequency from men with NGU than from controls.[17,26] In one study, HSV was isolated from 2 percent of 115 men with NGU, 6 percent of 53 men with gonorrhea, and 3 percent of 62 men without urethritis.[17] Cytomegalovirus was not isolated from any of 60 men with NGU, 28 men with gonorrhea, or 20 men without urethritis.[17] Multiple other attempts to isolate viruses from men with NGU have usually been unrewarding, although adenoviruses have repeatedly been isolated from men with urethritis in Perth.[68]

## Parasites and yeasts

*Trichomonas vaginalis* has been implicated in a surprisingly high proportion of NGU cases in the Soviet Union, India, and Africa and in a few surveys done in South America. This has not been the experience of most European countries or in North America. It remains possible that there are regional differences in the role of *T. vaginalis* in NGU. Future studies of the etiology of NGU in countries that report high rates of documented *T. vaginalis* should employ simultaneous cultures for both *T. vaginalis* and *C. trachomatis.*

The proportion of cases of NGU in which *T. vaginalis* was detected was small in four recent North American studies.[17,26,57,69] In one of these, however, 9 (11 percent) of 85 men with NGU demonstrated seroconversion or increased indirect hemagglutination titers to *T. vaginalis* (≥ 1:80) in paired sera.[69] The response of their urethritis to metronidazole was not determined.

In the first three studies,[17,26,57] yeasts were rarely detected, and although some men with yeast balanitis have symptoms of urethritis, yeasts are not a frequent cause of NGU.

### Nonsexually transmitted causes of NGU

The proportion of cases of NGU that are nonsexually transmitted has not been defined since the recognition of *C. trachomatis* as a cause of NGU. Bacterial urethritis may occur in association with urinary tract infection, bacterial prostatitis, urethral stricture, phimosis, and secondary to catheterization or other instrumentation of the urethra. Urethritis is also described with congenital abnormalities, chemical irritation, and tumors. Allergic etiologies have been postulated, but the supporting evidence is very meager. Similarly, there is no proof as yet that repeated stripping of the penis, masturbation, or use of caffeine, alcohol, too little or too much sexual activity, or eating of certain foods will result in urethritis. Stevens-Johnson syndrome may produce urethritis (Plate 3).

## EPIDEMIOLOGY

As discussed in Chapters 2 and 16, the incidence of NGU has surpassed that of gonococcal urethritis in men in the United States (where the incidence of NGU has been stable for several years, while that of gonococcal urethritis has been falling); and also in England in Wales (where the incidence of NGU continues to rise, while that of gonococcal urethritis is falling). To some extent the relative increase in number of cases of NGU is likely related to altered patterns of recognition and reporting,[70] but NGU is clearly more frequent than gonococcal urethritis.

In individual STD clinics the relative proportion of cases of urethritis that are nongonococcal has varied from 19 to 78 percent.[71] On college campuses, more than 85 percent of urethritis is nongonococcal.[72] Data on the rates of chlamydial and *U. urealyticum*-associated urethritis are not available.

For both gonorrhea and NGU, the peak age group affected is 20 to 24 years, followed by 15 to 19 years, and then by the 25- to 29-year-old group.

Some characteristics of men with gonorrhea and NGU differ, but not to the extent that the differences are diagnostic in individual cases. In a comparison between 113 men with NGU and 69 men with urethral gonorrhea, those with NGU were more often white, better educated, more likely to be students and less likely to be unemployed, members of a higher socioeconomic stratum, older at the age of first intercourse, and involved with fewer total sex partners.[17] Histories of previous gonorrhea were more frequent among men who had gonorrhea, while histories of NGU were more frequent among men with NGU.[17,73] There are no epidemiologic characteristics that will reliably separate *C. trachomatis*-negative NGU patients. Men with two or more previous episodes of NGU have a lower isolation rate of *C. trachomatis*[22] than those with one or no previous episode, but men with previous episodes of urethritis also have a lower isolation rate of *U. urealyticum*.[34]

## CLINICAL MANIFESTATIONS

## COMPARISON BETWEEN GONORRHEA AND NGU

The symptoms and signs of gonococcal and nongonococcal urethritis differ quantitatively, but not qualitatively, so that in an individual case it is impossible to make an absolute distinction between the two on clinical grounds. Both may cause urethral discharge, dysuria, or urethral itching. Frequency, hematuria, and urgency are infrequent with either infection. In one study, 71 percent of 185 men with gonorrhea, but only 38 percent of 214 men with NGU complained of both discharge and dysuria.[73] All but one man who had urethral gonorrhea had urethral discharge, but 19 percent of men with NGU did not. Discharges were more profuse and usually purulent in men with gonorrhea (Plate 1) but were generally mucoid in men with NGU (Plate 2). Especially with NGU, discharge may be detected only in the morning or noted as crusting at the meatus or as staining on underwear. Men with gonorrhea had a more abrupt onset and sought medical care sooner. More than three-fourths of the men who had gonorrhea, but less than one-half of those who had NGU sought treatment within 4 days of onset of symptoms.[73] The usual incubation period is also shorter with gonorrhea. Gonorrhea usually develops 2 to 6 days after exposure, whereas NGU generally develops between 1 and 5 weeks after the likely time of acquisition of infection, with a peak around 2 to 3 weeks. However, longer incubation periods for both infections are seen, and a significant proportion of both groups of men remain asymptomatic.

In urethritis caused by HSV, dysuria is usually severe, the urethral discharge is profuse and mucoid, and there may be localized urethral tenderness at the site of focal urethral ulceration. Regional lymphadenopathy and constitutional symptoms are common with primary HSV urethritis, probably even in the absence of penile lesions.

## ASYMPTOMATIC URETHRAL INFECTION

The importance of asymptomatic urethral gonococcal and chlamydial infection cannot be overstressed. In the studies listed in Table 52-2, the rate of isolation of *C. trachomatis* was usually low in asymptomatic men seen in STD clinics. However, as noted above, high rates of asymptomatic infection have been documented,[42] and just as with male partners of women with gonorrhea, male partners of women with *C. trachomatis* genital infections are frequently infected, and the infection is often asymptomatic. Among male contacts to infected women, Thelin et al. detected *N. gonorrhoeae* in 171 (78 percent) of 265 male contacts of women with gonorrhea, and *C. trachomatis* in 50 (53 percent) of 95 male contacts of women with *C. trachomatis*.[74] Only 50 percent of the male partners infected with either organism were symptomatic.[74] The possibility of asymptomatic infection in the male partner should be strongly considered if the female index case has cervicitis or pelvic inflammatory disease, has delivered an infant with a sexually transmitted disease, or has a positive diagnostic test for *C. trachomatis* or *N. gonorrhoeae*.

## COMPARISON BETWEEN *C. trachomatis*-POSITIVE AND *C. trachomatis*-NEGATIVE NGU

In cases of NGU, a clinical distinction between a *C. trachomatis*-positive and a *C. trachomatis*-negative infection is not possible

Some investigators report that men whose cultures are *C. trachomatis*-negative have more profuse and more purulent discharges,[17,24] but others have found the reverse.[22,28] In a study of men with and without NGU, *C. trachomatis* infection was associated with discharge but not dysuria, whereas *U. urealyticum* infection was associated with dysuria but not discharge.[26] However, in another study of symptomatic men with few or no PMN on urethral smear, isolation of *U. urealyticum* did not correlate with symptoms of dysuria.[75]

## IMPORTANCE OF AN OPTIMAL EXAMINATION

When urethritis is suspected clinically but a discharge is not detected on a routine visit, the patient should be examined in the morning after he has not voided overnight to enhance the likelihood of reaching a firm diagnosis.[76] In a study by Simmons in an STD clinic, 200 men with genitourinary symptoms in whom no firm diagnosis was made on the first visit were asked to return for reexamination in the morning prior to voiding. Among these men 108 new infections were diagnosed. Five had gonorrhea and 103 had NGU.[76]

Another study of symptomatic men with few or no PMN on urethral smear also showed the value of repeat examination after a longer interval without voiding.[75] Furthermore in that study, using the presence of pyuria as the criterion for urethritis, almost 80 percent of men with *C. trachomatis* were demonstrated to have urethritis. In contrast, only one-third of symptomatic men without *C. trachomatis* had pyuria documented at the initial or repeat visits.

## OTHER MANIFESTATIONS OF URETHRITIS

Other manifestations of urethritis are unusual. A very small proportion of patients with gonococcal or chlamydial urethritis will have conjunctivitis caused by *N. gonorrhoeae* or *C. trachomatis,* probably as a result of autoinoculation. Epididymitis develops infrequently today. Some patients with NGU present with Reiter's syndrome, or they develop it soon after their initial presentation. Inguinal lymphadenopathy is unusual and should suggest the possibility of HSV infection. Prostatic enlargement or tenderness is not usually present. In a study by Holmes et al.,[17] prostatic enlargement or tenderness was not significantly more common among patients with NGU (13 percent) than among those with gonorrhea or no urethritis (4 percent). If present, it was always of minimal severity. Symptoms of hematuria, chills, fever, frequency, hesitancy, nocturia, urgency, perineal pain, scrotal masses, postvoid dribbling, or genital pain other than dysuria or urethral pain are not typical of urethritis, and suggest the presence of other genitourinary abnormalities such as classic urinary tract infection, acute prostatitis, a flare-up of chronic prostatitis, or acute epididymitis or orchitis. Although it is said that in the preantibiotic era, prostatitis was a frequent complication of gonorrhea (see Chap. 54), this is not the case today.

## DIAGNOSIS

The diagnosis of gonorrhea simply requires demonstration of *N. gonorrhoeae* by Gram stain, culture, or a reliable nonculture technique. In contrast, diagnosis of NGU requires not only exclusion of urethral infection with *N. gonorrhoeae* but also demonstration of the presence of urethritis (Fig. 52-1, Table 52-4). Specific diagnostic tests for *C. trachomatis* and *U. urealyticum* are not always available (see Chaps. 26 and 74), and there is no alternative clinical or simple laboratory marker diagnostic of *C. trachomatis* or *U. urealyticum* infection. Consequently, arbitrary criteria are used to diagnose the presence of urethritis, but unfortunately these do not entirely correlate with the results of tests for *C. trachomatis.*

## CRITERIA FOR THE DIAGNOSIS OF URETHRITIS

For research purposes the criteria used for diagnosis of urethritis have usually included presence of urethral discharge and of 20 or more PMN in two or more of five random × 400 fields of the sediment of the first 10 to 15 ml of urine collected when the patient has not voided for 4 h or longer.[24] These criteria are undoubtedly too restrictive. In a study of men with minimal or no discharge, there was a definite bimodal distribution of the numbers of PMN in Gram-stained urethral specimens and in the first-voided urine; the presence of 15 or more PMN in any of five random × 400 fields of the sediment of the first-voided urine was correlated with a mean of more than four PMN/field in five × 1000 oil-immersion fields in Gram-stained specimens of urethral exudate, and either finding was regarded as abnormal.[77] Swartz et al. independently concluded that a mean of more than four PMN per oil-immersion field on urethral smear correlated with urethritis.[36] In that study, there was more of a continuum from normal to abnormal.

Subsequent studies among symptomatic men with minimal or no urethral discharge show similar strong correlations between the Gram stain and the first-voided urine sediment.[75] However, *C. trachomatis* was isolated from some men when neither the urethral Gram stain nor the first-voided urine sediment contained PMN. In many other *C. trachomatis*-positive men, only the urine or the smear, but not both, showed increased PMN. Isolation of *C. trachomatis* was more frequent from men with a positive urine alone than from men with a positive smear alone. In another study, Root et al. noted that 7 of 18 *C. trachomatis*-positive men had five or fewer PMN in "several representative fields" on urethral Gram stain.[41] Thus, use of smears or urines to provide objective evidence of urethritis is only a rough guide to the presence of urethral pathogens. Just as with gonorrhea, the inescapable conclusion is that a specific diagnostic test is necessary to exclude *C. trachomatis* infection in men with minimal or no evidence of urethritis.

Men who are symptomatic without objective evidence of urethritis should be examined in the morning without having voided overnight. The urethra should be stripped from the base to the meatus three or four times to detect urethral discharge. After obtaining urethral specimens, to detect PMNs in urine the first 10 to 15 ml of urine voided should be collected and centrifuged at 400 *g* for 10 min. All but 0.5 ml of the supernatant is decanted, and the sediment is resuspended in the residual urine. Sufficient sediment is placed on a slide to cover an area of approximately 1 $cm^2$, and a coverslip is placed over it. The area under the coverslip is examined at a magnification of × 400, and the number of PMN in each of five fields is enumerated. For Gram stain, any expressible urethral exudate can be obtained with a swab from the urethral meatus. When discharge is minimal or absent after an attempt to express discharge, a thin urethrogenital swab should be inserted 3 to 4 cm into the urethra. The patient should be warned that the procedure is painful and that the next urination will also be painful. The swab is then rolled gently back

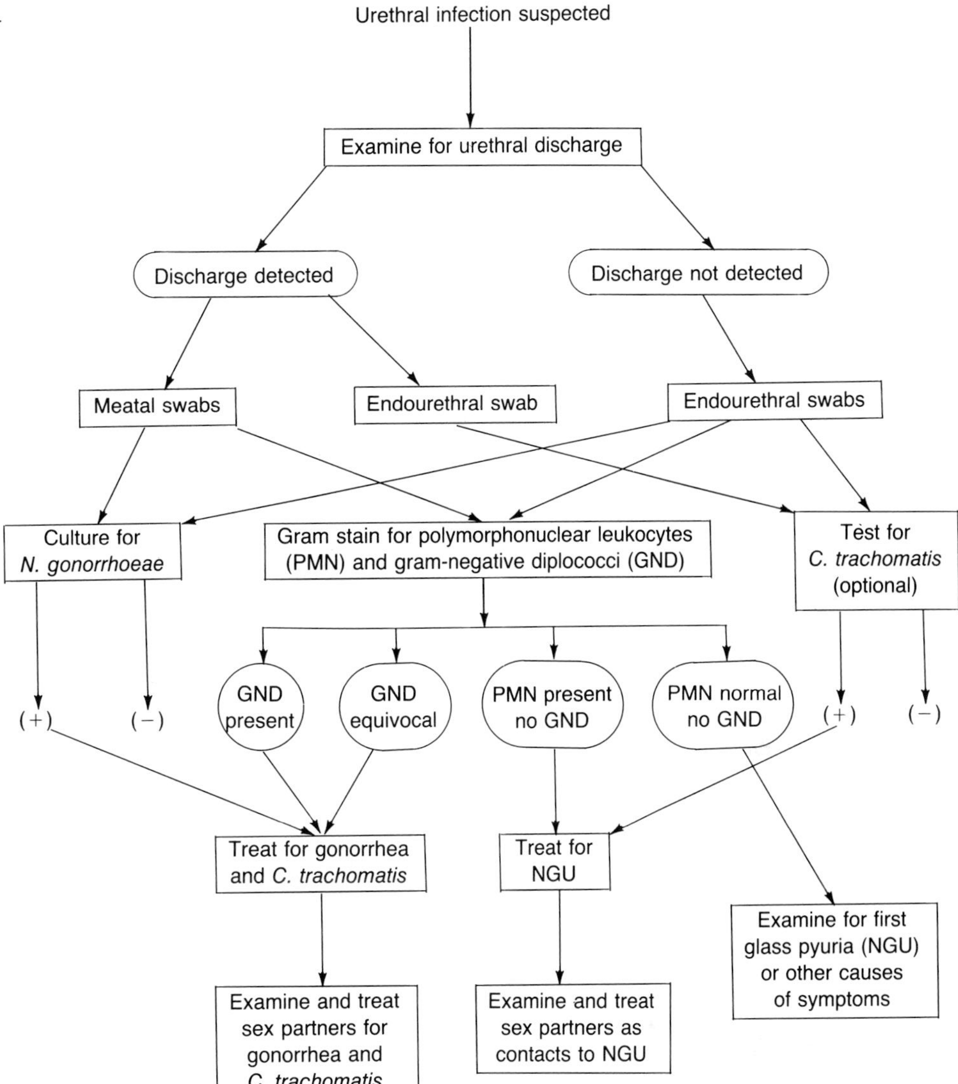


**Fig. 52-1.** Initial diagnosis and management in men with suspected urethritis.

**Table 52-4. Management of Urethritis**

1. Establish presence of urethritis
   *a.* Examine for urethral discharge
   *b.* Gram stain urethral discharge
   *c.* Examine first-voided urine if necessary
   *d.* Reexamine if necessary
2. Establish presence or absence of *N. gonorrhoeae*
   *a.* Gram stain
   *b.* Culture for *N. gonorrhoeae*
3. Diagnostic test for *C. trachomatis* (optional)
4. If gonorrhea, treat with
   *a.* Single-dose ceftriaxone 250 mg IM *plus*
   *b.* Seven days of tetracycline HCl 500 mg p.o. four times daily or doxycycline 100 mg p.o. twice daily
5. If NGU, treat with 7 days of tetracycline HCl 500 mg p.o. four times daily or doxycycline 100 mg p.o. twice daily
6. Treat partner(s) appropriately
7. Follow-up examinations (optional)
   *a.* 3–5 days after completing therapy for gonorrhea
   *b.* 2–4 weeks after completing therapy for NGU

and forth over a glass slide to cover an area approximately 1 $cm^2$. The slide is then stained with Gram's stain and scanned at a magnification of × 100. Areas that have the largest numbers of PMN are then examined under oil (× 1000), and the number of PMN in each of five fields is recorded. While the PMN are enumerated the slide should also be examined for gram-negative diplococci.

## LABORATORY DIFFERENTIATION BETWEEN GONORRHEA AND NGU

Although clinical suspicion that a patient with urethritis has either gonorrhea or NGU may be strong, the final distinction requires laboratory examination to determine if *N. gonorrhoeae* is present. The most rapid and least expensive procedure is microscopic examination of stained urethral exudate or material obtained with an endourethral swab. For experienced microscopists, the sensitivity and positive predictive value of the finding of typical gram-negative diplococci inside the PMN for the diagnosis of gonorrhea are close to 100 percent in men with urethritis (Plate 91). The specificity and negative predictive value of finding no evidence of typical or atypical gram-negative diplococci in ruling out gonorrhea are also close to 100 percent.[73] The presence of ≥ 5 PMN per oil-immersion field, with no evidence of gram-negative diplococci, is sufficient for the diagnosis of NGU (Plate 92). Thus, in a symptomatic case where the urethral smear contains increased numbers of PMN, gonorrhea can be differentiated from NGU at the initial visit and specific therapy can be given. When Gram-stained specimens are interpreted as being equivocal, with only extracellular typical or intracellular atypical gram-negative diplococci being detected, cultures for *N. gonorrhoeae* have been positive in 25 percent.[73] When the Gram-stained specimen is interpreted as being equivocal, or when an individual with expertise is not available to interpret the Gram's stain, cultures are necessary. Cultures are also necessary in cases that are positive by Gram stain when prior treatment has failed, when PPNG, CMRNG, or TRNG are prevalent or suspected on epidemiologic grounds, and when testing for cure. A strong argument can be made for performing a culture for *N. gonorrhoeae* in all men with urethritis, so that if *N. gonorrhoeae* is isolated, its susceptibility to penicillin and tetracycline can be evaluated.[4] In general these cultures for *N. gonorrhoeae* are performed on standard selective media containing antimicrobials including vancomycin (see Chap. 73). Since vancomycin-sensitive isolates may be frequent in some areas,[78] and overgrowth on nonselective media is unusual with male urethral specimens, nonselective media may be preferable. Ideally, cultures should be promptly inoculated and incubated at 36°C in increased carbon dioxide. When urethral exudate is present, it can be cultured, but when there is minimal exudate or when there is no exudate at all, a thin swab should be inserted at least 2 cm into the anterior urethra to obtain an adequate specimen. Although not desirable, recent micturition did not diminish the rate of isolation of *N. gonorrhoeae* in one study.[79] Special culture media to detect gonococcal L-forms are not generally considered useful. Tests for detection of gonococcal enzymes (e.g., oxidase), or of gonococcal lipopolysaccharide, are of interest, but their role in diagnosis of gonorrhea has not been established. Similarly, the detection of gonococcal antigens or DNA in exudates has been used for diagnosis of gonorrhea, but none of these nonculture techniques provides an isolate for susceptibility testing.

## DETECTION OF *C. trachomatis* AND *U. urealyticum*

Detection of *C. trachomatis* and *U. urealyticum* is impossible when diagnostic facilities are not available. Specific diagnosis of *C. trachomatis* urethritis usually requires cultures or detection by one of the newer nonculture techniques (see Chap. 74), although very occasionally serology is useful.[24] Because *C. trachomatis* is an intracellular parasite of columnar epithelial cells the preferable specimen is endourethral material rather than urethral exudate. As with gonorrhea, if *C. trachomatis* is isolated, the patient is considered to have a treatable infection, whether or not urethritis can be documented.

In men with obvious urethritis, the diagnostic yield of cultures for *U. urealyticum* from urethral swabs or first-voided urine is very similar. If urethritis is minimal or absent, an endourethral swab is preferable.[80] However, because *U. urealyticum* is isolated from many men who have no urethritis,[45] isolation of this agent from a male with urethritis does not mean that it is causing urethritis. Serology for *U. urealyticum* is not useful in the diagnosis of urethritis.

## THERAPY

### TREATMENT OF GONOCOCCAL URETHRITIS

Eradication of *N. gonorrhoeae* is not usually difficult, but current recommendations for treatment of gonorrhea in heterosexuals are to use a regimen that is active against both *N. gonorrhoeae* and *C. trachomatis*,[3] and there are no single-dose regimens that will reliably eradicate *C. trachomatis*.[75] Because of the increasing frequency of PPNG, CMRNG, and TRNG, the part of the regimen recommended for eradication for *N. gonorrhoeae* is frequently other than penicillin, ampicillin, or amoxicillin.[3,4] The specific treatment regimens to eradicate *N. gonorrhoeae* are discussed in more detail in Chap. 14 and in Refs. 3 and 4. The actual regimen chosen to eradicate *N. gonorrhoeae* will depend upon where the *N. gonorrhoeae* was acquired, what site of the body is involved, the antimicrobial susceptibility (if known), and whether or not the patient presents as a treatment failure. In some ways treatment for *N. gonorrhoeae* has become simpler, with the use of ceftriaxone, for which a single 250-mg IM injection will reliably eradicate *N. gonorrhoeae* from patients with uncomplicated infection.[81]

If ceftriaxone plus a tetracycline is used, the need for routine test of cure is minimal. If performed, the test of cure should be done 3 to 5 days after the end of treatment. If these cultures are positive, the isolates should be tested for susceptibility to penicillin and tetracycline, even though most failures are due to reinfection. Men who fail to respond to treatment with a penicillin or tetracycline or who have acquired gonorrhea in areas with high rates of PPNG (for example, the Philippines) should receive ceftriaxone 250 mg IM.

#### Use of treatment active against both *N. gonorrhoeae* and *C. trachomatis*

The recommendation for treatment of gonococcal urethritis in heterosexuals with a combination of a single-dose regimen active against *N. gonorrhoeae*, and a multiple-dose tetracycline regimen against *C. trachomatis* appears desirable[3,4] but is contentious for some. The advantages of a combined approach are that:

1. It maintains the traditional single-dose treatment for gonorrhea given to the patient when the patient is seen.
2. The regimen is effective against chlamydial infections.
3. It is effective for pharyngeal *N. gonorrhoeae* infection and usually for rectal *N. gonorrhoeae* infection.
4. It means that tetracycline-resistant *N. gonorrhoeae* are likely to be covered by the single-dose components of the regimen.
5. Potentially, this combined approach could also decrease the spread of resistant isolates of *N. gonorrhoeae*.

The disadvantages of the combined approach are that:

1. Although the approach has been shown to be effective in treatment of individuals with gonorrhea,[82] it has never been shown to be effective on a communitywide basis.
2. Approximately 80 percent of men and at least 50 percent of women with *N. gonorrhoeae* are given a multiple-day, multiple-dose regimen for *C. trachomatis* infection that they do not have.

3. The risk of secondary vulvovaginal candidiasis in women is increased.
4. Since test-of-cure cultures for *N. gonorrhoeae* must be delayed for at least 3 to 4 days after completion of the therapy, the time to test-of-cure cultures is prolonged.
5. There is an unknown potential for selection of resistant isolates of *C. trachomatis* if compliance is poor.
6. There is an unknown potential for masking *C. trachomatis* infections if compliance is poor.
7. There is an increased likelihood of giving a tetracycline to pregnant women.
8. The use of a tetracycline in conditions where it is not needed will likely contribute further to the rapid spread of tetracycline resistance in other genital pathogens.

The only single class of drugs on the market that has considerable activity against both *N. gonorrhoeae* and *C. trachomatis* are the tetracyclines. Prior to the increasing prevalance of TRNG, in many situations treatment with a tetracycline alone usually eradicated both *N. gonorrhoeae* and *C. trachomatis*. Such a regimen is no longer recommended. Activity of some of the new quinolones against both *N. gonorrhoeae* and *C. trachomatis* is promising,[83] so that it may again be possible to make recommendations using a single drug, even though multiple doses will still be required.

## TREATMENT OF NGU

Results of treatment for NGU are not as good as for gonorrhea, even though almost every antimicrobial in clinical usage has been tried. Tetracyclines, erythromycin, and a combination of sulfonamides and aminocylitols were recognized as being the most effective therapy in the 1950s. The basis for these observations has been clarified by subsequent research, because all three regimens are capable of eradicating *C. trachomatis*[20,24,43,84] and because tetracycline and erythromycin are also active against most strains of *U. urealyticum*, while spectinomycin eradicates *U. urealyticum* from the urethras of 60 to 70 percent of men.[24] Current recommendations for initial treatment of a previously untreated episode of NGU are to use 1 week of tetracycline 500 mg orally four times daily or doxycycline 100 mg orally twice daily.[3] Alternative choices when tetracyclines are not tolerated or are contraindicated are 7 days of an erythromycin base or stearate 500 mg orally four times daily or erythromycin ethylsuccinate 800 mg orally four times daily.

Tetracycline has been less expensive than doxycycline, but doxycycline requires less frequent administration, is generally better tolerated, has such a long half-life that even if some doses are missed the treatment is still likely to be effective, and is more active against *C. trachomatis* and *U. urealyticum* on a weight basis (but less doxycycline is given). However, for compliant patients, there are no data suggesting that doxycycline is more or less efficacious than tetracycline.

### Anticipated response to 1 week of treatment with a tetracycline

In compliant patients who are not reexposed to new or untreated partners, all but approximately 5 percent of men will show definite and often total improvement by the end of treatment. Among men who initially respond and are followed for 4 to 6 weeks posttreatment, 30 to 35 percent will have recurrence or incomplete resolution of pyuria.[34] About one-half of these men will have symptoms of urethritis. In compliant patients, the high rates of recurrent or incomplete resolution of urethritis are not due to failure to eradicate *C. trachomatis*. A report of a "positive" posttreatment test for *C. trachomatis* should raise several considerations. With a nonculture test there is a considerable likelihood that the result is a false-positive result. If, however, it is felt to be a true-positive result, it is highly likely that the male either did not take his medications or was reexposed to a new or untreated sexual partner. Tetracycline-resistant isolates of *C. trachomatis* have not yet been described.

### Difficulties in assessment of treatment for NGU

Although many studies of treatment of NGU have been performed, the optimal drug, dosage, and duration of therapy have not been determined. Tetracycline regimens reported to be efficacious range from a single 300-mg dose of doxycycline to 21 days of tetracycline or minocycline. However, assessment of the reported efficacy of various antimicrobial regimens is often difficult because (1) until the mid-1970s, most studies did not employ cultures for both *C. trachomatis* and *U. urealyticum*, (2) *C. trachomatis*-positive NGU responds differently from *C. trachomatis*-negative NGU, (3) manifestations may spontaneously disappear in some cases even without specific therapy, (4) patients frequently remain sexually active so that relapse cannot be distinguished from reinfection, (5) patients frequently default, (6) the appropriate duration of follow-up assessment of results is debatable, and (7) eradication of *C. trachomatis* and *U. urealyticum* does not ensure a lasting clinical cure.

### Duration of therapy

With short-term follow-up, tetracycline therapy has been consistently more effective than placebo.[19,43,85,86] Several investigators have concluded that long courses of antimicrobial therapy are more effective than short courses.[85,87,88] Holmes et al. showed that a 7-day course of tetracycline was more effective than a 4-day course,[85] and in an unblinded study John showed that 21 days were better than 10 days, which in turn were better than 5 days.[87] Thambar et al. concluded that 3 weeks of triple tetracycline was better than 1 week of therapy, but patients on the longer regimen had a much shorter follow-up after cessation of therapy—a critical problem, as discussed below.[88] In contrast to these studies, others have not found a significant difference with longer courses of therapy.[34,86,89] Grimble and Amarasuriya did not show any marked differences between results with 4- to 10-day regimens of several different tetracyclines.[86] Helmy and Fowler had essentially identical results in a double-blind comparison between tetracycline, 500 mg four times daily for 7 days, and 250 mg four times daily for 14 days, and the results were also similar to those of unblinded treatment with 4- and 21-day regimens.[89] Because the appropriate type or duration of therapy may vary between subgroups of NGU, future studies should incorporate cultures at least for *C. trachomatis* and *U. urealyticum*.

### Double-blind evaluation of two doses and two durations of therapy for NGU

A double-blind comparison of two doses and two durations of minocycline has been performed in a study which included cultures for *C. trachomatis* and *U. urealyticum*.[34] Overall, persistent or recurrent NGU within 6 weeks of initiation of therapy was seen in 32 percent of men. Prolonging therapy from 7 to 21 days delayed, but did not diminish, the rate of recurrence, and the use of 100 mg daily gave results which were as good as those obtained with twice daily therapy. The study showed that the critical determinant of response was the etiology of the NGU rather than the amount of drug given or the duration of therapy. Response to treatment was best in men infected with *C. trachomatis,* significantly worse in men infected with *U. urealyticum* alone, and significantly worse still in men from whom neither organism was initially isolated from urethral specimens. Of the men with persistent or recurrent NGU, none had *C. trachomatis* isolated in follow-up tests. In many cases the presence of *U. urealyticum* isolated at follow-up was probably related to resumption of sexual intercourse rather than failure of therapy to eradicate the organism. However, as mentioned earlier, persistence of *U. urealyticum* during and soon after therapy was associated with tetracycline-resistant *U. urealyticum,* and was correlated with persistence of urethritis.[48] This study showed that more than 7 days of treatment with minocycline did not appear justified for initial treatment of NGU. A subsequent study showed that 250 mg of tetracycline four times daily for 7 days was as effective as 500 mg of tetracycline four times daily for 7 days in eradicating both *C. trachomatis* and *U. urealyticum* and in treating NGU.[40] However, the higher daily dose is desirable for eradication of *N. gonorrhoeae* if present.[90] With the increasing spread of TRNG the additional benefit of using the higher daily dose may become less clear. Whether regimens employing a tetracycline for shorter than 7 days would be effective for eradicating *C. trachomatis* and *U. urealyticum,* and for producing similar clinical responses in NGU, is uncertain.

## Use of antimicrobials other than tetracyclines for NGU

Less experience is available with other antimicrobials. Erythromycin stearate, 500 mg twice daily for 2 weeks, effectively eliminated *C. trachomatis*[84] and should also be active against *U. urealyticum.* Erythromycin stearate 500 mg four times daily for 7 days (or equivalent doses of other forms of erythromycin) should also be effective. Erythromycin stearate, 250 mg four times daily for 7 days, resulted in failure to eradicate *C. trachomatis* from one-third of men with chlamydial urethritis.[75] Single-dose administration of any antimicrobial, including those used for gonorrhea, does not usually eradicate *C. trachomatis.* Trimethoprim-sulfamethoxazole is active but not synergistic against *C. trachomatis*[91] and is not active against *U. urealyticum.* Several of the new quinolones, especially ciprofloxacin and ofloxacin, have in vitro activity against *C. trachomatis,* with quite variable activity against genital mycoplasmas.[83] Norfloxacin has no activity in vivo against *C. trachomatis.*[92] Clinically, ciprofloxacin has been associated with frequent treatment failures in men with chlamydia-positive NGU.[93] More clinical data are required with the newer quinolones.

## Treatment of sex partners

As part of the management of urethritis, every attempt should be made to evaluate and treat the patient's sex partner(s). This procedure is widely accepted for partners of men with gonorrhea, and is equally appropriate for partners of men with NGU. It has not been clearly demonstrated that treatment of the partner diminishes the rate of recurrence of NGU in male partners, but even if the recurrence rate cannot be shown to be diminished, female partners need treatment for their own benefit. *C. trachomatis* is isolated from 30 to 60 percent of the female partners of men with gonococcal or nongonococcal urethritis[9,11,17,22,27,28,37,43] and has significant sequelae in women (Ref. 9, Chap. 16). Infected women constitute a major undiagnosed and untreated reservoir of *C. trachomatis* infection; control of the accelerating incidence of *C. trachomatis* infection is unlikely to be achieved without reduction of this reservoir of infection. In general, the same regimens used to treat males with urethritis can be used to treat their female partners.

## Management of recurrent or persistent NGU

Management of men with recurrent NGU represents one of the most difficult problems in venereology. The median time for such recurrences is about 2 weeks after completing therapy.[34] Most men with recurrences of NGU are culture-negative for both *C. trachomatis* and *U. urealyticum.* However, some recurrences after intercourse with untreated partners are *C. trachomatis*-positive, particularly if the recurrent urethritis develops several weeks after treatment. The initial step in management requires that the presence of urethritis again be documented to exclude patients with functional complaints or other disorders. The patient should be questioned about compliance and sexual intercourse or genital contact. When an exudate is present, it should be examined for *T. vaginalis* by culture or by mixing a drop of exudate with saline solution and looking for motile organisms; any exudate should be checked for fungi by adding 10 percent potassium hydroxide to a drop of exudate. In persistent (as opposed to recurrent) NGU, the possibility of herpes simplex virus urethritis should be reconsidered. Primary HSV urethritis typically lasts about 2 weeks. Urethral foreign bodies and periurethral fistula or abscess should be excluded by palpation. Cultures for *N. gonorrhoeae* and *C. trachomatis* should be repeated at least once. No firm guidelines for retreatment can be offered, since the cause of recurrent NGU is usually unknown, and since repeated courses of antimicrobials are often either unsuccessful or only result in transient benefit. However, since tetracycline-resistant *U. urealyticum* is a cause of persistent urethritis, treatment with a 1- to 2-week course of erythromycin, 500 mg four times daily, is reasonable if no other cause is detected at the examination. Such a regimen would also be expected to eradicate *C. trachomatis.* If both the male and female have taken their initial course of therapy correctly, the partner is not usually retreated.

Most men will improve again on the second course of therapy, but approximately 30 percent will have recurrence of symptoms. At that stage, unless urethritis is florid, there are some atypical features, or the man has been reexposed to a new or untreated partner, further antimicrobial therapy should be avoided. The following issues should be discussed with the male:

1. The likelihood of long-term sequelae such as infertility or cancer appears to be exceedingly low even in men who have recurrent urethritis after both therapies.
2. The risk of transmission of disease to partners is exceedingly low because these men do not have ongoing *C. trachomatis* infection, and other pathogens are usually not identified or are not important causes of sequelae in women.
3. Even if no treatment were given, symptoms would likely disappear over time in most of these men.
4. If the man has an ongoing monogamous sexual relationship, there is no need for further treatment of the partners if both have received an initial course of therapy active against *C. trachomatis.*

5. Most of these recurrences will arise independent of resumption of sexual activity, and these recurrences do not mean that the partner has been "unfaithful."
6. Persistent urethritis is not a presentation suggestive of AIDS.
7. Finally, as part of a general discussion with patients who have a sexually transmitted disease, men should be warned that one episode of urethritis does not provide immunity to subsequent episodes.

If the man has florid urethral discharge, or if symptomatic disease is prolonged and no cause is determined, treatment is often a 4- to 6-week course of a regimen such as tetracycline 500 mg four times daily, doxycycline 100 mg twice daily, or erythromycin 500 mg four times daily. Most men will improve on these regimens, but a proportion will have recurring symptoms. It is not known whether the prolonged course of therapy improves the ultimate outcome.

Patients who continue to have frequent recurrences or who have persistent urethritis that is unresponsive to antimicrobial regimens, or who have atypical features should undergo microbiological studies to detect prostatic infection according to the technique of Meares and Stamey.[94] These tests are usually negative, however. If no pathogen is detected by these studies, assessment of urine flow,[95] urethrography and, if necessary, urethroscopy should be performed to detect strictures, foreign bodies, or intraurethral lesions. This should definitely be performed in men with persistent or recurrent urethritis if there is any history of concurrent or past genital warts.

## PROGNOSIS

Although frequent in the preantimicrobial era, local complications of urethral gonorrhea are now unusual in developed countries. Epididymitis occurs in 1 to 2 percent, seminal vesiculitis is rare, and prostatitis and prostatic abscess are almost never seen. Other unusual complications include abscess of Tyson's glands, penile edema secondary to dorsal lymphangitis or thrombophlebitis, inflammation of the urethral wall including periurethral abscesses and fistula, and regional lymphadenitis. Urethral strictures secondary to urethritis rarely occur now in the developed countries but remain significant problems in certain areas of the world. Other complications include inflammation of other sites concurrently infected, for example, the rectum, and disseminated gonococcal infection.

NGU is generally a self-limited disease, and even without therapy the physical consequences to the individual are slight. One to two percent of both *C. trachomatis*-positive and *C. trachomatis*-negative men with NGU develop epididymitis, and another 1 to 2 percent develop conjunctivitis.[28] Urethritis is a manifestation of Reiter's syndrome, but it is unclear how frequently Reiter's syndrome develops as a consequence of NGU. In any case, 1 to 2 percent of men with urethritis will present to STD clinics with Reiter's syndrome or will rapidly develop it. Two recent studies indicate that the rate of development of Reiter's syndrome is not high in HLA-B27 positive men after initiation of therapy with a tetracycline for *C. trachomatis*-positive or *C. trachomatis*-negative NGU.[96,97] In one of the studies, however, men who were positive for *C. trachomatis* had more reactive arthritis than other men.[96] Although approximately 20 percent of men with NGU have an increased number of PMN leukocytes in expressed prostatic secretions,[17] development of prostatitis is rare. In contrast to the infrequent physical consequences, the psychological impact of persistent urethritis or frequent recurrences of urethritis may be great. A thorough discussion of the issues mentioned previously will usually greatly alleviate this distress.

## PREVENTION

Preventive measures offered by health care deliverers and health departments should include (1) the adequate recognition and treatment of patients with sexually transmitted diseases, (2) treatment of gonorrhea with regimens that will eradicate *C. trachomatis*, (3) improved contact tracing to detect and treat partners exposed to either *N. gonorrhoeae* or *C. trachomatis* infection, and (4) increased availability of adequate diagnostic facilities, especially for *C. trachomatis*. Although much progress has been made in understanding the immunobiology of these infections, effective vaccines are not presently available.

A sexually active individual can take three preventive measures. He can choose his partner carefully, use a condom, or take prophylactic antimicrobials. There is no way that one can determine by intuition that a prospective new partner is free of genital pathogens. Use of a condom probably diminishes transmission of many sexually transmitted diseases if properly used. Prophylactic antimicrobials are partially efficacious for prevention of urethritis (for example, 200 mg of minocycline or doxycycline soon after intercourse).[98] However, use of prophylactic antimicrobials for relatively benign and easily treated infections is probably seldom justified. Treatment doses rather than prophylactic doses should be used when the contact has proven infection.

# References


1 Shepard MC: The recovery of pleuropneumonia-like organisms from Negro men with and without nongonococcal urethritis. *Am J Syph Gonorrhea Vener Dis* 38:113, 1954.

2 Gordon FB, Quan AL: Isolation of the trachoma agent in cell culture. *Proc Soc Exp Biol Med* 118:354, 1965.

3 Centers for Disease Control: 1985 STD Treatment Guidelines. *MMWR* 34:75S, 1985.

4 Centers for Disease Control: Antibiotic-resistant strains of *Neisseria gonorrhoeae*. *MMWR* 36:1S, 1987.

5 Handsfield HH et al: Asymptomatic gonorrhea in men. Diagnosis, natural course, prevalence, and significance. *N Engl J Med* 290:117, 1974.

6 Crawford et al: Asymptomatic gonorrhea in men: Caused by gonococci with unique nutritional requirements. *Science* 196:1352, 1977.

7 Rice RJ et al: Chromosomally mediated resistance in *Neisseria gonorrhoeae* in the United States: Results of surveillance and reporting, 1983–84. *J Infect Dis* 153:340, 1986.

8 Knapp JS et al: Frequency and distribution in the United States of strains of *Neisseria gonorrhoeae* with plasmid-mediated, high level resistance to tetracycline. *J Infect Dis* 155:819, 1987.

9 Schachter J: Chlamydial infections. *N Engl J Med* 298:423, 490, 540, 1978.

10 Dunlop EMC et al: Chlamydial infection. Incidence in "nonspecific" urethritis. *Br J Vener Dis* 48:425, 1972.

11 Oriel JD et al: Chlamydial infection. Isolation of chlamydia from patients with non-specific genital infection. *Br J Vener Dis* 48:429, 1972.

12 Richmond SJ et al: Chlamydial infection. Role of chlamydia subgroup A in nongonococcal and postgonococcal urethritis. *Br J Vener Dis* 48:437, 1972.

13 Oriel JD et al: Infection with chlamydia group A in men with urethritis due to *Neisseria gonorrhoeae*. *J Infect Dis* 131:376, 1975.

14 Oriel JD et al: Minocycline in the treatment of nongonococcal urethritis: Its effect on *Chlamydia trachomatis*. *J Am Vener Dis Assoc* 2:17, 1975.
15 Schachter J et al: Are chlamydial infections the most prevalent venereal diseases? *JAMA* 231:1252, 1975.
16 Smith TF et al: Isolation of chlamydia from patients with urethritis. *Mayo Clin Proc* 50:105, 1975.
17 Holmes KK et al: Etiology of nongonococcal urethritis. *N Engl J Med* 292:1199, 1975.
18 Oriel JD et al: Chlamydial infection of the male urethra. *Br J Vener Dis* 52:46, 1976.
19 Prentice MJ et al: Non-specific urethritis. A placebo-controlled trial of minocycline in conjunction with laboratory investigations. *Br J Vener Dis* 52:269, 1976.
20 Bowie WR et al: Differential response to Chlamydial and Ureaplasma-associated urethritis to sulfafurazole (sulfisoxazole) and aminocyclitols. *Lancet* ii:1276, 1976.
21 Johannisson G et al: *Chlamydia trachomatis* infection and venereal disease. *Acta Derm Venereal (Stockh)* 57:455, 1977.
22 Alani MD et al: Isolation of *Chlamydia trachomatis* from the male urethra. *Br J Vener Dis* 53:88, 1977.
23 Vaughan-Jackson JD et al: Urethritis due to *Chlamydia trachomatis*. *Br J Vener Dis* 53:180, 1977.
24 Bowie WR et al: Etiology of nongonococcal urethritis. Evidence for *Chlamydia trachomatis* and *Ureaplasma urealyticum*. *J Clin Invest* 59:735, 1977.
25 Segura JW et al: Chlamydia and non-specific urethritis. *J Urol* 117: 720, 1977.
26 Wong JL et al: The etiology of nongonococcal urethritis in men attending a venereal disease clinic. *Sex Transm Dis* 4:4, 1977.
27 Paavonen J et al: Examination of men with nongonococcal urethritis and their sexual partners for *Chlamydia trachomatis* and *Ureaplasma urealyticum*. *Sex Transm Dis* 5:93, 1978.
28 Terho P: *Chlamydia trachomatis* in non-specific urethritis. *Br J Vener Dis* 54:251, 1978.
29 Terho P: *Chlamydia trachomatis* in gonococcal and postgonococcal urethritis. *Br J Vener Dis* 54:326, 1978.
30 Csango PA: *Chlamydia trachomatis* from men with nongonococcal urethritis. Simplified procedure for cultivation and isolation in replicating McCoy cell culture. *Acta Pathol Microbiol Scand Sect B* 86:257, 1978.
31 Ripa KT et al: *Chlamydia trachomatis* urethritis in men attending a venereal disease clinic: A culture and therapeutic study. *Acta Derm Venereol (Stockh)* 48:175, 1978.
32 Perroud HM, Miedzybrodzka K: Chlamydial infection of the urethra in men. *Br J Vener Dis* 54:45, 1978.
33 Bowie WR et al: Etiologies of postgonococcal urethritis in homosexual and heterosexual men: Roles of *Chlamydia trachomatis* and *Ureaplasma urealyticum*. *Sex Transm Dis* 5:151, 1978.
34 Bowie WR et al: Therapy for nongonococcal urethritis: Double-blind randomized comparison of two doses and two durations of minocycline therapy for nongonococcal urethritis. *Ann Intern Med* 95:306, 1981.
35 Smith TF et al: A comparison of genital infections caused by *Chlamydia trachomatis* and by *Neisseria gonorrhoeae*. *Am Soc Clin Pathol* 70:333, 1978.
36 Swartz SL et al: Diagnosis and etiology of nongonococcal urethritis. *J Infect Dis* 138:445, 1978.
37 Lassus A et al: Erythromycin and lymecycline treatment in Chlamydia-positive and Chlamydia-negative nongonococcal urethritis—A partner-controlled study. *Acta Derm Venereol (Stockh)* 59:278, 1979.
38 Coufalik ED et al: Treatment of nongonococcal urethritis with rifampicin as a means of defining the role of *Ureaplasma urealyticum*. *Br J Vener Dis* 55:36, 1979.
39 Taylor-Robinson D et al: *Ureaplasma urealyticum* and *Mycoplasma hominis* in chlamydial and non-chlamydial non-gonococcal urethritis. *Br J Vener Dis* 55:30, 1979.
40 Bowie WR et al: Tetracycline in nongonococcal urethritis. Comparison of 2 g and 1 g daily for 7 days. *Br J Vener Dis* 56:332, 1980.
41 Root TE et al: Nongonococcal urethritis: A survey of clinical and laboratory features. *Sex Transm Dis* 7:59, 1980.
42 Podgore JK et al: Asymptomatic urethral infections due to *Chlamydia trachomatis* in male U.S. military personnel. *J Infect Dis* 146:828, 1982.
43 Handsfield HH et al: Differences in the therapeutic response of Chlamydia-positive and Chlamydia-negative forms of nongonococcal urethritis. *J Am Vener Dis Assoc* 2(3):5, 1976.
44 DiGiacomo RF et al: Chlamydial infections of the male baboon urethra. *Br J Vener Dis* 51:310, 1975.
45 McCormack WM et al: Sexual experience and urethral colonization with genital mycoplasmas. A study in normal men. *Ann Intern Med* 78:696, 1973.
46 McCormack WM et al: The genital mycoplasmas. *N Engl J Med* 288:78, 1973.
47 Shepard MC: Quantitative relationship of *Ureaplasma urealyticum* to the clinical course of nongonococcal urethritis in the human male. *Colloq INSERM* 33:375, 1974.
48 Stimson JB et al: Tetracycline-resistant *Ureaplasma urealyticum*: A cause of persistent nongonococcal urethritis. *Ann Intern Med* 94:192, 1981.
49 Taylor-Robinson D et al: Human intraurethral inoculation of ureaplasmas. *Q J Med* 46:309, 1977.
50 Bowie WR et al: Genital inoculation of male *Macaca fascicularis* with *Neisseria gonorrhoeae* and *Ureaplasma urealyticum*. *Br J Vener Dis* 54:235, 1978.
51 Taylor-Robinson D et al: Urethral infection of chimpanzees by *Ureaplasma urealyticum*. *J Med Microbiol* 11:197, 1978.
52 Robertson JA, Stemke GW: Expanded serotyping scheme for *Ureaplasma urealyticum* strains isolated from humans. *J Clin Microbiol* 15:873, 1982.
53 Shepard MC, Lunceford CD: Serological typing of *Ureaplasma urealyticum* isolates from urethritis patients by an agar growth inhibition method. *J Clin Microbiol* 8:566, 1978.
54 Cracea E et al: Serotypes of *Ureaplasma urealyticum* isolated from patients with nongonococcal urethritis and gonorrhea and from asymptomatic urethral carriers. *Sex Transm Dis* 12:219, 1985.
55 Black FT: Modifications of the growth inhibition test and its application to human T-mycoplasmas. *Appl Microbiol* 25:523, 1973.
56 Stemke GW, Robertson JA: Problems associated with serotyping strains of *Ureaplasma urealyticum*. *Diagn Microbiol Infect Dis* 3:311, 1985.
57 Bowie WR et al: Bacteriology of the urethra in normal men and men with nongonococcal urethritis. *J Clin Microbiol* 6:482, 1977.
58 Fontaine EA et al: Anaerobes in men with urethritis. *Br J Vener Dis* 58:321, 1982.
59 Fontaine EA et al: Characteristics of a gram negative anaerobe isolated from men with non-gonococcal urethritis. *J Med Microbiol* 17:129, 1984.
60 Taylor-Robinson D et al: Urethral infection in male chimpanzees produced experimentally by *Mycoplasma genitalium*. *Br J Exp Pathol* 66: 95, 1985.
61 Sturm AW: *Hemophilus influenzae* and *Hemophilus parainfluenzae* in nongonococcal urethritis. *J Infect Dis* 153:165, 1986.
62 Barnes RC et al: Urinary tract infection in sexually active homosexual men. *Lancet* i:171, 1986.
63 Taylor CED et al: Serological response of patients with nongonococcal urethritis to causative organism of contagious equine metritis. *Lancet* i:700, 1979.
64 Hovelius B et al: *Staphylococcus saprophyticus* in the aetiology of nongonococcal urethritis. *Br J Vener Dis* 55:369, 1979.
65 Stamm W, Holmes KK: Personal communication.
66 Furness G et al: *Corynebacterium genitalium* (non-specific urethritis *Corynebacterium*): Biologic reactions differentiating commensals of the urogenital tract from the pathogens responsible for urethritis. *Invest Urol* 15:23, 1977.
67 Corey L et al: Genital herpes simplex virus infections: Clinical manifestations, course and complications. *Ann Intern Med* 98:958, 1983.
68 Harnett GB et al: Association of genital adenovirus infection with urethritis in men. *Med J Aust* 141:337, 1984.

69 Kuberski T: *Trichomonas vaginalis* associated with nongonococcal urethritis and prostatitis. *Sex Transm Dis* 7:135, 1980.

70 McCutchan JA: Epidemiology of venereal urethritis: Comparison of gonorrhea and nongonococcal urethritis. *Rev Infect Dis* 6:669, 1984.

71 Wiesner PJ: Selected aspects of the epidemiology of nongonococcal urethritis, in *Nongonococcal Urethritis and Related Oculogenital Infections*, D Hobson, KK Holmes (eds). Washington, DC, The American Society for Microbiology, 1977, p 9.

72 McChesney JA et al: Acute urethritis in male college students. *JAMA* 226:37, 1973.

73 Jacobs NF, Kraus SJ: Gonococcal and nongonococcal urethritis in men. Clinical and laboratory differentiation. *Ann Intern Med* 82:7, 1975.

74 Thelin I et al: Contact-tracing in patients with genital chlamydial infection. *Br J Vener Dis* 56:259, 1980.

75 Bowie WR: Treatment of chlamydial infections, in *Chlamydial Infections*, P-A Mårdh et al (eds). New York, Elsevier, 1982, p 231.

76 Simmons PD: Evaluation of the early morning smear investigation. *Br J Vener Dis* 54:128, 1978.

77 Bowie WR: Comparison of gram stain and first voided urine sediment in the diagnosis of urethritis. *Sex Transm Dis* 5:39, 1978.

78 Windall JJ et al: Isolation of vancomycin-susceptible gonococci. Abstract 323, 20th Interscience Conference on Antimicrobial Agents and Chemotherapy. New Orleans, September 22–24, 1980.

79 Judson FN et al: Recent micturition does not affect the detection of urethral gonorrhea. *Br J Vener Dis* 53:308, 1977.

80 Tarr PI et al: Comparison of methods for the isolation of genital mycoplasmas from men. *J Infect Dis* 133: 419, 1976.

81 Judson FN: Treatment of uncomplicated gonorrhea with ceftriaxone: A review. *Sex Transm Dis* 13:199, 1986.

82 Stamm WE et al: Effect of treatment regimens for *Neisseria gonorrhoeae* on simultaneous infection with *Chlamydia trachomatis*. *N Engl J Med* 310:545, 1984.

83 Wolfson JS, Hooper DC. The fluoroquinolones. Structure, mechanisms of action and resistance, and spectrum of activity in vitro. *Antimicrob Agents Chemother* 28:581, 1985.

84 Oriel JD et al: Comparison of erythromycin stearate and oxytetracycline in the treatment of nongonococcal urethritis: Their efficacy against *Chlamydia trachomatis*. *Scott Med J* 22:375, 1977.

85 Holmes KK et al: Studies of venereal diseases. III. Double-blind comparison of tetracycline hydrochloride and placebo in treatment of nongonococcal urethritis. *JAMA* 202:474, 1967.

86 Grimble AS, Amarasuriya KL: Nonspecific urethritis and the tetracyclines. *Br J Vener Dis* 51:198, 1975.

87 John J: Efficacy of prolonged regimens of oxytetracycline in the treatment of nongonococcal urethritis. *Br J Vener Dis* 47:266, 1971.

88 Thambar IV et al: Double-blind comparison of two regimens in the treatment of nongonococcal urethritis. Seven-day versus 21-day course of triple tetracycline (Deteclo). *Br J Vener Dis* 55:284, 1979.

89 Helmy N, Fowler W: Intensive and prolonged tetracycline therapy in non-specific urethritis. *Br J Vener Dis* 51:336, 1975.

90 Judson FN, Rothenberg R: Tetracycline in the treatment of uncomplicated male gonorrhea. *J Am Vener Dis Assoc* 3:56, 1976.

91 Johannisson G et al: Susceptibility of *Chlamydia trachomatis* to antibiotics in vitro and in vivo. *Sex Transm Dis* 6:50, 1979.

92 Bowie WR et al: Failure of norfloxacin to eradicate *Chlamydia trachomatis* in nongonococcal urethritis. *Antimicrob Agents Chemother* 30:594, 1986.

93 Arya OP et al: Evaluation of ciprofloxacin 500 mg twice daily for one week in treating uncomplicated gonococcal, chlamydial, and nonspecific urethritis in men. *Genitourin Med* 62:170, 1986.

94 Meares EM Jr, Stamey TA: Bacteriologic localization patterns in bacterial prostatitis and urethritis. *Invest Urol* 5:492, 1968.

95 Krieger J et al: Evaluation of chronic urethritis. Defining the role for endoscopic procedures. *Arch Intern Med* 148:703, 1988.

96 Keat AC et al: Role of *Chlamydia trachomatis* and HLA-B27 in sexually acquired reactive arthritis. *Br Med J* 1:605, 1978.

97 Bowie WR et al: Unpublished observations.

98 Harrison WO et al: A trial of minocycline given after exposure to prevent gonorrhea. *N Engl J Med* 300:1074, 1979.

# Chapter 53

# Acute epididymitis

Richard E. Berger

## DEFINITION AND HISTORY

The epididymis and vas deferens are derived from the wolffian system and mesonephric duct. The epididymis is a sausage-shaped structure positioned on the posterior aspect of the testicle. It consists of a single, delicate convoluted tubule 12 to 15 ft in length. The epithelium of the epididymis possesses stereocilia, which have no directional movement. The epididymis has been divided into six sections based on histological characteristics, which probably represent different functional capacities. Fluid and particulate matter are both secreted and absorbed by the epididymis. During passage through the epididymis sperm achieve motility and the potential to fertilize an ovum.

Inflammation of the epididymis causes pain and swelling which is almost always unilateral and usually relatively acute in onset. Monteggro in 1804 was probably the first to describe the gross pathology of epididymitis and differentiate it from orchitis. Despres in 1879 suggested that epididymitis was due to the retention of semen related to the pain of urethritis. Subsequently, specific infectious forms, such as tuberculous and gonococcal epididymitis, have been well recognized. With the advent of specific diagnostic criteria and effective antimicrobial therapy for gonorrhea and tuberculosis in the 1940s and 1950s, an increasing proportion of cases seen during the 1960s and 1970s were regarded as "idiopathic," often attributed to "straining" or reflux of sterile urine into the epididymis. However, recent studies have established the infectious etiology of most cases of epididymitis and the importance of sexually transmitted urethritis as a precursor of epididymitis.

Epididymitis is common, and it carries much morbidity in terms of suffering and loss of time from work. Because of epididymitis an estimated 634,000 patients sought treatment by American physicians in 1977.[1] In Great Britain, from 1963–1964, 13,600 claims were made for workman's compensation for epididymoorchitis.[2] Epididymitis has been shown to account for more days lost from service than any other disease in the military,[3] with over 20 percent of urologic admissions being due to epididymoorchitis.[4,5]

With improved understanding of the etiology of epididymitis, the diagnosis and management of this condition is becoming more rational, leading to decreased morbidity and possibly to prevention of recurrences. Epididymitis may occur as a complication of urethral infection with *Neisseria gonorrhoeae* or *Chlamydia trachomatis,* or of genitourinary infection with enteric gram-negative rods or *Pseudomonas aeruginosa.* It may also occasionally occur as a complication of systemic infection with various pathogens, including *Mycobacterium tuberculosis. Brucella* sp., *Streptococcus pneumoniae, Neisseria meningitidis, Treponema pallidum,* and various fungi. The proper management of these patients requires that an accurate etiologic diagnosis be established. The agent responsible must be identified, along with contributing factors which might lead to recurrence. In the case of epididymitis caused by *N. gonorrhoeae* or *C. trachomatis,* this would most certainly include treatment of the patient's sexual partners. In the case of epididymitis secondary to coliform urinary tract infection, primary genitourinary disease must be sought out and, if possible, corrected. The term *nonspecific epididymitis,* which has been used in the past to denote patients who have epididymitis associated with nonspecific urethritis or with no obvious infection, should generally be avoided. Only those cases for which no etiologic agent can be determined after a careful search for known pathogens should be referred to as "idiopathic" (Table 53-1).

## EPIDEMIOLOGY AND ETIOLOGY

### EPIDIDYMITIS ASSOCIATED WITH BACTERIURIA

In prepubertal children, epididymitis is frequently associated with coliform or pseudomonas infection of the genitourinary tract[6,7] (Table 53-2). These children often have predisposing structural or neurologic abnormalities. Gierup et al.[6] found that ten of 22 children who had epididymitis confirmed by surgical exploration had significant bacteriuria (e.g., $> 10^5$ *E. coli* per milliliter of urine). Prepubertal children had bacteriuria more often than postpubertal children. Pyuria with negative urine cultures occurred more often in older children. Cultures for *C. trachomatis* or *N. gonorrhoeae* were not performed, but these agents could be important among older boys who are sexually active. In a retrospective study, Gislason et al.[8] found that approximately two-thirds of boys with epididymitis were postpubertal, 29 percent had pyuria, but only 12.5 percent had urine cultures which yielded conventional pathogens. In adolescents with epididymitis, the age and sexual activity should be ascertained, as sexually transmitted pathogens may be important in such patients.

In postpubertal males less than 35 years of age, epididymitis is usually not attributable to coliforms, and the presence of *Pseudomonas aeruginosa* is unusual. In various series, from 0 to 35 percent of sexually mature young men with epididymitis have had infection with coliform bacteria or *Ps. aeruginosa.*[1,5,9,10] This low prevalence may be partially due to the low prevalence in this age group of structural disease predisposing an individual to urinary tract infections. Most males with congenital anomalies of the urinary tract have been discovered and treated surgically at an earlier age, while acquired structural or functional disorders of the male urinary tract, such as benign prostatic hypertrophy, develop later in life.[1] As shown in Table 53-3, 6 of 51 men less than 35 years of age in our series had coliform infection and 1 had infection with *Haemophilus influenzae.* All of those seven were homosexual men infected with gram-negative rods, who regularly practiced anal-insertive intercourse.[11] No pathogen was identified in the two additional homosexual men in this series, but all 9 homosexual men had many neutrophiles per 400×

**Table 53-1. Classification of Acute Epididymitis**

- I. Epididymitis due to infectious agents
  - A. Associated with urethritis
  - B. Associated with bacteriuria
  - C. Associated with systemic infections
- II. Epididymitis due to noninfectious causes
  - A. Associated with trauma
  - B. Associated with drugs (amiodarone)

**Table 53-2. Microbial Etiology and Predisposing Factors in Acute Epididymitis**

| Prepubertal children |
|---|
| *Usual etiology:* Coliforms, *Ps. aeruginosa* |
| *Unusual etiology:* Hematogenous spread from primary infected site |
| *Predisposing factors:* Underlying genitourinary pathology |
| **Men under 35** |
| *Usual etiology: C. trachomatis, N. gonorrhoeae* |
| *Unusual etiology:* Coliform or *Ps. aeruginosis, Mycobacterium tuberculosis* |
| *Predisposing factors:* Sexually transmitted urethritis |
| **Men over 35** |
| *Usual etiology:* Coliforms or *Ps. aeruginosa* |
| *Unusual etiology: N. gonorrhoeae, C. trachomatis, M. tuberculosis* |
| *Predisposing factors:* Underlying structural pathology or chronic bacterial prostatitis |

microscopic field on Gram stain of mid-stream urine. Drach[12] has previously noted that a history of anal intercourse was associated with chronic bacterial prostatitis. Barnes et al.[13] found that bacteriuria was more common among homosexual men than among heterosexual men in a venereal disease clinic population. Of those with bacteriuria, 61 percent had urethral discharge, presumably due to *E. coli* urethritis. Thus, we hypothesize that the occurrence of *E. coli* epididymitis in homosexual men may be due to more frequent exposure of the urethra to pathogenic enteric bacteria during anal intercourse. Although Stamey et al.[14] showed in 1971 that enteric pathogens isolated from the urine of women with urinary tract infections could be isolated from the urethra of their male sexual partners, coliform epididymitis appears to be uncommon in young heterosexual men.

In men over 35 years of age, up to 80 percent with epididymitis have coliform or *Ps. aeruginosa* urinary tract infection.[15] The high proportion of cases of epididymitis caused by coliform infections in older men may be due to the decreasing incidence of sexually transmitted disease and an increased incidence of acquired genitourinary abnormalities. These patients may have a history of prostastic calculi, recent urinary instrumentation, neurogenic bladder, benign prostatic hypertrophy, or chronic bacterial prostatis. We found only one of 17 patients over 35 years of age with epididymitis to have a sexually transmitted infection,[1] while 12 of the 17 had coliform or pseudomonas infection (Table 53-3). Almost one-half of the patients over 35 years of age had preexisting genitourinary pathology.

In military populations, epididymitis secondary to coliform bladder infections is unusual.[5,9,10,16,17] This may be due to the predominantly young age and absence of underlying urinary abnormalities in military populations. Mittemeyer[10] found underlying urinary abnormalities in only 3.4 percent of 610 patients with epididymitis. In Mittemeyer's study,[10] 70.1 percent were between the ages of 20 and 39; and in Shapiro's study,[9] 75 percent of the patients were between 18 and 32.

## EPIDIDYMITIS ASSOCIATED WITH URETHRITIS

Epididymitis caused by *N. gonorrhoeae* or *C. trachomatis* is rare in prepubertal children, but in postpubertal children, these organisms must be suspected. No study to date of postpubertal children with epididymitis has assessed the sexual history, or has utilized appropriate cultures for sexually transmitted organisms as well as for conventional uropathogens.

Sexually transmitted organisms are the most common cause of epididymitis in heterosexual men under the age of 35.[1,12] In the preantibiotic era, Pelouze[18] reported that epididymitis occurred in 10 to 30 percent of cases of gonorrheal urethritis. More recently, Watson[19] found that 16 percent of consecutive patients with epididymitis in a young military population had gonorrhea, although only 50 percent of those with gonorrhea had urethral discharge.

In our series of acute epididymitis, 28 (67 percent) of 42 men under 35 years of age had epididymitis secondary to *N. gonorrhoeae* or *C. trachomatis*. *N. gonorrhoeae* alone was isolated from the urethra from 9, *C. trachomatis* infection alone was found in 18, and both agents were recovered from one patient (Table 53-3). *C. trachomatis* was isolated as the sole pathogen from the epididymis in five of six men with *C. trachomatis* infection who underwent epididymal aspiration.

Characteristically, patients with epididymitis caused by *N. gonorrhoeae* or *C. trachomatis* are young and sexually active; they may have multiple sexual partners. Symptoms of urethritis may or may not be present. Nonetheless, even in patients who deny symptoms of urethritis, a urethral discharge may be expressible; a Gram-stained smear of an endourethral swab specimen may reveal $\geq 5$ polymorphonuclear leukocytes per $1000\times$ field; or urinalysis may reveal pyuria. Underlying urinary tract abnormalities usually are not found.

In our series,[1,11,15] 13 of 19 men with *C. trachomatis* epididymitis were referred from venereal disease clinics. Therefore, this could represent a biased population and could overestimate the proportion of cases actually associated with *C. trachomatis*. However, other studies[20–22] have confirmed our findings. Melekos and Asbach[22] found 9 of 17 (53 percent) men less than age 40 with acute epididymitis to be infected with *C. trachomatis*. Colleen and Mårdh[21] reported that 14 of 42 men less than 35

**Table 53-3. Etiology of Acute Epididymitis in 68 Consecutive Men**

| Etiology | Heterosexual men >35 years old ($n$ = 17) | Heterosexual men <35 years old ($n$ = 42) | Homosexual men <35 years old ($n$ = 9) |
|---|---|---|---|
| Coliforms, *Pseudomonas* | 12 | 0 | 6 |
| *N. gonorrhoeae* | 0 | 9 | 0 |
| *C. trachomatis* | 1 | 18 | 0 |
| *N. gonorrhoeae* plus *C. trachomatis* | 0 | 1 | 0 |
| *H. influenzae* | 0 | 0 | 1 |
| Trauma | 0 | 2 | 0 |
| Tuberculosis | 1 | 0 | 0 |
| Idiopathic | 3 | 12 | 2 |

SOURCE: Berger RE, Refs. 1, 11, and 15.

years old had *C. trachomatis* infection. Mulcahy et al.[20] isolated *C. trachomatis* from 65 percent of men less than age 35.

The argument has been popular that epididymitis in young men is caused by the reflux of sterile urine down the vas deferens during straining, producing sterile inflammation. The popularity of this theory may be partly due to the previous inability to recover a pathogenic organism from these patients. However, Shapiro[9] noted only 2 of 52 patients had a history of straining prior to the onset of epididymitis. Similarly, Mittemeyer[10] noted such a history in only 6.6 percent of his population. We studied two patients who had a history of strenuous lifting just before onset of epididymitis, and *C. trachomatis* was isolated from both of these patients.[15] Cathcart[23] reported that 12 of 14 cases of epididymitis with a history of "strain" also had urethral discharge. Although reflux of infected urine into the vas deferens may well be important in the production of epididymitis, reflux of sterile urine has not been shown to play an important role in causing epididymitis.

## MISCELLANEOUS CAUSES OF EPIDIDYMITIS

Epididymitis may occur in systemic tuberculosis. In Mittemeyer's military series, 0.8 percent of patients had epididymitis due to tuberculosis.[10] Halkier[24] reported that 75 percent of patients with renal tuberculosis had an episode of epididymitis. Ross[25] found the age of patients with tuberculous epididymitis to be between 20 and 40 years. Medlar[26] reported that no case of tuberculous epididymitis occurred without renal, prostate, or seminal vesicle involvement. Sixty-four percent of patients with tuberculous epididymitis had bilateral involvement, in contrast with epididymitis due to coliforms, *N. gonorrhoeae,* or *C. trachomatis,* which is nearly always unilateral.

Numerous other organisms which have been reported to cause epididymitis probably spread by a hematogenous route. These organisms include *Strep. pneumoniae,*[27] Brucella,[28] *N. meningitidis,*[29] *T. pallidum* and numerous other bacteria. Epididymitis may occur as a manifestation of disseminated fungal infections, such as histoplasmosis, coccioidomycosis, and cryptococcosis. Reports that sexually transmitted organisms such as *Trichomonas vaginalis* can cause epididymitis should be taken with caution, as the presence of one sexually transmitted organism may indicate the likelihood of the presence of others.

A new cause of epididymitis was reported by Gasparich et al.,[30] who reported a syndrome of epididymitis in 6 of 56 men taking the anti-arrhythmic drug amiodarone. Epididymal biopsy showed lymphocytic infiltration and fibrosis. Amiodarone levels in the epididymis were found to be 400 times higher than therapeutic blood levels in one patient. Reduction of the dosage of amiodarone resulted in resolution of epididymitis.

## CLINICAL MANIFESTATIONS AND DIAGNOSIS

In the patient with epididymitis secondary to coliform bacteria or pseudomonas, the clinical history suggests a urinary tract abnormality. In the infant, a history of urinary tract abnormalities in siblings may be significant. The child's parents should be asked about the quality of the urinary stream and history of hematuria. In the adult, a history of decreasing urinary stream, surgery on the urinary tract, or previous urinary tract infections may be important. In a patient with epididymitis secondary to sexually transmitted organisms, a history of urethral discharge or dysuria is helpful, and there usually is a history of recent sexual exposure. The patient with epididymitis secondary to tuberculosis will often have a prior history of pulmonary tuberculosis or a history of exposure.

Of 92 patients in the military service with epididymitis, one-third had a sudden onset, and two-thirds a gradual onset.[17] A history of lifting or straining on onset of pain is probably not significant in determining the etiology of the epididymitis or in its differentiation from other intrascrotal conditions. In addition to severe scrotal pain, the patient may also complain of inguinal pain.[15] In severe cases, with the cord acutely swollen, flank pain may result from obstruction of the ureter as it crosses over the spermatic cord.[18] A history suggestive of urinary infection may or may not be present.[17,31] We[1] found that only 1 of 10 patients with coliform infections, and only 6 of 14 patients with *C. trachomatis* infection had dysuria.

On examination, the scrotum on the involved side may be red and edematous. The degree of erythema may be greater in patients with coliform and gonococcal epididymitis than with *C. trachomatis* epididymitis. However, massive erythema and edema may occur even with *C. trachomatis* if left untreated. The testicle tends to ride in the normal position in the scrotum. The tail of the epididymis, which connects with the vas deferens, near the *lower* pole of the testes, is swollen first, and later swelling spreads to the head of the epididymis, near the upper pole of the testes. The groove between the epididymis and the testicle should be examined, as this will help to show whether the maximum swelling is in the testicle or the epididymis. The spermatic cord may be swollen and tender. If the patient has not recently voided, a urethral discharge may be present, but asymptomatic urethral infection without discharge is not uncommon. Watson[19] found that 50 percent of the cases due to *N. gonorrhoeae* did not have urethral discharge. If no spontaneous discharge is noted, the urethra should be stripped and again examined. Digital rectal exam may reveal abnormalities suggestive of prostatitis in some cases.[9,16]

Gram stain of the urethral swab specimen will usually indicate the presence of urethritis and establish with a high degree of certainty whether its etiology is gonococcal or nongonococcal. In our series,[1] the presence or absence of intracellular gram-negative diplococci on Gram stain or urethral smear correlated in all cases with the results of culture for *N. gonorrhoeae.* First-voided and midstream urine specimens should be examined for bacteria and white cells. Comparison of the urinary sediments in the first-voided urine and midstream urine may reveal whether pyuria is coming from the urethra or the bladder. Gram stain of uncentrifuged midstream urine can be used to presumptively establish the diagnosis of bacteriuria in cases of epididymitis secondary to coliform or pseudomonas infections. The presence of greater than 1 gram-negative rod per oil immersion field on Gram stain of one drop of unspun midstream urine is correlated with the presence of greater than $10^5$ coliforms or *Pseudomonas* sp. per milliliter of urine. Quantitative midstream urine culture for *N. gonorrhoeae* should nonetheless be obtained in all cases of acute epididymitis. In our series,[1] two-thirds of the cases of epididymitis not due to gram-negative rods or *N. gonorrhoeae* in men under 35 years of age were secondary to *Chlamydia trachomatis.* Obviously, urethral cultures for *C. trachomatis* are desirable if available.

In certain difficult cases, the etiologic diagnosis of epididymitis may be aided by the use of epididymal aspiration cultures.[32] These cultures may be useful in patients with (1) in-dwelling urethral catheters, (2) failure to respond to initial antimicrobial therapy, (3) epididymitis found on surgical exploration for torsion of the testicle, and (4) recurrent epididymitis in which the etiologic agent is uncertain. If the patient had received prior antimicrobial therapy and the urine is sterile, the organism responsible for epididymitis may only be obtainable from aspirate cultures. Patients with in-dwelling urethral catheters often have multiple organisms in the urine, and therapy may be best selected on the basis of the organism(s) found on epididymal aspiration.

## DIFFERENTIAL DIAGNOSIS OF ACUTE EPIDIDYMITIS

An algorithm for differential diagnosis and management of the patient with pain in the scrotal sac is presented in Fig. 53-1. Acute epididymitis always must be differentiated from torsion of the testicle. In infants and prepubertal children, torsion of the testicle is much more common than acute epididymitis, and any acute swelling of the scrotum must be presumed to be torsion of the testicle unless proved otherwise. Quinto[33] found that in pediatric patients only 12 of 158 with scrotal swelling had epididymitis. Children with epididymitis often have pyuria, whereas children with torsion generally do not have pyuria. Therefore, the absence of pyuria in boys with an acute scrotal condition should lead to immediate surgical exploration to perform detorsion and orchidopexy. Cases of suspected epididymitis in adolescents or young adults should be confirmed by Doppler and/or radionuclide scanning, since the incidence of torsion is also higher in this age group.

In consecutive cases of acute testicular swelling, Delvillar[34] noted that 11 of 13 patients under age 20 had torsion of the testicle. In contrast, of all patients from 20 to 30 years old, 10 percent had torsion of the testicle. Of 29 patients with acute epididymitis, only 8 were under age 20. Barker[35] also found that

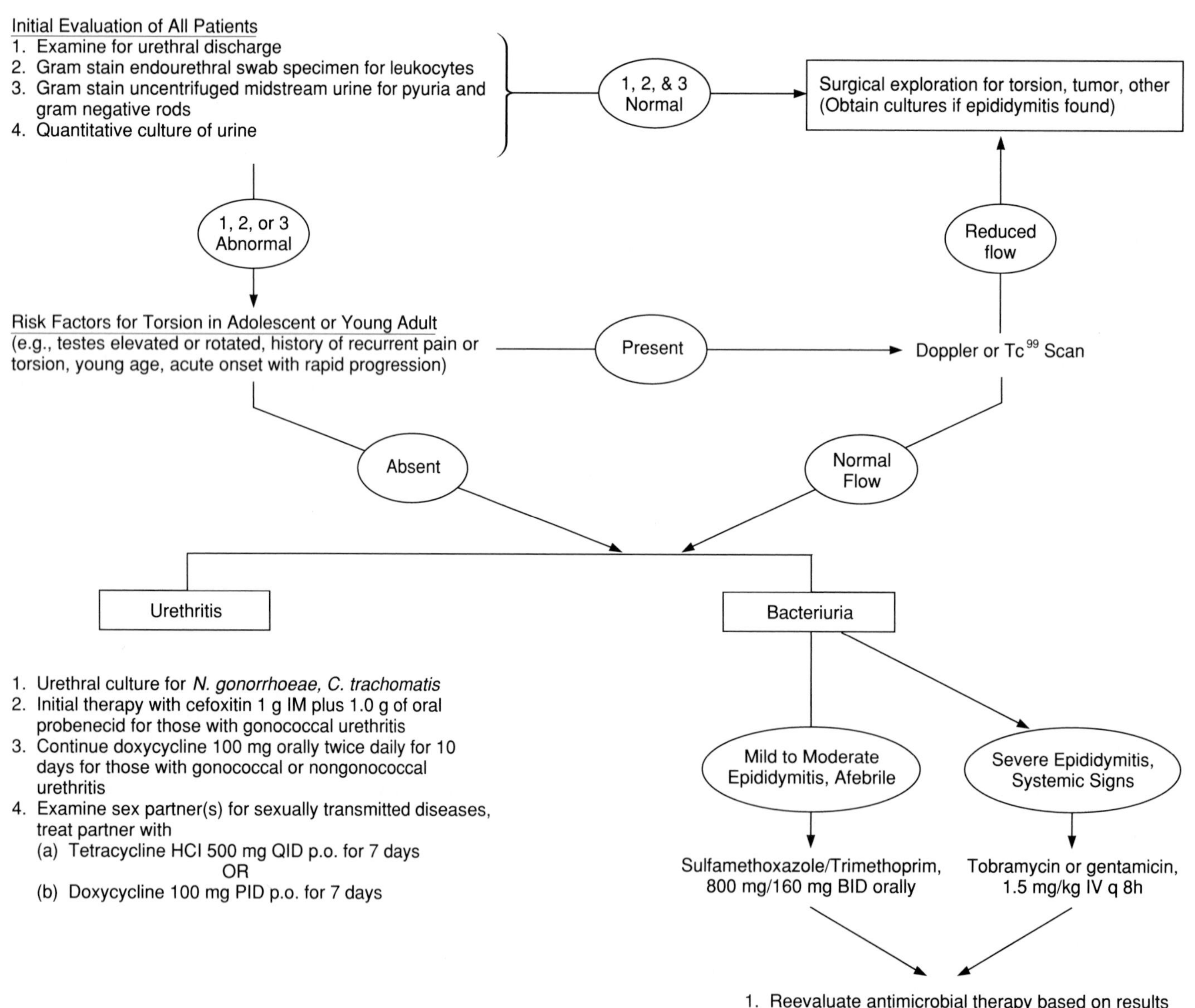


**Fig. 53-1.** Algorithm for the management of acute unilateral intrascrotal pain.

epididymitis was much more likely to be found in patients over 18 years of age than in patients less than 18 years of age, presumably because of increasing sexual activity and decreasing incidence of torsion with age. As sexual mores changed, however, and the age at first intercourse decreased, the incidence of epididymitis has increased in patients less than 18 years of age.

A history of previous scrotal pain is more common in torsion of the testicle than in epididymitis, presumably due to previous intermittent torsion. History of trauma to the testicle or of extreme exertion at the onset of pain may occur with either epididymitis or torsion of the testicle. Unless physical examination is performed early in the course of the acute scrotum, the physical examination in torsion and epididymitis may be very similar. Delvillar[34] noticed swelling of the testes in 28 percent of patients with epididymitis and in 77 percent of cases of torsion. On the other hand, swelling of the epididymis alone occurred in 59 percent of cases of epididymitis and in 15 percent of torsion. Differential diagnosis by physical exam therefore is helpful but not completely reliable. Figure 53-2*a* and *b*, showing the appearance of the testicle and epididymis at surgical exploration, illustrates why it may be difficult to distinguish epididymitis on physical examination in some cases. In torsion of the testicle, sometimes examination of the opposite testicle will reveal that the epididymis is anterior. This indicates that the congenital abnormality which allows torsion of the testicle may also be present on the opposite side and is a clue to the diagnosis of torsion. In torsion also, the testicle is often high into the scrotum, whereas in epididymitis this is not usually the case. In epididymitis, the cord in the inguinal canal may be quite tender, whereas in torsion tenderness is generally limited to the scrotal contents.

Examination of the urine and urethral smear is a very helpful procedure in differentiating epididymitis from torsion of the testicle as discussed above. Barker and Raper[35] noted that 31 of 32 patients with epididymitis had bacteriuria or pus cells in the urine, whereas none of 38 patients with torsion had bacteriuria or pyuria. In Doolittle's series,[36] 8 of 11 patients with epididymitis had pyuria, whereas none of 19 patients with torsion had pyuria. Urinary examination should include examination of first-voided urine, which would yield a higher quantity of white cells in patients with urethritis. In Madsen's series,[37] 49 of 50 patients with acute epididymitis had expressed prostatic secretions that were loaded with white blood cells. Although Madsen did not examine urethral smears routinely, the finding of clear evidence of urethritis on smear would eliminate the need for performing rigorous rectal examination in most cases. Some authors consider a rigorous rectal exam with epididymitis to be contraindicated because of the risk of exacerbating the symptoms or because of a possible risk of causing bacteremia in men with coliform or *Ps. aeruginosa* infection. Madsen reported no such exacerbations and neither did we in our series. However, we avoided prostatic

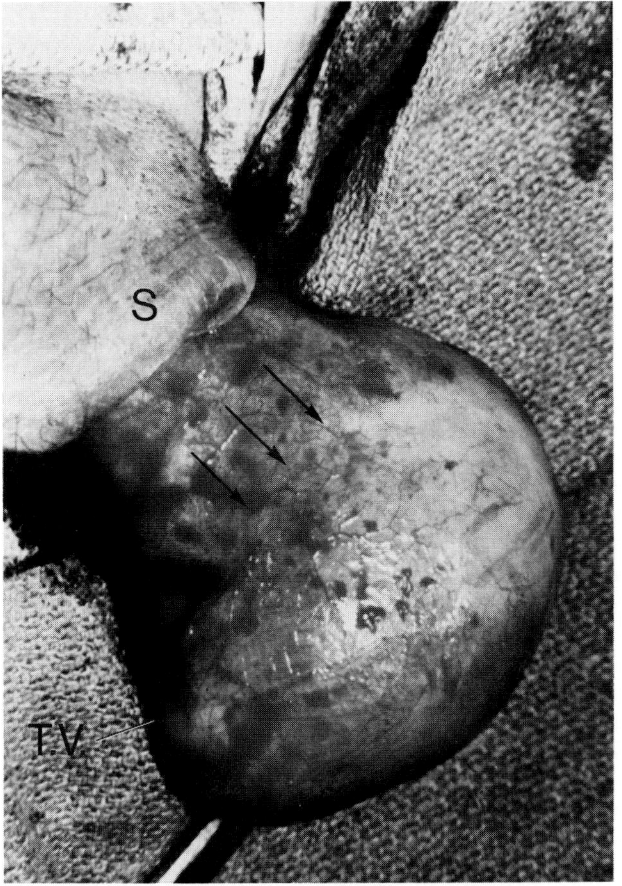


A

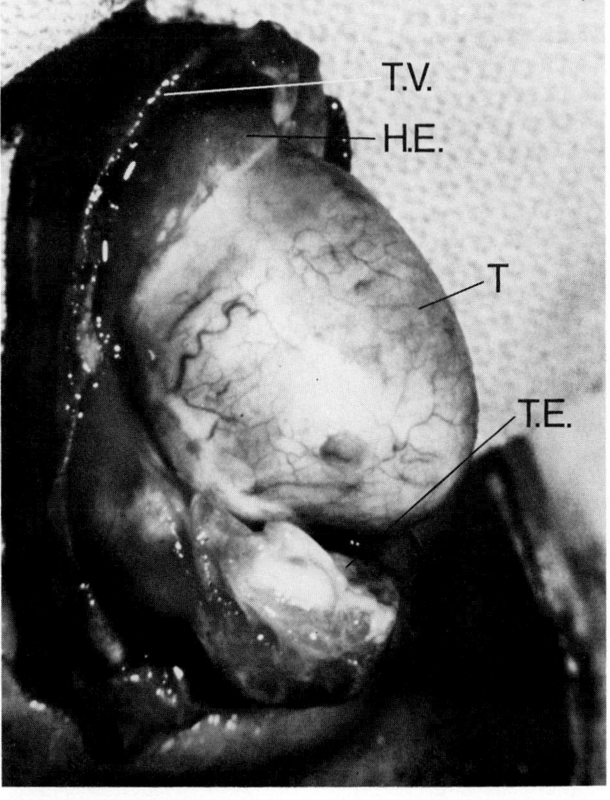


B

**Fig. 53-2** (*a*) View of surgical exploration of testicle and epididymis, which are pulled out of the scrotal sac. The testis and epididymis are surrounded by inflammatory hydrocele which fills the tunica vaginalis (TV) and obscures the groove (*arrows*) between the testes and epididymis. On physical examination, this could not be differentiated from torsion of the testes. (*b*) After the tunica vaginalis (TV), which formed the wall of the hydrocele, had been cut away, the acutely inflamed edematous epididymis with relatively normal-appearing testes can be seen. HE = head of the epididymis, TE = tail of the epididymis.

massages on older patients with suspected coliform or *Ps. aeruginosa* infection.[1]

The Doppler stethoscope is a useful tool in the differential diagnosis of torsion and epididymitis.[38] It shows increased blood flow to the acutely inflamed epididymis and decreased blood flow to a testicle which has undergone torsion, cutting off its blood supply. The opposite testicle is used as a control. Care must be performed in interpreting Doppler ultrasound examinations, as hyperemia surrounding a necrotic testicle may produce a false positive signal for epididymitis. Compression of the spermatic cord at the external ring will cause the Doppler pulse to disappear if blood flow is coming from the testicle, but not if it is coming from scrotal vessels. Similarly, a hydrocele surrounding an inflamed epididymis may produce a falsely decreased signal. The use of radionuclide testicular scanning is also based on a finding of increased blood flow in epididymitis (Fig. 53-3). In Holder's series,[39] 22 of 22 patients with acute epididymitis had increased blood flow and were correctly diagnosed. Abu-Sleiman et al.[40] found that a correct diagnosis could be made in 86 percent of cases. False positives were noted in hydroceles and false negatives in late torsions and patients with retracted scroti. Testicular tumor may also produce increased flow on testicular scan, resembling epididymitis.[41]

In all cases, unless the examiner can unequivocally rule out torsion of the testicle, scrotal exploration should be undertaken. After 4 h of torsion, there is a significant risk of irreversible testicular infarction. A "wait and see" attitude is never justified. We have encountered one patient who had simultaneous epididymitis and testicular torsion.

Another common and potentially disastrous mistake in diagnosis of acute epididymitis is to overlook a testicular carcinoma. The ages at which epididymitis and testicular tumors occur are similar, the peak age of testicular tumors being between the ages of 18 and 32. Approximately one-quarter of patients with testicular tumors present with testicular pain. Therefore, although the presentation of a painless testicular mass almost always indicates a testicular tumor, the presence of pain does not rule out a tumor. In the early stages of epididymitis, swelling is limited to the epididymis, and differentiation from testicular tumor usually is not difficult. However, as epididymitis progresses and the testicle becomes more involved, the limits of inflammation are not easily defined. Furthermore, a testicular tumor may invade the epididymis and thus, on physical exam, mimic exactly the findings of acute epididymitis. Reactive hydrocele formation may further limit the usefulness of physical examination. In testicular tumors, the urine and urethral smear should show no evidence of inflammation. *Failure of improvement in the size of swelling or pain in any young man being treated for epididymitis should lead to the suspicion that an incorrect diagnosis has been made. Scrotal exploration through an inguinal incision should be considered to rule out carcinoma of the testicle.* Transscrotal open or needle biopsy should never be performed when carcinoma of the testicle is suspected for fear of spreading tumor cells in the scrotal contents. Examination by ultrasound may be of value to confirm or deny the normalcy of the underlying testicular architecture.

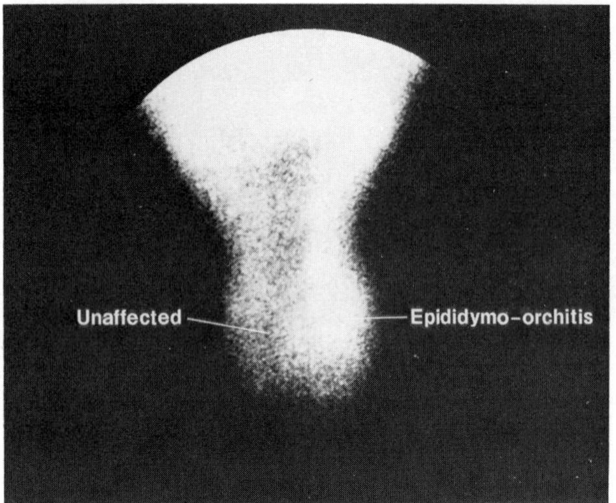


**Fig. 53-3.** Technetium radionuclide scan of patient with typical acute unilateral epididymoorchitis, showing increased uptake of $Tc^{99}$ on the affected side, with normal uptake on the unaffected side.

Other intrascrotal conditions which may occasionally present difficulties in diagnosis are presented in Table 53-4. Spermatocele and hydrocele are easily differentiated by transillumination. The scrotal varicosities of a varicocele disappear on assuming the supine position. A hernia protruding into the scrotum may sometimes present difficulties in diagnosis. However, this may be reducible as the patient lies down. Hernias are not transilluminable, and bowel sounds may occasionally be heard in the hernia contents.

## COMPLICATIONS OF ACUTE EPIDIDYMITIS

### SURGICAL COMPLICATIONS

Since the use of antibiotics, the incidence of surgical complications from epididymitis has decreased. From 1951 to 1955, Gartman[16] used few antibiotics and had a 30 percent incidence of surgical complications. From 1955 to 1959, he used antibiotics much more frequently and had an 8 percent incidence of surgical complications. He noted an overall 10.2 percent complication rate in idiopathic epididymitis, and a 16.2 percent rate when a definite pathogen was found in the urine or urethra.

The most serious local complications of epididymitis are abscess formation and infarction of the testicle. Both of these complications are clinically suggested by the failure of the patient to improve with appropriate bed rest and antibiotic therapy. Testicular infarction probably results from thrombosis of the spermatic vessels secondary to severe inflammation.[15] Gangrene of the testicle may take place while the epididymis remains viable (Fig. 53-4). Costas[42] suggested that the swollen spermatic cord may become compressed at the external ring and lead to vascular compromise of the testicle. In Gartman's[16] series, 3 of 310 cases resulted in gangrene of the testicle. Abscess may be suggested by a "cold" area in the middle of a "hot" area on radionuclide scan. In Mittemeyer's series,[10] 19 of 610 patients developed abscess formation which required surgical drainage. Treatment requires surgical drainage and probably orchiectomy. In Gartman's series,[16] 22 out of 310 patients developed hydroceles; however, only 11 of these failed to resolve after treatment of epididymitis and required surgical repair.

Recurrence of epididymitis usually reflects lack of adequate treatment, failure to identify factors predisposing to reinfection, and/or inadequate suppression of a source of chronic infection. We have found an unusually high rate of complications in homosexual men with coliform epididymitis. Of six such men, one developed a testicular abscess, one developed contralateral epididymitis, and two relapsed after initial treatment.[12]

Chronic epididymitis with chronic pain after the initial episode

Table 53-4. Common Differential Diagnosis of Acute Epididymitis in Adult Men

| | Usual age | Pain | Onset | Past history of pain | Spermatic cord tenderness | Scrotal tenderness | Transillumination | Decrease in swelling on lying down | Fever | Location of swelling | Urethritis, pyuria, bacteriuria | Activity on testicular scan | Blood flow on Doppler ultrasonic |
|---|---|---|---|---|---|---|---|---|---|---|---|---|---|
| Epididymitis | Any | Mild–severe | Gradual to sudden | Infrequent | Frequent | Severe | No | No | Frequent | Posterior to testes | Yes | ↑ | ↑ |
| Torsion of testes | < 30 | Severe | Sudden | Frequent | Infrequent | Severe | No | No | Infrequent | Testes* | No | ↓ | ↓ |
| Testes tumor | 18–32 | None–mild | Gradual | Infrequent | No | None–mild | No | No | No | Testes | No | ↑ or ↓ | Normal |
| Hydrocele | Any | None–mild | Gradual | Infrequent | No | None | Yes | No | No | Entire hemiscrotum | No | ↓ | Normal or ↓ |
| Spermatocele | Any | None–mild | Gradual | Infrequent | No | None | Yes | No | No | Above testes† | No | ↓ | Normal or ↓ |
| Varicocele | Any | None–mild | Gradual | Infrequent | No | None | No | Yes‡ | No | "Bag of worms" | No | Normal or ↑ | Normal§ |
| Hernia | Any | None–moderate | Gradual | Frequent | Frequent | None–mild | No | Yes¶ | No | Above testes | No | Normal | Normal |

*In torsion of testicle, epididymis of normal testicle may be anterior.
†Spermatocele may feel like "third testicle."
‡Varicocele should disappear on lying down.
§May get increased venous flow.
¶Hernia may be reducible on lying down.

developed in 15 percent of Mittemeyer's cases.[10] It is not clear whether this is related to persistence of bacteria in the epididymis or whether it is due to scarring or other factors. Chronic epididymitis is generally considered idiopathic and is notoriously unresponsive to antimicrobial therapy.

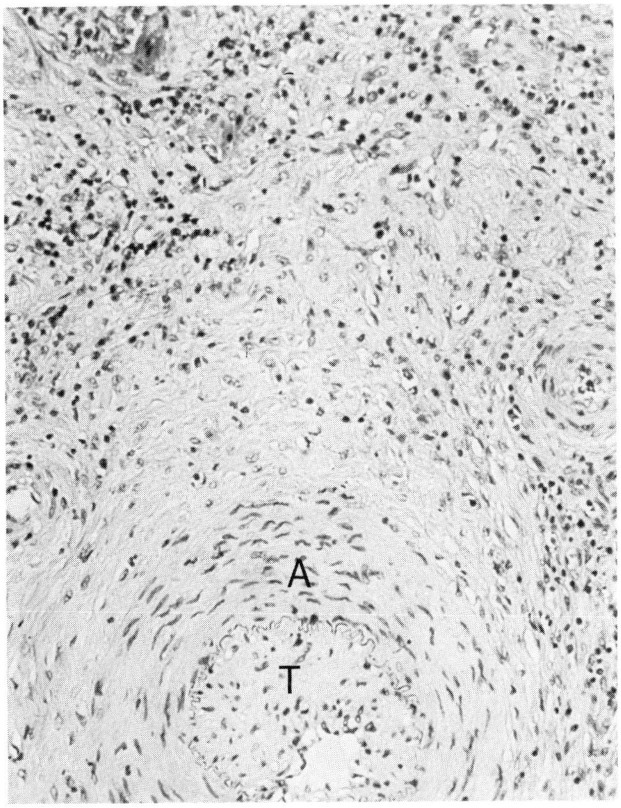

Fig. 53-4. Epididymal biopsy of orchiectomy specimen from a patient with acute epididymitis showing diffuse inflammatory infiltrate and organizing thrombus (T) within an arteriole (A).

## INFERTILITY

Another complication of acute epididymitis, although poorly documented, is decreased fertility. Patients with bilateral epididymitis and bilateral occlusion of the vas deferens or epididymis have virtually no potential for fertility. In some parts of sub-Saharan Africa where urethritis often goes untreated, epididymitis is a leading cause of male infertility.[43] Campbell[44] noted that 40 percent of patients with bilateral epididymitis secondary to gonorrhea were sterile. Pelouze[18] reported that, with only a history of gonococcal urethritis, 10.5 percent of patients had a history of involuntary infertility. With unilateral epididymitis, he reported a 23 percent incidence of male infertility. With bilateral epididymitis, he reported a 42 percent incidence of infertility. Gartman[16] reported that among 18 azoospermic men with normal testes biopsies and patent vas deferens, only four had histories of bilateral epididymitis, but all were found to have fine scars which transected the epididymal tubules. These data suggest that patients may have a subclinical form of epididymitis which may lead to asymptomatic scarring and decreased fertility. This intriguing observation may be analogous to the observation that among infertile women who have bilateral tubal obstruction (many of whom have serological evidence of past *C. trachomatis* infection), only about half have a past history of salpingitis (Chap. 63). Since sperm transit through the epididymis is known to be necessary for development of normal sperm function, it is possible that acute inflammation and damage to the epididymis could ultimately lead to decreased fertility even in the absence of occlusion of the epididymal tubules. Epididymal obstruction may be spontaneously reversible in some patients. Pelouze[18] reported one case who had a return of sperm and fertility after 5 years of apparent epididymal occlusion following gonococcal epididymitis. The inflammation in acute epididymitis is not limited to the epididymis but also involves the testicle. Wolin[5] found on testes biopsy during acute epididymitis that 20 of 28 patients had decreased spermatogenesis, and 9 of 28 had testicular inflammation. Nilsson[45] did aspiration biopsies on testicles in acute epididymitis and found that 16 of 22 showed inflammatory cells. Follow-up biopsy of these testicles after 2 to 3 years showed that five of nine had reduced or absent spermatogenesis. Bietz[46] found nonspecific toxic changes in the opposite testis 150 to 250 days following the onset of epididymitis. Both Tozzo[47] and we[1] have found low sperm counts in a high proportion of patients with acute epididymitis. Ludwig[48] followed 46 patients with unilateral epididymitis from 8 days to 1 year. He found initially that two-thirds had oligoesthenospermia. However, only 20 percent had long-term fertility disturbance as reflected in semen analysis, and only one had persisting sperm agglutinins after one year. In other unilateral conditions of the testicles, such as cryptorchidism and torsion of the testicle, decreased fertility has been demonstrated.[49,50] Whether unilateral testicular involvement in acute epididymitis can decrease fertility potential has not been definitively evaluated. Bandhauer[51] found that 9 of 48 men with acute unilateral epididymitis developed sperm agglutinins. Ingerslev et al.[52] found that 27 percent of men who had epididymitis developed serum antisperm agglutinating antibodies. We[53] have found that men without a history of clinical epididymitis, but with serological evidence of past exposure to *C. trachomatis,* have a significantly greater chance (50 percent) of having sperm autoantibody than do men without evidence of such exposure (16 percent).

## PATHOLOGY OF ACUTE EPIDIDYMITIS

The clinical manifestations of inflammation in acute epididymitis usually begin in the tail of the epididymis and spread to involve the rest of the epididymis and the testicle proper. Pelouze[18] noted in 98 percent of cases of epididymitis, the clinical course suggested that the epididymis was inflamed before the vas became inflamed. Early in the course of the disease, the epididymal ducts become distended with polymorphonuclear and mononuclear leukocytes which may actively phagocytize sperm.[54] The epithelium of the epididymis may be destroyed, and small abscesses form in the connective tissue, which is intensely hyperemic. In the stroma, lymphocytes may outnumber the polymorphonuclear leukocytes. Microabscesses may be present after 48 h.[54] Later on, the columnar epithelium of the epididymis may become squamoid in appearance and plasma cells more frequent. Cronquist[55] reported seven cases of epididymitis in which sperm penetrated the epithelium and basement lamina of the epididymis with a marked inflammatory reaction. In biopsies in acute epididymitis, Wolin[5] noted that 13 of 24 patients had epididymal tubular destruction with microabscesses and a predominance of polymorphonuclear leukocytes. However, in the remaining 11 cases, there was predominantly lymphocytic infiltration with no tubular involvement. Perivascular mononuclear cell infiltration was prominent in some of these cases. We have also noted mononuclear cell infiltrate in the epididymis of men with proven chlamydial infection.[56] As noted above, Wolin[5] and Nilsson et al.[45] described testicular inflammation. The latter reported that Sertoli's cells were vacuolated, with cloudy cytoplasm. Furthermore, the organism responsible for epididymitis was isolated from the testicle in four patients. After 2 to 7 months, repeat biopsies showed decreased inflammation with an increased proportion of lymphocytes, macrophages, and plasma cells. After 2 to 3 years, there was atrophy, which was proportional to the degree of initial inflammation.

In summary, available data suggest that most cases of acute epididymitis begin in the tail of the epididymis, with an acute intralumenal exudate, tubular epithelial damage, and subjacent microabsecesses. However, some cases show predominantly mononuclear and perivascular infiltration. Testicular involvement occurs and may lead to testicular atrophy. Unfortunately, these previous pathological studies have not employed comprehensive microbiological studies of etiology.

## EXPERIMENTAL PATHOLOGY

Moller[57] has reported a primate model of *C. trachomatis* epididymitis in Grivet monkeys. Injection of *C. trachomatis* down the vas deferens produced a marked infiltration with polymorphonuclear leukocytes and lymphocytes through all layers of the spermatic cord. In the epididymis, the ducts were also filled with exudate containing mostly leukocytes and polymorphonuclear leukocytes. They were able to isolate *C. trachomatis* from the vas deferens but were unable to isolate it from the epididymis. We[58] have used *Macaca nemistrina* as a primate model for chlamydial epididymitis, and after inoculation of *C. trachomatis* through the vas deferens, obtained mainly a mononuclear perivascular inflammation in the area of the epididymis. Lucchetta et al.[59] have developed a model for epididymitis caused by *E. coli* in the rat, and we have developed a similar model in the rabbit.[60] Both models show a marked decrease in spermatogenesis following epididymitis.

## ROUTE OF SPREAD OF INFECTION

The route of spread of infection to the epididymis has been a subject of much debate. Much of the controversy was spawned originally by the idea that "idiopathic" epididymitis was caused by "sterile" inflammation from urine refluxing down the vas deferens while straining with a full bladder. This theory had implications both for workman's compensation from results of injuries sustained while working, and for the military, where prevention of epididymitis and loss of time from service was of great importance. Currently, most cases of epididymitis are thought to be infectious in origin. Therefore, the route of spread to the epididymis may be more of academic interest, since the spread of naturally occurring infection from the urethra, bladder, or prostate does not carry the same legal implications as reflux of sterile urine caused by strenuous work.

Experimentally, infective epididymitis has been produced by inoculation and intralumenal spread.[57] On numerous occasions, it has been demonstrated that urine from the bladder can reflux into the ejaculatory ducts and into the vas deferens in patients undergoing prostatectomy or in those with serious urinary pathology. On the other hand, Kohler[61] was unable to produce reflux of radiographic contrast down the vas in patients recovering from acute epididymitis. Similarly, Herwig[62] was unable to demonstrate retrograde urination down the vas in patients with sterile urine. Pelouze[18] pointed out that the ejaculatory ducts contain no circular muscles, and for a peristaltic wave to carry urine in a retrograde fashion down the vas deferens, the seminal vesicle would have to first fill with urine and then contract and force the urine down into the epididymis. Inflammation of the seminal vesicle during acute epididymitis has been demonstrated by gallium scan.[63] We have noted grossly purulent semen in men who have epididymitis with minimal urethritis and no symptoms or signs attributable to prostatitis or seminal vesiculitis. Since the seminal vesicle is subject to the same intraabdominal pressures as the bladder, perhaps straining could force infected seminal vesicle contents down the vas and into the epididymis. Reflux of urine would therefore not be necessary to explain the sudden onset of epididymitis with straining in these patients. In men with prostate obstruction, Kendall[64] found positive vas cultures in only 15 percent of patients with positive urinary cultures *without* a catheter, but he found positive vas cultures in 36 percent of infected patients who had a urethral catheter in place. Orandi[65] performed preprostatectomy vas cultures and found that 32 of 67 patients with positive urine cultures also had positive vas cultures. He found none of 74 patients with negative urine cultures to have positive vas cultures. Reeves[66] ligated only one vas deferens in 505 preprostatectomy cases. He found a higher rate of epididymitis on the nonligated side. Perhaps a catheter or similar irritation from infection of the verumontanum may allow reflux of infected urine from the bladder down the vas deferens or lead to seminal vesiculitis with infection subsequently spreading to the epididymis.

Other theories have been proposed to explain how infection gets to the epididymis. Spread of organisms by continuity of surface down the vas has been questioned. Wesson[67] suggested that organisms could spread to the vas by means of lymphatics. He noted the frequent swelling of the spermatic cord in patients with epididymitis. Since the epididymis drains to hypogastric and iliac nodes and the prostate and seminal vesicles drain to the same area, spread by the way of lymphatic drainage was postulated. The lack of involvement of the testicle in some cases was attributed to the different lymphatic drainage of the two organs. Rolnick[68] suggested that the spread could advance along the sheath of the vas, since this sheath is a continuation of the sheath of the prostate and seminal vesicles. Infection which extended out of the prostate or seminal vesicles could thus travel along the sheath of the vas to the tail of the epididymis. Some infections, such as tuberculous, pneumococcal, fungal, and other infections, might well spread to the epididymis by a hematogenous route. However, this route is probably unusual for coliform or sexually transmitted organisms, since most often the offending organism can be found within the urethra or bladder.

## TREATMENT

Symptomatic treatment of the patient with epididymitis is always indicated. Scrotal elevation provides for maximum lymphatic and venous drainage. The patient should be placed at bed rest with the scrotum elevated on a towel between his legs. The use of constricting scrotal supports while the patient is supine often only holds the scrotal contents between the patient's legs in a dependent position. If the patient is standing, gravity prevents proper drainage of the tissues and may increase swelling. The patient should remain at bed rest until the scrotal contents are nontender. If the pain should return after ambulation, the patient should again return to bed rest and scrotal elevation.

In view of the microbial etiology of the vast majority of cases of epididymitis, antibiotics should never be withheld in this condition. Nilsson has provided evidence that antibiotic treatment is superior to placebo in patients with coliform epididymitis, as well as in patients without coliforms.[69] Appropriate antibiotics can be chosen on the basis of culture and Gram stain of the urine and urethra, as outlined in Fig. 53-1. In patients with bacteriuria, initiation of broad spectrum parenteral antimicrobial therapy (e.g., tobramycin) is recommended. However, if ambulatory therapy is used for afebrile patients with mildly or moderately severe epididymitis, trimethoprim-sulfamethoxazole or a quinolone antibiotic provides activity against most Enterobacteriaceae. The organism recovered from the urine is also responsible for epididymitis,[1,36] and therapy can be modified on the basis of susceptibility tests on the isolate from urine. In patients with in-dwelling urethral catheters who may have multiple organisms isolated from the urine and in patients who have been started on antibiotics who may have sterile urine, the use of epididymal aspiration cultures may identify the causal pathogen and provide needed antimicrobial sensitivity information.[32] Antibiotic treatment may need to be prolonged in some cases. We have isolated pathogenic organisms from the epididymis and testicular tissue for as long as 2 weeks after the beginning of appropriate antimicrobial therapy.

In patients with epididymitis associated with urethritis, cultures should initially be taken for both *N. gonorrhoeae* and *C. trachomatis*. Chlamydia can be isolated in approximately 20 percent of patients with gonorrhea, and is a cause of epididymitis in itself. Patients with gonorrhea should therefore preferably be treated with a regimen active against β-lactamase positive strains of *N. gonorrhoeae* (e.g., ceftriaxone 250 mg intramuscularly), followed by 10 days of oral doxycycline (100 mg twice daily for 10 days) or by tetracycline hydroxychloride (500 milligrams orally four times daily for 10 days) to adequately cover chlamydial infection.

In patients with epididymitis secondary to nongonococcal urethritis, therapy should be instituted with oral doxycycline, 100 mg twice daily, or with oral tetracycline, 500 mg four times daily for 10 days.

Drainage of testicular abscesses or orchiectomy is seldom necessary in patients who receive early therapy with bed rest, scrotal elevation, and appropriate antimicrobials.

Several nonantimicrobial treatments have been proposed for epididymitis. Smith found that patients with epididymitis had dramatic relief of pain after one or two injections of the spermatic cord with procaine hydrochloride. He noted that the relief of pain was not only immediate but lasted well beyond the period of local relief.[70] Kamat et al.[71] reported on three groups of patients. One group received antibiotics only, one group was treated with antibiotics plus oxyphenbutazone, and one group was treated with antibiotics plus infiltration of the spermatic cord with xylocaine hydrochloride. He found that patients treated with antibiotics plus oxyphenbutazone or antibiotics plus spermatic cord infiltration had quicker recovery than patients on antibiotics alone. His study was not blinded, however, and he did not report bacteriologic results. McClellan[72] found antibiotic treatment to be better than symptomatic treatment alone. He reported that the addition of paraenzyme or varidase also decreased the amount of swelling and percentage with residual chronic epididymitis. Lapides[73] found that 35 of 47 patients with acute epididymitis were relieved by oxyphenbutazone alone. He found decreased pain in these patients but no decrease in the amount of erythema or swelling. In a multicenter placebo study, Moore et al.[74] found that prednisone had no value as adjuvant to antibiotic therapy in the treatment of epididymitis. Thus, some clinicians believe that infiltration of the spermatic cord and the use of oxyphenbutazone in addition to antibiotics may increase the comfort of a patient. However, it is not clear whether these forms of treatment provide better symptomatic relief than the use of analgesics with antibiotics. The effect of such adjuvant therapy on the long-term sequelae of epididymitis is uncertain.

In patients in whom the etiologic agent is a sexually transmitted pathogen, treatment of epididymitis is not complete without treatment of the sexual partner(s). This, hopefully, will prevent recurrences in the patient as well as prevent disease in the partner. In the only study in which the sexual partners of patients with epididymitis were examined, mucopurulent cervicitis was found in one and pelvic inflammatory disease in two of eight women.[1]

In the treatment of a patient with acute epididymitis, the decision must be made as to whether to pursue radiologic or endoscopic evidence for intrinsic genitourinary disease. Svend-Hansen[75] found that, in patients under the age of 50, only 6 of 43 men had abnormal excretory urograms. All patients with abnormal findings in his study had symptoms suggestive of urologic disease. He concluded that in patients less than 50 years old, epididymitis in itself is not an indication for radiographic evaluation. This may well reflect the small proportion of cases of epididymitis which are due to underlying urinary tract infection with coliforms or *Ps. aeruginosa* in younger men and thus the lower prevalence of genitourinary abnormalities. Similarly, we[1] found no patient under the age of 35 years to have concurrent genitourinary pathology, whereas 7 of 12 patients over the age of 35 with coliform infection had underlying pathology. Certainly the presence of urethritis due to *N. gonorrhoeae* or *C. trachomatis* does not suggest that the patient has an underlying genitourinary problem. On the other hand, the presence of a coliform urinary infection in a male always requires investigation. Patients with epididymitis due to coliform or *Ps. aeruginosa* infection should also be evaluated after completion of antimicrobial therapy with four glass urine cultures for chronic bacterial prostatitis (see Chap. 54), as this may be a predisposing factor to recurrent epididymitis.

## References


1 Berger RE et al: Etiology, manifestations and therapy of acute epididymitis: Prospective study of 50 cases. *J Urol* 121:750, 1979.
2 Hanley HG: Non-specific epididymitis. *Br J Surg* 53:873, 1966.
3 Bormel P: Current concepts of the etiology and treatment of epididymitis. *Med Bull US Army, Europe* 20:332, 1963.
4 Heap G: Acute epididymitis attributable to Chlamydial infection: Preliminary report. *Med J Aust* I:718, 1975.
5 Wolin LH: On the etiology of epididymitis. *J Urol* 105:531, 1971.
6 Gierup J et al: Acute non-specific epididymitis in boys. *Scand J Urol Nephrology* 9:5, 1975.
7 Megalli M et al: Reflux of urine into ejaculatory ducts as a cause of recurring epididymitis in children. *J Urol* 108:978, 1972.
8 Gislason T et al: Acute epididymitis in boys: A five year retrospective study. *J Urol* 124:533, 1980.
9 Shapiro SR, Breschi LC: Acute epididymitis in Vietnam: Review of 52 cases. *Milit Med* 138:643, 1973.
10 Mittemeyer BT et al: Epididymitis: A review of 610 cases. *J Urol* 95:390, 1966.
11 Berger RE et al: Etiology and manifestations of epididymitis in young men: Correlations with sexual orientation. *J Infect Dis* 155:1341, 1987.
12 Drach GW: Sexuality and prostatitis: A hypothesis. *J Am Vener Dis Assoc* 3:87, 1976.
13 Barnes RC et al: Urinary tract infections in sexually active homosexual men. *Lancet* 1:171, 1986.
14 Stamey TA et al: Recurrent urinary infections in adult women. The role of introital enterobacteria. *California Med* 115:1, 1971.
15 Berger RE et al: *Chlamydia trachomatis* as a cause of acute "idiopathic" epididymitis. *N Engl J Med* 298:301, 1978.
16 Gartman E: Epididymitis: A reappraisal. *Am J Surg* 101:736, 1961.
17 Ross WM, Maynard JH: Nonspecific epididymitis in the military service. *US Armed Forces Med J* 8:841, 1957.
18 Pelouze PS: Epididymitis, in *Gonorrhea in the Male and Female,* PS Pelouze (ed). Philadelphia, Saunders, 1941, p 240.
19 Watson RA: Gonorrhea and acute epididymitis. *Milit Med* 144:785, 1979.
20 Mulcahy FM et al: Prevalence of chlamydial infection in acute epididymo-orchitis. *Genitourin Med* 63:16, 1987.
21 Colleen S, Mårdh P-A: Complicated infections of the male genital tract with emphasis on *Chlamydia trachomatis* as an etiologic agent. *Scand J Infect Dis* (suppl) 32:93, 1982.
22 Melekos MD, Asbach HW: Epididymitis: Aspects concerning etiology and treatment. *J Urol* 138:83, 1987.
23 Cathcart CW: Epididymitis from muscular strain followed by tuberculosis of epididymis. *Edinburg Med J* 26:152, 1921.
24 Halker E: *Treatment of Renal Tuberculosis with Chemotherapeutics.* Copenhagen, Nyt Nordisk Forlng Arnold Busk, 1956.
25 Ross JC et al: Tuberculosis epididymitis: A review of 170 patients. *Br J Surg* 48:663, 1961.
26 Medlar EM et al: Post-mortem compared with clinical diagnosis of genitourinary tuberculosis in adult males. *J Urol* 61:1078, 1949.
27 McDonald JH, Heckel NJ: Acute pneumococcal epididymitis. *Illinois Med J* 95:304, 1949.
28 Mitchell CJ, Huins TJ: Acute brucellosis presenting as epididymoorchitis. *Br Med J* 2:557, 1974.
29 Davis WH, Scardino PL: Meningitis presenting as epididymitis. *South Med J* 65:936, 1972.
30 Gasparich JP et al: Amiodarone-associated epididymitis in the absence of infection. *J Urol* 133:971, 1985.
31 Furness G et al: Epididymitis after the luminal spread of nsu corynebacteria and gram negative bacteria from the fossa navicularis. *Invest Urol* 11:486, 1974.
32 Berger RE et al: Clinical use of epididymal aspiration cultures in the management of selected patients with acute epididymitis. *J Urol* 124:60, 1980.
33 Quinto O: Swelling of scrotum in infants and children and nonspecific epididymitis. *Acta Chir Scand* 110:417, 1956.
34 Devillar RG et al: Early exploration in acute testicular conditions. *J Urol* 108:887, 1972.
35 Barker K, Raper RP: Torsion of the testis. *Br J Urol* 36:35, 1964.
36 Doolittle KH et al: Epididymitis in the prepubertal boy. *J Urol* 96:364, 1966.
37 Madsen PO: Acute epididymitis vs. torsion of spermatic in military service. *J Urol* 83:169, 1960.
38 Perri AJ et al: The Doppler stethoscope and the diagnosis of the acute scrotum. *J Urol* 116:598, 1976.
39 Holder LE et al: Testicular radionuclide angiography and static imaging: Anatomy, scintigraphic interpretation, and clinical indications. *Radiology* 125:739, 1977.
40 Abu-Sleiman R et al: Scrotal scanning: Present value and limits of interpretation. *Urology* 13:326, 1979.
41 Hankins AJ: Testicular torsion and epididymitis demonstrated by radionuclide angiograms and static imaging. *J Natl Med Assoc* 71:981, 1979.
42 Costas S, Van Blerk PJP: Incision of the external inguinal ring in acute epididymitis. *Br J Urol* 45:555, 1973.
43 Arya OP, Taber ST: Correlates of venereal disease and fertility in rural Uganda. Presented at the Medical Society for the Study of Venereal Diseases, Malta, April 1975.
44 Campbell MF: Surgical pathology of epididymitis. *Ann Surg* 88:98, 1928.
45 Nilsson S et al: Changes in the testis parenchyma caused by acute nonspecific epididymitis. *Fertil Steril* 19:748, 1968.
46 Bietz O: Fertilitatsuntersuchungen bei der unspezifischen Epididymitis. *Hautarzt* 10:134, 1959.

47 Tozzo PJ: Semen analysis in unilateral epididymitis. *NY J Med* 1:2769, 1968.
48 Ludwig VG, Haselberger J: Epididymitis und fertilitat: Behandlungsergebnisse bei akuter anspezifischer epididymitis. *Fortschr Med* o5:397, 1977.
49 Lipschultz LI et al: Testicular function after orchidopexy for unilateral undescended testicle. *N Engl J Med* 295:15, 1976.
50 Gartsch G et al: Testicular torsion: Late results with special regard to fertility and endocrine function. *J Urol* 124:375, 1980.
51 Bandhauer K, Marberger H: Spermagglutinins in diseases of epididymis. *5th World Congress Fertil Steril* 1966, p 781.
52 Ingerslev HJ et al: A prospective study of antisperm antibody development in acute epididymitis. *J Urol* 136:162, 1986.
53 Close CE et al: The relationship of infection with *Chlamydia trachomatis* to the parameters of male infertility and sperm autoimmunity. *Fertil Steril* 48:880, 1987.
54 Cunningham JH, Cook WH: The operative treatment and pathology of acute epididymitis. *J Urol* 7:139, 1920.
55 Cronquist S: Spermatic invasion of the epididymis. *Acta Pathol Microbiol Scand* 26:786, 1949.
56 Kiviat MD, Kiviat NB et al: *Chlamydia trachomatis* epididymitis diagnosed by fluorescent monoclonal antibody. *Urology* 30:395, 1987.
57 Moller BR, Mårdh P: Experimental epididymitis and urethritis in grivet monkeys provoked by *Chlamydia trachomatis. Fertil Steril* 34:275, 1980.
58 Berger RE et al: Epididymitis after the experimental inoculation of the nonhuman primate with *Chlamydia trachomatis*. Unpublished data.
59 Lucchetta R et al: Acute experimental *E. coli* epididymitis in the rat and its consequences on spermatogenesis. *Urol Res* 11:117, 1983.
60 Hackett RA et al: Experimental *E. coli* epididymitis in rabbits. *Urology*, in press.
61 Kohler FP: An inquiry into the etiology of acute epididymitis. *J Urol* 87:918, 1962.
62 Herwig KR et al: Response of acute epididymitis to oxyphenbutazone. *J Urol* 106:890, 1971.
63 Kiviat MD: Unpublished data.
64 Kendall AR: Rationale of prophylactic vasectomy. *J Urol* 89:712, 1963.
65 Orandi A et al: Vas culture, epididymitis and post-prostatectomy fever. *J Urol* 96:367, 1966.
66 Reeves JF et al: Prevention of epididymitis after prostatectomy by prophylactic antibiotics and partial vasectomy. *J Urol* 92:528, 1964.
67 Wesson MB: Epididymitis: Importance of determining etiology. *J Urol* 85:960, 1961.
68 Rolnick HC: Infections along the sheath of the vas deferens. *J Urol* 14:371, 1925.
69 Nilsson T, Fischer AB: Acute epididymitis: Investigation, etiology and treatment with doxycycline, in *Sexually Transmitted Disease* (Symposium Proceedings). Los Angeles, Science & Medicine Publishing, 1979, p 38.
70 Smith DR: Treatment of epididymitis by infiltration of spermatic cord with procaine hydrochloride. *J Urol* 46:74, 1941.
71 Kamat MH et al: Epididymitis: Response to different modalities of treatment. *J Med Soc NJ* 67:227, 1970.
72 McClellan DS et al: Effect of varidase on acute non-specific epididymitis. *J Urol* 84:6733, 1960.
73 Lapides J et al: Oxyphenbutazone therapy for mumps orchitis, acute epididymitis and osteitis pubis. *J Urol* 98:528, 1964.
74 Moore CA et al: Prednisone in the treatment of acute epididymitis: A cooperative study. *J Urol* 106:578, 1971.
75 Svend-Hansen H et al: The value of routine intravenous urography in acute epididymitis. *Int Urol Nephrology* 9:245, 1977.

# Chapter 54
# Prostatitis

Stig Colleen
Per-Anders Mårdh

## HISTORY

In the premicrobiological era urethral discharge was generally regarded as overproduction of semen, which was assumed to originate from the prostate. Though in most cases the condition resolved spontaneously, it was sometimes complicated by obstructive symptoms as a consequence of enlargement and altered consistency of the prostate during the healing process. The presumed association between urethritis and prostatic obstruction, benign or malignant, on the one hand and overproduction of semen on the other hand, may explain why physicians in former days warned that excessive *baccu et venere* in youth could result in urinary retention and uremia in old age.

By the end of the nineteenth century, prostatitis had been relatively well defined as an entity. It was then a frequent (20 to 40 percent) and feared complication of gonococcal urethritis. Gonococcal prostatitis could lead to septicemia, prostatic abscess, and fistula to the rectum, urethra, and perineal surface. The mortality in such complications approached 30 percent. If the inflammation subsided, chronic urgency, dysuria, and suprapubic pain could result. Sexual disturbances, often postejaculatory pain, were also seen.[1]

The advent of antibiotic therapy eliminated prostatitis as a life-threatening complication of acute urethritis. Gonococcal virulence may also have changed; nowadays, symptomatic prostatitis appearing in immediate association with acute urethritis is rare. Despite the availability of antibiotic treatment for infectious urethritis, however, the incidence of nonacute (chronic nonbacterial or idiopathic) prostatitis does not seem to have lessened in recent decades. The association, if any, between nonacute prostatitis and sexually transmitted diseases is not clear.

## ANATOMY AND PHYSIOLOGY OF THE PROSTATE

The prostate is a compound tubuloalveolar gland, consisting of periurethral (internal) and peripheral (external) groups of secretory units. With refined dissecting technique it is possible to identify paired dorsal, lateral, and median lobes in the adult prostatic gland.[2] The median lobes correspond to the coagulating gland of the rat.[3] The peripheral units empty into the urethra through a large number of orifices on either side of the verumontanum. The orifices have no sphincters. Secretion from the internal units enters the urethra in its entire circumference. These units seem to correspond to the urethral glands of Littré.

The supportive stroma of the prostate consists of elastic tissue with an abundance of smooth muscle. The gland is attached to the osseous pelvis by the puboprostatic ligaments and to the deep trigone by the transpiercing urethra. Contractions of the pelvic floor therefore affect the prostate[4] (see also Chap. 10).

The nervous control of the stromal and glandular component of the prostate is mediated by axons having cholinergic and noradrenergic endings and probably originating from the sympathetic outflow from T11 to L1. Sensations of prostatic pain are thought to be conveyed in the sympathetic supply or by afferents in the pelvic splanchnic nerves.[4]

The prostatic gland is one of the main contributors (30 to 40 percent of the total volume) to the seminal plasma. Its significance for fertility, however, is still obscure.

Some of the many substances isolated from prostatic secretion have attracted special interest: zinc, magnesium, calcium, citric acid, cholesterol, spermine, lysozyme, and acid phosphatase[5–8] (Table 54-1). Determination of these substances in seminal fluid has been utilized to indicate the functional state of the prostatic gland and to measure the prostatic contribution to the emission.

For proliferation and synthesis, the prostatic epithelium is dependent on androgens. Dihydrotestosterone is the trophic hormone. The prostate produces it by reduction of testosterone and from dehydroepiandrosterone and androstenedione trapped from the plasma. As the prostate is assumed to be the major consumer of testosterone, functional dropout of the prostate has been claimed to cause disturbances in the testicular-hypophyseal axis.[9]

## DEFINITIONS

From the histopathological viewpoint, prostatitis must be defined as an inflammatory reaction confined to the prostate. Histological study of prostatic sections from men without symptoms of prostatitis, however, shows a prevalence of inflammatory areas that increases with age.

Such inflammatory changes are usually confined to one or more excretory ducts. These ducts are dilated and filled with inspissated secretion and macrophages with phagocytized foamy material. The intensity of the inflammatory reaction may vary and both acute and chronic inflammatory changes may be present. Focal aggregation of lymphoid cells without ductal engagement is not considered to indicate prostatitis.[10]

Because of the focal character of the inflammatory lesions, transurethral, transperineal, or transrectal random biopsies often fail to confirm clinically suspected prostatitis. One consequence of the poor reliability of biopsy specimens has been doubt concerning the diagnostic possibilities in prostatitis.

Demonstration of inflammatory cells within the excretory ducts of the prostate forms the only reliable basis for the morphological diagnosis of prostatitis. This means that expressed prostatic fluid must be shown to contain pus cells. Failure to obtain prostatic secretion because of unsuitable collecting technique or inadequate instruction of the patient has tempted some

**Table 54-1. Concentration of Some Constituents of Expressed Prostatic Fluid**

| Compound | Concentration* | Reference |
|---|---|---|
| Zinc | 0.352 ± 0.048 g/liter | 5 |
| Magnesium | 0.120 ± 0.060 g/liter | 6 |
| Calcium | 1.200 ± 0.080 g/liter | 5 |
| Citric acid | 4.80 ± 26.9 g/liter | 5 |
| Cholesterol | 0.078 ± 0.013 g/liter | 5 |
| Spermine | 0.243 ± 0.025 g/liter | 7 |
| Lysozyme | 0.021 ± 0.006 g/liter | 8 |
| Acid phosphatase | 2.56 million IU per liter | 5 |

*Mean ± 2 SD.

**Table 54-2. Classification of Benign Painful Disorders of the Prostate Based on Findings in Expressed Prostatic Fluid**

| Nomenclature | Pathological culture findings* | Purulent prostatic fluid |
|---|---|---|
| Acute bacterial prostatitis | + | + |
| Chronic bacterial prostatitis | + | + |
| Nonbacterial prostatitis | − | + |
| Prostatodynia | − | − |

*The + denotes presence and the − denotes absence of common uropathogens.
SOURCE: GW Drach et al.[11]

clinicians to accept "characteristic" symptoms and/or palpatory findings as diagnostic criteria. This is probably the main reason why there is still much confusion concerning the diagnosis. Because of the lack of uniformity in terminology, a group of investigators[11] has suggested a classification of benign painful disease of the prostate based on morphological studies of prostatic fluid and cultures of urine and prostatic fluid sampled in a defined way (Table 54-2).

## ETIOLOGY

### INFECTIOUS PROSTATITIS

Infectious forms of prostatitis occur after puberty and progressively increase in incidence thereafter.[12] The causative microorganism may reach the prostate as an ascending urethral infection, by reflux of infected urine into the prostatic ducts or by lymphogenous or hematogenous spread. Canalicular spread seems to be most likely.

In urogenital tuberculosis in men, *Mycobacterium tuberculosis, M. bovis,* or rarely, other mycobacterial species, can almost always be isolated from semen or expressed prostatic fluid. In 20 percent of urogenital mycobacterial infections, these are the only specimens from which the causal agent can be recovered. Mycobacterial infection is a rare cause of prostatitis, however.

In introital coliform colonization of women, the same bacterial species can often be isolated from the urethra of their male consorts. Hence it is not surprising that species of coliforms isolated from urine in men with bacterial prostatitis are found in the vaginal secretion of their sexual partners.[13,14] Although coliforms can be spread by sexual intercourse, it is likely that defective host factors rather than characteristics of the pathogen are most essential in the pathogenesis of bacterial prostatitis. In *acute and chronic bacterial* prostatitis, urinary tract pathogens are causally involved, often *Escherichia coli,* though other Enterobacteriaceae such as *Proteus mirabilis* and various *Klebsiella* and *Pseudomonas* spp. may also be implicated. More than one species can often be simultaneously demonstrated in the prostatic secretion. The clinical course of this type of bacterial prostatitis is characterized by complicating recurrent infections of the urinary tract.

The etiologic role of gram-positive cocci in bacterial prostatitis is unclear. Enterococci, concomitant with gram-negative rods, may be associated with bacterial prostatitis. Coagulase-negative staphylococci, micrococci, and streptococci that occur as indigenous flora of the anterior urethra have been regarded as less likely etiologic agents, since they could not be isolated in a reproducible pattern in longitudinal studies of prostatitis.[15] Thus, gram-positive bacteria, with the possible exception of enterococci, can seldom be incriminated as causal agents in bacterial prostatitis.[16–18]

Recent unpublished studies from our departments have shown that *Staphylococcus saprophyticus,* a coagulase-negative, novobiocin-resistant species, is a common cause of urinary tract infection in males (as well as females). In contrast to women, the highest incidence of such infections in men is among the elderly. Our preliminary studies[19] did not indicate an etiologic role of *S. saprophyticus* in prostatitis. Bergman, Wedrén, and Holm (unpublished data) found *S. saprophyticus* in 12 (17 percent) of 71 men with assumed "chronic bacterial" prostatitis, with a peak in August and September (as in urinary tract infections in females). Seven of the 12 men had the greatest number of *S. saprophyticus* bacteria at the prostatic level, and the bacteria disappeared with treatment.

While it has been suggested that prostatitis is a common complication of urethritis due to sexually transmitted agents,[20] no reliable information supports this suggestion. However, evidence of previous gonococcal and/or chlamydial infection has been found in a small proportion (approximately 10 percent) of prostatitis cases.[19,21,22] In a number of such cases, gonococci were demonstrated by immunofluorescence tests of expressed prostatic fluid, though conventional cultures for gonococci had been negative. The history and serological studies indicated previous exposure to gonococci in most of these culture-negative patients. All of them had in the interval received antibiotics to which *Neisseria gonorrhoeae* is susceptible. In studies of *Chlamydia trachomatis,* neither cultures nor search for IgM and IgG microimmunofluorescent antibodies in serum and expressed prostatic fluid has indicated current or recent chlamydial infection in more than a small percentage of men with prostatitis. When there was serological evidence of exposure to *C. trachomatis,* the first symptoms were of urethritis rather than prostatitis. Epididymitis had also occurred in some of the patients.[22,23] Poletti et al.[23] claimed to have isolated *C. trachomatis* from biopsies of the prostate obtained by transrectal fine-needle aspiration in one-third of patients with symptoms suggestive of prostatitis and who had positive urethral cultures for this organism. The authors used noncentrifuged, cycloheximide-treated McCoy cells to recover the organisms, a method that has not been successful in the hands of others. Other authors have not been able to recover chlamydiae from prostatic biopsies.[24] Direct specimen antigen detection tests, i.e., ELISA and immunofluorescence tests, have not indicated a chlamydial etiology more often than did culture studies. In experimental infections in grivet monkeys, *C. trachomatis* produced urethritis, vasitis, and epididymitis, but not prostatitis.

Mårdh and Colleen[17] found *Mycoplasma hominis* in the urethra in 7 of 78 men with prostatitis but in none of 20 controls. However, this organism could not be isolated from semen or prostatic fluid. Serum antibodies to *M. hominis* could be demonstrated in only one culture-positive patient. Eradication of the organism was followed by only temporary relief of symptoms. *Ureaplasma urealyticum* occurs in the indigenous flora of the genitourinary tract and can be cultured from 40 to 80 percent of women of childbearing age. It can be isolated with the same frequency from the urethra of healthy young males and from patients with prostatitis.[21] *U. urealyticum* has been proposed as a cause of prostatitic infection; in this study, by using a segmental culture technique, *U. urealyticum* was isolated from 8.6 percent of inflamed prostates.[18] It was also recovered from the urethra in 55 percent of men with pus in expressed prostatic secretion. Of 108 controls, none was found to harbor *U. urealyticum* in the prostate, and in only 22 percent was the organism found in the urethra. In studies on patients with inflammatory disease of the prostate, $\geq 10^4$ colony-forming units (CFU) of *U. urealyticum* per ml of prostatic secretion was believed to favor an etiological relationship.[24] This would indicate an overall frequency of ureaplasma-associated prostatitis of 13.7 percent; a similar figure was obtained by others.[25]

## NONINFECTIOUS PROSTATITIS

The etiology of noninfectious forms of prostatitis (nonbacterial prostatitis, as defined by Drach et al.[11]) is obscure. The nomenclature might be slightly misleading since, as discussed below, different microorganisms can be etiologically involved. Though at present the term *idiopathic prostatitis* is not accepted, it would perhaps be a more accurate term to describe this condition. However, in this presentation we use the nomenclature proposed by Drach et al.[11]

The diagnosis is made by a process of exclusion when cultures have proved negative for assumed uropathogens. Obligate anaerobic bacteria, fungi, trichomonads, and viruses are among the other agents that have been tested for association with this condition. Thus, in 78 men with signs of nonbacterial prostatitis, *Candida albicans* was recovered from five and *Trichomonas vaginalis* from one, while cytomegalovirus and herpes simplex virus were never isolated. It seems scarcely possible, therefore, that all of the agents discussed above can account for more than isolated cases of prostatitis.[21,26–29]

*Reflux of sterile urine* into the efferent ducts of the prostate is commonly observed at micturition cystography in men with infraprostatic obstruction. Such reflux probably occurs also when there is no such obstruction, since crystallographic analysis of prostatic calculi has revealed constituents normally present in urine but not in prostatic secretion.[30] Although it is not known if urinary reflux may elicit an inflammatory reaction within the efferent ducts or may interfere with resistance against bacterial invasion, this mechanism has been discussed among possible causes of nonbacterial prostatitis.[31]

Prostatitis is frequently associated with benign hyperplasia of the prostate. It has been suggested that the nonpredictable course of obstructive symptoms in elderly men with benign prostatic enlargement may be partly ascribable to inflammatory changes in the gland elicited by *aseptic necrosis* of adenomatous foci.

Single cases of *allergic granulomatous prostatitis* have been reported among asthmatics and were thought to represent part of a systemic vascular disease, probably periarteritis nodosa, with fibrinoid necrosis. Biopsy specimens from the prostate showed histiocytic granulomas with eosinophils.[32]

Nonspecific *granulomatous prostatitis* was first reported by Tanner and McDonald in 1943.[33] The condition was found in 10 percent of surgically treated cases of prostatitis.[34] The condition occurs in elderly men, usually with obstructive symptoms. It is characterized by hard, ill-defined infiltrations. In the differential diagnosis, carcinoma of the prostate must be considered. The etiology of granulomatous prostatitis remains unknown. Transurethral resection is almost always curative. The patients are reported also to do well on steroids.[35]

Anxiety, psychosomatic problems, and mental stress are frequently experienced among patients with noninfectious prostatitis. Recent experimental data give some support for stress as a possible cause of noninfectious prostatitis. Such stimuli of short or long duration will provoke a reaction in the prostate of the rat resembling prostatitis in man.[36]

Although an increasing number of causes can be recognized when cases of nonbacterial prostatitis are subjected to careful study, the etiology in the majority remains obscure and presents a challenge to further research.

## EPIDEMIOLOGY

In 100 consecutive autopsies on men who had died suddenly in automobile accidents and from other causes, Boström[12] found that the prevalence of histological signs of prostatitis increased with age and was greatest when there was benign enlargement of the gland. Signs of prostatitis were present in 22 percent of the men younger than 40 years and in 60 percent of those above that age. In some studies[37] no correlation was found between histological signs of prostatitis and occurrence of pus cells in expressed prostatic fluid. These studies point to lack of awareness of the importance of examining repeated samples of prostatic fluid before the diagnosis is settled[21] rather than to absence of signs of inflammation in the drainage system of the prostatic gland.

In 156 urogenitally asymptomatic men who were either entering or leaving U.S. Army service, O'Shaughnessy and Parrino[38] found increased number of pus cells in expressed prostatic fluid, suggestive of prostatitis, in 38 percent. Other authors, however, have reported considerably lower figures for prevalence of prostatitis, often only 4 to 6 percent.[39]

The prevalence of clinically diagnosed prostatitis in a nonselected population is not known. Blacklock[40] reported an annual incidence of clinically diagnosed cases amounting to 0.1 percent in the Royal Navy.

Thus it is evident that prostatitis is a common disease and that it may or may not present symptoms.

## CLINICAL MANIFESTATIONS

*Acute bacterial prostatitis* is characterized by sudden chills, pyrexia, general malaise, bladder-outlet obstruction, frequency of micturition and, occasionally, acute retention. The nonacute conditions (i.e, *chronic bacterial prostatitis* and *nonbacterial prostatitis*) present with less fulminant symptoms. Though there may be no obviously prostatic symptoms in chronic bacterial prostatitis, the patients commonly have disturbances of bladder function such as increased frequency and urgency of micturition, dysuria, and postmicturition dribbling. A watery discharge is a less common complaint. Postejaculatory pain and hemospermia are more frequent in nonbacterial prostatitis, as is dull suprapubic pain that sometimes projects to the perineal area, the loins, the testes, and the penis.

Up to 3 percent of cases of nonspecific urethritis are reported to be complicated by other manifestations of Reiter's syndrome. The relative risk of such complications is increased tenfold in patients with tissue antigen HLA-B27.[41] Without exception, these complications of urethritis, which are generally associated with infection by sexually transmitted agents, are accompanied by prostatitis.[42]

## SEQUELAE

Sequelae of infection in the genitourinary tract may be causal factors in infertility. Orchitis complicating mumps and epididymitis complicating gonorrhea or tuberculosis can result in azoospermia and, hence, in sterility. Microorganisms whose effect, as far as is known, is less detrimental to the germinal epithelium or the genital duct system may interfere with the secretory functions of the accessory genital glands. Microbial elicitation of an immunologic response may reduce the motility and viability of spermatozoa. Thus, known urinary tract pathogens such as *E. coli, Proteus* ssp., *T. vaginalis,* and *C. albicans* can immobilize spermatozoa, and *E. coli* and *C. albicans* can cause spermatozoal agglutination. Many other indigenous constituents of the urethral flora possess none of these properties.[43,44] The concentration of microorganisms required to produce immobilization or agglutination of spermatozoa in vitro, however, is rarely, if ever, found in prostatic fluid except in cases of chronic bacterial prostatitis. Decreased sperm counts, increased percentage of tapering and immature forms, and reduced sperm motility have been found to correlate with occurrence of *U. urealyticum.*[45] However, *U. urealyticum* and *M. hominis* can be recovered in equal frequencies from infertile and fertile couples.[46]

In infection of the renal parenchyma, bacteria isolated from the urine are often antibody-coated.[47] Riedasch et al.[48] and Jones[49] found that bacterial prostatitis was also associated with antibody coating of bacteria isolated from ejaculate and urine. The presence of antibodies in secretion from the accessory genital glands is assumed to indicate a local immune response. In obstruction of the afferent pathways of the genital gland (epididymis or vas deferens), with or without infection, antibodies which can immobilize and/or agglutinate spermatozoa have been demonstrated in blood and in accessory genital gland secretions.[50] The prevalence of such antibodies was 2 to 3 percent in fertile men and was increased fivefold in infertile men.[51] The importance of prostatitis in eliciting this immune response is not known. However, spermatozoal antibodies have been demonstrated in serum by indirect immunofluorescence in 39 percent and with a microagglutination test in 10 percent of men with prostatitis, while the figures in matched controls were 5 and 0 percent.[52]

Zinc in ejaculated seminal plasma is bound by protein constituents in the genital secretions of the female recipient. Sperm motility and "capacitation" (acquisition of the ability to fertilize ova) are thereby evoked.[53,54] Biochemical changes induced by inflammatory reactions of the prostate may have an impact on fertility, though their relative importance is poorly understood. The normally high levels of zinc in prostatic fluid and seminal plasma are considerably reduced in prostatitis. This decreases sperm motility and induces higher basal activity of the spermatozoa than in men without prostatitis.[53]

That bacteria in the prostate can induce immunologic and/or biochemical changes leading to decreased motility and density of sperm remains a matter for conjecture.[55] The occurrence of morphologically abnormal spermatozoa is more difficult to explain.[56]

No hard evidence has yet been presented that incriminates an inflammatory reaction within the prostate as having an etiologic role in prostatic cancer. However, the observation of a higher prevalence of patients with a history of venereal disease and a greater sexual drive in individuals with cancer of the prostate has from time to time renewed the consideration of a sexually transmitted agent as a possible etiologic factor in prostatic cancer.[54,57]

## DIFFERENTIAL DIAGNOSIS

A number of conditions must be considered in the differential diagnosis of prostatitis. Similar bladder symptoms—urgency and frequency of micturition and postmicturition dribbling—occur with intravesical obstruction.

In elderly men, benign *prostatic hyperplasia* and *sclerotic bladder-neck obstruction* should be recognized by digital examination of the prostate and by endoscopy and urethroscopy. When pus cells are found in expressed prostatic secretion from men with suspected bladder-neck obstruction, the urinary flow should be measured. This will reveal any significant hindrance to outflow. Surgical treatment is then indicated. Inflammatory changes in the prostate should not be regarded as the cause of the symptoms in these cases unless urgency, pain, etc., persist despite postoperatively reestablished micturition.

*Urethral stricture,* in which urgency is the main complaint, can usually be relieved by surgery, though most patients with urethral stricture have concomitant prostatitis. In the preantibiotic era urethral stricture was one of the most prevalent complications of urethritis. In developing countries, a frequency of one out of seven males with gonorrhoea has recently been reported to develop urethral stricture.[58] Though the incidence of this disabling condition has decreased, 1.8 and 4.9 percent of patients with gonococcal and nongonococcal urethritis, respectively, developed urethral strictures in a study of the early sixties in central London.[59] More recent figures of less than 1 percent have been reported, yet urethritis still constitutes a major etiology in younger adult males offered reconstructive surgery for urethral stricture.[60–62] The preference of the gonococcus for secretory mucosal cells might reflect why strictures develop in the parts of the urethra carrying large numbers of glands, i.e., the very anterior and the entire posterior (bulbous) urethra.[63]

Once established, urethral stricture is a progressive condition[64] which sooner or later calls for urological correction. Although bouginage is the time-honored treatment, few patients are cured by this modality.[65] Most individuals subjected to this management face a lifetime of repetitive urologic contacts. Even in skillful hands the patient can develop recurrent urinary tract infections, calculi, or even septicemia. During the last few decades, operative techniques have been developed that seem to provide a chance for definite cure in the majority of cases. Thus, four out of five patients remain free of obstructive symptoms 5 years after the operation.[66]

*Bladder-neck dyssynergia,* which mainly affects younger men, seems to be a fairly infrequent malfunction of the lower urinary tract. It is characterized by urgency and frequency of micturition and postmicturition dribbling and sometimes by prostatitis. The diagnosis of bladder-neck dyssynergia is difficult to establish unless micturition urethrocystography and urinary flow measurements are performed.

Since perineal, as well as retropubic pain may be evoked by *anorectal disease,* proctoscopy should be included in the evaluation of patients with symptoms of prostatitis, especially if the symptoms are not relieved by bed rest.

Prostatic pain is generally aggravated when the patient is erect because the increased tension of the pelvic floor muscles leads to compression of the gland.[31] Increased tension of these muscles seems per se to be able to elicit pain from the perineal and suprapubic areas. In addition, stress on this muscular diaphragm can provoke urgency and frequency of micturition and often testicular pain. *Pelvic floor tension myalgia* (also known as levator ani syndrome, piriformis syndrome, diaphragma pelvis spastica, and coccygodynia) is typically aggravated by sitting, for instance, in an automobile. Objective evidence of the condition is limited to palpatory pain from the levator ani and short external rotators.[57,67] Expressed prostatic fluid contains no inflammatory cells. These patients benefit from neuromuscular retraining.[68,69]

Patients without signs of inflammatory prostatic disease but with vague symptoms from the urinary bladder, who complain mainly of pain and sexual dysfunction (i.e., pain on ejaculation, reduced libido, and impotence), may suffer from *prostatodynia.*[11] Urinary flow measurements should be made in these patients to exclude obstruction of the urinary tract.[70] This syndrome may present with typical symptoms of prostatic disease but no confirmatory objective evidence. A variety of conditions may underlie the symptoms, including psychiatric disturbance such as sexual difficulties produced by sex identity problems[71] and neurotic disorders.[72] Patients with these problems should not be dismissed with antibiotic or anti-inflammatory treatment; they should be managed in collaboration with psychiatric expertise. Unfortunately, use of the term prostatodynia focuses attention on the prostate as the origin of the symptoms, though this may not be the case.

## LABORATORY DIAGNOSIS

The only way in which the diagnosis of prostatitis can be objectively established is by microscopy of expressed prostatic fluid together with quantitative bacteriologic cultures of specimens from the urethra and the bladder and from expressed prostatic secretion.[73]

To obtain specimens for diagnosis, the patient should have a full bladder and be able to void on request. No other precautions are necessary in the circumcised man. In the uncircumcised man, the prepuce is retracted and the meatus is dried with a sterile sponge. The patient is asked to void. The first 10 ml (first voided bladder urine, or $VB_1$) and 10 ml from the midstream portion ($VB_2$) are collected in sterile test tubes for culture and microscopy. Micturition is interrupted before the bladder is empty, and the patient is instructed to adopt a knee-elbow position. The physician then massages the prostate and collects into a sterile petri dish the prostatic fluid (expressed prostatic secretion, or EPS) that drips from the urethral meatus. If no prostatic secretion appears, pressure applied along the entire urethra half a minute after the massage is ended will generally result in the expected amount of EPS. Finally, the patient is asked to empty his bladder and the first 10 ml of the voided urine ($VB_3$) is collected for analysis (Fig. 54-1).

This segmental culture technique[73] is believed to permit determination of the origin of the recovered microorganisms. Thus, if

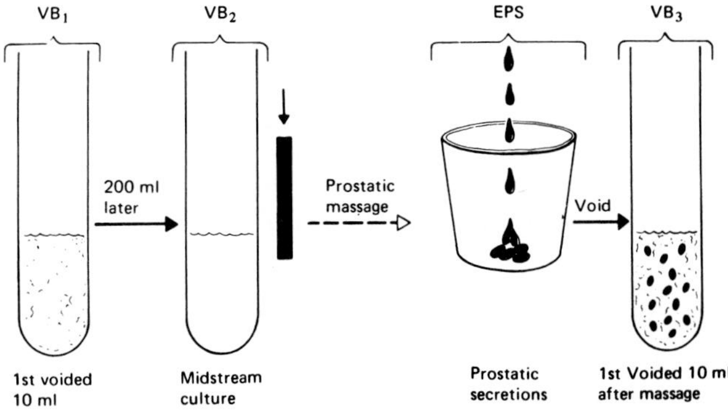


Fig. 54-1. Segmental culture of the lower urinary tract in the male. *(From EM Meares and TA Stamey.[73])*

the number of colony-forming units (CFUs) in $VB_1$ significantly exceeds the counts in $VB_2$, EPS, and $VB_3$, the urethra is assumed to be the microbial origin. When the CFUs in EPS and $VB_3$ are at least 10 times more numerous than in $VB_1$ and $VB_2$, the prostate is assumed to be colonized. Concomitant bacteriuria can be eliminated as an obstacle to the diagnosis of bacterial prostatitis by treatment with an appropriate antimicrobial substance, such as nitrofurantoin, which does not significantly penetrate the prostate. The patient is reexamined a few days after completion of the antimicrobial treatment.

The $VB_1$, $VB_2$, $VB_3$, and EPS should be sent chilled to the laboratory, where cultures are made with the calibrated loop technique: 0.1 ml of the specimen and an equal volume diluted 1:100 in saline are inoculated on blood agar plates and incubated overnight at 37°C. The numbers of CFUs are determined, and the concentration of bacteria in the original specimens can thereby be established.

The reliability of large amounts of pus cells in wet smears of EPS as a sign of prostatic inflammation has been questioned,[38] especially as Jameson[74] demonstrated increased numbers of leukocytes in specimens obtained soon after sexual stimulation and ejaculation (intercourse, masturbation, and nocturnal emission). After such stimulation, however, the leukocyte count only rarely approaches 20 per high-power ($\times 400$) microscopic field. In a carefully controlled study, Andersson and Weller[75] found significantly more leukocytes in EPS from men with symptoms of prostatitis than in EPS from controls without known genital disorders. The number of histiocytes [macrophages and oval fat bodies (Fig. 54-2)] per cubic millimeter of EPS from the prostatitis patients was eight times greater than in the controls. Moreover, there was correlation between the number of histiocytes and the intensity of symptoms reported by the patients. This study and others[21] indicated that a white blood cell (WBC) count of more than 1000 cells per cubic millimeter in EPS (i.e., $> 10$ WBCs per high-power field) is a sign of inflammation of the prostate. A high WBC concentration, however, is found also in patients with urethritis only. The presence of leukocyte aggregates, or rather of casts of pus cells, is mandatory for the diagnosis of prostatitis.

The poor correspondence in prostatitis between the cytological findings in semen and in EPS is probably ascribable to the focal involvement of the gland and poor drainage of the affected area at emission. The secretory function of the prostate as a whole is probably impaired in prostatitis, even though the inflammatory process may be focal. This is evidenced by diminution of constituents of semen which the healthy prostate secretes in high concentrations (e.g., zinc, magnesium, spermine, cholesterol, citric acid, and acid phosphatase).[7,76,77] The pH of prostatic fluid in healthy men is 6.5 to 6.8. In prostatitis the fluid tends to become alkaline and the pH may even approach 8.0 to 8.2.[78] Acidity is restored as the inflammatory reaction subsides.[79]

Antibacterial activity of prostatic fluid,[80] which has been reported against gram-negative as well as gram-positive bacteria,[81] is also affected by the secretory dysfunction in prostatitis. The concentration of lysozyme, which is particularly active against gram-positive bacteria, is likewise reduced in a percentage of patients with prostatitis.[82] The diminution in concentration or activity of constituents with antibacterial effect has led to speculations concerning compromised local resistance. If host-parasite relationships are disturbed, urethral commensals might act as pathogens.[83]

So far we do not know whether other conditions also may cause secretory dysfunction of the prostate. Consequently, the

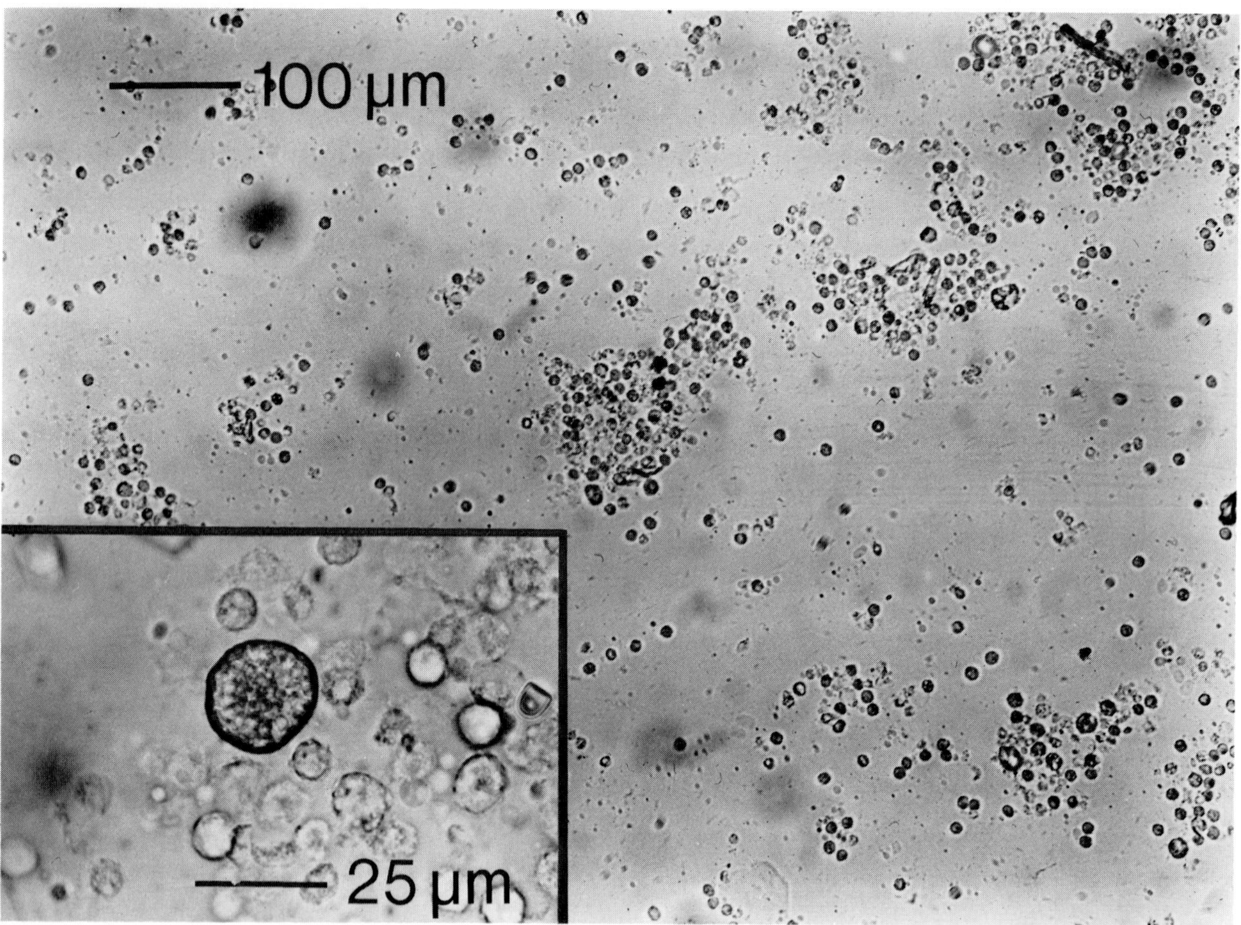


Fig. 54-2. Micrograph of an unstained specimen of expressed prostatic fluid originating from a patient with nonbacterial (idiopathic) prostatitis. Numerous leukocytes, lymphocytes, and plasma cells are found, with occasional casts. Inset visualizes a large macrophage with phagocytized foamy material (oval fat body).

diagnosis of prostatitis cannot as yet be based on chemical anayses of seminal fluid but must still rely on microscopic examination of EPS.

## MANAGEMENT

Bacterial prostatitis should be treated with antibiotics that are active against gram-negative organisms. The selected antibiotic must be able to penetrate to the focus of infection. To pass from the blood through the luminal lining of the prostatic epithelium and reach the draining ducts of the gland, a drug must be nonpolar (i.e., lipid-soluble) and uncharged. Antimicrobial agents in their undissociated state differ in these respects. Most are weakly acidic, though some are alkaline. Depending on the pK value of a specific agent, a variable amount is present as anions (in acidic agents) or cations (in basic agents). The relative proportion of a drug available in ionic and undissociated forms, however, is related not only to the pK of the drug, but also to the pH of the surrounding medium. There is a pH difference between blood (pH 7.4) and prostatic fluid (pH 6.8 to 7.2). This difference has been utilized to obtain enrichment of drugs in the excretory ducts of the prostate. Acidic agents will accumulate in an environment that is alkaline in comparison with blood, while basic agents will concentrate when the pH is below 7.4.

In a series of beautifully designed experiments on dogs, Stamey et al.[80] demonstrated a tenfold increased concentration of trimethoprim in prostatic fluid as compared with blood. Nevertheless, trimethoprim has not proved as useful as was originally hoped in the treatment of bacterial prostatitis. This disappointing experience may be related to a discrepancy in pH between fluid from the inflamed prostate in humans and the prostatic secretion in healthy dogs. The slightly acid pH of EPS in healthy men turns alkaline during inflammation.[84,85] If the pH of EPS is 8.2, a sixfold enrichment of an antimicrobial agent may be expected in the efferent ducts of the prostate, provided that this agent is less polar in the undissociated state and is an acid with pK less than 6.5 (Fig. 54-3). A basic agent that is lipid-soluble and has pK higher than 8.5 will give a prostatic concentration only one-fourth of that in the plasma. Recent data indicate that tetracyclines, erythromycin, and other macrolides and some sulfonamides can accumulate in the fluid in inflamed glands. This observation supports the theory of the distribution and kinetics of antimicrobial agents within the prostate.[86,87] In a carefully performed randomized study on men with recurrent urinary tract infections, Smith et al.[88] demonstrated better results with trimethoprim-sulfamethoxazole when treatment was extended from 10 days to 12 weeks, but this study also demonstrated the difficulty in eradicating infection when the prostate was infected.

Urinary tract infections associated with calculi cannot be eradicated unless the stones are removed. This maxim does not seem valid for calculi in the prostate. Most prostatic tissue specimens

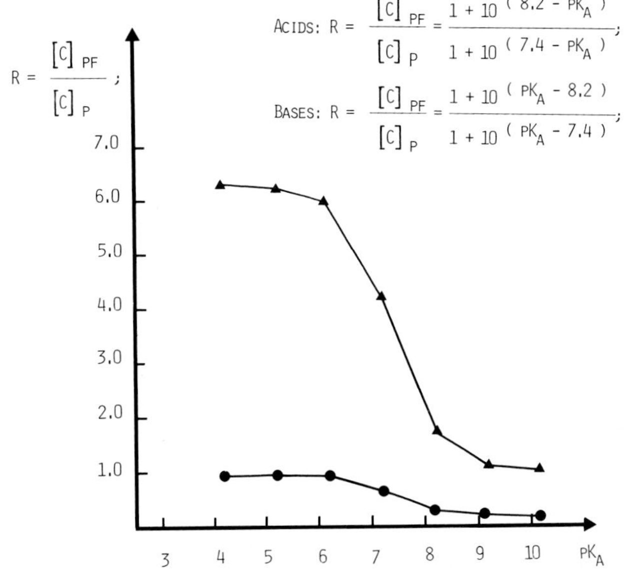


**Fig. 54-3.** Theoretical limits for antibiotic concentration ratio between prostatic fluid and blood plasma for acidic (*circle*) and basic (*triangle*) agents with different $pK_A$ values at postulated prostatic fluid pH of 8.2. Free exchange of the undissociated fraction of acid and base between the blood plasma and the prostatic secretion is assumed. R = ratio of total drug in prostatic fluid to blood plasma; C = total concentration of drug; PF = prostatic fluid; P = blood plasma.

from adults can be shown at microscopy to contain calculi. Pelvic x-ray examination reveals prostatic calculi in 13.6 percent of adult males.[89]

In chronic bacterial prostatitis accompanied by urinary tract infections which relapse repeatedly despite the use of antimicrobial agents (appropriately selected with regard to antibacterial spectrum and penetration ability), radical transurethral resection of the prostate is advised. The resection must include not only areas of benign hypertrophy, but also the main peripheral parts of the gland, where calculi usually lodge. With this single exception, surgical treatment of inflammatory conditions of the prostate nowadays has few advocates.

Total prostatectomy in bacterial or nonbacterial prostatitis must be rejected because of complications such as urinary incontinence and fistula and erectile dysfunction.

Antimicrobial treatment of acute bacterial prostatitis using a combination of an aminoglycoside and a β-lactam antibiotic or a tetracycline is usually successful in controlling the local infection. In nonacute infection of the prostate, Paulson and White[90] reported success with minocycline, an antibacterial agent that theoretically should reach appropriate concentrations in the prostate. The therapeutic results with this tetracycline drug, however, are less good in the nonacute than in the acute condition, despite the penetrating ability. This drug sometimes has unacceptable side effects such as dizziness.

Quinolone antibiotics should, on the basis of their lipid solubility and protein binding, reach therapeutic concentrations in prostatic secretion.[91,92] These drugs are active against many of the Enterobacteriaceae that can cause bacterial prostatitis.

Nitrofurantoin (100 mg per day) or trimethoprim (50 to 100 mg per day) will prevent bacteriuria, cystitis, and serious complications and will also diminish the symptoms.[83] The possibility of prostatic calculi as the source of bacteria in nonacute prostatitis must also be considered.

There are no generally accepted principles for treating nonbacterial prostatitis. According to the definition by Drach et al.,[11] bacterial prostatitis comprises only those cases that harbor gram-negative rods or enterococci in EPS. Patients with nonbacterial prostatitis can accordingly harbor organisms such as *M. hominis, U. urealyticum,* coagulase-negative staphylococci, and streptococci, whose pathogenicity in prostatitis is uncertain.

Antibiotic treatment of nonbacterial prostatitis seems in a considerable number of cases to be beneficial with regard to symptoms,[93] urodynamic changes,[70] and secretory function.[79] Because the etiologic significance of various microbes that can be isolated from EPS in patients with nonbacterial prostatitis is not clear, it may be warranted to offer these patients and their sexual consorts antibiotic treatment for 1 to 3 weeks. Tetracyclines or erythromycin may be used. If this treatment results in no improvement, however, one should not expect that continued medication with other antibiotics will be successful. When given information of the innocuous nature of their condition, most patients will accept minor symptoms. In symptomatic flare-up of the prostatitis, many patients report relief from hot sitz baths and bed rest.

Anticholinergics and tranquilizers usually benefit patients whose symptoms are dominated by urinary urgency and frequency, while anti-inflammatory drugs seem to be preferable when pain predominates. In patients with obstruction, alpha-receptor blocking agents have been recommended to achieve full relaxation of the autonomic part of the external sphincter.[31] Sexual or dietary restrictions are not nowadays regarded as therapeutic.

The use of prostatic massage to promote drainage of inflamed areas of the gland must be questioned. It can lead to acute bouts of synovitis, iridocyclitis, and conjunctivitis in patients who have previously experienced such complications.

Prostatodynia denotes many disparate conditions which produce symptoms mimicking those of prostatitis but which are associated neither with infection nor with noninfectious inflammatory processes in the prostate. In this chapter, prostatodynia has been discussed only as a differential diagnosis, and its treatment therefore is beyond the scope of this discussion.

## PREVENTION

Early and efficient treatment of urethritis may reduce the incidence of prostatitis. However, patients with nonbacterial prostatitis frequently have no history of symptomatic urethritis preceding the onset of characteristic symptoms of prostatitis. In order to prevent recurrence of prostatitis in men with bacteriologic evidence of genital infection, it may be advisable to also treat their sexual consorts, particularly if vaginal or cervical cultures reveal the same organism in both partners.

Recognized urinary tract pathogens (i.e., gram-negative rods) may be isolated from the prostate in both acute and chronic bacterial prostatitis. It is still not clear, however, if a primary infection with these microorganisms is the cause or if prostatic infection appears secondarily in a previously compromised prostate.

In bacterial as well as in nonbacterial prostatitis, the secretory function of the prostate is disturbed. Most components of the secretion appear in diminished concentrations, including the antimicrobial factor described by Fair and Cordonnier.[78] Whether or not the secretory function is restored by antibiotic treatment remains unknown, as does the relative importance of the prostatic secretion as a local resistance factor. Though the concept is speculative, it is tempting to assume that serious derangement of prostatic secretory function will increase susceptibility to urogenital infections. Clinical experience, however, does not unequivocally support such an assumption. Urinary tract infection in men is often combined with infection of the prostate. On the other hand, only a few patients with nonbacterial prostatitis develop bacteriuria.

The paucity of knowledge concerning the etiology of the condition is a hindrance to any firm recommendations for preventive measures.

## References


1 Finger E: *Die Blennorrhoe der Sexualorgane und Ihre Complicationen.* Leipzig und Wien, Franz Deuticke, 1901.
2 Tisell L-E, Salander H: The lobes of the human prostate. *Scand J Urol Nephrol* 9:185, 1975.
3 Prince D: Comparative aspects of the development and structure of the prostate. *Natl Cancer Inst Monogr* 12:1, 1963.
4 Blacklock NJ: Prostatic pain. *Br J Hosp Med* 20:80, 1978.
5 Diem K, Lentner C: *Scientific Tables,* 7th ed. Basel, Geigy, 1971.
6 Colleen S et al: Magnesium and zinc in seminal fluid of healthy males and patients with non-acute prostatitis with and without gonorrhoeae. *Scand J Urol Nephrol* 9:192, 1975.
7 Andersson RU, Fair WR: Physical and chemical determinations of prostatic secretion in benign hyperplasia, prostatitis and adenocarcinoma. *Invest Urol* 14:137, 1976.
8 Mårdh P-A, Colleen S: Lysozyme in seminal fluid of healthy males and patients with prostatitis and in tissues of the male urogenital tract. *Scand J Urol Nephrol* 8:179, 1974.
9 Yunda IF et al: Prostatitis and Pathospermie. *Dermatol Monatsschr* 164:564, 1978.
10 Drach GW, Kahonen PW: Prostatitis, in *Urologic Pathology: The Prostate,* M. Tannenbaum (ed). Philadelphia, Lea & Febiger, 1977, pp 157–170.
11 Drach GW et al: Classification of benign disease with prostatic pain: Prostatitis—prostatodynia? *J Urol* 120:266, 1978.
12 Boström K: Chronic inflammation of human male accessory sex glands and its effect on the morphology of the spermatozoa. *Scand J Urol Nephrol* 5:133, 1971.
13 Stamey TA: *Urinary Infections.* Baltimore, Williams & Wilkins, 1972.
14 Blacklock NJ: Anatomic factors in prostatitis. *Br J Urol* 46:47, 1974.
15 Meares EM: Differentiated diagnosis of prostatitis. *J Genitourinary Med* 1:43, 1979.
16 Meares EM: Bacterial prostatitis vs "prostatosis": A clinical and bacteriological study. *JAMA* 224:1372, 1973.
17 Mårdh P-A, Colleen S: Search for urogenital tract infections in patients with symptoms of prostatitis: Studies on aerobic and strictly anaerobic bacteria, mycoplasmas, fungi, trichomonads and viruses. *Scand J Urol Nephrol* 9:8, 1975.
18 Weidner W et al: *Ureaplasma urealyticum* bei chronischer unspezifischer Prostatourethritis. *Aktuel Urologie* 10:1, 1979.
19 Mårdh P-A et al: Role of *Chlamydia trachomatis* in non-acute prostatitis. *Br J Vener Dis* 54:330, 1978.
20 Chronic prostatitis, editorial. *Br Med J* 3:1, 1972.
21 Colleen S, Mårdh P-A: Studies on non-acute prostatitis: Clinical and laboratory finding in patients with symptoms of nonacute prostatitis, in *Genital Infections and Their Complications,* D Danielsson et al (eds). Stockholm, Almqvist & Wiksell, 1975, pp 121–131.
22 Grant JBF et al: The clinical presentation of *Chlamydia trachomatis* in a urological practice. *Br J Urol* 57:218, 1985.
23 Poletti F et al: Isolation of *Chlamydia trachomatis* from the prostatic cells in patients affected by nonacute abacterial prostatitis. *J Urol* 134:691, 1985.
24 Bruman H et al: Studies on the role of *Ureaplasma mealyticum* and *Mycoplasma hominis* in prostatitis. *J Inf Dis* 147:807, 1983.
25 Meseguer MA et al: Differential counts of *Ureaplasma urealyticum* in male urologic patients. Correspondence to the editor, comment and reply. *J Inf Dis* 149:659, 1984.
26 Vinje O et al: Laboratory findings in chronic prostatitis—with special reference to immunological and microbiological aspects. *Scand J Urol Nephrol* 17:291, 1983.
27 Meares EM: Prostatic syndrome. *J Urol* 123:141, 1980.
28 Ulstein M et al: Non-symptomatic genital tract infection and infertility, in *Human Semen and Fertility Regulation in Men,* ESE Hafez (ed). St Louis, Mosby, 1976, pp 355–362.
29 Deture FA et al: Herpes vires type 2: Study of semen in male subjects with recurrent infections. *J Urol* 120:449, 1978.
30 Sutor DJ, Wooley SE: The crystalline composition of prostatic calculi. *Br J Urol* 46:533, 1974.
31 Blacklock NJ: Prostatitis. *Practitioner* 223:318, 1979.
32 Kelalis PP. et al: Allergic granulomas of the prostate in asthmatics. *JAMA* 188:963, 1964.
33 Tanner FH, McDonald JR: Granulomatous prostatitis: Histologic study of group of granulomatous lesions collected from prostatic glands. *Arch Pathol* 36:358, 1943.
34 Kelalis PP et al: Granulomatous prostatitis. *JAMA* 191:111, 1965.
35 Bush I et al: Steroid therapy in nonspecific granulomatous prostatitis. *J Urol* 92:303, 1965.
36 Gatenbeck L: Stress stimuli and the prostatic gland—An experimental study in the cat. *Scand J Urol Nephrol* 20 (suppl):99, 1986.
37 Bourne CV, Frishette WA: Prostatic fluid analysis and prostatitis. *J Urol* 97:140, 1967.
38 O'Shaughnessy EJ, Parrino PS: Chronic prostatitis: Fact or fiction. *JAMA* 160:540, 1956.
39 Andersson RV, Weller C: Prostatic leucocytes studies in nonbacterial prostatitis (prostatosis). *J Urol* 121:292, 1978.
40 Blacklock NJ: Some observations on prostatitis, in: *Advances in the Study of the Prostate.* Marie Curie Foundation Workshop Conference. London, Heinemann, 1970, pp 37–55.
41 Kent AC et al: Role of Chlamydia trachomatis and HLA-B27 in sexually acquired relative arthritis. *Br Med J* 1:605, 1978.
42 Catterall RD: Uveitis, arthritis and non-specific genital infection. *Br J Vener Dis* 36:27, 1960.
43 del Porto GB et al: Bacterial effect on sperm motility. *Urology* 5:638, 1975.
44 Tegue NS et al: Interference of human spermatozoa motility by *Escherichia coli. Fertil Steril* 22:281, 1971.
45 Fowlkes DM et al: T-mycoplasmas and human infertility: Correlation of infection with alterations in seminal parameters. *Fertil Steril* 26:1212, 1975.
46 de Louvois J et al: Frequency of mycoplasmas in fertile and infertile couples. *Lancet* 1:1073, 1974.
47 Jones SR et al: Localization of urinary tract infections by detection of antibody-coated bacteria in urine sediment. *N Engl J Med* 290:591, 1974.
48 Riedasch GE et al: Antibody-coated bacteria in the ejaculate: A possible test for prostatitis. *J Urol* 118:787, 1977.
49 Jones SR: Prostatitis as cause of antibody-coated bacteria in urine. *N Engl J Med* 291:365, 1974.
50 Quesada EM et al: Genital infection and sperm agglutinating antibodies in infertile men. *J Urol* 99:106, 1968.
51 Halim A et al: The significance of antibodies to sperm in infertile men and their wives. *Br J Urol* 46:65, 1974.
52 Lunglmayor G, Stemberger H: Spermieantikörper und chronisch entzündliche Adnexaffection beim Mann. *Munch Med Wochenschr* 120:1603, 1978.
53 Lindholmer C. Elisasson R: The effect of albumin, magnesium and zinc on human sperm survival in different fractions of split ejaculate. *Fertil Steril* 25:424, 1974.
54 Caldamone AA, Cocket ATK: Infertility and genitourinary infection. *Urology* 12:304, 1978.
55 Schirren C, Zander HA: Genitalinfectionen des Mannes und ihre Auswirkung auf die Spermatozoen-motalität. *Med Welt* 1:45, 1966.

56 Kúsnik Z: Die Entzündungen der mänlichen Unfruchtbarkeit. *Z Urol* 59:767, 1966.
57 Steele R et al: Sexual factors in the epidemiology of cancer of the prostate. *J Chronic Dis* 24:29, 1971.
58 Kibukamusoke JW: Gonorrhoea and urethral stricture. *Br J Vener Dis* 41:135, 1965.
59 Dunlop EMC: Incidence of urethral stricture in male after urethritis. *Br J Vener Dis* 37:64, 1961.
60 Blandy JP et al: Urethroplasty in context. *Br J Urol* 48:697, 1976.
61 Brannan W et al: Free full thickness skin graft urethroplasty for urethral stricture: Experience with 66 patients. *J Urol* 115:677, 1976.
62 Wein AJ et al: Two-stage urethroplasty for urethral stricture disease. *J Urol* 118:392, 1977.
63 Singh M, Blandy JP: Pathology of urethral stricture. *J Urol* 115:673, 1976.
64 Beard DE, Goddyear WE: Urethral stricture: A pathological study. *J Urol* 59:619, 1948.
65 Blandy JP: Urethral stricture. *Postgrad Med J* 56:383, 1980.
66 Gardiner RA et al: One-stage island patch urethroplasty. *Br J Urol* 50:575, 1978.
67 Brühl P: Anogenital syndrome. *Int Urol Nephrol* 18:169, 1986.
68 Segura JW et al: Prostatitis and pelvic floor tension myalgia. *J Urol* 122:168, 1979.
69 Sinaki M et al: Tension myalgia of the pelvic floor. *Major Clin Proc* 52:717, 1977.
70 Buck AC: Disorders of micturition in bacterial prostatitis. *Proc R Soc Med* 68:508, 1975.
71 Nilsson IK et al: Relationship between psychological and laboratory findings in patients with symptoms of non-acute prostatitis, in *Genital Infections and Their Complications,* D Danielsson et al (eds). Stockholm, Almqvist & Wiksell, 1975, pp 133–144.
72 Junker H: Sind Patienten mit chronischer abakterieller Prostatitis Sexualneurasteniker? *Z Urol Nephrol* 63:273, 1970.
73 Meares EM, Stamey TA: Bacteriologic localization patterns in bacterial prostatitis and urethritis. *Invest Urol* 5:492, 1968.
74 Jameson RM: Sexual activity and the variations of the white cell count of prostatic secretion. *Invest Urol* 5:297, 1968.
75 Andersson RV, Weller WC: Prostatic secretion leucocyte studies in non-bacterial prostatitis (prostatosis). *J Urol* 121:292, 1979.
76 Eliasson R, Lindholmer G: Functions of the accessory organs, in *Human Semen and Fertility Regulation in Men,* ESE Hafez (ed). St Louis, Mosby, 1976, pp 44–50.
77 Boström K, Andersson L: Creatine phosphokinase relative to acid phosphatase, lactate dehydrogenase, zinc and fructose in human semen with special reference to chronic prostatitis. *Scand J Urol Nephrol* 5:123, 1971.
78 Fair WR, Cordonnier JL: The pH of prostatic fluid: Reappraisal and therapeutic implications. *J Urol* 120:695, 1978.
79 White MA: Change in pH of expressed prostatic secretion during the course of prostatitis. *Proc R Soc Med* 68:511, 1975.
80 Stamey TA et al: Antibacterial nature of prostatic fluid. *Nature* 218:444, 1968.
81 Mårdh P-A, Colleen S: Antibacterial activity of human seminal fluid. *Scand J Urol Nephrol* 9:17, 1975.
82 Mårdh P-A, Colleen S: Lysozyme in seminal fluid of healthy males and patients with chronic and subchronic prostatitis. *Scand J Urol Nephrol* 8:179, 1974.
83 Meares EM: Prostatitis syndromes: New perspectives about old woes. *J Urol* 123:141, 1980.
84 Winning DG et al: Diffusion of antibiotics from plasma in the prostatic fluid. *Nature* 219:139, 1968.
85 Pfau A et al: The pH of prostatic fluid in health and disease: Implications of treatment in chronic prostatitis *J Urol* 119:384, 1978.
86 Mobley DF: Erythromycin plus sodium bicarbonate in chronic bacterial prostatitis. *Urology* 3:60, 1974.
87 Oliveri RA et al: Clinical experience with Geocillin in the treatment of bacterial prostatitis. *Curr Ther Res* 25:415, 1979.
88 Smith JW et al: Recurrent urinary tract infections in men: Characteristics and response to therapy. *Ann Intern Med* 91:544, 1979.
89 Fox M: The natural history and significance of stone formation in the prostate gland. *J Urol* 89:716, 1963.
90 Paulson DF, White R deV: Trimethoprim sulfamethoxazole and minocycline hydrochloride in the treatment of culture proven bacterial prostatitis. *J Urol* 120:184, 1978.
91 Bologna M: Bacterial intraprostatic concentrations of Norfloxacin. *Lancet* ii:280, 1983.
92 Sabbaj J: Norfloxacin versus cotrimoxacle in the treatment of recurring urinary infections in men. *Scand J Infect Dis (suppl)* 48:48, 1986.
93 Colleen S, Mårdh P-A: Effect of metacycline treatment on non-acute prostatitis. *Scand J Urol Nephrol* 9:198, 1975.

# Chapter 55

# Proctitis, proctocolitis, enteritis, and esophagitis in homosexual men

Thomas C. Quinn
Walter E. Stamm

Anorectal infections with syphilis, gonorrhea, condyloma acuminatum, lymphogranuloma venereum (LGV), and granuloma inguinale (donovanosis) have been recognized for many years, but only recently have other common STD pathogens, such as herpes simplex virus (HSV) and non-LGV strains of *Chlamydia trachomatis*, been recognized as causing anorectal infection.[1–6] In addition, infections with pathogens that have traditionally been associated with food- or waterborne acquisition or with foreign travel (e.g., *Giardia lamblia, Entamoeba histolytica*, campylobacter, shigella, and hepatitis A) are now known to occur via sexual transmission in homosexual men.

Over the past several years, intestinal disorders in homosexual men have become even more complex with the recognition of opportunistic infections within the gastrointestinal tract of patients with AIDS.[7–9] Prominent among these infections are candida, cryptosporidium, isospora, *Mycobacterium avium-intracellulare,* and cytomegalovirus.[10–12] In addition, patients with AIDS have also been noted to have an increased incidence of gastrointestinal malignancies, including Kaposi's sarcoma and lymphoma.[7,13,14] This diverse array of infections and malignancies responsible for intestinal disease in homosexual men is a challenge to the clinician.

## DEFINITIONS

Anal and rectal infections represent increasingly frequent and complex problems seen by proctologists and in STD clinics. Because of the wide variety of pathogens that can infect the anorectal area and depending on the location of the infection, symptoms and clinical manifestations of these infections can vary widely. The normal anorectal anatomy is illustrated in Figs. 55-1 and 55-2. The perianal area up to the anal verge is lined by keratinized, stratified squamous dermal epithelium. Thus, perianal lesions caused by syphilis, HSV, granuloma inguinale, chancroid, and condyloma acuminatum generally resemble the corresponding lesions as they appear elsewhere in the genital area. The anal canal, which extends 2 cm from the anal verge internally to the anorectal (pectinate or dentate) line, is lined by epithelium which gradually changes from stratified squamous to stratified cuboidal epithelium, and is supplied with one of the richest networks of sensory nerve endings in the body. Infection of this area is commonly very painful and results in constipation and tenesmus (ineffectual straining to defecate) due to spasm of the anal sphincter muscle. The external hemorrhoidal venous plexus surrounds the anal verge.

At the anorectal line, the separation of the anal canal from the rectum is indicated by the longitudinal folds called the columns of Morgagni. The internal hemorrhoidal venous plexus occurs at the level of the columns of Morgagni. In this area the epithelium consists of transitional cuboidal cells, mucus-producing columnar cells, and blind-end crypts.

From the anorectal line cephalad, the rectum begins and is lined by columnar epithelium. The term *proctitis* refers to inflammation of the rectal mucosa. Symptoms include constipation, tenesmus, rectal discomfort or pain, hematochezia (passage of bloody stools), and a mucopurulent rectal discharge which is occasionally misinterpreted by the patient as diarrhea. Although stretching of rectal tissue causes pain, the area is insensitive to other direct stimuli such as rectal biopsy. Hence, infections which involve the

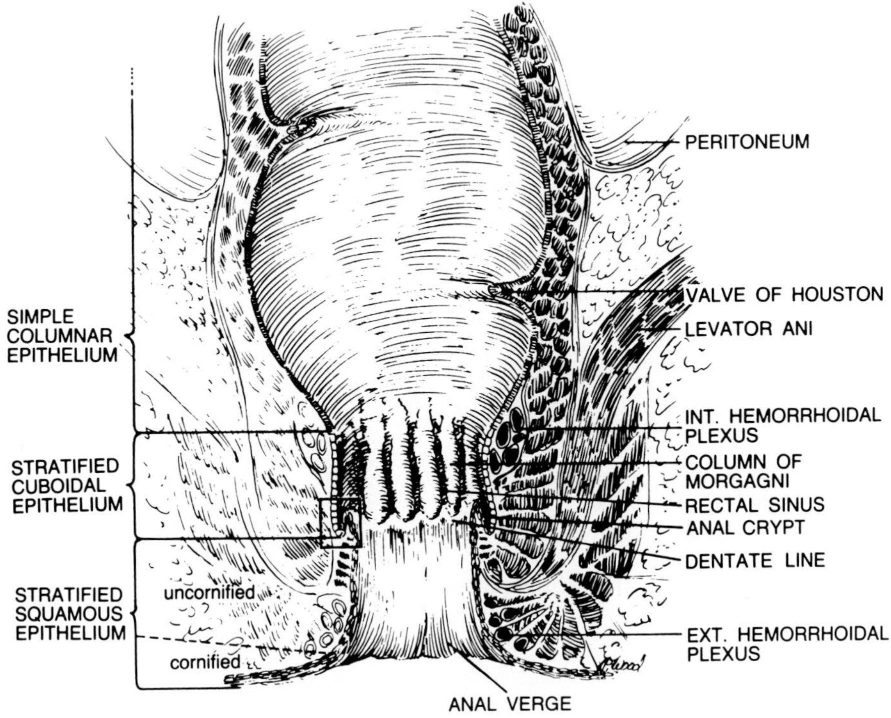


**Fig. 55-1.** Diagram of the rectum and anal canal, showing normal anal and rectal structures with the types of epithelium lining the anus and rectum. Box outlining the anal crypt is enlarged in Fig. 55-2.

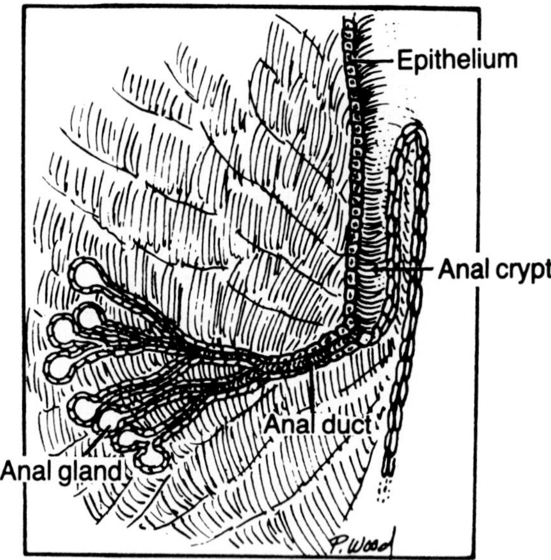


Fig. 55-2. Diagrammatic representation of the anal crypt. The anal crypts are located along the dentate line and consist of anal ducts which penetrate into muscle. These ducts are lined by both stratified squamous and mucus-secreting cells.

rectum but spare the anus are relatively painless. Sigmoidoscopic findings may range from normal mucosa with only mucopus present to diffuse inflammation of the mucosa with friability or discrete ulcerations. If these sigmoidoscopic findings are limited to the rectum, and further passage of the sigmoidoscope reveals normal mucosa above 15 cm, the condition is properly termed proctitis; if the mucosa is abnormal as high as the sigmoidoscope is passed, the condition probably represents *proctocolitis,* which could be confirmed by colonoscopy. Proctitis and proctocolitis generally have different infectious etiologies. Rectal biopsy provides histologic confirmation of proctitis, and findings may reveal nonspecific inflammation or changes highly suggestive of certain infections such as LGV, HSV, or syphilis.[15]

*Enteritis* is an inflammatory illness of the duodenum, jejunum, and/or ileum. Sigmoidoscopy shows no abnormalities. Infectious enteritis is usually contracted either by ingestion of pathogens present in feces-contaminated water or food or by certain sexual practices or other forms of human contact which result in fecal ingestion. Symptoms of enteritis consist of diarrhea, abdominal pain, bloating, cramps, and nausea. Additional symptoms may include flatulence, urgency, a mucous rectal discharge, and, in severe cases, melena. Systemic manifestations such as fever, saline depletion with orthostatic hypotension, acidosis, hypokalemia, malabsorption syndrome, weight loss, and myalgias may also be present.

*Esophagitis* is an inflammatory process of the esophagus which may or may not extend to involve the oral cavity. Infections of the esophagus are most commonly seen in immunocompromised individuals in whom opportunistic pathogens such as *Candida albicans,* cytomegalovirus, and herpes simplex virus infections proliferate and induce ulcerations. Symptoms of esophagitis typically consist of dysphagia and odynophagia. Esophograms may reveal dilatation and abnormal motility of the esophagus, and endoscopy frequently reveals either ulcerations or cottage cheese exudates depending upon the infecting organism.

The presence of fecal leukocytes as determined by Gram's stain or methylene blue stain of stool or rectal swabs usually implicates an inflammatory process but does not differentiate between various sites of involvement of the intestinal tract.

## ETIOLOGY AND EPIDEMIOLOGY

An enteric organism not requiring an intermediate host may be transmitted by the oral-anal or genital-anal routes.[16] Those pathogens which may cause gastrointestinal illness and which have been proved to be or have the potential to be sexually transmitted are shown in Table 55-1. Those enteric pathogens which are infectious at low inoculum size, such as shigella (10 to 100 organisms), *G. lamblia* (10 to 100 cysts), and *E. histolytica* (10 to 100 cysts), all occur commonly in homosexual men and are thought to be sexually transmitted, though the routes of transmission have not been defined. Hepatitis A virus appears to be transmitted by oral-anal sex.[17]

Sexual transmission of enteric pathogens which are shed in feces may be attributable to ingestion of feces during anilingus or during fellatio of a fecally contaminated penis or to direct intrarectal inoculation of organisms by a fecally contaminated penis. Anorectal infection with conventional STD pathogens in men is caused by rectal intercourse. The role of fomite transmission such as may occur with the shared use of unsterile equipment for rectal douching and colonic irrigation requires further study. An outbreak of amebiasis has been traced to use of unsterile equipment for colonic irrigation.[18]

In the pre-AIDS era, the role of homosexual transmission of certain enteric infections was recognized with increasing frequency.[19] For example, in San Francisco between 1975 and 1977 the reported cases of amebiasis, shigellosis, hepatitis A, and hepatitis B showed a marked predominance in males between the ages of 20 and 39. Many of these individuals acknowledged homosexual contact, including anilingus and fellatio. Fecal cultures of

**Table 55-1. Sexually Transmissible Causes of Intestinal or Anal Infections in Homosexual Men**

| |
|---|
| Bacterial pathogens |
| *Neisseria gonorrhoeae* |
| *Neisseria meningitidis* |
| *Chlamydia trachomatis* |
| *Haemophilus ducreyi* |
| *Calymmatobacterium granulomatis* |
| *Treponema pallidum* |
| Enteric bacterial pathogens |
| *Shigella* spp. |
| *Salmonella* spp. |
| *Campylobacter* sp. |
| Fungus |
| *Candida* spp.* |
| Protozoa |
| *Giardia lamblia* |
| *Entamoeba histolytica* |
| *Dientamoeba fragilis* |
| *Cryptosporidium* sp.* |
| *Isospora belli** |
| "Nonpathogenic" protozoans |
| Helminths |
| *Enterobius vermicularis* |
| *Strongyloides stercoralis* |
| Viruses |
| Herpes simplex virus |
| Cytomegalovirus* |
| Human papilloma virus |
| Human immunodeficiency virus |
| Hepatitis A and B viruses |

*Most commonly seen in HIV-infected men; not necessarily sexually transmitted.

homosexual contacts of men with shigella infection revealed that their contacts were often asymptomatic carriers of shigella of the same serotype. Similarly, several men with salmonella infection had had sexual relations with men who were asymptomatic carriers of the same serotype.[20] A marked predominance of men in this age group was reported for these infections in other parts of the United States as well.[21–25]

Heterosexuals could also be at risk for acquiring enteric infections by anilingus, and women can acquire anorectal STD by anal intercourse.[26] However, many sexually transmitted anorectal infections with *N. gonorrhoeae, C. trachomatis,* HSV, and human papilloma virus in women probably result from contiguous spread of infection from the genitalia (see below).

There are very few reports on the prevalence of anorectal infection with the above infectious agents in patients seen in the STD clinic setting. In a study of 260 homosexual men with anorectal symptoms, misnomered the "gay bowel syndrome," specific infections, including gonorrhea, syphilis, hepatitis, amebiasis, shigella, and LGV, were present in only 21 percent of the patients.[19] The remainder had condylomata acuminata, hemorrhoids, "nonspecific proctitis," and a variety of rectal conditions such as polyps, fissures, fistulas, perirectal abscesses, ulcers, and foreign bodies. However, in a more detailed microbiologic study of infectious agents in 119 homosexual men presenting to an STD clinic in the pre-AIDS era with anorectal and/or intestinal symptoms, specific anorectal or enteric infections with one or more pathogens were demonstrated in 80 percent.[27] In comparison, significantly fewer homosexual men without such symptoms who were seen in the same clinic were found to be infected with these pathogens. The prevalence of specific infections in each group is shown in Table 55-2. Prominent pathogens in patients with symptoms and signs of *proctitis* were *N. gonorrhoeae,* HSV, *C. trachomatis* (non-LGV), and *Treponema pallidum.* The only pathogen associated with symptoms and signs of enteritis was *G. lamblia. Campylobacter* sp., *C. trachomatis* (LGV), and *Shigella flexneri* were associated with evidence of proctocolitis (Table 55-3). In this study, 22 percent of symptomatic patients had multiple infections. For example, 48 percent of patients with anorectal gonorrhea were also found to have one or more

**Table 55-2. Infectious Pathogens Identified in 194 Homosexual Men with and without Anorectal or Intestinal Symptoms**

| Anorectal and intestinal pathogens* | Symptomatic group, % ($N = 119$) | Asymptomatic group, % ($N = 175$) |
|---|---|---|
| *Neisseria gonorrhoea* | 31 | 23 |
| Herpes simplex virus | 19† | 4 |
| *Chlamydia trachomatis* | 10 | 5 |
| *Treponema pallidum* | 5 | 1 |
| *Entamoeba histolytica* | 29 | 25 |
| *Giardia lamblia* | 14 | 4 |
| *Campylobacter jejuni/C. fetus fetus* | 7 | 3 |
| *Shigella flexneri* | 3 | 1 |
| *Clostridium difficile* cytotoxin | 3 | 1 |
| Enterovirus (Echovirus 11) | 3 | 1 |
| Patients with any of the above pathogens | 80† | 39 |
| Patients with more than one of the above pathogens | 22† | 4 |

*Other infectious agents identified were campylobacter-like organisms, nonpathogenic protozoans, *Candida albicans, Neisseria meningitidis, Ureaplasma urealyticum,* and *Mycoplasma hominis.*
†$P < .05$.
SOURCE: After TC Quinn et al.[27]

**Table 55-3. Microbiological and Symptomatic Correlates of Proctitis, Proctocolitis, and Enteritis among 65 Homosexual Men with Intestinal Symptoms Who Underwent Sigmoidoscopy to a Distance above 15 cm**

| | Proctitis: Sigmoidoscopic findings abnormal only below 15 cm ($N = 41$) | Proctocolitis: Sigmoidoscopic findings abnormal beyond 15 cm ($N = 15$) | Enteritis: Sigmoidoscopic findings normal ($N = 9$) |
|---|---|---|---|
| Sexually transmitted rectal pathogens | | | |
| *Neisseria gonorrhoeae* | 12 | 0 | 2 |
| Herpes simplex virus | 13 | 1 | 0 |
| *Chlamydia trachomatis* (non-LGV) | 8 | 1 | 0 |
| *Treponema pallidum* | 6 | 0 | 0 |
| Total with any rectal pathogen | 33* | 2 | 2 |
| Infectious causes of colitis | | | |
| *Campylobacter jejuni/C. fetus fetus* | 3 | 4 | 0 |
| *Shigella flexneri* | 0 | 2 | 0 |
| *Chlamydia trachomatis* (LGV) | 0 | 3 | 0 |
| *Entamoeba histolytica* | 5(26)† | 4(11) | 1(8) |
| *Clostridium difficile* cytotoxin | 1 | 1 | 0 |
| Total with any colitis pathogen | *8* | 9 | *1* |
| Infectious causes of inflammation limited to small intestine | | | |
| *Giardia lamblia* | 2(26) | 2(11) | 4(8) |
| Any three of the following four symptoms present: diarrhea, abdominal pain, bloating, nausea | 3 | 8 | 9† |
| Any three of the following four symptoms present: constipation, rectal discharge, anorectal pain, tenesmus | 38* | 7 | 0 |

*$P < .05$, by multiple logistic regression analysis.
† Figures in parentheses indicate the number of patients who submitted stools for examination for ova and parasites.
SOURCE: TC Quinn et al.[27]

additional pathogens present, and four or more pathogens were found in several patients. In the absence of a history of foreign travel, the demonstration of infections with multiple enteric pathogens, including "nonpathogenic" protozoa, should suggest sexual transmission. Histories of homosexual behavior have been recorded in other community outbreaks of shigellosis, giardiasis, and amebiasis.[23,24,28–30]

## IMPACT OF AIDS ON ENTERIC INFECTIONS IN HOMOSEXUAL MEN

The AIDS epidemic has dramatically altered the spectrum of enteric infections encountered in homosexual men. Table 55-4 compares homosexual men who attended the Seattle Sexually Transmitted Disease Clinic because of gastrointestinal or rectal symptoms in two time periods: 1980–1981 (considered pre-AIDS in Seattle) and 1983–1984. All these men were comprehensively evaluated for rectal and enteric pathogens using similar methods, and none in either group had overt clinical evidence of AIDS or ARC. The majority of the 1983–1984 group were seropositive for HIV; however, the proportion with a discoverable etiologic agent responsible for their symptoms declined from 80 percent in the earlier period to 66 percent in the 1983–1984 group. Significant decreases in the proportion of patients with gonococcal proctitis and with *E. histolytica* and campylobacter-like organisms were observed, while the occurrence of HSV proctitis significantly increased. These changes probably reflect a combination of factors, including less frequent acquisition of new infections due to implementation of safe-sex practices, more frequent gastrointestinal symptoms directly related to HIV infection of the gut, and more frequent reactivation of latent infections such as CMV and HSV and more frequent occurrence of infections such as candidiasis or cryptosporidiosis due to immunosuppression.

The gastrointestinal tract appears to be a major target organ in HIV infection.[7,31,32] In homosexual men, the intestinal tract is a primary site of inoculation, and some of the earliest symptoms originate at this site,[33–35] including fever, sweats, myalgias, arthralgias, anorexia, nausea, vomiting, and/or diarrhea. Many HIV-infected individuals later develop severe prolonged intestinal symptoms, frequently referred to as the diarrheal–weight loss syndrome. In many of these cases, the appearance of prolonged gastrointestinal symptoms was highly predictive of subsequent development of opportunistic infections and the eventual diagnosis of AIDS.[9,11]

The prevalence of gastrointestinal symptoms varies among different populations at risk for HIV infection. In developed countries, 40 to 50 percent of homosexual men with AIDS have a history of a clinical prodrome characterized by progressive weight loss of > 10 percent of the body weight and a diarrhea of unexplained origin,[9] while this clinical presentation is much less frequent among intravenous drug users, transfusion recipients, hemophiliacs, and heterosexual partners of other groups at risk for AIDS. In developing countries, gastrointestinal symptoms are observed in over 80 percent of AIDS patients, reflecting perhaps a greater exposure and susceptibility to gastrointestinal pathogens common to their specific geographic location.[36–38] Because of the frequency of gastrointestinal complaints in many of these patients, AIDS has been commonly referred to as "slim disease" in many developing countries.

Extensive microbiologic and gastrointestinal evaluations have been limited in HIV-infected individuals with gastrointestinal complaints. In limited studies, oral-esophageal candidiasis was evident in 80 percent of cases, cryptosporidiosis in 30 percent, isospora in 10 percent, and *Entamoeba histolytica, Strongyloides stercoralis, Giardia lamblia, Salmonella,* and *Mycobacteria* infections in approximately 5 to 10 percent of patients.[38–40] Evidence of cytomegalovirus infection of the gastrointestinal tract by culture of biopsy is evident in 30 to 50 percent of AIDS patients.[7,40,41] Overall, specific pathogens are frequently not identified in 25 to 50 percent of the patients with chronic diarrhea and HIV infection. Many of these patients have histologic evidence of cytomegalovirus infection at autopsy,[7,12,42] whereas others have nonspecific inflammation and evidence of chronic malabsorption, such as partial villus atrophy with crypt hyperplasia.[8,10,32,42] Malabsorption as demonstrated by abnormal xylose and C14-glycerol-tripalmitin absorption is relatively common in AIDS patients with gastrointestinal symptoms.[8,10]

## RECTAL GONORRHEA

In several studies reviewed by Klein et al.,[43] rectal gonorrhea has been documented in 30 to 50 percent of women with gonorrhea, although only 4 percent had positive rectal cultures alone. Rectal gonococcal infection in women may sometimes be attributable to rectal intercourse,[44,45] but in most cases there is no history of rectal intercourse[46,47] and the infection is thought to have resulted from contiguous spread of infected secretions from the vagina. The clinical manifestations of rectal gonococcal infection in women have not been well defined.

**Table 55-4. Comparison of Gastrointestinal Infections among Homosexual Men Attending the Seattle STD Clinic in Two Time Periods**

| | % of patients positive for each pathogen* | | |
|---|---|---|---|
| | 1980–1981 ($n$ = 119) | 1983–1984 ($n$ = 184) | $p$ value |
| *Neisseria gonorrhoeae* | 31 | 14 | $p$ = .0003 |
| HSV | 19 | 30 | $p$ = .05 |
| *Chlamydia trachomatis* | 10 | 14 | NS |
| *Treponema pallidum* | 5 | 6 | NS |
| *Entamoeba histolytica* | 29 | 15 | $p$ = .02 |
| *Giardia lamblia* | 14 | 7 | $p$ = .07 |
| *Campylobacter jejuni* | 7 | 7 | NS |
| Campylobacter-like organisms | 18 | 7 | $p$ = .005 |
| Shigella | 3 | 5 | NS |
| Any pathogen | 80 | 66 | $p$ = .02 |
| ≥ 2 pathogens | 22 | 19 | NS |
| HIV seroprevalence | 14 | 58 | $p$ < .001 |

*Data from TC Quinn et al.[27] and WE Stamm (personal communication).

The prevalence of rectal infection in the pre-AIDS era has been between 6 and 8 percent among homosexual men attending steam bathhouses[48,49] and between 13 and 45 percent among homosexual men seen at STD clinics.[44,47,50–52] In several studies, the rectum was more commonly found to be infected than the pharynx or urethra.[48,49] Men examined because they were identified as sexual contacts by homosexual men with gonococcal urethritis are usually found to have asymptomatic rectal gonorrhea, but in homosexual men attending an STD clinic who have not been named as gonorrhea contacts, rectal gonorrhea is more often symptomatic. The concept that rectal gonorrhea in homosexual men is usually asymptomatic is a misconception analogous to the old misconception that most women with gonorrhea do not develop symptoms. These misconceptions are based on sample biases in studies that used STD clinic populations. In such studies, men found to have rectal gonorrhea, like women found to have endocervical gonorrhea, were often asymptomatic chronic carriers called in to the clinic because they had been named as contacts of men with acute gonococcal urethritis. In a previous study in an STD clinic,[53] among men not named as gonorrhea contacts, *N. gonorrhoeae* was isolated from 11 of 23 with anorectal symptoms vs. 11 of 55 without anorectal symptoms ($p = 0.016$). Among 14 men named as gonorrhea contacts, however, 13 had no anorectal symptoms and 12 of the 13 had rectal gonorrhea. The proportion of gonococcal infections which are asymptomatic is much higher for rectal infections than for urethral infections in male homosexual STD clinic patients.[49,54] Thus, asymptomatic infection of the rectum constitutes the main reservoir of gonococcal infection in homosexual men.

When present, symptoms are usually mild and include constipation, anorectal discomfort, tenesmus, and a mucopurulent rectal discharge which may cause secondary skin irritation resulting in rectal itching and perirectal erythema.[3] Occasionally, the patient may only notice strands of mucus on his stool or small amounts of blood commonly mistaken for hemorrhoidal bleeding.

Findings during proctoscopy are also nonspecific and are limited to the distal rectum.[55–57] The most frequent finding is the presence of mucopus in the rectum. The rectal mucosa may appear completely normal or demonstrate generalized erythema with localized areas of easily induced bleeding primarily near the anorectal junction. Histologically, abnormal findings are especially prominent at the anorectal junction around the anal crypts and columns of Morgagni.[55,58] However, only limited histologic studies of gonococcal infection of the distal rectum have been conducted because of the hazards of biopsy of this area with its surrounding venous hemorrhoidal plexus. With gonococcal infection there is patchy disorganization and derangement of these mucus-secreting cells and an infiltration of neutrophils, plasma cells, and lymphocytes throughout the lamina propria.[55,56] These findings are not pathognomonic, and concomitant rectal infection with another pathogen may alter the proctoscopic and histopathologic findings.

Diagnosis is made by Gram's stain and culture of material obtained by swabbing the epithelial mucosa of the distal rectal area. In men with anorectal symptoms, the anoscope should be used to examine the rectum and obtain exudate for culture and Gram's stain. In a study of men with symptomatic rectal gonorrhea,[59] the sensitivity of Gram's stain of rectal exudate for identification of gonococci was 79 percent when obtained through an anoscope, compared to 53 percent for blindly obtained swabs. A positive smear, showing intracellular gram-negative diplococci, is usually reliable when the smear has been taken and analyzed properly, and therapy can be instituted while awaiting culture results. In men without anorectal symptoms, a sterile cotton swab can be inserted blindly 2 to 3 cm into the rectum. Cultures performed on material obtained in this way appear to be as sensitive as cultures performed on material obtained by anoscope.[60] The actual sensitivity of a single rectal culture for gonorrhea is unknown and probably is no greater than the estimated 80 percent sensitivity of a single endocervical culture in women. Most selective media used to isolate *N. gonorrhoeae* contain antimicrobials active against other bacteria (e.g., vancomycin and colistin). Since none of these antimicrobials inhibits swarming *Proteus* spp., which are often present in feces, trimethoprim is commonly added to inhibit *Proteus* in selective media used for rectal cultures.[61]

Treatment recommended for rectal gonorrhea in men consists of a single dose of ceftriaxone, 250 mg intramuscularly, or a single dose of spectinomycin hydrochloride, 2.0 g intramuscularly.[62] Both are highly effective for rectal gonorrhea with cure rates of up to 97 percent or more. The former is more effective for concomitant pharyngeal gonococcal infection, which commonly coexists with rectal infection in homosexual men.[63] Careful follow-up with posttreatment culture 10 days after therapy is essential. Penicillinase-producing *N. gonorrhoeae* (PPNG) may be responsible for drug failure in some patients, and spectinomycin or ceftriaxone are recommended for rectal infection with PPNG.[64] Ceftriaxone, an extended-spectrum cephalosporin with a long serum half-life, has been shown to be more active than penicillin G against beta-lactamase-positive and -negative strains of *N. gonorrhoeae*.[65] In a recent study, ceftriaxone was effective in 30 of 32 (94 percent) pharyngeal and 52 of 52 anorectal infections compared with 6 of 14 (43 percent) and 9 of 9, respectively, for spectinomycin.[65] Since ceftriaxone is so well tolerated and effective against anorectal infections and PPNG infections, it is the drug of choice for uncomplicated gonorrhea, particularly when homosexual men are treated and/or PPNG is prevalent. Treatment with 3.5 g of ampicillin plus 1.0 g of probenecid in a single oral dose or with oral tetracycline has been considerably less effective for rectal gonorrhea in homosexual men than for gonorrhea in heterosexuals.[64–66] A partial explanation for this difference is that gonococci isolated from rectal infections in homosexual men tend to be more resistant to penicillin and tetracycline than those isolated from heterosexuals; the types of gonococci involved in infection in homosexual men as determined by auxotyping tend to differ from the types which infect heterosexuals.[54] Also, gonococci isolated from homosexual men have the mtr mutation more often than gonococci isolated from heterosexual men,[67] perhaps because mtr mutants are less inhibited by fatty acids present in feces. Homosexual men with rectal gonococcal infection who have rectal symptoms should be followed closely, because the gonococcal infection may be coincidental rather than causal. If symptoms persist after therapy for gonorrhea, further evaluation is required for other agents such as HSV, chlamydia, enteric bacterial pathogens, and intestinal protozoans.

## ANORECTAL HERPES SIMPLEX VIRUS INFECTION

Although genital herpes infection is well recognized, and HSV is second only to *N. gonorrhoeae* in frequency of association with proctitis in homosexual men, there have been very few descriptions of anorectal herpetic infections.[5,68–70] A clinical description of anal herpes was recorded in 1736 by Astruc, physician to the king of France.[71] He stated, "[It is] observed in catamites and pathics, if they contract foul ulcers in the anus by the unnatural use of venery; from these ulcers they are tormented by a grievous inflammation upon the extremity of the rectum . . . hence the evacuation of the faeces becomes difficult and painful." Since then there have been only a few reports on anorectal herpes, suggesting that the disease is not common. However, 236 homosexual men with anorectal herpes were seen in one genitourinary medicine clinic in England over a 2-year period.[5] In two Seattle studies, HSV was cultured from the anorectal area from 32 and 20 percent of homosexual men with anorectal symptoms.[3,72] Data are not available on the risk of HSV anorectal infection in women.

Anorectal herpes is usually acquired by anal intercourse, although oral-anal contact with an individual who has HSV type 1 (HSV-1) infection of the mouth or lips presumably could lead to anorectal infection with HSV-1. In the Seattle studies, 37 of 39 isolates from the rectum were HSV type 2 (HSV-2) and the remaining two isolates were HSV-1.[3,72]

Clinically, herpes infection may involve the perianal areas, the anal canal, and/or the rectum. While symptoms are quite prominent in most cases, some individuals may be totally asymptomatic. In a study by Goldmeier,[70] 2 of 4 homosexual men with anorectal HSV infection were asymptomatic. In our study,[3] HSV was isolated from the anal canal from 3 of 75 asymptomatic homosexual men. Thus, asymptomatic anorectal HSV shedding may contribute to transmission of the infection to other individuals.

Anorectal HSV infections are typically characterized by severe, often debilitating anal pain, present in 94 percent of patients in one study.[72] Constipation, a nonspecific manifestation of proctitis, is usually present. The occurrence of constipation, anorectal pain, and urinary retention in a homosexual man strongly suggests herpetic proctitis.[3,73,74] Samarasinghe et al.[5] described 11 patients with herpetic proctitis, all of whom developed urinary difficulty of varying severity associated with sacral paresthesias, neuralgia, and impotence. Such symptoms are uncommon with HSV infection of the genitalia, which leads to latent infection of the $S_2$ and $S_3$ dorsal root ganglia. Urinary retention, constipation, and impotence in anorectal herpes are suggestive of a sacral radioculopathy, perhaps due to infection of lower-level sacral nerves and dorsal root ganglia; alternatively, urinary retention and constipation could be ascribed to a pain-induced reflex spasm of the anal and vesical sphincters caused by the severe anorectal pain associated with the syndrome. The dermatomic distribution of sacral dysesthesia or neuralgia has not been well characterized or compared in genital vs. anorectal herpes. Other symptoms of anorectal herpes include tenesmus, hematochezia, and rectal discharge. Constitutional symptoms such as fever, chills, malaise, and headache are common with primary anorectal HSV infection. Tender inguinal lymphadenopathy occurs in nearly one-half of men with primary anorectal herpes. Although initial attacks of genital herpes differ clinically from recurrent attacks (Chap. 35), initial and recurrent attacks of anorectal herpes have not yet been carefully compared. However, clinical experience suggests that recurrent anorectal attacks are often mild and rarely associated with constitutional symptoms.

Clinically, many infected individuals will not have any visible ulcerative perianal lesions but instead will present with ulcerative findings deep in the anal canal or involving the rectal mucosa.[3,72] When present externally, the initial lesion is a small vesicle or cluster of vesicles, each surrounded by a red areola. The vesicles soon rupture and may become confluent, particularly near or in the anal canal. With HSV infection of the rectum, the lower 10 cm of the rectum may appear edematous with discrete focal vesicular or ulcerative lesions occasionally present (Plates 73 and 74). The rectal mucosa is characteristically normal above this level, although we have occasionally seen involvement above 10 cm. Histological examination of rectal biopsies reveals acute nonspecific inflammation with focal ulcerative changes. The histologic findings which are characteristic of rectal herpes, though not found in all cases, are perivascular mononuclear cell infiltration, intranuclear inclusion bodies, and extensive nuclear debris (Fig. 55-3); multinucleated cells can also be seen occasionally but are not uniquely associated with this infection. Other rectal infections are commonly associated with HSV infection and may cause a more diffuse proctitis.

Diagnosis can often be made on clinical presentation on the basis of typical herpetic lesions externally or on the basis of proctitis with focal ulcerative changes of the distal rectum in a patient with severe anal pain, constipation, inguinal adenopathy, constitutional symptoms, and urinary retention. Cultures of external lesions, of rectal swabs, or of rectal biopsy are confirmatory. If viral cultures are not available, the clinical diagnosis can be confirmed by serology only if paired sera are collected and demonstrate seroconversion or a fourfold or greater rise in antibody titer.

The clinical course of an initial attack of anorectal herpes virus infection is self-limited, with manifestations usually resolving in 2 to 3 weeks. Secondary bacterial superinfections, which are uncommon in genital herpes, may be more common in anorectal herpes, although this has not been determined. Treatment includes analgesics and sitz baths, and one study suggests that oral acyclovir may be efficacious in shortening the duration of symptoms and viral shedding of anorectal herpes.[75] Recurrent anorectal infections do occur, but the temporal pattern and clinical manifestations of anorectal recurrences have not been well studied.

Progressive mucocutaneous herpes involving the anorectal area have also been described in patients with AIDS.[76] These infections cause severe large destructive ulcerations that progress unless antiviral therapy is initiated. Anecdotal reports suggest that severe mucocutaneous herpes in AIDS patients will respond to intravenous acyclovir but that recurrences frequently develop once therapy has stopped. Thus, it is recommended that for AIDS patients, intravenous acyclovir should be administered during an acute episode. The patient should then be placed on oral acyclovir 200 mg twice a day for up to 6 months for suppression of recurrences. In non-AIDS patients, this suppressive dose has been effective in preventing recurrences in up to 80 percent of cases,[77] and clinical experience suggests its effectiveness in AIDS patients as well.

## ANORECTAL SYPHILIS

As with other sexually transmitted diseases, the incidence of syphilis appears to be declining in homosexual men in industrialized countries, but a large percentage of early syphilis still occurs among homosexual men.[78] *Treponema pallidum* is commonly seen in its earliest infectious stages, with the primary anorectal lesion appearing 2 to 6 weeks after exposure by rectal intercourse. However, clinicians in the United States often fail to recognize anorectal chancres. Anorectal chancres have been recognized in 50 percent of the cases of primary syphilis in homosexual men in the United Kingdom but in only 15 percent of primary syphilis cases in homosexual men in the United States.[79] Consequently, early syphilis in homosexual men is diagnosed in the secondary

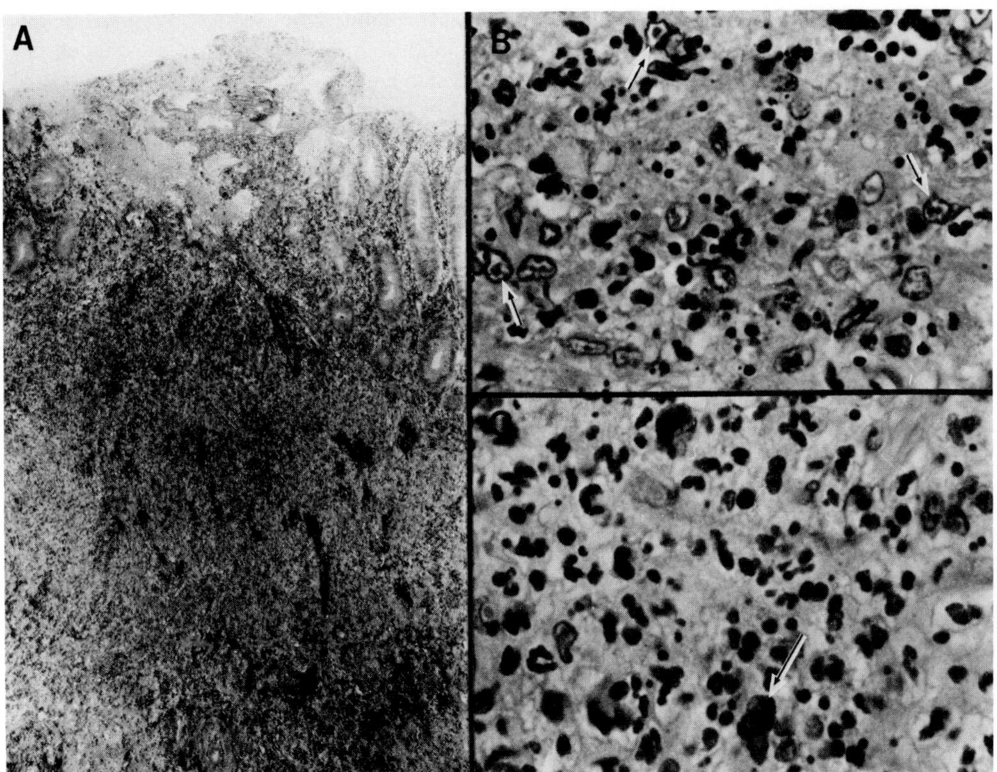


**Fig. 55-3.** Herpetic proctitis. (*a*) An ulceration and intense acute inflammation are present in the rectal mucosa. H&E stain, × 102 magnification. (*b*) Within this area of inflammation, intranuclear inclusions can be identified which are consistent with HSV infection (*arrows*), H&E stain, × 1360 magnification. (*c*) Multinucleated cells with a ground-glass appearance (*arrow*), a finding typical for HSV. H&E stain, × 1360 magnification. (*Courtesy of M. Schuffler.*)

or early latent stage much more often than in the primary stage. It is not certain what proportion of anorectal chancres are asymptomatic. Careful perianal examination can reveal unsuspected perianal chancres, while digital rectal examination and anoscopy may be required to detect asymptomatic chancres higher in the anal canal or rectum. When anorectal syphilis causes symptoms, it is commonly misdiagnosed as a traumatic lesion, fissure, or hemorrhoiditis.

Anorectal chancres due to syphilis have been recognized at least since the early 1900s. In 1925, Martin and Kallet found 20 patients (6.7 percent) with anorectal chancres among 300 proctologic cases.[80] Over the next 20 to 30 years there were several reports which stated that anorectal chancres represented 0 to 15 percent of extragenital chancres.[81–85] However, as STD clinicians have become more alert to the need of examining the anal area for chancres, the proportion of chancres found to involve the anorectal area has also increased.

Anorectal chancres usually appear within 2 to 6 weeks after exposure by rectal intercourse. As mentioned above, symptoms are commonly absent in the primary stage of anorectal syphilis, but when symptoms are present, they include mild anal pain or discomfort, constipation, rectal bleeding, and occasionally a rectal discharge. Primary anorectal syphilis may appear as single or multiple perianal ulcers or ulceration within the anal canal or rectum.[86–88] Within the rectum, secondary syphilis may cause discrete polyps,[85,86,89] smooth lobulated masses,[27,90–92] and mucosal ulcerations, as well as nonspecific mucosal erythema or bleeding.[93,94] In secondary syphilis, condylomata lata may be found near or within the anal canal. The term *condyloma latum* has generally been limited to morphologically characteristic lesions involving stratified squamous epithelium, and we therefore do not use the term to include lesions of the columnar epithelial mucosa of the rectum. It is probable that secondary syphilis frequently involves the gastrointestinal tract, particularly the stomach. The frequency with which the rectum is involved has not been compared in homosexual vs. heterosexual men. Late syphilis may involve any area of the gastrointestinal tract, and the involvement can range from infiltrative, constrictive, or polypoid masses within the stomach to lesions of the lower bowel.[95,96] However, most past descriptions of gastrointestinal syphilis should be interpreted cautiously since many of these lesions were ascribed to syphilis solely on the basis of serology, clinical responses to therapy, and compatible histology. Only a few reports have demonstrated *Treponema pallidum* in gastrointestinal lesions by silver stain or indirect immunofluorescence.[93,96]

Diagnosis of anorectal syphilis is based on serology, perirectal and digital rectal examination, and anoscopy. Detection of motile treponemes by dark field examination is useful for evaluation of perianal and anal lesions but may be less specific for rectal lesions, since nonpathogenic treponemes can be found in the intestine, although the number of species of nonpathogenic treponemes which have been described is greater in the mouth than in the intestine.[97] Biopsies of any rectal lesions or masses should be processed for silver staining, as well as routine histology, if syphilis is suspected. Although Nazemi et al.[93] described a case of syphilitic proctitis by demonstrating a spirochete on silver stain of a rectal biopsy, some investigators believe that silver stains are unreliable and recommend identification of *T. pallidum* by immunofluorescence using anti-*T. pallidum* antisera.[96,98,99] Figure 55-4 illustrates a positive immunofluorescent stain for *T. pallidum* in a rectal mass lesion found in a homosexual man who had secondary syphilis associated with anorectal pain and discharge.

In addition, the histopathology of anorectal syphilitic lesions is also quite characteristic. As shown in Fig. 55-5, a hematoxylin and eosin preparation of the same tissue shown in Fig. 55-4 demonstrates at low magnification a uniform infiltrate of mononuclear cells throughout the submucosa and lamina propria. At higher magnification, these are seen to be predominantly plasma cells, lymphocytes, and histiocytes. This degree of plasma cell infiltration is characteristic of gummas, syphilitic gastritis,

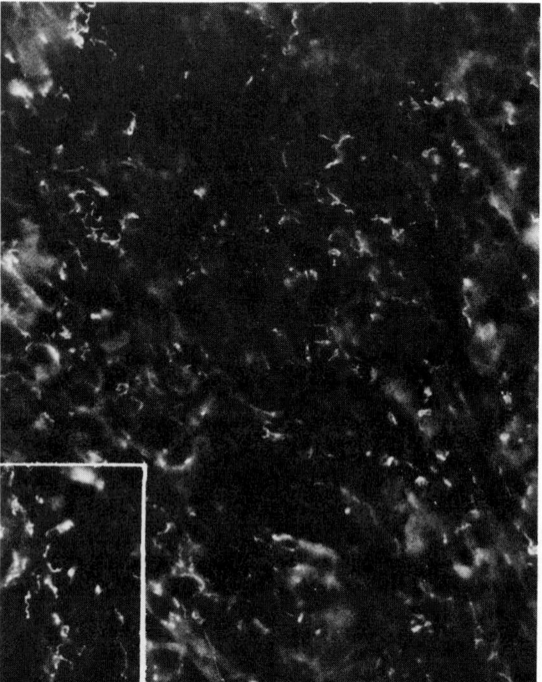

Fig. 55-4. Immunofluorescent staining for *Treponema pallidum* reveals numerous brightly stained organisms scattered throughout the mucosa and submucosa of a rectal biopsy from a patient with a rectal mass and secondary syphilis. (*Courtesy of S. Lukehart.*)

condylomata lata, and syphilitic chancres.[96,100] Presumably, this intense plasma cell infiltrate in early syphilis represents an immune response to the large number of treponemes demonstrated throughout the tissue by immunofluorescent antibody staining.[101]

The differential diagnosis of anorectal syphilis includes ulcers due to HSV infection, chancroid, granuloma inguinale, and LGV. They may be commonly misdiagnosed as anal fissures, fistulas, hemorrhoiditis, traumatic lesions, rectal polyps, condylomata acuminata, and even rectal carcinoma.[87,88,91,92] Indeed, there have been several reports of patients who underwent surgery for removal of lesions which were initially thought to be malignant but were later diagnosed as syphilitic lesions.[102]

Treatment for early syphilis is discussed in Chap. 20.

Benzathine penicillin, in a single dose of 2.4 IM, remains the treatment of choice for early syphilis. Penicillin-allergic patients may be treated with a 15-day course of tetracycline, 500 mg orally given 4 times daily. All sexual contacts should be screened and treated. Recent reports have suggested that the natural history of syphilis may be altered in patients with HIV infection. Consequently, very close follow-up of HIV-infected patients with syphilis is recommended following treatment with repeat serologies, and if indicated, repeat treatment on a regular basis.[103,104]

## *Chlamydia trachomatis* PROCTITIS

Intestinal involvement has been described in LGV infections, but only recently has non-LGV *C. trachomatis* infection of the rectum been recognized.[4,105,106] In a Seattle study, *C. trachomatis* was isolated by rectal culture from 24 (8.3 percent) of 288 randomized selected homosexual men and from 33 (21 percent) of 155 heterosexual women seen in an STD clinic.[107] Subsequent to that study, prevalence rates have decreased in Seattle and in other cities[107,108] but remain high in other areas. In a recent Baltimore study, *C. trachomatis* was isolated from the rectum of 9 percent

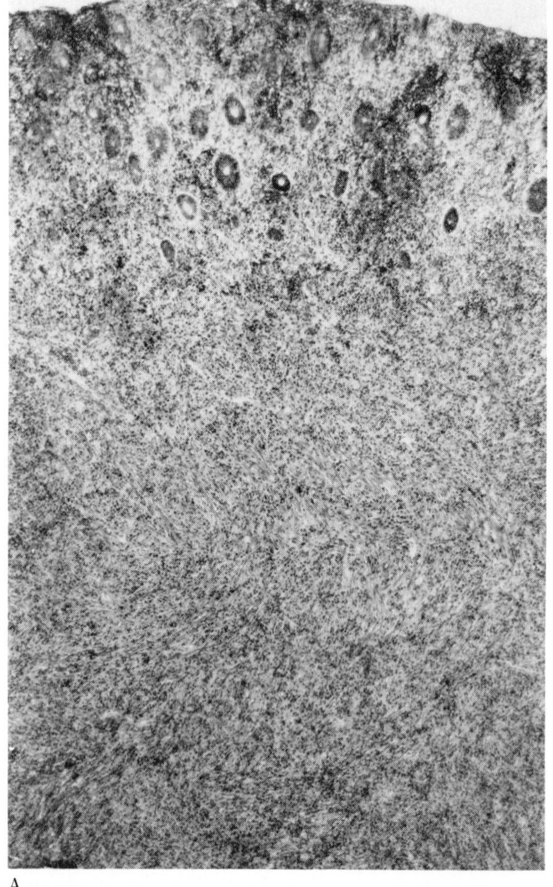

A

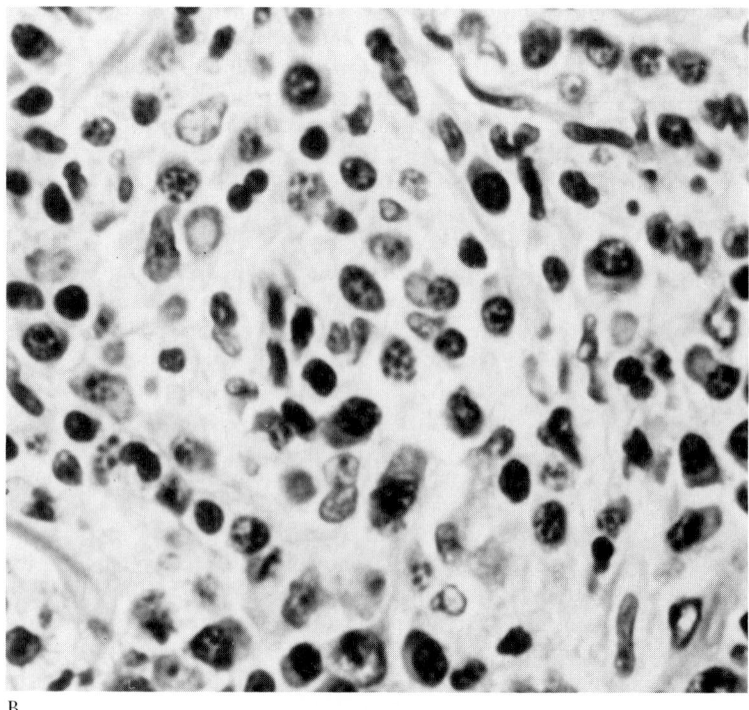

B

Fig. 55-5. Biopsy of a rectal mass from a patient with secondary syphilis. (*a*) An extensive uniform cellular infiltrate has replaced the submucosa and lamina propria and has disrupted the muscularis mucosa. (*b*) The infiltrate consists of plasma cells, histiocytes, and lymphocytes.

of 264 men attending an STD clinic (Quinn, unpublished data). In nearly all these studies, *C. trachomatis* was frequently associated with asymptomatic infection except for infections with LGV serovars which were more commonly associated with a severe proctocolitis. Since the clinical manifestations and histopathology of *C. trachomatis* rectal infections differ according to the infecting immunotype, these will be discussed separately.

Rectal infections with LGV immunotypes of *C. trachomatis* have been recognized since 1936.[109] Initially referred to as the anorectal syndrome of LGV, rectal involvement was generally believed to be a late manifestation of a genital infection: after contact with an infected individual, a transient papule or ulcer sometimes appeared on the genitalia, followed by systemic symptoms and prominent inguinal adenopathy. Without treatment, the infection progressed to destructive granulomatous lesions of the lymph nodes and lower intestinal tract, which progressed to the formation of fistulas, strictures, and perianal abscesses.[110,111] More recently, primary anal or rectal infections have been described in women and in homosexual men who practice anal intercourse. In this latter situation, rectal involvement is initially characterized by severe anorectal pain, a bloody mucopurulent discharge, and tenesmus. Inguinal adenopathy, which is characteristic of genital LGV, is often present.

In both secondary and primary anorectal LGV, sigmoidoscopy reveals diffuse friability with discrete ulcerations in the rectum that occasionally extend to the descending colon.[112,113] Strictures and fistulas may become prominent and can be easily misdiagnosed clinically as Crohn's disease or carcinoma.[110,111,114] Histologically, rectal LGV may also be confused with Crohn's disease. Commonly, there is diffuse inflammation throughout the mucosa and submucosa, as well as giant cells, crypt abscesses, and granulomas (Fig. 55-6). Due to these similarities, Crohn[115] and others[110,116,117] speculated about a possible relationship between the two disorders. Schuller et al.[118] later demonstrated antibody to LGV strains in over 70 percent of patients with Crohn's disease and in less than 2 percent of healthy controls. At least three subsequent studies have failed to document such a relationship.[119–121] However, in our own analyses of rectal biopsies from homosexual men with proctitis, histopathological findings were interpreted as consistent with Crohn's disease in two of three men from whom LGV immunotypes of *C. trachomatis* were isolated.[4] From these data, it appears that LGV infection should be suspected and ruled out in homosexual men with unexplained proctitis.[122]

The non-LGV immunotypes of *C. trachomatis* are less invasive than LGV and cause a mild proctitis characterized by rectal discharge, tenesmus, and anorectal pain.[3] Anal lesions have not been described. Many infected individuals may be asymptomatic and can be diagnosed only by routine culturing. Even in asymptomatic cases, a small number of fecal leukocytes are usually present. Sigmoidoscopy may be normal or may reveal mild inflammatory changes with small erosions or follicles in the lower 10 cm of the rectum.

Diagnosis of chlamydial proctitis is best made by isolation of *C. trachomatis* from the rectum, together with response to appropriate therapy. Direct FA staining of rectal secretions using monoclonal antibodies can also be used to make the diagnosis.[123,124] Serotyping by microimmunofluorescence[125] can differentiate LGV from non-LGV isolates. Serology is also useful for the diagnosis of LGV, particularly with the microimmunofluorescent (micro-IF) technique.[126] In consecutive cases of chlamydial proctitis, we have found titers of $\geq$ 1:512 (all with broad immunotype specificity consistent with LGV) in three of three men with rectal LGV and in none of eight men with non-LGV chlamydial proctitis.[4] However, Schachter[127] found that among men with anorectal symptoms selected on the basis of having a high titer of micro-IF antibody ($\geq$1:1000), four of six culture-positive men had non-LGV immunotypes isolated and the remaining two men had LGV immunotypes. Thus, the specificity of serodiagnosis of rectal LGV requires further study. Among men with non-LGV rectal chlamydial infection, serology has been less useful, since antibody titers are lower, and in the range of antibody titers commonly found in men who are culture-negative, presumably reflecting previous infection. Demonstration of a fourfold rise in antibody titer in paired sera provides stronger evidence of chlamydial infection than does demonstration of a single elevated titer.

Tetracycline or doxycycline are the drugs of choice for infection with *C. trachomatis*. We have used a 2- to 3-week course of tetracycline, 500 mg four times daily, for anorectal chlamydial

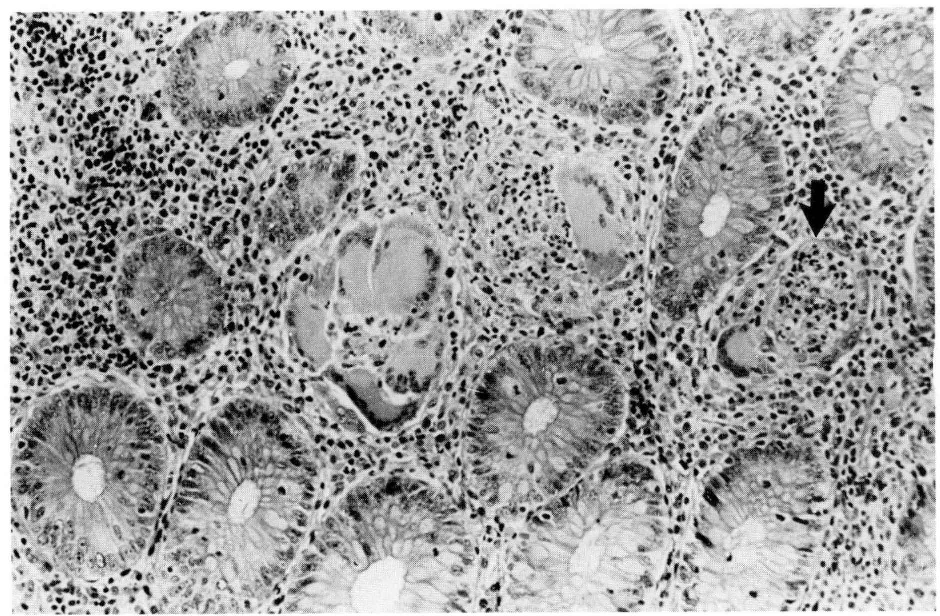

**Fig. 55-6.** Rectal biopsy from a patient with rectal LGV (*C. trachomatis*, LGV-2 immunotype). There is diffuse inflammation throughout the mucosa and submucosa. Giant cells, crypt abscesses (*arrow*), and granulomas are present.

infection with uniform success. Patients should be followed carefully with repeat sigmoidoscopy, particularly when there is any question about the differential diagnosis of LGV vs. inflammatory bowel disease.

## PROCTOCOLITIS AND ENTERITIS DUE TO ENTERIC PATHOGENS

Epidemiologic and anecdotal reports have implicated the sexual transmission of several enteric pathogens such as shigella, salmonella, and *Campylobacter jejuni*.[20–22,28,128–130] Since these organisms are described in depth in Chap. 41, we will only briefly review some of the clinical and epidemiologic data concerning the role of these pathogens in homosexual men with symptoms and signs of enteritis or proctocolitis.

Although several species of shigella are responsible for human disease, *S. sonnei* and *S. flexneri* account for most of the infections in the United States. Since shigella is highly infectious, transmission of the organism can occur rapidly and is commonly seen in children and travelers, in mental or penal institutions, and in localized outbreaks traced to contaminated food or water. The sexual transmission of shigella was recognized in 1972 when reports from San Francisco, and later from Seattle and New York, documented that 30 to 70 percent of patients with shigella were homosexual men.[21,25,128,131] Contact tracing demonstrated recovery of the same serotype from sexual partners, and no contaminated food or water source could be shown to be common to any of the cases.

Clinically, shigellosis presents with an abrupt onset of diarrhea, fever, nausea, and cramps. The diarrhea is usually watery but may contain mucus or blood. Sigmoidoscopy usually reveals an inflamed mucosa with friability *not* limited to the distal rectum, and histological examination shows diffuse inflammation with bacteria scattered through the submucosa and muscularis mucosa (Fig. 55-7). Diagnosis is made by culturing the organisms from the stool on selective media. Treatment is usually supportive, but antibiotics are of benefit in selected cases. Due to widespread development of resistance, selection of antibiotics should be based on regional antibiotic sensitivities. Since asymptomatic carriers of shigella exist, contact tracing is an important public health measure. Studies are needed on the value of tracing sexual contacts of homosexual men with shigellosis.

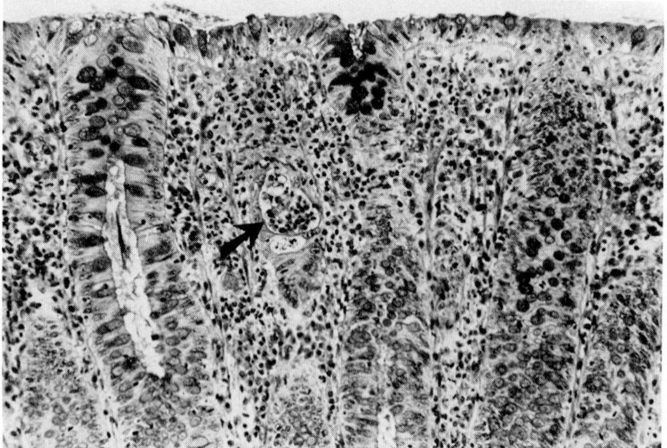

Fig. 55-7. Campylobacter colitis. The colonic mucosa is acutely inflamed, with polymorphonuclear leukocytes in the epithelium and lamina propria. A crypt abscess is also present (*arrow*). These findings are not specific for campylobacter and may be found in the acute colitis caused by other invasive pathogens. H&E stain, × 340 magnification. (*Courtesy of M. Schuffler.*)

*Campylobacter jejuni* is a curved gram-negative rod which has only recently been recognized as a common bacterial pathogen, isolated from 4 to 8 percent of patients with acute enteritis. This pathogen is generally acquired by ingestion of contaminated water or food or by close contact with infected animals.[132,133] Sexual transmission has been documented in animals and was suspected in early reported cases of human abortion,[134] and a few reports have recently addressed the possible sexual transmission of campylobacter in humans.[129,130,133,135] *Campylobacter* sp. or campylobacter-like organisms have been recovered from the stools from 24 percent of symptomatic homosexual men and 10 percent of asymptomatic homosexual men.[27] In a subsequent study performed in 1986 in Baltimore, campylobacter species were isolated from 4 percent of asymptomatic homosexual men, from 20 percent of homosexual men with intestinal symptoms, and from 9 percent of homosexual men with AIDS.[136] The most frequent isolates were *C. jejuni* followed by campylobacter-like organisms.

These studies have clearly documented the frequent occurrence of campylobacter-like organisms in homosexual men. In the AIDS era, campylobacter-like organisms have been recovered less often from rectal or stool cultures of homosexual men with diarrhea (Table 55-4) but have caused bacteremic illness in AIDS patients with fever.[137] Biochemical tests, morphology, and guanine-plus-cytosine content of whole-cell DNA have shown that these organisms are similar to but distinguishable from other species in the genus *Campylobacter*.[138] DNA homology studies show that most of these campylobacter-like organisms belong to two CLO groups that have been isolated from homosexual men with proctitis, proctocolitis, and/or enteritis. Even when isolated from asymptomatic homosexual men, these organisms are significantly correlated with the presence of polymorphonuclear leukocytes in rectal secretions, a finding that suggests clinical disease.[140] The two major CLO groups have been classified into two separate species, *Campylobacter cinadi* sp. *nov.* and *Campylobacter fennaelliae* sp. *nov.*[139]

Clinically, *C. jejuni* produces an acute diarrhea of several days duration with fever, chills, myalgias, and abdominal pain. Although the infection usually involves the small intestine, involvement of the colon and rectum has also been described.[140–143] We have isolated *C. jejuni* and campylobacter-like organisms predominantly in association with symptoms and sigmoidoscopic findings of proctocolitis. The sigmoidoscopic and rectal biopsy findings are nonspecific and similar to those described for shigellosis (Fig. 55-7). Fecal leukocytes are uniformly present, and diagnosis is confirmed by isolating the organisms from the stool by culture on selective media in a microaerophilic atmosphere.[132] Although the need for antimicrobial therapy has not been fully established in human campylobacter infection of the intestinal tract, treatment with erythromycin, 500 mg four times daily for 1 week, has been recommended for severely symptomatic cases.

There are several species of salmonella with more than 1700 different serotypes that cause a variety of clinical entities in humans. Only anecdotal reports have commented on the possible sexual transmission of salmonella; in one[22] *S. typhi* was recovered from the stools of homosexual men and the same serotype was recovered from asymptomatic sexual partners with whom no housing, food, or water was shared. These individuals presented with typhoid fever characterized by malaise, fever, abdominal pain, rash, and diarrhea. More recently, cases of *Sal-*

*monella enteritidis* have been reported with increasing frequency in AIDS patients.[144] These have included both homosexual men and AIDS patients from tropical areas such as Haiti or Central Africa.

Diagnosis is made by culturing the organisms from the stool on selective media. Treatment of typhoid fever must be individualized, depending on severity of symptoms and antibiotic sensitivity of the isolate. Since asymptomatic carriers are common and may be employed as food handlers in public establishments (as were the reported cases), tracing of sexual partners of infected individuals is particularly important.

## PARASITIC INFECTIONS

Although reports of cutaneous amebiasis of the penis, vulva, and cervix suggested sexual transmission of amebiasis,[145–147] it has only been within the last decades that sexual transmission of certain parasitic infections has been fully appreciated.[1,3,23,24] In 1972 it was suggested that *G. lamblia, Iodamoeba bütschlii, Dientamoeba fragilis,* and *Enterobius vermicularis* were sexually transmitted among homosexuals.[148–151] In two separate surveys in New York City, the prevalence of infection with giardiasis and/or amebiasis was between 30 and 40 percent in selected homosexual men.[23,24] The presence of infection correlated better with a history of anilingus than with travel history.[1,23] In Seattle, 25 percent of homosexual men we have studied with anorectal or intestinal symptoms have had either giardia, *E. histolytica* or both present in their stools.[27] *G. lamblia* was associated with symptoms of enteritis, while *E. histolytica* was equally common in symptomatic and asymptomatic men. In addition, mixed infections with a variety of intestinal parasites, including other protozoans and nematodes, have also been described in homosexual men.[3,148–150,152] Other protozoan intestinal infections may be seen in homosexual men with HIV infection, including *Cryptosporidium, Isospora,* and *Microsporidium.* These organisms have only recently been identified in humans. In immunocompetent individuals, these infections may cause self-limited diarrheal illnesses that resolve within two weeks with specific treatment, but in immunocompromised patients they may cause life-threatening diarrheal disease.[153]

The etiologic agent of amebiasis is *E. histolytica,* although *Dientamoeba fragilis* is believed by some authorities to be similarly pathogenic and closely related to *E. histolytica.*[154] Primarily a waterborne agent, sexual transmission may be responsible for the high prevalence of *E. histolytica* in certain communities. In 1977, 40 percent of all reported cases of amebiasis in the United States were from New York City. Eighty percent of these cases were located in Manhattan, and its large male homosexual community had the highest morbidity rate.[25] Similarly, in San Francisco, 89 percent of the reported cases of amebiasis were in males 20 to 39 years of age.[1] In a retrospective review of records of patients with *E. histolytica* infection seen at New York Hospital, Schmerin et al.[29] noted that 20 of 20 men who had not traveled were homosexual, while only 2 of 30 men with amebiasis who had traveled were homosexual. More recent studies have identified *E. histolytica* in 21 to 32 percent of selected homosexual male populations in North America and from 12 percent of homosexual men in the United Kingdom.[155–157]

Despite a positive wet prep exam, symptoms of amebiasis are often absent in homosexual men. When present, symptoms may vary from mild diarrhea to fulminant bloody dysentery. Extension of the infection to the liver, lung, or brain occurs rarely. Amebic proctocolitis causes diffuse inflammation and ulceration of the distal colon, often clinically indistinguishable from inflammatory bowel disease, shigellosis, and *C. jejuni* infection, and yersinia enterocolitis.[158,159]

There has been considerable recent debate about whether in most cases, *E. histolytica* actually causes illness in homosexual men who are positive by stool wet mount exam.[160] The prevalence of *E. histolytica* is approximately equal in symptomatic and asymptomatic groups of homosexual men,[27] and many of those who are symptomatic have other pathogens in addition to *E. histolytica.* Further, *E. histolytica* trophozoites have recently been divided into pathogenic and nonpathogenic zymodemes types using isoenzyme patterns.[156] Most *E. histolytica* strains isolated from homosexual men are the nonpathogenic zymodemes, which are not usually associated with gastrointestinal symptoms, invasive disease,[161] or a serological response.[162]

Diagnosis is based on the demonstration of *E. histolytica* in the stool or in a wet mount of a swab or a biopsy of rectal mucosal lesions. Occasionally, multiple fresh stool examinations are necessary to demonstrate the cysts or trophozoites of *E. histolytica.* Serology (indirect hemagglutination) is useful in acute amebic colitis because it is positive in 82 to 98 percent of infected patients.[163] Recommended treatment for symptomatic disease is with metronidazole, with or without diiodohydroxyquin,[164–166] as discussed further in Chap. 44.

*G. lamblia,* another frequent waterborne disease, also appears to be sexually transmitted through oral-anal contact. In a review of giardiasis in men seen at New York Hospital, 19 (22 percent) had not traveled recently and all were homosexual.[167] In 1977, Meyers et al. documented giardiasis in six of eight homosexual men who were sexual partners.[30] Giardiasis is typically an infection of the small intestine, although it is often found in association with amebiasis. Symptoms of giardiasis include diarrhea, abdominal cramps, bloating, and nausea. Multiple stool examinations are necessary to document infection with *G. lamblia.* Often, when stool examination has been negative, sampling of jejunal mucus by the Enterotest[168] or small bowel biopsy is necessary to confirm the diagnosis.

Quinacrine hydrochloride, 100 mg, or metronidazole, 250 mg three times a day for 7 days, is presently recommended in the United States, but both drugs are associated with a 10 to 15 percent failure rate.[166,169] Tinidazole, another 5-nitro imidazole available in Europe, may be more effective.[170] Follow-up stool examinations are particularly important in management of *G. lamblia* and *E. histolytica* infection. Examination of sex partners of homosexual men may be important in reducing the reservoir infection in the community.

Several reports have commented on the identification of *Enterobius vermicularis,* or pinworms, in homosexual men.[151,171] Although commonly found in children, adult pinworm infection in usually acquired by contact with an infected child or by sexual transmission via anilingus. Ova are deposited by the adult worm in the perianal area and are infective for several hours. Pruritus ani is a common symptom. Diagnosis is made by demonstrating the ova collected on cellophane tape from the anal area. Ova are rarely seen in stool examinations. Mebendazole, 100 mg twice a day for 2 days, or a single dose of pyrantel pamoate, 11 mg/kg orally, repeated once after 2 weeks, is usually effective and well tolerated.[166]

Although many helminth infections cannot be transmitted person to person because of their particular life cycle, *Strongyloides stercoralis* could be transmitted sexually since the infective filariform larvae are often found in the feces. However, there has been no published evidence as yet that this infection has been sexually transmitted.

Intestinal infection with three protozoan parasites, *Cryptosporidium, Isospora belli,* and *Microsporidium,* has been identified in homosexual men with AIDS.[172] Although there has been no documentation of sexual transmission of these parasites, this mode of transmission is highly suspect due to the relatively high frequency in homosexual men compared to other select populations with AIDS.

*Cryptosporidium* is a tiny (4 to 5 μm) protozoan parasite that primarily inhabits the microvillus region of epithelial cells. This parasite has been known to cause diarrhea in various animals, especially calves and other domestic animals.[173] In 1976, the first human infection with *Cryptosporidium* was reported, and until 1983 this pathogen was identified only in immunosuppressed patients.[174,175] In 1983, however, investigators reported identification of this parasite in immunocompetent persons exposed to infected calves.[153] The majority of these patients developed profuse diarrhea and abdominal cramps which were self-limited, subsiding in 7 to 10 days.

In AIDS, infection with *Cryptosporidium* and *Isospora belli,* another rare intestinal coccidian parasite, frequently results in prolonged watery diarrhea. The illness is characterized by intermittent episodes of abdominal cramps, bloating, and nausea in association with either steatorrhea or a profuse secretory diarrhea. Weight loss is usually profound and the infection is unresponsive to any therapeutic attempts to eradicate it or to sustain nutritional status.[172] The mechanism by which these organisms produce diarrhea remains unknown. Primarily parasites of the small bowel, *Cryptosporidium* or *Isospora* can be present throughout the small bowel, colon, or both in AIDS. Mucosal biopsies reveal the organisms clustered on the surface epithelial cells of the villi with little or no mucosal destruction, ulceration, or inflammation.

Diagnosis of either *Cryptosporidium* or *Isospora* can be rapidly established by a modified acid-fast stain or auramine stain of the stool, or by concentration and identification of the organisms by the sugar-flotation method.[176] Intestinal biopsies are also useful in confirming the diagnosis. Serological tests have been developed utilizing an indirect immunofluorescent test using serum from humans applied to tissue secretions of experimentally infected mice.[177] With these improved diagnostic techniques, the prevalence of *Cryptosporidium* and *Isospora* can be determined in the homosexual population and other populations at risk for infection.

Despite numerous attempts to treat symptomatic cryptosporidium and isospora infection in immunocompromised individuals, no drugs have been shown to be fully efficacious. In limited studies, the antiprotozoal drug spiromycin was reported to be effective in several AIDS patients with cryptosporidiosis,[178] but subsequent studies have not confirmed this finding. Unfortunately, there are no published reports evaluating the efficacy of spiromycin against cryptosporidiosis in animals, and preliminary results suggest that spiromycin does not inhibit cryptosporidial growth in tissue culture.

Treatment of isospora infection in immunocompetent individuals is rarely required, but the organism does respond in severe symptomatic cases to antifolates such as pyrimethamine and sulfadiazine.[179] As with cryptosporidiosis, no effective treatment has been identified for isospora infection in AIDS patients. Treatment with antifolates, including trimethoprim-sulfamethoxazole, may result in a decrease in symptomatic disease, but the organism is rarely eradicated. Another drug which may be of use in the treatment of this disease is amprolium, a quaternary organic base used as veterinary medicine for the treatment of *Eimeria* infection. Recently, the treatment of two cases suggested that amprolium may be a value in the treatment of *Isospora belli* infection, and possibly in cryptosporidiosis.[180] In a recent study,[181] furazoladone and trimethoprim-sulfamethoxazole were used in patients infected with *Isospora belli.* Two of three patients in this series had a relapse within weeks to months of treatment with these infections. These patients were then successfully retreated with a 4-week course of trimethoprim-sulfamethoxazole followed by chronic suppressive therapy. *Isospora belli* infection may be more effectively treated with antiprotozoan medication than cryptosporidiosis, but controlled trials are still required.

Intracellular protozoan organisms called microsporidia have recently been identified by electron microscopy of intestinal biopsies in several AIDS patients with enteritis.[182] The spores of microsporidia are only 1 to 2 μm in size and are not usually identified by routine stains of stool from infected patients. At present, it is not known whether this is a common infection of immunocompetent individuals or whether it causes disease only in immunocompromised individuals. Diagnosis currently depends upon electron microscopy of small intestinal biopsy which reveals the organisms in upper intestinal epithelial cells. The pathogenicity of these organisms is unknown and no drugs are known to be effective.

## ANORECTAL INFECTION WITH *Neisseria meningitidis*

The prevalence of *N. meningitidis* in the anorectum of homosexual men is estimated to be 2 to 4.5 percent.[183,184] In one series, 31 percent of rectal isolates from men which were initially presumed to be *N. gonorrhoeae* were identified as *N. meningitidis* by sugar utilization tests and fluorescent antibody tests.[185] However, the clinical significance of anorectal isolates of *N. meningitidis* is unknown. Most such infections are asymptomatic, but a report of several individuals with anorectal symptoms associated with recovery of only *N. meningitidis* from the rectum and of prompt response to therapy suggested that this organism may be pathogenic in the rectum.[173] Optimum therapy is not well defined. For symptomatic proctitis associated with *N. meningitidis* infection, we have used procaine penicillin G, 4.8 million units, plus 1.0 g of probenecid, particularly when no other pathogen has been identified. The need for treatment of asymptomatic anorectal colonization with *N. meningitidis* is even less clear. We currently do not treat asymptomatic rectal, pharyngeal, or urethral *N. meningitidis* colonization in homosexual or heterosexual individuals.

## CONDYLOMATA ACUMINATA

Anal warts are common in individuals who practice anal intercourse. In one series of 260 homosexual men seen by proctologists, 134 (51.5 percent) had anal warts.[19] These are caused by human papillomaviruses which are easily transmitted from person to person. They may occur anywhere in the anal or genital area but are particularly common in the anus in homosexual men. Of those individuals with warts in the above study,[19] 6 percent had them in the perianal area, 10.5 percent had them only in the anal canal, and 83.5 percent had them in both areas. They rarely if ever extend beyond the pectinate line into the rectum. Perianal condylomata acuminata appear as raised pink to brown papules, usually in clusters, and occasionally as large cauliflower-like masses.

Diagnostically, they should be differentiated from condylomata lata, the moist flat papules of secondary syphilis. These may be diagnosed by a reactive serology for syphilis and by a dark field demonstration of spirochetes in the lesions. Therapy of genital warts is discussed in Chap. 38. Topical podophyllin, commonly used for genital warts, is also effective in some cases of perianal and anal warts. Cryotherapy with liquid nitrogen applied with a swab or by focused spray is usually effective. Laser-beam therapy and surgical excision have been used in refractory cases.

Condyloma acuminata have the potential to undergo malignant transformation.[186] In one study, intraepithelial carcinoma developed in 9 homosexual men with anal warts, 6 of whom had histories consistent with AIDS. Therefore, these lesions, when they occur in high-risk individuals, deserve prompt excision and histologic examination if they recur. Recent studies have also suggested an increased incidence of cloacogenic anal carcinoma in homosexual men.[187] Prospective studies are currently underway to determine the association between these malignancies, papillomavirus, and HIV infection.

## MYCOBACTERIAL INFECTIONS

*M. avium-intracellulare* is an "atypical" mycobacterium that has been identified in severely immunocompromised patients, including homosexual men with AIDS.[10] The gastrointestinal tract and lymph nodes appear to be the most common organs infected by this organism. Infections of the intestinal tract frequently cause steatorrhea and malabsorption, and both the clinical and radiographic features of this disease may mimic Whipple's disease.[10,188] The main histologic features on small bowel biopsy include increased numbers of macrophages within the lamina propria which are filled with PAS-positive and acid-fast bacilli.

It has been postulated that the gastrointestinal symptoms of *M. avium-intracellulare* are due to defective macrophage processing of these pathogens, which lead to accumulation of macrophages and secondary malabsorption as seen in Whipple's disease. The defective T cell activation of macrophages has been proposed as a mechanism in the pathogenesis of Whipple's disease—an immunologic defect which is also characterized by depression of T cell function.[189] The characteristic difference seen in *M. avium-intracellulare* infection of AIDS patients is that severe lymphopenia, reduction of circulating helper-T cells, skin test anergy, and polyclonal hypergammaglobulinemia are not classically seen in Whipple's disease.

The diagnosis of *M. avium-intracellulare* infection is based on stool culture, acid-fast staining of the organism in the stool, and histologic examination of small bowel biopsy specimens. Blood cultures using special techniques for mycobacterial organisms are frequently positive in AIDS patients with disseminated *M. avium-intracellulare.*

Strains of *M. avium-intracellulare* vary widely in their in vitro susceptibility to chemotherapeutic agents. Most are highly resistant to antituberculous drugs, and current methods of treatment are unsatisfactory. Use of multiple drug regimens (3 to 8 drugs) for a long period of time has resulted in sputum conversion in patients with pulmonary disease, but without AIDS.[179] Of these, 15 to 23 percent have been reported to have a relapse during or after completion of therapy. No uniformly successful treatment has been reported in patients with intestinal infection with this organism.

## CYTOMEGALOVIRUS INFECTION

Esophageal and gastrointestinal infection with CMV is an exceedingly common finding among homosexual men with AIDS and in one autopsy series of AIDS patients was identified in 90 percent of cases.[7,12] In studies of the gastrointestinal tract in AIDS patients, CMV has been identified in either stool culture, rectal biopsy, or intestinal biopsy at time of autopsy in up to 50 percent of AIDS patients with intestinal symptoms. CMV infection of the gastrointestinal tract may be associated with esophagitis, esophageal ulcerations, enteritis, colitis, or proctitis. CMV most often presents as a diffuse colitis associated with abdominal pain and watery or bloody diarrhea.[190–192] Occasionally, patients with CMV intestinal symptoms may present clinically with a solitary intestinal ulcer, occasionally resulting in toxic dilatation, and rarely intestinal perforation.[193,194] Barium enema may show a picture of segmental colitis or pancolitis.[195] Sigmoidoscopy or colonoscopy frequently shows ulceration or, occasionally, violaceous lesions resembling Kaposi's sarcoma. Biopsy of these lesions reveals CMV vasculitis with CMV inclusions in endothelial cells, and acute hemorrhage and inflammation in the lamina propria. The presence of intranuclear inclusion bodies suggests that CMV is usually present in the tissue, but its role in disease pathogenesis remains unclear since its presence is documented in both inflamed and non-inflamed tissue. Marked involvement of endothelial cells can be associated with frank vasculitis and secondary mucosal ischemic changes.

Diagnosis of CMV infection is confirmed by histologic demonstration of intranuclear inclusion bodies or by viral cultures or intestinal biopsies. Systemic cytomegalovirus can be determined by viral culture of the white blood cell buffy coat or urine. New techniques using labeled nucleic acid probes and monoclonal antibodies have been effective in detecting CMV in tissue and other specimens.[196]

At present, there is no widely available effective therapy for CMV infection. However, new antiviral drugs against CMV such as 9-(1,3-dihydroxy-2-propoxymethyl)guanine (DHPG) have been developed in human clinical trials and have been initiated with promising results.[197–199] Cultures for CMV became negative during therapy, but relapses were common after therapy was discontinued. In some patients, substantial leukopenia developed during therapy but was readily reversed with discontinuation of the drug. Without treatment and with continued immunosuppression, CMV may result in intestinal complications such as intestinal perforation, toxic megacolon, and acalculous gangrenous colitis.[193,194,200,201]

## INTESTINAL SPIROCHETOSIS

Spirochetes other than *T. pallidum* were documented in the human intestinal tract as early as the nineteenth century. However, the pathologic and clinical significance of this condition remains unclear.[202] Recently, McMillan and Lee[203] reported the identification of intestinal spirochetes on biopsies of 36 of 100 homosexual men. There was no attempt to correlate symptoms with the presence or absence of spirochetes, and a comprehensive search for other pathogens in these patients was not carried out. More recent studies have identified intestinal spirochetosis by biopsy in 28 of 100 symptomatic homosexual men[15] and by culture in 13 (39 percent) of 33 symptomatic men and in 33 (16 percent) of 203 asymptomatic men.[41] Identification of spirochetes by culture was more commonly associated with symptoms of diarrhea than with symptoms of proctitis. Although these data are not definitive, they suggest that intestinal spirochetosis is more prevalent in homosexual men and that it may be associated with diarrhea.

Intestinal spirochetosis is readily diagnosed histologically by the presence of a prominent hematoxophilic band adjacent to the luminal surface of mucosal epithelial cells.[15] Morphologically distinct from *T. pallidum,* intestinal spirochetes can be demonstrated by dark field microscopy of fresh material or cultured anaerobically in selected medium.

Since the clinical significance of human intestinal spirochetosis remains in question, the treatment is controversial. No controlled trials have been undertaken to examine the efficacy of antibiotics and whether eradication of the spirochetes leads to resolution of symptoms. Anecdotal reports suggest that treatment with metronidazole 400 mg three times daily for 10 days is effective in eliminating spirochetes and may afford some symptomatic relief. Consequently, until adequate clinical antibiotic studies are performed, metronidazole should be recommended for the treatment of symptomatic human intestinal spirochetosis following the exclusion of other known pathogens. Treatment is not recommended for asymptomatic intestinal spirochetosis.

## ORAL-ESOPHAGEAL CANDIDIASIS

Oral candidiasis, or thrush, is one of the more common signs of AIDS. It appears early in the symptomatic prodrome of AIDS and is part of the AIDS-related complex.[9] In the absence of other underlying immunosuppressive diseases, the occurrence of thrush in a patient at risk for HIV or in association with chronic diarrheal-wasting syndrome is suggestive of HIV infection. Klein et al.[11] found that oral candidiasis in homosexual men was a predictor of underlying immunosuppression and incipient AIDS. In their study, 13 of 22 patients with oral candidiasis who were followed for 1 year acquired a major opportunistic infection or Kaposi's sarcoma. In contrast, none of 20 patients with generalized lymphadenopathy and immunodeficiency without oral candidiasis developed clinical evidence of AIDS.

Thrush is often associated with asymptomatic esophageal candidiasis. In a study by Tavitian et al.[204] 10 of 10 patients with AIDS and oral candidiasis were found to have esophageal candidiasis on endoscopy. Three of the 10 patients with esophageal candidiasis were symptom-free, whereas the remaining 7 were symptomatic. The authors concluded that the presence of oral candidiasis in patients with documented AIDS is invariably associated with esophageal candidiasis, which is often asymptomatic. Dilatation and abnormal motility of the esophagus on the esophagogram suggests the diagnosis of candidia esophagitis. The appearance of cottage cheese exudates is frequently seen on endoscopy, often in association with deep esophageal ulcerations.[7,32] Biopsies of these lesions typically reveal invasive hyphae in the mucosa and submucosa. High-risk patients with odynophagia or dysphagia should be carefully examined by endoscopy to ascertain if esophagitis is present and due to *Candida albicans.*

Oral candidiasis can often be controlled with nystatin 500,000 units swish-and-swallow 4 to 6 times daily. However, this regimen may be inadequate in the treatment of AIDS-associated esophageal candidiasis. Persistent oral candidiasis or oral-esophageal candidiasis should be treated with ketoconazole 200 mg twice daily or with intravenous amphotericin B in more severe cases. Even if treatment is successful, the infection tends to recur, and suppression with oral nystatin, clotrimazole, or ketoconazole is required.[179]

## OTHER PERIANAL SEXUALLY TRANSMITTED DISEASES

Donovanosis (or granuloma inguinale) is a chronic ulcerative disease which generally involves the skin and subcutaneous tissue of the genital, inguinal, and anal regions. Described in Chap. 25, donovanosis is believed to be caused by *Calymmatobacterium granulomatis,* a bacterium which multiplies within tissue histocytes and monocytes.

Donovanosis is rare in industrialized countries but relatively common in tropical and subtropical countries such as New Guinea, India, central Australia, and the Caribbean. The disease occurs more often in males than in females, and it is more common in homosexual than in heterosexual men. Although donovanosis is probably sexually transmitted, the exact mechanism of transmission is still debated. Perianal lesions occur predominantly among those who practice anal intercourse,[205,206] although the disease can also spread contiguously from the genital area to the anal region. Very little is known concerning involvement of the rectum or gastrointestinal tract. Within the perianal and anal area, the infection starts as a small, commonly pruritic papule and later ulcerates to form a granulomatous beefy-red ulcer. Opposing (kissing) lesions are common, and lesions can become hypertrophic and at that point will be similar in appearance to condylomata lata. Most of the lesions are painless. Lesions that are located in the anal canal may be associated with rectal bleeding and they may lead to stenosis of the anal canal.[205,207]

Diagnosis is based on demonstrating the intracellular organisms (Donovan bodies) on Giemsa-stained impression smears or sections of biopsies from a lesion. Treatment consists of tetracycline 2 g daily for 10 days or longer.

Chancroid occasionally causes perianal lesions in women and homosexual men. Although anorectal chancroid has not been well studied, it is likely that the painful lesions produced by *Haemophilus ducreyi* would most closely resemble herpetic lesions in the anorectal area, as in the genital tract. Diagnosis and therapy of anorectal chancroid are analogous to the management of genital chancroid.[208,209]

## ANORECTAL TRAUMA AND FOREIGN OBJECTS

Complications of anal intercourse include prolapsed hemorrhoids, fissures, rectal ulcers, tears, and foreign bodies.[19] Rectal tears and, occasionally, rectal perforation may be caused by rectal intercourse, by insertion of a closed fist and part of the forearm into the rectum, or by insertion of foreign bodies.[210,211] Typically, patients with anorectal trauma present with the acute onset of rectal bleeding or with signs of an "acute abdomen" if rectal perforation has occurred above the peritoneal reflection. Medical attention may be sought because the patient is unable to remove a foreign object. Retained foreign bodies have included vibrators, rubber phalluslike devices, bananas, bottles, apples, billiard balls, light bulbs, a Bermuda onion, and a variety of other unusual objects.[211]

Management of such cases is based on the clinical history, evidence of an acute abdomen, the degree of rectal trauma, and the type of retained object. If an object is present, digital and radiographic examination should confirm the position of the object. The object may be removed through a proctoscope with biopsy forceps, snare, or Foley catheter. Occasionally, local or general anesthesia may be required to remove a foreign body manually or with obstetric forceps.[211]

## DIFFERENTIAL DIAGNOSIS

Many agents that infect the gut in homosexual men cause similar pathology, and differentiation as to the causative agent is sometimes possible only by laboratory tests. Further, infection with several pathogens is not uncommon and overlapping symptoms make differentiation on clinical grounds even more difficult. However, characteristic features of some infections are helpful in narrowing the diagnostic possibilities. Use of the misnomer "gay bowel syndrome" should be discouraged, if for no other reason than that it encourages the lumping together of a large variety of problems which must be differentiated to allow a rational choice of therapy. It seems apparent that the majority of homosexual men with anorectal symptoms who consult an STD clinic have a specific infection, and diagnoses such as "gay bowel system," "nonspecific proctitis," or "trauma" are usually unwarranted unless specific infections are excluded. In general, it is clear that *proctitis* or discrete ulcerative lesions of the rectum are usually caused by conventional STD agents such as *N. gonorrhoeae*, *C. trachomatis*, HSV, and *T. pallidum* and are probably acquired by receptive rectal intercourse. Infections associated with *proctocolitis* are caused by enteric pathogens such as *E. histolytica*, *C. jejuni*, *Salmonella*, and *Shigella* sp., which may be acquired most often among homosexual men by anilingus. Symptoms of *enteritis*, without sigmoidoscopic evidence of *proctocolitis*, are most often attributable to *G. lamblia* infection in homosexually active men.[27]

In immunocompromised homosexual men with HIV infection, additional organisms should be considered, such as cryptosporidia, microsporidia, *Mycobacterium avium-intracellulare*, and cytomegalovirus. In these immunosuppressed patients, esophagitis may develop secondary to *Candida albicans*, herpes simplex virus, and cytomegalovirus.

The constellation of fever, severe anorectal pain, constipation, urinary retention, and sacral neuralgias in a patient with ulcerative rectal mucosa strongly suggests HSV infection. The presence of nonpainful anorectal ulcers, rectal polyps, or nonspecific anorectal symptoms in a patient with a rash should suggest the possibility of anorectal syphilis. LGV proctitis or proctocolitis should be considered in homosexual men who have severe anorectal symptoms such as hematochezia, rectal discharge, diarrhea, and fever and who may have severe ulcerative rectal mucosa with granulomas present on rectal biopsy. LGV should also be considered in homosexual men who are suspected to have Crohn's disease of the rectum. Since *N. gonorrhoeae* and non-LGV *C. trachomatis* cause nonspecific anorectal symptoms without symptoms of enteritis and result in nonspecific pathology of the lower rectum, these pathogens should be considered in most individuals who present with anorectal symptoms, have only mild proctitis on sigmoidoscopy, and acknowledge receptive anorectal intercourse.

Campylobacter, salmonella, and shigella should be suspected in those individuals with a history of acute diarrhea associated with bloody stools and fecal leukocytes, especially if sigmoidoscopic findings are not limited to the distal rectum and if stools are negative for ova and parasites. Giardia infection will more often cause diarrhea which is more chronic and nonbloody and is associated with nausea and bloating. *E. histolytica* infection presents with symptoms ranging from acute bloody diarrhea to chronic diarrhea with intermittent exacerbations.

A heavy concentration of *Candida albicans* in stool has been associated with pruritus ani or rectal itching in homosexual men in our studies, and topical and oral therapy with appropriate antifungal agents may be beneficial in such patients. The presence of perianal dermatitis with or without pustulae may suggest anorectal candidiasis. However, perianal erythema extending over an area of several centimeters in diameter is commonly associated with rectal discharge caused by a variety of agents and is not specific for anorectal candidiasis. When symptoms of proctitis or enteritis occur during or after antimicrobial therapy, *C. albicans* infection or pseudomembranous enterocolitis with *Clostridium difficile* infection should be considered.

When the patient is known to be immunocompromised secondary to HIV infection or AIDS, a more extensive evaluation for opportunistic infections should be undertaken. *Candida albicans*, herpes simplex virus, and cytomegalovirus should be evaluated in those patients with symptoms of esophagitis. Intestinal protozoans such as cryptosporidia, isospora, and microsporidia, as well as *Mycobacterium avium-intracellulare* and cytomegalovirus should be considered in those immunocompromised patients presenting with a diarrheal illness of a chronic nature ($>$ 2 to 3 weeks).

If no infectious etiology is demonstrated despite appropriate tests and a trial of antimicrobial therapy (see below) has no effect, then idiopathic inflammatory bowel disease, such as ulcerative colitis or Crohn's disease, should be considered. Because of clinical similarities between enteric infections (a common problem) and inflammatory bowel disease (much less common), all appropriate infectious agents should be ruled out before a diagnosis of inflammatory bowel disease is made. Additional noninfectious conditions that could be confused with enteric infections include radiation colitis, chemically induced colitis (due to drugs, gold therapy, soaps, lubricants, or other chemicals), and neoplasm.

## MANAGEMENT

The large number of infectious agents which cause enteric and anorectal infections in homosexual men necessitate a systematic approach to the management of these conditions. The medical history should attempt to differentiate among proctitis, proctocolitis, and enteritis and should assess the constellations of symptoms that suggest one or another likely infectious etiology. The history should also investigate types of sexual practices (see Chap. 6) and possible exposure to the pathogens known to cause proctitis, proctocolitis, or enteritis. Examination should include inspection of the anus, digital rectal examination, and anoscopy (avoiding or minimizing use of bacteriostatic lubricants, which might interfere with microbiological studies) to identify general mucosal abnormalities including easily induced bleeding and exudate, as well as discrete polyps, ulcerations, or fissures, which should be cultured and biopsied if appropriate. Anal warts are frequently detected, but if proctitis is present, therapy of these warts should usually be deferred until the proctitis is resolved.

Initial laboratory tests should include Gram's stain of any rectal exudate obtained with the use of an anoscope; if no exudate is seen, material should be obtained for Gram's stain from the rectal mucosa or from any abnormal-appearing stool. The demonstration of leukocytes provides objective evidence for the presence of an infectious or inflammatory disease. Cultures for *N. gonorrhoeae* should be obtained from the rectum, urethra, and pharynx, and if available, a rectal culture for *C. trachomatis* should be performed. A serological test for syphilis should be performed in all cases. If any external ulcers, rectal mucosal lesions, or suspected condylomata lata are seen, dark field examination of these lesions and a rapid plasma reagin test should be performed in the clinic. HSV cultures should be performed if ulcerative lesions are present, as recent studies indicate that HSV has become increasingly common as a cause of proctitis in the AIDS era and is not always associated with typical symptoms in HIV-positive patients. If proctocolitis is likely on the basis of either symptoms or sigmoidoscopic exam, then additional cultures for campylobacter, salmonella, and shigella and stool examination for *E. histolytica* are indicated.

If symptoms and signs suggest enteritis rather than proctitis or proctocolitis, then stool should be cultured for campylobacter and examined (in addition to jejunal aspirate, perhaps) for *G. lamblia*, cryptosporidia, and isospora. Cultures for salmonella, yersinia, and *V. parahemolyticus* and attempts to demonstrate *C. difficile* toxin or enterotoxigenic *E. coli* are sometimes indicated in homosexual men, as in heterosexual men and women, although these agents have not been found with more frequency in homosexual men.

If a diagnosis of gonorrhea is initially made by a positive Gram's stain (Plate 75) or if syphilis is confirmed by dark field examination or rapid plasma reagin serology, appropriate treatment with penicillin G should be instituted promptly. Similarly, anyone with sexual contact with a person with known gonorrhea, syphilis, or chlamydial urethritis should be treated appropriately on an epidemiologic basis after complete physical examination, while results of cultures for *N. gonorrhoeae* and serology for syphilis are pending. A presumptive diagnosis of HSV can often be made initially on clinical appearance alone or by history, but laboratory confirmation of suspected herpetic lesions is always desirable unless the clinical appearance of vesicular lesions is diagnostic. If the patient remains symptomatic and a careful search reveals no pathogen, or if the patient remains symptomatic despite appropriate therapy for any pathogen found or after empiric therapy, then the patient should be evaluated by a specialist for the possibility of inflammatory bowel disease or other diseases which are not sexually transmitted. In those patients found to be immunocompromised and infected with HIV, a more extensive evaluation of the intestinal tract is required. A careful oral examination should evaluate for the presence of thrush and/or oral lesions of Kaposi's sarcoma. Dysphagia or dynophagia may suggest the presence of esophageal candidiasis and/or esophageal involvement with cytomegalovirus or HIV infection. Systemic and/or abdominal lymphadenopathy and the presence or absence of gastrointestinal blood loss should suggest gastrointestinal neoplasms including Kaposi's sarcoma and gastrointestinal lymphomas. Careful radiographic examinations of the esophagus, small bowel, and colon, as well as endoscopy and colonoscopy may be warranted in these highly suspect patients. Stool examination should be carefully studied for the presence of cryptosporidia, isospora, and mycobacteria, as well as the other enteric pathogens described above. Intestinal biopsies may be obtained of suspicious

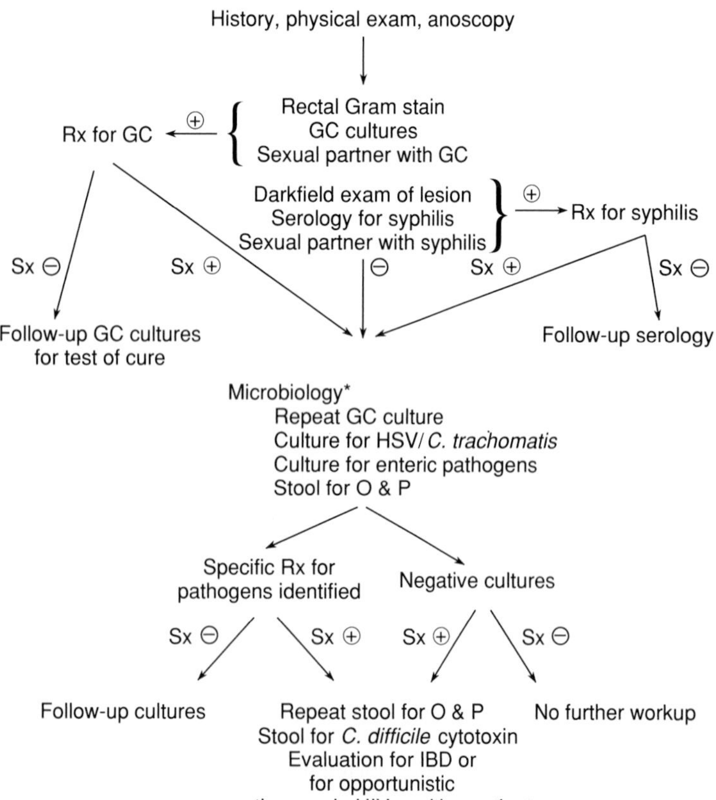


**Fig. 55-8.** Algorithm A: Evaluation and treatment of anorectal and/or intestinal symptoms in homosexual men. This algorithm emphasizes a full diagnostic evaluation and treatment for specific pathogens identified. Ideally, microbiological evaluation should be based on presenting symptoms and sigmoidoscopy findings. Rx = treatment, Sx = symptoms, GC = *N. gonorrhoeae*, O & P = ova and parasites, IBD = imflammatory bowel disease.

lesions and examined for cytomegalovirus, mycobacterium, intestinal protozoans, and other histologic features of infection or malabsorption.

Identification of any of the enteric pathogens should result in specific therapeutic regimens. Failure to respond to any specific antimicrobial regimens may represent drug resistance or, more commonly, the presence of additional pathogens, necessitating more comprehensive microbiologic and immunologic evaluation. If symptoms persist after eradication of infection or if no pathogens are identified, one must consider idiopathic inflammatory bowel disease, neoplastic lesions, or antibiotic resistant opportunistic infections, and institute diagnostic and therapeutic approaches to these diseases.

Because of the complexity of diagnosis and treatment of enteritis and proctitis in an STD population and the different levels of laboratory support at STD clinics and in office practice, we have outlined two algorithms. Algorithm A (Fig. 55-8) represents a systematic approach to diagnosis and treatment that is comprehensive and employs treatment only for identified pathogens. It basically represents a stepwise progression toward specific diagnosis and treatment of patient and exposed contacts. The major problem with this algorithm is that the microbiological evaluation is expensive and time-consuming, factors which may indirectly allow continued discomfort of the patient and transmission of the pathogen before final diagnosis and treatment.

Algorithm B (Fig. 55-9) is based on empirical therapy, which has the advantage of decreasing the cost of laboratory tests and provides immediate therapy to patients who may not return for follow-up visits. Such empirical therapy has recently been shown to produce more rapid resolution of the symptoms and signs of acute proctitis in homosexual men[212] than specific therapy. Empirical therapy has the disadvantage, however, of treating a patient before the diagnosis is known. In the study just cited, unrecognized HSV proctitis was the major reason for a failure of empiric therapy. The treatment may also convert the patient to an asymptomatic carrier, and most important, it interferes with the public health efforts to trace contacts of the patient who may harbor a specific pathogen. Such public health efforts would be possible only if a specific diagnosis were made in the patient.

Selection between these two methods of approach must be based on clinic and public health priorities, budget, laboratory support, and patient population. Alternative approaches will undoubtedly become preferable as more is learned about the etiology and epidemiology of enteritis, proctitis, and proctocolitis in homosexual men.

## PREVENTION

Because of the relatively high prevalence of asymptomatic anorectal carriage of pathogenic organisms in homosexual men, a concerted effort involving the clinician and public health authorities is necessary to control these infections. Examination and treatment of the sexual partners of homosexual men with STDs such as gonorrhea or syphilis is a conventional practice, yet similar management of the sexual contacts of homosexual men with enteric infection is not a routine procedure. Such an approach must be evaluated, not only for cases that come to medical attention through the STD clinic but also for those that are reported from other sources. We believe that when a specific pathogen is identified in a symptomatic homosexually active male patient, epidemiologic investigation of all sexual contacts within a time frame appropriate to the incubation period of the pathogen in question should be performed and appropriate diagnostic tests for the pathogen(s) involved should be obtained from the contacts. This is especially important for those agents which can be eliminated by treatment, such as gonorrhea, *C. trachomatis*, syphilis, and the enteric pathogens. Because of the intermittent nature of virus shedding, HSV cultures in sex partners of men with rectal HSV infection is frequently unrewarding. Most of the pathogens we have discussed should be reported to local public health workers, whose assistance in coordinating efforts to

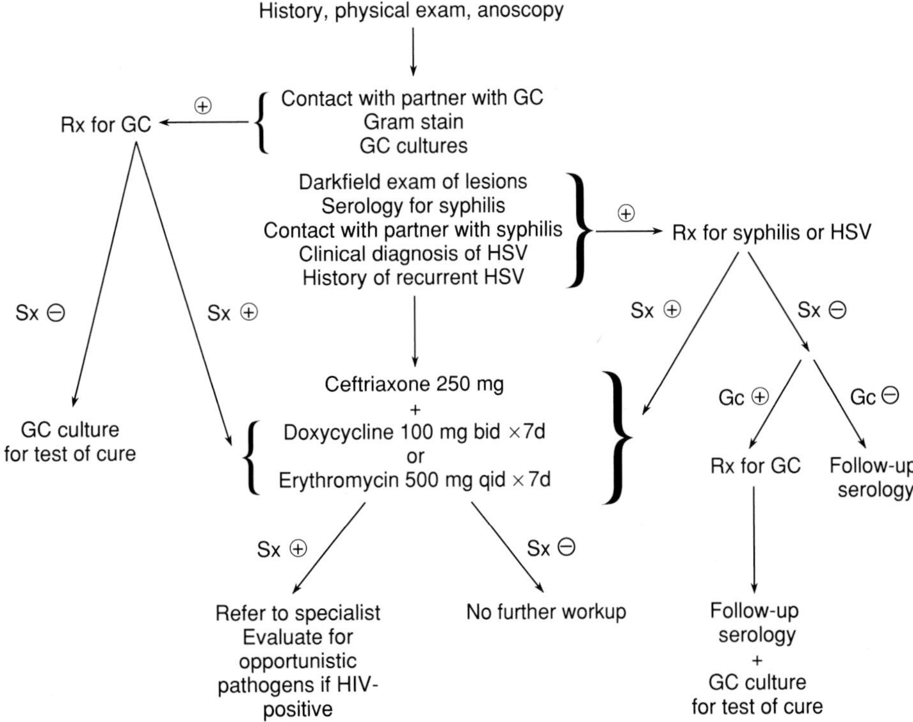


**Fig. 55-9.** Algorithm B: Evaluation and treatment of anorectal and/or intestinal symptoms in homosexual men. This algorithm emphasizes empirical therapy after an initial evaluation for gonorrhea and syphilis. Empirical therapy consists of intramuscular aqueous procaine penicillin, 4.8 million units, with 1.0 g of oral probenecid, followed by either doxycycline or erythromycin. If the patient remains symptomatic, he is referred for more complete evaluation. GC = *N. gonorrhoeae*, APPG = aqueous procaine penicillin G, Rx = treatment, Sx = symptoms.

identify and examine culture contacts is helpful. Household as well as sexual contacts should be screened for infection when investigating the spread of enteric pathogens. After the acute infection subsides or following therapy, repeat laboratory tests should be performed to detect possible development of a carrier state. Infected individuals should abstain from sexual practices which might spread infection, until repeat cultures are negative. Infected persons should also be educated regarding safe sex practices in the AIDS era.

Effective education of both physicians and patients about the different modes of transmission of these pathogens is necessary along with more reliable and available laboratory techniques for diagnosis of certain of them. Recognition of the importance of sexual transmission in the spread of these infections is a prerequisite to designing public health programs that will effectively prevent their spread in the community at large. In addition, recognition of the role that some of these pathogens (especially HSV and syphilis) may play in facilitating the spread of HIV infection provides added incentive for their prevention.[213,214]

## References


1 Dritz SK, Goldsmith RS: Sexually transmissible protozoal, bacterial and viral enteric infections. *Comp Ther* 6:34, 1980.
2 Dritz SK: Medical aspects of homosexuality, editorial. *N Engl J Med* 302:463, 1980.
3 Quinn TC et al: The etiology of anorectal infections in homosexual men. *Am J Med* 71:395, 1981.
4 Quinn TC et al: *Chlamydia trachomatis* proctitis. *N Engl J Med* 305:195, 1981.
5 Samarasinghe PL et al: Herpetic proctitis and sacral radiomyelopathy: A hazard for homosexual men. *Br Med J* 2:365, 1979.
6 Owen WF: Sexually transmitted diseases and traumatic problems in homosexual men. *Ann Intern Med* 92:805, 1980.
7 Gottlieb MS et al: The acquired immunodeficiency syndrome. *Ann Intern Med* 99:208, 1983.
8 Kotler DP et al: Enteropathy associated with the acquired immunodeficiency syndrome. *Ann Intern Med* 101:421, 1984.
9 Quinn TC: Gastrointestinal manifestations of human immunodeficiency virus, in *Current Topics in AIDS*, MS Gottlieb et al (eds). Chichester, Wiley, 1987, vol 1, p 155.
10 Gillin JS et al: Malabsorption and mucosal abnormalities of the small intestine in acquired immunodeficiency syndrome. *Ann Intern Med* 102:619, 1985.
11 Klein RS et al: Oral candidiasis in high-risk patients as the initial manifestation of the acquired immunodeficiency syndrome (AIDS). *N Engl J Med* 311:354, 1984.
12 Fauci AS et al: Acquired immunodeficiency syndrome: Epidemiologic, clinical, immunologic, and therapeutic consideration. *Ann Intern Med* 100:92, 1984.
13 Lozada F et al: Oral manifestations of tumors and opportunistic infection in AIDS: Findings in 53 homosexual men with Kaposi's sarcoma. *Oral Surg* 56:491, 1983.
14 Steinberg JJ et al: Small intestinal lymphoma in three patients with AIDS. *Am J Gastroenterol* 80:21, 1985.
15 Surawicz CM et al: Spectrum of rectal biopsy abnormalities in homosexual men with intestinal symptoms. *Gastroenterology* 91: 651, 1986.
16 Noble RC: *Sexually Transmitted Disease: Guide to Diagnosis and Therapy.* Garden City, NY Medical Examination Publishing Co, 1979, p 123.
17 Corey L, Holmes KK: Sexual transmission of hepatitis A in homosexual men: Incidence and mechanism. *N Engl J Med* 302:435, 1980.
18 Centers for Disease Control: Amebiasis associated with colonic irrigation: Colorado. *MMWR* 30:101, 1981.
19 Sohn N, Robilotti JG: The gay bowel syndrome: A review of colonic and rectal conditions in 200 male homosexuals. *Am J Gastroenterol* 67:478, 1977.
20 Dritz SK, Braff EH: Sexually transmitted typhoid fever. *N Engl J Med* 246:1359, 1977.
21 Bader M et al: Venereal transmission of shigellosis in Seattle-King county. *Sex Transm Dis* 4:89, 1977.
22 Drusin LM et al: Shigellosis: Another sexually transmitted disease? *Br J Vener Dis* 52:348, 1976.
23 William DC et al: High rates of enteric protozoal infections in selected homosexual men attending a venereal disease clinic. *Sex Transm Dis* 5:155, 1978.
24 Kean BH et al: Epidemic of amoebiasis and giardiasis in a biased population. *Br J Vener Dis* 55:375, 1979.
25 Felman YM, Ricciardi NB: Sexually transmitted enteric diseases. *Bull NY Acad Med* 55:533, 1979.
26 Bolling DR: Prevalence, goals and complications of heterosexual anal intercourse in a gynecologic population. *J Reprod Med* 19:120, 1977.
27 Quinn TC et al: The polymicrobial origin of intestinal infections in homosexual men. *N Engl J Med* 309:576, 1983.
28 Dritz SK et al: Patterns of sexually transmitted enteric diseases in a city. *Lancet* 2:3, 1977.
29 Schmerin MJ et al: Amebiasis: An increasing problem among homosexuals in New York City. *JAMA* 288:1386, 1977.
30 Meyers JD et al: Giardia lamblia infection in homosexual men. *Br J Vener Dis* 53:54, 1977.
31 Dworkin B et al: Gastrointestinal manifestation of the acquired immunodeficiency syndrome: A review of 22 cases. *Am J Gastroenterol* 80:774, 1985.
32 Cone LA et al: An update on the acquired immunodeficiency syndrome (AIDS). Associated disorders of the alimentary tract. *Dis Colon Rectum* 29:60, 1986.
33 Goedert JJ et al: Determinants of retrovirus HTLV-III and immunodeficiency conditions in homosexual men. *Lancet* ii:711, 1985.
34 Cooper DA et al: Acute AIDS retrovirus infection. *Lancet* i:537, 1985.
35 Ho DD et al: Primary human T-lymphotropic virus type III infection. *Ann Intern Med* 103:880, 1985.
36 Clumeck N et al: Acquired immune deficiency syndrome in African patients. *N Engl J Med* 310:429, 1984.
37 Pape JW et al: Characteristics of the acquired immune deficiency syndrome in Haitians. *N Engl J Med* 309:935, 1983.
38 Malebranche R et al: Acquired immunodeficiency syndrome with severe gastrointestinal manifestations in Haiti. *Lancet* ii:873, 1985.
39 Colebunders R et al: Persistent diarrhea, strongly associated with HIV infection in Kinshasa, Zaire. *Am J Gastroenterol* 82:859, 1987.
40 Smith PD et al: Intestinal infections in patients with the acquired immunodeficiency syndrome (AIDS). *Ann Intern Med* 108:328, 1988.
41 Laughon BE et al: Prevalence of enteric pathogens in homosexual men with and without acquired immunodeficiency syndrome. *Gastroenterology* 94:984, 1988.
42 Welch K et al: Autopsy findings in the acquired immunodeficiency syndrome. *JAMA* 252:1152, 1984.
43 Klein EJ et al: Anorectal gonococcal infection. *Ann Intern Med* 86:340, 1977.
44 Pariser H, Marino AF: Gonorrhea: Frequently unrecognized reservoirs. *South Med J* 63:198, 1970.
45 Bhattacharyya MN, Jephcott AE: Diagnosis of gonorrhea in women. *Br J Vener Dis* 50:109, 1974.
46 Heimans AL: Culture of gonococci from the rectum on Thayer and Martin's selective medium. *Dermatologica* 133:314, 1966.
47 Scott J, Stone AH: Some observations on the diagnosis of rectal gonorrhea in both sexes using a selective culture medium. *Br J Vener Dis* 42:103, 1966.
48 Judson FN et al: Screening for gonorrhea and syphilis in the gay baths: Denver, Colorado. *Am J Public Health* 67:740, 1977.
49 Merino HI, Richards JB: An innovative program of venereal disease case-finding, treatment and education. *Sex Transm Dis* 4:50, 1977.

50 British Cooperative Clinical Group: Homosexuality and venereal disease in the United Kingdom. *Br J Vener Dis* 49:329, 1973.
51 Owen RL, Hill JL: Rectal and pharyngeal gonorrhea in homosexual men. *JAMA* 220:1315, 1972.
52 McMillan A, Young H: Gonorrhea in the homosexual men. *Sex Transm Dis* 5:146, 1978.
53 Weisner PJ et al: Gonococcal anorectal infection, abstract. Eleventh Interscience Conference on Antimicrobial Agents and Chemotherapy, 1971.
54 Handsfield HH et al: Correlation of auxotype and penicillin susceptibility of *Neisseria gonorrhoeae* with sexual preference and clinical manifestations of gonorrhea. *Sex Transm Dis* 7:1, 1980.
55 Harkness AH: The pathology of gonorrhea. *Br J Vener Dis* 24:132, 1948.
56 Kilpatrick ZM: Gonorrheal proctitis. *N Engl J Med* 287:967, 1972.
57 Babb RR: Acute gonorrheal proctitis. *Am J Gastoenterol* 61:143, 1974.
58 Catterall RR: Anorectal gonorrhoea. *Proc R Soc Med* 55:871, 1962.
59 William DC et al: The utility of anoscopy in the rapid diagnosis of symptomatic anorectal gonorrhea in men. *Sex Transm Dis* 8:16, 1980.
60 Deheragoda P: Diagnosis of rectal gonorrhea by blind anorectal swabs compared with direct vision swabs taken via a proctoscope. *Br J Vener Dis* 53:311, 1977.
61 Seth A: Use of trimethoprim to prevent overgrowth by proteus in the cultivation of *Neisseria gonorrhoeae*. *Br J Vener Dis* 46:201, 1970.
62 Centers for Disease Control: Gonorrhea: CDC recommended treatment schedules, 1979. *MMWR* 28:13, 1979.
63 Karney WW et al: Spectinomycin versus tetracycline for the treatment of gonorrhea. *N Engl J Med* 296:889, 1977.
64 Washington AE et al: Treatment of sexually transmitted bacterial and protozoal enteric infections. *Rev Infect Dis* 4(suppl):S864, 1982.
65 Judson FN et al: Comparative study of ceftriaxone and spectinomycin for treatment of pharyngeal and anorectal gonorrhea. *JAMA* 253:1417, 1985.
66 Lebedeff DA, Hochman EB: Rectal gonorrhea in men: Diagnosis and treatment. *Ann Intern Med* 92:463, 1980.
67 Morse SA et al: Gonococcal membranes from homosexual men have outer membranes with reduced permeability to hydrophobic molecules. *Infect Immun* 37:432, 1982.
68 Waugh MA: Anorectal *Herpesvirus hominis* infection in man. *J Am Vener Dis Assoc* 3:68, 1976.
69 Jacobs E: Anal infections caused by herpes simplex virus. *Dis Colon Rectum* 19:151, 1976.
70 Goldmeier D: Proctitis and herpes simplex virus in homosexual men. *Br J Vener Dis* 56:111, 1980.
71 Hutfield DC: History of herpes genitalis. *Br J Vener Dis* 42:263, 1966.
72 Goodell SE et al: Herpes simplex virus proctitis in homosexual men: Clinical, sigmoidoscopic and histopathologic features. *N Engl J Med* 308:868, 1983.
73 Goldmeier D et al: Urinary retention and intestinal obstruction associated with ano-rectal herpes simplex virus infection. *Br Med J* 1:425, 1975.
74 Curry JP et al: Proctitis associated with herpesvirus hominis type 2 infection. *Can Med Assoc J* 119:485, 1978.
75 Rompalo AM et al: Oral acyclovir vs. placebo for treatment of herpes simplex virus proctitis in homosexual men. *Clin Res* 33:58A, 1985.
76 Siegal FP et al: Severe acquired immunodeficiency in male homosexuals, manifested by chronic perianal ulcerative herpes simplex lesions. *N Engl J Med* 305:1439, 1981.
77 Straus SE et al: Oral acyclovir to suppress recurring herpes simplex virus infections in immunodeficient patients. *Ann Intern Med* 100:522, 1984.
78 Carne CA et al: Prevalence of antibodies to human immunodeficiency virus, gonorrhoea rates, and changes sexual behavior in homosexual men in London. *Lancet* i:656, 1987.
79 Blount JH, Holmes KK: Epidemiology of syphilis and the nonvenereal treponematoses, in *The Biology of Parasitic Spirochetes*, RC Johnson (ed). New York, Academic, 1976, p 157.
80 Martin EG, Kallet HI: Primary syphilis of the anorectal region. *JAMA* 84:1556, 1925.
81 Downing JG: Incidence of extragenital chancres. *Arch Dermatol Syph* 39:150, 1939.
82 Wile UJ, Holman HH: A survey of sixty-eight cases of extragenital chancres. *Am J Syph* 25:58, 1941.
83 Jones AJ, Janis L: Primary syphilis of the rectum and gonorrhea of the anus. *Am J Syph* 28:453, 1944.
84 Smith D: Infectious syphilis of the anal canal. *Dis Colon Rectum* 6:7, 1963.
85 Smith D: Infectious syphilis of the rectum: Report of a case. *Dis Colon Rectum* 8:57, 1965.
86 Gluckman JB et al: Primary syphilis of rectum. *NY State J Med* 74:2210, 1974.
87 Samenius B: Primary syphilis of the anorectal region. *Dis Colon Rectum* 11:462, 1968.
88 Marino AWM: Proctologic lesions observed in male homosexuals. *Dis Colon Rectum* 7:121, 1964.
89 Wells BT et al: Rectal chancre: Report of a case. *AMA Arch Dermatol* 79:719, 1959.
90 Lieberman W: Syphilis of the rectum. *Rev Gastroenterol* 18:67, 1951.
91 Tar JD, Lugar RR: Early infectious syphilis: Male homosexual relations as a mode of spread. *Calif Med* 93:35, 1960.
92 Huburchak DR, Davidson H: Anorectal lesions and syphilitic hepatitis. *West J Med* 128:64, 1978.
93 Nazemi MM et al: Syphilitic proctitis in a homosexual. *JAMA* 231:389, 1975.
94 Akdamar K et al: Syphilitic proctitis. *Am J Dig Dis* 22:701, 1977.
95 Mitchell RD et al: Secretory and histologic changes after treatment of gastric syphilis. *Gastroenterology* 43:689, 1962.
96 Sachar DB et al: Erosive syphilitic gastritis: Darkfield and immunofluorescent diagnosis from biopsy specimen. *Ann Intern Med* 80:512, 1974.
97 Smibert RM: The spirochetes, in *Bergey's Manual of Determinative Bacteriology*, 8th ed, RE Buchanan, NE Gibbons (eds). Baltimore, Williams & Wilkins, 1974, p 167.
98 Yobs AR et al: Fluorescent antibody technique in early syphilis. *Arch Pathol* 77:220, 1967.
99 Jue R et al: Comparison of fluorescent and conventional darkfield methods for the detection of *Treponema pallidum* in syphilitic lesions. *Am J Clin Pathol* 47:809, 1967.
100 Johnson WC: Venereal diseases and treponemal infections, in *Dermal Pathology*, JH Graham et al (eds). New York, Harper & Row, 1972, p 371.
101 Quinn TC et al: Rectal mass caused by *Treponema pallidum:* Confirmation by immunofluorescent staining. *Gastroenterology* 82:135, 1982.
102 Drusin LM et al: The role of surgery in primary syphilis of the anus. *Ann Surg* 185:65, 1976.
103 Berry CD et al: Neurologic relapse after benzathine penicillin therapy for secondary syphilis in a patient with HIV infection. *N Engl J Med* 316:1587, 1987.
104 Tramont EC: Syphilis in the AIDS era (editorial). *N Engl J Med* 316:1600, 1987.
105 Dunlop EMC et al: Chlamydia infections: Incidence in nonspecific urethritis. *Br J Vener Dis* 48:425, 1972.
106 Goldmeier D, Darougar S: Isolations of *Chlamydia trachomatis* from throat and rectum of homosexual men. *Br J Vener Dis* 53:184, 1977.
107 Stamm WE et al: Chlamydia trachomatis proctitis in homosexual men and heterosexual women, in *Chlamydia Infections*, PA Mårdh, KK Holmes, DJ Oriel, P Piot, J Schacter (eds). Amsterdam, Elsevier Biomedical, 1982, p 111.
108 Jones RB et al: Chlamydia trachomatis from the pharynx and rectum of heterosexual patients at risk for genital infection. *Ann Intern Med* 102:757, 1985.

109 Bensaude R, Lambling A: Discussion on the aetiology and treatment of fibrous stricture of the rectum (including lymphogranuloma inguinale). *Proc R Soc Med* 29:1441, 1936.
110 Grace AW: Lymphogranuloma venereum. *Bull NY Acad Med* 17: 627, 1941.
111 Greaves AB: The frequency of lymphogranuloma venereum in persons with perirectal abscesses, fistula-in-ano, or both. *Bull WHO* 29:797, 1963.
112 Coutts WE et al: Digestive tract infection by the virus of lymphogranuloma inguinale. *Am J Dig Dis* 7:287, 1940.
113 Miles RPM: Rectal lymphogranuloma venereum. *Br J Surg* 45:180, 1957.
114 Levin I et al: Lymphogranuloma venereum: Rectal stricture and carcinoma. *Dis Colon Rectum* 7:129, 1964.
115 Crohn BB, Yarnis H: *Regional Ileitis*. New York, Grune & Stratton, 1958.
116 Rodaniche EC et al: The relationship between lymphogranuloma venereum and regional enteritis: An etiologic study of 4 cases with negative results. *Gastroenterology* 1:687, 1943.
117 Tomenius E et al: Positive Frei tests in 7 cases of morbus Crohn (regional ileitis). *Gastroenterologica* 99:369, 1963.
118 Schuller JL et al: Antibodies against chlamydia of lymphogranuloma-venereum type in Crohn's disease. *Lancet* 1:19, 1979.
119 Mårdh P-A et al: Lack of evidence for an association between infections with *C. trachomatis* and Crohn's disease, as indicated by micro-immunofluorescence antibody tests. *Acta Pathol Microbiol Scand [B]* 88:57, 1980.
120 Taylor-Robinson D et al: Low frequency of chlamydial antibodies in patients with Crohn's disease and ulcerative colitis. *Lancet* 1:1162, 1979.
121 Swarbrick ET et al: Chlamydia, cytomegalovirus and yersina in inflammatory bowel disease. *Lancet* 2:11, 1979.
122 Levine JS et al: Chronic proctitis in male homosexuals due to lymphogranuloma venereum. *Gastroenterology* 79:563, 1980.
123 Quinn TC et al: Screening for Chlamydia trachomatis infection in an inner-city population: A comparison of diagnostic methods. *J Infect Dis* 152:419, 1984.
124 Rompalo AM et al: Rapid diagnosis of Chlamydia trachomatis rectal infection by direct immunofluorescence staining. *J Infect Dis* 155: 1075, 1987.
125 Wang SP et al: A simplified method for immunological typing of trachoma-inclusion conjunctivitis-lymphogranuloma venereum organism. *Infect Immun* 7:356, 1973.
126 Wang SP et al: Simplified microimmunofluorescence tests with trachoma-lymphogranuloma venereum (*Chlamydia trachomatis*) antigens for use as a screening test for antibody. *J Clin Microbiol* 1:250, 1975.
127 Schachter J: Confirmatory serodiagnosis of lymphogranuloma venereum proctitis may yield false positive results due to other chlamydia infections of the rectum. *Sex Transm Dis* 8:26, 1981.
128 Dritz SK, Back AF: *Shigella* enteritis venerally transmitted, letter. *N Engl J Med* 291:1194, 1974.
129 Carey PB, Wright EP: *Campylobacter jejuni* in a male homosexual. *Br J Vener Dis* 55:381, 1979.
130 Quinn TC et al: Campylobacter proctitis in a homosexual male. *Ann Intern Med* 93:458, 1980.
131 William DC et al: Sexual transmitted enteric pathogens in male homosexual population. *NY State J Med* 77:2050, 1977.
132 Blaser MJ et al: Campylobacter enteritis: Clinical and epidemiologic features. *Ann Intern Med* 91:179, 1979.
133 Blaser MJ et al: Reservoirs for human campylobacteriosis. *J Infect Dis* 141:665, 1980.
134 Hood M, Todd JM: *Vibrio fetus:* A cause of human abortion. *Am J Obstet Gynecol* 83:506, 1960.
135 Simmers PD, Tabaqchali S: Campylobacter species in male homosexuals. *Br J Vener Dis* 55:66, 1979.
136 Laughon BE et al: Recovery of Campylobacter species from homosexual men. *J Infect Dis* 158:464, 1988.
137 Pasternak J et al: Bacteremia caused by Campylobacter-like organism in two male homosexuals. *Ann Intern Med* 101:339, 1984.
138 Fennell CL et al: Characterization of campylobacter-like organisms isolated from homosexual men. *J Infect Dis* 149S:58, 1984.
139 Totten PA et al: Campylobacter cinaedi (sp. nov.) and Campylobacter fennelliae (sp. nov.): Two new Campylobacter species associated with enteric disease in homosexual men. *J Infect Dis* 151:131, 1985.
140 Quinn TC et al: Infections with Campylobacter jejuni and Campylobacter-like organisms in homosexual men. *Ann Intern Med* 101: 187, 1984.
141 Blaser MJ et al: Acute colitis caused by *Campylobacter fetus* ss. *jejuni. Gastroenterology* 78:448, 1980.
142 Lambert ME et al: Campylobacter colitis. *Br Med J* 1:857, 1979.
143 Michalak DM et al: *Campylobacter fetus* ssp. *jejuni:* A cause of massive lower gastrointestinal hemorrhage. *Gastroenterology* 79: 742, 1980.
144 Smith PD et al: Salmonella typhimurium enteritis and bacteremia in the acquired immunodeficiency syndrome. *Ann Intern Med* 102:207, 1985.
145 Thomas JA, Antony AJ: Amoebiasis of the penis. *Br J Urol* 48:269, 1976.
146 Cooke RA: Cutaneous amoebiasis involving the anogenital region. *J Med Assoc Thai* 56:354, 1973.
147 Cohen C: Three cases of amoebiasis of the cervix uteri. *J Obstet Gynaecol Br Commonw* 80:476, 1973.
148 Abrahm PM: Snakes in the grass or, the worm turns on. *JAMA* 221:917, 1972.
149 Shookhoff HB: Parasite transmission. *JAMA* 222:1310, 1972.
150 Lynch V de P: Parasite transmission. *JAMA* 222:1309, 1972.
151 Waugh MA: Threadworm infestation in homosexuals. *Trans St Johns Hosp Dermatol Soc* 58:224, 1972.
152 Most H: Manhattan: A "tropic isle"? *Am J Trop Med Hyg* 17:333, 1968.
153 Current WL et al: Human cryptosporidiosis in immunocompetent and immunodeficient persons: Studies of an outbreak and experimental transmission. *N Engl J Med* 308:1252, 1983.
154 Faust EC et al: *Craig and Faust's Clinical Parasitology,* 8th ed. Philadelphia, Lea & Febiger, 1970, p 138.
155 Keyston JS et al: Intestinal parasitic infections in homosexual men: Prevalence, symptoms, and factors in transmission. *Can Med Assoc J* 123:512, 1980.
156 Sargeaunt PG et al: Entamoeba histolytica in male homosexuals. *Br J Vener Dis* 59:193, 1983.
157 Chin ATL, Gerken A: Carriage of intestinal protozoal cysts in homosexuals. *Br J Vener Dis* 60:193, 1984.
158 Pittman FE et al: Studies of human amebiasis: I. Clinical and laboratory findings in eight cases of acute amebic colitis. *Gastroenterology* 65:581, 1973.
159 Pittman FE et al: Studies on human amebiasis: II. Light and electron-microscopic observations of colonic mucosa and exudate in acute amebic colitis. *Gastroenterology* 65:588, 1973.
160 Goldmeier D et al: Is Entamoeba histolytica in homosexual men a pathogen? *Lancet* i:641, 1986.
161 Allason-Jones E et al: Entamoeba histolytica as a commensal intestinal parasite in homosexual men. *N Engl J Med* 315:353, 1986.
162 Sorvillo FJ et al: Amebic infections in asymptomatic homosexual men. Lack of evidence of invasive disease. *Public Health Briefs* 76: 1137, 1986.
163 Patterson M et al: Serologic testing for amoebiasis. *Gastroenterology* 78:136, 1980.
164 Kean BH: The treatment of amebiasis: A recurrent agony. *JAMA* 235:501, 1976.
165 Krogstad DJ et al: Current concepts in parasitology: Amebiasis. *N Engl J Med* 298:262, 1978.
166 Drugs for parasitic infections, editorial. *The Medical Letter* 21:105, 1979.
167 Schmerin MJ et al: Giardiasis: Association with homosexuality. *Ann Intern Med* 88:801, 1978.
168 Beal CB et al: A technique for sampling duodenal contents: Demonstration of upper small bowel pathogens. *Am J Trop Med Hyg* 19:349, 1970.

169 Wolfe MS: Current concepts in parasitology: Giardiasis. *N Engl J Med* 298:319, 1978.

170 Bakshi JS et al: How does tinidazole compare with metronidazole? *Drugs* 15(suppl 1):33, 1978.

171 McMillan A: Threadworms in homosexual males. *Br Med J* 1:367, 1978.

172 Centers for Disease Control: Cryptosporidiosis: Assessment of chemotherapy of males with AIDS. *MMWR* 31:589, 1982.

173 Tzipori S et al: An outbreak of calf diarrhea attributed to cryptosporidial infection. *Vet Res* 107:579, 1980.

174 Nime FA et al: Acute enterocolitis in a human being infected with the protozoan *Cryptosporidium*. *Gastroenterology* 70:592, 1976.

175 Weinstein L et al: Intestinal cryptosporidiosis complicated by disseminated cytomegalovirus infection. *Gastroenterology* 81:584, 1981.

176 Ma P, Soave R: Three-step stool examination for cryptosporidiosis in ten homosexual men with protracted watery diarrhea. *J Infect Dis* 147:824, 1983.

177 Campbell PN, Current WL: Demonstration of serum antibodies to *Cryptosporidium* sp. in normal and immunodeficient humans with confirmed infections. *J Clin Microbiol* 18:165, 1983.

178 Portnoy D et al: Treatment of intestinal cryptosporidiosis with spiramycin. *Ann Intern Med* 101:202, 1984.

179 Furio MM, Wordell CJ: Treatment of infectious complications of acquired immunodeficiency syndrome. *Clin Pharmacol* 4:539, 1985.

180 Veldhuyzenvan Van Zanten SJO et al: Amprolium for coccidiosis in AIDS. *Lancet* ii:345, 1984.

181 Whiteside ME et al: Enteric coccidiosis among patients with the acquired immunodeficiency syndrome. *Am J Trop Med Hyg* 33: 1065, 1984.

182 Dobbins WO, Weinstein WM: Electron microscopy of the intestine and rectum in acquired immunodeficiency syndrome. *Gastroenterology* 88:738, 1985.

183 Chapel TA et al: *Neisseria meningitidis* in the anal canal of homosexual men. *J Infect Dis* 136:810, 1977.

184 Judson FN et al: Anogenital infection with *Neisseria meningitidis* in homosexual men. *J Infect Dis* 137:458, 1978.

185 Carlson BL et al: Isolation of *Neisseria meningitidis* from anogenital specimens from homosexual men. *Sex Transm Dis* 7:71, 1980.

186 Howely PM: Papovaviruses: Search for evidence of possible association with cancer, in *Viruses Associated with Human Cancer,* LA Phillips (ed). New York, Marcel Dekker, 1983, p 256.

187 Daling JR et al: Correlates of homosexual behavior and incidence of anal cancer. *JAMA* 247:1988, 1982.

188 Stron RL, Gruminger RP: AIDS with Mycobacterium avium-intracellulare lesions resembling those of Whipple's disease. *N Engl J Med* 309:1323, 1983.

189 Gillin JS et al: Disseminated Mycobacterium avium-intracellulare infection in acquired immunodeficiency syndrome mimicking Whipple's disease. *Gastroenterology* 85:1187, 1983.

190 Knapp AB et al: Widespread cytomegalovirus gastroenterocolitis in a patient with AIDS. *Gastroenterology* 85:1399, 1983.

191 Gertler SL et al: Gastrointestinal cytomegalovirus infection in a homosexual man with severe acquired immunodeficiency syndrome. *Gastroenterology* 85:1403, 1983.

192 Meiselman MS et al: Cytomegalovirus colitis: Report of the clinical, endoscopic, and pathologic findings in two patients with the acquired immune deficiency syndrome. *Gastroenterology* 88:171, 1985.

193 Frank D, Raicht FF: Intestinal perforation associated with cytomegalovirus infection in patients with acquired immune deficiency syndrome. *Am J Gastroenterol* 79:201, 1984.

194 Kram HB et al: Spontaneous colonic perforation secondary to cytomegalovirus in a patient with acquired immune deficiency syndrome. *Crit Care Med* 12:469, 1984.

195 Balthazar EJ et al: Cytomegalovirus colitis in AIDS: Radiographic findings in 11 patients. *Radiology* 155:585, 1985.

196 Emanuel D et al: Rapid immunodiagnosis of cytomegalovirus pneumonia by bronchoalveolar lavage using human and murine monoclonal antibodies. *Ann Intern Med* 104:476, 1986.

197 Bach MC et al: 9-(1,3-dihydroxy-2-propoxymethyl) guanine for cytomegalovirus infection in patients with the acquired immunodeficiency syndrome. *Ann Intern Med* 103:318, 1985.

198 Masur H et al: Effect of 9-(1,3-dihydroxy-2-propoxymethyl) guanine on serious cytomegalovirus disease in eight immunosuppressed homosexual men. *Ann Intern Med* 104:41, 1986.

199 Collaborative DHPG Treatment Study Group: Treatment of serious cytomegalovirus infections with 9-(1,3 dihydroxy-2-propoxymethyl) guanine in patients with AIDS and other immunodeficiencies. *N Engl J Med* 314:801, 1986.

200 Blumberg RS et al: Cytomegalovirus and cryptosporidium associated acalculous gangrenous cholecystitis. *Am J Med* 76:1118, 1984.

201 Kavin H et al: Acalculous cholecystitic and cytomegalovirus infection in acquired immunodeficiency syndrome. *Ann Intern Med* 104:53, 1986.

202 Laughon BD, Quinn TC: Intestinal spirochetes, in *Enteric Infections,* MGJ Farthing, GT Keusch (eds). London, Chapman and Hall, 1989 (in press).

203 McMillian A, Lee FD: Sigmoidoscopic and microscopic appearance of the rectal mucosa in homosexual men. *Gut* 222:1035, 1981.

204 Tavitian A et al: Oral candidiasis as a marker for esophageal candidiasis in the acquired immunodeficiency syndrome. *Ann Intern Med* 104:54, 1986.

205 Marnell M: Donovanosis of the anus in the male: An epidemiologic consideration. *Br J Vener Dis* 34:213, 1955.

206 Goldberg J, Bernstein R: Studies on granuloma inguinale: VI. Two cases of perianal granuloma inguinale in male homosexuals. *Br J Vener Dis* 40:137, 1964.

207 Gould WM, Clark EE: Granuloma inguinale. *Cal Med* 104:392, 1966.

208 Marmar JL: The management of resistant chancroid in Vietnam. *J Urol* 107:807, 1972.

209 Kerber RE et al: Treatment of chancroid. *Arch Dermatol* 100:604, 1969.

210 Sohn N et al: Social injuries of the rectum. *Am J Surg* 134:611, 1977.

211 Barone JE et al: Perforations and foreign bodies of the rectum: Report of 28 cases. *Ann Surg* 184:601, 1977.

212 Rompalo AM et al: Empirical therapy for the management of acute proctitis in homosexual men. *JAMA* 260:348, 1988.

213 Holmberg SD et al: Prior herpes simplex virus type 2 infection as a risk factor for HIV infection. *JAMA* 259:1048, 1988.

214 Stamm WE et al: The association between genital ulcer disease and acquisition of HIV infection in homosexual men. *JAMA* 260:1429, 1988.

# Chapter 56
# AIDS-related malignancies

Paul A. Volberding

It is not unexpected that a broad range of malignancies has been seen in the setting of AIDS, considering the large population of HIV-infected individuals in the United States. Malignancies reported in HIV-infected individuals include squamous cell carcinomas of various sites, malignant melanoma, testicular cancers of all histologies, Hodgkin's disease, and primary hepatocellular carcinoma.[1] With the possible exception of Hodgkin's disease, minimal evidence exists that these cancers are caused by HIV-induced immune deficiency. However, a direct relationship with AIDS has been established for Kaposi's sarcoma (KS), primary central nervous system non-Hodgkin's lymphomas, and high-grade peripheral B-cell lymphomas. These malignancies in the presence of HIV infection are, in fact, diagnostic of AIDS.[2]

Although the etiology of these AIDS-associated tumors cannot be clearly defined, deficient immune surveillance, combined with viral reactivation and oncogenesis, is believed to play a significant role in their development. This chapter discusses the spectrum of HIV-related neoplasms, stressing their practical management from diagnosis to therapy.

## KAPOSI'S SARCOMA

### KS IN NON-AIDS POPULATIONS

A tumor first recognized and described by Moritz Kaposi[3] in the late 1800s, KS was rare in the United States before 1981, particularly in healthy young adults. When it did occur, it generally afflicted elderly men,[4] most commonly affecting the feet and lower extremities. This variant, now often referred to as classic KS, had an indolent course and was not accompanied by immunodeficiency. In the 1960s, KS was discovered to be a common malignancy in Central Africa, where some of its variants, although also present without underlying immune deficiency, were seen to be aggressive and infiltrating.

In the early 1970s, KS was reported to be associated with iatrogenic immunosuppression, generally in the setting of organ transplantation. It has been reported most commonly in renal allograft recipients[5] but also in patients with chronic immunosuppression resulting from treatment of various autoimmune diseases with corticosteroids.

## KAPOSI'S SARCOMA IN AIDS

### EPIDEMIOLOGY

KS, the first tumor to be linked with AIDS, occurs much more frequently in homosexual men than in heterosexual AIDS patients.[6,7] Because a very high incidence of coinfection with cytomegalovirus (CMV) occurs in homosexual men,[8] a cofactor relationship with this virus has been proposed. However, studies of cytomegalovirus in AIDS patients have not established a conclusive relationship to KS. Several epidemiologic and laboratory studies have investigated the possibility that recreational drugs, particularly inhaled nitrites or "poppers" used by at-risk populations, might be carcinogenic or immunosuppressive. Some studies have shown more frequent use of these drugs by AIDS patients diagnosed with KS,[9] but a conclusive cofactor relationship has not been demonstrated.

### HISTOPATHOLOGY

The histopathology of KS is characterized by a proliferation of abnormal vascular structures.[10] Three histologic variants have been reported: a spindle cell form, an anaplastic type, and a mixed cell form. In both the anaplastic and spindle cell variants, one cell population predominates. The spindle cell variant consists of bland, uniformly sized spindle cells[11] with rare mitoses, whereas the anaplastic form is characterized by disordered, malignant-appearing cells with frequent mitoses. Both these variants are uncommon in AIDS-related KS. The mixed cellular variant is by far the most common of the three seen in AIDS patients.[11] It is recognized by three features: (1) a proliferation within the tumor of vascular structures and slits, often lined by abnormally large, malignant-appearing endothelial cells; (2) a proliferation of surrounding spindle shaped cells; and (3) an extravasation of erythrocytes.

The cell of origin is controversial. Most agree that it is endothelial, but disagreement exists as to whether factor VIII antigen is expressed.[12,13]

### NATURAL HISTORY

The natural history of AIDS-related KS is variable and incompletely understood. Although occasional patients have had spontaneous remissions or long intervals without disease progression, others have persistent and often rapid progression. Patients with limited KS and no symptoms suggesting other underlying infectious disease (e.g., fevers, night sweats, weight loss) have a reasonably good 3-year survival expectancy. Usually, however, in the setting of HIV infection, KS patients have a rapid progression of their malignant disease, often with visceral involvement.

Predicting the clinical course for the newly diagnosed KS patient is difficult, but several factors are associated with disease progression and shorter survival:[14,15] previous opportunistic infections, night sweats, fever, weight loss, anemia, elevated erythrocyte sedimentation rate, low helper to suppressor T-cell ratio, an absolute helper cell count less than 100 cells/mm$^3$, and gastrointestinal or pulmonary KS. The best prognosis is seen in those patients who have only a few small nodular lesions, no previous serious infection, and no recent weight loss, fevers, or night sweats. Neither the site of cutaneous involvement nor the presence or absence of lymph node involvement appears to be particularly important prognostically. Visceral KS, however, does imply a poor prognosis.

### CLINICAL MANIFESTATIONS

#### Cutaneous KS

Most patients with AIDS-related KS have subcutaneous, painless, palpable, nonpruritic tumor nodules[15–18] or lymphatic involvement. Initial lesions on the face or in the oral cavity are typical, although they may begin in any site. Frequently, KS involves the plantar surface of the foot, but rarely the palms. The lesions are pigmented red to blue and are nonblanching; in deeper lesions the pigmentation may not be apparent. Exophytic tumor masses rarely occur in AIDS-related KS, but when they do, they can necrose, bleed, and when present on the feet or lower extremities can be moderately to severely painful. With advanced disease, plaques of coalesced lesions are common, especially over the medial aspect of the thigh. Lesions tend to be circular, but those on the back or around the neck can be linear, apparently following cutaneous lymphatic drainage. Other notable sites of disease include the tip of the nose, the region behind the ear, the conjunctiva, and the penis.

### Tumor plaques of KS

Often seen on the sole of the foot and the medial aspect of the thigh, tumor plaques are uncommon in other parts of the body. They are less common than discrete nodules but are seen more often than exophytic masses. Involvement of the superficial skin is common, but fixation to deeper structures and infiltration of underlying bone is rare. Plaques of tumor often cause chronic moderate pain.

### Lymphedema

This common sequela of AIDS-related KS[19] is not unexpected, since KS seems to arise from lymphatic endothelium. Lymphedema is often striking and is most typically seen in the face, where it causes disfiguration and can result in physical obstruction of vision and hearing. The lower extremities are also commonly affected, with associated scrotal and penile edema which can be striking and rapidly progressive. In both the face and the lower extremities lymphedema can occur out of proportion to the extent of cutaneous tumors, reflecting an obliteration of small cutaneous lymphatics.

## DIAGNOSIS

KS lesions are readily recognized. Most lesions are initially nodular and are pigmented red or purple, even early in the disease process. They are usually palpable, painless, and nonpruritic. Occasionally, especially in cases of rapidly progressing disease, surrounding ecchymosis is apparent. The differential diagnosis of KS includes other pigmented processes such as dermatofibromas, granuloma annulare, insect bite reactions, pyogenic granuloma, and stasis dermatitis.[20] AIDS-related KS is rare in populations other than homosexual men for as yet unexplained reasons. However, irrespective of risk group or clinical appearance, biopsy must be performed to establish a histologic diagnosis.

### Establishing a diagnosis

The biopsy can be performed at any site, but skin is most convenient. A small punch biopsy (2 to 4 mm) is usually adequate, but it is helpful to include unaffected adjacent skin in the punch specimen. Enlarged peripheral lymph nodes can also be biopsied, and even aspiration cytology has been used to diagnose KS.

In patients with a preexisting diagnosis of AIDS, typical appearing KS lesions may not require confirmation by biopsy. If a biopsy shows KS in a patient without previously established AIDS, an HIV serologic test, if positive, establishes the case as AIDS-related. If the serologic test is negative, the KS is not considered to be AIDS-related, even if the patient is a member of an AIDS risk group.

In the initial evaluation of a KS patient, tumor extent should be determined by a complete skin examination. The oral cavity should also be carefully examined. As many as one-third of patients with AIDS-related KS have oral involvement at the time of diagnosis.[21,22] KS lesions in the oral cavity commonly affect the mucosa of the hard and soft palate and, less commonly, the posterior pharyngeal wall or the tonsillar pillars.

Visceral involvement is common on AIDS/KS. The gastrointestinal tract is affected in as many as 50 percent of patients, even early in the course of the disease.[23–25] Thus, if unexplained gastrointestinal or pulmonary symptoms are present, endoscopy should be performed. Biopsies are diagnostic in only 23 percent of cases of gastrointestinal KS because the tumors are generally submucosal. Similarly, bronchoscopy should be performed if pulmonary involvement is suspected. Pulmonary KS is diagnosed by excluding the pulmonary opportunistic infections and by documenting the appearance of endobronchial KS lesions, appearing as small vascular nodules lining the tracheobronchial tree. Biopsy is usually not performed because of concerns about the possible risk of hemorrhage.

In all KS patients, associated symptoms such as fevers, night sweats, and weight loss should be recorded, and the patient's immunologic status, including T4 cell enumeration, assessed.

## THERAPY

The choice of therapy for AIDS/KS is problematic for several reasons. First, its natural history is highly variable and thus unpredictable. Second, there is no therapeutic agent to reverse the immune defect underlying the disease. Third, conventional and often used cytotoxic chemotherapy is controversial because it may further impair cellular immunity and thus increase the risk of infection. "Immunologic stimulators" have been largely ineffective and have the theoretic risk of further stimulating viral replication. Even effective antiviral agents may not lead to immune reconstruction in patients with established AIDS. Finally, as an accurate staging and prognostic classification system for this important disease has not as yet been validated, it has been difficult to select study subjects rationally or to objectively assess the results of clinical trials.

### Surgery

The usual role for surgery in KS is palliation of protuberant lesions that are uncomfortable or bleed with repeated friction against clothes or shoes. If the patient has only one or several such lesions, excision may be of temporary value. Repeated excision of lesions for the patient with slowly progressing KS is not a successful strategy over time, given the relentless progression typical of most AIDS/KS cases. Surgery is rarely needed for palliation of major visceral KS.

### Radiation therapy

Radiation therapy is highly useful in managing AIDS/KS.[26,27] The tumor is often locally symptomatic and is responsive to radiation. Although optimal dosing schedules have not been determined, 2500 to 3000 rad often induces prompt regression, and even lower doses are sometimes effective.[26,27] Radiation therapy is most useful for extensive intraoral or pharyngeal KS, painful cutaneous KS, especially on the feet, and lymphedema, especially of the face and lower extremities.

## Chemotherapy

Several research facilities in the United States are in the process of testing cytotoxic agents for activity and toxicity in the treatment of AIDS-related KS. Drugs found active to date include vinblastine, vincristine, etoposide (VP-16-213), and doxorubicin (Adriamycin).

**Vinblastine.** Previously found to be active in KS in the elderly,[29] vinblastine is also effective in AIDS/KS.[30] Administered as a weekly intravenous bolus, the initial dose is 4 mg per week and is increased gradually by 1 to 2 mg per week to maintain a total leukocyte count of 2500 to 3000 cells/mm$^3$. This regimen has resulted in an approximate 25 percent response rate, and an additional 50 percent of patients have had stable disease. The drug is convenient, relatively nontoxic, and minimally immunosuppressive. Response is not rapid, however, and therapy should be continued for at least 6 to 8 weeks. Additionally, many patients experience neutropenia to a degree that precludes longer-term effective doses of vinblastine.

**Vincristine (Alone or Alternated with Vinblastine).** This agent has been shown to be active in AIDS-related KS.[31] A 75 percent objective response rate, with no severe neurotoxicity, was reported in one study.[31] However, in trials conducted at the University of California, San Francisco (UCSF), and San Francisco General Hospital (SFGH), dose limiting peripheral neuropathy was observed. Thus, it must be used with caution, especially for patients with previous AIDS-related neurologic problems. Toxicity can be reduced by alternating this drug with vinblastine on a weekly basis.[32] In other cases, one drug can be used weekly until recovery from toxicity resulting from the other drug occurs. Vincristine can be used in KS patients with severe neutropenia or thrombocytopenia because it is nonmyelosuppressive.

**Etoposide (VP-16-213).** This drug may be more active than the vinca alkaloids in the treatment of AIDS/KS. Researchers in New York[33] reported a 76 percent response rate to etoposide. Patients received 150 mg of intravenous etoposide per m$^2$ of body surface, administered for 3 consecutive days every 3 to 4 weeks. The frequency and severity of toxicity were acceptable. Nausea was not reported, alopecia almost always occurred, and modest myelosuppression and stomatitis were frequent. Clinical trials of the newly available form of this drug are now being organized.

**Doxorubicin.** Useful in the treatment of non-AIDS-related soft tissue sarcomas, doxorubicin is also active in AIDS/KS. Studies have not been completed, but responses have been seen using frequent (weekly or biweekly) doses of 10 to 30 mg given as a slow intravenous bolus. Toxicity includes alopecia, nausea, and moderate myelosuppression. Severe vomiting is unusual. Cardiotoxicity is a potential concern and should be carefully sought given the underlying HIV-related myocarditis that has been reported.

**Combination Chemotherapy.** Initial trials using doxorubicin, bleomycin, and vinblastine have resulted in an overall response rate nearly equal to that using etoposide as a single agent. However, the rate of life-threatening opportunistic infections in early studies was higher than expected,[33] and because this combination may further damage the immune system, it has not been widely recommended. Recently, however, a trial of combined treatment with doxorubicin, bleomycin, and vincristine has begun, and early results suggest that this or similar combinations may ultimately prove valuable because they produce a more rapid tumor response than has been seen with single-agent chemotherapy.

## Biologic agents

**Alpha Interferon.** This agent was first tested in patients with AIDS/KS in the hope that its combined antineoplastic, antiviral, and immune modulating activities would prove beneficial. Early testing of recombinant and lymphoblastoid alpha interferons established antineoplastic activity in high doses (usually more than $20 \times 10^6$ units daily) using a variety of routes and schedules. Clinically significant immune potentiation was not detected, although serial CD4 cell counts were not often performed. Anti-HIV activity (now documented in vitro with alpha interferon) was not tested in these trials.

Although antineoplastic activity is present, inconvenience and toxicity have limited enthusiasm for alpha interferon as a routine agent for AIDS/KS. The drug must be used on a frequent (usually daily) schedule and is administered by parenteral injection in a dose that results in a flulike syndrome (fever, asthenia, anorexia) which many patients find unacceptable. Despite drawbacks, however, alpha interferon (and more recently also beta interferon) has features that require close consideration and further trials. Most significant is its anti-HIV activity and the probable absence of immune toxicity when compared with chemotherapeutic agents that have similar antineoplastic effectiveness. Clinical trials are underway to reexamine this agent's potential and to explore combinations of alpha interferon and azidothymidine in patients with AIDS/KS.

**Azidothymidine (AZT, Zidovudine, Retrovir).** This drug is probably not active as a direct antineoplastic agent in AIDS/KS but is often used in KS patients because of its established role in other parts of the HIV spectrum. In the initial phase I experience, some KS patients had partial tumor responses, while others had tumor progression. A separate study is being conducted in which KS patients with minimal disease are being treated with azidothymidine or placebo. Although results are still pending, many KS patients in the community are being treated with azidothymidine, not so much for its potential role as an antineoplastic agent as for its antiviral effect. Some of these patients also require chemotherapy for their KS, yet information is not yet available to allow accurate predictions of the results (toxicity and efficacy) of these combinations. It is expected that the myelosuppressive effect of azidothymidine would be accentuated by concomitant cytotoxic chemotherapy, and these agents should not be used together without very careful monitoring of patients.

# TREATMENT GUIDELINES

The decision to initiate therapy for AIDS-related Kaposi's sarcoma is difficult, since some patients with few lesions and without poor prognostic factors will do well for months to years without conventional treatment. On the other hand, many patients will have rapidly progressive disease and die either of KS itself or of opportunistic infections. Single-agent cytotoxic drugs, combinations of these drugs, as well as biologic approaches including antivirals, continue to be explored. The therapy of KS is an active area of investigation and will continue to be so for years to come. Where possible, patients should be treated in the context of one of these clinical trials. Meanwhile, some broad recommendations, as shown in Table 56-1, can be made.

### Minimal KS without poor prognostic factors

Patients with fewer than 15 cutaneous lesions, no previous serious infections, and no B symptoms can either be observed to document disease progression or given immediate chemotherapy with vinblastine alone, or vinblastine alternated with vincristine. KS patients with early disease are also better subjects for alpha interferon, since they have shown higher response rates and may tolerate side effects more easily.

### KS with poor prognostic factors

For patients with extensive tumor, rapid progression, B symptoms, or previous opportunistic infection, early treatment with chemotherapy (vinblastine, vinblastine alternated with vincristine, or doxorubicin) is recommended. More aggressive agents, including etoposide, can be considered, as well as combinations of agents.

### Lymphedema

Radiotherapy is recommended for palliation of tumor-associated lymphedema, delivered to generous treatment fields. Response is more gratifying for facial than for lower extremity edema.

### Pulmonary KS

Whole lung radiotherapy or more aggressive chemotherapy with etoposide, doxorubicin, or combination chemotherapy is recommended for this rapidly fatal manifestation of KS. Combination chemotherapy may include doxorubicin, bleomycin, and vincristine, although no such trials have yet been published.

**Table 56-1. Treatment of Kaposi's Sarcoma (KS)**

| Group | Recommendations |
|---|---|
| Minimal KS, no infections, fever, night sweats, or weight loss | Experimental immunomodulators and/or antiviral drugs; vinblastine sulfate, vincristine sulfate (alternating), other single-agent chemotherapy, investigational agents; expectant observation |
| Minimal KS, history of infections and/or fever, night sweats, or weight loss (B symptoms) | Vinblastine, vincristine (alternating), other single-agent chemotherapy, investigational agents |
| Advanced cutaneous KS, rapidly progressive KS, or pulmonary KS | Etoposide, low-dose doxorubicin hydrochloride, other single-agent chemotherapy, investigational agents, combination chemotherapy |
| KS with neutropenia or thrombocytopenia | Vincristine or bleomycin |
| Painful, bulky KS or lymphedema | Radiation therapy |

SOURCE: *JAMA* 257(10):1370, March 13, 1987. Copyright 1987, American Medical Association.

### Symptomatic oral involvement

When KS lesions are small, surgical excision, intralesional injection of dilute vinblastine, or laser excision should be considered, since these approaches avoid toxicity to normal mucosa. Radiotherapy is useful for large lesions. Complete or substantial partial tumor regression follows moderate dose (2000 rad) external beam radiation.[28] Toxicity of whole mouth radiotherapy (mucositis) has been significant but responds to local measures and resolves in 1 to 2 weeks.

## NON-HODGKIN'S LYMPHOMA

Since the first cases of high-grade non-Hodgkin's lymphoma (NHL) were reported in 1982,[34] many reports of aggressive lymphoma in patients at risk for AIDS have been published.[35,36] In June 1985, the Centers for Disease Control amended their case definition of AIDS to include patients with high-grade, B-cell non-Hodgkin's lymphoma in the setting of documented HIV infection.[37]

## NHL IN IMMUNODEFICIENT NON-HIV INFECTED POPULATIONS

NHL has been frequently seen in patients with primary immunodeficiency disorders such as the Wiskott-Aldrich syndrome or ataxia telangiectasia, diseases that are associated with abnormal cell-mediated immunity. Immunoblastic lymphoma has been the prevalent histologic pattern in these disorders,[38] and patients often have marked generalized lymphadenopathy for several years before the diagnosis of lymphoma. Lymph node biopsies often show a pattern of reactive hyperplasia.[38] Lymph node biopsies of postrenal transplant patients receiving treatment with immunosuppressive medications also show this pattern. These patients have a 35-fold increased risk of developing NHL, often in unusual sites.

Disease confined to the central nervous system has been observed in 33 percent of NHL associated with renal transplantation.[39] Lymphoproliferative disease may appear as a relatively benign polyclonal proliferation in renal transplant patients, or as an invasive and aggressive monoclonal large-cell non-Hodgkin's lymphoma.[40] A renal transplant recipient has been described in whom a high-grade immunoblastic lymphoma evolved from a polyclonal lymphoproliferative process.[41]

An etiologic role for Epstein-Barr virus (EBV) is supported by circumstantial evidence.[42] Serologic evidence suggests either acute or reactivation EBV infection in most patients with these disorders, and multiple copies of EBV genome have been identified within the cells of many of these lymphomas.

## NON-HODGKIN'S LYMPHOMA IN AIDS

AIDS-associated NHL bears a striking resemblance to that described associated with other immunodeficiency states. The histologic appearance of AIDS-associated lymphoma has included both the intermediate and high-grade large-cell varieties as well as the high-grade, small noncleaved cell variety (Burkitt's and non-Burkitt's lymphoma). Immunologically, these are B-cell malignancies. Epstein-Barr virus nuclear antigen (EBNA) has been identified in some of these tumors,[43] and most patients have shown evidence of previous EBV infection.[44] In addition, chromosomal translocations similar to those seen in patients with Burkitt's lymphoma are also seen in some patients with AIDS-associated Burkitt's-like lymphoma.[40,45,46]

Many of the patients described have had previous histories of persistent generalized lymphadenopathy (PGL). Lymph node biopsies in such patients generally reveal follicular hyperplasia. The development of a monoclonal surface immunoglobulin pattern in a lymph node cell suspension before the development of a high-grade lymphoma has been described in a patient with PGL whose lymph nodes showed a histologic pattern of follicular hyperplasia.[45] In 1984, Ziegler et al. published a report of their retrospective, multi-institutional study of 90 homosexual men with AIDS-associated NHL.[34] Of 77 patients diagnosed ante mortem, 33 had a prodrome of generalized lymphadenopathy, 15 had previous opportunistic infections, 9 had Kaposi's sarcoma, and 5 had both opportunistic infections and Kaposi's sarcoma before developing NHL. Similarly, of 14 homosexual patients with aggressive NHL reported by Kalter et al. at M.D. Anderson,[35] 8 had a preceding diagnosis of AIDS and 5 had ARC.

Extranodal sites of disease have been the rule in these patients. In Ziegler's series, all but two patients had evidence of extranodal disease; 42 percent of patients had central nervous system disease, and 33 percent had bone marrow involvement. Levine et al.[36] reported that 19 (86 percent) of 22 patients with high-grade B-cell lymphomas had disease in extranodal sites. These sites included the central nervous system in 7 patients and rectum in 3 patients.

High-grade B-cell non-Hodgkin's lymphomas confined to the central nervous system are also associated with AIDS. This diagnosis should be considered in any patient belonging to a risk group for AIDS who shows focal neurologic findings or evidence of increased intracranial pressure.

## THERAPY

Ziegler and his colleagues reported that 53 percent of 66 evaluable patients achieved complete response to combination chemotherapy, which is a response rate substantially lower than that reported in immunocompetent patients with the same high-grade lymphomas.[34] Fifty-four percent of the complete responders subsequently relapsed. Although prognosis was poor in all groups of patients, morbidity and mortality appeared to be directly related to the degree of previous HIV-related illness. Patients who were asymptomatic at the time of diagnosis showed the best treatment results. Those with a history of PGL fared less well, and only 2 of 21 patients with a previous AIDS diagnosis remained alive and well. Thirty-eight of 66 evaluable patients have died, half from progressive lymphoma and half from opportunistic infections.

In Kalter's series, 6 patients with diffuse large cell lymphoma responded poorly to therapy.[35] No patient had a complete response to chemotherapy, and all patients died within 6 months. In contrast, 7 patients who had undifferentiated lymphoma responded better to chemotherapy and survived longer; 3 patients remained alive at 19, 19, and 35 months.

Levine and colleagues, in their initial study, treated nine patients with methotrexate, bleomycin, doxorubicin, cyclophosphamide, dexamethasone, and leucovorin (M-BACOD).[36] Three of these achieved complete response and 2 were reported alive at 12 and 18 months after diagnosis. Seven patients were treated with either cytoxan, doxorubicin, vincristine, and prednisone (CHOP); or bleomycin, doxorubicin, cyclophosphamide, vincristine, and prednisone (BACOP). Two of these patients had complete responses, although 1 patient subsequently relapsed. In a subsequent update of their treatment results,[47] this institution now reports that 7 of 13 of those patients treated with M-BACOD attained complete remission. Two of these patients subsequently relapsed and 5 remained free of disease between 15 and 16 months after diagnosis. In contrast, only 3 of 9 patients who received a more aggressive, novel chemotherapeutic regimen achieved complete remission. The intensive regimen of combination chemotherapy was associated with significant risk of early death due to opportunistic infections.

Kaplan et al. have treated 60 patients with AIDS-associated non-Hodgkin's lymphoma at San Francisco General Hospital, where a recent and notable rise in the annual frequency of non-Hodgkin's lymphoma in patients at risk for AIDS has been observed. Patients were treated with a variety of standard chemotherapeutic regimens, radiation therapy alone, or with a novel chemotherapy protocol, COMET-A (cyclophosphamide, vincristine, methotrexate with leucovorin rescue, VP-16, and ARA-C). Karnofsky performance score (KPS) was the only factor significantly predictive of response. Sixty-seven percent of patients with a KPS of 70 percent or better achieved complete remission, whereas only 27 percent of patients with a KPS of less than 70 percent had a complete response to therapy. Absence of a previous AIDS diagnosis and a performance score of 70 percent or better were independently predictive of improved survival. No significant differences were noted in response or survival in patients treated with COMET-A compared with those treated with standard chemotherapy regimens (Kaplan et al., manuscript in preparation).

The prognosis for patients with primary central nervous system lymphoma is extremely poor. Most will die with recurrent disease within 1 year of diagnosis.[48]

In summary, the treatment of AIDS-related NHL with aggressive chemotherapy has resulted in a low complete response rate (33 to 50 percent), a high incidence of associated opportunistic infections, and high relapse and mortality rates.

# References


1 Volberding PA: Other cancers in AIDS, in *San Francisco General Hospital AIDS Knowledgebase,* PT Cohen et al (eds). Waltham, Massachusetts, Medical Society, 1988.

2 The case definition of AIDS used by CDC for national reporting (CDC reportable AIDS). Document 0312S. Centers for Disease Control, 1985.

3 Kaposi M: Idiopathisiches multiples pigmensarkom der haut. *Arch Dermatol Syph (Berl)* 4:265, 1872.

4 Safai B, Good RA: Kaposi's sarcoma: A review and recent developments. *CA* 31:2, 1981.

5 Harwood AR et al: Kaposi's sarcoma in recipients of renal transplants. *Am J Med* 64:759, 1979.

6 Guinan ME et al: Heterosexual and homosexual patients with acquired immunodeficiency syndrome: A comparison of surveillance, interview, and laboratory data. *Ann Intern Med* 1:213, 1984.

7 Haverkos HW, Drotman, DP: Prevalence of Kaposi's sarcoma among patients with AIDS [Letter]. *N Engl J Med* 313:1518, 1985.

8 Drew WL et al: Cytomegalovirus infection and abnormal T-lymphocyte subset ratios in homosexual men. *Ann Intern Med* 103:61, 1985.

9 Marmor M et al: Risk factors for Kaposi's sarcoma in homosexual men. *Lancet* 1:1083, 1982.

10 Reichert et al: Pathologic features of AIDS, in *AIDS: Etiology,*

*Diagnosis, Treatment and Prevention,* V De Vita et al (eds). Philadelphia, Lippincott, 1985, p 111.

11 Taylor JF et al: Kaposi's sarcoma in Uganda: A clinico-pathological study. *Int J Cancer* 8:122, 1971.

12 Dorfman R: Kaposi's sarcoma revisited. *Hum Pathol* 15:1023, 1984.

13 Beckstead JH et al: Evidence of the origin of Kaposi's sarcoma from lymphatic endothelium. *Am J Pathol* 119:294, 1985.

14 Cutler K et al: Prognostic indicators at presentation of Kaposi's sarcoma. *III International Conference on AIDS,* Washington, DC, 1985.

15 Mitsuyasu RT et al: Heterogeneity of epidemic Kaposi's sarcoma: Implications for therapy. *Cancer* (suppl) 57:1657, 1986.

16 Friedman-Kein AE et al: Disseminated Kaposi's sarcoma in homosexual men. *Ann Intern Med* 6:693, 1982.

17 Rogers MF et al: National case-control study of Kaposi's sarcoma and *Pneumocystis carinii* pneumonia in homosexual men: Part 2. Laboratory results. *Ann Intern Med* 99:151, 1983.

18 Volberding PA et al: Prognostic factors in staging Kaposi's sarcoma in the acquired immune deficiency syndrome. *Proc Am Soc Clin Oncol* 3:51, 1984.

19 Volberding P: Therapy of Kaposi's sarcoma in AIDS. *Semin Oncol* 11:60, 1984.

20 McNutt NS et al: Early lesions of Kaposi's sarcoma in homosexual men. An ultrastructural comparison with other vascular proliferations in skin. *Am J Pathol* 111:62, 1983.

21 Lozada F et al: Oral manifestations of tumor and opportunistic infections in the acquired immune deficiency syndrome: Findings in 53 homosexual men with Kaposi's sarcoma. *Oral Surg* 56:491, 1983.

22 Green T et al: Histopathologic spectrum of oral Kaposi's sarcoma. *Oral Surg* 58:306, 1984.

23 Reichert CM et al: Autopsy pathology in the acquired immune deficiency syndrome. *Am J Pathol* 112:357, 1983.

24 Rose H et al: Alimentary tract involvement in Kaposi's sarcoma: Radiographic and endoscopic findings in 25 homosexual men. *Am J Radiol* 139:661, 1982.

25 Friedman S et al: Gastrointestinal Kaposi's sarcoma in patients with acquired immunodeficiency syndrome: Endoscopic and autopsy findings. *Gastroenterology* 89:102, 1985.

26 Nobler MP et al: The impact of palliative irradiation on the management of patients with acquired immunodeficiency syndrome. *J Clin Oncol* 5:107, 1987.

27 El-Akkad S et al: Kaposi's sarcoma and its management by radiotherapy. *Arch Dermatol* 122:1396, 1986.

28 Harris JW, Reed TA: Kaposi's sarcoma in AIDS: The role of radiation therapy. *Ann Intern Med* 103:335, 1985.

29 Tucker S, Winkelmann R: Treatment of Kaposi's sarcoma with vinblastine. *Arch Dermatol* 112:958, 1976.

30 Volberding P et al: Vinblastine therapy for Kaposi's sarcoma in the acquired immunodeficiency syndrome. *Ann Intern Med* 103:335, 1985.

31 Mintzer D et al: Treatment of Kaposi's sarcoma and thrombocytopenia with vincristine in patients with acquired immunodeficiency syndrome. *Ann Intern Med* 102:200, 1985.

32 Kaplan L, Volberding P: Treatment of AIDS-related Kaposi's sarcoma with vincristine alternating with vinblastine. *Cancer* 70:1121, 1986.

33 Laubenstein L et al: Treatment of epidemic Kaposi's sarcoma with etoposide or a combination of doxorubicin, bleomycin and vinblastine. *Clin Oncol* 2:1115, 1984.

34 Ziegler et al: Non-Hodgkin's lymphoma in 90 homosexual men. Relation to generalized lymphadenopathy and the acquired immunodeficiency syndrome. *N Engl J Med* 311:565, 1984.

35 Kalter SP et al: Aggressive non-Hodgkin's lymphomas in immunocompromised homosexual males. *Blood* 66:655, 1985.

36 Levine et al: Retrovirus and malignant lymphoma in homosexual men. *JAMA* 254:1921, 1985.

37 Centers for Disease Control: Revision of the case definition of acquired immunodeficiency syndrome for notational reporting—United States. *MMWR* 373, 1985.

38 Frizzera G et al: Lymphoreticular disorders in primary immunodeficiencies. *Cancer* 46:692, 1980.

39 Hoover R, Fraumeni JF Jr: Risk of cancer in renal transplant recipients. *Lancet* 1:5, 1973.

40 Frizzera G et al: Polymorphic diffuse B cell hyperplasias and lymphomas in renal transplant recipients. *Cancer Res* 41:4262, 1981.

41 Hanto DW et al: Epstein Barr virus induced B cell lymphoma after renal transplantation. *Med Intell* 306:913, 1982.

42 Hanto et al: Clinical spectrum of lymphoproliferative disorders in renal transplant recipients and evidence for the role of Epstein Barr virus. *Cancer Res* 41:4253, 1981.

43 Ziegler JL et al: Outbreak of Burkitt's lymphoma in homosexual men. *Lancet* 2:631, 1982.

44 Lind SE et al: Malignant lymphoma presenting as Kaposi's sarcoma in a homosexual man with the acquired immunodeficiency syndrome. *Ann Intern Med* 102:388, 1985.

45 Levine et al: Development of B-cell lymphoma in homosexual men. *Ann Intern Med* 100:7, 1984.

46 Whang-Peng et al: Burkitt's lymphoma in AIDS: Cytogenic study. *Blood* 63:818, 1984.

47 Gill PS et al: AIDS-related malignant lymphoma: Results of prospective treatment trials. *J Clin Oncol* 5:1322, 1987.

48 Gill PS et al: Primary central nervous system lymphoma in homosexual men. *Am J Med* 78:742, 1985.

# Chapter 57

# Opportunistic infections in AIDS

Richard E. Chaisson
J. Louise Gerberding
Merle A. Sande

## INTRODUCTION

Individuals infected with the human immnodeficiency virus manifest a variety of chronic, progressive defects in cellular immunity (Chap. 29). In a substantial proportion, perhaps the majority, of infected persons the end stage of persistent HIV infection will be development of one or more opportunistic infections, most of which are diagnostic of AIDS by surveillance criteria used by the Centers for Disease Control and the World Health Organization. Deterioration of cellular immune competence has generally proceeded to an extreme degree by the time opportunistic diseases occur. Ultimate control of HIV-related opportunistic infections will rely on prevention or reversal of cellular immune dysfunction in persons infected by the virus. Nevertheless, the diagnosis and management of AIDS-related opportunistic infections remains a critical aspect of caring for patients with HIV infection.

AIDS-related opportunistic infections share several common features. First, the incidence of infection is greatly increased and relapses are common despite appropriate therapy. Second, atypical presentations of opportunistic infections are extremely common, e.g., *Pneumocystis carinii* pneumonia (PCP) with no radiographic abnormalities, dissemination of *Mycobacterium avium* complex, cryptococcal meningitis with an acellular cerebrospinal fluid, or bacteremic enteric infections. Third, the incidence of adverse reactions to drugs usually well tolerated by immunocompetent hosts is high, for reasons as yet unexplained. Finally, the mortality of AIDS-related opportunistic infections is high.

Complications of HIV infection involve almost every human organ system. However, pulmonary infections, central nervous system disorders, and infections of the gastrointestinal tract are the leading causes of AIDS-related morbidity and mortality. This chapter will review the clinical features, diagnosis, and management of opportunistic infections of these systems.

## PULMONARY OPPORTUNISTIC INFECTIONS

Patients with advanced HIV infection have a very high incidence of respiratory-tract infections. The relative frequency of pulmonary pathogens in AIDS patients with respiratory symptoms was reviewed by Murray and colleagues and is shown in Table 57-1.[1] In the United States, more than 60 percent of AIDS cases are diagnosed on the basis of *P. carinii* pneumonia, and an additional 20 percent of patients may develop PCP during the course of their illness. In addition to *P. carinii,* a variety of other organisms, including pyogenic bacteria, mycobacteria, fungi, and viruses, may produce respiratory illness in patients immunosuppressed by HIV. A decade-long decline in the incidence of tuberculosis in the United States has recently reversed, primarily because of HIV infection and AIDS. In San Francisco, a 60 percent increase in the number of cases of tuberculosis in American-born residents was observed between 1982 and 1987.[2] Tuberculosis cases in New York City increased by 36 percent between 1984 and 1986, most likely because of HIV infection.[3] Deaths caused by community-acquired pneumonias also increased in New York City in the early 1980s, primarily among IV drug users, the majority of whom are HIV-seropositive. Many hospitals have witnessed steady increases in tuberculosis and community-acquired pneumonias during the AIDS epidemic, as well. The overall impact of the HIV epidemic on the prevalence of pulmonary disease in endemic areas has been dramatic.

**Table 57-1. Relative Frequency of Pulmonary Disease in 441 Patients with AIDS.***

| Pathogen or disorder | Number of patients,% |
|---|---|
| *Pneumocystis carinii* | 85 |
| without other pathogen | 58 |
| with other pathogen | 27 |
| Cytomegalovirus | 11 |
| *Mycobacterium avium*-complex | 8 |
| *M. tuberculosis* | 3 |
| Legionella | 2 |
| Cryptococcus | 2 |
| Other | 1 |
| Other Infections | 21 |
| *M. avium*-complex | 8 |
| Cytomegalovirus | 5 |
| Pyogenic bacteria | 2 |
| Legionella | 2 |
| Fungi | 2 |
| Other | 2 |
| Kaposi's sarcoma | 8 |

*From Murray et al.[1]

## CLINICAL PRESENTATION

Pulmonary opportunistic infections in HIV-infected patients typically have an insidious onset, often preceded by prolonged periods of constitutional symptoms such as fevers, night sweats, and weight loss. A previous AIDS-related diagnosis is frequently reported. The majority of patients note the progressive onset of chest tightness, exertional dyspnea, dry cough, and fatigue, in addition to worsening constitutional symptoms. Sputum production, pleuritic chest pain, and rapid progression of symptoms may be experienced, often in association with infections caused by pyogenic organisms.[4] Physical examination usually reveals fever (38 to 40.5°) and tachypnea; oral candidiasis or hairy leukoplakia may be present. Chest examination often reveals only diffuse fine rales, or may be unremarkable. The remainder of the exam is often normal. Screening laboratory abnormalities are not usually helpful. The white blood cell count is frequently low with an absolute lymphopenia ($<1000/mm^3$) but may be normal or elevated in patients with bacterial pneumonia. A mild anemia may be present, and the erythrocyte sedimentation rate and the serum lactate dehydrogenase are usually elevated.[5] Further expeditious evaluation of the symptomatic patient with known or suspected HIV infection should aim to rapidly identify treatable pulmonary pathogens.

## DIAGNOSTIC WORKUP

A chest radiograph should be obtained on all patients with symptoms or signs of pulmonary disease. Diffuse interstitial infiltrates are the most common presentation of PCP, occurring in approximately 65 to 85 percent of patients with documented disease.[6,7] Other pathogens that can cause diffuse infiltrates are *M. tuberculosis*, pyogenic infections, CMV pneumonitis, or disseminated fungal infections. Focal infiltrates, often in a lobar, segmental, or subsegmental pattern, are commonly seen in patients with pyogenic pneumonias but may also be present in patients with PCP.[4,7] Upper-lobe infiltrates, with or without cavitation, may be seen in some HIV-infected patients with tuberculosis. Focal disease may also be present in patients with cryptococcal pneumonia or histoplasmosis. Mediastinal and hilar adenopathy is a rare finding in PCP and is not part of the lymphadenopathy syndrome. The usual causes of this pattern on the chest film are mycobacterial infections or lymphomas.[7] Diagnostic evaluation of isolated intrathoracic adenopathy can be made by peripheral lymph node biopsy, by mediastinoscopic approach to intrathoracic nodes, or by Wang needle biopsy via a bronchoscope. Pleural effusions are seen on the chest film of some patients with pyogenic pneumonias, disseminated CMV infection, or tuberculosis. The most common cause of pleural fluid accumulation in AIDS patients is pulmonary Kaposi's sarcoma, which can also be associated with diffuse infiltrates from tumor infiltration and hemorrhage.[8] Normal radiographs may be found in many patients, including 10 to 20 percent of patients with confirmed PCP. Further noninvasive evaluation of patients with a normal chest film is warranted.

## NONINVASIVE EVALUATION

Patients with normal chest radiographs may have significant pulmonary pathology that can be detected by several noninvasive tests. Determination of the arterial oxygen content is a useful measure that correlates well with chest radiographic findings. An exercise-induced increase in the alveolar-arterial oxygen difference (A-a$DO_2$) has a sensitivity of 85 to 90 percent for PCP, though this finding is nonspecific. Reduction in the membrane component of the diffusing capacity for carbon monoxide (DLCO) is another sensitive marker of PCP. More than 95 percent of patients with documented PCP have a reduction in the DLCO to <80 percent of predicted values.[9] Other tests of pulmonary function, including TLC and VC, are less sensitive indicators of pulmonary infection though often decreased in PCP. Use of the DLCO to evaluate patients with respiratory symptoms but normal chest radiographs is useful because the test may be performed expeditiously and at low cost. The presence of an increased A-a$DO_2$ following exercise or a low DLCO should prompt specific evaluation for *P. carinii*.

Gallium lung scanning is another useful noninvasive diagnostic test for pulmonary opportunistic infection.[10] Accumulation of any gallium at 48 to 72 h after injection is considered abnormal and has a 95 percent sensitivity for PCP. While diffuse uptake of gallium is the rule, focal accumulations can be seen in PCP, bacterial pneumonias, and tuberculosis. Lymphomas also take up gallium, and pulmonary involvement of an aggressive non-Hodgkin's lymphoma may result in a positive scan. The use of gallium scanning is constrained by the delay between injection and reading (2 to 3 days) and by cost. Patients with an abnormal gallium scan should have further evaluation to rule out pulmonary opportunistic infection.

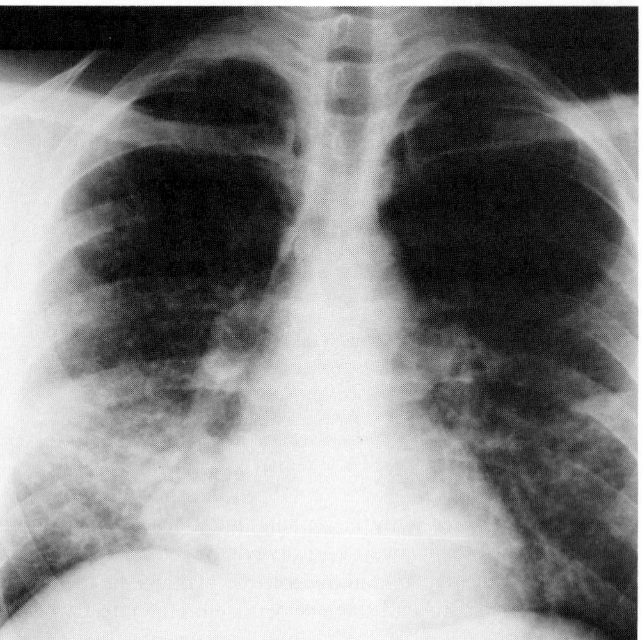

**Fig. 57-1.** Typical chest x-ray of patient with *Pneumocystis carinii* pneumonia showing bilateral, diffuse infiltration.

## SPECIFIC TESTS

The presence of radiographic or other noninvasive test abnormalities should be followed by the collection of the respiratory tract specimens needed to diagnose opportunistic infections. These include the following.

**Sputum Induction.** In experienced hands, examination of samples of induced sputum has high yield of diagnosing pulmonary pathogens in patients with AIDS.[11,12] Following an overnight fast and thorough mouth cleansing, patients inhale a mist of hypertonic saline generated by an ultrasonic nebulizer. Sputum samples induced by this technique are then digested, centrifuged, mounted on slides, and stained. Use of a modified Giemsa stain, silver methenamine, toluidine blue O, or an immunofluorescent monoclonal anti-*Pneumocystis* antibody stain reveals *P. carinii* in 60 to 90 percent of patients with PCP.[11,13] Sputum should also be Gram-stained and stained for acid-fast bacilli and cultured for bacteria, mycobacteria, fungi, and viruses. Use of sputum induction may reduce the need for bronchoscopy by 50 to 75 percent.

**Fiberoptic Bronchoscopy.** Fiberoptic bronchoscopy is an effective and safe technique to evaluate immunosuppressed patients with pulmonary disease. In particular, the use of bronchoalveolar lavage (BAL) results in a high diagnostic yield with low morbidity.[14,15] BAL specimens can be stained for *P. carinii*, as described above, and can be cultured for bacteria, mycobacteria, fungi, and viruses. The sensitivity of BAL for diagnosing PCP and mycobacterial infections is 95 to 99 percent. Transbronchial biopsy may increase the yield of bronchoscopy by permitting tissue stains. Approximately 10 percent of patients who have a transbronchial biopsy develop a pneumothorax, one-half of which require chest tube placement. In one series, the use of BAL and transbronchial biopsy had a yield of 100 percent for AIDS-related pulmonary disease.[14] In our institution, patients with suspected pulmonary infections who have a negative sputum induction undergo bronchoscopy with BAL. If no diagnosis is made, a repeat bronchoscopy with transbronchial biopsy is performed.[6]

## DIFFERENTIAL DIAGNOSIS

The AIDS patient with respiratory complaints may have one or more opportunistic infections or malignancies. The most frequent pulmonary opportunistic infection, by far, is *P. carinii* pneumonia.[16] *Pneumocystis* characteristically presents with a history of prodromal constitutional symptoms for several weeks with increasing respiratory symptoms and spiking fevers over several days. Occasionally PCP may present with an abrupt onset followed by rapid deterioration. Patients who have the acute onset of fever, productive cough, pleuritic chest pain, and dyspnea and who have focal radiographic infiltrates are most likely to have a community-acquired pyogenic infection.[4] Tuberculosis is more common in persons with an increased risk of prior infection with *M. tuberculosis* (e.g., persons from developing countries, intravenous drug users), and extrapulmonary disease sites are frequently noted. *M. avium* complex (MAC) is often isolated from the sputum of patients with PCP, but whether MAC causes pulmonary disease in AIDS patients is unclear. Likewise, CMV is isolated in the respiratory specimens of approximately 40 percent of patients with PCP, but the contribution that CMV makes to pulmonary disease is unknown. CMV pneumonitis can be suspected when no other pathogen is identified, when viral inclusions are found on biopsy specimens, and when cultures become positive in several days. Pulmonary cryptococcal infection may present with nonspecific respiratory symptoms and a focal nodule or cavity on chest x-ray. Serum cryptococcal antigen is often positive, and cultures of sputum or BAL specimens grow *Cryptococcus neoformans*. Histoplasmosis should be suspected in patients from endemic regions, and *Histoplasma capsulatum* may be identified by its characteristic appearance within pulmonary macrophages and by positive cultures. Pulmonary Kaposi's sarcoma is suspected in patients with other sites of tumor, who have pleural effusions on the chest radiograph, or who have lesions seen during bronchoscopy.[8] Nonspecific pneumonitis is a diagnosis of exclusion that is made when a complete diagnostic evaluation has been performed, when no pathogens are identified, and when biopsy specimens show inflammation and fibrosis. Lymphocytic interstitial pneumonitis (LIP) is more common in children with AIDS than in adults.[16] It may be diagnosed by transbronchial biopsy or open lung biopsy.

## THERAPY

### PCP

A number of drug therapies have been evaluated for the treatment of PCP. Pentamidine isoethionate is a diamidine that is active against *P. carinii* and was the mainstay of therapy in the pre-AIDS era. Pentamidine, when given in a single daily intravenous or intramuscular dose of 4 mg/kg, cures 70 to 80 percent of AIDS patients with PCP.[17–19] Adverse reactions to pentamidine occur frequently, however, and may limit the drug's usefulness. Commonly encountered toxicities include neutropenia, azotemia, and hepatitis.[17,18] Pentamidine is toxic to pancreatic islet cells and can result in significant dysglycemias, both hypo- and hyperglycemia.[20] Pancreatitis has been rarely reported, as have ventricular dysrhythmias.[21,22] Patients receiving pentamidine should be monitored closely for hematologic, renal, hepatic, and endocrine toxicity. Therapy should be altered when significant adverse reactions are noted. A recent study has examined the effect of lower dose pentamidine (3 mg/kg per day) in treating PCP in AIDS patients;[23] larger controlled studies are necessary before this can be recommended.

Trimethoprim-sulfamethoxazole (TMP-SMX) is also approved for the treatment of PCP and can be administered orally or intravenously at 15 to 20 mg/kg per day TMP and 75 to 100 mg/kg per day SMX in divided doses. Survival of patients with AIDS-related PCP treated with TMP-SMX is approximately 80 percent.[17] Like pentamidine, TMP-SMX is associated with significant toxicity in up to 60 percent of patients. Common adverse reactions are hyponatremia, neutropenia, nausea, hepatitis, rash, and drug fever. Rarely, renal insufficiency has been observed. Adverse reactions generally occur in the second and third weeks of therapy unless the patient has received treatment with TMP-SMX in the past.[17] Patients with significant adverse reactions should be placed on alternate therapy. Pentamidine and TMP-SMX have been compared in a randomized, nonblinded clinical trial in patients with AIDS and a first episode of PCP.[17] No significant differences in survival, clinical response, or incidence of adverse reactions were seen. More than 50 percent of patients assigned to each therapy were unable to complete a 21-day course because of adverse responses.

The high incidence of toxicity caused by pentamidine and TMP-SMX has prompted a search for less toxic agents for treating PCP.[23–25] Dapsone in combination with TMP is effective oral therapy for mild cases of PCP and is less toxic than TMP-SMX.[25] The efficacy of dapsone and TMP in more severe disease is unknown. Approximately 25 percent of patients treated with this regimen are unable to complete their course because of toxicity, including nausea, rash, hepatitis, and anemia. Dapsone use is associated with the development of methemoglobinemia; dapsone is also an oxidant which can precipitate hemolysis in an individual who is G6PD-deficient.

The delivery of pentamidine by aerosol has been investigated by AIDS-related PCP. Aerosolization of pentamidine particles by an ultrasonic nebulizer permits direct delivery of drug to the alveoli and minimizes systemic toxicity. In a pilot study, Montgomery and associates cured 13 of 15 patients with first episodes of PCP and a room air $PaO_2$ >55 mmHg with aerosolized pentamidine alone.[24] Airway toxicity may occur, but absorption of pentamidine from the lung is minimal. However, lack of systemic drug delivery can result in treatment failure for rare cases of extrapulmonary pneumocystosis.

Trimetrexate, a dihydrofolate reductase inhibitor, used in combination with sulfa drugs has been studied in treating primary episodes of PCP and patients with PCP that was refractory to conventional therapy.[18] The drug appears to hold promise as salvage therapy for patients unable to tolerate or not responding to standard therapy. However, relapse rates appear to be high shortly after drug discontinuation. Administration of folinic acid to prevent bone marrow toxicity is also required. Eflornithine (difluoromethylornithine) is a polyamine synthesis inhibitor that may have activity against *P. carinii*, though careful clinical trials are lacking.

The average time required for a clinical response, e.g., defervescence, improved arterial oxygen content, and resolution of dyspnea, is 5 to 8 days. A clinical failure is presumed for patients who deteriorate or fail to respond after 6 to 9 days of therapy. Patients who fail initial therapy have a high mortality (90 to 100 percent), though trimetrexate shows promise as a salvage regimen. Conversely, patients whose drug therapy is changed because of adverse reactions usually have a favorable outcome.

Following an episode of PCP, patients should be given maintenance therapy to prevent recurrences.[25–26] TMP-SMX given daily or thrice weekly is recommended for patients who have not developed adverse reactions during acute therapy. Aerosolized pentamidine maintenance is under study as a prophylactic regimen. Dapsone and sulfadoxine/pyrimethamine (Fansidar) have been used in uncontrolled series. Patients at risk for PCP, because of either other AIDS diagnoses or deteriorating cellular immune competence, should probably also receive prophylactic therapy, though clear criteria for initiating treatment have not been developed. One study of patients with AIDS-related Kaposi's sarcoma who had not had a major opportunistic infection showed a lower incidence of PCP and prolonged survival in subjects assigned to receive TMP-SMX compared with untreated subjects.[26]

Mycobacteria disease caused by *M. tuberculosis* responds well to standard antituberculosis drugs, even in AIDS.[2] Current recommended therapy is a combination of isoniazid (300 mg per day), rifampin (600 mg per day), ethambutol (15 to 25 mg/kg per day) or streptomycin (20 mg/kg per day), and pyrazinamide (25 mg/kg per day). After 2 months pyrazinamide is discontinued and three drugs are given for a total of 6 months, or 3 months following conversion of sputum cultures. Some authorities prefer longer treatment in HIV seropositives or AIDS patients, but prospective studies of tuberculosis in such patients have shown that conventional therapy may be adequate. Patients who have adverse reactions to antituberculosis treatment may be treated with fewer drugs for a longer period, e.g., 9 months of isoniazid and rifampin, 18 months of isoniazid and ethambutol. HIV-seropositive patients with a positive tuberculin skin test and no evidence of tuberculosis disease should receive prophylactic therapy with isoniazid for 6 to 9 months.

Atypical mycobacterial infections in AIDS patients are associated with significant morbidity, though the contribution that MAC makes to mortality is not known. Treatment of MAC is extremely difficult, as eradication of positive blood and tissue cultures is a rare outcome of therapy.[27] Therapy is sometimes undertaken for otherwise robust patients with symptomatic MAC disease in whom reversal of symptoms may lead to a good quality of life. A number of regimens have been suggested for treating MAC disease in AIDS patients, none of which has been proved effective. Agents with some in vitro activity against strains of MAC include rifabutin, clofazamine, ethambutol, the quinolone ciprofloxacin, and amikacin. The use of a combination of these agents has been recommended by Young as "induction therapy" in selected patients.[28] Patients who respond may be continued on drugs for life.

## PYOGENIC BACTERIA

Treatment of bacterial pneumonias in HIV seropositives can be effectively accomplished with a number of antimicrobial agents. Empiric therapy in a patient with suspected bacterial pneumonia should be with either TMP-SMX, which also will treat PCP, or with a second-generation cephalosporin such as cefuroxime, which covers both *Haemophilus influenzae* and *Streptococcus pneumoniae*. Ampicillin may be used in areas where the prevalence of beta-lactamase-producing strains of *H. influenzae* is known to be low. Definitive therapy for pneumococcal disease should be with penicillin G, a cephalosporin, or erythromycin. *H. influenzae* may be treated with ampicillin, amoxacillin plus clavulanic acid (Augmentin), TMP-SMX, or a cephalosporin, depending on the clinical setting and in vitro sensitivity of the isolate. Intravenous administration of antimicrobials is preferred initially, because of the high prevalence of bacteremic infections (85 percent).[4] Oral therapy may be substituted when a clinical response is achieved. Many patients with bacterial infections will relapse, despite appropriate therapy. Use of suppressive antibiotics is recommended for patients who have at least two episodes of bacteremia.

## CMV

CMV pneumonitis is difficult to document in AIDS patients because of the high yield of CMV in lung specimens of patients with PCP, most of whom respond to anti-*Pneumocystis* treatment alone. When CMV pneumonia is diagnosed, the experimental agent ganciclovir (DHPG) may be given. Responses have been described in variable proportions of treated patients, though experience is limited. The development of additional agents active against CMV [e.g., phosphonoformate (foscarnet)] may improve treatment of CMV pneumonitis.

## OPPORTUNISTIC INFECTIONS OF THE CENTRAL NERVOUS SYSTEM

Infections of the central nervous system (CNS) are common in patients with advanced HIV infection and for clinical purposes can be divided into two groups, those that affect the brain or spinal cord (encephalitis and abscesses) and those of the cerebrospinal fluid (meningitis). Diagnosis is simplified because only a few organisms produce the majority of disease, but therapy is complicated. Cure is rarely achieved by antimicrobial therapy alone, and maintenance or suppressive therapy is usually required to prevent relapse.

## INFECTIONS OF THE BRAIN (ENCEPHALITIS/ABSCESSES)

### Clinical presentation

When patients with advanced HIV infection present with headache, a change in mental status, or focal neurologic symptoms, a diagnosis of CNS toxoplasmosis should immediately be considered. In 3 to 5 percent of patients, toxoplasmic encephalitis constitutes the presenting illness of AIDS. The presentation is often vague and nonspecific. Headaches are usually present and described as dull and constant, but they may be severe and unresponsive to analgesics;[29] fever is present in less than 50 percent. An alteration in mental status occurs in two-thirds of patients and may vary from a personality change to confusion, lethargy, disorientation, and frank coma.[30] Focal neurologic abnormalities are found in one-third of patients and include hemiparesis, hemiplegia, neurosensory deficits, cerebellar tremor, homonymous hemianopia, diplopia, cranial nerve palsies, and blindness. Focal or major motor seizures occur in 15 to 30 percent.[29] Common generalized abnormalities include weakness, myoclonus, and ataxia. While involvement of other organ systems such as lung, heart, and muscle may be discerned at autopsy, patients rarely have symptoms referable to these systems.

While *Toxoplasma gondii* is by far the most common cause of encephalitis in the AIDS patient, other infectious and noninfectious causes may occur. Primary CNS lymphoma is the most common and may account for this complex of symptoms in 10 percent of AIDS patients.[31] A focal tuberculoma (*Mycobacterium tuberculosis*) becomes much more likely in patients with prior tubercular anergy and evidence of disseminated disease (e.g., Haitians, Africans, intravenous drug users). In one report of 420 patients, 52 had tuberculosis of some form and 10 of these patients had CNS involvement.[32] This type of involvement presents predominantly as cerebral abscess or tuberculomas.[33]

*Mycobacterium avium-intracellulare* has also been isolated from brain tissue, but its role in CNS disease has not been established. Rarely, focal abscesses may be caused by fungi; infections caused by cryptococcus, candida, and aspergillus have been seen, as have those caused by *Coccidioides immitis*. Bacterial brain abscesses do not appear to occur more frequently than in the general population, nor do those caused by *Nocardia asteroides*. Viral infections caused by papovavirus (progressive multifocal leukoencephalopathy), herpes simplex, and perhaps even the human immunodeficiency virus may occasionally present with focal disease.[34] In addition, there has been an increasing number of reports of toxoplasmic encephalitis that coexists with infections caused by other pathogens listed above.[29] Occasionally bacterial meningitis may present with focal neurologic signs without meningismus, especially when caused by *Listeria monocytogenes*.

## Diagnostic workup

Routine laboratory tests are of little value in establishing the diagnosis of toxoplasmic encephalitis. However, this disease is undoubtedly due to reactivation of latent infection, and thus the serologic tests for IgG antibody are usually positive and those for IgM invariably negative. Therefore, the absence of IgG antibody as measured by the Sabin-Feldman dye test or the immunofluorescence antibody test is strong evidence against a diagnosis of toxoplasmic encephalitis. Recent evidence suggests that intrathecal production of specific antibody to *T. gondii* may prove to be a useful diagnostic test for CNS infection.

When tuberculosis produces a mass lesion of the CNS, it is often a manifestation of disseminated disease involving the lungs, bone marrow, liver, and bloodstream. Examination of tissues from these organs may reveal the causative organisms. In addition, while anergy is common in AIDS patients with tuberculosis, 50 percent of patients in our series still had a positive skin test to 5 tu of intermediate-strength PPD (purified protein derivative).[2]

Lumbar puncture is of diagnostic value only insofar as to exclude other infections of the CSF. In 50 percent of patients with toxoplasmic encephalitis, the CSF protein level is slightly elevated, but glucose levels are normal, and 15 percent have a mild CSF lymphocytic pleocytosis. In some patients. *T. gondii* has been isolated by mouse inoculation of CSF.

**Imaging Studies.** Computerized axial tomography (CAT) scanning has proved extremely useful in diagnosing toxoplasmic encephalitis and is the most important diagnostic test. Typically, multiple, hypodense, ring-enhancing discrete lesions, often involving the basal ganglia, brainstem, or posterior fossa, are demonstrated (Fig. 57-2). Occasionally lesions are single or isodense, but, unlike those in patients with congenital toxoplasmosis, they are rarely calcified. Lymphomas, tuberculomas, and mycetomas caused by fungi are more likely to be seen on CAT scans as single lesions that involve the cerebral cortex. In patients with focal neurologic signs or evidence of intracranial hypertension, a CAT scan should be done prior to lumbar puncture.[35]

Occasionally the CAT scan is normal, but lesions may still be demonstrated by magnetic resonance imaging (MRI) scanning. It should be emphasized that both scanning techniques can be negative for discrete lesions in toxoplasmic encephalitis.

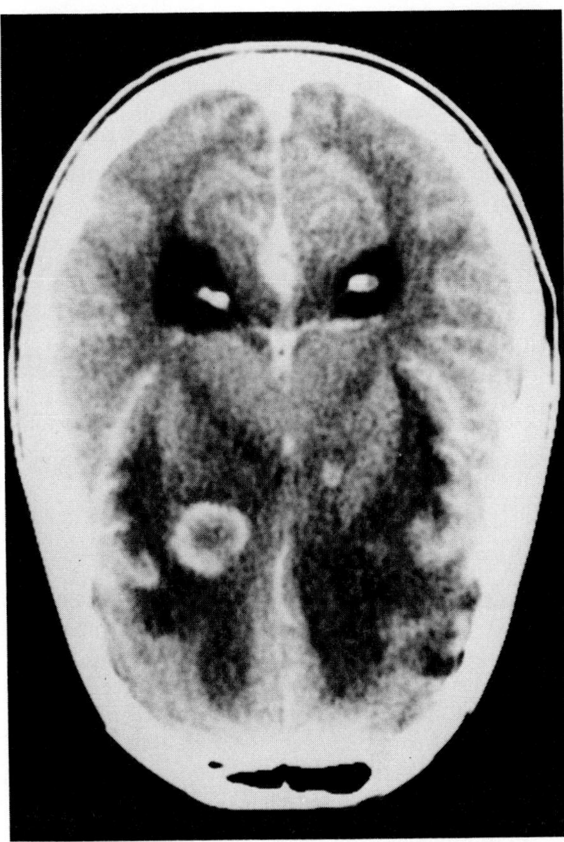

Fig. 57-2. Typical computed tomographic scan of patient with central nervous system toxoplasmosis showing ring-enhancing lesion.

**Brain Biopsy.** In patients with AIDS who have a positive IgG serology for toxoplasmal antibodies, focal neurologic findings, and multiple ring-enhancing lesions as seen by either CAT or MRI scanning technique, a presumptive diagnosis of toxoplasmosis can be made and medical therapy initiated. However, if the patient is atypical in presentation, has a negative serology, is in a high-risk group for other causes of focal CNS disease, or fails to respond to antitoxoplasmal therapy in 2 to 3 weeks, a brain biopsy should be performed.[35] Directed needle biopsy using a stereotaxic or CAT-scan-guided approach is recommended, and the tissue should be examined using both routine histopathologic and immunoperoxidase studies, as well as special stains for bacteria and fungi. Similarly, tissue should be cultured for aerobic and anaerobic bacteria, mycobacteria, and fungi. The number of organisms via needle biopsy may be small, and open excisional biopsy may eventually be necessary to establish the diagnosis.

## Therapy

At present the most effective therapy for toxoplasmic encephalitis in the AIDS patient is a combination of pyrimethamine (a dihydrofolate reductase inhibitor) and sulfadiazine or trisulfapyrimidine (a competitive inhibitor of dihydrofolate synthetase).[36] This combination acts synergistically against the infecting organisms by producing sequential blockade of folic acid metabolism. Dosages of 100 to 200 mg pyrimethamine (loading dose), then 75 to 100 mg per day orally *plus* 6 to 8 g sulfadiazine per day *plus* 10 to 50 mg folinic acid per day are recommended. However, this combination does not kill encysted toxoplasma, and, if therapy is discontinued, over 80 percent of patients will relapse, with the subsequent infection usually occurring in the same area of the brain as the initial infection. Thus, suppressive or maintenance therapy with the same combination in reduced dosages is recommended if it can be tolerated by the patient. In patients who cannot tolerate the sulfa drugs, clindamycin combined with pyrimethamine appears to be effective. To date these studies are anecdotal; clinical trials are ongoing.

## MENINGITIS

### Clinical presentation

The most common cause of meningitis in AIDS patients is *Cryptococcus neoformans*. Cryptococcal meningitis occurs in 5 to 10 percent of all patients with advanced HIV infection and is the presenting condition in 2 to 3 percent of patients. Cryptococcal meningitis may present either as an acute illness or in an indolent manner. Fever and persistent headache occur in 80 to 90 percent of cases, and when present in AIDS patients should always suggest the disease. Other signs that are typical of meningitis in the non-AIDS population are unusual: nausea and vomiting occur in less than 50 percent, meningismus in 30 percent, alteration in mental status or photophobia in 20 to 25 percent, and seizures or other focal neurologic findings in 10 percent.

Although *C. neoformans* is the most common cause of meningitis in patients with advanced HIV infection, other pathogens may also infect the CSF and the meninges. Disseminated pneumococcal infection occurs with a 50-fold increased frequency in AIDS patients and may produce a typical bacterial meningitis. Infection with *Haemophilus influenzae* may also occur. Meningitis caused by *Listeria monocytogenes* is surprisingly unusual, given the underlying defect in cellular immunity typical of HIV infection, but has occasionally been documented. As mentioned, disseminated tuberculosis is common in AIDS patients and is often accompanied by CNS involvement. Tuberculous meningitis is less common than a mass lesion (tuberculoma) but still needs to be considered in the differential diagnosis. *Mycobacterium avium*-complex organisms have been found in the CSF, but their relevance to clinical disease is controversial. Other fungi such as *Coccidioides immitis* and *Histoplasma* and some viruses, including herpes simplex and the human immunodeficiency virus, may invade the CSF. Involvement of the meninges with aggressive B-cell lymphoma may also produce an illness indistinguishable from meningitis.

### Diagnostic workup

Routine laboratory tests are of little value, although fungal culture of blood, sputum, or urine may occasionally yield *C. neoformans*. Extraneural cryptococcosis may accompany CNS disease and usually involves blood, bone marrow, the genitourinary tract, or the skin. Cryptococcal antigen in the blood can be detected in more than 95 percent of patients with cryptococcal meningitis, and elevated antigen titers may provide evidence of CNS infection. Titers of antibodies to cryptococcal antigen are typically very high, with a median of 1:400 (range, 1:4 to 1:100,000) being reported in one study.[37] Routine bacterial blood cultures will most likely be positive in cases of pneumococcal meningitis. Bacteremia was documented in 84 percent of AIDS patients with pneumococcal pneumonia at San Francisco General Hospital.[4]

A definitive diagnosis is most quickly established by examination of the CSF. The inflammatory response in cryptococcal meningitis is typically minimal.[38] In our study of 89 patients with cryptococcal meningitis the median cell count was 7 cells per cubic millimeter (range, 0 to 700) with greater than 90 percent lymphocytes. The median CSF glucose level was 47 mg per deciliter (range, 7 to 114), the median CSF protein level 54 mg per deciliter (range, 14 to 300). Seventy to eighty percent of these patients had a positive India ink preparation on direct smear of the CSF. Ninety-five percent had positive cryptococcal antigen titers (mean titer 1:177), and cultures were positive for the fungus in 99 percent of the patients.[39]

When the cryptococcal antigen test is negative, tuberculosis becomes a more likely diagnosis, but AFB smears of the CSF are rarely positive (approximately 10 percent in the non-AIDS population).[40] If examination of the CSF reveals a more intense inflammatory response with a predominance of polymorphonuclear leukocytes or a reduction in CSF glucose to levels less than 50 percent of simultaneous serum levels, a bacterial infection (e.g., infections caused by *Streptococcus pneumoniae*, *H. influenzae*, *L. monocytogenes*) should be strongly considered. Direct Gram stains of CSF are usually positive with pneumococcal and hemophilus infections, but *Listeria* is difficult to find when meningitis is caused by this gram-positive bacillus. Definitive diagnosis can be established by routine bacterial cultures.

**Imaging Studies.** Ideally, any patient with HIV infection and central neurologic dysfunction should first undergo CAT or MRI because of the possibility of a space-occupying lesion (see above). In patients with cryptococcal meningitis, imaging studies are usually normal or demonstrate nonspecific abnormalities such as cortical atrophy or ventricular enlargement. Occasionally AIDS patients with cryptococcal meningitis will have coexistent mass lesions (cryptococcomas).[37]

### Therapy

As with other opportunistic infections in patients with advanced HIV disease, therapy of cryptococcal meningitis is associated with high failure and relapse rates. No single regimen has been carefully evaluated for efficacy or toxicity, but most U.S. investigators use amphotericin (0.5 to 0.7 mg/kg per day) with or without 5-flucytosine (5FC, 75 to 100 mg/kg per day). Because of accelerated 5FC-associated bone marrow toxicity in AIDS patients, many clinicians use amphotericin alone. The bone marrow toxicity can probably be reduced by using lower doses of 5FC (less than 100 mg/kg per day) and maintaining serum levels between 50 and 100 μg/ml. There seems to be no improvement in response rate with the addition of the second drug.[39] Recent studies document about a 70 to 80 percent initial response to amphotericin, but up to 50 percent of patients will relapse if therapy is discontinued after 6 to 10 weeks.[38] Therefore, maintenance therapy with either amphotericin (1 mg/kg per week) or an imidazole is usually used. At San Francisco General Hospital maintenance therapy consisting of either amphotericin or ketoconazole (200 to 400 mg daily) was associated with a significant increase in survival as compared with survival of patients whose therapy was discontinued. Fluconazole, a new imidazole oral drug with increased activity against *Cryptococcus* and excellent penetration into the CSF, has been used successfully in Europe and is currently undergoing testing in the United States.

Bacterial meningitis in AIDS patients appears to respond to conventional antimicrobial therapy; suppressive or maintenance therapy is not required. The need for maintenance therapy after conventional therapy for HIV-infected patients with tuberculosis has not yet been established.

## GASTROINTESTINAL TRACT

The gastrointestinal tract is a major target organ system for both opportunistic and conventional pathogens in patients with AIDS and ARC. Distinguishing among the wide array of infections, solid tumors, and other malignancies likely to complicate HIV infection presents a difficult clinical challenge. Typical infections caused by conventional gastrointestinal pathogens, atypical presentations of conventional pathogens, and opportunistic infections must be included in the differential diagnosis of many gastrointestinal symptoms and signs. Some infections are more common in certain patient populations than are others; e.g., homosexual men with a history of multiple sexual partners are more likely to be infected with enteric bacterial pathogens and protozoa than are other patients. Evaluating the pathogenicity of a particular agent identified in culture is complicated by the frequent detection of more than one potential etiologic agent and the high prevalence of asymptomatic colonization with potential pathogens. For this reason, evidence of tissue invasion is required to definitively diagnose the etiology of diarrhea caused by many organisms.

Ideally, diagnostic and management strategies should be directed toward identifying specific treatable conditions with a minimum of morbidity. Although a careful history and physical examination will often localize the pathology to a specific site or organ, objective and often invasive studies usually are required to establish the etiology. The decision to include invasive procedures or extensive radiologic evaluation in the diagnostic approach should be based on a careful assessment of the severity of the patient's condition, the likelihood of identifying a treatable condition, and the overall impact of treatment on the patient's quality of life.

## INFECTIONS OF THE ORAL CAVITY

Oral infections are among the most common clinical manifestations of immunodeficiency in HIV disease. Often oral lesions are the first sign of HIV infection to be recognized by the patient and serve as the stimulus for seeking medical or dental consultation. Because most of these infections are associated with immunodeficiency, their presence is of significant prognostic importance to the patient and care provider. In many cases, development of oral opportunistic infection is the harbinger of impending progression to AIDS.

Painful white lesions in the oral mucosa are usually caused by *Candida albicans* infection. Pseudomembranous candidiasis (thrush) is one of the earliest clinical signs of immunodeficiency and is nearly ubiquitous in patients with severe immune impairment[41] (see Plate 61). Oral candidiasis may also present as red lesions on the tongue and palate (atrophic candidiasis), angular cheilitis, and bilateral white and red lesions on the buccal mucosa (chronic hypertrophic candidiasis).

Candidiasis must be distinguished from hairy leukoplakia (see below) and other white lesions of the oral mucosa (see Plate 62). The diganosis can be established by scraping the surface of lesions with a tongue depressor and examining the material obtained microscopically in a wet mount prepared with 10 percent potassium hydroxide. The presence of hyphae distinguishes infection from colonization. Fungal cultures are rarely indicated or helpful.

Treatment of oral candidiasis should be based on symptoms. Topical regimens [clotrimazole troches (10 mg 4 to 6 h) or nystatin vaginal tablets tid] provide symptomatic relief in most patients, although infection usually recurs or progresses when treatment is discontinued. Systemic therapy with oral antifungal agents (ketoconazole 200 mg qid to 200 mg bid) should be reserved for symptomatic patients with infections refractory to topical regimens.

Painless white plaques on the lateral margins of the tongue and other mucosal sites typify hairy leukoplakia, an oral condition unrecognized prior to the AIDS epidemic[42] (Plate 62). The lesions are usually raised and corrugated and can be easily confused with candidiasis. Biopsy and histopathologic examination is necessary to distinguish these lesions from other causes of leukoplakia.

Establishing a definitive diagnosis may be of substantial prognostic importance since hairy leukoplakia seems to be a reliable marker of moderate to severe immune dysfunction.[43] The appearance of this condition may immediately precede the development of AIDS. Diagnosing hairy leukoplakia in patients without a prior history of HIV infection should stimulate a search for evidence of HIV and immunodeficiency.

The etiology of hairy leukoplakia is not completely defined, but it appears to be a viral infection related to simultaneous Epstein-Barr virus and papillomavirus infection.[44] No treatment is of proved benefit. Fortunately the majority of lesions are asymptomatic.

A variety of viruses produce mucosal lesions in HIV-infected patients. The lesions of recurrent herpes simplex virus (HSV) gingivostomatitis are usually indistinguishable from those found in immunocompetent patients, although large ulcerations, secondary infections, and slow healing have been described.[45] Recurrent HSV involves only the keratinized oral epithelium (hard palate and gingiva) and therefore can be easily distinguished from recurrent oral apthous ulcers which involve nonkeratinized epithelium.[46] Virus cultures inoculated with fluid from a fresh unroofed vesicle will confirm the etiology in most cases. Diagnostic tests employing monoclonal antibodies can distinguish HSV type 1 from HSV type 2 but rarely contribute to clinical management.

Oral therapy with acyclovir (200 mg 5 times daily until all lesions have crusted) is effective in promoting healing of HSV. Parenteral acyclovir (5 mg/kg q 8 h IV with adjustment for renal function) should be reserved for patients with severe, refractory, nonhealing, or progressive disease. Chronic oral suppressive acyclovir therapy (200 mg tid to 400 mg bid) is usually efficacious for indolent or frequently recurring episodes, although resistant thymidine kinase-deficient strains may emerge.[47] If acyclovir resistance is documented, therapy should be temporarily discontinued.

Mucocutaneous varicella zoster virus (VZV) infection (shingles) in a trigeminal nerve distribution is another viral complication seen in immunodeficient HIV-infected patients (Plate 63). The oral lesions frequently coalesce to form large ulcers which may be extremely painful. The diagnosis is made on clinical grounds when typical dermatomal skin and mucosal lesions are seen in varying stages of development. However, dermatomal HSV can occasionally be confused with VZV. Because the treatment for these two infections differs (below), identifying the specific viral etiology is of some importance when treatment is required. Fluorescein-labeled monoclonal antibody techniques can rapidly identify VZV antigens in scrapings of the lesion.[48] Virus culture of VZV is not sensitive and is primarily performed to exclude HSV.

Severe zoster, ophthalmic zoster, and disseminated zoster should be treated with intravenous acyclovir (10 mg/kg q 8 h until lesions are crusted, with adjustment for renal function). Steroids for postherpetic neuralgia are of no proved benefit in AIDS and should be avoided.

Gingivitis is a recently recognized complication of HIV infection. In general, the severity of gingival inflammation parallels the severity of immunosuppression, although the exact microbial etiology of the condition has not been ascertained. Acute necrotizing ulcerative gingivitis is diagnosed clinically by the presence of severe gingival inflammation with ulcerations, bleeding, and halitosis.[46] Cervical lymphadenopathy may also be evident. The most severe form may be complicated by cellulitis and osteomyelitis. Treatment requires debridement. Mouth rinses containing dilute chlorhexidine may be effective.[46] The potential benefit of oral antibiotics for treatment or secondary prophylaxis has not been established.

Sexually transmitted diseases such as syphilis and gonorrhea produce oral symptoms and signs in HIV-infected patients identical to those in immunocompetent patients. Since these infections are prevalent in patients at risk for HIV, appropriate diagnostic tests should be performed whenever compatible history or clinical findings are present.

## ESOPHAGITIS

Esophagitis is suspected in patients who complain of odynophagia or dysphagia. Invasive *C. albicans* is the most common etiologic organism but herpes simplex and cytomegalovirus (CMV) ulcerations have been implicated. Esophageal candidiasis usually does not respond to topical antifungal agents but will improve with oral ketoconazole (200 to 600 mg qd). Amphotericin should be reserved for patients who fail oral treatment.[48]

An empiric trial of ketoconazole is a rational management strategy in patients with AIDS and mild to moderate symptoms, particularly when oral thrush is also present. Endoscopic biopsy is recommended to confirm the diagnosis when candidal esophagitis is the initial diagnostic criterion for AIDS. Brushings should be cultured for *Candida,* HSV, and CMV. The presence of these organisms in cultures is not sufficient proof of infection in the absence of tissue invasion on biopsy specimens. Double-contrast barium swallow radiograms is neither a sensitive nor a specific test for determining the etiology of esophagitis in this setting.

Herpes simplex esophagitis is diagnosed by the presence of shallow ulcerations or discrete vesicles. Tissue from the periphery of the lesions should be examined for the presence of epithelial cell invasion and nuclear changes. Cultures should also be obtained. Acyclovir (200 mg orally five times daily or 5 mg/kg q 8 h IV) will promote healing and resolution of symptoms.[49]

A diagnosis of CMV esophagitis is made when other etiologies are excluded and diffuse esophagitis or a single large necrotic ulceration is seen on endoscopy. Vasculitis is apparent in tissue biopsy samples. Cytomegalovirus esophagitis should never be diagnosed on the basis of culture alone since CMV is commonly detected as a commensual organism in HIV-infected patients. More than 50 percent of patients will respond to treatment with ganciclovir (10 to 15 mg/kg per day IV in 2 to 3 divided doses for 10 to 14 days), currently an investigational antiviral agent. Long-term maintenance with ganciclovir (4 to 7 mg/kg 5 to 7 days per week) is required in the vast majority of patients to prevent relapse.[49]

## HEPATOBILIARY INFECTIONS

Parenchymal liver disease in HIV-infected patients, manifested by hepatomegaly and sometimes jaundice, may be due to a large number of pathophysiologic processes including infection, lymphoma, Kaposi's sarcoma, and drug toxicity. The diagnostic evaluation should be directed toward excluding extrahepatic disease and identifying treatable conditions. Liver function tests, hepatitis B serologic tests, ultrasonography, and abdominal CT scanning will usually localize the problem but often fail to identify the specific etiology.

Liver biopsy is abnormal in nearly all patients with AIDS but only rarely identifies a specific etiology not evident elsewhere.[50] It is most useful for diagnosing symptomatic disease when a treatable etiology is suspected which has not been identified by less invasive measures.

*M. avium-intracellulare* is the most common infection associated with hepatic parenchymal disease in AIDS. Acid-fast bacilli identified in noncaseating granulomas accompanied by extreme elevations of alkaline phosphatase are clues to the diagnosis. *M. tuberculosis,* histoplasmosis, cryptococcosis, other fungal infections, and syphilis may also produce granulomatous lesions. Eosinophilic granulomas suggest drug-induced liver toxicity. Cytomegalovirus causes hepatitis in a small number of AIDS patients. Intranuclear inclusions and other histopathologic changes and not CMV culture results should be used to diagnose this infection. The efficacy of ganciclovir for CMV hepatitis has not been established.

Papillary stenosis with sclerosing cholangitis is a frequent cause of fever, abdominal pain, and extreme alkaline phosphatase elevation in AIDS patients.[51] Patchy dilation of intrahepatic and extrahepatic biliary ducts is seen on cholangiogram. Papillotomy during ERCP will relieve symptoms in many patients. The etiology of this condition is unknown, although opportunistic pathogens such as *Cryptosporidium, M. avium-intracelullare,* and cytomegalovirus are often cultured from the bile and intestinal tract in these patients.

## INTESTINAL INFECTIONS

Diarrhea and weight loss are found in more than 50 percent of patients with AIDS and are also frequently present in those with less severe clinical manifestations of immunodeficiency. The profound wasting which characterizes many severely ill AIDS patients is usually associated with diarrhea and may have a treatable etiology. The wide range of infections, neoplasms, and inflammatory processes which produce these symptoms presents a difficult problem to the clinician. However, as with other clinical syndromes in AIDS, the approach to the patient with diarrheal illness can be simplified by emphasizing the identification of treatable etiologies and avoiding unnecessary invasive procedures.

### Enteric bacterial pathogens

*Salmonella, Shigella,* and *Campylobacter* are more prevalent in homosexual men than in age-matched heterosexual men, even in the absence of evidence for immunodeficiency. Thus, these agents are the most frequent treatable causes of diarrhea in HIV-infected homosexual men. Symptoms range from mild diarrhea to severe dysentery. Bacteremia due to these enteric pathogens is common in febrile immunosuppressed HIV-infected patients, and blood cultures often help to establish an early diagnosis.[52]

Antimicrobial treatment of diagnosed enteric bacterial pathogens in HIV-infected patients is indicated. Parenteral therapy is recommended for initial management of bacteremic patients. Most will have a prompt symptomatic and microbiologic response to treatment. Long-term management is complicated by a high incidence of drug toxicity, relapses, recurrences, and emergence of resistant organisms. The rate of recurrences may be reduced in patients receiving suppressive doses of maintenance antibiotic therapy. The newer quinolones appear to be especially useful agents in this regard. Preliminary experience indicates that ciprofloxacin (750 mg orally bid) is an excellent empiric drug for diarrhea when *Salmonella, Shigella,* or *Campylobacter* enteritis is suspected.[53] AIDS and ARC patients receiving maintenance therapy (750 mg orally qd) have had few documented recurrences and minimal drug toxicity. Controlled clinical trials will be necessary to establish the utility of this approach in larger populations of patients and to evaluate the emergence of resistant organisms after long-term use.

## *C. difficile*-associated diarrhea

Pseudomembranous enterocolitis due to *C. difficile* cytotoxins should be considered in patients with diarrhea following antibacterial treatment. The sensitivity and specificity of identifying *C. difficile* toxin in stool specimens is disputed, but a positive test is strong evidence in favor of the diagnosis in a compatible clinical setting. Sigmoidoscopy to identify and biopsy pseudomembranes in the distal colon is useful when the diagnosis is uncertain and symptoms are severe. Oral treatment with vancomycin or metronidazole is usually effective if antibiotics can be discontinued. A trial of parenteral metronidazole in patients with extremely rapid intestinal transit times who fail oral reigmens may be of benefit.

## Parasitic infections

Protozoal infections are also common causes of diarrhea in HIV-infected patients. At least three stool specimens should be examined to identify ova or parasites. A saline wet mount of liquid stool may demonstrate trophozoites of *Entamoeba histolytica* or *Giardia lamblia*. Stool preserved in formalin or polyvinyl alcohol and stained with iron hematoxylin or trichrome often demonstrates the cysts of these organisms and can be used with formed stool where trophozoites are rarely detected. These infections respond to conventional therapeutic regimens. Extraintestinal amebiasis is distinctly uncommon in AIDS.

Immunosuppressed HIV-infected patients may be colonized with *Cryptosporidium,* but this organism is also associated with severe diarrhea and contributes to the wasting syndrome in many patients. Modified acid-fast stains for *Cryptosporidium* oocytes should be performed on stool from all patients with diarrhea. In cases of severe or persistent diarrhea of uncertain etiology, a mucosal biopsy may sometimes demonstrate *Cryptosporidium* when stool examinations are negative. Cryptosporidial infection in AIDS is refractory to therapy.[54] Numerous chemotherapeutic agents including metronidazole, quinidine-clindamycin, and pentamidine have been tried in an attempt to eradicate or suppress symptoms but have met with little success. Spiramycin, a macrolide antibiotic, has been useful in a small subset of patients and is relatively nontoxic. Supportive care directed toward decreasing intestinal motility, maintaining fluid and electrolyte balance, and parenteral alimentation is indicated.

Oocytes of *Isospora belli* and Charcot-Leyden crystals are also identified in AIDS patients with diarrhea. Multiple stool samples may be necessary to diagnosis isosporiasis when oocytes are shed intermittently. Trimethoprim-sulfamethoxazole is effective in eliminating symptoms in the majority of patients and appears to be effective in preventing recurrences in the minority of patients able to tolerate chronic administration.[55]

## Mycobacteria

*Mycobacterium avium-intracellulare* (MAI) often colonizes the colonic mucosa in AIDS patients and can be readily identified in acid-fast stains of stool. Presumptive diagnosis is confirmed by the presence of PAS-positive macrophages in biopsy specimens and by stool culture. MAI can be distinguished from Whipple's disease by acid-fast staining. The etiologic role of MAI in diarrheal disease in AIDS patients and the indications for treating MAI remain controversial.[56] Although many regimens have been evaluated, none have proved to be effective in altering long-term outcome. Some clinicians have had limited success in reducing symptoms of MAI infection in selected patients and advocate a trial of palliative therapy.

*M. tuberculosis* infection of the gut may be seen in AIDS patients with multisystem extrapulmonary infection and should be managed with conventional regimens.

## CMV infection

Discrete shallow ulcerations of the intestinal mucosa accompanied by submucosal hemorrhages and vasculitis suggest CMV infection.[56] Biopsies of the margins of lesions should be obtained for histopathologic evaluation and culture. As is true for other sites in the gastrointestinal tract, cytomegalovirus should not be considered etiologic on the basis of a positive culture in the absence of focal histopathology. In a minority of patients, large CMV ulcerations may lead to bowel necrosis and intestinal perforation.

Many patients with CMV colitis appear to respond to treatment with ganciclovir and may have extended symptom-free intervals when the drug is administered chronically.[57]

## HIV enteropathy

Small-bowel enteropathy due to HIV infection in the absence of other pathology has recently been reported. HIV has been identified by in situ hybridization in the lamina propria of small-bowel biopsy specimens.[58] Intracellular viruslike particles, lymphocytic infiltrates, nonspecific inflammatory changes, and villous atrophy have also been observed. Identification of HIV RNA in enterochromaffin cells has led to speculations that diarrhea in AIDS may be related to neurogenic peptide production. The response of this form of enteropathy to azidothymidine and other antiviral agents has not yet been systematically evaluated.

## Noninfectious causes of diarrhea in AIDS

Kaposi's sarcoma, carcinomas, lymphoma, and idiopathic inflammatory bowel disease produce clinical syndromes indistinguishable from infectious diarrhea in HIV-infected patients. Proctosigmoidoscopy is extremely valuable in diagnosing these disorders and is therefore recommended when an infectious etiology has not been established.

### Evaluation of diarrhea in HIV-infected patients

Systematic evaluation will often identify a treatable infectious cause of diarrhea in HIV-infected patients. Despite the tendency for recurrences, the majority of patients will respond to anti-infective therapy. Initial evaluation should include a thorough history and physical examination including anoscopy. Stool samples should be examined for fecal leukocytes and cultured for *Salmonella, Shigella,* and *Campylobacter*. If no etiology is determined from these tests, a stool for ova and parasites (including a modified acid-fast stain for *Cryptosporidium*) should be performed.

Invasive diagnostic procedures are often required to diagnose the etiology of diarrhea when stool examination is negative or when symptoms of proctocolitis are present. Proctosigmoidoscopy and colonoscopy allow direct visualization of the bowel mucosa and directed biopsy of focal lesions, and are extremely useful adjuvants to noninvasive modalities.

Small-bowel biopsy is indicated when stool evaluation and lower intestinal endoscopy fail to reveal a diagnosis, especially when symptoms suggest small-bowel involvement. Multiple biopsies can be obtained with either oral capsule techniques or fiberoptic endoscopy.

### PROCTITIS

Herpes simplex virus causes most cases of ulcerative proctitis in HIV-infected patients and can usually be diagnosed by direct IFA or by culture. Oral or parenteral therapy with acyclovir is usually efficacious, but recurrences are anticipated. Oral suppressive regimens are appropriate in patients with frequent or chronic indolent episodes. Chlamydial and gonococcal cultures should also be performed in sexually active homosexual patients with symptoms of proctitis (see Chap. 55).

## References


1 Murray JF et al: Pulmonary complications of the acquired immunodeficiency syndrome: Report of a National Heart, Lung, and Blood Institute Workshop. *N Engl J Med* 310:1682, 1984.

2 Chaisson RE et al: Tuberculosis in patients with the acquired immunodeficiency syndrome: Clinical features, responses to therapy, and survival. *Am Rev Respir Dis* 136:570, 1987.

3 Handwerger S et al: Tuberculosis and the acquired immunodeficiency syndrome at a New York City hospital: 1978–1985. *Chest* 91:176, 1987.

4 Gerberding JL et al: Recurrent bacteremic infection with *S. pneumoniae* in patients with AIDS virus infection. Programs and Abstracts of the 26th Interscience Conference on Antimicrobial Agents and Chemotherapy, American Society for Microbiology, 1986, p 177.

5 Medina I et al: Serum lactate dehydrogenase levels in *Pneumocystis carinii* pneumonia in AIDS: Possible indicator and predictor of disease activity. *Proc III Int Conf AIDS* 3:109, 1987.

6 Hopewell PC: Diagnosis of *Pneumocystis carinii* pneumonia, in *The Medical Management of AIDS*, MA Sande, PA Volberding (eds). Philadelphia, Saunders, 1988, p 177.

7 Curtis J et al: Noninvasive tests in the diagnostic evaluation for *P. carinii* pneumonia in patients with or suspected of having AIDS. *Am Rev Respir Dis* 133:A182, 1986.

8 Davis SD et al: Intrathoracic Kaposi sarcoma in AIDS patients: Radiographic-pathologic correlation. *Radiology* 163:495, 1987.

9 Coleman DL et al: Correlation between serial pulmonary function tests and fiberoptic bronchoscopy in patients with *Pneumocystis carinii* pneumonia and the acquired immune deficiency syndrome. *Am Rev Respir Dis* 129:491, 1984.

10 Coleman DL et al: Gallium lung scanning in patients with suspected pneumonia and the acquired immunodeficiency syndrome. *Am Rev Respir Dis* 130:1166, 1984.

11 Bigby T et al: The usefulness of sputum induction in the diagnosis of *Pneumocystis carinii* pneumonia in patients with the acquired immunodeficiency syndrome. *Am Rev Respir Dis* 135:422, 1986.

12 Pitchenik et al: Sputum examination for the diagnosis of *Pneumocystis carinii* pneumonia in the acquired immunodeficiency syndrome. *Am Rev Respir Dis* 133:226, 1986.

13 Kovacs JA et al: Diagnosis of *Pneumocystis carinii* pneumonia: Improved detection in sputum with use of monoclonal antibodies. *N Engl J Med* 318:589, 1988.

14 Broaddus VC et al: Bronchoalveolar lavage and transbronchial biopsy for diagnosis of pulmonary infections in patients with the acquired immunodeficiency syndrome. *Ann Intern Med* 102:747, 1985.

15 Coleman DL et al: Diagnostic utility of fiberoptic bronchoscopy in patients with *Pneumocystis carinii* pneumonia and the acquired immunodeficiency syndrome. *Am Rev Respir Dis* 128:795, 1983.

16 Centers for Disease Control: AIDS weekly surveillance report—United States. *MMWR* Oct 12, 1987.

17 Wharton JM et al: Trimethoprim-sulfamethoxazole or pentamidine for *Pneumocystis carinii* pneumonia in the acquired immunodeficiency syndrome: A prospective, randomized, controlled trial. *Ann Intern Med* 105:37, 1986.

18 Allegra CJ et al: Trimetrexate, a novel and effective agent for treatment of *Pneumocystis carinii* pneumonia in patients with the acquired immunodeficiency syndrome. *N Engl J Med* 317:978, 1987.

19 Millar AB: Respiratory manifestations of AIDS. *Br J Hosp Med* 39:204, 1988.

20 Stahl-Bayliss CM et al: Pentamidine-induced hypoglycemia in patients with the acquired immune deficiency syndrome. *Clin Pharmacol Ther* 39:271, 1986.

21 Zuger A et al: Pentamidine-associated fatal acute pancreatitis. *JAMA* 256:2383, 1986.

22 Loescher T et al: Severe ventricular arrhythmia during pentamidine treatment of AIDS-associated *Pneumocystis carinii* pneumonia (letter). *Infection* 15:455, 1987.

23 Conte JE Jr et al: Inhaled or reduced-dose intravenous pentamidine for *Pneumocystis carinii* pneumonia. *Ann Intern Med* 107:495, 1987.

24 Montgomery AB et al: Aerosolized pentamidine as sole therapy for pneumocystis pneumonia in patients with acquired immunodeficiency syndrome. *Lancet* II:480, 1987.

25 Masur H, Kovacs JA: Treatment and prophylaxis of *Pneumocystis carinii* pneumonia, in *The Medical Management of AIDS*, MA Sande, PA Volberding (eds). Philadelphia, Saunders, 1988, p 181.

26 Fischl MA et al: Safety and efficacy of sulfamethoxazole and trimethoprim chemoprophylaxis for *Pneumocystis carinii* pneumonia in AIDS. *JAMA* 259:1185, 1988.

27 O'Brien RJ et al: Rifabutin (ansamycin LM 427): A new rifamycin-S derivative for the treatment of mycobacterial diseases. *Rev Infect Dis* 9:519, 1987.

28 Young LS: *Mycobacterium-avium* complex infection. *J Infect Dis* 157:863, 1988.

29 Luft BJ, Remington JS: Toxoplasmic encephalitis. *J Infect Dis* 157:1, 1988.

30 Clement MJ et al: Clinical manifestations of toxoplasmosis in AIDS: Experience at UCSF-affiliated hospitals (in preparation).

31 De La Paz RL, Enzman D: Neuroradiology of acquired immunodeficiency syndrome, in *AIDS and the Nervous System*, ML Rosenblum et al (eds). New York, Raven, 1988.

32 Bishburg E et al: Central nervous system tuberculosis with acquired immunodeficiency syndrome and its related complex. *Ann Intern Med* 105:210, 1986.

33 Sunderman G et al: Tuberculosis as a manifestation of the acquired immunodeficiency syndrome. *JAMA* 256:362, 1988.

34 Price RW, Brew B: Management of the neurologic complications of HIV infection and AIDS, in *The Medical Management of AIDS*, MA Sande, PA Volberding (eds). Philadelphia, Saunders, 1988, p 111.

35 Gerberding JL: Diagnosis and management of cereberal toxoplasmosis in patients with acquired immunodeficiency syndrome, in *Contemporary Issues in Infectious Diseases*, vol 7: *Parasitic Infections*, JH Leech et al (eds). New York, Churchill Livingstone, 1988, p 271.

36 Israelski D, Remington JS: Toxoplasmic encephalitis in patients with AIDS, in *The Medical Management of AIDS*, MA Sande, PA Volberding (eds). Philadelphia, Saunders, 1988, p 193.

37 Zuger A et al: Cryptococcal disease in patients with AIDS. *Ann Intern Med* 104:234, 198.

38 Dismukes WE: Cryptococcal meningitis in patients with AIDS. *J Infect Dis* 157:624, 1988.

39 Chuck SL, Sande MA: Cryptococcal infections in patients with acquired immunodeficiency syndrome. Submitted to *N Engl J Med*, February 1989.

40 Kennedy DH, Fallon R: Tuberculous meningitis. *JAMA* 241:269, 1979.

41 Klein RS et al: Oral candidiasis in high-risk patients as the initial manifestation of the acquired immunodeficiency syndrome. *N Engl J Med* 311:354, 1984.

42 Hollander H et al: Hairy leukoplakia and the acquired immunodeficiency syndrome. *Ann Intern Med* 104:892, 1986.

43 Greenspan D et al: Relation of oral hairy leukoplakia to infection with the human immunodeficiency virus and the risk of developing AIDS. *J Infect Dis* 155:475, 1987.

44 Greenspan D et al: Oral "hairy" leukoplakia in male homosexuals: Evidence of association with both papillomavirus and a herpes-group virus. *Lancet* II:831, 1984.

45 Quinnan GV et al: Herpes simplex infections in the acquired immunodeficiency syndrome. *JAMA* 252:72, 1984.

46 Greenspan D: Oral manifestations of HIV infection and AIDS, in *The Medical Management of AIDS*, MA Sande, PA Volberding (eds). Philadelphia, Saunders, 1988, p 127.

47 Collins P: Viral sensitivity following the introduction of acyclovir. *Am J Med* 85:129, 1988.

48 Tavitian A et al: Ketoconazole-resistant *Candida* esophagitis in patients with acquired immunodeficiency syndrome. *Gastroenterology* 90:443, 1986.

49 Drew WL et al: Herpesvirus infections (caused by cytomegalovirus, herpes simplex virus, varicella-zoster virus): How to use ganciclovir (DHPG) and acyclovir, in *The Medical Management of AIDS*, MA Sande, PA Volberding (eds). Philadelphia, Saunders, 1988, p 271.

50 Schneiderman DJ et al: Hepatic disease in patients with acquired immunodeficiency syndrome. *Hepatology* 7:925, 1987.

51 Schneiderman DJ et al: Papillary stenosis and sclerosing cholangitis in the acquired immunodeficiency syndrome. *Ann Intern Med* 106: 546, 1987.

52 Celum C et al: Incidence of salmonellosis in patients with AIDS. *J Infect Dis* 156:998, 1987.

53 Jacobson MA et al: Ciprofloxacin therapy of breakthrough salmonella bacteremia in patients with the acquired immunodeficiency syndrome. *Ann Intern Med*, in press July 1989.

54 Navin TR, Hardy AM: Cryptosporidiosis in patients with AIDS. *J Infect Dis* 155:150, 1987.

55 DeHovitz JA et al: Clinical manifestations and therapy of *Isospora belli* infection in patients with the acquired immunodeficiency syndrome. *N Engl J Med* 315:87, 1986.

56 Cello JP: Gastrointestinal manifestations of AIDS, in *The Medical Management of AIDS*, MA Sande, PA Volberding (eds). Philadelphia, Saunders, 1988, p 141.

57 Koretz SH, Collaborative DHPG Treatment Study Group: Treatment of serious cytomegalovirus infections with 9-(1,3 dihydroxy-2-propoxymethyl) guanine in patients with AIDS and other immunodeficiencies. *N Engl J Med* 314:801, 1986.

58 Nelson JA et al: Human immunodeficiency virus detected in bowel epithelium from patients with gastrointestinal symptoms. *Lancet* I:259, 1988.

# Chapter 58

# Generalized rash

Eric Sandström
Philip Kirby

## INTRODUCTION

In general practice, cutaneous manifestations of STDs are important in the differential diagnosis of generalized rash. In the STD clinic, where multiple STDs often coexist in a single patient, a full clinical history and examination of the entire skin surface, including the oropharynx, not just that portion of the skin seen between the waist and the knees, may give valuable diagnostic clues. This is particularly true since the advent of human immunodeficiency virus (HIV) infection. In addition, some rashes, although not caused by sexually transmitted diseases, are frequently seen in the STD clinic. At times a skin biopsy will be of decisive help. Three- to 4-mm punch biopsies can be performed with minimal discomfort, without need for suturing. An attempt should be made to obtain samples of the most recent lesions as, with time, nonspecific reactions tend to blur the original histopathologic pattern.

The early syphilogists realized that not all rashes were caused by syphilis, and gradually accumulated an increased knowledge of other dermatologic disorders. Within dermatovenereology, the once dominant syphilis has declined in importance to a less prominent role as the "great imitator." Over the last few years the importance of venereology relative to the other aspects of dermatology is again increasing because of infections caused by HIV.

The differential diagnosis of generalized rashes in the STD clinic may be approached in many different ways, but for the nondermatologist, morphologic classification of lesions is most useful. An effort should be made to characterize the "primary lesion" in any rash, which is the initial alteration in the appearance of the skin before it is modified by external influences or time. In this way, a rash may be classified as "macular" if the primary alteration in the skin is in color without change in texture or surface contour. A "papular" rash consists of solid elevations in the skin surface irrespective of color or texture, while a "vesicular" or "pustular" rash is dominated by clear or purulent liquid material. After the primary lesion is characterized, secondary changes should be noted such as excoriation, superinfection, or the effects of prior attempts at therapy. The distribution of lesions of the skin should also be noted, as well as the orientation of individual lesions to one another, i.e., linear, grouped.

Syphilis continues to have a central position in any overview of skin rash in the context of STD. It is important to include syphilis in the differential diagnosis of a skin rash and to perform a serologic test for syphilis. Host responses to the spirochete result in a plethora of clinical manifestations (see Chap. 20) that often resemble other skin diseases. As outlined in Table 58-1, we will present a differential diagnosis of skin rashes by clinical appearance, emphasizing those which pose special problems in differentiation from syphilis, and then discuss cutaneous findings in HIV infection.

**Table 58-1. An Approach to Differential Diagnoses of Common Generalized Rashes, Based upon Lesion Morphology**

I. Differential diagnosis of macular and papular rash
   A. Roseolar rash of syphilis
   B. Viral exanthems
   C. Drug reaction
   D. Lyme disease
   E. Erythema multiforme
   F. Hepatitis B
   G. Toxic shock syndrome
   H. Scabies
II. Differential diagnosis of papulosquamous rash
   A. Psoriasis
   B. Lichen planus
   C. Pityriasis rosea
   D. Reiter's syndrome
   E. Dermatophytosis
   F. Atopic dermatitis
III. Differential diagnosis of pustules and crusts
   A. Syphilis
   B. Folliculitis/impetigo
   C. Pustular psoriasis
   D. "ID" reaction
   E. Ectoparasites
IV. Differential diagnosis of hypopigmentation
   A. Syphilis
   B. Vitiligo
   C. Tinea versicolor
   D. Postinflammatory hypopigmentation
V. Differential diagnosis of vasculitis
   A. Gonococcemia
   B. Meningococcemia
   C. Syphilis
VI. Dermatologic findings in human immunodeficiency virus infection
   A. Acute exanthem of HIV infection
   B. Cutaneous infection complicating HIV infection
      1. Bacterial infection
         a. *Mycobacterium avium-intracellulare*
         b. Impetigo
      2. Fungal infection
         a. Candidiasis
         b. Dermatophytosis
         c. Cryptococcosis
         d. Histoplasmosis
      3. Viral infection
         a. Herpes simplex
         b. Herpes zoster
         c. Molluscum contagiosum
         d. Oral hairy leukoplakia
   C. Dermatoses
      1. Seborrheic dermatitis
      2. Xeroderma
      3. Papular eruption of AIDS
      4. Eosinophilic pustular folliculitis
      5. Scabies
      6. Psoriasis
      7. Yellow nail syndrome
   D. Tumors
      1. Kaposi's sarcoma
      2. Squamous cell carcinoma

## DIFFERENTIAL DIAGNOSIS OF MACULAR AND PAPULAR RASH

The diffuse macular and papular *roseolar rash of early secondary syphilis* is well known (see Plates 42 to 45).[1] The lesions are often pale, minimally elevated papules and macules which require good lighting for visualization (preferably daylight) and are better seen after the skin (and the patient) become a little chilled. An important clue is the distribution, particularly on the palms and soles, where the lesions are often brownish. Lesions may be scaling and rarely pustular, but not vesicular or pruritic. There is always a more or less pronounced generalized lymphadenopathy.

*Viral exanthems* may resemble the rash of secondary syphilis but are often identified by their distribution, short duration, and association with febrile illness. Enterovirus infections may present with palmar and plantar lesions. In hand-foot-and-mouth disease, caused by Coxsackie virus, these are typically vesicular and associated with fever, sore throat, and mild gastrointestinal symptoms (which may also occur in secondary syphilis). The oral lesions may fuse to become large painful ulcers. The clinical course is relatively short (1 to 2 weeks) compared with the rash of secondary syphilis. The rashes of measles and rubella may also resemble the rash of secondary syphilis. In measles, the exanthem is preceded by a prodromal period of 2 to 4 days duration, characterized by fever, malaise, conjunctivitis, and upper respiratory symptoms. Gray-white papules on a red base are seen on mucosal surfaces, particularly the palate. The rash starts on the face (which is usually spared in syphilis) and gradually spreads to the trunk and extremities. It wanes over less than a week to brownish scaling macules. The exanthem of rubella also starts on the face after a mild prodrome of fever and conjunctivitis.

The typical morbilliform *drug reaction,* for example, due to ampicillin, can present problems in differential diagnosis. A febrile reaction, with chills and a morbilliform rash following ampicillin treatment of gonorrhea, could be induced by the drug but might also be due to the *Jarisch-Herxheimer reaction* in which there is a flare-up of an unnoticed rash of secondary syphilis in association with antitreponemal therapy. The latter typically occurs more rapidly (6 to 8 h) after the initiation of therapy than would be true for a drug reaction and is associated with constitutional symptoms that are often alarming to the unprepared patient. The morbilliform reaction to ampicillin is rarely associated with constitutional symptoms. The anaphylactic, urticarial reaction to penicillin is not easily confused with the Jarisch-Herxheimer reaction or with secondary syphilis.

The lesions of *erythema chronicum migrans* (Lyme disease) are slowly expanding annular plaques with central clearing and a slightly raised erythematous border, which may resemble lesions of secondary syphilis (Fig. 58-1). This disease is caused by the spirochete *Borrelia burgdorferi,* which is transmitted by tick bites. The lesions gradually enlarge over months to many decimeters in diameter, with no local symptoms. There may be several lesions and the palms and soles are usually spared. The infection can be complicated by meningitis or carditis (the second stage of Lyme disease) or by arthritis (the third stage).[2] The clinical and histologic presentation may be indistinguishable from *Sweet's syndrome.*[3] The patient often has a high persistent fever with pronounced neutrophilia. There is a rapid onset of dull-red nodules or plaque, especially on the forearms and neck. These persist for several weeks but respond rapidly to corticosteroids. The syphilitic erythema could take the form of *erythema nodosum,* and VDRL should be checked, in addition to work-ups for tuberculosis, sarcoidosis, drug reactions, or streptococcal infection.[4]

*Erythema multiforme* is not a disease per se but rather a reaction pattern of the skin that can have many causes, including viral and bacterial infections, drug reactions, collagen vascular disease, and carcinomas. In the most common papular form, lesions are dull red macules and papules that slowly enlarge to form the characteristic iris, or target lesions. Lesions are typically present on the backs of the hands, palms, forearms, feet, elbows, knees, and, less often, the trunk. More severe bullous forms may occur, affecting skin and mucous membranes (Fig. 58-2). The Stevens-Johnson syndrome is a distinct entity with sudden onset, marked constitutional symptoms, including fever, severe involvement of the oral, ocular, and genital epithelium, and pulmonary or renal disease. Erythema multiforme is often precipitated by recurrent herpes simplex virus infection, which may be subclinical. Oral acyclovir may prevent recurrences.[5]

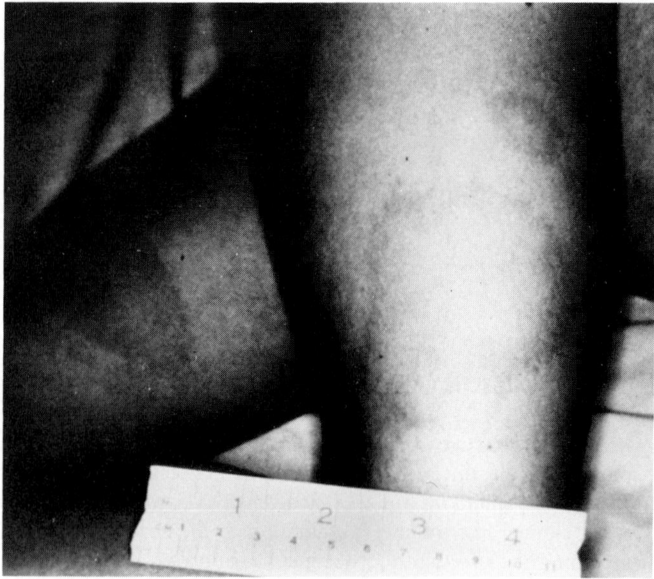

**Fig. 58-1.** Multiple annular plaques of erythema chronicum migrans occurring on the legs.

The prodromal or acute phase of *hepatitis B* may be complicated by dermatologic manifestations which may be protean (maculopapular, purpuric, scarlatiniform, vasculitis, etc.), but which are most often urticarial (Fig. 58-3).[6]

Although the patient with *toxic shock syndrome* most often will present in the emergency room, the physician treating STDs should be alert to the potential of toxin-producing staphylococci in tampons or other foreign bodies introduced into the vagina. The rash is of variable intensity and distribution, most commonly presenting as a diffuse macular erythema or a localized scarlatin-

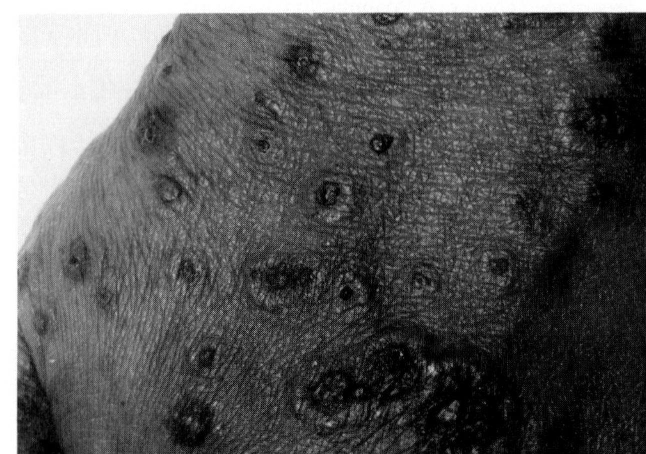

**Fig. 58-2.** Typical target lesions of erythema multiforme on the wrist and hand. These lesions have central vesicles.

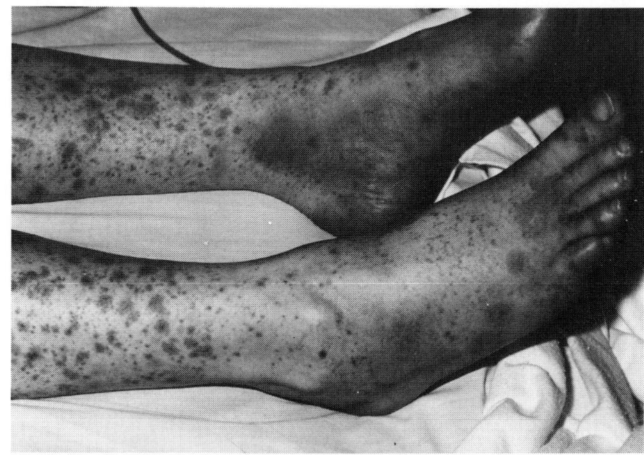

**Fig. 58-3.** Purpuric papules and vesicles of vasculitis on the legs of a female intravenous drug user with prodromal hepatitis B.

iform rash. Secondary desquamation may be limited to the fingertips or may extend to a widespread peeling of the palms, soles, and trunk. A rash (or desquamation about 2 weeks after onset), high fever, multisystem involvement (e.g., diarrhea, vomiting, myalgia), and hypotension are part of the case definition.[7] Shock was found in only 37 percent in a recent series. Inflammation of the conjunctiva, mouth, and vagina is usual, and renal, hepatic, hematologic, and CNS involvement may occur.[8]

In no case should pruritus be dismissed without an active search for *scabies* (see Plates 81 to 83). The clinical picture is frequently dominated by excoriated papules, and burrows are difficult to find. The distribution of lesions is often quite helpful, with involvement of the interdigital spaces, flexor surface of the wrists and forearms, axillary folds, nipples, buttocks, glans penis, and ankles.

## DIFFERENTIAL DIAGNOSIS OF PAPULOSQUAMOUS RASH

Some papular rashes have a scaling surface from their onset and are referred to as papulosquamous. This morphologic group of skin diseases includes a heterogeneous group of common and uncommon conditions, but secondary syphilis may mimic their clinical appearance closely (see Plates 46 and 56).

*Psoriasis* is a common disease of unknown etiology which affects 1 to 2 percent of the population. Psoriasis may start at any age and follows an unpredictable course in extent and time, ranging from a few transient plaques to a disseminated lifelong condition. Plaque-type psoriasis is most common and is characterized by oval or irregular plaques on the limbs and trunk that are one to several centimeters in diameter. On elbows, knees, and scalp, lesions typically have a thick, silvery scale; such lesions easily crack into fissures on joint movement. On the hands, lesions are less keratotic and may resemble eczema. In the flexures, hyperkeratosis is absent and psoriasis may resemble intertrigo or candidal infection. Penile lesions are well demarcated with thin scaling (see Chap. 60). Lesions tend to form in lines of skin trauma, showing the isomorphic response, or Koebner phenomenon. *Guttate psoriasis* (see Plate 56) is the variant which may be most difficult to differentiate from syphilis and which is not an infrequent presentation of psoriasis in young adults. Lesions are 2- to 20-mm rosy red papules which have little scale initially, although older papules have a waxy hyperkeratosis which may be scraped off leaving a smooth surface with punctate bleeding (Auspitz sign). Lesions are scattered more or less evenly over the body but spare the "typical" sites of psoriasis such as the elbows, knees, and nails and rarely affect the palms and soles. Guttate psoriasis is often precipitated by an asymptomatic infection with beta hemolytic streptococci. The diagnosis is usually clinical, but histopathology can be helpful in uncertain cases. Other variants of psoriasis may have prominent hyperkeratosis of the palms and soles and resemble Reiter's syndrome (see below), while still others may have pustules.

*Lichen planus* (see Plates 50 and 59) is another papulosquamous disease of uncertain etiology. The lesions of lichen planus are blue-red (violaceous), polygonal papules with a surface network of fine white lines (Wickham's striae). The lesions can be widely disseminated but are typically located on the flexor surface of the wrists and on the penis. The Koebner phenomenon is often prominent, and lesions may coalesce into annular forms. Approximately 50 percent of patients have oral lesions, most often as nondetachable white striations on the buccal mucosa. The onset of lichen planus is usually slow and the disease tends to resolve spontaneously over 9 to 18 months. Intense pruritus is typical and is especially associated with hypertrophic lesions. The histologic picture is diagnostic. Isolated lesions confined to the palms and soles may be difficult to differentiate from syphilis, psoriasis, or warts. In syphilis, as in lichen planus, papules may be arranged in small circles, although pruritus is rare.

*Pityriasis rosea* (see Plate 57) is thought to be caused by an infectious agent (virus?), although it is rare to find anyone with symptoms around the index case. Most cases occur in the winter months in persons 10 to 35 years of age. The first, and often largest "mother" lesion, often termed the "herald patch," is usually found on the thigh, upper arm, trunk, or neck. It is an initially well-defined bright-red papule covered by a thin scale. Being asymptomatic, it is often overlooked. After 5 to 15 days, crops of new lesions appear over a 7- to 10-day period. These lesions are oval in the direction of skin folds, pale red with a dull, yellow-brown center, and surrounded by a thin collarette of scale pointing toward the center of the papule. The rash is distributed over the trunk, upper arms, thighs, neck, and, infrequently, the face. There are no constitutional symptoms, but often a slight itch. The lesions fade after 3 to 6 weeks, and usually no therapy is required.

*Reiter's syndrome* (see Plates 67 to 69) is a reaction pattern to urogenital infections such as *Chlamydia trachomatis,* or to enteric infections such as *Shigella, Yersinia, Campylobacter,* or *Salmonella,* usually found in individuals with the HLA B27 genetic marker. It is diagnosed most often in young men and may be overlooked in females. An often unnoticed urethritis occurs 20 to 30 days after the initiating genital or enteric infection. About half of the cases develop mild conjunctivitis, and some develop anterior uveitis. A nonsuppurative polyarthritis involving the joints of the lower limbs and sacroiliac joints may dominate the clinical picture. Mucocutaneous lesions (keratoderma blenorrhagica) have been seen in 8 to 31 percent of cases, usually 2 to 3 months after the onset of the arthritis. The primary lesion is a dull red papule that rapidly forms a hyperkeratotic yellow surface. Lesions coalesce into plaques and may have a circinate collarette of scale. Pustular lesions may be seen. The plantar surface is most commonly involved, but lesions may be found on the dorsum of the feet, extensor surface of the legs, hands, fingers, nails, and scalp. On the penis, moist, red erosions merge to form a circinate balanitis in the uncircumcised male. Circinate vulvitis has been described. Oral lesions are seen in 10 to 15 percent of cases and include small vesicles that rapidly form superficial erosions, or a patchy erythema. Reiter's syndrome is often recurrent, without obvious relationship to new infections, although reinfection from untreated partners must be considered.[9]

*Dermatophyte fungal infection* and *erythrasma* of the genitocrural areas are discussed in Chap. 60, while *genital candidiasis* is discussed in Chap. 45. However, more generalized cutaneous involvement may be seen with each of these conditions, and dermatophyte infection may affect the nails (Fig. 58-4). Candida infection and erythrasma often involve other intertriginous sites, such as toe clefts, axillae, and intergluteal and submammary folds. Dermatophyte infection should be considered in the differential diagnosis of scaling rash of any site on the skin, and appropriate scrapings should be collected for KOH examination or culture.

*Atopic dermatitis,* or eczema, is a common, chronic, pruritic skin disease of uncertain etiology. Atopic dermatitis is often associated with a history of asthma and allergic rhinitis or conjunctivitis in the patient or family members. Although the onset of atopic dermatitis is typically between 2 and 6 months of age, it may be delayed until adolescence or later. The skin in atopic dermatitis is dry and pruritic and skin changes are usually dominated by the effects of chronic scratching, with lichenification, mild erythema, and fine scale in the flexures of the knees and elbows. In many adults, the eczema subsides except for persistent dry skin and a tendency for hand dermatitis. There is a potential for severe dissemination of *herpes simplex virus* infection (Kaposi's varicelliform eruption) in persons with active eczema. Prompt institution of antiviral therapy with acyclovir is important in this situation.[10,11]

## DIFFERENTIAL DIAGNOSIS OF PUSTULES AND CRUSTS

Pustular eruptions should always suggest infection with pyogenic bacteria, either as a primary problem or occurring as a secondary infection complicating some other skin disease. However, the differential diagnosis of pustular rash includes syphilis, inflammatory skin diseases such as psoriasis, and hypersensitivity reactions. The Gram stain of the contents of an intact pustule can sometimes provide a rapid means of distinguishing pyogenic infections from other etiologies of pustular lesions.

The pustular eruption of *secondary syphilis* (see Plate 42) is rare compared with the other skin manifestations of syphilis.[12] Lesions are initially erythematous papules which develop a central pustule and then break down into a persistent crusted erosion. Such lesions are typically found on the face and trunk. Dark field examination and serologic tests for syphilis can confirm the diagnosis.

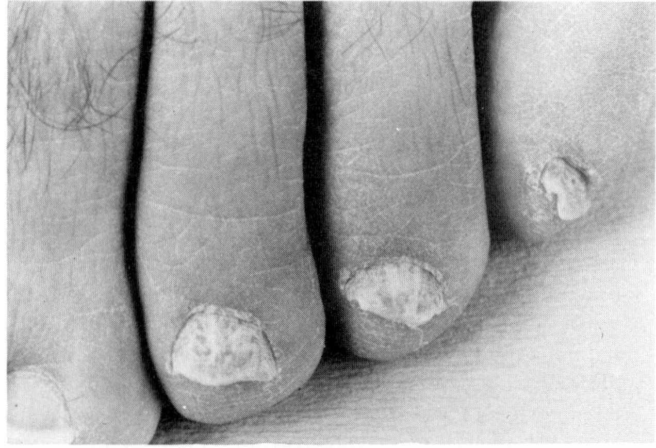

**Fig. 58-4.** Dermatophyte infection of the toenails, or onychomycosis.

*Staphylococcal folliculitis* is a common superficial infection, or pyoderma, caused by *Staphylococcus aureus* infection of hair follicles. Folliculitis is most common in conditions of heat, humidity, and poor hygiene, such as are found in the tropics. Certain diseases, such as diabetes mellitus, appear to be predisposing factors in folliculitis. Lesions are painful pustules surrounded by a narrow halo of erythema, and often showing a visible hair at their center. Older lesions may break down into crusted erosions. The scalp, forearms, buttocks, thighs, and beard are typical sites of involvement, but any area may be affected. Gram stain or culture of an intact pustule may help to confirm the diagnosis. Therapy involves oral antistaphylococcal antibiotics, and efforts to correct underlying dermatoses and improve hygiene.

Impetigo may be caused by either streptococci (90 percent of cases) or staphylococci (10 percent of cases), but the clinical appearance of lesions is different for each organism. *Streptococcal impetigo,* or impetigo contagiosa, caused by group A beta-hemolytic *Streptococcus pyogenes,* is most common in children and is quite contagious on skin-to-skin contact. Lesions begin as transient pustules on an erythematous base which quickly rupture into an expanding erosion covered with a characteristic "honey-colored" crust. Lesions typically occur on the exposed skin of the face and extremities but may complicate other skin diseases in any site. Poststreptococcal glomerulonephritis is a rare, but serious, complication of streptococcal impetigo. *Staphylococcal impetigo,* or bullous impetigo, is caused by specific phage types of *Staphylococcus aureus.* Staphylococcal impetigo is common in infancy but is also seen in adults in conditions of heat, humidity, and poor hygiene. Lesions are flaccid, thin-roofed vesicles and bullae which become cloudy and pustular over 1 to 2 days and rupture, leaving a dry, shiny, erythematous, "varnish-like" base. Lesions typically occur in the intertriginous areas of the axillae and groin and are pruritic, rather than painful. It is important to investigate if the impetigo was preceded by signs indicative of another, now disguised, skin disease—such as scabies or molluscum contagiosum. Oral therapy is preferred for impetigo, although topical cleansing and antibiotics may also be effective. Coinfections between streptococci and penicillinase-producing staphylococci are not uncommon.

*Pustular psoriasis* is an unusual variant of psoriasis which may mimic pyogenic infection, with acute onset, pustular skin lesions, and fever. Psoriasis is discussed above.

Some intense, immunologically mediated skin reactions may be associated with the poorly understood phenomenon of autosensitization, or the "id reaction." The reaction is commonly associated with inflammatory tinea pedis but may complicate a focal contact dermatitis. The id reaction is characterized by the development of a vesicular or pustular eruption at a site remote from the primary focus of inflammation. This typically occurs on the palms as pruritic vesicles which become pustules with time. In exceptional cases, id reactions may be generalized. Therapy is directed at the primary focus of inflammation as well as the "id reaction" and may include topical or systemic corticosteroids.

Infestation with any of the human *ectoparasites* (see Chaps. 41 and 42) induces a pruritic host response which is often manifested as excoriated papules. Secondary bacterial infection of these excoriated lesions is common and may obscure the characteristic lesions produced by the ectoparasites. The presence of an ectoparasite should be suspected whenever impetigo, folliculitis, or other pyoderma occurs in the distribution of an ectoparasite. Scalp infection should prompt a careful inspection for pediculosis capitis. Infection in the finger webs, wrists, buttocks, and ankles should suggest the possibility of scabies. Bacterial infection over the shoulders, flanks, waistline, and legs should prompt a search of the clothing for pediculosis corporis. In such cases, therapy should be directed at eliminating the ectoparasite as well as treating the bacterial infection.

## DIFFERENTIAL DIAGNOSIS OF HYPOPIGMENTATION

Skin lesions with partial or complete loss of cutaneous pigmentation are a common cause for dermatologic consultation. In most cases, hypopigmented lesions are macules which are visibly abnormal only because of their lack of color relative to the surrounding, normal skin.

The fading rash of *secondary syphilis* may leave hypopigmented macules on the back, neck, or genitalia (the necklace of Venus, or leucoderma syphiliticum).

*Vitiligo* is a condition which affects approximately 1 percent of the population and is caused by destruction of melanocytes by autoantibodies. Vitiligo starts before the age of 20 in about half of cases. Lesions are totally depigmented macules without any associated symptoms. Lesions are often symmetrically located around body orifices and areas which are normally hyperpigmented, such as the eyes, mouth, areolae, genitals, axillae, and crural folds. Lesions also occur in areas of frequent skin trauma, including the dorsum of the hands, feet, elbows, and knees. Less than 20 percent of patients regain pigmentation, and therapy is disappointing.

*Pityriasis versicolor,* or tinea versicolor, is a common superficial infection caused by the lipophilic yeast *Pityrosporum orbiculare,* or *P. ovale.* Men and women are equally affected, and the peak incidence is in the teens. Heat and sweating are thought to be contributing factors, and increased prevalence and extensive involvement is seen in the tropics. There are usually no local symptoms. Lesions are slightly hypopigmented or hyperpigmented compared with pigmented or nonpigmented normal skin respectively and may have very mild erythema. The lesions appear to be macules, but scraping the surface reveals the presence of delicate scale. The upper trunk is usually affected, with spread to the upper arms, axillae, neck, and upper abdomen. The diagnosis can be confirmed by examining scrapings in KOH for typical clusters of spherical spores and thick, short, curved mycelia. Topical antifungal creams or 2.5 percent selenium sulfide can clear the condition in temperate climates, but it tends to relapse.

*Postinflammatory hypopigmentation* follows healing of a large number of inflammatory skin conditions, including nummular and atopic dermatitis. The resulting hypopigmented macules are most prominent on tanned or black skin.

## DIFFERENTIAL DIAGNOSIS OF VASCULITIS

Vasculitis is a general term used to describe the local endothelial response to a variety of insults, which include immune complexes, cryoprecipitates, and direct invasion by viruses and bacteria. The pathogenesis includes endothelial damage, increased vascular permeability, fibrin deposition, invasion of leucocytes, and necrosis (i.e., necrotizing vasculitis). The local inflammation and hemorrhage produce the pathognomonic lesion of palpable purpura, which may progress to necrotic lesions and ulceration. Lesions are commonly found in areas of stasis and cooling, most often the lower legs (Fig. 58-3). In addition to cutaneous signs there are often fever, arthralgias, gastrointestinal symptoms, and other constitutional manifestations. Depending on the etiology, vasculitis may have an acute form with hemorrhagic, necrotic lesions which appear in crops and persist for 2 to 3 weeks, or a more indolent course in which purpura, maculoerythematous lesions, urticaria, and papules predominate and crops appear over months or years. Common causes of vasculitis include streptococcal infection, tuberculosis, persistent bacterial infection (such as dental abscess), drugs, malignancy, collagen vascular diseases, and pregnancy. It is important to exclude infectious causes before attempts are made to use corticosteroids.

*Gonococcal bacteremia* (see Plates 70 to 72) may produce skin lesions which suggest vasculitis (see Chap. 61), typically dull gray pustules on a blue-red base which are distributed over large joints, wrist, elbows, ankles, and knees. Meningococcemia may initially present with a very similar picture, requiring rapid intervention.[13] Cryoprecipitates that elicit a cutaneous vasculitis can form in *syphilis.*

## RASHES IN HIV INFECTION

In HIV infection, dermatological disorders are common. Skin disorders have been observed in 43 percent of patients with persistent generalized lymphadenopathy.[14] There are two distinct classes of skin lesions: those that are thought to be directly caused by HIV, and others (the majority) that are provoked by the subsequent immunological disorders. Among the latter, skin infections are prominent, but many common skin diseases in HIV infection remain idiopathic.

## ACUTE HIV INFECTION

In the *acute infection* (CDC group I HIV infection) a rash is often described together with fever, chills, tonsillitis, myalgia and arthralgia, and neurological symptoms that occur in varying combinations in about one-third of the patients, 1 to 6 weeks after acquiring the HIV infection. The rash is often morbilliform but may present as urticaria, vasculitis, or erythema multiforme. As the clinical condition improves over a couple of weeks, the skin clears. At presentation, serological tests for HIV are negative, but viral blood culture is usually positive and HIV p24 antigen can be detected in the serum. The clinical presentation is similar to infectious mononucleosis, which, however, is associated with exanthem in only 10 to 15 percent of the cases.[15]

## OTHER CUTANEOUS INFECTIONS COMPLICATING HIV INFECTION

### Bacterial infections

Although many infections can be precipitated by the HIV-induced immunodeficiency, *bacterial infections* are comparatively rare. This is true also for the skin. *Impetigo* may complicate eczemas, which are then difficult to treat. *M. avium-intracellulare* has been diagnosed in ill-defined macular discolored lesions on the forearms.[16]

### Fungal infections

In areas where the different pathogenic fungi are endemic, these may cause cutaneous manifestations. In cutaneous histoplasmosis

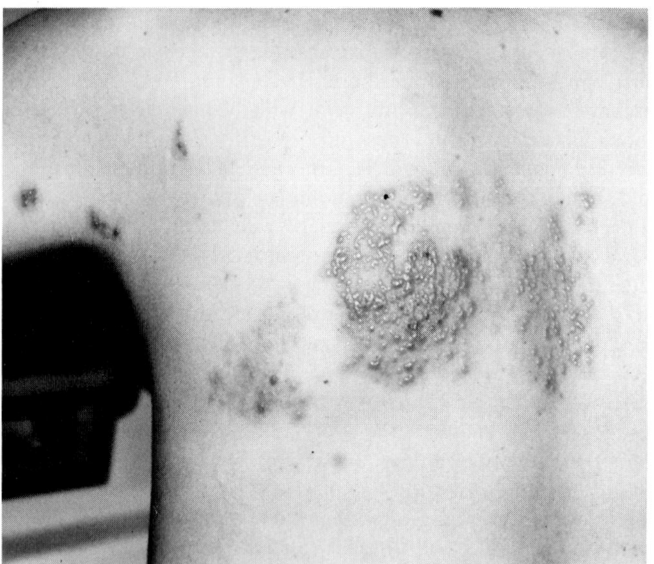

Fig. 58-5. Herpes zoster in a thoracic dermatome in a patient who was seropositive for HIV-1 infection, but otherwise asymptomatic.

and cryptococcosis, the clinical picture is often atypical in patients with HIV infection.[17,18]

*Oral thrush* is especially common (see Plate 61) and is a poor prognostic sign reflecting declining cellular immunity. The white, moderately adherent plaques often affect the hard palate, have a yellowish coloration and erythematous border. Not infrequently, erythema and superficial bleeding dominate the clinical picture with minimal development of plaques. When diagnosis is uncertain, scraping with a spatula and inspection in KOH will demonstrate massive presence of mycelium.

## Viral infections

The bulk of the complicating cutaneous infections are of viral origin. Most often recognized is *herpes zoster* (Fig. 58-5 and Plate 63), which carries the same prognostic weight as oral thrush, especially if it affects more than one dermatome and is severe or generalized.[19] The clinical diagnosis is usually easy. The zoster will respond to oral high-dose therapy with acyclovir (800 mg 5 times daily).

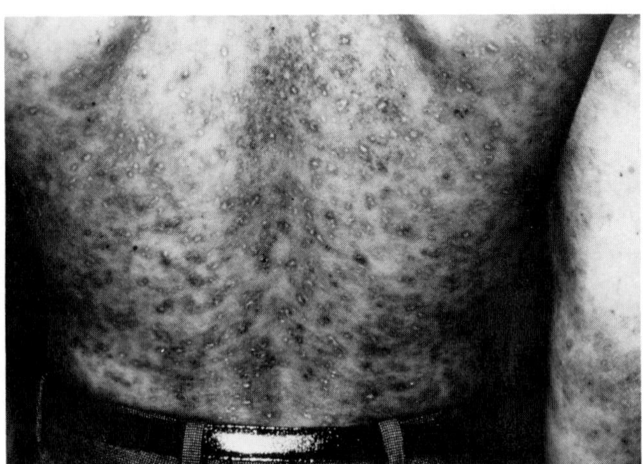

Fig. 58-6. Generalized, intensely pruritic dermatitis of recent onset in a man with AIDS. The skin is dry and lichenified, with scarring at sites of excoriation. The pathogenesis of such dermatitis is not defined, and empiric treatment currently often includes topical steroids with or without an oral antimicrobial such as erythromycin.

Nonhealing anal ulcers caused by *herpes simplex virus* have frequently been observed in HIV infection and are part of the case definition of AIDS, if present for 5 weeks or longer. Lesions caused by HSV have been reported to present as vesicular eruptions of the hands, as "chronic leg ulcers," or as multiple nonhealing lesions of the face.[20] Ulcers may also be caused by cytomegalovirus.

There have now been several reports of widespread *molluscum contagiosum* with a particular affinity to the face. The pale asymptomatic umbilicated papules are not morphologically altered, but giant molluscum may simulate basal cell carcinomas or kerato-acanthomas.[21]

On the sides of the tongue, the striate white, adherent lesions of *hairy leukoplakia* (Plate 62) are a pathognomonic sign of HIV infection. EB virus has been demonstrated in the lesions.[22]

## DERMATOSES

The most common dermatological disorder associated with HIV infection is morphologically similar to *seborrheic dermatitis* and is reported in up to 46 percent of AIDS patients.[23,24] Seborrheic dermatitis seems to be related to infection with *pityrosporon ovale*. The lesions tend to originate in the hairy skin and involve

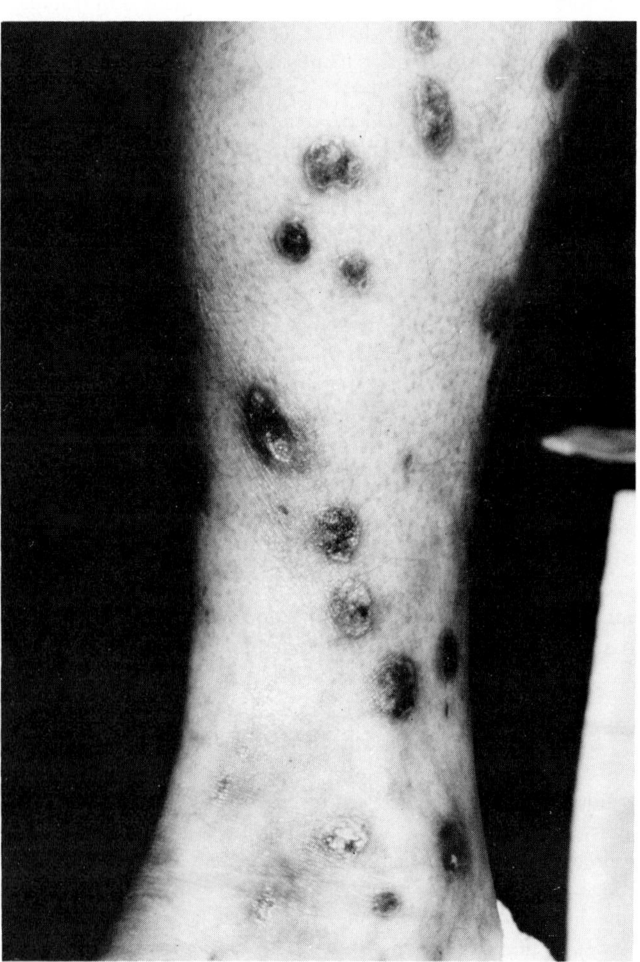

Fig. 58-7. Intense pruritis in this patient with AIDS and generalized dermatitis led to scratching, producing focal excoriations, and formation of nodules known as prurigo nodules, shown here on the lower leg.

the scalp and hairline, nasolabial furrows, sternum, interscapular region, and the flexures. They are dull or yellowish red in color and covered by greasy scales. On the trunk, the lesions are often small follicular red-brown papules covered by greasy scales. These lesions often coalesce to form circinate patches. In the flexures, seborrheic dermatitis presents as an intertrigo with an intense well-demarcated erythema and greasy scaling. External otitis and blepharitis are common. The course is variable, but often chronic. When not associated with HIV infection, seborrheic dermatitis is steroid-sensitive. Topical antifungal imidazoles (e.g., 2 percent ketoconazole cream) may be of help. However, treatment results are often disappointing in HIV disease. There is a fluid demarcation from this clinical presentation to *acneiform* eruptions at times with deep conglobate lesions in the face or on the trunk, or *folliculitis*. Necrotizing folliculitis is sometimes seen. More rarely there are pityriasiform lesions on the trunk.

The skin in HIV infection is often dry (*xeroderma*) and thin without clinical problems but may present with focal or generalized dermatitis, with erythema and scaling often with *pruritus* that is very difficult to manage (Figs. 58-6 and 58-7). Pruritic rashes are frequently seen in African AIDS patients and may be the presenting symptom (see Plate 66). *Acquired ichthyosis* is occasionally seen (Fig. 58-8).

Another cause of pruritus described in association with HIV infection is the chronic *papular eruption*. Two- to 5-mm skin-colored papules occur on the head, neck, and upper trunk. The condition is chronic but may wax and wane with time.[25]

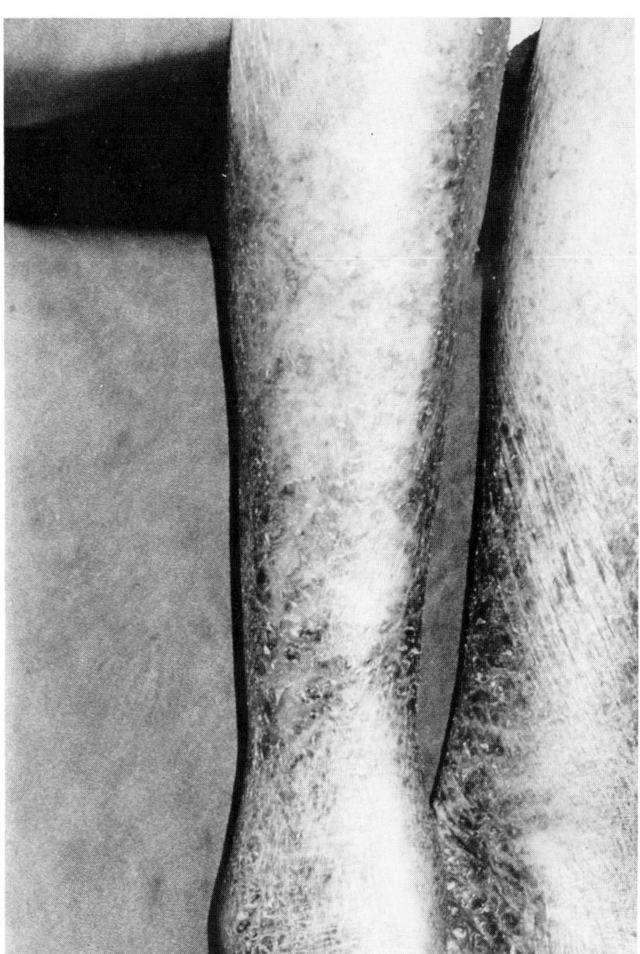

**Fig. 58-8.** Acquired ichthyosis on the legs of a man with AIDS.

Recently *eosinophilic pustular folliculitis* has been reported in AIDS patients. The lesions are 3 to 5 mm in diameter, with a flat hyperpigmented center and an active margin occupied by multiple tiny follicular pustules on erythematous papules combined with moderate pruritus. It typically affects the face, trunk, and proximal extremities.[26] Ultraviolet light treatments may be helpful in controlling symptoms.

*Scabies* may present with intense pruritus, but with unusual distribution of a generalized papulosquamous rash.[27]

*Psoriasis* in the setting of HIV infection is often difficult to manage, but there are now case reports suggesting that zidovudine might help.[28]

New *fungal infections* of the toenails have been observed as a bad prognostic sign in HIV infection. Yellow discoloration of nails has been described that does not strictly fall under the entity of "yellow nail syndrome" because of the lack of association with pulmonary disease.[29]

### TUMORS

In gay men, *epidemic Kaposi's sarcoma* has been particularly common for unknown reasons (see Chap. 56 and Plates 64 and 65). Other skin cancers, such as *malignant melanoma* and *squamous cell carcinoma*, may be more common in HIV infection, but this is not yet proved.

## References


1 Hira SH et al: Clinical manifestations of secondary syphilis. *Int J Dermatol* 26:103, 1987.
2 Burke WA et al: Lyme disease mimicking secondary syphilis. *J Am Acad Dermatol* 14:137, 1986.
3 Jordaan HF, Cilliers J: Secondary syphilis mimicking Sweet's syndrome. *Br J Dermatol* 115:495, 1986.
4 Silber TJ et al: Painful red leg nodules and syphilis. A consideration in patients with erythema nodosum. *Sex Transm Dis* 14:52, 1986.
5 Lemak MA et al: Oral acyclovir for the prevention of herpes associated erythema multiforme. *J Am Acad Dermatol* 15:50, 1986.
6 Rosen LB et al: Hepatitis B surface antigen positive skin lesions. *Am J Dermatopathol* 7:507, 1985.
7 Findlay RF, Odom RB: Toxic shock syndrome. *Int J Dermatol* 21: 117, 1982.
8 McKenna UG et al: Toxic shock syndrome, a newly recognized disease entity. *Mayo Clin Proc* 55:663, 1980.
9 Kousa M: Clinical observations on Reiter's disease with special reference to the venereal and non-venereal aetiology. Thesis. *Acta Derm Venereol (Stockh)* 58:81, 1978.
10 Bonifazi E et al: Role of some infectious agents in atopical dermatitis. *Acta Derm Venereol (Stockh)* 114:98, 1985.
11 Muelleman PJ et al: Eczema herpeticum treated with oral acyclovir. *J Am Acad Dermatol* 15:716, 1986.
12 Noppakun N et al: Pustular secondary syphilis. *Int J Dermatol* 26: 112, 1987.
13 Kingston MME, Mackey D: Skin clues in the diagnosis of life-threatening infections. *Rev Infect Dis* 8:1, 1986.
14 Gottlieb MS et al: The syndrome of persistent generalized lymphadenopathy. Experience with 101 patients. *Adv Exp Med Biol* 187:85, 1985.
15 Cooper DA et al: Acute AIDS retrovirus infection. *Lancet* i:537, 1985.
16 Penneys NS, Hicks: Unusual cutaneous lesions associated with acquired immunodeficiency syndrome. *J Am Acad Dermatol* 13:845, 1985.

17 Hazelhurst JA, Vismer HF: Histoplasmosis presenting with unusual skin lesions in acquired immune deficiency syndrome (AIDS). *Br J Dermatol* 113:345, 1985.
18 Rico MJ, Penneys NS: Cutaneous cryptococcosis resembling molluscum contagiosum in a patient with AIDS. *Arch Dermatol* 121:901, 1985.
19 Friedman-Kien AE et al: Herpes zoster: A possible early clinical sign for development of acquired immunodeficiency syndrome in high-risk individuals. *J Am Acad Dermatol* 14:1023, 1986.
20 Warner LC, Fisher BK: Cutaneous manifestations of the acquired immune deficiency syndrome. *Int J Dermatol* 25:337, 1986.
21 Katzman M et al: Molluscum contagiosum and the acquired immunodeficiency syndrome: Clinical and immunological details of two cases. *Br J Dermatol* 116:131, 1987.
22 Greenspan D et al: Oral "hairy" leukoplakia in male homosexuals: Evidence of association with both papilloma virus and a herpes-group virus. *Lancet* ii:831, 1984.
23 Soeprono FF et al: Seborrheic-like dermatitis of acquired immunodeficiency syndrome. *J Am Acad Dermatol* 14:242, 1986.
24 Eisenstat B, Wormser GP: Seborrheic dermatitis and butterfly rash in AIDS (letter). *N Engl J Med* 311:358, 1984.
25 James WD et al: A papular eruption associated with human T cell lymphotropic virus type III disease. *J Am Acad Dermatol* 13:563, 1985.
26 Soeprono FF et al: Eosinophilic pustular folliculitis in patients with acquired immunodeficiency syndrome. *J Am Acad Dermatol* 14:1020, 1986.
27 Sadick N et al: Unusual features of scabies complicating human T-lymphotropic virus type III infection. *J Am Acad Dermatol* 15:482, 1986.
28 Duvic M et al: Remission of AIDS-associated psoriasis with zidovudine (letter). *Lancet* ii:627, 1987.
29 Chernosky ME, Finley VK: Yellow nail syndrome and acquired immunodeficiency syndrome. *J Am Acad Dermatol* 14:844, 1986.

# Chapter 59

# Genital ulcer adenopathy syndrome

Peter Piot
Francis A. Plummer

Genital ulcerations are among the more complex clinical problems for physicians dealing with sexually transmitted diseases (STD). Their clinical presentation is diverse, multiple infections are common, their etiologic diagnosis is technically demanding, and their management has not been well evaluated for all causes. Genital ulceration can be defined as a genital lesion characterized by a defect in the epithelium of the skin or mucosa. Lymphadenopathy in the genital area is usually associated with genital ulceration but may also occur separately, as in lymphogranuloma venereum (LGV). The importance of genital ulcer disease has increased enormously with growing evidence that genital ulceration is a major risk factor for transmission of human immunodeficiency virus (HIV).

## EPIDEMIOLOGY

Genital ulcer adenopathy syndrome is rarely registered and reported as such. With the exception of syphilis, reporting of the various causes of genital ulceration is at best incomplete, because diagnostic tests for the etiologies of genital ulcer adenopathy syndrome other than syphilis are not widely available or are difficult. Even when all such tests are available, a specific microbiologic agent cannot be identified in 15 to 50 percent of cases (Table 59-1).[1–7] For all these reasons, epidemiological data on the genital ulcer adenopathy syndrome are very incomplete.

In the United States in 1987, 35,147 cases of primary and secondary syphilis, 4998 of chancroid, 303 of lymphogranuloma venereum, and 22 of donovanosis were reported. These equalled only 5.2 percent of the reported number of cases of gonorrhea for that year.[8] In England and Wales in 1982, genital ulcer disease was diagnosed in 2.2 percent of all patients treated in the National Health Service's STD clinics.[9]

Genital ulcerations are relatively more frequent in developing countries than in the industrialized world. Whereas in North America and Europe 1 to 5 percent of patients seen in STD clinics present with a genital ulcer, this may be the case for as many as 20 to 70 percent of clinic attenders in Africa and Asia.[10] The etiology of genital ulcer disease also shows striking geographic variability (Table 59-1). Genital herpes is by far the most common diagnosis in North America and Europe, whereas chancroid is particularly common in Africa, Asia, and Latin America. However, numerous outbreaks of chancroid have occurred since the early 1980s in North America, where chancroid is now reestablished as an endemic disease in several areas.[11–12] Lymphogranuloma venereum and donovanosis apparently occur mainly in geographical foci in the tropics. The proportion of STD patients who have genital ulcers, and the etiology of these ulcerations, may be influenced by several factors, such as the prevalence of other STD, the availability of diagnostic facilities, sexual practices and preference, cultural patterns of circumcision, and the role of prostitutes as a source of infection.

Risk factors for genital ulcer disease also vary by population and by etiology. In many countries, homosexual men account for a major proportion of syphilis cases, though the incidence in several homosexual populations, but not in heterosexuals, has drastically declined as a result of behavioral change during the AIDS epidemic.[13–14] Uncircumcised men are at higher risk for acquiring chancroid than circumcised men. In most countries, patients with chancroid belong to lower socioeconomic strata, and often indicate a prostitute as a source of infection.[11,12,15] Prostitutes seem to be a major reservoir of chancroid in several areas of the world.[16] Though LGV is usually an imported disease in Europe and North America, it has been a not uncommon cause of anorectal ulcers in homosexual men in the United States.[17]

Several cross-sectional and prospective studies in homosexual men and heterosexual men and women have demonstrated not only that genital ulcers enhance the susceptibility to HIV infection through sexual intercourse, but that individuals with a genital ulcer are more likely to transmit HIV.[18–21] This may partly explain why there is apparently more heterosexual spread of HIV in Africa than in North America and Europe. Because of this implication, genital ulcer disease should be considered a very high priority area in STD control programs.

**Table 59-1. Etiology of Genital Ulcerations among Consecutive Patients in Different Populations**

| | % of patients with diagnosis | | | | | | | |
|---|---|---|---|---|---|---|---|---|
| Diagnosis | Detroit (1)* N = 100 | Antwerp N = 100 | Johannesburg (2) N = 102 | Nairobi (3) N = 97 | Rwanda (4) N = 109 | Gambia (5) N = 104 | Papua New Guinea (6) N = 101 | Bangkok (7) N = 120 |
| Syphilis | 15 | 7 | 15 | 9 | 16 | 22 | 14 | 1 |
| Herpes | 37 | 61 | 8 | 4 | 15 | 6 | 0 | 10 |
| Chancroid | 0 | 5 | 58 | 62 | 18 | 52 | 0 | 36 |
| Lymphogranuloma venereum | 0 | 0 | 1 | 0 | 7 | 4 | 9 | 0 |
| Donovanosis | 0 | 0 | 1 | 0 | 0 | 0 | 22 | 0 |
| Mixed etiology | 5 | 3 | 3 | 2 | 8 | 44 | 37 | 2 |
| Other and unknown | 43 | 24 | 14 | 23 | 36 | 12 | 18 | 51 |

*The number in parentheses refers to the reference that is the source of the data.

## ETIOLOGY

The main microbial causes of genital ulceration include *Treponema pallidum*, herpes simplex virus, *Haemophilus ducreyi*, *Chlamydia trachomatis* serovars $L_1$, $L_2$, and $L_3$, and *Calymmatobacterium granulomatis*. Pyoderma, *Phthirus pubis*, *Entamoeba histolytica*, *Sarcoptes scabiei*, *Trichomonas vaginalis*, and nonsyphilis spirochetes may occasionally cause genital ulcer disease. It is not clear if *Neisseria gonorrhoeae* is a cause of genital ulceration, though it is a not uncommon isolate from such lesions. Fixed drug eruption, Behçet's and Reiter's syndromes, trauma, and malignancy should also be considered in the differential diagnosis (see Chap. 60).

## CLINICAL MANIFESTATIONS

Clinical features of the major causes of genital ulcer adenopathy syndrome are shown in Table 59-2. However, their clinical presentation frequently does not correspond to the typical picture as described in textbooks, and mixed infections are common. The use of local or systemic antibiotics, and of corticosteroid ointment, and the presence of a concomitant immunodeficiency may modify the classic pictures of genital ulcerations. Even clinicians experienced with the problem fail to achieve a correct clinical diagnosis in 22 to 50 percent of cases of genital ulcer.[22–24]

### Incubation period

The incubation period for herpes and chancroid is short (average of 2 to 7 days), whereas it may be longer for the other causes. Patients with adenopathy associated with LGV usually present after the initial lesion has healed, i.e., 2 to 6 weeks after exposure.

### Uncomplicated infection

**Genital Ulcers.** Most genital ulcers in the male are located in the coronal sulcus, and on the glans, prepuce, and shaft of the penis. Particularly in herpes and chancroid, the frenulum may be involved. When a condom has been used, lesions may be found at the basis of the shaft. Perianal and rectal locations may be found in women and homosexual men and should always be sought. Lesions may occur on the scrotum and extragenitally, particularly the lips and oropharynx. In women, lesions may occur on the labia, in the vagina and on the cervix, as well as on the fourchette and perianal area.

The number and size of lesions is variable, with usually one ulcer present in syphilis and LGV (if any), and multiple lesions occurring in herpes and chancroid. In the latter cases, they may coalesce giving an impression of a single, serpiginous lesion. Herpetic lesions are small, whereas those of chancroid and syphilis are usually larger.

The initial appearance of an ulcer may be vesicular, papular, or pustular. The lesions may have a regular (round, oval) or irregular shape, with demarcated or vague edges, which may be elevated, undermined, and/or erythematous. Deep, excavated ulcers are typically seen in chancroid, whereas herpes and erosive balanoposthitis yield the most superficial lesions. A purulent ulcer base is almost always found in chancroid. A syphilitic chancre often feels indurated, whereas a chancroidal ulcer is soft. Chancroid and herpes are painful and tender. Itching is often reported by patients with genital herpes.

**Lymphadenopathy.** In both men and women, the lymphatic drainage of the external genitalia is primarily to the inguinal nodes, but the femoral nodes may be involved as well. The inner two-thirds of the vagina and the cervix are drained to the sacral nodes. Genital lymphadenopathy is usually associated with a genital ulceration, with the latter usually appearing first. As for the ulcers, there is considerable overlap in the clinical characteristics of the adenopathy (Table 59-2). The lymphadenopathy may be bilateral or unilateral. Differential features include consistency of the nodes, fluctuance, location, aspect of the overlying skin, pain, and tenderness at palpation. In LGV several lymph nodes are usually involved. When inguinal and femoral nodes are involved, they may be divided by the inguinal ligament, producing the "groove" sign. This is considered pathognomonic for LGV, though it is occasionally seen in chancroid.[2] If a genital ulceration becomes secondarily infected with pyogenic bacteria, the characteristics of the adenopathy may reflect the secondary infection rather than the primary process.

Pseudobuboes occurring in donovanosis are granulomatous

**Table 59-2. Clinical Features of Genital Ulcers**

| | Syphilis | Herpes | Chancroid | Lymphogranuloma venereum | Donovanosis |
|---|---|---|---|---|---|
| Incubation period | 2–4 weeks (1–12 weeks) | 2–7 days | 1–14 days | 3 days–6 weeks | 1–4 weeks (up to 6 months) |
| Primary lesion | Papule | Vesicle | Papule or pustule | Papule, pustule or vesicle | Papule |
| Number of lesions | Usually one | Multiple, may coalesce | Usually multiple, may coalesce | Usually one | Variable |
| Diameter, mm | 5–15 | 1–2 | 2–20 | 2–10 | Variable |
| Edges | Sharply demarcated, elevated, round or oval | Erythematous | Undermined, ragged, irregular | Elevated, round or oval | Elevated, irregular |
| Depth | Superficial or deep | Superficial | Excavated | Superficial or deep | Elevated |
| Base | Smooth, nonpurulent | Serous, erythematous | Purulent | Variable | Red and rough ("beefy") |
| Induration | Firm | None | Soft | Occasionally firm | Firm |
| Pain | Unusual | Common | Usually very tender | Variable | Uncommon |
| Lymphadenopathy | Firm, nontender, bilateral | Firm, tender, often bilateral | Tender, may suppurate, usually unilateral | Tender, may suppurate, loculated, usually unilateral | Pseudoadenopathy |

nodules of the inguinal region which usually involve only the skin and subcutaneous tissue, but not the lymph nodes. Chronic nontender inguinal lymphadenopathy in the absence of a genital ulcer or associated with a persistent genital lesion is suggestive of a genital cutaneous malignancy or lymphatic malignancy. However, in the tropics a substantial proportion of adults may have inguinal adenopathy resulting from recurrent trauma and infection of the lower extremities.

**Complications and Sequelae.** Acute local complications include secondary infection, which may result in destructive or phagedenic ulceration, edema of the soft tissue (foreskin, labia minora), necrotic balanitis, paraphimosis, and phimosis. In chancroid and donovanosis, part or the whole of the glans penis may be lost.

The genitoanorectal syndrome of LGV includes a wide variety of severe late complications that may occur without preceding primary genital lesions or inguinal lymphadenopathy, and that result from lymphatic obstruction and fistulization (see Chap. 17). Donovanosis may be complicated by stenosis of urethral, vaginal, and anal orifices, deformation of the genitalia, and pseudoelephantiasis of the labia.

The lesions of primary syphilis and of genital herpes heal spontaneously with usually no scar within 6 weeks, and 1 to 3 weeks, respectively. If untreated, patients with syphilis progress to secondary syphilis. Recurrence of herpetic lesions is frequent in genital herpes.

Lesions of chancroid and donovanosis may gradually become very extensive, with considerable tissue and organ destruction. Satellite ulcers may occur in ruptured inguinal lymph nodes or in adjacent groin or gluteal folds in chancroid and in donovanosis. If untreated, chancroid will heal after approximately 5 weeks.[25]

## DIAGNOSIS

As noted above, the accuracy of a clinical diagnosis of genital ulcer adenopathy syndrome is often poor and may be not higher than 50 to 78 percent.[22–24] Nevertheless, a careful history and a thorough clinical observation may provide useful indications as to the etiology of the lesions, and lead to a presumptive diagnosis.

Because of the poor accuracy of a clinical diagnosis, genital ulcers should be investigated using all relevant laboratory tests available. In the industrialized world, these should include a dark field examination for *T. pallidum*, a culture for herpes simplex virus, and serologic tests for syphilis. Though in developing countries genital ulcers are more frequent and their etiology more complex, laboratory support is usually very limited or not available at all. In these parts of the world priority should be given to the diagnosis of syphilis, since this is potentially the most debilitating disease.

**Collection of Specimens.** The lesions should be washed with saline and dried with a swab or gauze, after which the lesion is squeezed between thumb and index finger until an exudate appears. This is collected for dark field microscopy using a spatula, loop, or coverslip. Specimens for culture of herpes simplex virus, *H. ducreyi* and *C. trachomatis* are collected after vigorous swabbing. Vesicles or pustules should also be swabbed or scraped, and cultured for herpes simplex virus. Aspiration of lymph nodes, particularly if they are fluctuant, may be necessary to demonstrate a causative organism in certain cases. This should always be performed through the intact skin to avoid fistula formation.

**Microscopy.** Dark field examination of the ulcer exudate remains the basis for the diagnosis of primary syphilis (Chap. 75). However, it requires considerable experience and a suitable microscope. If the initial result is negative, the examination should be repeated the following day. Spirochete-associated ulcerative balanoposthitis is common in the tropics and may make interpretation of dark field microscopy difficult.[26]

Smears and scrapings can be examined for herpes simplex virus infection by immunofluorescent and immunoperoxidase techniques, or by a Tzanck preparation (Chap. 77). Though they have a good sensitivity when the typical vesicles are present, the yield of these tests is lower for ulcers.

The validity of a Gram-stained smear for the diagnosis of chancroid is low, and therefore such a test is not recommended. The diagnosis of donovanosis is based on the demonstration of intracytoplasmic, encapsulated Donovan bodies in macrophages in Giemsa- or Wright-stained tissue smears and sections (Chap. 25 and Plate 96).

**Isolation of Causative Agent.** Virus isolation is the method of choice for the diagnosis of genital herpes, though its sensitivity decreases after the vesicles have ulcerated.

The diagnosis of chancroid should be supported by the isolation of *H. ducreyi* from an ulcer or bubo. Several satisfactory semiselective isolation media are now available, and in experienced hands the rate of isolation (sensitivity) with a single culture for *H. ducreyi* may be as high as 80 percent.[27,28]

Isolation of *C. trachomatis* LGV serovars $L_1$, $L_2$, or $L_3$ provides the proof of a diagnosis of LGV. Bubo aspirate is the most rewarding material for culture, but occasionally the organism can be isolated from the ulcer base, and also from rectal lesions (Chap. 17). However, bubo fluid may be toxic to cell cultures, resulting in an inconclusive test result.

**Table 59-3. Laboratory Tests for the Diagnosis of Genital Ulcer Adenopathy Syndrome**

| | Syphilis | Herpes | Chancroid | Lymphogranuloma venereum | Donovanosis |
|---|---|---|---|---|---|
| Microscopy | Dark field examination | Antigen detection | Gram stain has low sensitivity and specificity | Not available | Giemsa- or Wright-stained tissue smears and sections |
| Culture | Not available | Cell culture | Sensitive, selective media available | Cell culture | Not available |
| Serology | RPR/VDRL, FTA-ABS, MHA-TP | Rarely useful (primary herpes) | Experimental | Complement fixation and immunofluorescent antibody tests | Not available |

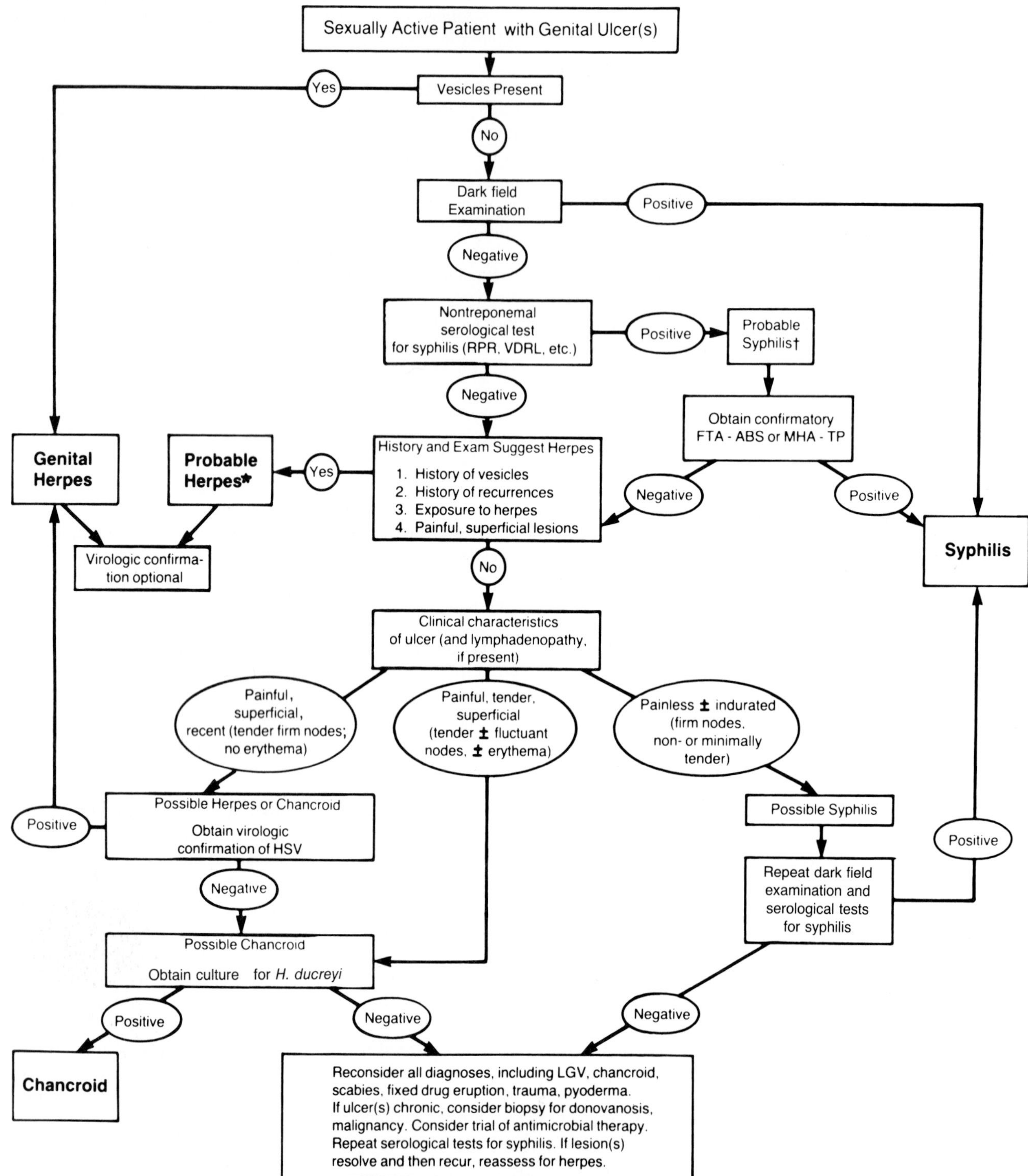


*Confirmation of probable herpes is desirable. If the confirmation test for herpes is negative, or if the course is atypical, reevaluate the diagnosis, repeat serological test for syphilis in 3 to 4 weeks, consider fixed drug eruption if there is history of recurrent lesions at the same time, and rule out herpes at the next recurrence.

†While awaiting the FTA-ABS test results, most clinicians would initiate syphilis therapy for patients having dark-field-negative, RPR-positive ulcers which resemble chancres.

**Fig. 59-1.** Algorithm for the diagnosis of genital ulcer-inguinal adenopathy syndromes in sexually active patients.

**Serology.** Serological tests for syphilis should always be part of the evaluation of a patient with genital ulcer adenopathy syndrome. Though a cardiolipin test (RPR, VDRL) may still be negative when a patient presents with a chancre, it will usually become positive during primary syphilis. The fluorescent treponemal antibody-absorption test (FTA-Abs) is more sensitive than a cardiolipin test but may reflect prior, treated syphilis (see Chap. 75 and 76 for an extensive discussion of syphilis serology). Though serologic tests for syphilis should not replace the dark field examination as the diagnostic standard for primary syphilis, they are valuable in clinical decision making when dealing with genital ulcer disease, and as a baseline quantitative test to document response to therapy.

Serum antibody to herpes simplex virus can be detected in a plethora of serological methods. However, serology appears useful in the diagnosis of primary herpes simplex virus infection only when a seroconversion or a fourfold or greater rise in antibody titer is observed between acute and convalescent sera. In addition, serological tests currently available to clinicians fail to distinguish between antibodies against virus types 1 and 2.

The complement-fixation test is the most commonly used test for the diagnosis of lymphogranuloma venereum. It becomes positive within 1 to 3 weeks after infection, and antibody titers of ≥1/64 are found in over half of the patients. Rising antibody titers are rarely observed because of the late presentation of the patients.[27,30] The titers in the microimmunofluorescence test are usually ≥1/512 in a broadly cross-reacting pattern.[29] Enzyme immune assays have become available for the serological diagnosis of chancroid but require further evaluation.[31,32]

**Differential Diagnosis.** An algorithm incorporating the major aspects of differential diagnosis of genital ulceration is given in Fig. 59-1. Ulcers not restricted to the genital area may indicate a nonvenereal origin such as Behçet's disease, erythema multiforme, and dermatitis herpetiformis.

As mentioned before, the clinical presentation of genital ulcer disease is often not typical, and any causative microorganism can produce the so-called typical picture of another pathogen (Figs. 59-2 and 59-3). Though vesicles are pathognomonic for herpes, most patients with genital herpes present later in the course of the disease, after the vesicles have ulcerated. For all other presentations of genital ulcer adenopathy syndrome, every effort should be made to use available laboratory tests to fully document their etiology. Simplified approaches for use in developing countries are discussed in Chap. 84.

The recent consumption of medication by the patient, and particularly a history of a similar lesion at the same anatomic site and associated with ingestion of the same medication, are suggestive or proof of fixed drug eruption. Frequent causes of fixed drug reactions include the tetracyclines and, less often, barbiturates and phenolphthalein laxatives.

## TREATMENT

There is no single antimicrobial agent active against all causes of the genital ulcer adenopathy syndrome, and treatment is best initiated after proper diagnosis. When antimicrobial therapy is started before a diagnosis is established, it is often preferable to use an antibiotic without activity against *T. pallidum*, such as trimethoprim/sulfamethoxazole, until syphilis is excluded on the basis of a proper dark field examination.

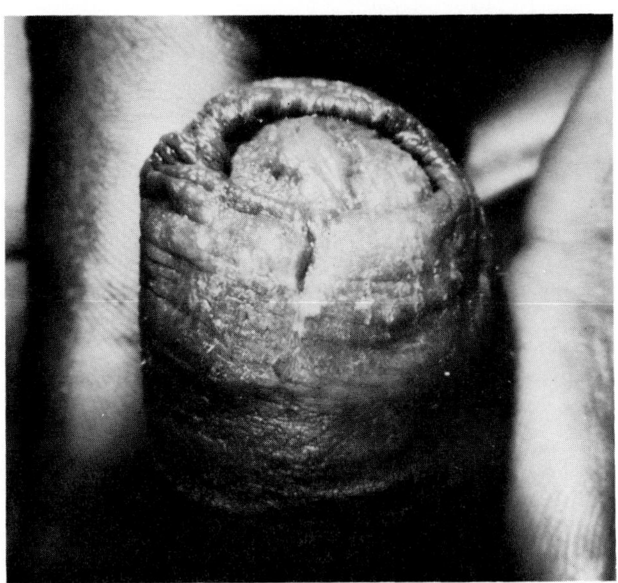

Fig. 59-2. Syphilis can mimic a fissured phimotic prepuce: *T. pallidum* identified by dark field microscopy.

The need for the treatment of secondary infections of an ulcer has not been firmly established, and it should be borne in mind that virtually all ulcers contain an abundant bacterial flora. In severe cases of apparent secondary infection, with a risk for phagedenic ulceration, a broad-spectrum systemic antimicrobial agent may be indicated. Topical antimicrobial therapy is not recommended. Necrotic material and purulent exudate should be removed by frequent application of warm-water compresses. If severe phimosis results in urinary retention, it may be necessary to make a dorsal slit incision of the prepuce.

Fluctuant buboes, which occur mostly in chancroid and LGV, should be aspirated, since they often do not respond well to antimicrobial therapy and may even become larger after successful

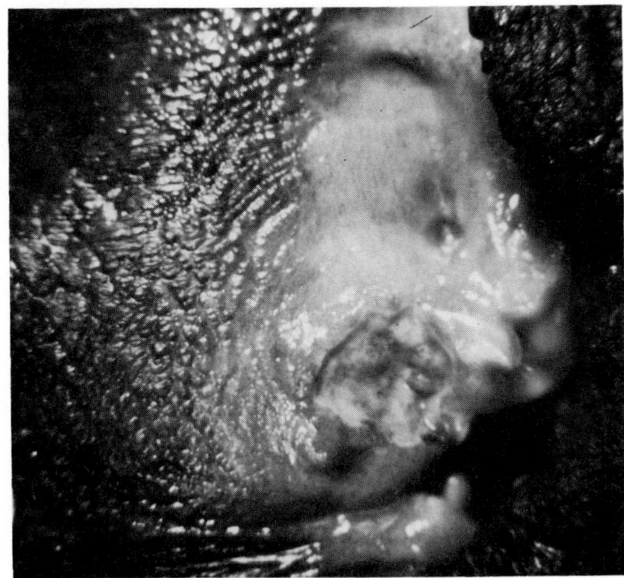

Fig. 59-3. Genital herpes simplex virus infection can mimic chancroid: HSV isolated in cell culture and *H. ducreyi* not isolated on sheep blood vancomycin agar from this exudative, painful, ulcerative lesion of the labium minus.

treatment of the associated ulcer. Aspiration should be performed through adjacent normal skin to avoid fistula formation. Repeated aspirations may be necessary. Incision and drainage are not indicated since the healing time will be longer and scarring more likely. Aspiration is best performed with a large-bore needle (16 or 18 gauge) and a large syringe or vacutainer (50 ml), because the bubo liquid is very viscous, and a strong negative pressure is needed to pull the exudate through the needle.

Specific therapy for the respective causes of genital ulcer adenopathy syndrome is discussed elsewhere in this book (Chapters 17, 20, 24, 25, and 35). Antimicrobial resistance is not a problem yet, except for *H. ducreyi,* which is multiresistant in many parts of the world.[33–35]

## References


1 Chapel TA et al: The microbiological flora of penile ulcerations. *J Infect Dis* 137:50, 1978.
2 Duncan MO et al: The diagnosis of sexually acquired genital ulcerations in black patients in Johannesburg. *S Afr J Sex Transm Dis* 1:20, 1981.
3 Nsanze H et al: Genital ulcers in Kenya: Clinical and laboratory study. *Br J Vener Dis* 57:378, 1981.
4 Bogaerts J et al: The etiology of genital ulceration in Rwanda. Submitted for publication. *Sex Transm Dis,* 1989, in press.
5 Mabey DCW et al: Aetiology of genital ulceration in the Gambia. *Genitourin Med* 63:312, 1987.
6 Vacca A, MacMillan LL: Anogenital lesions in women in Papua New Guinea. *Papua New Guinea Med J* 23:70, 1980.
7 Taylor DN et al: The role of *Haemophilus ducreyi* in penile ulcers in Bangkok, Thailand. *Sex Transm Dis* 11:148, 1984.
8 Centers for Disease Control: Sexually transmitted disease statistics 1987. Issue No. 136, Oct, 1988, Atlanta, GA.
9 Chief Medical Officer: Sexually transmitted diseases. Extract from the annual report of the Chief Medical Officer of the Department of Health and Social Security for the year 1983. *Genitourin Med* 61:204, 1985.
10 Piot P, Meheus A: Genital ulcerations, in *Clinical Problems in Sexually Transmitted Diseases,* D Taylor-Robinson (ed). Boston, Martinus Nyhoff Publishers, 1985, p 207.
11 Schmid GP et al: Chancroid in the United States. Reestablishment of an old disease. *JAMA* 258:3265, 1987.
12 Hammond GW et al: Epidemiologic, clinical, laboratory and therapeutic features of an urban outbreak of chancroid in North America. *Rev Infect Dis* 2:867, 1980.
13 Centers for Disease Control: Continuing increase in infectious syphilis—United States. *MMWR* 37:35, 1988.
14 Coutinho RA et al: Influence of special surveillance programmes and AIDS on declining incidence of syphilis in Amsterdam. *Genitourin Med* 63:210, 1987.
15 Plummer FA et al: Epidemiology of chancroid and *Haemophilus ducreyi* in Nairobi, Kenya. *Lancet* 2:1293, 1983.
16 D'Costa LJ et al: Prostitutes are a major reservoir of sexually transmitted diseases in Nairobi, Kenya. *Sex Transm Dis* 12:64, 1984.
17 Quinn TC et al: *Chlamydia trachomatis* proctitis. *N Engl J Med* 305:195, 1981.
18 Cameron DW et al: Female to male heterosexual transmission of HIV infection in Nairobi. Abstract MP 91, 3d International Conference on AIDS, Washington, DC, 1–5 June 1987.
19 Piot P et al: AIDS: An international perspective. *Science* 239:573, 1988.
20 Greenblatt RM et al: Genital ulceration as a risk factor for human immunodeficiency virus infection. *AIDS* 2:47, 1988.
21 Handsfield HH et al: Association of anogenital ulcer disease with human immunodeficiency virus infection in homosexual men. Abstract F1.6, 3d International Conference on AIDS, Washington, DC, 1–5 June 1987.
22 Chapel TA et al: How reliable is the morphological diagnosis of penile ulcerations? *Sex Transm Dis* 4:150, 1977.
23 Fast MV et al: The clinical diagnosis of genital ulcer disease in men in the tropics. *Sex Transm Dis* 11:72, 1984.
24 Plummer FA et al: Clinical and microbiologic studies of genital ulcers in Kenyan women. *Sex Transm Dis* 12:193, 1985.
25 Harp VC: Observations of chancroid therapy with and without sulfathiazole. *Am J Syph Gonorrhea Vener Dis* 30:361, 1946.
26 Piot P et al: Ulcerative balanoposthitis associated with nonsyphilitic spirochaetal infection. *Genitourin Med* 62:44, 1986.
27 Nsanze H et al: Comparison of media for the isolation of *Haemophilus ducreyi. Sex Transm Dis* 11:6, 1984.
28 Sottnek FO et al: Isolation and identification of *Haemophilus ducreyi* in a clinical study. *J Clin Microbiol* 12:170, 1980.
29 Perine PL et al: Diagnosis and treatment of lymphogranuloma venereum in Ethiopia. *Current Chemotherapy and Infectious Disease.* Washington, DC, American Society for Microbiology, 1980, p 1280.
30 Schachter J et al: Lymphogranuloma venereum. 1. Comparison of the Frei test, complement fixation test, and isolation of the agent. *J Infect Dis* 120:372, 1969.
31 Schalla WO et al: Investigation of clinically suspected cases of chancroid using a dot-immunobinding assay and immunofluorescence. *J Infect Dis* 153:879, 1986.
32 Museyi K et al: Use of an enzyme immunoassay to detect serum IgG antibodies to *Haemophilus ducreyi. J Infect Dis* 157:1039, 1988.
33 Schmid GP: The treatment of chancroid. *JAMA* 255:1757, 1986.
34 Taylor DN et al: Antimicrobial susceptibility and characterization of outer membrane proteins of *Haemophilus ducreyi* isolated in Thailand. *J Clin Microbiol* 21:442, 1985.
35 Slootmans L et al: Susceptibility of 40 *Haemophilus ducreyi* strains to 34 antimicrobial products. *Antimicrob Agents Chemother* 24:564, 1983.

# Chapter 60
# Other genital dermatoses

Ernst Stolz
Henk E. Menke
V. D. Vuzevski

Most skin diseases can also affect the genitals and genitocrural folds. Some diseases present with unusual features in these regions. Others are entirely or predominantly confined to the genitocrural region. Nonvenereal skin diseases which affect the genitals and genitocrural folds and which are reviewed in this chapter are summarized in Table 60-1.

Principles of diagnosis of skin diseases in the genitocrural region are not different from these principles in other parts of the skin. In making a dermatologic diagnosis, the following diagnostic steps are important:

1. A careful medical history, including questions about systemic and internal disease, family history, and use of systemic or local drugs.
2. A careful inspection of the skin in good light. Knowledge of the elementary dermatologic lesions is a prerequisite to accurate diagnosis.
3. Palpation of the skin, except for purulent, erosive, or ulcerative lesions.
4. Special diagnostic procedures. These are preeminent in modern dermatology and include punch biopsies for histologic and immunologic studies in noninfectious inflammatory diseases, benign tumors, and premalignant and malignant lesions, patch tests for the analysis of contact allergy, and microbial cultures and inspection under Wood's light for the diagnosis of fungal and bacterial diseases. Because of the importance and feasibility of histology in dermatologic diagnosis, characteristic histopathologic features of the noninfectious dermatologic conditions that can involve the genitalia are described in this chapter.

Treatment of skin diseases in the genitocrural region follows the general rules of dermatologic treatment. However, some drugs like dithranol (anthralin) and tar must be used carefully in the genitocrural area because of their irritating capacity for skin folds and mucosal membranes. Furthermore, it is also better either not to use potent fluorinated steroids in this region or to use such steroids for only a very limited period, because of side effects like atrophy of the skin and masking or promoting of infections. We strongly recommend hydrocortisone as the steroid of choice for the genitocrural region. For further detailed reading about the principles of diagnosis and treatment of skin diseases, we refer the reader to a textbook of dermatology.[5]

Apart from infectious diseases, the clinician should also consider inflammatory dermatoses, benign tumors, premalignant and malignant lesions which affect the genitals and genitocrural folds, and some developmental and congenital lesions which occur in these areas.

In the male patient, the examiner may encounter minor abnormalities affecting the median raphe, as well as cysts of various types, particularly at the penoscrotal junction or arising from

**Table 60-1. Nonvenereal Skin Diseases That May Affect the Genitals and Genitocrural Folds**

| |
|---|
| **Infectious diseases** |
| Fungal infections (dermatophytes) |
| Yeast infections |
| Erythrasma |
| **Inflammatory lesions** |
| Psoriasis |
| Seborrheic dermatitis |
| Lichen planus |
| Adverse drug reactions |
| Exanthemata |
| Urticaria |
| Exfoliative dermatitis |
| Erythema multiforme |
| Purpura |
| Lichenoid eruption |
| Fixed drug eruption |
| Eczema |
| Allergic contact |
| Primary irritant contact |
| Infectious |
| Atopic |
| Lichen sclerosus et atrophicus |
| Primary vulvar atrophy |
| Plasma cell balanitis/vulvitis |
| Nonvenereal sclerosing lymphangitis |
| Behçet's syndrome |
| Aphthosis |
| Hidradenitis suppurativa |
| **Benign tumors** |
| Epidermal tumors |
| Seborrheic keratosis |
| Fibroepithelial polyp |
| Epidermal appendages |
| Sebaceous gland |
| Sweat gland tumors |
| Syringoma |
| Hidradenoma papilliferum |
| Cysts |
| Epidermal cysts |
| Bartholin's gland cysts |
| Melanocytic tumors (moles) |
| Junctional nevus |
| Compound nevus |
| Intradermal nevus |
| Benign juvenile melanoma |
| Mesodermal tumors |
| Nodular fasciitis |
| Fibroma, lipoma, fibrolipoma |
| Angiokeratoma |
| Capillary nevus |
| Angiomatous nevus |
| Lymphangioma |
| Leiomyoma |
| **Premalignant lesions** |
| Erythroplasia of Queyrat |
| Lichen sclerosus et atrophicus |
| Multicentric pigmented Bowen's disease |
| **Malignant lesions** |
| Squamous cell carcinoma |
| Malignant melanoma |
| Other |

dysembryonic diverticula of the urethra. Profuse or enlarged sebaceous glands grouped together as a nevus comedonicus may also be present. A separate, frequently misdiagnosed entity is pearly penile papules or hairy penis or hirsutoid papillomas of the penis. These lesions are small, smooth, dome-shaped or hair-like papules involving the penile corona. They appear to be a physiological variant, symptomless and without functional significance. An incidence of 10 percent has been reported. They are chiefly detected between the ages of 20 and 50. They can be considered to represent angiofibromas. The patient with this harmless condition generally is afraid of having acquired venereal warts. On inspection the papules are found to be situated on the corona, particularly the anterior border, in one to three irregular rings, partly or completely encircling the glans. The papules are flesh-colored, white or red, and are from 1 to 3 mm broad and up to 3 mm in height. However, longer filiform lesions also occur. No treatment is necessary; only reassurance of the patient is required.

In the female patient, dermoid cysts at the perineal raphe and paraurethral cysts are both rare. Local or general dysplasia of the lymphatic system may manifest itself in childhood or young adult life.

All other developmental and congenital lesions in the male and female patient will be discussed under Benign Tumors.

## INFECTIOUS DISEASES

## DERMATOPHYTE INFECTIONS

Excessive perspiration and friction of the major intertriginous areas such as the groins predispose to superficial fungus infections. Dermatophyte infections of the genitals alone are not common, but dermatophyte infections of the genitocrural folds, sometimes associated with genital infections, occur frequently, in particular in the male patient. In general they are caused by *Trichophyton rubrum*, *T. mentagrophytes*, or *Epidermophyton floccosum*.

### Clinical features

Tinea of the intertriginous areas can be symmetrical but is often asymmetrical. In the crural region the lesions extend from the thighs toward the folds, forming erythematous scaly patches which later develop polycyclic borders (Fig. 60-1). The margin is usually active, showing papules and sometimes vesiculation and occasionally some crusting. There may be isolated peripheral annular lesions which can extend to the pubic area, the intergluteal fold, and the buttocks. Scratching may lead to lichenification. In milder forms there is only mild itching or no itching at all. In these cases the borders are less polycyclic, and follicular lesions are often present at the periphery. The course of intertriginous mycosis is chronic with a tendency to relapse in hot weather.

### Diagnosis

The laboratory diagnosis is based on routine microscopic examination looking for hyphae and spores in squamae taken from the border of a lesion in a 10% potassium hydroxide mount and on cultures using Sabouraud and Nickerson media.

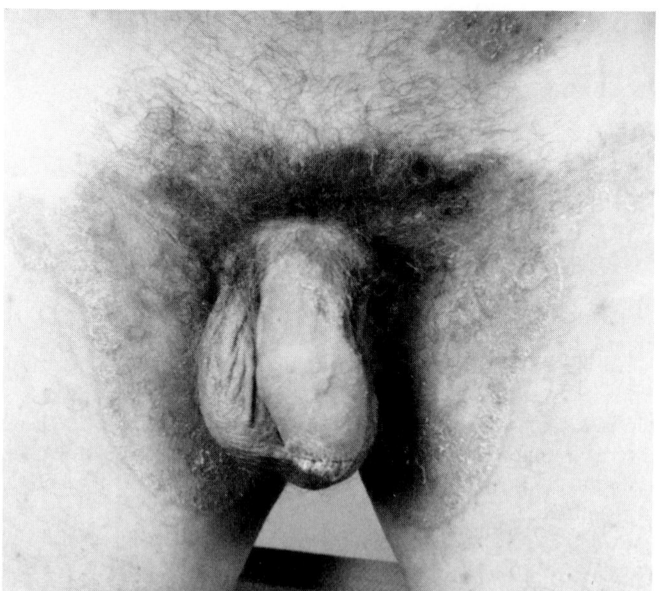

**Fig. 60-1.** Genitocrural dermatophyte infection. (*Courtesy of Dr. Philip Kirby, University of Washington.*)

### Differential diagnosis

The diagnosis of fungal infection is based on clinical features and laboratory test results. Dermatophyte infection in the genitocrural folds and on the genitals must be differentiated from psoriasis inversa, seborrheic dermatitis, yeast infections, and erythrasma.

### Treatment

Treatment can be divided into hygienic measures, topical therapy, and systemic therapy. Imidazole derivatives such as miconazole, isoconazole, econazole, clotrimazole, and bifonazole in an appropriate vehicle, for instance, a cream, are effective. Griseofulvin orally given in doses of 1 to 2 g daily for adults and 500 to 750 mg for children is an effective narrow-spectrum antifungal. If the micronized type is used, half this dosage is sufficient. Side effects are minor and usually gastrointestinal. The patient should be instructed to avoid sunlight as skin reactions may develop. Ketoconazole orally given in doses of 200 mg daily for adults and 100 mg for children is an effective broad-spectrum antifungal. Side effects are gastrointestinal complaints, nausea, headache, dizziness, anaphylactic reactions, exanthema, and pruritis. Hepatotoxicity with an incidence of 1 in 10,000 cases occurs mostly in patients with preexistent liver disease who are treated for more than 1 month. Treatment with topical medication, systemic therapy, or a combination of both should be continued until no clinical or laboratory signs of fungal infection are present.

## YEAST INFECTIONS

Yeast infections in the genital region are mostly caused by *Candida albicans* and *Torulopsis glabrata.* (Genital candidiasis is discussed fully in Chap. 45.)

Briefly, the symptoms of vulvovaginitis are pruritis, sometimes pain, and a whitish milky discharge. On inspection confluent red spots with whitish patches are seen. At the border small lesions

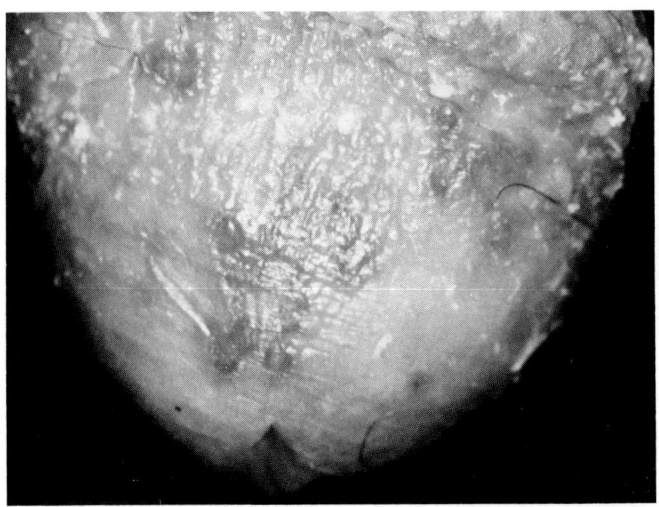

**Fig. 60-2.** *Candida* balanitis. (*Courtesy of Dr. Philip Kirby, University of Washington.*)

("islands in front of the coast") can be observed. The symptoms in balanoposthitis in the male (Fig. 60-2) are in general less severe. They consist of pruritus and red spots with whitish patches on the glans, prepuce, and shaft of the penis. The surface can become easily eroded. Frequently the genitocrural and anal folds are also involved.

The differential diagnosis of yeast infection is based on clinical features and laboratory test results. Yeast infection in the genitocrural folds and on the external genitals must be differentiated from psoriasis inversa, seborrheic dermatitis, fungal infections, and erythrasma.

## ERYTHRASMA

Erythrasma is a superficial, noninflammatory, and usually asymptomatic dermatosis, often affecting intertriginous areas. It is caused by a diphtheroid, *Corynebacterium minutissimum,* which infects the superficial portion of the stratum corneum. Erythrasma is exceedingly common in the tropics and subtropics. The genitocrural type is found usually in male patients.

### Clinical features

Round, oval, or irregular, well-outlined dry patches covered with fine desquamation may be visible. The patches run together forming a larger area with polycyclic borders. Young lesions are erythematous, and the older ones yellow or brownish; they look darker in pigmented skin. The sites of predilection are the intertriginous areas, such as the genitocrural area. Erythrasma is usually asymptomatic, but sometimes it may itch, especially in warm climates.

### Diagnosis

Wood's light reveals coral-red fluorescence, which is characteristic, though not constantly present. Preparations of scales, stained with Gram's, Giemsa's, or PAS stains and examined under oil immersion microscopy, show rodlike organisms, filaments, and coccoid forms. The filaments may be divided into segments and resemble chains of bacilli.

### Differential diagnosis

The diagnosis of erythrasma is based on clinical features including Wood's lamp examination and laboratory tests results. Erythrasma in the genitocrural folds must be differentiated from psoriasis inversa, seborrheic dermatitis, fungal infections, and yeast infections.

### Treatment

Treatment can be divided in hygienic measures, topical treatment, and systemic therapy. Imidazole creams like miconazole cream are effective. Erythromycin, as topical treatment or as oral treatment, is also very effective in the treatment of this condition.

## INFLAMMATORY LESIONS

## PSORIASIS

Psoriasis is a very common, genetically determined, erythematosquamous skin disease. Several factors such as trauma, streptococcal infections, and stress may provoke the disease in genetically predisposed persons. The association of psoriasis with HLA-B13 and HLA-B17 was made by Russell et al.[1] and White et al.[2] in 1972 and has been confirmed by many other investigators.

### CLINICAL FEATURES

The disease is clinically characterized by erythema, which is sharply demarcated from the surrounding, normal-looking skin, and by silvery-white scales that can vary in amount. The typical localizations are scalp, elbows, and knees, but the disease can occur anywhere on the body [see Fig. 60-3(*a*)], including the genitocrural region. In flexures such as are found in the groin, the scales are often completely absent. This is called *inversed psoriasis,* or *psoriasis des plis.* On the glans penis and labia majora, typical erythematosquamous psoriatic lesions may be seen.

### HISTOPATHOLOGY

The constant feature of psoriasis consists of irregular elongation of the rete ridges and thinning of the suprapapillary epidermis. The surface is covered by a parakeratotic horny layer. At places there are small collections of polymorphonuclear leukocytes (Munro microabscesses) in the stratum corneum or in the upper layers of the epidermis. The granular layer is usually absent. The dermal papillae show striking edema and contain dilated capillary loops. In the dermis there is a moderate mononuclear perivascular inflammatory infiltration [Fig. 60.3(*b*)].[3]

### DIFFERENTIAL DIAGNOSIS

The diagnosis of psoriasis is based on the typical clinical morphology of the lesions, combined with the histopathologic picture. Inverted psoriasis in the genitocrural folds must be differentiated from seborrheic dermatitis and intertrigo caused by

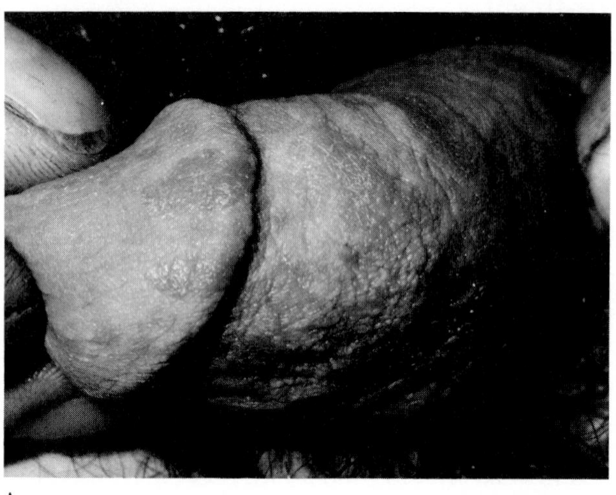

A

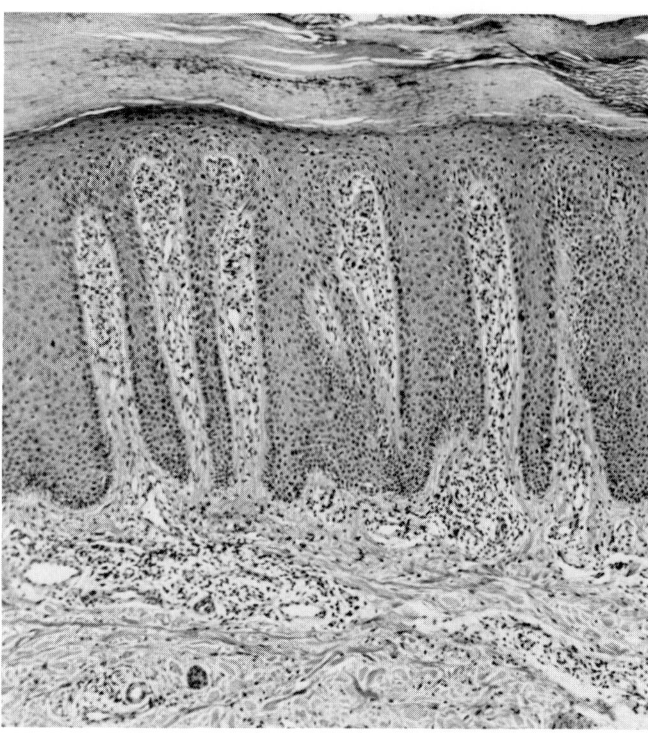

B

Fig. 60-3 (*a*) Penile psoriasis. Note well-demarcated papules of the glans, with minimal scales, which is typical of penile lesions. (*b*) Psoriasis.

*Candida* spp. or bacteria. Histopathologic studies and microbial cultures are helpful in differentiating between these disorders.

## TREATMENT

Local application of antipsoriasis drugs is effective in many cases. Because of their irritating capacity, tar preparations and dithranol should not be applied to the genitocrural region. Use of sulfur-containing pastes or hydrocortisone cream is a valuable means of treatment of genitocrural psoriasis. Systemic administration of cytotoxic drugs or PUVA (psoralen and ultraviolet A), currently widely used for the treatment of psoriasis, is not indicated in localized genitocrural psoriasis.

## SEBORRHEIC DERMATITIS

This is a very common erythematosquamous skin disease. The lesions are localized on the parts of the body that have the greatest concentration and activity of sebaceous glands.[4] The etiology is unknown, but it is assumed that this is a genetically determined disease.

## CLINICAL FEATURES

The typical locations of the lesions are the scalp, eyebrows, nasolabial fold, and sternum, but the lesions can be localized almost anywhere on the body. The disease is characterized by ill-defined pink-red erythematous lesions, covered with yellowish fatty scales. In the genitocrural region, seborrheic dermatitis can look different. Here it is characterized by red, sharply defined lesions, sometimes with a little scaling on the edges (Plate 49).

## HISTOPATHOLOGY

The histologic picture is consistent with a moderate irregular acanthosis (thickening of the stratum malpighii) and branching of the rete ridges. In addition there is focal and follicular parakeratosis (abnormal keratinization, with retention of nuclei in epidermal or adnexal keratinocytes), as well as areas of spongiosis (edema between keratinocytes) with microvesicle formations (Fig. 60-4).

## DIFFERENTIAL DIAGNOSIS

Diagnosis is based on a combination of clinical morphology and histopathologic studies. Seborrheic dermatitis in the genitocrural region must be differentiated from psoriasis and infective intertrigo.

## TREATMENT

Tar and sulfur are effective in seborrheic dermatitis, but corticosteroids are possibly the most active topical preparations. If the eruption becomes eczematous and is weeping, wet compresses are useful. If secondary microbial infection is suspected, it is advisable to add antimicrobials to the topical preparations.

## LICHEN PLANUS

Lichen ruber planus or lichen planus is a common papular skin disease of unknown cause. The principal hypotheses regarding its cause have been based on infectious (viral) origin, neurologic abnormalities, emotional stress, and autoimmunity.[5] Drugs such

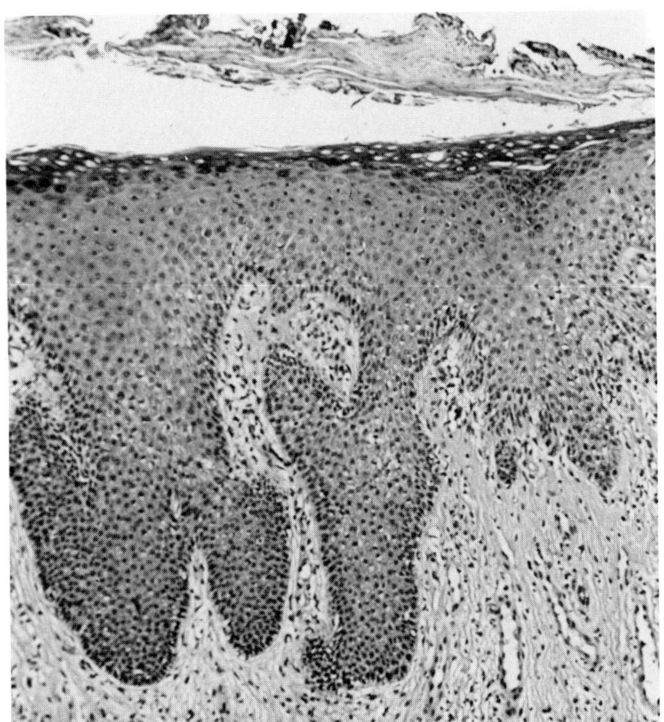

Fig. 60-4. Seborrheic dermatitis.

as bismuth, dapsone (diaminodiphenylsulfone, or DDS), phenothiazines, and arsenicals can cause a lichen planus-like eruption. Lichen planus, like eczema and urticaria, may possibly be a pattern reaction (*reaction cutanée*): many apparently completely unrelated causes can induce the same type of skin reaction.

## CLINICAL FEATURES

Lichen planus papules are flat and angular, violaceous and scaly (see Plate 59). On the surface there may be white dots or lines, known as Wickham's striae. The papules are often localized on extremities, but other localizations do occur. Although the eruption is very pruritic, one does not see excoriations. Koebner's isomorphic phenomenon (this is the induction of new lesions at the site of nonspecific trauma) is observed in lichen planus, as well as in psoriasis and eczema, in its active phases. Lichen planus is a self-limiting disease, often healing with hyperpigmentation and atrophy.

Involvement of the genitals is not rare [see Fig. 60-5(*a*) and Plate 50]. Sometimes the disease is confined to this region. In males, the glans penis is most often involved. The lesions may be typically papular, but annular configuration of the papules, white linear striae, or the atrophic variant of the disease may be seen. In females, the same type of lesions may involve the vulva. Marked atrophy may supervene here.

## HISTOPATHOLOGY

The papules of lichen ruber planus histologically reveal moderate to marked hyperkeratosis (increased thickness of the stratum corneum), focal increase of stratum granulosum, and irregular, sawtooth acanthosis (angular configuration of pointed, elongated rete ridges) of the epidermis. In the papillary dermis there is a bandlike inflammatory infiltration composed of lymphocytes and histiocytes in close proximity to the epidermis. Sometimes numerous hyaline-rounded bodies (Civatte's bodies) can be seen in the upper dermis [Fig. 60-5(*b*)].

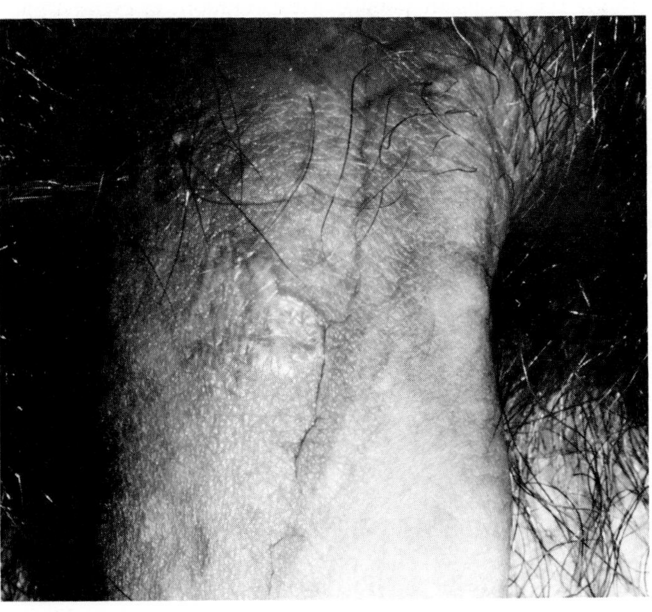

A

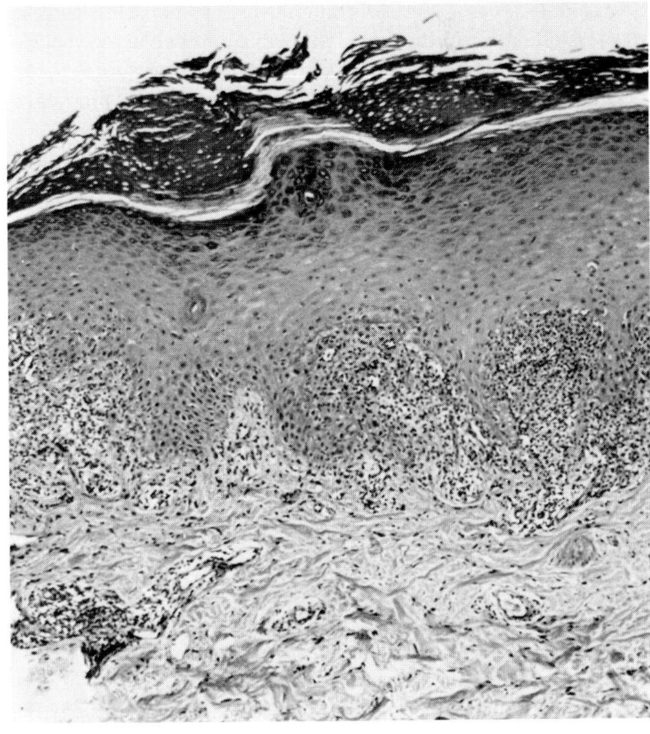

B

Fig. 60-5. (*a*) Lichen planus on the penile shaft. Note annular configuration. (*Courtesy of Dr. Philip Kirby, University of Washington.*) (*b*) Lichen planus.

## DIFFERENTIAL DIAGNOSIS

The papular form of the disease must be differentiated from papular secondary syphilis and drug-induced lichenoid eruptions. The atrophic variant must be differentiated from lichen sclerosus et atrophicus. A biopsy for histopathologic investigation is very rewarding in establishing a definite diagnosis of lichen planus.

## TREATMENT

One should remember that this is a self-limiting disease. Treatment is symptomatic. Drugs of choice are corticosteroids, either locally applied or systemically administered. Use of a hydrocortisone cream is to be preferred, but if this is not effective one should try a fluorinated steroid cream. Antihistamines given orally can sometimes give relief in cases with severe pruritis. Histamine is not involved in the pathophysiology of lichen planus, and therefore the antipruritic action of antihistamines in lichen planus is secondary to nonspecific sedation. Finally, aromatic retinoids, given orally in a dose of 1 mg per kilogram body weight, may be effective in recalcitrant cases.

## ADVERSE CUTANEOUS REACTIONS TO DRUGS

A drug eruption can be generalized or localized. If a localized eruption develops in the same place or places each time a particular drug is taken, this is called a fixed drug eruption. It is generally assumed that a drug reaction results from an allergic sensitization to the drug by previous exposure to the drug or to a cross-reacting immunochemically related compound. If the sensitization has been induced by external contact, leading to contact eczema, an eczematous reaction may develop when the same or a related drug is subsequently administered systemically. In practice it is often very difficult or impossible to prove in a given case that an immunologic process is involved in causing the drug eruption. Many reactions may have a nonimmunologic pharmacologic basis.[5]

## CLINICAL FEATURES

Several morphologic types of drug eruptions are recognized.[6] The most common types are

1. *Exanthematous eruptions* induced by, for example, penicillins, sulphonamides, chloramphenicol, and pyrazole derivatives (e.g., phenylbutazone).
2. *Urticaria* induced by, for example, penicillins, sulphonamides, chloramphenicol, tetracyclines, acetylsalicylic acid, and opiates.
3. *Exfoliative dermatitis* induced by, for example, streptomycin and pyrazole derivatives.
4. *Eczematous eruptions* induced by, for example, penicillins, streptomycin, sulphonamides, phenothiazine compounds, iodides, procaine, and other anesthetics.
5. *Erythema (exudative) multiforme, or Stevens-Johnson syndrome,* induced by, for example, sulphonamides, phenytoin and related anticonvulsants, pyrazole derivatives, barbiturates, penicillins, and carbamazepine.

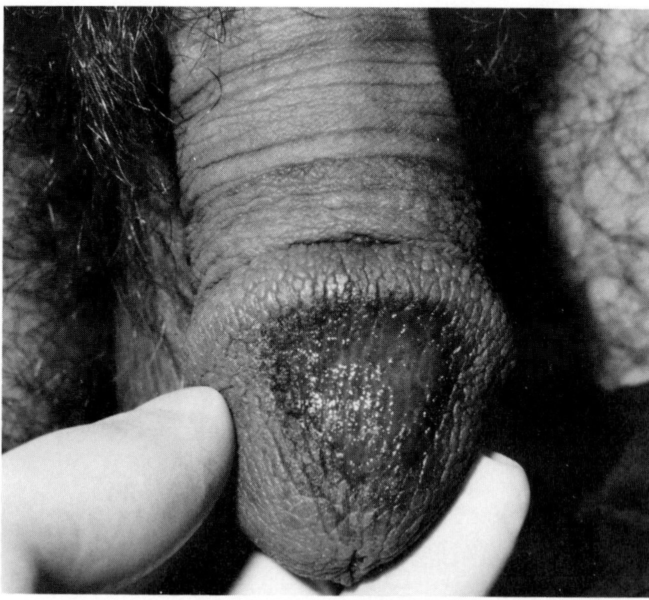

Fig. 60-6. Fixed drug eruption on glans penis, due to tetracycline ingestion. Note eroded surface and developing hyperpigmentation. (*Courtesy of Dr. Philip Kirby, University of Washington.*)

6. *Purpura* induced by, for example, pyrazole derivatives, sulphonamides, and acetylsalicylic acid.
7. *Lichenoid eruptions* induced by, for example, bismuth, dapsone (DDS), phenothiazines, and arsenicals.
8. *Fixed drug eruptions* induced by, for example, phenolphthalein, barbiturates, pyrazole derivatives, phenacetin, tetracycline, sulphonamides, and chlordiazepoxide (Fig. 60-6).

The genitals may be involved in generalized eruptions, and a fixed drug eruption may be confined to the genitals; so all types of drug reactions may be seen in this region. However, the most common types here are erythema multiforme and fixed drug eruption.

Erythema multiforme is a distinctive clinical and histologic reaction which can be precipitated by various agents, including drugs. The lesions are papular with a cyanotic or even purpuric center, or they are vesiculobullous with so-called iris or target lesions. Genital lesions are frequent and may present as balanitis, urethritis (see Plate 3), or vulvovaginitis. In many cases stomatitis and conjunctivitis occur.

Fixed drug eruptions are characterized by a reddish and pigmented plaque, which becomes edematous and sometimes bullous when active and hyperpigmented when inactive. The hyperpigmentation is probably of the postinflammatory type.

## HISTOPATHOLOGY

The histologic features of drug eruptions vary, according to the clinical type of reaction. The different histologic patterns will not be discussed here.

## DIFFERENTIAL DIAGNOSIS

The possibility of a drug reaction must always be considered in clinical dermatology, since drug eruptions mimic many skin diseases. This rule is also valid for dermatoses confined to the genitocrural region. The clinician must of course be acquainted with the morphologic patterns of drug eruptions,[6] and a careful case history is always indispensable. When a drug eruption is suspected, histologic studies are generally of limited help. Readministration of the drug is the most dependable test in demonstrating the responsible agent. However, this should not be done routinely; serious consequences may occasionally result.

## TREATMENT

Administration of the responsible drug should be stopped at once. Symptomatic treatment for a short time with antihistamines or steroids is sometimes necessary.

## ECZEMA

Eczema or eczematous dermatitis is basically a morphologic entity with characteristic clinical and histologic features. It can be regarded as a reaction pattern with multiple causes. A detailed classification of the clinical types of eczemas is difficult because of disputed nomenclature and multiple causes. The four major clinical etiologic types are: allergic contact eczema, primary irritant contact eczema, microbial or infective eczema, and atopic eczema. Although seborrheic dermatitis (or seborrheic eczema) has some features in common with eczematous dermatitis, it is generally regarded as a distinctive etiologic and clinical entity.

1. *Allergic contact eczema.* Allergic contact eczema is a response of the skin to contact with substances to which it is allergically sensitive. The allergens are "simple chemicals," with a relatively low molecular weight. The immunologic basis of allergic contact eczema is a delayed type hypersensitivity reaction [see Fig. 60-7(*a*)].
2. *Primary irritant contact eczema.* A primary irritant is a substance that in most people is capable, even at the first exposure, of causing cell damage if applied for sufficient time and in sufficient concentration. This damage produces an inflammatory response called the primary toxic reactions, the clinical manifestation of which is the primary irritant contact eczema.
3. *Microbial (infectious) eczema.* It is assumed that bacteria and fungi can induce an eczematous dermatitis.[7] This is not attributed to the specific pathogenic activities of the organisms. Evidence that the presence of bacteria is responsible for the persistence of the eczematous lesions is provided by the rapid response of some cases to an appropriate antibiotic. The mechanism of pathogenesis of this type of eczema, however, remains unclear.
4. *Atopic eczema.* Atopic eczema is a genetically determined disorder that may occur in association with asthma and hay fever in the same patient or family. Immunoglobulin E (IgE) appears to carry atopic skin-sensitizing activity.[8]

## CLINICAL FEATURES

Eczema is clinically characterized by polymorphism of the eruption. Acute eczema is characterized principally by erythema, papules, and vesicles; chronic eczema, by papules and lichenification. Other features common to eczematous lesions are scales, crusts, erosions, and fissures.

Eczema can be generalized or localized. The genitocrural region can be involved, and the eczematous dermatitis can be confined to this region. In all cases there is itching and often soreness.

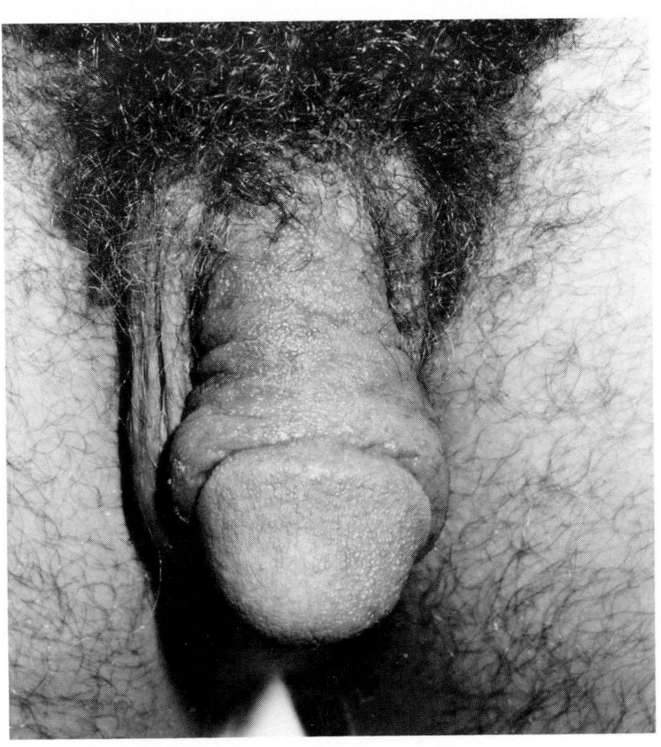

A

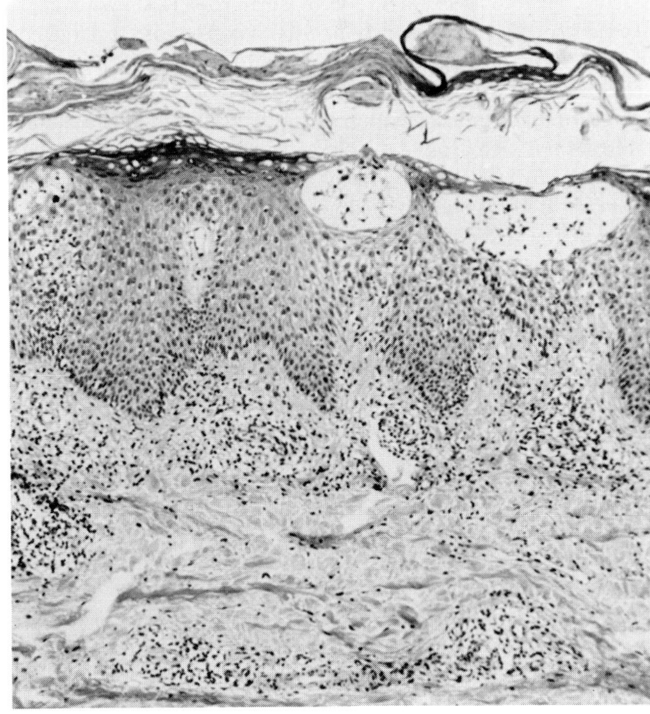

B

**Fig. 60-7.** (*a*) Acute allergic contact eczema, caused by handling mangoes. Note edema and reflection of light from small vesicles on the glans and shaft. (*Courtesy of Dr. Philip Kirby, University of Washington.*) (*b*) Acute allergic contact eczema.

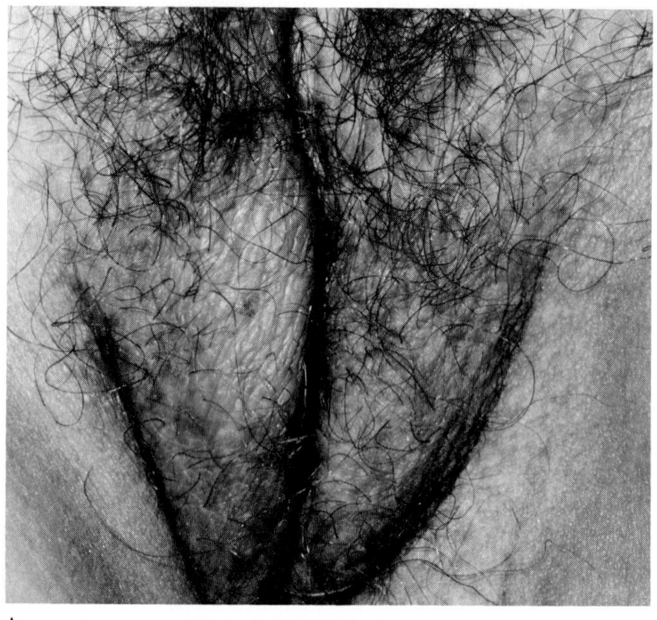

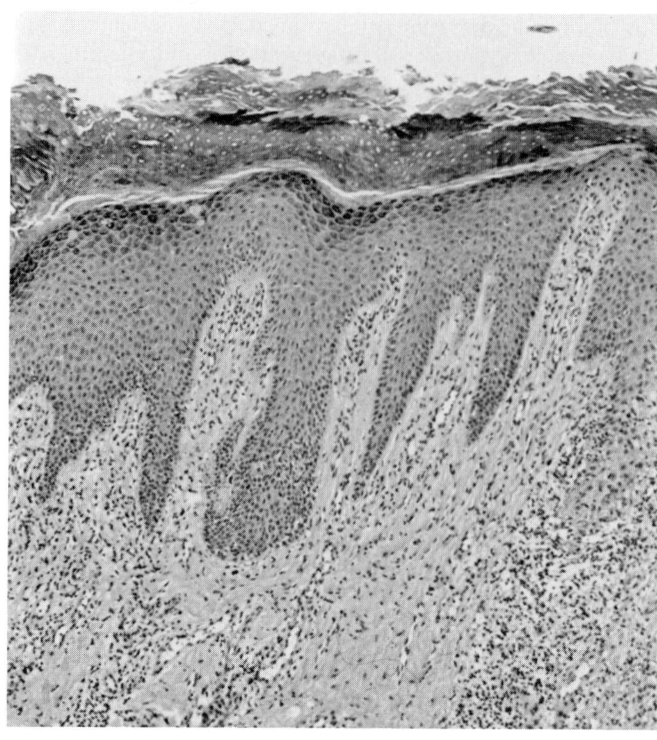

A B

Fig. 60-8. (*a*) Chronic eczema of right labia majora, showing pallor, lichenification, and hair loss associated with chronic scratching. (*Courtesy of Dr. Philip Kirby, University of Washington.*) (*b*) Chronic eczema.

## HISTOPATHOLOGY

A similar histologic picture is seen with the various type of eczema. Histologic examination of *acute* eczema shows a characteristic picture of severe spongiosis that gives rise to large epidermal vesicles containing serous exudate and inflammatory cells. There is a slight parakeratosis and moderate to severe edema of the dermis. Mononuclear perivascular inflammatory infiltration is seen around the blood vessels in the dermal papillae [Fig. 60-7(*b*)]. In *chronic* eczema [Fig. 60-8(*a*) and (*b*)] one encounters moderate to marked acanthosis with irregular lengthening of the rete ridges. There is marked hyperkeratosis associated with a pronounced granular layer. In the dermis there is patchy inflammatory infiltration composed of lymphocytes, histiocytes, and occasional eosinophil leukocytes.

## DIFFERENTIAL DIAGNOSIS

Generally the polymorphic character of the skin disorder easily leads to the clinical diagnosis of eczema. Histologic examination can give further support to this diagnosis. A carefully taken case history (ask for manifestations of atopy and use of local applications such as deodorant sprays, disinfectants, contraceptives, and antibiotics), patch tests, and microbial cultures are often necessary in making a definite diagnosis.

## TREATMENT

Treatment of eczema rests on removal of the cause, accompanied by suitable local symptomatic measures. In acute eczema, wet compresses (saline or potassium permanganate) are indicated; later, steroid creams together with an antimicrobial agent may be used. In chronic eczema, local application of steroids are indicated.

## LICHEN SCLEROSUS ET ATROPHICUS

Lichen sclerosus et atrophicus is an uncommon disease of unknown etiology with small white atrophic macules on the skin and atrophy of vulva, glans penis, and perianal skin. The disease is more common in women than in men, and can involve all ages, with as many as 50 percent of the cases beginning before puberty. In women, involvement of the genitals is known as kraurosis vulvae; in men as balanitis xerotica obliterans.

## CLINICAL FEATURES

Initially, the typical lesions are ivory-white, small, polygonal, flat but palpable lesions, each a few millimeters in diameter, often confluent. Later they become depressed, sclerotic, and typically atrophic. In females the vaginal introitus [Fig. 60-9(*a*)] and in males the urethral meatus is often constricted. In vulvar lesions pruritus is prominent.

## HISTOPATHOLOGY

The histopathology of lichen sclerosus et atrophicus is diagnostic of this entity and is characterized by marked hyperkeratosis associated with a severe atrophy of the epidermis. Sometimes there

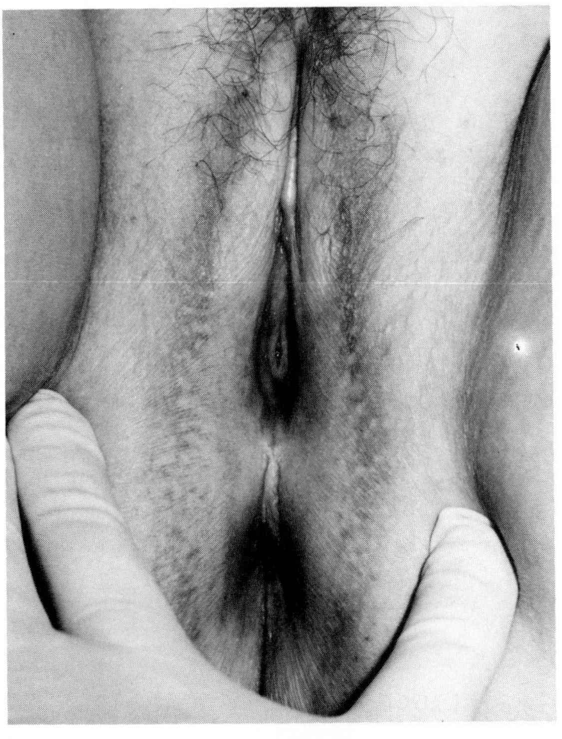

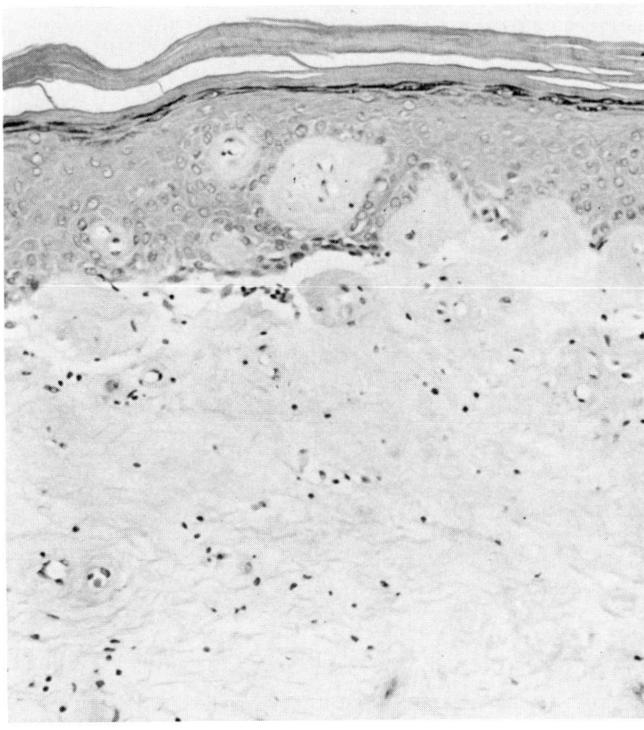

A B

**Fig. 60-9.** (*a*) Lichen sclerosus et atrophicus. Note shiny, pale, atrophic vulvar, perineal, and perianal skin, with surrounding hyperpigmentation. (*Courtesy of Dr. Philip Kirby, University of Washington.*) (*b*) Lichen sclerosus et atrophicus.

is liquefaction degeneration at the dermoepidermal junction. The papillary layer of the dermis reveals a striking edema and homogeneous appearance. Inflammatory infiltration of the dermis by lymphocytes and few histiocytes is very pronounced and confined to the reticular dermis [Fig. 60-9(*b*)].

## DIAGNOSIS

This condition must be differentiated from lichen planus and, in women, from primary atrophy of the vulva, and from senile atrophy of the vulva, which probably represents an exaggeration of physiological vulvar atrophy of elderly women.

## TREATMENT

Treatment is local application of hydrocortisone cream.

# PRIMARY ATROPHY OF THE VULVA

Primary atrophy of the vulva is a progressive sclerosing atrophy of the vulvovaginal mucosa of unknown etiology.

## CLINICAL FEATURES

The vulva, including the labia minora and clitoris (which may ultimately disappear), are sclerosed and atrophic. The labia majora are somewhat flattened. Subjectively, the vulva is sore or pruritic.

## HISTOPATHOLOGY

The epidermis is thin and flat, with normal or reduced keratinization, and directly under it and often in clumps there are inflammatory cells in the dermis. The elastic tissue is reduced or even absent.

## DIAGNOSIS

Early cases may be differentiated histologically from lichen sclerosus et atrophicus, but late cases cannot be distinguished from this condition. In fact it is suggested that in many cases primary atrophy is the end result of lichen sclerosus et atrophicus.[9]

## TREATMENT

Corticosteroid creams and a simple emollient are sometimes helpful.

# PLASMA CELL BALANITIS AND VULVITIS

This is a benign disorder of unknown etiology.[10] It may represent a reaction pattern to many diverse stimuli.

## CLINICAL FEATURES

A patch of erythema, sometimes slightly elevated, with a shiny, smooth, and moist surface is localized on the glans penis or inner

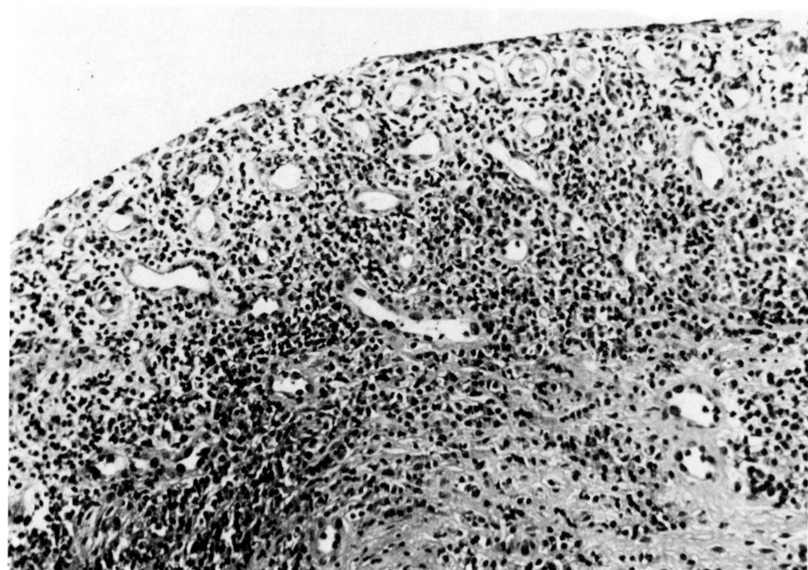

Fig. 60-10. Plasma cell vulvitis.

surface of the foreskin in males (Plate 51) and on the inner surface of the labia majora or minora in females.

## HISTOPATHOLOGY

The epithelium often appears thinned and may be even partially absent. The upper dermis contains a bandlike inflammatory infiltrate composed largely of plasma cells. In addition, the capillaries are dilated, and there may be deposits of hemosiderin.[3] (Fig. 60-10).

## DIAGNOSIS

Balanitis or vulvitis plasmocellularis must be differentiated from erythroplasia of Queyrat. A biopsy for histologic investigation is always indicated when these diagnoses are considered.

## TREATMENT

Treatment with hydrocortisone cream is successful in most cases.

# NONVENEREAL SCLEROSING LYMPHANGITIS

The etiology of this self-limiting, completely benign disorder is unknown. It is reported almost exclusively in males, but Stolz and van Kampen reported a case of sclerosing lymphangitis located on the vulva.[11]

## CLINICAL FEATURES

This symptomless disorder presents as a hard, cordlike thickening, usually lying just behind the corona of the glans penis.

## HISTOPATHOLOGY

The lymphatic vessels are sclerosed and hypertrophic with little inflammation.[5]

## TREATMENT

No treatment is needed; the condition resolves spontaneously.

# BEHÇET'S SYNDROME

Behçet's syndrome is a chronic progressive disease of unknown etiology and is characterized by recurrent ulcerations of the mouth and genitalia, iritis, multiple signs and symptoms in other organ systems, and papulopustules on the skin.

## CLINICAL FEATURES

The genital lesions are a small part of the whole picture. The ulcers are usually painful and variable in size and occur mainly on the labia majora and the scrotum (Plate 30).

## HISTOPATHOLOGY

The ulcers show nonspecific inflammatory changes with an infiltrate consisting of lymphocytes, histiocytes, and polymorphonuclear leukocytes. Vasculitis can be present.[3]

## DIAGNOSIS

In patients with recurrent painful ulcers on the genitals, Behçet's syndrome should be considered. The diagnosis is basically a clinical one. The condition must be differentiated from aphthosis and recurrent herpes simplex virus infection.

## TREATMENT

There is no specific treatment. Symptomatic treatment must be prescribed.

# APHTHOSIS

This is a common disorder characterized by recurrent ulcers in the mouth and rarely on the genitals. The etiology is unknown in most cases, although local recurrent trauma may cause recurrent aphthae; the syndrome of chronic cyclic neutropenia is a rare cause of recurrent aphthae.

## CLINICAL FEATURES

The ulcers are small (1 to 10 mm in diameter), shallow, with a grayish-white base, and they may be very painful. They generally occur in the mouth but are occasionally confined to the genitalia (vulva or scrotum).

## HISTOPATHOLOGY

The histologic features are the same as in Behçet's syndrome.[3]

## DIAGNOSIS

Aphthosis must be differentiated from recurrent herpes simplex and Behçet's syndrome.

## TREATMENT

Discomfort may be reduced with local application of steroids.

# HIDRADENITIS SUPPURATIVA

Hidradenitis suppurativa is a rather common inflammatory disorder of apocrine sweat glands with lesions in the axillae, groin, buttocks, and perianal region. The cause is unknown, but bacteria may play a role, as well as hormonal influences. The disorder is frequently associated with acne conglobata and perifolliculitis capitis.[5]

## CLINICAL FEATURES

The disease is characterized by painful nodules and, in a later stage, with the formation of abscesses, sinuses, and fistulas. Comedones are sometimes seen. Hidradenitis is a chronic disease that often has premenstrual flares.

## HISTOPATHOLOGY

Inflammatory changes are seen around hair follicles, with leukocytes and bacteria present. In a later stage, a foreign body reaction and scaling are found.[3]

## DIFFERENTIAL DIAGNOSIS

Other chronic inflammatory disorders such as lymphogranuloma venereum, actinomycosis, recurrent furunculosis, and Crohn's disease must be excluded.

## TREATMENT

Treatment is difficult and often not rewarding. Systemic use of antibiotics and steroids may be helpful. Small isolated lesions can be effectively treated with intralesional injection of a corticosteroid. In long-standing cases with sinuses and fistulas, surgery may offer a radical solution.

# BENIGN TUMORS

Any known tumor may on occasion be found at the penis, scrotum, or vulva. Benign tumors of the vagina are relatively rare. Benign tumors of the penis, scrotum, or vulva will be subdivided as outlined in Table 60-1.

## EPIDERMAL TUMORS

### Basal cell papilloma (seborrheic keratosis or seborrheic wart)

These keratoses are less common at the penis, scrotum, and vulva than elsewhere.

**Clinical Features.** The lesions are warty, pigmented, and flat. They are currently not regarded as being caused by papilloma virus.

**Histopathology.** The tumor is built up by an acanthotic, papillomatous, and hyperkeratotic epidermis. Most of the epidermal cells bear a resemblance to epidermal basal cells. Keratin-filled crypts often are numerous (Fig. 60-11).

**Differential Diagnosis.** The differential diagnosis includes melanocytic nevus, pigmented genital wart, pigmented basal cell carcinoma, and multicentric pigmented Bowen's disease.

**Treatment.** No treatment is required. For cosmetic reasons the warts can be removed by curettage, cautery, or cryosurgery.

### Fibroepithelial polyps (skin tags)

Skin tags are associated with obesity, moisture, dark skin coloring, and middle age. They are especially common in the genitocrural (and axillary) folds.

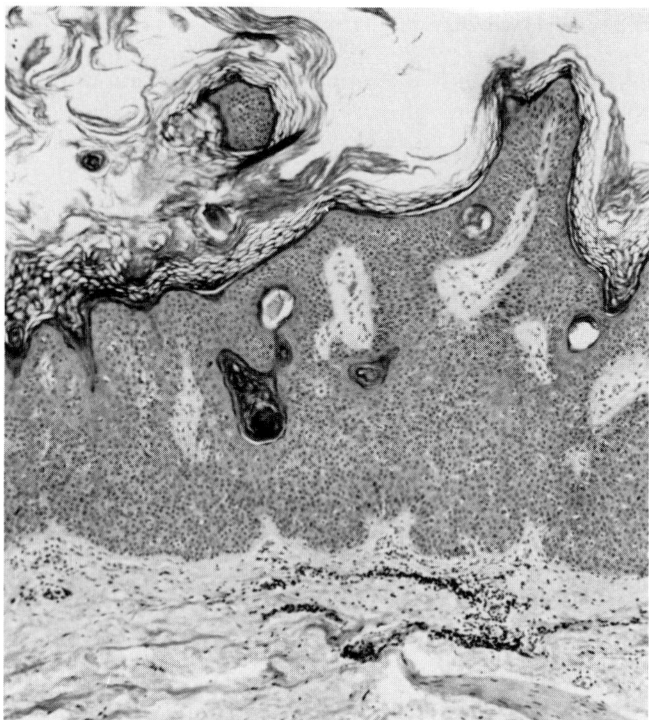

Fig. 60-11. Seborrheic keratosis.

**Clinical Features.** Skin tags are skin-colored, soft, pedunculated tags.

**Histopathology.** The skin tags are usually built up by acellular connective tissue and covered by normal or atrophic epidermis.

**Differential Diagnosis.** The lesions are unmistakable.

**Treatment.** There is no treatment. For cosmetic reasons the tags can be removed by cutting them with a pair of scissors or by curettage.

## TUMORS OF EPIDERMAL APPENDAGES

Benign tumors of epidermal appendages at the penis, scrotum, or vulva are rare.

### Sebaceous gland tumors

At the penis, scrotum, or vulva, yellowish-white nodules can be observed. They can be considered sebaceous retention cysts.

## SWEAT GLAND TUMORS

These tumors are rare. Two main types can be seen; one arises from the eccrine sweat ducts, the other arises from the apocrine sweat glands.

### Syringoma

Syringoma represents an adenoma of intraepidermal eccrine ducts. The tumor is more common in females than in males. It is more likely to appear at adolescence, and further lesions may develop during adult life. The front of the face and the chest and neck are the main areas affected. Involvement of the vulva is extremely rare; however, it seems likely that vulval lesions would be found if looked for in some patients with multiple syringomas.[9]

**Clinical Features.** Small dermal papules of flesh or yellowish color are seen. Sometimes they appear translucent; they vary in size from 2 to 5 mm.

**Histopathology.** Numerous cystic ducts are apparent, and they often terminate in epithelial strands. The eccrine origin of the tumor has been established by histochemical, enzymehistochemical, and electron microscopic examinations.

**Differential Diagnosis.** On the face, syringomas have to be differentiated from trichoepitheliomas.

**Treatment.** Usually, no treatment is necessary. For cosmetic reasons treatment by cautery can be considered.

### Hidradenoma papilliferum

This tumor occurs most often on the anogenital area of women, particularly on the vulva and the labia majora. The tumor arises from the apocrine sweat glands.

**Clinical Features.** The tumor is a solitary, firm or soft nodule with a diameter of 1 to 4 cm. Occasionally it ulcerates.

**Histopathology.** The tumor is located in the dermis. It is surrounded by a fibrous capsule and shows no connections with the overlying epidermis. The tumor is composed of cystlike lumens and papillary structures lined with an apocrine-type epithelium.

**Differential Diagnosis.** The tumor may be mistaken for a cyst, a polyp, an angioma, or a hemorrhoid.

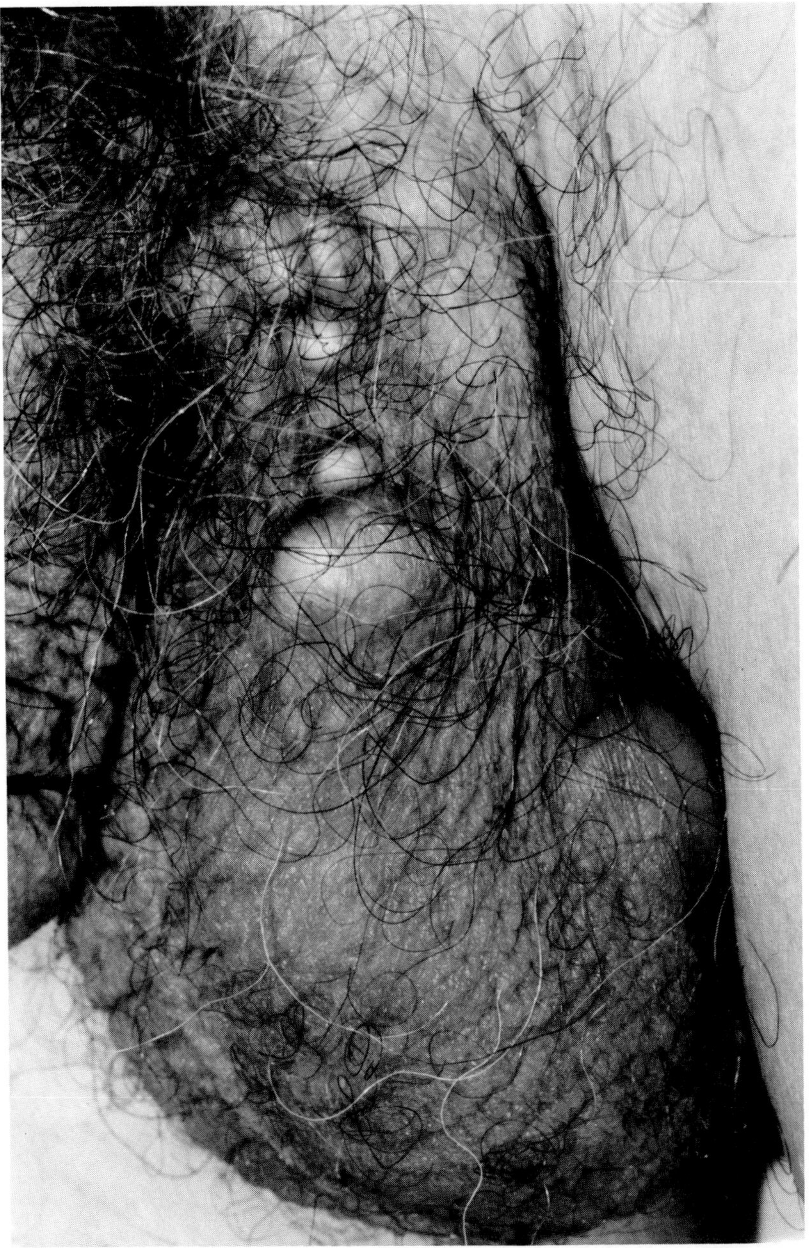

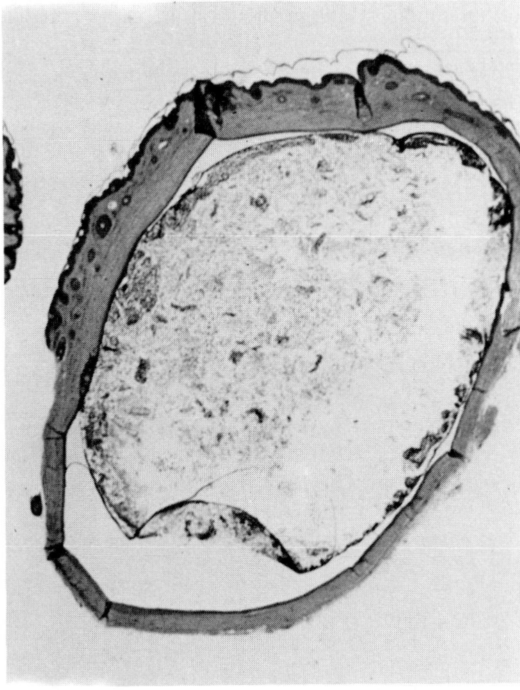

A B

Fig. 60-12. (*a*) Epidermal cysts of the scrotum (often called "sebaceous cysts," though few contain sebaceous elements). The pale color is characteristic. The most inferior cyst appears darker because it is inflamed. (*Courtesy of Dr. Philip Kirby, University of Washington.*) (*b*) Epidermal cysts.

**Treatment.** No treatment is required, but simple excision may be considered.

**Involvement of the Penis.** Ahmed and Jones[12] have reported an apocrine cystadenoma, or hidrocystoma, on the penis. The histogenesis of this tumor seems to be very similar to the histogenesis of hidradenoma papilliferum.

## CYSTS

Apart from cysts of developmental origin of several histopathologic types of the vagina and vulva and of the penis and scrotum, epidermal cysts can be observed in the female on the vulva, mainly the labia majora, and in the male on the penis and scrotum. In the female, cysts of Bartholin's gland deserve special attention.

### Epidermal cysts

These cysts follow traumatic implantation of an epidermal fragment. Generally, epidermal cysts are seen on the face, back, scalp, genitalia, fingers, and hands.

**Clinical Features.** These nontender tumors are tense. In general they are small, but they may become inflamed and reach large sizes [Fig. 60-12(*a*)]. Most cysts, however, reach a size of 1 to 5 cm in diameter.

**Histopathology.** The cysts lie in the dermis. The wall of the cyst is built up by true epidermis. Sometimes the wall shows marked atrophy. The cysts are filled with horny material arranged in laminated layers [Fig. 60-12(*b*)]. A ruptured cyst can cause a foreign-body reaction and may lead to a pseudocarcinomatous proliferation in remnants of the epithelial lining of the cyst.

**Differential Diagnosis.** Multiple nontender, tense tumors must be distinguished from multiple epidermoid cysts seen in Gardner's syndrome.

**Treatment.** Epidermal cysts can be easily excised or removed by curettage. Good results have also been reported by putting a needle in the cyst and aspirating the contents. This treatment must be repeated several times.

### Cysts of Bartholin's gland

Cysts result from obstruction in the main duct. The minor ducts and glandular acini also may be involved. The cysts may be uni- or multilobular. The obstruction can be caused by thick mucus or by congenital defects. Infection may follow. The cysts are mainly present in the reproductive years.

**Clinical Features.** The swelling is found in the posterior part of the labia majora. The diameter varies from 1 to 8 cm. In case of inflammation, the swelling can be tender if palpated.

**Differential Diagnosis.** Cysts of Bartholin's gland have to be distinguished from other benign tumors such as adenomas and hamartomas. Especially in postmenopausal women, neoplasia must be suspected.

**Treatment.** Excision or marsupialization of Bartholin's gland is recommended.

## MELANOCYTIC TUMORS (MOLES)

Melanocytic nevi may occur at any part of the penis, the scrotum, and the vulva. They have the same characteristics as melanocytic nevi elsewhere. They are uncommon in infancy, gradually increase in frequency during childhood, and increase sharply at adolescence. During old age their frequency drops.

### Clinical features

Melanocytic nevi have a wide range of clinical appearances. Pigmentation is usual, but not invariably present. Most of the lesions are relatively small. On histopathologic and clinical grounds, junctional nevi, compound nevi, and intradermal nevi can be distinguished. On the genitalia most nevi are of the junctional and intradermal nevus type. Occasionally, juvenile benign melanomas may occur.[9]

A junctional nevus is a flat, sometimes slightly raised area with a diameter of up to 1 cm. The color varies from light brown to brown black.

Compound nevi vary in form from a slightly raised plaque to a substantial papillomatous tumor. The form is elliptical or circular. Most lesions have a light-brown color [Fig. 60-13(*a*)]. A special compound nevus is the juvenile benign melanoma. This tumor arises predominantly in children. It is usually solitary and is encountered on the face and extremities. In most instances the lesion consists of a dome-shaped, hairless, small nodule, usually only a few millimeters in diameter. Because of the sparsity of melanin, the tumor has a reddish rather than a brown color.

Intradermal nevi may be domed, smooth-surfaced, hemispheric nodules. The diameter varies from 2 to 5 mm. The color varies from flesh-color to medium brown or exceptionally dark brown.

### Histopathology

Melanocytic nevi are composed of nevus cells, which, even though basically identical with melanocytes, differ from melanocytes by being arranged in clusters of nests and by not showing dendritic processes as best demonstrated by staining with silver.

In a *junctional nevus,* nevus cells are present as well-circumscribed nevus cell nests in the lower epidermis. The upper epi-

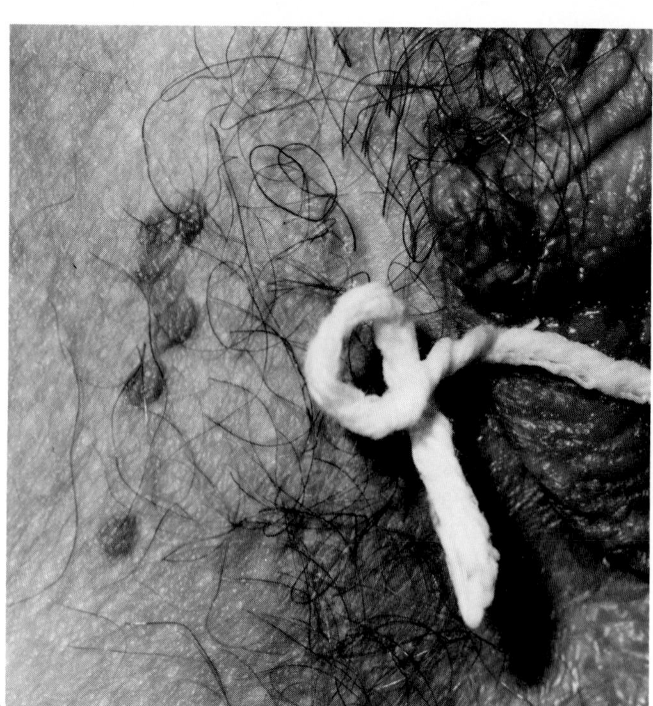


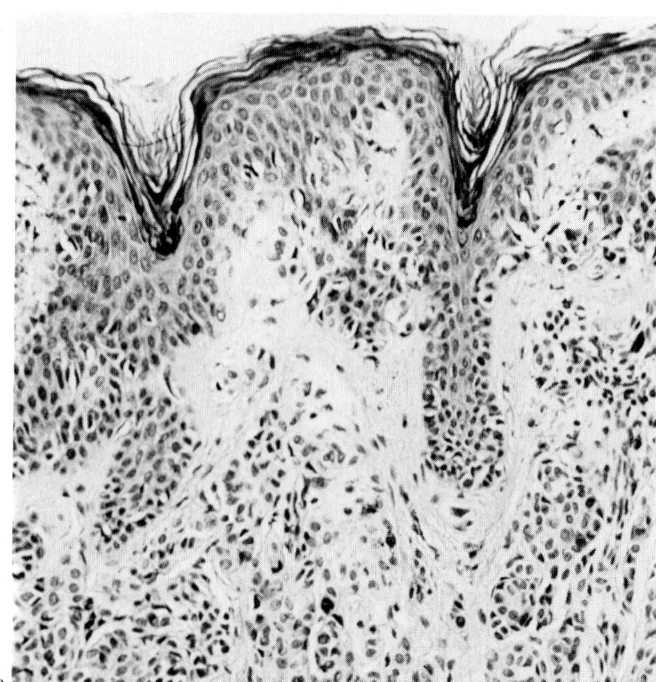


**Fig. 60-13.** (*a*) Compound nevi near the vulva. These multiple, tan, fleshy papules could be confused with warts. (*Courtesy of Dr. Philip Kirby, University of Washington.*) (*b*) Compound nevus.

dermis appears essentially normal. In addition, nests of nevus cells often lie beneath the epidermis but are still in contact with it and thus are in the stage of "dropping off." The nevus cells contain varying amounts of melanin and are cuboidal.

A *compound nevus* possesses features of both a junctional and an intradermal nevus. Nevus cell nests are seen in the epidermis, as well as dropping off from the epidermis into the dermis, and in the dermis. The nevus cells in the upper dermis contain a moderate amount of melanin, and the subepidermal cell nests contain little or no melanin. Contrary to the spindle-shaped cells in the subepidermal cell nests, the cells in the upper dermis are cuboidal [Fig. 60-13(*b*)].

*Intradermal nevus* shows no junctional activity. In the upper dermis there are nests and cords of nevus cells. Multinucleated nevus cells may be present. The nevus cell nests located in the upper dermis usually contain a moderate amount of melanin, but the nevus cells in the midportion and the lower dermis rarely contain melanin. In the midportion and the lower dermis, the nevus cells appear spindle-shaped.

*Benign juvenile melanoma* represents a compound nevus. The tumor is built up by spindle-shaped and large, oval multinucleated cells. Because of the pleomorphism of the cells and the frequent presence of an inflammatory infiltrate, the histologic picture often resembles that of a nodular malignant melanoma.

### Histogenesis

It seems established that nevus cells differ from Schwann cells but are identical with melanocytes.[3]

### Differential diagnosis

Melanocytic nevi must be distinguished from malignant melanomas. Other conditions which can sometimes simulate melanocytic nevi are vascular nevi, cutaneous mastocytosis, pigmented basal cell nevi and trichoepithelioma, seborrheic keratosis, pigmented basal cell carcinomas, histiocytomas, pyogenic granulomas, and Kaposi's sarcoma.

### Treatment

No treatment is required. For cosmetic reasons and in case the melanocytic nevi increase in size or are subject to friction, excision may be considered. Histopathologic examination of the excised mole is obligatory.

## MESODERMAL TUMORS

### Nodular fasciitis

This benign lesion is most common in the subcutaneous tissues; it may occur in any subcutaneous area and is also seen on the penis, the scrotum, and the vulva.

**Clinical Features.** Most frequently the patients complain of a subcutaneous lump of recent onset. The swelling is often tender and has a diameter of up to 2 cm. The most commonly affected sites are the upper extremities, especially the forearm. Generally, the lesion is solitary; however, multiple lesions have been described.

**Histopathology.** The lesion is found partially attached to the fascia from which it arises. It is ill-defined, and it may infiltrate into the underlying muscle. The nodule consists of numerous large, pleomorphic fibroblasts growing haphazardly in a stroma that often is highly vascularized and contains varying amounts of mucoid ground substance. Erythrocytes are also present outside the capillaries. Fibroblasts show a fair number of mitoses, but the mitoses do not appear atypical.

**Differential Diagnosis.** The lesion has to be distinguished from fibrosarcoma.[13]

**Treatment.** No treatment is necessary; the condition is self-limiting. If the patient complains, simple excision can be performed.

### Fibroma, lipoma, and fibrolipoma

These tumors may occur at the penis, scrotum, and vulva.

**Clinical Features.** The size is variable; generally these tumors are solitary.

**Histopathology.** In the dermis, loose fibrous tissue, fatty tissue, or a combination of both can be observed.

**Differential Diagnosis.** These tumors may resemble epidermoid cysts.

**Treatment.** No treatment is necessary; however, simple excision can be performed.

### Angiokeratoma

This tumor occurs in particular on the scrotum [Fig. 60-14(*a*)] but also may be seen on the penis and vulva. It occurs mainly in adult life.

**Clinical Features.** Small deep-red or blue-black papules may be seen on the scrotum, penis, and vulva. They occur also on the lower leg and foot and other sites of the body. In general they are a few millimeters in diameter. They are often multiple and grouped.

**Histopathology.** The tumor is covered by acanthotic and hyperkeratotic epidermis. Dilated capillaries are enclosed within the epidermis or are seen in the underlying connective tissue [Fig. 60-14(*b*)].

**Differential Diagnosis.** The solitary angiokeratoma must be distinguished from melanoma. Angiokeratoma of the scrotum, the penis, or the vulva may be a part of a rare hereditary disorder, angiokeratoma corporis diffusum universale (Anderson-Fabry disease).

**Treatment.** Small lesions may be destroyed with diathermy or laser. Larger lesions may be excised.

### Capillary nevus

Capillary nevi are congenital and persist during life. Usually they are unilateral.

**Clinical Features.** Capillary nevi are port-wine stained.

**Treatment.** Laser coagulation may be considered.

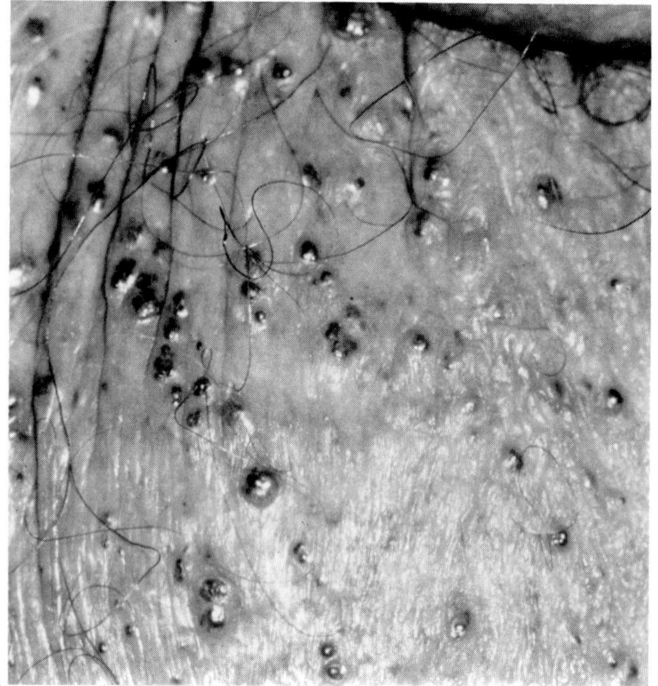
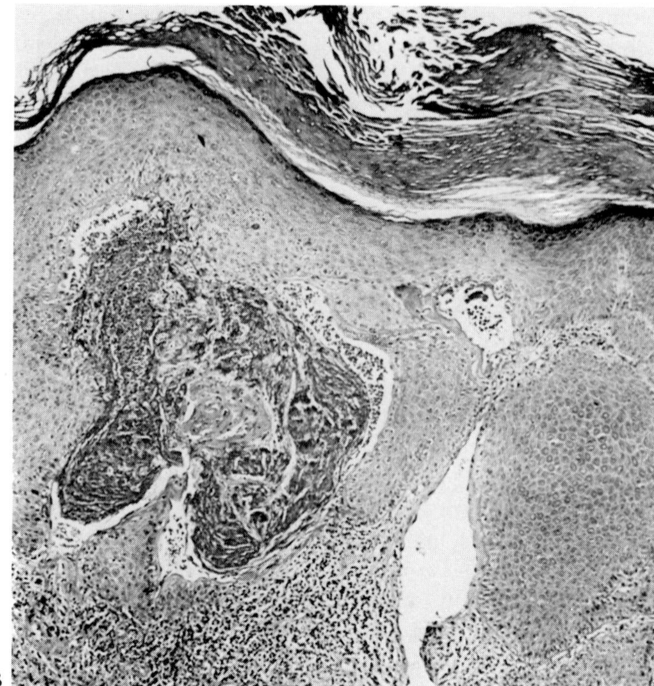

Fig. 60-14. (*a*) Angiokeratomas of the scrotum. (*Courtesy of Dr. Philip Kirby, University of Washington.*) (*b*) Angiokeratoma.

## Angiomatous nevus

Angiomatous nevi appear usually shortly after birth. They can be superficial, subcutaneous, or both.

**Clinical Features.** They appear as a bluish-red mass. The surface of the skin is often irregular.

**Histopathology.** In the dermis, dilated capillaries, endothelial proliferation, and cavernous spaces can be observed.

**Treatment.** Laser coagulation may be considered, particularly in superficial angiomatous nevi.

## Lymphangioma

Most lymphangiomas appear at birth or soon after. They vary in size and extent. Lymphangioma circumscriptum is the most common type of lymphangioma. It also may occur at the scrotum, penis, vulva, vagina, and perineum.

**Clinical Features.** Small deep vesicles resembling frog-spawn grouped together may be observed. Some vesicles may be blood-filled.

**Histopathology.** Cystic dilated lymph vessels lined by a single layer of endothelial cells are present in the dermis and even in the subcutaneous fat.

**Treatment.** Simple excision is often not sufficient. In these cases a deep excision is necessary.

## Leiomyoma (dartoic)

This rare tumor is derived from smooth muscle of the scrotum, the labia majora, and the nipples. It can occur at any age.

**Clinical Features.** Dartoic myoma presents itself as a dermal nodule. It usually is solitary. If stimulated by cold or touch, contractions may occur.

**Histopathology.** Within the dermis, bundles of smooth-muscle cells having an eosinophilic appearance can be observed.

**Differential Diagnosis.** Usually the tumor is not recognized clinically and diagnosis is made on histopathologic grounds.

**Treatment.** Dartoic leiomyomas can be removed by surgical excision.

# MALIGNANT TUMORS

# PREMALIGNANT LESIONS

## Erythroplasia of Queyrat

Erythroplasia is an intraepidermal carcinoma, histologically similar to Bowen's disease, situated on mucous membranes, particularly at the penis but also at the vulva. Erythroplasia may invade the dermis as squamous cell carcinoma.[14] The relationship of this condition to papilloma virus deserves further study.

**Clinical Features.** The lesions on the foreskin of the penis and the glans and the inner side of the vulva are red colored, glazed, and barely raised. They are well circumscribed and consist of irregularly shaped plaques (Plate 52). Ulceration and crusting may occur.

**Histopathology.** The surface may be denuded of stratum corneum and stratum granulosum. Parakeratotic scales or crusts may be present. The epidermis appears irregularly acanthotic. Epidermal cells are characterized by variation in cell and nuclear size, increased number of mitoses, and dyskeratotic and multinucleated cells (Fig. 60-15).

**Differential Diagnosis.** Erythroplasia must be distinguished from balanitis circumscripta, Zoon's balanitis, lichen planus, psoriasis, and circinate balanitis.

**Treatment.** In simple erythroplasia, excision or electron beam therapy are the treatments of choice. Topical therapy with 5-fluorouracil 5% in an ointment can be performed if therapy can be applied by the patient conscientiously.

### Lichen sclerosus et atrophicus

Lichen sclerosus et atrophicus has been presented above. Especially on mucous membranes, in particular on the vulva, the lesions have to be watched carefully for malignant degeneration.[5]

### Multicentric pigmented Bowen's disease

In recent years, many dermatologists have begun to differentiate Bowen's disease (usually a single genital lesion in people over age 50, associated with progression to invasive cancer) from multicentric pigmented Bowen's disease, also known as Bowenoid papulosis (multiple pigmented papules of the penis or vulva, occurring in young adults, with low risk of progression to invasive disease).

**Clinical Features.** The lesions are extensive and symmetrical. They appear as black spots or as velvety seborrheic warts (see Plate 53).

**Histopathology** Histologically, Bowen's disease and Bowenoid papulosis are indistinguishable, showing features of carcinoma in situ (see Chap. 48). The epidermis is irregularly hyperplastic. The epidermal cells are arranged in disorderly fashion. The cells are atypical, showing hyperchromatic nuclei. In addition there are numerous mitotic figures, multinucleated giant cells, and dyskeratotic cells (Fig. 60-16).

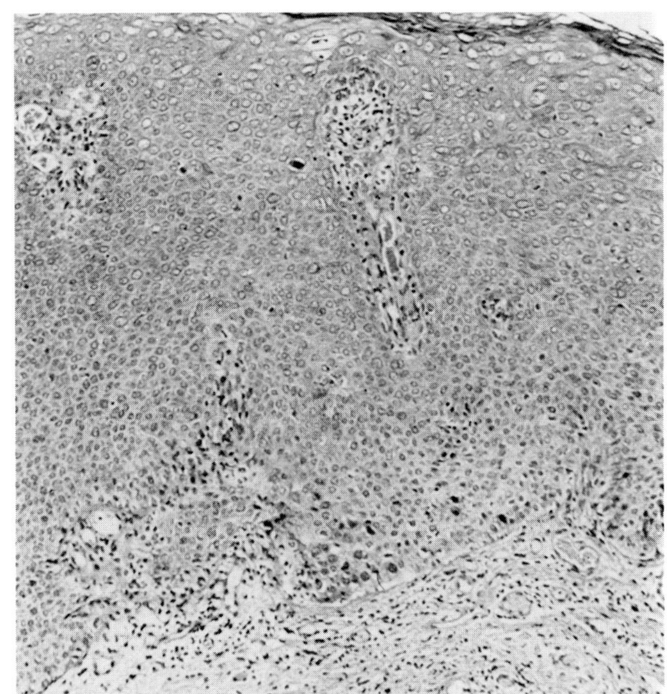

Fig. 60-15. Erythroplasia of Queyrat.

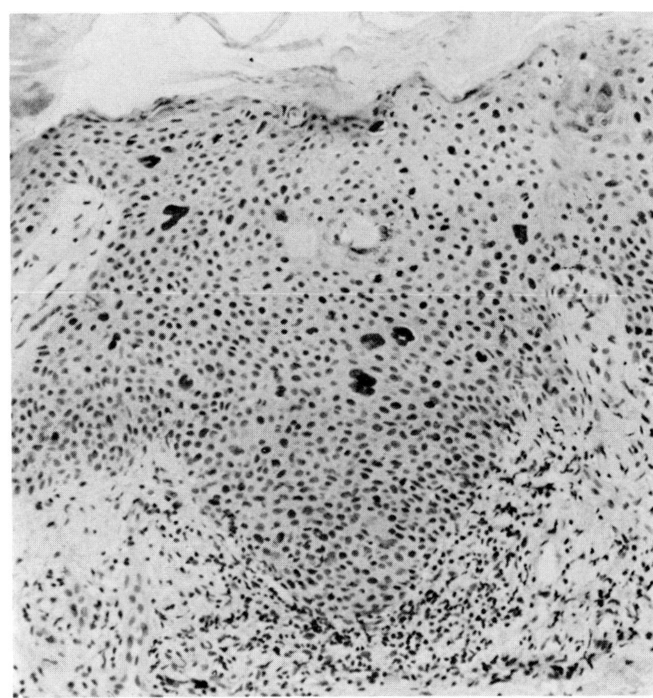

Fig. 60-16. Bowen's disease.

**Differential Diagnosis.** Bowen's disease must be distinguished from condylomata acuminata and seborrheic keratosis.

**Treatment.** Treatment with curettage, cautery, or liquid nitrogen and cryosurgery may be considered.

## MALIGNANT LESIONS

## SQUAMOUS CELL CARCINOMA

Squamous cell carcinoma of the vulva is not an uncommon tumor, although less than 5 percent of the malignancies of the female genital tract are on the vulva. Squamous cell carcinoma of the vulva can be postmenopausal. In these cases the tumor has usually been preceded by atrophy. In other, younger patients, preexistent Bowen's disease has preceded the carcinoma. Scrotal squamous cell carcinoma is much less common. It occurs in lower social classes and has been described in chimney sweepers. It is usually caused by carcinogens such as tar and similar substances. Penile squamous cell carcinoma is extremely rare in the circumcised.[5] Squamous cell carcinoma of the anus occurs with higher frequency in homosexual men than in heterosexual men.

### Clinical features

A lump or ulcer of variable size is very suspicious for carcinoma [Fig. 60-17(*a*); Plate 54]. Pruritus, bleeding, or soreness, especially in the female patient, may be additional symptoms.

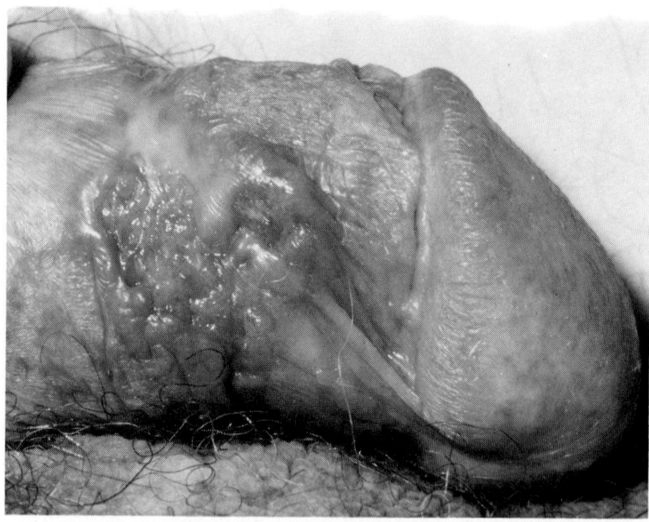

A

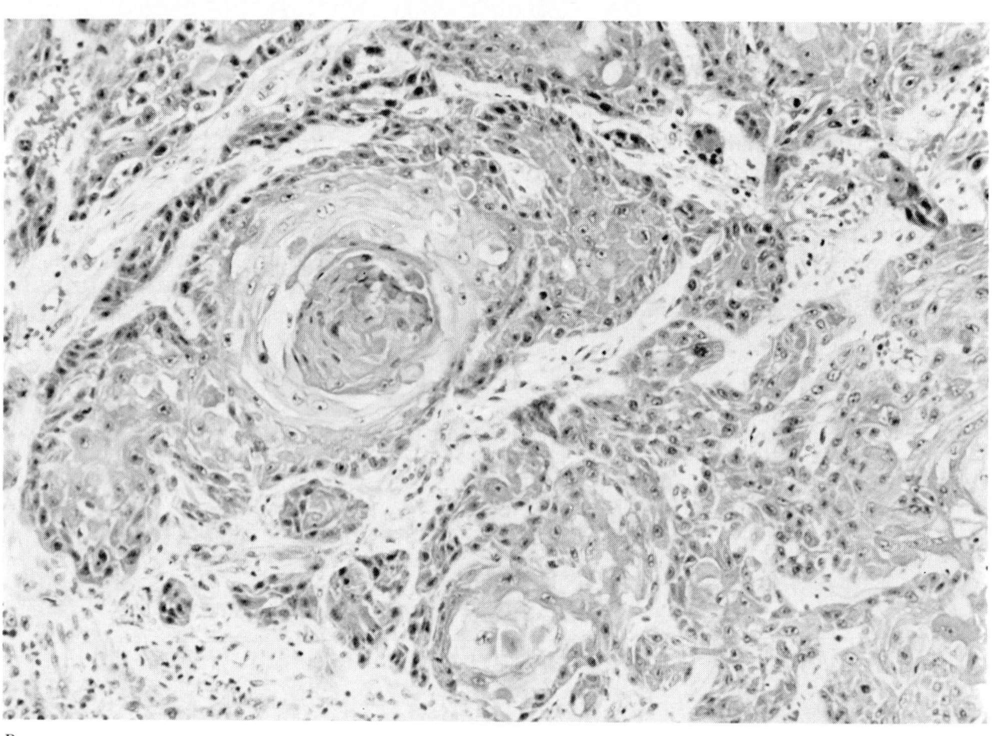

B

**Fig. 60-17.** (*a*) Squamous cell carcinoma of the penis. (*Courtesy of Dr. Philip Kirby, University of Washington.*) (*b*) Squamous cell carcinoma of the penis.

## Histopathology

Squamous cell carcinoma is characterized by irregular masses of epidermal cells that proliferate downward and invade the dermis. The tumor is composed of anaplastic squamous cells showing hyperchromasia of the nuclei, absence of desmosomes, mitotic figures, and keratinization of the individual cells. The cells of squamous cell carcinoma vary in shape and aspect. Well-differentiated polygonal cells with vesicular nuclei, prominent nucleoli, an abundant cytoplasm, and completely anaplastic cells may be present [Fig. 60-17(*b*)].

## Differential diagnosis

The tumor must be distinguished from keratoacanthoma and basal cell carcinoma.

## Treatment

Treatment of genital and anal squamous cell carcinomas is discussed in Chap. 48.

# MALIGNANT MELANOMA

This tumor is uncommon on the male genitalia; however, it represents about 10 percent of the malignant tumors of the vulva. About 3 percent of all malignant melanomas in the female occur on the vulva. Usually, the tumor arises in the skin from epidermal melanocytes and from the junctional component of a cellular nevus.[5]

Fig. 60-18. Malignant melanoma.

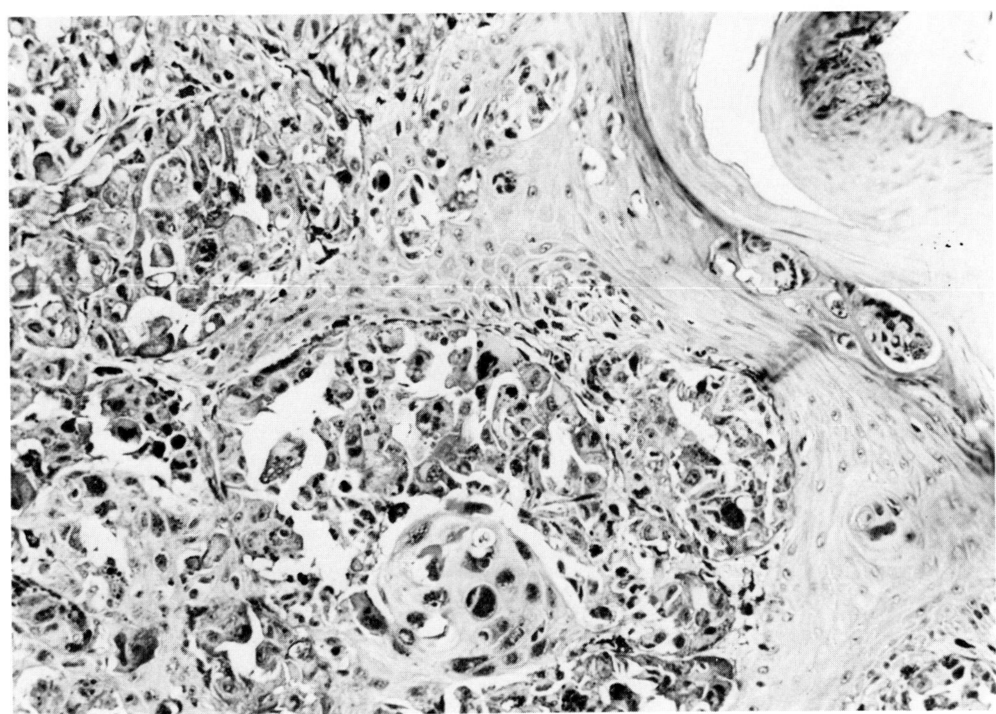

## Clinical features

The advanced lesion, if pigmented, can be diagnosed unmistakably. Smaller and amelanotic tumors are more difficult to recognize. A change in size and pigmentation of a preexisting mole, a reaction of inflammation, itching, bleeding, and crusting should raise suspicion of malignant melanoma.

## Histopathology

The histopathology can vary depending on the type of malignant melanoma. The tumor shows proliferation of atypical melanocytes present in the epidermis and invading the dermal layers. The tumor cells are usually round or polygonal with vesicular nuclei and prominent nucleoli. In addition, there is a dense inflammatory infiltration intermingled with the tumor cells (Fig. 60-18).

## Differential diagnosis

The tumor must be distinguished from a simple mole and from the pigmented basal cell carcinoma.

## Treatment

Malignant melanoma is usually treated by radical surgery and dissection of the regional lymph glands.

## OTHER MALIGNANT TUMORS

Carcinoma of Bartholin's gland is rare. Other malignant tumors such as extramammary Paget's disease and basal cell carcinoma, malignant hemangioendothelioma, Kaposi's sarcoma, fibrosarcoma, leiomyosarcoma, and undifferentiated sarcoma are uncommon on the genitalia and thus will not be discussed here.

# References


1 Russell TJ et al: Histocompatibility (HLA) antigens associated with psoriasis. *N Engl J Med* 287:738, 1972.
2 White S et al: Disturbance of HL-A antigen frequency in psoriasis. *N Engl J Med* 287:740, 1972.
3 Lever WF, Schaumberg-Lever G: *Histopathology of the Skin*. Philadelphia, Lippincott, 1983.
4 Davies TJM: Seborrheic eczema: An attempt to define the scope of the term. *Br J Dermatol* 64:213, 1952.
5 Rook A et al: *Textbook of Dermatology*. Oxford, Blackwell, 1986.
6 Bruinsma W: *A Guide to Drug Eruptions*. Amsterdam, *Excerpta Medica*, 1987.
7 Sutton RL: Infectious eczematoid dermatitis. *JAMA* 75:976, 1920.
8 Ishizaka K et al: Allergen-binding activity of IgE, IgG and IgA antibodies in sera from atopic patients. In vitro measurements of reaginic antibody. *J Immunol* 98:490, 1967.
9 Ridley CM: *The Vulva*. New York, Churchill, Livingstone, 1988.
10 Zoon JJ: Balanitis and vulvitis plasmacellularis. *Dermatologica* 111: 157, 1955.
11 Stolz E, van Kampen WJ: Sklerosiernde Lymphangitis des Penis, der Oberlippe und des Labium minus. *Hautarzt* 25:231, 1974.
12 Ahmed AE, Jones AW: Apocrine cystadenoma: A report of two cases occurring on the prepuce. *Br J Dermatol* 81:899, 1969.
13 Ahmed AE, Jones AW: Nodular fasciitis, editorial. *Lancet* 1:870, 1973.
14 Andrade R et al: *Cancer of the Skin: Biology-Diagnosis-Management*. Philadelphia, Saunders, 1976.

# Chapter 61

# Arthritis associated with sexually transmitted diseases

H. Hunter Handsfield
P. Scott Pollock

Acute arthritis is a common clinical problem, and in some settings disseminated gonococcal infection (DGI) and Reiter's syndrome together probably account for more than half of all new cases of acute nontraumatic arthritis in sexually active young adults.[1–3] The association of acute arthritis with urethritis in men was recognized repeatedly from antiquity through the eighteenth century, and gonococcal arthritis and nongonococcal venereal arthritis were recognized as distinct entities in the nineteenth and early twentieth centuries. The case described by Hans Reiter in 1916 was one of many such reports, and it is unclear why his name came to be associated with Reiter's syndrome. This syndrome was "rediscovered" and definitively described by Bauer and Engleman in 1942.[4] Gonococcal arthritis and Reiter's syndrome nevertheless were commonly confused until relatively recently, perhaps contributing to an apparent predominance of men over women in early reported series of gonococcal arthritis.

Reactive arthritis is the general term for inflammatory arthritis that follows a localized infection, which usually involves a mucosal surface.[5,6] Reiter's syndrome is reactive arthritis associated with various combinations of urogenital, ocular, and mucocutaneous inflammation, typically following a primary genital or lower gastrointestinal tract infection. It includes the disorders referred to as sexually acquired reactive arthritis, reactive spondyloarthropathy, reactive uroarthritis, postgonococcal arthritis, and postdysenteric arthropathy.[2,5,6] Reiter's syndrome and the other reactive arthritides occur predominantly in persons with the histocompatibility locus A B27 (HLA-B27) haplotype. Other sexually transmitted diseases associated with acute arthritis include syphilis, lymphogranuloma venereum, hepatitis B virus infection, human immunodeficiency virus infection, and rarely genital herpes, cytomegalovirus, and genital mycoplasma infections. Arthritis also may result from allergic reactions to drugs used in the treatment of sexually transmitted infections.

## DISSEMINATED GONOCOCCAL INFECTION

### ETIOLOGY AND PATHOGENESIS

*Neisseria gonorrhoeae* is the most common sexually transmitted pathogen that causes infective arthritis[1–3,7,8] and is among the most common causes of septic arthritis. Septic gonococcal arthritis with positive synovial fluid cultures accounts for some cases of DGI, but most patients present with sterile polyarthritis and experience clinical courses that often include early spontaneous resolution, features that suggest an immunologic pathogenesis.[9,10] Nevertheless, several lines of evidence indicate that this syndrome in fact results from direct synovial or periarticular infection. (1) Gonococcemia is common. Positive blood cultures occur in up to 50 percent of patients with polyarthritis who are examined within 2 days of onset; thus, the opportunity exists for synovial and periarticular seeding.[1,8,11–14] (2) Other common systemic manifestations of DGI, including cutaneous and visceral lesions, clearly are due to local infection.[8,9,14–17] (3) *N. gonorrhoeae* occasionally has been identified histologically or by immunochemical methods in apparently sterile synovial fluid or periarticular tissues of patients with DGI.[16,17] (4) The rapid response of polyarthritis to antimicrobial therapy, usually with complete resolution within 48 h, is consistent with a direct therapeutic effect.[8,11,12,14,18–21] (5) Searches for circulating immune complexes in patients with DGI have given conflicting results, and consumption of complement appears to be uncommon.[22–24] The question of pathogenesis, however, is not settled; immune-complex deposition or other immunologic mechanisms may play pathogenic roles in some patients. One study[25] suggested that an immune complex synovitis early in the course of DGI may predispose to later entry of circulating gonococci into the joint space. Other investigators[26] have hypothesized that peptidoglycan fragments from the gonococcal cell wall circulate from the site of a mucosal infection to initiate arthritis in the absence of viable gonococci. Host factors and characteristics of *N. gonorrhoeae* that predispose to dissemination are discussed in Chap. 13.

### EPIDEMIOLOGY

The overall risk of DGI in patients with gonorrhea has been estimated to be 0.5 to 3 percent, depending in part on the vigor with which it is sought and the local prevalences of specific strains of *N. gonorrhoeae*.[8,14,15] During the preantibiotic era, DGI was documented primarily in men, but studies in the 1960s and 1970s describe a female predominance of 78 to 97 percent.[11–14,27–29] A partial explanation for this change may be past misdiagnosis of Reiter's syndrome, until recently believed to be rare in women, as DGI. In addition, in the preantibiotic era, persistent genital infection was common in both men and women, but after effective therapy became available, men with uncomplicated gonorrhea were treated more promptly and thus may have had a lower risk of DGI than women. During the 1960s and 1970s, the evolution and spread of strains of *N. gonorrhoeae* with increased ability both to disseminate and to cause asymptomatic urethral infection in men (Chap. 13) may have resulted in a shift of the sex ratio back toward equality. For example, in a 1970 to 1973 series of 102 patients with DGI who underwent culture of all potentially infected mucosal sites regardless of symptoms and exposure history, 40 cases (39 percent) occurred in men.[1] Similarly, O'Brien et al.[8] documented 14 men (29 percent) among 49 patients with DGI. Gonococcal dissemination is relatively uncommon in homosexual men, because infection with the strains of *N. gonorrhoeae* that are most likely to disseminate is uncommon in this population (Chap. 13).[30]

### CLINICAL AND LABORATORY MANIFESTATIONS

Table 61-1 shows the distribution of the major clinical manifestations in 102 patients in the prospective series from Seattle.[1,3] In most series, signs of articular or periarticular inflammation have been present in approximately 80 percent of patients; an additional 10 to 15 percent who complained of arthralgias have lacked objective abnormalities. About 30 to 40 percent of patients present with monoarthritis, usually with overt synovial effusions; the remainder have multiple joint involvement.[1,3,8,11,14] The mean number of joints with objective inflammatory signs has

**Table 61-1. Major Presenting Clinical Manifestations in 102 Patients with Bacteriologically Confirmed DGI**

| | Number |
|---|---|
| Arthritis and dermatitis | 71 |
| Arthritis alone | 23 |
| Dermatitis alone | 7 |
| Endocarditis* | 1 |

*Without arthritis or dermatitis.
SOURCE: HH Handsfield et al.[1,3]

been between two and three joints per patient in almost all series. Although any joint may be affected, the wrists, knees, the small joints of the hands, and the ankles are the most frequently involved. Although tenosynovitis is characteristic, it does not reliably distinguish DGI from other acute arthritis syndromes.

The characteristic dermatitis (Fig 61-1; Plates 71 and 72) occurs in 50 to 75 percent of patients and consists primarily of papules, petechiae, pustules (often with a hemorrhagic component), and necrotic lesions in various stages of evolution, predominating on the extremities.[1,3,8,9,11–15] The number of skin lesions may range from 1 to over 100, although 90 percent of those with dermatitis have from 5 to 30 lesions.[1] Mild hepatitis has been reported in up to 50 percent of patients with DGI but usually is not clinically apparent.[1,3,14] Concurrent acute or chronic viral hepatitis may predispose to high fever and increased numbers of skin lesions.[1] Fever and leukocytosis each occur in only about 50 to 70 percent of patients with DGI.[1,3,8,13,14,29] As shown in Table 61-2, the primary genital, anorectal, or pharyngeal gonococcal infection is commonly asymptomatic in patients with DGI.[1,3,14]

## REITER'S SYNDROME

### ETIOLOGY AND PATHOGENESIS

The pathogenesis of reactive arthritis is poorly understood and undoubtedly is multifactorial. It is probable that a preceding infection serves as a trigger in a genetically predisposed host and that the disease may then persist or recur despite eradication of the infection.[2,5,6] Postulated triggering agents include *Chlamydia trachomatis, Shigella flexneri, Salmonella* spp., *Yersinia enterocolitica*, and *Campylobacter* spp, and perhaps *N. gonorrhoeae*, the genital mycoplasmas, or other organisms. The potential precipitating factors for reactive arthritis were reviewed recently.[30a]

In several studies, genital *C. trachomatis* infection has been documented in approximately 50 percent of men with sexually acquired Reiter's syndrome.[5,6,31,32] Antichlamydial antibody is

**Table 61-3. Comparison of Immune Responses in *Chlamydia*-Infected Men with Reiter's Syndrome and Nongonococcal Urethritis (NGU)**

| Disease | Antibody titer to *Chlamydia** | Lymphocyte transformation responses† *Chlamydia* | *Candida* |
|---|---|---|---|
| Reiter's syndrome | 1:69.7 | 33.2 ± 26.8 | 18.3 ± 13.1 |
| Nongonococcal urethritis | 1:24.5 | 13.4 ± 8.2 | 15.0 ± 9.9 |

*Geometric mean titer for the peak response ($N = 9$ for Reiter's syndrome, and $N = 26$ for NGU).
†Mean stimulation index (± SD) measured at the time of the peak response to the *Chlamydia* antigen. The *Candida* response was measured at the same time to serve as an antigen-specific control. ($N = 8$ for Reiter's syndrome, and $N = 24$ for NGU.)
SOURCE: DH Martin et al.[32]

even more common in these patients and usually is present in higher titer than in patients with uncomplicated chlamydial infection.[5,32] For example, Martin et al.[32] found higher prevalences and titers of antichlamydial antibodies in patients with Reiter's syndrome than in a control population of men with uncomplicated chlamydial urethritis (Table 61-3). These investigators also demonstrated higher lymphocyte transformation stimulation indexes with *C. trachomatis* antigen in patients with Reiter's syndrome than in the controls (Table 61-3).

A few reports have documented the occurrence of reactive arthritis after successful treatment of gonorrhea.[1,3,33–36] Often associated with postgonococcal urethritis, this syndrome is distinct from DGI and may be accompanied or followed by conjunctivitis or mucocutaneous lesions typical of Reiter's syndrome. Although simultaneous genital infection with *C. trachomatis* occurs in 20 to 40 percent of heterosexual patients with gonorrhea, infection with this organism has not been sought in most reported cases of postgonococcal arthritis. Martin et al.,[32] however, observed three patients who developed typical Reiter's syndrome following gonococcal urethritis and who lacked both culture and serologic evidence of chlamydial infection. Thus, *N. gonorrhoeae* itself may initiate some cases of Reiter's syndrome.

The failure to demonstrate an immune response to *C. trachomatis* in 25 percent of patients or to isolate any sexually transmitted organism from the urethras of one-third to one-half of those who had sexually acquired Reiter's syndrome or reactive arthritis[31,32] suggests that other infectious agents may cause the urethritis in some cases; *Ureaplasma urealyticum* is a possible candidate. In some cases of Reiter's syndrome the urethritis may be noninfective; this hypothesis is supported by the occurrence

**Table 61-2. Correlation of Genital Symptoms with Urethral or Endocervical Isolation of *N. gonorrhoeae* in 95 Patients with DGI**

| | Men (urethra) | | | Women (endocervix) | | |
|---|---|---|---|---|---|---|
| Clinical status* | Tested | *N. gonorrhoeae* isolated | Percent | Tested | *N. gonorrhoeae* isolated | Percent |
| Symptomatic | 13 | 11 | 85 | 31 | 29 | 94 |
| Asymptomatic | 24 | 11 | 46 | 27 | 18 | 67 |

*During the 14 days prior to onset of disseminated gonococcal infection. Symptomatic men gave histories of urethral discharge or dysuria; symptomatic women gave histories of vaginal discharge, dysuria, abnormal uterine bleeding, or abdominal pain.
SOURCE: HH Handsfield et al.[1,3]

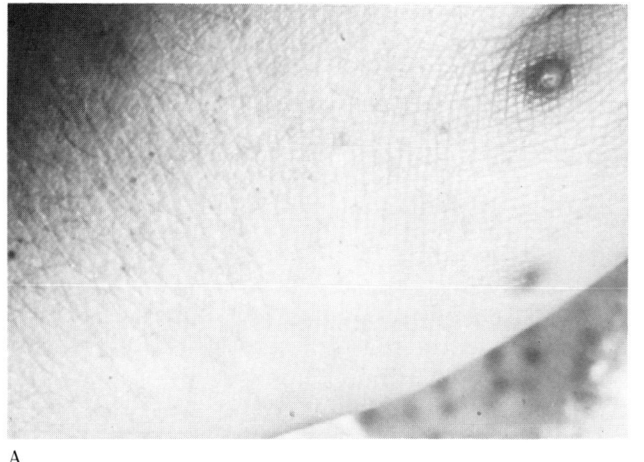
A

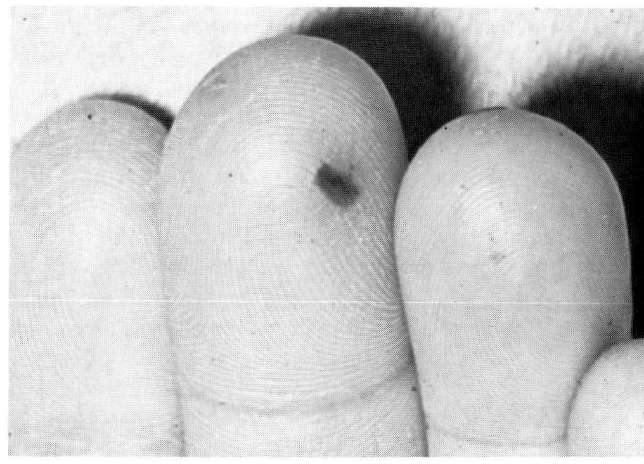
C

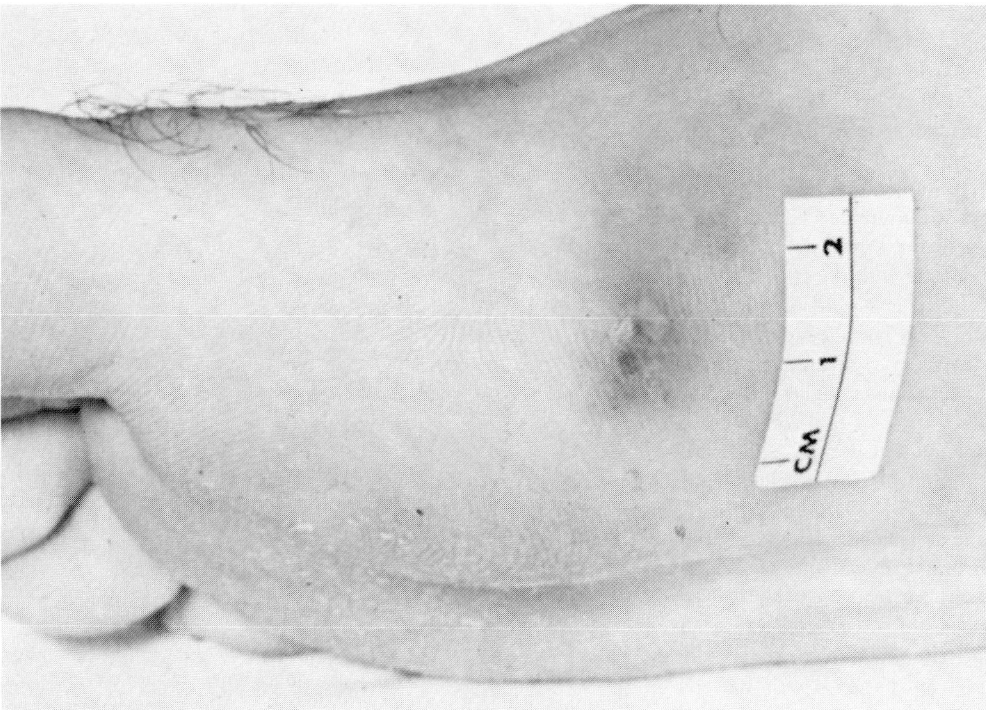

B

**Fig. 61-1.** Skin lesions in patients with disseminated gonococcal infection: (*a*) pustular and papular lesions of wrist and thumb; (*b*) large hemorrhagic pustule of foot; (*c*) petechial lesion of finger.

of urethritis in many patients with the postdysenteric form of the disease[5,37–39] and by recurrence of urethritis during late exacerbations of Reiter's syndrome in the absence of recent sexual contact.[3]

The mechanism by which infection or inflammation of a mucosal surface might initiate a sustained systemic illness is unknown. It is probable that genetically susceptible persons develop an exaggerated or aberrant immune response that results in the inflammatory manifestations of Reiter's syndrome.[5,39,40] The HLA-B27 haplotype is found in 70 to 80 percent of white patients with Reiter's syndrome[32,37,42,43] compared with 6 to 8 percent of whites in the general population; in blacks with Reiter's syndrome, the reported prevalence of HLA-B27 has varied from 15 to 75 percent,[44–46] compared with about 2 percent in blacks in the general population.[47] Nearly 70 percent of HLA-B27-negative patients with Reiter's syndrome, however, possess HLA antigens that cross react with B27.[44] It has been hypothesized[6,44] that HLA-B27 and related antigens may be linked to genes controlling the cellular immune responses to certain infectious agents, and that these genes cause an abnormal immune response to such agents. Alternatively, the theory of *molecular mimicry*[48,49] suggests that the HLA-B27 antigen may be immunologically cross-reactive with certain pathogens. The HLA-B27 haplotype is not the only determinant of disease expression, because no more than 25 percent of HLA-B27-positive individuals with nongonococcal urethritis (NGU) or shigellosis develop Reiter's syndrome. The initial manifestations of Reiter's syndrome and other forms of reactive arthritis tend to be more severe and the natural course more aggressive in persons with the HLA-B27 haplotype than in those without it.[5,41]

Conflicting reports exist on the potential role of direct dissemination of the triggering pathogen in causing the arthropathy and other inflammatory manifestations. Reports of isolation of *C. trachomatis* from the synovial fluid in Reiter's syndrome[50,51] were not confirmed in later studies,[52,53] including one from a laboratory that reported an earlier isolation.[50,52] Schumacher et al.[53a] reported finding ultrastructural evidence of chlamydial antigens in the synovium in Reiter's syndrome, and Keat et al. detected *C. trachomatis* by direct immunofluorescence with monoclonal antibody in synovial fluid or biopsy tissue in five of eight patients (seven men and one woman) with sexually acquired reactive arthritis[54] and in five of nine women with seronegative arthritis.[54a] Similarly, Granfors et al. recently documented the presence of *Yersinia enterocolitica* antigens in synovial fluid neutrophils or macrophages from 12 of 15 patients with reactive arthritis.[54b] Nevertheless, the role of direct synovial infection in pathogenesis is unclear, in part because antimicrobial therapy has no apparent clinical benefit.

Many immunologic phenomena have been associated with Reiter's syndrome, but their importance and pathogenic roles are unclear. Synovial fluid lymphocytes from patients with Reiter's syndrome may be more reactive than peripheral blood lymphocytes from the same patient when incubated with a variety of potential triggering agents, including *C. trachomatis, N. gonorrhoeae, U. urealyticum*, and various enteric organisms.[55,56] CD4-bearing (helper/inducer) lymphocytes outnumber CD8-positive (suppressor/cytotoxic) lymphocytes in the synovial fluid of patients with Reiter's syndrome, in contrast with the synovial fluid in rheumatoid arthritis.[57] However, Reiter's syndrome has developed in the presence of profound CD4 lymphocyte depletion associated with acquired immunodeficiency syndrome,[58] perhaps indicating that intact helper/inducer function is not central to the pathogenesis of reactive arthritis. The ratio of T to B lymphocytes is higher in synovial fluid from patients with Reiter's syndrome than in synovial fluid from normal controls.[59] The blastogenic response of circulating lymphocytes to *C. trachomatis*[32] or *Y. enterocolitica*[60] in Reiter's syndrome associated with these pathogens is elevated relative to the response in patients who have chlamydial or yersinial infections without reactive arthritis. The reactivity of synovial fluid lymphocytes also is greater than that of peripheral blood lymphocytes in Reiter's syndrome patients.[56] On the other hand, synovial fluid from patients with Reiter's syndrome inhibits responsiveness of autologous peripheral blood lymphocytes to the nonspecific mitogen phytohemagglutinin.[61]

Circulating IgA antibody levels are elevated in about 40 percent of patients with Reiter's syndrome, perhaps related to the initiating mucosal infection, and synovial fluid levels of polymeric IgA sometimes are elevated relative to those in serum.[62] Immune complexes of the IgG class are present in the blood of up to 76 percent of patients with Reiter's syndrome,[63] and synovial biopsies often reveal exudative synovitis with interstitial and intracellular deposits of IgG, IgA, and the third component of complement.[64,65] Nonetheless, the clinical features of the arthropathy and the usual absence of glomerulonephritis, vasculitis, and other manifestations of immune-complex deposition suggest that this mechanism is not central to the pathogenesis of reactive arthritis.

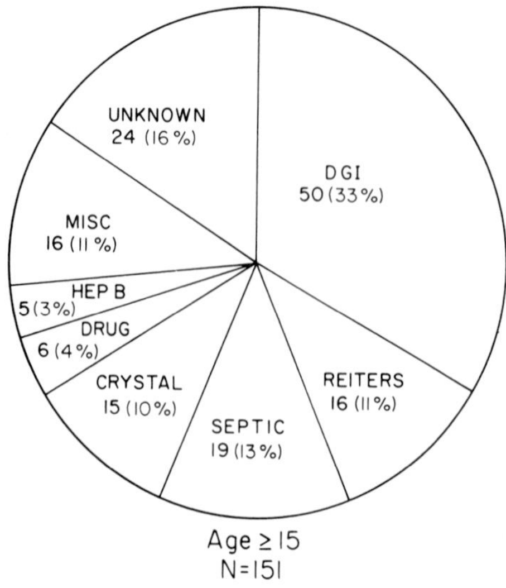


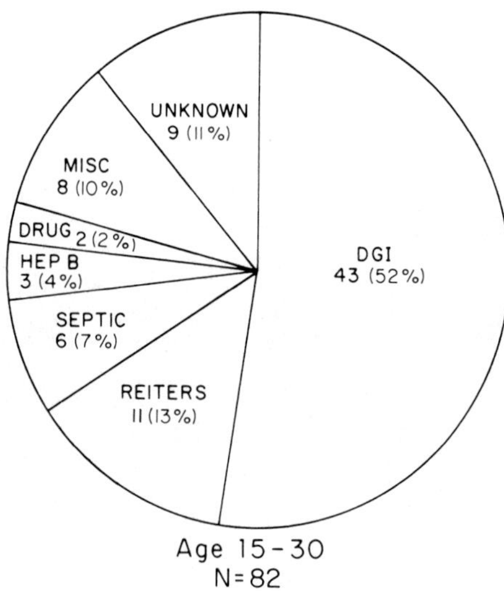


**Fig. 61-2.** Diagnoses in 151 consecutive adults (age ≥ 15 years) hospitalized in Seattle because of acute, nontraumatic arthritis of ≤ 14 days' duration. REITERS includes postgonococcal arthritis; DRUG denotes drug-induced arthritis; HEP B denotes hepatitis B infection. (*From HH Handsfield et al.*[1])

## EPIDEMIOLOGY

Epidemiologically, Reiter's syndrome is characterized by both an endemic form, usually sexually acquired, and a less common epidemic form, most often associated with enteric infection. Although endemic Reiter's syndrome commonly follows sexual contact with a new partner, clear evidence of sexual transmission of individual cases has been uncommon. One report[66] described the simultaneous occurrence of NGU and Reiter's syndrome in two HLA-B27-positive men after both had intercourse with the same woman. The dysenteric form of Reiter's syndrome typically follows an enteric infection with *S. flexneri*,[2,5,6,39,67] *Salmonella* spp.,[68,69] *Y. enterocolitica*,[70–72] or *C. jejuni*.[73] Although sexual transmission of dysenteric Reiter's syndrome has not been reported, such cases are likely to have occurred, because homosexual men are at increased risk for these infections (Chaps. 6, 27, 44).

The incidence and prevalence of Reiter's syndrome are uncertain and may vary geographically.[2,5,41] In the Seattle series,[1,3] the diagnosis was made in 16 (11 percent) of 151 consecutive adults hospitalized with acute nontraumatic arthritis and was second in frequency only to DGI as a cause of arthritis (Fig. 61-2). The overall risk of acquiring Reiter's syndrome has been estimated to be 1 to 3 percent, both for men with sexually transmitted

NGU[74,75] and for patients with acute shigellosis,[38] rising to as high as 20 to 25 percent for individuals with the HLA-B27 haplotype.[38,74]

Although postdysenteric Reiter's syndrome occurs in children, most patients are adults. The modal age of patients with sexually acquired Reiter's syndrome is in the fourth decade, compared with the third decade for patients with DGI and other sexually transmitted diseases. This may be due in part to the fact that some series included either patients whose Reiter's syndrome was not sexually acquired or patients with recurrent disease. Nevertheless, a true age-related predisposition to sexually acquired Reiter's syndrome cannot be excluded. In most series, 80 to 90 percent of patients with Reiter's syndrome have been white, with most of the remainder being black.[6,45,46,75] Differences in racial susceptibility remain poorly defined, since most studies did not report the racial compositions of the clinic population served. However, it is likely that blacks are less susceptible than whites, at least to the extent that the prevalence of the HLA-B27 haplotype is lower in blacks.

Dysenteric Reiter's syndrome has long been recognized to affect women only somewhat less commonly than men, with male/female ratios varying from 1:1 to 10:1 in various series.[5] By contrast, few women have been included in most series of sexually acquired reactive arthritis, accounting for only 20 (3.6 percent) of 557 cases summarized by Keat.[5] More recent studies, however, have documented greater numbers of affected women. Smith et al.[76] described 29 women whose clinical presentations, HLA haplotypes, and clinical courses were indistinguishable from those of men with Reiter's syndrome. In another series, 13 (52 percent) of 25 patients with Reiter's syndrome were women.[77] Yli-Kerttula et al.[78] documented associations of nonspecific rheumatic complaints and overt Reiter's syndrome in women with histories of salpingitis, gonorrhea, bacterial urinary tract infection, and trichomoniasis. These investigators also found high prevalences of musculoskeletal disorders in the sexual partners of men with Reiter's syndrome, suggesting that reactive arthritis may be common in women, and incidentally supporting sexual acquisition.[79] Other investigators have reported associations of salpingitis with radiologic evidence of sacroiliitis.[5,80]

Factors leading to past underdiagnosis may have included failure to recognize lower genital tract infection syndromes in women (Chap. 46), and the belief that Reiter's syndrome is rare in women may have been a self-fulfilling one that contributed to lack of recognition. Finally, many series of patients with Reiter's syndrome have drawn from predominantly male populations (e.g., from military installations, ships' companies, and Veterans Administration hospitals). Prospective studies with complete microbiological and immunologic evaluations and careful clinical examinations will be required to define the true sex distribution and other epidemiologic features of this disease.

## CLINICAL AND LABORATORY MANIFESTATIONS

The clinical manifestations of Reiter's syndrome include acute arthritis, lower urogenital tract inflammation, conjunctivitis, and mucocutaneous inflammatory lesions. Although it is uncommon for all these manifestations to be observed at the time of presentation, many patients eventually develop all four features, especially if HLA-B27 positive.[37,43,53] The frequencies of these manifestations at presentation and during follow-up are shown in Table 61-4. The articular, mucocutaneous, and ocular manifestations usually follow onset of urethritis or diarrhea by 1 to 4 weeks, although delays of several months occasionally are seen.[2,5,37,39,42]

### Urogenital inflammation

Patients with Reiter's syndrome frequently give histories of recent sexual contact with a new partner, followed by the development of urethritis that is clinically indistinguishable from uncomplicated NGU.[37,43] Gonococcal urethritis was found in 12 and 20 percent of patients in two series.[37,81] Some studies suggested that many patients had nonbacterial prostatitis,[35,37,82,83] but it is likely that prostatitis often was not differentiated from urethritis, cystitis, or other forms of lower urogenital tract inflammation. Urethritis occurs in up to 90 percent of patients with postdysenteric Reiter's syndrome[5,37,38,70,73] and has been documented in children[84] and sexually inactive adults with postdysenteric reactive arthritis. These observations imply an immunologic pathogenesis of urethritis, and various authors have cautioned that genital inflammation in Reiter's syndrome should not be assumed to be sexually acquired,[5,6] especially when reactive arthritis follows a gastrointestinal infection. Even in these cases, however, the possibility of sexual acquisition should be explored with the patient, and the sexual partner should be examined. Symptoms or signs of urethritis or pyuria were documented in 30 percent of the women in two studies,[76,77] but standardized criteria for lower genital tract inflammation (Chap. 46) were not applied, and the spectrum of urogenital inflammation in women with Reiter's syndrome remains to be established. Various studies[5,78–80] suggest that cervicitis, urethritis, cystitis, and salpingitis all may be important, but this issue requires more careful study.

**Table 61-4. Frequencies of Clinical Manifestations in Patients with Reiter's Syndrome**

| | Initial attack, percent* | Entire course, percent† |
|---|---|---|
| *Urogenital inflammation:* | | |
| Urethritis (criteria not specified) | 85 | 87 |
| Cervicitis (criteria not specified) | 71 | NA |
| *Arthritis:* | | |
| Monoarticular | 14 | 3 |
| Polyarticular | 81 | 86 |
| Arthralgia only | 0 | 9 |
| Sacroiliitis back pain | 49 | 21 |
| Heel pain | 40 | Not recorded |
| Tendonitis | 25 | 25 |
| Fusiform dactylitis ("sausage" digits) | 17 | Not recorded |
| *Ocular involvement:* | | |
| Conjunctivitis | 57 | 50 |
| Uveitis | 0 | 12 |
| *Mucocutaneous involvement:* | | |
| Balanitis/vulvovaginitis | 39 | 69 |
| Stomatitis | 31 | 17 |
| Keratodermia blennorrhagica | 21 | 18 |
| Nail changes | 9 | 16 |
| *Other:* | | |
| Cardiac | 0 | 9 |
| Neurologic | 1 | 2 |
| Diarrhea | 14 | 12 |

*Data from RF Wilkens.[43] ($N$ = 83).
†Data from M Kousa.[37] ($N$ = 173).

## Arthritis

A wide range of articular disease occurs. Asymmetrical polyarticular synovitis-tendonitis often is seen initially, followed by persistence in one or two joints. Tendon insertion sites (entheses) are common sites of inflammation, the basis for describing Reiter's syndrome as an enthesopathy.[41,85] Common enthesopathic sites include the insertion of the Achilles tendon and the plantar fascia. In one series,[37] 86 percent of patients with acute Reiter's syndrome had polyarticular involvement, and half of these patients had involvement of four or more joints. In the 557 cases of sexually acquired reactive arthritis summarized by Keat,[5] the mean number of affected joints was 2.8, and 91 percent of the patients had involvement of more than one joint. Arthritis typically begins in the distal weight-bearing joints (knees, ankles, feet), most commonly with knee effusions and fusiform dactylitis ("sausage digits") (Fig. 61-3). Sacroiliitis (Fig. 61-4) is common, occurring in up to 10 percent of cases acutely and in higher proportions of those with chronic Reiter's syndrome. It often is detected as a subclinical radiographic abnormality, especially in sexually acquired cases.[5,37,86]

In contrast to ankylosing spondylitis and other spondyloarthropathies, spinal involvement is uncommon in Reiter's syndrome. Radiographic evidence of sacroiliitis has been reported in association with chronic prostatitis[83] and salpingitis[80] without other manifestations of Reiter's syndrome; it remains to be determined whether this represents a variant of the disease.

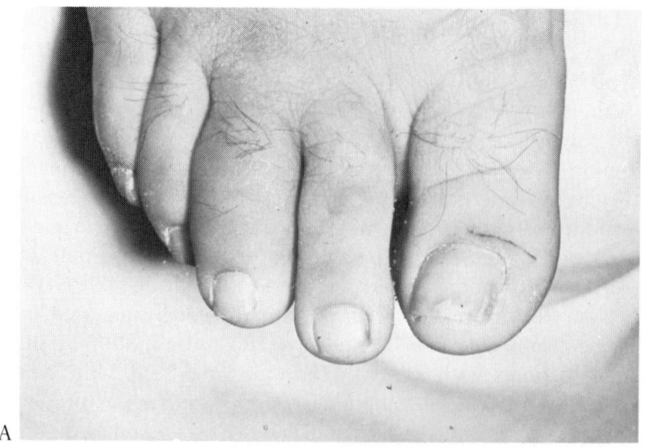

A

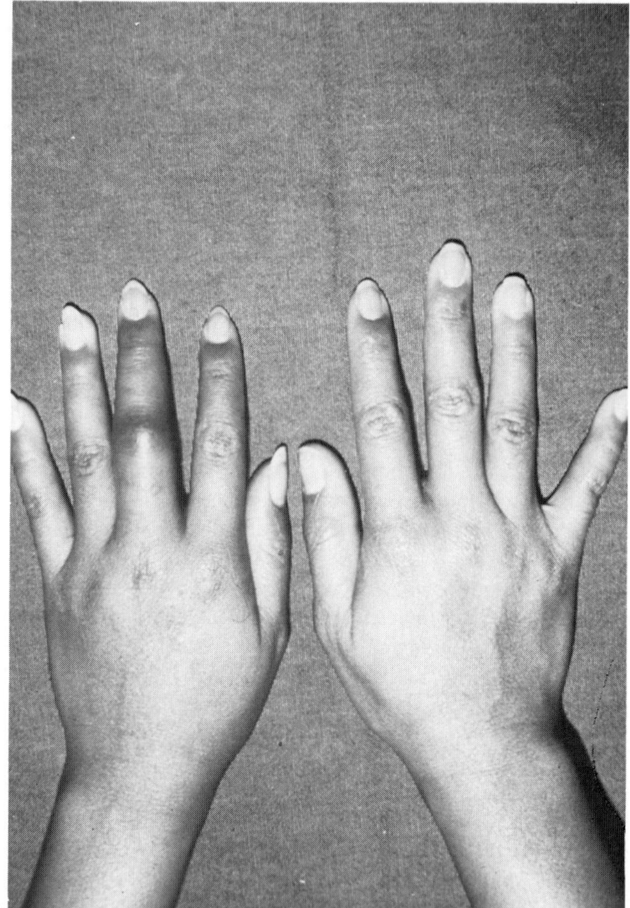

B

Fig. 61-3. Acute fusiform dactylitis in patients with Reiter's syndrome: (*a*) "sausage toe" involving middle toe; (*b*) "sausage finger" involving middle finger. (*Courtesy of RF Willkens.*)

## Mucocutaneous manifestations

Mucocutaneous lesions are common in sexually acquired Reiter's syndrome and reactive arthritis following shigellosis but have been reported infrequently in reactive arthritis associated with *Salmonella, Campylobacter*, or *Yersinia* infections.[5] These lesions usually are painless and are easily overlooked by the physician. Circinate balanitis is the most common cutaneous manifestation, typically occurring in 20 to 40 percent[5] and perhaps up to 85 percent[37] of men with the sexually acquired form of the syndrome. In uncircumcised men, this lesion appears as a painless, serpiginous, "geographic" dermatitis of the glans penis and is diagnostic of Reiter's syndrome (Plate 67). In circumcised men, circinate balanitis often takes the form of hyperkeratotic papules (Fig. 61-5) that closely resemble the other characteristic skin lesion, keratodermia blennorrhagica. Erosive vulvitis, perhaps the female equivalent of circinate balanitis, has been documented in some women with Reiter's syndrome.[86]

Lesions of keratodermia blennorrhagica (Fig. 61-6, Plate 68) begin as erythematous macules that gradually enlarge to form hyperkeratotic papules, sometimes with red halos and occasionally with central clearing. Keratodermia blennorrhagica resembles psoriasis, both macroscopically and histologically, and well-documented cases of Reiter's syndrome have progressed to become clinically indistinguishable from psoriatic arthritis.[3,5,6,41,87,88] Keratodermia blennorrhagica most commonly involves the plantar surfaces of the feet (Fig. 61-6), but may occur anywhere. Cutaneous manifestations have been reported to be more common (up to 20 percent of patients) in sexually acquired Reiter's syndrome than in the enteric form (no patients in the studies summarized by Keat).[5] However, this view has been challenged.[37]

In up to 20 percent of patients with Reiter's syndrome, especially those with the sexually acquired form, painless shallow ulcers occur on the palate, tongue, buccal mucosa, lips, tonsillar pillars, or pharynx (Fig. 61-7, Plate 69).[89] Nail involvement occurs in up to 10 percent of patients, manifested by thickening and brown-yellow discoloration due to subungual accumulation of hyperkeratotic material.[2,5,37] Erythema nodosum occasionally occurs in reactive arthritis following yersiniosis but apparently is rare in other forms of the disease.[5]

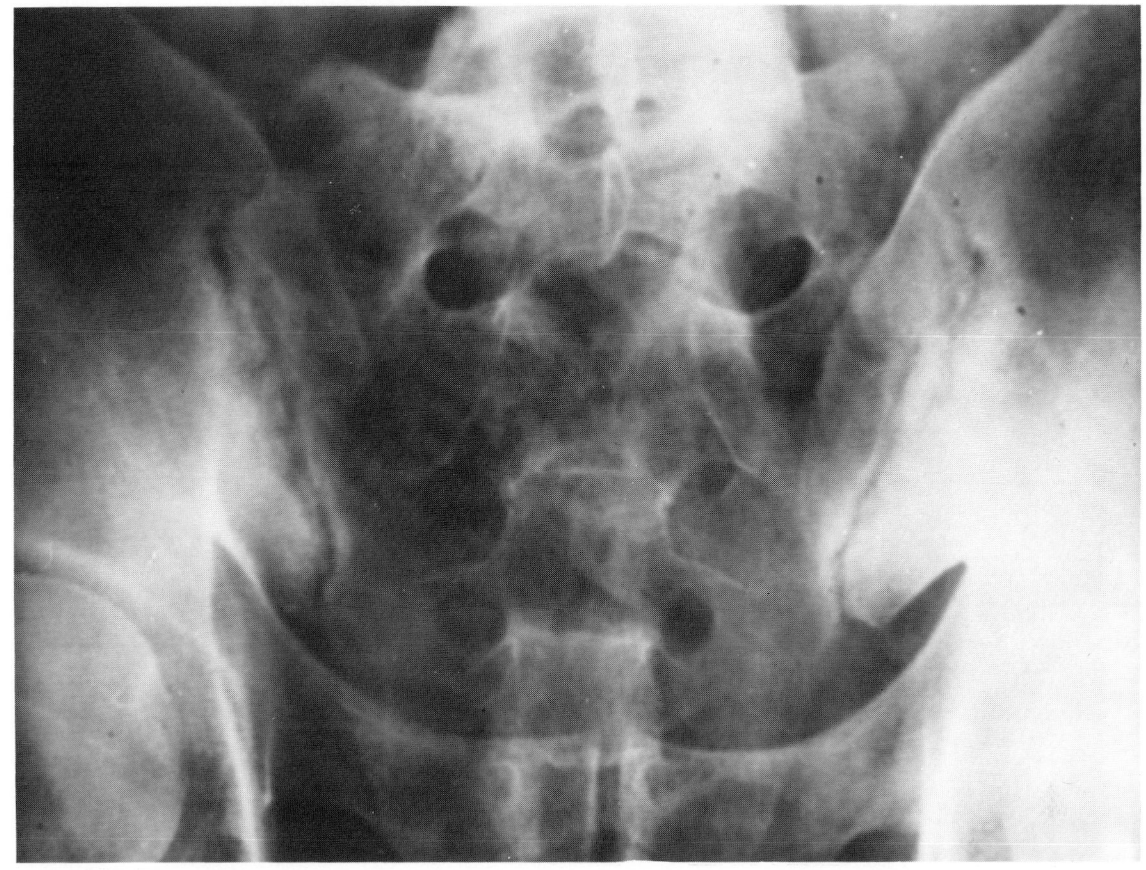

A

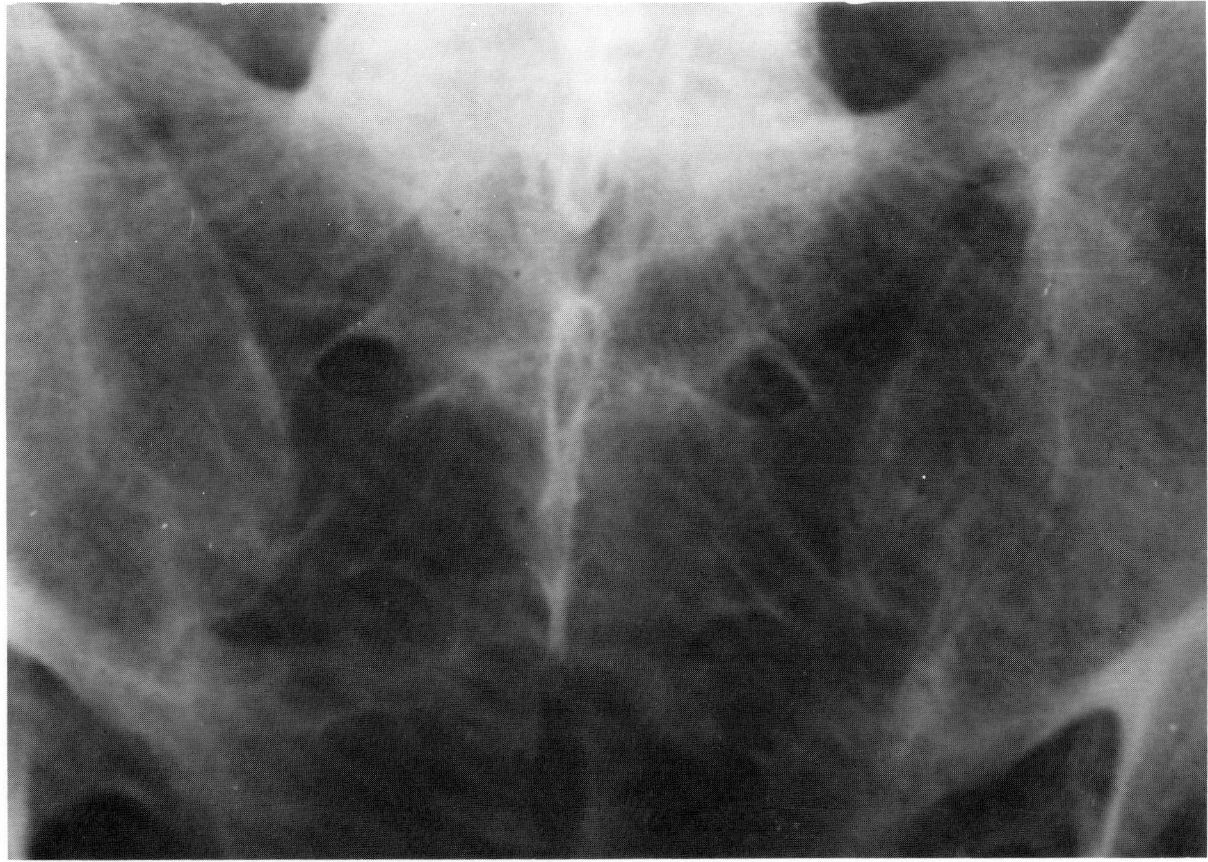

B

**Fig. 61-4.** Radiographs demonstrating bilateral sacroiliitis in patients with ankylosing spondylitis: (*a*) early sacroiliitis with subchondral bone resorption, sclerosis around joint, a "rosary bead" effect, and pseudo widening; (*b*) complete obliteration of sacroiliac joints with bony trabeculae across joints. (*From the Clinical Slide Collection of the Arthritis Foundation.*)

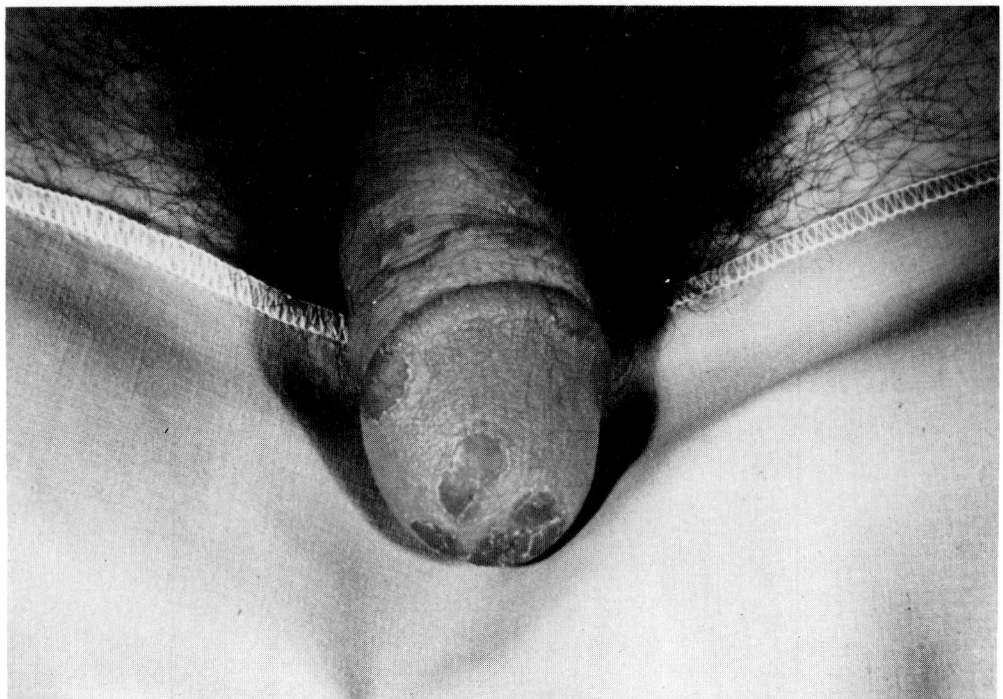

**Fig. 61-5.** Circinate balanitis in a circumcised man with Reiter's syndrome (see also Plate 67). (*Courtesy of RF Willkens.*)

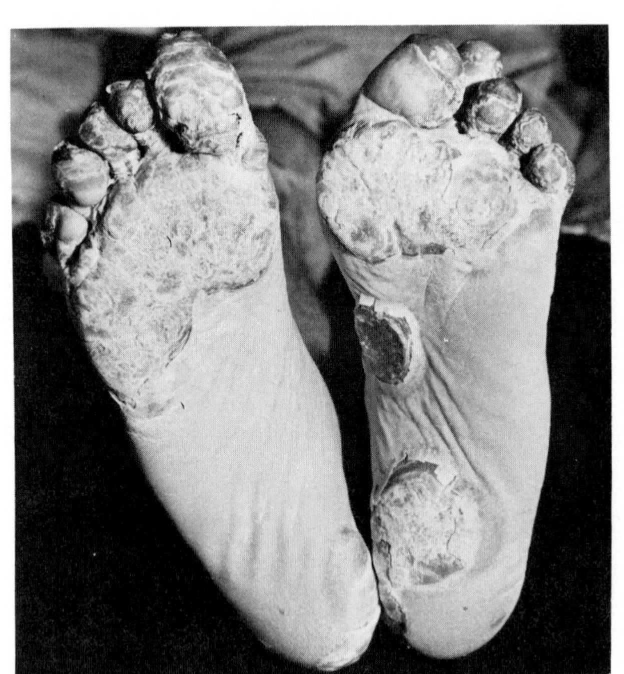

A

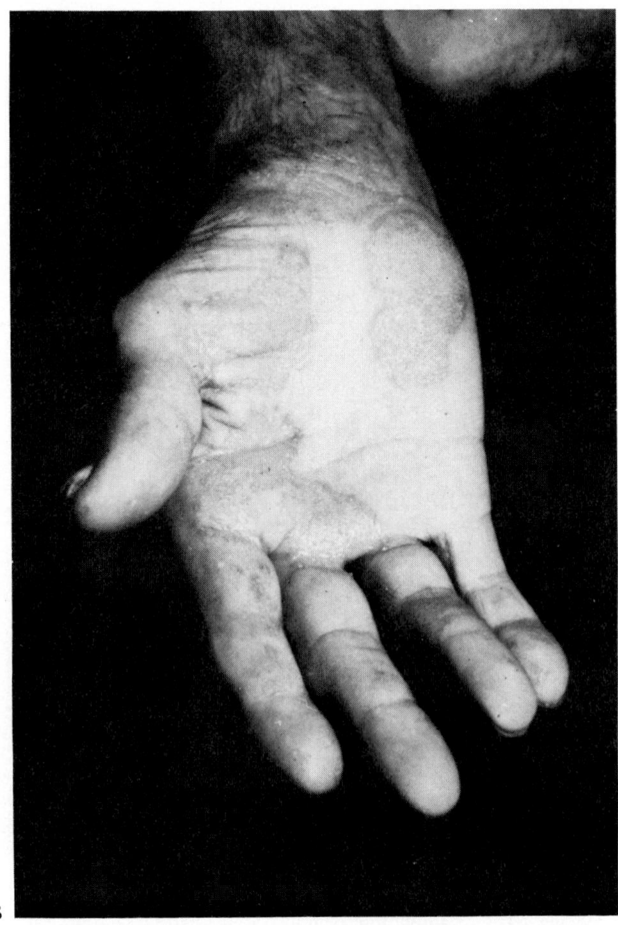

B

**Fig. 61-6.** Lesions of keratodermia blennorrhagica involving (*a*) the soles of the feet and (*b*) the palms (see also Plate 68). (*Courtesy of RF Willkens.*)

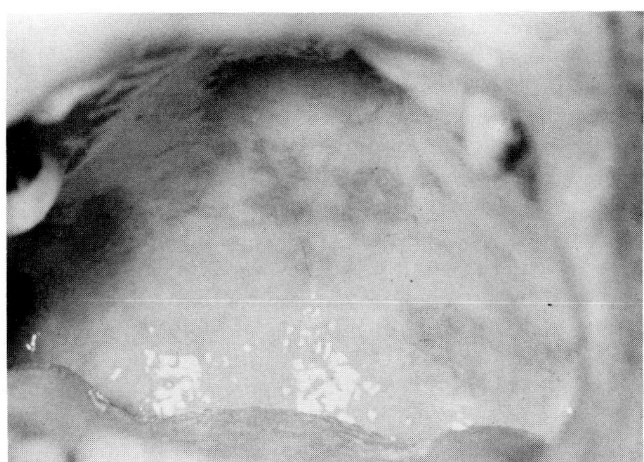

Fig. 61-7. Oral mucosal lesions in a patient with Reiter's syndrome (see also Plate 69).

## Ocular inflammation

Ocular manifestations occur in up to half of patients with acute sexually acquired Reiter's syndrome and up to 90 percent of cases following shigellosis.[5] Conjunctivitis, often sufficiently mild to escape detection in a cursory examination, is the most common ocular manifestation.[37] Although uncommon at presentation, iritis or more extensive uveitis ultimately develops in up to 10 percent of patients.[2,5,37,43]

## Other systemic manifestations

Other systemic manifestations are common in patients with acute Reiter's syndrome and include malaise, fever, anorexia, and weight loss; shaking chills are uncommon. Transient and usually benign electrocardiographic abnormalities, including atrioventricular conduction disturbances, ST-segment elevation or depression, and nonspecific T-wave changes, occur during 9 to 30 percent of acute episodes.[37,90] Complete heart block, myocarditis, pericarditis, acute aortitis with aortic valve incompetence, and congestive heart failure are rare but well-documented long-term sequelae, especially in sexually acquired cases.[91,92] Rare complications, each occurring in fewer than 1 percent of patients, include peripheral neuropathy, hemiplegia, meningoencephalitis, generalized lymphadenopathy, pleuritis, pneumonitis, thrombophlebitis, and amyloidosis.[2,37]

## Laboratory features

Several nondiagnostic laboratory abnormalities are common. The erythrocyte sedimentation rate exceeded 20 mm/h in 106 (60 percent) and 50 mm/h in 70 (40 percent) of 173 patients;[37] the degree of elevation did not correlate with disease activity. Mild inflammatory anemia and leukocytosis (up to 20,000 leukocytes per cubic millimeter) are common. Antinuclear antibodies, rheumatoid factor, cryoglobulins, C-reactive protein, or circulating immune complexes occasionally are present.[2,5,37]

Synovial fluid analysis is seldom specific, the results often mimicking those of septic arthritis. Leukocyte counts range from 500 to $>$ 50,000 per cubic millimeter and are $\geq$ 20,000 per cubic millimeter in about 50 percent of patients; differential counts usually demonstrate $\geq$ 90 percent neutrophils. Decreased viscosity, normal or elevated complement levels, decreased ratio of synovial fluid to serum complement concentration,[64] and elevated protein levels are common. Synovial fluid glucose levels usually are normal.

## Clinical course

Most initial episodes of acute Reiter's syndrome resolve completely within 2 to 6 months, but recovery was delayed for more than a year in 59 (34 percent) of 173 patients and indefinitely in a few cases.[5,37] The subsequent annual risk of recurrent acute episodes has been estimated to be about 15 percent.[2,5,37,75] Recurrences may be manifested by any of the clinical features, alone or in combination. Among 122 patients followed for a mean of 5.6 years, arthritis persisted or recurred in 83 percent, urethritis or cervicitis in 42 percent, ocular disease in 31 percent, circinate balanitis in 29 percent, and other mucocutaneous lesions in about 25 percent.[42] The severity of functional impairment caused by chronic Reiter's syndrome is controversial. In one series,[42] 34 percent of patients had sustained disease activity, almost 16 percent required a change of job, and 11 percent were disabled for further employment. Other investigators have reported similar rates of persistence or recurrence, but with minimal functional impairment.[93] Death from Reiter's syndrome is rare, occurring primarily as the result of aortic valve incompetence,[91,92] amyloidosis,[94] or complications of drug therapy.[37]

# OTHER ARTHRITIS SYNDROMES

## HEPATITIS B VIRUS INFECTION

The occurrence of articular symptoms early in the course of viral hepatitis was first reported by Robert Graves in 1843 and was "rediscovered" in the 1970s.[95–100] Although hepatitis B virus may invade the synovium,[96] several studies have confirmed the pathogenic role of immune-complex deposition in this syndrome. For example, complement levels are low in serum and synovial fluid during active joint inflammation and return to normal as the arthritis abates. Peak serum hepatitis B surface antigen (HBsAg) titers, synovial membrane and fluid viral antigen, and cryoprecipitates containing HBsAg, complement components, IgA, and complement-fixing IgG antibodies have all been detected during acute arthritis.[97–99]

Generalized arthralgias occur in up to 50 percent of patients during the prodrome of hepatitis B, and 10 to 20 percent of patients have overt polyarthritis, usually with symmetrical involvement of the hands, knees, ankles, shoulders, wrists, and feet.[95–100] An urticarial rash, usually involving the lower extremities, occurs in about 25 percent of patients with arthralgias and 50 percent of those with overt arthritis. The clinical picture closely parallels classic descriptions of serum sickness.[10] The onset of overt hepatitis usually coincides with resolution of the musculoskeletal and cutaneous manifestations, but many patients with hepatitis B are anicteric, and laboratory assessment of hepatic function and assay for HBsAg are indicated for all patients with acute polyarthritis, regardless of the presence or absence of jaundice or hepatomegaly.[100]

## SYPHILIS

A small minority (probably < 1 percent) of patients with secondary syphilis have overt osseous or synovial involvement.[101] Acute periostitis, sometimes mimicking acute arthritis, is the more common lesion, but at least some cases of true arthritis occur as the result of synovial invasion by *Treponema pallidum*, demonstrated by electron microscopy and dark field examination.[102] Indirect immunologic mechanisms nonetheless may be involved in some cases; complement consumption, circulating immune complexes, and immune-complex glomerulonephritis have all been documented in patients with primary, secondary, or congenital syphilis.[10,103] In late syphilis, acute or chronic arthritis usually is the result of direct spread from adjacent osteomyelitis or periostitis.[101] The Charcot joint is believed to be traumatic in origin, the indirect result of syphilitic neuropathy and, perhaps, of microvascular disease.[101,104,105] Although neuropathic joints almost always involve the lower extremities, a recent report documented multiple neuropathic joints in the upper limbs and spine of a patient whose occupation required heavy use of the upper body.[105] A case of vertebral syphilitic osteitis in an adult has been reported,[106] but it was unclear whether it was of neuropathic origin.

## LYMPHOGRANULOMA VENEREUM

Acute and chronic lymphogranuloma venereum (LGV) occasionally have been associated with a syndrome that resembles experimental serum sickness, including polyarthritis, rash, cryoglobulinemia, and circulating rheumatoid factor,[107–110] but direct measurements of circulating immune complexes have not been reported. It is uncertain whether direct synovial infection occurs; *C. trachomatis* antigen may have been demonstrated in synovial fluid of patients with LGV,[107] but isolation of the organism from synovial fluid has not been reported in this syndrome.

## HUMAN IMMUNODEFICIENCY VIRUS INFECTION

Rheumatic manifestations appear to occur frequently in persons with AIDS and earlier stages of human immunodeficiency virus (HIV) infection.[110a] Typical Reiter's syndrome and apparently limited forms of reactive arthritis are common in these patients, and have been documented both in HLA-B27-positive and -negative persons.[110b–d] Sjogren's syndrome with arthritis has been reported as well.[110e] Otherwise unexplained inflammatory arthritis has been attributed to HIV infection per se,[110e] but this is unproved. In a recent series of 101 patients with various stages of HIV infection, 72 had musculoskeletal manifestations.[110a] The most common of these was nonspecific generalized arthralgias (35 patients), followed by unexplained oligo- or polyarthritis (12 patients), Reiter's syndrome (10 patients), an apparently new syndrome of severe arthralgia involving one to four joints (10 patients), psoriatic arthritis (two patients), and arthritis associated with vasculitis (one patient). Septic arthritis due to various pathogens also has been reported in AIDS patients.

## OTHER DISEASES

*Mycoplasma hominis* rarely has caused septic arthritis,[111–113] often in association with postpartum fever and bacteremia. *U. urealyticum* is an occasional cause of acute monoarticular or polyarticular septic arthritis in patients with hypogammaglobulinemia.[114–117] Herpes simplex virus, Epstein-Barr virus, and cytomegalovirus infections rarely are associated with acute monoarticular arthritis, perhaps due to direct synovial infection, and with polyarthritis, probably related to circulating immune complexes.[118–122] Acute arthritis is a major manifestation of chronic meningococcemia and may also occur during or following acute meningococcemia, which rarely may be transmitted sexually;[123] the clinical picture may mimic that of DGI.[123–127] In addition, acute noninfective arthritis occasionally follows meningococcemia. This syndrome is not associated with HLA-B27 and probably is due to immune-complex deposition. Finally, therapy of sexually transmitted diseases with penicillin or other drugs occasionally causes allergic reactions manifested by serum sickness-like illnesses, with skin eruptions, arthralgias, or arthritis, associated with high concentrations of circulating immune complexes.[10]

## DIFFERENTIAL DIAGNOSIS

The differential diagnosis of acute arthritis is broad, but a large proportion of the cases are related to sexually transmitted infections. Figure 61-2 shows the diagnoses for 151 consecutive adults (age ≥ 15 years) who required hospitalization for acute, nontraumatic arthritis or tenosynovitis of ≤ 14 days' duration.[1,3] DGI was documented by isolation of *N. gonorrhoeae* from 38 patients (25 percent) and was suspected on the basis of clinical features and response to antibiotic therapy in 12 others (8 percent). Sixteen patients (11 percent) had Reiter's syndrome or postgonococcal arthritis; none of these had symptoms or signs of enteritis. None of five patients who had arthritis associated with acute hepatitis B gave histories of parenteral exposure, and two of six patients with arthritis attributed to drug reactions had been treated with penicillin or ampicillin for gonorrhea. Thus, 73 (48 percent) of the patients in this series had arthritis that was directly or indirectly related to a sexually transmissible infection. Among the subset of 82 patients ≤30 years of age, 43 (52 percent) had DGI and 58 (71 percent) were related to sexually transmissible infections. In more recent years, decreasing prevalences of the gonococcal strains most likely to disseminate probably have reduced the frequency of DGI in many geographic areas,[124] but the proportion of acute arthropathy that is directly or indirectly due to STD remains high. HIV infection should be ruled out in all sexually active persons who present with acute arthritis.

DGI and Reiter's syndrome are the two most common causes of sexually acquired arthritis, and both commonly present with a combination of arthropathy, dermatitis, and genitourinary inflammation. Therefore, the differentiation between these syndromes sometimes is considered difficult. Nevertheless, in most cases the correct diagnosis can be readily made on clinical grounds. The two syndromes are reliably differentiated from one another by their characteristic mucocutaneous lesions, if present. The presence of NGU, conjunctivitis, or radiographically confirmed sacroiliitis is almost always a feature of Reiter's syndrome rather than DGI.

Several surveys have documented differing predilections of DGI and Reiter's syndrome for various joints or groups of joints. However, as illustrated in Fig. 61-8, the overlap in affected joints may be considerable, and the pattern of joints involved is nonspecific, with the exceptions of sacroiliitis, typical fusiform dactylitis (Fig. 61-3), or calcaneal enthesopathy.[37,85] Although ten-

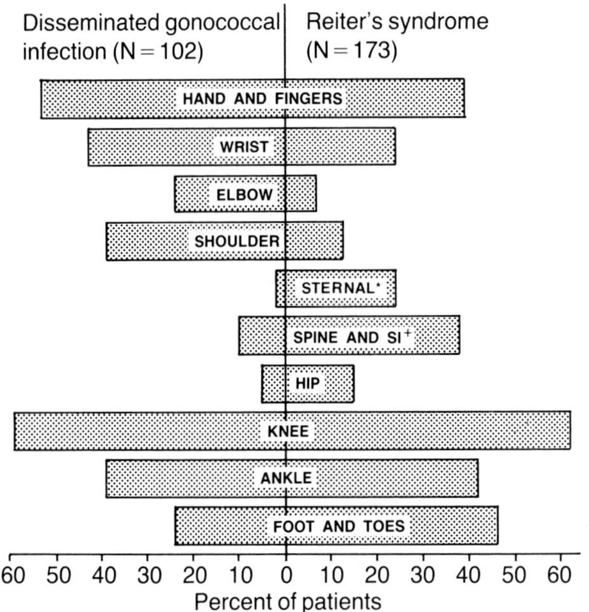


**Fig. 61-8.** Distributions of joints with arthritis in 102 patients with DGI[3] and 173 patients with Reiter's syndrome.[37] *Sternal includes the sternoclavicular joint. †SI denotes the sacroiliac joint.

osynovitis is often considered evidence for DGI, in our experience[1,3] tenosynovitis is a nonspecific finding that does not reliably distinguish DGI from Reiter's syndrome or other acute arthritides.

Genital, anorectal, or pharyngeal gonococcal infection can be identified in 70 to 80 percent of patients with DGI or in their sex partners but also has been documented in up to 20 percent of patients with acute Reiter's syndrome.[37] All potential mucosal sites of infection must be cultured, regardless of the presence or absence of local symptoms (Table 61-2). *N. gonorrhoeae* was identified by culture or by the direct fluorescent antibody test in blood, synovial fluid, or skin lesions of 52 (51 percent) of 102 patients with DGI in the Seattle series[1,3] and in 23 (47 percent) of 49 studied by O'Brien et al.[8] All recent sexual partners should also be examined, for diagnostic reasons as well as epidemiologic ones; DGI sometimes is confirmed bacteriologically only by detection of gonorrhea in a partner.[3,128] Similarly, *C. trachomatis* often can be isolated from the partners of patients with sexually acquired Reiter's syndrome.

Synovial fluid analysis and culture or specific antigen detection tests are important in identifying patients with crystal-induced arthritis and gonococcal or nongonococcal septic arthritis. Synovial fluid leukocyte counts are useful in establishing the presence of inflammation, but not in establishing its cause. Protein, glucose, and complement levels provide less specific information. Radiographs of peripheral joints, tests for serum uric acid levels, the erythrocyte sedimentation rate, and assays for rheumatoid factor, antinuclear antibodies, complement levels, and circulating immune complexes usually are not indicated as routine screening tests in acute arthritis, although they may be diagnostic in the appropriate clinical setting.

It has been argued that HLA typing is not diagnostically useful,[129] because the diagnosis of Reiter's syndrome is more reliably based on clinical criteria and the results of typing seldom affect therapy. On the other hand, a positive test may solidify an otherwise equivocal diagnosis of Reiter's syndrome.[130]

The diagnosis of DGI is unequivocal if *N. gonorrhoeae* is identified in blood, synovial fluid, a nongenital skin lesion, cerebrospinal fluid, or another nonmucosal site. The diagnosis also is secure if a mucosal gonococcal infection is documented in the presence of a typical clinical syndrome that responds promptly to appropriate antimicrobial therapy,[1,20] especially if other causes of acute arthropathy are excluded. In the absence of documented gonococcal infection in the patient, the diagnosis of DGI is probable if a typical clinical syndrome responds promptly to antibiotics.[20] The presence of gonorrhea in a sexual partner also supports the diagnosis.

The American Rheumatism Association defines Reiter's syndrome simply as an episode of peripheral arthritis of more than 30 days' duration occurring in association with urethritis or cervicitis.[43] Although apparently simplistic, these criteria will accurately classify the majority of patients with Reiter's syndrome. The occurrence of conjunctivitis or the typical mucocutaneous inflammatory lesions, documentation of the HLA-B27 haplotype, and clinical or radiologic evidence of sacroiliitis help to confirm the diagnosis. The pattern of joint involvement and other clinical and laboratory features serve to distinguish the reactive arthritides from rheumatoid arthritis and arthropathies due to immune-complex deposition.

Although most cases of DGI and Reiter's syndrome can be distinguished by the above criteria, neither set of criteria is completely satisfactory for the initial evaluation of patients presenting with acute arthritis, because the criteria for DGI require up to several days to obtain culture results and those for Reiter's syndrome may require a month or more of clinical observation. The algorithm in Fig. 61-9 illustrates a diagnostic approach to reach a tentative diagnosis at the time of presentation of a sexually active patient with acute arthritis. The algorithm is based on synovial fluid analysis for crystals and bacteria, the presence or absence of typical mucocutaneous lesions or conjunctivitis, and careful examination for urogenital inflammation and for evidence of gonococcal infection by Gram-stained smear. The algorithm does not supplant a careful history and physical examination; it represents the logic used in analyzing the results of the initial clinical and laboratory examinations, rather than a flow chart for their performance. For example, evaluation for genital inflammation is indicated for all patients, regardless of whether a probable diagnosis is reached prior to the relevant branching point. Finally, cultures and other late-arriving laboratory results and the clinical course will help to clarify the tentative diagnosis made using the algorithm and may result in reclassification or lead to other diagnoses.

If synovial fluid is obtained, examination for crystals by wet preparation and for bacteria by Gram stain should be performed; occasionally these will lead to an immediate diagnosis. If no synovial fluid is present or its analysis is nondiagnostic, the results of a careful examination of the skin are considered. The presence of typical papular, pustular, or hemorrhagic lesions in various stages of evolution, located primarily on the extremities, is strong evidence of DGI. Similarly, keratodermia blennorrhagica or circinate balanitis in the patient with acute arthritis are diagnostic of Reiter's syndrome. In the absence of typical skin lesions, the results of the evaluation for genital inflammation are considered. Gonococcal urethritis or cervicitis, identified by the presence of intracellular gram-negative diplococci, supports a tentative diagnosis of DGI, while the presence of nongonococcal genital tract inflammation implies Reiter's syndrome. For those individuals who lack both diagnostic mucocutaneous lesions and urogenital inflammation, conjunctivitis or iritis suggests Reiter's syndrome,

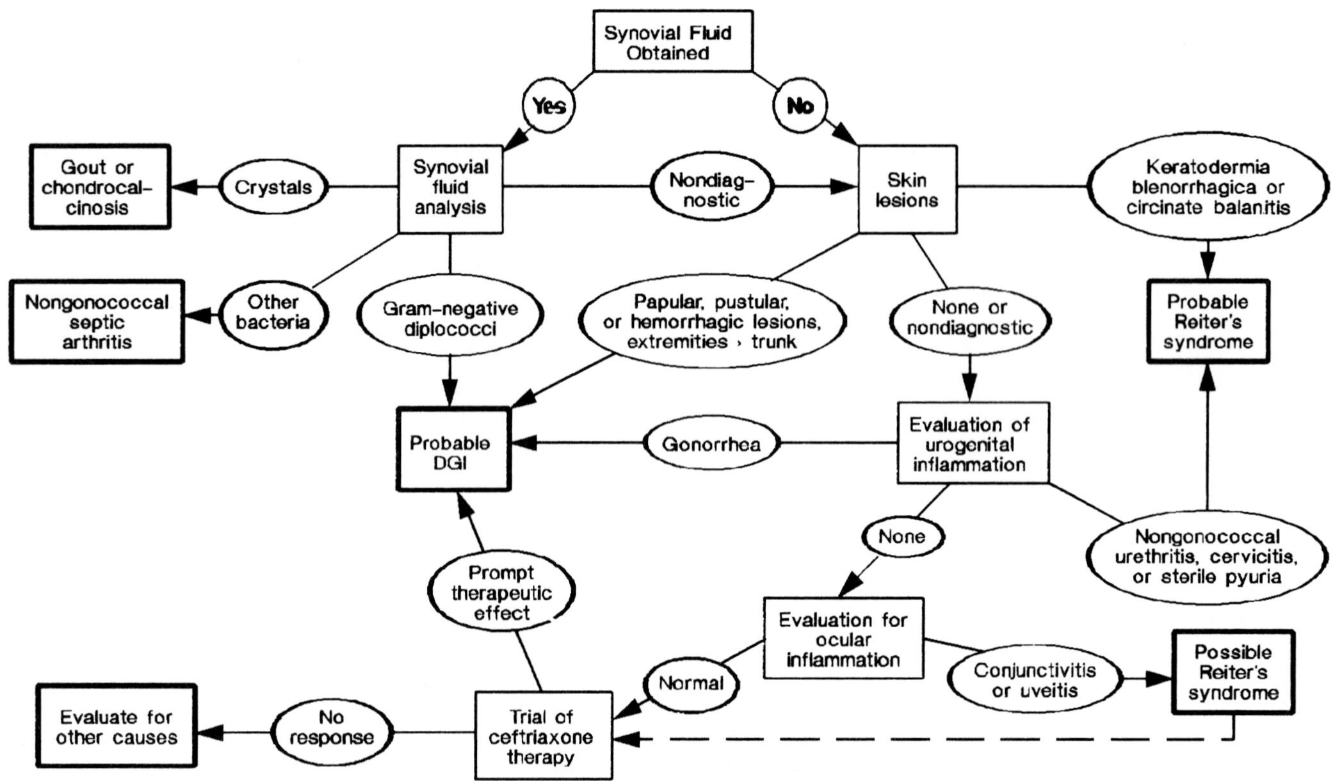


**Fig. 61-9.** Algorithm for the presumptive diagnosis of acute, nontraumatic arthritis in sexually active patients.

although absence of ocular inflammation is not diagnostically helpful. Regardless of the preliminary diagnosis, it is essential to obtain cultures or antigen-detection tests for *C. trachomatis* and cultures for *N. gonorrhoeae* from the cervix, urethra, and rectum, and for *N. gonorrhoeae* from the pharynx, blood, and synovial fluid. Finally, unless the initial evaluation reliably excludes DGI, a trial of antibiotic therapy is warranted; antibiotic-responsive, culture-negative acute arthritis in a sexually active person usually is due to this disease. Other potentially useful tests not reflected in the algorithm include HLA typing and radiologic or radionuclide imaging of the sacroiliac joints.

Failure of response to treatment at this point necessitates further evaluation for an acute presentation of a rheumatic disease such as rheumatoid arthritis or systemic lupus erythematosus. Blood cultures must be obtained prior to the therapeutic trial not only to detect gonococcemia but also to exclude infective endocarditis as a cause of arthritis. If monoarticular arthritis persists during continued observation, synovial biopsy may be required to exclude tuberculosis, fungal infection, or synovial tumor.

## MANAGEMENT

The treatment of DGI is discussed in Chap. 14. Ceftriaxone is now the mainstay of antibiotic therapy; bed rest, closed drainage of purulent synovial effusions, and anti-inflammatory drugs are adjuncts. In Reiter's syndrome, NGU or cervicitis should be treated as described in Chap. 16. Similarly, specific antimicrobial therapy should be administered if infectious enteritis is documented. However, treatment of the triggering infection has not been shown to affect the course of arthritis or the mucocutaneous manifestations, and the mainstay of treatment for Reiter's syndrome is administration of anti-inflammatory drugs. Indomethacin is the drug used most commonly (typically 75 to 150 mg daily in divided doses). However, several other nonsteroidal anti-inflammatory agents are effective for symptomatic control of the arthritis, and therapeutic trials with various drugs should be used as necessary to balance efficacy and tolerance in individual patients. Salicylates and corticosteroids are of little benefit for most patients. For fulminant cases resistant to these drugs, methotrexate or immunosuppressive agents (e.g., azathioprine) have been used with apparent success.

Arthritis due to hepatitis B virus infection is self-limited and usually does not require drug therapy, although symptoms may be ameliorated by transient use of aspirin or other nonsteroidal antiinflammatory drugs. Patients with arthritis due to syphilis, lymphogranuloma venereum, or other sexually transmitted infections should be treated with standard antibiotic regimens.

## PREVENTION

There are no specific measures to prevent sexually transmitted arthritis aside from those designed to prevent the precipitating causes. Patients with Reiter's syndrome should be advised of the ongoing risk and counseled to use condoms for future casual sexual contacts. Treatment of the sexual partners of patients with DGI or Reiter's syndrome is essential to prevent reinfection and may be important for prevention of recurrence of arthritis.

## References


1 Handsfield HH: Disseminated gonococcal infection. *Clin Obstet Gynecol* 18:131, 1975.

2 Calin A: Reiter's syndrome, in *Textbook of Rheumatology,* WN Kelly et al (eds). Philadelphia, Saunders, 1981, p 1033.

3 Handsfield HH et al: Unpublished data.

4 Bauer W, Engleman EP: A syndrome of unknown etiology characterized by urethritis, conjunctivitis, and arthritis (so-called Reiter's disease). *Trans Assoc Am Physicians* 57:307, 1942.

5 Keat A: Reiter's syndrome and reactive arthritis in perspective. *N Engl J Med* 309:1606, 1983.

6 Calin A: Seronegative spondyloarthritides. *Med Clin North Am* 70:323, 1986.

7 Manshady BM et al: Septic arthritis in a general hospital, 1966–1977. *J Rheumatol* 7:523, 1980.

8 O'Brien JP et al: Disseminated gonococcal infection: A prospective analysis of 49 patients and a review of pathophysiology and immune mechanisms. *Medicine* 62:395, 1983.

9 Shapiro L et al: Dermatohistopathology of chronic gonococcal sepsis. *Arch Dermatol* 107:403, 1973.

10 Williams RC: *Immune Complexes in Clinical and Experimental Medicine.* Cambridge, Harvard University Press, 1980.

11 Keiser H et al: Clinical forms of gonococcal arthritis. *N Engl J Med* 279:234, 1968.

12 Brandt KD et al: Gonococcal arthritis: Clinical features correlated with blood, synovial fluid and genitourinary cultures. *Arthritis Rheum* 17:503, 1974.

13 Gelfand SC et al: Spectrum of gonococcal arthritis: Evidence for sequential stages and clinical subgroups. *J Rheumatol* 2:83, 1975.

14 Holmes KK et al: Disseminated gonococcal infection. *Ann Intern Med* 74:979, 1971.

15 Barr J, Danielsson D: Septic gonococcal dermatitis. *Br Med J* 1:482, 1971.

16 Tronca E et al: Demonstration of *Neisseria gonorrhoeae* with fluorescent antibody in patients with disseminated gonococcal infection. *J Infect Dis* 129:583, 1974.

17 Rothschild BM, Schrank GD: Histologic documentation of gonococcal infection in the absence of a culturable organism. *Clin Rheumatol* 3:389, 1984.

18 Gantz NM et al: Gonococcal osteomyelitis: An unusual complication of gonococcal arthritis. *JAMA* 236:2431, 1976.

19 Garcia-Kutzbach A et al: Gonococcal arthritis: Clinical features and results of penicillin therapy. *J Rheumatol* 1:210, 1974.

20 Handsfield HH et al: Treatment of the gonococcal arthritis-dermatitis syndrome. *Ann Intern Med* 84:661, 1976.

21 Cooke CL et al: Gonococcal arthritis: A survey of 54 cases. *JAMA* 217:204, 1971.

22 Walker LC et al: Circulating immune complexes in disseminated gonorrheal infection. *Ann Intern Med* 89:28, 1978.

23 Ludivico CL, Myers AR: Survey for immune complexes in disseminated gonococcal arthritis-dermatitis syndrome. *Arthritis Rheum* 22:19, 1979.

24 Martin DA et al: Identification of immune complexes in synovial fluids and sera of patients with disseminated gonococcal infections (DGI) using the Raji cell assay. *Arthritis Rheum* 24:S74, 1981.

25 Manicourt DH, Orloff S: Gonococcal arthritis-dermatitis syndrome: Study of serum and synovial fluid immune complex levels. *Arth Rheum* 25:574, 1982.

26 Fleming RJ et al: Arthropathic properties of gonococcal peptidoglycan fragments: Implications for the pathogenesis of disseminated gonococcal disease. *Infec Immun* 52:600, 1986.

27 Holmes KK et al: The gonococcal arthritis dermatitis syndrome. *Ann Intern Med* 75:470, 1971.

28 Keefer CS, Spink WW: Gonococcal arthritis: Pathogenesis, mechanisms of recovery, and treatment. *JAMA* 109:1448, 1937.

29 Brogadir SP et al: Spectrum of the gonococcal arthritis-dermatitis syndrome. *Semin Arthritis Rheum* 8:177, 1979.

30 Handsfield HH et al: Correlation of auxotype and penicillin susceptibility of *Neisseria gonorrhoeae* with sexual preference and clinical manifestations of gonorrhea. *Sex Transm Dis* 7:1, 1980.

30a Editorial: Seronegative (reactive) arthropathy: Precipitating factors. *Lancet* 2:200, 1988.

31 Kousa M et al: Frequent association of chlamydial infection with Reiter's syndrome. *Sex Transm Dis* 5:57, 1978.

32 Martin DH et al: *Chlamydia trachomatis* infections in men with Reiter's syndrome. *Ann Intern Med* 100:207, 1984.

33 Rosenthal L et al: Aseptic arthritis after gonorrhea. *Ann Rheum Dis* 39:141, 1980.

34 Ford DK: Venereal arthritis. *Br J Vener Dis* 29:123, 1953.

35 Olhagen B: Chronic uropolyarthritis in the male. *Acta Med Scand* 168:339, 1960.

36 Cleuziou A et al: Reactive arthritis after gonococcal infection. *Rev Med Interne* 5:65, 1984.

37 Kousa M: Clinical observations on Reiter's disease with special reference to the venereal and nonvenereal aetiology: A follow-up study. *Acta Dermato Venereol (Stockh)* 58(suppl 81):1, 1978.

38 Calin A, Fries JF: An "experimental" epidemic of Reiter's syndrome revisited: Follow-up evidence on genetic and environmental factors. *Ann Intern Med* 84:564, 1976.

39 Paronen I: Reiter's disease: A study of 344 cases observed in Finland. *Acta Med Scand* 130(suppl 212):1, 1948.

40 Repo H et al: Exaggerated inflammatory responsiveness plays a part in the pathogenesis of HLA-B27 linked diseases: Hypothesis. *Ann Clin Res* 16:47, 1984.

41 Firestein GS, Zfaifler NJ: Reactive arthritis. *Annu Rev Med* 38:351, 1987.

42 Fox R et al: The chronicity of symptoms and disability in Reiter's syndrome. *Ann Intern Med* 91:190, 1979.

43 Willkens RF et al: Reiter's syndrome: Evaluation of preliminary criteria for definite disease. *Arthritis Rheum* 24:844, 1981.

44 Arnett FC et al: Cross-reactive HLA antigens in B27-negative Reiter's syndrome and sacroiliitis. *Johns Hopkins Med J* 141:193, 1977.

45 Khan MA et al: Low association of HLA-B27 with Reiter's syndrome in blacks. *Ann Intern Med* 90:202, 1979.

46 Good AE et al: HLA B27 in blacks with ankylosing spondylitis or Reiter's disease. *N Engl J Med* 194:166, 1976.

47 Khan MA et al: HLA-B27 in ankylosing spondylitis: Differences in frequency and relative risk in American blacks and Caucasians. *J Rheumatol* 4(suppl 3):39, 1977.

48 McDevitt HO, Bodmer WF: HLA, immune response genes and disease. *Lancet* 1:1269, 1974.

49 Zwillich SH, Lipsky PE: Molecular mimicry in the pathogenesis of rheumatic diseases. *Rheum Dis Clin North Am* 13:339, 1987.

50 Schachter J et al: Isolation of *Bedsoniae* from the joints of patients with Reiter's syndrome. *Proc Soc Exp Biol* 122:283, 1966.

51 Dunlop EMC et al: Infection by TRIC agent and other members of the Bedsonia group, with a note on Reiter's disease: III. Genital infection and diseases of the eye. *Trans Ophthalmol Soc UK* 86: 321, 1966.

52 Schachter J: Can chlamydial infections cause rheumatic disease? In *Infection and Immunology in the Rheumatic Diseases,* DC Dumonde (ed). Oxford, Blackwell, 1976, p 151.

53 Reiter's syndrome, editorial. *Lancet* 2:567, 1979.

53a Schumacher HR et al: Ultrastructural identification of chlamydial antigens in synovial membrane in acute Reiter's syndrome (abstract). *Arthritis Rheum* 29(suppl):115, 1986.

54 Keat A et al: *Chlamydia trachomatis* and reactive arthritis: The missing link. *Lancet* 1(8534):72, 1987.

54a Taylor-Robinson D et al: Evidence that *Chlamydia trachomatis* causes seronegative arthritis in women. *Ann Rheum Dis* 47:295, 1988.

54b Granfors K et al: Yersinia antigens in synovial-fluid cells from patients with reactive arthritis. *N Engl J Med* 320:216, 1989.

55 Ford DK et al: Cell-mediated immune responses of synovial mono-

nuclear cells to sexually transmitted, enteric, and mumps antigens in patients with Reiter's syndrome, rheumatoid arthritis, and ankylosing spondylitis. *J Rheumatol* 8:220, 1981.

56 Ford DK: Infectious agents in Reiter's syndrome. *Clin Exp Rheumatol* 2:273, 1983.

57 Nordstrom D et al: Synovial fluid cells in Reiter's syndrome. *Ann Rheum Dis* 44:852, 1985.

58 Winchester R et al: The co-occurrence of Reiter's syndrome and acquired immunodeficiency. *Ann Intern Med* 106:19, 1987.

59 Bjelle A, Tarnvik A: Lymphocytes of synovial fluid and peripheral blood in reactive arthritis. *Scand J Infect Dis* 24(suppl):58, 1980.

60 Brenner MB et al: In vitro T lymphocyte proliferative responses to *Yersinia enterocolitica* in Reiter's syndrome. *Arthritis Rheum* 27: 250, 1984.

61 Scher I et al: Selective inhibition of lymphocyte responsiveness to phytohemagglutinin in patients with Reiter's syndrome. *Clin Exp Immunol* 23:404, 1976.

62 Inman RD et al: Analysis of serum and synovial fluid IgA in Reiter's syndrome and reactive arthritis. *Clin Immunol Immunopathol* 43: 195, 1987.

63 Pereira AB et al: Detection and partial characterization of circulating immune complexes with solid-phase anti-C3. *J Immunol* 125: 763, 1980.

64 Yates DG et al: Complement activation in Reiter's syndrome. *Ann Rheumatol* 34:468, 1975.

65 Norton WL et al: Light and electron microscopic observations on the synovitis of Reiter's disease. *Arthritis Rheum* 9:747, 1966.

66 Paty JG: Reiter's syndrome: Occurrence in roommates. *Arthritis Rheum* 21:283, 1978.

67 Good AE, Schultz JS: Reiter's syndrome following *Shigella flexneri* 2a. *Arthritis Rheum* 20:100, 1977.

68 Jones RAK: Reiter's disease after *Salmonella typhimurium* enteritis. *Br Med J* 1:1391, 1977.

69 Warren CPW: Arthritis associated with *Salmonella* infection. *Ann Rheum Dis* 29:483, 1970.

70 Laitinen O et al: Relation between HLA-B27 and clinical features in patients with *Yersinia* arthritis. *Arthritis Rheum* 20:1121, 1977.

71 Ahvonen P: Human yersiniosis in Finland: II. Clinical features. *Ann Clin Res* 4:39, 1972.

72 Jacks JC: *Yersinia entercolitica* arthritis. *Pediatrics* 55:236, 1975.

73 van de Putte LBA et al: Reactive arthritis after *Campylobacter jejuni* enteritis. *J Rheumatol* 7:531, 1980.

74 Keat AC et al: The role of *Chlamydia trachomatis* and HLA B27 in sexually acquired reactive arthritis. *Br Med J* 1:605, 1978.

75 Csonka GW: The course of Reiter's syndrome. *Br Med J* 1:1088, 1958.

76 Smith DL et al: Reiter's disease in women. *Arthritis Rheum* 23:335, 1980.

77 Neuwelt CM et al: Reiter's syndrome: A male and female disease. *J Rheumatol* 9:268, 1982.

78 Yli-Kerttula UI et al: Urogenital involvements and rheumatic disorders in females: An interview study. *Clin Rheumatol* 4:170, 1985.

79 Vilppula AH et al: Musculoskeletal involvements in female sexual partners of males with Reiter's syndrome. *Clin Rheumatol* 2:347, 1983.

80 Hagenfeldt K, Szanto E: Sacroiliitis in women: A late sequela to acute salpingitis. *Am J Obstet Gynecol* 138:1039, 1980.

81 McCord WC et al: Acute venereal arthritis. *Arch Intern Med* 137: 858, 1877.

82 Catterall RD: Uveitis, arthritis and nonspecific genital infection. *Br J Vener Dis* 36:27, 1960.

83 Romanus R: Pelveospondylitis ossificans in the male and genitourinary infection. *Acta Med Scand* 280(suppl):53, 1963.

84 Singsen B et al: Reiter's syndrome in childhood. *Arthritis Rheum* 20:402, 1977.

85 Ball J: Enthesopathy of rheumatoid and ankylosing spondylitis. *Ann Rheum Dis* 30:213, 1971.

86 Daunt SD et al: Ulcerative vulvitis in Reiter's syndrome: A case report. *Br J Vener Dis* 58:405, 1982.

87 Russell AS et al: The sacroiliitis of acute Reiter's syndrome. *J Rheumatol* 4:293, 1977.

88 Moll JMH et al: Association between ankylosing spondylitis, psoriatic arthritis, Reiter's disease, the intestinal arthropathies and Behçet's syndrome. *Medicine* 53:343, 1974.

89 Montgomery MM et al: The mucocutaneous lesions of Reiter's syndrome and keratosis blennorrhagica. *Ann Intern Med* 51:99, 1959.

90 Rossen RM et al: A-V conduction disturbances in Reiter's syndrome. *Am J Med* 58:280, 1975.

91 Block SR: Reiter's syndrome and acute aortic insufficiency. *Arthritis Rheum* 15:218, 1972.

92 Paulus HE et al: Aortic insufficiency in five patients with Reiter's syndrome. *Am J Med* 53:464, 1972.

93 Butler MJ et al: A follow-up study of 48 patients with Reiter's syndrome. *Am J Med* 67:808, 1979.

94 Caughey DE et al: A fatal case of Reiter's disease complicated by amyloidosis. *Arthritis Rheum* 16:695, 1973.

95 Alarcon GS, Townes AS: Arthritis in viral hepatitis. *Johns Hopkins Med J* 132:1, 1973.

96 Schumacher HR, Gall EP, Arthritis in acute hepatitis and chronic active hepatitis. *Am J Med* 57:655, 1974.

97 Alpert E et al: The pathogenesis of arthritis associated with viral hepatitis: Complement-component studies. *N Engl J Med* 285:185, 1971.

98 Onion DK et al: Arthritis of hepatitis associated with Australia antigen. *Ann Intern Med* 75:29, 1971.

99 Wands JR et al: The pathogenesis of arthritis associated with acute hepatitis-B surface antigen-positive hepatitis. *J Clin Invest* 55:930, 1975.

100 Schumaker JB et al: Arthritis and rash: Clues to anicteric hepatitis. *Arch Intern Med* 133:483, 1974.

101 McEwen C, Thomas EW: Syphilitic joint disease. *Med Clin North Am* 22:1275, 1938.

102 Reginato AJ et al: Synovitis in secondary syphilis: Clinical, light, and electron microscopic studies. *Arthritis Rheum* 22:170, 1979.

103 Tourville DR et al: Treponemal antigen in immunopathogenesis of syphilitic glomerulonephritis. *Am J Pathol* 82:479, 1976.

104 Floyd W et al: The neuropathic joint. *South Med J* 52:563, 1959.

105 Fishel B et al: Multiple neuropathic arthropathy in a patient with syphilis. *Clin Rheumatol* 4:348, 1985.

106 Moran SM, Mohr JA: Syphilis and axial arthropathy. *South Med J* 76:1032, 1983.

107 Koteen H: Lymphogranuloma venereum. *Medicine* 24:1, 1945.

108 Hickam JB: Cutaneous and articular manifestations in lymphogranuloma venereum. *Arch Dermatol Syphil* 51:330, 1945.

109 Lassus A et al: Auto-immune serum factors and IgA elevation in lymphogranuloma venereum. *Ann Clin Res* 2:51, 1970.

110 Keat A et al: Chlamydial infection in the aetiology of arthritis. *Br Med Bul* 39:168, 1983.

110a Berman A et al: Rheumatic manifestations of human immunodeficiency virus infection. *Am J Med* 85:59, 1988.

110b Forster SM et al: Inflammatory joint disease and human immunodeficiency virus infection. *Br Med J* [Clin Res] 296:1625, 1988.

110c Rynes RI et al: Acquired immunodeficiency syndrome-associated arthritis. *Am J Med* 84:810, 1988.

110d Winchester R et al: The co-occurrence of Reiter's syndrome and acquired immunodeficiency. *Ann Intern Med* 106:19, 1987.

110e Ulirsch RC Jaffee ES: Sjogren's syndrome-like illness associated with the acquired immunodeficiency syndrome-related complex. *Hum Pathol* 18:1063, 1987.

111 Verinder DGR: Septic arthritis due to *Mycoplasma hominis*: A case report and review of the literature. *J Bone Joint Surg* 60B:224, 1978.

112 Taylor-Robinson D et al: The association of *Mycoplasma hominis* with arthritis. *Sex Transm Dis* 10(suppl):341, 1983.

113 McDonald MI et al: Septic arthritis due to *Mycoplasma hominis*. *Arthritis Rheum* 26:2044, 1983.
114 Taylor-Robinson D et al: *Ureaplasma urealyticum* in the immunocompromised host. *Pediatr Infect Dis* 5(suppl):S236, 1986.
115 Roifman CM et al: Increased susceptibility to *Mycoplasma* infection in patients with hypogammaglobulinemia. *Am J Med* 80:590, 1986.
116 Webster ADB et al: Mycoplasmal (Ureaplasma) septic arthritis in hypogammaglobulinemia. *Br Med J* 1:478, 1978.
117 Stuckey M et al: Identification of *Ureaplasma urealyticum* (T-strain mycoplasma) in patients with polyarthritis. *Lancet* 2:917, 1978.
118 Friedman HM et al: Acute monoarticular arthritis caused by herpes simplex virus and cytomegalovirus. *Am J Med* 69:241, 1980.
119 Sauter SVH, Utsinger PD: Viral arthritis. *Clin Rheum Dis* 4:225, 1978.
120 Brna JA, Hall RF Jr: Acute monoarticular herpetic arthritis. *J Bone Joint Surg* 66:623, 1984.
121 Remafedi G, Muldoon RL: Acute monoarticular arthritis caused by herpes simplex type I. *Pediatrics* 72:882, 1983.
122 Ray CG et al: Acute polyarthritis associated with active Epstein-Barr virus infection. *JAMA* 248:2990, 1982.
123 Keys TF et al: Endocervical *Neisseria meningitidis* with meningococcemia. *N Engl J Med* 285:505, 1971.
124 Rompalo AM et al: The acute arthritis-dermatitis syndrome: The changing importance of *Neisseria gonorrhoeae* and *Neisseria meningitidis*. *Arch Intern Med* 147:281, 1987.
125 Fam AG et al: Clinical forms of meningococcal arthritis: A study of five cases. *J Rheumatol* 6:567, 1979.
126 Loebl DH: Acute joint infection with *Neisseria meningitidis*: A case of mistaken identity. *Milit Med* 143:777, 1978.
127 Munoz AJ: Gonococcal and meningococcal arthritis. *Clin Rheum Dis* 4:169, 1978.
128 Mendelson J et al: Disseminated gonorrhea: Diagnosis through contact tracing. *Can Med Assoc J* 112:864, 1975.
129 Calin A: HLA-B27:To type or not to type. *Ann Intern Med* 92: 208, 1980.
130 Khan MA, Khan MK: Diagnostic value of HLA-B27 testing in ankylosing spondylitis and Reiter's syndrome. *Ann Intern Med* 96: 70, 1982.

Chapter 62

# Ocular manifestations of AIDS and other sexually transmitted diseases in the adult

Michael S. Insler
Linda C. Novak

## CHLAMYDIAL CONJUNCTIVITIS

In the adult, chlamydial conjunctivitis remains the most common type of ocular infection associated with sexually transmitted diseases. Although generally considered a benign disorder, adult chlamydial cervicitis may contribute significantly to infertility and ectopic pregnancy in women.

It has been estimated that *Chlamydia trachomatis* affects at least 3 million Americans a year.[1] From this it is conservatively estimated that 1 percent, or greater than 30,000, new cases of adult chlamydial conjunctivitis will be seen each year in the United States. Most patients are between 15 and 40, and over half of all individuals with chlamydial eye disease have genital infection.[2] Transmission of the disease in adults occurs from sexual partners with hand-to-eye contamination leading to ocular infection. Serotypes D to K are responsible for adult chlamydial conjunctivitis, while *C. trachomatis* serotypes A, B, and C are responsible for endemic trachoma.

Adult disease presents as a chronic follicular conjunctivitis (see Plate 11) with a foreign body sensation, tearing, redness, photophobia, and lid swelling. The conjunctivitis is often unilateral with a mucopurulent discharge. Frequently, a nontender preauricular node is present on the involved side. Corneal involvement occurs commonly, and the epithelial keratitis may be associated with superficial corneal vascularization, which distinguishes this condition from the corneal infiltrates seen in acute adenoviral infection. Cytological examination shows a mixed polymorphonuclear and mononuclear cellular response, and chlamydia can be detected by culture or direct immunofluorescence.

In adults, chlamydial conjunctivitis responds to systemic antimicrobial therapy, usually with doxycycline 100 mg twice daily for 7 to 14 days, or with equivalent dosages of other tetracyclines. Alternatively, erythromycin can be used in oral doses equivalent to 500 mg of the base given four times daily for 7 to 14 days. Sexual partners should also be treated with one of these regimens. Concurrent topical therapy with steroids in patients with associated mild anterior uveitis may decrease the symptoms associated with the infection.

## HERPES SIMPLEX VIRUS (HSV)

Ocular herpes is a leading cause of blindness due to corneal scarring and opacification. Both HSV type I and HSV type II are now considered important pathogens in adult ocular disease.[3–6]

A striking feature of adult HSV infection is the ability of the virus to remain dormant for periods of time and then to appear as recurrent episodes of infection, usually occurring at the same site. Upon stimulation the virus is reactivated at the ganglionic site and subsequently traverses the sensory nerve to the cornea, where it may be seen clinically as a dendrite which is pathognomonic for HSV infection (Fig. 62-1). While epithelial keratitis usually presents as a classic central, linear, branching ulcerated dendrite which stains with fluorescein, repeated infection may result in stromal disease or interstitial keratitis, a type of stromal infiltration associated with edema, necrosis, and subsequent neovascularization of the cornea.

The ocular disease produced by either HSV type I or type II is indistinguishable in the adult, although HSV type II may produce a more severe and prolonged disease with greater resistance to antiviral therapy.[7] Autoinoculation of the virus may be the most important means of spread to the eye in patients with genital herpes. The diagnosis of ocular disease is usually made by clinical observation with laboratory confirmation infrequently performed. Several antivirals are in use topically for epithelial disease, which usually resolves after a 10-day to 2 week course. Patients with stromal keratitis must weigh the risk benefit ratio of topical steroids together with concomitant therapy with the antivirals. The nonophthalmologist is forewarned against prescribing an antibiotic-steroid combination when HSV may be suspected as the cause of an acute or recurrent conjunctivitis or keratitis. Recurrent bouts of inflammation can result in permanent scarring requiring penetrating keratoplasty.[8]

## SYPHILIS

In the adult, interstitial keratitis, which is diffuse and bilateral, is seen in over 90 percent of cases with congenital syphilis.[9,10] The cornea has a stromal haze with infiltration (Fig. 62-2), and ghost vessels (Fig. 62-3) appear in the deepest layers of the cornea. The choroid and retina may be involved with postinflammatory pigmentary changes (Figs. 62-4 and 62-5).

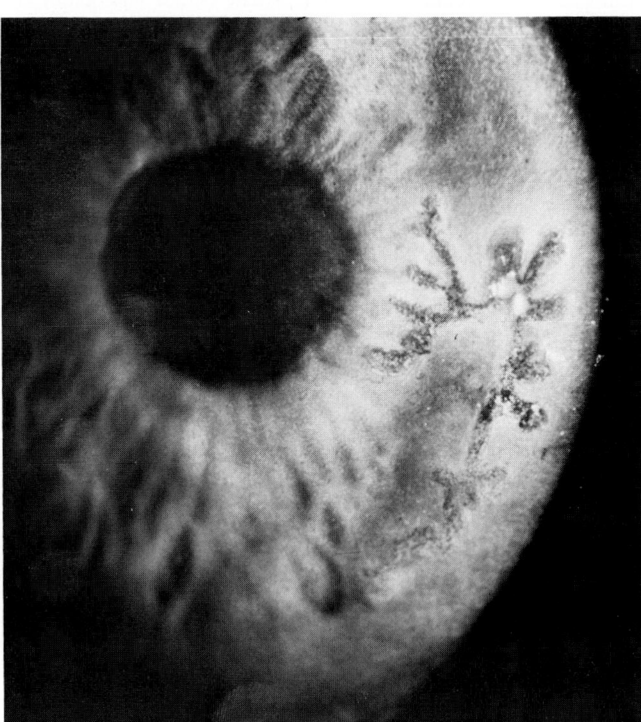

**Fig. 62-1.** Dendritic keratitis, which is characteristic of HSV infection.

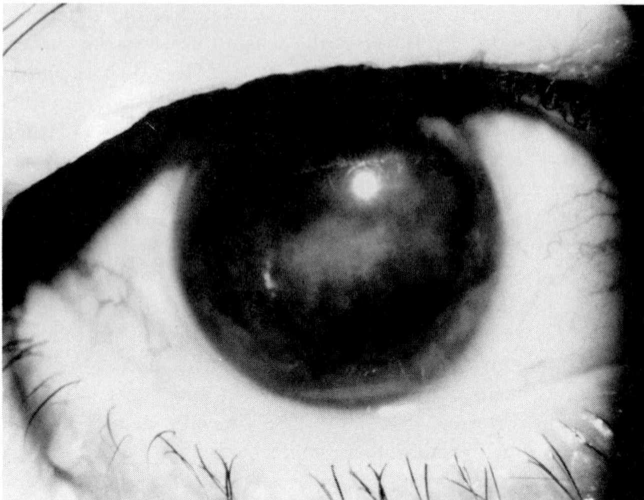

**Fig. 62-2.** Interstitial keratitis (old) due to congenital syphilis. Note patchy corneal clouding. (*Courtesy of J Chandler.*)

The diagnosis is usually based on the slit lamp appearance of the bilateral interstitial keratitis with a history of ocular inflammation occurring in childhood, together with a positive serologic examination.

The disease seen in the adult generally requires no treatment except a decision to perform keratoplasty (Fig. 62-6), which may or may not additionally involve cataract surgery. Systemic antibiotic therapy is indicated for untreated cases.

Other ocular manifestations of syphilis include chorioretinitis in secondary syphilis, and the classic pupillary abnormalities and optic atrophy of tertiary syphilis.[11,12]

## GONOCOCCAL CONJUNCTIVITIS

Gonococcal keratoconjunctivitis is a true ocular emergency because it can result in a severe, rapid ulcerative keratitis and corneal perforation.[13–15]

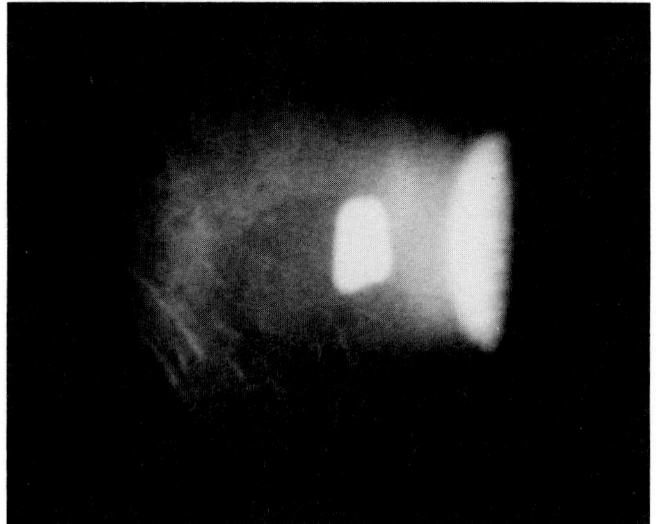

**Fig. 62-3.** Ghost vessels in the cornea due to old syphilitic interstitial keratitis, revealed by slit lamp examination. Ghost vessels are residual vessels from earlier keratitis, no longer perfused by blood. (*Courtesy of J Chandler.*)

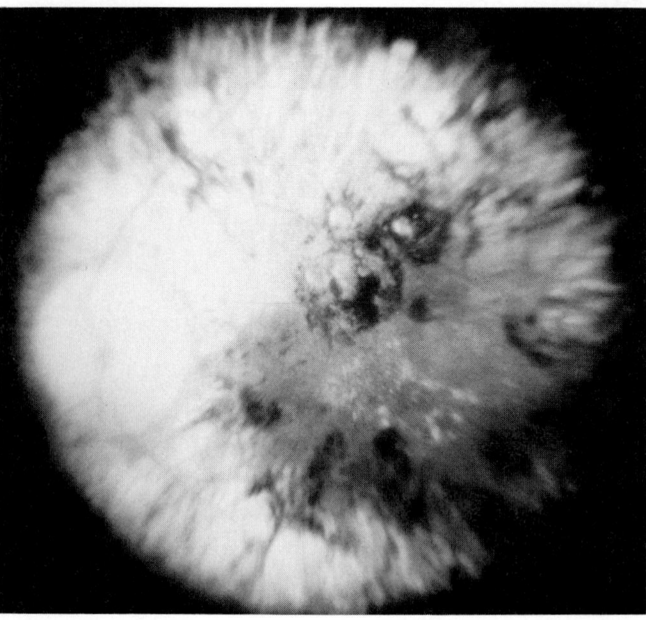

**Fig. 62-4.** Retinal scarring and pigmentary changes caused by healed syphilitic chorioretinitis. (*Courtesy of J Chandler.*)

A presumptive diagnosis of gonococcal conjunctivitis is based upon the finding of a hyperacute conjunctivitis (see Plate 9) associated with gram-negative diplococci. Most cases are believed due to inoculation of the conjunctiva with infected genital secretions. In adult patients with early ocular infection, systemic treatment with 250 mg of ceftriaxone intramuscularly is probably adequate, although experience is limited. Hospitalization is required with severe conjunctivitis and with corneal involvement, to permit frequent irrigation of the conjunctiva with saline to remove pus, together with parenteral administration of ceftriaxone in doses up to 1 g intravenously once daily. The optimal duration of parenteral treatment with ceftriaxone for gonococcal conjunctivitis has not been determined, but a 3- to 7-day course is probably adequate. Although not recommended by consultants to the Centers for Disease Control and the World Health Organization, the authors believe that topical penicillin G 100,000 units per ml should be used in conjunction with parenteral therapy for gonococcal conjunctivitis with corneal involvement.

## ACQUIRED IMMUNODEFICIENCY SYNDROME (AIDS)

Ocular manifestations of AIDS have assumed greater importance since the syndrome was first described in 1981.[16] Since that time, numerous investigators have conducted prospective and autopsy studies of the ophthalmic disorders most commonly associated with AIDS. From these studies the prevalence of abnormal ocular findings in AIDS patients has been found to range from 50 to 92 percent.[17–20]

While the clinical presentations of certain ophthalmic disorders in patients with AIDS may be different from the presentations in nonimmunocompromised individuals, their presentation in the AIDS patient remains relatively consistent. The ophthalmic manifestations may, therefore, be grouped into two major categories: noninfectious and infectious (Tables 62-1 and 62-2).[19] Neuro-ophthalmic complications result from both.

Noninfectious vascular disorders are the most common ophthalmic manifestation of AIDS. The prevalence of these le-

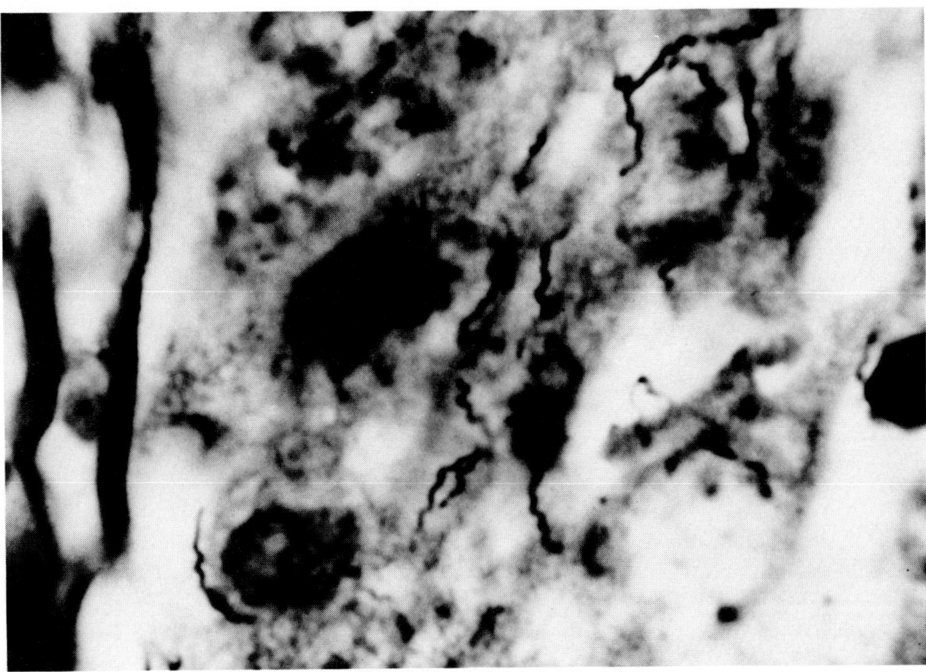

Fig. 62-5. *T. pallidum* demonstrated by silver stain in the retina in syphilitic chorioretinitis. (*Courtesy of J Chandler.*)

sions has been reported to range from 89 to 100 percent in autopsy studies.[18,19] The clinical appearance of these lesions varies from discrete areas of focal ischemia and hemorrhage to widespread areas of necrosis and atrophy.

Ophthalmic manifestations of opportunistic infection rarely present without evidence of systemic involvement. Cytomegalovirus (CMV) retinopathy, which is the most common opportunistic infection of the eye, is generally considered a late manifestation of systemic CMV infection.[17,21–23] Ocular involvement with the other opportunistic pathogens, such as in toxoplasmosis, is so infrequent that when ocular lesions occur with these infections, the presence of intracranial involvement or widespread systemic infection should be suspected.

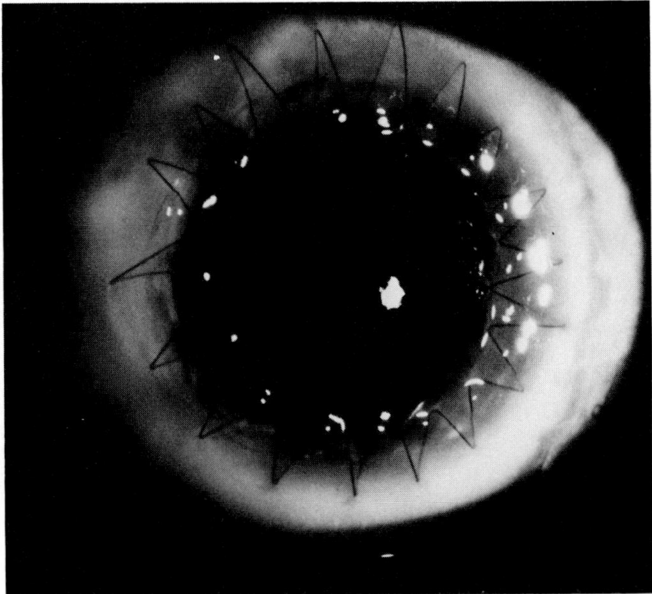

Fig. 62-6. Corneal transplant performed in a patient with interstitial keratitis due to syphilis. Note the remaining ring of cloudy scarring on the recipient cornea at the periphery of the donor graft.

The neuroophthalmic manifestations of AIDS are associated with viral and nonviral infections as well as with intracranial disease. Neoplasms and microvascular disorders less frequently result in neuroophthalmic abnormalities.

## NONINFECTIOUS MICROVASCULAR ABNORMALITIES

### Cotton wool spots

Cotton wool spots (CWS) are the most common ophthalmic lesion described in AIDS patients.[21–24] They have been reported in 42 to 71 percent of cases.[20,26] These lesions, however, are not specific for AIDS, but rather occur in a number of systemic diseases including hypertension and diabetes.[18–20,24,26]

Clinically they appear as single or multiple fluffy white opacities with indistinct borders located in the superficial retina (nerve fiber layer) along the vascular arcades (Fig. 62-7). They are asymptomatic and transient, lasting 4 to 6 weeks.[17–19,23–25,27]

At present the clinical significance of these lesions is not fully understood. Cotton wool spots have been found to be an isolated vascular abnormality in AIDS patients without apparent systemic infection, in addition to being found in patients with active or recent opportunistic infections.[18,20,22–24,27] They are not, however, thought to be a site of retinal infection, but rather a result of focal ischemia—a focal infarct in the nerve fiber layer.[17–19,22–24,27]

### Retinal hemorrhages

Retinal hemorrhage, another noninfectious microvascular disorder associated with AIDS, is encountered less frequently than CWS (8 to 40 percent of cases).[18,20,21] Similar to CWS, retinal hemorrhages are a transient and nonspecific finding which may also occur in a number of systemic diseases, such as diabetes, hypertension, collagen vascular disease, and renal failure.[18,22] Most commonly, they are either superficial flame-shaped hem-

Table 62-1. Ocular Disorders in AIDS

- I. Noninfectious Disorders
  - A. Vascular
    1. Cotton wool spots
    2. Microaneurysms
    3. Retinal hemorrhages
    4. Perivasculitis
    5. Ischemic retinopathy and bilateral acute retinal necrosis
  - B. Neoplastic
    1. Kaposi's sarcoma
    2. Burkitt's lymphoma
- II. Infections
  - A. Viral
    1. CMV (cytomegalovirus)
    2. Herpes simplex virus
    3. Herpes zoster virus
    4. Molluscum contagiosum
  - B. Protozoal
    1. Toxoplasmosis
    2. *Pneumocystis carinii*
  - C. Fungal
    1. *Cryptococcus neoformans*
    2. *Candida albicans*
    3. *Histoplasma capsulatum*
  - D. Bacterial
    1. *Mycobacterium avium* complex or *M. tuberculosis*
    2. Syphilis

orrhages lying within the posterior pole or deeper intraretinal blot-type hemorrhages found more anteriorly.[22] Their presence and distribution has been reported not to correlate with disease activity.[18,20]

## Perivasculitis

Perivasculitis is less common than CWS or retinal hemorrhages in noninfectious AIDS retinopathy and has been reported in only 3 percent of cases.[22] It also is a transient and nonspecific finding which may be associated with systemic as well as ophthalmic autoimmune disorders.

Clinically, the vasculitis, or sheathing of the retinal vessels, may range from a dense white sheathing of major vessels in the posterior pole to inconspicuous yellow-white patches along arterioles and venules.[22,24,28]

## Ischemic maculopathy and bilateral acute retinal necrosis

The least common of the microvascular abnormalities associated with AIDS is also the most visually incapacitating. Ischemic retinopathy and bilateral acute retinal necrosis are both characterized by a profound drop in visual acuity.

Ischemic maculopathy, found in 6 percent of patients,[21] is a focal ischemia of the macula. It has been characterized by retinal edema and macular star formation as well as by CWS.[21]

# NEOPLASMS

## Kaposi's sarcoma

Kaposi's sarcoma can involve the eye, as well as adnexal structures such as the eyelid and the orbit. The prevalence of ocular Kaposi's sarcoma ranges from 9 to 24 percent.[21,22] This represents primarily conjunctival Kaposi's sarcoma (Fig. 62-8), since it rarely presents on the eyelids and even less frequently in the orbit.[20,24,29–36] Although conjunctival Kaposi's sarcoma has been reported to occur without any prior cutaneous involvement, the ocular lesions usually develop after the appearance of the characteristic reddish-blue subcutaneous nodular skin lesions found elsewhere on the body.[22,32,36] Conjunctival lesions usually involve the inferior fornices or palpebral conjunctiva.[17,24,36] At this location a reddish or blue-black hemorrhagic subepithelial nodule or diffusely infiltrative lesion may occur simultaneously with a subconjunctival hemorrhage for which it may be mistaken.[17,22,24,36]

Bulbar involvement, while less frequent than conjunctival lesions, is more evident clinically.[33,34,36] A fleshy vascular mass or

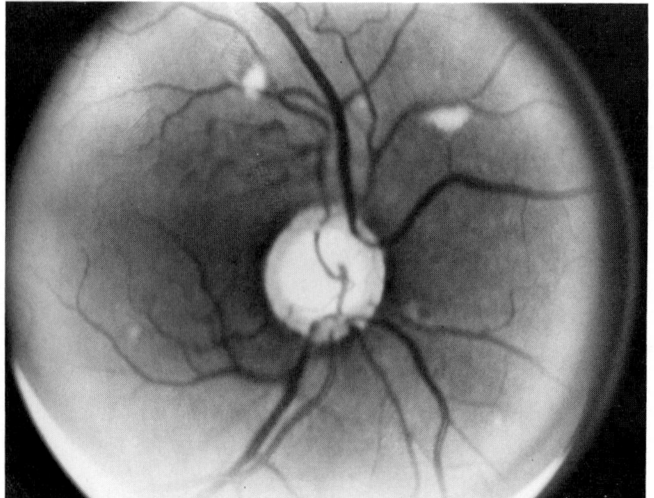

Fig. 62-7. Multiple cotton wool spots in a young homosexual man with HIV-1 infection.

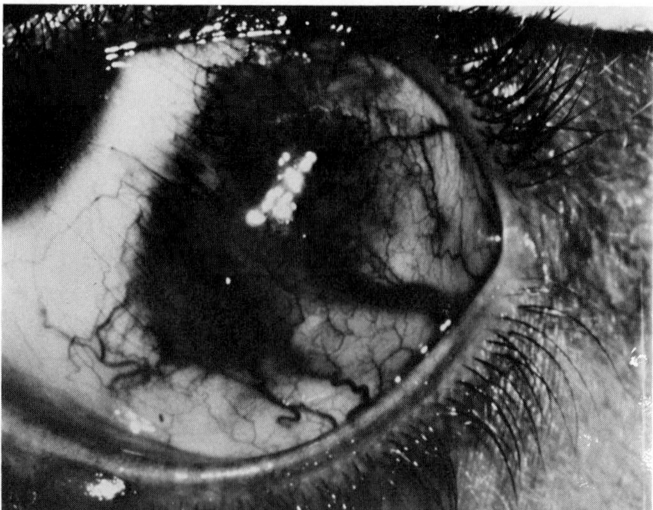

Fig. 62-8. Kaposi's sarcoma involving the conjunctiva in a man with AIDS. (*Courtesy of J Chandler.*)

**Table 62-2. Summary of Ocular Manifestations of AIDS**

| Disorder | Prevalence | Symptoms | Signs |
|---|---|---|---|
| I. Noninfectious microvascular disorders | | | |
| 1. Cotton wool spots | 42–71% | Asymptomatic<br>Transient<br>Nonspecific | Fluffy white opacity with borders along vascular arcades |
| 2. Retinal hemorrhages | 8–40% | Asymptomatic<br>Transient<br>Nonspecific | Superficial flame-shaped or blot hemorrhages |
| 3. Microaneurysms | 20% | Asymptomatic | Small dot hemorrhages |
| 4. Perivasculitis | 3% | Asymptomatic<br>Nonspecific | Sheathing of vessels |
| 5. Ischemic maculopathy | 6% | Decrease in visual acuity | Macular scar |
| II. Opportunistic Infections | | | |
| 1. Retina | | | |
| Cytomegalovirus | 4–53% | Decrease in acuity<br>Visual field defect | Granular white patch along vascular arcade with hemorrhage ("catsup and crumbled cheese fundus") |
| Toxoplasmosis | Rare | Decrease in acuity | Multifocal white lesion<br>Heavy vitreous haze |
| Others* | Rare | Decrease in acuity | Variable retinitis<br>Vitritis (systemic infection usually present) |
| 2. Ocular surface pathogens | | | |
| Herpes simplex virus | Rare | Decrease in visual acuity,<br>Red eye | Unilateral keratitis<br>Dendrite |
| Herpes zoster | Rare | Decrease in visual acuity,<br>Red eye | Vesicles on side of face<br>Keratitis<br>Uveitis |
| *C. albicans* | Rare | Decrease in visual acuity,<br>Red eye | Corneal ulcer |
| III. Neoplasms | | | |
| 1. Kaposi's sarcoma | 9–24% | No visual loss<br>Eyelid irregularity | Reddish conjunctival nodule or flat hemorrhage<br>Violaceous lid nodule |
| 2. Burkitt's lymphoma | Rare | Visual loss | Proptosis<br>Lid edema |

*Other: *M. avium*, HSV, varicella virus, *C. albicans*, *C. neoformans*.

hemorrhagic area of conjunctival thickening may be found next to the cornea with a clear zone of limbus intervening.[34]

The eyelid lesions present as a violaceous cutaneous nodule similar to that found on the extremities.[22] Complications such as ulceration and infection are more common in this location and lead to lid margin irregularities.[19]

Orbital Kaposi's sarcoma has not been documented histopathologically; however, bilateral periorbital lymphedema was described in one patient who died of disseminated Kaposi's sarcoma.[20,34]

Ocular lesions in patients who have Kaposi's sarcoma without opportunistic infection have not been reported to cause visual loss[17,37] Previously, treatment for the less virulent form of Kaposi's sarcoma in patients without AIDS involved external irradiation, excision, and cryotherapy and chemotherapy.[19,31,33,34,37] Kaposi's sarcoma associated with AIDS is radioresistant, but the response to systemic chemotherapy has been encouraging[31,32,37] (see Chap. 56).

## INFECTIONS

### Cytomegalovirus (CMV)

Prior to its association with AIDS, CMV chorioretinitis was a rare finding, with approximately 30 cases reported from 1959 to 1979.[27,37] These were associated with either renal transplantation or underlying malignancy. Since its association with AIDS, CMV retinitis is the most common opportunistic ophthalmic manifestation of AIDS, its prevalence ranging from 4 to 53 percent.[17-19,23,25,28] CMV retinitis is found more frequently in homosexuals with AIDS and is rarely encountered in heterosexual intravenous drug abusers with AIDS.[21,23,25]

The manifestations of CMV retinopathy are so characteristic that this diagnosis can be made clinically, even in the presence of negative CMV antibody titers.[23] Characteristically, CMV retinopathy is a necrotizing infection which involves all layers of the retina as well as the retinal pigment epithelium (RPE).[17,21,23,38]

Involvement of the choroid, however, is minimal. The lesions appear initially as scattered white granular patches within the posterior pole. They are usually found along the vascular arcade and may be associated with sheathing of the retinal vessels.[22,23,39] With time, these foci increase in size and become confluent (see Plate 12). This increase in size over serial examinations distinguishes foci of CMV from CWS.[17] Superficial and deep hemorrhages are found adjacent to these lesions so that the retina resembles a "crumbled cheese and tomato catsup fundus."[40] The infection usually terminates abruptly at the ora serrata,[19,21] however, it may involve the peripheral retina in an early asymptomatic stage.[41] The macula may be spared. These lesions progress slowly, taking a month or more to double in size. Resolution of these infiltrates is followed by full-thickness retinal necrosis which results in large zones of atrophy, retinal pigment epithelium atrophy, and pigment mottling.

CMV retinitis is the major cause of visual loss in AIDS.[17] With progression of CMV chorioretinitis, loss of retinal function occurs in 3 to 6 months.[17,21] In addition, visual field defects with absolute scotomas may occur in areas corresponding to excessive retinal atrophy.

Involvement of the optic nerve may occur and produce a profound decrease in visual acuity. The optic disk may be elevated with blurred margins and surrounded by retinal opacification and hemorrhage.[19,22,42] Retinal detachment is a late complication.[19,30,39,43]

Efforts to treat CMV retinitis with vidarabine, acyclovir,[17,23] immunomodulatory therapy[23], alpha and gamma interferon, and interleukin-2[17,23] have been disappointing and associated with unacceptable toxicity. Steroids[23] and antifungals[30] have also not proved useful. The most promising therapy for the treatment of CMV retinitis is an acyclic antiviral nucleoside, dihydroxypropoxymethylguanine (DHPG, ganciclovir), which is structurally similar to acyclovir.[39,42-44] Through selective phosphorylation, DHPG inhibits CMV DNA polymerase. It is more active than acyclovir against CMV in vitro.[38]

The use of DHPG has resulted in clinical improvement in 85 percent of patients with retinal involvement.[41,43,44] In addition, virologic clearing from throat, urine, and blood occurred in 82 percent of patients.[44] The clinical response is dose-dependent. Improvement in CMV retinitis has been noted with an induction of 2.5 mg/kg q 8 h,[41,47] whereas progression was noted at 1 mg/kg q 8 h.[47] The most adverse side effect was a reversible neutropenia.[43]

Relapses are common upon discontinuation of IV therapy, and these usually occur 2 to 6 weeks after discontinuation of intravenous DHPG therapy.[41,43] Reactivation is associated with clinical evidence of progression at the edges of old lesions as well as in areas of previously uninvolved retina.[41] Thus, DHPG is thought to be virostatic, and upon discontinuation of therapy, viral synthesis resumes. This was confirmed by electron microscopy, which demonstrated incomplete virions (empty capsids) in the nuclei of retinal cells of AIDS patients after treatment with ganciclovir.[38] The use of maintenance therapy[48] prevents reactivation in a significant number of patients.[41] If retinitis does recur, reinduction dosage of 2.5 mg/kg q 8 h for 10 days and a maintenance dosage of 5 mg/kg per day for 5 days per week may be employed.[41]

Other modes of delivery of DHPG, such as intravitreal injections, have also been tried. The rationale for this method is to circumvent the bone marrow suppression associated with intravenous ganciclovir as well as to increase penetration into the vitreous.[46] A dosage of 200 μg given in five injections over a 15-day period led to resolution of hemorrhage and vasculitis with RPE atrophy and pigment deposition. As with intravenous DHPG, intravitreal DHPG was also associated with relapse upon discontinuation of therapy. Remission occurred with the use of low-dose maintenance therapy of 200 mg per injection two times per week.[46]

## Toxoplasmosis

Toxoplasmosis is a common cause of posterior uveitis in the nonimmunosuppressed patient (most of these cases being congenitally acquired). However, ocular toxoplasmosis associated with AIDS is rarely encountered.[23,25,49,50] This is in contrast to CNS toxoplasmosis, which is a common opportunistic infection in AIDS.[46,50,51]

Characteristically, ophthalmic toxoplasmosis presents in adults as either a unilateral or a bilateral focal (or multifocal) necrotizing retinochoroiditis. Clinically, a heavy vitreous haze overlies a large confluent white lesion in the retina.[40,50] Scattered intraretinal hemorrhages may also be present. The active lesion in nonimmunosuppressed patients is usually at the border of a previous infection. In AIDS patients evidence of active inflammation may be present at the site of previous infection as well as in areas free of chorioretinal scars.[40,50] This suggests an acute infection. Anterior segment inflammation may also be present with keratic precipitates on the cornea and cells in the anterior chamber.

## NEUROOPHTHALMIC MANIFESTATIONS

The neuroophthalmic manifestations of AIDS, according to the American Uveitis Society, are (1) cranial nerve palsies, (2) visual field defects, (3) papilledema, (4) optic atrophy, and (5) visual loss of intracranial origin.[52]

Cranial nerve palsies in AIDS patients most commonly result from atypical aseptic meningitis.[53–57] The fifth, seventh, and eighth cranial nerves are most commonly involved. Cranial nerve palsies may be asymptomatic or associated with symptoms of diplopia, changes in lid position, ocular motility disorders, and abnormal head turning.[17]

Visual field defects may result from infections involving intracranial structures,[30] neoplasms, or infections involving the retina.[54] Hemianopsias have been reported to result from subacute encephalitis.[51] In addition, visual field defects with absolute scotomas have been reported to occur in areas of retinal atrophy in patients with CMV retinitis.[17,24,54]

Papilledema secondary to increased intracranial pressure may result from intracranial infections, or space-occupying lesions. In one series, Pepose described papilledema in 14 percent of cases of patients with AIDS.[21] *Cryptococcus neoformans* may cause papilledema as a result of meningeal involvement.[30,51]

Acute bilateral visual loss in AIDS may be secondary to syphilitic invasion of the retrobulbar optic nerve by *Treponema pallidum.*[55] Optic atrophy is the final result of invasion of the visual pathways.

## PREVENTION OF TRANSMISSION OF HIV BY OPHTHALMOLOGIC PROCEDURES

HIV has been detected in the tears, conjunctiva, cornea, iris, retina, and optic nerve.[56–58] While present evidence indicates that HIV is predominantly transmitted through infected bodily secretions or contaminated blood products in high-risk groups, recent reports of HIV transmission to health care workers has raised concern that transmission by other routes is theoretically possible. Infection control guidelines for ophthalmologists and eye care professionals are based on current recommendations issued by the CDC.[59] These include (1) hand washing with soap and water after any physical contact with blood or bodily excretions, (2) the use of gloves when contact with bodily fluids, mucous membranes, or open lesions is anticipated, or during invasive procedures, (3) extreme care and prompt disposal of needles and sharp instruments, and (4) use of protective eye wear to prevent accidental conjunctival inoculation with infected bodily fluids or contaminated irrigating solution during invasive procedures.[52,59] In addition, certain guidelines, pertinent to ophthalmologists, are recommended to minimize the risk of transmission through instruments that make direct contact with the eye, such as tonometer tips, ultrasound transducers, pachymeters, and contact lenses. These instruments should be disinfected for 5 to 10 min with (1) 3% hydrogen peroxide solution, (2) 0.5% sodium hypochloride (1:10 dilution of household bleach), or 70% isopropyl alcohol. Disinfection should be followed by rinsing with water and drying. Contact lenses should be disinfected after each use. Soft contact lenses may be heat-sterilized for at least 10 min by boiling (78 to 80°C, 172 to 176°F).[52,59] Commercially available hydrogen peroxide systems may also be used to disinfect soft contact lenses as well as polymethyl methacrylate and gas-permeable lenses. Effective sterilization of surgical instruments includes autoclaving, boiling for 15 minutes, and chemical sterilization.[52,59]

Serologic screening of potential corneal donors to detect antibodies against HIV is now performed routinely using the enzyme-linked immunosorbent assay (ELISA) of cadaveric sera. These tests have demonstrated a sensitivity of 94 to 97 percent and a 99 percent specificity, using cadaveric sera. False-negative results with ELISA testing may occur in individuals who have been recently infected. This underscores the importance of not only testing, but also obtaining a reliable medical history.[60]

Since 1986 all eye banks in the United States have attempted to screen potential donors of corneal tissue, and the Eye Bank Association has recommended that ELISA testing be performed on all high-risk donors.[61–63]

At this time, transmission of AIDS by contact with tears or through corneal transplantation has not been documented.[64]

The ocular manifestations of AIDS have diagnostic, prognostic, and therapeutic importance. Through increased awareness of these manifestations, it is hoped that the morbidity and mortality associated with AIDS may be reduced.

## References


1 Dawson CR: Eye disease with sexually transmitted chlamydia. *Ophthalmic Forum* 3:115, 1985.

2 Ronnerstam R et al: Prevalence of chlamydial eye infection in patients attending an eye clinic, a VD clinic, and in healthy persons. *Br J Ophthalmol* 69:385, 1985.

3 Oh JO et al: Acute ocular infection by type II herpes simplex virus in adults: Report of two cases. *Arch Ophthalmol* 93:1127, 1975.

4 Oh JO: Ocular infections of herpes simplex virus type II in adults, in *Viral Diseases of the Eye*, Darrell RW (ed). Philadelphia, Lea & Febiger, 1985, pp. 59–62.

5 Newman-Haefelin D et al: Herpes simplex virus type I and II in ocular diseases. *Arch Ophthalmol* 96:164, 1978.

6 Colin J et al: Ocular infection due to herpes simplex virus type II, in *Immunology and Immunopathology of the Eye*, AM Silverstein, GR O'Connor (eds). New York, Masson, 1978.

7 Chandler JW: Genital herpetic infections and their associations with ocular herpetic infections. *Ophthalmic Forum* 3:117, 1985.

8 Wilhelmus KR et al: Prognostic indications of herpetic keratitis: Analysis of a five year observation period after corneal ulceration. *Arch Ophthalmol* 99:1578, 1981.

9 Spicer WTH: Parenchymatous keratitis: Interstitial keratitis: Uveitis anterior. *Br J Ophthalmol Monogr* 1(suppl): 1924.

10 Oksala A: Studies on interstitial keratitis associated with congenital syphilis occurring in Finland. *Acta Ophthalmol* 30(suppl 38):1, 1952.

11 Loewenfield IE: The Argyll Robertson pupil, 1869–1969: A critical survey of the literature. *Surv Ophthalmol* 14:199, 1969.

12 McCrary JA III: The pupil in syphilis, in *Neuro-Ophthalmology*, JL Smith (ed). St. Louis, CV Mosby, 1972, vol 6, p. 164.

13 Thatcher RW: Treatment of acute gonococcal conjunctivitis. *Ann Ophthalmol* 10:445, 1978.

14 Thatcher RW et al: Gonorrheal conjunctivitis. *JAMA* 215:1494, 1971.

15 Ullman S et al: *Neisseria gonorrhoeae* keratoconjunctivitis. *Ophthalmology* 94:525, 1987.

16 Gottlieb MS et al: *Pneumocystis carinii* pneumonia and mucosal candidiasis in previously healthy homosexual men. *N Engl J Med* 305:1425, 1981.

17 Palestine AG et al: Ophthalmic involvement in acquired immunodeficiency syndrome. *Ophthalmology* 91:1092, 1984.

18 Newsome DA et al: Microvascular aspects of acquired immune deficiency syndrome retinopathy. *Am J Ophthalmol* 98:590, 1984.

19 Holland GN et al: Ophthalmic disorders associated with the acquired immunodeficiency syndrome, in *AIDS and Other Sexually Transmitted Diseases and the Eye,* MS Insler (ed). Orlando, Grune & Stratton, 1987, pps. 145–172.

20 Freeman WR et al: A prospective study of the ophthalmologic findings in the acquired immune deficiency syndrome. *Am J Ophthalmol* 97:133, 1984.

21 Pepose JS et al: Acquired immune deficiency syndrome: Pathogenic mechanisms of ocular disease. *Ophthalmology* 92:472, 1985.

22 Holland GN et al: Acquired immune deficiency syndrome: Ocular manifestations. *Ophthalmology* 90:858, 1983.

23 Friedman AH: The retinal lesions of the acquired immune deficiency syndrome. *Trans Am Ophthalmol Soc* 82:447, 1984.

24 Holland GN et al: Ocular disorders associated with a new severe acquired cellular immunodeficiency syndrome. *Am J Ophthalmol* 93:393, 1982.

25 Rosenberg PR et al: Acquired immunodeficiency syndrome: Ophthalmic manifestations in ambulatory patients. *Ophthalmology* 90:874, 1983.

26 Khadem M et al: Ophthalmologic findings in acquired immune deficiency syndrome (AIDS). *Arch Ophthalmol* 102:201, 1984.

27 Mines JA et al: Acquired immunodeficiency syndrome (AIDS): The disease and its ocular manifestations. *Int Ophthalmol Clin* 26:73, 1986.

28 Kestyln: Perivasculitis of the retinal vessels as an important sign in children with AIDS-related complex. *Am J Ophthalmol* 150:614, 1985.

29 Newman NM et al: Clinical and histologic findings in opportunistic ocular infections. Part of a new syndrome of acquired immunodeficiency. *Arch Ophthalmol* 101:396, 1983.

30 Hymes K et al: Kaposi's sarcoma in homosexual men. *Lancet* 2:598, 1981.

31 Friedman AH et al: Disseminated Kaposi's sarcoma in homosexual men. *Ann Intern Med* 96:693, 1982.

32 Lieberman PH et al: Kaposi's sarcoma of the bulbar conjunctiva. *Arch Ophthalmol* 88:44, 1972.

33 Howard GM et al: Kaposi's sarcoma of the conjunctiva. *Am J Ophthalmol* 104:420, 1975.

34 Nicholson DH et al: Epibulbar Kaposi's sarcoma. *Arch Ophthalmol* 96:95, 1978.

35 Macher AM et al: Multicentric Kaposi's sarcoma of the conjunctiva in a male homosexual with the acquired immunodeficiency syndrome. *Ophthalmology* 90:879, 1983.

36 Groopman JE et al: Recombinant alpha-2 interferon therapy for Kaposi's sarcoma associated with the acquired immunodeficiency syndrome, Atlanta. *Ann Intern Med* 100:671, 1984.
37 Pollard RB et al: Cytomegalovirus retinitis in immunosuppressed hosts: I. Natural history and effects of treatment with adenine arabinocide. *Ann Intern Med* 93:655, 1980.
38 Pepose JS et al: Pathologic features of cytomegalovirus retinopathy after treatment with the antviral agent ganciclovir. *Ophthalmology* 94:414, 1987.
38a Bloom JN, Palestine AG: The diagnosis of cytomegalovirus retinitis. *Ann Intern Med* 109:963, 1988
39 Henderly DE et al: Cytomegalovirus retinitis as the initial manifestation of the acquired immune deficiency syndrome. *Am J Ophthalmol* 103:316, 1987.
40 Schuman JS et al: Ocular effects in the acquired immune deficiency syndrome. *Mt Sinai J Med* 50:443, 1983.
41 Henderly DE et al: Cytomegalovirus retinitis response to therapy with ganciclovir. *Ophthalmology* 94:425, 1987.
42 Rosecan LR et al: Antiviral therapy for cytomegalovirus retinitis in AIDS with dihydroxy propoxymethyl guanine. *Am J Ophthalmol* 101:405, 1986.
43 Holland GN et al: Treatment of cytomegalovirus retinopathy with ganciclovir. *Ophthalmology* 94:815, 1987.
44 Devita VT et al: Developmental therapeutics of the acquired immunodeficiency syndrome. *Ann Intern Med* 106:568, 1987.
45 Egbert PR et al: Cytomegalovirus retinitis in immunosuppressed hosts: II. Ocular manifestations. *Ann Intern Med* 93:664, 1980.
46 Felsenstein D et al: Treatment of cytomegalovirus retinitis with 9-[-2-hydroxy-1-(hydroxymethyl) propoxymethyl] guanine. *Ann Intern Med* 103:377, 1985.
47 Henry K et al: Use of intravitreal ganciclovir (dihydroxy propoxymethyl guanine) for cytomegalovirus retinitis in a patient with AIDS. Am J Ophthalmol 103:17, 1987.
48 Jabs DA et al: Treatment of cytomegalovirus retinitis with ganciclovir. *Ophthalmology* 94:824, 1987.
49 Horowitz JL et al: CNS toxoplasmosis in acquired immunodeficiency syndrome. *Arch Neurol* 40:649, 1983.
50 Parke DW et al: Diffuse toxoplasmic retinochoroiditis in a patient with AIDS. *Arch Ophthalmol* 104:571, 1986.
51 Levy RM et al: Neurologic manifestations of the acquired immunodeficiency syndrome (AIDS): Experience at UCSF and review of the literature. *J Neurosurg* 62:475, 1985.
52 American Uveitis Society
53 Carne CA: ABC of AIDS: Neurological manifestations. *Br Med J* 294:1399, 1987.
54 Chiang M et al: Clinical pathologic correlations of ocular and neurologic findings in AIDS: Case report. *Ann Ophthalmol* 18:105, 1986.
55 Zambrano W et al: Acute syphilitic blindness in AIDS. *J Clin Neuro Ophthalmol* 7:1, 1987.
56 Salahuddin SV et al: Isolation of human T-cell leukemia/lymphotropic virus type III from the cornea. *Am J Ophthalmol* 101:149, 1986.
57 Doro S et al: Confirmation of HTLV-III in the cornea. *Am J Ophthalmol* 102:390, 1986.
58 Fujikawa LS et al: Human T-cell leukemia/lymphotropic virus type III in the conjunctival epithelium of a patient with AIDS. *Am J Ophthalmol* 100:507, 1985.
59 Francis DP et al: The prospects for and pathways toward a vaccine for AIDS. *N Engl J Med* 313:1586, 1985.
60 Woods SL et al: The acquired immune deficiency syndrome: Ocular findings and infection control guidelines. *Aust N Zealand J Ophthalmol* 14:287, 1986.
61 Pepose JS et al: The impact of the AIDS epidemic on corneal transplantation. *Am J Ophthalmol* 100:610, 1985.
62 Pepose JS et al: Screening cornea donors for antibodies against human immunodeficiency virus. Efficacy of ELISA testing of cadaveric sera and aqueous humor. *Ophthalmology* 94:95, 1987.
63 O'Day DM: The risk posed by HTLV-III infected corneal donor tissue. *Am J Ophthalmol* 101:246, 1986.
64 Pepose JS et al: Serologic markers after the transplantation of corneas from donors infected with the human immunodeficiency virus. *Am J Ophthalmol* 103:798, 1987.

# PART VII SEXUALLY TRANSMITTED DISEASES IN REPRODUCTION, PERINATOLOGY, AND PEDIATRICS

# Chapter 63

# Sexually transmitted diseases and infertility

Donald E. Moore
Willard Cates, Jr.

Sexually transmitted diseases (STDs) affect human fertility primarily through infections of the upper genital tract and their sequelae in women. Except for obstruction of the male epididymis or vas deferens (both rare events), sexually transmitted diseases rarely produce infertility in men. Therefore, this chapter will focus on infertility resulting from sexually acquired infections that produce salpingitis. Chapters 49 and 50 discuss the entities of acute and atypical pelvic inflammatory disease; we will focus on sequelae to these conditions.

## DEFINITIONS

Infertility is usually defined as the lack of recognized conception after 1 year of regular intercourse without the use of contraception. In the general population, the conception rate is 10 to 15 percent per cycle (Fig. 63-1), while in couples that have been infertile for 1 year, it is 5 to 6 percent per cycle.[1] If infertility has persisted for 2 or more years, the conception rate falls markedly to about 1 to 3 percent per cycle.[2,3] In one population-based study of infertile couples, pregnancy rates approached 75 to 80 percent 10 years after initial diagnosis. These long-term pregnancy rates were similar in women with primary vs. secondary infertility and relatively independent of the method of definition of infertility.[4]

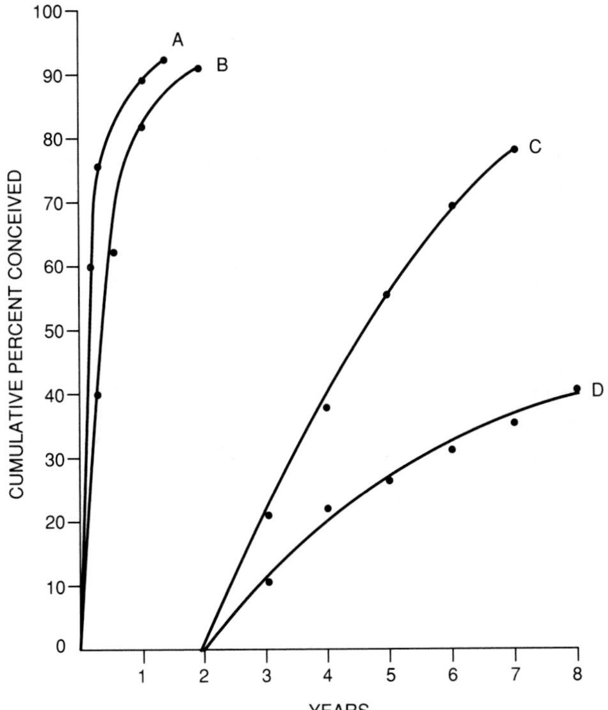


**Fig. 63-1.** The conception rates of a normal population of parous (*A*) and nulliparous (*B*) women are compared with the cumulative conception rates of apparently normal women with secondary infertility (*C*) and primary infertility (*D*). The *shaded area* represents the 67 percent confidence limits for the observations for both infertility groups. There were no conceptions before the 2- to 3-year interval in the infertile groups as this was part of the selection criteria for these patients. Used with permission of *Fertility and Sterility*.

Salpingitis is an inflammation of the epithelial surfaces of the fallopian tubes caused by active infection with one or more of a number of organisms, most of which are sexually transmitted and ascend along mucosal surfaces from the cervix to the endometrium to the salpinx and, in some women, to the peritoneum[5] (see Chap. 49). Pelvic inflammatory disease (PID) is used to describe the symptoms and signs associated clinically with acute salpingitis. However, only about two-thirds of patients with a clinical diagnosis of PID actually have visual evidence of acute salpingitis by laparoscopy.[6] In the United States, the diagnosis of PID usually is made without laparoscopy. Many women with salpingitis probably experience an asymptomatic or minimally symptomatic infection. In this chapter, we will use the term "silent salpingitis" (commonly called "silent PID") to describe this condition (see Chap. 50).

Tubal infertility refers to infertility caused by damaged fallopian tubes, which can result from salpingitis, endometriosis, pelvic surgery, or congenital causes. This chapter will discuss infertility only as it relates to salpingitis.

## HISTORY

A relationship between gonorrhea, PID, and tubal infertility was first reported in the preantibiotic era.[7,8] Upper genital tract infection, especially severe tubo-ovarian abscess, was a feared consequence of gonococcal infection, and rates of postgonococcal tubal obstruction of up to 70 percent were reported.[9] With the advent and use of penicillin in the 1930s and 1940s, both lower and upper genital tract infection caused by gonococci could be more effectively treated, and their sequelae were reduced.

The classic cohort studies of Weström and colleagues in Lund, Sweden[10] in the 1960s demonstrated the impact of STD and salpingitis on subsequent tubal infertility. These studies contributed data on such crucial topics as (1) the clinical difference between PID and salpingitis; (2) the importance of chlamydia (in addition to gonorrhea) as a cause of tubal infertility; (3) the effects of different risk factors on fertility; and (4) the effects of different antibiotic regimens used for treatment of acute PID upon fertility.

During the 1970s, the polymicrobial etiology of PID, and especially the role of *Chlamydia trachomatis,* became increasingly appreciated.[11,12] More recently, the influence of contraceptives on both PID and tubal factor infertility has become clearer. Intrauterine devices, especially the Dalkon shield, appeared to increase the risk of PID and infertility, whereas barrier methods—both mechanical and chemical—appeared protective.[13–15] Finally, an increased understanding of the role of silent salpingitis as a prelude to tubal obstruction has emerged from recent studies.[16]

## PREVALENCE OF TUBAL INFERTILITY

From demographic surveys conducted worldwide, two yardsticks have generally been used to measure the prevalence of infertility: (1) childlessness at older reproductive ages, and (2) the absence of recent pregnancies in noncontracepting sexually active couples.[17] Using these definitions, rates of infertility have ranged

**Table 63-1. Causes of Female Infertility, by Region**

| | % of cases associated with each cause | | | |
|---|---|---|---|---|
| Categories | Developed country | Africa | Asia | Latin America |
| No demonstrable cause | 40 | 16 | 31 | 35 |
| Bilateral tubal occlusion | 11 | 49 | 14 | 15 |
| Pelvic adhesions | 13 | 24 | 13 | 17 |
| Acquired tubal abnormalities | 12 | 12 | 12 | 12 |
| Anovulatory regular cycles | 10 | 14 | 9 | 9 |
| Anovulatory oligomenorrhea* | 9 | 3 | 7 | 9 |
| Ovulatory oligomenorrhea | 7 | 4 | 11 | 5 |
| Hyperprolactinemia | 7 | 5 | 7 | 8 |
| Endometriosis | 6 | 1 | 10 | 3 |
| Total† | 115 | 128 | 114 | 113 |

*Includes amenorrhea.
†Total greater than 100 percent due to the presence of more than one factor in some women.
SOURCE: Adapted from Ref. 20.

from 1 to 16 percent of couples, with considerable regional variation.[17]

The presence of tubal damage can be identified only in women who are evaluated by a specialist. In the United States, couples in the middle to upper classes are more likely to seek such evaluation, and thus the prevalence of tubal infertility in the entire population is probably underestimated. In Bristol, England, where medical care is less subject to this bias, an average of 1.2 couples per 1000 population annually requested infertility advice from a specialist.[18] At this rate, approximately 1 in 6 couples (with an average length of infertility of 2½ years) would seek help from a specialist at some time in their lives. Tubal damage was demonstrated in 14 percent of these infertile couples.

Internationally, the WHO multicenter study compared STD-related infertility in five different regions of the world.[19,20] Over 8000 infertile couples were enrolled in the study and over 6000 (71 percent) completed evaluation of the fallopian tubes. Almost two-thirds of infertility in African women was attributed to infection, including 40 percent with bilateral tubal occlusion and 24 percent with pelvic adhesions (Table 63-1). The prevalence of tubal occlusion in Africa was more than three times that of any other region. Developed countries had an 11 percent prevalence of tubal occlusion in infertile women. Non-African developing areas had higher rates of tubal occlusion than developed countries, though well below those of Africa.

Another approach to estimating the prevalence of tubal infertility utilizes extrapolation from the annual reported incidence of STDs. For example, approximately 3 million lower genital tract infections with chlamydia and/or gonorrhea occur in women each year in the United States.[21] Assuming 30 percent of these cause salpingitis,[22,23] and that 17 percent of salpingitis leads to tubal occlusion,[24] an estimated annual incidence of 125,000 cases of STD-related infertility occur each year. Converting these to cumulative numbers, we estimate that approximately 2 million reproductive-age women (range 200,000 to 2.7 million) currently have tubal occlusion in the United States. However, only about half may desire more children, and a smaller percentage will seek infertility services.[25]

While the above estimates are crude, they are internally consistent with the annually reported number of sexually transmitted infections, the number of ambulatory and hospitalized cases of PID, the number of infertility visits to private clinicians' offices, and the cross-sectional number of self-reported cases of PID and infertility in the American population of reproductive-age women.

## SALPINGITIS AND TUBAL INFERTILITY

Tubal infertility is generally the direct result of acute salpingitis. In long-term follow-up studies in Lund, Sweden, about 17 percent of women with laparoscopically documented acute salpingitis subsequently became infertile owing to tubal occlusion as compared with none of the control women with similar pelvic symptoms but noninflamed fallopian tubes (see Table 49-7).[10] The percentage of those who then became infertile was larger in older women (26 percent) and smaller in women who were using steroid contraceptives at the time of the acute infection (Chap. 49). The proportion who became infertile after a single episode of PID also varied directly with the severity of tubal inflammation (mild = 6

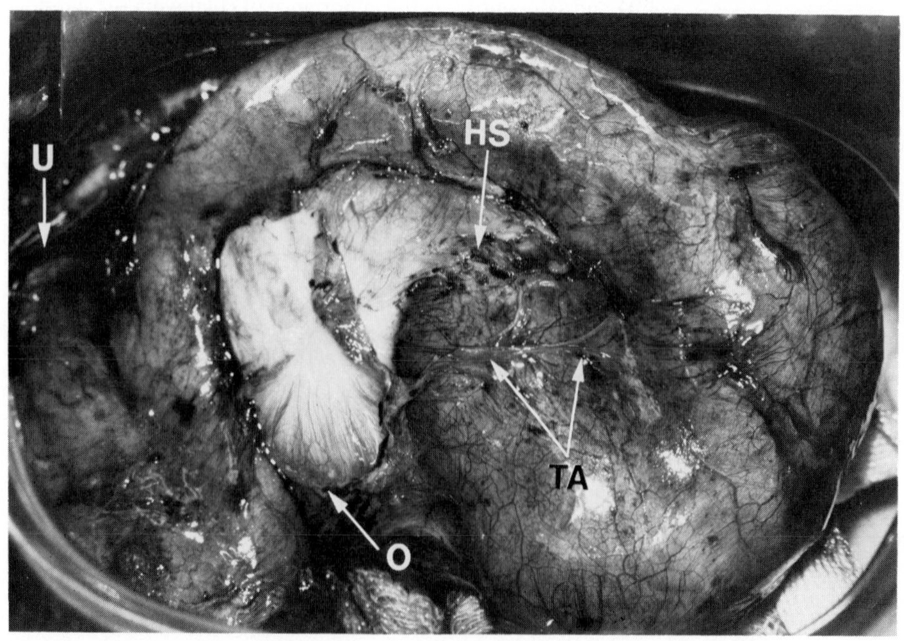


**Fig. 63-2.** Laparotomy view of large right hydrosalpinx (HS), 3 cm in diameter, in a 22-year-old infertile woman. Several tubal adhesions (TA) can be seen. Ovary (O) and uterus (U) are also indicated by arrows. The right hydrosalpinx was judged to be noncorrectable surgically, and the patient underwent right salpingectomy and left salpingostomy. *(Courtesy of Dr. Michael R. Soules, Department of Obstetrics and Gynecology, University of Washington.)*

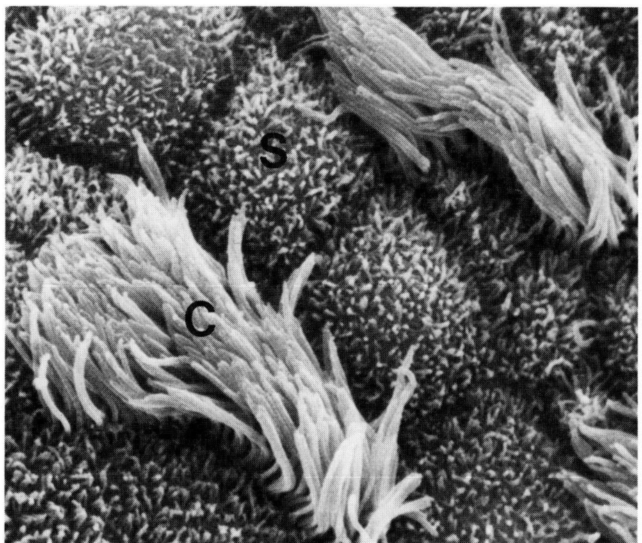


**Fig. 63-3.** Normal fallopian tube. Secretory cells (S) with abundant microvilli are surrounded by clumps of long, slender cilia (C) atop the ciliated cells. 4800× (*SEM provided by Dr. Dorothy L. Patton, Departments of Obstetrics and Gynecology and Biological Structure, University of Washington.*)

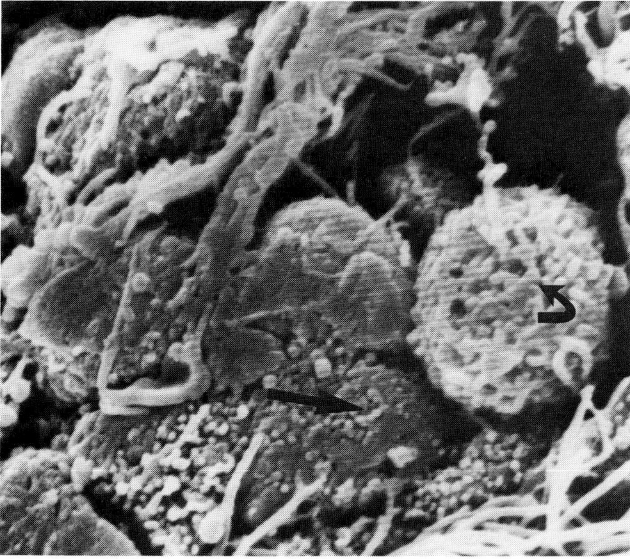

**Fig. 63-4.** Infertile fallopian tube following infection. Pronounced deciliation (*straight arrow*) of the ciliated cells and clubbing of the microvilli on the secretory (*curved arrow*) cells are evident in this biopsy taken from a distally occluded fallopian tube. 5200× (*SEM provided by Dr. Dorothy L. Patton, Departments of Obstetrics and Gynecology and Biological Structure, University of Washington.*)

percent, moderate = 13 percent, severe = 30 percent). Those women with symptomatic acute salpingitis who were taking steroid contraceptives generally had only mild tubal inflammation.[26] Women had an increasing risk of infertility with each episode of PID (one = 11 percent, two = 23 percent, three or more = 54 percent). Neither the type of antibiotic used for treatment of PID[24] nor the organism isolated (*Neisseria gonorrhoeae* vs. *C. trachomatis*)[26] made any discernible difference in subsequent infertility.

Most infertility following acute salpingitis presumably results from damaged fallopian tubes, since nearly all such women showed evidence of tubal obstruction by hysterosalpingography and/or surgery (see Fig. 63-2).[24] Further evidence that obstruction of the fallopian tubes and peritubal adhesions are the sequelae of acute salpingitis is derived from animal models, especially monkeys[27,28] and mice.[29] Although mechanical obstruction usually causes a hydrosalpinx, it leads to little residual damage.[30,31] In contrast, tubal infection with *C. trachomatis* results in necrosis of secretory cells and deciliation and eventually distal obstruction and hydrosalpinx (see Figs. 63-3 and 63-4).[32]

Women with bilaterally obstructed distal fallopian tubes are sterile and will not conceive unless the tubes are either surgically reopened or bypassed as in in vitro fertilization (IVF).[33] The overall pregnancy rate after microsurgical salpingostomy repair of the fallopian tubes is 23 percent (range 18 to 31) within 2 years of surgery,[33] or 9 to 10 percent per cycle with IVF.[34] Paterson[35] reported similar pregnancy rates between surgery and IVF in infertile women with distally obstructed fallopian tubes. The likelihood of pregnancy after surgical repair relates directly to the degree of damage before surgery, which can be divided into four prognostic groups (Fig. 63-5): (1) and (2) partial tubal obstruction (phimosis) or normal-appearing tubes with peritubal adhesions, associated with the best postoperative pregnancy rates; (3) complete distal obstruction with normal tubal diameters, with a reasonable pregnancy rate; and (4) complete distal obstruction with enlarged tubal diameters, with an unacceptability low pregnancy rate.[36] Also, no pregnancies were reported in women with both distal obstruction and thickened fallopian tube walls. The presence of either massive peritubal adhesions or dense adhesions that obscure ovarian or tubal borders with any of the above anatomic conditions probably worsens the prognosis.[37]

Despite surgical lysis of adhesions and establishment of tubal patency, subsequent fertility rates are low. This probably results from the severe cellular and subcellular damage observed along the entire length of both fallopian tubes. For example, the tubes of women undergoing surgical repair show marked deciliation. Physiologically, ciliary motion of such damaged epithelial cells is markedly reduced.[16] This marked reduction in ciliary activity is thought to be permanent, since it is not seen in mechanical obstruction of the fallopian tubes.[30,31] The cilia are thought to be the major mechanism by which the embryo is propelled through the tube.[38]

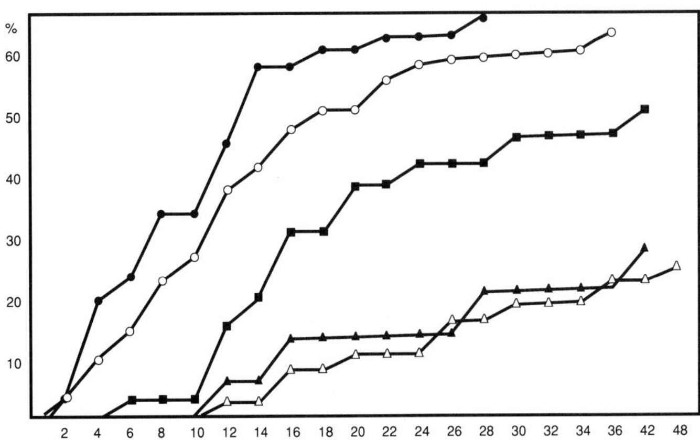


**Fig. 63-5.** Cumulative rate of pregnancy after microsurgery for distal tubal lesions. ●, Salpingolysis (n = 42). ○, Fimbrioplasty (n = 132). ■, Salpingostomy (n = 27) (degree II occlusion). ▲, Salpingostomy (n = 16) (degree III occlusion). △, Salpingostomy (n = 40) (degree IV occlusion). Used with permission of *Fertility and Sterility*.

## ETIOLOGY

All studies to date have found a strong association between STDs, PID, and tubal infertility. The cohort studies from Lund, Sweden, remain the best evidence for the link between salpingitis and infertility.[10] In addition, infertile women with a self-reported history of gonorrhea[39] or nonspecific STD or PID[21] were almost three times more likely to have tubal occlusion as a cause of their infertility. Similarly, among American women with a history of PID,[40] the proportion with fertility problems (44 percent) was twofold higher than among women without such a history (21 percent). This difference was found in both nulliparous and multiparous women.

Salpingitis associated with either *N. gonorrhoeae* or *C. trachomatis* has been causally related to subsequent tubal infertility.[24] Prospective studies show the fertility prognosis is poor for women suffering symptomatic PID caused by either gonococcal or chlamydial agents.[24,41–43] Gonorrhea has been related to tubal infertility in studies using self-reported cervical infections,[39] clinical diagnoses,[9] laparoscopically proved salpingitis,[44] and positive serology.[45,46] However, investigators from England have found gonococcal antibody less strongly associated with tubal occlusion (Table 63-2) than chlamydial antibody.[47,48]

The role that chlamydia plays in causing tubal infertility has been more exhaustively studied than gonorrhea.[49] Many investigators have examined the relationship between chlamydial serology and tubal infertility (Table 63-3). Investigators from at least 13 different cities around the world have documented that tubal occlusion is strongly associated with the presence of chlamydial antibody. When these studies are combined, 70 percent of women with tubal infertility had antibodies to chlamydia vs. 26 percent of control women (Table 63-3).

Despite the relatively benign symptoms and signs it produces, *C. trachomatis* apparently causes as much tubal inflammation—and ultimately tubal damage—as other agents.[63,64] The occurrence of severe tubal damage despite mild clinical signs is probably due to the more subacute nature of chlamydial salpingitis as compared with salpingitis caused by other organisms. This hypothesis is supported by the low prevalence of immunoglobulin M antibody to chlamydia among women with acute salpingitis.[63] As with trachoma, prolonged subacute chlamydial infection in the genital tract can lead to chronic inflammation and scarring in affected organs (Chap. 50).

Antibodies to *Mycoplasma hominis* occurred three times more often in women with tubal infertility than in other infertile women (36 percent vs. 11 percent).[47] Most women with peritubal adhesions had antibodies to *M. hominis,* consistent with findings that *M. hominis* in the monkey causes an exosalpingitis.[28] The effect that other organisms, or different combinations of organisms, have on tubal infertility awaits future studies.

## SILENT SALPINGITIS

Studies of tubal infertility have reported that 39 to 81 percent (median 63 percent) of cases had no history of symptoms or signs of PID (Table 63-3). Demographically, women with tubal infertility who have no history of PID are similar to women with the same diagnosis who had a PID history.[16] By electron microscopy and by assessment of mucosal ciliary activity, the two groups are identical. Both groups show severe ciliary denudation and decreased ciliary function of a similar degree.

An estimated 8 to 30 percent of women with cervical chlamydial infection will develop clinically apparent salpingitis if not treated with appropriate antibiotics.[23] The percentage that will develop silent salpingitis and tubal infertility is unknown. Although silent salpingitis is asymptomatic by the usual criteria, symptoms such as mild pelvic pain or abnormal uterine bleeding may signal ascending infection in some patients. In Paris, 12 percent of patients with tubal infertility had a past history of untreated mild pelvic pain.[58] Moreover in Seattle, 40 percent of women with cervicitis had endometritis demonstrated on biopsy; these women were either asymptomatic or had mild pelvic symptoms.[66] Uterine bleeding may also be an indication of endometritis.[65,66] Collectively, these data suggest that silent infection of the upper genital tract occurs frequently with *C. trachomatis.*

## PERSISTENCE OF ORGANISMS

Whether chlamydia or other microorganisms persist in the female genital tract for years after an initial episode of salpingitis is controversial. Since *C. trachomatis* produces chronic subclinical infection of the eye (trachoma) that may persist and reactivate during periods of immunosuppression, a similar situation might occur with chlamydial PID.[67–69]

Acute PID following hysterosalpingography (HSG) has been reported in 11 percent of women with obstructed or dilated fallopian tubes but not in women with normal tubes.[70–72] Prophylactic tetracycline, but not ampicillin, prevents acute PID after HSG. The isolation of *C. trachomatis* in these patients suggests that the PID following an HSG may be related to reactivation of chlamydial infection.[72] However, another possible explanation is that the damaged tubes may be structurally or immunologically incompetent in resisting inoculations of organisms.

**Table 63-2. Studies Comparing Chlamydial and Gonococcal Antibodies in Women with Tubal Infertility and Control Populations**

| Author, place (year) | Study populations | Chlamydial antibodies | | Gonococcal antibodies | |
|---|---|---|---|---|---|
| | | Percent | RR | Percent | RR |
| Mabey, Gambia (1985)[45] | Tubal infertility | 68 | 1.9 (1.2–3.1) | 68 | 2.4 (1.4–4.1) |
| | Pregnant women | 35 | 1.0 | 27 | 1.0 |
| Tjiam, Holland (1985)[46] | Tubal infertility | 21 | ∞ | 61 | $p < 0.01$ |
| | Infertile—normal tubes | 0 | 1.0 | 25 | |
| | Blood donors | 0 | 1.0 | 4 | |
| Robertson, Bristol, England (1987)[48] | Tubal infertility | 73 | 1.9 (1.3–2.9) | 2 | NS |
| | Infertile—normal tubes | 34 | 0.9 (0.5–1.5) | 3 | |
| | Barrier contraceptives | 25 | 0.7 (0.4–1.2) | 4 | |
| | Sterilization | 38 | 1.0 | 5 | |

**Table 63-3. Prevalence of Chlamydial Antibodies, of Positive Cultures for Chlamydia, and of Silent Salpingitis in Women with Tubal Infertility**

| Reference no., author, place, year | No. of cases | % with CT IgG abs | % with CT IgM abs | % with CT organisms* | % with silent salpingitis |
|---|---|---|---|---|---|
| 50. Moore, Seattle, 1982 | 33 | 73 | 3 | 0 | 45 |
| 51. Guderian, California, 1986 | 139 | 83 | — | — | 58 |
| 52. Quinn, Toronto, 1987 | 7 | 71 | — | — | — |
| 53. Brunham, Winnipeg, 1985 | 18 | 72 | 0 | 0 | 61 |
| 54. Kane, London, 1984 | 54 | 41 | 0 | 0 | 63 |
| 55. Jones, Indianapolis, 1982 | 77 | 60 | — | — | 81 |
| 47. Møller, Aarhus, 1985 | 22 | 36 | — | — | — |
| 56. Gump, Burlington, 1983 | 53 | 64 | — | 0.5 | 69 |
| 57. Conway, Bristol, 1984 | 48 | 75 | — | — | 75 |
| 58. Henry-Suchet, Paris, 1987 | 161 | 67 | — | 33 | 60 |
| 59. Anestad, Oslo, 1987 | 42 | 90 | 24 | 0 | 67 |
| 60. Punnonen, Turku, 1979 | 23 | 91 | — | 0 | 39 |
| 61. Battin, Los Angeles, 1984 | 16 | 94 | 0 | 0 | — |
| 62. Sellors, Ontario, 1988 | 43 | 75 | 21 | 6.3 | 69 |
| Total | 736 | 70 | 13 | 14 | 64 |

*See text for discussion of sites cultured.

The most direct but controversial evidence for persistence of chlamydia in the fallopian tubes is isolation of the organism from the upper genital tract in women with tubal infertility (Table 63-3). In Paris, women with tubal infertility often have a yellowish, viscous effusion in the pelvis which is reportedly culture-positive for CT.[58] In Indianapolis, CT has been isolated from the endometrium of 32 percent of women with tubal infertility.[73] Gump et al.[56] isolated CT organisms from the endometrium of 1 of 53 women with tubal infertility. Sellors et al.[62] were able to demonstrate chlamydial antigen with an immunochemical method in 1 of 16 tubal biopsy specimens in women with tubal factor infertility, despite negative endotubal cultures. In Oslo, serologic evidence of active infection was found; IgM antibody to CT was found in 24 percent of infertile women with tubal occlusion compared with 2 percent of controls.[59] However, six other centers have not been able to isolate chlamydia from women with tubal infertility using not only cervical cultures but also endometrial tissue[53,74] and tubal swabs.[50,53,54,59]

Differences in the populations studied may account for some of the differences in isolation rates in the studies just described. In Seattle, for example, infertile couples tend to be monogamous during their infertility years and they frequently use antibiotics for nonpelvic infections. In Paris, until recently most infertile couples had not received tetracycline for PID.[75] Furthermore, many continue to have more than one sexual partner. Differences in isolation techniques could also explain the differences. Further studies are clearly needed to resolve these important discrepancies.

## RISK FACTORS FOR TUBAL INFERTILITY

Several factors affect the likelihood of the progression of PID to tubal occlusion. The most important variable is the number of previous PID episodes.[24] Each new acute salpingitis episode approximately doubles the rate of postsalpingitis infertility (Chap. 49). Approximately 11 percent of women are infertile after a single episode of PID, 23 percent after two episodes, and over half after three or more episodes (see Table 49-7).[24]

Second, age affects the progression to tubal obstruction.[24] Women between ages 15 and 24 who develop salpingitis have less tubal damage than do older women. Even when the salpingitis is stratified by the number of episodes or by the severity of tubal inflammation, fewer young women in each stratum develop infertility.

Third, the severity of the pelvic inflammation, judged by laparoscopy, influences the fertility outcome. Women with severe inflammatory changes have fivefold higher rates of subsequent tubal infertility than those with mild disease;[44] women with moderate changes are in between.

Fourth, contraceptive choice also affects the likelihood of tubal infertility. Women using IUDs were found to have a higher risk of tubal factor infertility, with the Dalkon shield accounting for most of this risk.[13,14] Copper-containing IUDs had much lower risk of tubal infertility. Barrier methods of contraception—including both condoms and spermicides—provided protection against tubal infertility.[15] While the mechanical benefits of condoms provided only marginal protection, when coupled with the chemical benefits of spermicides, combination barrier methods provided a twofold protection against tubal infertility.

The relationship of oral contraceptive (OC) use to the risk of tubal infertility remains somewhat unclear. In one study, the use of oral contraceptives did not protect against tubal infertility, and OCs with higher levels of estrogen were associated with an increased risk of tubal infertility.[15] In contrast, a protective effect against acute PID has been reported by others[65,76–80] despite the fact that *C. trachomatis* cervicitis has been reported to be more prevalent in OC users.[65,81] Further studies are needed to clarify the relationship of OC use to acute PID and to its sequel tubal infertility.

Finally, smoking increases the risk of tubal infertility in nulligravid women and the risk appears dose-related.[82,83] Women who both smoked and used an IUD were at greater risk than women who had either risk alone. Former smokers had no increased risk. Smoking may impair immune defenses that prevent ascent of STD organisms to the fallopian tubes. Lymphocytes of smokers show decreased humoral and cell-mediated immunity in vitro.[84–86]

## PREVENTION

Preventing STD-related tubal infertility can take place on three levels—primary, secondary, and tertiary prevention. Primary prevention blocks acquisition of the infection, secondary prevention blocks progression of a lower genital tract infection to the upper genital tract, and tertiary prevention blocks the progression of upper genital tract infection to tubal obstruction and eventual infertility. Because of the excessive costs of treating "end stage" tubal infertility, investments in primary prevention have advantages over secondary and tertiary from the cost-benefit point of view.[87]

Primary prevention of STD has received a recent boost from the increased public awareness of the consequences of AIDS and HIV infections and is discussed in detail in Chaps. 88 to 90. Secondary prevention of tubal infertility also utilizes traditional STD control approaches (see Chap. 84). Tertiary prevention of STD-related infertility has been disappointing to date. Recent evidence indicates that the type of antibiotic treatment given for symptomatic PID has only a minimal impact on fertility outcome. In the Lund PID cohort, among women who were treated for PID with a variety of different antibiotic regimens, tubal infertility occurred among 10 to 13 percent regardless of the therapy used.[88] Antibiotic regimens that inhibited *N. gonorrhoeae, C. trachomatis,* or predominantly facultative anaerobes were associated with virtually identical tubal infertility rates. While most currently recommended antibiotic regimens cure acute PID,[89,90] these regimens may have a limited effect on tubal damage that already existed before treatment was started or they may not produce actual eradication of chlamydia despite apparently negative cultures after treatment.[42] This pessimistic picture is further complicated by the frequent use of inappropriate antibiotics to treat PID.[91–93]

It appears if we wish to have a sizable impact on STD-related tubal infertility, the infections will have to be prevented or treated before they reach the fallopian tubes.

## References


1 Lenton EA et al: Long-term follow-up of the apparently normal couple with a complaint of infertility. *Fertil Steril* 28:913, 1977.

2 Collins JA et al: Treatment-independent pregnancy among infertile couples. *N Engl J Med* 309:1201, 1983.

3 Collins JA: Pregnancy in infertile couples. Letter. *N Engl J Med* 310:1334, 1984.

4 Marchbanks PA et al and the Cancer and Steroid Hormone Study Group: Infertility: The effect of definition on prevalence. *Am J Epidemiol,* (in press).

5 Eschenbach DA: Acute pelvic inflammatory disease, in *Gynecology and Obstetrics,* JW Sciarra (ed). Philadelphia, Harper & Row, 1986, p 1.

6 Jacobson L, Weström L: Objectivized diagnosis of acute pelvic inflammatory disease. *Am J Obstet Gynecol* 105:1088, 1969.

7 Noeggerath E: Latent gonorrhea, especially with regard to its fertility in women. *Trans Am Gynecol Assoc* 1:292, 1976.

8 Brandt AM: *No Magic Bullet: A Social History of Venereal Disease in the United States Since 1880.* New York, Oxford University Press, 1985.

9 Falk V: Treatment of acute non-tuberculous salpingitis with antibiotics alone and in combination with glucocorticoids. *Acta Obstet Gynecol Scand* 44(suppl 6):85, 1965.

10 Weström L: Pelvic inflammatory disease: bacteriology and sequelae. *Contraception* 36:111, 1987.

11 Eschenbach DA et al: Polymicrobial etiology of acute pelvic inflammatory disease. *N Engl J Med* 293:166, 1975.

12 Mårdh P-A: An overview of infectious agents of salpingitis, their biology, and recent advances in methods of detection. *Am J Obstet Gynecol* 138:933, 1980.

13 Cramer DW et al: Tubal infertility and the intrauterine device. *N Engl J Med* 312:941, 1985.

14 Daling JR et al: Primary tubal infertility in relation to the use of an intrauterine device. *N Engl J Med* 312:937, 1985.

15 Cramer DW et al: The relationship of tubal infertility to barrier method and oral contraceptive use. *JAMA* 257:2446, 1987.

16 Patton DL et al: A comparison of the fallopian tube's response to overt and silent salpingitis. *Obstet Gynecol,* in press.

17 Sherris JD, Fox G: Infertility and sexually transmitted disease: A public health challenge. *Popul Rep* 4(L):L-114, 1983.

18 Hull MG et al: Population study of causes, treatment, and outcome of infertility. *Br Med J* 291:1693, 1985.

19 Cates W et al: Worldwide patterns of infertility: Is Africa different? *Lancet* ii:596, 1985.

20 World Health Organization: Infections, pregnancies, and infertility: Perspectives on prevention. *Fertil Steril* 47:964, 1987.

21 Cates W Jr: Epidemiology and control of sexually transmitted diseases: strategic evolution. *Infect Dis Clin N Am* 1:1, 1987.

22 Platt R et al: Risk of acquiring gonorrhea and prevalence of abnormal adnexal findings among women recently exposed to gonorrhea. *JAMA* 250:3205, 1983.

23 Stamm WE et al: Effect of treatment regimens for *Neisseria gonorrhoeae* on simultaneous infection with *Chlamydia trachomatis. N Engl J Med* 310:545, 1984.

24 Weström L: Influence of sexually transmitted diseases on sterility and ectopic pregnancy. *Acta Eur Fertil* 16:21, 1985.

25 Henshaw SK, Orr MT: The need and unmet need for infertility services in the United States. *Fam Plann Perspect* 19:180, 1987.

26 Svensson L et al: Infertility after acute salpingitis with special reference to *Chlamydia trachomatis. Fertil Steril* 40:322, 1983.

27 Patton DL et al: Host response to primary *Chlamydia trachomatis* infection of the fallopian tube in pig-tailed monkeys. *Fertil Steril* 40:829, 1983.

28 Møller BR et al: Experimental pelvic inflammatory diseases provoked by *Chlamydia trachomatis* and *Mycoplasma hominis. Obstet Gynecol* 138:990, 1980.

29 Swenson CE, Schachter J: Infertility as a consequence of Chlamydial infection of the upper genital tract in female mice. *Sex Transm Dis* 11:64, 1984.

30 Patton DL, Halbert SA: Mechanically-induced hydrosalpinz: Long-term oviductal dilation does not impair ciliary transport function. *Fertil Steril* 36:808, 1981.

31 Halbert SA, Patton DL: Hydrosalpinx: Effect of oviductal dilation on egg transport. *Fertil Steril* 35:69, 1981.

32 Patton DL et al: Distal tubal obstruction induced by repeated *Chlamydia trachomatis* salpingeal infections in pig-tailed macaques. *J Infect Dis* 155:1292, 1987.

33 Bateman BG et al: Surgical management of distal tubal obstruction—are we making progress? *Fertil Steril* 48:523, 1987.

34 Medical Research International. The American Fertility Society Special Interest Group: In vitro fertilization/embryo transfer in the United States: 1985 and 1986 results from the National IVF/ET Registry. *Fertil Steril* 49:212, 1988.

35 Paterson PJ: Indications for the treatment of tubal infertility patients by microsurgery or in vitro fertilization. *Aust NZ J Obstet Gynaecol* 24:262, 1984.

36 Donnez J, Casanas-Rouz F: Prognostic factors of fimbrial microsurgery. *Fertil Steril* 46:200, 1986.

37 Boer-Meisel ME et al: Predicting the pregnancy outcome in patients treated for hydrosalpinx: A prospective study. *Fertil Steril* 45:23, 1986.

38 McComb P, Gomel V: The effect of segmental ampullary reversal on the subsequent fertility of the rabbit. *Fertil Steril* 31:83, 1979.

39 Sherman KJ et al: Sexually transmitted diseases and tubal infertility. *Sex Transm Dis* 14:12, 1987.

40 Aral SO et al: Contraceptive use, pelvic inflammatory disease, and fertility problems among American women: 1982. *Am J Obstet Gynecol* 157:59, 1987.

41 Whittington WL et al: Infertility after pelvic inflammatory disease: report on American inner city women (Abstract 66). Presented at the International Society for STD Research, Atlanta, Georgia, August 3, 1987.

42 Plummer F et al: A comparison of doxycycline (DOX) and metronidazole (MET) with trimethaprim sulfametrol (TMP/SMT) and me-

tronidazole for treatment of pelvic inflammatory disease (PID): assessment of effect on infertility (Abstract 65). Presented at the International Society for STD Research, Atlanta, Georgia, August 3, 1987.

43 Brunham RC et al: Etiology and outcome of acute pelvic inflammatory disease. *J Infect Dis* 158:510, 1988.

44 Weström L: Effect of acute pelvic inflammatory disease on fertility. *Am J Obstet Gynecol* 121:707, 1975.

45 Mabey DCW et al: Tubal infertility in the Gambia: Chlamydial and gonococcal serology in women with tubal occlusion compared with pregnant controls. *Bull WHO* 63:1107, 1985.

46 Tjiam KH et al: Prevalence of antibodies to *Chlamydia trachomatis, Neisseria gonorrhoeae,* and *Mycoplasma hominis* in infertile women. *Genitourin Med* 61:175, 1985.

47 Møller BR et al: Serological evidence that chlamydiae and mycoplasmas are involved in infertility in women. *J Reprod Fertil* 73:237, 1985.

48 Robertson JN et al: Chlamydial and gonococcal antibodies in sera of infertile women with tubal obstruction. *J Clin Pathol* 40:377, 1987.

49 Cates W Jr: Sexually transmitted organisms and infertility: the proof of the pudding. *Sex Transm Dis* 11:113, 1984.

50 Moore DE et al: Increased frequency of serum antibodies to *Chlamydia trachomatis* in infertility due to distal tubal disease. *Lancet* ii:574, 1982.

51 Guderian AM, Trobough GE: Residues of pelvic inflammatory disease in intrauterine device users: A result of the intrauterine device or *Chlamydia trachomatis* infection? *Am J Obstet Gynecol* 154:497, 1986.

52 Quinn PA et al: Prevalence of antibody to *Chlamydia trachomatis* in spontaneous abortion and infertility. *Am J Obstet Gynecol* 156:291, 1987.

53 Brunham RC et al: *Chlamydia trachomatis:* Its role in tubal infertility. *J Infect Dis* 152:1275, 1985.

54 Kane JL et al: Evidence of chlamydial infection in infertile women with and without fallopian tube obstruction. *Fertil Steril* 42:843, 1984.

55 Jones RB et al: Correlation between serum antichlamydial antibodies and tubal factor as a cause of infertility. *Fertil Steril* 38:553, 1982.

56 Gump DW et al: Evidence of prior pelvic inflammatory disease and its relationship to *Chlamydia trachomatis* antibody and intrauterine contraceptive device use in infertile women. *Am J Obstet Gynecol* 146:153, 1983.

57 Conway D et al: Chlamydial serology in fertile and infertile women. *Lancet* i:191, 1984.

58 Henry-Suchet J et al: Microbiologic study of chronic inflammation associated with tubal factor infertility: Role of *Chlamydia trachomatis. Fertil Steril* 47:274, 1987.

59 Ånestad G et al: Infertility and chlamydial infection. *Fertil Steril* 48:787, 1987.

60 Punnonen R et al: Chlamydial serology in infertile women by immunofluorescence. *Fertil Steril* 31:656, 1979.

61 Battin DA et al: *Chlamydia trachomatis* is not an important cause of abnormal postcoital tests in ovulating patients. *Fertil Steril* 42:233, 1984.

62 Sellors JW et al: Tubal factor infertility: An association with prior chlamydial infection and asymptomatic salpingitis. *Fertil Steril* 49:451, 1988.

63 Gjonnaess H et al: Pelvic inflammatory disease: Etiologic studies with emphasis on chlamydial infection. *Obstet Gynecol* 59:550, 1982.

64 Svensson L et al: Differences in some clinical and laboratory parameters in acute salpingitis related to culture and serologic finding. *Am J Obstet Gynecol* 138:1017, 1980.

65 Wølner-Hanssen P: Personal communication, 1988.

66 Paavonen J et al: Prevalence and manifestations of endometritis among women with cervicitis. *Am J Obstet Gynecol* 152:280, 1985.

67 Yang Y-S et al: Reactivation of *Chlamydia trachomatis* lung infection in mice by cortisone. *Infect Immun* 39:655, 1983.

68 Wang S-P, Grayston JT: Trachoma in the Taiwan monkey, *Macaca cyclopis. Ann NY Acad Sci* 98:177, 1962.

69 Grayston JT: Personal communication, 1989.

70 Stumpf PG, March CM: Febrile morbidity following hysterosalpingography: Identification of risk factors and recommendations for prophylaxis. *Fertil Steril* 33:487, 1980.

71 Pittaway DE et al: Prevention of acute pelvic inflammatory disease after hysterosalpingography: Efficacy of doxycycline prophylaxis. *Am J Obstet Gynecol* 147:623, 1983.

72 Møller BR et al: Pelvic inflammatory disease after hysterosalpingography associated with *Chlamydia trachomatis* and *Mycoplasma hominis. Br J Obstet Gynecol* 91:1181, 1984.

73 Cleary RE, Jones RB: Recovery of *Chlamydia trachomatis* from the endometrium in infertile women with serum antichlamydial antibodies. *Fertil Steril* 44:233, 1985.

74 Cassell GH et al: Microbiologic study of infertile women at the time of diagnostic laparoscopy. *N Engl J Med* 308:502, 1983.

75 Henry-Suchet J: Personal communication, 1987.

76 Svensson L: Contraceptives and acute salpingitis. *JAMA* 251:2553, 1984.

77 Senanayake P, Kramer DG: Contraception and the etiology of pelvic inflammatory disease: New perspectives. *Am J Obstet Gynecol* 138:852, 1980.

78 Rubin GL et al: Oral contraceptives and pelvic inflammatory disease. *Am J Obstet Gynecol* 144:630, 1980.

79 Wølner-Hanssen P et al: Laparoscopic findings and contraceptive use in women with signs and symptoms suggestive of acute salpingitis. *Obstet Gynecol* 66:233, 1985.

80 Wølner-Hanssen P: Oral contraceptive use modifies the manifestations of pelvic inflammatory disease. *Br J Obstet Gynecol* 93:619, 1986.

81 Washington AE et al: Oral contraceptives, *Chlamydia trachomatis* infection and pelvic inflammatory disease. *JAMA* 253:2246, 1985.

82 Daling JR et al: Cigarette smoking and primary tubal infertility, in *Smoking and Reproductive Health,* PSG Publishing Company, Inc, 1987.

83 Phipps WR et al: The association between smoking and female infertility as influenced by cause of the infertility. *Fertil Steril* 48:377, 1987.

84 Hershey P et al: Effects of cigarette smoking on the immune system. Follow-up studies in normal subjects after cessation of smoking. *Med J Aust* 2:425, 1983.

85 Burton RC: Smoking, immunity, and cancer. *Med J Aust* 2:411, 1983.

86 Holt PG: Immune and inflammatory function in cigarette smokers. *Thorax* 42:241, 1987.

87 Potts M et al: STDs, IVF, and barrier contraception. *JAMA* 258:1729, 1987.

88 Weström L et al: Infertility after acute salpingitis: Results of treatment with different antibiotics. *Curr Ther Res* 26:752, 1979.

89 Goodrich JT: Pelvic inflammatory disease: Considerations related to therapy. *Rev Infect Dis* 4(S):S778, 1982.

90 Brunham RC: Therapy for acute pelvic inflammatory disease. A critique of recent treatment trials. *Am J Obstet Gynecol* 148:235, 1984.

91 Grimes DA et al: Antibiotic treatment of pelvic inflammatory disease, trends among private physicians in the United States, 1966 through 1983. *JAMA* 256:3223, 1986.

92 Gelphman KA et al: Pelvic inflammatory disease: Diagnosis and treatment patterns as reported by the providers (Abstract 185). Presented at the International Society for STD Research, Atlanta, Georgia, August 4, 1987.

93 Thompson SE et al: High failure rates in outpatient treatment of salpingitis with either tetracycline alone or penicillin/ampicilline combination. *Am J Obstet Gyneol* 152:635, 1985.

# Chapter 64

# Sexually transmitted diseases in pregnancy

Robert C. Brunham
King K. Holmes
Joanne E. Embree

As the spectrum of sexually transmitted diseases (STD) has broadened, the medical and social consequences of STD in pregnancy have become more apparent. Ectopic pregnancy, spontaneous abortion and stillbirth, prematurity, congenital and perinatal infection, and puerperal maternal infections represent outcomes of pregnancy in which sexually transmitted infectious agents play important etiologic roles. The incidence of many STDs has increased during the last two decades, and the number of pregnancies per year is also again increasing; the superimposition of the one factor upon the other can be expected to further amplify the effects of STD on pregnancy and neonatal morbidity.

In general, STD appears to pose a much greater problem in pregnant adolescents than in older pregnant women who are more sexually experienced and more likely to be involved in a stable monogamous sexual relationship at the time of conception. Adolescents have miscarriages more often than do older women—a difference which may be partly attributable to STD. Although the average age at which women first bear children is increasing, the average age that women first initiate sexual activity has decreased and teenage pregnancy remains common in many societies despite the availability of contraceptives. Among sexually active women, whether pregnant or nonpregnant, the prevalence of many STD agents, such as cytomegalovirus (CMV) and *Chlamydia trachomatis* is highest among adolescents. The younger the patient, the greater the likelihood that any given infection is a primary infection. Although immunity to most STD agents is not well defined, it is likely that in general, primary infections in a nonimmune host cause the greatest morbidity.

The two classic venereal agents, *Neisseria gonorrhoeae* and *Treponema pallidum*, have pronounced effects on pregnancy, but measures for the diagnosis and management of these infections in pregnancy are readily available and routinely employed where appropriate in at least developed countries. Introduction of such measures still remains a major achievable goal in many developing countries and in subpopulations who do not seek prenatal care in developed countries. Certain of the newly recognized STD pathogens such as *C. trachomatis*, group B streptococci (GBS), CMV, and herpes simplex virus (HSV-2) are even more common during pregnancy, are more difficult to diagnose and manage, and currently represent a greater dilemma to the obstetrician in all countries. Finally, the prevention of in utero, intrapartum, and postpartum transmission of human immunodeficiency virus (HIV) has become one of the greatest public health challenges of our time.

Although the pregnant host is more susceptible to the effects of certain lower genital tract infections such as *Candida albicans* or genital warts, it is the infections of the placenta, fetus, uterus, and tubes which make the effects of STDs on pregnancy particularly important. Infection prior to pregnancy can influence the process of implantation, causing ectopic pregnancy and infertility. Infections during pregnancy can produce spontaneous abortion, chorioamnionitis, prematurity, and congenital infection. Genital infections present at delivery can cause maternal puerperal infections and neonatal and infant infections.

Pregnancy modifies the manifestation of many STDs and presents unique problems for diagnosis and management. Some agents, such as *C. albicans*, produce disease more commonly during pregnancy; some, such as genital human papillomaviruses (HPV), have enhanced virulence; and some, such as GBS, produce disease mainly during the neonatal period. The susceptibility of the pregnant host to infection may be enhanced, owing either to alterations in host defense mechanisms or to changes in anatomic structure.

## ALTERATIONS OF HOST-PARASITE RELATIONSHIPS DURING PREGNANCY

Immunologic rejection of the fetus does not normally occur during pregnancy possibly in part because of suppression of maternal immunocompetence. Suppressed maternal immunocompetence may in turn affect the natural history of many infectious diseases. For instance, higher attack rates or more severe morbidity have been recorded for pneumococcal pneumonia,[1] smallpox,[2] influenza,[3] poliomyelitis,[4] candidiasis,[5] and malaria[6] in the pregnant host than in the nonpregnant host. Both the incidence and severity of viral hepatitis are increased in pregnancy.[7] Immunologically mediated diseases caused by infectious agents may lessen in severity during pregnancy; for example, in the preantibiotic era it was observed that symptomatic syphilis was ameliorated during pregnancy.[8] Animal studies also support the notion that pregnancy interferes with maternal defense mechanisms through immune suppression.[9,10]

The bases for alterations in host immune response are likely multifactorial. Humoral substances which potently suppress in vitro lymphocyte function are present in plasma from pregnant women.[11,12] T lymphocytes but not B lymphocytes are reduced in number in peripheral blood samples of pregnant women.[13] The decrease in T lymphocytes is entirely due to a decrease in the CD4+ T-helper subset, which is reduced nearly twofold compared with values found in nonpregnant women (543 ± 169 versus 1073 ± 441, CD4+ T lymphocytes per unit of peripheral blood $p < 0.001$). No significant change occurs in the number of CD8+ T lymphocytes. The decrease in CD4+ T lymphocyte number is maximal during the third trimester.

In a large number of women evaluated during and after pregnancy we have noted impairment in the in vitro lymphocyte transformation (LT) response to a number of microbial antigens and the phytohemagglutinin during pregnancy.[14] In vitro lymphocyte proliferation was significantly lower during pregnancy than in the postpartum period and was significantly lower for pregnant women than for nonpregnant women. Maximal suppression of the LT response was observed during the third trimester of gestation. Among women with current infection with *C. trachomatis*, the LT response was markedly suppressed in the third trimester in comparison with the LT response in the postpartum period or in nonpregnant women. These data support similar observations of suppressed LT response to microbial antigens made by Gehrz et al.[15] and may be due to reduced numbers of CD4+ T helper cells.

Factors other than immunosuppression may also contribute to the increased maternal susceptibility to certain infections during pregnancy. For example, excessive mortality from bacterial pneumonia during pregnancy has been attributed to altered pulmonary mechanics,[16] and the increased susceptibility to renal infection during pregnancy may be related to changes in ureterovesicular muscular tone induced by high levels of progesterone or to partial ureteral compression by the gravid uterus.

## ANATOMIC ALTERATIONS IN PREGNANCY

The anatomy of the genital tract changes dramatically during pregnancy. Figure 64-1 illustrates the relationship of the cervix and mucus plug, chorioamnion, and placental bed as seen in late pregnancy. Vaginal walls become hypertrophic and engorged with blood. The glycogen content of the vaginal epithelium increases, and the intravaginal pH significantly decreases during pregnancy.[17] These changes probably influence vaginal microbial flora. The cervix hypertrophies, and a larger area of columnar epithelium on the exocervix is exposed to microorganisms.[18] Similar cervical anatomic changes are evoked among nonpregnant women by oral contraceptives, and have been associated with an increased prevalence of infection with *C. trachomatis* and *N. gonorrhoeae*.[18] It is not certain whether the higher prevalence of chlamydial and gonococcal infection in nonpregnant women with cervical ectopy is due to increased susceptibility to infection or enhanced cervical shedding among previously infected women, or both. The increased area of cervical ectopy during pregnancy may also predispose the cervix to infection or reactivation of latent infection, but this has not been studied. The cervix secretes highly viscid mucus during pregnancy, forming the "mucus plug." This mucus is generally believed to limit the access of microorganisms into the uterus, but little research has been done to study the actual effectiveness of cervical mucus as a physical or antimicrobial barrier.[19]

Fetal growth is accommodated by uterine growth and by tremendous enlargement of uterine vessels. The risk of salpingitis decreases during pregnancy, especially after the twelfth week,[20] and the risk of choriamnionitis increases after the sixteenth week of gestation.[21] After the twelfth gestational week the uterine cavity becomes obliterated as the chorioamnion becomes juxtaposed with the decidua vera. The risk of infection of the uterine cavity and fallopian tubes is diminished by the elimination of this space.

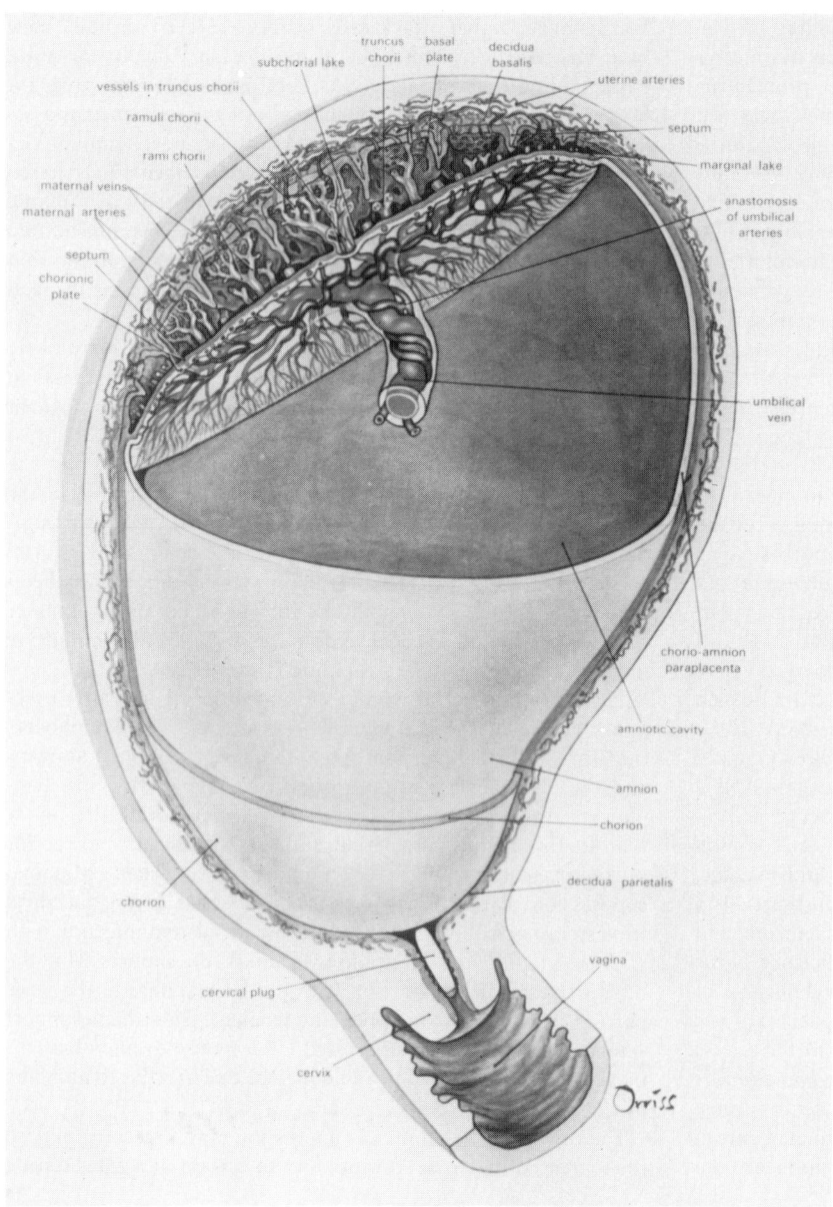


**Fig. 64-1.** The relationship within the gravid uterus of the mucus plug, fetal membranes (chorion and amnion), decidua, and placenta. (*From JD Boyd and WJ Hamilton, The Human Placenta, by permission.*)

By the sixteenth week the chorioamnion overlies the cervical os, which may be a factor in the increasing risk of chorioamnionitis during mid and late pregnancy.

The human placenta is of fetal origin and is directly perfused by maternal blood. The trophoblastic placental epithelium projects into the maternal vascular system. This trophoblastic layer regulates fetal uptake of many substances. Anatomically, two layers of trophoblastic epithelium are present, an inner multicellular stratified layer (cytotrophoblast or Langhan's layer) and an outer unicellular syncytial layer (syncytiotrophoblast). This is seen in Fig. 64-2. With advancing gestation Langhan's layer becomes less noticeable but does not completely regress. Lying within the stroma of the mature placenta are placental macrophages (Hofbauer cells) which act as a first line of fetal defense to transplacental infection.

## ALTERATIONS IN CERVICOVAGINAL MICROBIAL FLORA DURING PREGNANCY

The vaginal flora is a heterogeneous ecosystem of anaerobic and facultative bacteria.[22] Several studies have found that during pregnancy, *C. albicans* and the number of bacterial species present in the vagina decreases, particularly the number of anaerobic species, while the prevalence and the quantity of lactobacilli increase, and the rate of carriage of Enterobacteriaceae, GBS, and other facultative bacteria remains unchanged. Despite these data we feel that the effects of pregnancy on vaginal bacterial flora of current interest have not been well defined. The mechanisms which may promote the reported changes in vaginal flora might include changes in the vaginal pH, glycogen content, and vascularity of the lower genital tract, as described above. It has been proposed that these changes in flora provide a more benign milieu through which the fetus may pass during parturition.[22] Following delivery an increase in rates of isolation of *Escherichia coli* and *Bacteroides* species (which may promote puerperal endomyometrial infections) has been reported,[23] but this observation also requires confirmation.

## ECTOPIC PREGNANCY

Infertility and ectopic pregnancy are recognized consequences of salpingitis. Two sexually transmitted organisms, *N. gonorrhoeae* and *C. trachomatis*, produce the majority of cases of primary salpingitis (Chap. 49). The risk of ectopic pregnancy increases about tenfold after an initial episode of salpingitis. The incidence of ectopic pregnancy has tripled since 1970 in the United States, and this trend has also been observed in Sweden, Canada, and England. It is likely that this rising incidence of ectopic pregnancy is partly due to an increasing incidence of gonococcal and chlamydial infections, and of resulting tubal infections. Approximately 50 percent of operatively removed ectopic pregnancies are associated with histologic evidence of prior salpingitis.[24,25] One recent study correlated histology, *C. trachomatis* serology, and *C. trachomatis* cultures among 50 women with ectopic pregnancy.[26] Although no woman had *C. trachomatis* recovered from the fallopian tube, 22 percent had extensive subepithelial plasma cell infiltration in the tube and 47 percent had *C. trachomatis* antibody, with all women with plasma cell infiltration being seropositive. These data document an association of *C. trachomatis* infection with ectopic pregnancy. Based on these data Kosseim et al.[27] estimated that approximately 30 percent of cases of ectopic pregnancy were due to *C. trachomatis* infection.

## INTRAUTERINE INFECTION

Intrauterine infection can result from either hematogenous or ascending microbial spread. Other routes of spread such as extension from infection in areas adjacent to the uterus occur rarely, although spread from infected foci within the endometrium to the placenta may be important for some pathogens such as CMV. A hematogenous origin appears to be the major route of spread for organisms present in maternal blood, such as *T. pallidum*. Hematogenous infection initially involves the placenta, producing the characteristic pathologic lesion of villitis. Placental mononuclear phagocytes (Hofbauer cells) likely serve as the initial antimicrobial defense in this situation.

Ascending infection by microorganisms present in the cervix or vagina can occur through intact or compromised fetal membranes, producing the characteristic pathologic lesion of chorioamnionitis and the syndrome of amniotic fluid infection. The integrity of the chorioamnion and the antimicrobial activity of amniotic fluid likely serve as the first line of fetal defense in this situation.

## HEMATOGENOUS INFECTION

Only rarely does maternal bacteremia give rise to placental or fetal infection. The nature of the defense mechanisms responsible for protection of the developing placenta and fetus from bacteremic spread is not presently known. It appears that microbial

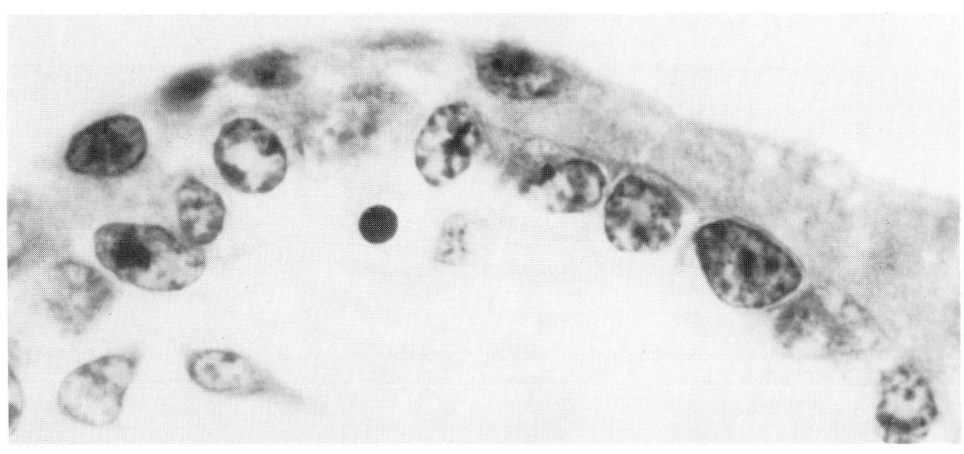

Fig. 64-2. Photomicrograph of the human trophoblast illustrating the outer (maternal) syncytiotrophoblast on the convex surface; and inner (fetal) cytotrophoblast or Langhan's layer. (*From JD Boyd and WJ Hamilton, The Human Placenta, by permission.*)

agents inhibited primarily by a cell-mediated immune response are more likely to establish placental infection than are agents inhibited primarily by a humoral immune response. This observation suggests either that pregnant women are most susceptible to systemic spread of those agents which are inhibited by cellular immunity, or that placental defense mechanisms are less effective against such microorganisms.

Microorganisms arrive at the placental bed within lymphocytes, monocytes, or neutrophils, or they may not be cell-associated. The pathogenesis of fetal infection with CMV is particularly interesting, since this virus is able to establish latent infection in human mononuclear cells. Productive infection may be recalled during alloreactivity of infected lymphocytes.[28] It may be that alloreactions between maternal lymphocytes and foreign paternal histocompatibility or other antigens on the placenta contribute to the pathogenesis of recurrent congenital CMV infection. A similar pathogenesis mechanism may exist for in utero transmission of HIV.

Fetal defense mechanisms during placental infection include placental macrophages and local production of immune factors such as antibody and lymphokines. The immune role of the trophoblast is unknown, but since this epithelium possesses Fc receptors for immunoglobulin and unique antigenic determinants and secretory products which regulate lymphocyte reactivity in vitro, an important effect on the immune response seems likely.[29] Placental histopathology following infection with *T. pallidum* serves to illustrate the range of responses detectable in this tissue. *T. pallidum* infected placentas are inappropriately large with focal proliferative villitis and vasculitis with areas of plasma cell infiltration and Langerhan's giant cell formation[30] (Fig. 64-3).

With hematogenous infection, placental infection generally precedes fetal infection, although theoretically it is possible for organisms to traverse the chorionic villi directly by pinocytosis or placental leaks or within maternal leukocytes. The fetal immune response to placental infection may be effective enough to limit infection to this site. Such circumscribed infection has been seen in cases of primary CMV[31] and in syphilis.[32] Often, however, spread from infected placental sites to the fetus occurs either by involvement of fetal blood vessels or by extension from placenta to fetal membranes with consequent infection of the amniotic fluid.

The manifestations of fetal infection depend to a great extent on the gestational age at which infection occurs. The STD agents capable of transplacental infection can produce similar effects. Abortion, stillbirth, prematurity, congenital disease, and persistent postnatal infection have all been described following infection with CMV, *T. pallidum*, and HSV. CMV also commonly causes developmental abnormalities.

## ASCENDING INFECTION: CHORIOAMNIONITIS AND AMNIOTIC FLUID INFECTION

Acute inflammation of the fetal membranes (chorioamnionitis) and umbilical cord (funisitis) is seen even more frequently than hematogenous placentitis, and is often associated with premature

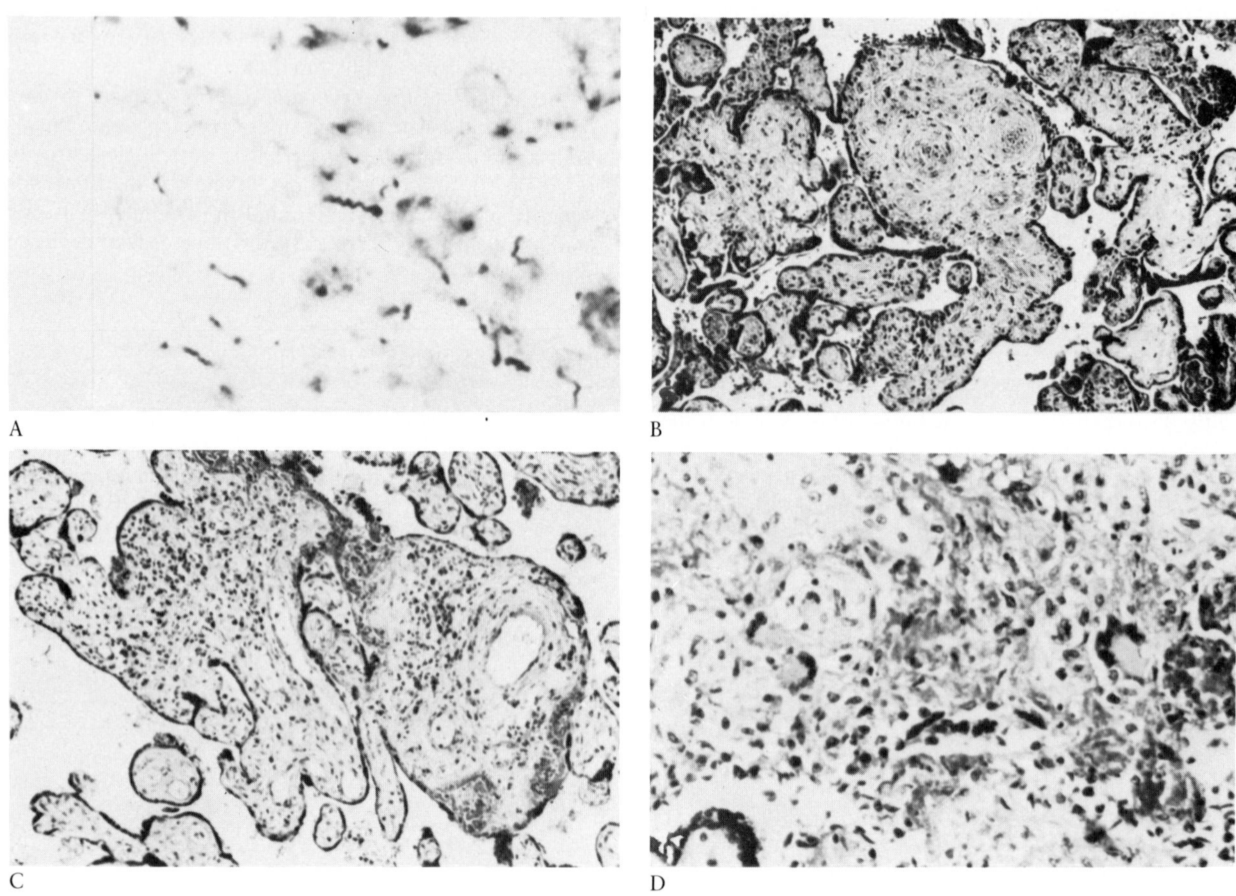


**Fig. 64-3.** Placental abnormalities of congenital syphilis. (*a*) Typical corkscrew morphology of *T. pallidum* (Warthin-Starry, ×2000 magnification). (*b*) Endovascular proliferation and villitis (H&E stain, ×150 magnification). (*c*) Villitis with plasma cell infiltration (H&E stain, ×300 magnification). (*d*) Proliferative villitis with granulomatous and giant cell formation (H&E stain, ×400 magnification). (*Courtesy of G. Altshuler.*)

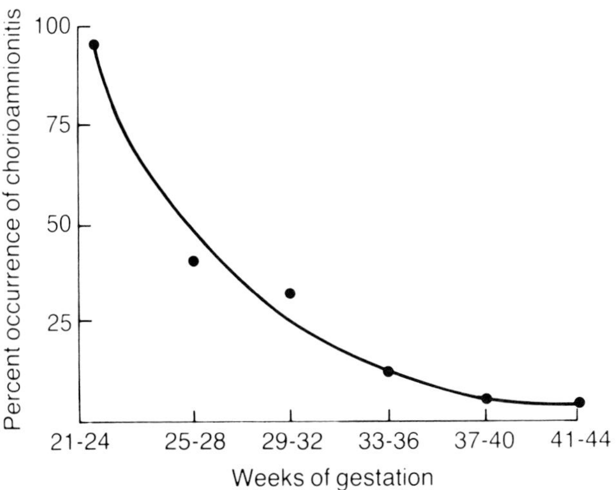


**Fig. 64-4.** Rate of chorioamnionitis among deliveries terminating at the stated intervals. The risk of chorioamnionitis is extremely high in very premature deliveries. (*From P Russell.*[21])

birth, prolonged rupture of membranes, intrapartum fever, and perinatal sepsis.

## Relationship of chorioamnionitis to prematurity and neonatal sepsis

Russell[21] clearly documented the correlation of acute chorioamnionitis with premature birth. Figure 64-4 illustrates the prevalence of chorioamnionitis by gestational age at delivery: chorioamnionitis was found in 95 percent of pregnancies <25 weeks' gestation, 35 to 40 percent of pregnancies from 25 to 32 weeks, 11 percent of pregnancies from 33 to 35 weeks, and 3 to 5 percent of term pregnancies. The mean birth weight of neonates in the chorioamnionitis group was significantly lower than in a control group without chorioamnionitis (2811 g versus 3320 g, $p < 0.001$). The lower birth weight of those with chorioamnionitis was appropriate for gestational age and not attributable to retarded intrauterine growth. Table 64-1 summarizes other findings found to be correlated with chorioamnionitis. Although chorioamnionitis frequently can be asymptomatic, especially when present near term, two-thirds of the group with chorioamnionitis had intrapartum fever, prolonged rupture of membranes, and/or premature labor.

Perinatal bacterial infections, especially those occurring within the first 48 h of life, are commonly acquired by ascending infection in utero. Russell[21] found evidence of neonatal sepsis in the first 48 h of life in almost one-quarter of neonates whose placentas showed chorioamnionitis; neonatal sepsis was rare in the absence of placental inflammation (Table 64-2). This study provides compelling data linking chorioamnionitis, prematurity, and perinatal sepsis.

Hillier et al.[33] recently reported a case control study in which chorioamnionitis was found in 61 percent of premature deliveries and 21 percent of control term deliveries (odds ratio 5.6, 95 percent CI = 2.1 to 15.6), and like Russell[21] found that the prevalence of chorioamnionitis was highest among those with the shortest gestations.

Naeye has examined the relationship of chorioamnionitis to perinatal mortality in several areas of the world.[34] As seen in Table 64-3, the rate of perinatal mortality during the study period was 30.4 per 1000 births in the United States, and was as high as 54.8 per 1000 in Durban, South Africa, and 69.4 per 1000 in Addis Ababa, Ethiopia. In all three areas amniotic fluid infection, reflecting chorioamnionitis, was the most frequent, single suspected cause of perinatal death, e.g., accounting for 25.9 to 33.4 percent of deaths due to a recognizable cause.

## Etiology of chorioamnionitis

The etiology of acute chorioamnionitis is in many cases unknown. Delayed delivery following rupture of membranes, sometimes called "prolonged rupture of membranes" (ROM), is an important correlate of acute chorioamnionitis, but most cases of chorioamnionitis are not associated with prolonged ROM antecedent event.[21] Up to 50 percent of cultures obtained from inflamed fetal membranes are sterile.[35] Limited microbiological studies have strongly linked *Ureaplasma urealyticum* to its etiology.[36] Hillier et al.[33] obtained swabs from the surfaces between the chorion and amnion, and isolated one or more microorganisms (usually *U. urealyticum*, *Mycoplasma hominis*, streptococci, *Gardnerella vaginalis*, or vaginal anaerobes such as *Mobiluncus* sp., *Bacteroides* sp., or Peptostreptococci) from 72 percent of women with chorioamnionitis compared with 22 percent of those without chorioamnionitis. The organism isolated from the chorioamnion resembled those found in the vagina of women with bacterial vaginosis, and in fact, positive chorioamnionic cultures were associated with bacterial vaginosis. Since microbial cultures of inflamed fetal membranes are often sterile, noninfectious causes such as meconium, anoxia, and decidual necrosis have also been proposed as eliciting inflammation within the membranes. However, studies in rabbits have clearly shown that only microorganisms are responsible for chorioamnionitis, and that the suspected chemical factors did not produce chorioamnionitis.[37]

Bacteria recovered from amniotic fluid of cases of chorioamnionitis include facultative organisms such as GBS, enteric gram-negative rods, *Haemophilus influenzae*, and strict anaerobic organisms such as peptococci, peptostreptococci, fusobacterium, and bacteroides species.[38–40] These infections are often polymicrobial, resembling the spectrum of organisms found in the upper genital tract of women with salpingitis or postpartum endometritis, and also include many of the organisms found in the vagina of women with bacterial vaginosis. It remains to be

**Table 64-1. Maternal Correlates of Acute Chorioamnionitis**

| | Control N = 388 | | Chorioamnionitis N = 392 | | |
|---|---|---|---|---|---|
| | Number | Percent | Number | Percent | *p* |
| Intrapartum fever | 71 | 18 | 202 | 52 | <0.001 |
| Prolonged rupture of membranes (delivery >24 h after ROM) | 4 | 1 | 66 | 17 | <0.001 |
| Delivery <36 weeks' gestation | 23 | 6 | 81 | 21 | <0.001 |
| None of the above | 298 | 77 | 134 | 34 | <0.001 |

SOURCE: From P Russell.[21]

**Table 64-2. Clinical Outcome of Neonate in Relation to Chorioamnionitis**

| | No sepsis | Sepsis with first 48 h | | | Sepsis occurring >48 h | Perinatal death |
|---|---|---|---|---|---|---|
| | | Possible | Probable | Proved | | |
| Chorioamnionitis ($N$ = 392) | 247 | 35 | 45 | 12 | 6 | 12% |
| Control ($N$ = 388) | 371† | 2 | 0 | 0 | 11 | 1% |
| $p$ | <0.001 | <0.001 | <0.001 | <0.001 | NS* | <0.001 |

*Nonsignificant.
†Note that the number 371 was misprinted as 271 in the original report.[21]
SOURCE: From P Russell.[21]

determined whether mixed anaerobic/facultative bacterial organisms found in the chorioamnion and in the amniotic fluid in association with chorioamnionitis is the primary cause of chorioamnionitis, or is secondary to necrosis or mechanical rupture of the membranes, or to other pathogens which primarily infect and compromise the integrity of the fetal membranes. Controlled trials of antimicrobial therapy for clinical chorioamnionitis may help address this issue.

Naeye has observed that chorioamnionitis is frequently associated with premature labor, even with labors lasting <8 h.[41] Only 15 percent of neonatal bacterial sepsis occurs in the setting of delayed delivery following rupture of membranes.[42] These observations in concert suggest that most cases of chorioamnionitis occur in the setting of intact membranes. Indeed, it is likely that chorioamnionitis can cause premature rupture of membranes, with delayed delivery after rupture as a result, rather than a cause of the chorioamnioinitis.

Chorioamnionitis is defined histologically by the presence of polymorphonuclear leukocytes in the membranes—usually within the chorion (N. Kiviat, personal communication); in some cases this acute inflammation is seen only on the fetal side of the discoid placenta. The migration of maternal polymorphonuclear leukocytes from the intervillous spaces or fetal PMN leukocytes through the amnion suggests transcervical infection of amniotic fluid rather than primary hematogenous infection.[43] Figure 64-5 diagrammatically illustrates the patterns and stages of the maternal and fetal inflammatory response to amniotic fluid infection. Figure 64-6 shows the opalescence of fetal membranes caused by PMN leukocytic infiltration in response to amniotic fluid infection.

Normal amniotic fluid has intrinsic antimicrobial activity which increases during the later weeks of gestation.[43a,44] Thus, chorioamnionitis is most common at early gestational ages, where amniotic fluid antimicrobial activity is lowest. Cases of chorioamnionitis occurring later, when amniotic antimicrobial activity is highest, are most often asymptomatic. Development of amniotic fluid infection may be related to reduced levels of antimicrobial activity in amniotic fluid.

The risk of chorioamnionitis is highest among nonwhite patients of low socioeconomic status who have not received prenatal care.[45,46] These demographic characteristics of patients with chorioamnionitis are similar to those of patients with sexually transmitted diseases.

**Table 64-3. Perinatal Death Rates (per 1000) from Selected Specific Disorders**

| Disorder | Perinatal mortality rate | | |
|---|---|---|---|
| | United States* | Ethiopia | South Africa |
| Amniotic fluid infection | 6.2† | 21.8 | 14.2 |
| Premature rupture membranes | 3.7 | 1.3 | 1.1 |
| Abruptio placentae | 3.9 | 5.5 | 8.1 |
| Congenital syphilis | 0.02 | 4.9 | 3.2 |
| All other defined causes | 9.1 | 32.0 | 28.2 |
| Idiopathic | 7.5 | 0.2 | |
| Total | 30.4 | 65.3 | 54.8 |

*Data collected during the Perinatal Collaborative Study 1959–1966.
†Perinatal mortality rate is defined as the death of fetus >20 weeks of gestational age or neonate ≤days of age per 1000 births.

## Coitus in pregnancy

Approximately 40 percent of women studied in Durban, in Addis Ababa, and in Seattle had intercourse during the last 2 weeks of their pregnancy.[47] Naeye reported that coitus during pregnancy was associated with low birth weight and with an increase in the perinatal mortality rate. Data shown in Table 64-4 reinterpret findings initially reported by Zachau-Christiansen and Ross in a study of over 9000 Danish pregnant women, and illustrates that coitus was associated with prematurity and excess fetal and neonatal deaths. The U.S. Collaborative Perinatal Project showed the perinatal mortality rate (PMR) to be two- to fourfold higher when women continued coitus until near delivery than when they were sexually inactive.[48] A large portion of the excess of perinatal deaths among those who had coitus was attributable to more frequent and severe amniotic fluid infections. At every gestational age, the proportion of fetuses and neonates dying with amniotic fluid infection was greater when coitus had occurred in the month before delivery. Abruptio placentae, the second most frequent cause of perinatal death in the collaborative study, was also 50 percent more frequent among sexually active than among sexually inactive pregnant women. Naeye has also observed seasonal variations both in sexual activity and in the PMR rates and that these are virtually synchronous, peaking in May, June, and July.[49] The incidence of gonococcal and chlamydial infections is also seasonal, peaking in August and September. Thus, it is interesting that Kelle and Nugent[50] observed an increase in perinatal mortality during July, August, and September, due mostly to an increase in infective causes of perinatal death.

Naeye has speculated that coitus may cause amniotic fluid infection by introduction of a new sexually transmitted pathogen, or by injury to the cervix or membranes, or because seminal fluid may increase cervical mucus penetrability to vaginal bacteria or may inactivate antibacterial systems in the vagina, cervix, fetal membranes, or amniotic fluid.

However, not all studies support the concept that coitus in late pregnancy is dangerous. Mills et al. reviewed nearly 11,000 pregnancies in Israel and observed no increased risk of low birth weight or perinatal death among women continuing coitus during the month prior to delivery when compared with women who

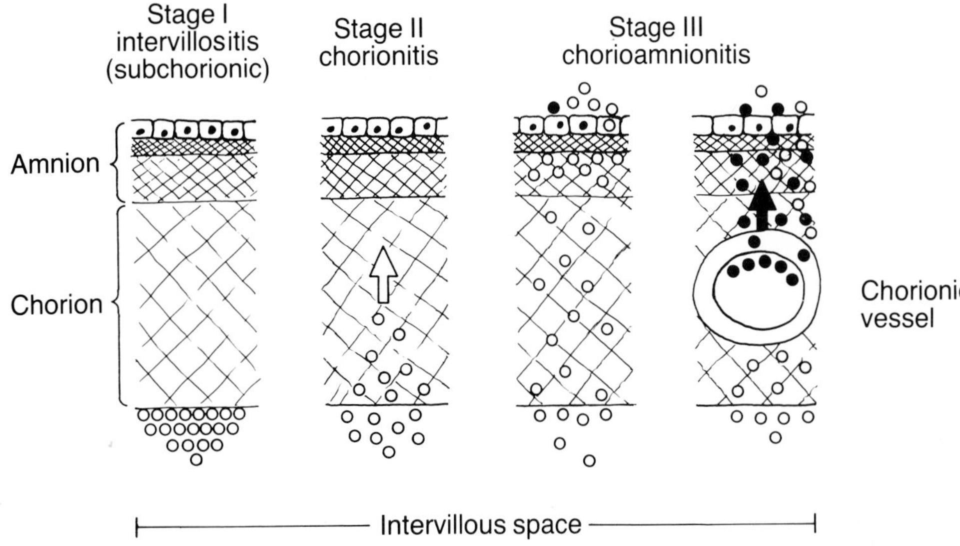


Fig. 64-5. The stages and patterns of maternal and fetal response to amniotic fluid infection. (*After W Blanc.*[43a])

abstained.[51] Reasons for these discordant findings are not readily apparent, but differences in time and population including the prevalence of STD in the populations studied may have influenced the results. Overall, the weight of evidence supports that coitus in pregnancy can be harmful and may be particularly so if the sexual partner harbors genital pathogens.

## FETAL WASTAGE AND PREMATURITY

Spontaneous abortion, stillbirth, and prematurity—all can be caused by infection. However, the proportion of these events attributable to infection is unknown. Spontaneous abortion, defined as the delivery of a previable fetus before the twentieth week of gestation and weighing less than 500 g, is a frequent outcome in pregnancy. It is estimated that 50 percent of fertilized ova fail to implant and of those that do implant, at least 15 to 30 percent subsequently abort.[52] Approximately half of the latter occur in the first trimester and half in the second.[53] This distinction is clinically useful since first trimester abortions are usually associated with phenotypic or chromosomal fetal abnormalities. Second trimester abortions and stillbirths (weight $>500$ g, gestation $\geq 20$ weeks) are more often associated with an otherwise normal fetus. Genital infections may thus be a relatively more important cause of fetal wastage in the second and third trimester than in the first trimester. Forty to 54 percent of pregnancies which terminated spontaneously in the second trimester have been associated with histologic evidence of chorioamnionitis.[21]

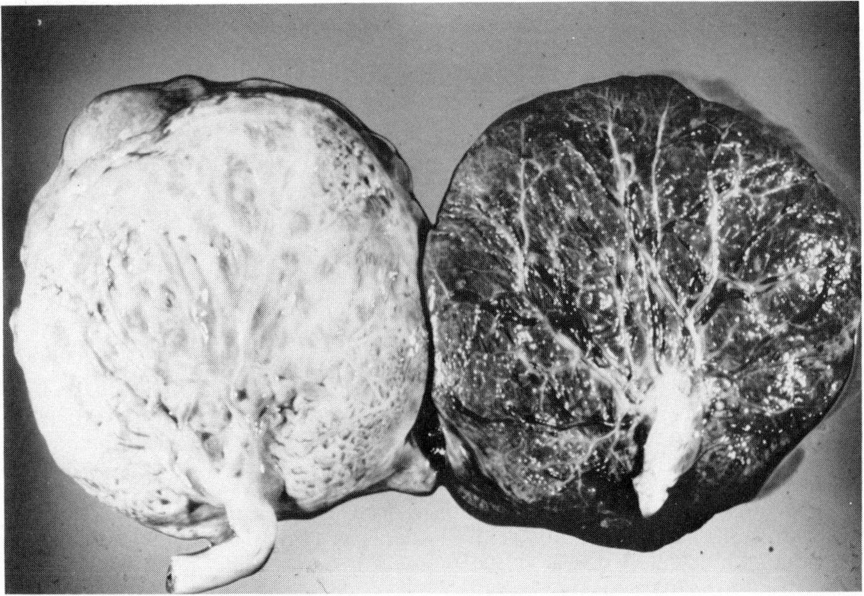

Fig. 64-6. Normal placenta contrasted with placenta showing gross appearance of chorioamnionitis. Opalescence of fetal membranes is due to polymorphonuclear infiltration of the chorioamnion. (*Figure provided by K Benirschke.*)

**Table 64-4. Association of Coitus with Prematurity and Increased Perinatal Mortality Rate**

| | Birth weight <2500 g per 1000 births | Perinatal mortality rate per 1000 births |
|---|---|---|
| No coitus | 127 | 49 |
| Discontinued coitus | | |
| First trimester | 187 ($p < 0.01$) | 67 |
| Second trimester | 192 ($p < 0.001$) | 100 ($p < 0.001$) |
| Third trimester | 169 ($p < 0.02$) | 71 ($p < 0.05$) |

SOURCE: From RL Naeye.[47]

Prematurity, defined as birth weight less than 2500 g, usually results from the birth of a preterm infant. However, a term baby can also weigh less than 2500 g as a result of intrauterine growth retardation. Both conditions have been associated with infectious agents. The proportion of cases of prematurity caused by infection versus that caused by noninfectious factors (e.g., diet, smoking, hypertension) remains to be defined. The previous section suggests that infection is relatively important.

Despite a remarkable decline in the perinatal mortality rate in the United States in the last three and one-half decades, the prematurity rate has remained essentially unchanged at approximately 6 to 8 percent (see Fig. 64-7).[54,55] Seventy to eighty percent of all perinatal deaths that are not attributable to congenital malformation occur following premature birth.[56] Since prematurity and perinatal mortality are so strongly linked, it appears that the decline in perinatal mortality achieved during the last three and one-half decades must be attributable to improvements in perinatal and neonatal care, more than to improvements in prematurity rates. The decline in perinatal mortality has thus been achieved as a result of enormously burgeoning costs of perinatal and neonatal intensive care. For instance, the cost of neonatal intensive care units in the United States in 1980 was $460 million. If neonates treated in these units had instead been delivered as healthy term infants, the cost savings would have been over $400 million.[34] The elucidation of treatable causes of prematurity will likely lead to preventive efforts which would further reduce the perinatal mortality rate and substantially decrease health care costs.

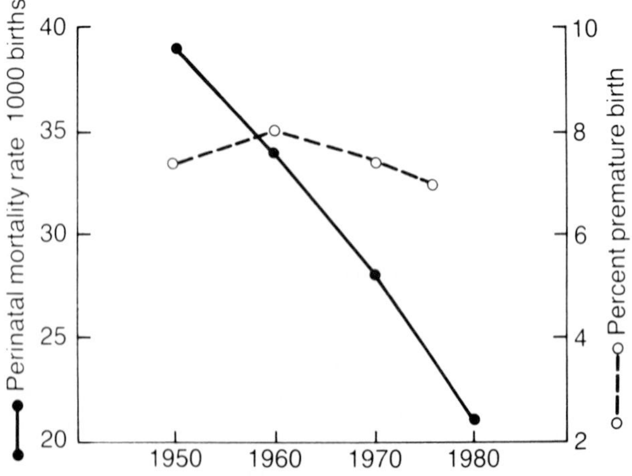


Fig. 64-7. Declining perinatal mortality rate which has occurred in the face of an unchanging prematurity rate in the United States. The perinatal mortality rate declined further to 10.7 per 100 live births for 1985, while the incidence of low birth weight (<2500 g) remained essentially unchanged at 6.8 per 100 live births for 1980 and 1985.

Intriguing data implicating infectious agents in prematurity were serendipitously derived from studies by Elder et al.[57] In the course of investigating the role of urinary tract infection in prematurity, 279 nonbacteriuric women seen prior to 32 weeks of gestation were alternately allocated to treatment with 6 weeks of oral tetracycline at 1 g per day or with placebo. The patients in both groups were of comparable age, gravidity, race, and marital status. As seen in Table 64-5, even in those without urinary infection, the tetracycline-treated group had significantly longer gestations, fewer premature liveborns, fewer episodes of postpartum fever, and fewer neonatal complications than the placebo-treated group. The salutary effect of tetracycline suggested the presence of unidentified tetracycline-susceptible microorganism(s) which contributed to prematurity.

In a subsequent treatment trial Kass et al.[58] randomized 148 women to erythromycin therapy given for 6 weeks in the third trimester or to placebo. Infants in the placebo group weighed less than infants in the treatment group (3187 g versus 3331 g, $p = 0.04$). More recently McGregor et al.[59] reported that women with preterm labor and cervical dilation had prolonged pregnancy when given adjunctive erythromycin treatment in comparison with a placebo-treated group. Because of the small size of the study group and the need to confirm this important finding, further placebo controlled treatment trials are necessary.

These effects of antibiotics on birth weights suggest that prematurity may result from unrecognized maternal infection, perhaps STDs involving the lower genital tract.[60] The fact that perinatal mortality rates and rates of birth weight <2500 g are approximately twice as high in blacks as in whites is consistent with racial differences in prevalence of a number of risk factors for these adverse pregnancy outcomes, including differences in rates of many STDs described below.

Two mechanisms by which lower genital tract infection might produce preterm labor have most often been suggested. One hypothesis is that microorganisms directly spread from the lower genital tract through the cervix to infect the lower pole of the chorioamnion resulting in localized chorioamnionitis, causing eventual premature ROM. Indeed premature ROM is noted in about 30 percent of preterm labors and frequently is accompanied by histologic evidence of inflammation.[41] In two studies, anaerobic bacteria were isolated from the cervix, more often from women with premature ROM than from control women.[61,62] Whether these associations reflect a causal association or a selective effect of amniotic fluid on vaginal flora is unknown. High priority should be given to comprehensive microbiologic and histologic study of premature ROM.

An alternate hypothesis[63] is that bacteria producing chorioamnionitis may induce preterm labor through activation of the prostaglandin-mediated parturition pathway. The current concept of the biochemical basis of labor suggests that arachidonic acid is released from precursors in fetal membranes by activated phospholipase $A_2$. Arachidonic acid is subsequently converted to active mediators of myometrial contraction, prostaglandins $E_2$ and $F_{2a}$.[64] This system is fully in place and susceptible to activation from early pregnancy onward. Bacteria which are common perinatal pathogens (e.g., *Bacteroides* spp., *Streptococcus agalactiae* (GBS), *Escherichia coli*) or which are commonly associated with amniotic fluid infection and/or bacterial vaginosis (Peptostreptococci, Fusobacterium, *Gardnerella vaginalis*) produce phospholipase $A_2$, the key enzyme activating this prostaglandin cascade. Speculation that either asymptomatic or symptomatic infection

Table 64-5. Effect of 6 Weeks of Oral Tetracycline Given Prior to 32 Weeks on Outcome of Pregnancy in 279 Nonbacteriuric Women

| Measurement | Tetracycline (*N* = 148) | | | Placebo (*N* = 131) | | | *p* |
|---|---|---|---|---|---|---|---|
| Gestation (weeks) | | | | | | | |
| Mean | 39.1 | | | 38.1 | | | <0.025 |
| Birth weight (g) | | | | | | | |
| Mean | 3277 | | | 3141 | | | NS* |
| | Number | | Percent | Number | | Percent | |
| Premature liveborn | 8 | | 5.4 | 20 | | 15.2 | <0.025 |
| Stillborn | 2 | | 1.4 | 1 | | 0.8 | |
| | Number | Total | Percent | Number | Total | Percent | |
| Premature rupture of membranes | 14 | 142 | 10 | 16 | 128 | 13 | NS |
| Postpartum fever | 8 | 142 | 6 | 15 | 129 | 12 | <0.001 |
| Neonatal resuscitation required | 11 | 140 | 8 | 24 | 125 | 19 | <0.005 |
| Respiratory distress | 1 | 140 | 1 | 9 | 125 | 7 | <0.05 |

*Nonsignificant.
SOURCE: HA Elder et al.[57]

of the maternal genital tract with any of these bacteria may precipitate preterm labor requires further study.[65]

## MATERNAL PUERPERAL INFECTION AS A COMPLICATION OF ANTENATAL STDs

### EPIDEMIOLOGY AND PATHOGENESIS

Puerperal endometritis, the most common maternal postpartum infection, can be divided into early infections occurring within the first 48 h after delivery and late infections occurring from 2 days to 6 weeks after delivery. Cesarean section greatly increases the risk of early postpartum infection. Without antimicrobial prophylaxis, 36 to 65 percent of women who undergo nonelective cesarean section develop infectious morbidity; women delivered by cesarean section are up to 20 times more likely to develop infectious morbidity than are women delivered vaginally. The high infection rate following cesarean section probably results from direct myometrial and peritoneal contamination by organisms present within the amniotic cavity at the time of cesarean section. Factors which increase microbial contamination of the uterus prior to or during delivery thus increase the risk of postpartum endometritis and puerperal sepsis. These factors include duration of labor, interval from rupture of membranes until delivery, chorioamnionitis, and number of vaginal examinations.

In developed countries, most postpartum infections are related to cesarean section. In developing countries where cesarean sections are less frequently performed and maternal STDs may be more prevalent, postpartum upper genital tract infections after vaginal delivery are approximately 10 times more common than in developed countries.[66]

### MICROBIAL ETIOLOGY OF POSTPARTUM ENDOMETRITIS AND PUERPERAL SEPSIS

Among women delivered vaginally in Nairobi, Kenya, Plummer et al.[66] noted that cervical gonococcal or chlamydial infection, prolonged labor (≥12 h), and low socioeconomic status were the major determinants of puerperal pelvic infection. Among women with gonococcal infection, gonococcal pelvic infection, and gonococcal ophthalmia neonatorum frequently occurred concomitantly. This association suggested that either uniquely virulent gonococcal strains were present or that shared host deficiency occurred in these mother infant pairs. In this study in Nairobi, Kenya, approximately 20 percent of mothers undergoing vaginal delivery developed postpartum pelvic infection and approximately 35 percent of cases were attributable to gonococcal and/or chlamydial infection.

Other microorganisms are undoubtedly involved in causing postpartum pelvic infections and puerperal sepsis and may be relatively more important causes in areas of low prevalence of maternal gonococcal and chlamydial infection. In particular, anaerobic bacteria (predominantly *Bacteroides* species, *Peptococci,* and *Peptostreptococci*). *M. hominis* have been incriminated in postpartum pelvic infections after vaginal delivery.[66a–68]

Wallace et al. isolated *M. hominis* from the blood of 10 to 15 percent of women with postpartum fever.[69] Women without antibody to *M. hominis* at the time of delivery had a higher rate of postpartum fever than women with antibody, and many febrile women acquired *M. hominis* antibody. None of the women with mycoplasmaemia was seriously ill; despite high temperatures, they had minimal uterine tenderness and no foul-smelling or purulent cervical discharge, and they rapidly improved following antibiotic administration.

The association of vaginal anaerobes and *M. hominis* with bacteria vaginosis suggests that bacterial vaginosis is a risk factor for puerperal infection after vaginal delivery. Similarly, early postpartum endometritis and bacteremia among women following cesarean delivery is usually due to the anaerobic and facultative bacteria of the cervicovaginal flora, predominantly but not exclusively those associated with bacterial vaginosis[70] (Table 64-6).

In contrast, late postpartum endometritis, occurring 2 days to 6 weeks after delivery, has been correlated with *C. trachomatis* infection. Wager et al.[71] found that approximately 30 percent of pregnant women with antepartum *C. trachomatis* developed puerperal infection. One-third of these cases had intrapartum fever attributed to chorioamnionitis, and two-thirds had late postpartum endometritis. Clinical manifestations of puerperal chlamydia endometritis, like those of nonpuerperal chlamydial endometritis and salpingitis, are generally mild. Patients are often afebrile, with mild uterine tenderness, and usually with no

**Table 64-6. Microorganisms Isolated from the Endometrium (via Triple Lumen Catheter) and from Blood from 55 Febrile Women with Early Postpartum Endomyometritis, 86 Percent of Whom Were Delivered by Cesarean Section**

| | Endometrium ($N = 55$) | | Blood ($N = 55$) | |
|---|---|---|---|---|
| Microorganism | Number | Percent | Number | Percent |
| Facultative: | | | | |
| *Gardnerella vaginalis* | 14 | 25 | 6 | 11 |
| *Streptococcus agalactiae* (group B) | 9 | 16 | 2 | 4 |
| Enterococcus | 7 | 13 | 1 | 2 |
| *Staphylococcus epidermidis* | 7 | 13 | 0 | |
| *Escherichia coli* | 6 | 11 | 0 | |
| *Streptococcus MG intermedius* | 5 | 9 | 1 | 2 |
| *Streptococcus sanguis* | 3 | 5 | 1 | 2 |
| Other Enterobacteriaceae | 2 | 4 | 0 | |
| *Staphylococcus aureus* | 1 | 2 | 0 | |
| Anaerobes: | | | | |
| *Bacteroides bivius* | 10 | 18 | 4 | 7 |
| *Peptococcus assacharolyticus* | 9 | 16 | 2 | 4 |
| Other bacteroides species | 7 | 13 | 4 | 7 |
| Peptostreptococcus species | 7 | 13 | 1 | 2 |
| Other peptococcus species | 5 | 9 | 3 | 5 |
| *Bacteroides fragilis* | 2 | 4 | 0 | |
| Mycoplasmas: | | | | |
| *Mycoplasma hominis* | 11 | 20 | 1 | 2 |
| *Ureaplasma urealyticum* | 38 | 69 | 2 | 4 |
| *Chlamydia trachomatis* | 2 | 4 | Not done | |
| Mixed | 30 | 55 | 5 | 9 |
| None | 4 | 7 | 37 | 67 |

SOURCE: K Rosene, D Eschenbach.[70]

adnexal tenderness. Such minimally symptomatic postpartum chlamydia infections may contribute to the high rate of chlamydia antibody among women with secondary infertility because of distal tube obstruction (see Chap. 65).

The frequency of involvement of the fallopian tubes during postpartum pelvic infection is unknown, as no laparoscopic studies have been reported. The observation of Platt et al.[66] that peritoneal infection (as assessed by culdocentesis) commonly accompanies postpartum pelvic infection suggests that fallopian tube infection may not be rare. Similarly the relationship of postpartum pelvic infection to secondary infertility due to tubal scarring is also unknown. Nevertheless secondary infertility, usually due to tubal obstruction, is a major problem in Africa,[72] where the prevalence rates of maternal gonococcal and chlamydial infection and the incidence rates of postpartum pelvic infection are very high.

## NEONATAL CONSEQUENCE OF STDs

Systemic perinatal bacterial infection is acquired in utero or during delivery in 1 to 5 per 1000 live births.[73] Perinatal bacterial infections are two to three times more common than are perinatal viral and protozoal infections. Presently about half of all neonatal bacterial infections in the United States are due to GBS, although marked regional variations occur. Temporal changes in the predominant pathogens found in perinatal infection have also occurred. The incidence of GBS neonatal infections has increased at several medical centers during the 1960s and 1970s, more or less in parallel with the increase in other STDs. Group A beta-hemolytic streptococci, *Staphylococcus aureus,* Enterobacteriaceae, and, most recently, anaerobes have also been important neonatal pathogens.

Neonatal STDs are discussed in detail in Chaps. 65 to 72. Table 64-7 summarizes the clinical manifestations and diagnostic findings which can occur with congenital or neonatal infection with STD agents.

## CONSEQUENCES, RECOGNITION, AND MANAGEMENT OF SPECIFIC SEXUALLY TRANSMITTED DISEASES DURING PREGNANCY

### SYPHILIS

#### Epidemiology and manifestations

A detailed clinical description of congenital syphilis is provided in Chap. 67. Untreated primary or secondary syphilis during pregnancy affects virtually 100 percent of fetuses, with 50 percent of such pregnancies resulting in premature delivery or perinatal death. Untreated early latent syphilis during pregnancy results in a 40 percent rate of prematurity or perinatal death. Ten percent of infants born to mothers with untreated late syphilis show signs of congenital infection, and the perinatal death rate is increased approximately tenfold. Whereas syphilis is rarely sexually transmissible longer than 2 years after acquisition, women with untreated syphilis apparently may remain infectious for their fetuses for many years, although the proportion of affected fetuses and the severity of fetal disease decrease with longer duration of untreated maternal infection.

In the preantibiotic era, syphilis was estimated to be an etiologic factor in as many as 40 percent of stillborn infants.[74] Presently syphilis is an uncommon cause of stillbirth in industrialized countries but remains a common cause in developing countries. Naeye noted that 0.2 percent of perinatal deaths were attribut-

Table 64-7. Clinical Manifestations of Neonatal Infection with Sexually Transmitted Agents Acquired In Utero or at Delivery

| | Microorganism | | | | | |
|---|---|---|---|---|---|---|
| Clinical sign | Cytomegalovirus | Herpes simplex virus | *Treponema pallidum* | Group B streptococci | *Chlamydia trachomatis* | *Neisseria gonorrhoeae* |
| Hepatosplenomegaly | + | + | + | + | − | − |
| Jaundice | + | + | + | + | − | − |
| Adenopathy | − | − | + | − | − | − |
| Pneumonitis | + | + | + | + | + + | − |
| Lesions of skin or mucus membranes: | | | | | | |
| Petechiae or purpura | + | + | + | + | − | + |
| Vesicles, ulcers | ? | + + | + | − | − | − |
| Maculopapular exanthem | − | + | + + | − | − | − |
| Lesions of nervous system: | | | | | | |
| Meningoencephalitis | + | + | + | + | − | + |
| Microcephaly | + + | + | − | − | − | − |
| Intracranial calcifications | + + | + | − | − | − | − |
| Bone lesions | + | + | + + | − | − | − |
| Joint lesions | − | − | + | − | − | + |
| Eye lesions: | | | | | | |
| Chorioretinitis | + | + | + | − | − | − |
| Conjunctivitis | − | + | − | − | + + | + + |

− = Finding rare or not present.
\+ = Finding occurs in neonates during infection.
\+ + = Finding has special diagnostic significance for this infection.
SOURCE: Modified from AJ Nahmias, AM Visintine.[192]

able to syphilis among over 50,00 pregnancies studied in the U.S. Collaborative Perinatal Project between 1959 and 1966.[75] From that time until 1978, the incidence of congenital syphilis in the United States steadily declined. However, since 1978, the incidence of primary and secondary syphilis in women of childbearing age has increased, particularly in women belonging to ethnic minorities, and this has been accompanied by an increase in congenital syphilis.[76] For example, from 1986 to 1987, the incidence increased 43 percent in black women and 24 percent in Hispanic women. In 1986, the incidence of reported congenital syphilis (about 1 per 1000 live births) was higher than in any of the previous 15 years, and in the latter half of 1987, the incidence of congenital syphilis increased a further 21 percent. Presently, approximately two cases of congenital syphilis occur for every 100 cases of primary and secondary syphilis detected in women in the United States. These increases have been regional, with major increases seen in Florida and California and New York City in the United States.[77,78] Congenital syphilis still remains a major problem in developing countries. In Addis Ababa, Ethiopia, congenital syphilis is the fifth and in Durban, South Africa, the fourth leading cause of perinatal death.[34] In a recent study of pregnant women in Zambia, serologic tests for syphilis were reactive in 43 percent of women who delivered stillborn babies, 19 percent who aborted, and 13 percent of normal women attending their first antenatal visit.[79]

Congenital syphilis is entirely preventable with appropriate case detection and treatment programs. In 1951, it was found that 50 percent of mothers of infants with congenital syphilis in Massachusetts had had inadequate or no prenatal care, 17 percent had failed to complete antibiotic therapy, and 12 percent had become infected after an initially negative prenatal serologic test for syphilis.[80] During the recent outbreak of congenital syphilis in Texas, 62 percent of mothers of infected infants had not received prenatal care.[77] The provision of adequate prenatal care to all pregnant women remains the foundation for prevention of congenital syphilis. Identification of women at high risk for syphilis (young unmarried women with multiple sexual partners) and rescreening these women later during pregnancy will reduce the incidence of congenital syphilis.

## Pathogenesis

Placental infection with *T. pallidum* occurs during maternal spirochetemia, which is intense until resolution of the secondary stage. After resolution of the initial and secondary stages, the prevalence and intensity of spirochetemia are unknown except during secondary relapses. Whether pregnancy promotes recrudescence of spirochetemia, accounting for the congenital infections which occasionally occur in late syphilis is uncertain. In the preantibiotic era, Moore observed that the manifestations of primary and secondary syphilis were particularly mild in the pregnant woman.[8] He speculated that pregnancy supplied "some substance which was able to suppress the manifestations of the disease." *T. pallidum* infection produces less evident pathology among pregnant rabbits that among nonpregnant rabbits.[81] Since many of the manifestations of adult and congenital syphilis are thought to have an immunologic basis, the milder manifestations of syphilis during pregnancy are consistent with a relative state of immunosuppression during pregnancy. However, students of syphilis during the antibiotic era have not been impressed with an effect of pregnancy on the manifestations of syphilis.

Once the infection reaches the placenta, fetal infection usually follows. Dippel showed that fetal infection with *T. pallidum* was not detectable until after 18 weeks of gestation.[74] He examined abortuses and stillbirths delivered between the fourteenth and twenty-eighth week of gestation from 67 syphilitic women for the presence of *T. pallidum* by Levaditi's staining of fetal tissue. None of the 12 abortuses between 14 and 17 weeks' gestation, 3 of 29 (10 percent) abortuses between 18 and 22 weeks' gestation, and 13 of 26 (50 percent) stillbirths between 23 and 28 weeks' gestation were found to be infected. On this basis, he proposed that a placental barrier, perhaps Langhan's epithelial layer of cytotrophoblast, protected the fetus from infection prior to the eighteenth week of gestation. The validity of this hypothesis has been challenged by Harter and Benirschke, who observed that fetal infection can occur as early as 9 weeks' gestation.[82] These authors identified five untreated syphilitic women who were to undergo first-trimester therapeutic abortion. Fetal and placental tissue was studied by silver stain and immunofluorescence for spirochetes and in two of the five cases fetal spirochetal infection was found. The authors comment on the paucity of organisms seen and the effort involved in their detection. Benirschke subsequently pointed out that although Langhan's layer becomes less apparent after the eighteenth week of gestation, it does not totally disappear.[83] Considered collectively, the data suggest that the fetus is susceptible to infection prior to the eighteenth week of gestation, but *T. pallidum* is more likely to be detectable in fetal tissue after the eighteenth week, for reasons not fully defined.

Silverstein has proposed that the lesions of congenital syphilis do not become manifest until early manifestations of fetal immunocompetence appear at about the sixteenth week of gestation.[84] He suggested that the pathogenesis of congenital syphilis may depend on the immune response of the fetus rather than on cytopathogenic effects of *T. pallidum.* This hypothesis (if true) may also explain why adequate therapy of maternal syphilis prior to the sixteenth week of gestation usually prevents fetal damage.

## Case detection

Congenital syphilis can be prevented by early prenatal diagnosis and treatment. Serology remains the most useful diagnostic test for syphilis in women. Signs or symptoms are confirmatory, but often are not demonstrable; of over 14,000 cases of early syphilis in women, only 11 percent had a primary lesion, 41 percent had secondary lesions, while 48 percent had no manifestations and were detected only by serology.[85]

Despite the low prevalence of maternal syphilis in many developed countries, cost-benefit analysis still favors prenatal first-trimester serologic screening.[86] For instance, in Norway with a 0.02 percent maternal prevalence rate, the benefit-cost ratio of the program was still 3.8. Only with an estimated prevalence of maternal syphilis of less than 1 per 20,000 would the costs of the screening program exceed the benefits. This analysis excluded the intangible benefit of screening which cannot be measured in economic terms. The U.S. Centers for Disease Control recommends serologic testing at the beginning of prenatal care and at delivery, with intermediate testing at the beginning of the third trimester (28 weeks) for high-risk women.[78]

There are many barriers to detection of syphilis early in pregnancy, including those which lead to delayed prenatal care, particularly in developing countries, and in poor and minority women in industrialized countries. Approximately one-fourth of pregnant women in the United States did not receive first-trimester prenatal care during 1985, with a disproportionately higher percentage among Medicaid recipients and uninsured women.[55] A recent publication outlines specific practical measures to improve early detection in pregnant women.[78] These measures include on-site pregnancy testing of women whose menstrual periods are late in STD clinics and drug-addiction programs; routine RPR testing whenever a positive pregnancy test is obtained in all pregnancy testing programs; and early testing by prenatal programs, before the regularly scheduled prenatal visit when the waiting time for the first scheduled visit is long.

## Treatment

A positive screening test should be further evaluated with a quantitative nontreponemal test (VDRL) and a confirmatory treponemal test such as the fluorescent treponemal antibody-absorption test (FTA-ABS) or the microhemagglutination *Treponema pallidum* (MHA-TP) test.

Women with a positive FTA-ABS test who do not have clear documentation of previous adequate treatment for syphilis require treatment. Women with an epidemiologic history of recent exposure to an individual with proved syphilis should be treated, regardless of serologic results.

It is not necessary to re-treat women who have had documented adequate treatment for previous syphilis as long as no evidence of serologic or clinical relapse exists. If clinical or serologic relapse or reinfection occurs, therapy should, of course, be reinstituted. If doubt exists about the adequacy of previous therapy, re-treatment should be given promptly.

Treatment of syphilis in the pregnant woman is generally the same as that of the nonpregnant patient and depends on the duration of infection and on the presence or absence of central nervous system involvement. Some authors warn against performing a lumbar puncture in the pregnant patient for fear of precipitating preterm labor. Such concern does not appear justified if the lumbar puncture is properly performed.

Recommended choice and schedules of antimicrobials for the various clinical forms of syphilis are found in Chaps. 20 to 23 and 67. Occasionally, pregnant women who develop a Jarisch-Herxheimer reaction after initiation of treatment for early syphilis have had precipitous onset of premature labor. We recommend hospitalization of women beyond 20 weeks' gestation who have early syphilis for close observation during initiation of therapy to permit fetal monitoring and early tocolytic therapy, if needed. Should penicillin allergy exist, no established recommendations for therapy are available. However, we recommended skin testing with penicillin G minor determinant mixture and penicylloyl polylysine. The great majority of patients with a past history of penicillin allergy will have negative (nonreactive) skin tests and can be safely treated with penicillin G. For pregnant women with positive immediate wheal and flare skin tests, desensitization can be rapidly achieved by oral administration of increasing doses of penicillin V. One desensitization schedule used in 15 pregnant women who had positive penicillin skin tests involved a starting oral dose of 100 units of penicillin V; the oral dose was doubled every 15 min, for a total of 14 doses, each diluted in 30 ml of water, given over a total elapsed time of 3 h and 45 min, with the final dose equal to 640,000 units.[87] Women were desensitized in hospital, with an intravenous line in place and a physician on hand at all times. After a further 30-min observation period, parenteral penicillin was begun. Five patients had evidence of allergic reaction, one requiring epinephrine. After completion of the procedure, full doses of parenteral penicillin therapy can be instituted. Failures to prevent congenital syphilis following treatment of the mother during pregnancy with erythromycin, tetracycline, and chloramphenicol were summarized by Thompson.[88] Available data suggest that the failure rate with erythromycin is unacceptably high. Certain cephalosporins show good treponemacidal activity, but clinical trials are required to prove their safety and efficacy for syphilis in pregnancy. Pregnant women treated for early syphilis should have monthly quantitative serologies throughout pregnancy. Those who do not show a fourfold drop in titer at 3 months, or who show a fourfold rise in titer should be retreated.

## GONORRHEA

The recognition that maternal gonococcal infection posed a threat to the newborn's sight motivated a major achievement of modern preventive medicine—Credé's prophylaxis. In the 1880s ophthalmia neonatorum was a frequent neonatal infection. In Credé's original series, 10 percent of newborns acquired ophthalmia neonatorum. Rothenberg estimated that the maternal gonococcal infection rate among patients studied by Credé must have approached the astounding figure of 30 percent.[89]

### Epidemiology

The reported prevalence of gonococcal infection among pregnant women shows wide variations, determined by differences in populations studied. Generally, studies of indigent populations in the United States have shown higher prevalence rates than studies from other industrialized countries, and rates in most of the developing world are higher than rates in developed countries. Risk factors for infection remain the same in pregnancy as in the nonpregnant state. In North America, gonococcal recovery rates are highest in young nonwhite unmarried mothers of low socioeconomic status, particularly in large cities. The Centers for Disease Control reported that of 1.7 million prenatal gonorrhea culture tests done during the period January 1979 to December 1979, approximately 3 percent were positive. More recently, isolates resistant to penicillin and other antibiotics have increased in frequency, raising therapeutic concerns. Despite a decreasing incidence of gonococcal infection in men in most industrialized countries (presumably owing to behavioral changes due to AIDS), in childbearing women having the characteristics described above, the prevalence rate of gonorrhea remains high.[90,91]

### Manifestations and pathogenesis

The manifestations and pathogenesis of gonococcal infection in the pregnant host have some unique features.[92] The rate of pharyngeal infection as the sole site of infection may be increased during pregnancy. In some studies, 15 to 35 percent of infected pregnant women have had *N. gonorrhoeae* isolated only from the throat and not from the endocervix or anal canal.[93,94] These findings suggest that endocervical cultures may be more apt to be falsely negative or the frequency of oral sexual activity relative to vaginal intercourse may be increased during pregnancy.

Pharyngeal colonization with gonococci may increase the risk of dissemination (Chaps. 14, 61), and some studies have suggested an increased risk of disseminated gonococcal infection (DGI) among pregnant women.[95]

The frequency of upper genital tract involvement following endocervical gonococcal infection during pregnancy is unknown. Among nonpregnant women, 10 to 20 percent with cervical gonorrhea have clinical evidence of pelvic inflammatory disease (PID), and up to 50 percent of women with recently acquired gonorrhea developed PID in one recent study.[96] Acute gonococcal PID appears to be a rare event during pregnancy. Positive prenatal cultures for *N. gonorrhoeae* are occasionally associated with fever and pain, and surgically verified cases of gonococcal salpingitis in pregnancy have been reported between 7 and 12 weeks' gestation (prior to obliteration of the endometrial cavity).[97]

Local cervical factors also may decrease the risk for ascending gonococcal infection in pregnancy. Serum progesterone concentrations are greatly increased in pregnancy and concentrations of progesterone 50 to 200 times that occurring during pregnancy are known to inhibit the growth of *N. gonorrhoeae* in vitro.[98] The menstrual cycle effects phenotypic changes in gonococci which may alter gonococcal virulence; the effects of pregnancy on phenotypic properties of *N. gonorrhoeae* have not been studied. Cervical mucus becomes impermeable to motile sperm (and perhaps to motile microorganisms) under the influence of progesterone.[99] Perhaps most importantly, after the twelfth week of gestation, the chorion attaches to the endometrial deciduae with obliteration of the intrauterine cavity, obstructing the route for ascending intraluminal spread of gonococci. All these factors may limit the spread of gonococci from the cervix to the endometrium and fallopian tubes during pregnancy.

We hypothesize that the chorioamnion itself may become the site of infection by ascending gonococci after the twelfth week of gestation. Among women hospitalized with gonococcal infection during pregnancy, in one study, 35 percent had septic abortion.[20] This observation has not subsequently been addressed. Remarkably little is known about the natural history of untreated maternal gonococcal infection and its relationship to outcome of pregnancy.

Several retrospective studies have analyzed the relationship of antepartum gonococcal infection to the course of late pregnancy. As reviewed elsewhere (Ref. 89 and in this chapter in the first edition [Chap. 67] of *Sexually Transmitted Diseases*), these studies have all shown an association with clinical infectious morbidity, such as premature delivery, premature or prolonged rupture of membranes, and chorioamnionitis.

Edwards et al.[100] matched 19 pregnant women who had intrapartum gonococcal infection to 41 uninfected controls on the basis of age, race, parity, socioeconomic status, and date of delivery. Patients with intrapartum gonococcal infection were significantly more likely than controls to have premature rupture of membranes, prolonged rupture of membranes, chorioamnionitis, and prematurity.

In noncontrolled studies of maternal gonococcal infection, Berstine reported that 32 percent of women with antenatal gonococcal infection had puerperal infectious morbidity.[101] A related observation can be found in a recent matched-pair analysis of 228 cases of endometritis among 4823 women following elective abortion.[102] These investigators found a threefold increased relative risk for endometritis in patients who had untreated gonococcal infection when compared with uninfected control subjects ($<0.05$).

In a recent study in Nairobi, Kenya, Plummer et al. found that postpartum upper genital tract infection (UGTI) was significantly correlated with intrapartum gonococcal and/or chlamydial infection.[66] Forty-seven percent of women with intrapartum gonococcal infection developed postpartum UGTI; approximately 22 percent of postpartum UGTI was attributable to gonococcal infection in this setting where the prevalence of maternal gonococcal infection was 6 percent.

These studies collectively provide convincing evidence that maternal gonococcal infection is detrimental to pregnancy. Gonococcal endocervicitis may cause premature ROM and chorioamnionitis by infecting the lower pole of the chorioamnion. The effect of gonococcal infection on early pregnancy is less well studied than its effect on late pregnancy, but early infection may cause septic abortion. Acute salpingitis also occurs during the first trimester, but very infrequently. Disseminated gonococcal infection may occur more frequently during pregnancy.

## Case detection and treatment

Because of these adverse effects on pregnancy and because of the risk for neonatal infection, detection of *N. gonorrhoeae* by screening cultures during the initial antenatal visit is justified in most populations.[103] Repeated culture at 36 to 38 weeks' gestation is also indicated among high-risk individuals (young, nonwhite, single, primigravida, low socioeconomic status, current or past STD, especially gonorrhea earlier in pregnancy). Nearly 40 percent of pregnant women with gonorrhea give a past history of gonorrhea; therefore, past history of gonorrhea is a strong indicator for repeated screening cultures. In patients with premature rupture of membranes, intrapartum fever, or septic abortion, an endocervical swab for Gram stain and culture for *N. gonorrhoeae* should also be obtained.

Uncomplicated gonorrhea in the pregnant patient can be treated with ceftriaxone, 250 mg, in a single intramuscular dose. In areas where penicillin-resistant strains represent less than 1 percent of all isolates, an acceptable alternative is aqueous procaine penicillin 4.8 million units injected intramuscularly at two sites, with 1.0 g of probenecid given by mouth. Tetracycline should not be used because of potential maternal and fetal toxic effects. Erythromycin can be added to treat possible coexisting *C. trachomatis* infections, in dosage discussed below. Reinfection after treatment is common. Reinfection rates of 11 to 30 percent have been reported despite efforts to treat partners. Contact tracing and treatment of sexual partners should be vigorously pursued. If sexual partner therapy is not accomplished, repeat monthly cultures are appropriate.

For complicated gonococcal infection in pregnancy (e.g., septic abortion, chorioamnionitis) we recommend treatment for several days with ceftriaxone or cefoxitin plus an antibiotic effective against possible coexisting chlamydial infections, as recommended for pelvic inflammatory disease (see Chap. 49).

## Neonatal gonococcal infection: Implications for management of gonorrhea in pregnancy

In a recent study in Kenya, 42 percent of 67 newborns not receiving ocular prophylaxis who were exposed to maternal gonococcal infection acquired gonococcal ophthalmia neonatorum.[104] In addition to this well-recognized neonatal manifestation of exposure to maternal gonorrhea, infection at other body sites can also occur. *N. gonorrhoeae* has been recovered from orogastric aspirate samples from approximately 30 percent of neonates born of infected mothers.[100,105] Extraocular sites of neonatal gonococcal infection may be associated with a higher risk of disseminated infection.

The risk of gonococcal amniotic fluid infection syndrome and gonococcal ophthalmia appears to be increased after prolonged rupture of membranes.[106,107] The failure of silver nitrate ocular prophylaxis to prevent gonococcal ophthalmia may result from in utero acquisition of *N. gonorrhoeae* in the setting of prolonged ROM.[108]

Gonococcal sepsis occurs in the newborn, although infrequently today. "Natural" gonococcal bactericidal antibody resides in the IgM fraction of serum and is absent from neonatal serum.[109] Whether neonates are at higher risk for gonococcal sepsis than are adults because of this is not established. More importantly, because neonates delivered of mothers with intrapartum gonococcal infection are more likely to be premature or to suffer prolonged labor, bacterial sepsis due to any etiology occurs more often.

**Table 64-8. Risk Estimates of Gonococcal Ophthalmia Neonatorum Following Various Types of Prophylaxis**

| Prophylaxis | Number of births | Risk estimate, % | Number of cases |
|---|---|---|---|
| Silver nitrate 1% | 831,737 | 0.063 | 526 |
| Tetracyclines | 49,666 | 0.012 | 66 |
| Erythromycin | 19,077 | 0.005 | 1 |
| Penicillin | 74,638 | 0.001 | 1 |
| Sulfonamides | 7,223 | 0.11 | 8 |
| Bacitracin | 6,311 | 0.25 | 16 |
| None | 171,240 | 0.038 | 65 |

SOURCE: R Rothenberg,[89] data compiled from 56 studies conducted since 1930. Use of different populations (e.g., low-risk populations may have been selected for no prophylaxis) precludes direct comparisons, but bacitracin and sulfonamide clearly appear to be ineffective.

For these various reasons ophthalmic prophylaxis alone will not prevent all the manifestations and complications of gonorrhea in the neonate. Diagnostic screening and early treatment of infected women during pregnancy represents the most effective means of preventing neonatal gonococcal infection, as well as preventing complications of pregnancy itself.

In addition, in areas where the prevalence of maternal gonococcal infection is greater than 1 percent or where maternal screening is not undertaken, ophthalmic prophylaxis is useful and should be required.[89] Rothenberg has provided risk estimates as derived from the literature for various forms of ophthalmic prophylaxis (see Table 64-8). The recommendations made by the Centers for Disease Control for the prevention of gonococcal ophthalmia neonatorum (now endorsed by the American Academy of Pediatrics) state that ophthalmic ointment or drops containing 1 percent tetracycline, 0.5 percent erythromycin, or 1 percent silver nitrate are effective and acceptable. The only randomized clinical trial of prophylaxis for gonococcal ophthalmia compared the effectiveness of 1 percent silver nitrate with 1 percent tetracycline ointment. Laga et al.[104,104a] found that both agents equally reduced the incidence of gonococcal ophthalmia between 83 and 93 percent when compared with a historical control group who did not receive prophylaxis. Both prophylactic agents were also highly effective against multiresistant *N. gonorrhoeae*.

Neonates born to mothers with documented untreated antepartum or intrapartum gonococcal infection are at high risk for infection and should receive parenteral antibiotics in standard curative dosage (see Chap. 65), in addition to topical ocular prophylaxis.

## *Chlamydia trachomatis* INFECTIONS

### Epidemiology

*C. trachomatis* infection rates for pregnant women have varied from 2 to 30 percent. Single marital status and young age, especially adolescence, are the major demographic correlates of chlamydial infections in pregnancy.

Whether pregnancy per se influences shedding of *C. trachomatis* from the cervix is unknown. The rate of isolation of *C. trachomatis* has been reported to be higher during the third trimester than during the first or second trimester.[110,111] However, women who sought prenatal care in the first trimester in these cross-sectional studies may have had a lower risk of STD than those who did not seek care until the third trimester. Shedding of chlamydia in pregnancy might be influenced by the development of ectopy which is positively correlated with *C. trachomatis* isolation in nonpregnant women, and/or by alteration of the immune response to the organism.

## Immune responses to *C. trachomatis* during pregnancy

During pregnancy the lymphocyte transformation LT response to *C. trachomatis* and other microbial antigens is significantly depressed, and a significant postpartum rise in the LT response occurs.[14] Whether the depressed cellular immunity influences susceptibility to shedding of *C. trachomatis* during pregnancy remains uncertain.

Maternal IgG antibody undergoes active transplacental transfer beginning as early as day 38.[112] The level of transfer remains fairly constant until the seventeenth week, at which time proportionate increases occur with advancing gestational age. Infants born to seropositive mothers with current or past *C. trachomatis* infection acquire antibody to this organism. Since about two-thirds of exposed neonates become infected (Chap. 66), it is clear that passively acquired antibody is not completely protective. The influence of maternal antibody on the risk of acquisition of infection or on the severity of disease is unknown.

The presence of antibody to *C. trachomatis* in breast milk or colostrum and the role of such colostral antibody in preventing or modifying neonatal chlamydial infection has not yet been evaluated.

## Influence of *C. trachomatis* on reproduction and pregnancy

In some areas, up to two-thirds of cases of tubal infertility have been attributed to *C. trachomatis* infection.[27] If incomplete blockage of fallopian tubes occurs with infection, there may be an increased risk of ectopic pregnancy. In one study, 10 of 17 (59 percent) of patients with a history of ectopic pregnancy had antibodies to *Chlamydia trachomatis*.[113] In another case control study, more women with ectopic pregnancy not related to intrauterine device or previous tubal ligation had antibodies to *C. trachomatis* than did women with uterine pregnancies [18/32 (56 percent) vs. 11/49 (22 percent), $p = 0.002$].[26] Kosseim et al.[27] estimated that approximately one-third of cases of ectopic pregnancy may be attributable to chlamydial infection.

Whether *C. trachomatis* infection can cause abortion is unknown. *C. psittaci* infection is an important cause of spontaneous abortion in lower mammals,[114] and Schachter reported that chlamydia were isolated from 4 of 22 first-trimester spontaneous abortuses in humans.[115] Further work on the relationship of chlamydial infection to abortion is needed.

The role of genital *C. trachomatis* infection in prematurity and in perinatal mortality is currently under active investigation. Examination of birth weights and gestational ages of infants with *C. trachomatis* infection has given conflicting results. Of infants with *C. trachomatis* ophthalmia neonatorum, 15 to 42 percent have had birth weights less than 2500 g.[107,116,117] A series of three separate studies at the University of Washington, each involving a different study design, have all shown a correlation of antenatal chlamydial infections with prematurity, defined by preterm delivery and/or low birth weight.[118,119,120] However, Frommell et al.[121] and Heggie et al.[122] found no association of antenatal *C. trachomatis* infection with prematurity. In a prospective study of 1365 pregnant women, Harrison et al.[123] observed no significant correlation of *C. trachomatis* infection with prematurity but did find a significantly increased risk of low birth weight and of premature rupture of membranes, and a shorter gestation among women with serologically defined *primary* infection with *C. trachomatis* than among other culture-positive women or among culture-negative women. Similarly, Berman et al.[124] followed the pregnancy and postpartum course of 1204 Navajo women, and in a subset of women with chlamydial infection, who had IgM antibody ($\geq$1:32) or IgG seroconversion to *C. trachomatis*, they observed a significantly increased risk for prematurity. The effect of such chlamydial infections on the total prematurity rate was modest. The association of premature birth with IgM seropositivity among *C. trachomatis* culture-positive women was confirmed in a recent study by Sweet et al.[125] Nineteen percent of IgM seropositive infected women delivered prematurely compared with 8 percent of IgM seronegative *C. trachomatis* culture-positive women ($p = 0.03$). The biologic basis for these serologic correlations among *C. trachomatis* infected women is not defined. Possibilities could include higher bacterial load and/or more extensive chlamydial infection in a relatively nonimmune host.

In an early study, Martin et al.[118] observed a study correlation of antenatal *C. trachomatis* infection not only with prematurity but also with perinatal mortality. The latter observation has not been confirmed in other studies.

Further prospective study of larger numbers of women is needed. A large multicenter study sponsored by the National Institute of Child Health & Human Development, still underway, should provide a more definitive assessment of the influence of *C. trachomatis* infection on pregnancy, and vice versa.

## The role of *C. trachomatis* in maternal puerperal morbidity

Thygeson noted in 1942 that 10 (26 percent) of 38 mothers whose infants had inclusion conjunctivitis developed puerperal infection.[126] Rees et al. reported that 19 (61 percent) of 31 mothers of infants with *C. trachomatis* conjunctivitis developed postpartum infection after discharge from hospital (13 to 38 days postpartum).[127]

Studies of pregnant women in Seattle and in Nairobi, Kenya, have confirmed that antepartum chlamydial infection, if not treated, is correlated with puerperal infection. Wager et al.[71] found that intrapartum fever (clinically ascribed to amnionitis) as well as late postpartum endometritis were both significantly correlated with untreated antepartum chlamydial infection (Table 64-9). Antenatal *C. trachomatis* infection was not associated with early postpartum fever which was in the majority of instances associated with cesarean section. Overall, among women who delivered vaginally, puerperal infectious morbidity occurred in 10 (34 percent) of 29 women with and in 23 (8 percent) of 300 without antenatal *C. trachomatis* infection ($p < 0.001$). Plummer et al.[66] recently reported from Nairobi that 24 percent of 183 women with intrapartum chlamydial infection developed postpartum upper genital tract infection (UGTI), a rate significantly greater than that observed in uninfected women (15 percent, $p = 0.02$). Chlamydial infection accounted for approximately 22 percent of postpartum UGTI in this setting; this may be representative of developing countries in Africa.

These studies collectively suggest that antepartum *C. tracho-*

**Table 64-9. Puerperal Infectious Morbidity in Patients with and without Antepartum *Chlamydia trachomatis* Infection, Who Were Matched for Demographic Characteristics and Parity**

| | *C. trachomatis* isolated ($N = 32$) | | *C. trachomatis* not isolated ($N = 350$) | | |
|---|---|---|---|---|---|
| Complication | Number | Percent | Number | Percent | |
| Intrapartum fever > 38°C | 3 | 9 | 5 | 1 | <0.025 |
| Early postpartum fever < 48 h | 1 | 3 | 26 | 7 | 0.06 |
| Late postpartum endometritis, 48 h to 6 weeks postpartum | 7 | 22 | 18 | 5 | <0.005 |
| Total infectious morbidity | 11 | 34 | 49 | 14 | <0.01 |

SOURCE: Wager et al.[71]

*matis* infection has an etiologic role in amnionitis and postpartum endometritis, although attempts have not generally been made to isolate *C. trachomatis* at the time these complications have occurred.

## Postabortal salpingitis

A syndrome related to postpartum pelvic infection is seen following therapeutic abortion. An excess rate of postabortal pelvic inflammatory disease has been seen among women with chlamydial infection at the time of the procedure.[128,129] Up to 60 percent of cases of postabortal PID may be attributable to chlamydial infection. In one study, the risk of postabortal PID among chlamydia-infected women was inversely related to serum antibody titers to chlamydia.[130] We recommend that women undergoing therapeutic abortion should be screened for chlamydial infection to prevent postabortal ascending infection.

## Current recommendations for diagnostic testing for chlamydial infection during pregnancy

The importance of detecting and treating chlamydial infection of the genital tract in pregnant women is certainly no less than in nonpregnant women. In fact, the unquestioned risk of intrapartum transmission to the neonate, and the growing evidence that chlamydial infections cause complications of pregnancy and postpartum pelvic infection, dictate that a very high priority be given to detecting and treating chlamydial infection in high-risk pregnant women. However, cell culture techniques currently available for isolation of *C. trachomatis* are highly tedious, labor-intensive, and expensive. Screening by culture of all antenatal patients would quickly overwhelm existing facilities. In the United States, the cost of culturing all pregnant women once for *C. trachomatis* would probably approach the entire allocation of federal funds for all STD control activities. Fortunately the development of antigen detection systems has substantially decreased the cost of identifying *C. trachomatis* infections and has made laboratory tests for *C. trachomatis* more widely available.

According to a recent cost-benefit analysis of ELISA diagnostic testing of nonpregnant women for *C. trachomatis,* benefit exceeded cost when the prevalence of infection exceeded 7 percent (Chap. 16). Cost-benefit analysis for pregnant women will require more definitive data on the risk and cost of pregnancy and puerperal morbidity attributable to chlamydial infection, but undoubtedly the cost-benefit ratio will be favorable at prevalence rates lower than 7 percent.[131] As a minimum preventive intervention at present we advocate selective diagnostic testing of pregnant women who are at high risk for chlamydial infection. Criteria for identifying women at high risk should be the same as for nonpregnant women, as outlined in Chap. 16. Screening should begin as early as possible during pregnancy.

## Treatment

Tetracyclines, the drugs of choice for *C. trachomatis* infection in nonpregnant adults, cannot be recommended for pregnant or nursing women. Erythromycin is considered the drug of choice in pregnant women. Among nonpregnant women, Oriel has reported that erythromycin stearate 500 mg orally twice daily for 2 weeks is as effective as tetracycline for the long-term eradication of chlamydia.[131a] Using erythromycin base in this dosage early in pregnancy, we have found treatment failures not infrequently, and higher daily dosage schedules were not well tolerated. Erythromycin estolate is probably contraindicated in pregnant women since 10 percent of pregnant women receiving the drug developed elevated serum glutamate oxaloacetate transaminase activity.[132a] Schachter et al.[133] reported that erythromycin ethylsuccinate 400 mg four times a day for 7 days given to pregnant women at approximately 36 weeks' gestation significantly reduced perinatal transmission of *C. trachomatis* from 50 percent among untreated mothers to 7 percent among treated mothers. Only 3 percent of pregnant mothers were intolerant of this regimen. Other agents with in vitro activity against *C. trachomatis* such as sulfonamides, chloramphenicol, trimethoprim-sulfamethoxazole, and rifampin are all contraindicated in pregnant women. While further clinical trials are needed to determine the efficacy and optimal dose and form of erythromycin for chlamydial infection in pregnant women, we recommend erythromycin ethylsuccinate 400 mg four times a day for 7 days for the treatment of chlamydial infection in pregnant women.

## Prevention of neonatal *C. trachomatis* infections

Hammerschlag et al.[132] reported that erythromycin ocular ointment was significantly more effective than 1 percent silver nitrate in preventing neonatal chlamydial conjunctivitis. Others have been unimpressed with the efficacy of topical erythromycin for this purpose.[133a] Laga et al.[104] evaluated the efficacy of 1 percent tetracycline ointment and 1 percent silver nitrate drops in the prevention of chlamydial ophthalmia. Both agents reduced the incidence of chlamydia conjunctivitis 68 to 77 percent in comparison with a historical control group of newborns who did not receive ocular prophylaxis. However, long-term follow-up of infants exposed to maternal chlamydial infection who received ocular prophylaxis revealed that 23 to 31 percent ultimately developed ocular *C. trachomatis* infection. Most of these infections were subclinical. As with gonococcal infection, the detection and treatment of chlamydial infection during pregnancy, together with ocular prophylaxis, would be preferable to neonatal ophthalmic prophylaxis alone.

## GROUP B STREPTOCOCCUS

### Epidemiology

Sexual transmission of group B streptococcus (GBS, *Streptococcus agalactiae*) is discussed in Chap. 69. GBS can be found as part of the vaginal flora of 5 to 25 percent of women. Only 1 in 50 to 1 in 100 neonates born to women with GBS vaginal colonization develop invasive disease, although 65 to 75 percent of exposed neonates become colonized.[134,135] Among nonpregnant women, GBS vaginal colonization is rarely associated with disease. Vaginitis and cervicitis have not been linked to this organism, but GBS is an occasional cause of pelvic inflammatory disease. Isolation rates are higher among young women (<20 years of age), are highest during the proliferative phase of the menstrual cycle, and are the same for pregnant as for nonpregnant women. Longitudinal studies of pregnant women have shown that approximately one-third or more are vaginal carriers of GBS at any time during pregnancy.[136] Among carriers, most appear to be intermittently colonized during pregnancy.[136,137] The risk of neonatal colonization with GBS is related more closely to the intrapartum culture status than to the antenatal or postnatal culture status.

### Influence of group B streptococcus on pregnancy and the neonate

Although the importance of GBS is greatest in neonatal infections, GBS has also been implicated in obstetric and puerperal complications. Regan et al.[138] reported that GBS colonization of the cervix at the time of parturition was significantly correlated with spontaneous ROM occurring 1 h or longer before onset of regular contractions, and with a threefold increase in preterm delivery at <32 weeks' gestation. Beargie et al.[139] noted that women from whom GBS was isolated prenatally had a five to tenfold excess rate of clinical amnionitis, postpartum endometritis, and neonatal sepsis when compared with the general obstetric population. As presented in Table 64-7, GBS was the second most common facultative bacterium isolated from the uterus or blood from febrile women with early postpartum endomyometritis in Seattle.

One to five cases of GBS neonatal sepsis per 1000 live births occur annually in the United States, accounting for about 3000 to 15,000 cases of neonatal sepsis per year. The mortality rate of neonatal GBS sepsis is 50 percent.[134,135] The manifestations of early-onset and late-onset disease in neonates are discussed in Chap. 69. Vertical transmission accounts for most early-onset disease, and early infection is significantly associated with premature birth, prolonged ROM, and maternal intra- and postpartum fever.[140,141] With late-onset disease, infection occurs after the first week of life; it is not associated with vertical transmission or with maternal obstetrical complications.[135]

The attack rate for GBS disease is only 1 to 2 percent among exposed neonates. Neonates at greatest risk have absent or low concentrations of maternal and neonatal serum antibody to GBS type-specific polysaccharide, are colonized by GBS in multiple anatomic sites, and have a high quantity of bacteria recovered from each site.[142,143] A high concentration of GBS in the vaginal flora is a risk factor for neonatal colonization[144] and perhaps for neonatal sepsis.

Since early-onset GBS infection in the neonate is associated with intrapartum fever, premature delivery, and prolonged ROM, amniotic fluid infection is a likely antecedent to many cases of early-onset infection. Eickoff observed that 40 percent of mothers who delivered neonates with GBS disease had clinical chorioamnionitis.[140] GBS may ascend from the vagina through the cervix to the chorioamniotic membrane, producing chorioamnionitis, amniotic fluid infection, rupture of membranes, and ineffective labor resulting in a prolonged interval from rupture of membranes until delivery. Alternatively, infection might also extend through membranes compromised by other factors. The presence of a high inoculum of vaginal GBS in a nonimmune host may favor the development of chorioamnionitis.

### Prevention of GBS disease

Antenatal culture screening for GBS and treatment of carriers has been proposed for prevention of GBS morbidity in the neonate and perhaps for prevention of obstetrical complications as well. The apparent prevalence of vaginal colonization is influenced by the type of screening cultures employed. Use of a selective medium to detect low concentrations of GBS increases the recovery of GBS from the vagina severalfold. However, the value of this enhanced sensitivity is questionable, since it may be more clinically relevant to detect those women in whom GBS is a predominant vaginal organism. Furthermore, both the intermittent nature of the carrier state and the high rate of recurrent infection after treatment is stopped severely limit the approach of antenatal treatment of carriers. It has been argued that even though recurrent infection is common after therapy during pregnancy, it might be feasible to detect and eradicate GBS for a "short but critical time period between 26 and 32 weeks, when a potential premature delivery would result in a viable neonate at highest risk for morbidity and death."[138,145] Indeed, this type of approach might also have merit for other infectious agents associated with premature ROM and preterm delivery, but until the relationship of various infectious agents to these complications has been sorted out by more comprehensive studies in which all infectious agents implicated in premature ROM and preterm delivery are sought simultaneously, there can be no strong rationale for antenatal treatment of GBS carriers at 26 to 32 weeks' gestation.

Intrapartum treatment of antenatal vaginal carriers of GBS is an alternative approach to prevent neonatal colonization by GBS.[146,147] At best, the predictive value of repeated prenatal screening of pregnant women for subsequent complications is 8 percent.[148] Thus, any program of this nature will treat a large number of women and infants unnecessarily. Boyer and Gotoff[149] demonstrated that ampicillin treatment of previously screened mothers who prenatally carried GBS and who presented with premature labor or prolonged ROM significantly reduced neonatal GBS colonization and prevented GBS bacteremia. A less expensive proposal was made by Minkoff and Mead,[150] who suggested that women presenting with premature labor should be treated with ampicillin while awaiting culture results. Newer methods of testing which could identify women with heavy GBS colonization within 5 h and who have premature ROM make this an attractive strategy.[151]

Another strategy would be to identify seronegative mothers and to antenatally immunize these women (see Chap. 69). It remains to be determined whether seronegative pregnant women will develop protective immunity in response to candidate GBS vaccines.

A final potential strategy would be prophylactic treatment of exposed neonates.[152,153] Siegel et al.[153] compared neonates who received parenteral penicillin with a similar group who received ocular instillation of tetracycline. Among the penicillin-treated group, the incidence of all serious bacterial disease due to penicillin-susceptible organisms, including GBS, was decreased; but the incidence of infection with penicillin-resistant pathogens increased during 1 of the 2 years of the study. Therefore, routine prophylactic treatment of all neonates with parenteral penicillin cannot currently be recommended for prevention of neonatal GBS disease.

## GENITAL MYCOPLASMAS

Many reproductive disorders have been ascribed to infection with the genital mycoplasmas. However, the ubiquity of these organisms and the high frequency of coinfection with other STD agents make it difficult to assess their etiologic roles in such disorders. In general, *M. hominis* has been associated with endometritis and postpartum fever while *U. urealyticum* has been correlated with amniotic fluid infection, chorioamnionitis, low birth weight, and prematurity. Their roles in infertility remain controversial.

Harwick et al.[154] detected *M. hominis* bacteremia in 8 percent of women with "septic" abortion vs. none of those with afebrile abortion. Serologic evidence of infection with *M. hominis* was found in 50 percent of septic abortions vs. 17 percent of afebrile abortions. These provocative data require confirmation, with studies of other relevant microbial species together with *M. hominis.*

Similar data link *M. hominis* to postpartum fever. Platt and colleagues,[67] in their follow-up study of 535 patients, found that 50 percent (14/28) of all postpartum fevers were associated with rises in titers of antibody to *M. hominis.* Positive genital colonization and low predelivery antibody titer to *M. hominis* were predictive of postpartum fever. Harrison et al.[123] also reported a significantly increased risk of postpartum endometritis/fever among women with antepartum *M. hominis* colonization who were delivered vaginally. However, only a small proportion of colonized women developed this complication. *M. hominis* has been isolated from amniotic fluid samples of women with signs of amnionitis,[155] and antibody responses to *M. hominis* have been detected in women with amniotic fluid infection.[156] However, almost invariably, another virulent organism was isolated in association with amniotic fluid infection, implying that *M. hominis* may be part of a mixed infection.

*Ureaplasma urealyticum* isolation from mothers, infants, and the placenta itself has been correlated with histopathological findings of chorioamnionitis with prematurity, and with perinatal death and neonatal morbidity. Kundsin et al.[157] isolated *U. urealyticum* from the chorionic surface of the placenta from 19 percent of pregnancies terminating in perinatal death, and from 27 percent which resulted in infants being admitted to a perinatal intensive care unit, as contrasted with 11 percent of placentas associated with normal full-term infants ($p < 0.005$ for both comparisons).

A number of studies have found a lower infant birth weight when there was genital colonization with *U. urealyticum.* Among vaginal carriers of *U. urealyticum,* those who demonstrate a significant rise in serum antibody titers to one of the serotypes of this organism at the time of parturition have a higher risk of delivering a low-birth-weight infant.[58] McCormack et al.[158] demonstrated that among pregnant women who were colonized with *U. urealyticum* erythromycin treatment in the third trimester was associated with a significantly higher infant birth weight, when compared with placebo treatment. Oddly, there was no effect of therapy started in the second trimester, and for those treated in the third trimester, the effect was limited to those who completed the 6 weeks of prescribed therapy. The recent large multicenter NICHHD Collaborative Study of vaginal infections in pregnancy has shown no benefit of erythromycin taken for up to 14 weeks, beginning at week 28, for vaginal colonization with *Ureaplasma* (DA Eschenbach et al., presented to the Society for Gynecologic Investigation, Baltimore, May 1988). Erythromycin is relatively ineffective in eradicating *U. urealyticum* from the vagina, probably because it has minimal antimicrobial activity at the acid pH of the vagina.

In Ethiopia, *U. urealyticum* was isolated as the sole agent from fetal lungs in 24 (8 percent) of 290 cases of perinatal death.[159] Twenty-two of these deaths occurred in utero, and all but one were associated with congenital pneumonia and chorioamnionitis. Eighteen of the 24 infected fetuses were born after 34 weeks' gestation, and in all, the initial obstetric event was labor rather than rupture of membranes. The authors suggest that most of these infections ascended through intact membranes to involve the amniotic fluid and fetus. Stagno et al.[160] also found *U. urealyticum* to be one of the commonest agents isolated from the nasopharynx of young infants with pneumonia; it was usually found in association with other STD agents.

Collectively these data are inconclusive regarding the role of antenatal colonization with *U. urealyticum* in chorioamnionitis, prematurity, and perinatal death. The etiologic role of this agent will remain uncertain until cohort or case control studies are completed in which other putative infectious causes of pregnancy morbidity, including other genital pathogens, are studied along with *U. urealyticum.*

### Current recommendations for management of genital mycoplasma infection during pregnancy

At present, antenatal serological studies or vaginal culture for either *U. urealyticum* or *M. hominis* are not recommended.

Postabortal and puerperal fever attributable to mycoplasma appear to be short-lived and relatively benign. Although a comprehensive diagnostic evaluation of women with postabortal and puerperal fever should include appropriate endometrial and blood cultures for *M. hominis,* this is infrequently done today except in clinical investigations. The tetracyclines are active against most strains of genital mycoplasmas, but the proportion of strains resistant to the tetracyclines is increasing, and tetracyclines may or may not be appropriate in the puerperal period. Erythromycin is active against *U. urealyticum* but not against *M. hominis,* while clindamycin is active against *M. hominis* but not against *U. urealyticum.*[161] Current evidence does not support the treatment of pregnant women colonized with *U. urealyticum* for prevention of prematurity.

## BACTERIAL VAGINOSIS

Bacterial vaginosis (BV) is characterized by a nonpurulent, homogeneous, malodorous vaginal discharge, by an increase in vaginal pH, by the presence of characteristic amines and organic acids in vaginal fluid, and by polymicrobial changes in vaginal flora, including a decrease in $H_2O_2$-producing facultative lactobacilli, and an increase in *Gardnerella vaginalis* and in several anaerobic species (Chap. 47).

The prevalence and natural history of BV do not appear to be dissimilar in pregnant and nonpregnant women.[162] However, BV and BV-associated microorganisms have been found to be correlated with amniotic-fluid-infection syndrome, prematurity, and puerperal infections. Edmunds[163] isolated *G. vaginalis* from the vagina from 71 percent of 45 women with and 31 percent of 26 without postpartum fever ($p = 0.001$). In 1979 at the University Hospital in Seattle, *G. vaginalis* was the most common isolate from blood and from the endometrium from women with postpartum fever and postpartum endometritis (Table 64-6). The relationship of BV to premature labor has been analyzed in a series of four studies at the University of Washington. Gravett et al.[164] initially found approximately a fourfold increase in premature onset of labor at ≥35 weeks' gestation among women with singleton pregnancies and intact membranes who had indirect evidence of BV, as determined by chromatographic analysis of vaginal fluids. In a separate prospective study of 534 pregnancies, the same group found that BV was significantly associated with premature rupture of membranes, preterm labor, and amniotic fluid infection but not with birth weight less than 2500 g.[119] Subsequently, Martius et al.[120] and Hillier et al.[33] have found a relationship of BV to preterm delivery and to chorioamnionitis and preterm delivery, respectively.

*G. vaginalis* has infrequently caused neonatal bacteremia, cutaneous abscess, and congenital pneumonia.[165] Anaerobes, however, may be relatively important in neonatal sepsis. Neonatal anaerobic sepsis is often associated with prematurity, amniotic fluid infection, and prolonged ineffective labor. Chow found that 26 percent of all cases of neonatal bacteremia observed at his institution were associated with anaerobes, with 1.8 episodes of anaerobic bacteremia per 1000 live births.[166] Anaerobic isolates were identified predominantly as bacteroides, peptococcus, and peptostreptococcus. The anaerobic flora associated with BV may provide a large inoculum and thus be associated with increased risk of anaerobic sepsis in the neonate.

### Case detection and management

At present BV is not generally treated during pregnancy since (1) the symptoms, if any, are well tolerated; (2) the possible relationship of BV to pregnancy morbidity has not been proved; (3) it has not been shown that treatment of BV during pregnancy reduces pregnancy or puerperal morbidity; and (4) the use of any drugs should be minimized in the pregnant woman. The diagnosis of BV can be made with reasonable accuracy by clinical examination or Gram stain of vaginal fluid (Chap. 47). The effect of treatment of BV during pregnancy on pregnancy and puerperal morbidity should be studied. In a pregnant woman who wants treatment for BV because of symptoms, use of amoxicillin can be considered (Chap. 47).

## CYTOMEGALOVIRUS INFECTION

Cytomegalovirus (CMV) is the commonest cause of congenital viral infection of the fetus and is the commonest infectious cause of mental retardation. The role of sexual transmission in the epidemiology of CMV is discussed in Chap. 36.

### Epidemiology of CMV infection during pregnancy

Several studies have shown increasing rates of isolation of CMV from pregnant women with advancing gestation. Women with the highest prevalence of CMV infection may tend to seek care only later in pregnancy. Stagno et al.[167] isolated CMV from nonpregnant women at the same rate as from demographically similar pregnant women studied in the third trimester, and suggested that lower rates of recovery in early pregnancy are actually due to suppression of CMV shedding in early pregnancy rather than to increased shedding in late pregnancy. Epidermal growth factor which interferes with the tissue culture isolation of CMV is present in urine during early pregnancy, and may artificially suppress recovery of CMV early in pregnancy.[168]

Reynolds et al.[169] found that young primiparous women are most likely to be cervical shedders of CMV. In one study 17 percent of women ≤14 years of age were culture-positive for CMV, compared with 0 percent of women ≥30 years of age.[167]

Most women from whom CMV is isolated during pregnancy have chronic or recurrent infection rather than primary infection. Depending on the serologic technique employed and the population studied, 50 to 90 percent of pregnant women have serum antibody to CMV. Stagno et al.[170,171] found that 36 percent of women in a middle- to high-income group and 77 percent of women in a low-income group were seropositive.

Among women who are seronegative at the beginning of pregnancy, primary infection occurs relatively frequently. As seen in Table 64-10, from 0.6 to 4.3 percent of seronegative women developed primary infection during pregnancy. At the present time primary CMV infection is undoubtedly many times more common than primary rubella infection during pregnancy.

Fetal, neonatal, and infant infections with CMV all occur frequently. Table 64-11 shows rates of congenital and infant infection in different settings. Congenital infection, as detected by isolation of CMV within the first week of life, occurred in 0.4 to 2.0 percent of liveborn infants studied in Western countries. Prevalence rates of CMV shedding increase during the first few months of life and peak between 3 and 9 months of age at rates ranging from 5.8 to 56 percent of all infants. High rates in some areas of the world seem independent of economic development.

Starr studied epidemiologic characteristics of mothers whose neonates developed congenital infection.[176] The mean maternal age of 19.0 ± 4.1 was significantly younger than that of the general population (22.9 ± 5.9, $p < 0.01$), and the frequency of primiparity (62 percent) was significantly greater than that of the general population (31 percent, $p < 0.01$). These data are also consistent with the concept that primary CMV infection during pregnancy was most likely to lead to congenital CMV infection. Stagno et al.[170] found in a prospective study that congenital CMV

**Table 64-10. Rate of Primary CMV Infection during Pregnancy**

| Series | Number of pregnancies | Number seronegative | Number with primary infection | | |
|---|---|---|---|---|---|
| | | | No. | Total | Percent |
| Monif et al.[173] | 6114 | 664 | 4 | 664 | 0.6 |
| Stern and Tucker[174] | 1040 | 347 | 11 | 254 | 4.3 |
| Griffiths et al.[172] | 5575 | 2387 | 14 | 1608 | 0.9 |
| Total | 12729 | 3398 | 29 | 2526 | 1.2 |

**Table 64-11. Rates of Congenital and Infant Infection with CMV**

| Country | Total number of infants | Percent shedding CMV according to age | | | | | | |
|---|---|---|---|---|---|---|---|---|
| | | At birth | 1 month | 2 months | 3 months | 6 months | 9 months | 12 months |
| Japan | 257 | – | 6 | 10 | 20 | 56 | 44 | 22 |
| Thailand | 140 | – | – | – | 38 | 55 | 18 | 15 |
| Guatemala | 109 | – | – | – | 23 | 42 | 40 | 35 |
| Finland | 148 | 2 | – | 16 | 32 | 36 | – | 39 |
| Sweden | 326 | 1 | 12 | – | – | – | – | 23 |
| England | 1395 | 0.4 | – | 1.8 | 3.2 | – | 5.8 | – |
| U.S., Seattle | 92 | 1 | 3 | – | 11 | 13 | – | 11 |
| U.S., Birmingham | 154 | 1.3 | 2 | 4 | 7 | 8 | 8 | 8 |

SOURCE: S Stagno et al.[175]

infections were attributable to primary maternal CMV infection in about half of the cases among high-income patients but were usually attributable to recurrent maternal infection among low-income patients. Importantly, primary maternal infections were significantly more likely than recurrent maternal infection to result in clinically apparent congenital CMV infection during the neonatal period when infection occurred within the first half of gestation.

## Manifestations in pregnant women and in the neonate

In the majority of pregnant women who develop primary CMV infection no recognized clinical illness is discerned. Starr could find no difference in the frequency or type of antenatal illness between 32 women who gave birth to congenitally infected infants and matched controls.[177] All but 1 of 14 primary CMV infections observed by Griffiths et al. in pregnant women were asymptomatic.[172] Heterophile-negative mononucleosis occasionally is recognized in a mother undergoing a primary infection, and Bell's palsy accompanying primary CMV infection has been described during pregnancy.[178]

Women with recurrent (nonprimary) CMV infections almost always have no recognizable clinical abnormality. Cervicitis has not been clearly linked to cervical CMV shedding, but Paavonen et al.[179] recently found a striking association between isolation of CMV from the cervix and the presence of colposcopically visualized immature metaplasia involving the zone of cervical ectopy (odds ratio for the association = 14.4, after adjustment for coinfections) among women attending an STD clinic. Thus, the presence of immature metaplasia could be examined as a risk factor for perinatal transmission of CMV. Isolate-positive women often have simultaneous shedding in the urine and milk, in addition to the genital tract.[167] However, attempts to recover CMV from white blood cells, or amniotic fluid from such women have not been successful. CMV has been isolated from placental tissue. Infected placentas may show chronic villitis with mononuclear or plasma cell infiltrates. Typical cytoplasmic inclusion bodies are not always seen.[180] Amniotic fluid infection, histological chorioamnionitis, and spontaneous abortion have not been recognized as manifestations of primary or recurrent maternal CMV infection.

Congenital infection is most common and often associated with early clinical manifestations among neonates born to nonimmune mothers who developed primary CMV infection during pregnancy. As seen in Table 64-12, among 37 pregnancies complicated by primary CMV infection in four separate studies, 16 (43 percent) were associated with congenital infections and nearly one-third of infants had clinical manifestations of CMV infection at birth or shortly thereafter.

Congenital infection is less common and much less often clinically apparent among neonates born to mothers with preexisting CMV infection. Stagno noted that seven (3.4 percent) of 208 seropositive women delivered congenitally infected neonates.[182] None of these neonates had apparent clinical involvement. Noting the high prevalence of seropositivity throughout the world, Stagno suggested that recurrent rather than primary infection during pregnancy may be the leading cause of intrauterine CMV infection. Stern et al.[174,183] concluded that cellular immunity may play a role in preventing intrauterine transmission of CMV. In their small study of women with primary CMV infection, they found that the eight women with positive lymphocyte transformation (LT) responses had unaffected infants in contrast to four congenitally infected infants born to the six women who had negative (LT) responses.

Clinical manifestations and prognosis of CMV infections in the child are described in (Chap. 70). Symptomatic congenital infection with CMV is characterized by hepatomegaly, splenomegaly, microcephaly, mental retardation, motor disability, jaundice, and petechiae. The mortality and long-term morbidity for such children are exceedingly high.[184] Often CMV-infected neonates are born prematurely and are of low birth weight. The birth weight may be inappropriately low for gestational age, suggesting intrauterine growth retardation.

**Table 64-12. Congenital CMV Infection among Infants of Mothers with Primary Infection during Pregnancy**

| Series | Number with primary CMV in mother | Number with congenital CMV infection | Number symptomatic |
|---|---|---|---|
| Monif et al.[173] | 4 | 4 | 2 |
| Stern and Tucker[174] | 11 | 5 | 1 |
| Gold and Nankervis[181] | 8 | 4 | 0 |
| Griffiths et al.[172] | 14 | 3 | 2 |
| Total | 37 | 16 (43%) | 5 (31%) |

Transplacental infection producing cytomegalic placentitis is well recognized and likely occurs during viremia associated with primary infection of the pregnant woman. When congenital CMV infection complicates nonprimary CMV infection during pregnancy, either transplacental or transcervical spread are possibilities.

Intrapartum CMV infection and infection during infancy and childhood occur much more frequently than does congenital infection. By the end of the first year of life 5 to 50 percent of infants have been infected. Intrapartum infection can result from exposure to maternal cervical CMV infection, while postpartum maternal-infant transmission can result from ingestion of infected maternal breast milk.[175] No short- or long-term ill effects are known to result from intrapartum or early postpartum CMV infection, but further study is necessary.

### Case detection and management

Although the incidence and clinical severity of congenital CMV infection are high following primary CMV infection during pregnancy, recommendations currently exist for early identification or seronegative pregnant women who are at risk for primary infections. Women who develop a viral-like illness during pregnancy should probably have serologic studies performed to exclude primary CMV, although most primary CMV infections in pregnancy are asymptomatic. Primary CMV infection if recognized in early pregnancy may be an indication for abortion since severe fetal involvement occurs in at least 31 percent of infants. Recurrent CMV infection in pregnancy is common, and no therapy exists. Gancyclovir is showing promise as an effective drug for CMV infections in AIDS patients and may be useful for primary CMV infection in early pregnancy or in infants with symptomatic CMV infection.[185] Further studies are needed to determine its safety and efficacy in pregnancy and in the newborn period.

Congenitally or perinatally infected infants often shed large amounts of the virus in saliva, respiratory secretions, and urine. Pregnant women should not be exposed to infants recognized to be shedding CMV.

## HERPES SIMPLEX VIRUS INFECTION

Herpes simplex virus (HSV) infection in pregnancy is of concern for two reasons: (1) primary HSV infection during pregnancy has been associated with an increased risk of spontaneous abortion and prematurity, and (2) maternal HSV at term is associated with life-threatening neonatal infection. Congenital infections are unusual.

### Epidemiology

The increase in incidence of genital HSV infection has been accompanied by an increase in neonatal HSV infection in some areas. The U.S. National Disease and Therapeutic Index Survey[186] showed a 15-fold increase in private physician consultations for genital herpes, and 8.8-fold increase in patient visits for newly diagnosed infections, from 1966 to 1984. In King County, Washington, the frequency of neonatal herpes rose from 2.6 to 11.9 cases per 100,000 live births between 1966 and 1981.[187] The point prevalence of HSV infection determined either cytologically or by culture among asymptomatic women seeking antenatal care is 0.5 to 1 percent. In the neonatal herpes simplex virus study, mothers of neonates acquiring HSV were most often young (mean age 21.2 years), white (63 percent), and primiparous (73 percent).[188]

### Natural history and manifestations of genital HSV infection during pregnancy

Primary genital infection with HSV is characterized by prolonged clinical illness, frequent systemic involvement indicating viremia, cervical infection, and high-titered viral shedding. These features distinguish primary from recurrent disease. Transplacental infection with HSV is recognized as a rare complication of viremia, and congenital infection with HSV occurs only rarely.[189]

As seen in Table 64-13, spontaneous abortion occurred in 54 percent of women with primary genital herpes occurring before 20 weeks' gestation, and low birth weight was seen in 35 percent of infants delivered by women who had primary genital herpes after 23 weeks of gestation.[190] These events may be attributable to either transplacental hematogenous infection or to ascending infection from the cervix. Histologic studies of the placenta and fetal membranes in such cases have not been reported.

More recently, Vontver et al. followed 80 pregnant women with a history of recurrent genital herpes, using repetitive clinical and virologic studies.[191] Fifty-six (70 percent) had at least one positive HSV culture during pregnancy. Ten had positive HSV cultures from the cervix, and 11 had positive vulvar cultures at a time when no lesions or symptoms were evident. The proportion with positive cultures did not change with advancing gestation. Twenty women (25 percent) had clinical or virologic evidence of recurrence within the week preceding delivery, but all had negative cervical and vulvar cultures 2 to 24 h prior to delivery. Only one neonate had a birth weight <2500 g, and the mean birth weight for the entire group was 3655 g. No neonatal disease occurred, although one neonate developed asymptomatic conjunctival infection with HSV. This study demonstrates the high recurrence rate of genital herpes during pregnancy, the fact that recurrences during pregnancy are no worse than recurrences in nonpregnant women, that recurrent genital herpes was not associated with prematurity, and that intrapartum transmission was uncommon. Although recurrences were frequent within the week prior to delivery, none were detectable intrapartum.

In contrast, primary genital HSV during pregnancy has substantial morbidity. Brown et al.[192] followed 29 women who

**Table 64-13. Risk of Spontaneous Abortion, Low Birth Weight, and Neonatal Infection in Primary vs. Recurrent Genital HSV Infection at Selected Times during Pregnancy**

| | Primary genital HSV | | | Recurrent genital HSV | | |
|---|---|---|---|---|---|---|
| | No. | Total | Percent | No. | Total | Percent |
| Spontaneous abortion* | 5 | 9 | 54 | 7 | 28§ | 25 |
| Birth weight < 2500 g† | 9 | 26 | 35 | 2 | 14 | 14 |
| Neonatal infection‡ | 3 | 6 | 50 | 1 | 23§ | 4 |

*Includes only cases diagnosed ≤ 20 weeks' gestation.
†Includes only cases diagnosed > 20 weeks' gestation.
‡Includes only cases diagnosed > 32 weeks' gestation and which were delivered vaginally.
§Includes cases of undetermined clinical type.
SOURCE: AJ Nahmias et al.[190]

acquired their first episode of genital herpes during pregnancy. Six infants (21 percent) developed severe perinatal morbidity (prematurity, intrauterine growth retardation, or neonatal HSV-2 infection). All six were born to mothers with a primary first episode of genital HSV infection; no infant born to a mother with a nonprimary first-episode infection had severe perinatal morbidity. Mothers with primary first-episode infection also more frequently shed HSV-2 asymptomatically from the cervix (10.6 percent per week) as compared with mothers with nonprimary first infection (0.5 percent per week, $p < 0.01$). Thus, infants born to women who acquire primary genital herpes during pregnancy are at high risk of HSV infection either due to premature labor at the time of the initial episode or subsequently because of exposure to asymptomatic cervical shedding of HSV-2.

## Risk of neonatal transmission

Most neonatal herpes simplex viral (HSV) infection is presumed to be due to intrapartum exposure to HSV-2 in the birth canal; up to 86 percent of HSV isolates from neonates are type 2. Few neonates are affected at birth, and most develop signs of infection in the second week of life. Up to one-half of neonates acquiring HSV infection have been exposed to mothers with primary infection occurring late in pregnancy. Whitley observed that 41 percent of neonates with HSV infection were <2500 g at birth, and that 51 percent lacked antibody to HSV in the initial serum sample.[188] Primary genital infection with HSV is likely the major risk factor for neonatal acquisition of HSV because of the large inoculum of virus present in the birth canal in primary maternal infection, the extensive cervical involvement, the absence of maternal antibody, and possible maternal viremia, all of which could contribute to the high risk of neonatal herpes in neonates born to mothers with primary genital herpes. Neonates born to mothers with recurrent HSV-2 infection appear to acquire protective immunity from the mother and are also at low risk of developing invasive disease.[191] Asymptomatic maternal genital HSV infection seems to be common among mothers of infants with perinatal HSV infection. Whitley observed that 70 percent of mothers with HSV-infected neonates had no signs or symptoms of HSV infection during pregnancy.[188] Only 38 percent of these mothers had a history of genital herpes or had sex partners with a history of genital lesions. This is consistent with recent unpublished studies from Atlanta and Seattle, which used improved serologic methods to differentiate antibodies to HSV-1 and HSV-2, and showed that only about one-third of individuals with antibody to HSV-2 actually give a past history suggestive of genital herpes.

In summary, the risk of perinatal morbidity with primary genital herpes during pregnancy is high, and probably includes spontaneous abortion, preterm delivery, intrauterine growth retardation, and neonatal HSV infection. Although the risk of neonatal infection is higher for primary maternal infections, up to 50 percent of neonatal infections may result from recurrent infection. Most of these infections arise from mothers who are not symptomatically shedding virus at the time of labor.

Whereas other neonatal viral infections are often subclinical, the majority of neonates with HSV infection have clinical manifestations of disease (see Chap. 70). The unique neonatal susceptibility to HSV infection which persists for several months following delivery is presumably related to a poor cellular immune response against HSV during this period.

The route of delivery and duration of rupture of membranes correlate with risk of neonatal infection among mothers who have genital herpes at term. Approximately 50 percent of neonates exposed to HSV during vaginal delivery acquired the disease. Cesarean section appeared to significantly reduce this risk if performed within 4 h of rupture of membranes, since only 1 (6 percent) of 16 neonates thus delivered acquired the disease.[192,192a] In cases where membranes had been ruptured for >4 h, nearly all exposed neonates acquired the disease (6 of 7), irrespective of the route of delivery.

## Case detection

Since it is not practical to perform routine screening cultures for HSV on all women throughout pregnancy, prevention of neonatal HSV infection currently rests on identifying high-risk women, on defining a strategy for clinical and virologic monitoring of this high-risk group, and on recognizing clinical manifestations of genital herpes in any woman near term. Whitley observed that 57 percent of mothers of neonates acquiring HSV had a history of HSV, a sex partner with genital lesions suggestive of HSV, or signs or symptoms of genital HSV infection during pregnancy.[188] The American Academy of Pediatrics recommends that women who have a history of recurrent genital HSV infection, with active disease during the current pregnancy, or whose sexual partners have proved genital HSV infection should be monitored during the last 6 weeks of pregnancy.[193] Unfortunately, Arvin et al.[194] reported that asymptomatic intrapartum shedding of HSV is not predictable from antepartum cultures for HSV. Furthermore, should inadvertent intrapartum neonatal exposure to HSV occur in a mother with asymptomatic HSV reactivation the risk of neonatal infection is less than 8 percent, much less than previously suspected.[191,191a] Cost-benefit analysis of weekly surveillance for asymptomatic HSV excretion in mothers near term has documented the extremely high cost of this program.[195] Analysis showed that screening of 3.6 million women would avert 11.3 neonatal deaths and 3.7 cases of severe retardation but 3.3 women would die as a result of cesarean delivery necessitated by culture results. The cost per case of neonatal HSV prevented was approximately $1.8 million.

## Management

Thus, we recommend the following approach. Clinicians should solicit and record in the prenatal record a history of genital herpes in the patient or her partner(s). These high-risk women should be observed carefully for clinical evidence of HSV reactivation and, in the absence of herpetic lesions during labor, should be delivered vaginally unless there are other indications for cesarean section. If recurrent herpetic lesions are present in the genital tract at the time of rupture of membranes or during labor, cesarean section may reduce the risk of neonatal infection, and should ideally be performed within 4 to 6 h after membrane rupture. At the time of delivery, women with a history of genital herpes or whose sex partner has a history should have a "sweep" culture of the vulva and cervix which is pooled for HSV culture, to identify potentially exposed neonates. Such infants, if clinically well, have a small risk of infection and should be followed closely. If clinical deterioration occurs or vesicular lesions develop, acyclovir can be started. These recommendations are similar, but not identical, to those offered by a group representing the Infectious Disease Society for Obstetrics and Gynecology.[196]

Although primary genital HSV infection in early pregnancy may cause spontaneous abortion, congenital infection is considered uncommon. For this reason therapeutic abortion is not recommended for pregnancies complicated by primary infection. If primary infection occurs at or near term, and genital herpetic lesions are present at time of rupture of membranes or during labor, there is general agreement that cesarean section should be performed if membranes have been ruptured for less than 4 h, although the American Academy of Pediatrics has recommended this time be increased to 12 h. We favor the latter recommendation. Infants born vaginally to mothers with primary infection are at particular risk of invasive disease. Consideration should be given to the early empiric use of acyclovir in this situation, although controlled trials of this approach are needed.

Hospital infection control procedures for protection of workers and other patients reflect the mode of transmission by direct contact or droplet. Patients with active lesions or who are culture-positive should have private rooms and bathrooms. Standard body substance isolation procedures should be followed with gowns and gloves used when handling contaminated articles; soiled linen and perineal pads should be handled as infected discharge and double-bagged.[197]

### Future developments in management of herpes during pregnancy

Acyclovir has become available for treatment for herpes simplex infections and has been successfully used in pregnancy to treat disseminated herpes infections.[198] Use of this agent for primary or recurrent infections near term to prevent transmission to the neonate needs study.

## HUMAN PAPILLOMAVIRUS

During the past decade, the number of office visits to physicians in the United States for condylomata acuminata, or genital warts, has dramatically increased.[199] Genital human papillomaviruses (HPV), the causative agents of genital warts and most cases of cervical intraepithelial neoplasia, are of concern in pregnancy for three reasons: (1) warts may rapidly enlarge with advancing gestation and mechanically obstruct labor, (2) the most common form of therapy, podophyllin application, is contraindicated during pregnancy, and (3) perinatal exposure may result in the development of laryngeal or genital papillomatosis in infancy or childhood. The worsening of cervical intraepithelial neoplasia (CIN) frequently observed during pregnancy may also be due to accelerated HPV replication.

### Epidemiology

Neonatal exposure probably occurs during birth by aspiration of contaminated cervical, vaginal, or vulvar material. During pregnancy, marked enlargement of genital warts may occur, associated with pronounced vascularity. During the puerperium, regression often follows. The mechanism underlying these changes is unknown but may relate to depression of maternal immunocompetence during pregnancy.

Laryngeal papillomatosis is the most frequent tumor of the larynx (Chap. 71). There is a bimodal age distribution with peaks in children between 2 and 5 years of age and in young adulthood. Twenty-eight percent of childhood cases were detected in infants under 6 months of age.[200] Studies using hybridization of labeled DNA probes prepared from various types of human papilloma virus, with cellular DNA from genital warts or from laryngeal papillomas, have shown that HPV types 6 and 11 account for the majority of genital warts and laryngeal papillomas.[201,202] There is a strong relationship between maternal genital warts during vaginal delivery and infant laryngeal papillomatosis.[203] History of condylomata acuminata can be obtained from over 50 percent of mothers whose infants develop laryngeal papillomas. Subclinical genital HPV infection is presumably responsible for most of the remainder. Perinatal transmission during vaginal delivery is the likely mode of spread, since children born by cesarean section seem to have a lower risk of acquiring the virus.[204] Anal-genital warts have been observed in infants and may also be related to maternal condylomata acuminata.[205] Papillomavirus DNA has also been detected in a small number of foreskins in normal newborn males.[206] The mode of acquisition in these cases is unclear.

### Case detection

A history of current or past genital warts may be useful in monitoring pregnant patients. Pregnant women with active or past genital warts should have Pap smears to detect CIN, and should be followed to detect recurrence or excessive growth of wart lesions.

### Treatment

In view of the potential complications of papillomavirus infection, removal of genital warts prior to delivery is desirable. The conventional techniques for treating genital warts in pregnancy include electrocoagulation, cryotherapy, and electrodesiccation. For large lesions, treatment of small areas in multiple sessions is recommended.[207–210] Ferenczy[210] has reported successful treatment of pregnant women using laser therapy with a failure rate of only 5 percent and relatively few complications. Since both maternal and neonatal deaths have resulted from podophyllin treatment of large vascular warts, this drug should not be used during pregnancy.

Cesarean section is not currently recommended to prevent neonatal exposure to papillomavirus. However, it may rarely be necessary in instances where extensive lesions obstruct the vaginal outlet.

## HUMAN IMMUNODEFICIENCY VIRUS (HIV)

With the high prevalence of HIV infection in women in some third world countries, and the increasing incidence of infection in women in North America and Europe, the effect of this virus upon pregnancy is increasing in importance. Although we have learned a great deal about HIV, we still know very little about its effect on pregnancy and pregnancy outcome, and this is the subject of current study for numerous research groups around the world.

### Maternal health

Women at greatest risk for HIV infection in North America include those who have received blood from an infected donor or who abuse intravenous (IV) drugs. However, as of 1988, nearly a third of U.S. women with AIDS were thought to have acquired it heterosexually, from men who abuse IV drugs, were bisexual, or were promiscuous heterosexuals.[211,212] A very small number of women have become infected through artificial insemination from an HIV-infected semen donor.[213] Whether pregnancy alters the natural history of HIV infection is still unknown. However, it is possible that the physiologic immune depression occurring during pregnancy might accelerate HIV infection, or transiently worsen the associated immunodeficiency. Preliminary results in IV-drug-abusing women in New York[214] have shown accelerated disease progression as measured by development of lymphadenopathy or oral thrush during pregnancy. This was not seen in the European multicenter study[215] or in a study from France.[216] However, in the latter study up to 25 percent of pregnant women were transiently p24-antigen-positive at delivery. Biggar et al.[217] found that patterns of immunosuppression were similar for HIV seropositive women and for HIV seronegative controls; however, the absolute number of CD4+ cells tended to be lower in seropositive women. The cohorts studied to date are small and further follow-up is necessary to confirm this impression. Other studies comparing seropositive and seronegative pregnant women have also shown slight progression in minor symptoms during pregnancy but no dramatic increase in development of AIDS.[218–220] It should be noted, however, that HIV seropositive pregnant women may have more infectious complications, such as gastroenteritis, pneumonia, pyelonephritis, and cellulitis, than do seronegative pregnant women[221] (M Braddick, unpublished data).

## Transmission of HIV from mother to the fetus and newborn

Prospective studies to date suggest that from 20 to 70 percent of infants exposed to a seropositive mother will acquire HIV infection.[222–228] However, the risk of perinatal transmission has varied widely and may be greater from symptomatic than from asymptomatic infected mothers. Problems have been encountered in confirming infection in exposed infants since all infants passively acquire maternal IgG antibodies against HIV. IgM antibody testing of cord blood has not yet proved reliable for predicting future serologic status of the exposed neonate. IgG titers may fall below detectable levels by 6 months only to reappear within a few months. In general, infants may have to be followed for 15 months to correctly determine their serologic status. Furthermore, antibody may be detected by one method but not by others; HIV antigen may be intermittently detected; and HIV can be isolated from blood of some seronegative infants even after 15 months of life. For the individual infant, multiple antibody, antigen, and viral isolation studies may therefore be necessary to determine whether infection has occurred. The detection of HIV-1 DNA by the polymerase chain reaction may be the optimal test.[223]

The relative frequency of in utero, intrapartum, and postpartum transmission from the mother is still uncertain. It is remarkable how slowly information on the clinical epidemiology of perinatal transmission of HIV has developed during the 1980s. At least some infants are infected prenatally, as suggested by the finding of HIV antigen in tissues from a neonate[229] who died at 20 days of age and from an aborted fetus.[230] Although a congenital syndrome considered characteristic of intrauterine HIV infection has been reported,[231] we have not yet seen evidence of this syndrome in a prospective case control study of HIV-exposed infants in Kenya. Cesarean section has not yet been found to prevent HIV transmission,[222] and the proportion of infants infected during birth is not known. Postnatal transmission may also occur via breast milk. Documented cases have occurred when the mother has been infected postpartum and seroconverted while breast feeding,[232] and HIV has been recovered from breast milk,[233] but the proportion of infected women who have HIV in breast milk is unknown. Nor is it known what added risk of transmission is imposed by breast feeding upon the infant who was already exposed in utero and at delivery. Breast milk is rich in IgA antibodies. Whether these are produced against HIV in breast milk in seropositive women, and whether they may neutralize the virus is unknown. In spite of these uncertainties, it seems wise to consider breast milk from a seropositive mother as potentially infectious.

## Treatment and prevention

Azidothymidine is the only effective treatment for the progressive immunodeficiency characterizing HIV infection. There has been limited experience with the drug during pregnancy. It is unknown whether the drug is embryotoxic. Whether AZT can prevent HIV transmission to the fetus is also unknown. Currently no antiviral agents have been evaluated for prevention of perinatal HIV transmission, nor has administration of gamma-globulin-containing antibodies to HIV been evaluated for this purpose.

## Case detection and prevention

One major issue involves screening of individuals for HIV infection. The Centers for Disease Control and the American College of Obstetricians and Gynecologists have recommended that pregnant women who are at increased risk for HIV infection should be counseled and tested.[234] Offering prepregnancy screening to women in high-risk groups would allow the high-risk woman to receive counseling and to decide to prevent pregnancy with contraception. Recent experience on the east coast of the United States has shown that the majority of pregnant women belonging to high-risk groups do not acknowledge high-risk behavior and refuse voluntary serologic testing, and these factors could also limit prepregnancy screening. IV-drug-abusing women in particular are difficult to access, and often noncompliant.

Screening women in the first trimester of pregnancy forces the decision regarding the recommendation of a therapeutic abortion. At present, no consensus has been reached as to whether abortion should be recommended to all seropositive women seen early in pregnancy. Screening all women in the first trimester of pregnancy might therefore have variable impact on the current pregnancy, though it should lead to counseling regarding avoidance of future pregnancies and avoidance of behaviors that could transmit the virus. The benefit-cost ratio would of course be highest in high-prevalence areas. Currently, data concerning the use of cesarean section to prevent perinatal HIV transmission are inconclusive.[222,231,235] Screening either cord blood or neonatal blood samples obtained on filter paper would allow early identification of HIV-exposed infants and an opportunity for counseling the infected women, regarding avoidance of future pregnancies and avoidance of other high-risk behaviors. Unfortunately, there is still no proved benefit of early intervention in HIV-exposed infants, although the possible benefit of prophylactic gamma globulin or prophylactic antimicrobial agents and of a heightened awareness of risk of infection cannot be ignored. Identification of seropositive women during pregnancy would permit counseling regarding avoidance of breast-feeding because of the potential for enteral transmission of HIV. Even this recommendation will likely prove unacceptable in the developing world because of the benefit of breast-feeding over bottle feeding in preventing infant mortality due to diarrhea. Thus we have the ironic contrast between the developed countries, where breast-feeding by HIV-positive mothers is considered contraindicated,

**Table 64-14. Potential Interventions Related to HIV Serologic Testing of the Pregnant Woman or of Cord Blood**

| | | |
|---|---|---|
| 1 | Therapeutic abortion | Important option |
| 2 | Cesarean section | Uncertain benefit |
| 3 | Counseling regarding future pregnancy | Important |
| 4 | Counseling regarding breast-feeding | Probably important |
| 5 | Usual conseling to avoid transmission of HIV | Important |
| 6 | Monitor infant immunosuppression, consider early prophylaxis, e.g., gamma globulin, antimicrobials (SMX-TMP), AZT | Uncertain benefits |
| 7 | Heightened awareness of risk or serious infection in the HIV-exposed child | Important |

and the developing countries, where bottle feeding, even by HIV-positive mothers, is currently still generally considered contraindicated.

In summary, there is no clear scientific or political consensus on many of the various potential interventions in HIV-positive pregnant women or HIV-exposed infants. However, a strong case can be made for active case detection programs for the following purposes: offering the option of therapeutic abortion, counseling against future pregnancy, counseling regarding breast-feeding, usual counseling to avoid transmission of HIV, and identification of exposed infants to permit early intervention and careful attention to vaccination (Table 64-14). Opponents of active case detection by serologic screening of pregnant women or cord blood are concerned about the societal risks of stigmatizing children as infected by HIV. Careful programs for patient counseling and confidentiality can reduce this risk.

Obviously, the major effort to prevent perinatal HIV infection must focus on reducing the incidence of HIV infection in all women, by education, prevention of IV-drug abuse, and avoiding high-risk sexual behavior. Breast milk donor programs, particularly where unpasteurized milk is used, and semen donor programs, like blood banks, should also screen their donors for HIV infection and high-risk practices. High-risk individuals should not donate. Antigen testing as well as antibody testing may eventually prove to be necessary in these settings. Finally, medical staff should be attentive to the increased physical and emotional needs of the pregnant and postpartum HIV-seropositive mothers, while still using precautions to prevent excess contact with blood and potentially infected body fluids, including amniotic fluid.[236]

## *Trichomonas vaginalis* VAGINITIS

Trichomonas vaginalis presents two problems unique to the pregnant host: (1) an association with puerperal maternal morbidity has been noted and (2) therapy with nitroimidazoles is not recommended during pregnancy, especially in the first trimester. Two early studies in the United States noted a 24 to 27 percent prevalence of *T. vaginalis* infection in pregnant women by microscopic examination of vaginal secretions.[237,238] A more recent study from Great Britain reported a 4 percent infection rate by culture among 868 third-trimester women.[239] Infection is significantly more common among blacks than among whites and significantly more common among women with gonorrhea.

Bland et al.[237] reported postpartum fever in 48 percent of 92 women with untreated antenatal trichomoniasis, compared with 25 percent of 110 women without trichomoniasis ($p = 0.001$). The difference was independent of race. These results, however, were not confirmed by Trussell et al.,[238] who noted postpartum fever in 8.5 percent of 223 women with trichomoniasis compared with 8.3 percent of 657 women without trichomoniasis. Further study of this issue is clearly needed. *T. vaginalis* might produce intra- or postpartum pelvic infections either on its own or through associated alterations in vaginal microbial flora. Quantitative increases in anaerobes commonly accompany vaginal infection with trichomonas (C Speigel et al., unpubished data), and it has been suggested that *T. vaginalis* may serve as a "vector" for the spread of other pathogens to the upper genital tract.[240]

Neonatal infection with *T. vaginalis* is detected infrequently and causes little morbidity. Because of estrogenic influence during pregnancy, the vaginal mucosa of female neonates is susceptible to infection or colonization with *T. vaginalis*. This is spontaneously reversed by 3 to 4 weeks postdelivery. The risk of neonatal infection with *T. vaginalis* overall is less than 1 percent, and among exposed neonates it is approximately 5 percent. Purulent vaginitis and urinary tract infection have been described as neonatal manifestations of infection.[241] Recently, *T. vaginalis* has been suspected as a cause of some cases of neonatal pneumonia.[241]

### Case detection

Whether pregnant women should undergo screening for *Trichomonas vaginalis* is unsettled, particularly in view of problems in therapy of infections detected early in pregnancy. Vaginal culture is more sensitive than direct microscopy of vaginal secretions, but *T. vaginalis* can be detected by microscopy in most women with symptomatic disease.[242] Vaginal fluid should be examined microscopically at any antenatal visit on all women with symptoms or signs of trichomonal vaginitis.

### Treatment

Nitroimidazoles are mutagens of bacteria and carcinogenic in some animals.[243] Studies which have examined the frequency of congenital defects in infants born to mothers treated during pregnancy with metronidazole[244,245] have not shown evidence of teratogenicity, although the numbers of patients examined precludes the exclusion of a small fetal risk. Metronidazole is probably safe in late pregnancy or postpartum, but treatment in early pregnancy should be deferred. Clotrimazole, used intravaginally, has reportedly been effective in some women with *T. vaginalis* vaginitis, and thus represents an alternative treatment.

## SUMMARY: APPROACH TO MANAGEMENT OF STDs IN PREGNANCY AND THE PERINATAL PERIOD

As an initial approach to the mangement of STD in pregnancy, a standard history concerning sexual behavior and past sexually transmitted diseases shold be obtained from all pregnant patients. Information on age, ethnicity, socioeconomic status, marital status, and health care behavior may also help identify those at highest risk of having STD. Specific questions, for example, should include (1) prior modes of contraception including IUD use; (2) previous history of gonorrhea, syphilis, vaginitis, genital warts, genital herpes, or pelvic inflammatory disease; (3) current sexual habits, number of current sexual partners (e.g., last 2 months), number of times of coitus per week, anticipated restriction of coital activity in pregnancy; (4) previous sexual experience (e.g., age at first coitus, lifetime number of sexual partners); and (5) intravenous drug abuse. Although it is not current practice to limit sexual activity during pregnancy, since data on the effects of coitus during pregnancy are conflicting, it may be wise to advise patients wishing to minimize risk that some studies have shown increased risk of prematurity and perinatal death with coital activity later in pregnancy. It may also be pointed out to such patients that sexual activity during pregnancy is quite variable but often declines as pregnancy progresses. Pregnant women should also be appraised of the particular risks of STD acquired during pregnancy.

Pregnant women in most populations should routinely undergo cervical screening culture for gonorrhea and serologic testing for syphilis. Those with a history of past gonococcal infection or who have more than one current sex partner should be screened again in late pregnancy with both tests, and in the United States it has been recommended that all women be tested for syphilis in late pregnancy. A routine screening test for *C. trachomatis* is indicated in pregnant women who have risk factors for chlamydial infection, as outlined in Chap. 16, especially in adolescents for whom the prevalence of chlamydial infection may exceed 25 percent. Schachter et al.[131] have argued that even culture testing (at $25 per test) is cost-effective in pregnant women when the prevalence of infection exceeds 6 percent. Tests for chlamydia should of course also be obtained from pregnant women with symptoms or signs consistent with chlamydial infection.

During pregnancy a number of clinical situations occur in which the patient should be evaluated for selected STDs. Dysuria, a common complaint in pregnancy, should not be attributed to urinary tract infection without excluding vaginitis, cervicitis, or urethritis as possible causes (see Chap. 46). Both gonorrhea and chlamydial infection can cause dysuria. Although it is not yet common practice, it seems advisable that women who suffer a syndrome consistent with cytomegalovirus (CMV) infection during pregnancy should be studied to exclude primary CMV infection in addition to other indicated studies. Women who have a history of genital herpes should be examined closely for recurrent clinical evidence of herpetic lesions late in pregnancy and during labor, as described above. Endocervical cultures for *N. gonorrhoeae* and *C. trachomatis* should be obtained from women at any stage of gestation who have signs of mucopurulent cervicitis or history of exposure to a sex partner with urethritis. Neonatal chlamydial conjunctivitis or pneumonia dictates examination and treatment of mother and father for chlamydial infection. It is to be emphasized that in the setting of neonatal STD, both parents must be interviewed, examined, and treated where appropriate. Women with otherwise unexplained complications such as septic abortion, premature labor, premature rupture of membranes, and intrapartum fever should be evaluated for sexually transmitted infection. Treatable infections (e.g., with *N. gonorrhoeae* and *C. trachomatis*) should always be excluded in women with these complications. Women with late-onset endometritis also should be evaluated for *C. trachomatis* infection.

Special surveillance of the neonate may be necessary when the mother is at high risk for STDs or develops puerperal infection or intrapartum fever. Such neonates may have to be closely monitored in the hospital for clinical evidence of sepsis and out of the hospital for evidence of ocular or respiratory infection.

Neonates exposed during delivery to HSV require especially close surveillance including frequent cultures from eye, throat, skin, rectum, and lesions, and antiviral treatment at the first clinical or virologic evidence of HSV infection.

Considerable controversy surrounds the use of neonatal ocular prophylaxis. To permit initial maternal-neonatal bonding, the American Academy of Pediatrics recommendations allow for prophylaxis to be delayed for up to 1 h following birth. Presently silver nitrate, erythromycin, and tetracycline ointment have all been recommended for the prevention of gonococcal ophthalmia neonatorum. An additional benefit of ocular prophylaxis may be the prevention of chlamydial conjunctivitis; the 1-h delay in applying prophylaxis may reduce the efficacy of prophylaxis for this purpose.

Neonatal prophylaxis for other STDs such as neonatal group B streptococcal disease and HSV requires further study. The efficacy of passive-active immunization for neonates exposed to hepatitis B has led to the recent recommendations that all women be tested early in pregnancy for HBsAg (later if clinically indicated), and that infants born to HBsAg-positive mothers receive both hepatitis B immunoglobulin, 0.5 ml intramuscularly, and hepatitis B vaccine in appropriate dosage[246] (Chap. 40).

In summary, as shown in Table 64-15, a spectrum of clinical events occurring during pregnancy is associated with infection by STD agents. The obstetric consequences of antepartum STD have been largely neglected until recently and, in fact, represent one

**Table 64-15. Disorders of Pregnancy and the Puerperium That Have Been Associated with Infection by STD Agents in One or More Studies**

| Clinical event | Associated STD agents |
|---|---|
| Ectopic pregnancy | Prior *C. trachomatis* infection; also, 50% of cases have histologic evidence of prior salpingitis |
| Spontaneous abortion | *N. gonorrhoeae, M. hominis, U. urealyticum,* herpes simplex virus |
| Posttherapeutic abortion–pelvic inflammatory disease | *C. trachomatis, N. gonorrhoeae* |
| Premature delivery, premature and prolonged rupture of membranes | *C. trachomatis, N. gonorrhoeae, Strep. agalactiae* (group B streptococci), bacterial vaginosis, *M. hominis, U. urealyticum, T. pallidum,* herpes simplex virus, cytomegalovirus |
| Amniotic fluid infection | Bacterial vaginosis, *Strep. agalactiae, N. gonorrhoeae* |
| Congenital abnormalities | CMV, HSV, HIV, *T. pallidum* |
| Intrauterine growth retardation | CMV, HSV, HIV, *T. pallidum* |
| Puerperal endomyometritis: | |
| Early (< 48 h postdelivery) | Bacterial vaginosis, *Strep. agalactiae, U. urealyticum, M. hominis, T. vaginalis* |
| Late (> 48 h postdelivery) | *C. trachomatis* |
| Perinatal: | |
| Stillbirth | *T. pallidum,* cytomegalovirus, *C. trachomatis* |
| Neonatal death, neonatal sepsis | *Strep. agalactiae,* herpes simplex virus, *N. gonorrhoeae, C. trachomatis* |

of the most important areas for future research on STD. Many studies have shown a relationship of individual STD agents to specific obstetric complications, as reflected by the large number of citations in this relatively selective review of STD in pregnancy. These individual studies are sometimes difficult to interpret, because coinfection with more than one STD agent is common, and STD infection itself may be associated with other noninfectious risk factors for obstetric morbidity. Primary infection with particular STD agents may carry a higher risk than chronic or recurrent infection with those same agents or less pathogenic STD agents. It may be that coinfection with multiple STD agents is synergistic or additive in causing obstetric morbidity. For example, primary infection with an agent such as *C. trachomatis*, *N. gonorrhoeae*, or HSV might produce chorioamnionitis and lead to premature rupture of membranes, which in turn might lead to a particularly high risk of amniotic fluid infection syndrome in the presence of bacterial vaginosis or trichomonal vaginitis, because of the increased concentration of anaerobic pathogens in the vagina in these types of vaginitis.

We must emphasize the underlying theme of this chapter: No study has yet been undertaken which has examined all the relevant STD agents simultaneously in relation to obstetric puerperal and perinatal morbidity, while controlling for sexual behavior and other risk factors which are associated with such morbidity. Definitive studies must include not only comprehensive antepartum maternal screening by culture with appropriate epidemiologic study design but also serologic testing to distinguish primary from recurrent infections, with histologic and microbiological examination of the placenta and membranes.

## References


1 Finland M: Pneumonia and pneumococcal infections with special reference to pneumococcal pneumonia. *Am Rev Respir Dis* 120:481, 1979.

2 Rao AR et al: Pregnancy and smallpox. *J Indian Med Assoc* 40:353, 1963.

3 Greenberg M et al: Maternal mortality in the epidemic of Asian influenza, New York, 1957. *Am J Obstet Gynecol* 76:897, 1958.

4 Siegel M, Greenberg M: Incidence of poliomyelitis in pregnancy. Its relation to maternal age, parity and gestational period. *N Engl J Med* 253:841, 1955.

5 Odds FC: Factors that predispose the host to candidosis, in *Candida and Candidosis,* FC Odds (ed). Baltimore, University Park Press, 1979, p 75.

6 Gilles HM et al: Malaria, anaemia and pregnancy. *Ann Trop Med Parasitol* 63:245, 1969.

7 Khuroo MS et al: Incidence and severity of viral hepatitis in pregnancy. *Am J Med* 70:252, 1981.

8 Moore JE: Studies on the influence of pregnancy in syphilis. I. The course of syphilitic infection in pregnant women. *Johns Hopkins Med Bull* 34:89, 1923.

9 Hodes HL: Effect of pregnancy upon immunity of mice vaccinated against St Louis encephalitis virus. *J Exp Med* 69:533, 1939.

10 Suzuki K, Tomasi TB: Immune responses during pregnancy. Evidence of suppressor cells for splenic antibody response. *J Exp Med* 150:898, 1979.

11 St Hill CA et al: Depression of cellular immunity in pregnancy due to a serum factor. *Br J Med* 1:513, 1973.

12 Stanley Y: Fetuin an inhibitor of lymphocyte transformation. *J Exp Med* 141:242, 1975.

13 Sridama V et al: Decreased levels of helper T cells. A possible cause of immunodeficiency in pregnancy. *N Engl J Med* 307:352, 1982.

14 Brunham RC et al: Depression of the lymphocyte transformation response to microbial antigens and to phytohemagglutinin during pregnancy. *J Clin Invest* 72:1629, 1983.

15 Gehrz RC et al: A longitudinal analysis of lymphocyte proliferative responses to mitogens and antigens during human pregnancy. *Am J Obstet Gynecol* 140:655, 1981.

16 Finland M: Pneumonia, in *Obstetric and Perinatal Infections,* D Charles, M Finland (eds). Philadelphia, Lea & Febiger, 1973, p 167.

17 Singer A: The uterine cervix from adolescence to the menopause. *Br J Obstet Gynaecol* 82:81, 1975.

18 Ayra OP et al: Epidemiological and clinical correlates of chlamydial infection of the cervix. *Br J Vener Dis* 57:118, 1981.

19 Moghissi KS: Composition and function of cervical secretion, in *Handbook of Physiology,* sec 7; *Endocrinology,* vol 2, Female Reproductive System, pt 2, RL Greep (ed). Washington, American Physiological Society, 1973, p 25.

20 Sarrell PM, Pruett KA: Symptomatic gonorrhea during pregnancy. *Obstet Gynecol* 32:670, 1968.

21 Russell P: Inflammatory lesions of the human placenta. I. Clinical significance of acute chorioamnionitis. *Am J Diagn Gynecol Obstet* 1:127, 1979.

22 Larsen B, Galask RP: Vaginal microbial flora: Practical and theoretic relevance. *Obstet Gynecol* 55(suppl 5):100S, 1980.

23 Goplerud CP et al: Aerobic and anaerobic flora of the cervix during pregnancy and the puerperium. *Am J Obstet Gynecol* 126:858, 1976.

24 Bone NC, Greene RR: Histologic study of uterine tubes with tubal pregnancy. *Am J Obstet Gynecol* 82:1166, 1961.

25 Novak E, Darner HL: Correlation of uterine and tubal changes in tubal gestation. *Am J Obstet Gynecol* 9:295, 1975.

26 Brunham RC et al: *Chlamydia trachomatis* infection in women with ectopic pregnancy. *Obstet Gynecol* 67:721, 1987.

27 Kosseim M, Brunham RC: Fallopian tube obstruction as a sequela to *Chlamydia trachomatis* infection. *Eur J Clin Microbiol* 5:584, 1986.

28 Olding LB et al: Pathogenesis of cytomegalovirus infection. I. Activation of virus from bone marrow–derived lymphocytes by *in vitro* allogenic reaction. *J Exp Med* 141:561, 1975.

29 McIntyre JA, Faulk WP: Antigens of human trophoblast. Effects of heterologous anti-trophoblast sera on lymphocyte responses *in vitro*. *J Exp Med* 149:824, 1979.

30 Russell P, Altshuler G: Placenta abnormalities of congenital syphilis. A neglected aid to diagnosis. *Am J Dis Child* 128:160, 1974.

31 Hayes K, Gibas H: Placental cytomegalovirus infection without fetal involvement following primary infection in pregnancy. *J Pediatr* 79:401, 1971.

32 Dorman HB, Sahyun PF: Identification and significance of spirochetes in the placenta. A report of 105 cases with positive findings. *Am J Obstet Gynecol* 33:954, 1937.

33 Hillier SL et al: Case control study of chorioamnionic infection and chorioamnionitis in prematurity. *N Engl J Med* 319:972, 1988.

34 Naeye R, Kissane JM: Perinatal diseases, a neglected area of the medical sciences, in *Perinatal Diseases,* RL Naeye et al (eds). International Academy of Pathology monograph. Baltimore, Williams & Wilkins, 1980, p 1.

35 Naeye R: Causes and consequences of chorioamnionitis. *N Engl J Med* 293:40, 1975.

36 Shurin PA et al: Chorioamnionitis and colonization of the newborn infant with genital mycoplasmas. *N Engl J Med* 293:5, 1975.

37 Lauweryns J et al: Intrauterine pneumonia. An experimental study. *Bio Neonate* 22:301, 1973.

38 Bobitt JR, Ledger WJ: Unrecognized amnionitis and prematurity: A preliminary report. *J Reprod Med* 19:8, 1977.

39 Miller et al: Bacterial colonization of amniotic fluid in the presence of ruptured membranes. *Am J Obstet Gynecol* 137:451, 1980.

40 Gibson M, Williams PP: *Haemophilus influenzae* amnionitis associated with prematurity and premature membrane rupture. *Obstet Gynecol* 52(suppl 1):70S, 1978.

41 Naeye RL, Peters EC: Causes and consequences of premature rupture of fetal membranes. *Lancet* 1:192, 1980.
42 Gluck L et al: Septicemia of the newborn. *Pediatr Clin North Am* 13:1131, 1966.
43 Schlievert P et al: Amniotic fluid antibacterial mechanisms: Newer concepts. *Semin Perinatol* 1:59, 1977.
43a Blanc W: Pathology of the placenta, membranes, and umbilical cord in bacterial, fungal and viral infection of man, in *Perinatal Diseases,* RL Naeye et al (eds). International Academy of Pathology monograph. Baltimore, Williams & Wilkins, 1980, p 67.
44 Larsen B, Galask RP: Host resistance to intra-amniotic infection. *Obstet Gynecol Surv* 30:675, 1975.
45 Naeye RL, Blanc WA: Relation of poverty and race to antenatal infection. *N Engl J Med* 283:555, 1970.
46 Naeye RL et al: Fetal and maternal features of antenatal bacterial infections. *J Pediatr* 79:733, 1971.
47 Naeye RL: Common environmental influences on the fetus, in *Perinatal Diseases,* RL Naeye (ed). International Academy of Pathology monograph. Baltimore, Williams & Wilkins, 1980, p 52.
48 Naeye RL: Coitus and associated amniotic-fluid infection. *N Engl J Med* 301:1198, 1979.
49 Naeye RL: Seasonal variations in coitus and other risk factors and the outcome of pregnancy. *Early Hum Dev* 4:61, 1980.
50 Keller CA, Nugent RP: Seasonal patterns in perinatal mortality and preterm delivery. *Am J Epidemiol* 118:689, 1983.
51 Mills JL et al: Should coitus late in pregnancy be discouraged? *Lancet* 1:136, 1981.
52 Biggers JD: *In vitro* fertilization and embryo transfer in human beings. *N Engl J Med* 304:336, 1981.
53 Harlap S et al: A prospective study of spontaneous fetal losses after induced abortions. *N Engl J Med* 301:677, 1979.
54 Bottoms SF et al: The increase in the cesarean birth rate. *N Engl J Med* 302:559, 1980.
55 CDC. Progress towards achieving the 1990 objectives for pregnancy and infant health. *MMWR* 37:405, 1988.
56 Rush RW et al: Contribution of preterm delivery to perinatal mortality. *Br Med J* 2:905, 1976.
57 Elder HA et al: The natural history of asymptomatic bacteriuria during pregnancy: The effect of tetracycline on the clinical course and the outcome of pregnancy. *Am J Obstet Gynecol* 111:441, 1971.
58 Kass EH et al: Genital mycoplasmas as a cause of excess premature delivery. *Trans Assoc Am Physicians* 94:261, 1981.
59 McGregor JA et al: Adjunctive erythromycin treatment for idiopathic preterm labor. Results of a randomized, double-blinded, placebo-controlled trial. *Am J Obstet Gynecol* 154:98, 1986.
60 Minkoff H: Prematurity: Infection as an etiologic factor. *Obstet Gynecol* 62:137, 1983.
61 Evaldson G et al: Microbiological findings in pregnant women with premature rupture of membranes. *Med Microbiol Immunol* 168: 283, 1980.
62 Creatsas G et al: Bacterial contamination of the cervix and premature rupture of membranes. *Am J Obstet Gynecol* 139:522, 1981.
63 Bejar R et al: Premature labor. II. Bacterial sources of phospholipase. *Obstet Gynecol* 57:479, 1981.
64 Huszar G, Naftolin F: The myometrium and uterine cervix in normal and preterm labor. *N Engl J Med* 311:571, 1984.
65 MacDonald P et al: From the National Institutes of Health: Summary of a workshop on maternal genitourinary infections and the outcome of pregnancy. *J Infect Dis* 147:596, 1983.
66 Plummer FA et al: Postpartum upper genital tract infections in Nairobi, Kenya: Epidemiology, etiology and risk factors. *J Infect Dis* 156:92, 1987.
66a Platt L et al: The role of anaerobic bacteria in postpartum endomyometritis. *Am J Obstet Gynecol* 135:814, 1979.
67 Platt R et al: Infection with *Mycoplasma hominis* in postpartum fever. *Lancet* 2:1217, 1980.
68 Harrison AR et al: Cervical *Chlamydia trachomatis* and mycoplasmal infections. Epidemiology and outcome. *JAMA* 250:1721, 1983.
69 Wallace RJ et al: Isolation of *Mycoplasma hominis* from blood cultures in patients with postpartum fever. *Obstet Gynecol* 51:181, 1978.
70 Rosene K et al: Polymicrobial early postpartum endometritis with facultative and anaerobic bacteria, genital mycoplasmas, and *Chlamydia trachomatis*: Treatment with piperacillin or cefoxitin. *J Infect Dis* 153(6):1028, 1986.
71 Wager GP et al: Puerperal infectious morbidity: Relationship to route of delivery and to antepartum *Chlamydia trachomatis* infection. *Am J Obstet Gynecol* 138:1028, 1980.
72 Cates W et al: Worldwide patterns of infertility: Is Africa different? *Lancet* 2:596, 1985.
73 Siegel JD, McCracken GH: Sepsis neonatorum. *N Engl J Med* 304:642, 1981.
74 Dippel AL: The relationship of congenital syphilis to abortion and miscarriage and the mechanisms of intrauterine protection. *Am J Obstet Gynecol* 47:369, 1944.
75 Naeye RL: Causes of perinatal mortality in the US collaborative perinatal project. *JAMA* 238:228, 1977.
76 CDC: Syphilis and congenital syphilis—United States, 1985–1988. *MMWR* 37:486, 1988.
77 Mascuta L et al: Congenital syphilis. Why is it still occurring? *JAMA* 252:1719, 1984.
78 CDC: Guidelines for the prevention and control of congenital syphilis. *MMWR* 37:S1:1, 1988.
79 Ratnam AV et al: Syphilis in pregnant women in Zambia. Presented at the First Sexually Transmitted Diseases World Congress, San Juan, Puerto Rico, 1981.
80 Fiumara NJ et al: The incidence of prenatal syphilis at the Boston City Hospital. *N Engl J Med* 247:48, 1952.
81 Brown WH, Pearce L: On the reaction of pregnant and lactating females to inoculation with *Treponema pallidum*—A preliminary note. *Am J Syph* 4:593, 1920.
82 Harter CA, Benirschke K: Fetal syphilis in the first trimester. *Am J Obstet Gynecol* 124:705, 1976.
83 Benirschke K: Syphilis—The placenta and the fetus. *Am J Dis Child* 128:142, 1974.
84 Silverstein AM: Congenital syphilis and the timing of immunogenesis in the human fetus. *Nature* 194:196, 1962.
85 Blount JH, Holmes KK: Epidemiology of syphilis and the nonvenereal treponematosis, in *The Biology of Parasitic Spirochetes,* RC Johnson (ed). New York, Academic, 1976, p 157.
86 Stray-Pederson B: Economic evaluation of maternal screening to prevent congenital syphilis. *Sex Transm Dis* 10:167, 1983.
87 Wendel GD Jr et al: Penicillin allergy and desensitization in serious infections during pregnancy. *N Engl J Med* 312:1229, 1985.
88 Thompson SE: Treatment of syphilis in pregnancy. *J Am Vener Dis Assoc* 3:159, 1976.
89 Rothenberg R: Ophthalmic neonatorum due to *Neisseria gonorrhoeae*: Prevention and treatment. *Sex Transm Dis* 6(suppl 2):187, 1979.
90 CDC: Declining rates of rectal and pharyngeal gonorrhea among men—New York City. *JAMA* 252:327, 1984.
91 Rice RJ et al: Gonorrhea in the United States 1975–1984: Is the giant only sleeping? *Sex Transm Dis* 14:83, 1987.
92 Goodrich JT: Treatment of gonorrhea in pregnancy. *Sex Transm Dis* 6:168, 1979.
93 Corman LC et al: The high frequency of pharyngeal gonococcal infection in a prenatal clinic population. *JAMA* 230:568, 1974.
94 Stutz DR et al: Oropharyngeal gonorrhea during pregnancy. *J Am Vener Dis Assoc* 3:65, 1976.
95 Holmes KK et al: Disseminated gonococcal infection. *Ann Intern Med* 74:979, 1971.
96 Platt R et al: Risk of acquiring gonorrhea and prevalence of abnormal adnexal findings among women recently exposed to gonorrhea. *JAMA* 23:3205, 1983.

97 Acosta AA et al: Intrauterine pregnancy and coexistent pelvic inflammatory disease. *Obstet Gynecol* 37:282, 1971.

98 Morse SA, Fitzgerald JJ: Effect of progesterone on *Neisseria gonorrhoeae*. *Infect Immun* 10:1370, 1974.

99 Moghissi KS: Cyclic changes of cervical mucus in normal and progestin-treated women. *Fertil Steril* 17:663, 1966.

100 Edwards L et al: Gonorrhea in pregnancy. *Am J Obstet Gynecol* 132:637, 1978.

101 Berstine JB, Bland GW: Gonorrhea complicating pregnancy and its relation to ophthalmia neonatorum. *Urol Cut Rev* 52:464, 1948.

102 Burkman RT et al: Untreated endocervical gonorrhea and endometritis following elective abortion. *Am J Obstet Gynecol* 126:648, 1976.

103 Goddeiris JH, Bronken TP: Benefit-cost analysis of screening. A comparison of tests for gonorrhea. *Med Care* 23:1242, 1985.

104 Laga M et al: Epidemiology of ophthalmia neonatorum in Kenya. *Lancet* 2:1145, 1986.

104a Laga M, Plummer FA, Piot P, et al: Prophylaxis of gonococcal and chlamydial ophthalmia neonatorum. A comparison of silver nitrate and tetracycline. *N Engl J Med* 318:653, 1988.

105 Handsfield HH et al: Neonatal gonococcal infection. I. Orogastric contamination with *Neisseria gonorrhoeae*. *JAMA* 225:697, 1973.

106 Rothbard MJ et al: Intrapartum gonococcal amnionitis. *Am J Obstet Gynecol* 121:565, 1975.

107 Armstrong JH et al: Ophthalmia neonatorum: A chart review. *Pediatrics* 57:884, 1976.

108 Thompson TR et al: Gonococcal ophthalmia neonatorum. Relationship of time of infection to relevant control measures. *JAMA* 228:186, 1974.

109 Schoolnik GK et al: Immunoglobulin class responsible for gonococcal bactericidal activity of normal human sera. *J Immunol* 122:1771, 1979.

110 Khurana CM et al: Prevalence of *Chlamydia trachomatis* in the pregnant cervix. *Obstet Gynecol* 66:241, 1985.

111 Harrison HR et al: The prevalence of genital *Chlamydia trachomatis* and Mycoplasmal infections during pregnancy in an American Indian population. *Sex Transm Dis* 10:184, 1983.

112 Githin D: Development and metabolism of the immune globulins, in *Immunologic Incompetence*, B Kagen, ER Stiehm (eds). Chicago, Year Book Medical, 1971, p 3.

113 Rowland GF, Moss TR: In vitro fertilization, previous ectopic pregnancy, and *Chlamydia trachomatis* infection. *Lancet* 2:830, 1985.

114 Page LA, Smith PC: Placentitis and abortion in cattle inoculated with Chlamydiae isolated from aborted human placental tissue. *Proc Soc Exp Biol Med* 146:269, 1974.

115 Schachter J: Isolation of Bedsoniae from human arthritis and abortion tissue. *Am J Ophthalmol* 63:1082, 1967.

116 Chandler JW et al: Ophthalmia neonatorum associated with maternal chlamydial infections. *Trans Am Acad Ophthalmol Otolaryngol* 83:302, 1978.

117 Rowe DS et al: Purulent ocular discharge in neonates: Significance of *Chlamydia trachomatis*. *Pediatrics* 63:628, 1979.

118 Martin DH et al: Prematurity and perinatal mortality in pregnancies complicated by maternal *Chlamydia trachomatis* infections. *JAMA* 247:1585, 1982.

119 Gravett MG et al: Independent associations of bacterial vaginosis and *Chlamydia trachomatis* infections with adverse pregnancy outcome. *JAMA* 256:1899, 1986.

120 Martus J et al: Relationships of vaginal lactobacillus sp., cervical *Chlamydia trachomatis*, and bacterial vaginosis to preterm birth. *Obstet Gynecol* 71:89, 1988.

121 Frommell GT et al: Chlamydial infection of mothers and their infants. *J Pediatr* 95:28, 1979.

122 Heggie AD et al: *Chlamydia trachomatis* infection in mothers and infants. *Am J Dis Child* 135:507, 1981.

123 Harrison HR et al: The epidemiology and effects of genital *C. trachomatis* and mycoplasmal infections in pregnancy. *JAMA* 250:1751, 1983.

124 Berman SM et al: Low birth weight, prematurity, and postpartum endometritis. Association with prenatal cervical *Mycoplasma hominis* and *Chlamydia trachomatis* infections. *JAMA* 257:1189, 1987.

125 Sweet RL et al: *Chlamydia trachomatis* infection and pregnancy outcome. *Am J Obstet Gynecol* 156:824, 1987.

126 Thygeson P, Stone W: Epidemiology of inclusion conjunctivitis. *Arch Ophthalmol* 27:91, 1942.

127 Rees E et al: Chlamydia in relation to cervical infection and pelvic inflammatory disease, in *Non-gonococcal Urethritis and Related Infections*, K Hobson, KK Holmes (eds). Washington, American Society for Microbiology, 1977, p 140.

128 Qvigstad E et al: Therapeutic abortion and *Chlamydia trachomatis* infection. *Br J Vener Dis* 58:182, 1982.

129 Moller BR et al: Pelvic infection after elective abortion associated with *Chlamydia trachomatis*. *Obstet Gynecol* 59:210, 1982.

130 Osser S, Persson K: Postabortal pelvic infection associated with *Chlamydia trachomatis* and the influence of humoral immunity. *Am J Obstet Gynecol* 150:699, 1984.

131 Schachter J, Grossman M: Chlamydial infections. *Annu Rev Med* 32:45, 1981.

131a Oriel JD, Ridgway GL: Comparison of erythromycin and oxytetracycline in the treatment of cervical infection by *Chlamydia trachomatis*. *J Infect* 2:259, 1980.

132 Hammerschlag MR et al: Erythromycin ointment for ocular prophylaxis of neonatal chlamydial infections. *JAMA* 244:2291, 1980.

132a McCormack WM et al: Hepatotoxicity of erythromycin estolate during pregnancy. *Antimicrob Agents Chemother* 12:630, 1977.

133 Schachter J et al: Experience with the routine use of erythromycin for chlamydial infections in pregnancy. *N Engl J Med* 314:276, 1986.

133a Bell TA et al: Comparison of ophthalmic silver nitrate solution and erythromycin ointment for prevention of natally acquired *Chlamydia trachomatis*. *Sex Transm Dis* 14:195, 1987.

134 Anthony BF, Okada DM: The emergence of group B streptococci in infections of the newborn infant. *Annu Rev Med* 28:355, 1977.

135 Baker CJ: Group B streptococcal infection. *Adv Intern Med* 25:475, 1980.

136 Anthony BF et al: Epidemiology of group B streptococcus: Longitudinal observations during pregnancy. *J Infect Dis* 137:524, 1978.

137 Ferrieri PA et al: Epidemiology of group B streptococcal carriage in pregnant women and newborn infants. *J Med Microbiol* 10:103, 1977.

138 Regan JA et al: Premature rupture of membrane, preterm delivery, and group B streptococcal colonization of mothers. *Am J Obstet Gynecol* 141:184, 1981.

139 Beargie R et al: Perinatal infection and vaginal flora. *Am J Obstet Gynecol* 122:31, 1975.

140 Eickhoff TC et al: Neonatal sepsis and other infections due to group B beta-hemolytic streptococci. *N Engl J Med* 271:1221, 1964.

141 Bobitt JR, Ledger WJ: Obstetric observations in eleven cases of neonatal sepsis due to group B beta-hemolytic streptococcus. *Obstet Gynecol* 47:439, 1976.

142 Baker CJ, Kasper KL: Correlation of maternal antibody deficiency with susceptibility to neonatal group B streptococcal infection. *N Engl J Med* 294:753, 1976.

143 Pass MA et al: Prospective studies of group B streptococcal infections in infants. *J Pediatr* 95:437, 1979.

144 Ancona FJ et al: Maternal factors that enhance the acquisition of group B streptococci by newborn infants. *J Med Microbiol* 13:273, 1980.

145 Thomsen AC et al: Antibiotic elimination of group B streptococci in urine in prevention of premature labor. *Lancet* 1:591, 1987.

146 Yow MD et al: Ampicillin prevents intrapartum transmission of group B streptococcus. *JAMA* 241:1245, 1979.

147 Merenstein GB et al: Group B beta-hemolytic streptococcus: Randomized controlled treatment study at term. *Obstet Gynecol* 55: 315, 1980.

148 Bobbitt JR et al: Perinatal complications in group B streptococcal carriers. A longitudinal study of prenatal patients. *Am J Obstet Gynecol* 151(6):711, 1985.

149 Boyer KM, Gotoff SP: Prevention of early-onset neonatal group B streptococcal disease with selective intrapartum chemoprophylaxis. *N Engl J Med* 314:1665, 1986.

150 Minkoff H, Mead P: An obstetric approach to the prevention of early onset group B β-hemolytic streptococcal sepsis. *Am J Obstet Gynecol* 154:973, 1986.

151 Morales WJ et al: Prevention of neonatal group B streptococcal sepsis by the use of rapid screening test and selective intrapartum chemoprophylaxis. *Am J Obstet Gynecol* 155:979, 1986.

152 Steigman AJ et al: Intramuscular penicillin administration at birth: Prevention of early onset group B streptococcal disease. *Pediatrics* 62:842, 1978.

153 Siegel JD et al: Single dose penicillin prophylaxis against neonatal group B streptococcal infection. *N Engl J Med* 303:769, 1980.

154 Harwick HJ et al: Mycoplasma hominis and abortion. *J Infect Dis* 121:260, 1970.

155 Blando JD et al: A controlled study of genital mycoplasmas in amniotic fluid from patients with intra-amniotic infection. *J Infect Dis* 147:650, 1983.

156 Gibbs RS et al: Further studies on genital mycoplasmas in intraamniotic infection. Blood cultures and serologic response. *Am J Obstet Gynecol* 154:716, 1986.

157 Kundsin RB et al: *Ureaplasma urealyticum* incriminated in perinatal morbidity and mortality. *Science* 213:474, 1981.

158 McCormack WM et al: Effect on birth weight of erythromycin treatment of pregnant women. *Obstet Gynecol* 69:202, 1987.

159 Tafari N et al: Mycoplasma T strains and perinatal death. *Lancet* 1:108, 1976.

160 Stagno S et al: Infant pneumonitis associated with cytomegalovirus, chlamydia, pneumocystis, and ureaplasma: A prospective study. *Pediatrics* 68:322, 1981.

161 Braun P et al: Susceptibility of genital mycoplasmas to antimicrobial agents. *Appl Microbiol* 19:62, 1970.

162 Paavonen J et al: Prevalence of nonspecific vaginitis and other cervicovaginal infections during the third trimester of pregnancy. *Sex Transm Dis* 13:5, 1986.

163 Edmunds PN: *Haemophilus vaginalis:* Its association with puerperal pyrexia and luecorrhoea. *J Obstet Gynecol Br Comm* 69:917, 1959.

164 Gravett MC et al: Preterm labour associated with subclinical amniotic fluid infection and with bacterial vaginosis. *Obstet Gynecol* 67:229, 1986.

165 Platt MS: Neonatal *Haemophilus vaginalis* infection. *Clin Pediatr* 10:513, 1971.

166 Chow AW et al: The significance of anaerobes in neonatal bacteremia: Analysis of 23 cases and review of the literature. *Pediatrics* 54:736, 1974.

167 Stagno S et al: Cervical cytomegalovirus excretion in pregnant and nonpregnant women: Suppression in early gestation. *J Infect Dis* 131:522, 1975.

168 Knox GG et al: Alteration of the growth of cytomegalovirus and herpes simplex virus type I by epidermal growth factor, a contaminant of crude human chorionic gonadotropin preparation. *J Clin Invest* 61:1635, 1978.

169 Reynolds DW et al: Maternal cytomegalovirus infection and perinatal infection. *N Engl J Med* 289:1, 1973.

170 Stagno S et al: Congenital cytomegalovirus infection: The relative importance of primary and recurrent maternal infection. *N Engl J Med* 306:945, 1982.

171 Stagno S et al: Primary cytomegalovirus infection in pregnancy. Incidence, transmission to fetus, and clinical outcome. *JAMA* 256:1904, 1986.

172 Griffiths PD et al: A prospective study of primary cytomegalovirus infection in pregnant women. *Br J Obstet Gynecol* 87:308, 1980.

173 Monif GRG et al: The correlation of maternal cytomegalovirus infection during varying stages in gestation with neonatal involvement. *J Pediatr* 80:17, 1972.

174 Stern H, Tucker SM: Prospective study of cytomegalovirus infection in pregnancy. *Br Med J* 2:268, 1973.

175 Stagno S et al: Breast milk and risk of cytomegalovirus infection. *N Engl J Med* 302:1073, 1980.

176 Starr JG et al: Inapparent congenital cytomegalovirus infection. Clinical and epidemiologic characteristics in early infancy. *N Engl J Med* 282:1075, 1970.

177 Starr JG: Cytomegalovirus infection in pregnancy. *N Engl J Med* 282:50, 1970.

178 Walters BNJ, Redman CWG: Bell's palsy and cytomegalovirus mononucleosis in pregnancy. *J R Soc Med* 77:429, 1984.

179 Paavonen J et al: Colposcopic manifestations of cervical and vaginal infections. *Obstet Gynecol Surv* 43:373, 1988.

180 Mostocefi-Zadeh M et al: Placental evidence of cytomegalovirus infection of the fetus and neonate. *Arch Pathol Lab Med* 108:403, 1984.

181 Gold E, Nankervis GA: Cytomegalovirus, in *Viral Infections of Humans,* AS Evans (ed). New York, Plenum, 1976, p 143.

182 Stagno S et al: Congenital cytomegalovirus infection. Occurrence in an immune population. *N Engl J Med* 296:1254, 1977.

183 Stern H et al: An early marker of fetal infection after primary cytomegalovirus infection in pregnancy. *Br Med J* 292:718, 1986.

184 Pass RF et al: Outcome of symptomatic congenital cytomegalovirus infection: Results of long-term longitudinal follow-up. *Pediatrics* 66:758, 1980.

185 Laskin O et al: Use of ganciclovir to treat serious cytomegalovirus infections in patients with AIDS. *J Infect Dis* 155:323, 1987.

186 Becker TM et al: Epidemiology of genital herpes infections in the United States. The current situation. *J Reprod Med* 31:359, 1986.

187 Sullivan-Bolyai J et al: Neonatal herpes simplex virus infection in King County, Washington. Increasing incidence and epidemiologic correlates. *JAMA* 250:3059, 1983.

188 Whitley RJ et al: The natural history of herpes simplex virus infection of mother and newborn. *Pediatrics* 66:489, 1980.

189 Sieber OF et al: *In utero* infection of the fetus by herpes simplex virus. *J Pediatr* 69:30, 1966.

190 Nahmias AJ et al: Perinatal risk associated with maternal genital herpes simplex virus infection. *Am J Obstet Gynecol* 100:825, 1971.

191 Vontver L et al: Recurrent genital herpes simplex virus infections in pregnancy: Infant outcome and frequency of asymptomatic recurrences. *Am J Obstet Gynecol* 143:75, 1982.

191a Prober CG et al: Low risk of herpes simplex virus infection in neonates exposed to the virus at the time of vaginal delivery to mothers with recurrent genital herpes simplex virus infection. *N Engl J Med* 316:240, 1987.

192 Brown ZA et al: Effects on infants of a first episode of genital herpes during pregnancy. *N Engl J Med* 317:1246, 1987.

192a Nahmias AJ, Visintine AM: Herpes simplex, in *Infectious Diseases of the Fetus and Newborn Infant,* JS Remington, JO Klein (eds). Philadelphia, Saunders, 1976, p 156.

193 American Academy of Pediatrics: Perinatal herpes simplex virus infections. *Pediatrics* 66:147, 1980.

194 Arvin AM et al: Failure of antepartum maternal cultures to predict the infant's risk of exposure to herpes simplex virus at delivery. *N Engl J Med* 315:796, 1986.

195 Binkin N et al: Preventing neonatal herpes. The value of weekly viral cultures in pregnant women with recurrent genital herpes. *JAMA* 251:2816, 1984.

196 Gibbs RS et al: Management of genital herpes infection in pregnancy. *Obstet Gynecol* 7:779, 1988.

197 Gibbs RS: Infection control of herpes simplex virus infections in obstetrics and gynecology. *J Reprod Med* 31:395, 1986.

198 Cox SM et al: Treatment of disseminated herpes simplex virus in pregnancy with parenteral acyclovir. A case report. *J Reprod Med* 31:1005, 1986.

199 CDC: Condyloma acuminatum—United States, 1966–1981. *MMWR* 32:306, 1983.

200 Cohen SR et al: Papilloma of the larynx and tracheobronchial tree in children: A retrospective study. *Ann Otol* 89:497, 1980.

201 Gissmann L et al: Human papillomavirus types 6 and 11 DNA sequences in genital and laryngeal papillomas and in some cervical cancers. *Proc Natl Acad Sci USA* 80:560, 1983.
202 Steinberg BM et al: Laryngeal papilloma virus infection during clinical remission. *N Engl J Med* 308:1261, 1983.
203 Hallden C, Majmundar B: The relationship between juvenile laryngeal papillomatosis and maternal condylomata acuminata. *J Reprod Med* 31:804, 1986.
204 Shah K et al: Rarity of cesarean delivery in cases of juvenile-onset respiratory papillomatosis. *Obstet Gynecol* 68:795, 1986.
205 De Jong A et al: Condyloma acuminata in children. *Am J Dis Child* 136:704, 1982.
206 Roman A, Fife K: Human papillomavirus DNA associated with foreskins of normal newborns. *J Infect Dis* 153:855, 1986.
207 Chamberlain MJ et al: Toxic effect of podophyllum application in pregnancy. *Br Med J* 1:391, 1972.
208 Young RL et al: The treatment of large condylomata acuminata complicating pregnancy. *Obstet Gynecol* 41:65, 1973.
209 Gorthey RL, Krembs MA: Vulvar condylomata acuminata complicating labor. *Obstet Gynecol* 4:67, 1954.
210 Ferenczy A: Treating genital condyloma during pregnancy with the carbon dioxide laser. *Am J Obstet Gynecol* 148:9, 1984.
211 Guinan ME, Hardy A: Epidemiology of AIDS in women in the United States 1981 through 1986. *JAMA* 257:2039, 1987.
212 Holmes KK, Kreiss J: Heterosexual transmission of human immunodeficiency virus: Overview of a neglected aspect of the AIDS epidemic. *J AIDS* 1:602, 1989.
213 Stewart GJ et al: Transmission of human T-cell lymphotropic virus type III by artificial insemination by donor. *Lancet* 2:581, 1985.
214 Schoenbaum EE et al: The effect of pregnancy on progression of HIV related disease. Presented at the 3rd International Conference on AIDS. Washington, DC, June 1–5, 1987. Abstract THP-140.
215 MacCallum LR et al: The effects of pregnancy on the progression of HIV infection. Presented at the IV International Conference on AIDS. June 12–16, 1988. Abstract 4032.
216 Berrebi A et al: The influence of pregnancy on the evolution of HIV infection. Presented at the IV International Conference on AIDS. June 12–16, 1988. Abstact 4041.
217 Biggar RJ et al: Helper and suppressor lymphocyte changes in HIV-infected mothers and their infants. Presented at the IV International Conference on AIDS, June 12–16, 1988. Abstract 4031.
218 Scott GB et al: Mothers of infants with HIV infection: Outcome of subsequent pregnancies. Presented at the 3rd International Conference on AIDS. Washington, DC, June 1–5, 1987. Abstract THP-91.
219 Goedert JJ et al: AIDS incidence in pregnant women, their babies, homosexual men and hemophiliacs. Presented at the 3rd International Conference on AIDS, Washington, DC, June 1–5, 1987. Abstract TP-56.
220 The New York Collaborative Study Group for Vertical Transmission of HIV: Human immunodeficiency virus (HIV) infection during pregnancy: A longitudinal study. Presented at the 3rd International Conference on AIDS, Washington, DC, June 1–5, 1987. Abstract TP-55.
221 Selwyn PA et al: Pregnancy outcomes and HIV infection in intravenous drug abusers. Presented at the 3rd International Conference on AIDS, Washington, DC, June 1–5, 1987. Abstract MP-156.
222 Brescianini C et al: HIV infection and AIDS in newborn babies of mothers positive for HIV antibody. *Br Med J* 294:610, 1987.
223 Laure F et al: Detection of HIV-1 DNA in infants and children by means of the polymerase chain reaction. *Lancet* 2:538, 1988.
224 Ryder RW et al: Perinatal HIV transmission in two African hospitals: One year follow-up. International Conference on AIDS, June 12–16, 1988. Abstract 4128.
225 Braddick M et al: Vertical transmission of HIV in Kenya. Presented at the 4th International Conference on AIDS, June 12–16, 1988. Abstract 5126.
226 Levy J et al: Prospective study of the vertical transmission of HIV. Presented at the 3rd International Conference on AIDS, Washington, DC, June 1–5, 1987. Abstract WP-80.
227 Peckham C: Consequences of HIV infection in pregnancy. Results from the European Collaborative Study. International Conference on AIDS, June 12–16, 1988. Abstract 4027.
228 Scott G et al: Probability of perinatal infections in infants of HIV-1 positive mothers. International Conference on AIDS, Washington, DC, June 12–16, 1988. Abstract 6583.
229 LaPointe N et al: Transplacental transmission of HIV-III virus. *N Engl J Med* 312:1325, 1985.
230 Jovaisas E et al: LAV/HTLV-III in 20 week fetus. *Lancet* 2:1129, 1985.
231 Marion K et al: Human T-cell lymphotrophic virus type III (HTLV-III) embryopathy. A new dysmorphic syndrome associated with intrauterine HTLV-III infection. *Am J Dis Child* 140:638, 1986.
232 Ziegler JB et al: Postnatal transmission of AIDS associated retrovirus from mother to infant. *Lancet* 1:896, 1985.
233 Thiry L et al: Isolation of AIDS virus from cell-free breast milk of three healthy virus carriers. *Lancet* 2:891, 1987.
234 Minkoff HL: Care of pregnant women infected with human immunodeficiency virus. *JAMA* 258:2714, 1987.
235 Chiodo F et al: Vertical transmission of HTLV-III. *Lancet* 1:739, 1986.
236 Mundy DC et al: Human immunodeficiency virus isolated from amniotic fluid. *Lancet* 2:459, 1987.
237 Bland PB et al: Vaginal trichomoniasis in the pregnant woman. *JAMA* 96:157, 1931.
238 Trussell RE et al: Vaginal trichomoniasis. Complement fixation, puerperal morbidity, and early infection of newborn infants. *Am J Obstet Gynecol* 44:292, 1942.
239 Bramley M: Study of female babies of women entering confinement with vaginal trichomoniasis. *Br J Vener Dis* 52:58, 1976.
240 Keith L et al: On the causation of pelvic inflammatory disease. *Am J Obstet Gynecol* 149:215, 1984.
241 Al-Salihi FL et al: Neonatal *Trichomonas vaginalis*. *Pediatrics* 53:196, 1974.
242 Fouts AC, Kraus SJ: *Trichomonas vaginalis:* Reevaluation of its clinical presentation and laboratory diagnosis. *J Infect Dis* 141: 137, 1980.
243 Goldman P: Metronidazole. *N Engl J Med* 303:1212, 1980.
244 Peterson WF et al: Metronidazole in pregnancy. *Am J Obstet Gynecol* 94:343, 1966.
245 Morgan J: Metronidazole treatment in pregnancy. *Int J Gynaecol Obstet* 15:501, 1978.
246 CDC: Prevention of perinatal transmission of hepatitis B virus: Prenatal screening of all pregnant women for hepatitis B surface antigen. *MMWR* 37:341, 1988.

Chapter 65

# Gonococcal diseases in infants and children

Laura T. Gutman
Catherine M. Wilfert

## GONOCOCCAL INFECTIONS IN CHILDREN

The worldwide epidemic of *Neisseria gonorrhoeae* infections has been widely publicized, but the increasing risk of infection in children has gained public recognition only slowly. In the United States, the age-specific incidences of gonococcal disease in children from birth to 9 years was rising until 1980. Since then the rates have plateaued and in this age range were 6.5/100,000 population in both 1980 and 1985. More gonococcal disease is reported in younger female children than in males, but an increase in the number of infected males occurs during the teens and early adult years.

Retrospective reviews and case reports based on detection of symptomatic infection provide us with the estimates of infection in preadolescent children and early adolescent youths. Presenting complaints of children who are subsequently established to have *N. gonorrhoeae* infection are primarily vaginal or urethral discharge, but some present for evaluation of sexual assault and a number of children have a variety of complaints not related to the genitalia. Gonococcal infection in prepubertal children is particularly important because it may be an indicator of child abuse. Identification of infection in children should lead to a search for adult contacts. Unfortunately, investigation of contacts of infected adults almost never includes children.

Gonococcal infections in children produce different clinical syndromes which are age-related. In addition, the means of acquisition of infection varies by age; thus, newborn gonococcal infection will be considered separately from *N. gonorrhoeae* in prepubertal children.

## MATERNAL AND PERINATAL *N. gonorrhoeae* INFECTION

Beginning in the 1970s, many health clinics encouraged the routine screening of sexually active women for gonorrhea. This is especially important during pregnancy, and rates of gonorrhea in pregnant women range from rare to about 10 percent. Teenagers in specific settings may have a high prevalence of gonorrhea, as evidenced by a study of girls in an adolescent obstetric clinic in whom the infection rate was 10 percent, and 28 percent of the girls were pregnant.[1] Recognition of gonorrhea early in pregnancy identifies a population at risk that should be followed sequentially throughout pregnancy. One prenatal clinic in North Carolina demonstrated a 30 percent reinfection rate by the time of delivery.

Gonococcal infections present several unique problems during pregnancy, some of which have important consequences for the fetus or neonate. Ascending infection of the upper genital tract may occur with gonococcal infection of pregnancy. From 10 to 20 percent of nonpregnant women with gonorrhea have had clinical evidence of pelvic inflammatory disease (PID) in most studies (see Chapter 49), and the rate increases in women with recently acquired gonorrhea. PID probably occurs less often in pregnant women with gonorrhea, although surgically verified gonococcal salpingitis has been reported between 7 and 12 weeks' gestation, prior to obliteration of the endometrial cavity.[2] Local factors may decrease the risk for ascending gonococcal infection during pregnancy. Cervical mucus becomes impermeable to motile sperm and possibly to microorganisms under the influence of progesterone. Most importantly, after the twelfth week of gestation the chorion attaches to the endometrial decidus with obliteration of the intrauterine cavity, obstructing the route for ascending intraluminal spread of gonococci.

The chorioamnion itself may become the site of ascending gonococcal infection after the twelfth week of gestation,[3,3a] and the clinical spectrum of symptomatic gonococcal infection in pregnant patients thus included septic abortion and premature rupture of membranes in 22 and 26 percent of cases in two studies.[4,5] Several other retrospective studies have analyzed the relationship of antepartum gonococcal infection to the course of late pregnancy. Charles et al.[6] reported that premature rupture of membranes occurred in 43 percent of 14 women with untreated gonorrhea at the onset of labor as opposed to 3 percent of 144 women with gonococcal infection that was identified and treated during pregnancy. Handsfield et al.[7] reported that prematurity and delayed delivery after rupture of membranes were significantly correlated with intrapartum gonococcal infection. Edwards et al. matched 19 pregnant women who had intrapartum gonococcal infection with 41 uninfected controls on the basis of age, race, parity, socioeconomic status, and date of delivery. Patients with intrapartum gonococcal infection were significantly more likely than controls to have chorioamnionitis, premature rupture of membranes, delayed delivery after rupture of membranes, and prematurity.[8]

The effects of untreated gonococcal disease of the mother on the health of the fetus and infant have been reviewed by several authors (see Table 65-1). In these six studies, rates of premature delivery were between 13 and 67 percent, of perinatal distress were 5 to 10 percent, and of perinatal deaths were 2 to 11 percent. The rates of apparently normal or term deliveries were only 35 to 77 percent of the reported pregnancies. The studies of Charles, Amstey, Edwards, and Handsfield included data concerning a comparison of the outcome of pregnancy of mothers who were not infected with *N. gonorrhoeae,* and the outcomes of uninfected mothers were significantly more favorable for the infant. In Amstey's study, the risk of these adverse outcomes was the same in women who were treated for gonorrhea during pregnancy as in those who were not treated prior to delivery.

These studies provided scant information on other associated conditions or genital infections. However, there is increasing evidence that many or most infections of the lower genital tract of women (including *M. hominis,*[10] *Ureaplasma urealyticum,*[11] and *Chlamydia trachomatis*[12,13]), if they occur during pregnancy, carry a significant burden of adverse outcomes to the pregnancy, including premature rupture of membranes, abortions, perinatal mortality, and prematurity.

A final demonstration of ascending infection of the fetus prior to delivery is found in a report of an infected stillborn infant who was found at autopsy to have multiple submucosal areas in the esophagus and upper respiratory tracts containing Gram-negative diplococci.[14] The location of the lesions indicated that infection

**Table 65-1. Outcome of Pregnancy in Mothers Who Were Infected with *N. gonorrhoeae* at Delivery**

| Outcome | Charles[6] ($n$ = 14) | Sarrell[4] ($n$ = 37) | Israel[9] ($n$ = 39) | Amstey*[5] ($n$ = 222) | Edwards*[8] ($n$ = 19) | Handsfield*[7] ($n$ = 12) |
|---|---|---|---|---|---|---|
| Normal or term infant | – | 13 (35%) | 30 (77%) | 142 (64%) | 7 (37%) | – |
| Aborted | – | 13 (35%) | 1 (2%) | 24 (11%) | – | – |
| Perinatal death | – | 3 (8%) | 1 (2%) | 15 (8%) | 2 (11%) | – |
| Premature | – | 6 (17%) | 5 (13%) | 49 (22%) | 8 (42%) | 8 (67%) |
| Perinatal distress | – | – | 2 (5%) | – | 2 (10%) | – |
| Premature rupture of membranes | 6 (43%) | 8 (21%) | – | 52 (26%) | 12 (63%) | 9 (75%) |

*Data is provided showing that the outcomes of pregnancies of mothers not infected with *N. gonorrhoeae* were significantly more favorable than for infected mothers.

had been contracted in utero during swallowing and respiration. There was also associated chorioamnionitis of the placenta.

## NEONATAL GONOCOCCAL OPHTHALMIA

An association of conjunctivitis in the newborn with vaginal discharge in the mother was noted by Quelimaltz in 1750, but gonococcal ophthalmia neonatorum was not recognized as a distinct entity until 1881. Inclusion conjunctivitis was subsequently differentiated from goncoccal ophthalmia by Lindner in 1909.

The incidences of various forms of neonatal gonococcal disease in exposed infants are listed in Table 65-2. Exposed infants who have had ocular silver nitrate prophylaxis have been reported to experience incidences of 0 to 5 percent, while exposed infants who have not had prophylaxis have had incidences of 2 to 30 percent. Oropharyngeal infection occurs in 35 percent of infants with gonococcal ophthalmia.

Ophthalmia neonatorum occurred in 1 to 15 percent of infants born in U.S. and European hospitals during the nineteenth century, and the great majority of cases were presumably gonococcal. In 1881, Credé reported the topical use of silver nitrate to prevent ophthalmia neonatorum.[23] Credé reported a reduction in the rate of ophthalmia neonatorum from 10 to 0.3 percent with his method of prophylaxis, which consisted of cleansing the eyes with ordinary water, after which the eyelids were held open and a single drop of 2 percent silver nitrate was instilled in each eye. This was later modified by substituting 1 percent silver nitrate in individual dispensers in place of the higher-strength solution. The prevention of ophthalmia neonatorum with increasing use of Credé's method was reflected in a reduction in the importance of this syndrome as a cause of blindness. In the United States, the proportion of new entrants to schools for the blind attributable to ophthalmia neonatorum decreased from 28 percent in 1908 to 11 percent by 1933. When sulfonamides and penicillin became available for antepartum care and for treatment of gonococcal ophthalmia neonatorum, the proportion of new entrants to schools for the blind with blindness attributable to ophthalmia neonatorum further decreased to 1 percent by 1950, and to less than 0.1 percent by 1959.[24]

## ETIOLOGY AND DIFFERENTIAL DIAGNOSIS

The resurgence of gonorrhea during the 1960s and 1970s was associated with a reappearance of gonococcal ophthalmia neonatorum in the United States[25–27] and in a report from Glasgow,[28] *N. gonorrhoeae* was the most common cause of ophthalmia neonatorum in children who required hospitalization for this condition. However, in most areas, gonococcal infection remains a relatively infrequent, albeit the most serious, cause of bacterial conjunctivitis in the newborn. Current data concerning the relative frequency of the various causes of ophthalmia neonatorum are available from a recent study in Seattle.[29] The causes of ophthalmia neonatorum in decreasing order of frequency are chemical conjunctivitis due to silver nitrate, followed by infections due to *C. trachomatis, Staphylococcus aureus, Hemophilus* sp., other respiratory tract bacteria such as pneumococci, herpes simplex, and *N. gonorrhoeae.* In developed countries, *C. trachomatis* is among the most common causes of neonatal conjunctivitis, and *N. gonorrhoeae* is among the least common.

A mild chemical conjunctivitis can be expected after instillation

**Table 65-2. Incidences of Neonatal Gonococcal Disease in Exposed Infants**

| Site of neonatal infection | Reported incidences of infection, % | Population | References |
|---|---|---|---|
| Conjunctiva | 5; 0; 2 | Exposed infants who had $AgNO_3$ ocular prophylaxis | Edwards[8]<br>Allen[15]<br>Armstrong[16] |
| | 2; 30 | Exposed infants who had no ocular prophylaxis | Rothenberg[17]<br>Fransen[18] |
| Orogastric fluid | 40; 26 | Infants of infected mothers | Handsfield[7]<br>Edwards[8] |
| Oropharynx | 43/122 (35) | Infants with gonococcal ophthalmia | Laga[19] |
| Disseminated disease as a proportion of all neonatal gonorrhea | 0–1 (rare) | Reported series of neonatal gonococcal disease | Folland[20]<br>Tomeh[21]<br>Wald[22]<br>Edwards[8]<br>Fransen[18] |

of 1 percent nitrate drops. Evidence of epithelial desquamation and polymorphonuclear leukocytic exudate appears usually within 6 to 8 h and disappears usually within 24 to 48 h.

Conjunctival infection caused by *N. gonorrhoeae* in the newborn usually produces an acute purulent conjunctivitis that appears from 2 to 5 days after birth (see Plate 7). However, the initial course is occasionally indolent, and onset can occur later than 5 days after birth,[16,27] perhaps because of partial suppression of infection by ophthalmic prophylaxis, because of small inoculum size, or because of strain-to-strain variations in gonococcal virulence. Cases with incubation periods up to 19 days have been reported after inoculation of the eye with contaminated urine,[30] and gonococcal conjunctivitis infection without any signs of inflammation has been detected by routine screening of neonates.[31] Chronic mild, intermittent gonococcal conjunctivitis of 3 months' duration has been reported in a 4-month-old child.[32] Prolonged incubation after perinatal acquisition is hard to distinguish from delayed onset due to postnatal acquisition. Therefore, *gonococcal infection must be ruled out in every case of conjunctivitis in infants,* regardless of severity or time of onset. At the opposite extreme, gonococcal ophthalmia neonatorum has also been detected at birth or during the first few hours of life in infants born after a prolonged interval between rupture of membrane and delivery,[33,16] and infection in utero may have also occurred in an infant who developed gonococcal ophthalmia following a cesarean section which was performed after membrane rupture.[33,34]

As already noted, the risk of disease in the newborn by *N. gonorrhoeae* may be increased by premature rupture of membranes and by prematurity.[16,35,36] Brown et al.[27] noted prematurity in 19 (83 percent) of 23 infants with gonococcal ophthalmia, perhaps because infants who are premature also often have been delivered after premature rupture of membranes, and therefore the infection was established before delivery. Ocular silver nitrate is not efficacious for therapy of established gonococcal ophthalmia.[16] Gonococcal ophthalmia neonatorum has been more common in male than in female infants in some studies.[27] In contrast, in older children gonococcal conjunctivitis is more common in girls, who usually have associated vulvovaginitis.

Although gonococcal conjunctivitis is usually less severe and less rapidly progressive in the newborn than in the adult, permanent corneal damage following gonococcal ophthalmia neonatorum was usual in the preantibiotic era. The infant typically develops tense edema of both lids, followed by chemosis and a progressively purulent and profuse conjunctival exudate, which literally pours or squirts out the lids when they are separated. If treatment is delayed, the infection extends beyond the superficial epithelial layers, reaching the subconjunctival connective tissue of the palpebral conjunctivae and more significantly, the cornea. Corneal complications include ulcerations that may leave permanent nebulae or may cause perforation and lead to anterior synechiae, anterior staphyloma, panophthalmitis (rarely), and loss of the eye. In the past, systemic spread occasionally caused peripheral manifestations of gonococcemia and death. Such local and systemic complications of gonococcal conjunctivitis are now rare in the newborn, if treatment is begun promptly, while the cornea is still intact.

In addition to ocular complications of neonatal gonococcal ophthalmia, the disease may spread locally, cause primary disease at other mucous membrane sites, or cause systemic disease. The ocular disease serves as a signal that the infant has been infected. Examples of extension of gonococcal disease beyond the eye include the observation that 35 percent of infants with gonococcal ophthalmia also yield *N. gonorrhoeae* from pharyngeal cultures[19] and the description of gonococcal meningitis[37] and arthritis[38] in infants with ophthalmia.

## GONOCOCCAL ARTHRITIS IN THE NEONATE

Septic arthritis has been the most commonly recognized manifestation of gonococcemia in the neonatal period. The association of arthritis in the newborn with ophthalmia neonatorum was noted by Lucas in 1885. Holt[39] reported 26 cases of gonococcal arthritis in children, including two infants who developed arthritis within the first month of life. One of these children also had ophthalmia neonatorum, most had no recognized focus, and rectal cultures were not taken. It is remarkable that ophthalmia neonatorum has also often been absent in subsequently reported cases of neonatal gonococcal arthritis. The primary focus of infection in most of the 53 infants with gonococcal arthritis reported by Cooperman[40] was uncertain; only one had ophthalmia neonatorum. All the females were said to have had vulvovaginitis, while several infants had proctitis. Bacteremia in some other cases has been attributed to infection of the mouth, nares, and umbilicus, while the source of bacteremia has been inapparent in many cases reported in the English language since the 1940s.[38,41–46]

The onset of clinical evidence of gonococcal arthritis in the newborn usually occurs from 1 to 4 weeks after delivery. One cannot distinguish between perinatal and postnatal acquisition of infection in most cases. The efficacy of ophthalmic prophylaxis, together with prompt recognition and treatment of gonococcal ophthalmia neonatorum when it occurs despite prophylaxis, may explain the absence of conjunctivitis in most cases of neonatal gonococcal arthritis reported since 1940. The pustular and necrotic skin lesions that characteristically appear during gonococcemia in the adult[47] have not yet been described in the newborn. The natural history of gonococcal arthritis in the infant is uncertain. Of the 53 cases described by Cooperman in newborns who were presumably infected by a single epidemic strain of *N. gonorrhoeae,* none had a fatal outcome, and permanent impairment of function was uncommon, even without antibiotic therapy.[48] In contrast, 14 of 26 cases that occurred in a series of outbreaks described by Holt[39] in 1905 were fatal.

Infants with neonatal gonococcal arthritis share several important characteristics with neonates whose arthritis is of other etiologies[49] (see Table 65-3). In particular, polyarticular involvement is the norm.[38] The primary presentation is refusal to move the involved limb, leading to the appearance of a paralytic process. Of particular concern is the difficulty in providing an early diagnosis of bacterial infection of the hip in neonates and young children. Inflammatory disease of the hip does not present

**Table 65-3. Presentations of Gonococcal Disease of the Newborn**

| |
|---|
| Associated mucosal sites: |
| Conjunctivitis, ophthalmia |
| Asymptomatic pyuria |
| Urethritis, vaginitis, proctitis, pharyngitis, rhinitis |
| Scalp abscess |
| Contaminated orogastric contents |
| Systemic findings: |
| Multiply involved joints |
| Pseudoparesis of involved joints |
| "Sepsis of the newborn" |
| Onset age 3–21 days |

with visible external swelling, and the hip joint capsule of an infant is relatively distensible so that pain on movement may fail to provide a diagnosis. Nevertheless, infants with bacterial infections of the hips have a high incidence of subsequent development of aseptic necrosis of the head of the femur, and the physician must examine the child with particular care for this condition. If the infant with gonococcal disease fails to show normal spontaneous movement of a leg, a full workup, often including arthrocentesis, is indicated.

## OTHER MANIFESTATIONS OF NEONATAL GONOCOCCAL INFECTION

Until recently, the recognized clinical spectrum of neonatal gonococcal infection essentially included only ophthalmia neonatorum and the systemic complications of gonococcemia, although other local forms of neonatal gonococcal infection such as vaginitis,[50] rhinitis,[51] anorectal infection,[18] funisitis, and urethritis[52] have also been reported. More recent are case reports of gonococcal scalp abscesses attributed to intrauterine fetal monitoring.[53–57]

*N. gonorrhoeae* may be an indirect or a direct cause of early neonatal sepsis in the absence of gonococcal arthritis. As noted, intrapartum gonococcal infection has been associated with premature delivery and premature rupture of membranes, which may lead to amniotic fluid infection with a variety of vaginal organisms capable of causing neonatal sepsis. Premature infants have increased susceptibility to sepsis. *N. gonorrhoeae* was the third most common pathogen (after *E. coli* and group B streptococci) recovered from nasogastric aspirates in one study, usually in association with suspected neonatal sepsis.[7] *N. gonorrhoeae* has been isolated from blood of newborn infants with clinical sepsis without arthritis.[57,38] The incidence of neonatal complications with *N. gonorrhoeae* will reflect, of course, the incidence of disease in that community and the success or failure of maternal screening and treatment programs.

## PREVENTION AND THERAPY OF NEONATAL GONOCOCCAL DISEASE

Prevention of ophthalmia neonatorum is a principal goal of medical care of the newborn. The optimal method is the prevention and treatment of the disease in the mother, so that exposure of the newborn does not occur. In this regard, it is recommended that endocervical cultures for gonorrhea should be taken in the first and third trimester, since women with gonorrhea in early pregnancy have a 30 percent incidence of recurrence during the pregnancy.[58]

Most states require eye prophylaxis of some form, and silver nitrate has been the single recommended agent for many decades. Because of the high incidence of chemical conjunctivitis with silver nitrate and the importance of eye contact in mother-infant bonding, there has been a recent increase in interest in other agents. For a summary of studies pertaining to this issue see the review of Rothenberg.[59] The most recent statement by the American Academy of Pediatrics states that effective prophylaxis may be given with topical installation of either 1% silver nitrate (in single-dose ampules), 1% tetracycline, or 0.5% erythromycin. It should be noted that chemical prophylaxis of the newborn conjunctivae provides excellent but not perfect protection. Silver nitrate does not provide effective therapy for an established infection, and some infants with failure of prophylaxis were born after prolonged rupture of the membranes, when the infection may already have been established.

Because of the increasing incidence of penicillinase-producing *N. gonorrhoeae* (PPNG), it is recommended that gonococcal isolates be routinely tested for penicillin sensitivity, penicillinase production, or both. This is particularly true for potentially serious gonococcal infection, including ocular infection. PPNG strains have already been implicated in gonococcal ophthalmia neonatorum, including reports from the United States. Some areas of this country have a particularly high incidence of resistant strains, and in these areas, all strains should be tested for penicillin sensitivity.

Although the sensitivities and the specificities of new and rapid methods for the diagnosis of gonococcal disease have been studied in adult gonococcal syndromes,[60] diagnosis by immunofluorescent methods or DNA hybridization in neonatal disease is as yet unstudied. Therefore, direct culture remains the method of choice for diagnosis of all forms of childhood gonorrhea. Conjunctival exudate should be directly examined by Gram stain for the presence of gram-negative intracellular bean-shaped diplococci typical of *N. gonorrhoeae;* for gram-negative coccobacilli typical of *Hemophilus* sp.; or for gram-positive cocci suggestive of infection with gram-positive pathogens. The presence of one or more polymorphonuclear leukocytes per oil immersion field in a conjunctival smear supports the diagnosis of conjunctivitis. Detection of typical gram-negative diplococci by Gram stain warrants the presumptive diagnosis of gonococcal conjunctivitis, although other *Neisseria* species, such as *N. meningitidis,* have also been associated with purulent ophthalmia neonatorum.

Conjunctival exudate should also be inoculated directly onto blood agar, MacConkey agar, and chocolate agar or Thayer-Martin medium (containing no more than 3 μg/ml of vancomycin) for recovery of *N. gonorrhoeae.* The latter medium should then be placed in a commercial carbon dioxide incubator or candle jar to provide an adequate concentration of carbon dioxide, and should then be incubated at 36°C. If gonococcal conjunctivitis is suspected on the basis of examination of the Gram-stained smear of conjunctival exudate, cultures for *N. gonorrhoeae* should also be obtained from the oropharynx and anal canal, since concomitant infection of these sites has been demonstrated in association with gonococcal ophthalmia neonatorum. Colonies resembling *N. gonorrhoeae* are further identified by Gram stain, positive oxidase test, and utilization of glucose but not maltose, sucrose, or lactose. Because of the social implications of the diagnosis of gonorrhea in a child, the laboratory should confirm the identification with at least one additional test (see Chapter 73).

## GONOCOCCAL DISEASE BEYOND INFANCY

### VAGINITIS

Excluding the neonatal period, gonococcal vaginitis is the most common form of gonorrhea in children. In contrast to adults, in prepubertal girls the nonestrogenized alkaline vaginal mucosa may be colonized and infected with *N. gonorrhoeae.* Gonococcal vaginitis is usually a mild disease, perhaps because it is restricted to the superficial mucosa. Prepubertal vaginitis has been attributed not only to *N. gonorrhoeae* but also to numerous irritative and infectious agents, such as pinworms, foreign bodies, streptococci, *T. vaginalis,* diphtheroids, and other bacteria.

The incidences of gonorrhea, genitourinary *Chlamydia,* and syphilis in several studies of children who were known to have

**Table 65-4. Prevalence of *Neisseria gonorrhoeae* in Abused or Sexually Active Children and Adolescents**

| Author, date, *Ref* | Age (years), sex | Infection | Number, % infected | Population | Special risk, etc. |
|---|---|---|---|---|---|
| Golden, 1984[1] | 12–17, F | *Chlamydia* | 19/186 (10.2%) | Adolescent* | Sexually active |
| | 12–17, F | *N. gonorrhoeae* | 18/186 (10%) | Adolescent* | Sexually active |
| | 12–17, F | *Syphilis* | 6/186 (3%) | Adolescent* | Sexually active |
| Ingram, 1984[61] | 1–12, F | *N. gonorrhoeae* | 10/50 (20%) | North Carolina | Known sexual contact or abuse |
| Fraser, 1983[62] | Adolescent, F | *N. gonorrhoeae* | 15/125 (12%) | Oklahoma | Sexually active |
| | Adolescent, F | *Chlamydia* | 10/125 (8%) | Oklahoma | Sexually active |
| DeJong, 1986[63] | 1–14, M and F | *N. gonorrhoeae* | 25/532 (4.7%) | Pennsylvania | Known sexual abuse |
| | 1–14, M and F | Venereal warts | 3.532 (0.7%) | Pennsylvania | Known sexual abuse |

*Obstetrics-Gynecology Center, New York.

been sexually abused or adolescents who were sexually active are tabulated in Table 65-4. Gonococcal vaginitis is the most frequently recognized of these. Not all children are symptomatic; Hein and associates[64] demonstrated a 7 percent prevalence of asymptomatic gonorrhea in sexually active adolescent females and a 1.9 percent rate in males. In prepubertal children also, asymptomatic disease is probably common, and is usually recognized when a child is undergoing an evaluation for suspected sexual abuse.[65] The majority of symptomatic children have vaginal itching and minor crusting discharge, may discolor the underwear, and have minimal to absent signs of systemic infection. Dysuria and polymorphonuclear leukocytes in the urine may accompany this infection. A Gram stain of the vaginal secretions may lead to diagnosis.[66]

A review of reported complications of 1232 cases of gonococcal vaginitis in the preantibiotic era revealed that 35 percent had urethritis, 19 percent had proctitis, and 6 percent had peritonitis.[67] Although ascending infection is uncommon, perhaps because of the lack of patency of the endocervix until age 9 or 10 years, it may result in salpingitis or peritonitis. Ten percent of girls with gonorrhea have signs compatible with peritonitis, including fever, diffuse abdominal pain, leukocytosis, and decreased bowel sounds, findings which are similar to those of appendicitis. For these reasons a perineal examination for vaginal irritation, discharge, or both is important prior to abdominal surgery in young girls.

## PELVIC INFLAMMATORY DISEASE AND SALPINGITIS

Vaginal infection of females who are adolescent or younger may progress to involve the fallopian tubes or may disseminate to the pelvis, leading to perihepatitis and pelvic inflammatory disease (PID). PID in adolescents is particularly likely to result in infertility and ectopic pregnancy, and PID is the single most common cause of infertility in young women. Between 1970 and 1980, the rate of ectopic pregnancies per 1000 live births in the United States increased from 4.8 to 14.5, and between 1975 and 1981 the rate of hospitalization for salpingitis of women 15 to 19 years of age was 4/100,000.[70]

The identification of the cause of PID is complicated by the difficulty of obtaining fallopian tube specimens prior to therapy. Most investigators believe that gonococcal infections are a very common cause of acute PID in adolescents, but not necessarily the only one. Other causes include *C. trachomatis, M. hominis,* and mixed aerobic and anaerobic flora, especially *Peptostreptococcus* and *Peptococcus* species.

Risk factors for PID and acute salpingitis have been shown to include young age at acquisition of gonococcal disease, a history of previous PID, multiple sexual partners, and use of an IUD for contraception. Approximately 15 percent of teenagers who develop gonorrhea will progress to PID.

Diagnosis of PID may be difficult, and the differential diagnosis in the adolescent includes numerous other conditions of the lower abdomen, including appendicitis, ectopic pregnancy, mesenteric adenitis, pyelonephritis, and septic abortion. Misdiagnosis of PID is common and is one of the more common causes of laparotomy. Recommendations by Shafer and associates[71] suggest that a clinical diagnosis of PID be supported by the presence of lower abdominal pain and tenderness with motion of the cervix, and adnexal tenderness. Fever, leukocytosis, elevated sedimentation rate, and adnexal mass on abdominal ultrasonography support the diagnosis but may be absent. Culdocentesis, if performed, may reveal evidence of purulent reaction in the peritoneal cavity. It is probable that the outcome for fertility is improved with prompt and vigorous therapy. Indications for hospitalization for therapy of PID including young age of patients (all adolescents) are listed in Table 65-5.

## URETHRITIS

Gonococcal urethritis in prepubertal males is much less common than is vaginitis in girls. When recognized, the disease is usually symptomatic and resembles gonococcal urethritis in the adult male. As with vaginitis, asymptomatic pyuria is a presentation with which the pediatrician should be familiar.[72] In children with gonorrheal infection of the genitourinary tract, concomitant anorectal and tonsillopharyngeal colonization is common. This colonization is usually asymptomatic as in adults, but may also be symptomatic.[73]

**Table 65-5. Indications for Hospitalization of Children with Suspected Salpingitis**

| |
|---|
| All adolescents |
| Diagnostic uncertainty |
| Failure to respond to prior regimen |
| Pregnancy |
| Fever, peritoneal signs |
| Adnexal mass |
| IUD use |
| Noncompliance with medical regimen |

## DISSEMINATED DISEASE

Gonococcal arthritis in older children resembles that of adults and may be accompanied by cutaneous lesions.[74] Multiple septic involvement of joints is not as common as in the newborn period, although a migratory polyarthritis may be part of the prodrome. However, there is typically a single, most severely affected joint and myositis and tenosynovitis may be prominent.

Treatment of gonococcal arthritis depends on prompt recognition of the disease. Cultures of all mucous membranes (nasopharynx, rectal, vaginal or endocervical, conjunctival), blood culture, and aspiration of the involved joint should be performed. In the newborn period, the gastric aspirate may be cultured to determine contamination from a maternal source. A history for an adult contact should be taken. If the contact has not responded to therapy, the possibility of a penicillinase-producing strain may be considered.

Each patient must be evaluated for the need for drainage of an involved joint. Since complete response to medical therapy may not occur for several days, most physicians attempt to avoid an open drainage procedure with needle aspirations if possible. An exception is purulent arthritis of the hips, in which early drainage may be necessary to prevent necrosis of the femoral head.

## OTHER FORMS OF GONOCOCCAL DISEASE

Other complications of gonorrhea are rarely if ever reported in the pediatric literature. Gonococcal sepsis, meningitis, endocarditis, myocarditis, and hepatitis occur in adults; they may be expected to occur in children and may be fatal.[74a] However, the pediatric experience with these conditions is too minimal for comment.

## GONORRHEA AS AN INDICATOR OF SEXUAL ABUSE IN CHILDREN

Gonorrhea in children other than newborns should be assumed to be sexually transmitted and is thus often an indicator of sexual abuse of the child. Among all STDs diagnosed in 744 children who were evaluated for suspected child abuse, gonorrhea was the single most common diagnosis, accounting for 7 to 20 percent of cases in these three studies.[76–78] Child abuse and STDs are discussed in greater detail in Chap. 72.

## TREATMENT

*Recommendations for therapy of childhood gonorrhea based on guidelines from the U.S. Centers for Disease Control are as follows:*

Pediatric patients encompass children from birth to adolescence. When a child is postpubertal or weighs more than 45.4 kg (100 lb), he or she should be treated with dosage regimens as defined for adults (see Chap. 14).

Studies of the efficacy of many therapeutic regimens for uncomplicated and complicated gonococcal infections of prepubertal children are sparse. The prevalence of penicillin-resistant *N. gonorrhoeae* continues to increase nationally. Because efficacious and prompt therapy has a profound effect on the outcomes of ophthalmic and systemic disease in infants and children, physicians may elect to treat all pediatric gonococcal disease with a regimen suitable for therapy of penicillin-resistant strains. In regions in which more than 3 percent of strains are penicillin-resistant, all children should be treated with those regimens.

## PREVENTION OF NEONATAL INFECTION

All pregnant women should have endocervical culture examinations for gonococci as an integral part of prenatal care at the first prenatal visit. A second culture late in pregnancy should be obtained from women who are at high risk of gonococcal infection.

### Routine prevention of gonococcal ophthalmia

1. One percent $AgNO_3$ (do not irrigate with saline, as this may reduce efficacy).
2. Ophthalmic ointments containing tetracycline, erythromycin, or neomycin are also probably effective.
3. Not recommended: Bacitracin ointment (not effective) and penicillin drops (sensitizing).

### Management of infants born to mothers with untreated gonococcal infection

The infant born to a mother with untreated gonorrhea should have orogastric and rectal cultures taken routinely and blood cultures taken if symptomatic. A term infant should receive aqueous crystalline penicillin G, 50,000 units intramuscularly or intravenously in a single dose. The preterm infant may receive 20,000 units aqueous crystalline penicillin G.

## NEONATAL DISEASE

*Gonococcal ophthalmia:* The patient should be hospitalized. Antimicrobial agents include aqueous crystalline penicillin G, 100,000 units/kg/24 h in four doses intravenously for 7 days *plus* frequent saline irrigations until the discharge ceases. Topical antimicrobial therapy is optional.

*Complicated infection:* Arthritis, abscess, and septicemia should be treated by hospitalization and administration of aqueous crystalline penicillin G, 75,000 to 100,000 units/kg/24 h in four doses, for a minimum of 7 days. Meningitis should be treated with aqueous crystalline penicillin G, 100,000 units/kg/24 h, divided into three or four intravenous doses a day and continued for at least 10 days.

## CHILDHOOD DISEASE BEYOND INFANCY

Gonococcal ophthalmia should be treated with hospitalization and by the administration of aqueous crystalline penicillin G, intravenously, 75,000 to 100,000 units/kg/24 h in four doses, or procaine penicillin G, intramuscularly, 75,000 to 100,000 units/kg/24 h in two doses for 7 days *plus* saline irrigations. Topical antibiotics alone are *not* adequate therapy of gonococcal ophthalmia. The source of the infection must be identified.

Uncomplicated vulvovaginitis and urethritis may not require hospitalization. Both may be treated at one visit by amoxicillin, 50 mg/kg plus probenecid, 25 mg/kg, both given orally. Alternative single-dose parenteral therapy is aqueous procaine penicillin G, 100,000 units/kg intramuscularly and probenecid, 25 mg/kg by mouth, although this regimen is discouraged because of the added trauma to the child. Topical and systemic estrogen therapy are of no benefit in vulvovaginitis. All patients should have follow-up cultures, and the source of infection should be identified, examined, and treated.

## ANORECTAL OR PHARYNGEAL GONOCOCCAL INFECTION

Treatment of anorectal and pharyngeal gonococcal disease in adults with oral amoxicillin has been less effective than with intramuscular penicillin. If the oral regimen is used for a child with this form of infection, repeat examinations with culture at 3 days and 2 weeks to ensure cure of the infection must be made. A repeat culture should also be taken in other forms of gonococcal disease in children.

## TREATMENT OF SALPINGITIS AND PELVIC INFLAMMATORY DISEASE

Coinfection with both chlamydia and gonococci is common in children as well as adults. In female adolescents, treatment of gonococcal cervicitis with drug regimens that are effective against gonococci but not chlamydia has led to a high incidence of residual salpingitis in females, and in males of urethritis, both of which are associated with continued disease due to *Chlamydia.*[70] Optimal therapy for known or possible coinfection with both diseases is not certain in adults and has also not been explored in children. The following regimen may be employed pending further data.[79] The reader is advised to look for recommendations in the reports from the CDC.

Penicillin, amoxicillin, ceftriaxone, and spectinomycin alone will all fail to eradicate *Chlamydia*. Trimethoprim-sulfamethoxazole (TMP-SMX), tetracycline, and erythromycin are effective in vitro and in many clinical forms of *Chlamydia* disease. The pediatrician may elect to treat the child with a combination of intramuscular penicillin or oral amoxicillin, or intramuscular ceftriaxone, and to add a 14-day course of TMP-SMX, erythromycin, or tetracycline orally.

## TREATMENT OF CHILDREN WHO ARE ALLERGIC TO PENICILLIN OR WHO ARE INFECTED WITH PENICILLINASE-PRODUCING *N. gonorrhoeae* OR CHROMOSOMALLY MEDIATED PENICILLIN-RESISTANT STRAINS

In these situations, the following regimens should be used:

Gonococcal conjunctivitis in newborns:
  Ceftriaxone, 50 mg/kg once
Gonococcal keratoconjunctivitis with corneal involvement:
  Ceftriaxone, 80 mg/kg/day IM for ≥3 days
*plus*
Oral erythromycin, 50 mg/kg/day for 14 days, if therapy for concomitant chlamydial disease is planned.

Children who are 8 years of age or older may receive tetracycline, 40 mg/kg/day orally in four divided doses for 7 days, if they are allergic to penicillin. Tetracycline is not effective in treatment of penicillinase-producing *N. gonorrhoeae.*

In areas where penicillin-resistant strains represent 3 percent or more of isolates, children with genitourinary gonorrhea should receive ceftriaxone, 125 mg IM, if the patient weighs less than 100 lbs, and 250 mg if larger. A test-of-cure is recommended for all children.

# References


1 Golden N et al: Prevalence of *Chlamydia trachomatis* cervical infections in female adolescents. *Am J Dis Child* 138:562, 1984.
2 Acosta AA et al: Intrauterine pregnancy and coexistent pelvic inflammatory disease. *Obstet Gynecol* 37:282, 1971.
3 Rothbard MJ et al: Intrapartum gonococcal amnionitis. *Am J Obstet Gynecol* 121:565, 1975.
3a Quinn PA et al: Chorioamnionitis: Its association with pregnancy outcome and microbial infection. *Am J Obstet Gynecol* 156:378, 1987.
4 Sarrell PM, Pruett KA: Symptomatic gonorrhea during pregnancy. *Obstet Gynecol* 32:670, 1968.
5 Amstey MS, Steadman KT: Symptomatic gonorrhea and pregnancy. *J Am Vener Dis Assoc* 3:14, 1976.
6 Charles AG et al: Asymptomatic gonorrhea in prenatal patients. *Am J Obstet Gynecol* 108:595, 1970.
7 Handsfield HH et al: Neonatal gonococcal infection. 1. Orogastric contamination with *Neisseria gonorrhoeae. JAMA* 225:697, 1973.
8 Edwards L et al: Gonorrhea in pregnancy. *Am J Obstet Gynecol* 132:637, 1978.
9 Israel KS et al: Neonatal and childhood gonococcal infections. *Clin Obstet Gynecol* 18:143, 1975.
10 Kass EH et al: Genital mycoplasmas as a cause of excess premature delivery. *Trans Assoc Am Physicians* 94:261, 1981.
11 Kundson RB et al: Association of *Ureaplasma urealyticum* in the placenta with perinatal morbidity and mortality. *N Engl J Med* 310:941, 1984.
12 Gravett MG et al: Independent associations of bacterial vaginosis and *Chlamydia trachomatis* infection with adverse pregnancy outcome. *JAMA* 256:1899, 1986.
13 Berman SM et al: Low birth weight, prematurity, and postpartum endometritis. Association with prenatal cervical *Mycoplasma hominis* and *Chlamydia trachomatis* infections. *JAMA* 257:1189, 1987.
14 Oppenheimer EH, Winn KJ: Fetal gonorrhea with deep tissue infection occurring in utero. *Pediatrics* 69:74, 1982.
15 Allen JH, Barrere LE: Prophylaxis of gonorrheal ophthalmia of the newborn. *JAMA* 141:522, 1949.
16 Armstrong JH et al: Ophthalmia neonatorum: A chart review. *Pediatrics* 57:884, 1976.
17 Rothenberg R: Ophthalmic neonatorum due to *Neisseria gonorrhoeae:* Prevention and treatment. *Sex Transm Dis* 6(suppl 2):187, 1979.
18 Fransen L et al.: Ophthalmia neonatorum in Nairobi, Kenya: The roles of *Neisseria gonorrhea* and *Chlamydia trachomatis. J Inf Dis* 153:862, 1986.
19 Laga M et al: Single-dose therapy of gonococcal ophthalmia neonatorum with ceftriaxone. *N Engl J Med* 315:1382, 1986.
20 Folland DS et al: Gonorrhea in preadolescent children: An inquiry into source of infection and mode of transmission. *Pediatrics* 60: 153, 1977.
21 Tomeh MO, Wilfert CM: Venereal diseases of infants and children at Duke University Medical Center. *North Carolina Med J* 34:109, 1973.
22 Wald ER et al: Gonorrheal disease among children in a University Hospital. *Sex Transm Dis* 7:41, 1980.
23 Forbes G, Forbes GM: Silver nitrate and the eyes of the newborn. *Am J Dis Child* 121:1, 1971.

24 Hatfield EM: Causes of blindness in school children. *Sight Sav Rev* 33:218, 1963.
25 Friendly DS: Gonococcal conjunctivitis in the newborn. *Clin Proc Child Hosp DC* 25:1, 1969.
26 Snowe RJ, Wilfert CM: Epidemic reappearance of gonococcal ophthalmia neonatorum. *Pediatrics* 51:110, 1973.
27 Brown WM et al: Gonococcal ophthalmia among newborn infants at Los Angeles County General Hospital, 1957–1963. *Public Health Rep* 81:926, 1966.
28 Smith JA: Ophthalmia neonatorum in Glasgow. *Scott Med J* 14:272, 1969.
29 Sandstrom KI et al: Diagnosis of neonatal purulent conjunctivitis caused by *Chlamydia trachomatis* and other organisms, in *Chlamydial Infections*, PA Mardh et al (eds). New York, Elsevier, 1982, pp 217–220.
30 Valenton MJ, Abendanio R: Gonorrheal conjunctivitis. *Can J Ophthalmol* 8:421, 1973.
31 Podgore JK, Holmes KK: Ocular gonococcal infection with minimal or no inflammatory response. *JAMA* 246:242, 1981.
32 Fivush B et al: Gonococcal conjunctivitis in a four-month-old infant. *Sex Transm Dis* 7:24, 1979.
33 Thompson TR et al: Gonococcal ophthalmia neonatorum. Relationship of time of infection to relevant control measures. *JAMA* 228:186, 1974.
34 Diener B: Cesarean section complicated by gonococcal ophthalmia neonatorum. *J Fam Pract* 13:739, 1981.
35 Dundas GHG: Ophthalmia neonatorum before birth. *Lancet* 1:122, 1921.
36 Pearson HE: Failure of silver nitrate prophylaxis for gonococcal ophthalmia neonatorum. *Am J Obstet Gynecol* 73:805, 1857.
37 Bradford WL, Kelley HW: Gonococcic meningitis in a newborn infant. *Am J Dis Child* 46:543, 1933.
38 Kohen DP: Neonatal gonococcal arthritis: Three cases and review of the literature. *Pediatrics* 53:436, 1974.
39 Holt LE: Gonococcus infections in children with especial reference to their prevalence in institutions and means of prevention. *NY Med J* 81:521, 1905.
40 Cooperman MB: Gonococcus arthritis in infancy. *Am J Dis Child* 33:932, 1927.
41 Parrish PP et al: Gonococcic arthritis of a newborn treated with sulfonamide. *JAMA* 114:241, 1940.
42 Jones JB, Ramsey RC: Acute suppurative arthritis of hip in children. *US Armed Forces Med J* 7:1621, 1956.
43 Sponzilli EE, Calabro JJ: Gonococcal arthritis in the newborn. *JAMA* 177:919, 1961.
44 Glaser S et al: Gonococcal arthritis in the newborn. *Am J Dis Child* 112:185, 1966.
45 Gregory JE et al: Gonococcal arthritis in an infant. *Br J Vener Dis* 48:306, 1972.
46 Kleiman MB, Lamb GA: Gonococcal arthritis in a newborn infant. *Pediatrics* 52:285, 1973.
47 Holmes KK et al: Disseminated gonococcal infection. *Ann Intern Med* 74:979, 1971.
48 Cooperman MB: End results of gonorrheal arthritis: Review of 70 cases. *Am J Surg* 5:241, 1928.
49 Gutman LT: Acute, subacute and chronic osteomyelitis and pyogenic arthritis in children. *Curr Probl Pediatr* 15:1, 1985.
50 Barton LL, Shuja M: Neonatal gonococcal vaginitis. *J Pediatr* 98: 171, 1981.
51 Kirkland H, Storer RV: Gonococcal rhinitis in an infant. *Br Med J* 1:263, 1931.
52 Hunter GW, Fargo ND: Specific urethritis (gonorrhea) in a male newborn. *Am J Obstet Gynecol* 38:520, 1939.
53 Plavidal FJ, Welch A: Gonococcal fetal scalp abscess: A case report. *Am J Obstet Gynecol* 127:437, 1977.
54 Reveri M, Krishnamurthy C: Gonococcal scalp abscess. *J Pediatr* 94:819, 1979.
55 Brook I et al: Gonococcal scalp abscess in a newborn. *South Med J* 73:396, 1980.
56 D'Auria A et al: Gonococcal scalp wound infection. *MMWR* 24:115, 1975.
57 Thadepalli H et al: Gonococcal sepsis secondary to fetal monitoring. *Am J Obstet Gynecol* 126:510, 1976.
58 Jones DED et al: Gonorrhea in obstetric patients. *J Am Vener Dis Assoc* 2:30, 1976.
59 Rothenberg R: Ophthalmia neonatorum due to *Neisseria gonorrhoeae:* Prevention and treatment. *Sex Transm Dis* 6:187, 1979.
60 Stamm WE: Diagnosis of *Neisseria gonorrhoeae* and *Chlamydia trachomatis* infections using antigen detection methods. *Diagn Microbiol Infect Dis* 4:93s, 1986.
61 Ingram DL et al: Vaginal *Chlamydia trachomatis* infection in children with sexual contact. *Pediatr Infect Dis* 3:97, 1984.
62 Fraser JJ et al: Prevalence of cervical *Chlamydia trachomatis* and *Neisseria gonorrhoeae* in female adolescents. *Pediatrics* 71:333, 1983.
63 DeJong AR: Sexually transmitted diseases in sexually abused children. *Sex Transm Dis* 13:123, 1986.
64 Hein K et al: Asymptomatic gonorrhea: Prevalence in a population of urban adolescents. *J Pediatr* 90:634, 1977.
65 Loney LC et al: Silent gonorrhea in siblings. *Missouri Med* 80:18, 1983.
66 Wald ER: Gonorrhea diagnosis by Gram stain in the female adolescent. *Am J Dis Child* 131:1094, 1977.
67 Benson RA, Weinstock E: Gonorrheal vaginitis in children. A review of the literature. *Am J Dis Child* 59:1083, 1940.
68 Eschenbach DA et al: Polymicrobial etiology of acute pelvic inflammatory disease. *N Engl J Med* 293:166, 1975.
69 Cates W: Sexually transmitted organisms and infertility: The proof of the pudding. *Sex Transm Dis* 11:113, 1984.
70 Washington AE et al: Hospitalization for pelvic inflammatory disease. *JAMA* 251:2529, 1984.
71 Shafer MAB et al: Acute salpingitis in the adolescent female. *J Pediatr* 100:339, 1982.
72 Dawar S, Hellerstein S: Gonorrhea as a cause of asymptomatic pyuria in adolescent boys. *J Pediatr* 81:357, 1972.
73 Abbott SL: Gonococcal tonsillitis-pharyngitis in a 5 year old girl. *Pediatrics* 52:287, 1973.
74 Angevine CD et al: A case of gonococcal osteomyelitis. A complication of gonococcal arthritis. *J Dis Child* 130:1013, 1976.
74a Pasquariello CA et al: Fatal gonococcal septicemia. *Pediatr Inf Dis* 4:204, 1985.
76 Rimsza ME, Niggemann EH: Medical evaluation of sexually abused children: A review of 311 cases. *Pediatrics* 69:8, 1982.
77 White ST et al: Sexually transmitted diseases in sexually abused children. *Pediatrics* 72:16, 1983.
78 Ingram DL et al: Vaginal *Chlamydia trachomatis* infection in children with sexual contact. *Pediatr Infect Dis* 3:97, 1984.
79 Burnakis TG, Hildebrandt NB: Pelvic inflammatory disease: A review with emphasis on antimicrobial therapy. *Rev Infect Dis* 8:86, 1987.

# Chapter 66

# Chlamydial infections in infants and children

H. Robert Harrison
E. Russell Alexander

The biology and the spectrum of adult infection by *Chlamydia trachomatis* are discussed in Chaps. 15 and 16. The infections considered in this chapter include neonatal inclusion conjunctivitis, infant pneumonitis, vaginitis, and otitis media.

## EPIDEMIOLOGY

### PREVALENCE AND TRANSMISSION

As with the gonococcus, the link between adult and infant chlamydial infections is vertical transmission from a cervically infected pregnant woman. Most genital isolates belong to serotypes D through K (see Chap. 15). Several published prospective studies of pregnant women have determined that about 2 to 37 percent carry *C. trachomatis* in their endocervix (Table 66-1), and that most of these are asymptomatic.

Other studies in clinic populations of pregnant women in New Orleans, Louisiana,[1] and Gallup, New Mexico (Gallup Indian Medical Center),[2] have determined prevalence rates of 22 to 26 percent. Prevalences up to 37 percent are seen in adolescent prenatal clinics.[3] It is clear that there is a wide range of prevalences depending upon the group studied, but a useful overall estimate of chlamydial infection in pregnancy would be 6 to 10 percent. Epidemiologically, the women with *C. trachomatis* infection tend to be younger, of lower socioeconomic status and gravidity, and more often unmarried and nonwhite. The infant is inoculated with organisms via passage through infected cervical secretions. Presumably, several sites (i.e., eye, nasopharynx, rectum, vagina) may be seeded independently. It is also possible that the infant directly aspirates infected secretions with the first breath. Even an infant delivered by cesarean section may be infected if the membranes have ruptured spontaneously prior to delivery. These proposed mechanisms of transmission are still somewhat speculative, since exact data are difficult to obtain. However, these mechanisms do explain instances of isolated site infection, such as isolated conjunctivitis, nasopharyngitis, pneumonia, or vaginitis, and of early infection in infants born to mothers with prolonged rupture of membranes.

## RISK ESTIMATES

### Conjunctivitis and pneumonia

Several studies have suggested that a substantial number of newborns are at risk to develop chlamydial infection (Table 66-1). In 1976, Chandler and Alexander performed a prospective study of 142 unselected pregnant women followed to the time of delivery.[4] Of these women, 18 (13 percent) had cervical chlamydial infection; of the infants born to infected women, 9 (50 percent) developed conjunctivitis and 12 (67 percent) had evidence of infection as demonstrated by the presence of serum antibody to *C. trachomatis* at 1 year of age. In a second study, Frommell and his colleagues[5] followed 340 pregnant women and their infants. Of these women, 30 (9 percent) had chlamydial infection; 12 of the 30 women were either lost to follow-up or refused participation. Of the 18 infants born to the remaining culture-positive women, 11 (61 percent) had culture or tear antibody evidence of conjunctival infection, 8 of 18 (44 percent) had clinical conjunctivitis, and 2 (11 percent) developed pneumonia. Schachter[6] followed 131 infants born to culture-positive women. Seventy-nine (60 percent) showed serologic evidence of infection. Culture-confirmed inclusion conjunctivitis occurred in 23 (18 percent) and pneumonia in 21 (16 percent). Additional studies (Table 66-1) have replicated these findings. Thus, several studies have estimated the attack rates to be 18 to 50 percent for conjunctivitis, 11 to 20 percent for pneumonia, and 60 to 70 percent for infection in infants born to women with cervical chlamydial infection. If one couples these data with a conservative estimate of 5 percent prevalence for chlamydial infection in the United States, the estimated incidence of clinical chlamydial conjunctivitis is then 18 to 25 cases per 1000 live births, and of chlamydial pneumonia 5 to 10 cases per 1000 live births. A total of 30 to 35 infants per 1000 live births may be infected, some asymptomatically with sequelae that are as yet unknown.

In addition to the above incidence figures, some prevalence and period prevalence data are available for that proportion of chlamydial pneumonitis that is severe enough to require hospitalization. Harrison and coworkers[7] found a period prevalence of 30 percent (9 of 30 patients) for chlamydial pneumonitis in hos-

**Table 66-1. Prospective Studies of Mothers and Infants for Chlamydia**

| | | | Positive infants† followed | | | |
|---|---|---|---|---|---|---|
| | | | | | Total infection | |
| Study | Location | Mothers,* positive/total | Conjunctivitis | Pneumonia | Culture | Seroconversion |
| Schachter[6] | San Francisco | 262/5531 (5%) | 23/131 (18%) | 21/131 (16%) | 47/131 (36%) | 79/131 (60%) |
| Chandler[4] | Seattle | 18/142 (13%) | 8/18 (44%) | — | — | 12/18 (67%) |
| Frommell[5] | Denver | 30/340 (9%) | 8/18 (44%) | 2/18 (22%) | 8/18 (44%) | 3/18 (33%) |
| Hammerschlag[70] | Boston | 6/322 (2%) | 2/6 (33%) | 1/6 (17%) | 4/6 (67%) | — |
| Hammerschlag[67] | Seattle | 67/572 (12%) | 12/36 (33%)‡ | 3/36 (8%)† | 22/36 (61%)‡ | — |
| Mårdh[71] | Lund | 23/273 (9%) | 5/23 (22%) | — | — | — |
| Datta[72] | Nairobi | 49/223 (22%) | 18/49 (37%) | 6/49 (12%) | — | — |

*Cultures taken from the cervix.
†Infants born to chlamydia-positive mothers.
‡Silver nitrate group only.

pitalized infants less than 6 months of age over a 6-month period. In a subsequent study[8] 10 of 47 infants (21 percent) under 6 months of age admitted to the hospital over a 5-year period with either bronchiolitis or pneumonia had retrospective serologic evidence of chlamydial disease. Stagno and colleagues[9] have also implicated *C. trachomatis* as the cause of pneumonitis in 25 percent of infants hospitalized between 1 and 3 months of age with pneumonitis. In a number of locations where prior prospective studies have been done, there is the perception that fewer infants are being seen with conjunctivitis and pneumonia, and, in particular, that fewer are being hospitalized. In some geographic areas there are decreases in adult chlamydia syndromes and in the prevalence of chlamydia in the cervices of pregnant women. There is also the perception that infants with a suggestion of conjunctivitis or lower respiratory tract disease are being treated immediately. The net result is that the overall morbidity due to this infection may be decreasing.

### Other infections

No risk data are available for chlamydial vulvovaginitis. It appears to occur sporadically in infants with accompanying inclusion conjunctivitis.[10] Others have reported vulvovaginitis in older children without a history of sexual contact.[11] Nevertheless, vulvovaginitis in prepubertal girls is frequent enough in sexually abused children[12] that this diagnosis must be considered in all cases. In sexual abuse cases, cell culture must be used as the primary diagnostic test, and at least for confirmation.[13] The role of *C. trachomatis* in otitis media is in the early stages of investigation and will be discussed below (see Clinical Manifestations).

Seroepidemiologic studies by Black,[14] San Joaquin,[15] and others[16] pointed out that there was significant seroconversion occurring in prepubertal children in diverse settings. This occurred at too young an age to be due to initiation of sexual activity. Furthermore, it is too frequent an occurrence to be attributed completely to sexual abuse. It was hypothesized that the antibody conversion was due to unrecognized respiratory infections, particularly as there was an association of pharyngitis with seroconversion in adults.[17] Of particular importance is the lack of recovery of *C. trachomatis* from the nasopharynx in either adults[17] or children.[18,19] A more plausible explanation has been put forward by Schachter.[37] He has suggested that the serologic conversion is not due to *C. trachomatis* but represents cross reactions in MIF to TWAR *(C. pneumoniae)* strains. Rettig[20] has confirmed this by reexamination of his prior study utilizing more careful MIF criteria and using TWAR and *C. trachomatis* antigens. He found that most of the antibody in childhood was, in fact, TWAR antibody. An additional hypothesis has been suggested by Persson[21] where spurious IgM responses to a number of antigens (including *C. trachomatis*) were observed in children with pharyngitis infected with EB virus.

## PATHOGENESIS AND PATHOLOGY

As was stated above, infants are probably inoculated during passage through an infected endocervical canal. One hypothesis of infection is that individual sites (eye, nasopharynx, lung, vagina) are inoculated independently. This makes sense on the basis of clinical observations, although a progressive infection (eye to nasopharynx to lung) by direct extension of infected secretions is also tenable.

A useful unifying concept is that, once transmitted to the infant, *C. trachomatis* infects and disrupts epithelial surfaces (conjunctivas, nasopharynx, airways, genital tract) but does not invade or destroy deep tissue or produce exotoxins. It is very probable that, as is true of ocular trachoma, the disease manifestations associated with infection seem to be a consequence of the host response to infection rather than the inherent destructiveness of the organism.

## CONJUNCTIVITIS

Following infection of the conjunctival epithelium, the initial host response consists of infiltration of the subepithelial tissues by a polymorphonuclear exudate followed by macrophages, lymphocytes, and plasma cells. This infiltration is manifested as thickened, diffusely red conjunctivae and by papillary hypertrophy of the upper tarsus. Since newborns have no lymphoid conjunctival layer, lymphoid follicles are not present. These germinal centers do not form until 3 to 6 weeks at the earliest in untreated cases.

Until 1966 it was generally thought that neonatal inclusion conjunctivitis was a benign disease with no chronic sequelae. Several studies[22–25] since then have indicated that chronic eye disease with changes similar to mild trachoma may occur. These changes consist of conjunctival scarring and superficial corneal vascularization around the limbus (micropannus). No lid deformities have been reported. This is significantly different from ocular trachoma, in which repeated reinfection (and bacterial superinfection) contributes to entropion (lid deformity) and trichiasis (turning in of eyelashes), both of which contribute to visual impairment. The differences in severity of outcome probably have more to do with multiple chlamydial reinfections and bacterial superinfection and perhaps with environmental factors such as dust and sunlight than with basic differences in organism virulence. In fact, in the monkey model, strains from genital and inclusion conjunctivitis sources have as much potential as, if not more than, the ocular trachoma strains to produce severe initial infection or pannus.[26]

## INFANT PNEUMONITIS

It is unclear whether chlamydial pneumonitis develops (1) from aspiration of infected cervical secretions at delivery, (2) from transmission down the respiratory tract from adjacent infected sites (conjunctivae and nasopharynx), (3) from postnatal aspiration of nasopharyngeal secretions, or (4) from all three mechanisms. Regardless of mechanism, however, a favorite locale for *C. trachomatis* infection appears to be the infant posterior nasopharynx. The organism can be cultured from this site when concurrent anterior nasopharyngeal, oropharyngeal, and conjunctival cultures are negative. Furthermore, organisms may be shed from the nasopharynx for prolonged periods of time in asymptomatic and symptomatic infants. Beem and Saxon,[27] in their classic description of the chlamydial pneumonitis syndrome, found that despite active examination only one-half of asymptomatic and symptomatic infants had clinical conjunctivitis and slightly more had conjunctival shedding of organisms. This was supported by the work of Harrison[7] and colleagues, who found that half of the infants with chlamydial pneumonitis had clinical findings or histories suggestive of conjunctivitis. However, by using the presence of tear antibody as an indicator of conjunctival infection, it was determined that 13 of the 14 infants with pneumonitis had tear antibody at admission for pneumonia.

The pathology of *C. trachomatis* infant pneumonitis has not been thoroughly elucidated. What is known has been gained from lung biopsy material in a few patients who underwent that procedure for diagnosis and from data obtained in animal models. Beem and Saxon[27] noted only an interstitial pneumonia without unusual histological features in two lung specimens obtained by open biopsy. They did not, however, recover organisms. Harrison and colleagues reported another case with similar lung biopsy histology, but again without recovery of *C. trachomatis*.[28] A number of other unpublished attempts to recover the organism at biopsy have been unsuccessful. Frommell[29] later isolated *C. trachomatis* and cytomegalovirus by culture from the lung biopsy of an infant with pneumonitis. Microscopic examination revealed a diffuse interstitial and alveolar infiltrate of monocytes and neutrophils. Intranuclear inclusions characteristic of cytomegalovirus infection were present in the tissue, while chlamydial inclusions could not be seen. Arth and his colleagues,[30] in another culture-positive lung biopsy specimen, found pleural congestion and nearly total alveolar and partial bronchiolar consolidation with a mononuclear exudate containing occasional eosinophils. No other pathogens were found by culture or microscopic examination. Again, no chlamydial inclusions were found in the tissue. Notably absent were significant interstitial or neutrophilic infiltrates.

## Animal models

Harrison and colleagues,[28] in an experimental model, induced chlamydial pneumonitis in two of three baboons. All three animals developed prolonged nasopharyngitis, including one that was not inoculated at that site; this development supports the observation that *C. trachomatis* infection appears to be favored at the nasopharynx. These investigators noted marked similarities in histopathology between the baboon lungs and a biopsy specimen from a human infant with chlamydial pneumonitis: (1) patchy and nodular areas of interstitial, peribronchiolar, and perivascular infiltration with lymphocytes, plasma cells, eosinophils, and neutrophils; (2) germinal centers within nodules; and (3) airway plugs of mucus and inflammatory cells that lead to atelectasis. In the baboons, inclusions were seen in airway tissue and chlamydia could be cultured from central but not peripheral lung tissue. However, they were neither seen nor cultured in high titer. The baboon experiments provided corroborative evidence for a *C. trachomatis*–produced pneumonitis and allowed more immunopathological investigation than had been available in human infants.

Even before the animal-model stimulus was provided by the discovery of *C. trachomatis*–induced human pneumonitis, the organism had been found to produce lung infection in mice. Graham[31,32] found that both lymphogranuloma venereum and oculogenital strains of *C. trachomatis* reliably induced pneumonitis in TO mice. This was characterized by early patchy consolidation with hyperactive airway epithelium, luminal exudate, and a peribronchiolar cellular infiltrate. Inclusions were found both in bronchiolar epithelial cells and in alveoli. By the fifth day after inoculation, alveolar and peribronchiolar exudates had become predominantly lymphocytic and histiocytic. Chen and Kuo[33] developed a model for *C. trachomatis* pneumonitis in Swiss-Webster white mice using intranasal inoculation. On pathological examination, the lungs showed congestion and patchy consolidation. Interstitial pneumonitis with intense infiltration of neutrophils was seen, with areas of alveoli filled by exudate. Bronchioles were spared even though they were often filled with the inflammatory exudate. Chlamydial inclusions were seen in the interstitium and in bronchial epithelial cells. Inflammation was most intense on days 2 and 3 after inoculation, gradually changed to mononuclear cells after day 3, and was gone by days 10 to 14. Organisms could be recovered from lung tissue on days 1 to 7, with highest yields on day 2. Antichlamydial antibody appeared between days 7 and 10 and was sustained. Furthermore, delayed hypersensitivity was present from days 5 to 21, with a maximum on day 7. Harrison and Lee[34] have developed a second mouse pneumonitis model using C57 black mice and a smaller intranasal dose. They too have found a patchy interstitial process with bronchial plugging and an early polymorphonuclear response changing to lymphocytes, plasma cells, and eosinophils. However, very little consolidation was seen, and the intensity of the acute response was not as great, which leads to the possibility that some of the acute changes seen in the Swiss-Webster mice were due to the direct toxic effect of the high-titer inoculum. In the C57 mice, organisms could be seen by immunofluorescence on days 3 to 6 in airways but not in interstitial space, and they could be recovered from tissue during that time. The lung infiltrates were maximal on days 7 to 10 and consisted predominantly of peribronchial infiltrates of mononuclear cells. By immunofluorescence, the mononuclear cells appear to be complement-, IgM-, and IgG-bearing lymphocytes. Antibody and cell-mediated immunity (CMI) to chlamydiae (as measured by blastogenic response of splenic lymphocytes to specific antigen) appeared on day 7. CMI was maximal on day 10.

In summary, despite minor differences, a consistent picture of the histopathology of chlamydial pneumonitis has emerged. Organisms infect the bronchial epithelium and replicate within it in a patchy fashion and perhaps also replicate within alveoli and interstitial spaces. The acute response is interstitial, alveolar, bronchial, and peribronchial, and predominantly polymorphonuclear, leading to some consolidation, interstitial thickening, plugging of airways, and atelectasis. The second stage of the response seems to be a combined humoral and cellular one with the appearance of antibody and mononuclear phagocytic cells, lymphocytes, plasma cells, and cell-mediated immunity. The response appears to reduce the growth of organisms, is maximal after organisms disappear, and persists for some time (in the baboons, 3½ weeks after infection). These results support the hypothesis that much of the prolonged pulmonary findings in infants are due to the host response.[34] The difficulty in recovering or seeing organisms in tissue (i.e., negative lung biopsies) may be due to the fact that tissue is obtained during the chronic phase when chlamydial replication has been limited by host defenses. It should also be noted that lung biopsies may be negative for the organism because the biopsies are peripheral whereas the focus of the disease is in the small airways.

## Role of other microorganisms

Another important question in chlamydial pneumonitis is that of mixed respiratory infection with another pathogen. In 41 infants with chlamydial pneumonitis, Tipple et al.[35] isolated cytomegalovirus from 9 infants (22 percent), respiratory syncytial virus from 4 infants (10 percent), as well as miscellaneous rhinoviruses (4 infants), adenovirus (1 infant), and enterovirus (1 infant). Of 19 infants observed, Harrison[7,8] demonstrated concurrent infection with respiratory syncytial virus in 3 (16 percent) and enterovirus and adenovirus in 1 infant each. Frommell et al.[29] saw cytomegalic inclusions in the lung biopsy of the infant on which they reported. Brasfield,[36] in studying pneumonitis in infants of less than 3 months, found other potentially pathogenic infections in half of them.

The high prevalence of cytomegalovirus infection in chlamydial pneumonia may be a consequence of the fact that both agents are sexually transmitted and often appear together in other epidemiologic situations. Frommell's data,[29] however, imply active coinfection, and the association certainly merits further study.

The presence of other viruses in these hospitalized patients is not entirely surprising. *C. trachomatis* pneumonitis is clearly a chronic illness (see below) with, in many cases, only mild to moderate symptoms and with respiratory dysfunction accompanying the high incidence of infant viral respiratory disease. It is plausible that acute or chronic viral coinfection will increase the respiratory dysfunction to the point where a mildly symptomatic infant requires hospitalization.

## OTHER INFECTIONS

Nothing is known of the pathogenesis or pathology of chlamydial otitis media, nor has the etiologic role of *C. trachomatis* been established, even though the organism has been recovered from ear fluid. For bronchiolitis, the pathogenesis would be similar to pneumonia. The infant vulvovaginitis that occurs presumably follows inoculation of the genital tract at delivery and has mechanisms of disease development similar to those found in conjunctivitis and pneumonia.

## SEROLOGIC RESPONSE TO INFECTION

Information about the antibody response to neonatal chlamydial infection has for the most part been gained using the microimmunofluorescence (micro-IF) test developed by Wang and coworkers.[38]

The serum antichlamydial IgM response is an early response to primary infection.[38] In 25 infants followed longitudinally, specific IgM antibody appeared, usually at low levels (<1:32), shortly after the development of clinical conjunctivitis and disappeared in a few weeks. In an additional 17 pneumonia cases, the specific IgM was present before clinical illness, reached a peak level (≥1:32) during the pneumonia, and fell over a 2-month period thereafter.[6] Schachter and colleagues[6] found the geometric mean of peak IgM titers in a small group of infants to be 1:28 in infants with conjunctivitis only, 1:48 in infants whose serum converted to specific IgM antibody but did not have clinical disease, and 1:448 in infants with pneumonitis.

The antichlamydial IgG titer usually does not change during conjunctivitis. In pneumonitis, however, there is generally a fourfold or greater rise in paired sera unless the maternal titer (and hence that of the infant) is initially high.[6] Elevated levels seem to persist, as Chandler and Alexander[4] found evidence of infection by serum IgG antibody at 1 year of age.

Several investigators have found the presence of tear antibody (antichlamydial antibody in conjunctival secretions) to be a useful indicator of conjunctivitis. However, this remains an area of controversy, since it is not clear whether this is purely local antibody or local plus serum antibody present in the inflammatory exudate.

## CLINICAL MANIFESTATIONS

### INCLUSION CONJUNCTIVITIS

Clinical findings generally appear between the fifth and the twelfth postnatal day. In many cases, the day of onset is difficult to ascertain since an early conjunctivitis due to silver nitrate is often present. In a study discussed earlier,[25] 38 infants were followed from birth for the development of clinical conjunctivitis. Of these infants, 14 had discharge on the first postnatal day and 6 more by the fourth day (20 of 38, or 53 percent). A further 8 infants showed illness between 10 and 13 days of age, 1 more infant during the third week. In Thygeson and Stone's classic study of 38 infants with inclusion conjunctivitis,[39] the average interval between birth and onset of symptoms was 7 to 8 days. In no case in their study was the interval less than 5 days, and in only a few cases was it greater than 10 days.

Clinical manifestations cover a wide spectrum from asymptomatic infection to severe purulent conjunctivitis. The first sign is usually a mucoid discharge that becomes progressively more purulent. The eyelids then become edematous, the palpebral conjunctivae become diffusely erythematous, and there is obliteration of the normal vascular pattern. The bulbar conjunctivae become inflamed, and papillary hypertrophy, primarily of the upper tarsal plate, is present. If the disease becomes prolonged, lymphoid follicles generally develop between 3 and 6 weeks of age (Plate 10). Untreated, active disease can remain for 3 to 12 months. However, study of several infants[25] has revealed that infection can persist for as long as 2 years postnatally.

It must be again stressed that inclusion conjunctivitis is not always a benign disease. Freedman[25] reported conjunctival scarring and superficial corneal vascularization in 10 infants in his series. These observations have since been confirmed by others.[22,24] Hence, prevention and proper treatment of inclusion conjunctivitis are of considerable public health importance. Nothing is known regarding transmission of disease within families and whether infected infants are a source for the infections that can be demonstrated seroepidemiologically in childhood.

### INFANT PNEUMONITIS

A possible association between infant pneumonitis and *C. trachomatis* was noted by Schachter,[40] who described an infant who developed pneumonitis at 52 days of age while on topical tetracycline for inclusion conjunctivitis. Sputum from the patient was heavily infected with *C. trachomatis*. However, the chlamydial pneumonia syndrome of infancy may have been described even earlier as the entity of pertussoid eosinophilic pneumonia. The initial 7 cases were reported by Botsztejn[41] in 1941, and another 12 by Biro[42] in 1960. Infants with this syndrome presented at 3 to 16 weeks of age with coughing spells, dyspnea, and minimal fever. Leukocytosis, eosinophilia, and bilateral pulmonary infiltrates were always present. The course was benign, with resolution of eosinophilia in less than 1 month and resolution of infiltrates in less than 2 months. Oetgen[43] recently described an additional 4 patients with this syndrome, all of whom had elevated serum IgM levels and 2 of whom had elevated IgG levels. This description is highly compatible with chlamydial disease. Following Schachter's report, the clinical syndrome of infant pneumonitis was elucidated largely through the work of Beem and his colleagues.[27] Age at diagnosis was typically 6 weeks, with the onset of gradually worsening symptoms at 2 to 3 weeks of age. Infants were afebrile and without systemic findings. Respiratory findings were documented by tachypnea and a distinctive cough pattern: a series of closely spaced staccato coughs, with no pertussis-like whoop. Partial nasal obstruction and some mucoid discharge were often noted. Tachypnea was commonly the chief abnormal physical finding, with respiratory rates of 50 to 70 breaths per minute. The chest radiograph revealed hyperexpansion with diffuse interstitial and patchy alveolar infiltrates (Fig. 66-1). Rales were the dominant auscultatory finding. Abnormal laboratory values consisted of consistently elevated serum IgG and IgM levels and a mild blood eosinophilia. Beem found that the illness often followed a protracted course; cough and tachypnea required weeks to clear, and rales and radiographic changes were present for over a month.[27]

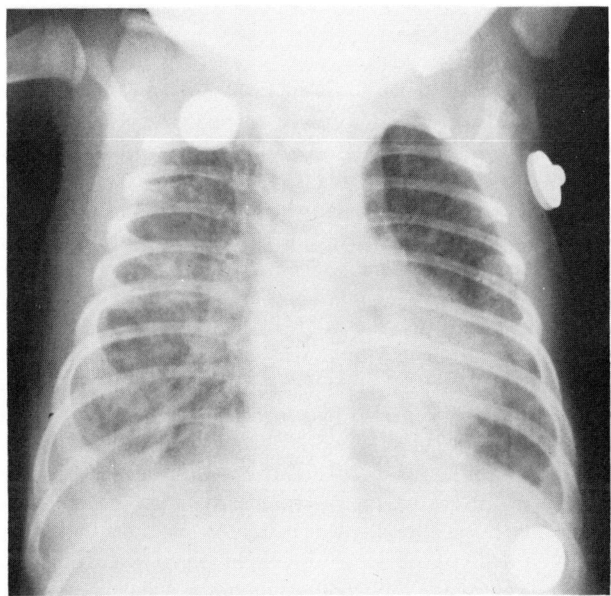

A

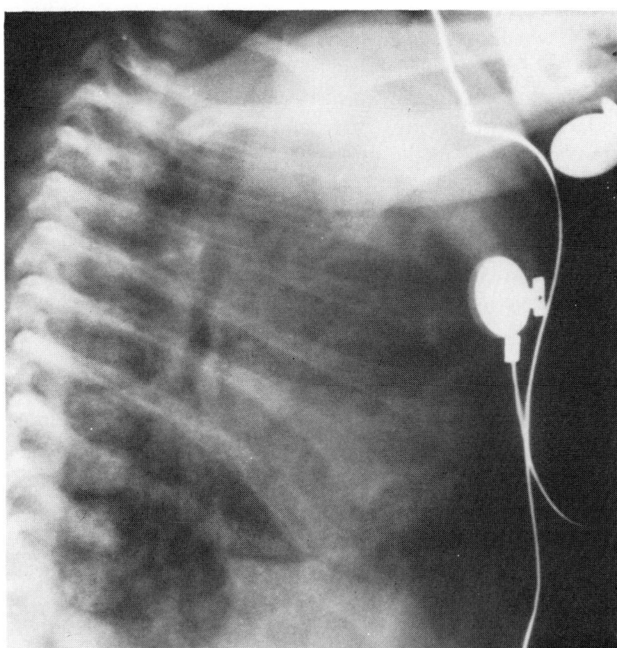

B

**Fig. 66-1.** (*a*) Anteroposterior and (*b*) lateral chest radiographs of a severely ill 1-month-old male infant with chlamydial pneumonitis. Diffuse interstitial infiltrates and hyperaeration with flattened diaphragms are prominent.

Beem's findings were corroborated and expanded by Harrison and his colleagues,[7] who compared 16 cases of *C. trachomatis* pneumonitis with 27 cases of pneumonitis not due to that agent. *C. trachomatis* was highly correlated with a history of cough and congestion of more than a week's duration, rales on auscultation, hyperinflation on x-ray, ≥400 eosinophils per cubic millimeter, and serum IgG ≥ 500 and IgM ≥ 110 mg/dl, respectively. Presentation for care occurred primarily at 3 to 11 weeks of age. Interestingly, conjunctivitis, wheezing, and diffuse interstitial radiographic infiltrates did not correlate with chlamydial illness in that study.

Tipple et al.[35] compared 41 infants with chlamydial pneumonitis to 15 infants with other types of afebrile pneumonia. Presentation for care at 4 to 11 weeks with a prolonged prodrome was highly associated with chlamydial pneumonitis. Staccato cough and wheeze were not correlated, although conjunctivitis and abnormal tympanic membranes (possibly due to otitis) were present significantly more often upon examination. Eosinophilia (≥300 eosinophils per cubic millimeter) and elevated immunoglobulin levels were again consistently present in cases of chlamydial disease.

In summary, a consistent clinical and laboratory picture of chlamydial pneumonitis has emerged (Tables 66-2 and 66-3). Infants typically present at 3 to 11 weeks of age with a prolonged history of cough and congestion. They need not have had previous clinical conjunctivitis (although that history should raise suspicion). They are usually afebrile and do not have significant systemic illness. Respiratory findings are dominated by cough, congestion, tachypnea, and rales. Although a pertussoid staccato cough is not necessarily a part of the clinical findings, such a cough should alert the physician to the possible diagnosis. Radiographs reveal hyperinflation with infiltrates (Fig. 66-1), and blood examination reveals eosinophilia and hyperimmunoglobulinemia. Untreated, the course may be protracted.

Data have been presented[8] which suggest that some fraction of infants (the proportion is as yet undetermined) will present with a clinical picture of bronchiolitis rather than pneumonitis. That is, wheezing and hyperinflation will be more prominent findings than cough, rales, and infiltrates.

## OTHER INFECTIONS

### Chronic respiratory disease resulting from infant infection

Some data suggest that chlamydial pneumonitis of infancy may be associated with chronic respiratory disease in childhood.[8] In a study investigating chronic sequelae of infant respiratory illness, admission sera from 47 infants less than 6 months of age, who were admitted to the hospital for acute lower respiratory disease between 1972 and 1977, were examined for evidence of chlamydial infection. Chlamydial pneumonitis was not being entertained as a diagnostic possibility during the period of the study, so the study was essentially double-blinded both at enrollment and throughout the follow-up period. The infants in the study received convalescent functional residual capacity (FRC) therapy during their hospitalization and yearly thereafter.

Table 66-2. Clinical Characteristics of Infant Pneumonitis

| | Infants | |
|---|---|---|
| | Chlamydia-positive total | Chlamydia-negative total |
| Presentation at 3–11 weeks | 53/57 (93%) | 19/42 (45%) |
| Prodrome more than 1 week | 45/57 (79%) | 17/42 (40%) |
| Conjunctivitis | 26/57 (46%) | 5/39 (13%) |
| Ear abnormalities | 24/41 (59%) | 0/15 (0%) |
| Staccato cough | 24/41 (59%) | 4/15 (27%) |
| Wheeze | 9/57 (16%) | 14/32 (44%) |
| Rales | 14/16 (88%) | 14/27 (52%) |

SOURCE: After Harrison[7] and Tipple.[35]

Of the 47 infants, 10 (21 percent) had antibody titers indicating acute, active infection with *C. trachomatis*. They were significantly younger than the other 37 infants, had more pneumonia (as opposed to bronchiolitis), and had significantly fewer viral etiologies identified (3 of 10 vs. 24 of 37, $p = 0.04$). All of these factors were consistent with chlamydial pneumonia syndrome.

The families of the 47 infants were given questionnaires to complete at the time of the infants' hospitalization and at the time of each annual follow-up visit. The questionnaires were used to determine histories of coughs and wheezing in the infants, as well as to determine histories for other family members of asthma, allergies, smoking, illness experiences, and several other factors. The FRC was analyzed for the infants as a measure of pulmonary function. The outcome measure employed was abnormal patient-months of reported symptoms (coughs, wheezing) or FRC divided by total patient-months of follow-up. On analysis, there was significantly more chronic cough and wheezing by history and abnormal FRCs in the chlamydial group than in the nonchlamydial group of infants. This association was not accounted for by family histories of asthma, smoking, allergies, emphysema, or chronic bronchitis or by histories of allergies, asthma, eczema, or hay fever in the children themselves.

These results should be looked upon with some caution and skepticism. They were derived from a small sample of infants hospitalized with moderate to severe illness; mild chlamydial disease may not have the same implications. There are two more studies which appear to confirm these findings. Weiss[44] showed diminution in respiratory function in a 7- to 8-year follow-up of some of Beem's original pneumonitis infants when he compared them with controls. Brasfield[36] showed abnormal pulmonary function in 60 percent of 25 infants with pneumonia caused by chlamydia, cytomegalovirus, pneumocystis, or ureaplasma. Whether or not this places such infants at increased risk of hyperactive airway disease in later childhood remains a debatable issue.[45]

Table 66-3. Laboratory Characteristics of Infant Pneumonitis

| | Infants | |
|---|---|---|
| | Chlamydia-positive total | Chlamydia-negative total |
| **Radiography** | | |
| Diffuse infiltrates | 47/57 (82%) | 20/42 (48%) |
| Hyperinflation | 47/57 (82%) | 15/42 (36%) |
| Eosinophilia | | |
| $>300/\text{mm}^3$ | 29/41 (71%) | 1/15 (7%) |
| $>400/\text{mm}^3$ | 12/16 (75%) | 3/27 (11%) |
| **Immunoglobulins** | | |
| IgG | | |
| Elevated | 38/41 (93%) | 3/15 (20%) |
| >500 mg/dl | 13/15 (87%) | 9/20 (45%) |
| IgM | | |
| Elevated | 41/41 (100%) | 8/15 (53%) |
| >110 mg/dl | 14/15 (93%) | 1/21 (5%) |
| IgA | | |
| Elevated | 34/41 (83%) | 4/15 (27%) |
| >30 mg/dl | 11/15 (73%) | 8/21 (38%) |

SOURCE: After Harrison[7] and Tipple.[35]

## OTITIS MEDIA

Tipple and her colleagues[35] reported isolation of *C. trachomatis* from the middle ear fluids of 3 of 11 infants with chlamydial pneumonia who had serous otitis media. However, the nasopharynx, a favorite site for chlamydial infection, is connected to the middle ear; true evidence of infection in terms of the presence of organisms, local antibody, and a serum response has been lacking. Hammerschlag[46] examined 68 children aged 9 months to 8 years, who underwent myringotomies for serous otitis media or recurrent acute otitis. She and her coworkers could not isolate *C. trachomatis* from any of the 68 middle ear effusions. The organism was, however, isolated from the nasopharynx of one 22-month-old girl who also had local antibody present. These results are supported by the work of Jones,[47] in whose series of 52 children aged 1 month to 11.9 years with persistent serous otitis media, *C. trachomatis* was not clearly found in any middle ear effusions. Local antibody was present in one child, and serum antibody in none of the 16 whose blood was tested. These two studies indicate that *C. trachomatis* is not a major agent in recurrent or persistent serous otitis media. A possible confounding factor here is that children with recurrent or persistent serous otitis media have usually had many previous courses of antibiotic therapy, which may have eliminated organisms in the middle ear fluid. Consequently, these studies may underestimate the role of *C. trachomatis* in middle ear disease.

In fact, in a third study, Chang and colleagues[48] have recovered *C. trachomatis* from the middle ear fluids of 2 of 11 children with acute otitis media, a 28-month-old and a 10-month-old; and from 1 of 14 children with recurrent otitis, a 6-year-old. Local and serum antibody data and nasopharyngeal culture results were not presented. In a retrospective case record study comparing infants born to infected vs. uninfected mothers, there was twice the rate of recurrent otitis media in exposed vs. unexposed infants during the first 6 months of life.[49] Since these studies were completed there has been little additional evidence to support otitis media as a significant sequela of infants' infection. In fact, larger prospective studies have not demonstrated such outcomes. This may be due to the increase in use of systemic erythromycin in infants with conjunctivitis or lower respiratory tract disease in the first 4 months of life.

## DIFFERENTIAL DIAGNOSIS OF CONJUNCTIVITIS AND PNEUMONITIS

### CONJUNCTIVITIS

Chemical conjunctivitis caused by silver nitrate prophylaxis and gonococcal ophthalmia neonatorum are the most common differential diagnostic possibilities in conjunctival inflammation in the first week of life. Silver nitrate prophylaxis usually causes marked lid swelling in the first 24 h of life but little discharge; the reaction is usually gone within 3 days. Gonococcal ophthalmia most often presents at 2 to 5 days of age with a copious yellow purulent exudate and marked lid edema. This illness has the worrisome potential of corneal invasion and rupture.

Other agents causing infant conjunctivitis include *Staphylococcus aureus, Streptococcus pneumoniae, Haemophilus influenzae,* and *Haemophilus aegyptius,* other gram-negative organisms such as *Klebsiella* and *Neisseria meningitidis,* and streptococci.[50,51] All of these have similar clinical findings: edema and erythema of the conjunctivas and purulent discharge. Gram's stain and bacterial culture of discharge are necessary for diagnosis.

*Staph. aureus* and enteric gram-negative organisms are usually nosocomially acquired, whereas the other organisms have been thought to be transmitted among family members. More recent evidence, however, suggests that *H. influenzae,* pneumococci, and streptococci are inhabitants of the genital tract and may be transmitted to the infant during delivery.

Another important consideration is viral infection. Herpes simplex virus, acquired by passage through the mother's infected genital secretions, may cause neonatal ophthalmia. Signs of meningitis, disseminated infection, or cutaneous herpes (vesicles) help to distinguish this infection from bacterial conjunctivitis, although vesicles have been occasionally reported in *H. influenzae* disease. As with gonococcal infections, herpetic eye infections have great potential for corneal damage. Finally, adenovirus type 8 has been reported as a cause of neonatal ophthalmia.[52] The infection was self-limited and occurred without scarring.

## PNEUMONITIS

Tipple[35] found respiratory syncytial virus, cytomegalovirus, and adenovirus in chlamydia-negative infants with afebrile pneumonia. Harrison's study[7] added nonpolio enteroviruses and parainfluenza type 3. Brasfield[36] has suggested that *Pneumocystis carinii* produces a clinical disease indistinguishable from those of *C. trachomatis* and cytomegalovirus.

Other agents that must be considered in infant pneumonitis, particularly in the presence of fever and systemic findings, include the influenza viruses (A and B) and the bacterial pathogens of infancy: group A and B beta-hemolytic streptococci, *S. aureus, Escherichia coli* and *Klebsiella* spp., *H. influenzae,* pneumococcus, and *N. meningitidis,* especially type Y. *Bordetella pertussis* infection is a very important consideration that cannot be overlooked. The current pertussis vaccine has an efficacy of only about 70 percent, even after a complete primary series; most infants presenting with possible chlamydial pneumonia are either not immunized or incompletely immunized. Pertussis can cause a similar cough (often subacute), may be afebrile, and may show hyperaeration and infiltrate on chest x-ray.

Tuberculosis and coccidioidomycosis must be considered in infant respiratory diseases, given appropriate exposures or residence in endemic areas. Finally, *Legionella pneumophilia* may occasionally cause pneumonitis in children less than 6 months of age and should be thought of in otherwise undiagnosed cases. There is generally little reason to be concerned about the lymphocytic interstitial pneumonia (LIP) associated with human immunodeficiency virus (HIV) and Epstein-Barr virus (EBV) infections, since chlamydial pneumonia is rare after 4 months of age and LIP is rare before 6 months of age, characteristically occurring after the first birthday. They also differ in that tachypnia, rather than staccato cough, appears at LIP onset, and the radiographic pattern is more diffuse in LIP.

Faced with a myriad of possibilities, clinicians generally rely on the degree of systemic illness, the findings of the chest radiograph (diffuse vs. local infiltrates, consolidation, effusion, hyperinflation, pneumatoceles, hilar adenopathy, etc.), the clinical picture, blood cultures, nasopharyngeal viral cultures, and nasopharyngeal fluorescent antibody and pertussis culture; direct tracheal aspirates (via laryngoscopy) and lung biopsy may be employed in refractory cases.

# DIAGNOSIS

## INCLUSION CONJUNCTIVITIS

Inclusion conjunctivitis of the newborn is perhaps the easiest of the chlamydial infections to diagnose. The principal method of diagnosis has been and remains, in most settings, the Giemsa-stained conjunctival smear (Plate 94). In this technique the eyelid is everted and conjunctival scrapings are taken, usually with a platinum spatula. Adequate epithelial cell preparations cannot be obtained with a swab. The scrapings are spread thinly on a microscope slide and stained with Giemsa stain. *C. trachomatis* inclusions are seen in the cytoplasm of conjunctival cells as a circumscribed group of blue or purple granules.[53] The inclusions frequently are adjacent to the nucleus and may replace much of the cell cytoplasm. In practice this technique requires experience in scraping the conjunctivas, preparing and staining the slide, and interpreting the smear. Often a prolonged and unhurried examination by an experienced technician is necessary.

A newer and more sensitive method for diagnosis is via culture of organisms in an in vitro cell culture system, with demonstration of the organism in the cell monolayer with an iodine or fluorescent antibody stain. These methods utilize a continuous cell monolayer, usually McCoy cells[54] or HeLa 229,[55] that have been treated with cycloheximide.[56] The second essential feature of the method is that the inoculum is centrifuged onto the cell monolayer (see Chaps. 15 and 74). In this procedure a vigorous conjunctival swab specimen obtained with a calcium alginate–tipped swab is placed in liquid transport medium, and an aliquot is inoculated in cell culture. The presence of chlamydial inclusions after 2 to 4 days of incubation is diagnostic. Experienced workers[57] have found cell culture techniques to be virtually 100 percent effective for diagnosis of neonatal inclusion conjunctivitis, whereas cytology is about 95 percent sensitive.

A third method of diagnosis is by antigen detection using either direct fluorescent antibody smears[51] or enzyme immunoassay.[58] Both are feasible and are only a little less sensitive than cell culture methods (although this is not well substantiated for these sites). In situations in which none of these techniques is available, practical diagnosis is made presumptively by suspecting chlamydial conjunctivitis on clinical grounds and excluding other bacterial etiologies via Gram's stain and culture. A culture for the gonococcus should be obtained in every case of neonatal conjunctivitis.

## PNEUMONITIS

Diagnosis of chlamydial pneumonitis has been made by isolation of the organism (in cell culture systems) from culture specimens of the nasopharynx,[7,27,35] tracheal aspirates,[7,40] and lung biopsy material.[29,30] More recently, antigen detection methods, by direct fluorescent antibody smear[59] or enzyme immunoassay,[58] have been used. In addition, serum antichlamydial antibody titers have been useful in diagnosing acute infection, especially in patients with prior antibiotic therapy, in whom cultures may be negative. The usual method is the micro-IF method of Wang,[38] which utilizes elementary bodies in yolk-sac suspension as antigen. With this method an acute IgM titer $\geq$ 1:32[7] has been highly correlated with chlamydial pneumonitis. Mahoney[60] evaluated a solid-phase enzyme immunoassay (EIA) for the measurement of IgM to *C. trachomatis*. This assay appears very useful in the diagnosis of infant pneumonia.

Both culture and serologic techniques require experienced laboratories. In the absence of readily available facilities, the diagnosis of chlamydial pneumonitis should be suspected in an infant with the clinical syndrome described in this chapter. The chest radiograph, the eosinophil count, and the serum IgG and IgM levels may be used as corroborating information. The concurrent presence of Giemsa-positive inclusion conjunctivitis also points to chlamydial etiology in an infant with pneumonitis. In addition, bacterial cultures and nasopharyngeal fluorescent antibody for pertussis should rule out other treatable pathogens.

## MANAGEMENT

### INCLUSION CONJUNCTIVITIS

Topical treatment of inclusion conjunctivitis with sulfonamide, tetracycline, or erythromycin ophthalmic preparations is no longer recommended for two reasons. They are often not applied correctly and they fail to eliminate nasopharyngeal carriage, and therefore do not decrease the risk of recurrent conjunctivitis or pneumonia. Therefore, the Centers for Disease Control[61] and the American Academy of Pediatrics[62] recommend oral erythromycin, 30 to 50 mg/kg of body weight per day in four divided doses for 2 weeks as initial therapy for chlamydia ophthalmia neonatorum.

### INFANT PNEUMONITIS

There are no controlled clinical trials of antibiotics vs. placebo (or no treatment) in the course of outcome of chlamydial pneumonitis. However, Beem and colleagues have utilized sulfisoxazole, 150 mg/kg per day, or erythromycin ethyl succinate, 40 mg/kg per day, for approximately 2 weeks in 32 infants.[63] All of the infants stopped shedding organisms and improved clinically soon after initiation of therapy, and none had clinical relapses. Improvement in symptoms usually began within 7 days of therapy, and progression to recovery was observed in 27 of 28 infants followed. This study suggests that both of the above regimens are successful. The recommendation of both the Centers for Disease Control[61] and the American Academy of Pediatrics[62] are for oral erythromycin therapy in the same dosage and duration as for ophthalmia neonatorum.

On occasion, infants with chlamydial pneumonitis may be severely hypoxemic[35] and exhibit marked respiratory distress. In these infants oxygen and, if necessary, mechanical ventilatory support are important supportive measures.

Since *C. trachomatis* is a sexually transmitted organism, the identification of an infant with conjunctivitis or pneumonitis implies the presence of one or possibly two infected parents. These individuals have the clear potential of further transmitting the organism among the sexually active adult population. Ideally, the parents of an infected infant should be cultured for *C. trachomatis* and, if positive, treated to eliminate infection. Although this is not routinely done because of difficulty, expense, and sensitivities it is an ideal that perhaps should be strived for.

## PREVENTION

If it is assumed that the majority of infant chlamydial infection (and subsequent disease) is a result of vertical transmission of the organism at delivery, then there are two theoretically optimal methods for preventive intervention to interrupt transmission. The first method would be simultaneous treatment of cervically infected mothers and their sexual partners with systemic antibiotics during the third trimester. The therapy must be effective for the mother and partner and nontoxic for the fetus. Of the three major antichlamydial drugs (erythromycins, sulfonamides, and tetracyclines), only the erythromycin derivatives are satisfactory. Podgore and associates have reported[64] preliminary results of a randomized third-trimester trial of erythromycin base vs. no treatment in cervix-positive women and their partners. Forty-seven women volunteered for the randomized study. Eleven had cesarean section deliveries and their infants remained uninfected. Fourteen infants born to twenty-two infected, untreated women developed chlamydial illness or infection: seven infants had conjunctivitis, one had pneumonia, two had asymptomatic nasopharyngeal infection, and four had asymptomatic antibody acquisition. This is in contrast to no infection or illness in fourteen infants of treated mothers. These results suggest that third-trimester therapy is the method of choice for prevention of infant disease. This approach has been supported in an uncontrolled study by Schachter.[65] Unfortunately cultures are expensive, time-consuming, and limited in availability. In addition, the group of women with the highest carriage rate of chlamydiae is the same group that has a high rate of pregnancies without prenatal care. In this group third-trimester prophylaxis is not a possibility even when diagnostic capabilities are available.

Up to now, ocular prophylaxis has been almost totally aimed at prevention of gonococcal ophthalmia, with silver nitrate as the drug of choice. Based upon review of large amounts of available data,[66] the Centers for Disease Control[61] and the American Academy of Pediatrics[62] have endorsed ointments containing 1% tetracycline or 0.5% erythromycin as alternative methods of eye prophylaxis. One study by Hammerschlag and coworkers[67] has compared the efficacy of erythromycin ointment vs. silver nitrate drops for prevention of neonatal inclusion conjunctivitis and/or respiratory chlamydial infection. Of 60 infants born to chlamydia-positive women, 36 received silver nitrate and 24 received erythromycin. Of the 36 infants who received silver nitrate, 12 developed chlamydial conjunctivitis, as compared to none of the 24 infants who received erythromycin ($p$ = 0.001). However, 10 of the 36 infants who received silver nitrate and 5 of the 24 infants who received erythromycin developed chlamydial nasopharyngeal infection, and 3 of the 10 and 1 of the 5, respectively, developed pneumonia. Thus, topical ocular erythromycin prophylaxis may prevent chlamydial conjunctivitis but does not appear to prevent the respiratory infections. Subsequent studies have not consistently shown the same protection. Laga in a large controlled trial in Kenya[68] showed a 77 percent reduction in the evidence of chlamydia ophthalmia when tetracycline prophylaxis was given but nearly as much (68 percent) when silver nitrate prophylaxis was used. Bell found erythromycin prophylaxis to be no more effective than silver nitrate. Hammerschlag recently found no difference between silver nitrate, erythromycin, and tetracycline prophylaxis.[73] In these instances the failures of antibiotic prophylaxis appear to be associated with late onset of conjunctivitis, suggesting that they are related to the failure of the method to eradicate nasopharyngeal carriage and reseeding of the conjunctiva. The reason for disparate results in different studies is not clear.

None of the eye prophylaxis regimens are adequate for prevention of nasopharyngitis or pneumonia. New approaches are needed in this area, as well as the development of faster and less expensive prenatal detection methods that will make third-trimester treatment possible.

## References


1 Martin DH et al: Risk factors for *Chlamydia trachomatis* in high risk populations of pregnant women, in *Chlamydia Infection,* D Oriel et al (eds). Cambridge, England, Cambridge University Press, 1986, p 189.

2 Berman S et al: Low birth weight, prematurity and post partum endometritis association with prenatal cervical *Mycoplasma hominis* and *Chlamydia trachomatis* infections. *JAMA* 257:1189, 1987.

3 Hardy PH et al: Prevalence of six sexually transmitted disease agents among pregnant inner city adolescents and pregnancy outcome. *Lancet* 2:333, 1984.

4 Chandler JW et al: Ophthalmia neonatorum associated with maternal chlamydial infections. *Trans Am Acad Ophthalmol Otolaryngol* 83:302, 1977.

5 Frommell GT et al: Chlamydial infections of mothers and their infants. *J Pediatr* 95:28, 1979.

6 Schachter J et al: Prospective study of perinatal transmission of *Chlamydia trachomatis. JAMA* 255:3374, 1986.

7 Harrison HR et al: *Chlamydia trachomatis* infant pneumonitis: Comparison with matched controls and other infant pneumonitis. *N Engl J Med* 298:702, 1978.

8 Harrison HR et al: *Chlamydia trachomatis* and chronic childhood lung disease. *Pediatr Infect Dis* 1:29, 1982.

9 Stagno S et al: Infant pneumonitis associated with cytomegalovirus, *Chlamydia, Pneumocystis,* and *Ureaplasma:* A prospective study. *Pediatrics* 68:322, 1981.

10 Dunlop EMC et al: Infection of the eye, genitalia, and rectum by a new serotype (type G) of TRIC agent: Clinical and laboratory aspects. *Br J Vener Dis* 49:301, 1973.

11 Dunlop EMC et al: Relation of TRIC agent to non-specific genital infection. *Br J Vener Dis* 42:77, 1966.

12 Fuster CD et al: Vaginal *Chlamydia trachomatis* prevalence in sexually abused prepubertal girls. *Pediatrics* 79:235, 1987.

13 Hammerschlag MR et al: False positive results with the use of chlamydia antigen detection tests in the evaluation of suspected abuse of children. *Pediatr Infect Dis* 7:11, 1988.

14 Black SB et al: Serologic evidence of chlamydial infection in children. *J Pediatr* 98:65, 1981.

15 San Joaquin VH et al: Prevalence of chlamydial antibodies in children. *Am J Dis Child* 136:425, 1982.

16 Schachter JS: Human *Chlamydia psittaci* infection, in *Chlamydia Infections,* D Oriel et al (eds). Cambridge, England, Cambridge University Press, 1986, p 311.

17 Komaroff AL et al: Serologic evidence of chlamydial and mycoplasmal pharyngitis in adults. *Science* 222:927, 1983.

18 Reed BD et al: Prevalence of *Chlamydia trachomatis* and mycoplasmic pneumoniae in children with and without pharyngitis. *J Fam Pract* 26:387, 1988.

19 Neinstein LS et al: Low prevalence of *Chlamydia trachomatis* in the oropharynx of adolescents. *Pediatr Infect Dis* 5:660, 1986.

20 Rettig PJ et al: Prevalence of antibody to *C. trachomatis, C. psittaci* and TWAR strain in pediatric sera. *Proc 1988 ICAAC* Los Angeles, CA, October 1988, p 212.

21 Persson K et al: Chlamydial respiratory infection in childhood and spurious immunoglobulin M. *Eur J Clin Microbiol* 5:581, 1986.

22 Mordhorst CH: Clinical epidemiology of oculogenital *Chlamydia* infection, in *Nongonococcal Urethritis and Related Infections,* D Hobson et al (eds). Washington, DC, American Society for Microbiology, 1977, p 126.

23 Goscienski PJ, Sexton RR: Follow-up studies in neonatal inclusion conjunctivitis. *Am J Dis Child* 124:180, 1972.

24 Forster RK et al: Late follow-up of patients with neonatal inclusion conjunctivitis. *Am J Ophthalmol* 69:467, 1970.

25 Freedman A et al: Infection by TRIC agent and other members of the bedsonia group; with a note on Reiter's disease: II. *Ophthalmia neonatorum* due to TRIC agent. *Trans Ophthalmol Soc* 86:313, 1966.

26 Alexander ER et al: Further characterization of TRIC agent strains of genital origin. *Rev Int Trach* 45:297, 1968.

27 Beem MO, Saxon EM: Respiratory-tract colonization and a distinctive pneumonia syndrome in infants infected with *Chlamydia trachomatis. N Engl J Med* 296:306, 1977.

28 Harrison HR et al: Experimental nasopharyngitis and pneumonia caused by *Chlamydia trachomatis* in infant baboons: Histopathologic comparison with a case in a human infant. *J Infect Dis* 139:141, 1979.

29 Frommell GT et al: Isolation of *Chlamydia trachomatis* from infant lung tissue. *N Engl J Med* 296:1150, 1977.

30 Arth C et al: Chlamydial pneumonitis. *J Pediatr* 93:447, 1978.

31 Graham DM: Growth and neutralization of the trachoma agent in mouse lungs. *Nature* 207:1379, 1965.

32 Graham DM: Growth and immunogenicity of *TRIC* agents in mice. *Am J Ophthalmol* 63:1173, 1967.

33 Chen W-J, Kuo C-C: A mouse model of pneumonitis induced by *Chlamydia trachomatis:* Morphologic, microbiologic, and immunologic studies. *Am J Pathol* 100:365, 1980.

34 Harrison HR et al: *Chlamydia trachomatis* pneumonitis in the C57BL/KsJ mouse: Pathologic and immunologic features. *J Lab Clin Med* 100:953, 1982.

35 Tipple MA et al: Clinical characteristics of the afebrile pneumonia associated with *Chlamydia trachomatis* infection in infants less than 6 months of age. *Pediatrics* 63:192, 1979.

36 Brasfield DM et al: Infant pneumonitis associated with cytomegalovirus, chlamydia, Pneumocystis and Ureaplasma. *Pediatrics* 79:76, 1987.

37 Schachter J et al: Prospective study of chlamydial infections in neonates. *Lancet* 2:377, 1979.

38 Wang S-P et al: Simplified microimmunofluorescence test with trachoma-lymphogranuloma venereum (*Chlamydia trachomatis*) antigens for use as a screening test for antibody. *J Clin Microbiol* 1:250, 1975.

39 Thygeson P, Stone W Jr: Epidemiology of inclusion conjunctivitis. *Arch Ophthalmol* 27:91, 1942.

40 Schachter J et al: Pneumonitis following inclusion blennorrhea. *J Pediatr* 87:779, 1975.

41 Botsztejn A: Die pertussoide, eosinophile pneumonie des sauglings. *Ann Paediatr (Basel)* 157:28, 1941.

42 Biro Z: Twelve more cases of interstitial pertussoid eosinophilic pneumonia in infants. *Helv Paediatr Acta* 15:135, 1960.

43 Oetgen WJ: Pertussoid eosinophilic pneumonia. Pulmonary infiltrates with eosinophilia in very young infants. *Chest* 71:492, 1977.

44 Weiss SG et al: Pulmonary assessment of children after chlamydial pneumonia of infancy. *J Pediatr* 108:659, 1987.

45 McConnachie KM et al: Normal pulmonary function measurements and airway reactivity in childhood after mild bronchiolitis. *J Pediatr* 107:54, 1985.

46 Hammerschlag MR et al: The role of *Chlamydia trachomatis* in middle ear effusions in children. *Pediatrics* 66:615, 1980.

47 Jones RB et al: Failure to demonstrate a major etiologic role for *Chlamydia trachomatis* in persistent serous otitis media, abstracted (no. 525). Read before the Twentieth International Conference on Antimicrobial Agents and Chemotherapy. Washington, DC, American Society for Microbiology, 1980.

48 Chang MJ et al: *Chlamydia trachomatis* in otitis media in children. *Pediatr Infect Dis* 1:95, 1982.

49 Schaefer C et al: Illnesses in infants born to women with *Chlamydia trachomatis* infection: A prospective study. *Am J Dis Child* 139:127, 1985.

50 Sandström KI et al: Microbial causes of neonatal conjunctivitis. *J Pediatr* 105:706, 1984.

51 Rapoza P et al: Assessment of neonatal conjunctivitis with a direct immunofluorescent monoclonal antibody stain for chlamydia. *JAMA* 255:3369, 1986.

52 Dawson CR et al: A family outbreak of adenovirus 8 infection (epidemic keratoconjunctivitis). *Am J Hyg* 72:279, 1960.

53 Yoneda C et al: Cytology as a guide to the presence of chlamydial inclusions in Giemsa-stained conjunctival smears in severe endemic trachoma. *Br J Ophthalmol* 59:116, 1975.

54 Wentworth BB, Alexander ER: Isolation of *Chlamydia trachomatis* by use of 2-iodo-2-deoxyuridine-treated cells. *Appl Microbiol* 27:912, 1974.

55 Kuo C-C et al: Primary isolation of TRIC organisms in HeLa 229 cells treated with DEAE-dextran. *J Infect Dis* 125:665, 1972.

56 Ripa KT, Mårdh P-A: Cultivation of *Chlamydia trachomatis* in cycloheximide-treated McCoy cells. *J Clin Microbiol* 6:328, 1977.

57 Schachter J, Dawson CR: Comparative efficiency of various diagnostic methods for chlamydial infection, in *Nongonococcal Urethritis and Related Infections,* D Hobson et al (eds). Washington, DC, American Society for Microbiology, 1977, p 337.

58 Hammerschlag MR et al: Comparison of enzyme immunoassay and culture for diagnosis of chlamydial conjunctivitis and respiratory infection in infants. *J Clin Microbiol* 25:2306, 1987.

59 Friis B et al: Rapid diagnosis of *Chlamydia trachomatis* pneumonia in infants. *Acta Pathol Microbiol Scand* (B) 92:139, 1984.

60 Mahony JB et al: Accuracy of immunoglobulin M immunoassay for diagnosis of chlamydial infections in infants and adults. *J Clin Microbiol* 24:731, 1986.

61 Centers for Disease Control: STD treatment guidelines. *MMWR* 34 (suppl):45, 1985.

62 American Academy of Pediatrics: Report of the Committee on Infectious Diseases. American Academy of Pediatrics, Illinois, 1988, p 152.

63 Beem MO et al: Treatment of chlamydial pneumonia in infancy. *Pediatrics* 63:198, 1979.

64 Podgore JK et al: Effectiveness of maternal third trimester erythromycin in prevention of infant *Chlamydia trachomatis* infection, abstracted (no. 524). Read before the Twentieth International Conference on Antimicrobial Agents and Chemotherapy. Washington, DC, American Society for Microbiology, 1980.

65 Schachter JS et al: Experience with the routine use of erythromycin for chlamydial infection in pregnancy. *N Engl J Med* 314:276, 1986.

66 Rothenberg R: *Ophthalmia neonatorum* due to *Neisseria gonorrhoeae. Sex Transm Dis* 6:187, 1979.

67 Hammerschlag MR et al: Erythromycin ointment for ocular prophylaxis of neonatal chlamydial infection. *JAMA* 224:2291, 1980.

68 Laga M et al: Prophylaxis of gonococcal and chlamydial ophthalmia neonatorum: A comparison of silver nitrate and tetracycline. *N Engl J Med* 318:653, 1988.

69 Bell TA et al: Comparison of ophthalmic silver nitrate solution and erythromycin ointment for prevention of natally acquired *Chlamydia trachomatis. Sex Transm Dis* 14:195, 1987.

70 Hammerschlag MR et al: Prospective study of maternal and infantile infection with *Chlamydia trachomatis. Pediatrics* 64:142, 1979.

71 Mårdh P-A et al: Colonization of pregnant and puerperal women and neonates with *Chlamydia trachomatis. Br J Vener Dis* 56:96, 1980.

72 Datta P et al: Infection and disease after perinatal exposure to *Chlamydia trachomatis* in Nairobi, Kenya. *J Infect Dis* 158:524, 1988.

73 Hammerschlag MR et al: Efficacy of neonatal ocular prophylaxis for the prevention of chlamydia and gonococcal conjunctivitis. *N Engl J Med* 320:769, 1989.

# Chapter 67
# Congenital syphilis

Kenneth F. Schulz
F. Kevin Murphy
Pisespong Patamasucon
André Z. Meheus

## HISTORY

### EARLY OBSERVATIONS

The transmission of syphilis to infants was recognized in the earliest medical writings on "the French disease." Among the first treatises on syphilis was that of Gaspar Torella written in 1497, within 4 years of the first known outbreaks of syphilis in Spain. Torella noted that syphilis was "often seen" in nursing children, infection first appearing on the face or in the mouth. Although early writers clearly recognized the possibility of congenital transmission,[1–3] their attention was focused on the wet nurse as harbinger of the disease. The first measure advocated for the prevention of congenital syphilis was proscription of the use of wet nurses who had the French disease, even if apparently cured. Ambroise Paré, the eminent French surgeon, displayed the same prejudice in a chapter on syphilis among his collected works.[4] Paré described a good family of Paris, all of whom allegedly were infected from a syphilitic wet nurse, even the nursing child's two siblings. He concluded by advocating that the nurse be whipped naked through the streets of the city!

Paracelsus first suggested that syphilis might be transmitted from father to son by heredity.[5] In 1565 Simon de Vallembert described a case in the first French text on pediatrics that suggested such "hereditary syphilis."[6] After apparent recovery from syphilis a goldsmith of Tours fathered several afflicted children over a 14-year period, although their mother remained unaffected.

In spite of several misconceptions in the nineteenth century about mechanisms of transmission of congenital syphilis, several important empirical observations were made. These were accorded, in that simpler time, the status of "laws." Colles' law (1837)[7] stated that syphilitic infants could transmit the disease to previously healthy wet nurses but never to their own mothers. Guiseppe Profeta's law (1865) stated that a healthy infant born to a syphilitic mother is immune to the disease. Kassowitz's law (1876) stated that the toll of a mother's syphilis on the baby diminishes in successive pregnancies, although both Paul Diday (1854)[8] and Jonathan Hutchinson (1865)[9] had made this observation earlier. The observations of Colles and Profeta illustrated the principle that infection confers immunity to reinoculation with syphilis. However, neither Colles nor Profeta understood their observations.

Daniel Defoe in *Moll Flanders* (1722)[10] seemed to understand the transmission of congenital syphilis well. Moll, recalling an encounter with a drunken baronet who had paid for her services, imagines the baronet's regret on arriving home to his family:

> how would he be trembling for fear he had got the pox, . . . how would he, if he had any principles of honour, abhor the thought of giving any ill distemper, if he had it, as for aught he knew he might, to his modest and virtuous wife, and thereby sowing the contagion in the life-blood of his posterity!

Nevertheless, the character of hereditary syphilis was not clarified totally until 1906, when the Wassermann test made it possible to demonstrate that transmission of syphilis to a fetus required an infected albeit sometimes asymptomatic mother.

### CLINICAL DESCRIPTIONS

Actual clinical descriptions of congenital syphilis were sparse during the sixteenth through the eighteenth century. Lenoir, in 1780, established a lying-in hospital in Paris for syphilitic mothers, the first such specialized care for either neonates or high-risk pregnancies. It was out of the large accumulated experience at this institution that Bertin wrote his classic monograph of congenital syphilis.[11] He recognized several cutaneous lesions; mucous membrane lesions involving eyes, nose, urethra, and anus; adenopathy; and bone lesions, including epiphysitis. Bertin and others recognized the importance of the skeletal examination, but many later authorities including Trousseau and Diday considered skeletal lesions rare in congenital syphilis. It would remain for a succession of bright new radiologists between 1900 and 1907 to prove that bony lesions could be demonstrated in infants with no other clinical lesions and were the most sensitive indication of clinical disease.

Parrot[12] and Wegner,[13] working without the benefit of x-rays, described clearly the osteochondritis of congenital syphilis, and Parrot went so far as to declare that every bone of the infantile syphilitic skeleton is affected. His name is applied both to the cranial nodes (hot cross bun skull) and to the pseudoparalysis which he described. However, Parrot, in his enthusiasm, believed that rickets was a later lesion of congenital syphilis, an error later corrected by the American, Robert Taylor.[14]

Jonathan Hutchinson's writings[15,16] dominated nineteenth century British clinical descriptions of congenital syphilis in the way that Diday's dominated the French literature. Hutchinson is best known for a clear description of the dental deformities[15] and their association with interstitial keratitis and deafness in late congenital syphilis. Diday's major text, originally published in 1854,[8] described most of the cutaneous and visceral manifestations of congenital syphilis known today and characterized the general appearance of the infant as that of "a little, wrinkled, pot-bellied old man with a cold in his head."

The risks of delivering a congenitally infected infant were well described in the Oslo study of untreated syphilis (from 1891 to 1910; see Chap. 19). Boeck observed that 26 percent of babies born to syphilitic mothers remained free of disease or recovered spontaneously with conversion to seronegativity, 25 percent were seropositive but remained clinically unaffected, and 49 percent displayed manifest disease.[17]

## PREVENTION

Fournier, a student of Diday, wrote a detailed treatise on prevention of congenital syphilis, originally published in 1858.[18] Fournier's concepts influenced premarital counseling for almost a century. He required before marriage, or before resumption of intercourse, that the syphilitic patient (1) have no active lesions, (2) wait 3 to 4 years after onset of disease, (3) wait at least 18 to 24 months after the last sign of disease, (4) that the form of syphilis not be grave, and (5) that an "adequate" course of potassium iodide and mercury be completed (3 to 4 years). After 1906, serological testing for syphilis was added as a further premarital requirement, a practice that persists from a period when the prevalence of syphilis was high and treatment wanting.

Three observations in rapid succession between 1903 and 1906 placed the infectious etiology and diagnosis of syphilis on a secure footing: the experimental transmission of the disease to apes by Roux and Metchnikoff, the microscopic demonstration of *Treponema pallidum* by Schaudinn and Hoffmann, and Wassermann's development of a complement fixation test for syphilis using syphilitic fetal liver as a source of antigen. Within a year Levaditi demonstrated both the presence of spirochetes in syphilitic fetal tissue and the equal suitability of uninfected liver as an antigen source for the Wassermann test. It was soon recognized that identification of cases of maternal syphilis by the Wassermann test and treatment of the mother, even with arsenicals, could prevent neonatal syphilis. Finally, with the introduction of penicillin in 1943 by Mahoney, the essential clinical tools for control of congenital syphilis were available.

## EPIDEMIOLOGY

### UNITED STATES AND EUROPE

The cause of congenital syphilis is not *T. pallidum* alone. The web of social and economic factors that permit syphilis in pregnancy to occur and to go untreated must be considered a part of the etiology. Penicillin is 98 percent effective in preventing congenital syphilis in babies born to treated mothers.[19,20] There was a dramatic decline in congenital syphilis incidence in the United States following the introduction of penicillin (Fig. 67-1) but the incidence began to rise again by 1959, despite the ready availability of inexpensive penicillin. It was not until 1978 that the incidence again reached the 1957 low of 3.8 cases per 100,000 live births, and incidence is once more rising. Penicillin alone is not enough.

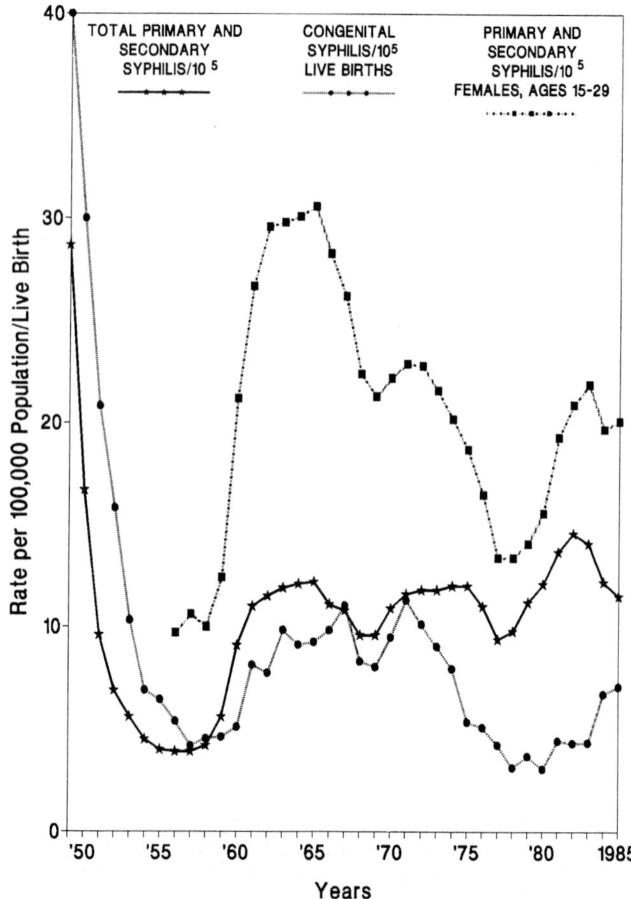


Fig. 67-1. Annual incidence of infant congenital syphilis compared to that of primary and secondary syphilis, United States, 1949 to 1985. The secular trend of incidence of infant congenital syphilis follows that of women in the childbearing age group by approximately 12 to 18 months. (*Courtesy of Joseph H. Blount, Division of Sexually Transmitted Diseases, Center for Prevention Services, CDC, US Public Health Service.*)

#### Incidence and prevalence prior to penicillin

Osler observed in 1917 that syphilis accounted for 20 percent of all stillbirths and 18 to 22 percent of infant deaths in the United States.[21] In Edinburgh, Browne (1922) found that 35 of 153 neonatal deaths were luetic in origin.[22] The overwhelming importance of perinatal syphilis in that period was a reflection of the prevalence of the disease in adults; 10 percent of women of the "hospital class" and 4.5 percent of umbilical cord blood samples in Glasgow's Royal Maternity & Women's Hospital had positive Wassermann tests.[23] School examinations in 1922 and 1923 in Plymouth indicated an 8 percent prevalence of manifest congenital syphilis among school age children. The prevalence of syphilis declined steadily between the wars, prenatal seropositivity falling to 1.8 percent in Glasgow, and from 12 to 4 percent in Kansas City between 1922 and 1937.[24] However, a 1936 U.S. Public Health Service survey indicated that 2 percent of U.S. children, and 5.6 percent of U.S. infants, were syphilitic, with striking disparities between whites and blacks (1.7 versus 12.2 percent) and between public and private patients (5.3 versus 1 percent). Investigations of families of an index case revealed latent or manifest syphilis in about one-fourth of family members.[25] A major upsurge in syphilis incidence during World War II in Europe and the United States was associated with a corresponding two- to three-fold increase in cases of congenital syphilis.[26] However, this effect was blunted somewhat in areas such as Glasgow, where comprehensive prenatal screening programs were already established.[25]

#### Syphilis and pregnancy

In the penicillin era in northern Europe and the United States, the prevalence of seropositivity in pregnancy is roughly 0.1 to 0.6 percent, after accounting for biological false-positive tests (0.08 to 0.22 percent) (Table 67-1). The prognosis for the outcome of pregnancy was studied by Harman (1917), who followed the obstetric events in 150 syphilitic women and 150 healthy women of similar social status[27] (Table 67-2). No impairment of subsequent ability to conceive was observed in the infected women, but 61.1 percent of their pregnancies were attended by accidents of pregnancy or birth of an infected child. Only 20.9 percent of pregnancies in healthy women were attended by complications. The risk of prematurity, perinatal death, and congenital syphilis is directly related to the stage of maternal syphilis during pregnancy. J. E. Moore believed that fetal infection occurred in 95 percent of cases of primary or secondary syphilis. In 59 cases of untreated maternal syphilis reviewed by Fiumara and colleagues (Table 67-3), all mothers with primary or secondary syphilis delivered a syphilitic, premature, or stillborn

**Table 67-1. Prevalence of Positive Serological Tests for Syphilis in Pregnancy**

| Period | Country | Population | Percent positive | Total tested |
|---|---|---|---|---|
| 1957–1958 | Norway | Nationalized maternal health clinics | 0.61 | 27,445 |
| 1959–1968 | U.K. | Queen Charlotte Hospital, London | 0.21* | 42,904 |
| 1966–1967 | U.K. | Bristol Public Health Laboratory | 0.13 | 35,912 |
| 1973–1974 | U.S. | Military dependents | 0.25 | 8,343 |
| 1982 | U.S. | Public hospital and clinics, Dallas | 1.0 | |

*Corrected for yaws; includes first visit serology only.

**Table 67-2. Prospective Observations of Obstetric Events in Syphilitic Women (1917)**

| Event | 150 syphilitic women | 150 controls |
|---|---|---|
| Pregnancies | 1001 | 826 |
| Miscarriages | 9.2% | 7.4% |
| Stillbirths | 8.0% | 2.1% |
| Infant deaths | 22.9% | 11.4% |
| Infant syphilis | 21.0% | 0.0% |
| Healthy child | 38.9% | 79.1% |

SOURCE: Harman.[27]

**Table 67-3. Outcome of Pregnancy in Relation to Stage of Maternal Syphilis**

| Outcome | Primary and secondary | Early latent | Late latent | Normal |
|---|---|---|---|---|
| Prematurity | 50% | 20% | 9% | 8% |
| Perinatal death | 0 | 20% | 11% | 1% |
| Congenital syphilis | 50% | 40% | 10% | 0 |
| Healthy child | 0 | 20% | 70% | 90% |

SOURCE: Fiumara et al.[28]

child, although only half of the children were manifestly syphilitic.[28] The rate of congenital syphilis and perinatal accidents dropped slightly in early latent syphilis. In late latent syphilis, 10 percent of the babies delivered had syphilis and 20 percent were stillborn or premature.

## Current incidence

The most useful congenital syphilis incidence figure is calculated as the number of cases under 1 year of age per 100,000 live births. The total reported cases gives a much larger and somewhat misleading numerator, because 85 percent of reported cases are late congenital syphilis; this included cases accumulated over as much as 5 to 10 years prior to the year of reporting, some of whom may have been previously reported. Infant cases, on the other hand, represent recent transmission and are a clearer representation of current disease activity.

The incidence of infantile congenital syphilis closely follows that of primary and secondary syphilis in women in the peak childbearing age group (15 to 29 years) (Fig. 67-1); this is also the peak age group in which early syphilis occurs. As men with male sexual partners accounted for an increasing share of syphilis morbidity, the ratio of male to female cases of infectious syphilis rose during the decade 1970–1979 (Fig. 67-2). The trend of infant congenital syphilis, accordingly, maintained a more steady decline than that of total primary and secondary syphilis. Nevertheless, 10 to 35 percent of gay men seen in STD clinics report female sexual partners;[29] it is therefore not surprising that in-

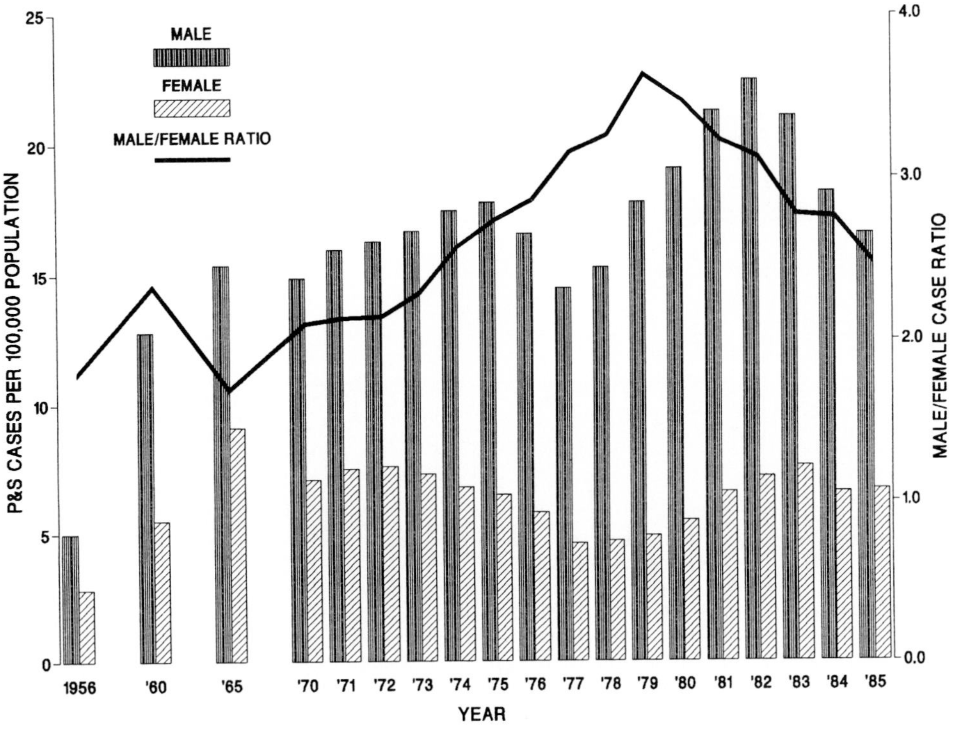

**Fig. 67-2.** Rising incidence of early infectious syphilis in men in the United States from 1970 to 1982 with a downtrend from 1982 to 1985. (*Courtesy of Joseph H. Blount, Division of Sexually Transmitted Diseases, Center for Prevention Services, CDC, US Public Health Service.*)

creasing incidence in this group was eventually followed by an upturn in early syphilis in women and their offspring by 1979 to 1981. With changing sexual behavior in male homosexuals due to the threat of AIDS, the male/female ratio of early syphilis cases has been decreasing since 1980 (Fig. 67-2).

Although the trend of infant congenital syphilis consistently follows that of female infectious syphilis, the numerical relationship between these two incidence figures is not constant (Fig. 67-3). An index of vertical transmission of syphilis can be calculated as the number of infant cases (under 1 year of age) per 1000 cases of female primary and secondary syphilis. The incidence curve for infant syphilis lags behind changes in that for infectious syphilis in 15- to 29-year-old women by approximately 1 year (Fig. 67-1).[26] This is taken into account in calculating a vertical transmission index (VTI) for syphilis: the number of cases of congenital syphilis under 1 year of age per 1000 cases of primary and secondary syphilis in women *in the preceding year*. The VTI can be seen as a reflection of the effectiveness of prevention of syphilitic births among a population of pregnant women who have or aquire syphilis in the year prior to delivery. As the proportion of women in the United States receiving early prenatal care improved, the number of infants born with congenital syphilis for every 1000 cases of female infectious syphilis also declined, at least through 1980 (Fig. 67-3). However, substantial increases in the VTI have been observed in recent years. Part of the increase observed in 1984 may be attributed to increased sensitivity of the surveillance system. The increases observed in 1985 and 1986, however, are not attributable to any change in reporting activity. The recent increases in congenital syphilis incidence and the VTI in the United States suggest that prenatal care is now becoming less adequate and underutilized.

## Demographic features

The demographic profile of women who deliver syphilitic babies resembles that of women with other STDs, as well as those who fail to seek adequate prenatal care (Table 67-4); they are more likely than the general population to be adolescent, unmarried, and black.[30]

Three studies have addressed the question of how congenital

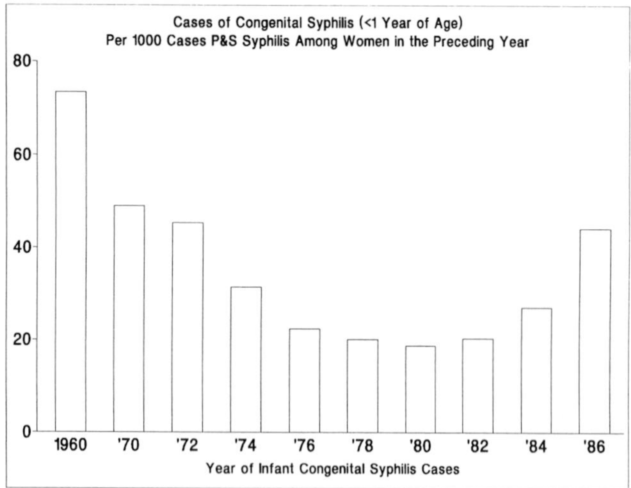


Fig. 67-3. Cases of infant congenital syphilis per 1000 cases of prior early infectious syphilis in women; this ratio reflects the efficacy of control efforts directed at women in the reproductive age group. (*Courtesy of Joseph H. Blount, Division of Sexually Transmitted Diseases, Center for Prevention Services, CDC, US Public Health Service.*)

**Table 67-4. Maternal Characteristics of Total Births and Syphilitic Births—United States, 1977**

| | General population* | Mothers of syphilitic infants† |
|---|---|---|
| Maternal age 19 or less | 19.3% | — |
| Maternal age 18 or less | — | 25.7% |
| Unmarried | 12.3% | 42.3% |
| Black | 16.3% | 60.1% |
| Primiparous | 48.0% | 40.5% |
| No prenatal care | 1.6% | 42.6% |

*National Center for Health Statistics, U.S. Department of Health and Human Services.[30]
†Kaufman et al.[31]

syphilis occurs in a population.[26,28,31] In general, the leading factor accounting for failure to prevent congenital syphilis was lack of prenatal care (about 30 percent). In the United States, one-third of the mothers of syphilitic babies who do receive prenatal care attend three or fewer clinical visits, and, overall, mothers of affected neonates average only six prenatal visits.[31] The general population of pregnant women in the United States averages 11 of the 13 visits recommended by the American College of Obstetrics & Gynecology.[32] The likelihood of seeking prenatal care is strongly associated with age, marital and socioeconomic status, rural residence, and low educational attainment.[32,33] Of unwed mothers, 16.2 percent receive late or no prenatal care, and this is significantly higher for white (18.9 percent) than for black (13.6 percent) mothers. Overall, black mothers are twice as likely to receive delayed or no care for their pregnancies.

## SUB-SAHARAN AFRICA

In parts of the world where traditional "venereal diseases" have not been controlled, such as sub-Saharan Africa, the problems associated with syphilis during pregnancy are strikingly reminiscent of those faced by the western world in the early 1900s. According to available data, the incidence of adverse outcomes attributed to syphilis in Africa are the highest in the world. In this section, we describe the seriousness and extent of these current public health problems in sub-Saharan Africa.

## Syphilis prevalence in pregnant women

Reported prevalences of syphilis seroreactivity in pregnant women attending antenatal clinics in Africa range from 4 to 15 percent (Table 67-5). Although these findings are consistently

**Table 67-5. Syphilis Seroreactivity Among Pregnant Women**

| Country | Reference | Seroreactive by VDRL or RPR, % |
|---|---|---|
| Central African Republic | Widy-Wirsky, D'Costa[36] 1980 | 10 |
| Ethiopia | Friedmann, Wright[34] 1977 | 13 |
| Ethiopia | Larsson, Larsson[35] 1970 | 15 |
| Mozambique | Liljestrand et al.[43] 1985 | 5–15 |
| Rwanda | De Clercq[37] 1982 | 4 |
| Swaziland | Meheus et al.[38] 1980 | 14 |
| Zambia | Ratnam et al.[39] 1980 | 15 |
| Zambia | Ratnam et al.[40] 1982 | 14 |
| Zambia | Hira[41] 1984 | 13 |
| Zambia | Watts et al.[42] 1984 | 15 |

high from country to country, they are probably underestimates. For example, specific treponemal tests in two of the studies yielded much higher prevalences than nontreponemal tests in the same women. Moreover, in Zambia, researchers analyzed the sensitivity of the RPR test and found a false-negative rate that ranged between 11 and 14 percent, leading them to conclude that the actual prevalence of syphilitic infection may be higher than reported based on this test.

One potential problem with the use of serologic tests to assess the prevalence of syphilis is that yaws and endemic syphilis can also cause seroreactivity. The countries referred to in Table 67-5, however, are not recognized as African foci of yaws or endemic syphilis.[42,44] Only two of the countries, Central African Republic and Rwanda, reported cases of yaws to WHO in the 1970s, and the numbers were relatively small.[44] Thus, these serologic findings likely reflect sexually transmitted syphilis infection rather than nonvenereal treponemal infections. Based on these studies from major African cities, as well as unpublished reports from other countries in Africa that demonstrate seroprevalences exceeding 10 percent, one can conclude that syphilis during pregnancy is prevalent throughout much of Africa.

## Effect of untreated syphilis on pregnancy outcome

An estimate of what happens to pregnancies that survive to the third trimester in syphilitic African women comes from earlier western-world data which appear to simulate present African conditions. One study was published in 1917 before effective syphilis treatment was available (Table 67-2), and the other was published in 1951 before modern syphilis control programs were operational (Table 67-6). These two prominent studies reported that about one-third of pregnancies yielded a nonsyphilitic infant.[27,45] The agreement between the two is quite remarkable, given the differences in time and in study populations. The older study resulted in a higher percentage of deaths and a lower percentage of syphilitic infants, presumably because an appreciable percentage of the syphilitic infants died during their first year of life. The more recent study only measured death during the neonatal period. Also, treatment of neonates in 1950 was more effective because of the availability of antibiotics, and, in addition, some women categorized as having untreated latent syphilis may have already received penicillin, since it was available in the late 1940s.

Early and late syphilis, when untreated, apparently produce a widely disparate impact on pregnancy outcome (Table 67-6). Assumptions regarding the early or late status of seroreactive women, therefore, are crucial to accurately estimating pregnancy outcomes in syphilitic pregnant women. In a study where early and late status was documented, 73 percent of the cases were classified as early syphilis.[45] In a recent report from Africa, quantitative RPR card test results were analyzed for seroreactive women. Seventy percent had a titer of $\geq$1:8, which corresponds to early untreated syphilis.[42] Thus, the distribution from the 1951 study seems to be roughly similar to current conditions in Africa, and we will apply its outcome distribution for all untreated pregnant women with syphilis to derive estimates of these outcomes for Africa.

## Congenital syphilis incidence

Data on congenital syphilis in Africa are not as abundant as on adult syphilis during pregnancy. A study in Zambia established that nearly 1 percent of the babies delivered at the University Teaching Hospital in Lusaka had signs of congenital infection at birth, and as many as 6.5 percent were seroreactive at birth and thus considered at risk.[46] These data are consistent with prior literature in that most congenital syphilis is not diagnosed until weeks or months after birth. In another study from Zambia, seroreactivity among infants under 6 months of age was 2.9 percent.[41] Within the first 6 months, 50 percent of seroreactive infants had two or more clinical features suggestive of early congenital syphilis and, of these, 60 percent required admission to the hospital. Moreover, the incidence of congenital syphilis may actually be much higher than reported here, since the RPR test was used and may have a false-negative rate ranging from 52 to 62 percent.[41]

Further confirmation of the incidence and morbidity associated with early congenital syphilis in Zambia comes from two treatment studies. Early congenital syphilis was diagnosed in 9 percent of admissions to one nursery ward[47] and in 8 percent of admissions to the intensive care unit.[48]

## Perinatal, neonatal, and infant deaths

The relationship between syphilis during pregnancy and stillbirths is well established. A recent case-control study from Zambia demonstrated a 28-fold increased risk (95 percent confidence interval, 12 to 63) in stillbirths among women with high-titer RPR card test seroreactivity.[42] This result is consistent with the 1951 study from the United States which showed that the relative risk of stillbirths for a mother with untreated early syphilis was 32 times greater than for a nonsyphilitic mother.[45] In pregnant women with untreated early syphilis, nearly 40 percent of pregnancies result in perinatal death; in pregnant women with untreated late syphilis over 20 percent result in perinatal death (Table 67-6).

In the University Teaching Hospital in Lusaka, Zambia, 42 percent of stillbirths were attributed to syphilis during pregnancy.[40] In Zambia, congenital syphilitic infection is implicated in 20 to 30 percent of the total perinatal infant mortality, which is 50 per 1000 births.[41] Thus 1 to 1.5 percent of all Zambian pregnancies that extend beyond 20 to 27 weeks end in death due to syphilis. Moreover, this underestimates the problem because postneonatal infant deaths are not included and because many stillborn infants do not have clinical evidence of congenital syphilis.

In Ethiopia, syphilis was the fourth most common cause of perinatal death, accounting for 10 percent of the approximately 70 perinatal deaths per 1000 births.[49] Also, studies found that

**Table 67-6. Effect of Untreated Syphilis on Outcome of Pregnancy, Philadelphia General Hospital, 1951[45]**

| Outcome of pregnancy | Untreated early syphilis, % | Untreated late syphilis, % | All untreated syphilis, % |
|---|---|---|---|
| Stillborn | 25 | 12 | 22 |
| Neonatal death | 14 | 9 | 12 |
| Syphilitic infant | 41 | 2 | 33 |
| Nonsyphilitic infant | 20 | 77 | 33 |

syphilis causes nearly 5 percent of all the postneonatal infant deaths.[49] Thus, at least 1 percent of Ethiopian pregnancies extending beyond 20 to 27 weeks end in a perinatal or postneonatal infant death due to syphilis. In absolute numbers, 15,000 fetal and infant deaths are directly attributable each year to syphilis in Ethiopia.[50]

### Spontaneous abortion

The most common outcome of syphilis during pregnancy is probably spontaneous abortions during the second and early third trimester. Most first trimester abortions are associated with phenotypic or chromosomal fetal abnormalities rather than infection. In Ethiopia, an estimated 5 percent of all pregnancies are lost each year through syphilis-induced abortions (75,000 pregnancy losses).[50] In Zambia, 19 percent of miscarriages were attributed to syphilis.[40] Again in Ethiopia, pregnant women who were found to be seroreactive to syphilis were five times more likely to have an abortion or stillbirth than women who were seronegative.[35] These data strongly point to spontaneous abortion as a major adverse outcome from syphilis during pregnancy. The precise magnitude, however, is especially difficult to measure in Africa, where women usually do not come for prenatal care until late in the third trimester. We estimate that of pregnancies which extend beyond 12 weeks' gestation, nonsyphilitic women have a spontaneous abortion rate of 15 percent and syphilitic women 50 percent. These estimates are consistent with what we know about spontaneous abortion and the pathogenesis of syphilis during pregnancy.[51–54]

### Model of outcomes of pregnancy in sub-Saharan Africa

To estimate adverse outcomes associated with syphilis in pregnancy, we assumed a 10 percent seroreactivity rate in pregnant women and followed 1000 women in a simple deterministic model (Table 67-7). We then compared the results from the model with actual reported data from Africa. The estimate that 5 percent of all pregnancies in Ethiopia are lost to spontaneous abortion caused by syphilis during pregnancy appeared to be plausible as the model yielded a consistent estimate of 3.5 percent. The model estimated that of pregnancies extending beyond 20 to 27 weeks, 1.7 percent would result in a perinatal death caused by syphilis. This was consistent with, though slightly higher than, the 1 to 1.5 percent estimates from Ethiopia and Zambia. Using the model, we estimated that 20 percent of perinatal deaths were caused by syphilis, which was consistent with the 10 to 30 percent reported from Zambia and Ethiopia. In the model, 2.1 percent of pregnancies that extended into the perinatal period resulted in infants with syphilis, which was consistent with results from Zambia of 1 percent with signs of congenital syphilis at birth and 2.9 to 6.5 percent seroreactive at birth or shortly thereafter.

**Table 67.7. Reproductive Outcome Model Assuming 10% Seroreactivity in 1000 Pregnant Women**

| | Seroreactive | Nonseroreactive |
|---|---|---|
| Pregnancies | 100 | 900 |
| Pregnancies lost to spontaneous abortion in the second or early third trimester | 50 (50%) | 135 (15%) |
| Excess spontaneous abortions due to syphilis | 35 | — |
| Pregnancies extending beyond 20 to 27 weeks | 50 | 765 |
| Perinatal deaths | 17 (34%) | 54 (7%) |
| Excess perinatal deaths due to syphilis | 14 | — |
| Syphilitic infants | 17 | — |

### Conclusions on syphilis during pregnancy in Africa

Africa in the 1980s faces problems associated with syphilis during pregnancy similar in severity and magnitude to those faced by the western world in the early 1900s. The prevalence of syphilis seroreactivity among pregnant women in many parts of Africa is at least 10 percent. Assuming that prevalence, 3 to 4 percent of pregnancies that extend beyond 12 weeks will spontaneously abort because of syphilis; 1 to 2 percent of pregnancies that extend beyond 20 to 27 weeks will end in perinatal or infant death because of syphilis; and 1 to 2 percent of pregnancies that extend beyond 20 to 27 weeks will yield an infant with syphilis. Therefore, an aggregate of 5 to 8 percent of pregnancies surviving past 12 weeks, i.e., 50 to 80 percent of those in seroreactive women, will have an adverse outcome caused by syphilis. We recommend commitment of resources to STD control initiatives in Africa and additional research into the cost-effectiveness of different prevention and control strategies.

## PATHOLOGY AND PATHOGENESIS

The fundamental histological lesions of both congenital and acquired syphilis are vasculitis and its consequences, necrosis, and fibrosis.[55–58] The pattern of histopathology seen in congenital syphilis depends on the gestational age at the time of infection and, to a lesser degree, on the tissue examined. Unlike the staged histopathology of acquired syphilis, the full range of these lesions is seen in *neonatal* syphilis as part of a single syndrome. While spirochetes are distributed widely throughout the tissue, inflammation is seen preferentially, though not exclusively, around small vessels. Initial granulocytic infiltrates are replaced by infiltrating lymphocytes and plasma cells. In the vessel, this may be followed by intimal hyperplasia. Although obliterative endarteritis is a classic lesion, any small vessel may be involved, including veins, capillaries, and lymphatic vessels. Three tissue reactions are usually attributed to vasculitis: (1) focal ischemic necrosis, (2) fibrosis, and (3) gummas. Fibrosis may be relatively fine in character or may substantially distort and replace parenchyma. Microscopic gummas are common, especially in skin, mucous membranes, bone, and liver. These typically consist of a thin peripheral rim of mononuclear cell infiltration, central coagulation ("gummy" necrosis), and fibrosis, but any of these three features may predominate.

The pathology of *fetal* syphilis depends on the gestational age at which the abortus is examined.[58,59] Until recently[60] it was a commonly held obstetric principle that infection of the fetus does not occur before 18 weeks. This belief was supported by Dippel's series and his review of more than 200 fetal autopsies culled from the literature.[61] He found no cases of an infected abortus prior to 18 weeks, and the proportion of abortuses that were infected rose steadily with advancing gestation to a peak at 8 months. He argued that the probability of fetal infection simply increased with increasing duration of exposure. In 1938 Beck and Dailey proposed that the prominence of the Langhans' cell layer of the cytotrophoblast prior to midgestation explained the rarity of early transplacental infection, and its regression thereafter left the fetus vulnerable to spirochetal invasion.[62] Dippel noted that only 19 percent of syphilitic abortuses showed delayed regression of the Langhans' layer, whereas 50 percent of uninfected abortuses had an intact Langhans' layer.[61] All of these studies were performed on spontaneously aborted fetuses, which were usually macerated and exhibited a selective bias for late gestation.

In 1976 Harter and Benirschke found syphilis in much earlier stages of pregnancy, examining fetuses of five women with untreated latent syphilis undergoing therapeutic abortions.[60] Using both Warthin-Starry silver stains and immunofluorescence, they were able to demonstrate spirochetes in two fetuses, 9 and 10 weeks gestation, with Langhans' cell layers intact. In these two cases the organisms were remarkably sparse and inflammation was absent. The absence of inflammation in early fetal syphilis has been noted by others.[56,59] The best-studied early fetal infection is rubella, in which no inflammatory response is seen in the first trimester and relatively little is seen thereafter until the perinatal period.[63,64] First-trimester syphilis may not be appreciated, because the fetus is incapable of an inflammatory response before 18 to 20 weeks. In the absence of typical lesions, treponemes are not routinely sought.

Even in the latter part of gestation, the major fetal pathology consists of retarded growth of parenchymal cells and fibrosis[58,65] rather than inflammation; however, small perivascular inflammatory foci begin to appear in parenchyma, and a lymphocytic infiltrate appears in marrow. Abundant mononuclear infiltrates are found after 24 weeks.[66] The fibrosis is fine and diffuse, particularly affecting liver, pancreas, bone, and lung.

## THE PLACENTA

The inflammatory changes in the placenta are often more striking than those of the fetus; these changes include (1) focal proliferative villitis with necrosis and focal infiltrations of maternal lymphocytes and plasma cells, and (2) endothelial and adventitial proliferation of villous vessles, leading to obliteration. In addition, however, (3) the villi are immature, large, clubbed, and crowded; (4) there is extensive stromal hyperplasia; and (5) occasionally there is multiple small ("miliary") gummata.[58,67,68] The placenta ultimately exhibits diffuse fibrosis as its most prominent feature and is large, firm, and pale, weighing up to one-third of fetal weight. Spirochetes seem to be less numerous in the placenta than in the fetus.

## TEETH

The late dental consequences of neonatal syphilis are abnormalities of form, structure, and size: there is apical notching, the amelodentinal junction is irregular, enamelization is defective, and the affected teeth are small. The pathogenesis of dental stigmata has been a longstanding controversy. Although Hutchinson himself at first regarded the changes as a part of the syndrome of mercurial stomatitis, he subsequently attributed them to trophic changes.[15,16] Early difficulty in conforming the presence of spirochetes in developing dental tissue contributed to the notion that hypoplasia and malformation were due to the general nutritional state of syphilitic infants, to local impairment of nutrition due to endarteritis, or even to rickets.[57] Indeed, as Hutchinson emphasized, it is the first (6-year) molars and central incisors of the permanent set that are specifically affected. These begin to calcify just before and just after birth, respectively. Therefore, perinatal injury would be expected to produce malformation of these teeth, particularly if a disturbed process of calcification is the major mechanism of pathogenesis. However, from 1932 to 1953, a series of observations suggested that direct invasion of the developing permanent tooth and the resulting inflammation are the cause of dental stigmata.[69]

The tooth is formed by mesenchymal protrusion into an ectodermal tooth bud, which invaginates to receive it (Fig. 67-4). A dental papilla of mesenchymal origin gives rise to an outer layer of odontoblasts that ultimately produce dentin abutting the ectodermal enamel organ. An enamel epithelium on the inner aspect of the enamel organ consists of ameloblasts that ultimately produce a layer of enamel rods, lining the outer aspect of the dentin. Interactions between ameloblasts and the underlying mesenchymal odontoblasts initiate the apposition of enamel and dentin. This is followed by calcification of both enamel and dentin and finally by eruption.

When the jaws of newborn infants dying of congenital syphilis

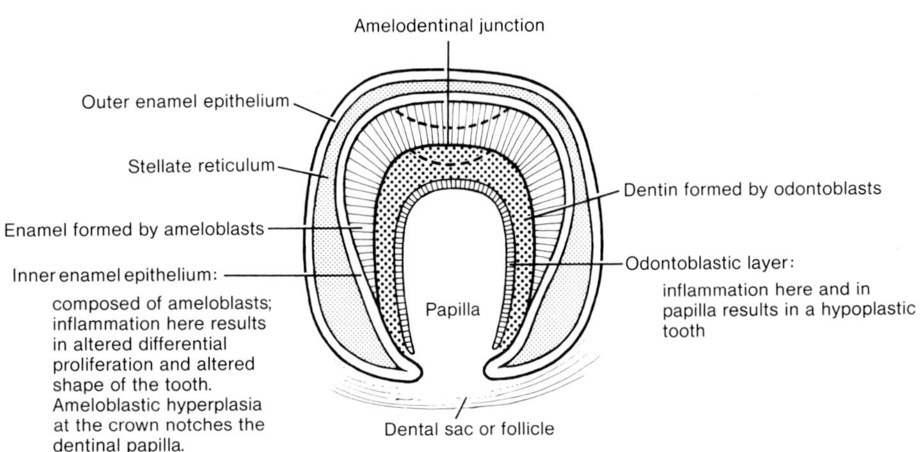


**Fig. 67-4.** Development of the permanent incisor, illustrating the effect of treponemal infection or morphogenesis.

are examined, the tooth germs of the permanent teeth are inflamed and spirochetes can be found throughout the enamel organ and dental papilla. There is endarteritis and perivascular inflammation in the dental papilla, and spirochetes are found in vessel walls. This results in a complex pathological process culminating in a failure to lay down enamel at the center of the notch and an irregular amelodentinal junction in the mature tooth. Radiographs of syphilitic incisors suggest that the irregular amelodentinal junction is the internal counterpart to the external deformity. The impaired growth of the dentinal papilla, on the other hand, is the precursor of the small size of the incisors and first molars.

Syphilis affects morphodifferentiation and apposition, rather than the later stage of calcification as in rickets. However, like vitamin D deficiency during the preeruptive period, congenital syphilis primarily affects the permanent incisors and first molars. This undoubtedly contributed to the historical confusion of the disease with rickets. Whether deciduous teeth are affected may depend upon whether infection takes place prior to 18 weeks gestation, by which time deciduous teeth are fully formed. There are no consistent abnormalities of shape in deciduous teeth, but when affected, they are misshapen and hypoplastic. The permanent teeth that develop later than the central incisors and first molars are much less commonly affected. If the mesenchymal progenitor cells have been destroyed in the newborn period, later developing permanent teeth may be missing.

## BONE

Characteristic bony lesions are present in 97 percent of autopsied infants by 6 months of age.[58] Membranous bones are less involved than endochondrial (long) bones, in which the pathological process is concentrated at the metaphyseal-epiphyseal junction. Grossly, an irregular yellow line is found at the zone of provisional calcification.[70] When membranous bone is involved, it is generally as a focal periostitis, which leads to exostosis and osteoporosis at the site. A perivascular inflammatory infiltrate is found in both types of bone, which erodes the trabeculae and eventually gives way to fibrosis.[71,72] A debate persists regarding the relative importance of inflammatory and trophic influences ("syphilitic dystrophy") on the production of these lesions.[73,74] Caffey attributes the transverse striping of the metaphyses to nutrition and argues that any severe disease of the fetal and neonatal period may produce it.[73] Others have made careful pathoradiological correlations, describing the sequential development of an "osteochondritis."[75,76] When fully developed, the epiphyseal plate is destroyed, the end of the diaphysis is destroyed, and fragments of bone and cartilage separate from the bone to produce a "pseudo-Charcot's joint." The diaphysis acquires a worm-eaten appearance resembling fibrocystic disease. Marrow is trapped between thick layers of periosteum, and islands of cartilage are trapped within metaphyseal bone. Epiphyseal ossification centers are usually spared.

In surviving infants, healing occurs over the first 6 months, usually without residual lesions, and seems little influenced by penicillin.[20,77] This suggests that much of the pathogenesis of these lesions may be trophic rather than directly infectious, and that the severely ill infant who comes to autopsy may not be representative of the survivors whom radiologists and clinicians most commonly encounter. Marked inflammation and exuberant fibrosis may be hallmarks of more profoundly affected infants, but in a larger context may be atypical.

## CLINICAL MANIFESTATIONS

Traditionally, congenital syphilis has been divided into two clinical syndromes. Those features that typically appear within the first 2 years of life comprise early congenital syphilis. Those features that occur later than 2 years, most often near puberty, comprise late congenital syphilis.

## EARLY CONGENITAL SYPHILIS

Most syphilitic infants lack manifestations at birth.[25,78–81] As a consequence, where routine umbilical cord blood screening for syphilis is not performed, the opportunity for diagnosis may be delayed until the patient is seen weeks later for such nonspecific complaints as rhinitis, pneumonia, or failure to thrive.[82,83] In two-thirds of cases, the early clinical signs of congenital syphilis begin to appear in the third to the eighth week of life; in nearly all cases, within 3 months.[82,84] Neonates who are born with manifest syphilis are usually severely affected and carry a worse prognosis. These few are the infants who are most likely to display the classic picture of marasmic syphilis: the "wizened, pot-bellied, hoarse old man with withered brown skin and runny fissured nose . . . senescent decrepitude in miniature."[25] Multiple organ system involvement is universal in congenitial syphilis at autopsy[85] and is apparent in the clinical syndrome as well. A number of signs in an earlier era were very suggestive of syphilis, especially when seen together (e.g., snuffles, certain skin eruptions, pseudoparalysis, and epitrochlear lymphadenopathy).[78] Marfan considered snuffles, palmar and plantar bullae, splenomegaly, pseudoparalysis, and cutaneous syphilids to form a diagnostic pentad (cited in Ref. 82); recently, Bueno suggested a triad of the first three of these signs.[86] However, none can be considered entirely pathognomonic.

### Prematurity and intrauterine growth retardation

In the era before penicillin, syphilis accounted for as many as a third of premature births.[87] Approximately 20 percent of babies born to mothers with early latent syphilis in turn are premature in the absence of a syndrome of congenital syphilis, and half of those born to women with infectious syphilis are either premature or stillborn.[28]

Intrauterine growth retardation is a commonly cited feature of congenital syphilis.[88–90] Established concepts of syphilitic effects on bone growth[74] and modern case reports[83,91,92] support this view. However, until recently there were no clear criteria for distinguishing between premature infants and those who are small for gestational age. Furthermore, Naeye's study of 36 syphilitic perinatal deaths[65] seemed to show that, in contrast to rubella and cytomegalovirus infections, *T. pallidum* infection did not affect fetal growth. The difficulty is compounded by the fact that gestational syphilis disproportionately affects the same population in which idiopathic fetal growth retardation is most prevalent.

### The mononuclear phagocyte system

Syphilis was once the most common cause of hepatosplenomegaly in infancy.[93] Hepatosplenomegaly occurs in approximately half the cases of early manifest congenital syphilis[74,81,85,91,92,94–96] (Table 67-8). Hepatomegaly may occur as an isolated manifestation,[95] but splenomegaly rarely occurs except associated with an enlarged liver. Both hepatic and splenic enlargement are caused by subacute inflammation and by compensatory extramedullary hematopoiesis.[85,97] In addition, hypersplenism (as well as hemolysis and thrombocytopenia) may contribute to spleen size.[82,98]

Little is known about clinical liver tests in congenital syphilis. Serum transaminases may be evaluated. Jaundice occurs in about 30 percent of cases; the hyperbilirubinemia may be due to either indirect or direct and indirect bilirubin, depending on the relative contributions of syphilitic hepatitis and hemolysis. Hepatosplenomegaly may require more than a year to resolve following treatment, and cirrhosis may be the cause of death despite treatment.[95]

Generalized lymphadenopathy is found in 20 to 50 percent of cases.[20,91,99,100] The nodes are firm, rubbery, and nontender. Epitrochlear adenopathy, found in 20 percent of those with adenopathy, is considered especially characteristic of congenital syphilis.[82,88,99,101] In 1935 Ingraham reported this sign to be 51 percent specific as an indication of syphilis before the age of 2 months;[102] it may have much less specificity today.

## Mucocutaneous lesions

The earliest sign of congenital syphilis, occurring 1 to 2 weeks before the rash, is a nasal discharge (Fig. 67-5). It was reported in 68 to 86 percent of older series,[20,57,84] but has been much less common in recent years (Table 67-8).[95,99] The discharge is initially watery and indistinguishable from that of viral or allergic rhinitis but then becomes progressively thicker and purulent and then hemorrhagic. Resulting nasal obstruction interferes with feeding. Ulceration leads to deeper involvement, including chondritis with necrosis, and eventually to the septal perforation or saddle nose deformity of late congenital syphilis. Extension into the throat produces laryngitis and either a hoarse or aphonic cry.

The varied panoply of cutaneous lesions in congenital syphilis resembles that of acquired secondary syphilis. They occur in 30 to 60 percent of infant cases. The most common lesion is a large round pink macule that fades to a dusky or coppery hue, lasts 1 to 3 months without treatment, and leaves a residual pigmentation.[25,82] These lesions are typically distributed over the back, perineum, extremities, palms, and soles, sparing the anterior trunk, and develop slowly over a period of weeks. They may be covered with a fine, silvery scale and may mingle with indurated plaques of similar size and color. A variety of papular and maculopapular eruptions may be seen. The corymbiform lesion consists of a grouped papule around a large central plaque, like a "hen and chicks"; annular lesions occur but are less common

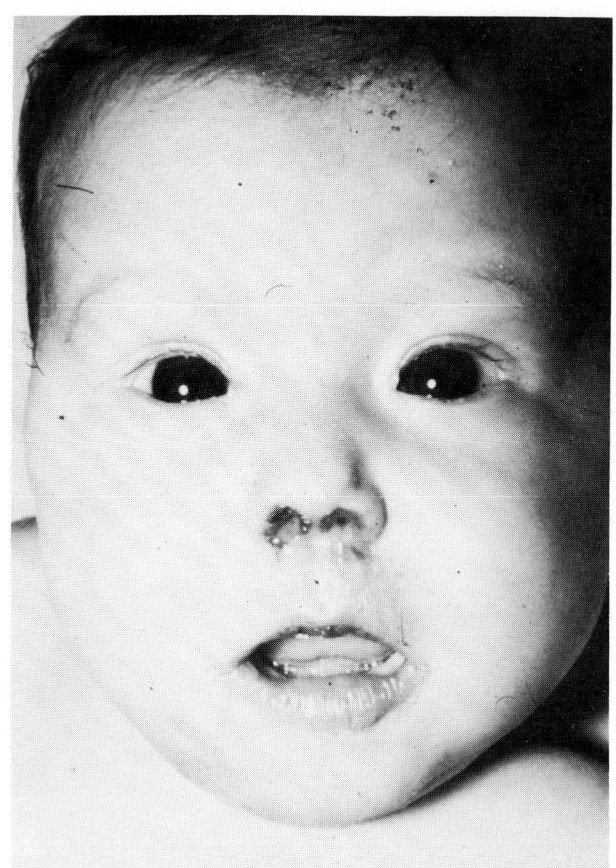

**Fig. 67-5.** Snuffles: a persistent, often sanguinous, nasal discharge. Treponemes abound in the discharge, providing a definitive means of diagnosis. (*Courtesy of C Ginsburg.*)

than in acquired secondary syphillis.[24] The general skin color of affected infants has an earthen or "café au lait" tint.[25,82] Purpura and petechiae may appear when thrombocytopenia is severe; as a response to anemia, cutaneous extramedullary hematopoiesis produces the "blueberry muffin" rash, just as in other congenital infections.

The vesiculobullous eruption is highly distinctive, when present.[82] Intraepidermal edema leads to spongiotic midepidermal blisters that are most prominent on the palms and soles; the blister fluid, under dark field examination, swarms with active spirochetes.[58] When the bullae rupture, they leave a macerated, dusky red surface that readily dries and crusts (Fig. 67-6). Even in the absence of frank bulla formation, desquamation is common

**Table 67-8. Clinical Presentations of Early Congenital Syphilis, Selected Series Since 1960**

| | Total number | Hepatomegaly | Splenomegaly | Anemia | Jaundice | Skin rash | Petechiae | Snuffles | Abnormal bone x-ray | Lymphadenopathy | Pseudoparalysis | Ref. |
|---|---|---|---|---|---|---|---|---|---|---|---|---|
| | 15 | 13/15 | 15/15 | 13/15 | 6/15 | 11/15 | 8/15 | — | 6/7 | — | — | 94 |
| | 18 | 17/18 | 14/18 | 7/18 | 6/18 | 6/18 | — | 3/18 | 13/15 | — | 1/18 | 95 |
| | 102 | 21/102 | 21/102 | 13/102 | 21/102 | 21/102 | — | 11/102 | 43/102 | — | 16/102 | 74 |
| | 16 | 16/16 | 16/16 | 8/16 | 7/16 | 8/16 | 4/16 | 8/16 | 11/16 | 6/16 | — | 85 |
| | 21 | 12/21 | 12/21 | — | — | 12/21 | — | 11/21 | 21/21 | — | 21/21 | 81 |
| | 6 | 2/6 | 4/6 | 4/6 | 1/6 | 2/6 | — | 1/6 | — | 1/6 | 3/6 | 91 |
| | 10 | 10/10 | 10/10 | — | — | 5/10 | — | 2/10 | — | — | — | 92 |
| | 24 | 18/24 | 12/24 | 15/22 | 13/24 | 9/22 | 10/23 | 9/21 | 14/17 | — | — | 96 |
| *Total* | 212 | 104/212 | 104/212 | 60/179 | 54/181 | 74/210 | 22/54 | 45/194 | 108/178 | 7/22 | 41/147 | |
| *Percent* | | 51 | 49 | 34 | 30 | 35 | 41 | 23 | 61 | 32 | 28 | |

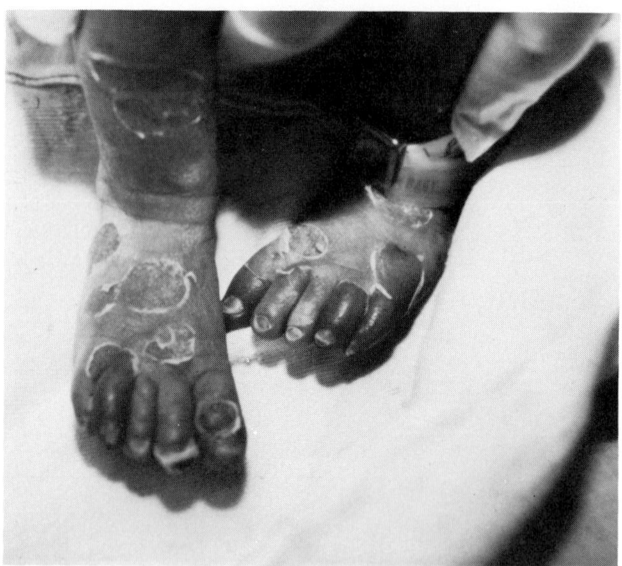

**Fig. 67-6.** Typical bullae and desquamation of congenital syphilis. (*Courtesy of C Ginsburg.*)

and may be generalized or confined to the periungual areas of fingers and toes. Palmar and plantar desquamation is preceded by subcutaneous edema underlying a shiny erythema and sometimes accompanied by shedding of the nails.[24,25] Paronychia also leads to narrow, atrophic nails, producing a claw-nail deformity, particularly of the fourth and fifth digits. The hair may be brittle and sparse; infantile alopecia, especially affecting the eyebrows, is considered very suggestive of syphilis.[25]

The face, perineum, and intertriginous sites are particular targets of syphilitic lesions that may be eczematoid, impetiginous, or even gangrenous (Fig. 67-7).[24,25,82] The facial eruption preferentially affects the middle third of the face, from the medial portions of the supraorbital ridges in the chin.[103] At the nares, lips, and anus, the initial lesions may be indistinguishable from the mucous patches of secondary syphilis but then become deeply fissured and hemorrhagic, leading to Parrot's radial scars of late congenital syphilis, known as rhagades.[25] Mucous patches are also found on the tongue and palate.

Condylomata lata affect the same mucocutaneous and intertriginous areas and are raised, flat, moist verrucae that are seen in recurrences of untreated congenital syphilis.[25] They are seen typically toward the end of the first year of life,[24] and together with the furuncle of Barlow may be regarded as an intermediate manifestation between early and late congenital syphilis. The syphilitic furuncle is a deep violaceous nodule, usually on the upper outer thigh and occurring after 9 months and before 3 years of age.[25]

## Skeletal involvement

Among syphilitic infants under 1 year of age studied by Nabarro,[25] over 30 percent had physical and over 80 percent had radiographic evidence of osteochondritis. In a recent series from Texas, 70 percent of infants with probable or definite congenital syphilis had osteochondritis,[104] which is similar to many other recent reports (Table 67-8).

With the exception of rare cases of dactylitis and cranial nodules, the physical signs of skeletal syphilis in infants are limited to the signs of epiphysitis, including the pseudoparalysis of Parrot. Epiphyses of the radius, femur, humerus, and fibula are involved in descending order of frequency. There may be periarticular swelling, and the end of the bone is tender on passive motion of the adjacent joint. When the proximal humerus is affected, the arm hangs in flaccid immobility, internally rotated with the forearm in pronation. However, pain elicited by passive motion of shoulder and development of the condition after birth distinguish this pseudoparalysis from intrapartum brachial plexus injury. When the femur is involved, the leg is held in rigid flexion. Dactylitis (tender, fusiform swelling of the fingers) was observed in 2 to 6 percent of older series,[57] but has been uncommon in recent experience, probably because it was typically seen in recurrences of untreated congenital syphilis.[25] Osteitis of the skull, particularly of the central margins of the occipital and parietal bones, produces softening (craniotabes) that indents[82] or yields on pressure "like stiff parchment."[25] Parrot's nodes are focal, bilateral, frontoparietal swellings, typically separated by a cruciform furrow.

Roentgenographic methods have been used diagnostically in congenital syphilis for more than 80 years (Table 67-8). Because the radiographic changes are relatively specific, the x-ray has rivaled serology in importance in the past.[78] These changes sometimes occur before the venereal disease reaction level (VDRL) test is positive, and indeed the diagnosis can be made in utero. The proliferative and destructive changes in bone tissue produce an appearance of increased density alternating with rarefaction on

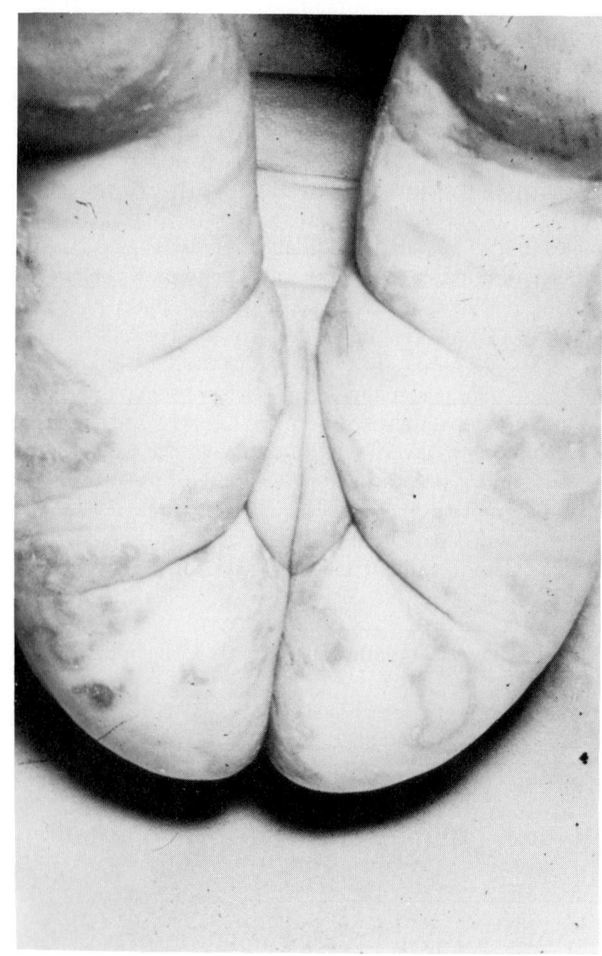

**Fig. 67-7.** Scaling, annular serpiginous rash of infant syphilis. (*Courtesy of C Ginsburg.*)

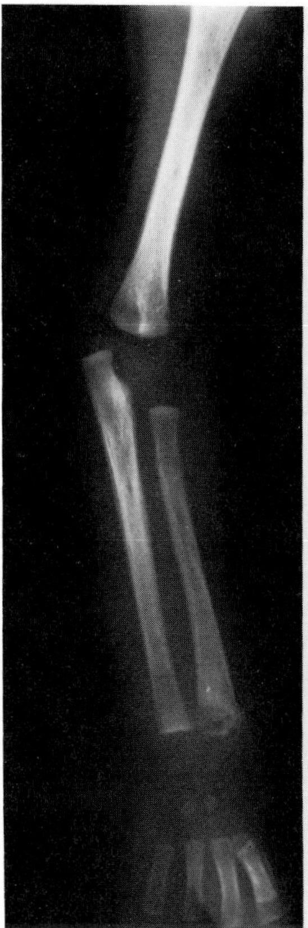
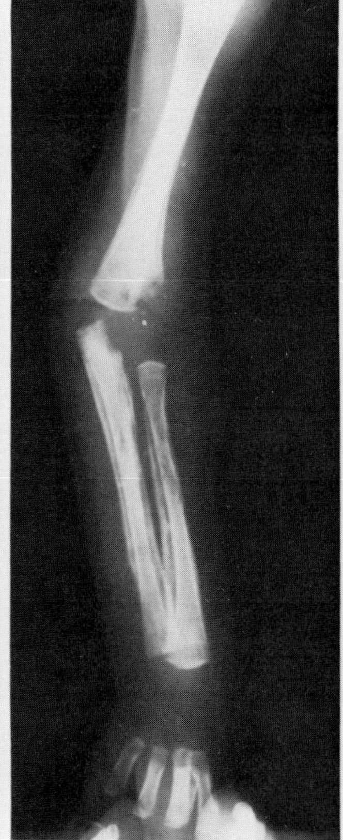
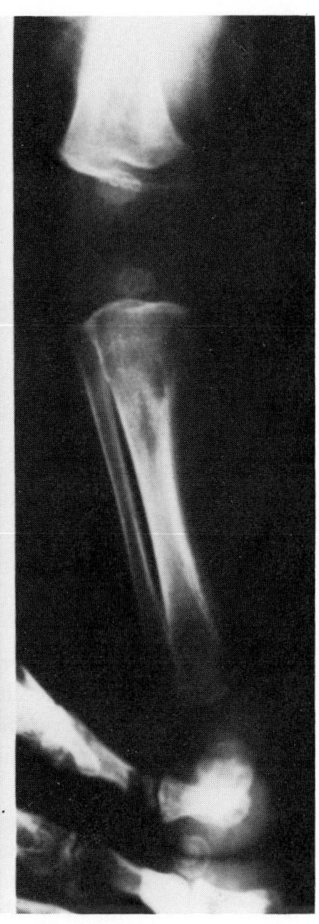

**Fig. 67-8.** (*Left*) Focal metaphyseal destruction of the lateral aspect of the distal radius; faint metaphyseal banding of distal ulna; longitudinal lines of rarefaction and density extend into the ulnar diaphysis proximally. (*Middle*) Extensive mottling of diaphysis and periostitis. Dense periosteal new bone formation encasing ulna and radius (periosteal cloaking); complete encasement is called the *sarcophagus sign*. Focal lateral metaphyseal defect of distal humerus; erosion of sigmoid notch of ulna (Levin's sign). (*Right*) Focal metaphyseal defect of proximal tibia (Wimberger's sign). (*Courtesy of G Currarino.*)

x-ray.[75,105] Radiographic changes are most readily observed in the areas of rapid bone growth, such as in the provisional zone of calcification and in the periosteum (Fig. 67-8). Syphilitic osteochondritis requires approximately 5 weeks to become roentgenographically demonstrable, while periostitis requires 16 weeks. This corresponds to the clinical observation that osteochondritis is usually manifest perinatally, whereas periostitis is sometimes not seen until 4 to 5 months later.[102] When both lesions are present perinatally, it suggests that the baby was infected during the second trimester;[106] the combination of these lesions makes a diagnosis of syphilis very likely. When periostitis is present alone, it usually means that an earlier osteochondritis has already healed. Although single bone lesions can occur,[107] such a finding should suggest another diagnosis.

A skeletal survey is mandatory when congenital syphilis is in the differential diagnosis. Widespread lesions involve multiple, symmetrical sites of the long bones and occasionally involve the cranium, spine, and ribs. The tibia and ulna are most commonly followed by fibula, radius, humerus, and femur. Lower extremities are more commonly affected than upper extremities; the femur is more often affected distally, the tibia and humerus proximally.[25]

The earliest changes occur in the metaphysis, consisting of a transverse sawtooth radiodense band below the epiphyseal plate; this widened and enhanced zone of provisional calcification is accompanied by an underlying zone of osteoporosis, evident as a radiolucent band. A series of alternating dense and lucent bands may extend into the diaphysis.[72] This process may be followed by radiolucent mottling and finally fragmentation of the metaphysis itself. Focal defects with cortical destruction may be seen on the lateral aspect of the metaphysis; in the tibia, such lesions occur on the medial aspect of the proximal metaphysis and are usually bilateral, giving rise to the distinctive "cat bite" or Wimberger's sign in 21 percent of infant syphilis.[108] Erosion of the sigmoid notch of the ulna may be of similar significance.[77] The cat bite sign is also seen in hyperparathyroidism, infantile generalized fibromatosis, and bacterial osteomyelitis, but cat bite sign in the infant is most suggestive of syphilitic osteitis. Later, longitudinal lines of rarefaction may also extend into the diaphysis; in serial array, these linear lucencies resemble a "celery stick," a sign also seen in rubella and cytomegalovirus infection.[72] Irregular, patchy focal lucencies may appear in the diaphysis, sometimes containing sequestra that invite confusion with suppurative osteomyelitis.[109] The epiphysis is relatively spared of radiographic changes, except that it may separate as a result of minor trauma. Fractures through the degenerating metaphysis occur readily, followed by exuberant callus formation, resulting in a cap over the metaphysis called the "bucket handle" sign.[108] Periostitis is found in 71 percent of infant syphilis[108] and consists of multiple layers of periosteal new bone formation ("onion peel periosteum") in response to diaphyseal inflammation; when exuberant, this process leads to hypertrophic "periosteal cloaking" of the bone, with layers of marrow trapped between layers of subperiosteal bone,[25] thus encasing the entire shaft and producing a radiographic "sarcophagus sign" (Fig. 67-8).

## Hematologic manifestations

The major hematologic features of early congenital syphilis are anemia, leukocytosis or leukopenia, and thrombocytopenia. Whitaker et al. found anemia to be the most common laboratory finding in 24 cases (96 percent).[98] It is Coombs' test–negative normochromic and normocytic or macrocytic anemia with increased polychromasia and often striking reticulocytosis and erythroblastosis.[25] Severe anemia may be associated with replacement of marrow by syphilitic granulation tissue in luetic osteitis[25,110] or with maturation arrest in the erythroblastoid line.[111] Autoimmune hemolysis, however, is a more common mechanism[98,111] and may be associated with cryoglobulinemia, macroglobulinemia, or circulating immune complexes.[112–115] Hemolysis may persist for some time following treatment and can be sufficient, if prolonged or complicated by bleeding, to lead to iron deficiency anemia. Paroxysmal nocturnal hemoglobinuria is seen in late congenital syphilis, long after resolution of early acute hemolysis.

Neutrophilic leukocytosis occurs in over 70 percent of cases, and congenital syphilis is one of the classic causes of leukemoid reactions in infancy.[116] A few infants are leukopenic. Up to 80 percent of syphilitic infants exhibit monocytosis.[117]

Thirty percent of babies with syphilis develop significant thrombocytopenia.[94,98] Bleeding complications occur in 60 percent of those who are thrombocytopenic. Thrombocytopenia is associated with decreased megakaryocyte formation in some but not all cases and is therefore believed to be due primarily to diminished platelet survival.[94,98] Platelet consumption might be mediated by adherent immune complexes, antiplatelet antibody, or hypersplenism.

### Nephropathy

Syphilitic nephrotic syndrome in infancy is an uncommon complication that has nevertheless been recognized since the end of the nineteenth century.[103] Nephrosis was found in 5 percent of cases of infant syphilis at the Hospital for Sick Children, London, between 1917 and 1939,[25] which is similar to recent series;[72,111] glomerulonephritis, with hematuria and cylindruria, is less common.[118] Evidence of nephrotic syndrome appears at 2 to 3 months of age with the onset of edema, ascites, hypoproteinemia, and proteinuria. Either proliferative or membranous glomerulitis may be found; epimembranous deposits of immune complexes, composed primarily of IgG, are found in the glomeruli, as well as IgM and IgA.[113–115, 119]

### Central nervous system involvement

Abnormal cerebrospinal fluid findings are present in 40 to 60 percent of infant patients with syphilis.[20,25,57,99] These include lymphocytosis of up to several hundred cells per cubic millimeter, increased protein, and positive serology. Central nervous system involvement is ten times more common among white than among black infants with syphilis.[57] Manifest neurosyphilis does not appear until the third to sixth month of life; 5 to 15 percent of infant syphilitics were affected in the prepenicillin era,[89,99,101] but these cases are now rarely seen. The neurosyphilitic syndromes described in early congenital syphilis essentially represent diverse clinical expressions of a single pathogenic process, meningovascular syphilis. Acute syphilitic meningitis, with meningismus, bulging fontanelles, and intractable vomiting, carried a grave prognosis but is very responsive to penicillin.[88] Patients who survived this syndrome untreated or inadequately treated were usually left with obstructive hydrocephalus, seizure disorders, and impaired intellectual development. Cerebrovascular accidents occur in the neonatal period, probably as a combined consequence of cerebral arteritis and thrombocytopenia.[94] Untreated neurosyphilis can lead to a chronic meningovascular process that results in hydrocephalus, cranial nerve palsies, and cerebral infarction late in the first year.

### Ocular involvement

Three ocular lesions are associated with early congenital syphilis: chorioretinitis, glaucoma, and uveitis. Syphilitic chorioretinitis typically produces a "salt and pepper" pattern of pigmentary patches at the periphery of a granular fundus.[120] Proptosis, blepharospasm, corneal clouding and edema, and excessive tearing should suggest the possibility of glaucoma. Uveitis usually occurs as an extension of choroiditis. Interstitial keratitis and optic neuritis have been described in infantile syphilis,[25] but are generally regarded as lesions of late congenital syphilis.

### Other manifestations

Syphilitic pneumonitis or pneumonia alba is usually present in fatal cases but is otherwise uncommon. Radiographically it produces a patchy interstitial pattern (Fig. 67-9). Diarrhea in early congenital syphilis may be due to either pancreatitis with malabsorption or direct involvement of the intestinal mucosa. Approximately 10 percent of infants dying of syphilis have myocarditis.[121] The clinical importance of myocardial involvement in living infants is unknown; there is no convincing evidence of myocardial sequelae in surviving adolescents and adults with congenital syphilis.

## LATE CONGENITAL SYPHILIS

Eighty percent of children ultimately diagnosed as having congenital syphilis pass through the early stage undetected.[31] At one time, half of the children with late congenital syphilis had manifest lesions at the time of diagnosis.[122] Inadvertent partial treatment associated with management of other intercurrent infections seems to have so greatly modified the expression of the disease that classic syndromes of late congenital syphilis are now rare, in spite of a persistent incidence of infant syphilis. Late congenital syphilis in the child or adolescent corresponds to tertiary syphilis in the adult. Although the cardiovascular system is relatively spared in the child, the target organs are otherwise similar: bone and soft tissue, eyes, ears, and the central nervous system. In late syphilis of either adult or child, more indolent, gummatous lesions supplant the dense lymphocytic and histiocytic infiltrates of early syphilis, and manifest lesions often represent the irreversible end stage of healed prior inflammation. The distinctive lesions of late congenital syphilis are the stigmata, which are malformations that occur because of prior infection at a critical period of growth and development and, presumably, at a relatively immature stage of immunologic development. Thomas grouped the clinical elements of late congenital syphilis into either stigmata or inflammatory or hypersensitivity reactions.[123]

### Malformations (stigmata)

Chondritis and focal osteitis in infancy may lead to craniofacial malformations, which classic writers on congenital syphilis found so fascinating. The most common is frontal bossing, which occurs in some form in 30 to 87 percent of symptomatic cases.[57,82,99,124,125] Involvement of the parietal bone produces squaring of the cranium or occasionally a "hot cross bun" deformity. Other variations of this malformation include supraor-

Fig. 67-9. Syphilitic pneumonitis ("pneumonia alba") in this infant consists of a patchy interstitial infiltrate. Long bone involvement in the same x-ray is highly suggestive of congenital syphilis.

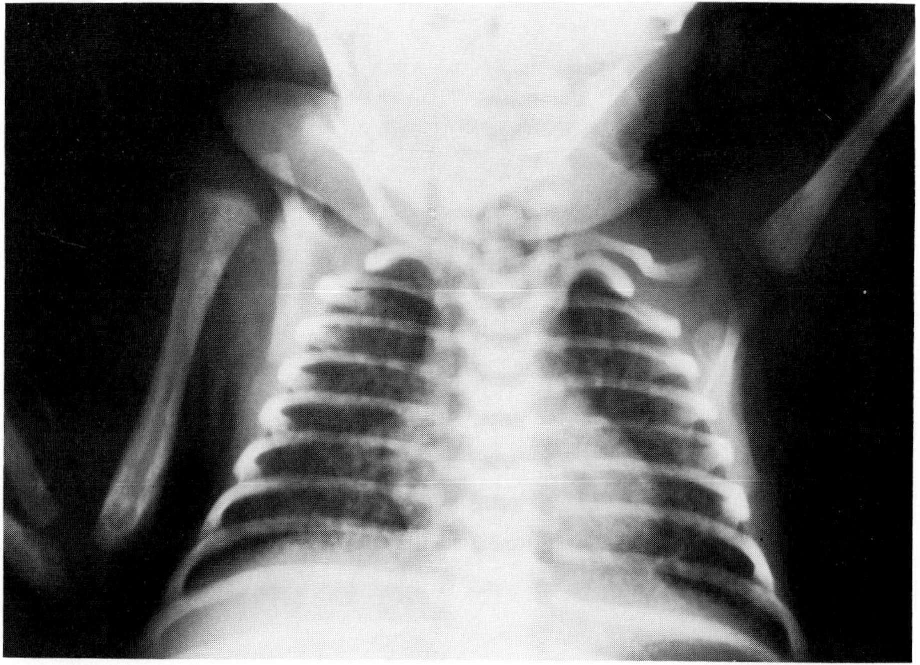

bital thickening (Olympian or beetled brow), a high cranium or "tower skull," and with parietal bossing alone, a sloping skull.[24] Robinson attributed the absence of bossing among his own cases to the disappearance of rickets.[126] By ascribing cranial bossing to associated, unrecognized rickets, he revived the nineteenth century confusion between rickets and congenital syphilis. Since bossing was common in the only other modern series of cases,[125] the controversy may outlive the disease.

Deep necrotizing nasal chondritis in infancy produces a collapsed saddlenose deformity in 10 to 30 percent of patients with late congenital syphilis.[82,99] Involvement of adjacent structures may also lead to a short maxilla and a high palatal arch. The resulting facies has a flat, "dished out" look, with a relatively prominent mandible. Circumoral radiating furrows (rhagades) complete the syphilitic facies in 5 to 10 percent. Laryngeal scarring may leave the child hoarse.[25]

Sequelae of periostitis of long bones affect primarily the tibia, clavicle, and scapula, in that order. Anterior bowing of the tibia (saber shin) occurred in 30 to 40 percent of older series but is now uncommon[125,126] (Fig. 67-10). Particularly in these children, recurrent acute periostitis of the tibia, ulna, fibula, or femur sometimes followed trauma or febrile illness, and might be heralded by local tender nodules resembling erythema nodosum.[25] Thickening of the clavicle in its medial third is called Higoumenakis' sign and occurs preferentially on the side of the patient's handedness.[82] Robinson doubted its authenticity as a sign of syphilis.[126] Affected scapulae assume a scaphoid shape, concave medially.

**Hutchinson's Teeth.** Hutchinson's description of characteristic dental malformations before the Pathological Society of London in 1857 represented the first recognition of late sequelae of infant syphilis and was received with "expressions of incredulity." He described small canines and incisors which were widely spaced and peg- or screwdriver-shaped; were tapered from the gingival bases toward a notched biting edge; and were rough, dull, and dirty gray in color due to insufficient enamel (Fig. 67-11). These changes most often affect the upper central incisors but may affect the upper, lower, and lateral incisors. They are changes of

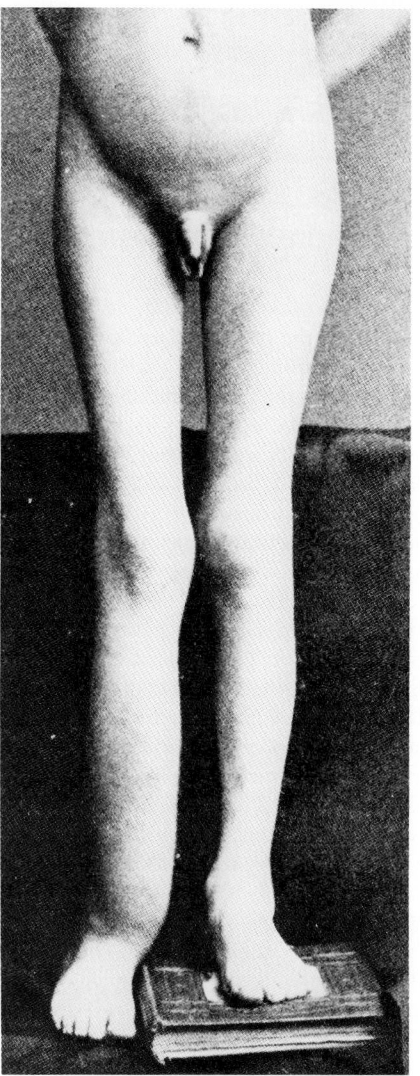

Fig. 67-10. Tibial thickening (saber shin) due to periostitis in late congenital syphilis; one of Hutchinson's cases. (*From J Hutchinson.*[16])

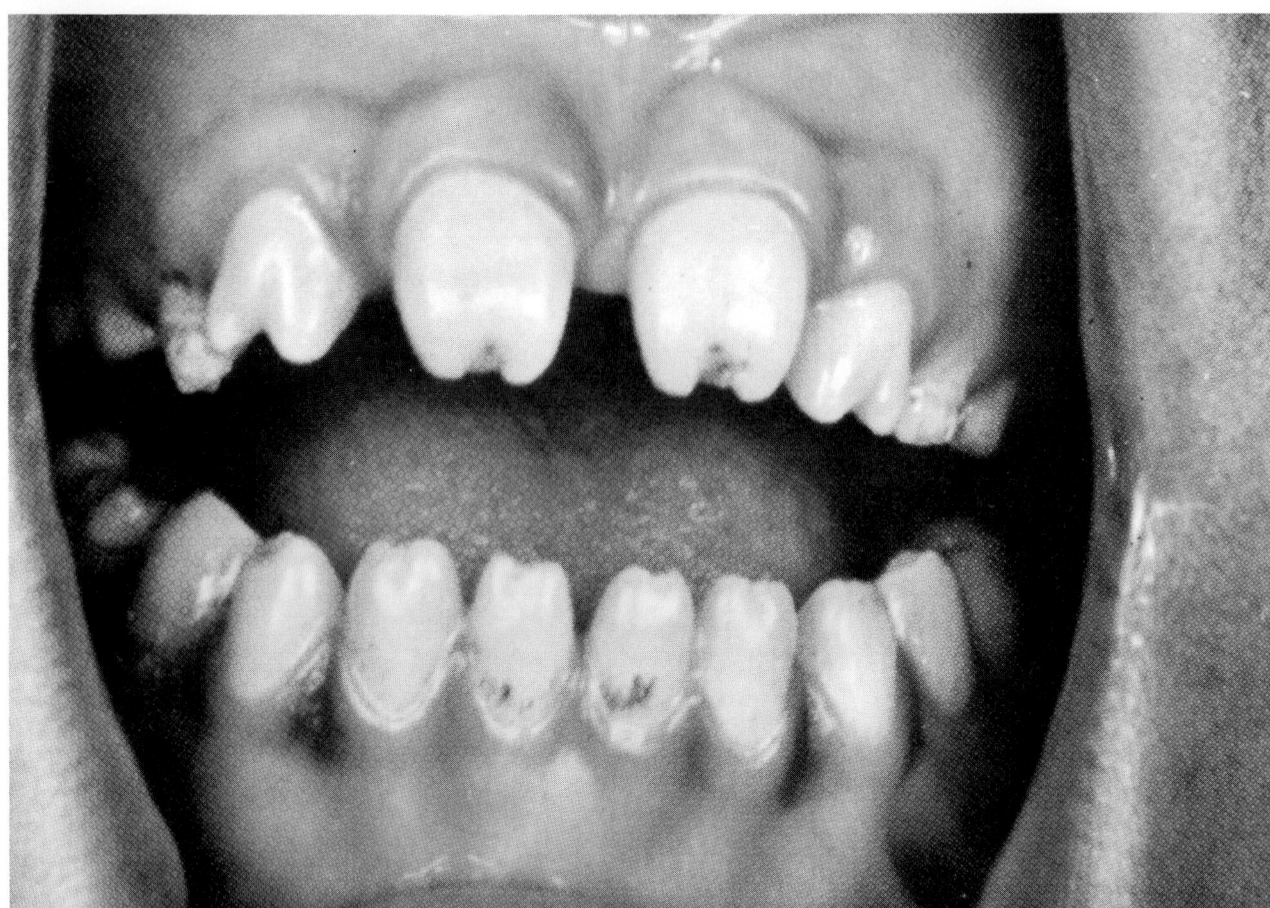

**Fig. 67-11.** Hutchinson's teeth: the upper and lower incisors are conical, tapered toward the apex, and notched; the canine teeth are hypoplastic and poorly enamelized. (*From RA Colby et al, Color Atlas of Oral Pathology, Philadelphia, Lippincott, 1971.*)

the permanent, not the deciduous teeth, although the latter are believed to be more prone to caries than normal in late congenital syphilis. In the first year of life, the diagnosis can be made by x-ray of the unerupted central incisors.[127] Variations of the classic Hutchinson tooth occur; the lower incisors may have parallel sides and lack a notch but are otherwise small, round, and spaced, resembling little tombstones or top hats projecting from the gum.[25] The upper incisors are sometimes pointed (cannibal teeth) rather than notched.[24] The proportion of congenital syphilitic children reported to have typical dental deformities has varied according to the age and race of the patients studied and strictness of diagnostic criteria. At the Hospital for Sick Children, Great Ormond Street, 55 percent had dental dystrophies, but only 15 percent had fully developed Hutchinson's teeth.[25] Jeans and Cooke made similar observations and noted that typical deformities occurred almost entirely in white and rarely in black children.[57] Robinson found such "characteristic" teeth in 1 of 450 normal children,[126] illustrating the importance of requiring more than mere notching for the diagnosis.

**Mulberry Molars.** Henry Moon described more completely the molars whose peculiar "tubercular projections" Hutchinson had mentioned; the characteristic 6-year (first lower) molars are dome-shaped with diminutive cusps arrayed in a tight circle at the top of the dome (Fig. 67-12). Moon's molars have been variously likened to a mulberry, a *bouton de fleur,* a cow's udder, or a string purse. Poorly enamelized, they are highly prone to decay and are rarely present beyond puberty; they are strongly indicative of congenital syphilis when found.

## Inflammatory lesions

**Interstitial Keratitis.** Interstitial keratitis, when accompanied by neural deafness and typical teeth, forms Hutchinson's triad, which remains undeniably strong evidence of congenital syphilis when found. Taken alone, keratitis is the most common late manifestation (20 to 50 percent).[82,126] The onset, between 5 and 16 years of age, is announced by unilateral photophobia, pain, excess tearing, and blurred vision. Neovascularization may be so marked as to give the cornea a "salmon patch" appearance. The second eye is involved within 2 months in 80 to 90 percent of patients. Keratitis occurs more commonly in females than males and pursues a self-limited, sometimes relapsing course that ends in corneal clouding (syphilitic nebulae) or secondary glaucoma. Chorioretinitis and iritis may be found, but less commonly than in congenital syphilis of infancy.

**Deafness.** Deafness is the least common of Hutchinson's triad. The primary lesion is osteochondritis affecting the otic capsule and leading to cochlear degeneration. The ossicles occasionally may be affected, so that an associated conduction defect does not exclude syphilis as a cause of sensorineural hearing loss. Karmody and Schuknecht distinguished between the abrupt onset of bilateral deafness without vertigo in childhood and a more gradual

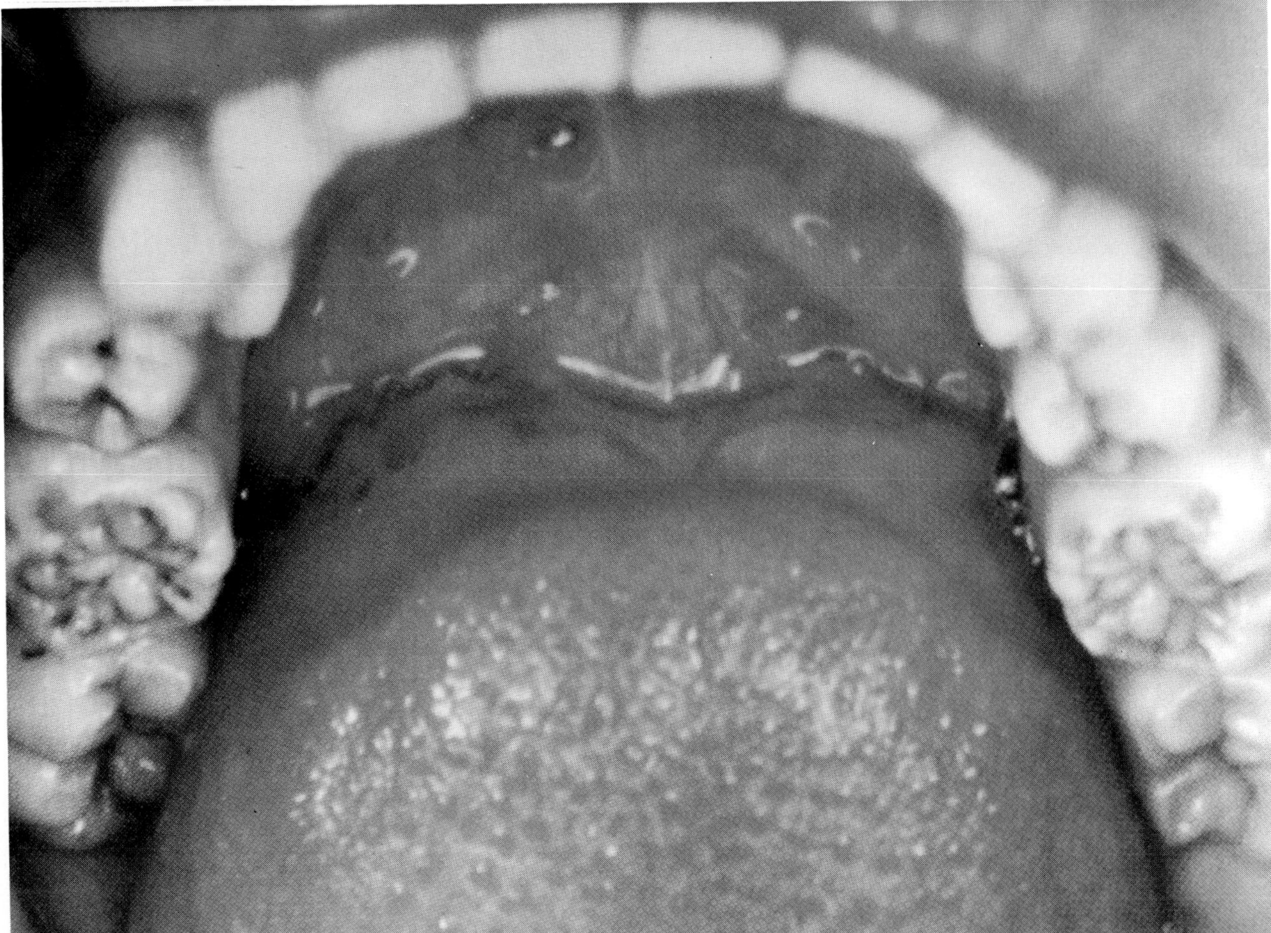

Fig. 67-12. Mulberry molars: the 6-year molars are dome-shaped with a circle of small nob-shaped cusps at the apex. (*From RA Colby et al, Color Atlas of Oral Pathology, Philadelphia, Lippincott, 1971.*)

asymmetric pattern in adults associated with tinnitus and vertigo.[128] Congenital leutic involvement of the otic capsule leads to fibrous adhesion between the medial surface of the stapedial foot plate and the membranous labyrinth (vestibulofibrosis). The result is Hennebert's positive "fistula sign without a fistula"; this consists of nystagmus and vertigo, despite an intact tympanic membrane, when positive and negative pressure are alternately applied to the external canal. Once considered a classic sign of syphilis, Hennebert's sign also occurs in Ménière's disease and vestibular Schwannoma.[129] Hearing loss begins at high frequencies and often progresses to complete bilateral loss of cochlear and vestibular function.

**Clutton's Joints.** Between the ages of 8 and 15, 1 to 3 percent of children with congenital syphilis develop symmetrical, painless swelling of the knees (occasionally elbows), with preservation of mobility, often following trauma.[130,131] Adjacent bone erosion (von Gie joint) is rarely seen. Synoviocentesis reveals 10,000 to 30,000 leukocytes, predominantly lymphocytes. This hydrarthrosis is believed due to perisynovitis and resolves spontaneously over several months.

**Palatal Deformations.** Gummata of the palate, throat, and nasal septum begin in late childhood or even adulthood as a gray, sharply defined "mucous patch." These lead painlessly to perforation of the septum and of the soft palate, usually in the midline. Deep ulcers of the throat and tongue occur in a similar fashion.

**Neurosyphilis.** As many as one-fourth to one-third of patients over the age of 2 years have asymptomatic neurosyphilis.[99] Symptomatic neurosyphilis, on the other hand, is quite rare, is usually delayed until adolescence, and fits the adult patterns of tabes dorsalis, syphilitic encephalitis (general paresis), and local gummata. Juvenile paresis is the most common of these, occurring in 1 to 5 percent of congenital syphilitics, and is generally more severe than the acquired variety.[25,99,126] It typically begins around puberty with deteriorating school performance, bizarre behavior, emotional inappropriateness, and inattention. Over the ensuing 6 to 12 months, the child develops ataxis, tremor, and dysarthria; half of these patients have a seizure disorder, and nearly all have pupillary findings.[132,133] Sequelae of untreated neurosyphilis in infancy were once common, including hydrocephalus, convulsive disorders, and cranial neuropathies.

**Paroxysmal Cold Hemoglobinuria.** Late congenital and acquired syphilis were once the leading cause of paroxysmal cold hemoglobinuria.[134] Only half of these syphilitic patients had other manifestations of disease. About 8 h following immersion of hands or feet into ice water (Rosenbach test) or other cold exposure, the patient experiences a myalgic, shaking chill and voids dark red or black urine. Many of the syphilitic cases have associated Raynaud's phenomenon.[25] The Coombs' test, Donath-Landsteiner (cold hemolysin) test, and VDRL are all positive. In the syphilitic cases, the attacks cease following penicillin therapy.

## DIAGNOSIS

The general features of syphilis serology and of dark field and fluorescent microscopy are discussed in Chaps. 75 and 76. There are special problems in the diagnosis of syphilis in mother, fetus, and infant, however. Pregnancy itself occasionally produces biological false-positive nontreponemal tests, but a confirmatory treponemal test will resolve this issue.[135] Although false-positive fluorescent tremponemal antibody-absorption (FTA-ABS) tests are reported in pregnancy,[136,137] this is rare if their performance is confined to patients with positive nontreponemal tests. Women who have previously received standard therapy for syphilis are sometimes believed to be "serofast" when a VDRL is subsequently positive in the prenatal clinic. However, women who have previously had syphilis are at greater risk than others of acquiring syphilis again. The only means of distinguishing between the serofast and the reinfected patient is by retreatment and serological follow-up. All pregnant women with a positive nontreponemal and confirmatory treponemal test should be treated.

The fetus before 4 months of gestation may show relatively little inflammatory reaction to infecting organisms. Therefore, if dark field or fluorescence microscopy is confined to those with signs of inflammation, the diagnosis will routinely be missed in first-trimester abortuses. The liver is a particularly rich site of treponemal proliferation and should be routinely examined at fetal autopsy in cities with a high incidence of early syphilis.

## CRITERIA FOR DIAGNOSIS IN THE INFANT

### Definite congenital syphilis: Visualization of *T. pallidum*

Criteria for the modern diagnosis of syphilis in an infant have been proposed and are classified as definite, compatible, or unlikely (Table 67-9). A *definite* diagnosis requires demonstration of *T. pallidum* in a lesion by dark field examination, immunofluorescence, or histological examination (e.g., silver stain). Sadly, this degree of clinical certainty is achieved uncommonly, and nearly all reported cases fall into the compatible (63 percent) or unlikely (36 percent) categories. With reasonable care and follow-up, it should be possible to make at least a compatible diagnosis in nearly all cases. Dark field microscopy or immunofluorescence should be performed whenever nasal discharge, mucous patches, vesiculobullous lesions, or condylomata are present. Treponemes abound in such lesions, so definitive diagnosis can be achieved in most cases that exhibit these signs.

### Compatible congenital syphilis: Serodiagnosis

When treponemes cannot be demonstrated, the diagnosis rests essentially on serology. A positive nontreponemal test confirmed by a treponemal test [FTA-ABS or microhemagglutination-*T. pallidum* (MHA-TP)] should be regarded as due to syphilis until proved otherwise. Three clinical circumstances sometimes give rise to diagnostic confusion, however: the recently treated mother, the apparently "serofast" mother, and the seronegative infant or mother. In the first two instances, the difficulty is distinguishing between passively transferred maternal IgG antibody and fetal antibody produced in response to continuing active infection. Two tests have been suggested for this purpose, the total IgM determination and the FTA-ABS (IgM) test to detect IgM antitreponemal antibody.

**Table 67-9. Congenital Syphilis Diagnostic Classification**

*Definite/Confirmed*
- Identification of *T. pallidum* by dark field microscopy, fluorescent antibody, or other specific stains in specimens from lesions, autopsy material, placenta, or umbilical cord

*Compatible (formerly "probable" or "possible")*
- A reactive serological test for syphilis (STS) in a stillborn

*OR*
- A reactive STS in an infant whose mother had syphilis during pregnancy and was not adequately treated, regardless of symptoms in the infant

*OR*
- A reactive VDRL test in cerebrospinal fluid

*OR*
- A reactive STS in an infant with any of the following signs: snuffles, condyloma lata, osteitis, periostitis or osteochondritis, ascites, skin and mucous membrane lesions, hepatitis, hepatomegaly, splenomegaly, nephrosis, nephritis, hemolytic anemia

*OR*
- Fourfold or greater rise in titers* of nontreponemal tests (VDRL or RPR) and a confirmed treponemal test (FTA-ABS or MHA-TP) over a 3-month interval

*OR*
- A reactive treponemal test or nontreponemal test that does not revert to nonreactive in 6 months

*Unlikely*
- Infants who never had a reactive STS

*OR*
- Infants whose treponemal tests revert to nonreactive within 6 months

*OR*
- Asymptomatic live-born infants whose mothers were treated for syphilis during pregnancy and subsequently experienced a fourfold or greater fall in titer *provided* the infant's own STS is also fourfold or lower than the maternal titer at the time of treatment

*"Fourfold rise in titer," "fourfold fall in titer," and other similar phrases refer to changes in serum titers of at least 2 dilutions (2 "tubes"), e.g., from 1:2 to 1:8 (and the reverse), or from 1:4 to 1:16 (and the reverse), or from 1:32 to 1:8 (and the reverse).

SOURCE: MMWR, Vol. 37, No. S-1, Centers for Disease Control, U.S. Public Health Service, U.S. Department of Health and Human Services, Jan. 15, 1988.

**Neonatal IgM Levels.** IgM does not cross the placenta and is actively synthesized by the third-trimester fetus in response to infection. Elevated umbilical cord blood IgM (>20 mg/dl) has therefore become a useful, though nonspecific, indicator of neonatal infection.[138–140] IgM is elevated in 88 percent of neonates with congenital infections of all kinds, though less frequently in rubella. The prevalence of infection among neonates with an elevated IgM is 34 percent, which is 42-fold greater than the general population of newborns. Contamination of umbilical cord blood with maternal IgM due to placental leaks may account for some elevated levels but can be detected by simultaneous measurement of IgA or by repeating the IgM determination in 3 to 4 days.[140] In congenital infection, IgM will exceed IgA level, whereas maternal contamination will produce an IgA level in excess of IgM, reflecting the ratio in maternal blood. Maternal IgM will disappear rapidly from neonatal blood after birth, whereas IgM elevation persists in the face of infection. Within 5 days of birth, IgM levels normally rise in response to bacterial colonization. Therefore IgM must exceed 50 mg/dl after this period to be considered elevated; nevertheless 87 percent of infected infants in the first month of life exhibit such elevations. An elevated infant IgM level in combination with positive nontreponemal and treponemal tests creates a strong presumption of syphilis. Normal IgM levels may be seen in congenital syphilis, however, especially if the patient is small and premature.

**IgM-FTA-ABS Test.** In 1968 Scotti and Logan reported an FTA-ABS test for IgM antibody against *T. pallidum* as a means of distinguishing infant from maternal antibody.[141] The test is very sensitive in babies with symptomatic syphilis at birth, but only 60 to 80 percent sensitive when onset of disease is delayed.[142] There are further difficulties with the specificity of the test. Placental leaks must be excluded by repeating the test or concurrently measuring IgA levels. In addition, any congenital infection associated with elevated IgM (especially toxoplasmosis) may elicit an IgM anti-IgG from the fetus that results in a false-positive FTA-ABS (IgM) test.[143] For these reasons the FTA-ABS (IgM) test cannot yet be recommended for diagnosis of congenital syphilis.

**Serial Observation.** A strategy recommended by some authorities for distinguishing maternal from infant antibody in the asymptomatic infant is to follow the baby's titer. An infant's titer due to maternal antibody should fall fourfold within 2 months and disappear by 6 months of life; a stable or rising titer indicates active infection. Leaving asymptomatic infants untreated for such a diagnostic purpose is obviously undesirable, and this approach should be reserved for babies whose mothers have been treated *during* pregnancy and in whom reinfection during pregnancy can be reasonably excluded by an appropriate serological response and prompt treatment of sexual partners. For asymptomatic seropositive infants who do not meet these criteria, an alternative is to treat at birth or upon discovery and to retest by treponemal serology at 3 to 6 months. If the treponemal test is still positive, the baby may be reported as a case; if the nontreponemal test also remains positive, the baby should be retreated.

Additional cases can be more confidently diagnosed if clinical evaluation is thorough (Table 67-10). Up to 80 percent have cerebrospinal fluid pleocytosis. A positive cerebrospinal fluid VDRL is found in 50 percent of cases but may be attributed to maternal antibody.[144] Bone findings are highly characteristic and occur in 50 to 80 percent of infant cases, often when no other manifestations of syphilis are present; if left untreated, virtually all infants develop radiographic evidence of disease by the sixth to twelfth week of life.

Affected infants can be born to seronegative mothers who have incubating syphilis or late latent syphilis. Accordingly, infants whose mothers develop syphilis in the postpartum period should be treated expectantly. Mothers who acquire syphilis late in pregnancy, even if seropositive themselves, may give birth to seronegative infants who are nevertheless at risk of developing syphilis in the ensuing 2 months. Such infants should be treated without benefit of diagnosis, unless the mother has been adequately treated prior to the delivery.

Diagnosis of syphilis in the neonate or older child clearly is not easy in the absence of direct visualization of *T. pallidum*. Correct diagnosis requires thorough knowledge of the differential diagnosis. For convenience, we have listed the common problems in differential diagnosis of early (infantile) congenital syphilis (Table 67-11) and late stigmata (Table 67-12).

**Table 67-10. Clinical Criteria for Infant Syphilis**

| Major | Minor |
|---|---|
| Condylomata lata | Perioral fissures |
| Osteochondritis or periostitis (symmetric metaphyseal lesions) | Characteristic rash, especially vesiculobullous eruption |
| Snuffles or hemorrhagic rhinitis | Mucous patches |
| Vesiculobullous eruption, other causes excluded | Hepatomegaly or splenomegaly |
| | Generalized lymphadenopathy |
| | Central nervous system signs or cerebrospinal fluid pleocytosis |
| | Hematologic signs (hemolysis or thrombocytopenia) |
| | Nonimmunologic hydrops |
| | Pseudoparalysis |
| | Nephrotic syndrome or glomerulonephritis |

SOURCE: *After Kaufman et al,[31] and Ingall and Norins.[88]*

**Table 67-11. Differential Diagnosis of Infant Congenital Syphilis**

| | Other causes |
|---|---|
| Vesiculobullous eruption | Toxic epidermal necrolysis |
| | Staphylococcal infection (Ritter's disease) |
| | Pseudomonas sepsis |
| | Sepsis due to listeria, group B streptococci, *Haemophilus influenzae* type B |
| | Viral infection: herpes simplex, varicella, vaccinia, cytomegalovirus (CMV) |
| | Candidiasis |
| | Hereditary: epidermolysis bullosa, urticaria pigmentosa, porphyria, Letterer-Siwe, dermatitis herpetiformis |
| Hepatosplenomegaly (with or without lymphadenopathy, cutaneous hematopoiesis, and hematologic abnormalities) | Erythroblastosis |
| | Other congenital infections: sepsis, CMV, rubella, herpes simplex, toxoplasmosis, varicella, hepatitis |
| | Biliary atresia, choledochal cyst |
| | Metabolic disorders: galactosemia, cystic fibrosis, mucopolysaccharidosis |
| Hydrops fetalis | Erythroblastosis |
| | α-Thalassemia |
| | Congestive heart failure |
| | Neuroblastoma |
| | Congenital nephrotic syndrome: lupus, microcystic disease, renal vein thrombosis |
| | Congenital infection: CMV, toxoplasmosis, hepatitis |
| Pseudoparalysis of Parrot | Erb's palsy |
| | Osteomyelitis |
| Wimberger's sign (focal metaphyseal defects) | Osteomyelitis |
| | Infantile generalized fibromatosis |
| Metaphyseal lesions | Hyperparathyroidism |
| Celery stick diaphysis | Rickets, rubella, CMV, tuberculosis |
| Higoumenakis' sign | Rubella |
| Pathological fractures | Healed clavicular fracture |
| Periostitis | Battered child syndrome |
| | Melorheostosis, Caffey's infantile cortical hyperostosis |

**Table 67-12. Differential Diagnosis of Late Congenital Syphilis**

| Syndrome | Features |
|---|---|
| Ectodermal dysplasia (Marshall's syndrome) | Conical pointed incisors, saddle nose, frontal bossing, sparse hair or alopecia, cataracts, sensorineural deafness |
| Enamel hypoplasias | Defects of incisors consist of deep horizontal grooves; small hypoplastic teeth, sometimes with apical notching |
| Rubella | Dental hypoplasia with small, peg-shaped teeth |
| Erythroblastosis | Enamel hypoplasia, but predominantly affects deciduous crowns |
| Dental fusion | Developmental fusion of adjacent incisors may produce a round notched tooth resembling Hutchinson's incisor |
| Cogan's syndrome | Interstitial keratitis and vestibuloauditory symptoms |
| Rickets | Periostitis and deformities; anterior bowing of tibia, frontal bossing |

## TREATMENT

In all cases of maternal syphilis the goal should be to prevent congenital syphilis by treating the mother, and thereby the fetus, as early in pregnancy as possible. Initial reports suggested that prenatal treatment of syphilis with penicillin virtually always prevented congenital disease.[145] However, failures of three kinds occur in 1 to 2 percent of pregnant women treated with penicillin:[146–148] (1) An already severely diseased fetus may be aborted shortly after therapy. (2) The mother may be reinfected (or possibly relapse) before delivery. (3) The mothers treated within 2 weeks of delivery may still deliver affected newborns. Dental abnormalities are entirely prevented by treatment during pregnancy or within the first 3 months of life.

A rare complication of penicillin therapy noted in early studies is "placental shock" (i.e., the precipitation of labor during a Jarisch-Herxheimer reaction).[146] Accordingly, treatment of secondary syphilis in pregnancy should be monitored with care. There is no evidence that altering the dosage schedule affects the risk of spontaneous abortion. Many of these early reactions may have been secondary to impurities in the penicillin preparations of that era.[146] Less than 1 percent of women (0.7 percent) previously treated with adequate doses of penicillin deliver babies with congenital syphilis in subsequent pregnancies; most of these represent reinfections. Therefore it is not necessary to retreat such women routinely at each pregnancy, if they are seronegative and have not delivered a syphilitic child subsequent to treatment.[149]

There is no satisfactory alternative to penicillin in the treatment of syphilis in pregnancy. For women allergic to penicillin, erythromycin has been recommended.[150] However, the failure rate for adults treated with standard doses of erythromycin is 13 to 30 percent,[151] and it has never been evaluated in a controlled or randomized fashion or in latent syphilis. Most of the studies of erythromycin used the estolate salt, which is currently regarded as too hepatotoxic for clinical use, and other salts produce lower serum levels and may be less effective. Furthermore fetal blood levels achieved with erythromycin are only 6 to 20 percent of maternal levels.[152] Only eight cases of syphilis in pregnancy with erythromycin treatment have been reported,[149,153] of whom five have delivered babies with congenital syphilis. Schroeter and others[154] alluded to five cases treated successfully without documentation. In one case, two successive courses of erythromycin failed to cure the mother; in other cases the mother, but not the fetus, was cured. Those who recommend erythromycin in pregnancy advise routine treatment of the newborn with penicillin, recognizing that the fetus has not been adequately treated.

Tetracycline is the only alternative regimen that has been proved effective for the treatment of syphilis. However, it is not recommended in pregnancy because of dental staining and hypoplasia and because of the hazard of hepatotoxicity when given intravenously in pregnancy. Very few pregnant patients with syphilis have been treated with cephalosporins, and these may produce allergic reactions in patients allergic to penicillin.

In our view the only satisfactory management of syphilis in allergic pregnant patients consists of skin testing followed by desensitization of the reactors by the oral method of Parker and his colleagues.[155] In the combined experience of Parker[155] and Sullivan et al.,[156] 65 patients who required penicillin for various indications were managed in this way without anaphylaxis, although 25 to 30 percent had urticaria not requiring cessation of therapy. Two orally desensitized patients required cessation of penicillins for endocarditis, one for hemolytic anemia and the other for nephritis. The oral method appears to be safer than intradermal desensitization, but should be carried out with emergency equipment ready at the bedside, and no deviation from the described protocol should be permitted.[156]

Since allergy does not pose a problem in the neonatal period, penicillin is the only drug that requires consideration for infant congenital syphilis. The major consideration is whether the baby has central nervous system involvement, since a conventional regimen of benzathine penicillin G does not produce detectable penicillin levels in cerebrospinal fluid.[157] Neurosyphilis was shown by Platou[20] to be more resistant to therapy; the clinical significance of this observation is unclear, since clinical trials of the higher doses of penicillin currently in standard usage have not been done. Infants with evidence of central nervous system involvement should therefore be treated with daily intramuscular procaine penicillin G at 50,000 units per kilogram of body weight per day for 10 days. Therapy with a single injection of 50,000 units per kilogram of body weight of benzathine penicillin G should be used only in infants known to have normal cerebrospinal fluid.

Following treatment at birth, serological tests should be obtained at 3, 6, and 12 months.[150] The majority of reagin tests will become nonreactive at 3 months, nearly all by 6 months.[145] Infants treated later may require a year before the VDRL or similar test is nonreactive. Clinical and serological relapses are extremely rare after penicillin treatment of congenital syphilis, suggesting that "relapses" in adults are, in fact, reinfections after all. Virtually 100 percent of infants so treated, with the exception of those severely ill babies who die acutely, will be clinically and serologically cured.[45]

Most patients treated after 2 years of age do not revert to seronegativity, but a fourfold drop in titer should be seen. No specific recommendation has been made for treatment of late congenital syphilis, but a longer duration of therapy, as in late adult syphilis, seems prudent. In patients without central nervous system involvement, this should consist of 50,000 units per kilogram of body weight (up to the adult dose of 2.4 million units) weekly for 3 weeks. Tetracycline causes dental staining up to 8 years of age, but should be offered to penicillin-allergic patients, if such staining is acceptable. If not, oral desensitization should be considered. Erythromycin has not been evaluated in late congenital syphilis and would be expected to be substantially less effective than penicillin. Patients with late congenital syphilis should be followed with twice-yearly reagin tests for at least 3 years after treatment.

Mucocutaneous lesions in infants clear rapidly following penicillin. Osseous lesions heal slowly, resolving in 3 to 4 months, as would be expected without treatment. In late congenital syphilis, progression of eighth nerve deafness is arrested but hearing is not restored by treatment.[145] Interstitial keratitis is not affected by penicillin. The adjunctive use of steroids has been associated with improvement of both of these conditions but has not been critically evaluated.[158–160] The best treatment of these lesions is prevention.

## PREVENTION

When cases of congenital syphilis are reviewed, the reasons for failure of prevention that emerge include faulty public health procedures and policy and occasionally faulty clinical judgment. For instance, 30 to 60 percent of cases are accounted for by delay of prenatal care until too late to prevent congenital syphilis, either to the third trimester or to delivery itself. Even among women who attend prenatal clinic, the VDRL is sometimes omitted, accounting for 12 percent of recent cases in the United States. In addition, when syphilis is discovered in pregnancy, sufficient priority is not always given to the case to assure full and adequate therapy.

When a mother is seronegative, the assumption may be made that she will remain so throughout pregnancy, whereas infection subsequent to an initially negative VDRL (or incubating at the time of the test) accounts for 31 percent of cases.

It is sometimes assumed that women previously treated for syphilis are seropositive because they are "serofast"; however, some are seropositive because of reinfection or treatment failure, and these account for 3 to 5 percent of cases of unprevented congenital syphilis. Serofastness can only be established by demonstrating a stable titer following *re*treatment, and cannot be assumed.

## STRATEGIES FOR PREVENTION

### Case detection

The lines of public health defense against congenital syphilis can be seen as a series of demographic circles around the fetal population at risk (Fig. 67-13). The first line of defense is the treatment of cases of primary and secondary syphilis and case detection through contact investigations. This activity is aimed at reducing the total number of cases of early syphilis by preventive therapy of sexual contacts. The fewer the total number of cases of primary and secondary syphilis, the fewer the number of cases that joins the pool of early and late latent syphilis, and therefore the fewer latent syphilitics among women in the childbearing age group.

Women may acquire syphilis during pregnancy, in effect, bypassing subsequent lines of defense, particularly if the screening VDRL has already been drawn. This eventuality can only be prevented by (1) reducing early infectious syphilis morbidity in the general population and (2) rescreening high-risk women in the third trimester, a kind of redoubt against cases that breech primary preventive defenses. High-risk women should generally include those attending public clinics or those who are of low income, single, or report more than one STD. Specific criteria should be more inclusive in urban settings or in regions of the

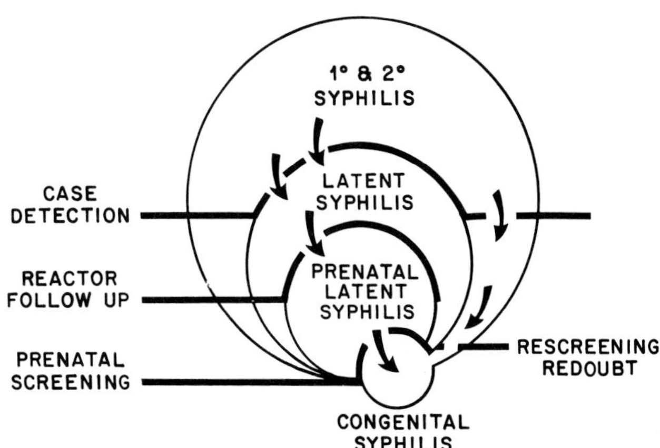


**Fig. 67-13.** Sequential lines of defense against congenital syphilis consist of: (1) case detection to decrease the population of transmitters of early syphilis, (2) reactor follow-up to decrease the residual pool of latent syphilis, and (3) the last line of defense, prenatal screening. In addition, a redoubt is needed to protect the flank (i.e., rescreening to detect acquisition of syphilis during pregnancy).

country with high syphilis morbidity, such as the southeastern and middle Atlantic regions, and may be less strict in rural areas in states with low syphilis morbidity.

### Follow-up of positive serologies

The second line of defense is follow-up of positive serological tests reported to the health department by clinical laboratories, supplemented by routine screening of special populations. By assuring adequate therapy of cases so detected, this strategy is designed to reduce the pool of latent syphilis and thereby the proportion of women who begin gestation with latent syphilis. This "reactor follow-up" effort also identifies some cases of infectious syphilis. Accessible populations known to have a substantial prevalence of seropositives include routine admissions to hospitals, jail populations, and registrants in selected public clinics and emergency rooms. In the United States, 2.2 percent of hospital admission serologies are positive; at New York Hospital, a tertiary care center, it is 3.7 percent; at county hospitals in Atlanta and Dallas, 7 to 10 percent.[161,162] Only about 50 percent of these are biological false positives. The yield of premarital syphilis screening is, by contrast, low (0.02 percent), and its contribution of total reported cases is marginal (2.1 percent of reported latent syphilis in the United States).[163] However, premarital screening is the only broad population-based survey of the age group at highest risk of acquiring syphilis; as such it not only recovers cases in childbearing women that would otherwise be missed, but also provides potentially useful data for assessing secular trends in syphilis prevalence.[164]

### Prenatal screening

Routine prenatal screening is the last major line of defense against congenital syphilis. Four states still do not mandate it, although they require the less productive premarital screening test. It is not enough to require prenatal screening: it must be performed, and quality control of prenatal care is required to assure full screening.

Consultants to the World Health Organization have recently elaborated a managerial strategy for improving maternal and child health services called the "risk approach," which can be adapted to include detection of mothers at special risk of syphilis or of defaulting prenatal care. The vertical transmission index can be used in regions of high syphilis morbidity to test the efficacy of prenatal screening. Indices above 20 to 25 should prompt evaluation of maternal health care delivery.

Clearly a major challenge for the public health of children is to extend prenatal care to all pregnancies. Such an achievement, if combined with case investigation, reactor follow-up, and targeted screening, could not only eradicate congenital syphilis, but could also substantially reduce total infant and maternal mortality from a multiplicity of causes.

## References


1 Mettler CC: *History of Medicine.* Philadelphia, Blakiston, 1947.
2 Goodman H: *Notable Contributions to the Knowledge of Syphilis.* New York, Froben Press, 1943.
3 Dennie CC: *A History of Syphilis.* Springfield, Charles C Thomas, 1962.
4 Paré A: *The Works,* T Johnson (trans). London, J Hindmarsh, 1691 (originally published in Paris, 1575).
5 Paracelsus: *The Hermetic and Alchemical Writings of Aureolus Philippus Theophrastus Bombast of Hohenheim, called Paracelsus the Great,* AE Waite (trans). London, 1894.
6 de Vallembert S: *Cinq Livres, de la Manière de Nourrir et Gouverner les Enfans dès leur Naissance.* Poitiers, Marnefs and Bouchetz, 1565.
7 Colles A: *Practical Observations on the Venereal Disease and on the Use of Mercury.* London, Sherwood, Gilbert and Piper, 1837.
8 Diday PE: *A Treatise on Syphilis in Newborn Children and Infants at the Breast,* G Whitley (trans). New York, Wm Wood and Co, 1883 (originally published in Paris, 1854).
9 Hutchinson J: *A Clinical Memoir on Certain Diseases of the Eye and Ear Consequent on Inherited Syphilis.* London, 1863.
10 Defoe D: *Moll Flanders.* New York, Modern Library, 1950.
11 Bertin M: *Traité de la Maladie Vénérienne Chez les Enfants Nouveau-nés, les Femmes Enceintes et les Nourrices, etc.* Paris, Gabon, 1810.
12 Parrot J: *La Syphilis Herreditaire et la Rachitis.* Paris, Masson, 1886.
13 Wegner FRG: Ueber hereditare Knochensyphilis bei jungen Kindern. *Virchows Arch* 50:305, 1870.
14 Taylor RW: *Syphilitic Lesions of the Osseous System in Infants and Young Children.* New York, Wm Wood and Co, 1875.
15 Hutchinson J: Clinical lecture on heredito-syphilitic struma: And on the teeth as a means of diagnsois. *Br Med J* 1:515, 1861.
16 Hutchinson J: *Syphilis.* London, Cassell, 1909.
17 Danholt N et al: The Oslo study of untreated syphilis: A restudy of the Boeck-Brunsgaard material concerning the fate of syphilitics who receive no specific treatment. *Acta Derm Venereol* 34:34, 1954.
18 Fournier A: *Syphilis and Marriage,* PA Morrow (trans). Lectures delivered at the St. Louis Hospital, Paris. New York, Appleton and Co, 1881.
19 Ingraham NR, Beerman H: The present status of penicillin in the treatment of syphilis in pregnancy and infantile congenital syphilis. *Am J Med Sci* 219:433, 1950.
20 Platou RV: Treatment of congenital syphilis with penicillin. *Adv Pediatr* 4:39, 1949.
21 Osler W: The anti-venereal campaign. *Trans Med Soc Lond* 40:290, 1917.
22 Browne FJ: Neonatal death. *Br Med J* 2:590, 1922.
23 Cruickshank JT: Maternal syphilis as a cause of death of the foetus and of the newborn child. *Medical Research Council Special Report Series* no 82, 1924.
24 Dennie CC, Pakula SF: *Congenital Syphilis.* Philadelphia, Lea & Febiger, 1940.
25 Nabarro D: *Congenital Syphilis.* London, E Arnold, 1954.
26 Laird SM: Elimination of congenital syphilis. *Br J Vener Dis* 35:15, 1959.
27 Harman N: *Staying the Plague.* London, Methuen, 1917.
28 Fiumara N et al: The incidence of prenatal syphilis at the Boston City Hospital. *N Engl J Med* 247:48, 1952.
29 Judson F et al: Comparative prevalence rates of sexually transmitted diseases in heterosexual and homosexual men. *Am J Epidemiol* 112:836, 1980.
30 National Center for Health Statistics, U.S. Department of Health and Human Services: *Vital Statistics of the US, 1977.* Vol I, *Natality.* U.S. Government Printing Office, 1981.
31 Kaufman RE et al: Questionnaire survey of reported early congenital syphilis. *Sex Transm Dis* 4:135, 1977.
32 Taffel S: *Prenatal Care in the US, 1969–75.* Ser 21, no 33. Data from the National Vital Statistics System. US Department of Health, Education, and Welfare Publication no PHS 78-1911, 1978.
33 Wallace HM et al: *Maternal and Child Health Practices.* Springfield, Charles C Thomas, 1973.
34 Friedmann PS, Wright DJM: Observations on syphilis in Addis Ababa. 2. Prevalence and natural history. *Br J Vener Dis* 53:276, 1977.
35 Larsson Y, Larsson V: Congenital syphilis in Addis Ababa. *Ethiop Med J* 8:163, 1970.
36 Widy-Wirsky R, D'Costa J: Maladies transmises par voie sexuelle dans une population rurale en Centrafrique, in Rapport final, 13[e] Conference technique, OCEAC, Yaounde, Cameroon, 1980, p 651.
37 De Clercq A: Problèmes en obstétrique et gynécologie, in *Santé et maladies au Rwanda,* A Meheus et al (eds). Bruxelles, Administration Générale de la Cooperation au Developpement, 1982, p 627.
38 Meheus A et al: Genital infections in prenatal and family planning attendants in Swaziland. *East Afr Med J* 57:212, 1980.
39 Ratnam AV et al: Sexually transmitted diseases in pregnancy women. *Med J Zambia* 14:75, 1980.
40 Ratnam AV et al: Syphilis in pregnant women in Zambia. *Br J Vener Dis* 58:355, 1982.
41 Hira SK: Epidemiology of maternal and congenital syphilis in Lusaka and Copperbelt Provinces of Zambia. Republic of Zambia, Lusaka, Zambia, 1984, p 1.
42 Watts TE et al: A case-control study of stillbirths at a teaching hospital in Zambia, 1979–80: Serological investigations for selected infectious agents. *Bull WHO* 62:803, 1984.
43 Liljestrand J et al: Syphilis in pregnant women in Mozambique. *Genitourin Med* 61:355, 1985.
44 Report of a WHO Scientific Group: Treponemal infections. World Health Organization Technical Report Series 674, World Health Organization, Geneva, 1982, p 14.
45 Ingraham NR: The value of penicillin alone in the prevention and treatment of congenital syphilis. *Acta Derm Venereol* 31 (suppl 24): 60, 1951.
46 Hira SK et al: Congenital syphilis in Lusaka—II. Incidence at birth and potential risk among hospital delivered infants. *East Afr Med J* 59:306, 1982.
47 Hira SK et al: Conegnital syphilis in Lusaka—I. Incidence in a general nursery ward. *East Afr Med J* 59:241, 1982.
48 Bhat GJ et al: Congenital syphilis in Lusaka—III. Incidence in neonatal intensive care unit. *East Afr Med J* 59:374, 1982.
49 Naeye RL et al: Causes of perinatal mortality in an African City. *Bull WHO* 55:63, 1977.
50 Bishaw T et al: Prevention of congenital syphilis, in *Proceedings of the Third African Regional Conference on Sexually Transmitted Diseases,* H Nsanze et al (eds). Basle, Switzerland, Ciba Geigy, 1983, p 148.
51 Biggers JD: In vitro fertilization and embryo transfer in human beings. *N Engl J Med* 304:336, 1981.
52 Miller JF et al: Fetal loss following implantation: A prospective study. *Lancet* i:554, 1980.
53 Poland BJ, Carr DH: Abortion: Pathogenesis, cytogenetics, in *Perinatal Medicine: The Basic Science Underlying Clinical Practice,* GW Chance (ed). Baltimore, Williams and Wilkins, 1976, p 48.
54 Brunham RC et al: Sexually transmitted diseases in pregnancy, in

*Sexually Transmitted Diseases,* KK Holmes et al (eds). New York, McGraw-Hill, 1984, p 782.
55 Fraser JF: The pathology of congenital syphilis. *Arch Dermatol Syph* 38:491, 1920.
56 Hoffmann E: Congenital syphilis in light of 30 years' investigation of the spirochete and 25 years' experience with salvarsan. *J Pediatr* 9:569, 1936.
57 Jeans PC, Cooke JV: *Prepubescent Syphilis.* New York, Appleton-Century, 1930.
58 Stowens D: *Pediatric Pathology.* Baltimore, Williams & Wilkins, 1959.
59 Ekehorn G: Syphilis fetuum: A critical study of the syphilitic endometritis of the secundines, and of the presences, nature, functions and development of the antibody producing tissues of the fetal organism. *Acta Med Scand (Suppl)* 12:1, 1925.
60 Harter CA, Benirschke K: Fetal syphilis in the first trimester. *Am J Obstet Gynecol* 124:705, 1976.
61 Dippel AL: The relationship of congenital syphilis to abortion and miscarriage and the mechanism of intrauterine protection. *Am J Obstet Gynecol* 47:369, 1944.
62 Beck AC, Dailey WT: Syphilis in pregnancy, in Syphilis. *Pub Am Assoc Adv Sci* 6:101, 1938.
63 Driscoll SG: Histopathology of gestational rubella. *Am J Dis Child* 118:49, 1969.
64 Tondury G, Smith DW: Fetal reubella pathology. *J Pediatr* 68:867, 1966.
65 Naeye RL: Fetal growth with cogential syphilis. *Am J Clin Pathol* 55:228, 1971.
66 Silverstein AM, Lukes R: Fetal response to antigenic stimulus: Plasmacellular and lymphoid reactions in the human fetus to intrauterine infection. *Lab Invest* 11:918, 1962.
67 McCord JR: Syphilis of the placenta. The histologic examination of 1,085 placentas of mothers with strongly positive Wassermann reactions. *Am J Obstet Gynecol* 28:743, 1934.
68 Russell P, Altschuler G: Placental abnormalities of congenital syphilis. *Am J Dis Child* 128:160, 1974.
69 Bradlaw R: The dental stigmata of prenatal syphilis. *Oral Surg* 6:147, 1953.
70 Turnbull HM: Recognition of congenital syphilis inflammation of the long bones. *Lancet* 1:1239, 1922.
71 Park EA, Jackson DA: The irregular extensions of the end of the shaft in the x-ray photograph in congenital syphilis, with pertinent observations. *J Pediatr* 13:748, 1938.
72 Cremin BJ, Fisher RM: The lesions of congenital syphilis. *Br J Radiol* 43:333, 1970.
73 Caffey J: *Pediatric X-Ray Diagnosis.* Chicago, Year Book, 1978.
74 Engest A et al: On the significance of growth in the roentgenological skeletal changes in early congenital syphilis. *Am J Radiol* 69:542, 1953.
75 Pendergrass EP, Bromer RS: Congenital bone syphilis. Preliminary report: Roentgenologic study with note on the histology and pathology of the condition. *Am J Roent Ther* 22:1, 1929.
76 McLean S: The roentgenographic and pathologic aspects of congenital osseous syphilis. *Am J Dis Child* 41:130, 1931.
77 Levin E: Healing in congenital osseous syphilis. *Am J Radiol* 110:591, 1970.
78 Ingraham NR: The diagnosis of infant congenital syphilis during the period of doubt. *Am J Syph Neurol* 19:547, 1935.
79 Brown JW, Moore BM: Congenital syphilis in the United States. *Clin Pediatr (Phila)* 2:220, 1963.
80 Mamunes P et al: Early diagnosis of neonatal syphilis: Evaluation of a gamma M-fluorescent treponema antibody test. *Am J Dis Child* 120:17, 1970.
81 Bwibo NO: Congenital syphilis. *East Afr Med J* 48:185, 1971.
82 Stokes JH: *Modern Clinical Syphilology.* Philadelphia, Saunders, 1934.
83 McDonald R: Congenital syphilis has many faces. *Clin Pediatr (Phila)* 9:110, 1970.
84 Findlay L: *Syphilis in Childhood.* Oxford, Oxford Medical Publications, 1919.
85 Oppenheimer DH, Hardy JB: Congenital syphilis in the newborn infant: Clinical and pathological observations in recent cases. *John Hopkins Med J* 129:63, 1971.
86 Bueno M et al: Congenital syphilis. *Paediatrician* 8:17, 1979.
87 Woody NC et al: Congenital syphilis: A laid ghost walks. *J Pediatr* 64:63, 1963.
88 Ingall D, Norins L: Syphilis, in *Infectious Diseases of the Fetus and Newborn Infant,* J Remington, JO Klein (eds). Philadelphia, Saunders, 1976.
89 Budell JW: Treatment of congenital syphilis. *J Am Vener Dis Assoc* 3:168, 1982.
90 Rathbun KC: Congenital syphilis. *Sex Transm Dis* 10:93, 1983.
91 Teberg A, Hodgman JE: Congenital syphilis in the newborn. *Calif Med* 118:5, 1973.
92 Tan KL: The re-emergence of early congenital syphilis. *Acta Paediatr Scand* 62:661, 1973.
93 Sylvester PH: Observations on congenital syphilis. *So Med J* 193:392, 1925.
94 Freiman I, Super M: Thrombocytopenia and congenital syphilis in South African Bantu infants. *Arch Dis Child* 41:87, 1966.
95 Saxoni F et al: Congenital syphilis: A description of 18 cases and re-examination of an old but ever-present disease. *Clin Pediatr (Phila)* 6:687, 1967.
96 Murphy K, Patamasucon P: unpublished data, 1981.
97 Brooks SEH: Hepatic ultrastructure in congenital syphilis. *Arch Pathol Lab Med* 102:502, 1978.
98 Whitaker TA et al: Hematological aspects of congenital syphilis. *J Pediatr* 66:629, 1965.
99 Wile U, Mundt LK: Congenital syphilis: A statistical study with special regard to sex incidence. *Am J Syph Gon Vener Dis* 26:70, 1942.
100 Roberts MH: Congenital syphilis. *Am J Dis Child* 45:461, 1933.
101 Hill RM, Knox JM: Syphilis, in *Brennerman's Practice of Pediatrics.* New York, Harper & Row, 1970.
102 Ingraham NR: The lag phase in early congenital osseous syphilis: A roentgenographic study. *Am J Med Sci* 191:819, 1936.
103 Still FG: Hereditary Syphilis, in *System of Syphilis,* Vol I, D'A Power, JK Murphy (eds). Oxford, Oxford University Press, 1909.
104 Masola A: personal communication, 1983.
105 Whipple DV, Dunham EC: Congenital syphilis. I: Incidence, transmission and diagnosis. *J Pediatr* 12:386, 1938; II: Prevention and treatment. *J Pediatr* 13:101, 1938.
106 Rosen EU, Solomon A: Bone lesions in early congenital syphilis. *S Afr Med J* 50:135, 1976.
107 Dzebolo NN: Congenital syphilis: An unusual presentation. *Radiology* 136:372, 1980.
108 Solomon A, Rosen E: The aspect of trauma in the bone changes of congenital lues. *Pediatr Radiol* 3:176, 1975.
109 Solomon A, Rosen E: Focal osseous lesions in congenital lues. *Pediatr Radiol* 7:36, 1978.
110 Josephs HW: Anemia of infancy and early childhood. *Medicine* 15:307, 1936.
111 Sartain P: The anemia of congenital syphilis. *So Med J* 58:27, 1965.
112 Marchi AG et al: An isolated case of congenital luetic cryoglobulinemia. *Minerva Pediatr* 18:1155, 1966.
113 Kaplan BS et al: The glomerulopathy of congenital syphilis—an immune deposit disease. *J Pediatr* 81:1154, 1972.
114 Wiggelinkhuizen J et al: Congenital syphilis and glomerulonephritis with evidence for immune pathogenesis. *Arch Dis Child* 48:375, 1973.
115 Losito A et al: Membranous glomerulonephritis in congenital syphilis. *Clin Nephrol* 12:32, 1979.
116 Hilts SV, Shaw CC: Leukemoid blood reactions. *N Engl J Med* 249:434, 1953.
117 Karayalcin GM et al: Monocytosis in congenital syphilis. *Am J Dis Child* 131:782, 1977.
118 Yampolsky J, Mullins DF: Acute glomerular nephritis in an infant with congenital syphilis. *Am J Dis Child* 69:163, 1945.
119 Hill LL et al: The nephrotic syndrome in congenital syphilis: An immunopathy. *Pediatrics* 49:260, 1972.

120 Contreras R, Pereda J: Congenital syphilis of the eye with lens involvement. *Arch Ophthalmol* 96:1052, 1978.
121 McCulloch H: Congenital syphilis as a cause of heart disease. *Am Heart J* 6:136, 1930.
122 Platou RV, Kometani JT: Penicillin therapy of late congenital syphilis. *Pediatrics* 1:601, 1948.
123 Thomas EN: *Syphilis: Its Course and Management.* New York, Macmillan, 1949.
124 Cooperative Clinical Group: Late prenatal syphilis. *Arch Dermatol* 35:563, 1937.
125 Fiumara N, Lessel S: Manifestations of late congenital syphilis: An analysis of 271 patients. *Arch Dermatol* 102:78, 1970.
126 Robinson RCV: Congenital syphilis. *Arch Dermatol* 99:599, 1969.
127 Putkonen T, Paatero YV: X-ray photography of unerupted permanent teeth in congenital syphilis. *Br J Vener Dis* 37:190, 1961.
128 Karmody CS, Schuknecht HF: Deafness in congenital syphilis. *Arch Otolaryngol* 83:44, 1966.
129 Nadol JB: Positive Hénnébert's sign in Ménière's disease. *Arch Otolaryngol* 103:524, 1977.
130 Clutton HH: Symmetrical synovitis of the knee in hereditary syphilis. *Lancet* 1:391, 1886.
131 Gray SM, Philp T: Syphilitic arthritis. *Ann Rheum Dis* 22:19, 1963.
132 Kauder JV, Solomon HC: Juvenile paresis. *Am J Med Sci* 166:545, 1923.
133 Meninger WC: *Juvenile Paresis.* Baltimore, Williams & Wilkins, 1936.
134 MacKenzie GM: Paroxysmal cold hemoglobinuria: A review. *Medicine* 8:159, 1929.
135 Boak R et al: Biologic false positive reactions for syphilis in pregnancy as determined by the Treponema pallidum immobilization test. *Surg Gynecol Obstet* 101:751, 1955.
136 Buchanan CS, Haserick JR: FTA-ABS test in pregnancy: A probably false positive reaction. *Arch Dermatol* 102:322, 1970.
137 Drew FL, Saradria JL: False-positive FTA-ABS in pregnancy. *J Am Vener Dis Assoc* 1:165, 1975.
138 Alford CA: Immunoglobulin determination in the diagnosis of fetal infection. *Pediatr Clin North Am* 18:99, 1971.
139 Alford CA et al: Subclinical central nervous system disease of neonates: A prospective study of infants born with increased levels of IgM. *J Pediatr* 75:1165, 1969.
140 Miller MJ et al: Quantitation of cord serum IgM and IgA as a screening procedure to detect congenital infection: Results in 5006 infants. *J Pediatr* 75:1287, 1969.
141 Scotti AT, Logan L: A specific IgM antibody test in neonatal congenital syphilis. *J Pediatr* 73:242, 1968.
142 Kaufman RE et al: The FTA-ABS (IgM) test for neonatal congenital syphilis: A critical review. *J Am Vener Dis Assoc* 1:79, 1974.
143 Reimer CG et al: The specificity of fetal IgM: Antibody or antiantibody? *Ann NY Acad Sci* 254:77, 1975.
144 Thorley JD et al: Passive transfer of antibodies of maternal origin from blood to cerebrospinal fluid in infants. *Lancet* 1:651, 1975.
145 Idsoe O et al: Penicillin in the treatment of syphilis. *Bull WHO* 47(suppl):6, 1972.
146 Ingraham NR: Prevention and treatment of prenatal syphilis. *Am J Med* 5:693, 1948.
147 Jackson FR et al: Use of aqueous benzathine penicillin G in the treatment of syphilis in pregnant women. *Am J Obstet Gynecol* 83:1389, 1962.
148 Hardy JB et al: Failure of penicillin in a newborn with congenital syphilis. *JAMA* 212:1345, 1970.
149 Thompson S: Treatment of syphilis in pregnancy. *J Am Vener Dis Assoc* 3:159, 1976.
150 Centers for Disease Control: Sexually transmitted diseases treatment guidelines—1982. *MMWR* 31:33, 1982.
151 Elliott WC: Treatment of primary syphilis. *J Am Vener Dis Assoc* 3:128, 1976.
152 Philipson A et al: Transplacental passage of erythromycin and clindamycin. *N Engl J Med* 288:1219, 1973.
153 Hashisaki P et al: Erythromycin failure in the treatment of syphilis in a pregnant woman. *J Am Vener Dis Assoc* 10:36, 1983.
154 Schroeter AL et al: Treatment for early syphilis and reactivity of serologic tests. *JAMA* 221:471, 1972.
155 Parker CW: Allergic drug responses: Mechanisms and unsolved problems. *CRC Crit Rev Toxicol* 1:61, 1972.
156 Sullivan TS et al: Desensitization of patients allergic to penicillin using orally administered beta-lactam antibiotics. *J Allergy Clin Immunol* 69:275, 1982.
157 Kaplan M, McCracken GH Jr: Clinical pharmacology of benzathine penicillin G in neonates with regard to its recommended use in congenital syphilis. *J Pediatr* 82:1069, 1973.
158 Morrison AW: Management of severe deafness in adults. *Proc R Soc Med* 62:959, 1969.
159 Hahn RD: *Proceedings of the World Forum on Syphilis and Other Treponematoses.* U.S. Government Printing Office, 1964.
160 Rasmussen DH: The treatment of syphilis. *Surv Ophthalmol* 14:184, 1969.
161 Drusin LM et al: Epidemiology of infectious syphilis at a tertiary hospital. *Arch Intern Med* 139:901, 1979.
162 Henderson RH: Routine serological testing for syphilis recommended for all hospital inpatients. *JAMA* 226:212, 1973.
163 Felman Y: Repeal of mandated premarital tests for syphilis: A survey of state health officers. *Am J Public Health* 71:155, 1981.
164 Kingon R, Wiesner PJ: Premarital syphilis screening: Weighing the benefits. *Am J Public Health* 71:160, 1981.

# Chapter 68

# HIV infections in infants and children

Arye Rubinstein

## DEFINITION AND DIFFERENTIAL DIAGNOSIS

The case definition for pediatric HIV infection has been modified several times coinciding with the broadening of our understanding of the clinical spectrum of the disease. The first case definition developed by the Centers for Disease Control (CDC), Atlanta, Georgia, mainly took notice of the definitive identification of opportunistic infections (OI). While OIs are an important feature of HIV infection in children, they represent end-stage disease. Opportunistic infections eventually appear in many HIV-infected children but are the presenting symptoms in only a small percentage. In 1983, a large group of HIV-infected children was identified with a more favorable outcome than in infants with OI. These children exhibited a progressively incapacitating lung disease, termed lymphoid interstitial pneumonitis (LIP) or pulmonary lymphoid hyperplasia (PLH). The PLH/LIP syndrome complex was recognized and included in the revised CDC case definition for pediatric AIDS of 1985.[1] Subsequently, newly developed serologic and virologic tests have demonstrated, as expected, that the spectrum of HIV infection in children ranges from indeterminate infection to asymptomatic infection and finally to a broad constellation of clinical syndromes of variable gravity. These new insights were incorporated in the 1987 CDC case definition,[2] as outlined in Table 68-1.

The latest classification system (Table 68-1) includes the class P-0, or "indeterminate" infection. Class P-0 includes perinatally exposed infants and children up to 15 months of age who may have serum antibodies to HIV, indicating in utero exposure to an infected mother, but who cannot be classified as definitively being HIV-infected. In one instance, we were unable to determine the actual status of HIV infection until the age of 23 months. This period of indeterminate infection may be a difficult period for both parents and medical personnel.

**Table 68-1. Classification of HIV Infection in Children**

Class P-0. Indeterminate infection
Class P-1. Asymptomatic infection
  Subclass A. Normal immune function
  Subclass B. Abnormal immune function
  Subclass C. Immune function not tested
Class P-2. Symptomatic infection
  Subclass A. Nonspecific findings
  Subclass B. Progressive neurologic disease
  Subclass C. Lymphoid interstitial pneumonitis
  Subclass D. Secondary infectious diseases
    Category D-1. Specified secondary infectious diseases listed in the CDC surveillance definition for AIDS
    Category D-2. Recurrent serious bacterial infections
    Category D-3. Other specified secondary infectious diseases
  Subclass E. Secondary cancers
    Category E-1. Specified secondary cancers listed in the CDC definition for AIDS
    Category E-2. Other cancers possibly secondary to HIV infection
  Subclass F. Other diseases possibly due to HIV infection

The indeterminate infection is, however, not the only differential diagnostic difficulty in the pediatric age group. Multiple conditions can simulate HIV infection in an infant, and the diagnosis of HIV infection can only be made after other conditions with an associated immune deficiency such as congenital immune deficiencies and congenital infections are excluded.[3] Congenital immundeficiencies, including B cell defects, T cell defects, and severe combined immunodeficiencies, can generally be identified by a characteristic set of immunological aberrations which are nonprogressive in nature. The same applies to congenital infections such as cytomegalovirus, rubella, and toxoplasmosis. In most non-HIV congenital infections, the associated immune deficiency is static or transient and limited in terms of the secondary infecting agents seen.[4] It must be recognized that the immunodeficiency in HIV-infected pregnant women can result in reactivation of a variety of latent infections including cytomegalovirus and toxoplasmosis. These women may thus transmit to their fetus the AIDS virus, another congenital infection, or both. For example, newborns with concomitant HIV and congenital cytomegalovirus (CMV) infection have been described. Conversely, infants may be infected only by cytomegalovirus with all the usual associated clinical symptoms but also have passively acquired material antibodies to HIV. Under these circumstances, the most sophisticated immunological and virological methodologies may fail to define the actual status of the HIV infection in the first months or year of life. Moreover, HIV-uninfected babies born to IV-drug-abusing mothers may exhibit a transient immune deficiency in the first year of life characterized by recurrent upper respiratory infections and oral thrush.[5] This immune deficiency, which is probably related to maternal drug abuse, presents with transiently low lymphocyte mitogenic responses to phytohemagglutinin and low T4/T8 cell ratios, both of which can also be observed in HIV-infected children. For all these reasons, the diagnosis of HIV infection in the first and second year of life may be extremely difficult to establish with certainty.

## LABORATORY DIAGNOSIS OF HIV INFECTION IN INFANTS

The performance, accuracy, sensitivity, and specificity of currently available serological and virological tests for HIV are reviewed in Chap. 79. However, there are a variety of problems in the evaluation and interpretation of test results as they pertain to the pediatric age group.[6] Especially in infants, the sensitive serological tests which measure antibodies to a host of HIV antigens are far less specific than viral cultures. The value of serological testing is compromised by two phenomena unique to this age group: (1) maternal antibodies to HIV cross the placenta and are detectable in the cord blood of both HIV-infected and HIV-uninfected newborns; (2) humoral immunity is often compromised in perinatal infection, leading to deficient host antibody responses to a variety of antigens, including HIV antigens. Maternal HIV antibodies that cross the placenta may persist in HIV-uninfected infants for up to 16 months. A positive serology in this age group is therefore not necessarily indicative of infection. Conversely, we observed a false-negative serology in a 21-month-old HIV-infected infant. Because of their HIV-associated B cell defect, a prolonged "antibody-negative window period" frequently occurs in HIV-infected infants. An early diagnosis of HIV infection in infants must therefore rely heavily on laboratory tests other than routine serology. These tests include the measurement of specific IgM antibodies,[7] specific IgG subclasses (especially early IgG3 antibodies),[8] and in vitro antibody production to HIV antigens.[9] The ultimate proof of infection, however, rests with the detection of virus or viral particles. Goudsmit et al.[10] found a good correlation of HIV antigenemia with both subsequent antibody production and the onset of symptoms in children and adults. HIV antigenemia preceded the presence of antibodies by several weeks.[10] In another study[11] of nine children who had no specific HIV antibodies, active HIV infection was documented by the presence of P-24 core HIV antigen in the plasma. This is, however, not always the case. In adults, HIV antigens generally appear shortly after infection and are present transiently; their reappearance forewarns clinical deterioration.[10] The latter also seems to be the case in children. However, the presence of HIV antigens in cord blood does not necessarily indicate active fetal infection. It has yet to be determined if the occasional presence of HIV antigens in cord bloods of HIV "uninfected" newborns is due to transplacental passive transfer of HIV antigens or to an "abortive infection." Most recently, an HIV detection method has been developed that utilizes the amplification of viral genes by the polymerase chain reaction (PCR). The PCR can detect a few viral copies in tissues, but its specificity and sensitivity has yet to be determined for newborns and infants.

Various nonspecific immunological parameters may also be helpful in raising suspicion of active HIV infection in infants.[3] Early detection of diminished lymphocyte mitogenic response to pokeweed mitogen and to phytohemagglutinin, as well as low thymic hormones in the absence of a zinc deficiency are highly suggestive of HIV infection. Polyclonal hypergammaglobulinemia with poor specific antibody responses is also quite unique and suggestive of an active HIV infection. A hypergammaglobulinemia can often be detected in the first months of life; marked IgG and IgD elevations are characteristic.[3]

## THE SPECTRUM OF DISEASE

The complexity of the CDC case definition for pediatric AIDS clearly demonstrates that HIV infection in the child has a wide spectrum ranging from an asymptomatic stage to severe disease. In adults, about 3 to 6 percent of infected individuals develop the full-blown syndrome annually. Presently, it is estimated that the ratio of asymptomatically HIV-infected adults to adults with AIDS is 20:1 to 30:1. Prospective studies in HIV-infected pregnant women and in their offspring indicate that the manifestation of disease in children is different.[3,6] Most children become symptomatic by the age of 2 years. Of several hundred HIV-positive children attending our clinics, only six remained asymptomatic at the age of 6 years. None of these asymptomatic children had intact immunity, suggesting that clinical disease is imminent. In an Italian multicenter study, 132 of 135 children considered to have acquired perinatal infection from seropositive mothers had symptoms.[12] On the other hand, the European Collaborative Study in which 271 children born to HIV-infected mothers were evaluated prospectively for a little over 1 year seems to indicate a more favorable short-term outcome. Most of the 271 children remained clinically well. However, for the 24 HIV-infected children over 15 months of age, the outcome was poor; only 33 percent remained asymptomatic.[13] Longer prospective follow-ups of HIV-infected neonates are therefore necessary to document the actual incidence of asymptomatic disease.

Among symptomatic children, two main disease patterns are observed: those with and those without early onset of OI. Children who develop an OI early have a poor outlook and usually do not survive beyond 2 years of age. Conversely, children with the LIP/PLH complex rarely develop opportunistic infections early in life. Unfortunately, many children in the latter group still develop OI before school age. According to Blanche et al.,[14] an improved prognosis is predicted by the demonstration of normal in vitro and in vivo antigenic responses, and by the presence of specific antibody production to various immunizations and to several HIV proteins. These children may survive to school age.

## EPIDEMIOLOGY

In November 1987, a study of cord bloods in New York State showed that the highest prevalence of positive HIV serology was in New York City.[15] At some hospitals in Brooklyn[16] and in the Bronx cord blood antibody prevalence ranged between 2.5 and 4 percent. Assuming a transmission rate of 30 to 40 percent,[17] this suggests that 0.75 to 1.6 percent of all newborns in the Bronx are HIV-infected. Initially, the underlying risk factors in HIV-infected babies varied by geographic area. On the east coast of the United States, the main risk factor for pediatric AIDS was an HIV-infected mother, while on the west coast the predominant risk factor was transfusion of HIV-contaminated blood in the neonatal period. This picture has changed since the introduction of serological screening of blood donors. Presently, the epidemic in children nationwide parallels the rate of infection in women of childbearing age. In the United States as a whole, less than 7 percent of all AIDS patients are women, but in the pediatric AIDS epicenter of the Bronx, 23 percent of all adult AIDS patients are women. The major risk factors for these women are intravenous drug abuse and sexual promiscuity. Until 1985, the majority of HIV-infected mothers were intravenous-drug abusers. Presently, more than a third of all mothers of HIV-infected children in the Bronx are not IV-drug abusers. These women appear to have acquired the disease via heterosexual contact, but the risk factors of their sexual partners are often unknown. In recent surveys,[16,18] up to half of all HIV-infected women did not acknowledge previous high-risk activities, while the remainder admitted to promiscuity, IV-drug abuse, or heterosexual contact with a male who is a known drug user.

The epidemiology of pediatric AIDS in Europe is similar to that in the United States.[12,13] In the eight European Collaborative studies of 264 HIV-infected pregnant women, 85 percent of the women and a further 7 percent of sexual partners had a history of intravenous-drug abuse.[13] Perinatal HIV infection occurred in 32.6 percent of children born to seropositive mothers in one study[12] and in at least 24 percent in the other study.[13]

In Africa, the male to female ratio among adult AIDS patients approaches unity, and consequently, the proportion of HIV-infected infants is much higher than in the Western world.[19] In Kigali 35 percent of all AIDS patients are children as compared with a little over 1 percent in the United States. The outcome of the disease in Africa is extremely poor, with a 38 percent mortality rate at up to 6 months follow-up.[19,20]

There is ample evidence to incriminate in utero HIV transmission. Virus has been detected in 13- to 20-week fetuses in specimens of neural tissue and thymus. The virus has also been grown from cord blood. The described fetal AIDS syndrome, with multiple midline facial dysmorphic features, is also suggestive of in utero infection.[21] Intrapartum infection of the baby during labor and delivery may also occur through exposure to maternal blood and genital secretions. Such transmission has, however, not been documented yet. HIV infection is also present in babies born via cesarian section. The prospective European studies[12,13] failed to establish a significant independent risk from vaginal delivery.

Other routes of infection have been described, but their contribution to the epidemic in children is negligible. As described above, infection of infants and children via contaminated blood transfusions is now rare where blood screening is performed.[22] Isolated cases of HIV infection via breast milk feeding have been described.[6,23] In these cases, the mothers were HIV-infected postpartum by a blood transfusion and then breast-fed their babies. In the United States as well as in Europe and in Africa, prenatal or perinatal transmission appears to be the major route of HIV infection. In Africa, 85 percent of HIV-infected children are born to seropositive women, 8 percent have a history of transfusion, and 7 percent have no risk factors.[19,20] Medical injections have been implicated as a risk factor in HIV-infected children in Zaire.[24]

Although HIV is present in tears, saliva, urine, and stool, horizontal spread from an infected child to other children or to a caretaker has not been clearly documented. In one instance of apparent transmission from a child to his mother, the mother served as a nurse and had extensive unprotected contact with a variety of body secretions, with an open surgical wound, and with intravenous lines and blood. Transmission by bites has been considered highly unlikely, but in one case reported from West Germany seems to be the only risk factor.[25] Lastly, sexual abuse is a possible mode of transmission to children but has so far been documented only in isolated cases.

## CLINICAL PRESENTATION

A wide range of symptoms has been described in HIV-infected children. During the initial phases of the epidemic, the most frequently described causes of morbidity were various bacterial infections, the PLH/LIP syndrome complex, and neurodevelopmental disorders. As the epidemic has progressed, neurodevelopmental disorders have undoubtedly become the most commonly observed abnormality (Table 68-2). Up to 93 percent of all HIV-infected children have a documented neurological or developmental abnormality.[26] Encephalopathy and dementia may be observed long before any infectious complication is noted.

**Table 68-2. Frequent Clinical Syndromes in HIV-Infected Children**

| |
|---|
| Neurodevelopmental delay, encephalopathy, microcephaly |
| Recurrent bacterial and viral infections |
| Pulmonary lymphoid hyperplasia (PLH), lymphoid interstitial pneumonitis (LIP) complex |
| Lymphadenopathy, hepatosplenomegaly |
| Failure to thrive |
| Recurrent or chronic diarrhea |
| Salivary gland swelling |
| Opportunistic infections |
| Hematologic changes (leukopenia, thrombocytopenia, anemia) |

Acquired microcephaly, cognitive deficits, and bilateral pyramidal tract disease are frequent. Lymphomas of the central nervous system, cerebrovascular accidents, and central nervous system infections have been documented in 15 percent of children.[26]

One of the most unique presentations of HIV infection in children is the pulmonary lymphoid hyperplasia/lymphoid interstitial pneumonitis (PLH/LIP complex), which is found in about 25 percent of all symptomatic HIV-infected children. Its onset is insidious, leading to slowly progressive hypoxia, respiratory failure, and digital clubbing. The PLH/LIP complex is often accompanied by salivary gland enlargement and generalized lymphadenopathy. Chest x-rays (Fig. 68-1) are characterized by 1- to 5-mm nodules distributed throughout the lungs.[27–29] Epstein-Barr virus DNA has been found in lung biopsies of patients with PLH/LIP[27,30] and may cause this syndrome. PLH/LIP can generally be distinguished from PCP on the basis of clinical symptoms and simple laboratory tests (Table 68-3).

HIV-associated lymphadenopathy in newborns and infants is often being overlooked. Small but palpable lymph nodes in a newborn may be the first clue of an HIV infection. Histologically, a marked follicular hyperplasia with abundant B cells is characteristic.

Most acute morbidity in children with HIV infection is due to infectious complications. Among the opportunistic infections *Pneumocystis carinii* pneumonia (PCP) is the most common.[27,29] This infection can appear as early as in the first weeks of life and, in contradistinction to PLH/LIP, is characterized by an acute onset with fever, respiratory distress, and hypoxia (Table 28-3). The definitive diagnosis requires identification of the causative organism, usually by flexible bronchoscopy with bronchoalveolar lav-

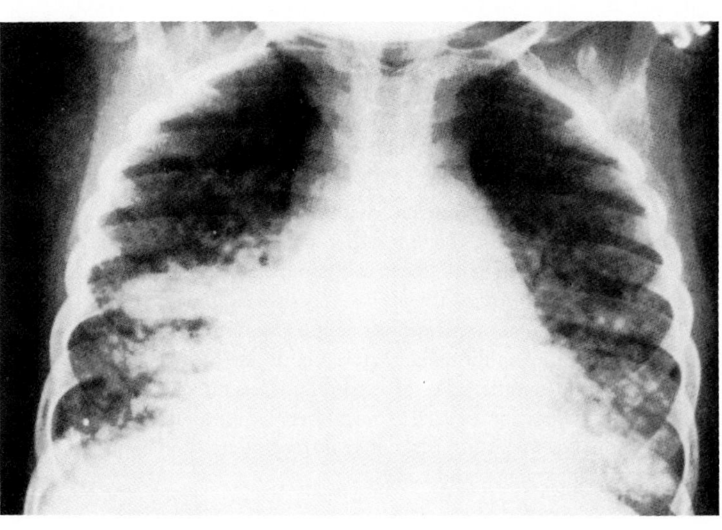

**Fig. 68-1.** Chest radiograph shows a diffuse nodular pattern with evidence of mediastinal and hilar lymph node enlargement typical of pulmonary lymphoid hyperplasia/lymphoid interstitial pneumonitis complex. In addition, there is bilateral lower lobe consolidation caused by acute and chronic superimposed infection.

**Table 68-3. Characteristic Features of *Pneumocystis carinii* Pneumonia and Pulmonary Lymphoid Hyperplasia/ Lymphocytic Interstitial Pneumonitis**

| Symptoms | PLH/LIP* | PCP |
|---|---|---|
| Acute onset | − | + |
| Insidious onset | + | Seldom |
| Fever | − | + |
| Tachypnea with retractions | Late | Early, acute |
| Hypoxia | Late | Early, severe |
| Diminished breath sounds | − | + |
| Wheezes | Rare | + |
| Rhonchi | − | + |
| Digital clubbing | + | − |
| Nodular roentgenographic pattern | + | − |
| Salivary gland enlargement | + | − |
| Generalized lymphadenopathy | + + | + |
| Isomorphic serum lactate dehydrogenase elevation | + | + + |
| Elevated serum IgG | + + | + |
| Bronchoalveolar lavage: increased lymphocytes, T8 cells | + | − |
| Tissue: | | |
| HIV genome | + | − |
| Epstein-Barr virus genome | + | − |

*PLH/LIP = pulmonary lymphoid hyperplasia/lymphocytic interstitial pneumonitis; PCP = *Pneumocystis carinii* pneumonia.

age. Bronchoalveolar lavage can be performed safely in children under the age of 1 year and is an effective alternative diagnostic technique[29,31] to open lung biopsy. Its diagnostic efficacy has been further improved by the simultaneous use of silver methenamine stains, toluidene blue D stains, and fluorescent staining with monoclonal antibodies to *P. carinii* antigens.[32] The diagnostic value of serum antibodies to *P. carinii* antigens has not yet been determined in children.

Other pulmonary infections that should be considered are various bacterial pneumonias, *Mycobacterium avium-intracellulare, Candida albicans,* cytomegalovirus, histoplasmosis, cryptococcosis, measles, varicella, herpes virus, and respiratory syncytial virus. Respiratory syncytial virus infection usually presents as an acute febrile illness with cough, dyspnea, and hypoxia.[33] An asthmoid component with hyperinflation of the lungs and a diffuse interstitial infiltrate on chest x-ray are typical. Measles and varicella pneumonitis can be life-threatening and are characterized by dyspnea, rapidly progressive hypoxia, and diffuse reticulonodular interstitial changes.

As mentioned earlier, the oftentimes recurrent and overwhelming bacterial infections in pediatric AIDS patients are due mainly to the underlying early B cell defect. In spite of polyclonal hypergammaglobulinemia, these children mount poor antibody responses to primary and booster challenges with various immunogens.[34] Consequently, they present clinically like patients with agammaglobulinemia, with the most common pathogens being *Streptococcus pneumoniae, Staphylococcus* species, *Haemophilus influenzae,* and *Neisseria meningitis.* These organisms often cause sepsis. Nontyphoid salmonella bacteremia occurs in 5 to 10 percent of all symptomatic HIV-infected infants. Acute and chronic gastroenteritis may be caused by a variety of organisms other than salmonella, including *M. avium-intracellulare,* cryptosporidium, cytomegalovirus, and candida.

## MANAGEMENT OF CHILDREN WITH HIV INFECTION

### IMMUNIZATIONS

Policies for immunization of HIV-infected children are dictated by the poor antibody responses to vaccines and by the potential increased risk of adverse reactions. Redfield et al.[35] described a military recruit with an asymptomatic HIV infection and subclinical T cell deficiency who became symptomatic and had disseminated vaccinia infection after receiving the customary battery of immunizations (including smallpox vaccine). Serious complications to live virus vaccines have been previously reported in immunodeficient recipients, including patients with agammaglobulinemia. For example, oral polio vaccine (OPV) associated paralytic poliomyelitis in the United States occurs predominantly after primary and secondary immunization of immunodeficient individuals. A severe underlying T cell deficiency may pose a potentially serious health threat to the HIV-infected child and to HIV-infected adult family members after immunization with live virus vaccines. The limited experience to date with attenuated live poliomyelitis and measles vaccines in HIV-infected children has not yet demonstrated unusual complications, with one exception related to measles vaccine.[36] The Advisory Committee on Immunization Practices has therefore suggested that (Table 68-4) although OPV should be replaced by a killed vaccine, live MMR immunization can be given at 15 months of age to asymptomatic and symptomatic children.[37] We are still hesitant in using measles vaccine in symptomatic and severely T cell–deficient children with AIDS. Moreover, some investigators raised the possibility that multiple immunizations (live or killed) may increase HIV replication via activation of latently infected helper T cells, but convincing evidence that immunizations accelerate the disease course is lacking. One should also not develop a false sense of complacency when caring for HIV-infected children who have received their immunizations. Even though they may initially develop an immune response to the immunization, this response wanes in most children with time and may leave them unprotected against the respective organism.

**Table 68-4. Recommendations for Routine Immunization of HIV-Infected Children—United States, 1988**

| | HIV infection | |
|---|---|---|
| Vaccine | Known asymptomatic | Symptomatic |
| DTP | Yes | Yes |
| OPV | No | No |
| IPV | Yes | Yes |
| MMR | Yes | Should be considered |
| Hib | Yes | Yes |
| Pneumococcal | No | Yes |
| Influenza | No | Yes |

DTP = diphtheria and tetanus toxoids and pertussis vaccine
OPV = oral attenuated poliovirus vaccine, containing poliovirus types 1, 2, and 3
IPV = inactivated poliovirus vaccine, containing poliovirus types 1, 2, and 3
MMR = live measles, mumps, and rubella viruses in a combined vaccine
Hib = *Haemophilus influenzae* type b conjugate vaccine

## PREVENTION OF INFECTION

The humoral and cellular immune deficiency associated with HIV infection in infants renders them susceptible to a wide range of microorganisms. As mentioned earlier, the predominant morbidity is initially related to the B cell defect with resultant recurrent and often life-threatening bacterial infections. Preliminary studies also suggest that recurrent infections may contribute to an acceleration of the immune attrition. It is therefore imperative that the focus of our attention is placed not only on early diagnosis and aggressive treatment of each infection but also on strategies for infection prevention. Two approaches to prevention of infection have been investigated: the use of prophylactic antibiotics and "passive" immunization using intravenous gammaglobulin (IVGG). Treatment trials with daily doses of antibiotics such as penicillin, ampicillin, or trimethoprim-sulfamethoxazole (TMP-SMX) were not beneficial or at best inconclusive. The main problems encountered with this type of antimicrobial chemoprophylaxis were noncompliance, incomplete coverage of potential infectious microorganisms, and development of resistant strains. Intravenous gammaglobulin on a biweekly schedule of 300 mg/kg[38] or 400 mg/kg[39] does not seem to have these disadvantages. In addition, it provides a broader range of protection that includes both bacterial and nonbacterial infections, including potentially serious infections such as chickenpox and measles. Over a period of 2 years of IVGG treatment, the incidence of bacteremia and sepsis decreased from 76 percent in the control group to 7 percent in IVGG-treated children. Moreover, IVGG seems to delay immunological attrition.[38] The use of IVGG in B cell–deficient but asymptomatic HIV-infected children has not yet been evaluated.

## PROPHYLAXIS FOR SPECIFIC INFECTIONS

*Pneumocystis carinii* pneumonia (PCP) is the infection with the greatest morbidity and mortality in both children and adults. In adults, various prophylactic regimens have been utilized to prevent the first infection or to delay recurrence of infection, including pyrimethamin and sulfadoxine, dapsone,[40,41] trimethoprim-sulfamethoxazole (TMP-SMX) on a daily or intermittent schedule,[42] and aerosolized pentamidine.[43] In children little experience has yet been gained with these regimens. It must be remembered that even a single dose of dapsone may cause profound hemolysis in G6PD-deficient children. G6PD levels should therefore be measured before dapsone treatment is used. In addition, although the pulmonary toxicity of aerosolized pentamidine seems to be mild, its effect is only local, and extrapulmonary infection in children may progress with this regimen. TMP-SMX prophylaxis is often accompanied by an increase in candidal infections that need to be treated, or by rash or marrow suppression. Sulfadoxine is an attractive alternative treatment that should be tested in children since it has also an effect on toxoplasmosis. It has recently been shown that prenatal spiramycin treatment of pregnant women at risk for congenital toxoplasmosis reduces the severity of the manifestations of the disease in their babies.[44] In the future, similar strategies will be attempted in HIV-infected pregnant women with reactivated toxoplasmosis, cytomegalovirus, or other infections in order to avert infection of the fetus.

## TREATMENT OF SPECIFIC INFECTIONS

**Bacterial Infection.** The HIV-infected child with sepsis may not always present with the characteristic acute septic picture. Yet seemingly benign bacterial infections can suddenly become fulminant and irreversible. It is therefore recommended that any HIV-infected febrile child should be evaluated for potentially being bacteremic. In addition, aggressive antimicrobial treatment should be instituted early. We usually initiate treatment with ampicillin or a cephalosporin in febrile children. Toxic-appearing children are hospitalized and treated with combinations of multiple intravenous antibiotics. Antibiotics are selected according to the circumstances and later are adapted to the sensitivities of cultured organisms. Salmonella isolates in acute and chronic gastroenteritis in HIV-infected children frequently develop antibiotic resistance, and their successful eradication is not always possible. As a result of this, recurrences are not uncommon.

***Pneumocystis carinii* Pneumonia.** Early detection and initiation of therapy markedly improves chances of survival. Chances of survival of the first bout of *P. carinii* infection are greatest in patients with intact or nearly cell-mediated immunity.[45] TMP-SMX and pentamidine are the mainstays of treatment. TMP-SMX (20 mg of trimethoprim per kilogram of body weight per day and 100 mg of sulfamethoxazole per kilogram per day q 6 h) is administererd for 3 weeks. The outcome of therapy is commonly not affected by the route of administration. TMP-SMX can be given orally if compliance, absorption, and tolerance are not problems. We still prefer to initiate therapy by the intravenous route in symptomatic patients. A slow response to therapy is common. However, if no improvement or worsening is noticeable by 4 to 6 days, it is recommended that treatment with intravenous (or deep intramuscular) pentamidine isethionate (4 mg per kilogram of body weight per day in one dose) be initiated for 2 weeks. TMP-SMX can result in leukopenia, thrombocytopenia, rash, hepatitis, or fever requiring its discontinuation. Pentamidine has its own side effects in children. When given intramuscularly, it appears to cause sterile abscesses more frequently in children than in adults. In addition, pentamidine can cause severe azotemia (especially in children with underlying HIV nephropathy), leukopenia, thrombocytopenia, hepatitis, hypotension, hypoglycemia, and diabetes mellitus.[42,46] In children, little experience is available with newer modes of treatment such as the combination of dapsone and trimethoprim[47] and intravenous or oral trimetrexate with leucovorin rescue.

**Fungal Infections.** For cryptococcosis, amphotericim B is the drug of choice; experience with fluconazole is limited. Occasionally improvement can be obtained with oral ketoconazole (5 to 8 mg/kg per day). Candidiasis presenting as oral thrush can be treated with the topical use of nystatin or clotrimazole. For more extensive or invasive disease, ketoconazole (5 to 8 mg/kg per day for 7 to 14 days) or intravenous amphotericin may be required.

**Disseminated *Mycobacterium avium-intracellulare* (MAI).** The known toxicity and poor outcome associated with combination chemotherapy for this disease (ansamycin, isoniazid, clofazimine, cycloserine, ethambutol, etc.) often influences physicians to forgo any treatment.

## VIRAL INFECTIONS

**Cytomegalovirus.** Only disseminated infection should be treated aggressively. Culturing of cytomegalovirus from the stool and urine is not indicative of disseminated infection, since positive cultures occur also in healthy HIV-uninfected children. The diagnosis of cytomegalovirus colitis can usually be established only by tissue biopsy. Treatment with gancyclovir (DHPG) 10 mg (7.5 to 15 mg)/kg per day[48] is effective in colitis and retinitis. Lifelong treatment (5 mg/kg per day) 5 days a week is required to avoid clinical relapse. The same treatment appears to be much less effective for cytomegalovirus pneumonitis. Foscarnet at doses of 60 mg/kg IV g 8 h for 14 days has been used in some cases, especially for serious cytomegalovirus retinitis.

**Varicella.** Pneumonitis is often fatal, even in children with nearly intact T cell functions. Varicella in the HIV-infected child may initially present with an apparently benign course which by day 3 to 7 suddenly takes an irreversible and progressive course. We therefore recommend treatment of varicella with acyclovir as early as possible in all HIV-infected children. In some instances, the vesicular rash will recur for months and long-term acyclovir therapy is required to control the disease.

**Measles.** Pneumonia due to measles also has a grim prognosis. Treatment with aerosolized ribavirin should be attempted, although its effectiveness has yet to be evaluated.

**Respiratory Syncytial Virus (RSV).** Airway infection often responds to a 3- to 5-day course of aerosolized ribavirin.[33]

**Mucocutaneous Herpes (HSV) Infection.** HSV infection of the mucous membranes is often responsive to oral acyclovir. However, for extensive disease acyclovir must be administered intravenously at a dose of 15 mg/kg. Herpes zoster has been observed in young children with AIDS. For severe disease, intravenous acyclovir at doses of up to 30 mg/kg are effective.

**Antiretroviral Therapy.** Preliminary studies with azidothymidine (AZT, Zidovudine) in children have been inconclusive. In one study, children treated intravenously with 0.9 to 1.4 mg/kg/h experienced clinical improvement as expressed by weight gain, decreased lymphadenopathy and hepatosplenomegaly, improvement of neuropsychological deficits, and an increase of CD4-positive cells. The side effects of AZT were tolerable.[49] Conversely, oral AZT at doses of 180 mg/m$^2$ q 6 h appears to be less effective than continuous infusion therapy. The incidence of bacterial infections does not decrease in AZT-treated children. A combined trial of AZT and IVGG is therefore being evaluated. As yet, there is little experience with other antiretroviral drugs in children.

Presently, treatment trials with antiviral agents are being conducted in symptomatic and asymptomatic children. In some instances, AZT has been administered to HIV-infected pregnant women as early as at the twenty-eighth week of gestation. The benefit of early institution of AZT is as yet unknown.

## TREATMENT OF THE PLH/LIP COMPLEX

Corticosteroids seem to be beneficial without having any serious side effects even in long-term alternate-day treatment. In general, prednisone at doses of 1 to 2 mg/kg is administered daily for 2 to 4 weeks until an increase in $Pa_{O_2}$ above 70 is noted. Subsequently, an alternate-day regimen is implemented at a dose that stabilizes the $Pa_{O_2}$ levels. Chest x-rays and $Pa_{O_2}$ levels may return to normal.[50] After discontinuation of long-term (1 to 2 years) alternate-day corticosteroids, often no recurrence of symptoms occurs. However, in some cases a rapid reemergence of pulmonary disease within days of discontinuation of treatment is observed.

## IMMUNOPOTENTIATION

Various immunoreconstitutive methods have been evaluated in adults and in children without any lasting benefit. A transient benefit from immunopotentiation may be followed by an accelerated clinical deterioration.[51] It has been postulated that immunopotentiation may be accompanied by activation of T cells and enhancement of HIV replication. The latter was suggested with thymic hormone treatment[51] but not with interleukin-2. Combination therapies using antiviral drugs and immunopotentiation are the rational approaches for future trials.

## References


1 Centers for Disease Control: Revision of the case definition of the acquired immunodeficiency syndrome for national reporting—US. *MMWR* 34:373, 1985.
2 Centers for Disease Control: Classification system for HIV infection in children under 13 years of age. *MMWR* 36:225, 1987.
3 Rubinstein A: Pediatric AIDS. *Curr Probl Pediatr* 16:7, 1986.
4 Gehrz RC et al: Cytomegalovirus infection in infancy: Virological and immunological studies. *Clin Exp Immunol* 47:27, 1982.
5 Culver KW et al: Lymphocyte abnormalities in infants born to drug abusing mothers. *J Pediatr* 111:230, 1987.
6 Novick B, Rubinstein A: Editorial review: AIDS the Paediatric Perspective. *AIDS* 1:3, 1987.
7 Bedaria G et al: HIV IgM antibodies in risk groups who are seronegative on ELISA testing. *Lancet* 2:570, 1986.
8 Pyun KH et al: Perinatal infection with HIV. Specific antibody responses of the neonate. *N Engl J Med* 317:611, 1987.
9 Amadori A et al: In vitro production of HIV-specific antibody in children at risk of AIDS. *Lancet* 1:852, 1988.
10 Goudsmit J et al: Antigenemia and antibody titers to core and envelope antigens in AIDS, ARC and subclinical HIV infection. *J Infect Dis* 133:558, 1987.
11 Borkowsky W et al: HIV infection in infants negative for anti HIV by ELISA. *Lancet* 1:1168, 1987.
12 Italian Multicenter Study: Epidemiology, clinical features and prognostic factors of pediatric HIV infection. *Lancet* 11:1043, 1988.
13 The European Collaborative Study. Mother-to-child transmission of HIV infection. *Lancet* 11:1039, 1988.
14 Blanche S et al: Longitudinal study of 18 children with perinatal LAV/HTLV-III infection: Attempt at prognostic evaluation. *J Pediatr* 109:965, 1986.
15 Novick LF et al: HIV seroprevalence in newborn infants in New York State. IV International Conference on AIDS, Abstract 7221, 1988.
16 Landesman S et al: Serosurvey of HIV infection in parturients. *JAMA* 258:2701, 1987.
17 Rubinstein A, Bernstein L: The epidemiology of pediatric AIDS. *Clin Immunol Immunopathol* 40:115, 1986.
18 Quinn TC et al: HIV infection among patients attending clinics for sexually transmitted diseases. *N Engl J Med* 318:197, 1988.
19 Lepage P, Van de Perre P: Clinical manifestation of AIDS in infants and children. *Bailliere's Clin Trop Med Commun Dis* 3 (1):89, 1988.
20 Lepage P, Van de Perre P: Strategies in the identification and control of HIV infected women in Africa, in *AIDS in Children, Adolescents*

*and Heterosexual Adults*, AJ Schinazi-Nahmias (ed). New York, Elsevier, pp 214–215, 1988.

21 Marion R et al: The fetal AIDS syndrome score: Correlation between severity of dysmorphism and age at diagnosis of immunodeficiency. *Am J Dis Child* 141:429, 1987.

22 Peterman TA et al: Estimating the risk of transfusion associated with AIDS and HIV infection. *Transfusion* 27:371, 1987.

23 Ziegler JB et al: Postnatal transmission of AIDS associated retrovirus from mother to infant. *Lancet* 1:896, 1985.

24 Lepage P et al: Are medical injections a risk factor for HIV infection in children? *Lancet* II:1103, 1986.

25 Wahn V et al: Horizontal transmission of HIV infection between two siblings. *Lancet* 2:694, 1986.

26 Belman A et al: Pediatric AIDS, neurologic syndromes. *Am J Dis Child* 142:29, 1988.

27 Rubinstein A et al: Pulmonary disease in children with acquired immune deficiency syndrome and AIDS-related complex. *J Pediatr* 108:498, 1986.

28 Joshi VV, Oleske JM: Pulmonary lesions in children with the acquired immunodeficiency syndrome: A reappraisal based on data in additional cases and follow-up study of previously reported cases (letter). *Hum Pathol* 17:641, 1986.

29 Rubinstein A et al: Pulmonary disease in infants and children. *Clin Chest Med* 9:3, 1988.

30 Andiman WA et al: Opportunistic lymphoproliferations associated with EBV DNA in infants and children with AIDS. *Lancet* 2:1390, 1985.

31 Bye BR et al: Diagnostic bronchoalveolar lavage in children with AIDS. *Pediatr Pulmonol* 3:425, 1987.

32 Gill VJ et al: Detection of Pneumocystis carinii by fluorescent antibody stain using a combination of three monoclonal antibodies. *J Clin Microbiol* 25:1837, 1987.

33 Chandwani S et al: Clinical features of respiratory syncitial virus infection in HIV infected children. Third International Conference on AIDS, Washington, DC, 1987.

34 Bernstein L et al: Defective humoral immunity in pediatric AIDS. *J Pediatr* 107:352, 1985.

35 Redfield RR et al: Disseminated vaccinia in a military recruit with HIV disease. *N Engl J Med* 316:673, 1987.

36 Von Reyn CF et al: HIV infection and routine childhood immunizations. *Lancet* 2:669, 1987.

37 ACIP revised recommendations for measles-mumps-rubella vaccination in HIV-infected children. *Vaccine Bull* July 1988.

38 Calvelli TA, Rubinstein A: Intravenous gammaglobulin in infant AIDS. *Pediatr Infect Dis* 5:207, 1986.

39 Schaad UB et al: Intravenous immune globulin in symptomatic paediatric HIV infection. *Eur J Pediatr* 147:300, 1988.

40 Fischl M et al: Fansidar prophylaxis of Pneumocystis carinii pneumonia in AIDS. *Ann Intern Med* 105:629, 1986.

41 Glatt A et al: Treatment of infection associated with human immunodeficiency virus. *N Engl J Med* 318:1439, 1988.

42 Fischl M et al: Safety and efficacy of sulfamethoxazole and trimethoprim chemoprophylaxis for Pneumocystis carinii pneumonia in AIDS. *JAMA* 259:1185, 1988.

43 Montgomery AB et al: Aerosolized pentamidine as sole therapy for Pneumocystis carinii pneumonia in patients with AIDS. *Lancet* 2:480, 1987.

44 Daffos F et al: Prenatal management of 746 pregnancies at risk for congenital toxoplasmosis. *N Engl J Med* 318:271, 1988.

45 Bernstein L et al: Prognostic factors and life expectancy in children with AIDS and Pneumocystis carinii pneumonia. *Am J Dis Child* 1989.

46 Falloon J et al: Human immunodeficiency virus infection in children. *J Pediatr* 114:1, 1989.

47 Leoung GS et al: Dapsone-trimethoprim for Pneumocystis carinii pneumonia in AIDS. *Ann Intern Med* 105:45, 1986.

48 Jacobson MA, Mills J: Serious cytomegalovirus disease in AIDS: Clinical findings, diagnosis and treatment. *Ann Intern Med* 108:584, 1988.

49 Pizzo PA et al: Effect of continuous intravenous infusion of zidovudine (AZT) in children with symptomatic HIV infection. *N Engl J Med* 319:889, 1988.

50 Rubinstein A et al: Corticosteroid treatment for pulmonary lymphoid hyperplasia in children with AIDS. *Pediatr Pulmonol* 4:13, 1988.

51 Rubinstein A et al: Circulating thymulin and thymosin $\alpha_1$ activity in pediatric AIDS (in vivo and in vitro studies). *J Pediatr* 109:422, 1986.

# Chapter 69

# Group B streptococcal infections

Harry R. Hill

## HISTORY

The recognition of group B streptococci as a major cause of perinatal morbidity and mortality as well as an organism capable of being spread by a venereal route has come about largely in the past 50 years. Such organisms were first associated with problems in the dairy industry, where they were found to cause bovine mastitis.[1,2] Strains isolated from bovine and dairy sources which were designated *Streptococcus agalactiae* fell into Lancefield's group B on the basis of precipitin reactions between acid extracts of these organisms and hyperimmune rabbit antiserum.[3] Subsequently, group B streptococci were isolated from the urogenital tract of both healthy and postpartum women with or without fever.[4] Fry[5] of London and Hill and Butler[6] of Australia in 1938 and 1940, respectively, reported fatal cases of human puerperal infections due to group B organisms. Nevertheless, most cases of puerperal sepsis were caused by group A strains, so many microbiologists continued to discount the importance of *S. agalactiae.*

In 1961 Hood et al.[7] reported a high incidence (5 to 6 percent) of colonization with group B streptococci in pregnant females seen at Charity Hospital in New Orleans. Furthermore, group B organisms were isolated from 24 percent of a group of patients who experienced marked difficulty during pregnancy and from 9.7 percent of brains of dead fetuses and stillborn infants. Approximately 37 percent of pregnant women from whom the organism was isolated had significant complications such as abortion, perinatal death, premature birth, or severe neonatal illness. Subsequently, Eickhoff et al.[8] reported that group B streptococci were the most frequent cause of neonatal sepsis from July 1, 1962, through June 30, 1963, at Boston City Hospital. Moreover, strains of this group were also frequently isolated from infections in diabetic individuals and from cases of pyelonephritis. Franciosi et al.[9] confirmed the importance of these organisms in neonatal infections in Denver, Colorado, and suggested the occurrence of two distinct forms of neonatal disease: an *early-onset septicemic* form and a *late-onset meningitic* variety. They also presented the first data indicating probable venereal transmission of group B streptococci, since the organism could often be cultured from the urethra of spouses of colonized females. Barton et al.[10] and Baker et al.[11] simultaneously described additional cases of neonatal meningitis due to these agents.

Subsequently, a host of clinical reports, epidemiological studies, and immunologic investigations relating to group B streptococci have appeared in the literature. In most studies, group B streptococci have been found to be the first or second leading cause of neonatal sepsis and meningitis.[7–12] Urogenital colonization of pregnant and nonpregnant females has ranged from approximately 4 percent to as high as 29 percent.[9,12,13,14,15] Moreover, neonatal disease is estimated to occur in from 1.3 to 5.4 neonates per 1000 live births per year.[16] In infants who are "heavily" colonized with group B streptococci, the attack rate may be as high as 50 per 1000.[17] It has been estimated that approximately 7500 early-onset and 2400 late-onset cases of group B neonatal infection occur annually[16] and approximately 5000 infants per year die of group B streptococcal infection in the United States. The annual economic burden of perinatal infections due to group B streptococci has been estimated at $700 million.[18] These organisms almost certainly also cause abortions and stillbirths as well as serious infections in postpartum women, diabetics, and other immunocompromised hosts; their significance as a major human pathogen is apparent.

## BIOLOGY OF THE ORGANISM

### MICROBIOLOGY

#### Colonial morphology and hemolytic activity

A number of morphologic and biochemical characteristics help differentiate group B streptococci from organisms of Lancefield's other groups. Colonies on sheep blood agar plates are somewhat more gray and mucoid appearing than group A organisms. Furthermore, β hemolysis is less pronounced and appears in a narrow zone around colonies. Strains of nonhemolytic group B streptococci have been isolated from human sources, which serves to complicate the laboratory identification of these pathogens. Roe et al.[19] reported that up to 36 percent of group B streptococci produced only α hemolysis when incubated aerobically on sheep blood agar plates. Anaerobic incubation for prolonged periods of time still resulted in 18 percent of the strains being α-hemolytic. Although other centers have not reported such a high incidence of these unusual strains,[16] this problem must be kept in mind.

#### Pigment production

From 85 to 97 percent of strains of group B organisms produce pigmentation which is nonextractable with a variety of agents including water, methanol, ethanol, acetone, diethyl ether, petroleum ether, or alcoholic potassium hydroxide.[20] The pigmentation, which is usually light red in color, is localized to a membranous fraction of the cell and may be similar to a carotenoid. It is best detected with special media prepared as described by Merritt and Jacobs[21] but can be seen in stabs or punctures made into a columbia-based agar.

#### Hippuricase activity

An important biochemical characteristic of group B streptococci that is quite useful in laboratory identification is the ability to hydrolyze hippuric acid to benzoic acid and glycine. Over 95 percent of strains have hippuricase activity that can be detected in a test that can be completed within 2 h.[22,23] The procedure consists of inoculating a large loop of group B streptococci into a 0.4-ml aliquot of 1% aqueous sodium hippurate. The solution is then incubated for 2 h at 37°C, and the resulting glycine is detected with 0.2 ml of a triketohydrindene hydrate (Ninhydrin) solution. Hippurate-positive strains produce a deep-purple color with the triketohydrindene hydrate reagent after 10 min of additional incubation. Strains of groups A, C, D, G, and F are negative for this activity.[23]

### CAMP factor production

Another means of identifying group B streptococci depends upon the production of an interesting factor first described by Christie, Atkins, and Munch-Petersen.[24] The name, CAMP factor, is derived from the initials of these authors and is not related to cyclic adenosine monophosphate, as was incorrectly implied in a review.[16] *CAMP factor* is an extracellular, diffusible product of group B organisms which, when combined with staphylococcal β-lysin, produces a markedly enhanced zone of hemolysis on sheep blood agar plates. A simple screening test for CAMP factor production can be carried out by streaking strains of group B streptococci at right angles to a strain of β-lysin-producing staphylococci.[25] A flamelike zone of exaggerated hemolysis is produced in the area where the streaks cross and the two diffusible products mix. Darling[25] has indicated that all strains of group B streptococci produce the CAMP factor; this results in a visible flame-shaped reaction within 18 h of aerobic incubation. Some group A strains are also positive but only when incubated under anaerobic conditions. Most other groups of streptococci fail to produce CAMP factor. Brown et al.[26] have demonstrated that hyperimmune rabbits and experimentally infected cows produce antibody to the factor that is capable of neutralizing its activity. The role that this factor alone, or in combination with staphylococcal toxin(s), has in the pathogenesis of group B disease remains to be determined.

### Neuraminidase production

Hayano and Tanaka[27] first demonstrated that group B streptococci produce a sialidase (neuraminidase) that is active against a preparation of bovine submaxillary gland sialomucin. Subsequently, Milligan et al.[28] have demonstrated production of this enzyme by a number of group B strains grown under a variety of different cultural conditions. Neuraminidase production is most often observed in type III group B strains. Most but not all strains from infected infants (42 of 65 strains) elaborate the enzyme.[29] The role of neuraminidase production in the pathogenesis of group B disease needs to be examined more closely, as does the possibility that other toxic extracellular factors are produced by these organisms.

### Sensitivity of bacitracin and other antibiotics

Susceptibility to low-concentration (0.04 units) bacitracin disks is a characteristic of group A streptococci. Although many hospital laboratories make a presumptive diagnosis of a group A infection on the basis of demonstrable sensitivity to this agent, approximately 2 to 6 percent of group B strains also are sensitive to bacitracin.[16,30] Thus, this test alone cannot be used to exclude the presence of group B organisms.

Group B streptococci are susceptible to penicillin G, ampicillin, cephalothin, and erythromycin but are often resistant to tetracycline.[30] Despite the uniform sensitivity of group B streptococci to penicillin and ampicillin, relapses and treatment failures are not uncommon. Schauf et al.[31] have studied antibiotic killing curves using group B organisms and ampicillin with or without gentamicin. In these in vitro studies, bacterial killing is complete with ampicillin alone only after 10 to 24 h of incubation. More rapid killing of these strains (less than 4 h) occurred in every instance in which gentamicin was included with ampicillin in the incubation mixture. Kim and Anthony[32] have described penicillin-tolerant strains of group B streptococci. Approximately 4 percent of 100 strains they tested persisted in the presence of penicillin levels 16 times greater than the minimal inhibitory concentrations. Thus, group B strains may be relatively more resistant to the bactericidal activity of the penicillins and require a combination of an aminoglycoside plus penicillin for rapid and effective killing. Synergism between ampicillin and gentamicin has also been demonstrated in experimental meningitis due to group B streptococci in rabbits.[33]

### Comparative performance of identification methods

Jokipii and Jokipii[30] compared the three most common presumptive identification tests for group B streptococci, i.e., (1) the CAMP test, (2) hippurate hydrolysis, and (3) pigment production, using 371 clinical isolates of these organisms. Positive identification was obtained in 95.0 percent of the CAMP tests, 96.1 percent of the hippurate hydrolysis tests, and 97.3 percent of the pigment production tests. A combination of any two tests was positive in identifying over 99.8 percent of strains. Rapid antigen tests for the identification and detection of group B streptococci will be discussed later.

## SEROLOGIC CLASSIFICATION GROUP AND TYPING

Lancefield[34] has reviewed the serologic classification of group B streptococci and pointed out that the previous classification of these organisms, based on cultural and biochemical tests, often yielded overlapping results or exceptions to the criteria for identification. Thus, classification based upon serologic reactions has a decided advantage. In contrast to group A streptococci, which have a group-specific cell wall polysaccharide (C substance) and protein type-specific antigens (M and T proteins), group B streptococci have at least two polysaccharide antigens associated with the cell. The group-specific C substance common to all group B strains consist of rhamnose, *N*-acetylglucosamine, and galactose; rhamnose is the most important immunodeterminant.[35] Since this determinant is also present in the group G polysaccharide, cross-reactions are observed. The second category of major polysaccharide antigens of group B streptococci are probably capsular polysaccharides, which can be demonstrated in acid or saline washes of these organisms. On the basis of serologic reactions to these polysaccharides, group B strains can be classified into four types: Ia, Ib, II, and III. Although most human strains (97 percent) can be classified by this system, bovine strains are much less likely to react with antisera raised against these substances. Subsequently, Wilkinson has defined an additional type (Ic)[36] on the basis of the presence of a protein which is shared by types Ib and Ic. The Ic strains share the major polysaccharide-typing antigen with Ia strains. Thus, Ic strains react with antisera raised against Ia (polysaccharide) and Ib (protein) organisms. In addition to these antigens, Ia, Ib, and Ic strains also share a minor polysaccharide determinant which is termed the Iabc polysaccharide.[37] An R antigen like that observed in type 28, group A streptococci has also been detected in some type III and non-typeable group B strains. The functions of these antigens, as well as their role in the pathogenesis of group B disease, are discussed under Immunology and Pathogenesis, below. Table 69-1 details the serologic reactions expected when capillary precipitin tests are performed with hydrochloric acid (HCl), trichloroacetic acid (TCA), or saline extracts of the various types and with hyper-

Table 69-1. Serologic Reactions of Group B Streptococci

| | Rabbit antiserum prepared against | | | | | |
|---|---|---|---|---|---|---|
| Extract of type | Ia | Ib | Ic | II | III | R |
| Ia | + | − | + | − | − | − |
| Ib | − | + | + | − | − | − |
| Ic | + | + | + | − | − | − |
| II | − | − | − | + | − | − |
| III | − | − | − | − | + | ± |
| II/Ic | − | + | + | + | − | − |
| III/Ic | − | + | + | − | + | − |
| Nontypeable | − | − | − | − | − | ± |

immune rabbit antiserum. Recently, strains possessing both the II polysaccharide and the Ibc protein have been isolated with increasing frequency.[36] Less commonly, strains sharing the III polysaccharide and the Ibc protein have also been observed.

## IMMUNOCHEMISTRY

Determining the chemical composition of the typing polysaccharides and proteins of group B streptococci has become the subject of intense investigation because a protective vaccine would most likely be composed of these substances, at least in part. Lancefield[34] pointed out that different methods of extraction resulted in polysaccharide preparations of different chemical and serologic composition. Extraction of organisms with hot HCl results in a degraded polysaccharide antigen of smaller molecular weight (15,000 to 50,000) capable of absorbing some but not all precipitin and mouse protective antibodies from hyperimmune rabbit serum. In contrast, mild extraction with TCA in the cold results in a larger-molecular-weight polysaccharide that removes most precipitin and protective antibodies. Saline or water extracts were also found to contain this less-degraded, native antigen. The type II antigen extracted with water was found to contain sialic acid (17.5%), galactose (3.12%), glucose (20.0%), *N*-acetylglucosamine (9.2%), and amino acids (4.5%) and to have a molecular weight of 5 million.[35,37] In contrast, the hot HCl extracts contain no sialic acid. TCA or neutral buffer extracts of types Ia, Ib, and II strains yield antigens consisting of galactose, glucosamine, glucose, and sialic acid.[37] The neutral buffer extracts of type III strains contain these components plus two additional sugars, heptose and mannose. It appears that the TCA- or neutral-buffer-extracted antigens possess two antigenic specificities: one directed at the heat-labile sialic acid component, and one directed at the core antigen present in the hot HCl extracts. Wilkinson[38] has indicated that the Ia precipitin reactions are best inhibited by *N*-acetylglucosamine, while Ib reactions are most responsive to inhibition by glucosamine.

The Ibc protein antigen is not related to the R antigen or the M or T antigens of group A streptococci. The Ibc protein antigen has two determinants, one susceptible to pepsin and trypsin and the other sensitive to pepsin but not trypsin.[39] Acrylamide gel electrophoresis of the Ibc protein antigen reveals 13 bands, all of which react with hyperimmune rabbit antiserum.

Extensive work has been carried out by Kasper et al.[40,41] and by Baker et al.[42] on the immunochemistry of the type III group B streptococcal polysaccharide. These studies have defined a *core antigen* consisting of galactose, glucose, and glucosamine. In addition, neutral buffer extraction yields a larger molecule containing up to 24% sialic acid. These *native antigens* are serologically distinct from the core antigen in having determinants ending in sialic acid, while the core antigen terminates in β-digalactopyranose. Interestingly, the core antigen of the type III group B streptococcus cross reacts with the type 14 pneumococcal polysaccharide.[43]

## IMMUNOLOGY AND PATHOGENESIS

### OPSONIC AND PROTECTIVE STUDIES IN ANIMALS

Lancefield and Freimer[44,45] have shown that homologous type-specific but not group B–specific rabbit antisera protect mice against challenge with type Ia, Ib, Ic, and II organisms. Antibodies directed at both the polysaccharide and protein-typing antigens appear to confer protection in this animal model. Absorption of the antiserum with hot HCl extracts of the homologous organisms removes some but not all protective activity against the homologous type strain. Absorption with cold TCA extracts of the organisms removes more of this activity, but generally some remains. Employing several assays of opsonic activity, Hemming et al.[46] showed that homologous-type hyperimmune rabbit antiserum promotes phagocytic uptake of types Ia, II, and III group B streptococci. Furthermore, the classic complement pathway contributes significantly to opsonization of these strains. Subsequently, Shigeoka et al.[47] found that these strains do not activate the alternative pathway in antibody-deficient serum. Although Edwards et al.[48] reported that type III strains can trigger the alternative pathway when homologous-type antibody is present in the sera, all seem to agree that antibody is required for opsonization of at least type II and III strains.

Anthony[49] has reported that rabbit sera containing antibody to the Ia or Ib carbohydrates or the Ibc protein promoted uptake of Ia, Ib, and Ic strains by macrophage monolayers. In contrast to these findings and those of Hemming et al.,[46] Baker et al.[50] have recently suggested that Ia strains do not require antibody for opsonization. Further clarification is needed on this point.

Animal studies of group B disease, including mice,[44,45] neonatal rats,[43,51] and chick embryos,[52] have generally indicated that rabbit hyperimmune antiserum is capable of protecting animals from challenge with the homologous type of group B streptococci. Moreover, neonatal animals often develop marked neutropenia and depletion of bone marrow granulocyte reserves during fatal group B infection.[53] Treatment of such animals with type-specific antibody and/or transfusion of functional leukocytes is capable of prolonging life and improving survival rates in most cases.[51] Immunotherapy of group B disease would appear, therefore, to be feasible in the future. The development of means for providing active or passive immunotherapy may not be as simple as previously thought, however. Shigeoka et al.[54] reported that some strains of type Ia, II, and III group B streptococci are extremely resistant to opsonization by most antibody-containing sera. Moreover, these opsonin-resistant strains appear to be more virulent in neonatal animals.[55] Similar results were observed by Fischer et al.,[56] who found that extremely high antibody concentrations were required for opsonization of some group B strains. The reason for the increased virulence and resistance to opsonization by some strains remains to be determined, but it may be related to additional antiphagocytic factors,[57] adverse effects of streptococcal products on phagocytes, or the release of soluble toxins. One potential candidate for such a product is the neuraminidase mentioned previously. Neuraminidase production is more common in isolates from cases of group B disease than in isolates from asymptomatic cases.[29] Moreover, neuraminidase production is more common in type III strains, which tend to be more invasive and to produce the majority of cases of meningitis. The role of neuraminidase in interactions of group B streptococci with antibody or phagocytes needs to be determined.

Other toxins may play a role in the pathogenesis of group B disease. Since the clinical, radiographic, and pathologic picture in group B neonatal infection so closely mimics that seen in hyaline membrane disease,[58,59] it is tempting to speculate that these organisms produce a toxin(s) that directly affects pulmonary tissue. Recently, Rojas et al.[60] have reported that a toxic material derived from group B streptococci was capable of producing a granulocytopenic response in sheep that resulted in pulmonary sequestration of granulocytes. Furthermore, the toxic material caused an early phase of pulmonary hypertension and a late phase of increased lung permeability. Indomethacin, a prostaglandin synthetase inhibitor, prevented the pulmonary hypertension but did not modify the granulocytopenic response. Hellerqvist and coworkers[61] have indicated that the interaction of cellular receptors with mannosyl phosphodiester groups plays a critical role in the pathophysiologic response to this group B streptococcal toxin. Recently, we[62] have found that the type III specific antigen, in the presence of plasma, enhances the interaction of endothelial cells with polymorphonuclear leukocytes which could contribute to the capillary plugging, endothelial damage, and increased lung lymph flow observed in group B streptococcal pneumonia. Thus, toxic streptococcal products acting alone or through normal inflammatory mediators may contribute to the pathogenesis of this fulminant disease.

## HUMAN IMMUNITY TO GROUP B STREPTOCOCCI

### Opsonic activity and type-specific antibody levels

Baker and Kasper presented data on a radioactive antigen-binding assay (RABA) for detecting antibody to a broadly reactive type III group B streptococcal antigen at the Lancefield Society meetings in Washington, D.C., in 1975. At that same meeting Hemming and Hill described an opsonic assay for group B streptococcal types Ia, II, and III that was based upon the generation of chemiluminescence by neutrophils exposed to opsonized, but not unopsonized, group B streptococci. Subsequently, Baker and Kasper[63] indicated that the prevalence of antibody to the broadly reactive type III antigen, which contained group B determinants as well as type-specific ones, was lower in mothers of infected infants (0 of 7) than in mothers of infants who became colonized but were not infected (22 of 29). Hemming et al.[46] later reported that opsonic activity to the patient's own infecting strain was usually lacking (0 of 13) in neonates who developed group B disease due to types Ia, II, and III group B organisms. This was in contrast to a 56 and 78 percent prevalence of antibody in 18 mothers and their infants who were colonized but the infants of whom did not show evidence of disease. Opsonic activity was shown to cross the placenta and appear in approximately equal levels in the mother and infant. Interestingly, discrepancies in opsonic requirements were often noted between stock strains and those isolated from infected patients. Serum containing opsonic activity and antibody against one strain of a given serotype often would not opsonize another strain of the same serotype.[46,54] Stewardson-Krieger et al.[64] reported that sera from adult women often contained opsonic activity for type Ia group B streptococci and were capable of protecting mice from challenge with these organisms. Baker and Kasper[65] later indicated that infants convalescing from group B disease usually lacked antibody (0 of 10) to the broadly reactive type III group B antigen employed in their RABA. In contrast, four adults developed antibody to this antigen following invasive infection.

Wilkinson and Jones[66] developed another radioimmunoassay technique for measuring group B streptococcal antibody levels in human sera. Their procedure, which employed both HCl- and TCA-extracted antigens, showed little cross-reactivity with group B determinants such as the one used by Baker and Kasper.[63,65] Employing her more specific assay, Wilkinson[67] was unable to show an association between susceptibility to disease and low-to-absent antibody levels as measured by her RABA. A similar lack of correlation between type-specific antibody concentrations and risk of infection was observed by Rote et al.,[68] who employed an enzyme-linked immunoabsorbent assay (ELISA) for antibodies directed against types II and III TCA-extracted antigen. Although Edwards et al.[69] reported a close correlation between antibody levels to type III group B streptococci as determined by RABA and opsonophagocytic activity, others have failed to observe this uniform association.[54,56,57,70] Human sera possessing antibody directed against the type-specific polysaccharide of one type may not, in fact, protect against or act as an opsonin for all strains of the same serotype. The enhanced virulence of these "resistant" strains has been related to the presence of higher cell-associated levels of sialic acid containing type-specific antigen.[71–73]

### Phagocyte number and function in group B infection

Group B streptococcal invasive disease occurs almost exclusively in immunocompromised hosts, including newborns, diabetics, and patients with liver or renal disease.[8] Each of these patient groups has been found to have abnormalities in the number or functional activity of their phagocytic cells. Inasmuch as opsonization and phagocytosis appear to represent the most important host defense parameters for clearing the body of group B streptococci, the cellular portion of the acute inflammatory response represents a critical factor in protection. Several workers have noted a marked neutropenia and depletion of bone marrow granulocyte reserves in human neonates and experimental animals with group B streptococcal infection.[53,74,75] Recently, Christensen et al.[74] have demonstrated that experimental group B streptococcal infection in neonatal rats also leads to a diminution in the number of marrow, unipotent, granulocytic stem cells and their proliferative rate. These facts, plus the profound defect in polymorphonuclear neutrophil leukocyte (PMN) chemotaxis observed in almost all neonates and the decreased bactericidal activity and metabolic activity reactions observed in PMNs of stressed neonates,[76] probably contribute significantly to the susceptibility of neonates to invasive group B disease. Thus, antibody deficiency cannot be accepted as the only important determinant of susceptibility to group B streptococcal infection. Further studies are needed to define the role of phagocytes (including PMN, monocytes and macrophages, and lymphocytes) in protecting humans from invasive group B disease.

## EPIDEMIOLOGY

### COLONIZATION RATES

Numerous investigations have documented high asymptomatic colonization rates for group B streptococci in pregnant and nonpregnant females and in males. In general, detection of these high rates has depended upon the use of multiple cultures at different sites and the utilization of selective broth media containing antibiotics.[16] Cervicovaginal colonization in females has ranged from 4.6 percent to as high as 28 percent, while pharyngeal cultures may be positive in from 5 to 12 percent.[16,17,36] Vulvar and periurethral cultures in females are more often positive than cervical cultures. Badri et al.[77] found a higher incidence of rectal colonization in pregnant females and suggested that the gastrointestinal tract is the primary site of colonization with these organisms. Other studies, however, have suggested that males and females are more often colonized at the urethra.[16,78,79] Dillon and coworkers[80] in a prospective study of 2540 pregnant females found that the intestinal tract was the primary site of acquisition. Thus, in screening for either urethral or vaginal group B streptococcal carriage, cervical and anorectal cultures should be obtained. In general, pregnancy does not affect the carrier rate; rates are similar during the first, second, or third trimester.[16] Sexually active females have a higher colonization rate than virgins, and patients attending a venereal disease clinic are more likely to be colonized than those attending medical clinics.[16] There is a high urethral colonization rate (50 percent) in spouses of colonized females[9] and in heterosexual and homosexual males (up to 22 percent). These considerations suggest that venereal spread is an important mode of transmission of these organisms. The studies suggesting or documenting such spread are summarized in Table 69-2.

Anthony et al.[81] observed a significantly lower colonization rate in females of Mexican-American descent. Preliminary studies in the author's laboratory suggest that such individuals have a higher incidence of antibodies to types II and III group B streptococcal polysaccharide antigens. Vogel et al.,[82] employing an indirect fluorescent antibody technique, have observed low levels of type-specific and protective antibodies in a predominately black population of females of lower socioeconomic status in Chicago. Gray and coworkers[83] found a low prevalence of antibody to the type II group B streptococcal polysaccharide in uncolonized (2 percent) and colonized mothers (37 percent). Infants who developed disease with this serotype often (50 percent) lacked antibody to the type II antigen. In 6 of 23 infected patients, however, the antibody level exceeded 2 μg/ml. Thus, antibody deficiency alone clearly does not explain all neonatal group B streptococcal disease.

Carriage of group B streptococci may be chronic (36 percent), intermittent (15 percent), transient (20 percent), or indeterminant (29 percent).[81] Cultures taken during the first to third trimester of pregnancy have some usefulness in predicting which women will be colonized at delivery. Boyer and colleagues[84] have indicated that approximately 67 percent of prenatal carriers of group B streptococci remain positive at the time of delivery. Approximately 8.5 percent of women who are culture-negative during the first, second, or third trimester, in contrast, become positive by the time of delivery. Among 10 infants in their study who developed early-onset group B streptococcal disease, 8 (80 percent) were born to mothers who had positive vaginal or rectal cultures for this organism during pregnancy. This has made prophylactic treatment of mothers in order to prevent group B disease in their offspring a promising possibility.[85,86]

## ACQUISITION OF GROUP B STREPTOCOCCI BY THE FETUS AND NEWBORN

Studies have indicated that the vertical transmission rate of group B streptococci from colonized mother to infant at or near birth is quite high (65 to 72 percent).[16,36,81] Such colonization undoubtedly occurs during passage of the infant through the birth canal in most cases. Early-onset neonatal infection has been reported, however, in the absence of ruptured membranes in patients delivered by cesarean section.[8,87] Thus, at least some cases of disease result from ascending infection with passage of micro-

**Table 69-2. Studies Relating to Possible Venereal Transmission of Group B Streptococci**

| Study findings | Reference |
|---|---|
| **Evidence suggesting or consistent with venereal transmission** | |
| Urethral cultures were positive from 45 percent of the husbands of 18 vaginally positive women. | Franciosi et al: *J Pediatr* 82: 707, 1973 |
| Only 5.6 percent of 90 male convicts without a history of sexual relations for 6 months were positive. | |
| Of 14 vaginally positive women with positive spouses, therapy of both partners resulted in persistently negative cultures in 13. | |
| The overall frequency of group B streptococcal colonization was 31.7 percent in 41 patients with gonococcal infection versus 19 percent in 526 controls. | Christensen et al: *Acta Pathol Microbiol Scand* [B] 82: 470, 1974 |
| Group B streptococcal colonization in 499 college women was increased in: | Baker et al: *J Infect Dis* 135: 392, 1977 |
| Sexually experienced women (20 percent vs 7.1 percent; $p < 0.02$) | |
| Women with an intrauterine device (50 percent vs. 18.6 percent; $p < 0.001$) | |
| Women 20 years of age or younger (21.4 percent vs. 14.8 percent; $p < 0.05$) | |
| The isolation rate of group B streptococci from genitourinary cultures was higher (32 percent) among patients from dermatovenereological wards than from gynecological patients (21.1 percent) or normal individuals (18.0 percent). | Jensen and Andersen: *Scand J Infect Dis* 11: 199, 1979 |
| **Evidence not supporting venereal transmission** | |
| No relationship was found between isolation of gonorrhea and group B streptococci from 757 men and women attending a venereal disease clinic. | Wallin and Forgsren: *Br J Vener Dis* 51: 401, 1975 |
| The presence of group B streptococci in urogenital cultures could not be related to promiscuity. | |
| Group B colonization in college women could not be related to: | Baker et al: *J Infect Dis* 135: 392, 1977 |
| The number of sexual partners | |
| A history of venereal disease | |

organisms through intact membranes. The mechanism of this type of spread is entirely unknown.

In spite of the high colonization rate in pregnant females and a high incidence of vertical transmission of the organism to the neonate, the attack rate for neonatal disease in colonized infants is usually said to be approximately 1 to 2 percent. Pass et al.[87] reported a much higher attack rate (8 percent) for neonatal disease in infants who were heavily colonized and had positive cultures from three or more sites. Those with only one or two positive-culture sites were at no greater risk than uncolonized infants. These studies have now been extended and indicate that the attack rate among infants who are heavily colonized may be as high as 50 per 1000 live births.[17] Thus, quantitative bacteriology may be required to identify those infants at most risk for developing invasive group B disease.[17,87,88]

Nosocomial transmission of group B streptococci has also been suggested as an important means of spread of these organisms.[16,36,87,88] A high colonization rate has been reported in nursery and hospital personnel,[9,16] and direct spread within infant cohorts has been documented by phage typing.[88] In most cases, however, infants who are infected at the time of birth have heavier colonization than those who acquire the organisms from a nosocomial source. This may account for the lower attack rate of late-onset infection compared to early-onset disease. In all likelihood, late-onset infection probably can result from initial colonization at the time of delivery, colonization from nosocomial sources, or even infection acquired in the home from asymptomatic contacts. Dillon and coworkers[17] have recently reported that 10 of 21 infants with late-onset infection were actually colonized at birth; 6 had heavy colonization. Thus, the main source of infection still appears to be the mother's urogenital or gastrointestinal tract, even in late-onset disease.

## SEROTYPES ASSOCIATED WITH DISEASE

Initial reports suggested that the early-onset form of group B disease was often caused by type I organisms.[9] Subsequent studies, however, have shown an almost equal breakdown of types in the septicemic form of the disease.[36] A striking preponderance of type III organisms has been observed in the late-onset meningitic variety of the disease seen in neonates. The reason for the invasiveness of this particular type in neonates is unknown, but it may be related to the elaboration of neuraminidase, which is more common in type III strains.[28,29] In contrast to the propensity of type III strains to cause neonatal meningitis, type II organisms are more commonly found in association with meningitis in adults.[36] The reason for these differences is also not known at present.

## CLINICAL MANIFESTATIONS AND SEQUELAE

### DISEASE IN ADULTS

Genitourinary colonization in the adult male or female is usually asymptomatic. On occasion, however, the presence of group B streptococci may be associated with signs and symptoms of vaginitis, cervicitis, urethritis, cystitis, pyelonephritis, and even balanitis.[8,9,16,36,78,89] As mentioned, more invasive infections in adults usually occur only in:[8,90,91]

Immunocompromised patients, such as diabetics, who frequently develop cellulitis, pyelonephritis, or bacteremia due to this agent;
Patients with renal failure with or without obstructive disease, who suffer pyelonephritis and sepsis;
Patients with alcoholic liver disease;
Patients on corticosteroids;
Patients with skull fractures or mastoiditis, who may develop meningitis.

Puerpural sepsis with meningitis or other complications may occur in women during the immediate postpartum period. In at least one study, group B streptococci were the most frequent blood culture isolates from postpartum women.[16] Patients with malignancy, especially those receiving chemotherapeutic drugs, are apparently at increased risk of group B streptococcal infection. Endocarditis may occur, especially in patients with underlying heart disease.

### NEONATAL DISEASE

#### Early-onset infection

Early-onset group B streptococcal infection usually becomes clinically apparent within the first 72 h of life[36] (Table 69-3). Although several investigators have used various time intervals to differentiate early- from late-onset infection (2 to 14 days), no sharp demarcation exists. Over 70 percent of the cases occur within the first 3 days; the incidence falls off drastically over the next 3 to 4 months. Most of the initial symptomatology in this most fulminant form of the disease is related to the respiratory tract and to bacteremia.[9,16,36,58,87,88] Respiratory distress may develop at birth and often is indistinguishable clinically and radiographically from hyaline membrane disease (HMD).[58] In general, however, patients with group B streptococcal infection have better lung compliance than those with HMD, are more likely to suffer from shock and apnea, and may have gram-positive cocci in gastric or tracheal aspirates. Patients with this form of the disease are often low-birth-weight infants whose mothers had obstetrical complications such as premature delivery, placental complications, or peripartum febrile courses (Table 69-3). At autopsy, findings include congested hemorrhagic lungs with or without small pleural effusions, infiltration of alveolar spaces with bacteria and leukocytes, and the presence of typical hyaline membranes.[16,36,57,58] The mortality rate in this form of the disease ranges from 30 to 50 percent.

#### Late-onset infection

There is not a clear definition of when late infection occurs.[36] Onset is generally not as fulminant as in early infection, and the major presenting manifestations are related to meningitis in 80 percent of the cases (Table 69-3). In one recent series of late-onset cases, 15 of 21 patients had sepsis rather than meningitis as a predominant presenting manifestation. Other sites of involvement are quite varied and include cellulitis, otitis media, conjunctivitis, osteomyelitis, and asymptomatic bacteremia. In general, infection cannot be related to obstetrical complications in the mother. Initial colonization of the infant may be from maternal, nosocomial, or community sources. As mentioned, however, approximately one-half of the late-onset cases occur in infants who are colonized at birth.[17] The mortality rate in late-onset disease is somewhat lower (generally around 15 to 25 per-

Table 69-3. Findings Associated with Neonatal Group B Streptococcal Disease*

| Characteristic | Early onset | Late onset |
|---|---|---|
| Incidence per 1000 live births | 3.0–4.2 | 0.5–1.0 |
| Presence of maternal complications, percent | 92 | 19 |
| Prematurity | 50 | 10 |
| Premature bursting of amniotic sac | 59 | 0 |
| Chorioamnionitis | 17 | 0 |
| Perinatal fever | 59 | 14 |
| Time of onset, days | 0–3 | >7 |
| Clinical findings, percent | | |
| Respiratory distress | 90–100 | 10–15 |
| Apnea | 80–90 | 10–15 |
| Shock | 50–60 | 10–15 |
| Fever | 30–40 | 80–90 |
| Jaundice | 15–20 | 15–20 |
| Coma | 50–60 | 20–25 |
| Bulging fontanelle | 5–10 | 60–70 |
| Meningitis | 30 | 80 |
| Positive cultures, percent | | |
| Cerebrospinal fluid | 20–30 | 80–90 |
| Blood | 80–90 | 90–95 |
| Other sites | 85–90 | 10–15 |
| Mortality, percent | 30–50 | 15–25 |
| Neurologic sequelae, percent | — | 50 |

*Approximate incidence of findings is taken from a large number of clinical and epidemiological reports given in the References.

cent) but significant sequelae, including cranial nerve deficits, subdural effusions, blindness, and abnormal hypothalamic function, occur in up to 50 percent of survivors.[16,36]

## DIAGNOSIS

The diagnosis of group B streptococcal infection in the symptomatic adult patient with evidence of urethritis, vaginitis, cervicitis, or urinary tract infection is based on simple culture techniques and, as described previously, the use of selective broth media containing antibiotics. In general, however, patients with group B colonization are entirely asymptomatic and cultures for this organism are often not obtained. Attempts to document colonization should include use of selective broth media, and cultures should be taken from multiple sites, including the cervix, urethra, and anorectal area.

The diagnosis of early-onset group B streptococcal infection should be suspected in any neonate with respiratory distress and especially in individuals with apnea or shock and without a decrease in lung compliance.[92] Gram stain examinations of gastric or tracheal aspirates may be quite helpful in increasing the level of suspicion that group B streptococci are involved. Neutrophilia or neutropenia are also quite common. Multiple cultures should be obtained from blood, tracheal aspirates, external ear, umbilicus, and rectum. In 1975 Hill et al.[93] demonstrated that soluble group B streptococcal antigen could be detected in broth filtrates and in infected body fluids by counterimmunoelectrophoresis (CIE). Rhodes and Hall[94] subsequently demonstrated that approximately one-half of early-onset cases of group B disease had detectable antigenuria when examined by CIE. Additional reports by Stechenberg et al.[95] and by Jacobs et al.[96] showed that approximately 95 percent of cases of group B disease can be diagnosed by CIE, if blood, cerebrospinal fluid, and concentrated urine samples are examined. Recent studies suggest that latex agglutination may be an even more sensitive method for detecting group B antigen in body fluids.[97] Ingram and coworkers[98] have indicated that group B streptococcal antigen can be demonstrated with commercially available latex agglutination reagents in up to 100 percent of cases of early-onset infections if serum, urine, and CSF are examined. Latex agglutination reagents have also been used in attempts to rapidly identify colonized women admitted in labor. Up to 85 percent of heavily colonized females can be quickly identified with this technique.[99] Immunofluorescent staining procedures for group B streptococci have also been developed but are not widely used.[100]

## MANAGEMENT

Management of group B streptococcal disease is less than optimal at present since clinical diagnosis is often delayed[58] and, despite appropriate antimicrobial therapy, the morbidity and mortality rates are still quite high. Group B streptococci are quite sensitive to penicillin, ampicillin, and a variety of other antibiotics, although not at the same extremely low levels as group A streptococci. In spite of demonstrable in vitro resistance of these organisms to aminoglycosides, there does appear to be a significant synergistic bactericidal effect between aminoglycosides and penicillin or ampicillin. In view of treatment failures and recurrences of group B disease in neonates treated with penicillins, McCracken[101] recommended that therapy be instituted with 250,000 units of penicillin per kilogram of body weight per day or 200 mg per kilogram body weight per day of ampicillin plus an aminoglycoside (gentamicin, amikacin, or kanamycin). Although clinical data are not yet available on the efficacy of such therapy, it seems wise to employ the combination initially, until the patient is stabilized and cerebrospinal fluid or other body fluids become culture-negative. Therapy can then be continued with penicillin or ampicillin alone for 10 days (bacteremia), 3 weeks (meningitis or arthritis), or 4 weeks (osteomyelitis or endocarditis).[16]

Passive immunotherapy of group B disease in the compromised neonate must also be considered. Shigeoka et al.[102] reported that transfusion of fresh whole blood containing opsonic antibody into neonates with early-onset disease increased survival to 100 percent, compared with a rate of 50 percent in infants who received blood that lacked antibody. Subsequently, Santos et al.[51] showed that experimental animals with group B infection could be protected by the administration of opsonic antibody and/or the transfusion of functional adult leukocytes. These investigators have also shown that a modified immune serum globulin for intravenous use can protect neonatal rats from group B infection.[70] Recent data from Europe[103] suggest that the administration of immune globulin intravenous (IGIV) to premature infants may result in an increase in the survival rate. Randomized double-blind studies are currently underway to determine the true efficacy of such therapy.

Studies from Italy[104] and the United States[105–107] have suggested that granulocyte transfusions may be of significant value in altering morbidity and mortality from neonatal sepsis, including that due to group B streptococci. This was especially true if the infants were neutropenic and had depletion of their marrow stores of mature neutrophil precursors. Additional studies are needed, however, to ascertain the safety of such therapy and especially to rule out (1) leukocyte aggregation in the lungs, (2) the appearance of graft-versus-host disease in the neonate, or

(3) the transmission of viral agents in the blood products. These preliminary results suggest, however, that passive immunotherapy with leukocytes and/or opsonic antibody may turn out to be the ultimate therapy for neonatal group B disease.[75]

## PREVENTION

### ANTIBIOTIC PROPHYLAXIS

#### Treatment of the carrier state

Eradication of the maternal carrier state by antibiotic therapy would seem to be a simple means of preventing group B disease in neonates. Unfortunately, the problem is not a straightforward one. Using oral penicillin, Hall et al.[85] treated 27 pregnant women who had group B colonization. A significant reduction in colonization was noted within 3 weeks of such therapy, but at the time of delivery the group B colonization rate was not different from that of an untreated control group. Other studies indicated that male spouses are often colonized and that they also should be treated if reinfection is to be prevented.[9] A group of infectious disease experts have pointed out, however, that we have little data on (1) whom to treat to eradicate group B carriage; (2) how to treat such individuals; (3) when to treat them during pregnancy, because cultures during early pregnancy do not predict accurately who will be positive at term; and (4) what effect such treatment will have on the incidence of disease due to group B streptococci or other agents.[108] Furthermore, successful antibiotic therapy of the carrier of group B streptococci may be impossible since the gastrointestinal tract appears to be the major reservoir of infection.[80]

#### Prevention of intrapartum transmission

Yow et al.[109] first attempted intrapartum prophylaxis of group B streptococcal disease by treating 34 colonized women with intravenous ampicillin during labor. None of these women delivered colonized infants, as opposed to 58 percent of 24 women who were not given such antibiotics. Boyer and Gotoff[86] have greatly expanded these studies showing that selective intrapartum prophylaxis of colonized mothers at high risk (premature delivery, prolonged rupture of the membranes, or intrapartum fever) with ampicillin significantly lowered group B streptococcal colonization rates and disease in their offspring. Such therapy would not, of course, affect earlier complications of pregnancy such as premature delivery, stillbirth, or abortion. In addition, a large number of women would have to receive this intensive and expensive therapy to prevent one case of neonatal disease if the case/carrier ratio is 100:1, as stated.[16] Adverse reactions to the antibiotics will also have to be considered, although only one case of urticaria was noted in a mother in their series.[86]

#### Prophylactic antibiotic therapy of the neonate

Steigman et al.[110] indicated in 1975 that they had seen no cases of documented group B disease in over 120,000 deliveries in which the infants had received 50,000 units of aqueous penicillin intramuscularly for gonococcal ophthalmic prophylaxis. Although subsequent authors questioned these data, a large controlled trial of single-dose penicillin prophylaxis was initiated.[111] In this study 18,738 neonates received either 25,000 or 50,000 units of aqueous penicillin G intramuscularly (depending upon their weight) or tetracycline ophthalmic drops for gonococcal prophylaxis. The mean colonization rate for mothers in both groups was 27 percent. Infants who received penicillin had a much lower colonization rate with group B streptococci than did untreated infants. The overall rate for group B disease was also decreased in the treated neonates. There was, however, an increase in infections due to penicillin-resistant organisms in the treated group during one of the years of the study. Subsequent studies by Pyati and coworkers[112] in infants less than 2000 g at birth failed to show that prophylactic penicillin had any effect on group B streptococcal disease. In their study, 21 of 24 patients had blood cultures that were positive at the time (1 h) that the antibiotics were administered. Thus, in these premature infants, infection was most likely acquired prenatally and was manifest at or before antibiotics could be administered. Additional studies in different medical centers are needed to confirm the efficacy of this approach and to determine if penicillin prophylaxis does result in a shift in the microbial pathogens in neonatal infection.

### ACTIVE IMMUNIZATION

The development of an effective vaccine for prevention of group B disease is complicated by a number of factors. First, the vaccine will have to be administered to the mother if neonatal disease is to be prevented. Second, the vaccine will have to protect against all five types of group B streptococci, each of which is capable of causing the fulminant early-onset form of disease. Third, such a vaccine may also have to provide activity against strain-specific virulence factors.[54,55,56,113] Additional problems include (1) the need to vaccinate essentially all women of childbearing age, many of whom are in lower socioeconomic classes and may be hard to reach in a vaccine program, and (2) the possibility that immunization may not be capable of providing protective immunity to infants of less than 34 weeks' gestation, who receive little immunoglobulin by placental transfer. Thus, a number of very serious problems will have to be overcome before such a vaccine can be put into routine use. At present, two groups are concentrating on the development of such a vaccine.[114–117] One is employing a neutral-buffer-extracted type III polysaccharide preparation,[115,116] while the other is employing a natural antigen released into broth cultures by actively multiplying microorganisms.[114] Both groups have demonstrated rises in type-specific antibody levels as determined by RABA and an ELISA following immunization of humans. Native type Ia, II, and III polysaccharides have been shown to be safe and nontoxic and to elicit antibody production in 65, 95, and 70 percent of adults, respectively.[117] Additional studies are underway to determine if such vaccines will be effective in raising type-specific antibody levels in human neonates and preventing group B streptococcal disease. Venereologists, infectious disease specialists, obstetricians, and pediatricians will undoubtedly follow closely the progress of these potential vaccines. Because of the problems mentioned, however, eradication or marked reduction in the number of cases of group B disease by such a vaccine seems unlikely in the near future.

## References


1 Brown JH et al: Hemolytic streptococci of the beta type in certified milk. *J Infect Dis* 38:381, 1926.

2 Litte RB, Plastridge WN: *Bovine Mastitis*. New York, McGraw-Hill, 1946.

3 Lancefield RC: Microprecipitin-technic for classifying hemolytic streptococci, and improved methods for producing antisera. *Proc Soc Exp Biol Med* 38:473, 1938.
4 Lancefield RC, Hare R: Serological differentiation of pathogenic and nonpathogenic strains of hemolytic streptococci from parturient women. *J Exp Med* 61:335, 1935.
5 Fry RM: Fatal infections by haemolytic streptococcus group B. *Lancet* 1:199, 1938.
6 Hill AM, Bulter HM: Haemolytic streptococcal infections following childbirth and abortion: Clinical features, with special reference to infections due to streptococci of groups other than A. *Med J Aust* 1:293, 1940.
7 Hood M et al: Beta hemolytic streptococcus group B associated with problems of the perinatal period. *Am J Obstet Gynecol* 82:809, 1961.
8 Eickhoff TC et al: Neonatal sepsis and other infections due to group B beta-hemolytic streptococci. *N Engl J Med* 271:1221, 1964.
9 Franciosi RA et al: Group B streptococcal neonatal and infant infections. *J Pediatr* 82:707, 1973.
10 Barton LL et al: Group B beta-hemolytic streptococcal meningitis in infants. *J Pediatr* 82:719, 1973.
11 Baker CJ et al: Suppurative meningitis due to streptococci of Lancefield group B: A study of 33 infants. *J Pediatr* 82:724, 1973.
12 Baker CJ, Barrett FF: Transmission of group B streptococci among parturient women and their neonates. *J Pediatr* 83:919, 1973.
13 Baker CJ et al: The influence of advancing gestation on group B streptococcal colonization in pregnant women. *Am J Obstet Gynecol* 122:820, 1975.
14 Beachler CW et al: Group B streptococcal colonization and antibody status in lower socioeconomic parturient women. *Am J Obstet Gynecol* 133:171, 1979.
15 Baker CJ et al: Vaginal colonization with group B streptococcus: A study in college women. *J Infect Dis* 135:392, 1977.
16 Baker CJ: Group B streptococcal infections. *Adv Intern Med* 25:475, 1980.
17 Dillon HC et al: Group B streptococcal carriage and disease: A 6 year prospective study. *J Pediatr* 100:365, 1987.
18 Boyer KM, Gotoff SP: Prevention of early-onset neonatal group B streptococcal disease with selective intrapartum chemoprophylaxis. *N Engl J Med* 314:1665, 1986.
19 Roe MH et al: Nonhemolytic group B streptococcal infections. *J Pediatr* 89:75, 1976.
20 Merritt K, Jacobs N: Characterization and incidence of pigment production by human clinical group B streptococci. *J Clin Microbiol* 8:105, 1978.
21 Merritt K, Jacobs N: Improved medium for detecting pigment production by group B streptococci. *J Clin Microbiol* 4:379, 1976.
22 Facklam RR et al: Presumptive identification of group A, and B, streptococci. *Appl Microbiol* 27:107, 1974.
23 Hwang M, Ederer GM: Rapid hippurate hydrolysis method for presumptive identification of group B streptococci. *J Clin Microbiol* 1:114, 1975.
24 Christie R et al: A note on a lytic phenomenon shown by group B streptococci. *Aust J Exp Biol Med Sci* 22:1977, 1944.
25 Darling CL: Standardization and evaluation of the CAMP reaction for the prompt, presumptive identification of *Streptococcus agalactiae* (Lancefield group B) in clinical material. *J Clin Microbiol* 1:171, 1975.
26 Brown J et al: CAMP factor of group B streptococci: Production, assay, and neutralization by sera from immunized rabbits and experimentally infected cows. *Infect Immun* 9:377, 1974.
27 Hayano S, Tanaka A: Sialidase-like enzymes produced by group A, B, C, G and L streptococci and by *Streptococcus sanguis*. *J Bacteriol* 97:1328, 1969.
28 Milligan TW et al: Extracellular neuraminidase production by group B streptococci. *Infect Immun* 18:189, 1977.
29 Mattingly SJ et al: Extracellular neuraminidase production by clinical isolates of group B streptococci from infected neonates. *J Clin Microbiol* 12:633, 1980.
30 Jokipii AMM, Jokipii L: Presumptive identification and antibiotic susceptibility of group B streptococci. *J Clin Pathol* 29:736, 1976.
31 Schauf V et al: Antibiotic-killing kinetics of group B streptococci. *J Pediatr* 89:194, 1976.
32 Kim KS, Anthony BJ: Penicillin tolerance in group B streptococci isolated from infected neonates. *J Infect Dis* 144:411, 1981.
33 Scheld WM et al: Synergy between ampicillin and gentamicin in experimental meningitis due to group B streptococci. *J Infect Dis* 146:100, 1982.
34 Lancefield RC: Cellular antigens of group B streptococci, in *Streptococci and Streptococcal Diseases,* LW Wannamaker, JM Matsen (eds). New York, Academic, 1972, p 57.
35 Curtis SN, Krause RM: Antigenic relationships between groups B and G streptococci. *J Exp Med* 120:629, 1964.
36 Wilkinson HW: Group B streptococcal infection in humans. *Annu Rev Microbiol* 32:41, 1978.
37 Baker CJ: Summary of the workshop on perinatal infections due to group B streptococcus. *J Infect Dis* 136:137, 1977.
38 Wilkinson HW: Immunochemistry of purified polysaccharide antigens of group B streptococcal types Ia, Ib, and Ic. *Infect Immun* 11:845, 1975.
39 Wilkinson HW, Eagon RG: Type-specific antigens of group B type Ic streptococci. *Infect Immun* 4:596, 1971.
40 Kasper DL et al: Immunochemical characterization of native polysaccharides from group B streptococcus: The relationship of the type III and group B determinants. *J Immunol* 121:1096, 1978.
41 Kasper DL et al: Immunodeterminant specificity of human immunity to type III group B streptococcus. *J Exp Med* 149:327, 1979.
42 Baker CJ et al: Immunochemical characterization of the "native" type III polysaccharide of group B streptococcus. *J Exp Med* 143:258, 1976.
43 Fischer GW et al: Demonstration of opsonic activity and in vivo protection against group B streptococci type III by *Streptococcus pneumoniae* type 14 antisera. *J Exp Med* 148:776, 1978.
44 Lancefield RC, Freimer EH: Type-specific polysaccharide antigens of group B streptococci. *J Hyg (Camb)* 64:191, 1966.
45 Lancefield RC: Multiple mouse-protective antibodies directed against group B streptococci. *J Exp Med* 142:165, 1975.
46 Hemming VG et al: Assessment of group B streptococcal opsonins in human and rabbit serum by neutrophil chemiluminescence. *J Clin Invest* 58:1379, 1976.
47 Shigeoka AO et al: Role of antibody and complement in opsonization of group B streptococci. *Infect Immun* 21:34, 1978.
48 Edwards MS et al: The role of specific antibody in alternative complement pathway-mediated opsonophagocytosis of type III, group B streptococcus. *J Exp Med* 151:1275, 1980.
49 Anthony BF: Immunity to the group B streptococci: Interaction of serum and macrophages with types Ia, Ib, and Ic. *J Exp Med* 143:1186, 1976.
50 Baker CJ et al: Antibody independent classical pathway (CP)-mediated opsonophagocytosis (OP) of type Ia group B streptococci. *Pediatr Res* 15:591, 1981.
51 Santos JI et al: Functional leukocyte administration in protection against experimental neonatal infection. *Pediatr Res* 14:1408, 1980.
52 Tieffenberg J et al: Chicken embryo model for type III group B beta-hemolytic streptococcal septicemia. *Infect Immun* 19:481, 1978.
53 Christensen RD et al: Circulating and storage neutrophil changes in experimental type II group B streptococcal sepsis. *Pediatr Res* 14:806, 1980.
54 Shigeoka AO et al: Strain specificity of opsonins for group B streptococci types II and III. *Infect Immun* 23:438, 1979.
55 Santos JI et al: Strain differences in virulence of group B streptococci. *Pediatr Res* 16:347, 1982.
56 Fischer GW et al: Quantitative protection studies in a suckling rat model of group B streptococcal sepsis, abstracted. *Pediatr Res* 15:609, 1981.
57 Hill HR et al: Neonatal cellular and humoral immunity to group B streptococci. *Pediatrics* 64S:787, 1979.

58 Hemming VG et al: Pneumonia in the neonate associated with group B streptococcal septicemia. *Am J Dis Child* 130:123, 1976.
59 Katzenstein A et al: Pulmonary changes in neonatal sepsis due to group B hemolytic streptococcus: Relation to hyaline membrane disease. *J Infect Dis* 133:430, 1976.
60 Rojas J et al: Pulmonary vascular and granulocyte response to group B streptococcal (GBS) toxin. *Pediatr Res* 15:619, 1981.
61 Hellerqvist CG et al: Molecular basis for group B beta-hemolytic streptococcal disease. *Proc Natl Acad Sci USA* 84:51, 1987.
62 McFall TL et al: Effect of group B streptococcal type-specific antigen on PMN function and PMN-endothelial cell interaction. *Pediatr Res* 21:517, 1987.
63 Baker CJ, Kasper DL: Correlation of maternal antibody deficiency with susceptibility to neonatal Group B streptococcal infection. *N Engl J Med* 294:753, 1976.
64 Stewardson-Kreiger PB et al: Perinatal immunity to group B β-hemolytic streptococcus type Ia. *J Infect Dis* 136:649, 1977.
65 Baker CJ, Kasper DL: Immunological investigation of infants with septicemia or meningitis due to group B streptococcus. *J Infect Dis* 136:598, 1977.
66 Wilkinson HW, Jones WL: Radioimmunoassay for measuring antibodies specific for group B streptococcal types Ia, Ib, Ic, II and III. *J Clin Microbiol* 3:480, 1976.
67 Wilkinson HW: Detection of group B streptococcal antibodies in human sera by radioimmunoassay: Concentration of type-specific antibodies in sera of adults and infants infected with group B streptococci. *J Clin Microbiol* 7:194, 1978.
68 Rote NS et al: Enzyme-linked immunosorbent assay for group B streptococcal antibodies. *Infect Immun* 27:118, 1980.
69 Edwards MS et al: Opsonic specificity of human antibody to the type III polysaccharide of group B streptococcus. *J Infect Dis* 140: 1004, 1979.
70 Santos JI et al: Protective efficacy of a modified immune serum globulin in experimental group B streptococcal infection. *J Pediatr* 99: 873, 1981.
71 Shigeoka AO et al: Assessment of the virulence factors of group B streptococci. I. Correlation with sialic acid content. *J Infect Dis* 147: 857, 1983.
72 Klegerman ME et al: Type-specific capsular antigen in association with virulence in late-onset group B streptococcal type III disease. *Infect Immun* 44:124, 1984.
73 Yeung MK, Mattingly SJ: Biosynthetic capacity of type-specific antigen synthesis determines the virulence of serotype III strains of group B streptococci. *Infect Immun* 44:217, 1984.
74 Christensen RD et al: Blood and marrow neutrophils during experimental group B streptococcal infection: Quantification of the stem cell, proliferative, storage and cirulating pools. *Pediatr Res* 16:549, 1982.
75 Hill HR: Phagocyte transfusion—Ultimate therapy of neonatal disease? *J Pediatr* 98:59, 1981.
76 Shigeoka AO, Santos JI: Functional analysis of neutrophil granulocytes from healthy, infected, and stressed neonates. *J Pediatr* 95: 454, 1979.
77 Badri MS et al: Rectal colonization with group B streptococcus: Relation to vaginal colonization of pregnant women. *J Infect Dis* 135:308, 1977.
78 Jensen ME, Andersen BL: The prevalence of group B streptococci in human urogenital secretions. *J Infect Dis* 11:199,1979.
79 Christensen KK et al: Rectal colonization with group B streptococci: Relation to urogenital carriage. *Scand J Infect Dis* 10:291, 1978.
80 Dillon HC Jr et al: Anorectal and vaginal carriage of group B streptococci during pregnancy. *J Infect Dis* 145:794, 1982.
81 Anthony BF et al: Epidemiology of group B streptococcus: Longitudinal observations during pregnancy. *J Infect Dis* 137:524, 1978.
82 Vogel LC et al: Prevalence of type-specific streptococcal antibody in pregnant women. *J Pediatr* 96:1047, 1980.
83 Gray BM et al: Seroepidemiological studies of group B streptococcus type II. *J Infect Dis* 151:1073, 1985.
84 Boyer KM et al: Selective intrapartum chemoprophylaxis of neonatal group B streptococcal early-onset disease. II. Predictive value of prenatal cultures. *J Infect Dis* 148:802, 1983.
85 Hall RT et al: Antibiotic treatment of parturient women colonized with group B streptococci. *Am J Obstet Gynecol* 124:630, 1976.
86 Boyer KM, Gotoff SP: Prevention of early-onset neonatal group B streptococcal disease with selective intrapartum chemoprophylaxis. *N Engl J Med* 26:1665, 1986.
87 Pass MA et al: Prospective studies of group B streptococcal infections in infants. *J Pediatr* 95:437, 1979.
88 Anthony BF et al: Epidemiology of the group B streptococcus: Maternal and nosocomial sources for infant acquisitions. *J Pediatr* 95: 431, 1979.
89 Brook I: Group B beta-hemolytic streptococci causing balanitis. *South Med J* 73:1095, 1980.
90 Reinarz JA, Sanford JP: Human infections caused by nongroup A or D streptococci. *Medicine (Baltimore)* 44:81, 1965.
91 Lerner PI: Meningitis caused by streptococcus in adults. *J Infect Dis* 131:59, 1975.
92 Ablow RC et al: A comparison of early-onset group B streptococcal neonatal infection and the respiratory-distress syndrome of the newborn. *N Engl J Med* 294:65, 1976.
93 Hill HR et al: Rapid identification of group B streptococci by counterimmunoelectrophoresis. *J Clin Microbiol* 1:188, 1975.
94 Rhodes PG, Hall RT: Countercurrent immunoelectrophoresis (CIE) of urine: A rapid diagnostic tool for group B streptococcal (GBS) sepsis in the neonate. *J Pediatr* 91:833, 1977.
95 Stechenberg BW et al: Countercurrent immunoelectrophoresis in group B streptococcal disease. *Pediatrics* 64:632, 1970.
96 Jacobs RF et al: Detection of streptococcal antigen by counterimmunoelectrophoresis. *Am J Clin Path* 75:203, 1980.
97 Bromberger PI et al: Rapid detection of neonatal group B streptococcal infections by latex agglutination. *J Pediatr* 96:104, 1980.
98 Ingram DL et al: Detection of group B streptococcal antigen in early-onset and late-onset group B streptococcal disease with the Wellcogen Strep B latex agglutination test. *J Clin Microbiol* 16:656, 1982.
99 Wald ER et al: Rapid detection of group B streptococci directly from vaginal swabs. *J Clin Microbiol* 25:573, 1987.
100 Romero R, Wilkinson HW: Identification of group B streptococci by immunofluorescence staining. *Appl Microbiol* 28:199, 1974.
101 McCracken GH Jr, Feldman WE: Editorial comment. *J Pediatr* 89: 203, 1976.
102 Shigeoka AO et al: Blood transfusion in group B streptococcal sepsis. *Lancet* 1:636, 1978.
103 Sidiropolous D et al: Immunoglobulin supplementation in prevention or treatment of neonatal sepsis. *Pediatr Infect Dis* 5:S193, 1986.
104 Laurenti F et al: Polymorphonuclear leukocyte transfusion for the treatment of sepsis in the newborn infant. *J Pediatr* 98:118, 1981.
105 Christensen R et al: Granulocyte transfusions (GT) increase survival in neonates with sepsis and neutrophil depletion, abstracted. *Pediatr Res* 15:608, 1981.
106 Cairo MS et al: Improved survival of newborns receiving leukocyte transfusions for sepsis. *Pediatrics* 74:887, 1984.
107 Laing IA et al: Polymorphonuclear leukocyte transfusion in neonatal septicaemia. *Arch Dis Child* 58:1003, 1983.
108 Eickhoff TC et al: The issue of prophylaxis of neonatal group B streptococcal infections. *J Pediatr* 83:1097, 1973.
109 Yow MD et al: Ampicillin prevents intrapartum transmission of group B streptococcus. *JAMA* 241:1245, 1979.
110 Steigman AJ et al: Does intramuscular penicillin at delivery prevent group B beta hemolytic streptococcal disease of the newborn infant? *J Pediatr* 87:496, 1975.
111 Siegel JD et al: Single-dose penicillin prophylaxis against neonatal group B streptococci infections. *N Engl J Med* 303:769, 1980.
112 Pyati SP et al: Penicillin in infants weighing two kilograms or less with early-onset group B streptococcal disease. *N Engl J Med* 308: 1383, 1983.

113 Ferrieri P et al: Production of bacteremia and meningitis in infant rats with group B streptococcal serotypes. *Infect Immun* 27:1023, 1980.
114 Carey RB et al: Soluble group and type-specific antigens from type III group B streptococcus. *Infect Immun* 28:195, 1980.
115 Baker CJ et al: Immunogenicity of polysaccharides from type III group B streptococcus. *J Clin Invest* 62:1107, 1978.
116 Baker CJ et al: Influence of preimmunization antibody levels on the specificity of the immune response to related polysaccharide antigens. *J Exp Med* 303:173, 1980.
117 Baker CJ, Kasper DL: Group B streptococcal vaccines. *Rev Infect Dis* 7:458, 1985.

Chapter 70

# Herpesvirus infection in the neonate and children

Sergio Stagno
Richard J. Whitley

## CONGENITAL AND PERINATAL CYTOMEGALOVIRUS INFECTIONS

### INTRODUCTION

Cytomegaloviruses (CMV) comprise a group of agents in the herpesvirus family known for their ubiquitous distribution in humans and in numerous other mammals. Both in vivo and in vitro, the infection is highly species-specific and results in a characteristic cytopathology consisting of large (cytomegalic) inclusion-bearing cells with an "owl's eye" appearance.[1] The first description of these cells containing intranuclear and cytoplasmic inclusions dates from 1881 when Ribbert found them in the kidneys of a stillborn infant with congenital syphilis.[2] In 1954, Smith succeeded in propagating murine CMV in explant cultures of mouse embryonic fibroblasts.[3] Utilization of similar techniques led to the independent isolation of human CMV shortly thereafter by Smith,[4] Rowe et al.,[5] and Weller et al.[6] The term cytomegalovirus was proposed in 1960 by Weller, Hanshaw, and Scott to replace the names cytomegalic inclusion disease and salivary gland virus which were misleading, since the virus usually involved other organs and the term salivary gland virus had been used to designate unrelated agents obtained from bats.[7]

The propagation of CMV in vitro led to the rapid development of serologic methods such as neutralization and complement fixation. Using these antibody assays and viral isolation, several investigators quickly established that human CMV was a significant pathogen.[8,9] The natural history of human CMV infection is very complex. Following a primary infection, viral excretion (occasionally from several sites) persists for weeks, months, or even years before becoming latent. Episodes of recurrent infection with renewed viral shedding are common, even years after primary infection. These episodes of recurrent infection are most often due to reactivation of latent viruses, but reinfections with an antigenically diverse strain of CMV are also possible. In most cases, CMV infections are subclinical. However, while infection during pregnancy may be without consequences for the mother, it can have serious repercussions for the fetus. Even though most immune compromised hosts tolerate CMV infections relatively well, in some instances it can cause disease of diverse severity, and can be life-threatening.

### EPIDEMIOLOGY

#### General

Humans are the only reservoir for CMV.[1] The infection is endemic and without seasonal variation.[9] Climate does not affect the prevalence of infection, and there are no known vectors in the natural transmission cycle. Seroepidemiologic surveys have found CMV infection in every human population that has been tested.[8,9] The prevalence of antibody to CMV increases with age, but according to geographic and ethnic and socioeconomic backgrounds, the patterns of acquisition of infection vary widely among populations.[10] In general, the prevalence of CMV infection is higher in developing countries and among the lower socioeconomic strata of developed nations. These differences are particularly striking during childhood. For instance, in Africa and the South Pacific the rate of seropositivity was 95 to 100 percent among preschool children, while similar surveys in Great Britain and in the United States have generally found that less than 20 percent of preschool children are seropositive.

The level of immunity among women of childbearing age, which is an important factor in determining the incidence and significance of congenital and perinatal CMV infection, also varies widely in different populations. In the United States and western Europe, several reports indicate that seropositivity rates in young women range from less than 50 to 85 percent.[13,70] In contrast, in the Ivory Coast,[12] Japan,[13] and Chile[14] the rate of seropositivity is greater than 90 percent by the end of the second decade of life. Prospective studies of pregnant women in the United States indicate that the rate of CMV acquisition for childbearing age women of middle to higher socioeconomic background is approximately 2 percent per year, while it is 6 percent among women of lower socioeconomic background.[15]

The modes of transmission from person to person are incompletely understood, and several features of CMV infection make it difficult to study modes of acquisition.[11] In the majority of individuals, CMV infections are subclinical, including those acquired in utero and during the perinatal period. Virus excretion persists for years following congenital, perinatal, and early postnatal infections. Prolonged viral shedding is also a feature of primary infection in older children and adults. These infected persons continue to expose other susceptible people. Since recurrent infections are fairly common, intermittent excretion of virus can be anticipated in a significant proportion of seropositive adults. It is clear that a large reservoir of CMV exists in the population at all times. Transmission occurs by direct or indirect person-to-person contact. Sources of virus include urine, oropharyngeal secretions, cervical and vaginal secretions, semen, milk, tears, and blood.[16–19]

CMV is not very contagious since the spread of infection appears to require close or intimate contact with infected secretions. As indicated, the prevalence of CMV infection and the risk of seroconversion are higher for populations of low socioeconomic status, presumably a reflection of such factors as crowding, sexual practices, and increased exposure to infants and toddlers.[20–23]

Group care of children as practiced in some developing countries, in Israeli kibbutzim, and in day care centers in industrialized nations facilitate the horizontal spread of CMV.[24,25] Sarov et al. compared the prevalence of antibodies to CMV in urban Jewish children, children in a kibbutz, and Bedouin children.[24] In a kibbutz children live under highly hygienic standards and socioeconomic conditions. By the second year of life, 76 percent of children in a kibbutz were seropositive, while only 44 percent and 54 percent of urban Jewish children and Bedouin children, respectively, were seropositive. Moreover in the kibbutz, by the second year of life, 87 percent of those children who sleep in children's houses with their peers were seropositive, in contrast to 69 percent of those sleeping at home. For urban children, the higher prevalence of CMV was significantly associated with crowding but not with sex, place of residence, educational level, or country of origin of the parents. In urban Jewish children, a significant rise in seropositivity occurred while the children attended nurseries. In contrast, in Bedouin children a significant rise in seropositivity occurred between the ages of 5 and 8 years when they first attended school. These increases in the rates of seropositives clearly illustrate the importance of horizontal transmission.

Similar findings were reported by Pass et al. in children of middle to upper income background in a day care center in the United States.[25] In a group of 70 children whose ages ranged from 3 to 65 months, they found a 51 percent rate of CMV excretion in urine and saliva. The lowest rate of excretion occurred in infants less than 1 year of age (9 percent) and the highest rate (88 percent) among toddlers in their second year of life. There were 12 children excreting CMV whose mothers were seronegative, indicating that their infection was not perinatally acquired. Cytomegalovirus was isolated from plastic toys that had been mouthed by children known to be excreting virus, suggesting that this is a potential vehicle for transmission of CMV.[25] The highest rate of infection was noted in children between the ages of 1 and 2 years. These children walked, exhibited constant oral behavior, commonly came into close contact with one another, and shared toys. Transmission from infected urine, though possible, was unlikely as the children under 2 years had not begun toilet training. The fact that the infection rate was lowest in infants under 12 months of age suggests that spread through aerosols or transmission by employees is very unlikely, at least in the setting of the day care center. The findings of Pass et al. have been confirmed by other investigators.[26,27]

These observations in day care centers and in kibbutzim indicate that as children become mobile and engage in close interpersonal contact, CMV can be expected to spread rapidly among them. With the changes in child rearing practices now occurring in the United States and the resurgence of breast feeding, significant changes in the epidemiology of CMV can be expected within the next decades.

An important issue is whether children excreting CMV can become a source of infection for susceptible child care personnel and parents, particularly women of childbearing age. Transmission of CMV from an infant to his mother and from an infant to a pregnant aunt with subsequent transmission to her infant has been confirmed with restriction endonuclease mapping of CMV DNA.[28,29] Recent seroepidemiologic studies suggest that parents often acquire CMV from their children who became infected outside the family.[30–33] Pass et al.[34] and Adler et al.[35] have presented compelling evidence for transmission of CMV from children excreting CMV to seronegative parents. Pass et al. did a longitudinal serologic follow-up study of seronegative parents whose children attended day care and of seronegative parents whose children did not attend day care.[34] The study revealed that 14 of 67 seronegative parents with children in day care centers acquired CMV, as compared with none of 31 serosusceptible parents whose children did not attend day care. More significant, all 14 parents of the day care group who seroconverted had a child who was shedding CMV in saliva or urine. In fact, seroconversion occurred in 14 of 46 parents of children who shed CMV, as compared with none of 21 whose children did not excrete CMV. The highest risk of seroconversion (45 percent) was for parents with a child shedding CMV who was 18 months of age or less at enrollment.

Fomites may also play some role in transmission, as CMV has been shown to retain infectivity for hours on plastic surfaces, and CMV has been isolated from randomly selected toys and surfaces in a day care center.[36,37]

## Maternal infection and vertical transmission

Because maternal CMV infection is the origin of congenital infections and of most perinatal infections, it is important to review the relevant issues that pertain to vertical transmission. As used here, vertical transmission implies mother-to-infant transmission.

**Congenital Infection.** Congenital infection is assumed to be the result of transplacental transmission. In the United States, congenital CMV infection occurs in between 0.2 and 2.2 percent (average 1 percent) of all newborn infants. The natural history of CMV infection during pregnancy is particularly complex and has not been fully explained. Infections such as rubella and toxoplasmosis cannot serve as models. With these infections, transmission in utero occurs only as a result of a primary infection acquired during pregnancy, while the in utero transmission of CMV can occur as a consequence of both primary and recurrent infections.[12,38] Far from being a rare event, congenital infection resulting from recurrent CMV infection has been shown to be quite common, especially in highly immune populations. The initial clue was provided by three independent reports of congenital CMV infections that occurred in consecutive pregnancies.[39–41] In all three instances, the first infant was severely affected or died and the second born in each case was subclinically infected. More convincing evidence came from a prospective study of women known to be seroimmune before conception.[38] The rate of congenital CMV infection was 1.9 percent among 541 infants born to these seropositive women. Clearly these congenitally infected infants were not infected as a result of primary maternal CMV infection since all of the mothers were known to have been infected with CMV from one to several years before the onset of pregnancy. Schopfer et al. found that in an Ivory Coast population in which virtually all inhabitants are infected in childhood, the prevalence of congenital CMV infection was 1.4 percent.[12] This remarkable phenomenon of intrauterine transmission that occurs in the presence of humoral immunity has been attributed to reactivation of endogenous virus. This unique characteristic (intrauterine transmission in immune women) accounts for the high incidence of congenital CMV infection in populations with the highest rate of seropositivity.[42] At present, it is impossible to define by either virologic or serologic markers which patient may reactivate CMV, neither is it possible to define the time of intrauterine transmission with such reactivation during pregnancy. The sites from which CMV reactivates to produce congenital infection are not known and are likely inaccessible to sampling during pregnancy. Although CMV excretion is a relatively common event during and after pregnancy, simple isolation of virus from the cervix or urine or both is a poor indicator of the risk of intrauterine infection.[18,43,44]

Virus can be shed at variable rates from single or multiple sites following primary or recurrent infections in both pregnant and nonpregnant women. Sites of excretion include the genital tract, cervix, urinary tract, pharynx, and breast milk. In one study of pregnant women, virus was excreted most commonly from the cervix (8.6 percent) and in decreasing order from the urinary tract (3.9 percent) and the throat (1.8 percent).[42] Of 37 specimens of amniotic fluid and 108 buffy coat specimens of heparinized blood, CMV was isolated twice from buffy coats but not from the amniotic fluids. In the immediate postpartum period, viral shedding into breast milk occurred in 14.4 percent of the patients. The rates of cervical and urinary tract shedding in nonpregnant women are comparable with those found in pregnant cohorts of similar demographic and socioeconomic characteristics.[42] In general, rates of cervical shedding range from 5.2 percent for nonpregnant women drawn from private practice or family planning clinics to 24.5 percent among women attending a sexually transmitted disease clinic.[12,18,20,21,45]

Pregnancy per se has no discernible effect on the overall prevalence of viral shedding. However, gestational age has a significant influence on the rate of CMV excretion. The findings from four large investigations are summarized in Table 70-1. These studies included populations of various ethnic and socioeconomic backgrounds. On the average the prevalence of excretion increased from 2.6 percent in the first trimester to 7.6 percent near term. In three of the four studies, the rate of viral shedding in the first trimester was significantly lower. This phenomenon was initially interpreted as an indication that pregnancy enhances productive CMV infection in the genital tract. It was assumed that the lower rate seen during the first trimester was similar to the frequency in the nonpregnant state. As discussed, however, in controlled studies the prevalence of genital tract infection in nonpregnant women is comparable with that found in pregnant women near term, and the majority of pregnant women who shed virus near term are seropositive before the onset of excretion.[46] A more reasonable explanation is that productive CMV infection is significantly suppressed in early gestation and, as the suppressive effect wanes with advancing pregnancy, viral shedding resulting from reactivation steadily increases. It has been speculated that this phenomenon may have teleological significance for the protection of the fetus from viral infection during the critical early months of gestation.

The rates of CMV excretion in the genital and urinary tract of women are inversely related to age after puberty. In one study, the rate of genital CMV excretion fell from 15 percent in girls between 11 and 14 years of age to undetectable levels in women 31 years and older.[47] From a peak of 8 percent in the younger group, urinary excretion fell to zero in women 26 years and older. No CMV excretion occurred from either site in postmenopausal women.

The transient depression of cellular immune responses to CMV antigens during the second and third trimesters is yet another peculiar aspect of the relationship between CMV and the pregnant human host. Gehrz and collaborators first described this phenomenon in a small group of seropositive pregnant women and showed that depressed CMV-specific lymphocyte proliferative responses returned to levels found in early pregnancy by 90 to 120 days postpartum.[48] They did not observe a generalized depression of cellular immunity since numbers of T lymphocytes, T-cell proliferative responses to other mitogens, and serum antibody titers remained unchanged during the study period. None of these mothers shed virus during the period of depressed cellular immune response, nor did they transmit the infection to their infants. In a more recent article, Stern et al. studied the lymphocyte transformation response in pregnant women with recent primary CMV infection and found that the eight patients with a positive response gave birth to uninfected babies, while four of the six who showed negative responses gave birth to congenitally infected babies.[49] These findings suggest that cellular immunity plays a part in preventing intrauterine infection and that its depression following primary CMV infection during pregnancy may lead to fetal infection. The reasons for the changes in blastogenic response that occur during pregnancy have not been defined, but immunosuppressive factors such as IgG alloantibodies, alpha fetoprotein, and human chorionic gonadotropin have been incriminated during pregnancy.

**Perinatal Infection.** In contrast to the poor correlation that exists between CMV excretion during pregnancy and congenital infection, there is good correlation between maternal shedding in the genital tract and milk and perinatal acquisition. In one study,[19] the two most efficient sources of transmission in the perinatal period were infected breast milk (which resulted in a 63 percent rate of perinatal infection) and the infected genital tract, particularly in late gestation, which was associated with transmission in 57 percent of the cases (natal infection). Viral shedding from the pharynx and urinary tract of the mother late in gestation and during the first months postpartum has not been associated with perinatal transmission.

There is considerable variability in perinatal transmission of CMV throughout the world.[19] The age of the mother and her prior experience with CMV, which in turn influence the frequency of viral excretion into the genital tract and breast milk, are certainly important factors. Younger seropositive women who breast feed are at a greater risk for transmitting virus in early infancy, especially in lower socioeconomic groups. It is remarkable that in Japan, Guatemala, Finland, and Thailand, where the rates of CMV excretion within the first year of life are extremely high (39 to 56 percent), the practice of breast feeding is almost universal, and the majority of women of childbearing age are seroimmune for CMV.

## Sexual transmission

In general, in developing areas of the world, 90 to 100 percent of the population is infected during childhood, even as early as 5 years of age. Sexual transmission in these populations plays a minor role as a source of primary CMV infection, and its importance in reinfection is unclear. In developed countries, the infection is acquired at a lower rate and in some population

**Table 70-1. Rates of Isolation of CMV from the Cervix According to Length of Gestation**

| | Trimester | | |
|---|---|---|---|
| | 1 | 2 | 3 |
| Place | +/Total (%) | +/Total (%) | +/Total (%) |
| Sendai, Japan | 0/30 (0) | 6/62 (9.7) | 17/61 (28) |
| Seattle, Washington* | 4/120 (3.3) | — | 1/50 (2) |
| Pittsburgh, Pennsylvania† | 0/29 (0) | 3/60 (5) | 2/23 (8.7) |
| Najavo Reservation, Arizona | 1/14 (7.1) | 3/23 (13) | 4/26 (15.4) |
| Birmingham, Alabama‡ | 4/147 (2.7) | 25/546 (4.6) | 117/1691 (6.9) |
| Total | 9/340 (2.6) | 37/691 (5.4) | 141/1851 (7.6) |

*Caucasian, middle class.
†Low-income black and middle-class caucasian.
‡Low income, predominantly black.
SOURCE: S Stagno et al: *Clin Obstet Gynecol* 25:571, 1982.

groups there is a marked increase in prevalence of infection after puberty.

Several lines of evidence indicate that sexual transmission of CMV is at least partly responsible for this increase in seroprevalence. CMV is frequently recovered from semen and cervical secretions.[17,18] Increased seroprevalence of CMV and excretion of virus has been found in women attending sexually transmitted disease clinics and in young male homosexuals.[20–23,50] Chretien et al. reported a cluster of cases with CMV mononucleosis that occurred in sex partners but not in persons who shared living quarters but did not engage in sexual contact.[23] Handsfield et al. showed that, in two pairs of sex partners with CMV infections attending a sexually transmitted disease clinic, strains of virus were identical by restriction endonuclease analyses of DNA.[51] Evidence has also been provided for sexual transmission in less promiscuous populations.[22,23,51] Among the many variables investigated, a significant correlation was found between seropositivity to CMV and greater numbers of lifetime sexual partners and past or present infection with *Chlamydia trachomatis.* Although the evidence for sexual transmission of CMV is thus compelling, the fact that CMV is frequently shed in saliva indicates that oral contact may also be an important route of transmission.

## Transmission via transfusion of blood and blood products

Nosocomial CMV infection is an important hazard of blood transfusion and organ transplant. In compromised hosts such as small premature newborns and bone marrow transplant recipients, transfusion acquired CMV has been associated with serious morbidity and even fatal infection. The association between the acquisition of CMV infection and blood transfusion was first suggested in 1960 by Kreel et al., who described a syndrome characterized by fever and leukocytosis occurring 3 to 8 weeks after open heart surgery.[52] Reports that followed expanded the syndrome to include fever, atypical lymphocytosis, splenomegaly, rash, and lymphadenopathy.[53–60] The term "postperfusion mononucleosis" was then proposed. Prospective studies incriminated blood transfusion as the major risk factor and demonstrated that while the clinical syndrome occurred in approximately 3 percent of the patients receiving transfusion, inapparent acquisition of CMV infection occurred in 9 to 58 percent. It has been estimated that blood donors capable of transmitting CMV range from 2.5 to 12 percent. In a study of seronegative children receiving blood for cardiac surgery, the risk of acquiring CMV was calculated to be 2.7 percent per unit of blood.[56] There is a significant correlation between the risk of acquisition of CMV by seronegative patients and the total volume of blood transfused. In one study, the incidence of primary infection increased from 7 percent among patients receiving one unit of blood to 21 percent among those that received greater than 15 units.[57] Recent studies have demonstrated that seronegative immunocompromised patients receiving prophylactic white blood cell (WBC) transfusions from multiple donors (of whom 50 percent are expected to be seropositive) are also at increased risk of acquiring CMV.[61]

The observation that two newborn infants who received large volumes of fresh blood subsequently developed symptomatic CMV infections led McCracken et al. to suggest an association between blood transfusion and clinically apparent postnatal CMV infection.[62] Subsequent reports indicated an association between postnatal CMV infection and exchange transfusions. With exchange transfusions, the probability of a seropositive infant receiving seropositive blood becoming infected is 20 percent, while for a seronegative infant receiving seropositive blood, the probability is 50 percent.[63] This remarkably high incidence after exchange transfusions is most likely due to the fact that infants who receive the transfusions usually receive large volumes (150 to 200 ml/kg) of fresh whole blood from a single donor. Intrauterine transfusions were implicated by King-Lewis and Gardner as the source of CMV in two pregnant women who subsequently seroconverted and whose infants developed viruria between 2 and 8 weeks of postnatal life.[64] Pass et al. reported that the risk of CMV infections in newborn infants was significantly greater for infants (13 of 37) receiving blood from donors with complement fixation titers to CMV greater than 1/8 than for those (2/28) receiving blood from donors with titers of less than 1/8.[65]

Two prospective studies have presented compelling evidence that seropositive blood is the source of acquired CMV in neonates undergoing multiple transfusions. In the study of Yeager et al., 10 of 74 infants of seronegative mothers who were exposed to one or more seropositive blood donors acquired CMV. The risk of infection increased to 24 percent for patients who received more than 50 ml of packed red cells from at least one seropositive donor.[66,67] The use of solely seronegative blood completely eliminated the acquisition of CMV by seronegative infants.[67] A subsequent study by Adler confirmed these findings and proved further that significant risk factors for transmission of CMV and subsequent disease included transfusions from multiple seropositive donors, lack of passively acquired maternal antibody to CMV, and low birth weight (less than 1250 g).[53,68]

## Transmission to hospital workers

Because hospital workers are often women of childbearing age, there has been concern about occupational risk through contact with patients shedding CMV.[31,69–75] Yeager reported a higher seroconversion rate for neonatal (4.1 percent per year) and pediatric nurses (7.7 percent per year) than for nonnurse hospital employees (0 percent), but these differences were not statistically significant.[70] Friedman et al. noted higher seroconversion rates in a pediatric hospital among workers with patient contact compared with those without such contact.[70] Although the difference in rates was not statistically significant, when "high-risk" employees (intensive care nurses and an IV team) were compared with others, a significantly higher rate of CMV infection was found in the former. Dworsky studied nurses in newborn nurseries and other health care workers and found no difference when the seroconversion rate in these women was compared with that of a large group of pregnant women in the community.[31] Balfour and Balfour measured incidence of CMV infection among transplant/dialysis nurses, neonatal intensive care nurses, student nurses, and a control group;[71] neither the initial rate of seropositivity nor the annual seroconversion rate differed significantly among any of the groups. Their annualized seroconversion rate of 1.84 percent was very close to rates determined for middle-income pregnant women in Birmingham, Alabama.[15]

The risk for hospital personnel is a function of the prevalence of CMV excretion among patients, the prevalence of seronegative health care workers, and the degree of their exposure to infected patients. In general, among hospitalized infants and children, viruria occurs in approximately 1 percent of newborn infants, 13 to 30 percent of premature infants hospitalized for 1 month or longer, and 5 to 10 percent of older infants and toddlers. On the other hand, age, race, and, to some extent, sex, influence the prevalence of seronegative hospital personnel.

Working with hospitalized children will inevitably lead to contact with a child shedding CMV. However, it is important that workers who develop primary infection not assume that their occupational exposure or contact with a specific patient is the source of infection. Two case reports illustrate this point well. Yow et al.[76] and Wilfert et al.[77] described health care workers who acquired CMV while pregnant and after attending a patient known to be excreting CMV. In each of these reports, restriction endonuclease analysis of DNA from CMV isolates indicated that the source of CMV for the worker and her aborted fetus was not the patient under suspicion. Adler et al. used restriction enzyme methods to study CMV strains from 34 newborns and a nurse who seroconverted. All 35 strains were different, supporting the conclusion that nosocomial spread of CMV to workers or among newborns was not occurring in their nursery.[74] Although hospital workers, particularly those who attend children or immunocompromised patients, will likely have occupational exposure to CMV, there is no convincing evidence that their risk of infection is increased. There is little information about the risk of CMV acquisition by house officers and medical students. In one study, the annual rate of seroconversion for 25 seronegative pediatric residents was 2.7 percent, which differed little from nursery nurses (3.3 percent) but was higher than the risk (0.6 percent) for 89 serosusceptible students completing their clinical rotations.[31]

## PATHOGENESIS

### Routes of transmission

Many women acquire or reactivate CMV infection during pregnancy, but only a minority transmit the virus to their fetuses causing acute and/or long-term morbidity in a small number of offspring. Generalized cytomegalic inclusion disease of the newborn is almost always the result of primary maternal infection.[15] Even so, clinically apparent infection occurs in less than 15 percent of the infected newborns. Fetal damage following recurrent maternal infection is clearly uncommon.[78,79] Although not clearly established, intrauterine infection is assumed to result from maternal viremia with subsequent placental infection and hematogenous dissemination to the fetus. Since intrauterine transmission occurs in only 30 to 40 percent of pregnant women with primary CMV infection, a mechanism(s) which is not understood but which is generally referred to as the placental barrier must operate to prevent fetal infection.

In immune pregnant women with recurrent infection, it is difficult to postulate that congenital infection results from cell-free virus in plasma causing placental infection with subsequent spread to the fetus. In this circumstance, the virus could evade the immune system within leukocytes,[80] or local reactivation of infection within the endometrium, myometrium, or cervical canal could occur.

### Pathogenic mechanisms

Once intrauterine infection has occurred, the incidence of harmful effects is higher than at any other time in life, with the exception of severely immunocompromised patients. The clinical manifestations of congenital CMV infection are very different from the signs and symptoms associated with infection acquired at delivery or soon after, even in immature infants, suggesting the importance of the intrauterine environment itself.

Why some infants are severely affected and others remain free of symptoms is not clear. The most obvious, but not necessarily the most important, pathogenic mechanism is continuous viral replication in affected organs. Longitudinal studies have demonstrated that excretion of CMV into urine and saliva persists for years. It is likely that chronic viral replication also occurs at other sites that are less accessible to virologic examination. Many cells are susceptible to the direct cytocidal effect of CMV, but differences in the intrinsic susceptibility of various tissues to CMV-mediated injury may determine the frequency with which different organs are involved during the course of CMV infection. Low-grade persistent or latent infection with a slow turnover of infected cells may not elicit cytopathic changes, yet specific antigens have been identified in various tissues by means other than histopathologic staining. Another possible factor is vasculitis, which may occur in utero or after birth. Infants with serious congenital CMV who die soon after birth usually have disseminated intravascular coagulopathy.[81] Proliferating endothelial cells within inflamed tissue are susceptible to CMV infection.

Injury mediated by immunologic factors has also been studied. The humoral immune system of infected infants is generally intact and responds normally to antigenic stimulation.[42] Early after birth, symptomatic congenitally infected infants have an accelerated development of IgG and IgM. Their specific antibody response is substantial and prolonged, regardless of the serologic assay used or the nature of the infection—symptomatic, subclinical, active, or latent.[82] Unfortunately, available serologic data offer no clues that explain a propensity for symptomatic infection. At a molecular level, studies of CMV polypeptides immunoprecipitated by IgG antibodies have demonstrated that in symptomatic infants the appearance of precipitating antibodies is delayed until 12 months of age.[83] However, when a humoral immune response develops, antibodies to viral polypeptides are precipitated in greater numbers and for longer periods.[84] This sustained humoral immune response to congenital infection occurs in the presence of persistent viral replication, thereby resulting in the formation of immune complexes. During the first year of life, immune complexes circulate in a large proportion of infants with congenital infection.[85] The molecular weight of these immune complexes is higher in symptomatic infants than in asymptomatic infants. In a few fatal symptomatic cases, deposition of immune complexes in renal glomeruli has been demonstrated.

Perinatal infection results mainly from recurrent (mostly reactivated) infection in immune women. However, transplacental maternal antibody protects only 50 percent of exposed infants from becoming infected.[18] The ensuing infection, although chronic, remains subclinical in the vast majority of infants, indicating that the passive transfer of maternal antibody is more protective for virulence than for transmission. Studies show transfusion-acquired infection is more virulent in seronegative than in seropositive infants irrespective of underlying diseases or gestational age.

Congenitally and perinatally infected infants have also been noted to have impaired specific cell-mediated immunity as assessed by the lymphocyte transformation response to CMV antigen (LTR).[48,86–89] This test measures only the recognition, not the effector function, of T-lymphocytes and does not require other techniques like the use of syngeneic target cells. Another defect consistently observed is the inability of the lymphocytes of these infants to induce interferon production in vitro when challenged with CMV antigens. The impairments are not a reflection of a generalized disturbance, since it is restricted to a blastogenic response to CMV and is highly virus-specific. CMV-infected patients who have antibodies to herpes simplex virus, for example, have a normal blastogenic response to this virus.[87] Infants with impaired LTRs respond normally to both killed and live vaccines. Furthermore, the number of T cells, the response to phytohemagglutinin, and the proportions of helper and suppressor subpopulations of T lymphocytes are normal. The impairment has no relation to the clinical presentation and outcome, but it is more intense and longer-lasting in patients with symptomatic CMV infection. As patients grow older, the impairment disappears, together with viral replication. It is possible that subtle alterations of host defense mechanisms could contribute to disease, in conjunction with persistent viral replication.

Gehrz et al. showed that in a small group of seropositive pregnant women during the second and third trimesters, there was a transient depression of the blastogenic response.[48] This abnormality was not a reflection of a generalized defect of cell-mediated immunity, and moreover none of the women with LTRs excreted CMV during the period of abnormality, nor did they transmit the infection in utero. In a more recent study, Stern et al.[49] found that women with recently acquired CMV infection who had depressed LTRs had a greater risk of delivering a congenitally infected infant.

### Nature of maternal infection

The nature of the maternal infection is a major pathogenetic factor for congenital CMV infection. Primary infections are more likely to be transmitted to the fetus and are likely to cause more fetal injury than recurrent infections.[90] Intrauterine transmission following primary infection occurs in approximately 30 to 40 percent of cases. Current information suggests that gestational age has no apparent influence on the risk of transmission of CMV in utero.[15] However, several studies suggest that infection at an earlier gestational age produces the worst outcome.[15]

Congenital infection may also result from recurrences of infection.[12,38–41] A recurrence is used here to represent either reactivation of infection or reinfection with the same or a different strain of CMV during pregnancy. Evidence to date indicates that despite the inability of maternal immunity to prevent transmission of this virus to the fetus, congenital infections that result from recurrent infections are less likely to affect the offspring than those resulting from primary infections.[15] The risk of congenital CMV infection resulting from a recurrence of infection during pregnancy ranges from a high of 1.5 percent for an American population of low socioeconomic background to 0.19 percent for women of middle or upper socioeconomic extraction in the United States[15] or from Britain[91] and Sweden.[78]

In recurrent infection, it is likely that preexisting immunity partially inhibits the occurrence of viremia. Maternal IgG antibodies are transmitted to the fetus but their precise role has not been elucidated. It is conceivable that cellular immunity may be more important than humoral immunity. One case of severe fetal infection has been reported following therapeutic immunosuppression of a mother known to have been seropositive before conception.

### Perinatal infection

Naturally acquired perinatal CMV infections result from exposure to infected maternal genital secretions at birth or to breast milk during the first months of postnatal life. The presence of CMV in these two sites may be the result of either primary or recurrent maternal infection. Iatrogenic CMV infections are acquired predominantly from transfusions of blood or blood products and breast milk from CMV-infected donors. Exposure to CMV in the maternal genital tract has resulted in a 30 to 50 percent rate of perinatal infection. During delivery the infant is literally bathed in genital secretions which may contain high titers of CMV. The transmission from mother to infant via breast milk occurs in 30 to 70 percent if nursing lasts for over 1 month. Following ingestion, CMV infection is presumably established at a mucosal surface (buccal, pharyngeal, or esophageal mucosa) or in the salivary glands for which CMV is known to have a special tropism.

Transmission of CMV by blood transfusion is more likely to occur when larger quantities of blood are transfused. The failure to isolate CMV from the blood or blood elements of seropositive healthy blood donors suggests that the virus exists in a latent state, presumably within leukocytes. It has been suggested that following transfusion, when infected cells encounter the allogeneic stimulus, CMV becomes reactivated. Recent studies with DNA hybridization as a method to detect CMV in peripheral blood leukocytes support this hypothesis.[92,93] With DNA-RNA hybridization using a probe for CMV immediate early gene products, it was possible to identify CMV-specific message in the peripheral blood leukocytes of normal healthy seropositive adults.[94] These results indicate that DNA hybridization is more sensitive than standard tissue culture procedures for detecting viremia. It is likely that hybridization procedures may one day be used to identify which donors have a high risk of transmitting the virus.

## CLINICAL MANIFESTATIONS

### Congenital infection

**Symptomatic Infection.** *Acute manifestations:* Cytomegalic inclusion disease, or CID, is characterized by involvement of multiple organs, in particular the reticuloendothelial and central nervous system (CNS), with or without ocular and auditory damage. Weller and Hanshaw defined the abnormalities found most frequently in infants with symptomatic congenital infection as hepatomegaly, splenomegaly, microcephaly, jaundice, and petechiae.[95] As illustrated in Table 70-2, a combination of petechiae, hepatosplenomegaly, and jaundice is the most frequently noted presenting sign. In addition, the magnitude of the prenatal insult is noted by the occurrence of microcephaly with or without cerebral calcification, intrauterine growth retardation, and prematurity.[96] Inguinal hernia in males and chorioretinitis with or without optic atrophy are less common. Occasionally clinical findings include hydrocephalus, hemolytic anemia, and pneumonitis. Among the most severely affected infants, mortality may be as high as 30 percent.[96] Most deaths occur in the neonatal period. Mortality during the neonatal period is usually due to multiorgan disease with severe hepatic dysfunction, bleeding, disseminated intravascular coagulation, and secondary bacterial infections. When death occurs after the first month but during the first year, it is usually due to progressive liver disease with severe failure to thrive. Death after the first year is usually restricted to the severely neurologically handicapped children and is due to malnutrition, aspiration pneumonia, and overwhelming infections.

*Hepatomegaly:* This sign, along with that of splenomegaly, is probably the most common abnormality found in the newborn period in infants born with symptomatic congenital CMV infection.[97] Liver function tests are often abnormal but usually not markedly so. The persistence of hepatomegaly is variable. In some infants liver enlargement disappears by the age of 2 months. In others, significant enlargement persists throughout the first year of life. However, massive hepatomegaly extending beyond the first 12 months of life is uncharacteristic of CID.

*Splenomegaly:* Enlargement of the spleen is especially frequent in congenital CMV infections.[97] It may be the only abnormality present at birth. In some instances splenomegaly and a petechial rash coexist as the only manifestations of the disease. Occasionally the enlargement is such that the spleen may be felt 10 to 15 cm below the costal margin. Splenomegaly usually persists longer than hepatomegaly.

*Jaundice:* Jaundice is a common manifestation of CID. The pattern of hyperbilirubinemia may take several forms, ranging from high levels on the first day to undetectable jaundice on the first day with gradual elevation of the bilirubin level to clinically apparent jaundice.[97] In some instances jaundice is a transient phenomenon, beginning on the first day and disappearing by the end of the first week. More often, however, it tends to persist beyond the time of physiologic jaundice. Occasionally transient jaundice may occur in early infancy with pronounced elevation of bilirubin levels during the third month. Bilirubin levels are high in both the direct and indirect components. Characteristically, the direct component increases after the first few days of life and may constitute as much as 50 percent of the total bilirubin level. It is rare for the indirect bilirubin component to rise high enough to require exchange transfusion, but this has been reported.[97]

*Petechiae and purpura:* There is evidence that CMV has a direct effect on the megakaryocytes of the bone marrow that results in a depression of the platelets and a localized or generalized petechial rash.[97] In some patients the rash is purpuric in character, not unlike that observed in the expanded rubella syndrome. Unlike the latter infection, however, pinpoint petechiae are a more common manifestation of congenital CMV infection. The rash is rarely present at birth but often appears within a few hours thereafter; it may be transient, disappearing within 48 h. The petechiae may be the only clinical manifestation of CMV infection. More often, however, enlargement of the liver and spleen is associated. The petechiae may persist for weeks after birth. Crying, coughing, the application of a tourniquet, a lumbar puncture, or restraints of any kind may result in the appearance of petechiae even months after birth. Platelet counts in the first week of life range from less than 10,000 to 125,000, with a majority in the 20,000 to 60,000 range. Some infants with petechial rashes do not have associated thrombocytopenia.

*Microcephaly:* Microcephaly, usually defined as a head circumference of less than the fifth percentile, was found in 14 of 17 patients with CID studied by Medearis in 1964.[98] In a subsequent study of 34 patients with congenital CMV infection, all of whom were symptomatic by 2 weeks of age, we documented microcephaly in 17 (50 percent).[96] In a more recent examination of 64 surviving patients who were born with symptomatic CMV infection, 32 (50 percent) were microcephalic. Not all infants with microcephaly continue to have head circumferences of less than the fifth percentile. This is especially true if the head measurement is close to the fifth percentile in an infant of low birth weight.[97] If intracranial calcifications are present, the growth of the brain is invariably impaired. Occasionally microcephaly is followed by obstruction of the fourth ventricle and subsequent hydrocephalus. Unlike toxoplasmosis, the presence of calcification is an indication that the infant will have at least moderate and probably severe mental retardation.

*Ocular defects:* The principal abnormality related to the eye in CMV infection is chorioretinitis, with strabismus and optic atrophy being uncommon.[97] Microphthalmia, cataracts, retinal necrosis and calcification, blindness, anterior chamber and optic disk malformations, and pupillary membrane vestige have also been described in association with generalized congenital CID. In spite of this, the presence of abnormalities such as microphthalmia and cataracts is strong presumptive evidence that the disease process is not caused by CMV. Chorioretinitis occurs in approximately 14 percent of infants born with symptomatic congenital infection.[96] Although chorioretinitis occurs less frequently in symptomatic congenital CMV than in congenital toxoplasmosis, CMV chorioretinitis cannot be differentiated from the lesions produced by toxoplasmosis on the basis of location or appearance.[99] Both *Toxoplasma gondii* and cytomegalovirus can induce central retinal lesions. Chorioretinitis caused by CMV differs from that caused by toxoplasmosis in that it rarely progresses postnatally, becoming inactive in early infancy.

**Table 70-2. Clinical Findings in 34 Newborns with Congenital CMV Infection, All of Whom Were Symptomatic by 2 Weeks of Age**

| Abnormality | Positive/total examined (%) |
|---|---|
| Petechiae | 27/34 (79) |
| Hepatosplenomegaly | 25/34 (74) |
| Jaundice | 20/32 (63) |
| Microcephaly* | 17/34 (50) |
| Small for gestational age† | 14/34 (41) |
| Prematurity‡ | 11/32 (34) |
| Inguinal hernia | 5/19§ (26) |
| Chorioretinitis | 4/34 (12) |

*Less than tenth percentile based upon Colorado Intrauterine Growth Charts, for premature newborns (Lubechenco et al.) or more than 2 SD below mean for term babies based upon Nelhaus.
†Weight less than tenth percentile for gestational age.
‡Gestational age less than 38 weeks.
§Males.
Reproduced from RF Pass, S Stagno, GJ Myers, CA Alford: *Pediatrics* 66:758, 1980.

*Fetal growth retardation:* Intrauterine growth retardation, occasionally severe, was reported in 41 percent of 34 patients with symptomatic congenital CMV infection, while prematurity occurred in 34 percent.[96] Infants with asymptomatic congenital infection in general show no IUGR or prematurity, and CMV cannot be considered an important cause of either condition.

*Pneumonitis:* Pneumonitis, a common clinical manifestation of CMV infection following bone marrow and renal transplants in adults, is not usually a part of the clinical presentation of congenital CMV infection in newborn infants. In the author's experience, diffuse interstitial pneumonitis occurs in less than 1% of congenitally infected infants, even when the most severely affected cases are considered. As will be discussed in greater detail later, CMV-associated pneumonitis is more likely to develop in infants with perinatally acquired CMV infections.

*Dental defects:* It is now apparent that congenital CMV infections are also associated with a distinct defect of enamel which thus far seems to affect mainly primary dentition.[101] This defect is more severe in children with the symptomatic form of the infection than in those born with asymptomatic infections. Clinically, this defect appears on all or nearly all of the teeth and is characterized by generalized yellowish discoloration. The enamel is opaque, moderately soft, and tends to chip away from dentin. Affected teeth tend to wear down rapidly and may be the basis for the rampant dental caries frequently seen in these children. Microscopic examination showed generalized brown to yellow discoloration with marked incisal attrition and excessive secondary dentin formation. Biochemical studies have not been performed.

*Deafness:* Sensorineural deafness is probably the most common handicap caused by congenital CMV infection. Medearis was the first investigator to call attention to the presence of deafness in symptomatic congenitally infected infants.[98] Subsequent reports confirmed this association and provided evidence that CMV can also cause sensorineural hearing loss in children with subclinical infection.[99,104–106]

CMV can replicate in many structures of the inner ear as noted by typical CMV-induced cytopathology in the Reissner's membrane, stria vascularis, semicircular canals or by CMV-specific immunofluorescence in the organ of Corti and neuromas of the eighth nerve.

Because hearing is not commonly assessed within the first month of life, it is difficult to say how many congenitally infected infants, whether symptomatic or not, are born with hearing impairments. This handicap, however, becomes significant in infancy and early childhood. In general, the frequency and severity of the hearing impairment is worse in patients with symptomatic infection. Of 64 surviving patients with symptomatic CMV infection we have prospectively followed over the past 20 years, 49 have had adequate audiometric evaluations and 30 of them (61 percent) suffer from some degree of hearing impairment. Among the 267 patients with subclinical infection, 216 have received at least one adequate audiometric evaluation and 11 (5.1 percent) manifest some degree of hearing loss. The sensorineural hearing loss is bilateral in over half the cases and of significant magnitude (50 to 100 dB) to produce serious difficulties with verbal communication and learning. Another alarming characteristic is that in nearly half the cases the hearing impairments have either developed or become severe after the first year of life. Although in most cases the deterioration of hearing occurs within the first 2 to 3 years of life, we have documented its onset between 5 and 14 years of age in four cases.

*Congenital anomalies:* There are reports suggesting an association between CMV and congenital anomalies involving various organs.[97] Most of the studies are retrospective or in the form of single case reports. To date, with the exception of inguinal hernias occurring in males, anomalies of the first brachial arch, and a defect of tooth enamel that becomes apparent when teeth erupt, there is little evidence that CMV can be considered a teratogen.[97,101] Anatomical defects and abnormalities such as microcephaly, spastic quadriplegia, generalized hypotonia, and microphthalmia do occur in connection with congenital CMV infection, but they are not an indication of a teratogenic effect of CMV.

*Long-Term Outcome:* The clinical manifestations of symptomatic congenital CMV infection are highly variable. It is clear that the infection is usually not recognized in infants, especially when minor signs such as failure to thrive, mild splenomegaly, and neonatal jaundice occur. In some cases, psychomotor retardation, neurologic dysfunction, hearing loss, and other delayed complications may take years to identify. The medical significance of congenital CMV derives primarily from the adverse effects that this infection has on the developmental potential of children. The likelihood of survival with normal intellect and hearing following symptomatic congenital CMV infection is small.[62,95,98,105] The most common complications are mental retardation, microcephaly, chorioretinitis, optic atrophy, seizures, paraparesis, diplegia, hearing loss, language delay, and learning disabilities (Table 70-3).

**Table 70-3. Outcome for Patients Presenting at Birth with Symptomatic or Asymptomatic Congenital CMV Infection**

| Complication | 92 symptomatic cases (%) | 267 asymptomatic cases (%) |
|---|---|---|
| Fatal | 30 | 0 |
| Microcephaly | 48 | 4 |
| Psychomotor retardation neuromuscular disorder | 70 | 4 |
| Hearing loss | 59 | 5 |
| Unilateral | 30 | 64 |
| Bilateral | 70 | 36 |
| Stable | 43 | 64 |
| Progressive | 57 | 36 |
| Chorioretinitis or optic atrophy | 14 | 2 |
| Dental defects | 27 | 4 |
| Serious bacterial infections | 4 | 5 |
| Total with one or more complications | 92 | 6 |

**Asymptomatic Infection.** As indicated in the previous section, nearly 90 percent of infants with congenital CMV infections have no early clinical manifestations and their long-term outcome is much better. Nevertheless, there is now solid evidence derived from controlled prospective studies that at least 5 percent, and perhaps as many as 15 percent, are at risk for developing a multitude of developmental abnormalities, such as sensorineural hearing loss, microcephaly, motor defects such as spastic diplegia or quadriplegia, mental retardation, chorioretinitis, and dental defects. These abnormalities usually become apparent within the first 2 years of life.[99,102,103,106,107] Table 70-3 illustrates results based on our prospective longitudinal study of 267 patients with asymptomatic congenital infection and followed by using serial clinical, psychometric, audiometric, and visual assessments. Follow-up studies of patients with inapparent congenital CMV infection have also been done by Kumar et al.,[106] Saigal et al.,[103] Melish and Hanshaw,[102] and Pearl et al.[108] In general their findings resemble the results of our study presented in Table 70-3.

In summary, these observations underscore the need for longitudinal follow-up of patients with congenital CMV infection regardless of its clinical presentation at the outset. Careful assessments of perceptual functions (hearing, visual acuity), psychomotor development, and learning abilities must be made in order to recognize the full impact of CMV. With early identification of a problem corrective measures can be instituted to reduce psychosocial and learning problems.

**Public Health Significance.** Considering an average incidence of 1 percent and a birth rate of 3½ million per annum, approximately 35,000 infants are born each year with congenital CMV infection. Of these, as many as 3500 present with signs and symptoms of infection (CID). About 700 of them can be expected to die within the first year and nearly 2500 of the survivors will develop handicaps. Another 3000 or so among the subclinically infected will develop significant hearing and mental deficits. In addition to the personal and family suffering associated with these conditions, the cost to society for caring for all these children must run into the millions of dollars annually.

## Perinatal infection

In order to establish the diagnosis of perinatal CMV infection, one must first exclude congenital infection by showing absence of viral excretion during the first 2 weeks of life. The incubation period of perinatal CMV infection ranges between 4 and 12 weeks. Although the quantity of virus excreted by infants with perinatal infection is less than that seen with intrauterine acquisition, the infection is also of a chronic nature, with viral excretion persisting for years.[81] The vast majority of infants with naturally acquired perinatal infections remain asymptomatic. Asymptomatic perinatal CMV infection in term and otherwise healthy infants does not appear to have an adverse effect on growth, perceptual functions, or motor or psychosocial development.

CMV has been incriminated as a cause of pneumonitis in infants less than 4 months of age.[98,100,109] CMV-associated pneumonitis is clinically and radiographically indistinguishable from other causes of afebrile pneumonia such as *C. trachomatis*, respiratory syncytial virus, *Pneumocystis carinii, Ureaplasma urealyticum*, parainfluenza viruses, influenza viruses, adenoviruses, enteroviruses, and so on. Clinically, patients with CMV-associated pneumonitis have an afebrile course with tachypnea, apnea, cough (sometimes paroxysmal), coryza, nasal congestion, intercostal retractions, and roentgenographic evidence of diffuse lower airway obstruction (air trapping, thickened bronchial walls with prominent pulmonary markings and varying degrees of atelectasis). Expiratory wheezing is unusual. Laboratory findings include elevated levels of one or more serum immunoglobulins (especially IgM, 66 percent), leukocytosis of greater than 12,000 white blood cells per $mm^3$ (59 percent), and absolute eosinophilia. The median time of hospitalization is 17 days. Some infants require oxygen therapy and ventilatory assitance. Long-term follow-up of patients with pneumonitis associated with CMV and other respiratory pathogens provides evidence that significant mortality and morbidity do occur irrespective of the etiologic agent involved.[110] Seven of 205 (3.4 percent) patients enrolled died. Morbidity among the survivors was characterized by recurrent wheezing (46 percent of the patients), hospitalizations with exacerbations of pulmonary problems (16 percent), persistently abnormal chest roentgenograms 12 months after discharge (15 percent), and abnormal pulmonary function (60 percent of patients tested at mean age of 5 years).

In premature and sick term infants, naturally acquired CMV infection may pose a greater risk. Yeager et al. found that premature infants weighing less than 1500 g at birth who acquired CMV from a maternal source often developed hepatosplenomegaly, neutropenia, lymphocytosis, and thrombocytopenia coinciding with the onset of virus excretion. Frequently, these patients required longer treatment with oxygen.[111] In a later prospective study, Paryani et al. suggested that there may be a propensity for an increased incidence of neuromuscular impairments, particularly in premature infants with onset of CMV excretion during the first 2 months of life.[112] However, sensorineural hearing loss, chorioretinitis, and microcephaly occurred with similar frequency in both groups.

Transfusion-acquired perinatal CMV infection can cause significant morbidity and mortality, particularly in premature infants with a birth weight of less than 1500 g born to CMV seronegative mothers.[63–68] The syndrome of posttransfusion CMV infection in premature newborn infants has been characterized by Ballard and coworkers[113] and consists of deterioration of respiratory function, hepatosplenomegaly, unusual gray pallor with disturbing septic appearance, both an atypical and absolute lymphocytosis, thrombocytopenia, and hemolytic anemia. The syndrome was more severe in low-birth-weight infants and occurred approximately 4 to 12 weeks posttransfusion, at a time when the infants were progressing satisfactorily. Although the course of the disease was generally self-limited (lasting from 2 to 3 weeks), death occurred in 20 percent of the sick infants. Subsequent work by Yeager[67] and Adler[53] has confirmed these observations. Yeager demonstrated that the risk of infection is related to the serologic status of the donor and that these infections could be prevented by transfusing seronegative newborns with blood from seronegative donors.

## TREATMENT AND PREVENTION

### Chemotherapy

A small number of systemically administered antiviral agents have been used in therapeutic trials of CMV infection, mostly in immunosuppressed patients, normal adults with mononucleosis syndrome, and infants with symptomatic congenital infection.[114–119] Most trials with idoxuridine, 5-fluor-2′ deoxyuridine, cytosine arabinoside, adenine arabinoside, acyclovir, leukocyte interferon, interferon stimulators, transfer factor, or combinations of these agents have proved very disappointing in the treatment of symptomatic infections. During therapy these compounds cause reductions in the amount of virus excreted but the effect is short-lived. With the exception of vidarabine and acyclovir, drug-related toxicity is a significant problem. Thus far it has been impossible to verify clinical efficacy in any of these studies. Besides the fact that suppression of viral replication was only transient, other confounding factors are the wide spectrum of disease resulting from congenital infection, its unpredictable natural course, the fact that many patients had incurred irreversible damage before birth, and the lack of controls.

The most recent addition to the aramamentarium is 9-(1, 3 dihydroxypropoxymethyl) guanine (DHPG) which in preliminary studies has proved partially effective in the treatment of CMV retinochoroiditis and pneumonitis in immunosuppressed transplant patients.[117] No controlled studies of treatment of congenital CMV infection are yet available. However, because of the high frequency of systemic toxicity, it is unlikely that DHPG will ever be used very extensively to treat congenital or perinatal CMV infections. In summary, the treatment of established CMV disease with antivirals has yielded little or no clinical benefit and is complicated by moderate to severe toxicity. There is as yet no safe, effective treatment for symptomatic congenital or perinatal CMV infections.

### Passive immunization

Hyperimmune plasma and globulin have been used with some success as prophylaxis for primary CMV infection in immunosuppressed transplant patients.[118,120,121] In seronegative renal transplant recipients, intravenous CMV-Ig decreased the severity of CMV infection. In bone marrow transplant patients, results of several trials have demonstrated that the prophylactic use of CMV-Ig prevents CMV infection or reduces the severity of disease. It is unlikely that passive immunoprophylaxis will ever work for treatment of congenital infections, since the cases are identified weeks and months after infection occurred in utero. It might work, however, as a means of preventing primary CMV infection and disease associated with transfusion-acquired infections in premature infants. No controlled studies are available.

### Vaccines

Two live attenuated vaccines have been developed and undergone efficacy trials in both immune and susceptible normal individuals and renal transplant recipients.[122,123] Immunization of susceptible kidney transplant patients with Towne strain, live attenuated CMV vaccine significantly reduced the morbidity of primary CMV infection although it did not prevent acquisition of infection. No evidence was found of reactivation of vaccine virus when the patients were immunosuppressed.[124] An important reason to develop a CMV vaccine is to prevent the serious consequences of congenital infection. A candidate vaccine should therefore prevent primary infection in pregnant women without inducing latent infection. In a very small study of 22 young females immunized with the AD169 attenuated strain followed up for 8 years, antibody and lymphocyte antigenic response induced by the vaccine disappeared in 50 percent of the cases.[124,125] In eight women immunized at different intervals prior to pregnancy congenital infection was not detected. Although this and the Towne strain vaccines have not been shown to reactivate, the possibility that reactivations might occur during pregnancy with transmission to the fetus raises concern about their use, even in vaccine trials.

### Prevention

In general, CMV is not very contagious and its horizontal transmission requires close direct contact with infected material, namely, secretions that contain the virus and less likely, fomites.[25–37,42,55,90] With the exception of a few small studies that were designed to prevent infection via blood and blood products and grafted organs, no broad-based strategies for preventing the transmission of this virus have been tested.[55,67,68,126] Although there are still no effective means of preventing congenital CMV infection, or most perinatally acquired CMV infections, a few common-sense recommendations can be made.

**Pregnant Women.** An average of 2 percent of susceptible pregnant women acquire CMV infection during pregnancy in the United States; the majority have no symptoms and only 40 percent of the episodes result in fetal infection. Because there is no effective drug therapy and the risk of fetal morbidity is low, several investigators have concluded that routine serologic screening of pregnant women searching for primary CMV infections during pregnancy is of limited value.[91,127,128]

Primary CMF infection should be suspected in pregnant women with symptoms compatible with a heterophil-negative, mononucleosis-like syndrome. At present there are no reliable means to determine whether intrauterine transmission has occurred following symptomatic or subclinical primary infection or to assess the relatively small number of fetuses at risk of disease. Thus, there is inadequate information to serve as a basis for recommendations regarding termination of pregnancy after a primary CMV infection.[90] Similarly, there is no information regarding how long conception should be delayed after primary infection.

The data on which to base recommendations for prevention of congenital CMV infection after recurrent maternal infection are even more inadequate. At present, there are no techniques for identifying women with reactivation of CMV that result in intrauterine transmission. Since the risk of transmission is very low and the risk of fetal disease even lower, women known to be seropositive before conception do not need to be virologically or serologically tested, nor do they need to be unduly worried about the very low risk of transmitting the virus to the fetus.

The principal sources of CMV infection among women of childbearing age are exposure to children excreting CMV and sexual contacts. Sexual transmission of CMV can probably be prevented by barrier methods (condoms, spermicides) that reduce the transmission of more common sexually transmitted infections, although no data have been published to specifically assess the effectiveness of such methods for CMV. Concerning the risk from exposure to children, those at greatest risk are susceptible pregnant mothers of CMV-infected children who attend day care centers.[25,26,34,36,37] Hand washing and simple hygienic measures that are routine for hospital care can be recommended, but it is unrealistic to expect many mothers to comply.

Although hospital workers do not appear to be at increased risk for CMV infection,[31,32,69–71,73–75] personnel who work in day care centers certainly are.[25,26,34,36,37] In the hospital, routine infection control procedures such as hand washing and gloving should make nonparenteral acquisition of CMV less likely than in the community. Since the majority of patients who shed CMV are asymptomatic and unrecognized, universal precautions should be emphasized to prevent transmission from unrecognized infected patients as well as from known CMV-excreting patients. In the day care setting, where hygiene is difficult at best, preventive measures may be more difficult to implement. Although there is still debate about the need for routine screening of female hospital personnel and day care workers, I believe it should be recommended for potentially childbearing women whose occupation exposes them to CMV. Those found seropositive can be strongly reassured. Those found to be serosusceptible should be provided with information and reassured that common-sense measures such as hand washing and avoiding contact with secretions should prevent acquisition of CMV.[129] Attempts to identify all CMV-excreting patients or children in the workplace so that seronegative workers can avoid contact with them is totally unreasonable.

## NEONATAL HERPES SIMPLEX VIRUS INFECTIONS

### HISTORY

Infections caused by herpes simplex viruses have been recognized since the era of the ancient Greeks. Greek scholars defined the word *herpes* to mean to creep or crawl in reference to the visualized skin lesions. The Greek historian Herodotus associated mouth ulcers and lip vesicles with fever[130] and called this event *herpes febrilis*. Genital herpetic infections were first described by a physician to the eighteenth century French court, Astruc.[131] Over the ensuing two centuries, the infectious nature of herpes simplex viruses was delineated. The transmissability of these viruses was unequivocally established by passage of virus from lip and genital lesions of humans to either the cornea or the scarified skin of the rabbit.[132]

Only fifty years ago, the first written descriptions of neonatal herpes simplex virus infections were attributed nearly simultaneously to Hass, when he described the histopathologic findings of a fatal case, and to Batignani, who described a newborn child with herpes simplex keratitis.[133,134] Subsequently, histopathologic descriptions of the disease demonstrated a broad spectrum of involvement in infants.

In the mid 1960s, Nahmias and Dowdle demonstrated two antigenic types of herpes simplex virus.[135] The differentiation of herpes simplex virus into two types resulted in the development of viral typing methods, which were critical in clarifying the epidemiology of these infections. Herpes simplex virus infections "above the belt," primarily of the lip and oropharynx, were found in most cases to be caused by herpes simplex virus type 1. Those infections "below the belt," particularly genital infections, were usually caused by herpes simplex virus type 2. With the finding that both genital herpes infections and neonatal herpes simplex virus infections were most often caused by herpes simplex virus type 2, a natural cause-and-effect relationship developed between these two disease entities. This causal relationship was strengthened by the finding of viral excretion in the maternal genital tract at the time of delivery, suggesting that acquisition of the virus by the infant occurs by contact with infected genital secretions during birth.

Over the past 15 years, our knowledge of the epidemiology, natural history, and pathogenesis of neonatal herpes simplex virus infections has expanded greatly. The development of antiviral therapy represents a significant advance in the management of infected children, providing the opportunity to decrease mortality and improve the morbidity associated with these infections. Of all the herpesvirus infections, neonatal herpes simplex virus infection represents the one which should be most amenable to prevention and treatment because it is acquired most often at birth rather than early in gestation. As our knowledge of the epidemiology of herpes simplex virus infections has increased, it has become apparent that there are modes of infection other than contact with infected maternal genital infections during delivery. Postnatal acquisition of herpes simplex virus type 1 has been documented from nonmaternal sources. These issues, as well as the management of hospital personnel with herpes simplex virus infections, will be the focus of this section. The changing presentation of neonatal herpes simplex virus infection, particularly the increasing difficulty of diagnosing infection, and the success of antiviral therapy will be stressed.

## EPIDEMIOLOGY OF NEONATAL HSV INFECTION

### Nature of infection

Transmission of herpes simplex virus most often occurs in association with intimate, personal contact. Virus must come in contact with mucosal surfaces or abraded skin for infection to be initiated. After viral replication at the site of infection, either an intact virion or the nucleocapsid is transported by neurons to the ganglia where latency is established. Infection with HSV-1, generally limited to the oropharynx, can be transmitted by respiratory droplets or through direct contact of a susceptible individual with infected secretions (such as virus-containing labial vesicular fluid). Acquisition often occurs during childhood.

Primary herpes simplex virus type 1 infection in the young child is usually asymptomatic. If present, clinical illness is manifested by gingivostomatitis. Primary infection in young adults has been associated with pharyngitis and with a mononucleosis-like syndrome. Like other herpesvirus infections, seroprevalence studies have demonstrated that acquisition of herpes simplex virus type 1 infection is related to socioeconomic factors. Antibodies, indicative of past infection, are found early in life among individuals of lower socioeconomic groups and are presumed to be the consequence of crowded living conditions which provide a greater opportunity for direct contact with infected individuals. As many as 75 to 90 percent of individuals from lower socioeconomic populations develop antibodies by the end of the first decade of life. In comparison, in middle and upper middle socioeconomic groups only 30 to 40 percent are seropositive by the middle of the second decade of life.[136–139] A declining seroprevalence of herpes simplex virus type 1 may account, in part, for the increased clinical awareness of herpes simplex virus type 2 infections, since herpes simplex virus type 1 antibodies may be partially protective against type 2 infection.[140,141]

Because infections with herpes simplex virus type 2 are usually acquired through sexual contact, antibodies to this virus are rarely found until adolescence. There is then a progressive increase in seroprevalence with herpes simplex virus type 2 in all populations. As with herpes simplex virus type 1 infections, the risk of acquisition of infection with herpes simplex virus type 2 appears related to socioeconomic factors. Until recently, the precise seroprevalence of antibodies to herpes simplex virus type 2 had been difficult to determine because of cross-reactivity with herpes simplex virus type 1 antigens. Utilizing less specific serologic assays, as many as 50 to 60 percent of lower socioeconomic populations have antibodies to herpes simplex virus type 2. In contrast, 10 to 20 percent of individuals in higher socioeconomic groups are seropositive.[142,143] Recently, seroepidemiologic studies performed by Dr. A. Nahmias in Atlanta utilizing a type-specific assay for herpes simplex virus type 2 (glycoprotein G-2) identified antibodies in 35 percent of middle-class women receiving care through an Atlanta health maintenance organization.[144]

### Maternal infection

The epidemiology and clinical nature of genital HSV infection do not appear to be greatly influenced by pregnancy. Infection during gestation can manifest in a variety of ways. The most serious but fortunately uncommon problem encountered with herpes simplex infections during pregnancy is that of widely disseminated disease. Infection has been documented to involve multiple visceral sites, in addition to cutaneous dissemination.[145–150] In a limited number of cases, dissemination after primary oropharyngeal or genital infection has led to such severe manifestations of disease as necrotizing hepatitis with or without thrombocytopenia, leukopenia, disseminated intravascular coagulopathy, and encephalitis. Although only a small number of patients have suffered from disseminated infection, the mortality among these pregnant women is reported to be greater than 50 percent. Fetal deaths have also occurred in more than 50 percent of cases, although mortality did not necessarily correlate with the death of the mother. Surviving fetuses were delivered by cesarean section either during the acute illness or at term and none had evidence of neonatal herpes simplex virus infection.

Localized genital infection is the most common form of herpes simplex virus infection during pregnancy. Overall, prospective investigations utilizing cytologic and virologic screening indicate that genital herpes occurs with a frequency of about 1 percent at any time during gestation.[151] Most of these infections have been considered recurrent in nature. Those factors which influence the frequency of both primary and recurrent infection in pregnancy are not well defined.

Maternal primary infection prior to 20 weeks gestation in a proportion of women has been associated with spontaneous abortion.[152,153] While the original estimate of spontaneous abortion following a symptomatic primary infection during gestation was thought to be as high as 25 percent, it is likely that this calculation is erroneously high because of the very small number of women followed. Unfortunately, precise data, indicating the true risk of spontaneous abortion following primary infection during gestation, are not available. Infection which develops later in gestation was not associated with the termination of pregnancy.[153–155]

The frequency of herpes simplex virus recurrences during gestation should be of concern for women with a known history of infection. Transmission of infection to the fetus is most frequently related to the actual shedding of virus at the time of delivery. Since herpes simplex virus infection of the fetus is usually the consequence of contact with infected maternal genital secretions at the time of delivery, the determination of viral excretion at this time is of utmost importance. The actual incidence of viral excretion at delivery has been suggested to be 0.01 to 0.39 percent for all women, irrespective of past history, as was summarized by Nahmias and reported by others.[151,156–159]

Several prospective studies have evaluated the frequency and nature of viral shedding in pregnant women with a known history of genital herpes. In a predominantly white, middle-class population, documented recurrent infection occurred in 84 percent of pregnant women.[158] Moreover, asymptomatic viral shedding occurred in at least 12 percent of the recurrent episodes. Viral shedding from the cervix occurred in only 0.56 percent of symptomatic infections and 0.66 percent of asymptomatic infections. These data are similar to those obtained in other populations.[157,159] The incidence of cervical shedding in asymptomatic pregnant women has been reported to be as high as 3 percent.[155] However, the observed rate of shedding among asymptomatic pregnant women has varied more than that among nonpregnant women (from 0.2 to 7.4 percent), depending upon the study population and trial design.[155,157,159–162] Overall, these data indicate that the frequency of cervical shedding is low, rendering the risk of transmission of virus to the infant similarly low when the infection is recurrent in nature.[151] The frequency of shedding does not appear to vary by trimester during gestation.[155,163] Overall, no increased incidence of premature onset of labor is apparent in these prospective studies. Regardless, given the high seroprevalence of infection, a significant degree of protection for the fetus must exist or else the incidence of neonatal disease should be significantly higher. Importantly, most infants who develop neonatal disease are born to women who are completely asymptomatic at the time of delivery and have neither a past history of genital herpes nor a sexual partner reporting a genital vesicular rash.[151,162–164] These women account for 60 to 80 percent of all women whose infected children develop infection.

Recently, an analysis of women delivering children who developed neonatal herpes simplex virus infection has been summarized.[164] Only 27 percent of these women had either a history of or evidence of recurrent lesions indicative of herpes simplex virus infection during the current pregnancy. Furthermore, only half of these women reported genital herpes simplex virus infection in their sexual partners. The majority of women were without signs or symptoms of genital herpetic infection.

## Factors which influence transmission of infection to the fetus

The type of maternal genital infection at the time of delivery probably influences the frequency of neonatal acquisition of infection. The duration and quantity of viral excretion and the time to total healing vary with primary, initial (first episode at the nonprimary site) and recurrent (herpes simplex virus types 1 and 2) maternal genital infection.[165,166] As discussed previously, primary infection is associated with larger quantities of virus replicating in the genital tract (>$10^6$ viral particles per 0.2 ml of inoculum) and a period of viral excretion which may persist for an average of 3 weeks. In contrast, virus is shed for an average of only 2 to 5 days and at lower concentrations (approximately $10^2$ to $10^3$ per 0.2 ml of inoculum) in women with recurrent genital infection. The difference in the natural history of primary and recurrent disease is likely a major factor which influences the frequency of transmission and, perhaps, the severity of neonatal disease.

Paralleling the type of maternal infection, the mother's antibody status to herpes simplex virus at delivery appears to be an additional factor which also influences the severity of infection as well as the likelihood of transmission. Transplacental maternal neutralizing antibodies appear to have a protective, or at least an ameliorative, effect on acquisition of infection for babies inadvertently exposed to virus.[156,167,168] Maternal primary infection late in gestation may not result in significant passage of maternal antibodies across the placenta to the fetus. It should be noted that the distinction between symptomatic and asymptomatic disease whether primary, initial, or recurrent remains poorly defined at present in relation to the risks of transmission of infection to the infant.

The duration of ruptured membranes has also become an important indicator of risk for acquisition of neonatal infection. Observations by Nahmias and colleagues indicate that prolonged rupture of membranes (greater than 6 h) increases the risk of acquisition of virus, probably the consequence of ascending infection from the cervix.[151,153] Based on this observation, it is recommended that women with active genital lesions at the time of onset of labor be delivered by cesarean section, as will be discussed below. The potential benefits of cesarean section beyond 6 h of ruptured membranes may be demonstrated, but this has not been proved at the present time. However, it should be recognized that infection of the newborn has occurred in spite of delivery by cesarean section.[164,169]

A final note regarding factors which can influence disease transmission relates to in utero monitoring for fetal distress. It should be recognized that fetal scalp monitors can be a site of inoculation of virus, and may increase the risk of neonatal herpes simplex virus infection.[170,171] Such devices are contraindicated in women with a history of recurrent genital herpes simplex virus infections.

## Incidence of newborn infection

The estimated rate of neonatal herpes simplex virus infection is approximately 1 in 2000 to 1 in 5000 deliveries per year.[151] A progressive increase in the number of cases of neonatal herpes simplex virus infection has been noted in some areas with rates approaching 1 in 1500 deliveries.[172] Neonatal herpes simplex virus infection occurs far less frequently than genital herpes simplex virus infections in the adult childbearing population. It should be noted that several countries do not appear to recognize a significant number of cases of neonatal herpes simplex infection in spite of the high prevalence of antibodies to herpes simplex virus type 2. Serologic studies in central Africa indicate that women have a high frequency of antibodies to herpes simplex virus type 2, but the first case of neonatal herpes was reported only relatively recently.[173,174] The United Kingdom presents a similar dilemma. Genital herpetic infection is relatively common in the United Kingdom, but very few cases of neonatal herpes simplex virus infection are recognized in that country. Overall, the United States has approximately 3.5 million deliveries a year and an estimated 700 to 1000 cases of neonatal infection.

## Times of transmission of infection

Herpes simplex virus infection of the newborn can be acquired at one of three times: in utero, during birth, or postnatally. The mother is the source of infection for the first two routes of transmission. For postnatal acquisition of herpes simplex virus infection, the mother may be the source of infection from a genital or nongenital site, or other environmental or patient sources of virus can lead to infection of the child. Nevertheless, a maternal source should be suspected when herpetic lesions are discovered promptly after the birth of the child or when the baby's illness is caused by herpes simplex virus type 2. While intrapartum transmission accounts for 85 to 90 percent of cases, the other two routes must be recognized and identified in a child with suspect disease for both public health and prognostic purposes.

While it was originally presumed that intrauterine infection resulted in either a totally normal baby or premature termination of gestation,[153] it has become apparent that intrauterine acquisition of infection can lead to the clinical symptomatology of congenital infection.[157,175–177] Utilizing stringent diagnostic criteria (namely, identification of infected babies within the first 48 h of life who have virologic confirmation of infection) and excluding other pathogens with similar clinical findings such as congenital cytomegalovirus infection, rubella, syphilis, or toxoplasmosis, over 70 babies have been identified in the world's literature to date with symptomatic congenital disease.[177] The manifestations of disease in this group of children range from neurologic abnormalities to simply the presence of skin vesicles at the time of delivery.

Intrauterine infection can occur as a consequence of either transplacental or ascending infection. Examination of the placenta in cases of neonatal herpes thought to be the consequence of in utero transmission has helped to clarify the route of transmission. A placenta showing evidence of necrosis and inclusions in the trophoblasts suggests a transplacental route of infection[178–180] and can result in a baby with hydraencephaly at birth or may be associated with spontaneous abortion following intrauterine herpes simplex viremia. Virus has been isolated from the products of conception in such circumstances.[178] Histopathologic evidence of chorioamnionitis, suggestive of ascending infection, has been identified as an alternative route for in utero infection as compared with transplacental spread.

Risk factors associated with intrauterine transmission are not known. However, both primary and recurrent maternal infection can result in infection of the fetus in utero. While it might be convenient to assume that only primary maternal infection is associated with transmission of virus in utero, it has been documented that women with recurrent genital infection can transmit herpes simplex virus to the fetus as well, leading to disease.

The second, and most common, route of infection is that of intrapartum contact of the fetus with infected maternal genital secretions. Approximately 80 to 90 percent of infected babies acquire herpes simplex virus infection by this route. Those factors which favor intrapartum transmission of infection have been described above.

The third route of transmission is postnatal acquisition. Even though herpes simplex virus type 1 has been associated with genital lesions, postnatal transmission of herpes simplex virus has been increasingly suggested because 15 to 20 percent of neonatal herpes simplex virus infections are caused by this virus type.[151] In fact, more recent data from the National Institutes of Allergy and Infectious Diseases, NIAID, Antiviral Study Group indicate that the frequency of babies with neonatal herpes simplex virus type 1 infections has increased to nearly 30 percent.[164] This observation, in light of the recognition that genital herpes simplex virus type 1 infections appear to account for only approximately 5 to 15 percent of all genital herpes simplex virus infections, creates greater concern for postnatal acquisition of infection.

Relatives and hospital personnel with orolabial herpes may be a reservoir of virus for infection of the newborn. The recent documentation of postnatal transmission of herpes simplex virus has focused attention on such sources of virus for neonatal infection.[181–189] Postnatal transmission from mother to child has been documented. Maternal-infant postpartum transmission has been reported as a consequence of nursing on an infected breast.[185–188] Furthermore, father-to-baby transmission has been documented.[189]

Many individuals asymptomatically excrete herpes simplex virus from the oropharynx and, therefore, can provide a source of infection for the newborn. The occurrence of fever blisters in various groups of adults has ranged from 16 to 46 percent.[190,191] Population studies in two hospitals indicated that 15 to 34 percent of hospital personnel had a past history of nongenital herpetic lesions.[192–194] In both hospitals surveyed, at least 1 in 100 individuals had a recurrent cold sore each week. No cases of neonatal herpes simplex virus infection were documented in these nurseries.[192,195] However, the demonstration in other studies of identical viruses (utilizing restriction endonuclease analyses of viral DNA) in babies with different mothers leaves little doubt as to the possibility of spread of virus in a high-risk nursery.[182,184] The sources of virus and vectors for transmission have been inadequately studied. The potential legal implications for herpes simplex virus infections acquired in a nursery are obvious. There is significant variation in the United States regarding both the concern for nosocomial transmission of infection in the hospital as well as infection control policies for its prevention.

Various individuals and committees have recommended that personnel with cold sores not work in the nursery. If such a policy were followed, the estimated medical costs would be nearly 20 million dollars annually in the United States if calculated just on the basis of estimates of lost work days.[194] Likely, vigorous handwashing procedures and continuing education of personnel in newborn nurseries has helped contribute to the low frequency of transmission in this environment. The existence of a herpetic whitlow in staff providing patient care should preclude direct patient contact, irrespective of nursing unit.

## IMMUNOLOGIC RESPONSE

The host response of the newborn to herpes simplex virus must be distinguished from that of older individuals. Impairment of host defense mechanisms has been implicated as a cause of the increased severity of some infectious agents in the fetus and the newborn. Factors which must be considered in defining host response include the mode of transmission of the agent (viremia versus mucocutaneous infection), time of acquisition of infection, and the potential of increased virulence of certain strains, although this last point remains purely speculative. Two broad issues are of relevance—protection of the fetus by transplacental antibodies and definition of host response of the newborn.

Host responses to herpes simplex virus infection may well influence the acquisition of disease, severity of infection, and the host resistance to the development, maintenance, and reactivation of herpes simplex virus.[196–198] Clearly, humoral immunity does not prevent either recurrences or exogenous reinfection. Thus, it is not surprising that transplacentally acquired antibodies from the mother are not totally protective against newborn infection. The key issue, then, is to what extent these antibodies are protective and whether specific antibody classes confirm greater protection than others. Transplacentally acquired neutralizing antibodies seem to either prevent or ameliorate infection in exposed newborns.[167,168] Nevertheless, the presence of antibodies at the time of clinical presentation with disease does not appear to influence the subsequent outcome.[162,164,199]

Infected newborns produce IgM antibodies, as detected by immunofluorescence, specific for herpes simplex virus within the first 3 weeks of infection. These antibodies increase rapidly in titer during the first 2 to 3 months and may be detectable for as long as 1 year after infection. The most reactive immunodeterminants include the viral surface glycoproteins, particularly gD. Humoral antibody responses have been studied recently using immunoblot technology.[199,200] These studies indicate that the severity of infection correlates directly with the number of antibody bands to defined polypeptides. Children with more limited infection, namely, infection of the skin, eye, and/or mouth, have fewer antibody bands as compared with those children with disseminated disease. It has been suggested that the quantity of neutralizing antibodies in babies with disseminated infection is lower.[200]

Of particular interest is the recent observation that antibodies to the alpha gene product responsible for initiating viral replication (alpha-4) are predictive of long-term neurologic outcome. These antibodies probably reflect the extent of viral replication. A regression analysis which compared neurologic impairment with the quantity of these antibodies demonstrated that increased antibodies to alpha-4 are predictive of the child at risk for severe neurologic impairment.[199]

Cellular immunity has been considered important in the host response to primary herpetic infections. Newborns with herpes simplex virus infections have a delayed T-lymphocyte proliferative response compared with older individuals.[200] Most infants studied in a recent evaluation had no detectable T-lymphocyte responses to herpes simplex virus 2 to 4 weeks after the onset of clinical symptoms.[200,201] This observation had been made previously by other investigators where delayed blastogenic responses to herpes simplex virus have been observed.[201,202] The delayed response to T-lymphocyte antigens in children who have disease localized to the skin, eye, or mouth at the onset of disease may be an important determinant of the frequency of disease progression.[200,203]

Infected newborns have decreased production of alpha interferon in response to herpes simplex virus antigen when compared with adults with primary herpes simplex virus infection.[200] The importance of interferon alpha on the maturation of host responses, particularly the elicitation of natural killer cell responses, remains to be defined. Lymphocytes from infected babies have decreased responses to gamma interferon generation during the first month of life.[200,204,205] Taken together, these data indicate that the newborn has a delayed immune response in terms of both cell-mediated immunity and lymphokine generation.

Antibodies plus complement and antibodies with killer lymphocytes, monocytes, macrophages, or polymorphonuclear leukocytes will lyse herpes simplex virus infected cells in vitro.[206] Antibody-dependent cell-mediated cytotoxicity is an important component of the development of host immunity to infection.[207] However, the total population of killer lymphocytes in the newborn is lower than that in older individuals. Thus, certain cell-mediated immune factors do appear relevant in neonatal disease. Both the type and quantity of antibodies present as well as the immaturity of monocyte and macrophages of human neonates are of greater importance than in adults.[208–215] These findings are supported by animal model data.[213–215]

## NEONATAL INFECTION

### Pathogenesis

Following direct exposure, the newborn will either limit viral replication to the portal of entry (namely, the skin, eye, or mouth) or viral replication will progress and cause more serious disease, including involvement of the brain (causing encephalitis) or multiple other organs. Host mechanisms responsible for control of progression of viral replication at the site of entry are unknown. For central nervous system disease, it is possible that intraneuronal transmission of viral particles provides a privileged site which may be immune to circulating humoral and cell-mediated defense mechanisms. Thus, transplacental maternal antibodies may be of less value under such circumstances. In contrast, disseminated infection may be the consequence of viremia or secondary to extensive cell-to-cell spread as occurs with pneumonitis following aspiration of infected secretions.

### Clinical presentation

The clinical presentation of babies with neonatal herpes simplex virus infection is a direct reflection of the site and extent of viral replication. Neonatal herpes simplex virus infection is almost invariably symptomatic and frequently lethal. Although reported cases of asymptomatic infection in the newborn exist, they are most uncommon, and long-term follow-up of these children to document absence of subtle disease or sequelae has not been carefully performed. Classification of newborns with herpes simplex virus infection is mandatory for prognostic and therapeutic considerations. Babies with congenital infection should be identified within the 48 to 72 h following birth. Those babies who are infected intrapartum or postnatally can be divided into three categories: (1) disease localized to the skin, eye, or mouth; (2) encephalitis with or without skin, eye, and/or mouth involvement; and (3) disseminated infection which involves multiple organs, including central nervous system, lung, liver, adrenals, skin, eye, and/or mouth. Historically, babies with neonatal herpes simplex virus infection were classified as having localized or disseminated disease with the former group being subdivided into those with skin, eye, or mouth disease versus those with central nervous system infection. However, this classification system understates the significant differences in outcome according to each category,[216] and the revised classification system will be used here. The prospectively acquired data obtained through the NIAID Collaborative Antiviral Study Group will be reported here.

### Intrauterine infection

In the most severely afflicted group of babies, intrauterine infection is apparent at birth and is characterized by a triad of findings, including skin vesicles or skin scarring, eye disease, and the far more severe manifestations of microcephaly or hydranencephaly. Often chorioretinitis alone or in combination with other eye findings, such as keratoconjunctivitis, is a component of the clinical presentation. Serial ultrasound examination of the mothers of those babies infected in utero has demonstrated the presence of hydranencephaly. Chorioretinitis alone can be a presenting sign and should alert the pediatrician to the possibility of this diagnosis, albeit HSV infection is a less common cause than other congenital infections. Severe disease can follow acquisition of infection virtually at any time in gestation. The frequency of occurrence of these manifestations has been estimated to be between 1 in 100,000 to 1 in 200,000 deliveries.[177]

A small group of children will have skin or eye lesions which are present at the time of delivery. These children are frequently born to women who have had prolonged rupture of membranes, sometimes for as long as 2 weeks prior to delivery. The babies have no other findings of invasive multiorgan involvement, chorioretinitis, encephalitis, or evidence of other diseased organs. The prognosis for successful antiviral therapy in this group of babies is far better than in the children who are born with hydranencephaly.

## Disseminated infection

Table 70-4 summarizes the disease classification of 291 babies with neonatal herpes simplex virus from the NIAID Collaborative Antiviral Study Group. Babies with disseminated infection have the worst prognosis in terms of both mortality and morbidity. Children with disseminated infection usually present to tertiary care centers for therapy between 9 and 11 days of life. However, signs of infection are usually present on an average of 4 to 5 days earlier. This group of babies has historically accounted for approximately one-half to two-thirds of all children with neonatal herpes simplex virus infection. The principal organs involved following disseminated infection are the liver and adrenals. However, infection can involve multiple other organs including the larynx, trachea, lungs, esophagus, stomach, lower gastrointestinal tract, spleen, kidneys, pancreas, and heart. Constitutional signs and symptoms include irritability, seizures, respiratory distress, jaundice, bleeding diatheses, shock, and frequently the characteristic vesicular exanthem which is often considered pathognomonic for infection. The vesicular rash, as described below, is particularly important in the diagnosis of herpes simplex virus infection. However, over 20 percent of children having disseminated infection will not develop skin vesicles during the course of their illness.[164,217] In the absence of skin vesicles, the diagnosis becomes exceedingly difficult, since the other clinical signs are often vague and nonspecific, mimicking those of neonatal sepsis. Mortality in the absence of therapy exceeds 80 percent; all but a few survivors are impaired. The most common cause of death in babies with disseminated disease is either herpes simplex virus pneumonitis or disseminated intravascular coagulopathy.

Evaluation of the extent of disease is imperative, as with all cases of neonatal herpes simplex virus infection. The clinical laboratory should be utilized to define hepatic enzyme elevation (SGOT and CGT), direct hyperbilirubinemia, neutropenia, thrombocytopenia, and bleeding diatheses, among others. In addition, chest roentgenograms, abdominal x-rays, electroencephalography, and computed tomography of the head all can be judiciously and serially employed to determine the extent of disease. The radiographic picture of herpes simplex virus lung disease is characterized by a diffuse, interstitial pattern which progresses to a hemorrhagic pneumonitis. Not infrequently, pneumitosis intestinalis can be detected when gastrointestinal disease is present.

Encephalitis appears to be a common component of this form of infection, occurring in about 60 to 75 percent of children.

**Table 70-4. Demographic and Clinical Characteristics of Infants Enrolled in NIAID Collaborative Antiviral Study**

| | Disease classification | | |
|---|---|---|---|
| | Disseminated | CNS | SEM |
| No. babies (%) | 93 (32) | 96 (33) | 102 (35) |
| Male/female | 54/39 | 50/46 | 51/51 |
| Race: caucasian/other | 60/33 | 73/23 | 76/26 |
| Premature (<36 weeks) | 33 (35) | 20 (21) | 24 (24) |
| Gestational age: | 36.5 ± 0.4 | 37.9 ± 0.4 | 37.8 ± 0.3 |
| Enrollment age | 11.6 ± 0.7 | 17.4 ± 0.8 | 12.1 ± 1.1 |
| Maternal age | 21.7 ± 0.5 | 23.1 ± 0.5 | 22.8 ± 0.5 |
| Clinical findings: | | | |
| Skin lesions | 72 (77) | 60 (63) | 86 (84) |
| Brain involvement | 69 (74) | 96 (100) | 0 (0) |
| Pneumonia | 46 (49) | 4 (4) | 3 (3) |
| Mortality:* 1 year | 56 (60) | 13 (14) | 0 (0) |
| Neurologic impairment of survivors: | | | |
| Total | 15/34* (44) | 45/81† (56) | 10/93† (11) |
| Ara-A | 13/26† (50) | 25/51† (49) | 3/34† (9) |
| Acyclovir | 1/6† (17) | 18/27† (67) | 4/51† (8) |
| Placebo | 1/2† (50) | 2/3† (67) | 3/8† (38) |

*Irrespective of therapy.
†Denominators vary according to number with follow-up available.

Cerebrospinal fluid examination and use of noninvasive neurodiagnostic tests, as defined below, will help assess the extent of brain disease.

## Encephalitis

Infection of the central nervous system alone or in combination with disseminated disease presents with the findings indicative of encephalitis in the newborn. Overall, nearly 90 percent of babies with dissemination or encephalitis have evidence of acute brain infection. Brain infection can occur either as a component of multiorgan disseminated infection or as encephalitis with or without skin, eye, and mouth involvement. Nearly one-third of all babies with neonatal herpes simplex virus infection have only the encephalitis component of disease. The pathogenesis of these two forms of brain infection is most likely different. Babies with disseminated infection probably seed the brain by a blood-borne route, resulting in multiple areas of cortical hemorrhagic necrosis. In contrast, babies who present with encephalitis alone are likely to develop brain disease as a consequence of retrograde axonal transmission of virus to the central nervous system. Two pieces of data support this contention. First, babies with disseminated disease have documented viremia and are hospitalized earlier in life (at 9 to 10 days versus 16 to 17 days) than those with isolated encephalitis. Second, babies with encephalitis are more likely to receive transplacental neutralizing antibodies from their mothers, which may not prevent intraneuronal transmission of virus to the brain.

The clinical manifestations of encephalitis, either alone or in association with disseminated disease, include seizures (both focal and generalized) lethargy, irritability, tremors, poor feeding, temperature instability, bulging fontanelle, and pyramidal tract signs. While babies with disseminated infection often have skin vesicles in association with brain infection, the same is not true for the baby with encephalitis alone. The latter group of children have skin vesicles in only 60 percent of cases at any time in the disease course.[164,217–219] Cultures of cerebrospinal fluid yield virus in 25 to 40 percent of all cases. Anticipated findings on cerebrospinal fluid examination include pleocytosis and proteinosis (as high as 500 to 1000 mg/dl). While a few babies with central nervous system infection demonstrated by brain biopsy have been reported to have no abnormalities of their cerebrospinal fluid, this occurs very rarely. Serial cerebrospinal fluid examination is useful diagnostically as the infected child with brain disease will demonstrate progressive increases in the CSF protein content. The importance of cerebrospinal fluid examinations in all infants is underscored by the finding that even subtle changes have been associated with significant developmental abnormalities. Electroencephalography and computed tomography can be very useful in defining the presence of central nervous system abnormalities.[222] Death occurs in 50 percent of babies with localized central nervous system disease who are not treated and is usually related to brain stem involvement. With rare exceptions, survivors are left with neurologic impairment.[217,219]

The long-term prognosis, following either disseminated infection or encephalitis, is poor. As many as 50 percent of surviving children have some degree of psychomotor retardation, often in association with microcephaly, hydranencephaly, porencephalic cysts, spasticity, blindness, chorioretinitis, or learning disabilities. It is unclear at this time whether visceral or central nervous system damage can be progressive after initial clearance of the viral infection, a possibility suggested by long-term assessment of children with skin, eye, or mouth disease[151,164,220] and more recently, in a group of babies with more severe disease.[221]

Despite the presumed difference in pathogenesis, the clinical manifestations of encephalitis alone are virtually identical to those which occur with brain infection in disseminated cases. Only two of three babies with encephalitis will develop a vesicular rash characteristic of herpes simplex virus infection. Thus, a newborn with pleocytosis and proteinosis of the cerebrospinal fluid but without a rash can easily be misdiagnosed as having a bacterial or other viral infection unless herpes simplex virus infection is carefully considered. In such circumstances, a history of genital lesions in the mother or her sexual partner may be very important in suggesting herpes simplex virus as a cause of illness.

### Skin, eye, and/or mouth infection

Infection localized to the skin, eye, and/or mouth is associated with lower mortality, but it is not without significant morbidity. When infection is localized to the skin, the presence of discrete vesicles remains the hallmark of disease. Clusters of vesicles often appear initially on the presenting part of the body which was in direct contact with the virus during birth. With time, the rash can progress to involve other areas of the body as well. Vesicles occur in 90 percent of children with skin, eye, and/or mouth infection. Children with disease localized to the skin, eye, or mouth generally present at about 10 to 11 days of life. Those babies with skin lesions invariably will suffer from recurrences over the first 6 months (and longer) of life, regardless of whether therapy was administered or not. Although death is not associated with disease localized to the skin, eye, and/or mouth, approximately 30 percent of these children eventually develop evidence of neurologic impairment.[154,164,222]

Vesicles usually erupt from an erythematous base and are usually 1 to 2 mm in diameter. They can progress to larger bullous lesions greater than 1 cm in diameter. While discrete vesicles on various parts of the body are usually encountered, crops and clusters of vesicles have also been described. For most babies with neonatal herpes simplex virus infection localized to the skin, eye, and/or mouth, the vesicular skin rash involves multiple and often distant cutaneous sites. However, a limited number of babies have had infection of the skin limited to one or two vesicles and no further evidence of cutaneous disease. This group of babies warrants careful evaluation because many have developed encephalitic involvement when antiviral therapy was not administered. Other manifestations of skin lesions have included a zosteriform eruption.

Infections involving the eye may manifest as keratoconjunctivitis or, later, chorioretinitis. The eye can be the only site of herpes simplex virus involvement in the newborn.[218] These children present with keratoconjunctivitis or, surprisingly, evidence of microphthalmia and retinal dysplasia. In the presence of persistent disease and no therapy, chorioretinitis can result, caused by either herpes simplex type 1 or 2.[223–225] Keratoconjunctivitis, even in the presence of therapy, can progress to chorioretinitis, cataracts, and retinal detachment. Cataracts have been detected on long-term follow-up in three infants with proved perinatally acquired herpes simplex virus infections.[226]

Localized infection of the oropharyngeal cavity is found in approximately 10 percent of neonates with herpes simplex virus infection.

Long-term neurologic impairment including spastic quadriplegia, microcephaly, and blindness has been encountered in children whose disease appeared localized to the skin, eye, and/or mouth. Important questions regarding the pathogenesis of delayed-onset neurologic debility are raised by such clinical observations. Despite normal clinical examinations in these children, neurologic impairment has become apparent between 6 months and 1 year of life. The clinical presentation occurs in a manner similar to that associated with congenitally acquired toxoplasmosis or syphilis.

### Subclinical infection

The question of subclinical infection has been raised on numerous occasions. While it has been suggested that two newborns had evidence of herpes simplex virus infection proved by culture isolation of virus but without evidence of symptoms, it has been difficult to document such cases through the serial evaluation in over 1000 infants evaluated in multiple centers around the United States. Because of the propensity of the newborn to develop disease, any evidence of infection should be considered potentially serious and an indication for antiviral therapy.

## DIAGNOSIS

### Clinical evaluation

The clinical diagnosis of neonatal herpes simplex virus infection has become increasingly difficult because of the apparent decrease in the incidence of skin vesicles as an initial component of disease presentation. A variety of other infections of the newborn can masquerade as neonatal herpes simplex virus infections, including hyaline membrane disease, intraventricular hemorrhage, necrotizing enterocolitis, and various ocular or cutaneous disorders. Bacterial infections of newborns can mimic neonatal herpes simplex virus infection. It is not uncommon for some babies infected by herpes simplex virus to also experience a concomitant bacterial infection, particularly those caused by the group B streptococcus, *Staphylococcus aureus, Listeria monocytogenes,* and gram-negative bacterial infections.

As with other vesicular rashes, alternative causes of such exanthems should be excluded. Such diseases include varicella-zoster virus infection, enteroviral disease, and disseminated cytomegalovirus infection. With the aforementioned clinical findings in a child presenting to the hospital during the first 3 weeks of life, serious consideration to neonatal herpes simplex virus infection must be given. The presence of skin vesicles provides a natural site for attempted isolation of virus in order to rapidly determine if the etiology of the vesicular rash is herpes simplex virus as opposed to varicella-zoster virus. Simultaneously, serologic specimens and other virologic cultures should be obtained to exclude other common causes of perinatal infection, including toxoplasmosis, cytomegalovirus infection, rubella, and syphilis. Such cutaneous disorders as erythema toxicum, neonatal melanosis, or acrodermitis enteropathica often confuse physicians who suspect neonatal herpes simplex virus infections. Lesions associated with these diseases can be rapidly distinguished from those caused by herpes simplex virus by the presence of eosinophils on a Wright stain of a tissue scraping and by appropriate viral cultures.

The most difficult clinical diagnosis to make is that of herpes simplex encephalitis, as nearly 40 percent of children with central nervous system infection will not have a vesicular rash at the time of clinical presentation. Herpes simplex virus infection of the central nervous system should be suspected in the child who has evidence of acute neurologic deterioration with the onset of seizures and in the absence of intraventricular hemorrhage and metabolic causes. Serial increases in cerebrospinal fluid cell counts and protein concentrations, negative bacterial cultures of the cerebrospinal fluid, and negative CSF antigen studies help suggest the diagnosis of herpes simplex virus infection of the central nervous system. A maternal genital culture or history of genital herpes in either the mother or a sexual partner reinforces the suspicion of neonatal herpes simplex virus infection. As noted previously, noninvasive neurodiagnostic studies can be used to define the sites of involvement.

### Laboratory assessment

Every effort should be made to confirm infection by viral isolation, the definitive diagnostic method. If skin lesions are present, a scraping of skin vesicles should be transferred in appropriate virus transport media to a diagnostic virology laboratory. Clinical specimens should be shipped on ice for inoculation into appropriate cell culture systems (see Chapter 77). Shipping of specimens and their processing should be expedited. In addition to skin vesicles, other sites from which virus may be isolated include the cerebrospinal fluid, stool, urine, throat, nasopharynx, and conjunctivae. It may also be useful in infants with evidence of hepatitis or other gastrointestinal abnormalities to obtain duodenal aspirates for herpes simplex virus isolation. The virologic results of cultures from these sites along with clinical findings should be used in conjunction with clinical findings to establish a disease classification. Typing of a herpes simplex virus isolate may be done by one of several techniques (see Chapter 77).

In contrast to other neonatal infections, serologic diagnosis of HSV infection is not of great clinical value. Therapeutic decisions can *not* await the results of serologic studies. Further, the inability of the commonly available serologic assays to distinguish between antibodies to herpes simplex virus type 1 and 2 as well as to denote the presence of transplacentally acquired maternal IgG, as opposed to endogenously produced antibodies, makes the assessment of the neonate's antibody status difficult during acute infection. Serial antibody assessment may be useful if a mother without a prior history of herpes simplex virus infection has a primary infection late in gestation and transfers very little or no antibody to the fetus.

## TREATMENT

### Background

Since most babies acquire HSV infection at the time of delivery or shortly thereafter, successful antiviral therapy should decrease mortality and improve long-term outcome. Inherent in this presumption is the recognition that diagnosis shortly after the onset of clinical illness is essential, as is the case with other perinatally acquired infections. It has been documented that children presenting with disease localized to the skin, eye, and/or mouth can progress to either involvement of the central nervous system or disseminated infection in approximately 70 percent of cases.[162] When such events occur, the likelihood of an adequate outcome, even with established drugs, is not optimal as many of these children will either die or be left with significant neurologic impairment. Such factors must be considered in the development of any treatment strategy.

### Antiviral therapy

In a collaborative study, the use of vidarabine in infants with disseminated or localized central nervous system disease was associated with a decline in mortality rate from 75 to 40 percent (Fig. 70-1).[220] When outcome was examined according to each of the three disease classifications (Fig. 70-2), the best therapeutic result was achieved in babies with either encephalitis or skin, eye, and/or mouth infection. Mortality was decreased from nearly 90 percent in babies with disseminated infection to approximately 70 percent with therapy. For babies with encephalitis, mortality was decreased from 50 to 15 percent. Approximately 30 percent of children with either encephalitis or disseminated infection were reported as functioning normally at 1 year of life. Finally, following skin, eye, and/or mouth infection severe neurologic impairment was decreased from 30 to 10 percent with therapy.[163,220] Notably, there is no enhanced therapeutic benefit for mortality or morbidity if the dosage of vidarabine is increased.[163]

Therapy with vidarabine is most efficacious if instituted early.

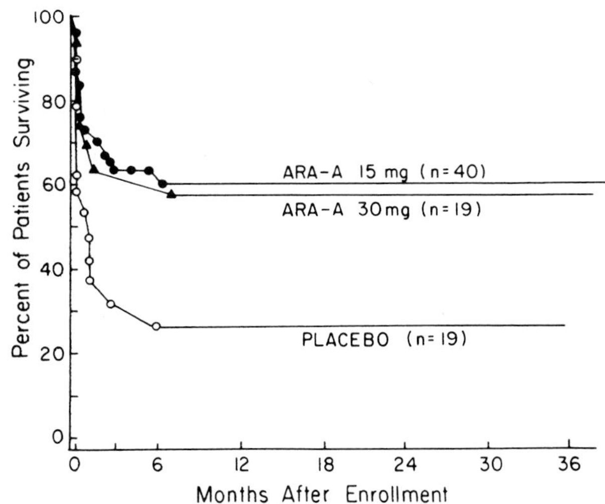


**Fig. 70-1.** Survival of babies with neonatal herpes simplex virus infections—encephalitis and disseminated infections—according to therapeutic regimen. *(Reproduced by permission of Pediatrics 72:778, 1983.)*

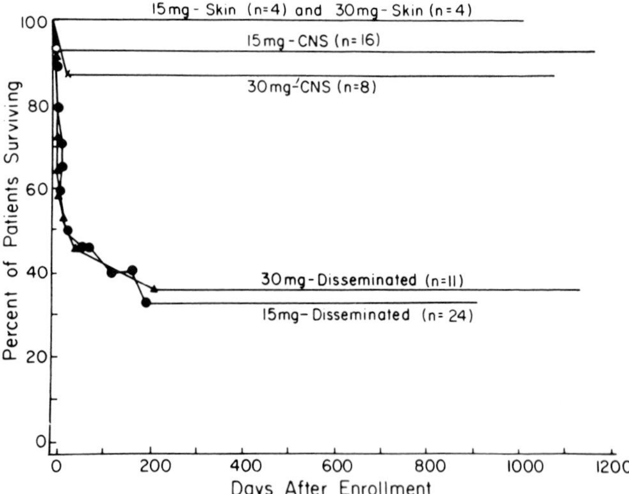


Fig. 70-2. Survival of babies with neonatal herpes simplex virus infection according to disease classification and vidarabine dosages. *(Reproduced by permission of Pediatrics 72:778, 1983.)*

Recognizing that disease is often present in these babies for 4 or 5 days, a window for administration of therapy earlier in life does exist. This point must be reiterated as earlier therapeutic intervention for any microbial infection will lead to improved outcome, particularly when a vital organ such as the brain is involved. Furthermore, when therapy is instituted early, fewer children will progress from localized skin involvement to more serious forms of infection. Therapy decreases the frequency of progression. For those infants receiving vidarabine at doses of 15 or 30 mg/kg/day, progression occurred in approximately 20 and 5 percent of infected babies, respectively.[163,218]

Vidarabine can be given intravenously in dosages of 15 to 30 mg/kg/day over a 12-h period for 10 to 14 days. At these dosages, there is no evidence of significant toxicity. Because a significantly lower percentage of babies receiving 30 mg/kg/day progress to more serious forms of illness, this higher dose is recommended. In some circumstances, longer periods of therapy may be indicated. Approximately 2 percent of infants treated for 10 to 14 days appear to have recurrence of infection leading to central nervous system disease.[163,220] Whether this clinical event is actually recurrence of disease or simply progression of the original infection remains poorly documented. However, these infants require the reinstitution of therapy. Of note, it has been suggested that progressive encephalitic disease can occur.[221]

Acyclovir, a relatively new antiviral compound presently undergoing extensive clinical trials, is activated by the thymidine kinase induced by herpes simplex virus and acts as competitive inhibitor of herpes simplex virus DNA polymerase.[227] It is a DNA chain terminator. Acyclovir has been established as efficacious for the treatment of primary genital herpes simplex infection when administered by intravenous, oral, and topical routes.[228–230] Furthermore, the oral and intravenous administration of acyclovir to the immunocompromised host decreases both the frequency of reactivation following immunosuppression and disease duration.[231,232] Acyclovir is superior to vidarabine for the treatment of herpes simplex encephalitis.[233] Because this compound is a selective inhibitor of viral replication, it has a low frequency of side effects. Acyclovir has become a preferred treatment for all herpes simplex virus infections in spite of the lack of published data to indicate utility for neonatal HSV infection.

Acyclovir has been administered to a limited number of infants with neonatal HSV.[234,235] The NIAID Collaborative Antiviral Study Group is currently completing its evaluation of the relative value of vidarabine versus acyclovir for the treatment of neonatal herpes simplex virus infection.[236] Three aspects of this study are worthy of note. First, there does not appear to be a difference in either mortality or morbidity for infected babies treated with either of these two drugs. Specifically, the mortality for babies with disseminated infection 1 year after therapy for acyclovir and vidarabine is 65 and 40 percent, respectively ($p = 0.123$), for encephalitis 15 percent for both treatment groups, and for disease localized to the skin, eye, and/or mouth, no baby died. Furthermore, there are no differences in either adverse effects or laboratory evidence of toxicity.[236] Second, the overall morbidity for all treatment groups shows no statistically significant difference when comparing vidarabine with acyclovir recipients. Third, regardless of therapeutic agent employed, there has been a significant increase in the number of babies who return to normal function. Of the babies enrolled, over 40 percent have disease localized to the skin, eye, and/or mouth.[164] This represents a threefold increase in babies with skin, eye, and/or mouth involvement as compared with previous studies and historical data. The number of babies with encephalitis has remained constant at about 30 percent while the number of babies with disseminated disease has decreased to 20 percent. The overall mortality is 19 percent and morbidity for this group of infants is significantly reduced from previous studies (Fig. 70-3). This change in the clinical spectrum of neonatal herpes simplex virus infection and the associated improved outcome is most likely related to earlier diagnosis and institution of antiviral therapy, thereby preventing

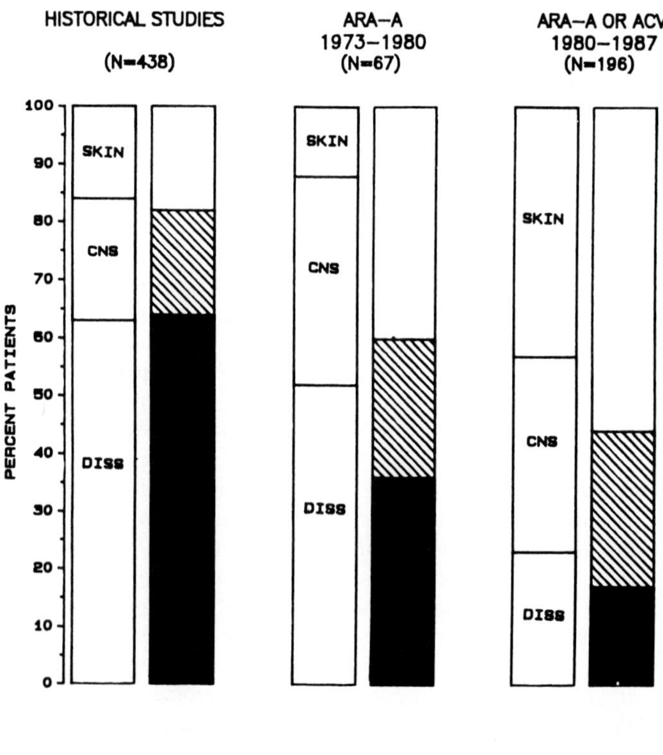


Fig. 70-3. Changing presentation and outcome of neonatal herpes simplex virus infections. The historical data were derived from babies who did not receive a therapeutic drug as previously reported by Dr. A. J. Nahmias. *(From RJ Whitley in Infectious Diseases of the Fetus and Newborn, JS Remington et al (eds). Philadelphia, Saunders, in press. Reproduced with permission of the publisher.)*

progression of disease from skin, eye, and/or mouth to more severe disease. Available data indicate that therapy was begun an average of 3 days earlier for this group of infants.[164] However, the mean duration of disease for all children, irrespective of disease classification, entered into these studies was 4 to 5 days. Thus, therapy can be instituted even earlier in the disease course than is currently occurring.

Infants with ocular involvement caused by herpes simplex virus should receive topical antiviral medication in addition to parenteral therapy. At the present time, few safety and tolerance data are available for topical ophthalmic antiviral drugs. In older patients, viroptic (trifluorothymidine) has the greatest antiviral activity and is the treatment of choice for herpes simplex virus infection of the eyes. Vidarabine ophthalmic and Stoxil (idoxuridine) have been utilized for a longer period of time. There is more experience regarding their safety in both adults and children, but they are less active.

During the course of therapy, careful monitoring is important in order to assess therapeutic response. Even in the absence of clinical evidence of encephalitis, the central nervous system should be examined serially for prognostic purposes. Evaluation of certain hepatic (increased SGPT or SGOT) and bone marrow parameters (decreased platelets) may indicate viral involvement of these organs or drug toxicity.

As for all drugs, a consideration of the therapeutic index for a ratio of efficacy to toxicity is important. Experience with vidarabine and acyclovir, thus far, has indicated little toxicity when used appropriately. However, the possibility of both acute and long-term toxicity should be considered in any child receiving parenteral antiviral therapy and assessed by serially evaluating bone marrow, renal, and hepatic function. The potential for long-term harm from these drugs remains to be defined. Since these compounds act at the level of DNA replication, physicians responsible for follow-up of these children should be aware of the possibility of mutagenic or even teratogenic effects which may not appear until decades later. A recent topic of intense debate is the possibility of the development of viral resistance to a drug; the clinical significance remains to be defined.

Since the child with neonatal herpes simplex virus infection, particularly with skin vesicles, will excrete virus in large quantities, isolation of the newborn is important in order to decrease the potential for nosocomial transmission of infection.

### Other therapeutic approaches

At present there is no indication that administration of immune globulin or hyperimmune globulin is of value in therapy of neonatal herpes simplex virus infection. While a series of studies have suggested that high levels of transplacental neutralizing antibodies will ameliorate neonatal herpes simplex virus infections[167,168] at the time of presentation with clinical disease, the presence or absence of antibodies does not influence the subsequent course of infection.[164] At present no other form of therapy is useful for treating neonatal herpes simplex virus infection. Various experimental modalities including BCG, interferon, immune modulators, and immunization have been used, but none have produced demonstrable effects.

## LONG-TERM MANAGEMENT OF INFECTED BABIES

With the advent of antiviral therapy, an increasing number of newborns who suffer from herpes simplex virus infection are surviving and require careful long-term follow-up. Three areas of follow-up warrant attention from a medical standpoint. First, it is not infrequent that parents of children with neonatal herpes simplex virus infection have significant guilt feelings. A once stable marriage can suffer and require interventive support from psychologists, psychiatrists, or marriage counselors. The family physician or pediatrician in this situation can provide a supportive role of great value to the family. Second, the most common complications of neonatal herpes simplex virus infection include neurologic and ocular sequelae which are detected only on long-term follow-up. Therefore, it is necessary that these children receive serial long-term evaluations from qualified pediatric specialists in these areas. These should include neurodevelopmental, ophthalmalogic, and hearing assessments. Third, the skin vesicles present in a majority of children at the time of onset of clinical illness or later during the acute course of infection recur with time. These vesicles provide a potential reservoir for transmission of infection to other children who have direct contact with these infants. The increasing use of day care for children in this country, including children surviving neonatal herpes simplex virus infections, has stimulated many questions concerning how these children should receive care. Certainly, there is some risk that children with recurrent herpes simplex virus skin lesions will transmit the virus to other children in this environment. The most reasonable recommendation in this situation appears to be simply to cover the lesions to prevent direct contact with them. It is much more likely that herpes simplex virus type 1 will be present in the day care environment in the form of symptomatic or asymptomatic gingivostomatitis. In both cases, virus is present in the mouth and pharynx, so that the frequent exchange of saliva and other respiratory droplets that occurs among children in this setting makes this route of transmission much more likely. Education of day care workers and the general public concerning herpesvirus infections, their implications, and the frequency with which they occur would do much to calm fears and correct common misconceptions concerning infections with this virus.

## PREVENTION

### Background

In spite of the progress that has been made over the last 15 years in the development of antiviral therapy for treatment of neonatal herpes simplex virus infection, the best approach is that of prevention. It is not surprising that because of the attention of the lay press to the devastating outcome of neonatal herpes, many women with known genital herpetic infection elect to be delivered by cesarean section rather than undergo the potential risks of exposure of the fetus to the virus at the time of vaginal delivery. As a consequence, an unnecessarily high frequency of cesarean infections is believed to occur in these individuals. All individuals involved in the care of pregnant women and their offspring should individualize the care of mother and child to optimize patient management. Advisory committees have recommended genital cultures of all women with a history of herpes beginning at 34 to 36 weeks in gestation and continuing weekly until delivery.[237,238] If cultures are positive within a week of delivery or lesions are present, cesarean section is indicated. Despite these measures, some cases will occur.[164,169]

Several questions regarding the value of cesarean section in the prevention of neonatal herpes simplex virus infections remain unresolved. While surgical abdominal delivery has been associated with the decreased transmission of infection when membranes are ruptured less than 4 h, cesarean section has not proved efficacious when membranes are ruptured for longer periods of time. Nevertheless, it has been recommended that when membranes are ruptured up to 24 h, cesarean section will be of value. It should be emphasized that while these recommendations are predicted upon logic, no data from adequately performed clinical trials are available.

For women with a past history of genital herpes simplex virus infection, a careful vaginal examination at presentation to the delivery suite is of paramount importance. While visualization of the cervix is often difficult, speculum examination for documentation of recurrent lesions is extremely important and should be attempted in these women. A culture for herpes simplex virus obtained at the time of delivery may be of great importance in establishing whether transmission of infection to the fetus is likely.

Both cost-benefit analyses and recent prospective studies have questioned the culture screening practice described above.[239] In spite of recommendations for screening prior to delivery, the crucial time to determine viral excretion is at the onset of labor. As recently proved, predelivery cultures are not predictive of those women who will excrete virus when in labor.[240] The fact that predelivery cultures not only fail to predict the woman who excretes virus at delivery but are also an unnecessarily large health care cost burden places their value in further question. Thus, alternative management approaches will have to be developed.

Clearly, identifying the woman who excretes herpes simplex virus at delivery and then optimizing either prophylactic protocols with safe and acceptable antivirals or delivery by cesarean section is the optimal way to manage genital infection at the time of delivery. Unfortunately, at present only isolation of virus in tissue culture will document the excretion of virus. Alternative rapid non-culture-based diagnostic approaches are being developed in order to expedite identification of women at risk for delivering an infected baby.[241] Nevertheless, many obstetrical services are resorting to culture of either mother or baby at the time of delivery or 24 h postpartum to identify those at greatest risk.

For infections which occur in the first half of gestation, no specific recommendations regarding the termination of pregnancy can be made at this time. It appears that the frequency of infection acquired in utero is approximately 1 in 200,000 deliveries and can occur as a consequence of either maternal primary or recurrent infection. Nevertheless, detailed prospective studies to document this occurrence have yet to be performed. Thus, no specific recommendation regarding termination of pregnancy with such findings can be made.

Serious forms of neonatal herpes simplex virus infections will continue to be associated with significant mortality and morbidity, even with acyclovir or vidarabine therapy. As a consequence, some investigators have suggested that acyclovir may be useful in preventing the occurrence of neonatal herpes simplex virus infections in infants who are delivered unknowingly through an infected birth canal. The prophylactic use of acyclovir has also been suggested in pregnant women who have a history of genital lesions, but there are no data to establish the value of prophylactic therapy for the newborn.

Suppressive therapy of genital herpes in women with a known history of recurrent infection may pose a significant but undefined risk to the fetus. Suppressive therapy of the woman with recurrent genital herpes may not prove efficacious. It has already been established from the suppressive trials of acyclovir in individuals with frequently recurrent genital herpes that reactivation of virus can occur in spite of the administration of 200 mg of acyclovir three times daily.[242,243] It is not unreasonable to think that such an event could occur in women who take acyclovir for suppressive therapy for recurrent genital herpes simplex virus infection during the last 4 weeks of gestation. Furthermore, the pharmacokinetics and metabolism of acyclovir in the human fetus is totally unknown at the present time. The possibility of acyclovir fetal nephrotoxicity creates a potential risk of drug administration which must be considered. In addition, it must be recognized that the women who are at greatest risk for delivering babies who develop neonatal herpes simplex virus infection are those least likely to have a history of recurrent genital herpes simplex virus infection.

## Management of high-risk women and their offspring

Infants delivered either vaginally or by cesarean section when membranes are intact to mothers who have no evidence of active genital herpetic infection are at low risk for acquiring neonatal herpes simplex virus infection. These children need no special evaluation in the nursery other than initial isolation until results of maternal genital cultures are available. With negative maternal genital cultures, these children can be discharged at the time the mother leaves the hospital.

Infants delivered vaginally to mothers with active genital herpes should be isolated if medically possible, and appropriate cultures obtained between 24 and 48 h after delivery. These cultures should be repeated at 2- to 3-day intervals during the period of time when infection is usually detectable—the first 4 weeks of life, but especially the first 2 weeks. Sites from which virus should be sought include eye, oro-/nasopharynx, and suspect lesions. These recommendations should serve only as guidelines until formal data are available. It should be emphasized that if any site is positive, a thorough virologic and clinical examination must be performed and therapy instituted. Other sites to be considered for viral isolation include the cerebrospinal fluid, urine, and buffy coat of the blood. In addition, neurodiagnostic evaluation by electroencephalogram and a computed tomographic scan, if indicated, is essential. In the absence of skin lesions and questionable central nervous system involvement, the value of a diagnostic brain biopsy should be considered.

## Postnatal infection

**Isolation of Mother from Baby.** An issue of frequent concern is whether the mother with active genital herpes simplex virus infection at delivery should be isolated from her child after delivery. Women with recurrent orolabial herpes simplex infection as well as cutaneous herpes simplex infections at other sites (breast lesions) are at similar risk for transmission of virus to their newborn. The risks presented to the newborn by other family members, medical personnel, and friends remain unknown but are low and do not justify removal of personnel from the nursery at this time. Since transmission occurs by direct contact with the virus, appropriate precautions by the mother, including careful hand washing before touching the infant, should prevent the necessity of separation of mother and child. Similarly, breast feeding is contraindicated only if the mother has vesicular lesions involving the breast. We do not isolate babies born to infected women unless they themselves become infected. Hospitalization is not prolonged in the uninfected child.

**Parental Education.** At the time of discharge, it is essential to educate parents with known recurrent herpetic infection regarding the possibility that their child may become infected. The parental stigma of a diagnosis of genital herpes and the monitoring procedures associated with evaluating the newborn can create excessive fear and anxiety in the family. The parents and responsible family members must be educated in order to relieve anxiety and provide prompt access to the health care delivery system should evidence of infection appear. Information regarding infection should include an overview of herpes simplex virus infection, the risks associated with transmission of infection to the newborn, the necessity for monitoring, the anticipated consequences of positive and negative viral cultures, planned approaches to treatment, and the potential for postnatal acquisition of infection at home.

**Hospital Staff.** At many institutions, a policy which requires transfer or provision of medical leave for nursing or other personnel in nurseries with a labial herpes simplex virus infection is impractical and causes an excessive burden in those attempting to provide adequate care. Temporary removal of personnel with cold sores has been advocated on some clinical services. As noted previously, individuals with herpetic whitlows carry a high risk of viral shedding. These individuals should be removed from care of newborns at risk for acquiring neonatal herpes simplex virus infection since even gloves may not prevent transmission of infection. Education regarding the risk of transmission of virus and the importance of hand washing when lesions are present should be repeatedly emphasized to health care workers. In addition, hospital personnel should wear masks when active lesions are present.

## CONCLUSION

Neonatal herpes simplex virus infection remains a life-threatening infection for the newborn in the United States today. With an increasing incidence of genital herpes and an increase in the incidence of neonatal herpes simplex virus infections, it is important that pediatricians, neonatologists, obstetricians, and family practitioners continue to maintain a high index of suspicion in infants whose symptoms may be compatible with herpes simplex virus infections so that early identification leads to prompt treatment. Hopefully, over the next decade, the development of safe and efficacious vaccines as well as a better understanding of factors associated with transmission of virus from mother to baby will allow ultimate prevention of neonatal herpes simplex virus infection.

### ACKNOWLEDGMENTS

The cytomegalovirus portion of this chapter was supported in part by grants from the National Institutes of Health, NICHD (HD10699), and General Clinical Research Center (M01 RR0032). Dr. Whitley is indebted to the members of the National Institute of Allergy and Infectious Diseases Collaborative Antiviral Study Group for their support and assistance in developing the database which provided the basis for this report, in particular Drs. C.A. Alford, Jr., and A.J. Nahmias. In addition, he is exceedingly grateful for the assistance of S. Burks, S. Byrd, and S. Culberson for preparation of this document.

Studies performed by Dr. Whitley and reported in this chapter were supported in part by research grant RR-032 from the Division of Research Resources, National Institutes of Health, grant CA-13148 from the National Cancer Institute, a contract, N01-AI-62554, from the Development and Applications Branch from the National Institute of Allergy and Infectious Diseases, and a grant from the state of Alabama.

## References

1 Weller TH: The cytomegaloviruses: Ubiquitous agents with protean clinical manifestations. *N Engl J Med* 285:203, 1971.

2 Ribbert H: Über protozoenartigen Zellen in der Nireeines syphilitischen Neugeboren und in der Parotis von Kindren. *Zentralbl Allg Pathol* 15:945, 1904.

3 Smith MG: Propagation of salivary gland virus of the mouse in tissue culture. *Proc Soc Exp Biol Med* 86:435, 1954.

4 Smith MG: Propagation in tissue cultures of a cytopathogenic virus from human salivary gland virus (SGV) disease. *Proc Soc Exp Biol Med* 92:424, 1956.

5 Rowe WP et al: Cytopathogenic agent resembling salivary gland virus recovered from tissue cultures of human adenoids. *Proc Soc Exp Biol Med* 92:418, 1956.

6 Weller TH et al: Isolation of intranuclear inclusion-producing agents from infants with illnesses resembling cytomegalic inclusion disease. *Proc Soc Exp Biol Med* 94:4, 1957.

7 Weller TH et al: Serologic differentiation of viruses responsible for cytomegalic inclusion disease. *Virology* 12:130, 1960.

8 Krech U et al: *Cytomegalovirus Infections of Man.* Basel, Karger, 1971, p 28.

9 Gold E, Nankervis GA: Cytomegalovirus, in *Viral Infections of Humans: Epidemiology and Control,* AS Evans (ed). New York, Elsevier, 1976, pp 143–161.

10 Alford CA et al: Epidemiology of cytomegalovirus, in *The Human Herpesviruses: An Interdisciplinary Perspective,* A Nahmias, W Dowdle, R Schinazi (eds). New York, Elsevier, 1981, pp 159–171.

11 Gold E, Nankervis GA: Cytomegalovirus, in *Viral Infections of Humans: Epidemiology and Control,* AS Evans (ed). New York, Plenum, 1982, pp 167–186.

12 Schopfer K et al: Congenital cytomegalovirus infection in newborn infants of mother infected before pregnancy. *Arch Dis Child* 53:536, 1978.

13 Numazaki Y et al: Primary infection with human cytomegalovirus: Virus isolation from healthy infants and pregnant women. *Am J Epidemiol* 91:410, 1970.

14 Vial P et al: Serological screening for cytomegalovirus, rubella virus, herpes simplex virus, hepatitis B virus and toxoplasma gondii in two populations of pregnant women in Chile. *Bol Of Sanit Panam* 99(5): 528, 1985.

15 Stagno S et al: Primary cytomegalovirus infection in pregnancy: Incidence, transmission to fetus and clinical outcome. *JAMA* 256:1904, 1986.

16 Hayes K et al: Cytomegalovirus in human milk. *N Engl J Med* 287:177, 1972.

17 Lang DJ, Krummer JF: Cytomegalovirus in semen: Observations in selected populations. *J Infect Dis* 132:472, 1975.

18 Reynolds DW et al: Maternal cytomegalovirus excretion and perinatal infection. *N Engl J Med* 289:1, 1973.

19 Stagno S et al: Breast milk and the risk of cytomegalovirus infection. *N Engl J Med* 302:1073, 1980.

20 Jordan MC et al: Association of cervical cytomegaloviruses with venereal disease. *N Engl J Med* 288:932, 1973.

21 Willmott FE: Cytomegalovirus in female patients adding a VD clinic. *Br J Vener Dis* 51:278, 1975.

22 Drew WL et al: Prevalence of cytomegalovirus infection in homosexual men. *J Infect Dis* 143:188, 1981.

23 Chandler SJ et al: The epidemiology of cytomegaloviral infection in women attending a sexually transmitted disease clinic. *J Infect Dis* 152:597, 1985.

24 Sarov B et al: Prevalence of antibodies to human cytomegalovirus in urban, kibbutz, and Bedouin children in Southern Israel. *J Med Virol* 10:195, 1982.

25 Pass RF et al: Cytomegalovirus infection in a day care center. *N Engl J Med* 307:477, 1982.

26 Adler SP et al: Cytomegalovirus transmission among children attending a day care center. *Pediatr Res* 19:285A, 1985.

27 Murph JR et al: The prevalence of cytomegalovirus infection in a midwest day care center. *Pediatr Res* 19:205A, 1985.

28 Dworsky ME et al: Cytomegalovirus transmission within a family. *Pediatr Infect Dis* 3:236, 1984.

29 Spector SA, Spector DH: Molecular epidemiology of cytomegalovirus infection in premature twin infants and their mother. *Pediatr Infect Dis* 1:405, 1982.

30 Yeager AS: Transmission of cytomegalovirus to mothers by infected infants: Another reason to prevent transfusion-acquired infections. *Pediatr Infect Dis* 2:295, 1983.

31 Dworsky ME et al: Occupational risk for primary cytomegalovirus infection. *N Engl J Med* 309:950, 1983.

32 Stagno S et al: Factors associated with primary cytomegalovirus infection during pregnancy. *J Med Virol* 13:347, 1984.

33 Taber LH et al: Acquisition of cytomegaloviral infections in families with young children: A serological study. *J Infect Dis* 151:948, 1985.

34 Pass RF et al: Increased rate of cytomegalovirus infection among parents of children attending day care centers. *N Engl J Med* 314:1414, 1986.

35 Adler SP: Molecular epidemiology of cytomegalovirus: Evidence for viral transmission to parents from their children infected at a day care center. *Clin Res* 34:348A, 1986.

36 Hutto C et al: Isolation of cytomegalovirus from toys and hands in a day care center. *J Infect Dis* 154:527, 1986.

37 Faix RG: Survival of cytomegalovirus on environmental surfaces. *J Pediatr* 106:649, 1985.

38 Stagno S et al: Congenital cytomegalovirus infection: Occurrence in an immune population. *N Engl J Med* 296:1254, 1977.

39 Embil JA et al: Congenital cytomegalovirus infection in two siblings from consecutive pregnancies. *J Pediatr* 77:417, 1970.

40 Stagno S et al: Congenital cytomegalovirus infection (C-CMV): Consecutive occurrence with similar antigenic viruses. *Pediatr Res* 7:141, 1973.

41 Krech U et al: Congenital cytomegalovirus infection in siblings from consecutive pregnancies. *Helv Paediatr Acta* 26:355, 1971.

42 Stagno S et al: Maternal cytomegalovirus infection and perinatal transmission, in *Clinical Obstetrics and Gynecology,* GE Knox (ed). Philadelphia, Lippincott, 1982, pp 563–576.

43 Stern H, Tucker SM: Prospective study of cytomegalovirus infection in pregnancy. *Br Med J* 2:268, 1973.

44 Nankervis A et al: Primary infection with cytomegalovirus during pregnancy. *Pediatr Res* 8:487, 1974.

45 Gump DW et al: Contraception and cervical colonization with mycoplasmas and infection with cytomegalovirus. *Fertil Steril* 26:1135, 1975.

46 Stagno S et al: Cervical cytomegalovirus excretion in pregnant and nonpregnant women: Suppression in early gestation. *J Infect Dis* 131:522, 1975.

47 Knox GE et al: Comparative prevalence of subclinical cytomegalovirus and herpes simplex virus infections in the genital and urinary tracts of low income, urban women. *J Infect Dis* 140:419, 1979.

48 Gehrz RC et al: Cytomegalovirus-specific humoral and cellular immune response in human pregnancy. *J Infect Dis* 143:391, 1981.

49 Stern H et al: An early maker of fetal infection after primary cytomegalovirus infection in pregnancy. *Br Med J* 292:718, 1986.

50 Chretien JH et al: Venereal causes of cytomegalovirus mononucleosis. *JAMA* 238:1644, 1977.

51 Handsfield HH et al: Cytomegalovirus infection in sex partners: Evidence for sexual transmission. *J Infect Dis* 151:344, 1985.

52 Kreel I et al: A syndrome following total body perfusion. *Surg Gynecol Obstet* 111:317, 1960.

53 Adler SP: Transfusion-associated cytomegalovirus infections. *Rev Infect Dis* 5:977, 1983.

54 Seaman AJ, Starr A: Febrile postcardiotomy lymphocytic splenomegaly: A new entity. *Ann Surg* 156:956, 1962.

55 Onorato IM et al: Epidemiology of cytomegalovirus infections: Recommendations for prevention and control. *Rev Infect Dis* 7:479, 1985.

56 Armstrong JA et al: Cytomegalovirus infection in children undergoing open-heart surgery. *Yale J Biol Med* 49:83, 1976.

57 Prince AM et al: A serologic study of cytomegalovirus infections associated with blood transfusions. *N Engl J Med* 284:1125, 1971.

58 Rinaldo CR et al: Interaction of cytomegalovirus with leukocytes from patients with mononucleosis due to cytomegalovirus. *J Infect Dis* 136:667, 1977.

59 Stevens DP et al: Asymptomatic cytomegalovirus infection following blood transfusion in tumor surgery. *JAMA* 211:1341, 1970.

60 Kaariainen L et al: Rise of cytomegalovirus antibodies in an infectious mononucleosis-like syndrome after transfusion. *Br Med J* 1:1270, 1966.

61 Lang DJ et al: Reduction of postperfusion cytomegalovirus infections following the use of leukocyte depleted blood. *Transfusion* 17:391, 1977.

62 McCracken GJ et al: Congenital cytomegalic inclusion disease: A longitudinal study of 20 patients. *Am J Dis Child* 117:522, 1969.

63 Kumar A et al: Acquisition of cytomegalovirus infection in infants following exchange transfusion: A prospective study. *Transfusion* 20:327, 1980.

64 King-Lewis PA, Gardner SD: Congenital cytomegalic inclusion diseases following intrauterine transfusion. *Br Med J* 2:603, 1969.

65 Pass MA et al: Evaluation of a walking donor blood transfusion program in an intensive care nursery. *J Pediatr* 89:646, 1976.

66 Yeager AS: Transfusion-acquired cytomegalovirus infection in newborn infants. *Am J Dis Child* 128:478, 1974.

67 Yeager AS et al: Prevention of transfusion-acquired cytomegalovirus infection in newborn infants. *J Pediatr* 98:281, 1981.

68 Adler SP et al: Cytomegalovirus infections in neonates due to blood transfusions. *Pediatr Infect Dis* 2:114, 1983.

69 Yeager AS: Longitudinal, serological study of cytomegalovirus infections in nurses and in personnel without patient contact. *J Clin Microbiol* 2:448, 1975.

70 Friedman HM et al: Acquisition of cytomegalovirus infection among female employees at a pediatric hospital. *Pediatr Infect Dis* 3:233, 1984.

71 Balfour CL, Balfour HH: Cytomegalovirus is not an occupational risk for nurses in renal transplant and neonatal units. *JAMA* 256:1909, 1986.

72 Stagno S et al: Congenital cytomegalovirus infection: The relative importance of primary and recurrent maternal infection. *N Engl J Med* 306:945, 1982.

73 Brady MT et al: Cytomegalovirus infection in pediatric house officers: Susceptibility and risk of primary infection. *Pediatr Res* 19:179A, 1985.

74 Adler SP et al: Molecular epidemiology of cytomegalovirus in a nursery: Lack of evidence for nosocomial transmission. *J Pediatr* 108:117, 1986.

75 Demmler GJ et al: Nosocomial transmission of cytomegalovirus in a children's hospital. *Pediatr Res* 20:308A, 1986.

76 Yow MD et al: Use of restriction enzymes to investigate the source of a primary CMV infection in a pediatric nurse. *Pediatrics* 70:713, 1982.

77 Wilfert CV et al: Restriction endonuclease analysis of cytomegalovirus DNA as an epidemiological tool. *Pediatrics* 70:717, 1982.

78 Ahlfors K et al: Congenital cytomegalovirus infection and disease in Sweden and the relative importance of primary and secondary maternal infections. *Scand J Infect Dis* 16:129, 1984.

79 Rutter D et al: Cytomegalic inclusion disease after recurrent maternal infection. *Lancet* 2:1182, 1985.

80 Griffiths PD: Cytomegalovirus, in *Principles and Practice of Clinical*

*Virology,* AJ Zuckerman, JE Banatvala, JR Pattison (eds). New York, Wiley, 1987, pp 75–109.
81 Stagno S et al: Congenital and perinatal cytomegaloviral infections. *Semin Perinatol* 7:31, 1983.
82 Stagno S et al: Comparative serial virologic and serologic studies of symptomatic and subclinical congenitally and natally acquired cytomegalovirus infections. *J Infect Dis* 132:568, 1975.
83 Britt WJ, Auger D: Antibody reactivity against CMV envelope proteins in infants with symptomatic and subclinical congenital infection. Program and Abstracts, 25th ICAAC 908, 1985.
84 Pereira L et al: Cytomegalovirus infected cell polypeptides immune precipitated by sera from children with congenital and perinatal infections. *Infect Immun* 39:100, 1983.
85 Stagno S et al: Immune complexes in congenital and natal cytomegalovirus infections of man. *J Clin Invest* 60:838, 1977.
86 Pass RF et al: Specific cell mediated immunity and the natural history of congenital infection with cytomegalovirus. *J Infect Dis* 148:953, 1983.
87 Pass RF et al: Specific lymphocyte blastogenic responses in children with cytomegalovirus and herpes simplex virus infections acquired early in infancy. *Infect Immun* 34:166, 1981.
88 Reynolds DW et al: Specific cell-mediated immunity in children with congenital and neonatal cytomegalovirus infection and their mothers. *J Infect Dis* 140:493, 1979.
89 Starr SE et al: Impaired cellular immunity to cytomegalovirus in congenitally infected children and their mothers. *J Infect Dis* 140:500, 1979.
90 Stagno S, Whitley RJ: Herpesvirus infections of pregnancy. *N Engl J Med* 313:1270, 1985.
91 Griffiths PD, Baboonian C: A prospective study of primary cytomegalovirus infection during pregnancy: Final report. *Br J Obstet Gynaecol* 91:307, 1984.
92 Martin DC et al: Cytomegalovirus viremia detected by molecular hybridization and electron microscopy. *Ann Intern Med* 100:222, 1984.
93 Spector SA, Spector DH: The use of DNA probes in studies of human cytomegalovirus. *Clin Chem* 31:1514, 1985.
94 Schrier RD et al: Detection of human cytomegalovirus in peripheral blood lymphocytes in a natural infection. *Science* 230:1048, 1985.
95 Weller TH, Hanshaw JB: Virologic and clinical observations on cytomegalic inclusion disease. *N Engl J Med* 266:1233, 1962.
96 Pass RF et al: Outcome of symptomatic congenital cytomegalovirus infection: Results of long-term longitudinal follow-up. *Pediatrics* 66:758, 1980.
97 Hanshaw JB, Dudgeon JA (eds): *Viral Diseases of the Fetus and Newborn.* Philadelphia, Saunders, 1978.
98 Medearis TN: Observations concerning human cytomegalovirus infection and disease. *Bull Johns Hopkins Hosp* 114:181, 1964.
99 Stagno S et al: Auditory and visual defects resulting from symptomatic and subclinical congenital cytomegaloviral and toxoplasma infections. *Pediatrics* 59:669, 1977.
100 Stagno S et al: Infant pneumonitis associated with cytomegalovirus, chlamydia, pneumocystis and ureaplasma—A prospective study. *Pediatrics* 68:322, 1981.
101 Stagno S et al: Defects of tooth structure in congenital cytomegalovirus infection. *Pediatrics* 69:646, 1982.
102 Melish ME, Hanshaw JB: Congenital cytomegalovirus infection: Developmental progress of infants detected by routine screening. *Am J Dis Child* 126:190, 1973.
103 Saigal S et al: The outcome in children with congenital cytomegalovirus infection: A longitudinal follow-up study. *Am J Dis Child* 136:896, 1982.
104 Williamson WD et al: Symptomatic congenital cytomegalovirus: Disorders of language, learning and hearing. *Am J Dis Child* 136:902, 1982.
105 Berenberg W, Nankervis G: Long-term follow-up of cytomegalic inclusion disease of infancy. *Pediatrics* 37:403, 1970.
106 Kumar ML et al: Inapparent congenital cytomegalovirus infection: A follow-up study. *N Engl J Med* 288:1370, 1973.
107 Reynolds DW et al: Inapparent congenital cytomegalovirus infection with elevated cord IgM levels: Causal relationship with auditory and mental deficiency. *N Engl J Med* 290:291, 1974.
108 Pearl KN et al: Neurodevelopmental assessment after congenital cytomegalovirus infection. *Arch Dis Child* 61:232, 1986.
109 Whitley RJ et al: Protracted pneumonitis in young infants associated with perinatally acquired cytomegaloviral infection. *J Pediatr* 89:16, 1976.
110 Brasfield DM et al: Infant pneumonitis associated with cytomegalovirus, chlamydia, pneumocystis and ureaplasma: Follow-up. *Pediatrics* 79:76, 1987.
111 Yeager AS et al: Sequelae of maternally derived cytomegalovirus infections in premature infants. *Pediatrics* 102:918, 1983.
112 Paryani SG et al: Sequelae of acquired cytomegalovirus infection in premature and sick term infants. *J Pediatr* 107:451, 1985.
113 Ballard RB et al: Acquired cytomegalovirus infection in preterm infants. *Am J Dis Child* 133:482, 1979.
114 Alford CA: Chronic intrauterine and perinatal infections, in *Antiviral Agents and Viral Diseases of Man,* 2d ed, GJ Galasso, RA Buchanan (eds). New York, Raven, 1984, pp 433–486.
115 Ho M: Treatment and prevention of cytomegalovirus infection, in *Cytomegalovirus Biology and Infection: Current Topics in Infectious Disease,* WB Greenough, TC Merigan (eds). New York, Plenum, 1982, pp 205–213.
116 Plotkin SA et al: Prevention and treatment of cytomegalovirus infection, in *The Human Herpesviruses: An Interdisciplinary Perspective,* A Nahmias, W Dowdle, R Schinazi (eds). New York, Elsevier, 1981, pp 403–413.
117 Collaborative DHPG Treatment Study Group: Treatment of serious cytomegalovirus infections with 9-(1, 3-dihydroxy-2-propoxymethyl) guanine in patients with AIDS and other immunodeficiencies. *N Engl J Med* 314:801, 1986.
118 Meyers JD: Prevention and treatment of cytomegalovirus infections with interferons and immune globulins. *Infection* 12:143, 1984.
119 Dworsky ME et al: Therapeutic approaches to the control of cytomegalovirus infections, in *CMV: Pathogenesis and Prevention of Human Infection,* SA Plotkin, S Michelson, JS Pagano, F Rapp (eds). New York, Alan R Liss, 1984, vol 20, pp 65–85.
120 Bowden RA et al: Cytomegalovirus immune globulin and seronegative blood products to prevent primary cytomegalovirus infection after marrow transplantation. *N Engl J Med* 314:1006, 1986.
121 Condie RM, O'Reilly RJ: Prevention of cytomegalovirus infection in bone marrow transplant recipients by prophylaxis with an intravenous, hyperimmune cytomegalovirus globulin, in *CMV: Pathogenesis and Prevention of Human Infection,* SA Plotkin, S Michelson, JS Pagano, F Rapp (eds). New York, Alan R Liss, 1984, pp 327–344.
122 Elek SD, Stern H: Development of a vaccine against mental retardation caused by cytomegalovirus infection in utero. *Lancet* 1:1, 1974.
123 Plotkin SA et al: Candidate cytomegalovirus strain for human vaccination. *Infect Immun* 12:521, 1975.
124 Plotkin S et al: *CMV: Pathogenesis and Prevention of Human Infection.* New York, Alan R Liss, 1984.
125 Stern H: Live cytomegalovirus vaccination of healthy volunteers: eight-year follow-up studies, in *CMV: Pathogenesis and Prevention of Human Infection,* SA Plotkin, S Michelson, JS Pagano, F Rapp (eds). New York, Alan R Liss, 1984, pp 263–269.
126 Brady MT et al: Use of deglycerolized red blood cells to prevent posttransfusion infection with cytomegalovirus in neonates. *J Infect Dis* 150:334, 1984.
127 Peckham CS et al: Cytomegalovirus infection in pregnancy: Preliminary findings from a prospective study. *Lancet* 1:1352, 1983.
128 Hunter K et al: Prenatal screening of pregnant women for infections due to cytomegalovirus, Epstein-Barr, herpes, rubella and Toxoplasma gondii. *Am J Obstet Gynecol* 145:269, 1983.
129 Pass RF, Stagno S: Cytomegalovirus, in *Hospital Acquired Infection in the Pediatric Patient,* L Donowitz (ed). Baltimore, Williams and Wilkins, 1988, p 174.

130 Mettler C: *History of Medicine*. Philadelphia, Blakiston, 1947, p 356.
131 Astruc J: *De Morbis Venereis Libri Sex*. Paris, G Cavelier, 1736, p 361.
132 Gruter W: Das herpesvirus, seine atiologische und klinische bedeutung. *Munch Med Wochenschr* 71:1058, 1924.
133 Hass M: Hepatoadrenal necrosis with intranuclear inclusion bodies: Report of a case. *Am J Pathol* 11:127, 1935.
134 Batignani A: Conjunctivite da virus erpetico in neonato. *Boll Ocul* 13:1217, 1934.
135 Nahmias AJ, Dowdle W: Antigenic and biologic differences in herpesvirus hominis. *Prog Med Virol* 10:110, 1968.
136 McClung H et al: Relative concentrations in human sera of antibodies to cross-reacting and specific antigens of herpes simplex virus types 1 and 2. *Am J Epidemiol* 104:192, 1976.
137 Smith IW et al: The incidence of herpesvirus hominis antibodies in the population. *J Hyg (Camb)* 65:395, 1967.
138 Wentworth BB, Alexander ER: Seroepidemiology of infections due to members of the herpesvirus group. *Am J Epidemiol* 94:496, 1971.
139 Nahmias AJ et al: Antibodies to herpesvirus hominis types 1 and 2 in humans. *Am J Epidemiol* 91:539, 1970.
140 Allen WP, Rapp F: Concept review of genital herpes vaccines. *J Infect Dis* 145:413, 1982.
141 Brown ZA et al: Effects on infants of a first episode of genital herpes during pregnancy. *N Engl J Med* 317:1246, 1987.
142 Stavraky KM et al: Sexual and socioeconomic factors affecting the risk of past infections with herpes simplex virus type 2. *Am J Epidemiol* 118:109, 1983.
143 Mann SL et al: Prevalence and incidence of herpesvirus infections among homosexually active men. *J Infect Dis* 149:1026, 1984.
144 Nahmias AJ et al: Prevalence of herpes simplex virus (HSV) type-specific antibodies in a USA prepaid group medical practice population. Sixth International Meeting of the International Society for STD Research, London, England, 1985.
145 Flewett TH et al: Acute hepatitis due to herpes simplex virus in an adult. *J Clin Pathol* 22:60, 1969.
146 Anderson JM, Nicholls MWN: Herpes encephalitis in pregnancy. *Br Med J* 1:632, 1972.
147 Goyette RE et al: Fulminant herpesvirus hominis hepatitis during pregnancy. *Obstet Gyneol* 43:191, 1974.
148 Young EJ et al: Disseminated herpesvirus infection: Associated with primary genital herpes in pregnancy. *JAMA* 235:2731, 1976.
149 Hensleigh PA et al: Systemic herpesvirus hominis in pregnancy. *J Reprod Med* 22:171, 1979.
150 Peacock JE, Sarubbi FA: Disseminated herpes simplex virus infection during pregnancy. *Obstet Gynecol* 61:13, 1983.
151 Nahmias AJ et al: Herpes simplex, in *Infectious Diseases of the Fetus and Newborn Infant,* JS Remington, JO Klein (eds). Philadelphia, Saunders, 1983, p 638.
152 Hutto C et al: Intrauterine herpes simplex virus infections. *J Pediatr* 110:97, 1987.
153 Nahmias AJ et al: Perinatal risk associated with maternal genital herpes simplex virus infection. *Am J Obstet Gynecol* 110:825, 1971.
154 Grossman JH et al: Management of genital herpes simplex virus infection during pregnancy. *Obstet Gynecol* 58:1, 1981.
155 Harger JH et al: Characteristics and management of pregnancy in women with genital herpes simplex virus infection. *Am J Obstet Gynecol* 145:784, 1983.
156 Tejani N et al: Subclinical herpes simplex genitalis infections in the perinatal period. *Am J Obstet Gynecol* 135:547, 1978.
157 Bolognese RJ et al: Herpesvirus hominis type II infections in asymptomatic pregnant women. *Obstet Gynecol* 48:507, 1976.
158 Vontver LA et al: Recurrent genital herpes simplex virus infection in pregnancy: Infant outcome and frequency of asymptomatic recurrences. *Am J Obstet Gynecol* 143:75, 1982.
159 Rattray MC et al: Recurrent genital herpes among women: Symptomatic versus asymptomatic viral shedding. *Br J Vener Dis* 54:252, 1978.
160 Adams HG et al: Genital herpetic infection in men and women: Clinical course and effect of topical application of adenine arabinoside. *J Infect Dis* 133:151, 1976.
161 Guinan ME et al: The course of untreated recurrent genital herpes simplex infection in 27 women. *N Engl J Med* 304:759, 1981.
162 Whitley RJ et al: The natural history of herpes simplex virus infection of mother and newborn. *Pediatrics* 66:489, 1980.
163 Whitley RJ et al: Neonatal herpes simplex virus infection: Follow-up evaluation of vidarabine therapy. *Pediatrics* 72:778, 1983.
164 Whitley RJ et al: Changing presentation of neonatal herpes simplex virus infection. *J Inf Diseases* 158:109–116, 1988.
165 Corey L et al: Genital herpes simplex virus infections: Clinical manifestations, course and complications. *Ann Intern Med* 98:958, 1983.
166 Corey L: The diagnosis and treatment of genital herpes. *JAMA* 248:1041, 1982.
167 Yeager AS et al: Relationship of antibody in outcome in neonatal herpes simplex virus infections. *Infect Immun* 29:532, 1980.
168 Prober CG et al: Low risk of herpes simplex virus infections in neonates exposed to the virus at the time of vaginal delivery to mothers with recurrent genital herpes simplex virus infections. *N Engl J Med* 316:240, 1987.
169 Stone KM et al: Neonatal herpes—Results of one year's surveillance. Abstract 515, Interscience Conference on Antimicrobial Agents and Chemotherapy, 1985.
170 Parvey LS, Chien LT: Neonatal herpes simplex virus infection introduced by fetal monitor scalp electrode. *Pediatrics* 65:1150, 1980.
171 Kaye EM, Dooling EC: Neonatal herpes simplex meningoencephalitis associated with fetal monitor scalp electrodes. *Neurology* 31:1045, 1981.
172 Sullivan-Bolyai J et al: Neonatal herpes simplex virus infection in King County, Washington: Increasing incidence and epidemiologic correlates. *JAMA* 250:3059, 1983.
173 Adam E et al: Seroepidemiologic studies of herpesvirus type 2 and carcinoma of the cervix. *Uganda J Natl Cancer Inst* 48:65, 1972.
174 Templeton AC: Generalized herpes simplex in malnourished children. *J Clin Pathol* 23:24, 1970.
175 Florman AL et al: Intrauterine infection with herpes simplex virus: Resultant congenital malformations. *JAMA* 225:129, 1973.
176 South MA et al: Congenital malformation of the central nervous system associated with genital type (type 2) herpesvirus. *J Pediatr* 75:8, 1969.
177 Baldwin S et al: Intrauterine HSV infection. *J Teratology,* in press, 1987.
178 Garcia A: Maternal herpes simplex infection causing abortion: Histopathologic study of the placenta. *O Hospital* 78:1266, 1970.
179 Witzleben CL, Driscoll SG: Possible transplacental transmission of herpes simplex infection. *Pediatrics* 36:192, 1965.
180 Gagnon A: Transplacental inoculation of fatal herpes simplex in the newborn. *Obstet Gynecol* 31:682, 1968.
181 Light IJ: Postnatal acquisition of herpes simplex virus by the newborn infant: A review of the literature. *Pediatrics* 63:480, 1979.
182 Linnemann CC et al: Transmission of herpes simplex virus type 1 in a nursery for the newborn: Identification of viral isolates by DNA "fingerprinting." *Lancet* 1:964, 1978.
183 Light IJ: Postnatal acquisition of herpes simplex virus by the newborn infant: A review of the literature. *Pediatrics* 63:480, 1979.
184 Hammerberg O et al: An outbreak of herpes simplex virus type 1 in an intensive care nursery. *Pediatr Infect Dis* 2:290, 1983.
185 Sullivan-Bolyai JZ et al: Disseminated neonatal herpes simplex virus type 1 from a maternal breast lesion. *Pediatrics* 71:455, 1983.
186 Dunkle LM et al: Neonatal herpes simplex infection possibly acquired via maternal breast milk. *Pediatrics* 63:150, 1979.
187 Kibrick S: Herpes simplex virus in breast milk. *Pediarics* 64:390, 1979.
188 Yeager AS et al: Transmission of herpes simplex virus from the father to neonate. *J Pediatr* 103:905, 1983.
189 Douglas JM et al: Acquisition of neonatal HSV-1 infection from a paternal source contact. *J Pediatr* 103:908, 1983.
190 Rawls WE, Campione-Piccardo J: *The Human Herpesviruses: An*

*Interdisciplinary Perspective.* A Nahmias, W Dowdle and R Schinazi (eds). New York, Elsevier, 1981, p 137.

191 Nahmias AJ, Josey WE: *Viral Infections of Humans.* A Evans (ed). New York, Plenum, 1981, p 351.

192 Hatherley LI et al: Herpesvirus in an obstetric hospital. Asymptomatic virus excretion in staff members. *Med J Aust* 2:273, 1980.

193 Schreiner R et al: Maternal oral herpes: Isolation policy. *Pediatrics* 63:247, 1979.

194 Hatherley LI et al: Herpes virus in an obstetric hospital: Herpetic eruptions. *Med J Austr* 2:205, 1980.

195 Hatherley LI et al: Herpes virus in an obstetric hospital. Prevalence of antibodies in patients and staff. *Med J Aust* 2:325, 1980.

196 Notkins AL: Immune mechanisms by which the spread of viral infections is stopped. *Cell Immunol* 11:478, 1974.

197 Lopez C: *The Herpesviruses. Immunobiology and Prophylaxis of Human Herpesvirus Infections.* B Roizman and C Lopez (eds). New York, Plenum, 1985, vol 4, p 37.

198 Pakes JE et al: Lymphocyte reactivity contributes to protection conferred by specific antibody passively transferred to herpes simplex virus-infected mice. *Infect Immun* 29:642, 1980.

199 Kahlon J, Whitley RJ: Antibody response of the newborn after herpes simplex virus infection. *J Infect Dis* 158:925, 1988.

200 Sullender WM et al: Humoral and cell-mediated immunity in neonates with herpes simplex virus infection. *J Infect Dis* 155:28, 1987.

201 Rasmussen L, Merigan TC: Role of T-lymphocytes in cellular immune responses during herpes simplex virus infection in humans. *Proc Natl Acad Sci USA* 75:3957, 1978.

202 Pass RF et al: Specific lymphocyte blastogenic responses in children with cytomegalovirus and herpes simplex virus infections acquired early in infancy. *Infect Immun* 34:166, 1981.

203 Chilmonczyk BA et al: Characterization of the human newborn response to herpesvirus antigen. *J Immunol* 134:4184, 1985.

204 Burchett SK et al: Ontogeny of neonatal mononuclear cell transformation and interferon gamma production after herpes simplex virus stimulation. *Clin Res* 34:129, 1986.

205 Taylor S, Bryson YJ: Impaired production of interferon by newborn cells in vitro is due to a functionally immature macrophage. *J Immunol* 134:1493, 1985.

206 Rouse BT: *The Herpesviruses. Immunobiology and Prophylaxis of Human Herpesvirus Infections,* B Roizman and C Lopez (eds). New York, Plenum, 1985, vol 4, p 103.

207 Kohl S et al: Normal function of neonatal polymorphonuclear leukocytes in antibody-dependent cellular cytotoxicity to herpes simplex virus infected cells. *J Pediatr* 98:783, 1981.

208 Kohl S et al: Human neonatal and maternal monocyte-macrophage and lymphocyte mediated antibody dependent cytotoxicity to herpes simplex infected cells. *J Pediatr* 93:206, 1978.

209 Zisman B et al: Selective effects of anti-macrophages. An analysis of the cell virus interaction. *J Exp Med* 133:19, 1971.

210 Trofatter KJ et al: Growth of type 2 herpes simplex virus in newborn and adult mononuclear leukocytes. *Intervirology* 2:117, 1979.

211 Mintz H et al: Age dependent resistance of human alveolar macrophages to herpes simplex virus. *Infect Immun* 28:417, 1980.

212 Lopez C et al: Marrow dependent cells depleted by Sr mediate genetic resistance to herpes simplex virus type 1 infection in mice. *Infect Immun* 28:1028, 1980.

213 Armerding D, Rossiter H: Induction of natural killer cells by herpes simplex virus type 2 in resistant and sensitive inbred mouse strains. *Immunobiology* 158:369, 1981.

214 Hirsch MS et al: Macrophages and age-dependent resistance to herpes simplex virus in mice. *J Immunol* 104:1160, 1970.

215 Kohl S et al: Protection of neonatal mice against herpes simplex viral infection by human antibody and leukocytes from adult, but not neonatal humans. *J Immunol* 127:1273, 1981.

216 Nahmias A et al: *Advances in Pediatrics,* I Schulman (ed). Chicago, Year Book Medical Publishers, 1970, p 186.

217 Arvin AM et al: Neonatal herpes simplex infection in the absence of mucocutaneous lesions. *J Pediatr* 100:715, 1982.

218 Whitley RJ, Hutto C: Neonatal herpes simplex virus infections. *Pediatr Rev* 7:119, 1985.

219 Yeager AS, Arvin AM: Reason for the absence of a history of recurrent genital infections in mothers of neonates infected with herpes simplex virus. *Pediatrics* 73:188, 1984.

220 Whitley RJ et al: Vidarabine therapy of neonatal herpes simplex virus infection. *Pediatrics* 66:495, 1980.

221 Gutman LT et al: Herpes simplex virus encephalitis in children: Analysis of cerebrospinal fluid and progressive neurodevelopmental deterioration. *J Infect Dis* 154:415, 1986.

222 Mizrahi EM, Tharp BR: A unique electroencephalogram pattern in neonatal herpes simplex virus encephalitis. *Neurology* 31:164, 1981.

223 Nahmias A et al: Eye infections. *Surv Ophthalmol* 21:100, 1976.

224 Nahmias A, Hagler W: Ocular manifestations of herpes simplex in the newborn. *Int Ophthalmol Clin* 12:191, 1972.

225 Reersted P, Hansen B: Chorioretinitis of the newborn with herpes simplex type 1:Report of a case. *Acta Ophthalmol* 57:1096, 1979.

226 Cibis A, Burde RM: Herpes simplex virus induced congenital cataracts. *Arch Ophthalmol* 85:220, 1971.

227 Elion GB et al: Selectivity of action of an antiherpetic agent 9-(2-hydroxyethoxymethyl) guanine. *Proc Natl Acad Sci USA* 74:5716, 1977.

228 Corey L et al: Treatment of primary first-episode genital herpes simplex virus infections with acyclovir: Results of topical, intravenous and oral therapy. *J Antimicrob Chemother* 12:79, 1983.

229 Bryson YJ: Treatment of first episode genital herpes simplex virus infections with oral acyclovir. A randomized double blind controlled trial in normal subjects. *N Engl J Med* 308:916, 1983.

230 Corey L et al: A trial of topical acyclovir in genital herpes simplex virus infections. *N Engl J Med* 306:1313, 1982.

231 Saral R et al: Acyclovir prophylaxis of herpes simplex virus infections. A randomized double blind, controlled trial in bone marrow transplant patients. *N Engl J Med* 305:63, 1981.

232 Meyers JD et al: Multicenter collaborative trial of intravenous acyclovir for treatment of mucocutaneous herpes simplex virus infection in the immunocompromised host. *Am J Med* 73(1A):229, 1981.

233 Whitley RJ et al: Vidarabine versus acyclovir therapy of herpes simplex encephalitis. *N Engl J Med* 314:144, 1986.

234 Yeager AS: Use of acyclovir in premature and term neonates. *Am J Med* 73:205, 1982.

235 Hintz M et al: Neonatal acyclovir pharmacokinetics in patients with herpesvirus infections. *Am J Med* 73:210, 1982.

236 Whitley RJ et al: Vidarabine versus acyclovir therapy of neonatal herpes simplex virus, HSV, infection. *Pediatr Res* 20:323, 1986.

237 American Academy of Pediatrics, Committee on Fetus and Newborn and Committee on Infectious Diseases: Perinatal herpes simplex virus infections. *Pediatrics* 66:147, 1980.

238 Grossman JH et al: Management of genital herpes simplex virus infection during pregnancy. *Obstet Gynecol* 58:1, 1981.

239 Binkin NJ et al: Preventing neonatal herpes: The value of weekly viral cultures in pregnant women with recurrent genital herpes. *JAMA* 251:2816, 1984.

240 Arvin AM et al: Failure of antepartum maternal cultures to predict the infant's risk of exposure to herpes simplex virus at delivery. *N Engl J Med* 315:796, 1986.

241 Richman D: *Immunobiology and Prophylaxis of Human Herpesvirus Infections.* B Roizman and C Lopez (eds). New York, Raven, 1986.

242 Douglas JM et al: A double-blind study of oral acyclovir for suppression of recurrences of genital herpes simplex virus infection. *N Engl J Med* 310:1551, 1984.

243 Straus SE et al: Suppression of frequently recurring genital herpes: A placebo-controlled, double-blind trial of oral acyclovir. *N Engl J Med* 310:1545, 1984.

# Chapter 71

# Recurrent respiratory papillomatosis

Haskins K. Kashima
Keerti Shah
Matthew Goodstein

## INTRODUCTION

Recurrent respiratory papillomatosis (RRP) designates benign epithelial growths, papillomata, occurring in the respiratory tract at widely scattered areas. The growths are histologically benign but are clinically characterized as exhibiting patterns of regrowth, hence the designation "recurrent."

The syndrome of recurrent respiratory papillomatosis is most frequently identified on the basis of laryngeal tumors which cause hoarseness and upper airway obstructive symptoms. The common sites of papillomatous growths include the nasal vestibule, the nasopharyngeal surface of the soft palate, the midsection of the laryngeal surface of epiglottis, the true vocal cords, the subglottis (undersurface of the true cords), carina, bronchi and bronchioles, particularly at the sites of bifurcation, and the peripheral lung fields. Isolated papilloma of the oral cavity occurring on the palate, tonsils, tongue dorsum, and the buccal mucosa are not usually considered together with the recurrent respiratory papillomatosis.

Recurrent respiratory papillomatosis occurs among two distinct age groups. At least half the cases are designated *juvenile onset,* and manifest symptoms shortly after birth, during infancy, and in the preschool years. Newly diagnosed cases may occur as late as 12 to 13 years of age; it is most unusual to diagnose new cases between the age of 12 and 20 years. *Adult onset* RRP occurs after age 20 years and peak incidence is during the third and fourth decades, but new cases are diagnosed in patients as old as 60 and 70 years of age. Juvenile onset disease, particularly during the first several years of life, is the most florid and troublesome and, for this reason, the syndrome has been designated as juvenile laryngeal papillomatosis. Inasmuch as half of the cases occur in adulthood, however, the preferred terminology is recurrent respiratory papillomatosis.[1]

## HISTORY

The essential features of laryngeal papillomata, encompassing the clinical and histologic appearance as well as the tendency to recur, was recognized by Sir Morrell Mackenzie (1871). The first reference of "warts" in the throat is ascribed to Marcellus Donatus in the early seventeenth century. The first reported case in the United States was by J.C. Cheeseman in 1817.

Virchow, Mackenzie, and others attributed the papillomatous growths to chronic inflammation and catarrh, whereas Fauvel (1876) identified excessive voice use as the primary factor in the development of these lesions.[2] A report by Dunbar Roy in 1902 incriminated alcohol and tobacco, in addition to voice abuse, as important factors in the development of papillomata. Roy, in addition, recognized that papillomata occurred in adults as well as in children and considered that these might have differing etiologies. Baumgarten [cited by Roy, 1902] speculated that maternal gonorrheal discharge at birth could have etiologic relevance.

Recognition of the similarity of laryngeal papillomata, condyloma acuminata, and epidermal verrucae is attributed to Buck (1853) [cited by Webb, 1956]. A similar finding was advanced by Thost (1890) [cited by Geopfert, 1982].[3] Jadasshon in 1895 identified the filterable virus as the causative agent for skin warts. Victor Egon Ullman performed a series of experiments using cell-free filtrate of laryngeal papilloma and succeeded in producing papillomas on his own arm and on the arm of an associate.[4]

The history of the treatment of respiratory papillomatosis begins with the first successful per oral excision of laryngeal papillomata by Koderik (1750). Surgical excision by thyrotomy was first performed by Brauers in 1883.[5] Subsequent development and perfection of the laryngoscope caused Mackenzie to advocate endoscopic excision as the most effective means for papilloma removal, surpassing the more invasive methods of thyrotomy and laryngofissure. Endoscopic excision has been the cornerstone of therapy, and the major improvements have been the utilization of the operating microscope and of the surgical laser.[6,7] Surgical excision, even with additional refinements, has not been successful in total eradication of this troublesome disorder. A wide variety of agents have been used including "causticum, sanguinaria, thuja, belladonna, calcerea phosph, conium silicea."[6] Podophylum has enjoyed long-standing favor as an adjuvant to surgical excision.[8,9] This agent has proven efficacy in condyloma acuminata, but its adverse reactions have included growth stimulation of papilloma and possible carcinogenicity in mice, raising a note of caution in the use of this agent.[10]

Crowe and Breitstein (1922) advocated the careful use of radium in the treatment of papillomatosis, particularly in adults. Subsequent experience with the use of irradiation therapy led to the recognition of growth disturbance in the laryngeal cartilages of pediatric patients and, more importantly, the risk of malignant degeneration in previously benign laryngeal papillomatosis.[11]

During the 1980s the use of biological modifiers, notably interferon, was found effective in numerous pilot studies. In the United States two major multiinstitutional randomized studies have been completed, and the preliminary review of the data corroborates the favorable findings noted in the earlier studies (see below).

Historical review of respiratory papillomatosis is instructive in that the recognition and definition of this unique disorder led to the early suspicion of a probable viral etiology. Within the past decade a viral etiology for this syndrome has been firmly established and treatment options are under intense investigation.

## EPIDEMIOLOGY

Laryngeal papilloma is recognized as the commonest benign neoplasm in the larynx. One of every 1000 children examined in the Throat Department at the Massachusetts General Hospital was reported to have laryngeal papilloma.[12] Ono (1957) reported one of every 1544 children examined at Keio University in Tokyo, Japan, had papilloma.[13] On the basis of a USA mail survey with a 62 percent response rate, it was estimated that 1500 new cases of recurrent respiratory papillomatosis were diagnosed in the

United States in 1976, an average of 7.1 new cases per million population.[14] No pattern of racial predominance is recognized at this time.

Buck in 1853 and Hajek in 1956[15] are generally credited as having described maternal condyloma in association with a newborn subsequently diagnosed as having respiratory papillomatosis. Hajek's case is particularly noteworthy in that the condylomata in the mother underwent spontaneous regression shortly after childbirth; this pattern of rapid growth and regression without doubt accounts for the failure to recognize the probable association of these two conditions. In recent years there has been increasing recognition of the relevance of maternal condyloma to respiratory papillomatosis.[16,17] Presently 30 to 50 percent of juvenile onset recurrent respiratory papillomatosis occurs in a setting of maternal condylomata.

It is not irrelevant that in our own clinical population 20 percent of patients with juvenile onset RRP are adopted. This conforms to the recognized pattern of the disorder occurring predominantly in the first-born child and when the mother is young, frequently a teenager. An additional finding of considerable interest is that there is no documentation of siblings having respiratory papillomatosis.[18] The wider availability of sensitive and accurate testing methods, including human papillomavirus (HPV) typing of the RRP lesion and specimens from the mother's birth canal, may provide more conclusive evidence on the mechanism of transmission. Among adult onset RRP patients, it has been presumed that this is a sexually transmitted disorder, but epidemiological verification has not been published.

The prevalence of genital HPV infection among sexually active women of childbearing age is estimated to be 14 to 16 percent, based on DNA analysis of cervical scrapings.[19] One-third of the HPV infections were typed HPV-6 or HPV-11. Of the 3.5 million live births occurring in the United States annually, 175,000 pregnancies would occur in women with HPV infection if it is assumed that 5 percent of the women are infected with HPV-6 or HPV-11. Presently 20 percent of deliveries are performed by caesarean section so that 140,000 of the foregoing pregnancies would be delivered vaginally.[20] On the basis of the crude estimates of new cases of papillomatosis diagnosed annually, the risk of an offspring developing papillomatosis can be estimated to be as great as 1 in 80 or as low as 1 in 1500. The best estimate would be that the risk of developing papillomatosis may be in the range of 1 in 400 pregnancies occurring in the mother with genital condyloma. The factors accounting for this apparent discrepancy between the numbers developing infection from those at risk may be attributable to features of the genital tract infection, including the time of acquisition of infection, status of treatment, and host immune factors. In a similar manner, the host immune status of the newborn as well as the period of exposure (time in labor, premature rupture of membranes, and other obstetrical considerations) may be decisive.

In a recent review, combining the clinical experiences from two major medical centers, 1 of 109 patients with juvenile onset recurrent respiratory papillomatosis was found to have been delivered by cesarean section. Hence, the recommendation for cesarean section in mothers with condylomata is not 100 percent protective of their offspring developing respiratory papillomatosis.

The relevance of the host immune status is underscored in the reports of papillomavirus infections, including skin warts and respiratory papilloma, occurring in individuals whose immune status is compromised as a result of immune suppression for organ transplantation or while receiving cancer chemotherapy.

## ETIOLOGY

The viral etiology for respiratory papillomatosis has been long suspected. Precise identification of HPV as the primary etiologic agent[21] (primarily HPV-6 and HPV-11) was achieved simultaneously in several laboratories. HPV types 6 and 11 are also implicated as the causative agents in genital condylomata. Specific subtypes of HPV-6 have been correlated with the extent of spread and severity of disease; HPV-6C, in particular, identifies the subset of patients with the most severe spread of disease, including into the trachea and lungs.[22]

HPV-6, -13, and -16 were identified in papilloma of the oral cavity.[23]

## PATHOGENESIS

Utilizing immunochemical and immunohistologic techniques of high sensitivity and specificity, the presence of HPV in tissue sections of respiratory papilloma is demonstrable. Inasmuch as the identical HPV types are associated with genital condyloma, it has been commonly assumed that viral transmission occurs at the time of delivery. The observed low rate of clinical respiratory papillomatosis (described in the section on History) is imperfectly understood. Cases of self-limited papillomatosis, manifested only by hoarseness, are undoubtedly undiagnosed. It has been speculated that some cases of neonatal and infantile asphyxia may be attributable to papillomatous growths in the airway. Because of the small size of the infant larynx and airway, even the smallest papilloma deposit could produce hoarseness or airway obstruction.

Adult onset recurrent respiratory papillomatosis has been presumed to occur on basis of sexual contact, namely, oral-genital exposure. In some cases of papillomatosis initially diagnosed in adulthood, a lifelong history of hoarseness suggests the possibility that the initial viral transmission may have occurred at childbirth and remained dormant until adulthood.

Transmission of viral infection through infected oropharyngeal secretions is rare. There are no documented cases of papillomatosis occurring in family members who have been constantly exposed to secretions from patients with papillomatosis. There are, however, numerous anecdotal reports of surgeons who have developed warty growths on the face and upper body, presumably from exposures occurring at the time of surgical excisions.

## CLINICAL MANIFESTATIONS

Juvenile onset papillomatosis is diagnosed on the basis of hoarseness, usually present from the time of birth. Upper airway obstructive symptoms of varying severity are aggravated during intercurrent upper respiratory tract infection, and the initial presentation may be as an airway emergency (Fig. 71-1). Endoscopic excision of the papillomatous growths is effective in the majority of patients. Others experience rapid regrowth of papilloma so that endoscopic excisions may require repetition at as often as weekly intervals so that as many as 100 or more endoscopic excisions are necessary to maintain a safe and adequate airway.

The intervals between operations are generally lengthened as the patient enters puberty due to the combined result of laryngeal enlargement and reduced rate of papilloma regrowth. It has been long recognized that a certain proportion of patients undergo

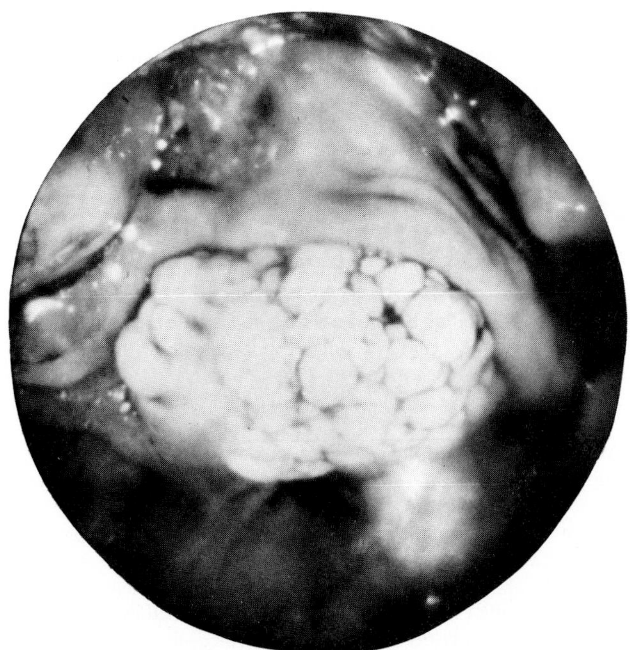

**Fig. 71-1.** Clinical view of the larynx showing impaction of the laryngeal vestibule by typical papillomatous growths.

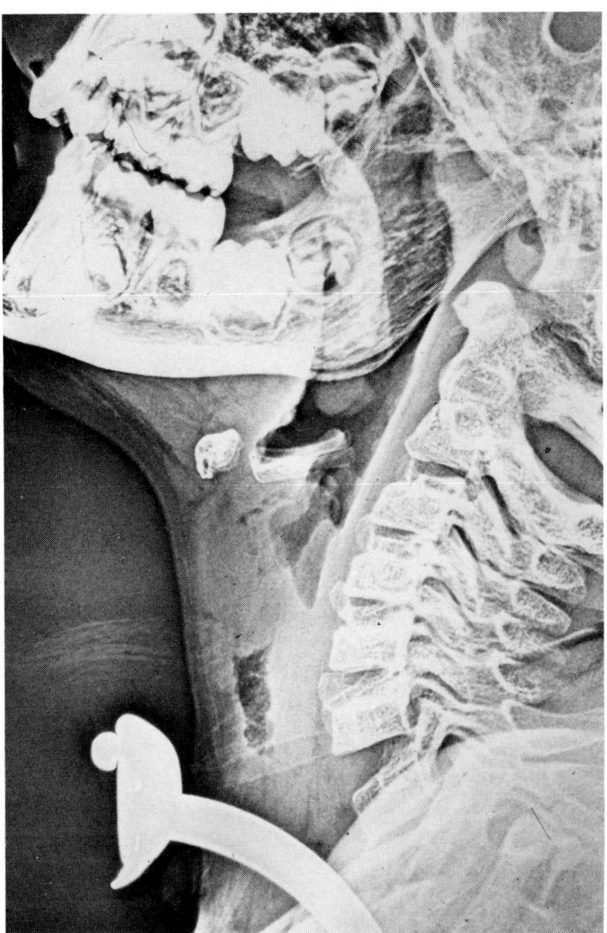

**Fig. 71-2.** Neck xeroradiogram showing total laryngeal obstruction by papilloma. The trachea is narrowed by nodular papillomatous growths. Tracheostomy bypasses the obstruction.

spontaneous remission at or about puberty. An undetermined proportion of patients, however, will continue to experience papilloma regrowth, and the lesions may extend from the larynx into the trachea, to the bronchi, and eventually to the lungs (Fig. 71-2).[24] The risk of extension into the trachea and lower respiratory tract appears to be increased in patients who have had tracheotomy performed; hence, experienced laryngologists advocate repeated and meticulous endoscopic excision and the avoidance of tracheotomy.

Among the adult onset papillomatosis patients the usual initial symptom is persistent hoarseness. The clinical evaluation may suggest a benign polyp, but histologic examination of the excised specimen reveals the growth to be a papilloma. In a small proportion of the adult onset patients widespread papillomatosis occurs. In patients who have this aggressive clinical course, we have identified HPV-6C to be the etiologic agent.

In a small proportion of patients, estimated to be in the range of 3 to 5 percent, squamous cell carcinoma has been observed.[25,26] Irradiation therapy and tobacco usage have been implicated as factors predisposing to malignant transformation in respiratory papillomatosis.[27]

The issue of spontaneous remission of respiratory papillomatosis is unsettled. In 1964, Majoros reported that a 56-year review of 77 patients at the Mayo Clinic disclosed that 85 percent of 77 patients became "free of disease."[28] Holinger, Bjork, and Weber, in reviewing separate clinical experiences, agreed that adult onset respiratory papillomatosis patients were more likely to attain remission than juvenile onset patients.[29,30] However, Dedo and Jackler described 10 patients with a *normal* indirect laryngoscopic examination in whom the presence of papilloma was found upon suspension microlaryngoscopy on the following day.[31] Steinberg has demonstrated the presence of HPV DNA in histologically normal laryngeal epithelium, examined in biopsies from patients with papillomatosis elsewhere in the respiratory tract.[32] These reports underscore the necessity to accept the report of complete remission from papillomatosis with caution.

## DIAGNOSIS

The diagnosis of papillomatosis is established on the basis of histologic examination of the biopsy specimen (Fig. 71-3). The papillomas have characteristic clinical appearance of multinodular growths with a small subepithelial vascular tuft. The lesions may be sessile and widespread or exophytic and arising from a narrow stalk. Varying degrees of epithelial atypia have been observed, and these cases require careful follow-up examinations and repeat biopsies. Inasmuch as malignant transformation has been noted in the larynx, trachea, and lungs, the specimens obtained at each operation should be carefully separated to identify their source so that any histologic change of concern can be precisely identified as to their tissue of origin.

## ANTIMICROBIAL SUSCEPTIBILITY AND TREATMENT

The clinical course of recurrent respiratory papillomatosis is predictably unpredictable. Accordingly, the evaluation as to the efficacy of any treatment modality requires objective and reproducible description and staging.

A long list of escharotics, antimitotic agents, hormonal preparations, and antibiotics have been proposed but ultimately proved to be ineffective. Autogenous vaccines, prepared from the patient's own lesions, were used by Holinger with variable bene-

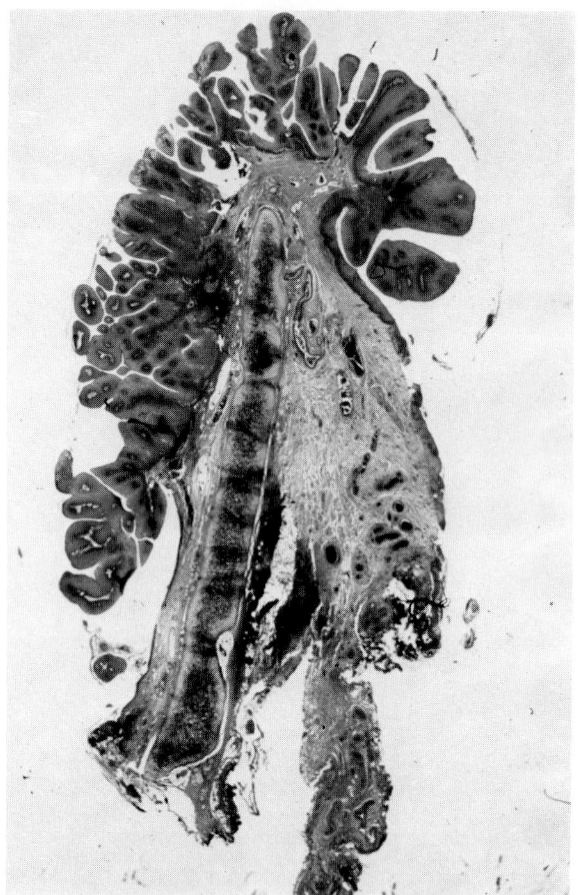

**Fig. 71-3.** Mid-sagittal histologic section of the epiglottis (shown in Fig. 71-1). The papillomatous growths arise from the laryngeal surface of the epiglottis.

fit.[33] Gross and Hubbard reported favorable responses in 9 of 22 patients receiving autogenous vaccine.[34] Leventhal (1985) reviewed the published experience of chemotherapeutic agents in papillomavirus infections.[35]

Haglund and colleagues reported 7 patients with RRP treated with interferon. Their promising results in studies at the Karolinska Institute stimulated numerous pilot studies, all reporting favorable outcome, including complete remission of short duration.[36] Two multiinstitutional randomized studies have been completed in the United States and corroborate the findings from these earlier studies.[37–40]

The major questions remaining to be answered are the identification of the subgroup of patients most likely to be benefited, the duration of clinical remission and response, the optimum dose and duration of interferon administration, and the long-term or delayed effects of use of these or similar agents.

## PREVENTION

The identification of the etiologic agent and its optimum management in women of childbearing age requires detailed study. Neither the specific clinical lesion (whether cervical, vaginal, or vulvar) or the cofactors predisposing to increased risk of developing papillomatosis have been identified. Given the present state of indefinite knowledge regarding the prevalence of recurrent respiratory papilloma, the precise risk of developing papillomatosis cannot be defined. The risk rates as presently estimated do not justify the recommendation for delivery by cesarean section, particularly given the several instances in which papillomatosis has developed in children delivered by cesarean section.

## References


1 Strong MS et al: Recurrent respiratory papillomatosis: Management with the $CO_2$ laser. *Ann Otol Rhinol Laryngol* 85:508, 1976.
2 Webb WW: Papillomata of the larynx. *Laryngoscope* 66:871, 1956.
3 Goepfert H et al: Leukocyte interferon in patients with juvenile laryngeal papillomatosis. *Ann Otol Rhinol Laryngol* 91:431, 1982.
4 Ullman EV: On the aetiology of the laryngeal papilloma. *Acta Otolaryngol* 5:317, 1923.
5 Mackenzie M: *Essay on Growths of the Larynx: With Reports on an Analysis of 100 Consecutive Cases Treated by the Author.* Philadelphia, Lindsay and Blakiston, 1981.
6 Cohen SR et al: Papilloma of the larynx and tracheobronchial tree in children. *Ann Otol Rhinol Laryngol* 89:497, 1980.
7 Clemente MA: Microchirurgia com laser na papillomatose respiratoria recomente estudio clinico e experimental. Doctoral Thesis, Faculty of Medicine, Porto Medical College, Portugal, 1978. As cited by Strong MS, et al: Recurrent respiratory papillomatosis: Management with the $CO_2$ laser. *Ann Otol Rhinol Laryngol* 85:508, 1976.
8 Holinger PH et al: Laryngeal papilloma, in review of etiology and therapy. *Laryngoscopy* 78:1462, 1968.
9 Hollingsworth JB et al: Treatment of juvenile papilloma of the larynx with resin of podophylum. *Arch Otolaryngol* 52:82, 1950.
10 Szpunar J: Laryngeal papillomatosis. *Acta Otolaryngol* 63:68, 1967.
11 Walsh TE, Beamer PR; Epidermoid carcinoma of the larynx occurring in 2 children with carcinoma of the larynx. *Laryngoscope* 60:1110, 1950.
12 Clark JP: Papilloma of the larynx in children. *Trans Am Laryngol Assoc* 27:185, 1905.
13 Ono J et al: The etiology of papilloma of the larynx. *Ann Otol Rhinol Laryngol* 66:1119, 1957.
14 Strong MS et al: Recurrent respiratory papillomatosis, in *Laryngotracheal Problems in the Pediatric Patient,* GB Healy et al (eds). Springfield, IL, Charles C Thomas, 1979.
15 Hajek EF: Contribution to the etiology of laryngeal papilloma in children. *J Laryngol Otol* 70:166, 1956.
16 Quick CA et al: The etiology of laryngeal papillomatosis. *Laryngoscope* 88:1789, 1978.
17 Cook TA et al: Laryngeal papilloma: Etiologic and therapeutic considerations. *Ann Otol Rhinol Laryngol* 82:649, 1973.
18 Kashima HK: Unpublished observations, 1987.
19 Lorincz A et al: Correlation of cellular atypia in human papillomavirus DNA sequences in exfoliated cells of the uterine cervix. *Obstet Gynecol* 68:508, 1986.
20 Shah K et al: Rarity of cesarean delivery in cases of juvenile-onset respiratory papillomatosis. *Obstet Gynecol* 68:795, 1986.
21 Mounts P et al: Viral etiology of juvenile- and adult-onset squamous papilloma of the larynx. *Proc Natl Acad Sci USA* 79:5425, 1982.
22 Mounts P, Kashima H: Association of human papillomavirus subtype and clinical course in respiratory papillomatosis. *Laryngoscope* 94:28, 1984.
23 Naghashfar Z et al: Infection of the oral cavity with genital tract papillomaviruses. *Papillomaviruses: Molecular & Clinical Aspects,* 1985, pp 155–163.
24 Weiss MD, Kashima HK: Tracheal involvement in laryngeal papillomatosis. *Laryngoscope* 93:45, 1983.
25 Jackson C, Jackson CL: *The Larynx and Its Diseases.* Philadelphia, Saunders, 1937.
26 Bjork H, Teir H: Benign and malignant papilloma of the larynx in adults. *Acta Otolaryngol* 47:95, 1957.
27 Solomon D et al: Malignant transformation in non-irradiated recurrent respiratory papillomatosis. *Laryngoscope* 95:900, 1985.

28 Majoros M et al: Papilloma of the larynx in children. *Am J Surg* 108:470, 1964.
29 Holinger PH et al: Papilloma of the larynx: A review of 109 cases with a preliminary report of oreomycin therapy. *Ann Otol Rhinol Laryngol* 59:547, 1950.
30 Bjork H, Weber C: Papilloma of the larynx. *Acta Otolaryngol* 46: 499, 1956.
31 Dedo HH, Jackler RK: Laryngeal papilloma: Results of treatment with the $CO_2$ laser and podophyllum. *Ann Otol Rhinol Laryngol* 91:425, 1982.
32 Steinberg BM et al: Laryngeal papillomavirus infection during clinical remission. *N Engl J Med* 388:1261, 1983.
33 Holinger PA et al: Studies of papilloma of the larynx. *Ann Otol Rhinol Laryngol* 71:443, 1962.
34 Gross CW, Hubbard R: Management of juvenile laryngeal papilloma: Further observations. *Laryngoscope* 84:1090, 1974.
35 Leventhal B, Kashima H: Chemotherapy of papillomavirus infection, in *UCLA Symposia on Molecular and Cellular Biology, New Series,* PM Howley et al (eds). New York, Alan R Liss, 1985, pp 235–248.
36 Haglund S et al: Interferon therapy in juvenile laryngeal papillomatosis. *Arch Otolaryngol* 107:327, 1981.
37 Kashima HK, Papilloma Study Group: Interferon Alfa-N1 (Welleferon) in juvenile onset recurrent respiratory papillomatosis: Results of a randomized study in twelve collaborative institutions. *Laryngoscope,* 98:334–340, 1988.
38 Healy GB et al: Treatment of recurrent respiratory papillomatosis with human leukocyte interferon. *N Engl J Med* 319:401, 1988.
39 Leventhal BG et al: Randomized surgical adjuvant trial of Interferon Alfa-N1 (Wellferon) in recurrent papillomatosis. *Arch Otolaryngol* 114:1163, 1988.
40 Kashima H et al: Carcinoma ex Papilloma: Histologic and virologic studies in whole-organ sections of the larynx. *Laryngoscope* 98:619, 1988.

# Chapter 72
# Child sexual abuse and STD

Carole Jenny

## INTRODUCTION

Child sexual abuse occurs commonly. Although its exact incidence and prevalence are unknown, it is estimated that at least one in four girls and one in ten boys will be molested before age 16. Over 50,000 cases are reported each year in the United States.[1,2] Statistics from other countries show similar frequencies of occurrence.[3–5]

When sexually transmitted diseases (STD) occur in children, sexual abuse must be considered a "rule out" diagnosis. Except for chancroid, every STD that occurs in adults has also been reported in children.[6] Since sexual abuse is deleterious to the psychological health of children, cases of STD in children should be carefully investigated to determine the nature of the child's contact with infectious microorganisms.

In children who are known to be abused, estimates of the prevalence of STD vary depending on the criteria and microbiological tests used for diagnosis, the age range of the children examined, and the underlying prevalence of disease in the community where the children were studied. Table 72-1 lists STD found in surveys of sexually abused children and their frequencies of occurrence. Controlled studies of STD in abused and nonabused children are listed in Table 72-2.

## HISTOLOGY AND PHYSIOLOGY OF THE GENITAL TRACT IN CHILDREN

The genital tract of prepubertal girls provides a different microclimate for STD pathogens than that of postmenarchal females.[21] The vagina of young girls is lined with a thin, atrophic columnar epithelium. The pH is 6.5 to 7.5, higher than that found in adults. The cervix does not have active mucus-secreting glands, and the normal female child will not have a demonstrable vaginal discharge.

After puberty, the vaginal wall is lined with a thick, stratified squamous epithelium containing glycogen. The vagina is normally acid (pH less than 4.5), and cervical glands secrete varying amounts of mucus. The epithelium of the cervical canal is columnar.[21] Because of the presence of columnar epithelium in the child's vagina, some STD pathogens such as *Neisseria gonorrhoeae* and *Chlamydia trachomatis* that infect the cervix of adult women will cause vaginitis in children. The high vaginal pH may also increase a child's susceptibility to infection.

Similar differences in the histology of the genital tract of boys as compared with adult males have not been reported. STD in male children probably occurs less frequently than in female children because male children have less exposure to STD pathogens owing to their lower incidence of sexual abuse.[22]

## MODES OF TRANSMISSION OF STD IN CHILDREN

Determining the sources of infection with STD pathogens in children is often difficult. Much of the existing literature reporting STD in children does not reflect a consideration that the disease may have been acquired through sexual contact.

**Table 72-1. STD Reported in Surveys of Sexually Abused Children**

| Reference | Ages | Number of Subjects | Disease* | Number Tested | No. (%) positive |
|---|---|---|---|---|---|
| Tilelli 1980[7] | 2–16 yr | 130 | GC | 103 | 3 (2.9%) |
| DeJong 1982[8] | 6 mo–17 yr | 142 | GC | 142 | 2 (1.4%) |
| Rimsza 1982[9] | 2 mo–17 yr | 311 | GC | 285 | 21 (7.4%) |
| | | | TP | 104 | 0 (0%) |
| Groothuis 1983[10] | < 13 yr | 16 | GC | 11 | 5 (45.4%) |
| Khan 1983[11] | < 13 yr | 113 | GC | 71 | 14 (19.7%) |
| White 1983[12] | < 13 yr | 409 | GC | 176 | 47 (26.7%) |
| | | | TP | 108 | 6 (5.5%) |
| | | | TV | 21 | 4 |
| | | | HPV | | 3 |
| Grant 1984[13] | 8 mo–17 yr | 157 | GC | | 12 |
| | | | HPV | | 2 |
| | | | HSV | | 1 |
| DeJong 1986[14] | 6 mo–13 yr | 532 | GC | 532 | 25 (4.7%) |
| | | | BV | | 3 |
| | | | HPV | | 3 |
| | | | HSV | | 1 |
| | | | TP | 532 | 1 (0.2%) |
| Fuster 1987[15] | 1–12.5 yr | 50 | CT | 47 | 8 (17%) |
| | | | GC | 49 | 0 (0%) |

*GC = *N. gonorrhoeae*
TP = *T. pallidum*
TV = *T. vaginalis*
HPV = human papilloma virus (anogenital warts)
HSV = herpes simplex virus (genital)
BV = bacterial vaginosis
CT = *C. trachomatis*

**Table 72-2. STD Found in Sexually Abused Children Compared with Controls**

| | | Number | | | % positive | | |
|---|---|---|---|---|---|---|---|
| Reference | Ages, years | Abused | Controls | Disease* | Abused | Controls | P† |
| Hammerschlag 1984[16] | 2–14 | 51 | 43 | CT | 3.9 | 6.9‡ | |
| | | | | GC | 9.8 | | |
| Hammerschlag 1985[17] | 2–13 | 31 | 23 | BV | 29 | 4.3 | |
| Ingram 1986[18] | 1–12 | 124 | 90 | CT | 8.9 | 1.1 | <.02 |
| | | | | GC | 15.3 | 0 | |
| Bartley 1987[19] | 1–11 | 137 | 119 | GV | 14.6 | 4.2 | <.01 |
| Hammerschlag 1987[20] | 2–14 | 50 | 40 | MH | 38 | 22 | NS |
| | | | | MH—rectum | 23 | 8 | < |
| | | | | MH—vagina | 34 | 17 | <.10 |
| | | | | UU | 45 | 25 | NS |
| | | | | UU—rectum | 19 | 3 | <.025 |
| | | | | UU—vagina | 30 | 8 | <.025 |

*CT = *C. trachomatis*
GC = *N. gonorrhoeae*
BV = bacterial vaginosis
GV = *G. vaginalis*
MH = *M. hominis*
UU = *U. urealyticum*
†*P* = probability value of statistical significance (NS = not significant).
‡Two of three controls positive for *C. trachomatis* had previous sexual abuse history.

Four factors make it difficult to determine modes of transmission of STD in children:

1. The magnitude of the problem of child sexual abuse only recently has been recognized. Before Henry Kempe's historic speech on child sexual abuse to the American Academy of Pediatrics in 1977,[23] the fact that STD in children were likely to be a manifestation of abuse was not appreciated by many practitioners and researchers.
2. Often children are reluctant to report sexual abuse because of fear of retaliation from the abuser or because of feelings of guilt or embarrassment. In addition, they may be unable to report because of a lack of verbal skills. Histories given by caretakers may be unreliable because the child has not informed them of the abuse, or because of the caretaker's involvement in the abuse. A high percentage of abused children have been found to be abused by family members.
3. It is conceivable that diseases which are transmitted only by sexual contact in adults may be nonsexually transmitted in children. Even in normal, healthy families, children have much more intimate contact with family members than most adults would ever have with people who are not their sexual partners. Young children frequently sleep and bathe with their parents[24] and share household objects such as towels and toothbrushes with others. This degree of intimacy in normal, nonabusive households raises the possibility that STD are not necessarily sexually transmitted in all instances.
4. Some STD in children can be acquired before birth, during birth, or through breast feeding.[25] It is often difficult to differentiate perinatal infection from infection acquired through sexual abuse.

Accurately determining the mode of transmission of STD pathogens in children requires the examiner to have an open mind and willingness to consider the possibility of sexual or nonsexual transmission.

## Sexual versus nonsexual transmission of STD in children

***Neisseria gonorrhoeae.*** Although *N. gonorrhoeae* can infect an infant during birth, asymptomatic infection has not been shown to persist after the neonatal period. Only one case of nonsexual transmission of genital *N. gonorrhoeae* is documented in adults,[6] involving two patients in a military hospital who shared a urinal. *N. gonorrhoeae* has been shown to survive for 20 and 24 h, respectively, in infected secretions on towels and handkerchiefs.[26] However, cultures from toilet seats in public restrooms and venereal disease clinics have failed to yield *N. gonorrhoeae*.[27,28] The paucity of reported cases indicates that nonsexual transmission is rare in adults.

In children diagnosed with gonococcal pharyngeal, genital, and anorectal infections, histories of sexual abuse are commonly obtained.[29–33] When gonorrhea is diagnosed in a child, it is important to culture household contacts for the disease. Other infected adults and children are commonly found in the child's environment.[34,35]

***Chlamydia trachomatis.*** *C. trachomatis* infects infants during vaginal delivery, causing conjunctivitis and pneumonia during the neonatal period.[36,37] Some infants will not manifest positive cultures until several weeks after birth, probably because of the suppression of infection by maternal antibody.[38] Carriage of *C. trachomatis* from birth has been documented for up to 28 months in the nasopharynx, 55 weeks in the rectum, and 53 weeks in the vagina, and may persist for longer periods of time.[39]

Acquisition of *C. trachomatis* infection during childhood is suggested by an increasing prevalence of antibody to the organism between birth and 15 years of age.[40,41] However, this has not been a consistent finding in all studies of antibody prevalence, and in part could be due to cross-reacting antibody of the recently described TWAR chlamydia strain.[42,43] *C. trachomatis* has been implicated in the pathogenesis of some cases of upper respiratory tract disease, otitis media, and myocarditis, as well as pneumonia and conjunctivitis after infancy.[44] Although the importance of the organism as a cause of these infections is unclear, such infections could account for the increasing prevalence of antibody during childhood.

Alternatively, acquisition of chlamydial antibody during childhood could reflect sexual abuse. The prevalence of culture-proved *C. trachomatis* vaginal and rectal infections has been found to be significantly more common in sexually abused children than in controls.[18] Since *C. trachomatis* infections of the adult genitalia and rectum are clearly sexually transmitted,[45] a similar mode of transmission is likely to occur in children.

**Trichomonas vaginalis.** *T. vaginalis* has been shown to be present in the nasopharynx and vagina of newborns born to infected mothers.[46,47] Sexual transmission in prepubertal children has been infrequently reported.[48] The prepubertal vagina does not provide a favorable environment for the organism.

Trichomonads have been isolated from droplets of water splashed from toilets containing urine from infected individuals.[49] However, there are no documented cases of adults becoming infected from fomites. Since trichomonal infections in children are so uncommon, the possibility of easy spread through fomites is unlikely.

**Herpes Simplex Virus (HSV).** The acquisition of genital HSV by children should raise the possibility of sexual abuse.[50] Infection by either type I or type II virus can occur in the genital area.

HSV can survive in fomites for 2 h on latex gloves and toilet seats, 24 h on a speculum, and 72 h on gauze.[51] Fomite transmission of the disease, however, is considered unlikely.[52] Transmission requires direct contact of viable virus with either a mucus membrane or an abraded skin surface on the individual who is becoming infected.

Children have been shown to transmit HSV from symptomatic or asymptomatic infections in their mouths to their genital area.[53] Sexual transmission through child abuse is also well documented.[54]

Other viruses and bacteria can cause lesions in the genital area of children which resemble herpes simplex.[53] Viral cultures should be carefully obtained from the base of such lesions. Any herpes virus found should be typed (I or II). Viral cultures may not detect the virus after crusting of vesicles occurs. Obtaining sera for HSV I and HSV II antibodies acutely and 6 weeks after the infection can be helpful in documenting the acquisition of HSV.

**Condyloma Acuminatum.** Genital and anal warts are caused by human papilloma virus (HPV). Certain types of HPV are thought to cause genital, anal, and cervical warts, including types 6, 11, 16, 18, and 31.[55] There is little evidence that common warts on other parts of the body can cause anal or genital warts by "autoinoculation."[56] Condylomata acuminata in children have been shown to be caused by the same type of HPV which causes anogenital warts in adults.[57]

The sexual transmission of condyloma acuminatum is well documented.[56,58] Skin-to-skin contact between individuals is thought to be necessary for infection to be transmitted. Perinatal transmission is also known to occur.[59] Condyloma acuminatum in the first year of life in the absence of sexual abuse can be considered to be the result of infection through contact with the virus during delivery.

The time after birth at which the onset of lesions can no longer be attributed to perinatal infection is unknown. Virus is known to exist in tissues in a latent state,[60] at which time no lesions can be seen. Even after warts begin to develop, many smaller warts cannot be visualized without the use of acetic acid and colposcopy.[61]

A potential "model" of the pathogenesis of childhood condylomata is the development of laryngeal warts in children. These warts are thought to be caused by perinatal infection with genital-type HPV.[62] Most children develop these warts in the first year of life, but clinically obvious infection can occur up to 5 years of age. However, small, asymptomatic lesions might be present earlier and not recognized.

At least 50 percent of children with anal or genital warts have histories of sexual abuse.[63,64] The presence of the warts should thus raise the suspicion of abuse.

**Gardnerella vaginalis.** *G. vaginalis* is considered a sexually transmitted organism in adults.[65] The organism has been found to be more prevalent in sexually active adolescent males and females.[66,67] It is also more commonly found in sexually abused children than in controls.[19] Clinical evidence of bacterial vaginosis, a mixed infection of *G. vaginalis* and other microorganisms, has also been described in abused children.[17]

Most studies of *G. vaginalis* in children and adolescents show that a small proportion of the nonabused or non-sexually-active subjects will also carry the organism.[17,19,66–68] Although the organism is not pathognomonic of abuse, its presence should raise the index of suspicion that abuse might have occurred.

**Human Immunodeficiency Virus (HIV).** Infection with HIV has been reported as a sequela of sexual abuse.[69] The frequent occurrence of microtrauma from abusive sexual activities with children could lead to a portal of entry for the virus from infected adults. The Centers for Disease Control have not identified sexual abuse as a common cause of clinical AIDS. The frequency of transmission of HIV via sexual abuse of children is not known.

**Syphilis.** Syphilis is rarely reported as a complication of sexual abuse.[70] The diagnosis of syphilis outside the neonatal period is likely to be caused by sexual contact.

**Molluscum Contagiosum.** Although molluscum contagiosum has been identified as a sexually transmitted disease in adults, the frequent occurrence of the disease in young children indicates it is easily spread by casual contact.[71] In many children with molluscum, a careful history will reveal the presence of lesions on other parts of the body before genital lesions were noted.

## DIAGNOSIS AND TREATMENT OF STD WITH SUSPECTED CHILD ABUSE

### SCREENING FOR STD IN ABUSED CHILDREN

The diagnosis of an STD in a child should suggest the possibility of sexual abuse. The child should be carefully evaluated with that in mind. To confirm the diagnosis of abuse, however, requires a careful review of the child's history, physical examination, and social situation. If the diagnosis of sexual abuse is made, laws in most jurisdictions mandate reporting to child protection agencies. The safety, health, and welfare of the child should be the practitioner's primary concern. The following general considerations should guide the evaluation:

1. Many institutions have a service that is particularly skilled in the interview and examination of children suspected of having experienced sexual abuse. This may be a child protection team within the pediatric department or a person or group in gynecology. This group, if available, should be involved in the workup from the first contact.
2. If the child is symptomatic, all available and appropriate cultures and examination should be completed before the child is begun on therapy. For example, if the child has conjunctivitis, cultures of other mucosal areas should be taken before therapy is started.
3. All culture and examination samples must be thoroughly and clearly labeled, and delivery to the appropriate laboratory must be ensured by personal delivery if necessary. The results may be required for legal proceedings.
4. If sexual abuse is documented by the presence of spermatozoa, an STD, or by social history, the child must be placed in a secure environment pending investigation and social and legal disposition.
5. The majority of children who have been the victims of sexual abuse will not have specific physical findings to confirm the diagnosis. Subtle findings such as bruising may be present, but the physical examination is likely to reveal no abnormality. However, the absence of abnormalities on physical examination does not make a diagnosis of sexual abuse unlikely. Oral sexual contact is a common form of abuse, as are fondling and external genital contact.
6. The presence of multiple STDs in a child may indicate that the child has been abused by multiple persons.

Table 72-3 shows the recommendations from the CDC for screening for STD in sexually abused children.[72] The CDC protocol advises obtaining cultures from anus, pharynx, and either female vagina or male urethra. Screening cultures are indicated because over 50 percent of gonococcal infections found in abused children are asymptomatic. Thirty percent have been found in orifices not specifically reported by the children to have been involved in abusive sexual activity.[14] Children often tend to minimize or do not understand the extent of abuse and are likely to underreport the types of sexual activity that occur.

**Table 72-3. CDC Recommendations for Screening for STD in Sexually Abused Children**

Females:
1. Culture pharynx, anal canal, and vagina for *Neisseria gonorrhoeae.*
2. Culture pharynx, vagina, and rectum for *Chlamydia trachomatis.*
3. Examine urine and culture vagina for *Trichomonas vaginalis.*
4. If inflammation is present, obtain herpes simplex cultures from vagina, rectum, urethra, or eye area.
5. Obtain serologic test for syphilis.
6. Examine for venereal warts.
7. Examine for vaginitis with a wet mount for clue cells.
8. Examine for pregnancy if appropriate.

Males:
1. Culture pharynx, rectum, and urethra for *Neisseria gonorrhoeae.*
2. Culture rectum, pharynx, and urethra for *Chlamydia trachomatis.*
3. Obtain herpes simplex culture from areas of the genital tract which show inflammation.
4. Obtain serologic test for syphilis.
5. Examine for venereal warts.

Follow-up cultures at 2 weeks and serology at 6 weeks are required in cases of acute assault or molestation.
SOURCE: Ref. 72.

Any positive culture for *N. gonorrhoeae* should be confirmed by a reference laboratory. A false-positive diagnosis of gonorrhea because of the misidentification of nonpathogenic *Neisseria* species can cause unnecessary difficulties for children and their families.[73] In addition, noncultural tests for gonorrhea should not be used in suspected child abuse cases because of their lesser sensitivity and specificity.

The advisability of an initial serology for syphilis followed by a repeat test 6 weeks after the first visit is questionable owing to the low yield of such tests in children. A survey of 80 physicians attending a national meeting showed that only 25 positive tests for syphilis had been obtained in over 49,000 abused children tested.[74] All but one of the infected children had also been found to have other STD. Because of the low incidence of true positives, the benefit of syphilis screening in sexually abused children has been questioned. On the other hand, the diagnosis of secondary syphilis in a child would be difficult because of the common occurrence of generalized viral exanthems and the low index of suspicion of syphilis in children. A single serology at a 6-week follow-up visit should be sufficient and will spare the child a second phlebotomy.[75]

Rapid diagnostic tests for *C. trachomatis* using either monoclonal antibodies in direct immunofluorescent stains or enzyme-linked immunoassays are not sufficiently sensitive or specific in low-risk populations to be used in sexually abused children to screen for chlamydial infections.[15,76] The higher than acceptable level of false-negative and -positive test results limits their usefulness as medical-legal tests. Cultures should be used to screen for chlamydial infections if child sexual abuse is suspected.

The sensitivity of the test commonly used for the diagnosis of trichomoniasis (the saline wet mount) is low compared with culture.[77] Wet mounts have been shown to diagnose only 60 percent of culture-proved *T. vaginalis* infections. In sexually abused children, the use of culture rather than wet mount would probably increase the frequency of diagnosis of trichomoniasis.

*Gardnerella vaginalis* resembles other coryneform bacteria commonly found in the vaginal flora of children. Using a media selective for *G. vaginalis* will increase the accuracy of identification of the organism.[78]

Screening for other STD, such as HIV virus infection and hepatitis B, may be indicated, especially if the offender is known to be seropositive or to be in a "high risk" group for such infections. The clinical presentation of the child may also indicate that more extensive testing is needed.

If offenders are identified in cases where children are found to have STD, efforts should be made to culture the alleged offender to validate the mode of transmission of the disease. Matching microorganisms in the victim and offender can provide corroborative evidence of abuse and can usually be presented in criminal or civil trials.

## PROPHYLACTIC ANTIBIOTICS

Prophylactic antibiotics are not generally indicated when sexual abuse of children is suspected. The infection rate in children is sufficiently low such that prophylactic treatment will prevent few infections. In addition, the risk of complications from STD in children is low. Very few cases of pelvic inflammatory disease or peritonitis in prepubertal children have been documented,[79,80] perhaps because the immature cervix presents a barrier to the ascending spread of infection. Epididymitis and other upper genital tract infections of male children are also unusual and are rarely caused by STD pathogens.[81,82] Since STD are not likely to cause severe illness in children, their value as corroborative evidence of molestation exceeds the risk to the child of not treating prophylactically.

The treatment of individual diseases is discussed in other chapters.

## References


1 Russell DEH: *Sexual Exploitation: Rape, Child Sexual Abuse, and Workplace Harassment.* Beverly Hills, Sage Publications, 1984, p 177.

2 Peters SD et al: Prevalence, in *A Sourcebook on Child Sexual Abuse,* D Finkelhor (ed). Beverly Hills, Sage Publications, 1986, p 15.

3 Sexual offenses against children: Report of the Committee on Sexual Offenses against Children and Youth, Ottawa, Minister of Justice and Attorney General of Canada, Canadian Government Publication J 2-50/1984E, 1984.

4 Baker T: Report on a reader survey: Child sexual abuse, "19" confidential survey. Unpublished manuscript, London, St. George's Hospital, 1983.

5 Ronstrom A: Sexual abuse of children in Sweden: Perspectives on research, interventions, and consequences. Unpublished manuscript, 1985.

6 Neinstein LS et al: Nonsexual transmission of sexually transmitted diseases: An infrequent occurrence. *Pediatrics* 74:67, 1984.

7 Tilelli JA et al: Sexual abuse of children. *N Engl J Med* 302:319, 1980.

8 DeJong AR et al: Sexual abuse of boys. *Am J Dis Child* 136:990, 1982.

9 Rimsza ME, Niggemann EH: Medical evaluation of sexually abused children: A review of 311 cases. *Pediatrics* 69:8, 1982.

10 Groothuis JR et al: Pharyngeal gonorrhea in young children. *Pediatr Infect Dis* 2:99, 1983.

11 Khan M, Sexton M: Sexual abuse of young children. *Clin Pediatr* 22:369, 1983.

12 White St et al: Sexually transmitted diseases in sexually abused children. *Pediatrics* 72:16, 1983.

13 Grant LJ: Assessment of child sexual abuse: Eighteen months' experience at the Child Protection Center. *Am J Obstet Gynecol* 148:617, 1984.

14 DeJong AR: Sexually transmitted diseases in sexually abused children. *Sex Transm Dis* 13:123, 1986.

15 Fuster CD, Neinstein LS: Vaginal *Chlamydia trachomatis* prevalence in sexually abused prepubertal girls. *Pediatrics* 79:235, 1987.

16 Hammerschlag MR et al: Are rectogenital chlamydial infections a marker of sexual abuse in children? *Pediatr Infect Dis* 3:100, 1984.

17 Hammerschlag MR et al: Nonspecific vaginitis following sexual abuse in children. *Pediatrics* 75:1028, 1985.

18 Ingram DL et al: Childhood vaginal infections: Association of *Chlamydia trachomatis* with sexual contact. *Pediatr Infect Dis* 5:226, 1986.

19 Bartley DL et al: *Gardnerella vaginalis* in prepubertal girls. *Am J Dis Child* 141:1014, 1987.

20 Hammerschlag MR et al: Colonization of sexually abused children with genital mycoplasmas. *Sex Transm Dis* 14:23, 1987.

21 Wald ER: Gynecologic infections in the pediatric age group. *Pediatr Infect Dis* 3:S10, 1984.

22 Sexual abuse and sexually transmitted diseases in children. *Can Med Assoc J* 134:1272, 1986.

23 Kempe CH: Sexual abuse, another hidden pediatric problem: The 1977 C. Anderson Aldrich lecture. *Pediatrics* 62:382, 1978.

24 Rosenfeld AA et al: Familial bathing patterns: Implications for cases of alleged molestation and for pediatric practice: *Pediatrics* 79:224, 1987.

25 Frau LM, Alexander ER: Public health implications of sexually transmitted diseases in pediatric practice. *Pediatr Infect Dis* 4:453, 1985.

26 Srivastava AC: Survival of gonococci in urethral secretions with reference to the nonsexual transmission of gonococcal infection. *J Med Microbiol* 13:593, 1980.

27 Gilbaugh JH, Fuchs PC: The gonococcus and the toilet seat. *N Engl J Med* 301:91, 1972.

28 Rein MF: Nonsexual acquisition of gonococcal infection (letter). *N Engl J Med* 301:1347, 1979.

29 Branch G, Paxton P: A study of gonococcal infections among infants and children. *Public Health Rep* 80:347, 1965.

30 Folland DS et al: Gonorrhea in preadolescent children: An inquiry into source of infection and mode of transmission. *Pediatrics* 60: 153, 1977.

31 Farrell MK et al: Prepubertal gonorrhea: A multidisciplinary approach. *Pediatrics* 67:151, 1981.

32 Ingram DL et al: Sexual contact in children with gonorrhea. *Am J Dis Child* 136:994, 1982.

33 Silber TJ, Controni G: Clinical spectrum of pharyngeal gonorrhea in children and adolescents. *J Adolesc Health Care* 4:51, 1983.

34 Alexander WJ et al: Infections in sexual contacts and associates of children with gonorrhea. *Sex Transm Dis* 11:156, 1984.

35 Nair P et al: *Neisseria gonorrhoeae* in asymptomatic prepubertal household contacts of children with gonococcal infection. *Clin Pediatr* 25:160, 1986.

36 Rowe DS et al: Purulent ocular discharge in neonates: Significance of *Chlamydia trachomatis. Pediatrics* 63:628, 1979.

37 Beem MO, Saxon EM: Respiratory-tract colonization and a distinctive pneumonia syndrome in infants infected with *Chlamydia trachomatis. N Engl J Med* 296:306, 1975.

38 Bell TA et al: Delayed appearance of *Chlamydia trachomatis* infections acquired at birth. *Pediatr Infect Dis* 6:928, 1987.

39 Bell TA et al: Chronic *Chlamydia trachomatis* infections in infants, in *Chlamydial Infections,* JD Oriel (ed). Cambridge, Cambridge University Press, 1986, pp 305–308.

40 Black SB et al: Serologic evidence of chlamydial infection in children. *J Pediatr* 98:65, 1981.

41 San Joaquin VH et al: Prevalence of chlamydial antibodies in children. *Am J Dis Child* 136:425, 1982.

42 Grayston JT et al: Seroepidemiology of *Chlamydia trachomatis* infection, in *Chlamydial Infections,* PA Mardh et al (eds). New York, Elsevier, 1982.

43 Burney P et al: The epidemiology of chlamydial infections in childhood: A serological investigation. *Int J Epidemiol* 13:491, 1984.

44 Rettig PJ: Infections due to *Chlamydia trachomatis* from infancy to adolescence. *Pediatr Infect Dis* 5:449, 1986.

45 Schachter J: Chlamydial infections. *N Engl J Med* 298:428, 1978.

46 Blattner RJ: *Trichomonas vaginalis* infection in a newborn infant. *J Pediatr* 71:608, 1967.

47 Al-Salihi FL et al: Neonatal *Trichomonas vaginalis.* Report of three cases and a review of the literature. *Pediatrics* 53:196, 1974.

48 Jones JG et al: *Trichomonas vaginalis* infection in sexually abused girls. *Am J Dis Child* 139:846, 1985.

49 Burgess JA: Trichomonas vaginalis infection from splashing in water closets. *Br J Vener Dis* 39:248, 1963.

50 Kaplan KM et al: Social relevance of genital herpes simplex in children. *Am J Dis Child* 138:872, 1984.

51 Larson T, Bryson YJ: Fomites and herpes simplex virus [letter]. *J Infect Dis* 151:746, 1985.

52 Douglas JM, Corey L: Fomites and herpes simplex virus: A case for nonvenereal transmission? *JAMA* 250:3093, 1983.

53 Nahmias AJ et al: Genital infection with herpes-virus hominis types 1 and 2 in children. *Pediatrics* 42:659, 1968.

54 Gardner M, Jones JG: Genital herpes acquired by sexual abuse of children. *Pediatrics* 104:243, 1984.

55 Chuang T-Y: Condylomata acuminata (genital warts): An epidemiologic view. *J Am Acad Dermatol* 16:376, 1987.

56 Oriel JD: Natural history of genital warts. *Br J Vener Dis* 47:1, 1971.
57 Rock B et al: Genital tract papillomavirus infection in children. *Arch Dermatol* 122:1129, 1986.
58 Barrett TJ et al: Genital wart: A venereal disease. *JAMA* 154:333, 1954.
59 Patel R, Groff DB: Condyloma acuminata in childhood. *Pediatrics* 50:153, 1972.
60 Ferenczy A et al: Latent papillomavirus and recurring genital warts. *N Engl J Med* 313:784, 1985.
61 Carpiniello V et al: Magnified penile surface scanning in diagnosis of penile condyloma. *Urology* 28:190, 1986.
62 Bennett RS, Powell KR: Human papillomaviruses: Association between laryngeal papillomas and genital warts. *Pediatr Infect Dis* 6:229, 1987.
63 Genital warts and sexual abuse in children. *J Am Acad Dermatol* 11:529, 1984.
64 Shelton TB et al: Condylomata acuminata in the pediatric patient. *J Urol* 135:548, 1986.
65 Pheifer TA et al: Nonspecific vaginitis: Role of *Haemophilus vaginalis* and treatment with metronidazole. *N Engl J Med* 298:1429, 1978.
66 Chambers CV et al: Microflora of the urethra in adolescent boys: Relationships to sexual activity and nongonococcal urethritis. *J Pediatr* 110:314, 1987.
67 Shafer MA et al: Microbiology of the lower genital tract in postmenarchal adolescent girls: Differences by sexual activity contraception, and presence of nonspecific vaginitis. *J Pediatr* 107:974, 1985.
68 Bump RC et al: Sexually transmissible infectious agents in sexually active and virginal asymptomatic adolescent girls. *Pediatrics* 77: 488, 1986.
69 Leiderman IZ, Grimm KT: A child with HIV infection [letter]. *JAMA* 256:3094, 1986.
70 Ginsburg CM: Acquired syphilis in prepubertal children. *Pediatr Infect Dis* 2:232, 1983.
71 Bargman H: Is genital molluscum contagiosum a cutaneous manifestation of sexual abuse in children [letter]? *J Am Acad Dermatol* 14:847, 1986.
72 1985 STD treatment guidelines. *MMWR* 34(4S):34, 1985.
73 Whittington WL et al: Incorrect identification of *Neisseria gonorrhoeae* from infants and children. *Pediatr Infect Dis J* 7:3, 1988.
74 Bayes J: Criteria for doing serologic tests for syphilis in suspected child sexual abuse. Presented at the American Academy of Pediatrics, San Francisco, 1987.
75 Yeager TD, Altemeir WA: Assessment of routine serology in evaluation of child sexual abuse. *Am J Dis Child* 141:370, 1987.
76 Rettig PJ: Chlamydial infections in pediatrics: Diagnostic and therapeutic considerations. *Pediatr Infect Dis* 5:158, 1986.
77 Krieger JN et al: Diagnosis of trichomoniasis: Comparison of conventional wet mount examination with cytological studies, culture, and monoclonal antibody staining of direct specimens. *JAMA* 259:1223, 1988.
78 Totten PA et al: Selective differential human blood bilayer media for isolation of *Gardnerella (Hemophilus vaginalis)*. *J Clin Microbiol* 15:141, 1982.
79 Fuld GL: Gonococcal peritonitis in a prepubertal child. *Am J Dis Child* 115:621, 1968.
80 Burry VF: Gonococcal vulvovaginitis and possible peritonitis in prepubertal girls. *Am J Dis Child* 121:536, 1971.
81 Gialason T et al: Acute epididymitis in boys: A 5 year-retrospective study. *J Urol* 124:533, 1980.
82 Likitnukul S et al: Epididymitis in children and adolescents. A 20-year retrospective study. *Am J Dis Child* 141:41, 1987.

# PART VIII Diagnostic Testing for Selected Sexually Transmitted Diseases: Guidelines for Clinicians

# Chapter 73

# *Neisseria gonorrhoeae*

Per-Anders Mårdh
Dan Danielsson

The diagnosis of gonorrhea should be confirmed by demonstration of the causative organism, i.e., *Neisseria gonorrhoeae,* by microscopy and/or culture.[1,2,3] Recently introduced methods involve the demonstration of gonococcal antigens, e.g., by enzyme immunoassays[4,5] or techniques based on DNA hybridization,[6,7] although their clinical values remain to be established. The use of serological methods to demonstrate serum antigonococcal antibodies has also been suggested[8,9,10] but has so far remained of less importance.[11]

In this chapter we describe and discuss the relative value of laboratory diagnostic methods in uncomplicated or complicated gonococcal infections. For optimal results it is essential to have a solid knowledge of the biologic characteristics of *N. gonorrhoeae* and of the broad clinical spectrum of infections caused by this organism, matters that are elucidated and discussed in Chaps. 13,14, and 65.

## CULTURE VERSUS MICROSCOPY OF STAINED SMEARS

By the current use of enriched and selective media the gonococcus can no longer be considered difficult to grow. Even though microscopy of stained smears of urethral or cervical secretions is of great value in making a presumptive diagnosis of gonorrhea and documenting the presence or absence of inflammation, cultural methods have remained important in controlling gonorrhea for a number of reasons. First, identifying men and women with asymptomatic gonorrhea may be difficult by microscopy. Every second woman with gonorrhea may be asymptomatic, as is every fourth to fifth male (see Chap. 14). Second, cultural methods help to identify penicillinase-producing *N. gonorrhoeae* (PPNG), first recognized in 1976[12,13,14,15] and now spreading worldwide,[16,17] and chromosomally mediated penicillin-resistant (MIC > 2.5 mg/1) or multiresistant gonococcal strains[18,19] now being reported as common in several geographic areas.[20,21] Third, cultural methods are important for test of cure after treatment.

### Sensitivity, specificity, and predictive values of positive and negative tests

In order to correctly evaluate any diagnostic method, including laboratory techniques to diagnose gonorrhea, the sensitivity, specificity, and predictive values of positive (PVP) and of negative tests (PVN) of the methods are important to establish. As outlined by Galen and Gambino,[22] these statistical terms should be applied for any diagnostic method to identify diseased or infected people within a given population. Table 73-1 demonstrates how this statistical method can be applied to evaluate the efficiency of culture as a method for the diagnosis of gonorrhea. Accordingly, *sensitivity* is defined as the number of positive cultures/the true number of infected persons *(A/A + C); specificity* as the number of negative cultures/the number of noninfected persons *(D/B + D);* PVP as the number of positive cultures of persons with disease/the number of all positive cultures (i.e., true positives + false positives) *(A/A + B);* PVN as the number of negative cultures of healthy persons/the number of all negative cultures (i.e., true negatives + false negatives) *(D/C + D).* In the ideal situation all these four parameters should be 1 (or 100 percent). However, this never holds true in any laboratory diagnostic method. Recommended diagnostic tests for all these parameters however, should be as close as possible to 1 (100 percent).

It has been the objective for reference groups and centers in the United States, the United Kingdom, and the Scandinavian countries as well as by WHO[1,2,23,24] to establish reference methods for the laboratory diagnosis of gonorrhea.

Culture procedures are still the method of choice in the diagnosis of gonorrhea; PVP is 100 percent and specificity (with the recommended confirmatory tests used correctly) is 100 percent, whereas the sensitivity will be dependent on the viability and the ability of present gonococci to grow on the culture media used. Under optimized conditions the sensitivity may be 90 to 95 percent, and the PVN very close to 100 percent.[25] Thereby it follows that when the efficiency of any new test is subjected to evaluation, the yield must be compared with that of the cultural method used under optimized conditions in order to be able to establish the sensitivity, specificity, PVP, and PVN of the test (Table 73-2).

The efficiency of any diagnostic method will be dependent on the prevalence of disease in the particular study population. In a population with a low prevalence of disease—for example, in a group with 1 percent of gonorrhea—using a diagnostic method

**Table 73-1. Method for the Calculation of Sensitivity, Specificity, and the Predictive Values of Positive and Negative Results of a Diagnostic Method Used to Diagnose People with Disease (in this Case Gonorrhea)**

| Diagnostic method (culture for gonococci) | People (patients) subjected to testing: Gonorrhea | People (patients) subjected to testing: Not gonorrhea | Total |
|---|---|---|---|
| Positive result | *A* | *B* | *A + B* |
| Negative result | *C* | *D* | *C + D* |
| Total | *A + C* | *B + D* | *A + B + C + D* |

| | | |
|---|---|---|
| Sensitivity of the method | Positive culture / True number of people with gonorrhea | = $\frac{A}{A + C}$ |
| Specificity of the method | Negative culture / True number of people without gonorrhea | = $\frac{D}{B + D}$ |
| Predictive value of a positive (PVP) culture | Positive culture of people with gonorrhea / Number of all positive cultures (true positives = *A*; false positives = *B*) | = $\frac{A}{A + B}$ |
| Predictive value of a negative (PVN) culture | Negative culture of people without gonorrhea / Number of all negative cultures (true negatives = *D*; false negatives = C) | = $\frac{D}{C + D}$ |

Adapted from Galen and Gambino.[22]

**Table 73-2. Method for Calculation of the Sensitivity, Specificity, and the Predictive Values of Positive (PVP) and Negative (PVN) Results of an Alternative Diagnostic Test for the Laboratory Diagnosis of Gonorrhea**

| Alternative diagnostic method (antigen detection or DNA hybridization) | Reference method (culture under optimal conditions) Positive | Negative | Total |
|---|---|---|---|
| Positive results | $A$ | $B$ | $A + B$ |
| Negative results | $C$ | $D$ | $C + D$ |
| Total | $A + C$ | $B + D$ | $A + B + C + D$ |
| Alternative method | | | |
| Sensitivity | | | $\frac{A}{A + C}$ |
| Specificity | | | $\frac{D}{B + D}$ |
| PVP | | | $\frac{A}{A + B}$ |
| PVN | | | $\frac{D}{C + D}$ |
| Overall agreement of the two methods | | | $\frac{A + D}{A + B + C + D}$ |

The alternative method, e.g., antigen detection or DNA-hybridization, is compared with the reference method (in this case culture performed under optimal conditions).

with a sensitivity of 90 percent and a specificity of 99 percent, the PVP will only be 50 percent, whereas the PVN will be 99.9 percent. However, in a population with a prevalence of 10 percent gonorrhea when using a diagnostic method with a sensitivity of 90 percent and a specificity of 98 percent, the PVP will be 91 percent and the PVN 98.9 percent. Obviously, it is of great importance to be aware of these interrelations, not the least when selecting laboratory methods for screening programs for gonorrhea, and for the evaluation of the relative value of new diagnostic methods as compared with the standard reference method.

## COLLECTION, TRANSPORT, AND STORAGE OF SPECIMENS TO BE TESTED

### Sampling site

Table 73-3 shows a compilation of the sampling sites in uncomplicated or complicated gonorrhea in males and females with regard to sexual preference. The sampling techniques are thoroughly discussed in Chap. 14. The special problems faced in sampling from infants and children are considered in Chap. 65.

### Specimen collection and sampling technique

Specimens from the urethra, the cervical os, the Bartholin's glands, the anal canal, the oropharynx, and the conjunctivae (see Table 73-3) can be collected by the aid of sterile cotton-tipped swabs or with a bacteriologic loop or blunt curette for ("bedside") inoculation directly on gonococcal culture media, or with specially prepared (charcoal-treated) samplings swabs (see below) for transport of the sample to the laboratory in nonnutritive transport media.[3,26,27] For both methods, the following sampling techniques are recommended.

**Table 73-3. Compilation of Sampling Sites for Culture of Gonococci in Specimens from Males and Females, Newborns, Infants, and Children**

| Patient category | Primary sampling site | Additional sites |
|---|---|---|
| Men: | | |
| Heterosexual | Urethra | Oropharynx if practicing cunnilingus<br>Urethral secretion after prostatic massage |
| Homosexual/bisexual | Urethra<br>Anal canal (rectum)<br>Oropharynx | Urethral secretion after prostatic massage |
| Women | Cervical os | Urethra and anal canal. Oropharynx if practicing fellatio. Bartholin's glands if bartholinitis |
| Men and women with disseminated gonococcal infection (DGI) | As above | Blood<br>Joint fluid (if present)<br>Skin lesions |
| Newborns with ophthalmia | Conjunctivae | Mother: cervix, urethra, and anal canal |
| Infants and children | See Chap. 65 | |

Anal canal is the only positive site in 4 to 6 percent of females with gonorrhea.[29]
Blood for culture gives a low diagnostic yield.[30,31]
Acute and convalescent sera for demonstrating an immune response.
Smears on glass slides of material from skin lesions for immunofluorescent staining.[30,31]

Urethral samples from men are collected by introducing the sampling swab approximately 1 to 2 cm up into the urethra, where it is gently rotated before withdrawal. The swab can be moistened in saline before use in order to facilitate its introduction. Alternatively, the mucosa of the anterior urethra is scraped by a sterile blunt curette or a sterile (cool) bacteriological loop. To increase the chance of recovering gonococci the patient should not have voided for at least a couple of hours before sampling, particularly men without discharge. Urethral samples from women are collected by stripping the urethra from the vagina toward the orifice in order to express exudate, which is collected on a sampling swab when it appears at the orifice. For both men and women, it is considered important to let the swab remain in the urethra for some seconds to allow secretion to be absorbed.

In order to collect samples from the cervix, a speculum is introduced into the vagina. The speculum may be moistened with warm water before use. Gynecologic exploration creme should not be used since many such cremes may contain ingredients lethal to gonococci. The vaginal wall and the cervix are carefully inspected and material is taken from the lateral vaginal fornix for preparation of a wet smear for microscopy (see also Chap. 46). Excess cervical mucus should be removed with a cotton ball held in a ring forceps. A sampling swab is introduced in the cervical canal and moved from side to side before withdrawal after 10 to 30 s. To increase the diagnostic yield by approximately 5 percent, a second specimen can be collected from the endocervical canal.[28]

If the hymen is intact, samples are collected from the vaginal orifice. Vaginal samples may also be collected from the posterior vaginal fornix, but this is not recommended as a standard procedure.

Rectal samples are collected by introducing a sterile swab 3 to 4 cm into the rectum. Preferably a proctoscope is used (see Chap. 14 for details of this sampling technique). The anal canal is the only positive site in 4 to 6 percent of women with gonorrhea.[29]

Oropharyngeal specimens are collected by streaking the swab over the posterior pharynx and the tonsils, and also by pressing the tip of the swab against tonsillar crypts. This technique has been considered especially efficient.

In patients with a suspected disseminated gonococcal infection (DGI) urogenital, oropharyngeal, and rectal (in women and in homosexual men) specimens should always be collected since a combination of such samples will give the best diagnostic yield (positive in about 90 percent of cases). Additional specimens to establish the diagnosis are blood for conventional blood culture, joint fluid and materials from skin lesions, and acute and convalescent sera to demonstrate an active immune response. Blood culture specimens should be collected as soon as the diagnosis of DGI is suspected, since the percentage of patients with positive blood cultures declines rapidly after the onset of symptoms and signs of DGI. The medium employed must support growth of gonococci. If sodium polyanetholsulfonate (SPS) is used as anticoagulant in the blood culture medium, it may interfere with the recovery of some gonococcal strains. Joint fluid is aspirated from possibly infected joints, transported to the laboratory in a capped syringe or in a sterile tube for Gram stain and culture, or inoculated directly in blood culture bottles. Materials from skin lesions are scraped off with a sterile lancet or scalpel, smeared on a glass slide, and sent to the laboratory for examination with fluorescent labeled antigonococcal antibodies. In the hands of experienced laboratories the last mentioned method is, next to culture or genitourinary specimens, the most sensitive diagnostic test in DGI cases.[30,31] Culture of skin lesions usually gives negative results.

The prerequisites and the special techniques used for sampling specimens from the endometrium, the fallopian tubes, and the cul-de-sac in etiologic studies of endometritis and pelvic inflammatory disease are described in Chaps. 49 and 50.[32] The special sampling techniques in etiologic studies of epididymitis and prostatitis are described in Chaps. 53 and 54.[32]

## Inoculation of specimens on growth media bedside, storage and transport

Gonococci are highly susceptible to environmental influences (oxidation, desiccation, heat, etc.). They may occur in low numbers in the clinical specimens and they also need $CO_2$ for their initial growth in vitro. Specimens inoculated on nutritive media bedside must therefore be handled properly at the office, and transported to the laboratory in a manner that preserves viability.

For bedside inoculation, solid gonococcal culture medium should be used. These plates must be less than 2 to 3 weeks old, kept in sealed plastic bags in the refrigerator to prevent drying, and brought to room temperature before being inoculated. The specimen swab is rolled over one-third to one-half of the agar surface, after which the remainder surface is crossed-streaked with a sterile bacteriologic loop or swab. The agar plates are incubated within 20 to 30 min at 35 to 36°C in an atmosphere of 4 to 6 percent $CO_2$. This atmosphere is most easily achieved with the candle extinction jar technique, the method of choice for STD clinics that do not possess a $CO_2$-regulated incubator. A candle extinction jar may be arranged by using any jar with a lid and placing a candle on the plates before closing the lid. An optimal $CO_2$-atmosphere is achieved when the candle is extinguished by the lack of oxygen. A moistened blotting paper may be placed in the bottom of the jar to ensure high humidity. For maximum recovery and survival of gonococci the plates should be incubated at 35 to 36°C for 18 to 24 h before transfer to the local laboratory. On arrival the plates can be incubated for an additional 24 h before reading the plates.

It has been well documented that direct plating in the patient care area onto freshly prepared and well-stored culture media is the most sensitive means to diagnose gonococcal infections.[33,34] Alternatives to this technique are bedside inoculation on nutritive (growth) transport systems or "culture kits" such as the JEMBEC plate,[35,36] the Bio-Bag (Marion Scientific, Kansas City, MO), and the Gono-Pak system (Nasco, Modesto, CA). The JEMBEC plate is a rectangular polystyrene dish with a removable cover and a molded inner well into which a $CO_2$-generating tablet (composed of sodium bicarbonate and citric acid) can be placed after inoculation of the medium. The plates contain selective gonococcal culture media and must be stored in the office as indicated above for conventional culture plates. In the Bio-Bag and Gono-Pak systems the plates are after inoculation placed in individual ziplocked plastic bags, each of which contains a $CO_2$-generating tablet or ampoule. Moisture evaporated from the medium during incubation is sufficient to activate the tablet to generate a suitable $CO_2$-atmosphere. For maximum recovery and survival of gonococci, the JEMBEC plates or the plastic bags with agar plates are incubated at 35 to 36°C for 18 to 24 h before transfer to the laboratory. The plates may be delivered by mail. On arrival at the laboratory, the plates can be handled in the same way as described for bedside inoculation with the use of the candle extinction jar method.

Quality control has been an occasional problem, and some kits perform less well with samples from "bacteriologically complicated" sites, i.e., the pharynx and the rectum. The choice of transport and/or culture-kit system must be made in the light of local requirements and circumstances. The lifetime of the kits employed must be checked before use. It is advisable to have the local laboratory perform quality-control comparisons periodically.

## Transport of specimens in nonnutritive transport media

Specimens for gonococcal culture may be transported to the laboratory on Amie's medium[26] or on modified Stuart's medium[27] which are both nonnutritive transport media. These media can also be used for other kinds of clinical specimens. The nonnutritive transport media have the advantage of being simple to use and are relatively inexpensive and easy to store. They have a long shelf life, even at room temperature. They have greatly facilitated, for public health clinics, private physicians, emergency rooms, various types of hospital wards, etc., the taking of specimens for culture diagnosis of gonorrhea. If the specimens reach the laboratory within 24 h, the sensitivity may only be 5 to 10 percent lower than bedside inoculation using the candle extinction jar method.[33] However, the sensitivity may be less than 50 percent if the specimens are delayed in transit to the laboratory for 2 days or more. Thus rapid transfer of specimens to the laboratory is essential.

Precautions must be taken for the sampling swabs used for transport of gonococcal specimens in nonnutritive media since swabs may be toxic for gonococci, both cotton, wooden, and metal sticks. To prevent the toxic effect of wooden sticks, they must be boiled in 0.2*M* phosphate buffer, pH 7.2, for 5 to 10 min to eliminate the toxic resins present in certain types of wood.[3] Metal sticks are not recommended. The cotton-tipped

Table 73-4. Modified Stuart's Medium

Bacto agar: 20 g
Thioglycollate: 2 ml
Sodium glycerophosphate (20% w/v): 1000 ml
$CaCl_2$ (1% w/v): 20 ml
Methylene blue (0.1% w/v): 4 ml
Distilled water: 1900 ml

Dissolve the thioglycollate in distilled water. Suspend the agar in the solution and adjust the pH of the mixture to 7.2. Add the sodium glycerophosphate and calcium chloride solutions and adjust the pH to 7.4. Add the methylene blue solution. Heat to boiling and distribute the medium into tubes to a height of at least 8 cm. Sterilize by autoclaving at 121°C for 20 min

SOURCE: B Gästrin and LO Kallings.[27]

sampling stick should be treated with charcoal. The carbon particles will absorb fatty acids and other toxic compounds present in the cotton of the sampling swab, in the sample itself, and in most types of agar. Thus the cotton-tipped wooden stick is treated with medical charcoal (20 g dissolved in 1000 ml distilled water) by dipping the cotton-tipped sampling swab in the solution. The treated swab is air-dried and autoclaved at 120°C for 15 min. Sampling swabs treated in that way are commercially available.

Amie's[26] and the modified Stuart's media[27] (Table 73-4) are based on the principle of being nonnutritive and having a low redox potential to prevent oxidation, achieved by the addition of thioglycollate to the medium. Reduced methylene blue (which in a reduced state is colorless) is added as a marker of the redox potential being sufficiently low. When the redox potential rises, the methylene blue will become oxidized and turns blue. Transport tubes should be stored in the dark, since an irreversible color change of methylene blue will take place if the medium is stored in the light. Test tubes with Stuart's medium should not be used if the medium has turned blue for more than two-thirds of the height of the medium.

## CULTURE MEDIA AND ISOLATION

### Media formulations and preparation

Several commercial media are available, most of which give satisfactory results. They usually consist of a phosphate buffered peptone-starch agar base (Difco, BBL GC-agar base; Oxoid Columbia agar) to which is added hemoglobin or horse blood, a defined supplement (IsoVitaleX) or yeast dialysate, and horse or pig serum (Table 73-5). Two, three, or even four antibiotics may be added at the recommended concentrations (Table 73-6). The widely used modified Thayer-Martin (MTM) and Martin-Lewis (ML) media[37,38] contain no serum in their original version. However, it is the experience of most laboratories involved in quality controls that the addition of horse or pig serum is necessary to stimulate growth of fastidious gonococcal strains,[34,39,40] most of which have the auxotrophic markers $Arg^-/Hyg^-/Ura^-$ and belong to serogroup WI (see Chap. 13). We therefore strongly recommend that serum is added as suggested in the recipe of Table 73-5. The use of hemoglobin or heated horse blood may be optimal. The New York City (NYC) medium,[39] which is widely used in certain parts of the United States, contains hemolyzed horse erythrocytes, yeast dialysate, and horse plasma in place of hemoglobin and defined supplement in the MTM and ML media.

Table 73-5. Modified Thayer-Martin's Medium for *Neisseria gonorrhoeae**

**Composition of Gc agar base, grams per liter distilled water**

Peptone: 15
Dipotassium phosphate ($K_2HPO_4$): 4
Monopotassium phosphate ($KH_2PO_4$): 1
Cornstarch: 1
Sodium chloride: 5
Agar: 10

**Preparation of medium**

1. Suspend 36 g of dehydrated Gc agar base in 500 ml of distilled water, heat to boiling under frequent agitation.
2. Prepare 500 ml of a 2% (w/v) suspension of dehydrated hemoglobin. Autoclave both suspensions at 121°C (15 lb) for 15 min.
3. Cool to 50°C.
4. Mix aseptically 500 ml of the Gc agar base and 500 ml of the hemoglobin solution. Keep the temperature at 50°C!
5. Add aseptically the antibiotic solution prepared so the final concentration will be 12.5 μg nystatin, 7.5 μg colistin, 3.0 μg vancomycin, and 5 μg trimethoprim per milliliter.
6. Reconstitute the IsoVitaleX enrichment by adding aseptically to the lyophilized constituents sterile rehydrating fluid (10 ml). Shake to obtain complete solution.
7. Add aseptically 10 ml of the IsoVitaleX solution and 100 ml horse or pig serum to 1000 ml medium.
8. Mix gently (but thoroughly) and pour the medium into sterile petri dishes. Store it at 4°C.

*See also Refs. 33, 37, 40.
Thayer-Martin's selective agar medium for culture of gonococci is based on commercially available Gc agar base (BBL, Difco) to which hemoglobin (BBL, Difco), IsoVitaleX enrichment (BBL), and a mixture of nystatin, colistin, vancomycin, and trimethoprim is added. (BBL = Baltimore Biological Laboratory)
*Note:* Horse or pig serum is also added.

NYC medium is translucent, which facilitates the selection of oxidase positive colonies and inspection of the plates under a stereomicroscope. It also supports the growth of *Mycoplasma hominis* and *Ureaplasma urealyticum*.

Some gonococcal strains, usually of auxotype $Arg^-/Hyg^-/Ura^-$ (see also below), are susceptible to the concentration of vancomycin used in MTM and ML media (3 to 4 mg/l medium) and will therefore not be recovered on selective media using the

Table 73-6. Amounts of Antimicrobial Agents Present in Three Common Media Used for the Isolation of Pathogenic *Neisseria*

| | | Concentrations, mg/l | | |
|---|---|---|---|---|
| Antimicrobial | Function | MTM* | NYC† | SBL‡ |
| Vancomycin | Inhibits gram-positive bacteria | 3 | 2 | 1.5 |
| Colistin | Inhibits gram-negative bacteria | 7.5 | 5.5 | 7.5 |
| Trimethoprim lactate | Inhibits swarming *Proteus* | 5 | 3 | 5 |
| Nystatin | Inhibits some yeasts | 12.5 | | |
| Amphotericin B | Inhibits some yeasts | | 1.2 | |

*Modified Thayer-Martin's medium.
†New York City Medium.
‡Concentrations usually used in Sweden and other Scandinavian countries.

drug.[25,34,41] Most of these problems are solved by using lower concentrations of vancomycin, e.g., 2 mg/l in the NYC medium and 1.5 mg/l in the media used and recommended in, for example, the Scandinavian countries. A medium containing lincomycin instead of vancomycin has also been suggested.[25,41] Some gonococcal strains are also susceptible to trimethoprim but seldom to the concentrations used.[40] The number of gonococcal strains susceptible to the concentrations of the antimicrobials used will vary in different geographic areas with time. The prevalence of such strains can be evaluated by periodically including nonselective culture media (no antibiotics) or media containing only trimethoprim together with the selective medium.

Liquid media that allow growth of most strains of *N. gonorrhoeae* have been described.[42] Improved recovery from clinical specimens was reported by selective enrichment and detection by immunological methods.[43]

## Incubation conditions and colony growth

An incubation temperature of 35 to 36°C, a high humidity, and an atmosphere of 4 to 6 percent $CO_2$ are optimal for growth of *N. gonorrhoeae*. Incubated plates should be inspected after 24 to 28 h with the use of a stereomicroscope but should be kept for another overnight incubation before being read and discarded.

The colony size may vary considerably, and those representing $Arg^-/Hyg^-/Ura^-$ strains are often the smallest, whereas those representing prototrophic or proline dependent strains are generally much larger.

Colonies of different morphology type occur. In primary cultures, colonies of types T1 and T2, according to the nomenclature by Kellogg and coworkers,[44] dominate. These designations correspond to the piliated transparent ($P^+Op^-$) and piliated opaque ($P^+Op^+$) colony type, respectively, according to the nomenclature by Swanson[45] (see also Chap. 13). Colonies of types T1 and T2 convert on passage on artificial media to T3 and T4 (nonpiliated opaque and nonpiliated transparent, respectively). These colony morphology types are most easily recognized on the medium described by Kellogg et al. which is translucent and easy to use for inspection of the colonies under a stereomicroscope. This medium cannot, however, be used for the primary isolation of gonococci from clinical specimens.

## Identification

**Oxidase Test and Presumptive Identification.** The oxidase reaction can be used to aid the search for gonococcal colonies in mixed cultures. A drop of tetramethyl- or dimethyl-paraphenylene-diamine is poured over suspected gonococcal colonies which quickly (within 10 s, though slower with the dimethyl reagent, which is more toxic) turn pink and then dark blue. False-positive reactions may be seen with oxidase-negative organisms after a longer interval of the reagent on the colonies. The test can also be made on a piece of blotting paper when material from a suspected gonococcal colony is rubbed on a spot previously impregnated with the reagent. The oxidase reagent kills the gonococcus relatively rapidly. Thus subculture may be necessary when only a few suspected colonies are detected before the oxidase test can be performed.

Fresh oxidase reagent should be prepared daily from a stock solution (Table 73-7).

It should be remembered that all other species of *Neisseria* and bacteria of a number of other genera, including *Moraxella, Branhamella, Eikenella, Kingella,* and *Pseudomonas,* are also oxidase-positive.[34,46] A Gram stain of oxidase-positive colonies is therefore essential. In urogenital specimens, oxidase-positive organisms forming characteristic colonies containing gram-negative diplococci may be given the presumptive diagnosis of gonococci. Further confirmatory testing is strongly recommended because of the risk of misinterpretations. This risk is considerable when gonococci are searched for in specimens collected from extragenital sites.

**Table 73-7. Reagent for Tests of Oxidase Production by Gonococci**

*Stock solution:*
Dissolve 1 g tetramethyl-paraphenylene-diammonium-dichloride ($C_{10}H_{18}Cl_2N_2$) in 4 ml distilled water and add ethanol (96% v/v) up to 100 ml. Store the solution in darkness
*Ready-to-use solution:*
Mix before use 1 part of the stock solution and 2 parts of distilled water

## Confirmatory identification by biochemical reactions

*N. gonorrhoeae* are oxidase-positive, gram-negative diplococci with the capacity to degrade glucose but not maltose, sucrose, fructose, or lactose. Carbohydrate degradation tests are the reference confirmatory tests to differentiate gonococci from other *Neisseria* spp. and related organisms. *N. meningitidis* degrade glucose and maltose, *N. lactamica* glucose, maltose, and lactose, while apathogenic *Neisseria* spp. degrade glucose, maltose, sucrose, and fructose or none of these carbohydrates.[34,46] DNase and superoxol tests may be used to distinguish *Branhamella catarrhalis* from pathogenic and nonpathogenic *Neisseria* species.[47]

Some other characteristics of the different *Neisseria* spp. and related bacteria are shown in Table 73-8.

Carbohydrate degradation tests can be performed in a number of different ways, for example, by growing gonococci on carbohydrate-containing media, with preformed enzyme tests,[2] radiometric detection,[48] chromogenic enzyme substrate systems,[49] and similar tests.

**Carbohydrate Degradation Tests on Solid Medium.** A considerable number of more or less complicated media formulations have been devised for such tests, probably reflecting the difficulties encountered, particularly with some gonococcal strains that grow poorly on the media. Many laboratories have preferred to use the modified cystine-tryptic digest agar-base (modified CTA) medium (Table 73-9), which consists of CTA with an agar concentration of 1.5 percent and a carbohydrate concentration of 2 percent.[50] The medium is tubed on slants. The CTA test battery commonly includes glucose, maltose, sucrose, fructose, and lactose. Ortho-nitrophenyl-beta-D-galactosidase (ONPG) tests may substitute for lactose. Heavy inocula of pure cultures are needed, and when performed properly, identification can usually be made within 24 h. CTA tests should not be incubated in $CO_2$ atmosphere since this affects pH and therefore the test results. Failures with the proper identification may be due to (1) poor growth; (2) contamination of the culture with other bacteria; (3) use of other than reagent-grade carbohydrates, for example, maltose containing too much glucose. Difficulties are particularly met with poorly growing AHU strains. Moreover, strict aerobes (like the *Neisseria* organisms) produce less acid

Table 73-8. Characteristics of *Neisseria* and *Branhamella* Species

| | Utilization of | | | | | Reduction of | | Other characteristics | | |
|---|---|---|---|---|---|---|---|---|---|---|
| | Glucose | Maltose | Lactose | Fructose | Sucrose | Nitrate | Nitrite | Growth at 22°C | Oxidase | Catalase |
| *N. gonorrhoeae* | + | − | − | − | − | ∓ | ∓ | − | + | + |
| *N. meningitidis* | + | + | − | − | − | ∓ | *v* | − | + | + |
| *N. lactamica** | + | + | + | − | − | ∓ | + | *v* | + | + |
| *N. flavescens* | ∓ | ∓ | ∓ | ∓ | ∓ | + | + | + | + | + |
| *N. subflava* | + | + | ∓ | *v* | *v* | ∓ | + | *v* | + | + |
| *N. sicca* | + | + | ∓ | + | + | ∓ | + | *v* | + | + |
| *N. mucosa* | + | + | ∓ | + | + | + | + | + | + | + |
| *B. catarrhalis* | ∓ | ∓ | ∓ | ∓ | ∓ | − | − | + | + | − |

*ONPG positive = production of β-galactosidase.
NOTE: ∓ = positive in few instances; *v* = variable.

Table 73-9. Media for Testing Carbohydrate Utilization by *Neisseria gonorrhoeae**

**Composition of basic CTA medium, grams per liter distilled water†**

Cystine: 0.5
Typticase peptone: 20.0
Agar: 15.0
Sodium chloride: 5.0
Sodium sulfite: 0.5
Phenol red: 0.017

**Preparation of medium**

1. Suspend the components in distilled water.
2. Mix thoroughly and heat gently with frequent agitation, until the solution is complete.
3. Sterilize by autoclaving at 115 to 118°C (not over 12 lb steam pressure) for 15 min.
4. Cool to 50°C.
5. Add aseptically suitable volumes of 20% (w/v) filter-sterilized, reagent-grade carbohydrate solution (glucose, maltose, lactose, fructose, and sucrose) to obtain a final concentration of 2% of the carbohydrates.
6. Adjust the pH of the mixture to 7.3.
7. Dispense aseptically in screw-capped tubes.
8. Allow medium to solidify in a slanted position.
9. Store at 4°C with tightly closed screw caps.

**Composition of basic modified oxidation-fermentation (MOF) medium, grams per liter of distilled water**

Proteose peptone no. 3 (Difco): 2.0
NaCl: 5.0
$K_2HPO_4$: 0.3
Agar: 3.0
Phenol red: 0.017

**Preparation of medium**

1. Dissolve reagents and sterilize at 121°C for 15 min.
2. Filter sterilize carbohydrate solutions and add to give a final concentration of 1% (w/v).
3. Adjust pH to 7.2.
4. Dispense medium aseptically in 2.5 ml volumes in sterile test tubes.
5. Basic medium can be stored at 4°C for several months and at room temperature for several weeks before use.

*See Ref. 50.
†The basic medium is available from BBL.
SOURCE: Based on data from Dr. Joan Knapp (personal communication).

from degradation of carbohydrates than fermentative organisms. Many *Neisseria* spp. also produce ammonia from peptone, which might neutralize acid produced from utilization of carbohydrates.

Hugh and Leifson[51] modified the CTA medium by reducing the concentration of protein relative to carbohydrate so that less ammonia is produced. This medium was further altered by Knapp to produce a modified oxidation-fermentation medium (MOF, Table 73-9), which appears to be preferable to CTA for carbohydrate utilization tests of *Neisseria*. The medium is simple to prepare and may be stored for several months at 4°C. The test tubes should be inoculated by a single stab. Incubation is for 18 to 24 h at 35 to 36°C without added $CO_2$. Reactions can often be read after 4 to 8 h incubation.

**Rapid Carbohydrate Degradation Tests.** Non-growth-requiring methods to differentiate *Neisseria* spp. are used by many laboratories.[2] Basically, a very dense suspension (corresponding to 5 to 10 percent) of suspected gonococci is added to lightly buffered salt solutions containing the carbohydrates to be tested and phenol red. The tests depend on preformed enzyme in the inoculum and not on growth in the medium. The test is economic and results are available within 1 to 4 h. The carbohydrates used may include glucose, maltose, sucrose, and fructose. The ONPG test is routinely included for identification of *N. lactamica*.[34,46] It is of great importance to use reagent-grade maltose (<0.25 percent of glucose), which is commercially available.

Minitek (BBL) is an alternative to the rapid degradation test.[52] It uses paper disks impregnated with high concentrations of appropriate carbohydrates that are placed in individual wells of a plastic plate. A small volume of a heavy suspension of the organisms is prepared in broth and is pipetted into each disk-containing well. Plates are incubated without $CO_2$ and observed hourly. Most reactions occur within 4 h; the remainder are read after overnight incubation.

Recently, tests have become available that use conventional biochemical reactions and bacterial enzyme substrates to identify and differentiate *Neisseria* and *Branhamella* spp. The API NeIdent panel (Analytab Products, Inc., Plainview, NY) consists of 11 miniaturized conventional and chromogenic enzyme substrates.[53] The RapID NH system (Innovative Diagnostics Systems, Inc., Decatur, GA) is a plastic cuvette containing substrate for 12 tests, which can be read after 4 h.[49] Conventional tests and two aminopeptidase substrate tests are included in the system, which can also be used for identification of *Haemophilus* spp. The two mentioned kits have given satisfactory results in comparative studies, but more experience from routine use is needed.

**The BACTEC Method.** The BACTEC *Neisseria* Differentiation Kit[48] (Johnston Laboratories) is a possibility for users of the BACTEC radiometric instrument for blood cultures. Three vials in the kit contain small volumes of $^{14}C$-labeled glucose, maltose, and fructose in deionized water. The vials should be heavily inoculated with a suspension of the organisms under test and read in the BACTEC machine after 3 h incubation. The instrument detects $^{14}CO_2$ evolved from the vials due to degradation. An ONPG test is performed to detect betagalactosidase in order to identify *N. lactamica*. The BACTEC method is highly sensitive and may identify strains of gonococci that do not produce detectable acid in growth-dependent identification systems.[48] However, some strains of apathogenic *Neisseria* spp. that do not degrade glucose in conventional tests may yield a low-positive glucose reading in the BACTEC system.

**Comments on Biochemical Confirmatory Tests.** There are several pitfalls with these test systems. Failures are mainly due to (1) impure culture; (2) too small an inoculum; (3) use of nonreagent-grade carbohydrates, especially maltose that often contains various amounts of glucose; (4) use of pH, buffer, and indicator that may not be optimal for the test. There are usually no problems with the identification of gonococcal strains isolated from urogenital specimens, but occasionally problem strains are met. Attention must especially be paid to assumed gonococcal strains from extragenital sites. For these isolates usually more than one confirmatory test method must be used. Problem strains should be sent to reference laboratories and be labeled with a presumptive diagnosis until the final identification result is obtained.

## Confirmatory identification by serological tests

**Immunofluorescence (IF).** Direct IF tests with polyclonal rabbit antigonococcal antibodies, appropriately absorbed, were previously widely used for identification of gonococci. Though very few problems are encountered with urogenital isolates, these reagents give cross-reactions with other *Neisseria* spp.[54] and are no longer recommended as confirmatory tests. If used they should be considered as presumptive tests. Recently, fluorescent labeled monoclonal mouse antigonococcal antibodies have given highly specific and reproducible results.[55] Extensive experience from routine laboratory use is, however, still lacking.

**Coagglutination (CoA).** The basic principle for the coagglutination test is the ability of protein A-containing *Staphylococcus aureus* (Cowan I staphylococci) to bind IgG molecules via the Fc fragment.[56] If the test is performed with antigonococcal antibodies, and reagent staphylococci are mixed with gonococci, a CoA lattice is formed within less than 2 min, well visible to the naked eye (Fig. 73-1). It is highly essential that the antibodies used have a defined specificity. The original CoA tests for identification and confirmation of *N. gonorrhoeae* were based on absorbed polyvalent rabbit antigonoccal antibodies.[57] These have now been replaced by mouse monoclonal antibodies against epitopes of protein I of the major outer membrane protein of the gonococcus (see also Chap. 13). A commercial kit (Pharmacia Diagnostics, Uppsala, Sweden) contains two vials with reagent staphylococci that react with serogroup WI and WII/III gonococci, respectively, and one vial with negative control reagent.[58] A similar diagnostic kit is manufactured by Gono Gen Tek (Micro-Media Systems, Potomac, MD).

The coagglutination test is simple to perform, and no sophisticated equipment is needed. Suspected colonies to be tested are suspended to about 1 percent in saline, boiled for 3 to 5 min, cooled, and tested as a slide agglutination with results available within a couple of minutes. The test does not discriminate between PPNG and nonPPNG strains. However, nonPPNG serogroup WI strains have until now usually been fully susceptible to penicillin G, ampicillin, cephalosporins, and tetracyclines.[59]

The coagglutination test is rapid and simple and has a high specificity. CoA tests are also an excellent adjunct to biochemical tests of extragenital isolates that are, as mentioned, better subjected to at least two confirmatory tests, preferably the combination of a biochemical and a serological test, such as CoA.

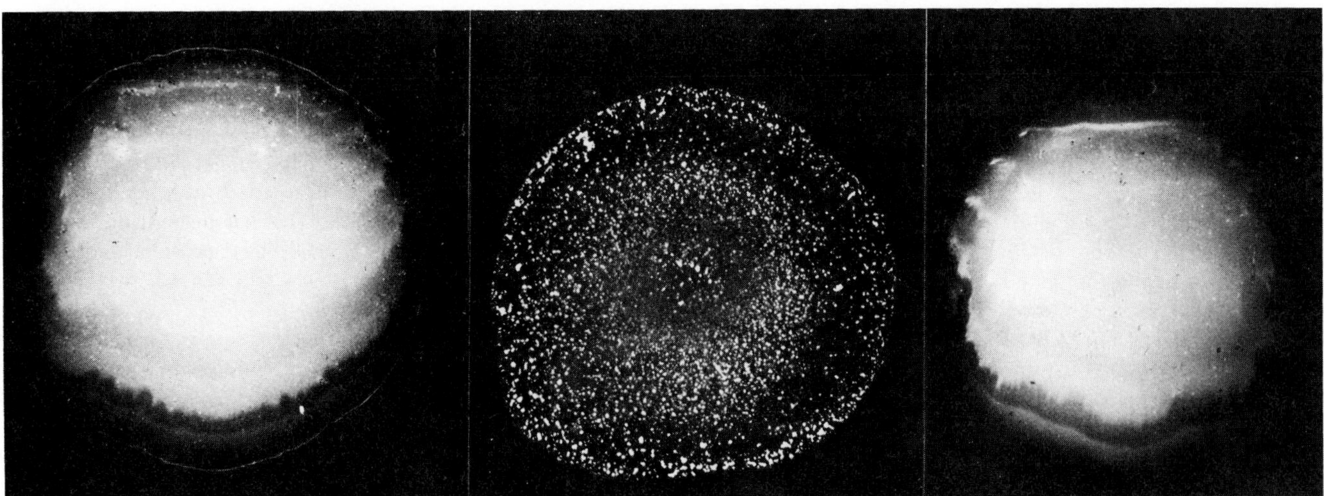

**Fig. 73-1.** Positive coaggulation test for *Neisseria gonorrhoeae* (*center*) with reagents for serogroup WI. Negative reaction with control reagent (*left*) and negative reaction with reagents for serogroup WII/III (*right*).

## ANTIBIOTIC SENSITIVITY TESTING

The policy of antibiotic susceptibility testing of gonococci varies in different countries or even between laboratories within one and the same state or country. An increasing number of PPNG strains as well as an alarming number of strains with chromosomal resistance to several antibiotics indicate that antibiotic susceptibility tests of freshly isolated strains of gonococci now ought to be performed on a routine basis. Present practice generally includes only periodic monitoring of susceptibility patterns. However, it is advisable to test *all* isolates for betalactamase production, especially from cases of treatment failure. The prevalence and relative incidence of PPNG strains is sufficiently high in most countries to warrant such routine testing.

### Test for betalactamase production

Test for betalactamase production of the gonococcus should be performed on all isolates.[3,17,34,60] This production can be mediated by different R plasmids[17,61] (see Chap. 13).

The chromogenic cephalosporin test for betalactamase production[62] is probably the most convenient test method. It is sensitive and specific and performs as well as the iodometric test.[63] Ten milligrams of the chromogenic cephalosporin (Nitrocefin) are dissolved in 1 ml of dimethyl sulfoxide (DMSO). The mixture is diluted in phosphate-buffered solution (PBS), pH 7.0, to a cephalosporin concentration of 500 μg/ml. The solution is yellow. In larger volumes it may appear orange. The solution is stable at 4°C for several weeks. The substance should not be allowed contact with eyes and skin. Tests with Nitrocefin may be performed on a piece of blotting paper previously soaked with a drop of the cephalosporin solution, giving a wet spot with a diameter of 0.5 to 1 cm. If the tested strain produces betalactamase, the cephalosporin solution changes color from yellow-orange to red-purple within 1 to 2 min. Tests can also be made in microtitration plates and in small test tubes.

### Minimum inhibitory concentration (MIC) determinations

Antibiotic susceptibility tests of gonococci are faced with several inherent problems, many of which are due to the complex growth requirements of *N. gonorrhoeae*. The *agar dilution method* is the reference method for MIC determinations of gonococci.[2,19,63] The *agar disk diffusion* test is much less accurate.[19] Benzylpenicillin and tetracycline may be used as a first-line selection with the addition of ampicillin, spectinonmycin, cefuroxim (or equivalent cephalosporin), and erythromycin in the second line. The medium recommended is shown in Table 73-10. Twofold dilutions of the drugs should be used in determining the MIC, which should be expressed as μg/ml or mg/l. When the stock solutions are prepared, the amount of drugs used should be based on the active portion of the compound. The stock solutions should be sterilized by membrane filtration (0.22 μm) and stored at −20°C until use (and never refrozen). The ready-to-use medium can be stored for 2 weeks at 4°C provided the petri dishes are kept in sealed plastic bags (see Table 73-10).

The inoculum is grown overnight on gonococcal medium (without antibiotics), suspended in saline (or phosphate buffered saline) with 0.1 percent Tween 80 (vol/vol) to a density corresponding to ca. $10^8$ colony-forming units (CFU) per ml = McFarland No. 2. The suspension is then further diluted in trypticase soy broth (TSB) to $10^7$ CFU/ml. Volumes of 1 μl (containing $10^4$ CFU) are delivered on the plates using a multipoint inoculator or a plastic loop calibrated to hold 0.001 ml. One agar plate without antibiotics is inoculated for control of growth and purity of the inoculum. The plates are left so the inoculum will dry before incubating the plates for 18 to 24 h in 4 to 6 percent $CO_2$ atmosphere as described above. The MIC is considered the lowest dilution of antibiotics resulting in no visible growth as judged by the naked eye.

**Table 73-10. Medium for Gonococcal Antibiotic Susceptibility Testing**

1 Prepare Proteose no. 3 agar (Difco) according to directions of the manufacturer.
2 Prepare a 2% hemoglobin (Difco) solution. Let the hemoglobin solution soak overnight at 4 to 8°C to obtain a smooth suspension. Autoclave the solution.
3 Place the agar hemoglobin solution to cool in a 50°C water bath. Decant the hemoglobin solution in the agar medium.
4 Add 1% IsoVitaleX (BBL).

To 9 parts of the cooled medium (48 to 50°C), 1 part of antibiotic solution is added. The mixture is poured into 9-cm petri dishes which are filled with 25 ml antibiotic-containing medium. The ready-to-use medium can be stored for 2 weeks at 4°C provided the petri dishes are kept in heat-sealed plastic bags or are carefully taped. A non-antibiotic-containing control plate should be used in each test as control.

SOURCE: Biddle et al.[60]

Reference control strains of *N. gonorrhoeae* with known MIC should preferably be included, e.g., strains with chromosomal resistance to a number of antibiotics. Such strains can generally be obtained from the national reference laboratory or from WHO. The MIC for benzylpenicillin of the WHO reference strains III, V, and VII are 0.01, 0.1, and 1.0 mg/ml, respectively.[63] The strains with chromosomal resistance have MIC for penicillin and tetracycline of 4 mg/l or more.

Many laboratories find the agar plate dilution method too cumbersome to be used on a routine basis. They therefore prefer using disk diffusion tests for screening antibiotic susceptibility with a selection of antibiotic disks, usually benzylpenicillin, ampicillin, tetracycline, spectinomycin, and cefuroxime or equivalent cephalosporin. The inoculum in disk diffusion tests should be prepared from a plate inoculated with up to 10 representative colonies from the primary plate. The growth of the secondary plate is suspended in saline or TSB to a concentration of ca. $10^5$ CFU/ml, with which the agar plate is seeded. The plate is allowed to dry for up to 5 min before the disks are applied. The plates are incubated for 24 h before being read. The inhibition zones should be measured with a caliper or millimeter ruler. The zones obtained are dependent on, among other things, the medium used, the amount of medium in the petri dish, and the concentrations of the antibiotic disks. This has made it difficult to reproduce translated MIC obtained via regression lines with the agar plate dilution method, which, as described, has its inherent problems.

Though the disk diffusion method is simple, there is no general agreement how to define standard cutoff points and regression lines that can be generally used. It is therefore recommended that each laboratory using disk diffusion as a routine screening test makes up its own regression curves. The emergence of gonococcal strains with chromosomal resistance to antibiotics has made it important for periodic monitoring of the susceptibility at least of selected strains of *N. gonorrhoeae*. This should be made in laboratories receiving large numbers of gonococcal specimens or organized on a national or even international level. Continuous information from the clinicians about the occurrence of treatment failures is important.

## GONOCOCCAL TYPING

Among all methods that have been used to differentiate strains of *N. gonorrhoeae,* auxotyping[64,65] and serological classification by coagglutination[66,67] have received the greatest attention. Both methods have been used extensively to define a number of strain-specific differences in gonococcal virulence and to study the epidemiology of gonorrhea. Recently restriction enzyme analyses of gonococcal chromosomal DNA have also been used to differentiate gonococcal strains.[68,69]

### Auxotyping

A method for auxotyping of gonococci was developed by Catlin[64] (see also Chap. 13) employing a chemically defined protein-free medium, called the NEDA medium. It supports growth of most gonococci. By omitting amino acids, e.g., proline, arginine, or methionine, the nitrogenous bases, e.g., uracil and hypoxanthine, and vitamins, e.g., thiamine, one at a time or in combinations and examining the growth of gonococci, it is possible to divide the isolates into distinct groups according to their nutritional requirements. In this way the auxotype pattern is determined by the requirement of the strain. The auxotyping pattern is indicated by, for example, $Pro^-$ for proline; $Arg^-/Hyx^-/Ura^-$ for arginine, hypoxanthine, and uracil. Gonococci able to grow on all media of an auxotyping set are called prototrophic (Prot or Zero). Most gonococcal strains belong to one of the five most common auxotypes as exemplified in Table 73-11.[59,65,71] A large number of odd and occasionally occurring auxotypes can be found in most surveys. Thus more than 35 auxotypes have been identified by testing various collections of clinical isolates.

Strain-specific characteristics are associated with certain auxotypes; e.g., nonPPNG AHU strains are highly susceptible to penicillins[59,67] and may be resistant to the bactericidal activity of normal human serum. Such strains occur significantly more often in patients with DGI[70] or in those with asymptomatic gonorrhea. There is also great geographic variation in the distribution of various auxotypes (Table 73-11), and temporal changes occur.[59,65,71]

Auxotyping is a powerful tool for epidemiological studies and for characterizing virulence, especially if combined with serological classification and with other markers, e.g., plasmid markers, restriction enzyme patterns. Unfortunately, it is laborious to perform auxotyping. It is desirable that one or more laboratories on a national reference level can offer auxotyping for periodic monitoring of the auxotypes occurring in a given geographic area, to help with the characterization of strains, as in forensic or legal situations.

**Table 73-11. Auxotyping of *Neisseria gonorrhoeae.* Frequencies and Geographic Distribution of the Most Common Auxotypes in Three Investigations**

| Auxotypes | Milwaukee* 251 isolates, % | Stockholm† 166 isolates, % | Swedish survey‡ 245 isolates, % |
|---|---|---|---|
| Prototrophic | 25.5 | 15.7 | 28.4 |
| $Pro^-$ | 33.8 | 12.8 | 18.8 |
| $Arg^-$ | 17.5 | 1.9 | 3.3 |
| $Arg^-/Hyx^-/Ura^-$ | 9.6 | 40.0 | 19.2 |
| $Pro^-/Arg^-/Hyx^-/Ura^-$ | 2.0 | 6.0 | 16.7 |

*Carifo and Catlin.[65]
†Moberg.[71]
‡Danielsson et al.[59]

### Serological classification

In 1980, Sandström and Danielsson[66] described the basis for serological classification of gonococci by coagglutination. With the help of specific polyclonal rabbit antigonococcal antibodies, laboratory strains and clinical isolates were separated into three main serogroups designated WI, WII, and WIII. The distinction was based on differences in the antigens of protein I of the major outer membrane protein. By peptide mapping, two principal PI molecules designated A and B were demonstrated.[72] WI strains possessed antigens of PI/A, while WII/III strains had antigens of PI/B. Monoclonal antibodies were developed against epitopes of PI/A and PI/B, respectively.[73] Most strains of serogroups WI and WII/III reacted with more than one of the monoclonals against PI/A and PI/B. Two sets of six monoclonals in each were selected. The reaction pattern observed with a particular strain was designated "serovar" to denote a variety, serologically defined by these monoclonal antibodies.[67]

Serological classification by coagglutination with the available sets of monoclonal antibodies has proved to be a powerful tool to characterize clinical isolates with regard to auxotype, antibiotic susceptibility, restriction endonuclease pattern, plasmid contents, clinical disease syndromes, virulence characteristics, and geographic distribution.[59,67,69,74–76] Classification by this method is feasible for monitoring clinical, epidemiological, and laboratory studies. The tests are easy to perform and show good reproducibility between laboratories, which indicated stability of the epitopes of protein I. A great diversity of serovars has been detected. There is a genetic linkage between serogroup/serovar specificity and antibiotic susceptibility.[77] In a study of in vitro transformation of chromosomal DNA mutations to increased resistance to penicillin, cotransformation of serogroup and serovar specificity was obtained. On some occasions transformants appeared with new serovar specificities, which was interpreted to be due to chromosomal recombinations that may well occur in the clinical situation with increased resistance to penicillin.[78]

## DIRECT SPECIMEN ANTIGEN DETECTION METHODS AS ALTERNATIVE OR COMPLEMENTARY DIAGNOSTIC TECHNIQUES

The development of enzyme immunoassays as well as immunofluorescence and DNA hybridization techniques has contributed to improvement of the laboratory diagnosis of many infectious diseases. Compared with culture, these methods might in principle have one or more of the following advantages for the diagnosis of gonococcal infections: rapidity, sensitivity, specificity, suitability for automation (to process large numbers of specimens), and solving transport problems for remote clinics and settings.

The test principles and current experience of methods for direct specimen antigen detection tests and for serum antibody tests for laboratory diagnosis of gonorrhea, including their cost-effectiveness, will be discussed below.

## ANTIGEN DETECTION

### Direct immunofluorescence (IFL)

This technique was first applied in the late fifties and early sixties for serological demonstration of gonococcal organisms in smears of urethral and cervical secretions. It was named direct fluorescent antibody test (FAT) for gonorrhea.[79] A specific diagnosis was arrived at within less than 1 h, it was considered a potential tool for specific diagnosis of gonorrhea at the office level. However, its sensitivity was inferior to culture, and it was expensive and much more laborious than a Gram's stain. In order to increase the sensitivity, an enrichment procedure was developed, the so-called Deacon's delayed FAT.[80] Urethral or cervical secretion collected with a cotton-tipped swab was inoculated onto the surface of a gonococcal culture medium slant, which was then incubated at 36°C in $CO_2$-atmosphere overnight (12 to 18 h). The swab, which was left in the tube, was used to make a smear on a glass slide stained with labeled antigonococcal antibodies and examined under a fluorescence microscope. Nonspecific reactions with protein A-containing staphylococci were blocked by adding normal rabbit serum or rhodamine labeled anti *Staphylococcus aureus* globulin to the antigonococcal conjugate, or by using fluorochrome labeled F(ab′)2 fragments.[54] Cross-reactions with other *Neisseria* spp. were controlled by absorption of the conjugates.[54] This was tedious and expensive, and with the introduction of selective gonococcal culture media, Deacon's delayed FAT was not competitive.[81] Moreover, the method did not allow antibiotic sensitivity testing, a general and inherent problem with antigen detection of pathogenic bacteria. IFL tests were used as a confirmatory test alternative to carbohydrate degradation, however. Some laboratories still use the IFL technique as a complementary test to culture for certain diagnostic purposes, for example, to demonstrate gonococci in smears of skin lesions in DGI, as discussed above. With the advent of fluorochrome labeled monoclonal mouse antigonococcal antibodies a reevaluation of direct IFL tests for the diagnosis of gonorrhea seems to be justified since many of the specificity problems with polyclonal antibodies are eliminated with the monoclonals.[55]

### Solid-phase enzyme immunoassays

A solid-phase enzyme immunoassay for detection of gonococcal antigen (Gonozyme) was introduced on the market in the early 1980s (Abbott Laboratories, North Chicago) as the first commercial antigen detection test for gonococci. It was adapted for testing urethral or cervical secretions. Cervical or urethral secretions collected with swabs (prepared by the manufacturer and called STD-EZE for the cervix, STD-PEN for the male urethra) are transported in the EIA transport tube containing 200 μl transport medium for delivery to the laboratory, where it is subjected to the following working sequence:

1. Dilution buffer (1 ml) is added to the tube with the swab submerged for 10 to 15 min to elute collected material. This is further enhanced by vortexing the tube for 3 cycles of 15 s each.
2. 200 μl of the specimens and controls are added to appropriate wells of a reaction tray. A treated bead is added to each well. The tray is incubated for 60 min at 37°C, after which the liquid is aspirated and the bead washed 4 times.
3. Polyclonal antigonoccal antibodies are added and left to react for 60 min at 37°C, after which the antibody dilution is aspirated and the bead washed 4 times.
4. Horseradish peroxidase labeled sheep antirabbit antibodies are added and left to react with the antigen-antibody complex on the bead for 60 min at 37°C, followed by aspiration of the liquid and washing of the bead 4 times.
5. The beads are then transferred to tubes (properly identified) to which are added an enzyme substrate, 300 μl of o-phenylenediamine (OPD) containing hydrogen peroxide. The mixture is left to react for 30 min at room temperature. A yellow-orange color develops in proportion to the quantity of gonococcal antigen absorbed by the bead.
6. Absorbance of the color is determined in a spectrophotometer at 492 nm and the results are compared with those of positive and negative controls. The cutoff value for a negative test is calculated, and specimens giving absorbance values greater than the cutoff level are considered positive for the occurrence of *N. gonorrhoeae*.

The Gonozyme test has been evaluated with regard to sensitivity, specificity, and predictive values for positive and negative tests in males and females representing high or low prevalence groups for gonorrhea (>15 and <10 percent respectively). Culture has been used as the reference method. Data from some of these comparative studies[4,5,82,83,84] have been compiled in Table 73-12.

The prevalences of gonorrhea of the study populations have varied from 12 to 67 percent for the males and from 4 to 28 percent for the females, respectively. The overall agreements between the EIA test and culture have varied from 91.7 to 100 percent for male samples and from 87.4 to 99.3 percent for those from females. Correspondingly, sensitivities ranged from 83.3 to 100 percent for male and from 73.1 to 100 percent for female samples; specificities from 96.3 to 100 percent for male and from 87.8 to 100 percent for female samples; PVP from 66.7 to 100 percent for males and from 29.2 to 100 percent for female samples; PVN from 89.4 to 100 percent for male and 94.6 to 100 percent for female samples. EIA performed better in males than in females in all the studies cited in Table 73-12. It is notable, however, that the prevalence of gonorrhea was higher in the males than in the females studied. It should be noted that the PVP was low in females with a prevalence of gonorrhea of less than 7 percent. In the majority of the cited studies PVN was high (usually >97 percent) (see also Chap. 82).

### Advantages and disadvantages of EIA versus culture and indirect microscopy

The EIA may be considered an alternative or complementary test to traditional diagnostic techniques in gonorrhea. Some important objections against its general use, however, concern clinical, diagnostic, epidemiological, medicolegal, and cost-effectiveness aspects.

Extragenital specimens, i.e., rectal specimens in women, pharyngeal specimens in patients practicing fellatio or cunnilingus, and rectal and pharyngeal specimens in homosexuals are advisable for test. The currently used Gonozyme test is adapted only for urethral and cervical specimens. Antibiotic sensitivity determinations including tests for betalactamase production of gonococcal strains cannot be performed, a drawback if only Gonozyme tests are performed.

As shown in Table 73-12, the sensitivity of the current Gonozyme ranges from 73 to 100 percent, better in males than in females, as compared with culture (considered to have an 85 to 95 percent sensitivity). The test is more sensitive than microscopy of stained cervical smears, being in the range of 40 to 60 percent.

Table 73-12. Enzyme Immunoassay (EIA) versus Results of Culture. Compilation of Data from Studies with Gonozyme Used for the Detection of Gonococcal Antigen in Specimens from the Urethra of Males and the Cervix of Females

| Authors | Patient groups No. tested | Prevalence % | Overall agreement, % | Sensitivity, % | Specificity, % | PVP % | PVN % |
|---|---|---|---|---|---|---|---|
| *Males:* | | | | | | | |
| Aardoom et al.[4] | 52 | 67 | 67 | 90–100* | 90–100* | 100 | 100 |
| Danielsson et al.[5] | 101 | 12 | 93.1 | 83.3 | 94.4 | 66.7 | 97.7 |
| Hofmann and Petzoldt[82] | 526 | 23 | 99.2 | 98.3 | 99.5 | 98.3 | 99.5 |
| | 261† | 12 | 99.2 | 100 | 99.1 | 93.8 | 100 |
| Schachter et al.[83] | 117 | 64 | 94.9 | 93.3 | 100 | 100 | 89.4 |
| | 151 | 30 | 98 | 95.6 | 99.1 | 97.7 | 98.1 |
| Stamm et al.[84] | 1171 | 16 | 97.4 | 94 | 98 | 90 | 99 |
| *Females:* | | | | | | | |
| Aardoom et al.[4] | 54 | 28 | 88.9 | 60–98 | 76–97 | 75 | 94.6 |
| | 102 | 12 | 96 | 62–100 | 91–99 | 78.6 | 98.9 |
| Danielsson et al.[5] | 150 | 7 | 99.3 | 90.9 | 100 | 100 | 99.3 |
| Hofmann and Petzoldt[82] | 464 | 10 | 93.8 | 88.6 | 94.3 | 61.9 | 98.8 |
| | 220† | 7 | 98.6 | 93.7 | 99 | 88.2 | 99.5 |
| | 548‡ | 6 | 87.4 | 81.3 | 87.8 | 29.2 | 98.7 |
| | 345†‡ | 4 | 95.8 | 77.4 | 96.5 | 46.2 | 99.1 |
| Schachter et al.[83] | 171 | 14 | 90.6 | 87 | 91.2 | 60.6 | 97.8 |
| Stamm et al.[84] | 723 | 15 | 95.6 | 76 | 99 | 88 | 96 |

*95% confidence intervals are given as probability percentages.
†Modified Gonozyme.
‡Prostitutes.
PVP and PVN = predictive values of positive and negative tests.

The sensitivity of stained smears of males with symptomatic urethritis is in the range of 95 to 97 percent, i.e., equal to the current Gonozyme test.

The specificity of the EIA antigen detection test is more important since it is not a confirmatory test. Analysis of culture-negative but EIA-positive results has indicated that false positives may occur. From a medicolegal point of view a positive Gonozyme should therefore be followed by culture. Schachter and colleagues[83] have pointed out that screening with antigen detection for the sensitivity (89 percent) and specificity (98 percent) of a hypothetical population of 10,000 women with a 1 percent prevalence of gonococcal infection would have correctly identified 87 out of 100 culture-proved infected women, missing 13 and falsely labeling 205 women as positive. Since culture also has a sensitivity less than 100 percent, 5 to 10 of these 205 women might have been missed by culture. The PVP of a positive EIA in the discussed hypothetical population was 29.8 percent, which is similar to the results arrived at by Hofmann and Petzoldt[82] in females with a prevalence of gonorrhea of 4 to 6 percent and by Stamm and colleagues[84] in men who had a prevalence of 2 percent.

It is documented that the loss of positive gonococcal cultures is considerable for specimens delivered and kept for 2 days or more in transport medium.[33] Stamm and colleagues[84] showed that the EIA results were not affected by transport or by refrigerator storage for 14 to 26 days. Antigen detection tests are definitely valuable for clinics and settings at remote distances from diagnostic laboratories.

## General comments and cost-effectiveness

Antigen detection tests might sometimes be complementary to traditional methods since they are not affected by transport, ongoing antibiotic treatment, or the presence of vancomycin-sensitive strains. Rapidity is an often recurring word in discussion of the specific diagnosis of infectious diseases. Antigen detection is more rapid than culture but considerably less rapid than examination of a stained smear. The availability of a Gram's stain for males with symptomatic urethritis with results in 10 min will probably not alter empiric handling and treatment. This is further magnified by the fact that it takes 4 to 5 h to complete the whole Gonozyme test cycle whether 5 to 10 or 50 to 100 specimens are tested. A low-volume laboratory would be likely to batch the specimens to minimize cost, and the benefit of rapidity would be lost.

Thomas and colleagues[85] have made a cost comparison of Gram's stain, culture, and Gonozyme in a low- (< 100 specimens per month) and a moderate-volume laboratory (>400 to 700 specimens per month). Applying their figures to a hypothetical group of 100 females with an assumed prevalence of 1 percent of gonorrhea (which today is common in many countries in screening situations), the cost would be $181.71 for culture and $692.71 for EIA (screening plus culture since EIA is not confirmatory). The "hands-on time" for the negative specimens by culture is generally very short, whereas for EIA the assay time is independent of whether the assay is positive or negative.

## Genetic transformation and DNA hybridization

Jaffe and associates[86] described a diagnostic test to detect gonococcal DNA in patient specimens by genetic transformation of temperature-sensitive recipient test strains. They applied the technique to detect gonococcal DNA in mailed clinical specimens since the test was not dependent on live organisms. It might therefore be a potential test where transport is a practical problem. It has no advantage over antigen detection tests, however, since it does not discriminate between betalactamase- and non-betalactamase-producing strains.

Recently, Totten and coworkers[6] described a DNA-hybridization technique to detect *N. gonorrhoeae* directly in clinical specimens using the 2.6-megadalton (MDa) gonococcal cryptic plasmid as a radiolabeled probe. Briefly, nitrocellulose papers were inoculated with male urethral exudate, treated with NaOH to lyse cells and denature DNA, washed in buffers, treated with pronase and chloroform to lower background radioactivity, and heated for 2 h in a vacuum oven at 80°C. The filters were then soaked in prehybridization solution for 1 h at 42°C. The radiolabeled probe was denatured by heating at 100°C for 10 min and suspended in a hybridization solution. The solution was overlayered onto the inoculated nitrocellulose papers which were wrapped in plastic and incubated at 42°C overnight. The next morning, excess hybridization solution was removed by rinsing in buffers. The nitrocellulose filters were dried and exposed to x-ray film at −70°C for 1 to 3 days, followed by developing of the film. A positive reaction showed up as a black spot on the film overlayering the area on the nitrocellulose paper where the urethral discharge had been placed.

The technique[6] detected as few as 100 colony-forming units of *N. gonorrhoeae* or as little as 0.1 pg of purified gonococcal plasmid DNA, and it was highly specific. They studied 130 men with urethritis. Sixty-three (89 percent) of 71 who had cultures positive for *N. gonorrhoeae* were also positive by DNA hybridization. All 42 men whose urethral cultures were negative were also negative by DNA hybridization. Five of six gonococcal isolates from patients who were positive by culture but negative by hybridization lacked the cryptic plasmid. This is an expected finding, since 10 percent of large strain collections of *N. gonorrhoeae* lack the cryptic plasmid.

The described DNA-hybridization method[6] was further developed by Perine and associates[7] who used both the 2.6-MDa cryptic plasmid and the 4.4-MDa betalactamase plasmid as radiolabeled probes for direct detection of gonococci and for distinction of betalactamase plasmid-carrying gonococci in urethral exudates from men with urethritis. Men from four African and two Asian countries were tested. The sensitivity and specificity of the two DNA probes were compared with isolation and biochemical tests for betalactamase production (chromogenic cephalosporin test). Of the 216 urethral specimens, 180 were positive for *N. gonorrhoeae* by DNA probe and culture, 27 were negative in both tests, and 9 gave discordant results. Compared with culture and chromogenic cephalosporin tests the sensitivity and the specificity of the DNA probe were 99 and 93 percent and those of the betalactamase probe assay 91 and 96 percent, respectively. Ninety gonococcal strains were examined for plasmids; all contained the 2.6-MDa plasmid, 29 possessed a 3.2-MDa betalactamase plasmid, and 18 had a 4.4-MDa betalactamase plasmid. It was concluded that the sensitivity of the DNA probes was comparable with that of culture for the diagnosis of gonorrhea and with the chromogenic cephalosporin tests for detection of betalactamase.

In principle, DNA hybridization would doubtless be an attractive noncultural method for the diagnosis of gonorrhea. A specimen can be sent in an envelope on a piece of nitrocellulose paper. The technique has the advantage over antigen detection test and Gram's stain of allowing the identification of PPNG strains. It seems to have a sensitivity equal to culture, but so far it seems to have been evaluated only in males with symptomatic urethritis. Perine and coworkers[7] mentioned that it was less sensitive for detection of gonococci in cervical and rectal samples than in urethral ones. False-negative test results are obtained with gonococcal strains that lack the 2.6-MDa cryptic plasmid. Moreover, it is likely that specimens from the cervix, the rectum, and the pharynx (unlike those from the male urethra) can contain a sufficient number of organisms other than *N. gonorrhoeae,* such as *Haemophilus influenzae* or *Escherichia coli,* that may contain betalactamase-encoding plasmids that would react with the gonococcal betalactamase plasmid probe. In its present stage, DNA hybridization cannot compete with traditional culture because of its low sensitivity in female gonococcal infections and because the turnaround time is even longer than for culture. Using probes labeled with other markers may improve the sensitivity. Significantly sped up time for performing the test is also needed.

## Serological tests

The complement fixation (CF) test was the first test in general use for the serodiagnosis of gonorrhea (cf. Refs. *1,87*). Novel tests appeared in the 1970s and 1980s, including a modified CF test,[88] latex agglutination,[89] indirect IFL,[90] tests for antibodies against pili antigens with radio immunoassay (pili-RIA),[8] indirect hemagglutination (pili-IHA),[9] and ELISA (pili-ELISA).[10] More recently, Western blotting technique (immunoblotting) has been applied to detect class-specific antibodies against antigens characterized by SDS polyacrylamide gel electrophoresis.[91]

Two main approaches are featured when evaluating serologic tests for gonorrhea; (1) for *diagnostic purposes,* i.e., for establishing the presence of gonorrhea in a patient with compatible symptoms or recent exposure for gonorrhea; (2) for *case detection,* i.e., routine testing for gonorrhea among patients examined for some other purpose.

The reported serological tests have usually had high sensitivities. However, the prevalence of gonorrhea in the patient population, cross-reactive antibodies to antigens of other *Neisseria* spp. as well as to species of other bacterial genera, and antibody persistence from past infections are some of the major factors influencing sensitivity, specificity, PVP, and PVN of serological tests for gonorrhea. Thus in a population of patients with DGI (all of whom have gonorrhea), the PVP would be 100 percent. Among patients with pelvic inflammatory disease, 40 to 50 percent of whom may have gonorrhea, the PVP would be at least 40 to 50 percent. Among female STD patients, 20 percent of whom may have gonorrhea, the PVP would be at least 40 percent, even if the test is not discriminatory but sensitive enough to detect antibodies. However, among patients having a low prevalence (<2 percent) of gonorrhea, the PVP has been shown to be very low (10 percent) with the most specific and sensitive tests (pili-RIA).[11] In fact, some of the advocated tests were just somewhat more discriminatory than history of gonorrhea.

Efforts have been made to identify unique gonococcal antigens that would be useful in case detection of asymptomatic gonorrhea with a serodiagnostic test. However, there are still problems in distinguishing serum antibodies due to current or past infection on the basis of analyzing a single serum specimen. An examination of paired sera to demonstrate changes in antibody patterns is the rule for most serodiagnostic tests. This may be accomplished in patients with DGI, PID, or other complications compatible with gonorrhea but is difficult to perform in screening situations for case detection. Thus serological tests of gonorrhea may be useful as an adjunct to culture of acute gonorrhea, but not for gonorrhea case detection.

# References

1 Reyn A: Laboratory diagnosis of gonococcal infections. *Bull WHO* 32:449, 1965.

2 Kellogg DS et al: Laboratory diagnosis of gonorrhea, in *Cumitech 4,* S Marcus, JC Sherris (eds). Washington DC, American Society for Microbiology, 1976.

3 Mårdh P-A: Bacteria, chlamydiae, and mycoplasmas, in *Sexually Transmitted Diseases,* KK Holmes et al (eds). New York: McGraw-Hill, 1984, p 829.

4 Aardoom HA et al: Detection of *Neisseria gonorrhoeae* antigen by a solid phase enzyme immunoassay. *Br J Vener Dis* 58:359, 1982.

5 Danielsson D et al: Diagnosis of urogenital gonorrhoea by detecting gonococcal antigen with a solid phase enzyme immunoassay (Gonozyme). *J Clin Pathol* 36:674, 1983.

6 Totten PA et al: DNA hybridization technique for the detection of *Neisseria gonorrhoeae* in men with urethritis. *J Infect Dis* 148:462, 1983.

7 Perine PL et al: Evaluation of a DNA-hybridization method for detection of African and Asian strains of *Neisseria gonorrhoeae* in men with urethritis. *J Infect Dis* 152:59, 1985.

8 Buchanan TM et al: Quantitative determination of antibody to gonococcal pili. Changes in antibody levels with gonococcal infection. *J Clin Invest* 52:2896, 1973.

9 Reimann K, Lind I: An indirect haemagglutination test for demonstration of gonocococal antibodies using gonococcal pili as antigen. I. Methodology and preliminary results. *Acta Pathol Microbiol Scand* Sec C 85:115, 1977.

10 Young H, Low AC: Serological diagnosis of gonorrhoea: Detection of antibodies to gonococcal pili by enzyme linked immunosorbent assay. *Med Lab Sci* 38:41, 1980.

11 Holmes KK et al: Is serology useful in gonorrhea? A critical analysis of factors influencing serodiagnosis, in *Immunobiology of Neisseria gonorrhoeae,* GF Brooks et al (eds). Washington, American Society for Microbiology, 1978, p 370.

12 Phillips I: Beta-lactamase producing penicillin resistant gonococcus. *Lancet* ii:656, 1976.

13 Ashford WA et al: Penicillinase producing *Neisseria gonorrhoeae. Lancet* ii:657, 1976.

14 Centers for Disease Control: Penicillinase-producing *Neisseria gonorrhoeae. MMWR* 25(33):261, 1976.

15 Percival A et al: Penicillinase producing gonococci in Liverpool. *Lancet* ii:1379, 1976.

16 Centers for Disease Control: Global distribution of penicillinase producing *Neisseria gonorrhoeae* (PPNG). *MMWR* 32:1, 1982.

17 Adler MW: Epidemiology and treatment of penicillinase-producing *Neisseria gonorrhoeae,* in *Recent Advances in Sexually Transmitted Diseases,* JD Oriel, JRW Harris (eds). London, Churchill Livingstone, 1986, p 23.

18 Centers for Disease Control: Penicillin resistant gonorrhea—North Carolina. *MMWR* 32:273, 1983.

19 Faruki H et al: A community-based outbreak of infection with penicillin-resistant *Neisseria gonorrhoeae* not producing penicillinase (chromosomally mediated resistance). *N Engl J Med* 313:607, 1985.

20 Ison CA et al: Chromosomal resistance of gonococci to antibiotics. *Genitourin Med* 63:239, 1987.

21 Tapsall JW et al: Chromosomally mediated intrinsic resistance to penicillin of penicillinase producing strains of *Neisseria gonorrhoeae* isolated in Sydney: Guide to treatment with Augmentin. *Genitourin Med* 63:305, 1987.

22 Galen RS, Gambino RS: Screening for gonorrhoea. How the model defines essential criteria for an efficient screening test, in *Beyond Normality: The Predictive Value and Efficiency of Medical Diagnosis,* New York, Wiley, 1975.

23 Wilkinson AE: Cultural methods for the diagnosis of gonorrhoea, in *Gonorrhoea. Epidemiology and Pathogenesis,* FA Skinner et al (eds): FEMS Symposium No. 2, London, Academic, 1977, p 17.

24 WHO Scientific Group: *Neisseria gonorrhoeae* and gonococcal infections. *Technical Report Series 616,* World Health Organization, Geneva, 1978.

25 Lind I: The laboratory diagnosis of gonorrhoea, in *Recent Developments in Laboratory Identification Techniques,* R Facklam et al (eds). Amsterdam, Excerpta Medica, 1979, p 3.

26 Amie CR: A modified formula for the preparation of Stuart's Transport Medium. *Can J Public Health* 58:296, 1967.

27 Gästrin B, Kallings LO: Improved methods for gonococcal sampling and examination. *Acta Pathol Microbiol Scand* 74:362, 1968.

28 Schmale JD et al: Observation on the culture diagnosis of gonorrhea in women. *JAMA* 210:312, 1969.

29 Dans PE, Judson F: The establishment of a venereal disease clinic: II. An appraisal of current diagnostic methods in uncomplicated urogenital and rectal gonorrhea. *J Am Vener Dis Assoc* 1:107, 1975.

30 Holmes KK et al: The gonococcal arthritis-dermatitis syndrome. *Ann Intern Med* 75:470, 1971.

31 Barr J, Danielsson D: Septic gonococcal dermatitis. *Br Med J* 1:482, 1971.

32 Mårdh P-A et al: Sampling, specimen handling, and isolation techniques in the diagnosis of genital chlamydial and other genital infections. *Sex Transm Dis* 8:280, 1981.

33 Danielsson D et al: Culture diagnosis of gonorrhoea—A comparison between two standard laboratory methods and a commercial gonococcal culture kit. *Acta Dermatol Venereol* 58:69, 1978.

34 Morello JA et al: *Neisseria* and *Branhamella,* in *Manual of Clinical Microbiology,* 4th ed, EG Lennette et al (eds). Washington DC, American Society for Microbiology, 1985, p 176.

35 Martin JE, Jackson RL: A biological environment chamber for culture of *Neisseria gonorrhoeae. J Am Vener Dis Assoc* 2:28, 1975.

36 Jephcott AE et al: Improved transport and culture system for the rapid diagnosis of gonorrhoea. *Br J Vener Dis* 52:250, 1976.

37 Thayer JD, Martin JE: Improved medium selective for cultivation of *N. gonorrhoeae* and *N. meningitidis. Health Lab Reports* 81:559, 1966.

38 Martin JE, Lewis JS: Anisomycin: Improved antimycotic activity in modified Thayer-Martin medium. *Public Health Lab* 35:53, 1977.

39 Faur YC et al: A new medium for the isolation of pathogenic *Neisseria* (NYC medium). I. Formulations and comparisons with standard media. *Health Lab Sci* 10:44, 1973.

40 Mårdh P-A et al: An effective, simplified medium for the culture of *Neisseria gonorrhoeae. Sex Transm Dis* 5:10, 1978.

41 Brorson JE et al: Vancomycin-sensitive strains of *Neisseria gonorrhoeae:* A problem for the diagnostic laboratory. *Br J Vener Dis* 49: 452, 1973.

42 Soltesz LV, Mårdh P-A: Serum-free liquid medium for *Neisseria gonorrhoeae. Curr Microbiol* 4:45, 1980.

43 Lue YA et al: Improved recovery of *Neisseria gonorrhoeae* from clinical specimens by selective enrichment and detection by immunological methods. *Sex Transm Dis* 7:165, 1980.

44 Kellogg DS et al: *Neisseria gonorrhoeae.* I. Virulence genetically linked to clonal variation. *J Bacteriol* 85:1274, 1963.

45 Swanson J: Cell wall outer membrane variants of *Neisseria gonorrhoeae,* in *Immunobiology of Neisseria gonorrhoeae,* GF Brooks et al (eds). Washington, American Society for Microbiology, 1978, p 130.

46 Vedros NA: *Neisseria,* in *Bergey's Manual of Systematic Bacteriology,* NR Krieg (ed). Baltimore/London, Williams & Wilkins, 1984, vol 1, p 290.

47 Ahmed F et al: Characterization of *Branhamella catarrhalis* and differentiation from *Neisseria* species in a diagnostic laboratory. *J Clin Pathol* 40:1369, 1987.

48 Strauss RR et al: Comparison of a radiometric procedure with conventional methods for identification of Neisseria. *J Clin Microbiol* 7:419, 1978.

49 Robinson MJ, Oberhofer TR: Identification of pathogenic *Neisseria* species with the RapID NH system. *J Clin Microbiol* 17:400, 1983.

50 Reddick A: A simple carbohydrate fermentation test for the identification of pathogenic *Neisseria. J Clin Microbiol* 2:72, 1975.

51 Hugh R, Leifson E: The taxonomic significance of fermentative versus oxidative metabolism of carbohydrates by various gram negative bacteria. *J Bacteriol* 66:24, 1963.

52 Morse SA, Bartenstein L: Adaptation of the Minitek system for the rapid identification of *Neisseria gonorrhoeae. J Clin Microbiol* 3:8, 1976.

53 Janda WM et al: Use of the API NeIdent system for identification of pathogenic *Neisseria* spp and *Branhamella catarrhalis. J Clin Microbiol* 19:338, 1984.

54 Danielsson D, Forsum U: Diagnosis of *Neisseria* infections by defined immunofluorescence. Methodologic aspects and applications. *Ann NY Acad Sci* 254:334, 1975.

55 Laughon BE et al: Fluorescent monoclonal antibody for confirmation of *Neisseria gonorrhoeae* cultures. *J Clin Microbiol* 25:2388, 1987.

56 Kronvall G: A rapid slide-agglutination method for typing pneumococci by means of specific antibody adsorbed to protein A-containing staphylococci. *J Clin Microbiol* 6:187, 1973.

57 Danielsson D, Kronvall G: Slide agglutination method for the serological identification of *Neisseria gonorrhoeae* with anti-gonococcal antibodies adsorbed to protein A-containing staphylococci. *Appl Microbiol* 27:368, 1974.

58 Carlson BL et al: Phadebact monoclonal GC OMNI test for confirmation of *Neisseria gonorrhoeae. J Clin Microbiol* 25:1982, 1987.

59 Danielsson D et al: Epidemiology of gonorrhoea: Serogroup, antibiotic susceptibility and auxotype patterns of consecutive gonococcal isolates from 10 different areas of Sweden. *Scand J Infect Dis* 15:33, 1983.

60 Biddle JW et al: Disc agar diffusion and microbial susceptibility tests of beta-lactamase producing *Neisseria gonorrhoeae. J Antibiot (Tokyo)* 31:352, 1978.

61 Cannon JG, Sparling PF: The genetics of gonococcus. *Annu Rev Microbiol* 38:11, 1984.

62 O'Callaghan CH et al: Novel method for detection of beta-lactamases by using a chromogenic cephalosporin substrate. *Antimicrob Agents Chemother* 1:283, 1972.

63 Reyn A et al: Susceptibility testing of *Neisseria gonorrhoeae* to antimicrobial agents: Recommended methods and use of reference strains, WHO/VDT/80. 423, Geneva, Switzerland, 1980.

64 Catlin W: Nutritional profiles of *Neisseria gonorrhoeae, Neisseria meningitidis* and *Neisseria lactamica* in chemically defined media and the use of growth requirement of gonococcal typing. *J Infect Dis* 128: 178, 1973.

65 Carifo K, Catlin BW: *Neisseria gonorrhoeae* auxotyping: Differentiation of clinical isolates based on growth responses on chemically defined media. *Appl Microbiol* 26:223, 1973.

66 Sandström E, Danielsson D: Serology of *Neisseria gonorrhoeae*. Classification with co-agglutination. *Acta Pathol Microbiol Scand* Sec B 88:27, 1980.

67 Knapp JS et al: Serological classification of *Neisseria gonorrhoeae* with use of monoclonal antibodies to gonococcal outer membrane protein I. *J Infect Dis* 150:44, 1984.

68 Falk ES et al: Restriction endonuclease fingerprinting of chromosomal DNA of *Neisseria gonorrhoeae. Acta Pathol Microbiol Scand,* Sec B 92:271, 1984.

69 Falk ES et al: Phenotypic and genotypic characterization of penicillinase producing strains of *Neisseria gonorrhoeae. Acta Pathol Microbiol Scand,* Sec B 93:91, 1985.

70 Knapp JS, Holmes KK: Disseminated gonococcal infections caused by *Neisseria gonorrhoeae* with unique nutritional requirements. *J Infect Dis* 132:204, 1975.

71 Moberg I: Auxotyping of gonococcal isolates, in *Genital Infections and Their Complications,* D Danielsson et al (eds). Stockholm, Almqvist & Wiksell International, 1975, p 271.

72 Sandström EG et al: Serology of *Neisseria gonorrhoeae:* Co-agglutination serogroups WI and WII/III correspond to different outer membrane protein I molecules. *Infect Immun* 38:462, 1982.

73 Tam MR et al: Serological classification of *Neisseria gonorrhoeae* with monoclonal antibodies. *Infect Immun* 36:1042, 1982.

74 Whittington L et al: Serological classification of *Neisseria gonorrhoeae:* Uses at the community level, in *The Pathogenic Neisseria,* GK Schoolnik et al (eds). Washington DC, American Society for Microbiology, 1985, p 20.

75 Coghill DV, Young H: Serological classification of *Neisseria gonorrhoeae* with monoclonal antibody coagglutination reagents. *Genitourin Med* 63:225, 1987.

76 Dillon DV JR et al: Auxotypes, plasmid contents, and serovars of gonococcal strains (PPNG and non-PPNG) from Jamaica. *Genitourin Med* 63:225, 1987.

77 Bygdeman S et al: Genetic linkage between serogroup specificity and antibiotic resistance in *Neisseria gonorrhoeae. Acta Pathol Microbiol Scand* Sec B 90:243, 1982.

78 Danielsson D et al: Recombination near antibiotic resistance locus penB results in antigenic variation of gonococcal outer membrane protein I. *Infect Immun* 52:529, 1986.

79 Deacon WE et al: Indentification of *Neisseria gonorrhoeae* by means of fluorescent antibodies. *Proc Soc Exp Biol Med* 101:322, 1959.

80 Deacon WE et al: Fluorescent antibody tests for detection of the gonococcus in women. *Public Health Rep* 75:125, 1960.

81 Lucas JB et al: Diagnosis and treatment of gonorrhea in the female: *N Engl J Med* 276:1454, 1967.

82 Hofmann H, Petzoldt D: Nachweis von Gonokockenantigen mit einem Enzymimmunoassay (Gonozyme). Ergebnisse met dem ursprünglichen und dem modifizierten Testverfahren. *Hautarzt* 36:675, 1985.

83 Schachter J et al: Enzyme immunoassay for diagnosis of gonorrhoea. *J Clin Microbiol* 19:57, 1984.

84 Stamm WE et al: Antigen detection for the diagnosis of gonorrhea. *J Clin Microbiol* 19:399, 1984.

85 Thomas JG et al: Multicenter clinical trial and laboratory utilization of an enzymatic detection method for gonococcal antigens. *An J Clin Pathol* 86:71, 1986.

86 Jaffe HW et al: Diagnosis of gonorrhea using a genetic transformation test on mailed clinical specimens. *J Infect Dis* 146:275, 1982.

87 Sandström E, Danielsson D: A survey of gonococcal serology, in *Genital Infections and Their Complications,* D Danielsson et al (eds). Stockholm, Almqvist & Wiksell International, 1975, p 253.

88 Danielsson D et al: Serologic investigation of the immune response in various types of gonococcal infection. *Acta Derm Venereol* (Stockholm) 52:467, 1972.

89 Wallace R et al: The bentonite flocculation test in assay of *Neisseria* antibody. *Can J Microbiol* 16:655, 1970.

90 Gaafar HA, D'Arcangelis DC: Fluorescent antibody test for the serological diagnosis of gonorrhea. *J Clin Microbiol* 3:438, 1976.

91 Lammel CJ et al: Antibody-antigen specificity in the immune response to infection with *Neisseria gonorrhoeae. J Infect Dis* 152:990, 1985.

# Chapter 74
# *Chlamydia trachomatis*

Walter E. Stamm
Per-Anders Mårdh

*C. trachomatis* causes trachoma (chronic keratoconjunctivitis) as well as acute conjunctivitis and keratitis, urethritis, cervicitis, endometritis, salpingitis, perihepatitis, epididymitis, and lymphogranuloma venereum (LGV). Reiter's disease is often associated with *C. trachomatis* infection as well. In all of these infections, asymptomatic carriers are common and can be identified only through specific diagnostic testing, usually culture or a direct antigen detection test (see Chap. 16).

Since chlamydia are obligate intracellular parasites, they can multiply only in living eukaryotic cells, where they produce intracytoplasmic inclusions. For the isolation of chlamydiae, certain lines of tissue culture cells have proved more useful than others. However, the technical difficulty and cost of chlamydia cultures have limited their availability in many parts of the world. The lack of a sensitive, specific test for diagnosis and screening has been a major factor contributing to the chlamydia epidemic. Recent advances in simplifying cell culture techniques have made cultures more widely available.[1,2] Culture results may be significantly improved by irradiation of the host cells or by exposing them to various cytostatic agents. Centrifugation and treatment with DEAE-dextran both increase the uptake of chlamydia by tissue culture cells. Inclusions of *C. trachomatis* contain glycogen and stain with iodine, in contrast to those of *C. psittaci*. However, the use of fluorescein-conjugated monoclonal antibodies improves the sensitivity of cell culture and reduces the need for a second passage.[1] The use of microtiter plates rather than small vials and coverslips has also made it possible to process larger numbers of specimens per unit cost.

Finally, the development of ELISA tests and direct immunofluorescence staining of cervical and urethral smears for chlamydia using monoclonal antibodies, as well as other antigen diagnostic detection methods, has finally allowed specific chlamydia diagnostic testing to be done where cell cultures aren't available.

## ISOLATION TECHNIQUE

### Tissue culture cells and tissue culture medium

McCoy cells were once considered to be human synovial cells but, probably because of contamination, are now considered mouse fibroblasts (L cells). This is the most widely used cell line for the isolation of *C. trachomatis*. Some laboratories use HeLa 229 cells and DEAE-dextran treatment with excellent results[3] while others use baby hamster kidney cells (BHK 21). In a comparative study of different tissue culture media, we found RPMI 1640 to be the most suitable basic medium, using McCoy cell cultures. The composition of a complete cell culture medium is shown in Table 74-1.

**Table 74-1. Growth and Maintenance Medium for McCoy Cells to Be Used for the Isolation of *C. trachomatis***

*Growth medium:*
RPMI 1640 (Flow Ltd.): 500 ml
Fetal calf serum (inactivated): 50 ml
Glutamine (200 mmol/ml): 5 ml
Gentamicin (20 mg/ml): 1.4 ml
Final pH 7.4

*Maintenance medium:*
RPMI 1640 (Flow Ltd.): 500 ml
Fetal calf serum (inactivated): 25 ml
Glucose (0.11 g/ml): 25 ml
Glutamine (200 mmol/ml): 5 ml
Amphotericin B (Squibb) (250 μg/ml): 5.6 ml
Gentamicin (1000 μg/ml): 5.6 ml
Final pH 7.4

### Irradiation of tissue culture cells

Irradiation pretreatment of cell cultures improves the sensitivity of culture.[4] The cells should be exposed to 4000 to 6000 rads, 6 to 10 days before being used for specimen inoculation. After irradiation, the cells become nonreplicating giant cells. For the most part, the greater convenience and safety of cytostatic agents for this purpose has led to the abandonment of irradiation.

### Pretreatment of tissue-culture cells using cytostatics and DEAE-dextran

*Cycloheximide* is a glutaramide antibiotic which reduces the metabolic activity of eukaryotic cells. The antibiotic is added to the culture medium at a concentration of approximately 2 μg/ml (depending on the source and batch of the drug used) simultaneously with the specimen inoculation.[5] The optimal concentration of cycloheximide must be titrated for each new batch of drug used. The different steps in the culture technique using cycloheximide treatment of the McCoy cells are shown in Tables 74-2 and 74-3.

**Table 74-2. Passage of McCoy Cells from Roux Bottles to Test Tubes to Be Used for Chlamydial Cultures**

1. Check (under a stereomicroscope using inversed light) that the cells have multiplied and have formed an almost confluent cell sheet, and that the cells are in good condition.
2. Pour off the cell culture medium and wash the cells three times in phosphate-buffered saline, pH 7.2.
3. Add 2 ml trypsin-versene solution (2.5 ml trypsin + 50 ml versene). Pour off the solution and check that cells remain in the bottle.
4. Add 10 ml cell-tissue culture medium per bottle (volume 250 ml).
5. Shake the bottle so the cells loosen from the glass surface.
6. Transfer 0.5 ml cell suspension and 10 ml fresh tissue culture medium to a Roux bottle to maintain the cell line.
7. Transfer the remaining medium to a new bottle and add fresh medium in a volume corresponding to a cell density of $2 \times 10^5$ cells per ml. Using a 250 ml Roux bottle, cells for approximately 50 vials (containing 1 ml medium) can be prepared.
8. Incubate cells for 1 day at 37°C, when they are generally ready to use.
9. The McCoy cells should be passaged each third day of incubation at 37°C.

**Table 74-3. Technique for the Isolation of *C. trachomatis*, Using Cycloheximide-Treated McCoy Cells**

1. Pass $2.0 \times 10^5$ McCoy cells to flat-bottomed plastic tubes with a coverslip and incubate at 37°C for 24 h.
2. Exchange tissue culture medium with 0.5 ml specimen in transport medium (Table 74-4) plus 0.5 ml maintenance (Table 74-1).
3. Centrifuge at least 4000 *g* for 1 h at 35°C.
4. Incubate 2 h at 37°C.
5. Exchange specimen/medium with 2 ml fresh tissue maintenance medium (Table 74-1) containing 2 μg/ml cycloheximide.
6. Incubate for 72 h at 37°C.
7. Fix coverslips in methanol for 10 min.
8. Stain cells with 5% iodine solution for 10 min.
9. Transfer cells to 2.5% iodine solution for staining for another 10 min.
10. Place coverslip on a glass slide on which is a solution of one part glycerol and one part of 5% iodine solution.

SOURCE: Modified from KT Ripa and P-A Mårdh.[5]

IUdR (5-iodo-2-deoxyuridine) pretreatment of McCoy cells is another means of increasing the susceptibility of McCoy cells to *C. trachomatis* infection.[6] Three days before the McCoy cells are inoculated with the clinical specimen, 25 μg/ml of IUdR is added per milliliter of cell culture medium. However, different sources of IUdR vary widely in their activity and thus titration experiments should be performed when introducing new batches of IUdR.

*Cytochalasin B* and mitomycin C are other cytostatic drugs that have been recommended for pretreatment of cells used for chlamydial isolation.[7,8] At present, however, these compounds are less widely used than cycloheximide.[9] Like IUdR, they require that the cells be pretreated for 3 days before clinical samples can be inoculated in the cell culture.

*DEAE-dextran* (molecular weight approximately $2 \times 10^6$) transforms the physicochemical properties of the surface of HeLa 229 cells, which enhances attachment and phagocytosis of TRIC agents of *C. trachomatis*.[3] When using McCoy cells, treatment with DEAE also increases the chlamydial inclusion count, though the count is lower than when McCoy cells are treated with cycloheximide.

## Comparative studies on the sensitivity of different cell treatment methods

Cycloheximide has proved to be the most sensitive method for pretreatment of McCoy cell cultures.[7] The method has the advantage of using fresh (1-day-old) cells, and it yields excellent inclusion counts. It also avoids the need of an irradiation source (i.e., x-ray equipment or a $^{60}$Cobalt gun). While some have claimed that cycloheximide-treated tissue cell cultures are more susceptible to superinfection as well as to toxic compounds in the samples, this has not been our experience.

## Centrifugation

For primary isolation, centrifugation of cell cultures inoculated with chlamydiae is required in order to obtain optimal culture results. At centrifugation forces of 3000 to 6000 *g*, the organisms are pelleted onto the cell monolayer, thus increasing the chlamydiae-cell contact. Experimental studies indicate that centrifugation at this force for 1 h, using a centrifuge maintained at 35 to 36°C, gives a satisfactory inclusion count. At a centrifugation force of 2500 *g*, the isolation rate of chlamydiae from clinical specimens was lower than at 3000 to 6000 *g*.[10] The use of temperatures higher than 37°C also can be deleterious. Use of higher centrifugation forces causes several problems (including lack of test tubes that can stand such forces) and results in only an approximately 5 percent increase in the recovery rate compared with 3000 to 6000 *g*.

## Staining of inclusions

In all isolation methods, chlamydial inclusions develop within 48 to 72 h of incubation at 36°C and can be identified using Giemsa, iodine, or immunofluorescence staining. Giemsa staining is not widely used for purposes of routine isolation because the inclusions are more difficult to visualize. Iodine staining produces dark brown inclusions that are readily seen against a yellow background. This method has been widely used and is quite effective, particularly when cell cultures are grown on coverslips in vials.[11] When iodine staining is used in microtiter systems (see below), a second passage is generally required to achieve optimal sensitivity.[12]

An important advance in culturing *C. trachomatis* has been the use of fluorescein-conjugated monoclonal antibodies to identify chlamydial inclusions in infected monolayers.[13,14] Compared with iodine or Giemsa staining, this method identifies three- to eightfold more inclusions and, using the microtiter method, results in an increased sensitivity in specimens from both men and women.[12] More importantly, immunofluorescence staining greatly increases the sensitivity of the initial inoculation and makes it unnecessary to perform a second passage, thus making results available and reducing the cost of the culture method.[13]

Recently, an immunoperoxidase staining method was also shown to be an effective means of identifying inclusions in cell culture.[15]

All of these staining methods require experience in order to differentiate inclusions from artifacts.

## Microtiter plates vs. coverslip vials

Recent studies have demonstrated that growing cell monolayers in 96-well microtiter plates rather than on coverslips in glass vials greatly simplifies the processing of large numbers of specimens and reduces the cost per culture.[16,17] In patients with infections characterized by ≥10 inclusion-forming units (IFU) per coverslip, the microtiter method and the coverslip-vial method are essentially equal in terms of sensitivity.[16] In patients whose infections are characterized by lower inclusion counts, the larger volume of inoculation in the coverslip-vial method (200 vs. 100) results in a higher recovery rate using the latter method[18] (W.E. Stamm, unpublished data). Thus, the microtiter plate method is most sensitive in clinical settings such as STD clinics where the majority of infections are symptomatic and are characterized by higher inclusion counts. Twenty-four- and 48-well microtiter plates permit a larger inoculum to be used and may further improve the sensitivity of the microtiter method.

## Passage

Whether the sensitivity of culture increases greatly after a passage (that is, disruption of the initial monolayer after 48 to 72 h with subsequent inoculation of this material onto a fresh monolayer for another 48 to 72 h) seems to depend in part on the precise method used. Using a microtiter method with iodine staining we have found that passage adds 15 to 20 percent to the sensitivity of the method.[11] In contrast, when monoclonal IF staining is used, the sensitivity is not increased even after five passages. Schachter and Martin have reported similar findings in vial system.[19] In contrast, Jones reports a marked increase in yield using a microtiter system and monoclonal IF staining.[20] Each laboratory should evaluate the incremental yield attributable to passage when optimizing their method.

## SAMPLING

### Sampling devices

Sampling, particularly from the male urethra, requires the use of a thin sampling stick to avoid causing pain and mucosal lesions. When choosing a sampling swab, its toxic properties for chlamydiae must also be considered.[21–23] In comparative studies using experimentally infected transport medium, some lots of swabs tipped with calcium alginate were more toxic to chlamydiae than other swabs tested. In addition, the glue used to attach cotton or other materials to the stick may be toxic to chlamydiae.[22] The least toxic type of swab was a cotton-tipped metal stick (ENT, Medical Wire & Equipment). Dacron and rayon-tipped plastic swabs were also comparatively nontoxic. Sampling swabs with shafts of wood from various commercial sources differed in their toxicity (Fig. 74-1), but many were toxic to chlamydia.

Sampling devices other than swabs can also be used to obtain specimens for chlamydial culture, but most are less widely used and less acceptable to patients. Thus, plastic or wire loops have been satisfactorily used to collect urethral specimens. Curettes or other "scraping" devices collect excellent specimens, often increasing the sensitivity of the culture, but are painful and poorly tolerated by patients. A device for collecting cervical specimens, the cytobrush, is a small brush on a wire shaft. Samples collected with the cytobrush have excellent cellularity and improve both direct FA and culture results.[23]

### Sampling sites

Since chlamydia is an intracellular pathogen, specimens should contain as many epithelial cells as possible. For urethral specimens, the sample swab is introduced 2 cm into the male or female urethra and is rotated and withdrawn. Such sampling results in a significantly higher isolation frequency than samples from the urethral meatus. To obtain specimens from the cervix, a large cotton-tipped swab should first be used to remove external secretions from the exocervix. A specimen should then be obtained by inserting a swab 1 to 2 cm into the cervical os, rotating it, and withdrawing it. The swabs used for cervical specimens are generally larger in size than those for urethral samples.

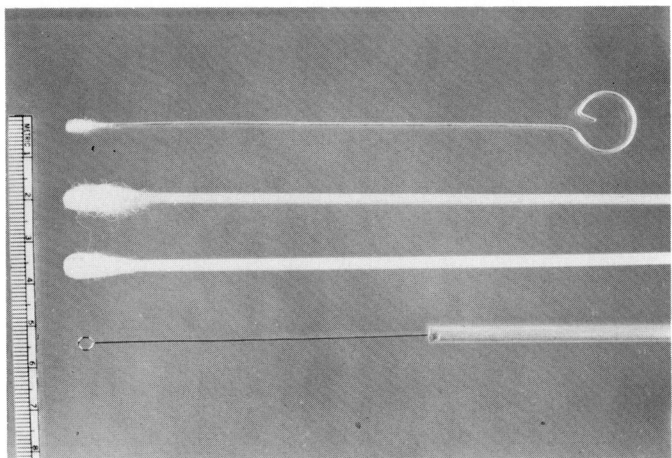

**Fig. 74-1.** Swabs for useful urogenital cultures. (*Top to bottom*) Calcium-alginate-tipped wire, cotton-tipped wood, rayon-tipped plastic, platinum wire loop. (*From HH Handsfield et al, N Engl J Med, 1973.*)

It is advisable to study both urethral and cervical samples from females if the laboratory has the capacity, since 15 to 20 percent more chlamydia-positive patients can be identified. Bacterial overgrowth and cytopathogenic effects are also greater problems with cervical samples, which is another reason why concomitant urethral samples may be of benefit.

In sampling from the *eye,* the eyelid is lifted and preferably everted and the sampling swab is rubbed over the mucosa. The sampling should be rather "active," that is, with vigorous rubbing. If a chlamydial eye infection is suspected, especially when studying infants, samples should also be collected for direct microscopy (Plate 94). In chronic chlamydial eye infections (trachoma), chlamydial cultures from the eye are often negative.

To collect *nasopharyngeal* samples, the swab is introduced through the nostrils to the pharyngeal wall before withdrawal. Such sampling may be difficult in neonates, which is why washing of the posterior pharynx with saline through a baby feeding catheter has been recommended. Pharyngeal samples from neonates may be positive for chlamydiae, even when cultures from the eyes are negative.[24]

Rectal specimens should be collected with the same type of swab used for cervical specimens. Specimens are best collected via anoscopy, with direct visualization of erythematous, friable mucosa and areas of mucopus from which samples can be obtained. Alternatively, a swab can be inserted 2 cm into the rectum, rotated, and withdrawn. Since rectal specimens frequently cause contamination or cytotoxicity, many labs sonicate the specimen before inoculating it.

At most sites of infection, the yield in culture correlates with the number of epithelial cells in the sample. In addition, the use of multiple samples produces a higher yield.[25]

### Transport medium

A sucrose buffer (2-SP)[11,26] should be used for transportation of chlamydial samples for culture. The formula for the buffer is given in Table 74-4. The addition of antimicrobials such as gentamicin, amphotericin B, and vancomycin is essential. Using this transport medium, the percentage of cell cultures invalidated by nonspecific cytopathogenic effects and/or bacterial or fungal overgrowth can be kept below 1 percent for cervical and urethral specimens.

**Table 74-4. Transport Medium for *C. trachomatis***

*Composition of transport medium:*
Sucrose buffer: 100 ml
Fetal calf serum: 10 ml
Gentamicin: 2 mg
Amphotericin: 0.5 mg
Vancomycin: 10 mg

*Preparation of the sucrose buffer:*
Dissolve 68.5 g sucrose in distilled water. Add 2.1 g $K_2HPO_4$ dissolved in 60 ml of distilled water and 1.1 g $KH_2PO_4$ disolved in 40 ml of distilled water. Mix the salt solutions and add distilled water up to 1000 ml. Boil for 30 min. The transport medium can be stored in the refrigerator for approximately 2 weeks and at −20°C for months.

SOURCE: Modified from FB Gordon et al.[26]

Specimens should be refrigerated as soon as possible after collection and should remain refrigerated throughout the period of transport. Since the number of viable elementary bodies in a refrigerated specimen begins to decline substantially after 24 h, the specimen should be delivered and inoculated by that time. If longer transport or storage is anticipated prior to inoculation, the specimen should be frozen at −70°C.

## DIRECT MICROSCOPY

Elementary bodies (EB) of *Chlamydia* are approximately 0.3 μm in diameter and stain purple or bluish with Giemsa's and red with Macchiavello's stain. Reticulate bodies (RB) (measuring 0.5 to 1.0 μm), which are the replicating unit in eukaryotic cells, stain blue using these dyes. The EB is round to oval and smaller and more electron-dense than the RB. Gram stain cannot be used to detect EB and RB because chlamydiae are gram-negative and do not take counterstain. Intracytoplasmatic inclusions of *C. trachomatis* stain dark purple with Giemsa's stain and brown with iodine solution. However, microscopy of clinical genital samples using these methods has a low sensitivity compared with cultures, particularly in asymptomatic, nonacute cases, and are thus not recommended. The presence of mucus, debris, other microorganisms and a low number of infected cells all contribute to difficulties in the diagnosis of a chlamydial infection by microscopy. In other situations, however, such as in acute chlamydial eye infections, microscopy is of great diagnostic value.[27]

Early reports suggesting that cervical chlamydial infections could be detected by visualizing inclusions on routinely stained Papanicolaou smears have not been corroborated by comparative studies versus culture.[28]

## ANTIGEN DETECTION METHODS

Despite the simplification of chlamydia culture procedures, the rigorous transport conditions needed to maintain viability and the small number of laboratories with cell culture facilities have limited *C. trachomatis* cultures to larger centers. Noncultural methods for detection of *C. trachomatis* antigen in infected secretions are now available. Two general approaches to antigen detection have been taken: (1) direct immunofluorescence staining of smears using monoclonal antibodies and (2) detection of chlamydial antigen eluted from swabs and measured by enzyme-linked immunoassay (ELISA) with polyclonal or monoclonal antibodies.[29] DNA probes have also been studied but aren't yet available commercially.[1,2]

The use of fluoresceinated species-specific monoclonal antibodies to *C. trachomatis* makes it possible to reliably identify extracellular elementary bodies in infected secretions.[30] Compared with previously used polyclonal antibodies, monoclonal antibody staining markedly reduces nonspecific background staining and reliably identifies chlamydial elementary bodies rather than the much larger but less frequently seen intracellular inclusions.

Antigen detection tests have generally been evaluated by comparsion with *C. trachomatis* cultures. Tables 74-5 and 74-6 summarize selected studies that have compared antigen detection methods with *C. trachomatis* cultures for the diagnosis of uncomplicated urethral and cervical infections.[31–54] Either the Microtrak (Syva Company, Palo Alto, California) direct immunofluorescence test or the Chlamydiazyme enzyme immunoassay (Abbott Laboratories, North Chicago, Illinois) was used, since these are the only two assays that have been extensively evaluated to date. Using the direct immunofluorescence assay in males with symptoms or signs of urethritis, a median sensitivity of 92 percent and specificity of 97 percent was achieved (Table 74-5). The test has not been evaluated in low-risk, asymptomatic males. In high-risk populations of women in whom the prevalence of infection was 15 to 26 percent, the median sensitivity was 90 percent (range 88 to 99 percent) and the median specificity was 95 percent (range 89 to 99 percent) (Table 74-3). In other populations of women, primarily women attending family planning clinics or prenatal clinics with a prevalence of infection between 9 and 11 percent, the test's sensitivity decreased (median 77 percent). This decrease most likely results from the greater number of asymptomatic infections, which are usually characterized by fewer inclusion-forming units, in such populations. The direct immunofluorescence test has not been adequately studied in truly low prevalence groups of women. Most discrepancies between culture and the direct immunofluorescence test occur in specimens with fewer than 20 inclusion-forming units in culture.

Using the ELISA test, the median sensitivity in men with overt urethritis was 79 percent (Table 74-6). Median specificity was 97 percent. The sensitivity of the ELISA test fell markedly in men without clinical evidence of urethritis (Table 74-6). In women, the sensitivity of the ELISA approximated that of the direct immunofluorescence test in high-risk women seen in sexually transmitted disease clinics, and appeared to be higher than the direct immunofluorescence test in populations of women in the intermediate prevalence range.

Two published studies have directly compared the direct immunofluorescence test and ELISA with culture and with each other.[50,54] Chernesky found the direct immunofluorescence test to be more sensitive in males and the ELISA to be more sensitive

**Table 74-5. Reported Experience with the Direct Immunofluorescence Test in 11 Studies*†**

| | Sensitivity | Specificity | Positive predictive value | Negative predictive value |
|---|---|---|---|---|
| Men: | | | | |
| Symptomatic population | 92 (90–100) | 97 (72–99) | 87 (82–93) | 98 (95–100) |
| Asymptomatic population | NA | NA | NA | NA |
| Women: | | | | |
| High-prevalence population | 89 (89–98) | 98 (89–99) | 90 (68–97) | 98 (98–100) |
| Intermediate-prevalence population | 79 (61–96) | 98 (94–99) | 79 (65–93) | 98 (94–99) |

*Based on Refs. 31–39, 41–42.

†Median (range) in percentages.

Reproduced with permission from Stamm WE: Diagnosis of *Chlamydia tachomatis* genitourinary tract infections. *Ann Intern Med* 108:710, 1988.

**Table 74-6. Reported Experience with Enzyme Immunoassay in Eight Studies*†**

| | Sensitivity | Specificity | Positive predictive value | Negative predictive value |
|---|---|---|---|---|
| Men: | | | | |
| Symptomatic population | 79 (70–95) | 97 (96–100) | 93 (84–100) | 90 (89–94) |
| Asymptomatic population | 49 (48–50) | 95 (90–100) | 85 (69–100) | 88 (79–98) |
| Women: | | | | |
| High-prevalence population | 90 (70–98) | 97 (86–98) | 84 (61–94) | 98 (97–99) |
| Intermediate-prevalence population | 89 (82–96) | 97 (93–98) | 73 (45–80) | 98 (98–99) |

*Based on Refs. 43–50.
†Median (range) in percentages.
Reproduced with permission from Stamm WE: Diagnosis of *Chlamydia trachomatis* genitourinary tract infections. *Ann Intern Med* 108:710, 1988.

in females.[50] The two tests were equivalent in specificity in his study. Taylor-Robinson and coworkers reported the direct immunofluorescence test to be sensitive and specific as compared with culture[54] but found the ELISA test to have a low sensitivity in both men and women (approximately 60 and 70 percent, respectively), and a low specificity in women (approximately 90 percent).

## SELECTION OF THE APPROPRIATE LABORATORY TEST

Selection of the most appropriate laboratory test for detection of *C. trachomatis* depends upon local availability and expertise, the prevalence of infection in the test population, and the intended purpose of the test. Isolation in cell culture remains the most sensitive and specific test and thus should be used where it is available and where transport conditions, cost, and other logistical factors permit its use. Because of their high specificity, cell cultures may be of greatest value in screening low-risk populations. In populations of women in which the prevalence of infection exceeds 10 percent, both the direct smear test and the ELISA provide alternative diagnostic methods with satisfactory sensitivity and specificity, rapid turnaround time, and simplified transport conditions. The direct smear test is best suited to laboratories handling relatively small numbers (<30) of specimens per day. The test requires a high-quality fluorescence microscope and an experienced technician, and is somewhat labor-intensive. It allows continuous monitoring of specimen quality and, in experienced hands, a very high specificity. As with all immunofluorescence procedures, however, the endpoint is subjective, and both false-positive and false-negative results occur with inexperienced microscopists. The test can be used for rectal[55] and for eye infections[40,56–58] as well as for urethral and cervical infections.

The ELISA test, by virtue of automation and batching, is better suited to laboratories doing larger numbers of tests (>50 per day). The test requires less technical expertise and has an objective (optical density) endpoint. Disadvantages of the test include the inability to monitor specimen quality, nonspecificity (particularly in cervical infections), and a low sensitivity in male urethral infections. Second-generation ELISA tests, including some that can be done in a doctor's office and require only 30 min to perform, are now being marketed. However, the sensitivity and specificity of these tests are not presently established. Ultimately each laboratory should determine the test best suited to its capabilities and to the needs of the population served.

## IMMUNOTYPING OF *Chlamydia trachomatis*

For many years, determination of the immunotype (A, B, Ba, C to K, $L_1$ to $L_3$) of isolated strains of *C. trachomatis* could be performed only by micro-IF tests. As this is a laborious procedure, and few clinical laboratories possess suitable antigens for micro-IF tests (see below), immunotyping was rarely done.

More recently batteries of serovar-specific and subspecies-specific monoclonal antibodies have been developed that have greatly simplified immunotyping.[60] Both micro-IF and dot-ELISA systems have been used.[60,61] These methods are primarily of research interest, however, as serotyping has little clinical utility at this time.

## ANTIBIOTIC SUSCEPTIBILITY TESTING

*C. trachomatis* are susceptible in cell culture systems to a large number of antibiotics, particularly broad spectrum antibiotics (see Chap. 16).

To evaluate the activity of an antimicrobial against *C. trachomatis*, twofold dilutions of antibiotic are added to the medium in tissue-cell cultures infected with a standard inoculum of *C. trachomatis*. High concentrations of *C. trachomatis* are toxic for the host cell, which is why concentrations of approximately $10^4$ inclusion-forming units (IFU) per milliliter should be used. After 48 h, the cultures are studied for the presence of inclusions. Direct IF staining is preferable to other methods as aberrant inclusion forms (frequently induced by antibiotics) can be recognized. The MIC is the lowest concentration of antibiotics that completely inhibits the development of inclusions when the incubated medium is passaged to fresh cultures. The $IC_{50}$ is the concentration of antibiotics reducing the inclusion count by 50 percent compared with control cultures without antibiotic. For tetracycline, MIC values of 0.25 to 1.0 μg/ml and $IC_{50}$ values of 0.05 to 0.25 μg/ml have been reported.[59] Although strains of *C. trachomatis* with a decreased susceptibility to erythromycin (MICs of more than 0.5) have been detected, emergence of drug resistance to erythromycin or tetracycline in clinical isolates is as yet unreported.

## SEROLOGY

### Genus-specific antibodies

Antibodies to a group antigen of *Chlamydia*, that is, an antigen shared by *C. trachomatis*, *C. psittaci*, and the TWAR strains, can be detected by CF tests.[62] The CF test is the only widely available serological test for *Chlamydia* at present. The test can be used to help diagnose cases of psittacosis, ornithosis, and lymphogranuloma venereum, but is of rather limited diagnostic value in the diagnosis of most sexually transmitted chlamydial infections (see Chap. 16). For CF tests, egg-grown antigens may be used. To detect antibodies to the group antigen, radioisotope precipitation and hemolysis-in-gel and ELISA techniques have also been described, but are little used.

## Immunotype-specific antibodies

Immunotype-specific antibodies to *C. trachomatis* may be detected by the use of micro-IF tests. The micro-IF technique was introduced for detection of chlamydial antigens[63] but can also be employed for detection of immunotype-specific antibodies to *C. trachomatis*. Immunoglobulin classes of such antibodies may also be determined.

**Table 74-7 Preparation of Chlamydial Antigen for Microimmunofluorescence Tests**

*Preparation of test antigen from yolk-sac-grown organisms:*

1. Inject 0.5 ml of a dilution of highly infectious sample of *Chlamydia* into the yolk sac of 6- to 8-day-old embryonated hen's eggs. Incubate the eggs at 37°C. Examine the eggs daily under a candle light. Eggs that die within 72 h are rejected.
2. When half of the eggs have died, the yolk sacs of the surviving eggs are harvested.
3. A piece (1 to 2 $mm^2$) of the yolk sac, close to the umbilicus, is removed, crushed with tweezers, and smeared on a glass slide. The slide is fixed by heat and stained by the Macchiavello or Giemsa method. The slide is read under the oil-immersion lens of the dark field microscope (× 1000). The elementary bodies (EB) are seen as cherry-red particles (yellow-green with Giemsa) on the background of yolk-sac tissue, which stains blue.
4. Yolk sacs from eggs producing numerous EB are selected for antigen production. Egg yolk material should be removed as much as possible. The infected yolk sacs are kept frozen at −80°C until use.
5. Weigh the yolk sac from which antigen is to be prepared. A 40% (w/v) suspension of the yolk sac in phosphate-buffered saline (PBS), pH 7.2, is prepared.
6. The yolk sac is ground either by a mortar and pestle, by a Tenbroeck tissue grinder, or by shaking with glass beads, and 0.01 *M* PBS is added to make a 40% (w/v) yolk-sac suspension.
7. Centrifuge the suspension at 900*g* for 15 min at 4°C.
8. Avoid the surface layer of fat and the bottom layer of gross debris, but collect the in-between layer suspension and centrifuge again at 900*g* for 15 min.
9. The suspension devoid of fat and gross debris is then transferred to a 40-ml centrifuge tube, and PBS is added to fill the tube.
10. Mix and centrifuge at 20,000*g* at 4°C for 45 min.
11. Collect the pellet, which consists of relatively pure EBs. PBS is added to make a 40% suspension.
12. Centrifuge the suspension at 900*g* for 10 to 15 min to remove any gross debris.

*Immunization for production of antisera:*

1. Dilute the antigen preparation (from step 11, above) to give a 1% suspension in PBS.
2. Inoculate 5-week-old mice intravenously with 0.5 ml of the suspension.
3. Immunizations are made 7 days apart. The mice are exsanguinated 3 days after the second immunization. The blood is collected and sera separated.

SOURCE: S-P Wang; unpublished research.

During recent years, various modifications of the micro-IF technique have been described in order to simplify the laborious testing procedure.[64] Pools of antigens may be prepared from different immunotypes of *C. trachomatis* that have been grown in embryonated hen's egg or in HeLa 229 cell cultures. Some workers[65] use pools containing antigens of immunotypes of ABC, DEFGHIK, and $LGF_1$ to $LGF_3$ (based on the concept of epidemiologic distribution), while others use other pools (i.e., CJ, A, H, I, $KL_3$, B, ED, $L_1L_2$, and GF) (based on the relatedness of cross-reactions).

Recent studies suggest that antibodies cross-reacting with *C. trachomatis* may be produced during and after infection with TWAR chlamydia strains.[66] The antigens shared by these strains are group-specific (LPS). The micro-IF test should theoretically distinguish TWAR antibodies from *C. trachomatis* infections by demonstrating a serovar-specific antibody rise for *C. trachomatis*. Nevertheless, considerable experience may be necessary before a reader can accurately distinguish these patterns.[67] The LPS antigens shared by TWAR and by *C. psittaci* also explain why cases of TWAR pneumonia have been considered cases of ornithosis when the diagnostic test used was a complement-fixation test based on the LPS antigen.

Antigen for the micro-IF test can be produced in embryonated hen's egg as described in Table 74-7. In the micro-IF method, the different antigens are placed as small dots close to each other on a glass slide by means of an old-fashioned fountain pen. The dots are placed in a pattern on the slide so that they can be easily found by means of the coordinator screws of the microscope (Fig. 74-2). By having the different antigens on one glass slide, the intensity of positive immunofluorescence reactions can easily be compared, which is essential in determining immunotype-specific antibodies. The various steps in the micro-IF test procedure are shown in Table 74-8.

The laborious preparation of antigens has also resulted in attempts to simplify the methodology. Thus, glass slides on which experimentally infected tissue cell cultures have been grown have been employed as antigen. Broadly reacting elementary body antigen of a single immunotype (i.e., $L_2$) has also been employed. This cross-reacts with most (95 percent) high-titer antisera of *C. trachomatis*.[68]

## Interpretation of micro-IF test for *C. trachomatis* antibodies

Up to 60 to 80 percent of STD clinic patients have antibodies to *C. trachomatis,* as do 25 to 40 percent of female contacts of male NGU patients and 25 to 75 percent of chlamydia culture-negative males with NGU. Much of this antibody has resulted from previous infections. In conformity with serological tests in general, a micro-IF test should be interpreted as indicative of a current infection when a fourfold or greater change in the titer of IgG antibodies can be demonstrated, or when IgM antibody is found. These criteria can also be used for a seronegative patient developing antibodies during the course of the disease.

The diagnostic value of a single high titer of antichlamydial antibodies of any Ig class or of a stable high titer is uncertain. However, the presence of a high titer of IgM (i.e., ≥ 1:128) and/or IgG (i.e., ≥ 1:2048) antibodies to *C. trachomatis* strongly suggests an acute infection. Most experimental animal studies indicate that the occurrence of serum IgM antibodies is related to recent infection. In experimental studies in monkeys, IgM antibodies to *C. trachomatis* had disappeared and only IgG antibodies persisted after 5 weeks.[69] In humans, some studies indi-

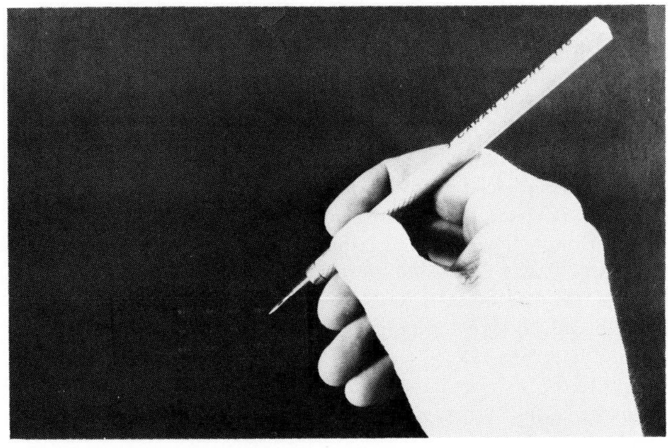

A

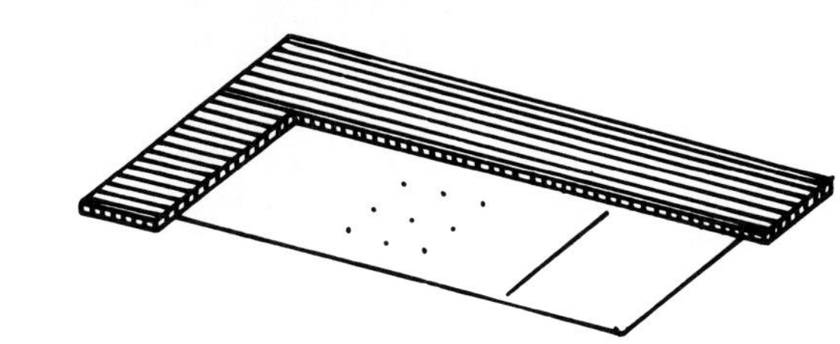

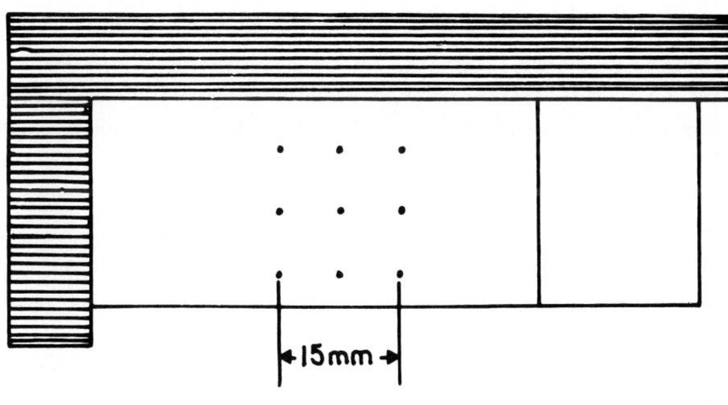


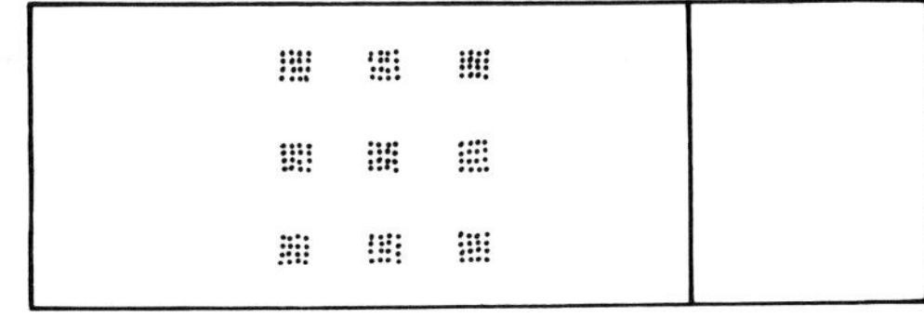

B

**Fig. 74-2.** (*a*) Application of antigen using a pen and a template and (*b*) pattern for application of antigen dots on glass slides for microimmunofluorescence tests. (*Courtesy of S-P Wang.*)

cate, however, that IgM antibodies to *C. trachomatis* may persist for years and that IgG antibodies to the organism may often be demonstrated years after infection. It is unknown whether treatment with antibiotics influences the persistence of specific antibodies.

Maternal IgG antibodies to *C. trachomatis* can be demonstrated in infants but disappear within months. Chlamydiae antibodies start to appear again at 5 years of age or later. It is not known by which route(s) children are infected or whether antibody reactivity in this group of individuals represents cross-reactions with other antigens (perhaps TWAR strains, for example). It has also been argued that *C. trachomatis* antibodies may be the result of polyclonal B cell stimulation.[70]

**Table 74-8 Method to Perform Microimmunofluorescence Antibody Tests for Detection of Antibodies to Chlamydiae**

1. Antigens of different immunotypes (or pools thereof) are applied onto acid-washed glass slides. A template (see Fig. 74-2*A*) is placed under the slide for guidance of antigen placement. The antigens are placed on slides according to the marking by the aid of a fine pen (see Fig. 74-2*B*). The antigen spots should be located close together, so that the intensity of the fluorescence from the different antigen spots can easily be compared. When thawed, the antigens should be shaken to assure a homogeneous suspension, before being applied. Yolk-sac antigens, or antigens prepared of homogenates of highly infected HeLa 299 cells diluted in normal yolk-sac suspensions, can be used.
2. The slides are air-dried for 30 min and fixed in acetone for 10 to 15 min in room temperature. They can then be stored at −20°C for up to 6 months before use (or when stored for longer periods of time, at −80° C).
3. Twofold serum dilutions (using 0.05 ml) are made and applied to the slides with a bacterial loop or Pasteur pipette.
4. Incubate at 37°C for 30 min in a moist chamber.
5. Wash (using a forceps) each slide by dips and drains: four changes in phosphate-buffered saline (PBS), pH 7.2, and three changes in distilled water. Air-dry slides at room temperature.
6. Apply fluorescein isothiocyanate-labeled anti-immunoglobulin (IgM, IgG, or IgA) and as counterstain rhodamine-conjugated bovine albumin on the antigen spots. Dilutions to be used depend on preparations used.
7. Incubate slides at 37°C for 30 min and wash again as described in step 5, above.
8. Mount slides with coverslip and glycerol (in TRIS buffer, pH 8). The slides can be read immediately or kept in the refrigerator for a few days without losing too much fluorescence.
9. Study slide under a fluorescence microscope. Use filter combination recommended by microscope producer. Monocular observation is made using a 10× ocular 50× objective lens. A 4× objective lens is used to locate the antigen dots.
10. The highest serum dilution resulting in definite fluorescence of the elementary bodies is considered the serum titer to that particular antigen. Only fluorescence associated with evenly distributed elementary bodies is considered positive.

SOURCE: S-P Wang; unpublished research.

Among patients with laparoscopic signs of acute salpingitis and who are culture-positive from the fallopian tube for *C. trachomatis,* antibodies to *C. trachomatis* may be absent or may be present in low or high stationary titers, or a significant change in titer of IgM and/or IgG antibodies may occur.[71] In such patients, cervicitis probably often precedes the tubal infection, during which time an antibody response may be induced. Once the infection ascends from the cervix, the period of primary antibody response may have already passed. Previous genital infection, including salpingitis, and previous exposure to *C. trachomatis* are common in this group of patients. This may explain why IgM antibodies are not particularly common in salpingitis patients, including those who are culture-positive from the tubes. However, in patients with deep-sited chlamydial infections (e.g., pneumonia and salpingitis), IgM titers up to 256 to 512 may occur and high IgG titers are often found. There is great individual variation in the titer rise and persistence of antichlamydial antibodies in patients with acute salpingitis.[72]

Antibodies to *C. trachomatis* occur less often and generally in lower titers in males than in females (similar to other STD agents).

## References


1 Stamm WE: Diagnosis of *Chlamydia trachomatis* genitourinary tract infections. *Ann Intern Med* 108:710, 1988.

2 Mårdh P-A et al: *Chlamydia.* New York, Plenum, 1988.

3 Kuo C-C et al: Primary isolation of TRIC organisms in HeLA 229 cells treated with DEAE-dextran. *J Infect Dis* 125:665, 1972.

4 Darougar S et al: Simplified irradiated McCoy cell culture for isolation of chlamydiae, in *Trachoma and Related Disorders,* RL Nichols (ed). Amsterdam, Exerpta Medica, 1971, p 63.

5 Ripa KT, Mårdh P-A: Cultivation of *Chlamydia trachomatis* in cycloheximide-treated McCoy cells. *J Clin Microbiol* 6:328, 1977.

6 Wentworth BB, Alexander ER: Isolation of *Chlamydia trachomatis* by use of 5-iodo-2-deoxyuridine-treated cells. *Appl Microbiol* 27:912, 1974.

7 Sompolinsky D, Richmond S: Growth of *Chlamydia trachomatis* in McCoy cells treated with cytochalasin B. *Appl Microbiol* 28:912, 1974.

8 Woodland RM et al: Sensitivity of mitomycin-C treated McCoy cells for isolation of *Chlamydia trachomatis* from genital specimens. *Eur J Clin Microbiol* 6:653, 1987.

9 Evans RT, Taylor-Robinson D: Comparison of various McCoy cell treatment procedures used for the detection of *Chlamydia trachomatis. J Clin Microbiol* 10:198, 1979.

10 Reeve P et al: Laboratory procedure for the isolation of *Chlamydia trachomatis* from the human genital tract. *J Clin Pathol* 28:910, 1975.

11 Schachter J: Chlamydial infections. *N Engl J Med* 298:428, 490, 540, 1978.

12 Mårdh P-A et al: Sampling, specimen handling, and isolation techniques in the diagnosis of chlamydial and other genital infections. *Sex Transm Dis* 4:280, 1981.

13 Stamm WE et al: Detection of *Chlamydia trachomatis* inclusions in McCoy cell cultures with fluorescein-conjugated monoclonal antibodies. *J Clin Microbiol* 17:666, 1983.

14 Stephens RS et al: Sensitivity of immunofluorescence with monoclonal antibodies for detection of *Chlamydia trachomatis* inclusions in cell culture. *J Clin Microbiol* 16:4, 1982.

15 Mahoney JB et al: Detection of chlamydial inclusions in cell culture or biopsy tissue by alkaline-phosphatase anti-alkaline phosphatase staining. *J Clin Microbiol* 25:1864, 1987.

16 Yoder BL et al: Microtest procedure for isolation of *Chlamydia trachomatis. J Clin Microbiol* 13:1036, 1981.

17 McComb DE, Puzniak CI: Micro cell culture method for isolation of *Chlamydia trachomatis. Appl Microbiol* 28:727, 1974.

18 Schachter J: Immunodiagnosis of sexually transmitted diseases. *Yale J Biol Med* 58:443, 1985.

19 Schachter J, Martin DH: Failure of multiple passages to increase chlamydial recovery. *J Clin Microbiol* 25:1851, 1987.

20 Jones RB et al: Effect of blind passage and multiple sampling on recovery of *Chlamydia trachomatis* from urogenital specimens. *J Clin Microbiol* 24:1029, 1986.

21 Mårdh P-A, Zeeberg B: Toxic effect of sampling swabs and transportation test tubes on the formation of intracytoplasmatic inclusions of *Chlamydia trachomatis* in McCoy cell cultures. *Br J Vener Dis* 57:628, 1978.

22 Soltecz LV: Toxic effect of sampling materials on the reproduction of *Chlamydia trachomatis* in McCoy cell cultures. In *Proceedings of European Society for Chlamydial Research.* 1st Meeting, Stockholm, Almquist and Wiksell, 1989, p 259.

23 Ciotti RA et al: Detecting *Chlamydia trachomatis* by direct immunofluorescence using a Cytobrush sampling technique. *Genitourin Med* 64:245, 1988.

24 Stenberg K et al: Colonization of the nasopharynx in cases of chlamydial conjunctivitis. In *Proceedings of European Society for Chlamydia Research.* 1st Meeting, Stockholm, Almquist and Wiksell, 1989, p 129.

25 Singal SS et al: Isolation of *C. trachomatis* from men with urethritis: Relative value of one vs two swabs. *Sex Transm Dis* 13:50, 1986.

26 Gordon FB et al: Detection of Chlamydia (Bedsonia) in certain infections of man: I. Laboratory procedures: Comparison of yolk-sac and cell culture for detection and isolation. *J Infect Dis* 120:451, 1969.

27 Schachter J, Dawson CR: Comparative efficiency of various diagnostic methods for chlamydial infection, in *Nongonococcal Urethritis and Related Disorders,* KK Holmes, D Hobson (eds). Washington, DC, American Society for Microbiology, 1974, p 795.

28 Spence MR et al: A correlative study of Papanicolaou smear, fluorescent antibody, and culture for the diagnosis of *Chlamydia trachomatis. Obstet Gynecol* 68:691, 1986.

29 Stamm WE: Diagnosis of *Neisseria gonorrhoeae* and *Chlamydia trachomatis* infections using antigen detection methods. *Diagn Microbiol Infect Dis* 4:93S, 1986.

30 Tam MR et al: Culture-independent diagnosis of *Chlamydia trachomatis* using monoclonal antibodies. *N Engl J Med* 310:1146, 1984.

31 Stamm WE et al: Diagnosis of *Chlamydia trachomatis* infections by direct immunofluorescence staining of genital secretions. A multicenter trial. *Ann Intern Med* 101:638, 1984.

32 Teare EL et al: Conventional tissue culture compared with rapid immunofluorescence in identifying *Chlamydia trachomatis* in specimens from patients attending a genitourinary clinic. *Genitourin Med* 61:739, 1985.

33 Quinn TC et al: Screening of *Chlamydia trachomatis* infection in an innercity population: A comparison of diagnostic methods. *J Infect Dis* 152:419, 1985.

34 Thomas BJ et al: Sensitivity of detecting *Chlamydia trachomatis* elementary bodies in smears by use of a fluorescein labelled monoclonal antibody: Comparison with conventional chlamydial isolation. *J Clin Pathol* 37:812, 1984.

35 Lipkin ES et al: Comparison of monoclonal antibody staining and culture in diagnosing cervical chlamydial infection. *J Clin Microbiol* 23:114, 1986.

36 Uyeda CT et al: Rapid diagnosis of chlamydial infections with the Microtrak Direct Test. *J Clin Microbiol* 20:948, 1984.

37 Shafer MA et al: Evaluation of fluorescein-conjugated monoclonal antibody test to detect *Chlamydia trachomatis* endocervical infections in adolescent girls. *J Pediatrics* 108:779, 1986.

38 Ridgway GL et al: Comparison of methods for detecting *Chlamydia trachomatis. J Clin Pathol* 39:232, 1985.

39 Francis RA, Abbas AMA: The Syva "Microtrak" stains: Their use in a routine laboratory. *J Clin Pathol* 38:236, 1985.

40 Mårdh PA et al: Comparison of two tests in the diagnosis of chlamydial conjunctivitis, in *Abstracts of the 5th International Symposium on Rapid Methods and Automation in Microbiology and Immunology,* Florence, November 4–6, 1987, p 228.

41 Forbes BA et al: Evaluation of a monoclonal antibody test to detect chlamydia in cervical and urethral specimens. *J Clin Microbiol* 23:1136, 1986.

42 Foulkes SJ et al: Comparison of direct immunofluorescence and cell culture for detection of *Chlamydia trachomatis. Genitourin Med* 61:255, 1985.

43 Amortegui AJ, Meyer MP: Enzyme immunoassay for detection of *Chlamydia trachomatis* from the cervix. *Obstet Gynecol* 65:523, 1985.

44 Howard LV et al: Evaluation of Chlamydiazyme for the detection of genital infections caused by *Chlamydia trachomatis. J Clin Microbiol* 23:329, 1986.

45 Van Ulsen J et al: Solid-phase enzyme immunoassay for detection of *Chlamydia trachomatis. Eur J Clin Microbiol* 4:397, 1986.

46 Mumtaz G et al: Enzyme immunoassay for the detection of *Chlamydia trachomatis* antigen in urethral and endocervical swabs. *J Clin Pathol* 38:740, 1985.

47 Jones MF et al: Detection of *Chlamydia trachomatis* in genital specimens by the Chlamydiazyme test. *J Clin Microbiol* 20:465, 1984.

48 Hambling MH, Kurtz JB: Preliminary evaluation of an enzyme immunoassay test for the detection of *Chlamydia trachomatis. Lancet* i:53, 1985.

49 Ryan RW et al: Rapid detection of *Chlamydia trachomatis* by an enzyme immunoassay method. *Diagn Microbiol Infect Dis* 5:225, 1986.

50 Chernesky MA et al: Detection of *Chlamydia trachomatis* antigens by enzyme immunoassay and immunofluorescence in genital specimens from symptomatic and asymptomatic men and women. *J Infect Dis* 154:141, 1986.

51 Smith JW et al: Diagnosis of chlamydial infection in women attending antenatal and gynecologic clinics. *J Clin Microbiol* 25:868, 1987.

52 Wiesmeier E et al: Detection of *Chlamydia trachomatis* infection by direct immunofluorescence staining of genital secretions. *Obstet Gynecol* 69:347, 1987.

53 Baselski VS et al: A comparison of nonculture-dependent methods for detection of *Chlamydia trachomatis* infections in pregnant women. *Obstet Gynecol* 70:47, 1987.

54 Taylor-Robinson D et al: Evaluation of enzyme-immunoassay (Chlamydiazyme) for detecting *Chlamydia trachomatis* in genital tract specimens. *J Clin Pathol* 40:194, 1987.

55 Rompalo AM et al: Rapid diagnosis of *Chlamydia trachomatis* rectal infection by direct immunofluorescence staining. *J Infect Dis* 155: 1075, 1987.

56 Mabey DCW, Booth-Mason S: The detection of *Chlamydia trachomatis* by direct immunofluorescence in conjunctival smears from patients with trachoma and patients with ophthalmia neonatorum using a conjugated monoclonal antibody. *J Hyg* 96:83, 1986.

57 Bell TA et al: Direct fluorescent monoclonal antibody stain for rapid detection of infant *Chlamydia trachomatis* infections. *Pediatrics* 74:224, 1984.

58 Rapoza PA et al: Assessment of neonatal conjunctivitis with a direct immunofluorescent monoclonal antibody stain for chlamydia. *JAMA* 255:3369, 1986.

59 Johannison G et al: Susceptibility of *Chlamydia trachomatis* to antibiotics in vitro and in vivo. *Sex Transm Dis* 6:50, 1979.

60 Wang SP et al: Immunotyping of *Chlamydia trachomatis* with monoclonal antibodies. *J Infect Dis* 152:791, 1985.

61 Barnes RC et al: Rapid immunotyping of *Chlamydia trachomatis* with monoclonal antibodies in a solid-phase enzyme immunoassay. *J Clin Microbiol* 22:609, 1985.

62 Dkir SP et al: Immunochemical studies on chlamydial group antigen (presence of 2-keto-3-deoxycarbohydrate as immunodominant group). *J Immunol* 109:116, 1972.

63 Wang S-P: A microimmunofluorescence method: Study of antibody response to TRIC organisms in mice, in *Trachoma and Related Disorders Caused by Chlamydial Agents*, RL Nichols (ed). Amsterdam, Excerpta Medica, 1971, p 273.

64 Treharne JD et al: Modification of the microimmunofluorescence test to provide a routine serodiagnostic test for chlamydial infection. *J Clin Pathol* 30:510, 1977.

65 Wang S-P et al: Serodiagnosis of *Chlamydia trachomatis* infection with the micro-immunofluorescence test, in *Nongonococcal Urethritis and Related Disorders*, KK Holmes, E Hobson (eds). Washington, American Society for Microbiology, 1977, p 237.

66 Schachter J: *Chlamydia psittaci*—"Reemergence of a forgotten pathogen." *N Engl J Med* 315:189, 1986.

67 Schachter J: Human *Chlamydia psittaci* infection, in *Chlamydial Infections*. New York, Cambridge University Press, 1986, p 311.

68 Saikku P, Paavonen J: Single-antigen immunofluorescence test for chlamydial antibodies. *J Clin Microbiol* 8:119, 1978.

69 Ripa KT et al: Experimental salpingitis in grivet monkeys provoked by *Chlamydia trachomatis*. *Acta Pathol Microbiol Scand* [B] 87:65, 1979.

70 Gray J et al: Antibody response to *Chlamydia trachomatis* in sera of children; a seroepidemiological study. *Eur J Clin Microbiol* 5:576, 1986.

71 Svensson L et al: Acute salpingitis with *Chlamydia trachomatis* isolated from the fallopian tubes: Clinical, cultural and serological findings. *Sex Transm Dis* 8:51, 1981.

72 Puolakkainen M et al: Persistence of chlamydial antibodies after pelvic inflammatory disease. *J Clin Microbiol* 23:924, 1986.

# Chapter 75
# Syphilis

Sandra A. Larsen
Elizabeth F. Hunter
Ernest T. Creighton

Syphilis is a chronic infection with diverse clinical manifestations that occur in distinct stages. Each stage has a particular testing requirement. Microscopic examination methods are the tests of choice for the primary stage or whenever syphilitic lesions are present. During the secondary and subsequent stages, serologic methods are the more frequently used diagnostic procedures.

Laboratory diagnostic procedures for syphilis have existed from the early 1900s. Yet, since the pathogenic treponemes, *Treponema pallidum*, subspecies *pallidum*, subspecies *pertenue*, and subspecies *endemicum*, and *T. carateum*, are morphologically, serologically, and chemically indistinguishable, none of the current diagnostic procedures are subspecies-specific.

## DEVELOPMENT OF DIAGNOSTIC TESTS

### Microscopy

Direct microscopic examination of lesion material permits the most definitive diagnosis of treponemal infection. Microscopic examination of treponemes in stained tissue sections was described in 1910, and the dark field method became a routine diagnostic procedure in 1923. The application of the fluorescent antibody technique to dark field preparation was described in 1964[1] and later modified for use with paraffin-embedded tissue sections.[2]

### Nontreponemal serologic tests

The Wassermann test reported in 1906 by Wassermann, Neisser, and Bruck[3] was the first of the nontreponemal (reagin) serologic tests for diagnosing infection with *Treponema pallidum*. Soon, many tests were developed, each with its own modification of the basic lipoidal antigen (an alcoholic extract of liver or other animal organs). The earliest tests were based on the complement fixation procedure of Bordet and Gengou.[4] Later, precipitin and flocculation tests were developed in an attempt to simplify test procedures. The antigen was a crude alcoholic extract of beef heart, and standardization was difficult. Often, these tests were unreliable because of lack of control both in antigen sensitivity and specificity and in test procedures.

In 1941, Pangborn[5] isolated and purified serologically reactive substances, i.e., cardiolipin and lecithin, from beef heart muscle. The use of more purified chemical components to prepare the antigens increased the sensitivity and specificity of nontreponemal tests.

### Treponemal serologic tests

Although *T. pallidum* was identified in 1905 by Schaudin[6] as the causative agent of syphilis, it was not until 1949 that the first serologic test, the *Treponema pallidum* immobilization (TPI) test, that used the pathogenic treponeme as antigen was described.[7] As with the nontreponemal tests, an array of treponemal tests was later developed. Each new test represented an attempt to develop a test that was specific, sensitive, and less complicated to perform than the existing tests.

## SPECIMEN COLLECTION AND TRANSPORT

## MICROSCOPIC EXAMINATION

### Dark field microscopy

The ideal specimen for dark field examination is serous fluid rich in *T. pallidum* and free of red blood cells and other lesion constituents. In collecting specimens from external lesions, the lesion should be cleaned with 0.9 percent sterile saline and gently abraded to provoke oozing. The lesion exudate may be collected directly on a microscope slide, transferred by a sterile bacteriologic loop to a slide, or collected on a cover slip which is then inverted on a microscope slide. Skin lesions that are healing also warrant examination. These lesions should be abraded with scalpel or needle tip, or the fluid may be collected from the lesion by injecting a drop or two of sterile saline into the base of the lesion and then aspirating the fluid. Internal vaginal and cervical lesions require visualization with a bivalve speculum. The lesion should be cleaned and abraded and the exudate collected with a sterile bacteriologic loop. Collection of material from enlarged lymph nodes requires sterilization of the skin over the node, injection of 0.2 ml or less of sterile saline into the node with maceration of the tissue, and then aspiration of the fluid. Mucous membrane lesions usually present little problem. Material may be collected from oral cavity lesions if care is taken in cleaning the lesion.

Specimens for dark field microscopy should not be transported. Any appreciable delay in the examination of a specimen may result in questionable findings, since motility of the organism is critical to identification. If more than one slide has been prepared, the additional slides should be kept in a moist chamber until read to prevent drying.

### Direct fluorescent antibody tests

The collection methods described for dark field microscopy are applicable to the direct fluorescent antibody test for *T. pallidum* (DFA-TP). However, slides and/or cover slips are air-dried and heat-fixed or air-dried and fixed with acetone or 10 percent methanol before staining. For the DFA-TP, lesion material may also be collected in heparinized, microhematocrit capillary tubes, sealed with plasticine or like material, and stored at 4 to 8°C until slides are prepared. If specimens are to be mailed to a reference laboratory for staining, smears prepared on microscope slides should be air-dried only and mailed without being fixed. Specimens in capillary tubes should be properly packaged for mailing and may be mailed without refrigerant.

Paraffin-embedded biopsy or autopsy material may also be examined by DFA-TP. Tissues are fixed in 10 percent neutral-buffered formalin for at least 24 h at room temperature. The tissues are then dehydrated, cleared, and infiltrated with paraffin on an automatic tissue processor. Tissue blocks may be stored at room temperature and mailed without refrigerant.

## SEROLOGIC TESTS

Specimens for serologic tests are collected by venipuncture into dry tubes without anticoagulant. After the blood has clotted, the serum is separated by centrifugation at 1500 to 2000 r/min for 5 min. If the serologic test is not to be performed immediately, the serum is removed from the clot. Serum may be stored at 4 to 8°C for several days or frozen; however, repeated freezing and thawing of specimens should be avoided.

## CULTURE

Specimens for in vivo isolation of *T. pallidum* can be collected from lesions in heparinized, microhematocrit capillary tubes, immediately placed in cryovials, frozen, and transported in liquid nitrogen. On arrival at the reference laboratory, the lesion material is dispersed in saline and injected intratesticularly into rabbits. After 11 to 28 days or at orchitis, treponemes are harvested from testicles and passed to a second animal. More than one passage may be required to achieve sufficient numbers of treponemes to produce orchitis.

Limited success has been achieved in growing treponemes in tissue cell culture.[8] To date, subculture has not been successful.

## DIAGNOSTIC TESTS

Tests that have been evaluated by the *Guidelines for Evaluation and Acceptance of New Syphilis Serology Tests for Routine Use*[9] are listed according to their status and type in Table 75-1.

## DIRECT MICROSCOPIC EXAMINATION

Dark field microscopy and the DFA-TP are considered standard tests for syphilis. Dark field microscopy[10] is the test of choice when the patient has moist lesions. A diagnosis of syphilis in the primary and secondary stages can be made by demonstrating *T. pallidum* in suspected lesions or regional lymph nodes by this means. Additionally, dark field microscopy is used to rule out syphilis as the cause of lesions associated with other sexually transmitted diseases such as herpes simplex, chancroid, and lymphogranuloma venereum.

To perform a satisfactory dark field examination, one needs the proper microscopic equipment, adequate training, a good specimen, and perseverence.[11a] *T. pallidum* is recognized by its morphologic characteristics: length 6 to 14 μm, thickness 0.25 to 0.30 μm, spiral amplitude 0.5 to 1.0 μm, and characteristic movement. It may be necessary to examine several slides before treponemes are found.

The DFA-TP test[2,11] is a practical alternative to direct dark field examination when smears cannot be examined immediately and when examining oral lesions. The lesion material fixed to the slide is stained with fluorescein-labeled anti-*T. pallidum* globulin. The test offers the advantage of specifically detecting *T. pallidum*, thereby eliminating confusion with other spiral organisms, especially in oral lesions. In addition, motile organisms are not required. This test is applicable to the identification of *T. pallidum* in tissues as well.

While the earliest and empirically most specific means of diagnosing syphilis, provided that the diseases yaws, bejel, and pinta are excluded, is through direct microscopic examination, precautions must be taken in test interpretation. The demonstration of treponemes with characteristic morphology and motility for *T. pallidum* by dark field microscopy or reactive DFA-TA results constitutes a positive diagnosis of syphilis in primary, secondary, early congenital, and infectious relapse stages, regardless of the outcome of serologic testing. However, a failure to find the organism does *not* exclude a diagnosis of syphilis. Failure to demonstrate *T. pallidum* from typical lesions may be due to the age or condition of the lesion, treatment of the patient either locally or systemically before the specimen was taken, and most commonly, poor technique in collecting and reading the specimen.[12]

**Table 75-1. Diagnostic Tests for Syphilis**

| |
|---|
| **Standard status tests** |
| *Nontreponemal:* |
| Venereal Disease Research Laboratory (VDRL) Slide |
| Unheated serum reagin (USR) |
| Rapid plasma reagin (RPR) 18-mm Circle Card |
| Automated reagin test (ART) |
| Reagin screen test (RST) |
| *Treponemal:* |
| Fluorescent treponemal antibody absorption (FTA-ABS) |
| Microhemagglutination assay for antibodies to *T. pallidum* (MHA-TP) |
| Dark field microscopy |
| Direct fluorescent antibody test for *T. pallidum* (DFA-TP) |
| Hemagglutination treponemal test for syphilis (HATTS) |
| Fluorescent treponemal antibody-absorption double-staining (FTA-ABS DS) |
| **Provisional status tests** |
| *Treponemal:* |
| Syphilis Bio-Enzabead |
| *Nontreponemal:* |
| Toluidine red unheated serum test (TRUST) |

## NONTREPONEMAL TESTS

The nontreponemal tests for syphilis in use today are flocculation tests using cardiolipin, lecithin, and cholesterol as antigen. The basic antigen formula used in most tests is that of the Venereal Disease Research Laboratory (VDRL) test, which contains 0.03 percent cardiolipin, 0.9 percent cholesterol, and sufficient lecithin to produce standard reactivity, usually 0.21 ± 0.01 percent.[13] Modifications of VDRL antigen have been made by stabilizing the suspension and by adding various visualization agents. All these tests can be used for initial screening and to follow treatment of the patient,[14–16] and all are similar in sensitivity and specificity.

All nontreponemal tests measure antilipid IgG and IgM antibodies formed by the host in response to lipid from the treponemes' cell surfaces.[17] Because of either the lipid nature of the antigen or some unusual property of the antibody, the antigen-antibody complex remains suspended in these tests and flocculation rather than agglutination or precipitation occurs.

All nontreponemal tests are performed in a similar manner. The test antigen is mixed with the patient's serum on a solid matrix, rotated for a specified number of minutes, and read. Two of the tests, the VDRL slide (Fig. 75-1) and the unheated serum reagin (USR),[10] are microscopic flocculation tests. On the basis of antigen cost, the VDRL slide test is probably the least expensive of the nontreponemal tests and is the only standard status test that can be used with CSF. The major disadvantage of the

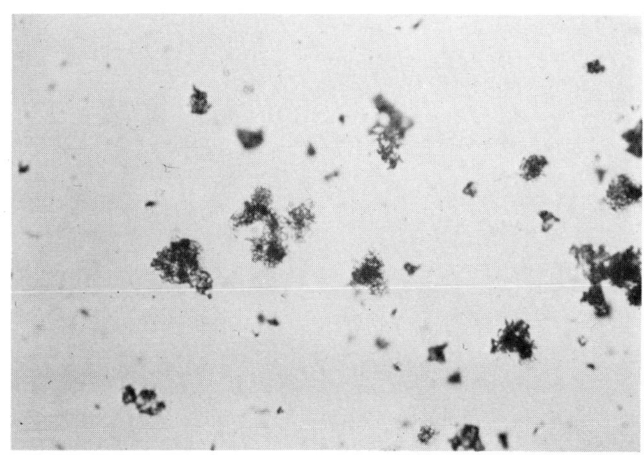

Fig. 75-1. Nonreactive (*left*) and reactive (*right*) VDRL slide tests.

VDRL test is that the VDRL antigen suspension must be prepared fresh daily. The USR test antigen is only slightly more expensive than the VDRL slide test antigen. The antigen in the USR test is stabilized, thereby omitting the need for daily preparation of antigen suspension and disposal of unused antigen at the end of a day's testing. As the name implies, the sera for this test do not need to be heated. The only apparent disadvantage of the USR is that either glass slides with paraffin rings must be prepared or reusable ceramic ring slides must be cleaned for use in the test as with the VDRL slide test.

The antigen used in the rapid plasma reagin (RPR) 18-mm circle card test[10] is a stabilized suspension to which sized charcoal particles have been added. The antigen is not attached to these particles, but the charcoal is trapped in the lattice formed by the antigen-antibody combination when reactive serum is tested. Thus the reaction can be seen without the aid of a microscope. Such tests are known as macroscopic flocculation tests. The RPR card test is performed on the Brewer diagnostic 18-mm circle card,[18] a disposable plastic-coated card, using unheated sera (Fig. 75-2).

Another macroscopic card test is the reagin screen test (RST).[19] In place of charcoal, this test employs a stabilized antigen stained with the lipid-soluble diazo dye Sudan Black B. The RST can be used with both serum and plasma. The plasma should be from blood collected in tubes containing anticoagulant and tested within 48 h after the blood is drawn.

The toluidine red unheated serum test (TRUST)[20,21] is another macroscopic flocculation test. In the TRUST, uniform particles of the azo pigment toluidine red are added to the basic stabilized antigen to aid in the visualization of reactive serum, much as charcoal does in the RPR card test. The test is performed on a disposable plastic-coated card similar to the Brewer[18] diagnostic 18-mm circle card. The antigen can be easily prepared in the central laboratory, with little expense for basic materials and equipment. The test is also available commercially.

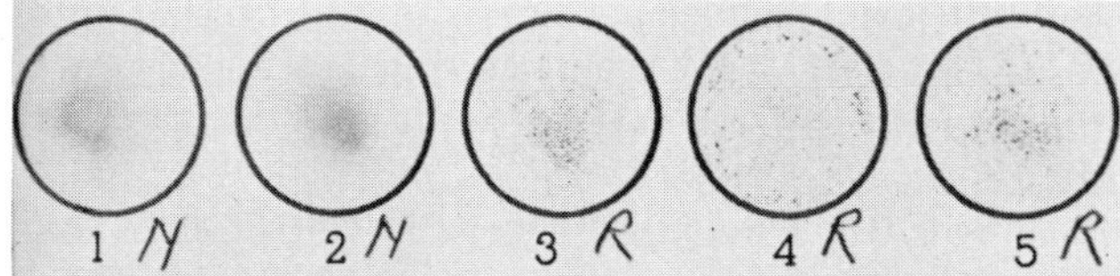


Fig. 75-2. Rapid plasma reagin 18-mm circle card test showing two nonreactive (1 and 2) and three reactive (3, 4, and 5) tests.

Most nontreponemal tests are reported as either reactive or nonreactive. The two exceptions are the USR and VDRL tests, which have a weakly reactive report. Quantitative results are usually reported as the reciprocal of the dilution, for example, 4 dils rather than 1:4. Problems in nontreponemal test performance can be avoided if the instructions for test performance, reagent control, and general quality control are carefully followed. The use of plasma or cord serum in the card tests may cause particular problems in reading results. Improperly collected specimens can appear as minimally reactive.

False-positive results occur in the general population at a rate of 1 to 2 percent regardless of the nontreponemal test used.[22–24] In populations of IV drug users, more than 10 percent of the sera may give false-positive results. As a rule, 90 percent of the false-positive titers are less than 1:8, but low titers are also seen in latent and late syphilis. In low-risk populations, all reactive test results should be confirmed by a treponemal test since over 50 percent of the reactive nontreponemal tests may be false-positive in such populations.

## TREPONEMAL TESTS

Currently four treponemal tests are considered standard tests for syphilis (Table 75-1): the fluorescent antibody absorption (FTA-ABS), the FTA-ABS double staining (DS), the microhemagglutination assay for antibodies to *T. pallidum* (MHA-TP), and the hemagglutination treponemal test for syphilis (HATTS). All the treponemal tests use *T. pallidum,* subspecies *pallidum,* as the antigen, all are based on the detection of antibodies directed against treponemal cellular components, and all are designed as confirmatory tests. These sensitive, specific, and relatively inexpensive tests have replaced the TPI test as a routine clinical test procedure.[25]

The FTA-ABS test (Fig. 75-3) is an indirect immunofluorescent antibody test.[10,26] A serum for testing must first be diluted 1:5 in sorbent, an extract of Reiter treponeme cultures, to remove antibodies to nonpathogenic treponemes present in the serum of most presumed-normal individuals. Next the serum is placed on the microscope slide to which the antigen, a suspension of *T. pallidum* organisms, has been fixed. Finally the conjugate, fluorescein-labeled antihuman globulin, is added. Presence of an-

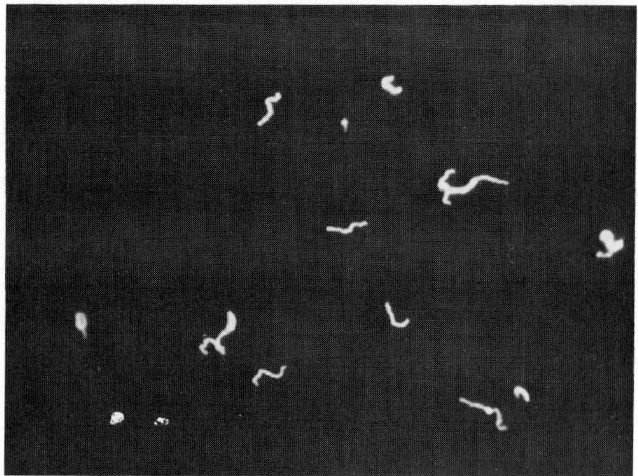

Fig. 75-3. Positive fluorescent treponema antibody absorption test.

tibody in the patient's serum is indicated by fluorescence. The FTA-ABS test is extremely sensitive and must be well controlled. The 1 + reading standard control and correct conjugate dilution are critical elements to the reliability and reproducibility of the test's results.

The FTA-ABS DS test[27] is designed specifically for use with newer fluorescent microscopes that have incident rather than transmitted illumination. The test is the basic FTA-ABS test with the addition of a contrasting fluorochrome-labeled counterstain for *T. pallidum* as a final staining step in the standard FTA-ABS procedure. The counterstain eliminates the need to use transmitted light to locate treponemes that are not stained with the antihuman IgG fluorochrome-labeled conjugate. The test also eliminates errors in the standard procedure that are caused by improper alignment of the dark field condenser. The current procedure includes the use of rhodamine-labeled primary reagent and a fluorescein-labeled counterstain.

Laboratories that are not already equipped with a fluorescent microscope may find the MHA-TP[28,29] a less expensive and less complex alternative for confirmatory testing. The MHA-TP is a qualitative hemagglutination test using tanned, formalinized sheep red cells as the carrier for the *T. pallidum* antigen. The patient's serum is first diluted in absorbing diluent containing sheep red cell and bovine red cell membranes, normal rabbit testicular extract, Reiter treponeme sonicate, normal rabbit serum, and stabilizers. Serum is tested both with cells sensitized with *T. pallidum* and with unsensitized sheep red blood cells. Although the MHA-TP test is easier to perform than the FTA-ABS test and has fewer variables, the test is less sensitive in primary syphilis,[23,30,31] and heterophile reactions with unsensitized cells may occur.

The HATTS[24] is similar to the MHA-TP, but in the HATTS, glutaraldehyde-stabilized erythrocytes are used as carriers for the *T. pallidum* antigen. Serum for testing in the HATTS is diluted in sorbent (the same sorbent as for the FTA-ABS test) before testing with both sensitized and unsensitized red cells. Like the MHA-TP, the HATTS is relatively insensitive in the early primary stage of syphilis, and heterophile reactions may occur. However, the HATTS, like the MHA-TP, provides a convenient confirmatory test for syphilis in laboratories that are not equipped for fluorescent procedures or that have to test many specimens in a short time.

Enzyme immunoassay methods have been heralded as the model test systems for present-day immunologic procedures. The first application of the enzyme-linked immunosorbent assay (ELISA) to the area of syphilis serology was in 1975.[32] Since that time, several ELISAs for syphilis have been described.[33–37] In 1984, the first commercially available ELISA for the serodiagnosis of syphilis received recognition as a provisional status test. This test, the syphilis Bio-Enzabead, uses *T. pallidum* subspecies *pallidum* as the antigen fixed to ferrous metal beads.[38] Control beads coated with normal rabbit testicular extract are used to determine nonspecific reactions. The detection system consists of horseradish peroxidase-conjugated antihuman IgG as the second antibody and 2,2′-azino-di(3-ethyl-2,3-dihydro-6-benzthiazoline-sulfonate) as the enzyme substrate. Recent studies[39–42] have shown the Bio-Enzabead to be comparable in sensitivity and specificity to the FTA-ABS test and MHA-TP.

Treponemal test misinterpretation most often results from the misuse of the treponemal tests as screening procedures. About 1 percent of the general population have false-positive results in the treponemal tests, although the specificity of the FTA-ABS test has been increased with a change in the reporting system.[43] The borderline reading, which has been eliminated, had less than a 5 percent association with the diagnosis of syphilis. While the FTA-ABS test is the most sensitive of all the tests, it is also the test with the greatest possibility for laboratory error. Alterations in dilution of conjugate,[44] improper use of multicircle slides,[45] improper matching of individual components, and improper alignment of the microscope can all contribute to an incorrect result.

## NEW DIAGNOSTIC TESTS

Two categories of syphilis remain for which specific standard status serodiagnostic tests need to be developed. These categories are congenital syphilis and neurosyphilis. While research directed toward understanding the pathogenicity of *T. pallidum* has resulted in the cloning of various antigenic determinants[46–48] and the production of monoclonal antibody,[49,50] no diagnostic tests based on these products have yet reached the U.S. market. Recently, an IgM capture method[51] has been applied to the diagnosis of both early and congenital syphilis (Mercia Diagnostics Limited, Surrey, England). This system uses an anti-human IgM antibody to capture patient IgM. The patient's syphilis IgM antibody is then traced with *T. pallidum* antigen labeled with the enzyme horseradish peroxidase. In clinical trials, the IgM capture procedure has been compared with patient history and the FTA-ABS IgM test[52] using fractionated serum (19S) with excellent correlation (Mercia Diagnostics, personal communication). Although the FTA-ABS IgM test for diagnosing congenital syphilis has been criticized for lack of sensitivity and specificity,[53] when the test is used with fractionated serum it appears to be both sensitive and specific[54] for the diagnosis of congenital syphilis. Many of the problems ascribed to the IgM FTA-ABS test may be related to the quality of the reagents used[55] and not to the basic principle of the test. The ELISA procedures and the FTA-ABS test have been modified for use with CSF for diagnosing both symptomatic and asymptomatic neurosyphilis with limited success.[56–58] However, as with congenital syphilis, a test that can be considered a standard diagnostic procedure other than the VDRL test for CSF is not available.

As clinical trials and evaluations are completed in the near future, a new generation of immunodiagnostic tests for syphilis should appear that combine recombinant treponemal antigens and variations of the ELISA, such as dot immunobinding.[59,60]

## QUALITY CONTROL

In the United States, uniformity of tests for syphilis has been achieved through a program including personnel training, laboratory consultation, reagent control, proficiency testing programs, and publications of detailed standard test procedures that now has run for many years. Although the progression from investigational test status to standard test status can be long and tedious for the developer of a new test, it provides for a thorough evaluation of tests under a variety of test conditions.

Quality control measures in syphilis serology[10] are designed to ensure reliable and reproducible test results both within a laboratory and among laboratories. Strict adherence to test protocols and the use of standardized reagents and controls will eliminate most technical errors. Quality control measures that are essential for reliable and reproducible results are:

1. Clean, well-lighted, and temperature-controlled laboratories. Special attention must be paid to temperature ranges for the flocculation tests (23 to 29°C).
2. Equipment, instruments, and glassware that meet protocol specifications and that have periodic maintenance.
3. Clean glassware and plastic ware.
4. Test procedures that have been selected on the basis of applicability to the physician's need and to the qualifications of the personnel performing the tests.
5. Up-to-date techniques that are available for immediate reference and that are followed without modification.
6. Careful and precise measurements of specimens and reagents. This includes periodic testing of safety pipetting devices for accuracy.
7. Periodic, within-laboratory check readings to maintain uniform reading levels among laboratory personnel.
8. Strict control of reagents. This includes (*a*) adequate testing of new lots of reagents for standard reactivity, (*b*) proper preparation, labeling, and storage of reagents, and (*c*) adequate documentation of the preparation of new lots of reagents, control sera, and the date they are first routinely used.
9. Control sera with established reactivity patterns for each test performed. These controls should be similar to the test specimens and include a reactive, an intermediate, and a nonreactive test pattern. Each time a serologic test is performed, the controls must be included to monitor day-to-day consistency.
10. Acceptable test specimens. Specimens should not be grossly hemolyzed or chylous and should be labeled as to plasma or serum and heated or unheated. CSF specimens with even minute traces of blood are unsuitable for testing.
11. Daily worksheets that include space for specimen number, results of all tests performed, controls, reagents identification, room temperature, and the laboratorian's initials.
12. Careful scrutiny of report forms and test records for clerical errors.
13. Periodic interlaboratory checks, which may include proficiency testing programs.
14. Participation of laboratorians in basic and refresher training courses.

Reference reagents and sera for quality control and training are available through state health departments, the Centers for Disease Control, and World Health Organization Reference Laboratories.

## USE AND INTERPRETATION OF SEROLOGIC TESTS FOR SYPHILIS

All serum samples submitted for the diagnosis of syphilis should be tested in a nontreponemal test. Reactive nontreponemal tests may indicate past or present infection with pathogenic treponemes that may or may not have been adequately treated. Likewise, a reactive test may also be false-positive. A nonreactive test may be interpreted as no current infection or an effectively treated infection. A nonreactive test does not rule out incubating-stage syphilis, however. Generally a fourfold increase in titer indicates infection, reinfection, or treatment failure; whereas a fourfold decrease in titer indicates adequate therapy. Nontreponemal test misinterpretation most often results from the failure to recognize the variation of plus or minus 1 endpoint titer, inherent in most serologic tests, or the failure to establish the true reactivity of the test. A particular error that leads to misinterpretation is using more than one nontreponemal test to follow treatment. The same nontreponemal test used initially should be used for subsequent quantitative testing, since up to a fourfold difference in endpoint titers can occur with certain sera in various nontreponemal tests.

Use of treponemal serologic tests should be reserved for confirmation of nontreponemal tests and for patients with symptoms suggesting late syphilis regardless of the nontreponemal test results. A reactive treponemal test usually indicates past or present infection with pathogenic treponemes. For the majority of cases, once the treponemal tests are reactive they remain reactive for a lifetime. However, when treatment is begun early in primary syphilis, about 10 percent of these patients will test nonreactive within 2 years after treatment.[14] Generally a nonreactive test indicates no past or present infection. The treponemal test, however, may be nonreactive for incubating-stage syphilis. Treponemal test misinterpretation most often results from the misuse of the test as a screening procedure; about 1 percent of the general population tests false-positive.

## PRIMARY SYPHILIS

For primary stage syphilis a direct microscopic examination should be performed either as a dark field or as a DFA-TP. A positive test plus typical lesions indicate need for treatment. When dark field examination is not available, a reactive nontreponemal test from sera of patients with typical lesions usually indicates the need for treatment. The reactive nontreponemal test should be quantitated. The FTA-ABS test or MHA-TP should be performed when the lesion is suspect and the nontreponemal test reactive. Treponemal serologic tests are not recommended in the absence of a reactive nontreponemal test. If the initial nontreponemal test is nonreactive, as approximately 30 to 50 percent will be, then the patient should have a repeat reagin test at 1 week, 1 month, and 3 months. Nonreactive nontreponemal tests over the 3 months exclude the diagnosis of syphilis as the cause of the lesion.

## SECONDARY SYPHILIS

Demonstration of *T pallidum* in lesion or lymph nodes by dark field microscopy or DFA-TP is diagnostic of secondary syphilis. Patients with typical lesions and reactive reagin test titers of greater than 1:16 are considered to have secondary syphilis. Nearly all patients with secondary syphilis have reactive nontreponemal tests. Less than 2 percent of sera from these patients will give a nonreactive "rough" appearance or weakly reactive results due to the prozone phenomenon. Upon dilution, these sera will have titers of 1:16 or greater. Patients with atypical findings and/or nontreponemal test titers lower than 1:16 should have repeat nontreponemal tests and a confirmatory treponemal test.

## LATENT SYPHILIS

Patients with reactive nontreponemal and treponemal tests in the absence of clinical and historical findings are said to have latent syphilis. False-positive test results may be exluded through repetition of the test immediately and at 6-month intervals. There is an increased incidence of false-positive nontreponemal results in patients over 60 years old and in younger patients with lupus and other autoimmune (collagen) diseases.

A patient is categorized as having early latent syphilis if the serologic tests of that patient are known to have been nonreactive within the previous year or if symptoms suggestive of primary or secondary syphilis were present during that time. Other patients are considered to have late latent syphilis and should be evaluated for potential asymptomatic neurosyphilis. The nontreponemal test may be nonreactive in approximately 20 percent of these cases.

## NEUROSYPHILIS

Examination of the cerobrospinal fluid (CSF) is suggested whenever the duration of syphilis is unknown or late syphilis is suspected. The diagnostic aids for defining asymptomatic neurosyphilis are (1) a reactive serum nontreponemal and/or treponemal test, (2) $\geq 5$ white cells per cubic millimeter of CSF and/or at least 45 mg/dl of total protein in the CSF, and (3) a reactive CSF VDRL test. Some patients with neurosyphilis do not have increased numbers of cells in the CSF and do not have a reactive CSF VDRL test.

## CONGENITAL SYPHILIS

Neonatal congenital syphilis is definite if *T. pallidum* is demonstrated by direct examination of nasal discharge or skin lesion material. A rising nontreponemal test titer in serial bleedings from the infant monthly over an 8-month period is also diagnostic. Conversely, the diagnosis of congenital syphilis can be ruled out if the treponemal test is nonreactive after 8 months.

## PREGNANCY

Prenatal care should begin with a serologic test for syphilis and end with a serologic test for syphilis. In high-risk populations, intermediate testing at the beginning of the third trimester (28 weeks) should be included. Irrespective of reports of false positive results in both the nontreponemal and treponemal tests,[61,62] expectant mothers should be treated if nontreponemal and treponemal tests are reactive and if a prompt and thorough evaluation of the cause of a possible false-positive result cannot be ensured. In pregnancy there is a tendency for nontreponemal titers remaining from previous treatment to increase nonspecifically, which may be confused with the diagnosis of reinfection. Patients for whom adequate treatment for syphilis in the past is documented need not be retreated unless dark field positive lesions are present or the increase in titer is greater than or equal to fourfold or a history of recent sexual exposure to a person with early syphilis exists.

## PREVIOUSLY TREATED SYPHILIS

Patients previously treated for syphilis must either test dark field positive or there must be a fourfold, two doubling dilution, increase in the quantitative nontreponemal test titers to establish a new diagnosis of syphilis.

## CONTACTS OF SYPHILIS PATIENTS

Sexual partners of patients with early syphilis should have a nontreponemal test for syphilis performed. Usually, partners with reactive nontreponemal serology and a reactive follow-up treponemal test should be treated.

## FOLLOW-UP TREATMENT

To follow the efficacy of therapy, a quantitative nontreponemal test should be performed on the patient's serum drawn at 3-month intervals for at least 1 year. With adequate treatment for primary and secondary syphilis, there should be at least a fourfold decline in titer by the third or fourth month and an eightfold decline in titer by the sixth to eighth month.[63] For most patients treated for early syphilis, the titer declines until little or no reaction is detected after the first year.[16] Patients treated in the latent or late stages may show a more gradual decline in titer,[15] and low titers may persist in approximately 50 percent of these patients after 2 years of observation.[64]

As with all serologic tests, those used to diagnose syphilis are not infallible. The sensitivity, specificity, and predictive values of the serologic tests are discussed in Chap. 76. When laboratory results contradict the physician's opinion or the patient's history, a repeat specimen should be submitted. The diagnosis of syphilis must include serologic tests as well as careful history and a thorough physical examination.

## ANTIMICROBIAL SUSCEPTIBILITY TESTING

In the past, the most commonly used methods for testing the susceptibility of *T. pallidum*, subspecies *pallidum*, to various antimicrobial agents have been either rather crude or extremely involved. The simplest methods[65] consisted of adding various doses of antibiotics to static suspensions of *T. pallidum* and then observing loss of motility or of virulence during short-term incubation. In vivo antimicrobial studies, although necessary, are usually quite involved and may result in only a qualitative answer. Recently, chamber implants in rabbits have permitted the measurement of tissue levels of various antimicrobials (Rice et al., personal communication). More recently, Norris and Edmondson[66] described the use of the tissue culture systems of Fieldsteel et al.[8] as a means to determine minimal inhibitory and bactericidal concentrations of antimicrobial agents against *T. pallidum*, subspecies *pallidum*.

## COINFECTION WITH HUMAN IMMUNODEFICIENCY VIRUS (HIV)

The effect of coinfection of syphilis and HIV at this writing is poorly understood. Several reports of individual cases have appeared[67–69] which indicate that neurologic involvement attributable to syphilis may occur during primary or secondary syphilis and perhaps even in patients treated with the recommended regimen of penicillin. Both failure of an RPR card test titer to fall after treatment and failure of antibodies to syphilis to appear with infection have been noted.[70] Thus concurrent infections with HIV and syphilis confuse the diagnosis of both diseases. Polyclonal B-cell activation is presumed to be responsible for the maintenance of titer after treatment. However, because of other alterations in the immune response of the host, the possibility exists that treponemal proliferation may be unhampered by natural cellular immunity and the current recommended therapeutic regimens may not be sufficient to eliminate this increased number or organisms.[71]

# References


1 Yobs AR et al: Fluorescent antibody technique in early syphilis. *Arch Pathol* 77:220, 1964.

2 Hunter EF et al: Immunofluorescent staining of *Treponema* in tissues fixed with formalin. *Arch Pathol Lab Med* 108:878, 1984.

3 Wassermann A et al: Eine serodiagnostische Reaktion bei Syphilis. *Dtsch Med Wochenschr* 32:745, 1906.

4 Bordet J, Gengoi O: Sur l'existence de substances sensibilisatrice dan la plupart des serums antimicrobiens. *Ann Inst Pasteur* 15:289, 1901.

5 Pangborn MC: A new serologically active phospholipid from beef heart. *Proc Soc Exp Biol Med* 48:484, 1941.

6 Schaudin F: Fur Kenntniss der Spirochaete pallida. *Dtsch Med Wochenschr* 31:1665, 1905.

7 Nelson RA Jr, Mayer NM: Immobilization of *Treponema pallidum* in vitro by antibody produced in syphilitic infection. *J Exp Med* 89: 369, 1949.

8 Fieldsteel AH et al: Cultivation of virulent *Treponema pallidum* in tissue culture. *Infect Immun* 32:908, 1981.

9 Centers for Disease Control: *Guidelines for Evaluation and Acceptance of New Syphilis Serology Tests for Routine Use, 1977.*

10 Manual of Tests for Syphilis, 1969. Public Health Service Publication no. 411, 1969.

11 Kellogg DS: The detection of *Treponema pallidum* by a rapid, direct fluorescent antibody darkfield (DFATP) procedure. *Health Lab Sci* 7:34, 1970.

11a Larsen SA et al: Syphilis, in *Sexually Transmitted Diseases,* KK Holmes et al (eds). New York, McGraw-Hill, p 875.

12 Daniels KC, Ferneyhough HS: Specific direct fluorescent antibody detection of *Treponema pallidum. Health Lab Sci* 14:164, 1977.

13 Manual for Tests for Syphilis, 1964. Public Health Service Publication no 411, 1964.

14 Schroeter AL et al: Treatment of early syphilis and reactivity of serologic tests. *JAMA* 221:471, 1972.

15 Fiumara NJ: Treatment of early latent syphilis of less than one year's duration. *Sex Transm Dis* 5:85, 1978.

16 Fiumara NJ: Treatment of primary and secondary syphilis. Serological response. *JAMA* 243:2500, 1980.

17 Matthews HM et al: Unique lipid composition of *Treponema pallidum* (Nichols virulent strain). *Infect Immun* 24:713, 1979.

18 Portnoy J et al: Rapid plasma reagin card test for syphilis and other treponematoses. *Pub Health Rep* 77:645, 1962.

19 March RW, Stiles GE: The reagin screen test: A new reagin card test for syphilis. *Sex Transm Dis* 7:66, 1980.

20 Kasatiya SS, Lambert NG: Color-coded antigen for the automated reagin test for syphilis. *Appl Microbiol* 28:317, 1974.

21 Pettit DE et al: Toluidine red unheated serum test (TRUST). A non-treponemal test for syphilis. *J Clin Microbiol* 18:1141, 1983.

22 Cohen P et al: Serologic reactivity in consecutive patients admitted to a general hospital. *Arch Intern Med* 124:364, 1969.

23 Jaffe HW et al: Hemagglutination tests for syphilis antibody. *Am J Clin Pathol* 70:230, 1978.

24 Wentworth BB et al: Comparison of a hemagglutination treponemal test for syphilis (HATTS) with other serologic methods for the diagnosis of syphilis. *Sex Transm Dis* 5:103, 1978.

25 Rein MF et al: Failure of the *Treponema pallidum* immobilization test to provide additional diagnostic information about contemporary problem sera. *Sex Transm Dis* 7:101, 1980.

26 Hunter EF et al: An improved FTA test for syphilis, the absorption procedure (FTA-ABS). *Pub Health Rep* 79:410, 1964.

27 Hunter EF et al: Double-staining procedure for the fluorescent treponemal antibody absorption (FTA-ABS) test. *Br J Vener Dis* 55:105, 1979.

28 Rathlev T: Haemagglutination tests utilizing antigens from pathogenic and apathogenic *Treponema pallidum. Br J Vener Dis* 43:181, 1967.

29 Cox PM et al: Further studies of a quantitative automated hemagglutination assay for antibodies to *Treponema pallidum. Public Health Lab* 29:43, 1971.

30 Shore RN: Haemagglutination tests and related advances in serodiagnosis of syphilis. *Arch Dermatol* 109:854, 1974.

31 Dyckman JD et al: Reactivity of microhemagglutination, fluorescent treponemal antibody absorption, and venereal disease research laboratory tests in primary syphilis. *J Clin Microbiol* 12:629, 1980.

32 Veldekamp J, Visser AM: Application of the enzyme-linked immunosorbent assay (ELISA) in the serodiagnosis of syphilis. *Br J Vener Dis* 51:227, 1975.

33 Hardy PH et al: An enzyme linked immunospecific assay for the diagnosis of syphilis. Presented in part at the American Society for Microbiology in Las Vegas, May 18, 1978.

34 Pedersen NS et al: Serodiagnosis of syphilis by an enzyme-linked immunosorbent assay for IgG antibodies against the Reiter treponema flagellum. *Scand J Immunol* 15:341, 1982.

35 Pope V et al: Evaluation of the microenzyme-linked immunosorbent assay with *Treponema pallidum* antigen. *J Clin Microbiol* 15:630, 1982.

36 Farshy CE et al: Four-step enzyme linked immunosorbent assay for detection of *Treponema pallidum* antibody. *J Clin Microbiol* 21: 387, 1985.

37 Chen J et al: Treponemal antibody-absorbent enzyme immunoassay for syphilis. *J Clin Microbiol* 23:876, 1986.

38 Smith KO, Gehle WD: Magnetic transfer devices for use in solid phase radioimmunoassays and enzyme-linked immunosorben assays. *J Infect Dis* 136:S329, 1977.

39 Stevens RW, Schmitt ME: Evaluation of an enzyme-linked immunosorben assay for treponemal antibody. *J Clin Microbiol* 21:399, 1985.

40 Moyer NP et al: Evaluation of the Bio-EnzaBead Test for syphilis. *J Clin Microbiol* 25:619, 1987.

41 Burdash NM et al: Evaluation of the syphilis Bio-EnzaBead assay for the detection of treponemal antibody. *J Clin Microbiol* 25:808, 1987.

42 Larsen SA et al: Review of the standard tests for syphilis and evaluation of a new commercial ELISA, the syphilis BioEnzaBead test. *J Clin Lab Anal* 1:300, 1987.

43 Larsen SA et al: Staining intensities in the fluorescent treponemal antibody-absorption (FTA-Abs) test: Association with the diagnosis of syphilis. *Sex Transm Dis* 13:221, 1986.

44 Dans PE et al: The FTA-Abs test: A diagnostic help or hindrance? *South Med J* 70:312, 1977.

45 Hunter EF et al: Problems affecting performance of the fluorescent treponemal antibody-absorption test for syphilis. *J Clin Microbiol* 9:163, 1979.

46 Peterson, KM et al: Isolation of a *Treponema pallidum* gene encoding immunodominant outer envelope protein P6, which reacts with sera from patients at different stages of syphilis. *J Exp Med* 164: 1160, 1986.

47 Norgard MV et al: Cloning and expression of the major 47-Kilodalton surface immunogen of *Treponema pallidum* in *Escherichia coli. Infect Immun* 54:500, 1986.

48 Stamm LV et al: Identification and preliminary characterization of *Treponema pallidum* protein antigens expressed in *Escherichia coli. Infect Immun* 41:709, 1983.

49 Moskophidis M, Muller F: Monoclonal antibodies to immunodominant surface-exposed protein antigens of *T. pallidum. Eur J Clin Microbiol* 4:473, 1985.

50 Norgard MV et al: Sensitivity and specificity of monoclonal antibodies directed against antigenic determinants of *Treponema pallidum* Nichols in the diagnosis of syphilis. *J Clin Microbiol* 20:711, 1984.

51 Duermeyer W et al: A new principle for the detection of specific IgM antibodies applied to an ELISA for hepatitis A. *J Med Virol* 4: 25, 1979.

52 Scotti AT, Logan L: S specific IgM angibody test in neonatal congenital syphilis. *J Pediatr* 73:242, 1968.

53 Kaufman RE et al: The FTA-ABS (IgM) test for neonatal congenital syphilis, a critical review. *J Am Vener Dis Assoc* 1:79, 1974.

54 Muller F: Review specific immunoglobulin M and G antibodies in the rapid diagnosis of human treponemal infections. *Diagn Immunol* 4:1, 1986.

55 Hunter EF et al: Immunoglobulin specificity for the fluorescent treponemal antibody absorption test conjugate. *J Clin Microbiol* 4:338, 1976.

56 Lee JB et al: Detection of immunoglobulin M in cerebrospinal fluid from syphilis patients by enzyme-linked immunosorbent assay. *J Clin Microbiol* 24:736, 1986.

57 Muller F et al: Demonstration of locally synthesized immunoglobulin M antibodies to *Treponema pallidum* in the central nervous system of patients with untreated neurosyphilis. *J Neuroimmunol* 7: 43, 1984.

58 Larsen SA et al: Cerebrospinal fluid serologic test for syphilis. Treponemal and nontreponemal tests, in *Advancia in Sexually Transmitted Diseases,* R Morisset, E Kurstak (eds). The Netherlands, VNW Science Press, 1986, p 157.

59 Ijsselmuiden OE et al: Enzyme-linked immunofiltration assay for rapid serodiagnosis of syphilis. *Eur J Clin Microbiol* 6:281, 1987.

60 Hensel U et al: Sodium dodecyl sulfate-polyacrylamide gel electrophoresis immunoblotting as a serological tool in the diagnosis of syphilitic infections. *J Clin Microbiol* 21:82, 1985.

61 Buchanan CS, Haserick JR: FTA-ABS test in pregnancy a probable false positive reaction. *Arch Dermatol* 102:322, 1970.

62 Thorton JG et al: False positive results of tests for syphilis and outcome of pregnancy: A retrospective case-control study. *Br Med J* 295:355, 1987.

63 Brown ST et al: Serological response to syphilis treatment: A new analysis of old data. *JAMA* 253:1296, 1985.

64 Fiumara NJ et al: Serologic responses to treatment of 128 patients with late latent syphilis. *Sex Transm Dis* 6:243, 1979.

65 Rein MF: Biopharmacology of syphilis. *Sex Transm Dis* 3:109, 1976.

66 Norris SJ, Edmondson DG: Use of an *in vitro* culture system to determine the minimal inhibitory and bactericidal concentrations of antimicrobial agents against *Treponema pallidum* subspecies pallidum (Nichols strain). *Antimicrob Agents Chemother* 32:68, 1988.

67 Johns DR et al: Alteration in the natural history of neurosyphilis by concurrent infection with the human immunodeficiency virus. *N Engl J Med* 316:1569, 1987.

68 Berry CD et al: Neurologic relapse after benzathine penicillin therapy for secondary syphilis in a patient with HIV infection. *J Engl J Med* 316:1587, 1987.

69 Zaidman GW: Neurosyphilis and retrobulbar neuritis in a patient with AIDS. *Ann Ophthalmol* 18:260, 1986.

70 Hicks et al: Seronegative secondary syphilis in a patient infected with the human immunodeficiency virus (HIV) with Kaposi sarcoma. *Ann Intern Med* 107:492, 1987.

71 Tramont EC: Syphilis in the AIDS era. *N Engl J Med* 316:1600, 1987.

Chapter 76

# Management of the reactive syphilis serology

Harold W. Jaffe
Daniel M. Musher

The use of serologic testing for the diagnosis of syphilis continues on a large scale. For example, in 1977 an estimated 43 million serologic tests for syphilis were done in the United States, of which about 1.5 million were reactive. Follow-up of 164,480 persons with reactive tests by health departments led to the reporting of 51,411 newly identified syphilis infections.[1] All health workers engaged in patient care should therefore have some familiarity with the use of these tests.

In this chapter we will review the clinical use of serologic tests for syphilis in adult patients. Readers interested either in the use of these tests for the diagnosis of congenital syphilis in children or in the details of laboratory testing procedures should consult Chaps. 67 and 75, respectively.

## SENSITIVITY, SPECIFICITY, AND PREDICTIVE VALUE

Basic to the optimal use of any diagnostic test is an understanding of the concepts of sensitivity and specificity. The *sensitivity* of a diagnostic test for a particular disease is measured by the proportion of persons with the disease who have a positive test. Conversely, *specificity* is measured by the proportion of persons without the disease who have a negative test. The relative sensitivity or specificity of one test as compared with another may vary with the proficiency of laboratory personnel. For example, the fluorescent treponemal antibody absorption (FTA-ABS) test for syphilis is intrinsically more sensitive than the Venereal Disease Research Laboratory (VDRL) slide test, but it is also more difficult to do. (Tests are described below.) In laboratories with inexperienced personnel, small errors in the performance of the FTA-ABS test may cause it to appear less sensitive than the VDRL test.

Once the sensitivity and specificity of a diagnostic test for a particular disease have been established, the test can be used to determine the probability that an individual has the disease. The *predictive value* of a test (also called posterior or posttest probability) is the probability that a person with a positive test actually has the disease.[2] Predictive value is measured by the proportion of positive results that are true positives [true positives/(true positives + false positives)] and is influenced by disease prevalence.

Predictive value is most easily understood by an example. Assume that the FTA-ABS test has a sensitivity of 100 percent and a specificity of 99 percent. If the test were used to screen 1000 persons from the general population, in which the prevalence of syphilis might be 1 percent, 10 true-positive and 10 false-positive results would be obtained. However, different results are obtained if the test is applied to a population with a high disease prevalence, such as a group already known to have reactive VDRL tests. With a population of 1000 such persons, in which the prevalence of syphilis might be 50 percent, the FTA-ABS test would give 500 true-positive and 5 false-positive results. By applying the FTA-ABS test to a high- rather than a low-prevalence population, its predictive value improves from 50 percent, no better than coin tossing, to 99 percent.

## TYPES OF TESTS

### NONTREPONEMAL TESTS

Nontreponemal tests are designed to test serum for the presence of antibody that reacts with a cardiolipin-lecithin antigen. This antigen, usually derived from beef heart, is a normal component of human tissue and comprises a small percentage of the lipid components of *Treponema pallidum*. In addition to the VDRL slide test, nontreponemal tests given standard technique status (see Chap. 75) by the Centers for Disease Control's Bureau of Laboratories include the unheated serum reagin (USR) test, and the rapid plasma reagin (RPR) (18-mm circle) card test, plus its automated version, the automated reagin test (ART).[3,4] A newer test now given provisional technique status is the reagin screen test (RST).[5] In all of these tests, antibody to cardiolipin is detected by measuring the flocculation of an antigen suspension; flocculation is seen with a microscope in the VDRL and USR tests and is macroscopic in the other tests. At present, most laboratories in the United States do either the RPR card test or the VDRL slide test.

The characteristics of all the currently used nontreponemal tests are quite similar. All are relatively inexpensive and easy to do. All have sensitivities similar to that of the VDRL test (Table 76-1). Compared with the FTA-ABS test, the nontreponemal tests are somewhat less sensitive in primary and late syphilis. Sensitivity data for all the tests in latent syphilis should be interpreted with caution, since diagnosis of these cases without the use of serologic criteria may be difficult. Nontreponemal tests can be quantified, and measuring serial titers is useful in assessing serologic response to therapy of early syphilis (see below).

All of the nontreponemal tests are occasionally reactive in sera from persons who have not had treponemal diseases. In studies in which the tests have been used to screen general populations for syphilis, the nonspecificity of these tests is usually 1 percent or less.[11–13] In some patient groups, however, the probability that these tests will be false-positive is much higher.[14–16] Nontreponemal tests may be transiently false-positive after a variety of acute febrile illnesses, after immunizations, and during pregnancy. Chronic false-positive tests, usually defined as persisting

**Table 76-1. Percent Sensitivity of Serologic Tests in Untreated Syphilis**

| | Stage of disease | | | |
|---|---|---|---|---|
| | Primary | Secondary | Latent | Late |
| VDRL slide test | 59–87 | 100 | 73–91 | 37–94 |
| FTA-ABS test | 86–100 | 99–100 | 96–99 | 96–100 |
| MHA-TP | 64–87 | 96–100 | 96–100 | 94–100* |

*Includes some patients whose treatment status is unknown.

SOURCES: References 6 to 10 and Bureau of Laboratories, Centers for Disease Control, Atlanta, GA, unpublished data.

for at least 6 months, occur most often in chronic infections (such as lepromatous leprosy), in autoimmune diseases (such as lupus erythematosus and Hashimoto's thyroiditis), and in narcotic addiction. When false-positive tests occur, their titer is usually low, e.g., a VDRL titer of no more than 1:8.[15]

## TREPONEMAL TESTS

Treponemal tests detect an antibody that reacts with antigenic component of pathogenic members of the genus *Treponema*. The *Treponema pallidum* immobilization (TPI) test, at one time the standard treponemal test in the United States, is now done in only a few research laboratories. For many years the FTA-ABS test[3] was the treponemal antibody test in use in the United States. In this test, a serum sample, previously diluted in a "sorbent" made from the nonpathogenic Reiter treponeme, is layered on a slide to which *T. pallidum* has been fixed. Fluorescein-labeled antibody to human gamma globulin is added, and fluorescence of the treponemes indicates the presence of antitreponemal antibodies to the serum. Since the FTA-ABS test requires fluorescence microscopy, it is relatively difficult and expensive to do.

Two newer treponemal tests have been given technique status: the microhemagglutination assay for *T. pallidum* (MHA-TP)[12] and the hemagglutination treponemal test for syphilis (HATTS).[13] The MHA-TP test has recently been given technique status (Chap. 75). Using these methods, serum is tested for antibodies which agglutinate erythrocytes that have been coated with *T. pallidum* antigen. Sheep erythrocytes are used in the MHA-TP test; turkey erythrocytes are used in the HATTS test. Both tests are easier and less expensive to do than the FTA-ABS test (see Chap. 75).

In general, treponemal tests are more sensitive than the nontreponemal tests. The FTA-ABS test is highly sensitive in all stages of syphilis (Table 76-1). The hemagglutination tests, as illustrated with the MHA-TP test, are somewhat less sensitive in primary disease. Since all of the treponemal tests tend to remain reactive despite syphilis therapy, they should not be used in assessing serologic response to treatment.

By virtue of their names, one expects that treponemal tests are more specific for syphilis than the nontreponemal tests. This, however, is not always so. Like the nontreponemal tests, treponemal tests are reactive in approximately 1 percent of healthy persons with no history or findings of syphilis.[12,13,17] These apparently false-positive results are often transient; their cause is unknown. All serologic tests for venereal syphilis, both treponemal and nontreponemal, are also reactive in persons with nonvenereal treponematoses. The major problem with specificity is that, once positive, treponemal tests remain so for life. Thus a single positive test accurately reflects prior exposure to *T. pallidum* but does not indicate that an infection is currently present. In this sense, a positive VDRL reaction is more specific for diagnosing an active case of syphilis.

False-positive treponemal tests rarely occur in association with other underlying illnesses. Lupus erythematosus, of both systemic and discoid varieties, has definitely been associated with false-positive MHA-TP tests.[18,19] For the FTA-ABS test, the false-positive fluorescence pattern may be either homogeneous or "beaded," a pattern in which fluorescence is limited to a few portions of the fixed treponeme.[18] Beaded FTA fluorescence produced with sera from lupus patients is apparently caused by the binding of antinuclear antibodies in the test serum to treponemal DNA, which has extruded through the wall of the treponeme.[20] False-positive MHA-TP tests occur in drug-induced lupus.[21,22] False-positive MHA-TP tests occur in infectious mononucleosis, due to the presence of heterophile antibody, and have also been reported for patients with lepromatous leprosy.[23]

## USE OF SEROLOGIC TESTS FOR SYPHILIS

### SCREENING FOR SYPHILIS

Much of the use of serologic tests for syphilis is in the screening of people who have no history or findings of syphilis. Such testing is appropriate for persons who are likely to have had multiple sex partners for short periods of time and patients seen for sexually transmited diseases other than syphilis. Routine serologic screening should also be used for pregnant women as a means of preventing congenital syphilis. Since the fetus may be infected as early as the ninth week of gestation, such testing should be done during the first trimester.[24] Women thought to be at high risk for syphilis should be rescreened during the third trimester.[25]

The use of serologic tests to do widespread screening for syphilis is somewhat controversial. Although most states mandate premarital serologic testing, such testing is expensive and only rarely identifies persons with infectious syphilis.[26] However, premarital testing may have other benefits, such as the detection of latent disease and the prevention of late complications.[27] The benefits of routine serologic testing of hospital inpatients are also controversial.[28] The entire problem of serologic tests for syphilis in asymptomatic patients has recently been reviewed.[29,30]

By virtue of their low cost and simplicity, nontreponemal tests are the most appropriate screening tests for syphilis. However, as previously discussed, a reactive test result in a low-prevalence population will have a low predictive value; many of the positive results will be false-positive. To decrease the chance of misdiagnosing syphilis, a second serum sample should be obtained from a patient with an unexpectedly reactive nontreponemal test. This serum should be tested again with a nontreponemal test, and, if reactive, it should then be tested with a treponemal test. Using the treponemal tests in this way gives them a high predictive value; almost all positive results will be true positives. For pregnant patients, any additional serologic testing should be done as quickly as possible so that a therapeutic decision can be made without delay.

### PATIENTS WITH LESIONS

For patients with moist lesions of primary and secondary syphilis, dark field microscopy is the diagnostic method of choice. When dark field examination is either not available or a negative result has been obtained in a lesion that might be syphilitic, serologic tests are useful in the evaluation of such patients.

The findings of a clinically suspicious lesion and a reactive nontreponemal test have a high predictive value in primary and secondary syphilis; routine confirmation with a treponemal test is usually not necessary. In primary syphilis, nontreponemal tests may be nonreactive in approximately one-fourth of the cases. Since the sensitivity of these tests increases with the duration of untreated disease, a second serum sample should be obtained 1 to 2 weeks after an initially nonreactive result. Although the FTA-ABS test is more sensitive than the nontreponemal tests in primary syphilis, delays inherent in obtaining an FTA-ABS test result usually negate the advantage of higher test sensitivity. Nontreponemal tests are virtually 100 percent sensitive in secondary syphilis. If the possibility of a prozone phenomenon can be excluded, a nonreactive result in any of the nontreponemal tests essentially excludes the diagnosis of secondary syphilis.

## PATIENTS WITH SYMPTOMATIC LATE SYPHILIS

Any patient having signs or symptoms suggesting late syphilis should have a serum test for syphilis. Since the nontreponemal tests are relatively insensitive in this stage of disease, either an FTA-ABS test or a hemagglutination test should be done. Those patients suspected of having symptomatic neurosyphilis must also have a cerebrospinal fluid (CSF) examination done as part of their diagnostic evaluation (see below).

## SEROLOGIC RESPONSE TO THERAPY

In accord with CDC recommendations, all patients treated for syphilis should have quantitative nontreponemal tests done 3, 6, and 12 months after treatment. An additional test at 24 months is recommended for patients treated for syphilis of more than 1 year's duration.

Patients treated for early syphilis (primary, secondary, and latent syphilis of less than 1 year's duration) should show a serologic response to therapy.[31,32] The titer of the tests should decrease, and in most cases the tests will become negative. In one study of the recommended treatment schedules, 97 percent of patients with seropositive primary syphilis and 76 percent of those with secondary syphilis had nonreactive VDRL tests 2 or more years after treatment.[31] The time needed to attain seronegativity is generally proportional to the duration of untreated disease (see Chap. 20).

Failure to observe a serologic response after therapy of early syphilis or the occurrence of a fourfold (i.e., two-tube) or greater titer rise in any treated syphilis patient may be due to one of several causes. The most likely cause is reinfection. All patients who have not had the anticipated serologic response to therapy should be examined for signs of early syphilis and should be interviewed to elicit the names of sexual contacts. If either clinical evidence of reinfection or infected contacts are found, the patient should be re-treated for early syphilis. Another possible cause would be the occurrence of an event associated with false-positive nontreponemal tests. For example, if a patient treated for syphilis receives an immunization or has a febrile illness, his or her test titer may transiently increase. A final possible cause would be the occurrence of a true treatment failure. Although currently recommended treatment schedules for early syphilis appear to be highly effective,[33,34] optimal schedules for syphilis of more than 1 year's duration are less well established. Patients who appear to be true treatment failures should have a CSF examination done to exclude asymptomatic neurosyphilis and then should be retreated with schedules recommended for syphilis of more than 1 year's duration.

Because each of the nontreponemal tests may show a slightly different titer of reactivity on the same serum sample, the tests should not be used interchangeably in following serologic response to therapy. For example, the titer of the RPR test tends to be higher than that of the VDRL test.[35] Switching from the VDRL test to the RPR test during posttreatment serologic evaluation may produce an apparent titer rise and thus may cause unnecessary concern about reinfection or treatment failure.

## CEREBROSPINAL FLUID EXAMINATION

CSF examination is an essential part of the diagnostic evaluation of all syphilis patients with unexplained neurologic abnormalities. Such abnormalities are rare in primary and secondary syphilis, although the prevalence of syphilitic infection in AIDS has greatly complicated the interpretation of such symptoms. CSF examination is needed only for those unusual patients in whom syphilis must be distinguished from other causes of meningitis or papillitis.[36] In syphilis of longer duration, CSF examination is mandatory to distinguish late symptomatic neurosyphilis from the many other diseases with similar clinical presentations.

For syphilis patients without neurologic abnormalities, CSF examination is needed only if the results of the examination might affect therapy. Such examination is unnecessary in early syphilis, because treatment results are good despite the high frequency of CSF "abnormalities" (elevated cell count or protein concentration, reactive serologic test for syphilis) during this stage of the disease.[33,34,37] For patients with syphilis of more than 1 year's duration, the need for CSF examination is an unsettled issue. The central question is whether the treatment schedules recommended for all such patients are adequate for those with asymptomatic neurosyphilis. Because the efficacies of these treatment schedules are not clearly established,[38,39] CSF examination is desirable in all patients with syphilis of more than 1 year's duration, particularly those who are allergic to penicillin.

All patients treated for neurosyphilis, either symptomatic or asymptomatic, should have posttreatment CSF examinations done to assess response to therapy. Six months after adequate therapy, patients should have a normal CSF cell count and, if initially elevated, a decreased CSF protein concentration.[40] CSF nontreponemal serologic tests may or may not return to nonreactivity. Repeat examinations should be done at 6-month intervals until findings have stabilized.

At present, the standard CSF serologic test for syphilis is the VDRL slide test. With very rare exceptions, this test is specific for neurosyphilis.[41] However, a negative result does not exclude the diagnosis of central nervous system syphilis. The low sensitivity of these tests has been most clearly shown in patients with tabes dorsalis.[42]

To increase the sensitivity of the CSF examination for syphilis, some authors have recommended using the FTA test, with or without absorption;[43,44] however, the meaning of a reactive CSF-FTA test remains unclear. In one study, 5 of 15 syphilitic patients with no other evidence of neurosyphilis had reactive CSF-FTA tests.[45] The CSF reactivity in these cases may have been due to the diffusion of immunoglobulins from serum into CSF. Contamination of CSF with minute amounts of FTA-ABS–reactive blood has also been reported to cause false-positive CSF-FTA tests.[46] At present, syphilitic patients with unexplained neurologic abnormalities should not be assumed to have neurosyphilis solely on the basis of a reactive CSF-FTA test. Detecting IgM that reacts in a treponemal test such as FTA-ABS or MHA-TP may be diagnostic of neurosyphilis;[47] this technique is still regarded as experimental. The management of neurosyphilis is discussed in more detail in Chap. 21.

## MANAGEMENT OF PATIENTS WITH UNEXPECTEDLY REACTIVE TESTS

A common problem in clinical practice is the management of patients with unexpectedly reactive serologic tests for syphilis.

This situation, which excludes those patients with signs of early syphilis or a well-documented history of past treponemal infection, occurs most often with elderly patients who may have a reactive nontreponemal test in the course of care for other medical problems.

The first step in the diagnostic evaluation of such patients is the exclusion of a false-positive test result. As previously outlined, the nontreponemal test should be repeated on a second serum sample, and, if the nontreponemal test is reactive, the serum should be subjected to a treponemal test. The findings of reactive nontreponemal and treponemal tests should be considered presumptive evidence of treponemal infection. In rare cases, such as in patients with lupus erythematosus, both types of tests may be falsely positive. However, all such patients should be carefully evaluated for treponemal disease before a diagnosis of false-positive serology is made.

In taking a history for treponemal disease, the clinician should consider the possibilities both of syphilis, either congenital or acquired, and of nonvenereal treponematosis. Unfortunately, such a history is often unreliable. Patients, particularly elderly patients, may be reluctant to discuss a previous syphilis infection. In these cases, a request to a local or state health department for a search of syphilis treatment records may be useful. Nonvenereal treponematoses do not confer complete immunity to syphilis. Therefore, a history of nonvenereal treponemal infection does not exclude the possibility of syphilis.[48]

Examination of patients with unexpectedly reactive tests should focus on late signs of congenital or acquired syphilis. Signs of congenital syphilis, such as interstitial keratitis or tooth deformities, may be subtle and require referral to an appropriate subspecialist for complete evaluation.[49,50] Chest x-ray and CSF examination may be needed for the evaluation of possible cardiovascular syphilis or neurosyphilis.

Even after taking a careful history and doing a physical examination, the clinician may still not be sure if an individual patient has syphilis. Whether to treat such patients is a difficult decision. However, with the exception of very elderly patients or patients with underlying fatal illnesses, these patients should probably be treated for syphilis, using schedules recommended for syphilis of more than 1 year's duration. The advantage of decreasing the possibility of disease progression appears to outweigh the risk of an adverse reaction to treatment. Any treatment should be carefully documented so that the same questions do not arise the next time the patient is found to have a reactive serologic test for syphilis.

## SYPHILIS SEROLOGY AND AIDS

Preliminary data from our laboratory (R. Baughn, unpublished observations) suggest that serologic tests for syphilis may give results that are difficult to interpret in patients with AIDS. This problem is unresolved at the time this chapter is completed (September, 1988).

# References


1 Centers for Disease Control: *STD Fact Sheet*, 34th ed, US Department of Health, Education, and Welfare Publication (CDC) 79-8195, p 10.

2 McNeil BJ et al: Primer on certain elements of medical decision making. *N Engl J Med* 293:211, 1975.

3 Centers for Disease Control: *Manual of Tests for Syphilis*, US Department of Health, Education, and Welfare Publication (CDC) 78-8347, 1969.

4 McGrew BE et al: Automation of a flocculation test for syphilis. *Am J Clin Pathol* 50:52, 1968.

5 March RW, Stiles GE: The reagin screen test: A new reagin card test for syphilis. *Sex Transm Dis* 7:66, 1980.

6 Communicable Disease Center: *Serology Evaluation and Research Assembly, 1956–1957*, US Department of Health, Education, and Welfare Publication 650.

7 Deacon WE et al: Fluorescent treponemal antibody-absorption (FTA-ABS) test for syphilis. *JAMA* 198:156, 1966.

8 Aho K et al: Late complications of syphilis: A comparative epidemiological and serological study of cardiovascular syphilis and various forms of neurosyphilis. *Acta Derm Venereol* (Stockh) 49:336, 1969.

9 Coffey EM et al: Evaluation of the qualitative and automated quantitative microhemagglutination assay for antibodies to *Treponema pallidum*. *Appl Microbiol* 24:26, 1972.

10 Lesinski J et al: Specificity, sensitivity, and diagnostic value of the TPHA test. *Br J Vener Dis* 50:334, 1974.

11 Cohen P et al: Serologic reactivity in consecutive patients admitted to a general hospital. *Arch Intern Med* 124:364, 1969.

12 Jaffe HW et al: Hemagglutination tests for syphilis antibody. *Am J Clin Pathol* 70:230, 1978.

13 Wentworth BB et al: Comparison of a hemagglutination treponemal test for syphilis (HATTS) with other serologic methods for the diagnosis of syphilis. *Sex Transm Dis* 5:103, 1978.

14 Moore JE, Mohr CF: Biologically false positive serologic tests for syphilis: Type, incidence, and cause. *JAMA* 150:467, 1952.

15 Tuffanelli DL et al: Fluorescent treponemal-antibody absorption tests: Studies of false-positive reactions to tests for syphilis. *N Engl J Med* 276:258, 1967.

16 Catterall RD: Presidential address to the MSSVD: Systemic disease and the biologic false positive reaction. *Br J Vener Dis* 48:1, 1972.

17 Goldman JN, Lantz MA: FTA-ABS and VDRL slide test reactivity in a population of nuns. *JAMA* 217:53, 1971.

18 Kraus SJ et al: Fluorescent treponemal antibody-absorption test reactions in lupus erythematosus. *N Engl J Med* 282:1287, 1970.

19 Shore RN, Faricelli JA: Borderline and reactive FTA-ABS results in lupus erythematosus. *Arch Dermatol* 113:37, 1977.

20 Strobel PL, Kraus SJ: An electron microscopic study of the FTA-ABS "beading" phenomenon with lupus erythematosus sera, using ferritin-conjugated antihuman IgG. *J Immunol* 108:1152, 1972.

21 Monson RAM: Biologic false-positive FTA-ABS test in drug-induced lupus erythematosus. *JAMA* 224:1028, 1973.

22 Anderson B, Stillman MT: False-positive FTA-ABS in hydralazine-induced lupus. *JAMA* 239:1392, 1978.

23 Garner MF et al: The *Treponema pallidum* haemagglutination (TPHA) test in biological false positive and leprosy sera. *J Clin Pathol* 26:258, 1973.

24 Harter CA, Benirschke K: Fetal syphilis in the first trimester. *Am J Obstet Gynecol* 124:705, 1976.

25 Ingall D et al: Syphilis, in *Infectious Diseases of the Fetus and Newborn Infant*, JS Remington, JO Klein (eds). Philadelphia, Saunders, 1988.

26 Felman YM: Repeal of mandated premarital tests for syphilis: A survey of state health officers. *Am J Public Health* 71:155, 1981.

27 Kingon RJ, Wiesner PJ: Premarital syphilis screening: Weighing the benefits. *Am J Public Health* 71:160, 1981.

28 Henderson RH: Routine serological testing for syphilis recommended for all hospital inpatients. *JAMA* 226:212, 1973.

29 Musher DM: Evaluation and management of an asymptomatic patient with a positive VDRL reaction, in *Current Clinical Topics in Infectious Diseases*, JS Remington, MN Swartz (eds). New York, McGraw-Hill, 1987, p 147.

30 Hart E: Syphilis tests in diagnostic and therapeutic decision making. *Ann Intern Med* 104:368, 1986.

31 Schroeter AL et al: Treatment of early syphilis and reactivity of serologic tests. *JAMA* 221:471, 1972.

32 Fiumara NJ: Treatment of early latent syphilis of less than one year's duration. *Sex Transm Dis* 5:85, 1978.
32 Fiumara NJ: Treatment of primary and secondary syphilis: Serological response. *JAMA* 243:2500, 1980.
33 Elliott WC: Treatment of primary syphilis. *J Am Vener Dis Assoc* 3:128, 1976.
34 Brown ST: Treatment of secondary syphilis. *J Am Vener Dis Assoc* 3:136, 1976.
35 Falcone VH et al: Evaluation of rapid plasma reagin (circle) card test. *Public Health Rep* 79:491, 1964.
36 Stokes JH et al: *Modern Clinical Syphilology*, 3d ed. Philadelphia, Saunders, 1944, p 609.
37 Hahn RD, Clark EG: Asymptomatic neurosyphilis: A review of the literature. *Am J Syph Gonor Vener Dis* 30:305, 1946.
38 Rothenberg R: Treatment of neurosyphilis. *J Am Vener Dis Assoc* 3:153, 1976.
39 Greene BM et al: Failure of penicillin G benzathine in the treatment of neurosyphilis. *Arch Intern Med* 140:1117, 1980.
40 Dattner B et al: Criteria for the management of neurosyphilis. *Am J Med* 10:463, 1951.
41 Madiedo G et al: False-positive VDRL and FTA in cerebrospinal fluid. *JAMA* 244:688, 1980.
42 O'Leary PA et al: Cooperative clinical studies in the treatment of syphilis: Tabes dorsalis. *Vener Dis Inform* 19:367, 1938.
43 Escobar MR et al: Fluorescent antibody tests for syphilis using cerebrospinal fluid: Clinical correlation in 150 cases. *Am J Clin Pathol* 53:886, 1970.
44 McGeeney T et al: Utility of the FTA-ABS test of cerebrospinal fluid in the diagnosis of neurosyphilis. *Sex Transm Dis* 6:195, 1979.
45 Jaffe HW et al: Tests for treponemal antibody in CSF. *Arch Intern Med* 138:252, 1978.
46 Davis LE, Sperry S: The CSF-FTA test and the significance of blood contamination. *Arch Neurol* 6:68, 1979.
47 Muller F: Specific immunoglobulin M and G antibodies in the rapid diagnosis of human treponemal infections. *Diagn Immunol* 4:1, 1986.
48 Yaws or syphilis, editorial. *Br Med J* 1:912, 1979.
49 Robinson RCV: Congenital syphilis. *Arch Dermatol* 99:599, 1969.
50 Fiumara NJ, Lessell S: Manifestations of late congenital syphilis. *Arch Dermatol* 102:78, 1970.

# Chapter 77
# Herpes simplex virus

Kenneth H. Fife
Lawrence Corey

A basic principle of medicine is the need to establish a specific etiologic diagnosis. This is critical because of the importance of understanding the natural history and spectrum of the disease and, in the case of infectious diseases, of isolating and identifying the causative agent. Knowledge of the etiology provides the physician and patient with information about the prognosis of the disease, and helps guide the selection of therapies that may alter the course of the disease. In sexually transmitted disease (STD), mixed infections are common and the identification of all agents involved is essential.

In the past, the laboratory diagnosis of viral diseases has received little attention because of the scarcity of diagnostic virology laboratories, the relative difficulty of identifying viral agents, the time required for viral culture and serology, and the relative lack of specific treatments. Over the last few years, this situation has changed. Currently, diagnostic virology laboratories have been established in many areas and are providing an increasing number of clinicians with access to viral cultures. In addition, newer diagnostic methods, many of which can be conducted in less sophisticated laboratories, are also widely available and make rapid diagnosis of many viral diseases possible. We have now entered the era of effective antiviral chemotherapy and it is almost certain that our therapeutic options will continue to increase in the future. Viral STDs are major targets of efforts to develop effective antiviral therapies; thus, accurate diagnosis of these conditions will continue to be important. This chapter discusses the laboratory methods used in the diagnosis of herpes simplex virus infections.

## THE AGENT

Genital herpes simplex virus (HSV) infection accounts for approximately 5 percent of all visits to STD clinics in the United States. In western industrialized nations, HSV is the most common etiologic agent in genital ulcerations.[1–3] It is also the most frequent agent isolated from homosexual men who present with nongonococcal proctitis.[4,5] In most studies, HSV has been isolated from the urethra from approximately 2 percent of men with nongonococcal urethritis. In studies in which HSV isolations are routinely performed in patients attending STD clinics, this virus has been isolated from the cervix in 3 to 8 percent of women and from the urethra of 1.5 to 5 percent of men. Many patients from whom HSV is isolated are asymptomatic (see Chap. 35).

HSV is a member of the herpes group of viruses, agents characterized by their ability to become latent as well as demonstrate persistent infection. For a more complete discussion of the biology and pathogenesis of this organism, the reader should consult Chap. 34.

HSV is intermittently excreted from the genital tract, usually (but not always) in association with cutaneous or mucosal lesions. HSV has not been demonstrated to be latent in the epithelium of the genital tract but is latent in the sacral nerve root ganglia which innervate the genital region.[6,7] When latent in sacral ganglionic tissue, specialized techniques such as cocultivation or in situ hybridization must be utilized in order to demonstrate latent virus. The ability to isolate virus from infected cells in the genital tract is indicative of the infectious or lytic cycle of this agent. In many patients, HSV can be isolated from the genital tract in the absence of overt signs or symptoms of disease. While asymptomatic HSV infection can result in transmission of the infection to sexual partners or newborn infants, detailed studies of the infectivity of HSV during symptomatic or asymptomatic periods of infection are not available. Only about 50 percent of source contacts of patients who present with primary genital herpes report the presence of lesions at the time of sexual contact.[8,9]

Although antigenic differences among HSV isolates had been suspected for some time, it was not until 1967[10,11] that the two distinct types of HSV, viz., HSV-1 and HSV-2, were convincingly demonstrated by kinetic neutralization tests using antibodies prepared in rabbits against standard laboratory strains of HSV. Antisera against the homologous viral type more rapidly neutralized that virus than antibody raised against the heterologous virus.

## ANATOMIC SITES OF INFECTION

HSV can be isolated from many anatomic sites; the site of infection depends upon the source of inoculation, age of the patient, and immune status of the host. Table 77-1 illustrates common and uncommon sites of infection with HSV. HSV-1 tends to cause oropharyngeal disease, and HSV-2 tends to cause genital disease; however, each virus is capable of causing disease in both locations and produces clinically indistinguishable manifestations.

Primary genital infection with HSV is often associated with multiple sites of infection, for example, the external genitalia, cervix, urinary tract, pharynx, conjunctiva, and occasionally the central nervous system. In contrast, recurrent genital herpes is usually localized to the genital area.[12] Occasionally, HSV has been isolated from seminal and prostatic fluids and from the endometrium and fallopian tubes. In immunosuppressed patients, reactivation of genital herpes and dissemination of disease to distant cutaneous sites or visceral organs, such as liver, lung, and brain, may occasionally occur. In neonates, virus may be localized to the skin and conjunctiva, may spread through peripheral nerves into the central nervous system, or may disseminate through the bloodstream to visceral organs such as liver, adrenal glands, and lung.

## RELATIONSHIP BETWEEN STAGE OF LESION AND ABILITY TO ISOLATE THE VIRUS

The ability to demonstrate virus or viral antigen varies over the course of the disease.[13] Characteristically, lesions progress from the maculopapular stage to vesicles, pustules, then ulcerate, and finally crust. Eventually, most lesions will heal and completely reepithelialize without scarring. Studies of oral-labial as well as genital HSV disease indicate that the titer of virus in lesions will vary over the course of infection. Viral titers are highest in the vesicular and pustular stages of the disease and decrease over the course of the infection.[13,14] Primary genital herpes is typically associated with higher viral titers and longer duration of viral shedding than nonprimary first episodes of genital infection. The

**Table 77-1. Tissues and Secretions Infected by Herpes Simplex Virus Types 1 and 2**

| | HSV-1 | HSV-2 |
|---|---|---|
| *Skin*: | | |
| Face | + + + + | + |
| Trunk | + + + | + + |
| Extremities | + + + | + + |
| External genitalia | + + | + + + + |
| Oral cavity | + + + + | + + |
| Lips | + + + + | + |
| *Eye*: | | |
| Conjunctiva/cornea | + + + + | + |
| Lens, choroid, retina* | + + | + + |
| *Viscera*: | | |
| Larynx, trachea* | + | ? + |
| Lung parenchyma* | + | + |
| Esophagus* | + + | * |
| Pancreas,* liver/spleen,* heart,* kidney/adrenals* | + | + |
| *Urogenital*: | | |
| Bladder | + | + + |
| Urethra | + | + + + |
| Anal canal | + | + + + |
| Seminal vesicles/prostate | ? | + |
| Cervix | + + | + + + + |
| Vaginal mucosa | + | + + |
| Endometrium | + | + |
| Fallopian tubes | + | + + |
| *Central nervous system*: | | |
| Brain | + + | + * |
| Meninges, cerebrospinal fluid | + | + + |
| *Ganglia*: | | |
| Trigeminal | + + + + | + ? |
| Sacral | + | + + + + |
| Sympathetic or parasympathetic | + + | + + |
| *Others*: | | |
| Lymph nodes, placenta, bone marrow, leukocytes | + | + |

*Seen most frequently in immunocompromised or neonatal patients.

nonprimary first episode of genital infection is the first episode of HSV-2 in a person having had prior HSV-1 infection. In addition, first episodes of genital herpes (either primary or nonprimary) tend to have a more prolonged pattern of viral shedding than recurrent genital disease.[15] It should be remembered, however, that the duration and severity of genital herpes episodes vary widely among individuals and even within a single individual over time.[12]

Table 77-2 illustrates the results of viral isolation procedures according to stage of lesion in patients with initial and recurrent infection. While HSV can be isolated from over 90 percent of vesicular or pustular lesions, the isolation of virus is markedly reduced in the ulcerative and crust stages of disease. In addition, the duration of viral excretion from ulcerative lesions is longer in patients with initial as compared with patients with recurrent disease.[12] HSV can be isolated from ulcerative lesions in 82 percent of initial disease patients compared with 42 percent in recurrent disease patients.[13,15] These data are important in interpreting the results of all isolation and antigen detection techniques used in the laboratory for the diagnosis of herpes. Thus, for example, in a patient with a history compatible with past genital HSV infection who presents with an ulcer of 4 days' duration, the lack of isolation of HSV from the lesion does not rule out HSV as the initiating cause. In a recent study of 103 patients with suspected genital HSV, virus was isolated in only 56 percent. Follow-up of the originally culture-negative patients revealed subsequent episodes of genital lesions from which HSV was isolated in over 80 percent.[15] Thus, in some cases, multiple specimens must be submitted to confirm the diagnosis of genital herpes.

**Table 77-2. Viral Isolation and Stage of Disease in Genital HSV Infection (Percent HSV Culture-Positive Lesions)**

| Maculopapular (*N*=9) | Vesicle (*N*=136) | Pustule (*N*=68) | Ulcer (*N*=132) | Crust (*N*=93) |
|---|---|---|---|---|
| 25 | 94 | 87 | 70 | 27 |

## LABORATORY DIAGNOSIS

The laboratory diagnosis of HSV infection relies on the cultivation of virus from infected secretions or tissues or the demonstration of compatible viral cytopathology, viral antigen, viral particles, or viral nucleic acid sequences in infected areas. Commonly used techniques include (1) isolation of the virus in tissue culture; (2) demonstration of characteristic pathological alterations, such as giant cells or cells with intranuclear inclusions in biopsies or lesion smears; (3) demonstration of viral antigen by immunologic methods, such as immunofluorescence (IF) or immunoperoxidase (IP); (4) demonstration of viral particles in infected secretions, for example, by electron microscopy; or (5) demonstration of viral DNA in clinical specimens. Although the serological response to HSV infection can be useful in some clinical situations (e.g., primary infection), serology is generally less informative in the acute setting and is discussed separately.

### Acquisition and transport of samples for isolation studies

HSV is an obligate intracellular parasite, and although some extracellular virus will be present in lesions, the most predictable way to obtain intact virus is to collect infected cells. This can be done by vigorously rubbing lesions with a cotton- or Dacron-tipped swab. Vesicular fluid contains as many as $10^9$ HSV particles per milliliter[14,16] (usually $10^6$ to $10^7$ plaque-forming units per milliliter) and should be collected whenever possible. Vesicles can be opened with a small-gauge needle or a cotton-tipped swab. When the lesions are large enough, the vesicular fluid should be aspirated. Many STD clinics use calcium alginate swabs for obtaining urethral and cervical samples; however, it has been shown that HSV is inactivated upon storage in the presence of calcium alginate swabs.[17] Cotton or Dacron swabs should be employed. A small Dacron-tipped swab on a wire or plastic shaft (Dacroswab, Inolex Co.) has in our experience been especially useful in patients with single or multiple small lesions. Commercially available swab/transport sets can be used but some contain large swabs which may make sampling of small lesions difficult. HSV infection of the cervix usually involves squamous rather than columnar epithelium. Thus, when obtaining specimens from the cervix, one should also swab the exocervix as well as the endocervical canal.

After the sample has been obtained, the swab should be immediately placed in an appropriate transport medium for storage until the culture is set up (see Appendix). The swab should not be allowed to dry. The transport medium should be a nutrient solution containing antibiotics to inhibit bacterial growth and buffers to maintain a neutral pH. Examples of such media include Hank's balanced salt solution, nutrient broth,[18] and sucrose phosphate gelatin broth used for the transport of samples to be cultured for *Chlamydia trachomatis*.[19] If an appropriate transport medium is not available, sterile distilled water can be substituted with only small losses of yield. HSV will remain viable in an appropriate transport medium for 48 to 96 h at 4°C although there is a slight ongoing loss of titer with time.[20] One commercially available Chlamydia transport medium (Chlamydiaport, Scott Laboratories) has been reported to maintain HSV with minimal loss of titer for several days at room temperature (22°C).[21] The virus will be viable for years upon storage at −70°C. Herpes group viruses (and many other viruses) are rapidly inactivated at −20°C.[22,23] Thus, a specimen should never be frozen in an ordinary freezer. Specimens for viral isolation should be held at 4°C until they can be inoculated onto tissue culture. If a delay of more than 48 h is anticipated between the time the specimen is obtained and the time it arrives in the laboratory, the specimen should be frozen on dry ice (−70°C), if possible.

## Isolation

The ability to identify HSV by growth in cultured cells has been considered the "gold standard" by which other tests are measured. These methods are still considered the most reliable and several modifications of the basic method have been introduced which may improve the speed of isolation.

**Standard Viral Cultures.** HSV will grow in a variety of tissue culture cells of both human and animal origin.[24] Human diploid fibroblast cell lines such as human embryonic tonsil (HET), embryonic lung (HEL), embryonic kidney (HEK), and amnion cells are often used. Commonly used animal cells include rabbit kidney, guinea pig embryo, continuous African green monkey kidney (Vero) cells, and baby hamster kidney (BHK) cells. All these cell lines are used because of their ease of handling, their ability to maintain viability for relatively long periods of time, and their easily recognized cytopathic changes seen after HSV infection. These characteristics plus local availability are probably the most important determinants in choosing a cell culture system for the isolation of HSV. Each of the cell lines mentioned has its advocates and all have sufficient sensitivity for the isolation of HSV.[25] There is some evidence to suggest that rabbit kidney and guinea pig embryo cells are more sensitive than standard fibroblast cell lines such as MRC-5 or WI-38.[26]

The typical cytopathic effect (CPE) seen after HSV infection of Vero cells is shown in Fig. 77-1. The earliest change seen is some rounding of the cells, and this change usually occurs in several areas of the cell monolayer. The cells will later become swollen and refractile and will eventually die and become detached from the surface of the culture vessel. The average replication time of HSV is 12 to 18 h.[27] With a large inoculum, a CPE can be seen as early as 18 to 24 h after infection. In a laboratory in which cultures are routinely examined for CPE daily, the median time from inoculation of HSV to development of a CPE is 2 to 3 days. In many studies, 80 percent of positive specimens are identified by 4 days and 95 percent within 7 days. Low-titer specimens or specimens from episodes of asymptomatic shedding may take longer to show a CPE, so cultures for HSV should be observed for 10 to 14 days for maximum sensitivity.

Isolates can be confirmed as HSV by neutralization using type-specific antisera, by immunologic methods such as immunofluorescence (IF), or by nucleic acid hybridization. In general, all specimens exhibiting a suspected CPE should be confirmed by one of these tests. For the IF method, cells from cultures exhibiting a CPE are scraped off the glass. The cells are spotted onto glass well slides and fixed in acetone. Fluorescein-conjugated anti-HSV antiserum is added. The slides are washed and examined for specific IF. If human diploid fibroblasts, such as WI-38, are used, a fast-growing cytomegalovirus (CMV) may exhibit CPE similar to HSV. Measurement of growth in differential cell lines may help differentiate HSV from CMV (e.g., HSV will grow in Vero, HeLa, rabbit kidney, and BHK cells, but CMV will not). Similarly, in some cell lines adenovirus will occasionally produce a cytopathic effect that may be similar to HSV. Adenoviruses may be differentiated from HSV by neutralization, by specific IF tests, or by agglutination of erythrocytes.

**Modifications of the Standard Culture Technique.** Although HSV exhibits typical CPE much more rapidly than many other viruses, especially CMV, several approaches have been used

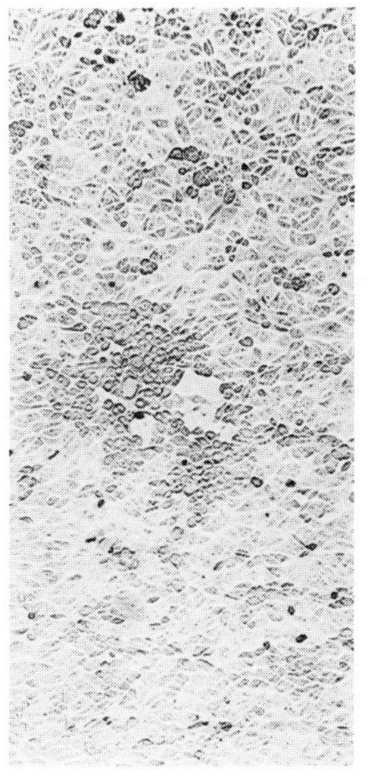

A

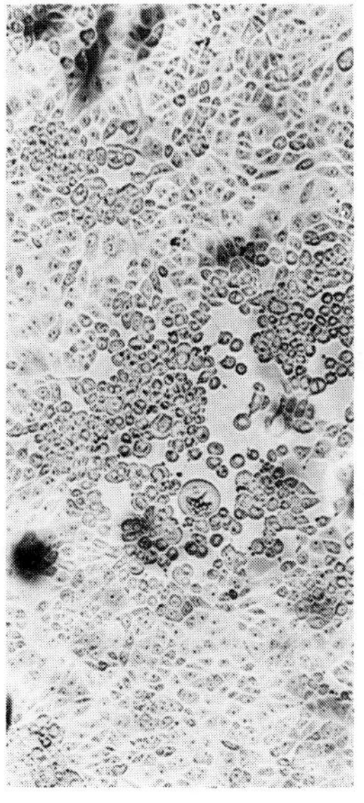

B

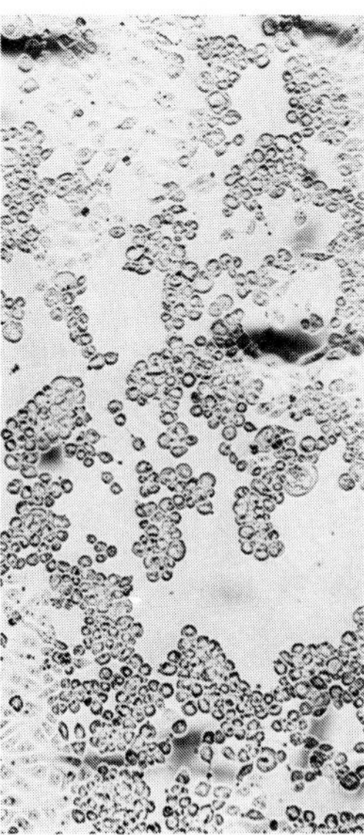

C

**Fig. 77-1.** Cytopathic effects of HSV in monkey kidney (Vero) cells. Note the slight rounding of the cells early after infection (A), followed by more extensive rounding and giant cell formation (B), and finally by universal rounding and cell death (C).

to enhance the speed with which HSV can be identified in tissue culture. One such approach combines culture and immunologic detection by inoculating cells growing on microscope slides with the specimen to be tested, incubating the culture for 24 (or 48) h, and removing the slide and staining with antibody to HSV. The slides are evaluated by immunofluorescent, immunoperoxidase, or biotin-avidin immunodetection assays. The cultured cells will usually contain detectable HSV antigens before CPE is evident. Depending on the detection system used, 65 to 100 percent of specimens positive by standard culture (i.e., after up to 10 to 14 days of incubation) are detected by various versions of this system.[28–34] Most studies suggest these assays are about 90 percent sensitive for specimens taken from genital lesions. One disadvantage of this method is that the virus is destroyed by the detection system so that the isolate cannot be saved for further analysis unless a parallel culture is set up for harvesting. The variability in reported sensitivity suggests that any laboratory utilizing such a system should carefully standardize it against conventional viral culture to provide the clinician with local estimates of sensitivity.

Another approach to improving the speed of the standard culture technique is the use of centrifugal inoculation of cells in culture. In this method, small vials or microwells in plates with cultured cells growing on cover slips at the bottom are inoculated with the specimen by centrifugation, thus improving the efficiency of infection. Because HSV is a rapidly growing virus, this increase in the number of cells in the culture which are infected permits much more rapid detection of CPE. This method can also be combined with immunologic detection techniques for greater speed and accuracy.[35,36] However, not all laboratories have been able to achieve the sensitivity of standard culture with this method.[37]

Cocultivation has been used to demonstrate virus in latently infected tissues such as ganglia.[6,7,38] In this method, the tissue specimen is manually minced and dispersed with trypsin. These cells are then either mixed with a suspension or susceptible cells (e.g., diploid fibroblasts) or added to a monolayer culture of susceptible cells. Such cultures often require weeks to months of observation and multiple passages before viral growth is apparent.

## Rapid diagnostic tests

There are a number of situations in which the diagnosis of HSV infections needs to be confirmed within a matter of hours rather than days. Several rapid diagnostic methods are available to detect the presence of HSV, including cytologic, immunologic, electron microscopic, and DNA hybridization techniques.

**Cytologic Diagnosis of Mucocutaneous HSV Infection.** Cells in lesions caused by HSV show cytopathic changes similar to those described above for tissue culture cells. The cells will become enlarged and intranuclear inclusions will develop. Fusion of cells to form multinucleated giant cells will also occur (Fig. 77-2; see also Plate 29). Scraping of oral-labial or genital HSV lesions and staining of the cells by Papanicolaou or Wright-Giemsa (Tzanck preparation) stains is a rapid, inexpensive, and simple test for the detection of infections caused by the herpes group of viruses.[39–41] It should be remembered that the examination of these stained smears does not discriminate between

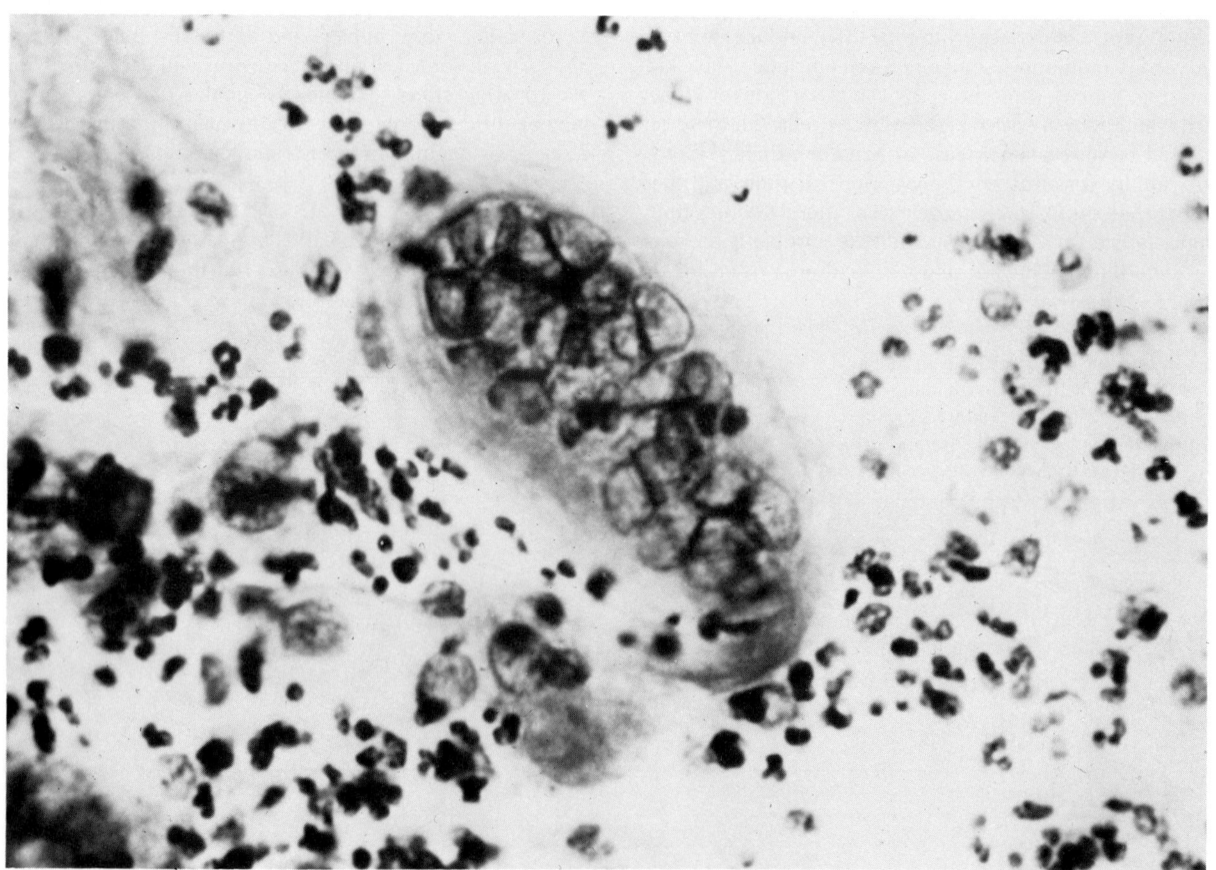

Fig. 77-2. Cytological preparation (Pap smear) of lesion demonstrating a multinucleated giant cell: cervical scraping from a woman with HSV cervicitis.

HSV and varicella-zoster (VZ) virus. CMV rarely produces vesicular lesions. More specific techniques, such as IF or viral isolation, can be used to differentiate HSV from VZ infections when necessary. VZ infection of the genital area is uncommon among immunocompetent patients between 15 and 40 years of age, the population in whom genital HSV infections most commonly occur. However, VZ infection is frequently seen in individuals infected with the human immunodeficiency virus, type 1 (HIV-1), and because the dose and type of antiviral chemotherapy differ between HSV and VZ, these two agents must be differentiated from each other.

In studies comparing viral isolation and cytology for the diagnosis of mucocutaneous HSV infection, cytologic screening has been a specific but often insensitive test when applied to genital lesions. Depending on the stage of the lesion and training of the observer, cytologic examination may detect 30 to 80 percent of culture-positive lesions. The authors recently studied 35 women with documented cervical HSV infection and found that cytologic evidence of HSV by Papanicolaou staining was present in only 51 percent. Cytological examination of cells from lesions or cervical secretions thus appears to have good specificity but low sensitivity.

**Antigen Detection.** Detection of HSV antigen by immunologic techniques is currently the most commonly used rapid diagnostic method. One such method uses fluorescein-conjugated anti-HSV antibodies in the direct immunofluorescence (IF) test.[42,43] In this technique cells are removed from a suspicious lesion either by vigorously swabbing the area or by scraping with a scalpel or needle. If a swab is used, it may then be placed into an appropriate transport medium. In the laboratory the cells are concentrated and spotted onto glass slides. If scrapings are made, they should be immediately placed on glass slides. The cells are fixed in cold acetone, washed, and incubated with anti-HSV antibody conjugated with fluorescein isothiocyanate. After further washing, the slide is examined under a fluorescence microscope for the presence of intracellular fluorescence. Although some experience in distinguishing background fluorescence from specific fluorescence is needed for accurate interpretation, this technique is relatively easy to learn. Positive and negative controls consisting of HSV-infected and uninfected cells are included in each assay for improved accuracy. If monoclonal antibodies are utilized, typing of the virus can be performed at the same time (see below). The major factor limiting the utility of this method is the number of cells present in the specimen to be studied. If the specimens studied contain a sufficient number of cells, the sensitivity of the direct IF test for detection of HSV in genital lesions is between 70 and 95 percent compared with culture.[13,15] In specialized clinics, where personnel are trained in collecting specimens for the IF test, up to 90 percent of specimens obtained from genital lesions are adequate. In a routine viral diagnostic laboratory, where specimens are received from numerous practitioners throughout the Seattle area, we found that adequate specimens were obtained in approximately 70 percent of submitted samples.

Some specimens are positive by IF but negative by culture. Although these are usually considered false-positive IF tests, one study showed that in 82 percent of patients with a positive IF and a negative culture, HSV was subsequently isolated from later cultures.[15] These results suggest that IF (or other antigen-detection methods), if done by an experienced laboratory with appropriate controls, may be more sensitive than culture in some situations.

Another immunologic technique for the detection of HSV antigen is the use of immunoperoxidase (IP) staining.[44] This method has the advantage of utilizing light rather than fluorescence microscopy. Specimens are prepared in a manner similar to that for the direct IF test. The anti-HSV antibodies may be polyclonal (e.g., prepared in rabbits) or monoclonal. After the slide is treated with anti-HSV antibody, anti-rabbit or anti-mouse globulin conjugated with horseradish peroxidase is added. The sample is then treated with diaminobenzidine, which reacts with the peroxidase enzyme and deposits a reddish-brown color where the antibody has bound. This slide is then examined under a light microscope for the presence of reddish-brown granules. Most studies have shown similar sensitivities and specificities of the two immunostaining methods.[45] In both the IF and IP methods, the use of monoclonal antibodies in place of polyclonal rabbit antisera will generally improve the specificity by reducing nonspecific binding of the antiserum while maintaining a sensitivity comparable with the polyclonal reagents.[46–48] Obviously, the problem of specimen adequacy remains.

Another antibody-based rapid method to diagnose HSV infections is the enzyme-linked immunosorbent assay (ELISA). To perform this test, a reaction vessel such as a plastic tube or well is coated with antibody to HSV and the specimen to be tested for the presence of HSV is added to the well. If HSV is present in the specimen, it will be bound to the antibody. After washing, a second anti-HSV antibody (prepared in a different animal species from that used to coat the tube) is added to the tube, and this will bind to the HSV. After further washing, an antiglobulin directed at the second anti-HSV antibody is added. This last antibody is conjugated to an enzyme such as alkaline phosphatase. After additional washing, *p*-nitrophenyl phosphate is added. This compound is split by alkaline phosphatase, and the products of the reaction cause a color change in the solution. The test can be read qualitatively by visual inspection or quantitatively in a spectrophotometer. Studies using ELISA for the detection of HSV in clinical specimens suggest that ELISA has a sensitivity similar to that of the IF and IP methods (i.e., 70 to 90 percent compared with viral isolation).[49–53] Recently, a commercially available ELISA system has been reported to be as sensitive as virus isolation for detection of HSV in mucosal ulcers.

**Electron Microscopy.** Demonstration of herpes virus particles in vesicular lesions by electron microscopy has been advocated as a rapid diagnostic technique. Its utility is, however, limited by the specialized equipment required and the apparent low sensitivity of this technique in genital herpes. For example, Brown et al.[54] demonstrated HSV by electron microscopy of genital lesion material in only 2 of 27 patients from whom HSV was isolated. In selected cases (e.g., in neonatal infection or review of biopsied brain tissue) electron microscopy can be a useful adjunct to viral isolation for the diagnosis of HSV infection.

**Viral DNA Detection.** Another approach to rapid identification of HSV in clinical specimens is to apply DNA hybridization technology. The introduction of nonradioactive DNA probes has made this approach more feasible in standard diagnostic virology laboratories. Cells from clinical specimens are spotted onto slides and fixed in much the same way as for antibody staining. The fixed cells are then treated with formamide to denature the viral (and cellular) DNA and are incubated with cloned segments of HSV DNA which contain biotin covalently linked to the DNA. The cloned HSV DNA forms double-stranded DNA hybrids with any HSV DNA in the cells and is not removed by subsequent washing steps. The presence of the bound biotinylated DNA is detected by incubation with avidin which has been conjugated with peroxidase, followed by incubation with a peroxidase substrate and examination by light microscopy. The high specificity of the DNA-DNA hybridization reaction coupled with the high affinity of avidin for biotin yield a sensitivity and specificity comparable with immunofluorescence methods.[55,56]

### Typing of HSV isolates

Once the presence of HSV is established by one of the preceding methods, it is often useful to determine if the isolated virus is HSV-1 or HSV-2. Although the clinical disease is usually the same, prognostic information such as the probability of subsequent recurrence may be gained by typing (see Chap. 35). Historically, biological differences between the two serotypes such as differential growth in primary chick embryo fibroblast cultures[57–59] or the size of pocks produced on the chorionic membranes of embryonated hen's eggs[60] were used for typing. These methods have been largely supplanted by more sophisticated immunologic and molecular techniques.

**Immunologic Typing.** For differentiation between HSV-1 and HSV-2, most laboratories utilize an immunologic technique (e.g., IF, IP, ELISA) that employs monoclonal antibodies made against prototype strains.[18,44,61] Several monoclonal antibody preparations, including some already conjugated to fluorescein isothiocyanate or horseradish peroxidase, are commercially available. The assays are performed as described earlier using cells infected in vitro. Almost all isolates can be confirmed and typed in this manner.[46–48] The monoclonal typing antisera have a virtually 100 percent correlation with other methods such as restriction endonuclease cleavage patterns (see below).[62] When polyclonal antisera are used for typing, type assignment is based on the intensity of the reaction (staining, absorbance, cytolysis, or reduction of infection), assuming that the reaction is more intense with the homologous than with the heterologous antiserum. However, the considerable cross-reactivity between HSV-1 and HSV-2 can make differentiation between the two types difficult.[63] Cross-adsorbing a monospecific antiserum with the heterologous virus type may help remove cross-reacting antibodies, but it may also greatly decrease the sensitivity. Because there are several good type-specific monoclonal antibody preparations now available, these have largely supplanted the older "type-specific" polyclonal reagents used previously.

**Molecular Techniques for Typing.** The molecular methods rely on the fact that the DNA genomes of the two HSV types exhibit only about 45 percent DNA sequence homology.[64] These methods are more reliable than the use of polyclonal antibodies but they are also more cumbersome. They have been used as the "gold standard" for establishing the reliability of the monoclonal antibody typing systems. The most commonly used molecular typing method is the restriction endonuclease mapping technique. This method uses restriction endonucleases purified from various bacteria. These enzymes recognize specific nucleotide sequences in DNA and cleave the DNA at these sequences. The cleavage products can then be separated by size in a gel electrophoresis system; the pattern of fragments on the gel will be unique for any unique piece of DNA such as a viral genome. The pattern generated by cleavage of HSV-1 DNA with any one of several restriction endonucleases is different from that of strains of HSV-2 (Fig. 77-3). This procedure can be carried out by infecting cells in microwells with the virus to be tested in the presence of $^{32}P$ orthophosphate to label the DNA.[65] This is done under conditions where the bulk of the label goes into viral DNA. After CPE has developed, the cells are lysed, and the DNA is partially purified and then treated with ribonuclease. The preparation is digested with the desired restriction endonuclease and subjected to electrophoresis on an agarose gel. The fragments are then located by autoradiography. This method is probably too cumbersome and expensive to be used for routine typing of HSV, but it can be helpful in cases where immunologic methods have given equivocal or conflicting results.

Another use for the restriction endonuclease mapping technique is in identification of strain variation within each type of HSV. It has been found that there are minor variations in the DNA sequence of different isolates of HSV-1 and HSV-2, and that no two epidemiologically different HSV-1s are likely to be identical.[66,67] The same is true for HSV-2. Because of this, the "fingerprints" of the DNA of different isolates of HSV-1 (or HSV-2), digested with the same restriction endonuclease, will be slightly different. The differences are not as pronounced as those between HSV-1 and HSV-2 but they are reproducible. This method allows one to follow a particular strain as it is transmitted between individuals.[68,69]

## ANTIVIRAL SUSCEPTIBILITY TESTING

Routine determination of the susceptibility of HSV isolates to antiviral agents is usually not necessary. However, in selected cases, especially immunosuppressed patients or patients with HIV-1 infection who have received multiple courses of antivirals, drug-resistant strains may emerge. There is currently no standardized methodology for determining antiviral susceptibility for HSV isolates. Most methods currently in use rely on the ability of an antiviral drug to protect a cell culture from HSV-induced cytopathology. The plaque reduction assay is the most widely used test of this type.[70] In this assay, a known amount of HSV is used to infect a set of monolayer cell cultures which are then incubated in the presence of varying concentrations of an antiviral drug. After several days, the number of infectious foci (plaques) are counted for each culture and are plotted against the corresponding drug concentration. The concentration of drug which reduces the number of plaques by 50 percent (the $ID_{50}$) is then calculated from the plot.

A variation of this test which is faster and more amenable to automation is the dye exclusion technique.[71] Cells in microwell cultures are infected with HSV in the presence of varying concentrations of the antiviral drug and are incubated for 72 h. At that time, the medium is removed and neutral red dye is added. This dye is taken up by viable (uninfected) cells but not by cells injured by HSV infection. After washing the wells, the dye is extracted from the cells with ethanol and the amount of extracted dye is quantitated spectrophotometrically. By plotting the optical density of the extract against the drug concentration, an $ID_{50}$ can again be calculated. Although the $ID_{50}$ values calculated by these (and other) methods often differ from each other, the relative values of different antiviral agents and different HSV isolates are comparable. More standardization of these laboratory methods is needed so that the results obtained in different laboratories can be compared and the breakpoint between sensitive and resistant strains can be ascertained. For the antiviral drug acyclovir, an $ID_{50}$ of $>3$ μg/ml is generally felt to indicate a resistant strain.

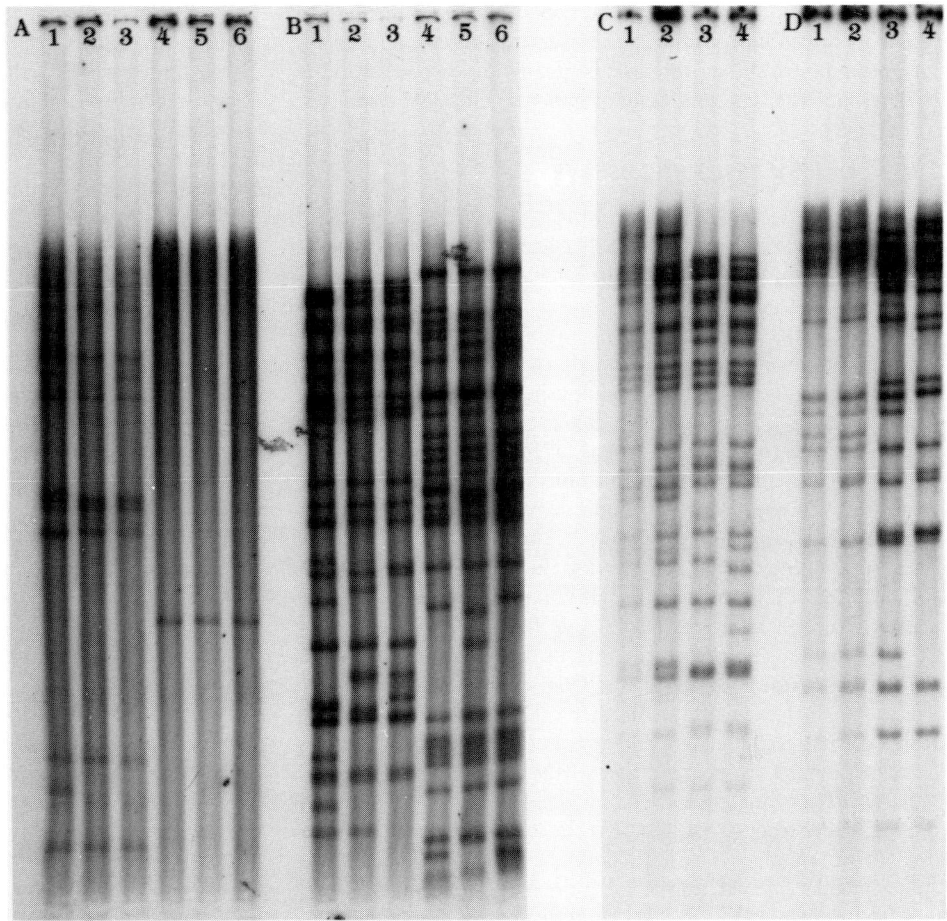


Fig. 77-3. Restriction endonuclease cleavage of HSV DNA for typing and for strain identification. (*A*) Lanes 1 to 6 show the size of DNA fragments after digestion of DNA from six genital HSV isolates with Hpa I. (*B*) The same six isolates are shown digested with BamH-1. Isolates 1, 2, and 3 are HSV-1 and isolates 4, 5, and 6 are HSV-2. Note the striking difference in pattern between the two types, especially with Hpa-1. Also note that each of the HSV-1 and HSV-2 isolates appears to have slightly different digestion patterns with both enzymes; these different patterns suggest strain differences. (C) Lane 1 is the pattern of an isolate (HSV-1) from a baby who died of disseminated neonatal herpes. Lane 2 is the pattern of an isolate obtained from a breast lesion of the baby's mother, and lanes 3 and 4 are HSV-1 isolates from unrelated patients. DNA from each isolate was digested with BamH-1. (*D*) The same isolates 1 to 4 are shown digested with Kpn-1.

Note that with both enzymes the pattern seen with the mother's isolate is identical to that of the baby. (*C* and *D* are adapted from Ref. 69.)

## SEROLOGIC TESTING FOR HSV ANTIBODIES

The appropriate use of HSV antibody testing often poses a confusing issue to the clinician, because of the variety of antibody assays available, the inability of many of the most widely utilized serologic assays to effectively discriminate between HSV-1 and HSV-2 antibodies, and the inadequacy of serologic assays for predicting disease recurrence or transmission. Serologic assays for HSV may be utilized to document past infection with HSV. Acute and convalescent sera can be utilized to retrospectively determine first-episode infection.

Recent studies have shown the insensitivity and lack of specificity of the clinical history in documenting past genital herpes; two-thirds of persons who possess antibodies to HSV-2 are asymptomatic.[72–75] As such, HSV antibody testing is the only effective way to document past infection with either HSV-1 or HSV-2. Accumulated evidence in animals and humans has indicated that persons who are seropositive to HSV possess latent ganglionic virus and have the potential to develop either symptomatic recurrences or have asymptomatic excretion of virus. Thus, serologic testing is the most cost-effective way to identify the asymptomatic carrier of HSV infection.

Until recently, the major limitation to HSV antibody testing has been the inability to differentiate between the antibody response to HSV-1 and HSV-2 infection. While numerous antibody detection systems for defining HSV antibodies have been developed, including complement fixation, neutralization, passive hemagglutination, immunofluorescence, immunoperoxidase, radioimmunoassay, ELISA, and various cytotoxicity assays, these assays use prototype HSV isolates as antigen sources and don't discriminate well between the two virus types. They are, however, useful for differentiating HSV seronegative from HSV seropositive persons or for documenting recent seroconversion after primary infection. Many of these assays are quantitative but there is little evidence correlating antibody titer with protection from disease recurrence or transmission. In fact, persons who have frequent recurrences of HSV tend to have the highest antibody titers.[76] The one major exception is in infants exposed to mothers shedding HSV at birth. Infants who have low levels of neutralizing antibody to HSV in cord blood appear to be more prone to acquire neonatal HSV than similarly exposed infants with higher neutralizing antibody titers.[77,78]

### Determining HSV antibody subtypes by serologic methods

Differentiation of HSV antibody type has been attempted by comparing antibody titers with prototype strains of each of the types. These assays tend to be accurate in determining type specificity when one is infected with only one of the HSV subtypes. For example, a young adult who developed primary genital HSV-1 might exhibit HSV neutralizing antibody titers in convalescent phase sera of 1:128 to HSV-1 and 1:8 to HSV-2. An HSV-2 infected person would exhibit nearly equal antibody titers to each of the prototype agents. The major targets of serum antibodies are, however, the surface glycoproteins.[79,80] Most of the immunogenic epitopes on the surface glycoproteins are common to both HSV types.[81] Thus, in persons with prior HSV-1 infection who then acquire HSV-2, a concomitant rise in antibodies to both HSV-1 and HSV-2 infection occurs making discrimination between the antibody response to the two viral types difficult. The recent identification of type-specific surface proteins and assays for antibodies to these proteins has greatly improved our ability to determine the type specificity of patients' anti-HSV responses.

## Types of HSV serologic assays

The following sections provide a brief review of the assays used to detect anti-HSV antibody. Each assay has its own strengths and weaknesses. Not all assays are available in all laboratories.

**Neutralization.** HSV neutralizing antibodies can be detected by the prevention of viral cytopathic effect (CPE) or by plaque reduction.[82] Titration of sera is accomplished in these tests by using serial dilutions of sera against a fixed challenge dose of virus. The serum titer to each virus type is taken as the highest dilution inhibiting cytopathic effect. A ratio of the antibody titers to the two virus subtypes is used to indicate whether the patient has been infected with HSV-1 or HSV-2. This ratio is calculated by the formula [(log titer to HSV-2)/(log titer to HSV-1)] × 100. A II/I ratio less than 85 indicates HSV-1 infection, while a ratio greater than 100 indicates HSV-2 infection.[10,82,83] This method of subtyping is valid only if the titer of the working dilutions of the two virus stocks (as calculated from the back titer assay) are within $10^{0.5}$ of each other. Another calculation can be utilized which calculates the relative potency of neutralization and factors in any difference in working titer of the stock viruses. The formula is: $pN = [\log(c - a - 0.16)] + T + 0.638$, where $c$ is the log of the stock virus titer, $a$ is the log of the dilution factor used to obtain the working titration, and $T$ is the 50 percent endpoint titer calculated as ($\log_2$ of the dilution yielding 50 percent neutralization) × (0.301). A difference in the potency of neutralization of HSV-1 and HSV-2 ($pN_1 - pN_2$) greater than 0.5 indicates prior HSV-1 infection; a value $<0.05$ indicates prior HSV-2 infection.[82] Before the development of the type-specific glycoprotein and Western blot assays, neutralization assays were the standard with which the specificity of most HSV antibody assays were compared. Recent studies comparing these newer assays with neutralization testing indicate good specificity for the neutralization assays when the $pN_1 - pN_2$ values are $<0.05$ or $>0.5$, but poor specificity for sera with $pN_1 - pN_2$ values between 0.05 and 0.5.[82a,82b]

**Hemagglutination Tests.** Passive hemagglutination using tanned sheep erythrocytes sensitized with HSV-1 or HSV-2 and antigen capture passive hemagglutination using monoclonal antibodies also have demonstrated good correlation with microneutralization.[84] Infected cell proteins are used to sensitize tanned sheep red blood cells (RBC) which are then reacted in microtiter plate wells with serial serum dilutions for 2 to 3 h. The antibody titer is the serum dilution where agglutinated cells produce a thin layer which covers 80 percent or more of the bottom of the well. Separate endpoints are recorded for cells sensitized with type 1 and type 2 antigen.

**Complement Fixation.** Complement-fixing antibodies can also be detected and titrated in human sera. The complement-fixation assay is not useful in discriminating HSV subtypes.[85] Antibodies detected by this test usually can be demonstrated in human serum within 2 weeks of the onset of infection.

**Cytotoxicity Tests.** Cytotoxic antibody assays are based upon the antibody-mediated lysis of HSV-infected target cells in the presence of complement.[86] A sensitive technique, the antibody-dependent cell-mediated cytotoxicity (ADCC) assay, amplifies the cytotoxicity endpoint (in most cases measured by release of $^{51}$Cr from target cells) by the addition of primed killer cells.[87] Antibody reactivity is limited to IgG directed against antigens expressed on the infected cell surface.

**Immunoassays.** Indirect fluorescent antibody (IFA) staining of HSV-infected cells can be used to detect antibody to cell surface and internal HSV proteins. Serum dilutions are added to infected cells, and binding is detected with a fluorescein-conjugated antihuman globulin. The dilution at which 50 percent of the cells show fluorescence is taken as the titer. IFA titers correlate well with neutralizing antibody titers. Solid-phase enzyme immunoassay (EIA) and radioimmunoassay (RIA) tests have also been described using a variety of conditions and antigens. EIA and RIA tests are more sensitive than microneutralization and can detect antibody within 1 week of the onset of symptoms. A wide range of neutralizing and complement-fixing antibody titers have been found with a given EIA titer suggesting variable reactivity in biologic tests and, perhaps, different subsets of antibodies all of which are detected by binding assays such as EIA.[88,89] The type specificity of most commercially available EIA and IFA assays has not been rigorously established.

**Precipitating Antibodies.** Gel diffusion and crossed immunoelectrophoresis have also been used to evaluate serologic response to HSV. Precipitating antibodies are primarily directed against the viral glycoproteins.

**Protein-Specific Serologic Assays.** The most promising approach to typing HSV antibodies has involved the use of type-specific antigens. Recently, several novel proteins specific for HSV-1 and HSV-2 have been defined.[90,91] One of the most helpful is a glycoprotein called gG, a minor component of the HSV envelope. Antibodies directed at gG-1 (gG of HSV-1) or gG-2 (gG of HSV-2) have been shown to be highly specific for viral subtype, and antibody assays to these proteins can accurately discriminate between either past HSV-1 or HSV-2 infection or both.[92–95] Purification of these proteins by immunoaffinity binding, by helix pomatia chromatography, or by hydroxylapatite chromatography has been described.[94]

One format for the detection of anti-gG antibodies is the immunodot enzyme assay. Immunoaffinity purified gG-1 and gG-2 antigen preparations are made; their concentration is optimized and antigen spotted in 1.0-μl volumes onto nitrocellulose disks which have been placed into 96-well microtiter plates. Test serum (100 μl) is diluted 1:50 in buffer, added to duplicate wells, and incubated overnight, and the disks are washed. A standard ELISA detection format is then utilized. The disks are dried in the dark overnight, then examined visually for color change appearing as a bluish-purple dot in the center of the disk. These new type-specific assays are ideal for identifying individuals with past HSV infection. However, it takes 6 to 8 weeks after infection for anti-gG-1 or anti-gG-2 to be identified using this method.[82b]

The drawback to the gG assay has been the difficulty of obtaining and quality-controlling the purified antigen. Alternative approaches to detecting anti-gG-1 and anti-gG-2 have been developed involving either immunoprecipitation of crude infected-cell lysates or the reaction of serum with electrophoresed, nitrocellulose-bound proteins, the Western blot assay.[82,82b,92–94]

**Western Blot Assay (WBA).** For the WBA, HSV antigen is prepared from fibroblasts infected with $10^7$ $TCID_{50}$ per ml of HSV-1 or HSV-2. The cells are lysed in an 8 percent sodium

**Table 77-3. Interpretation of Western Blot Banding Patterns**

| Observed bands* | Interpretation |
|---|---|
| No bands, or weak bands to nonviral proteins as determined by comparison with banding patterns on strips reacted with known, negative sera | Seronegative |
| A predominance of binding to the HSV-1 strip and, if binding is present on the HSV-2 strip, no reactivity with gG-2 bands | HSV-1 antibody |
| A predominance of binding to the HSV-2 strip including reactivity with gG-2 | HSV-2 antibody |
| Full complement of bands on both the HSV-1 and HSV-2 strips, including reactivity with both gG-1 and gG-2 | HSV-1 + HSV-2 antibody |

*If complex patterns appear which are different from those described, cross-adsorption experiments may be required (see text).

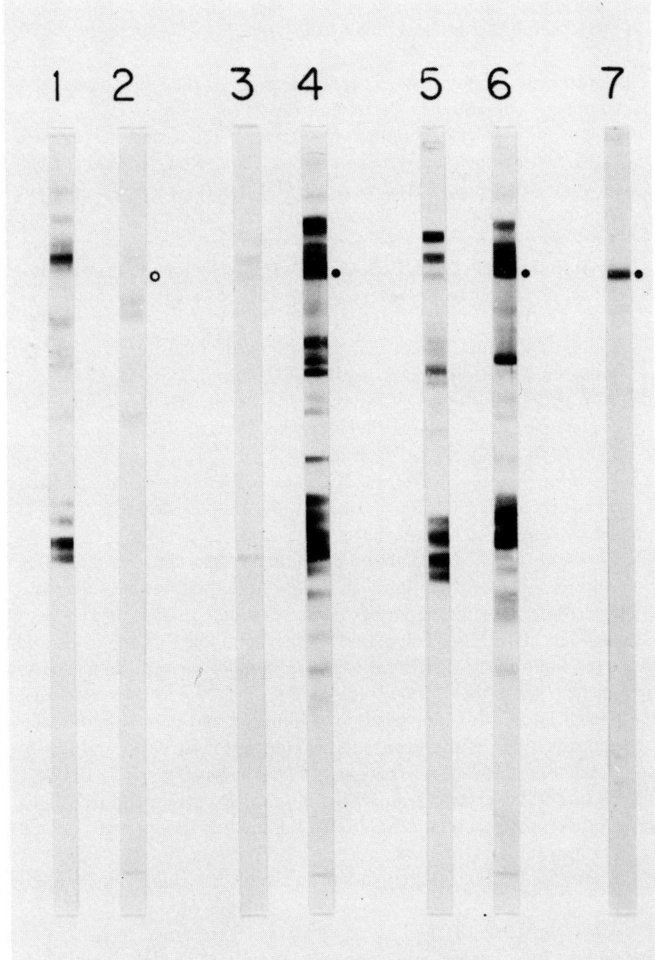


**Fig. 77-4.** Detection of specific antibody response to HSV-1 and HSV-2 by Western blot analysis. Western blots prepared with HSV-1-infected cell lysates (lanes 1, 3, and 5) or HSV-2-infected cell lysates (lanes 2, 4, and 6) were reacted with sera from a patient with primary genital HSV-1 (lanes 1 and 2), a patient with primary genital HSV-2 (lanes 3 and 4), or a patient with active recurrent genital HSV-2 and a history of HSV-1 mucocutaneous infection (lanes 5 and 6). Monoclonal antibody to gG-2 was reacted with an HSV-2-containing nitrocellulose paper strip (lane 7) to localize this protein. Note that the gG-2 band appears only on those HSV-2 strips which have been reacted with serum which contains HSV-2 antibodies (solid circles). HSV-1 antibody does not bind to gG-2 (lane 2, open circle). *(Reproduced from Ref. 82b, with permission.)*

dodecyl sulfate (SDS), 10 percent 2-mercaptoethanol buffer, the proteins denatured by boiling for 2 min, and the lysate is electrophoresed into 9 percent discontinuous polyacrylamide gels. After electrophoresis, the proteins are transferred to nitrocellulose (NC) which can then be cut into strips and stored. Human sera are diluted in buffer (1:100), 10 μl of sera is added to each strip, and the strips are extensively washed. Peroxidase conjugated antihuman IgG is then added followed by peroxidase substrate (4-chloro-1-naphthol). Sera are reacted with two strips containing either HSV-1 or HSV-2 proteins. The interpretation of the resulting patterns is shown in Table 77-3.

Atypical reactivity on either HSV-1 or HSV-2 strips or equivalent reactivity on each strip without a clear gG-2 band on the HSV-2 strip is considered to be an equivocal result. Sera giving these results are adsorbed against both HSV-1 and HSV-2 antigens and rerun against both HSV-1 and HSV-2 strips. After adsorption, the presence of HSV-2 antibody can be determined if bands occur only on the HSV-2 strip after the serum has been adsorbed with HSV-1-coupled sepharose. Type 1 HSV antibody can be detected by the presence of bands on only the HSV-1 strip after adsorption with HSV-2 coupled sepharose. The presence of both HSV-1 and HSV-2 antibodies is detected by the appearance of bands on both the HSV-1 strip (after HSV-2 adsorption) and the HSV-2 strip (after HSV-1 adsorption). A typical Western blot profile demonstrating sera with reactivity to HSV-1, HSV-2, and both HSV-1 and HSV-2 is shown in Fig. 77-4.

The WBA has been shown to have somewhat increased sensitivity over tests using purified gG-1 or gG-2 in recognizing early seroconversion. This increased sensitivity is due to the fact that patients seroconvert to gG relatively late after infection. Seroconversion to HSV-2 in patients with prior HSV-1 antibody is also more sensitive because of the ability of the WBA to detect antibodies to other HSV-2 antigens.

## SUMMARY

Knowledge of the availability and use of laboratory tests for HSV is an important facet of the clinical management of HSV-infected patients. When patients present with symptomatic disease, especially genital lesions, use of diagnostic techniques to isolate virus or demonstrate viral antigen or DNA is the quickest and cheapest approach to confirm the diagnosis. As many genital lesions are "atypical," these viral-isolation or antigen-detection methods may markedly increase the clinical acumen of clinicians. HSV serologic assays can be utilized to discriminate seronegative from seropositive persons. To identify those with past HSV-2 infection, newly developed type-specific assays should be utilized.

## APPENDIX: PREPARATION OF TRANSPORT MEDIA FOR VIRAL ISOLATION

Either of the two preparations that follow is adequate for transporting specimens for isolation of HSV (and most other viruses).

### HANK'S BALANCED SALT SOLUTION (HBSS) WITH ANTIBIOTICS*

1. Mix 1 liter of 1X HBSS in sterile distilled water.
2. Adjust pH to 6.7 to 6.9 with $Na_2HCO_3$.

*After Lennette, *Diagnostic Procedures,* 4th ed.

3. Add the following:
   *a.* Nystatin (Mycostatin), 5 ml (10,000 units per milliliter), or amphotericin B (Fungizone), 5 mg/ml.
   *b.* Gentamicin, 10 ml (1000 μg/ml).
   *c.* Penicillin G, $10^6$ units (final concentration in HBSS, 1000 units per milliliter.)
   *d.* Polymyxin B sulfate, 50 ml (10,000 units per milliliter) (optional).
4. Dispense 1.5 ml medium aseptically in 1-dram vials. (Shelf life of medium is 3 months at −20°C.)

## VEAL INFUSION BROTH (VIB)*

1. Dissolve the following:
   *a.* VIB (Difco), 25 g, into 1000 ml deionized distilled water. Autoclave at 121°C and 15 lb pressure for 15 min.
   *b.* Gelatin, 25 g, in 100 ml hot distilled water. Autoclave, as in *a,* in 20-ml aliquots.
2. Mix autoclaved VIB and one aliquot of gelatin and allow to cool.
3. Add the following:
   *a.* Penicillin G, $10^6$ units.
   *b.* Amphotericin B (Fungizone), 10 ml (5 mg/ml), or nystatin (Mycostatin), 1 ml (25,000 units per milliliter).
   *c.* Gentamicin, 10 ml (1000 μg/ml).
4. Dispense 1.5 ml medium aseptically in 1-dram vials.
5. Freeze at −20°C for storage. (Shelf life for complete viral transport medium is 1 year at −20°C; for VIB, 6 months at 4°C; and for 25% gelatin, 6 months at 4°C.)

## References


1 Chapel T et al: The microbiological flora of penile ulcerations. *J Infect Dis* 137:50, 1978.
2 Friedrich EG et al: The vulvar clinic: An eight year appraisal. *Am J Obstet Gynecol* 135:1036, 1979.
3 Corey L, Holmes KK: Genital herpes simplex virus infections: Current concepts in diagnosis, therapy, and prevention. *Ann Intern Med* 98:973, 1983.
4 Quinn TC et al: Etiology of anorectal infections in homosexual men. *Am J Med* 71:395, 1981.
5 Goodell SE et al: Herpes simplex virus proctitis in homosexual men. *N Engl J Med* 308:868, 1983.
6 Baringer JR: Recovery of herpes simplex virus from human sacral ganglions. *N Engl J Med* 291:828, 1974.
7 Stevens JG: Latent herpes simplex virus and the nervous system. *Curr Top Microbiol Immunol* 70:31, 1975.
8 Mertz GJ et al: Frequency of acquisition of first-episode genital infection with herpes simplex virus from symptomatic and asymptomatic source contacts. *Sex Transm Dis* 12:33, 1985.
9 Rooney JF et al: Acquisition of genital herpes from an asymptomatic sexual partner. *N Engl J Med* 314:1561, 1986.
10 Pauls FP, Dowdle WR: A serologic study of Herpesvirus hominis strains by microneutralization tests. *J Immunol* 98:941, 1967.
11 Dowdle WR et al: Association of antigenic type of Herpesvirus hominis with site of viral recovery. *J Immunol* 99:974, 1967.
12 Corey L et al: Genital herpes simplex virus infections: Clinical manifestations, course, and complications. *Ann Intern Med* 98:958, 1983.
13 Moseley RC et al: Comparison of viral isolation, direct immunofluorescence, and indirect immunoperoxidase for the detection of genital herpes simplex virus infection. *J Clin Microbiol* 13:913, 1981.


*VIB with 0.5% gelatin, 5 μg/ml amphotericin B (Fungizone), 1000 units penicillin per milliliter, and 10 μg/ml gentamicin per milliliter.


14 Smith KO, Melnick JL: Recognition and quantitation of herpes virus particles in human vesicular lesions. *Science* 137:543, 1962.
15 Lafferty WE et al: Diagnosis of herpes simplex virus by direct immunofluorescence and viral isolation from samples of external genital lesions in a high-prevalence population. *J Clin Microbiol* 25:323, 1987.
16 Overall JC Jr: Dermatologic diseases, in *Antiviral Agents and Viral Diseases of Man*, GJ Galasso et al (eds). New York, Raven, 1979, p 305.
17 Crane LR et al: Incubation of swab materials with herpes simplex virus. *J Infect Dis* 141:531, 1980.
18 Nahmias A et al: Rapid identification and typing of herpes simplex virus types 1 and 2 by a direct immunofluorescence technique. *Appl Microbiol* 22:455, 1971.
19 Warford AL et al: Sucrose phosphate glutamate for combined transport of chlamydial and viral specimens. *Am J Clin Pathol* 81:762, 1984.
20 Yeager AS et al: Storage and transport of cultures for herpes simplex virus, type 2. *Am J Clin Pathol* 72:977, 1979.
21 Barnard DL et al: Suitability of new Chlamydia transport medium for transport of herpes simplex virus. *J Clin Microbiol* 24:692, 1986.
22 Ash RJ, Barnhart ER: Optimal cooling and warming rates in the preservation of herpes simplex virus (type 2). *J Clin Microbiol* 2:270, 1975.
23 Anderca I, Iftimovici M: Practical aspects of the storage of herpes simplex virus samples. *Rev Roum Med-Virol* 30:5, 1979.
24 Rawls WE: Herpes simplex virus types 1 and 2 and herpes virus Simiae, in *Diagnostic Procedures for Viral, Rickettsial and Chlamydial Infections*, EH Lennette, NJ Schmidt (eds). Washington, American Public Health Association, 1979, p 309.
25 McSwiggan DA et al: Comparison of the sensitivity of human embryo kidney cells, HeLa cells, and WI-38 cells for the primary isolation of viruses from the eye. *J Clin Pathol* 28:410, 1975.
26 Landry ML et al: Comparison of guinea pig embryo cells, rabbit kidney cells, and human embryonic lung fibroblast strains for isolation of herpes simplex virus. *J Clin Microbiol* 15:842, 1982.
27 Roizman B, Furlong D: The replication of herpesviruses, in *Comprehensive Virology*, vol 3, H Frenkel-Conrat, RR Wagner (eds). New York, Plenum, 1974, p 281.
28 Nerurkar LS et al: Detection of genital herpes simplex infections by a tissue culture-fluorescent-antibody technique with biotin-avidin. *J Clin Microbiol* 17:149, 1983.
29 Fayram SL et al: Comparison of cultureset to a conventional tissue culture-fluorescent-antibody technique for isolation and identification of herpes simplex virus. *J Clin Microbiol* 18:215, 1983.
30 Hayden FG et al: Comparison of the Immulok Cultureset kit and virus isolation for detection of herpes simplex virus in clinical specimens. *J Clin Microbiol* 18:222, 1983.
31 Sewell DL et al: Comparison of Cultureset and Bartels Immunodiagnostics with conventional tissue culture for isolation and identification of herpes simplex virus. *J Clin Microbiol* 19:705, 1984.
32 Nerurkar LS et al: Comparison of standard tissue culture, tissue culture plus staining, and direct staining for detection of genital herpes simplex virus infection. *J Clin Microbiol* 19:631, 1984.
33 Rubin SJ, Rogers S: Comparison of Cultureset and primary rabbit kidney cell culture for the detection of herpes simplex virus. *J Clin Microbiol* 19:920, 1984.
34 Phillips LE et al: Retrospective evaluation of the isolation and identification of herpes simplex virus with Cultureset and human fibroblasts. *J Clin Microbiol* 22:255, 1985.
35 Gleaves CA et al: Detection and serotyping of herpes simplex virus in MRC-5 cells by use of centrifugation and monoclonal antibodies 16 h postinoculation. *J Clin Microbiol* 21:29, 1985.
36 Pruneda RC, Almanza I: Centrifugation-shell vial technique for rapid detection of herpes simplex virus cytopathic effect in vero cells. *J Clin Microbiol* 25:423, 1987.
37 Woods GL, Mills RD: Conventional tube cell culture compared with centrifugal inoculation of MRC-5 cells and staining with monoclonal antibodies for detection of herpes simplex virus in clinical specimens. *J Clin Microbiol* 26:570, 1988.

38 Stevens JG, Cook ML: Latent herpes simplex virus in spinal ganglia of mice. *Science* 173:843, 1971.
39 Naib ZM: Exfoliative cytology of viral cervicovaginitis. *Acta Cytol* 10:126, 1966.
40 Nahmias AJ et al: Genital herpes simplex infection: Virologic and cytologic studies. *Obstet Gynecol* 29:395, 1967.
41 Barr RJ et al: Rapid method for Tzanck preparations. *JAMA* 237:1119, 1977.
42 Biegeleisen JZ et al: Rapid diagnosis of herpes simplex virus infections with fluorescent antibody. *Science* 129:640, 1959.
43 Gardner PS et al: Rapid diagnosis of Herpesvirus hominis infections in superficial lesions by immunofluorescent antibody technique. *Br Med J* 4:89, 1968.
44 Benjamin DR: Rapid typing of herpes simplex virus strains using the indirect immunoperoxidase method. *Appl Microbiol* 28:568, 1974.
45 Schmidt NJ et al: Comparison of direct immunofluorescence and direct immunoperoxidase procedures for detection of herpes simplex virus antigen in lesion specimens. *J Clin Microbiol* 18:445, 1983.
46 Balachandran N et al: Identification and typing of herpes simplex viruses with monoclonal antibodies. *J Clin Microbiol* 16:205, 1982.
47 Goldstein LC et al: Monoclonal antibodies to herpes simplex viruses: Use in antigenic typing and rapid diagnosis. *J Infect Dis* 147:829, 1983.
48 Nowinski RC et al: Monoclonal antibodies for diagnosis of infectious diseases in humans. *Science* 219:637, 1983.
49 Adler-Storthz K et al: Biotin-avidin-amplified enzyme immunoassay for detection of herpes simplex virus antigen in clinical specimens. *J Clin Microbiol* 18:1329, 1983.
50 Ziegler T et al: Solid-phase enzyme-immunoassay for the detection of herpes simplex virus antigens in clinical specimens. *J Virol Methods* 7:1, 1983.
51 Morgan MA, Smith TF: Evaluation of an enzyme-like immunosorbent assay for the detection of herpes simplex virus antigen. *J Clin Microbiol* 19:730, 1984.
52 Land SA et al: Rapid diagnosis of herpes simplex virus infections by enzyme-linked immunosorbent assay. *J Clin Microbiol* 19:865, 1984.
53 Clayton AL et al: Factors influencing the sensitivity of herpes simplex virus detection in clinical specimens in a simultaneous enzyme-linked immunosorbent assay using monoclonal antibodies. *J Med Virol* 17:275, 1985.
54 Brown ST et al: Sensitivity and specificity of diagnostic tests for genital infection with Herpesvirus hominis. *Sex Transm Dis* 6:10, 1979.
55 Fung JC et al: Comparison of the detection of herpes simplex virus in direct clinical specimens with herpes simplex virus-specific DNA probes and monoclonal antibodies. *J Clin Microbiol* 22:748, 1985.
56 Langenberg A et al: Detection of herpes simplex virus DNA from genital lesions by in situ hybridization. *J Clin Microbiol* 26:933, 1988.
57 Figueroa ME, Rawls WE: Biological markers for differentiation of herpes virus strains of oral and genital origin. *J Gen Virol* 4:259, 1969.
58 Lowry SP et al: Investigation of plaque formation in chick embryo cells as a biological marker for distinguishing herpes virus type 2 from type 1. *J Gen Virol* 10:1, 1971.
59 Wentworth BB, Zablotney SL: Efficiency of plating on chick embryo cells and kinetic neutralization of Herpesvirus hominis strains. *Infect Immun* 5:377, 1972.
60 Nahmias AJ, Dowdle WR: Antigenic and biologic differences in Herpesvirus hominis. *Prog Med Virol* 10:110, 1968.
61 Vestergaard BF, Grauballe PC: ELISA for herpes simplex virus (HSV) type-specific antibodies in human sera using HSV type 1 and type 2 polyspecific antigens blocked with type heterologous rabbit antibodies. *Acta Pathol Microbiol Scand* 87:261, 1979.
62 Peterson E et al: Typing of clinical herpes simplex virus isolates with mouse monoclonal antibodies to herpes simplex virus types 1 and 2: Comparison with type-specific rabbit antisera and restriction endonuclease analysis of viral DNA. *J Clin Microbiol* 17:92, 1983.
63 Fife KH et al: Incorrect typing of herpes simplex virus isolates by direct immunofluorescence. *J Infect Dis* 148:338, 1983.
64 Kieff ED et al: Genetic relatedness of type 1 and type 2 herpes simplex virus. *J Virol* 9:738, 1972.
65 Lonsdale DM: A rapid technique for distinguishing herpes simplex virus type 1 from type 2 by restriction enzyme technology. *Lancet* i:849, 1979.
66 Hayward GS et al: Anatomy of herpes simplex virus DNA: Strain differences and heterogeneity in the locations of restriction endonuclease cleavage sites. *Proc Natl Acad Sci USA* 72:1768, 1975.
67 Roizman B: The structure and isomerization of herpes simplex virus genomes. *Cell* 16:481, 1979.
68 Buchman TG et al: Restriction endonuclease fingerprinting of herpes simplex virus DNA: A novel epidemiological tool applied to a nosocomial outbreak. *J Infect Dis* 138:488, 1978.
69 Sullivan-Bolyai JZ et al: Disseminated neonatal herpes simplex virus type 1 from a maternal breast lesion. *Pediatrics* 71:455, 1983.
70 Crumpacker CS et al: Resistance to antiviral drugs of herpes simplex virus isolated from a patient treated with acyclovir. *N Engl J Med* 306:343, 1982.
71 McLaren C et al: In vitro sensitivity to acyclovir in genital herpes simplex viruses from acyclovir-treated patients. *J Infect Dis* 148: 868, 1983.
72 Corey L, Spear PG: Infections with herpes simplex viruses. *N Engl J Med* 314:749, 1986.
73 Nahmias AJ et al: Prevalence of herpes simplex virus (HSV) type-specific antibodies in a USA prepaid group medical practice population (abstract). 6th International Meeting of the International Society for STD Research, Brighton, England, July 31–August 2, 1985.
74 Blackwelder WC et al: A population study of herpesvirus infections and HLA antigens. *Am J Epidemiol* 115:569, 1981.
75 Stavraky KM et al: Sexual and socioeconomic factors affecting the risk of past infections with herpes simplex virus type 2. *Am J Epidemiol* 118:109, 1983.
76 Reeves WC et al: Risk of recurrence after first episodes of genital herpes: Relation to HSV type and antibody response. *N Engl J Med* 305:315, 1981.
77 Yeager AS et al: Relationship of antibody to outcome in neonatal herpes simplex virus infections. *Infect Immun* 29:532, 1980.
78 Yeager AS, Arvin AM: Reasons for the absence of a history of recurrent genital infections in mothers of neonates infected with herpes simplex virus. *Pediatrics* 73:188, 1984.
79 Eberle R, Mou S-W: Relative titers of antibodies to individual polypeptide antigens of herpes simplex virus type 1 in human sera. *J Infect Dis* 148:436, 1983.
80 Ashley RL et al: Humoral immune response to HSV-1 and HSV-2 viral proteins in patients with primary genital herpes. *J Med Virol* 27:153, 1985.
81 Spear PG: Glycoproteins specified by herpes simplex virus, in *The Herpesviruses*, vol 3, B Roizman (ed). New York, Plenum, 1984, p 315.
82 Nahmias AJ et al: Antibodies to herpesvirus hominis types 1 and 2 in humans. *Am J Epidemiol* 92:539, 1970.
82a Bernstein D et al: Serologic analysis of first episode nonprimary genital herpes simplex virus infection. *Am J Med* 77:1055, 1984.
82b Ashley RL et al: Comparison of Western blot and gG-specific immunodot enzyme assay for detecting HSV-1 and HSV-2 antibodies in human sera. *J Clin Microbiol* 26:662, 1988.
83 Stadler H et al: Herpes simplex virus neutralization: A simplification of the test. *J Infect Dis* 131:430, 1975.
84 Fucillo DA et al: Herpesvirus hominis types 1 and 2: A specific micro-indirect hemagglutination test. *Proc Soc Exp Biol Med* 122: 735, 1970.
85 Wentworth BB, Alexander ER: Seroepidemiology of infections due to members of the herpesvirus group. *Am J Epidemiol* 94:496, 1971.
86 Subramanian T, Rawls WE: Comparison of antibody-dependent cellular cytotoxicity and complement-dependent antibody lysis of herpes simplex virus-infected cells as methods of detecting antiviral antibodies in human sera. *J Clin Microbiol* 5:551, 1977.

87 Kohl S et al: Kinetics of human antibody responses to primary genital herpes simplex virus infection. *Intervirology* 18:164, 1981.

88 Fortier B et al: Comparison of an ELISA technique with quantal microneutralization test for serotyping of HSV-1 or HSV-2 infected patients. *J Virol Methods* 11:11, 1982.

89 Denoyel GA et al: Enzyme immunoassay for measurement of antibodies to herpes simplex virus infection: Comparison with complement fixation, immunofluorescent-antibody, and neutralization techniques. *J Clin Microbiol* 11:114, 1980.

90 Marsden HS et al: Characterization of the 92000 dalton glycoprotein induced by herpes simplex virus type 2. *J Virol* 50:547, 1984.

91 Roizman B et al: Identification and preliminary mapping with monoclonal antibodies of a herpes simplex virus type 2 glycoprotein lacking a known type 1 counterpart. *Virology* 122:242, 1984.

92 Coleman MAR et al: Determination of herpes simplex virus type-specific antibodies by enzyme-linked immunosorbent assay. *J Clin Microbiol* 18:287, 1983.

93 Lee FK et al: Detection of herpes simplex virus type 2-specific antibody with glycoprotein G. *J Clin Microbiol* 22:642, 1985.

94 Svennerhold B et al: Herpes simplex virus type-selective enzyme-linked immunosorbent assayy with helix pomatia lectin-purified antigens. *J Clin Microbiol* 19:235, 1984.

Chapter 78

# Human papillomavirus detection tests

Attila T. Lörincz

The detection and classification of human papillomavirus (HPV) infection presents unique problems to physicians and clinical laboratory personnel. Cytologists and colposcopists working in concert can usually detect and diagnose characteristic HPV-associated lesions. They cannot, however, ascertain or predict accurately the HPV type present, especially in low-grade cervical intraepithelial neoplasia (CIN). These lesions may contain any one (or combination) of 15 or more HPV types, many with distinct disease associations[1–7] (also see Chap. 37). Furthermore, tissue from 10 percent or more of women with cytologically normal cervices contain HPV DNA. These cases may represent latent HPV infection or an HPV-associated lesion that was missed by cytology.[8–11] A subset of these cases may progress to CIN and cancer; thus accurate diagnosis of HPV infection is desirable. Because HPV does not duplicate in cell cultures, the only reliable way at present to detect and type HPV infection is nucleic acid hybridization.

## COLLECTION, TRANSPORT, AND STORAGE OF SPECIMENS

### TISSUE BIOPSIES

There are many different anatomic sites which can be infected by HPV (see Chaps. 37 and 38). These are amenable to sampling by biopsy followed by nucleic acid hybridization or immunocytochemical analysis.

When possible, biopsies should be bisected and one-half fixed and embedded in paraffin for a permanent record. Fresh tissue destined for HPV analysis should be quickly frozen on dry ice and stored at −70°C to prevent destruction of the cells and their contents.[3,4,6] Tissue fragments approximately 3 mm$^3$ are sufficient for several hybridization tests.

### EXFOLIATED CELLS

Exfoliated cells may be obtained with swabs, scrapers, or aspirators (see Chap. 48). These devices reliably provide a good yield of cells from the vagina and cervix. Generally, samples which are suitable for a Pap smear are also suitable for HPV testing. Cervical samples should contain squamous cells from the transformation zone. Additional cells from the endocervical canal and the vaginal wall can be included or tested separately if deemed necessary. Collected material should be frozen or analyzed as soon as possible. Transport and storage may be handled in a fashion similar to biopsies.[8–11]

A sample-stabilizing solution available from Life Technologies, Inc. (Gaithersburg, MD), allows storage of exfoliated cells for at least 2 weeks at room temperature and for prolonged periods at 4° to −20°C. These samples are suitable for nucleic acid hybridization analysis by dot blot or Southern blot.

## LABORATORY DETECTION OF HPV

Laboratory detection of HPV and determination of HPV type is not amenable to classical or common diagnostic procedures such as electron microscopy, cell culture, or immunological methods. Despite extensive experimental attempts, HPV virions cannot be grown in vitro.[12] Although immunological methods are available for detection of antigens common to all HPV,[13] diagnostically useful HPV antigens are typically not detectable in high-grade lesions or latent infections.[14]

In the 1980s, sophisticated nucleic acid hybridization techniques were introduced for detecting and typing HPV.[1–4] Several different methods are currently in use (reviewed in Ref. 15). Of these, Southern blot analysis[16] has proved to be one of the most sensitive and reliable, albeit one of the most difficult and time-consuming.

## PROCESSING OF SAMPLES

### Tissue biopsies

**Fresh Tissues.** Large tissue samples are usually cut or crushed into pieces of approximately 1 mm or smaller. This can be achieved by cutting sections with a cryostat. Representative sections can then be examined by histopathology to confirm the diagnosis of the permanent sections.[6] Tissues can also be minced finely with a blade or scissors,[17] ground in sand,[18,19] or fragmented by mechanical devices.[20] Biopsies up to approximately 3 mm$^3$ in size can be processed without fragmentation (Ref. 21, personal observations).

Partly homogenized tissues are usually digested in a solution of protease and detergent (usually proteinase K and sodium dodecyl sulfate). Samples are incubated in digest buffer with agitation at 37 to 65°C for a few hours to overnight. The exact time, temperature, or nature of the digestion buffer does not appear critical.[17,18,21] Some procedures call for an RNase step,[17,18] but we have found this unnecessary. In fact, in dot-blot-type assays performed using nylon filters, HPV RNA may add to the DNA signal. Nucleic acids are usually partially purified by phenol/chloroform extraction and ethanol precipitation.[22] Some investigators have omitted the protease digestion and have extracted powdered tissues directly with phenol/chloroform.[20] Nucleic acid pellets should be washed several times with ice-cold ethanol (to remove residual phenol which could interfere with subsequent restriction enzyme digestion), dried, and then resuspended in some suitable buffer such as TE [10 mM Tris HCl, 1 mM EDTA, pH 8.0[22]] at a DNA concentration of approximately 1 mg per ml (a 3-mm$^3$ piece of cervical tissue can yield up to 50 μg of DNA, Kiviat personal communication). The purified DNA should be stored at 4°C, or for long periods at −20 to −70°C. Care must be taken to prevent contamination with extraneous matter that can introduce nucleases which can degrade sample DNA.

**Embedded Tissues.** Sections 3 to 5 μm thick are cut with a microtome[23–26] and placed onto acid-washed slides which may be precoated with a number of different reagents to aid in the retention of the sections. The tissue sections can be tested for nucleic acids by in situ hybridization[23–26] or can be used for the immunodetection of HPV common antigen using a kit available from DAKO (Santa Barbara, CA) or with antisera prepared and used as previously described.[13]

## Exfoliated cells

Cells obtained with swabs or scrapers can be eluted into a digestion buffer containing protease and detergent. Wood or cotton should not remain in contact with the buffer any longer than necessary to recover cells because these materials may release compounds which inhibit restriction endonuclease action. Cells can also be washed out of the swabs or scrapers with phosphate buffered saline, pelleted, and resuspended in digestion buffer.[8] Cells in aspirates are pelleted by centrifugation and resuspended in digestion buffer.[21] Digestion of cells, extraction, and precipitation of nucleic acids are performed as described for tissues.

Samples to be analyzed by filter in situ hybridization are not digested. Instead, $1 \times 10^5$ to $5 \times 10^5$ cells suspended in phosphate buffer are filtered directly onto nitrocellulose filters.[10] In a variation of this procedure, a special suction instrument is used to wash cells off the cervix and to deposit them directly onto filters.[27]

## ANALYSIS OF SAMPLES

### Dot blots

This is one of the simplest and fastest HPV detection tests and is well suited for analysis of large numbers of samples[11,15,28,29] The ViraPap and ViraType HPV detection and typing kits (Life Technologies, Inc.) are based on the dot-blot format. For most diagnostic purposes, DNA is the target; however, RNA can also be detected. The basic dot-blot procedure is shown in Fig. 78-1*a*. DNA must be denatured prior to fixation on the filters. This is accomplished by heating above the DNA melting temperature (Tm) or by incubating at pH >13 for a few minutes (0.1 to 0.5*M* NaOH). To bind DNA to nitrocellulose filters, the samples must be neutralized and adjusted to approximately 1*M* NaCl. Neutralization is not necessary for nylon filters. Many detergents in-

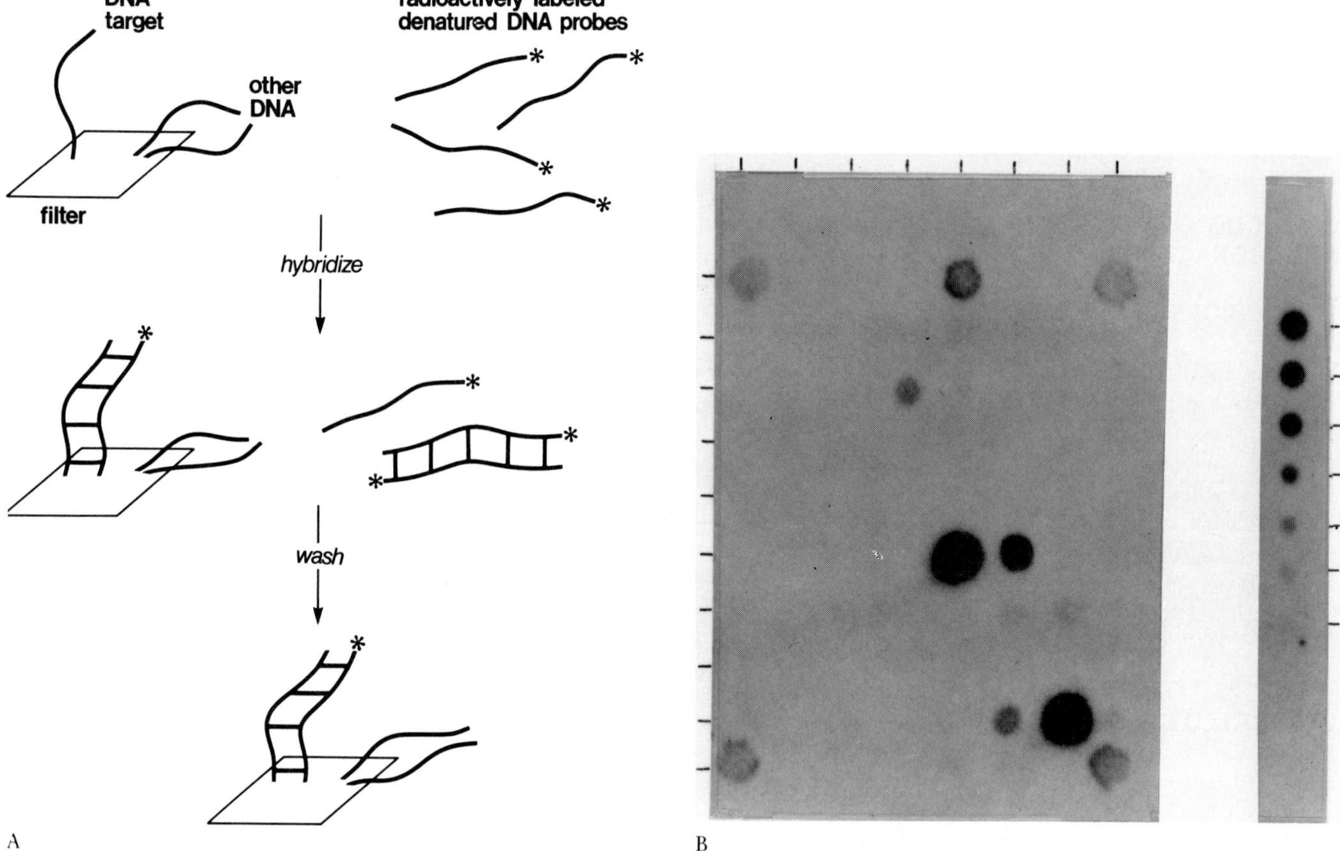


Fig. 78-1. (*a*) Detection of DNA targets by dot-blot hybridization. (*From Lorincz.*[15]) Typically, total DNA is extracted from samples, denatured to separate the strands, and immobilized on a filter by spotting or filtration with a vacuum manifold. The filter is prehybridized with a blocking solution to prevent nonspecific sticking of probes to the filter.[22,29] A solution of radioactively labeled single-stranded probes is then incubated with the filter to allow the formation of hybrids. After hybridization the filter is washed at a carefully chosen temperature to remove non-specifically-bound probes. In the example shown the sample contains target DNA and hence radioactivity is retained on the filter. These areas of radioactivity can be visualized with x-ray film.[22] (*b*) Autoradiographs of a typical dot-blot test containing 76 samples of exfoliated cervical cells, following a 12-h exposure at −70°C with intensifying screens. After extraction and purification, the sample DNAs were spotted onto a nitrocellulose filter in a grid pattern. The filter was hybridized with a DNA probe mixture of HPV types 16, 18, and 31 at Tm −25°C and washed at Tm −10°C. The four corner dots were HPV 16 DNA reference points; other positions (indicated by the marks) contained samples. Shown on the right is a 12-h autoradiograph of a hybridization control. These DNA samples were applied to the filter with a vacuum manifold. It contained, from top to bottom, 200 pg, 50 pg, 20 pg, 5 pg, 2 pg, 1 pg, and 0.2 pg of HPV 16 DNA. The HPV 18 and HPV 31 controls also run in this experiment are not shown.

terfere with the binding of nucleic acids to filters. They can be removed from samples by organic extractions with phenol or chloroform. DNA samples (1 to 5 μg) can be applied to filters by spotting small volumes (≤10 μl) onto dry filters. Larger sample volumes can easily be accommodated using vacuum manifolds because the liquid is sucked through the filter and nucleic acids bind as they contact the filter surface. An often-encountered problem with suction manifolds is that certain samples (especially crude lysates) filter slowly. This is much less of a problem with phenol-extracted samples or with alkaline samples.

Either nitrocellulose or nylon filters can be employed. Nitrocellulose, however, is easily torn, becomes brittle with use, and leaches nucleic acids (DNA or RNA), which limits its usefulness to three or four different probings. In contrast, nylon membranes are resistant to tearing, and leaching of nucleic acids is also much reduced. We have reprobed Hybond-N filters (Amersham, Arlington Heights, IL) as many as ten times with minimal losses of signal strength.

**Probes.** Nucleic acid probes in hybridization tests are the analogs of antibodies in immunological tests. Under carefully controlled conditions, probes recognize and bind only to single-stranded regions of complementary DNA or RNA targets. The probes can be labeled with radioisotopes,[22,31] haptens, or fluors.[32] Thus when probes bind to their targets, such as HPV DNA on a filter, they can be detected by autoradiographic (Fig. 78-1*b*), colorimetric, or other methods.[15,22,32] The most sensitive and specific probes are labeled with radioisotopes. Although nonradioactive detection methods have improved greatly they still cannot match radioisotopic methods in quality of results.[23,26,33]

DNA probes can be prepared by propagation of cloned sequences in plasmid vectors such as pBR322. Probe sequences should always be purified from the vector plasmid sequences by gel electrophoresis[22] because clinical samples often contain DNA homologous to vector sequences,[8] which can generate false-positive results. The purified DNA can then be labeled by nick translation or random primers.[22,31] Oligonucleotide DNA probes can be made synthetically.[29] These probes suffer from poor sensitivity because of the relatively small target size they recognize and thus are not particularly useful for the routine detection of HPV in clinical samples.

RNA probes have a number of advantages over DNA probes. One advantage is that a net output of probes 10- to 50-fold in excess of the input DNA can be generated. In contrast, nick translation converts unlabeled DNA templates into labeled probes, resulting in no net synthesis. Carefully prepared RNA probes are also practically free of cross-reactive vector sequences, obviating the need for electrophoretic purification. Although RNA probes are more sticky (adsorb nonspecifically) than DNA probes, the use of RNase A to destroy unhybridized RNA gives superior specificity. This is especially true with crude samples where the use of DNA probes can sometimes produce false-positive results (personal observations). To take full advantage of RNA probes the antisense strand should be used to enable the detection of both DNA and RNA targets. A disadvantage of RNA probes is that they are unsuitable for low-stringency hybridizations (see below).

To prepare RNA probes, it is necessary to clone the nucleotide sequences of interest into special vectors downstream from promoters specifically recognized by RNA polymerases of bacteriophage SP6, T7, or T3.[34,35] Radiolabeled RNA is prepared by incubating DNA templates with the specific RNA polymerase in the presence of radioactive nucleotide substrates.

**Hybridizations and Washes.** It is of utmost importance to rigorously control the stringency conditions during hybridization and washing of filters.[15,35] Excessively high stringency may give no signal where one would otherwise be detected. Alternatively, stringency conditions which are too low will give unreliable HPV-type data because all HPV types cross-react to some degree.[2–5] There are many different hybridization and wash conditions.[2,4,7,11,17,18,21] Fortunately it is possible to calculate the Tm of any perfectly matched DNA-DNA and RNA-DNA duplexes under most conditions.[29,35]

For most routine diagnostic applications, it is appropriate to use high-stringency conditions to detect only those HPV types identical with or very closely related to the probe(s). To maximize hybridization kinetics, probes are usually incubated with filters at 25°C below the temperature at which 50 percent of DNA duplexes denature (Tm − 25°C).[35] At probe concentrations of 50 to 100 ng/ml, the time of incubation may be as short as 2 h in the presence of kinetic enhancers such as dextran sulfate[22,29,35] but need not be longer than 14 to 16 h in their absence. Washes at Tm − 25°C allow significant cross-reactivity between different HPV types. Hence, it is advisable to perform several washes (4 washes of 20 min each) at 10°C below the melting temperature (Tm − 10°C) to reduce cross-reactivity to a minimum. Probe cross-reactivity can manifest itself in the guise of samples positive for multiple HPV types.

Under low-stringency conditions (approximately Tm − 35°C or less) the extensive cross-reactivity existing between many HPV types can be used to advantage in Southern-blot analysis (see below) to detect new types of HPV for which homologous probes are unavailable. Low-stringency hybridizations of dot blots, however, cannot be trusted because human DNA will also cross-react with HPV probes at Tm − 35°C.

## Filter in situ hybridization

This test has features of both a dot blot and an in situ procedure.[10] It facilitates the rapid analysis of samples by omitting extensive digestion and purification steps. Approximately $10^5$ exfoliated cells are filtered directly onto nitrocellulose disks using a vacuum manifold. The filters are treated with sodium hydroxide to disrupt the cells and to liberate and denature their DNA. The filters are neutralized and baked to immobilize the nucleic acids to their surfaces. Hybridizations and washes are performed according to standard procedures.

## Southern blots

Southern demonstrated in 1975 that mixtures of DNA fragments separated according to size by gel electrophoresis could subsequently be denatured and transferred to nitrocellulose filters.[16] The DNA on these filters could then be reacted with nucleic acid probes to enable the detection of specific fragments of DNA (Fig. 78-2).

It is typical to analyze 5 to 20 μg of total DNA per lane. As little as 0.5 μg per lane can be analyzed; however, this increases the chances of false-negative results. For detecting HPV, best results are obtained if samples are first digested with one or more restriction endonucleases; preferably with restriction enzymes such as *Pst* I which give distinctive patterns for different HPV types.[37] Although analysis of undigested samples is less laborious,[18,36] it is also less informative and, consequently, less accurate. Samples simply can be treated with a "stop mix" after completion of the digest and directly loaded onto agarose gels for

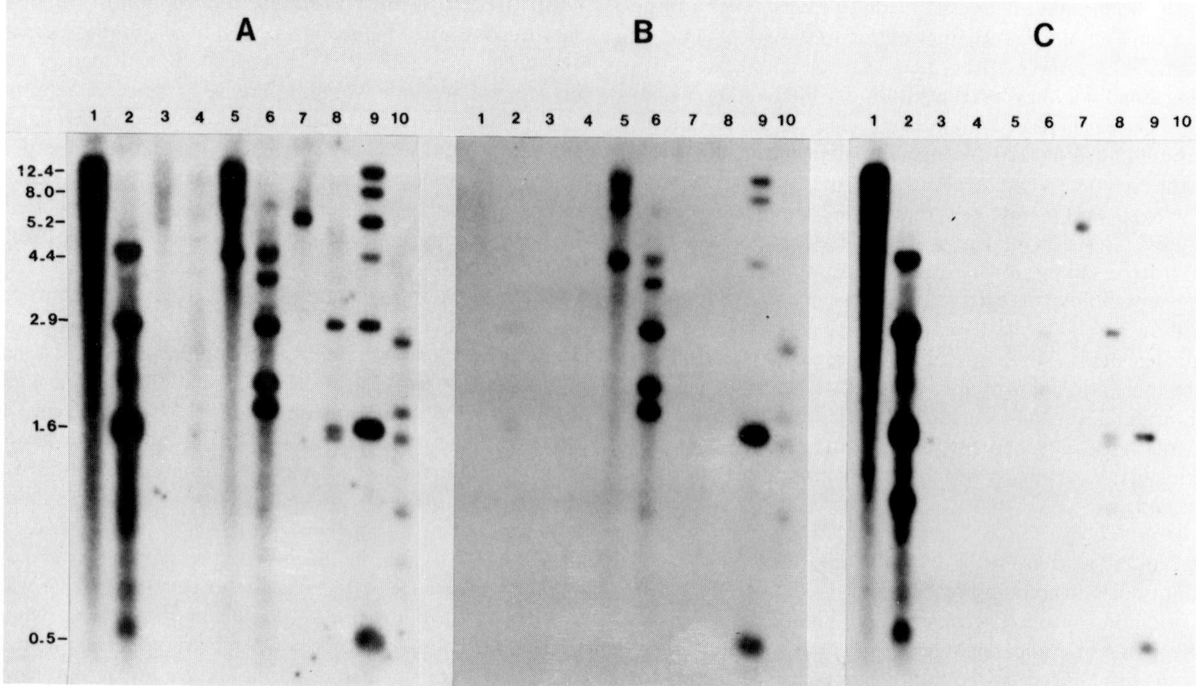


**Fig. 78-2.** Southern-blot analysis of cervical cancers. (*From Lorincz.*[6]) Total DNA was purified from five different cervical cancers, digested with *Bam*H I (lanes 1,3,5, and 7) or *Pst* I (lanes 2,4,6,8, and 10) and electrophoresed in a 1% agarose gel. DNA from the gel was blotted onto nitrocellulose and probed with $^{32}$P-labeled HPV 11 and HPV 16 at Tm −35°C (*panel A*). After autoradiography the probes were stripped from the filter which was then reprobed at Tm −10°C with HPV 16 (*panel B*). Finally, the filter was reprobed at Tm −10°C with HPV 31 (*panel C*). The cancers were determined to contain the following HPV types: 1 (lanes 1 and 2), HPV 31; 2 (lanes 3 and 4), HPV negative; 3 (lanes 5 and 6), HPV 16; 4 (lanes 7 and 8), HPV 31; and 5 (lane 10), HPV 16. Lane 9 contained molecular-size markers, whose sizes are shown to the left of panel A.

electrophoresis.[22] Many conditions for gel electrophoresis and transfer to filters are available.[22,29] It matters little which of these is used as long as good resolution of DNA fragments in the 0.5- to 10-kb range is achieved.

Southern-blot filters may be hybridized and washed at a variety of stringencies depending on the specific requirements. High-stringency conditions (Tm −10°C), like those described for dot blots, are best for routine diagnostic procedures. Low-stringency conditions (Tm −35°C to Tm −40°C) are less sensitive—with these conditions lowest background noise is obtained using nitrocellulose filters; however, these conditions enable detection (and subsequent cloning) of HPV types absent from the probe mix.

A variation of the standard Southern blot has been used occasionally for analyzing clinical samples. In this "reverse Southern blot" procedure, cloned HPV DNAs are immobilized on filters and the purified DNAs from clinical samples are labeled and used as probes.[11,38] A positive reaction is characterized by an autoradiographic signal from one or more of the immobilized DNAs.

## In situ hybridization

As its name implies, in situ hybridization detects DNA or RNA molecules within cells or within relatively intact macromolecular structures (reviewed in Refs. 26 and 33). Fixed tissues analyzed by this method provide good histological detail (Fig. 78-3). Routinely fixed and embedded tissues can be analyzed by in situ hybridization, obviating the requirement for fresh tissues. Several variations on the basic method have been published.[23–25,39–41] Detection of HPV by in situ hybridization is usually performed on tissue sections, but the use of exfoliated cells also has been reported.[42]

After sections are placed onto glass slides the tissues are deparaffinized in xylene and rehydrated through graded concentrations of ethanol. There are many different in situ procedures. Some procedures call for acetylation of tissues[24,25] to reduce background; others contain an HCl treatment to improve signal,[23,29] while yet others contain both HCl treatment and acetylation.[41] Tissues may be treated with a mild detergent followed by protease[25] or alternatively by protease digestion alone.[23,24,39,41] Many investigators postfix the tissues with paraformaldehyde.[23,25,39] This may improve signal by preventing some renaturation of DNA. After processing, the sections are usually dehydrated in graded alcohols, hybridized, and washed using conditions similar to those for filter tests. In a recently published procedure,[40] which omitted most of the usual processing steps, deparaffinized sections were boiled to denature target DNA and were probed using radioactive RNA.

## SEROLOGY

A few reports describe the detection of anti-HPV antibodies in sera. In one study,[43] antibodies cross-reactive to bovine papillomavirus type 2 antigens (derived from disrupted bovine warts) were detected in 93 percent of patients with cervical cancer, in 95 percent with anogenital condylomas, and in 60 percent with

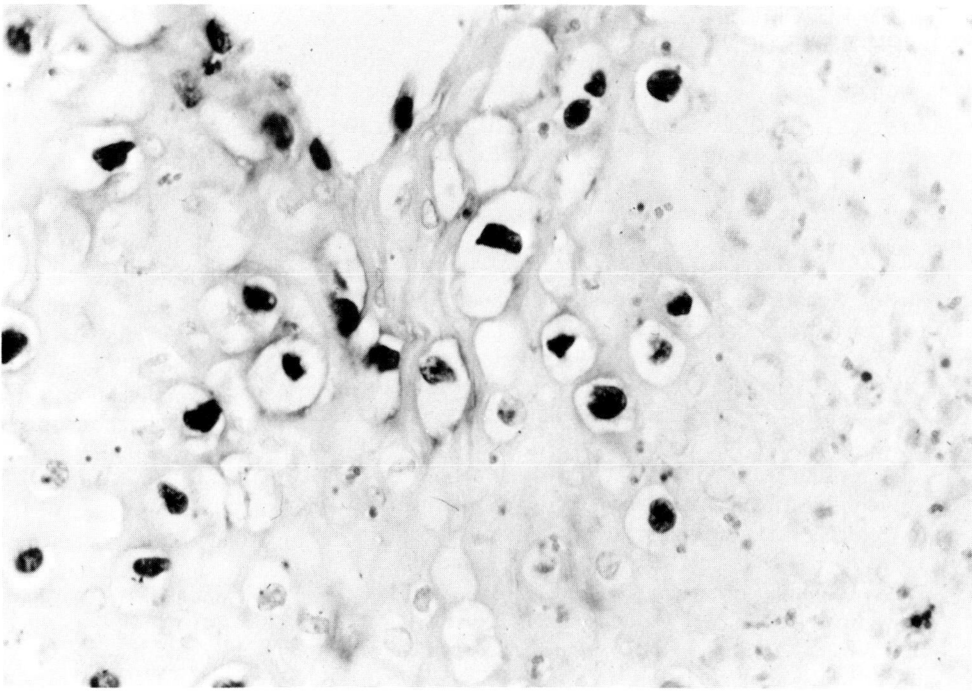

**Fig. 78-3.** HPV 6 infection of a vulvar condyloma demonstrated by in situ hybridization. (*Courtesy of M. Hammer.*) The tissue was sectioned and hybridized with biotinylated HPV 6 probe. The darkly staining nuclei of many koilocytotic cells are positive for HPV 6. Other sections from this condyloma were hybridized with HPV types 16, 18, and 31; these gave negative results.

CIN. In contrast, none of the controls (normal children and adults) were positive. Other studies have shown positive serological results using a variety of antigens such as disrupted BPV 2 warts,[44] genetically engineered recombinant HPV 6 LI proteins (Ref. 45; Jenison and Galloway personal communication), and HPV 16 E4 proteins (Gissmann personal communication). Generally, a higher percentage of sera from patients with condylomas or CIN, or from patients attending colposcopy clinics, showed positivity (≤80 percent) than controls (≤30 percent). All reactivities seen to date appear to be non-type-specific. Present serological tests are still too insensitive and nonspecific to be useful for screening or epidemiological studies; however, with the construction of more refined HPV type-specific antigens through genetic engineering or other methods, it may be possible to develop assays with suitable sensitivity and specificity.

## TEST SELECTION

There is no type of test which is optimal for every situation. Dot blots and filter in situ hybridizations are simple, inexpensive, and fast. However, as commonly performed in most research laboratories they can generate results with great variability in quality. Southern-blot analysis, on the other hand, is difficult, expensive, and time-consuming. Results can take days or even weeks to obtain. This method, however, should always be used to verify novel procedures or controversial data because of its exceptional accuracy.

An optimally performed Southern blot using restriction enzyme digestion and carefully controlled hybridization and wash conditions, will rarely, if ever, give a false-positive HPV result. This cannot be said for other methods. Spurious hybridization would not, for example, generate a characteristic *Pst* I pattern for HPV 31 as shown in Fig. 78-2. Southern-blot analysis is also highly sensitive. The detection of as little as one HPV genome per 20 human cells is possible, but requires $^{32}$P-labeled probes of high specific activity (≥3 × $10^8$ dpm/μg) and autoradiographic exposures of weeks (personal observations).

Reverse Southern-blot tests are at least 10-fold less sensitive and are also less specific than Southern blots.[11,38] Because the test samples are used as probes, there are fewer probe molecules; hence, hybridization is slower and the signal lower. In addition spurious hybridization data are not as readily recognized because of the lack of restriction enzyme patterns.

Dot blots can be more sensitive than Southern blots; however, a major disadvantage is that dot blots lack internal controls analogous to restriction enzyme patterns of Southern blots, and thus false-positive results are difficult to recognize.[11,15,28,29] These can arise from a number of sources, such as: (1) nonspecific sticking of DNA probes to sample components, which is especially troublesome with crude lysates; (2) cross-reactivity between probes and non-HPV nucleotide sequences such as human DNA or vector-like sequences; (3) cross-reactivity between HPV sequences; and (4) autoradiographic artifacts which sometimes appear as dots on x-ray film. Many of these problems can be eliminated through careful quality control during reagent preparation and optimization of procedures, as, for example, with the ViraPap method noted earlier.

Filter in situ hybridization shares many of the features of dot blots.[10] It is quick and easy to perform but is prone to false-positives for the same reasons as dot blots. In addition, in our hands filter in situ hybridization is somewhat less sensitive than regular dot blots.

In situ hybridization is suitable for analyzing paraffin-embedded tissues. Most protocols are technically more demanding than some of the simple filter tests. Highly sensitive procedures utilizing RNA probes have been developed.[24,40] Radiolabeled probes offer greater sensitivity and specificity, but nonradioactive probes are easier to use.[23,26,33] Although in situ tests are widely regarded as highly accurate, there have been no carefully controlled and sufficiently large studies performed correlating in situ to Southern-blot hybridization to fully assess the quality of in situ tests.

## DETAILED RECOMMENDATIONS FOR HPV DETECTION

All hybridization tests must be carefully monitored to detect erroneous results. There are many ways in which false-negative results can occur. For example, the sample may be taken or stored improperly, the hybridization may fail, and so on. If a false-negative result is suspected, a new sample should be taken a few weeks later and reanalyzed. Every laboratory test must be accompanied by positive and negative controls. Positive controls consist of banks of samples containing known amounts of HPV DNA which are included in each analysis to ensure that signal generation is working properly. There are two types of positive controls: (1) sensitivity controls (range approximately 1 to 100 pg) and (2) cross-reactivity controls (several hundred picograms of various types of HPV DNAs). If a test fails to detect 1 pg of HPV DNA, it is not sufficiently sensitive (personal observation). Cross-reactivity controls are required when HPV-type information is sought. Controls performed with low concentrations of potentially cross-reactive DNAs are not valid, because clinical samples may contain hundreds of picograms of HPV DNA. At this level unrelated HPV types can show extensive cross-reactivity, especially if stringency is not properly regulated. Negative controls are samples which are known to be free of HPV DNA or which mimic as closely as possible true negative clinical samples. Several of these should be run with each batch of tests; if any are positive the entire set of test results should be suspect.

The clinical relevance of a positive HPV DNA result in the absence of a demonstrated lesion is still uncertain. If no lesion is detectable by colposcopy or on cytology (1) the HPV DNA may be derived from a latent infection; (2) the lesion may be extremely small and well hidden; or (3) the lesion may be located elsewhere in the genital tract.[8–11] Alternatively, the Pap smear may be falsely negative due either to missampling or misreading. Our own studies (Ref. 8 and unpublished) suggest that an apparently normal Pap smear is much more likely to be falsely negative if the sample is HPV positive than if it is HPV negative. Therefore, in the absence of other evidence of CIN or condylomas, women who are HPV positive deserve follow-up cytology and colposcopy when appropriate, especially if the samples are positive for HPV types strongly associated with cervical cancer, such as types 16, 18, or 35.[2,3,5] Knowledge of HPV type may be useful in cases of borderline abnormalities detected by Pap smear; with these it is often difficult to decide if there is a need for treatment. In contrast, obvious lesions containing HPV DNA (regardless of type) are presently treated identically to those which are HPV-negative because for individual patients it is not possible to guarantee that any given condylomatous or neoplastic lesion is totally benign. Additional large studies are needed, however, to clarify further the optimal use of HPV tests in the clinical setting.

## FUTURE DIRECTIONS

Commonly used tests are technically demanding and slow. The most sensitive and reliable methods utilize radiolabeled probes which present special problems in the clinical laboratory. Simpler nucleic acid tests are being developed. Sandwich hybridization[46] is one novel method which may simplify future HPV testing. Another procedure called the polymerase chain reaction (PCR) has generated excitement, as it has the power to amplify DNA sequences many-thousand-fold.[47] The method requires a knowledge of the nucleotide sequences flanking the target DNA in order to generate oligonucleotide primers of 20 to 25 bases which mediate cycles of DNA synthesis. The target DNA is selectively amplified through repeated cycles of denaturation, primer hybridization, and primer extension with either DNA polymerase 1 (Klenow fragment) on the thermo-tolerant DNA polymerase *Taq* 1. The target DNA concentration increases almost exponentially, and after 30 cycles over 100,000 copies of target DNA can be achieved. The target DNA is then detected by one of the conventional methods such as dot blot, Southern blot, or even gel electrophoresis and ethidium staining of the DNA fragments. PCR has been used to detect HPV 16 and HPV 18 DNA in single sections of paraffin-embedded tissue biopsies from CIN or cervical cancer, [48] and in samples of normal cervical cells.[49] The L1 region of the HPV genome seems to be a particularly good region for PCR amplification as it is one of the most conserved regions, and a carefully chosen pair of primers may be able to detect all HPV types. A potential problem with PCR may be its extremely high sensitivity. It is prone to false-positives due to laboratory contamination of even a few copies of target DNA. Although most laboratory contamination can be eliminated by careful procedure, contamination of samples in the physician's office is another possibility. The utility of PCR in HPV detection must be assessed by studies which focus particularly on the clinical relevance of very low levels of HPV DNA.

# References


1 Gissmann L et al: Human papillomavirus types 6 and 11 DNA sequences in genital and laryngeal papillomas and in some cervical cancers. *Proc Natl Acad Sci USA* 80:560, 1983.

2 Durst M et al: A papillomavirus DNA from a cervical carcinoma and its prevalence in cancer biopsy samples from different geographic regions. *Proc Natl Acad Sci USA* 80:3812, 1983.

3 Boshart M et al: A new type of papillomavirus DNA, its presence in genital cancer biopsies and in cell lines derived from cervical cancer. *EMBO J* 3:1151, 1984.

4 Lorincz AT et al: Cloning and characterization of the DNA of a new human papillomavirus from a woman with dysplasia of the uterine cervix. *J Virol* 58:225, 1986.

5 Lorincz AT et al: A new type of papillomavirus associated with cancer of the uterine cervix. *Virology* 159:187, 1987.

6 Lorincz AT et al: Oncogenic association of specific human papillomavirus types with cervical neoplasia. *J Natl Cancer Inst* 79:671, 1987.

7 Beaudenon S et al: A novel type of human papillomavirus associated with genital neoplasias. *Nature* 321:246, 1986.

8 Lorincz AT et al: Correlation of cellular atypia and human papillomavirus deoxyribonucleic acid sequences in exfoliated cells of the uterine cervix. *Obstet Gynecol* 68:508, 1986.

9 Toon PG et al: Human papillomavirus infection of the uterine cervix of women without cytological signs of neoplasia. *Br Med J* 293:1261, 1986.

10 Wagner D et al: Identification of human papillomavirus in cervical smears by deoxyribonucleic acid *in situ* hybridization. *Obstet Gynecol* 64:767, 1984.

11 Fife KH et al: Symptomatic and asymptomatic cervical infections with human papillomavirus during pregnancy. *J Infect Dis* 156:904, 1987.

12 Broker T, Botchan M: Papillomaviruses: Retrospectives and prospectives, in *Cancer Cells* 4, *DNA Tumor Viruses,* MT Botchan et al (ed). New York, Cold Spring Harbor Laboratory, 1986, p 17.

13 Jenson AB et al: Immunologic relatedness of papillomaviruses from different species. *N Natl Cancer Inst* 64:495, 1980.

14 Guillet G et al: Papillomaviruses in cervical condylomas with and without associated cervical intraepithelial neoplasia. *J Invest Dermatol* 81:513, 1983.

15 Lorincz AT: Detection of human papillomavirus infection by nucleic acid hybridization, in *Obstetrics and Gynecology Clinics of North*

*America*, R Reid (ed). Philadelphia, Saunders, 1987, vol 14, p 451.

16 Southern EM: Detection of specific sequences among DNA fragments separated by gel electrophoresis. *J Mol Biol* 98:503, 1975.

17 Yoshikawa H et al: Occurrence of human papillomavirus types 16 and 18 DNA in cervical carcinomas from Japan: Age of patients and histological type of carcinomas. *Jpn J Cancer Res* 76:667, 1985.

18 Crum C et al: Cervical papillomaviruses segregate within morphologically distinct precancerous lesions. *J Virol* 54:675, 1985.

19 zur Hausen H et al: EBV DNA in biopsies of 20 Burkitt tumors and anaplastic carcinomas of the nasopharynx. *Nature* 228:1056, 1970.

20 Krieg P et al: The simultaneous extraction of high-molecular-weight DNA and of RNA from solid tumors. *Anal Biochem* 134:288, 1983.

21 Burke RD et al: Human papillomavirus infection of the cervix detected by cervicovaginal lavage and molecular hybridization: Correlation with biopsy results and Papanicolaou smear. *Am J Obstet Gynecol* 154:982, 1986.

22 Maniatis T et al: *Molecular Cloning: A Laboratory Manual.* New York, Cold Spring Harbor Laboratory, 1982, p 1.

23 Crum CP et al: *In situ* hybridization analysis of HPV 16 DNA sequences in early cervical neoplasia. *Am J Pathol* 123:174, 1986.

24 Stoler MH, Broker TR: *In situ* hybridization detection of human papillomavirus DNAs and messenger RNAs in genital condylomas and a cervical carcinoma. *Hum Pathol* 17:1250, 1986.

25 Ostrow RS et al: Detection of human papillomavirus DNA in invasive carcinomas of the cervix by *in situ* hybridization. *Cancer Res* 47: 649, 1987.

26 Nagai N et al: Detection of papillomavirus nucleic acids in genital precancers with the *in situ* hybridization technique. *Int J Gynecol Pathol* 6:366, 1987.

27 Schneider A et al: Papillomavirus infection of the lower genital tract: Detection of viral DNA in gynecological swabs. *Int J Cancer* 35:443, 1985.

28 Pater MM et al: Human papillomavirus types 16 and 18 sequences in early cervical neoplasia. *Virology* 155:13, 1986.

29 Meinkoth J, Wahl G: Hybridization of nucleic acids immobilized on solid supports. *Anal Biochem* 138:267, 1984.

30 Chromczynski P, Qasba PK: Alkaline transfer of DNA to plastic membrane. *Biochem Biophys Res Commun* 122:340, 1984.

31 Rigby PJW et al: Labelling deoxyribonucleic acid to high specific activity *in vitro* by nick translation with DNA polymerase 1. *J Mol Biol* 113:237, 1977.

32 Leary JJ et al: Rapid and sensitive colorimetric methods for visualizing biotin labeled DNA probes hybridized to DNA or RNA immobilized on nitrocellulose: Bio blots. *Proc Natl Acad Sci USA* 80:4045, 1983.

33 Moench TR: *In situ* hybridization. *Mol Cell Probes* 1:195, 1987.

34 Little PFR: Application of plasmids containing promoters specific for phage-encoded RNA polymerases, in *DNA Cloning III. A Practical Approach*, DM Glover (ed). Washington DC, IRL Press, 1987, p 1.

35 Hames BD, Higgins SJ: *Nucleic Acid Hybridization. A Practical Approach.* Washington DC, IRL Press, 1985, p 3.

36 Okagaki T et al: Identification of human papillomavirus DNA in cervical and vaginal intraepithelial neoplasia with molecularly cloned virus-specific DNA probes. *Int J Gynecol Pathol* 2:153, 1983.

37 Lorincz AT et al: Characterization of human papillomaviruses in cervical neoplasias and their detection in routine clinical screening, in *Banbury Report* 21: *Viral Etiology of Cervical Cancer*, H zur Hausen, T Peto (eds). New York, Cold Spring Harbor Laboratory, 1986, p 225.

38 de Villiers E-M et al: Papillomavirus DNA in human tongue carcinomas. *Int J Cancer* 36:575, 1985.

39 Beckmann AM et al: Detection and localization of human papillomavirus DNA in human genital condylomas by *in situ* hybridization with biotinylated probes. *J Med Virol* 16:265, 1985.

40 Schneider A et al: Distribution pattern of human papilloma virus 16 genome in cervical neoplasia by molecular *in situ* hybridization of tissue sections. *Int J Cancer* 39:717, 1987.

41 Gupta J, Shah KV: Human papillomaviruses in genital tissue: Examination by immunohistochemistry and *in situ* DNA hybridization, in *Herpes and Papilloma Viruses. Their Role in the Carcinogenesis of the Lower Genital Tract*, G DiPaolo et al (eds). New York, Raven, 1986, p 199.

42 Gupta JW et al: Detection of human papillomavirus in cervical smears. A comparison of *in situ* hybridization, immunocytochemistry and cytopathology. *Acta Cytol* 31:387, 1987.

43 Baird PJ: Serological evidence for the association of papillomavirus and cervical neoplasia. *Lancet* 2:17, 1983.

44 Beiss BK et al: Host immune responses to genital and laryngeal human papillomavirus infections, in *Cancer Cells 5*, *Papillomaviruses*, BM Steinberg et al (eds). New York, Cold Spring Harbor Laboratory, 1987, p 387.

45 Li C-CH et al: Identification of the human papillomavirus type 6b LI open reading frame protein in condylomas and corresponding antibodies in human sera. *J Virol* 61:2684, 1987.

46 Ranki M et al: Sandwich hybridization as a convenient method for detection of nucleic acids in crude samples. *Gene* 21:77, 1983.

47 Saiki RK et al: Enzymatic amplification of β-globin genomic sequences and restriction site analysis for diagnosis of sickle cell anemia. *Science* 230:1350, 1985.

48 Shibata DK et al: Detection of human papilloma virus in paraffin-embedded tissue using the polymerase chain reaction. *J Exp Med* 167:225, 1988.

49 Shibata DK et al: Detection of human papillomavirus in normal and dysplastic tissue by the polymerase chain reaction. *Lab Invest* 59:555, 1988.

# Chapter 79

# Immunodiagnosis of human immunodeficiency virus infections

Lynn Goldstein

## INTRODUCTION

The etiologic agent of acquired immunodeficiency syndrome (AIDS) is a retrovirus now known as human immunodeficiency virus (HIV).[1,2] Membership in this group of viruses is expanding. At the moment, there are two fully characterized types; HIV-1 is the major isolate responsible for the world pandemic, and HIV-2, which is distinct from HIV-1, has been isolated from AIDS patients in West Africa.[3–5] The detection of HIV infection is not necessarily synonymous with AIDS, as individuals infected with HIV may develop a spectrum of clinical syndromes, including asymptomatic infection (70 percent), lymphadenopathy (20 percent), AIDS-related complex (ARC) and full-blown AIDS (10 percent).[6] Identification of infected individuals is usually determined by the presence of antibody reactive with the retrovirus.[7,8] This antibody response to the virus has been shown to be indicative of infection, since virus can be isolated from the majority of HIV seropositive individuals.[9,10]

An estimated 1 to 2 million people in the United States currently are infected with HIV, and at least 300,000 have clinical symptoms.[6] Patients present throughout the spectrum of the illness, from an asymptomatic carrier state, with nonspecific general complaints such as fatigue and weight loss, or with more severe and disabling illnesses. Generally, the clinical suspicion of an AIDS diagnosis is not very difficult given the appropriate signs, symptoms, and a history of membership in a high-risk group for HIV infection; homosexual-bisexual male, intravenous drug user, recipient of multiple blood product transfusions, heterosexual contact with a high-risk or HIV seropositive partner, native of certain areas of Central Africa or Haiti, prostitute from certain urban areas, or child born to parents who are members of these risk groups. A major challenge arises when diagnosing HIV infection in the asymptomatic individual who has atypical signs and symptoms, or who denies membership in a high-risk group. Current approaches to immunodiagnosis of HIV infection are outlined in Table 79-1.

## ANTIBODY DETECTION

### ENZYME IMMUNOASSAYS

Enzyme immunoassays were first developed to detect HIV antibodies in infected potential blood donors.[7,8,11] These tests have now been adopted for screening high-risk groups for HIV infections.[12,13] Following the initial screening procedure, more specific tests confirm the diagnosis.

To understand the basis for serologic testing, a brief review of the HIV antigens is helpful. HIV has three major structural genes—*gag, pol,*and *env*—each of which codes for one or more proteins expressed in infected cells or in the mature virus (see Chap. 28). The *gag* gene encodes the major core proteins, including p55, a precursor polypeptide of 55 kilodaltons, which is cleaved to form p24 and p18. The *pol* gene encodes three proteins: p66 and p51, both known to have reverse transcriptase activity, and the nuclease-integrase, p31. The *env* gene encodes a precursor glycoprotein of 160 kilodaltons, gp160, which is cleaved into the surface glycoprotein gp120 and the transmembrane protein gp41. HIV-infected persons produce a spectrum of antibodies to all or some of these proteins.

A prototype enzyme immunoassay procedure is shown in Fig. 79-1. The test detects antibodies to multiple viral proteins, since a whole virus lysate is used as the target antigen. The antigen is produced from virus grown and purified from established human tissue culture T cell lines such as H9 or CEM.[2,14] Serum samples are incubated with the viral lysate, and antibody to HIV is detected with enzyme-labeled antihuman antibody and substrate. Serum samples that the enzyme immunoassay shows to be "initially reactive" are repeat tested in duplicate to rule out technical errors in test performance. If either repeat test is positive, the sample is considered "repeatably reactive." To rule out false-positive enzyme immunoassay results, these reactive specimens are then tested by a confirmatory method.

Clinical studies have shown that the enzyme immunoassay procedure has greater than 99 percent sensitivity and specificity in both low-risk blood donors and high-risk populations.[12–16] The predictive value of a positive result, however, varies with the population tested owing to differences in prevalence of the infection in low- and high-risk populations. The sensitivity of the test is defined as the probability that a person who has antibody to HIV will be positive in the test. Specificity is the probability that a person who does not have antibody to HIV will be negative in

**Table 79-1. Immunodiagnosis of HIV Infection**

1. *Enzyme Immunoassays*
   - Widely available and the primary diagnostic test
   - Defined sensitivity and specificity
   - Sensitivity and specificity may be improved with recombinant viral proteins and synthetic peptides
   - Positive predictive value varies with prevalence of exposure in the population and usually requires confirmatory testing by Western blot, immunofluorescence, or radioimmunoprecipitation
2. *Confirmatory Methods*
   - Western blot most widely accepted
   - Radioimmunoprecipitation and immunofluorescence are alternative methods
   - Sensitivity and specificity may vary owing to laboratory methodology and test interpretation
3. *Second-Generation Tests*
   - Use recombinant DNA technology or chemically synthesized peptides
   - May have improved sensitivity and specificity
   - Major immunodominant region defined within the *env* gene glycoprotein
4. *Antigen Detection*
   - Investigational
   - Undefined sensitivity and specificity for clinical specimens
   - Solid-phase radioimmunoassay and enzyme immunoassay usually detect >50 pg of p24 antigen/ml of serum; requires confirmation by p24 antigen neutralization

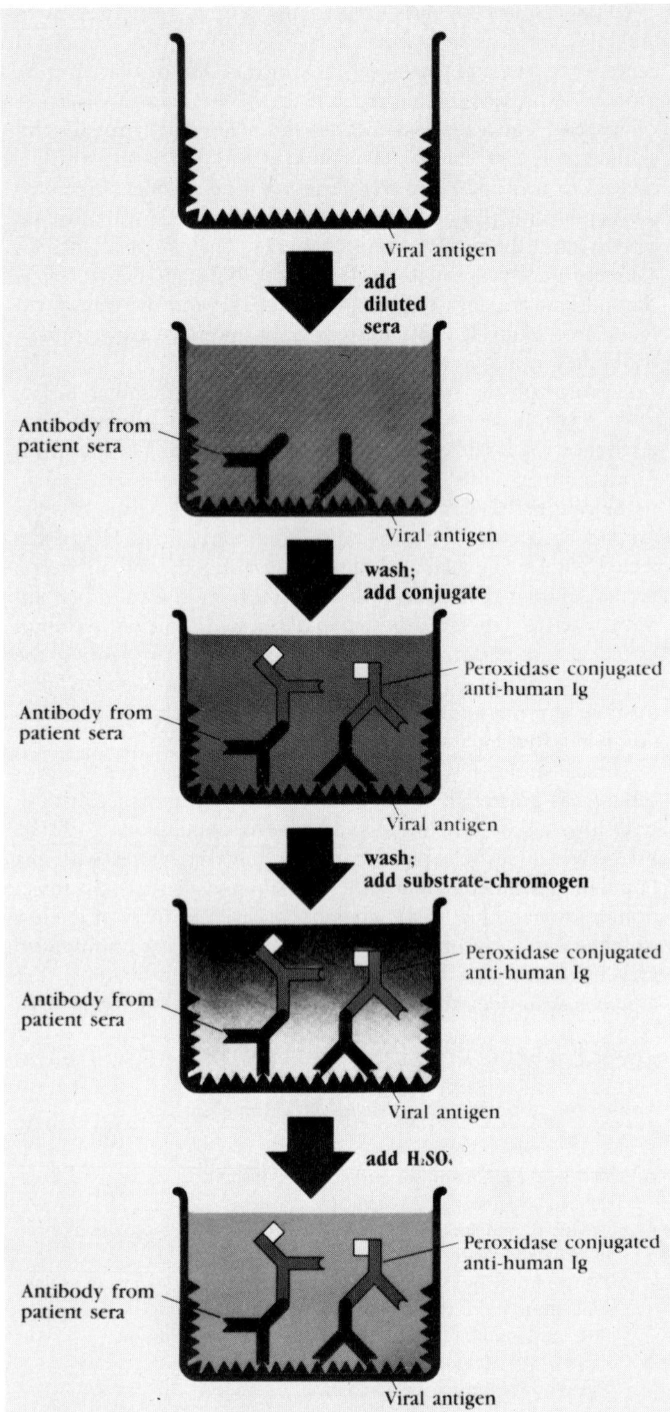


**Fig. 79-1.** A prototypical enzyme immunoassay procedure. (1) The purified, inactivated virus is absorbed onto wells of a microwell plate. (2) Samples to be tested are diluted in sample diluent and added to each well, incubated with the adsorbed antigen, and washed. If antibodies to the virus are present, they bind to antigen and are removed by washing. (3) The conjugate reagent, peroxidase-labeled goat antihuman immunoglobulin, is then added to the wells and will bind to the antibody-antigen complex, if present. Unbound conjugate is removed by a wash step. (4) Next, chromogen reagent is added to the plate and allowed to incubate. A blue or blue-green color develops in proportion to the amount of antibody bound to the antigen-coated plate. (5) The addition of acid stops the enzyme reaction, resulting in a color change to yellow. The optical absorbance of controls and specimens is determined with a spectrophotometer with wavelength set at 450 nm.

the test. The predictive value of a positive test is the probability that a person has antibody to HIV when the test is positive. For example, the Genetic Systems LAV enzyme immunoassay was tested on 9703 serum and plasma samples from blood donation centers from cities considered both high- and low-risk for HIV infection.[14] In this population, 21 specimens were repeatably reactive and 14 of 21 were positive by a confirmatory method, demonstrating 100 percent sensitivity and 99.9 percent specificity. The predictive value of a positive enzyme immunoassay result in this population with low prevalence (<1 percent) of disease thus was 67 percent. In studies from 1414 patients from a high-risk group, the sensitivity of the enzyme immunoassay compared with the confirmatory method was 99.9 percent (875 positive/876 confirmatory positive) and the specificity was 99.9 percent (537 negative/538 confirmatory negative). Since this population had a high prevalence of infection (66 percent), the enzyme immunoassay's positive predictive value was 99.9 percent.[13] In general, it is important to have a bimodal distribution of nonreactive and reactive results (that is, no "gray area" of overlap between reactives and nonreactives) independent of the population tested to achieve maximum sensitivity and specificity in the enzyme immunoassay.

Compared with other test formats, the enzyme immunoassay has the advantages of sensitivity, specificity, and ease of automation for time and cost reductions. Several problems can occur with the procedure, however, that may give false-positive or false-negative results. False-positive results are most often due to reactions to some specific cellular antigens in the cell line used to produce the virus.[17,18] Circulating antibodies to HLA, nuclear, and other cellular antigens can be seen in patients with autoimmune disease, lymphoproliferative disorders, in multiparous women, and in people who have received multiple transfusions. False-negative results may be due either to diminished antibody associated with late-stage disease, or to the lack of detectable antibody soon after initial infection.

Current enzyme immunoassay screens are designed to detect antibody to HIV-1. They do not reliably detect antibody to HIV-2 in blood from all persons with HIV-2 infection because HIV-1 and HIV-2 exhibit only limited antigenic cross-reactivity mostly between *gag* and *pol* proteins. Current enzyme immunoassays for HIV-1 detect between 42 and 96 percent of HIV-2 infections.[19]

## CONFIRMATORY TESTS

Following enzyme immunoassay screening, repeatably reactive specimens are tested by a confirmatory method to assure the specificity of the reaction.[20,21] Confirmatory methods include those that detect antibody to individual viral proteins, such as Western blot or radioimmunoprecipitation, and those that use infected cultured cells to detect antibody, such as immunofluorescence.[22–24]

The Western blot, shown in Fig. 79-2, is the most commonly used method to confirm specific antibody responses to HIV viral proteins. Purified HIV viral proteins are electrophoresed in sodium dodecyl sulfate gels and transferred to nitrocellulose paper. The paper is then incubated with the serum sample, and specific antibody is detected with an enzyme-conjugated, antihuman antibody and enzyme substrate. Most human sera that contain antibodies to the virus react with a constellation of viral proteins representing envelope (gp160, 120, gp41) or core (p55, p31, p24, p18) or both (lane g, Fig. 79-2). Using conservative criteria, serum specimens which show reactions to both the viral glycoproteins

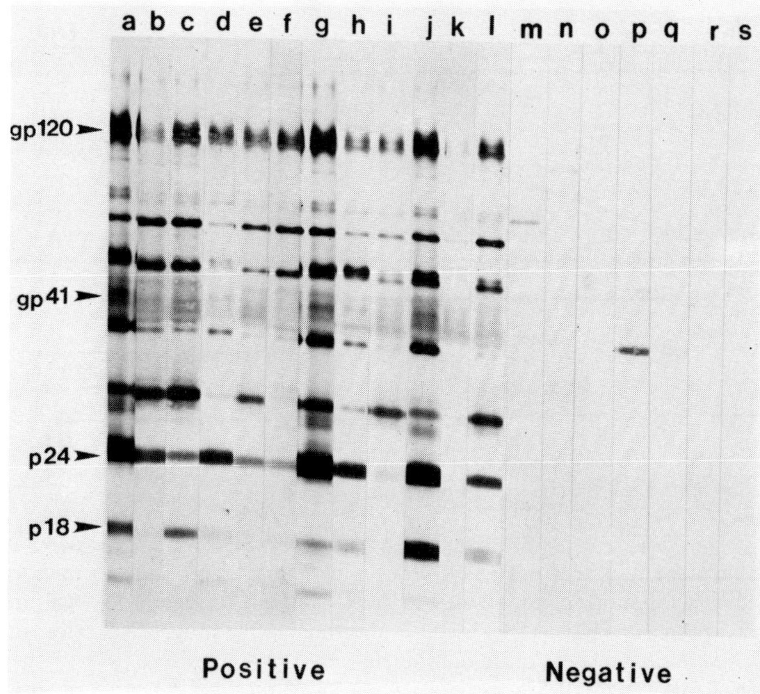


Fig. 79-2. Western blot of sera positive and negative for antibody to specific HIV viral proteins. Purified HIV viral proteins are electrophoresed on gels, transferred to paper, and antibody is detected by an enzymatic assay. Sera positive for antibody to HIV react with glycoproteins (gp160, 120, 41) or core proteins (p55, p34, p24, p18) or both, as demonstrated in lanes a–l. Sera negative for antibody to HIV do not react with HIV viral proteins, as demonstrated in lanes m–s.

and the core proteins are considered positive for antibody to HIV. Specimens which show no reactions or reactions to nonviral proteins are considered negative for antibody to HIV and represent false-positive results by enzyme immunoassay. A small percentage of sera reacts only with single-core proteins (p24, p18, or p55). The specificity of antibodies to a single-core protein of HIV and the significance of these reactions is uncertain; therefore, this reaction pattern is called atypical or indeterminant.

The Western blot has demonstrated greater than 99 percent sensitivity and specificity, but the procedure is time-consuming, labor-intensive, and subjective. The method is less sensitive for detection of antibodies to the viral glycoproteins (gp120, gp41) and very sensitive for antibodies to viral core proteins (p24). The Western blot's use to confirm enzyme immunoassay results is especially important in populations with a low prevalence of infection. In some high-risk populations, the predictive value of a positive enzyme immunoassay result is greater than 99 percent and a confirmatory method may not be necessary.

Radioimmunoprecipitation is another method that detects antibody to specific viral proteins.[22] HIV viral proteins are radiolabeled with amino acids, and lysates are incubated with the serum sample. Following washing procedures, the radiolabeled proteins binding to the antibodies are electrophoresed on sodium dodecyl sulfate gels and detected by autoradiography. This procedure is less adaptable to a clinical laboratory than the Western blot but may be more sensitive in detecting viral glycoproteins.

Immunofluorescence is a third method of detecting HIV antibody.[25,26] A serum sample is incubated with HIV-infected cells fixed to microscope slides. Specific antibody is detected by fluorescein-labeled, antihuman antibody, and positive cells are visualized using the fluorescence microscope. The method has been demonstrated to be as sensitive and specific as the Western blot in laboratories experienced with this technique. It is relatively simple and inexpensive, but it can be subjective and is not widely available.

## SECOND-GENERATION TESTS

To develop more sensitive and specific tests for HIV, second-generation assays have used recombinant DNA technology or synthetic peptide chemistry to detect antibodies to specific viral proteins. Viral glycoproteins encoded by the *env* gene (gp41) and core proteins from the *gag* gene (p24) have been expressed in *Escherichia coli* and have been used in enzyme immunoassay and Western blot assay formats.[27–34] The recombinant proteins from the *env* region, in particular those encoding the carboxy terminus of gp120 and amino terminus of gp41, have shown greater than 99 percent sensitivity. The immunodominant regions of the viral glycoprotein are presented in Fig. 79-3. Analysis of recombinants from the *gag* gene show that the immune response has more diverse reactivity, compared with that in the *env* region. Therefore, recombinants in the *gag* region show approximately 80 percent sensitivity for anti-p24 antibodies compared with Western blot.[35]

An alternative approach is to use chemically synthesized peptides representing immunodominant regions of the viral proteins.[36–40] Viral peptides have been synthesized using the Merrifield solid-phase method from viral protein sequences representing both *env* and *gag* genes. It has been demonstrated that a 25 amino acid sequence from the gp41 protein of the virus has greater than 99 percent sensitivity and represents the major immunodominant epitope reactive with patient sera (Fig. 79-3).[36,37] Synthetic peptides from the corresponding region of HIV-2 have also been used in sensitive and specific immunoassays for HIV-2 infection.[41] Synthetic peptides may be more sensitive and specific than the recombinant proteins because they are not contaminated by bacterial or mammalian cell proteins.

Both recombinant proteins and synthetic peptides offer the advantages of cost, safety, and manufacturing reliability. They also may be more sensitive and specific because the target antigens do not contain cellular contaminants present in many enzyme im-

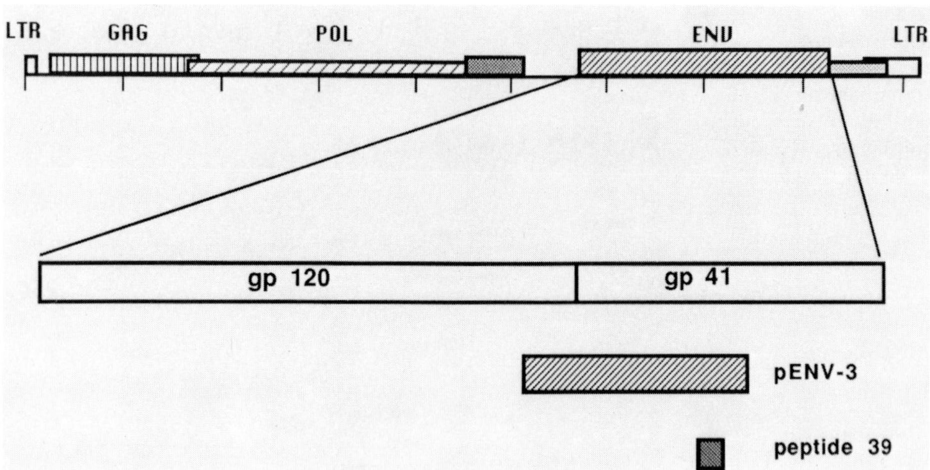


**Fig. 79-3.** Viral glycoproteins from the *env* gene produced by recombinant DNA technology and chemical peptide synthesis. The immunodominant regions are represented by the recombinant protein (penv3) and the synthetic peptide (peptide 39).

munoassay tests that use whole viral lysates. In addition, individual viral antigens can be used to detect antibody to separate viral proteins. This may be useful in determining the prognosis of seropositive people, since individuals with AIDS-related complex (ARC) and AIDS appear to have a lower titer and lower prevalence of anti-*gag* (p24) antibodies. A disadvantage of these antigens may be that they differ from the native protein because they contain only a portion of the gene product and are denatured proteins. Finally, these synthetic antigens offer the sensitivity and specificity to be used in rapid tests (less than 30 min) which are simple to perform, economical, and stable.[31,42]

## ANTIBODY RESPONSE TO HIV INFECTION

Persons infected with HIV develop antibody to the virus within 4 to 12 weeks of infection as detected in currently available enzyme immunoassays.[43,44] In one report, antibody to the virus was not detected for up to 6 to 14 months.[45] The initial antibody response is directed to the core proteins (p24) as evaluated by Western blot and to the glycoproteins (gp160, gp41) as evaluated by radioimmunoprecipitation, recombinant DNA technology, and synthetic peptides.[15] A majority of infected people then develop antibody to all of the viral proteins including core proteins and glycoproteins. In longitudinal studies it has been shown that the antibody response to the glycoproteins remains stable throughout the disease course, while the antibody response to the p24 core protein tends to decline.[46–50]

Antibodies can be detected in a variety of body fluids from infected persons, including blood, saliva, cerebrospinal fluid, and cervical secretions.[51–53] Detection of antibodies in blood remains the most sensitive method.

## ANTIGEN DETECTION

### ANTIGEN IMMUNOASSAYS

Third-generation tests have been developed that detect HIV viral antigen.[35,54] These assays utilize an antigen detection immunoassay format in which specific anti-HIV antibody (monoclonal or polyclonal) is used to capture HIV antigen. Enzyme-labeled, anti-HIV antibody and enzyme substrate are then used to detect the antibody-antigen complex. Current assays detect the p24 core antigen.[55] These tests can be used to detect antigen during viral culture, replacing the tedious method of monitoring for reverse transcriptase, the viral enzyme[55,56] (see Chapter 80).

The tests also have been used to detect antigen in serum specimens.[54–57] A theoretical profile of antigen and antibody detection in infected persons is represented in Fig. 79-4. Studies show that very early after infection, antigen is present for a short time in the serum before circulating antibody develops. This may correlate with an acute clinical syndrome characterized by fever, rash, myalagia-arthralgias, and pharyngitis[58–60] (see Chapter 30). The "window" of antigen ranges from 2 weeks to 2 months or more after acquiring infection. The level of antigen present during this time may fluctuate. Following the development of serum antibody, the presence of antigen is absent or variable in infected patients. Subsequently, more people who have ARC and AIDS have detectable serum p24 antigen than do healthy, seropositive people.[57,61] The relationship between the presence of p24 antigen, HIV recovery from plasma, and the lower titer of antibody to p24 in patients with AIDS or ARC remains to be determined.[62–65] It has been suggested, however, that the presence of p24 antigen may indicate a poorer clinical prognosis.[61] It has been reported that persons treated with the HIV antiviral drug zidovudine (formerly known as azidothymidine or AZT) may show a reduced amount of circulating antigen.[66] The antigen test, therefore, may be useful to monitor patients on antiviral chemotherapy. Finally, the presence of antigen in cerebrospinal fluid has been associated with progressive encephalopathy in AIDS patients.[67] Therefore, detection of antigen may correlate with particular clinical syndromes and may be useful for differential diagnosis.

## HIV TESTING IN CLINICAL PRACTICE

### THE DIAGNOSTIC SETTING

The following example demonstrates how a variety of HIV diagnostic tests may be used clinically. A patient reports fatigue and weight loss to a physician. After taking a medical history, the physician determines that the patient is a member of a high-risk group for HIV infection. Following consent, the patient's serum is tested for antibody to HIV by enzyme immunoassay. If the serum is repeatably reactive to enzyme immunoassay, it is then tested by Western blot to confirm the presence of specific anti-

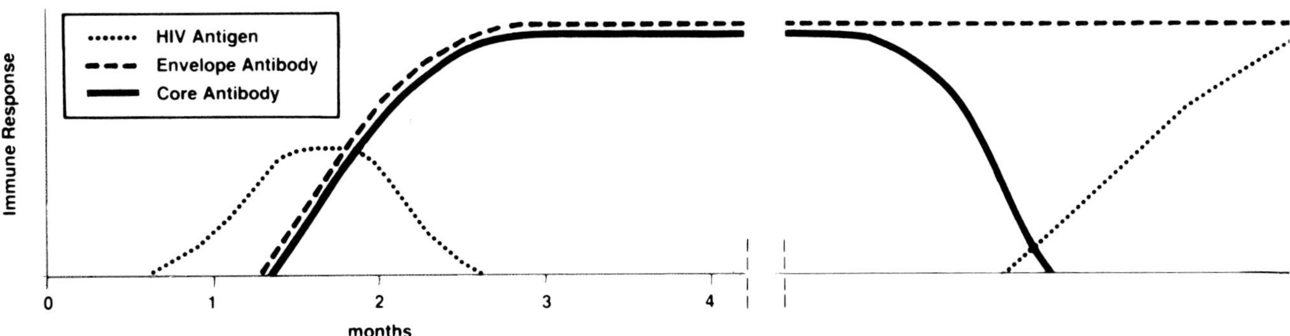


Fig. 79-4. Hypothetical time course for occurrence of specific serum markers following HIV infection. Viral antigen (p24) appears early, followed by antibody to envelope and core proteins. As the disease progresses, antibody to the core protein (p24) declines and viral antigen appears.

body to HIV viral proteins. If positive, the patient is then counseled and followed for changes in clinical status. In the future, it is likely that such patients may be tested for specific antibody to the core protein p24 using second-generation assays, or for the presence of the p24 core antigen. If there is a lower titer of antibody to p24 or if antigen is present in serum, the patient may need closer monitoring for disease progression. A patient treated with anti-HIV chemotherapy may be monitored for drug efficacy by assays for the presence of viral antigen or viral nucleic acid.

## INTERPRETATION OF HIV ANTIBODY TEST RESULTS

Current screening programs for HIV antibody use a sequence of tests. This starts with a repeatably reactive enzyme immunoassay followed by a more specific assay, such as a Western blot. The sensitivity of immunoassays is greater than 99 percent; therefore, the probability of a false-negative result is remote except very early in infection before antibody is detectable. The specificity of the currently licensed antibody tests is greater than 99 percent. Confirmatory tests are intended to distinguish the false-positive results of enzyme immunoassays from those that truly represent HIV infection. A positive confirmatory test is now considered to be conclusive evidence for HIV infection.

The Western blot is the most commonly used confirmatory test in the clinical laboratory and is highly specific when strict criteria are used for interpretation. When routine Western blot confirmation was initiated in 1985, a band indicating antibody to the p24 core protein was regarded as evidence of infection. It has now been shown that apparent bands in this region represent artifacts and are not specific for HIV infection.[68–70] In order to distinguish reactions to the p24 band which represent artifact from those that represent the early antibody response to HIV, it has been suggested that the Western blot be repeated in 1 to 2 months. If the reaction is due to HIV infection, antibodies to the other viral proteins, including the glycoprotein, should be present at that time. In the future, Western blots may be replaced by highly specific second-generation tests which distinguish true HIV infections from false-positive antibody reactions.[31]

Ideally, the probability that a testing sequence will be falsely positive in a low-incidence population ranges from less than 1 in 100,000 to an estimated 5 in 100,000.[71] Currently, clinical laboratories should establish quality-control procedures and participate in performance evaluations in order to assure consistent quality in performance of HIV tests.

## GUIDELINES FOR HIV ANTIBODY TESTING

Serologic testing to confirm HIV infection has two important functions: to establish a diagnosis and to decrease transmission of the virus. The presence of antibody indicates current infection even though no clinical symptoms may be present for years. Most of the infected persons in the United States are unaware that they are infected with HIV. HIV antibody tests, combined with counseling, may modify behavior and encourage low-risk sexual practices.[72]

To assist the clinician in deciding who would most benefit from serologic testing, Table 79-2 outlines the current U.S. Public Health Service guidelines for HIV antibody testing.[72] These guidelines may be subdivided into those recommendations that

**Table 79-2. Guidelines for HIV Antibody Testing**

Decrease Transmission:
1. All blood and organ (including semen) donors
2. Persons who consider themselves at risk for HIV infection
3. Persons with a sexually transmitted disease
4. Intravenous drug abusers
5. Persons who received blood transfusions between 1978 and 1985
6. Women of childbearing age with identifiable risk for infection (also those planning surrogate motherhood)
7. Persons planning marriage where the seroprevalence is 0.1 percent or greater
8. Male and female prostitutes
9. Persons admitted to hospitals in those age groups deemed to have a high prevalence of HIV infection
10. Persons in correctional institutions (and perhaps institutions for chronic psychiatric care where regulation of sexual activity may be difficult and segregation may be necessary to protect seronegative persons)

Diagnosis:
1. Generalized lymphadenopathy
2. Unexpected dementia or encephalopathy
3. Chronic unexplained fever
4. Chronic unexplained diarrhea
5. Unexplained weight loss or wasting syndrome
6. Tuberculosis
7. Chronic candidiasis
8. Kaposi's sarcoma
9. Primary lymphoma of the brain
10. Generalized herpes virus infection affecting a patient greater than 1 month old

directly assist with decreasing HIV transmission and those that help the clinician to diagnose HIV infection. In certain instances it may be necessary to increase the scope of testing, and these suggestions should prompt the clinician to search for a history of high-risk group membership and to obtain consent for HIV antibody testing. For early HIV infection (which could present as either an acute mononucleosis-like syndrome or acute aseptic meningitis), repeated serologic testing at 6, 9, and 24 weeks may be necessary because of the delayed antibody response to HIV infection. Repeated testing in neonates is also necessary because of the presence of maternal antibody for up to 15 months. Although AIDS remains, for the most part, a clinical diagnosis, it is unusual under current clinical practice for a diagnosis to be made without prior HIV serology.

## SUMMARY

Persons with HIV infection develop antibodies to several HIV-encoded proteins. The enzyme immunoassay currently used for screening blood donations and patient specimens detects antibody to multiple viral antigens, and demonstrates greater than 99 percent sensitivity and specificity. In populations having a high prevalence of infection (66 percent), the predictive value of a repeatably positive enzyme immunoassay is greater than 99 percent. However, in populations where the prevalence of infection is low (less than 1 percent), such as blood donors, the predictive value of a repeatably positive enzyme immunoassay is only about 60 percent. Other, more specific methods—such as Western blot, immunofluorescence assay, or radioimmunoprecipitation—are used to confirm the presence of antibody to individual viral proteins in serum specimens that are repeatably positive by enzyme immunoassay.

Second-generation tests for antibody to individual, specific viral proteins encoded by *env* and *gag* genes use either recombinant proteins produced in bacteria or chemically synthesized peptides. These tests are more specific than current enzyme immunoassays and are cheaper and safer to produce. Additionally, detection of antibodies to individual proteins may be important in monitoring disease progression. Third-generation assays have been developed to detect viral antigen or viral RNA and DNA. Detection of viral antigen may be important early in infection, late in disease, and during antiviral chemotherapy.

Future development of laboratory tests for HIV detection must take into account the recent isolation and characterization of HIV-2 and other HIV types from Africa. Because HIV-1 and HIV-2 exhibit only limited antigenic cross-reactivity, blood infected with HIV-2 may not be detected by current enzyme immunoassay screens that are based on detection of HIV-1 antibodies.

## References

1 Barre-Sinoussi F et al: Isolation of a T-lymphotropic retrovirus from a patient at risk for acquired immune deficiency syndrome (AIDS). *Science* 220:868, 1983.

2 Gallo RC et al: Isolation of human T-cell leukemia virus in acquired immune deficiency syndrome (AIDS). *Science* 220:865, 1983.

3 Clavel F et al: Isolation of a new human retrovirus from West African patients with AIDS. *Science* 233:343, 1986.

4 Clavel F et al: Human immunodeficiency virus type 2 infection associated with AIDS in West Africa. *N Engl J Med* 316:1180, 1987.

5 Barin F et al: Serological evidence for virus related to simian T-lymphotropic retrovirus III in residents of West Africa. *Lancet* ii:1387, 1985.

6 Curran JW et al: The epidemiology of AIDS: Current status and future prospects. *Science* 229:1352, 1985.

7 Brun-Vezinet F: Detection of IgG antibodies to lymphadenopathy-associated virus in patients with AIDS or lymphadenopathy syndrome. *Lancet* i:1253, 1984.

8 Sarngadharan MG: Antibodies reactive with human T-lymphotropic retroviruses (HTLV-III) in the serum of patients with AIDS. *Science* 224:506, 1984.

9 Gallo RC et al: Frequent detection and isolation of cytopathic retroviruses (HTLV-III) from patients with AIDS and at risk for AIDS. *Science* 224:500, 1984.

10 Salahuddin SZ et al: Isolation of infectious human T-cell leukemia lymphotropic virus type III (HTLV-III) from patients with acquired immunodeficiency syndrome (AIDS) or AIDS-related complex (ARC) and from healthy carriers: A study of risk groups and tissue sources. *Proc Natl Acad Sci USA* 82:5530, 1985.

11 Weiss SH et al: Screening test for HTLV-III (AIDS agent) antibodies. *JAMA* 253:221, 1985.

12 Carlson JR et al: AIDS serology testing in low and high-risk groups. *JAMA* 253:3405, 1985.

13 Handsfield HH et al: Screening and diagnostic performance of enzyme immunoassay for antibody to lymphadenopathy-associated virus. *J Clin Microbiol* 25:879, 1987.

14 Peetom F and the Cooperative Study Group: Use of an enzyme immunoassay for detection of antibody to human immunodeficiency virus in low risk populations. *Transfusion* 26:536, 1986.

15 Saah AJ et al: Detection of early antibodies in human immunodeficiency virus infection by enzyme-linked immunosorbent assay, Western blot, and radioimmunoprecipitation. *J Clin Microbiol* 25:1605, 1987.

16 Reesink HW et al: Evaluation of six enzyme immunoassays for antibody against human immunodeficiency virus. *Lancet* ii:483, 1986.

17 Sayers MH et al: HLA antibodies as a cause of false-positive reactions in screening enzyme immunoassays for antibodies to human T-lymphotropic virus type III. *Transfusion* 26:113, 1986.

18 Ameglio F et al: Antibodies reactive with nonpolymorphic epitopes on HLA molecules interfere in screening tests for the human immunodeficiency virus. *J Infect Dis* 156:1034, 1987.

19 Denis F et al: Efficacy of five enzyme immunoassays for antibody to HIV in detecting antibody to HTLV-IV. *Lancet* i:324, 1987.

20 Centers for Disease Control: Provisional public health service interagency recommendations for screening donated blood and plasma for antibody to the virus causing acquired immunodeficiency syndrome. *MMWR* 34:1, 1985.

21 Esteban JI et al: Importance of Western blot analysis in predicting infectivity of anti-HTLV-III/LAV positive blood. *Lancet* ii:1083, 1985.

22 Goldstein L et al: Genetic Systems enzyme immunoassay for the detection of antibody to lymphadenopathy associated virus (LAV/HTLV III), in *Medical Virology V*, LM dela Maza, EM Peterson (eds). Lawrence Erlbaum Assoc, Hillsdale, NJ 1986, p 287.

23 Gallo D et al: Comparison of detection of antibody to the acquired immune deficiency syndrome virus by enzyme immunoassay, immunofluorescence, and Western blot methods. *J Clin Microbiol* 23:1049, 1986.

24 Carlson JR: Comparison of indirect immunofluorescence and Western blot for detection of anti-human immunodeficiency virus antibodies. *J Clin Microbiol* 25:494, 1987.

25 Sandstrom EG et al: Detection of human anti-HTLV-III antibodies by indirect immunofluorescence using fixed cells. *Transfusion* 25: 308, 1985.

26 Kaminsky LS et al.: High prevalence of antibodies to acquired immune deficiency syndrome (AIDS)-associated retrovirus (ARV) in AIDS and related conditions but not in other disease states. *Proc Natl Acad Sci USA* 82:5535, 1985.

27 Chang NT et al: An HTLV-III peptide produced by recombinant DNA is immunoreactive with sera from patients with AIDS. *Nature* 315:151, 1985.

28 Thorn RM et al: Enzyme immunoassay using a novel recombinant polypeptide to detect human immunodeficiency virus *env* antibody. *J Clin Microbiol* 15:1207, 1987.

29 Certa U et al: Subregions of a conserved part of the HIV gp41 transmembrane protein are differentially recognized by antibodies of infected individuals. *EMBO J* 5:3051, 1986.

30 Palker TJ et al: A conserved region at the COOH terminus of human immunodeficiency virus gp120 envelope protein contains an immunodominant epitope. *Proc Natl Acad Sci USA* 84:2479, 1987.

31 Burke DS et al: Diagnosis of human immunodeficiency virus infection by immunoassay using a molecularly cloned and expressed virus envelope polypeptide. *Ann Intern Med* 106:671, 1987.

32 Kanner SB et al: Human retroviral *env* and *gag* polypeptides: Serologic assays to measure infection. *J Immunol* 137:674, 1986.

33 Shoeman RL et al: Comparison of recombinant human immunodeficiency virus *gag* precursor and *gag/env* fusion proteins and a synthetic *env* peptide as diagnostic reagents. *Anal Biochem* 161:370, 1987.

34 Cabradilla CD et al: Serodiagnosis of antibodies to the human AIDS retrovirus with a bacterially synthesized *env* polypeptide. *Bio/Technology* 4:128, 1986.

35 Allain J-P et al: Serological markers in early stages of human immunodeficiency virus infection in haemophiliacs. *Lancet* ii:1233, 1986.

36 Cosand WL: Synthetic antigen for the detection of AIDS-related disease. U.S. Patent 4,629,783, December 16, 1986.

37 Wang JJG et al: Detection of antibodies to human T-lymphotropic virus type III by using a synthetic peptide of 21 amino acid residues corresponding to a highly antigenic segment of gp41 envelope proteins. *Proc Natl Acad Sci USA* 83:6159, 1986.

38 Smith RS et al: Antibody to a synthetic oligopeptide in subjects at risk for human immunodeficiency virus infection. *J Clin Microbiol* 25:1498, 1987.

39 Gnann JW et al: Diagnosis of AIDS by using a 12-amino acid peptide representing an immunodominant epitope of the human immunodeficiency virus. *J Infect Dis* 156:261, 1987.

40 Gnann JW et al: Fine mapping of an immunodominant domain in the transmembrane glycoprotein of human immunodeficiency virus. *J Virol* 61:2639, 1987.

41 Gnann JW et al: Synthetic peptide immunoassay distinguishes HIV type 1 and HIV type 2 infections. *Science* 237:1346, 1987.

42 Carlson JR et al: Rapid, easy, and economical screening test for antibodies to human immunodeficiency virus. *Lancet* i:361, 1987.

43 Cooper DA et al: Antibody response to human immunodeficiency virus after primary infection. *J Infect Dis* 155:1113, 1987.

44 Gaines H et al: Antibody response in primary human immunodeficiency virus infection. *Lancet* i:1249, 1987.

45 Ranki A et al: Long latency precedes overt seroconversion in sexually transmitted human-immunodeficiency-virus infection. *Lancet* ii:589, 1987.

46 Kalyanaraman VS et al: Antibodies to the core protein of lymphadenopathy-associated virus (LAV) in patients with AIDS. *Science* 225: 321, 1984.

47 Schüpbach J et al: Antibodies to HTLV-III in Swiss patients with AIDS and pre-AIDS and in groups at risk for AIDS. *N Engl J Med* 312:265, 1985.

48 Pan L-Z et al: Patterns of antibody response in individuals infected with the human immunodeficiency virus. *J Infect Dis* 155:626, 1987.

49 Steimer KS et al: Differential antibody responses of individuals infected with AIDS-associated retroviruses surveyed using the viral core antigen $p25^{gag}$ expressed in bacteria. *Virology* 150:283, 1986.

50 Groopman JE et al: Serological characterization of HTLV-III infection in AIDS and related disorders. *J Infect Dis* 153:736, 1986.

51 Parry JV et al: Sensitive assays for viral antibodies in saliva: An alternative to tests on serum. *Lancet* 72, 1987.

52 Archibald DW et al: Antibodies to human immunodeficiency virus in cervical secretions from women at risk for AIDS. *J Infect Dis* 156: 240, 1987.

53 Resnick L et al: Intra-blood-brain-barrier synthesis of HTLV-III-specific IgG in patients with neurologic symptoms associated with AIDS or AIDS-related complex. *N Engl J Med* 313:1498, 1985.

54 Goudsmit J et al: Expression of human immunodeficiency virus antigen (HIV-Ag) in serum and cerebrospinal fluid during acute and chronic infection. *Lancet* ii:177, 1986.

55 Wittek AE et al: Detection of human immunodeficiency virus core protein in plasma by enzyme immunoassay. *Ann Intern Med* 107: 286, 1987.

56 Feorino P et al: Comparison of antigen assay and reverse transcriptase assay for detecting human immunodeficiency virus in culture. *J Clin Microbiol* 25:2344, 1987.

57 Goudsmit J et al: Antigenemia and antibody titers to core and envelope antigens in AIDS, AIDS-related complex, and subclinical human immunodeficiency virus infection. *J Infect Dis* 155:558, 1987.

58 Ho DD et al: Primary human T-lymphotropic virus type III infection. *Ann Intern Med* 103:880, 1985.

59 Cooper DA et al: Acute AIDS retrovirus infection: Definition of a clinical illness associated with seroconversion. *Lancet* i:537, 1985.

60 Kessler HA et al: Diagnosis of human immunodeficiency virus infection in seronegative homosexuals presenting with an acute viral syndrome. *JAMA* 258:1196, 1987.

61 Allain JP et al: Long-term evaluation of HIV antigen and antibodies to p24 and gp41 in patients with hemophilia. *N Engl J Med* 317: 1114, 1987.

62 Kenny C et al: HIV antigen testing. *Lancet* i:565, 1987.

63 Baillou A et al: Human immunodeficiency virus antigenemia in patients with AIDS and AIDS-related disorders: A comparison between European and Central African populations. *J Infect Dis* 156:830, 1987.

64 Gaines H et al: HIV antigenaemia and virus isolation from plasma during primary HIV infection. *Lancet* i:1317, 1987.

65 Lange J, Goudsmit J: Decline of antibody reactivity to HIV core protein secondary to increased production of HIV antigen. *Lancet* i:448, 1987.

66 Chaisson RE et al: Significant changes in HIV antigen level in the serum of patients treated with azidothymidine. *N Engl J Med* 315: 1610, 1986.

67 Goudsmit J et al: Intra-blood-brain barrier synthesis of human immunodeficiency virus antigen and antibody in humans and chimpanzees. *Proc Natl Acad Sci USA* 84:3876, 1987.

68 Biberfeld G et al: Blood donor sera with false-positive Western blot reactions to human immunodeficiency virus. *Lancet* 289, 1986.

69 Burke DS, Redfield RR: False-positive Western blot tests for antibodies to HTLV-III. *JAMA* 256:347, 1986.

70 Courouće A-M et al: False-positive Western blot reactions to human immunodeficiency virus in blood donors. *Lancet* ii:921, 1986.

71 Meyer KB, Pauker SG: Screening for HIV: Can we afford the false positive rate? *N Engl J Med* 317:238, 1987.

72 Public Health Service guidelines for counseling and antibody testing to prevent HIV infection and AIDS. *MMWR* 36:509, 1987.

Chapter 80

# Isolation of human immunodeficiency virus

James R. Carlson
Myra B. Jennings

## INTRODUCTION

The first isolation of the human immunodeficiency virus (HIV)[1] by Barré-Sinoussi et al.[2] in 1983 identified the etiologic agent of acquired immunodeficiency syndrome (AIDS). The further development and application of this technique to clinical studies has fulfilled the modern equivalent of the postulates of Koch: HIV has been isolated from most patients with AIDS;[3–6] antibodies to HIV have been shown to develop in temporal association with the onset of HIV infection and AIDS;[7] HIV infection and AIDS have been transmitted from an infected person, blood donor, to an uninfected person, blood recipient;[8,9] and isolation of the same virus from both donor and recipient has been accomplished. HIV isolation has been applied to other clinical studies involving diagnosis of infection[10–12] and as an end point for testing antiviral drugs.[13] HIV isolation has also proved useful for the collection and characterization of field isolates of HIV[14] for comparative studies and as a method for the discovery of new human and animal retroviruses.[15,16]

The laboratory methods for the isolation of HIV are primarily research methods and have remained unstandardized. The purpose of this chapter is to describe a basic method for HIV isolation and review the performance characteristics, variations, and clinical applications of this new laboratory method. Serologic methods for diagnosis of HIV infection, which are more broadly used for general clinical purposes, are described in Chap. 79.

## LABORATORY SAFETY

The highest priority in the retrovirology laboratory should be the safety of laboratory personnel. Good microbiological technique and the use of appropriate safety equipment are essential for protection of personnel and the immediate laboratory environment. Laboratory technique, safety equipment, and facility design are the three critical considerations of safe handling of infectious agents.[17]

Basic points of laboratory technique are: (1) Protect skin and mucous membranes from contact with contaminated material by wearing gloves (two pairs are recommended), masks, laboratory gown, and eye protection. (2) Use a biological safety cabinet for all work with HIV cultures and materials. (3) Avoid the use of needles and sharp objects that could lead to accidental puncture wounds. (4) Use plastic pipettes and labware. Eliminate the use of glass objects. (5) Use mechanical pipetting devices. Do not mouth pipet. (6) Baseline serum samples for all laboratory personnel should be collected and stored, and all personnel should be tested periodically for HIV antibody.

Safety equipment should include centrifuges equipped with safety cups or sealed rotors to prevent aerosols during centrifugation of infectious materials. Biological safety cabinets must be provided for the manipulation of cultures and infectious materials. Class II vertical laminar-flow biological safety cabinets provide protection for both the operator and the materials. Horizontal-flow clean benches do not provide protection for the laboratory worker and must not be used for work with infectious materials.

Protection of the environment and personnel external to the laboratory is also of utmost importance, and this is accomplished by the combination of facility design and operational practices. Ideally, the laboratory should be separated from areas which are open to unrestricted traffic flow, and passage through two sets of doors is required for entry into the laboratory from access corridors or other adjoining areas. In addition, an autoclave for decontaminating laboratory wastes should be available, preferably within the laboratory.

HIV is inactivated by a number of disinfectants.[18] The use of disinfectants is recommended only for decontamination of work surfaces and equipment which cannot be autoclaved.

Policies for biosafety containment should be reviewed at frequent intervals and an ongoing educational program should be implemented for new employees or persons working with concentrated HIV for the first time.[19]

## IN VITRO METHOD FOR HIV ISOLATION

### SPECIMEN

HIV causes a systemic infection and has been isolated from a variety of body fluids and tissues including peripheral blood,[3,4,5,6,8,9,20] bone marrow,[6] lymph nodes,[2] semen,[21,22] genital secretions from women,[23,24] tears,[25] saliva,[26,27] brain and nerve tissue and cerebrospinal fluid (CSF),[28] placenta tissue,[29] and plasma.[6]

Tables 80-1, 80-2, 80-3, and 80-4 list the basic methods and reagents for HIV isolation. HIV isolation can be best accomplished by cultivation of the test specimen with phytohemagglutinin (PHA)-stimulated normal peripheral blood mononuclear cells (PBMCs) in the presence of T-cell growth factor, interleukin-2 (IL-2), to stimulate the growth of T-cell subsets, and polybrene to facilitate the attachment of HIV to donor cells.[2,5,20] The cultures are monitored for HIV using assays for reverse transcriptase (RT) (Table 80-5)[30,31,32] and specific HIV antigen p24.[33,34,35,36]

## SPECIMEN COLLECTION AND TRANSPORT

HIV has been most commonly isolated from peripheral blood. Blood can be collected by venipuncture in heparinized tubes and transported directly to the virology laboratory for HIV isolation. Specimens should be transported at 25°C (not refrigerated or frozen) and, as with any clinical virology specimen, delivered as rapidly as possible. Studies at the University of California at Davis, however, have demonstrated that a 24 h delay, when the specimen remains at 25°C, does not significantly diminish the sensitivity of HIV isolation (Table 80-6).[37] Both the time to detection of HIV and rates of isolation were equal when same-day processing was compared with a 24 h delay in processing. Handling and delays caused by commercial, overnight, transport de-

**Table 80-1. Procedure for HIV Isolation from Peripheral Blood Mononuclear Cells (PBMCs)**

1. Fresh peripheral blood[2,5,20]
   *a.* Peripheral blood mononuclear cells (PBMCs) from aseptically collected heparinized blood are separated by Ficoll-Hypaque gradient centrifugation (density 1.077)
   *b.* The separated test PBMCs are washed several times with lymphocyte preparation medium to remove the Ficoll-Hypaque (Table 80-2)
   *c.* The viable cell concentration is determined by trypan blue exclusion
   *d.* The cell concentration is adjusted to $1 \times 10^6$ cells/ml in PHA stimulation medium (Table 80-2)
   *e.* Cells are incubated for 3–4 days at 37°C in a humidified, 5% $CO_2$ atmosphere
   *f.* PHA-stimulated test PBMCs are added to PHA-stimulated PBMCs from a seronegative donor at a ratio of 1:3, and the total cell concentration is adjusted to $2 \times 10^6$ cells/ml in HIV growth medium (Table 80-2)
   *g.* The cultures are tested two times a week for reverse transcriptase activity (Table 80-5), HIV antigen (p24), and examined microscopically for giant cell formation. (Cultures are replenished with additional PHA-stimulated seronegative donor PBMCs if cell concentration appears to be decreasing or with more HIV growth medium if cell density increases)
2. Frozen peripheral blood mononuclear cells[20]
   *a.* After PBMCs are separated by Ficoll-Hypaque gradient centrifugation, the PBMCs are resuspended in RPMI-1640 with 50% fetal bovine serum (inactivated at 56°C for 30 min) and 10% DMSO
   *b.* The PBMCs are slowly frozen at −60°C and stored at −190°C
   *c.* To initiate culture for HIV, the frozen PBMCs are rapidly thawed at 36°C and prepared for PHA stimulation (step 2*b*, above)
3. Lysed PBMCs[20]
   *a.* Lyse either frozen or fresh PBMCs by freeze-thaw and then process as in step 1f, above

livery services did not adversely affect the sensitivity of HIV isolation from heparinized peripheral blood specimens.

An alternate method that avoids the limitations associated with fresh blood specimens is the use of frozen PBMCs (Table 80-1).[20] The disadvantage of this method is that the collection site must

**Table 80-2. Reagents for HIV Isolation Procedure**

1. Lymphocyte preparation medium:
   RPMI-1640 supplemented with gentamicin 5 μg/ml
2. PHA stimulation medium:
   RPMI-1640 supplemented with 10% fetal bovine serum
   gentamicin 5 μg/ml
   β-mercaptoethanol $5 \times 10^{-5}$ *M*
   Hepes buffer 10 m*M*
   PHA-P (Difco) 5 μg/ml
3. HIV growth medium:
   RPMI-1640 supplemented with 10% fetal bovine serum
   gentamicin 5 μg/ml
   antihuman interferon alpha (sheep) (ICN Immunobiologicals)
   Polybrene (Sigma) 1 μg/ml
   1% IL-2 (human interleukin-2) (Cellular Products)
   β-mercaptoethanol $5 \times 10^{-5}$*M*
4. Ficoll-Hypaque (density 1.077):
   Histopaque 1077-(Sigma 1077–1) or lymphocyte separation medium (LSM) (Litton Bionetics 8410–01)
5. Trypan blue (Flow Laboratories):
   0.5% in 0.85% sodium chloride

**Table 80-3. Method for the Preparation of Peripheral Blood Mononuclear Cells**

1. PBMCs are separated by Ficoll-Hypaque from a buffy coat obtained at the blood donor center from an HIV and hepatitis B serology negative donor
2.* Wash PBMCs in lymphocyte preparation medium by low-speed centrifugation
3. Cell concentration is adjusted to $2 \times 10^6$ cells/ml in PHA-stimulation medium (Table 80-2)
4. Culture for 3 days as in step 1*e*, Table 80-1
5. Add to test PBMCs for cocultivation

*Seronegative donor PBMCs can be frozen for later use as in step 2, Table 80-1.

be equipped for separating and freezing PBMCs. This method, however, at least in the initial report, has been shown to be as sensitive as the use of fresh specimens for the isolation of HIV (See Sensitivity of HIV Isolation Methods, below).

In general, aseptically collected fluids from sites not contaminated with normal microbial flora can be cultured directly with PHA-stimulated seronegative donor PBMCs. For example, CSF,

**Table 80-4. Methods for Processing Specimens Other than Peripheral Blood for HIV Isolation**

1. Semen[22]
   *a.* Dilute specimen 1:10 in RPMI-1640 with 20% fetal calf serum
   *b.* Separate cells by Ficoll-Hypaque (density 1.077 g/ml)
   *c.* Cultivate with PHA-stimulated seronegative donor PBMCs in HIV growth medium
   *d.* Culture and monitor for HIV, as in Table 80-1
2. Genital secretions from women[23,24]
   *a.* Vaginal secretions are collected with a cotton swab. Cervical samples can be collected with a glass rod or by scraping with a wooden spatula and added to lymphocyte preparation medium
   *b.* Clarify specimen by centrifugation and filter supernatant (0.45 μ)
   *c.* Supernatant may be added directly to PHA-stimulated seronegative donor PBMCs
   *d.* Cells from centrifuged pellet are cultivated with PHA-stimulated PBMCs; supernatant is removed and filtered (0.45 μ) before adding to fresh PHA-stimulated PBMCs
   *e.* Culture and monitor for HIV, as in Table 80-1
3. Saliva[26]
   *a.* Dilute specimen 1:2 in HIV growth medium and incubate at 37°C for 2 h
   *b.* Centrifuge (1000 *g*) for 10 min and collect supernatant
   *c.* Filter supernatant (0.45 μ)
   *d.* Add filtered supernatant to PHA-stimulated seronegative donor PBMCs
   *e.* Culture and monitor for HIV, as in Table 80-1
4. Tears[25]
   *a.* Collect tear samples (about 15 μl) with sterile Schirmer's filter paper strips as for a routine tear function test
   *b.* Add tear sample to PHA-stimulated seronegative donor PBMCs
   *c.* Culture and monitor for HIV as in Table 80-1
5. Cerebrospinal fluid[28]
   *a.* Cultivate specimen directly (or filter 0.45 μ to remove cells) with PHA-stimulated seronegative donor PBMCs
   *b.* Culture and monitor for HIV as in Table 80-1
6. Tissues[28,29]
   *a.* Homogenize tissue by grinding and pass supernatant through a 0.45 μ filter
   *b.* Add filtered homogenate to PHA-stimulated seronegative donor PBMCs
   *c.* Culture and monitor for HIV as in Table 80-1

Table 80-5. Method for Reverse Transcriptase Assay

1. Pellet HIV from clarified cell culture fluid by centrifugation at 100,000 *g* for 60 min
2. Discard supernatant fluid
3. Add disruption mixture to the pellet to disrupt the virions and release the reverse transcriptase enzyme
4. Add template primer (poly rA:oligo dT), $MgCl_2$, and $^3$H-thymidine triphosphate to the disrupted virus. Incubate at 37°C for 60 min
5. Add cold 10% trichloroacetic acid and 0.1*M* sodium pyrophosphate to precipitate the reverse transcriptase-synthesized DNA
6. Add mixture to glass fiber or Whatman No. 1 filters. Rinse with 10% TCA and then 95% ethanol
7. Add filters to vials containing scintillation fluid. Count in beta scintillation counter. The presence of reverse transcriptase enzyme is indicated by the incorporation of $^3$H-thymidine triphosphate into TCA-precipitable DNA

tears, and plasma samples can be cultured in this manner. In contrast, specimens from sites with normal flora, e.g., saliva, genital secretions from women, must be centrifuged and filtered before culturing in cell culture. Semen is a more difficult specimen to culture because it is toxic to tissue culture cells. Attempts to isolate HIV from semen should be directed at the cells that must be diluted and separated from the fluid portion of the specimen. HIV has been isolated from both cells and the cell-free filtrates of genital secretions of women[23] and CSF.[28] Tissue should be processed as a homogenate,[28,29] and the filtrate of the homogenate can be cultivated directly with the PHA-stimulated PBMCs.

## CULTURE METHODS

Fresh or frozen PBMCs from peripheral blood are stimulated with PHA and then cocultivated with PHA-stimulated seronegative donor PBMCs for 4 to 6 weeks. Other types of specimens are cultivated directly with PHA-stimulated seronegative donor PBMCs for the same period of time. The cultures are maintained by the addition of fresh media and/or PHA-stimulated seronegative PBMCs and are monitored for HIV. HIV is detected in culture by the production of RT (Table 80-5) and the production of specific HIV antigen p24. Other methods of detection that include electron microscopy,[28] immunofluorescence microscopy,[5] and molecular probes[38] have been used for the confirmation of HIV in culture, but these research methods are not yet sufficiently convenient for routine use.

Table 80-6. Evaluation of Same Day versus Overnight Delay in Processing of Whole Heparinized Blood Specimens for HIV Isolation

| | Time (days) to isolation of HIV | |
|---|---|---|
| Specimen | Less than 8 h delay | Greater than 18 h delay |
| 1 | 12 | 7 |
| 2 | 15 | 11 |
| 3 | 19 | 14 |
| 4 | 19 | 18 |
| 5 | Negative | Negative |
| 6 | 41 | 43 |
| 7 | 15 | 11 |
| 8 | 19 | 14 |
| 9 | 11 | 13 |
| 10 | 11 | 10 |
| 11 | 14 | 17 |
| 12 | 14 | 13 |
| 13 | 12 | 11 |
| 14 | 8 | 13 |
| Average | 15 days | 14 days |

## Detection of HIV in culture

**Reverse Transcriptase Assay.** Reverse transcriptase enzyme is a DNA polymerase unique to retroviruses, including HIV and related viruses. Reverse transcriptase enzyme is necessary for the incorporation of radiolabeled nucleotides into a DNA polymer from an RNA template, and demonstration of reverse transcriptase is an indication of a retrovirus in a culture. The enzyme is detected by adding a mixture of a synthetic homopolymer template, oligonucleotide primer, radiolabeled nucleotides, and $MgCl_2$ to disrupted virions, and measuring the radiolabeled nucleotides incorporated into trichloroacetic acid (TCA)-precipitable material. It is necessary, however, to distinguish between retroviral reverse transcriptase and cellular DNA polymerase.[20] This is accomplished by testing with a polyriboA:oligodeoxyT template-primer mixture, which is preferentially used by the virion reverse transcriptase enzyme and polydeoxyA:oligodeoxyT template-primer mixture which is preferentially used by the cellular polymerase.

**HIV Antigen Assay.** Enzyme immunoassays (EIA) for the detection of HIV antigens in tissue culture supernatants have been reported as research methods.[35,36] A number of tests are commercially available for this purpose,[33,34] and other tests are in development. These EIAs are useful not only for the detection of HIV antigens in tissue culture supernatants but also for the detection of HIV antigens in plasma and other body fluids from HIV-infected people (see Chap. 79).[39,40,41]

The basic assay is a solid-phase, sandwich-type EIA. Polyclonal or monoclonal antibodies to HIV are used as the capture and probe antibodies and an enzyme-labeled second antibody conjugate is used to identify the presence of HIV antigen in the supernatant or specimen. One manufacturer, Abbott, has increased the specificity of the assay by including a "neutralization" test in the method.

In studies at the University of California at Davis, antigen assays were shown to be more sensitive than RT for the detection of HIV in culture. In the examples shown in Table 80-7 for 11 consecutive cultures, there was complete agreement between methods for negative and positive final results, but the antigen assays were positive earlier than reverse transcriptase assay results for all but one of the positive cultures. These data are in agreement with recently published results for 34 positive cultures that were tested in parallel.[33] The antigen assays were positive several days (range, 3 to 9 days; average, 5.9 days) before the RT assays were positive (range, 7 to 16 days; average, 9.6 days). In addition, the specificity of the antigen assay was demonstrated by negative reactivity to HTLV-I, HTLV-II, varicella zoster virus, Epstein-Barr virus, cytomegalovirus, herpes simplex I and adenovirus type 5 cultures, as well as common, uninfected continuous T-cell lines. Cross-reactivity to HIV-2 and the simian immunodeficiency virus (SIV) has been demonstrated in preliminary studies at the University of California at Davis.

If the question is only the presence or absence of HIV, the HIV antigen assays offer a more efficient alternative to RT assays for detection of HIV in culture. The antigen assays are standardized and easy to perform. For those research and reference laborato-

Table 80-7. Comparison of HIV Antigen Assay and Reverse Transcriptase Assay for the Detection of HIV in Culture Supernatants

| Culture No. | Time (days) to detection of HIV: Antigen assays* No. 1 | Antigen assays* No. 2 | Reverse transcriptase assay |
|---|---|---|---|
| 1 | 15 | 15 | 22 |
| 2 | —† | — | — |
| 3 | 12 | 12 | 12 |
| 4 | — | — | — |
| 5 | 11 | 11 | 18 |
| 6 | 21 | 21 | 28 |
| 7 | — | — | — |
| 8 | — | — | — |
| 9 | — | — | — |
| 10 | 10 | 10 | 13 |
| 11 | 27 | 24 | 30 |

* Two different commercial antigen assays were used for detection of HIV antigen.
† Negative at 35 days in culture.

ries interested in identifying other human retroviruses, RT assays must be performed alongside antigen assays since a negative antigen assay with a positive RT might indicate a retrovirus other than HIV-1, HIV-2, or SIV.

## SENSITIVITY OF HIV ISOLATION METHODS

The sensitivity of HIV isolation is dependent on the method and the specimen source. The relative sensitivity of a method can be determined by comparing the time to detection of HIV in positive cultures and the rate of isolation within risk groups and other clinical categories of HIV-infected people. Thorough comparative studies of HIV isolation methods have not been completed primarily because culture isolation methods are labor-intensive and expensive.

Table 80-8 illustrates the time to detection of HIV in culture for methods used by the AIDS Virus Diagnostic Laboratory at the University of California at Davis, as well as data from two other reports.[5,20] For the methods using fresh PBMCs, at least 80 percent of the positive cultures were detected by reverse transcriptase assay within the first 3 weeks of culture. If the antigen assay for HIV detection is used, this time period would probably be reduced.[33] At least equal or shorter times to isolation were achieved by the use of frozen or fresh PBMCs that were lysed before cultivation.[20]

Table 80-9. HIV Isolation Rates from Studies Using Peripheral Blood from Seropositive Subjects

| Specimen type | Clinical symptoms | No. positive/ No. tested | Reference |
|---|---|---|---|
| Fresh PBMCs | + | 77/128 (60%) | University of California, Davis |
| | – | 14/42 (33%) | |
| | + | 86/129 (67%) | 5 |
| | – | 4/12 (33%) | |
| Frozen PBMCs* | + | 12/15 (80%) | 20 |
| | – | 11/12 (92%) | |
| Frozen, lysed PBMCs* | + | 11/15 (73%) | |
| | – | 12/12 (100%) | |
| Fresh PBMCs* | + | 6/8 (75%) | |
| | – | 7/9 (78%) | |
| Fresh, lysed* | + | 7/8 (88%) | |
| | – | 6/9 (67%) | |

*Split specimens.

Table 80-9 compares the sensitivity of HIV isolation for methods using peripheral blood specimens. Overall, the method described by Gallo et al.[20] appears to be the most sensitive. This sensitivity was particularly demonstrated for the asymptomatic group in which isolation rates of 67 to 100 percent were achieved compared with 33 percent in the other studies.

In Table 80-10 the sensitivity of HIV isolation for specimens other than peripheral blood is compared. HIV is a systemic disease and the virus is found in a variety of body tissues and fluids, but peripheral blood appears to be the specimen from which HIV may be most readily isolated. In addition, isolation of HIV from plasma,[32] filtered CSF,[28] and vaginal or cervical secretions[23] shows that viability of HIV does not require cell association.

## ROLE OF HIV ISOLATION IN CLINICAL STUDIES

HIV isolation from blood, semen, and female genital secretions has provided essential data in determining the role of these fluids in transmission of disease and confirms previous epidemiological observations about HIV transmission routes.[42] In the absence of epidemiological data to implicate tears[25] and saliva[26,27] in disease transmission, the isolation of HIV from these fluids has added to the characterization of HIV infection as systemic. HIV isolation has verified the etiology of clinical observations such as dementia and peripheral neuropathy,[28] and provided critical information about the pharmacokinetic requirements for potential antiviral agents, i.e., that they must penetrate the blood-brain barrier.

Table 80-8. Comparison of HIV Isolation Methods: Time to Detection with Reverse Transcriptase Assay of Positive Cultures from Peripheral Blood

| Study | Specimen type | No. of positive cultures | Cumulative percent positive cultures detected by RT by day: ≤15 | ≤21 | ≤28 | >28 |
|---|---|---|---|---|---|---|
| University of California, Davis | Fresh | 99 | 57 | 84 | 94 | 100 |
| Ref. 5 | Fresh | >160 | 64 | 85 | 100 | — |
| Ref. 20 | Frozen* | 23 | 57 | 79 | 96 | 100 |
| | Frozen* | 23 | 61 | 91 | 100 | — |
| | Fresh* | 13 | 69 | 84 | 100 | — |
| | Fresh, lysed* | 13 | 62 | 93 | 100 | — |

*Split samples.

**Table 80-10. HIV Isolation from Specimens Other than Peripheral Blood**

| Specimen Type | No. positive/ No. tested | References |
|---|---|---|
| Semen | 3/3 (100%) | 21,22 |
| Contemporaneous peripheral blood | 1/1 (100%) | |
| Genital secretions from women | 10/23 (44%) | 23,24 |
| Contemporaneous peripheral blood | 14/21 (67%) | |
| Saliva | 8/18 (44%) | 26 |
| Contemporaneous peripheral blood | 28/50 (56%) | |
| Tears | 1/7 (14%) | 25 |
| Cerebrospinal fluid | 19/37 (51%) | 28 |
| Brain | 10/14 (71%) | |
| Lymph node | 5/5 (100%) | 2,6 |
| Bone marrow | 1/6 (17%) | 6 |
| Plasma | 3/6 (50%) | 6 |

HIV isolation is seldom useful as a diagnostic test, however, since serological methods are more sensitive indicators of HIV infection (See Chap. 79).[5,20] Nonetheless, isolation of virus may be useful in infants from seropositive mothers where transplacentally transmitted maternal antibody prevents serological confirmation of HIV infection.[10,11] Because HIV isolation methods are not 100 percent sensitive, only a positive result can be considered definitive.

Ideally, HIV isolation should be used as an end point in any study to assess the *in vivo* efficacy of antiviral drugs. However, in the recent trials of azidothymidine (AZT) (see Chap. 30), HIV isolation proved not to be a sensitive indicator of drug efficacy.[13] Isolation of HIV occurred in both placebo and treatment groups after initiation of AZT, even though the treatment group demonstrated increased survival times. For AZT, it appears that titration of circulating HIV p24 antigen is a more sensitive indicator of *in vivo* antiviral efficacy.[41] This may reflect the fact that HIV isolation from PBMCs is at best only semiquantitative. This is not to say, however, that as newer drugs become available for study, HIV isolation will not be useful as a biological end point. In addition, HIV isolation may prove useful in staging or categorizing cohorts for drug and immunotherapeutic studies; e.g., isolation or lack of isolation from the peripheral blood or central nervous system may be used to define certain treatment groups.

HIV isolation has produced a number of field strains that will provide critical information about the biology of HIV infection as molecular and virological data are correlated with clinical studies. Characterization of field isolates will also provide valuable information about how broad or narrow antiviral agents or vaccines must be.

Finally, the application of HIV isolation will be useful in the search for new human and animal retroviruses.[15,16] The isolation of new human retroviruses will help define new epidemics while the isolation of new animal retroviruses will aid in the development of new models to describe the human disease.

## FUTURE DIRECTIONS

Although HIV infections can usually be detected by serology and frequently confirmed by HIV isolation, sensitive and potentially quantitative methods for the detection of the viral genome must be developed. Such methods would be useful for diagnosis and as an end point for antiviral studies. Methods for the detection of HIV sequences have used Southern blotting[43] and in situ hybridization methods,[44] and although they provide useful data they have lacked sensitivity.

A recent advance that may prove to be both sensitive and adaptable to quantitation is a new nucleic acid amplification procedure,[38] polymerase chain reaction (PCR), that uses two primers of known sequence positioned 10 to 300 base pairs apart that are complementary to the plus and minus strands of target DNA. After denaturation of the target DNA and annealing of the primers, template-directed incorporation of deoxynucleoside triphosphates occurs with the addition of the Klenow fragment of *Escherichia coli* DNA polymerase I, or the heat-stable *Taq* polymerase. Since the newly synthesized DNA strands may serve as templates themselves, repeated cycles of denaturation, primer annealing, and extension result in an exponential increase of copies of the region flanked by the primers. This procedure has demonstrated a 220,000-fold amplification of a 110-base-pair region of the beta-globin gene[45] and has identified HIV sequences in both established cell lines harboring HIV and cells cultured from PBMCs, semen mononuclear cells, and semen supernatants of AIDS or ARC patients. The sensitivity appears greater than either Southern blotting or detection of RT. A recent report suggests that this method may be more sensitive than virus isolation for detection of the HIV genome in some clinical specimens.[46] Further evaluation and applications of this method await the development and general availability of automated instrumentation.

## References


1 Coffin J et al: What to call the AIDS virus? *Nature* 225:840, 1984.
2 Barré-Sinoussi F et al: Isolation of a T-lymphotropic retrovirus from a patient at risk for acquired immune deficiency syndrome (AIDS). *Science* 220:868, 1983.
3 Levy JA et al: Isolation of lymphocytopathic retroviruses from San Francisco patients with AIDS. *Science* 225:840, 1984.
4 Gallo RC et al: Frequent detection and isolation of cytopathic retroviruses (HTLV-III) from patients with AIDS and at risk for AIDS. *Science* 224:500, 1984.
5 Levy JA, Shimabukuro J: Recovery of AIDS-associated retroviruses from patients with AIDS or AIDS-related conditions and from clinically healthy individuals. *J Infect Dis* 152:734, 1985.
6 Markham PD et al: Advances in the isolation of HTLV-III from patients with AIDS and AIDS-related complex and from donors at risk. *Cancer Res* (suppl) 45:4588s, 1985.
7 Esteban JI et al: Importance of western blot analysis in predicting infectivity of anti-HTLV-III positive blood. *Lancet* ii:1083, 1985.
8 Feorino PM et al: Transfusion associated acquired immunodeficiency syndrome: Evidence for persistent infection in blood donors. *N Engl J Med* 312:1293, 1985.
9 Feorino PM et al: Lymphadenopathy associated virus infection of a blood donor-recipient pair with acquired immunodeficiency syndrome. *Science* 225:692, 1984.
10 Mok JQ et al: Infants born to mothers seropositive for human immunodeficiency syndrome virus. Preliminary findings from a multicenter European study. *Lancet* i:1164, 1987.
11 Borkowsky W et al: Human-immunodeficiency-virus infections in infants negative for anti-HIV by enzyme-linked immunoassay. *Lancet* i:1168, 1987.
12 Jaffe HW et al: Persistent infection with human T-lymphotropic virus type III/lymph-adenopathy associated virus in apparently healthy homosexual men. *Ann Intern Med* 102:627, 1985.
13 Fischl MA et al: The efficacy of 3′-azido-3′-deoxythymidine (azi-

dothymidine) in the treatment of patients with AIDS and AIDS-related complex: A double-blinded placebo-controlled trial. *N Engl J Med* 317:185, 1987.

14 Weiss RA et al: Variable and conserved neutralization antigens of human immunodeficiency virus. *Nature* 324:572, 1986.

15 Clavel F et al: Isolation of a new human retrovirus from West African patients with AIDS. *Science* 233:343, 1986.

16 Desrosiers RC, Letvin NL: Animal models for AIDS. *Rev Infect Dis* 9:438, 1987.

17 US Department of Health and Human Services: Biosafety in microbiological and biomedical laboratories. Publ (CDC) 84-8395, Washington, DC, Government Printing Office, 1984.

18 Martin LS et al: Disinfection and inactivation of human T lymphotropic virus type III/lymphadenopathy-associated virus. *J Infect Dis* 152:400, 1985.

19 Weiss SH et al: Risk of human immunodeficiency virus (HIV-1) infection among laboratory workers. *Science* 239:68, 1988.

20 Gallo D et al: Comparative studies on use of fresh and frozen peripheral blood lymphocyte specimens for isolation of human immunodeficiency virus and effects of cell lysis on isolation efficiency. *J Clin Microbiol* 25:1291, 1987.

21 Zagury D et al: HTLV-III in cells cultured from semen of two patients with AIDS. *Science* 226:449, 1984.

22 Ho DD et al: HTLV-II in the semen and blood of a healthy homosexual man. *Science* 226:451, 1984.

23 Wofsy CB et al: Isolation of AIDS-associated retrovirus from genital secretions of women with antibodies to the virus. *Lancet* i:527, 1986.

24 Vogt MW et al: Isolation of HTLV-III/LAV from cervical secretions of women at risk for AIDS. *Lancet* i:525, 1986.

25 Fujikawa LS et al: Isolation of human T-lymphotropic virus type III from the tears of a patient with the acquired immunodeficiency syndrome. *Lancet* ii:529, 1985.

26 Groopman JE et al: HTLV-III in saliva of people with AIDS-related complex and healthy homosexual men at risk for AIDS. *Science* 226:447, 1984.

27 Ho DD et al: Infrequency of isolation of HTLV-III virus from saliva in AIDS. *N Engl J Med* 313:1606, 1985.

28 Ho DD et al: Isolation of HTLV-III from cerebrospinal fluid and neural tissues of patients with neurologic syndromes related to the acquired immunodeficiency syndrome. *N Engl J Med* 313:1493, 1985.

29 Hill WC et al: Isolation of acquired immunodeficiency syndrome virus from the placenta. *Am J Obstet Gynecol* 157:10, 1987.

30 Rey et al: Characterization of the RNA dependent DNA polymerase of a new human T lymphotropic retrovirus (lymphadenopathy associated virus). *Biochem Biophys Res Commun* 121:126, 1984.

31 Spira TJ et al: Micromethod for assaying reverse transcriptase of human T-cell lymphotropic virus type III/lymphadenopathy-associated virus. *J Clin Microbiol* 25:97, 1987.

32 Hoffman AD et al: Characterization of the AIDS-associated retrovirus reverse transcriptase and optimal conditions for its detection in virions. *Virology* 147:326, 1985.

33 Feorino P et al: Comparison of antigen assay and reverse transcriptase assay for detecting human immunodeficiency virus in culture. *J Clin Microbiol* 25:2344, 1987.

34 Newell AL et al: Antigen test versus reverse transcriptase assay for detecting HIV. *Lancet* ii:1146, 1987.

35 McDougal JS et al: Immunoassay for the detection and quantitation of infectious human retrovirus, lymphadenopathy-associated virus (LAV). *J Immunol Methods* 76:171, 1985.

36 Higgins et al: Detection and differentiation by sandwich enzyme-linked immunosorbent assay of human T-lymphotropic virus type III/lymphadenopathy-associated virus and acquired immunodeficiency syndrome-associated retrovirus clinical isolates. *J Clin Microbiol* 24:424, 1986.

37 Carlson JR et al: Adequacy of overnight transport for the recovery of AIDS retroviruses from whole blood specimens. Abstract, Interscience Conference on Antimicrobial Agent and Chemotherapy, New Orleans, LA, 1986.

38 Kwok S et al: Identification of human immunodeficiency virus sequences by using in vitro enzymatic amplification and oligomer cleavage detection. *J Virol* 61:1690,1987.

39 Goudsmit J et al: Expression of human immunodeficiency virus antigen (HIV-Ag) in serum and cerebrospinal fluid during acute and chronic infection. *Lancet* ii:177, 1986.

40 Allain J-P et al: Long-term evaluation of HIV antigen and antibodies to p24 and gp41 in patients with hemophilia. Potential clinical importance. *N Engl J Med* 317:1114, 1987.

41 Chaisson RE et al: Significant changes in HIV antigen level in the serum of patients treated with azidothymidine. *N Engl J Med* 315:1610, 1986.

42 Friedland GH, Klein RS: Transmission of the human immunodeficiency virus. *N Engl J Med* 317:1125, 1987.

43 Shaw GM et al: Molecular characterization of human T-cell leukemia (lymphotropic) virus type III in the acquired immune deficiency syndrome. *Science* 226:1165, 1984.

44 Harper MH et al: Detection of lymphocytes expressing human T-lymphotropic virus type III in lymph nodes and peripheral blood from infected individuals by in situ hybridization. *Proc Natl Acad Sci USA* 83:772, 1986.

45 Saiki RK et al: Enzymatic amplification of beta-globin genomic sequences and restriction site analysis for diagnosis of sickle anemia. *Science* 230:1350, 1985.

46 Ou C-Y et al: DNA amplification for direct detection of HIV-1 in DNA of peripheral blood mononuclear cells. *Science* 239:295, 1988.

Chapter 81

# HIV diagnostic testing: ethical, legal, and clinical considerations

Sheldon H. Landesman
Jack A. DeHovitz

## INTRODUCTION

The HIV antibody test is useful to physicians in the care of infected individuals and for prevention of HIV transmission. How best to utilize the test for these purposes has been controversial from the day it appeared on the horizon.

The concerns that prompted the sharp, sometimes acrimonious debate about the test sprang from fears that improper disclosure or use of test information would result in loss of job or housing, denial of health or life insurance, decreased access to health care, social discrimination, or loss of sexual partners. Because of these concerns, the debate surrounding use of this diagnostic blood test has left the traditional medical arena and entered the political, ethical, and legal realms.[1–19] Therefore, an understanding of the appropriate use of the HIV test requires not only a sound knowledge of its meaning, but also a broad view of the social ramifications of testing and its dual role in disease prevention and care of the HIV-infected individual.

In the following text, several issues regarding the test will be discussed. First is a summary of evolving concepts of the utility and appropriateness of HIV testing. This section provides perspective on the current recommendations for HIV testing. It also highlights the central ethical dilemma faced by an HIV-positive person. This first section is followed by a discussion of (1) who should be tested, (2) management of the asymptomatic HIV-positive patient, and (3) the ethical and legal implications of testing.

## A SUMMARY OF ARGUMENTS FOR AND AGAINST HIV TESTING

When HIV testing first became available, there were strong feelings among civil libertarians and gay advocacy groups that the test should be avoided because it (1) was uninterpretable, (2) was not medically relevant, (3) would have severe and adverse social consequences, and (4) was not necessary to protect the public health.[19] Many of the initial reasons for opposing the test have disappeared with time and experience.

## INTERPRETATION OF THE TEST

Concerns regarding interpretation of a positive test were legitimate in 1985; at that time we had little knowledge of its true meaning. At this time (1989), however, we have a better idea of what the test means and can give a patient reasonably accurate information relative to the diagnostic and prognostic meaning of a positive test.

The HIV antibody test is a highly sensitive assay for detection of antibodies against HIV (see Chap. 79). When used in conjunction with a confirmatory test, it is also very specific.[20] A person with a confirmed positive test is infected and potentially infectious to others for life. Infection with HIV is communicable through sexual intercourse, blood exchange, and from mother to offspring.[21] The chronic infectious status of an HIV-positive individual raises serious ethical and legal concerns for patient and physicians alike.

Once infected with HIV, nearly all persons experience a progressive, time-dependent, apparently irreversible destruction of their immune system. This destruction can best be assessed by serial measurement of T4 cells. The end result of this immune destruction has been defined as AIDS.

## MEDICAL RELEVANCE OF TESTING

The second rationale put forth to avoid testing was that it would not benefit the person being tested because of the absence of effective therapy. Changing medical practice related to care of HIV-infected individuals has weakened this rationale greatly. The development of zidovudine (azidothymidine, AZT) as partially effective therapy for HIV infection,[22] the use of prophylactic regimens to prevent *Pneumocystis carinii* pneumonia (PCP) in immunologically compromised HIV-infected persons,[23,24] the need to screen positive persons for tuberculosis (TB),[25,26] and possible modification of treatment regimens for HIV-infected persons with syphilis[27–29] all create a legitimate argument for accrual of significant medical benefit to a patient who is discovered to be HIV-positive.

Another major benefit of knowing if one is HIV-positive relates to reproductive options. Given the 20 to 40 percent probability of an HIV-infected woman passing the infection to her offspring, it is obviously useful for a woman of childbearing age to know if she is infected before she gets pregnant or early in pregnancy.[30–34] Even if a woman does not alter her reproductive behavior, the knowledge of seropositivity allows for better monitoring and care of her HIV-exposed infant.

## SOCIAL CONSEQUENCES OF TESTING

The central concern of those who advocate limited use of the HIV test relates to the social consequences that would ensue if other persons or organizations (governmental or private) had knowledge of who was HIV-positive. Loss of jobs, housing, insurance, and health care and sexual or social isolation are real consequences of indiscriminate use of or inappropriate dissemination of HIV test results.[1–4,8–11] Concerned individuals fear that the coercive powers of the state, exercised in the past in attempts to control other communicable or venereal diseases, would be indiscriminately applied to HIV-positive persons.[2–4,10,19,35] To some extent, these concerns are legitimate. A positive test bars entry into the military, Peace Corps, and several other governmental positions. Insurance companies are reluctant to insure HIV-infected persons, and cases of job and housing discrimination against known AIDS patients or asymptomatic HIV-positive persons are not uncommon. Laws proposing quarantine, mandatory testing, and severe curtailment of civil liberties have been put forth in many state legislatures.[1–4,13,35]

## PUBLIC HEALTH BENEFITS OF TESTING

The argument that the test was unnecessary for public health purposes was based on the belief that change in behavior could be accomplished by education alone and was not dependent on test knowledge. This argument, put forth most strongly by members of the gay community, has some justification in that the rate of infection in the gay community has decreased sharply in the last several years. Nonetheless, several studies have shown that knowlege of positivity contributes to a decrease in sexual behaviors known to transmit the virus.[5,36–39]

Among intravenous drug abusers the impact of knowing one's serological status is more complex. Studies by Des Jarlais and colleagues document behavior change among seropositive drug users who have information about how AIDS is transmitted. The change is primarily limited to a decrease in needle sharing, not sexual behavior.[40]

Despite the belief of many that testing programs may not significantly change behavior or alter transmission, health officials have come to the conclusion that targeted testing programs carried out in conjunction with counseling can provide a public health benefit by decreasing transmission of HIV.[5,41–43] The greatest benefit of testing would be the identification of positives or at-risk populations, followed by the development of supportive environments that would lead to lifelong behavior modification (i.e., avoidance of behavior that transmits the virus). This public health benefit has yet to be fully realized.

## BEING HIV-POSITIVE: DIFFICULT CHOICES, UNPALATABLE OPTIONS

Within the arguments stated above, what are the ethical issues related to use of the HIV test? A central problem, rarely discussed in the literature, is the situation that confronts an HIV-positive individual. If individuals behave in an ethical manner, they will inform their partners of their status, and a mutual decision on the nature of their sexual relationship will be made. Often the sexual relationship will end as a consequence of informing a partner about seropositivity. If a seropositive person does not inform his or her partner, then clearly the individual is violating the partner's rights and placing the partner at risk. Regardless of the type of sexual behavior a person participates in, all persons have the right to know if their partner is infected. This then is the dilemma faced by seropositive persons. If HIV-positive persons act responsibly to inform their partners, they may have no partners. If positive persons do not tell their partners, they are putting other persons at risk for acquiring a lifelong, potentially fatal disease.

Behavior modification that decreases transmission of HIV can only be accomplished on a voluntary basis. This is due to the private, consensual, and pleasurable nature of sexual and social acts that spread the virus. Infected people may have to choose between denial of pleasure for themselves and placing others at risk for infection and illness.

The goal of any testing program is thus to encourage HIV-positive people or people at high risk to change their behavior even when the behavior change may have adverse effects on their social or sexual practices. This can be done only if the HIV test and the accompanying counseling are seen as a useful act with clear benefits to the tested individual and to society, and there is minimal social damage to the individual offered testing. Only if counseling and testing are done within the above context will their ultimate utility in slowing transmission of HIV and improving care of HIV-infected individuals be realized.

## WHO SHOULD BE TESTED FOR HIV

The decision whether or not to test a patient for HIV should be part of the evaluation of any new patient. HIV testing encompasses both medical and public health indications.[42,43] Medically, HIV testing is indicated in the evaluation of patients who present with symptoms of other infections suggestive of HIV disease. Public health indications take into consideration the important role that counseling and testing play in the prevention of HIV transmission.

## MEDICAL INDICATIONS

There are several medical indications for HIV testing. A primary indication for testing is the presence of symptomatology suggestive of HIV disease. Specifically, the test is a useful diagnostic tool for evaluating patients with selected signs and symptoms such as generalized lymphadenopathy, unexplained weight loss, persistent diarrhea, or oral candidiasis (see Chap. 30). Other early manifestations of HIV infection that should prompt consideration of HIV testing include oral hairy leukoplakia, molluscum contagiosum, or other cutaneous viral disease such as herpes zoster infection or severe herpes simplex infection.

As more is learned about the manifestations of HIV infection, the spectrum of disease associated with HIV-induced immunosuppression is expanding. Pneumonia due to *Streptococcus pneumonia* or *Haemophilus influenzae*[44] and bacterial endocarditis occur more frequently in HIV-infected individuals, especially in intravenous-drug addicts. At our own institution, a large increase in both of these conditions has been noted coincident with the epidemic of HIV disease (L. Mandel, personal communication). Consequently, individuals with a history of high-risk behavior and these infections should be offered HIV counseling and testing.

Increasingly, *Mycobacterium tuberculosis* infection is being recognized as an HIV-associated process. While extrapulmonary tuberculosis in the presence of laboratory evidence of HIV infection currently meets the Centers for Disease Control (CDC) case definition for AIDS, pulmonary infection alone does not.[45] Currently, it appears that one-third to one-half of HIV-associated tuberculosis is confined to the lungs. Almost all of these cases are thought to represent reactivation of latent *M. tuberculosis* infection acquired in the past. Since persons infected with both HIV and the tubercle bacillus are at high risk for severe clinical tuberculosis, the CDC currently recommends that all patients with tuberculosis—regardless of disease location—be routinely counseled and tested for HIV antibody.[25,43,46]

In addition to assisting in the diagnosis and management of HIV-associated infections, use of the HIV antibody test as an aid to early detection of infection may enable the patient to benefit from new methods for prevention of opportunistic infections. Combining HIV testing with lymphocyte enumeration may prevent some of the more common secondary infections. For example, patients with $CD4^+$ cell counts of less than 200/mm$^3$ have a high probability of developing PCP. These patients may be appropriate candidates for regimens which have been shown to prevent PCP infection such as trimethoprim-sulfamethoxazole, aerosolized pentamidine, or dapsone.[23,24] Identification of asymptomatic HIV-infected patients can also serve to prevent tuberculosis. Individuals who are HIV- and PPD-positive should receive isoniazid (INH) for 9 to 12 months.[25,43,46]

Finally, HIV testing can be used to fulfill the criteria for a diagnosis of AIDS.[45] A positive HIV antibody test in the setting of a number of disease states (for example, disseminated coccidioidomycosis, isosporiasis, extrapulmonary TB, HIV encephalopathy, salmonella bacteremia) meets the current CDC case definition of AIDS. While this can certainly assist in the management of the patient's illness, it can also be useful in many localities for obtaining medical and social welfare benefits.

## PUBLIC HEALTH INDICATIONS

Counseling and testing programs for HIV play an important role in the prevention of HIV transmission. Knowledge of serostatus in conjunction with counseling provides information on risk reduction that may reduce HIV transmission. This will usually hold true independent of what one's ultimate serostatus is.[5,36–39] Consequently, physicians should attempt to identify those individuals with a history of high-risk behavior. Clinicians must become comfortable in nonjudgmentally inquiring about a patient's drug and sexual history in order to determine whether HIV testing is indicated. Some patients may be aware that they are at risk. With others, carefully phrased questions focusing on specific behaviors or knowledge of partners' behaviors will better identify risk.

The Public Health Service recommendations for groups that should be offered HIV counseling and testing are discussed below.[43] It is these groups, at highest risk for infection, in whom counseling and testing may be most beneficial in reducing transmission of HIV.

### Targeted populations for testing program

Perhaps at highest risk are those individuals in the major risk categories: men who have sex with men, males and females with a history of intravenous drug use, and sex partners of these two groups. All these individuals, if identified, should be routinely counseled and offered testing for HIV antibody.

All persons seeking treatment for a sexually transmitted disease in any health care setting, including the offices of private physicians, should be routinely counseled and offered testing for HIV antibody. Studies in this country have now documented rates of 5 to 7 percent seropositivity in patients seen in STD clinics in New York City and Baltimore.[47,48] Additionally, at our own institution, we have seen a 15 percent seropositivity rate among women hospitalized with pelvic inflammatory disease (H. Minkoff, personal communication). Seroprevalence rates are lower (1.3 percent) in Detroit, a city less severely affected by the epidemic.[49] Sexually transmitted diseases rarely travel alone, and infection with a single STD must be considered in itself a risk factor that increases the probability of a person being HIV-positive. Sexually transmitted disease clinics provide an additional opportunity to educate individuals in high-risk groups who may not utilize specific HIV-prevention programs. Finally, there is a natural linkage in the message of risk reduction for the traditional STDs and HIV.

Persons with multiple sexual partners or partners with risk factors are at increased risk of acquiring HIV. This is especially true in the inner cities where there are many HIV-infected sexually active addicts. Consequently, persons with multiple sex partners or partners with known risk factors should be offered HIV counseling and testing.

Male and female prostitutes should be counseled and tested and made aware of the risks of HIV infection to themselves and others. Prostitutes who are HIV antibody–positive should be encouraged to discontinue the practice of prostitution.

In addition, individuals who received blood or blood products between 1979 and 1985 (prior to the use of HIV antibody screening of all blood products) should be offered HIV counseling and testing. This is of particular concern for those individuals who received large numbers of units of blood collected from areas with a high incidence of HIV infection.

### HIV testing of women

All women of childbearing age with identifiable risks for HIV infection should be routinely offered counseling and testing for HIV antibody, regardless of the health care setting. Additionally, women who are living in communities or were born in countries where there is a known high prevalence of infection should be offered testing. The utilization of women's health care providers in identifying high-risk populations and providing counseling and testing is of critical importance in any preventive strategy. This group of health care professionals sees large numbers of women at high risk for HIV disease.

Pregnant women living in high-prevalence communities, particularly minority women living in inner city areas on the east coast, have a high rate of infection with HIV.[50–53] All should be offered counseling and testing without regard to stated risk. These women, who live in close social and sexual contact with infected drug-abusing heterosexual men, have a high rate of seropositivity. In New York City, 2 percent of women delivering in a Brooklyn hospital were seropositive.[51] Overall, one in 61 women delivering in the entire city of New York is seropositive.[52] In Boston, 0.8 percent of women delivering in an urban inner city hospital were infected.[50]

The rate of infection among these women will surely grow with time. The HIV infection rate in STD clinics and the steady pool of infected intravenous drug users provide a reservoir of infection that will be transmitted to women with increasing frequency. Currently, the majority of HIV-infected women acquire their infection through intravenous-drug use. This will change, as the number of women infected through heterosexual contact is certain to rise.

Physicians who care for pregnant women should be guided by local seroprevalence rates when developing policies for HIV testing. The microblot method developed by Hoff makes it possible for all states to determine the seroprevalence in each locale and hospital.[50] We recommend that hospitals or locales with relatively high rates of HIV infection (a positivity rate of about 0.5 percent or more) offer HIV testing to all pregnant women whether or not a risk factor is evident. For areas of lower prevalence (about 0.2 percent) a more targeted approach may be useful. In these populations counseling and testing of women with an identified risk may be more cost- and time-efficient. For populations with intermediate seroprevalence, the decision on how to proceed should be left to the local obstetrical and public health authorities.

Similar guidelines can be developed for family planning and abortion services. It should be emphasized that testing of women at high risk is more beneficial if done *prior* to pregnancy. Testing during pregnancy, while useful, leaves seropositive women with equally unpalatable options: pregnancy termination or a high risk of birthing an infected child.

Testing of pregnant women serves several purposes. First, it allows women to fully exercise their reproductive options by providing them with knowledge of all relevant risks to themselves and their offspring. Even if the woman decides to continue a pregnancy after being told she is seropositive, as the majority of women do, there are still material benefits from testing that accrue to the woman and her child.[34]

Knowledge of serostatus and T cell enumeration permits optimal management of the HIV-infected pregnant woman, and may allow for avoidance of serious infections that may place the woman and child at risk. Symptoms of PCP can easily be confused with third trimester pregnancy-associated shortness of breath if serostatus is unknown. At our own institution, we have noted an increased rate of serious infections (opportunistic infections and abscesses) in previously asymptomatic pregnant women with CD4$^+$ cell counts under 300/mm$^3$.

Additional benefits in identifying seropositive pregnant women include advice to refrain from breast feeding, selection of the appropriate types of vaccination for infants, and alerting pediatricians to the potential of early infection in an HIV-exposed infant.

## CLINICAL MANAGEMENT OF ASYMPTOMATIC SEROPOSITIVE INDIVIDUALS

The identification and management of seropositive individuals should proceed with two goals: decreasing the incidence of HIV-associated infections and providing education that reduces the possibility of further HIV transmission.[42] Consequently, the determination that an individual is seropositive should direct the clinician to develop a specific assessment with regard to the history, physical examination, and laboratory evaluation. Once this initial evaluation is complete, the focus will shift to determining the appropriate therapeutic and preventive interventions.

The initial review of systems should attempt to determine the presence of clinical manifestations of HIV-induced immunosuppression. Most of these manifestations, if confirmed, will indicate that the patient has substantial immune impairment. Specific questions should be directed at assessing signs and symptoms such as low-grade fever, fatigue, changes in cough pattern, decreased tolerance to physical exercise, gastrointestinal disturbances, weight loss, or visual disturbances.

The physical examination may be helpful in determining the stage of disease. Specific attention should be paid to the presence of hairy leukoplakia of the tongue, presence of skin lesions consistent with Kaposi's sarcoma, evidence of retinitis, or the presence of oral thrush—all findings that are highly suggestive of advanced HIV infection. Other physical findings suggestive of symptomatic HIV infection include onycholysis, retinal cotton-wool spots, extrainguinal lymphadenopathy, herpes lesions, and organomegaly.

There are a number of laboratory tests that can provide useful information in the initial evaluation of patients with HIV disease. A complete blood count is essential and can detect a variety of abnormalities that occur with HIV infection. These include anemia, lymphopenia, and granulocytopenia. Asymptomatic but severe thrombocytopenia is not uncommon in HIV-infected individuals.

Perhaps the most useful laboratory evaluation of the HIV-infected patient is enumeration of T-lymphocyte subsets. Quantification of the CD4$^+$ (T4 helper/inducer) lymphocytes is more useful than the ratio of CD4$^+$ to CD8$^+$. HIV infection in the setting of a depressed CD4$^+$ cell count is highly suggestive of severe HIV-induced immunosuppression.

HIV-infected patients should always have a tuberculin skin test. If the patient is PPD negative, controls should be placed to determine whether the patient is anergic. Any patient with a positive PPD should be started on a prophylactic course of isoniazid (INH).

Serologic evaluations for *Toxoplasma gondii,* syphilis, and hepatitis B are recommended. Positive serology for *Toxoplasma* may be an important predictor in the subsequent development of symptomatic disease. In addition, patients with risk factors for HIV infection are often at risk for syphilis and hepatitis B. There is also evidence that the natural history of syphilis is accelerated in HIV-positive individuals.[28,29,54]

Finally, medical evaluation is an opportunity for educational intervention. The education should include information about the disease, its prognosis, and possible interventions. Patients should be given a clear explanation about how HIV is transmitted and how to prevent its transmission. Patients who are sexually active must be advised about the possibility of transmitting the virus to their partners during intercourse. Women must also receive information on the implications of seropositivity for present or future pregnancies. Since psychosocial support is so critical to patients with HIV disease, the office visit also gives the clinician the opportunity to provide the patient with a list of appropriate community resources that provide such support. Finally, it is important to counsel other family members as well as sexual partners about the disease and its transmission.

The frequency of follow-up of the HIV-infected patient should depend on the patient's clinical status and the stage of the disease. The progression of this chronic lifelong disease does not follow a clear, well-defined path. Patients should understand the potential course of disease, and have an increased awareness of the subtle signs and symptoms that may be early indicators of progressive disease. Signs such as increasing fatigue, low-grade fever, changes in cough patterns, or weight loss may be early indicators of opportunistic infections.

The asymptomatic HIV-infected patient with a CD4$^+$ cell count of approximately 500/mm$^3$ can be monitored every 3 to 6 months. Those patients with mild or vague symptoms and fewer CD4$^+$ cells may need more frequent follow-up, while individuals with hairy leukoplakia or thrush should be monitored every 4 weeks. Specific prophylaxis for PCP should be considered at $\leq$ 200 CD4$^+$ cells/mm$^3$.

## ETHICAL AND LEGAL CONSIDERATIONS OF HIV TESTING

HIV testing poses difficulties for the physician and patient in four areas: (1) informed consent, (2) confidentiality, (3) duty to warn, and (4) access to care and duty to treat.

### INFORMED CONSENT

Informed consent is required for procedures or treatments that are associated with significant risks to the patient or are experimental in nature. Informed consent requires that the patient has the capacity to reason and to understand the information provided. It also assumes that decisions are voluntary and made without coercion, and that all risks and benefits of a particular intervention and alternative treatments are explained.[55–57]

Shortly after the HIV test was licensed, some states mandated written informed consent for testing. The requirement for written informed consent prior to HIV testing was unusual: except for assays or tests that screen for genetic defects, written informed consent is generally not required for blood tests.

Over the last several years public policies concerning written informed consent for HIV testing have undergone nuanced changes. A recent modification is the introduction of the term "routine counseling and testing." As defined by the CDC branch of the Public Health Service, "routine counseling and testing" is "a policy to provide these services to all clients after informing them that testing will be done." Included in this policy pronouncement is the statement that "except where testing is required by law, individuals have the right to decline to be tested without being denied health care or other services."[43] These same guidelines emphasize the importance of the counseling component to any testing program that seeks to decrease transmission and provide good medical care.

Despite these recommendations, many locales and hospitals mandate neither informed consent nor pre- and posttest counseling. A recent study by Henry et al. documented the fact that one-third to one-half of hospitals required neither informed consent nor risk-reduction counseling to accompany HIV testing.[58]

The legal implications of the informed consent controversy are unclear. In part, physicians must be guided by local administrative and statutory requirements. Violation of written informed consent regulations in states where it is required can result in heavy civil penalties. This is currently the case in New York, California, and several other states. In many states and municipalities, the law is unclear: hospital guidelines are administrative in nature and only "recommend" certain procedures.[58] In many hospitals guidelines do not exist at all. In these situations, the physician or health care provider must be guided by the commonsense objectives of any HIV counseling and testing programs, i.e., to diagnose HIV disease and to prevent transmission of the virus. With these clear objectives in mind, HIV testing should be performed within the following framework:

1. Testing should be voluntary except where required by law.
2. Both pre- and posttest counseling should be provided to those seeking HIV testing. The extent of the pretest counseling may vary greatly with the population being offered the test. For pregnant women, especially those who are intravenous-drug users, extensive pretest counseling is useful. This population may have a very difficult time in receiving information that they are test-positive. Extensive pretest counseling in this setting may mitigate some of the negative and even counterproductive effects of testing these patients.[59]

   Patients in STD clinics generally require less pretest counseling than pregnant women or drug addicts. Nonetheless, an investment in pretest counseling combined with a supportive attitude toward taking the test is useful in identifying HIV-infected persons and providing risk-reduction information. The HIV-positive patient should then be given a full medical evaluation and provided with ongoing medical and psychologic care. The long-term provision of medical and social service support to the ambulatory HIV-positive patient is essential if the twin objectives of caring for the infected and preventing new infections are to be achieved.
3. Informed consent should be secured in a manner consistent with local or state laws. If no policy on informed consent exists, then the physician should, at a minimum, follow the PHS guidelines: inform the patient about the test, provide some pretest counseling, and give the patient the option to refuse. Medical care should be provided regardless of whether the test is performed.
4. Those being tested should be informed as to how the confidentiality of their test result will be protected. They should be made aware of who will have access to results and the possible consequences of misuse of test results, especially with regard to health and life insurance. Issues of confidentiality and discrimination should be discussed with the patient, although some of the consequences are unknown risks. The patient should be made aware of the availability of anonymous testing, where appropriate.
5. Test results should be given in person, preferably by the same person who provided pretest counseling.
6. Information should be recorded in compliance with existing state and local laws. Some states prohibit HIV results from appearing in medical charts. Other states, e.g., New York State, require that the results of an HIV test, when performed within a hospital setting, be placed in the chart. In general, results of tests done within the hospital setting should be placed in the hospital medical record. In this manner, other health care providers who see the chart for medical reasons will have access to this important medical information. As noted above, the patient should be informed of who will have access to the information.

## CONFIDENTIALITY

Confidentiality between physician and patient has never been absolute. Reporting of communicable or venereal disease,[60] gunshot wounds, and suspected child abuse are a few examples wherein information obtained within patient-doctor relationships is revealed to government agencies or third parties. The limits of doctor-patient confidentiality were clearly enunciated in *Whalen v. Roe*, where the Supreme Court held that "Disclosures of private medical information to doctors, to hospital personnel, to insurance companies, and to public health agencies are often an essential part of modern medical practice even when the disclosure may reflect unfavorably on the character of the patient. Requiring such disclosures to a representative of the State having responsibility for the health of the community does not automatically amount to an impermissible invasion of privacy."[61] The court also held that the parties receiving the private medical information must be capable of keeping the information confidential; otherwise they cannot receive it.

Confidentiality is further eroded by judicial decisions that are creating a legal obligation for a physician toward a third party who may be endangered by the patient.[62] This duty to protect a third party at risk might include warning that party, and is discussed in detail in the subsequent section. Confidentiality is also compromised by the needs of third party payers, social service agencies, and quality assurance staff to review medical records in the performance of their assigned functions. Within the hospital itself, confidentiality is limited by the needs of multiple health care providers to have all information relevant to the provision of care.

Who should have access to HIV test results given the large number of individuals, agencies, and companies that have a legitimate need for this information? Policies and procedures for confidentiality should be guided by the goals of any counseling and testing program: care of the infected and decreasing transmission of the virus. Stated simply, confidentiality must be protected to the extent that it optimizes patient care and encourages people to seek counseling and testing.

With this principle in mind a reasonable set of guidelines for confidentiality of HIV test results would be as follows:

1. Patients tested as part of hospital or medical clinic evaluation should have their results placed in the medical records. The rationale for this recommendation is that information concerning a person's serostatus is important for the interpretation and management of many conditions, especially if the patient is seropositive. Many people do not see a single health care provider for all aspects of their care. Other health care providers who may be seeing the patient for the first time require access to this important medical information if opti-

mal care is to be delivered to the patient. A good example is the pregnant woman who knows she is positive and develops shortness of breath, a common symptom in the third trimester of pregnancy. Interpretation of this symptom is very different in an HIV-positive patient, compared with an HIV-negative patient. Obstetricians may easily miss PCP and leave the mother and infant at serious risk if they do not know the serostatus of the woman.

Similar examples exist across the entire spectrum of HIV-associated illness. Many infectious diseases associated with HIV have subtle or atypical presentations which can easily be missed if the physician is not aware of the patient's seropositivity. One important caveat relative to test results being entered into the medical record is that the patient should always be informed at the time of testing that results will become part of the medical record, and who will have access to those results.

Testing for HIV infection has little role in prevention of nosocomial transmission of the virus. A more prudent approach is to universally apply recommended blood and body fluid precautions to all patients.

2. Insurance companies may legitimately access hospital records containing HIV serology results, especially if the purpose is to provide for payment of HIV-related illness. Patients who request their health insurance to pay for such care should provide written authorization for release of the record. Similarly, social service agencies that provide direct services to HIV-infected individuals will need access to the medical record prior to awarding the requested social service support.
3. The issue of access to medical records containing HIV serostatus becomes more complex when a person receives health care from a company-funded health care plan or HMO. In this situation, the employer could theoretically access HIV test results and use a positive test to deny employment or change the employee's job. Under these circumstances the physician should be aware of company policy with regard to HIV-positive employees. The physician should be alert to potential misuse of test results in these circumstances, and in some cases may recommend that the patient be tested at an off-site, non-company-related health facility.
4. As a general rule, HIV test results, regardless of where they are recorded, should be provided to third parties only on a "need to know" basis.[16] This includes health care providers who are directly serving the patient, insurance companies paying for their care, and social agencies, including foster care agencies, that may be caring for an infected child.

Reinforcement of the traditional concept of doctor-patient confidentiality is critical to ensuring appropriate release of HIV test results. Information provided for provision of care or social services is not for general distribution. Repeated emphasis of the concept that confidential information is given in confidence, and for the sole purpose of assisting in patient care, is essential if HIV testing is to be useful in provision of care and acquisition of services. Releasing test results for purposes other than patient care or clearly defined public health reasons should be viewed as a clear breach of the doctor-patient relationship, and should be punished according to applicable statutes and administrative regulations.

## DUTY TO WARN

Do physicians have a legal obligation to inform the sexual partner of their seropositive patient that the patient is HIV-positive? The previous section discussed release of HIV test results for the benefit of patients. What about circumstances where release of this information is for the benefit of third parties at risk, and not the patient? This circumstance is most often encountered when asymptomatic persons are identified as HIV-positive.

Although there is relevant previous case law, a case decided in California in 1976 forms a significant part of the legal basis for a physician's responsibility to a third party at risk.[62] *Tarasoff* concerned a psychiatrist who was held liable for failing to notify the girlfriend of his patient, after the patient voiced violent intentions toward the woman. The patient subsequently murdered his girlfriend, and her family prevailed in a lawsuit against the psychiatrist for failure to exercise reasonable care to protect the foreseeable victim from a probable danger.[62]

As stated by the California Supreme Court in the *Tarasoff* decision, "the protected privilege (doctor-patient) ends where the public peril begins."[10,62] The *Tarasoff* decision, and subsequent cases based on *Tarasoff*, may place physicians at legal peril if they do not fulfill their duty to take action to protect a third party who is clearly endangered by a patient. In relation to HIV disease, this means that the physician or health care provider may have a legal duty to warn the sexual partner of an HIV-positive person.

What does the physician do with a positive patient who refuses to inform a partner? What defines a partner—a single sexual contact, a month-long relationship, a consenting spouse, a previous partner? What of future partners? The American Medical Association (AMA) adopted a position on duty to warn at their June 1988 meeting, which supports the notion that physicians have an obligation to warn third parties at risk of acquiring HIV from an infected partner.[63] However, is a physician who knowingly violates the confidentiality of the patient also legally liable? The answer to this question will vary with each case, although the law suggests that physicians are permitted and perhaps expected to violate doctor-patient confidentiality when necessary to protect an endangered third party. When specifically provided for by state law, the reporting of known contacts (e.g., spouses) to public health authorities may provide legal immunity to the disclosing physician. In other states, however, any disclosure may run counter to prevailing statutes. Thus, knowledge of local statutes and regulations is essential.

Physicians and health providers caught in the above situations may decide to violate patient confidentiality and warn the sexual partner of their patient. However, violation of patient confidentiality in order to protect a third party must be viewed as the last step in a lengthy process designed to secure the active cooperation of the patient. The physician should violate the physician-patient relationship and warn the third party only when voluntary means fail. He or she may want to seek advice from legal or public health authorities before doing so.

Physicians should first try to educate the patient and convince them to tell their partner. Alternatively, they can offer their own services to tell the partner alone or have the couple come in together. Another option is to provide the name of the partner to the health department and have a department caseworker inform and educate the third party. Whatever method is chosen to inform the partner, the name of the infected patient need not and should not be revealed unless agreed upon by the HIV-infected individual.

The HIV-infected patient also has legal and ethical responsibilities. Societal and ethical norms require that an HIV-infected person inform his or her sexual partner of their seropositivity. If the HIV-infected individual has unprotected intercourse with an unknowing and seronegative partner, ethical and in some cases legal norms (civil and criminal) are violated.[4,10,17] Case law related to other communicable or sexually transmitted diseases, e.g., genital herpes and syphilis, suggests that liability may be incurred or quarantine authority may be invoked when sexual transmission of HIV occurs in the above described circumstance.[1,10,17,65–67] Several states, including Florida and Idaho, have identified the act of knowingly or willfully exposing another to the HIV virus as a crime. Other jurisdictions, relying on existing laws, have brought manslaughter or attempted murder charges against persons who willfully engage in acts that could transmit the virus.[1,4,10,17]

Successful prosecution of these cases is difficult for a variety of legal reasons.[1–4,10,17] Nonetheless, the social climate in the country is changing rapidly and large segments of the population and their representatives view transmission of the virus to an unsuspecting partner as morally reprehensible and criminally negligent. This is reflected increasingly in attempts at the state level to declare such transmission criminal in nature.

## ACCESS TO CARE AND DUTY TO TREAT

Individuals who are HIV-positive are fearful of being denied appropriate medical treatment because physicians and other health care workers are concerned about acquiring HIV infection from them. The estimated probability of acquiring HIV from a puncture wound with a needle contaminated with HIV-positive blood is 1:200 to 1:300.[68] For doctors who work in hospitals with many AIDS patients, this risk has real meaning. The CDC has issued specific guidelines designed to decrease nosocomial acquisition of HIV.[69] All physicians should become familiar with these recommendations.

Most physicians have maintained that they will operate on and care for HIV-infected patients provided they can take extra precautions on those patients known to be HIV-positive. Nonetheless, there is lingering doubt among many HIV-infected individuals that this is the case. The original statement of the AMA council on Ethical and Judicial Affairs, issued in 1986 stated:

> Physicians and other health professionals have a long tradition of tending to patients affected with infectious diseases with compassion and courage. However, not everyone is emotionally able to care for patients with AIDS. If the health professional is unable to care for their patients with AIDS that individual should be removed from the case. Alternative arrangements for care of the patient must be made.[70]

This statement is not encouraging, and a reader could easily infer that there is little commitment to treat infected individuals. Further, it allows for physicians to reject HIV-infected patients if the physician is emotionally unable to provide care. This exception is broad enough to encompass almost any situation. Legally, physicians are not required to treat patients except in limited situations like emergencies. The AMA code specifically states, "A physician is not required to accept as patients all who apply to him for treatment. He may arbitrarily refuse to accept a patient."[71]

In late 1987, because of criticism directed at its initial position, the AMA Council on Ethical Judicial Affairs affirmed that a physician may not ethically refuse to treat a patient with HIV disease, if the patient's condition is within the physician's current realm of competence, solely because the patient has AIDS or is infected with HIV.[72]

As noted by Annas,[18] the revised AMA statement did not say that physicians must care for HIV-infected persons but made refusal to provide care unethical if such care was within the physician's realm of competence and refusal was based solely on HIV status. Even this statement, clearly stronger than its predecessor, is incomplete. Officials of the AMA have made it clear that physicians who don't want to take care of AIDS patients will be considered "incompetent" to treat and they will be excused.[73] According to AMA Vice President James Sammona, this exemption includes physicians with a "psychological hang-up" that impairs their abilities to care for HIV-infected patients.[18] As stated by Annas, "This reduces the AMA position to a statement that a physician must treat an AIDS patient if the doctor wants to care for an AIDS patient."[18]

The Infectious Diseases Society of America and the American College of Physicians have enunciated a positive ethical responsibility for physicians to care for HIV-infected patients. They state, in a revised document published in August 1988, "that physicians, other health care professionals and hospitals are obligated to provide competent and human care for all patients, including patients with AIDS and AIDS related conditions as well as HIV infected patients with unrelated medical problems. The denial of appropriate care to any patient for any reason is unethical."[74]

Other powerful influences on physician behavior toward HIV-infected patients include state licensing boards, employer contracts, and hospital bylaws. Most state licensing boards have not clarified the legal obligation of licensees to render proper care to HIV-positive individuals: board policies vary from state to state.

Many employer contracts and hospital bylaws state that refusal to care for HIV-infected patients is discriminatory and could be punishable by loss of job or staff privileges. This is often the case in hospitals with many AIDS patients. Legal actions in response to "refusal to treat" situations are rare. Most often they are resolved by quiet diplomacy, with the outcome not always favoring the patient. The major federal antidiscrimination statute for the handicapped (section 504 of the Federal Rehabilitation Act of 1973), its application to HIV-infected individuals as interpreted by the U.S. Justice Department, and a major case associated with the statute (*Arline v. School Board of Nassau County, Florida*) have little impact on the physician's responsibility to treat.[75,76] The ultimate impact of section 504 in preventing employment or housing discrimination is not yet clear, but it is not likely to strongly influence physician behavior. The effect of applicable state handicapped nondiscrimination laws may vary widely among different states.

Physicians have no legal obligation to treat HIV-infected patients except in certain defined and limited areas. However, strong statements by professional societies, state licensing boards, medical schools, and hospital can change a "no duty rule" into a "professional duty to treat."[9,18]

Despite the small risk of nosocomial acquisition of HIV, many physicians and other health care workers have continued to care for AIDS patients. In doing so, they exemplify the highest ideals of the caring professions and serve as a model for us all.

## CONCLUSIONS

1. HIV counseling, testing, and programs must be directed toward two goals—providing care for the infected and decreasing transmission of the virus.
2. This goal can best be accomplished by targeted counseling and testing of "at-risk populations" in an environment that provides optimal medical and psychological care to the infected, protects them from discriminatory acts, and supports them in making the difficult behavioral changes needed for their protection and the protection of others.

3. Applicable laws and administrative regulations concerning HIV testing and counseling vary widely among different states. Responsible physicians should be aware of laws and regulations affecting their practice, in order to protect their patients and reduce their own liability.
4. Voluntary and active participation on the part of the infected or "at-risk" individual is critical to achievement of these aims. Provisions for informed consent before testing, confidentiality of records, equal access to care, and strong antidiscrimination laws are keys to their participation.

## References


1 Gostin L et al: A review of AIDS regulatory policy in the United States: *Law Med Health Care* 15:1, 1987.
2 Curran W et al: AIDS: Legal and policy implications of the applications of traditional disease control measures. *Law Med Health Care* 15:27, 1987.
3 Hermann HJ: Liability related to diagnosis and transmission of AIDS. *Law Med Health Care* 15:36, 1987.
4 Field M: AIDS and criminal law. *Law Med Health Care* 15:46, 1987.
5 Cates W Jr et al: HIV counseling and testing: Does it work. *Am J Public Health* 78:394, 1988.
6 Steinbrook R et al: Ethical dilemmas in caring for patients with acquired immunodeficiency syndrome. *Ann Intern Med* 103:787, 1985.
7 Gostin L et al: AIDS screening, confidentiality and duty to warn. *Am J Public Health* 77:361, 1988.
8 Nolan K (ed): AIDS: The responsibilities of health professions. *Hastings Cent Rep,* April/May 1988.
9 Freedman B: Health professions, codes and the right to refuse to treat HIV infectious patients. *Hastings Cent Rep,* April/May 1988, p 20.
10 Dickens BM: Legal rights and duties in the AIDS epidemic. *Science* 239:580, 1988.
11 Walters L: Ethical issues in the prevention and treatment of HIV infection and AIDS. *Science* 239:597, 1988.
12 Bayer R et al: HIV antibody screening: An ethical framework for evaluating proposed programs. *JAMA* 256:1768, 1986.
13 Gostin L et al: Legal control measures for AIDS: Reporting requirements, surveillance quarantine and regulation of public meeting places. *Am J Public Health* 77:214, 1987.
14 Parmet WE: AIDS and the limits of discrimination. *Law Med Health Care* 15:62, 1988.
15 Osborn JE: AIDS: Politics and science. *N Engl J Med* 318:444, 1988.
16 American Hospital Association (AHA), Special Committee on AIDS/HIV Infection Policy. AIDS/HIV infection policy: Ensuring a safe hospital environment, 1987.
17 Mills M et al: The acquired immunodeficiency syndrome: Infection control and public health law. *N Engl J Med* 314:931, 1986.
18 Annas GJ: Legal risks and responsibilities of physicians in the AIDS epidemic. *Hastings Cent Rep,* April/May 1988, p 26.
19 Bayer R: *Private Acts, Social Consequences: AIDS and the Politics of Public Health.* New York, Free Press, 1989. (This book provides an excellent description of the social, political, and ethical arguments that took place around the issue of HIV testing.)
20 Burke DS et al: Measure of false positive rate in screening program for human immunodeficiency virus infections. *N Engl J Med* 319:961, 1988.
21 Friedland GR et al: Transmission of the human immunodeficiency virus. *N Engl J Med* 317:1125, 1987.
22 Fischl MA et al: The efficacy of Azidithymidine (AZT) in the treatment of patients with AIDS and AIDS related complex. *N Engl J Med* 317:185, 1987.
23 Metroka CE et al: Successful chemoprophylaxis for pneumocystis carinii pneumonia with dapsone in patients with AIDS and ARC. Presented at the Third International Conference on AIDS, June 1–5, 1987.
24 Bernard EM et al: Clinical trials with aerosol pentamidine for prevention of *Pneumocystis carinii* pneumonia. *Clin Res* 35:468A, 1987.
25 CDC: Diagnosis and management of mycobacterial infection and disease in persons with HTLV-III/LAV infection. *MMWR* 35:448, 1986.
26 Glatt AE et al: Treatment of infections associated with human immunodeficiency virus. *N Engl J Med* 318:1439, 1988.
27 Tramont EC: Syphilis in the AIDS era. *N Engl J Med* 316:1600, 1987.
28 Johns DR et al: Alteration in the natural history of neurosyphilis by concurrent infection with the human immunodeficiency virus. *N Engl J Med* 316:1569, 1987.
29 Berry CD et al: Neurologic relapse after benzathine penicillin therapy for secondary syphilis in a patient with HIV infection. *N Engl J Med* 316:1587, 1987.
30 Mendez H et al: Human immunodeficiency virus (HIV) infection in pregnant women and their offspring. *Pediatr Res* 21:418A, 1987.
31 Abrams E et al: The New York City Collaborative Study Group for Maternal Transmission of Human Immunodeficiency Virus (HIV): Longitudinal study of infants born to women at risk for AIDS. IV International Conference on AIDS, Stockholm, Sweden, 1988:442. Abstract 7258.
32 Mok JQ et al: Infants born to mothers seropositive for human immunodeficiency virus. *Lancet* i:1164, 1987.
33 The European Collaborative Study: Mother to child transmission of HIV infection. *Lancet* ii:1039, 1988.
34 Feinkind L et al: HIV in pregnancy. *Clin Perinatol* 15:189, 1988.
35 State AIDS Reports: Number 3 May/June 1988. Published by the State AIDS Policy Center of the Intergovernmental Health Policy Project of George Washington University.
36 Schechter MT et al: Patterns of sexual behavior and condom use in a cohort of homosexual men. *Am J Public Health* 78:1535, 1988.
37 Van Griensven GJP et al: Impact of HIV antibody testing on changes in sexual behavior among homosexual men in the Netherlands. *Am J Public Health* 78:1575, 1988.
38 Fox R et al: Effect of HIV antibody disclosure on subsequent sexual activity in homosexual men. *AIDS* 1:241, 1988.
39 Coates TJ et al: Behavioral consequences of AIDS antibody testing among gay men. *JAMA* 258:1189, 1987.
40 Des Jarlais et al: HIV infection among intravenous drug users: Epidemiology and risk reduction. *AIDS* 1:67, 1987.
41 CDC: Additional recommendations to reduce sexual and drug abuse-related transmission of human T-lymphotropic virus type III/lymphadenopathy-associated virus. *MMWR* 35:152, 1986.
42 Francis DP et al: The prevention of acquired immunodeficiency syndrome in the United States. *JAMA* 257:1357, 1987.
43 CDC: Public Health Service guidelines for counseling and antibody testing to prevent HIV infection and AIDS. *MMWR* 36:509, 1987.
44 Polsky B et al: Bacterial pneumonia in patients with the acquired immunodeficiency syndrome. *Ann Intern Med* 104:38, 1986.
45 CDC: Revision of the CDC surveillance care definition for acquired immunodeficiency syndrome. *MMWR* 36 (suppl. 15):15, 1987.
46 American Thoracic Society/CDC: Mycobacterioses and the acquired immunodeficiency syndrome. *Am Rev Respir Dis* 136:492, 1987.
47 Quinn JC et al: Human immunodeficiency virus infection among patients attending a sexually transmitted disease clinic. *N Engl J Med* 318:197, 1988.
48 Chaisson MA et al: HIV infection in persons attending a sexually transmitted disease clinic in New York City. Presented at the 27th Interscience Conference on Antimicrobial Agents and Chemotherapy, New York, Oct. 4–7, 1987.
49 Sienko DG: Screening for HIV infection in sexually transmitted disease clinics. *N Engl J Med* 319:242, 1988 (letter).
50 Hoff R et al: Seroprevalence of human immunodeficiency virus among child bearing women: estimation by testing samples of blood from newborns. *N Engl J Med* 318:525, 1988.
51 Landesman S et al: Serosurvey of human immunodeficiency virus infection on parturients. *JAMA* 258:2701, 1987.
52 Lambert B: One in 61 babies in New York City has AIDS antibodies, study says. *New York Times,* Jan. 13, 1988, p A1.
53 Donegan DS: HIV seroprevalence rate at the Boston City Hospital. *N Engl J Med* 319:653, 1988 (letter).
54 Recommendations for diagnosing and treating syphilis in HIV infected patients. *MMWR* 37:600, 1988.

55 Meisel A et al: What we do and do not know about informed consent. *JAMA* 246:2463, 1981.

56 Miller LJ: Informed consent. *JAMA* 240:2100, 2347, 2556, 2661, 1980.

57 Lynne J: Informed consent: An overview. *Behav Sci Law* 1:29, 1983.

58 Henry K: Human immunodeficiency virus antibody testing: A description of practices and policies at U.S. infectious disease teaching hospitals and Minnesota hospitals. *JAMA* 259:1819, 1988.

59 James ME: HIV positivity diagnosed during pregnancy: Psychosocial characterization of patients and their adaptation. *Gen Hosp Psychiatry* 10:309, 1988.

60 Brandt A: *No Magic Bullet: A Social History of Venereal Disease in the United States Since 1880.* New York, Oxford, 1985.

61 *Whalen v. Roe,* 429 U.S. 589, 602 (1977).

62 *Tarasoff v. Regents of University of California.* 551 P. 2d 334 (Cal. 1976).

63 Adopted by House of Delegates, American Medical Association, Annual Meeting, June 1988.

64 *Hoffman v. Blackmon,* 241 So. 2d 752 (Fla. App. 1970). Also *Wojcik v. Aluminum Co. of America,* 18 Misc. 2d 740. 183 N.Y.S. 2d 351, 357–358 (1959).

65 Prentice RA et al: Liability for transmission of herpes: Using traditional tort principles to encourage honesty in sexual relationships. *J Contemp Law* 11:67, 1984.

66 *Simonsen v. Simonsen,* 177 N.W. 831 (Neb. 1920).

67 *Kathleen K. v Robert B. California Reporter* 1984; 198:273-7 Court of Appeal, Second District.

68 Marcus B et al: Surveillance of health care workers exposed to blood from patients infected with the human immunodeficiency virus. *N Engl J Med* 319:1118, 1988.

69 CDC: Recommendations for prevention of HIV transmission in health care settings. *MMWR* 1987 36:2S (suppl).

70 AMA, Council on Ethical and Judicial Affairs: Statement on AIDS, December 1986.

71 AMA: *Medicolegal Forms with Legal Analysis.* Chicago, AMA, 1973, p 1.

72 AMA Council on Ethical and Judicial Affairs: Ethical issues involved in the growing AIDS crisis, December 1987.

73 Refusing care of AIDS patients: New policies and admissions emerge. *Hosp Ethics* January/February 1988, p 5.

74 Health Policy Committee of American College of Physicians and the Infectious Disease Society of America: The acquired immune deficiency syndrome (AIDS) and infection with the human immunodeficiency virus (HIV). *J Infect Dis* 158:273, 1988.

75 *Arline v. School Board of Nassau County, Florida* 772 F 2d 759 (11th Cir, 1985).

76 Memorandum of Charles Cooper, Assistant Attorney General, Office of Legal Counsel, re: Application of Section 504 of Rehabilitation Act to persons with AIDS, AIDS related complex or infection with the AIDS virus, June 20, 1986. See also revision of memorandum wherein the initial position of the Justice Department was reversed (e.g., persons with HIV infection would now be considered handicapped). Revised memorandum delivered to White House Counsel on Oct. 14, 1988.

## ACKNOWLEDGMENTS

This work was supported by grants from the New York State AIDS Institute (815332A and C001720) and the National Institute of Child Health and Human Development (25714) and a subcontract from Research Triangle Institute (0225703722) and Westat Inc. (study of the natural history of HIV infection in pregnant women and their offspring).

The authors wish to acknowledge the invaluable assistance of Peter Gillette, M.D., and Susan Holman, R.N., M.S., for their review and comments on the manuscript and Karen Murray, who worked tirelessly in typing and correcting the document.

Chapter 82

# Necessary laboratory support at the peripheral, regional, and national levels in developing countries

Ewe-Hui Sng

The etiologic agents responsible for sexually transmitted diseases (STD) may cause variable clinical manifestations, and multiple agents may give rise to similar syndromes. Consequently it is often not possible to establish the correct diagnosis by clinical features alone. Laboratory support is necessary to enable the clinical and health officer to manage and control sexually transmitted diseases in a rational manner.

## DEVELOPMENT OF A LABORATORY SERVICE

Unfortunately most developing countries do not have sufficient resources to provide the necessary laboratory support. Even in those countries with some form of laboratory organization the development has often been uncoordinated, and facilities are concentrated in certain institutions at the expense of those peripheral clinics where most of the patients are seen. The net result is that many patients are managed without accurate diagnosis and treatment is often given either inadequately or wrongly. In view of rising health costs and new technologies, and as STD agents become more widespread, there is urgent need for laboratory services to be developed and used more rationally.

Although the difficulties encountered in each developing country are not always the same, most problems have common features, and certain basic principles are applicable to most. Adequate provisions and proper management of resources are two key factors. Inadequate funding is often the result of negligence in monitoring the size and nature of the problem. A special effort must be made to gather and present the necessary data to decision makers. Such data may be obtained from existing clinics, hospitals, and laboratories or from a pilot survey.

The concept of development, however, is not limited to the creation or enlargement of a budget. It also involves making the best use of resources. Laboratory administrators should have a clear concept of the role that the laboratory should play in patient management, epidemiology, control, and research activities. The major areas that require emphasis for development are considered in the light of the objectives of the health service.

The emergence of human immunodeficiency virus (HIV) infection must lead developing countries to further stress the importance of developing good laboratory management, comprehensive staff training programs, and efficient communication systems for the laboratory organization.

## ORGANIZATION

Most laboratories supporting STD clinics have both specific functions and an overall role. The immediate purpose often is the management of patients by helping to establish the etiologic diagnosis, determining the drug of choice, testing for cure, and assisting in the epidemiologic management of contacts. However, laboratories can also play an important element in control programs. To fulfill these functions, it is desirable to have a laboratory organization comprised of a central laboratory and a network of regional and peripheral laboratories to provide a diagnostic service and a means for continuous surveillance. The aim is for the laboratory to provide service at the level required, with minimal cost, and in the shortest time possible. The details of the laboratory network will vary in different countries, but a consideration of certain factors should be made in planning the distribution of the laboratories:

- The level of disease in the community should be of sufficient magnitude to warrant the facilities. In many developing countries HIV and chlamydial infections, syphilis, and gonorrhea are highly prevalent and they lead to serious sequelae. High priority should be accorded to them.
- Adequate staff and funds should be available to maintain the laboratory. Sharing of facilities with other laboratories will reduce the resources needed.
- The laboratory should be conveniently located for patients or suitable for the receipt of specimens and the dispatch of reports to clinics within the area. It should also be located so that it is possible to receive supervision from and make referrals to larger laboratories. This will be determined by a number of factors such as the transport system, telephone, and postal services. The use of electronic data communication can greatly facilitate such activities.
- Every attempt should be made to integrate the laboratory service with the primary health care clinics. Particular attention should be paid to blood banks, prenatal and gynecologic clinics, besides clinics frequented by STD patients.

The organization consists of a system of laboratories spreading outward with progressive decrease in the levels of sophistication to cover a wide area. In order that the various laboratories provide an effective and reliable service, it is essential that the units are functionally linked. Peripheral units should be able to refer problems beyond their capabilities to intermediate-level laboratories at a higher level. Similarly, supervision and supplies can be provided by intermediate laboratories to more peripheral ones. Judicious use of simple means of communication, such as a motorcycle or telephone, can improve access to laboratories and reduce delay in the reporting of results.

## SELECTION OF LABORATORY TESTS

Although most laboratories will employ a number of different tests, the range that is available is rapidly increasing. The types of investigations which a laboratory can offer will depend on the level of its competence and a combination of various factors. Laboratories should generally develop tests which are simple to perform and for which the running cost is low. However, in a number of situations the choice is not easy. Before any test is implemented, a careful consideration of the following principles is recommended, since the introduction of an inappropriate test is wasteful:

- The purpose of the test should be consonant with the role of the laboratory.

- The more prevalent and serious the disease, the greater will be the necessity for a test.
- The disease should preferably be treatable or controllable.
- The result of the test is likely to influence treatment or to require the institution of preventive measures.
- The requirements to perform the test should be consistent with the level of resources available to the laboratory.
- No other laboratory in the area should be better able to perform the service.
- The test is not being developed at the expense of some other function of higher priority.

The laboratory should be sufficiently dynamic to adapt to changing circumstances. This may occur as a result of new problems emerging, such as HIV infection. A new pattern of disease may take place, requiring new emphasis, such as the increasing significance of chlamydial (nongonococcal) urethritis in relation to gonorrhea in certain countries. New technologies may provide improved tests, which will enable laboratories to enlarge their capabilities in both quantitative and qualitative terms.

## FUNCTIONS OF LABORATORIES AT DIFFERENT LEVELS

Conceptually, the laboratory service may be regarded as a three-tier system, each with its own level of competence and responsibilities. This will provide a rational division of work on a local, regional, and national basis. A summary of the different levels of competence is given in Table 82-1.

## PERIPHERAL LEVEL

The bulk of patients with STDs have traditionally been seen either by private practitioners or in government outpatient clinics. Nowadays, increasing numbers are also being seen at specialist (pediatric, surgical, etc.) clinics. Laboratories which service these clinics have an important role which larger laboratories at a higher level are unable to fulfill. They offer a speedy service which is vital to patient compliance. In many instances patients can be seen, investigated, and treated in one visit. They do not need to make a return visit for the results of the investigations. It is usually optimal for such laboratories to be polyvalent in function, serving a number of different health facilities. Laboratories and clinics of this level are important stations for the collection of specimens for more centralized laboratories.

Facilities at this level are generally limited. The equipment should be simple to operate, rugged, and easy to maintain. The major instrument is usually a microscope. One person usually will be expected to perform various investigations in microbiology, hematology, and biochemistry. If the laboratory is sited in a remote area, more is expected of the staff. They will need to be skillful not only in maintenance but also in the repair of equipment. The organization of such a basic health laboratory has been described in a manual by the World Health Organization[1].

The types of investigations performed in such laboratories are usually limited to microscopy and tests which are supplied in the form of kits. The standard tests are a Gram stain microscopy for gonorrhea and nongonococcal urethritis, darkfield microscopy for syphilis, and wet smear microscopy for clue cells (in the absence of pus cells) for bacterial vaginosis. Wet smear microscopy should also be available for pathogens such as *Trichomonas vaginalis* and *Candida spp*. The ability of the microscopist to recognize *C. trachomatis* inclusions regularly is limited to acute eye infections. Microscopy for chancroid and donovanosis should best be carried out by laboratories where these are encountered regularly. If transport is efficient, it may be possible for some laboratories to provide growth-transport medium for the culture of *N. gonorrhoeae*. However, because of its cost and delay compared with microscopy, the test should be used selectively (e.g., asymptomatic females).

Syphilis serology requires the practice of proper quality control for reliable results (see also Chap. 75). In localities where syphilis is prevalent and larger laboratories are not within easy reach, the local laboratory may have to undertake the responsibility. In such situations it is preferable to use a test like the Rapid Plasma Reagin (RPR) 18-mm Circle Card Test. Several similar tests are now commercially available. Compared with the standard Venereal Disease Research Laboratory (VDRL) slide test, they are simpler to perform, and less equipment is necessary. Problems which are beyond the competence of the staff should be referred to the nearest regional laboratory where there are more extensive facilities.

## INTERMEDIATE LEVEL

Laboratories at this level often have several different functions to fulfill. They should be a key element in most control programs. Compared with peripheral units, each laboratory has a far larger capacity to contribute to implementation of many control programs planned on a regional basis. They are a vital link between the peripheral units and the national laboratory in the overall organization. Many of them are regional or state health laboratories. Many of the investigations at this level are also undertaken by government or university hospital laboratories.

A wide range of investigations is available. These may be more sensitive and specific than those offered by the peripheral units. The main feature is the ability to prepare the necessary media for a culture service. Ideally for the diagnosis of gonorrhea, each laboratory should be in a position to supply prepared culture plates to clinics and smaller laboratories in the region for direct inoculation of specimen. Such a service is especially important in areas where gonorrhea is a major problem. The emergence of penicillinase-producing *N. gonorrhoeae* (PPNG) has necessitated this not only for females but also for males. In the tropics the inoculated culture plate may be kept in a carbon dioxide–enriched environment at ambient temperature for up to 5 h[2] with a good isolation rate. Our experience indicates that this may be extended up to 24 h with minimal loss[3]. The network of a culture system for peripheral units, which do not possess their own incubators, is therefore determined by the time that it takes to transport the culture plates, enclosed in a carbon dioxide–enriched environment, to the regional laboratory.

If bacteriologic medium cannot be supplied, a number of commercial transport and growth systems may be used. (See also Chap. 73.) They vary in their performance (toxicity being a problem), shelf life, and cost, and laboratories should carefully assess which will best meet their needs. Nonnutrient holding systems like Stuart's medium or one of its modifications have generally given variable results. They are more satisfactory in temperate than in tropical climates. While an overnight transit time may result in slight loss in a colder climate[4], the loss is over 50 percent in Singapore after a similar period. In the tropics, transit time should probably not exceed 6 h[5].

**Table 82-1. Levels* of Laboratory Diagnostic Support for STD**

| Etiological agents | Peripheral laboratories | Intermediate laboratories | Central laboratories |
|---|---|---|---|
| *N. gonorrhoeae* | Direct smear, with Gram's stain | Isolation<br>Identification<br>Screening for β-lactamase | Test for β-lactamase<br>Antibiotic susceptibility test<br>Antigen detection by EIA† |
| *C. trachomatis* | Smear (eye only) with Giemsa's stain | LGV, CF test<br>Histopathology (LGV)†<br>Isolation in some intermediate labs<br>Direct FA† or EIA† in some intermediate labs | Isolation<br>Serotyping<br>Micro-IF antibody† test<br>Antigen detection by direct FA† or EIA† |
| *M. hominis* | | Isolation<br>Identification | Serology<br>Antibiotic susceptibility test |
| *G. vaginalis* | Wet mount ("clue cells") | Isolation<br>Identification | |
| *T. vaginalis* | Wet mount | Acridine orange FM†<br>Isolation | Antibiotic susceptibility test |
| *C. albicans* | Smear, KOH preparation | Isolation<br>Identification | Antibiotic susceptibility test |
| *T. pallidum* | Dark field microscopy<br>RPR card† test | Nontreponemal test<br>MHA-TP† or equivalent | FTA-ABS test† |
| *H. ducreyi* | Direct smear, with Gram's stain | Isolation<br>Presumptive identification | Confirmatory identification<br>Antibiotic susceptibility test |
| β-hemolytic streptococci Group B | Direct smear, with Gram's stain | Isolation<br>Identification | Typing |
| *C. granulomatis* | Direct impression smear | Histopathology | Confirmatory identification |
| Human immunodeficiency virus | | Serology by PA†, FAb†, or ELISA† in some intermediate labs | Confirmation with recombinant antigen or WB†<br>Antigen detection by EIA† |
| Herpes simplex virus | Cytology (Pap† or Tzanck smear) | Direct FA† or immunoperoxidase<br>CF test†<br>Isolation in some intermediate labs | Isolation<br>Typing<br>Type-specific serology |
| Human papilloma-virus | Cytology (Pap† smear) | Histopathology | Genotyping by DNA† probes |

*Intermediate and central level laboratories should be able to perform all tests available at lower level laboratories plus any additional tests for the corresponding level.

†*Abbreviations*: CF test: complement fixation test; DNA: deoxyribonucleic acid; EIA: enzyme immunoassay; ELISA: enzyme-linked immunosorbent assay; FA: immunofluorescence for antigen; FAb: immunofluorescence for antibody; FM: fluorescent microscopy; FTA-ABS: fluorescent treponemal antibody-absorption; LGV: lymphogranuloma venereum; MHA-TP: microhemagglutination, *Treponema pallidum*; Micro-IF: microimmunofluorescence for antibody; PA: gelatin-particle agglutination; Pap: Papanicolaou staining of cells; RPR: rapid plasma reagin, 18-mm circle; WB: Western blot.

Presumptive identification of the gonococcus will usually suffice for anogenital specimens. However, those laboratories servicing homosexual populations may need to consider specific identification in view of the increased percentage of meningococci found in these sites. The use of rapid methods will enable such confirmation to be made with minimum delay. Several methods are available for the detection of PPNG strains which have a high prevalence in many developing countries. The acidometric methods are cheap and simple and enable rapid detection of β-lactamase.

Syphilis serology should consist of both nontreponemal and treponemal tests. (See also Chap. 75.) The VDRL slide test is used by most laboratories for reason of cost, though there are several other alternative tests, like the RPR Card tests, which are technically simpler and which require less equipment (see above)[6].

Certain laboratories have developed the expertise to culture *C. trachomatis*, which is a major etiologic agent of genital infections and sequelae thereof in developing and developed countries. Its isolation is influenced by several factors, such as types of swab used[7], number of specimens taken, transportation conditions, method for detecting inclusions, and number of subcultures carried out. The current direct specimen antigen detection systems are generally less sensitive than the culture method. Because of this and cost, they are probably more suitable for the identification of risk groups than for routine diagnostic use.

Other pathogens, such as *Mycoplasma hominis*, may also be identified at intermediate laboratories.

The spread of the HIV has added a new dimension to the problem of STD. Laboratories in developing countries will have to develop facilities to at least protect their blood supplies and provide a basic diagnostic service. Several good tests are available (see Chap. 79). In our hands, a gelatin-particle agglutination system[8] has given levels of sensitivity and specificity comparable with the ELISA systems. It is simple to perform and is suitable for laboratories with limited facilities.

Intermediate-level facilities should be available to as many clinics as possible. The use of Stuart's transport medium for herpes simplex virus[9] will extend the network of clinics. Similarly, acridine orange fluorescent microscopy[10] will enable many clinics to send dried smears to a regional laboratory for examination.

## CENTRAL LEVEL

Tertiary-level laboratories are generally well equipped and have specialized staff who may be able to perform sophisticated tests. Tissue culture techniques and electron microscopy are often employed. These laboratories are usually set up as national research or reference centers by the federal or national governments. In the organization of the laboratory service, a center of excellence should be identified and developed to provide leadership in the laboratory framework. Such a national laboratory has the responsibility to manage the laboratory organization and to ensure an efficient service. A key element in the setup is to appoint a laboratory manager who is well versed in management skills.

One of the functions of a central laboratory is to provide a service for diagnostic problems. Some of these investigations, such as the Western blot test for HIV or the microimmunofluorescence test for chlamydial serology, may not be carried out at intermediate level because of lack of facilities or expertise. Others, like the fluorescent treponemal antibody absorption (FTA-ABS) test may not be developed at a lower level because simpler alternatives are available or because there are too few specimens for such tests. Since many of the tests are costly, they are usually performed only on selected cases.

Research activities are undertaken by many laboratories. The main thrust of many central laboratories is to undertake research aimed at problem solving. This includes the development of simpler and less costly methods for investigations. The use of a filter paper method for the collection and dispatch of dried blood should be further explored. This will bring technology to a wider range of laboratories and clinics. Another important aspect of this activity is the evaluation of new tests. Since many of the new tests are studied under ideal conditions, only a field trial will reveal their practicability.

A national laboratory also serves as a resource center for expertise and supplies. It is important to provide comprehensive training programs for all levels of staff to ensure that they are maximally utilized. Senior staff may visit local laboratories to advise on problems and to provide supervision. Central purchasing permits items to be purchased at lower cost. Adequate stocks may be kept to ensure continuous supply. Repairs of equipment may be undertaken by a central pool of workers.

A laboratory investigation usually involves a number of activities. No matter how reliable a test may be, there are always several areas where things can go wrong. It is the responsibility of the national laboratory to design and manage a quality assurance program. Such a program is especially important for developing countries since many of the laboratories rely on locally prepared reagents, facilities may be inadequate to keep reagents at proper temperatures, staff may not have received adequate training, etc. No program is foolproof, and a balance between reliability and cost should be determined when designing a program.

In many control programs the national laboratory has the role of coordinating the activities of various laboratories to ensure that the objectives of the programs are met at moderate cost. The necessary assistance in the form of staff, training, and supplies is provided by the national laboratory.

## UTILIZATION OF LABORATORY SERVICES

The utilization of laboratory services embodies a chain of events that are linked together for a common goal. Although the reliability of a test is determined to a large extent by the quality of the laboratory, several external factors usually influence the result of an investigation. The physician ordering the investigation is responsible for several of these factors. Physicians should therefore be conversant with certain aspects, such as the selection of the tests, collection (types of swab, sampling sites, etc.) and handling of specimens, and the interpretation of test results. Such information may not be readily available to many users in developing countries. Laboratory managers should embark on educational programs for users.

No one test will detect everyone who has a particular disease (100 percent sensitive), and exclude everyone without that disease (100 percent specific). The predictive value of a test is based only on the probability that a person with a positive or negative test result actually has or does not have the disease. The predictive value is dependent not only on the sensitivity and specificity of the test but also on the prevalence of the disease in the population tested. For example, if a test with a sensitivity and specificity of 99 percent is used to screen a population of 100,000 with a 1 percent disease prevalence, then 990 of the 1000 infected persons will be detected. At the same time 990 of the 99,000 uninfected persons will give false-positive results. The predictive value of the positive result is only 50 percent. If the same test is used on a population with 10 percent disease prevalence, the predictive value of a positive result increases to 92 percent. The greater the disease prevalence, the higher will be the predictive value. A high predictive value for a positive result will reduce the difficulty in interpretation. High disease prevalence in the population being tested can be assured if the tests are used selectively.

Even in the preparation of a simple smear, errors can occur if the smear is prepared too thickly, or a rupturing of the cells can take place if the smear has been prepared too vigorously. In a more complex system, such as in the culture of the gonococcus, there are more areas for mistakes. These may include the nature of the medium (its basic composition and antibiotics used), its quality (whether it is outdated, dried, or contaminated), the number and variety of sites for sample collection, the care used in collecting samples, the quality of streaking, whether the culture plates have been placed in a carbon dioxide–enriched environment within 2 h[11], the amount of time involved in transporting the culture, and the experience of the staff. (See also Chap. 73.)

Constant feedback between the clinical and laboratory services is essential. The physician should report any deficiency to the laboratory, e.g., delay in receiving a report, or an erroneous result. A simple check on the sensitivity of the culture system can be made by comparing the culture results with microscopy. Similarly the laboratory staff should inform the clinician of any defect, such as improper streaking which they may have detected. The object is to ensure that patients are treated promptly and that waste is kept at a minimum.

## COST IMPLICATIONS OF LABORATORY SUPPORT FOR SCREENING

Population screening has always been one of the strategies to control STDs. Traditionally this has included examining premarital individuals, pregnant women, workers in certain occupations, immigrants, blood donors, and prostitutes. The presence of HIV infection has led many to advocate widespread screening programs. Screening activity is not cheap, and planners of such programs should be aware of the cost implications of laboratory support in these activities, as well as the problems with false-positive results.

All programs have some deficiencies inherent in the laboratory test system adopted. Although the effort to solve a diagnostic problem may involve the use of several effective but expensive procedures, the test system for screening should be simple and

**Table 82-2. Cost Analysis of Two Test Systems for the Detection of Gonorrhea in 1000 Females**

| Test system | Smear* | | | | | Culture† | | | | |
|---|---|---|---|---|---|---|---|---|---|---|
| Prevalence, % | 1 | 5 | 10 | 25 | 50 | 1 | 5 | 10 | 25 | 50 |
| *a*. Screening cost | 1000DS‡ | 1000DS | 1000DS | 1000DS | 1000DS | 1000DC‡ | 1000DC | 1000DC | 1000DC | 1000DC |
| *b*. Number of laboratory positives | 24.8 | 44 | 68 | 140 | 260 | 14 | 49.8 | 94.5 | 228.8 | 452.5 |
| *c*. Number of cases detected | 5 | 25 | 50 | 125 | 250 | 9 | 45 | 90 | 225 | 450 |
| *d*. Cost to detect per case ($a \div c$) | 200DS | 40DS | 20DS | 8DS | 4DS | 111DC | 22.2DC | 11.1DC | 4.4DC | 2.2DC |
| *e*. Management cost for laboratory positives | 24.8M§ | 44M | 68M | 140M | 260M | 14M | 49.8M | 94.5M | 228.8M | 452.5M |
| *f*. Total cost per case detected $(a + e) \div c$ | 200DS + 4.96M | 40DS + 1.76M | 20DS + 1.36M | 8DS + 1.12M | 4DS + 1.04M | 111DC + 1.56M | 22.2DC + 1.11M | 11.1DC + 1.05M | 4.4DC + 1.02M | 2.2DC + 1.01M |

*Smear: sensitivity, 50%; specificity, 98%.
†Culture: sensitivity, 90%; specificity, 99.5%.
‡D: cost to investigate one person by smear (DS) or culture (DC).
§M: cost to manage a person whose laboratory test was positive, inclusive of test of cure by culture.

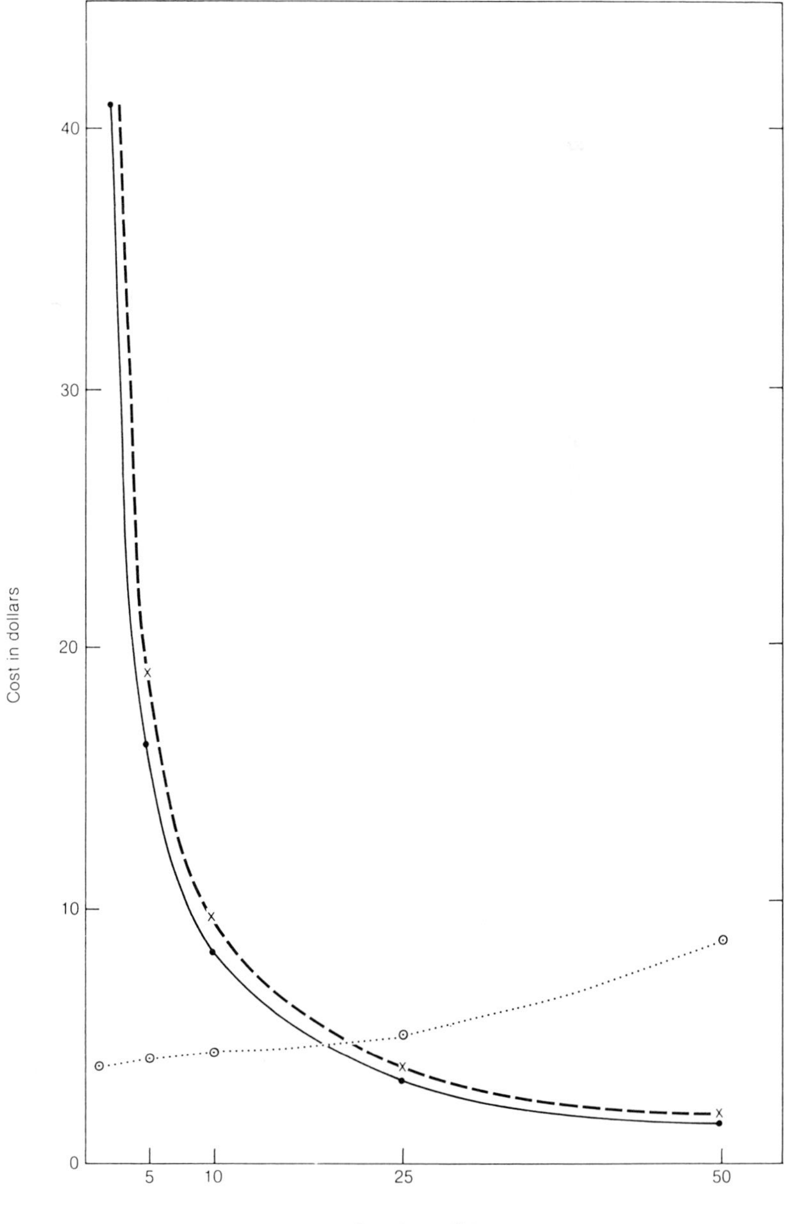


**Fig. 82-1.** Cost-effectiveness of detecting gonorrhea by smear and culture of anogenital specimens. Cost per case of gonorrhea detected by smear (*solid line*) and by culture (*dashed line*). *Dotted line*: Cost of managing a laboratory-positive person at which the cost to detect (and manage) per true positive was the same by either microscopy or culture. The cost of a smear examination was estimated at 41 cents, while that of a gonococcal culture was 86 cents.

inexpensive. Cost is usually the limiting factor. As a result the proportion of cases, say for gonorrhea, detected per given period of time, is limited by factors such as the number of sites examined per person at each visit or the frequency of visits by each person. The selection of a sound option is sometimes not simple, and it may be necessary to use quantitative methods to assess the various alternatives. The use of the following smear-vs.-culture example should illustrate some of the principles involved.

Table 82-2 analyzes the cost of detecting gonorrhea in a hypothetical population of 1000 females by smear or culture. The sensitivity for the culture system assumes a combination of endocervical and rectal cultures. Although either system may be used for screening, culture is always used as a test of cure in the management of a person who has a positive laboratory test. By adding the cost to screen (item *a*) the population to the cost of managing (item *e*) the laboratory positives, and by dividing the total cost by the number of true positives (cases) detected (item *c*), we can compare the cost-effectiveness of the two test systems (item *f*).

The cost-effectiveness of either system will vary in different places, depending on such factors as the cost of labor and supplies, certain technical factors and other "hidden costs" which contribute to the values of D (the cost to investigate one person by smear, DS, or by culture, DC) and M (the cost to manage a laboratory positive person, inclusive of test of cure by culture). Hidden costs varies in different countries, and is probably less in developing countries. In Singapore the cost per endocervical smear examination (DS) is 41 cents, while the culture cost (DC) per person is 86 cents. Figure 82-1 shows the comparative diagnostic costs of the two systems to detect one true positive for different levels of disease prevalence. Though the cost for a smear examination is much less than that for culture, the difference between the diagnostic cost-effectiveness of the two systems is not much because of the greater efficiency of the culture system. The cost-effectiveness of both systems is dependent on disease prevalence. Therefore, in the face of limited resources, screening effort should preferably be concentrated on high-prevalence groups. When the prevalence rate is below 5 percent, the cost escalates so rapidly that it is probably not cost-effective to screen such a population, unless epidemiologic data strongly suggest otherwise.

Looking at the problem in a broader perspective, the choice of a test system influences the management cost as well. Using the following formula, it is possible to calculate the value of M at which the total cost (diagnostic plus management) per true positive for either system is the same:

$$200\ \mathrm{DS} + 4.96\mathrm{M} = 111\ \mathrm{DC} + 1.56\ \mathrm{M}$$

(at 1 percent disease prevalence)

By determining the M value of equivalence for various disease prevalence rates, we can plot a graph as shown in Fig. 82-1. If the cost of managing a patient whose test was positive at a given disease prevalence rate is higher than the M value of equivalence, then the total amount (diagnostic plus management) required per case detected is less for the culture than for the smear method. If the M value is below the line of equivalence, then the reverse is preferable. The example shows that it may be more cost-effective to adopt a test system for screening which superficially appears to be costly. Careful assessment of the variables is advisable in selecting the laboratory support system for population screening (see also Chap. 73), in particular in developing countries with very limited economic resources and poorly developed laboratory support.

## References


1 World Health Organization: *Manual of Basic Techniques for a Health Laboratory*. Geneva, WHO, 1980.

2 Westbrook WG III: Delay and inhibition of growth of *Neisseria gonorrhoeae* in vitro. Relationship of delayed incubation, penicillinase production, urine culture and self-treatment. *Br J Vener Dis* 56:83, 1980.

3 Sng EH et al: The recovery of *Neisseria gonorrhoeae* from clinical specimens. Effects of different temperatures, transport times, and media. *Sex Transm Dis* 9:74, 1982.

4 Danielsson D, Johannisson G: Culture diagnosis of gonorrhea. A comparison of the yield with selective and non-selective gonococcal culture media inoculated in the clinic and after transport of specimens. *Acta Derm Venereol* 53:75, 1973.

5 Kandhari KC et al: Viability of *N. gonorrhoeae* in transport media. *Indian J Med Res* 60:1418, 1972.

6 Sng EH et al: Evaluation of a low cost, macroscopic nontreponemal test for syphilis using reuseable supplies. *Singapore Med J* 27:410, 1986.

7 Mårdh P-A, Zeeberg B: Toxic effect of sampling swabs and transportation test tubes on the formation of intracytoplasmatic inclusions of *Chlamydia trachomatis* in McCoy cell cultures. *Br J Vener Dis* 57:268, 1981.

8 Yoshida T et al: A novel agglutination test for the human immunodeficiency virus antibody: A comparative study with enzyme-linked immunosorbent assay and immunofluorescence. *Jpn J Cancer Res* 17:1211, 1986.

9 Rodin P et al: Transport of herpes simplex virus in Stuart's medium. *Br J Vener Dis* 47:198, 1971.

10 Hipp SS et al: Screening for *Trichomonas vaginalis* infection by use of acridine orange fluorescent microscopy. *Sex Transm Dis* 6:235, 1979.

11 Chapel TA et al: The effect of delaying incubation in a $CO_2$-enriched environment on gonococci. *Health Lab Sci* 13:45, 1976.

# PART IX PHARMACOLOGY

Chapter 83

# Pharmacology of drugs used in venereology

Teresa A. Tartaglione
Mary E. Russo

The clinical pharmacology of the oral and parenteral antimicrobial agents used most commonly in the treatment of sexually transmitted diseases is discussed in this chapter. Indications for use, modes of action, antimicrobial sensitivity patterns, and mechanisms of drug resistance are briefly presented; pharmacokinetics, adverse reactions, and drug interactions are discussed in more depth. Newer agents are reviewed, including the combinations of amoxicillin/clavulanic acid and ampicillin/sulbactam, cefotetan, ceftriaxone, and the quinolone antibiotics. Additionally, the antiretroviral agents used for treatment of human immunodeficiency virus infections are discussed. For recommended regimens and dosages, the reader is referred to specific chapters on the relevant infection.

## PENICILLINS

### INDICATIONS

The major indications for using the penicillins in venereology are infections caused by *Neisseria gonorrhoeae* and *Treponema pallidum*. Penicillin remains the drug of choice for treatment of syphilis. While there is no evidence that *T. pallidum* has developed resistance to penicillins, both chromosomal and plasmid-mediated resistance to penicillin among *N. gonorrhoeae* has become a problem worldwide (see Chaps. 13, 14). Less frequent uses of the penicillins include treatment of group B streptococci, *Salmonella*, or *Shigella* in geographic areas where the latter remain sensitive to amoxicillin. Newer combinations of penicillins and β-lactamase inhibitor compounds (ampicillin/sulbactam or amoxicillin/clavulanic acid) may have a role in selected infections.

### MODE OF ACTION

The concept that penicillins inhibit the last step in cell wall synthesis is an overly simplistic one. Because of their structural similarities to portions of the cell wall mucopeptide of multiplying bacteria, the penicillins bind to specific membrane proteins or murein-synthesizing enzymes such as transpeptidase, and disrupt cell growth and metabolism. Structural differences between the various penicillins determine their relative affinity for a particular penicillin-binding protein, resulting in diverse morphological effects upon the bacterium. In some bacteria, inhibition of cell growth results in lysis and immediate death, while in other bacteria, interference with cell wall growth is only inhibitory and not lethal to the organism.

### SPECTRUM OF ACTIVITY

Patterns of in vitro sensitivity of the penicillins against selected sexually transmitted disease pathogens are constantly changing. An increase in penicillinase-producing *N. gonorrhoeae* strains has been recognized in the United States since 1981 (see Chaps. 14, 73). In general, penicillinase-producing strains produce a zone of inhibition ≤23 mm on Kirby-Bauer disk testing,[1] and the MIC for penicillin G is usually ≥2.0 μg/ml.

The in vitro sensitivities of non-PPNG *N. gonorrhoeae* are divided into two groups based upon the MIC.[1–7] For penicillin G, the first modus is seen within the MIC range of 0.004 to 0.06 μg/ml (the corresponding zone of inhibition around the 10-IU Kirby-Bauer disk for penicillin G is ≥ 34 to 56 mm). Organisms with these sensitivities are considered very susceptible. The second modus is within 0.03 to 2.0 μg/ml and is designated an intermediate or relatively resistant group. Penicillin G, ampicillin, and amoxicillin have the greatest in vitro activity. Dicloxacillin and related agents demonstrate little in vitro activity.

Sodium clavulanate, a microbial metabolite of *Streptomyces clavuligaris*, irreversibly inhibits certain beta-lactamases in vitro and also has some endogenous antibacterial activity against gonococci.[2,8] When subinhibitory concentrations (0.5 μg/ml) of this agent are used in combination with penicillin G, ampicillin, or amoxicillin, the MICs of these antibiotics were decreased more than 32-fold from > 8 to 0.25 μg/ml. Sodium clavulanate does not affect the MICs against penicillin of non-beta-lactamase-producing strains of *N. gonorrhoeae*. Similar findings have been reported for ampicillin/sulbactam combinations.[9]

Treponemicidal levels for penicillin G are 0.005 to 0.01 μg/ml or 0.23 IU/ml.[10,11] Minimal data are available on the other penicillins.

### MECHANISM OF RESISTANCE

Bacteria acquire resistance to the penicillins by two major mechanisms: chromosomal mutation and acquisition of plasmids. Mutations occur spontaneously, and selective antibiotic pressure secondary to antibiotic use leads to emergence and spread of resistant mutants.[5]

Penicillinase production, mediated by plasmids, results in hydrolysis of the beta-lactam bond and complete loss of antibiotic activity (high-level resistance). In addition to penicillinase production, plasmids can also mediate penicillin resistance by altering the target sites which bind various penicillins.

### BIOPHARMACEUTICS AND PHARMACOKINETICS

Table 83-1 summarizes the most useful biopharmaceutic and pharmacokinetic information on the penicillins.

#### Absorption

The oral absorption of penicillins ranges from 15 to 80 percent, with penicillin G the lowest because of its acid lability and amoxicillin the highest. Only 30 to 50 percent of most of the oral penicillins reach the systemic circulation. Absorption from intramuscular sites is very good.

**Table 83-1. Biopharmaceutic and Pharmacokinetic Data on Various Penicillins, Cephalosporins, and Cephamycins**

| Drug | Half-life, h | | Total peak serum concentrations, µg/ml | Major route of elimination (minor route) |
|---|---|---|---|---|
| | Normal | Renal failure | | |
| **Penicillins** | | | | |
| Amoxicillin | 0.9–2.3 | 5–20 | IM 500 mg = 8–10<br>PO 500 mg = 8–10<br>3.0 g = 23 | Renal<br>(hepatic) |
| Ampicillin | 1.5 | 7–20 | IV push 500 mg = 35<br>IM 500 mg = 8<br>PO 500 mg = 3–7 | Renal<br>(hepatic) |
| Cloxacillin | 0.4–0.6 | 0.8 | PO 500 mg = 7–14 | Hepatic<br>(renal) |
| Dicloxacillin | 0.5–0.9 | 1–1.6 | PO 500 mg = 15–18 | Renal<br>(hepatic) |
| Penicillin G | 0.5 | 6–20 | IV 1 million units = 20<br>PO 500 mg = 1.5–2.7<br>Benzathine 2.4 µM ≤ 1.0<br>Procaine 4.8 µM + probenecid = 23 | Renal<br>(hepatic) |
| **Cephalosporins or cephamycins** | | | | |
| Cefaclor | 0.6–0.9 | 2.3–2.8 | 23–35 (PO) | Renal (53–70%) |
| Cefoperazone | 1.8–2 | 2.5 | 100–125 (IV) | Biliary (75%) |
| Cefotaxime | 1.1 | 2.5 | 10–15 (IM)<br>40 (IV) | Renal (75%)<br>Metabolism (40%) |
| Cefotetan | 3–4.6 | 12–35 | 255 (IV) | Renal (90%) |
| Cefoxitin | 0.7 | 13–22 | 22 (IM)<br>56–110 (IV) | Renal (90–99%) |
| Ceftriaxone | 6.2–8.0 | ND | 151 (IV) | Renal (60%)<br>Biliary (40%) |
| Cefuroxime | 1.1–1.4 | 15–22 | 32–40 (IM)<br>90–144 (IV) | Renal (91–96%) |
| Cephalexin | 0.9 | 5–30 | 31–40 (PO) | Renal (85–99%) |

SOURCE: Compiled from Refs. 12, 18, 19, 30, 31.

Peak serum concentrations of the penicillins usually occur at 1 or 2 h after oral dosing and 30 to 60 min after intramuscular administration. Doubling the dose will double the serum concentration. By 4 to 6 h after oral therapy, serum levels are quite low for most of the penicillins. When ampicillin is administered in a dose of 3.5 g with 1.0 g of probenecid, mean peak levels of 22 µg/ml at 2 h and 1 µg/ml at 10 to 12 h are achieved. A dose of 3.0 g amoxicillin achieves peak levels similar to the ampicillin and probenecid combination, but they decline to about 1 µg/ml by 8 h.[12] Concomitant administration of probenecid increases the peak to 35 µg/ml at 3 h with levels $>$ 10 µg/ml maintained at 8 h.[13] Both of these dosages maintain bactericidal levels for susceptible *N. gonorrhoeae* over 5 to 12 h.[14,15] The pharmacokinetics of both ampicillin and amoxicillin are unaltered when combined with sulbactam or clavulanic acid, respectively. Absorption of amoxicillin is not appreciably affected by food.

Of the repository forms of penicillin G given intramuscularly, the levels achieved with aqueous procaine penicillin G (APPG) are higher but less prolonged than with benzathine penicillin G. A dose of 4.8 million units of APPG with 1.0 g probenecid yields peak levels of 23 µg/ml in 3 h. Levels of 5 µg/ml are still seen at 12 h, and detectable levels can be measured for more than 24 h.[12] Benzathine penicillin G administration results in prolonged, low concentrations, usually $<1$ µg/ml, which is less than the MIC of penicillin G for some gonococci but is above the MIC for all strains of *T. pallidum*. Since *T. pallidum* multiplies approximately every 30 h, syphilis cannot be cured with a single dose of shorter-intermediate-duration repository forms of penicillin. The dose of benzathine penicillin recommended for early syphilis is 2.4 million units, which maintains treponemicidal levels for 3 to 4 weeks.[11]

## Distribution

Penicillins are widely distributed in the body, including interstitial, pleural, pericardial, ascitic, and synovial fluids and inflamed bone. The penicillins cross the placental barrier, and concentrations in the fetus and amniotic fluid can be demonstrated in the second and third trimesters. Because of their lipid insolubility, the penicillins penetrate the blood-brain and blood-aqueous barriers poorly unless these areas are inflamed. Concurrent administration of probenecid increases the concentration of penicillins in the cerebrospinal fluid (CSF) and eye by impairing the activity of the organic anion pump in the choroid plexus and ciliary body, respectively. Benzathine penicillin G achieves CSF concentrations of less than 0.0005 mg/ml, raising doubts as to its effectiveness in treating neurosyphilis (see Chap. 21).[16,17]

Protein binding of the penicillins ranges from 20 percent for ampicillin and amoxicillin to 96 percent for dicloxacillin.[18] However, it is not clear to what extent protein binding affects the efficacy of the penicillins.

## Metabolism and excretion

The penicillins are largely excreted unchanged via glomerular filtration and tubular secretion by the kidneys. Tubular secretion is the pathway interfered with by probenecid. For this reason, doses and dosage intervals for most of the penicillins should be adjusted in patients with renal insufficiency who are being treated with extended therapy.[19]

## ADVERSE REACTIONS

Adverse effects to short-term penicillin therapy as in the treatment of uncomplicated gonorrhea include hypersensitivity reactions, gastrointestinal complaints, procaine toxicity, and local reactions at the site of injection (Table 83-2). Additionally, in patients with syphilis, the Jarisch-Herxheimer reaction (JHR) can occur. In large-scale national surveys done to characterize the reactions found in patients treated for uncomplicated gonorrhea or syphilis,[20,21] the risk of side effects (excluding JHR and local reactions) was ≤2 percent. The most common problems were nausea, vomiting, urticaria, or wheezing. In the National Gonorrhea Therapy Monitoring study of almost 7000 patients, urticaria, wheezing, or rash occurred in 0.81 percent of the patients given either APPG or ampicillin and probenecid. There were no life-threatening reactions, and only 0.18 percent of the patients experienced procaine toxicity. In a 1969 national survey of penicillin reactions among patients in venereal disease clinics, only 0.66 percent of over 27,000 patients experienced a reaction. The most frequent side effect was urticaria, followed by vertigo and syncope, maculopapular rash, pruritus, gastrointestinal distress, angioneurotic edema, and procaine reactions. Additionally, intramuscular procaine penicillin G was associated with a 5 percent incidence of allergic reactions compared with only 0.3 percent following oral penicillin G.

**Table 83-2. Adverse Reactions to Various Penicillins**

| Side effect | Penicillin most commonly implicated |
|---|---|
| Jarisch-Herxheimer reaction | All penicillins |
| Allergic reactions | All penicillins |
| Neurologic toxicity | Procaine penicillin G<br>All penicillins, especially with high doses in renal failure or concomitant use of probenecid |
| Electrolyte disturbances, especially with high doses in renal failure | $Na^+$ of $K^+$ penicillin G contain 1.7 meq $Na^+$ and $K^+$, respectively, per 1 million units<br>Carbenicillin and ticarcillin contain about 5 meq $Na^+$ per gram<br>Azlocillin, mezlocillin, and piperacillin contain about 1.8 meq $Na^+$ per gram |
| Diarrhea | Ampicillin |
| Pseudomembranous colitis | Ampicillin, carbenicillin |
| Hematologic reactions, such as hemolytic anemia (high doses), neutropenia, thrombocytopenia, decreased platelet function (high doses) | All penicillins, especially decreased platelet function with carbenicillin in the doses used |
| Drug fever | All penicillins |
| Nephropathy, especially interstitial nephritis | All penicillins, especially methicillin |
| Elevated liver function tests | Nafcillin, oxacillin, carbenicillin |
| Skin rashes | "Ampicillin" maculopapular rash; all penicillins |
| Thrombophlebitis | Nafcillin |
| Nerve and muscle injury | Intramuscular penicillin administration |

SOURCE: Compiled from Ref. 18.

### Penicillin allergic reactions

Anaphylactic reactions occur in about 0.004 to 0.04 percent of patients given penicillin parenterally, with a mortality rate of 1 to 2 deaths per 100,000. In the 1973 national survey of venereal disease clinics, a history of previous penicillin allergy was an important factor in determining which patients were most likely to exhibit a hypersensitivity reaction. Approximately 12.8 percent of the patients with a positive history reacted when they were subsequently inadvertently given penicillin, whereas only 0.6 percent of the patients who never received penicillin or had the drug in the past with no sequelae developed an allergic reaction.[20]

Penicillin-allergic reactions can be classified as immediate, accelerated, or delayed (Table 83-3), and by their Gell and Coombs typing pattern.[22] The prototype of the type 1 reaction is anaphylaxis, although some forms of urticaria are also included in this category. This reaction is mediated by IgE antibodies formed against the minor antigenic determinants of penicillin breakdown products, including penicilloic acid, penicillenic acid, panamaldate, penicillenic disulfide, and penicillamine. IgE is also formed against the penicilloyl-protein conjugate or major determinant of penicillin degradation. However, it usually does not cause an immediate hypersensitivity reaction since IgG is also synthesized against penicilloyl and acts as a blocking antibody to IgE. The type 2 reaction is a cytotoxic response mediated by IgG. In this case, one of the metabolic products of penicillin binds covalently to an endogenous substrate such as the red cell membrane, and forms a hapten. Penicillin-induced hemolytic anemia is an example of this response. The type 3 reaction is immune complex–mediated. Here, circulating antigen-antibody complexes lodge in vessel walls, fix complement, and initiate tissue damage. Serum sickness and some forms of urticaria are in this class. The last typing pattern, type 4, is a cell-mediated response as exemplified by penicillin-induced contact dermatitis and interstitial nephritis.

In general, treatment of anaphylactic reactions requires the maintenance of a patent airway and administration of oxygen and epinephrine.[22] The use of corticosteroids, antihistamines, volume replacement, and pressor agents may be indicated in selected cases. The accelerated and delayed reactions usually subside upon discontinuation of the drug. For immune complex– and cellular-mediated reactions, steroids may be beneficial.

**Table 83-3. Characteristics of Penicillin Allergic Reactions**

| Time | Characteristics |
|---|---|
| | **Immediate reaction** |
| 2–20 min after administration | Diffuse (giant) urticaria; laryngeal edema; wheezing, rhinitis; hypoxia; hypotension; tachycardia; nausea; vomiting; abdominal pain; diarrhea; rigors; vascular collapse |
| | **Accelerated reaction** |
| 30 min to 48 h after administration | Urticaria; laryngeal edema (infrequently) |
| | **Delayed reaction** |
| Usually greater than 3 days after administration | Skin rashes (erythema, urticaria, exfoliative dermatitis, Stevens-Johnson syndrome, fixed drug eruption, contact dermatitis, bullous eruptions); serum sickness; hematologic reactions; lupuslike syndrome; vasculitis; drug fever; hepatitis; nephropathy |

### Ampicillin rash

The so-called ampicillin rash is described as a nonallergic macular or maculopapular rash appearing in the trunk and spreading peripherally.[23] It is not associated with urticaria. The lesions may coalesce or eventually become purpuric. The rash usually begins 4 or more days (median 9 days) after starting ampicillin and may occur after treatment is discontinued. The median duration of the reaction is 6 days. It does not become worse if therapy is continued, and in fact, may resolve. The rash may or may not reappear if ampicillin is subsequently administered. Diarrhea is more common in patients who develop the rash and some of these patients have fever. The incidence of the ampicillin rash is about 7 percent as compared with a 2 to 3 percent incidence of true allergic rashes to penicillin. Groups that are at high risk for developing this reaction include patients with viral respiratory tract infections (17 percent as compared with a 7 percent incidence in nonviral cases) and mononucleosis (60 to 100 percent vs. 1 to 3 percent with other penicillins), patients with lymphatic leukemia (90 percent), and patients on allopurinol therapy (22 percent compared with an 8 percent incidence for allopurinol alone and 7 percent for ampicillin alone). It is possible that hyperuricemia is a predisposing cause in the last two groups. The specific mechanism responsible for the rash is not known.

### Jarisch-Herxheimer reaction (JHR)

The JHR is a self-limited reaction consisting of transient fever, chills, malaise, myalgias, headache, leukocytosis with lymphopenia, and exacerbation of syphilitic lesions[24] that occurs within the first 2 to 24 h of starting antimicrobial treatment for syphilis. This reaction is discussed in detail in Chap. 20.

### Procaine toxicity

Two types of reactions to procaine penicillin have been described.[25,26] The first involves onset of extreme anxiety and a sensation of "impending doom" almost immediately after intramuscular administration of APPG. Some patients experience hallucinations, disorientation, and depersonalization or psychosis. This is generally a self-limited reaction occurring in about 0.1 to 0.3 percent of the patients, and usually abates within 15 to 30 min. The reaction is probably a result of direct CNS procaine toxicity since high levels of free procaine can be detected in the serum of some patients after intramuscular administration. Some patients exhibiting this reaction may have reduced procainesterase activity resulting in decreased degradation of procaine.[27]

The second reaction is similar, but hyperventilation, convulsions, fever, hypertension, tachycardia, and vomiting may also be present. In severe cases, hypotension and cardiovascular collapse occur. This is usually secondary to inadvertent intravenous administration of procaine penicillin. The reaction may be due to microembolization of procaine to the lungs and brain, although direct toxicity may also play a role.

These reactions are not allergic in nature. Patients should be restrained and reassured. More severe reactions can be managed by supportive care and appropriate treatment of convulsions and cardiopulmonary problems.

## DRUG INTERACTIONS

At the dosage schedules used in venereology, interactions between penicillins and other drugs are rare, as summarized in Table 83-4.

## CEPHALOSPORINS AND CEPHAMYCINS

## INDICATIONS

Cefuroxime, cefotetan, and all of the third-generation cephalosporins are exceptionally active against *N. gonorrhoeae* in vitro and, unlike the first-generation cephalosporins (e.g., cephalothin, cefazolin), are not destroyed by gonococcal beta-lactamases. Of these agents, both cefoxitin and ceftriaxone have been highly effective in the treatment of uncomplicated gonorrhea, including cases caused by penicillinase-producing strains.[28] The unusually long half-life (6 to 8 h) and exquisite sensitivity of the gonococcus

**Table 83-4. Potential Interactions between Various Beta-Lactam Antibiotics and Other Drugs**

| Drug | Interaction mechanism | Most implicated β-lactam |
|---|---|---|
| Tetracyclines | Interaction of a bacteriostatic agent (tetracycline) with a bactericidal antibiotic may result in antagonism. Clinical significance uncertain | All |
| Neomycin | Decrease absorption | Phenoxypenicillins |
| Aminoglycosides | In patients with renal failure, in vivo inactivation of both antibiotics may occur. | Carbenicillin/ticarcillin, penicillin G |
| | Increased nephrotoxicity clinical significance unknown | Cephalosporins |
| Antacids | Decrease absorption; questionable significance | Oral agents |
| Urine-glucose tests | False-positive glucose results may occur with copper-reduction tests (Clinitest) when large doses of penicillins are administered. Recommend use of glucose oxidase tests (Testape) | All |
| Allopurinol | Increased incidence of rash due to unknown mechanisms | Ampicillin |
| Probenecid | Decrease tubular secretion resulting in increased serum and tissue levels | All |
| Sulfonamides | Decrease absorption | Oxacillin |
| Oral contraceptives | Decrease effectiveness of birth control pills | Ampicillin |
| Nonsteroidal anti-inflammatory agents | Inhibit tubular secretion of penicillin | All |
| Ethanol | Antibuse-like reaction | Cefoperazone, cefotetan, moxalactam |

to ceftriaxone have made it very useful for single-dose therapy of uncomplicated gonorrhea.

Cefoxitin continues to be used in the treatment of pelvic inflammatory disease (PID) because of a broad spectrum of activity against *N. gonorrhoeae,* many anaerobes, and facultative gram-negative rods. Cefotetan may also find a role in the treatment of PID, but few studies have been completed to date. However, neither drug is active against *C. trachomatis* and thus both are used in combination with doxycycline.

Resistance to the penicillins has not yet been reported for *T. pallidum.* Thus, alternative drugs are needed only in patients with penicillin allergy. Ceftriaxone has been as effective as penicillin G in treating experimental syphilis in rabbits, but further data are required in humans.

## MODE OF ACTION

As described above, the antimicrobial effects of the cephalosporins and cephamycins are similar to those of the penicillins. Variations accounting for different spectrums of activity are probably related to specific beta-lactam-binding proteins on some bacteria reacting to one antibiotic and not another.

## SPECTRUM OF ACTIVITY

Many of the second- and third-generation cephalosporins and cephamycins have in vitro activity against penicillinase- and nonpenicillinase-producing *N. gonorrhoeae* and other pathogens associated with venereal infection.

## MECHANISM OF RESISTANCE

Mechanisms of resistance to the cephalosporins and cephamycins are similar to that described for the penicillins, including chromosomal mutation and plasmid-mediated resistance. Plasmids can code for resistance by producing enzymes that destroy cephalosporins. However, cefoxitin, cefotetan, and many third-generation cephalosporins are not hydrolyzed by the TEM-type beta-lactamase R plasmids in *N. gonorrhoeae.*[29]

## BIOPHARMACEUTICS AND PHARMACOKINETICS

### Absorption

Although cefaclor, cephalexin, cefadroxil, and cephradine are all well absorbed by mouth (75 to 100 percent), none are used for the treatment of STD.[30,31] Other cephalosporins are not well absorbed orally and must be administered parenterally.

### Distribution

Distribution of the cephalosporins into most body tissues is very good. In humans, placental transfer of cephalothin, cephacetrile, cefazolin, and cephaloridine results in fetal concentrations that approximate 50 percent of the maternal levels.[30] Cefuroxime and most third-generation cephalosporins except cefoperazone penetrate the meninges in the presence of inflammation and achieve bactericidal CSF concentrations. Ceftriaxone or cefotaxime would be useful agents in central nervous system infections caused by penicillinase-producing *N. gonorrhoeae.* Penetration of all cephalosporins into pleural and synovial fluids is very good.[30] Third-generation cephalosporins also penetrate well into the aqueous humor of the eye. In contrast, vitreous penetration is poor. Bile concentrations are very high for all cephalosporins, with maximum levels being achieved with cefoperazone.

### Metabolism and excretion

The major route of elimination for most cephalosporins is the kidneys via glomerular filtration and tubular secretion. Dosage adjustments are necessary in patients with renal insufficiency who are given extended therapy.[19] Probenecid inhibits the tubular secretion of the cephalosporins as well as the penicillins.

## ADVERSE REACTIONS

The cephalosporins cause adverse reactions similar to the penicillins, probably owing to similar chemical structures. Allergic reactions have occurred in approximately 5 percent of patients receiving cephalosporins.[32] About 6 to 9 percent of the patients who are allergic to penicillin exhibit a hypersensitivity to the cephalosporins.[33] However, immunological studies have found cross-reactivity in up to 20 percent of penicillin-allergic patients.[34] This is in part due to cross-allergenicity, but it is also secondary to the fact that atopic individuals exhibit multiple allergies and may have independently acquired cephalosporin hypersensitivity.[35] Hypersensitivity reactions are not associated with any particular cephalosporin. Patients with a history of a mild or temporary distinct penicillin reaction appear to be at low risk of developing a cephalosporin allergic reaction.

Renal failure, both acute and chronic, has been associated with the cephalosporins.[36] High doses of cephalothin have caused acute tubular necrosis, whereas standard doses (8 to 12 g per day) have been nephrotoxic in patients with preexisting renal disease.[37] Interstitial nephritis has been observed, especially in individuals greater than 60 years of age.

Thrombophlebitis is a frequent side effect during intravenous therapy. Cephalothin is implicated more than the newer cephalosporins.[38] Diarrhea and pseudomembranous colitis have been reported with most cephalosporins. Hematologic abnormalities such as hemolytic anemia, leukopenia, and thrombocytopenia occur rarely.[33] Bleeding secondary to hypoprothrombinemia and platelet dysfunction has been observed with several beta-lactams.[39] High doses of moxalactam (> 6 g per day), cefoperazone (> 4 g per day), and cefotetan (>4 g per day) are highly associated with this phenomenon, possibly because of the *N*-methylthioethyltetrazole (NMTT) side chains shared by these three drugs.[40] This problem is particularly frequent in the elderly, malnourished, and renal-insufficient patient populations. The FDA recommends that 10 mg of vitamin K be administered simultaneously at the start of therapy and then once per week during treatment. Bleeding times should be monitored closely when prolonged therapy is given.

# TETRACYCLINES

## INDICATIONS

The tetracyclines are among the most widely used antibiotics in venereology. Since they are the drugs of choice for *C. trachomatis* and *Mycoplasma* infections, the tetracyclines are indicated for nongonococcal urethritis, epididymitis, cervicitis, and salpingitis. Tetracyclines may also be used in syphilis in penicillin-allergic patients and for chancroid caused by tetracycline-susceptible strains of *Haemophilus ducreyi*. They should not be used in penicillinase-resistant *N. gonorrhoeae* infections since there is a high incidence of cross-resistance with the penicillins. Tetracyclines may be used for selected cases of shigellosis or *C. jejuni* enteritis and with metronidazole for treatment of *Entamoeba histolytica* intestinal infections.

## MODE OF ACTION

The tetracyclines inhibit bacterial synthesis by reversibly binding to the 30-S ribosomal subunit, which interferes with subsequent binding of aminoacyl-tRNA to its adjacent acceptor site on the mRNA ribosome complex. Protein synthesis is thus inhibited. Higher concentrations may cause alterations in the bacterial cell membrane, resulting in leakage of nucleotides from the cell, and may also inhibit mammalian protein synthesis.

## SPECTRUM OF ACTIVITY

Organisms are generally considered sensitive to tetracycline if the MIC is $\leq 1$ μg/ml, intermediate in sensitivity for MICs between 1 and 5 μg/ml, and resistant at MICs $> 5$ μg/ml. For minocycline and doxycycline, resistance is usually suspected if MICs are $> 2$ to 3 μg/ml. Differences in sensitivities between the other available tetracyclines are minor. In general, tetracyclines have in vitro activity against *N. gonorrhoeae, C. trachomatis, Ureaplasma urealyticum,* and *H. ducreyi.*

Clinical data demonstrate that *T. pallidum* is susceptible to the tetracyclines. Approximately 70 to 90 percent of group B streptococci and up to 50 to 70 percent of *Salmonella* and *Shigella* spp. demonstrate resistance.[41–44] Although *Campylobacter* spp. are very sensitive to the tetracyclines, in particular minocycline, resistant isolates are being found in some countries.[45]

## MECHANISM OF RESISTANCE

Both chromosomal mutations and plasmid-mediated resistance to tetracyclines have been described. Predominantly, resistance occurs by preventing accumulation of the antibiotic within the cell, because either the influx transport system is impaired and/or the cell increases elimination of the antibiotic. Resistance demonstrated by group B streptococci, *N. gonorrhoeae,* and *Salmonella* and *Shigella* spp. can occur by either of these mechanisms.[7,46]

## BIOPHARMACEUTICS AND PHARMACOKINETICS

Since doxycycline is now available as a generic product at a low cost, it should generally be used as the preferred tetracycline because of its twice daily dosing schedule, lower frequency of side effects, and relative safety in renal failure. Although some other compounds demonstrate better absorption (e.g., minocycline), they are more expensive and cause more side effects than generic doxycycline hydrochloride. Triple tetracycline does not appear to have an advantage over other tetracyclines.

### Absorption

Absorption of the tetracyclines varies from 30 to 100 percent in the fasting state and occurs primarily in the proximal small bowel (Table 83-5). Food and other compounds impair absorption of most tetracyclines.

Peak serum concentrations of the tetracyclines after oral administration usually occur 1 to 2 h after ingestion but may occur as long as 4 h later (Table 83-5). After intramuscular injection, peak levels are achieved in about 1 h. However, since absorption after IM injection is erratic and severe pain is produced on injection, this route is not recommended.[47]

### Distribution

The tetracyclines penetrate well into most body fluids and tissues, including pleural, ascitic, and synovial fluids, cord serum, and maxillary sinuses. Lower concentrations are found in saliva, tears, and sputum. About 10 to 20 percent of the serum concentrations of most tetracyclines penetrate the normal blood-brain barrier. Minocycline, followed by doxycycline, is more lipophilic than the other tetracyclines and exhibits the greatest tissue penetration, especially into the brain, eyes, and intestinal epithelium.[47] Minocycline achieves tissue concentrations approaching, and in many cases, exceeding serum levels. Prostate tissue levels of doxycycline may reach 60 percent of the serum concentration and peritoneal fluid levels are about 75 percent of the serum levels.

Protein binding of the tetracyclines ranges from 30 to 95 percent. These antibiotics are bound to bone, teeth, and neoplasms and cause yellow discoloration in these tissues. Whether these binding properties affect therapeutic efficacy is unknown.

### Metabolism and excretion

Most of the tetracyclines are eliminated primarily by the kidneys. Exceptions to this include chlorotetracycline and minocycline, which are primarily metabolized by the liver, and doxycycline, which is excreted in the feces.

## ADVERSE REACTIONS

Since most treatment regimens for STDs that utilize tetracyclines consist of multiple-dose regimens over a period of 1 or 2 weeks, side effects are frequent.[47]

### Gastrointestinal effects

Gastrointestinal reactions (nausea, vomiting, epigastric distress) occur in about 10 percent of patients receiving 2 g per day of tetracycline. They are most likely due to direct irritation of the bowel by unabsorbed drug, although even compounds with the greatest absorption may still cause side effects. Administration of food often ameliorates these symptoms but may decrease drug absorption. Doxycycline produces fewer gastrointestinal side effects than the other agents. Although doxycycline is primarily excreted in the feces, it is in a chelated form and has little effect on the fecal flora. About 40 to 50 percent of patients taking therapeutic doses of minocycline complain of nausea. It is unclear whether this is from gastrointestinal irritation or vestibular toxicity. Esophageal ulceration has been rarely reported following

Table 83-5. Biopharmaceutic and Pharmacokinetic Data on Various Tetracyclines

| Tetracyclines | Half-life, h: Normal | Half-life, h: Renal failure | Absorption, % | Peak serum concentrations, μg/ml | Major route of elimination (minor route) |
|---|---|---|---|---|---|
| Chlorotetracycline | 5–7 | 7–11 | 30 | PO 500 mg = 7<br>IV over 15–20 min 500 mg = 35 | Hepatic |
| Demelocycline | 10–15 | Increased | 66 | PO 500 mg = 2.5<br>IV over 15–20 min 500 mg = 22 | Renal (hepatic) |
| Doxycycline | 14–25 | 15–36 | 93 | PO 200 mg = 3–6.7<br>IV over 30 min 200 mg = 4 | Feces (hepatic) |
| Methacycline | 8–14 | 44 | 58 | PO 300 mg = 1–2 | Renal (hepatic) |
| Minocycline | 12–17 | 12–21 | 95 | PO 200 mg = 0.7–4.5<br>IV over 30 min 100 mg = 8.8 | Hepatic (renal, feces) |
| Oxytetracycline | 9–10 | 47–66 | 58 | PO 500 mg = 2.3–3<br>IV over 15–20 min 500 mg = 5 | Renal (hepatic) |
| Tetracycline hydrochloride | 6–10 | 57–108 | 77 | PO 500 mg = 3.8–5<br>IM 250 mg = 2<br>IM 330 mg* = 1.77<br>IV over 15–20 min 500 mg = 7.5 | Renal (hepatic) |

*Tetracycline phosphate complex.
SOURCE: Compiled from Refs. 19 and 47.

tetracycline and doxycycline administration; patients reportedly took their medication prior to going to bed with little to no fluid.[48] Diarrhea is a common complaint and appears to be associated with poor absorption; it is usually reversible upon discontinuation of the drug. Pseudomembranous colitis and staphylococcal enterocolitis have also been reported.[49]

Suprainfections such as oral candidiasis and vaginal moniliasis often occur in patients on tetracycline therapy, but the use of nystatin or clotrimazole in combination with the tetracyclines is not routinely recommended.

## Skin and allergy

Hypersensitivity reactions, although rare (≤ 0.5 percent), may include anaphylaxis, urticaria, periorbital edema, fixed drug eruptions, and morbilliform rashes. Photosensitivity reactions are reported primarily with demeclocycline, although any of the tetracycline agents can cause this reaction. It is a "phototoxic" dermatitis consisting of erythema on the sun-exposed areas of the skin. Severe reactions may result in the formation of edema, papules, vesiculation, and onycholysis.

## Vestibular Disturbances

Vestibular disturbances, consisting of dizziness, vertigo, ataxia, and tinnitus, occur most often with minocycline and are more common in women. About 70 to 90 percent of patients who develop this reaction are affected within 24 to 48 h of the onset of treatment with minocycline. Symptoms are completely reversible within several days of drug discontinuation.

## Hepatotoxicity

Tetracyclines are hepatotoxins which produce fatty infiltration of the liver, probably secondary to tetracycline-induced inhibition of the synthesis of proteins required to remove lipid compounds from the liver. Risk factors for steatosis include daily intravenous doses greater than 1 g, renal failure, serum concentrations greater than 16 μg/ml, and pregnancy. Women in their last trimester may be at greater risk. Toxicity ranges from mild elevation of liver function tests to severe hepatic insufficiency with jaundice, acidosis, and shock. Fatalities have been reported.

## Nephrotoxicity

Patients with renal insufficiency should not receive tetracyclines since their antianabolic effect produces an additional nitrogen load for the kidneys to excrete. Since this is dose-dependent, accumulation of the tetracyclines in renal failure will exacerbate the problem. Minocycline, doxycycline, and chlorotetracycline have a lesser effect on nitrogen retention since they are mainly excreted by nonrenal mechanisms. However, they are still catabolic and caution should be exercised when using them. If tetracyclines are given in renal failure, the dosages should be reduced to minimize toxicity.[19] Chlorotetracycline, doxycycline, and possibly minocycline do not accumulate in renal failure and dosage adjustments are not necessary.

Nonoliguric renal failure has occurred with the tetracyclines in conjunction with so-called acute fatty liver in pregnancy.

Administration of outdated oral tetracyclines has been associated with renal tubular damage (the Fanconi syndrome). This probably occurred because of the acid excipient in the formulation, which degraded the antibiotic during storage. Since many preparations no longer contain the acid, this reaction is now relatively uncommon.

Finally, demeclocycline can cause a nephrogenic diabetes insipidus by inhibiting the action of antidiuretic hormone (ADH) in the kidneys. The polyuria which occurs is dose-dependent and vasopressin-resistant.

## Pigmentation of teeth

Tetracyclines are permanently deposited in calcifying areas of teeth, causing a gray-brown to yellow discoloration in the permanent teeth of children between the ages of 4 months and 6 years when mineralization takes place. Anterior deciduous teeth are mineralized from the fourteenth week in utero to 2 to 3 months after birth. Discoloration is more likely after the twenty-fifth week of gestation. The magnitude of effect is proportional to dose and number of treatment courses given.[50] For this reason, tetracyclines should be avoided, if possible, during pregnancy and in children less than 8 years of age.

### Bone growth

Tetracyclines are deposited in bone during the twelfth week of gestation. They are later resorbed, resulting in a temporary inhibition of skeletal growth. Rapid reversal of this effect is seen upon discontinuation of the antibiotic.

## DRUG INTERACTIONS

Food decreases the absorption of the tetracyclines by 50 percent or more in many patients. Exceptions are doxycycline and minocycline, which are adequately absorbed when given with food. Iron salts chelate the tetracyclines in the gastrointestinal tract, resulting in poor absorption. Antacids containing high concentrations of calcium, aluminum, or magnesium complex with tetracyclines and thus decrease absorption. Tetracyclines should be administered 1 to 2 h before or after meals, iron supplementation, and antacid therapy.

# SPECTINOMYCIN

## INDICATIONS

Spectinomycin is used in uncomplicated (nonpharyngeal) *N. gonorrhoeae* infections, especially in patients with histories of penicillin hypersensitivity, treatment failure, or suspected penicillin-resistant strains.

## MODE OF ACTION

Spectinomycin inhibits protein synthesis by binding to the 30-S ribosomal subunit. Unlike its structural analogue streptomycin, it does not cause misreading of the polyribonucleotide code. Some evidence suggests that the surface morphology of the gonococcus is changed after exposure to spectinomycin, resulting in altered cytoplasmic membrane proteins. This causes osmotic lysis of the cell and organism death.

## SPECTRUM OF ACTIVITY

Approximately 99 percent of gonococcal isolates tested by McCormack and Finland in 1975 were inhibited by ≤ 6.3 μg/ml.[51] In other series, 97.8 to 100 percent of over 2000 isolates were inhibited by ≤ 20 μg/ml.[6] Resistance of *N. gonorrhoeae* to spectinomycin was rarely observed prior to 1982.[52,53] More recently, highly resistant strains of *N. gonorrhoeae* have been isolated with increasing frequency (8 percent), especially in Korea.[54] These strains were also beta-lactamase producers. At least 10 cases of gonococci resistant to spectinomycin have been reported in the United States.[55] Spectinomycin lacks significant in vitro activity for *T. pallidum* or *C. trachomatis* but it has some effectiveness against *U. urealyticum* and *Gardnerella vaginalis*.[56–58]

## MECHANISMS OF RESISTANCE

The major mechanism of resistance to spectinomycin is one-step chromosomal mutation, which alters the ribosome such that the antibiotic cannot bind to it.

## BIOPHARMACEUTICS AND PHARMACOKINETICS

Spectinomycin is poorly absorbed from the gastrointestinal tract but is well absorbed after intramuscular injection. After a 2-g intramuscular dose, serum concentrations of about 100 μg/ml are achieved at 1 h. Detectable levels can be measured for up to 8 h. Penetration into saliva is poor and unpredictable, thereby explaining the ineffectiveness of spectinomycin in eradicating pharyngeal *Neisseria*. Spectinomycin is primarily excreted unchanged by the kidneys with an elimination half-life of 1 h.[51]

## ADVERSE REACTIONS

Side effects after single-dose administration of spectinomycin are minimal, including occasional reports of transient dizziness, fever, chills, gastrointestinal discomfort, headache, insomnia, and urticaria occurring in from < 1 to 5 percent of those treated. Discomfort at the site of deep intramuscular injection occurs in about 20 percent of the patients. Prolonged treatment with spectinomycin for 3 weeks did not show any further toxicities.[21,51,59]

The safety of spectinomycin in pregnancy has not been established. Neither maternal nor fetal toxicity has arisen in treated cases, but third-generation cephalosporins now represent another alternative for patients with a history of penicillin allergy other than anaphylaxis.

# ERYTHROMYCIN AND OTHER MACROLIDES

## INDICATIONS

Erythromycins are among the drugs of choice for chancroid, and are considered second- and third-line antibiotic choices for many STDs. They are recommended in nongonococcal urethritis for patients who are allergic to the tetracyclines, in *C. trachomatis* infection in pregnant women, and for syphilis in penicillin-allergic patients. Erythromycins are also indicated in neonatal conjunctivitis or other pediatric infections caused by *C. trachomatis* since tetracyclines and sulfonamides are usually avoided in children. They are good alternatives to penicillin for group B streptococcal infections in penicillin-allergic patients. *Campylobacter* sp. infections also respond to the erythromycins. Donovanosis and lymphogranuloma venereum have been treated successfully with erythromycin in a small number of cases.[60,61] Erythromycin treatment of gonorrhea is not reliably effective, most often because of high-level resistance.[62]

## MODE OF ACTION

Erythromycin and other macrolide antibiotics reversibly bind to bacterial ribosomes at the 50-S subunit, interfering with bacterial growth by inhibiting protein synthesis.

## SPECTRUM OF ACTIVITY

Erythromycin demonstrates in vitro activity against *N. gonorrhoeae, C. trachomatis*, Campylobacter sp., *T. pallidum*, and *U. urealyticum*. Erythromycin may be bacteriostatic or bactericidal depending on drug concentration, bacteria species, phase of growth, and inoculum size. Additionally, erythromycin (a weak base) has markedly decreased activity in environments with a low pH (i.e., the vagina).

## MECHANISM OF RESISTANCE

Resistant bacteria usually result from mutations in ribosomal structure which prevents binding of the erythromycins to the target site. Plasmid-mediated resistance is also reported but is less common. A characteristic feature of the macrolide antibiotics is "dissociated" resistance. Since only one macrolide can bind to the ribosome, bacteria resistant to one macrolide exhibit in vitro resistance to others if they are tested in the presence of the initial drug. However, the latter drugs may in fact be active in vivo. This type of resistance can also be demonstrated with chloramphenicol, clindamycin, and other antibiotics that bind to the 50-S ribosomal subunit.

## BIOPHARMACEUTICS AND PHARMACOKINETICS

### Absorption

Erythromycins exhibit variable absorption following oral administration (Table 83-6). Absorption of erythromycin is particularly variable in pregnant women, and serum levels may be lower in this population.[63] Between 18 and 45 percent of an oral dose is bioavailable; only the base is biologically active. Erythromycin base is inactivated by gastric acids, whereas the esters and ester salts are more acid-stable. The base is usually administered as an enteric-coated or film-coated tablet that is absorbed in the upper portion of the small intestine. Erythromycin base, the stearate salt (absorbed as the base), and the ethylsuccinate salt [absorbed as both the inactive ester and the active free base (55 percent) after hydrolysis in the intestine] appear to be better absorbed in the fasting state. However, other reports indicate that the stearate and ethylsuccinate preparation have enhanced bioavailability with food.[64,65] Erythromycin base is also marketed as a capsule containing enteric-coated granules which may provide more consistent absorption.[66] The estolate form is less affected by acid and food, and produces serum levels that consist of both free base (20 to 30 percent) and estolate (70 to 80 percent).

### Distribution

Erythromycin penetrates well into most body tissues, achieving levels well above the MICs of common gram-positive organisms in sinus fluid, aqueous humor, and middle ear fluid. Concentrations in tonsillar tissue are 12.5 to 65 percent of simultaneous serum concentration.[67] Erythromycin also penetrates into prostatic fluid, where levels are approximately 40 percent of the serum concentrations. Cerebrospinal fluid penetration is variable; concentration without inflammation ranges from 0 to 2 percent, compared with 5 to 10 percent during meningitis.[68] Placental transfer of erythromycin is poor and fetal serum levels are approximately 1 percent of maternal serum concentrations.[69] Poor placental transfer together with the variable absorption in pregnancy severely limits the usefulness of this drug for treatment of syphilis in penicillin-allergic pregnant women. Erythromycins are excreted in breast milk.

### Metabolism and excretion

Erythromycin is metabolized in the liver by *N*-demethylation to inactive metabolites, most of which have not been identified. Erythromycin estolate dissociates in the upper intestine, liberating the propanoate ester, which is inactive. This is absorbed and partially hydrolyzed in the blood to the free, microbiologically active base. From 1 to 5 percent of the drug is excreted in the urine unchanged when administered orally, and from 12 to 15 percent when given parenterally.[68] The inactive metabolites are also eliminated via the kidney. After an oral dose, significant amounts of the drug are recovered in the feces, probably representing both unabsorbed drug as well as biliary excretions of drug.

The normal serum elimination half-life of erythromycin is 1.4 h, which is prolonged to 5 h in end-stage renal disease.[19]

**Table 83-6. Biopharmaceutic and Pharmacokinetic Data on Various Macrolide Antibiotics**

| Macrolide antibiotics | Half-life, h: Normal | Half-life, h: Renal failure | Peak serum concentrations, μg/ml | Major route of elimination (minor route) |
|---|---|---|---|---|
| Erythromycin base | 0.8–3.0 | 4.8–6.0 | 0.3–1.0† (250 mg PO) | Metabolism (biliary 1.5%, renal 1–5%) |
| Erythromycin estolate | * | * | 1.4‡ (250 mg PO) | Metabolism (biliary 0.04–0.22%; renal 1–5%) |
| Erythromycin ethylsuccinate | * | * | 1.5‡ (500 mg PO) | Metabolism (renal 2–15%) |
| Erythromycin gluceptate | 1.5 | 5.0 | 3–7 (200 mg IV) | Metabolism (renal 12–15%) |
| Erythromycin lactobionate | 1.9–2.4 | 2.1–7.0 | 3.4 (200 mg IV) | Metabolism (renal 12–15%) |
| Erythromycin stearate | 1.7 | 5.5 | 0.4–0.8 (250 mg PO fasting)<br>0.4–1.8 (500 mg PO fasting)<br>0.1–0.4§ (500 mg PO after food) | Metabolism (renal 1–5%) |

*Similar to erythromycin base.
†Somewhat high levels reported for enteric-coated products following multiple doses.
‡Total drug (inactive ester plus free base).
§One study noted higher levels (to 2.8 μg/ml) following a meal.
SOURCE: Compiled from Refs. 19 and 68.

Peritoneal dialysis or hemodialysis are not effective in removing erythromycin.

## ADVERSE REACTIONS

Macrolides are among the safest of antimicrobials. Although serious side effects are rare, less severe but bothersome ones may be quite frequent.

### Gastrointestinal side effects

Gastrointestinal irritation is the most common adverse effect with erythromycin and often limits use of these drugs. Nausea, vomiting, and diarrhea occur in up to 10 to 20 percent of patients and appear to be dose-related. Pseudomembranous colitis has been reported infrequently following erythromycin therapy.[70] Superinfection of the gastrointestinal tract or vagina with *Candida* species may occur.

### Hepatotoxicity

The most significant serious adverse effect is hepatotoxicity, which is more common with erythromycin estolate,[71–73] but it is also reported with erythromycin ethylsuccinate,[74] lactobionate,[75] and other forms of erythromycin. Hepatotoxicity reactions may be induced by erythromycin estolate in as many as 2 to 4 percent of patients, usually after ≥ 14 days of therapy. The toxicity appears to be idiosyncratic and may be a hypersensitivity reaction.[72,76] Subsequent exposures usually produce renewed symptoms rapidly, sometimes after only one or two doses of drug. The syndrome usually begins with nausea, vomiting, and abdominal pain followed by jaundice, fever, and abnormal liver function studies that are consistent with cholestatic hepatitis. Laboratory changes include increased transaminases and eosinophilia. Total and direct bilirubin and alkaline phosphatase are generally elevated two to three times normal. As many as 10 percent of pregnant women have developed elevated serum transaminases when given erythromycin estolate for 6 weeks.

### Miscellaneous

Allergic reactions are uncommon and the incidence of skin reactions is only about 0.3 percent. Ototoxicity has been reported with both intravenous and oral use of erythromycin but appears to be more common with parenteral administration. Hearing loss is reversible if the drug is discontinued and recovery usually occurs at the same rate at which the loss occurred.[77] This reaction may be more common in elderly patients with renal impairment. Intramuscular erythromycin is painful, and sterile abscesses may occur. Thrombophlebitis may occur following intravenous administration and can be avoided with adequate volumes (≥ 250 ml) and prolonged infusion times (≥ 45 min). It appears to be dose-related since almost every patient receiving a 1-g dose every 6 h developed the reaction.[78]

## DRUG INTERACTIONS

Antagonism may occur if erythromycin is administered with chloramphenicol or clindamycin because of in vitro competitive ribosomal binding, but there is little need for concurrent use of these antibiotics.

Clinical observations have shown that erythromycin increases the serum concentration of theophylline. Patients who are given both of these drugs should be monitored for theophylline toxicity.[79]

## SULFONAMIDES AND TRIMETHOPRIM

## INDICATIONS

Sulfonamides alone or trimethoprim-sulfamethoxazole are usually second- or third-line antibiotics in treating a variety of venereal diseases including gonorrhea, chlamydial urethritis or cervicitis, chlamydial conjunctivitis, chancroid, lymphogranuloma venereum, and donovanosis. These agents are not effective against *U. urealyticum*.[80] Data concerning efficacy of trimethoprim-sulfamethoxazole (TMP-SMZ) against *N. gonorrhoeae* are conflicting, in part because of regional differences in susceptibility to this combination; these data are summarized in Chap. 13. Trimethoprim alone is not effective for gonorrhea, and in recent years, failure rates have exceeded 60 percent when sulfonamides were used alone.[81,82]

Sulfonamides alone are alternatives to the tetracyclines or erythromycins in infections caused by *C. trachomatis*. The addition of trimethoprim does not produce meaningful synergy against chlamydia. Sulfonamides are not recommended in premature infants or those less than 2 months of age who have chlamydia infection because of the risk of kernicterus.

## MODE OF ACTION

The sulfonamides and trimethoprim interfere with DNA synthesis by affecting consecutive steps in the formation of purines. Sensitive bacteria are unable to utilize exogenous folic acid and must synthesize it from *para*-aminobenzoic acid (PABA). The sulfonamides are structurally similar to PABA and compete for the enzyme dihydrofolic acid synthetase, which converts PABA to dihydrofolic acid. Higher animals that are unable to synthesize PABA utilize preformed folate and are therefore unaffected by the drug. Trimethoprim inhibits dihydrofolic acid reductase, the enzyme responsible for reducing dihydrofolic acid to tetrahydrofolic acid. This enzyme is required by humans as well, but trimethoprim has 50,000 to 100,000 times the inhibitory effect on the bacterial enzyme as compared with the mammalian enzyme. Combinations of sulfamethoxazole and trimethoprim act synergistically to produce bactericidal effects on susceptible bacteria.[83,84]

## SPECTRUM OF ACTIVITY

Sulfisoxazole is the usual drug used in disk sensitivity studies, although sensitivities for the sulfonamides are interchangeable. Sulfonamides alone or in combination with trimethoprim are not usually active against *T. pallidum*,[85] *U. urealyticum*,[80] or *C. fetus*.[45]

## MECHANISMS OF RESISTANCE

Resistance to sulfonamides most often occurs because of mutation, resulting in either excessive microbial production of PABA[86] or structural change in a folic acid synthesizing enzyme which decreases its affinity for sulfonamide.[87] Other mechanisms of resistance include R plasmids, which encode production of drug-resistant enzymes and decreased bacterial cell permeability to sulfonamides.

Trimethoprim resistance may occur by chromosomal mutation or by plasmid-mediated genetic exchange. Resistant strains of *N. gonorrhoeae* have altered affinities for dihydrofolate reductases or altered permeability of the cell envelope to trimethoprim.

## BIOPHARMACEUTICS AND PHARMACOKINETICS

### Absorption

Most sulfonamides are rapidly absorbed from the gastrointestinal tract following oral administration (Table 83-7). Approximately 70 to 100 percent of an oral dose is absorbed,[88] and peak serum concentrations are achieved 2 to 4 h following an oral dose. Parenteral therapy (only sulfadiazine and sulfamethoxazole) results in similar levels.

Trimethoprim is well absorbed after oral administration and peak levels are achieved in approximately 2 to 4 h.[89] Coadministration with a sulfonamide does not affect the rate or extent of absorption.

The administration of the combination of TMP-SMZ in a ratio of 1:5 results in the serum concentration ratio of approximately 1:20, respectively.[89,90] Intravenous administration yields peak levels similar to oral dosing.[91]

### Distribution

Sulfonamides are widely distributed throughout body fluids and tissue.[92–94] They penetrate into ocular, peritoneal, pleural, and synovial fluids and reach concentrations of 50 to 80 percent of serum levels. CSF concentrations range between 10 and 80 percent of simultaneous serum levels. Sulfonamides achieve only very low levels in vaginal secretions but do cross the placenta and are found in fetal blood and amniotic fluid.[95]

Trimethoprim is also widely distributed.[94,96,97] Antibiotic concentrations in saliva exceed simultaneous serum concentrations. Unlike the sulfonamides, high drug levels are also found in vaginal secretions and prostatic fluids. Lower levels, however, have been observed in men with chronic prostatitis.[98,99] Bactericidal concentrations are achieved in the CSF.[100] Trimethoprim has been detected in human breast milk and does cross the placenta (approximately 15 percent of maternal blood levels).[101]

### Metabolism and excretion

The sulfonamides are metabolized primarily in the liver by $N^4$-acetylation and to a lesser extent by $N^4$-oxidation and glucuronidation. The extent of metabolism ranges from 5 to 40 percent. The metabolites are not active but are potentially toxic. Both the active sulfonamide and inactive metabolites are excreted in the urine by glomerular filtration and tubular secretion. Approximately 30 to 90 percent of an oral dose can be recovered from the urine. Excretion also occurs through bile, saliva, and sweat.[92] Plasma half-lives vary widely and are inversely related to lipid solubility but are not associated with the degree of protein binding. Urine pH affects the excretion of sulfonamides.[102] Alkalinization increases the amount of ionized drug which is excreted rather than reabsorbed by the tubules. Acidification may decrease solubility of the drugs and precipitate crystalluria.

Urinary excretion is the major route of elimination of trimethoprim.[91,103] Approximately 40 to 60 percent of an oral dose and 42 to 75 percent of an intravenous dose is excreted unchanged. Unlike sulfamethoxazole, acidification of the urine increases the rate of trimethoprim excretion. Ten percent of the drug is eliminated as inactive metabolites. Hydroxylation is the major metabolite, and five inactive metabolites have been identified thus far. Biliary excretion is only a minor excretory route.[104] The serum half-life in healthy adults is 9 to 11 h.

Dosage adjustments are necessary for sulfonamides and trimethoprim in patients with renal insufficiency.[19]

## ADVERSE REACTIONS

### Sulfonamides

Adverse reactions to the sulfonamides are numerous and range in severity from mild to fatal. Hypersensitivity reactions are by far the most common.[105] Allergic rashes usually occur 7 to 10 days after initial therapy but recur rapidly with subsequent exposures. The risk of allergic rash is increased with higher daily doses. Maculopapular or urticarial rashes are the most common, but severe reactions such as erythema nodosum, exfoliative der-

**Table 83-7. Biopharmaceutic and Pharmacokinetic Data on Various Sulfonamides and Trimethoprim**

| | Half-life, h | | | | |
|---|---|---|---|---|---|
| Antibiotic | Normal | Renal failure | Total peak serum concentrations, μg/ml | Protein binding, % | Major route of elimination (minor route) |
| Sulfadiazine | 10–12 | 34 | 40–60 μg/ml (3–4 g PO) | 45 | Renal (metabolism 15–40%) |
| Sulfadoxine | 100–230 | ND* | 50–75 μg/ml [free drug (2 g PO)] | 80–98 | Renal |
| Sulfamethoxazole | 9–12 | 20–28 | 60 μg/ml (1.2 g PO) | 70 | Renal 30–50% (metabolism 60%) |
| Sulfisoxazole | 3–7 | 6–12 | 110 μg/ml (2 g PO)<br>250 μg/ml (4 g PO)<br>233.7 μg/ml (4.8 g PO) | 92 | Renal 50–70% (metabolism 30–35%) |
| Trimethoprim | 8–15 | 24 | 2 μg/ml (160 mg PO)<br>3 μg/ml (240 mg PO)<br>9.2 μg/ml (960 mg PO)<br>1.4 μg/ml (100 mg IV) | 40–70 | Renal 40–75% (metabolism 10%; biliary) |

*ND = not done in studies reviewed.

SOURCE: Compiled from Refs. 19, 88–91, 103.

matitis, and Stevens-Johnson syndrome may occur.[106–108] The latter are rare but much more frequent with the long-acting sulfonamides. Photosensitization is also reported with these drugs.

Blood dyscrasias associated with sulfonamides include agranulocytosis, thrombocytopenia, aplastic anemia, hemolytic anemia, and megaloblastic anemia. Agranulocytosis is rare with the agents used today. Hemolytic anemia may occur in patients with glucose-6-phosphate dehydrogenase deficiency.

Renal damage is a concern with sulfonamide therapy (especially sulfadiazine and sulfathiazole) but has decreased considerably with the use of newer, short-acting, and more soluble drugs.[105] The damage is usually secondary to precipitation of the drug in the tubules resulting in crystalluria. Interstitial nephritis infrequently occurs with the sulfonamides and is considered a hypersensitivity reaction.[109]

Hepatotoxicity occurs rarely.[110] Sulfonamides displace bilirubin from albumin-binding sites and may result in kernicterus in the newborn, and thus should be avoided in pregnant women near term.

### Trimethoprim and trimethoprim-sulfamethoxazole

Gastrointestinal side effects occur in approximately 5 percent of patients taking TMP-SMZ. Symptoms seen include loss of appetite, nausea, vomiting, abdominal cramps, and diarrhea. This effect is dose-related, and a maximum daily dose of 480 mg of trimethoprim is usually recommended.[89]

Skin rashes may occur and are usually attributable to the sulfonamide, but trimethoprim alone, in doses exceeding 2000 mg daily, is also associated with rash. Increased frequency and intensity of rash have been observed in patients with acquired immunodeficiency syndrome.[111]

Reversible renal impairment has been associated with the use of TMP-SMZ. Toxicity may occur from accumulation of conjugated metabolites of sulfamethoxazole.

Temporary rises in serum creatinine have been reported in subjects with normal renal function receiving TMP.[112] Trimethoprim appears to compete for tubular secretion of creatinine, and an increase in serum creatinine results.[113]

Inhibition of folate metabolism by trimethoprim is normally insignificant in humans. However, TMP-SMZ may cause megaloblastic anemia in uremic patients[114] and may aggravate preexisting megaloblastic anemia. Subjects with a folic acid or vitamin $B_{12}$ deficiency are susceptible. Neutropenia and thrombocytopenia resulting from concurrent use of TMP-SMZ and azothioprine have recently been described in renal allograft patients[115] and in bone marrow transplant patients. Megaloblastic hematopoiesis induced by azothioprine may potentiate TMP-SMZ-induced myelosuppression.

## DRUG INTERACTIONS

Sulfonamides displace warfarin, methotrexate, and phenytoin from protein-binding sites, resulting in higher concentrations of free drug. Sulfonamides also inhibit the metabolism of warfarin, thiopental, phenytoin, and oral hypoglycemic agents. The interactions which are most often clinically relevant include enhanced hypoprothrombinemia with warfarin, methotrexate toxicity, and hypoglycemia with tolbutamide. Appropriate monitoring and dosage adjustments should be made in patients who are treated with these drug combinations.

# CHLORAMPHENICOL

## INDICATIONS

Chloramphenicol is effective in severe salmonellae and shigellae infections such as septicemia. Chloramphenicol is sometimes used in salpingitis and is active against several STD pathogens but is usually considered a second- or third-line drug because of its toxic potential.

## MODE OF ACTION

Chloramphenicol inhibits bacterial protein synthesis by binding to the 50-S ribosomal subunit. The transpeptidation reaction which occurs at the ribosome acceptor site is inhibited.

## SPECTRUM OF ACTIVITY

Organisms are usually considered sensitive to chloramphenicol when MICs are $\leq$ 5.0 μg/ml. Organisms that are not inhibited by 25 μg/ml are considered resistant. Few bacteria fall into the intermediate range.

## MECHANISM OF RESISTANCE

Resistance to chloramphenicol is uncommon. When it is present, however, it is usually mediated by plasmids coding for chloramphenicol acetyltransferase, an inactivating enzyme. Nonenzymatic, plasmid-mediated resistance to chloramphenicol occurs infrequently because of alterations to bacterial cell permeability. Reductions in chloramphenicol's binding affinity to the ribosome may also result in bacterial resistance.

## BIOPHARMACEUTICS AND PHARMACOKINETICS

### Absorption

Chloramphenicol is rapidly and completely absorbed from the gastrointestinal tract. The oral suspension is formulated as a palmitate ester and is hydrolyzed in the duodenum by pancreatic lipases to active chloramphenicol, which is then absorbed, reaching therapeutic concentrations in 1 to 2 h. Doubling the dose will double the serum level. Chloramphenicol succinate ester is rapidly hydrolyzed within the body to active drug-producing concentrations that are 70 percent of those obtained with the palmitate ester.[116] Serum concentrations of 5 to 12 μg/ml are achieved following a 1-g intravenous dose. Administration of equivalent doses of the succinate ester by the intramuscular and oral route demonstrates that after 2 h, IM injection achieves only about one-half the serum levels obtained orally. This suggests delayed or inadequate hydrolysis of the succinate ester in the muscle depot. Serum levels can be followed to ensure peak concentrations between 10 and 25 μg/ml when chloramphenicol is used to treat serious infections.[117]

### Distribution

Chloramphenicol penetrates well into body fluids and tissues,[117] with serum protein binding ranging from 30 to 60 percent. It crosses the placenta, and fetal concentrations are about 30 to 80 percent of the maternal serum levels. Passage into breast milk is variable. It penetrates the central nervous system, including lumbar and ventricular fluid, regardless of meningeal inflammation. It diffuses readily into the tissues of the eye. The drug is also found in saliva and semen.

### Metabolism and excretion

Chloramphenicol is primarily metabolized in the liver by glucuronyl transferase to inactive conjugates which are then excreted by the kidneys. Conjugated metabolites are secreted in the bile and feces. Only 5 to 10 percent of chloramphenicol is excreted unchanged in the urine by glomerular filtration. The elimination half-life of chloramphenicol is 2 to 3 h in patients with normal renal and hepatic function. In renal failure the half-life is relatively unchanged.[117] The half-life increases to 4 to 6 h in cirrhosis, and doses should be adjusted according to serum concentrations.[118]

## ADVERSE REACTIONS

The most toxic reaction associated with chloramphenicol is bone marrow suppression: irreversible, idiopathic, aplastic anemia and reversible, dose-related hematopoietic toxicity.[117,119,120]

### Irreversible aplastic anemia

The incidence of chloramphenicol-induced aplastic anemia is 1 in 40,000, with a mortality rate in excess of 50 percent. It is unrelated to dose and duration of therapy, although it usually occurs weeks to months after discontinuation of the drug. It is postulated that the *para*-nitrosulfathiazole group of chloramphenicol is responsible for inhibition of thymidine incorporation into DNA, resulting in hypoplasia for all three hematopoietic cell lines. Pancytopenia is most common. Selective red cell aplasia, leukopenia, or thrombocytopenia are infrequent. It is recommended that twice weekly complete blood counts be obtained throughout the course of chloramphenicol therapy. The drug should be discontinued if the white count drops to less than $2500/mm^3$.

### Reversible bone marrow suppression

This reaction is predictable, reversible, dose-dependent, and more common at serum concentrations of chloramphenicol $> 25$ μg/ml or in patients receiving greater than 4 g per day. The mechanism for this effect is thought to be inhibition of mitochondrial protein synthesis secondary to suppression of ferrochelatase, an enzyme that catalyzes hemoglobin synthesis. Early signs of toxicity include increased serum iron, decreased reticulocyte count, increased myeloid/erythroid ratio in the bone marrow, and vacuolization and maturation arrest of erythroid and myeloid precursors. These occur within the first week. Decreased hemoglobin and mild thrombocytopenia occur within 1 and 2 weeks. Neutropenia is seen infrequently. These effects reverse themselves within 7 to 10 days after discontinuation of the drug.

### Other side effects

Gray baby syndrome can occur in newborns and premature infants who are treated with large doses of chloramphenicol.[117] Because of their immature glucuronyl transferase activity, chloramphenicol cannot be adequately metabolized. High serum concentrations may cause abdominal distention, vomiting, pallor, cyanosis, circulatory collapse, and even death. Serum levels should be monitored closely in these infants and in those who are receiving breast milk. This syndrome has also been observed in toddlers and after accidental cases of adult overdose.

Other side effects associated with chloramphenicol are infrequent and include optic and peripheral neuritis, gastrointestinal distress, hypersensitivity reactions, hearing loss, and hemolytic anemia in patients with glucose-6-phosphate dehydrogenase deficiency. Herxheimer-like reactions during the treatment of syphilis have been observed. Pseudomembranous or staphylococcal enterocolitis occur rarely.

## DRUG INTERACTIONS

Chloramphenicol can potentiate the effects of phenytoin, tolbutamide, cyclophosphamide, ethanol, warfarin, and possibly other oral anticoagulants by inhibiting or competing with the metabolism of these agents.[117] Phenobarbital can decrease the serum concentrations of chloramphenicol by enzyme induction.

# METRONIDAZOLE AND OTHER NITROIMIDAZOLES

## INDICATIONS

Metronidazole is a 5-nitroimidazole antibiotic that is effective in the treatment of *Trichomonas vaginalis* vaginitis, nonspecific vaginitis, giardiasis, and amebiasis.

## MODE OF ACTION

The mode of action of metronidazole has not been fully elucidated. It is postulated that under anaerobic conditions, the nitro group and the imidazole ring on metronidazole act as electron acceptors. They compete with ferredoxin, an electron-transfer protein endogenous to the organisms being treated. This results in inhibition of the evolution of hydrogen gas, chemical reduction of metronidazole, and interaction of the free radicals so produced with DNA. Nucleic acid synthesis is disrupted with subsequent cell death.[121] This reaction does not occur in an aerobic environment because oxygen reduces the uptake of metronidazole into bacteria and protozoa.

## SPECTRUM OF ACTIVITY

Metronidazole has no activity against *N. gonorrhoeae, C. trachomatis,* or most facultative gram-negative rods. Evaluation of in vitro sensitivity of *T. vaginalis* depends upon the laboratory testing conditions since susceptibility is altered by environmental factors and inoculum size.[122,123] Aerobically cultured organisms have higher MICs than the same organisms cultured anaerobically.

## MECHANISM OF RESISTANCE

Development of resistance to metronidazole is rare, but resistant strains of *T. vaginalis* have been reported.[122,123] Resistance has also been reported for other anaerobes. Philips et al. demonstrated decreased uptake of metronidazole in *Bacteroides bivius*–resistant isolates.[124] The rate of metronidazole reduction was also found to be lower when compared with a sensitive strain. Plasmids coding for resistance have not been demonstrated.

## BIOPHARMACEUTICS AND PHARMACOKINETICS

### Absorption

Metronidazole is rapidly and almost completely absorbed orally.[125,126] Peak serum concentrations usually occur in 30 to 60 min. Food appears to delay absorption. A 2-g single dose results in peak levels of 40 μg/ml of metronidazole. Concentrations of 32 and 5.7 μg/ml are maintained at 6 and 24 h, respectively. With multiple-dosing regimens of metronidazole, a peak level of 13.5 μg/ml is reached after 250 mg every 8 h for 2 days.[127]

Based on minimum inhibitory and bactericidal concentration data, a large single oral dose of these compounds yields adequate antibiotic levels over 6 h for *T. vaginalis* and *G. vaginalis* and most strains of *C. fetus*. Intravenous doses (15 mg/kg) result in mean peak and trough steady-state plasma concentrations of 25 and 18 μg/ml, respectively.

### Distribution

Metronidazole is widely distributed in the body and is found in saliva, breast milk, cerebrospinal fluid, bile, and abscess fluid. Lower concentrations are found in bone, semen, embryonic tissue, and the placenta.

### Metabolism and elimination

Metronidazole is metabolized to five major hydroxy and acid metabolites in the liver. Both types of metabolites are antibacterial against some anaerobes. The acid metabolite achieves only very low levels in the serum. The ratio of hydroxy metabolite to parent compound is about 0.03 to 0.3.

Metronidazole and its metabolites are primarily eliminated in the urine (60 to 80 percent of the dose). From 6 to 15 percent (notably hydroxymetabolite) is excreted in the feces. Only 8 percent of metronidazole is excreted unchanged by the kidneys. The elimination half-life of metronidazole is 7 to 9 h. It is not known whether accumulation of the metabolites of metronidazole in renal insufficiency causes a greater incidence of side effects. Hemodialysis effectively removes metronidazole and its metabolites. Patients with hepatic dysfunction, even in the absence of renal disease, probably require dosage modification. However, no good guidelines are currently available.

## ADVERSE REACTIONS

Most adverse reactions to metronidazole are minor and self-limited.[128] They include gastrointestinal complaints (nausea, abdominal pain, rarely vomiting or diarrhea), metallic or bitter taste, ataxia, vertigo, headaches, drowsiness, and depression. Metronidazole should be used cautiously in patients with a history of seizures or other central nervous system disorders. Urticaria and pruritis occur infrequently. Peripheral neuropathy has been reported in patients on long-term high-dose therapy. This effect is reversible upon discontinuation of the drug, although sensory changes have persisted in a few patients for months. Vaginal and urethral burning may occur. The urine can be colored a reddish brown from excretion of an azo metabolite. Occasionally *Candida* and *C. difficile* superinfections have been noted. However, pseudomembranous colitis is rare as the drug has been shown to be effective therapy for this condition. A transient reversible neutropenia has also been reported in a few cases.

The two most concerning and controversial problems with the 5-nitroimidazoles are mutagenicity and carcinogenicity.[129,130]

### Mutagenicity

Metronidazole increases the mutation rate in bacterial chromosomes in vitro. The development of mutant colonies of *Salmonella typhimurium* (Ames test) after exposure to urine from patients treated with a 10-day course of 750 mg metronidazole has gained attention because of a proposed correlation between *S. typhi* mutagenicity and carcinogenicity in animals.[131] However, if a nitroreductase minus mutant of *S. typhimurium* is used, metronidazole has no mutagenic activity, suggesting that the reduction product(s) and not the parent compound are responsible for mutagenicity. It appears that protozoa, anaerobic bacteria, some capnophilic bacteria, facultative anaerobes, and fungi are capable of reducing metronidazole to its mutagenic derivatives. Eukaryotic organisms have little nitroreductase activity, thereby minimizing the quantity of reduction product(s) formed. Thus, the Ames test cannot be extrapolated to a mammalian system. Additionally, there are no human data corroborating these results.

Evaluation of 1469 pregnancies in women who received metronidazole, of which 206 were in their first trimester, demonstrated no increase in the number of abortions, malformations, or stillbirths as compared with women not taking the drug.[132] Studies evaluating the effect of metronidazole on chromosome aberrations in humans have produced conflicting results.[133] but from these data it is difficult to suggest a mutagenic effect for metronidazole in humans. Additional studies are necessary to evaluate the potential teratogenicity of metronidazole in humans. At present, metronidazole should be avoided during pregnancy, especially during the first trimester.

### Carcinogenicity

A carcinogenic potential for metronidazole was noted when Rustia and Shubik demonstrated increased adenocarcinomas of the lung and malignant lymphomas in mice fed a powdered diet containing 0.06 to 0.05 percent of the bulk as metronidazole.[134] The survival rate, however, was not different between the control and treated groups. An increase in hepatocarcinomas, mammary tumors, and other neoplasms has also been reported in rats. Studies in hamsters, however, have been negative. Two small studies in humans have not found a significant increase in cancers among women given the drug with the exception of uterine cancer.[135,136] However, women with trichomonas infections have a higher incidence of uterine cancer than women without trichomoniasis regardless of whether they ingest metronidazole. When this is taken into consideration, no increase in cancers of any type has been associated with metronidazole.

## DRUG INTERACTIONS

Some patients who ingest ethanol while taking metronidazole experience a "disulfiram reaction." Symptoms include nausea, flushing, palpitations, and tachycardia. This reaction is caused by inhibition of the metabolism of ethanol and acetaldehyde by metronidazole. Patients given metronidazole should avoid alcohol during and for 1 day after its use.

Metronidazole enhances the hypoprothrombinemic effect of the racemic mixture of warfarin.[137] This interaction is stereospecific for the more potent S(-) entantiomorph. Inhibition of warfarin metabolism is thought to be the mechanism. Patients on warfarin therapy who are receiving multiple doses of metronidazole may need to have their anticoagulant dose reduced.

## QUINOLONES

### INDICATIONS

The quinolones are promising new drugs that may be useful alternatives in the treatment of some sexually transmitted infections. Specifically, *N. gonorrhoeae* (including penicillinase producers), enteric pathogens such as *Salmonella* spp., *Shigella* spp., and *Campylobacter* sp., and *Gardnerella vaginalis* are very susceptible to the fluoroquinolones (usually with MICs of less than 1 μg/ml). Both norfloxacin and ciprofloxacin given as single oral doses successfully cure > 95 percent of penicillin-resistant and penicillin-sensitive gonococcal strains.[138] Although earlier reports suggested that norfloxacin and ciprofloxacin had in vitro activity against *C. trachomatis*, clinical findings in the treatment of chlamydial urethritis using these compounds have been inconsistent.[139,140] Many strains of *S. saprophyticus* are inhibited in vitro by the quinolones, but anaerobic organisms and most streptococci are not. Data are lacking on the activity of quinolones against *T. pallidum*. Only two quinolones, norfloxacin and ciprofloxacin, are currently approved for use in the United States. Several others are in clinical trials, including ofloxacin, enoxacin, and pefloxacin, and preliminary studies suggest that some of these compounds will be effective against *C. trachomatis* infections.

### MODE OF ACTION

The antibacterial activity of the quinolones results from inhibition of bacterial DNA gyrase,[141] an enzyme consisting of A and B subunits, which controls supercoiling of DNA. The A subunits produce single-strand incisions on the bacterial chromosome and then reseal the chromosome after supercoiling; subsequently the B subunits introduce negative superhelical twists by an energy-dependent process. Bactericidal activity appears to involve inhibition of the resealing process. The single-stranded DNA is left exposed with ultimate degradation of chromosomal DNA. The resulting disruption of cellular metabolism may lead to (1) premature cell division; (2) delayed cell division; or (3) complete failure of cell division and ultimate cell lysis. Other postulated mechanisms of action include prevention of DNA gyrase binding to the DNA molecule and mutation of the DNA gyrase B subunit.

### MECHANISMS OF RESISTANCE

The exact mechanisms of resistance to fluoroquinolones have not been elucidated. One likely mechanism is mutation of bacterial DNA gyrase, resulting in a change in the target site of the antibiotic.[141] Mutations in the A subunit result in high-level resistance. Subunit B mutation appears to confer low-level resistance and correlates with permeability of the bacteria to nalidixic acid. Development of single-step, high-level resistance as was seen with nalidixic acid has not been observed with the newer fluoroquinolones. Although resistance to nalidixic acid can be associated with modest cross-resistance to other quinolones, this is of little clinical significance since the new derivatives have much greater activity.

### SPECTRUM OF ACTIVITY

All of the newer quinolones are manyfold more active than nalidixic acid and related compounds such as cinoxacin and oxolinic acid against most enteric gram-negative bacilli. In general, ciprofloxacin has greater activity than norfloxacin. The quinolones are bactericidal; MBC values are only slightly higher than MIC values for most organisms. Inoculum size does not significantly influence sensitivity patterns, although a pH effect has been observed. Most quinolones lose substantial activity at a pH below 5.5; optimal activity occurs between pH 7.5 and 8.[142]

### BIOPHARMACEUTICS AND PHARMACOKINETICS

#### Absorption

Table 83-8 summarizes the pharmacokinetic properties of the fluoroquinolones. Following oral administration, maximum serum concentrations of most quinolones occur between 1 and 2 h. Peak concentrations following single oral doses of norfloxacin (400 mg) range from 1.3 to 1.6 μg/ml.[143] Higher doses were not found to consistently produce proportionally higher serum levels; delayed absorption appears to explain this phenomenon. Accumulation of norfloxacin following multiple oral doses does not occur. Following 250, 500, and 750 mg oral ciprofloxacin doses, mean peak levels range from 1.0 to 1.5, 1.5 to 3.0, and 3.5 to 4.0 μg/ml, respectively.[144] Oral bioavailability for both agents is

**Table 83-8. Biopharmaceutic and Pharmacokinetic Data on Various Fluoroquinolones**

| Quinolone | Half-life, h: Normal | Half-life, h: Renal failure | Total peak serum concentrations, μg/ml | Protein binding, % | Major route of elimination (minor route) |
|---|---|---|---|---|---|
| Norfloxacin | 2–4 | 6–7 | 1–2 (400 mg PO) | 14 | Renal |
| Ciprofloxacin | 4–5 | 8–12 | 1.3–1.4 (250 mg PO) | 30–40 | Renal |
| | | | 2.6–2.9 (500 mg PO) | | |
| | | | 3.4–4.2 (750 mg PO) | | |
| Ofloxacin | 6–7 | 20–50 | 10–12 (600 mg PO) | 6 | Renal |
| Enoxacin | 6–7 | 15–30 | 3–4 (600 mg PO) | 32–38 | Renal |
| Pefloxacin | 10–12 | NA | 6 (400 mg PO) | 20–30 | Hepatic (renal) |

SOURCE: Compiled from Refs. 143–148, 158–160.

estimated to be approximately 70 percent. Absorption is delayed by food and antacids, and thus it is advised that these antibiotics be taken at least 1 or 2 h before or after meals or antacids. Antacids also appear to decrease the extent of absorption.

Linear relationships between serum concentrations and dose have been observed following oral ofloxacin in doses from 100 to 600 mg.[145,146] Mean peak levels following single 200-, 400-, and 600-mg doses were approximately 2.6, 5.0, and 6.8 μg/ml, respectively. Some degree of accumulation is observed with the higher dose (600 mg twice daily). Unlike norfloxacin and ciprofloxacin, food had little influence on ofloxacin absorption. In a comparative pharmacokinetic study, ofloxacin achieved higher maximum concentrations (2.3 μg/ml) compared with ciprofloxacin (1.1 μg/ml) and norfloxacin (0.8 μg/ml) when each was given as a single 200-mg dose.[147]

### Distribution

All of the fluoroquinolones are distributed widely in body fluids. Protein binding to albumin is low for norfloxacin, ciprofloxacin, and ofloxacin at 14, 30, and 20 percent, respectively. Norfloxacin has been detected in tonsillar tissue, maxillary sinus mucosa, vaginal tissue, cervix tissue, salpinges, ovaries, renal cortex, and the gallbladder wall at concentrations about that achieved in serum.[148] Concentrations higher than those achieved in serum have been reported in both common duct and gallbladder bile, liver tissue, and renal medulla. Little drug was detected in amniotic fluid and umbilical serum, with no detectable drug in breast milk. A significant amount of drug (28 percent) appears in the feces.

Ciprofloxacin is concentrated in the bile and prostate.[149,150] Therapeutic concentrations are found in female pelvic tissue, sputum, bone, and peritoneal fluid.[151–154] Following 200 mg IV q 12 h for 3 doses, a CSF level of 0.8 μg/ml was measured.[155] It is unknown if ciprofloxacin penetrates into breast milk.

Ofloxacin tissue concentrations exceeded serum levels in the lung, gallbladder, and bile and were at least equivalent to serum in the prostate, genitourinary tract, lacrimal fluid, and saliva, and lower than serum in sputum.[156] Umbilical cord serum and amniotic fluid concentrations were bactericidal in 11 pregnant women. Concentrations in breast milk measured 0.4 to 2.0 μg/ml in 6 women several days following delivery.[157]

## METABOLISM AND EXCRETION

Six metabolites of norfloxacin have been identified; less than 10 percent of a given dose appears in the urine.[148] Ciprofloxacin has been shown to have four urinary metabolites of varying activity (30 to 40 percent). At least two metabolites of ofloxacin appear in the urine; 3.5 percent of the dose as desmethylofloxacin and minute amounts of ofloxacin *N*-oxide.[156]

The fluoroquinolones have relatively long serum half-lives, 3 to 4 h for norfloxacin and ciprofloxacin, 6 to 7 h for ofloxacin and enoxacin and 10 to 11 h for pefloxacin.[143–145] Percent of drug eliminated unchanged in the urine by 24 h is approximately 27, 30, and 73 percent for norfloxacin, ciprofloxacin, and ofloxacin, respectively. Renal clearance of norfloxacin, ciprofloxacin, and ofloxacin exceeds glomerular filtration, thus implying tubular secretion. This has been confirmed by the fact that probenecid reduces urinary recovery of these drugs. In patients with moderate impairment of liver function, norfloxacin's pharmacokinetics were not found to be impaired.

The serum half-life of norfloxacin and ciprofloxacin are moderately reduced in patients with serum creatinine clearance between 30 and 80 mg/min. With advanced renal dysfunction, elimination half-life increased to 6.5 and 8.6 for norfloxacin and ciprofloxacin, respectively.[158,159] Hemodialysis does not appear to significantly effect the pharmacokinetics of norfloxacin and ciprofloxacin.[158,159] Ofloxacin's half-life has been reported to increase to 37 h when the glomerular filtration rate was $< 5$ ml/min.[160] Renal clearance is directly correlated with creatinine clearance. In patients on continuous ambulatory peritoneal dialysis (CAPD) with peritonitis, half-life was only mildly altered.[161] Hemodialysis also failed to alter ofloxacin's elimination half-life.[160]

## ADVERSE REACTIONS

Prolonged use of nalidixic acid and early quinolone derivatives such as oxolinic acid and cinoxacin were associated with frequent and severe reactions involving many organ systems, including the central nervous system (pseudotumor cerebri) and ophthalmologic toxicities. Photosensitivity, previously associated with nalidixic acid, has not occurred with these newer agents. The newer fluoroquinolones do not appear to cause significant side effects. When reactions do occur, drug discontinuation is rarely necessary.

In over 1200 patients treated with norfloxacin 800 mg orally per day, side effects were reported in less than 5 percent.[148] Gastrointestinal disorders accounted for the majority of side effects (2 to 4 percent), with nausea and vomiting seen most frequently. Headache, lightheadness, and drowsiness were the most common neurologic effects. Dermatologic side effects, mainly skin rashes, were rarely observed (0.3 percent). Less frequent side effects included abdominal pain, diarrhea, anorexia, drowsiness, insomnia, joint swelling, and tendonitis. Several patients reported a "bitter or metallic" aftertaste. Abnormal laboratory values have been reported infrequently (0.01 percent); most often mild elevations in liver transaminases have been noted.[148] Crystalluria has been reported in patients receiving high doses (1200 to 1600 g per day). This reaction has not been observed with standard treatment doses.

In worldwide trials, ciprofloxacin has had an overall incidence of adverse experiences of 6.4 percent.[162] Similar to norfloxacin, gastrointestinal disturbances were most frequently reported. Transient elevations in liver enzymes have been observed. Ophthalmologic examinations performed prior to and following therapy revealed no significant changes.

Ofloxacin's incidence of side effects appears to be very low (3.3 percent) among 1600 patients treated in phases II to IV trials.[156] Gastrointestinal symptoms were seen in 2.6 percent, followed by central nervous system reactions at 0.9 percent and hypersensitivity reactions of 0.5 percent. Most of the reported events occurred within 3 days of drug initiation. More recent experience among at least 1.5 million treated patients revealed that neurologic side effects were the most prevalent reactions, including headache, insomnia, or restlessness.[156] Hallucinations or psychotic reactions were occasionally observed in elderly patients with high fever. Significant changes in laboratory indices have not been observed.

Although degeneration of cartilage was observed in young animals treated with nalidixic acid, there are few clinical data to indicate development of cartilage erosions in adults or in young children who have received the new fluoroquinolones. Transient reports of arthralgia have appeared in the literature mainly in older children and adults. However, at this time, the newer quinolones should not be used in the treatment of sexually transmitted diseases in children or in pregnant females. Their use in nursing mothers is debatable; further studies regarding excretion into breast milk are needed.

## DRUG INTERACTIONS

The most significant interaction reported to date with the newer quinolones is interference with theophylline metabolism. Wijnands and colleagues in 1984 noted nausea and vomiting associated with significantly increased theophylline serum concentrations in 8 of 10 patients also receiving enoxacin (600 mg bid).[163] The mechanism of this effect appears to be inhibition of theophylline metabolism at the cytochrome P-450 site. In a comparative interaction study with normal volunteers, enoxacin and ciprofloxacin were found to decrease theophylline clearance by 64 and 30 percent, respectively.[164] The 4-oxo metabolite has been hypothesized to be responsible for the reduced theophylline clearance; enoxacin is more extensively metabolized to the 4-oxo metabolite than ciprofloxacin. In the same study, ofloxacin was not found to alter the pharmacokinetics of theophylline. Other studies have confirmed that ofloxacin does not share this drug interaction.[165] More recently, norfloxacin has been observed to interact with theophylline derivatives, although the clinical significance is uncertain.[166,167]

Antacids containing aluminum and magnesium cations significantly decrease the absorption of the quinolone antibiotics. This reaction is a direct result of chelation. Gastrointestinal absorption of ofloxacin was decreased in 7 healthy volunteers receiving concurrent aluminum hydroxide gel.[168] Peak serum concentrations and AUC were reduced from 1.4 to 0.5 μg/ml and 5.4 to 2.2 mg/l h, respectively. Thus, in patients receiving antacids (containing these cations) and requiring antibacterial therapy, the quinolones may prove less effective. The patient should be instructed to take antacids 1 h prior to or 2 h following quinolone administration.

## PROBENECID

### INDICATIONS

Probenecid in combination with the penicillins increases the serum concentrations of the latter and is utilized in the treatment of gonorrhea. This drug is primarily a uricosuric used in the treatment of hyperuricemia and gout.[169]

### MODE OF ACTION

Probenecid inhibits the renal tubular secretion of the penicillins and cephalosporins, resulting in higher serum concentrations and longer half-lives of the antibiotics. It can also increase the amount of free drug by displacing these compounds from protein-binding sites, and it interferes with the active organic anion pump in the choroid plexus and the ciliary body, thereby increasing cerebrospinal fluid levels and eye concentrations of the antibiotics.

### BIOPHARMACEUTICS AND PHARMACOKINETICS

Probenecid is well absorbed orally. About 90 percent of the drug is protein-bound. Probenecid is eliminated mainly via metabolism to both active and inactive metabolites. Both the parent compound and metabolites are eliminated by the kidneys. The elimination half-life of the parent compound is 6 to 12 h.[169]

The serum concentrations of penicillin G are approximately doubled with concomitant administration of probenecid. The extent to which the other penicillins, cephalosporins, and quinolones are affected depends upon their degree of renal elimination.

### ADVERSE REACTIONS

The side effects of probenecid in patients who do not have hyperuricemia or gout are minor. They include gastrointestinal complaints in 8 to 18 percent of patients and hypersensitivity reactions in about 5 percent.[169] Anaphylactoid reactions have been reported in a few cases.[170] Because of the very short-term administration of probenecid in venereology, the risk of urate stone formation or the precipitation of gouty arthritis in patients with hyperuricemia or gout is unlikely to occur. Probenecid can increase the toxicity of the penicillins and cephalosporins if high doses of the antibiotics are used or if patients have renal insufficiency.

## ANTIVIRAL DRUGS

### ACYCLOVIR

#### Indications

Acyclovir [9-(2-hydroxyethoxymethyl)guanine] is a purine nucleoside analogue with greatest activity against herpes simplex virus types 1 and 2 (HSV-1 and HSV-2). Therapeutic efficacy of oral acyclovir in the treatment of primary genital HSV infections and in suppression of recurrent infections is well established.[171–173] Topical preparations are not as efficacious.

#### Mode of Action

Acyclovir exerts its effect through inhibition of viral DNA synthesis. It is first metabolized intracellularly to a monophosphate derivative by virus-coded thymidine kinase and subsequently phosphorylated to the di- and triphosphate derivatives by cellular enzymes. The triphosphate compound inhibits viral DNA synthesis by acting as a competitive inhibitor and false substrate for the viral DNA-polymerase enzyme. Since acyclovir is preferentially taken up and converted to its active form by HSV-infected cells, it has a lower potential for toxicity in uninfected normal host cells.

#### Spectrum of activity

In vitro sensitivity tests for acyclovir are difficult to evaluate since viral susceptibility tests are not standardized. Acyclovir concentrations causing 50 percent reduction in plaque formation range from 0.02 to 0.2 μg/ml for HSV-1 and 0.2 to 0.4 μg/ml for HSV-2.[174] However, there may be tenfold variations in these data depending on whether the results are from dye-uptake or plaque-reduction methods.

## Mechanism of Resistance

Resistance of HSV to acyclovir has been demonstrated in tissue culture systems. The most common cause of resistance is the formation of mutants which are deficient in thymidine kinase, thereby preventing conversion of acyclovir to its active form. There may be a reduction in virulence in such mutants in mice and in humans.[175] A second, less common mechanism for resistance is alteration of the DNA polymerase locus. Finally, a third mechanism for resistance is altered substrate specificity of viral thymidine kinase such that the enzyme no longer recognizes acyclovir as the substrate. The clinical significance of the emergence of resistant viruses is controversial.

## Biopharmaceutics and Pharmacokinetics

Following oral administration, only 15 to 30 percent of acyclovir is bioavailable and this appears to decrease with increasing doses.[176] However, the concentrations achieved are well above the MICs for HSV-1 and HSV-2. Peak concentrations of about 0.6 and 0.9 μg/ml were reached between 1 and 4 h after oral 200- and 400-mg doses, respectively. Steady-state peak concentrations averaged 1.4 μg/ml (range 0.9 to 1.8) in adults receiving 200 mg orally five times per day.[177] Peak concentrations after a 1-h intravenous infusion of 2.5, 5.0, 10.0, and 15.0 mg/kg were 3.7 to 4.5, 8.3, 14.6, and 22.7 μg/ml, respectively. Plasma concentrations have been low (range $< 0.01$ to 0.3 μg/ml) in patients receiving topical acyclovir for herpes zoster.[178] Acyclovir penetrates the blood-brain barrier and achieves viricidal concentrations in the CSF.[179] Distribution of the drug into the saliva and vaginal fluid has been reported.[180]

The elimination half-life in patients with normal renal function ranges from 2.2 to 5.0 h. Since the majority of the drug is excreted unchanged in the urine, the half-life is longer in patients with renal insufficiency (19.5 h in anuric patients).[179] The renal clearance of acyclovir is about three times the creatinine clearance, which indicates that it is eliminated by glomerular filtration and tubular secretion. About 15 percent is excreted as 9-carboxymethoxymethylguanine or minor metabolites (8.5 to 14 percent over 14 h).[179]

## Adverse reactions

Adverse reactions to acyclovir are minimal and those which have been reported are mild and reversible in nature. Extravasation of the intravenous formulation results in irritation, pruritus, edema, and erythema. Reversible encephalopathic changes have been observed in approximately 1 percent of patients receiving intravenous medication and are characterized by lethargy, tremors, confusion, hallucinations, delirium, seizures, and coma.[181] Other reported adverse reactions include increased serum creatinine and liver transaminases, decreased white blood cell count, and gastrointestinal disturbances. Acyclovir may crystallize in the kidneys; therefore, patients should be kept well hydrated. Oral acyclovir is associated with less frequent side effects, most notably nausea and headache.

Topical acyclovir may cause transient burning when applied to genital lesions; this appears more common in female patients and during first episodes.[178]

Although acyclovir demonstrated some mutagenic activity in vitro, no effects were found in eukaryotic systems.[182,183] Furthermore, no significant immunosuppressive activity or teratogenicity has been observed in animal or humans.[184] Safety in the pregnant female has not been studied.

# ANTIVIRAL CHEMOTHERAPY FOR HUMAN IMMUNODEFICIENCY VIRUS

The complex biology of the human immunodeficiency virus (HIV), the fact that it infects a wide variety of cells and anatomic sites, and its ability to both latently and productively infect lymphocytes and neuronal cells present enormous challenges for any chemotherapeutic agent. Multiple strategies to inhibit HIV may be needed. This section focuses on current strategies to treat HIV infection and provides guidelines for the use of zidovudine, the only FDA-approved antiretroviral.

## Mode of action

The replicative ("life") cycle of HIV follows a set pattern of virus attachment, entry into the host cell, virus uncoating, viral replication, and virus assembly and release from the cell. Each step represents a potential target for antiviral attack (Fig. 83-1).

Inhibition of attachment or entry of HIV into a cell has theoretical appeal because such a strategy would prevent development both of latent and of productive infection. Attachment can be inhibited by human monoclonal antibodies directed against the cell receptors (T4 molecules) to which the virus attaches.[185,186] Compounds that block the cell receptor or alter the virus envelope glycoprotein by which the virus attaches to the cell receptor are undergoing clinical investigation.[187–189] Peptide T, a 10-amino-acid peptide, binds to a region on the T4 molecule and appears to prevent HIV from entering cells.[188] AL 7,2,1 is a combination of fatty acids which are taken up by infected cells and alter the composition of the virus envelope glycoprotein, resulting in inhibition of HIV replication in vitro.[190] Soluble $CD_4$ has been shown to bind strongly with viral protein gp120 and prevent syncytium formation in cell cultures.[189,191] A more familiar agent, dextran sulfate, has been shown in vitro to have an inhibitory effect on HIV and to prevent binding of HIV to T lymphocytes.[192,193] Pharmacokinetic and toxicity studies are under way in humans.

After attachment and entry, the next step that could be inhibited is the intracellular uncoating of the virus. No compounds that inhibit this viral process have yet entered clinical trials. However, several compounds have been developed that inhibit the subsequent processes in viral replications, which involve viral RNA and DNA replication. Reverse transcriptase is a viral enzyme that is essential to HIV replication but has no essential mammalian cell function. Inhibition of reverse transcriptase, therefore, acts selectively on retroviruses. Zidovudine (formerly known as azidothymidine or AZT) appears to be the prototype of compounds with this mechanism of action.[194,195]

Other potential targets for inhibiting HIV replication include viral integration into the host cell DNA, posttranscription processing of viral messenger RNA, and assembly and release of the virus. Several HIV gene products (tat-III and trs-art) enhance viral replication but not cellular DNA replication. Inhibitors of these gene products may decrease the number of infectious virions circulating in the body, but none have been developed to date. Finally, the antiretroviral effect of interferon appears to be on the release of HIV from infected cells.[196] Clinical trials of interferon as a single agent for HIV treatment have been disappointing thus far.

Antiviral combinations may be more effective than a single antiviral agent alone, especially if the drugs have different mechanisms of action and appear additive or synergistic in vitro and/ or in animal models. Combination chemotherapy with antiviral

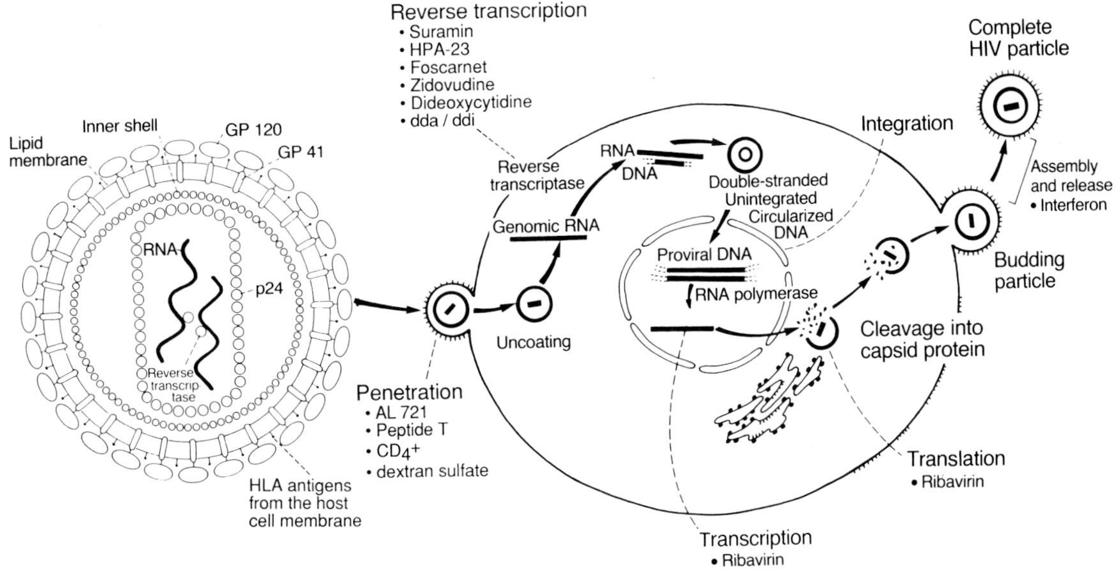


**Fig. 83-1.** Schematic diagram of possible sites of action of antiviral agents against the human immunodeficiency virus type III. (*Adapted and reproduced with permission from* Clinical Pharmacy *6:927, 1987.*)

agents and immune modulators (e.g., interferon, interleukin-2) also has been proposed.

## SELECTED ANTI-HIV AGENTS

The most extensively tested of the antiviral compounds that inhibit HIV in vitro are summarized in Table 83-9. In nearly all in vitro systems tested, HIV replication resumes when the antiviral drug is removed from HIV-infected cells, indicating that the drugs inhibit productive viral replication but don't cure the cell of latently infected provirus. This implies that chronic administration of these drugs will be required. Because HIV is usually present in the central nervous system in most infected persons, antiviral drugs for HIV infection must be able to cross the blood-brain barrier.

## SURAMIN

Suramin, an agent used to treat East African trypanosomiasis and onchocerciasis, was the first drug reported to have in vitro activity

**Table 83-9. In Vitro Inhibition of HIV**

| Agent | Anti-HIV concentration | Achievable serum level | Action |
|---|---|---|---|
| Suramin[197] | Suppress 50 μg/ml, inhibit 100–1000 μg/ml | > 100 μg/ml with 1 g IV dose | RT inhibition* |
| Ribavirin[209] | Suppress 10–100 μg/ml | 1–3 μg/ml | RT inhibition |
| HPA-23[207] | $ID_{50}$† 30 μg/ml | — | RT inhibition |
| Foscarnet[214] | Suppress 132 μM, inhibit 680 μM | 100–450 μM | RT inhibition |
| Zidovudine[219,220] | < 0.13–2.7 μg/ml | 0.5–3 μg/ml | RT inhibition; DNA chain termination |
| AL721[190] | $ED_{50}$‡ 100 μg/ml<br>$ED_{90}$§ 1000 μg/ml | — | Alteration of viral envelope |
| Dideoxycytidine[225] | 0.1–0.5 μg/ml | 0.02–0.4 μg/ml | RT inhibition; DNA chain termination |

*RT = reverse transcriptase.
†$ID_{50}$ = median infective dose, being that amount of pathogenic microorganisms which will produce infection in 50 percent of test subjects.
‡$ED_{50}$ = median effective dose, a dose that produces effects in 50 percent of a population.
§$ED_{90}$ = median effective dose, the dose that produces effects in 90 percent of the population.
SOURCE: Reproduced with permission; Tartaglione TA, Collier AC: Development of antiviral agents for the treatment of human immunodeficiency virus infection. *Clin Pharm* 6:927, 1987.

**Table 83-10. Pharmacokinetic Properties of Several Anti-HIV Agents**

| Agent | Dose (route) | Peak serum concentration | Bioavailability | Elimination half-life normal renal function | Mode of elimination | CSF penetration |
|---|---|---|---|---|---|---|
| Suramin[202] | 1 g (IV) | > 100 μg/ml | Poor | 44–54 days | Renal | Minimal |
| Ribavirin[211] | 600–2400 mg (IV)<br>600–2400 mg (PO) | 10–40 μg/ml<br>1–3 μg/ml | 10% | 2 h (beta)<br>36 h (gamma) | Extensively metabolized | Yes |
| HPA-23[208] | 1–3.3 mg/kg (IV) | — | Poor | 2–3 h | Renal (15–50%) | Unknown |
| Foscarnet[216] | 20 mg/kg/24 h (IV) | 250–500 μM | Poor | 6 h | Renal | Yes |
| Zidovudine[203,221] | 200–250 mg q 4 h (IV)<br>200–250 mg q 4 h (PO) | 1.5–3.0 μg/ml<br>1–2 μg/ml | 70% | 1.1 h | Hepatic (75%) | Yes |
| ddC[226] | 0.03 mg/kg (IV)<br>0.25 mg/kg (IV) | 0.02–0.06 μg/ml<br>0.2–0.4 μg/ml | 30–80% | 1.0 h | Renal | Yes |

SOURCE: Reproduced with permission; Tartaglione TA, Collier AC: Development of antiviral agents for the treatment of human immunodeficiency virus infection. *Clin Pharm* 6:927, 1987.

against HIV through reverse transcriptase inhibition.[197,198] The main pharmacokinetic properties of suramin are summarized in Table 83-10.

Clinical trials of suramin for HIV treatment were undertaken in early 1984. Although isolation of HIV from peripheral blood lymphocytes was transiently decreased[199–201] on therapy, side effects were frequent and severe and included adrenal insufficiency in 23 percent of treated patients. As there was not clinical or immunologic improvement or reduction in the frequency of opportunistic infections,[202–206] suramin, as currently administered, cannot be recommended as effective therapy for HIV infection.

## HPA-23

Ammonium 21-tungsto-9 antimoniate (HPA-23) inhibits reverse transcriptase in vitro at concentrations of approximately 30 μg/ml.[207] However, despite phase I trials initiated 2 years ago, little is known about its potential antiviral effects or its pharmacology. The drug is poorly absorbed orally, elimination half-life is short (2 to 3 h), and its penetration into the cerebrospinal fluid is unknown (Table 83-10).[208]

In France, 47 patients have received intravenous doses of HPA-23 ranging from 50 to 200 mg per day, with some evidence of in vivo inhibition of HIV replication. However, 33 of the 47 developed thrombocytopenia and many had hepatic transaminase elevations. Little observable clinical improvement was noted. These limited data suggest HPA-23 is fairly toxic and lacks dramatic antiviral effects.

## RIBAVIRIN

Ribavirin is a synthetic purine nucleoside that is active in vitro against a broad spectrum of DNA and RNA viruses, including HIV. Ribavirin's mechanism of action is not completely understood, though it is a competitive inhibitor of reverse transcriptase and interferes with viral mRNA synthesis.[209,210] Pharmacokinetic parameters can be found in Table 83-10.[211]

Trials of systemic ribavirin in HIV infection were initiated in early 1985. Men with HIV infections tolerated ribavirin well; a reversible reduction in hemoglobin was its major toxic effect. In a controlled trial involving 163 patients with generalized lymphadenopathy, 107 patients received either 600 or 800 mg of ribavirin orally once per day, and 56 received placebo. Initial reports indicated that 18 percent of placebo recipients progressed to AIDS, versus 11 percent of the recipients of 600 mg of ribavirin and none of the recipients of 800 mg.[212] However, it appears that the placebo and 600-mg groups had a lower number of circulating T4 cells prior to entry, a parameter known to markedly affect the rate of progression to AIDS. When data were stratified by T4 count, there was no evidence that ribavirin decreased progression of disease in patients with HIV-associated lymphadenopathy. A similar trial in patients with ARC showed no significant short-term benefit of ribavirin.[213]

## PHOSPHONOFORMATE

Trisodium phosphonoformate hexahydrate (PFA, foscarnet) was first synthesized in 1924 and is structurally related to pyrophosphate. PFA inhibits a wide range of DNA and RNA polymerases, including those of all herpes viruses (herpes simplex virus, cytomegalovirus, Epstein-Barr virus, and varicella zoster virus), hepatitis B virus, and HIV.[214] Specifically, PFA appears to interact with nucleic acid polymerases at the site where pyrophosphate is released during elongation of the DNA or RNA chain.[215] PFA inhibits HIV reverse transcriptase at concentrations (approximately 1 μM of PFA) that do not affect cell DNA synthesis.[214]

PFA is currently available only as an intravenous product. It has been tested in humans most extensively as a topical drug for herpes simplex virus infections and as intravenous therapy in immunosuppressed patients with severe cytomegalovirus infection. In the latter studies, a dosage of 20 mg/kg/24 h was administered as a continuous infusion. An estimated serum elimination half-life of 6 h should permit intermittent dosing.[216] PFA appears to penetrate into the cerebrospinal fluid in patients with and without meningeal inflammation (Table 83-10).

Pilot studies with PFA in patients with AIDS and ARC are under way in both the United States and Europe. Preliminary results indicate some clinical improvement, return of delayed-type hypersensitivity, and negative cultures for the virus during therapy in several patients.[217,218] Clinical trials with PFA administered daily as an intermittent intravenous infusion started in the United States in late 1988.

## ZIDOVUDINE (ZDV, AZIDOTHYMIDINE OR AZT)

### Indications

The Food and Drug Administration (FDA) approved ZDV in March 1987 for management of adult patients with AIDS and advanced ARC who have a history of *Pneumocystis carinii* pneumonia or an absolute T4 lymphocyte count of less than 200/mm$^3$ in their peripheral blood. The recommended starting dose is 200 mg orally every 4 h around the clock, with dosage adjustment frequently required during the course of therapy as dictated by toxicity.

## Mode of action

Zidovudine (ZDV) is a clinically effective inhibitor of HIV reverse transcriptase and is marketed under the name Retrovir. ZDV is a thymidine analogue in which the 3' hydroxy (-OH) group is replaced by an azido ($NH_3$) group. At concentrations of 0.13 μg/ml or less, ZDV inhibits 90 percent of detectable HIV replication in vitro.[219,220] In vivo, ZDV is converted by cellular enzymes to a triphosphate form (ZDV-TP) that is subsequently utilized by HIV reverse transcriptase (Fig. 83-2). When ZDV-TP is incorporated into the growing DNA chain of HIV, the DNA chain is terminated.

## Biopharmaceutics and pharmacokinetics

A series of pharmacokinetic studies of oral ZDV showed that serum concentrations averaged 0.62 μg/ml (range 0.05 to 1.46 μg/ml) following chronic oral administration of 250 mg (3 to 5.4 mg/kg) every 4 h.[221] Following oral administration, ZDV bioavailability is approximately 70 percent due to drug metabolism in its first pass through the liver (Table 83-10). Plasma protein binding is 24 to 38 percent. ZDV's mean terminal half-life is approximately 1.1 h. Renal clearance of ZDV is estimated to be 400 ml/min/70 kg, approximately 20 percent of total body clearance. The 5'-glucuronide conjugate of ZDV (glucuronyl-ZDV) is a major inactive plasma and urinary metabolite. Glucuronyl-ZDV is rapidly cleared from plasma with a half-life of approximately 1 h. Accumulation of G-ZDV has been noted in end-stage renal disease,[222] but the clinical significance of this observation is uncertain. The cerebrospinal fluid/plasma concentration ratio was 0.15 in one patient 1.8 h following a 2 mg/kg oral dose.[210] Two to four hours after a 5 mg/kg intravenous dose, the ratio was 0.64. Unpublished data from the University of Washington revealed that viricidal CSF concentrations were not achieved in the majority of persons with AIDS ($n$ = 26) receiving chronic oral ZDV from 600 to 1200 mg per day.

## Adverse reactions

ZDV has been associated with serious side effects. Granulocytopenia and anemia necessitated dose reduction or drug discontinuation in 49 of the 143 (34 percent) patients in a phase III study.[223] Blood transfusions were required for 31 percent of the patients receiving ZDV and for 11 percent of those on placebo. In general, decreases in hemoglobin and neutrophils occurred during the second month of therapy and appeared to be reversible if the dose was decreased or the drug discontinued. Other side effects reported with ZDV include rashes, pruritus, nausea, headache, mild confusion, and other neurotoxicities.[224] Complaints of headache or confusion may precede severe neurotoxicity and should be monitored closely.

Hematologic parameters should be carefully monitored at least every 2 weeks; reductions in hemoglobin may occur as early as 2 to 4 weeks, whereas granulocytopenia often is not observed until weeks 6 to 8. Patients whose hemoglobin concentration drops to $< 7.5$ g/dl should have ZDV discontinued until the hemoglobin value is at least 9.5 g/dl. We recommend that patients

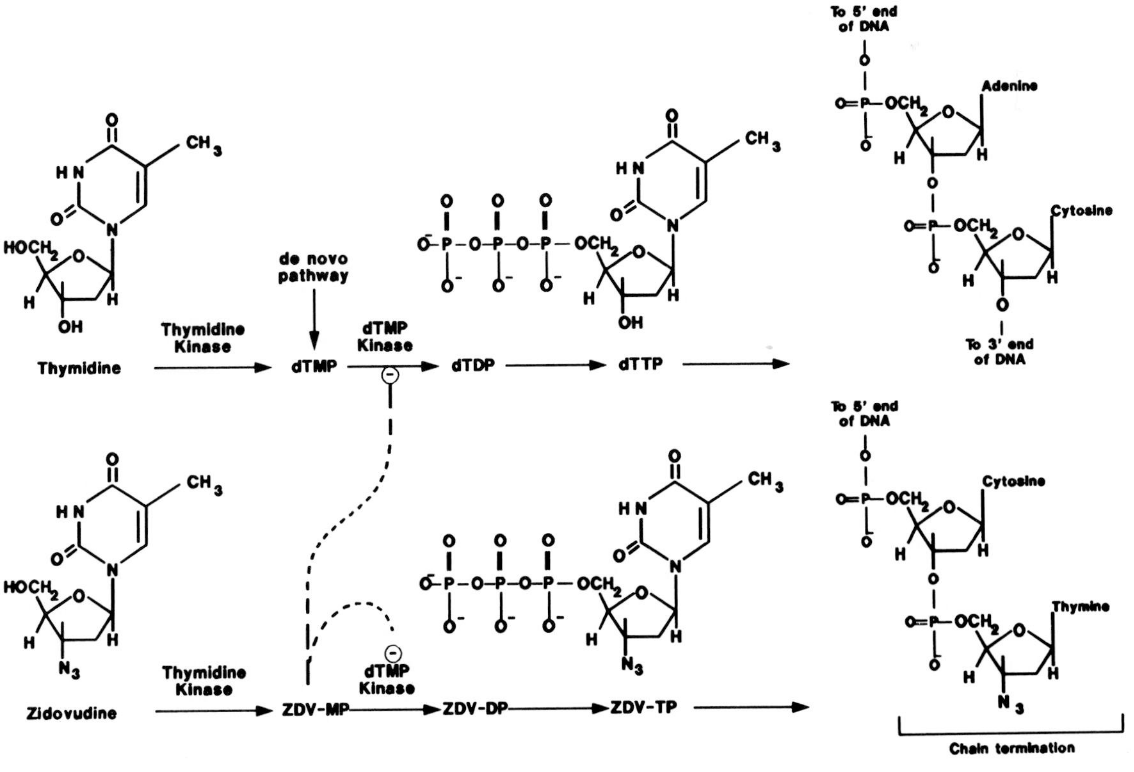

Fig. 83-2. Intracellular metabolism of zidovudine and thymidine and postulated mechanism of inhibition of HIV replication by dideoxynucleoside triphosphates. (*Reproduced with permission from* The New England Journal of Medicine, *316:557, 1987.*)

not be transfused at this time unless their cardiovascular status is compromised or their hemoglobin concentration fails to improve by at least 1 g/dl within 7 days of ZDV discontinuation. If transfusion is performed, ZDV may be restarted in 7 days if the hemoglobin concentration has stabilized. In either case, ZDV should be restarted at half the initial dose (for example, 100 mg q 4 h). If a patient continues to exhibit low or falling hemoglobin concentrations, we currently continue the medication if transfusion requirements are less than four units every 21 days or if the hemoglobin concentration does not fall below 6.5 g/dl on two consecutive episodes at least 1 week apart despite blood transfusions. If persistent life-threatening anemia develops (Hgb < 6.5 g/dl), we discontinue ZDV permanently. This occurs in 10 to 20 percent of persons. For other severe ZDV-induced toxicities, including granulocytopenia (white blood count 500 to 750/mm$^3$), we discontinue ZDV until baseline values return. ZDV is then restarted at 100 mg q 4 h. If severe toxicity resumes, we recommend discontinuing ZDV permanently.

### Drug interactions

Limited information is available regarding the interaction of other drugs with ZDV. Coadministration of ZDV with agents that produce hematologic, nephrotoxic, or cytotoxic effects (e.g., dapsone, pentamidine, amphoteracin B, flucytosine, vincristine, vinblastine, adriamycin, interferon) may potentiate the risk of toxicity. To date, only probenecid has been shown to increase ZDV blood levels. Acetaminophen, rifampin, cimetidine, ranitidine, flurazepam, indomethacin, probenecid, and other drugs which may competitively inhibit glucouronidation should be avoided. Acetaminophen used concomitantly with ZDV originally was thought to enhance the risk of marrow suppression; however, reanalysis refuted this observation.[223] Because of uncertainties regarding drug interactions, it is recommended that persons with AIDS receiving many chronic medications be followed at regional centers or by specialists experienced with the clinical presentations of AIDS and the complications of ZDV therapy. Additionally, ZDV and ribavirin have been shown to be antagonistic in vitro (see below).

## DIDEOXYCYTIDINE

2', 3'-Dideoxycytidine (ddC) is another nucleoside analogue similar in structure to ZDV which in some in vitro systems appears to be a more potent inhibitor of the replication and cytopathic effect of HIV than ZDV. Dideoxycytidine is currently under clinical investigation. Concentrations ranging from 0.5 (1.0 μg/ml) to 2 μM (0.425 μg/ml) of ddC have been shown to inhibit HIV growth and to prevent the expression of the p24 core protein in T-cell lines with ddC.[225] Preliminary data from a phase I trial demonstrated plasma concentrations of 0.1 to 0.3 μM and 1 to 2 μM following a single 1-h intravenous infusion of 0.03 mg/kg and 0.25 mg/kg, respectively (Table 83-10).[226] The elimination half-life of ddC is approximately 1 h. ddC appears to be completely absorbed in both fasting and nonfasting states. Of significance is ddC's ability to cross the blood-brain barrier.

Patients with AIDS or ARC are currently being enrolled in phase 1 clinical trials.[226] Transient increases in absolute T4 counts and reduction of p24 antigen have been observed. Side effects observed so far include painful peripheral neuropathy, rashes, fever, aphthous stomatitis, thrombocytopenia, LDH elevation, and anemia. The neuropathy appeared after 6 to 14 weeks of treatment and resolved several months after ddC discontinuation. A small number of patients have received ddC alternating weekly with zidovudine for a minimum of 6 months. Preliminary results indicate that this alternating regimen was better tolerated at the lower doses compared with ZDV alone. Furthermore, sustained elevations in T-cell counts have been observed.

## NEWER AGENTS

Several novel anti-HIV agents have recently been developed and are just entering clinical trials. These include ampligen, castanospermine, and phosphorothiate analogues of oligodeoxynucleosides. Ampligen is mismatched double-stranded RNA which in vitro protects lymphoblastoid cells from HIV infection; much of its effect might be as a potent interferon inducer.[227] Eleven patients with ARC or AIDS have received this drug in doses ranging from 200 to 250 mg twice weekly for 12 to 16 weeks with half the dose given subsequently as maintenance therapy.[228] Skin test anergy returned for all patients, and lymphadenopathy was resolved in three of five patients. Virologic changes, including reduction in p24 antigen, were observed in 9 of 11 patients. T4 cell numbers increased in three patients and were stable in the others. No patient showed side effects. One patient died following an episode of *Pneumocystis carinii* pneumonia after 7 weeks of ampligen therapy. Ampligen's future is uncertain, since the FDA recently deemed the drug ineffective.

Castanospermine exerts an anti-HIV effect by altering the env glycoprotein of HIV and decreasing gp120 production, thus altering the T4 molecule.[229] The drug appears to inhibit lymphocyte synctium formation by the virus and may therefore be useful in slowing the depletion of T4 cells, which is thought to be possibly attributable to synctium formation. Phosphate analogues of nucleosides inhibit HIV in vitro by preventing normal synthesis of viral DNA.[230] Preclinical testing of these analogues is now under way.

## COMBINATIONS OF ANTIRETROVIRALS: SYNERGISM AND ANTAGONISM

Several combinations of antivirals have demonstrated additive, synergistic, or antagonistic effects for inhibition of HIV. Studies suggest that combinations of drugs may have enhanced clinical efficacy and may inhibit HIV replication at concentrations that can be more easily achieved and are better tolerated in vivo. Additionally, such combinations may prevent selection of drug-resistant HIV mutants. Presently, however, there is no evidence correlating synergy in vitro with enhanced clinical outcome.

The interactions between ZDV and interferon and between ZDV and the antiviral acyclovir have stimulated interest in HIV combination therapy. In vitro, both these drugs enhance ZDV's inhibition of HIV.[231,232] The mechanism of acyclovir-ZDV synergism is unknown; however, because acyclovir is a well-tolerated drug with minimal hematologic toxicity, its use with ZDV appears encouraging. Alpha interferon prevents release of infectious viruses and, hence, inhibits HIV at a different stage in the viral replication process than ZDV. Additionally, suramin, ddC, lymphoblastoid interferon, and foscarnet have been found to be synergistic with ZDV in vitro.[233]

Not all antivirals are additive or synergistic. This fact is illustrated by the in vitro antagonistic effects between ZDV and ribavirin.[234] Ribavirin appears to increase deoxythymidine triphosphate levels which, in turn, cause feedback inhibition of thymidine kinase. This reduces phosphorylation of ZDV to ZDV-TP. These data also suggest ribavirin should not be used in vivo with ZDV or similar derivatives except under investigational conditions. The clinical importance of the in vitro antagonism of ZDV and ribivirin requires clarification. On a more positive note, ribavirin has been shown to be synergistic in vitro with PFA.[235]

## References


1 Hall WH et al: Comparative susceptibility of penicillinase-positive and -negative *Neisseria gonorrhoeae* to 30 antibiotics. *Antimicrob Agents Chemother* 15:562, 1979.

2 Piot P et al: Antibiotic susceptibility of *Neisseria gonorrhoeae* strains from Europe and Asia. *Antimicrob Agents Chemother* 15:535, 1979.

3 Vanhoof R et al: In-vitro activity of antimicrobial agents against *Neisseria gonorrhoeae* in Brussels. *Br J Vener Dis* 54:309, 1978.

4 Meheus A et al: Activity in vitro of ten antimicrobial agents against *Neisseria gonorrhoeae:* A study of the correlation between the sensitivities. *Br J Vener Dis* 52:329, 1976.

5 Thornsberry C et al: Patient variables associated with penicillin resistance in *Neisseria gonorrhoeae. Antimicrob Agents Chemother* 14:327, 1978.

6 Seth AD et al: Sensitivity of *Neisseria gonorrhoeae* to antibiotics in London (1976–78). *Br J Vener Dis* 55:325, 1979.

7 Platt DJ: Prevalence of multiple antibiotic resistance in *Neisseria gonorrhoeae. Br J Vener Dis* 52:384, 1976.

8 Miller JM et al: Inhibition of beta-lactamase in *Neisseria gonorrhoeae* by sodium clavulanate. *Antimicrob Agents Chemother* 14:794, 1978.

9 Kim J-H et al: Treatment of infections due to multiresistant *Neisseria gonorrhoeae* with sulbactam/ampicillin. *Rev Infect Dis* (suppl 5) 8:S599, 1986.

10 Eagle H et al: The effective concentrations of penicillin in vitro and in vivo from streptococci, pneumococci, and *Treponema pallidum. J Bacteriol* 59:625, 1950.

11 Idsoe O et al: Penicillin in the treatment of syphilis. *Bull WHO* 47(suppl):6, 1972.

12 Eisenstein BI: Effective treatment of gonorrhoea. *Drugs* 14:57, 1977.

13 Barbhaiyo R et al: Clinical pharmacological studies of amoxicillin: Effect of probenecid. *Br J Vener Dis* 55:211, 1979.

14 Rajan VS et al: Inactivation of gonococci by procaine penicillin in vivo. *Br J Vener Dis* 54:398, 1978.

15 Jaffe HW et al: Pharmacokinetic determinants of penicillin cure of gonococcal urethritis. *Antimicrob Agents Chemother* 15:587, 1979.

16 Mohr JA et al: Neurosyphilis and penicillin levels in cerebrospinal fluid. *JAMA* 236:2208, 1976.

17 Dunlop EMC et al: Penicillin levels in blood and CSF achieved by treatment of syphilis. *JAMA* 241:2538, 1979.

18 Barza M: Antimicrobial spectrum, pharmacology and therapeutic use of antibiotics: 2 Penicillins. *Am J Hosp Pharm* 34:57, 1977.

19 Bennett WM et al: Drug therapy in renal failure: Dosing guidelines for adults 1. Antimicrobial agents, analgesics. *Ann Intern Med* 93(part 1):62, 1980.

20 Rudolph AH, Price EV: Penicillin reactions among patients in venereal disease clinics: A national survey. *JAMA* 223:499, 1973.

21 Jaffe HW et al: National gonorrhea therapy monitoring study: Adverse drug reactions. *J Am Vener Dis Assoc* 3:29, 1976.

22 Fellner MJ: Penicillin allergy 1976: A review of reactions, detection and current management. *Int J Dermatol* 15:497, 1976.

23 Croydon EAP et al: Prospective study of ampicillin rash: Report of a collaborative study group. *Br Med J* 1:7, 1973.

24 Aronson IK, Soltani K: The enigma of the pathogenesis of the Jarisch-Herxheimer reaction. *Br J Vener Dis* 52:313, 1976.

25 Galpin JE et al: Pseudoanaphylactic reactions from inadvertent infusion of procaine penicillin G. *Ann Intern Med* 81:358, 1974.

26 Green RL et al: Elevated plasma procaine concentrations after administration of procaine penicillin G. *N Engl J Med* 291:223, 1974.

27 Downham II TF et al: Systemic toxic reactions to procaine penicillin G. *Sex Transm Dis* 5:4, 1978.

28 Handsfield HH et al: Dose-ranging study of ceftriaxone of uncomplicated gonorrhea in men. *Antimicrob Agents Chemother* 20:839, 1981.

29 Percival A et al: Penicillinase-producing gonococci in Liverpool. *Lancet* 2:1379, 1976.

30 Nightingale CH et al: Pharmacokinetics and clinical use of cephalosporin antibiotics. *J Pharm Sci* 64:1899, 1975.

31 Lode H et al: Comparative pharmacokinetics of cephalexin, cefaclor, cefadroxil, and CGP 9000. *Antimicrob Agents Chemother* 16:1, 1979.

32 Weistein L, Kaplan K: The cephalosporins: Microbiological, chemical, and pharmacological properties and use in chemotherapy of infection. *Ann Intern Med* 72:729, 1970.

33 Dash CH: Penicillin allergy and the cephalosporin. *J Antimicrob Chemother* 1(suppl):107, 1975.

34 Levine B: Antigenicity and cross-reactivity of penicillins and cephalosporins. *J Infect Dis* 128(suppl):S364, 1973.

35 Petz LD: Immunologic cross-reactivity between penicillins and cephalosporins: A review. *J Infect Dis* 137(suppl):74, 1978.

36 Barza M: The nephrotoxocity of cephalosporins: An overview. *J Infect Dis* 137(suppl):60, 1978.

37 Pasternack DP et al: Reversible nephrotoxicity associated with cephalothin therapy. *Arch Intern Med* 135:599, 1975.

38 Inagaki J, Bodey JP: Phlebitis associated with cephalosporins: Cephapirin versus cephalothin. *Curr Ther Res* 15:37, 1973.

39 Bank NU et al: Hematologic complications associated with beta-lactam antibiotics. *Rev Infect Dis* 5(suppl 2):S380, 1983.

40 Andrassy K et al: Hypoprothrombinemia caused by cephalosproins (letter). *J Antimicrob Chemother* 15:133, 1985.

41 Anthony BF, Concepcion NF: Group B *Streptococcus* in a general hospital. *J Infect Dis* 132:561, 1975.

42 Baker CJ et al: Antimicrobial susceptibility of group B streptococci isolated from a variety of clinical sources. *Antimicrob Agents Chemother* 10:128, 1976.

43 Barros F et al: In vitro antibiotic susceptibility of salmonellae. *Antimicrob Agents Chemother* 11:1071, 1977.

44 Byers PA et al: Antimicrobial susceptibilities of shigellae isolated in Houston, Texas, in 1974. *Antimicrob Agents Chemother* 9:288, 1976.

45 Vanhoof R et al: Susceptibility of *Campylobacter fetus* ssp. *jejuni* to twenty-nine antimicrobial agents. *Antimicrob Agents Chemother* 14:553, 1978.

46 Chun D et al: Drug resistance and R-plasmids in *Salmonella typhi* isolated in Korea. *Antimicrob Agents Chemother* 11:209, 1977.

47 Wilson WR: Tetracyclines, chloramphenicol, erythromycin, and clindamycin. *Mayo Clin Proc* 52:635, 1977.

48 Winckler K. Tetracycline ulcers of the oesophagus: Endoscopy, histology, and roentgenology in two cases, and review of the literature. *Endoscopy* 13:225, 1981.

49 Gorbach SL et al: Anaerobic infections. *N Engl J Med* 290:1289, 1974.

50 Grossman ER et al: Tetracycline and permanent teeth: The relationship between doses and tooth color. *Pediatrics* 47:567, 1971.

51 McCormack WM, Finland M: Spectinomycin. *Ann Intern Med* 84:712, 1976.

52 Reyn A et al: Spectinomycin hydrochloride (Trobicin) in the treatment of gonorrhea: Observation of resistant strains of *Neisseria gonorrhoeae. Br J Vener Dis* 49:54, 1973.

53 Thornsberry C et al: Spectinomycin-resistant *Neisseria gonorrhoeae. JAMA* 237:2405, 1977.

54 Zenilman JM et al: Spectinomycin-resistant gonococcal infections in the United States, 1985–1986. *J Infect Dis* 156:1002, 1987.

55 Spectinomycin-resistant penicillinase-producing *Neisseria gonorrhoeae. MMWR* 32:51, 1983.

56 Davies J et al: Inhibition of protein synthesis by spectinomycin. *Science* 149:1096, 1965.

57 Word ME: The bactericidal action of spectinomycin on *Neisseria gonorrhoeae. J Antimicrob Chemother* 3:323, 1977.

58 Virtanen S: Sensitivity of *Haemophilus vaginalis* (*Corynebacterium vaginale*) to oleandomycin and spectinomycin. *Pathol Microbiol* 42:36, 1975.

59 Duaneic A et al: Comparison of spectinomycin hydrochloride and aqueous procaine penicillin G in the treatment of uncomplicated gonorrhea. *Antimicrob Agents Chemother* 6:512, 1974.

60 Ginsburg CM, Eichenwald HF: Erythromycin: A review of its use in pediatric practice. *J Pediatr* 89:872, 1976.

61 Willcox RR: How suitable are available pharmaceuticals for the treatment of sexually transmitted diseases? 2. Conditions presenting as sores or tumors. *Br J Vener Dis* 53:340, 1977.

62 Brown ST et al: Comparison of erythromycin base and estolate in gonococcal urethritis. *JAMA* 238:1371, 1977.

63 Philipson A et al: Erythromycin and clindamycin absorption and elimination in pregnant women. *Clin Pharmacol Ther* 19:68, 1976.

64 McCracken GH Jr et al: Pharmacologic evaluation of orally administered antibiotics in infants and children: Effect of feeding on bioavailability. *Pediatrics* 62:738, 1978.

65 Malmborg A: Effect of food on absorption of erythromycin. A study of two derivatives, the stearate and the base. *J Antimicrob Chemother* 5:591, 1979.

66 McDonald PJ et al: Studies on absorption of a newly developed enteric-coated erythromycin base. *J Clin Pharmacol* 17:601, 1977.

67 Ginsburg CM et al: Concentrations of erythromycin in serum and tonsil: Comparison of the estolate and ethyl-succinate suspensions. *J Pediatr* 89:1011, 1976.

68 Steigbigil NH: Erythromycin, lincomycin and clindamycin, in *Principles and Practice of Infectious Diseases*, JL Mandell et al (eds). New York, Wiley, 1985, p 226.

69 Philipson A et al: Transplacental passage of erythromycin and clindamycin. *N Engl J Med* 288:1219, 1973.

70 Gantz NM et al: Pseudomembranous colitis associated with erythromycin. *Ann Intern Med* 91:866, 1979.

71 Gilbert FI: Cholestatic hepatitis caused by esters of erythromycin and oleandomycin. *JAMA* 182:1048, 1962.

72 Cacace LG et al: Erythromycin estolate induced hepatotoxicity report of a case and review of the literature. *Drug Intell Clin Pharm* 11:22, 1977.

73 McCormack WM et al: Hepatotoxicity of erythromycin estolate during pregnancy. *Antimicrob Agents Chemother* 12:630, 1977.

74 Viteri AL et al: Erythromycin ethyl succinate–induced cholestasis. *Gastroenterology* 76:1007, 1979.

75 Moran D: Personal communication.

76 Tolman KG et al: Chemical structure of erythromycin and hepatotoxicity. *Ann Intern Med* 81:58, 1974.

77 Mintz U et al: Transient perceptive deafness due to erythromycin lactobionate. *JAMA* 225:1122, 1973.

78 Meade III RH: Drug therapy reviews: Antimicrobial spectrum, pharmacology, and therapeutic use of erythromycin and its derivates. *Am J Hosp Pharm* 36:1185, 1979.

79 Kozak PP et al: Administration of erythromycin to patients on theophylline. *J Allergy Clin Immunol* 60:149, 1977.

80 Bowie WR et al: Differential response of chlamydial and ureaplasma-associated urethritis to sulphafurazole (sulfisoxazole) and aminocyclitols. *Lancet* 2:1276, 1976.

81 Csonka GW, Knight GJ: Therapeutic trial of trimethoprim as a potentiator of sulphonamides in gonorrhoea. *Br J Vener Dis* 43:161, 167.

82 Wright DJM, Grimble AS: Sulfamethoxazole combined with 2, 4-diaminopyrimidines in the treatment of gonorrhea. *Br J Vener Dis* 46:34, 1970.

83 Stolz E et al: Potential of sulfamethoxazole by trimethoprim in *Neisseria gonorrhoeae* strains. *Chemotherapy* 23:65, 1977.

84 Rein MF et al: Sulfamethoxazole trimethoprim synergism for *Neisseria gonorrhoeae. Antimicrob Agents Chemother* 17:247, 1980.

85 Svindland HB: Treatment of gonorrhoeae with sulfamethoxazole trimethoprim: Lack of effect concomitant syphilis. *Br J Vener Dis* 49:50, 1973.

86 Landy M et al: Increased synthesis of p-aminobenzoic acid associated with the development of resistance in *Staph. aureus. Science* 97:265, 1943.

87 Wolf B et al: Genetically modified folic acid synthesizing enzymes in Pneumococcus. *Biochemistry* 2:145, 1940.

88 Gleckman R et al: Drug therapy reviews: Trimethoprim-sulfamethoxazole. *Am J Hosp Pharm* 36:893, 1979.

89 Fass RJ et al: Pharmacokinetics and tolerance of a single twelve-tablet dose of trimethoprim (960 mg)-sulfamethoxazole (4800 mg). *Antimicrob Agents Chemother* 12:102, 1977.

90 Bergan T, Brodwall EK: The pharmacokinetic profile of cotrimoxazole. *Scand J Infect Dis* 8:542, 1976.

91 Bushby SRM, Hitchings GH: Trimethoprim, a sulphonamide potentiator. *Br J Pharmacol Chemother* 33:72, 1968.

92 Newbould BB, Kilpatrick R: Long-acting sulphonamides and protein-binding. *Lancet* 1:887, 1960.

93 Madsen ST et al: Antibacterial activity of long-acting sulphonamides. *Acta Med Scand* 173:707, 1963.

94 Stamey TA, Condy M: The diffusion and concentration of trimethoprim in human vaginal fluid. *J Infect Dis* 131:261, 1975.

95 Sparr RA et al: Maternal and newborn distribution and excretion of sulfamethoxypyridazine (Kynex). *Obstet Gynecol* 12:131, 1958.

96 Eatman FB et al: Blood and salivary concentrations of trimethoprim-sulfamethoxazole in man. *J Pharmacokinet Biopharm* 5:615, 1977.

97 Madsen P et al: Prostatic tissue and fluid concentrations of trimethoprim and sulfamethoxazole. *Urology* 8:129, 1976.

98 Winningham DG et al: Diffusion of antibiotics from plasma into prostate fluid. *Nature* 219:139, 1968.

99 Meares EM Jr: Prostatitis: Review of pharmacokinetics and therapy. *Rev Infect Dis* 4:475, 1982.

100 Greene BM et al: Trimethoprim-sulfamethoxazole and brain abscess. *Ann Intern Med* 82:812, 1975.

101 Pater RB et al: Clinical pharmacokinetics of co-trimoxazole (trimethoprim/sulfamethoxazole). *Clin Pharmacokinet* 5:405, 1980.

102 Williams DM et al: Renal clearance of sodium sulphadimidine in normal and uraemic subjects. *Lancet* 2:1058, 1968.

103 Bach MC et al: Absorption and urinary excretion of trimethoprim, sulfamethoxazole, trimethoprim-sulfamethoxazole: Results with single doses in normal young adults and preliminary observations during therapy with trimethoprim-sulfamethoxazole. *J Infect Dis* 128:S584, 1973.

104 Reider J: Excretion of sulfamethoxazole and trimethoprim into human bile. *J Infect Dis* 128:S574.

105 Appel GB, Neu HC: The nephrotoxicity of antimicrobial agents: 3. *N Engl J Med* 296:784, 1977.

106 Taylor GML: Stevens-Johnson syndrome following the use of an ultra long-lasting sulphonamide. *S Afr Med J* 42:501, 1968.

107 Kauppin K: Cutaneous reactions to drugs, with special reference to severe bullous mucocutaneous eruptions and sulphonamides. *Acta Derm Venereol (Stockh)* 52(suppl 68):1, 1972.

108 Weinstein L: Erythema nodosum. *DM* 21:21, 1969.

109 Linton AL et al: Acute interstitial nephritis due to drugs: Review of the literature with a report of nine cases. *Ann Intern Med* 93:735, 1980.

110 Duyovne CA et al: Sulfonamide liver injury: Review of the literature and report of a case due to sulfamethoxazole. *N Engl J Med* 277:785, 1967.

111 Gordin FM: Adverse reactions to trimethoprim-sulfamethoxazole in patients with the acquired immunodeficiency syndrome. *Ann Intern Med* 100:495, 1984.

112 Shouval D et al: Effect of co-trimoxazole on normal creatinine clearance. *Lancet* 1:244, 1978.

113 Berglund F et al: Effect of trimethoprim-sulfamethoxazole on the renal excretion of creatinine in man. *J Urol* 114:802, 1975.

114 Yuill GM: Megaloblastic anemia due to trimethoprim-sulfamethoxazole therapy. *Postgrad Med J* 49:100, 1973.

115 Bradley PP et al: Neutropenia and thrombocytopenia in renal allograft recipients treated with trimethoprim-sulfamethoxazole. *Ann Intern Med* 93:560, 1980.

116 Kauffman RE et al: Relative bioavailability of intravenous chlor-

amphenicol succinate and oral chloramphenicol palmitate in infants and children. *J Pediatr* 99:963, 1981.
117 Meissner HC, Smith AL: The current status of chloramphenicol. *Pediatrics* 64:348, 1979.
118 Azzollini F et al: Elimination of chloramphenicol and thiamphenicol in subjects with cirrhosis of the liver. *Int J Clin Pharmacol* 6:130, 1972.
119 Oski FA: Hematologic consequences of chloramphenicol therapy, editorial. *J Pediatr* 94:515, 1979.
120 Keiser G: Co-operative study of patients treated with thiamphenicol: comparative study of patients treated with chloramphenicol and thiamphenicol. *Postgrad Med J* 50(suppl 5):143, 1979.
121 Edwards DI, Matheson GE: The mode of action of metronidazole against *Trichomonas vaginalis*. *J Gen Microbiol* 63:297, 1970.
122 Meingassner JG, Thurner J: Strain of *Trichomonas vaginalis* resistant to metronidazole and other 5-nitroimidazoles. *Antimicrob Agents Chemother* 15:254, 1979.
123 Forsgen A, Forssman L: Metronidazole-resistant *Trichomonas vaginalis*. *Br J Vener Dis* 55:351, 1979.
124 Philips I et al: The antimicrobial susceptibility of anaerobic bacteria in a London teaching hospital. *J Antimicrob Chemother* 8:17, 1981.
125 Wood BA, Munro AM: Pharmacokinetics of tinidazole and metronidazole in women after single large oral doses. *Br J Vener Dis* 51:51, 1975.
126 Schwartz DE, Jeunet F: Comparative pharmacokinetic studies of ornidazole and metronidazole in man. *Chemotherapy* 22:19, 1976.
127 Wheeler LA et al: Use of high-pressure liquid chromatography to determine plasma levels in metronidazole and metabolites after intravenous administration. *Antimicrob Agents Chemother* 13:205, 1978.
128 Anjaneyulu R et al: Single-dose treatment of trichomonal vaginalis: A comparison of tinidazole and metronidazole. *J Int Med Res* 5:438, 1977.
129 Koch-Weser J: Metronidazole. *N Engl J Med* 303:1212, 1980.
130 Finegold SM: Metronidazole. *Ann Intern Med* 93:585, 1980.
131 Legator MS: Detection of mutagenic activity of metronidazole and niridazole in body fluids of humans and mice. *Science* 188:1118, 1975.
132 Shepard TH, Fantel AG: Is metronidazole teratogenic? *JAMA* 237:1617, 1977.
133 Hartley-Asp B: Mutagenicity of metronidazole, letter. *Lancet* 1:275, 1979.
134 Rustia M, Shubik P: Induction of lung tumors and malignant lymphomas in mice by metronidazole. *J Natl Cancer Inst* 48:721, 1972.
135 Beard CM et al: Lack of evidence for cancer due to use of metronidazole. *N Engl J Med* 301:519, 1979.
136 Friedman GD: Cancer after metronidazole, letter. *N Engl J Med* 302:519, 1980.
137 O'Reilly RA: The steroselective interaction of warfarin and metronidazole in man. *N Engl J Med* 295:354, 1976.
138 Crider SR et al: Treatment of penicillin-resistant *Neisseria gonorrhoeae* with oral norfloxacin. *N Engl J Med* 311:137, 1984.
139 Loo PS et al: Single dose ciprofloxacin for treating gonococcal infections in men. *Genitourin Med* 61:302, 1985.
140 Ishigami J et al: Efficacy of norfloxacin (Am-715) for the treatment of acute urethritis. *Chemotherapy* 30:1349, 1982.
141 Wolfson JS et al: The fluoroquinolones: Structure, mechanisms of action and resistance, and spectra of activity in vitro. *Antimicrob Agents Chemother* 28:581, 1985.
142 Borobio MV et al: Effect of inoculum, pH, and medium of the activity of ciprofloxacin against anaerobic bacteria. *Antimicrob Agents Chemother* 25:342, 1984.
143 Swanson BN et al: Norfloxacin disposition after sequentially increasing oral doses. *Antimicrob Agents Chemother* 23:284, 1983.
144 Tartaglione TA et al: Pharmacokinetics and tolerance of ciprofloxacin after sequential increasing oral doses. *Antimicrob Agents Chemother* 29:62, 1986.
145 Dagrosa EE et al: Multiple-dose pharmacokinetics of ofloxacin, a new broad spectrum antimicrobial agent. *Clin Ther* 8:632, 1986.
146 Ichihara N et al: Phase I study on DL-8280. *Chemotherapy* 32 (suppl 1):118, 1984.
147 Beermann D et al: Comparative pharmacokinetics of three new quinolone carboxylic acid antibiotics after oral administration in healthy volunteers. *J Clin Pharmacol* 24:403, 1984.
148 Holmes B et al: Norfloxacin: A review of its antibacterial activity, pharmacokinetic properties and therapeutic use. *Drugs* 30:482, 1985.
149 Boerema JBJ et al: Ciprofloxacin distribution in prostatic tissue and fluid after oral administration. *Chemotherapy* 31:13, 1985.
150 Brogard TM et al: Comparison of high-pressure liquid chromatography and microbiological assay for the determination of biliary elimination of ciprofloxacin in humans. *Antimicrob Agents Chemother* 28:311, 1985.
151 Fong IW et al: Ciprofloxacin concentrations in bone and muscle after oral dosing. *Antimicrob Agents Chemother* 29:405, 1986.
152 Segev S et al: Penetration of ciprofloxacin into female pelvic tissues. *Eur J Clin Microbiol* 5:207, 1986.
153 Lockley MR et al: Intraperitoneal penetration of ciprofloxacin. *Eur J Clin Microbiol* 5:209, 1986.
154 Bergogne-Berezin E et al: Penetration of ciprofloxacin into bronchial secretions. *Eur J Clin Microbiol* 5:197, 1986.
155 Wolff M et al: Diffusion of ciprofloxacin into the CSF of patients with purulent meningitis (abstract). *Program and Abstracts of the 26th Interscience Conference on Antimicrobial Agents and Chemotherapy*. New Orleans, 1986:184.
156 Monk JP et al: Ofloxacin: A review of its antibacterial activity, pharmacokinetic properties and therapeutic use. *Drugs* 33:346, 1987.
157 Matsuda S et al: Experimental and clinical studies of DL-8280 in the field of obstetrics and gynecology. *Chemotherapy* 32(suppl):900, 1984.
158 Fillastre JP et al: Pharmacokinetics of norfloxacin in renal failure. *J Antimicrob Chemother* 14:439, 1984.
159 Boelaert J et al: The pharmacokinetics of ciprofloxacin in patients with impaired renal function. *J Antimicrob Chemother* 16:87, 1985.
160 Fillastre JP et al: Ofloxacin pharmacokinetics in renal failure. *Antimicrob Agents Chemother* 31:156, 1987.
161 Chan MX et al: Concentrations of ofloxacin in sera and peritoneal fluid of patients on continuous ambulatory peritoneal dialysis. Abstract. International Symposium on New Quinolones, Geneva, 1986.
162 Arcieri G et al: Clinical experience with ciprofloxacin in the U.S.A. *Euro J Clin Microbiol* 5:220, 1986.
163 Wijnands WJA et al: Enoxacin raises plasma theophylline concentrations. *Lancet* 2:108, 1984.
164 Wijnands WJA et al: The influence of quinolone derivatives on theophylline clearance. *Br J Clin Pharmacol* 22:677, 1986.
165 Fourtillan JB et al: Pharmacokinetics of ofloxacin and theophylline alone or in combination. *Infection* 14(suppl):67, 1986.
166 Bowles SK et al: Effect of norfloxacin on theophylline pharmacokinetics at steady state. *Antimicrob Agents Chemother* 32:510, 1988.
167 Sano M et al: Comparative pharmacokinetics of theophylline following two fluoroquinolones co-administration. *Eur J Clin Pharmacol* 32:431, 1987.
168 Matsumoto K et al: In vitro, pharmacokinetic and clinical studies of DL-8280, a new oxazine derivative. *Chemotherapy* 32(suppl)1:509, 1984.
169 Mangini RJ: Drug therapy reviews: Pathogenesis and clinical management of hyperuricemia and gout. *Am J Hosp Pharm* 36:497, 1979.
170 Hillecke NA: Acute anaphylactoid reaction to probenecid. *JAMA* 193:740, 1965.
171 Corey et al: Intravenous acyclovir for the treatment of primary genital herpes. *Ann Intern Med* 98:914, 1983.
172 Bryson YJ et al: Treatment of first episode of genital herpes simplex virus infection with oral acyclovir. *N Engl J Med* 308:916, 1983.
173 Mindel A et al: Intravenous acyclovir treatment for primary genital herpes. *Lancet* 1:697, 1982.

174 Schaeffer HJ et al: 9-(2-hydroxyethoxymethyl) guanine activity against viruses of the herpes group. *Nature* 272:583, 1978.
175 Crumpacker CS et al: Resistance to antiviral drugs of herpes simplex virus isolated from patients treated with acyclovir. *N Engl J Med* 306:343, 1982.
176 Laskin OL: Clinical pharmacokinetics of acyclovir. *Clin Pharmacokinet* 8:187, 1983.
177 Bryson YJ et al: Treatment of first episodes of genital herpes simplex virus infections. *N Engl J Med* 306:1313, 1982.
178 Corey L et al: Genital herpes simplex virus infections: Current concepts in diagnosis, therapy, and prevention. *Ann Intern Med* 98:973, 1983.
179 Blum RM et al: Overview of acyclovir pharmacokinetic disposition in adults and children. *Am J Med* 73(suppl):186, 1982.
180 Van Dyke RB et al: Pharmacokinetics of orally administered acyclovir in patients with herpes progenitalis. *Am J Med* 73(suppl):172, 1982.
181 Keeney RE: Acyclovir tolerance in humans. *Am J Med* 73(suppl):176, 1982.
182 Steele RW et al: Comparative in vitro immunotoxicology of acyclovir and other antiviral agents. *Infect Immun* 28:957, 1980.
183 McGuffin RW et al: Lack of toxicity of acyclovir to granulocyyte progenitor cells in vitro. *Antimicrob Agents Chemother* 10:471, 1980.
184 Quinn RP et al: Effect of acyclovir on various murine in vivo and in vitro immunologic assay systems. *Am J Med* 73(suppl):62, 1982.
185 Dalgleish AG et al: The CD4 (T4) antigen is an essential component of the receptor for the AIDS retrovirus. *Nature* 312:763, 1984.
186 Klatzmann D et al: The lymphocyte T4 molecule behaves as the receptor for human retrovirus LAV. *Nature* 312:767, 1984.
187 Pert CB et al: Octapeptides deduced from the neuropeptide receptor-like pattern of antigen $T_4$ in brain potently inhibit human immunodeficiency virus receptor binding and T-cell infectivity. *Proc Natl Acad Sci USA* 83:9254, 1986.
188 Wetterberg L et al: Peptide T in treatment of AIDS. *Lancet* i:159, 1987.
189 Smith DH et al: Blocking of HIV-1 infectivity by a soluble secreted form of the $CD_4$ antigen. *Science* 238:1704, 1987.
190 Sarin PS et al: Effect of a novel compound (AL 721) on HTLV-III infectivity in vitro (letter). *N Engl J Med* 313:1289, 1985.
191 Clapham PR et al: Soluble $CD_4$ neutralizes infectivity and syncytia of HIV-1, HIV-2 and SIV. Paper presented to the Fourth International Conference on AIDS. Stockholm, Sweden, June 1988.
192 Ueno R et al: Dextran sulphate, a potent anti-HIV agent in vitro having synergism with zidovudine. *Lancet* i:1379, 1987.
193 Mitsuya H et al: Dextran sulfate suppression of viruses in the HIV family: Inhibition of virion binding to $CD_4$+ cells. *Science* 240:646, 1988.
194 Baltimore D: Viral RNA-dependent DNA polymerase. *Nature* 226:1209, 1970.
195 Temin HM, Mizutani S: RNA-dependent DNA polymerase in virions of rous Sarcoma virus. *Nature* 226:1211, 1970.
196 Vogt M, Hirsch MS: Prospects for the prevention and therapy of infections with the human immunodeficiency virus. *Rev Infect Dis* 8:9991, 1986.
197 Mitsuya H et al: Suramin protection of T cells in vitro against infectivity and cytopathic effect of HTLV-III. *Science* 226:172, 1984.
198 De Clerq E: Suramin: A potent inhibitor of the reverse transcriptase of RNA tumor viruses. *Cancer Lett* 8:9, 1979.
199 Broder S et al: Effects of suramin on HTLV-III/LAV infection presenting as Kaposi's sarcoma or AIDS-related complex: Clinical pharmacology and suppression of virus replication in vivo. *Lancet* 2:627, 1985.
200 Rouvroy D et al: Short term results with suramin for AIDS-related conditions. *Lancet* 1:878, 1985.
201 Busch W et al: Suramin treatment for AIDS. *Lancet* 2:1247, 1985.
202 Cheson BD et al: Suramin therapy in AIDS and related diseases: Initial report of the U.S. Suramin Working Group. Paper presented to the Second International Conference on AIDS. Paris, France, June 23, 1986.
203 Saimot AT et al: Long term administration of suramin to AIDS patients: Effects on LAV/HTLV-III replication and clinical outcome. Paper presented to the Second International Conference on AIDS. Paris, France, June 23, 1986.
204 Mildvan D et al: Suramin treatment in AIDS complicated by opportunistic infections (AIDS-OI). Paper presented to the Second International Conference on AIDS. Paris, France, June 23, 1986.
205 Wolfe PR et al: Suramin in AIDS and ARC: Results of a pilot toxicity/efficacy study. Paper presented to the Second International Conference on AIDS. Paris, France, June 23, 1986.
206 Kaplan LD et al: Failure of suramin as treatment for AIDS. Paper presented to the Second International Conference on AIDS. Paris, France, June 23, 1986.
207 Dormont D et al: Inhibition of RNA-dependent DNA polymerases of AIDS and SAIDS retroviruses by HPA-23 (ammonium-21-tungsto-9-antimoniate). *Ann Virol* 136E:75, 1985.
208 Kornhauser DM et al: Pharmacokinetics of intravenous HPV-23. Paper presented to the 26th Interscience Conference on Antimicrobial Agents and Chemotherapy. New Orleans, LA, Sept 28, 1986.
209 McCormick JB et al: Ribavirin suppresses replication of lymphadenopathy-associated virus in culture of human adult T-lymphocytes. *Lancet* 2:1367, 1984.
210 Gilbert BE, Knight V: Biochemistry and clinical application of ribavirin. *Antimicrob Agents Chemother* 30:201, 1986.
211 Catlin OH et al: $^{14}$C-ribavirin: Distribution and pharmacokinetics studies in rats, baboons and man, in *Ribavirin: A Broad Spectrum Antiviral Agent*, NA Smith, W Kirkpatrick (eds). New York, Academic, 1980, p 83.
212 Mansell PWA et al: Ribavirin delays progression of the lymphadenopathy syndrome (LAS) to the acquired immune deficiency syndrome (AIDS). Paper presented to the Third International Conference on AIDS. Washington, DC, June 2, 1987.
213 Vernon A, Schulof RS: Serum HIV core antigen in symptomatic ARC patients taking oral ribavirin or placebo. Paper presented to the Third International Conference on AIDS. Washington DC, June 2, 1987.
214 Sandstrom EG et al: Inhibition of human T-cell lymphotropic virus type III *in vitro* by phosphonoformate. *Lancet* 1:1480, 1985.
215 Öberg B: Antiviral effects of phosphonoformate (FPA, foscarnet sodium). *Pharmacol Ther* 19:387, 1983.
216 Farthing CF et al: Pilot study on the treatment of AIDS and ARC patients with intravenous foscarnet. Paper presented to the Second International Conference on AIDS. Paris, France, June 23–25, 1986.
217 Farthing CF et al: Phosphonoformate (foscarnet): A pilot study in AIDS and AIDS-related complex. *AIDS* 1:21, 1987.
218 Gaub J et al: The effect of foscarnet (phosphonoformate) on human immunodeficiency virus isolation, T-cell subsets and lymphocyte function in AIDS patients. *AIDS* 1:27, 1987.
219 Mitsuya H et al: BW A509U blocks HTLV-3 infection of T lymphocytes in culture. Paper presented to the 25th Interscience Conference on Antimicrobial Agents and Chemotherapy. Minneapolis, MN, Sept 29, 1985.
220 Furman PA et al: Selective inhibition of HTLV-3 by BW A509U. Paper presented to the 25th Interscience Conference on Antimicrobial Agents and Chemotherapy. Minneapolis, MN, Sept 29, 1985.
221 Blum MR et al: Pharmacokinetics of azidothymidine (AZT) following intravenous and oral administration. Paper presented to the Second International Conference on AIDS. Paris, France, June 23, 1986.
222 Deray G et al: Pharmacokinetics of zidovudine in a patient on maintenance hemodialysis. *N Engl J Med* 319:1606, 1988.
223 Richman DD et al: The toxicity of azidothymidine (AZT) in the treatment of patients with AIDS and AIDS-related complex. *N Engl J Med* 307:192, 1987.
224 Hagler DNA, Frame PT: Azidothymidine neurotoxicity. *Lancet* 2:1392, 1986.
225 Mitsuya H, Broder S: Inhibition of the in vitro infectivity and cytopathic effect of HTLV-III/LAV by 2′,3′-dideoxynucleosides. *Proc Natl Acad Sci USA* 83:1911, 1986.
226 Yarchoan R et al: Phase I studies of 2,′3′-dideoxycytidine in severe

human immunodeficiency virus infection as a single agent and alternating with zidovudine. *Lancet* i:76, 1988.

227 Mitchell WM et al: Mismatched double-stranded RNA (ampligen) protects target cells from HIV infection and reduces the concentration of 3′-azido-3′ deoxythymidine (AZT) required for virus-static activity. Paper presented to the Third International Conference on AIDS. Washington, DC, June 2, 1987.

228 Henrigues HF et al: Ampligen therapy for HIV-related immunodeficiency. Paper presented to the Third International Conference on AIDS. Washington, DC, June 2, 1987.

229 Walker BD et al: Anti-HIV properties of castanospermine. Paper presented to the Third International Conference on AIDS. Washington, DC, June 2, 1987.

230 Matsukura M et al: Phosphorothioate analogs of oligodeoxynucleotides: Novel inhibitors of replication and cytopathic effects of HTLV-III/LAV (human immunodeficiency virus) in vitro. Paper presented to the Third International Conference on AIDS. Washington, DC, June 2, 1987.

231 Hartshorn KL et al: Synergistic inhibition of human immunodeficiency virus by azidothymidine and recombinant alpha A interferon. *Antimicrob Agents Chemother* 31:168, 1987.

232 Mitsuya H et al: Rapid in vitro systems for assessing activity of agents against HTLV-III/LAV, in *AIDS, Modern Concepts and Therapeutic Challenges*, S Broder (ed.) New York, Marcel Dekker, 1987, p 303.

233 Vogt MW et al: Synergism and antagonism in vitro among various antiviral drugs in the treatment of HIV infections. Paper presented to the Third International Conference on AIDS. Washington, DC, June 2, 1987.

234 Vogt et al: Ribavirin antagonizes the effect of azidothymidine on HIV replication. *Science* 235:1376, 1987.

235 Walker R et al: Therapy of AIDS patients with early Kaposi's sarcoma with 3′-azido-3′deoxythymidine. Paper presented to the Third International Conference on AIDS. Washington, DC, June 2, 1987.

# PART X CONTROL OF SEXUALLY TRANSMITTED DISEASES

# Chapter 84

# Strategies for development of sexually transmitted diseases control programs

Willard Cates, Jr.
André Meheus

Few fields of medicine are more dynamic than sexually transmitted diseases (STDs). For instance, in the United States during the past decade, this discipline has evolved from one emphasizing the traditional venereal diseases of gonorrhea and syphilis to one concerned with the bacterial and viral syndromes associated with *Chlamydia trachomatis*, herpes simplex virus (HSV), and human papillomavirus (HPV) to one preoccupied with the fatal systemic infections caused by human immunodeficiency virus (HIV).[1–3] Awareness of health and economic importance of STD complications and late sequelae has also increased considerably during the last decade. These complications include adverse outcomes of pregnancy for mother and newborn, neonatal infections, infertility, and genital cancers, in particular carcinoma of the cervix uteri.

This expanded spectrum of infection and responsibilities has been a two-edged sword. On the one hand, it has stretched limited resources allocated to prevention and control of STD quite thin; on the other, it has accelerated the acceptance of constructive new approaches to reducing STD transmission among high-risk groups. This chapter will describe current strategies for controlling STD, with a special emphasis on approaches to planning for a continually changing public health environment.

## DETERMINANTS OF STD CONTROL PROGRAMS

Factors which influence STD control are complex since they involve interactions of (1) the health care system, (2) governmental structures, (3) the public's interest in STD, and (4) resources available for prevention and control programs. First, health care systems vary from country to country. In the developed world, STD services are provided by different combinations of public and private facilities. In the United States, clinical care for STD is estimated to be equally divided between that offered by local health department clinics and that available from private physicians (Chaps. 87 and 93). In Europe, a more centralized system of STD care is organized around the specialty of venereology and genitourinary medicine.[4]

In developing countries, limited health resources have not allowed widespread STD clinical services to be available.[5] Physicians are mainly working in hospital settings, from the district level up to national reference (teaching) hospitals; these facilities cater to health problems of only 10 to 30 percent of the population. If countries have a private medical system, this is available to only a tiny fraction of the population.[6] As a result, third world STD care has been delivered generally in peripheral health units and has been based on simplified clinical algorithms. (See Chap. 86.)

Second, different tiers of government frequently have complementary responsibilities for STD control.[7] For example, in the United States, the Centers for Disease Control (CDC), a federal agency, coordinates STD control strategies and provides technical assistance for implementation. State health departments have the statutory responsibility for control of STD, which includes disease reporting and program evaluation. Local health departments are charged with providing direct clinical services which include diagnosis, treatment, patient counseling, and sex partner referral activities.[8] In the United Kingdom, similar clinical structures exist at central, regional, and district levels to deliver STD services.[1] In developing countries,[7] health services are also organized into a clinical hierarchy with relatively little coordination (Table 84-1).

Third, public interest in STD has varied unpredictably. In recent years, AIDS has catapulted the field of STD into a major national and international issue. Indeed, fear of STD has become the number one health concern among the American population,[9] ahead of cancer and heart disease. Similar reactions have occurred in Europe, fueled by national media campaigns. Public awareness of the link between sexually transmitted HPV and cervical, anal, vulvar, and penile cancer has not yet arisen. If this message gets across to the public, demand for further STD prevention and control will undoubtedly arise. Because the public's perception of the STD problem influences both policy makers and program planners, it has a strong effect on the resources available for STD control.

Finally, governmental funding influences the magnitude and range of strategies for STD control. In the United States, after adjusting for effects of inflation, the peak year for federal grant funding of STD control programs was 1947. By 1988, the aggregate amount for STD control (excluding AIDS) had declined to one-third its post World War II level.[2] In developing areas, the situation is worse; STD control is frequently low on the public health resources priority list. Several simultaneous approaches are necessary to gain resource leverage on the range of sexually transmitted infections: (1) lessons learned in primary prevention of HIV transmission must be rapidly applied to other STD; (2) resources from other government programs, namely, education, mental health, family planning, and maternal and child health, must be marshaled to complement STD funds; and (3) the private medical community must commit itself to the prevention and control of STD as a basic part of primary care.[3]

**Table 84-1. The Organization of Health Services in Many Developing Countries**

| Health facility | Type of personnel |
|---|---|
| Ministry of health | Senior administrative/policy staff |
| National reference hospital | Medical specialists, laboratory experts and technicians |
| Regional hospital | Some medical specialists and laboratory technicians |
| District hospital | Mostly general medicine only, laboratory technicians |
| Health center | Paramedics with variable supervision by physicians; laboratory auxiliaries |
| Dispensary | Paramedical or auxiliary workers only |
| Community | Community health workers |

SOURCE: Adapted from Arya OP, Bennett FJ: Role of the medical auxiliary in the control of sexually transmitted diseases in a developing country. *Br J Vener Dis* 52:116, 1976.

**Table 84-2. Approaches to Developing Strategies for STD Control**

| Approach | Components |
|---|---|
| 1. Making assumptions | Political and social |
| | Organism and syndrome |
| | Diagnosis and treatment |
| | Demography and behavior |
| | Communications and data |
| 2. Estimating public health importance | Surveillance |
| | Cost-benefit analysis |
| 3. Targeting priority groups | Risk markers |
| | Age |
| | Race |
| | Geography |
| | "Core" populations |
| | Prostitutes |
| | IV drug users |
| | Migrant workers |

Because of these complexities, the approaches to controlling STD frequently overlap.[10,11] While STD control strategies are described here as systematic, sequential, and ordered, they are in reality interdependent activities. Thus, the variety of intervention strategies should take place simultaneously, and most STD interventions are less effective on their own than when combined with one or more others.

## PLANNING STRATEGIES

Planning for STD control programs involves making assumptions about the future, estimating the public health importance of the problem, and targeting STD resources to key priority groups (Table 84-2).

## MAKING ASSUMPTIONS

A difficult, yet essential, step in strategic planning is agreeing on assumptions about future trends; by definition, assumptions are speculative—more hunch than science. For purposes of discussion, we provide examples of assumptions used in addressing national and international STD priorities; these are not comprehensive but instead serve to highlight typical factors which must be considered:

1. Political and social
   - Political pressure will increase to justify programs on economic grounds rather than on technical feasibility or humanitarian grounds. The economic burden of STD will need to be clearly documented.
   - Most countries will have to consider resource trade-offs when they attempt to get into new STD program areas; thus, they may have to build new programs at the expense of traditional public health activities. The ability and interest of individual countries and regions to meet this responsibility will vary.
   - Continued tension will be felt between (1) those who favor an expansion in the use of regulatory approaches to public health, particularly in regulating exposure to HIV, and (2) those who oppose regulatory mechanisms for public health programs, regardless of effectiveness. With STD, regulatory approaches to limit human behavior will be considered.
   - STD will become increasingly viewed as an international issue rather than solely an internal domestic concern of each country.
2. Organisms and syndromes
   - HIV, and its sequelae AIDS, will continue as the STD of primary importance, with spread outside of the initial risk groups.
   - In developed countries, moderate levels of early syphilis will rise, as resources are directed to other STD. In developing countries, syphilis and chancroid will continue as important symptomatic STD. The interaction of syphilis and other genital ulcer diseases with HIV transmission and progression will become a critical problem.
   - Upward trends in the prevalence of other viral STD, especially HSV and HPV, will persist. The association of HPV with neoplasia will be increasingly recognized in both the developed and developing world.
   - The upward trend in *Chlamydia trachomatis* will persist, with chlamydia continuing as the most prevalent bacterial STD in both the developed and developing world.
   - Resistant strains of gonorrhea—penicillinase producing *Neisseria gonorrhoeae* (PPNG) and chromosomally mediated resistant *Neisseria gonorrhoeae* (CMRNG)—will increase as a percentage of total gonorrhea. Gonococcal conjunctivitis in the newborn will become a blinding disease of major importance in developing countries if no adequate control measures are taken.
   - Awareness of the seriousness and costs (both human and financial) of STD sequelae will increase—infertility, ectopic pregnancy, adverse pregnancy outcome, neonatal infections, neoplasia, immune deficiencies, and central nervous system degeneration.
3. Diagnosis and treatment
   - Resources dedicated to HIV research will pay diagnostic and therapeutic dividends for other STD.
   - Less expensive and cumbersome diagnostic methods for chlamydia and viral STD will be developed.
   - In syphilis serology, sensitive and practical methods for the detection of treponema-specific antibodies of the different immunoglobulin classes will be developed.
   - Relatively expensive antiviral therapies will become available, but their potential long-term adverse effects will be of increasing concern. Moreover, the emergence of resistant viral organisms will need to be monitored.
   - Surgical diagnostic and therapeutic technology will become more applicable to managing primary STD infections, particularly HPV.
   - A wider spectrum of STD vaccines will be developed, especially for viral infections, which will pose challenges for broad distribution to high-risk adult populations.
   - Antibiotic and antiviral abuse will increase, in both the developing and the developed world, as black markets arise to meet increasing demand.
4. Demography and behavior
   - Rates of STD will remain high in adolescent populations, despite increasing emphasis to change sexual behavior in this group.
   - Primary preventive behaviors will be increasingly emphasized for all STD, especially for the viral organisms, until such time as therapies and vaccines become available.
   - Condoms and other barrier methods of contraception will become of crucial importance to primary prevention efforts.
   - Compliance problems with STD therapy will increase be-

cause of more complex, multidose therapeutic approaches and a shift from injections to oral medication (fear of HIV transmission through contaminated needles, particularly in developing countries).
 - Educational systems will be challenged to provide adequate STD education in school curricula. Despite increasing public support for STD and sex education in schools, this topic will continue to generate intense controversy.
5. Communications and data
 - Simplification of computer technology will provide greater opportunities for using STD data worldwide.
 - Continued technological advances will allow wider information sharing among health professionals and educators. The public will become increasingly knowledgeable about STD.

## ESTIMATING PUBLIC HEALTH IMPORTANCE

Until STDs are recognized by policy makers as an important public health problem, only limited resources will be allocated for their control. Moreover, when resources are scarce, their epidemiology cannot be studied fully—consequently program managers encounter difficulties in describing the importance of STD and have problems in efficiently using the sparse available resources.

One of the first steps of planning for STD control is to establish which STD is important in a particular country.[10] Prevalence surveys provide a good start; formal surveillance systems are even better. This process will help to focus efforts of the staff during preliminary planning and will reveal priority issues of STD control to decision makers (Chaps. 85 and 86). Regarding specific STD, current international interest in AIDS and HIV will be invaluable as an STD "attention getter." However, the "other STDs" cause sizable morbidity. For example, gonorrhea is important not only because it leads to infertility and blindness,[12] but also because the infection is resistant to the available inexpensive antimicrobial drugs.[13] Similarly, in Africa, syphilis is a priority STD because (1) it is a common cause of pregnancy wastage,[14] (2) it can be prevented with proved intervention approaches,[15] and (3) genital ulcers may be an important cofactor for heterosexual HIV transmission.[16–18]

The economic consequences of STD may be used to persuade fiscally oriented decision makers that these problems are of considerable importance to public health. The cost of these diseases results from both direct and indirect measures.[19] Direct costs include the care for patients with both uncomplicated and complicated diseases. The indirect costs include productivity losses resulting from sick leave, disabilities, or premature death. In the United States, the costs of PID attributed to STD amounted to nearly $2.4 billion in 1985.[20] For a Central African country, the medical costs related to gonorrhea alone were estimated to take 17 percent of the budget for medicines and 4.3 percent of the overall health budget (M Jancloes, unpublished observations). Insufficient data are available in most countries on which to base such a calculation, but approximations are possible.

In countries where STD are accompanied by socially important consequences, emphasis on these particular issues will be relevant.[21] The importance of these diseases in causing infertility, fetal wastage, neonatal death, and disabilities in children such as blindness should be emphasized.[14] Data linking particular diseases to these outcomes may need to be strengthened and more widely publicized. In addition, the chronic pain, disability, and PID-related deaths which affect women and interfere with their contribution to a healthy family unit should be highlighted.[22]

## TARGETING PRIORITY GROUPS

An underlying epidemiologic principle is that diseases are not evenly distributed throughout populations. As a result, some groups are of greater importance to STD control efforts than others, and inerventions should focus on these target populations.[23] Recent identification of "core groups" of disease transmitters provides empiric demonstration that a subgroup of infected persons is responsible for the perpetuation of a disease within a community.[24,25]

Priority groups may be categorized on the basis of risk markers (Chap. 2)—age, gender, and ethnic group.[26] Descriptions that also include place of residence or occupation may be even more helpful in designing interventions.[27] Such information is relatively simple to collect and generally less stigmatizing. In addition, control activities that can be aimed at one particular area of a city or at specific work groups, e.g., the military or students, are usually more effectively implemented.[28–30] Pregnant women are a special priority group because of the risk of vertical transmission of STD and adverse pregnancy outcome for mother and/or newborn. Other characteristics that may be used to identify priority groups include their sexual and health care–seeking behavior.

## INTERVENTION STRATEGIES—DIRECT CONTROL ACTIVITIES

Two recent World Health Organization publications have addressed the key interventions to reduce STD.[10,11] These components include both direct control activities and indirect support processes essential to providing a foundation of human skills and technological efficiency (Table 84-3).

**Table 84-3. STD Intervention Strategies—Examples of Applications**

| Strategy | Examples |
|---|---|
| 1. Control activities | |
| *a.* Health education | STD patient education<br>School AIDS/STD curricula<br>Media advertisements |
| *b.* Disease detection | Screening priorities<br>Diagnostic algorithms |
| *c.* Appropriate treatment | Isolate monitoring<br>Treatment guidelines<br>Prophylactic treatment |
| *d.* Partner notification | Interviewing techniques<br>Partner follow-up |
| *e.* Clinical services | Patient protocols<br>Management protocols |
| 2. Support components | |
| *a.* Medical training | Model STD centers<br>Medical school curricula |
| *b.* Managerial training | Graduated supervision<br>Networking skills |
| *c.* Research | Basic and applied needs<br>Private liaison |
| *d.* Information systems | Microcomputer application<br>Surveillance potential |

## HEALTH EDUCATION AND PROMOTION

Health education messages are, in general, an integral part of STD intervention activities. Specific community health education efforts, if presented properly, can supplement other strategies by encouraging primary preventive behaviors before infection occurs in healthy persons at risk (Chap. 90). Traditionally, "scare tactics" based on judgmental messages have not been an effective method of changing behavior.[31] In fact, stigmatizing infected individuals by widespread social disapproval may even hinder disease control through delaying care.

To have the greatest chance of success, behavior modification approaches must promote and reinforce individual decision making. For example, messages which emphasize "safer" sexual practices may have already had an impact. In 1982 in the United States, because of increasing concern with genital herpes, over half of unmarried persons who believed themselves at risk reported changing their sexual behavior to avoid this disease.[32] Moreover, behavior changes among homosexual men in response to concern about AIDS have simultaneously affected other STD trends in the United States and Europe.[33–36]

Health education interventions also affect secondary prevention, by reducing risks of complications in those already infected and by limiting the transmission of infection after symptoms appear. Recent experience with use of videotapes to promote such actions as follow-up cultures, treatment compliance, and condom use have been encouraging, at least for short-term behaviors.[37] These messages are generally given to STD patients as they are being counseled about the appropriate actions they should take both to ensure a cure and to prevent a reinfection (Chap. 88).

School sex education courses to increase students' knowledge of the full spectrum of STD are widely taught in Europe.[38] Moreover, they have recently been encouraged in the United States by the Surgeon General.[39] Unfortunately, past heritage of teaching about "VD" in U.S. high schools has generally consisted of didactic biomedical lectures concentrating only on syphilis and gonorrhea. Moreover, when delivered in health science rather than sex education texts, the information failed to stress appropriate preventive behaviors.[40] To correct this situation, prototype school curriculum materials for both teachers and students in grades 6 through 12, based on a self-instructional format and emphasizing behavioral messages, have been developed and field tested.[41] These will facilitate systematic AIDS and STD education in family life and sex education courses throughout the country. Sex education for the young is no less a priority in many developing settings, particularly in the cities of the third world, where unwanted pregnancy, abortions, and STD are immense health problems in adolescents.[42]

For specific questions about STD by the general public, national hotlines for both STD and AIDS can provide relevant information to interested persons. In 1987 in the United States, almost 58,000 calls were answered on the STD hotline. Over 30,000 persons requested referral to confidential medical services in either the public or private sector.[43] The response to the AIDS hotline was even more dramatic. In the first 3 months of 1987, an average of 50,000 callers per month received taped messages and over 20,000 per month requested operator calls.[44] Knowing where to turn for STD treatment and AIDS information plays a crucial role in preventing both transmission and complications and is a major component of community education efforts.

In the future, those concerned with preventing STD need to make better use of the mass media to convey effective health promotion messages. Awareness of AIDS and herpes is widespread throughout the world largely because of the attention given these conditions by the media. In developed countries, teenagers are a special audience for the broadcast media; they spend an average of 23 hours a week listening to radio or watching television.

Messages should be aired to encourage condom use in high-risk settings or to publicize hotline numbers for further questions.[45] In developing countries, communication through radio is important. For instance, Uganda has 3 million radio sets (population of 16 million) and messages such as "love carefully" by the National AIDS Control Program and "love faithfully" by the Uganda Catholic Medical Bureau can be widely broadcasted (L Ochero, personal communication).

## DISEASE DETECTION

Early disease detection is crucial to STD intervention strategies.[46] Case-finding methods include clinical diagnosis based on symptoms and signs, confirmatory laboratory diagnostic testing in patients with symptoms or signs suggestive of an STD, targeted testing in individuals at high risk for having STD, broad screening without regard to likelihood of STD, and examination of sex partners of individuals with STD.

Accurate diagnosis is the intervention cornerstone for the early detection strategies of STD control. Whether for making specific diagnoses in those with symptoms, or for screening of persons without symptoms, diagnostic tests for STD should ideally be rapid, inexpensive, simple, and accurate. The usual considerations for assessing diagnostic techniques—sensitivity, specificity, and predictive value—have a slightly different interpretation for STD control than for screening of chronic conditions, largely because STD treatment is generally shorter and safer than therapy for other conditions.[47] Moreover, curing bacterial STD in one individual frequently prevents disease in others. Consequently, achieving high sensitivity by reducing false negatives takes on an increased importance because missed cases (1) place the infected person at continued risk of more serious complications and (2) result in further disease dissemination.

Achieving high specificity by reducing false positives is generally less important from the public health perspective when treatment is associated with minimal morbidity, cost, and inconvenience.[19] From the perspective of the individual "diagnosed" as having an STD, however, the human and emotional costs of erroneously stigmatizing anyone means specificity cannot be neglected. Also, the public health costs of interviewing and tracing large numbers of partners of patients with false-positive tests would drain limited STD resources.

Advances in laboratory techniques have led to most of the major initiatives in STD control. Serologic capabilities improved syphilis case finding,[48] and selective culture media allowed gonorrhea screening and diagnostic testing.[49] Development of more rapid and less expensive immunodiagnostic tests for chlamydia have stimulated guidelines for controlling these infections.[50] Finally, the availability of the HIV antibody tests has appropriately shifted the focus of public health efforts away from the surveillance of AIDS cases to the determination of the larger number of asymptomatic infected persons.[51]

## APPROPRIATE TREATMENT

Once the diagnosis is suspected, treatment should be inexpensive, simple, safe, and effective. Early and adequate treatment of patients and their sexual partners is an effective means of preventing the spread of STD in the community and STD complications in the individual. To promulgate successful treatment regimens for specific diagnoses, both the U.S. Public Health Service and the World Health Organization have established treatment recommendations as a standard part of their control strategy. Initially, these recommendations covered syphilis and gonorrhea, but during the 1980s they have expanded to include 18 other sexually transmitted organisms and syndromes.[52,53] Achieving consensus among groups of clinicians and public health physicians expert in STD therapy has proved a useful approach to establishing treatment guidelines which are applicable to diverse communities.

Selective prophylactic (preventive or epidemiological) treatment also has a major role in STD control strategies (Chap. 91). In certain instances, waiting to confirm the specific diagnosis prior to initiating therapy is inappropriate. Rather, based on epidemiological indications, antibiotics should be administered to high-risk individuals when the diagnosis is considered likely, even without clinical signs of infection and before proof of infection by laboratory methods.[54] Thus, selected groups of patients with a high likelihood of infection are identified by epidemiological analyses—usually because of history of exposure—and treated before confirmation of their infection status. This interrupts the chain of transmission and prevents complications which might occur between the time of testing and treatment, ensures treatment for infected individuals with false-negative laboratory tests, and guarantees treatment for those who might not return when notified of positive tests.

The benefits of this approach are generally thought to outweigh the costs of treating a percentage of uninfected persons, especially those exposed to gonorrhea, syphilis, or chlamydial infection. Most recently, this approach of selective preventive treatment has effectively limited outbreaks of PPNG and chancroid in metropolitan areas.[55,56] The same philosophy underlies the recommendation for giving tetracycline concurrently with penicillin to patients with confirmed gonococcal infection, since a relatively high proportion are liable to be harboring coexistent *C. trachomatis*.[57,58]

## SEX PARTNER REFERRAL AND PATIENT COUNSELING

Traditionally, STD control programs have assumed, with some justification, that patients play relatively passive roles in disease control and prevention (Chap. 91). Reluctance to confront one's sex partner with sexual transgressions is part of the human condition. Thus, efforts to identify and ensure treatment of sexual partners have emphasized active intervention by the health providers to interview the patient, to locate the named individuals, and to assure that these individuals are evaluated and treated.[59] The privacy of the original patients and their sex partners is rigorously protected.[15,60] During recent years, however, this process of active intervention has been modified in many settings to include a more simplified approach. Instead of relying solely on the health worker, the patient is often encouraged to assume responsibility for locating and referring all of his or her sexual partners (Chap. 88).

This self-referral method actively involves patients in the disease control effort, is inexpensive, is normally acceptable to patients, and reserves scarce staff time for other activities.[61] Potential shortcomings of patient referral methods, however, include: (1) limited effectiveness, (2) difficulty in evaluating its outcomes, and (3) nonproductivity with noncompliant patients.

Under most circumstances, some form of simplified self-referral of partners will be among the most cost-beneficial approaches to STD control. More active control tracing by the health provider is more expensive; therefore, this system is increasingly being restricted to high-yield cases or to high-risk "core" environments (Chap. 89).[29,62] Special situations where this more costly strategy has been useful include: (1) introduction of a serious disease (e.g., syphilis or PPNG infection) into a community previously unaffected; (2) men and women with repeated STD infections; (3) female consorts of infectious syphilis cases; and (4) STD infections in children.

A further shift in this disease-control strategy focuses on counseling (e.g., educating) patients to facilitate changes in their behavior (Chap. 88). The traditional focus on partner tracing—assurance that sexual partners are brought to treatment—has been expanded to encourage changing patient behaviors. The behaviors sought include: (1) responding to disease suspicion by promptly seeking appropriate medical evaluation, (2) taking medications as directed, (3) returning for follow-up tests, (4) assuring examination of sexual partners, (5) avoiding sexual exposure while infectious, and (6) preventing exposure by using protection in high-risk settings. In light of the HIV epidemic, these behavioral messages have taken on a new urgency; their evaluation and refinement may lead to improved knowledge regarding behavior-modification approaches.

## STD CLINICAL SERVICES

Adequate clinical management of patients and their partners is still the most effective measure for STD control. However, clinical services vary widely in different settings and are often inadequate at providing appropriate care for patients with STD (Chap. 87). Whether patient care is provided by experts at special STD clinics with sophisticated laboratory support or by primary clinicians with limited laboratory facilities (Chap. 93), the objectives of clinical management are the same: (1) to determine the most likely etiology of the patient's complaint, (2) to provide appropriate treatment for that condition, (3) to detect other STD, (4) to ensure patient follow-up for test of cure after treatment, (5) to manage properly those patients who failed treatment, (6) to educate patients to reduce their risk of further disease acquisition or transmission and to return if symptoms recur, and (7) to encourage identifiable sexual partners to attend for appropriate evaluation and treatment. Thus, all key STD control strategies are contained in the microcosm of providing clinical services.

Public STD facilities are relegated to a lower-class status in most countries. Recent control efforts have sought to upgrade the physical appearance and the patient capacity, to improve the utilization of clinic facilities, and to improve patient care within these clinics.[63] For example, a type of time management known as patient flow analysis may lead to more efficient use of existing staff resources.[64] A redistribution of room use may provide greater privacy for patients during interviews and examination. Hours of clinic operation should include evening or early morning hours to improve services for employed patients.

Some countries have a well-established network of public clinics that integrate the various aspects of good patient management, such as diagnosis, treatment and counseling, contact tracing, and health education, and regularly provide health authorities with data on STD incidence and on patient characteristics.[1,4]

The content of clinical care is an important determinant of outcome. Because the STD field has become so complex, clinical services benefit from systematic approaches. To assist midlevel practitioners (e.g., physician's assistants and nurse practitioners) as well as physicians in training in making diagnoses and providing adequate treatment, standardized patient management protocols have been widely used in the developed and developing worlds.[5,11,65] These protocols summarize typical clinical presentations, criteria for diagnosis, appropriate treatment recommendations, and practical prevention points. They are useful in both public and private health care settings.[66]

## INTERVENTION STRATEGIES—SUPPORT COMPONENTS

### MEDICAL TRAINING

Medical schools throughout the world have been slow to respond to the increasing magnitude of the STD problem. For example, in 1980, less than one in six American medical schools had a specific STD clinic available for STD training.[67] Moreover, during the past 15 years, clinical instruction in STD in United States medical schools had apparently declined, averaging less than 1 hour per student in 1980. A survey conducted in 1985 showed some improvement, but still only one in five medical schools provided even half its students with STD clinical training.[68] Paradoxically, this occurred just when American physicians need STD training the most; the majority enter specialties requiring knowledge of STD diagnosis and treatment. In 1987, nearly two-thirds of first-year residents chose such STD-related specialties as internal medicine, pediatrics, obstetrics and gynecology, family practice, emergency medicine, and dermatology.[69,70] Without training in STD problems, the medical community cannot be effectively mobilized to support control programs.

Thus, an integral part of recent STD control strategies has been to train health care providers in the rapidly changing field of STD. This training must involve all specialties affecting STD control—clinicians, laboratory workers, managers, field investigators, and health educators. For each group, both formal education systems and ongoing inservice training opportunities are essential.

The training initiatives have taken several approaches. To respond to immediate needs, clinical guidelines were developed to assist STD facilities to improve patient management.[63] National and international STD treatment recommendations are regularly updated to reflect changing diagnostic capabilities, antibiotic susceptibilities, and pharmacological innovations.[52,53]

To create a cadre of medically qualified clinicians who have a career commitment to the STD discipline, interest in this field must be developed early during clinical training. These individuals could subsequently establish their own STD academic programs, thus multiplying the effect of the training efforts.

Physicians interested in STD will need to complement their traditional diagnostic and therapeutic skills with training in additional sciences—psychology, sociology, and epidemiology. Regarding psychosocial training, the increasing emphasis on behavioral factors in STD control is part of the general growing awareness in medicine of the importance of behavior in both producing and preventing disease.[71] The role of lifestyle in STD is obvious; the transition from curable bacterial STD to incurable viral STD makes it particularly important that physicians shift their emphasis toward education of individuals to voluntarily modify their behavior.

### MANAGERIAL TRAINING

Administration of a comprehensive STD control program frequently benefits from management skills. In the United States, STD managers often begin as case workers at the clinic and in the community—interviewing and counseling patients, locating individuals, and motivating them to seek examination and/or treatment. After several years' experience, they generally become supervisors of STD programs in states or major cities with high STD morbidity. Thus, a career system evolves which is capable of attracting skilled people with field experience into public health management.

To be effective, STD administrators have to rely on a spectrum of public and private health agencies to achieve their widening objectives.[72] Trained to coordinate activities among clinical, laboratory, and community institutions, the instinct for networking should be part of the STD specialist's fabric. Future efforts to control HIV will require communication with colleagues in drug treatment centers, mental health, maternal and child health, gynecology, occupational health, and other disciplines not traditionally aligned with communicable disease. This foundation will further broaden the knowledge necessary for both STD control and other fields of public health.

### RESEARCH

Both basic and applied research are crucial to STD control. Major changes in intervention strategy have accompanied the introduction of new antibiotics (e.g., penicillin), the development of better detection methods (e.g., selective enriched media for the isolation of *N. gonorrhoeae*), the identification of resistant organisms (e.g., PPNG), and the recognition of high-risk groups (e.g., homosexuals, patients with repeat infections, women with PID). Most STD research is supported by international and national research organizations, although an increasing amount is funded either by voluntary organizations concerned with the magnitude of the STD problem or by pharmaceutical firms or medical diagnostic companies aware of the potential market for diagnostic or therapeutic products for STD. STD control strategies will benefit from closer cooperation between those public and private groups conducting research. The limited resources available to study the expanding list of sexually transmitted organisms and syndromes require both focusing on those areas most likely to influence STD control and avoiding wasteful duplication of research efforts.[73] Moreover, only through close liaison among researchers will we determine if results gained under controlled laboratory settings can be transferred to real life field operations. The rapid transfer of the latest control technology from research circles to medical practice will depend on cooperation among the team of STD professionals.

### INFORMATION SYSTEMS

The supervisory and policy-making responsibilities of STD professionals demand that they become computer literate, since STD control programs have entered the computer age. To successfully carry out STD control responsibilities, programs must collect, collate, analyze, and utilize data from patient medical records, disease intervention documents, laboratory results, and treatment outcomes. When STD clinic record systems are manually maintained, such systems are cumbersome, often inefficient, and difficult to link. Records of services provided at one source may not be available to other nearby locations except by telephone.

Many countries, as resources permit, have installed computer systems to improve the operational capabilities of STD control programs. This allows more effective data processing for the three levels of STD control—at the local level for individual case management, at the regional level for overall program evaluation, and at the national level for comprehensive disease surveillance.

Use of computers for surveillance will allow STD control programs to expend resources more efficiently. By processing data quickly and analyzing disease trends, the program can identify outbreaks and commit resources to control them. Using epidemiologic skills, STD patterns can be broken down by time, place, and person. Therefore, target groups will be identified, and STD program priorities can be redirected so the resources are maximized. For example, recent syphilis increases in the United States have occurred primarily in heterosexual, minority, inner-city populations.[74]

## CONCLUSION

STD control programs have been, and will continue to be, at the cutting edge of public health management. Strategies to prevent transmission of organisms spread by intimate human contact must remain flexible to adapt to social, technical, clinical, financial, and political realities. Both basic STD control activities (health education, disease detection, appropriate treatment, partner notification, STD clinical services) and support components (medical training, managerial training, research, information systems) must be carefully integrated to achieve maximum effect. Strategic planning is a process which seeks to set priorities, identify weaknesses, and build on the strengths of existing STD control efforts. Over the next 5 years, the specter of HIV infection and AIDS will dominate the STD horizon. Interest in and resources committed to preventing AIDS will also provide a unique opportunity for STD officials to make further inroads on controlling the other STD.

# References


1 Morton RS: Control of sexually transmitted diseases today and tomorrow. *Genitourin Med* 63:202, 1987.
2 Cates W Jr: Epidemiology and control of sexually transmitted diseases: Strategic evolution. *Infect Dis Clin North Am* 1:1, 1987.
3 Horsburgh CR et al: Preventive strategies in sexually transmitted diseases for the primary care physician. *JAMA* 258:814, 1987.
4 Caterall RD: Education of physicians in the sexually transmitted diseases in the United Kingdom. *Br J Vener Dis* 52:97, 1976.
5 Meheus AZ: Practical approaches in developing nations, in *Sexually Transmitted Diseases*, KK Holmes et al (eds). New York, McGraw-Hill, 1984, p 998.
6 Meheus A, Piot P: Provision of services for sexually transmitted diseases in developing countries, in *Recent Advances in STD,* JD Oriel, JRW Harris (eds). Edinburgh, Churchill Livingston, 1986, pp 261–272.
7 Arya OP, Bennett FJ: Role of the medical auxiliary in the control of sexually transmitted diseases in a developing country. *Br J Vener Dis* 52:116, 1976.
8 Cates W Jr et al: Control of sexually transmitted disease: View from the United States. *Br J Vener Dis* 60:322, 1984.
9 The Gallup Organization: The New York poll. *New York Newsday*, June 16, 1987, p 1.
10 World Health Organization and Pan American Health Organization: *Control of Sexually Transmitted Diseases.* Geneva, Switzerland, World Health Organization, 1985.
11 World Health Organization: *WHO Expert Committee on Venereal Diseases and Treponematoses, Sixth Report.* Geneva, Switzerland, World Health Organization, 1986.
12 Barnes RC, Holmes KK: Epidemiology of gonorrhea—Current perspectives. *Epidemiol Rev* 6:1, 1984.
13 Zenilman JM et al: *Neisseria gonorrhoeae*: An old enemy rearms. *Infect Dis Med Let Obstet Gynecol* 7:2, 1986.
14 Schulz KF et al: Pregnancy loss infant death and suffering: The legacy of syphilis and gonorrhea in Africa. *Genitourin Med* 63:320, 1987.
15 Kaufman RE et al: Current trends in syphilis. *Public Health Rev* 3:175, 1974.
16 Cameron DW et al: Female to male heterosexual transmission of HIV infection in Nairobi (abstract MP91:25). III International Conference on AIDS, Washington, DC, 1987.
17 Greenblatt RM et al: Genital ulceration as a risk factor for human immunodeficiency virus infection in Kenya (abstract ThP68:174). III International Conference on AIDS, Washington, DC, 1987.
18 Potterat JJ: Does syphilis facilitate sexual acquisition of HIV? *JAMA* 258:473, 1987.
19 Cates W Jr, Holmes KK: Sexually transmitted diseases, in *Maxcy-Rosenau Public Health and Preventive Medicine*, 12 ed, JM Last, J Fielding, J Chin (eds). East Norwalk, CT, Appleton-Century-Crofts, 1986, p 257.
20 Washington AE et al: The economic cost of pelvic inflammatory disease. *JAMA* 255:1735, 1986.
21 Meheus A et al: Determinants of infertility in Africa. *Afr J Sex Transm Dis* 2:31, 1986.
22 Grimes DA: Deaths due to sexually transmitted diseases. *JAMA* 255:1727, 1986.
23 Cates W Jr: Priorities for sexually transmitted diseases in the late 1980s and beyond. *Sex Transm Dis* 13:114, 1986.
24 Hethcote HW, Yorke JA: *Gonorrhea Transmission Dynamics and Control.* Berlin, West Germany, Springer-Verlag, 1984.
25 Rothenberg RB: The geography of gonorrhea: Empirical demonstration of core group transmission. *Am J Epidemiol* 117: 688, 1983.
26 O'Reilly KR, Aral SO: Adolescents and sexual behavior. *J Adolesc Health Care* 6:262, 1985.
27 Brooks FG et al: Repeated gonorrhea: An analysis of importance and risk factors. *J Infect Dis* 137:161, 1978.
28 Alvarez-Dardet C, Marquez S, Perera EJ: Urban clusters of sexually transmitted diseases in the City of Seville, Spain. *Sex Transm Dis* 12:166, 1985.
29 Potterat JJ et al: Gonorrhea in street prostitutes: Epidemiologic and legal implications. *Sex Transm Dis* 6:58, 1979.
30 Coutinho RA et al: Influence of special surveillance programmes and AIDS on declining incidence of syphilis in Amsterdam. *Genitourin Med* 63:210, 1987.
31 Brandt AM: *No Magic Bullet: A Social History of Venereal Disease in the United States since 1880.* New York, Oxford University Press, 1985.
32 Aral SO et al: Genital herpes: Does knowledge lead to action? *Am J Public Health* 75:69, 1985.
33 Judson FN: Fear of AIDS and gonorrhea rates in homosexual men. *Lancet* ii:159, 1983.
34 Handsfield HH: Decreasing incidence of gonorrhea in homosexually active men—Minimal effect on risk of AIDS. *West J Med* 143:469, 1985.
35 Schultz S et al: Declining rates of rectal and pharyngeal gonorrhea among males—New York City. *MMWR* 33:295, 1984.
36 Carne CA et al: Prevalence of antibodies to human immunodeficiency virus, gonorrhea rates and changed sexual behavior in London. *Lancet* i:656, 1987.
37 Solomon MZ, DeJong W: Recent sexually transmitted disease prevention efforts and their implications for AIDS health education. *Health Ed Q* 13:301, 1986.
38 World Health Organization: Sex and family planning: How we teach the young. *Report on a study by B. Lewin. Public Health in Europe No. 23*, Regional Office for Europe, Copenhagen, 1984, p 170.
39 Koop E: *The Surgeon General's Report on AIDS.* Washington, DC, US Public Health Service, 1986.

40 Kroger F, Yarber WL: STD content in school health textbooks: An evaluation using the worth assessment procedure. *J School Health* 54:41, 1984.
41 Yarber WL: *STD: A Guide for Young Adults.* Reston, VA, American Alliance for Health, Physical Education, Recreation, and Dance, 1985.
42 *Sunday Nation.* Sex education: A ten-tenths cure. Nairobi, August 20, 1978.
43 Division of Sexually Transmitted Diseases, Centers for Disease Control: *Annual Report 1986.* Atlanta, GA, December 10, 1986.
44 Rosenberg MJ et al: What the public wants to know: The national AIDS hotline (abstract T6.3:56). III International Conference on AIDS, Washington, DC, 1987.
45 Greydanus DE: Should the media advertise contraceptives? *Am J Dis Child* 135:687, 1981.
46 Henderson RH: Control of sexually transmitted diseases in the United States—A federal perspective. *Br J Vener Dis* 53:211, 1977.
47 Hart G: Role of preventive methods in the control of venereal disease. *Clin Obstet Gynecol* 18:243, 1975.
48 Baumgartner L et al: *The eradication of syphilis. A task force report.* Washington, DC, Department of Health, Education, and Welfare, 1962.
49 Brown ST, Wiesner PJ: Problems and approaches to the control and surveillance of sexually transmitted agents associated with pelvic inflammatory disease in the United States. *Am J Obstet Gynecol* 138:1096, 1980.
50 Centers for Disease Control: Chlamydia trachomatis Infections: Policy Guidelines for Prevention and Control. *MMWR* 34(suppl no. 35), 1985.
51 Curran JW et al: The epidemiology of AIDS: Current status and future prospects. *Science* 229:1352, 1985.
52 Centers for Disease Control: 1985 STD Treatment Guidelines. *MMWR* 34(suppl no. 45), 1985.
53 World Health Organization: Unpublished WHO document DDT/83.433. Geneva, Switzerland, World Health Organization, 1983.
54 Hart G: Epidemiologic treatment for syphilis and gonorrhea. *Sex Transm Dis* 7:149, 1980.
55 Handsfield HH et al: Epidemiology of penicillinase-producing *Neisseria gonorrhoeae* infections, analysis by auxotyping and serogrouping. *N Engl J Med* 306:950, 1982.
56 Blackmore CA et al: An outbreak of chancroid in Orange County, California: Descriptive epidemiology and disease-control measures. *J Infect Dis* 151:840, 1985.
57 Stamm WE et al: Effect of treatment regimens for *Neisseria gonorrhoeae* on simultaneous infection with *Chlamydia trachomatis.* *N Engl J Med* 310:545, 1984.
58 Washington AE et al: Cost-effectiveness of combined treatment for endocervical gonorrhea. *JAMA* 257:2056, 1987.
59 Ennes H, Bennett TG: The contact-education interview: Its functions, principles, and techniques in venereal disease contact investigation. *Am J Syph Vener Dis* 29:647, 1945.
60 Fichtner RR et al: Syphilis in the United States, 1967–1979. *Sex Transm Dis* 10:77, 1983.
61 Potterat JJ, Rothenberg RB: The casefinding effectiveness of a self-referral system for gonorrhea: A preliminary report. *Am J Public Health* 67:174, 1977.
62 Rothenberg RB: The geography of syphilis: A demonstration of epidemiologic diversity, in *Advances in Sexually Transmitted Diseases, Diagnosis and Treatment*, R Morrisett, E Kourstak (eds). Utrecht, The Netherlands, VNU Sciences Press, 1986, p 125.
63 Centers for Disease Control: *Quality Assurance Guidelines for STD Clinics—1986.* Atlanta, Georgia, Centers for Disease Control, 1986.
64 Graves JL et al: Computerized patient flow analysis of local family planning clinics. *Fam Plann Perspect* 13:164, 1981.
65 Spagna VA, Prior RB: *Sexually Transmitted Disease: A Clinical Syndrome Approach.* New York, Marcel Dekker, 1985.
66 World Health Organization: Simplified approaches for sexually transmitted diseases (STD) control at the primary health care (PHC) level. Unpublished WHO Document WHO/VDT/85.437 (1985).
67 Stamm WE et al: Clinical training in venereology in the United States and Canada. *JAMA* 248:2020, 1982.
68 Guinan ME: Survey of states regarding STD training in medical schools, 1985, in *Dear Colleague Letter*, W Cates Jr., October 1, 1986.
69 Rosenblatt RA et al: The content of ambulatory medical care in the United States. *N Engl J Med* 309:892, 1983.
70 American Medical Association: Medical education in the United States, 1986–1987. *JAMA* 258:1034, 1987.
71 Relman AS: Encouraging the practice of preventive medicine and health promotion. *Public Health Rep* 97:216, 1982.
72 Rowe MJ, Ryan CC: *AIDS—A Public Health Challenge (State Issues, Policies, and Programs).* Washington, DC, Intergovernmental Health Policy Project, 1987.
73 National Institute of Allergy and Infectious Diseases: Sexually Transmitted Diseases: 1986 NIAID Study Group Summary and Recommendations. Washington, DC, National Institutes of Health, 1987.
74 Centers for Disease Control: Increases in primary and secondary syphilis—United States. *MMWR* 36:393, 1987.

# Chapter 85

# Evaluation of sexually transmitted diseases control programs in industrialized countries

Gavin Hart
Michael W. Adler
Andrzej Stapinski
Tomasz F. Mroczkowski
Paul J. Wiesner

## INTRODUCTION

International experts formulated a framework for developing and evaluating STD control programs.[1] This framework was adopted in Chap. 84 to depict strategies for development of STD control. We also will use it to critically evaluate current STD control programs in industrialized countries. Optimal control programs do not exist. Current programs can be evaluated in terms of planning, intervention strategies, support components, and implementation (Table 85-1).

Our intent is to provide examples of program evaluation by comparing programs in several countries using similar criteria whenever possible.

## COMPARING CONTROL PROGRAMS

By any criteria, comparing STD control programs in different countries is severely limited. Even among countries with similar affluence and lifestyle, enormous variation exists in the background against which STDs occur and are managed. For instance, the organization and funding of health services are very different in the United States, United Kingdom, and Poland. In some countries, ethnic minorities may have a dominant influence on STD control; these populations may have a totally different living environment and interaction with health services than the majority of the population (e.g., rural aborigines in Australia and illegal immigrants in the southern United States). Differences within large countries may be so great that presenting a national description is misleading.

Few countries have documented their STD programs, and even fewer document the detail adequate for the foregoing framework. Documented descriptive accounts are often oversimplified and minimize inadequacies within a system. The perspective of a national leader or central office professional may be different from that of regional staff or front-line workers. The adequacy of a system may be viewed differently by doctors, paramedical staff, or the clients using the system.

Finally, STD programs change over time. This is particularly true at the present because a global epidemic of HIV infection has altered public perceptions of STD, reinvigorated some programs, and almost decimated others.

Against this background of subjectivity, few published evaluations have provided objective outcome measures of program performance. In recent years, quality control within laboratories and evaluation of clinical processes have provided valuable information, but assessment of field activities and disease transmission within general populations is more difficult.

Notwithstanding these difficulties, we have assembled information from the published literature and personal communication on several countries to which we have had greatest access: Australia, Poland, United Kingdom, and United States. For each of these countries, we discuss the available information on the resources allocated to STD control, the measures of morbidity, and the current STD control program.

Proper management of a program ensures that its objectives are achieved. Evaluation of program processes should also be undertaken. Adequate evaluation which compares actual outcomes with the intended objectives is rarely undertaken.

**Table 85-1. Framework for Evaluating STD Control Programs[1]**

I. Planning:
  A. Estimating the importance of STDs
  B. Establishing priorities
  C. Considering sociologic factors
II. Intervening:
  A. Decreasing risky sexual exposure
  B. Preventing infection by prophylaxis
  C. Detecting and curing infections
  D. Limiting complications through:
    1. Health promotion
    2. Disease detection
    3. Treatment programs
    4. Counseling and contact tracing
III. Support components:
  A. Specialized centers
  B. Information systems
  C. Professional training
  D. Laboratory services
IV. Implementation

## AUSTRALIA

### BACKGROUND

In Australia, STD control programs are operated by individual states with minimal federal coordination. The state programs are similar; this description focuses on South Australia unless otherwise specified. In 1984/1985, Australia spent 7.2 percent of the gross domestic product on health. In South Australia, 1 percent of the health budget was spent on public health and 4.3 percent of that was spent on STD control[2] (Table 85-2).

In 1985, syphilis and gonorrhea rates were 15.8 per 100,000 and 48 per 100,000, respectively. However, over 75 percent of syphilis occurs in rural aborigines, who comprise less than 2 percent of the total population. Although not quantified, cases of congenital syphilis occur every year. Pelvic inflammatory disease (PID) is perceived as a major problem by venereologists throughout Australia, but its importance is not appreciated by other health professionals or the general public. The actual impact of PID on Australian society has not been quantified. One report

**Table 85-2. Comparative Information for Evaluation of STD Control in Selected Countries**

| | Australia | Poland | United Kingdom | United States |
|---|---|---|---|---|
| Estimated proportion GNP* for health expenditures | 0.07 | 0.02 | 0.07 | 0.11 |
| Crude estimate† GNP for STD care and control | 0.00003 | 0.00002 | ? | 0.00003 |
| Reported rates (per 100,000): | | | | |
| Gonorrhea | 48 | 20 | 142 | 400 |
| Early syphilis | 16 | 3.2 | 1.8 | 12 |

*GNP = gross national product.

†Estimates use data available prior to large increases for expenditures for HIV infections (see text).

suggests that ectopic pregnancy has doubled between 1971 and 1980, in association with a similar increase in STDs in women.[3]

Over 1000 AIDS cases had been reported in Australia by October 1988. Sixty percent of cases occurred in Sidney, and 90 percent of these arose from homosexual activity. In South Australia, 70 percent of diagnosed HIV infections have resulted from homosexual activity and 20 percent from intravenous-drug use.

## PLANNING

No adequate studies have quantified the impact of STDs on the general population. As noted above, the aboriginal population has accounted for most cases of syphilis, with documented incidence rates up to 23 percent per year in some communities and up to 60 percent per year in some age groups.[4] Donovanosis and gonorrhea[5] are also common among aborigines. Homosexual behavior is another major risk indicator, being associated with increased rates of syphilis, gonorrhea, and AIDS. Most cases of the other STDs occur in a large and less well-defined segment of the population, with the majority being unmarried and aged 15 to 25.

The general Australian population has a relatively high health awareness and compliance. Most individuals with STD present within a few days of the development of symptoms, follow-up rates are over 70 percent, and compliance with therapy is usual. Individuals increasingly request screening following unprotected intercourse with new partners. In contrast, the health service interaction with many rural aborigines and drug users is less positive. Because of cultural and lifestyle factors, most STDs in rural aborigines are detected through screening instigated by the health service; adequate follow-up occurs in a minority of cases.

Health service delivery to aborigines has been improved in the past decade[6] by the appointment of community-based aboriginal health workers and by extensive involvement with community leaders. These initiatives have primarily benefited time-limited efforts such as communitywide screening but have been less effective in improving day-to-day health care delivery. Targeted clinical and counseling services have also been organized by homosexual professionals and are generally acceptable to the homosexual community.

## INTERVENTION STRATEGIES

Providing clinical services is the main intervention strategy. Although most STDs are probably managed at government-run clinics, private practitioners see large numbers of patients. Clinic facilities have been generally mediocre, and recruiting adequate staff at all levels has been difficult. In recent years, new clinics have been commissioned in two states, and staffing has improved.

Negligible resources have been allocated to health promotion activities. Patient information pamphlets are provided to clinic patients, and this service has been expanded to private practitioners through the auspices of a local pharmaceutical company. Occasional seminars are conducted for high school students and nurses. STD services have been highlighted in television documentaries, but no organized public information programs exist. Recently a sexual health toll-free hotline has been established for disseminating information to the public.

Case finding is the major disease-detection process in urban areas. Large screening programs for syphilis have been undertaken in rural aboriginal communities, and all aborigines over 15 have been screened at least once (and many several times) in three states. Antenatal screening of nonaboriginal women is universal, and congenital syphilis virtually never occurs. Aboriginal screening programs aim to test women twice in pregnancy, but breakdown in this system, even in city hospitals, results in regular cases of congenital syphilis.

A national treatment program does not exist, but each state has treatment regimens fairly similar to those of the Centers for Disease Control. A handbook for medical students produced by the National Health and Medical Research Council provides guidelines for national uniformity.[7]

Partner notification and counseling services associated with specialized STD centers are available for both clinic patients and those seen by private practitioners. Unfortunately, this staff is usually provided with inadequate training and support; moreover, the systems used have never been adequately evaluated. Active provider referral focuses on syphilis and gonorrhea, although investigation of steady partners of those with chlamydia infection, warts, and trichomoniasis can occur.

In Australia, the major problems related to HIV infection control are service organization and confidential testing. In most states HIV programs are fully integrated with general STD services, which facilitates both efficiency and effectiveness. Strong opposition to confidential testing by some community lobby groups has hindered the control of HIV infection.

## SUPPORT COMPONENTS

A specialized STD central clinic provides a statewide coordinating role. An operations manual covering all aspects of STD control provides guidelines for STD clinic operations as well as for other types of clinics and private practitioners throughout the state. Patient information handouts are also provided for these other clinical facilities. This center is also the focus for all information and training activities.

Both a laboratory and medical notification system exists for gonorrhea, syphilis, and chlamydia. The purpose of the laboratory system is to monitor medical notification and to contact the attending doctor rapidly when such notification is not forthcoming. By this mechanism, complete ascertainment of cases diagnosed through laboratory services occurs. A few doctors (who may see substantial numbers of patients) avoid the notification system by not using laboratory services.

A small group of private practitioners participate in a sentinel surveillance system monitoring 12 diseases each year, and other STDs have been assessed on an annual basis within this system. Only two laboratories perform diagnostic tests for chlamydia, enabling simple monitoring of chlamydia screening activity and yield.

A computerized clinic case record system (STD Clinic Resource Utilization System) commenced in 1987 and provides a detailed analysis of test performance, screening yields, and other process data from clinic patients. The partner notification system is computerized (Syphilis, Chlamydia, and Gonorrhea Surveillance System), enabling further evaluation of process measures. Statistics on AIDS are compiled from compulsory notifications whereas a computerized system (Systematic Inventory of Diagnosed Aids-carriers) is used for informally compiling a data base on HIV infection. Unfortunately guidelines for diagnosing and reporting gonorrhea and syphilis differ among the states, and have changed over time.

Professional training has always been suboptimal. Undergraduate training comprises seminars and practical experience for final year students. In the past, no postgraduate training has been available in Australia; thus many practitioners obtain the venereology diploma in England. Few STD practitioners in Australia have relevant specialist qualifications. A Master of Medicine course in venereology commenced at the University of Sydney in 1987, and venereology training as a component of an MPH program is proposed in Adelaide. No adequate training exists for STD case workers and counselors. They often have a nursing or social work background and are given introductory instruction on an individual program basis.

Laboratory services are provided by the microbiology laboratory associated with the STD clinic, as well as several large government and private laboratories. The Australian gonococcal surveillance program monitors antibiotic sensitivity throughout the states and facilitates exchange of information about gonococcal laboratory techniques by workers throughout Australia. No formal proficiency testing program exists, although the serology section of the major government laboratory had participated in the Centers for Disease Control program for many years. Considerable variation occurs in the serology results of different laboratories.

### IMPLEMENTATION

Because of limited resources, the STD control emphasis has been placed on providing a major clinic in each state, with little planned intervention on a population basis. General practitioner liaison and rudimentary partner notification/counseling services have been the major focus of extra clinic activities. No adequate evaluation of the control process has been documented.

Beginning in the mid-1970s, intensive syphilis control programs were initiated among rural aborigines in three states. This strategy, involving repeated annual screening of the total population, public relations activities, and management guidelines for all levels of health workers, reduced the prevalence of syphilis and prevented any transmission in one community for one year.[4] However, owing to limited resources, this strategy could not be sustained and has been replaced by one emphasizing antenatal screening and testing through the primary health care system.

## POLAND

### BACKGROUND

In Poland, free medical care is provided to every citizen in a socialized health care system. In response to alarmingly high rates of early syphilis and gonorrhea, the Institute of Venereology was established within the Warsaw Medical Academy in 1969 and given nationwide responsibility for STD control in the country. By 1986, the rate of early symptomatic syphilis fell to 3.1 per 100,000 (6 percent of the 1969 rate) as did the gonorrhea rate to 26.5 per 100,000 (18 percent of the 1969 rate). These changes have probably resulted from a comprehensive multidirectional STD control program. By November 1988, 83 cases of AIDS (and 3 deaths) were recorded in Poland.

In 1986, 2 percent of the gross national income in Poland was spent on health care. Based on consultation with several provincial STD clinic directors, we estimate that less than 0.1 percent of the total health care expenditure is spent on STDs.

Poland has 575 dermatovenereologic outpatient clinics; forty-nine are at the provincial level and the remainder at the local level. The provincial clinics are responsible for collection of epidemiologic data on STDs, quality assurance of the clinical care, and STD education. These clinics report quarterly to the Institute of Venereology on the number of cases of syphilis and gonorrhea and, since 1979, nongonococcal urethritis. The vast majority of STD patients are treated in public clinics and hospitals; private practice is a small percentage of all health care services.

No separate STD speciality exists in Poland. Clinic physicians are either first- or second-degree specialists of dermatovenereology or residents in training for this specialty. Generally, patients with both skin and STD problems are seen by the same physicians at the same clinic.

### PLANNING

Statistical data from Poland are considered accurate; however, an unknown proportion of cases go unreported. No formal cost-benefit studies from Poland have been conducted. Because of the sizable decrease in the rates of reportable STDs, it has been increasingly difficult to sustain attention to the STD problem by either local medical authorities or the general public. Thus, adequate resources to conduct an optimal program have been hard to obtain. However, recently, concern for the viral STDs (HSV, HPV), and the appearance of HIV infections, has resulted in increased funding.

Since the beginning of the program, specific populations have been identified as the risk groups for certain STDs. Syphilis and gonorrhea have been more common in the urban population, among unmarried people in the 19 to 25 age range,[8,9] and among prostitutes.[10] NGU appears to occur most often in men of the 25 to 30 age group. The male with NGU is more likely to be married and better educated than the male with gonorrhea.[11,12]

Alcohol abuse is thought to be an important factor stimulating promiscuity and increasing the risk of acquiring STDs.[8] Recently, homosexuals and drug abusers have been recognized as risk groups, not only for AIDS but also for other STDs; they have been the subject of recently introduced screening programs for various STDs.

## INTERVENTION STRATEGIES

Five major interventions (quality assurance of clinical services, contact tracing, screening of prostitutes, focused screening of specific populations, and health education) have been in place with varying emphasis since 1969.[13] Formal evaluations of each intervention differed in degree and clustered in the 1970s. The backbone of the national control continues to be the network of clinics.

A sample of the clinics underwent sociomedical evaluation[14] and were found by both former patients and people who have never had STDs to be acceptable. The existing network of clinics, though sufficient in number, has areas for improvement. While clinic hours seem plentiful, facilities vary a great deal—from well-equipped ones, located in modern buildings, to poorly equipped clinics in buildings requiring modernization. More than a third of the clinics have difficulties in recruiting highly qualified staff, and although the total number of dermatovenereologists working in Poland is probably adequate, their distribution is uneven.

STD education is an important element of the control program in Poland, but few data examine its effectiveness. Health promotion has been conducted among all social groups, with an emphasis on young people (Fig. 85-1). Surveys of knowledge of STDs among different segments of the society helped direct the development of appropriate educational materials.[15,16]

In 1972, 13.5 million copies of printed material were distributed free of charge by the Institute of Venereology. In recent years, owing to budget cuts and lower demand, the annual number of copies distributed ranged from 3 to 4 million. The institute has also produced and distributed 15 (20-min) movies and 50 animated cartoons (1 to 2 min) on STDs for use in movie theaters before the projection of the feature movie, a series of slides and audiocassettes for teachers or health educators, and a special STD and basic human sexuality educational manual for all school libraries. Every grammar school graduate is given a brochure containing information on STDs, including AIDS. In 1985, before the first case of HIV infection was detected in Poland, AIDS was included in the STD educational materials. The effectiveness of these different forms of STD health education has been difficult to evaluate.[15]

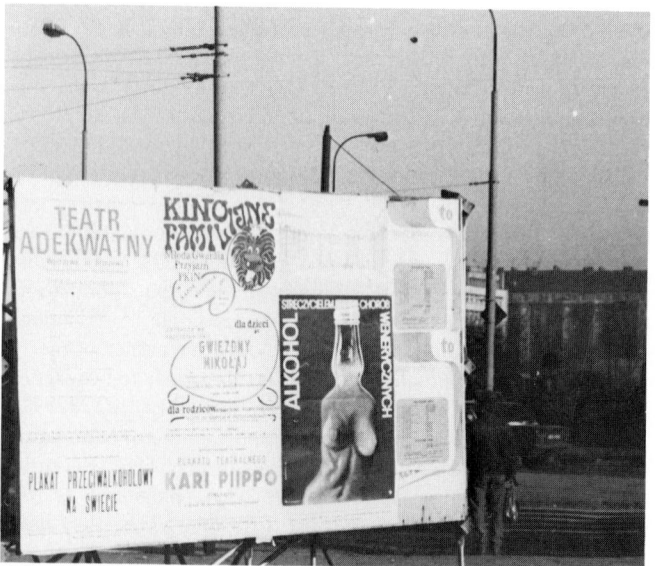


Fig. 85-1. Street poster in Warsaw stressing association between alcohol and STDs.

Mass screening for syphilis is common. The number of blood specimens tested increased from 3.7 million in 1969 to 9.8 million in 1986. About one-third of the population between 15 and 65 years of age is screened every year. Screening of selective groups was abandoned as being too complex and costly. Instead, syphilis serologic tests are performed on blood specimens obtained for other purposes: in all adult hospitalized patients, during the physical checkups of schoolchildren and students and periodic checkups among a variety of professions, pregnant women, blood donors, people applying for new jobs, army draftees, and persons under arrest. By this screening, about 40 percent of syphilis cases (mainly early latent and late latent syphilis) are detected each year. Formal cost-benefit analysis of screening has not been done.

Screening for gonorrhea is much less common. The Institute of Venereology has recommended that each woman between 15 and 65 years of age examined by a gynecologist in the health system should be tested for gonorrhea by culture. Many new laboratories have been established, existing ones have been better equipped, and many laboratory personnel have been trained to perform gonococcal cultures. Despite clear recommendations issued by the Ministry of Health, mass screening for gonorrhea in women has never materialized because gynecologists could not be convinced of its importance. It is unknown whether a more epidemiologically focused recommendation could have been followed.

Since 1987, several risk groups have been selected for mandatory HIV testing. These include prostitutes tested every 6 months, foreign students tested after first arrival to Poland, drug abusers known to medical authorities tested every 6 months, and blood donors. Homosexuals are strongly encouraged to obtain frequent HIV testing but there is no mandatory screening for them.

Pelvic inflammatory disease (PID) has not been well documented. Gynecologists do not often report cases and often do not perform bacteriological evaluations prior to the administration of antibiotics. Prostitution, particularly in big cities, has been an important factor influencing STD control. No special legal regulations restrict prostitution.[8] In several big cities, special clinics for prostitutes were established. Systematic screening and treatment of these women decreased the prevalence of gonorrhea from approximately 50 percent in 1970 to 18 percent in 1983, and the prevalence of syphilis from 18 percent to a fraction of a percent in the same time period.[8,10] Constant screening of prostitutes appears to be necessary to keep these STDs at a relatively low level.

Diagnostic and treatment methods are nationally standardized through the network of clinics. The Institute of Venereology has developed diagnostic, treatment, and follow-up guidelines which are periodically updated. Deviations from the recommendations are possible, but they have to be noted on the patient's chart with appropriate justification.

Detection of the source of infection through partner notification is inadequate. Interviewing, counseling, and partner notification services are the responsibility of the clinics. Because of a belief that patients will be open with physicians, physicians obtain the information about sexual partners. Trained clerks perform the basic field work of contacting and referring sexual partners for examination and treatment. The results have always been poor, and in 1986, the average number of partners named by patients was 0.84 for syphilis and 0.58 for gonorrhea. Epidemiological treatment is strongly recommended, is reportable, is commonly applied in both syphilis and gonorrhea, and is credited as a major factor in the reduction of disease.

The contribution of each of the five major interventions to the decline in STD morbidity in recent years is unknown.

## SUPPORT COMPONENTS

The Institute of Venereology in Warsaw is the central institution coordinating all STD control activities in Poland. It is supported by those medical academies that participate in STD research and training programs. The crucial role of the 49 provincial clinics cannot be overemphasized. Each provincial clinic monitors the quality of work in its local clinics and has a register office which verifies reported STD cases. Each provincial clinic is also responsible for partner notification within its territory and for notifying clinics in other provinces of partners outside its jurisdiction.

STD training for medical undergraduates is provided in all 11 medical academies. It consists of lectures, clinical, and abridged experience for the fourth-year student. Twenty hours out of 90 devoted to dermatovenereology is spent on STD teaching. Postgraduate training is provided by the Institute of Venereology and, to some extent, by other medical academies. During the 10-day STD update courses given by the institute, 70 to 120 dermatovenereology specialist residents are trained every year. The dermatovenereology specialty in Poland has two degrees. Postgraduate training of physicians in other specialties in STD, as well as training of nurses or other health care providers, is suboptimal. Special emphasis is being made with only limited success to train gynecologists in appropriate STD control.

Laboratory services are heavily invested in syphilis testing. The current policy gives preference to the large, well-equipped laboratories and elimination of the small ones. Testing for gonorrhea needs to be improved. The number of laboratories capable of performing cultures increased from 19 to 200 in recent years. Although they perform 350,000 cultures every year, many more could be performed. Infections caused by *Chlamydia trachomatis* can be identified by culture in four laboratories in the country; several others can identify chlamydia with the chlamydiazyme or direct immunofluorescence tests.

## IMPLEMENTATION

Sizable reduction in the incidence of syphilis and gonorrhea in Poland might indicate that all components have been successfully implemented. However, despite the existing antenatal screening for syphilis, about 10 cases of congenital syphilis are reported each year. Periodic review of skin and STD clinics reveals a variety of errors, e.g., poor specimen collection, inadequate testing for PID, poor partner identification, inadequate tracing, and delays in the reporting system. In summary, constant monitoring of the quality of work performed by the clinics, high-quality laboratory work, implementation of epidemiologic treatment, and mass screening for syphilis and gonorrhea appear to be key factors in the control of STDs in Poland. Balanced STD education has attempted to keep the public alerted.

## UNITED KINGDOM

## BACKGROUND

A universal National Health Service (NHS) has been in existence since 1948. However, even prior to this, a free and confidential service existed for sexually transmitted diseases (STDs). The magnitude and urgency of the health problems represented by these diseases gained enough recognition in the early part of the twentieth century for the government to set up a Royal Commission on the Venereal Diseases in 1916.[17] They recommended the establishment of an open-access medical service, but it was not really until the inception of the NHS in 1948 that a properly coordinated and comprehensive service came into being. Now 230 STD clinics exist in the United Kingdom. The specialty has been renamed Genito Urinary Medicine (GUM).

Currently 7 percent of the GNP is spent on the Health Service. Within this it is not possible to identify the amount spent on the control program for STDs. The workload in departments of GUM, expressed as total numbers of cases seen, has increased ever since 1916. For example, in the last 15 years the number of cases has risen threefold and now amounts to 702,000 new cases a year seen in the 230 departments. The most recent rates of reported syphilis and gonorrhea show a continuing decline, which first started in the late 1940s and 1970s, respectively. The rate for syphilis currently stands at 1.8 per 100,000 population and for gonorrhea at 142. Pelvic inflammatory disease (PID) continues to increase, and in England and Wales the number of cases of acute PID admitted to hospitals has doubled in the last 20 years. The only routine data on PID come from hospitals. The number of hospitalized cases in 1985 (latest available figures) reached 16,390. Physicians in GUM and gynecologists are the two major groups treating women with PID. Many of the patients with PID diagnosed in STD clinics are managed on an outpatient basis. At one central London clinic, 92 percent of women with PID were not hospitalized.[18] These outpatients do not appear in the routinely published figures for PID; thus the problem is substantially larger than suggested by the number of cases hospitalized per year.

Congenital syphilis is now rare. The latest figures (1986) showed a total of nine cases.

## PLANNING

All STD clinics report the number of cases seen per year by diagnoses and sex to the department of health. This allows for monitoring of trends over time. United Kingdom data on the national incidence of the whole range of STD are probably the most complete and accurate available internationally. Within the United Kingdom, most patients with STD symptoms will consult one of the 230 specialized clinics, as a result of either self-referral or partner notification action. However, patients could still choose to be seen outside the clinic service by their general practitioner (primary care physician) or by a private practitioner. Other agencies could be used by women, such as family planning, antenatal, and gynecology clinics. Unfortunately, the United Kingdom has no requirement that doctors seeing patients with an STD outside a clinic must report cases.

In the past, surveys have been carried out in gynecology, antenatal, and family planning clinics to provide crude estimates of the prevalence of certain STDs. These studies were limited to specific age groups and those who had opted to seek medical care. To some extent the varying rates reported in these types of studies reflect these demographic and consulting differences and not "true" differences in disease prevalence. Since the women studied represented only one part of the total population at risk of contracting an STD, the findings could not be related to a defined population at risk and correct incidence or prevalence rates could not be obtained. An attempt has been made to overcome these problems by population-based studies that attempt to identify asymptomatic and symptomatic patients and those seeking care as well as those not doing so. Such an approach has shown that the proportion of women with infections such as gonorrhea not receiving care in the United Kingdom is low.[19]

## INTERVENTION STRATEGIES

The major platform for STD control has been through the network of 230 clinics mentioned previously. Currently 120 consultant physicians staff these clinics in the United Kingdom. These clinics are all attached to hospitals and are part of the National Health Service (NHS).[20] Patients can walk in off the street and refer themselves. This direct access reduces delays and hopefully makes it easier for patients to be seen. Thus, patients pay no fee to the physician and, unlike in other sectors of the NHS, the patient does not make any contribution toward drugs prescribed. The STD clinical services are also provided free of charge to visitors from abroad.

The physicians in charge of the clinics are fully trained in venereology (genitourinary medicine). Other junior medical staff work in the clinics, and each clinic also employs trained nurses, health advisers (to notify partners), and clerical staff.

This system appears to be sophisticated and is often used as a model for other countries. However, good as it undoubtedly is, little is known about how it actually functions and how the quality of service varies throughout the United Kingdom. For example, we have little idea of what processes are used in achieving any given diagnosis or what criteria are used to notify the Department of Health. Moreover, unlike the United States, no firm guidelines exist concerning diagnostic procedures and treatment schedules.

A survey in England and Wales was carried out to evaluate the existing clinic system.[21–27] The study was designed to collect information on the diagnostic and reporting criteria used by consultants in charge of clinics and to compare current treatment and management policies. It was hoped that the survey findings would allow individual clinicians to judge their own practices and standards against those of their peers and would provide the basis for the development of an improved and, possibly, a more rational service. Information was sought on clinic facilities and on the diagnostic, treatment, and reporting criteria in use for a number of different diseases.

The survey of STD clinics indicated that facilities and diagnostic tests were not always used in an optimal way. For example, in some clinics serological tests for syphilis were carried out singly or in inappropriate combinations, were not repeated at all, or were repeated within 3 months of the patient's initial exposure. Some physicians were not taking samples from the correct anatomic sites or carrying out the appropriate tests to establish a diagnosis, whereas others were carrying out unnecessary tests. Wide discrepancies existed in the criteria used both to make positive diagnosis of various diseases and also to report them. Finally, the treatment of patients for a given disease varied throughout England and Wales and was often inappropriate. For example, 17 different routine treatment schedules were used for male patients with gonorrhea, and 15 for female patients. Some antibiotics were not appropriate, and the dosage for some of the efficacious preparations was inadequate.

Genitourinary medicine is a medical specialty in its own right. Physicians specializing in this branch of medicine initially need 3 years of training in general medicine after registration.[28] After this, they embark on their specialist training within a formal department of genitourinary medicine attached to a medical school and associated teaching hospital. This specialist training may last up to 4 years, after which the individual would be in a position to run his or her own department. Genitourinary medicine in the United Kingdom has been a Cinderella specialty, which to some extent has been reflected in the quality of entrants to the specialty and the lack of political influence for change from within its own ranks. This has started to change within the last decade. The specter of infection with human papilloma virus and human immunodeficiency virus (HIV) has greatly speeded up this process.

The British government has realized the need to control HIV infection and AIDS through STD control programs. They have made special financial allocations, mainly within London, to STD clinics with a heavy load of HIV. While current resources are not enough to modernize the whole GUM service in the manner required, recent increases do provide a unique opportunity to achieve major developments in controlling all STDs, including HIV.

Within clinics, support services are provided by trained nurses of both sexes, laboratory staff, health advisers, clerical staff, and, increasingly, clinical psychologists for HIV infection and AIDS. Partner notification is conducted by health advisers working within each clinic and responsible to the consultant in charge. Workers are selected on the basis of personality, maturity, and at least 3 years of training in a related discipline such as nursing or social studies.[29]

The activities of health advisers in STD include partner notification, record keeping, education of individual patients about their disease, educating other health workers, provision of social guidance to patients, and professional liaison both within the clinic and with health advisers in other clinics.

Health education on a national basis is the responsibility of the Health Education Authority (HEA), previously called the Health Education Council. It produces a range of pamphlets and educational materials on STDs for the general public. Concern about the AIDS epidemic has overcome the rather ambivalent approach toward STD education. Changes have been dramatic, and the British public has received extensive and explicit information about AIDS. For example, every household in the United Kingdom received a pamphlet about the disease at the beginning of 1987, and the public is regularly shown detailed instructions on how to use condoms on their television screens.

## SUPPORT COMPONENTS

The larger, more modern clinics serve as a general model for others. All clinics are supported by laboratories either on site or elsewhere within the hospital. Verification of serology and cultures can be obtained at reference laboratories. The specialty has its own learned society—the Medical Society for the Study of Venereal Diseases. Frequent meetings are held on a monthly basis from September to May. This, plus the production of the journal *Genitourinary Medicine*, allows for a regular exchange of information on both a formal and informal basis.

All medical undergraduates receive some training in the specialty. Unfortunately, as with clinic facilities and clinical management, this is variable. All 25 medical schools in the United

Kingdom teach undergraduates; the time devoted to the subject ranges from 10 to 24 h.[30] Specialist training has been mentioned previously. Research into the STDs is poorly developed. This is changing; the establishment of the first Professor of Genito Urinary Medicine at London's Middlesex Hospital Medical School in 1979, and the concern over AIDS, has infused STD research with heightened interest.

Postgraduate courses in the subjects are held once a year in Liverpool and twice in London. They last 3 months and are primarily intended for overseas graduates. The course is followed by a written and clinical examination and viva, following which the successful student is awarded a diploma. Six-month courses in STDs for qualified nurses are provided in three centers. They are primarily for nurses working in, and wishing to remain within, the specialty.

Health advisers in STD undertake a basic 5-day residential training course. They have their own society, the Society of Health Advisers in Sexually Transmitted Diseases, and hold an annual conference. A detailed manual provides guidelines for their work.[31]

## IMPLEMENTATION

The 1978 survey of United Kingdom STD facilities provided a detailed description of the processes involved in clinics throughout the country. As indicated earlier, the survey demonstrated suboptimal clinical practices involving specimen collection, diagnostic criteria, and treatment regimes. The possibility of conducting clinic audits has been discussed but not yet implemented.

## UNITED STATES

## BACKGROUND

The goal of STD control programs within the United States is to prevent the incidence and consequences of STD. Specific strategies are implemented in a complex interaction of governmental levels and private medical practice and in the absence, until recently, of a dominant professional discipline primarily devoted to STD.[32] In a typical year the United States expended about 11 percent of its gross national product (GNP) on health,[33] mostly for treatment of illness; an estimated 0.00003 of the GNP was spent on STD control and services[34] (Table 85-2). In response to the epidemic of HIV infection, national annual expenditures for prevention of this infection now exceed 500 million dollars.

Recent rates of reported cases of gonorrhea exceed 400 per 100,000 population and early syphilis rates are about 12 per 100,000 population (Chap. 2). Congenital syphilis cases still occur and have recently increased to exceed 400 cases per year. Viral STDs have risen rapidly between the 1960s and 1980s.

Recently, the country has been racked by an uncontrolled epidemic of HIV infection in which more than 46,000 persons have died of AIDS, and an estimated 1.25 million persons are infected with HIV. The epidemic of HIV infection has consumed public and professional attention, obscuring the recognition of an ongoing epidemic of HSV infections, HPV infection (and associated risk of cervical cancer), chlamydial infections, a resurgence of syphilis, and the STD consequences of pelvic inflammatory disease and ectopic pregnancy.

## PLANNING

Publications beginning in the 1930s have documented the impact of STDs on the American population.[35] Interpretation of reported STD morbidity in the United States has always been plagued by problems of diagnostic inaccuracy and underreporting. Nevertheless, available surveillance data reveal STD trends, help identify high-risk groups, and are heavily referenced in planning documents at the federal, state, and large city levels (Chaps. 2 and 84). Sophisticated modeling and cost-benefit and epidemiologic analysis have been produced.[36] Surveillance and epidemiologic studies of behavioral determinants of STD risk have been undertaken. Recent methodologic developments have been stimulated by the epidemic of HIV infection and await application to broader populations to help in planning STD control in the United States. Minorities, urban populations, prostitutes, homosexual men, unmarried young people, and older single people are at particular risk of STD in the United States (Chap. 2).

Most high-risk populations tend to receive their STD services in public clinics, whereas low-risk populations can afford to use private medical care. Anecdotal accounts suggest that in some communities, prostitutes and homosexual men use private medical practitioners for STD treatment. Thus the majority of STD is probably diagnosed and treated by private physicians who individually see relatively few cases and therefore have low diagnostic suspicion (Chap. 93). On the other hand, high-risk groups contain core populations who are efficient transmitters of the disease but are treated in public clinics where diagnostic quality has been quite variable (Chaps. 87 and 91).

At the national level, a considerable investment in planning occurs, including the explicit statement of national STD objectives and model standards for care.[37] States and localities have followed suit, but a recent summary of public health in the United States suggests that these national objectives and standards are not consistently pursued at local levels.[38]

## INTERVENTION STRATEGIES

Since the 1950s, at the national level, considerable emphasis in STD control has been on partner notification and epidemiologic treatment.[32] Clinical services in public STD clinics have historically been weak owing to poorly trained staff, antiquated facilities, and limited resources. Private physicians have been trained in medical schools that have offered almost no STD-related clinical curriculum.[39] This has improved somewhat in recent years owing to a national STD training program[40] and expanded STD research in medical schools and associated teaching. Recently, behavioral emphasis stimulated by the HIV epidemic has probably raised the level of sophistication of STD counseling services. Quality-assurance protocols for clinical services have been promulgated and incorporated into program audits.[41] Adequate studies to permit a nationwide or statewide estimate of the quality of clinical services have not been documented. Special surveys of private practice have shown reasonable compliance with treatment standards.

Health promotion, including sex education, has received a steadily increasing emphasis in STD control in the United States. Even prior to the HIV epidemic, quality-assurance guidelines for STD education, national and state STD hotlines, and episodic intensive media campaigns were undertaken. The HIV epidemic has vastly accelerated this interest, initially rejuvenated by the

1982 herpes scare. Because of concern about HIV, health promotion events unprecedented for STD (and for most other health risks) have occurred: a massive national media campaign, a mailing of explicit information about sexual matters and personal STD prophylaxis to every American household, and advertisement of condoms.[42] The status of STD education in schools has also been greatly enhanced. Evaluations of the behavioral effectiveness of these and other campaigns are incomplete but suggest some impact (Chaps. 89 and 90).

Case finding and screening have always held a special emphasis for STD control in the United States.[35] A long history of serologic screening for syphilis was followed in the 1970s by a massive gonococcal screening program, and in the 1980s millions of people have been tested for serologic evidence of HIV infection. In each instance, formidable logistical barriers were overcome to implement case detection in all medical sectors. Cost-effectiveness was limited by the low prevalence in screened populations. Moreover, STD control effectiveness has been compromised by failure to screen high disease transmitters frequently enough, limited resources for adequate follow-up, and in the case of HIV infection, the absence of effective treatment.[32]

For more than two decades, the Centers for Disease Control or its predecessor have developed and disseminated guidelines for treatment of STD. This model program is described in detail by WHO and recommended to those developing a national STD control program.[1] The treatment guidelines have focused on an expanding list of STDs and their consequences. Summaries of these guidelines inform the day-by-day routine of public STD clinics and eventually influence the standard of practice for private medicine.

Partner notification and counseling activities (Chaps. 91 and 88) recently have been extended to partners of patients with HIV infection with hopes of both detecting new cases and also preventing spread to uninformed others. Training of "disease intervention specialists" (STD caseworkers) is formal, elaborate, and high priority to the national and state programs. In recent years, the training has evolved to a complex and sophisticated approach (Chap. 88).

## SUPPORT COMPONENTS

The Centers for Disease Control is the major federal agency influencing STD control. This agency has no direct clinical responsibilities, and in many states, a recognized clinical expert or specialized clinic does not exist. However, in an increasing number of states, academic clinical facilities have influenced STD control through their training or research activities. Referral of patients for uncomplicated STD is uncommon, as a specific STD specialty does not exist.

As noted earlier, simplified patient management protocols are promoted and assurance of quality is guided through appropriate documents for public clinics.[41] Site visits by experts help review status of current STD programs and make recommendations for improvements.

Statistical and epidemiologic expertise is abundant in the United States as compared with other countries. Such activities are supported by an increasing network of sophisticated computer-based information systems. In addition, laboratory capabilities for many STDs are expanding, but cost prohibits screening for certain viral diseases. Many have called for more chlamydial culture capability. Laboratory proficiency testing for *Neisseria gonorrhoeae* cultures and syphilis serology were available without charge at the Centers for Disease Control until the mid-1980s when the laboratory proficiency testing (PT) program was stopped. Presently a PT program of more limited scope is offered by private professional associations but the value of its use to STD control is unknown. A national laboratory performance-evaluation program that enrolls more than 1400 laboratories continues for HIV serologies.[43]

## IMPLEMENTATION

Our judgment regarding implementation of the program in the United States is particularly subjective because of the size and diversity of the country. These judgments are recorded in Table 85-3.

## CONCLUSIONS

As we attempt general conclusions, we reemphasize the cautions (stated at the beginning of this chapter) about attempting to compare the STD control programs of different countries. One striking conclusion stands out (Table 85-2). Despite a remarkably similar expenditure on STD services, at least as measured by the percentage of gross national product, the rates of selected and comparably measured, treatable and preventable STD are distinctly dissimilar. Apparently, similar expenditures are not associated with similar rates of disease. Why is this? In our judgment the three most plausible reasons are differences in the

**Table 85-3. Summary Comparison of Emphasis[1] and Subjective Evaluation[2,3] of STD Control Programs**

| | Australia | Poland | United Kingdom | United States |
|---|---|---|---|---|
| Planning: | | | | |
| Estimating importance | △1 N | □5 Y | □2 N | ○5 Y |
| Setting priorities | △3 N | □4 Y | △1 N | □4 Y |
| Considering social factors | □3 N | □4 N | △1 N | △3 ? |
| Intervening: | | | | |
| Health promotion | △2 N | □5 Y | □2 N | □3 ? |
| Disease detection | △4 N | △3 Y | □2 N | □5 Y |
| Treatment programs | □4 N | ○5 Y | ○5 Y | □4 Y |
| Counseling, partner notification | □3 N | □5 Y | □5 Y | □5 Y |
| Support components: | | | | |
| Specialized centers | △3 ? | ○5 ? | ○5 Y | △3 Y |
| Information systems | □5 ? | □4 ? | ○3 ? | ○5 Y |
| Professional training | □5 ? | ○5 Y | ○5 ? | □3 ? |
| Laboratory services | □3 ? | □3 Y | □4 ? | □4 ? |
| Implementation* | □ N | ○ ? | ○ ? | □ ? |

1. Degree of emphasis placed by the program on the component: 1 = low, 3 = moderate, 5 = high.
2. Authors' judgment of programs' achievement of quality and quantity of components: △ = minimal, □ = moderate, ○ = substantial.
3. Authors' judgment based upon some form of formal evaluation: Y = yes, N = no, ? = uncertain.

*Overall degree to which emphasized objectives are judged to be met by the authors.

behavior of the populations, differences in the system of health care delivery, and differences in the appropriateness, effectiveness, and implementation of STD control strategies. It is the last of these three that is the focus of this chapter (Table 85-3). For each country, we indicate the degree of emphasis on and the quality and actual implementation of STD control components. The judgment is ours, and we indicate whether or not that judgment is based upon a formal evaluation. Finally, risking reputation and friendship, we make a judgment as to the evidence that the overall emphasized objectives are met.

We preface general conclusions about each country's efforts with a statement about how the HIV epidemic confuses this evaluation. In each of the countries, the epidemic of HIV infection has highlighted the public awareness and political visibility of STD in general. Expenditures have increased, dramatically in some countries, but it is too early for formal evaluations to determine the overall effect of increased resources on the HIV infection rates and STD control in general. Additionally, the pattern of emphasis upon individual components with the overall STD control programs further complicates evaluation. The hope is that full public commitment and adequate resource allocation will lead to balanced and effective programs—a hope that remains to be evaluated and documented.

For the United States, the resources devoted to STD control appear to have been insufficient to overcome the barriers of a complex health care and political system and of a mobile, sexually active society; therefore, STD rates are relatively high. For the United Kingdom, rates of treatable STD are relatively low, reflecting a long tradition of specialty-run STD clinics serving a relatively homogeneous population, but the future threats of HIV and other viral STDs require increased resources and an extension of innovative health education strategies to traditional as well as new STDs. For Australia, an organized approach to STD control is just beginning and will require investment in epidemiologic analysis and a sustained outreach to minority populations. Perhaps Poland has the most comprehensive and consistently balanced program that takes full advantage of public medical care, an enlightened approach to prostitution, and substantial commitment to health education.

In the future, countries should invest in program evaluation, document the results for others, and show how change based on data can prevent STD. Then the judgments in this chapter would not be so subjective.

## References


1 *Control of Sexually Transmitted Diseases.* Geneva, World Health Organization, 1985. ISBN 924151989.

2 *Perspectives on Health.* Adelaide, South Australian Health Commission, 1985. ISBN 0730800881.

3 Siskind V: Ectopic pregnancy in Queensland, 1971–1980. *Med J Aust* 142:672, 1985.

4 Hart G: Syphilis control in populations previously exposed to yaws. *Int J Epidemiol* 11:181, 1982.

5 Melbourne J, Handke G: STD screening in a remote aboriginal community. *Communicable Dis Intelligence* 82/10:2, 1982. STD surveillance, *WHO Weekly Epidemiol Rec* 57(29):220, 1982.

6 Soong FS: The role of aboriginal health workers as cultural brokers: Some findings and their implications. *Aust J Soc Issues* 18(4):268, 1983.

7 National Health and Medical Research Council: *Handbook on Sexually Transmitted Diseases.* Canberra, 1981. ISBN 0644019972.

8 Stapinski A: Zwalczanie kily i rzezaczki w Polsce. Warszawa, PZWL, 1979.

9 Stapinski A: Fight against syphilis and gonorrhea in Poland during 1970–1975 (summary in English).

10 Stapinski A, Seliborska Z: Value of smear examination and culture on Biocult = Gc trans-grow medium in the diagnosis of gonorrhea in prostitutes (summary in English). *Przegl Dermatol* 70:379, 1983.

11 Stapinski A, Mroczkowski TF: Epidemiology of nongonococcal urethritis in Poland. *Przegl Dermatol* 72:182, 1985.

12 Stapinski A et al: Epidemiology of nongonococcal urethritis. Authors' experience. *Przegl Dermatol* 72:43, 1985.

13 Towpik J: New campaign against venereal disease in Poland. *Br J Vener Dis* 49:144, 1973.

14 Kelus J, Stapinski A: The present forms of venereal disease medical service in public opinion (summary in English). 13 Konferencja Naukowa Sekcji Wenerologicznej Polskiego Towarzystwa Dermatologicznego, Warszawa, PZWL, 1977, p 149.

15 Kelus J et al: Evaluation of VD education program for youth (summary in English). *Przegl Dermatol* 64:299, 1977.

16 Kelus J: Social and behavioral aspects of venereal disease. *Br J Vener Dis* 49:167, 1973.

17 Adler MW: The terrible peril—a historical perspective on the venereal diseases. *Br Med J* 281:206, 1980.

18 Adler MW: Trends for gonorrhoea and pelvic inflammatory disease in England and Wales and gonorrhoeas in a defined population. *Am J Obstet Gynecol* 138:901, 1980.

19 Adler MW et al: Sexually transmitted diseases in a defined population of women. *Br Med J* 283:29, 1981.

20 Catterall RD: The British Service for patients with sexually transmitted diseases. *Health Trends* 15(4):82, 1983.

21 Adler MW et al: Facilities and diagnostic criteria in sexually transmitted disease clinics in England and Wales. *Br J Vener Dis* 54:2, 1978.

22 Adler MW: Diagnostic, treatment and reporting criteria for gonorrhoea in sexually transmitted disease clinics in England and Wales. 1: Diagnosis. *Br J Vener Dis* 54:10, 1978.

23 Adler MW: Diagnostic, treatment and reporting criteria for gonorrhoea in sexually transmitted disease clinics in England and Wales. 2: Treatment and reporting criteria. *Br J Vener Dis* 54:15, 1978.

24 Belsey EM, Adler MW: Current approaches to the diagnosis of herpes genitalis. *Br J Vener Dis* 54:115, 1978.

25 Adler MW: Diagnostic, treatment and reporting criteria for non-specific genital infection in sexually transmitted disease clinics in England and Wales. 1: Diagnosis. *Br J Vener Dis* 54:422, 1978.

26 Adler MW: Diagnostic, treatment and reporting criteria for non-specific genital infection in sexually transmitted disease clinics in England and Wales. 2: Treatment and reporting criteria. *Br J Vener Dis* 54:428, 1978.

27 O'Connor BH, Adler MW: Current approaches to the diagnosis, treatment and reporting of trichomoniasis and candidosis. *Br J Vener Dis* 54:52, 1979.

28 Catterall RD: Education of physicians in the sexually transmitted diseases in the United Kingdom. *Br J Vener Dis* 52:97, 1976.

29 Thin RN: Health advisers (contact tracers) in sexually transmitted disease. *Br J Vener Dis* 60:269, 1984.

30 Adler MW: Survey of medical undergraduate training in genitourinary medicine. *Genitourin Med* 62:405, 1986.

31 Hunter I et al: *Handbook on Contact Tracing in Sexually Transmitted Diseases.* London, Health Education Council, 1980.

32 Cates W: Epidemiology and control of sexually transmitted diseases in *Sexually Transmitted Diseases,* Felman (ed). New York, Churchill Livingstone, 1986, pp 1–22.

33 Health Issuance Association of America: *HIAA Health Trends Chartbook.* Health Care Financing Administration, HHS, 1988, p 5.

34 Public Health Agencies: Expenditures and Source of Funds. *Public Health Foundation Publication* 103, September 1987, derived from p 24.

35 Paran T: *Shadow on the Land: Syphilis.* New York, Reynal Hitchcock, 1937.

36 Hethcote HW, Yorke JA: Lecture Notes in Biomathematics, Gonorrhea Transmission Dynamics and Control, 1984.

37 *The 1990 Health Objectives for the Nation: A Midcourse Review.* Public Health Service, U.S. Department of Health and Human Services, 1986.

38 *The Future of Public Health.* Institute of Medicine, 1988.

39 Stamm WE et al: Clinical training in venereology in the United States and Canada. *JAMA* 248:2020, 1982.

40 Margolis S: Initiation of the sexually transmitted disease prevention/training clinic program. *Sex Transm Dis* 8:87, 1981.

41 Centers for Disease Control: *Quality Assurance Guidelines for STD Clinics.* Atlanta, Centers for Disease Control, 1982.

42 Centers for Disease Control: *National AIDS Information and Education Program.* Atlanta, Centers for Disease Control, 1987.

43 Schalla EO et al: Role of the Centers for Disease Control in monitoring the quality of laboratory testing for human immunodeficiency virus infection. *Clin Microbiol Newsletter* 10(20):156, 1988.

# Chapter 86

# Development of prevention and control programs for sexually transmitted diseases in developing countries

André Meheus
Kenneth F. Schulz
Willard Cates, Jr.

## SEXUALLY TRANSMITTED DISEASES (STD)—A MAJOR PUBLIC HEALTH PROBLEM

The epidemiology of sexually transmitted diseases (STD) in developing countries differs greatly from the situation in industrialized nations[1–4] (Chaps. 2 and 85). First, the rates of STD overall are a much more frequent health problem in both rural and urban areas of developing countries. For example, STD are among the top five causes of consultation at health services in many African countries (Table 86-1). Ranking of STD would be even higher if age-specific consultation rates (15 to 44 years) were available. High STD incidence and prevalence rates are found in specific population groups. For example, prostitutes and their clients are an important high-risk group for STD infection and transmission, while male homosexuals are not a significant group.[5–6]

Second, among the STD, genital ulcer disease occurs at a higher relative frequency.[7–11] The so-called tropical STD, in particular chancroid, and to a lesser degree lymphogranuloma venereum and granuloma inguinale, are major causes of genital ulcers. Syphilis is roughly 10-fold higher while genital herpes accounts for a smaller proportion of ulcerative disease.

Third, the incidence of STD complications and sequelae is also much higher, related to a lack of resources for adequate diagnosis and treatment. Major complications and sequelae are adverse pregnancy outcome for mother and newborn, neonatal and infant infections, infertility in both sexes, ectopic pregnancy, urethral stricture in males, blindness in infants due to gonococcal ophthalmia neonatorum and in adults due to gonococcal keratoconjunctivitis, and genital cancers, in particular cancer of the cervix uteri and penile cancer.[12–17]

**Table 86-1. Most Important Causes of Morbidity in Cameroon, 1986–1987: Cases Declared by Health Care Institutions, All Age Groups[50]**

| | 1986 | 1987 |
|---|---|---|
| Malaria | 496,663 | 671,608 |
| Intestinal helminths | 230,409 | 279,791 |
| STD | 98,518 | 122,133 |
| Gonorrhea | 82,049 | 110,994 |
| Diarrhea | 94,075 | 141,623 |
| Amebiasis | 24,126 | 32,718 |
| Measles | 20,236 | 13,142 |
| Onchocerciasis | 18,272 | 30,366 |

Fourth, the epidemiology of the acquired immunodeficiency syndrome (AIDS) is markedly different from that in Western countries: heterosexual contact is the predominant transmission mode of human immunodeficiency virus (HIV).[18,19] The epidemic is increasing rapidly in those population groups which have a high level of sexual activity with multiple partners. Evidence is accumulating that other sexually transmitted diseases, in particular genital ulcers, enhance HIV transmission.[20–23]

Although the health and economic consequences of STD remain enormous, many governments and international donor agencies have ignored the real magnitude of the STD problem until recently. Unfortunately, a fatal sexually transmitted infection, AIDS, was needed to alert worldwide decision makers and the community alike to the STD problem and to generate resources for the control of these infections. For optimal efficiency, the epidemiological picture outlined above indicates that AIDS prevention should be closely linked or integrated with comprehensive STD control. Separating AIDS and the other STD in national control programs creates a false dichotomy which detracts from the commonality of intervention strategies.[24]

## GENERAL PRINCIPLES FOR STD CONTROL

STD control has two main aims:[25] (1) to interrupt the transmission of infection and (2) to prevent the development of complications and sequelae.

These aims can be accomplished by (1) reducing exposure to infection by educating persons at risk to reduce number of sex partners and avoid sexual intercourse with persons who have a high probability of being infected; (2) preventing infection by promoting the use of condoms or other prophylactic barriers; (3) detecting and curing disease by implementing disease detection activities, providing adequate diagnostic and treatment facilities, and promoting health-seeking behavior; (4) limiting complications and further transmission of infection by providing early and appropriate treatment for symptomatic and asymptomatic patients and their sex partner(s), and through counseling.

Guidelines for the development of comprehensive national STD control programs have been elaborated by the World Health Organization.[26,27] Owing to the increasing importance of the incurable viral STD, in particular the fatal condition of AIDS, primary prevention strategies currently receive much higher priority than a decade ago. Priority activities of an STD control program in developing countries now include:[4]

1. Health promotion to change sexual behavior and adopt "safer sex" practices.
2. Adequate management of patients with STD and their sex partner(s).
3. Screening for HIV, gonorrhea, and syphilis in high-risk groups known to have a high prevalence of infection. If this strategy cannot be implemented, epidemiological treatment might be considered.
4. Case finding for syphilis, and eventually gonorrhea, in antenatal populations.
5. Ocular prophylaxis to prevent gonococcal ophthalmia neonatorum.

Any primary prevention efforts to reduce risky sexual behaviors will have spin-off effects on all STD, including HIV. In addition, the traditional interventions of secondary prevention and adequate management directed to bacterial STD will have a threefold effect: first, to decrease transmission of bacterial STD within communities; second, to reduce the reproductive sequelae of those STD; and third, especially through controlling genital ulcers, to slow the HIV epidemic.[23]

## SURVEILLANCE SYSTEM

Health planners require convincing evidence of the magnitude and seriousness of the problems posed by STD to justify the allocation of an appropriate share of scarce resources.[28] In the past, poor data collection contributed to the low political awareness of STD. However, because considerable resources are now allocated to AIDS/STD prevention to decrease risk-taking sexual behavior, evaluation systems are necessary. Surveillance of STD incidence (for example, gonorrhea, chancroid, or syphilis) is a sensitive indicator of whether health promotion efforts are working.

### Clinician reporting

A variety of clinicians, from the nurse, medical assistant, or general practitioner at the primary health care level up to the STD specialist in more sophisticated health care settings, treat patients suffering from STD and can potentially report STD cases. The reporting system must be simple and provide feedback to the clinicians. The degree of detail of the information to be gathered must be adapted to the degree of sophistication and to the interest of the clinician. A simple clinician reporting form can be used in settings without access to complex diagnostic tests (Fig. 86-1). The form yields data by syndrome (urethral discharge, vaginal discharge, genital ulcer, etc.) and by sex. Eventually age grouping can be obtained by using different forms (age under 15, 15 to 19, 20 to 29, 30 and above).

The reporting system should provide an estimate of the incidence of STD in the population and a projection of drug supplies needed. The form is especially adaptable for health services that use standardized STD management protocols, such as flowcharts or algorithms that were proposed by the World Health Organization.[25] The first column of the form yields data that allow an assessment of STD trends; the second and third columns provide information on the effectiveness of the STD case management protocols.

### Laboratory reporting

The laboratory may provide an adjunct to clinician reporting. The number of positive STD isolates and/or positive serological tests gives a cross-check on cases reported. The number of total specimens processed is a useful indicator of overall activity.

### Sentinel surveillance

Sentinel systems can be used to identify biases in the routine reporting system. They can also provide an alternative to routine reporting, since periodic surveillance efforts might be less costly than developing and maintaining a routine system.

Sentinel surveillance is the identification of representative health care facilities that can collect reliable STD data and report them to the program. Sentinel facilities could include randomly chosen health facilities, such as private practitioners, outpatient departments, special clinics (e.g., for students, military) and STD clinics where they exist.

### Periodic surveys

Periodic ad hoc surveys can include etiological studies or epidemiological surveys. Background on the etiological categories of patients with STD syndromes such as urethral discharge, vaginal discharge, genital ulcers, pelvic inflammatory disease, or ophthalmia neonatorum are essential in the design and adaptation of STD management protocols.

Cross-sectional sample surveys from either the general population or in subgroups (for instance, pregnant women) yield prevalence data on STD useful for planning interventions and evaluating their impact on STD. Serosurveys are a major tool in HIV surveillance; combining them with serological markers for other STD should be attempted.[29]

Clinician __________ Week (month) __________ Year __________
Location __________

| Syndrome | No. of Patients Treated/ Initial Visit | No. of Patients Treated/ Follow-up Visit | No. of Patients Referred |
|---|---|---|---|
| Urethral discharge | | | |
| Balanitis | | | |
| Swollen scrotum | | | |
| Vaginal discharge | | | |
| Pelvic inflammatory disease | | | |
| Conjunctivitis in newborn | | | |
| Genital ulcer | Men:<br>Women: | Men:<br>Women: | Men:<br>Women: |
| Bubo | Men:<br>Women: | Men:<br>Women: | Men:<br>Women: |
| Other STD | Men:<br>Women: | Men:<br>Women: | Men:<br>Women: |

**Fig. 86-1.** Weekly (monthly) clinician STD notification form.

## HEALTH EDUCATION

The growing importance of incurable viral STD, particularly HIV infection, has tremendously increased the importance of health education in changing behaviors toward safer sex practices.[27]

Major efforts must be directed toward specific target groups, including adolescents, STD patients and contacts, prostitutes and their clients, the military, students, long-distance truck drivers, and others.[30] Methods of communication such as mass media, manuals for primary and secondary schools, posters, and leaflets are important. As many children drop out of school and adult illiteracy might be high (especially among women), other methods of communication must be used, such as radio messages, meetings, discussions, drama, songs, and pictures.[31] Religious and cultural sensitivities should be considered and both the target group and community leaders should be involved in the development of the messages.

The rapid spread of HIV infection has made sexual behavior change urgent. In some areas, however, skepticism has prevailed as to the possibility to do so. For instance, group health education did not increase condom acceptability, which remained at about 40 percent, among community leaders in Uganda.[32] Conversely, STD/AIDS education was successful in increasing condom use among military populations in Central Africa, which in turn led to decreased STD; condom use also increased significantly in Nairobi prostitutes following a health promotion and condom distribution program.[33]

## CLINICAL SERVICES

Primary health care settings provide most STD clinical services in developing countries.[25,34] These include a clinic, hospital, private office, health post, drugstore, or any other facility ensuring some privacy for the patient-clinician encounter. Adequate clinical management of STD cases by the clinician encompasses (1) detecting or ruling out disease, (2) giving treatment if necessary (3) counseling the patient on STD prevention through change of risky sexual behavior, (4) advising the patient to comply with treatment, (5) ensuring that the patient's sex partner(s) are treated, and (6) screening for other STD including HIV infection.

The confidence which a patient has in the health service is determined by the effectiveness of management of his or her STD at the first consultation. A practical approach to clinical care in primary health care settings includes:[4]

1. The presenting symptoms and signs define the health problem to be solved. The diagnosis must be based on the history, physical examination, and simple laboratory tests, if available.
2. Laboratory investigations should be performed routinely only if they are important to decide the management of the health problem.
3. Correct management should take less than 5 min.
4. The choice of treatment should be rational, and treatment regimens standardized.
5. Referral of patients should be exceptional, preferably less than 5 percent of the total.

Many developing countries reserve the more expensive treatments for penicillin-resistant gonorrhea for the referral level of care. They provide primary health care settings with penicillin only, even if prevalence of resistant strains is 20 percent or more. This is a bad policy, because primary health care workers evidently have at least 20 percent failures of gonorrhea management, not because of incompetence but because of lack of the efficacious drug. The official health sector is thus discredited, and patients turn to quacks and alternative treatment sites where they do not receive the comprehensive management needed.

In many developing countries STD referral is a real problem owing to lack of time, distance to travel, or financial and sociocultural barriers between peripheral and more sophisticated levels of care. Therefore, practical, useful guidelines for simplified approaches to STD control, such as simple management protocols, are of the utmost importance.[25,35]

### Problem-oriented approach to STD management

Patients with STD in developing countries generally present in their acute stages as one of the following syndromes:

- Urethral discharge
- Gynecologic complaints such as vaginal discharge, dysuria, or low abdominal pain
- Genital ulceration
- Inguinal bubo
- Swollen scrotum
- Conjunctivitis in the newborn

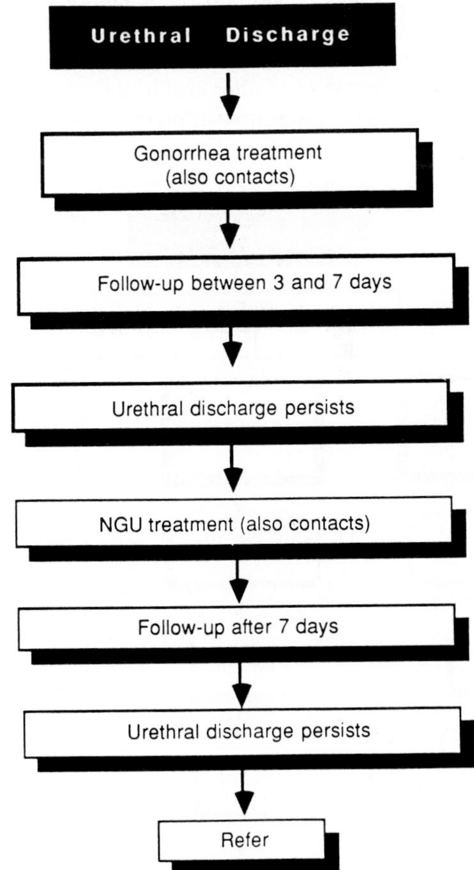


**Fig. 86-2.** Urethral discharge case management in settings in which urethral discharge is mainly due to gonococcal infection (e.g., where local surveys show above 80 percent of cases are gonorrhea).*

*Figs. 86-2, 3, and 4 show STD case management protocols reformatted by the Program for International Training in Health (INTRAH), University of North Carolina, Chapel Hill, from the unpublished document WHO/VDT/85.437.

STD management protocols have been developed and evaluated during the last 5 years. The general principles for the design of these protocols have been outlined.[25] The most important are knowledge of the local etiology of the health problem, information on the laboratory tests available for diagnosis (sensitivity, specificity, cost, operational value in local circumstances), and treatment efficacy. The standardization of treatment is essential, and this can be established by controlled and uncontrolled clinical trials, knowledge of antimicrobial sensitivity patterns, information from neighboring countries, or international recommendations.[27] Furthermore, the current STD care practices and policies in the community should be assessed, and the intended users of the protocols should be clearly defined. Once a protocol has been designed for a country, it is desirable to test and evaluate its performance in a small demonstration or pilot project.

As examples, Figs. 86-2 and 86-3 outline a management protocol for urethral discharge in a setting with and without a microscope, and Fig. 86-4 outlines a protocol for pelvic inflammatory disease in a setting where no gynecological examination of the patient is possible.

### Patient counseling and partner notification

Counseling can be provided to both those individuals with STD and also their partners (Chap. 88). By definition, persons with STD are at high risk for repeat infections and HIV because of their sexual behavior. Counseling these high-risk individuals provides an ideal opportunity to offer health education on lowering the risks of acquisition and transmission of STD in a one-on-one, non-judgmental, confidential setting. This may also be a useful opportunity to provide other information on relevant topics, such as family planning, to a sexually active group (Chap. 92).

In addition, treatment of the sexual partner(s) of STD infected individuals is central to STD prevention and control (Chap. 91). This not only prevents reinfection by their regular sexual partner(s) but also reduces the likelihood of further STD transmission throughout the population. Partner notification can consist of either patient referral or provider referral. Patient referral is simpler, less expensive, but might be less effective. Provider referral is more effective, but labor-intensive; thus, it is usually reserved for specific high-yield circumstances.

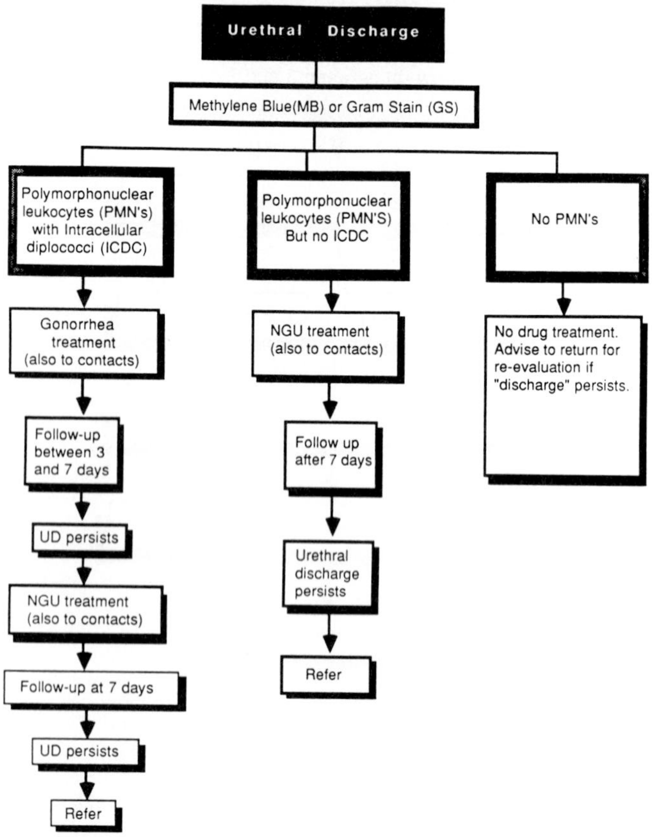

Urethral Discharge

Methylene Blue(MB) or Gram Stain (GS)

Polymorphonuclear leukocytes (PMN's) with Intracellular diplococci (ICDC)

Gonorrhea treatment (also to contacts)

Follow-up between 3 and 7 days

UD persists

NGU treatment (also to contacts)

Follow-up at 7 days

UD persists

Refer

Polymorphonuclear leukocytes (PMN'S) But no ICDC

NGU treatment (also to contacts)

Follow up after 7 days

Urethral discharge persists

Refer

No PMN's

No drug treatment. Advise to return for re-evaluation if "discharge" persists.

**Fig. 86-3.** Urethral discharge case management (laboratory available).

## EARLY DETECTION OF STD

Detection programs for STD usually are designed to reach asymptomatic individuals. Therefore, laboratory tests should be available in sufficient quantity and must be checked regularly for quality of performance. Cost-effectiveness and possible operational problems should be evaluated before the introduction of routine STD detection programs.[4,36,37]

Cost-effectiveness of the detection program can be increased by concentrating on high-risk individuals, who can be identified based on presence of symptoms, presence of clinical signs such as cervicitis, or an epidemiological risk profile. Among pregnant women in Nairobi, for example, risk factors for gonorrhea were being single and residing in a particular area of town.[12,38]

## MASS TREATMENT

Under certain circumstances, such as high prevalence of STD, insufficient or nonexistent laboratory facilities, and highly mobile populations, mass treatment (i.e., treatment without diagnosis) of high-risk groups could be considered.[27] Occasional or more regular mass treatment of prostitutes for a number of STD is done in some countries, but the strategy remains controversial owing to insufficient data on its impact.

Prostitutes play a major role in STD transmission in the tropics, evidently now also in HIV infection[39–41] (Chap. 7). STD infection, particularly genital ulcers, increases chances of HIV transmission more than fivefold. Regimens that could be considered, since they are effective against chancroid and gonorrhoea, are, for instance, spectinomycin 2 g or ceftriaxone 250 mg as a single dose intramuscularly, or sulphamethoxazole/trimethoprim (320 mg/80 mg) 10 tablets once a day for two days. Data from Nairobi have shown that if prostitutes are treated every 3 weeks for gonorrhea, at least two-thirds of infections are prevented.[5]

### Ocular prophylaxis at birth

The incidence of gonococcal ophthalmia neonatorum is estimated between 1 to 5 percent in many developing countries. In 20 to 80 percent of these cases this is due to a PPNG.[12,42] Thus, antibiotics such as kanamycin, cefotaxime, or ceftriaxone have to be administered instead of penicillin to cure the full-blown infection.[43–46]

As these drugs may not be available in many settings, gonococcal ophthalmia neonatorum again is an important cause of

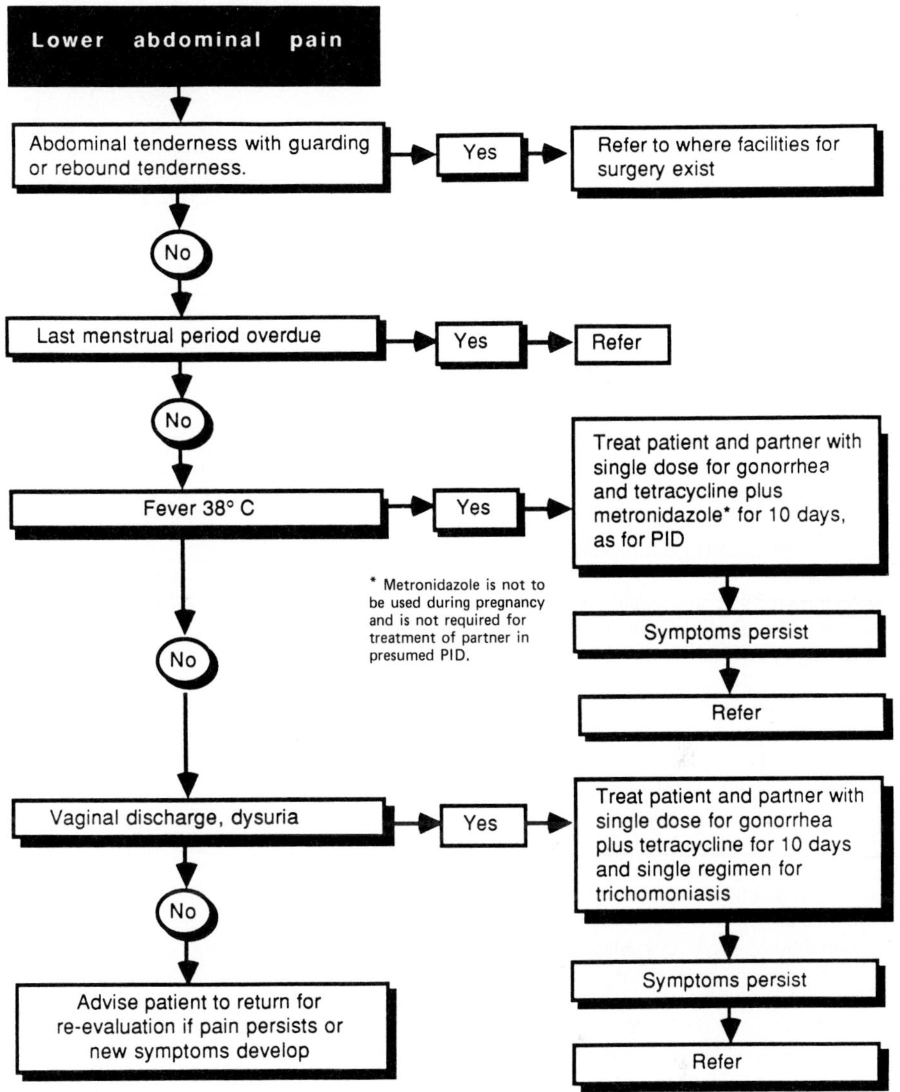


**Fig. 86-4.** Pelvic inflammatory disease (PID) management in cases where only taking a history and external palpation of patient are possible.

blindness in neonates and children. The most cost-effective prevention strategy is ocular prophylaxis directed against the gonococcus, and this must be applied to all newborns immediately at birth. The choice of method is between silver nitrate 1% eye drops in single-dose wax ampoules or tetracycline 1% ointment; both are effective.[47–49]

## SUMMARY

STD are causing enormous public problems in the world, but especially in developing countries. Not only is the emergence of a new STD epidemic, HIV, adding to and compounding the problems, but we are now learning that other STD facilitate transmission of HIV. STD prevention and control programs must now be initiated in the developing world. If implemented, at the very least, treatment and prevention of STD would be occurring with programs that should have been begun years ago; moreover, at current expectations, prevention of new HIV transmission would also be occurring as a consequence.

## References

1 Arya OP, Lawson JB: Sexually transmitted diseases in the tropics. Epidemiological, diagnostic, therapeutic and control aspects. *Trop Doct* 7:51, 1977.
2 Osoba AO: Sexually transmitted diseases in tropical Africa. *Br J Vener Dis* 57:89, 1981.
3 Piot P, Meheus A: Epidemiologie des maladies sexuellement transmissibles dans les pays en developpement. *Ann Soc Belge Med Trop* 63:87, 1983.
4 Meheus A, Piot P: Provision of services for sexually transmitted diseases in developing countries, in *Recent Advances in STD,* JD Oriel, JRW Harris (eds). Edinburgh, Churchill Livingston, 1986, pp 261–272.
5 D'Costa L et al: Prostitutes are a major reservoir of sexually transmitted diseases in Nairobi, Kenya. *Sex Transm Dis* 12:64, 1985.
6 Arya OP, Bennett FJ: Venereal disease in an elite group (university students) in East Africa. *Br J Vener Dis* 43:275, 1967.
7 Nsanze H et al: Genital ulcers in Kenya: Clinical and laboratory study. *Br J Vener Dis* 57:378, 1981.
8 Duncan MO et al: The diagnosis of sexually acquired genital ulcerations in black patients in Johannesburg. *S Afr J Sex Transm Dis* 1:20, 1981.

9 Thirumoorthy T et al: Purulent penile ulcers of patients in Singapore. *Genitourin Med* 62:253, 1986.

10 Meheus A et al: Etiology of genital ulcerations in Swaziland. *Sex Transm Dis* 10:33, 1983.

11 Mabey DCW et al: Aetiology of genital ulceration in the Gambia. *Genitourin Med* 63:312, 1987.

12 Laga M et al: Epidemiology of ophthalmia neonatorum in Kenya. *Lancet* ii:1145, 1986.

13 Schulz KF et al: Pregnancy loss, infant death and suffering: The legacy of syphilis and gonorrhea in Africa. *Genitourin Med* 63:320, 1987.

14 Cates W Jr et al: Worldwide patterns of infertility: Is Africa different? *Lancet* ii:596, 1985.

15 Brown ST et al: STD control in less developed countries: The time is now. *Int J Epidemiol* 14:505, 1985.

16 Schwab L, Tizazu T: Destructive epidemic *N. gonorrhoeae* keratoconjunctivitis in African adults. *Br J Ophthalmol* 69:525, 1985.

17 Kestelyn P et al: Gonorrheal keratoconjunctivitis in African adults. *Sex Transm Dis* 14:191, 1987.

18 Piot P et al: AIDS: An international perspective. *Science* 239:573, 1988.

19 Carael M et al: Human immunodeficiency virus transmission among heterosexual couples in Central Africa. *AIDS* 2:201, 1988.

20 Simonsen JN et al: Human immunodeficiency virus infection among men with sexually transmitted diseases. Experience from a center in Africa. *N Engl J Med* 319:274, 1988.

21 Greenblatt RM et al: Genital ulceration as a risk factor for human immunodeficiency virus infection. *AIDS* 2:47, 1988.

22 Potterat JJ: Does syphilis facilitate sexual acquisition of HIV? *JAMA* 258:473, 1987.

23 Kreiss J et al: Role of sexually transmitted diseases in transmitting human immunodeficiency virus. *Genitourin Med* 64:1, 1988.

24 Cates W: The "Other STD." Do they really matter? *JAMA* 259:3606, 1988.

25 World Health Organization: Simplified approaches for sexually transmitted diseases (STD) control at the primary health care (PHC) level. Unpublished WHO Document WHO/VDT/85.437, 1985.

26 World Health Organization and Pan American Health Organization: Control of sexually transmitted diseases. Geneva, Switzerland, World Health Organization, 1985.

27 World Health Organization: WHO Expert Committee on Veneral Diseases and Treponematoses, Sixth Report. Geneva, Switzerland, World Health Organization, 1986.

28 Willcox RR: VD education in developing countries—A comparison with developed countries. *Br J Vener Dis* 52:88, 1976.

29 Dondero TJ et al: Monitoring the Levels and Trends of HIV infection: The Public Health Service's HIV Surveillance Program. *Public Health Rep* 103:213, 1988.

30 Leslie-Harwit M, Meheus A: Information may be their only defense. *World Health* July 1988, p 16.

31 Bennett FJ: Control of sexually transmitted diseases in the tropics and developing countries, in *Sexually Transmitted Diseases in the Tropics,* AO Osoba (ed).*Bailliere's Clinical Tropical Medicine and Communicable Diseases* 2:223, 1987.

32 Konde-Lule JK: Group health education against AIDS in rural Uganda. *World Health Forum* 9:384, 1988.

33 Ngugi EN et al: Prevention of transmission of human immuno-deficiency virus in Africa: Effectiveness of condom promotion and health education among prostitutes. *Lancet* ii:887, 1986.

34 Arya OP, Bennett FJ: Role of the medical auxiliary in the control of sexually transmitted diseases in a developing country. *Br J Vener Dis* 52:116, 1976.

35 Meheus AZ: STD-Control—Practical approaches in developing nations, in *Sexually Transmitted Diseases,* KK Holmes et al (eds). New York, McGraw-Hill, 1984, p 998.

36 Hart G: Screening to control infectious diseases: Evaluation of control programme for gonorrhoea and syphilis. *Rev Infect Dis* 2:701, 1975.

37 Meheus A: *Sexually Transmitted Pathogens in Mother and Newborn—Strategies for Control.* New York Academy of Sciences, 1988, in press.

38 Fransen L et al: Parents of infants with ophthalmia neonatorum: A high risk group for sexually transmitted diseases. *Sex Transm Dis* 12:150, 1985.

39 Van de Perre P et al: Female prostitutes: A risk group for infection with human T-cell lymphotropic virus type III. *Lancet* ii:524, 1985.

40 Kreiss JK et al: AIDS virus infection in Nairobi prostitutes. Spread of the epidemic to East Africa. *N Engl J Med* 314:414, 1986.

41 Mann JM et al: HIV infection and associated risk factors in female prostitutes in Kinshasa, Zaire. *AIDS* 2:249, 1988.

42 Meheus A: Gonorrhoea, in *Sexually Transmitted Diseases in the Tropics,* Osoba AO (ed). *Bailliere's Clinical Tropical Medicine and Communicable Diseases* 2:17, 1987.

43 Fransen L et al: Single dose kanamycin therapy of gonococcal ophthalmia neonatorum. *Lancet* ii:1234, 1984.

44 Latif AS et al: Management of gonococcal ophthalmia neonatorum with single-dose kanamycin and ocular irrigation with saline. *Sex Transm Dis* 15:108, 1988.

45 Laga M et al: Single-dose therapy of gonococcal ophthalmia neonatorum with ceftriaxone. *N Engl J Med* 315:1382, 1986.

46 Lepage P et al: Single-dose cefotaxime cures gonococcal ophthalmia neonatorum. *Br J Ophthalmol* 72:518, 1988.

47 World Health Organization: *Conjunctivitis of the Newborn—Prevention and Treatment at the Primary Health Care Level.* Geneva, 1986.

48 Laga M et al: Prophylaxis of gonococcal and chlamydial ophthalmia neonatorum: Silver nitrate versus tetracycline. *N Engl J Med* 318:653, 1988.

49 Dillon HC: Prevention of gonococcal ophthalmia neonatorum. *N Engl J Med* 315:1414, 1986.

50 OCEAC: Activités de surveillance épidémiologique en République du Cameroun. *Bull Liais Doc Oceac* 83:87, 1988.

# Chapter 87

# Clinical facilities for sexually transmitted diseases control

Franklyn N. Judson

The keystone of a community sexually transmitted diseases (STD) control program is the STD clinic. Important supporting activities such as sex education for teenagers, screening for infection, and tracing contacts will be impaired if patients are reluctant to seek care at a clinic. Clinics should be able to deliver diagnostic and treatment services that are convenient, sensitive, competent, and cost-effective. The actual mix of services will depend upon the clinic's location, patient population, level of personnel training, and financial resources. This chapter will pay special attention to how a program can maximize STD control while minimizing costs.

Whether developing a new clinic or improving an existing one, the following factors deserve careful consideration (Table 87-1) and will help to determine clinic acceptance and effectiveness.

## THE PHYSICAL PLANT

Some STD clinics are physically grim, disorganized, and poorly maintained. This is rarely necessary. The facility may be anything from a single room shared with other types of patients to a multiroom specialty clinic seeing hundreds of patients a day, but it should be located as close as is practical to the population at greatest risk of STD. Signs directing patients to the clinic should be clearly displayed and the clinic telephone number(s) cross-referenced in the city directory under both clinic name and "venereal diseases." Sign-in and examination rooms should be comfortable and provide privacy.

Care of the physical plant promotes acceptance by patients as well as respect for themselves, the clinic staff, and the facility. It is usually possible with even a modest budget to assure that the interior is well-lit, clean, and cheerful. Paint, curtains, wall decorations, and colorful durable plastic chairs are inexpensive. Proper heating and air conditioning are desirable, but expensive.

## CLINIC HOURS

Operating hours should take into account the living patterns of patients and daily variations in demand for services. In most European and North American countries hours should span two work shifts, providing daytime and evening services. In Denver, this is accomplished by two separate clinics with complementary schedules. Mondays may require longer hours while Saturday morning clinics may be poorly attended.

**Table 87-1. Factors to Be Considered When Developing or Improving a Clinic for Sexually Transmitted Diseases (STD)**

| |
|---|
| Physical plant |
| Hours of operation |
| Clinic personnel |
| Organization of patient flow |
| Patients' records, clinic statistics, data processing |
| Diagnostic tests |
| Treatments |
| Patient referrals |
| STD education |
| Community outreach |
| Quality control |

## CLINIC PERSONNEL

Ideally all patients potentially infected with STD should be evaluated by physicians with a specific training in STD (genitourinary medicine in the United Kingdom). Owing to both high cost and limited availability of these specialists, this will not be possible in many countries. Nonetheless, a high-quality care system can be built around a physician's assistant (PA) model[1–3] in which a single physician serves as consultant while supervising and reviewing the work of three to six assistants. Because nursing schools do not offer adequate clinical training in STD, the background qualifications for assistants should depend less on formal degrees and more on work experience and personal qualities. The most important qualities are the ability to relate quickly and effectively to a wide variety of patients, intelligence, a friendly and positive mental attitude, flexibility, and a willingness to work hard. This opens employment opportunities to many capable individuals who otherwise might be excluded from the STD health care field.

The PA is trained on the job to follow physician-designed protocols. With good supervision a PA should become proficient within 2 or 3 months in caring for 80 to 90 percent of STD problems. Critical to proper PA performance is the understanding that when a clinical problem falls outside the dictums of the protocol or is otherwise confusing, the attending physician must be consulted.

Rigid job descriptions should not prevail. When needed, PAs should be willing and able to perform other key clinic functions such as signing in patients, drawing blood, and carrying out routine diagnostic tests. Indeed, in less-developed countries it may be necessary for the PA, or "barefoot doctor," to perform all clinic functions, often without physician supervision. STD training centers of the United States and Europe can be used to improve and accelerate the training process for physicians and their assistants.

Other clinic personnel may include secretaries and laboratory technicians. The personal qualities desirable in PAs are equally applicable to them.

## ORGANIZATION OF PATIENT FLOW

Of the many factors that determine patients' satisfaction with their care, none is more important than waiting time. Despite the variable and unpredictable patient loads inherent in walk-in-type clinics, waiting time can be greatly reduced by maintaining an efficient flow of patients from sign-in to discharge.

Efficient flow requires that clinic staff remain flexible in their assignments and adhere to certain work principles. The first principle holds that "no one dawdles while a patient waits," and the second that tasks ancillary to patient care such as compiling statistics, transcribing test results, and training sessions are put aside during peak clinic loads. As examples, an unoccupied PA assigned to examine patients may be asked to help draw bloods or retrieve patient records, or a secretary compiling statistics may be needed temporarily to operate a second sign-in station.

Flow should be organized so that patients waiting for completion of test results do not occupy examination rooms. PAs can use the interim time to initiate evaluations of further patients. The Denver Metro STD Clinic appoints a PA, known affectionately as the clinic "whip," to assume first-line responsibility for adjusting the work force to minute-by-minute changes in patient load and flow.

Mondays may require longer clinic hours and an "all hands on deck" approach in which staff vacations and elective tasks are deferred. Test-of-cure and other appointed visits can be scheduled for predictably less busy days and hours. By these means, long and decompensating patient waits are anticipated and avoided; the clinic is busy but the waiting room is empty.

## PATIENT RECORDS, CLINIC STATISTICS, DATA PROCESSING

A patient record system should permit: (1) rapid retrieval of previous information about patients; (2) efficient recording of a clinical data base; (3) efficient communication of test results to patients; (4) periodic output reports (statistics); and (5) easily monitored internal quality control. This requires a minimum of three paper documents: a patient clinic card, a daily patient log, and a patient chart.

As patients arrive, they are assigned sequential identification numbers (beginning with 1) for the day. The numbers assure the order in which they will be seen and their anonymity with regard to other patients. They will identify all test results. It is understood that a number system may not be acceptable to "mixed" clinics that also see non-STD patients.

A sign-in secretary dates and numbers a clinic card and enters the patient's name and number into the log (Table 87-2). The log will be used to record test results, to report them to patients when they call in, or, in the case of positive HIV results, to schedule counseling, to initiate tracing of patients with positive tests who do not call in, and to tabulate routine clinical statistics. The data items shown in Table 87-3 can be tabulated daily and added over time to generate monthly, semiannual, and annual reports.

**Table 87-2. Useful Data Items for a Daily Patient Log**

1. Date
2. Sequential patient number for the date
3. Name
4. Age
5. Sex
6. Ethnic group
7. Results of tests for HIV infection
8. Results of serologic test(s) for syphilis
9. Results of gonorrhea culture(s) by site
10. Results of other tests such as Pap smears, *Chlamydia* cultures and/or antigen, herpesvirus cultures, and hepatitis B virus antibody and/or antigen
11. Diagnosis
12. Treatment (date completed)
13. Date patient due to call in for test results
14. Date patient due to return for treatment, counseling, and/or further diagnostic tests
15. Remarks

**Table 87-3. Useful Statistics for Monthly and Annual Clinic Reports Which Can Be Tabulated from Daily Patient Log or from the Clinic's Stand-Alone Computer**

1. Patient visits by age, sex, sexual preference, and ethnic group
2. Patients tested for HIV and percent positive by age, sex, and risk behavior group
3. Patients treated for gonorrhea by age, sex, sexual preference, and ethnic group
4. Persons treated epidemiologically for gonorrhea by sex and rates of gonococcal infection
5. Patients treated for syphilis by age, sex, sexual preference, ethnic group, and stage
6. Persons treated epidemiologically for syphilis
7. Sex-specific prevalence rates for nongonococcal urethritis, trichomoniasis, candidiasis, nonspecific vaginitis, pelvic inflammatory disease, herpes genitalis, scabies, pediculosis, genital warts, molluscum contagiosum, dermatitis, other diagnosis, no diagnosis (or no illness)

Lastly, a current visit form is initiated which comprises the most important part of the patient chart. The example shown (Fig. 87-1) may not be ideal for all facilities but has performed well in the Denver Metro STD Clinic over the past 10 years and is suitable for automated data processing.[4] It efficiently guides the PA (or physician) through reason for attending, review of symptoms, relevant sexual history, use of contraception, limited obstetric and gynecologic history, history of STD, history of drug use and allergy, genital examination, ordering of diagnostic tests, recording of immediate tests results (Gram stains, dark field examinations, etc.), assessment of problems and plan for therapy. Rigorous completion of the clinic visit form provides a comprehensive STD clinical data base and facilitates review by the attending physician of the PA's ability to follow instructions and solve problems.

Declining cost and greatly enhanced performance of microcomputers have brought stand-alone automated clinic record systems and sophisticated statistical analysis within reach of most full-service STD clinics in the developed world. The form shown in Fig. 87-1 has been redesigned (Fig. 87-2) to permit rapid optical scanning and automated data entry into a personal computer that has an 8086 Intel CPU and 60 megabytes of hard-disk memory. The scanner can also be used by the attending physician to preedit charts of patients seen by PAs for protocol errors. A single 20-megabyte hard disk is sufficient to store all the data generated by 20,000 patient visits.

## DIAGNOSTIC TESTS

The effectiveness of a clinic to control STD depends upon its effectiveness to detect STD. Unfortunately, a constantly expanding list of increasingly sophisticated diagnostic tests creates a difficult dilemma for a clinic manager who must husband scarce resources. This section considers the applicability of common tests for STD to clinics of different funding levels and sophistication. It makes recommendations on how to achieve the highest diagnostic rates for the lowest costs. Other chapters detail technical aspects of the tests.

In Table 87-4, clinic resources are arbitrarily divided into three

NAME DMHC No. DATE

**REASON FOR ATTENDING**

☐ Asympt. Check-up ☐ Premarital ☐ VSR
☐ Contact to ____
☐ Suspect ☐ Established ____
☐ Referred by sex partner ____
☐ Follow-up for: ____
☐ Other ____

| NO | YES | DESCRIBE |
|---|---|---|
| ☐ Discharge | ☐ | |
| ☐ Dysuria | ☐ | |
| ☐ Lesion (G) | ☐ | |
| ☐ Lesion (XG) | ☐ | |
| ☐ Rash | ☐ | |
| ☐ Itching | ☐ | |
| ☐ Abdm. Pain | ☐ | |
| ☐ Other: | ☐ | |

**PHYSICAL EXAM** ☐ None

| NO | YES | DESCRIBE |
|---|---|---|
| ☐ Discharge | ☐ | |
| ☐ Lesion (G) | ☐ | |
| ☐ Lesion (XG) | ☐ | |
| ☐ Rash | ☐ | |
| ☐ Abn Nodes | ☐ | |
| ☐ Other | ☐ | |

| NL | ABN |
|---|---|
| ☐ Vulva | ☐ |
| ☐ Vagina | ☐ |
| ☐ Cervix | ☐ |
| ☐ Bimanual | ☐ |
| ☐ Rebound | ☐ |
| ☐ Other | ☐ |

**SEXUAL HISTORY**

Last exposure (days ago) ____
Preference ☐ M ☐ F ☐ Both
Number in past month ____
Site(s): ☐ Vaginal
Active: ☐ Oral ☐ Anal
Passive: ☐ Oral ☐ Anal

**CONTRACEPTION** ☐ None

☐ Condom ☐ Diaphragm
☐ IUD ☐ Pill
☐ Other: ____

**OBSTETRIC HISTORY**

Gr ____ Para ____ Ab ____ LMP ____

**PREVIOUS STD** ☐ None ☐ Other: ____

☐ GC ☐ Herpes ☐ Warts
☐ Syphillis ☐ Candida ☐ Scabies
☐ NGU ☐ Trich ☐ Crabs ☐ PID

**CURRENT MEDICATIONS**

Antibiotics? ☐ No ☐ Yes
Specify ____
Other Drugs? ☐ No ☐ Yes
Specify ____
IV Drug Use? ☐ No ☐ Yes
Specify ____

**ALLERGIES**

Penicillin ☐ No ☐ Yes
Specify ____
Asthma and/or Hay Fever ☐ No ☐ Yes

**LABORATORY**

Gram Stain ☐ None

| SITE | RESULT |
|---|---|
| ____ | ____ |
| ____ | ____ |

Gonorrhea Cultures ☐ None

☐ Urethra ☐ Pharynx
☐ Rectum ☐ Cervix

☐ RPR: ____
☐ VDRL
☐ FTA-ABS
☐ Dark Field: ____
☐ KOH: ____
☐ Wet Prep: ____
☐ Other ____

**ASSESSMENT**

**PLAN**

RTC ____
Cards ____

DC 118 (Rev. 4/76) DHH

**Fig. 87-1.** Visit form used by the Denver Metro STD Clinic to guide the clinician through an orderly encounter with patients and the recording of relevant STD information.

levels: Level I: "barefoot doctors" working in rural areas of a less-developed country without a reliable source of electricity for incubators or refrigerators. A light microscope and stains for urethral exudates are available. Level II: some clinics in big cities of less-developed countries as well as most clinics in developed countries. Electricity, incubators, and refrigerators are available. Level III: the occasional clinic in less-developed countries with access to reference laboratories and most clinics in developed countries affiliated with university research centers or which have access to reference laboratories.

## HUMAN IMMUNODEFICIENCY VIRUS INFECTIONS

AIDS is predominantly a sexually transmitted disease which demands a central control role for STD clinics and programs. HIV testing and counseling should be routinely offered to all patients and actively encouraged for any patient with continuing high-risk behavior who has not tested positive within the past 3 months. Technically, testing could be available through any clinical service which can draw blood and transport it to a central

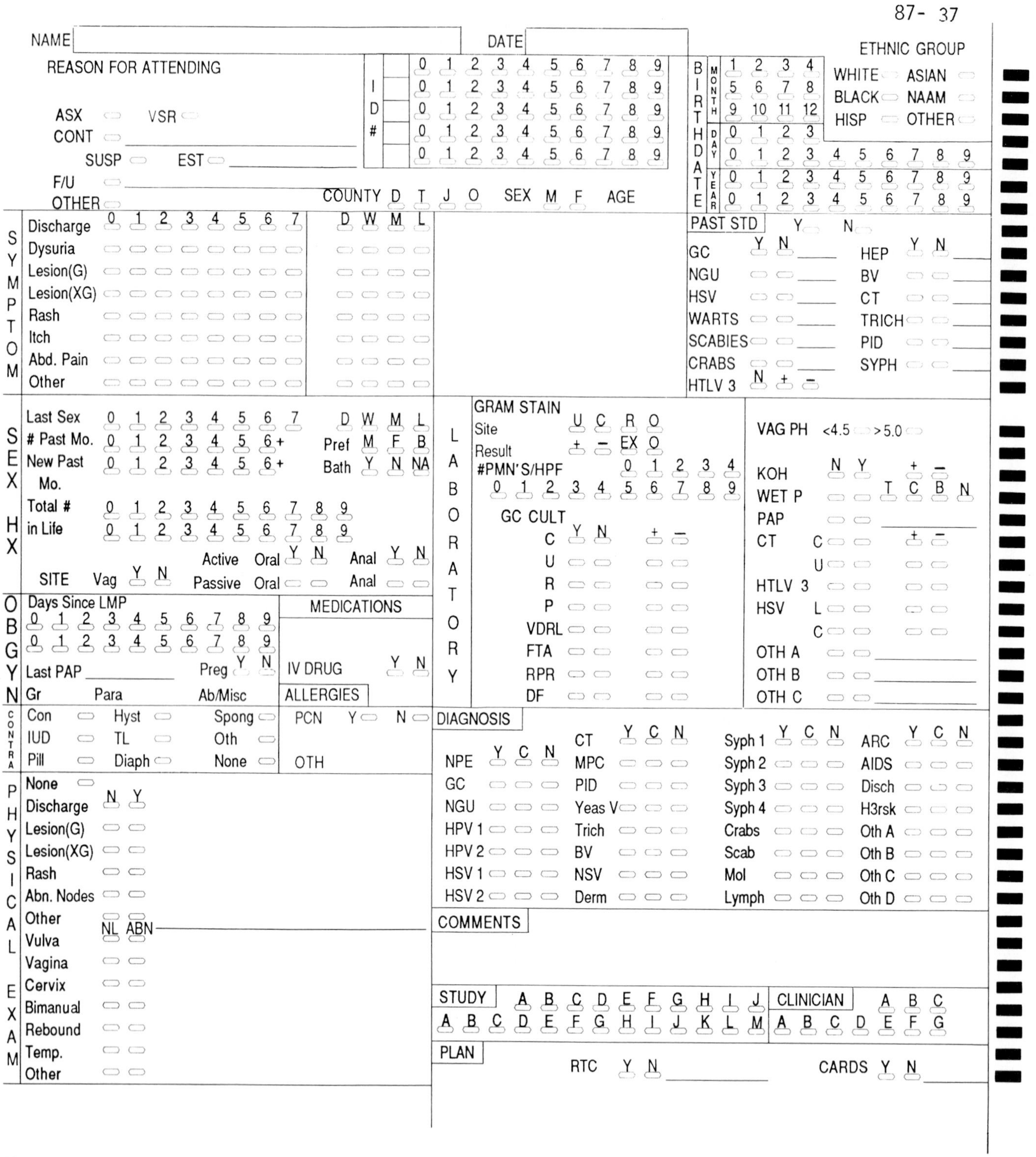

87- 37

NAME | DATE | ETHNIC GROUP: WHITE, ASIAN, BLACK, NAAM, HISP, OTHER

REASON FOR ATTENDING: ASX, VSR, CONT, SUSP, EST, F/U, OTHER

ID #: 0 1 2 3 4 5 6 7 8 9 (five rows)

BIRTH DATE: MONTH 1 2 3 4 5 6 7 8 9 10 11 12; DAY 0 1 2 3 / 0 1 2 3 4 5 6 7 8 9; YEAR 0 1 2 3 4 5 6 7 8 9 / 0 1 2 3 4 5 6 7 8 9

COUNTY D T J O   SEX M F   AGE

SYMPTOM (0 1 2 3 4 5 6 7; D W M L): Discharge, Dysuria, Lesion(G), Lesion(XG), Rash, Itch, Abd. Pain, Other

PAST STD Y N: GC, NGU, HSV, WARTS, SCABIES, CRABS, HTLV 3 (N + −); HEP, BV, CT, TRICH, PID, SYPH

SEX HX: Last Sex 0 1 2 3 4 5 6 7 (D W M L); # Past Mo. 0 1 2 3 4 5 6+; New Past Mo. 0 1 2 3 4 5 6+; Pref M F B; Bath Y N NA; Total # in Life 0 1 2 3 4 5 6 7 8 9 / 0 1 2 3 4 5 6 7 8 9; SITE Vag Y N; Active Oral Y N; Anal Y N; Passive Oral; Anal

OBGYN: Days Since LMP 0 1 2 3 4 5 6 7 8 9 / 0 1 2 3 4 5 6 7 8 9; Last PAP; Preg Y N; Gr; Para; Ab/Misc

MEDICATIONS; IV DRUG Y N; ALLERGIES: PCN Y N; OTH

CONTRA: Con, IUD, Pill, Hyst, TL, Diaph, Spong, Oth, None

LABORATORY: GRAM STAIN — Site U C R O; Result + − EX O; #PMN'S/HPF 0 1 2 3 4 / 0 1 2 3 4 5 6 7 8 9; GC CULT Y N + −: C, U, R, P; VDRL; FTA; RPR; DF

VAG PH <4.5 >5.0; KOH N Y + −; WET P T C B N; PAP; CT C U (+ −); HTLV 3; HSV L C; OTH A; OTH B; OTH C

PHYSICAL EXAM: None; Discharge N Y; Lesion(G); Lesion(XG); Rash; Abn. Nodes; Other; NL ABN: Vulva, Vagina, Cervix, Bimanual, Rebound, Temp., Other

DIAGNOSIS (Y C N): NPE, GC, NGU, HPV 1, HPV 2, HSV 1, HSV 2; CT, MPC, PID, Yeas V, Trich, BV, NSV, Derm; Syph 1, Syph 2, Syph 3, Syph 4, Crabs, Scab, Mol, Lymph; ARC, AIDS, Disch, H3rsk, Oth A, Oth B, Oth C, Oth D

COMMENTS

STUDY A B C D E F G H I J / A B C D E F G H I J K L M; CLINICIAN A B C / A B C D E F G

PLAN: RTC Y N; CARDS Y N

Fig. 87-2. Patient visit data form designed for optical scanning and automated data entry into a stand-alone clinic microcomputer.

laboratory. Practically, cost and transportation restraints may exclude the "barefoot doctor" from HIV testing until rapid serologic tests for the field are developed. During 1987, the Denver Metro STD Clinic tested and counseled nearly 5000 patients which represented approximately one-third of new clinic visits and nearly one-half of the 10,000 HIV tests provided by the Denver Public Health Department.

Wherever protections of confidentiality can be assured, HIV test results should be reported with patient identifiers to public health officials. This permits accurate assessment of the HIV epidemic, patient follow-up (about 15 percent of patients do not return for their test results), and notification (duty to warn) of partners who are unlikely otherwise to learn that they were exposed.

**Table 87-4. Approximate Sensitivity, Cost, and Appropriate Clinic Level(s) for Diagnostic Tests Commonly Used to Detect Sexually Transmitted Diseases**

| Disease | Diagnostic test | Approximate sensitivity | Approximate cost* | Appropriate clinic level |
|---|---|---|---|---|
| HIV infection | Serum antibody (ELISA) | 0.95–0.99 | \$2–\$5 | II, III |
| Gonorrhea: | | | | |
| Urethra | Stained smear | 0.95–0.98 | \$0.50–\$1 | I, II, III |
| | Culture | 0.95–0.98 | \$1–\$2 | II, III |
| Cervical | Stained smear | 0.50–0.60 | \$0.75–\$1.5 | II, III |
| | Culture | 0.80–0.95 | \$1–\$2 | II, III |
| Anorectal | Culture | <0.90 | \$1–\$2 | II, III |
| Pharyngeal | Culture | <0.90 | \$1–\$4 | II, III |
| Nongonococcal urethritis | Stained smear | 0.95–0.98 | \$0.50–\$1 | I, II, III |
| Chlamydia infection: | | | | |
| Urethral | Culture | 0.80–0.90 | \$15–\$30 | III |
| | Antigen detection | 0.75–0.80 | \$4–\$6 | II, III |
| Cervical | Culture | 0.75–0.90 | \$15–\$30 | III |
| | Antigen detection | 0.75–0.80 | \$4–\$6 | II, III |
| Trichomoniasis, vaginal | Saline wet prep | 0.50–0.75 | \$0.50–\$1 | I, II, III |
| | Culture | 0.85–0.90 | \$5–\$15 | III |
| Yeasts, vaginal | 10% KOH preparation | 0.50–0.75 | \$0.50–\$1 | I, II, III |
| | Culture | 0.95 | \$2–\$5 | II, III |
| Genital herpes | Cytological smear | 0.25–0.50 | \$2–\$4 | II, III |
| | Culture | 0.85–0.95 | \$25–\$35 | III |
| Syphilis | Dark field microscopy | † | \$2–\$3 | II, III |
| | Reagin (nontreponemal) | 0.70–1.00† | \$2–\$5 | I, II, III |
| | FTA-ABS (treponemal) | 0.85–1.00† | \$5–\$7 | II, III |
| | MHA-TP (treponemal) | 0.50–1.00† | \$3–\$5 | II, III |
| Cervical dysplasia | Pap smear | 0.85–0.90 | \$5–\$15 | I, II, III |

* Approximate costs are stated in United States currency and based on estimated of 1987 technician labor and supply costs in the United States. Actual charges for diagnostic tests may greatly exceed actual costs.
† Varies according to syphilis stage.

## GONORRHEA

Symptomatic gonococcal urethritis in men is most efficiently diagnosed by staining a smear of urethral exudate, a technique that should be about 98 percent sensitive.[5] Gram's method is frequently used in clinics of the developed world, but safranin, alone, or methylene blue may be equally sensitive and are more appropriate for clinicians practicing in isolated areas. A culture adds considerable cost and little diagnostic yield (about 2 percent) but is employed by many clinics when the stained smear is negative. Now that tetracycline is included in the treatment of men with either gonococcal or nongonococcal urethritis and their female contacts, the only practical value of the culture is to monitor gonococcal antimicrobial resistance trends.

The site of choice for obtaining specimens from women suspected of having gonorrhea is the endocervix. Gram-stained smears are, however, relatively insensitive (30 to 60 percent)[5] and their interpretation is difficult and time-consuming. Nonetheless, they are indicated when a high risk of infection exists, as in the presence of pelvic inflammatory disease, endocervical mucopurulent discharge, or a history of contact to gonorrhea. In these situations a positive smear may permit earlier diagnosis and treatment, thereby reducing complications and further spread of infection.

A culture on selective medium is essential to properly diagnose gonorrhea in most women. Owing to inoculum effect, either an anal canal or a second endocervical culture will add about 5 percent to the sensitivity of a single endocervical culture. This can be accomplished at lowest cost by combining two endocervical specimens on opposite sides of the same culture plate.[6]

With the possible exception of mucopurulent anorectal discharges, stained smears of anorectal or pharyngeal specimens are too nonspecific for routine use. The diagnosis of gonococcal infection of these sites requires cultures on selective medium. Single anorectal or pharyngeal cultures are of undetermined sensitivity but likely well below 90 percent. Because pharyngeal infection is not often spread to others, is rarely symptomatic, and is often self-limited[7] and because pharyngeal isolates must be confirmed as *Neisseria gonorrhoeae* by expensive additional tests, a strong argument can be made for omitting routine cultures of this site in level I and II clinics.

Transport systems (e.g., Transgrow, Jembec) would seem to offer gonorrhea culturing capabilities to level I clinics. Unfortunately, they are expensive, use fresh medium with a shelf life that is particularly short in tropical climates and need to be preincubated and delivered to a processing laboratory within 48 h in order to achieve acceptable sensitivity.[8] The disease control potential of transport media is therefore limited. The best solution may lie in incubators which do not require electricity. Based upon current cost and performance considerations, I do not feel that commercially available antigen detection systems (e.g., enzyme immunoassay, direct fluorescent microscopy) can provide an answer to the transport problem at this time.

## NONGONOCOCCAL URETHRITIS AND CHLAMYDIA INFECTIONS

Nongonococcal urethritis (NGU) ranks as the most common sexually transmitted disease of men. In the majority of clinics its diagnosis is one of exclusion made by the failure to detect "typical" intracellular diplococci on a stained smear of urethral exudate. To the extent that tetracycline is the regimen of choice for most NGU cases of undetermined etiology, this is satisfactory.

*Chlamydia trachomatis* has become recognized as the cause of 40 to 50 percent of NGU[9] and could be the most common of all sexually transmitted pathogens (Chap. 16). Although a few level III clinics perform *Chlamydia* cultures, routinely on men with NGU and on women, cultures remain expensive ($15 to $30), technically complex, and of uncertain sensitivity. Antigen detections systems utilizing enzyme immunoassays or fluorescent staining have made specific testing for chlamydial infections technically possible in most clinics. Unfortunately, they are not inexpensive and are somewhat less sensitive than well-performed cultures (e.g., relative sensitivities of 80 to 95 percent in women and in men with NGU).

## TRICHOMONIASIS

Trichomoniasis is an extremely common STD (Chap. 43) that causes a great deal of discomfort but few serious complications. Accordingly, no country has a designated control program for *Trichomonas vaginalis*. A reasonable goal for clinics is to detect and treat for the lowest cost as many women with trichomoniasis and their sexual partners as is possible.

Diagnosis by clinical presentation is insufficiently sensitive and specific;[10,11] thus a saline wet prep or culture is desirable. Of the two, the wet prep is by far the simplest and least costly; however, it may detect no more than 50 percent of cases.[10,11] Wet preps perform better in symptomatic than in asymptomatic infections. An alternative to on-site wet mounts is the fixation preparation of slides to be transported to a central laboratory for staining by acridine orange or Papanicolaou methods.[12] They could be used by "barefoot doctors" but are more costly and inconvenient and require a second patient visit. Although the most sensitive, screening women or men with trichomonal cultures is not often clinically practical. The culture technique is highly labor-intensive and for best results requires special modification of established media,[10] such as Diamonds or Feinberg-Whittington, which are not widely available.

## YEAST INFECTIONS

Yeasts, particularly *Candida albicans,* are often present on human genitalia. Although vaginal yeast infections are frequently asymptomatic and rarely sexually acquired, STD clinics must be prepared to diagnose and treat them. Of symptoms associated with vaginal yeast infections, only vulvar pruritis is somewhat specific, but it is found in no more than half of women with positive cultures.[13]

Yeasts can be identified in vaginal fluid or scrapings by saline wet preparations, stained smears, or 10 percent KOH preparations; however, none of these techniques is more than 50 percent sensitive when compared with cultures. KOH preparations are 10 to 15 percent more sensitive than saline wet preparations and are able to detect the majority of symptomatic women. They are the budget-minded diagnostic method of choice for all clinic levels.

Of the many culture media that will grow yeasts, dextrose-peptone agar (Sabourauds) is the commonly accepted diagnostic standard. We believe that few clinics should expend scarce resources on cultural identification of asymptomatic yeast infections. Speciation of fungal isolates has little impact on therapy and is of value only in research studies.

## BACTERIAL VAGINOSIS

The microbial etiology of bacterial vaginosis is complex and incompletely understood.[14] Typical diagnostic criteria[14] include: first, vaginal secretions negative by microscopical examination for yeast and *T. vaginalis* and second, two or more of the following: homogeneous quality of secretions; pH > 4.5; presence of "clue" cells; and release of a "fishy" amine odor on addition of 10 percent potassium hydroxide (Chap. 47). These methods are readily available at most clinics.

## GENITAL HERPES

Symptomatic genital herpes simplex virus (HSV) infections are seen with high frequency in STD, dermatology, and gynecology clinics. During 1987, genital herpes was the most commonly diagnosed open lesion at the Denver Metro STD Clinic. Herpetic lesions were ten times more common than primary syphilis in men and seventeen times more common in women. High rates of genital HSV infections and their serious acute and chronic complications (Chap. 35) emphasize the need for diagnostic services.

In spite of effective suppressive therapy with acyclovir, control measures for genital herpes are limited to early diagnosis and patient education aimed at promoting behavioral changes that will reduce the risk of further viral transmission. Unfortunately, this will miss the majority of HSV infections, since most are asymptomatic or ignored symptomatic. Cultures for HSV are expensive and not practical for level I and II clinical facilities. Cytologic smears necessitate stocking additional stains and are only 25 to 50 percent sensitive, while newer antigen detection systems are more sensitive but not yet adequately evaluated or widely available (Chap. 77). However, with experience, physicians and PAs can reliably diagnose most genital herpes infections by physical examination and distinguish between primary infection and recurrences by history.[15,16]

## SYPHILIS

The diagnosis of syphilis and its proper staging usually require the application of many informational sources including risk factors for infection, clinical history, physical findings, and the results of dark field microscopy and/or serologic tests.[17,18] Level I facilities will not have microscopes equipped to perform dark field examinations; in some countries this can be accomplished by performing smears of syphilitic lesion expressate for transportation to a central laboratory and direct fluorescent antibody staining. The "barefoot doctor" will be able to diagnose most cases of early, infectious syphilis by careful integration of epidemiological, historical, and physical findings with the results of a field reagin test (e.g., RPR Card Test). The cardiolipin antigen for this test is stable at 56°C for at least 2 months.

Costs of detecting new cases of syphilis can be minimized by concentrating serology screening resources on defined clinic groups at high risk of infection. Clinics should attempt to estimate risk factors for the populations they serve. Owing to fear of AIDS, the majority of new cases of infectious syphilis in the United States are no longer in homosexual men. Recently, large increases in syphilis incidence have been reported for urban, poor, heterosexual, black and Hispanic men and women. In northern Europe "heroin prostitutes" are another high-risk group. The Denver Metro STD clinic screens these patients every time they come to clinic. Conversely, white heterosexual men and women rarely are found to have syphilis and are tested routinely only if they have not been seen within 6 months or give a history of prostitution or IV-drug use.

FTA-ABS and MHA-TP tests are useful for confirming all cases of syphilis but have their greatest utility in late latent and late stages.[17] With the possible exception of microautomated MHA-TP, they should not be used for routine screening.

## GENITAL WARTS, MOLLUSCUM CONTAGIOSUM, SCABIES, PEDICULOSIS PUBIS, PELVIC INFLAMMATORY DISEASE

Although examination of genital wart biopsy material, staining of the molluscum "central core," microscopic examination of oil preparation scrapings of excoriated scabetic papules (less than 10 percent sensitive), and cultures of peritoneal fluid aspirates from women with pelvic inflammatory disease (PID) have been well studied, they are impractical for most clinics, and a diagnosis will need to be made on clinical grounds.

## LYMPHOGRANULOMA VENEREUM, CHANCROID, GRANULOMA INGUINALE

As a result of more extensive experience with lymphogranuloma venereum, chancroid, and granuloma inguinale, the well-trained "barefoot doctor" will be able to outperform STD specialists in the developed world who seldom see these diseases and must depend on laboratory tests that are not readily available and/or are not fully proved.

## CERVICAL DYSPLASIA

Women who develop cervical cancer share many risk factors with women who attend STD clinics including early age of coitus, multiple sex partners, a high prevalence of antibodies to herpes simplex virus type 2, and evidence of cervical infection with certain types of HPV. Accordingly, STD clinics are logical places to screen higher-risk women for the cervical dysplasia that antedates carcinoma. Even "barefoot doctors" could fix endocervical smears for later staining and reading by a central laboratory. The major problems are cost ($5 to $15 per test), a high rate of unreadable smears which need repeating, and poor patient follow-up.

In summary, the "barefoot doctor" will be able to adequately diagnose about 80 to 90 percent of all cases of STD. From the standpoint of controlling serious STD, the main deficiencies will occur in the diagnosis of asymptomatic gonorrhea, subclinical HIV infections, asymptomatic chlamydial infections, and the late stages of syphilis.

## TREATMENT

Although prohibited by the pharmacy laws of some countries, the overall costs to society of controlling STD will be minimized and patient compliance maximized if treatment and prevention supplies are given at the clinic. Clinics can usually buy antibiotics and condoms in large quantities at reduced rates (e.g., less than $0.06 per condom). Antibiotics can then be efficiently packaged and/or dispensed by clinic personnel under a physician's supervision and license.

Many clinics will not have the financial resources to provide all treatment services. As a compromise, the Denver Metro STD Clinic has elected to treat without charge all cases of gonorrhea, pelvic inflammatory disease, epididymitis, NGU, trichomoniasis, syphilis, genital warts, and their contacts. Prescriptions are issued for treatment of yeast vaginitis, scabies, and pediculosis pubis.

Treatment of STD has been categorized as personal prophylaxis,[19,20] epidemiologic,[21] and postdiagnostic.

## PERSONAL PROPHYLAXIS

Personal prophylaxis for STD consists of the following: restricting sexual activities, using mechanical barriers impervious to microbes, applying local agents that destroy microbes, and taking systemic chemotherapy before or soon after sexual exposure.

Avoiding sexual contact with unknown persons or with persons thought to be promiscuous minimizes the risk of contracting STD. Unfortunately, the likelihood of markedly influencing sexual behavior of high-risk patients appears to be small.

The condom is the most common form of mechanical prophylaxis. Undamaged latex condoms have been shown in vitro to provide an effective physical barrier against most sexually transmitted agents and can be made safer yet by the addition of a backup microbicidal chemical barrier such as a lubricant or ointment containing no less than 5.5 percent nonoxynol-9.[22] Although acceptance rates vary according to gender, sexual preference, and sociologic factors, condom use by all STD clinic patients has increased dramatically during the AIDS epidemic. For example, only 3 percent of gay men attending the Denver Metro STD clinic in 1981–1983 used condoms at all, but 61 percent used them in 1986–1987.[22] We recommend that STD clinics encourage the use of condoms by offering them free of charge, along with proper instructions, to all patients who might benefit. Instructions should include the warning that condoms can never provide absolute protection against any STD. At $0.056 per condom, the budget impact is small even for the Denver Metro STD Clinic, which distributed 35,000 in 1987.

Local prophylactic measures such as soap and water, douching, contraceptive foams, jellies or creams, chemotherapeutics, and antibiotics have been tried. Most studies in which these methods were evaluated were uncontrolled, and the results are contradictory.[19,20] Factors critical to the success of local prophylaxis may include the extent of drug application, the regularity of use, and the timing of application (preexposure or postexposure).

Systemic chemotherapy is the most effective form of prophylaxis against syphilis, gonorrhea, and chancroid.[20,21] Nonetheless, there remain several concerns about this practice. It does not protect against all STD; the drugs often are not used properly; the risks of toxic and allergic drug reactions are increased; and resistant microorganisms may be given a selective advantage. Systemic chemotherapy, however, may be indicated in situations where diagnostic procedures are poor or absent, the opportunity to contract STD is high, and follow-up of patients is impossible. With the exception of promoting the use of condoms, clinics have little else to offer as proved personal prophylaxis.

## EPIDEMIOLOGIC TREATMENT

Epidemiologic treatment refers to treatment when the diagnosis is likely on behavioral, clinical, or epidemiologic grounds but before the results of confirmatory tests, if any, are known.[22] Because it short-circuits the time required to complete diagnostic tests, this type of treatment is a potent clinic weapon for reducing the duration of infection and thus the risk of further transmission. Epidemiologic treatment has been used successfully in the control of gonorrhea and syphilis. It is also widely practiced on contacts of NGU, proved chlamydial infections, and trichomonal vaginitis. Each clinic should devise protocols governing epidemiologic treatment that carefully weigh local risk factors for having STD against the risks of adverse effects from treatments.

## POSTI IAGNOSTIC TREATMENT

Most patients with STD will be treated after diagnosis. The details of treatments are discussed in chapters on each specific disease. For clinics deciding which chemotherapeutic regimens to use, it is important to consider cure rates, ease of administration, duration of treatment, patient compliance (clinic administered single dosing has the advantage of 100 percent patient compliance), adverse effects, cost, microbiological spectrum, stability at ambient temperature, and the rates at which STD coexist. For the "barefoot doctor" and other level I practitioners, generic tetracycline will be the single most useful drug to stock. However, in areas of Southeast Asia and Africa, care must be taken to monitor periodically for gonorrhea treatment efficacy as background chromosomally mediated resistance to tetracycline and some other antibiotics is relatively high.

The potential STD control benefits of curing coexisting infections with a single chemotherapeutic regimen should not be underestimated. This is particularly true for *C. trachomatis*, which can be isolated from about 25 percent of men with gonococcal urethritis and 45 percent of women with endocervical gonorrhea.[23] Specific diagnosis of chlamydial infection still is relatively difficult and costly. Treating heterosexual men and women with gonorrhea with a regimen which includes 7 days of tetracycline (500 mg four times a day) will help to reduce the patient reservoir of *Chlamydia* at little additional cost.

Patients treated for gonorrhea should be instructed to return for a test-of-cure. This will permit an ongoing comparison of treatment results as well as early awareness of increasing resistance to or adverse effects of antimicrobial agents. Posttreatment visits may not be indicated for STD which are less serious and/or lack clear-cut determinants of cure.

## PATIENT REFERRALS

An STD clinic should function as an integral part of an overall health care delivery system. Success in this area can be measured by the extent to which other health care providers utilize the clinic for consultations and patient referrals. The clinic should be viewed as a community resource for current information on recommended diagnostic tests and treatments and for resolution of complicated STD clinical problems. It should not be viewed as a repository for obstreperous and/or proverty-stricken patients.

In like manner, the STD clinic should carefully develop its professional relationships with private practitioners in the community and, where possible, with other related subspecialty clinics. In some areas, close relationships with family planning clinics have benefited both STD and contraceptive practices (Chap. 90). Among the subspecialties most frequently referred to by the Denver Metro STD Clinic are dermatology, obstetrics and gynecology, psychiatry, urology, and proctology. The proper indication for a referral is a patient problem that exceeds the capability of the clinic. However, the broader the clinic's capability and willingness to diagnose and attend to certain other conditions easily confused with STD (e.g., minor dermatoses, uncomplicated cystitis, minor psychosexual concerns), the more patients will be likely to return to the clinic when afflicted with serious STD and the more effective the clinic will be in controlling STD.

## STD EDUCATION

In theory, effective community education could play a major role in control programs. Preferably, fundamentals of STD education will be taught to all 14- to 16-year-old students during sex education components of health education courses. In practice, education often fails to modify human behavior in ways that will prevent disease.[24]

Nonetheless, clinics are in a favored position to positively influence health behavior of the population at risk because concern about STD is at a maximum when patients are sick and/or anxious. This is the time for clinicians to take full advantage of the patient's focused attention and use it to communicate in concise, nonmedical language: what the disease is, how it is spread, how to treat the disease, what type of follow-up is necessary, what to tell sexual partners, and how to avoid getting the disease again. In addition, summary information sheets on each disease may help to reinforce these points.

Training and education of health care providers are functions that need to be integrated into most level III clinics, particularly when they are affiliated with university medical centers. The control value from improving STD health care delivered by practicing physicians, nurses, PAs, and laboratory technicians deserves priority consideration.

## CLINIC OUTREACH

Model clinics will not be content to operate as passive health care islands, forming narrow impressions of the epidemiology of STD in the community based upon the patients who elect to come through their doors. Rather, they will attempt to reach out into the community to identify segments of the population at high risk of infections and to understand how disease is maintained in the population.

This may consist of active tracing of partners of patients with repeated infections, serious complications (e.g., pelvic inflammatory disease), difficult to treat infections (e.g., penicillinase-producing *N. gonorrhoeae*), or deadly infections (e.g., HIV). It may also consist of prevalence studies to locate epidemiologically defined groups that would benefit from out-of-clinic periodic case detection services. This approach has been used successfully in a poor black area of Denver experiencing a high rate of gonorrhea, in Denver's steam baths where homosexual men are at high risk of having HIV infections, gonorrhea, hepatitis B, and syphilis,[25] and in the Netherlands where women attending abortion clinics and heroin prostitutes are likely to have many STDs.

Outreach that establishes cooperative programs through primary care physicians (Chap. 93), family planning clinics (Chap. 90), adolescent medicine clinics, gay health care centers, AIDS projects, school-based clinics, substance treatment centers, jails, and any other facilities likely to see persons at risk of STD is desirable. Finally, clinic personnel can make a valuable contribution to STD education in the schools. Students appreciate learning about STD from clinicians who have firsthand professional experience, and clinicians appreciate the variety and prestige associated with teaching.

## QUALITY CONTROL

A clinic may evaluate the quality of its services by a number of different methods. The most important factors that contribute to quality are the proper selection and training of personnel. For clinics using PAs, it is best that charts be reviewed by the attending physician for completeness and internal logic within 30 min of the patient visit. This ensures that details of the patient encounter are still memory-fresh. Periodically, PAs should also be monitored while seeing patients. Less direct measures of the performance of a physician or PA include the percent of their patients who return for a test-of-cure visit as well as the rates at which partners appear at the clinic for evaluation.

The clinic census should be representative of the local population at risk of STD with respect to age, gender, sexual preference, race, and socioeconomic status. The reasons of underrepresentation of a high-risk group should be sought. Clinic attendance and disease rates should move in response to community secular trends in STD morbidity.

Quality control of treatments and diagnostic tests depends initially on adherence to process recommendations regarding refrigeration and/or shelf life of antibiotics, culture medium, and test reagents. More important are outcome measurements. Among these are the percent of patients who are properly followed up and found cured for each treatment regimen and, whenever possible, the level of agreement between different diagnostic tests for the same disease. Level II and III facilities will be able to determine the relative performance of various serologic tests in proved cases of clinical syphilis. Some clinics may participate in proficiency testing programs which employ sera of unstated reactivity sent periodically to a central laboratory.

All level II and III clinics should develop methods for comparing results of Gram-stained smears and cultures for *N. gonorrhoeae*. This is the only practical way to continuously monitor the quality of gonorrhea diagnostic techniques which begins with medium production and ends with transmittal of results to patients.[5] When Gram stains and cultures are recorded by the performing clinician, it also is possible to identify clinician-specific defects in culture or Gram-staining techniques.

In recent years quality-control efforts have received assistance from two additional sources. One is the computerized clinic record system (Fig. 87-2), which can monitor most of the foregoing quality measures more efficiently than a hand tabulation system. The other is the Centers for Disease Control "Quality Assurance Guidelines for Clinical Services" and on-site STD program review procedures. The "guidelines" provide an excellent framework with which to evaluate an STD clinic's strengths and weaknesses but must be interpreted in a flexible manner to allow for local differences in clinic structure, staff composition, patient characteristics, and disease incidence.

## References


1 Sox HC et al: The training of physicians' assistants. The use of a clinical algorithm system for patient care, audit of performance and education. *N Engl J Med* 288:818, 1973.

2 Greenfield S et al: Efficiency and cost of primary care by nurses and physicians' assistants. *N Engl J Med* 298:305, 1978.

3 Sox HC: Quality of patient care by nurse practitioners and physicians' assistants: A ten-year perspective. *Ann Intern Med* 91:459, 1979.

4 Rothenberg RB, Judson FN: Strategic planning system for control of venereal disease: Record-keeping in a clinic for treatment of sexually-transmitted diseases. *Sex Transm Dis* 6:1, 1979.

5 Judson FN: A clinic-based system for monitoring the quality of techniques for the diagnosis of gonorrhea. *Sex Transm Dis* 5:141, 1978.

6 Judson FN, Werness BA: Combining cervical and anal-canal specimens for gonorrhea on a single culture plate. *J Clin Microbiol* 12:216, 1980.

7 Hutt DM, Judson FN: Epidemiology and treatment of oropharyngeal gonorrhea. *Ann Intern Med* 104:655, 1986.

8 Phillips I: Assessment of transport and isolation methods for gonococci. *Br J Vener Dis* 56:390, 1980.

9 Holmes KK et al: Etiology of nongonococal urethritis. *N Engl J Med* 292:1199, 1975.

10 Fouts AC, Kraus SJ: *Trichomonas vaginalis*: Reevaluation of its clinical presentation and laboratory diagnosis. *J Infect Dis* 141:137, 1980.

11 Spence MR et al: The clinical and laboratory diagnosis of *Trichomonas vaginalis* infection by use of acridine orange fluorescent microscopy. *Sex Transm Dis* 7:168, 1980.

12 Krieger JN et al: Diagnosis of trichomoniasis. Comparison of conventional wet-mount examination with cytologic studies, cultures, and monoclonal antibody staing of direct specimens. *JAMA* 259:1223, 1988.

13 Oriel JD et al: Genital yeast infections. *Br Med J* 4:761, 1972.

14 Spiegel CA et al: Anaerobic bacteria in nonspecific vaginitis. *N Engl J Med* 303:601, 1980.

15 Corey L, Holmes KK: Genital herpes simplex virus infections: Current concepts in diagnosis, therapy, and prevention. *Ann Intern Med* 98:973, 1983.

16 Corey L et al: Genital herpes simplex virus infections: Clinical manifestations, course, and complications. *Ann Intern Med* 98:958, 1983.

17 Lee TJ, Sparling PF: Syphilis. An algorithm. *JAMA* 242:1187, 1979.

18 Hart G: Syphilis tests in diagnostic and therapeutic decision making. *Ann Intern Med* 104:368, 1983.

19 Stone KM et al: Primary prevention of sexually transmitted diseases. A primer for clinicians. *JAMA* 255:1763, 1986.

20 Hart G: Role of preventive methods in the control of venereal disease. *Clin Obstet Gynecol* 18:243, 1975.

21 Hart G: Epidemiologic treatment for syphilis and gonorrhea. *Sex Transm Dis* 7:152, 1970.

22 Judson FN et al: In vitro evaluations of condoms with and without nonoxynol 9 as physical and chemical barriers against *C. trachomatis*, herpes simplex virus type 2, and human immunodeficiency virus. *Sex Transm Dis*, 1988 (in press).

23 Judson FN: The importance of coexisting syphilitic, chlamydial, mycoplasmal and trichomonal infections in the treatment of gonorrhea. *Sex Transm Dis* 6:112, 1979.

24 Judson FN: How to control gonorrhea: The view of a local public health officer. *Sex Transm Dis* 6:231, 1979.

25 Judson FN et al: Screening for gonorrhea and syphilis in the gay baths—Denver, Colorado. *Am J Public Health* 67:740, 1977.

# Chapter 88

# Patient counseling and behavior modification

William Parra
D. Peter Drotman
Karolynn Siegel
Karin Esteves
Timothy Baker

Radical changes in the way both patients and clinicians respond to sexually transmitted diseases (STDs) have occurred in the short interval since the first edition of this book was published. The most dramatic changes have resulted from the public health challenges posed by the human immunodeficiency virus (HIV) infections and their most severe manifestation, acquired immunodeficiency syndrome (AIDS). The most significant impact of AIDS in patient care, especially STD patient care, has been the consistent emphasis on effective patient counseling. As a result of the sobering consequences of AIDS, patients and health care providers alike have come to recognize the enormous direct benefits that can be realized from effective efforts to change behaviors.

However, the transition from knowledge of prevention methods to implementation of corresponding behavioral changes which reduce the potential of becoming infected remains difficult for many persons at risk. The psychological, social, and medical reasons for this are manifold, but the challenge is clear for counselors who struggle with these issues: counseling must, in essence, attempt to modify human behavior.

The main reasons for the high incidence rates of STD are behavioral[1] and include the behavior of: (1) individuals who contract and transmit STD, (2) health personnel who manage these diseases, and (3) national, state, and community leaders who provide the technical guidance and appropriate the financial support required for the success of control programs. An increasing awareness in recent years of the importance of psychosocial factors (Chaps. 5, 9, 89, 90) in STD control[2] has underscored the importance of the behavior of patients who contract STD for reducing the incidence of STD. Quality assurance guidelines for disease intervention specialists (counselors) in STD control programs, published by the Centers for Disease Control (CDC), clearly regard the patient as a key resource who must be actively recruited to assist in disease-prevention efforts.[3] Historically, syphilis contact tracing strongly emphasized aggressive efforts of public health personnel to elicit the identity of, locate, diagnose, and treat sex partners. Unfortunately, patients were relegated to relatively passive roles in disease prevention and control activities. The recognition of viral STDs such as genital herpes, hepatitis B, and HIV infection helped change this view in the 1980s and highlighted the importance of the patient's role in reducing disease transmission. More than ever, change of the patient's sexual behavior is now regarded as an essential element in the prevention and ultimate control of STD.[2,4] There is growing recognition of the value of using knowledge from the social and behavioral sciences in influencing lifestyle choices, reinforcing positive health habits, and promoting the adoption of health-promoting behavior.[5]

The wider scope of recognized STDs in the 1980s precipitated the development of a flexible and comprehensive patient counseling model that responds to the varied needs of patients with different infections. This led to the gradual replacement of disease-specific with behavior-specific approaches. Patient behavior became the focus. Not only was this approach more directly associated with patient counseling goals but it also simplified the role of the counselor. The complexity of the psychosocial issues associated with AIDS, however, could not be addressed by any existing STD approach. As a result, this chapter separates HIV counseling from other STD. Any STD patient should be viewed as potentially HIV-infected or at least at increased risk for HIV infection. By adopting this viewpoint, counselors and clinicians will be taking a major step forward in AIDS prevention and STD risk reduction.

## GENERAL STD COUNSELING

The goal of patients counseling is patient compliance with several important behaviors. *Compliance* is defined as the extent to which the patient follows through with prescribed treatment regimens and other instructions for the management or cure of a disease or infection and with advice on changing sexual behavior leading to the prevention of infection and disease.[6] This implies the transfer of knowledge as well as the added dimension of inducing, persuading, or otherwise motivating patients to prevent the future risk of infection.[7]

Effective counseling is not easy for many medical conditions, even under the best of circumstances. However, it may be even more difficult with STD patients because much of the burden of morbidity is borne by poorer and less well educated members of society. These groups often feel alienated and powerless over events in their lives[8] and frequently are made up of minority racial and ethnic groups. This is true with AIDS patients as well. Blacks and Hispanics have been more likely to have contracted AIDS than whites.[9] The probability that a patient will comply with treatment- and prevention-related recommendations is generally recognized to be determined by a complex range of factors, including health beliefs, psychological characteristics, and social conditions. The AIDS epidemic has heightened the level of concern of STD patients in general and those who perceive themselves at risk for HIV infection particularly.

Although many behavioral messages may be given patients within the context of STD counseling, five principal messages are discussed in this chapter. They are as follows:

1. Take oral medication as directed (when applicable).
2. Return for follow-up tests (when applicable).
3. Ensure examination of sex partners.
4. Reduce risk by
   *a.* Abstaining from any sexual activity until follow-up test.
   *b.* Abstaining from any sexual activity whenever symptoms appear.
   *c.* Using condoms in risky or unknown settings.
5. Respond immediately and appropriately to infection or disease suspicion.

Counselors can address these matters in whatever order best fits the needs of the patient as long as they consider (1) which message is most important to the patient, (2) which message is most important for the patient, (3) how much time is available, and (4) how the time can be most effectively used to achieve the best results. Logically, patients may respond to messages most pertinent to their own cure first, next to the cure of those closest to them, and finally to their longer-term health status and the health of others. The most successful counselors tailor the messages to the needs of the patient. For example, "cure" is mainly applicable to bacterial and parasitic STD and would thus be inappropriate as a counseling concept for viruses such as herpes, hepatitis B, or HIV. Specific messages to stress for each STD are listed in Table 88-1.

**Table 88-1. Sexually Transmitted Disease Counseling Summary**

| Disease and biologic agents | Behavioral messages to emphasize |
|---|---|
| Chlamydial infections<br>Nongonococcal urethritis (NGU) | Understand how to take any prescribed oral medications. If tetracycline is prescribed, take it 1 h before or 2 h after meals and avoid dairy products, antacids, iron or other mineral-containing preparations, and sunlight. Return for test-of-cure or evaluation 4–7 days after completion of therapy, or earlier if symptoms persist or recur. Refer sexual partner(s) for examination and treatment. Avoid sex until patient and partner(s) are cured. Use condoms to prevent future infections |
| Mucopurulent cervicitis (MPC) | Understand how to take any prescribed oral medications. If tetracycline is given, take it 1 h before or 2 h after meals, and avoid dairy products, antacids, iron or other mineral-containing preparations, and sunlight. Return for reevaluation 4–7 days after completion of therapy, or earlier if symptoms persist or recur. Refer sexual partner(s) for examination and treatment. Avoid sex until patient and partner(s) are cured. Use condoms to prevent future infections |
| Gonorrhea | Understand how to take any prescribed oral medications. If tetracycline is prescribed, take it 1 h before or 2 h after meals and avoid dairy products, antacids, iron or other mineral-containing preparations, and sunlight. Return for test-of-cure 4–7 days after completing therapy. Refer sexual partners for examination and treatment. Avoid sex until patient and partner(s) are cured. Return early if symptoms persist or recur. Use condoms to prevent future infections |
| Pelvic inflammatory disease (PID) | Understand how to take any prescribed oral medications. If tetracycline is given, take it 1 h before or 2 h after meals and avoid dairy products, antacids, iron or other mineral-containing preparations, and sunlight. Return 2–3 days after initiation of therapy for progress evaluation. Return for test-of-cure 4–7 days after completing therapy. Refer sexual partner(s) for evaluation and treatment. Avoid sexual activity until patient and partner(s) are cured. If an IUD is used, consult with family planning physician. Use condoms to prevent future infections |
| Vaginitis | Understand how to take or use any prescribed medications. Avoid alcohol until 3 days following completion of metronidazole therapy. Continue taking vaginally administered medications even during menses. Return if problems not cured or if it recurs. Use condoms to prevent trichomonas infections |
| Genital warts | Return for weekly or biweekly treatment and follow up until lesions have resolved. Partners should be examined for warts. Abstain from sex or use condoms during therapy |
| Herpes genitalis | Keep involved area clean and dry. Since both initial and recurrent lesions shed high concentrations of virus, patients should abstain from sex while symptomatic. An undetermined but presumably small risk of transmission also exists during asymptomatic intervals. Condoms may offer some protection. Annual Pap smears are recommended. Pregnant women should make their obstetricians aware of any history of herpes |
| Syphilis | Understand how to take any prescribed oral medications. If tetracycline is given, take it 1 h before or 2 h after meals, and avoid dairy products, antacids, iron or other mineral-containing preparations, and sunlight. Return for follow-up serologies 3, 6, 12, and 24 months after therapy. Refer sexual partner(s) for evaluation and treatment. Avoid sexual activity until patient and partner(s) are cured. Use condoms to prevent future infections |
| Chancroid | Assure examination and treatment of sexual partner(s) as soon as possible. Return weekly or biweekly for evaluation until the infection is entirely healed. Use condoms to prevent future infections |
| Pediculosis pubis | Clothing and linen should be disinfected by washing them in hot water, by dry cleaning them, or by removing them from human exposure for 1–2 weeks. Avoid sexual or close physical contact until after treatment. Assure examination of sexual partners as soon as possible. Return if problem is not cured or recurs |
| Scabies | Clothing and linen should be disinfected by washing them in hot water, by dry cleaning them, or by removing them from human exposure for 1–2 weeks. Avoid sexual or close physical contact until after treatment. Assure examination of sexual partners as soon as possible. Return if problem is not cured or recurs |
| Hepatitis B | The frequency of clinical follow-up is determined by symptomatology and the results of liver function tests. Hepatitis B immune globulin (HBIG) and hepatitis B vaccine are available. Both are protective against hepatitis B infection |
| Enteric infections | Follow dietary and medical regimens. Avoid oral-anal contact at least until infection is cleared. Refer sexual partner(s) for examination. Avoid sex until patient and partner(s) are cured. Return early if symptoms persist or recur |
| AIDS (acquired immunodeficiency syndrome) and HIV infection | Sexual contact with individuals who have had sex with multiple or anonymous partners increases risk of infection and should be avoided. For individuals who choose to initiate a new sexual relationship with a person at increased risk for HIV or who maintain casual sexual relationships, sexual practices should be limited to those that do not permit any exchange of blood or bodily secretions. Condoms should be used consistently. Fisting is strongly discouraged. Do not inject illicit drugs. If such practices continue, do not share needles and syringes. Do not use inhalant nitrates ("poppers"). These have been implicated as a cofactor for Kaposi's sarcoma |

SOURCE: Ref. 22.

## TAKE MEDICATION AS DIRECTED

The difference between the oral medication regimen the clinician prescribes and the one the patient actually follows may be distressingly great. In general, clinicians not only overestimate patient compliance but also cannot reliably predict which of their patients will comply.[10] Estimates of rates of compliance vary widely, regardless of treatment regimens prescribed and diseases treated. However, an axiom which summarizes many studies states that one-third of patients always take their medicine as directed, one-third sometimes do, and one-third seldom or never do.[11] In addition, compliance with short-term medication regimens has been found to decline rapidly from one day to the next.[12]

Several studies have shown that reasons for noncompliance are: side effects;[13] complexity of the regimen;[11,14] and communication failure between health care provider and patient.[15] Many patients simply do not understand or retain the instructions given by the health care provider. In one clinical setting, only about one-half of the information provided to patients could be recalled within 5 minutes after it was communicated.[16]

The most obvious consequence of noncompliance is possible treatment failure resulting in further spread of the infection as well as complications for the patient. Additional or modified regimens to correct apparent treatment failure incur further costs and possible health problems caused by the treatments themselves.[17] Several investigations have attempted in vain to define factors that could reliably characterize the noncomplier;[18,19] unfortunately and surprisingly, few significant differences were found between defaulters and compliers.

The quality of the clinician-patient relationship has been judged to be a critical factor in compliance. Satisfaction with treatment and resulting compliance are greater when patients' expectations have been fulfilled, the clinician has responded to their concerns, responsive information about their conditions has been provided, and sincere concern and empathy have been shown.[20] Many studies have confirmed that compliance improves if more attention is paid by the health care staff to the instructions provided to patients.[21] When clinicians informed patients why their medication should be taken in the prescribed doses and duration, compliance significantly improved.

When new or complex information is offered, the clinician may wish to evaluate comprehension by asking the patient to repeat essential elements of the message, particularly the specific actions required by the treatment plan. Written instructions should be provided whenever possible in order to reinforce oral communication. The written instructions should be individualized[20] and include information about both the benefits and the side effects of medications.

The following key points should be included in the patient–health care provider interaction to ensure that medication is taken as prescribed:[3]

1. Emphasize the need for taking all the medication, regardless of symptoms and even after they resolve, and why the medication should not be shared with others.
2. Establish a specific medication schedule
   *a.* What time the patient will take the oral medication.
   *b.* What the patient will do if a dose is missed.
   *c.* What to do if the patient feels the medication is not working or is causing side effects.
3. Review contraindications and potential side effects.
4. Identify and discuss potential compliance problems.

Communication rivals diagnosis and management as one of the prime responsibilities of a clinician. Patient compliance in the management of STD is so important that all staff members including nurses and counselors should convey similar messages in different forms, without being patronizing or excessively repetitive. It is important that patients be motivated to assume at least some responsibility for their own health.[19]

In summary, the entire staff should be organized to communicate in clear, uncomplicated terms what the patient is to do or not do concerning treatment. The staff should

1. Provide the results of all tests.
2. Discuss the patient's disease and emphasize its importance.
3. Review the medication and explain why it is used.
4. Specify how much medication to take and when to take it.
5. Suggest what to do when doses are missed.
6. Review the expected outcome of treatment.
7. Inform the patient of the potential side effects and what to do about them.
8. Describe behaviors and conditions that will enhance efficacy and reduce or avoid side effects of treatment (for example, taking tetracycline "on an empty stomach," the interaction of metronidazole and alcohol).
9. Describe symptoms of and suggest appropriate responses to apparent treatment failure.
10. Provide information on whom to contact when new questions arise.
11. Encourage the patient to raise any questions or concerns and provide clear, candid responses.
12. Provide in written form the information detailed above (points 1 to 10).

## RETURN FOR FOLLOW-UP TESTS

During the last decade, test-of-cure (TOC) cultures have been reevaluated by the CDC[22] which found the importance of this procedure to the management of specific STD to vary. For example, because most men with gonorrhea respond to therapy with the rapid disappearance of signs and symptoms, this response to therapy seemingly could predict successful treatment and eliminate the need for further TOC evaluations. Recent data indicate that men who are initially symptomatic and become asymptomatic after therapy do in fact have a small chance (2 percent) of remaining infected.[23] Since the original symptomatic group is large, the men who become asymptomatic but remain infected after therapy, although proportionally small in number, still constitute almost one-half of all treatment failures.[23] These men may be a more important source of gonorrhea transmission than are symptomatic men, who would be more likely to reduce or cease sexual activity and seek treatment.[24–27]

Improving the quality of communication between the health care provider and the STD patient can lead to increased return rates. An Atlanta clinic tripled its return rates for gonorrhea TOC evaluations after implementing an innovative series of activities.[28] After the study ended, rates returned to their original level. Whether the improvement was due to the specific strategies employed or to the reactive effects of the providers' awareness of the ongoing study (sometimes called the "Hawthorne effect") is a matter for speculation.[28] The investigators concluded that if health care providers are never taught, do not understand, and are not reminded that appropriate communication with patients is a prerequisite to compliance, then patient indifference and noncompliance are the inevitable result.

To summarize, TOC cultures are evolving as a control effort for several STDs (see Table 88-1). In clinics where resources are limited, posttreatment cultures for all patients are not feasible and policies for TOC evaluations must be based on cost-effectiveness analysis. In areas where TOC evaluations can be encouraged, clinicians and disease intervention specialists can enhance the likelihood of improving patient return rates[3] as follows:

1. Review the medical purpose of TOC evaluations.
2. Negotiate appointment date and time.
3. Emphasize the need to avoid unprotected sex until the retest is negative.
4. Identify and discuss potential compliance problems.
5. Provide in written form information detailed above (items 1 to 3).

## ENSURE EXAMINATION OF SEX PARTNERS

Identification and timely referral of sex partners (Chap. 91) can reduce reinfection rates among STD patients since reinfections in a large portion of men and women can be traced to the person who was the source of the original infection.[29–31]. Although sex partner referrals by health provider staff (sometimes referred to as "contact tracing") were recommended for "priority" STD patients in the past, recent CDC guidelines take a different, more flexible approach. Guidelines for the prevention and control of *Chlamydia trachomatis* infections, for example, indicate that the sex partners of these patients should be referred for medical care through the efforts of individual patients or through the health provider staff.[32] Attempts must be made to capitalize on patients' knowledge of, and influence with, their own sex partners.

In addition to deciding who on the staff should provide sex partner referral counseling, health care providers must determine the most useful methods for such referrals. AIDS and the growing volume of priority STD cases necessitate increased patient participation in sex partner referrals,[3] with decisions based on public health importance of the STD, availability of effective intervention or prevention, and cost-benefit analysis rather than on tradition. Three methods are commonly used (Table 88-2):

1. *Self-referral* is an economical method for the referral of sex partners in relatively low priority situations. The patient assumes full responsibility for notifying all sex partners in need of medical assessment. The health professional gathers no identifying information. Although this is frequently seen as a last resort method, its benefits may be underestimated. Data from one study indicate that a carefully implemented and monitored self-referral system can match the effectiveness of other referral methods.[33] More studies are needed to test these approaches with HIV infections. A successful self-referral system can save considerable time and expense.
2. *Contract referral* assumes that patients can effectively communicate referral messages for medical evaluation to at least some sex partners. This system is recommended for "priority" situations which require monitoring of sex partner referral efforts by health provider staff. Patients can elect the option of referring some or all of their sex partners; the remaining partners are contacted by health provider staff. For obvious reasons, a contract referral system must be applied selectively to be effective. A patient who is disinterested, lacking in communication skills, or hostile toward some sex partners is not a suitable candidate for this referral effort. The counselor assists patients in deciding how to present information to sex partners to elicit the desired results. The clinic staff helps patients understand why they can and should participate in the process, as well as emphasizing that *partners must be examined promptly (usually within 24 to 48 hours)*. Patients must be aware that action by health personnel remains an option for ineffective referrals. The staff of the medical facility elicits identifying and locating information on each sex partner to monitor the examination and epidemiologic treatment of sex partners and to contact sex partners who do not comply with the referral.

The health provider retains responsibility for ensuring that all who have been exposed are adequately examined. The counselor has information in trust and has an obligation to follow up unsuccessful referrals. Failure may be due to the patient's change of mind or lack of understanding of the referral plan, the sex partner's failure to execute the plan presented, or the sex partner's choice of seeking care elsewhere. Allowing patients to refer sex partners to appropriate medical care affords both partners the opportunity to discuss the disease. Such discussions allow a patient to know when consorts have had a medical assessment and thus avoid the potential for reinfection.

**Table 88-2. Referral Options for the Examination of Sexual Partners**

| Procedure | Description | Advantages | Disadvantages |
|---|---|---|---|
| Self-referral | Total patient responsibility; no identification of sex partners requested; appointment cards are provided to patient for distribution to sex partners | Reduces cost. Requires less personnel time | Difficult to evaluate. Some patients may be disinterested, lack communication skills, or be hostile toward some sex partners |
| Contract referral | Health care professional provides patient the option of having partners referred by health care personnel or by themselves within specified time period. Option is provided only if the patient appears to be interested, responsible, and able. Identification of sex partners required | A monitoring system assures that epidemiologic treatment is applied. Reduces cost. Encourages patient participation | Lacks anonymity. Patient may not comply, requiring health department to intervene and lose time in the referral process |
| Health provider referral | Health care provider assumes total responsibility for referral of sex partners | Maintains patient anonymity. Permits monitoring by health department. Ensures application of epidemiologic treatment | Increases cost. Discourages patient participation |

3. The *health provider referral* was used almost exclusively with priority patients until the scope of the STD problem made this method too expensive to apply. The disease intervention specialist elicits identifying and locating information on all sex partners from the patient and assumes full responsibility for referring these persons for medical assessment. The patient is not involved in the process and is not advised of the outcome of the effort. This approach provides a high degree of confidentiality as well as accountability for measuring the success of individual referrals but strongly depends on staff and fiscal resources. Despite this dependence, a recent study has shown that this method can be an efficient way of locating patients and/or individuals who are at risk of infection.[34] The use of trained investigators for the referral of sexual partners to chlamydial infections was found to be a cost-effective approach in terms of dollars spent. However, patients who assume no responsibility for solving their own health problems gain no experience for subsequent situations.

In summary, health provider staff involved in the process of patient referral should[3]

1. Assess the patient's response and determine the patient's concern regarding sex partners.
2. Determine the patient's capability to participate in sex partner referral.
3. Describe the methods of sex partner referral that are available.
4. Determine the method of referral for each sex partner.
5. Establish time limits for the referral of sex partners by the patient.
6. Recommend that the patient abstain from any sexual activities with others until they are medically assessed and counseled. As an adjunct, reinforce this final item by restating it in any written material provided to the patient.

## REDUCE RISK

Risk-reduction counseling for STDs now entails considerably less controversy than in the past. As the range of STDs has expanded to include viral pathogens, the possibility of cure through prompt treatment has shrunk accordingly, thus increasing dependence on the promotion of risk-reduction techniques. In addition, the concept of "safer sex" has captured worldwide interest with the advent of HIV infection.

Yet many people at risk for HIV infection have misperceived the risk or denied its existence.[35–37] Most models of health behavior indicate that a perception of personal vulnerability or susceptibility to a disease is a necessary precondition for persons to consider adopting preventive actions. As a result, a patient whose history of infection is likely to create a perception of susceptibility may be more motivated to adopt preventive measures to reduce risk of HIV infection. Likewise, those who are HIV antibody positive may have an even greater incentive to adopt measures that both prevent HIV transmission and protect against the acquisition of other STD pathogens. Although the natural history of HIV infection is still being resolved, there are preliminary indications that bacterial, viral, or protozoal infections, many of them sexually transmitted, may stimulate the replication of the virus and accelerate and exacerbate the progression of HIV infection to clinical disease.[38,39] However, the relationship between past infection with another STD and perceived vulnerability to AIDS is by no means a simple one. Some STD patients who have a pattern of multiple partners and have managed to avoid HIV infection may conclude that they possess some "resistance" to the virus or that members of their network of sex partners are not infected. Under these circumstances, the motivation to adopt risk reduction measures may be low.

Conflicting opinions exist on the specific value of preventive techniques as well as the likelihood of their sustained use among groups at high risk of acquiring STDs. Few comparative studies have been done.[40–42] Most of the reported studies have failed to use adequate controls; as a result, their findings are difficult to interpret. Techniques that are successful in preventing some STDs may not be effective with others. Moreover, even a prophylactic method of known effectiveness may have little preventive value if used improperly or inconsistently.[43]

In general, four methods of prophylaxis can be used to prevent or reduce the risk of STD: one social and three personal methods (local, systemic, and mechanical). Social prophylaxis, in the early part of this century, represented the principal strategy for controlling STD and consisted of community suppression of prostitution and promotion of "family life"; prostitutes and their clients were considered the major source of venereal infections.[44] Today, the effectiveness of this approach is questionable since the proportion of STD attributed to prostitutes is not significant and Western societies have met with limited success in suppressing prostitution (Chap. 7). Despite changing sexual standards and practices in America,[45–47] abstinence and fidelity remain the only proved methods of avoiding STD, including AIDS. From a pragmatic perspective, however, the limitations of abstinence and fidelity as a universal control strategy are obvious.

Local prophylaxis includes washing hands and perineum with soap and water, urinating after coitus, and applying topical chemical antiseptic or antibiotic agents. Although some local prophylaxis may eradicate or inactivate some STD pathogens,[48–50] problems often arise in application, consistent use, and timing. Compounding these problems, many products for local prophylaxis lack specific instructions for their correct use. Another obstacle to use of local prophylactic agents is availability. Appropriate agents must be readily available and regularly used with any penetrative sexual act with an infected partner. Too few sexually active persons seem willing to comply with the rigid behavioral requirements for effective local prophylaxis. Moreover, neither washing nor postcoital urination is a reliable prophylactic measure.[51] Furthermore, infection may develop at other sites.[43,52]

Antibiotics can be effective if used as systemic prophylaxis in smaller doses than are needed to cure established bacterial infections. Systemic antibiotics are unique in that they may abort infections when administered after exposure. Systemic prophylaxis was effective in trials conducted decades ago by the armed forces.[53–55] However, the potential for sexually transmitted agents to develop antimicrobial resistance has deterred a recommendation for widespread use of this prophylaxis.[56–61] In addition, no single preparation protects against all STDs.

Barrier methods of prophylaxis, such as the condom, appear to be highly effective in preventing the transmission of many STDs (Chap. 92) including HIV infection when used properly.[21,41,49,62–66] However, although epidemiologic condom study results are generally encouraging, they must be interpreted with caution. Individuals who consistently use condoms may differ from those who do not. Most studies have not compared users and nonusers regarding demographic variables, specific sexual practices (particularly the use of condoms in anal intercourse), frequency of sexual activity, frequency of exposure to infected partners, use of other prophylactic measures, and mechanical adequacy of condom use.[42]

Latex condoms should be promoted for STD prevention rather than natural membrane condoms, which have tiny pores through which some smaller viruses conceivably might pass.[65] No data exist on the breakage rate or on whether condoms made of thicker latex are less likely to tear than "superthin" ones are.[67] Nonoxynol-9-containing spermicides may be a useful protective adjunct to condoms since this substance has been shown to inactivate HIV and several other STD pathogens,[68] although the use of spermicides as an STD prevention agent with condoms has not been evaluated as such in people. To maximize their effectiveness, explicit information on condoms and how to use them, as outlined in Table 88-3, should be provided.

A major challenge with condoms has been motivating sexually active adults to use them. Clinicians, nurses, health educators, counselors, and other staff members must be taught how to persuade patients to recognize their risk and to use condoms regularly.[69] Initial expressions of negative attitudes by patients do not necessarily deter condom use. In fact, directly confronting the disadvantages of condom use may result in increased use.[70]

Prevention, as well as risk-reduction counseling, involves more than simply promoting condom use (Tables 88-1 and 88-3). Patients need to know which sexual practices reduce the potential risk of infection (Table 88-4). Patients should be counseled on such social skills as negotiating sexual limits with their partners and clarifying unsafe and safer sex practices. Counselors need to adopt a nonjudgmental attitude in discussing lifestyles and lifestyle changes. Recommendations for making abrupt, unrealistic changes may produce only short-term results. The patient must find these messages acceptable and attainable.[71]

Concern about AIDS prevention has apparently increased condom use patterns among some groups. Sales of condoms have increased significantly in both New York City and San Francisco,[72] cities with large homosexual and singles communities, with women customers accounting for the biggest increase. Additionally, homosexual and bisexual men in San Francisco report having considerably reduced both the number of nonsteady sexual partners as well as the specific sexual practices associated with increased risk of HIV infection, especially receptive anal intercourse.[73–76]

**Table 88-3. Instructions for Condom Users**

For maximum protection, condoms must be used correctly. Health workers should not assume that people know how to use condoms. All condom users should receive very clear and explicit instructions:

Use a condom every time you have intercourse.
Always put the condom on the penis before intercourse begins.
Put the condom on when the penis is erect.
Do not pull the condom tightly against the tip of the penis. Leave a small empty space—about 1 or 2 cm—at the end of the condom to hold semen. Some condoms have a nipple tip that will hold semen.
Unroll the condom all the way to the bottom of the penis.
If the condom breaks during intercourse, withdraw the penis immediately and put on a new condom.
After ejaculation, withdraw the penis while it is still erect. Hold onto the rim of the condom as you withdraw so that the condom does not slip off.
Use a new condom each time you have intercourse. Throw used condoms away.
If a lubricant is desired, use water-based lubricants such as contraceptive jelly. Lubricants made with petroleum jelly may damage condoms. Do not use saliva because it may contain virus.
Store condoms in a cool, dry place if possible.
Condoms that are sticky or brittle or otherwise damaged should not be used.

SOURCE: Ref. 106.

**Table 88-4. Gradient from Higher to Lower Risk of HIV Transmission by Sexual Contact with an Infected Sexual Partner**

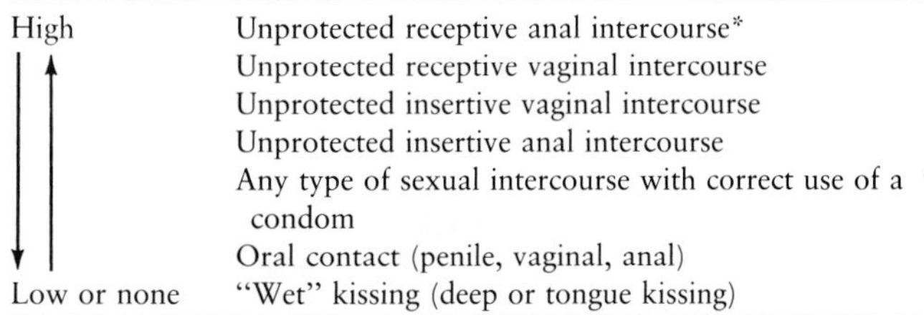

| Risk | Practice |
|---|---|
| High | Unprotected receptive anal intercourse* |
| | Unprotected receptive vaginal intercourse |
| | Unprotected insertive vaginal intercourse |
| | Unprotected insertive anal intercourse |
| | Any type of sexual intercourse with correct use of a condom |
| | Oral contact (penile, vaginal, anal) |
| Low or none | "Wet" kissing (deep or tongue kissing) |

*Although "fisting" has been found to be highly associated with HIV infection,[75] it is assumed that the relative risk of this sexual practice is high when it is followed by unprotected receptive anal intercourse. As a result, it has not been included as a separate item in this table.
SOURCE: Ref. 107.

Whether these behavioral changes in homosexual men will be sustained over time is not known, but preliminary HIV seroprevalence data indicate rapid and profound declines in percentages of uninfected gay men who were acquiring HIV infection in large U.S. cities in the late 1980s.[77] Knowledge of the guidelines for avoiding transmission of HIV, for some, however, is not sufficient to induce the desired behavior changes. In a study of gay men in San Francisco, respondents unanimously regarded the prevention of HIV infection as an important personal goal; however, half indicated that in the future they intended to engage in anal sex with the exchange of semen as often or more often than before despite generally high levels of awareness concerning safer sex recommendations.[78] These persons will need to be studied more intensively, and appropriate health promotion programs will have to be implemented, an important challenge for public health workers. STDs such as gonorrhea, syphilis, and genital herpes should be viewed as evidence of behavioral risk for HIV infection and an indication for counseling intervention. By the end of 1987, syphilis incidence had declined markedly in gay men in most urban areas, but, at the same time, had reached peak levels not recorded since 1951 in heterosexuals and minorities.[79] Routinely offering HIV antibody testing in STD clinics and making confidential counseling readily available will be a useful step in expanding the opportunities for risk-reduction counseling.[80]

Patients should be provided with an opportunity to consider alternative lifestyles that reduce their risk of future infection. Clinicians and other staff members should stress the following key points:[3]

1. Present options tailored to the patient's sexual lifestyle.
2. Emphasize reducing future risk by
   *a.* Abstaining from any sexual activity until follow-up test.
   *b.* Abstaining from any sexual activity whenever symptoms appear.
   *c.* Using condoms in any risky or unknown settings.
3. Provide written information detailed above (item 2).

## RESPOND TO DISEASE SUSPICION

Unfortunately, a common response to illness—even STDs—is to "wait and see" if the symptoms persist or subside.[81] Recent data indicated that men with primary syphilis who sought medical care on their own waited an average of over 2 weeks after the initial appearance of lesions. A review of STD clinic visits of over 12,700 patients revealed that after controlling for previous STD in symptomatic heterosexual men, blacks sought treatment sooner than did whites after becoming symptomatic with gonorrhea or nongonococcal urethritis.[82]

The symptoms of many STDs can be inconspicuous or mild, especially for women. Health providers should encourage patients to seek medical evaluation after having unprotected sex (intercourse without a condom) with someone who is known to have or is suspected of having an STD. Although patients should be taught to recognize symptoms as a signal to seek immediate medical care, it is even more important to stress that STDs in both men and women may be asymptomatic. HIV infections may be asymptomatic for years. Because lack of symptoms is an unreliable guide to freedom from infection, periodic examinations should be encouraged for persons involved in high-risk practices.

A prompt response to symptoms can contribute significantly to disease prevention and control. A study of gonorrhea transmission in Des Moines, Iowa,[83] suggested that if the duration of response to symptoms for heterosexual patients were reduced by an average of 1 day, the number of cases of reported gonorrhea would have declined within a year by approximately 8 percent. The results of this study have potential implications for national control programs. Sufficient importance has not been given to health promotion strategies and to patients' responses. Positive reinforcement by medical personnel can decrease the delay in the patient's response time for subsequent infections. For their future reference, health providers should ensure that patients[3]

1. Recognize the major signs and symptoms of common STD.
2. Understand that asymptomatic infections are common.
3. Pursue prompt medical evaluation of signs and symptoms or of exposure to known or suspected STD.
4. Abstain from sexual activity while symptoms are present or while suspicion of infection exists.
5. Bring or refer sex partner(s) for evaluation and counseling.
6. Retain this information by reinforcing, through the provision of the information above (items 1 to 5) in written form.

## AIDS COUNSELING

The importance of patient counseling is dramatically evident with HIV infection. In the absence of safe and effective treatment or vaccine, the best hope today for controlling the AIDS epidemic is to educate the public about the seriousness of the threat, the ways the virus is transmitted, and the practical steps each person can take to avoid acquiring or spreading it.[84] Counseling persons who are at risk of acquiring HIV infection and offering HIV antibody testing are important components of that strategy. The primary public health purpose of counseling is to induce behavior changes to minimize the risk of HIV infection and transmission.[85] This can best be achieved not only by motivating individuals to modify their behavior, but by creating social acceptance for safe behavior and reinforcing it whenever possible.

The development of serologic tests for detecting evidence of HIV infection provided a scientific tool for both studying and controlling the AIDS epidemic. Although its first use was in blood banks, HIV antibody testing has served as an adjunct to preventive counseling services, ranging from pretest counseling to the counseling of those affected by AIDS, including the patient, family, and partners. AIDS counseling is an extremely important and complex process that should, indeed must, be addressed by all health care professionals.[86]

Reasonable guidelines for HIV antibody testing and counseling are that[85,87]

1. They are recommended routinely to clients or patients by knowledgeable health professionals when indicated for medical or public health purposes.
2. They are available to persons seeking self-initiated testing.
3. The testing is done after appropriate counseling and receipt of information that allows specific consent to be given.
4. Specific verbal or written consent is obtained.
5. The procedures are conducted confidentially or anonymously.
6. Posttest counseling should increase the person's understanding of the significance of HIV infection and knowledge of what behavior modification is necessary to avoid infection, if uninfected, or to avoid transmission to others, if infected.

In addition, patient counseling may require more than just addressing the immediate crisis. Ancillary referral resources (medical, psychosocial, social, and/or supportive) should also be made available to the individual to assist in the long-term adjustment to infection.[88]

In general, for STD counselors to become AIDS counselors does not require learning an entirely new set of skills, but it does differ in the following ways:

1. *Population counseled.* Counseling services provided to STD patients are usually limited to persons already diagnosed with an STD listed as reportable in the state where the diagnosis is made. Counseling at HIV antibody testing sites, however, is provided to at least four categories of persons: (*a*) persons voluntarily requesting the serologic test; (*b*) persons in the posttesting phase, including those found to be HIV negative; (*c*) persons diagnosed with AIDS; and (*d*) the family members, friends, or sex partners of those infected with HIV or affected by AIDS.
2. *Supportive counseling.* HIV and other STD counseling both depend heavily on exposure and risk-reduction counseling as a primary public health goal. However, AIDS counseling also aims to maintain the social, emotional, and physical health of persons affected by the virus or by AIDS itself. As a result, AIDS counselors must develop a wide range of skills and be prepared to arrange specific referrals and ongoing patient care services.
3. *Sex partner notification.* Bacterial STD counseling normally emphasizes sex partner referral for testing and education as a pivotal intervention strategy in preventing reinfection and further disease transmission in the community. Without effective therapeutic regimens, this procedure isn't generally emphasized in the counseling of HIV antibody positive persons, although many public health officials believe a sizable benefit could be realized.[89] CDC guidelines indicate that sexual partners and those who share needles with HIV-infected persons are at risk for HIV infection and should be routinely tested for HIV antibody.[87] With appropriate education and motivation of the infected and susceptible sexual partners to eliminate or reduce their risky behavior, further transmission could be prevented.

## PRETEST COUNSELING

Counseling before testing is essential in moderate- to high-prevalence settings,[87] since a person requesting this service should have a reasonable understanding of the medical and social implications of HIV infection before providing consent. The benefits and potential consequences of testing should be explored with each individual wishing to be tested. Although it has not yet been determined whether the individual is in fact infected, pretest counseling can emphasize that the sexual transmission of HIV can be prevented if precautions are taken. The need for precautions, however, depends on whether the individual or his or her sex partners are infected. If neither is infected, no precautions are needed as long as each can be certain that the relationship is exclusively monogamous. A single negative test should not be interpreted as evidence that the patient is not infected if high-risk behavior has occurred within the previous 6 months, and counseling should emphasize continued prevention measures until any necessary follow-up testing is completed. If one partner is infected, the most certain way to avoid transmission is to abstain from sexual intercourse.[80] If both are infected, it is not known whether continued reexposure with the virus causes the disease to progress in persons infected with HIV.[80] Finally, if the infection status of a sex partner is unknown, it is wise to assume that the partner could be infected and thus avoid sexual contact where mucous membranes may be exposed to bodily fluids.[86] In general, the same methods that prevent passing the virus on to others also prevent infection from occurring in a person who is not infected.[89]

The ability of health departments, hospitals, and other health care providers to ensure confidentiality of patient information and the public's confidence in that ability is crucial to increasing the number of persons requesting or willing to undergo counseling and testing for HIV antibody.[85] Most U.S. public health agencies concur it is possible to conduct antibody testing with reasonable assurance that confidentiality can be maintained.[90] If, however, confidentiality cannot be ensured, procedures allowing anonymity should be available as an option for persons who would otherwise not be tested.[85]

Finally, persons need to consider what means of social support they will have if they are infected. Will they be able to obtain sufficient support from family members or friends and who among these will keep the information confidential? They may wish to establish contact with community support groups receiving the test results.

In summary, pretest counseling should

1. Establish the patient's risk behaviors for HIV infection.
2. Provide risk-reduction counseling.
3. Provide details on the meaning and implication of test results.
4. Help the patient prepare a plan for dealing with the information provided by the test, including assessing the patient's support system and coping resources and informing the patient of community resources for seropositive and seronegative persons.

## POSTTEST COUNSELING

Posttest counseling should be provided to all persons who take the serologic test. One-on-one counseling can enhance the effects of health promotion programs on behavior modification. This procedure is best handled by trained professionals, face-to-face and not by letter or telephone. Most persons with a negative serologic test result may be motivated to take precautions to remain seronegative although others may conclude that their sexual practices have been safe or that they are somehow immune to infection.[85] In particular, the latter group should be counseled to reduce risk of future infection by observing the following:[91]

1. Reduce the number of sex partners. A stable, mutually monogamous relationship with an uninfected person eliminates any new risk of sexually transmitted HIV infection.
2. Protect themselves during sexual activity with any possibly infected person by taking appropriate precautions to prevent contact with the person's blood, semen, and cervical or vaginal secretions. Anal sex should be emphasized as the sexual behavior of highest risk. In particular, receptive anal sex (for men and women) with an infected person may result in virus transmission. Although the efficacy of condoms in preventing infection with HIV is still under study, consistent use of condoms with spermicides containing nonoxynol-9 should reduce transmission of HIV.
3. For intravenous drug abusers, enroll or continue in programs to eliminate use of intravenous substances. Unsterilized needles must never be used and no apparatus should be shared. For those who cannot be dissuaded from intravenous drug use, participation in any needle exchange program that may be available should be strongly encouraged or needle/syringe decontamination techniques should be taught.

In addition, a negative antibody test may not ensure freedom from infection because of the 6 to 12 week lag time between infection and the appearance of antibodies.[91] Persons with an initial negative test may need to consider a second test a few months later to monitor their serologic status if they have been recently exposed to an infected or high-risk sex partner less than 3 to 4 months before the most recent negative test. The validity of any subsequent testing will be based on the avoidance of any new exposures. Otherwise, future monitoring will be required.

Those who are seropositive but asymptomatic require counseling to enable them to prevent further transmission and to come to terms with their infection. Although learning of one's infection can be profoundly distressing, it provides the opportunity to emphasize the necessary adoption of safer sexual behavior to prevent future transmission.

In addition, those who are infected with HIV often require emotional support, social services, and health care. Although these individuals may not face the threat of imminent death, they will confront the possibility of progression to frank AIDS. Changing established sex practices or drug habits—likely to prolong their own lives as well as protect others—becomes the focus of intense psychological concern.[92]

A sense of hopelessness and despair is common, especially in the first few weeks following notification. Many patients will develop an initial sense of doom. Suicidal ideas and gestures may occur and succeed in some instances. Counselors should be prepared to make referrals to appropriate psychosocial resources in the community.

Patients should also be counseled on the importance of carefully limiting discussions on their antibody status to a select number of people; unfortunate consequences have resulted, especially when too many, or thoughtless, people are told.

Seropositive women of childbearing age should understand the risks and implications of mother-to-infant transmission of HIV. Evidence indicates the high risk (25 to 50 percent)[90] of fetal transmission and infant infection, although the transmission may depend on the timing of the mother's HIV infection, the mother's immunological status, and other possible factors.[93] In addition, the infected mother may have an increased likelihood of developing AIDS when pregnancy occurs in association with HIV infection.[94] For these reasons, infected women should be advised of means to avoid pregnancy. All HIV-positive women should be referred for family planning services. The identification of HIV-infected pregnant women as early in pregnancy as possible is important to enable optimal management of the pregnancy, to plan medical care for the infant, and to provide counseling about family planning and future pregnancies.[85]

Seropositive people should be counseled to prevent further transmission of HIV by taking the following steps:

1. Inform prospective sex partners of their own infection with HIV. Sexual abstention is the only option that would eliminate all risk of sexually transmitted HIV infection.
2. Take appropriate precautions (e.g., avoiding, in particular, anal sex) to prevent the sexual partner from coming into contact with the infected person's blood, semen, or cervical or vaginal secretions. Although the efficacy of using condoms to prevent infection with HIV is still under study, consistent use of condoms should reduce transmission of HIV.
3. Inform previous sex partners and any persons with whom needles were shared of their potential exposure to HIV and encourage them to seek counseling or testing.
4. For intravenous drug abusers, needles and other equipment must never be shared.
5. Refrain from sharing toothbrushes, razors, or other items that could become contaminated with blood.
6. Do not donate blood, plasma, body organs, breast milk, tissues, or semen.
7. Avoid pregnancy and use family planning services.
8. Clean and disinfect contaminated surfaces in accordance with previous CDC recommendations.[95]

## COUNSELING OF PERSONS WITH AIDS

AIDS is the severest manifestation of HIV infection; it occurs in adults typically after 3 or more years of infection have passed. Ideally, persons diagnosed with AIDS will have known of the risk for developing this syndrome for some time, although even then the emotional implications of a potential diagnosis for these patients can be enormous. Physicians should inform the patient directly as soon as possible after the diagnosis is confirmed, providing a clear, frank, and sensitive explanation of what the patient can expect. Although wide variation in the progression has been observed in patients with the same clinical diagnosis, meeting the criteria for an AIDS diagnosis as defined by CDC has resulted in death in at least three-quarters of reported cases within 2 years of diagnosis.[96] Persons with AIDS will feel uncertain about the future and wonder how this condition will affect the way they live, the risk they may pose to others, and the risk others may pose to them. Risk-reduction advice concerning safer sex and infection control represents essential elements for counseling persons diagnosed as having AIDS just as it is for all other HIV-infected persons. Although patients may need to face the future with a hopeful outlook, they should be encouraged to consult with their physicians rather than seeking out unproved "miracle" cures they may hear about. The patient should be told that massive efforts are underway to find an effective treatment. Information concerning how to learn about available treatment and experimental drug trials should be provided to the patient.

Even for counselors accustomed to discussing serious or fatal diseases with patients, the differences between AIDS and most other diseases need to be considered:

1. HIV is potentially transmissible throughout the time a person is infected; moreover, it appears the older the infection the greater the likelihood of transmission.[97] Permanent lifestyle changes can eliminate or reduce the potential for infecting others. These changes, although difficult, must be encouraged, and the patient must be assured that some personal control over the future is possible by avoiding unsafe sexual practices and intravenous drug abuse.[92]
2. Because of ignorance, a diagnosis of AIDS can result in fear of abandonment or outright rejection by loved ones, family, friends, and even health professionals, resulting in social isolation, and leaving the patient without the emotional or financial support required during this important period. Guilt may even cause them to attempt to terminate important social and/or familial linkages, creating unnecessary social and domestic disruption. The patient may suffer from fear about infecting others or of being infected with opportunistic organisms by others. These anxieties may be manifested in sexual dysfunction and social withdrawal or even hostility. Persons who have recently been diagnosed with HIV infection or AIDS require psychological support, and the many community support groups that have been formed to meet this need may prove of great benefit. Initially, these persons may find joining a support group too frightening. Instead, more informal social settings may provide the structures needed for the patient to resist the tendency to remain isolated.[92]
3. The natural history of AIDS is frequently marked by intermittent development of unusual and severe illnesses. As a result, each new illness represents a major psychologic stress. This pattern of intermittent illnesses is often progressive and additive, leading to the physical and emotional exhaustion of the patient.[98]

A person diagnosed with AIDS must be made aware of and encouraged to adopt guidelines for sexual behavior that avoid HIV transmission as well as the risk of subsequent opportunistic diseases. In addition, these guidelines should reduce the potential for other STD which may be much more serious than usual because of existing immunodeficiency.[99]

In summary, counseling of persons with AIDS should

1. Encourage limiting sexual activity to an established and informed partner, avoiding any practices which entail the exchange of semen, vaginal or cervical secretions, or blood, especially insertive anal sex.
2. Inform the patient, as well as any partner, of the necessity for fidelity.
3. Provide information on cleaning and disinfection procedures.
4. Provide referral services to community support groups established to meet the needs of persons with AIDS.
5. Include information on how to learn about experimental drug trials.
6. Provide, in written form, information detailed above (items 1 to 5).

## COUNSELING OF FAMILY, PARTNERS, AND FRIENDS

As with any potentially terminal illness or condition, AIDS and HIV infection create a crisis not only for the patients but also for those close to them. At a minimum, patients must be strongly encouraged to notify their sex or needle-sharing partners of their potential exposure. These individuals should be counseled and encouraged to be tested. If the HIV antibody test is negative, recent sex partners may be advised to repeat the test within several months to allow time for the antibodies to be detected. In addition, the partners should be encouraged to monitor their own health status by consulting their physicians, especially if they choose not to be tested, if they are seropositive, or if they continue to engage in sex with the patient. This is true even if safer sex practices are continued, since these may still carry some risk of infection.

The patient's family and friends who have neither had sexual contact nor shared needles with the patient should be reassured that they could not have become infected as a result of casual contact with the patient. Indeed, they should be made aware that the patient is likely to be extremely sensitive to indications that these family members and friends are withdrawing and are afraid of close contact. Fear of abandonment and isolation is frequently extremely pronounced in terminally ill patients and can be even further exaggerated in AIDS patients because of the stigma attached not only to the disease but to certain population groups associated with it. In fact, the attitudes of some health care providers toward these groups may constitute a major barrier to the provision of optimal care.[100–102]

In most instances, the partners of other family members and friends will react to the news of the patient's diagnosis with grief. Most people have come to recognize that an AIDS diagnosis will almost certainly result in death. Despite this, the counselor should try to forestall a premature initiation of the mourning process by keeping the family and patient focused on prevention and treatment issues. The availability of treatments and experimental protocols and the possibility of extending the patient's survival time should all be discussed.

However, the family, partners, and friends will eventually need to be prepared for the patient's functional and cognitive decline. As death nears, referral for more intensive grief counseling may be appropriate. Agencies offering support groups for caretakers of AIDS patients can be a particularly valuable resource.

Because of the continuous growth and change in our understanding of HIV-associated conditions, the continually changing treatment options, and the extensive (often sensational) media coverage of AIDS and related conditions, the counselor will need to ensure that some arrangement for continuing communication with the patient, the family, partners, and friends about these issues is available. Support groups, community voluntary organizations, and AIDS information services can serve this purpose.

In summary, the counseling of family, partners, and friends should

1. Encourage abstinence or the adoption of sexual practices between the established partner and the AIDS patient that do not entail the exchange of semen, vaginal or cervical secretions, or blood.
2. Inform the established partner of the necessity for abstinence or fidelity.
3. Reassure family and friends that infection is not possible through casual contact with the person with AIDS.
4. Provide information on cleaning and disinfection procedures.
5. Provide referral services to community programs established to meet the needs of persons with AIDS.
6. Include information on how to learn about experimental drug trials.
7. Provide, in written form, information detailed above (items 1 to 6).

## CONCLUSION

Many authorities have stressed that education will be the primary means of AIDS prevention in the 1990s.[103–105] Counseling is an emotionally charged and psychologically challenging intervention strategy. When one discusses AIDS with HIV-infected persons and those at risk, major life events and issues, such as sex, love, relationships, family, and death, are involved. Many people, particularly young adults, are not accustomed to dealing with some of these issues or even discussing them. The counselor will be indispensable in helping people discuss these issues while maintaining the primary goal of counseling: behavior modification to decrease the risk of disease transmission.

The same behaviors that prevent HIV transmission prevent the transmission of other STD as well. If our AIDS prevention efforts are fruitful, we can expect reduced prevalence for all STDs. Although AIDS prevention counseling contains elements familiar to experienced STD counselors, it requires greater depth, sensitivity, and skills. Training will be needed by many to improve their capacity to provide counseling to troubled individuals. Training will also be needed to increase the quality of and the opportunities for counseling services. The ultimate control of AIDS and prevention of HIV infection will depend in large part on how widely available counseling services are and how well counselors meet their challenges.

## References


1 Hart G: Sexually transmitted diseases, in *Carolina Biology Readers*, JJ Head (ed). Burlington, NC, Carolina Biological Supply Co, 1976.
2 Cates W: Priorities for sexually transmitted diseases in the late 1980s and beyond. *Sex Transm Dis* 13:114, 1986.
3 Centers for Disease Control: Quality assurance guidelines for managing the performance of disease intervention specialists in STD control. Department of Health and Human Services Publication 00-4608, Atlanta, 1985.
4 Centers for Disease Control: Guidelines for STD Control Program Operations, US Department of Health and Human Services Publication 00-4715, Atlanta, 1985.
5 Green LW: Modifying and developing health behavior. *Annu Rev Public Health* 5:215, 1984.
6 Benfari RC et al: Behavioral interactions and compliance to treatment regimens. *Annu Rev Public Health* 2:431, 1981.
7 Institute of Medicine, National Academy of Sciences: *Confronting AIDS: Directions for Public Health, Health Care, and Research*. Washington, DC, National Academy Press, 1986.
8 Chilman SC: A biological-psychological view of adolescent sexuality, in *Adolescent Sexuality in a Changing American Society*. US Department of Health, Education and Welfare, Public Health Service, National Institutes of Health, Bulletin 80-1426, 1980, p 33.
9 Centers for Disease Control: Prevention of human immunodeficiency virus (HIV) infection among ethnic/racial minority populations in the United States. Department of Health and Human Services, Atlanta, Aug 5, 1987, p 10 (Draft).
10 Sackett DL, Snow JC: The magnitude of compliance and non-compliance, in *Compliance in Health Care*, RB Haynes et al (eds). Baltimore, Johns Hopkins University Press, 1979, p 11.
11 Podell RN: Physicians guide to compliance in hypertension, in *Health Promotion and Consumer Health Education*. New York, Prodist, 1976, p 209.
12 Sackett DL, Haynes RB: *Compliance with Therapeutic Regimens*. Baltimore, Johns Hopkins University Press, 1976, p 293.
13 Evans L, Spelman M: The problem of non-compliance with drug therapy. *Drugs* 25:63, 1983.

14 Blackwell B: The drug regimen and treatment compliance, in *Compliance in Health Care,* RB Haynes et al (eds). Baltimore, Johns Hopkins University Press, 1979, p 144.
15 Morris LA, Halperin JA: Effects of written drug information on patient knowledge and compliance: A literature review. *Am J Public Health* 69:47, 1979.
16 Ley P: The measurement of comprehensibility. *J Inst Health Educ* 11:17, 1973.
17 Becker MH: Patient adherence to prescribed therapies. *Med Care* 23:539, 1985.
18 Stimson GV: Obeying doctors orders: A view from the other side. *Soc Sci Med* 8:97, 1974.
19 Haynes RB: A critical review of the "determinants" of patient compliance with therapeutic regimens, in *Compliance with Therapeutic Regimens.* Baltimore, Johns Hopkins University Press, 1976, p 26.
20 Eraker SA et al: Understanding and improving patient compliance. *Ann Intern Med* 100:258, 1984.
21 Svarsted B: The doctor-patient encounter: An observational study of communication and outcome. Doctoral dissertation, Madison, University of Wisconsin, Department of Sociology, 1974.
22 Centers for Disease Control: Sexually Transmitted Diseases Summary 1986. Department of Health and Human Services Publication 00-3380, Atlanta.
23 Schmid GP et al: Symptomatic response to therapy of men with gonococcal urethritis: Do all need posttreatment cultures? *Sex Transm Dis* 14:37, 1987.
24 Handsfield HH et al: Asymptomatic gonorrhea in men: Diagnosis, natural course, prevalence and significance. *N Engl J Med* 290:117, 1974.
25 Barnes RC, Holmes KK: Epidemiology of gonorrhea: Current perspectives. *Epidemiol Rev* 6:1, 1984.
26 Potterat JJ, King RD: A new approach to gonorrhea control: The asymptomatic man and incidence reduction. *JAMA* 245:578, 1981.
27 Potterat JJ et al: Disease transmission by heterosexual men with gonorrhea: An empiric estimate. *Sex Trans Dis* 14:2, 1987.
28 Kroger F: Compliance strategies in a clinic for treatment of sexually transmitted diseases. *Sex Transm Dis* 7:178, 1980.
29 Study of epidemiologic methods for control of gonorrhea reinfections, Louisville, Kentucky, 1976–1981. Atlanta, US Department of Health and Human Services, Public Health Service, Centers for Disease Control, Contract 200-76-0639, 1979.
30 Tucker CW: Gonorrheal recidivism in Richland County, South Carolina. South Carolina Department of Health and Environmental Control, Centers for Disease Control, Venereal Disease Control Division, Contract 200-76-0672, 1977.
31 Riley C: Milwaukee study of female recidivists. Unpublished study, 1976–1978, personal communication.
32 Centers for Disease Control: *Chlamydia trachomatis* Infections. Policy Guidelines for Prevention and Control. US Department of Health and Human Services Publication 00-4770, Atlanta, 1985.
33 Potterat JJ, Rothenberg RB: The casefinding effectiveness of a self-referral system for gonorrhea: A preliminary report. *Am J Public Health* 67:174, 1977.
34 Katz BP, Danos CS: Efficiency and cost-effectiveness of field follow-up for patients with *Chlamydia trachomatis* infection in a sexually transmitted diseases clinic. *Sex Transm Dis* 15:11, 1988.
35 Bauman LJ, Siegel K: Misperception among gay men of the risks for AIDS associated with their sexual behavior. *J Appl Soc Psychol* Special issue: Acquired Immune Deficiency Syndrome (AIDS) 17:329, 1987.
36 Siegel K, Gibson WC: Barriers to the modification of sexual behavior among heterosexuals at risk for acquired immunodeficiency syndrome. *NY State J Med* 88:66, 1988.
37 Centers for Disease Control, National Center for Health Statistics Advanced Data: AIDS knowledge and attitudes for October 1987: Provisional data from the National Health Interview Survey. March 9, 1988.
38 Quinn TC et al: Serologic and immunologic studies in patients with AIDS in North America and Africa. The potential role of infectious agents as cofactors in human immunodeficiency virus infection. *JAMA* 257:2619, 1987.
39 Nabel G, Baltimore D: An inducible transcription factor activates expression of human immunodeficiency virus in T cells. *Nature* 326:711, 1987.
40 Darrow WW, Wiesner PJ: Personal prophylaxis for venereal disease. *JAMA* 233:444, 1975.
41 Stone KM et al: Primary prevention of sexually transmitted diseases. A primer for clinicians. *JAMA* 255:1763, 1986.
42 Stone KM et al: Personal protection against sexually transmitted diseases. *Am J Obstet Gynecol* 155:180, 1986.
43 Hart G: The role of preventive methods in the control of venereal disease. Atlanta, US Department of Health, Education and Welfare, Public Health Service, Centers for Disease Control, 1975.
44 Darrow WW: Approaches to the problem of venereal disease prevention. *Prev Med* 5:165, 1976.
45 Nass GD et al: *Sexual Choices.* Monterey, CA, Wadsworth, 1981, p 144.
46 *Teenage Pregnancy: The Problem That Hasn't Gone Away.* New York, The Alan Guttmacher Institute, 1981, p 9.
47 Hofferth SL et al: Premarital sexual activity among U.S. teenage women over the past three decades. *Fam Plann Perspect* 19:46, 1987.
48 Porter HH et al: Social diseases at the crossroads. *J Okla State Med Assoc* 32:54, 1939.
49 Singh B et al: Studies on the development of a vaginal preparation providing both prophylaxis against venereal disease and other genital infections and contraception: II. *In vitro* effect of vaginal contraceptive and noncontraceptive preparation of *Treponema pallidum* and *Neisseria gonorrhoeae. Br J Vener Dis* 48:57, 1972.
50 Singh B et al: Studies on the development of a vaginal preparation providing both prophylaxis against venereal disease and other genital infections and contraception: III. *In vitro* effect of vaginal contraceptive and selected vaginal preparations of *Candida albicans* and *Trichomonas vaginalis. Contraception* 5:401, 1972.
51 Wittkower ED, Cowan J: Some psychological aspects of sexual promiscuity. *Psychosom Med* 6:287, 1944.
52 Burgess JA: Gonococcal tysonotis without urethritis after prophylactic post-coital urination. *Br J Vener Dis* 47:40, 1971.
53 Eagle H: Prevention of gonorrhea with penicillin tablets. *Public Health Rep* 63:1411, 1948.
54 Joses M: Sulfathiazole prophylaxis of gonorrhea and chancroid. *US Nav Med Bull* 40:113, 1942.
55 Moore JE: Oral penicillin in the prophylaxis of syphilis. *Am J Syph Gonorrhea Vener Dis* 36:585, 1952.
56 Barrett-Connor E: The prophylaxis of gonorrhea. *Am J Med Sci* 269:4, 1975.
57 Guthe T: Prevention of venereal infections. *Bull WHO* 19:405, 1958.
58 Thayer JD, Moore MD: Gonorrhea: Present knowledge, research and control efforts. *Med Clin North Am* 48:755, 1964.
59 Rudolph AH, Price EV: Penicillin reactions among patients in venereal disease clinics: A national survey. *JAMA* 223:499, 1973.
60 Harrison WO et al: Prevention of gonorrhea. Paper presented at the Interscience Conference on Antimicrobial Agents and Chemotherapy, Washington, DC, Sept 19, 1973.
61 Sparling PF: Antibiotic resistance in *Neisseria gonorrhoeae. Med Clin North Am* 56:1133, 1972.
62 Hart G: The impact of prostitution on Australian troops at war. Doctoral thesis, South Australia, Adelaide University, 1974.
63 McCormack WM et al: Sexual experience and urethral colonization with genital mycoplasmas. *Ann Intern Med* 78:696, 1973.
64 Berger GS et al: Prevalence of gonorrhea among women using various methods of contraception. *Br J Vener Dis* 51:307, 1975.
65 Centers for Disease Control: Condoms for prevention of sexually transmitted diseases. *MMWR* 37:133, 1988.
66 Conant M et al: Condoms prevent transmission of AIDS-associated retrovirus. *JAMA* 255:1706, 1986.

67 Goldsmith MF: Sex in the age of AIDS calls for common sense and "condom sense." *JAMA* 257:2261, 1987.
68 Hicks DR et al: Inactivation of LAV/HTLV-III infected cultures of normal human lymphocytes by nonoxynol-9 in vitro. *Lancet* 2:1422, 1985.
69 Rogers EM: *Diffusion of Innovations*. New York, Free Press, 1962.
70 Darrow WW: Attitudes toward condom use and the acceptance of venereal disease prophylactics, in *The Condom: Utilization in the United States,* 1974. US Department of Health, Education and Welfare, Public Health Service, Reprint 00-2634.
71 Carr GS, Gee G: AIDS and AIDS-related conditions: Screenings for populations at risk. *Nurse Pract* 11:25, 1986.
72 Menzies HD: Back to a basic contraceptive. *New York Times,* Section 3, January 5, 1986.
73 Centers for Disease Control: Self-reported changes in sexual behaviors among homosexual and bisexual men from the San Francisco City Clinic cohort. *MMWR* 36:187, 1987.
74 Jaffe HW et al: The acquired immunodeficiency syndrome in a cohort of homosexual men: A six-year follow-up study. *Ann Intern Med* 103:210, 1985.
75 Darrow WW et al: Risk factors for HIV infections in homosexual men. *Am J Public Health* 77:479, 1987.
76 McKusick L et al: Reported changes in the sexual behavior of men at risk for AIDS, San Francisco 1982–1984—the AIDS Behavioral Research Project. *Pubic Health Rep* 100:622, 1985.
77 Centers for Disease Control: Human immunodeficiency virus infection in the United States. *MMWR* (suppl.): 18, 1987.
78 Research and Decisions Corporation: *Designing an Effective AIDS Prevention Campaign Strategy for San Francisco: Results from the First Probability Sample of an Urban Gay Male Community*. San Francisco, Research and Decisions Corporation, 1984.
79 Centers for Disease Control: Continuing increases in infectious syphilis—United States. *MMWR* 37:35, 1988.
80 Peterman TA, Curran JW: Sexual transmission of human immunodeficiency virus. *JAMA* 256:16, 1986.
81 Suchman EA: Stages of illness and medical care. *J Health Soc Behav* 6:114, 1965.
82 Kramer MA et al: Self-reported behavior patterns of patients attending a sexually transmitted disease clinic. *Am J Public Health* 70:997, 1980.
83 Orduna BC: Time delays critical to gonorrhea control. *Polk County Medical Bulletin (Iowa)* 51:79, 1980.
84 *AIDS: Information/Education Plan to Prevent and Control AIDS in the United States.* US Public Health Service, March 1986.
85 Centers for Disease Control: Recommended additional guidelines for HIV Antibody counseling and testing in the prevention of HIV infection and AIDS. April 30, 1987.
86 Drotman DP, Peterman TA: Your patients need your help to prevent AIDS. *Medical Aspects of Human Sexuality,* April 1987.
87 Public Health Service guidelines for counseling and antibody testing to prevent HIV infection and AIDS. *MMWR* 36:31, 1987.
88 Ostrow DG et al: Mental health and behaviorial correlates of HIV antibody testing in a cohort of gay men. Paper presented at the IV International Conference on AIDS, Stockholm, June 1988.
89 Francis DP, Chin J: The prevention of acquired immunodeficiency syndrome in the United States. An objective strategy for medicine, public health, business, and the community. *JAMA* 257:1361, 1987.
90 Centers for Disease Control: Conference on the role of AIDS virus antibody testing in the prevention and control of AIDS. February 24–25, 1987.
91 Centers for Disease Control: Additional recommendations to reduce sexual and drug abuse-related transmission of human-T lymphotropic virus type III/lymphadenopathy-associated virus. *MMWR* 35:152, 1985.
92 Coping with AIDS. Psychological and social considerations in helping people with HTLV-III infection. US Department of Health and Human Services, National Institute of Mental Health, Office of Scientific Information, Rockville, Maryland.
93 World Health Organization: Breast-feeding/breast milk and human immunodeficiency virus (HIV). *Wkly Epidem Rec* 62:241, 1987.
94 Centers for Disease Control: Recommendations for assisting in the prevention of perinatal transmission of human T-lymphocytes type III/lymphadenopathy-associated virus and acquired immunodeficiency syndrome. *MMWR* 34:721, 1985.
95 Centers for Disease Control: Summary: Recommendations for preventing transmission of infection with human T-lymphotropic virus type III/lymphadenopathy-associated virus in the workplace. *MMWR* 34:682, 1985.
96 Centers for Disease Control: AIDS Weekly Surveillance Report—United States. July 27, 1987, Atlanta.
97 Goedert J et al: Heterosexual transmission of human immunodeficiency virus (HIV): Association with severe T4-cell depletion in male hemophiliacs. Paper presented at the III International Conference on AIDS, Washington, DC, June 1987.
98 Abrams DI et al: Routine care and psychosocial support of the patient with the acquired immunodeficiency syndrome. *Med Clin North Am* 70:707, 1986.
99 Miller D, Green J: Psychological support and counselling for patients with acquired immune deficiency syndrome (AIDS). *Genitourin Med* 61:273, 1985.
100 Lewis CE et al: AIDS-related competence of California's primary care physicians. *Am J Public Health* 77:7, 1987.
101 Kelly JA et al: Stigmatization of AIDS patients by physicians. *Am J Public Health* 77:7, 1987.
102 Darrow WW: A framework for preventing AIDS. *Am J Public Health* 77:7, 1987.
103 Koop CE: Surgeon General's report on acquired immune deficiency syndrome. US Public Health Service.
104 Centers for Disease Control: Results of a Gallup poll on acquired immunodeficiency syndrome—New York City, United States, 1985. *MMWR* 34:513, 1985.
105 World Health Organization: Fortieth World Health Assembly: Document A40/5 WHO Special Programme on AIDS. Report by the Director General, May 1987.
106 Instructions for condom users. *Population Reports Series* L:6, XIV:3, p L-274, 1986. The Johns Hopkins University, Baltimore.
107 World Health Organization: Prevention of sexual transmission of human immunodeficiency virus (HIV): Management and counseling. (In preparation.)

# Chapter 89

# Behavioral intervention and the individual

William B. Carter
Terence C. Gayle
Sharon Baker

*If it is our serious purpose to understand the thoughts of a people, the whole analysis of experience must be based upon their concepts, not ours.*

Franz Boaz[1]

## INTRODUCTION

In this chapter we examine two promising theoretical perspectives for designing behavior interventions—value expectancy theories and social learning theory. The approaches are based on a well-established body of knowledge in the psychological literature, and currently represent the state of the art in predicting behavior and behavioral intervention design.[2,3] Both of these approaches assume the perspective of the individual and provide a theoretical framework for exploring the anatomy of subjective domain underlying specific behaviors. The content of these models, in large part, is based on the issues and concerns individuals confront as they consider changing or maintaining their behavior.

While these approaches assume the perspective of the individual, they are not limited to a single person. In assembling the content of a model, an attempt is made to represent fairly the issues and concerns of individuals from a target population about a specific behavior. The model content is therefore designed to represent the issues and concerns of a target population. The model content is then tailored to a specific individual in a second step, where weights are assigned by each individual to each content issue that reflect that individual's beliefs and values. The validity of the model is assessed in terms of its accuracy in predicting the behavior of individuals in the target population.

Since sexual decisions happen in a dyadic context, factors external to the individual make a substantial contribution to sexual practices. Some investigators[4] have argued that sexual behavior cannot be adequately explained without modeling the decisions of both members of the dyad. Here, we will argue as others have[5] that behaviors are governed by the individual's cognitive perceptions of both internal and external factors, and that these models are appropriate for understanding decisions about sexual practices. Thus, the impact of another person's influences on the individual's decision is represented in terms of the individual's perception of its role and influence. We further propose that these models can also be applied to a variety of populations, that they provide a reasonably accurate prediction of voluntary health behavior, and that they suggest specific decision-related dimensions for developing behavioral intervention strategies. These dimensions are compatible with and can be readily incorporated by social learning theory approaches to provide a framework for examining the dynamics of the behavior change process and the maintenance of positive or protective health behavior over time.

In the first two sections that follow, we will examine some of the important background issues in modeling the behavior of individuals, with an emphasis on value expectancy models and examples of their application to health-related behavior. The next two sections provide a brief introduction to social learning theory, and an example of how social learning theory can be integrated into the relapse-prevention model. In the final section, we discuss how value expectancy theories can be integrated into the relapse-prevention model, the implications of these approaches, and future research topics.

## RISK STATUS: A MATTER OF INDIVIDUAL CHOICE

The success of the majority of sexually transmitted disease (STD) prevention programs depends on the voluntary cooperation of individuals in specific high-risk groups as well as those in the general population. The AIDS epidemic has certainly brought STDs more to the forefront as a public health concern. In contrast to most other communicable diseases, the widespread use of vaccines or early prophylaxis seems unlikely in the near future. Primary prevention for STDs is based on the individual adoption of "protective sex" including abstinence, monogamy, nonpenetration, or the use of barrier methods such as condoms.

The potential effectiveness of behavior change to reduce STD transmission is reflected by recent reductions in the number of cases of syphilis and gonorrhea reported among gay men.[6–9] In Seattle and surrounding King County, Washington, for example, infection rates among homosexual men have decreased dramatically since information about the sexual transmission of AIDS has been available and methods of protected sex have been widely publicized.[10] Many gay men made changes in response to seeing the impact of AIDS in their community. While AIDS has made incursions into high-risk heterosexual populations (persons using IV drugs, their partners, and individuals who buy and sell sexual favors) in this country, the opportunity still exists to prevent it from spreading as extensively in this group. This can only be accomplished by persuading at-risk individuals to make major behavior changes, thereby reducing the transmission of all sexually transmitted infections.

Risk status for STDs depends almost exclusively on an individual's behavioral choices. Increasing adherence to protective sexual practices depends on our ability to (1) identify those individuals who are likely to have difficulty following these practices, and (2) develop effective strategies for promoting protective sexual practices. Characteristics that may be used to identify groups of persons who potentially may have difficulty practicing protective sex (e.g., sociodemographic characteristics, sexual preferences, IV-drug use) provide little insight into the actual "causes" of practicing unsafe sex. The effectiveness of strategies developed to promote protective sex depends on (1) understanding the natural history of the target behavior; (2) identifying salient and potentially modifiable cognitive and behavioral "causes" or determinants; and (3) designing and implementing effective strategies to modify these determinants and enhance the practice of protective sex.

## IDENTIFYING BEHAVIORAL DETERMINANTS

### DETERMINANTS IDENTIFIED FROM THE LITERATURE

Despite the fact that behavior change is the only viable means of preventing most sexually transmitted infections, efforts directed at behavior change have lagged far behind those directed at medical diagnosis and treatment.[11] Recent reviews[4,12] have suggested that most research on the behavioral aspects of STD has focused on sociodemographic and knowledge variables. However, sociodemographic data do not explain behavior or suggest methods of intervention. Years of health education research have shown that, although knowledge is necessary and useful, it is not sufficient for behavior change.[13,14]

Several investigators have explored the relationship between personality characteristics and the acquisition of sexually transmitted disease.[15–18] The results of these studies have suggested that there may be differences along some dimensions measured by the depression, schizophrenia, psychasthenia, hysteria, and psychopathic scales of the MMPI, and on measures of locus of control[16] or relationship with parents, attitudes toward homosexuality, and sex-role variables.[18] Yet others have found that psychiatric disorders, delinquent or other abnormalities of personality, and abnormal sexual attitudes do not predict STD.[17] As in most investigations of the relationship between relatively global characteristics and specific behaviors, the magnitude of these relationships is very modest[17] and often of little predictive value. Furthermore, the personality characteristics identified are relatively stable and are likely to be immutable. Thus, they may be of use in helping to identify population subgroups at risk for certain behaviors, but they will be of little value in designing behavioral interventions.

## CHOOSING THE TARGET BEHAVIOR AND TARGET POPULATION

The development of any predictive model of behavior begins with careful determination of behaviors that need intervention and appropriate target groups. Clinical evidence or data regarding the risk of a clinic population of interest may be principal data sets for identifying target groups. In some cases the choice will be clear-cut. For example, three high-risk groups account for 91 percent of AIDS cases nationwide [gay and bisexual males (66 percent), gay and bisexual male IV-drug users (8 percent), and nongay IV-drug users (17 percent)]. These risk groups reflect the two most common modes of transmission of HIV: sexual and parenteral.

Since the natural history of the behavioral change process may vary for each behavior, the predictive power of a model is considerably improved if the focus is on a specific behavior or at least a homogeneous class of behaviors. For example, an attempt to predict whether gay men continue to engage in "unsafe sex" would be difficult not only because of the multiple personal meanings the term "unsafe sex" might have, but also because there may be different determinants for each of the high-risk practices, such as unprotected genital-anal, oral-anal, and oral-genital sex. Unless exploratory interviews with target group members reveal substantial overlap in attitudes and beliefs concerning these different sex practices, each behavior should be modeled separately. While there are limitations due to the heterogeneity within each target group, there is usually sufficient overlap to allow the emergence of salient beliefs common to most of the group members. However, the behavioral determinants identified for, say, gay and bisexual men, may not be generalizable to members of other heterogeneous target groups such as heterosexual adolescents and young adults, IV-drug users, or men who frequent prostitutes.

## A BEHAVIORAL MODEL: VALUE EXPECTANCY THEORIES

Few attempts have been made to systematically model individuals' decisions about sexual practices. The approaches that have been attempted have used the health belief model (Chap. 9).[19,20] While it has been widely applied to studies of asymptomatic health behavior (e.g., tuberculosis screening, vaccinations, and utilizing preventive dental care) and to studies of sickness, sick role, and compliance behavior,[21] the explanatory power of the health belief model has been very modest. Research findings from attempts to validate this model have been variable and often not replicated. Furthermore, as currently formulated, the health belief model does not specify how the model components are interrelated or how they act to determine behavior. Nor does it offer much flexibility or sensitivity to complex issues that may confront an individual considering a specific health action or to variations in cognitions that may occur across different but related behaviors.

In the psychological literature several other theoretical approaches have shown promise in predicting behavior.[22–26] In these approaches, behavior is viewed as the endpoint of a chain of psychological events that begins with an evaluation of the possible consequences associated with each action under consideration. On the basis of this evaluation, an action is chosen and becomes the course that the decision maker intends to follow. Subsequent events permitting, this intention is carried out by performance of the chosen action. With substantial variation, this chain-of-events model is the basis for what are collectively called expectancy theories.[27] For the most part, specific content (outcomes or consequences of target behaviors) is not specified by the model itself or a priori by the researchers, but rather is derived empirically for each behavior from the target population. Expectancy theories fully specify the interrelationships among outcomes and provide an operational methodology for combining individuals' evaluations of these outcomes to predict behavior.

The value expectancy models described here do not attempt to describe how people make decisions. Rather, they provide a method for operationally defining and systematically assessing the elements of a decision to perform a specific behavior. The end product of these efforts is to identify the most important beliefs and attitudes, for subsequent use in behavioral interventions.

Expectancy theories have a long history in psychological research areas pertaining to attitude formation and decision making,[2,3] and leadership, learning, motivation, personality, and social power.[27] In fact, the health belief model shares a common historical origin with expectancy theories but has never been theoretically or operationally defined in a fashion consistent with this approach.

Modern expectancy theories have evolved from two areas of research: social-psychological investigations of the relationships between attitudes, beliefs, and behaviors,[24] and from behavioral decision theory.[28] These approaches have many common characteristics,[29] and both approaches have provided strong and valid behavioral prediction in a variety of settings. Each approach may have relative advantages in given settings. For example, behavioral decision models provide the following for each individual: (1) judgments of relative importance for each outcome associated with the behavior in question, (2) a direct behavioral prediction for these alternative courses of action, and (3) decision aids in helping individuals resolve complex health decisions.

By contrast, the value expectancy model developed by Fishbein and Ajzen[24] combines individuals' judgments using multiple regression to provide a behavioral prediction for groups rather than for individuals. This model also has a normative component in addition to beliefs and values. This component assesses people's perception of what significant other persons think they should do, and the degree of influence these beliefs are likely to have on the choice of the action in question.

## USING THE PRODUCTS OF VALUE EXPECTANCY MODELS TO DESIGN HEALTH BEHAVIOR INTERVENTIONS

Recent studies[30–33] have successfully utilized a value expectancy model to improve influenza vaccination rates among elderly and/or chronically ill patients (persons at risk for influenza complications) in ambulatory care settings. Influenza and related complications are the fifth leading cause of death for older persons, yet national surveys indicate that only 20 percent of this population obtain flu shots in any given year.[34] Carter et al.[30–32] found that a flu shot decision model correctly predicted vaccination behavior for 82 percent of the more than 700 patients who participated in the study. More importantly, the model differentiated "flu shot takers" and "nontakers" along several attitudinal dimensions that suggested specific content areas for a clinic intervention. An intervention based on this information was found to nearly double vaccination rates (64 percent versus 34 percent for the control group) when administered for the first time. When the intervention is repeated annually for several years, vaccination rates have been found to increase to 80 percent. The intervention was found to generalize to other settings[32] and other patient populations.[33]

Of particular interest here are a number of applications of expectancy theories to sexual decision making including decisions about abortion,[35,36] birth planning intentions,[22,23,29,37,38] and Lamaze childbirth intentions[39] and contraceptive decision making.[40–46] The proportion of variance accounted for in people's stated intentions to use contraceptive methods by attitudes and norms is typically quite high. Intention to use birth control pills is correlated with attitude toward use and norms about using of .89 for college students[43] and .86 for married women.[38] Moreover, examination of the specific belief strengths and outcome evaluations for women who did and did not choose to use birth control pills demonstrate which beliefs were most salient to choosing to use or not to use this method. Among college students, for example, both users and nonusers agreed that birth control pills are inexpensive and convenient and would enable them to regulate birth intervals and family size. Those who did not intend to use birth control pills have a number of negative beliefs about pills not held by those who intended to use them: that they lead to major side effects and birth defects, and would have detrimental effects on sexual morals. Knowledge of such differences can suggest the content of specific attitude-change interventions that would be most likely to be effective.

## PROSPECTS OF APPLYING VALUE EXPECTANCY MODELS TO STD PREVENTION

The authors are currently conducting two other studies that are attempting to apply these models to protected sex. The first is a recently completed study[47] that examined an STD clinic population's attitudes toward condom use using the value expectancy model developed by Fishbein.[24] The study examined two specific behavioral intentions, intention to use condoms to prevent STD with a steady partner and intention to use condoms with new or infrequent partners. The content of the survey was determined by interviews with STD clients to identify their beliefs about the outcome of using condoms as well as to identify the people whose opinions were most likely to influence their decision.

The first phase of this study examined the extent to which survey responses about sexual practices are influenced by an individual's tendency to respond in a socially desirable manner. In this study, social desirability did not significantly affect responses to the survey instrument. In phase two, the survey was given to over 1000 clients. More than 80 percent returned usable surveys. The obtained sample was quite representative of the clinic population, and preliminary analyses suggest that salient beliefs differ across subgroups of the clinic population and across situations. For gay men, the most important predictors of intentions to use condoms with a steady partner were the belief that one's health care provider thinks that one should use condoms with a steady partner, and the belief that using condoms will decrease the individual's sexual pleasure. In contrast, the belief that condoms were an effective means of preventing STD and embarrassment about buying condoms were the most important predictors with new or occasional partners.

A different set of beliefs was most salient for heterosexual women, and here, too, belief importance differed for consideration of using condoms with a new versus a steady partner. The most important predictors of use of condoms with a steady partner were perceptions of their health care provider's norms, perceptions of their partner's norms, beliefs about the effect of condoms on their own sexual pleasure and their partner's sexual pleasure, and belief that condoms interrupt sex. Heterosexual women's intentions to use condoms with a new partner also rested on their perceptions of their healthcare provider's norms, but embarrassment and the problem of not having condoms available when they were needed were the other salient concerns. Examination of the outcome and normative beliefs of various subsets of this clinic population will provide useful information for the design of interventions that address the most critical beliefs of each group.

A second study currently in progress[48] is examining whether a value expectancy decision modeling approach will be useful for predicting whether gay and bisexual men at risk for AIDS abstain from high-risk sex practices. The model was developed by interviewing a diverse group of 58 gay or bisexual men to determine salient factors affecting their choices to refrain from unprotected anal and oral sex. Thus, the content of the decision model was obtained entirely from the comments of the target group members. This "ethnographic" interview process yielded 12 outcome categories that fall within three general areas: (1) health concerns (physical, psychological, and concern for partner's health); (2) issues related to sexual pleasure (e.g., sexual release, physical/sensory sensations); and (3) relationship issues (e.g., intimacy, rejection, need to satisfy partners). Up to this time, 53 at-risk men have completed the decision questionnaire. The model has predicted intention of future abstention from unsafe sex with an overall accuracy of 79 percent. Furthermore, the model differentiated persons with different sexual practices along attitudinal dimensions that might be useful in designing future behavioral interventions. We hope that this empirically derived lay decision model may be useful also in allowing clinicians and their at-risk gay and bisexual patients to determine which personal beliefs and values are most important in the adoption of protective sex practices.

## SELF-EFFICACY AND SOCIAL LEARNING THEORY

Other theories of behavior have incorporated two distinct components: cognitive processes and the performance of a behavior. This approach argues that while cognitive factors like knowledge, beliefs, and attitudes have important influences on behavior, they alone cannot always explain the full range of a person's actions. It is not uncommon, for example, for people to act consciously in ways that are detrimental to their personal health. People continue to smoke, or drink and eat excessively even though they are aware of the many dangers. These inconsistencies suggest that other variables may need to be added to approaches that seek to explain complex behaviors.

Self-referent thoughts, like I can or cannot do a particular behavior, may mediate the relationship between attitudes and beliefs and action. This kind of self-referent is called self-efficacy,[49] which is described as "judgments about how well one can organize and execute courses of action required to deal with prospective situations that contain many ambiguous, unpredictable, and often stressful elements" (Ref. 50, pp. 201, 202).

Social learning theory provides a more general framework for viewing the role of self-efficacy in psychological functioning. In social learning theory, behavior is viewed as reciprocally determined by the relationship between people, by behavior, and by the environment. The individual's actions help produce the environmental conditions that affect subsequent actions, and the experience generated by actions helps determine what people think. In this model people's perceptions of self-efficacy are learned not only from their own experiences, but from observations of others, from social persuasion, and from judgments of their own physiological capabilities. In social learning theory, self-efficacy plays a major role in explaining an individual's choices of activities, the level of effort expended, and persistence with any activities in the face of obstacles or aversive experiences.[51]

A recent review of the research in five health areas—smoking cessation, pain management, eating disorders, cardiac rehabilitation, and adherence to medical regimens—suggests that self-efficacy is a good predictor of successful behavior change in a variety of applications.[52] In the case of smoking cessation, for example, perceived self-efficacy for abstinence from smoking reliably predicts who will remain abstinent and who will relapse across different treatment programs and populations. It appears to be a better predictor than the amount of physiological dependence, coping history, motivation to quit, confidence in treatment rationale, or expectancies concerning rewards of smoking.

Finally, the major principles of value expectancy theory are also included in social learning theory.[53] Cognitive processes, similar in concept to those described previously, play a key role by mediating behavior change. Furthermore, beliefs about the outcomes of performing a specific behavior, the principal focus of value expectancy theories, are viewed as important determinants of behavior in social learning theory.[49] While no one has fully operationalized a value expectancy approach within the context of a social learning theory application, such an aggregation may substantially enhance our understanding of behavior change.

## STRATEGIES FOR MAINTAINING POSITIVE BEHAVIOR CHANGE

### THE DYNAMICS OF BEHAVIOR CHANGE

The cornerstone of most problem behaviors is the inability to maintain positive behavior over the long run. The approaches and applications we have examined thus far reflect a snapshot of a decision at one point in time for a given individual. Obviously decisions are dynamic, and values are likely to change over time; thus it is useful to introduce this dynamic process as we broaden our perspective of individual decision making.

A model of the stages of smoking cessation provides a useful framework for understanding the dynamics of most behavior change.[54] According to this model, behavior change proceeds through distinct stages: (1) precontemplation, not currently considering behavior change (e.g., "I don't intend to change my sexual practices during the next year."), (2) contemplation, considering making a behavior change (e.g., "Do I want to have only protected sex?"), (3) decision, making the decision to change (e.g., "I'm going to use condoms."), (4) action, initiating efforts directed at actually changing behavior, (5) maintenance (e.g., "I haven't had unprotected sex for one week."), and (6) relapse.

Selecting a strategy to change a target problem behavior will depend, in large part, on the complexity of the behavior. Any behavior which is an integral part of an individual's lifestyle and/or has a physical addiction will be considerably more difficult to change than an occasional activity. In addition, different strategies may be required to facilitate behavior change during different stages.[55] For example, persuasive communications designed to educate and change attitudes may be the most helpful interventions at the precontemplation and contemplation stages, whereas, depending on the complexity of the behavior, behavioral therapy using stimulus control and coping skills may be most helpful during the behavior change stage.

### RELAPSE PREVENTION

**Overview of the Theoretical Approach.** Relapse prevention is a behaviorally based self-control program designed to teach individuals how to anticipate and cope with the difficulties of maintaining behavior change over time. When an individual attempts to change any major behavior, lapses or setbacks are likely to occur frequently. The key to whether an individual is able to change or maintain positive behavior change in the long run depends, in large part, on how successfully these lapses are handled in order to prevent them from leading to complete relapses. Among the cognitive-behavioral approaches that have been adapted to behavior change interventions, relapse-prevention programs are the most comprehensive and are at least as effective as the best other approaches in changing behavior.

The theoretical model for relapse prevention is based on a cognitive-behavioral approach derived from social learning theory and self-control theory.[56] While it was originally developed as a behavioral maintenance program for addictive behaviors, it can be applied either in the form of a specific maintenance strategy to prevent relapse (e.g., to prevent a recent ex-smoker from returning to habitual smoking) or as a general program of lifestyle change (e.g., to teach people how to achieve a balanced lifestyle and to prevent the formation of unhealthy habits).

**Intervention Strategies.** The behavioral approach used to change and maintain behavior in the relapse-prevention model encompasses[54] the stages of behavior change in three major phases of treatment that emphasize: (1) exploring issues that influence behavioral decisions and enhancing motivation and commitment to change, (2) identifying high-risk situations, and (3) building and maintaining self-control. Below, we will briefly summarize the intervention process which has been described in detail in Ref. 55. This approach is supervised by a therapist and can be applied to individuals or small groups.

The goal of phase I, exploring issues that influence behavioral decisions and enhancing motivation and commitment to change, is to help an individual make a firm decision to implement a plan of behavior change. To reach this goal, clients are asked to list positive and negative consequences that they believe will result, in the short and long term, from the decision to maintain their current behavior or to change that behavior. The resulting decision matrix is similar to the decisional balance sheet developed by Janis and Mann[57] and to the decision model derived empirically from the initial exploratory interview phase of value expectancy modeling.

Self-image (e.g., perceptions of self and life with and without the behavior) and past experiences (successes and failures in previous attempts to change the behavior) are discussed and positive counterarguments (e.g., one of the predictors of success is the number of prior attempts to change) are provided in an attempt to raise self-confidence. Finally, an attempt is made to set the expectations for the treatment process (e.g., difficulty of change, need to develop skills to cope with stress/urges, recognize early warning signs of relapse, and to prepare for possible backsliding.

The goal of phase II, enhancing self-efficacy, is to assist individuals to engage in active behavior change. The emphasis in this phase is on learning to recognize situations where they will be at risk for the problem behavior and acquiring skills to cope with those situations. During this phase behavior is monitored with diaries, and self-efficacy and coping skills are assessed. While specific instruments are not currently available for assessing self-efficacy and coping skills associated with sexual practices, role playing can be used as an alternative assessment strategy. In this procedure, clients are asked to respond to high-risk situations enacted with a therapist or other clients.

Skills training is a vital component of phase II and is central to the relapse-prevention approach. Individuals are encouraged to maintain a "lifestyle balance" between activities one feels they should do (shoulds) and those they would like to do (wants). Identifying desirable behaviors that might be used to replace the problem behavior are emphasized. In addition, considerable emphasis is placed on problem solving and developing effective coping skills to deal with high-risk situations. High-risk scenarios might include being with certain partners or being under the influence of alcohol or drugs during sexual encounters. For example, a recent cross-sectional study of gay men in San Francisco in 1984 and 1985 shows a positive association between continued high-risk sex behavior and use of drugs and alcohol during sex.[58] In skills training, clients would discuss how they view this situation and suggest ways of responding to it and the consequences of different responses. A therapist may suggest alternatives and then model them for the group. Then, each client would choose an alternative, rehearse it, and receive feedback. After each person has rehearsed, the group summarizes how to generate an effective coping response in this situation. This process gives each individual a chance to learn and practice a range of coping strategies.

The goal of phase III, building self-control, is to teach skills that will be useful in maintaining behavior change over the long term. The procedures used in this phase are similar to those described above, but the focus is on control of urges, coping with setbacks and lapses to prevent them from becoming full-blown relapses, and incorporating these changes into a more balanced general lifestyle.

Researchers at the University of Washington are currently developing and testing a relapse-prevention intervention for gay and bisexual men who seek help with self-control around unsafe sex.[59]

## IMPLICATIONS AND FUTURE RESEARCH NEEDS

### INTEGRATING VALUE EXPECTANCY AND RELAPSE-PREVENTION MODELS

The most effective strategy for inducing behavior change through public communication[60] or through intensive behavior change programs like relapse prevention is to address specific behavior-related issues and concerns of the target population. In almost all cases, however, this information has not been collected in any systematic fashion. The value expectancy models provide a systematic method for collecting this information as well as information related to the variations that may occur across the behavior change continuum.

#### Decision Aids for Clinical Settings

One practical implication of the ideas developed in this chapter for clinicians working in STD settings is the need to be frank and highly specific about sex behaviors when discussing risk reduction guidelines with patients. The use of a decision balance sheet approach during the course of a safe sex counseling session could be a potentially useful approach to systematically explore and clarify patients' values and beliefs about target behaviors and determine the personal consequences of change. In other clinical settings, information derived from belief modeling can be incorporated into teaching aids and client handouts.

#### Adapting Behavior Change Programs to Large Populations

Franz Boaz's[1] insight into understanding an individual's experience is extremely relevant to today's efforts in health promotion. The effectiveness of most behavior change strategies depends on this very simple principle. One inherent problem with programs like relapse prevention from a public health perspective is that they can only be applied to a small number of persons. Future research is needed to find ways of adapting these procedures so that they can be distributed on a larger scale. Promising attempts have been made to adapt relapse prevention to self-help smoking programs.[61] Value expectancy approaches may be useful to future development of these programs by providing content issues that are representative of a larger population.

## References


1 Boaz F: Recent anthropology. *Science* 98:311, 1943.
2 McGuire WJ: The vicissitudes of attitudes and similar representational constructs in twentieth century psychology. *Eur J Soc Psychol* 16:89, 1986.
3 Cooper J, Croyle RT: Attitudes and attitude change. *Annu Rev Psychol* 35:395, 1984.
4 Darrow WW, Pauli ML: Health behavior and sexually transmitted diseases, in *Sexually Transmitted Diseases*, KK Holmes et al (eds). New York, McGraw-Hill, 1984, p 65.
5 Marlatt GA: Cognitive assessment and intervention procedures for relapse prevention, in *Relapse Prevention*, GA Marlatt and JR Gordon (eds). New York, Guilford, 1985, p 201.
6 Handsfield HH: Decreasing incidence of gonorrhea in homosexually active men—Minimal effect on risk of AIDS. *West J Med* 143:469, 1985.
7 Judson FN: Fear of AIDS and gonorrhea rates in homosexual men. *Lancet* 2:159, 1983.

8 Schultz S et al: Declining rates of rectal and pharyngeal gonorrhea among males—New York City. *MMWM* 33:295, 1984.
9 Aral SO, Holmes KK: Epidemiology of sexually transmitted diseases, in *Sexually Transmitted Diseases,* KK Holmes et al (eds). New York, McGraw-Hill, 1984.
10 Seattle/King County Department of Public Health: *Communicable Disease Control.* Seattle, King County, 1987.
11 Stone KM et al: Primary prevention of sexually transmitted diseases: A primer for clinicians. *JAMA* 255:1763, 1986.
12 Darrow WW, Siegel K: Preventive health behavior, in *Sexually Transmitted Diseases,* 2d ed, KK Holmes et al (eds). New York, McGraw-Hill, 1984.
13 Bates IJ, Winder AE: *Introduction to Health Education.* Palo Alto, Mayfield, 1984.
14 Aral SO et al: Genital herpes: Does knowledge lead to action? *Am J Public Health* 75:69, 1985.
15 Gravitz MA: Personality correlates of venereal disease experience. *J Am Soc Psychosomatic Dentistry Med* 20:20, 1973.
16 Hayes J, Prokop CK: Sociopsychiatric characteristics of clinic patrons with repeat gonorrhea infections. *J Am Vener Dis Assoc* 3:43, 1976.
17 Fulford KWM et al: Social and psychological factors in the distribution of STD in male clinic attenders. *Br J Vener Dis* 59:381, 1983.
18 Ross MW: Predictors of partner number in homosexual men: Psychosocial factors in four societies. *Sex Transm Dis* July–September:119, 1984.
19 Rogers RW, Mewborn CR: Fear appeals and attitude change: Effects of a threat's noxiousness, probability of occurrence, and the efficacy of coping responses. *J Pers Soc Psychol* 34:54, 1976.
20 Simons KJ, Das A: An application of the health belief model toward educational diagnosis for VD education. *Health Educ Q* 11:403, 1984.
21 Becker MH et al: Selected psychosocial models and correlates of individual health-related behaviors. *Med Care* 15 suppl:27, 1977.
22 Beach LR et al: Developing and testing a decision aid for birth planning decisions. *Organizational Behav Hum Perf* 24:19, 1976.
23 Beach LR et al: Subjective expected utility and the prediction of birth-planning decisions. *Organizational Behav Hum Perf* 24:18, 1979.
24 Fishbein M, Ajzen I: *Beliefs, Attitudes, Intention and Behavior: An Introduction to Theory and Research.* Reading, MA, Addison-Wesley, 1975.
25 Triandis HC: Values, attitudes and interpersonal behavior, in *Nebraska Symposium on Motivation,* HE Howe, Jr (ed). Lincoln, NE, University of Nebraska Press, 1980.
26 Bentler PM, Speckart G: Models of attitude-behavior relations. *Psychol Rev* 86:452, 1979.
27 Lawler EE: *Pay and Organizational Effectiveness: A Psychological View.* New York, McGraw-Hill, 1971.
28 Edwards W: Behavioral decision theory. *Annu Rev Psychol* 12:473, 1961.
29 Davidson A, Beach LR: Error patterns in the prediction of fertility behavior. *J Appl Soc Psychol* 37:1364, 1981.
30 Carter WB et al: Developing and testing a decision model for predicting influenza vaccination compliance. *Health Serv Res* 20:897, 1986.
31 Carter WB et al: The flu shot study: Using multiattribute utility theory to design a vaccination intervention. *Organizational Behav Hum Decision Making* 38:378, 1986.
32 Carter WB: *A Test of Influenza Vaccination Program Effectiveness in VA Settings.* Final Report for HSR&D Grant Number IIR #82-091. Washington, DC, Health Services Research and Development, Veterans Administration, 1987.
33 Westbrook L et al: Test of an influenza vaccination compliance program in an HMO clinic setting. Final Report, Center for Health Studies, Group Health Cooperative of Puget Sound, Seattle, WA.
34 *Promoting Health/Preventing Disease: Objectives for the Nation.* Washington, DC, Government Printing Office, 1980.
35 Smetana J, Adler N: Understanding the abortion decision: A test of Fishbein's value × expectancy model. *J Population* 2:338, 1979.
36 Smetana J, Adler N: Fishbein's value × expectancy model: An examination of some assumptions. *Personality Soc Psychol Bull* 6:89, 1986.
37 Crawford TJ, Boyer R: Salient consequences, cultural values, and childbearing intentions. *J Appl Soc Psychol* 15:16, 1985.
38 Davidson AR, Jaccard JJ: Population psychology: A new look at an old problem. *J Personality Soc Psychol* 37:1073, 1975.
39 Lowe RH, Frey JD: Predicting Lamaze childbirth intentions and outcomes: An extension of the theory of reasoned action to a joint outcome. *Basic Appl Soc Psychol* 4:353, 1983.
40 Adler NE, Kegeles SM: Understanding adolescent contraceptive choice: An empirical test. Paper presented at the American Psychological Association Meetings, New York, 1987.
41 Cohen J et al: An extended expectancy-value approach to contraceptive alternatives. *J Population* 1:22, 1978.
42 Davidson AR, Morrison DM: Predicting contraceptive behavior from attitudes: A comparison of within- versus across-subjects procedures. *J Personality Soc Psychol* 45:997, 1983.
43 Jaccard JJ, Davidson AR: Toward an understanding of family planning behaviors: An initial investigation. *J Appl Soc Psychol* 2:228, 1972.
44 Jorgensen SR, Sosnstegard JS: Predicting adolescent sexual and contraceptive behavior: An application and test of the Fishbein model. *J Marriage Family* 46:43, 1984.
45 McCarty D: Changing contraceptive usage intention: A test of the Fishbein model of intention. *J Appl Soc Psychol* 11:192, 1981.
46 Werner PD, Middlestadt SE: Factors in the use of oral contraceptives by young women. *J Appl Soc Psychol* 9:537, 1979.
47 Baker S et al: An application of the Fishbein model for predicting behavior intentions to a sexually transmitted disease clinic population. In preparation.
48 Gayle TC et al: A decision model to predict whether gay and bisexual men will abstain from unsafe anal and oral sex. (Research in progress) Department of Psychiatry and Behavioral Sciences, University of Washington, RP-10.
49 Bandura A: Self-efficacy: Toward a unifying theory of behavior change. *Psychol Rev* 84:191, 1977.
50 Bandura A: Self-referent thought: A developmental analysis of self-efficacy, in *Social Cognitive Development: Frontiers and Possible Futures,* JH Flavel, L Ross (eds). Cambridge, Cambridge University Press, 1981, p 200.
51 Bandura A: Self-efficacy mechanism in human agency. *Am Psychol* 37:122, 1982.
52 O'Leary A: Self-efficacy and health. *Behav Res Ther* 23:437, 1985.
53 Schunk DH, Carbonari JP: Self-efficacy models, in *Behavioral Health: A Handbook of Health Enhancement and Disease Prevention,* JD Matarazzo et al (eds). New York, Wiley-Interscience, 1984, p 230.
54 Prochaska JO, DiClemente CC: Stages and processes of self-change of smoking: Toward an integrative model of change. *J Consulting Clin Psychol* 51:390, 1983.
55 Curry SG, Marlatt GA: Building self-confidence, self-efficacy and self-control, in *Treatment and Prevention of Alcohol Problems: A Resource Manual,* WM Cox (ed). New York, Academic, 1987.
56 Marlatt GA, Gordon JR: *Relapse Prevention: Maintenance Strategies in the Treatment of Addictive Behaviors.* New York, Guilford, 1980.
57 Janis IL, Mann L: *Decision Making.* New York, Free Press, 1977.
58 Stall R et al: Alcohol and drug use during sexual activity and compliance with safe sex guidelines for AIDS: The AIDS Behavioral Research Project. *Health Educ Q* 13:359, 1986.
59 Roffman R et al: Relapse Prevention Training Project. School of Social Work, University of Washington, Seattle, WA Project sponsored by AIDS Prevention Project, Seattle/King County Department of Public Health and the Centers for Disease Control. Work in progress.
60 McGuire WJ: Public communication as a strategy for inducing health-promoting behavior change. *Prev Med* 13:299, 1984.
61 Curry SG et al: A comparison of alternative theoretical approaches to smoking cessation and relapse. *Health Psychol* 7:545, 1988.
chology, University of Washington, Seattle, WA Prepublication manuscript.

# Chapter 90

# Behavioral change using interventions at the community level*

Thomas J. Coates
Ruth M. Greenblatt

## INTRODUCTION

The least common denominator of any sexually transmitted disease intervention program is individual behavior change. This is true whether the intervention is aimed at encouraging the use of condoms, increasing access to case contacts, or advancing compliance with treatment regimens. However, the community provides the macroscopic context for any intervention program targeted to individuals. Communities can be groups defined by behavior (sexual orientation, IV drug use), by identification (of ethnicity, sexual identity), by geographic boundaries, or by places where individuals are available for education (schools, prisons).

The initiation and maintenance of behavior change, especially when the behavior is personally sensitive and laden with societal value (as is sexual behavior) depends in large part on community support. Decrements in the incidence of gonorrhea and syphilis that occurred during World War I, when support for STD interventions was high, and the resurgence of these diseases after the war (when community support for STD control programs waned) are good examples of the effect of community attitudes and policy on disease control.[1,2]

The determinants of health-diminishing and health-promoting behaviors exist within each community. For example, the behavior of peers, acceptance of various forms of sexual expression, and approaches to education are community factors that may influence the prevalence of any given behavior among individuals in a community. The nature and success of an intervention as well as the prevalence and recognition of the behaviors that health-promoting interventions are intended to change are influenced in large part by the community. STD intervention programs often focus on disease control through individual case finding, possibly by persons who are not part of an individual's community.[3-7] The case finding approach is limited because it may be difficult to identify every sexual contact of persons with STDs, treatment may not be available, treatment failure may occur and not be identified, and behavior change is not guaranteed among identified cases in effectiveness. On a theoretical basis, prevention of STDs can be best accomplished by the avoidance of sexual behaviors which permit transmission of pathogens.

The failure to sustain beneficial behavior change is a major shortcoming of most intervention programs; the recurrence of unhealthful behaviors is the most common cause of failure and produces the greatest challenge to the development of new interventions.[8,9] In its simplest formulation, behavior change requires information, motivation, skills, and an environment which supports healthful behaviors.[10,11]

Community-based approaches to behavior change are aimed at providing individuals with information and skills to change behavior through channels of influence indigenous to the community, and simultaneously at providing a supportive social environment that encourages appropriate behaviors.[12,13] An individual is much more likely to initiate and maintain healthful behavior when (1) a variety of avenues are used to inform and motivate; (2) specific strategies are used to teach skills (e.g., how to use condoms, how to inform a partner of an illness) needed for low-risk activities; (3) specific health-diminishing behaviors become less socially accepted in a community; (4) perceived social sanctions regarding unhealthy behaviors are persistent, inescapable, and provided on a sufficiently regular basis; and (5) sources of resistance to behavior change and comprehension of the intervention message are addressed.[14]

In any community, a finite number of ways exist to inform, motivate, and teach skills. We provide one schema to reduce the risk of sexually transmitted disease (STD) transmission, using resources available to a typical community (Table 90-1). In this example, media (both general and directed at specific subgroups in the communities) are especially influential in teaching about the health risks asssociated with specific behaviors.[15,16] The media can also motivate behavior change by providing examples of individuals experiencing injury as a result of specific behaviors (thereby increasing the perception of personal susceptibility). The media can also teach skills through modeling those skills and provide information about both prevailing and desired community norms. Information, motivation, and skills training can occur through a variety of existing avenues including schools, workplace, health care systems, churches, organizations, and clubs.

Community-based behavior change efforts are also designed to create structures and systems which will maintain the practice of health-promoting behaviors, including explicit changes in policies and the perceptions of normative behavior (Table 90-1). These provide one avenue for ensuring a context in which individuals will be reminded that the healthier alternative is preferred according to community standards and norms.

Finally, the design and implementation of community change programs require a balance between "exogenous" and "endogenous" resources.[17] Organization which emanates from an agency outside the community (e.g., a health department or university-based group) is termed exogenous, while that which arises from within the community is termed endogenous. The temporal sequence for the activities is generally one in which the initial surge of activity originates from exogenous sources but is then replaced by increasing collaboration and finally by takeover from endogenous sources. Change may require ideas and technology from the outside, but adoption, maintenance, and adaptation require the explicit collaboration of individuals and agencies from within the community.

## THEORETICAL FORMATIONS

The development of community organization for health behavior change draws on several theoretical formulations of behavior change, including social learning models,[18] communication-persuasion models,[19] the health belief model,[20] and attitude change model. In addition, we have recently unified elements from these and other models onto an AIDS risk reduction model (ARRM).[21] The ARRM is based on the premise that to avoid disease, people

*Preparation of this manuscript was supported in part by NIMH/NIDA AIDS Center Grant No. MH42459.

Table 90-1. Coordinated Community-Based Program to Reduce STD: An Example

| Intervention channel | Public education | Behavior change resources | Policy changes |
|---|---|---|---|
| Media | Increase awareness of problem | 1. Teach about how to use prophylaxis<br>2. Model skills for prophylaxis | Publicize policy changes re availability of diagnostic, treatment, or educational resources |
| Health care | Inrease skills in detection, treatment, and reference | Improve skills in taking sexual histories and in prevention promotion | Seminars and consultations to improve access to treatment, availability of prophylaxis, "destigmatization" of STDs |
| Schools | Education about STD prevention, diagnosis, and treatment | Skill training in small groups | 1. School clinics<br>2. Policies promoting sex education |
| Work sites | 1. Education about STD prevention, diagnosis, and treatment<br>2. Media and other events to promote awareness<br>3. Pamphlets available | Skill training in small groups | 1. Release time to attend family planning clinics<br>2. Explicit sexual education allowed and encouraged |
| Non-profit and voluntary organizations | Presentations at meetings, schools, work sites, continuing medical education | 1. Skill training<br>2. Free materials for other relevant community agencies | 1. Destigmatization of STDs<br>2. Availability of free resources for others who can benefit |
| Hotline | Oral and written information | Telephone counseling | 1. Reference to community agencies<br>2. Information on local laws and policies |

engaging in high-risk activities first must perceive that their sexual behavior places them at risk for HIV infection and related morbidity and mortality. After their sexual behavior is seen as a problem, individuals must be willing to commit themselves to changing their behavior. This process may require deciding if the behaviors can be altered and whether the benefits of change outweigh the costs. After making a commitment to change one's behavior, individuals need skills for help in changing. Support may be sought from self-help strategies (e.g., friends, family), or professional helpers (e.g., physicians, mental health professionals, clergy). Similarly, skills training may occur through a variety of mediated, formal, and informal sources.

Social networks and community norms influence each step in the behavior change process. The ability to perceive sexual behavior as problematic depends upon knowledge of risky sexual activities, and the belief in personal susceptibility. Networks and norms can influence how the individual labels the risky behavior by (1) influencing the person's level of health knowledge, (2) funneling people toward appropriate health decisions by providing sanctions for continuance of high-risk activities, and (3) the presence in the environment of individuals whose high-risk behavior leads to disease. Social networks and community norms can also inhibit an individual from labeling behavior as a problem. The fear of being stigmatized for admitting socially undesirable behavior may decrease an individual's willingness to perceive their behavior as problematic. If a health-diminishing behavior has acquired political or fiscal value within a community, the community may support continued engagement in the activity despite awareness of health risk. An example of this phenomenon was the response of the San Francisco gay community to information regarding the risks of sexual intercourse with multiple male partners. The community was unable to agree to censure this high-risk activity because it was seen by some gay members as part of their identity.[22]

The second step in the process of changing health-diminishing behavior involves reaching a firm decision to make behavioral changes and committing strongly to that decision. Influencing the process of commitment to change are (1) an individual's analysis of the costs (e.g., reduced pleasure) of changing, (2) analysis of the benefits of changing (e.g., will using condoms reduce chances of infection?), and (3) perceived self-efficacy (can I perform the actions that will lead to change and obtain the outcomes I want?). Social factors and community norms have considerable influence on the cost-benefit analysis and on self-efficacy. Friends, for example, may inform us of how much they enjoyed using condoms or how easy it is to implement using condoms in their sexual relationships. Other social conditions that foster change are those that reinforce expectations that change will be beneficial and not too costly. In addition, belief in the ability to accomplish change may be augmented by providing an opportunity for observing that people with whom we identify can accomplish change successfully.

Once committed to the task of reducing a risk behavior, the individual must take action. This requires that the individual has the necessary skills to take action. The ability to engage a sexual partner in behaviors which do not permit the transmission of STDs depends upon the ability to communicate verbally about sexual issues and desires. Sexual communication abilities are essential in reaching success in changing sexual behaviors and can be taught.

Other theories which have been relied upon for the development of community-based health behavior change programs are diffusion theory and community self-development models. Diffusion theory[23,24] states that communication leading to persuasion and learning flows through natural social networks. Community self-development models posit that community residents and organizations must collaborate with agencies advocating change to achieve successful maintenance of change. Such collaborations become more difficult to achieve as the cultural gap between community and agency increases, as may occur with international programs.

Social marketing[25] techniques are needed to produce a message and mode of dissemination that are appropriate and effective within the context of their use. These techniques include development of a marketing plan, message design, use of mass media, consideration of cultural and organizational obstructions, consensus building, and packaging. Design of the message is crucial to the social marketing scheme. The message needs to be relevant to the target audience and include content as determined by the goals of the intervention program and what is comprehensible to the target audience. Resistance points, which are defined as "behavioral constraints that act as barriers to desired behavior change," must be resolved by the message. Examples of resistant points include cultural practices and beliefs, habits, or limits in acceptance of authority. For example, in family planning campaigns around the world, the rate of diffusion of contraception innovations has sometimes stalled because of the taboo nature of the practices and communication about them. This may also be true of safe sex innovations within certain cultural groups in the United States.[11] Format is chosen to produce the maximum distribution and to be considered credible by the target audience. Mass media are frequently the best mode of message delivery, including in the developing world where radio communication is often the most influential means of communication. Persistence of the intervention program over long periods of time with an orderly presentation of the components of the message produces the greatest effect on community attitudes and norms as well as the most enduring behavior change.

**Table 90-2. Variables Relevant to Analysis of Behavioral Determinants Derived from the ARRM**

| |
|---|
| Perception of Morbid Event as Problematic |
| Perception of Associated Behavior as Problematic |
| Knowledge of Behaviors Involved in Disease Transmission |
| Perceived Susceptibility |
| Perceived Norms |
| Aversive Emotional States Associated with Problem Behavior |
| **Decision to Change** |
| Perceived Costs of Low- vs. High-Risk Behaviors |
| Perceived Benefits of Low- vs. High-Risk Behaviors |
| (Response Efficacy, Enjoyment) |
| Self-Efficacy |
| Perceived Norms |
| **Taking Action** |
| Information/Help-Seeking Behavior |
| Skills in Healthful Sexual Behavior |
| Sexual Communication Skills |
| Perceived Norms |

## IMPLICATIONS OF THESE MODELS FOR THE DEVELOPMENT OF COMMUNITY-BASED BEHAVIOR CHANGE PROGRAMS

**Principle 1: The Achievement of Health Behavior Change Requires Information on the Prevalence of Health-Diminishing Behaviors in Specific Communities.** This information is essential in order to determine how to intervene in a given community. Community-based programs cannot proceed without formative evaluation (or sound marketing research) to identify the prevalence and determinants of high-risk behaviors for specific communities. Determinants should focus on key markers (e.g., age, income, acculturation, sex, education) that allow the identification of subgroups at risk for health-diminishing behavior, as well as a range of psychological, social, and environmental variables that may be related to such behavior.

**Principle 2: Determinants of Health-Diminishing Behavior Must Be Assessed for Specific Communities. Several Levels of Factors Associated with This Behavior Must Be Addressed Simultaneously in Assessing Determinants of High-Risk Behaviors.** Assessment of the determinants of health-diminishing behavior and essential components in behavior change programs should include all levels of variables, for example, appreciating that a STD is a problem and understanding that the behavior which transmits the STD is problematic and necessary for behavior change (Table 90-2). For some individuals, the presence of STDs may convey a sense of masculinity. Because they are treatable, STDs such as gonorrhea or chlamydia may be considered insignificant.

**Principle 3: The Religious, Economic, Legal, and Policy Norms and Regulations of the Community Must Be Analyzed to Determine the Extent That They Foster or Inhibit Health-Promoting Behavior.** These analyses are essential to determine the social climate in which community interventions take place. A systematic detailed analysis of community organizations, leadership, and social and political structures permits an important understanding of community change dynamics. This analysis is needed to identify the capacity for change and the resources that can be tapped in the change program. Special care in this analysis may be required when intervention programs are intercultural in scope.

**Principle 4: Achieving Behavior Change Requires Maximizing Opportunities for the Provision of Knowledge, Skills Training, and, If Indicated, for Changing Community Norms.** Behavior change objectives are reached through systematic, organized, and continuous community interventions which use multiple channels of communication to teach information, motivate, develop skills and modify community norms. The objective is to inform, motivate, and teach each individual in as many ways as possible and preferably through channels already existing in the community. Each community contains formal and informal structures that can be encouraged to support behavior change efforts. Formal structures include the health care delivery system, the public health system, legal systems, schools, workplaces, voluntary health organizations, organized neighborhood groups, churches, and media. Informal structures include the existing leadership structure of the community, ethical standards, environmental constraints or opportunities, and individuals and organizations committed to the task of change but not usually associated with the specific behaviors which are the target of interventions. Examples of the latter could include civic and fraternal organizations.

**Principle 5: Each Avenue of Influence in a Given Community Needs to Be Analyzed to Determine Its Utility in Informing, Motivating, and Teaching Skills** (Table 90-1). For example, the media can provide information and also influence attitudes and norms in the community through coverage of specific behaviors. Face-to-face strategies might be particularly useful in skills development by providing opportunities for individuals to observe and practice with corrective feedback. Health service organizations (hospitals, and outpatient settings; physicians, dentists, pharmacists, nurses) can be especially potent because they reach large numbers of individuals and because they are perceived to be authoritative with regard to health issues. Providers can promote acceptance of behavior change campaigns, put behavior change on the agenda of individual patents, motivate for behavior change by relating patient problems and symptoms to health-diminishing behaviors, and give opportunities for skills training.

**Principle 6: Communication Leading to Persuasion and Learning Flows Best through Natural Social Networks.**[23,24] This principle is derived directly from diffusion theory. Application of this principle requires analysis and understanding of these networks so that teaching and training opportunities can be maximized. Opinion leaders within systems are needed as collaborating allies to achieve adequate adoption of the health innovations being advocated. Leaders (both formal and informal) need to be identified and recruited to assist in the health behavior change effort. Explicit attention needs to be devoted to encouraging and enhancing interpersonal communication as a stimulant to behavior change.

**Principle 7: Specific Strategies Need to Be Enacted to Identify and Modify Prevailing Community Norms.** Intervention strategies should generate positive peer group influence and social support for health behavior change. An important lesson from diffusion theory is that the generation of interpersonal communication should be an explicit goal of the community educational program. Long-term maintenance of changes in any community depend upon the change in social norms when social support for behavior change becomes diffuse and widespread.

**Principle 8: Both Formative and Summative Evaluation Strategies Are Needed.** Formative evaluation methods are used to determine the needs of the community and the impacts of specific program elements on the community. For example, in the Stanford Five-City Project, formative evaluation included audience needs analysis, audience segmentation, program design, program testing, message design pretesting, community event analysis, and media event analysis. In addition, it is important to identify a number of steps in the process of community change and to measure each of these steps. It is important to evaluate the success of achieving stable and meaningful change in community practices that may run on its own momentum. Summative evaluation methods include independent surveys of knowledge, attitudes, and behaviors, and physiological and disease endpoints.

**Principle 9: The Project Needs to Be Viewed as a Collaborative Venture between the Exogenous Group and the Community (the Endogenous Group).**[17,23] Diffusion theory's central theme is that external resources will instigate change and provide technical assistance. Endogenous resources will provide ready avenues for change programs, and also adopt and adapt the programs to meet the needs of the community. Ultimately, these endogenous resources will take over and manage the change and maintenance process. In many respects, the change process might be facilitated if the endogenous group increases its involvement and ownership of the program itself.

**Principle 10: The Project Needs to Progress through Planned Stages That Adhere to These 10 Principles.** Project phasing should proceed through planning, initial analyses, preparation of program modules and their implementation, turnover of the project to endogenous resources, and final evaluation of the outcomes of the project in terms of morbidity and mortality (Table 90-3).

**Table 90-3. Phases in Community Behavior Change Programs**

**A. Planning**

1. *Initial planning:* clarification of research goals, identifying target groups and resistance points, developing message, testing materials, assembling multidisciplinary intervention and research team, obtaining community support, recruitment of key community leaders, proposal preparation and funding.
2. *Final project planning:* complete community recruitment, identifying community organizers (change agents), establishment of expert groups for survey design and education development, setting specific goals and objectives, assembling planning guides
3. *Prefield studies:* assessment of components to community intervention, designation of needed prefield studies, implementation and evaluation of results

**B. Formative Evaluation**

Audience needs analysis, audience segmentation, program design, program testing, message design and pretesting, community event analysis, media event analysis

**C. Prefield Studies**

Pretests of survey instruments and development of education methods

## ADVANCES IN COMMUNITY INTERVENTIONS

## CARDIOVASCULAR DISEASE RISK-REDUCTION TRIALS

Community-based intervention methodology advanced considerably in trials in cardiovascular disease and cancer risk reduction. Trials have been conducted simultaneously in the United States, Finland, Australia, Switzerland, and the Federal Republic of Germany. Other comprehensive programs are underway in Portugal, Italy, the German Democratic Republic, Yugoslavia, Cuba, and the Peoples Republic of China.[17]

For example, the Stanford Three-Community Study[27] compared two communities which received media-based health education programs with a third community which served as a no treatment control. Material that was widely distributed included weekly newspaper columns, bus cards, billboards, 50 different television spots, three hours of television programming time, and 100 radio spots and several hours of radio program time. In one of the intervention communities, a small sample of individuals who were assessed to be at high risk received supplementary face-to-face instruction. This group received 25 h of instruction with special attention to skills training and the generation of social support. Evaluation of the program was based on annual assessments of cohorts in each of the two intervention communities and a third no-treatment control community. The communities that were exposed to the mass-media-only campaign reduced cardiovascular risk (as computed from a composite risk score for cardiovascular disease) by approximately 25 percent; those exposed additionally to the intensive instruction reduced risk by approximately 30 percent. Risk reduction in the community that was provided with mass media education was comprised almost equally of reduced hypertension, blood cholesterol, and decreased cigarette use. Among the individuals who received intensive instruction, additional change seen in decreased cigarette use. Changes were reasonably well maintained during a third year of decreased education, especially for the intensively instructed group.[28]

The Stanford Five-Community Project[26] began in 1978 and

will continue into the 1990s. The Five-Community Project differs from the Three-Community Project in that the two communities selected for education were much larger, the education program was more complex and extensive, and a community organizing program was devised to create a cost-effective and long-lasting program of community health. The efficacy of this program is being assessed by comparing the results of the four independent sample surveys and cohort sample surveys in the two treatment communities with the results of those surveys in three reference communities. Epidemiologic surveillance of morbidity and mortality will occur in all five communities simultaneously.

The National Cancer Institute (NCI) examined the results of these multifactor risk-reduction trials with a specific emphasis on the problem of heavy smoking (>25 cigarettes per day).[29] This examination was undertaken because of an important observation that as the prevalence of smoking in the community decreases, those individuals who continue to smoke are significantly more likely to be classified as "heavy smokers." While heavier smokers are generally less successful than lighter smokers in many kinds of smoking cessation programs (including clinic-based programs and those delivered by health care providers), preliminary data from community trials suggested that when smoking cessation efforts were well incorporated into the community and provided sustained social influences that promote cessation, heavier smokers quit at rates almost equal to those of light and moderate smokers.[30]

For example, the Austrialian North Coast Program[31] used a design similar to the Stanford Three-Community Study and measured effect on independent population samples. This study demonstrated a 15 percent net reduction in smoking. Early data from the Stanford Five-City Project demonstrated a 26.5 percent quit rate among smokers in the two intervention communities during the first 3.5 years of intervention compared with 18.6 percent in the control communities. Preliminary data from the Minnesota Heart Health Program[30] suggested that a large proportion of smokers can be recruited to participate in cessation activities and that heavy smokers can be recruited successfully and aided in quitting. In fact, heavy smokers in these studies quit smoking at rates almost equal to those of light and moderate smokers.

Given this success, the NCI began the Community Intervention Trial for Smoking Cessation[29] to test the best cessation methodologies developed in smaller clinical trials in a synergistic community-based setting. The trial is designed to determine if community-based approaches with interventions organized and delivered by existing community structures and groups can reach and involve a large proportion of smokers in successful cessation efforts. The design includes 11 pairs of communities which are matched by size and demographics by pair. Communities within each pair will be randomized to either an intervention or comparison condition. Results from current cessation trials are providing numerous strategies for inclusion in this trial (and hence can be regarded as prefield studies for this larger trial). Programs offered by physicians and dentists, media programs supported by the community, school-based prevention programs that also involve parents, self-help cessation services offered in communitywide settings, and communitywide smoke-free mobilization efforts appear encouraging. Through high levels of community involvement, persistent and inescapable smoking cessation influences will be provided. Especially important is the focus on providing smoke-free policies at work sites, health care settings, schools, and public facilities.

## COMMUNITY-BASED INTERVENTION FOR FAMILY PLANNING AND REDUCTION IN UNWANTED PREGNANCY

A community-based education program in South Carolina attempted to reduce the occurrence of unintended pregnancy among never-married teens and preteens.[32] Achievement of these goals involved postponement of initial intercourse and the consistent use of contraception among those who chose to become sexually active. The program was modeled on the Stanford community intervention model. Community recognition of the problem was followed by the creation of advisory groups, community intermediaries, and a mechanism for needs and resource assessment. Community agencies, teachers, religious leaders, and parents were involved in all phases of the project.

Intervention programs were targeted at parents, teachers, ministers, and representatives of churches, community leaders, and children enrolled in the public school system. The program goals involved the development of decision-making and interpersonal communication skills, self-esteem enhancement, and understanding of human reproductive anatomy, physiology, and contraception. Two-thirds of the district teachers, administrative staff, and special services personnel completed courses aimed at the above objectives. These teachers introduced sex education in all grades (K through 12) and subject areas. Where there was no specific sex education course, elements were integrated into other relevant curricula. Clergy, church leaders, and parents were continually recruited to attend minicourses that addressed the educational objectives. Program staff used the local media to create additional opportunities to promote the program objectives. Organizations seeking a speaker were encouraged to use the program resources.

Magnet events were used to raise community awareness. The estimated rates of pregnancy per 1000 female population for females aged 14 to 17 years in the county's western portion declined remarkably since the beginning of the intervention. The changes were statistically significant when compared with three sociodemographically similar counties and also with the eastern portion of the county. At the beginning of the intervention, the portion of the county that received intervention reported 54.1 pregnancies for females aged 14 to 17 per 1000 females; this declined to 25.1 at the end of the intervention program. The three comparison counties reported rates of 46.0, 60.2, 53.7, and 54.9, which were essentially unchanged since baseline.

## COMMUNITY AIDS RISK-REDUCTION INTERVENTIONS

Behavior changes among the gay and bisexual communities in San Francisco have been dramatic, remarkable in their scope, and sustained. Over 50 percent of the men practiced unprotected anal intercourse in 1984. By 1987, less than 10 percent practiced unprotected receptive and less than 5 percent practiced unprotected insertive intercourse.[33,34] Changes have not been nearly so dramatic among heterosexuals in San Francisco,[35,36] adolescents,[37] or gay and bisexual men elsewhere.[38] While it is not possible to determine the precise elements for the dramatic changes in high-risk populations in San Francisco, the city used many of the elements we have described in formulating and implementing its AIDS risk-reduction campaigns. In addition to media, instruction and skill training through various channels (health care providers, the workplace, special groups), principles of diffusion theory were used to increase the rate of peer communication and to generate public commitment to change. San Francisco sponsored the STOP AIDS project,[38] a powerful one-time evening-long peer-led discussion entailing scrutiny of norms sanctioning high-risk behaviors. Community organizing techniques were used to bring individuals into the program. Basic messages involved empowerment, action, and support. Theories of behavior change in concert with social marketing strategies were used to define the needs of a community and build an intervention designed to penetrate into the community.

## CONCLUSIONS

Using approaches we have described, it should be possible to analyze any community and to build a strong base to modify the risk STD behaviors of large population segments. The success with specialized community interventions with cardiovascular, cancer, and unplanned pregnancy risk reduction calls for empirical trials of these techniques with sexually transmitted diseases other than HIV.

# References


1 Brandt A: *No Magic Bullet.* New York, Oxford University Press, 1985.

2 Cutler JC, Arnold RC: Venereal disease control by health departments in the past: Lessons for the present. *Am J Public Health* 78:372, 1988.

3 Judson FN: How to control gonorrhea: The view of a local public health officer. *Sex Transm Dis* July–September: 231, 1978.

4 Hart G: Screening to control infectious diseases: Evaluation of control programs for gonorrhea and syphilis. *Rev Infec Dis* 2:701, 1980.

5 Wiesner P, Parra WC: Sexually transmitted diseases: Meeting the 1990 objectives—A challenge for the 1980s. *Public Health Rep* 97: 409, 1982.

6 Meheus AZ: Surveillance, prevention, and control of sexually transmitted agents associated with pelvic inflammatory disease. *Am J Obstet Gynecol* 138:1064, 1980.

7 Potterat JJ, King RD: A new approach to gonorrhea control: The asymptomatic man and incidence reduction. *JAMA* 245:578, 80, 1981.

8 McGuire WJ: The myth of massive media impact: Savagings and salvagings, in *Public Communication and Behavior,* G Comstock (ed). New York, Academic, 1986, vol 1, pp 175–257.

9 Pechacek TF: Modifications of smoking behavior, in *Smoking and Health: A Report of the Surgeon General.* Diter Publication PHS 79-50066. Washington, DC: Government Printing Office, 1979.

10 McKusick L et al: The AIDS epidemic: A model for developing intervention strategies for reducing high risk behavior in gay men. *Sex Transm Dis* 12:229, 1985.

11 Communication Technologies. A report on designing an effective AIDS prevention campaign strategy for San Francisco: Results from Fourth Probability. Sample of an urban gay male community. San Francisco Communication Technologies, 1982.

12 Farquhar JW et al: Community studies of cardiovascular disease prevention, in *Prevention of Coronary Heart Disease,* W Kaplan, J Stamler (eds). Philadelphia, Saunders, 1983.

13 Green LW, McAlister AL: Main intervention to support health behavior: Some theoretical perspective and practice reflections. *Health Educ Q* 11:322, 1984.

14 Coates TJ: Preventing AIDS: Strategies for primary and secondary prevention. *J Consult Clin Psychol,* in press.

15 McGuire WJ: Public communication as a strategy for inducing health-promoting behavior change. *Prev Med* 13:299, 1984.

16 Flay BR: Man, media and smoking cigarettes: A critical review. *Am J Public Health* 77:153, 1987.

17 Farquhar JW et al: Education and communication studies, in *Oxford Textbook of Public Heath,* WW Holland, R Detels, G. Knox (eds). Oxford, London, Oxford University Press, 1985, vol 3, pp 207–221.

18 Bandura A: *Social Learning Theory.* Englewood Cliffs, NJ, Prentice-Hall, 1977.

19 Green LW et al: *Health Education Planning: A Diagnostic Approach.* Palo Alto CA, Mayfield Publishing, 1980.

20 Ajzen I, Fishbein M: *Understanding Attitudes and Predicting Social Behavior.* Englewood Cliffs, NJ, Prentice-Hall, 1980.

21 Catania J et al: The CAPS AIDS Risk Reduction Model (AARM). Submitted for publication, Center for AIDS Prevention Studies. Health Education Quarterly, in press.

22 Shilts R: *And the Band Played On.* New York, Saint Martins Press, 1987.

23 Rogers EM: *Diffusion of Innovation.* New York, Free Press, 1983.

24 Rogers EM, Kincaid DC: *Communication Network: Toward a New Paradigm for Research.* New York, Free Press, 1981.

25 Manoff RK: *Social Marketing: New Imperative for Public Health.* New York, Praeger, 1985.

26 Farquhar JW: The community-based model of lifestyle intervention trials. *Am J Epidemiol.* 108:103, 1978.

27 Farquhar JW et al: Community education for cardiovascular health. *Lancet* 1:1191, 1977.

28 Meyer AJ et al: Skills training in a cardiovascular health education campaign. *J Consult Clin Psychol* 48:129, 1980.

29 National Cancer Institute: Community Intervention Trial for Smoking Cessation. Bettesdame, NCI, 1988.

30 Blackburn H, Pechacek T: Smoking cessation and the Minnesota Heart Health Program, in Proceedings of the Fifth World Congress on Smoking and Health, D Nashbakken (ed). 1986.

31 Egger G et al: Results of a large scale media antismoking campaign in Australia: North Coast "Quit for Life" programme. *Br Med J* 287: 1125, 1983.

32 Vincent M et al: Reducing adolescent pregnancy through school and community-based education. *JAMA* 257:3382, 1987.

33 Ekstrand ML, Coates TJ: Prevalence and change in AIDS high risk behavior among gay and bisexual men. Paper presented at the IV International Conference on AIDS, Stockholm, June 1988.

34 Winkelstein W et al: Sexual practice and risk of infection by the human immunodeficiency virus. *JAMA* 257:321, 1987.

35 Guydish J, Coates TJ: Changes in AIDS-related high-risk behavior among heterosexual men. Paper presented at the IV International Conference on AIDS, Stockholm, June 1988.

36 McKusick L et al: AIDS prevention education in the high school: Result of a study of California USA Adolescents. Paper presented at the IV International Conference on AIDS, Stockholm, June 1988.

37 Coates TJ et al: Changes in high risk behavior among gay and bisexual men since the beginning of the AIDS epidemic. Report prepared for the Office of Technology Assessment, 1988.

38 Puckett S, Bye L: The Stop AIDS Program. Unpublished manuscript, San Francisco, 1988.

# Chapter 91

# Strategies for management of sex partners

Richard B. Rothenberg
John J. Potterat

Because sex is the unifying event in sexually transmitted diseases, tools for STD control must consider social and behavioral factors more prominently than for other communicable infections. Indeed, the standard methods of public health—immunization, mass chemoprophylaxis, environmental modification—are either inappropriate or not yet available. Our current armamentarium rests on our underdeveloped understanding of social and personal interaction.

We can educate (Chap. 88); we can screen large numbers of individuals (Chap. 84); we can provide acceptable diagnostic and treatment services (Chap. 87). One major tool, however, consists of the extraordinary act of asking perfect strangers their best-guarded secrets: with whom they have sex, when, how often, and in what ways. More remarkable, they frequently tell us. This approach must be keyed to a coherent theory of disease transmission and to a detailed understanding of clinical and sociological factors.

## GENERAL BACKGROUND

The historical perspective on national control strategies and the management of sex partners in the United States was succinctly summarized by Henderson in 1977.[1] Until 1972 national policy was concerned with syphilis only. Largely through the efforts of Dr. Thomas Parran,[2] public and official awareness fostered the establishment of rapid treatment centers during and after World War II. The belief that syphilis eradication was imminent led to premature dismantling of the federal program in the late 1950s. Sustained resurgence of syphilis and other STDs in the late 1950s and early 1960s[3] stimulated a redetermination of public policy,[4] with primary focus on the provision of case investigation and contact tracing services. A cadre of "public health advisers" was developed and has been the personnel cornerstone for federal STD control efforts in the United States.

While public policy for the STDs in the United States focused on diagnosed patients and their contacts, a different choice was made in Great Britain.[5] The establishment of venereology as a distinct speciality (rather than an offshoot of dermatology, as it is in much of Western Europe) and the creation of a strong, decentralized "special clinic" system have been the hallmarks of the British approach. As in most other medical fields, the senior consultants in venereology make their own clinical and epidemiologic decisions and do not rely on a strong central agency, as is the case in the United States, for guidelines vis-à-vis treatment recommendations, control strategies, clinic protocols, or outreach efforts.

## PARTNER TRACING

Partner ("contact") tracing, formerly referred to as "the epidemiologic process",[6] remains a cornerstone of management for syphilis and gonorrhea in the United States. The partner interview process has endured because it can be an effective control and investigative tool.[7–17] Limited resources in most areas preclude the interviewing and counseling of all STD cases and/or the field follow-up of the partners they name. Judicious focus on those who contribute disproportionately to disease transmission maximizes efficiency.[16–18] In establishing priorities, consideration must be given to the reliability of self-referral behavior. Self-referral of contacts may work well with certain populations,[13] but poorly with some groups deemed important in disease endemicity.[17] A mixed effort may be appropriate in some instances.

When interviewing cannot be performed, all patients with sexually transmitted disease should at least be offered epidemiologic information about their infection, including relevant detail on disease transmission, asymptomatic carriage, critical time periods of infectiousness, and the consequences of not informing sexual partners and of premature resumption of sexual activity. Considering the frequent coexistence of sexually transmitted infections, encouragement of sexual partner referral may be an effective screening tool.

Much of the technical detail and statistical evaluation in the United States concerning the contact tracing process has appeared only as unpublished documents.[19] A complicated management scheme has evolved for interviewing patients with syphilis and gonorrhea, recording pertinent information, ensuring timely field investigation of contracts and clinical follow-up of selected patients, and assessing effectiveness both through a variety of contact indices and also through uniform reporting of results. These procedures are monitored in a number of periodic publications available through the Public Health Service, Centers for Disease Control.

In contrast, British activity, while no less thoughtful, has been less intense, less formal, and usually not aggregated (except for morbidity reports) on a national level. Nonetheless, several schemes for contact referral have been in continuous operation for many years[20,21] and even antedate those in the United States. While forms and procedures differ and bear the linguistic stamp of their respective origins, the content and intent are substantially similar.[22–24]

In sum, both sides of the Atlantic offer a clear consensus that a basic strategy in the management of sex partners includes identifying them and bringing them to medical examination. As noted, the limitation to this approach is resource availability.

## EPIDEMIOLOGIC TREATMENT

Considerable difference of opinion exists, however, about how to deal with sex partners who come for medical care. Soon after the general introduction of antibiotics, it was established that simple, effective single-dose therapy was available for both syphilis and gonorrhea. Furthermore, it became apparent that prevention was possible, i.e., that treatment after exposure to, but before clinical manifestations of, syphilis could "abort" the disease.[25] The concept of treatment before diagnosis pits the clinical importance of accurate diagnosis against the primacy of public health prevention.[26,27] Seven key factors provide a useful framework for decision making: (1) risk of infection, (2) seriousness of disease, (3) difficulties in diagnosis, (4) effectiveness of treatment, (5) side effects, (6) likelihood of spread if procedure is not used, and (7) facilities for observation.[28,29] Application of this framework to a disease such as syphilis provides a coherent picture for determining the use of epidemiologic treatment: Syphilis is a "very serious" disease of "medium (9 to 30 percent)" infectivity, for which diagnosis is often "delayed." Treatment is "very effective" with "few, if any" side effects. The likelihood of spread is variable, but as high as "62.1 percent in regular consorts." Default rates are also variable, but as high as "81 percent."

The arguments for and against epidemiologic treatment are clouded by a number of other terms in common use which bear an imprecise relationship to the temporal sequence of sexual exposure, infection, development of symptoms, diagnosis, treatment, and/or transmission.[30,31]

The following definitions establish a more precise relationship to the moment of public health intervention:

*Preventive*—treatment administered prior to a diagnosis in an asymptomatic sex partner, who is subsequently demonstrated to have been infected.

*Prophylactic*—treatment administered prior to diagnosis in an asymptomatic sex partner who is subsequently found to be uninfected.

*Abortive*—treatment given to a sex partner found to be infected but not yet symptomatic.

*Presumptive*—treatment based on clinical presentation (signs and symptoms) for which laboratory confirmation is not yet available.

The first two terms are invoked for the asymptomatic patient prior to diagnosis, the third for the asymptomatic patient after diagnosis. In a sense, all these are epidemiologic, a term which simply refers to consideration of nonclinical data in the decision to intervene. These distinctions provide precision in assessing the impact of intervention. The epidemiologist can provide the clinician with data on the aggregate consequences of individual treatment decisions.

Opponents of epidemiologic treatment have stressed that diagnosis should precede treatment, that premature treatment may preclude diagnosis, and that "epi-treatment" leads to indiscriminant antibiotic use and results in substandard medical evaluation. While recognizing the possibility of these unwelcome concomitants to epidemiologic treatment, current proponents couch the argument in public health terms: use must be predicated on quantitative assessment of risk. Infected sex partners who are "epi-treated" may not have contracted disease from the original patient interviewed but may be infected because they are part of a high-risk milieu.[30] Thus, epidemiologic treatment could also be offered to similar high-risk groups, implying that contact with a known case is a convenient marker, but not the only one. Rather, a spectrum of risk exists among subgroups of "suspects" (nonsexual contact of infected patients) and "associates" (individuals named by uninfected person).[31]

The need for risk assessment is even more graphically illustrated by gonorrhea infection rates in a variety of groups in an STD clinic setting.[32] The prevalence of gonorrhea during a 6-month period ranged from 0.8 percent among men requesting premarital exams to 65.1 percent among women who were established contacts to gonorrhea. They point to a number of logical discrepancies in the use of "epi-treatment." Several subgroups not recommended for epidemiologic treatment had higher rates of infection than others to whom "epi-treatment" is routinely offered. Although the issue for gonorrhea can sometimes be resolved by Gram's stain, the problem of where to draw the line remains.

Decision analysis (Chap. 3) may provide some guidance. By quantifying the interaction of initial risk, the sensitivity and specificity of diagnosis, the likelihood of complications and spread, of default, of drug reaction, and of adverse psychosocial effects, it was estimated that 12 to 30 percent of women and 4 to 13 percent of men seeking care as sex partners would be infected in the absence of epidemiologic treatment.[33] Another decision analysis determined that the optimal strategy for managing women who are asymptomatic contacts to men with gonorrhea is to obtain a culture, treat, and follow up sexual partners if the culture is positive.[34] But other, less quantitative issues must be weighed in the balance as well: (1) the relative ethics of treating uninfected individuals compared with preventing clinical illness and disease transmission, and (2) the absolute level of disease in a group compared with the propensity of that group to transmit.[35]

Complexities aside, epidemiologic treatment is usually given to sex partners of men and women with syphilis and gonorrhea in the United States. In Great Britain as well,[36–38] 85 percent of STD clinics use some form of epidemiologic treatment. Moreover, British consultants who provided care to 89 percent of all female cases used epidemiologic treatment.[39,40] One unwelcome concomitant, however, is that substantial misreporting of gonorrhea may result from epidemiologic treatment.

## SPECIFIC DISEASES

Enunciation of a strategy for seeking the sex partners of infected individuals and offering them epidemiologic treatment presents formidable problems in view of the huge numbers of potential infectees. Decisions must be made concerning which disease and which patient-contact clusters have the greatest potential for complications and continued transmission. These decisions rest on an understanding of the epidemiologic distinctions among STDs and on a theoretical basis for persistent endemicity.

## GONORRHEA

With about 1 million cases of gonorrhea reported annually in the United States, the need for targeting control efforts is obvious, and a sound theoretical basis is required. A number of models have been proferred to explain the epidemiology of gonorrhea. For example, in a nonmathematical approach, it was postulated that endemicity is maintained through a finely balanced equilibrium which required continued reintroduction of gonorrhea into defined groups.[41] In a deterministic model which projected gonorrhea prevalence in the presence or absence of control efforts, key parameters were transmissibility, frequency of contact, and duration of infection.[42,43]

Perhaps the most important of these models[44] proposed that gonorrhea endemicity is maintained through the existence of small, definable, stable groups (core groups) with high prevalence. These core groups represent a small portion (2.5 percent or less) of those at risk for gonorrhea, but they are directly or indirectly responsible for most cases. A more comprehensive mathematical treatment of this model,[45] based on sexual interaction among subpopulations and the duration of infectiousness, demonstrated the importance of core-noncore interactions, and the key role of "saturation" (sexual contact between infected individuals).

A number of recent studies have provided empirical validation of the notion of core groups. Each of the 12 Standard Metropolitan Statistical Areas in upstate New York contained a central core area (with 50 percent of cases) surrounded by an adjacent area (30 percent of cases) and by a peripheral area.[46] A decreasing gradient in gonorrhea case rates radiated from the core outward, and the relative risk of gonorrhea in some of the core areas was 20-fold higher than in peripheral areas. In Colorado Springs, Colorado, a core group with definable sociodemographic characteristics and close social aggregation was identified.[47] In Seville, Spain,[48] urban clustering of gonorrhea cases occurred in certain districts, which were also foci for syphilis, chlamydial infection, and all STDs taken together.

The importance of core groups is reflected in the number of days of potential infectivity which core group members with gonorrhea generate in their contacts.[49] The total of such days, summed over all members of a subgroup, represents the "force of infectivity" exerted by that group. This serves as an epidemiologic surrogate for the duration-of-infectiousness parameter in transmission models.[45] Though it helps delineate areas of intense transmission, infectious patient days may not be directly correlated with yearly gonorrhea rates.[50]

Intrinsic to the concept of core groups is that some individuals must have a "reproduction rate" of greater than one. (The term "reproduction rate" is borrowed from ecologic analysis. As used in the context of infectious disease dynamics, it refers to the ability of an infectious case to reproduce itself, and should not be confused with its more common use in reproductive health.) This implies that the average number of infected contacts per case is a weighted average of those with two or more (transmitters who may be in core groups) and those with one (nontransmitters). Since 1973,[19] the national average has been fewer than 0.5 infected contacts per case. With allowance for less than perfect efficiency in case finding, this suggests that nontransmitters predominate. If the core group theory is valid, the appropriate control strategy would be to focus contact tracing efforts on transmitters in the core areas, in an attempt to bring the reproductive rate to less than one.

Several epidemiologic observations support the notion of definable groups that are important in transmission. The contacts of women with gonococcal pelvic inflammatory disease (GPID) are often high-level transmitters,[17] as are the women with GPID themselves, prostitutes,[51] and patients with repeated gonorrhea.[52,53] Targeting such groups has shed light on the role of the asymptomatic male in gonorrhea transmission.[18] In Colorado Springs, almost three-fifths of the contacts of women with GPID were asymptomatic. This represents the high end of the spectrum, but, among men examined as contacts, 20 to 40 percent of those found to have had gonorrhea were asymptomatic (Table 91-1). The importance of asymptomatic gonorrhea in men may have been underestimated because of earlier work,[11,12,54] which argued against the utility of interviewing women with gonorrhea. Those earlier studies included a larger number of women who were themselves named as contacts by men with gonococcal urethritis. Intensive interviewing of special groups of women, on the other hand, may lead to identification of transmitters who are remote (i.e., 2 or more months since last contact) and asymptomatic. Continued endemicity should indeed result from continued sexual activity by individuals who are unaware of their infection.

Direct validation of the core group theory—and its implication for focused intervention—at the community level is more difficult, in view of the many social forces that may influence the outcome. Some direct and indirect evidence has accumulated, however. A substantial decrease in gonorrhea occurrence in Colorado Springs during a 30-month period of intensive targeting.[16–18] A 20 percent decline in gonorrhea occurred at Whitechapel (London) during the 1960s,[55] concomitant with the introduction of contact tracing, compared with an increase of 33 percent in England and Wales for the interval. Similarly, the decrease in gonorrhea in Sheffield[56] for the period 1977–1983 far exceeded that for England as a whole. This was attributed in part to the greater intensity and efficiency of contact tracing efforts. Though neither of the two latter studies was consciously focused on core groups, both acknowledge their attempt to deal with those at higher risk. In the United States, a number of studies are now in progress which are using the core group theory as an approach to disease control.

The notion of core group transmission is further supported by epidemiologic observations on the spread of penicillinase-producing *Neisseria gonorrhoeae* (PPNG).[57] In a large outbreak in Liverpool in 1976,[58] cases were noted to have occurred primarily in two inner city districts. In a more recent analysis of PPNG transmission in Miami, Florida, cases were clustered in small inner city areas, with a diminishing risk outward from the center. After introduction, the subsequent growth or disappearance of PPNG in a community may well be dependent on its presence among core transmitters of gonorrhea.[57]

Whatever the underlying theory, however, a control strategy must be comprehensive and multifaceted. Widespread screening for gonorrhea in the United States, begun in 1972, may have played a major role in halting the increase in gonorrhea four years

**Table 91-1. Observed Proportions of Asymptomatic Men with Gonorrhea**

| Study | Men with gonorrhea, No. | Asymptomatic | | How ascertained |
|---|---|---|---|---|
| | | No. | % | |
| Pariser et al., 1964[63] | 43 | 26 | 60 | Recent contacts to clinic cases |
| Pederson et al., 1970[54] | 19 | 5 | 26 | Contacts, not previously treated |
| Marino et al., 1972[11] | 280 | 82 | 29 | Contacts of clinic cases |
| Blount, 1972[12] | 124 | 48 | 39 | Contacts of family planning cases |
| Wallin, 1974[64] | 92 | 21 | 23 | Contacts of clinic cases |
| Portnoy et al., 1974[65] | 63 | 27 | 43 | Contacts of clinic cases |
| Handsfield et al., 1974[66] | 59 | 40 | 68 | From 2628 "normals" |
| Nielson et al., 1975[67] | 89 | 13 | 15 | Patients in clinic |
| Dunlop et al., 1976[68] | 19 | 7 | 37 | Contacts of clinic cases |
| Gilstrap et al., 1977[14] | 63 | 14 | 22 | Contacts of PID |
| John and Donald, 1978[69] | 203 | 50 | 24 | Patients in clinic |
| Braff and Wibbelsman, 1978[70] | 70 | 25 | 36 | Patients in clinic |
| Volkin et al., 1979[15] | 34 | 11 | 32 | Contacts of PID |
| Phillips et al., 1980[16] | 65 | 32 | 49 | Contacts of recent repeaters |
| Potterat et al., 1980[17] | 86 | 51 | 59 | Contacts of PID |
| Phillips et al., 1980[16] | 123 | 84 | 68 | Contacts of routine discoveries |

later. Though now less important as a general strategy, there may well be a place in specific programs for screening of special groups. In addition, contact investigation and followup activities should incorporate some of the innovative procedures that have been introduced in recent years: special education modules, use of nontraditional sites such as gay bathhouses, renovation in actual interview technique, and the increased use of a contact slip or self-referral system, with transfer of responsibility for contact referral to the patient.[13,24,60–62] Better use can be made of information related to social milieu (so-called cluster information), as well as pursuit of infection in suspects or associates.

## SYPHILIS

The principles for managing syphilis patients and their contacts have been based on empirical models of syphilis transmission:[6,71]

1. Interviewing and reinterviewing every reported case of early syphilis for sexual contacts.
2. Intensive effort by field workers to locate and offer medical examination with minimal time period so that further spread of disease is reduced.
3. Counseling and blood testing of social-sexual peers who are possibly involved in an infectious chain (cluster procedure).
4. "Epidemiologic" treatment of all sexual contacts to persons with infectious syphilis.

In support of these tenets, essentially unchanged for many years, a coherent body of management tools has been developed, including special forms, a "lot" system for linking cases and contacts, and a system of training and interviewing techniques. Unfortunately, these techniques for syphilis control have not been rigorously tested.

National contact indices (the number of infected contacts identified per index case), first described by 1948,[9] have been consistently available for syphilis since 1969.[19] As with gonorrhea, it is difficult to make a case for an impact of the control program from these raw data. At best, a consistency of performance seems apparent over the years. Circumscribed effectiveness, based on local application of these techniques, is not well documented. In addition, over the past decade, a growing preponderance of syphilis has occurred in homosexual men. Since a significant portion of their sexual activity is anonymous, the contact interviewing system is less effective in this group.

A number of outreach efforts have been attempted, similar to those outlined for gonorrhea. Procedures such as screening for STD at bathhouses catering to homosexual men have met with varied success,[19,72] none has addressed the fundamental issue of alteration in personal behavior. At present, the general approach might include augmentation of intensive interviewing and case management with periodic screening and increased patient participation (i.e., self-referral). Some evidence exists that core groups also play a role in syphilis transmission,[73] and the targeted approach to core syphilis transmission may apply.

## CHLAMYDIAL SYNDROMES

The past decade has witnessed burgeoning interest in the biology of *Chlamydia trachomatis* (see Chaps. 15 and 16).[74] Its role in a variety of genitourinary syndromes and the advisability of case follow-up have now become apparent. A study performed prior to the general availability of culture techniques[75] indicated that sex partner follow-up may be efficacious in diagnosing disease and interrupting transmission. With the dissemination of inexpensive culture methods, a number of studies have investigated the cost-effectiveness of routine culture. Despite the fact that chlamydia may not be as readily transmissible as gonococci,[76] routine culturing appears to be cost-effective for patients undergoing routine gynecologic evaluation,[77] as well as for women attending a clinic for sexually transmitted diseases.[78] Field follow-up of asymptomatic individuals who are culture-positive for *C. trachomatis*, though a labor-intensive process, appears to be the most efficient method for follow-up and to be cost-effective as well.[79]

The profile for epidemiologic treatment, described earlier,[27,28] offers an affirmation of the advisability of such treatment when applied to chlamydial infection (see Table 91-2). Diagnostic techniques, coupled with effective methods for field follow-up, make the arguments for intense programmatic efforts in chlamydia control far more compelling.[80]

## OTHER SEXUALLY TRANSMITTED DISEASES

The profile for epidemiologic treatment[27,28] is equally applicable to other diseases, not just for decision making about what groups to treat, but in planning an overall program as well. Unfortunately, data are, for the most part, embryonic and few definitive statements can be made.

Assessment of trichomoniasis, for example, suggests the utility of treating sexual partners, primarily to prevent the patient's reexposure. This does appear to be standard practice, with the patient often acting as medication courier. The same technique is used for treating partners and household contacts of individuals with scabies and crabs. Selected male sex partners of patients with candidiasis (Chap. 45) and with bacterial vaginosis (Chap. 47) may be shown to be infected, but blanket treatment of sex partners is usually not indicated. A recommendation to use epidemiologic treatment for the prevention of these STDs must await more data.

Some of the most exciting developments in the field of sexually

**Table 91-2. Profile for Epidemiologic Treatment: Chlamydia**

| Factors | Assessment | Reported figures |
|---|---|---|
| Risk of infection | Medium–high | 65% in women; 52.6% in men |
| Seriousness of disease | Low to medium | Complications: PID, epididymitis, inclusion conjunctivitis, pneumonia |
| Difficult in diagnosis | Moderate | No convenient lab test emerging |
| Effectiveness of treatment | Good | Up to 90% or greater eradication of organisms |
| Side effects | Minimal | As low as 5–10% with tetracycline |
| Likelihood of spread if procedure not used | Probably high | Variable; not yet specifically studied |
| Facilities for observation | Variable | High default rates likely |

transmitted disease have been the implications of recent epidemiologic research on the viral STDs. Considerable strides have been made, for example, in defining relapse vs. reinfection for herpes simplex virus infections, in describing the biological subtypes and the risk of infection with autologous versus heterologous strains, and in developing chemotherapeutic agents with systemic and possibly local potency against the herpes virus (Chap. 35). This will, in the near future, have significant implications for the treatment and follow-up of sex partners to individuals with herpes infections. Similarly, the development of a highly effective vaccine against hepatitis B has altered the approach to exposed and unexposed contacts.

## ACQUIRED IMMUNODEFICIENCY SYNDROME (AIDS)

As detailed elsewhere (Chaps. 28–32), AIDS has become the primary focus of STD control in the United States. To date, no published data on partner notification are available and routine screening of individuals, either voluntary or mandatory, is passionately debated. Both of these major methods for STD control—in particular, contact notification—raise important social and epidemiologic issues.

On the social side, considerable concern exists about the perceived potential for abrogation of civil liberties and for adverse economic and social consequences. The use of contact notification, with identification of individuals and the attendant record keeping, offers an opportunity for realization of these concerns. In addition, the absence of an interventive tool (e.g., vaccine, epidemiologic treatment) attenuates the value of universal application of contact tracing.[81] This limitation may be countered, however, by the potential for individual targeting of risk-reduction educational efforts—particularly for those who do not perceive themselves at risk.

On the epidemiologic side, however, an understanding of the dynamics of transmission of AIDS, analogous to work that has been done in gonorrhea and syphilis, depends on data available only through contact investigation. Considerable effort has been invested in creating predictive models of the AIDS epidemic.[82,83] These methods are statistically based and, though they provide the needed forecasts, are couched in the inherent uncertainty for using prior history to forecast the future. Models which use the biology and epidemiology of transmission, however, while less effective for short-term prediction, have a theoretical underpinning that is not linked to the shape of the epidemic curve. Effective use of such an approach requires information on the frequency of new sexual partners, the number, variety, and characteristics of sexual contact, and the duration of infectiousness.[84]

Contact notification, even if limited in scope and duration, can provide information on the parameters of interest and may be possible in a context which avoids direct conflict with issues of social concern. Several state health departments[85,86] have initiated programs of HIV antibody testing at selected sites, with pre- and posttest counseling of subjects, and the offer of epidemiologic follow-up for their sex partners. As expected, a substantial proportion of sex partners (14 to 17 percent) were positive for HIV antibody, but perhaps more important is demonstration of a secure and confidential mechanism for improved targeting of risk-reduction efforts. It is likely that testing will become more widespread as biologic understanding and social technology improve. This will hopefully provide a better understanding of the dynamics of AIDS transmission as well.

## References


1 Henderson RH: Control of sexually transmitted diseases in the United States—A federal perspective. *Br J Vener Dis* 53:211, 1977.
2 Parran T: *Shadow on the Land.* New York, Reynal & Hitchcock, 1937.
3 Schamberg IL: Syphilis and Sisyphus. *Br J Vener Dis* 39:87, 1963.
4 Baumgartner L et al: *The Eradication of Syphilis, A Task Force Report.* Department of HEW, PHS, 1962.
5 King A: The life and times of Colonel Harrison. *Br J Ven Dis* 50:391, 1974.
6 Kaufman RE et al: Current trends in syphilis. *Public Health Rev* 3:175, 1974.
7 *V.D. Epidemiology Report* 12, September 1973, HEW, PHS, CDC.
8 Ennes H, Bennett TG: The contact-education interview: Its functions, principles and techniques in venereal disease contact investigation. *Am J Syph Vener Dis* 29:647, 1945.
9 Ishrant AP, Kahn HA: Statistical indices used in the evaluation of syphilis contact investigation. *J Vener Dis Info* 29:1, 1948.
10 Johnson EW et al: An evaluation of gonorrhea case finding in the chronically infected female. *Am J Epidemiol* 90:438, 1969.
11 Marino AF et al: Gonorrhea epidemiology—Is it worthwhile? *Am J Public Health* 62:713, 1972.
12 Blount JH: A new approach for gonorrhea epidemiology. *Am J Public Health* 62:710, 1972.
13 Potterat JJ, Rothenberg RB: The case-finding effectiveness of a self-referral system for gonorrhea: A preliminary report. *Am J Public Health* 67:174, 1977.
14 Gilstrap LC et al: Gonorrhea screening in male consorts of women with pelvic infection. *JAMA* 238:956, 1977.
15 Volkin LBV et al: Epidemiologic follow-up of patients with gonococcal pelvic inflammatory disease. *Sex Transm Dis* 6:267, 1979.
16 Phillips L et al: Focused interviewing in gonorrhea control. *Am J Public Health* 70:705, 1980.
17 Potterat JJ et al: Gonococcal pelvic inflammatory disease: Casefinding observations. *Am J Obstet Gynecol* 138(2):1101, 1980.
18 Potterat JJ, King RD: A new approach to gonorrhea control. The asymptomatic man and incidence reduction. *JAMA* 245:578, 1981.
19 Division of Sexually Transmitted Diseases, Centers for Disease Control, Atlanta, GA.
20 Burgess JA: A contact tracing procedure. *Br J Vener Dis* 39:113, 1963.
21 Wigfield AS: 27 years of uninterrupted contact tracing: The "Tyneside Scheme." *Br J Vener Dis* 48:37, 1972.
22 Satin A: A record system for contact tracing. *Br J Vener Dis* 53:84, 1977.
23 Satin A, Mills A: Measuring the outcome of contact tracing. 1: A description of the patient and contact population studied. *Br J Vener Dis* 54:187, 1978.
24 Mills A, Satin A: Measuring the outcome of contact tracing. 2: The responsibilities of the health worker and the outcome of contact investigations. *Br J Vener Dis* 54:192, 1978.
25 Alexander LJ et al: Abortive treatment of syphilis. *Am J Syph Gonorrhea Vener Dis* 33:429, 1949.
26 King AJ: For and against treatment before diagnosis. *Br J Vener Dis* 30:13, 1954.
27 Willcox RR: Treatment before diagnosis in venereology. *Br J Vener Dis* 30:7, 1954.
28 Willcox RR: "Epidemiologic" treatment in non-venereal and in treponemal diseases. *Br J Vener Dis* 49:107, 1973.
29 Willcox RR: "Epidemiologic" treatment in venereal disease other than syphilis. *Br J Vener Dis* 49:116, 1973.
30 Hart G: Epidemiologic treatment of syphilis. *J Am Vener Dis Assoc* 3 (suppl):1977, 1976.
31 Hart G: Epidemiologic treatment for syphilis and gonorrhea. *Sex Transm Dis* 7:149, 1980.
32 Judson FN, Maltz AB: A rational basis for the epidemiologic treatment of gonorrhea in a clinic for sexually transmitted diseases. *Sex Transm Dis* 5:89, 1978.

33 Johnson RE: Epidemiologic and prophylactic treatment of gonorrhea: A decision analysis review. *Sex Transm Dis* 2(suppl):159, 1979.
34 Turshen IJ et al: Decision analytic approach to the management of gonorrhea contacts. *Sex Transm Dis* 11(3):137, 1984.
35 Wiesner PJ: Epidemiologic and prophylactic treatment of gonorrhea: A decision analysis review. *Sex Transm Dis* 5:120, 1978.
36 Adler MW et al: Facilities and diagnostic criteria in sexually transmitted disease clinics in England & Wales. *Br J Vener Dis* 54:2, 1978.
37 Adler MW: Diagnostic treatment & reporting criteria in sexually transmitted disease clinics in England and Wales: 1. Diagnosis. *Br J Vener Dis* 54:10, 1978.
38 Adler MW: Diagnostic treatment & reporting criteria in sexually transmitted disease clinics in England and Wales: 2. Treatment & reporting criteria. *Br J Vener Dis* 54:15, 1978.
39 Kelson MC et al: Practices in STD clinics in England and Wales. *Br J Vener Dis* 57:221, 1981.
40 Belsey EM. Epidemiological treatment of gonorrhea and non-specific genital infection in female sexual contacts. *Br J Vener Dis* 58:113, 1982.
41 Willcox RR: Importance of "feedback" in gonorrhea control. *Br J Vener Dis* 41:287, 1965.
42 Reynolds GH, Chan YK: A control model for gonorrhea. *Bull Inst Int Statist* 106:264, 1975.
43 Kramer MA, Reynolds GH: The evaluation of a gonorrhea vaccine and other gonorrhea control strategies on basis of computer simulation model. Presented at 108th Annual Meeting, APHA, Detroit, October 1980.
44 Yorke JA et al: Dynamics and control of the transmission of gonorrhea. *Sex Transm Dis* 5:51, 1978.
45 Hethcote HW, Yorke JA: Gonorrhea transmission dynamics and control. Berlin, Springer-Verlag, 1984.
46 Rothenberg RB: The geography of gonorrhea. Empirical demonstration of core group transmission. *Am J Epidemiol* 117:688, 1983.
47 Potterat JJ et al: Gonorrhea as a social disease. *Sex Transm Dis* 12(1):25, 1985.
48 Alvarez-Dardet C et al: Urban clusters of sexually transmitted disease in the city of Seville, Spain. *Sex Transm Dis* 12(3):166, 1985.
49 Rothenberg RB, Potterat JJ: Temporal and social aspects of gonorrhea transmission: the force of infectivity. *Sex Transm Dis* 15:88, 1988.
50 Talbot MD: Relation between incidence of gonorrhea in Sheffield and efficiency of contact tracing: A paradox? *Genitourin Med* 62:377, 1986.
51 Potterat JJ et al: Gonorrhea in street prostitutes: Epidemiologic and legal implications. *Sex Transm Dis* 6:58, 1979.
52 Brooks FG et al: Repeated gonorrhea: An analysis of importance and risk factors. *J Infect Dis* 137:161, 1978.
53 Noble RC et al: Recidivism among patients with gonococcal infection presenting to a venereal disease clinic. *Sex Transm Dis* 4:39, 1977.
54 Pederson AHB, Harra WD: Follow-up of male and female contacts of patients with gonorrhea. *Public Health Rep* 85:997, 1970.
55 Dunlop EMC et al: Improved tracing of contacts of heterosexual men with gonorrhea. *Br J Vener Dis* 47:192, 1971.
56 Talbot MD, Kinghorn GR. Epidemiology and control of gonorrhea in Sheffield. *Genitourin Med* 61:230, 1985.
57 Rothenberg RB, Voigt R: Epidemiologic aspects of PPNG control. submitted, *Sex Transm Dis.*
58 Arya OP et al: Epidemiology of penicillinase-producing Neisseria gonorrhoeae in Liverpool from 1977 to 1982. *J Infect* 8:70, 1984.
59 Zenilman JM et al: Penicillinase-producing Neisseria gonorrheae (PPNG) in Miami. Etiologic role of core group transmitters and the illicit use of antibiotics. Presented at 25th Interscience Conference on Antimicrobial Agents and Chemotherapy, New Orleans, LA. 28 September–1 October, 1986.
60 Jamison H, Mueller DP: Patient initiative and responsibility: The potential effect on treatment and control of disease; the case of gonorrhea. *Soc Sci Med* 13A:303, 1979.
61 Judson FN, Wolf FC: Tracing and treating contact of gonorrhea patients in a clinic for sexually transmitted diseases. *Public Health Rep* 93:460, 1978.
62 Winfield J, Latif AS: Tracing contacts of person with sexually transmitted diseases in a developing country. *Sex Transm Dis* 12(1):5, 1985.
63 Pariser H et al: Asymptomatic gonorrhea in the male. *South Med J* 67:688, 1964.
64 Wallin J: Gonorrhea in 1972: A 1-year study of patients attending the VD unit in Uppsala. *Br J Vener Dis* 51:41, 1975.
65 Portnoy J et al: Asymptomatic gonorrhea in the male. *Can Med Assoc J* 110:169, 1974.
66 Handsfield HH et al: Asymptomatic gonorrhea in men. *N Engl J Med* 290:117, 1974.
67 Nielson R et al: Asymptomatic male and female gonorrhea. *Acta Derm Venereol* 55:449, 1975.
68 Dunlop EMC et al: Gonorrhea in the asymptomatic patient: Presentation and the role of contact tracing for heterosexual men and women for homosexual men. *Infection* 4:125, 1976.
69 John J, Donald WH: Asymptomatic urethral gonorrhea in men. *Br J Vener Dis* 54:322, 1978.
70 Braff EH, Wibbelsman CJ: Asymptomatic gonococcal urethritis in selected males. *Am J Public Health* 68:799, 1978.
71 Brown WJ et al: *Syphilis and Other Venereal Disease.* Cambridge, Harvard University Press, 1970, pp. 36–57.
72 Judson FN et al: Screening for gonorrhea and syphilis in the gay baths—Denver CO. *Am J Public Health* 67:740, 1977.
73 Rothenberg RB. The geography of syphilis: A demonstration of epidemiologic diversity, in *Advances in Sexually Transmitted Diseases, Diagnosis and Treatment,* R Morisett, E Kourstak (eds). Utrecht, Netherlands, VNU Sciences Press, 1986, pp 125–133.
74 Bowie WR: Etiology and treatment of nongonococcal urethritis. *Sex Transm Dis* 5:27, 1978.
75 Thelin I et al: Contact-tracing in patients with genital chlamydial infection. *Br J Vener Dis* 259, 1980.
76 Lyche E et al: The risk of transmission of genital chlamydia trachomatis infection is less than that of genital *Neisseria gonorrhoeae* infection. *Sex Transm Dis* 7(1):6, 1980.
77 Phillips RD et al: Should tests for chlamydia trachomatic cervical infection be done during routine gynecologic visits? *Ann Intern Med* 107:188, 1987.
78 Nettleman MD et al: Cost-effectiveness of a culturing for Chlamydia trachomatis. *Ann Intern Med* 105:189, 1986.
79 Katz BP et al: Efficiency and cost-effectiveness of field followup for patients with chlamydia trachomatis infection in a sexually transmitted disease clinic. *Sex Transm Dis,* in press.
80 1985 STD Treatment Guidelines. *MMWR Suppl* 34(45):1, 1985.
81 Gostin L, Curran WJ: AIDS screening, confidentiality, and the duty to warn. *Am J Public Health* 77(3):361, 1987.
82 Duong QP, MacNeil IB: Methodologies for forecasting the incidence of AIDS. Manuscript in preparation.
83 Liu KJ et al: A model-bases approach for estimating the mean incubation period of transfusion-associated acquired immunodeficiency syndrome. *Proc Natl Acad Sci USA* 83:3051, 1986.
84 May RM, Anderson RM: Transmission dynamics of HIV infection. *Nature* 326:137, 1987.
85 Virginia State Department of Health. Unpublished data.
86 Colorado State Department of Health. Unpublished data.

# Chapter 92

# Family planning and sexually transmitted diseases

David A. Grimes
Willard Cates, Jr.

The relationship between family planning methods and sexually transmitted diseases (STDs) is suddenly front-page news. Once the province of a small number of health professionals with interests in these related fields,[1] fertility control and its impact on STD have achieved national prominence because of the acquired immunodeficiency syndrome (AIDS) epidemic.

In part because of the mandate of the U.S. Surgeon General, condoms, long recognized as effective for contraception, should play a pivotal role in strategies to prevent transmission of AIDS. Indeed, the growing viral STD epidemic in the United States has rendered traditional containment strategies for control of treatable bacterial STD largely ineffective. In addition to AIDS, two other viral STDs fall in this category. Herpes simplex virus (HSV) infections can be recurrent and socially debilitating, and acyclovir offers only suppression or palliation for selected patients. Human papilloma virus (HPV) infections are far more frequent than HSV infections and have been linked with genital neoplasia. Topical treatment of HPV infections is often ineffectual, since the virus can infect adjacent, normal-appearing tissue.

The impact of family planning methods on the transmission and clinical course of STDs extends beyond viral STDs to encompass a broad range of important infections. This chapter reviews this relationship with a focus on the protection against STDs afforded by barrier methods, the relationship between IUDs and pelvic inflammatory disease (PID), the impact of oral contraceptives on STDs, and the effect of female sterilization on the risk of PID. The chapter also documents the unmet need for family planning services among STD patients and vice versa, and it outlines contraceptive strategies for couples at different stages of life.

## BARRIER CONTRACEPTIVES

### CONDOMS

Condoms protect against transmission of STDs by preventing direct contact with semen, genital discharge, some genital lesions, or infectious secretions. To be effective, condoms must be applied prior to genital contact and used consistently, and they must remain intact.

A growing number of laboratory studies confirm that condoms provide an impervious barrier to most STD pathogens. In experimental transmission models, condoms have been shown to be effective barriers against HSV type II,[2–4] *Chlamydia trachomatis*,[3] cytomegalovirus,[5] and human immunodeficiency virus (HIV).[6]

"Natural" condoms, made of sheep intestinal membrane, may not be as effective as synthetic condoms. Latex condoms have been reported to be impermeable to high concentrations of hepatitis B surface antigen (HBsAg) particles, while "natural" condoms of sheep intestine are not.[7] The larger intact virus particle (HBV) passed through "natural" condoms as well.[8] This permeability may relate to the size of pores in the intestinal membranes. HIV may also pass through "natural" condoms.[9,10] Thus, limited data suggest that "natural" condoms may offer less protection than latex condoms.

In human studies reviewed previously,[11] condoms have been found to confer protection against gonorrhea, urethritis from *Ureaplasma urealyticum*, and PID (Table 92-1). In an Irish cross-

**Table 92-1. Efficacy of Condom Use in Preventing Sexually Transmitted Diseases**

| Study | Study design | Study population | Outcome | Measure of effect | 95% confidence interval |
|---|---|---|---|---|---|
| Pemberton et al., 1972[12] | Cross-sectional | Males, STD clinic, Belfast | Urethral gonorrhea | 0.51 | 0.33–0.80 |
| | | | Nongonococcal urethritis | 1.20 | 0.90–1.59 |
| McCormack et al., 1973[14] | Cross-sectional | Male college volunteers, United States | Urethral T-mycoplasma colonization | 0.33 | 0.16–0.68 |
| Darrow, 1973[19] | Cohort | STD clinic attendees, California | Urethral gonorrhea | 0.34 | 0.10–1.13 |
| Hart, 1974[15] | Cohort | Australian soldiers, Vietnam | Self-reported venereal diseases | 0.00* | |
| Barlow, 1977[13] | Cross-sectional | Males, STD clinic, London | Urethral gonorrhea | 0.25 | 0.11–0.59 |
| | | | Nongonococcal urethritis | 0.85 | 0.69–1.07 |
| Hooper et al., 1978[20] | Cohort | Naval crewmen, Far East | Urethral gonorrhea | 0.00† | |
| Kelaghan et al., 1982[16] | Case-control | Hospitalized women, United States | Pelvic inflammatory disease | 0.6 | 0.4 –0.9 |
| Austin et al., 1984[17] | Case-control | Females, STD clinic, Alabama | Cervical gonorrhea | 0.87 | 0.64–1.19 |
| Syrjanen et al., 1984[18] | Case-control | Females, obstetrics & gynecology clinic, Finland | Cervical human papilloma virus infection | 1.35 | 0.72–2.78 |
| Cramer et al., 1987[21] | Case-control | Infertility patients, United States | Tubal infertility | 0.7‡ | 0.5 –1.1 |
| | | | | 0.5§ | 0.2 –0.9 |
| Fischl et al., 1987[22] | Cohort | Spouses of AIDS patients, Florida | HIV antibody seroconversion | 0.12 | 0.04–0.38 |
| Mann et al., 1987[23] | Cross-sectional | Prostitutes, Zaire | HIV antibody | 0.00‖ | |

SOURCE: Updated from Stone et al., 1986.[11]
* $p < 0.0001$, Fisher's exact test (none of 55 condom users were infected; 26 of 96 using no prophylaxis were infected).
† $p < 0.1$, Fisher's exact test (none of 29 condom users were infected; 51 of 498 nonusers were infected).
‡ Condoms without spermicide.
§ Condoms with spermicide.
‖ $p = 0.046$ by Fisher's exact test (none of 8 frequent condom users were infected; 26 of 77 less frequent users were infected).

sectional study of men attending an STD clinic for the first time, condom users were significantly less likely to be infected with gonorrhea than were nonusers.[12] A similar study from England[13] showed an even stronger protection against gonorrhea.

Among asymptomatic college men in Boston, regular use of condoms afforded significant protection against colonization with *Ureaplasma urealyticum;* this effect persisted despite the number of sexual partners.[14] Among Australian soldiers returning from Vietnam, those who had used condoms were significantly less likely to have reported having had an STD than were those who had not;[15] however, substantial methodologic flaws limit the interpretation of this study.

Women are protected by condoms as well. In a large, multicenter case-control study in the United States,[16] women who relied on condoms for contraception had a significantly lower risk of being hospitalized for PID than did women who used no contraception. In another case-control study based in an Alabama STD clinic, women whose partners had used condoms in the past 3 months had a lower risk of gonorrhea than did women whose partners had not used condoms;[17] this difference, however, was not statistically significant. A Finnish case-control study[18] found no protective effect of condoms against HPV infections of the cervix when the histories of women with HPV infections were compared with histories of women with normal Pap smears. However, women with HPV infections were at higher risk of infection than were control women, which probably masked any protective effect.

Two cohort studies have also reported a protective effect. In one,[19] men attending an STD clinic were given free condoms, then examined 3 months later. Those who always used condoms had less risk of gonorrhea than did men who never used them, although the difference was not statistically significant. In the other study,[20] seamen who reported using condoms while in port had a lower risk of acquiring gonorrhea than did seamen not using condoms; this difference, however, was not statistically significant, and information bias may have influenced these results.

Three more recent studies corroborate the protective effect of condoms. In a large, multicenter, case-control study of tubal infertility[21] in the United States, condom use alone was associated with a 30 percent reduced risk of infertility (not statistically significant). However, when condom plus spermicide had been used for contraception, the protection increased to 50 percent, which was statistically significant. In a longitudinal study of the spouses of AIDS patients in Florida, use of condoms was related to a marked reduction in the risk of HIV seroconversion.[22] Finally, in a study of prostitutes in Zaire, frequent use of condoms was associated with a significant reduction in the risk of HIV antibody presence in the prostitutes as compared with those prostitutes using condoms less frequently.[23] Taken together, these clinical studies suggest that the protective effect of condoms against many STDs is real and clinically important.

## OTHER BARRIER CONTRACEPTIVES

Several studies have described a protective effect for other barrier contraceptives (Table 92-2). In some studies, however, the authors did not distinguish between condoms and diaphragms. Another limitation to the interpretation of these studies is that the diaphragm is nearly always used with a spermicide, which has a protective effect itself, as described below. In two cross-sectional studies, one in a family planning clinic[24] and the other in an STD clinic,[25] the risk of cervical gonorrhea was lower (though not significantly so) among barrier users. In contrast, a large multicenter case-control study[16] found significant protection against hospitalization for PID among diaphragm users. Another case-control study in an STD clinic[17] found more than a 50 percent reduction in cervical gonorrhea among diaphragm users, though this difference was not statistically significant. In a large, multicenter case-control study of tubal infertility,[21] diaphragm use was associated with a 50 percent reduction in this condition, a highly significant difference.

Barrier contraceptives may also confer protection against cervical neoplasia. That cervical neoplasia has the epidemiologic features of an STD has been known for years,[26] and recent attention has focused on several subtypes of HPV as potential etiologic agents. Two British case-control studies[27,28] have shown a strong protective effect of barrier contraceptives against cervical neoplasia.

## SPERMICIDES

In vitro studies have shown that contraceptive spermicides kill or inactivate a host of STD pathogens. The most commonly used spermicidal agent in the United States is nonoxynol-9, a nonionic surfactant that damages the cell walls of sperm—and STD pathogens. Laboratory tests have documented activity against *Neisseria gonorrhoeae,*[29–31] *Trichomonas vaginalis,*[30] herpes simplex virus,[32,33] HIV,[34] and *Treponema pallidum.*[29] *Ureaplasma urealyticum*[35] also is inactivated by spermicides. Reports on the effect of spermicides on *Chlamydia trachomatis* are conflicting: three[36–38] found that nonoxynol-9 inactivated chlamydial organisms, while a fourth[39] found no such effect.

**Table 92-2. Efficacy of Contraceptive Barrier Use in Preventing Sexually Transmitted Diseases in Women**

| Study | Study design | Study site | Barrier | Outcome | Measure of effect | 95% confidence interval |
|---|---|---|---|---|---|---|
| Berger et al., 1975[24] | Cross-sectional | Family planning clinic, Louisiana | Condom/ diaphragm, foam | Cervical gonorrhea | 0.53 | 0.18–1.59 |
| Kelaghan et al., 1982[16] | Case-control | 16 hospitals, United States | Diaphragm | Pelvic inflammatory disease | 0.4 | 0.2 –0.7 |
| Austin et al., 1984[17] | Case-control | STD clinic, Alabama | Diaphragm | Cervical gonorrhea | 0.45 | 0.12–1.67 |
| Quinn and O'Reilly, 1985[25] | Cross-sectional | STD clinic, Tennessee | Condom/ diaphragm | Cervical gonorrhea | 0.11 | 0.08–0.17 |
| Cramer et al., 1987[21] | Case-control | Infertility centers, United States | Diaphragm | Tubal infertility | 0.5 | 0.3 –0.7 |

SOURCE: Updated from Stone et al., 1986.[11]

**Table 92-3. Efficacy of Spermicides in Preventing Sexually Transmitted Diseases in Women**

| Study | Study design | Study site | Spermicide | Outcome measure | Measure of effect | 95% confidence interval |
|---|---|---|---|---|---|---|
| Cutler et al., 1979[40] | Randomized clinical trial | STD clinic, Pennsylvania | Nonoxynol-9 | Cervical gonorrhea | 0.11 | 0.02–0.55 |
| Rendon et al., 1980[41] | Randomized clinical trial | Outpatient clinic, Mexico | Phenylmercuric acetate | Cervical gonorrhea | 0.30 | 0.08–1.14 |
| | | | Nonoxynol-9 | Cervical gonorrhea | 0.60 | 0.21–1.73 |
| Cole et al., 1980[42] | Community trial | STD clinic, Florida | Phenylmercuric acetate | Cervical gonorrhea | 0.51 | 0.32–0.80 |
| Jick et al., 1982[43] | Case-control | Health maintenance organization, Seattle | Octoxynol or nonoxynol-9 | Cervical gonorrhea | 0.13 | 0.04–0.40 |
| Kelaghan et al., 1982[16] | Case-control | 16 hospitals, United States | Not specified | Pelvic inflammatory disease | 0.7 | 0.4 –1.4 |
| Austin et al., 1984[17] | Case-control | STD clinic, Alabama | Not specified | Cervical gonorrhea | 0.90 | 0.47–1.73 |
| Quinn and O'Reilly 1985[25] | Cross-sectional | STD clinic, Tennessee | Not specified | Cervical gonorrhea | 0.39 | 0.31–0.50 |
| Cramer et al., 1987[21] | Case-control | Infertility centers, United States | Not specified | Tubal infertility | 1.0 | 0.6 –1.8 |
| Rosenberg et al., 1987[45] | Randomized clinical trial | Prostitutes, Bangkok | Nonoxynol-9 in sponge | Cervical gonorrhea | 0.31 | 0.16–0.60 |
| | | | | Cervical *C. trachomatis* infection | 0.67 | 0.42–1.07 |
| Louv et al., 1988[44] | Randomized clinical trial | STD Clinic, Alabama | Nonoxynol-9 | Cervical gonorrhea | 0.76 | 0.59–0.98* |
| | | | | Cervical *C. trachomatis* infection | 0.78 | 0.64–0.96* |

*90% confidence interval.
SOURCE: Updated from Stone et al., 1986.[11]

Clinical studies provide further support for a protective effect of spermicides (Table 92-3). Two large randomized trials,[40,41] albeit with methodologic flaws, found a powerful protective effect against cervical gonorrhea. One community-based trial[42] also noted significant protection against this infection. In two large case-control studies, protection was found against cervical gonorrhea[43] and PID,[16] although the latter was not statistically significant. In an STD clinic population, another group of investigators[17] observed a small reduction in the risk of cervical gonorrhea, while in another STD clinic,[25] significant protection against this infection was noted. In a large, multicenter case-control study of tubal infertility,[21] spermicide used alone had no impact on this outcome. When combined with a mechanical barrier, a powerful protective effect resulted (50 percent reduction).

Finally, two recent investigations support the clinical efficacy of spermicides in protecting against STDs. In Alabama, regular use of nonoxynol-9 by women attending an STD clinic reduced cervical gonorrhea by 24 percent and cervical chlamydial infections by 22 percent.[44] Likewise, in Thailand, use of the contraceptive sponge impregnated with spermicide by women at high risk of STDs showed strong protection against cervical gonorrhea and less protection against infection with *Chlamydia trachomatis*. On the other hand, vaginal infection with *Candida albicans* was more likely in sponge users, although this difference was not significantly different.[45]

These research findings, however, may not be directly applicable to public health practice. Under well-financed, carefully controlled situations, the efficacy of methods for primary prevention of infection or pregnancy represents a best case scenario.[46] However, in less ideal circumstances—where knowledge, sustained behavior change, cost of method, availability of method, etc., provide practical hurdles—these methods are less effective. For example, in preventing pregnancy, the "lowest expected" failure rate for condoms is 3 percent, the "lowest reported" rate is 4 percent and the "typical" rate is 10 percent.[46] For spermicides, the equivalent estimates are 3, 0, and 21 percent, respectively.

## INTRAUTERINE DEVICES

The potential link between IUD use and the development of PID is one of the most important and controversial topics in contemporary contraception. As of mid-1980, 16 studies[47] had all found an increased risk of PID among IUD users, with the increase ranging from two- to ninefold. The consistency of these findings strongly suggested a causal association.

Growing evidence suggests that the association between IUD use and PID has been overestimated. Several persistent methodologic flaws in early studies of the IUD and PID contributed to this overly pessimistic assessment. First, women using barrier or oral contraceptives served as the comparison group in many studies. As noted previously, since these methods reduce the risk of PID, such comparisons artifactually elevate the apparent risk associated with IUD use.

Second, PID is notoriously difficult to diagnose, and the diagnosis often rests on highly subjective symptoms and signs that are difficult to assess. Since the putative association between IUD use and PID has been known to physicians since at least the 1960s, this knowledge made overdiagnosis of PID in IUD users highly likely. An IUD user with a cluster of signs and symptoms would be more likely to be diagnosed as having PID then would a woman with similar complaints but without an IUD. This relative overdiagnosis of PID among IUD users would also inflate the risk estimate.

Since mid-1980, a number of large, more sophisticated studies[48–55] have revised our understanding of the IUD-PID association (Table 92-4). By adjusting the comparison groups to

Table 92-4. Summary of Recent Studies Concerning Intrauterine Devices and Pelvic Inflammatory Disease

| Authors | Location | No. of cases | Relative risk | 95% confidence interval | Comment |
|---|---|---|---|---|---|
| Paavonen and Vesterinen[48] | Helsinki, Finland | 144 | 2.1 | 1.2– 3.5 | Standardized for effect of parity. Referent group: women not using IUDs or OCs |
| Burkman et al.[49] | 16 U.S. hospitals | 1447 | 1.6 | 1.2– 2.0 | Adjusted for the effect of age, race, parity, no. of partners, frequency of coitus. Referent group: women not using contraception |
| Kaufman et al.[50] | U.S. and Canadian hospitals | 155 | 8.6 | 5.3–13.8 | Standardized for effect of age. Referent group: women using contraception but never an IUD |
| Lee et al.[51] | 16 U.S. hospitals | 657 | 1.9 | 1.5– 2.4 | Adjusted for effect of education. Referent group: women not using contraception |
| Witoonpanich et al.[52] | 12 centers worldwide | 608 | 11.5 | 3.6–36.2 | Nulliparous women in developed country; Referent group: women not using contraception, no prior IUD use |
| | | | 4.1 | 1.2–15.1 | Parous women in developed country |
| | | | 2.3 | 1.4– 3.9 | Parous women in developing country |
| Westrom[53] | Lund, Sweden | 571 | 1.5 | 1.2– 1.9 | Referent group: sexually active women not using contraception |
| Vessey et al.[54] | 17 clinics, England and Scotland | 42 | 10.5 | 5.4–32 | Standardized for effect of age. Referent group: women using contraception other than IUD |

SOURCE: Ref. 55.

include women using no method of contraception,[49,51,53] the risk of PID associated with IUD use dropped below 2.0. In contrast, in those studies where the comparison groups included women using methods which protected against PID,[48,50,52,54] the risks were much higher.

Current evidence suggests that the increased risk of PID associated with IUD use centers around the time of insertion. In other words, contamination of the endometrial cavity at insertion appears responsible for IUD-related PID, and not the device itself. Although numerous studies[55] have noted an inverse relationship between risk of PID and duration of IUD use, the NIH-CDC study[51] has provided the most explicit estimate. When Dalkon shield users were excluded, the relative risk associated with other IUDs was highest in the first month after insertion (3.8), lower in months 2 to 4 (1.7), and not significantly elevated above baseline (1.1) at 5 months and beyond. A randomized clinical trial[56] of prophylactic administration of doxycycline at the time of IUD insertion has found benefit from prophylaxis, which lends further support to the concept that bacterial contamination of the endometrium at insertion incites most cases of IUD-related PID.

Are some IUDs associated with a higher risk of PID than others? Because of the infrequency of IUD-related PID and because of the limited size of most studies, data are insufficient to distinguish statistically between IUDs, with one exception.[55] The NIH-CDC study[51] found the risk of PID with the Dalkon shield to be five times that of other devices. In addition, the risk of PID associated with the Dalkon shield remained elevated beyond 4 months of use, which may be related to the design of its multifilament string.

Does use of an IUD lead to an increased risk of primary tubal infertility? Two case-control studies (Table 92–5) suggest yes, but with qualifications. In a multicenter study conducted in Boston,[57] women who had used IUDs in the past had a twofold increased risk. In a companion study from Seattle,[58] the relative risk was 2.6. Of note, however, is the finding that among women who had used copper IUDs and who had had only one sexual partner, there was no increase in the risk of tubal infertility.

Thus, a large number of studies have indicated an increased risk of PID among IUD users. In studies[53,57,58] with objective outcome measures (e.g., laparoscopy or hysterosalpingogram), the relative risk is much lower (1.5 to 2.6) than previous estimates. Even these revised estimates may be exaggerated because of the influence of selection bias and confounding.

## ORAL CONTRACEPTIVES

Oral contraceptives (OCs) have an array of noncontraceptive health benefits, and protection against PID is one of this method's most important health benefits. Studies from Europe and the United States[53,59,60] have revealed about a 50 percent reduction in the risk of being hospitalized for PID as compared with women

Table 92–5. Summary of Recent Studies Concerning Intrauterine Devices and Tubal Infertility

| Authors | Location | No. of cases | Relative risk | 95% confidence interval | Comment |
|---|---|---|---|---|---|
| Cramer et al.[57] | 7 U.S. and Canadian centers | 283 | 2.0 | 1.5–2.6 | Primary tubal infertility as outcome, adjusted or matched for multiple factors. Referent group: women not using contraception |
| Daling et al.[58] | King County, Washington | 159 | 2.6 | 1.3–5.2 | Primary tubal infertility as outcome, adjusted or matched for multiple factors. Referent group: women with no prior IUD use |

SOURCE: Ref. 55.

who are sexually active but who do not use contraception. In a large, multicenter case-control study from the United States,[61] the protection was observed only among women who had been using oral contraceptives for more than 12 months. In this group, there was a 70 percent reduction, a highly significant finding. Past use of pills conferred no protection.

The mechanism for the protective effect remains speculative. The progestin component of combination OCs makes the cervical mucus thick and relatively impenetrable to sperm. If PID stems from pathogens carried passively to the upper genital tract by sperm,[62] then changes in cervical mucus composition or immunologic properties might account for this protection. An alternative explanation relates to the decreased menstrual blood loss associated with pill use. About 90 percent of women with patent fallopian tubes experience retrograde menstruation; this flow of potentially contaminated material into the tubes may initiate PID. In pill users, the inoculum introduced into the tubes may be smaller because of reduced menstrual blood loss. Regardless of the mechanism, the protective effect appears to be real and clinically important.

Use of OCs also seems to modify the course of PID favorably. As judged by laparoscopic examination, women with PID who were using OCs had milder inflammation than did women not using OCs.[63] Among women with chlamydial salpingitis, use of OCs was protective against Fitz-Hugh-Curtis syndrome. In addition, pill users had a significantly lower titer of antibodies agains *C. trachomatis* than did nonusers.[64] While the mechanism(s) remains unknown, there is some evidence that sex steroids modify immunologic function.

All the news about OCs and STDs has not been favorable, however. A review published in 1985[65] startled the medical community by noting that the majority of studies found an increased risk of cervical infection with *C. trachomatis* among users of OCs as compared with nonusers. Other recent studies[66,67] have not confirmed an increased risk of chlamydial cervicitis among OC users. If there is an association between OC use and cervical infection with *C. trachomatis*, it may be mediated through the cervical ectropion commonly induced by OCs. In one study,[68] *C. trachomatis* was isolated more frequently among women with ectropion than among women without ectropion, regardless of the method of birth control used.

Could an increased risk of chlamydial cervicitis translate into an increased risk of chlamydial PID and subsequent infertility? Thus far, limited data have not confirmed this fear. In a large population-based study with meticulous evaluation,[69] OC use was associated with a significant reduction in the risk of chlamydial PID, although the protective effect was not as strong as that for gonorrheal PID. As noted before, OC users tend to have milder infection with *C. trachomatis*, as manifested by antibody response. Moreover, primary tubal infertility is not increased among former users of OCs, as might be expected if their use led to an increased risk of either overt or silent chlamydial PID.[21]

## TUBAL STERILIZATION

Tubal sterilization protects against PID, but this protection is not complete. Most cases of PID are thought to arise from ascent of pathogens from the cervix via the endometrial cavity; hence, disrupting the continuity of this passage should prevent inoculation of the fallopian tubes. Since the classic study of Falk,[70] other authors[71,72] have noted the scarcity of PID seen among women after tubal sterilization. This protection is not absolute, however. Small numbers of cases of PID[73] and tubo-ovarian abscess[74] continue to be reported. In some cases involving group A beta-hemolytic streptococci, ascent to the tubes may occur through the parametrial tissue.[75]

## ABORTION

Women who have cervical infection with either *N. gonorrhoeae* or *C. trachomatis* have an increased risk of endometritis after induced abortion. The risk appears to be at least tripled with either organism.[76–78] A number of studies suggest that use of prophylactic antibiotics around the time of abortion reduces the risk of infection by one-half to two-thirds.[79–81] In settings where preoperative screening for infection with these organisms is not feasible, a brief perioperative course of an antibiotic such as doxycycline seems both safe and cost-effective.[79]

## OVERLAPPING NEEDS FOR SERVICES

In many health departments, family planning and STD clinical services are organizationally separated (Chap. 87). Largely because of the categorical nature of their funding, most publicly supported family planning and STD clinics function as independent entities rather than one coordinated reproductive health unit. In contrast, the women being served by these clinics frequently have health needs which overlap. For example, in family planning clinics, recent risk assessment surveys have found approximately one-quarter of women report behaviors which put them at increased risk for HIV and the other STDs.[82] In STD clinics, upward of half of reproductive-age, sexually active women report using no method of contraception,[83] despite most having histories of both STDs and unintended pregnancies.

These overlapping needs provide each field with a unique opportunity to deliver more broad-based reproductive health care.[84,85] In part, this collaboration was initiated in the early 1970s, when family planning clinics became crucial allies for the federal gonorrhea control program.[85,86] By 1982, half of all women receiving family planning services were simultaneously screened for STDs, primarily gonorrhea; this screening appropriately targeted those women who had the highest STD risks.[87] Moreover, efforts to screen for chlamydia in family planning settings have also been productive, especially when selective criteria are applied—e.g., age younger than 24, more than one sexual partner in the past 2 months, or signs of cervical infection.[67,88] In Seattle,[67] women with one or more risk factors who attended a family planning clinic were three times more likely to have chlamydial infections than those without risk factors. As a result, regional chlamydia control programs delivered in family planning settings have been established using resources for both categorical family planning and STD programs.

Likewise, STD clinics increasingly have been willing to provide rudimentary contraceptive services. As emphasized earlier, the condom has been a mainstay of STD primary prevention. Even before recent concerns with incurable viral STDs, increasing the use of condoms was a major STD 1990 Objective for the Nation, as formulated by the U.S. Public Health Service.[89] The Surgeon General's report on AIDS increased attention on the condom and provided necessary impetus to overcome the moratorium on advertising condoms in the media. Unfortunately, even though the gay community has apparently increased the use of condoms,[90,91] the core heterosexual STD population still has not widely adopted their use. For example, in one DeKalb County (Georgia) STD clinic, only 12 percent of patients counseled to use condoms to prevent recurrent STD reportedly complied with this recommendation.[92] However, as emphasized above, use of other mechanical and chemical contraceptives may also be of value in reducing risks of STDs. Diaphragms and spermicides may play a wider role in upcoming efforts to prevent STDs.

## FUTURE DIRECTIONS

What are future directions for family planning and STD fields? The specter of HIV infection and AIDS will undoubtedly dominate our public health considerations. Evidence suggests that more women of childbearing age will become infected with HIV through heterosexual transmission of the virus.[93] Indeed, the prevalence of HIV antibodies in women of reproductive age may be higher than many would suspect. In Brooklyn, New York, 2.5 percent in a study of 527 postpartum women at a municipal hospital were positive for HIV antibody.[94] In Boston, the rate of seropositivity at birth among inner city hospitals was 1.5 percent.[95] In Jacksonville, Florida, nearly 1 percent of consecutive prenatal patients were HIV seropositive.[96]

These concerns have led to increased interest among family planning specialists to begin a program of AIDS prevention in family planning clinics. CDC has recommended that all family planning clinics should offer at least AIDS education, counseling on HIV risks, and infection control and patient referral services. Other HIV-prevention services such as risk assessment, counseling about HIV-antibody testing, and actually administering the tests themselves could also be provided.[97] As resources increase to allow for additional AIDS prevention activities in family planning settings, spinoff educational efforts directed to the other STDs would also be indicated. Clearly family planning and STD will overlap even more in the future.

## CONTRACEPTIVE STRATEGIES TODAY

"Safe sex" today has at least two meanings: protection against unwanted pregnancy and protection against STD. For single persons, abstinence from sexual activity protects against both outcomes. For couples, assumed to be sexually active, contraception is fundamentally important for both.

For couples whose families are not completed, OCs remain the most popular and effective method of reversible contraception in the United States. While OCs confer protection against PID, they may increase the risk of chlamydial cervicitis. Hence, for couples that are not mutually monogamous, addition of a barrier method, such as a condom, will help reduce the risk of STD as well as unplanned pregnancy.

Barrier methods are substantially less effective in preventing conception than are OCs, yet they offer important protection against STDs. To maximize protection against both unwanted pregnancy and STD, a barrier method should be used in conjunction with a spermicide. Until more data are available, use of "natural" membrane condoms should be considered potentially less effective in blocking disease transmission than use of latex condoms.

For couples whose families are complete, male or female sterilization is the most popular method of contraception in the United States. While these operations protect against upper genital tract infections in sterilized persons of both sexes, they confer no protection against lower genital tract infections. An alternative to sterilization is the IUD, an excellent method for selected women. Epidemiologic data suggest that white women older then 25 years who have only one sexual partner and who have coitus less than five times per week can be expected to have very little risk of PID. That risk may be reduced further by a single oral dose of doxycycline at the time of IUD insertion, although this observation awaits corroboration. For couples not mutually monogamous, a barrier method plus spermicide should be recommended.

Because both barrier and chemical prophylaxis are coitally dependent, their efficacy in preventing either infection or unplanned pregnancy relies to a greater extent on human initiative than do coitally independent methods. Behavioral changes—among them increased condom use—by gay men in response to AIDS prevention recommendations have been associated with decreases in other STD, including rectal gonorrhea and syphilis.[98,99] Unfortunately, to date, despite the publicity, core heterosexual STD populations have not reported the same magnitude of condom use and have not experienced decreases in the traditional STD.

## CONCLUSION

The marriage of the disciplines of family planning and STD is destined to be a fruitful one. "Strange bedfellows"[1] no longer, these related fields are growing increasingly intertwined in research and in clinical practice. Already, the needs for sex education, family planning services, and STD prevention and treatment overlap substantially. In the years ahead, health care workers who are knowledgeable and skilled in these disciplines will give broader meaning to the term "reproductive health."

# References


1 Cates W Jr.: Sexually transmitted diseases and family planning. Strange or natural bedfellows? *J Reprod Med* 29:317, 1984.

2 Smith L et al: Efficacy of condoms as barriers to HSV-2 and gonorrhea: An in vitro model, in *Program and Abstracts of the First Sexually Transmitted Diseases World Congress*. San Juan, Puerto Rico. Latin American Union Against Venereal Diseases, 1981.

3 Judson FN et al: In vitro tests demonstrate condoms provide an effective barrier against *Chlamydia trachomatis* and herpes simplex virus, in *Program and Abstracts of the Fifth International Meeting of the International Society for Sexually Transmitted Diseases Research*. Seattle, International Society for Sexually Transmitted Diseases, 1983.

4 Conant MA et al: Herpes simplex virus transmission: Condom studies. *Sex Transm Dis* 11:94, 1984.

5 Katznelson S et al: Efficacy of the condom as a barrier to the transmission of cytomegalovirus. *J Infect Dis* 150:155, 1984.

6 Conant M et al: Condoms prevent transmission of AIDS-associated retrovirus. *JAMA* 255:1706, 1986.

7 Minuk GY et al: Condoms and hepatitis B virus infection. *Ann Intern Med* 104:584, 1986.

8 Minuk GY et al: Condoms and prevention of AIDS. *JAMA* 256:1443, 1986.

9 Goldsmith M: Sex in the age of AIDS calls for common sense and "condom sense." *JAMA* 257:2261, 1987.

10 Van de Perre P et al: The latex condom, an efficient barrier against sexual transmission of AIDS-related viruses. *AIDS* 1:49, 1987.

11 Stone KM et al: Personal protection against sexually transmitted diseases. *Am J Obstet Gynecol* 155:180, 1986.

12 Pemberton J et al: Socio-medical characteristics of patients attending

a VD clinic and the circumstances of infection. *Br J Vener Dis* 48:391, 1972.

13 Barlow D: The condom and gonorrhoeae. *Lancet* 2:811, 1977.

14 McCormack WM et al: Sexual experience and urethral colonization with genital mycoplasmas: A study in normal men. *Ann Intern Med* 78:696, 1973.

15 Hart G: Factors influencing venereal infection in a war environment. *Br J Vener Dis* 50:68, 1974.

16 Kelaghan J et al: Barrier-method contraceptives and pelvic inflammatory disease. *JAMA* 248:184, 1982.

17 Austin H et al: A case-control study of spermicides and gonorrhea. *JAMA* 251:2822, 1984.

18 Syrjanen K et al: Sexual behavior of women with human papillomavirus (HPV) lesions of the uterine cervix. *Br J Vener Dis* 60:243, 1984.

19 Darrow WW: Innovative health behavior (Dissertation). Atlanta, GA, Emory University, 1973.

20 Hooper RR et al: Cohort study of venereal disease. I. The risk of gonorrhea transmission from infected women to men. *Am J Epidemiol* 108:136, 1978.

21 Cramer DW et al: The relationship of tubal infertility to barrier method and oral contraceptive use. *JAMA* 257:2446, 1987.

22 Fischl MA et al: Evaluation of heterosexual partners, children, and household contacts of adults with AIDS. *JAMA* 257:640, 1987.

23 Mann J et al: Condom use and HIV infection among prostitutes in Zaire. *N Engl J Med* 316:345, 1987.

24 Berger GS et al: Prevalence of gonorrhea among women using various methods of contraception. *Br J Vener Dis* 51:307, 1975.

25 Quinn RW, O'Reilly KR: Contraceptive practices of women attending the sexually transmitted disease clinic in Nashville, Tennessee. *Sex Transm Dis* 12:99, 1985.

26 Kesseler II: Human cervical cancer as a venereal disease. *Cancer Res* 36:783, 1976.

27 Harris RWC et al: Characteristics of women with dysplasia or carcinoma in situ of the cervix uteri. *Br J Cancer* 42:359, 1980.

28 Wright NH et al: Neoplasia and dysplasia of the cervix uteri and contraception: A possible protective effect of the diaphragm. *Br J Cancer* 38:273, 1978.

29 Singh B et al: Studies on the development of a vaginal preparation providing both prophylaxis against venereal disease and other genital infections and contraception. *Br J Vener Dis* 48:57, 1972.

30 Bolch OH Jr, Warren JC: In vitro effects of Emko on *Neisseria gonorrhoeae* and *Trichomonas vaginalis*. *Am J Obstet Gynecol* 115:1145, 1973.

31 Cowan ME, Cree GE: A note on the susceptibility of *N. gonorrhoeae* to contraceptive agent Nonyl-P. *Br J Vener Dis* 49:65, 1973.

32 Singh B et al: Virucidal effect of certain chemical contraceptives on type 2 herpesvirus. *Am J Obstet Gynecol* 126:422, 1976.

33 Asculai SS et al: Inactivation of herpes simplex viruses by nonionic surfactants. *Antimicrob Agents Chemother* 13:686, 1978.

34 Hicks DR et al: Inactivation of HTLV-III/LAV-infected cultures of normal human lymphocytes in vitro. *Lancet* 2:1422, 1985.

35 Amortegui AJ et al: The effect of chemical intravaginal contraceptives and betadine on *Ureaplasma urealyticum*. *Contraception* 30:135, 1984.

36 Benes S, McCormack WM: Inhibition of growth of *Chlamydia trachomatis* by nonoxynol-9 in vitro. *Antimicrob Agents Chemother* 27:724, 1985.

37 Kelly JP et al: In vitro activity of the spermicide nonoxynol-9 against *Chlamydia trachomatis*. *Antimicrob Agents Chemother* 27:760, 1985.

38 Amortegui AJ, Myer MP: The in vitro effect of chemical intravaginal contraceptives on *Chlamydia trachomatis*. *Contraception* 36:481, 1987.

39 Kappus EW, Quinn TC: The spermicide nonoxynol-9 does not inhibit *Chlamydia trachomatis* in vitro. *Sex Transm Dis* 13:134, 1986.

40 Cutler JC et al: Vaginal contraceptives as prophylaxis against gonorrhea and other sexually transmissible diseases. *Adv Planned Parent* 12:45, 1977.

41 Rendon AL et al: A controlled, comparative study of phenylmercuric acetate, nonoxynol-9 and placebo vaginal suppositories as prophylactic agents against gonorrhea. *Curr Ther Res* 27:780, 1980.

42 Cole CH et al: Vaginal chemoprophylaxis in the reduction of reinfection of women with gonorrhoeae. *Br J Vener Dis* 56:314, 1980.

43 Jick H et al: Vaginal spermicides and gonorrhea. *JAMA* 248:1619, 1982.

44 Louv WC et al: A clinical trial of nonoxynol-9 as a prophylaxis for cervical *Neisseria gonorrhoeae* and *Chlamydia trachomatis* infections. *J Infect Dis* 158:518, 1988.

45 Rosenberg MJ et al: Effect of the contraceptive sponge on chlamydial infection, gonorrhea, and candidiasis. A comparative clinical trial. *JAMA* 257:2308, 1987.

46 Trussell J, Kost K: Contraceptive failure in the United States: A critical review of the literature. *Stud Fam Plann* 18:237, 1987.

47 Senanayake P, Kramer DG: Contraception and the etiology of pelvic inflammatory disease: New perspectives. *Am J Obstet Gynecol* 138:852, 1980.

48 Paavonen J, Vesterinen E: Intrauterine contraceptive device use in patients with acute salpingitis. *Contraception* 22:107, 1980.

49 Burkman RT, Women's Health Study: Association between intrauterine device and pelvic inflammatory disease. *Obstet Gynecol* 57:269, 1981.

50 Kaufman DW et al: The effect of different types of intrauterine devices on the risk of pelvic inflammatory disease. *JAMA* 250:759, 1983.

51 Lee NC et al: Type of intrauterine device and the risk of pelvic inflammatory disease. *Obstet Gynecol* 62:1, 1983.

52 Witoonpanich P et al: PID associated with fertility regulating agents. *Contraception* 30:1, 1984.

53 Westrom L: Incidence, prevalence, and trends of acute pelvic inflammatory disease and its consequences in industrialized countries. *Am J Obstet Gynecol* 138:880, 1980.

54 Vessey MP et al: Pelvic inflammatory disease and the intrauterine device: Findings in a large cohort study. *Br Med J* 282:855, 1981.

55 Grimes DA: Intrauterine devices and pelvic inflammatory disease: Recent developments. *Contraception* 36:97, 1987.

56 Sinei SKA et al: Preventing IUD-related pelvic infection: The efficacy of prophylactic doxycycline at insertion (submitted for publication).

57 Cramer DW et al: Tubal infertility and the intrauterine device. *N Engl J Med* 312:937, 1985.

58 Daling JR et al: Primary tubal infertility in relation to the use of an intrauterine device. *N Engl J Med* 312:937, 1985.

59 Eschenbach DA et al: Pathogenesis of acute pelvic inflammatory disease: Role of contraception and other risk factors. *Am J Obstet Gynecol* 128:838, 1977.

60 Royal College of General Practitioners Oral Contraception Study: *Oral Contraceptives and Health*. New York, Pitman, 1974.

61 Rubin GL et al: Oral contraceptives and pelvic inflammatory disease. *Am J Obstet Gynecol* 144:630, 1982.

62 Friberg J et al: *Chlamydia trachomatis* attached to spermatozoa recovered from the peritoneal cavity of patients with salpingitis. *J Reprod Med* 32:120, 1987.

63 Svensson L et al: Contraceptives and acute salpingitis. *JAMA* 251:2553, 1984.

64 Wølner-Hanssen P: Oral contraceptive use modifies the manifestations of pelvic inflammatory disease. *Br J Obstet Gynaecol* 93:619, 1986.

65 Washington AE et al: Oral contraceptives, *Chlamydia trachomatis* infection, and pelvic inflammatory disease. *JAMA* 253:2246, 1985.

66 McCormack WM et al: Infection with *Chlamydia trachomatis* in female college students. *Am J Epidemiol* 121:107, 1985.

67 Handsfield HH et al: Criteria for selective screening for *Chlamydia trachomatis* infection in women attending family planning clinics. *JAMA* 255:1730, 1986.

68 Harrison HR et al: Cervical *Chlamydia trachomatis* infection in university women: Relationship to history, contraception, ectopy, and cervicitis. *Am J Obstet Gynecol* 153:244, 1985.

69 Wølner-Hanssen et al: Laparoscopic findings and contraceptive use

in women with signs and symptoms suggestive of acute salpingitis. *Obstet Gynecol* 66:233, 1985.

70 Falk HC: Interpretation of the pathogenesis of pelvic infection as determined by cornual resection. *Am J Obstet Gynecol* 52:66, 1946.

71 Hajj SN: Does sterilization prevent pelvic infection? *J Reprod Med* 20:289, 1978.

72 Vessey M et al: Tubal sterilization: Findings in a large prospective study. *Br J Obstet Gynaecol* 90:203, 1983.

73 Vermesh M et al: Acute salpingitis in sterilized women. *Obstet Gynecol* 69:265, 1987.

74 Edelman DA, Berger GS: Contraceptive practice and tuboovarian abscess. *Am J Obstet Gynecol* 138:541, 1980.

75 Grimes DA: Nongonococcal pelvic inflammatory disease. *Clin Obstet Gynecol* 24:1227, 1981.

76 Burkman RT et al: Untreated endocervical gonorrhea and endometritis following elective abortion. *Am J Obstet Gynecol* 126:648, 1976.

77 Osser S, Persson K: Postabortal pelvic infection associated with *Chlamydia trachomatis* and the influence of humoral immunity. *Am J Obstet Gynecol* 150:699, 1984.

78 Westergaard L et al: Significance of cervical *Chlamydia trachomatis* infection in postabortal pelvic inflammatory disease. *Obstet Gynecol* 60:322, 1982.

79 Grimes DA et al: Prophylactic antibiotics for curettage abortions. *Am J Obstet Gynecol* 150:689, 1984.

80 Park TK et al: Preventing febrile complications of suction curettage abortion. *Am J Obstet Gynecol* 152:252, 1985.

81 Darj E et al: The prophylactic effect of doxycycline on postoperative infection rate after first-trimester abortion. *Obstet Gynecol* 70:755, 1987.

82 Donovan P: AIDS in family planning clinics: Confronting the crisis. *Fam Plann Perspect* 19:111, 1987.

83 Upchurch DM et al: Contraceptive needs and practices among women attending an inner city STD clinic. *Am J Public Health* 77:1427, 1987.

84 Bureau of Community Health Services: *Guidelines for Health Promotion and Disease Prevention Services in Reproductive Health Care Settings*. Washington, DC, Rockville, Maryland, 1981.

85 Cates W Jr: Epidemiology and control of sexually transmitted diseases: Strategic evolution. *Infect Dis Clin North Am* 1:1, 1987.

86 Brown ST, Wiesner PJ: Problems and approaches to the control and surveillance of sexually transmitted agents associated with pelvic inflammatory disease in the United States. *Am J Obstet Gynecol* 138:1096, 1980.

87 Aral SO et al: Screening for sexually transmitted diseases by family planning providers: Is it adequate and appropriate? *Fam Plann Perspect* 18:255, 1986.

88 Schachter J et al: Screening for chlamydial infections in women attending family planning clinics. *West J Med* 138:375, 1983.

89 Public Health Service: *Promoting Health/Preventing Diseases: Objective for the Nation*. Washington, DC: US Department of Health and Human Services, 1980.

90 McKusick L et al: Reported changes in the sexual behavior of men at risk for AIDS, San Francisco, 1982–1984—The AIDS behavioral research projects. *Public Health Rep* 100:622, 1985.

91 Martin JL: The impact of AIDS on gay males sexual behavior patterns in New York City. *Am J Public Health* 77:578, 1987.

92 Whittington WL et al: Condom practices in STD patients with recurrent infections. Personal communication, September 1, 1987.

93 Guinan ME, Hardy A: Epidemiology of AIDS in women in the United States: 1981–1986. *JAMA* 257:2039, 1987.

94 Landesman S et al: Sero-survey of human immunodeficiency virus infection in parturients: Implications for human immunodeficiency virus testing programs of pregnant women. *JAMA* 255:2701, 1987.

95 Grady GF et al: HIV seropositivity in newborns: A novel method for estimating the prevalence of infection in childbearing women. Presented at the III International Conference on AIDS, Washington, DC, June 4, 1987. Abstract ThP.175.

96 Kaunitz AM et al: Prenatal care and HIV screening. *JAMA* 258:2693, 1987.

97 Centers for Disease Control: Public Health Service guidelines for counseling and antibody testing to prevent HIV infection and AIDS. *MMWR* 36:509, 1987.

98 Judson FN: Fear of AIDS and gonorrhea rates in homosexual men. *Lancet* ii:159, 1983.

99 Handsfield HH: Decreasing incidence of gonorrhea in homosexually active men—Minimal effect on risk of AIDS. *West J Med* 143:469, 1985.

# Chapter 93

# The primary care physician and sexually transmitted diseases control

Alfred O. Berg

Diagnostic and management strategies and physician responsibilities appropriate for sexually transmitted diseases (STDs) in specialized centers often require modification for primary care practice. Data concerning STDs as encountered in noninstitutional primary care practice in the United States are few; this chapter highlights many issues in urgent need of more research. The complementary responsibilities of primary care and specialist physicians are emphasized as they interact around issues of STD management in a community.

## DEFINING PRIMARY CARE

Primary care is first-contact care, comprehensive in scope, continuous in duration, and offering the generalist rather than the specialist perspective. Most primary care in the United States is provided in ambulatory settings in solo and small group fee-for-service practices.[1] However, economic pressures are remodeling the practice of primary care medicine, with more service delivered in larger group practices, managed health care systems (HMOs, IPAs, PPOs, and other capitated plans), and hospital-owned outpatient departments. Each setting has unique implications for the recognition and management of sexually transmitted diseases.

Family physicians and general practitioners provide 37 percent of all office-based ambulatory care in the noninstitutionalized civilian population in the United States. Internal medicine accounts for approximately 12 percent of ambulatory care overall, general pediatrics 10 percent, and obstetrics and gynecology 9 percent.[2] Many ambulatory visits to internists and obstetrician-gynecologists, and some visits to pediatricians are for specialized (secondary or tertiary care) services, while nearly all the care provided by general and family practitioners is primary care. In fact, the exact proportions of ambulatory care provided within each specialty that is primary care, and the contribution that each specialty makes to the total of all primary care are not known.

## EPIDEMIOLOGY OF STDS IN PRIMARY CARE

The incidence of sexually transmitted diseases in the United States can only be crudely estimated from the available data. Most reported cases are generated from publicly operated specialized clinics in major cities, but data from Seattle have suggested that the majority of cases are seen in private ambulatory practice.[3] Moreover limited survey data imply that many more patients are seen than reported by private physicians in the primary care medical specialties.[4,5] In comparing survey responses and direct chart reviews from primary care practices, however, one study suggested that respondents tend to overstate the number of cases actually seen.[6] Underdiagnosis and undertreatment, rather than underreporting, by primary care physicians are thought to minimize overall estimates of incidence, in addition to causing unnecessary morbidity and contributing to the spread of infection.[7]

The presentation, diagnosis, management, and outcome of sexually transmitted diseases vary by individual patient characteristics (see Chaps. 46–62). The same characteristics influence patients' choices of physicians. It is therefore not surprising that primary care practices and STD clinics experience differences in the incidence, presentation, and follow-up of patients with STDs. As discussed in Chap. 2, patients with STDs are more likely to be adolescents, racial minorities, homosexual men, singles of both sexes, and the poor, all groups underrepresented in typical primary care practices.

Sexually transmitted diseases, exluding vaginitis, accounted for only 0.7 percent of all ambulatory visits, in data from the 1980–1981 National Ambulatory Medical Care Survey (NAMCS). This overall percentage differed among primary care specialties: obstetrics and gynecology 1.8 percent, general and family physicians 0.6 percent, general internal medicine 0.2 percent. Although the age range of children seen by some general pediatricians is expanding into the third decade of life, the diagnosis and management of STDs remains an exceedingly small proportion of the general pediatrician's practice (0.1 percent).[8]

Few studies have attempted to establish the prevalence of specific STDs in typical primary care practices. Excluding vaginitis, all sexually transmitted diseases combined accounted for only 1 percent of over 100,000 patient encounters in a group of primary care practices in the Pacific Northwest serving approximately 30,000 patients, distributed as follows: gonorrhea 0.3 percent, chlamydia 0.4 percent, and herpes 0.3 percent.[9] A Seattle study of 204 symptomatic and asymptomatic women screened in a family medicine residency practice found 1 percent with gonorrhea and 4 percent with chlamydia, all in the symptomatic group.[10] For comparison, CDC data from 1984 showed 878,556 reported cases of gonorrhea in the population of 236 million, for an incidence of approximately 0.4 percent.[11] Directly comparable data on chlamydia and genital herpes are not available.

In summary, available data regarding the incidence and prevalence of STDs in primary care practice are presumed to be underestimates, but by unknown amounts. By whatever measure, however, sexually transmitted diseases are uncommon in many primary care practices, and rare in some. This low frequency has important implications for case finding, diagnosis, management, and follow-up.

## CASE FINDING AND DIAGNOSIS IN PRIMARY CARE

The fundamental problem with case finding and diagnosis in primary care arises from the low prevalence of STDs in a typical practice. Although studies fully exploring the performance of diagnostic tests for STDs in primary care settings do not exist, even highly accurate diagnostic tests are likely to falter when applied in the low-prevalence populations typical of primary care practice. For example, a screening test with 95 percent sensitivity and 95 percent specificity, when applied to a population with underlying disease prevalence of 1 percent (a not unreasonable average for herpes, gonorrhea, or chlamydia in primary care practice) will yield approximately 60 positives per 1000 individuals screened, 50 of which will be false-positives; and one patient with disease will be missed. Thus although the negative predictive value of such a test would be greater than 99.9 percent, the positive predictive value would be only 20 percent. A case-finding protocol using such a test would be costly, especially with the expense of evaluating each positive test to determine whether it is a false-positive. Further, the psychological costs of inappropriate labeling, however short-lived, of patients with initially but falsely positive tests cannot be discounted.[12]

Understandably, diagnostic tests are first studied in high-prevalence populations typical of a public STD clinic. However, the success of a diagnostic method in the public STD clinic may not guarantee success in ambulatory primary care. Frustration with false positives and false negatives—especially in practices with the lowest prevalences of STDs—leads to lower test use and consequent lower rates of diagnosis, an inevitable spiral with serious implications for overall STD control in a population. Clearly, studies documenting performance of diagnostic tests in primary care practices are needed.

## MANAGEMENT STRATEGIES IN PRIMARY CARE

Antibiotic protocols developed in specialized centers for treating STDs have not had the problem of questionable applicability to primary care practice. No published studies have suggested that treatment failures are more common in primary care practice. If anything, medication regimens developed in the high-prevalence and often medically complicated STD clinic populations may overtreat the same usually uncomplicated condition seen in a suburban primary care practice.

Differences in follow-up strategies between primary and specialty care have not been well studied. Primary care physicians believe that their patients have both less complicated disease and higher rates of compliance with therapeutic regimens (with resulting higher rates of cure), and thus may not be as aggressive in arranging the recommended test-for-cure follow-up of some STDs (e.g., gonorrhea). Whether such beliefs are warranted is unknown.

The development of inexpensive yet effective management strategies is likely to become more important with the proliferation of prepaid managed health care systems. These new financing arrangements provide economic incentives to minimize diagnostic testing, to find the least costly yet effective antibiotic regimens, and to limit unnecessary follow-up visits and testing. Little research to date has focused on cost containment in the detection and treatment of STDs.

## PREVENTIVE STRATEGIES IN PRIMARY CARE

Primary care physicians are uniquely situated to participate in the prevention of sexually transmitted diseases, since they are both the physicians who see patients for periodic examinations and the physicians to whom many individuals turn first when a medical problem arises. Opportunities for prevention are present in each patient encounter, regardless of the stated reason for visit.

The United States Preventive Services Task Force has considered strategies to prevent STDs in primary care.[13] Each general and disease-specific recommendation for STDs was based on the quality of the available evidence before the task force assigned a final graded recommendation (Table 93-1). Several of the recommendations are arguable in degree (e.g., opinion supporting higher recommendation levels on barrier methods of general prevention[14] and on syphilis serology in pregnant women), but the task force remains open to new research findings that may make modifications necessary in the guidelines in future years.

Among the general recommendations from the task force, epidemiologic treatment has the highest grade of evidence and level of recommendation. Contact tracing, disease reporting, use of barrier methods, and patient education are less highly recommended. Primary care physicians share responsibility with all physicians for implementing the general recommendations.

Disease-specific recommendations from the task force cover gonorrhea, syphilis, chlamydia, HIV infection, hepatitis A, genital warts, and neonatal herpes (Table 93-1). Screening cultures and serologic testing are strongly recommended only in high-risk groups. Specific criteria outlining the characteristics of asymptomatic women at high risk for chlamydia (and reasonable for gonorrhea as well) include at least two of the following: (1) women less than 25 years of age, (2) three or more sexual partners in the preceding year, (3) intercourse with a new partner in the preceding 2 months, or (4) purulent cervical exudate or cervical friability.[15] Using these criteria, screening by primary care physicians may be tailored to the risk of the individual patient rather than applied indiscriminately to patients who may be at negligible risk.

## SPECIAL PRIMARY CARE RESPONSIBILITIES

The characteristics of primary care (first-contact, comprehensive, continuous) translate into special opportunities and responsibilities for primary care practitioners when managing patients with sexually transmitted diseases. Responsibilities for prevention—many shared with specialist physicians—are discussed above; three other responsibilities will be addressed here: reporting requirements, partner treatment, and patient and partner follow-up.

The underreporting of STDs from primary care has already been discussed. With increasing reliance on central laboratories for diagnostic testing this problem may be on the wane, since such laboratories are often required by statute to report cases of notifiable disease. Notifiable diseases vary from state to state; among STDs only syphilis, gonorrhea, and AIDS are notifiable in all states.[11] Primary care physicians, like all other physicians, should keep informed about local reporting requirements and should cooperate with public health officials in reporting important but optionally notifiable disease when asked to do so.

Partner treatment is particularly appropriate and feasible in many primary care practices in which the physician may already be caring for the index patient's sexual partner. Difficulties arise when both members of a presumably mutually faithful sexual relationship are patients of a single physician, and one of the patients develops a sexually transmitted disease that discloses sexual activity outside the relationship. The physician's role may be complicated by legal requirements for reporting and by the possibility of litigation from the "injured" partner if full disclosure is not made. Scrupulous attention to patient confidentiality coupled with skills in medical ethics, family counseling, and knowledge of referral resources are all essential to the physician dealing with this potentially destructive predicament. Physician responsibility in such situations is evolving rapidly as new ethical guidelines and case law define acceptable alternatives.

Patient and partner follow-up may be enhanced in the primary care setting by the longitudinal relationship between patient and physician over time. This long-term relationship should enhance the primary physician's ability to inquire about and deal with potentially embarrassing issues surrounding sexuality and STDs, especially if both partners are cared for by the same physician.

**Table 93-1. Recommendations for Prevention of Sexually Transmitted Diseases**

| Disease | Intervention | Grade of evidence* | Recommendation† |
|---|---|---|---|
| General recommendations | Epidemiologic treatment | I | A |
| | Contact tracing | II-2 | B |
| | Disease reporting | III | B |
| | Barrier methods | II-3 | B |
| | Patient education | III | C |
| Gonorrhea: | | | |
| Gonococcal ophthalmia neonatorum | Erythromycin ophthalmic ointment, postpartum | I | A |
| | Culture of pregnant women | III | C |
| Gonorrhea | Culture of high-risk group members | II-1 | A |
| Syphilis: | | | |
| Syphilis | Epidemiologic treatment of sexual contacts of established infection | I | A |
| | VDRL testing of high-risk group members | II-3 | B |
| Congenital syphilis | VDRL testing of pregnant women | II-3 | Risk group B<br>No risk group C |
| HIV infection | HIV antibody testing | III | Risk group B<br>No risk group C<br>Pregnant women B |
| | Use of heat-treated blood products | II | A |
| | Blood and needle precautions for persons exposed to infected secretions | II | A |
| Hepatitis A | Immune serum globulin | I | A |
| Genital warts | Physical examination of risk group members | III | C |
| Neonatal herpes | Caesarean section in women with active genital herpes during labor | III | B |
| Chlamydia trachomatis: | | | |
| Ophthalmia neonatorum | Erythromycin eye ointment | I | A |
| Neonatal chlamydial infection | Culture screening of pregnant women | III | Risk group B |

*Effectiveness of interventions:
I: Evidence obtained from at least one properly randomized controlled trial.
II-1: Evidence obtained from well-designed controlled trials without randomization.
II-2: Evidence obtained from well-designed cohort or case-control analytic studies, preferably from more than one center or research group.
II-3: Evidence obtained from multiple time series studies with or without the intervention. Dramatic results in uncontrolled experiments could also be regarded as this type of evidence.
III: Opinions of respected authorities, based on clinical experience, descriptive studies, or reports of expert committees.
†Classification of recommendations:
A: There is good evidence to support the recommendation that the condition be specifically considered in a periodic health examination.
B: There is fair evidence to support the recommendation that the condition be specifically considered in a periodic health examination.
C: There is poor evidence regarding the inclusion of the condition in a periodic health examination, but recommendations may be made on other grounds.
SOURCE: Horsburgh CR et al: Preventive strategies in sexually transmitted diseases for the primary care physician. *JAMA* 258:814, 1987 (with permission).

Patient compliance with therapeutic regimens is assumed by many primary care physicians to be higher in primary care than in the STD clinic setting, but no data are available to support this assumption. Primary care physicians should be as meticulous as their STD specialist colleagues in aggressively following up their patients treated for sexually transmitted disease.

## SPECIALIST RELATIONSHIPS WITH PRIMARY CARE PHYSICIANS

The relationship between primary care physicians and specialist physicians practicing in STD clinics should be one of respect and collegiality, although this is not always the case. Primary care physicians may not receive timely information from STD clinics concerning their patients who may be seen there, nor do they always feel that the special practice challenges of primary care physicians are respected by STD specialists. Specialists may be consulted by some patients inadequately or inappropriately treated in primary care practices and may generalize their experience to a negative view of all physicians practicing outside specialized centers. As with most misunderstandings, conflicts between primary care and specialist physicians are best resolved by improving opportunities for personal contact and communication.

Specialist STD physicians should make sure that local primary care practitioners are kept informed of diagnostic criteria, reporting requirements, treatment protocols, recommendations for follow-up, and opportunities for enrolling patients in research protocols. Short newsletters, reports in the local medical society bulletin, direct mailings, and continuing education courses are commonly used and effective in transmitting the necessary information. Specialist physicians should be scrupulous in informing (with the patient's consent, of course) the primary physician of the diagnosis, treatment, and planned follow-up for any patients of the primary physician seen in the STD clinic. Primary care physicians should have quick telephone access to specialized advice regarding patients who are being seen in the office, with ready consultation and referral available for patients with more complex or unusual problems.

Primary care physicians should pay attention to information coming from the STD specialists and should develop office systems so that timely reporting of notifiable disease and patient and partner follow-up occurs. Primary care physicians should remain flexible in allowing for epidemiologic treatment and contact tracing where appropriate in their practices. Finally, primary care physicians need to be aware of their inevitable knowledge and skill limitations in the rapidly changing field of STDs, consulting readily with their specialist colleagues whenever substantive questions of diagnosis, treatment, or follow-up arise.

## RESEARCH IMPLICATIONS

Primary care physicians generally see the majority of patients with STDs in the United States, yet little research has been performed and disseminated to these practitioners concerning current STD prevention, diagnostic testing, treatment strategies, and follow-up in the primary care setting.

More research conducted within primary care settings is needed. The low frequency with which sexually transmitted diseases are seen in most office settings argues for the conduct of research in very large practices or in practice networks. Two settings for primary care research in STDs are promising: health maintenance organizations (HMOs) and practice-based research networks.

The characteristics of patient populations seen in large HMOs may approximate those of the overall population in a given geographic area. Since these HMOs have virtually complete capture of medical care utilization, laboratory testing, and diagnosis, research on the epidemiology of STDs might profitably be carried out in such settings.

Practice-based research networks are a new and promising development for research in primary care. By aggregating data from a number of individual primary care practices, such networks should be able to address questions regarding relatively uncommon events, including STDs. The Dartmouth COOP[16] and the Ambulatory Sentinel Practice Network[17] are two examples of such networks in the United States that are beginning to realize the potential for collaborative office-based research, but sexually transmitted diseases have not yet been studied.

## References


1 McLemore T, Koch H: 1980 summary: National ambulatory medical care survey: NCHS advance data. Hyattsville, MD: Office of Health Research, Statistics, and Technology, 1982, DHHS Publication no. (PHS)82-1250.

2 Rosenblatt RA et al: The content of ambulatory medical care in the United States. *N Engl J Med* 309:892, 1983.

3 Gale JL, Hinds MW: Male urethritis in King County, Washington, 1974–75: I. Incidence. *Am J Public Health* 68:20, 1978.

4 Curtis AC: National survey of venereal disease treatment. *JAMA* 186:152, 1963.

5 Fleming WL et al: National survey of venereal disease treated by physicians in 1968. *JAMA* 211:1827, 1970.

6 Eisenberg MS, Wiesner PJ: Reporting and treating gonorrhea: Results of a statewide survey in Alaska. *J Am Vener Dis Assoc* 3:79, 1976.

7 Hinds MW, Gale JL: Male urethritis in King County, Washington, 1974–75: II. Diagnosis and treatment. *Am J Public Health* 68:26, 1978.

8 Hart G: Unpublished data from the National Ambulatory Medical Care Survey, Department of Family Medicine, University of Washington, personal communication.

9 Schneeweiss RA: Unpublished data from the Network Information Management System, Department of Family Medicine, University of Washington, personal communication.

10 Berg AO et al: Establishing the cause of genitourinary symptoms in women in a family practice. *JAMA* 251:620, 1984.

11 Centers for Disease Control. Annual summary 1984: Reported morbidity and mortality in the United States. *MMWR* 32(54):1986.

12 Haynes RB et al: Increased absenteeism from work after detection and labelling of hypertensive patients. *N Engl J Med* 299:741, 1978.

13 Horsburgh CR et al: Preventive strategies in sexually transmitted diseases for the primary care physician. *JAMA* 258:814, 1987.

14 Koop CE: Surgeon general's report on acquired immune deficiency syndrome. *JAMA* 256:2784, 1986.

15 Handsfield HH et al: Criteria for selective screening of *Chlamydia trachomatis* infection in women attending family planning clinics. *JAMA* 255:1730, 1986.

16 Nelson EC et al: The cooperative information project: A sentinel practice network for service and research in primary care. *J Fam Pract* 13:641, 1981.

17 Green LA et al: The Ambulatory Sentinel Practice Network: Purpose, methods, and policies. *J Fam Pract* 18:275, 1984.

# PART XI SPECIAL MEDICAL, LEGAL, AND SOCIAL ISSUES

Chapter 94

# Legal aspects of STD control: Public duties and private rights

Edward P. Richards
Donald C. Bross

## INTRODUCTION

The practice of public health is a legal as well as medical specialty. Within the context of traditional public health concerns, especially with regard to disease control, official public health activities must be based on law.[1] Vaccinations, pasteurization of milk, restaurant sanitation, and the control of typhoid carriers are all public health measures that depend on statutory authority. Since the legal authority to identify and treat the members of high-risk core groups is basic to STD control,[2] STD control depends on understanding public health law.

This chapter outlines a broad view of legal strategies for the control of STDs. It is a guide for both lawmakers and those charged with enforcing existing laws. To the authors' knowledge, no single jurisdiction employs the full range of legal control strategies for STDs. In the United States, for example, most states have repudiated some very customary STD control measures for HIV infection. The legal foundation of control programs for STDs has frequently been influenced by shortsighted political expediency. This shortsightedness has led to the questionable situation of a rich country that has large numbers of medical practitioners such as the United States tolerating 2 million cases of gonorrhea a year. It is now predicted that tolerating a few hundred thousand cases of HIV infection each year may cripple even the United States.[3]

## LEGAL THEORIES

A central role of a nation is to protect its citizens from harms that they, individually, are unable to fend off.[4] Nations with Anglo-American legal systems discuss this right in terms of parens patriae, police powers, and other formulations that recognize the authority of the state to protect its citizens, even from themselves. Since these labels have less meaning in nations that do not have Anglo-American legal systems, we will discuss legal roles from a more general human rights perspective.

## PROTECTION FROM SELF

A nation may choose to act as a parent and prevent citizens from harming themselves. Laws against suicide, such as India's attempts to outlaw the ritual suicide of widows, are the clearest example of this protection from self-harm. While some cultures view this protection from self as contrary to their societal norms, many endorse it as a valid concern for protecting society by preserving its productive citizens. The greatest consensus on necessity to prevent self-harm is the protection of minors from personally harmful behavior such as smoking and drinking.

## PROTECTION FROM OTHER CITIZENS

A nation may choose not to protect its citizens from themselves without creating a serious threat to public order. A nation must, however, exercise a police function to protect citizens from other citizens. Again, the basic motivation of this protection is the preservation of the nation itself, with the citizen's individual welfare a secondary concern. The crime which best illustrates this motivation is mayhem,[5] which was the crime of injuring a person so that he would not be an effective soldier. The mayhem law protected individual citizens from injury, both the immediate injury and the possibility of future injury derivative of the inability to protect oneself, but the intent was to protect the king's ability to raise an army.

Criminal laws and disease control laws have the objective of protecting individuals from the threat posed by other citizens. While these laws are primarily concerned with outward-directed behavior, they also restrict an individual's inward-directed behavior as necessary to preserve order in society. An individual may consent to be neither the victim of a criminal act nor the carrier of a communicable disease. In both instances the protection of the individual is secondary to the protection of society.

## PROTECTION FROM OTHER NATIONS

Nations must be secure from the threats posed by other nations. These threats may be military, demographic, economic, or environmental.[6] Infectious disease is an environmental threat. National borders have proved very permeable to disease.[7] The Black Plague destroyed the fabric of European society, and the diseases carried by western missionaries and sailors did more to destroy indigenous cultures than did their religion and materialism. While the threat of HIV has yet to become a source of significant international friction, countries with low HIV infection rates and homogeneous populations are already limiting the immigration of HIV carriers.

Disease control programs are also fundamental to maintaining an army in the field. It has only been in the last 75 years that munitions have outstripped disease as a killer of soldiers. STDs have been the hallmark of military campaigns for the last 1000 years. Even in the United States, serious attempts at controlling gonorrhea and syphilis have grown out of a concern with military readiness.[8] The same is true of HIV infection. The earliest systematic HIV testing in the United States has been of military personnel and recruits. This testing is based on the premise that soldiers with HIV infection would compromise the effectiveness of the military. While the heterosexual transmission of HIV is a serious public health issue, the United States' preoccupation with military preparedness may transform the spread to prostitutes around military installations into a national security issue.

## THE NATURE OF PUBLIC HEALTH LAWS

Public health authority must be broad and flexible to meet the challenges of new diseases and new knowledge about old diseases. Until recently this was the rule. Even in the United States, with its suspicion of unconstrained public authority, state laws generally gave health officers the authority to do whatever was necessary to protect the public health. Courts might limit actions that did not further the public health,[9] but it was considered prudent to err on the side of too much power rather than too little.

It seems obvious that the citizens of a nation will vest discretionary power in public health officials in proportion to the citizenry's fear of communicable diseases. In the United States and other industrialized countries, the fear of communicable diseases has diminished since the polio epidemics of the 1950s.[10] An uncritical belief in medical technology, combined with a focus on individual rights rather than societal duties, has reduced the public's fear of communicable diseases and desire to support public health authority.

This diminished fear of communicable diseases is reflected in the changing nature of public health laws in the United States. Older statutes specify the broad outlines of disease control programs, leaving the specific details, such as which diseases will be reported, within what time frame, in what form, and how the infected individuals will be managed, to the discretion of the health officer. The health officer may then promulgate administrative regulations to detail the specifics of the disease control strategies. These administrative regulations give notice of a citizen's obligations but may be quickly changed to reflect changes in disease dynamics. While the courts have always placed some limits on public health authority, it was recognized that there was an overriding public interest in disease control. Current statutes, particularly those that have been passed since the recognition of the AIDS epidemic,[11] tend to subrogate the public interest in disease control to interests in personal privacy.

Unlike other classes of laws, public health laws are not concerned with the state of mind of the infector or infectee. Public health laws seek to regulate and prevent harm, not to punish wrongdoers or compensate victims. Since they do not involve the criminal justice system and do not generate fees to support private litigation, public health laws are the poor stepchildren of the legal system. Until recently they have been all but ignored by legal scholars. Any area that does not generate extensive litigation is invisible to legal scholars because academic legal research is confined to that small universe of legal cases decided by appeals courts, preferably the United States Supreme Court or the highest legal tribunal in other countries.

In the United States this has not been benign neglect. Legal scholars have assumed that since most public health cases are old, they must have been implicitly overruled by later civil rights decisions. Quite the contrary is true. The United States Supreme Court has repeatedly affirmed the right of states to restrict the actions of persons who pose a threat to the public health or safety.[12] In the case of public health laws, the lack of appellant decisions reflects the breadth of the power of the states, not the absence of that power.[13]

## OTHER LEGAL REMEDIES

In addition to public health law remedies, many STD control problems may trigger criminal and other civil law remedies. In Anglo-American legal systems, the application of these alternate remedies is dependent on the state of mind of the parties involved in the transmission of the disease. An HIV carrier may be a murderer or an innocent sexual partner, depending on his or her state of mind when having intercourse. STDs may be transmitted intentionally, knowingly, recklessly, negligently, stupidly, unknowingly, or uncontrollably. These states of mind are generally irrelevant to public health law. Pursuant to public health law, a person who is spreading a dangerous disease such as drug-resistant tuberculosis may require isolation without personal culpability for his or her actions.[14]

## CRIMINAL LAW

A carrier who transmits the disease knowingly or recklessly could be subject to criminal prosecution for endangering the infectee. The state of mind of the infectee is not relevant, because the criminal law recognizes acceptance of risk only in certain limited contexts, mostly involving sports such as boxing. While one may consent to sex, few people consent to catching gonorrhea. Even if a person does consent to catch gonorrhea, this consent violates the public policy of discouraging the transmission of communicable diseases. To manifest the requisite intent, carriers must know or have reason to know that they have the disease, the methods of transmission, and the methods of preventing transmission. If there is no criminal intent, there is no crime, irrespective of the fate of the infectee.[15]

Physicians and other health care workers may violate criminal laws when caring for communicable disease carriers. The most common violation is failing to comply with disease reporting laws. In some circumstances, there are also laws governing other aspects of the patient's care. These may mandate the method of treatment (prophylaxis for ophthalmia neonatorum), require the patient to be tested for a venereal disease (syphilis serologies in pregnant women), require the patient to be counseled in methods of preventing the spread of the disease, or sanction the physician for violating the patient's confidences.

As matter of course, physicians are not prosecuted for breaking public health laws. Detection of the offense, proof of the offense, and willingness to prosecute complicate enforcing a disease control law. Obviously, few societies will approve the jailing of a physician who fails to report a case of STD. This reflects both the low priority accorded public health law enforcement and the high social status of physicians. The traditional difficulty in enforcing constant compliance with a reporting law[16] has led reporting laws to be seen primarily as a goal, with sanctions available in cases of willful or wanton disregard of the standard or where full reporting becomes so urgent that a "crackdown" is warranted.

As a practical matter, the most effective criminal sanction for a physician who violates a public health law is probably a small fine ($100 to $1000) which can be imposed by a public health officer. Letting health officers write tickets obviates the need to involve prosecutors and the criminal justice system. A small, sure penalty is much more effective than the usual more severe but never enforced sanctions. Short-term, intensive efforts to acquire data are more likely to increase reporting to optimal levels than any program relying solely on a statute. The writing of tickets may be combined with time-limited crackdowns to optimize compliance with STD reporting.[17,18]

Treating public health laws as goals rather than "real" laws may either reflect or reinforce the view that stopping the transmission of a disease is not very important. This view may change with HIV. If a physician's failure to report an HIV carrier is seen as causing the deaths of innocent persons, society may choose to be more severe with physician law breakers. This is most likely if an HIV carrier sought treatment for other, more recently acquired STDs that should indicate to the physician the patient's dangerousness.

## MENTAL HEALTH LAW

As with criminal law, mental health law is concerned with states of mind. Unlike criminal law, personal culpability is usually not an issue. Persons who are unable to understand the consequences of their actions, or do not appreciate these consequences, may be legally restrained if the actions pose a threat to themselves or others. Mentally ill HIV carriers could be committed under the mental health laws if they engaged in prostitution secondary to their mental illness.[19] They would be endangering the health of others, but would not be mentally able to appreciate this risk. If they could appreciate their actions, they would be subject to prosecution for the criminal act of prostitution.

## TORT LAW

Tort law is the private law remedy in which the injured person sues to recover monetary compensation from the person or entity who caused the injury. While most countries have some type of private law system, torts are a uniquely American institution. In the United States, attorneys may prosecute a case for a percentage of the ultimate recovery. These contingent fees open the courts to persons who are not wealthy. More importantly, as a policy matter, the United States encourages private law compensation rather than state-financed medical and disability programs.

Because tort law is a private remedy, the state of mind of both the infector and the infectee is in issue. Unlike criminal law, in which consent is not an issue, one may assume the risk of a communicable disease, just as one assumes the risk of smoking cigarettes. However, one must understand the risks and voluntarily assume them. For example, knowing one's partner is an HIV carrier does not imply that one has enough knowledge to know how it is spread. A person who knowingly assumes the risk of the disease may not sue the infector or others for compensation.

The United States has well-articulated liability theories that will be applied to the three types of communicable disease compensation cases: (1) infectees suing infectors, (2) infectees suing physicians for failing to warn them that a patient of the physician was a disease carrier, and (3) patients suing their physicians for medical malpractice. There have already been cases awarding compensation for infecting an unsuspecting person with an STD and for malpractice in treating an STD.[20] While there are not yet any reported cases involving a failure to warn of a patient with an STD, this will rapidly change as more "innocent" persons discover that they have been infected with HIV. These lawsuits will be particularly effective in states such as Colorado that attempt to control the spread of HIV through traditional disease control measures.[1,21] A physician who fails to report HIV in a state that attempts to warn persons at risk will be sued for negligence per se: the tort remedy for breaking a law. These are difficult lawsuits to defend against because the reporting law sets the standard of behavior.

In the United States and a few other countries, a private physician must obtain voluntary patients' informed consent before treating them for an STD. The proposed treatment should be explained in layman's language, and alternative treatments, potential benefits, and the risks should be discussed. Since treatment regimens for most STDs are fairly well established, the main concern will be reactions to antibiotics and the need to stress the limited efficacy for treatments for viral diseases such as herpes simplex virus type T2 and HIV.

In some states, state legislatures have been persuaded to require that physicians also obtain informed consent for HIV tests.[22] This has led many physicians to tell the patient the political risks of being tested (discrimination, etc.), while ignoring the medical risks of not being tested. Since failing to perform a medically indicated test is malpractice,[23] the physician must carefully document that the patient was told the medical risks of not being tested, including spreading the disease to others. If the physician has reason to believe that a patient has HIV but refuses to be tested, that patient should be reported to the public health officials.

Private law remedies are very important in the United States. While few people actually sue physicians, the threat of litigation causes third parties such as insurance companies and peer review committees to monitor and enforce compliance with litigation-driven norms. In countries that do not have contingent fees or a well-funded patient litigation fund, private law remedies will not be effective. Countries that have well-developed regulatory systems for the licensing of physicians will have better results by making violations of public health laws a ground for the loss of the medical license.

## PUBLIC HEALTH LAW STRATEGIES

The HIV epidemic has made it fashionable to decry the effectiveness of public health laws. Many factors influenced syphilis control efforts in the United States between 1912 and 1964, and STD control efforts worked best with stringent social controls, less individual freedom, and more centralized control of programs.[24] In nations where there is no consensus on how to control STDs, it must be recognized that laws alone may have little effect. It is frequently noted that laws to control prostitution, whether for disease control or other purposes, may be totally ignored.[17,25–27] Yet, where an effective program of control over STD and prostitutes is dropped, the ensuing rise in STD cautions against ruling out legal interventions to control STDs.[28]

Even homogeneous or tightly controlled societies may find that commerce with the outside world, e.g., in the form of activities by tourists, sailors, or prostitutes, requires specific controls, regulation, or legislation. As one example, tourists in some northern European countries have been found responsible for as much as 20 to 25 percent of early syphilis.[28] As another example, the success in reducing STDs reported by Polish authorities during the 1970s depended in part on such methods as screening of prostitutes in seaports, towns, and industrial centers and in contact tracing,[29] activities that must be legislated in societies with less centralized forms of government.

Just as public health cannot be practiced without the force of law, public health laws must be based on science to be effective. This scientific knowledge is of two types: technical knowledge about the spread and prevention of the disease, and knowledge about the risk calculus of the disease. Technical knowledge establishes the universe of possible control measures. The risk calculus determines which control measures will be most resource-effective in the given situation. In its simplest form, risk calculus is the qualitative determination of a risk factor $R$ that reflects the threat that a given disease poses to society. This risk calculus is a method of integrating knowledge about the pathology and epidemiology of a disease into a form that may be used for establishing disease control policy.

## GENERAL RISK CALCULUS

The risk factor $R$ for a disease is determined by the severity $S$ of the disease, its transmissibility $T$, and the number of persons at risk $P$:

$$R = S\,T\,P$$

Severity may range from very low (the common cold) to high (HIV). Transmissibility may range from *gonorrhea* (high) to leprosy (extremely low). The population at risk may range from the entire population (a new strain of influenza) to all sexually active individuals (gonorrhea) to persons with defects in their immune systems (*Pneumocystis carinii* pneumonia).

It is obvious that variables such as the time frame of the spread and progression of the disease will disproportionately affect $R$. Diseases that spread rapidly and cause immediate illness are recognized as a great threat to society because they can overwhelm the health care system. The obviousness of the threat prompts the mobilization of the resources necessary to contain the threat. HIV is more insidious because it spreads relatively rapidly, but the infection is disassociated from symptomatic illness and death by many years. HIV has the same potential for overwhelming societal resources as more acute illnesses, but it can be ignored in the short term because the societal consequences of the illness lag the spread of the illness.

The higher $R$, the greater the threat to the citizens and the stability of the nation. In nations such as the United States with a constitutional mandate to balance individual and societal rights, the balance will shift away from individual rights with increasing $R$. In nations with different forms of government, the value of $R$ should be used by the sovereign as guide to the need for intrusive disease control measures and the application of state resources to disease control.

## RISK CALCULUS FOR GONORRHEA

Gonorrhea is an extremely common disease, which makes it readily susceptible to statistical analysis. Yet for all of the understanding of the epidemiology of gonorrhea, it is still a scourge, causing significant morbidity from pelvic inflammatory disease and sterility (Ref. 2, p. 5). This is true despite the ease with which gonorrhea is treated. Gonorrhea is also a useful model for the transmission of other STDs. Political considerations aside, there are parallels between the epidemiology of HIV and gonorrhea. For these reasons, insights from the risk calculus of gonorrhea should be useful in evaluating legal strategies for the control of all STDs.

Gonorrhea is a disease at endemic equilibrium. This is a stable equilibrium, in that the disease is sufficiently far from the extinction point that incremental changes in the resources available for gonorrhea control result in proportional changes in gonorrhea incidence (Ref. 2, p. 27). The gonorrhea equilibrium is rapidly responsive in that changes in sexual behaviors or control resources are reflected in changes in gonorrhea rates in less than 2 months. Gonorrhea is under control, in the sense that the United States has chosen to allocate only enough resources to gonorrhea control programs to set the equilibrium point at approximately 2 to 3 million cases a year. Assuming that this resource allocation has been rationally determined, it reflects the amount of money that the United States is willing to invest in a disease that poses the risk to society ($R$) of gonorrhea.

A significant characteristic of gonorrhea epidemiology, from a legal perspective, is that it is a disease whose incidence and prevalence in the general population are driven by a core group of carriers. While there is mixing between this core group and the general population, it is the incidence and prevalence of gonorrhea in the group that determines gonorrhea dynamics (Ref. 2, p. 38). Thus, core group members pose a disproportionate threat to the community, justifying legal strategies that disproportionately focus on members of this group. These strategies are good law precisely because they flow from good science.

Core group transmission is possible for diseases that do not induce immunity, thus allowing members of a subpopulation to remain infectious. This is possible for gonorrhea because core group members cycle between uninfected (susceptible) and infected. This results in what is termed a susceptible-infected-susceptible dynamic (Ref. 2, p. 13). Since infection with gonorrhea renders a person infectious essentially at once, the probability that a core group member will be infectious at a given time is determined by two intervals: the delay between infection and treatment, and the delay between treatment and reinfection. Increased numbers of sexual partners in a given time increases the reinfection rate; asymptomatic disease increases the delay between infection and treatment.

Since the critical factor for core group transmission is that core group members remain infectious, infectious HIV carriers form a core group because the disease is untreatable. This is similar to a gonorrhea carrier who is always immediately reinfected after treatment: the probability that he is infectious $I$ at any given time approaches unity, while susceptibility $S$ approaches zero.

## IDENTIFYING CORE GROUP MEMBERS

The identification of core group members is a sociological as well as epidemiologic task. It is the demographics of these core group members that raise legal questions. For example, the following factors are correlated with gonorrhea transmission: age, race, marital status, socioeconomic status, and urban residence (Ref. 2, p. 36). Each of these factors is a legally troubling classification, yet epidemiologically they are a necessary part of the characterization of a gonorrhea core group member. STD control policy decisions must balance the use of such classifications and the public health benefits of more efficiently identifying core group members. Demographic factors are valuable in determining which groups to target for control measures, but core-group-oriented control measures depend on identifying infected individuals. Individual identification depends on screening and contact tracing.

## SCREENING

Screening is the process of testing persons for evidence of disease. Screening may be universal, or it may be based on identified risk factors. In this sense, contact tracing is a subset of the general class of screening strategies. Because gonorrhea is spread by a core group, screening of the general population is not as effective as screening persons with certain risk factors for gonorrhea infection. For example, previous infection with gonorrhea increases the probability that a given person is a core group member. Seeking out and testing these previously infected persons is rescreening: "rescreening is approximately four times as effective per number of individuals tested as screening in reducing incidence. The intuitive reason why rescreening is more effective than screening is that since rescreened individuals were infected before, they are more likely to be infectious again when rescreened" (Ref. 2, p. 41).

Thus for gonorrhea, limited screening resources are best spent monitoring the infectious status of known core group members. To the extent that there are privacy concerns about screening, the legal rationale for rescreening known core group members is stronger than the rationale for de novo screening of the general population. Rescreening for the purpose of determining infectiousness may be obviated for HIV infection by maintaining a roster of known carriers. In HIV control, resources are most efficiently expended on the de novo screening of persons at demographic risk of HIV and the tracing of contacts of known infectives.

Screening for STDs has been legislated for many specified population subgroups, including prostitutes, newborns, and marriage license applicants. Since theoretical models show that gonorrhea "adjusts rapidly to changes in social behaviors, medical treatment, and control programs," screening programs must be able to respond to local conditions. Enabling legislation should provide general authority for screening, while allowing public health officials to determine the specific form of the programs.

The identification and cooperation of high-risk groups raises several legal issues. Repeaters,[30] prostitutes, homosexuals, young people, and "travelers" or "transients" of many kinds are usually included among groups at greater risk for STD.[31] Identification of some groups, such as prostitutes and military personnel, can be relatively easy. Screening of other groups, such as homosexuals, students, and professional travelers, can be hampered by identification problems or the overinclusiveness of the definition in terms of appropriate indices of suspicion. Administratively, this problem can create unacceptable costs and inefficiencies, while legally it may lead to attacks on statutes or regulations for "overbreadth" or "vagueness." However, when there is epidemiologic evidence that a person may be a disease carrier, the courts will even support testing that person involuntarily.

## CONTACT TRACING

Contact tracing may be viewed as screening based on the risk factor of contact with an infectious individual. Contact tracing (or investigation) seeks to identify contacts of known infectives and encourage them to be treated as soon as possible. It may also be used to identify recalcitrant carriers so that they may be legally persuaded to seek treatment. Contact tracing has proved invaluable in elucidating subpopulation dynamics. For example, the discovery that a select group of males experienced high rates of asymptomatic gonorrhea resulted from tracing the infection of children under 5 with gonorrhea to pimps.[32] Contact tracing is a highly leveraged activity because it deals with persons known to be at highest risk for infection. Since the probability of transmitting gonorrhea to a contact is high, sexual contact with a gonorrhea carrier is justification for treatment without further testing.[33]

Contact tracing deals with two classes of individuals. Infectees are persons who have acquired the disease but have not passed it on. If the sexual contacts of gonorrhea carriers are viewed as a network, then pure infectees would be dead ends with no contacts after the contact that infected them. Infectors are persons with at least two contacts, the person that infected them and person that they infected. In practical terms, infectees are the persons that an infector names as contacts, and an infector is a person named by an infectee as the infecting contact. (This is based on the anecdotal information that persons can identify the person who infected them.)

For gonorrhea, it is estimated that each infectee contact traced and cured reduces the incidence by 5.3 persons. Each infector traced and cured is estimated to reduce the incidence by 12.3 people (Ref. 2, p. 44). This difference is accounted for by the increased probability that an infector will be a core group member. While contact tracing infectors is more efficient than tracing infectees, even contact tracing infectees (or not differentiating between infectors and infectees) is a very effective strategy for gonorrhea control.

Contact tracing in gonorrhea control reduces the incidence of gonorrhea by reducing the time between infection and treatment, particularly for otherwise asymptomatic cases. Given that there is no treatment for HIV infection, it has been argued that there is no legal justification for tracing HIV carriers. This ignores three factors that are masked by the easy treatability and high transmissibility of gonorrhea. First, since HIV is less infectious than gonorrhea, contact tracing can warn persons as yet uninfected that they are being exposed to HIV by one of their partners. Second, for persons who do not know that they are infected, it provides an early warning so that they may take measures to protect their loved ones. These self-imposed restrictions will be most critical for women of childbearing potential. Third, contact tracing allows the identification of the small but epidemiologically significant number of persons with HIV who act in a socially irresponsible manner. This is critical for HIV precisely because it is an untreatable, fatal disease. If a person is repeatedly named as a contact, the nation must consider restricting that person for the safety of society. The legal justification for restriction would be greater for HIV as an untreatable, fatal disease than for almost any treatable disease.

## DISEASE REPORTING

Disease epidemiology must be the basis of all disease control strategies. Conversely, epidemiologic information for STDs is frequently impossible to collect without legal persuasion. This problem is most acute in countries such as the United States where most medical care is delivered by unregulated private practitioners. In general, private physicians will not voluntarily provide the state with information about their patients.[34]

The importance of incidence, prevalence, and population data makes compulsory reporting of STDs the logical foundation for an STD control program. Such legislation should recognize the three functions served by reporting: (1) statistical assessment of disease dynamics, (2) direct disease control interventions, and (3) discharge of the physician's duty to warn persons at risk of contracting a disease from the patient. High-quality data on disease dynamics may be obtained by large-scale statistical surveys of randomly sampled practitioners, without requiring routine individual disease reports. This type of survey is expensive and time-consuming, making it virtually impossible to detect short-term changes in disease dynamics. Statistically sampled surveys also fail to address the duty to warn, which requires the identification of individual infected patients. Requiring the reporting of each infected individual is essential for maintaining the contact tracing programs that serve to warn persons at risk of contracting a communicable disease.

Requiring individual reporting of STDs does not assure adequate epidemiologic data. The most effective approach is a combination of mandated reporting with health department polling of the designated practitioners most likely to diagnose and treat STDs. Many physicians do not comply with their statutory reporting duties but will supply information on request.

## INVOLUNTARY TESTING AND TREATMENT

When an individual is identified as epidemiologically at risk for STDs, the courts have repeatedly upheld involuntary examinations and treatment.[35] For example, the high prevalence of gonorrhea in pregnant women has led to the legal requirement that all persons attending a birth provide prophylaxis for ophthalmia neonatorum. These laws are most effective when they carefully distinguish between punishment and restriction. A health hold, ordered by a public health official, is an allowable restriction. Detaining a person in the same facility for the same period of time as a punishment would be a constitutionally improper punishment. Reserving this authority to health officers is a safeguard against possible excesses. It protects the general public by assuring that health matters are not delegated to police officials. Finally, it protects the public health officer by preventing improper delegation or supervision of health duties.[34]

## RESTRICTION OF INDIVIDUALS

Isolation and quarantine are venerable techniques of public health officials.[36] The use of confinement in the case of STDs, however, seems to have little practical use. Unlike many diseases, intimate contact is required for the spread of STDs. In effect, drawing a blood sample or administering an antibiotic under medically indicated circumstances is a less restrictive means of state intervention in the control of STDs than isolation.

The fatal and untreatable nature of HIV infection may force attention to isolation as a remedy in rare cases. Depending on the factual situations which arise with HIV infection, for example, associated dementia or an independent mental illness, the courts may well have to consider mental health law and public health law measures for isolating an individual with HIV who is clearly a danger to others or who is gravely disabled and unable to obtain treatment.

Given that isolation is a very restrictive approach to STD control, some comparable mechanism which will ensure participation in examinations and agreements not to expose others is needed. The alternative of health hold orders should be considered. As used here, health hold order means a specific order issued by an authorized public health official to a named individual to cooperate with examination, treatment, or to behave within certain limits necessary to protect the public health.[37] Such an order could be appealed to the courts in a confidential proceeding. The health hold also might be in the form of a voluntary agreement subject to enforcement by court order, and result in a very brief detention for examination or a "show cause" contempt proceeding if the voluntary agreement is not likely to be kept or in fact is not being kept. Health holds might also be administered conveniently to persons detained in institutional settings for alleged sexual crimes. Health authorities can avoid having the health hold used for nonhealth matters, such as to compel cooperation in criminal matters, by focusing strictly on what is required for individual and epidemiologic treatment of STD.

## IMMUNIZATIONS

Currently the only STD with an effective vaccine is hepatitis B. Physicians should strongly recommend this vaccine to all patients at risk of infection with hepatitis B virus (HBV), especially health care workers. Lawmakers should require all third party payers to pay for the vaccine and should consider mandating the screening of pregnant women for the virus. If a pregnant woman is infected, the law should require that her baby be vaccinated.[38] Since approximately 60 percent of the babies of these women (estimated to be at least 3500 per year in the United States) will become chronic HBV carriers, with the high attendant risk of liver cancer, this is an extremely cost-effective control measure. Given that most of these babies are currently not detected because physicians do not comply with the guidelines for screening, HBV may pose nearly as serious a medical malpractice threat as HIV infection.

If a vaccine were available for gonorrhea, mathematical modeling predicts that the highest leveraged use of the vaccine would be to immunize known core group members. Combined with acute treatment, this would take known effective carriers out of the SIS cycle. This strategy would be the same for other treatable STDs. For untreatable STDs, such as HIV, the best strategy would be to immunize uninfected persons at demographic risk first, then expand the program to all potential sexually active individuals.

## PROTECTION OF CARRIERS

Historically, disease carriers have felt the wrath of their fellow countrymen. In biblical times, the archetypical act of Christian charity was to suffer a leper. In a modern society, a prime role of law is to protect disease carriers from the unfounded fears of their fellow citizens. This is a quid pro quo for society's imposition of disease control measures.

HIV infection has focused attention on discrimination in jobs, education, and insurance. The U.S. Supreme Court has ruled that damage to certain bodily systems, even if caused by a communicable disease, is a "handicap" under the United States law which forbids employment discrimination against individuals who are deemed handicapped but otherwise qualified to work.[39] Given the increasing evidence that all HIV carriers have some level of immune system compromise (a statutorily defined handicap), this law will apply to HIV carriers. An HIV-infected employee may continue to work until dementia or other HIV-related illness renders him or her unfit to continue in the job.[40]

Other United States laws prevent children infected with communicable disease from being segregated or excluded from school unless they pose a health risk to other children.[41] These laws would prevent children with HIV infection from being excluded from schools, absent clear and substantial risk, perhaps in the person of a child with a history of biting or an older, sexually aggressive child.

Preventing discrimination is important to encouraging persons to cooperate with public health laws, but this may cause a perverse effect in the United States by increasing the cost and thus decreasing the availability of health insurance for employees. Many smaller employers, who do not have the financial leverage to negotiate competitive health insurance rates, are expected to drop group health plans out of fear of economic ruin. Antidiscrimination laws must be paired with public funds to pay the costs, or they will only exacerbate existing problems in paying for health care.

## THE ROLE OF TRANSNATIONAL STANDARDS

Despite the devastation of gonorrhea and other endemic STDs, heads of state and international lawyers have, until recently, ignored the issue of international disease control laws and treaties. This is ironic because admiralty law agreements on quarantine are among the oldest examples of international agreements. HIV has again focused the attention of the international community on disease control measures. Countries with little documented HIV infection want to test foreigners and exclude those with HIV. Countries with high levels of HIV, such as the United States, resist the testing and exclusion of their citizens from other countries but test and exclude persons from other countries attempting to become citizens of the United States.[42]

Industrialized countries criticize developing countries, particularly those in Africa, for not facing their HIV problems. Yet these same industrialized countries fail to apply basic disease control measures to their own citizens. Developing countries fail to act for lack of resources and a fear of being stigmatized in the world community. Industrialized countries fail to act in part out of a highly developed sensitivity to the rights of individuals. If industrialized countries are to provide leadership in HIV control, they must apply the same laws and control strategies to HIV that they do to other equally dangerous communicable diseases.

## PUBLIC EDUCATION

In most of the United States, and in many other countries, public education has been substituted for HIV disease control measures. Education may take a generation or more to have effects on sexual behavior. Adolescents in an environment with high levels of AIDS were found not to be particularly informed about AIDS despite massive local publicity.[43] Older studies have demonstrated that even if techniques like condoms are readily available and the importance of their use is understood generally, many problems interfere with their effective use.[44]

The role of law in sex-related education is to require schools, communications networks, and other organizations to provide nonjudgmental, sexually appropriate information to children and adolescents. Religious and other groups have successfully prevented the passage of laws mandating this type of education in the United States. Given that the incremental effects of education on sexual behavior have little effect on limiting the transmission of HIV among core group members,[45] countries with limited disease control resources should consider whether it is desirable to pass laws that commit these resources primarily to public education.

## CONCLUSIONS

Effective laws to control STDs are based on accurate understanding of available resources, legal and cultural traditions, and intelligent shaping of legislation to meet sound, and probably narrow, disease control goals. Laws to mandate the reporting of STDs, the screening of persons at greatest risk, and the tracing of the contacts of disease carriers must be the first priority of lawmakers concerned with controlling STDs. Personal privacy and liberty must be protected to the greatest extent possible, consistent with the protection of society from STDs. As demonstrated by the contrast between the risk calculus for gonorrhea and for HIV infection, the milder the disease, the more it can be tolerated for the sake of preserving personal liberties.

Public and private professionals involved in STD control must conform their actions to laws governing diagnosis, treatment, reporting, quarantine, and isolation. Law is an effective device in the control of STDs to the extent that it is wielded as one tool in a comprehensive prevention, diagnosis, treatment, and management strategy. Many traditions of public health and legal precedents are valuable standards against which responses to new conditions such as HIV infection must be measured.

## References


1 Richards EP: Communicable Disease Control in Colorado: A Rational Approach to AIDS, 65 U Denver Law Review (1988), in press.
2 Hethcote HW, Yorke JA: *Gonorrhea Transmission Dynamics and Control,* 1984. Extensions of HIV dynamics are drawn from work in progress at the University of Denver and the Colorado Department of Health.
3 Bloom DE, Carliner G: The economic impact of AIDS in the United States. *Science* 239:604, 1988.
4 Hobbes T: *Leviathan,* 1651.
5 Blackstone W: *Commentaries on the Laws of England,* Book the Fourth, 1769.
6 International Nuclear Safety Advisory Group, Summary Report on the Post-Accident Review Meeting on the Chernobyl Accident, 1 (Safety Series No. 75-INSAG-1, IAEA 1986).
7 Syphilis, a synopsis, Public Health Service Publication 1660, 1968.
8 Cutler JC, Arnold RC: Venereal Disease Control by Health Departments in the Past: Lessons for the Present. *Am J Public Health* 78:372, 1988.
9 *Yick Wo v. Hopkins,* 118 U.S. 356 (1886).
10 Wain H: *A History of Preventive Medicine,* 1970.
11 California Health and Safety Code sec. 195 et seq., 1985.
12 *United States v. Salerno,* 107 S.Ct. 2095 (1987); *Hilton v. Braunskill,* 107 S.Ct. 2113 (1987); *Schall v. Martin,* 467 U.S. 253 (1984).
13 *City of New York v. New Saint Mark's Baths,* 130 Misc.2d 911, 497 N.Y.S.2d 979 (Supp. 1986).
14 *State v. Snow,* 324 S.W.2d 532 (1959); *Moore v. Draper,* 57 So.2d 648 (1952).
15 *United States v. Moore,* United States Court of Appeals, Eighth Circuit, No. 87-5422, Decided May 24, 1988.
16 Rothenberg R et al: Reporting of gonorrhea by private physicians: A behavioral study. *Am J Public Health* 70983, 1980.
17 Taha Oma et al: Study of STD's in patients attending venereal disease clinics in Khartoum, Sudan. *Br J Vener Dis* 55:313, 1979.
18 Trends in Child Protection Laws. Denver: Education Commission of the United States, 1977.
19 Price RW et al: The brain in AIDS: Central nervous system HIV-1 infection and AIDS dementia complex. *Science* 239:586, 1988.
20 Molien v. Kaiser Foundation Hospitals, 616 P.2d 813 (1980); *B.N. v. K.K.,* 538 A.2d 1175 (Md. 1988).
21 Colo. Rev. Statutes, sec. 25-4-1401, et seq. (Supp. 1987).
22 Guide to Public Health Practice: AIDS Confidentiality and Anti-Discrimination Principles, Association of State and Territorial Health Officials, March 1988.
23 *Truman v. Thomas,* 27 Cal.3d 336, 165 Cal. Rptr. 308 (1980).
24 Anderson OW: *Syphilis and Society: Problems of Control in the United States, 1912–1964.* Center for Health Administration Studies, Health Information Foundation, Research Series 22. University of Chicago Press, 1965.

25 Rajan VS: Sexually transmitted diseases on a tropical island. *Br J Vener Dis* 54:141, 1978.
26 Blair HI: The venereal disease problem in a women's federal reformatory. *Am J Syph Gonorrhea Vener Dis* 30:165, 1946.
27 Wilcox RR: Prostitution and venereal disease. *Br J Vener Dis* 38:37, 1962.
28 Morton RS, Harris JRW: *Recent Advances in Sexually Transmitted Diseases.* Edinburgh, Churchill-Livingstone, 1975.
29 Towpik J: Critical evaluation of the venereal disease control campaign in Poland 1970. *Br J Vener Dis* 55:127, 1979.
30 Brooks GF et al: Repeated gonorrhea: An analysis of importance and risk factors. *J Infect Dis* 137:161, 1978.
31 Antal G-M et al: *Social and Health Aspects of Sexually Transmitted Diseases.* Geneva Work Health Organization, 1977.
32 John J. Potterat, personal communication, November 5, 1987.
33 Willcox RR: "Epidemiological" treatment in non-venereal and in treponemal diseases. *Br J Vener Dis* 49:107, 1973.
34 Potterat JJ et al: Gonorrhea in street prostitutes: Epidemiologic and legal implication. *Sex Transm Dis* 6:58, 1979.
35 *Reynolds v. McNichols,* 488 F.2d 1378 (10th Cir. 1973).
36 *People v. Victor,* 398 P.2d 391 (1965); *Ex Parte Woodruff,* 210 P.2d 191 (Crimm App. 1949); *Ex Parte Kilbane,* 67 N.E.2d 22, 22-23 (1945); *People v. Robertson,* 302 Ill. 422 (1922).
37 *Application of Halko,* 246 Cal. App. 2d 553, 54 Cal. Rptr. 661 (1966).
38 Prevention of Perinatal Transmission of Hepatitis B Virus: Prenatal Screening of all Pregnant Women for Hepatitis B Surface Antigen. *MMWR* 37:341, 1988.
39 *School Board of Nassau County v. Arline* 107 S. Ct. 1123 (1987).
40 Tuberculosis and acquired immunodeficiency syndrome. *MMWR* 36:785, Dec. 11, 1987; Richards EP: AIDS Dementia. Prev. Law Rptr. 7 (#3):23 (1988).
41 *New York State Association for Retarded Children v. Carey,* 612 F.2d 633 (1979).
42 Voss KE: Re-evaluating alien exclusion in light of AIDS, *Dickenson J Int Law* 6:119, 1987.
43 DiClemente RJ et al: Adolescents and AIDS: A survey of knowledge, attitudes and beliefs about AIDS in San Francisco. *Am J Public Health* 76(12):1443, 1986.
44 Darrow WW, Wiesner PJ: Personal prophylaxis for venereal diseases. *JAMA* 233(5):444, 1975.
45 Fineberg HV: Education to prevent AIDS: Prospects and obstacles. *Science* 239:592, 1988.

# Chapter 95

# Sexual assault and STD

Carole Jenny

Sexual assault is defined as acts of sexual intimacy performed without the consent of the victim through use or threat of use of force, or when the victim is unable to give consent because of physical or mental disability.[1]

Sexually transmitted diseases are the most common medical problems complicating sexual assault. In a recent Seattle study, 56 percent of female victims were found to have an STD at their initial or follow-up medical visits.[2] STD diagnosed at the time of a sexual assault can add to the emotional problems experienced by victims, whether or not the disease was acquired as a result of the assault. In addition, victims often express severe anxiety about the possibility of contracting an STD from the assailant. This anxiety can accentuate the emotional trauma they experience, aggravate any posttraumatic stress, and delay their recovery.

## INCIDENCE AND PREVALENCE OF SEXUAL ASSAULT

Exact statistics on the incidence and prevalence of sexual assault are unknown. In 1985, 87,340 rapes were reported to police in the United States.[3] The U.S. rate is many times higher than that of other western countries.[4] In a study of 930 randomly selected San Francisco households, 24 percent of adult women reported having experienced a sexual assault.[5] Although sexual assault of males is probably less common, no comparable study has been done to determine its prevalence.

Any statistics collected by law enforcement agencies are low estimates of the occurrence of assault, since many victims are reluctant to report the crime.[6] Because sexual assaults occur commonly, medical practitioners who treat STD are likely to see sexual assault victims in their practices.

## FACTORS AFFECTING THE RISK OF STD AFTER SEXUAL ASSAULT

Several factors make the diagnosis and treatment of STD in victims of sexual assault different from other sexual relationships.[7] Although sometimes well known to the victim, often the assailant is a stranger or casual acquaintance. Since the health status of the offender is likely to be unknown, it is difficult to estimate the risk of contracting an STD in any individual case. Moreover, male sex offenders may be at higher risk for STD than the general population. In surveys of sexual behaviors of sex offenders, they report multiple sexual behaviors that would expose them to sexually transmitted organisms, including sexual contact with numerous consenting and nonconsenting male and female partners.[8]

Often, sexual assault victims are seen after a single episode of sexual contact. Little is known about the infectivity of various STDs after a single episode of intercourse, although the relative infectivity of some organisms has been determined.[9] This makes it difficult to estimate the risk of contracting an STD after assault.

In addition, it is difficult to determine if an STD diagnosed after a sexual assault predated the assault or was a result of the assault. Even if a positive culture is obtained shortly after the assault, it is possible that the culture represents bacteria or viruses found in infected semen rather than a previously undiagnosed asymptomatic infection. With some organisms such as herpes simplex virus, changes in antibodies to the organism in the victim's sera can be monitored to discover whether or not the infection was recently acquired.[10] Reliable tests for immune responses to many sexually transmitted organisms do not exist, as in the case of *Neisseria gonorrhoeae*. Others, such as *Chlamydia trachomatis*, are difficult to interpret in relation to the acquisition of repeated infections.

The site of the assault may also affect the likelihood of contracting an STD. For example, because of their predisposition for cervical columnar epithelium, *N. gonorrhoeae* and *C. trachomatis* would be more readily transmitted by vaginal intercourse than by anal or oral intercourse, while human immunodeficiency virus (HIV) would be more likely to be transmitted by anal intercourse.[11]

An increased incidence of postassault infections was found in women who had been assaulted by more than one assailant.[12] However, a later prospective study did not find the same association with number of assailants.[13]

Finally, whether or not the male assailant ejaculates during a sexual assault will affect the likelihood of the victim's contracting an STD. A survey of sexual functioning during episodes of assault reported by male sex offenders in prisons showed that 34 percent were sexually dysfunctional.[14] Sexual problems prohibiting intromission and ejaculation decrease the victim's risk of STD or pregnancy resulting from the assault.

## EPIDEMIOLOGY OF SEXUAL ASSAULT

The epidemiology of sexual assault is similar to the epidemiology of STD. Several risk factors have been defined which are the same for both conditions:

*Age.* Young people are at increased risk of sexual assault. The highest incidence occurs in older adolescents and young adults.[15]

*Marital status.* Single people report sexual assault in disproportionately high numbers.[15] Some of these assaults are "date rapes" that occur after social encounters.

*Socioeconomic status.* Sexual assault is more frequently reported among low-income populations.[16] Poor people are more likely to live in unsafe or overcrowded housing, to live in high-risk neighborhoods, and to have less safe means of transportation.

*Race.* All studies of sexual assault done to date report a higher incidence in minorities. Noncaucasian women report sexual assault twice as frequently as caucasian women.[16]

*Seasonality.* More sexual assaults occur during the summer months than during other times of the year. Fewest occur during the winter months.[17]

The above factors are somewhat interrelated. For instance, young people and minorities are more likely to be poor. Young people are also more likely to be single. All these factors may also be affected by different rates of reporting of sexual assault to law enforcement agencies. People are more likely to report rape if they believe the reporting leads to arrest and conviction of the offender.[18] Different group's perceptions of the effective-

**Table 95-1. Cases of Gonorrhea Found on Initial Evaluation of Sexual Assault Victims**

| Authors | Location | Dates of study | Number of victims | % with gonorrhea |
|---|---|---|---|---|
| Hayman et al. | Washington, DC | 9/65–6/69 | 2190 | 2.4* |
| Kaufman et al. | Albuquerque, NM | ? | 50 | 6.0 |
| Everett et al. | Oklahoma City, OK | 8/73–7/74 | 117 | 12.0 |
| Soules et al. | Denver, CO | 7/74–11/74 | 110 | 9.0 |
| Evard et al. | Providence, RI | 6/30–7/76 | 126 | 4.5 |
| Corey et al. | Seattle, WA | 1976 | 297 | 3.7 |
| Tintinalli et al. | Royal Oak, MI | 7/80–12/80 | 375 | 5.0 |
| Foster et al. | London, GB | 1984 | 46 | 6.5 |
| Jenny et al. | Seattle, WA | 3/85–4/86 | 204 | 6.0 |

*Diagnosis by cervical Gram stain.
SOURCES: Refs. 19, 23, 12, 24, 25, and 2.

ness of the law enforcement could lead to different rates of reporting.

In summary, sexual assault victims are more likely to be young, single, female members of minority groups who have a low income. Many of the same factors have been identified as risk factors for STD. These epidemiologic factors reinforce the need for careful evaluation for STD as part of the medical care of sexual assault victims.

## DATA ON SPECIFIC DISEASES AFTER VAGINAL SEXUAL ASSAULT OF FEMALES

All studies done to date on STD after sexual assault have looked at vaginally assaulted females.[2,12,19–25] No data exist on STD in assaulted males or after anal or oral assault. In addition, no studies have attempted to determine the frequency of STD resulting from the rape instead of preexisting STD or STD acquired after the rape. Treatment with prophylactic antimicrobials and low rates of medical follow-up after assault also make the determination of risk of STD difficult.

Each study will be influenced by the underlying prevalence of disease in the population in the community at the time the data were collected. Most studies have examined the prevalence of gonorrhea and syphilis. Limited data are available on viral STD or vaginitis in this group.

*Gonorrhea.* The rate of cervical infections with *Neisseria gonorrhoeae* detected after sexual assault in female victims in nine studies varied from 2.4 to 12 percent (Table 95-1). The weighted average of the prevalence of gonorrhea in the eight studies where cultures were obtained is 5.9 percent (78/1325). Rates of gonorrhea at follow-up of previously culture-negative victims were 2.6 and 6.6 percent in retrospective chart reviews[12,26] and 2.9 percent in a prospective study.[2] This suggests that the chance of contracting gonorrhea after a sexual assault is low.

*Syphilis.* Rates of positive serologic tests for syphilis in eight studies of sexual assault victims ranged from zero to 4.2 percent.[2,12,19–24] The weighted average of the results of these studies was 3.0 percent (105/3469). Most of these studies did not differentiate between previously treated and newly diagnosed cases of syphilis. Three studies looked at syphilis serologies at follow-up visits. None of these showed any changes from negative to positive serologies.[2,12,26]

*Chlamydia.* Two studies of *Chlamydia trachomatis* infections in female rape victims have been done. In Seattle, 10.1 percent (20/198) of women were found to be infected when examined immediately after their assault.[2] At follow-up, the rate of infection in women whose initial cultures were negative and who had not had prophylactic antibiotics was 1.5 percent.[2] In London, the infection rate was 13 percent (6/46), although patients were examined up to 1 year after the assault.[25]

*Vaginitis.* Three studies have shown the rates of trichomonal vaginitis (TV) and bacterial vaginosis (BV) at initial examinations of female rape victims to be as high as or higher than the infection rates the *N. gonorrhoeae* or *C. trachomatis*.[2,12,25] *Candida albicans* infections were found less frequently.[12,25] The rates of BV and TV are even higher at sexual assault follow-up visits (Table 95–2).

*Viral STD.* Studies show the prevalence and rate of acquisition of viral STD is low in rape victims (Table 95-3). Only 1.6 percent of 193 sexual assault victims in 1976 acquired primary genital herpes.[12] In 1985–1986 in Seattle, none of 31 sexually assaulted victims had acquired HIV antibody at follow-up. Concern about these diseases in sexual assault victims is great because of the serious and incurable nature of AIDS and genital herpes. These studies suggest that the victim is unlikely to become infected with HIV or HSV because of sexual assault.

Rates of abnormal Papanicolaou (Pap) smears of the cervix in sexual assault victims were reported in three studies, ranging from 3.5 to 27.2 percent.[2,25,27] Some of these abnormalities were undoubtedly caused by human papillomavirus (HPV) infections. In addition, 2.1 percent of rape victims examined in London up to 1 year after sexual assault had clinically obvious condyloma acuminatum.[25]

In summary, STDs are frequently diagnosed in rape victims. *N. gonorrhoeae* and *C. trachomatis* are less frequently found than trichomoniasis and bacterial vaginosis. Syphilis and viral STD are rarely reported after assault. Genital herpes and HIV infections are not likely to be contracted during a sexual assault, but the threat of these infections creates severe anxiety for victims. STD

**Table 92-2. Vaginitis Diagnosed in Sexual Assault Patients at Follow-up Examinations**

| | Corey et al | | Jenny et al | |
|---|---|---|---|---|
| | Number | Percent | Number | Percent |
| Bacterial vaginosis | 13/193 | 6.7 | 29/109* | 26.6* |
| Trichomonal vaginitis | 12/193 | 6.2 | 27/109† | 24.7† |
| Candidal vaginitis | 12/193 | 6.2 | | |

*Diagnosed by wet mount and/or Gram stain.
†Diagnosed by wet mount and/or culture.
SOURCES: Refs. 12 and 2.

Table 93-3. Viral STD in Sexual Assault Victims

| | HSV* | CMV† | HIV‡ | Condyloma acuminatum |
|---|---|---|---|---|
| Corey et al., follow-up | 1.6% | — | — | — |
| Foster et al., initial | — | — | — | 2.1% |
| Jenny et al.: | | | | |
| Initial | 2.4% | 7.6% | 0.8% | — |
| Follow-up | 0.0% | 14.9% | 0.0% | — |

*Herpes simplex virus diagnosed by culture.
†Cytomegalovirus diagnosed by culture.
‡Antibody to human immunodeficiency virus by ELISA and Western blot (blind testing on unlabeled sera).
SOURCES: Refs. 12, 25, and 2.

after assault is common enough to warrant a thorough diagnostic work-up for STD as part of a sexual assault evaluation.

## STD AS EVIDENCE IN SEXUAL ASSAULT CASES

Sexually transmitted diseases are often a factor in sexual assault cases tried in courts of law in the United States. STDs have been recognized by criminal courts as proof that sexual contact has occurred, especially where the victim is a child or young adolescent.[28] STD as evidence of rape has been upheld when both the defendant and the victim were infected with the same disease.[29–32] Even when a child victim was infected without evidence that the accused rapist was infected, the Alabama Court of Appeals held that "such . . . evidence was competent to show the corpus delicti" (that a crime had been committed).[33]

When an STD is found in the victim and is thought to be the result of sexual contact with the accused, positive cultures or blood tests for antibodies from the defendant can be helpful as corroborative evidence. The collection of those specimens, however, must be done without violating the defendant's rights. Compulsory physical examinations and blood tests for diagnosis of a sexually transmitted disease without permission of the accused or without a court order to obtain such evidence were once held by some courts to violate witnesses' immunity from testifying against themselves.[34,35] A ruling in 1893 said "that an accused person cannot be compelled to exhibit those portions of his body which are usually covered, for the purpose of securing his identification, or in other ways affording evidence against him."[35]

However, under the modern federal rules of evidence for criminal proceedings, cultures, blood tests, and physical examinations for STD can be done on the defendant after court hearings are held before a judge to determine "probable cause" that evidence will be recovered. The defendant's fourth amendment rights to protection from unreasonable search and seizure must be respected.[36]

The interpretation of STD evidence requires a thorough knowledge of the epidemiology, natural course of infection, infectivity, and response to treatment of the STD in question. For instance, if a victim is found to be infected with an STD at the time of a rape, the accused may not become infected after a single act of intercourse. Negative cultures obtained from the defendant will not necessarily prove he did not commit the crime.

When positive cultures are obtained from both the victim and the assailant, matching the organisms for various biologic properties can be useful in linking the assailant to the crime. In three cases, strains of *N. gonorrhoeae* from both molested children and their alleged assailants were matched for auxotypes and serovars.[37] In each case, the organisms were the same between the victim-offender pairs, and the biologic characteristics of the organisms were used as corroborative evidence. Such matching can be used if the characteristics studied are stable from generation to generation in in vivo and in vitro systems. Potentially, DNA restriction mapping could provide very specific matching of organisms to trace the path of transmittal between sexual partners.[38]

## DIAGNOSIS AND TREATMENT OF STD IN VICTIMS OF SEXUAL ASSAULT

### DIAGNOSTIC TESTS FOR STD

Five diagnostic tests for STD after sexual assault are recommended by the Centers for Disease Control (see Table 95–4).[39] A follow-up visit at 7 days postassault is recommended. However, a 2-week follow-up visit would be less likely to miss acquired chlamydial infections.

Given the frequency of STD in these patients, other tests may be indicated if available. Additional tests for trichomoniasis such as culture or monoclonal antibody stains will increase the yield of infections diagnosed. The standard wet amount is a relatively insensitive diagnostic method for this organism, and will probably miss 40 percent of infection.[40]

It is extremely important to emphasize to victims the importance of a follow-up examination for evidence of new infections. Even if prophylactic antimicrobials are used, it is impractical to treat for the entire spectrum of infections which might occur. Prophylactic antimicrobials may give the patient a false sense of security regarding other STDs which may have been acquired during the assault. Special care should be taken to explain the reasons why follow-up evaluations are necessary.

Other diagnostic tests may be indicated depending on the situation. If the offender is known to be in a high-risk group for AIDS or hepatitis B, the appropriate serologic test for those diseases can be done. Many victims are now requesting tests for HIV antibody. Testing should be done only after counseling the patient about the implications of positive or negative tests.[41]

Although no studies have been done on the incidence of STD in male victims after sexual assault, screening tests for *N. gonorrhoeae*, *C. trachomatis*, and syphilis should be done as they are for female victims. Other tests to be done should depend on the risk of infection given the nature of the assault and assailant, and on the patient's symptoms postassault.

Table 95-4. Recommended Diagnostic Tests for STD in Sexual Assault Victims

Initial visit

1. Cultures for *N. gonorrhoeae* from any potentially infected sites
2. If available, cultures for *C. trachomatis* from any infected sites
3. Examinations of vaginal specimens for *T. vaginalis* by wet mount and, if available, by culture
4. A serologic test for syphilis
5. A sample of serum to be frozen and saved for future testing

Follow-up

1. Repeat above except for syphilis serology and frozen serum at 7 days
2. Syphilis serology at 6 weeks

SOURCE: Ref. 39.

## THE USE OF PROPHYLACTIC ANTIBIOTICS

Current CDC recommendations do not call for the routine use of prophylactic antimicrobials but suggest that each patient be evaluated individually.[39] Prophylaxis may be indicated if the patient is not likely to return for follow-up or if the patient is extremely anxious about the possibility of contracting an STD.

Prophylactic regimens should be effective against both *N. gonorrhoeae* and *C. trachomatis* because of the potentially serious nature of their complications. Amoxicillin combined with probenecid or ceftriaxone alone can be used to protect against *N. gonorrhoeae*, depending on the nature and extent of antimicrobial resistant organisms found in the community. Tetracycline or doxycycline are effective against *C. trachomatis*. Although trichomoniasis and bacterial vaginosis are commonly found after sexual assault of females, no prophylactic regimen of low risk and toxicity has been tested against these infections.

More importantly, prophylaxis is no substitute for careful follow-up for STD and/or unwanted pregnancy after sexual assault. At a follow-up visit, the patient's physical and emotional status can be evaluated, and appropriate treatment or referral can be offered. Good medical care after assault can help alleviate some of the patient's anxieties and fears, and can help him or her return to a more normal functional status.

## References


1 Rodabaugh BJ, Austin M: *Sexual Assault*. New York, Garland STPM Press, 1981, pp 6–10.

2 Jenny C et al: STD in victims of sexual assault. Presented at ISSTDR, Atlanta, GA, 1987.

3 US Department of Justice: *Uniform Crime Reports for the United States*. Washington, DC, Government Printing Office, 1985.

4 Schiff AF: Rape in other countries. *Med Sci Law* 11:3, 1971.

5 Russell DEH: *Sexual Exploitation: Rape, Child Sexual Abuse, and Workplace Harassment*. Beverly Hills, CA, Sage, 1985, p 35.

6 Holmstrom LL: The criminal justice system's response to the rape victim, in *Rape and Sexual Assault*, AW Burgess (ed). New York, Garland Publishing, 1985, pp 189–191.

7 Glaser JB et al: Sexually transmitted diseases in victims of sexual assault. *N Engl J Med* 315:625, 1986.

8 Abel GG et al: Self-reported sex crimes of nonincarcerated paraphiliacs. *J Interpersonal Violence* 2:3, 1987.

9 McCutchan JA: Epidemiology of venereal urethritis: Comparison of gonorrhea and nongonococcal urethritis. *Rev Infect Dis* 6:669, 1984.

10 Nahmias AJ et al: Antibodies to herpesvirus hominis types 1 and 2 in humans: Patients with genital infections. *Am J Epidemiol* 91:539, 1970.

11 Winkelstein W et al: Sexual practices and risk of infection by the human immunodeficiency virus: The San Francisco Men's Health Study. *JAMA* 257:321, 1987.

12 Corey L et al: Sexually transmitted diseases after sexual assault. Unpublished data.

13 Hooton TM et al: Evaluation of criteria for antimicrobial prophylaxis after sexual assault. Presented at ISSTDR, Atlanta, GA, August 1987.

14 Groth AN, Burgess AW: Sexual dysfunction during rape. *N Engl J Med* 297:764, 1977.

15 Amir M: *Patterns in Forcible Rape*. Chicago, University of Chicago Press, 1971, pp 51–52.

16 *Report to the Nation on Crime and Justice: The Data*. Washington, DC, US Department of Justice, NCJ–87068, 1983, p 20.

17 Katz S, Mazur MA: *Understanding the Rape Victim: A Synthesis of Research Findings*, New York, Wiley, 1979, pp 132–133.

18 Lizotte AJ: The uniqueness of rape: Reporting assaultive violence to the police. *Crime Delinquency* 31:169, 1985.

19 Hayman CR, Lanza C: Sexual assault on women and girls. *Am J Obstet Gynecol* 109:480, 1971.

20 Kaufman A et al: Follow-up of rape victims in a family practice setting. *South Med J* 69:1569, 1976.

21 Everett RB, Jimerson GK: The rape victim: A review of 117 consecutive cases. *Obstet Gynecol* 50:88, 1977.

22 Soules MR et al: The spectrum of alleged rape. *J Reprod Med* 20:33, 1978.

23 Evard JR, Gold EM: Epidemiology and management of sexual assault victims. *Obstet Gynecol* 53:381, 1989.

24 Tintinalli JE, Hoelzer M: Clinical findings and legal resolution in sexual assault. *Ann Emerg Med* 14:447, 1985.

25 Forster GE et al: Incidence of sexually transmitted diseases in rape victims during 1984. *Genitourin Med* 62:267, 1986.

26 Hayman CR et al: Rape in the District of Columbia. *Am J Obstet Gynecol* 113:91, 1972.

27 Seltzer VL et al: Abnormal Papanicolaou smears found in victims of sexual assault. *J Reprod Med* 20:233, 1978.

28 Annot., Rape—What constitutes penetration? 76 ALR 3d 163, 1977.

29 *Poe v State*, 95 Ark 172, 129 SW 292, 1910.

30 *Long v State*, 84 Ga App 638, 66 SE 2d 837, 1951.

31 *State v Mason*, 152 Minn 306, 189 NW 452, 1922.

32 *State v Oliver*, 78 ND 398, 49 NW 2nd 564, 1951.

33 *Malone v State*, 37 Ala App 432, 71 So 99, 1953.

34 *State v Horton*, 247 Mo 663, 153 SW 1051, 1912.

35 *State v Nordstrom*, 7 Wash 506, 35 P 382, 1853.

36 *Schmerber v California*, 384 US 757, 16 L Ed 2d 908, 86 S CT 1826, 1966.

37 Morse SA et al: Use of auxotype/serovar classification of *Neisseria gonorrhoeae* isolates for forensic purposes. Unpublished manuscript.

38 Peterson E et al: Typing of clinical herpes simplex virus isolates with mouse monoclonal antibodies to herpes simplex virus types I and II: Comparison with type-specific rabbit antisera and restriction endonuclease analysis of viral DNA. *J Clin Microbiol* 17:92, 1983.

39 Centers for Disease Control: *1985 STD Treatment Guidelines*, Atlanta, 1985.

40 Krieger JN et al: Diagnosis of trichomoniasis: Comparison of conventional wet mount examination with cytological studies, culture, and monoclonal antibody staining of direct specimens. *JAMA* 259:1223 1988.

41 Public Health Service guidelines for counseling and antibody testing to prevent HIV infection and AIDS. *MMWR* 36:509, 1987.

# EPILOGUE FUTURE DIRECTIONS

# Epilogue
# Future directions

King K. Holmes
Per-Anders Mårdh
P. Frederick Sparling
Paul J. Wiesner
Willard Cates, Jr.
Stanley M. Lemon
Walter E. Stamm

## HOW DID THE CURRENT SITUATION DEVELOP?

During the first half of the 20th century, important directions in venereology included the social hygiene movement, the development of improved diagnostic tests through microbiologic research, and the development of effective antimicrobials for gonorrhea and syphilis. After World War II, the incidence of gonorrhea and syphilis fell in every developed country, and the specialty of dermatovenereology all but disappeared in most. In the United States, for example, local public health departments assumed the role of "mopping up" the remaining cases of venereal disease, which seemed to be retreating to pockets of high incidence in indigent populations in large cities and in the South. Few countries—England and Wales being notable exceptions—maintained an active academically based venereology specialty.

However, demographic and behavioral changes, among others, were occurring that ultimately led to a resurgence not only of gonorrhea and syphilis but also to epidemics of a panoply of other sexually transmitted infections and to a growing contribution by sexual transmission to the spread of infections not previously regarded as venereal diseases. These changes included the emergence of growing numbers of adolescent and young adult baby-boomers, the advent of effective oral contraception, and increasingly permissive attitudes toward sexual freedom dating back at least to World War I and culminating in the sexual revolution and the gay liberation movement during the 1960s and 1970s.

As a result, the gonorrhea epidemic of the 1960s was followed by epidemic rates of syphilis in homosexual men, and this was followed in turn by recognition of epidemic increases in genital chlamydial infection and genital herpes during the 1970s. By the late 1970s, sexual transmission was recognized as an important route of transmission of hepatitis B, cytomegalovirus, and various enteric infections. Clinical epidemiological research intensified on the relationship of STD to infertility, to morbidity of pregnancy and the puerperium, to perinatal infection, and to genital cancers. When the incidence of gonorrhea began to decline during the 1970s in all developed countries, and the incidence of syphilis leveled off or began to fall in many countries, it appeared that public health measures were working, at least for control of the curable STDs. However, the recognition of AIDS as a fatal sexually transmitted viral syndrome has irrevocably changed the direction of future work on STDs.

In contemplating future directions in the STD field, these past events underscore the influence of social and demographic forces, of unanticipated biomedical advances (e.g., improved diagnosis, therapy, and oral contraceptives), and the possibility of unanticipated ecological phenomena (e.g., the explosive spread of HIV in homosexual men, in intravenous drug users, and in urban heterosexual populations of many countries). They reveal the extent to which we can and cannot predict future changes in this field.

## STD DURING THE AIDS ERA

Unprecedented efforts have been brought to bear during the 1980s on studying molecular mechanisms of HIV infection, and on behavioral interventions for primary prevention of HIV infection.

As health education and individual counseling have been developed for primary prevention, these have initially focused on reduction of high-risk sexual behavior among homosexual men and on providing information about AIDS and HIV infection to the general public. Substantial risk reduction by homosexual men has been well documented and, although not equally impressive in all regions, is responsible for dramatic reductions among homosexual men in the incidence not only of HIV infection but also of other STDs, such as syphilis, gonorrhea, and acute hepatitis B. We have also witnessed a marked shift in the pattern of intestinal infections in this group.

Among heterosexuals in developed countries, the decline in the incidence of gonorrhea has accelerated during the mid-1980s, a fact suggestive of sexual behavior changes in some heterosexuals during the AIDS era. It is hoped that such trends may also presage a decline in the incidence of the incurable viral STDs.

## RISE OF STD IN THE INNER CITY: CONTRACTION OF THE EPIDEMIC AROUND AN EXPANDING CORE

Unfortunately, in North America these encouraging trends have been limited to those middle class populations most likely to respond early to health education. In certain black, Hispanic, Native American, and Native Canadian populations, incidence rates of gonorrhea and chlamydial infection are not falling, and rates of syphilis and chancroid have actually increased rapidly during the past few years in cities and even in rural areas.

Several socioeconomic factors contribute to the epidemic spread of bacterial STD and of HIV as well in inner city populations. These include the sustained relatively high birth rates in ethnic minority groups, which result in a growing proportion of these populations in the 15- to 29-year-old age group; the continuing disintegration of family and social structures; and worsening poverty in inner cities. These trends contribute to the current "crack" cocaine epidemic, which began in the Caribbean and in North America in the mid-eighties and is now spreading to other continents, and to the increasing inability of public health programs to meet the growing need for diagnostic and treatment services for STDs in the inner cities.

As rates of the treatable bacterial STDs fall rapidly in the white middle class population—in homosexual men as well as in heterosexuals—as they rise rapidly in inner city minority groups, the relative contribution of the latter groups to the maintenance and spread of STD grow. Within inner city ethnic minority populations, those involved in prostitution or sex-in-exchange-for-drugs appear to be especially important as core transmitters of easily treatable STDs such as gonorrhea, syphilis, and chancroid, and probably for such other STDs as HIV and hepatitis B virus infection as well. Thus, clearer definition and interruption of the factors responsible for such practices and for spread of STD within and from STD core groups is a matter of urgent and high priority.

## THE ROLE OF RESEARCH

Clearly, basic and applied research continues to contribute at an increasingly rapid pace to improved understanding of the pathogenesis and immunobiology of STD. The most important practical consequence to date of research in the basic sciences has been the development of improved diagnostic tests and improved treatments for STDs. STDs have figured prominently in the early applications of biotechnology for improved diagnostics; and in important applications of new pharmaceutical agents—particularly beta lactams, quinolones, macrolides, and the new antiviral agents. However, curative therapies are still needed for the incurable viral STDs, such as HIV, HPV, HSV-2, and hepatitis B. Although an intensive research effort is focused on creating vaccines for several STDs (gonorrhea, syphilis, HSV, HIV, and others), no new vaccine for a major STD is on the immediate horizon. It nonetheless remains necessary to press for continued research to develop STD vaccines—not only for HIV but for the other major STDs as well. Basic research is needed on sexual and drug use behaviors in representative samples of the general population, in different cultures, and in high-risk groups; on determinants of high-risk behaviors; and on the comparative efficacy of innovative behavioral interventions. Finally, epidemiologic methodology has been increasingly important in defining patterns of transmission of STDs and in defining the risk factors for their transmission and for the development of preventable complications; in defining the role of STD pathogens in important human diseases; and in conducting clinical trials of new diagnostics, therapeutics, and prevention strategies, including vaccines.

Unfortunately, we have failed to use the one available STD vaccine (that for hepatitis B) in a way that prevents its sexual transmission, which is the major known route of transmission of hepatitis B virus in developed countries. Clearly, the behavioral and policy issues regarding utilization of such vaccines require closer attention. Thus, the recommendations for improved use of available methods are very relevant today—not only for the use of the hepatitis B vaccine but also for the use of many other effective tools for primary and secondary prevention of STD. These recommendations have been provided in several recent documents.[1–3]

## WHAT METHODS WORK FOR STD CONTROL, AND HOW CAN WE USE AVAILABLE METHODS MORE EFFECTIVELY?

The importance of behavioral intervention to reduce high-risk sexual behavior in ethnic minority groups is increasingly apparent. Moreover, improved health care-seeking behavior is both attainable and important, particularly for control of bacterial STD.

In addition to those primary prevention strategies which are already having a measurable impact on reducing the incidence of HIV infection and other STD in homosexual men, the secondary prevention strategies available for control of curable STD include the appropriate use of laboratory diagnosis and the treatment of infected patients and their sexual contacts. These strategies have clearly been highly effective in controlling gonorrhea, syphilis, chancroid, and trichomoniasis in developed countries. Furthermore, in Sweden, in King County, Washington, and elsewhere where public funds have been provided to implement chlamydia control programs, the proportion of screening cultures for *Chlamydia trachomatis* that are positive has been steadily falling among females. It appears that programs to control genital chlamydial infection can be as effective as programs to control the other curable STDs. The failure of public health departments to obtain resources to develop chlamydia control programs has been particularly frustrating.

It is ironic that, while expenditures for health education, for partner notification, and for counseling to improve health care-seeking behavior are increasing, many public STD clinics have not kept up with the growing demand for clinical health care services. Thus, in many major cities, patient waiting times are getting longer, and growing numbers of infected patients are turned away. In England, efforts to upgrade genitourinary medicine clinic facilities and to increase clinical staff are being made. In the United States, such efforts appear to vary markedly at the local public health level: in recent years some clinics have greatly expanded their clinic hours and staff and have provided new clinical services for STDs to increased numbers of patients, while other clinics have reallocated their resources to HIV testing and counseling and have, in effect, decreased services for diagnosis and treatment of other STDs. It seems evident that many public health programs have failed to provide increased services for diagnosis and treatment to match the increasing funding for primary prevention through behavioral intervention and that this programmatic imbalance is at least partly responsible for a gradual but continuing shift of patient care services for STDs from the public to the private sector. More balanced allocation of resources is appropriate. Why should we spend more to improve health care-seeking behavior and partner notification when clinics are turning patients away?

The greatest challenge today for those involved in STD is to design and implement primary and secondary prevention programs for impoverished populations in developing countries and in the inner cities of developed countries. What is needed is the political will to develop national STD program priorities, goals, and strategies, and also to allocate sufficient resources to implement those strategies needed to achieve the program goals. In all countries, AIDS and STD programs must be coordinated in the context of an evolving national program for AIDS and STD, and these programs should make the maximum use possible of existing health infrastructures, including STD clinics, family planning clinics, and maternal and child health clinics. Many of these facilities urgently require upgrading and expansion, and they must substantially re-orient activities so as to include primary prevention of STD through modification of sexual behavior and promotion of the use of condoms. All of these clinics should offer diagnosis and treatment of STD and testing and counseling for HIV, where possible.

In Asia, Latin America, and, particularly, in Africa, control of certain STDs, such as gonorrhea and chlamydial infection, will ultimately depend on the development and use of more cost-effective diagnostic tests for detection of subclinical infection. In these regions, programs for primary prevention deserve higher priority. Even in these developing regions, however, secondary prevention of syphilis, chancroid, and trichomoniasis, is possible now through early diagnosis and treatment, using available cost-effective methods. Since syphilis, chancroid, and trichomoniasis, as well as genital chlamydial infection and HSV-2 infection have been implicated as risk factors for transmission of HIV, innovative programs for control of these infections should receive high priority for rapid development, implementation, and evaluation in all countries.

## WHO IS RESPONSIBLE FOR PREVENTION AND MANAGEMENT OF STD?

Currently, the responsibility of various components of the health care system for prevention and management of STD and HIV infection is not completely settled. The task of dealing with STDs clinically was taken up during the 1960s and 1970s by a variety of medical disciplines, among them public health and preventive medicine, dermatology, gynecology, pediatrics and adolescent medicine, and—particularly in North America—infectious diseases. The need for clinical specialists with expertise in managing AIDS and other STDs has subsequently grown, even as the pivotal role of the primary care clinician in managing these problems has become increasingly obvious. We believe that all primary care physicians should be able to manage most manifestations of STDs, including AIDS. Moreover, they should be able to take a sexual history and establish risk of exposure to STDs. They should initiate notification of sexual partners and request assistance from public health agencies or specialists for difficult or unusual problems. Despite recent emphasis on such training for medical students, residents, and practicing physicians, these goals are largely unmet. Thus, public health agencies should provide expertise and services for diagnosis, treatment, partner notification, and counseling for STDs to all who need it, and they should provide expert consultation and training to physicians and students. When the lines of patients waiting to be registered at STD clinics begin to lengthen, and patients are turned away, the public health system has failed to cope with even the most elementary aspects of the problem. We must acknowledge and correct the failure of society and of politicians to support the basic needs for public health in general[4] and for STD control in particular.

What should be the role of public clinics in the management of HIV infection? We believe that wherever possible, they should perform pretest counseling, HIV testing, and comprehensive posttest clinical evaluation of seropositive patients. The latter will result in the most effective counseling of these individuals and will allow appropriate referrals to primary care physicians. Although medical care for persons living with AIDS should be largely in the private sector in many countries, funding of public AIDS clinics is now needed in most major cities.

## ROLE OF OTHER HEALTH CARE SPECIALISTS AND EDUCATORS IN STD CONTROL

Other health care providers are greatly underutilized in dealing with STDs. Pharmacists, for example, have the opportunity to encourage primary prevention through education and promotion of condom use at the local level in their own communities. In developing countries, where pharmacists may provide initial diagnosis and treatment to a large proportion of patients with STDs, they can be even more effectively utilized in STD control programs. The content of public health training for pharmacists thus deserves close examination. Nurse clinicians provide much of the direct medical care for patients in public clinics in North America and are the principal participants in federally funded regional clinical STD training programs in the United States. Their role in the management of persons with AIDS—for whom adequate numbers of primary care physicians have been difficult to find—is now being assessed.

Professionals trained in the behavioral sciences should be better utilized by having them participate in behavioral intervention with the individual high-risk patient. The most appropriate training and experience for behavior intervention specialists in the STD field should be determined. With the growing importance of disease prevention in general, and with modification of sexual and drug use behaviors being in the vanguard of behavioral research, training in public health and behavioral sciences must be combined to develop a new cadre of preventive medicine professionals.

Innovative programs for prevention of high-risk sexual behaviors, STDs, and drug use must clearly deal with adolescents in a variety of settings, including schools, churches, and community organizations. As with other social skills, those skills needed to cope with high-risk sexual experiences must be taught before risky sexual experiences are "imprinted." Adolescent peers can be moved to support postponing sexual intercourse and to support the routine use of condoms during sexual intercourse. For the foreseeable future, the major strides in preventing STD-related morbidity and mortality will depend on widespread use of interventions designed for those who are entering their sexually formative years.

## References

1 *Control of Sexually Transmitted Diseases.* World Health Organization, Geneva, 1985.

2 WHO Expert Committee on Venereal Diseases and Treponematoses, Sixth Report. *Tech Report Series 736.* World Health Organization, Geneva, 1986.

3 Turner, CF, Miller HG, Moses LE, National Research Council: *AIDS, Sexual Behavior and Intravenous Drug Use.* National Academy Press, 1989.

4 Institute of Medicine: *The Future of Public Health.* Washington, D.C.: National Academy Press, 1988.

# APPENDIX 1989 SEXUALLY TRANSMITTED DISEASES TREATMENT GUIDELINES

Appendix

# 1989 Sexually transmitted diseases treatment guidelines*†

## TABLE OF CONTENTS



*U.S. Department of Health and Human Services
Public Health Service
Division of Sexually Transmitted Diseases
Center for Prevention Services
Centers for Disease Control
Atlanta, Georgia 30333

†The use of trade names and commercial sources is for identification purposes only and does not constitute endorsement by the Public Health Service or by the Department of Health and Human Services

## ABBREVIATIONS USED IN THIS PUBLICATION

| | |
|---|---|
| ACIP | Advisory Committee on Immunization Practices |
| AIDS | Acquired immunodeficiency syndrome |
| BV | Bacterial vaginosis |
| CDC | Centers for Disease Control |
| CMRNG | Chromosomally mediated resistant *Neisseria gonorrhoeae* |
| CMV | Cytomegalovirus |
| CSF | Cerebrospinal fluid |
| DGI | Disseminated gonococcal infection |
| DIS | Disease Intervention Specialist |
| ELISA | Enzyme-linked immunosorbent assay |
| FTA-ABS | Fluorescent treponemal antibody absorbed |
| HBIG | Hepatitis B immune globulin |
| HBsAg | Hepatitis B surface antigen |
| HIV | Human immunodeficiency virus |
| HPV | Human papillomavirus |
| HSV | Herpes simplex virus |
| IM | Intramuscularly |
| IV | Intravenous or intravenously |
| LGV | Lymphogranuloma venereum |
| MHATP | Microhemagglutination assay for antibody to *Treponema pallidum* |
| MPC | Mucopurulent cervicitis |
| NGU | Nongonococcal urethritis |
| PID | Pelvic inflammatory disease |
| PPD | Purified protein derivative |
| PPNG | Penicillinase-producing *N. gonorrhoeae* |
| RPR | Rapid plasma reagin |
| STD | Sexually transmitted disease(s) |
| TCA | Trichloroacetic acid |
| TRNG | Tetracycline-resistant *N. gonorrhoeae* |
| VDRL | Venereal Disease Research Laboratory |
| ZDV | Zidovudine |

## INTRODUCTION

These guidelines for treatment of sexually transmitted diseases (STD) were established after consultation with a group of outside experts and staff of the Centers for Disease Control (CDC). These guidelines represent their best judgment based on the available efficacy data, practical applicability to the majority of clinical situations, and cost. These recommendations should not be construed as rules, but rather as a source of clinical guidance within the United States. The guidelines focus on the STD treatment and counseling of individual patients and do not address other community services and interventions which may play roles in STD prevention. Clinical and laboratory diagnosis are briefly alluded to when appropriate in the context of therapy.

## EXPERT CONSULTANTS

King K. Holmes, M.D., Ph.D. (Co-Chair), University of Washington School of Medicine

P. Frederick Sparling, M.D. (Co-Chair), University of North Carolina School of Medicine
Jorge D. Blanco, M.D., Texas Tech University Medical School
Gail Bolan, M.D., San Francisco Department of Public Health and UCSF School of Medicine
Virginia Caine, M.D., Bellflower Clinic, Indianapolis
Margaret Hammerschlag, M.D., State University of New York Health Science Center at Brooklyn
Edward W. Hook III, M.D., Johns Hopkins University School of Medicine and Baltimore City Health Department
Robert B. Jones, M.D., Ph.D., University of Indiana School of Medicine
Franklyn N. Judson, M.D., Denver Department of Health
William M. McCormack, M.D., State University of New York Health Science Center at Brooklyn
Richard C. Reichman, M.D., University of Rochester School of Medicine
Allan R. Ronald, M.D., University of Manitoba Health Science Center (Winnipeg)
A. Eugene Washington, M.D., Stanford University School of Medicine
Richard J. Whitley, M.D., University of Alabama School of Medicine
M. Lynn Yonekura, M.D., UCLA School of Medicine

## LIAISON OBSERVERS

Sandra Adamson Fryhofer, M.D., Atlanta, Georgia, American College of Physicians
H. Hunter Handsfield, M.D., Seattle-King County Department of Public Health, University of Washington; Infectious Disease Society of America
William R. Bowie, M.D., University of British Columbia; Canadian Laboratory Centre for Disease Control
Kenneth Noller, M.D., University of Massachusetts; American College of Obstetrics and Gynecology
Peter L. Perine, M.D., Uniformed Services University of Health Sciences

## STAFF, CENTERS FOR DISEASE CONTROL

Willard Cates, Jr., M.D., M.P.H., Director, Division of Sexually Transmitted Diseases, Center for Prevention Services
E. Russell Alexander, M.D., Chief, Epidemiology Research Branch, Division of Sexually Transmitted Diseases, Center for Prevention Services
STD Treatment Guidelines 1989 Project—Jonathan M. Zenilman, M.D., Coordinator; Contributors: Robert C. Barnes, M.D.; Yvonne T. Green, M.S.N., Stephen J. Kraus, M.D.; Joseph G. Lossick, D.O., M.S.; John S. Moran, M.D.; Allyn K. Nakashima, M.D.; Thomas A. Peterman, M.D., M.Sc.; Herbert B. Peterson, M.D.; Robert T. Rolfs, Jr., M.D.; George P. Schmid, M.D.; Sandra K. Schwarcz, M.D; Katherine M. Stone, M.D.; Kathleen Toomey, M.D.; M.P.H.; William L. Whittington; Paul Zenker, M.D., M.P.H. Editor: Martha S. Mayfield. Staff: Sandra W. Bowden, Garrett K. Mallory.

## USER'S GUIDE

STDs and their therapies have been categorized by etiologic agent, where possible. Some syndromes overlap; for example, urethritis may be caused by *Neisseria gonorrhoeae* or *Chlamydia trachomatis*. The following table (Table 1) correlates disease syndromes with etiologic organisms and directs the user to the appropriate section in this document.

**Table 1**

| Symptoms/Signs | Organism/ Syndrome | Document Section | Page |
|---|---|---|---|
| **Infections in Men** | | | |
| Urethritis | *N. gonorrhoeae* | Gonorrhea | A-13 |
| | *C. trachomatis* | Chlamydia | A-16 |
| | Herpes simplex virus (HSV) | Herpes (primary) | A-11 |
| | *Mycoplasma hominis* | Nongonococcal urethritis (NGU) | A-16 |
| | *Ureaplasma urealyticum* | NGU | A-16 |
| | Uncharacterized | NGU | A-16 |
| Epididymitis | | See specific section | A-17 |
| **Infections in Women** | | | |
| Cervicitis | *N. gonorrhoeae* | Gonorrhea | A-13 |
| | *C. trachomatis* | Chlamydia | A-16 |
| | HSV | Herpes | A-11 |
| Mucopurulent cervicitis (MPC) | | See specific section | A-17 |
| Pelvic inflammatory disease (PID) | | See specific section | A-17 |
| Vaginal infections | *Trichomonas vaginalis* | Trichomoniasis | A-19 |
| | *Candida albicans* | Candida infections | A-19 |
| | Bacterial vaginosis (BV) | See specific section | A-20 |
| Perinatal infections | *Treponema pallidum* | Syphilis | A-7 |
| | *N. gonorrhoeae* | Gonorrhea | A-13 |
| | *C. trachomatis* | Chlamydia | A-16 |
| | HSV | Herpes | A-11 |
| | BV | BV | A-20 |
| | Candida | Candida infections | A-19 |
| | *T. vaginalis* | Trichomoniasis | A-19 |
| | Human immunodeficiency virus (HIV) | HIV | A-6 |
| | Human papillomavirus (HPV) | Genital warts | A-12 |
| | Hepatitis B | Hepatitis B | A-20 |
| | Cytomegalovirus (CMV) | Cytomegalovirus | A-21 |
| **Infections in Both Men and Women** | | | |
| Genital ulcer disease | *T. pallidum* | Syphilis | A-7 |
| | *Haemophilus ducreyi* | Chancroid | A-6 |
| | HSV | Herpes | A-11 |
| | *C. trachomatis* | Lymphogranuloma venereum (LGV) | A-11 |
| Genital warts | Human papillomavirus (HPV) | Genital warts | A-12 |
| Enteric infection | | See specific section | A-18 |
| Proctitis (See also enteric infections) | *N. gonorrhoeae* | Gonorrhea | A-13 |
| | *C. trachomatis* | Chlamydia | A-16 |
| | *T. pallidum* | Syphilis | A-7 |
| | HSV | Herpes | A-11 |

| Symptoms/Signs | Organism/ Syndrome | Document Section | Page |
|---|---|---|---|
| Proctitis (*cont.*) | Other | See enteric infection section | A-18 |
| Ophthalmic disease (See specific section for general prevention) | *N. gonorrhoeae* | Gonorrhea | A-13 |
| | *C. trachomatis* | Chlamydia | A-16 |

## CLINICIAN GUIDELINES AND PUBLIC HEALTH CONSIDERATIONS

Control of STD is based on four major concepts: First, education of those at risk on the modes of disease transmission and means to reduce the risk of transmission; second, detection of asymptomatically infected individuals and persons who are symptomatic but unlikely to seek diagnostic and treatment services; third, effective diagnosis and treatment of those who are infected; fourth, evaluation, treatment, and counseling of sex partners of persons with an STD. Although this document deals largely with clinical aspects of STD control, it must be stressed that in most cases, primary prevention of STD is based on changing the sexual behaviors which put patients at risk.

## CLINICAL CONSIDERATIONS

For persons requesting health services for evaluation of an STD, appropriate care consists of the following components (the temporal order of the interventions may vary depending on the specific case and diagnosis):

History
Medical and behavioral risk assessment
Physical examination
Laboratory investigations
Diagnosis
Curative or palliative therapy
Counseling and education:
  Present episode of STD
  Prevention of future episodes
Reporting of case when required
Sex partner identification, notification, and evaluation
Clinical follow-up when appropriate

Persons who are seeking health care services for other reasons, but who are at risk for acquisition of STD,* should undergo the following as part of their routine health care:

STD risk assessment
Directed physical examination based on elicited symptoms
Screening for asymptomatic infections

In special situations, such as prenatal visits and in women undergoing legally induced abortion, screening for STD may have greater impact in preventing complications of STD. For specific recommendations in cases of sexual assault or child abuse, see page A-21.

Specific guidelines for screening in each situation are beyond the scope of this document. However, whenever possible, the following laboratory screening tests for STD should be available:

HIV antibody test (screening + confirmatory test)
Syphilis serology (nontreponemal test + treponemal confirmatory test)
Culture for *N. gonorrhoeae*
Culture or antigen test for *C. trachomatis*
Pap smear (if not done within the past year)
Light microscopy for gram stain, wet mounts of vaginal secretions
Dark-field microscopy for *T. pallidum*

Diagnosis of an STD should be considered a "sentinel event" reflecting unprotected sexual activity. Patients with one STD are at high risk for having others. Therefore, patients should be closely evaluated for other STD infections. This includes syphilis and HIV serology (if not performed within the previous 3 months), gonorrhea and chlamydial testing from appropriate anatomic sites, and physical examination. Women wishing to prevent unplanned pregnancy and who are not using contraception should be counseled about contraception services; ideally, contraceptives and pregnancy testing should be available at the same facility providing STD services. Annual Pap smear evaluation should also be available.

## PRIMARY PREVENTION

Clinics and practitioners who treat patients with STD should have resources available to educate patients about risk assessment and behavioral choices. Behavioral assessment is an integral part of the STD history, and patients should be counseled on methods to lower their risk of acquiring STD, including abstinence, careful selection of partners, use of condoms and spermicides, and periodic examination. Specific recommendations for behavioral assessment and counseling are beyond the scope of these treatment guidelines.

### Condoms and spermicides

Condoms and spermicides should be available in any facility providing clinical STD services. Instruction in proper use should also be provided. Although condoms do not provide absolute protection from any infection, if properly used, they should reduce the risk of infection. Recommendations for proper use of condoms (Table 2) have been made by CDC and other public health organizations (adapted from *MMWR* 1988;37:133–7).

## SPECIAL POPULATIONS

### Pregnant women

Intrauterine or perinatally transmitted STD can have fatal or severely debilitating effects on the fetus. Routine prenatal care should include an assessment for STD which in most cases includes serological screening for syphilis and hepatitis B, testing for chlamydia, and gonorrhea culture (see specific sections for management of clinical disease). Prenatal screening for HIV is indicated in all patients with risk factors for HIV, or with a high-risk sexual partner; some authorities recommend HIV screening in all pregnant women.

Practical management issues are discussed in the sections per-

*Persons at higher risk for STD include: sexually active persons who are under age 25, those who have had multiple sexual partners within the past 6 months, and those with a past history of STD. In addition, prostitutes and those having sexual contact with prostitutes, users of illicit drugs, and inmates of detention centers have increased rates of STD and should be evaluated when seeking medical care.

**Table 2. Recommendations for Use of Condoms**

1. Latex condoms should be used because they may offer greater protection against HIV and other viral STDs than natural membrane condoms.
2. Condoms should be stored in a cool, dry place out of direct sunlight.
3. Condoms in damaged packages or those that show obvious signs of age (e.g., those that are brittle, sticky, or discolored) should not be used. They cannot be relied upon to prevent infection or pregnancy.
4. Condoms should be handled with care to prevent puncture.
5. The condom should be put on before any genital contact to prevent exposure to fluids that may contain infectious agents. Hold the tip of the condom and unroll it onto the erect penis, leaving space at the tip to collect semen, yet ensuring that no air is trapped in the tip of the condom.
6. Only water-based lubricants should be used. Petroleum- or oil-based lubricants (such as petroleum jelly, cooking oils, shortening, and lotions) should not be used because they weaken the latex and may cause breakage.
7. Use of condoms containing spermicides may provide some additional protection against STDs. However, vaginal use of spermicides along with condoms is likely to provide still greater protection.
8. If a condom breaks, it should be replaced immediately. If ejaculation occurs after condom breakage, the immediate use of spermicide has been suggested. However, the protective value of post-ejaculation application of spermicide in reducing the risk of STD transmission is unknown.
9. After ejaculation, care should be taken so that the condom does not slip off the penis before withdrawal; the base of the condom should be held throughout withdrawal. The penis should be withdrawn while still erect.
10. Condoms should never be reused.

taining to specific diseases. Pregnant women and their sexual partners should be questioned about STD and counseled about possible neonatal infections. Pregnant women with primary genital herpes infection, hepatitis B, primary CMV infection, or Group B streptococcal infection may need to be referred to an expert for management. In the absence of lesions or other evidence of active disease, tests for HSV and cesarean delivery are *not* routinely indicated in women with a history of recurrent genital herpes infection during pregnancy. Routine HPV screening is not recommended. For a fuller discussion of these issues, as well as for infections not transmitted sexually, refer to "Guidelines for Perinatal Care" (second edition, 1988), jointly written and published by the American Academy of Pediatrics and the American College of Obstetrics and Gynecology.

## Children

Management of cases of STD in children requires close cooperation between the clinician, laboratory, and child-protection authorities. Investigations, when indicated, should be initiated promptly. Some diseases, such as gonorrhea, syphilis, and chlamydia, if acquired after the neonatal period, are almost 100 percent indicative of sexual contact; in other diseases, such as HPV infection and vaginitis, the association with sexual contact is not so clear (see "Sexual Assault and STD," p. A-21).

## Patients with Multiple Episodes of STD ("Repeaters")

These patients have a disproportionately high rate of STD and should be targeted for intensive counseling on methods to reduce risk. More research is needed into methods of behavior modification in these patients, including the role of outreach and support services. In many cases, periodic call-back for STD evaluation may be indicated.

## STD core groups

In most areas, populations of core STD transmitters account for the majority of STD morbidity. Although substantial regional variation occurs, in most urban areas the core groups are comprised largely of ethnic minority populations with low levels of education and socioeconomic attainment. In many such environments, illicit drug use and prostitution are common. Core groups are often geographically limited, permitting definition of core geographic areas as well as populations. STD programs should evaluate the occurrence of STD in their jurisdictions to define core populations and core areas for targeted education, screening, clinical outreach, call-back reexamination programs, and other control measures.

## Illicit drug users

STD appears to be increasingly linked to illicit drug use. Illicit drug users may be at higher risk for sexual behaviors that put one at risk for STDs. In addition, illicit drug users account for an increasing proportion of HIV infections. Further research is needed into the behaviors associated with drug use and STD, particularly to facilitate behavioral and clinical interventions targeted at drug users. Outreach programs in the community and in cooperation with drug treatment programs should be considered.

## Prison and detention populations

Residents of short-term correctional and detention facilities often have high prevalence rates of STD. Screening and treatment for infections that are highly prevalent in the community should be provided for all inmates. In many situations, screening and treatment in the prison population is central to effective STD control. In addition, for many patients, correctional health services may be only opportunity for interaction with health care providers.

## Patients with HIV infection and STD

The management of patients with STD who are coinfected with HIV presents complex clinical and behavioral issues. Because of its effect on the immune system, HIV may alter the natural histories of many STDs, and the effect of antimicrobial therapy. Close clinical follow-up is imperative. STD infection in patients with and without HIV is a sentinel event, often indicating continued unprotected sexual activity. Further patient counseling is indicated in these situations.

## STD reporting and confidentiality

Disease surveillance activities, which include the accurate identification and timely reporting of STDs, form an integral part of successful disease control. Reporting assists local health authorities in identifying sexual contacts who may be infected (see next section). Reporting is also important for assessing morbidity trends.

Reporting may be provider- and/or laboratory-based. Cases should be reported in accordance with local statutory requirements, and in as timely a manner as possible. Clinicians who are unsure of local reporting requirements are encouraged to seek advice through their local health departments or state STD program.

STD reports are held in strictest confidence; in many jurisdictions they are protected by statute from subpoena. Before any follow-up of a positive STD test is conducted by STD program representatives, these personnel consult with the provider to verify the diagnosis and treatment. Most local health departments offer STD partner notification and follow-up services for selected STD.

### Management of sex partners and partner notification

Clinical guidelines for sex partner management are included in each disease section.

Breaking the chain of transmission is crucial to STD control. Further transmission and reinfection are prevented by referral of sex partners for diagnosis and treatment. Patients should ensure that their sex partners, including those without symptoms, are referred for evaluation. Partners of patients with STD should be examined; treatment should not be provided for partners who are not examined, except for rare exceptions such as when the partner is at a site remote from medical care. Appropriate referral for sexual partners should be provided if care will not or cannot be provided by the initial health-care provider. Disease Intervention Specialists (DIS), who are public health professionals trained in STD management, can assist patients and practitioners in this process through interviewing and confidential field outreach procedures. Local and state health departments offer DIS referral services. Physicians and other community health personnel are encouraged to use DIS services to ensure complete case management. Health department managers should allocate DIS resources based on local morbidity patterns, outbreak situations, and available resources.

### Medical resources

Health care providers caring for STD patients should ensure that medical resources for the following are available either on site or through referral:

1. Medical evaluation and treatment facilities for HIV-infected patients.
2. Hospitalization facilities for patients with complicated STD infection, such as PID and disseminated gonococcal infection (DGI).
3. Medical, pediatric, infectious disease, dermatologic, and gynecological/obstetrical referral services.
4. Family planning services.
5. Substance abuse treatment services.

## AIDS AND HIV INFECTION IN THE GENERAL STD SETTING

The acquired immunodeficiency syndrome (AIDS) is a late manifestation of infection with human immunodeficiency virus (HIV). Most people infected with HIV remain asymptomatic for long intervals. HIV infection is most often diagnosed using HIV antibody tests. Detectable antibody usually develops within 3 months of infection. A confirmed positive antibody test means that a person is infected with HIV and is capable of transmitting the virus to others. Although a negative antibody test usually means a person is not infected, antibody tests cannot rule out infection from a recent exposure. If antibody testing is related to a specific exposure, the test should be repeated 3 and 6 months after the exposure.

Antibody testing for HIV begins with a screening test, usually an enzyme-linked immunosorbent assay (ELISA). If the screening test is positive, it is followed by a more specific confirmatory test, most commonly the Western blot assay. New antibody tests are being developed and licensed which are either easier to perform or more accurate. Positive results from screening tests must be confirmed before being considered definitive.

The time between infection with HIV and development of AIDS is extremely variable, ranging from a few months to 10 or more years. Most people who are infected with HIV will eventually develop some symptoms related to their infection. In one cohort study, 48 percent of a group of gay men have developed AIDS with 10 years of infection, but additional AIDS cases are expected among those who have remained AIDS-free for over 10 years.

Therapy with zidovudine (ZDV—previously known as azidothymidine) has been shown to benefit persons in the later stages of disease (AIDS or AIDS-related conditions along with a CD4 [T4] lymphocyte count less than 200/mm$^3$). Serious side effects, usually anemias and cytopenias, have been common during therapy with ZDV; therefore, patients taking ZDV require careful follow-up in consultation with physicians who are familiar with ZDV therapy. Clinical trials are currently evaluating ZDV therapy for persons with asymptomatic HIV infection to see if it decreases the rate of progression to AIDS. Other trials are evaluating new drugs or combinations of drugs for persons with different stages of HIV infection, including asymptomatic infections. The complete therapeutic management of HIV infection is beyond the scope of this document.

## PREVENTING THE SEXUAL TRANSMISSION OF HIV

Currently the only way to prevent AIDS is to prevent the initial infection with HIV. Prevention of sexual transmission of HIV can be ensured with certainty in only two situations: sexual abstinence, or choosing only sexual partners who are not infected with HIV.

Many HIV-infected persons are asymptomatic and are unaware that they are infected. Therefore, without an antibody test, it is difficult to know who is infected. AIDS case surveillance and HIV seroprevalence studies allow estimation of risk for persons in different areas; however, these population estimates may have a limited impact on an individual's sexual decisions. Although knowledge of antibody status is desirable before initiating a sexual relationship, this information may not be available. Therefore, individuals initiating a sexual relationship should be counseled about using sexual practices that reduce the risk of HIV transmission.

Sexual practices may influence the likelihood of HIV transmission during sexual contact with an infected partner. Women who practice anal intercourse with an infected partner are apparently more likely to acquire infection than women who have only vaginal intercourse. The relative risk of transmission by oral-genital contact is probably somewhat lower than the risk of transmission by vaginal intercourse. Other STD or local trauma that breaks down the mucosal barrier to infection would be expected to increase the risk of HIV transmission. Condoms supplement natural barriers to infection and therefore reduce the risk of HIV transmission (see "Clinician Guidelines and Public Health Considerations," p. A-3).

## WHEN TO TEST FOR HIV

**Voluntary, confidential, HIV antibody testing should be done routinely when the results may contribute either to the medical management of the person being tested or to the prevention of further transmission.**

Testing for medical management is important for persons with symptoms of HIV-related illnesses or with diseases such as syphilis, chancroid, herpes, or tuberculosis, for which a positive test result might affect the recommended diagnostic evaluation, treatment, or follow-up. HIV counseling and testing for persons with STD is a particularly important part of an HIV prevention program, because patients who have acquired STD have demonstrated their potential risk for acquiring HIV.

Because no vaccine or cure is available, HIV prevention requires behavior changes by people at risk for transmitting or acquiring infection. Therefore, patient counseling must be an integral part of any HIV testing program in an STD clinic. Counseling should be done both before and after HIV testing.

## PRETEST COUNSELING

**Pretest counseling should include assessment of the patient's risk for HIV infection and measures to reduce that risk.**

Intravenous (IV) drug users should be advised to stop using drugs; if they cannot stop they should not share needles; if needle-sharing continues, injection equipment should be cleaned with bleach between uses. Sexually active persons who have multiple partners should be advised to consider sexual abstinence or enter a mutually monogamous relationship with a partner who has also been tested for HIV. Condoms should be used consistently if either or both partners are infected or have other partners. Similarly, heterosexuals with STD other than HIV should be encouraged to bring their partners in for HIV testing and to use condoms if they are not in a mutually monogamous relationship with an uninfected partner.

## POSTTEST COUNSELING AND EVALUATION

**Persons who have negative HIV antibody tests should be told their test result by a person who understands the need to reduce unsafe sexual behaviors and can explain ways to modify sexual practices to reduce risks.**

Antibody tests cannot detect infections that occurred in the several weeks prior to the test (see above). People who have negative tests should understand that the negative result does not signify protection from acquiring infection. They should be advised about the ways the virus is transmitted and how to avoid infection. Their partners' risks for HIV infection should be discussed, and partners who may be at risk should be encouraged to be tested for HIV.

**Persons who test positive for HIV antibody should be told their test result by a person who is able to discuss the medical, psychological, and social implications of HIV infection. Routes of HIV transmission and methods to prevent further transmission should be emphasized.**

Risks to past sexual and needle-sharing partners of HIV antibody positive patients should be discussed, and they should be instructed in how to notify their partners and to refer them for counseling and testing. If they are unable to notify their partners or if it cannot be ensured that their partners will seek counseling, physicians or health department personnel should assist, using confidential procedures, to ensure that the partners are notified. Infected women should be advised of the risk of perinatal transmission (see below), and methods of contraception should be discussed and provided. Additional follow-up, counseling, and support systems should be available to facilitate behavior change among HIV antibody-positive persons.

## PERINATAL INFECTIONS

Infants born to women with HIV infection may also be infected with HIV; this risk is estimated to be 30 to 40 percent. The mother may be asymptomatic and her HIV infection not recognized at delivery. Infected neonates are usually asymptomatic and currently HIV infection cannot be readily or easily diagnosed at birth. (A positive antibody test may reflect passively transferred maternal antibodies and must be followed over time to determine if neonatal infection is present.) Infection may not become evident until 12 to 18 months of age. All pregnant women with a history of STD should be offered HIV counseling and testing. Recognition of HIV infection in pregnancy permits health care workers to inform patients about the risks of transmission to the infant and the risks of continuing pregnancy.

## ASYMPTOMATIC HIV INFECTIONS

As more HIV-infected persons are identified, primary health care providers will need to assume increased responsibility for these patients. Most internists, pediatricians, family practitioners, and gynecologists should be qualified to provide initial evaluation of HIV-infected individuals and follow-up of those with uncomplicated HIV infection. These services should be available in all public health clinics.

**Health care professionals who identify HIV-positive patients should provide posttest counseling; medical evaluation (either on site or by referral)—including a physical examination, complete blood count, lymphocyte subset analysis, syphilis serology, and a purified protein derivative (PPD) skin test for tuberculosis. Psychosocial counseling resources should also be available.**

All clinics and providers should establish and maintain contacts with resources in their regions for persons concerned about HIV infection, and should refer patients when necessary. Possible resources for referral include counseling services, support groups, social workers, physicians, and clinics.

## DISEASES CHARACTERIZED BY GENITAL ULCERS OR INGUINAL LYMPHADENOPATHY

In the United States, most patients with genital ulcers have genital herpes, syphilis, or chancroid. Inguinal lymphadenopathy is common in these infections. More than one of these diseases may be present in an individual patient. Patients who have genital ulcers may be at increased risk for HIV infection.

Diagnosis based only on history and physical examination is often inaccurate. Thus, evaluation of most persons with genital ulcers should include one or more of the following:

1. Dark-field examination or direct immunofluorescence test for *T. pallidum*.
2. Serologic test(s) for syphilis.
3. Culture or antigen test for HSV.
4. Culture for *H. ducreyi*.

## CHANCROID

Because of recent spread of *H. ducreyi*, chancroid has become an important STD in the United States. Its importance is enhanced by the knowledge that outside the United States chancroid has been associated with increased infection rates for HIV. Chancroid must be considered in the differential diagnosis of any patient with a painful genital ulcer. Painful inguinal lymphadenopathy is present in about half of cases.

### Recommended regimen

- **Erythromycin base 500 mg orally 4 times a day for 7 days,**

*or*

- **Ceftriaxone 250 mg IM in a single dose.**

### Alternative regimen

- **Trimethoprim/sulfamethoxazole 160/800 mg (one double-strength tablet) orally 2 times a day for 7 days.**
  *Comment:* The susceptibility of *H. ducreyi* to this combination of antimicrobial agents varies throughout the world; clinical efficacy should be monitored, preferably in conjunction with monitoring of susceptibility patterns.

*or*

- **Amoxicillin 500 mg plus clavulanic acid 125 mg orally 3 times a day for 7 days.**
  *Comment:* Not evaluated in the United States.

*or*

- **Ciprofloxacin 500 mg orally 2 times a day for 3 days.**
  *Comment:* Although a regimen of 500 mg orally once has been effective outside the United States, based on pharmacokinetics and susceptibility data, 2- or 3-day regimens of the same dose may be prudent, especially in patients coinfected with HIV.

### Management of sex partners

Sexual partners, within the 10 days preceding onset of symptoms is an infected patient, whether symptomatic or not, should be examined and treated with a recommended regimen.

### Follow-up

If successfully treated, ulcers due to chancroid symptomatically improve within 3 days and objectively improve (evidenced by resolution of lesions and clearing of exudate) within 7 days after institution of therapy. Clinical resolution of lymphadenopathy is slower than that of ulcers and may require needle aspiration (through healthy, adjacent skin), even during successful therapy. Patients should be followed until healing of the ulcer is complete. Because of the epidemiologic association with syphilis, serological testing for syphilis should be considered within 3 months after therapy.

### Treatment failures

If no clinical improvement is evident by 7 days after therapy, the clinician should consider whether antimicrobials were taken as prescribed; the *H. ducreyi* causing infection is resistant to the prescribed antimicrobial; the diagnosis is correct; coinfection with another STD agent exists, or the patient is also infected with HIV. Preliminary information indicates that patients coinfected with HIV do not respond to antimicrobial therapy as well as patients not infected with HIV, especially when single-dose treatment is used. Antimicrobial susceptibility testing should be performed on *H. ducreyi* isolated from patients who do not respond to recommended therapies.

## SYPHILIS

### General principles

**Serologic Tests.** Dark-field examinations and direct fluorescent antibody tests on lesions or tissue are the definitive methods for diagnosing early syphilis. Presumptive diagnosis is possible using two types of serologic tests for syphilis: (1) treponemal (e.g., fluorescent treponemal antibody absorbed [FTA-ABS], microhemagglutination assay for antibody to *T. pallidum* [MHATP], etc.) and (2) nontreponemal (e.g., venereal disease research laboratory [VDRL], rapid plasma reagin [RPR], etc.). Neither test alone is sufficient for diagnosis. Treponemal tests, once positive, usually remain so for life, regardless of treatment or disease activity. Treponemal antibody titers do not correlate with disease activity and should be reported as positive or negative. Nontreponemal test antibody titers tend to correlate with disease activity, usually rising with new infection and falling after treatment. Nontreponemal antibody test results should be reported quantitatively, and titered out to a final end point, rather than reported as greater than an arbitrary cutoff (e.g., >1:512). In describing changes in nontreponemal test results, a fourfold change in titers is equivalent to a two-dilution change—e.g., from 1:16 to 1:4, or from 1:8 to 1:32.

Sequential serologic tests on a patient should use the same test (e.g., VDRL or RPR) and be run by the same laboratory. The VDRL and RPR are equally valid, but RPR titers are often slightly higher than VDRL titers and therefore are not comparable.

No one test can accurately diagnose neurosyphilis. Cerebrospinal fluid (CSF) tests should include cell count, protein, and VDRL (not RPR). The CSF leukocyte count is usually elevated (>5WBC/mm$^3$) when neurosyphilis is present and is a sensitive measure of the efficacy of therapy. VDRL is the standard test for CSF; *when positive* it is considered *diagnostic* of neurosyphilis. However, it may be negative when neurosyphilis is present and cannot be used to rule out neurosyphilis. Some experts also order an FTA-ABS; this may be less specific (more false positives) but is highly sensitive. The positive predictive value of the CSF-FTA-ABS is low, but this test, *when negative*, provides evidence *against* neurosyphilis.

**Penicillin Therapy.** Penicillin is the preferred drug for treatment of syphilis. Penicillin is the only proven therapy for which there is wide experience for neurosyphilis or syphilis during pregnancy. For patients with penicillin allergy, skin testing, with desensitization if necessary, should be done. Sample guidelines for skin testing and desensitization are included (see Appendix to this section, p. A-10). However, the minor determinant mixture for penicillin is not currently available commercially.

**Jarisch-Herxheimer Reaction.** The Jarisch-Herxheimer reaction is an acute febrile reaction, often accompanied by headache, myalgia, and other symptoms, that may occur after any therapy for syphilis, and patients should be so warned. Jarisch-Herxheimer reactions are more common in patients with early syphilis. Antipyretics may be recommended, but there are no proven methods for preventing this reaction. Pregnant patients, in particular, should be warned that early labor may occur.

### Persons exposed to syphilis (epidemiologic treatment)

Sexual partners of someone diagnosed with infectious syphilis within the last 90 days should be evaluated clinically and serologically for evidence of syphilis. If no indication of infection exists, they should be preventively treated with a regimen recommended for early syphilis. Patients who have other STDs may also have been exposed to syphilis and should have a serologic test for syphilis. The dual therapy regimen currently recommended for gonorrhea (ceftriaxone and doxycycline; see p. A-13) probably effectively treats incubating syphilis. If a different non-penicillin antibiotic regimen is used, the patient should have a repeat serologic test for syphilis in 3 months.

## Early syphilis: primary and secondary syphilis and early latent syphilis (less than 1 year duration)

### Recommended Regimen

- **Benzathine penicillin G, 2.4 million units IM, in one dose.**

### Alternative Regimen for Penicillin-Allergic Patients

- **Doxycycline, 100 mg orally 2 times a day for 2 weeks.**

*or*

- **Tetracycline, 500 mg orally 4 times a day for 2 weeks.**

Doxycycline and tetracycline are equivalent therapies. There is less clinical experience with doxycycline, but compliance is better. In patients who cannot tolerate doxycycline or tetracycline, three options exist:

1. If follow-up or compliance cannot be ensured, the patient should have skin testing for penicillin allergy and be desensitized if necessary.
2. If compliance and follow-up are ensured, **erythromycin, 500 mg orally 4 times a day for 2 weeks,** can be used.
3. Preliminary data suggest that **ceftriaxone, 250 mg IM once a day for 10 days,** is curative; but careful follow-up is mandatory.

**Follow-Up.** Treatment failures can occur with any regimen. Patients should be reexamined clinically and serologically at 3 months and 6 months. If nontreponemal antibody titers have not declined fourfold by 6 months (by 3 months with primary or secondary syphilis), or if signs or symptoms persist and reinfection has been ruled out, patients should have a CSF examination and be re-treated appropriately. HIV-infected patients should have follow-up serologic testing at 1, 2, 3, 6, 9, and 12 months.

**Lumbar Puncture in Early Syphilis.** CSF abnormalities are common in adults with early syphilis. Despite the frequency of these CSF findings, very few patients develop neurosyphilis using the treatment regimens described above. Therefore, unless clinical signs and symptoms of neurologic involvement exist, such as optic, auditory, cranial nerve, or meningeal symptoms, lumbar puncture is not recommended for routing evaluation of early syphilis. This recommendation also applies to immunocompromised and HIV-infected patients, since no clear data currently exist to show that these patients need increased therapy (see p. A-10).

**HIV Testing.** All syphilis patients should be encouraged to be counseled and tested for HIV.

## Late latent syphilis (greater than 1 year duration), gummas, and cardiovascular syphilis

All patients should have a thorough clinical examination. Ideally, all patients with syphilis of greater than 1 year's duration should have CSF examination, however performance of lumbar puncture can be individualized. In older (>50 years) asymptomatic individuals, the yield of lumbar puncture is relatively low; however, CSF examination is clearly indicated in specific situations (Table 3).

### Recommended Regimen

- **Benzathine penicillin G, 7.2 million units total, administered as 3 doses of 2.4 million units IM, given 1 week apart for 3 consecutive weeks.**

If patients are allergic to penicillin, alternate drugs should be used only after CSF examination has excluded neurosyphilis. Penicillin allergy is best determined at present by careful history taking, but skin testing may be used if the major and minor determinants are available (see Appendix, p. A-10).

### Alternative Regimen

- **Doxycycline, 100 mg orally 2 times a day for 4 weeks.**

*or*

- **Tetracycline, 500 mg orally 4 times a day for 4 weeks.**

*Note:* If CSF examination is performed and reveals findings consistent with neurosyphilis, patients should be treated for neurosyphilis (see next section). Some experts also treat cardiovascular syphilis with a neurosyphilis regimen.

**Follow-Up.** Quantitative nontreponemal serologic tests should be repeated at 6 months and 12 months. If titers increase fourfold, or if an initially high titer (≥1:32) fails to decrease, of if the patient develops signs or symptoms attributable to syphilis, the patient should be evaluated for neurosyphilis and retreated appropriately.

**HIV Testing.** All syphilis patients should be encouraged to be counseled and tested for HIV antibody.

## Neurosyphilis

Central nervous system disease may occur during any stage of syphilis. Clinical evidence of neurologic involvement (optic and auditory symptoms, cranial nerve palsies, etc.) warrants CSF examination.

### Recommended Regimen

- **12–24 million units aqueous crystalline penicillin G daily, 2–4 million units every 4 hours IV, for 10–14 days.**

### Alternative Regimen (If Outpatient Compliance Can Be Ensured)

- **2.4 million units procaine penicillin IM daily, and probenecid, 500 mg orally 4 times a day, both for 10–14 days.**

Many authorities recommend addition of benzathine penicillin, 2.4 million units IM weekly for three doses after completion of these neurosyphilis treatment regimens. No systematically collected data have evaluated therapeutic alternatives to penicillin. Patients who cannot tolerate penicillin should be skin tested, and desensitized if necessary, or managed in consultation with an expert.

**Follow-Up.** If an initial CSF pleocytosis was present, CSF examination should be repeated every 6 months until the cell count is normal. If it has not decreased at 6 months, or is not normal by 2 years, retreatment should be strongly considered.

**HIV Testing.** All syphilis patients should be encouraged to be counseled and tested for HIV antibody.

## Syphilis in pregnancy

**Screening.** Pregnant women should be screened early in pregnancy. Seropositive pregnant women should be considered infected unless treatment history and sequential serologic antiboby titers are clearly documented. In populations in which prenatal care utilization is not optimal, RPR card screening and treatment should be performed at the time pregnancy is detected. In areas of high syphilis prevalence, or in patients at high risk, screening should be repeated in the third trimester and again at delivery.

**Treatment.** Patients should be treated with the penicillin regimen appropriate for the woman's stage of syphilis. Tetracycline and doxycycline are contraindicated in pregnancy. Erythromycin should not be used because of the high risk of failure to cure infection in the fetus. Pregnant women with histories of penicillin allergy should first be carefully questioned regarding the validity of the history. They should then be skin tested and either treated with penicillin or referred for desensitization (see Appendix, p. A-10). Women who are treated in the second half of pregnancy are at risk for premature labor and/or fetal distress if their treatment precipitates a Jarisch-Herxheimer reaction. They should be advised to seek medical attention if they notice any change in fetal movements or have any contractions. Stillbirth is a rare complication of treatment; however, since therapy is necessary to prevent further fetal damage, this concern should not delay treatment.

**Follow-Up.** Monthly follow-up is mandatory so that retreatment can be given if needed. The antibody response should be appropriate for the stage of disease.

**HIV Testing.** All syphilis patients should be encouraged to be counseled and tested for HIV antibody.

## Congenital syphilis

**A. Who Should Be Evaluated.** Infants should be evaluated if they were born to seropositive (nontreponemal test confirmed by treponemal test) women who:

1. Have untreated syphilis; *or*
2. Had syphilis which was treated in pregnancy but:
   a. less than 1 month before delivery; *or*
   b. with a non-penicillin regimen; *or*
   c. with the appropriate penicillin regimen but without the expected decrease in nontreponemal antibody titers following penicillin therapy; *or*
3. Do not have a well-documented history of syphilis treatment; *or*
4. Have a well-documented history of treatment before pregnancy but had insufficient serologic follow-up during pregnancy to assess disease activity.

*An infant should not be released from the hospital until the serologic status of its mother is known.*

**B. Evaluation of the Infant.** The clinical and laboratory evaluation of infants born to women described above in **A.** should include:

1. A thorough physical examination for evidence of congenital syphilis.
2. Nontreponemal antibody titers.
3. CSF analysis for cells, protein, and VDRL.

**Table 3. Indications for CSF Examination in Adults with Latent Syphilis Present for More than One Year**

| |
|---|
| Neurologic signs or symptoms |
| Treatment failure (see p. A-9) |
| Serum nontreponemal titer $\geq$1:32 |
| Other evidence of active syphilis (aortitis, gumma, iritis) |
| Non-penicillin therapy planned |
| Positive HIV antibody test |

4. Long bone x-rays.
5. Other test as clinically indicated (e.g., chest x-ray).
6. If possible, FTA-ABS on the purified 19S-IgM.of serum (e.g., separation by Isolab columns).

**C. Therapy Decisions.** Infants should be treated if they have:

1. Any evidence of active disease (physical examination or x-ray); *or*
2. A reactive CSF-VDRL; *or*
3. An abnormal CSF finding (white blood cell count >5/mm$^3$ or protein >50 mg/dl) irrespective of CSF serology; *or*
4. Quantitative nontreponemal serologic titers which are fourfold (or greater) higher than their mother; *or*
5. Positive FTA-ABS-19S-IgM antibody, if performed, *or*
6. A mother who has untreated syphilis.

**D. Treatment.** Treatment should consist of: **100,000–150,000 units/kg of aqueous crystalline penicillin G daily (administered as 50,000 units/kg IV every 8–12 hours)** *or* **50,000 units/kg of procaine penicillin daily (administered once IM) for 10–14 days. If more than 1 day of therapy is missed, the entire course should be restarted. All symptomatic neonates should also have an ophthalmologic examination.**

If all conditions described above in **C.** are negative, so that the infant does not meet the criteria for intensive therapy but did need evaluation (i.e., met the criteria in **A.**), and if close follow-up cannot be ensured, then **50,000 units/kg of benzathine penicillin G should be given IM as a one-time dose.**

**E. Follow-Up.** Seropositive untreated infants must be closely followed at 1, 2, 3, 6, and 12 months. Nontreponemal antibody titers should be decreasing by 3 months of age and should have disappeared by 6 months of age. If these titers are found to be stable or increasing, the child should be reevaluated and fully treated. Treponemal antibodies may be present up to 1 year of age. If they are present beyond 1 year, the infant should be treated for congenital syphilis.

Treated infants should also be followed to ensure decreasing nontreponemal antibody titers. Treponemal tests should not be used since these may remain positive despite effective therapy if the child was infected. Infants with documented CSF pleocytosis should have this reexamined every 6 months or until the cell count is normal. If the cell count is still abnormal after 2 years, or if a downward trend is not present at each examination, the infant should be re-treated. The CSF-VDRL should also be checked at 6 months; if it is still reactive, the infant should be retreated.

**F. Therapy of Older Infants and Children.** After the newborn period, children discovered to have syphilis should have a CSF examination. Any child who is thought to have congenital syphilis, or who has neurologic involvement, should be treated with **200,000–300,000 units/kg/day of aqueous crystalline penicillin in divided doses for 10–14 days.** Older children with definite acquired syphilis, a normal neurologic examination, and normal CSF findings, may be treated with one dose of **benzathine penicillin G, 50,000 units/kg IM, up to the adult dose of 2.4 million units.** Children with a history of penicillin allergy should be skin tested, and desensitized if necessary (see Appendix, below). Follow-up should be performed as described previously.

**G. HIV Testing.** In cases of congenital syphilis, the mother should be encouraged to be counseled and tested for HIV, and, if her test is positive, the infant should be referred for follow-up.

## Syphilis in HIV-infected patients

### Diagnosis

1. All sexually active patients with syphilis should be encouraged to be counseled and tested for HIV, because of the frequency of association of the two diseases and because of its relevance to clinical assessment and management.
2. Neurosyphilis should be considered in the differential diagnosis of neurologic disease in HIV-infected persons.
3. When clinical findings suggest that syphilis is present, but serologic tests are negative or confusing, alternative tests, such as biopsy of lesions, dark-field examination and direct fluorescent antibody staining of lesion material, should be employed.
4. In cases of congenital syphilis, the mother should be encouraged to be counseled and tested for HIV, and, if her test is positive, the infant should be referred for follow-up.

### Treatment and Follow-Up

1. Penicillin regimens should be used whenever possible for all stages of syphilis in HIV-infected patients. Skin testing to confirm penicillin allergy and desensitization may be employed if minor and major determinants are available (see Appendix, below).
2. No change in therapy for early syphilis for HIV-coinfected patients is recommended. However, experts disagree on this issue; some authorities advise CSF examination and/or treatment with a regimen appropriate for neurosyphilis for all patients coinfected with syphilis and HIV, regardless of the clinical stage of syphilis. In all cases, careful follow-up is necessary to ensure adequacy of treatment.
3. HIV-infected patients treated for syphilis should be followed clinically and with quantitative nontreponemal serologic tests (VDRL, RPR) at 1, 2, 3, 6, 9, and 12 months after treatment. Patients with early syphilis whose titers fail to decrease four-fold within 6 months should undergo CSF examination and be re-treated. In such patients, CSF abnormalities could be due to HIV-related infection, neurosyphilis, or both. STD clinics and others providing STD treatment should ensure adequate follow-up.

## Appendix

**Management of Patients with Histories of Penicillin Allergy.** Currently, no proven alternative therapies to penicillin are available for treating neurosyphilis, congenital syphilis, or syphilis in pregnancy. Therefore skin testing, with desensitization if indicated, is recommended for these patients.

**Skin Testing.** Skin testing is a rapid, safe, and accurate procedure (see below). It is also productive: 90 percent of patients with a history of "penicillin allergy" have negative skin tests and can be given penicillin safely. The other 10 percent with positive skin tests have an increased risk of being truly penicillin allergic and should undergo desensitization. Clinics involved in STD management should be equipped and prepared to do skin testing or should establish referral mechanisms to have skin tests performed.

Skin testing is quick; four determinants, along with positive and negative controls, can be placed and read in an hour (see Table 4). Skin testing is also safe, if properly performed. The determinant antigens should be diluted 100-fold for use in patients who have had a severe, life-threatening reaction in the past year; these patients should be tested in a controlled environment such as a hospital setting. Other patients can be skin-tested safely in a physician-staffed clinic.

**Table 4. Penicillin Allergy Skin Testing (adapted from Beall*)**

*Note:* If there has been a severe generalized reaction to penicillin in the past year, the antigens should be diluted 100-fold, and patients should be tested in a controlled environment. Both major and minor determinants should be available for the tests to be interpretable. The patient should not have taken antihistamines in the previous 48 hours.

Reagents
- Major Determinants:
  - Benzylpenicilloyl-polylysine (major, Pre-Pen [Taylor Pharmacal Co., Decatur, Illinois], $6 \times 10^{-5}$M)
- Benyzylpenicillin ($10^{-2}$M or 6000 U/mL
- Minor determinants:
  - Benzylpenicilloic acid ($10^{-2}$M)
  - Benzylpenicilloic acid ($10^{-2}$M)
- Positive control (histamine, 1.0 ug/mL)
- Negative control (buffered saline solution)
- Dilute the antigens 100-fold for preliminary testing if there has been an immediate generalized reaction within the past year.

Procedure
- Epicutaneous (scratch or prick) test: apply one drop of material to volar forearm and pierce epidermis without drawing blood; then examine for 20 minutes; if there is no significant wheal (4 mm or greater) proceed to intradermal test
- Intradermal test: inject 0.02 ml *intradermally* with a 27-gauge short-bevelled needle; observe for 20 minutes.

Interpretation
- For the test to be interpretable, the negative (saline) control must elicit no reaction and the positive (histamine) control must elicit a positive reaction.
- Positive test: a wheal greater than 4 mm in mean diameter to any penicillin reagent; erythema must be present
- Negative test: the wheals at the site of the penicillin reagents are equivalent to the negative control
  - Indeterminate: all other results.

*Beall GN: Immediate hypersensitivity reactions to Beta-lactam antibiotics. *Ann Intern Med* 1987; 107:105–9.

**Desensitization.** Patients who have a positive skin test to one of the penicillin determinants can be desensitized. This is a straightforward, relatively safe procedure. It can be done orally or intravenously; while the two approaches have not been compared, oral desensitization is thought to be safer, and is also simpler and easier. Desensitization should be done in a hospital setting because serious IgE-mediated allergic reaction, although unlikely, can occur. Desensitization can be completed in 4 hours, after which the first dose of penicillin is given (see Table 5). STD programs should have a referral center where patients with positive skin tests can be desensitized. After desensitization, patients must be maintained on penicillin.

Table 5. Oral-Desensitization Protocol (from Wendel‡)

| Dose* | Penicillin V Suspension (units/ml) | Amount† | | Cumulative dose (units) |
|---|---|---|---|---|
| | | ml | units | |
| 1 | 1000 | 0.1 | 100 | 100 |
| 2 | 1000 | 0.2 | 200 | 300 |
| 3 | 1000 | 0.4 | 400 | 700 |
| 4 | 1000 | 0.8 | 800 | 1500 |
| 5 | 1000 | 1.6 | 1600 | 3100 |
| 6 | 1000 | 3.2 | 3200 | 6300 |
| 7 | 1000 | 6.4 | 6400 | 12,700 |
| 8 | 10,000 | 1.2 | 12,000 | 24,700 |
| 9 | 10,000 | 2.4 | 24,000 | 48,700 |
| 10 | 10,000 | 4.8 | 48,000 | 96,700 |
| 11 | 80,000 | 1.0 | 80,000 | 176,700 |
| 12 | 80,000 | 2.0 | 160,000 | 336,700 |
| 13 | 80,000 | 4.0 | 320,000 | 656,700 |
| 14 | 80,000 | 8.0 | 640,000 | 1,296,700 |

Observation period: 30 minutes before parenteral administration of penicillin.

*Interval between doses, 15 minutes; elapsed time, 3 hours and 45 minutes; cumulative dose, 1.3 million units.

†The specific amount of drug was diluted in approximately 30 ml of water and then given orally.

‡Reprinted with permission from *The New England Journal of Medicine* 1985; 312:1329–32.

## LYMPHOGRANULOMA VENEREUM

Lymphogranuloma venereum (LGV) is caused by *C. trachomatis* (LGV serovars). Inguinal lymphadenopathy is the most common clinical manifestation. Diagnosis is often made clinically and may be confused with chancroid. LGV is not currently a common cause of inguinal adenopathy in the United States.

### Treatment of LGV: genital, inguinal, or anorectal

#### Recommended Regimen

- **Doxycycline 100 mg orally 2 times a day for 21 days.**

#### Alternative Regimen

- **Tetracycline 500 mg orally 4 times a day for 21 days**

*or*

- **Erythromycin 500 mg orally 4 times a day for 21 days**

*or*

- **Sulfisoxazole 500 mg orally 4 times a day for 21 days or equivalent sulfonamide course**

## GENITAL HERPES SIMPLEX VIRUS INFECTIONS

Genital herpes infection is a viral disease which may be chronic and recurring and for which no known cure exists. Systemic acyclovir treatment provides partial control of the symptoms and signs of herpes episodes, and accelerates healing, but does not eradicate the infection nor affect the subsequent risk, frequency, or severity of recurrences after the drug is discontinued. Topical therapy with acyclovir is substantially less effective than therapy with the oral drug.

### First clinical episode of genital herpes

#### Recommended Regimen

- **Acyclovir 200 mg orally 5 times a day for 7–10 days or until clinical resolution occurs.**

### First clinical episode of herpes proctitis

#### Recommended Regimen

- **Acyclovir 400 mg orally 5 times a day for 10 days or until clinical resolution occurs.**

### Inpatient therapy

For patients with severe disease or complications necessitating hospitalization.

#### Recommended Regimen

- **Acyclovir 5 mg/kg body weight IV every 8 hours for 5–7 days or until clinical resolution occurs.**

### Recurrent episodes

Most episodes of recurrent herpes do not benefit from therapy with acyclovir. In severe recurrent disease, some patients who are able to start therapy at the beginning of the prodrome or within 2 days of onset of lesions may benefit from therapy, although this has not been proven.

- **Acyclovir 200 mg orally 5 times a day for 5 days**

*or*

- **Acyclovir 800 mg orally 2 times a day for 5 days.**

### Daily suppressive therapy

Daily treatment reduces frequency of recurrences by at least 75 percent among patients with frequent (more than six per year) recurrences. Safety and efficacy have been clearly documented among persons receiving daily therapy for up to 3 years. Acyclovir-resistant strains of HSV have been isolated from persons receiving suppressive therapy, but have not been associated with treatment failure among immunocompetent patients. After 1 year of continuous daily suppressive therapy, acyclovir should be discontinued to reassess the patient's recurrence rate.

- **Acyclovir 200 mg 2 to 5 times a day***

*or*

- **Acyclovir 400 mg 2 times a day**

### Genital herpes in HIV-infected patients

The need for higher-than-standard doses of oral acyclovir in HIV-infected, but immunocompetent patients, has not been established. Immune status, not HIV infection alone, is the likely predictor of a disease severity and response to therapy. Case reports strongly suggest that patients with clinical immunodeficiency have a more severe clinical course of anogenital herpes than do immunocompetent patients, and some centers are using increased doses of acyclovir in patients with immunodeficiency. However, neither the need for nor the proper increased dosage of acyclovir has been conclusively established. Immunocompromised as well as immunocompetent hosts who fail initial therapy may benefit from an increased dosage of acyclovir.

*Dosage must be individualized for each patient.

The indications for suppressive therapy in immunocompromised patients, and the dose required, are controversial. Clinical benefits to the patient must be weighed against the potential for selecting HSV strains that are resistant to acyclovir. Patients who fail therapy for a recurrence because of resistant strains of HSV should be managed in consultation with an expert.

### Acyclovir in pregnant patients

The safety of systemic acyclovir therapy in pregnant women has not been established. In the presence of life-threatening maternal HSV infection (e.g., disseminated infection that includes encephalitis, pneumonitis, and/or hepatitis) acyclovir administered IV is probably of value. In pregnant women without life-threatening disease, systemic acyclovir treatment *should not* be used to treat recurrent genital herpes episodes or as suppressive therapy to prevent reactivation near term.

### Perinatal infections

Most mothers of infants who acquire neonatal herpes lack histories of clinically evident genital herpes. The risk of transmission to the neonate from an infected mother is highest among women with primary herpes infection near the time of delivery, and is low among women with recurrent herpes. The results of viral cultures during pregnancy do not predict viral shedding at the time of delivery; such cultures are not routinely indicated.

At the onset of labor, all women should be carefully questioned about symptoms and examined. Women without symptoms or signs of genital herpes infection or prodrome may be delivered vaginally. In women who have a history of genital herpes, or have a sex partner with genital herpes, cultures of the birth canal at delivery may be helpful in decisions about neonatal management. Infants delivered through an infected birth canal (proven by culture or presumed by observation of lesions) should be cultured and followed carefully. Although insufficient data exist to recommend the use of acyclovir in asymptomatic infants, some experts presumptively treat infants who were exposed to HSV at delivery. Herpes cultures should be obtained from infants before therapy; positive cultures obtained 24 to 48 hours, or more, after birth indicate active viral infection.

### Counseling and management of sex partners

Patients with genital herpes should be told about the natural history of their disease with emphasis on the potential for recurrent episodes. Patients should be advised to abstain from sexual activity while lesions are present. Sexual transmission of HSV has been documented during periods without recognized lesions. Suppressive treatment with oral acyclovir will reduce the frequency of recurrences, but does not totally eliminate viral shedding. Genital herpes (and other diseases causing genital ulcers) has been associated with an increased risk of acquiring HIV infections. Therefore, the use of condoms should be encouraged during all sexual exposures. Sex partners of patients with genital herpes may benefit from evaluation, if they have genital lesions. However, evaluating asymptomatic partners has little value for preventing transmission of HSV.

The risk of fetal infection should be explained to all patients—male and female—with genital herpes. Women of childbearing age with genital herpes should be advised to inform their clinicians of their history during any future pregnancy.

## INFECTIONS OF EPITHELIAL SURFACES

## GENITAL WARTS

Exophytic genital and anal warts are caused by certain types (most frequently types 6, 11) of HPV. Other types sometimes present in the anogenital region (most commonly types 16, 18, and 31) have been found to be strongly associated with genital dysplasia and carcinoma. For this reason, atypical, pigmented, or persistent warts should be biopsied. All women with anogenital warts must have an annual Pap smear, as should any woman with a history of STD.

Some subclinical HPV infections may be detected by Pap smear and colposcopy. Application of acetic acid may also detect otherwise subclinical lesions, but false-positive tests occur. Tests for the detection of HPV-DNA are now widely available. The clinical utility of these tests in managing of individual patients is not known. Therefore, therapeutic decisions should not be made on the basis of these HPV-DNA tests.

No therapy has been shown to eradicate HPV. HPV has been demonstrated in adjacent tissue after laser treatment of HPV-associated cervical intraepithelial neoplasia and after attempts to eliminate subclinical HPV by extensive laser vaporization of the anogenital area. The benefit of treating subclinical HPV infection has been demonstrated and recurrence is common. The effect of genital wart treatment on HPV transmission and the natural history of HPV is unknown. *Therefore, the goal of treatment is removal of the warts and the amelioration of signs and symptoms, not the eradication of HPV.*

Expensive therapies, toxic therapies, and procedures that result in scarring should be avoided. Sexual partners should be examined for evidence of warts and other STD. Patients with anogenital warts should be made aware that they are contagious to uninfected sexual partners. The use of condoms is recommended to help reduce transmission.

In most clinical situations, cryotherapy with liquid nitrogen or cryoprobe is the treatment of choice for external genital and perianal warts. Cryotherapy is nontoxic, does not require anesthesia, and if used properly, does not result in scarring. Podophyllin, trichloroacetic acid (TCA), and electrodesiccation/electrocautery are alternative therapies. Because of its relatively low efficacy, high incidence of toxicity, and high cost, treatment with interferon cannot be recommended.

The carbon dioxide laser and conventional surgery are useful in the management of extensive warts, particularly in those patients who have not responded to cryotherapy; these alternatives are not appropriate for treatment of limited lesions. Like more cost-effective treatments, these therapies do not eliminate HPV and are associated with significant rates of clinical recurrence.

### Pregnant patients and perinatal infections

Cesarean delivery for prevention of transmission of HPV infection to the newborn is not indicated. However, in rare instances, cesarean delivery may be indicated for women with genital warts if the pelvic outlet is obstructed or if vaginal delivery would result in excessive bleeding.

Genital papillary lesions have a tendency to proliferate and to become friable during pregnancy. Many experts advocate removal of visible warts during pregnancy, although data are limited.

HPV can cause laryngeal papillomatosis in infants. The route of transmission (transplacental, birth canal, or postnatal) is unknown. Hence, the preventive value of cesarean delivery is unknown. The perinatal transmission rate is also unknown, although it must be very low, given the relatively high prevalence of genital warts and the rarity of laryngeal papillomas. Neither routine HPV screening tests nor cesarean delivery are indicated to prevent transmission of HPV infection to the newborn.

## Treatment recommendations

### External Genital/Perianal Warts

**RECOMMENDED REGIMEN**

- **Cryotherapy with liquid nitrogen or cryoprobe.**

**ALTERNATIVE REGIMEN**

- **Podophyllin 10–25% in compound tincture of benzoin.** Limit the total volume of podophyllin solution applied to <0.5 ml per treatment session. Thoroughly wash off in 1–4 hours. Treat <10 cm$^2$ per session. Repeat applications at weekly intervals. Biopsy and switch to cryotherapy if the wart persists after three treatments. Mucosal warts are more likely to respond than highly keratinized warts on the penile shaft, buttocks, and pubic areas. *Contraindicated in pregnancy.*
- **Trichloroacetic Acid (85%).** Apply only to warts; powder with talc or sodium bicarbonate (baking soda) to remove unreacted acid. Repeat application at weekly intervals.
- **Electrodesiccation/Electrocautery.** Electrodesiccation is contraindicated in patients with cardiac pacemakers, or for lesions proximal to the anal verge. Extensive or refractory disease should be referred to an expert.

**Cervical Warts.** For women with cervical warts, dysplasia must be excluded before treatment is begun. Management should therefore be carried out in consultation with an expert.

### Vaginal Warts

**RECOMMENDED REGIMEN**

- **Cryotherapy with liquid nitrogen.** (The use of a cryoprobe in the vagina is not recommended because of the risk of vaginal perforation and fistula formation.)

**ALTERNATIVE REGIMEN**

- **Trichloroacetic acid (80–90%).** Apply only to warts; powder with talc or sodium bicarbonate (baking soda) to remove unreacted acid. Repeat application at weekly intervals.
- **Podophyllin 10–25% in compound tincture of benzoin.** Treatment area must be dry before removing speculum. Treat <2 cm$^2$ per session. Repeat application at weekly intervals. *Contraindicated in pregnancy.* Extensive or refractory disease should be referred to an expert.

### Urethral Meatus Warts

**RECOMMENDED REGIMEN**

- **Cryotherapy with liquid nitrogen.**

**ALTERNATIVE REGIMEN**

- **Podophyllin 10–25% in compound tincture of benzoin.** Treatment area must be dry before contact with normal mucosa, and podophyllin must be washed off in 1–2 hours. *Contraindicated in pregnancy.* Extensive or refractory disease should be referred to an expert.

### Anal Warts

**RECOMMENDED REGIMEN**

- **Cryotherapy with liquid nitrogen.** Extensive or refractory disease should be referred to an expert.

**ALTERNATIVE REGIMEN**

- **Trichloroacetic acid (80–90%).**
- **Surgical removal.**

### Oral Warts

**RECOMMENDED REGIMEN**

- **Cryotherapy with liquid nitrogen.**

**ALTERNATIVE REGIMEN**

- **Electrodesiccation/electrocautery.**
- **Surgical removal.** Extensive or refractory disease should be referred to an expert.

# GONOCOCCAL INFECTIONS

Treatment of gonococcal infections in the United States is influenced by the following trends: (1) the spread of infections due to antibiotic-resistant *N. gonorrhoeae,* including penicillinase-producing *N. gonorrhoeae* (PPNG), tetracycline-resistant *N. gonorrhoeae* (TRNG), and strains with chromosomally mediated resistance to multiple antibiotics; (2) the high frequency of chlamydial infections in persons with gonorrhea; (3) recognition of the serious complications of chlamydial and gonococcal infections; and (4) the absence of a fast, inexpensive, and highly accurate test for chlamydial infection.

All gonorrhea cases should be diagnosed or confirmed by culture to facilitate antimicrobial susceptibility testing. The susceptibility of *N. gonorrhoeae* to antibiotics is likely to change over time in any locality. Therefore, gonorrhea control programs should develop a program of regular antibiotic sensitivity testing of a surveillance sample of *N. gonorrhoeae* isolates as well as all isolates associated with treatment failure.

Because of the wide spectrum of antimicrobial therapies effective against *N. gonorrhoeae,* these guidelines are *not* intended to be a comprehensive list of all possible treatment regimens.

## Treatment of adults

**Uncomplicated Urethral, Endocervical, or Rectal Infections.** Single-dose efficacy is a major consideration in choosing an antibiotic regimen to treat *N. gonorrhoeae.* Another important concern is coexisting chlamydial infection, documented in up to 45 percent of gonorrhea cases in some populations. Until universal testing for chlamydia with quick, inexpensive, and highly accurate tests becomes available, it is generally more cost-effective to treat presumptive chlamydial infections in all persons with gonorrhea. Simultaneous treatment of all gonorrhea infections with antibiotics effective against both *C. trachomatis* and *N. gonorrhoeae* may lessen the possibility of gonorrhea treatment failure due to antibiotic resistance.

### Recommended Regimen

- **Ceftriaxone 250 mg IM once**

*plus*

- **Doxycycline 100 mg orally 2 times a day for 7 days.**

Some authorities prefer a dose of **125 mg ceftriaxone IM** because it is less expensive and can be given in a volume of only **0.5 ml,** which is more easily administered in the deltoid muscle. However, the **250 mg dose is recommended because it may delay the emergence of ceftriaxone-resistant strains.** At this time, both doses appear highly effective for mucosal gonorrhea at all sites.

### Alternative Regimens

For patients who cannot take ceftriaxone, the preferred alternative is:

- **Spectinomycin 2 g IM,** in a single dose (followed by doxycycline). Other alternatives, for which experience is less extensive, include **ciprofloxacin 500 mg orally once; norfloxacin 800 mg orally once; cefuroxime axetil 1 g orally once with probenecid 1 g, cefotaxime 1 g IM once; and ceftizoxime 500 mg once.** All of these regimens are followed by **doxycycline 100 mg orally, twice daily for 7 days.** If infection was acquired from a source proven *not* to have penicillin-resistant gonorrhea, a penicillin such as **amoxicillin 3 g orally with 1 g probenecid followed orally by doxycycline** may be used for treatment.

Doxycycline or tetracycline alone is no longer considered adequate therapy for gonococcal infections but is added for treatment of coexisting chlamydial infections.

**Tetracycline** may be substituted for **doxycycline;** however, compliance may be worse since **tetracycline must be taken at a dose of 500 mg 4 times a day between meals while doxycycline is taken at a dose of 100 mg 2 times a day without regard to meals.** Moreover, at current prices, **tetracycline** is not significantly less expensive than generic **doxycycline.**

For patients who cannot take a tetracycline (e.g., pregnant women), erythromycin may be substituted (**erythromycin base or stearate at 500 mg orally 4 times a day for 7 days or erythromycin ethylsuccinate, 800 mg orally 4 times a day for 7 days**). See "Chlamydial Infections" (p. A-16) for further information on management of chlamydial infection.

## Special considerations

All patients diagnosed with gonorrhea should have a serologic test for syphilis and should be offered confidential counseling and testing for HIV infection. The majority of patients with incubating syphilis (those who are seronegative and have no clinical signs of syphilis) may be cured by any of the regimens containing β-lactams (e.g., **ceftriaxone**) or **tetracyclines.**

Spectinomycin and the quinolones (ciprofloxacin, norfloxacin) have not been shown to be active against incubating syphilis. Patients treated with these drugs should be followed with a serologic test for syphilis in 1 month.

Patients with gonorrhea and documented syphilis and gonorrhea patients who are sex partners of syphilis patients should be treated for syphilis as outlined in "Syphilis" (p. A-7) as well as for gonorrhea.

Some practitioners report that mixing 1% lidocaine (without epinephrine) with ceftriaxone reduces the discomfort associated with the injection. No adverse reactions have been associated with use of lidocaine diluent.

## Management of sex partners

Persons exposed to gonorrhea within the preceding 30 days should be examined, cultured, and treated presumptively.

## Follow-up

Treatment failure following combined ceftriaxone/doxycycline therapy is likely to be rare; therefore, a follow-up culture ("test-of-cure") is not essential. In many instances, a more cost-effective strategy may be to reexamine with culture 1 to 2 months after treatment ("rescreening"); this strategy will detect both treatment failures and reinfections. Patients should be advised to return for examination if any symptoms persist at the completion of treatment.

## Treatment failures

Persistent symptoms after treatment should be evaluated by culture for *N. gonorrhoeae,* and any gonococcal isolate should be tested for antibiotic sensitivity. Symptoms of urethritis may also be caused by *C. trachomatis* and other organisms associated with nongonococcal urethritis (see "Nongonococcal Urethritis," p. A-16). Additional treatment for gonorrhea should be **ceftriaxone, 250 mg, followed by doxycycline.** Infections occurring after treatment with one of the recommended regimens are commonly due to reinfection rather than treatment failure and indicate a need for improved sex-partner referral and patient education.

## Pharyngeal gonococcal infection

Patients with uncomplicated pharyngeal gonococcal infection should be treated with **ceftriaxone 250 mg IM once.** Patients who cannot be treated with ceftriaxone should be treated with **ciprofloxacin 500 mg orally as a single dose.** Since experience with this regimen is limited, such patients should be evaluated with repeat culture 3 to 7 days after treatment.

## Treatment of gonococcal infections in pregnancy

Pregnant women should be cultured for *N. gonorrhoeae* (and tested for *C. trachomatis* and syphilis) at the first prenatal care visit. In women at high risk of STD, a second culture for gonorrhea (as well as tests for chlamydia and syphilis) should be obtained late in the third trimester.

### Recommended Regimen

- **Ceftriaxone 250 mg IM once**

*plus*

- **Erythromycin base* 500 mg orally 4 times a day for 7 days.**

Pregnant women allergic to β-lactams should be treated with **spectinomycin 2.0g IM once (followed by erythromycin).** Follow-up cervical and rectal cultures for *N. gonorrhoeae* should be obtained 3–7 days after completion of treatment.

Ideally, pregnant women with gonorrhea should be treated for chlamydia on the basis of chlamydial diagnostic studies. If chlamydial diagnostic testing is not available, then treatment for chlamydia should be given. **Tetracyclines** (including **doxycycline**) and the **quinolones** are contraindicated in pregnancy because of the possibility of adverse effects on the fetus. Treatments for pregnant patients with chlamydial infection and acute salpingitis are described in their respective sections (pp. A-16 and A-17).

***Erythromycin stearate 500 mg or erythromycin ethylsuccinate 800 mg or equivalent may be substituted for erythromycin base.**

## Disseminated gonococcal infection (DGI)

Hospitalization is recommended for initial therapy, especially for those who cannot reliably comply with treatment, have uncertain diagnoses, or have purulent synovial effusions or other complications. Patients should be examined for clinical evidence of endocarditis or meningitis.

### Recommended Regimens—DGI Inpatient

- **Ceftriaxone 1 g, IM or IV, every 24 hours**

*or*

- **Ceftizoxime 1 g, IV, every 8 hours**

*or*

- **Cefotaxime 1 g, IV, every 8 hours.**

Patients who are allergic to β-lactam drugs should be treated with **spectinomycin 2 g IM every 12 hours.**

When the infecting organism is proven to be penicillin-sensitive, parenteral treatment may be switched to **ampicillin 1 g every 6 hours (or equivalent).**

Patients treated for DGI should be tested for genital *C. trachomatis* infection. If chlamydial testing is not available, the patients should be treated empirically for coexisting chlamydial infection.

Reliable patients with uncomplicated disease may be discharged 24 to 48 hours after all symptoms resolve and complete therapy (for a total of 1 week of antibiotic therapy) with an oral regimen of **cefuroxime axetil 500 mg 2 times a day** *or* **amoxicillin 500 mg with clavulanic acid 3 times a day** *or*, if not pregnant, **ciprofloxacin 500 mg 2 times a day.**

## Meningitis and endocarditis

Meningitis and endocarditis caused by *N. gonorrhoeae* require high-dose IV therapy with an agent effective against the strain causing the disease, such as **ceftriaxone 1–2 g IV every 12 hours.** Optimal duration of therapy is unknown, but most authorities treat patients with gonococcal meningitis for 10 to 14 days and with gonococcal endocarditis for at least 4 weeks. Patients with gonococcal nephritis, endocarditis or meningitis, or recurrent DGI should be evaluated for complement deficiencies. Treatment of complicated DGI should be undertaken in consultation with an expert.

## Adult gonococcal ophthalmia

Adults and children over 20 kg with nonsepticemic gonococcal ophthalmia should be treated with **ceftriaxone 1 g IM once.** Irrigation of the eyes with saline or buffered ophthalmic solutions may be useful adjunctive therapy to eliminate discharge. All patients must have careful ophthalmologic assessment including slit-lamp exam for ocular complications. Topical antibiotics alone are not sufficient therapy and are unnecessary when appropriate systemic therapy is given. Simultaneous ophthalmic infection with *C. trachomatis* has been reported and should be considered in patients who do not respond promptly.

## Gonococcal infections of infants and children

Child abuse should be carefully considered and evaluated (see "Sexual Assault and Abuse of Children," p. A-22) in any child with documented gonorrhea.

## Treatment of infants born to mothers with gonococcal infection

Infants born to mothers with untreated gonorrhea are at high risk of infection (e.g., ophthalmia and DGI) and should be treated with a single injection of **ceftriaxone (50 mg/kg IV or IM, not to exceed 125 mg). Ceftriaxone** should be given cautiously to hyperbilirubinemic infants, especially premature infants. Topical prophylaxis for neonatal ophthalmia is not adequate treatment for documented infections of the eye or other sites.

## Treatment of infants with gonococcal infection

Infants with documented gonococcal infections at any site (e.g., eye) should be evaluated for DGI. This evaluation should include a careful physical examination, especially of the joints, as well as blood and CSF cultures. Infants with gonococcal ophthalmia or DGI should be treated for 7 days (10 to 14 days if meningitis is present) with one of the following regimens:

- **Ceftriaxone 25–50 mg/kg/day in a single daily dose**

*or*

- **Cefotaxime 25 mg/kg 2 times a day.**

**Alternative Regimen.** Limited data suggest that uncomplicated gonococcal ophthalmia in infants may be cured with a single injection of **ceftriaxone (50 mg/kg up to 125 mg).** A few experts use this regimen in children who have no clinical or laboratory evidence of disseminated disease.

If the gonococcal isolate is proven to be susceptible to penicillin, **crystalline penicillin G may be given. The dose is 100,000 units/kg/day given in 2 equal doses (4 equal doses per day for infants more than 1 week old). The dose should be increased to 150,000 units/kg/day for meningitis.**

Infants with gonococcal ophthalmia should receive eye irrigations with buffered saline solutions until discharge has cleared. Topical antibiotic therapy alone is inadequate. Simultaneous infection with *C. trachomatis* has been reported and should be considered in patients who do not respond satisfactorily. Therefore, the mother and infant should be tested for chlamydial infection.

## Gonococcal infections of children

Children who weigh 45 kg or more should be treated with adult regimens. Children who weigh less than 45 kg should be treated as follows:

**Recommended Regimen.** For uncomplicated vulvovaginitis, cervicitis, urethritis, pharyngitis, and proctitis:

- **Ceftriaxone 125 mg IM once.**

Patients who cannot tolerate ceftriaxone may be treated with:

- **Spectinomycin 40 mg/kg IM once.**

Children 8 years of age or older should also be given **doxycycline 100 mg 2 times a day for 7 days.** All patients should be evaluated for coinfection with syphilis and *C. trachomatis.* Follow-up cultures are necessary to ensure that treatment has been effective.

Bacteremia or arthritis should be treated with **ceftriaxone 50 mg/kg (maximum 1 g) once daily for 7 days. For meningitis, the duration of treatment is increased to 10 to 14 days and the maximum dose is 2 g.**

## PREVENTION OF OPHTHALMIA NEONATORUM

Instillation of a prophylactic agent into the eyes of all newborn infants is recommended to prevent gonococcal ophthalmia neonatorum and is required by law in most states. While all regimens proposed below effectively prevent gonococcal eye disease, their efficacy in preventing chlamydial eye disease is not clear. Furthermore, they do not eliminate nasopharyngeal colonization with *C. trachomatis*. Treatment of gonococcal and chlamydial infections in pregnant women is the best method for preventing neonatal gonococcal and chlamydial disease.

### Recommended regimen

- **Erythromycin (0.5%) ophthalmic ointment,**

*or*

- **Tetracycline (1%) ointment,**

*or*

- **Silver nitrate (1%).**

One of these should be instilled into the eyes of every neonate as soon as possible after delivery, and definitely within 1 hour after birth. Single-use tubes or ampules are preferable to multiple-use tubes.

The efficacy of tetracycline and erythromycin in the prevention of TRNG and PPNG ophthalmia is unknown, though because of the high concentrations of drug in these preparations, both are probably effective. Bacitracin is *not* a recommended regimen.

## CHLAMYDIAL INFECTIONS

Culture and non-culture methods for diagnosis of *C. trachomatis* are now available. Appropriate use of these diagnostic tests is strongly encouraged, especially for screening asymptomatic high risk women in whom infection would otherwise be undetected. However, in clinical settings where testing for chlamydia is not routine or available, treatment often is prescribed on the basis of clinical diagnosis or as co-treatment for gonorrhea (see "Gonococcal Infections," p. A-13). We also recommend that clinic settings perform periodic surveys to determine local chlamydial prevalence in patients with gonorrhea. Priority groups for chlamydia testing, if resources are limited, are high-risk pregnant women, adolescents, and women with multiple sexual partners.

Results of chlamydial tests should be interpreted with care. The sensitivity of all currently available laboratory tests for *C. trachomatis* tests is substantially less than 100 percent; thus, false-negative tests are possible. Although the specificity of non-culture tests have improved substantially, false-positive test results may still occur with non-culture tests. Chlamydial infections may remain asymptomatic for extended periods of time.

### Treatment of uncomplicated urethral, endocervical, or rectal *C. trachomatis* infections

#### Recommended Regimen

- **Doxycycline 100 mg orally 2 times a day for 7 days**

*or*

- **Tetracycline 500 mg orally 4 times a day for 7 days.**

#### Alternative Regimen

- **Erythromycin base 500 mg orally 4 times a day or equivalent salt for 7 days**

*or*

- **Erythromycin ethylsuccinate 800 mg orally 4 times a day for 7 days.**

If erythromycin is not tolerated due to side effects, the following regimen may be effective:

- **Sulfisoxazole 500 mg orally 4 times a day for 10 days or equivalent.**

### Test-of-cure

Because antimicrobial resistance of *C. trachomatis* to recommended regimens has not been observed, test-of-cure evaluation is not necessary when treatment has been completed.

### Treatment of *C. trachomatis* in pregnancy

Pregnant women should undergo diagnostic testing for *C. trachomatis, N. gonorrhoeae,* and syphilis, if possible, at their first prenatal visit and, for women at high risk, during the third trimester. Risk factors for chlamydial disease during pregnancy include: young age (<25 years old), past history or presence of other STD, a new sex partner within the past 3 months, and multiple sex partners. Ideally, pregnant women with gonorrhea should be treated for chlamydia on the basis of diagnostic studies, but if chlamydial testing is not available, then treatment should be given because of the high likelihood of co-infection.

#### Recommended Regimen

- **Erythromycin base 500 mg 4 times a day for 7 days.**

If not tolerated, the following regimens are recommended:

#### Alternative Regimen

- **Erythromycin base 250 mg 4 times a day for 14 days**

*or*

- **Erythromycin ethylsuccinate 800 mg 4 times a day for 7 days**

*or*

- **Erythromycin ethylsuccinate 400 mg 4 times a day for 14 days.**

#### Alternative If Erythromycin Cannot Be Tolerated

- **Amoxicillin 500 mg orally 3 times a day for 7 days, limited data exist for this regimen.**

**Erythromycin estolate** is contraindicated during pregnancy as drug-related hepatoxicity can occur when the drug is administered in pregnancy.

### Sex partners of patients with *C. trachomatis* infections

Sex partners of patients with *C. trachomatis* infection within the past 30 days should be tested for *C. trachomatis*. If testing is not available, they should be treated with the appropriate antimicrobial regimen.

## BACTERIAL STD SYNDROMES

## NONGONOCOCCAL URETHRITIS

In men with urethral symptoms, nongonococcal urethritis (NGU) is diagnosed by Gram stain demonstrating abundant polymorphonuclear leukocyte without intracellular gram-negative diplococci.

*C. trachomatis* has been implicated as the etiology of NGU in about 50 percent of cases. Other organisms which cause 10 to 15 percent of cases include *Ureaplasma urealyticum, T. vaginalis,* and herpes simplex virus. The etiology of the remaining cases is unknown.

### Recommended regimen

- **Doxycycline 100 mg orally 2 times a day for 7 days**

*or*

- **Tetracycline 500 mg orally 4 times a day for 7 days.**

### Alternative regimen

- **Erythromycin base 500 mg orally 4 times a day or equivalent salt for 7 days**

*or*

- **Erythromycin ethylsuccinate 800 mg orally 4 times a day for 7 days.**

If high dose **erythromycin** schedules are not tolerated, the following regimen is recommended:

- **Erythromycin ethylsuccinate 400 mg orally 4 times a day for 14 days**

*or*

- **Erythromycin base 250 mg orally 4 times a day or equivalent salt for 14 days.**

## Management of sex partners

Sex partners of men with NGU should be evaluated for STD and treated with an appropriate regimen based on the evaluation.

## Recurrent NGU unresponsive to conventional therapy

Recurrent NGU may be due to lack of compliance with an initial antibiotic regimen, to reinfection due to failure to treat sex partners, or to factors which are currently undefined. If noncompliance or reinfection cannot be ruled out, repeat **doxycycline** (**100 mg orally 2 times a day for 7 days**) *or* **tetracycline** (**500 mg orally 4 times a day for 7 days**).

If compliance with the initial antimicrobial agent is likely, treat with **erythromycin base** (**500 mg orally 4 times a day for 7 days**) *or* **erythromycin ethylsuccinate** (**800 mg orally 4 times a day for 7 days**).

If objective signs of urethritis continue after adequate treatment, these patients should be evaluated for evidence of other causes of urethritis and referred to a specialist.

## MUCOPURULENT CERVICITIS

The presence of mucopurulent endocervical exudate often suggests mucocorpulent cervicitis (MPC) due to chlamydial or gonococcal infection. Presumptive diagnosis of MPC is made by the finding of mucopurulent secretion from the endocervix, which may appear yellow when viewed on a white cotton-tipped swab (positive swab test). Patients with MPC should have Gram stain and culture for *N. gonorrhoeae,* test for *C. trachomatis,* and a wet mount examination for vaginitis.

### Recommended regimen

- **If *N. gonorrhoeae* is found on Gram stain or culture of endocervical or urethral discharge, treatment should be given as recommended for uncomplicated gonorrhea in adults including cotreatment for chlamydial infection.**
- **If *N. gonorrhoeae* is not found, treatment should be given as recommended for chlamydial infection in adults.**

## Management of sex partners

Sex partners of women with MPC should be evaluated for STD and treated with an appropriate regimen based on the evaluation.

## EPIDIDYMITIS

In sexually active heterosexual men less than 35 years of age, epididymitis is most likely caused by *N. gonorrhoeae* or *C. trachomatis.* Patients should have urethral smear for Gram stain and culture for *N. gonorrhoeae* and *C. trachomatis* and a urine culture. Empiric therapy based on the clinical diagnosis is recommended before culture results are available.

### Recommended regimen

- **Ceftriaxone 250 mg IM**

*and*

- **Doxycycline 100 mg 2 times a day for 10 days.**

## PELVIC INFLAMMATORY DISEASE

## Proposed treatment guidelines

Pelvic inflammatory disease (PID) comprises a spectrum of inflammatory disorders of the upper genital tract in women. PID may include endometritis, salpingitis, tubo-ovarian abscess, and pelvic peritonitis. Sexually transmitted organisms, especially *N. gonorrhoeae* and *C. trachomatis,* are implicated in the majority of cases; however, endogenous organisms, such as anaerobes, gram-negative rods, streptococci, and mycoplasmas may also be etiologic agents of disease.

A confirmed diagnosis of salpingitis and more accurate bacteriologic diagnosis is made by laparoscopy. Since laparoscopy often is not available, the diagnosis of PID is often based on imprecise clinical findings and culture of antigen tests from the lower genital tract.

Guidelines for the treatment of PID have been designed to provide flexibility in therapeutic choices. Because PID therapy has traditionally covered likely etiologic pathogens, treatment is empiric and broad-spectrum. Antimicrobial coverage should include *N. gonorrhoeae, C. trachomatis,* gram-negatives, anaerobes, Group B streptococcus, and the genital mycoplasmas. Few data demonstrate that effective treatment of the pyogenic process of the upper genital tract is more likely to decrease the incidence of long-term complications such as tubal infertility and ectopic pregnancy.

Ideally, as for all intra-abdominal infections, hospitalization is recommended whenever possible, and particularly when: (1) the diagnosis is uncertain; (2) surgical emergencies such as appendicitis and ectopic pregnancy cannot be excluded; (3) a pelvic abscess is suspected; (4) the patient is pregnant; (5) the patient is an adolescent, (the compliance of adolescent patients with therapy is unpredictable, and the long-term sequelae of PID may be particularly severe in this group); (6) severe illness precludes outpatient management; (7) the patient is unable to follow or tolerate an outpatient regimen; (8) the patient has failed to respond to outpatient therapy; or (9) clinical follow-up within 72 hours of starting antibiotic treatment cannot be arranged. Many experts recommend that all patients with PID be hospitalized to initiate treatment with parenteral antibiotics.

The prescribing clinician's familiarity with a treatment regimen, institutional availability, cost-control efforts, patient acceptance, and regional differences in bacterial resistance must be taken into account in the selection of antibiotics.

We stress that these treatment regimens are only recommendations and that the specific antibiotics named are merely examples. Treatment of PID will continue to be broad spectrum and empiric until more definitive studies are performed.

### In-patient treatment

One of the following:

#### Recommended Regimen A

- **Cefoxitin 2 g IV every 6 hours,** *or* **Cefotetan*** **IV 2 g every 12 hours**

*plus*

- **Doxycycline 100 mg every 12 hours orally or IV.**

The above regimens are given for at least 48 hours after the patient clinically improves.

After discharge from hospital, continue:

- **Doxycycline orally 100 mg 2 times a day for 10–14 days total.**

#### Recommended Regimen B

- **Clindamycin IV 900 mg every 8 hours**

*plus*

- **Gentamicin loading dose (2.0 mg/kg) plus maintenance (1.5 mg/kg) every 8 hours**

The above regimens are given for at least 48 hours after the patient improves. After discharge from hospital, continue:

- **Doxycycline 100 mg orally 2 times a day for 10–14 days total.**

Continuation of **clindamycin, 450 mg orally, 5 times daily, for 10 to 14 days,** may be considered as an alternative. Continuation of medication after hospital discharge is important for the treatment of possible *C. trachomatis* infection. **Clindamycin** has more complete anaerobic coverage. Although limited data suggest **clindamycin** is effective for treatment of *C. trachomatis* infection, **doxycycline** remains the treatment of choice for chlamydial disease. When *C. trachomatis* is strongly suspected or confirmed as an etiologic agent, **doxycycline** is the preferable alternative. In such instances, **doxycycline therapy** may be started during hospitalization if initiation of therapy prior to hospital discharge is thought likely to improve patient compliance.

### Rationale

Clinicians have extensive experience with both the cefoxitin/doxycycline and clindamycin/aminoglycoside combinations. Each of these regimens provides broad coverage against polymicrobial infection. Cefotetan has properties similar to those of cefoxitin and requires less frequent dosing. Fewer clinical data are currently available on third-generation cephalosporins (ceftizoxime, cefotaxime, ceftriaxone), although many authorities believe they are effective. Doxycycline administered orally has bioavailability similar to that of the IV formulation and may be given if normal gastrointestinal function is present.

While experimental studies suggest that aminoglycosides may not be optimal treatment for gram-negative organisms within abscesses, clinical studies suggest that they are highly effective in the treatment of abscesses when administered in combination with clindamycin.

Although short courses of aminoglycosides in healthy young women usually do not require serum-level monitoring, many practitioners may elect to monitor levels.

### Ambulatory management of PID

#### Recommended Regimen

- **Cefoxitin 2 g IM plus Probenecid, 1 g orally concurrently** *or* **equivalent cephalosporin,** *or* **ceftriaxone 250 mg IM**

*plus*

- **Doxycycline 100 mg orally 2 times a day for 10–14 days.**

#### Alternative Regimen for Patients Who Do Not Tolerate Doxycycline

- **Erythromycin, 500 mg orally 4 times a day for 10–14 days.**

This regimen, however, is based on limited clinical data.

### Rationale

These empiric regimens provide broad spectrum coverage against the common etiologic agents of PID. Parenteral β-lactam antibiotics are recommended in all cases. The cephalosporins are effective in the treatment of gram-negative organisms, including enteric rods, anaerobic organisms, and gonococci.

Although decreased susceptibility of gonococci to cefoxitin has been recently noted, treatment failure has not yet been a clinical problem. Patients who do not respond to therapy within 72 hours should be hospitalized for parenteral therapy. Doxycycline provides definitive therapy for chlamydial infections. Patients treated on an ambulatory basis need to be monitored closely and reevaluated in 72 hours.

**Management of Sex Partners.** Sex partners of women with PID should be evaluated for STD. After evaluation, sex partners should be empirically treated with regimens effective against *N. gonorrhoeae* and *C. trachomatis* infections.

## SEXUALLY TRANSMITTED ENTERIC INFECTIONS

Sexually transmitted gastrointestinal syndromes include proctitis, proctocolitis, and enteritis. With the exception of rectal gonococcal infection, these syndromes occur predominantly in homosexual men who participate in receptive anal intercourse. Evaluation should include additional diagnostic procedures, such as anoscopy or sigmoidoscopy, stool examination, and culture.

*Proctitis* is inflammation limited to the rectum (the distal 10 to 12 cm), and is associated with anorectal pain, tenesmus, constipation, and discharge. *N. gonorrhoeae, C. trachomatis,* and HSV are the most common sexually transmitted pathogens involved. In patients coinfected with HIV, herpes proctitis may be especially severe.

*Proctocolitis* is associated with symptoms of proctitis plus diarrhea and/or abdominal cramps, and the colonic mucosa is

*Other cephalosporins such as **ceftizoxime, cefotaxime,** and **ceftriaxone** which provide adequate gonococcal, other facultative gram-negative, and anaerobic coverage, may be utilized in appropriate doses.

inflamed proximal to 12 cm. Etiologic organisms include *Campylobacter jejuni, Shigella* spp., amebiasis, and, rarely, *T. pallidum* or *C. trachomatis* (often LGV serovars). Cytomegalovirus may be involved in patients coinfected with HIV.

*Enteritis* in homosexual men usually results in diarrhea without signs of proctitis or proctocolitis. In otherwise healthy patients, *Giardia lamblia* is most commonly implicated. In patients also coinfected with HIV, cytomegalovirus, *Mycobacterium avium-intracellulare, Salmonella* spp., *Cryptosporidium* and *Isospora* must be considered. Special stool preparations are required to diagnose giardiasis or cryptosporidiosis. Additionally, some cases of enteritis may be a primary effect of HIV infection.

All patients with sexually transmitted enteric infections should be counseled and tested for HIV infection.

### Treatment

Treatment recommendations for all enteric infections are beyond the scope of these guidelines. However, acute proctitis of recent onset in an individual who has recently practiced unprotected receptive anal intercourse is most often sexually transmitted. Such patients should be examined by anoscopy, and should be evaluated for infection with *N. gonorrhoeae, C. trachomatis,* HSV, and *T. pallidum.* Treatment can be based on specific etiologic diagnosis or can be empiric.

#### Empiric Treatment for Sexually Transmitted Proctitis

RECOMMENDED REGIMEN

- **Ceftriaxone 250 mg IM** *plus* **doxycycline 100 mg orally 2 times a day for 7 days provides adequate treatment for gonorrhea and chlamydial infection.**

## VAGINAL DISEASES

### TRICHOMONIASIS

In almost all patients, trichomoniasis is a sexually transmitted infection. Diagnosis is usually made by direct microscopic visualization (wet prep) or by culture. Diagnosis by cervical cytology or fixed preparation should be confirmed by direct visualization or culture. Symptomatic and asymptomatic patients should be treated.

### Treatment

#### Recommended Treatment

- **Metronidazole 2 g orally in a single dose.**

#### Alternative Treatment

- **Metronidazole 500 mg twice daily for 7 days.**

If failure occurs with either regimen the patient should be retreated with **metronidazole 500 mg twice daily for 7 days.** If repeated failure occurs, the patient should be treated with a single **2 g dose of metronidazole daily for 3 to 5 days.**

Cases of further culture-documented treatment failure in which reinfection has been excluded should be managed in consultation with an expert. Evaluation of such cases should include determination of the susceptibility of *Trichomonas vaginalis* to **metronidazole.**

### Treatment of sexual partners

- **Sexual partners should be treated with either the single dose or the 7-day metronidazole regimen.**

### Trichomoniasis during pregnancy

**Metronidazole** is contraindicated in the first trimester of pregnancy and its safety in the rest of pregnancy is not established. However, no other adequate therapy exists. For patients with severe symptoms after the first trimester, treatment with **2 g metronidazole in a single dose** may be considered.

### VULVOVAGINAL CANDIDIASIS

Generally not considered a sexually transmitted disease, vulvovaginal candidiasis is frequently diagnosed in women presenting with genital symptoms. Treatment with antibiotics predisposes women to the development of vulvovaginal candidiasis.

### Treatment

Many effective treatment regimens exist, but 3- and 7-day regimens are superior to a single-dose therapy.

**Recommended Treatment.** Examples of effective regimens include the following:

- **Miconazole nitrate** (**vaginal suppository 200 mg**), **intravaginally at bedtime for 3 days**

*or*

- **Clotrimazole** (**vaginal tablets 200 mg**), **intravaginally at bedtime for 3 days**

*or*

- **Butaconazole** (**2% cream 5 g**), **intravaginally at bedtime for 3 days**

*or*

- **Teraconazole 80 mg suppository or 0.4% cream, intravaginally at bedtime for 3 days.**

#### Alternative Treatment

- **Miconazole nitrate** (**vaginal suppository 100 mg or 2% cream 5 g**), **intravaginally at bedtime for 7 days**

*or*

- **Clotrimazole** (**vaginal tablets 100 mg or clotrimazole 1% cream 5 g**), **intravaginally at bedtime for 7 days.**

*Comment:* Nystatin and single-dose therapy are less effective than the recommended therapies and are not recommended.

### Treatment failure

Patients with recurrent infections should have their infection documented by culture. Systemic therapy is usually not indicated. Patients with frequent unexplained infections should be evaluated for predisposing conditions (especially HIV infection) and should be referred to an expert for care.

### Treatment of sexual partners

Treatment of sex partners is not necessary unless candidal balanitis (which responds to local anticandidal preparations) is present.

### Candidiasis during pregnancy

Treatment is the same as in non-pregnant patients.

## BACTERIAL VAGINOSIS (BV)

Bacterial vaginosis (BV) (formerly called non-specific vaginitis, *Haemophilus*-associated vaginitis, or *Gardnerella*-associated vaginitis) is the clinical result of alterations in the vaginal microflora. Clinical diagnosis is made when three or four criteria (homogeneous discharge, pH >4.5, positive amine odor test, or presence of clue cells) are present. Diagnosis can also be made using Gram stain. Asymptomatic infections are common. Many authorities do not recommend treatment for asymptomatic infection.

### Treatment

#### Recommended Treatment

- **Metronidazole 500 mg orally, 2 times a day for 7 days.**

#### Alternate Treatment

- **Clindamycin 300 mg orally, 2 times a day for 7 days.**

### Treatment of male partners

No clinical counterpart of BV is recognized in the male, and treatment of the male sexual partner has not been shown to be beneficial for the patient or the male partner.

### BV in pregnant patients

In pregnancy, recent studies suggest that BV may be a factor in premature rupture of membranes and premature delivery; thus, close clinical follow-up of pregnant women with BV is essential. These studies require confirmation, however, and intervention studies have not been conducted. Until such studies have been conducted, routine treatment appears to be unnecessary and treatment of pregnant women with BV should be at the option of the physician.

**Metronidazole** is contraindicated in the first trimester of pregnancy, and its safety in the rest of pregnancy is not established. Thus, treatment with **clindamycin 300 mg orally twice daily for 7 days is recommended.**

## MISCELLANEOUS DISEASES

## VIRAL HEPATITIS

Sexual contact is currently the most frequent reported mode of hepatitis B virus transmission in the United States. Delta hepatitis also can be transmitted sexually. Persons at high risk for sexual transmission of hepatitis B include homosexual men, heterosexual men and women with multiple partners, and sex partners of intravenous drug abusers. Immunity to hepatitis B also confers immunity to delta hepatitis. Sexual transmission of hepatitis A is unimportant except in cases where sexual practices include fecal-oral contact. The extent of sexual transmission of nonA-nonB hepatitis is currently uncertain.

Etiologic diagnosis of viral hepatitis is made by serological testing. Most cases of acute viral hepatitis are asymptomatic. Although no specific therapy is available for viral hepatitis, specific vaccination and post-exposure prophylaxis strategies are of proven efficacy in preventing hepatitis B. Although expensive, the costs of these strategies must be measured against the morbidity associated with hepatitis B and delta hepatitis, which in many cases include chronic hepatic disease and cirrhosis. Post-exposure immune serum globulin prophylaxis is indicated for contacts of patients with hepatitis A and perhaps nonA-nonB hepatitis. The following recommendations are for hepatitis B prophylaxis.

### Hepatitis B prevention

**Vaccination** is recommended for all persons with multiple sexual partners within the preceding 6 months. IV drug users, homosexual/bisexual men, and residents of correctional or long-term care facilities, persons seeking treatment for STD, and prostitutes should also be vaccinated. Both plasma-derived and recombinant vaccines are safe and effective. Among groups at high risk for hepatitis B (such as homosexual men), pre-vaccination screening for antibody to hepatitis B is cost effective. Testing in moderate-groups (such as heterosexual persons with STD) is usually not indicated.

#### Hepatitis B Vaccination

- **Hepatitis B Vaccine (several FDA-approved recombinant or plasma-derived preparations are available) in dosages as recommended by the manufacturer. The vaccination series requires an initial visit and two follow-up visits.**

Vaccine should *not* be administered in the gluteal (buttocks) or quadriceps (thigh) muscle. Following vaccination, testing for antibody response is not routinely indicated unless the patient is infected with HIV.

### Post-exposure prophylaxis

Prophylactic treatment with hepatitis B immune globulin should be considered in the following situations: Sexual contact with a patient who has active hepatitis B or who develops hepatitis B; sexual contact with a hepatitis B carrier (blood test positive for hepatitis B surface antigen). Prophylactic treatment for sexual exposure should be given within 14 days of sexual contact. Assay for preexisting immunity to HBV may be cost effective in individuals from populations at high risk for HBV.

#### Recommendation for Post-Exposure Prophylaxis

- **Hepatitis B immune globulin (HBIG) .06 ml/kg, IM in a single dose**

*followed by*

- **Initiation of hepatitis B vaccine series as described above.**

### Perinatal infections

Pregnant women with HBV infection can transmit hepatitis B to their infants at delivery. Infants infected at birth are at high risk for developing chronic hepatitis B infection. This can be prevented by administering HBIG and hepatitis B vaccine to the infant. Therefore, all pregnant women should be screened during their first obstetrical visit for the presence of HBsAg. If this is positive, their newborns should be given HBIG *as soon as possible* after birth, and subsequently should be immunized with hepatitis B vaccine.

Hepatitis guidelines are updated periodically by the Advisory

Committee on Immunization Practices (ACIP), and are published in *MMWR* and secondary outlets. Reference to the most current ACIP recommendations is advised.

Persons at risk for sexual transmission of hepatitis B are also at risk for acquiring HIV and other STD. HIV coinfection reduces the humoral response to HB vaccine.

## CYTOMEGALOVIRUS

Cytomegalovirus (CMV) is a common infection in pregnant women, and 0.5 to 2 percent of all infants are congenitally infected, although most of those are only mildly affected. Another 5 to 10 percent of infants are perinatally infected; these infections are without known sequelae. The risk of severe congenital disease (retardation, deafness, visual problems) is highest when primary CMV infection occurs during pregnancy, although recurrent CMV may also cause severe congenital infection. Because severe congenital infection occurs before delivery, and because CMV infection is widespread, the route of delivery should not be influenced by viral shedding. No accepted routine therapy exists for either maternal or neonatal infection.

## ECTOPARASITIC INFECTIONS

### Pediculosis pubis

#### Recommended Regime

- **Permethrin (1%) creme rinse applied to affected area and washed off after 10 minutes**

*or*

- **Pyrethrins and piperonyl butoxide applied to the affected area and washed off after 10 minutes**

*or*

- **Lindane 1 percent shampoo applied for 4 minutes and then thoroughly washed off. (Not recommended for pregnant or lactating women.)**

Patients should be reevaluated after 1 week if symptoms persist. Re-treatment may be necessary if lice are found or eggs are observed at the hair-skin junction. Clothing or bed linen that may have been contaminated by the patient within the past 2 days should be washed/or dried by machine (hot cycle in each), or dry cleaned.

**Special Considerations.** Pediculosis of the eyelashes should be treated by the application of **occlusive ophthalmic ointment to the eyelid margins, 2 times a day for 10 days,** to smother lice and nits. **Lindane** or other drugs should not be applied to the eyes.

**Sex partners should be treated as above.**

### Scabies

#### Recommended Regimen (Adults and Older Children)

- **Lindane (1%) 1 oz of lotion or 30 g of cream applied thinly to all areas of the body from the neck down and washed off thoroughly after 8 hours. (Not recommended for pregnant or lactating women.)**

#### Alternative Regimen

- **Crotamiton (10%) applied to the entire body from the neck down for 2 nights and washed off thoroughly 24 hours after the second application.**

**Infants, Children 2 Years or Less, Pregnant and Lactating Women.** In these groups lindane is contraindicated. The **crotamiton** regimen should be used.

**Contacts.** Sex partners and closed household contacts should be treated as above.

**Special Considerations.** Pruritus may persist for several weeks after adequate therapy. A single re-treatment after 1 week may be appropriate if there is no clinical improvement. Additional weekly treatments are warranted only if live mites can be demonstrated.

Clothing or bed linen that may have been contaminated by the patient within the past 2 days should be washed and dried by machine (hot cycle in each), or dry cleaned.

## SEXUAL ASSAULT AND STD

Recommendations are limited to the identification and treatment of sexually transmitted infections. Sensitive management of potential pregnancy and of physical and psychological trauma are of great importance and should be addressed, but are beyond the scope of these guidelines. Victims of sexual assault are evaluated both to provide necessary medical services and to identify and collect forensic evidence. Although some information may be useful for the medical management of a victim, this information may not be admissible in court.

Some STDs, such as gonorrhea and syphilis, are almost exclusively transmitted sexually and may be useful markers of sexual assault. Trichomoniasis and BV are both commonly found after assault, but both have high prior prevalence in most populations, which limits their utility as markers of assault. Non-culture tests have lower sensitivity and specificity than culture techniques.

## SEXUAL ASSAULT

Any sexually transmissible agents, including HIV, may be transmitted during an assault. Few data exist on which to establish the risk of an assaulted person's acquiring an STD. The risk of acquiring gonococcal and/or chlamydial infections appears to be highest. Inferences about STD risk may be based on the known prevalences of these diseases in the community. If the suspected assailant is identified, that individual should be evaluated for STD to the extent possible under the law.

The presence of STD within 24 hours of the assault may represent prior infection and not assault-acquired disease. Furthermore, some syndromes, such as BV, may be non-sexually transmitted.

### Evaluation

**The initial evaluation of the victim for STD should be performed, if possible, within 24 hours of the assault and should include the following (see also subsection of test selection and specimen handling, p. A-22):**

- **Cultures for *N. gonorrhoeae* and *C. trachomatis* from specimens from any sites of penetration or attempted penetration.**
- **Collection of a blood sample for a serologic test for syphilis and for storage of a serum sample for possible future testing. Serologic testing for HIV and hepatitis B infection should be considered.**

- **For women, examination of vaginal specimens for *T. vaginalis* and for evidence of BV.**
- **Pregnancy tests.**

Follow-up evaluations should be scheduled after 14 to 21 days, to repeat studies other than those for syphilis and viral STDs. A third visit may be scheduled at 8 to 12 weeks to repeat initial serologic studies, including tests for antibodies to syphilis and/or hepatitis B, and/or HIV.

### Treatment

Treatment should be given for any infection identified on examination or for any infection identified in the assailant. Although the risk of infection is frequently low, use of presumptive treatment is controversial. Some experts recommend presumptive treatment for all victims of sexual assault, while some reserve presumptive treatment for special circumstances, for example, when follow-up examination of the victim cannot be ensured, or when treatment is specifically requested by the patient. Although no regimen provides coverage for all potential pathogens, the following regimens should be effective against gonorrhea, chlamydia, and, most likely, syphilis.

#### Empiric Regimen for Victims of Sexual Assault

- **Ceftriaxone, 250 mg, given IM,**

*to be followed by either*

- **Doxycycline 100 mg orally 2 times a day for 7 days**

*or*

- **Tetracycline HCl 500 mg orally 4 times a day for 7 days.**

## SEXUAL ASSAULT AND ABUSE OF CHILDREN

In general, the identification of a sexually transmissible agent from a child beyond the neonatal period suggests sexual abuse. However, exceptions do exist, for example, rectal and genital infection with *C. trachomatis* in young children may be due to persistent perinatally acquired infection, which may persist for up to 3 years. In addition, BV and genital mycoplasmas have been identified in both abused and non-abused children. A finding of genital warts, while suggestive of assault, is too nonspecific without other evidence of abuse. Where the only evidence of sexual abuse is the isolation of an organism or the detection of antibodies, findings should be carefully confirmed. Incorrect test results have led to inappropriate and traumatic sexual abuse investigations.

### Evaluation

In sexually abused children, the prevalence of STD appears relatively low; in most studies, *C. trachomatis* is the most frequently isolated organism. Sexually abused children are best managed by a team of professionals experienced in dealing with the many needs of the child. Although testing for the diseases appropriate for children (Table 6) is essentially the same as for adults, the special needs of children must be taken into account.

### Recommended evaluation in case of suspected child abuse/assault

- **Since a child's report of assault may not be complete, specimens for culture for *N. gonorrhoeae* and *C. trachomatis* should be collected from the pharynx and rectum as well as from the vagina (girls) or urethra (boys).**

**Table 6. Recommended Laboratory Procedures at Initial and Follow-up Evaluation of Sexually Abused Children (Prepubertal)**

| |
|---|
| Gram stain of any genital or anal discharge* |
| Culture for *N. gonorrhoeae*† |
| Culture for *C. trachomatis*† |
| Wet preparation of vaginal secretion for trichomonads, clue cells, and the presence of an amine odor when mixed with KOH‡ |
| Culture of lesions for herpes simplex virus (HSV) |
| Serologic test for syphilis |
| Serologic test for human immunodeficiency virus (HIV)§ |
| Frozen serum sample |

*Note:* Syphilis and HIV serology should be repeated in 12 weeks. All other tests should be repeated 10–14 days after the initial examination.

*Care should be taken in the interpretation of results of any Gram stain of anal discharge.

†Cultures of pharynx, rectum, and vagina/urethra should be done.

‡Females only; vaginal pH testing is not recommended because of a lack of known standard in children.

§Testing for HIV should be based upon the prevalence of infection and on suspected risk.

- **Internal pelvic examinations usually should not be performed unless indicated by the presence of a foreign body or by trauma.**
- **Follow-up visits should be scheduled so as to minimize trauma to the child; for asymptomatic children, an initial visit and one at 8 to 12 weeks may be sufficient.**
- **In cases of continuing abuse, the alleged offender may be available for medical evaluation. In such instances, care for the child may be modified when results of the evaluation of the offender are known.**

### Treatment

Treatment prior to diagnosis is not indicated, unless there is evidence that the assailant is infected. Presumptive treatment following assault may be given if the victim or victim's family requests it, or if follow-up examination of the victim cannot be ensured.

### Test selection and specimen handling

When a sexually transmitted agent is identified from a sexually abused adult or child, that laboratory result may be required to be admissible to pending legal action. Isolation of gonorrhea and chlamydia organisms by culture, and their confirmation by recognized techniques, is the necessary standard. All presumptive isolates of *N. gonorrhoeae* from children should be confirmed by at least two tests that use different principles, e.g., biochemical, enzyme substrate, or serologic. Direct specimen antigen detection tests or DNA probe tests are *not recommended* for use on specimens from any victim of sexual abuse. These tests may be used to diagnose *C. trachomatis* in adults only in those areas where culture is not available. Results of non-culture tests may be used to guide medical management but should not be used for forensic purposes. The potential for an inaccurate result is greatest in children, and non-culture tests are not recommended at anytime in the evaluation of sexual assault or sexual abuse in children. Isolates should be stored at −70°C for possible future studies, and the use of a reference laboratory should be considered. Expert laboratory consultations are recommended for testing as well as for chain of evidence issues.

# INDEX

# INDEX

Page references in italics indicate tables; page references in boldface indicate illustrations.

# Drug Interactions for Antimicrobial Agents Used Commonly for Sexually Transmitted Diseases*

| STD Agent | Interacting Drug | Interaction/Mechanism | Clinical Significance |
|---|---|---|---|
| *Acyclovir* | Zidovudine | Severe drowsiness and lethargy (two reports); mechanism unknown | Not clinically significant |
| *Cephalosporins* | *See* Table 83-4 (p. 996) | | |
| *Chloramphenicol, Thiamphenicol* | Penicillins | Antagonism; interferes with bactericidal effect | Little with therapeutic doses |
| | Phenobarbital | Increased phenobarbital levels and decreased chloramphenicol levels; competitive metabolic pathways | Monitor levels of both drugs |
| | Phenytoin | Increased levels of phenytoin; inhibits phenytoin metabolism | Monitor phenytoin levels |
| | Rifampin | Decreased chloramphenicol levels; enhanced metabolism of chloramphenicol | Monitor chloramphenicol levels |
| | Sulfonylureas | Enhanced hypoglycemic effect; impaired metabolism | Monitor serum glucose |
| | Warfarin | Enhanced anticoagulant effect; decreased vitamin K production by bacteria or prothrombin by liver or decreased metabolism of the anticoagulant | Low unless dicumarol used instead of warfarin |
| *Ciprofloxacin* | Antacids | Decreased clinical effect of ciprofloxacin; decreased bioavailability due to binding of aluminum and magnesium to ciprofloxacin | Avoid use together |
| | Theophylline | Theophylline toxicity; decreased clearance of theophylline by inhibition of demethylation metabolism pathway | Monitor theophylline levels especially in older patients |
| *Erythromycin* | Carbamazepine | Inhibits hepatic metabolism of carbamazepine | Carbamazepine toxicity has been reported |
| | Clindamycin | Antagonism; competes for same ribosomal binding site | Uncertain |
| | Cyclosporine | Increased cyclosporine levels; inhibition of cyclosporine clearance | Monitor cyclosporine levels |
| | Digoxin | Increased digoxin levels; alteration of gut flora—increased absorption? | Monitor digoxin levels |
| | Theophylline | Increased theophylline levels/toxicity; inhibits theophylline metabolism | Monitor theophylline levels |
| | Warfarin | Potentiation of anticoagulant effects; inhibition of warfarin metabolism | Monitor PTs |
| *Metronidazole* | Barbiturates | Decreased clinical response; increased metabolism of metronidazole | Increase metronidazole doses |
| | Cimetidine | Increased metronidazole toxicity; inhibition of metronidazole metabolism | Monitor for toxicity |
| | Disulfiram | Psychosis and confusion; inhibition of aldehyde dehydrogenase | Avoid combination |
| | Phenytoin | Increased phenytoin serum concentration; inhibition of phenytoin metabolism | Monitor levels |
| | Warfarin | Increased anticoagulant effect; inhibition of S(-) isomer metabolism | Monitor PTs |
| *Penicillin* | *See* Table 83-4 (p. 996) | | |

*Compiled by Teresa Tartaglione, Pharm.D.